WHAT'S NEW?

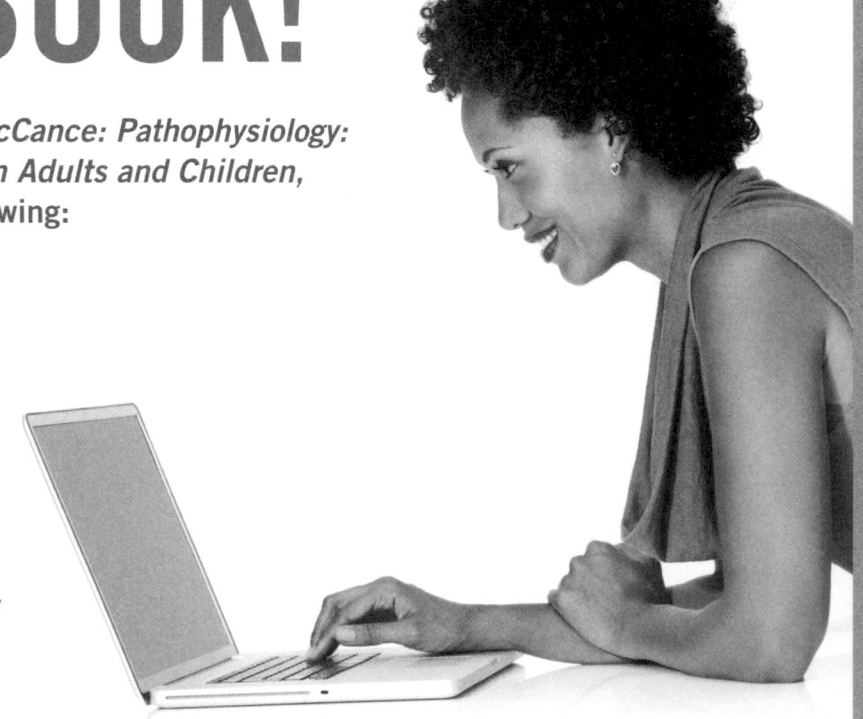

PATHOPHYSIOLOGY

THE BIOLOGIC BASIS FOR DISEASE IN ADULTS AND CHILDREN

ABOUT THE COVER IMAGE

The bean shaped image is bacteria, *Neisseria gonorrhoeae*, which causes gonorrhea. Gonorrhea is a very common sexually transmitted infection and is sometimes called the *clap* or the *drip*. It is especially prevalent for teens and young adults. Gonorrhea is spread through vaginal, anal, and oral sex. It can infect the vagina, penis, cervix, anus, urethra, throat, and rarely, eyes. If a mother has gonorrhea it can spread to a baby during birth. People often have no symptoms and do not know they are infected until they get tested. It can lead to serious health problems and even infertility if untreated. Gonorrhea can be cured with the right treatment. Treatment is by antibiotics, and all sexual partners need testing and treatment. Some strains of gonorrhea resist antibiotics and have become more challenging to treat.

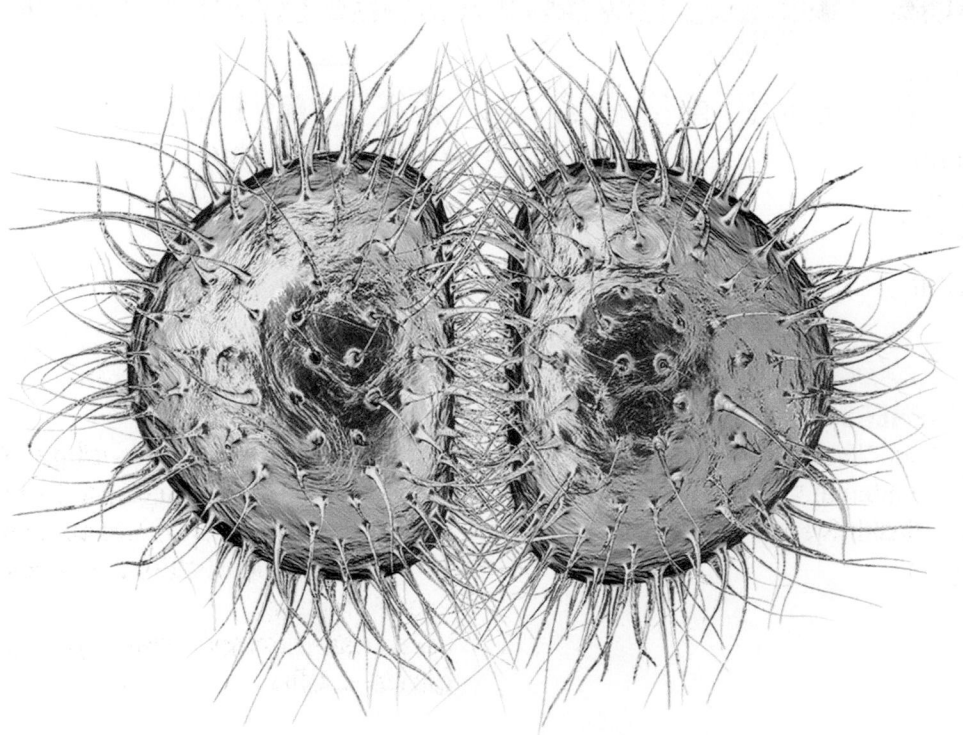

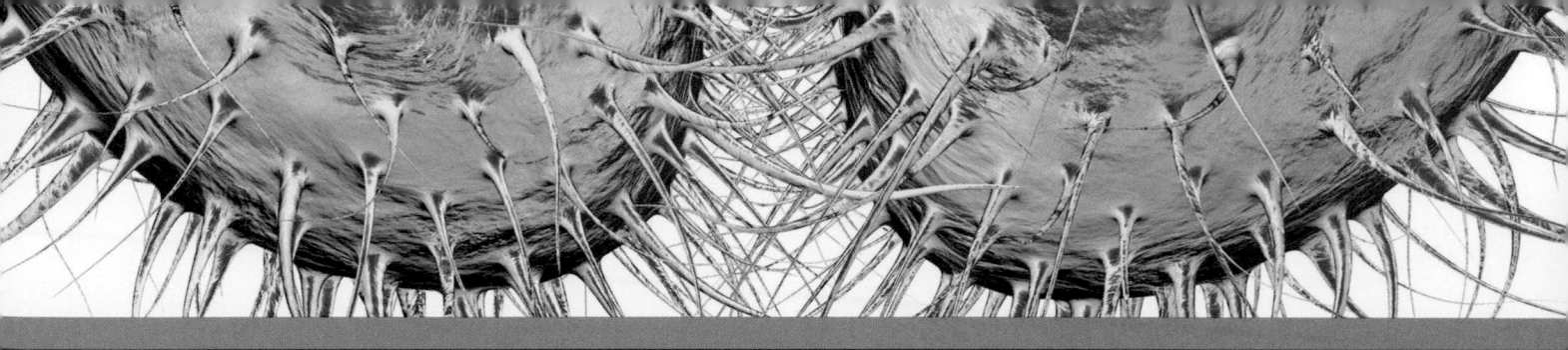

PATHOPHYSIOLOGY

THE BIOLOGIC BASIS FOR DISEASE IN ADULTS AND CHILDREN

Eighth Edition

KATHRYN L. McCANCE, MS, PhD
Professor Emeritus
College of Nursing
University of Utah
Salt Lake City, Utah

SUE E. HUETHER, MS, PhD
Professor Emeritus
College of Nursing
University of Utah
Salt Lake City, Utah

SECTION EDITORS

VALENTINA L. BRASHERS, MD, FACP, FNAP
Professor of Nursing and Woodard Clinical Scholar
Attending Physician in Internal Medicine
University of Virginia Health System
Charlottesville, Virginia

NEAL S. ROTE, PhD
Academic Vice-Chair and Director of Research,
   Department of Obstetrics and Gynecology
University Hospitals Case Medical Center
William H. Weir, MD Professor of Reproductive Biology
   and Pathology
Case Western Reserve University, School of Medicine
Cleveland, Ohio

ELSEVIER

with more than 1200 illustrations

ELSEVIER

3251 Riverport Lane
St. Louis, Missouri 63043

PATHOPHYSIOLOGY: THE BIOLOGIC BASIS FOR DISEASE IN ADULTS AND CHILDREN, EIGHTH EDITION

ISBN: 978-0-323-58347-3

Previous editions copyrighted 2014, 2010, 2006, 2002, 1998, 1994, and 1990.

Executive Content Strategist: Kellie White
Content Development Specialists: Jennifer Wade, Karen C. Turner
Publishing Services Manager: Jeffrey Patterson
Senior Production Manager: Mary Pohlman
Design Direction: Ashley Miner, Margaret Reid

Printed in Canada.

Last digit is the print number: 9 8 7 6 5 4 3

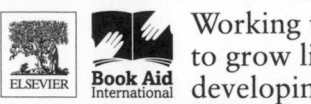

Rose A. Urdiales Baker, PhD, PMHCNS-BC
Assistant Lecturer
School of Nursing
College of Health Professions
University of Akron
Akron, Ohio

Barbara J. Boss, RN, PhD, CFNP, CANP
Professor Emeritus of Nursing
University of Mississippi Medical Center
Jackson, Mississippi

Valentina L. Brashers, MD, FACP, FNAP
Professor of Nursing and Woodland Clinical Scholar
Attending Physician in Internal Medicine
University of Virginia Health System
Charlottesville, Virginia

Russell J. Butterfield, MD, PhD
Assistant Professor
Departments of Pediatrics and Neurology
University of Utah School of Medicine
Salt Lake City, Utah

Dennis J. Cheek, RN, PhD, FAHA
Abell-Hanger Professor of Gerontological Nursing
Harris College of Nursing and Health Sciences
Texas Christian University
Fort Worth, Texas

Margaret F. Clayton, PhD, FNP, APRN-BC
Assistant Professor
University of Utah College of Nursing
Salt Lake City, Utah

Susanna G. Cunningham, BSN, MA, PhD, FAAN, FAHA
Professor
School of Nursing
University of Washington
Seattle, Washington

Kathleen E. Danhausen, CNM, MSN, MPH
Instructor of Clinical Nursing
Vanderbilt University
Nashville, Tennessee

Sara J. Fidanza, MS, RN, CNS-BC, CPNP-BC
Digestive Health Institute Advanced Practice Nurse
Children's Hospital Colorado
Aurora, Colorado

Diane P. Genereux, PhD
Broad Institute of MIT and Harvard
Cambridge, Massachusetts

Todd C. Grey, MD
Chief Medical Examiner-Retired
Office of the Medical Examiner
State of Utah
Salt Lake City, Utah

Mary Fran Hazinski, RN, MSN, FAAN, FAHA, FERC
Professor
Vanderbilt University School of Nursing
Assistant
Departments of Surgery and Pediatrics
Vanderbilt University School of Medicine
Clinical Nurse Specialist
Monroe Carell, Jr. Children's Hospital at Vanderbilt
Nashville, Tennessee

Leslie W. Hopkins, DNP, APRN-BC, FNP-BC, ANP-C
Assistant Professor
Adult Gerontology Primary Care Nurse Practitioner
   Academic Director
Vanderbilt University School of Nursing
Nashville, Tennessee

Robert E. Jones, MD, FACP, FACE
Medical Director
Utah Diabetes Center
Professor of Medicine
University of Utah School of Medicine
Salt Lake City, Utah

Lynn B. Jorde, PhD
Mark and Kathie Miller Presidential Professor and Chair
Department of Human Genetics
University of Utah School of Medicine
Salt Lake City, Utah

Lauri A. Linder, PhD, APRN, CPON
Associate Professor
University of Utah College of Nursing
Clinical Nurse Specialist
Cancer Transplant Center
Primary Children's Hospital
Salt Lake City, Utah

Linda L. Martin, DNP, RN, CFNP
Associate Professor of Professional Nursing
Harris College of Nursing and Health Sciences
Texas Christian University
Fort Worth, Texas

Sue Ann McCann, MSN, RN, DNC
Photopheresis/Cutaneous T-cell Lymphoma
   Research Coordinator
Department of Dermatology
University of Pittsburgh Medical Center
Pittsburgh, Pennsylvania

McCall G. McDaniel, MD
Pediatric Orthopaedic Surgeon
Bone and Joint Clinic
St. Tammany Parish Hospital
Covington, Louisiana

Mary A. Mondozzi, MSN, BSN, RN, WCC
Burn Center Education/Outreach Coordinator
The Paul and Carol David Foundation Burn Institute
Akron Children's Hospital
Akron, Ohio

Stephen E. Morris, MD, FACS
Professor of Surgery
Director, University of Utah Health Burn Center
University of Utah Department of Surgery
Salt Lake City, Utah

Noreen Heer Nicol, PhD, RN, FNP, NEA-BC
Associate Professor
College of Nursing
University of Colorado, Anschutz Medical Campus
Aurora, Colorado

Jennifer K. Peterson, MS, RN, CCNS
PhD Candidate
Sue and Bill Gross School of Nursing
University of California, Irvine
Congenital Heart Clinical Program Director
Miller Children's & Women's Hospital
Long Beach, California

Julia C. Phillippi, PhD, CNM, FACNM
Assistant Professor
Nurse-Midwifery
Vanderbilt University School of Nursing
Nashville, Tennessee

Nancy Pike, PhD, RN, CPNP-AC, FAAN
Associate Professor
UCLA School of Nursing
Nurse Practitioner, Cardiothoracic Surgery
Children's Hospital
Los Angeles, California

Geri C. Reeves, PhD, APRN, FNP-BC
Assistant Professor
Vanderbilt University School of Nursing
Nashville, Tennessee

Patricia Ring, RN, MSN, PNP, BC
Renal/Voiding Improvement Program
Children's Hospital of Wisconsin
Milwaukee, Wisconsin

George W. Rodway, PhD, APRN
Associate Professor of Clinical Nursing
University of California—Davis School of Nursing
Sacramento, California

Neal S. Rote, PhD
Academic Vice-Chair and Director of Research, Department
   of Obstetrics and Gynecology
University Hospitals Case Medical Center
William H. Weir, MD Professor of Reproductive Biology
   and Pathology
Case Western Reserve University, School of Medicine
Cleveland, Ohio

Sharon Sables-Baus, PhD, MPA, RN, PCNS-BC, CPPS, FAAN
Associate Professor
The College of Nursing and School of Medicine
Department of Pediatrics
University of Colorado, Anschutz Medical Campus
Aurora, Colorado

Benjamin A. Smallheer, PhD, RN, ACNP-BC, FNP-BC, CCRN, CNE
Lead Faculty Adult-Gerontology Acute Care Nurse
   Practitioner Program
Duke University School of Nursing
Durham, North Carolina

Lorey K. Takahashi, PhD
Professor
Psychobiology Laboratory
University of Hawaii
Honolulu, Hawaii

Marcella R. Woiczik, MD
Associate Professor
Department of Orthopaedics
University of Utah
Pediatric Orthopaedic Surgeon
Shriner's Intermountain Unit
Salt Lake City, Utah

The authors also would like to thank the following previous edition contributors.

Kristen Lee Carroll, MD
Chief of Staff
Medical Staff/Orthopedics
Shriners Hospital for Children
Professor of Orthopedics
University of Utah
Salt Lake City, Utah
Chapter 46

Christy L. Crowther-Radulewicz, RN, MS, CRNP
Nurse Practitioner
Orthopedic Surgery
Anne Arundel Orthopedic Surgeons
Annapolis, Maryland
Chapter 45

Lynne M. Kerr, MD, PhD
Associate Professor
Department of Pediatrics
Division of Pediatric Neurology
University of Utah Medical Center
Salt Lake City, Utah
Chapters 15, 20, 46

†**Nancy E. Kline, PhD, RN, CPNP, FAAN**
Director, Nursing Research, Medicine
Patient Services/Emergency Department
Boston Children's Hospital
Boston, Massachusetts
Chapters 14, 31

Anna L. Schwartz, PhD, FNP-BC, FAAN
Associate Professor
School of Nursing
Northern Arizona University
Flagstaff, Arizona
Chapter 30

---

†Deceased.

Dawn Binns, RN, MSN
Faculty, Emergency Nursing Specialty
British Columbia Institute of Technology
Burnaby, British Columbia, Canada

Janet Czermak Russell, MA, MS, DNP, ACNS-BC
Associate Professor of Nursing
Essex County College
Newark, New Jersey

David J. Derrico, RN, MSN, CNE
Clinical Assistant Professor
University of Florida College of Nursing
Gainesville, Florida

Janice S. Dorman, PhD, MSHyg
Professor
Department of Health Promotion & Development
University of Pittsburgh, School of Nursing
Pittsburgh, Pennsylvania

Julie Eggert, PhD, GNP-BC, AGN-BC, AOCN(R), FAAN
Professor and Coordinator
Healthcare Genetics Doctoral Program, School of Nursing
College of Behavioral, Social and Health Sciences
Clemson University
Clemson, South Carolina;
Advanced Genetics Nurse, Cancer Risk Screening Program
Bon Secours St. Francis Cancer Center
Greenville, South Carolina

Charlene Beach Gagliardi, RN, BSN, MSN
Assistant Professor of Nursing
Mount Saint Mary's University
Los Angeles, California

Diane P. Genereux, PhD
Staff Scientist
Broad Institute of MIT and Harvard
Cambridge, Massachusetts

Sandra Kaminski, MS, PA-C
Physician Assistant
VA NJ Healthcare System
East Orange, New Jersey;
Adjunct Faculty
Pace University Physician Assistant Program
Manhattan, New York

Lori L. Kelly, RN, MSN, MBA
Associate Professor of Nursing
Aquinas College
Nashville, Tennessee

Kathryn Kennedy, MSN, ENC(C)
Program Head Emergency Nursing Specialty
British Columbia Institute of Technology
British Columbia, Canada

Stephen D. Krau, PhD, RN, CNE
Associate Professor
School of Nursing
Vanderbilt University Medical Center
Nashville, Tennessee

Josef Kren, ScD, PhD
Professor
Department of Biomedical Sciences
Bryan College of Health Sciences
Lincoln, Nebraska

Kayla R. Kroschel, CRNA, ARNP, MSNA
Certified Registered Nurse Anesthetist
Naples, Florida

Debora A. Lawson, DC, PhD
Adjunct Professor
College of Nursing
University of Missouri, St. Louis
St. Louis, Missouri

Dale Maughan, RN, MSN, PhD
Associate Professor of Nursing
Utah Valley University
Orem, Utah

Vikki McCleary, PhD, LRD
Associate Professor
Physician Assistant Studies
University of North Dakota School of Medicine and
    Health Sciences
Grand Forks, North Dakota

Gillian Meyers, RN, BSN
Oregon Health and Science University
Portland, Oregon

Katrina Dawn Miller, MSN, RN, CNL
Clinical Coordinator and Instructor
School of Nursing
Aquinas College
Nashville, Tennessee

Jason Mott, PhD, RN, CNE
Assistant Professor
University of Wisconsin Oshkosh College of Nursing
Oshkosh, Wisconsin

Jack Pennington, PhD
Professor of Nursing
Barnes Jewish College at Washington University
   Medical Center
St. Louis, Missouri

Patricia A. Rouen, PhD, FNP-BC, RN
Professor
Family Nurse Practitioner
McAuley School of Nursing
University of Detroit Mercy
Detroit, Michigan

Kathy Smith-Stillson, PhD, RN
Professor, Affiliate Faculty
Nursing and Biology
Colorado Christian University
Northglenn, Colorado;
Regis University
Denver, Colorado

Dr. Duncan Sproul
Cancer Research UK Career Development Fellow
Medical Research Council Human Genetics Unit and
   Edinburgh Cancer Research Centre
Medical Research Council Institute of Genetics and
   Molecular Medicine
University of Edinburgh
Edinburgh, United Kingdom

Kim Webb, MN, RN
Adjunct Nursing Professor
Pioneer Technology Center
Ponca City, Oklahoma

PREFACE

Pathophysiology incorporates basic, translational, and clinical research to advance understandings of disease and dysfunction. The study of pathophysiology involves many biomedical sciences and a wide range of research activities. Multiple aspects of cellular physiology are progressing rapidly, generating vast amounts of data to understand. The information expansion involves a greater understanding of the behavior of individual cells, their neighboring microenvironment, and the molecules that not only make up those cells but also communicate with their surroundings. Importantly, the forward movement of biomedical sciences occurs within the context of social, economic, and political processes that determine how disease is defined, experienced, and treated.

Interdisciplinary research has led to significant advancements in genetics, epigenetics, cell signaling and communication, control of cell behavior, metabolism, and cell fate. Knowledge about normal cell structures, function, and signaling pathways is at the forefront of translational science and foundational to the understanding of pathophysiology. Cells are nimble and respond to changes in their environment. Advancements in tools to observe cells are providing new understanding of cellular processes, including how cells function and prioritize their activities, monitor their environment, move, differentiate, and regenerate. For disease, conditions of cells under stress—for example, when stem cells become corrupted—help to define restorative activities that are lost. An important emerging goal is to learn what biologic *switches* restore function and reprogram the cell for normal function. Advances in the molecular mechanisms of disease, particularly cell signaling, genetic directives, and immune and metabolic modulators are providing an understanding of individual differences in disease risk, biologic markers, diagnostic strategies, and personally tailored treatment.

Although these advancements have created an ever-increasing state of excitement, they have also created the problem of how students, teachers, and clinicians can cope with the expanding new information. Translating and compressing these data into simplified discussions for students and clinicians is challenging. Our approach in this book has been to present an organized, logical sequence of content based on current literature and research reports with understandable explanations and accompanied by illustrations and summary tables. The primary focus is on pathophysiology, and there is less emphasis on the evaluation and treatment that is found in clinical management textbooks. As in previous editions, the following is a list of our specific goals for the textbook:

- Draw attention to differences in etiology, epidemiology, pathophysiology, clinical manifestations, and treatment according to sex and age.
- Pay careful attention to presentations of emerging new data on controversial topics.
- Integrate health promotion and disease prevention by updating risk factors, explaining certain relationships between nutrition and disease, and referencing screening recommendations and other therapeutic approaches.

ORGANIZATION AND CONTENT: WHAT'S NEW IN THE EIGHTH EDITION

The book is organized into two parts. Part One presents the cellular and tissue responses common to disease. Normal organ system structure and function and the pathophysiology of disease, organized by body systems, are presented in Part Two. All content has been reviewed and updated with extensive new references, revised figures, and one new chapter.

Part One: Central Concepts of Pathophysiology: Cells and Tissues

Part One begins with an in-depth study of the cell and progresses to cover the underlying processes of disease. Concepts covered include cell signaling and cell communication processes; genes and common genetic diseases; epigenetics and disease; fluid, electrolyte, and acid-base balance; inflammation, cytokines and their biologic functions, and normal and altered immunity; infection, stress, coping, and immunity; and tumor biology, epidemiology of cancer, and cancer in children. Particularly important revisions and updated additions to Part One include the following:

- Content on cellular organelles, the plasma membrane, cell signaling, and communication (Chapter 1)
- Content on agents of cell injury, oxidative stress, apoptosis, autophagy, and aging (Chapter 2)
- Chapter on epigenetics and disease (Chapter 6)
- Content on normal innate and adaptive immunity (Chapters 7 and 8)
- Content on alterations of immunity and inflammation (Chapter 9)
- Content on infection (Chapter 10)
- Reorganization of content on stress and disease (Chapter 11)
- Extensive revisions and reorganization of tumor biology and invasion and metastases (Chapter 12)
- Extensive revisions and reorganization of epidemiology of cancer (Chapter 13)

Part Two: Pathophysiologic Alterations: Organs and Systems

Part Two is a systematic survey of diseases within body systems. Each unit focuses on a specific body system and begins with an anatomy and physiology chapter to provide a basis of comparison for understanding the alterations created by disease. A brief summary of normal aging is included at the end of the section on anatomy and physiology. The discussion of each disease in the alterations chapters is developed in a logical manner that begins with an introductory paragraph on etiology and epidemiology, followed by pathophysiology, clinical manifestations, and evaluation and treatment, which are set off with icons. Separate chapters are dedicated to pediatric pathophysiology, and sensitivity is paid to sex and age. Chapter 23 is a new chapter on Obesity and Disorders of Nutrition. Especially significant revisions and updated additions to Part Two include the following:

- Information on pain syndromes and sleep disorders (Chapter 16)
- Content on concepts of alterations in consciousness, memory, and delirium syndromes; new information related to Parkinson disease; amyotrophic lateral sclerosis; Huntington disease; and the dementias, including Alzheimer disease (Chapter 17)
- Molecular mechanisms of traumatic brain and spinal cord injury, stroke and headache syndromes, and multiple sclerosis (Chapter 18)
- Updated content on schizophrenia, mood disorders, and anxiety (Chapter 19)
- Cerebral palsy, seizure disorders, and pediatric brain tumors (Chapter 20)
- Extensive updates on diabetes mellitus, insulin resistance, and thyroid and adrenal gland disorders (Chapter 22)

- A new chapter on obesity and disorders of nutrition with summaries of the eating disorders and starvation (Chapter 23)
- Extensively rewritten material on female reproductive disorders including cancers, benign breast diseases, and breast cancer (Chapter 25)
- A separate chapter on male reproductive disorders and cancer with extensive updating and reorganization (Chapter 26)
- Reorganization and extensive updating of sexually transmitted infections (Chapter 27)
- Bone marrow, blood cell formation, and hemostasis (Chapter 28)
- Revised content on alterations of leukocyte, lymphoid, and hemostatic function (Chapter 29)
- Extensively rewritten chapter on the anatomy and physiology of the cardiovascular and lymphatic systems (Chapter 32)
- Extensively updated coverage of atherosclerosis, endothelial injury and dysfunction, coronary artery disease, myocardial infarction, and heart failure (Chapter 33)
- Immune mechanisms of asthma; chronic lung disease; and updates for respiratory tract infection, pulmonary hypertension, pulmonary embolism, and lung cancers (Chapters 36)
- Major updates for childhood asthma, respiratory distress syndrome, cystic fibrosis, lung infections, and sudden infant death syndrome (Chapter 37)
- Kidney stones, urinary tract infection, glomerulopathies, acute and chronic renal failure, and bladder and kidney tumors (Chapter 39)
- Urinary tract infection and renal failure in children (Chapter 40)
- Gastroesophageal reflux disease, peptic ulcer disease, irritable bowel syndrome, inflammatory bowel disease, colon cancer, and hepatitis (Chapter 42)
- New information on gluten-sensitive enteropathy, necrotizing enterocolitis, infections of the intestine, and liver disease in children (Chapter 43)
- Updated content on alterations of the musculoskeletal system (Chapter 44)
- Pressure ulcers, dermatitis and psoriasis, scleroderma, and melanoma (Chapter 47)
- Childhood atopic dermatitis, skin infections, and immune drug reactions (Chapter 48)
- Extensive updating and reorganization of content on septic shock, multiple organ dysfunction syndrome, and burns for adults and children (Chapters 49 and 50)

FEATURES TO PROMOTE LEARNING

Ease of learning has been enhanced by designing a number of features that guide and support understanding, including:
- *Chapter Outlines* for each chapter
- *Consistent Headings with Icons* to underscore the consistent treatment of each disease—Pathophysiology, Clinical Manifestations, and Evaluation and Treatment
- More than 70 *What's New?* boxes that review the most current research and clinical developments; a list of these is included on the inside front cover
- *Nutrition & Disease* boxes to emphasize nutrition as a health promotion strategy that may alter disease risk or pathogenesis
- End-of-chapter *Summary Review* sections that summarize the content in each chapter and serve as built-in content review guides
- Boldface *Key Terms* with end-of-chapter term lists and page numbers for rapid access
- A comprehensive *Glossary* with approximately 1000 terms to help students with the often-difficult terminology related to pathophysiology

ART PROGRAM

The art program is extensive and has received as much attention and revision as the narrative. Nearly 100 new or revised full-color illustrations were created and strategically placed throughout the textbook. Also included are many new high-quality, full-color photographs of clinical manifestations, pathologic specimens, and clinical imaging techniques. The combination of illustrations, algorithms, and photographs and the use of color for tables and boxes allow clarification for complex concepts and the emergence of easily recognized essential information.

ANCILLARIES

For Students

On **Evolve**, at http://evolve.elsevier.com/McCance/, students can access Evolve-only figures, tables, and boxes, 570 review questions, 100 animations to help students master the text content, 26 case studies with questions and answers, and downloadable chapter summaries documents for each chapter.

The **Study Guide** includes a variety of question styles, aiming to help the diverse way students learn. Question types include the following:
- Choose the Correct Words
- Complete These Sentences
- Categorize These Clinical Examples
- Explain the Pictures
- Teach These People about Pathophysiology
- Plus many more…

Answers are found in the back of the Study Guide for easy reference for students.

For Instructors

The **Evolve Instructor Resources** for this textbook provide the following teaching aids:
- Image Collection with all of the approximately 1200 figures from the text
- PowerPoint lecture slides for each chapter (approximately 3300 slides and 440 images total), including integrated Audience Response Questions in each chapter (218 total), and integrated case studies at the end of each unit (15 total)
- Teach for Nurses Instructor's Manual, broken down by chapter, detailing the resources available to instructors for their lesson planning, and including unique case studies and class activities they can share with students
- Test Bank in ExamView with 1560 questions (in multiple choice and multiple response formats) with answers, rationales, and textbook page references

Evolve is an Internet-based learning environment that works in coordination with the text. This resource enables you to publish your class syllabus, outline, and lecture notes; set up "virtual office hours" and e-mail communication; share important dates and information through the online class calendar; and encourage student participation through chat rooms and discussion boards. Free with qualified adoption. Contact your sales representative or visit http://evolve.elsevier.com for more information about integrating **Evolve** into your curriculum.

ACKNOWLEDGMENTS

The enormous task of keeping this book current and readable greatly depends on our contributors; new writers have joined our team for this edition. We thank them for their knowledge and tremendous labor of reviewing relevant literature, synthesizing it, and writing and revising chapters to make them highly readable for others. Our section editors are Neal Rote and Tina Brashers, and we thank them for their tireless editing, writing, and development of new art. Neal managed the immunity, infection, and cancer biology chapters. Tina managed the endocrine, pulmonary, and cardiovascular alterations chapters. Both Neal and Tina are exceptional teachers and have a special ability to integrate, simplify, and illustrate the complex content of pathophysiology. Always motivated to *really* help students and clinicians, we are grateful to you both. In addition, Tina Brashers, Linda Turchin, and Amber Ballard developed modules for the Online Review Course. There were also many faculty and clinicians who provided critiques of content revision, and we appreciate their insight and recommendations.

We extend gratitude to those who contributed to the book supplements. Linda Felver has thoroughly updated the resourceful Study Guide. Thank you Linda for very astute edits. For the Evolve website, Joanna Cain updated the review questions and PowerPoints. Meg Blair updated and revised the Test Bank. Melanie Cole revised the Teach for Nurses Instructor's Manual. Also thank you to Joanna Cain who aided in the update of the glossary. Thank you all for your help.

Sue Meeks is the leader of our manuscript management team. Her "behind the scenes" work is extensive and complex and completed with tireless effort, insight, and humor. Every edition is monumental work—and she retypes and recounts endlessly—and unruffled. She coordinates transfer of the manuscript between editors, contributors, and reviewers. For more than 32 years she has provided unwavering dedication to excellence and detail, keeping us sane and on track. As always, you have our deepest appreciation for your continuing skill and patience.

Our production team and editorial staff at Elsevier deserve special recognition. Karen Turner and Jennifer Wade are our Content Development Specialists. This job is key. Karen monitored and suggested edits with an eagle eye and was especially helpful with illustrations. Her questions were thoughtful and critically timed. Jennifer Wade helped keep things moving along so we didn't lose sight of our goals. Beth Welch and Kristin Landon, our copyeditors, were thorough, consistent, and vital for getting the manuscript ready for publication. Thank you all for the top-notch quality of work. Executive Content Strategist Kellie White helped with the overall planning and production of the book and all the business needed for contributors, designers, artists, and other editors. This is a big job, and Kellie made sure that we had all resources necessary to complete this book. Thank you, Kellie.

The production manager for a book of this size and complexity of content has an enormous responsibility. The Senior Project Manager was Mary Pohlman. From copy edit to final page proofs with unremitting attention, Mary was masterful. Her persistent diligence was noteworthy and kept us on schedule. Thank you, Mary. The design of the interior portion of the book was in the capable hands of Ashely Miner and we are especially pleased with the layout, dynamic colors, and presentation of pedagogy. She also coordinated the work that went into creating the striking cover design. Thank you, Ashley.

The newly drawn and revised artwork for this edition was completed by Graphic World. The art is key and challenging, and our initial drawings are often pathetic. Graphic World assisted with the conceptual arrangements, labels, and beautiful colors.

We also thank the Department of Dermatology at the University of Utah School of Medicine, which provided numerous photos of skin lesions. Thanks to Dr. John Hoffman for the PET scan images of non–small cell lung cancer.

We are grateful to the many colleagues and friends at the University of Utah Health Sciences Center for their assistance with references and consultation on content. Special thanks are given to students, particularly nursing and other health science students, for the e-mails and phone calls we receive. Your questions are vital to guide us in our efforts to prepare a clear and up-to-date manuscript with much visual impact.

Sincerely and with great affection we thank our families, especially John, Mae, and Dorothy. Although disentangling certain data is inconvenient at times, we thank those committed to increasing patient-centered quality care, safety, and satisfaction.

Kathryn L. McCance
Sue E. Huether

The word root "patho" is derived from the Greek word *pathos,* which means suffering. The Greek word root "logos" means discourse or, more commonly, system of formal study, and "physio" pertains to functions of organisms. Generally, pathophysiology is the systematic study of the functional changes in cells, tissues, and organs altered by disease and/or injury. Important, however, is the inextricable component of suffering.

Knowledge of cellular biology as well as anatomy and physiology and the various organ systems of the body is an essential foundation for the study of pathophysiology. To understand pathophysiology the student must also use principles, concepts, and basic knowledge from other fields of study, including biology, genetics, immunology, pathology, and epidemiology. A number of terms are used to focus the discussion of pathophysiology; they may be used interchangeably at times, but that does not necessarily indicate that they have the same meaning. These terms are reviewed in Table I-1.

Pathophysiology is one of the most important bridging sciences between preclinical and clinical courses for students in the health sciences, and it requires in-depth study at an early stage in the curriculum. The definitions or conceptual models of pathophysiology that we carry in our minds influence what we do with our observations and the rationale that we provide for our actions. Therefore, the clinician must understand that although pathophysiology is a science, it also designates suffering in people; the clinician should never lose sight of this aspect of its definition.

As students study clinically-related sciences, they learn to recognize and categorize disease. From the formulation of a differential diagnosis one understands the different *clinical manifestations,* the signs, and the symptoms of certain pathologies. These understandings structure further investigations, treatment plans, and evaluation. The interaction of these activities determines clinical outcomes and treatment success. Still, the concept of disease can be inherently ambiguous and elusive; many pathologies remain hidden and resist easy classification. One should appreciate that the naming and diagnosing of diseases involve evaluative judgments as well as scientific fact, and that the process is as much a social endeavor as it is a scientific one. Some diseases, such as tuberculosis, identify a highly specific causative or etiologic agent or process. Others, such as Alzheimer disease or arthritis, indicate pathologic changes of unclear cause. There is considerable need for more research to validate mental health diagnoses. In addition, syndromes and functional disorders simply describe multiple symptoms and signs that frequently occur together. Does commonality exist in all of these labels? The answer is "yes" and "no" and depends on our conception of health and disease. In the strictest sense, objective scientific facts help us know if an individual is healthy or suffering from disease and disability. A critical question remains: "Are we living longer, healthy lives as well as longer lives?" The fraction of the United States population aged 65 and over has increased. Older Americans are living longer, and the proportion of life spent with disability is changing. A recent finding for people 65 years and older was that the proportion of life spent with disability decreased, but this finding was not shared among the younger, aging population. In the young, researchers speculate that the increase in disability with aging may have resulted from change in emphasis on mental health, the rise in autism and attention deficit hyperactivity disorder, and the changing patterns of drug use overtime.[1] More studies related to these questions need to be done.

An individual's conception of disease is based on personal beliefs and histories, professional and lay healers who interact with that individual, and society at large. Each idea or construct has the power to influence other ideas and constructs, and each relationship has the ability to shape the way disease is understood and experienced.[2] Although a discerning mind is key, education for collaboration and tolerance of uncertainty or ambiguity is necessary for the changing science and understanding of disease.

Pathophysiology has had great success in explaining the mechanisms and clinical manifestations associated with infectious diseases. Syndromes of unclear etiology, such as chronic fatigue syndrome or fibromyalgia, have proven to be troublesome. Even more difficult are multifactorial conditions, such as atherosclerosis or type 2 diabetes mellitus, where several interacting factors contribute to the etiology. Learning how interacting factors relate to one another to increase morbidity or actually cause disease contributes to an appreciation of how emerging concepts revolutionize current understandings. One revolution in thought that has driven intensive research is that low levels of chronic inflammation cause or contribute to many diseases.

The language that clinicians use to discuss diseases and their manifestations is powerful. Lives are altered by a few words uttered by a clinician in a white coat or uniform. "AIDS," "cancer," and "heart attack"

TABLE I-1	TERMS AND DEFINITIONS RELATED TO PATHOPHYSIOLOGY
Pathology	Study of structural alterations in cells, tissues, and organs that help to identify the cause of disease
Pathogenesis	Pattern of tissue changes associated with the development of disease
Etiology	Study of the cause(s) of disease and/or injury
Idiopathic	Diseases with no identifiable cause
Iatrogenic	Diseases and/or injury as a result of medical intervention
Clinical manifestations	Signs and symptoms
Nosocomial	Diseases acquired as a consequence of being in a hospital environment
Diagnosis	Naming or identification of a disease
Prognosis	Expected outcome of a disease
Acute disease	Sudden appearance of signs and symptoms lasting a short time
Chronic disease	Develops more slowly, lasting a long time or a lifetime
Remissions	Periods when clinical manifestations disappear or diminish significantly
Exacerbations	Periods when clinical manifestations become worse or more severe
Sequelae	Any abnormal conditions that follow and are the result of a disease, treatment, or injury

have become culturally ingrained symbols that portend an individual's future. Although some futures are determined by scientific evidence, others are determined by subjective experience.[3] For example, a person diagnosed with a familial disease may ask, "Will I suffer like my mother did?" This questioning influences individuals' suffering.

In conclusion, pathophysiology—the understanding of disease—requires descriptive evidence as well as an evaluative component regarding suffering and the language we use to describe it. Combining objective and subjective perspectives requires new conceptual models that take into account the complex interactions among the body, mind, environment, and spirit.

REFERENCES

1. Crimmins EM, Zhang Y, Saito Y: Trends over 4 decades in disability-free life expectancy in the United States. *Am J Public Health* 106(7):1287–1293, 2016.
2. Magid C: Developing tolerance for ambiguity. *JAMA* 285(1):88, 2001.
3. Goldstein J: In the twilight: life in the margins between sick and well. *JAMA* 285(1):92, 2001.

CONTENTS

PART TWO: Pathophysiologic Alterations: Organs and Systems, 433

UNIT V The Neurologic System

Central Concepts of Pathophysiology: Cells and Tissues

CHAPTER

1

Cellular Biology

Kathryn L. McCance

evolve WEBSITE

CHAPTER OUTLINE

All body functions depend on the integrity of cells. Therefore, an understanding of cellular biology is intrinsically necessary for an understanding of disease. An overwhelming amount of information is revealing how cells behave as a multicellular "social" organism. At the heart of cellular biology is cellular communication ("cellular crosstalk")—how messages originate and are transmitted, received, interpreted, and used by the cell. This streamlined conversation between, among, and within cells maintains cellular function and specialization. Intercellular signals allow each cell to determine its position and specialized role. Cells must demonstrate a "chemical fondness" for other cells and their surrounding environment to maintain the integrity of the entire organism. When they no longer tolerate this fondness, the conversation breaks down and cells either adapt (sometimes altering function) or become vulnerable to isolation, injury, disease, or even death.

PROKARYOTES AND EUKARYOTES

Living cells generally are divided into two major classes—eukaryotes and prokaryotes. The cells of higher animals and plants are eukaryotes, as are the single-celled organisms fungi, protozoa, and most algae. Prokaryotes include cyanobacteria (blue-green algae), bacteria, and rickettsiae. Prokaryotes traditionally were studied as core subjects of molecular biology. Current emphasis is on the eukaryotic cell; much of its structure and function has no counterpart in bacterial cells.

Eukaryotes (*eu* = good; *karyon* = nucleus; also spelled "eucaryotes") are larger and have more extensive intracellular anatomy and organization than do prokaryotes. Eukaryotic cells have a characteristic set of membrane-bound intracellular compartments, called *organelles,* that includes a well-defined nucleus. Prokaryotes contain no organelles, and their nuclear material is not encased by a nuclear membrane. Prokaryotic cells are characterized by lack of a distinct nucleus.

Besides having structural differences, prokaryotic and eukaryotic cells differ in chemical composition and biochemical activity. The *nuclei* of prokaryotic cells carry genetic information in a single circular chromosome, and they lack a class of proteins called *histones,* which in eukaryotic cells bind with deoxyribonucleic acid (DNA) and are involved in the supercoiling of DNA (see Fig. 1.2). We now understand that the loops and coiling of DNA are important for many diseases. Eukaryotic cells have several chromosomes. Protein production, or synthesis, in the two classes of cells also differs because of major structural differences in ribonucleic acid (RNA)–protein complexes. Other distinctions include differences in mechanisms of transport across the outer cellular membrane and differences in enzyme content.

CELLULAR FUNCTIONS

Cells become specialized through the process of differentiation, or maturation, so that some cells eventually perform one kind of function and other cells perform other functions. Cells with a highly developed function, such as movement, often lack some other property, such as hormone production, which is more highly developed in some other type of specialized cell.

The eight chief cellular functions follow:
- *Movement.* Muscle cells can generate forces that produce motion. Muscles that are attached to bones produce limb movements, whereas those that enclose hollow tubes or cavities move or empty contents when they contract. For example, the contraction of smooth muscle cells surrounding blood vessels changes the diameter of the vessels; the contraction of muscles in walls of the urinary bladder expels urine.
- *Conductivity.* Conduction as a response to a stimulus is manifested by a wave of excitation, an electrical potential that passes along the surface of the cell to reach its other parts. Conductivity is the chief function of nerve cells.
- *Metabolic absorption.* All cells take in and use nutrients and other substances from their surroundings. Cells of the intestine and the kidney are specialized to carry out absorption. Cells of the kidney tubules reabsorb fluids and synthesize proteins. Intestinal epithelial cells reabsorb fluids and synthesize protein enzymes.
- *Secretion.* Certain cells, such as mucous gland cells, can synthesize new substances from substances they absorb and then secrete the new substances to serve as needed elsewhere. Cells of the adrenal gland, testis, and ovary can secrete hormonal steroids.
- *Excretion.* All cells can rid themselves of waste products resulting from the metabolic breakdown of nutrients. Membrane-bound sacs

(lysosomes) within cells contain enzymes that break down, or digest, large molecules, turning them into waste products that are released from the cell.
- *Respiration.* Cells absorb oxygen, which is used to transform nutrients into energy in the form of adenosine triphosphate (ATP). Cellular respiration, or oxidation, occurs in organelles called *mitochondria.*
- *Reproduction.* Tissue growth occurs as cells enlarge and reproduce themselves. Even without growth, tissue maintenance requires that new cells be produced to replace cells that are lost normally through cellular death. Not all cells are capable of continuous division.
- *Communication.* Communication is vital for cells to survive as a society of cells. Pancreatic cells, for instance, secrete and release insulin necessary to signal muscle cells to absorb sugar from the blood for energy. Constant communication allows the maintenance of a dynamic steady state.

STRUCTURE AND FUNCTION OF CELLULAR COMPONENTS

Fig. 1.1 shows a "typical" eukaryotic cell. It consists of three components: an outer membrane called the *plasma membrane,* or *plasmalemma;* a fluid filling called cytoplasm; and the intracellular "organs," or *organelles,* which are membrane bound and include the nucleus. Researchers are astounded by the advances in microscopy and computer software that allow resolution to the nanoscale—cells seem to come "alive" with the molecular world more visible. Understanding structure and function will reveal, for example, how the cell responds to mechanical forces or emerges from different gene expression patterns. The overall impact on biology is huge.[1]

Nucleus

The nucleus, which is surrounded by the cytoplasm and generally is located in the center of the cell, is the largest membrane-bound organelle. Two pliable membranes comprise the nuclear envelope (Fig. 1.2, *A*). The nuclear envelope is pockmarked with pits, called nuclear pores, in which nuclear pore complexes (NPCs) are positioned that allow molecules to move between the nucleus and the cytosol (see Fig. 1.2, *A, B, and D*). The outer membrane is continuous with membranes of the endoplasmic reticulum (see Fig. 1.1). The inner membrane encloses the nucleus. The nucleus contains the nucleolus, a small, dense structure composed largely of RNA; most of the cellular DNA; and the DNA-binding proteins, the histones, that regulate its activity. The DNA chain in eukaryotic cells is so extensive that the risk of breakage is high. Therefore, the histones binding to DNA cause DNA to fold into chromosomes (Fig. 1.2, *C*). The wrapping of DNA into tight packages of chromosomes is essential for cell division in eukaryotes.

The primary functions of the nucleus are cell division and control of genetic information. Other functions include the replication and repair of DNA and the transcription of the information stored in DNA. Genetic information is transcribed into RNA, which can be processed into messenger, transport, and ribosomal RNA and introduced into the cytoplasm, where it directs cellular activities. Most of the processing of RNA occurs in the nucleolus.

Cytoplasmic Organelles

Cytoplasm is an aqueous solution (cytosol) that fills the cytoplasmic matrix—the space between the nuclear envelope and the plasma membrane. The cytosol represents about half the volume of a eukaryotic cell. It contains thousands of enzymes involved in intermediate metabolism and is crowded with ribosomes that make proteins. The cytosol

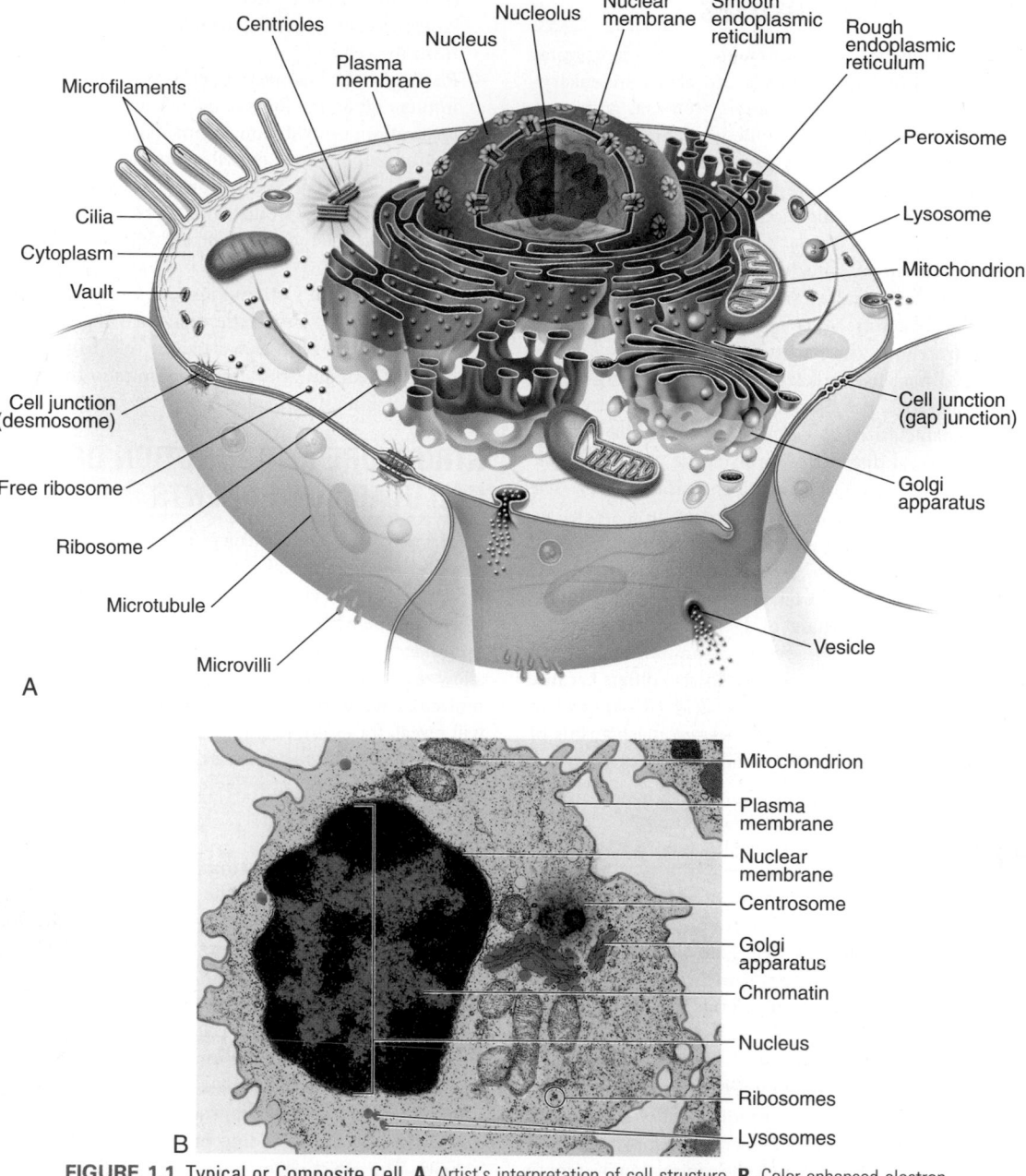

FIGURE 1.1 Typical or Composite Cell. A, Artist's interpretation of cell structure. **B,** Color-enhanced electron micrograph of a cell. Both show the many mitochondria known as the "power plants of the cell." Note, too, the innumerable dots bordering the endoplasmic reticulum. These are ribosomes, the cell's "protein factories." (**B** courtesy A. Arlan Hinchee. From Patton KT, Thibodeau GA: *Anatomy & physiology,* ed 9, St Louis, 2016, Mosby.)

is the main site for protein synthesis and degradation. Newly synthesized proteins remain in the cytosol if they lack a sorting signal for transport to a cell organelle.[2] The organelles suspended in the cytoplasm are enclosed in biologic membranes, which enables them to simultaneously carry out functions that require different biochemical environments. These functions, many of which are directed by coded messages carried from the nucleus by RNA, include synthesis of proteins and hormones and their transport out of the cell, isolation and elimination of waste products from the cell, metabolic processes, breakdown and disposal of cellular debris and foreign proteins (antigens), and maintenance of cellular structure and motility. Also, the cytosol functions as a storage unit for fat, carbohydrate, and secretory vesicles.

Ribosomes

Ribosomes are RNA-protein complexes (nucleoproteins) that are synthesized in the nucleolus and secreted into the cytoplasm through pores in the nuclear envelope called nuclear pore complexes (NPCs). These tiny ribosomes may float free in the cytoplasm or attach themselves to the outer membranes of the endoplasmic reticulum (see Fig. 1.1, *A*). Their chief function is to provide sites for cellular protein synthesis. Newly formed ribosomes synthesize a "recognition sequence," or signal, like an address on a letter. Signal recognition particles (SRPs) in the cytosol bind to the ribosome after recognizing the SRP. *Ribophorins,* receiver proteins found on the rough sections of the endoplasmic reticulum (ER), act as the "address" site or binding site. The developing

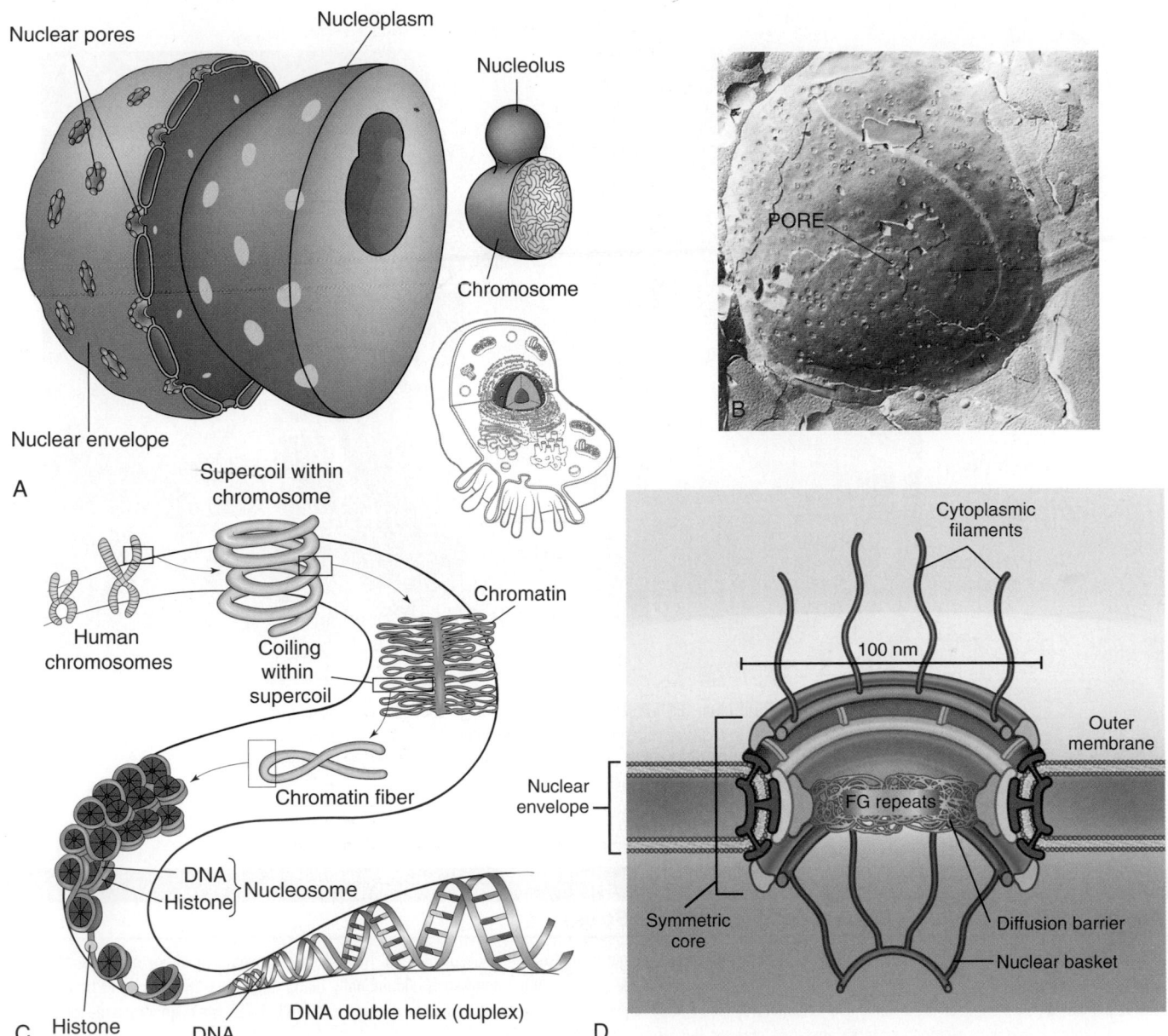

FIGURE 1.2 The Nucleus. The nucleus is composed of a double membrane, called a nuclear envelope, that encloses the fluid-filled interior, called nucleoplasm. The chromosomes are suspended in the nucleoplasm (illustrated here much larger than actual size to show the tightly packed DNA strands). Swelling at one or more points of the chromosome, shown in **A,** occurs at a nucleolus where genes are being copied into RNA. The nuclear envelope is studded with pores. **B,** The pores are visible as dimples in this freeze etch of a nuclear envelope. **C,** Histone-folding DNA in chromosomes. **D,** Nuclear pore complex. (**B** from Raven PH, Johnson GB: *Biology,* St Louis, 1992, Mosby. **D** adapted from *The scientist: infographic: the nuclear pore complex.* Available at http://www.the-scientist.com/?articles. view/articleNo/47560/title/Infographic-The-Nuclear-Pore-Complex/.)

protein threads its way through the ER membrane into the lumen. The SRP is removed and the new protein chain is folded into its final conformation.

Endoplasmic Reticulum

The **endoplasmic reticulum (ER)** (*endo* = within; *plasma* = cytoplasm; *reticulum* = network) is a membrane factory that specializes in the synthesis and transport of the protein and lipid components of most of the cell's organelles. It consists of a network of tubular or saclike channels (cisternae) that extend throughout the cytoplasm and are continuous with the outer nuclear membrane (Fig. 1.3). The folded

membranes that comprise the cisternae of the endoplasmic reticulum may be *rough* (granular) or *smooth* (agranular). The **rough endoplasmic reticulum (rER)** is rough because ribosomes and ribonucleoprotein particles are attached to it (see Fig. 1.3). Some of the proteins synthesized by these ribosomes remain in the ER, and others are used to construct membranes of other organelles (the Golgi complex, lysosomes, peroxisomes, and the nucleus) and of the cell itself. Importantly, the ER is responsible for much of a cell's protein synthesis and folding, and a new role for the ER is sensing cellular stress (see *What's New?* Endoplasmic Reticulum, Protein Folding, and ER Stress). Understanding mechanisms of cellular stress will aid diagnosis and treatment of disease.

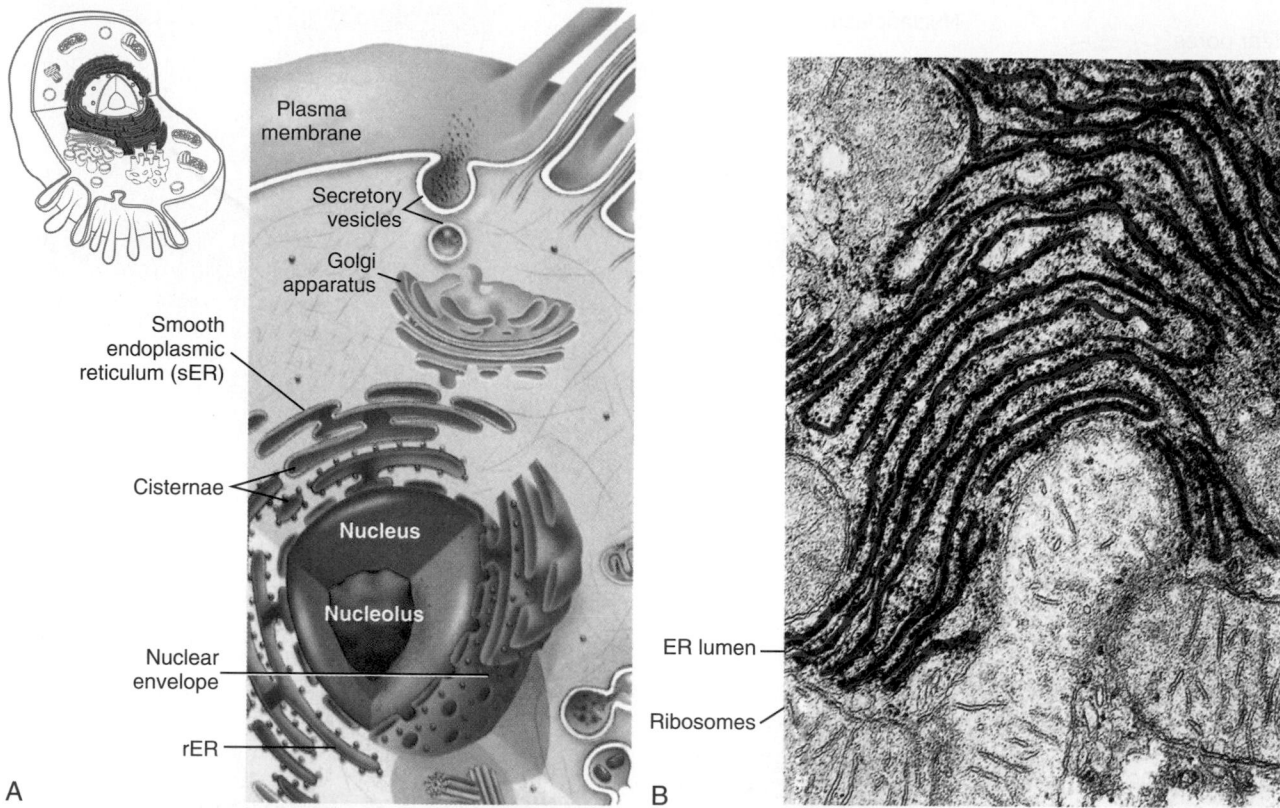

A

B

FIGURE 1.3 Endoplasmic Reticulum (ER). **A,** The ER consists of rough endoplasmic reticulum *(rER)* arranged into ribosome-coated cisternae and vesicles of smooth endoplasmic reticulum *(sER)*. **B,** Electron micrograph of rough and smooth ER. (**B** courtesy Kelloes C, Farmer M: Center for Advanced Ultrastructural Research, University of Georgia. From Lindsay DT: *Functional human anatomy,* St Louis, 1996, Mosby.)

WHAT'S NEW?

Endoplasmic Reticulum, Protein Folding, and ER Stress

Protein folding in the endoplasmic reticulum (ER) is critical for us. As the biologic workhorses, proteins perform vital functions in every cell. To do these tasks, proteins must fold into complex three-dimensional structures (see figure). Most secreted proteins *fold* and are modified in an error-free manner, but ER or cell stress, mutations, or random (stochastic) errors during protein synthesis can decrease the folding amount or the rate of folding. Pathophysiologic processes, such as viral infections, environmental toxins, and mutant protein expression, can perturb the sensitive ER environment. Natural processes also can perturb the environment, such as the large protein-synthesizing load placed on the ER. These perturbations cause the accumulation of immature and abnormal proteins in cells, leading to **ER stress**. Fortunately, the ER is loaded with protective ways to help folding, for example, protein so-called *chaperones* that facilitate folding and prevent the formation of off-pathway types. Because specialized cells produce large amounts of secreted proteins, the movement or flux through the ER is tremendous. Therefore, misfolded proteins not repaired in the ER are observed in some diseases and can initiate apoptosis or cell death. It has recently been shown that the endoplasmic reticulum mediates intracellular signaling pathways in response to the accumulation of unfolded or misfolded proteins; collectively, the adaptive pathways are known as the **unfolded-protein response (UPR)**. Investigators are studying UPR-associated inflammation and how the UPR is coupled to inflammation in health and disease. Specific diseases include Alzheimer disease, Parkinson disease, prion disease, amyotrophic lateral sclerosis, diabetes mellitus, and sepsis. Additionally being studied is ER stress and how it may accelerate age-related dysfunction. Overall, the ER is a major organelle for protein quality control.

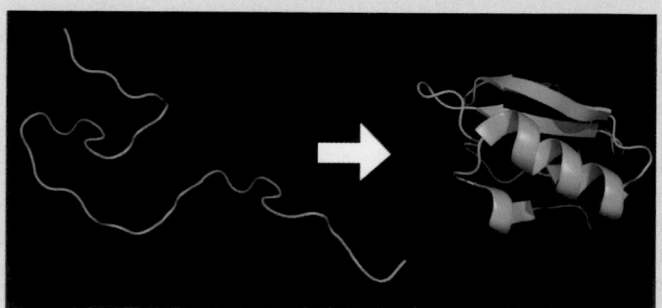

Protein Folding

Each protein exists as an unfolded polypeptide *(left)* or a random coil after the process of translation from a sequence of mRNA to a linear string of amino acids. From amino acids interacting with each other they produce a three-dimensional structure called the folded protein *(right)* that is its native state.

Data from Alberts B et al: *Molecular biology of the cell,* ed 6, New York, 2015, Garland Science; Brodsky J, Skach WR: *Curr Opin Cell Biol* 23:464–475, 2011; Jäger R et al: *Biol Cell* 104(5):259–270, 2012; Khan MM, Yang VVL, Wang P: *Shock* 44(4):294–304, 2015; Shah SZ et al: *J Mol Neurosci* 57(4):529–537, 2015.

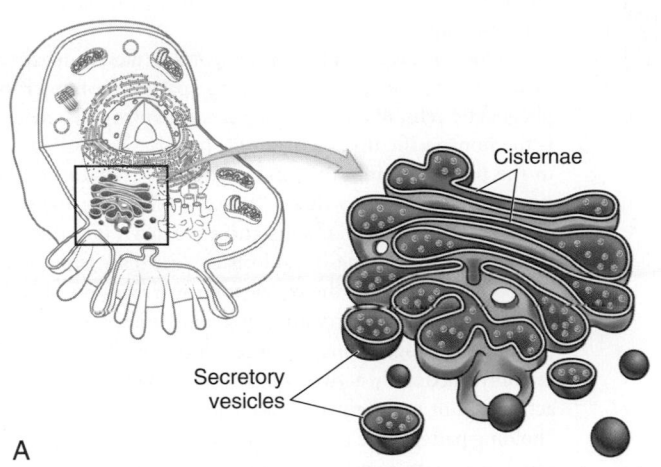
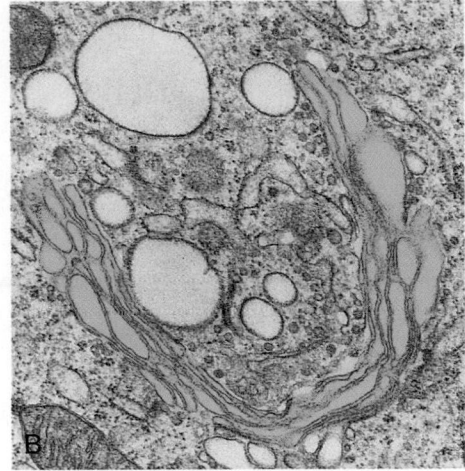

Cisternae

Secretory
vesicles

A

B

FIGURE 1.4 Golgi Complex. A, Schematic representation of the Golgi complex showing a stack of flattened sacs, or cisternae, and numerous small membranous bubbles, or secretory vesicles. **B,** Transmission electron micrograph showing the Golgi complex highlighted with color. (**B** Courtesy Charles Flickinger, University of Virginia.)

Smooth endoplasmic reticulum (sER) does not contain ribosomes or ribonucleoprotein particles (see Fig. 1.1). Rather, membranous surfaces of the smooth endoplasmic reticulum contain enzymes involved in the synthesis of steroid hormones and are responsible for a variety of reactions required to remove toxic substances from the cell. The endoplasmic reticulum communicates with the Golgi complex and interacts with other organelles, particularly lysosomes and peroxisomes.

Golgi Complex

The Golgi complex (or Golgi apparatus) is a network of flattened, smooth membranes and vesicles frequently located near the nucleus of the cell (Fig. 1.4). Proteins from the endoplasmic reticulum are processed and packaged into small membrane-bound sacs or vesicles called secretory vesicles, which collect at the end of the membranous folds of the Golgi bodies—called cisternae (like a stack of pita breads). The secretory vesicles then break off from the Golgi complex and migrate to a variety of intracellular and extracellular destinations, including the plasma membrane. The vesicles fuse with the plasma membrane, and their contents are released from the cell. The best-known vesicles are those that have coats made largely of the protein clathrin and are called *clathrin-coated vesicles.* They bud from the Golgi complex on the outward secretory pathway and from the plasma membrane on the inward endocytic pathway. Newly synthesized ER proteins are carried from the Golgi network to *endosomes* by clathrin-coated transport vesicles before progressing to lysosomes. Many molecules, including lipids, proteins, glycoproteins, and enzymes of lysosomes, pass through the Golgi complex at some stage in their maturation. The Golgi complex is a refining plant and directs traffic (e.g., protein, polynucleotide, polysaccharide molecules) in the cell[2] (Fig. 1.5).

Lysosomes

Lysosomes (*lyso* = dissolution; *soma* = body) are membrane-enclosed organelles (saclike) filled with enzymes that digest macromolecules and defunct intracellular organelles and particles engulfed from outside the cell by endocytosis (see Fig. 1.1, *A*). They contain more than 60 digestive enzymes called hydrolases, which catalyze bonds in proteins, lipids, nucleic acids, and carbohydrates. Hydrolases function optimally at an acidic pH. Lysosomes function as the intracellular digestive system

(Fig. 1.6, *A*). Lysosomal enzymes are capable of digesting most cellular constituents completely to their basic components, such as amino acids, nucleotides, and carbohydrates. Transport proteins in the lysosome membrane carry these final components to the cytosol where the cell can reuse or excrete them. Recent data have radically shifted the view that lysosomes are not just trash cans and recycling agents but have established a *central role* of the lysosome in nutrient-dependent signal transduction for cellular adaptation.[3] The newly discovered signaling function cooperates with the known degradative role of the lysosome to mediate basic cellular functions, such as nutrient-sensing metabolic adaptation, and quality control of proteins and organelles.[3] Complex transcriptional programs control the synthesis, composition, and quantity of lysosomes and regulate their activity to match the evolving needs of the cell. Alterations in these essential functions are central to the pathophysiology of an expanding range of conditions and include storage diseases, neurodegenerative diseases, and cancer.[3] Lysosomes maintain cellular health because of efficient removal of toxic cellular components, removal of useless organelles, termination of signal transduction, and maintenance of metabolic homeostasis. Aging can lead to progressive loss of lysosomal efficiency and decline of the regenerative capacity of organs and tissues.[4] Lysosomes are key signaling hubs of a sophisticated network for cellular adaptation, and the network includes ion and nutrient transporters, protein kinases and phosphatases, and transcription factors and transcriptional regulators.[3] Altogether these components integrate functions, such as nutrient abundance, energy levels, and cell stressors, and translate them into instructions that regulate cellular metabolism toward either proliferation or inactivity.[3] The signaling functions have far-reaching implications for metabolic regulation in health and in disease.

The lysosomal membrane acts as a protective shield between the powerful digestive enzymes within the lysosome and the cytoplasm, preventing their leakage into the cytoplasmic matrix. Disruption of the membrane by various treatments or cellular injury leads to a release of the lysosomal enzymes, which can then react with their specific substrates, causing *cellular self-digestion.* Lysosomal abnormalities are involved in a number of conditions that involve cellular injury and death.

Lysosomal storage diseases (LSDs) may be the result of a genetic defect or lack of one or more lysosomal enzymes. For example, the lack

include (1) endocytosis, (2) phagocytosis, (3) macropinocytosis, and (4) autophagy (Fig. 1.6, *A*).

Endocytosis is the uptake of macromolecules from extracellular fluid; phagocytosis is engulfment of large particles or microorganisms in phagocytic cells, like macrophages and neutrophils; macropinocytosis is the nonspecific uptake of fluids, membrane, and particles attached to the plasma membrane; and autophagy (self-eating) begins in the cytosol and is used to digest cytosol and ineffectual organelles[2] (see Chapter 2). Extracellular substances are taken into the cell and encapsulated in a membrane-bound vesicle (see discussion on endocytosis). Lysosomes merge with the vesicle to form a digestive vacuole. Lysosomes remain fully active by maintaining a low internal pH. They do this by pumping hydrogen ions into their interiors. The hydrolytic enzymes are only maximally active at acidic pH values. Lysosomes that are not active do not maintain such an acidic internal pH. Lysosomes in this "holding pattern" are called primary lysosomes. When a primary lysosome fuses with a vacuole or other organelle, its pH decreases and the hydrolytic enzymes become activated. When it becomes active, it is called a secondary lysosome, or heterophagosome (Fig. 1.6, *B*).

As cells complete their life span and die, lysosomes digest the resultant debris or obsolete parts by autophagy. Lysosomes involved in this process, which is called autodigestion, are called autolysosomes, or autophagosomes (Fig. 1.6, *A* and *B*). In living cells, cellular debris is encapsulated within a vesicle that reacts with a lysosome to complete its degradation. Autophagy promotes homeostasis because it involves continuous biosynthesis and cell turnover. Therefore, autophagy plays a crucial role in health. Defects in autophagy may challenge disposal mechanisms from removing microbes, unnecessary protein aggregates, and abnormal proteins, resulting in contributions to disease ranging from infectious disorders to neurodegeneration and cancer.

Products of autophagy (and of phagocytosis) pass out of the lysosome and are reused by the cell. Indigestible material is stored in vesicles called residual bodies, whose contents are actively expelled from the cell (see Fig. 1.6). High concentrations of lipids may accumulate within the residual bodies and remain there for a long time. The lipids are eventually oxidized, and a pigmented substance containing polyunsaturated fatty acids and proteins accumulates in the cell. This pigmented substance, termed *lipofuscin*, is often called "age pigment" or "age spots," and is noted in older individuals.

Peroxisomes

Peroxisomes (microbodies) are membrane-bound organelles that contain several oxidative enzymes such as *catalase* and *urate oxidase*. These oxidative enzymes can detoxify compounds and fatty acids. Similar to lysosomes in microscopic appearance, peroxisomes are larger and oval or irregular in shape. Like mitochondria, peroxisomes are major sites of oxygen utilization. Peroxisomes are so named because they usually contain enzymes that use oxygen to remove hydrogen atoms from specific substrates in an oxidative reaction that produces hydrogen peroxide (H_2O_2). Hydrogen peroxide is a powerful oxidant, potentially destructive if it accumulates or escapes from peroxisomes. Catalase, an antioxidant enzyme, uses the H_2O_2 to oxidize a variety of other substrates—phenols, formic acid, formaldehyde, and alcohol—by the peroxidative reaction:

$$H_2O_2 + R^1H_2 \rightarrow R^1 + 2H_2O$$

Thus the breakdown of H_2O_2 yields H_2O and O_2 (see discussion of free radicals in Chapter 2). Peroxisomes also have an important role in the synthesis of specialized phospholipids necessary for nerve cell myelination. Such reactions are important in detoxifying various wastes within the cell or foreign components that enter the cell, such as ethanol. Impairment of peroxisomes can lead to disease.

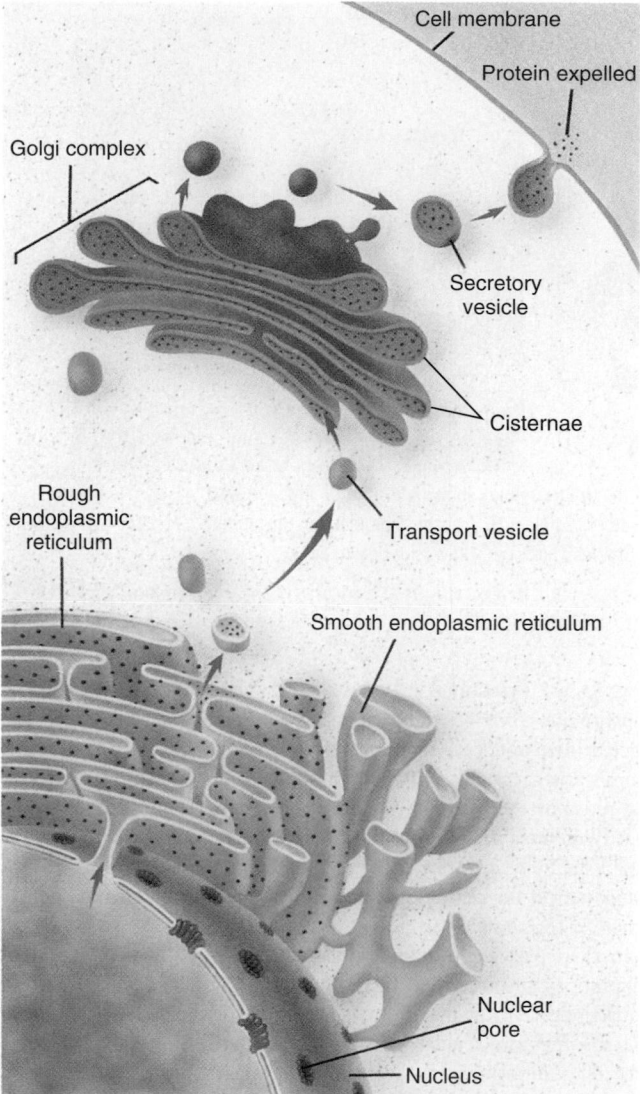

FIGURE 1.5 How the Internal Membrane System of a Cell Packages a Protein for Export. The instructions for making a protein that is destined for export from a cell, such as a digestive enzyme made by a pancreas cell, are first transcribed from DNA by RNA in the nucleus. The RNA then leaves the nucleus through a nuclear pore and proceeds to a ribosome located on the rough endoplasmic reticulum (rER). There, it provides instructions for the correct sequence of amino acids for synthesizing that particular digestive enzyme. When enzyme synthesis is complete, the enzyme travels through the ER and is then encapsulated in a transport vesicle. The transport vesicle fuses with a Golgi body, releasing the enzyme. In the Golgi complex the enzyme is further modified and is then shunted to the flattened stacks, or cisternae. There, the enzyme waits for a secretory vesicle, which will carry it to the perimeter of the cell, the cell membrane. The secretory vesicle membrane then fuses with the cell membrane, and the enzyme is released outside the cell. (From Raven PH, Johnson GB: *Understanding biology*, ed 3, Dubuque, IA, 1995, Brown.)

of lysosomal α-1,4-glucosidase leads to an accumulation of glycogen in lysosomes known as *Pompe disease*. Tay-Sachs disease is characterized by an accumulation of GM2 ganglioside (a lipid) in lysosomes as a result of the deficiency or absence of lysosomal hexosaminidase A. In gout, undigested uric acid accumulates within lysosomes, damaging the lysosomal membrane. Subsequent enzyme leakage results in cell death and tissue injury. Four pathways of degradation in lysosomes

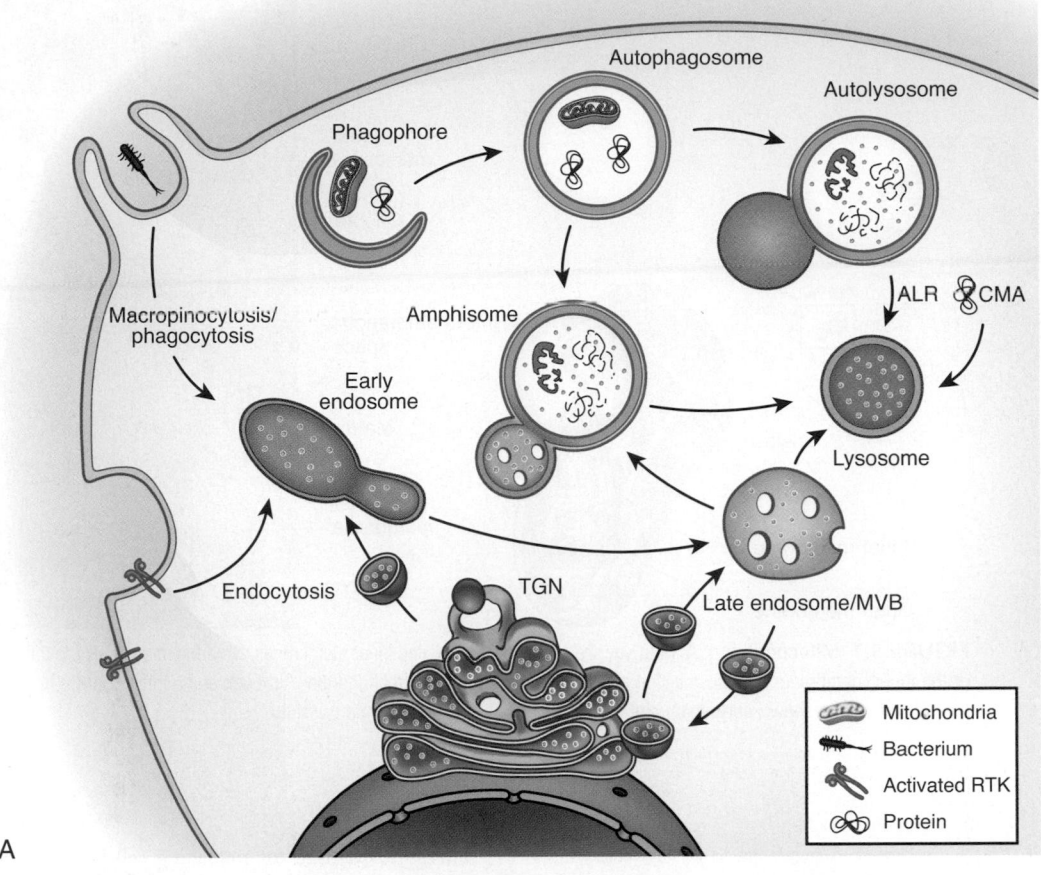

A

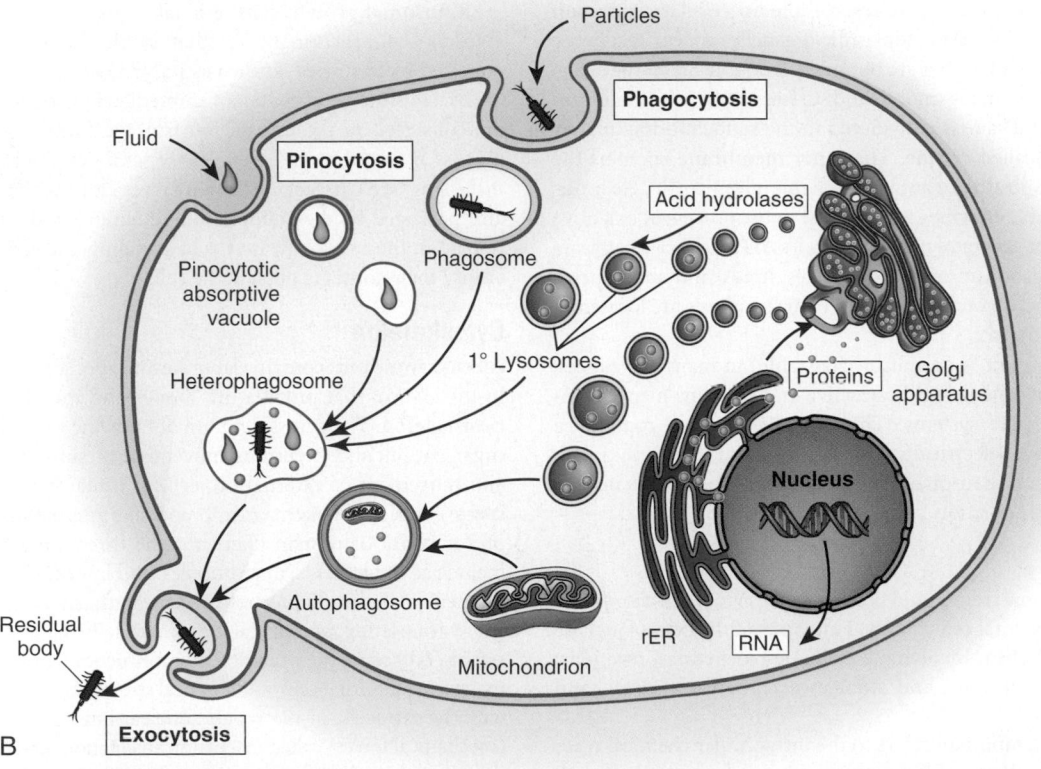

B

FIGURE 1.6 Endolysosomal System and Four Pathways to Degradation in Lysosomes. **A,** Endolysosomal system. **B,** Four pathways to degradation in lysosomes and in all pathways the final step is fusion with lysosomes. *ALR,* Autophagic lysosomal reformation; *CMA,* chaperone-mediated autophagy; *MVB,* multivesicular body; *TGN,* trans-Golgi network; *rER,* rough endoplasmic reticulum. (**A** adapted from Perera RM, Zoncu R: *Annu Rev Cell Dev Biol* 2016 Aug 2 [Epub]; **B** from Damjanov L: *Pathology for the health professions,* ed 4, Philadelphia, 2012, Saunders.)

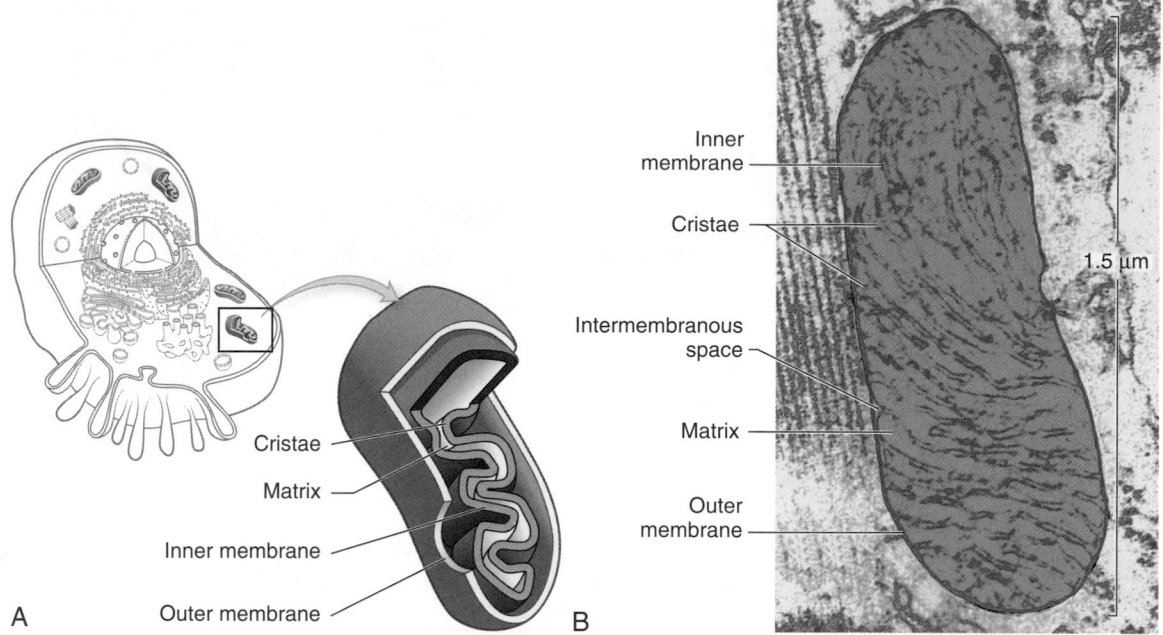

FIGURE 1.7 Mitochondrion. **A,** Cutaway sketch showing outer and inner membranes. Note the many folds (cristae) of the inner membrane. **B,** Transmission electron micrograph of a mitochondrion. Although some mitochondria have the capsule shape shown here, many are round or oval. (**B** Courtesy Brenda Russell.)

Mitochondria

Mitochondria (*mito* = thread; *chondros* = granule), organelles found in large numbers in most cells, are responsible for cellular respiration and energy production. These cytoplasmic organelles appear as spheres, rods, or filamentous bodies that are bound by a double membrane (Fig. 1.7). The outer membrane is smooth and surrounds the mitochondrion itself; the inner membrane is convoluted in the mitochondrial matrix to form partitions called cristae. The inner membrane contains the enzymes of the respiratory chain—the name given to the electron-transport chain. These enzymes are essential to the process of oxidative phosphorylation that generates most of the cell's ATP. Metabolic pathways involved in the metabolism of carbohydrates, lipids, and amino acids and special pathways involving urea and heme synthesis are located in the mitochondrial matrix.

The outer membrane is permeable (passable) to many substances, but the inner membrane is highly selective and contains many trans-membranous transport systems. The inner membrane contains a transporter to move electrically charged calcium (calcium ions). Mitochondria contain their own DNA that codes for enzymes needed for oxidative phosphorylation.

Cytosol

Cytosol is the gelatinous, semiliquid portion of the cytoplasm accounting for about 55% of the total cell volume. Functions of the cytosol include intermediary metabolism involving enzymatic biochemical reactions; ribosomal protein synthesis; and storage of carbohydrates, fat, and secretory vesicles.

Intermediary metabolism refers to the intracellular chemical reactions that include synthesis, degradation, and transformation of small organic molecules (e.g., simple sugars, fatty acids, and amino acids). All intermediary metabolism occurs in the cytoplasm or that portion of the cell interior not occupied by the nucleus—with most of the metabolism being accomplished in the cytosol. These reactions enable energy to be used for managing cellular activities and for providing substrates to maintain cell integrity.

Ribosomal protein synthesis takes place in free ribosomes in the cytosol. Cytosolic ribosomes that synthesize identical proteins are collected in "factories" known as polyribosomes.

Excess stored nutrients not immediately used for ATP production are converted in the cytosol into storage forms; for example, excess glucose is stored as glycogen. These temporary masses are known as *inclusions* (see Chapter 2). Secretory vesicles that have been processed and packaged by the endoplasmic reticulum and Golgi complex also remain in the cytosol. By means of signaling, the vesicles transport and empty their contents outside the cell.

Cytoskeleton

All eukaryotic cells contain elaborate and specialized internal structures in the cytosol that provide the "bones and muscles" of the cell—the cytoskeleton. The cytoskeleton maintains the cell's shape and internal organization, and it permits movement of substances within the cell and movement of external projections (cilia or microvilli; flagella in sperm) outside the plasma membrane. The internal skeleton is composed of a network of protein filaments; the three main types of filaments include actin filaments, microtubules, and intermediate filaments. These filaments collectively promote cell strength, shape, and movement.

By translating mechanical forces and deformations into biochemical signals, cells sense their physical environment including the extracellular matrix, neighboring cells, and physical stress. The cytoskeleton is involved with the extracellular matrix and nuclear interior in force transmission (mechanical forces) called mechanotransduction. Mechanotransduction describes the cellular processes that translate mechanical stimuli into biochemical signals, allowing cells to adapt to their surroundings. Cell stresses, however, that involve adaptations of mechanotransduction are associated with several alterations and diseases including loss of hearing, cardiovascular disease, muscular dystrophy, and cancer.

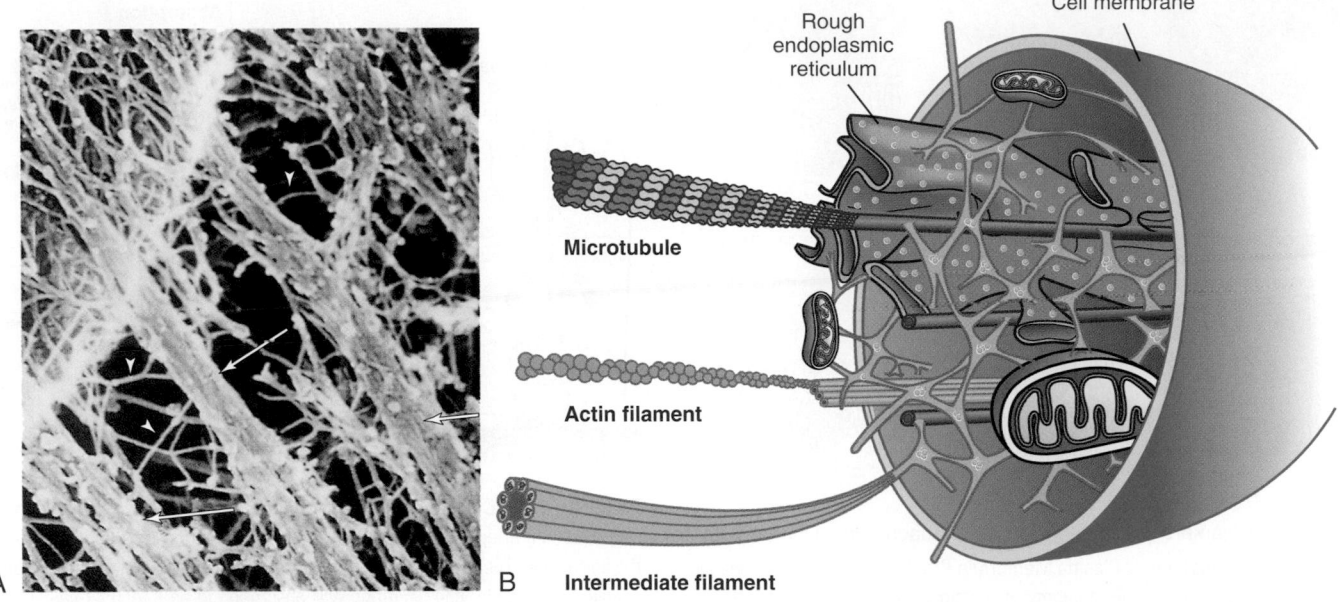

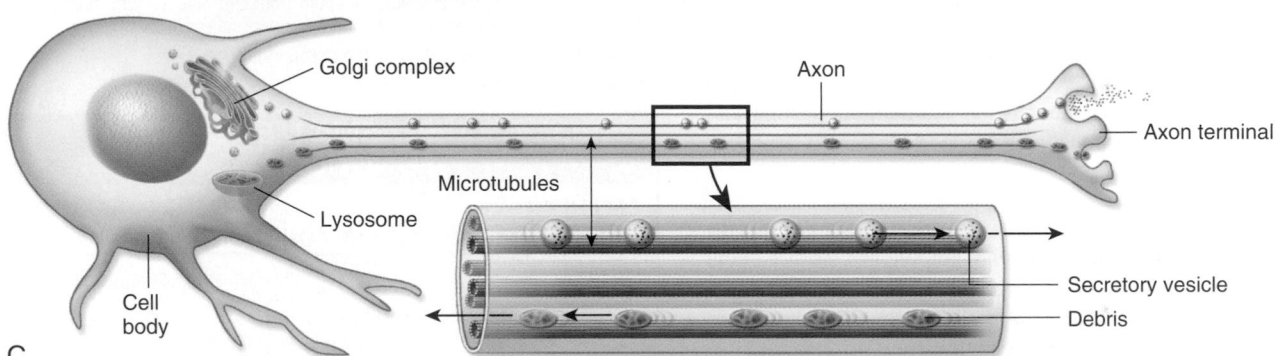

FIGURE 1.8 Cytoskeleton. **A,** Electron micrograph of a portion of the cell's internal framework. Arrowheads mark the intermediate filaments, and the complete arrows mark the microtubules. **B,** Artist's interpretation of the cell's internal framework. Note that the "free" ribosomes and other organelles are not really free at all. **C,** Microtubules are necessary for maintaining an asymmetrical cell shape, such as that of a nerve cell. In addition, specific chemicals are released from the terminal end of the axon to influence neural transmission. (**A** and **B** from Patton KT, Thibodeau GA: *Anatomy & physiology,* ed 6, St Louis, 2007, Mosby.)

Microtubules are small, hollow, cylindrical, unbranched tubules made of protein. When found together, microtubules exhibit rigidity, unlike the rest of the cytoplasm. Microtubules thus add strength to the cell's structure (Fig. 1.8, *A, B*). Within the cell, microtubules support and move organelles from one part of the cytoplasm to another, facilitate transport of impulses along nerve cells, and have roles in the inflammatory and immune responses and hormone secretion (Fig. 1.8, *C*). Microtubules are also involved in the external movement, or motility, of some cells.

Microtubules are arranged in the thickened base, or basal body, of a protrusion from the cell's plasma membrane. This arrangement occurs in the basal bodies of sperm flagella and the cilia of certain other cells. The long, whiplike flagella enable the movement of sperm cells. Cilia usually move substances past the cell, which remains stationary. For example, cilia on cells lining the respiratory tract move together to "beat" mucus toward the throat so it can be removed by coughing.

While the cell is not in the process of division, only a few microtubules are assembled; cellular division (mitosis) or defense (phagocytosis) does, however, induce a cycle of rapid assembly and disassembly. Microtubules involved in cellular division are arranged in a **centriole**. Centrioles always consist of nine bundles containing three microtubules each.

During division, the pairs of centrioles split and migrate to opposite poles of the cell.

Actin filaments (microfilaments) are smaller fibrils that generally occur in bundles rather than as single entities (Fig. 1.8, *B*). They are concentrated in the cell *cortex,* just beneath the plasma membrane.[2] The cortical actin network is a major driver for many cell functions including cell movement, endocytosis, and maintenance of cell and tissue shape. Actin filaments link the interior of the cell to adjacent cells through cell junctions.

In addition, microfilaments are necessary for regulating cell growth and drive the pinching of one cell into two.[2] Cellular locomotion depends on contractile properties that involve both microtubules and actin filaments. The actin cytoskeleton in motile cells has recently been described as a "wave of excitation" that may account for the spontaneous migration of cells.[5]

Intermediate filaments are braided, ropelike fibers made of several filament proteins. The different filaments form a mesh called the nuclear lamina beneath the inner nuclear membrane, creating a protective chamber for the cell's DNA.[2] Other types crisscross the cytoplasm, promoting mechanical strength. In epithelial tissue these filaments bridge

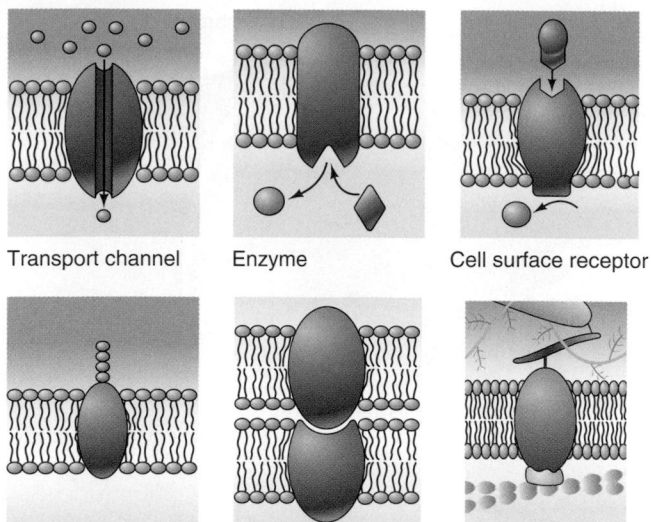

Transport channel   Enzyme   Cell surface receptor

Cell surface markers   Cell adhesion   Attachment of cytoskeleton

FIGURE 1.9 Functions of Plasma Membrane Proteins. The plasma membrane proteins illustrated here show a variety of functions performed by the different types of plasma membranes. (From Raven PH, Johnson GB: *Understanding biology*, ed 3, Dubuque, IA, 1995, Brown.)

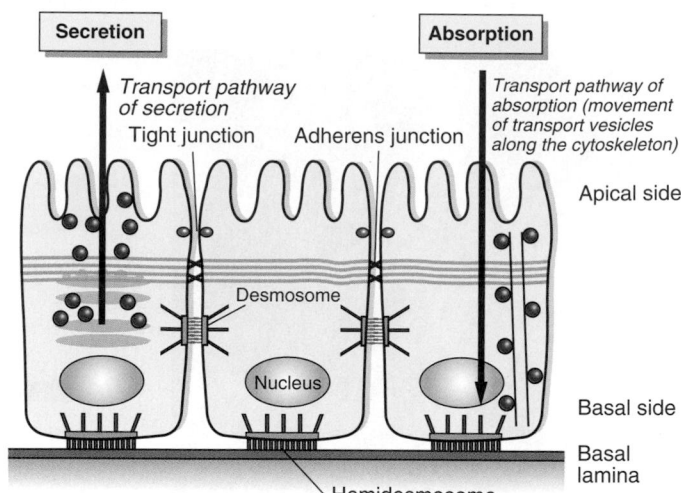

FIGURE 1.10 Cell Polarity of Epithelial Cells. A schematic of cell polarity (cell direction) of epithelial cells. Shown are the directions of the basal side and the apical side. The organelles and cytoskeleton are also arranged directionally to enable, for example, cell secretion and absorption in an intestinal cell. The red circles represent cellular content. (Adapted from Life Science web textbook, The University of Tokyo.)

the cytoplasm from one cell junction to another, supporting and strengthening the sheet of epithelium.[2]

Plasma Membranes

Membranes define the cell's boundaries. Whether they surround the cell or enclose an intracellular organelle, membranes are crucial to normal physiologic function because they control the composition of the space, or compartment, they enclose. They can allow or exclude various molecules, and because of selective transport systems, they can move molecules in or out of the space (Fig. 1.9). By controlling the movement of substances from one compartment to another, membranes exert a powerful influence on metabolic pathways. Directional transport is facilitated by polarized domains, distinct apical and basolateral domains. The direction of cells—**cell polarity**—maintains normal cell and tissue structure for numerous functions, most importantly transport of nutrients in and out of the cell, and becomes altered with diseases such as cancer (Fig. 1.10). In addition to these functions, the plasma membrane has an important role in cell-to-cell recognition. For example, protein receptors for hormones and for other chemical signals are associated with the membrane and act as markers that identify a cell to its neighbors. Other functions of the plasma membrane include assistance with cellular mobility and maintenance of cellular shape (Table 1.1).

Membrane Composition

The main components of cell membranes are lipids and proteins. The basic structure of cell membranes is the **lipid bilayer**, composed of two continuous opposing leaflets and proteins that span the bilayer or interact with the lipids on either side of the two leaflets (Fig. 1.11). The lipid bilayer provides the basic fluid structure of the membrane and is mostly an impermeable barrier to water-soluble molecules. Individual lipid molecules can diffuse readily throughout their own monolayer. Most membrane proteins span the lipid bilayer and mediate most of the functions of the membrane including transport of molecules across the membrane and ATP synthesis[2] (see Fig. 1.9).

Historically, the plasma membrane was described as a fluid lipid bilayer composed of a *uniform* lipid distribution with inserted moving

TABLE 1.1	PLASMA MEMBRANE FUNCTIONS
CELLULAR MECHANISM	**MEMBRANE FUNCTIONS**
Structure	Usually thicker than the membranes of intracellular organelles Containment of cellular organelles Maintenance of relationship with cytoskeleton, endoplasmic reticulum, and other organelles Outer surfaces in many cells are not smooth but are studded with cilia or even smaller cylindrical projections called microvilli; both are capable of movement; caveolae are also outer indentations Maintenance of fluid and electrolyte balance
Protection	Barrier to toxic molecules and macromolecules (proteins, nucleic acid, and polysaccharides) Barrier to foreign organisms and cells
Activation of cell	Hormones (regulation of cellular activity) Mitogens (cellular division) Antigens (antibody synthesis) Growth factors (proliferation and differentiation)
Transport	Diffusion and exchange diffusion Endocytosis (pinocytosis and phagocytosis); receptor-mediated endocytosis Exocytosis (secretion) Active transport
Cell-to-cell interaction	Communication and attachment at junctional complexes Symbiotic nutritive relationships Release of enzymes and antibodies to extracellular environment Relationships with extracellular matrix

Modified from King DW, Fenoglio CM, Lefkowitch JH: *General pathology: principles and dynamics,* Philadelphia, 1983, Lea & Febiger.

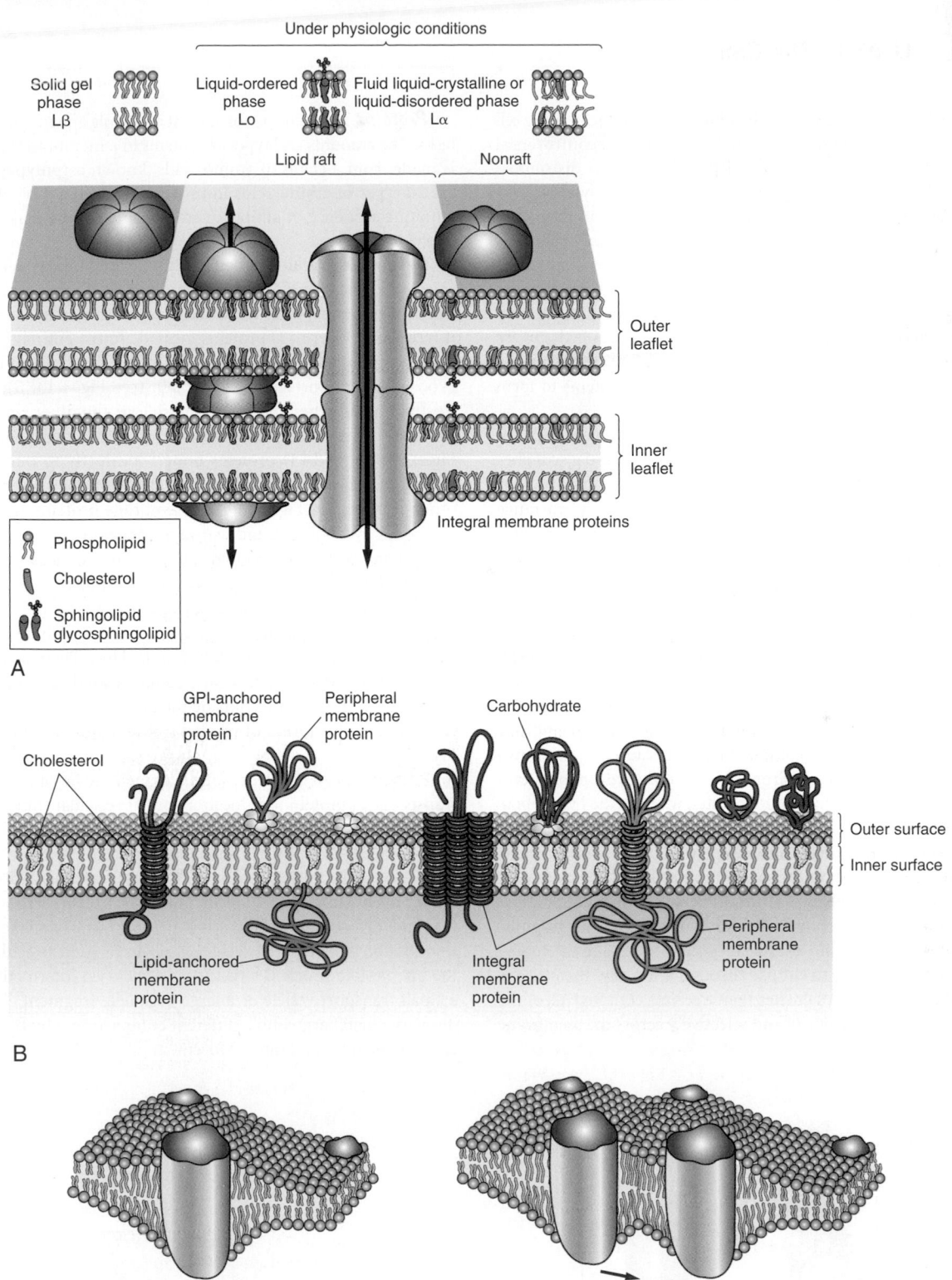

FIGURE 1.11 Lipid Bilayer Membranes. A, Concepts of biologic membranes have markedly changed in the last two decades, from the classic fluid mosaic model to the current model that lipids and proteins are not evenly distributed but can isolate into microdomains, differing in their protein and lipid composition. An example of a microdomain is lipid rafts (colored yellow). Rafts are dynamic domain structures composed of cholesterol, sphingolipids, and membrane proteins important in different cellular processes. Various models exist to clarify the functions of domains. The three major phases of lipid bilayer organization include a solid gel phase (e.g., with low temperatures), a liquid-ordered phase (high temperatures), and a fluid liquid-crystalline (or liquid-disordered) phase. **B,** Some membrane-associated proteins are integrated into the lipid bilayer; other proteins are loosely attached to the outer and inner surfaces of the membrane. Transmembrane proteins protrude through the entire outer and inner surfaces of the membrane, and they can be attracted to microdomains through specific interactions with lipids. Interaction of the membrane proteins with distinct lipids depends on the hydrophobic thickness of the membrane, the lateral pressures of the membrane (mechanical force may shift protein channels from an open to a closed state), the polarity or electrical charges at the lipid-protein interface, and the presence on the protein side of amino acid side chains. Important for pathophysiology is the proposal that protein-lipid interactions can be critical for correct insertion, folding, and orientation of membrane proteins. For example, diseases related to lipids that interfere with protein folding are becoming more prevalent. **C,** Investigators are studying the cooperative behavior of lipids, membrane fluctuations, and domains that influence protein organization and consequently protein function. Here a perturbed region develops around an integral protein. **D,** Two proteins are attracted because of the sharing of a perturbed region of the lipid bilayer. *GPI,* glycophosphatidylinositol. (Adapted from Bagatolli LA et al: *Prog Lipid Res* 49[4]:378–389, 2010; Contreras F-X et al: *Cold Spring Harb Perspect Biol* 3[6]:pii:a004705, 2011; Cooper GM: *The cell—a molecular approach,* ed 2, Washington, DC, 2000, Sinauer Associates; Defamie N, Mesnil M: *Biochim Biophys Acta* 1818[8]:1866–1869, 2012.)

proteins. Whether lipid molecules in the plasma membrane in *living* cell membranes segregate into domains called **lipid rafts** is a controversial topic. It is known that many lipids and proteins are not distributed uniformly but are seen to concentrate in a *temporary*, dynamic way assisted by protein-protein interactions that enable transient formation of domains or lipid rafts.[2] Organization of lipid rafts in living cells may be important for cell communication where protein assemblies convert extracellular signals into intracellular signals.[2] Larger assemblies of clusters are *caveolae*, flask-shaped invaginations thought to form from lipid rafts and to be important for endocytosis. Carbohydrates are mainly associated with plasma membranes, where they are chemically combined with lipids to form **glycolipids** and with proteins to form **glycoproteins**.

Lipids. Cell membranes may contain many different lipid classes, but in animals the main ones are phospholipids, cholesterol, and glycolipids. The most abundant lipids are phospholipids. Phospholipids are key for repairing the membrane—they tend to spontaneously rearrange themselves to avoid a tear (free edge with water) by folding on themselves and forming a sealed compartment.[2] Inositol phospholipids are a subclass of phospholipids important for cell signaling because in the cytosolic lipid leaflet of the bilayer they respond to extracellular signals. Lipids along with protein assemblies act as "molecular glue" for the structural integrity of the membrane. Each lipid molecule is said to be polar, or amphipathic. An **amphipathic molecule** is one in which one part is **hydrophobic** (uncharged, or "water fearing") and another part is **hydrophilic** (charged, or "water loving") (Fig. 1.12). The membrane spontaneously organizes itself into a bilayer because of these two incompatible solubilities. The hydrophobic region (hydrophobic tail) of each lipid molecule is protected from water, whereas the hydrophilic region (hydrophilic head) is immersed in it. The bilayer's structure accounts for one of the essential functions of the plasma membrane: it is impermeable to most water-soluble molecules (molecules that dissolve in water) because they are insoluble in the oily core region. The bilayer serves as a barrier to the diffusion of water and hydrophilic substances while allowing lipid-soluble molecules, such as oxygen (O_2) and carbon dioxide (CO_2), to diffuse through it readily. Because the bilayer is fluid at temperatures greater than freezing, components of the cellular environment move slowly and selectively across the membrane all the time.

Proteins. Proteins perform most of the plasma membrane's specific tasks. The amounts and types of proteins in a membrane vary. A **protein** is made from a chain of amino acids, known as **polypeptides**. There are 20 types of amino acids in proteins, and each type of protein has a unique sequence of amino acids. Proteins are the major workhorses of the cell.

Membrane proteins associate with the lipid bilayer in different ways (Fig. 1.13) including (1) **transmembrane proteins** extending across the bilayer and exposed to an aqueous environment on both sides of it (see Fig. 1.13, *A*); (2) proteins located almost entirely in the cytosol and associated with the cytosolic half of the lipid bilayer by an α helix exposed on the surface of the protein (see Fig. 1.13, *B*); (3) proteins existing outside the bilayer, on one side or the other, and attached to the membrane by one or more covalently attached lipid groups (see Fig. 1.13, *C*); and (4) proteins bound indirectly to one or the other bilayer membrane face and held in place by their interactions with other proteins (see Fig. 1.13, *D*).[2] Membrane proteins are amphiphilic, with both hydrophobic and hydrophilic regions.

Proteins exist in densely folded molecular configurations rather than straight chains; so an excess of hydrophilic units is at the surface of the molecule and an excess of hydrophobic units is inside. Membrane proteins, like other proteins, are synthesized mainly by ribosomes in the cytosol and then travel, called *trafficking*. Their fate depends on their amino acid sequence, which contains **sorting signals** that direct their delivery to locations outside the cytosol or to organelle surfaces.[2] A simplified illustration of protein traffic within a cell is presented in Fig. 1.14.

Proteins move from one compartment to another by (1) gated transport, (2) protein translocation, or (3) vesicular transport. In **gated transport** selective gates direct the movement of proteins and RNA molecules between the cytosol and the nucleus through nuclear pore complexes in the nuclear envelope[2]. In **protein translocation** *transmembrane protein translocators* directly transport proteins across a membrane from the cytosol to a different distinct location. To snake through the translocator, the protein molecule usually unfolds. In **vesicular transport**, the bubble-like vesicle is a membrane-enclosed intermediate of either a small transport vesicle or a large organelle fragment. These vesicles discharge their cargo into a different compartment by fusing with that compartment's membrane.[2] Movement of soluble proteins from the ER

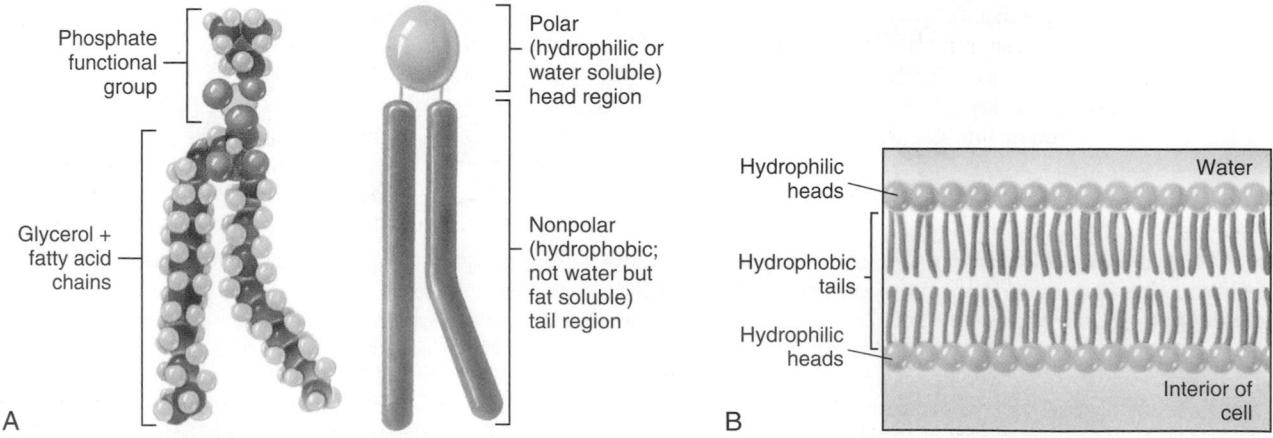

FIGURE 1.12 Structure of a Phospholipid Molecule. A, Each phospholipid molecule consists of a phosphate functional group and two fatty acid chains attached to a glycerol molecule. **B,** The fatty acid chains and glycerol form nonpolar, hydrophobic "tails," and the phosphate functional group forms the polar, hydrophilic "head" of the phospholipid molecule. When placed in water, the hydrophobic tails of the molecule face inward, away from the water, and the hydrophilic head faces outward, toward the water. (From Raven PH, Johnson GB: *Understanding biology,* ed 3, Dubuque, IA, 1995, Brown.)

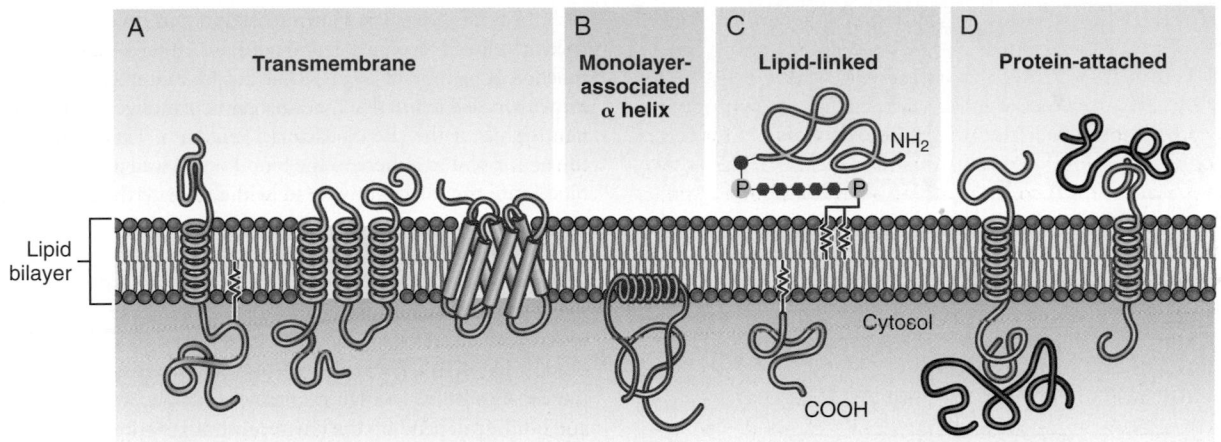

FIGURE 1.13 Proteins Attach to the Plasma Membrane in Different Ways. A, Transmembrane proteins extend through the membrane as a single α helix, as multiple α helices, or as a rolled-up barrel-like sheet called a β barrel. **B,** Some membrane proteins are anchored to the cytosolic side of the lipid bilayer by an amphipathic α helix. **C,** Some proteins are linked on either side of the membrane by a covalently attached lipid molecule. **D,** Proteins are attached by weak noncovalent interactions with other membrane proteins. (**D** adapted from Alberts B: *Essential cell biology,* ed 4, New York, 2014, Garland.)

to the Golgi apparatus occurs by vesicular transport. Those proteins that lack a sorting signal remain in the cytosol permanently. Trafficking places unique demands on membrane proteins for folding, translocation, and stability. Thus, much research is now being done to understand misfolded proteins, for example, as a cause of disease (see *What's New?* Endoplasmic Reticulum, Protein Folding, and ER Stress).

Proteins facilitate transport across membranes by serving as receptors, enzymes, or transporters. Proteins act as (1) recognition and binding units (receptors) for substances moving in and out of the cell; (2) pores or transport channels for various electrically charged particles called *ions* or *electrolytes* and specific carriers for amino acids and monosaccharides; (3) specific enzymes that drive active pumps that promote concentration of certain ions, particularly potassium (K^+), within the cell while keeping concentrations of other ions, for example, sodium (Na^+), below concentrations found in the extracellular environment; (4) cell surface markers, such as glycoproteins (proteins attached to carbohydrates), that identify a cell to its neighbor; (5) cell adhesion molecules (CAMs), or proteins that allow cells to hook together and form attachments to the cytoskeleton for maintaining cellular shape; and (6) catalysts of chemical reactions, for example, conversion of lactose to glucose. Membrane proteins are key components of energy transduction, converting chemical energy into electrical energy, or electrical energy into either mechanical energy or synthesis of ATP.[6]

The interaction of plasma membrane proteins with lipids is complex and is the subject of much research. The role of proteins in the onset and progression of disease is important because they govern communication between cells through enzymatic, transport, and recognition-receptor functions in cellular physiology.

Protein regulation in a cell: Proteostasis. Proteostasis (or proteome [complete collection of cell proteins] homeostasis) is a state of cell balance of the processes of protein synthesis, folding, and degradation. Proteostasis is vital to cellular health. The cellular protein pool is in constant change or flux. The number of copies of a protein in a cell depends on how quickly it is made and how long it survives or is broken down. The system of protein homeostasis is adaptable and defined by the "proteostasis" network comprised of ribosomes (makers); chaperones (helpers); and two protein breakdown systems or proteolytic systems, lysosomes and the ubiquitin-proteosome system (UPS). The molecular

chaperones called *heat-shock proteins (hsp)* are important and are so named because they increase after cells are exposed to elevated temperature (proteotoxic stress). The increase in hsp is part of a feedback system that responds to an increase in misfolded proteins and helps these proteins refold. These chaperones also facilitate transportation and ubiquitination or tagging the protein with a small molecule, *ubiquitin,* that signals the protein to the proteasome for degradation.[7] Together, all of these systems regulate protein homeostasis under a large variety of conditions including nutrient supply variation, oxidative stress, cellular differentiation, temperature changes, heavy metal ion presence, and other stresses.[8] Malfunction or failure of the proteostasis network is associated with human disease (Fig. 1.15).

Proteases are enzymes that cause the breakdown of proteins. Certain proteases can be tethered to cell membranes. Proteases are involved in the physiologic regulation of essential processes by participating in a tightly orchestrated sequence of events termed a proteolytic cascade. Four major proteolytic cascades with disease relevance are candidates for treatment modalities, including (1) cell death or caspase-mediated apoptosis, (2) the blood coagulation cascade, (3) degrading membrane enzymes or matrix metalloproteinase cascade, and (4) the complement cascade. Some proteases within a proteolytic cascade act as initiators; others are involved in amplification and propagation and execution. Understanding the various steps involved is crucial for designing drug interventions. Dysregulation of proteases features prominently in many human diseases, including cancer, autoimmunity, and neurodegenerative disorders.

Carbohydrates

The short chains of sugars or carbohydrates *(oligosaccharides)* contained within the plasma membrane are generally bound to membrane proteins (glycoproteins) and lipids (glycolipids). Long polysaccharide chains attached to membrane proteins are called *proteoglycans.* All of the carbohydrate on the glycoproteins, proteoglycans, and glycolipids is located on the outside of the plasma membrane, and the carbohydrate coating is called the *glycocalyx* (or cell coat). The glycocalyx helps protect the cell from mechanical damage.[2] Additionally, the layer of carbohydrate gives the cell a slimy surface that assists the mobility of other cells, like leukocytes, to squeeze through the narrow spaces.[2] The functions of

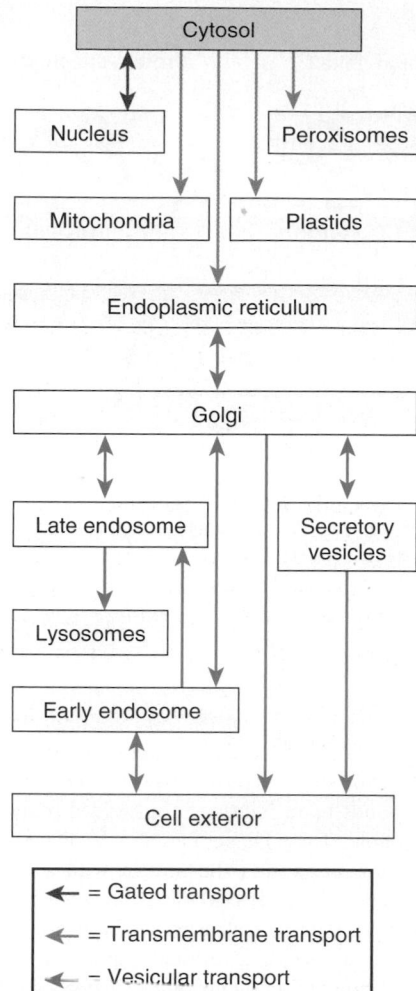

FIGURE 1.14 Simplified "Roadmap" of Protein Traffic. Proteins can move from one compartment to another by gated transport *(red)*, transmembrane transport *(blue)*, or vesicular transport *(green)*. Sorting signals direct a protein's movement through the cell and determine its final destination. The trip begins with synthesis of a protein on a ribosome in the cytosol and ends when the protein reaches the final destination. A sorting signal is required either for retention at an intermediate station *(boxes)* or for exit from the station or compartment. (Adapted from Alberts B: *Essential cell biology*, ed 4, New York, 2014, Garland.)

carbohydrates are more than protection and lubrication and include specific cell-cell recognition and adhesion. Intercellular recognition is a function of membrane oligosaccharides; for example, the transmembrane proteins, called *lectins* that bind to a particular oligosaccharide, recognize neutrophils at the site of bacterial infection. This recognition allows the neutrophil to adhere to the blood vessel wall and migrate from the blood into the infected tissue to help eliminate the invading bacteria.[2]

Cellular Receptors

Cellular receptors are protein molecules on the plasma membrane, in the cytoplasm, or in the nucleus that are capable of recognizing and binding with specific smaller molecules called **ligands** (Latin *ligare,* "to bind") (Fig. 1.16). The region of a protein that associates with a ligand is called its **binding site.** Hormones, for example, are ligands. Recognition and binding depend on the chemical configuration of the receptor and its smaller ligand, which must fit together somewhat like pieces of a jigsaw puzzle. Binding selectively to a protein receptor with high affinity to a ligand depends on formation of weak, noncovalent interactions—hydrogen bonds, electrostatic attractions, and van der Waals attractions—and favorable hydrophobic forces.[2] Numerous receptors are found in most cells, and ligand binding to receptors activates or inhibits the receptor's associated signaling or biochemical pathway.

Although the chemical nature of both ligands and the receptors to which they bind differs, receptors are classified on the basis of their location and function (see Cellular Communication and Signal Transduction). Cellular type determines overall cellular function, but plasma membrane receptors determine which ligands a cell will bind with and how the cell will respond to binding with each. For example, the ability of a hormone or a neurotransmitter to stimulate a cell is regulated by the specificity and number of receptors present on the plasma membrane. Specific processes also control intracellular mechanisms. Hormone binding, for example, depends on special messenger molecules that regulate protein synthesis within the cell (see Chapter 21). Neurotransmitters also operate by causing special messengers to react with specific receptors.

Receptors for different drugs are found on the plasma membrane, in the cytoplasm, and in the nucleus. Membrane receptors have been found for certain anesthetics, opiates, endorphins, enkephalins, antibiotics, cancer chemotherapeutic agents, digitalis, and other drugs. Membrane receptors for endorphins, which are opiate-like peptides isolated from the pituitary gland, are found in large quantities in pain pathways of the nervous system (see Chapters 15 and 16). With binding, the endorphins (or drugs like morphine) change the cell's permeability to

FIGURE 1.15 Protein Homeostasis System and Outcomes. A main role of the protein homeostasis network *(proteostasis)* is to minimize protein misfolding and protein aggregation. The network includes ribosome-mediated protein synthesis, chaperone (folding helpers in the ER) and enzyme-mediated folding, breakdown systems of lysosome and proteasome-mediated protein degradation, and vesicular trafficking. The network integrates biologic pathways that balance folding, trafficking, and protein degradation depicted by arrows *b, d, e, f, g, h,* and *i.* (Adapted from Lindquist SL, Kelly JW: *Cold Spring Harb Perspect Biol* 3[12]:pii:a004507, 2011.)

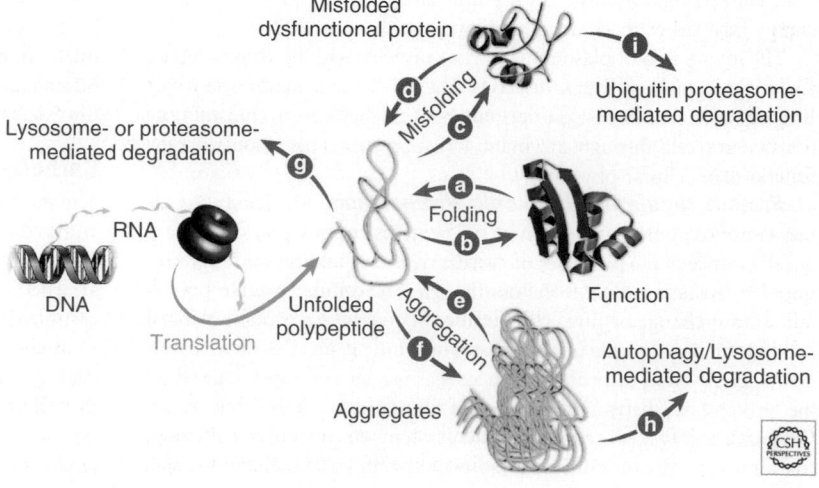

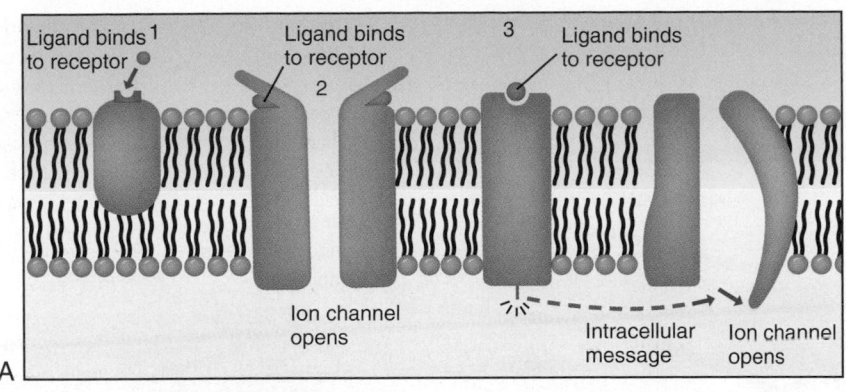

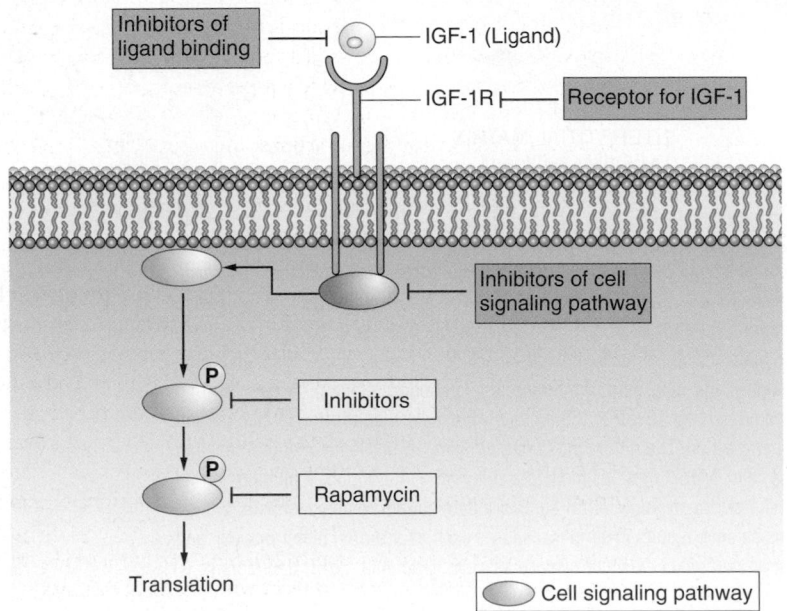

FIGURE 1.16 Cellular Receptors. (**A**) **1,** Plasma membrane receptor for a ligand (here, a hormone molecule) on the surface of an integral protein. A neurotransmitter can exert its effect on a postsynaptic cell by means of two fundamentally different types of receptor proteins; **2,** channel-linked receptors, and **3,** non–channel-linked receptors. Channel-linked receptors are also known as ligand-gated channels. (**B**) Example of ligand-receptor interaction. Insulin-like growth factor 1 (IGF-1) is a ligand and binds to the insulin-like growth factor 1 receptor (IGF-1R). With binding at the cell membrane the intracellular signaling pathway is activated, causing translation of new proteins to act as intracellular communicators. This pathway is important for cancer growth. Researchers are developing pharmacologic strategies to reduce signaling at and downstream of the IGF-1R, hoping this will lead to compounds useful in cancer treatment. *P,* phosphate group from ATP.

ions, increase the concentration of molecules that regulate intracellular protein synthesis, and initiate molecular events that modulate pain perception.

Receptors for infectious microorganisms, or antigen receptors, bind bacteria, viruses, and parasites. Antigen receptors on white blood cells (lymphocytes, monocytes, macrophages, granulocytes) recognize and bind with antigenic microorganisms and activate the immune and inflammatory responses (see Chapters 7 and 8).

CELL-TO-CELL ADHESIONS

Cells are small and squishy, *not* like bricks. They are enclosed only by a flimsy membrane, yet the cell depends on the integrity of this membrane for its survival. How can cells be combined together strongly, with their membranes intact, to form a muscle that can lift this textbook? Plasma membranes not only serve as the outer boundaries of all cells but also allow groups of cells to be held together robustly, in **cell-to-cell adhesions,** to form tissues and organs. Once arranged, cells are held together by three different means: (1) the extracellular matrix, (2) cell adhesion molecules in the cell's plasma membrane, and (3) specialized cell junctions.

Extracellular Matrix and Basement Membrane

Cells can be bound together by attachment to one another or through the **extracellular matrix (ECM;** also including the basement membrane),

which the cells secrete around themselves. The ECM is an intricate meshwork of interstitial fibrous proteins embedded in a watery, gel-like substance composed of complex carbohydrates (Fig. 1.17). A specialized type of extracellular matrix is called the **basement membrane** (also known as the **basal lamina**). This sheet of matrix molecules is very thin, tough, and flexible; lies beneath epithelial cells; and surrounds individual muscle cells, fat cells, and Schwann cells (which wrap around peripheral nerve cell axons) (Fig. 1.18). The extracellular matrix is like glue; however, it does provide a pathway for diffusion of nutrients, wastes, and other water-soluble traffic between the blood and tissue cells. Overall, the matrix helps regulate cell growth, movement, and differentiation. Specifically, the major functions of the ECM include (1) mechanical support, (2) control of cell proliferation, (3) formation of a scaffold for tissue regeneration, and (4) establishment of tissue microenvironments (Box 1.1). Interwoven within the matrix are three groups of **macromolecules:** (1) fibrous structural proteins, including collagen and elastin; (2) a diverse group of adhesive glycoproteins, such as fibronectin; and (3) proteoglycans and hyaluronic acid.

Collagen forms cable-like fibers or sheets that provide tensile strength or resistance to longitudinal stress. Collagen breakdown, such as occurs in osteoarthritis, destroys the fibrils that give cartilage its tensile strength.

Elastin is a rubber-like protein fiber most abundant in tissue that must be capable of stretching and recoiling, such as the lungs.

Fibronectin, a large glycoprotein, promotes cell adhesion and cell anchorage. Reduced amounts have been found in certain types of

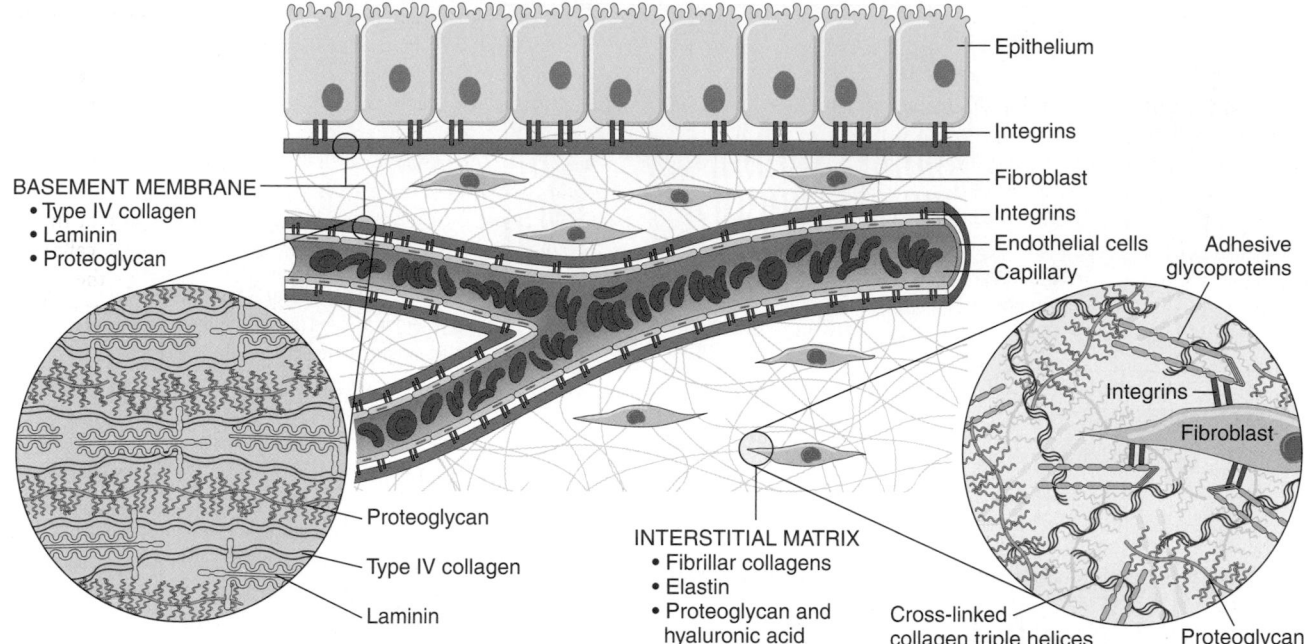

BASEMENT MEMBRANE
- Type IV collagen
- Laminin
- Proteoglycan

Epithelium

Integrins

Fibroblast

Integrins

Endothelial cells

Capillary

Adhesive glycoproteins

Integrins

Fibroblast

Proteoglycan

Type IV collagen

Laminin

INTERSTITIAL MATRIX
- Fibrillar collagens
- Elastin
- Proteoglycan and hyaluronic acid

Cross-linked collagen triple helices

Proteoglycan

FIGURE 1.17 Extracellular Matrix. Tissues are not just cells but also extracellular space. The extracellular space is an intricate network of macromolecules called the *extracellular matrix (ECM)*. The macromolecules that constitute the ECM are secreted locally (by mostly fibroblasts) and assembled into a meshwork in close association with the surface of the cell that produced them. Two main classes of macromolecules include proteoglycans, which are bound to polysaccharide chains called glycosaminoglycans; and fibrous proteins (e.g., collagen, elastin, fibronectin, and laminin), which have structural and adhesive properties. Together the proteoglycan molecules form a gel-like ground substance in which the fibrous proteins are embedded. The gel permits rapid diffusion of nutrients, metabolites, and hormones between the blood and the tissue cells. Matrix proteins modulate cell-matrix interactions including normal tissue remodeling (which can become abnormal, for example, with chronic inflammation), embryogenesis, wound healing, and angiogenesis. Disruption of this balance results in serious diseases such as arthritis, tumor growth, and others. (From Kumar V et al: *Robbins & Cotran pathologic basis of disease,* ed 9, Philadelphia, 2015, Saunders.)

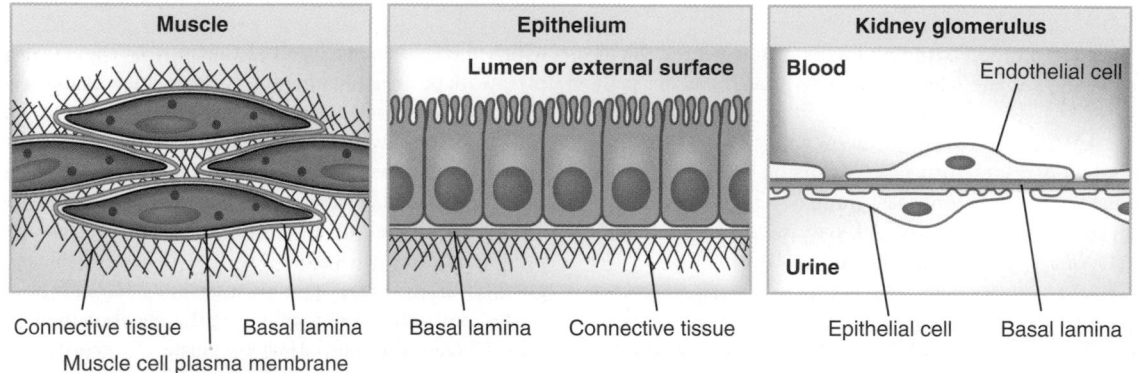

Muscle	Epithelium	Kidney glomerulus
	Lumen or external surface	Blood Endothelial cell
Connective tissue Basal lamina Muscle cell plasma membrane	Basal lamina Connective tissue	Urine Epithelial cell Basal lamina

FIGURE 1.18 Three Ways Basement Membranes (Basal Laminae) Are Organized. Basal laminae *(yellow)* surround certain cells like skeletal muscle cells, underlie epithelia, and occur between two cell sheets (kidney glomerulus). (Adapted from Alberts B: *Essential cell biology,* ed 4, New York, 2014, Garland.)

cancerous cells; this allows cancer cells to travel or metastasize to other parts of the body.

The extracellular matrix is secreted by **fibroblasts** ("fiber formers"), local cells that are present in the matrix. The matrix and the cells within it are known collectively as *connective tissue* because they connect cells together to form tissues and organs. Human connective tissues are enormously varied. They can be hard and dense, like bone; flexible, like tendons or the dermis of the skin; resilient and shock-absorbing, like

cartilage; or soft and transparent, like the jelly-like substance that fills the eye. In all these examples, the majority of the tissue is composed of extracellular matrix, and the cells that produce the matrix are scattered within it like raisins in a pudding[9] (see Fig. 1.17).

The matrix is not just passive scaffolding for cellular attachment; it also helps regulate the functions of the cells within which it interacts. The matrix helps regulate cell growth, movement, and differentiation.

Cell Adhesion Molecules (CAMs)

Cell adhesion molecules (CAMs) are cell surface proteins that bind the cell to an adjacent cell and to components of the extracellular matrix (ECM). CAMs include four protein families: the integrins, the cadherins, the selectins, and immunoglobulin (Ig) superfamily. Integrins are a major class of receptors within the ECM and regulate cell-ECM interactions with collagen, fibronectin, vitronectin, and fibrinogen. Cadherins are Ca^{++}-dependent glycoproteins and have a unique pattern of tissue distribution, for example, epithelial (E-cadherin). Selectins are a family of proteins that bind certain carbohydrates, for example, mucins. The immunoglobulin superfamily CAMs (IgSF CAMs) bind integrins or other IgSF CAMs.

Specialized Cell Junctions

Cells in direct physical contact with neighboring cells are often linked together at specialized regions of their plasma membranes called cell junctions. Cell junctions are classified by their function: (1) to hold cells together, forming a tight seal (tight junctions); (2) to provide strong mechanical attachments (adherens junctions, desmosomes, hemidesmosomes); (3) to provide a special type of chemical communication, for example, inorganic ions and small water-soluble molecules to move from the cytosol of one cell to the cytosol of another cell, such as those causing an electrical wave (gap junctions); and (4) to maintain apico-basal polarity of individual epithelial cells (tight junctions) (Fig. 1.19). Overall, cell junctions make the epithelium leak-proof (mediating mechanical attachment of one cell to another), allow communicating tunnels, and maintain cell polarity.

Cell junctions can be classified as symmetrical and asymmetrical. Symmetrical junctions include tight junctions (zonula occludens), the belt desmosome (zonula adherens), desmosomes (macula adherens), and gap junctions also called intercellular channel or communicating junctions.[10] An asymmetrical junction is the hemidesmosome (see Fig. 1.19). Together the zones between epithelial cells—typically consisting of the zonula occludens, the zonula adherens, and the macula adherens—form the junctional complex. Desmosomes unite cells either by forming continuous bands or belts of epithelial sheets or by developing button-like points of contact. Desmosomes also act as a system of braces to maintain structural stability. Tight junctions are barriers to diffusion, prevent the movement of substances through transport proteins in the plasma membrane, and prevent the leakage of small molecules between the plasma membranes of adjacent cells. Gap junctions are clusters of communicating tunnels or connexons that allow small ions and molecules to pass directly from the inside of one cell to the inside of another. Connexons are hemichannels that extend outward from each of the adjacent plasma membranes (see Fig. 1.19, C).

The junctional complex is a highly permeable part of the plasma membrane. Its permeability is controlled by a process called gating, which depends on concentrations of calcium ions in the cytoplasm. Increased cytoplasmic calcium concentration causes decreased permeability at the junctional complex. Gating is an important cellular defense mechanism because it enables uninjured cells to seal themselves off from injured neighbors. Damaged cells release calcium, which travels through the junctional complex and increases calcium levels in neighboring cells, causing damaging effects. The increased calcium concentration decreases the permeability of the junctional complexes of the neighboring cells, which form a relatively impermeable wall around the injured area (see Chapter 2).

CELLULAR COMMUNICATION AND SIGNAL TRANSDUCTION

Cells need to communicate with each other to maintain a stable internal environment, or homeostasis; to regulate their growth and division and their development and organization into tissues; and to coordinate their functions. Cells communicate by using hundreds of kinds of signal molecules; however, cells communicate in three main ways: (1) they display plasma membrane–bound signaling molecules (receptors) that affect the cell itself and other cells in direct physical contact (Fig. 1.20, A); (2) they affect receptor proteins *inside* the target cell and the signal molecule has to enter the cell to bind with them (Fig. 1.20, B); and (3) they form protein channels (gap junctions) that directly coordinate the activities of adjacent cells (Fig. 1.20, C). Alterations in cellular communication affect disease onset and progression. In fact, if a cell is unable to perform gap junctional intercellular communication, it is hypothesized that normal growth control and cell differentiation are compromised, favoring cancerous tumor development. Secreted chemical signals involve communication at a distance. Primary modes of intercellular signaling are contact-dependent, paracrine, hormonal, neurohormonal, and neurotransmitter (Fig. 1.21).

Contact-dependent signaling requires cells to be in close membrane-membrane contact. In paracrine signaling, cells secrete local chemical mediators that are quickly absorbed, destroyed, or immobilized. Paracrine signaling usually involves different cell types; however, cells also may produce signals that they, themselves, respond to, which is called autocrine signaling (see Fig. 1.21). For example, cancer cells use this form of signaling to stimulate their survival and proliferation. Hormonal signaling involves specialized endocrine cells that secrete chemicals called hormones (e.g., thyroid-stimulating hormone); hormones are released by one set of cells and travel through the tissue and through the bloodstream to produce a response in other sets of cells. In neurohormonal signaling, hormones (e.g., angiotensin II) are released into the blood by neurosecretory neurons. Like endocrine cells, neurosecretory neurons release blood-borne chemical messengers, whereas ordinary neurons secrete short-range neurotransmitters into a small, discrete space (i.e., synapse). Neurons communicate directly with the cells they innervate by releasing chemicals or neurotransmitters at specialized junctions called chemical synapses; the neurotransmitter diffuses across the synaptic cleft and acts on the postsynaptic target cell (see Fig. 1.21). Many of these same signaling molecules are receptors used in hormonal, neurohormonal, and paracrine signaling. The

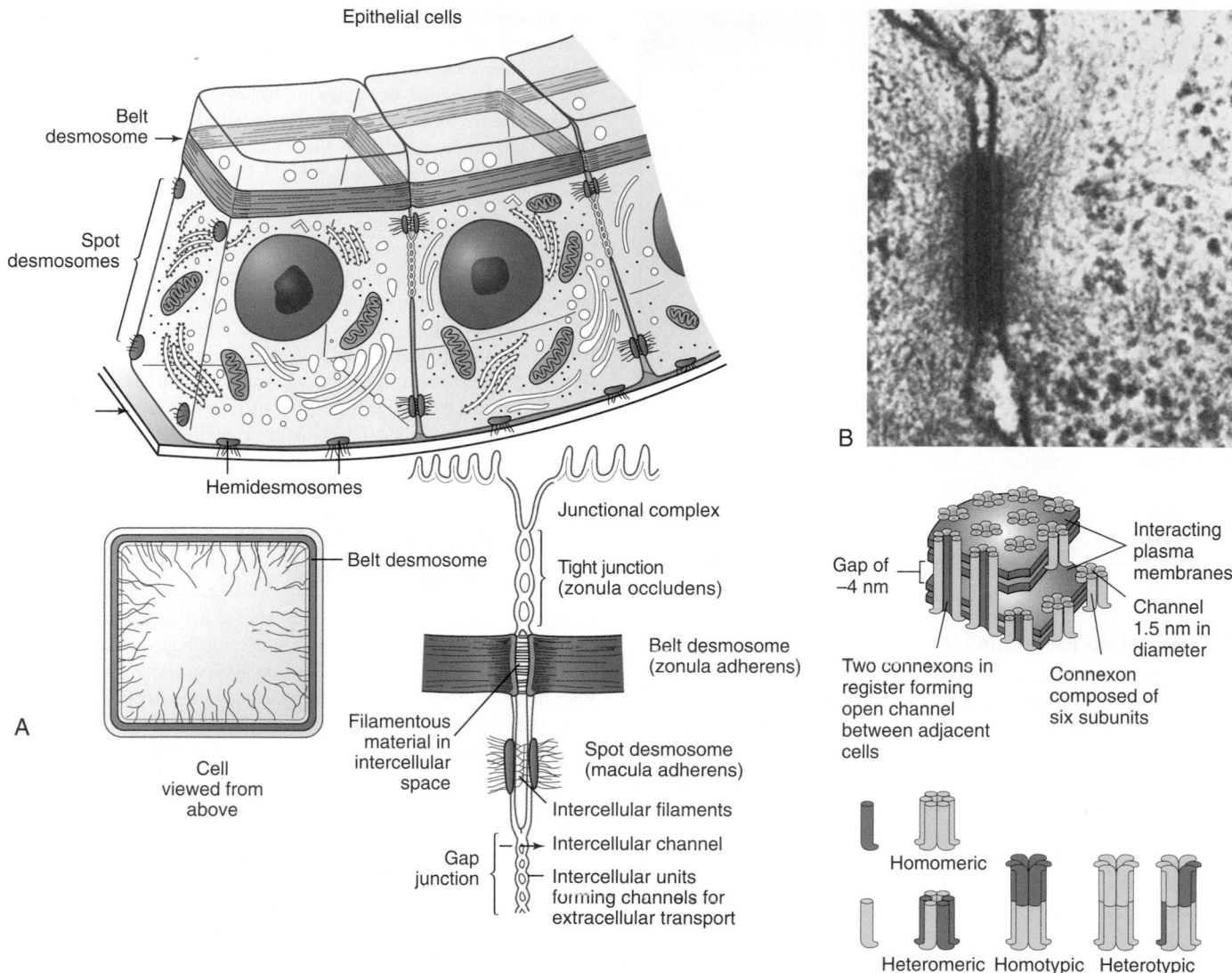

FIGURE 1.19 Types of Cell Connections. **A,** Schematic drawing of a belt desmosome between epithelial cells. This junction, also called *zonula adherens,* encircles each interacting cell. The spot desmosomes and hemidesmosomes, like the belt desmosomes, are adhering junctions. This tight junction is an impermeable junction that holds cells together but seals them in such a way that molecules cannot leak between them. The gap junction, as a communicating junction, mediates the passage of small molecules from one interacting cell to the other. **B,** Electron micrograph of desmosomes. **C,** Connexons. (**A** and **B** from Raven PH, Johnson GB: *Biology,* St Louis, 1992, Mosby. **C** from Alberts B et al: *Molecular biology of the cell,* ed 5, New York, 2008, Garland.)

important differences lie in the speed and selectivity with which the signals are delivered to their targets.[2]

Plasma membrane receptors belong to one of three classes that are defined by the signaling (transduction) mechanism used. Table 1.2 summarizes these classes of receptors.

Signal Transduction

Signal transduction involves incoming signals or instructions from extracellular chemical messengers (ligands) that are conveyed to the cell's interior for execution. Cells respond to external stimuli by activating a variety of **signal transduction pathways**, which are communication pathways, or signaling cascades (Fig. 1.22). Signals are passed between cells when a particular type of molecule is produced by one cell—the **signaling cell**—and received by another—the **target cell**—by means

of a **receptor protein** that recognizes and responds specifically to the signal molecule (Fig. 1.22, *A* and *B*). In turn, the signaling molecules activate a path of intracellular protein kinases that results in responses, such as grow and divide, survive, or differentiate (Fig. 1.22, *C* and *D*). If deprived of appropriate signals, most cells undergo a form of cell suicide known as *programmed cell death,* or *apoptosis.*

Signal transduction pathways, or relay chains, of intercellular signaling molecules have several important functions (see Fig. 1.22):

1. They physically *transfer* the signal from the place at which it is received to some other part of the cell where the response is expected.
2. They *amplify* the signal received, making it stronger; this is caused by a multiplying effect in the pathways; for example, binding of one ligand molecule to a receptor activates a number of adenylyl cyclase molecules.

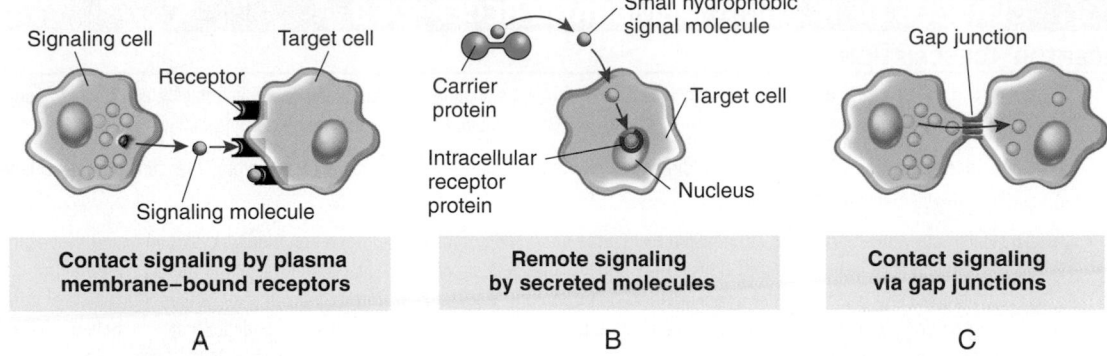

FIGURE 1.20 Cellular Communication. Three ways in which cells communicate with one another. (**B** adapted from Alberts B et al: *Molecular biology of the cell,* ed 5, New York, 2008, Garland.)

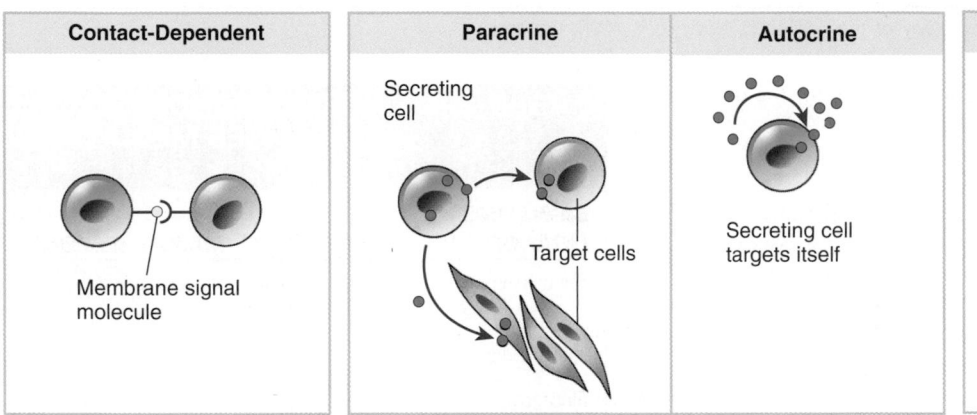
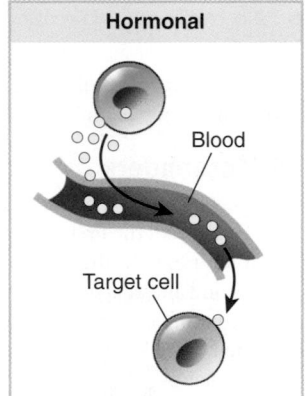

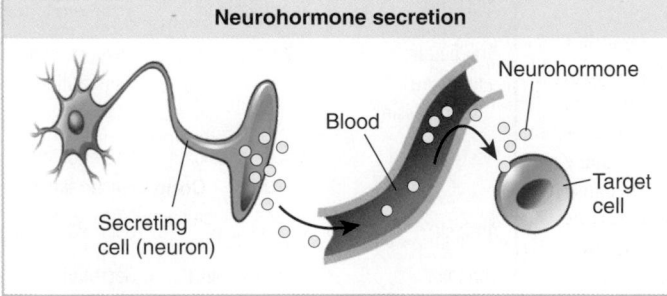
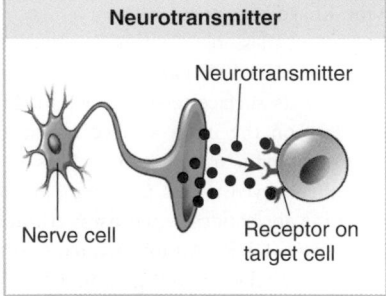

FIGURE 1.21 Primary Modes of Chemical Signaling. Five forms of signaling mediated by secreted molecules. Hormones, paracrines, neurotransmitters, and neurohormones are all intercellular messengers that accomplish communication between cells. Autocrines bind to receptors on the same cell. Not all neurotransmitters act in the strictly synaptic mode shown; some act in a contact-dependent mode as local chemical mediators that influence multiple target cells in the area.

3. They *distribute* the signal so that it influences several processes in parallel; at any step in the pathway, the signal can *diverge* and be relayed to several different intracellular targets, creating branches in the flow and causing a complex response (see Fig. 1.22).

4. Last, the signal can be *modulated* by other interfering factors prevailing inside or outside the cell.

Two general responses from binding of the extracellular signaling messenger (i.e., ligand), or **first messenger**, to the membrane receptors occur: (1) opening or closing specific channels in the membrane to regulate the movement of ions into or out of the cell, and (2) transferring the signal to an intracellular messenger, or **second messenger**, which in turn triggers a cascade of biochemical events within the cell.

Extracellular Messengers and Channel Regulation

Membrane channels, or "gates," can open and close depending on the circumstances of the first messenger. Opening and closing occur because of conformational changes (shaping) of the proteins that form the channels—blocking the channel (closing) or permitting passage through it (opening). Channel opening and closing can be initiated in one of three ways: (1) by binding of a ligand to a specific membrane receptor that is closely associated with the channel (for example, G proteins); (2) by making changes in the electrical current in the plasma membrane, altering the flow of Na^+ and K^+; and (3) by stretching or other mechanical deformation of the channel. Fig. 1.23 summarizes ways by which

TABLE 1.2   CLASSES OF PLASMA MEMBRANE RECEPTORS

TYPE OF RECEPTOR	DESCRIPTION
Channel linked	Also called ligand-gated channels; involves rapid synaptic signaling between electrically excitable cells. Channels open and close briefly in response to neurotransmitters, changing ion permeability of plasma membrane of postsynaptic cell.
Catalytic	Once activated by ligands, function directly as enzymes. Composed of transmembrane proteins that function intracellularly as tyrosine-specific protein kinases.
G-protein linked	Indirectly activate or inactivate plasma membrane enzyme or ion channel; interaction mediated by guanosine triphosphate (GTP)–binding regulatory protein (G protein). When activated, a chain of reactions occurs that alters the concentration of intracellular messengers, such as cyclic adenosine monophosphate (cAMP) and calcium, or signaling molecules. Behaviors of other target proteins are also altered. May also interact with inositol phospholipids, which are significant in cell signaling, and molecules involved in the inositol-phospholipid transduction pathway. A G-protein–linked receptor activates the enzyme phosphoinositide-specific phospholipase, which in turn generates two intracellular messengers: (1) inositol triphosphate (IP$_3$) releases Ca^{++}, and (2) diacylglycerol remains in the plasma membrane and activates protein kinase C. Protein kinase C further activates various cell proteins. Several different plasma membrane receptors are known to use the inositol-phospholipid transduction pathway.

Data from Alberts B et al: *Molecular biology of the cell*, ed 5, New York, 2008, Garland.

extracellular messengers regulate channel function for the other two methods of controlling channels.

Second Messengers

Many ligands cannot enter their target cells to cause the desired intracellular response. Instead, the first messengers, or ligands, issue orders by binding with receptors on the surface membrane, triggering a "pass it on" signal. Second messengers are generated in large numbers when the membrane-bound enzyme is activated, and they then rapidly diffuse away from their source, broadcasting the signal throughout the cell (Fig. 1.24). Remember, most cell surface receptor proteins belong to one of three large classes: ion channel–linked receptors, G-protein–linked receptors, or enzyme-linked receptors.

The two major second-messenger pathways are **cyclic adenosine monophosphate (cyclic AMP, cAMP)** and Ca^{++}. In the cAMP pathway, binding of the ligand to its surface receptor eventually activates the enzyme adenylyl cyclase on the inner surface of the membrane. A membrane-bound "middleman," a **G protein**, acts as an intermediary between the receptor and adenylyl cyclase. G proteins are named because they are bound to guanine nucleotides—**guanosine triphosphate (GTP)** or **guanosine diphosphate (GDP)**. An unactivated G protein consists of a complex of alpha (α), beta (β), and gamma (γ) subunits, with a GDP molecule bound to the α subunit. The cAMP pathway with G proteins is summarized in Fig. 1.24.

Instead of cAMP, some cells use Ca^{++} as a second messenger. In this pathway, binding of the first messenger to the surface receptor eventually leads, by means of G proteins, to activation of the enzyme phospholipase C, an enzyme protein effector (an ion channel for an enzyme) that is bound to the inner side of the membrane. Fig. 1.25 summarizes the Ca^{++} second-messenger pathway. The cAMP and Ca^{++} pathways frequently overlap in triggering a specific cellular response. For example, cAMP and Ca^{++} can influence each other. Calcium-activated calmodulin can regulate adenylyl cyclase and thus influence cAMP; conversely, cAMP-dependent kinase may phosphorylate and thereby change the activity of Ca^{++} channels or carriers. In some instances, both Ca^{++} and cAMP regulate the same intracellular protein. In a few cells, **cyclic guanosine monophosphate (cyclic GMP, cGMP)** serves as a second messenger similar to the cAMP pathway. For example, cGMP is the signal transduction pathway involved in vision. Some cellular responses mediated by cAMP and phospholipase C are summarized in Table 1.3. Major types of receptors and signal transduction pathways are contained in Table 1.4.

TABLE 1.3   HORMONE-INDUCED CELL RESPONSES MEDIATED BY cAMP

SIGNALING LIGANDS	TARGET TISSUE	MAJOR RESPONSE
Epinephrine	Heart	Increase in heart rate and force of contraction
Epinephrine, ACTH	Muscle	Breakdown of glycogen
Glucagon	Fat	Breakdown of fat
ACTH	Adrenal gland	Secretion of cortisol
Antidiuretic hormone (vasopressin)	Kidney	Increase in retention of water; promotion of fluid balance
Acetylcholine	Pancreas; smooth muscle	Secretion of amylase; contraction
Antigen	Mast cells	Secretion of histamine
Thrombin	Blood platelets	Secretion of serotonin and platelet-derived growth factor; aggregation of platelets

ACTH, Adrenocorticotropic hormone; *cAMP*, cyclic adenosine monophosphate.

A large number of human disorders involve problematic signaling in cells. Cancer, for example, results from genetic mutations leading to the overactivity of proteins in signal relaying pathways that normally induce the cells to divide. Affected proteins cause cells to behave as if other cells were constantly telling them to reproduce, even when no such orders were sent. Signal blockers are already in use against tumors.

CELLULAR METABOLISM

All the chemical tasks of maintaining essential cellular functions are referred to as **cellular metabolism**. The energy-using process of metabolism is called **anabolism** (*ana* = upward), and the energy-releasing process is known as **catabolism** (*cata* = downward). Metabolism provides

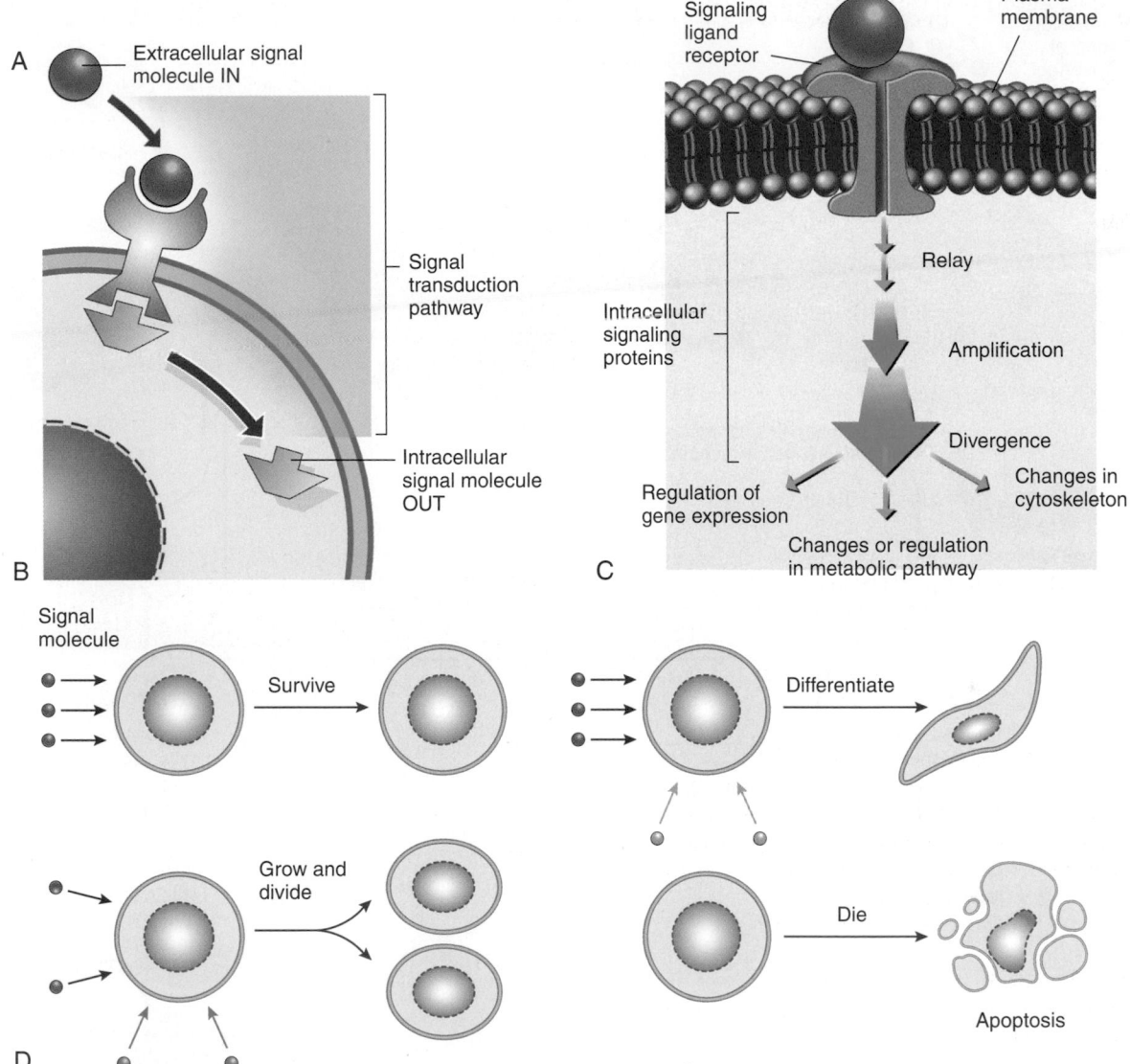

FIGURE 1.22 Schematic of a Signal Transduction Pathway. Like a telephone receiver that converts an electrical signal into a sound signal, a cell converts an extracellular signal (**A**) into an intracellular signal. **B** and **C,** An extracellular signal molecule (ligand) binds to a receptor protein located on the plasma membrane, where it is transduced into an intracellular signal. This process initiates a signaling cascade that relays the signal into the cell interior, amplifying and distributing it en route. Amplification is often achieved by stimulating enzymes. Steps in the cascade can be modulated by other events in the cell. **D,** Different cell behaviors rely on multiple extracellular signals.

the cell with the energy it needs to synthesize (produce) cellular structures.

Dietary proteins, fats, and starches are hydrolyzed in the intestinal tract into amino acids, fatty acids, and glucose, respectively. These constituents are then absorbed, circulated, and taken up by the cell, where they may be used for various vital cellular processes, including the production of ATP. The process by which ATP is produced is one example of a series of reactions called a **metabolic pathway**. A metabolic pathway involves several intermediate steps whose end products are not always detectable. A key feature of cellular metabolism is the directing of biochemical reactions by protein catalysts, or enzymes. Most biochemical reactions in a pathway are catalyzed by a specific enzyme. Each enzyme has a high affinity for a **substrate**—a specific substance that is converted to a product of the reaction.

Role of Adenosine Triphosphate

Best known about ATP is its role as a universal "fuel" *inside* living cells. This fuel or energy drives biologic reactions necessary for cells to function. For a cell to function it must be able to extract and use the chemical energy contained within the structure of organic molecules. When 1 mole (mol) of glucose is metabolically broken down in the presence of oxygen into carbon dioxide (CO_2) and water (H_2O), 686 kilocalories (kcal) of energy are released. In a test tube this energy is released as heat. Because a cell cannot transform heat into work, chemical energy, rather than heat, is created by metabolism. The chemical energy lost by one molecule is transferred to the chemical structure of another molecule by an energy-carrying or energy-transferring molecule, such as ATP. The energy stored in ATP can be used in a variety of energy-requiring reactions and in the process is generally converted to adenosine

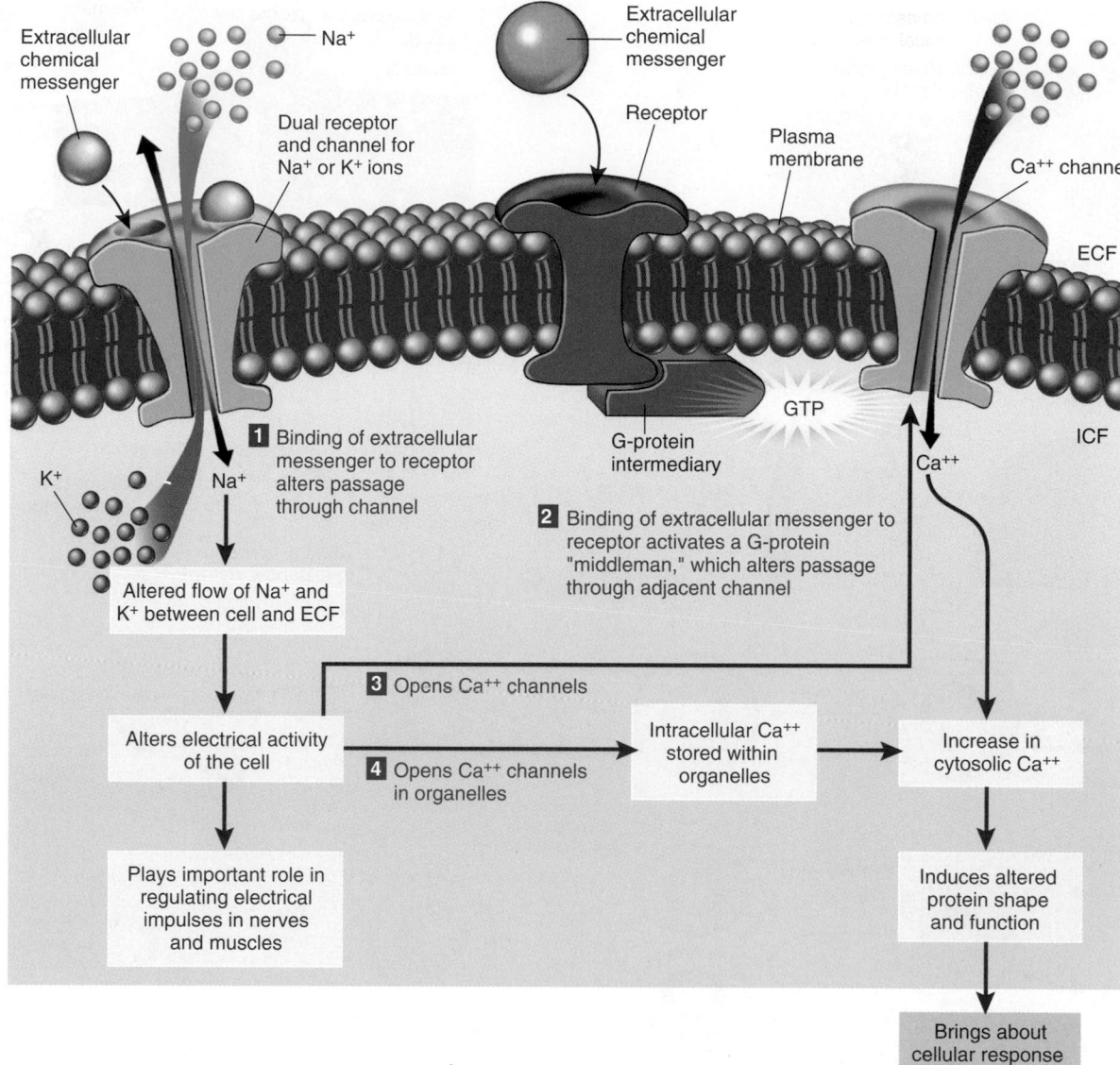

FIGURE 1.23 How Extracellular Messengers Regulate Channel Function. Binding of an extracellular messenger to a dual receptor/channel brings about a quick opening or closing of ion channels, such as Na⁺ or K⁺ channels, which generate electrical impulses **(1)**. A transient opening of membrane Ca⁺⁺ channels occurs when binding of an extracellular messenger to a receptor activates a G-protein intermediary, which alters a nearby ion channel, such as a Ca⁺⁺ channel **(2)**. A transient opening of Ca⁺⁺ channels also occurs indirectly in response to electrical impulses produced by extracellular messenger–induced changes in Na⁺ and K⁺ channels **(3)**. Release of Ca⁺⁺ from intracellular stores results when Ca⁺⁺ channels in organelles open in response to electrical impulses **(4)**. An increase in cytosolic Ca⁺⁺ concentration arising from pathways **2, 3,** or **4** causes a change in the shape and function of specific intracellular proteins to produce the desired cellular response. *ECF,* Extracellular fluid; *GTP,* guanosine triphosphate; *ICF,* intracellular fluid. (Redrawn with permission from Sherwood L: *Human physiology,* ed 3, ©1997 Brooks/Cole, a part of Cengage Learning, Inc. Reproduced by permission from www.cengage.com/permissions.)

diphosphate (ADP) and inorganic phosphate (Pi). The energy available as a result of this reaction is about 7 kcal/mol of ATP. In addition to its use in synthesis (anabolism) of organic molecules, ATP is used by the cell for muscle contraction and active transport of molecules across cellular membranes. The function of ATP is not only to *store* energy but also to *transfer* it from one molecule to another. Energy is stored by molecules of carbohydrate, lipid, and protein, which, when catabolized, transfer energy to ATP.

Food and Production of Cellular Energy

The process of catabolism of the proteins, lipids, and polysaccharides found in food can be divided into the following three phases (Fig. 1.26).

Phase 1: **Digestion.** Large molecules are broken down into their smaller subunits—proteins into amino acids, polysaccharides into simple sugars, and fats into fatty acids and glycerol. These processes occur outside the cell by the action of secreted enzymes.

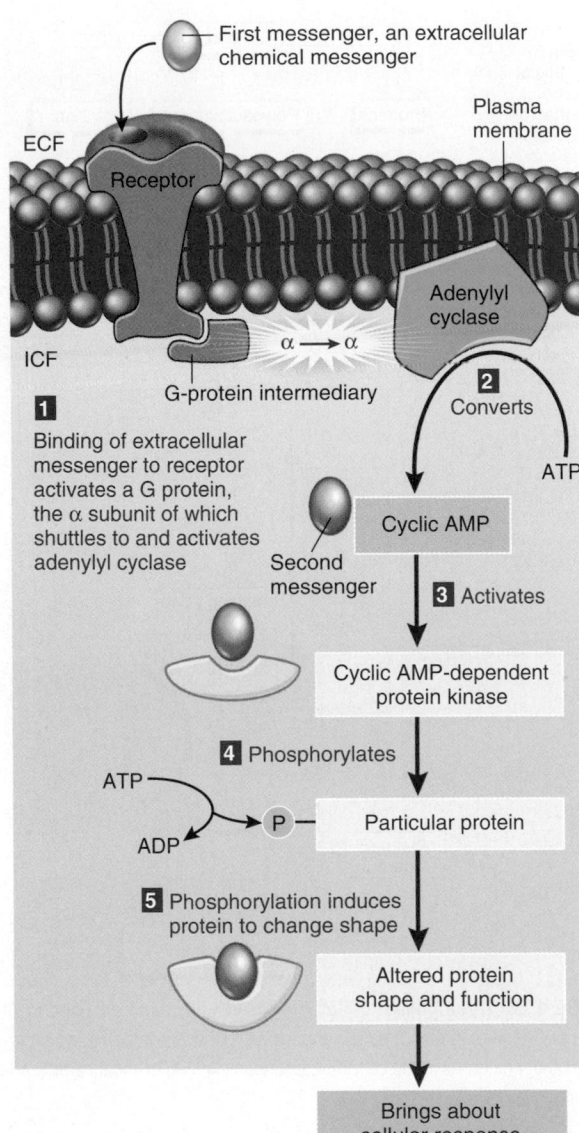

FIGURE 1.24 Extracellular Messenger and Activation of the cAMP Second-Messenger System. The first messenger, or binding of an extracellular chemical messenger to a surface membrane receptor, activates the membrane-bound enzyme adenylyl cyclase by means of a G-protein intermediary **(1),** which in turn converts intracellular ATP into cAMP **(2).** cAMP is an intracellular second messenger, triggering the cellular response by activating the cAMP-dependent protein kinase **(3),** which in turn phosphorylates **(4),** and therefore modifies **(5)** a specific intracellular protein. The altered protein then directs the cellular response dictated by the extracellular messenger. *ADP,* Adenosine diphosphate; *AMP,* adenosine monophosphate; *ATP,* adenosine triphosphate; *ECF,* extracellular fluid; *ICF,* intracellular fluid. (Redrawn with permission from Sherwood L: *Human physiology,* ed 3, 1997, Brooks/Cole, a part of Cengage Learning, Inc. Reproduced by permission from www.cengage.com/permissions.)

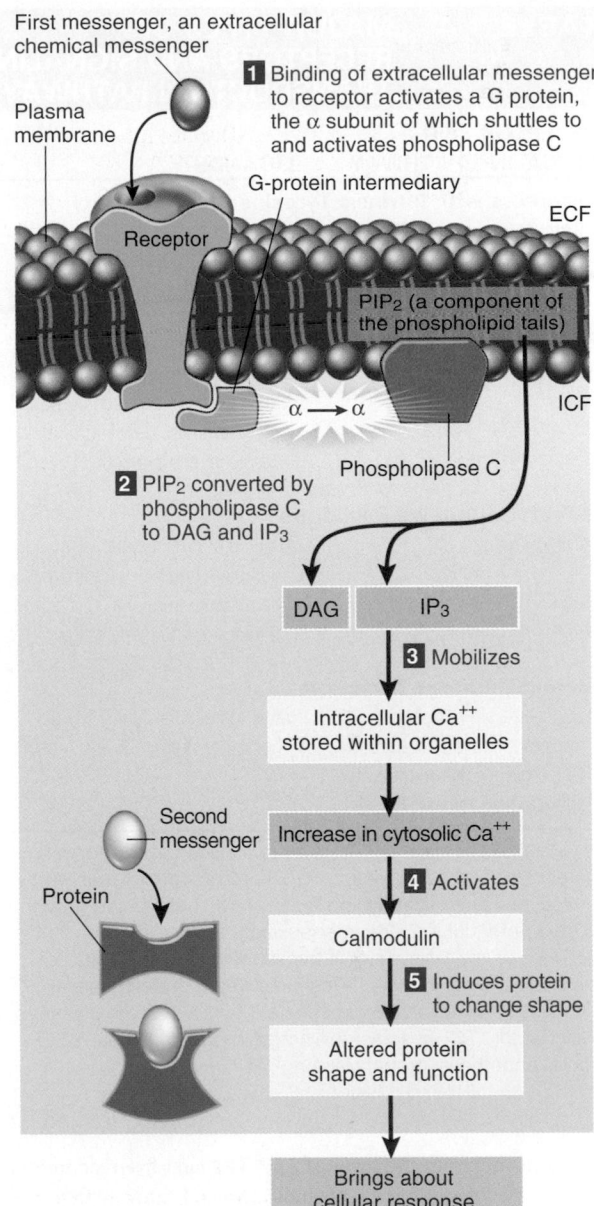

FIGURE 1.25 Extracellular Messenger and Activation of the Calcium Second-Messenger System. Binding of an extracellular messenger to a membrane receptor activates the membrane-bound enzyme phospholipase C by means of a G-protein intermediary **(1).** Phospholipase C converts phosphatidylinositol biphosphate *(PIP$_2$)* into diacylglycerol *(DAG)* and inositol triphosphate *(IP$_3$)* **(2).** IP$_3$ then mobilizes Ca^{++} stored within organelles **(3).** Ca^{++}, as a second messenger, activates calmodulin **(4),** causing a change in the shape and function of a specific intracellular protein to produce the cellular response **(5).** *ECF,* Extracellular fluid; *ICF,* intracellular fluid. (Redrawn with permission from Sherwood L: *Human physiology,* ed 3, 1997, Brooks/Cole, a part of Cengage Learning, Inc. Reproduced by permission from www.cengage.com/permissions.)

Phase 2: **Glycolysis** and **oxidation.** The small molecules enter cells and are further broken down in the cytoplasm. Most of the sugars are converted into pyruvate. Pyruvate then enters mitochondria and is converted to the acetyl groups of acetyl coenzyme A (acetyl CoA). Acetyl CoA, like ATP, releases energy when it is hydrolyzed. The most important part of phase 2 is the lysis (splitting) of glucose, known as

glycolysis (Fig. 1.27). Glycolysis produces a net of two molecules of ATP per glucose molecule through the process of oxidation, or the removal and transfer of a pair of electrons. This process, often called **oxidative cellular metabolism,** involves 10 biochemical reactions. In reactions 1 through 5, glucose is converted to two, three-carbon aldehyde compounds (glyceraldehyde-3-phosphate [G3P]), which

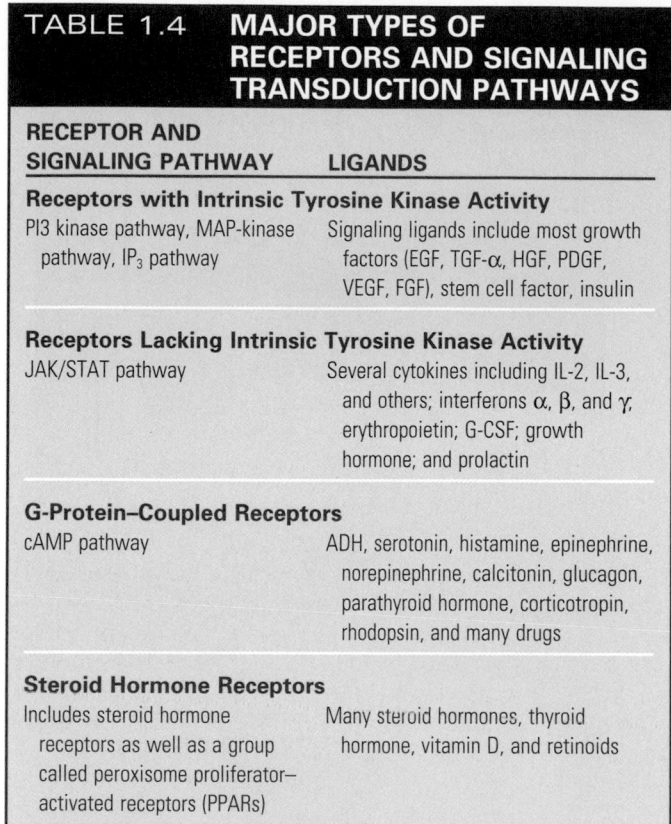

TABLE 1.4	MAJOR TYPES OF RECEPTORS AND SIGNALING TRANSDUCTION PATHWAYS	
RECEPTOR AND SIGNALING PATHWAY	**LIGANDS**
Receptors with Intrinsic Tyrosine Kinase Activity	
PI3 kinase pathway, MAP-kinase pathway, IP₃ pathway	Signaling ligands include most growth factors (EGF, TGF-α, HGF, PDGF, VEGF, FGF), stem cell factor, insulin
Receptors Lacking Intrinsic Tyrosine Kinase Activity	
JAK/STAT pathway	Several cytokines including IL-2, IL-3, and others; interferons α, β, and γ; erythropoietin; G-CSF; growth hormone; and prolactin
G-Protein–Coupled Receptors	
cAMP pathway	ADH, serotonin, histamine, epinephrine, norepinephrine, calcitonin, glucagon, parathyroid hormone, corticotropin, rhodopsin, and many drugs
Steroid Hormone Receptors	
Includes steroid hormone receptors as well as a group called peroxisome proliferator–activated receptors (PPARs)	Many steroid hormones, thyroid hormone, vitamin D, and retinoids

ADH, Antidiuretic hormone; *cAMP*, cyclic adenosine monophosphate; *EGF*, epidermal growth factor; *FGF*, fibroblast growth factor; *G-CSF*, granulocyte colony–stimulating factor; *HGF*, hepatocyte growth factor; *IL-2, IL-3*, interleukin-2 and interleukin-3; *IP₃*, inositol triphosphate; *JAK/STAT*, Janus kinase-signal transducers and activators of transcription; *MAP-kinase*, mitogen-activated protein kinase; *PI3*, phosphatidylinositol-4,5-bisphosphate 3-*kinase*; *PDGF*, platelet-derived growth factor; *TGF-α*, transforming growth factor-alpha; *VEGF*, vascular endothelial growth factor.

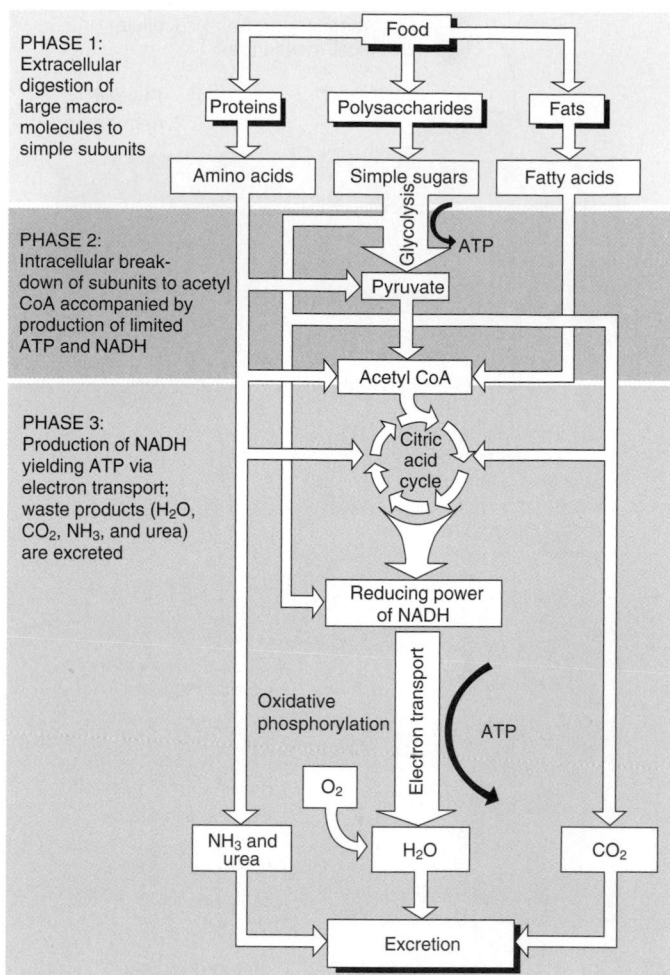

FIGURE 1.26 Three Phases of Catabolism, Which Lead from Food to Waste Products. These reactions produce adenosine triphosphate (ATP), which is used to drive other processes in the cell. *CoA*, Coenzyme A; *NADH*, nicotinamide adenine dinucleotide.

require energy in the form of ATP. The next five reactions convert G3P molecules into pyruvate molecules and generate four molecules of ATP for each two molecules of G3P. In addition, two molecules of nicotinamide adenine dinucleotide (NAD) are further oxidized to produce four more molecules of ATP. After subtracting two molecules of ATP to drive the reactions, the net yield is six ATP molecules for each molecule of glucose.

Phase 3: Citric acid cycle (Krebs cycle, tricarboxylic acid cycle). Most of the ATP is generated during this final phase. It begins with the citric acid cycle and ends with oxidative phosphorylation. About two thirds of the total oxidation of carbon compounds in most cells is accomplished during this phase. The major end products are carbon dioxide (CO_2) and two dinucleotides—reduced nicotinamide adenine dinucleotide (NADH) and the reduced form of flavin adenine dinucleotide ($FADH_2$)—which transfer their electrons into the electron-transport chain.

Oxidative Phosphorylation

Oxidative phosphorylation occurs in the mitochondria and is the mechanism by which the energy produced from carbohydrates, fats, and proteins is transferred to ATP. During the breakdown (catabolism) of foods, many of the reactions involve the removal of electrons from various intermediates. These reactions generally require a coenzyme (a nonprotein carrier molecule), such as nicotinamide adenine dinucleotide (NAD), to transfer the electrons and thus are called **transfer reactions**.

Molecules of NAD and flavin adenine dinucleotide (FAD) transfer electrons they have gained from the oxidation of substrates to molecular oxygen, O_2. The electrons from reduced NAD and FAD, NADH and $FADH_2$, respectively, are transferred to a series of carrier molecules (the **electron-transport chain**) on the inner surfaces of the mitochondria with the release of hydrogen ions. Some carrier molecules are a group of brightly colored iron-containing proteins known as **cytochromes** that accept a pair of electrons. These electrons eventually combine with molecular oxygen. If oxygen is not available to the electron-transport chain, ATP will not be formed by the mitochondria. Instead, an anaerobic (without oxygen) metabolic pathway synthesizes ATP. This process, called **substrate phosphorylation**, or **anaerobic glycolysis**, is linked to the breakdown (glycolysis) of carbohydrate (Fig. 1.28).

Because glycolysis occurs in the cytoplasm of the cell, it provides energy for cells that lack mitochondria. However, as noted, glycolysis also provides energy to the cell when oxygen delivery is insufficient or delayed (e.g., with strenuous exercise). The reactions in anaerobic glycolysis involve the conversion of glucose to pyruvic acid (pyruvate) with the simultaneous production of ATP. With the glycolysis of one molecule of glucose, two ATP molecules and two molecules of pyruvate

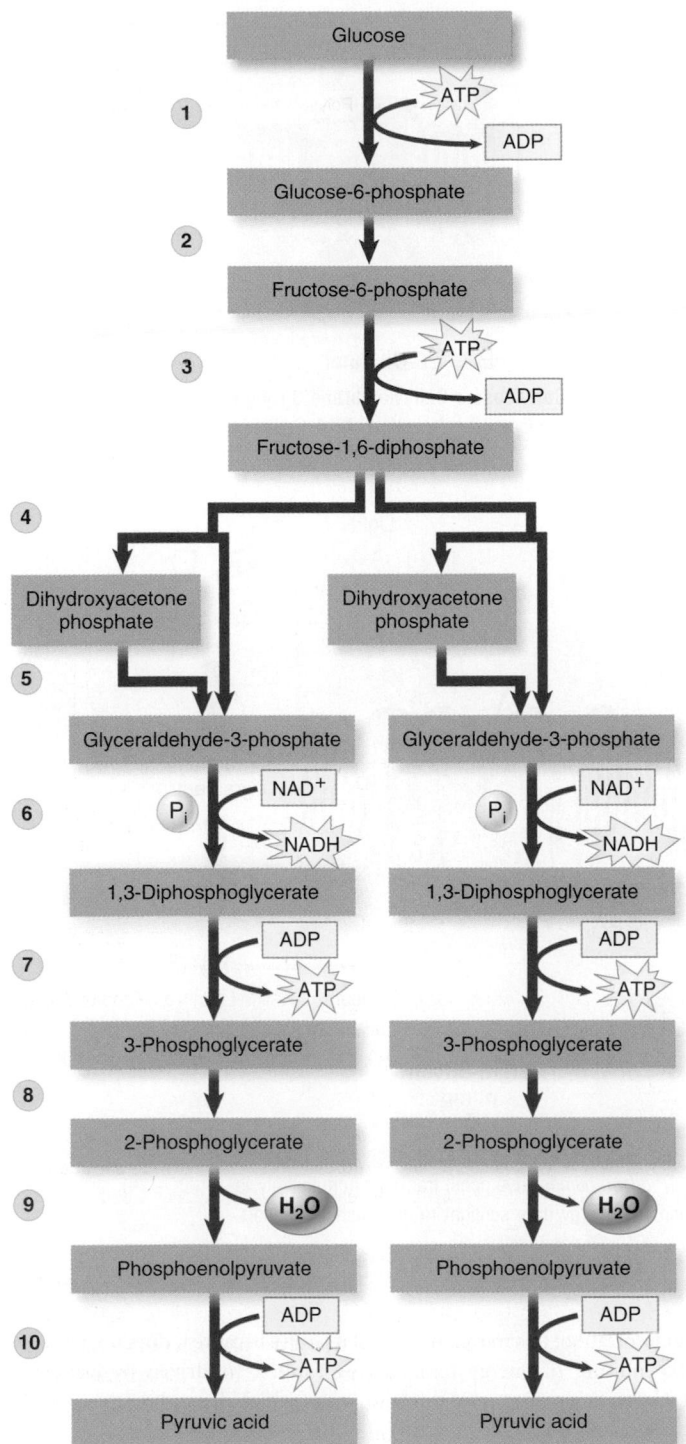

FIGURE 1.27 Glycolysis. Each of the numbered reactions is catalyzed by a different enzyme. At step **4**, a six-carbon sugar is broken down to give two, three-carbon sugars, so that the number of molecules at every step after this is doubled. Reactions **5** and **6** are the reactions responsible for the net synthesis of adenosine triphosphate *(ATP)* and reduced nicotinamide adenine dinucleotide *(NADH)* molecules. *ADP*, adenosine diphosphate; *Pᵢ*, three phosphate groups. (From Patton KT, Thibodeau GA: *Anatomy & physiology*, ed 9, St Louis, 2016, Mosby.)

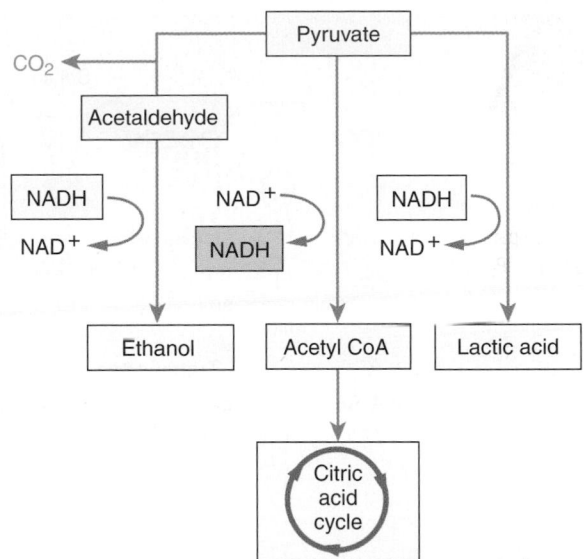

FIGURE 1.28 What Happens to Pyruvate, the Product of Glycolysis? In the presence of oxygen, pyruvate is oxidized to acetyl coenzyme A *(acetyl CoA)* and enters the citric acid cycle. In the absence of oxygen, pyruvate instead is reduced, accepting the electrons extracted during glycolysis and carried by reduced nicotinamide adenine dinucleotide *(NADH)*. When pyruvate is reduced directly, as it is in muscle, the product is lactic acid. When CO_2 is first removed from pyruvate and the remainder reduced, as it is in yeasts, the product is ethanol.

are liberated. If oxygen is present, the two molecules of pyruvate move into the mitochondria, where they enter the citric acid cycle.

If oxygen is absent, pyruvate is converted to lactic acid, which is released into the extracellular fluid (see Fig. 1.28). Elevated lactate level is indicative of tissue hypoxia or low oxygen concentration. The conversion of pyruvic acid to lactic acid is reversible; therefore, once oxygen is restored, lactic acid is quickly converted back to either pyruvic acid or glucose. The anaerobic generation of ATP from glucose, through the reactions of glycolysis, is not as efficient as the aerobic generation of ATP. The addition of an oxygen-requiring stage to the catabolic process (stage 3) provides cells with a much more powerful method for extracting energy from food molecules.

MEMBRANE TRANSPORT: CELLULAR INTAKE AND OUTPUT

Cell survival and growth depend on the constant exchange of molecules with their environment. Cells continually import nutrients, fluids, and chemical messengers from the extracellular environment and expel metabolites or the products of metabolism and end products of lysosomal digestion. Cells also must regulate ions in their cytosol and organelles. Simple diffusion across the lipid bilayer of the plasma membrane occurs for such important molecules as O_2 and CO_2. However, the majority of molecule transfer depends on specialized **membrane transport proteins** that span the lipid bilayer and provide private thoroughfares for select molecules.[2] Membrane transport proteins occur in many forms and are present in all cell membranes.[2] Transport by membrane transport proteins is sometimes called **mediated transport**. Most of these transport proteins allow selective passage, for example, Na+ but not K+ or K+ but not Na+. Each type of cell membrane has its own transport proteins that determine which solute can pass into and out of the cell or organelle.[2] The two main classes of membrane transport proteins are *transporters* and *channels*. These transport proteins differ in the type of **solute**—small

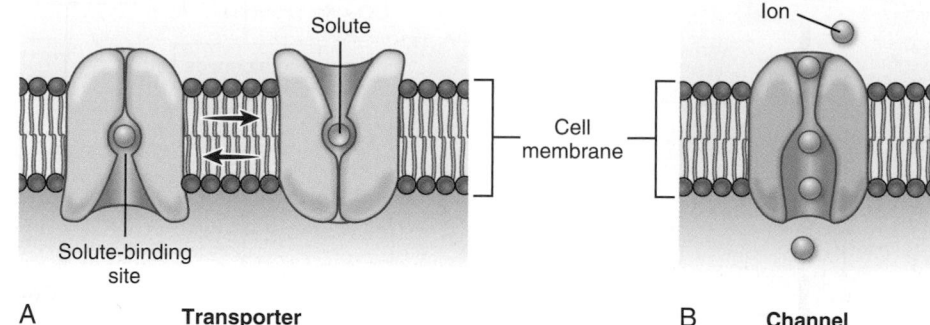

FIGURE 1.29 Inorganic Ions and Small, Polar Organic Molecules Can Cross a Cell Membrane through Either a Transporter or a Channel. (Adapted from Alberts B: *Essential cell biology,* ed 4, New York, 2014, Garland.)

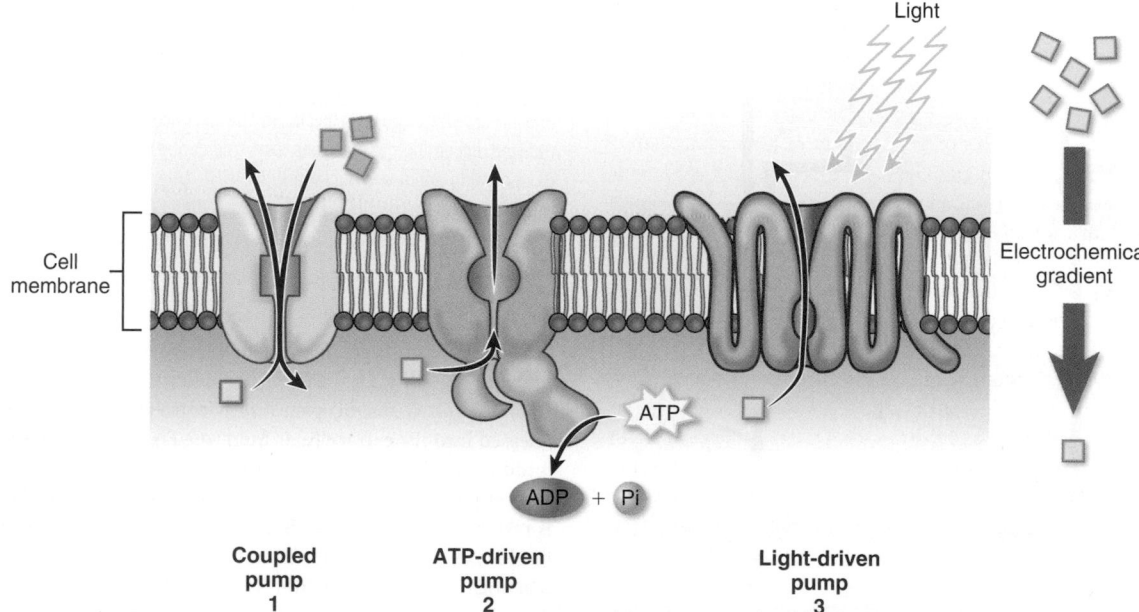

FIGURE 1.30 Pumps Carry Out Active Transport in Three Ways. **1,** *Coupled pumps* link the uphill transport of one solute to the downhill transport of another solute. **2,** *ATP-driven pumps* drive uphill transport from hydrolysis of ATP. **3,** *Light-driven pumps* are mostly found in bacteria and use energy from sunlight to drive uphill transport. (Adapted from Alberts B: *Essential cell biology,* ed 4, New York, 2014, Garland.)

particles of dissolved substances—they transport. A **transporter** is specific, allowing only those ions that fit the unique binding sites on the protein (Fig. 1.29, *A*). A transporter undergoes conformational changes to enable membrane transport. A **channel**, when open, forms a pore across the lipid bilayer that allows ions and selective polar organic molecules to diffuse across the membrane (see Fig. 1.29, *B*). Transport by a channel depends on the size and electrical charge of the molecule. Some channels are controlled by a gate mechanism that determines which solute can move into it. Ion channels are responsible for the electrical excitability of nerve and muscle cells and play a critical role in the membrane potential.

The mechanisms of membrane transport depend on the characteristics of the substance to be transported. In **passive transport**, water and small, electrically uncharged molecules move easily through pores in the plasma membrane's lipid bilayer (see Fig. 1.29). This process occurs naturally through any semipermeable barrier. Molecules will easily flow "downhill" from a region of high concentration to a region of low

concentration; this movement is called *passive* because it does not require expenditure of energy or a driving force. It is driven by osmosis, hydrostatic pressure, and diffusion, all of which depend on the laws of physics and do not require life.

Other molecules are too large to pass through pores or are ligands bound to receptors on the cell's plasma membrane. Some of these molecules are moved into and out of the cell by **active transport**, which requires life, biologic activity, and the cell's expenditure of metabolic energy (see Fig. 1.29). Unlike passive transport, active transport occurs across only living membranes that have to drive the flow "uphill" by coupling it to an energy source. Movement of a solute against its concentration gradient occurs by special types of transporters called *pumps* (see Fig. 1.29). These transporter pumps must harness an energy source to power the transport process. Energy can come from ATP hydrolysis, a transmembrane ion gradient, or sunlight (Fig. 1.30). The best-known is the Na^+-K^+–dependent adenosine triphosphatase (ATPase) pump (see Fig. 1.34). It continuously regulates the cell's volume by

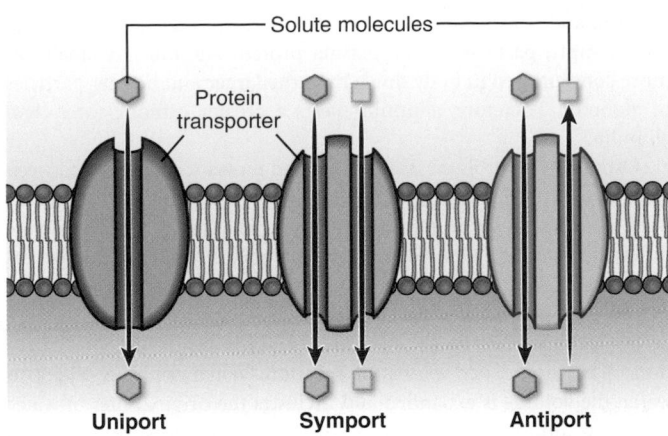

FIGURE 1.31 Mediated Transport. Illustration shows simultaneous movement of a single solute molecule in one direction *(Uniport)*, of two different solute molecules in one direction *(Symport)*, and of two different solute molecules in opposite directions *(Antiport)*.

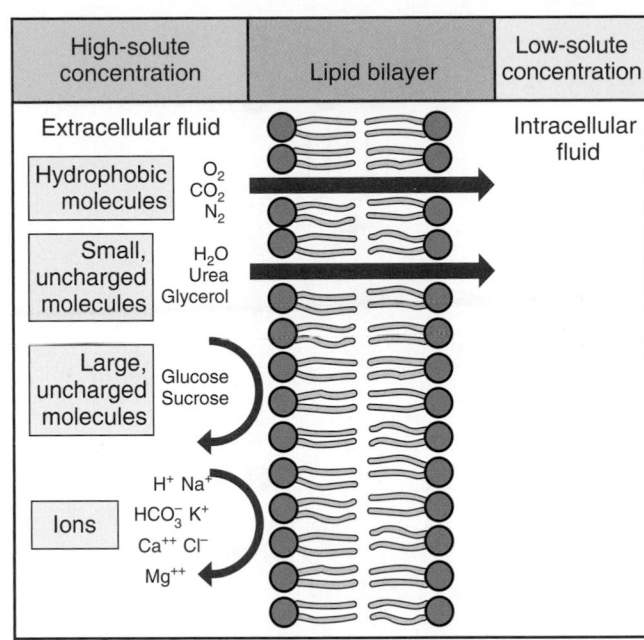

FIGURE 1.32 Passive Diffusion of Solute Molecules Across the Plasma Membrane. Oxygen, nitrogen, water, urea, glycerol, and carbon dioxide can diffuse readily down the concentration gradient. Macromolecules are too large to diffuse through pores in the plasma membrane. Ions may be repelled if the pores contain substances with identical charges. If the pores are lined with cations, for example, other cations will have difficulty diffusing because the positive charges will repel one another; diffusion can still occur, but it occurs more slowly.

controlling leaks through pores or protein channels and maintaining the ionic concentration gradients needed for cellular excitation and membrane conductivity. The maintenance of intracellular K^+ concentrations is required also for enzyme activity, including enzymes involved in protein synthesis. Large molecules (macromolecules), along with fluids, are transported by endocytosis (taking in) and exocytosis (expelling). Receptor-macromolecule complexes enter the cell by means of receptor-mediated endocytosis.

Mediated transport systems can move solute molecules singly or two at a time. Two molecules can be moved simultaneously in one direction (a process called **symport**, for example, sodium-glucose in the digestive tract) or in opposite directions (called **antiport**, for example, the sodium-potassium pump in all cells), or a single molecule can be moved in one direction (called **uniport**, for example, glucose) (Fig. 1.31).

Electrolytes as Solutes

Body fluids are composed of two types of solutes: **electrolytes**, which are electrically charged and dissociate into constituent **ions** when placed in solution; and nonelectrolytes, such as glucose, urea, and creatinine, which do not dissociate. Electrolytes account for approximately 95% of the solute molecules in body water. Electrolytes exhibit **polarity** by orienting themselves toward the positive or negative pole. Ions with a positive charge are known as **cations** and migrate toward the negative pole, or cathode, if an electrical current is passed through the electrolyte solution. **Anions** carry a negative charge and migrate toward the positive pole, or anode, in the presence of electrical current. Anions and cations are located in both the intracellular fluid (ICF) and the extracellular fluid (ECF) compartments, although the concentration of particular ions varies depending on their location. For example, Na^+ is the predominant extracellular cation, and K^+ is the principal intracellular cation. The difference in ICF and ECF concentrations of these ions is important to the transmission of electrical impulses across the plasma membranes of nerve and muscle cells (see Chapter 3).

Electrolytes are measured in milliequivalents per liter (mEq/L) or milligrams per deciliter (mg/dL). Milliequivalents per liter indicate the number of electrical charges per unit volume of fluid. The term *milliequivalent* thus indicates the chemical-combining activity of an ion, which depends on the electrical charge, or valence, of its ions. In abbreviations, valence is indicated by the number of plus or minus signs. Monovalent ions, or ions with one charge, include sodium (Na^+),

chloride (Cl^-), and potassium (K^+). Divalent ions, which have two charges, include calcium (Ca^{++}) and magnesium (Mg^{++}). One milliequivalent of any cation can combine chemically with 1 mEq of any anion; one monovalent anion will combine with one monovalent cation. Divalent ions combine more strongly than monovalent ions. To maintain electrochemical balance, one divalent ion will combine with two monovalent ions (e.g., $Ca^{++} + 2\ Cl^- = CaCl_2$).

Passive Transport: Diffusion, Filtration, and Osmosis

Diffusion. Diffusion is the movement of a solute molecule from an area of greater solute concentration to an area of lesser solute concentration. This difference in concentration is known as a **concentration gradient**. Particles in a solution move randomly in any direction. If the concentration of particles in one part of the solution is greater than that in another part, the particles distribute themselves evenly throughout the solution. According to the same principle, if the concentration of particles is greater on one side of a *permeable membrane* than on the other side, the particles diffuse spontaneously from the area of greater concentration to the area of lesser concentration until equilibrium is reached. The higher the concentration on one side, the greater the diffusion rate. The overall effect of diffusion is the passive movement of particles "down" a concentration gradient, that is, from an area of high concentration to an area of low concentration.

The diffusion rate is influenced by differences of electrical potential across the membrane. Because the pores in the lipid bilayer are often linked with Ca^{++}, other cations (e.g., Na^+ and K^+) diffuse slowly because they are repelled by positive charges in the pores.

The rate of diffusion of a substance depends also on its size (diffusion coefficient) and its lipid solubility (Fig. 1.32). Usually the smaller the molecule and the more soluble it is in oil, the more hydrophobic or nonpolar it is and the more rapidly it will diffuse across the bilayer.

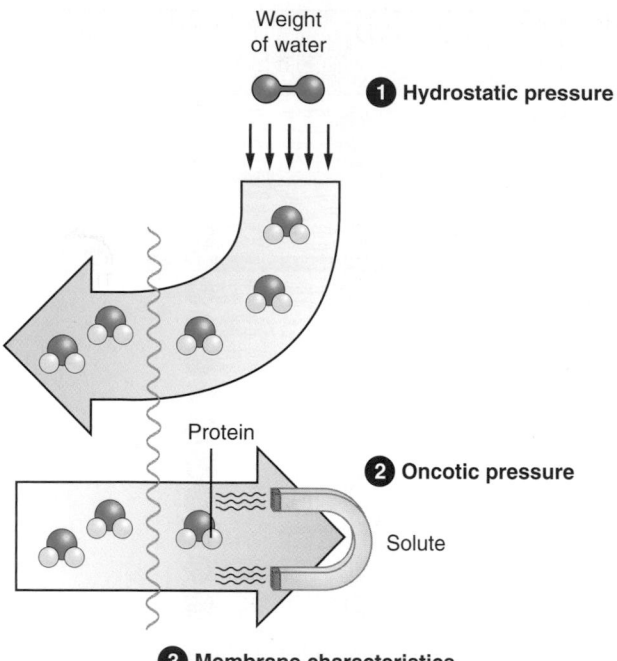

Weight of water

1 **Hydrostatic pressure**

Protein

2 **Oncotic pressure**

Solute

3 **Membrane characteristics**

FIGURE 1.33 Hydrostatic Pressure and Oncotic Pressure in Plasma. **1,** Hydrostatic pressure in plasma. **2,** Oncotic pressure exerted by proteins in the plasma usually tends to *pull* water into the circulatory system. **3,** Individuals with low protein levels (e.g., starvation) are unable to maintain a normal oncotic pressure; therefore, water is not reabsorbed into the circulation and, instead, causes body edema.

Oxygen, carbon dioxide, and the steroid hormones are all examples of nonpolar molecules. Water-soluble substances, such as sugars and inorganic ions, diffuse very slowly, whereas uncharged lipophilic ("lipid-loving") molecules, such as fatty acids and steroids, diffuse rapidly. Ions and other polar molecules generally diffuse across cellular membranes more slowly than lipid-soluble substances.

Water readily diffuses through biologic membranes because water molecules are small and uncharged. Although the mechanism is not known with certainty, the dipolar structure of water allows it to cross rapidly through the regions of the bilayer containing the lipid head groups. Lipid head groups constitute the two outer regions of the lipid bilayer.

Filtration: Hydrostatic pressure. Filtration is the movement of water and solutes through a membrane because of a greater pushing pressure (force) on one side of the membrane than on the other side. Hydrostatic pressure is the mechanical force of water pushing against cellular membranes (Fig. 1.33, *1*). In the vascular system, hydrostatic pressure is the *blood pressure* generated in vessels by the contraction of the heart. Blood reaching the capillary bed has a hydrostatic pressure of 25 to 30 mmHg, which is sufficient force to push water across the thin capillary membranes into the interstitial space. Hydrostatic pressure is partially balanced by osmotic pressure, whereby water moving *out* of the capillaries is partially balanced by osmotic forces that tend to *pull* water *into* the capillaries. Water that is not osmotically attracted back into the capillaries moves into the lymph system.

Osmosis. Osmosis is the movement of water "down" a concentration gradient, that is, across a semipermeable membrane from a region of higher water concentration to a region of lower water concentration. For osmosis to occur, the membrane must be more permeable to water than to solutes and the concentration of solutes must be greater so that water moves more easily. Osmosis is directly related to both hydrostatic

pressure and solute concentration but *not* to particle size or weight. For example, particles of the plasma protein albumin are small but more concentrated in body fluids than the larger and heavier particles of globulin. Therefore, albumin exerts a greater osmotic force than globulin.

Osmolality controls the distribution and movement of water between body compartments. The terms *osmolality* and *osmolarity* are often used interchangeably in reference to osmotic activity, but they define different measurements. Osmolality is a measure of the number of milliosmoles per kilogram (mOsm/kg) of water, or the concentration of molecules per *weight* of water. Osmolarity is a measure of the number of milliosmoles per liter (mOsm/L) of solution, or the concentration of molecules per *volume* of solution. When solute is added to water, the volume is expanded and includes the original liter of water plus the volume occupied by the solute particles. In measuring osmolarity, the volume of water is therefore reduced by an amount equal to the volume of added solute (also see Chapter 3).

In solutions that contain only dissociable substances, such as Na^+ and Cl^-, the difference between the two measurements is negligible. In considering all the different solutes in plasma (e.g., proteins, glucose, lipids), however, the difference between osmolality and osmolarity becomes more significant. In plasma less of the plasma weight is water, and the overall concentration of particles is therefore greater. The osmolality will be greater than the osmolarity because of the smaller proportion of water. Osmolality is thus the preferred measure of osmotic activity in clinical assessment of individuals.

The normal osmolality of body fluids is 280 to 294 mOsm/kg. The osmolality of intracellular and extracellular fluid tends to equalize and therefore provides a measure of body fluid concentration and thus the body's hydration status. Hydration is also affected by hydrostatic pressure because the movement of water by osmosis can be opposed by an equal amount of hydrostatic pressure. The amount of hydrostatic pressure required to oppose the osmotic movement of water is called the osmotic pressure of the solution. Factors that determine osmotic pressure are the type and thickness of the plasma membrane, the size of the molecules, the concentration of molecules or the concentration gradient, and the solubility of molecules within the membrane. Examples of movement of water in relation to hydrostatic and osmotic forces occur in the glomerulus of the kidney and in the capillaries of the microcirculation.

Effective osmolality is sustained osmotic activity and depends on the concentration of solutes remaining on one side of a permeable membrane. If the solutes penetrate the membrane and equilibrate with the solution on the other side of the membrane, the osmotic effect will be diminished or lost. For example, urea is a small solute that readily diffuses across cellular membranes. Solutions containing urea rapidly lose their effective osmolality because they rapidly equilibrate. Solutes too large to pass through the membrane thus sustain an effective osmolality, meaning that they enhance osmotic activity. Plasma proteins are examples of molecules that provide effective osmolality because they normally do not cross cellular membranes.

Plasma proteins also influence osmolality because they have a negative charge (see Fig. 1.33). The principle by which the plasma protein charge influences osmolality is known as *Gibbs-Donnan equilibrium,* and it affects the distribution of ions across cellular membranes. Gibbs-Donnan equilibrium occurs when fluid in one compartment contains small, diffusible ions such as Na^+ and Cl^-, together with large, nondiffusible charged particles, such as plasma proteins. Because the body tends to maintain an electrical equilibrium, the nondiffusible protein molecules cause asymmetry in the distribution of small ions. Anions such as Cl^- are thus driven out of the cell or plasma, and cations such as Na^+ are attracted. The protein-containing compartment will maintain a state of electroneutrality, but the osmolality will be higher. The overall osmotic effect of colloids, such as plasma proteins, is called the **oncotic pressure**, or **colloid osmotic pressure**.

Tonicity describes the effective osmolality of a solution. (The terms *osmolality* and *tonicity* may be used interchangeably.) Solutions, then, have relative degrees of tonicity. An **isotonic solution** (or isosmotic solution) has the same osmolality or concentration of particles (285 mOsm/kg) as the ICF or ECF. Diarrhea, for example, is loss of isosmotic fluid from the gastrointestinal tract. As a result, ECF volume decreases but there is no change in ECF osmolarity. Examples of isotonic solutions include 5% dextrose in water and normal (0.9%) saline solution. A **hypotonic solution** has a lower concentration and is thus more dilute than body fluids. Water is a hypotonic solution. Consequently, water is osmotically pulled into the cells, causing cells to swell or burst. A **hypertonic solution** has a concentration greater than 285 to 294 mOsm/kg. An example of a hypertonic solution is 3% saline solution. Water can be pulled out of the cells by a hypertonic solution, so the cells shrink. The concept of tonicity is important when correcting water and solute imbalances by administering different types of replacement solutions.

Active transport of Na⁺ and K⁺. The active transport system for Na^+ and K^+ is found in virtually all mammalian cells. The Na^+-K^+ antiport system (Na^+ moving out of and K^+ moving into the cell) uses the direct energy of ATP to move these cations. The transporter protein is an enzyme, adenosine triphosphatase (ATPase). ATPase has a requirement for Na^+, K^+, and Mg^{++} ions. The concentration of ATPase in plasma membranes is directly related to Na^+-K^+ transport activity. Approximately 60% to 70% of the ATP synthesized by cells, especially muscle and nerve cells, is used to maintain the Na^+-K^+ transport system. Excitable tissues (e.g., muscle and nerve tissues) have a high concentration of Na^+-K^+ ATPase, as do other tissues that transport significant amounts of Na^+, for example, kidneys and salivary glands. For every ATP molecule hydrolyzed, three molecules of Na^+ are transported out of the cell, whereas only two molecules of K^+ move into the cell. The process leads to an electrical potential and is called *electrogenic,* with the inside of the cell more negative than the outside. The exact mechanism for transport of Na^+ and K^+ across the membrane is uncertain. One proposal is that ATPase induces the transporter protein to undergo several conformational changes, causing Na^+ and K^+ to move short distances (Fig. 1.34). The conformational change creates a lowering affinity for Na^+ and K^+ to the ATPase transporter, resulting in the release of the cations after transport.

The sarcoplasmic reticulum of heart muscle and skeletal muscle has an ATP-dependent Ca^{++} active transport system that regulates the Ca^{++} levels in the cell's cytoplasm, which in turn regulates muscle contraction and relaxation cycles. The Ca^{++} transport system depends on ATPase activity and is similar to that of Na^+-K^+ ATPase.

The transport of sugars and amino acids across the plasma membrane depends on the simultaneous movement (symport) of Na^+ or Na^+-dependent transport (see Fig. 1.31). Na^+-dependent symport occurs primarily in the plasma membrane of epithelial cells of the kidney tubules and intestines. The transport of glucose is not directly dependent on the hydrolysis of ATP; however, the Na^+ gradient is ATP dependent, and thus ATP is indirectly involved in glucose transport.

The epithelial cells that line the intestines depend on Na^+ to transport various amino acids. Similarly, the uptake of Cl^- by the small intestine depends on Na^+ symport and antiport mechanisms for the secretion of Ca^{++} from the cell.

Table 1.5 summarizes the major mechanisms of transport through pores and protein transporters in the plasma membranes. Many disease states are caused or manifested by loss of these membrane transport systems.

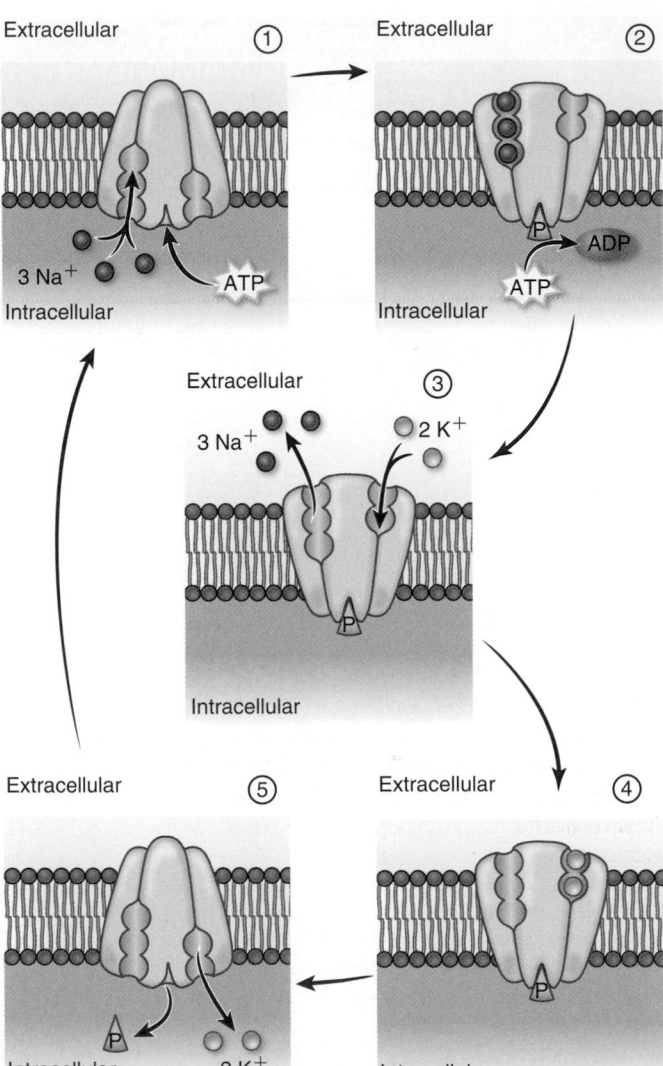

FIGURE 1.34 Active Transport and the Sodium-Potassium Pump. 1, Three Na^+ ions bind to sodium-binding sites on the carrier's inner face. **2,** At the same time, an energy-containing adenosine triphosphate *(ATP)* molecule produced by the cell's mitochondria binds to the carrier. The ATP dissociates, transferring its stored energy to the carrier. **3** and **4,** The carrier then changes shape, releases the three Na^+ ions to the outside of the cell, and attracts two potassium *(K⁺)* ions to its potassium-binding sites. **5,** The carrier then returns to its original shape, releasing the two K^+ ions and the remnant of the ATP molecule to the inside of the cell. The carrier is now ready for another pumping cycle.

Transport by Vesicle Formation
Endocytosis

Endocytosis is a cellular internalizing process where a section of the plasma membrane enfolds substances from outside the cell, invaginates (folds inward), and separates from the plasma membrane, forming an **endocytic vesicle** that moves into the inside of the cell (Fig. 1.35, *A*). Endocytosis mediates cellular uptake of receptor-ligand complexes, nutrients and their carriers, extracellular matrix components, bacteria, viruses, cell debris, and sometimes even other cells.[2] Endocytosis regulates the composition of the plasma membrane in response to changes in the extracellular environment, counterbalances exocytosis, and maintains homeostasis.

TABLE 1.5   MAJOR TRANSPORT SYSTEMS IN MAMMALIAN CELLS*

SUBSTANCE TRANSPORTED	MECHANISM OF TRANSPORT	TISSUES
Sugars		
Glucose	Passive: protein channel	Most tissues
	Active: symport with Na$^+$	Small intestines and renal tubular cells
Fructose	Passive	Intestines and liver
Amino Acids		
Amino acid–specific transporters	Coupled channels	Intestines, kidney, and liver
All amino acids except proline	Active: symport with Na$^+$	Liver
Specific amino acids	Active: group translocation	Small intestine
	Passive	
Other Organic Molecules		
Cholic acid, deoxycholic acid, and taurocholic acid	Active: symport with Na$^+$	Intestines
Organic anions (e.g., malate, α-ketoglutarate, glutamate)	Antiport with counter–organic anion	Mitochondria of liver cells
ATP-ADP	Antiport transport of nucleotides; can be active	Mitochondria of liver cells
Inorganic Ions		
Na$^+$	Passive	Distal renal tubular cells
Na$^+$/H$^+$	Active: antiport, proton pump	Proximal renal tubular cells and small intestines
Na$^+$/K$^+$	Active: ATP driven, protein channel	Plasma membrane of most cells
Ca^{++}	Active: ATP driven, antiport with Na$^+$	All cells, antiporter in red cells
H$^+$/K$^+$	Active	Parietal cells of gastric cells secreting H$^+$
Cl$^-$/HCO$_3^-$ (perhaps other anions)	Mediated: antiport (anion transporter–band 3 protein)	Erythrocytes and many other cells
Water	Osmosis passive	All tissues

*NOTE: The known transport systems are listed here; others have been proposed. Most transport systems have been studied in only a few tissues, and their sites of activity may be more limited than indicated.

ADP, Adenosine diphosphate; ATP, adenosine triphosphate.
Data from Alberts B et al: *Molecular biology of the cell,* ed 5, New York, 2008, Garland; Devlin TM, editor: *Textbook of biochemistry: with clinical correlations,* ed 3, New York, 1992, Wiley; Raven PH, Johnson GB: *Understanding biology,* ed 3, Dubuque, IA, 1995, Brown.

Depending on the size of the cargoes and other factors, binding of ligands on the cell surface activates appropriate intracellular mechanisms that then trigger changes in membrane shape to mediate their cell entry (Fig. 1.36). Endocytosis can be subdivided into four different categories: (1) clathrin-mediated endocytosis, (2) caveolae-mediated endocytosis, (3) macropinocytosis, and (4) phagocytosis. Over time, however, these categories may change.

Because most cells continually ingest fluid and solutes by **pinocytosis**, the terms *pinocytosis* (cell ingestion of extracellular fluid and its contents and bits of the plasma membrane) and *endocytosis* are often used interchangeably. **Micropinocytosis** is the taking up of specific macromolecules by invagination of the cell membrane, which is then pinched off, forming a small vesicle in the cytoplasm. In micropinocytosis the vesicle containing fluids, solutes, or both, fuses with a lysosome, and lysosomal enzymes digest them for use by the cell. **Macropinocytosis** is when a large fluid-filled vesicle or *macropinosome* is pinched off from the cell membrane and brought into the interior of the cell (gulping rather than sipping). Macropinocytosis is an important pathway for antigen presentation by specialized antigen presenting cells.[11] In **phagocytosis** the large molecular substances are engulfed by the plasma membrane and enter the cell so that they can be isolated and destroyed by lysosomal enzymes. Substances that are not degraded by lysosomes are isolated in residual bodies and released by the cell by exocytosis. Both pinocytosis and phagocytosis require metabolic energy and often involve binding of the substance with plasma membrane receptors before membrane invagination and fusion with lysosomes in the cell.

Clathrin-mediated endocytosis. Ligand binding to *some* plasma membrane receptors leads to clustering, aggregation, and immobilization of the receptors in specialized areas of the membrane called **coated pits** (Fig. 1.37). The pits, which are coated with a complex of proteins and cytosolic bristle-like structures (or clathrin), deepen and enfold (invaginate), internalizing ligand-receptor complexes and forming clathrin-coated vesicles (CCVs). This internalization process is not completely understood, called **clathrin-mediated endocytosis** (also **receptor-mediated endocytosis**), is rapid and enables the cell to ingest large amounts of specific ligands, for example, low-density lipoprotein, growth factors, and antibodies, without ingesting large volumes of extracellular fluid. After the coated pits pinch off from the plasma membrane, they quickly shed their coat and fuse with an endosome. An **endosome** is a vesicle pinched off from the plasma membrane from which their contents can be recycled to the plasma membrane or sent to lysosomes for digestion (see Fig. 1.37). Additionally, clathrin is required for the internalization of pumps and transporters for ions and small nutrients to maintain homeostasis and synaptic transmission in neurons.[12] The ingested material is processed by lysosomal enzymes inside the cell.

Caveolae-mediated endocytosis. The outer surface of the plasma membrane is dimpled with tiny flask-shaped pits (cavelike) called caveolae. Caveolae are also called **microdomains. Caveolae** are cholesterol- and glycosphingolipid-rich microdomains where the protein caveolin is thought to be involved in several processes, including transportation and endothelial cell functions, membrane repair, uptake of various cell surface receptors, protection against lipotoxicity, and mechanotransduction.[13] Caveolae are present in most mammalian cell types and are abundant in endothelial and smooth muscle cells, adipocytes, and fibroblasts.[14] Caveolae-mediated endocytosis has been implicated in the endocytosis of simian virus 40 (SV40), papillomavirus (wart causing), and cholera. Additionally, evidence is accumulating that these microdomains are important in regulating endothelial cell functions mainly because they compartmentalize various signaling molecules.[14]

Clathrin- and caveolin-independent endocytosis. Some proteins or small molecules enter cells by clathrin- and caveolin-independent

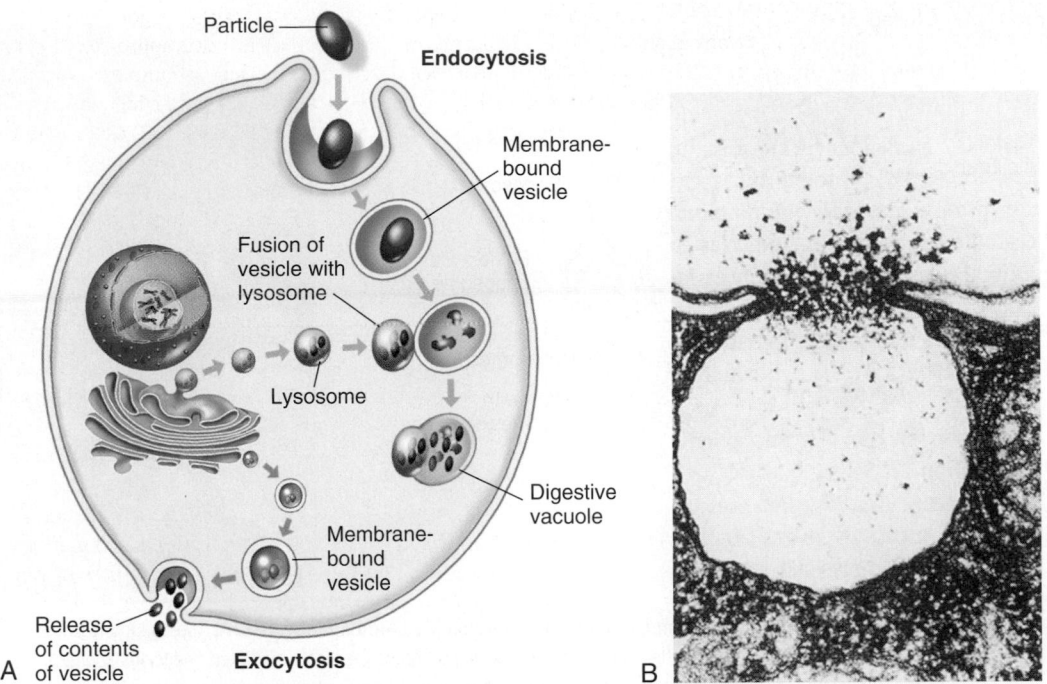

FIGURE 1.35 Endocytosis and Exocytosis. **A,** Endocytosis and fusion with lysosome and exocytosis. **B,** Electron micrograph of exocytosis. (**B** from Raven PH et al: *Biology,* ed 8, New York, 2008, McGraw-Hill.)

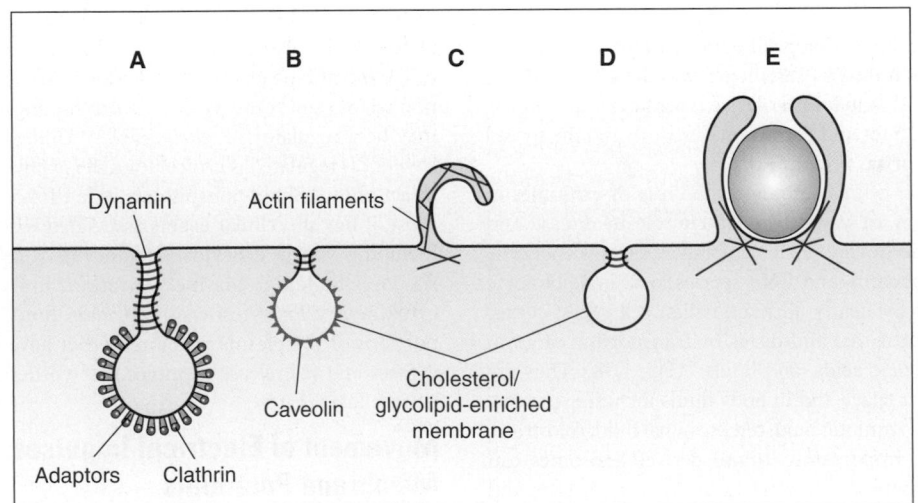

FIGURE 1.36 Multiple Pathways of Endocytosis. The pathways of endocytosis depend on the class of cargo (receptors, ligands, and lipid-associated molecules), the mechanism of vesicle formation (coats, GTPases, and dynamin), and the size of the endocytic vesicle that eventually pinches off into the cytoplasm. **A,** *Clathrin-mediated endocytosis* (CME) uses adaptor proteins that link cargo proteins to the clathrin scaffold, forming the endocytic vesicle. **B,** *Caveolae,* formed by caveolin proteins, are adorned in cholesterol, sphingolipids, and glycolipids that are believed concentrated in membrane microdomains. **C,** During *macropinocytosis* fluid-phase uptake is dependent on actin-driven membrane protrusions that enclose the extracellular fluid and fuse with the plasma membrane. **D,** Some cargoes associate with membrane microdomains that eventually are internalized in a clathrin- and caveolin-independent manner. Different modes of internalization are distinguished by their dependence on dynamin, a membrane-remodeling GTPase. **E,** *Phagocytosis* mediates internalization by membrane protrusions formed around large, ligand-coated molecules. (Adapted from Krauss M, Haucke V: *Rev Physiol Biochem Pharmacol* 161:45–66, 2011.)

pathways (see Fig. 1.36, *C* and *D*).[12] These routes are defined and classified by their requirements for dynamin during fission, and the regulatory roles of guanosine triphosphatases (GTPases). The mechanism by which internalization occurs is not known but is thought to be dependent on cargo concentration and membrane curvature.

Much new research in the past decade has shown extracellular vesicles as important mediators of intercellular communication involved in biologic signaling to mediate a diverse number of biologic processes.[14] Extracellular vesicles play a key role in the regulation of normal physiology, such as stem cell number, tissue repair, immune surveillance, and

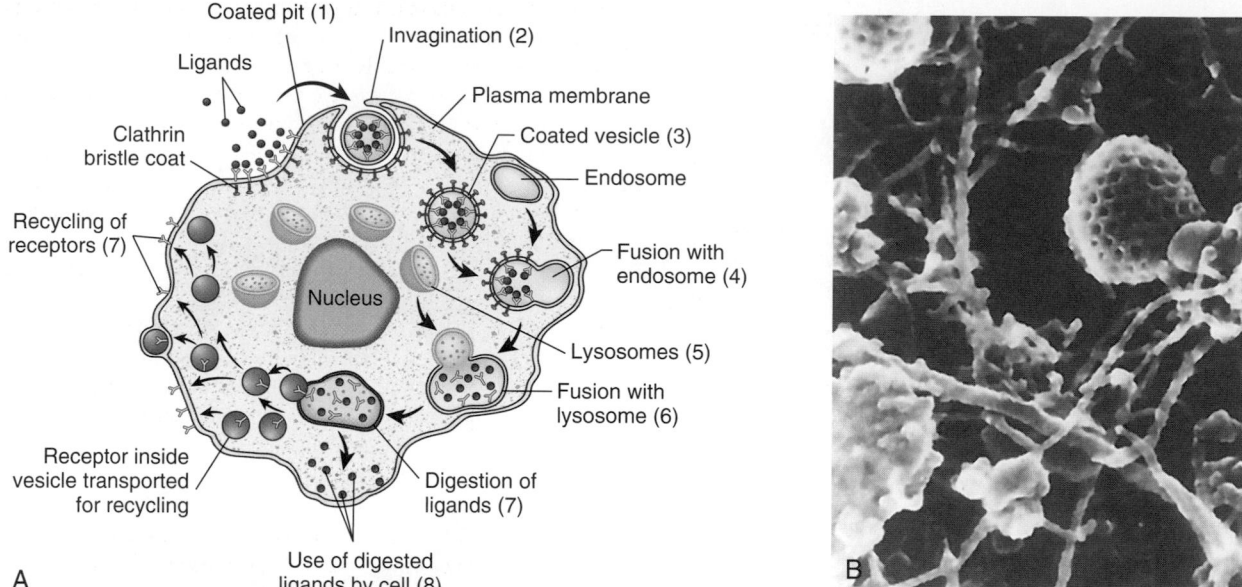

FIGURE 1.37 Ligand Internalization by Means of Receptor-Mediated Endocytosis. **A,** The ligand attaches to its surface receptor (through the bristle coat or clathrin coat) and, through receptor-mediated endocytosis, enters the cell. The ingested material fuses with a lysosome and is processed by hydrolytic lysosomal enzymes. Processed molecules can then be transferred to other cellular components. **B,** Electron micrograph of a coated pit showing different sizes of filaments of the cytoskeleton (×82,000). (**B** from Erlandsen SL, Magney JE: *Color atlas of histology,* St Louis, 1992, Mosby.)

blood coagulation, and in the pathology of many diseases. Extracellular vesicles have been tightly linked to carcinogenesis; the dissemination of viruses such as HIV-1, amyloid-β–derived peptides, and alpha-synuclein (linked to Alzheimer and Parkinson diseases); and the spread of abnormal cell surface prion protein PrP^C.[15]

A new advancement in cellular biology is the role of exosomes in understanding the biology of vesicles and their role in disease and therapeutic potential. **Exosomes** are small membrane vesicles of endocytic origin containing lipid, protein, and RNA species in a single biologic unit. Exosomes, secreted by nearly all mammalian cell types, confer messages between cells, proximal and distal, by transporting cargo in the form of proteins, nucleic acids, and lipids[16] (Fig. 1.38). They are present in the intracellular space and in body fluids including plasma, saliva, urine, plural ascites, amniotic fluid, cerebrospinal fluid, colostrum, breast milk, and semen. Importantly, tumor-derived exosomes can prepare a favorable microenvironment at future metastatic sites and mediate nonrandom patterns of metastasis.[17] Investigators have defined a specific group of integrins expressed on tumor-derived exosomes, distinct from tumor cells, which dictate exosome adhesion to specific cell types and ECM molecules in particular organs. Recent data show that the actin cytoskeletal regulatory protein *cortactin* promotes exosome secretion.[18] Thus, exosomes may be important not only to predict metastatic propensity but also to determine organ sites of future metastasis[17] (see Chapter 12).

Exocytosis

In eukaryotic cells, secretion of macromolecules almost always occurs by exocytosis (see Fig. 1.35, *B*). **Exocytosis** is the discharge or secretion of material from the intracellular vesicles at the cell surface. For example, to secrete macromolecules of insulin across plasma membranes, insulin-producing cells store and package insulin molecules in intracellular vesicles, which fuse with the plasma membrane and open to the extracellular space, or matrix, releasing the insulin. Not all secreted substances are secreted into the extracellular matrix. Some

adhere to the plasma membrane and are thought to replace segments of the membrane lost through endocytosis or diffuse into the blood to nourish or signal other cells. Research findings suggest membrane lipids may be a regulator of exocytosis.[19,20] Understanding how the *exocyst complex* is regulated is critical for diverse physiological processes.[21] The intact phospholipid phosphoinositide PI(4,5)P$_2$ plays a critical role in most, if not all, cellular events associated with the plasma membrane, including vesicle exocytosis, endocytosis, cell adhesion, phagocytosis, viral budding, enzyme activation, ion channel regulation, and cytokinesis.[22] Exocytosis has two main functions: (1) replacement of portions of the plasma membrane that have been removed by endocytosis, and (2) release of molecules synthesized by the cells into the extracellular matrix.

Movement of Electrical Impulses: Membrane Potentials

All body cells are electrically polarized, with the inside of the cell more negatively charged than the outside. The difference in electrical charge, or voltage, is known as the **resting membrane potential** and is about −70 to −85 millivolts. The difference in voltage across the plasma membrane is a result of the differences in the ionic composition of ICF and ECF. Sodium ions have a greater concentration in the ECF, and potassium ions have a greater concentration in the ICF. The concentration difference is maintained by the active transport of Na$^+$ and K$^+$ (the sodium-potassium pump), which transports sodium outward and potassium inward (Fig. 1.39). Because the resting plasma membrane is more permeable to K$^+$ than to Na$^+$, K$^+$ can diffuse easily from its area of higher concentration in the ICF to its area of lower concentration in the ECF. Because Na$^+$ and K$^+$ are both cations, the net result is an excess of anions inside the cell, resulting in the resting membrane potential.

Nerve and muscle cells are excitable and can change their resting membrane potential in response to electrochemical stimuli. Changes in resting membrane potential convey messages from cell to cell. When a nerve or muscle cell receives a stimulus that exceeds the membrane

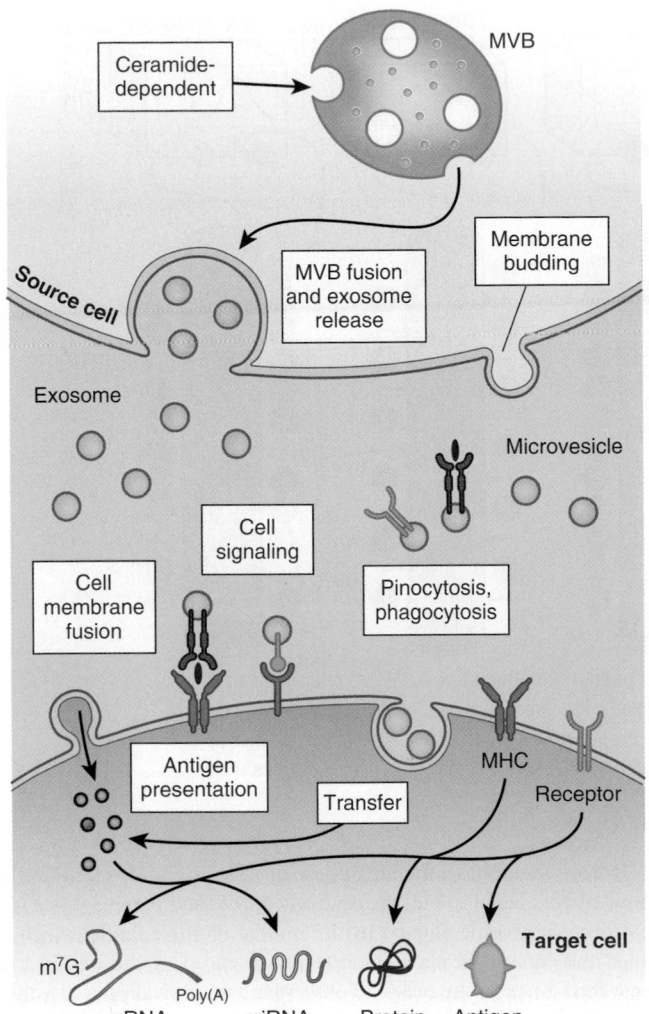

FIGURE 1.38 Exosomes and Cellular Functions. Exosomes are vesicles of endocytic origin formed from the inward budding of the multivesicular body (MVB) membrane. Exosomes undergo cargo sorting to generate exosomes of certain biochemical compositions. Exosomes are secreted following the fusion of MVBs with the cell membrane. Extracellular vesicles are regarded as signaling moieties (signalosomes) for many biologic processes. They are involved in antigen presentation and transfer of both major histocompatibility complex (MHC) molecules and antigens and are thereby involved in immune regulation. Extracellular vesicles can directly activate cell surface receptors from protein and lipid ligands, transfer receptors, or deliver effectors, including transcription factors, oncogenes, and infectious particles, into recipient cells. Various RNA species, including mRNAs and small regulatory RNAs (e.g., microRNAs [miRNAs] and noncoding RNAs), are contained in extracellular vesicles and delivered to appropriate recipient cells. The same properties of extracellular vesicles that are important for normal physiology can lead to their involvement in pathologic conditions. For example, extracellular vesicles can support tumor growth and tumor-related pathologies by inducing unwanted immune tolerance, spreading oncogenes, switching on angiogenic programs, and promoting metastases. For autoimmune diseases, vesicles can induce immune responses toward self-antigens. Vesicles can mediate transfer of prion proteins and toxic protein aggregates that modulate the progression of neurodegenerative diseases; vesicle transfer-bound viral material has been implicated in HIV-1 infection. Because of their involvement in disease progression, extracellular vesicles may be targets for therapeutic intervention as well as disease biomarkers. (Adapted from Andaloussi SEL et al: *Nat Rev Drug Discov* 12:347–357, 2013.)

threshold value, there is a rapid change in the resting membrane potential known as the **action potential**. The action potential carries signals along the nerve or muscle cell and conveys information from one cell to another. When a resting cell is stimulated through voltage-regulated channels, the cell membranes become more permeable to sodium. There is a net movement of sodium into the cell, and the membrane potential decreases, or "moves forward," from a negative value (in millivolts) to zero. This decrease is known as **depolarization**. The depolarized cell is more positively charged, and its polarity is neutralized.

To generate an action potential and the resulting depolarization, a critical value known as the **threshold potential** must be reached. Generally this occurs when the cell has depolarized by 15 to 20 millivolts. When the threshold is reached, the cell will continue to depolarize with no further stimulation. The sodium gates open, and sodium rushes into the cell, causing the membrane potential to reduce to zero and then become positive (depolarization). The rapid reversal in polarity results in the action potential.

During **repolarization** the negative polarity of the resting membrane potential is reestablished. As the voltage-gated sodium channels begin to close, voltage-gated potassium channels open. Membrane permeability to sodium decreases, and potassium permeability increases, with an outward movement of potassium ions. The sodium gates close, and with the outward movement of potassium, the membrane potential becomes more negative. The Na^+-K^+ pump then returns the membrane to the resting potential by pumping potassium back into the cell and sodium out of the cell.

During most of the action potential, the plasma membrane cannot respond to an additional stimulus. This time is known as the **absolute refractory period** and is related to changes in permeability to sodium. During the latter phase of the action potential, when permeability to potassium increases, a stronger-than-normal stimulus can evoke an action potential, known as the **relative refractory period**.

When the membrane potential is more negative than normal, the cell is in a *hyperpolarized* (less excitable) state. A larger-than-normal stimulus is then required to reach the threshold potential and generate an action potential. When the membrane potential is more positive than normal, the cell is in a *hypopolarized* (more excitable than normal) state, and a smaller-than-normal stimulus is required to reach the threshold potential. Changes in the intracellular and extracellular concentration of ions or a change in membrane permeability can cause these alterations in membrane excitability. Understanding the mechanisms of ion movement and membrane excitability led to the discovery of calcium blocking agents for heart disease and migraine.

CELLULAR REPRODUCTION: THE CELL CYCLE

The most fundamental task for the generation of life is cellular reproduction. "The only way to make a new cell is to duplicate a cell that already exists."[2] The continuity of life depends on constant rounds of cell growth and division. The cycle of repeated duplication and division is called the **cell cycle** (Fig. 1.40, *A*). Humans must make millions of cells every second to just survive.[2]

Reproduction of gametes (sperm and egg cells) occurs through a process called *meiosis*, described in Chapter 4. The reproduction, or division, of other body cells (somatic cells) involves two sequential phases: **mitosis**, or nuclear division, and **cytokinesis**, or cytoplasmic division (Fig. 1.40, *B*). These two phases occur in close succession, with cytokinesis beginning toward the end of mitosis. Before a cell can divide, however, it must double its mass and duplicate all its contents. Most of the work of preparing for division occurs during the growth phase, called **interphase**. The cell cycle drives the alternation between mitosis and interphase in all tissues with cellular turnover.

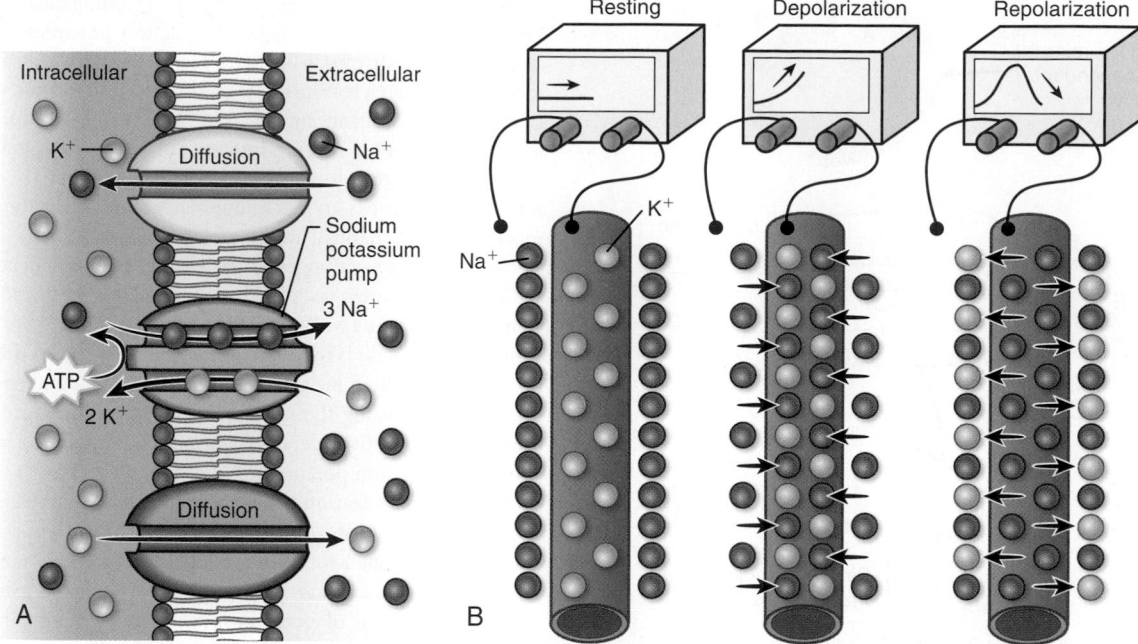

FIGURE 1.39 Sodium-Potassium Pump and Propagation of an Action Potential. **A,** Concentration difference of sodium *(Na⁺)* and potassium *(K⁺)* intracellularly and extracellularly. The direction of active transport by the sodium-potassium pump is also shown. **B,** The left diagram represents the polarized state of a neuronal membrane when at rest. The middle and right diagrams represent changes in sodium and potassium membrane permeabilities with depolarization and repolarization.

Most of the early work on the cell cycle was limited to microscopic observation of mitosis and cytokinesis. Interphase was considered the "resting stage" of the cell. With recent technologic advances a considerable amount has been learned about the interphase part of the cell cycle. During interphase many important processes are taking place as the cell produces DNA, RNA, protein, lipids, and other substances; and each pair of **chromosomes** (paired organelles that carry genetic information) makes exact copies of themselves.

The four designated phases of the cell cycle are (1) the G_1 phase (G = gap), which is the period between the M phase and the start of DNA synthesis; (2) the **S phase** (S = synthesis), in which DNA is synthesized in the cell nucleus; (3) the G_2 **phase**, in which RNA and protein synthesis occurs, the period between the completion of DNA synthesis and the next phase (M); and (4) the **M phase** (M = mitosis), which includes both nuclear and cytoplasmic division (Fig. 1.41).

Phases of Mitosis and Cytokinesis

Interphase (the G_1, S, and G_2 phases) is the longest phase of the cell cycle. During interphase the chromatin consists of very long, slender rods that are jumbled together in the nucleus. Late in interphase, strands of **chromatin** (the substance that gives the nucleus its granular appearance) begin to coil, causing them to shorten and thicken.

The M phase of the cell cycle, mitosis and cytokinesis, begins with **prophase**, the first appearance of chromosomes. As the phase proceeds, each chromosome is seen as two identical halves called **chromatids**, which lie together and are attached at some point by a spindle attachment site called a **centromere**. (The two chromatids of each chromosome, which are genetically identical, are sometimes called *sister chromatids.*)

The nuclear membrane, which surrounds the nucleus, disappears. Spindle fibers are microtubules formed in the cytoplasm. **Spindle fibers** radiate from two centrioles located at opposite poles of the cell. The role of the spindle fibers is to pull the chromosomes to opposite sides of the cell.

During **metaphase**, the next phase of mitosis and cytokinesis, the spindle fibers begin to pull the centromeres of the chromosomes. The centromeres become aligned in the middle of the spindle, which is called the **equatorial plate** (or **metaphase plate**) of the cell. In this stage chromosomes are easiest to observe microscopically because they are highly condensed and arranged in a relatively organized fashion in the two-dimensional equatorial plate.

Anaphase begins when the centromeres split and the sister chromatids are pulled apart. The spindle fibers shorten, causing the sister chromatids to be pulled, centromere first, toward opposite sides of the cell. When the sister chromatids are separated, each is considered to be a chromosome. Thus the cell has 92 chromosomes during this stage. By the end of anaphase, 46 chromosomes are lying at each side of the cell. Barring mitotic errors, each of the 2 groups of 46 chromosomes is identical to the original 46 chromosomes present at the start of the cell cycle.

During **telophase**, the final stage, a new nuclear membrane is formed around each group of 46 chromosomes, the spindle fibers disappear, and the chromosomes begin to uncoil. Cytokinesis causes the cytoplasm to divide into roughly equal parts during this phase. At the end of telophase, two identical diploid cells, called *daughter cells,* have been formed from the original cell.

The Cell Cycle Control System

Various features of the cell cycle differ from one cell type to another including the length of time to complete certain functions. Most of the variability in cell cycle length in the adult body occurs during the time the cell spends in the G_1 or G_0 phase of the cell cycle. This length of time is different than the brief time a cell takes to progress from the beginning of the S phase through mitosis—typically 12 to 24 hours. Cells are capable of disassembly of their cell cycle control system and can withdraw from the cycle to a nondividing state called G_0. The reversibility of the G_0 state varies in different types of cells. For example, most of the neurons and skeletal muscle cells are in a

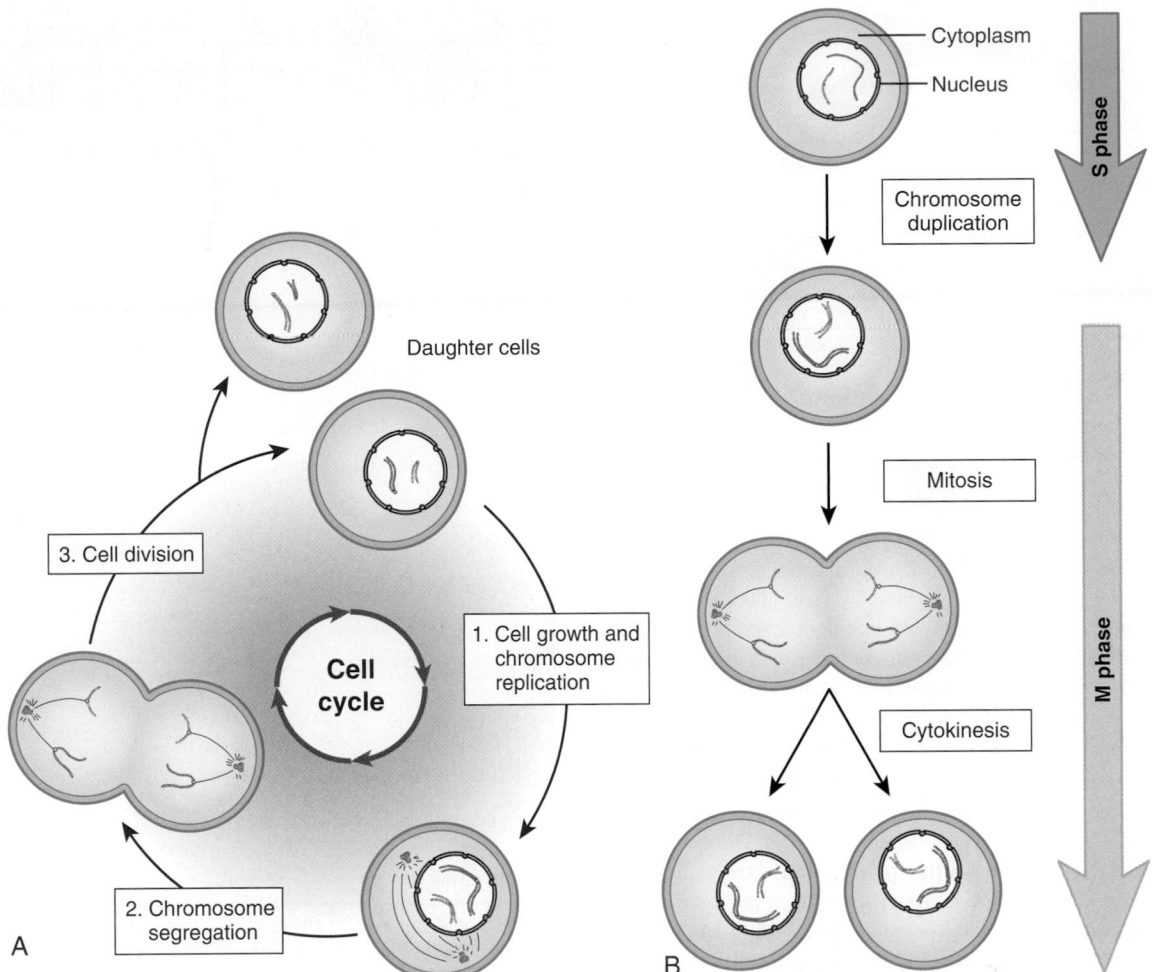

FIGURE 1.40 The Cell Cycle. **A,** Simplified figure of schematic cell with one green chromosome and one yellow chromosome to show how two genetically identical daughter cells are produced in each cycle. **B,** Cell cycle events: mitosis and cytokinesis. (Adapted from Alberts B et al: *Molecular biology of the cell,* ed 6, New York, 2015, Garland Science.)

terminally differentiated G_0 state; with their cell cycle control system disassembled, the molecular regulatory switches (Cdks and cyclins, see following text) become permanently turned off and cell division rarely occurs.[2]

In eukaryotic cells, the basic organization of the cell cycle is mainly the same.[2] The **cell cycle control system** triggers the essential events of the cell cycle. The system operates like a timer that triggers the constant sequence of events. Although early embryonic divisions are independent of feedback controls, in most cells the control system responds to feedback (information) from the processes it controls. For example, if some malfunction occurs with DNA synthesis, signals are sent to the control system to delay progression to the M phase.[2] Such delays allow repair and prevent progression of cellular disasters.

The cell cycle control system works because of a connected series of biochemical switches that either activate or inhibit cell events. Two classes of *switches* or regulatory molecules that determine a cell's progress through the cell cycle are cyclin-dependent kinases (Cdks) and cyclins (Fig. 1.42).

Cyclin-dependent kinases (Cdks) are protein kinases and their functions rise and fall as the cell moves through the cycle. The rise and fall leads to cyclical changes in phosphorylation of intracellular proteins that start or regulate the events of the cell cycle. Many enzymes

and other proteins regulate the different Cdks and the most important are proteins called **cyclins**.[2] Cdk activity is dependent on binding of cyclins (*cyclin-Cdk complexes*). For example, activation of S-phase cyclin-Cdk complexes (s-Cdk) initiates the S phase. Without cyclin, Cdk is inactive. Binding of *Cdk inhibitor proteins (CKIs)* inactivates cyclin-Cdk complexes. Two other essential enzyme complexes that regulate the cell cycle control system are the APC/C and SCF ubiquitin ligases, which promote ubiquitylation (process of marking for destruction) and subsequent destruction of various proteins that modulate the cell cycle (see Fig. 1.42).

Control of Cell Division and Cell Growth: Mitogens, Growth Factors, and Survival Factors

The size of an organ depends on the total number of cells and cell size. Cell number depends on the total quantity of cell division and cell death. Organ size and body size are determined by three main processes: cell growth, cell division, and cell survival.[2] These processes are tightly regulated by intracellular programs and extracellular signal molecules. The signal molecules that regulate growth, division, and survival are usually soluble proteins, proteins bound to cells, or components of the extracellular matrix. The molecules can be divided into three main classes: (1) mitogens, (2) growth factors, and (3) survival factors.

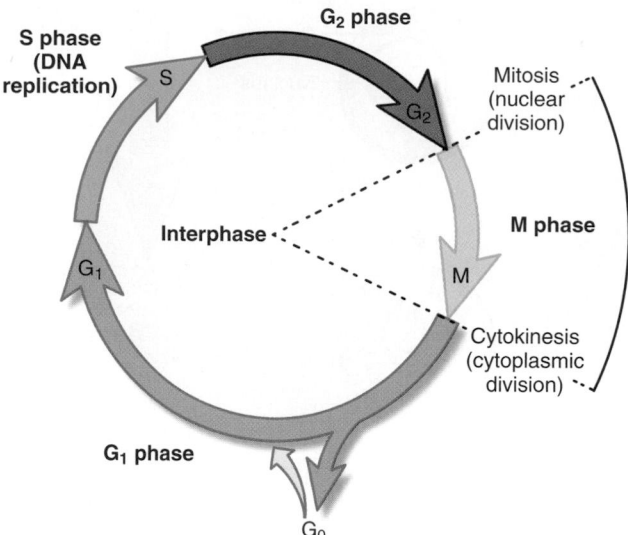

FIGURE 1.41 Four Phases of the Cell Cycle. The four phases of the cell cycle are gap 1 (or G_1, presynthesis), S (DNA synthesis), G_2 (premitotic), and M (mitotic phase). Not a main phase of the cell cycle but a specialized nondividing state called G_0 refers to cells where the cell cycle control system is disassembled (various cyclin-dependent kinases and cyclins are permanently turned off), and cell division rarely occurs.

A **mitogen** is a substance that induces or stimulates mitosis (cell division). For a cell to proliferate it must receive an extracellular signal, or mitogen, from other cells, usually neighboring cells. Mitogens relieve intracellular braking mechanisms that block progress through the cell cycle by triggering a wave of G_1/S-Cdk activity.[2] One of the first mitogens to be identified was *platelet-derived growth factor (PDGF)*. Importantly, when blood clots, platelets that exist in the clot are stimulated to release the contents of their secretory vesicles such as PDGF. Liberated PDGF helps stimulate blood clotting at sites of tissue damage to prevent excessive bleeding. PDGF can stimulate many cell types including smooth muscle cells, neuroglial cells, and fibroblasts. In addition to cell division, PDGF and other mitogens can stimulate cell growth, differentiation, migration, and survival.[2]

Mitogens interact with cell receptors to activate multiple intracellular signaling pathways. A major pathway through the GTPase is **Ras**, which leads to activation of a mitogen-activated protein kinase *(MAP kinase)* cascade (Fig. 1.43). Eventually, this cascade leads to the production of transcription regulatory proteins including MYC. **Myc** is very important because it activates many genes involved in cell growth and is under investigation as a contributor to cancer cell stemness.[23] Tumors appear to be "addicted" to Myc (proto-oncogene), and the persistence of many human cancers requires sustained Myc activation.[24] Activation of Myc leads to increases in expression of many *delayed-response genes* including those that increase G_1-Cdk activity, causing phosphorylation of a molecular ON-OFF switch, the **retinoblastoma (Rb) susceptibility protein**. In its unphosphorylated (or hypophosphorylated) state, RB prevents cells from replicating by forming a tight inactive complex with the transcription factor **E2F** (Fig. 1.44). Phosphorylation of RB eliminates the "brakes" (by reducing binding to E2F proteins) and the liberated E2F proteins then activate other target genes, promoting cell cycle progression and cell replication.

Growth factors (also called *cytokines*) stimulate an increase in cell mass or cell growth by promoting the synthesis of proteins and other macromolecules and inhibiting their degradation. Table 1.6 includes examples of mitogens and growth factors. Cells that are starved of growth factors come to a halt after mitosis and enter the arrested, or G_0, state

TABLE 1.6	EXAMPLES OF MITOGENS AND GROWTH FACTORS AND THEIR ACTIONS
GROWTH FACTOR	**PHYSIOLOGIC ACTIONS**
Platelet-derived growth factor (PDGF)	Stimulates proliferation of connective tissue cells and neuroglial cells
Epidermal growth factor (EGF)	Stimulates proliferation of epidermal cells and other cell types
Insulin-like growth factor 1 (IGF-1)	Collaborates with PDGF and EGF; stimulates proliferation of fat cells and connective tissue cells
Insulin-like growth factor 2 (IGF-2)	Collaborates with PDGF and EGF; stimulates proliferation of fat cells and connective tissue cells
Transforming growth factor-beta (TGF-β)	Stimulates or inhibits response of most cells to other growth factors; regulates differentiation of some cell types (e.g., cartilage)
Fibroblast growth factor (FGF)	Stimulates proliferation of fibroblasts, endothelial cells, myoblasts, and other cell types
Interleukin-2 (IL-2)	Stimulates proliferation of T lymphocytes
Nerve growth factor (NGF)	Promotes axon growth and survival of sympathetic and some sensory and CNS neurons
Hematopoietic cell growth factors (IL-3, GM-CSF, M-CSF, G-CSF, erythropoietin)	Promotes growth of white and red blood cells

CNS, Central nervous system; *CSF*, colony-stimulating factor; *G*, granulocyte; *GM*, granulocyte-macrophage; *M*, macrophage.

of the cell cycle. **Survival factors** promote cell survival by suppressing the type of programmed cell death called *apoptosis* (see Chapter 2).

DNA Damage Response: Blocks Cell Division

The **DNA damage response** occurs when DNA is damaged and several protein kinases are recruited to the site of damage and start a signaling pathway that stops the progression of the cell cycle, or **cell cycle arrest** (Fig. 1.45). Importantly, the cell cycle control system detects DNA damage and arrests the cycle at two points: (1) at Start, which prevents entry into the S phase; and (2) at the G_2/M transition, stopping entry into mitosis. DNA damage initiates a signaling pathway by activating one of a pair of protein kinases called **ataxia-telangiectasia mutated (ATM)** and **ataxia-telangiectasia and rad-3 (ATR)** (see Fig. 1.45).

TISSUES

The body is made up of four levels of organization: cells, tissues, organs, and systems. Cells of common structure and function are organized into **tissues**, of which there are four primary types: *muscle, neural, epithelial,* and *connective* tissue.

Tissue Formation

To form tissues, cells must exhibit intercellular recognition and communication, adhesion, and memory. Specialized cells sense their environment through signals, such as growth factors, from other cells. This type of communication ensures that new cells are produced only when and where they are required. Different cell types have different adhesion molecules in their plasma membranes, sticking selectively to other cells

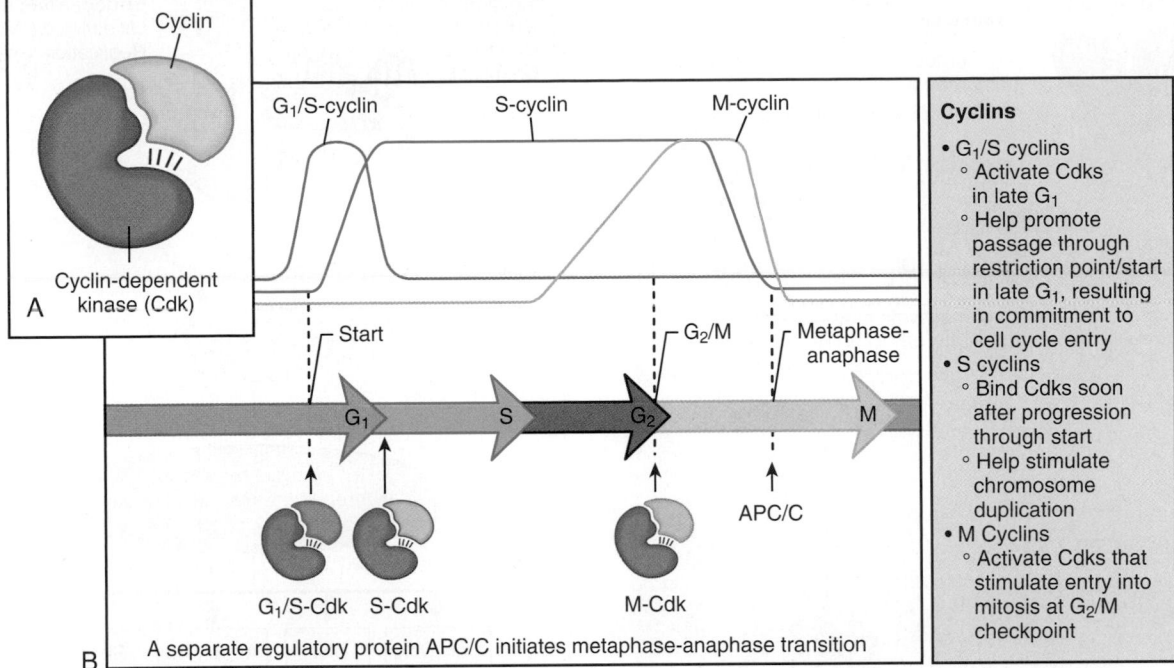

FIGURE 1.42 Cell Cycle Control System. **A,** Key components or protein kinases of the cell cycle control system are cyclin-dependent kinases (Cdks) and cyclins. Cyclin forms a complex with Cdk. **B,** Cyclin-Cdk complexes of the cell cycle control system. *APC/C,* Anaphase promoting complex. (Adapted from Alberts B et al: *Molecular biology of the cell,* ed 6, New York, 2015, Garland Science.)

of the same type. They also can adhere to extracellular matrix components. Strength can occur because of the extracellular matrix and the strength of the cytoskeleton with cell-cell adhesions to neighboring cells. Cells have memory because of specialized patterns of gene expression evoked by signals that acted during embryonic development. Memory allows cells to autonomously preserve their distinctive character and pass it on to their progeny.[2]

Form generation, or *morphogenesis,* that cells undergo to assemble into tissues and organs with different shapes and sizes is less well understood than the processes of gene expression and induced signaling that result in cell-type specialization.[2] The underlying molecular mechanisms are complex. Fully specialized or terminally differentiated cells that are lost are generated from committed proliferating *precursor cells* or transit amplifying cells; and they, in turn, have been derived from a smaller number of stem cells.[2] **Stem cells** are cells with the potential to develop into many different cell types during early development and growth. A stem cell itself is not terminally differentiated; it can divide without limit, and when it divides each daughter cell has a choice. The daughter cell either can remain a stem cell or can move on a course that commits it to terminal differentiation.[2] Two ways a stem cell can produce daughter cells with different fates are asymmetrical division and independent choice, as shown in Fig. 1.46.

In many tissues, stem cells serve as an internal repair and maintenance system dividing indefinitely. These cells can maintain themselves over very long periods of time, called **self-renewal,** and can generate all the differentiated cell types of the tissue, or **multipotency.** This stem cell–driven tissue renewal is very evident in the epithelial lining of the intestine, stomach, blood cells, and skin, which is continuously exposed to environmental factors. Tissue renewal and repair, however, do not always depend on stem cells.[2] For example, enlargement and renewal of insulin-producing cells in the pancreas occur by simple duplication of existing insulin-producing cells. In the liver, differentiated hepatocytes can divide throughout life and significantly increase their division rate

when needed. At the extreme opposite end of this spectrum, some tissues, like the ear and the eye, do not undergo any turnover and are not renewable—once lost, forever lost.[2]

Types of Tissues
Epithelial Tissue

Epithelial tissue covers most internal and external surfaces of the body. Epithelial cells are closely joined and are attached to a basement membrane or lamina (extracellular matrix), which provides a supporting layer and separates the epithelium from underlying connective tissue (see Table E 1.1 on Evolve). Because of its variety of locations, epithelial tissue has several diverse functions, including protection, absorption, secretion, and excretion. For example, the epidermis provides a protective barrier between the host and the outside environment, and the linings of the internal body organs help absorb substances into the body, excrete waste products, and secrete substances into body cavities.

Epithelial cell surfaces differ according to their location and function. Epithelial cells that line body cavities and blood vessels are smooth, whereas other epithelial cells have tiny cytoplasmic projections called **microvilli** on their free surfaces. Microvilli considerably increase a cell's surface area and are found on cells whose main functions are absorption and secretion, such as the epithelial cells lining the digestive tract. **Cilia,** which are hairlike projections that propel mucus, pus, and dust particles out of the body, characterize cells lining the respiratory passages.

Epithelial tissue is classified in two ways: (1) according to the number and arrangement of cell layers and (2) according to cell shape. Epithelium that is formed by a single layer of cells, all of which are in contact with the basement membrane, is called **simple epithelium. Stratified epithelium** has two or more layers of cells, and only the deepest layer is in contact with the basement membrane. Tissue that appears to consist of several cellular layers but is actually a single layer with all cells contacting the basement membrane is called **pseudostratified epithelium.**

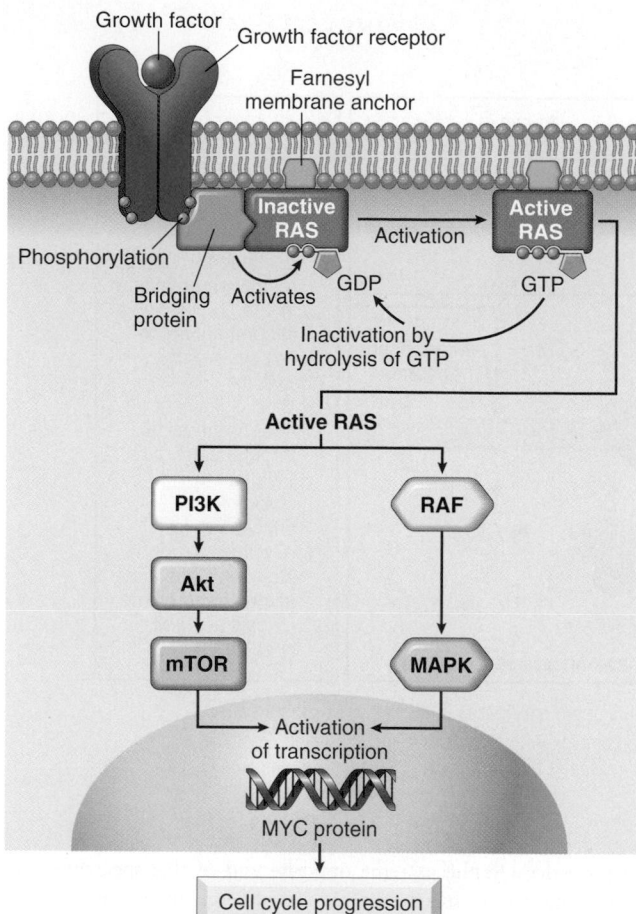

FIGURE 1.43 Signaling Cascade RAS, MAPK, MYC. Binding of a ligand (growth factor) causes a chain of reactions of proteins in the cell that relays a signal to the DNA in the nucleus and results in transcription of MYC protein. The pathway includes many protein kinases acting as "on/off" switches by adding phosphate groups to neighboring proteins. Mutations in RAS can lead to increased proliferation common in cancers. (From Kumar et al: *Robbins & Cotran pathologic basis of disease,* ed 9, Philadelphia, 2015, Saunders.)

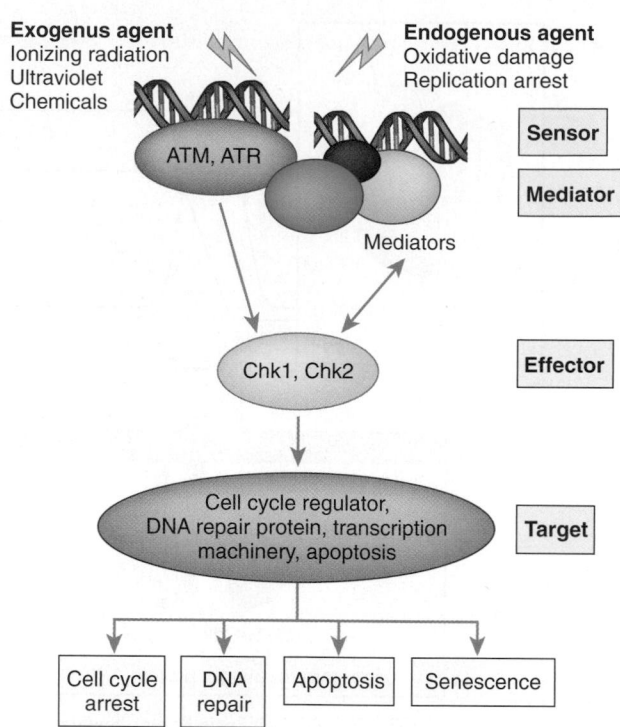

FIGURE 1.45 DNA Damage Response. In response to DNA damage the first kinase at the damaged site is either ATM or ATR, depending on the injurious agent. Protein kinases Chk1 and Chk2 are then recruited and activated. (Although not shown in the figure, these kinases result in phosphorylation of the transcription regulatory protein p53.) Mdm2 is a protein that acts as a ubiquitin ligase (enzyme involved in the ligation [binding] step of ubiquitylation), which targets p53 for destruction by proteasomes.[2] Phosphorylation of p53 blocks its binding to Mdm2, causing p53 to accumulate to high levels, which stimulates transcription of numerous genes, including the gene that encodes protein 21. p21 binds G_1/S-Cdk and S-Cdk complexes, causing arrest of the cell cycle in G_1. The arrest prevents entry into mitosis. Several cell fates can occur including DNA repair, apoptosis or cell death, and senescence (not capable of dividing). *ATM*, ataxia-telangiectasia mutated; *ATR*, ataxia-telangiectasia and rad-3. (Adapted from Yun J: *Molecular signal transduction laboratory*, Busan, South Korea, 2009, Dong-A University. http://web.donga.ac.kr/yunj/page01.htm.)

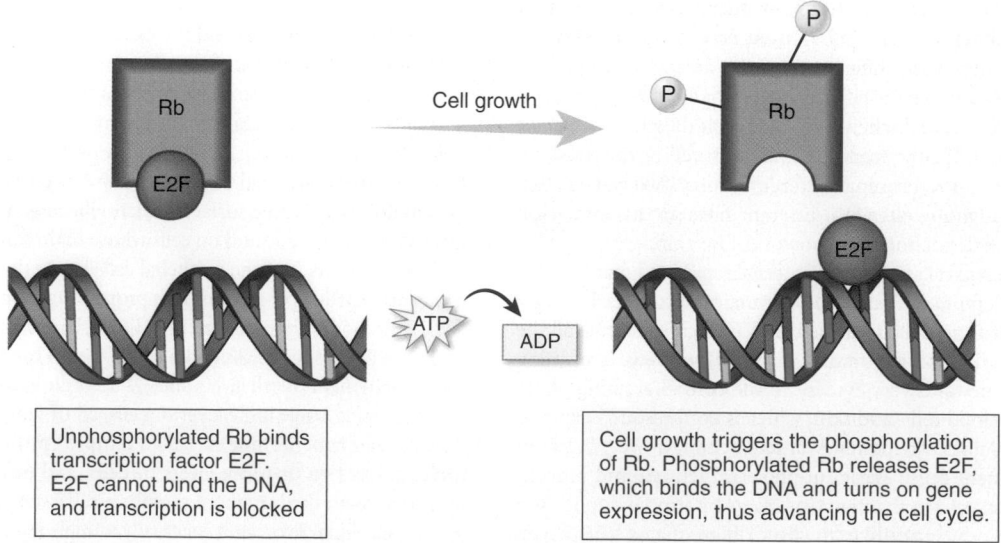

FIGURE 1.44 Rb Master Regulator of Cell Cycle. *P,* Phosphate group from ATP. (Adapted from OpenStax, Control of the Cell Cycle. *OpenStax CNX.* http://cnx.org/contents/69b8e2ee-f350-4202-8085-878c433e1cd5@6.)

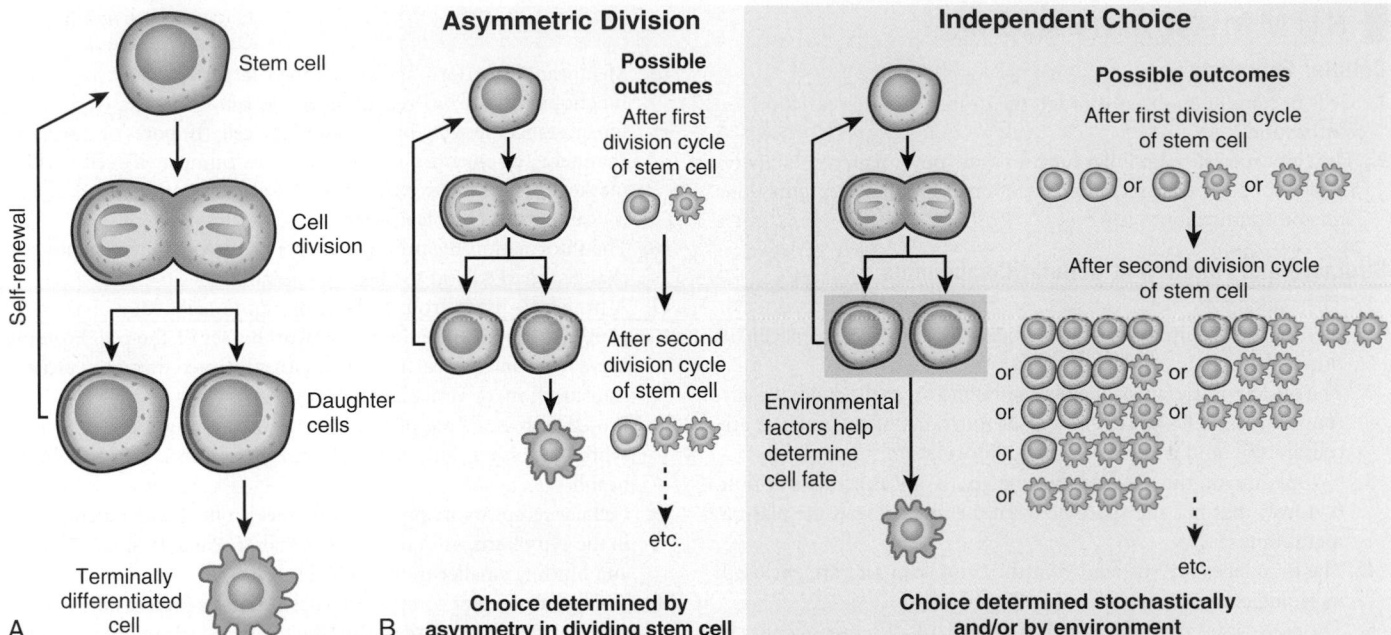

FIGURE 1.46 Stem Cell and Asymmetrical Division and Independent Choice Theory. **A,** When a stem cell divides, each daughter cell can either remain a stem cell or proceed to become terminally differentiated. Frequently, a daughter cell that becomes terminally differentiated undergoes additional cell divisions before terminal differentiation. **B,** Emerging understandings have defined two ways a stem cell can produce daughter cells with different fates: (1) asymmetrical division and (2) independent choice. Asymmetrical division gives a clone one stem cell plus an increasing number of differentiating cells proportional to the number of cell divisions. The independent-choice strategy has more variability or possibilities. These possibilities are subject to the cell's environment, sometimes called a stochastic or random occurrence. (Adapted from Alberts B et al: *Molecular biology of the cell,* ed 6, New York, 2015, Garland Science.)

Three basic cell shapes are found in epithelium: squamous, cuboidal, and columnar. **Squamous cells** are flat and thin; **cuboidal cells** are as high as they are wide and thus appear square in vertical sections; and **columnar cells** are taller than they are wide and appear rectangular in vertical sections. Overall classifications of epithelial tissue, which take into account both the number of cell layers and the cell shape, are summarized in Table E 1.1 on Evolve.

Connective Tissue

Connective tissue varies considerably in structure and function but is most common as the framework on which epithelial cells cluster to form organs. Other functions include binding various tissues and organs together, supporting them in their locations, and serving as storage sites for excess nutrients.

In contrast to epithelial tissue, connective tissue is characterized by an abundant extracellular matrix that surrounds few cells. The extracellular matrix is composed of ground substance and fibers. **Ground substance** is a homogeneous mass that varies in consistency from fluid to semisolid gel. Fibers are produced by connective tissue cells (fibroblasts) found within the ground substance. The three types of fibers are collagenous (white), elastic (yellow), and reticular. **Collagenous fibers** are formed of bundles of smaller fibers appearing as wavy bands under the microscope. These fibers are composed of the protein collagen and are strong and inelastic. **Elastic fibers** are long, branching fibers composed of a protein called *elastin* that enables the fibers to return to their original length after stretching. Elastin occurs not only as fibers but also as membranes, particularly the membranes of blood vessels. **Reticular fibers** are thin, short, branching fibers that form an inelastic network made from a collagen-like protein called *reticulum*. Reticular fibers form the internal framework (stroma) to which the epithelial cells of glands are attached. They are found in loose connective tissue,

generally in bone marrow and in the **parenchyma** (i.e., the essential substance of an organ rather than its framework) of the liver, spleen, and lymph nodes.

Connective tissues are classified according to the consistency (e.g., loose, dense) of the ground substance and the type and organization of the fibers within it. Table E 1.2 on Evolve summarizes the characteristics of connective tissues.

Muscle Tissue

Muscle tissue is composed of long, thin cells or fibers called *myocytes*. Myocytes are highly contractile. The three types of muscle tissues are skeletal, cardiac, and smooth (see Table E 1.3 on Evolve). (Muscles are discussed in detail in Chapter 44.)

Neural Tissue

Neural tissue is composed of highly specialized cells called *neurons*, which receive and transmit electrical impulses very rapidly across junctions called synapses. **Synapses** are points of functional contact between neurons. At synapses, impulses pass from neuron to neuron or from a neuron to a muscle cell while chemical messengers called *neurotransmitters* are released. The total number of neurons is fixed at birth, and replacement is impossible thereafter.

Different types of neurons have special characteristics that depend on their distribution and function within the nervous system. All neurons, however, are composed of the following parts: (1) a cell body, (2) a single axon, and (3) one or more dendrites (see Fig. 15.1). The cell body contains special cytoplasmic structures, as well as microtubules, actin filaments, Golgi complex, lysosomes, and lipofuscin. The axons and dendrites can be very long. Generally, the axon conducts nerve impulses away from the cell body, and dendrites conduct nerve impulses toward the cell body.

SUMMARY REVIEW

Cellular Functions

1. Cells become specialized through the process of differentiation, or maturation.
2. The eight specialized cellular functions are movement, conductivity, metabolic absorption, secretion, excretion, respiration, reproduction, and communication.

Structure and Function of Cellular Components

1. The eukaryotic cell consists of three general components: the plasma membrane, the cytoplasm, and the intracellular organelles.
2. The nucleus is the largest membrane-bound organelle and is usually found in the cell's center. The chief functions of the nucleus are cell division and control of genetic information.
3. Cytoplasm, or the cytoplasmic matrix, is an aqueous solution (cytosol) that fills the space between the nucleus and the plasma membrane.
4. The organelles are suspended in the cytoplasm and are enclosed in biologic membranes.
5. The endoplasmic reticulum (ER) is a network of tubular channels (cisternae) that extends throughout the outer nuclear membrane. It specializes in the synthesis and transport of protein and lipid components of most of the organelles. Importantly, the ER is responsible for protein folding and sensing cell stress.
6. The Golgi complex is a network of smooth membranes and vesicles located near the nucleus. The Golgi complex is responsible for processing and packaging proteins into secretory vesicles that break away from the Golgi complex and migrate to a variety of intracellular and extracellular destinations, including the plasma membrane.
7. Lysosomes are saclike structures that originate from the Golgi complex and contain digestive enzymes. These enzymes are responsible for digesting most cellular substances completely to their basic components, such as amino acids, fatty acids, and carbohydrates. A newly understood role of lysosomes is nutrient-dependent signal transduction. The signaling function cooperates with the known degradative role to mediate basic cell functions, such as nutrient sensing, metabolic adaptation, and quality control of proteins and organelles.
8. Four pathways of degradation in lysosomes include endocytosis, phagocytosis, macropinocytosis, and autophagy.
9. Peroxisomes are similar to lysosomes but contain several oxidative enzymes, such as catalase and urate oxidase.
10. Mitochondria are found in great numbers in most cells and are responsible for cellular respiration and energy production. The enzymes of the respiratory chain (electron-transport chain), found in the inner membrane of the mitochondria, generate most of the cell's ATP.
11. The cytosol or liquid portion of the cytoplasm has several functions including intermediary metabolism involving enzymatic biochemical reactions; ribosomal protein synthesis; and storage of carbohydrates, fat, and secretory vesicles.
12. The cytoskeleton is the "bone and muscle" of the cell. The internal skeleton is composed of a network of protein filaments including microtubules and actin filaments (microfilaments).
13. The plasma membrane encloses the cell and, by controlling the movement of substances across it, exerts a powerful influence on metabolic pathways.
14. The plasma membrane is a bilayer of lipids and proteins. The basic structure of the cell membrane is the lipid bilayer.
15. Membrane functions are determined largely by proteins. These functions include (a) recognition and binding units (receptors) for substances moving in and out of the cell; (b) pores or transport channels; (c) enzymes that drive active pumps; (d) cell surface markers, such as glycoproteins; (e) cell adhesion molecules; and (f) catalysts of chemical reactions.
16. The information regarding concepts of biologic membranes has changed markedly in the last two decades.
17. A protein is made from a chain of amino acids known as polypeptides. Proteins are the major workhorses of the cell. Proteins move from one compartment to another by gated transport, protein translocation, or vesicular transport.
18. Proteostasis is a state of cell balance of the processes of protein synthesis, folding, and degradation. Proteostasis is vital to cellular health.
19. Cellular receptors are protein molecules on the plasma membrane, in the cytoplasm, or in the nucleus that are capable of recognizing and binding smaller molecules, called *ligands*.
20. The ligand-receptor complex initiates a series of protein interactions, causing adenylyl cyclase to catalyze the transformation of cellular ATP to messenger molecules that stimulate specific responses within the cell.
21. The carbohydrate contained within the plasma membrane is generally bound to membrane proteins.

Cell-to-Cell Adhesions

1. Cell-to-cell adhesions are formed on plasma membranes, thereby allowing the formation of tissues and organs. Cells are held together by three different means: (a) the extracellular membrane, (b) cell adhesion molecules in the cell's plasma membrane, and (c) specialized cell junctions.
2. The extracellular matrix includes three types of protein fibers: collagen, elastin, and fibronectin. The matrix helps regulate cell growth and differentiation.
3. The basement membrane is a thin layer of connective tissue underlying the epithelium of many organs. It is also called the basal lamina.
4. Cell adhesion molecules (CAMs) are cell surface proteins that bind to an adjacent cell and to components of the extracellular matrix. CAMs include four main protein families: the integrins, the cadherins, the selectins, and the immunoglobulin (Ig) superfamily.
5. The three main types of cell junctions are desmosomes, tight junctions, and gap junctions.

Cellular Communication and Signal Transduction

1. Cells communicate in three main ways: (a) they display plasma membrane–bound signaling molecules (receptors) that affect the cell itself and other cells in direct physical contact; (b) they activate receptor proteins inside the target cell, and the signal molecule has to enter the cell to bind to them; and (c) they form protein channels (gap junctions) that directly coordinate the activities of adjacent cells.
2. Primary modes of intercellular signaling are contact-dependent, paracrine, hormonal, neurohormonal, and neurotransmitter.
3. Signal transduction involves signals or instructions from extracellular chemical messengers that are conveyed to the cell's interior for execution.
4. Signal transduction pathways (signaling cascades, relay chains) have several important functions, including physically transferring the signal around the cell, amplifying the signal, distributing the signal, and modulating the signal.

▌ SUMMARY REVIEW—cont'd

5. Two important second-messenger pathways are cAMP and Ca^{++}.
6. G protein is an intermediary between the receptor and adenylyl cyclase.
7. Phospholipase C, an enzyme protein effector, is bound to the inner side of the membrane.

Cellular Metabolism

1. The chemical tasks of maintaining essential cellular functions are referred to as *cellular metabolism.* Anabolism is the energy-using process of metabolism, whereas catabolism is the energy-releasing process.
2. ATP functions as an energy-transferring molecule. Energy is stored by molecules of carbohydrate, lipid, and protein, which, when catabolized, transfer energy to ATP.
3. Oxidative phosphorylation occurs in the mitochondria and is the mechanism by which the energy produced from carbohydrates, fats, and proteins is transferred to ATP.

Membrane Transport: Cellular Intake and Output

1. Cell survival and growth depend on the constant exchange of molecules with their environment. Simple diffusion across the lipid bilayer of the plasma membrane occurs for important moles, such as O_2 and CO_2.
2. The majority of molecule transfer depends on specialized membrane transport proteins that span the lipid bilayer and provide private thoroughfares for select molecules.
3. The two main classes of membrane transport proteins are transporters and channels.
4. Water and small, electrically uncharged molecules move through pores in the plasma membrane's lipid bilayer in the process called *passive transport.*
5. Passive transport does not require the expenditure of energy; rather, it is driven by the physical effects of osmosis, hydrostatic pressure, and diffusion.
6. Larger molecules and molecular complexes (e.g., ligand-receptor complexes) are moved into the cell by active transport, which requires expenditure of energy (by means of ATP) by the cell.
7. Two types of solutes exist in body fluids: electrolytes and nonelectrolytes. Electrolytes are electrically charged and dissociate into constituent ions when placed in solution. Nonelectrolytes do not dissociate when placed in solution.
8. Diffusion is the passive movement of a solute from an area of higher solute concentration to an area of lower solute concentration.
9. Hydrostatic pressure is the mechanical force of water pushing against cellular membranes.
10. Osmosis is the movement of water across a semipermeable membrane from a region of lower solute concentration to a region of higher solute concentration.
11. The amount of hydrostatic pressure required to oppose the osmotic movement of water is called the *osmotic pressure* of the solution.
12. The overall osmotic effect of colloids, such as plasma proteins, is called the *oncotic pressure* or *colloid osmotic pressure.*
13. Mediated transport can be passive or active. Mediated transport includes the movement of two molecules simultaneously in one direction (symport) or in opposite directions (antiport), or the movement of a single molecule in one direction (uniport).
14. Endocytosis is a cellular internalizing process where a section of the plasma membrane enfolds substances from outside the cell, invaginates, and separates from the plasma membrane forming a vesicle that moves inside the cell.

15. Endocytosis can be subdivided into four categories: (1) clathrin-mediated endocytosis, (2) caveolae-mediated endocytosis, (3) macropinocytosis, and (4) phagocytosis. Over time, however, these categories may change.
16. A new advancement in cellular biology is the role of exosomes in understanding the biology of vesicles and their role in disease. Exosomes are small membrane vesicles of endocytic origin containing lipid, protein, and RNA species in a single biologic unit. They are secreted by nearly all mammalian cell types and confer messages between cells.
17. Exocytosis is the discharge of secretion of material from the intracellular vesicles at the cell surface. Exocytosis has two main functions: replacement of portions of the plasma membrane that have been removed by endocytosis and release of molecules synthesized by the cells into the extracellular matrix.
18. Pinocytosis is a type of endocytosis in which fluids and solute molecules are ingested through formation of small vesicles.
19. Phagocytosis is a type of endocytosis in which large particles, such as bacteria, are ingested through formation of large vesicles, called *vacuoles.*
20. All body cells are electrically polarized, with the inside of the cell more negatively charged than the outside. The difference in voltage across the plasma membrane is the resting membrane potential.
21. When an excitable (nerve or muscle) cell receives an electrochemical stimulus, cations enter the cell, causing a rapid change in the resting membrane potential known as the *action potential.* The action potential "moves" along the cell's plasma membrane and is transmitted to an adjacent cell. This is how electrochemical signals convey information from cell to cell.

Cellular Reproduction: The Cell Cycle

1. The continuity of life depends on constant rounds of cell growth and division.
2. Cellular reproduction in body tissues involves mitosis (nuclear division) and cytokinesis (cytoplasmic division).
3. Only mature cells are capable of division. Maturation occurs during a stage of cellular life called *interphase* (growth phase).
4. The cell cycle is the reproductive process that begins after interphase in all tissues with cellular turnover. The four phases of the cell cycle are (1) the **G_1 phase** (G = gap), which is the period between the M phase and the start of DNA synthesis; (2) the **S phase** (S = synthesis), in which DNA is synthesized in the cell nucleus; (3) the **G_2 phase**, in which RNA and protein synthesis occurs, the period between the completion of DNA synthesis and the next phase (M); and (4) the **M phase** (M = mitosis), which includes both nuclear and cytoplasmic division.
5. The M phase (mitosis) involves four stages: prophase, metaphase, anaphase, and telophase.
6. The mechanisms that control cell division depend on the integrity of genetic, epigenetic, and protein growth factors.
7. Two classes of switches or regulatory molecules that determine a cell's progress through the cell cycle are cyclin-dependent kinases (Cdks) and cyclins.
8. Organ size and body size depend on cell growth, cell division, and cell survival.
9. A mitogen is a substance that induces or stimulates mitosis.
10. Growth factors stimulate an increase in cell mass or cell growth by promoting the synthesis of proteins and other macromolecules and inhibiting their degradation.

SUMMARY REVIEW—cont'd

11. The DNA damage response occurs when DNA is damaged and several protein kinases are recruited to the site of damage and start a signaling pathway that stops the progression of the cell cycle called cell cycle arrest.

Tissues

1. Cells of one or more types are organized into tissues, and different types of tissues compose organs. Organs are organized to function as tracts or systems.
2. To form tissue, cells must exhibit intercellular recognition and communication, adhesion, and memory.
3. The four basic types of tissues are epithelial, muscle, neural, and connective tissues.
4. Stem cells are cells with the potential to develop into many different cell types during early development and growth. Stem cells serve as an internal repair and maintenance system dividing indefinitely. Tissue repair and renewal does not always depend on stem cells.
5. Epithelial tissue covers most internal and external surfaces of the body. The functions of epithelial tissue include protection, absorption, secretion, and excretion.
6. Connective tissue binds various tissues and organs together, supporting them in their locations and serving as storage sites for excess nutrients.
7. Muscle tissue is composed of long, thin, highly contractile cells or fibers called *myocytes*. Muscle tissue that is attached to bones enables voluntary movement. Muscle tissues in internal organs enable involuntary movement, such as the heartbeat.
8. Neural tissue is composed of highly specialized cells called *neurons* that receive and transmit electrical impulses very rapidly across junctions called *synapses*.

KEY TERMS

Absolute refractory period, 35
Actin filament (microfilament), 11
Action potential, 35
Active transport, 28
Amphipathic molecule, 14
Anabolism, 22
Anaerobic glycolysis, 26
Anaphase, 36
Anion, 29
Antiport, 29
Ataxia-telangiectasia and rad 3 (ATR), 38
Ataxia-telangiectasia mutated (ATM), 38
Autocrine signaling, 19
Autodigestion, 8
Autolysosome (autophagosome), 8
Autophagy, 8
Basal lamina, 17
Basement membrane (basal lamina), 17
Binding site, 16
Cadherin, 19
Catabolism, 22
Cation, 29
Caveolae, 32
Cell adhesion molecule (CAM), 15
Cell cycle, 35
Cell cycle arrest, 38
Cell cycle control system, 37
Cell junction, 19
Cell polarity, 12
Cell-to-cell adhesion, 17
Cellular metabolism, 22
Cellular receptor, 16
Centriole, 11
Centromere, 36
Channel, 28
Chemical synapse, 19
Chromatid, 36
Chromatin, 36
Chromosome, 36
Cilia, 39
Cisternae, 7
Citric acid cycle (Krebs cycle, tricarboxylic acid cycle), 26
Clathrin, 7
Clathrin-mediated endocytosis (receptor-mediated endocytosis), 32
Coated pit, 32
Collagen, 17
Collagenous fiber, 41
Colloid osmotic pressure, 31

Columnar cell, 41
Concentration gradient, 29
Connexon, 19
Contact-dependent signaling, 19
Cristae, 10
Cuboidal cell, 41
Cyclic adenosine monophosphate (cyclic AMP, cAMP), 22
Cyclic guanosine monophosphate (cyclic GMP, cGMP), 22
Cyclin, 37
Cyclin-dependent kinase (Cdk), 37
Cytochrome, 26
Cytokinesis, 35
Cytoplasm, 3
Cytoplasmic matrix, 3
Cytoskeleton, 10
Cytosol, 3
Depolarization, 35
Desmosome, 19
Differentiation, 3
Diffusion, 29
Digestion, 24
DNA damage response, 38
E2F, 38
Effective osmolality, 30
Elastic fiber, 41
Elastin, 17
Electrolyte, 29
Electron-transport chain, 26
Endocytic vesicle, 31
Endocytosis, 31
Endoplasmic reticulum (ER), 5
Endosome, 32
Equatorial plate (metaphase plate), 36
ER stress, 6
Eukaryote, 3
Exocytosis, 34
Exosome, 34
Extracellular matrix (ECM), 17
Fibroblast, 18
Fibronectin, 17
Filtration, 30
First messenger, 21
G_1 phase, 36
G_2 phase, 36
G_0 phase, 36
G protein, 22
Gap junction, 19
Gated transport, 14

Gating, 19
Glycolipid, 14
Glycolysis, 25
Glycoprotein, 14
Golgi complex (Golgi apparatus), 7
Ground substance, 41
Growth factor, 38
Guanosine diphosphate (GDP), 22
Guanosine triphosphate (GTP), 22
Homeostasis, 19
Hormonal signaling, 19
Hydrolase, 7
Hydrophilic, 14
Hydrophobic, 14
Hydrostatic pressure, 30
Hypertonic solution, 31
Hypotonic solution, 31
Immunoglobulin superfamily CAM (IgSF CAM), 19
Inner membrane, 10
Integrins, 19
Intermediary metabolism, 10
Intermediate filament, 11
Interphase, 35
Ion, 29
Isotonic solution, 31
Junctional complex, 19
Ligand, 16
Lipid bilayer, 12
Lipid raft, 14
Lysosome, 7
Macromolecule, 17
Macropinocytosis, 32
Mechanotransduction, 10
Mediated transport, 27
Membrane protein, 14
Membrane transport proteins, 27
Metabolic pathway, 23
Metaphase, 36
Microdomain, 32
Micropinocytosis, 32
Microtubule, 11
Microvilli, 39
Mitochondria, 10
Mitogen, 38
Mitosis, 35
M phase, 36
Multipotency, 39
Myc, MYC, 38
Neurohormonal signaling, 19

■ KEY TERMS—cont'd

Neurotransmitter, 19
Nuclear envelope, 3
Nuclear pore, 3
Nuclear pore complexes (NPCs), 3
Nucleolus, 3
Nucleus, 3
Oncotic pressure (colloid osmotic pressure), 31
Osmolality, 30
Osmolarity, 30
Osmosis, 30
Osmotic pressure, 30
Outer membrane, 10
Oxidation, 25
Oxidative cellular metabolism, 25
Oxidative phosphorylation, 26
Paracrine signaling, 19
Parenchyma, 41
Passive transport, 28
Peroxisome (microbody), 8
Phagocytosis, 32
Pinocytosis, 32
Polarity, 29
Polypeptide, 14
Polyribosome, 10
Primary lysosome, 8
Prokaryote, 3
Prophase, 36
Protease, 15

Protein, 14
Protein translocation, 14
Proteolytic, 15
Proteolytic cascade, 15
Proteostasis (proteome), 15
Pseudostratified epithelium, 39
Ras, 38
Receptor protein, 20
Relative refractory period, 35
Repolarization, 35
Residual body, 8
Respiratory chain, 10
Resting membrane potential, 34
Reticular fiber, 41
Retinoblastoma (Rb) susceptibility protein, 38
Ribosomal protein synthesis, 10
Ribosome, 4
Rough endoplasmic reticulum (rER), 5
Second messenger, 21
Secondary lysosome (heterophagosome), 8
Secretory vesicle, 7
Selectins, 19
Self-renewal, 39
Signal transduction, 20
Signal transduction pathway, 20
Signaling cell, 20
Simple epithelium, 39
Smooth endoplasmic reticulum (sER), 7

Solute, 27
Sorting signal, 14
S phase, 36
Spindle fiber, 36
Squamous cell, 41
Stem cell, 39
Stratified epithelium, 39
Substrate, 23
Substrate phosphorylation (anaerobic glycolysis), 26
Survival factor, 38
Symport, 29
Synapse, 41
Target cell, 20
Telophase, 36
Threshold potential, 35
Tight junction, 19
Tissue, 38
Tonicity, 31
Transfer reaction, 26
Transmembrane protein, 14
Transporter, 28
Ubiquitination, 15
Unfolded-protein response (UPR), 6
Uniport, 29
Vesicular transport, 14

REFERENCES

1. Bourzac K: Cell imaging: beyond the limits. *Nature* 526(7574):S50–S54, 2015.
2. Alberts B, et al: *Molecular biology of the cell*, ed 6, New York, 2015, Garland Science.
3. Perera RM, Zoncu R: The lysosome as a regulatory hub. *Annu Rev Cell Dev Biol* 32:17.1–17.31, 2016.
4. Rodriguez-Navarro JA, et al: Inhibitory effect of dietary lipids on chaperone-mediated autophagy. *Proc Natl Acad Sci USA* 109:E705–E714, 2012.
5. Katsuno H, et al: Actin migration driven by directional assembly and disassembly of membrane-anchored actin filaments. *Cell Rep* 12(4):648–660, 2015.
6. Vinothkumar KR, Henderson R: Structures of membrane proteins. *Q Rev Biophys* 43:65–158, 2012.
7. Dai C, Sampson SB: HSF1: guardian of proteostasis in cancer. *Trends Cell Biol* 26(1):17–28, 2016.
8. Amm I, et al: Protein quality control and elimination of protein waste: the role of the ubiquitin proteosome system. *Biochim Biophys Acta* 1843:182–196, 2014.
9. Alberts B, et al: *Essential cell biology*, ed 4, New York, 2013, Garland.

10. Kierzenbaum AL, Tres LT: *Histology and cell biology: an introduction to pathology*, ed 3, St Louis, 2011, Elsevier.
11. Liu Z, Roche PA: Macropinocytosis in phagocytes: regulation of MHC class-II–restricted antigen presentation in dendritic cells. *Front Physiol* 6:1, 2015.
12. Krauss M, Haucke V: Shaping membranes for endocytosis. *Rev Physiol Biochem Pharmacol* 161:45–66, 2012.
13. Johannes L, et al: Building endocytic pits without clathrin. *Nat Rev Mol Cell Biol* 16(5):311–321, 2015.
14. Sowa G: Caveolae, caveolins, cavins, and endothelial cell function: new insights. *Front Physiol* 2:120, 2012.
15. Andaloussi SEL, et al: Extracellular vesicles: biology and emerging therapeutic opportunities. *Nat Rev Drug Discov* 12:347–357, 2013.
16. Munson P, Shukla A: Exosomes: potential in cancer diagnosis and therapy medicines. *Medicines (Basel)* 2(4):310–327, 2015.
17. Hoshino A, et al: Tumour exosome integrins determine organotropic metastasis. *Nature* 527(7578):329–335, 2015.

18. Sinha S, et al: Cortactin promotes exosome secretion by controlling branched actin dynamics. *J Cell Biol* 214(2):197–213, 2016.
19. Ammar MR, et al: Lipids in regulated exocytosis: what are they doing? *Front Endocrinol (Lausanne)* 4:125, 2013.
20. He B, et al: Exo 70 interacts with phospholipids and mediates the targeting of the exocyst to the plasma membrane. *EMBO J* 26(18):4053–4065, 2007.
21. Wu B, Guo W: the exocyst at a glance. *J Cell Sci* 128(16):2957–2964, 2015.
22. Martin TFJ: PI(4,5)P2-binding effector proteins for vesicle exocytosis. *Biochim Biophys Acta* 1851(6):785–793, 2015.
23. Kumar V, Abbas A, Fausto N: *Robbins & Cotran pathologic basis of disease*, ed 9, Philadelphia, 2015, Saunders.
24. Gabay M, Li Y, Feisher DW: MYC activation is a hallmark of cancer initiation and maintenance. *Cold Spring Harb Perspect Med* 4(6):1–13, 2014.

CHAPTER

2

Altered Cellular and Tissue Biology: Environmental Agents

Kathryn L. McCance, Todd C. Grey, George W. Rodway

CHAPTER OUTLINE

Injury to cells and their surrounding environment, called the *extracellular matrix*, leads to tissue and organ injury. Although the normal cell is restricted by a narrow range of structure and function, it can *adapt* to physiologic demands or stress to maintain a steady state called *homeostasis*. Adaptation is a reversible, structural, or functional response to both normal or physiologic conditions and adverse or pathologic conditions. For example, the uterus adapts to pregnancy—a normal physiologic state—by enlarging. Enlargement occurs because of an increase in the size and number of uterine cells. In an adverse condition, such as high blood pressure, myocardial cells are stimulated to enlarge by the increased work of pumping. Like most of the body's adaptive mechanisms, however, cellular adaptations to adverse conditions are

usually only temporarily successful. Severe or long-term stressors overwhelm adaptive processes and cellular injury or death ensues. Altered cellular and tissue biology can result from adaptation, injury, neoplasia, accumulations, aging, or death.

Knowledge of the structural and functional reactions of cells and tissues to injurious agents, including genetic defects, is key to understanding disease processes. Cellular injury can be caused by any factor that disrupts cellular structures or deprives the cell of oxygen and nutrients required for survival. Injury may be reversible (*sublethal*) or irreversible (*lethal*) and is classified broadly as chemical, hypoxic (lack of sufficient oxygen), free radical, unintentional or intentional, and immunologic or inflammatory. Cellular injuries from various causes have different clinical and pathophysiologic manifestations. Stresses from metabolic derangements may be associated with intracellular *accumulations* and include carbohydrates, proteins, and lipids. Sites of cellular death can cause accumulations of calcium resulting in *pathologic calcification*. Cellular death is confirmed by structural changes seen when cells are stained and examined with a microscope. The most important changes are nuclear; clearly, without a healthy nucleus, the cell cannot survive. The two main types of cell death are *necrosis* and *apoptosis*, and nutrient deprivation can initiate *autophagy* that results in cell death.

Cellular aging causes structural and functional changes that eventually lead to cellular death or a decreased capacity to recover from injury. Mechanisms explaining how and why cells age are not known, and distinguishing between pathologic changes and physiologic changes that occur with aging is often difficult. Aging clearly causes alterations in cellular structure and function, yet *senescence*—growing old—is both inevitable and normal.

CELLULAR ADAPTATION

Cells adapt to their environment to escape and protect themselves from injury. An adapted cell is neither normal nor injured—its condition lies somewhere between these two states. Adaptations are reversible changes in cell size, number, phenotype, metabolic activity, or functions of cells.[1] However, cellular adaptations are a common and central part of many disease states. In the early stages of a successful adaptive response, cells may have enhanced function; thus, it is hard to differentiate a pathologic response from an extreme adaptation to an excessive functional demand. The most significant adaptive changes in cells include atrophy (decrease in cell size), hypertrophy (increase in cell size), hyperplasia (increase in cell number), and metaplasia (reversible replacement of one mature cell type by another less mature cell type or a change in the phenotype). Dysplasia (deranged cellular growth) is not considered a true cellular adaptation but rather an atypical hyperplasia. These changes are shown in Fig. 2.1.

Atrophy

Atrophy is a decrease or shrinkage in cellular size. If atrophy occurs in a sufficient number of an organ's cells, the entire organ shrinks or becomes atrophic. Atrophy can affect any organ, but it is most common in skeletal muscle, the heart, secondary sex organs, and the brain (Fig. 2.2). Atrophy can be classified as *physiologic* or *pathologic*. **Physiologic atrophy** occurs with early development. For example, the thymus gland undergoes physiologic atrophy during childhood. **Pathologic atrophy** occurs as a result of decreases in workload, use, pressure, blood supply, nutrition, hormonal stimulation, and nervous stimulation. Individuals immobilized in bed for a prolonged time exhibit a type of skeletal muscle atrophy called **disuse atrophy**. Aging causes brain cells to become atrophic and endocrine-dependent organs, such as the gonads, to shrink as hormonal stimulation decreases. Whether atrophy is caused by normal physiologic conditions or by pathologic conditions, atrophic cells exhibit the same basic changes.

The atrophic muscle cell contains less endoplasmic reticulum (ER) and fewer mitochondria and myofilaments (part of the muscle fiber that controls contraction) than does the normal cell. In muscular atrophy caused by nerve loss, oxygen consumption and amino acid uptake are rapidly reduced. The mechanisms of atrophy include decreased protein synthesis or increased protein degradation, or both. The degradation of proteins occurs mainly by the ubiquitin-proteosome pathway (see Chapter 1).

Atrophy as a result of malnutrition may activate ubiquitin ligases that target the proteins for degradation in proteasomes. The accelerated protein degradation may be a mechanism responsible for catabolic conditions, including cancer cachexia. Atrophy is often accompanied by a "self-eating" process called *autophagy* inducing **autophagic vacuoles**. These vacuoles are membrane-bound vesicles within the cell that contain cellular debris—small fragments of mitochondria and ER—and hydrolytic enzymes. Atrophic change causes a rapid increase in hydrolytic enzymes, which are isolated in autophagic vacuoles to prevent uncontrolled cellular destruction. Thus the vacuoles proliferate as needed to protect the uninjured organelles from the injured organelles and are eventually

FIGURE 2.1 Adaptive Alterations in Simple Cuboidal Epithelial Cells.

Nucleus

Basement membrane

Normal

Atrophy

Hypertrophy

Hyperplasia

Metaplasia

Dysplasia

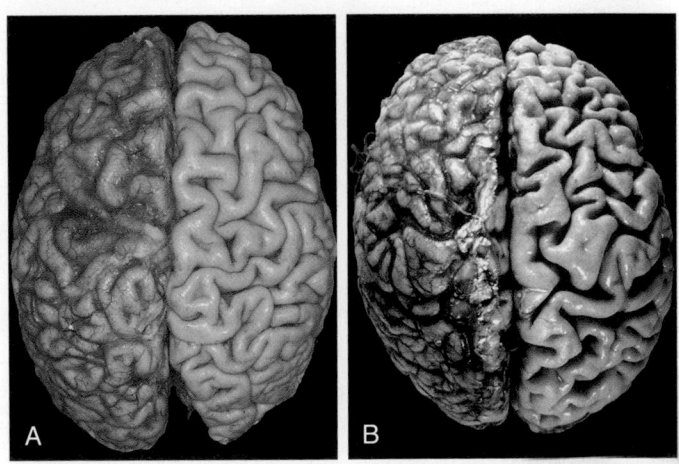

FIGURE 2.2 Atrophy. **A,** Normal brain of a young adult. **B,** Atrophy of the brain in an 82-year-old male with atherosclerotic disease. Atrophy of the brain is a result of aging and reduced blood supply. Note that loss of brain substance narrows the gyri and widens the sulci. The meninges have been stripped from the right half of each specimen to reveal the surface of the brain. (From Kumar V, Abbas A, Aster J: *Robbins & Cotran pathologic basis of disease,* ed 9, Philadelphia, 2015, Saunders.)

taken up and destroyed by lysosomes. Certain contents of the autophagic vacuole may resist destruction by lysosomal enzymes and persist in membrane-bound residual bodies. An example of this is granules that contain **lipofuscin**, the yellow-brown age pigment. Lipofuscin accumulates primarily in liver cells, myocardial cells, and atrophic cells.

Hypertrophy

Hypertrophy is an increase in the size of cells that consequently increases the size of the affected organ. Much of the knowledge on hypertrophy is from studies of the heart. The cells of the heart and kidneys are particularly responsive to enlargement. Hypertrophy can be *physiologic* or *pathologic*. **Physiologic hypertrophy** is the result caused by increased demand, stimulation by hormones (e.g., atrial natriuretic peptide hormone), and growth factors (e.g., IGF-1). Physiologic hypertrophy in skeletal muscle occurs in response to heavy work. Muscular hypertrophy tends to diminish if the excessive workload diminishes. Pregnancy is an example of physiologic hypertrophy and hormone-induced uterine enlargement.

Pathologic hypertrophy results from chronic hemodynamic overload, for example, from hypertension or heart valve dysfunction. A focus of much research is the molecular basis of cardiac hypertrophy because it can progress to maladaptive states, including dysrhythmias, heart failure, and sudden death.

The triggers for cardiac hypertrophy include two types of signals: *mechanical signals,* such as stretch, and *trophic signals,* such as growth factors and vasoactive agents (Fig. 2.3). The stretch mechanical sensors are triggered from increased workload. These sensors, themselves, can increase production of growth factors (e.g., IGF-1) and vasoactive factors (e.g., angiotensin II).[1] The signals from these membrane sensors activate complex signaling pathways, including the phosphoinositide 3-kinase (PI3K)/AKT pathway and G-protein–coupled receptors. Transcription factors are activated from the signaling pathways to increase synthesis of muscle proteins.[1] Initial enlargement of the heart is caused by dilation of the cardiac chambers, is short-lived, and is followed by increased synthesis of cardiac muscle proteins allowing muscle fibers to do more work. The nucleus also is hypertrophic and exhibits increased synthesis of deoxyribonucleic acid (DNA). The increase in cellular size is associated with an increased accumulation of protein in the cellular components (plasma membrane, ER, myofilaments, mitochondria) and *not* with an increase in the amount of cellular fluid. With time cardiac hypertrophy is characterized by extracellular matrix remodeling and increased growth of adult myocytes. Prolonged cardiac hypertrophy progresses to contractile dysfunction, decompensation, and finally heart failure. Heart failure is a leading cause of mortality worldwide. One area of investigation is microRNAs (miRNAs) that regulate target gene expression post-transcriptionally. In mice, the miRNA 212-/132 family regulates cardiac hypertrophy and autophagy in cardiomyocytes.[2,3] Remodeling of cardiac tissue occurs after cardiac stress and can progress to heart failure and death. Investigators are studying the formation of cardiac fibrosis caused by increased activity of cardiac fibroblasts leading to excessive extracellular matrix production. Noncoding RNAs (ncRNAs) as gene regulators is one focus of study for cardiac fibrosis and therapeutic targets.[4]

Hyperplasia

Hyperplasia is an increase in the number of cells in an organ or tissue resulting from an increased rate of cellular division. Hyperplasia occurs as a response to injury that results when the injury has been severe and prolonged. The main mechanism for hyperplasia is the production of growth factors, which stimulate the remaining cells (after cell loss or injury) to synthesize new cell components and, ultimately, to divide. Another mechanism is increased output of new cells from tissue stem cells. For example, if liver cells are compromised, new cells can regenerate

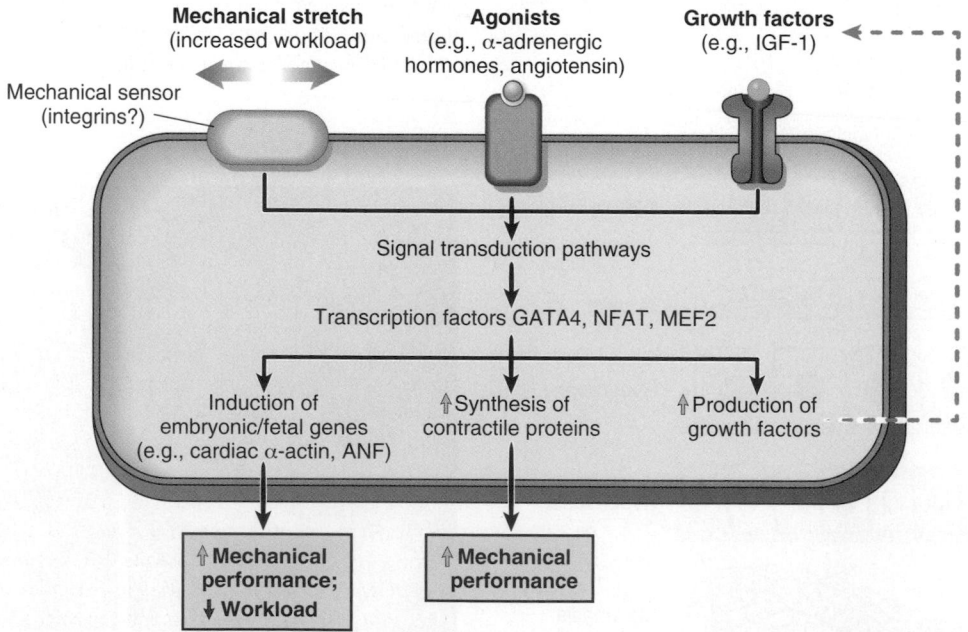

FIGURE 2.3 **Mechanisms of Myocardial Hypertrophy.** Mechanical sensors appear to be the main stimulators for physiologic hypertrophy. Other stimuli possibly more important for pathologic hypertrophy include agonists (initiators) and growth factors. These factors then signal transcription pathways whereby transcription factors then bind to DNA sequences, activating muscle proteins that are responsible for hypertrophy. These pathways include induction of embryonic/fetal genes, increased synthesis of contractile proteins, and production of growth factors. *ANF,* atrial natriuretic factor; *IGF-1,* insulin-like growth factor-1. (From Kumar V, Abbas A, Aster J: *Robbins & Cotran pathologic basis of disease,* ed 9, Philadelphia, 2015, Saunders.)

from intrahepatic stem cells.[1] Although hyperplasia and hypertrophy have distinct processes, they can occur together and the specific mechanism is unknown. Hyperplasia can be *physiologic* or *pathologic*.

Two types of normal, or physiologic, hyperplasia are compensatory hyperplasia and hormonal hyperplasia. **Compensatory hyperplasia** is an adaptive mechanism that enables certain organs to regenerate. For example, removal of part of the liver leads to hyperplasia of the remaining liver cells (hepatocytes) to compensate for the loss. Even with removal of 70% of the liver, regeneration is complete in about 2 weeks. The liver can renew itself by simple duplication of fully differentiated cells.[5] Hepatocytes usually live a year or more; and then, through a very slow rate of cell division, they renew themselves. If large numbers of hepatocytes are lost from surgery or injury, a burst of cell division occurs from the surviving hepatocytes—rapidly replacing the lost tissue.[5] Much is unknown about stem cell activation and hepatocyte renewal in severe forms of liver injury.

Significant compensatory hyperplasia occurs in epidermal and intestinal epithelia, hepatocytes, bone marrow cells, and fibroblasts. An example of compensatory hyperplasia is a **callus**, or thickening, of the skin as a result of hyperplasia of epidermal cells in response to a mechanical stimulus. Another example is the response to wound healing as part of the inflammation process (see Chapter 7).

Hormonal hyperplasia occurs chiefly in estrogen-dependent organs, such as the uterus and breast. After ovulation, for example, estrogen stimulates the endometrium to grow and thicken for reception of the fertilized ovum. If pregnancy occurs, hormonal hyperplasia, as well as hypertrophy, enables the uterus to enlarge.

Pathologic hyperplasia is the abnormal proliferation of normal cells and can occur as a response to excessive hormonal stimulation or the effects of growth factors on target cells (Fig. 2.4). Hyperplastic cells are identified by pronounced enlargement of the nucleus, clumping of chromatin, and the presence of one or more enlarged nucleoli. The most common example is pathologic hyperplasia of the endometrium, which is caused by an imbalance between estrogen and progesterone levels with relative increases of estrogen. Pathologic endometrial hyperplasia, which causes excessive menstrual bleeding, is under the influence of regular growth-inhibition controls. If these controls fail, hyperplastic endometrial cells can undergo malignant transformation. Benign prostatic hyperplasia is another example of pathologic hyperplasia and results from changes in hormone balance. In both of these examples, if the hormonal imbalance is corrected hyperplasia regresses.[1]

Dysplasia: Not a True Adaptive Change

Dysplasia refers to abnormal changes in the size, shape, and organization of mature cells. Dysplasia is not considered a true adaptive process but

is related to hyperplasia and is often called **atypical hyperplasia**. Dysplastic changes are mostly found in epithelia. The architecture of the dysplastic tissue can be disorderly. Importantly, the term *dysplasia* is *not* cancer and may not progress to cancer. Dysplasias that do not involve the entire thickness of epithelium may be completely reversible.[1] Removal of the inciting stimulus, for example, certain hormonal stimuli, in mild to moderate dysplasia that does not involve the entire epithelium may be reversed.[1] When dysplastic changes penetrate the basement membrane it is considered a preinvasive neoplasm and is known as *carcinoma in situ*.

Metaplasia

Metaplasia is the reversible replacement of one mature cell type (epithelial or mesenchymal) by another, sometimes less differentiated, cell type. It is found in association with tissue damage, repair, and regeneration.[1] At certain times, the adaptive replacement cell type may be more suitable to the changed conditions in the surrounding environment. For example, gastroesophageal reflux damages squamous epithelium of the esophagus, and the adapted change or replacement by glandular epithelium may better tolerate the acidic environment.[1] Usually, however, the change is not beneficial. In the long-term cigarette smoker, the chronic irritation from the smoke causes the normal ciliated columnar epithelial cells of the trachea and bronchi to become replaced by stratified squamous epithelial cells (Fig. 2.5). The newly formed squamous epithelial cells do not secrete mucus or have cilia, causing loss of a vital protective mechanism. Bronchial metaplasia can be reversed if the inducing stimulus, usually cigarette smoking, is removed. If the inducing stimulus is persistent, it can initiate malignant transformation in the metaplastic epithelium.

Metaplasia develops from a reprogramming of stem cells existing in most epithelia or of undifferentiated **mesenchymal** (tissue from embryonic mesoderm) **cells** present in connective tissue. These precursor cells mature along a new pathway because of signals generated by cytokines and growth factors in the cell's environment. The mechanism of metaplasia is, therefore, *not* the result of a change in the phenotype of an already differentiated cell type.[1]

CELLULAR INJURY

Injury to cells and to extracellular matrix (ECM) leads to injury of tissues and organs ultimately determining the structural patterns of disease. Loss of function derives from cell and ECM injury and cell death. Cellular injury occurs if the cell is "stressed" or unable to maintain homeostasis in the face of injurious stimuli or cell stress. Injured cells may recover (**reversible injury**) or die (**irreversible injury**). Injurious stimuli include chemical agents, lack of sufficient oxygen (hypoxia), free radicals, infectious agents, physical and mechanical factors, immunologic reactions, genetic factors, and nutritional imbalances. Types of cellular injury and their responses are summarized in Table 2.1 and Fig. 2.6.

Cell injury and cell death often result from exposure to toxic chemicals, infections, physical trauma, and hypoxia. The mechanisms causing chemical and hypoxic injury are perhaps the best understood. Both of these mechanisms can lead to disruption of selective permeability (i.e., transport mechanisms) of the plasma membrane; reduction or cessation of cellular metabolism; lack of protein synthesis; damage to lysosomal membranes with leakage of destructive enzymes into the cytoplasm; enzymatic destruction of cellular organelles; cellular death (exhibited by nuclear changes); and phagocytosis of the dead cell by cellular components of the acute inflammatory response. The extent of cellular injury depends on the type, state (including level of cell differentiation and increased susceptibility to fully differentiated cells),

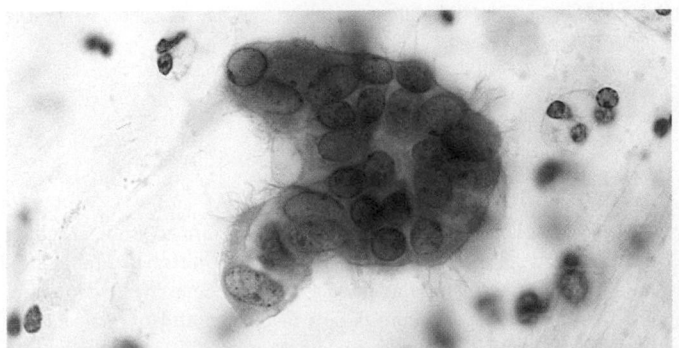

FIGURE 2.4 Hyperplasia of Bronchial Epithelium (Bronchial Brush). (From Damjanov I, Linder J: *Anderson's pathology*, ed 10, St Louis, 1996, Mosby.)

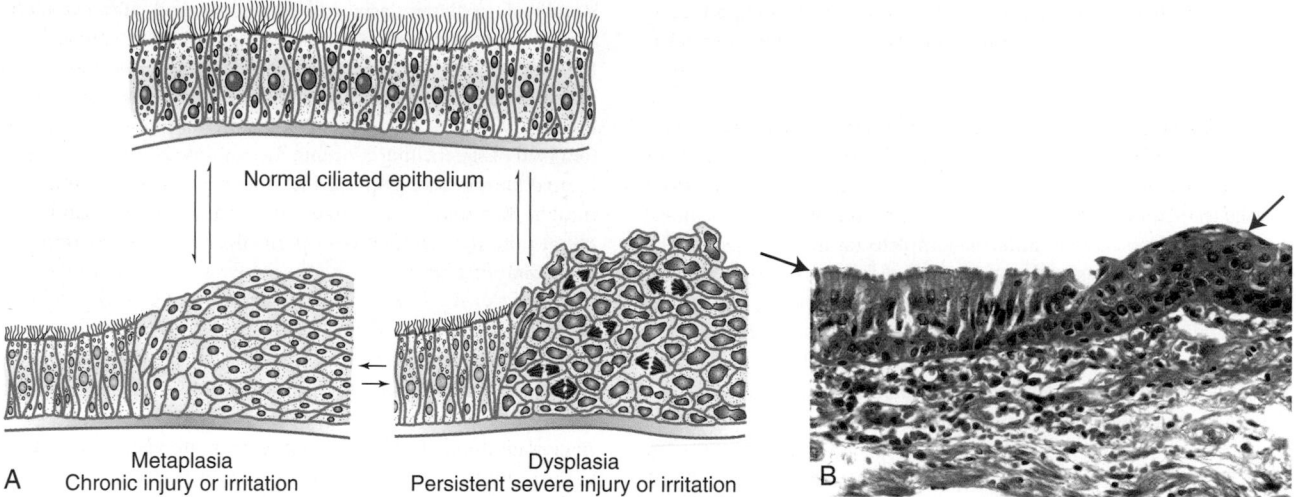

FIGURE 2.5 Reversible Changes in Cells Lining the Bronchi. **A,** Normal ciliated epithelium, metaplasia, and dysplasia. **B,** Histologic slide with upper left *(black arrow)* normal columnar epithelium and basement membrane, and upper right *(red arrow)* squamous metaplasia. (**B** from Kumar V, Abbas A, Fausto N: *Robbins & Cotran pathologic basis of disease,* ed 8, Philadelphia, 2007, Saunders.)

TABLE 2.1	PROGRESSIVE TYPES OF CELL INJURY AND RESPONSES
TYPE	**RESPONSES**
Adaptation	Atrophy, hypertrophy, hyperplasia, metaplasia
Active cell injury	Immediate response of "entire" cell
Reversible	Loss of adenosine triphosphate (ATP), swelling of cell, detachment of ribosomes, autophagy of lysosomes
Irreversible	"Point of no return" structurally when severe vacuolization of mitochondria occurs and Ca^{++} moves into the cell, including mitochondrial membrane damage
Necrosis	Common type of cell death with severe cell swelling and breakdown of organelles
Apoptosis, a type of programmed cell death	Cellular self-destruction for elimination of unwanted cell populations
Chronic cell injury (subcellular alterations)	Persistent stimuli response may involve only specific organelles or cytoskeleton (e.g., phagocytosis of bacteria)
Accumulations or infiltrations	Water, pigments, lipids, glycogen, proteins
Pathologic calcification	Dystrophic and metastatic calcification

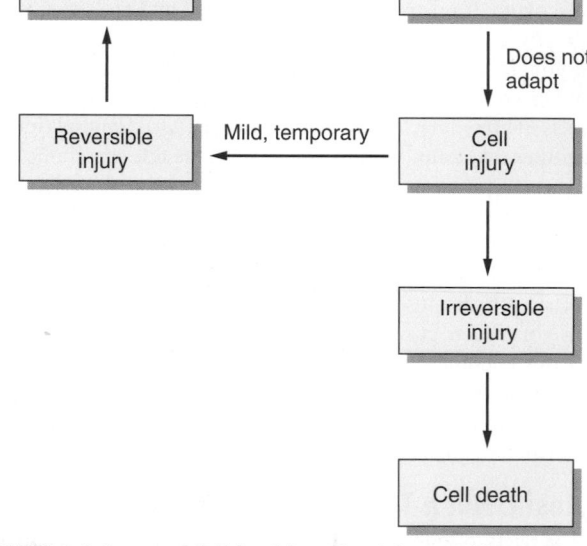

FIGURE 2.6 Stages of Cellular Adaptation, Injury, and Death. The normal cell responds to physiologic and pathologic stresses by adapting (atrophy, hypertrophy, hyperplasia, metaplasia). Cell injury occurs if the adaptive responses are exceeded or compromised by injurious agents, stress, and mutations. The injury is reversible if it is mild or transient, but if the stimulus persists the cell suffers irreversible injury and eventually death.

and adaptive processes of the cell, as well as the type, severity, and duration of the injurious stimulus. Two individuals exposed to an identical stimulus may incur varying degrees of cellular injury. Modifying factors, such as nutritional status, can profoundly influence the extent of injury. The precise "point of no return" that leads to cellular death is a biochemical puzzle, and the exact mechanisms responsible for the transition from reversible to irreversible cellular damage are being debated.

General Mechanisms of Cell Injury

Common biochemical mechanisms are important to understanding cell injury and cell death regardless of the injuring agent (Table 2.2). These mechanisms include adenosine triphosphate (ATP) depletion, mitochondrial damage, accumulation of oxygen and oxygen-derived free radicals, membrane damage (depletion of ATP), protein folding defects, DNA damage defects, and calcium level alterations (Fig. 2.7). Examples of cell injury are (1) ischemic and hypoxic injury, (2) ischemia-reperfusion injury, (3) oxidative stress or accumulation of oxygen-derived free radicals–induced injury, and (4) chemical injury.

Ischemic and Hypoxic Injury

Hypoxia, or lack of sufficient oxygen, is the single most common cause of cellular injury (Fig. 2.8). Hypoxia can result from a reduced amount of oxygen in the air, loss of hemoglobin or hemoglobin function, decreased production of red blood cells, consequences of respiratory and cardiovascular system diseases, and poisoning of the oxidative enzymes (cytochromes) within the cells. The most common cause of hypoxia is ischemia (reduced blood supply). Hypoxia can induce inflammation, and inflamed lesions can become hypoxic (Fig. 2.9).

Ischemic injury is often caused by gradual narrowing of arteries (arteriosclerosis) and complete blockage by blood clots (thrombosis). Progressive hypoxia caused by gradual arterial obstruction is better tolerated than the sudden acute anoxia (total lack of oxygen) caused by a sudden obstruction, such as can occur with an embolus (a blood clot or other plug in the circulation). An acute obstruction in a coronary artery can cause myocardial cell death (infarction) within minutes if the blood supply is not restored, whereas the gradual onset of ischemia usually results in myocardial adaptation. Myocardial infarction and stroke, which are common causes of death in the United States, generally result from atherosclerosis (a type of arteriosclerosis) and consequent ischemic injury.

Cellular responses to hypoxic injury in heart muscle have been extensively studied. Within 1 minute after blood supply to the myocardium is interrupted, the heart becomes pale and has difficulty contracting normally. Within 3 to 5 minutes the ischemic portion of the myocardium ceases to contract. The abrupt lack of contraction is caused by a rapid decrease in mitochondrial phosphorylation, which results in insufficient adenosine triphosphate (ATP) production. Lack of ATP leads to an increase in anaerobic metabolism, which generates ATP from glycogen when there is insufficient oxygen. When glycogen stores are depleted, even anaerobic metabolism ceases.

A reduction in ATP levels causes the plasma membrane's sodium-potassium (Na^+-K^+) pump and sodium-calcium exchange to fail, which leads to an intracellular accumulation of sodium and calcium, resulting in cellular swelling and diffusion of potassium out of the cell. Because all cells are bathed in a fluid rich in calcium ions, cell membrane damage allows rapid movement of calcium intracellularly. The movement of water and ions into the cell causes early dilation of the ER. Dilation causes the ribosomes to detach from the rough ER, resulting in reduced protein synthesis. With continued hypoxia, the entire cell becomes markedly swollen, with increased concentrations of sodium, water, and chloride and decreased concentrations of potassium. These disruptions are reversible if oxygen is restored. If oxygen is not restored, however, there is vacuolation (formation of vacuoles or cytoplasmic small cavities) within the cytoplasm, swelling of lysosomes, and marked swelling of the mitochondria resulting from mitochondrial membrane damage. Continued hypoxic injury with accumulation of calcium subsequently activates multiple enzyme systems, including proteases, nitric oxide synthase, phospholipases, and endonuclease. These activations result in cytoskeleton disruption, membrane damage, inflammation, DNA

TABLE 2.2	COMMON MECHANISMS IN CELL INJURY AND CELL DEATH
THEME	**COMMENTS**
ATP depletion	Loss of mitochondrial adenosine triphosphate (ATP) and decreased ATP synthesis; results include cellular swelling, decreased protein synthesis, decreased membrane transport, and lipogenesis, all changes that contribute to loss of integrity of the plasma membrane (see text)
Oxygen and oxygen-derived free radicals	Lack of oxygen is key in progression of cell injury in ischemia (reduced blood supply); activated oxygen species (free radicals, H_2O_2, O_2^-, NO) cause destruction of cell membranes and cell structure
Intracellular calcium and loss of calcium steady state	Normally intracellular cytosolic calcium concentrations are very low; ischemia and certain chemicals cause an increase in cytosolic Ca^{++} concentrations; sustained levels of Ca^{++} continue to increase with damage to plasma membrane; Ca^{++} causes intracellular damage by activating a number of enzymes (see text)
Defects in membrane permeability	Early loss of selective membrane permeability found in all forms of cell injury (see text)

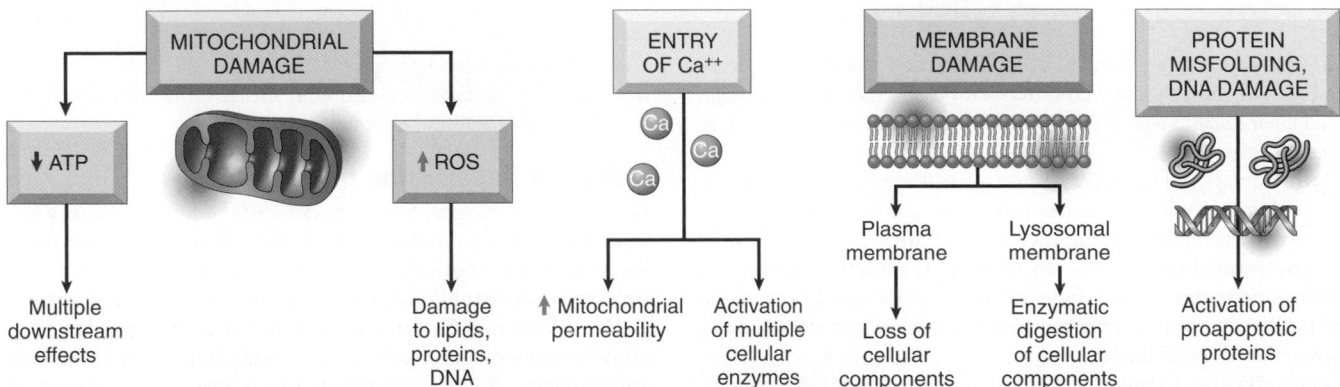

FIGURE 2.7 Example of Biochemical Mechanisms and Damage in Cell Injury. *ATP,* Adenosine triphosphate; *ROS,* reactive oxygen species. (Adapted from Kumar V, Abbas A, Aster J: *Robbins & Cotran pathologic basis of disease,* ed 9, Philadelphia, 2015, Saunders.)

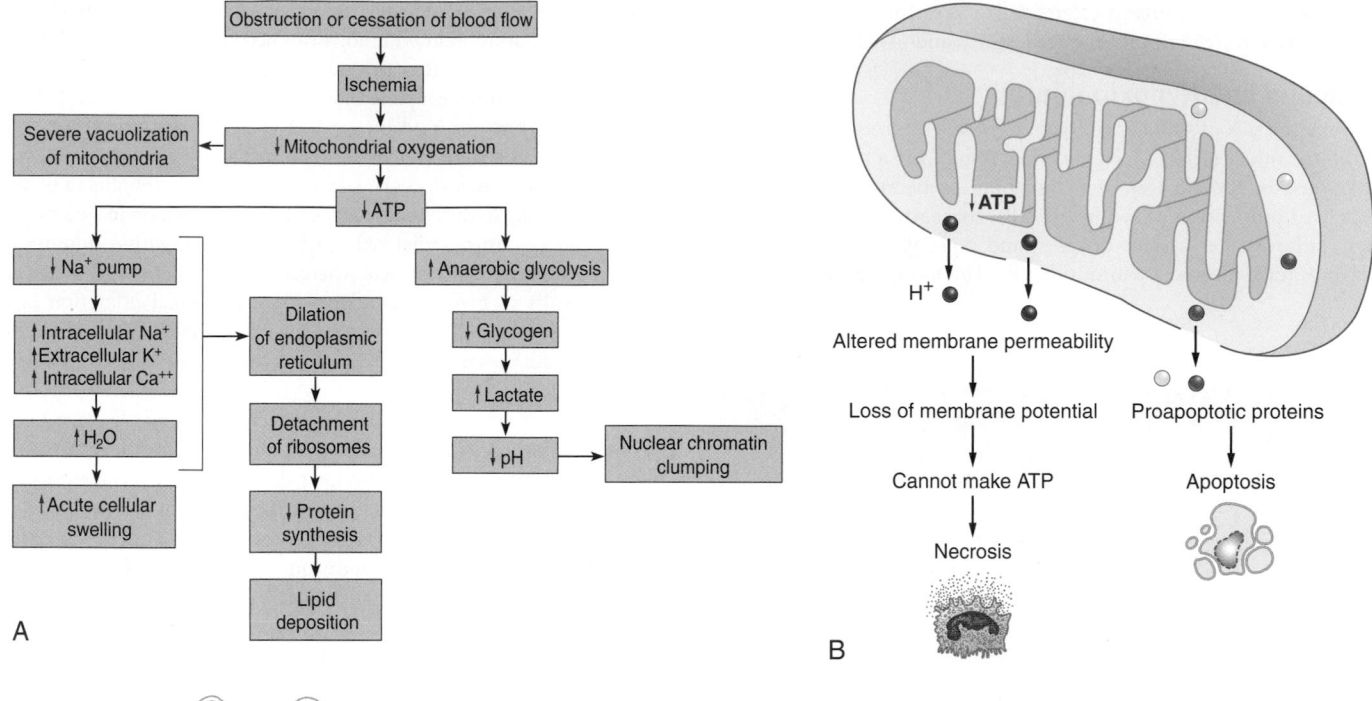

A

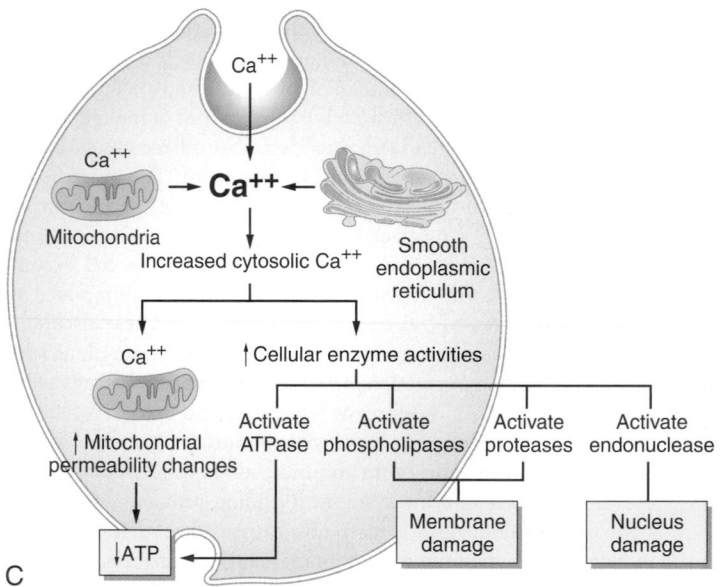

C

FIGURE 2.8 Hypoxic Injury Induced by Ischemia. A, Consequences of decreased oxygen delivery or ischemia with decreased ATP. The structural and physiologic changes are reversible if oxygen is delivered quickly. Significant decreases in ATP concentration result in cell death, mostly by necrosis. **B,** Mitochondrial damage can result in changes in membrane permeability, loss of membrane potential, and a decrease in ATP production. Between the outer and inner membranes of the mitochondria are proteins that can activate the cell's suicide pathways, called *apoptosis.* **C,** Calcium ions are critical mediators of cell injury. Calcium ions are usually maintained at low concentrations in the cell's cytoplasm; thus, ischemia and certain toxins can initially cause an increase in the release of Ca^{++} from intracellular stores and later an increased movement (influx) across the plasma membrane. *ATP,* Adenosine triphosphate; *ATPase,* enzyme.

and chromatin degradation, ATP depletion, and eventual cell death (see Figs. 2.8 and 2.30). Structurally, with plasma membrane damage, extracellular calcium readily moves into the cell and intracellular calcium stores are released.

Intracellular calcium results in the activation of enzymes that can further damage membranes, proteins, ATP, and nucleic acids. The increased permeability of the membrane causes continued loss of proteins, essential coenzymes, and ribonucleic acids. In addition, the substrates necessary to reconstitute ATP are lost. Increased intracellular calcium levels activate cell enzymes (caspases) that promote cell death by apoptosis (see Fig. 2.36).

Acid hydrolases from leaking lysosomes are activated in the reduced pH of the injured cell and they digest cytoplasmic and nuclear components. Leakage of intracellular enzymes into the peripheral circulation provides a diagnostic tool for detecting tissue-specific cellular injury

and death using blood samples; for example, the contractile protein troponin from cardiac muscle is found after myocardial injury and liver transaminases are found after hepatic injury.

Ischemia-Reperfusion Injury

Restoration of oxygen, however, can cause additional injury called **reperfusion (reoxygenation) injury.** Reperfusion injury results from the generation of highly reactive oxygen intermediates (oxidative stress), including hydroxyl radical (OH•), superoxide O_2^-, and hydrogen peroxide (H_2O_2). These radicals can all cause further membrane damage and mitochondrial calcium overload. The white blood cells (neutrophils) are especially affected with reperfusion injury, including neutrophil adhesion to the endothelium.

Reperfusion is a serious complication and an important mechanism of injury in instances of tissue transplantation and in myocardial, hepatic,

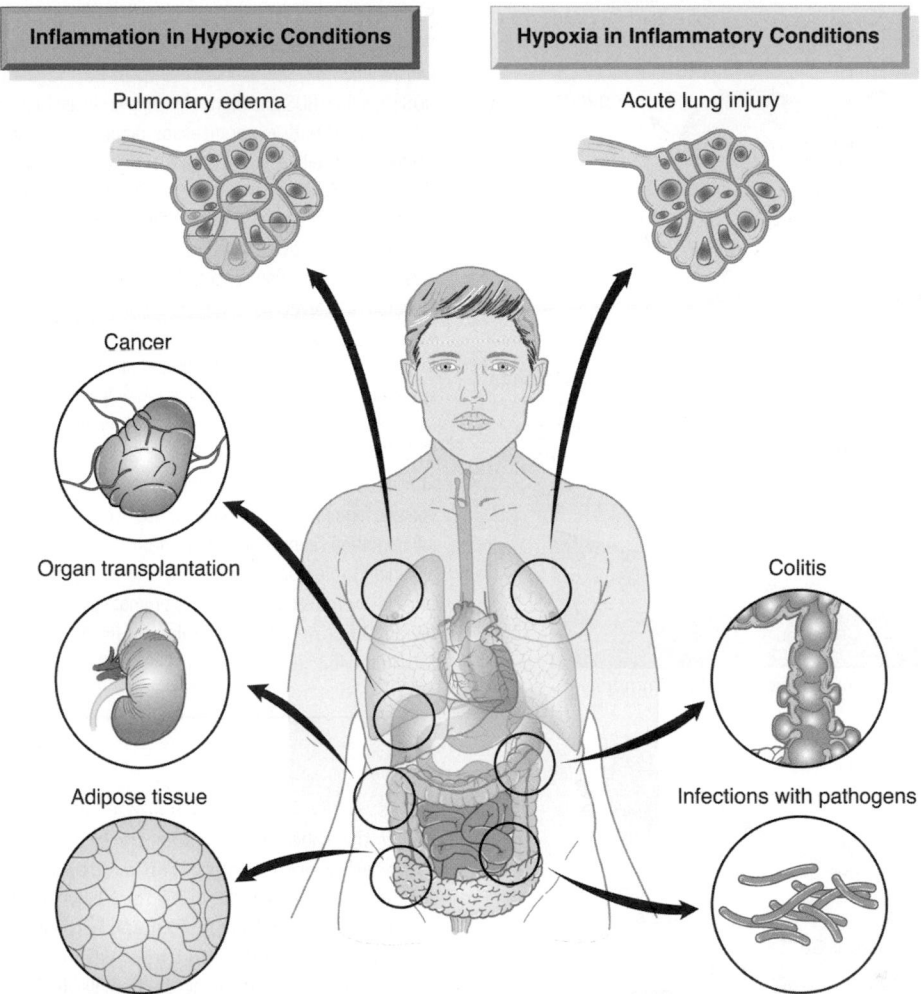

FIGURE 2.9 Hypoxia and Inflammation. Shown is a simplified drawing of clinical conditions characterized by tissue hypoxia that causes inflammatory changes *(left)* and inflammatory diseases that ultimately lead to hypoxia *(right).* These diseases and conditions are discussed in more detail in their respective chapters. (Adapted from Eltzschig HK, Carmeliet P: *N Engl J Med* 364:656–665, 2011.)

intestinal, cerebral, renal, and other ischemic syndromes, including stroke.[6,7] Xanthine dehydrogenase, an enzyme that normally uses oxidized nicotinamide adenine dinucleotide (NAD+) as an electron acceptor, is converted during reperfusion with oxygen to xanthine oxidase. During the ischemic period, excessive ATP consumption leads to the accumulation of the purine catabolites hypoxanthine and xanthine, which upon subsequent reperfusion and influx of oxygen are metabolized by xanthine oxidase to make *massive* amounts of superoxide and hydrogen peroxide. These radicals can all cause membrane damage and mitochondrial calcium overload.[8] Cardiac ischemia and reperfusion injury cause excessive reactive oxygen species (ROS), pH alterations, osmotic changes, gap junction changes, inflammatory signaling, and calcium overload of the mitochondria. These changes, especially rapid restoration of intracellular pH, lead to the opening of a large conductance pore on the mitochondrial membrane called the *mitochondrial permeability transition pore* (MPTP) with massive escape of ATP and solutes leading to cell death activation (apoptosis).[6,9] These changes also lead to irreversible cardiomyocyte hypercontracture.[10] Cardioprotection from ischemia/reperfusion injury is an important focus of much research. Other potential and current treatments include use of antioxidants, blockage of inflammatory mediators, and inhibition of apoptotic pathways.

Free Radicals and Reactive Oxygen Species

It is now widely accepted that inherent reactive oxygen species (ROS) from aerobic metabolism play a crucial biologic role not just in various diseases but also for normal cellular communication and cell function (Fig. 2.10). ROS reversibly modulates many intracellular signaling pathways.[11] ROS are increasingly implicated in various cell fates and signal transduction pathways.[11] ROS-dependent signaling involves the reversible oxidation and reduction of specific amino acids; reactive cysteine (Cys) residues are most frequently targeted.[11] ROS can affect protein functions through several mechanisms, including regulation of protein expression, posttranslational modifications, and alteration of protein stability. The outcome effects of these mechanisms include regulating protein stability, increasing and decreasing protein function, altering protein location, and altering protein-protein interaction (Fig. 2.11).

Reduction-oxidation (redox)–dependent regulation and the roles of ROS encompass both normal physiologic and pathologic roles. These expanding roles include proliferation and differentiation, immune function, stem cell self-renewal, tumor progression, autoimmunity, stem cell exhaustion, senescence, and longevity (see Fig. 2.11). These topics

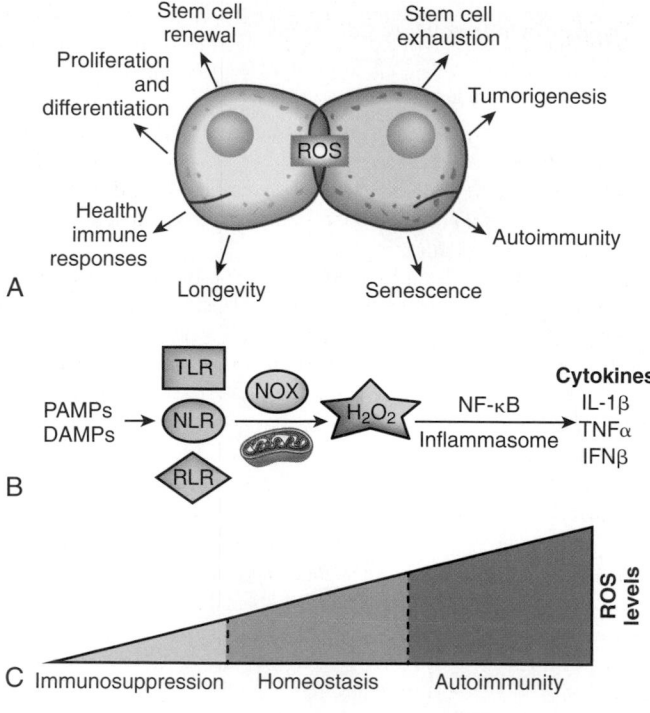

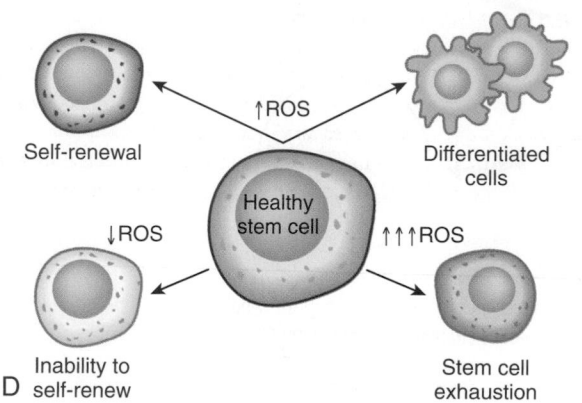

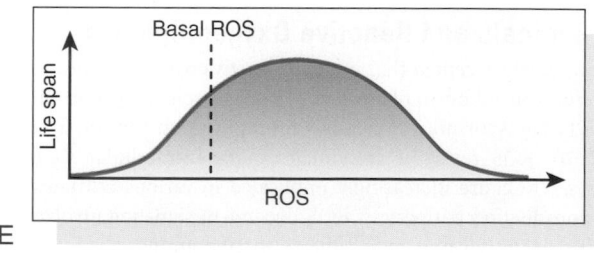

FIGURE 2.10 Physiologic and Pathologic Roles of Redox Biology and Reactive Oxygen Species. **A,** Summary figure of expanding roles of redox biology and reactive oxygen species (ROS). **B,** ROS regulation of inflammation requires ROS signaling. ROS and redox signaling is crucial to understand because inflammation is associated with many diseases processes. Common patterns associated with pathogens or cell damage (PAMPS or DAMPS) activate immune surveillance receptors (TLR, NLR, RLR), which increase ROS from NAPDH oxidase (NOX) enzymes and mitochondria. The release of proinflammatory cytokines (IL-1β, TNF-α, IFNβ) depends on ROS. **C,** Low levels of ROS maintain a normal immune system. Decreasing ROS levels inhibit activation or normal immune responses resulting in immunosuppression. Elevated ROS levels contribute to autoimmunity increasing the release of proinflammatory cytokines and proliferation of some adaptive immune cells. **D,** Moderate levels of ROS are required for proper stem-cell differentiation and renewal through activation of signaling pathways. ROS levels that are elevated lead to stem-cell exhaustion and premature aging through activation of signaling pathways. **E,** Increased ROS levels are not always detrimental to life span. Slight increases in ROS can drive signaling pathways that counter the normal aging process; conversely, high levels of ROS can cause hyperactive signaling pathways that promote inflammation, cancer and cell death, and an accelerated aging phenotype. The expanding roles of redox biology and ROS present challenges for understanding the use of pro-oxidant therapy to promote physiologic ROS responses or antioxidant therapy to prevent ROS pathologies. (From Schieber M, Chandel NS: *Curr Biol* 24:R453–R462, 2014.)

makes the molecule unstable; the molecule becomes stabilized either by donating or by accepting an electron from another molecule. When the attacked molecule loses its electron, it becomes a free radical. Therefore it is capable of injurious chemical bond formation with DNA, RNA, proteins, lipids, and carbohydrates—many are key molecules in membranes and nucleic acids. Free radicals are difficult to control and initiate chain reactions. With low chemical specificity and high reactivity, free radicals can react with most molecules in their proximity.

Reactive oxygen species (ROS) are chemically reactive molecules from molecular oxygen formed as natural oxidant species in cells during mitochondrial respiration and energy generation. The intracellular sources of oxidants are numerous and include (1) cellular organelles with mitochondria (thought to be the largest contributor), ER (particularly during endoplasmic stress), and peroxisomes; (2) NADPH oxidases (NOX enzymes); and (3) other enzymes (Fig. 2.12).[11] From oxidative phosphorylation, mitochondria utilize oxygen to generate ATP from organic fuel molecules and in the process produce ROS.[12]

An important mechanism of membrane damage is injury induced by free radicals, especially by a disturbance in the balance between the production of ROS and antioxidant defenses called oxidative stress (Fig. 2.13). Oxidative stress can be caused by an increase of different reactive species or a depletion of antioxidant defense, or both, and results in detrimental oxidation of different molecules including proteins, lipids, nucleic acids, and others. Oxidative stress can activate several intracellular signaling pathways because ROS can modulate enzymes and transcription factors. This process is an important mechanism of cell damage in many conditions, including cell injury, cancer, certain degenerative diseases (e.g., Alzheimer disease), and aging. ROS can mediate posttranslational modifications of molecules involved in intracellular signaling networks and regulate normal signaling components, a process called redox signaling. Although ROS have been appreciated for their damage-promoting, detrimental effects, there is now a greater understanding of their roles as signaling molecules.[12]

are discussed in relevant sections in the textbook, and some aspects of redox signaling are included here with the main emphasis on cell injury.

Cell injury produced by free radicals, particularly reactive oxygen species, is an important mechanism of cell damage in many conditions including chemical and radiation injury, ischemia-reperfusion injury (induced with restoration of blood flow in ischemic tissue), microbial killing by phagocytes (rapid bursts), and cellular aging.[1] A free radical is any molecular species capable of independent existence that contains a single unpaired electron in an outer orbit. Having one unpaired electron

Free radicals are generated within cells in several ways: (1) reduction-oxidation reactions (redox reactions) in normal metabolic processes, such as respiration; (2) absorption of extreme energy sources (e.g., ultraviolet light, radiation); (3) enzymatic metabolism of exogenous chemicals, drugs, and pesticides; (4) the process of transition metals (i.e., iron and copper) donating or accepting free electrons during intracellular reactions and activating the formation of free radicals, such as in the Fenton reaction (Fig. 2.14); and (5) nitric oxide (NO) acting as an important chemical mediator and can act as a free radical. NO is a colorless gas and an intermediate in many reactions generated by endothelial cells, neurons, macrophages, and other cell types. It can be converted to peroxynitrite anion ($ONOO^-$), NO_2, and NO_3^- (Table 2.3). All biologic membranes contain redox systems important for cell defense, for example, inflammation.

Emerging data indicate that ROS play roles in the initiation and progression of cardiovascular alterations associated with hypertension, hyperlipidemia, diabetes mellitus, ischemic heart disease, chronic heart failure, and sleep apnea.[13-15] ROS generation is thought to lead to vascular endothelial injury and consequently atherosclerosis. Upregulation of adhesion molecule production in the endothelium can be accomplished by ROS, which diminishes nitric oxide (NO) synthase activity and promotes NO breakdown. This disturbance of the vascular environment presumably causes a reduction of endothelial-dependent vasodilation.[16] Such reduction in endothelium-dependent vasodilation has been demonstrated through intraarterial infusion of vasoactive agents. Specific mechanisms by which ROS control endothelial function and vascular tone and pathophysiologic consequences include inflammation, hypertrophy, proliferation, apoptosis, fibrosis, angiogenesis, and vascular remodeling resulting in endothelial dysfunction.[14] Emerging is a better understanding of increased oxidative stress and elevation of ROS in diabetes and hypertension that can lead to dysrhythmia.[15] Oxidative stress-induced arrhythmia can lead to sudden death, and a summary of these mechanisms includes the effect on ion channels, effect on intracellular Ca^{++}, effect on myocyte conduction velocity, and activation of fibrosis with an effect on the extracellular matrix.[17]

Development of the placenta during pregnancy is interrelated to oxygen concentration.[18] ROS can regulate gene transcription and affect

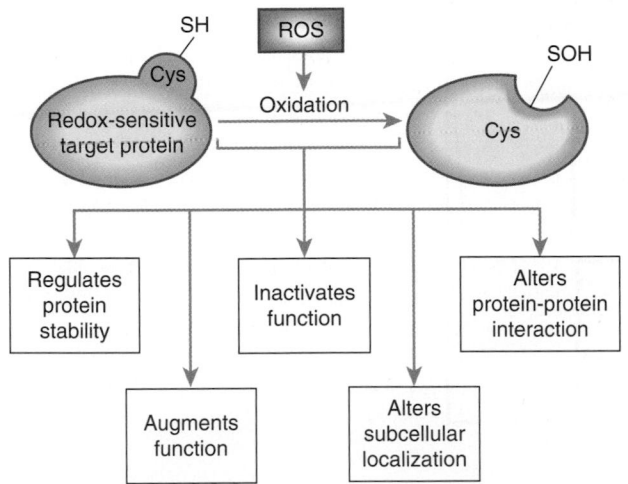

FIGURE 2.11 Redox-Dependent Signaling: Biologic Mechanisms and Consequences. The oxidation and reduction (redox) of sensitive targets or proteins with cysteine (Cys) residues provide a mechanism to rapidly and reversibly alter protein function. Cys residues can function as redox-dependent "switches." Oxidation of Cys residues (SH[thiol]) to SOH (sulfenic acid) leads to alterations in the redox-sensitive target that result in many effects on protein stability, activity, and protein-protein interaction. (Adapted from Homstrom KM, Finkel T: *Nat Rev* 15[6]:411–421, 2014).

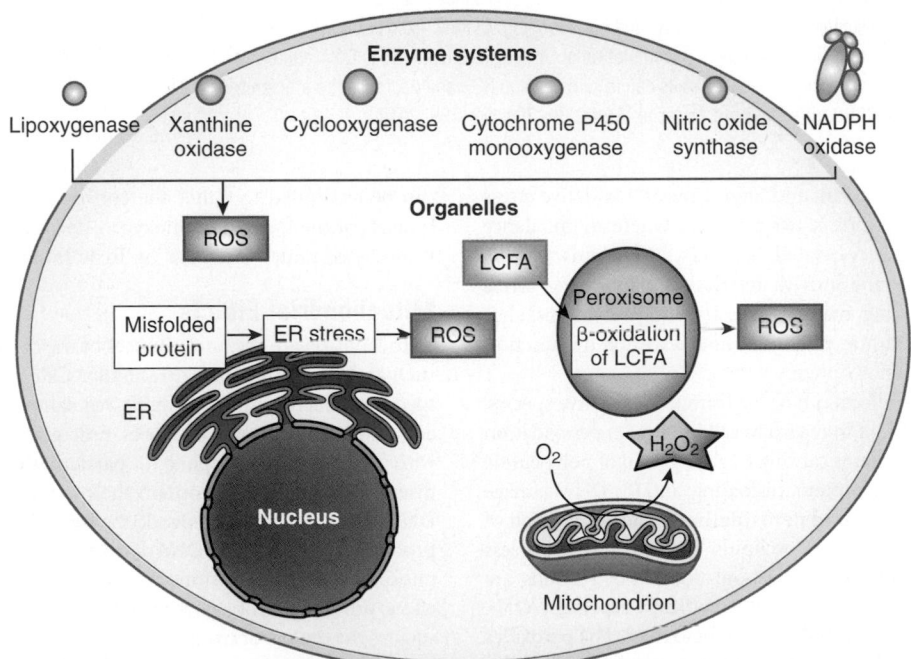

FIGURE 2.12 Intracellular Sources of ROS and Sites of Generation of ROS From Mitochondria. The intracellular sources of reactive oxygen species (ROS) include some organelles: mitochondria, endoplasmic reticulum (ER) (particularly ER stress), and peroxisomes (metabolizing long-chain fatty acids [LCFAs]). As part of the enzymatic reaction cycles, various enzymes generate ROS, including oxidases and oxygenases. H_2O_2, Hydrogen peroxide; *NADPH*, nicotinamide adenine dinucleotide phosphate. (Adapted from Homstrom KM, Finkel T: *Nat Rev* 15[6]:411–421, 2014).

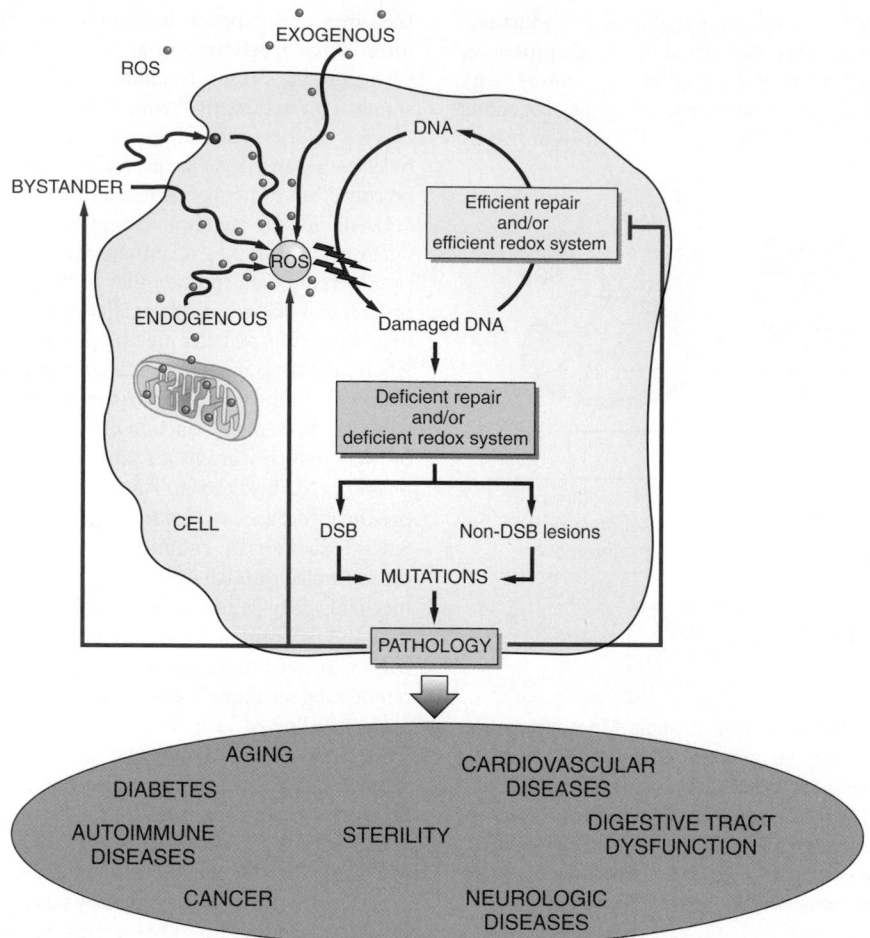

FIGURE 2.13 Oxidative Stress in Human Pathogenesis. Reactive oxygen species (ROS) have a role in a wide variety of diseases and age-related diseases including cancer, neurologic disease, type 2 diabetes, autoimmune and cardiovascular diseases, infertility, and normal aging. Chronic exposure to ROS and decreased DNA repair can result in persistent DNA mutations. Accumulation of DNA lesions can lead to DNA double strand breaks *(DSBs)* and disease onset/progression. Diseased cells can in turn develop ROS and decrease the efficiency of the DNA repair mechanism. (Adapted from Sedelnikova OA et al: *Mutat Res* 704:152–159, 2010.)

trophoblast proliferation, invasion, and angiogenesis. Oxidative stress influences autophagy and apoptosis, two processes where an imbalance seems to be linked to pregnancy-related disorders, such as miscarriage, preeclampsia, and intrauterine growth restriction.[18] Oxidative stress observed in maternal smoking, maternal obesity, and preeclampsia has been associated with aberrant angiogenesis and placental dysfunction resulting in adverse pregnancy outcomes.[19,20]

Although wide-ranging effects can occur from these reactive species, three are particularly important in regard to cell injury: (1) peroxidation of lipids; (2) alterations of proteins causing fragmentation of polypeptide chains that can lead to loss and protein misfolding; and (3) DNA damage causing mutations (Fig. 2.15). **Lipid peroxidation** is the destruction of unsaturated fatty acids. Fatty acids of lipids in membranes possess double bonds between some of the carbon atoms. Such bonds are vulnerable to attack by oxygen-derived free radicals, especially OH•. The lipid-radical interactions themselves yield peroxides. The peroxides instigate a chain reaction resulting in membrane, organelle, and cellular destruction. Because of the increased understanding of free radicals, a growing number of diseases and disorders have been linked either directly or indirectly to these reactive species (Box 2.1).

Table 2.4 summarizes methods that contribute to inactivation or termination of free radicals. The toxicity of certain drugs and chemicals can be attributed to either the conversion of these chemicals to free radicals or the formation of oxygen-derived metabolites.[7] This process is discussed under Chemical or Toxic Injury.

Mitochondrial Effects

Mitochondria are the powerhouses of the cell involved in key functions such as ATP production, intracellular Ca^{++} regulation, reactive oxygen species production and scavenging, regulation of apoptotic cell death, and activation of the caspase proteases. Emerging is the role of mitochondria with autophagy (mitophagy), particularly with neurodegenerative diseases. Mitochondria contain their own DNA called **mitochondrial DNA (mtDNA)** and can encode the central proteins involved in energy production. Because mtDNA encodes enzymes involved in oxidative phosphorylation, mutations affecting these genes exert their damaging effects primarily on organs most dependent on oxidative phosphorylation, such as the central nervous system, skeletal muscle, cardiac muscle, liver, and kidneys.[1] New is emerging information that mitochondria act as a central environmental sensor (see *What's New?* Mitochondria May Have a Central Role in Mediating Environmental Changes and Genomic Responses). Mitochondria can be damaged by ROS and by increases of cytosolic Ca^{++}. During normal metabolism, the mitochondria are the greatest source and target of ROS (see previous discussion in section Free

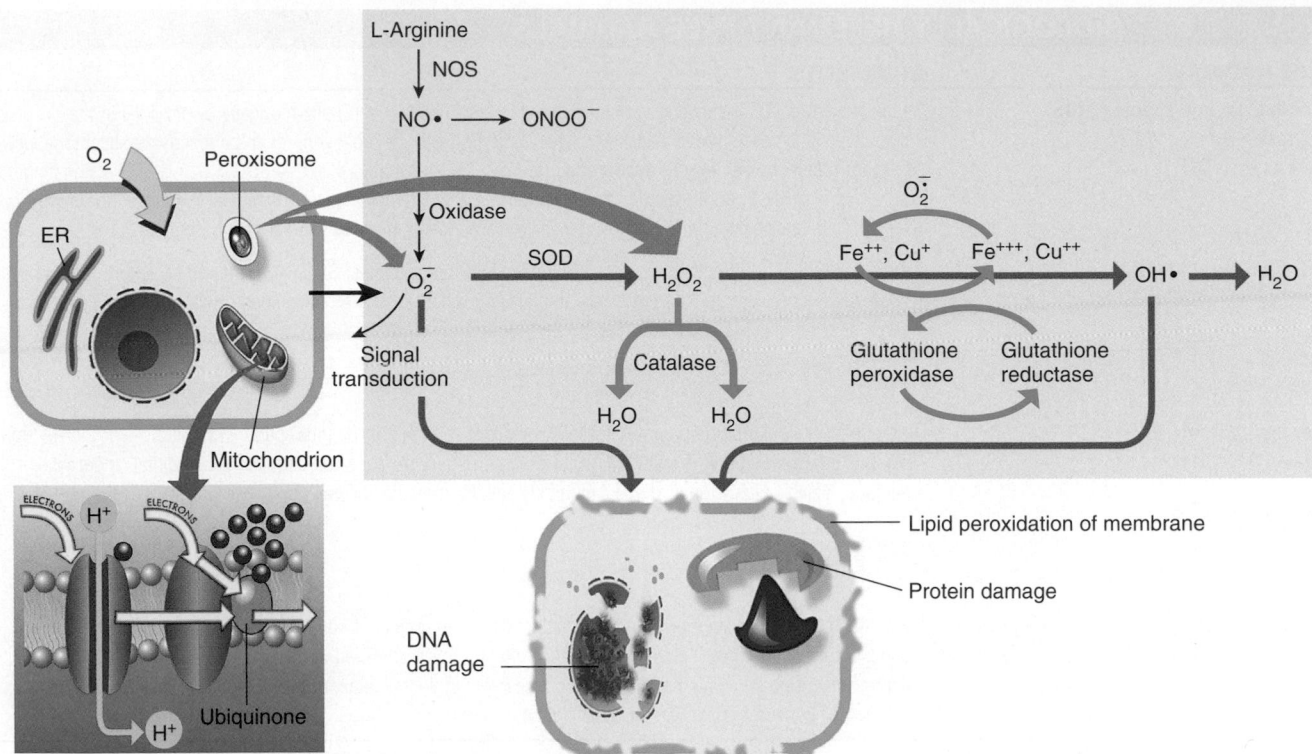

FIGURE 2.14 Generation of Reactive Oxygen Species (ROS) and Antioxidant Mechanisms in Biologic Systems. Mitochondria have four sites of entry for electrons coming into the electron-transport system: one for reduced nicotinamide adenine dinucleotide (NADH) and three for the reduced form of flavin adenine dinucleotide (FADH$_2$). These pathways meet at the small, lipophilic molecule ubiquinone (coenzyme Q), at the beginning of the common electron-transport pathway. Ubiquinone transfers electrons in the inner membrane, ultimately enabling their interaction with O$_2$ and H$_2$ to yield H$_2$O. In so doing, the transport allows free energy change and the synthesis of 1 mol of adenosine triphosphate (ATP). With the transport of electrons, free radicals are generated within the mitochondria. ROS (H$_2$O$_2$, OH•, and O$_2^-$ and nitric oxide [NO]) act as physiologic modulators of some mitochondrial functions but also may cause cell damage. O$_2$ is converted to superoxide (O$_2^-$) by oxidative enzymes in the mitochondria, endoplasmic reticulum (ER), plasma membrane, peroxisomes, and cytosol. O$_2$ is converted to H$_2$O$_2$ by superoxide dismutase (SOD) and further to OH• by the Cu^{++}/Fe^{++} Fenton reaction. Superoxide catalyzes the reduction of Fe^{++} to Fe^{+++}, thus increasing OH• formation by the Fenton reaction. H$_2$O$_2$ is also derived from oxidases in peroxisomes. The NO• (radical) is produced by the oxidation of one of the terminal guanido-nitrogen atoms of L-arginine. Depending on the microenvironment, NO can be converted to other reactive nitrogen species including the highly reactive peroxynitrite (ONOO$^-$). Both OH• and ONOO$^-$ are very reactive and can modify cellular macromolecules and cause toxicity. The less reactive molecules O$_2^-$ and H$_2$O$_2$ can serve as cellular signaling molecules. The major antioxidant enzymes include SOD, catalase, and glutathione peroxidase. (Data from Dröge W: *Physiol Rev* 82:47–95, 2002; Buetler TM, Krauskopf A, Ruegg UT: *News Physiol Sci* 19:120–123, 2004.)

Radicals and Reactive Oxygen Species and Fig. 2.12). Usually the number of ROS is reduced by intracellular antioxidant enzymes, including superoxide dismutase (SOD), glutathione peroxidase, and catalase; as well as antioxidant molecules, such as glutathione and vitamin E. ROS, however, contribute to mitochondria dysfunction and are related to many human diseases and aging. In pathologic conditions, the large numbers of ROS overwhelm the balance by antioxidants. This inefficiency of antioxidants is even more serious in mitochondria because mitochondria in most cells lack catalase.[21] Consequently, the excessive production of hydrogen peroxide and eventually hydroxyl radicals (OH•) in mitochondria will damage lipid, proteins, and mtDNA, which then causes cells to die.[21] Mitochondrial oxidative stress has been implicated in heart disease, Alzheimer disease, Parkinson disease, prion diseases, and amyotrophic lateral sclerosis (ALS), as well as aging itself.[22,23] Accumulating evidence shows ROS are important for cell proliferation and survival.[24] Dysfunction of autophagy may result in abnormal mitochondrial function and

oxidative or nitrative (i.e., reactive nitrogen species) stress. Investigators have provided new understanding of how autophagy of mitochondria (also known as *mitophagy*) is controlled, and the impact of autophagic dysfunction on cellular oxidative stress. Impaired mitochondrial function, oxidative stress, accumulation of protein aggregates, and autophagic stress are common in many diseases.[25] Additionally, investigators are trying to identify the polypeptides (i.e., proteomes) directly involved in diseases associated with mitochondrial dysfunction.

Chemical or Toxic Injury Mechanisms

Humans are exposed to thousands of chemicals that have inadequate toxicologic data.[26] The given societal considerations of time, cost, and reduced animal use have increased the need to develop new methods for toxicity testing. To meet this public health need, many agencies have

TABLE 2.3   BIOLOGICALLY RELEVANT FREE RADICALS

FREE RADICAL	COMMENTS
Reactive oxygen species (ROS) Superoxide O_2^- $O_2 \rightarrow$ oxidase O_2^-	Generated either (1) directly during autooxidation in mitochondria or (2) enzymatically by enzymes in the cytoplasm, such as xanthine oxidase or cytochrome P-450; once produced, it can be inactivated spontaneously or more rapidly by the enzyme superoxide dismutase (SOD): $O_2^- + O_2^- + 2H^+ \rightarrow SOD\ H_2O_2 + O_2\ O_2^-$; a signaling molecule in growing or differentiating tissue, including hypertrophy, can alter cellular responses to growth factors and vasoconstrictor hormones; increasing levels of O_2^- may lead to apoptosis (see Fig. 2.11)
Hydrogen peroxide (H_2O_2) $O_2^- + O_2^- + 2H \rightarrow SOD\ H_2O_2 + O_2$ *or* Oxidases present in peroxisomes O_2 peroxisome $O_2^- \rightarrow SOD\ H_2O_2$	Generated by SOD or directly by oxidases in intracellular peroxisomes; SOD is considered an antioxidant because it converts superoxide to H_2O_2; catalase (another antioxidant) can then decompose H_2O_2 to $O_2 + H_2O$; H_2O_2 can serve as a cellular signaling molecule
Hydroxyl radicals (OH•) $H_2O \rightarrow H• + OH•$ *or* $Fe^{++} + H_2O_2 \rightarrow Fe^{+++} + OH• + OH^-$ *or* $H_2O_2 + O_2^- \rightarrow OH• + OH^- + O_2$	Generated by the hydrolysis of water caused by ionizing radiation or by interaction with metals—especially iron (Fe) and copper (Cu); iron is important in toxic oxygen injury because it is required for maximal oxidative cell damage; OH• is highly reactive and can modify cellular macromolecules and cause toxicity
Nitric oxide (NO) $NO• + O_2^- \rightarrow ONOO^- + H^+$ ↑↓ $OH• + NO_2 \leftrightharpoons ONOOH \rightarrow NO_3^-$	NO by itself is an important mediator that can act as a free radical; it can be converted to another radical—peroxynitrite anion ($ONOO^-$), as well as $NO_2•$ and NO_3^-; NO is formed in neuronal cells, where it modulates neurotransmission; in endothelial cells as a modulator of vessel relaxation; and in neutrophils and macrophages as a factor in vessel relaxation and inactivation of pathogens

Data from Kumer V, Abbas A, Aster J: *Robbins & Cotran pathologic basis of disease*, ed 8, Philadelphia, 2010, Saunders; Buetler TM, Krauskopf A, Ruegg UT: *News Physiol Sci* 19:120–123, 2004.

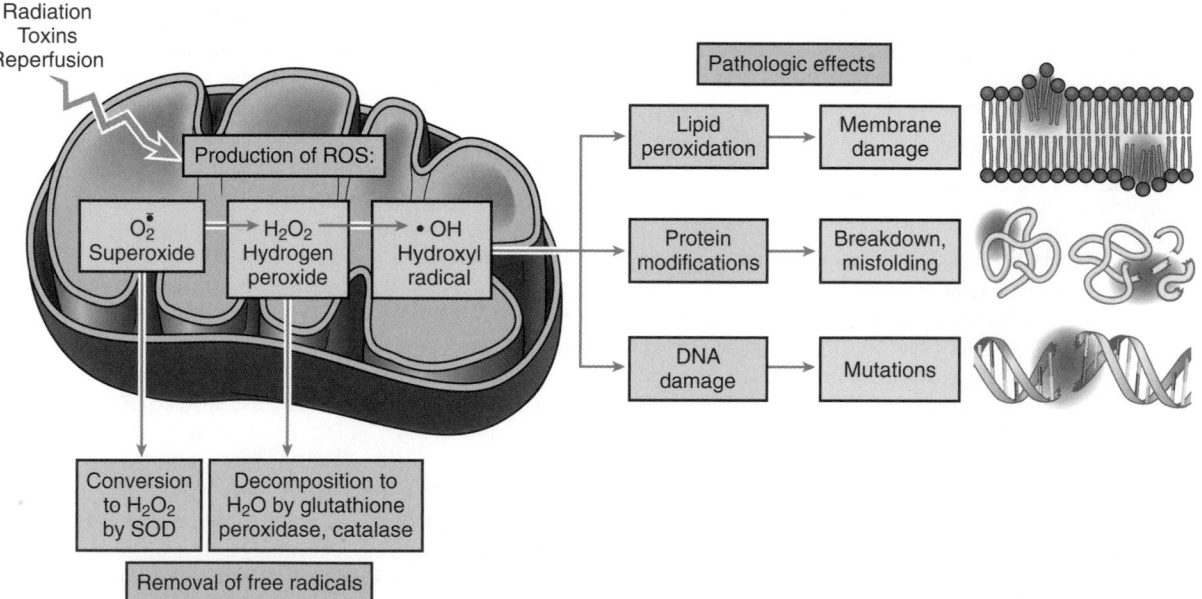

FIGURE 2.15 Role of Reactive Oxygen Species in Cell Injury. The production of reactive oxygen species (ROS) can be initiated by many cell stressors, such as radiation, toxins, and reperfusion of oxygen. Free radicals are removed by normal decay and enzymatic systems. ROS accumulate in cells because of insufficient removal or excess production leading to cell injury, including lipid peroxidation, protein modifications, and DNA damage or mutations. *SOD,* Superoxide dismutase. (Adapted from Kumar V, Abbas A, Aster J: *Robbins & Cotran pathologic basis of disease*, ed 9, Philadelphia, 2015, Saunders.)

partnered to investigate how chemicals interact with biologic systems. Advances in molecular and systems biology, computational toxicology, and bioinformatics have increased the development of powerful new tools.

The systems biology approach includes delineation of toxicity pathways that may be defined as cellular response pathways that when disturbed are expected to result in adverse health effects. Using this model of testing, investigators proposed screening and classifying compounds using a "cellular stress response pathway." Components or mechanisms of these pathways include oxidative stress, heat shock response, DNA damage response, hypoxia, ER stress, mental stress,

WHAT'S NEW?

Mitochondria May Have a Central Role in Mediating Environmental Changes and Genomic Responses

Mitochondria may be key sensors of environmental changes. Changes in the environment would affect mitochondrial bioenergetics and alter the production of high-energy mitochondrial molecules. High-energy molecules produced by mitochondria modify the cytoplasmic signaling proteins and epigenomic proteins that regulate nuclear DNA (nDNA) expression. These changes may reprogram gene expression, altering expressions of nDNA-derived and mitochondrial DNA–derived (mtDNA-derived) proteins that act in and on the mitochondria. More simply, mitochondrial physiologic states determined by mtDNA variation sense environmental changes and send specific signals to the nucleus to produce the ideal gene-expression response. These responses influence mitochondrial function, affecting energetic homeostasis and ultimately health, longevity, and disease.

Data from Latorre-Pellicer A et al: *Nature* 535(7613):561–565, 2016; Wallace DC: *Nature* 535:498–500, 2016.

inflammation, and osmotic stress. Many chemicals have already been classified under these mechanisms.

Humans are constantly exposed to a variety of compounds termed **xenobiotics** (Greek *xenos*, "foreign"; *bios*, "life") that include toxic, mutagenic, and carcinogenic chemicals (Figs. 2.16 and 2.17). Some of these chemicals are found in the human diet. Many xenobiotics are toxic to the liver (hepatotoxic). The liver is the initial site of contact

TABLE 2.4   METHODS CONTRIBUTING TO INACTIVATION OR TERMINATION OF FREE RADICALS

METHOD	PROCESS
Antioxidants	Endogenous or exogenous; either blocks synthesis or inactivates (e.g., scavenges) free radicals; includes vitamin E, vitamin C, cysteine, glutathione, albumin, ceruloplasmin, transferrin
Enzymes	Superoxide dismutase*, which converts superoxide to H_2O_2; catalase* (in peroxisomes) decomposes $H_2O_2\bullet$; glutathione peroxidase* decomposes $OH\bullet$ and H_2O_2

*These enzymes are important in modulating the cellular destructive effects of free radicals, also released in inflammation.

for many ingested xenobiotics, drugs, and alcohol, making this organ most susceptible to chemically induced injury. The toxicity of many chemicals results from absorption through the gastrointestinal tract after oral ingestion. A main cause for withdrawing medications from the market is hepatotoxicity. Dietary supplements, for example, chaparral and ma huang, are potent hepatotoxins.[27] Other common routes of exposure for xenobiotics are absorption through the skin and inhalation. The severity of chemically induced liver injury varies from minor liver injury to acute liver failure, cirrhosis, and liver cancer.

The liver as the principal site for xenobiotic metabolism, called *biotransformation*, converts the lipophilic xenobiotics to more hydrophilic forms for efficient excretion. Biotransformation, however, also can produce short-lived unstable highly reactive chemical intermediates that can lead to adverse effects.[28] These harmful intermediates are called **toxicophores**. The intermediates include electrophiles, nucleophiles, free radicals, and redox-active reactants. An **electrophile** (electron lover) is an atom or molecule attracted to electrons and accepts a pair of electrons to make a covalent bond. This process creates a partially or fully charged center in electrophilic molecules.[28] A **nucleophile** is an atom or molecule that donates an electron pair to an electrophile to make a chemical bond. All chemical species with a free pair of electrons can act as nucleophiles. Nucleophiles are strongly attracted to positively charged regions in other chemicals and can be oxidized to free radicals and electrophiles.[28] In general, the majority of all *reactive* chemical species are electrophilic because the formation of nucleophiles is rare.[28] The generation of these excess reactive chemical species leads to molecular damage in liver cells. These reactive intermediates can interact with cellular macromolecules, such as proteins and DNA, forming protein adducts and DNA adducts, or can react directly with cell structures to cause cell damage. Adduct formation can lead to adverse conditions including disruption in protein function, excess formation of fibrous connective tissue (fibrogenesis), and activation of immune responses.[28] The identity of proteins modified by xenobiotics can be found in the resource known as the *reactive metabolite target protein database*.[29] The body has two major defense systems for counteracting these effects: (1) detoxification enzymes and their cofactors and (2) antioxidant systems. Phases of detoxification include Phase I enzymes, such as cytochrome P-450 (CYP) oxidases, which are the most important oxidative reactions (see Fig. 2.16, *B*). Other Phase I detoxification enzymes include those for reduction and hydrolysis. In Phase II detoxification, conjugation enzymes, such as glutathione (GSH), detoxify reactive electrophiles and produce polar metabolites that cannot diffuse across membranes. Most conjugation enzymes are located in the cytosol. Phase III detoxification

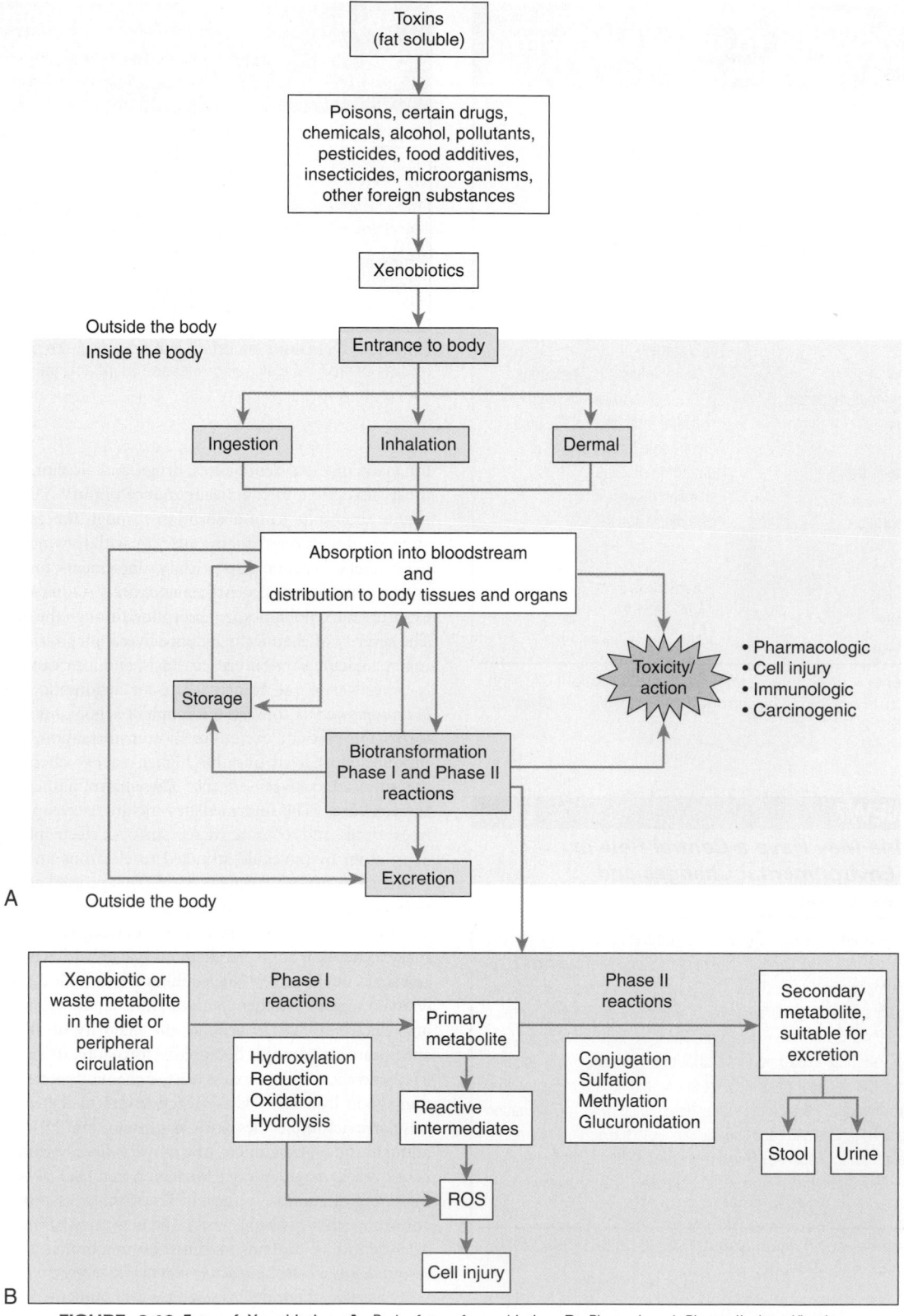

FIGURE 2.16 Fate of Xenobiotics. A, Body fate of xenobiotics. **B,** Phase I and Phase II detoxification reactions.

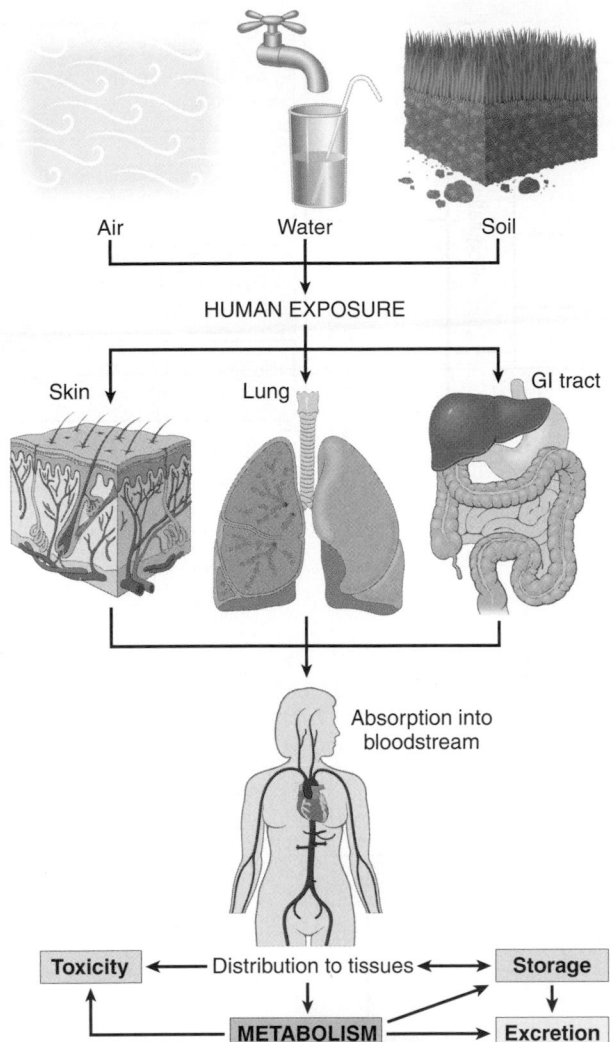

Air   **Water**   **Soil**

HUMAN EXPOSURE

Skin   **Lung**   **GI tract**

Absorption into
bloodstream

Toxicity ← Distribution to tissues ⇄ **Storage**

METABOLISM → **Excretion**

FIGURE 2.17 Human Exposure to Pollutants. Pollutants contained in air, water, and soil are absorbed through the lungs, gastrointestinal (GI) tract, and skin. In the body they may act at the site of absorption but are generally transported through the bloodstream to various organs where they can be stored or metabolized. Metabolism of xenobiotics may result in the formation of water-soluble compounds that are excreted, or a toxic metabolite may be created by activation of the agent. (From Kumar V, Abbas A, Aster J: *Robbins & Cotran pathologic basis of disease*, ed 9, Philadelphia, 2015, Saunders.)

is often called the *efflux transporter system* because enzymes remove the parent drugs, metabolites, and xenobiotics from cells. The liver has the highest supply of biotransformation enzymes of all organs and, therefore, has the key role in protection from chemical toxicity.[28] Fig. 2.18 is a summary of chemically induced liver injury.

Chemical injury begins with a biochemical interaction between a toxic substance and the cell's plasma membrane, which is ultimately damaged, leading to increased permeability. Not all the mechanisms causing chemically induced membrane destruction are known; however, the two general mechanisms include (1) *direct toxicity* by combining with a molecular component of the cell membrane or organelles and (2) *conversion to toxic intermediates or metabolites*, such as reactive free radicals and membrane lipid peroxidation. Lipid peroxidation is the oxidative degradation of lipids. In this process free radicals "steal" electrons from the lipids in cell membranes resulting in cell damage.

Chemical Agents Including Drugs

Numerous chemical agents cause cellular injury. Minute amounts of some, such as arsenic and cyanide, can rapidly destroy enough cells to cause death of the individual. Long-term exposure to air pollutants, insecticides, and herbicides can cause cellular injury (see Fig. 2.17). Carbon monoxide, carbon tetrachloride, and social drugs, such as alcohol, can significantly alter cellular function and injure cellular structures. Over-the-counter and prescribed drugs can cause cellular injury, sometimes leading to death. The abuse of and addiction to opioids, such as heroin, morphine, and prescription pain relievers, is a serious global problem that affects the health, social, and economic welfare of all societies.[30] It is estimated that between 26.4 million and 36 million people abuse opioids worldwide.[31] In 2012, it was estimated that 2.1 million people in the United States suffer from substance use disorders related to prescription opioid pain relievers, and an estimated 467,000 people were addicted to heroin.[32] The leading cause of child poisoning is medications. Acetaminophen (known as *paracetamol* outside the United States), commonly used as an analgesic, is one of the most common causes of poisoning worldwide. Drug-induced acute liver failure accounts for about 20% of liver failure in children and a higher percentage in adults.[33]

The use of some plants and the consumption of different fruits have played basic roles in human health care, and diverse scientific investigations have indicated that beneficial effects can be attributed to the presence of chemical compounds called *phytochemicals*. Examples of natural products being investigated include some fruits (grapefruit, cranberries, schisandra, and grapes) and plants (cactus pear [nopal] and cactus pear fruit, chamomile, silymarin, and spirulina), resin (propolis), carrot, eleuthero root (Siberian ginseng), ginger root, ginkgo leaf, grape seed/skin, kudzu root, milk thistle seed (silymarin), rosemary leaf, and turmeric.[34,35] Accidental or suicidal poisonings by chemical agents cause numerous deaths. The injurious effects of some of these agents—lead, carbon monoxide, ethyl alcohol, and mercury—exemplify common cellular injuries.

Air Pollution

The world's largest single environmental health risk is air pollution.[36] Household air pollution and ambient air pollution were responsible for 5.5 million deaths worldwide in 2013 (Fig. 2.19). From WHO data, every year 4.3 million deaths occur from exposure to indoor air pollution and 3.7 million deaths to outdoor air pollution.[36] **Air pollution** is contamination of the indoor or outdoor environment by any chemical, physical, or biologic agent that modifies natural characteristics of the atmosphere.[36] Indoor air pollution (household) occurs when people cook and heat their homes using solid fuels (i.e., wood, charcoal, coal, dung, crop wastes) on open fires or traditional stoves. These inefficient practices produce high levels of household air pollution with fine particles and carbon monoxide.[36] In poorly ventilated houses, smoke in and around the house can greatly exceed acceptable levels for fine particles. These exposures are particularly high for women and young children.

By reducing air pollution levels, countries can lower the burden of disease from stroke, heart disease, lung cancer, and chronic and acute respiratory diseases, including asthma.[36] As a leading cause of morbidity and mortality worldwide, several studies have found that long-term particulate matter air pollution exposure is associated with cardiovascular disease (CVD) morbidity and mortality.[37,38] About 88% of premature deaths occurred in low- and middle-income countries; the greatest numbers occur in the WHO Western Pacific and South-East Asia regions. Reducing outdoor emissions from household coal and biomass energy systems, agricultural waste incineration, forest fires, and certain agroforestry activities (e.g., charcoal production) would reduce key rural and peri-urban air pollution sources in developing regions.[36] Reducing

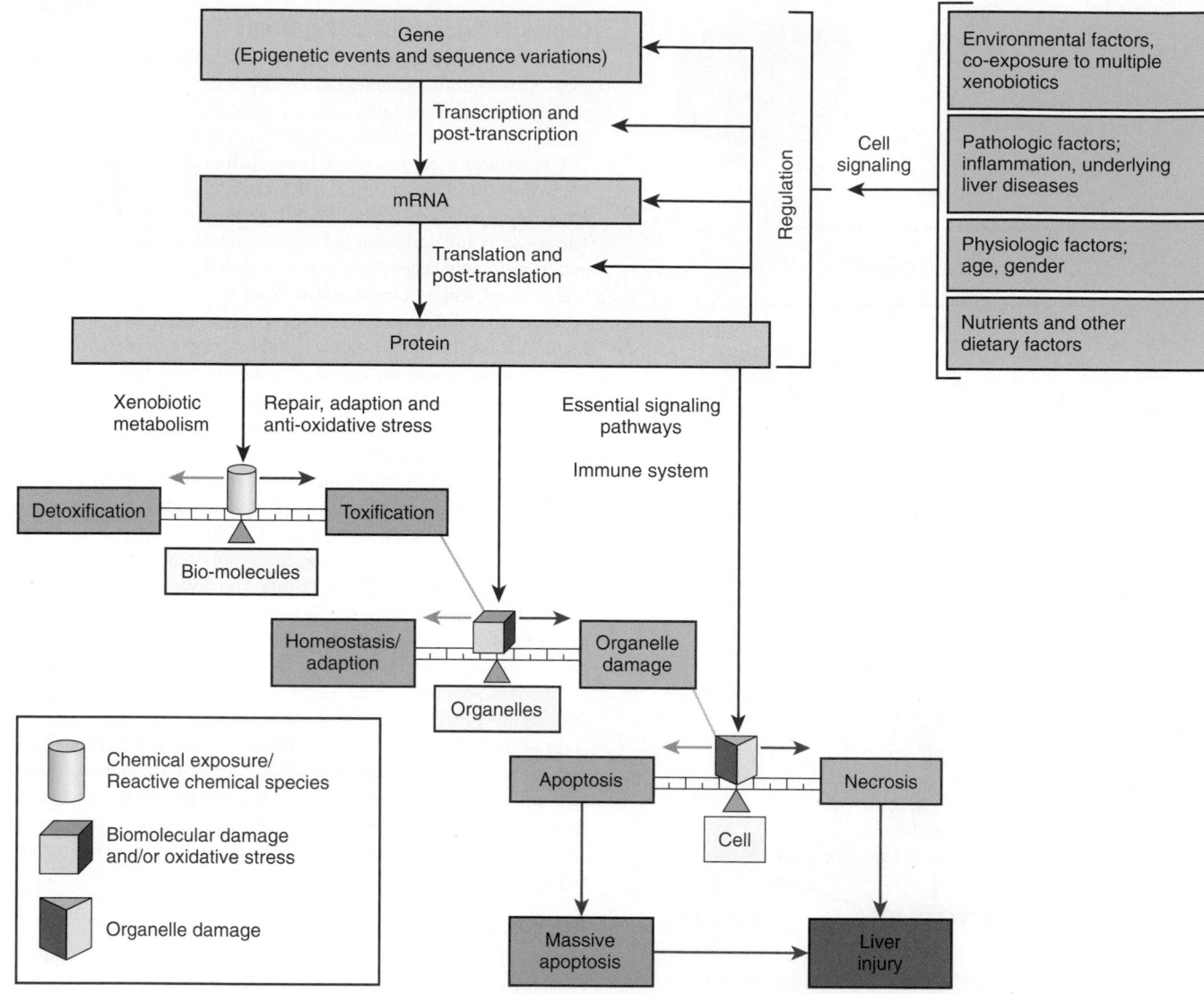

FIGURE 2.18 Chemical Liver Injury. Liver injury is a result of genetic, environmental, biologic, and dietary factors. Certain chemicals can form toxic or chemically reactive metabolites. The risk of liver injury also can increase with increasing doses of a toxicant. Xenobiotic enzyme induction can lead to altered metabolism of chemicals, and drugs can either inhibit or induce drug-metabolizing enzymes. These changes can lead to greater toxicity. The dose at the site of action is controlled by the Phase I to III xenobiotic metabolites, and metabolizing enzymes are encoded by numerous different genes. Therefore, the metabolism and toxicity outcomes can vary greatly among individuals. Additionally, all aspects of xenobiotic metabolism are regulated by certain transcription factors (cellular mediators of gene regulation). Overall, the extent of cell damage depends on the balance between reactive chemical species and protective responses aimed at decreasing oxidative stress, repairing macromolecular damage, or preserving cell health by inducing apoptosis or cell death. Significant clinical outcomes of chemical-induced liver injury occur with necrosis and the immune response. Covalent binding of reactive metabolites to cellular proteins can produce new antigens (haptens) that initiate autoantibody production and cytotoxic T-cell responses. Necrosis, a form of cell death, can result from extensive damage to the plasma membrane with altered ion transport, changes of membrane potential, cell swelling, and eventual dissolution. Altogether the pathogenesis of chemically induced liver injury is determined by genetics, environmental factors, and other underlying pathologic conditions. Green arrows are pathways leading to cell recovery; red arrows indicate pathways to cell damage or death; black arrows are pathways leading to chemically induced liver injury. (Adapted from Gu X, Manautou JE: *Exp Rev Mol Med* 14:e4, 2013.)

outdoor air pollution decreases emissions of CO_2 and short-lived climate pollutants, for example, black carbon particles and methane. These actions would contribute to mitigating climate change.

Various types of studies all support the finding that prompt and sustained health benefits can come from improved air quality.[39] The Environmental Protection Agency (EPA) has identified the following six pollutants as "criteria" air pollutants: carbon monoxide, lead, nitrogen oxides, photochemical oxidants, ground-level ozone particle pollution known as *particulate matter*, and sulfur oxides.[40] Table 2.5 defines each of the criteria pollutants.

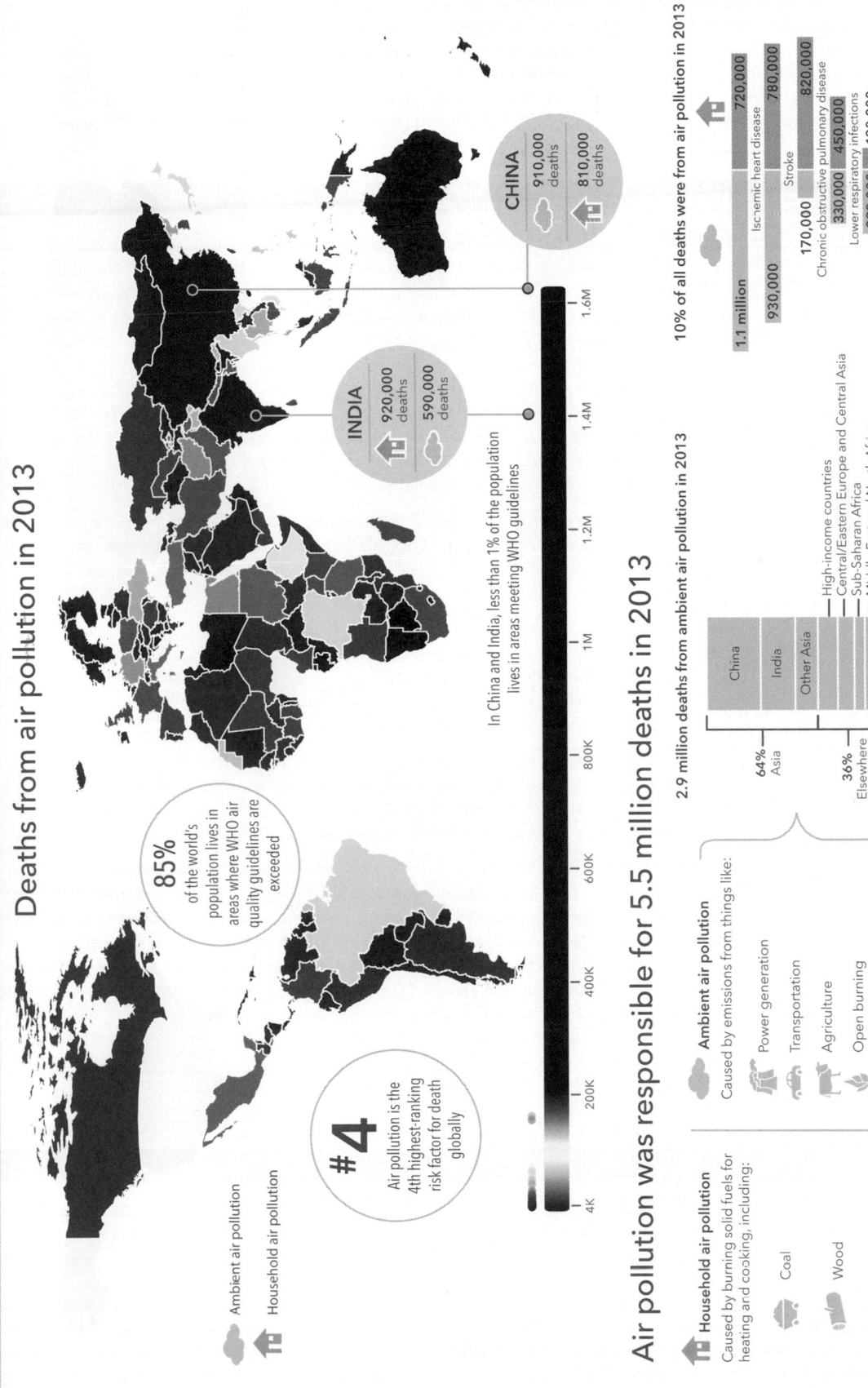

FIGURE 2.19 Global Burden of Air Pollution. (From Brauer M et al: *Environ Sci Technol* 50[1]:79–88, 2016; Forouzanfar MH et al: *Lancet* 386[10010]:2287–2323, 2015.)

Heavy Metals as Environmental Pollutants

Heavy metals most commonly associated with harmful effects in humans include lead, mercury, arsenic, and cadmium. Investigators are studying the involvement of metals in DNA repair mechanisms, tumor suppressor functions, and interference with signal transduction pathways.

Lead. Lead (Pb) is a heavy toxic metal ubiquitous in older homes (built before 1978), the environment, and the workplace. Lead may be found in hazardous concentrations in food, water, and air and it is one of the most common overexposures found in industry.[41] Despite efforts to reduce exposure through government regulation, lead exposure still persists in homes, the environment, and the workplace for many people, and lead toxicity is still a primary hazard to children (see *What's New?* CDC Update: Primary Prevention of Lead Exposures for Children).

Although Pb was removed from paint in the United States in 1978, many homes in the United States still contain leaded paint, and chipped

TABLE 2.5	EPA CRITERIA OF AIR POLLUTANTS
POLLUTANT	CRITERIA
Carbon monoxide (CO)	Colorless, odorless gas emitted from combustion processes. Although the majority of CO emissions come from mobile sources, those who (1) breathe air polluted by gasoline engines or defective furnaces and appliances; (2) work in occupations such as coal mining, firefighting, welding, or engine repair; and (3) smoke cigarettes, cigars, or pipes are at risk for CO exposure. At highest risk for CO poisoning are unborn babies, infants, and people with chronic heart disease, respiratory disease, and anemia. Harm from CO is from reduction of oxygen delivery to organs, such as the heart and brain, and at very high levels can cause death. CO can reduce the oxygen-carrying capacity of the blood. Minute amounts of CO can produce significant percentages of **carboxyhemoglobin** (carbon monoxide bound with hemoglobin [COHb]). Other mechanisms may include disruption of cellular oxidative processes, binding to myoglobin and hepatic cytochromes, and lipid peroxidation of brain lipids. Individuals with several types of heart disease are at increased risk for the effects of CO and can cause them to have ischemia and angina when exercising or under increased stress.
Particle pollution/particulate matter (PM)	PM is a complex mixture of extremely small particles and liquid droplets that get into the air. Inhalation of these particles can affect the heart and lungs and cause serious health effects. Particles less than 10 micrometers in diameter pose the greatest health problems. Fine particles ($PM_{2.5}$) are the main cause of haze or reduced visibility. Most particles form in the atmosphere as a result of reactions of chemicals from power plants, industries, and automobiles.
Ozone	Ground-level ozone is not emitted directly into the air but is created by chemical reactions between oxides of nitrogen (NOX) and volatile organic compounds (VOCs) in the presence of sunlight. The main sources of NOX and VOC are from emissions from industrial facilities and electrical utilities, motor vehicle exhaust, gasoline vapors, and chemical solvents. Breathing ozone can trigger a variety of health effects, particularly for children, the elderly, and people with lung diseases, such as asthma. Ground-level ozone can have harmful effects on vegetation and ecosystems.
Sulfur dioxide (SO_2)	SO_2 is one of a group of gases called *sulfur oxides* (SOx). All of the group of gases are harmful but most important is SO_2. Short-term exposure to SO_2 can cause respiratory system dysfunction and difficulty breathing. Children, the elderly, and those who suffer from asthma are most sensitive. High concentration of SO_2 can lead to SOx that can form small particles. These particles can contribute to PM pollution, harm trees and plants, and may penetrate deep in the lungs, causing additional health concerns.
Nitrogen dioxide (NO_2)	NO_2 is one of a group of highly reactive gases known as *nitrogen oxides* (NOX). NOX forms quickly from emissions from cars, trucks and buses, power plants, and off-road equipment. In addition to forming ground-level ozone, NO_2 is linked with several adverse respiratory effects, including airway inflammation. NOX can react with ammonia and other compounds to form small particles. These particles can penetrate deeply in the lungs and worsen respiratory tract diseases, such as emphysema and bronchitis, aggravate existing heart disease, and lead to hospital admissions and premature death. Those at greatest risk from ozone are individuals who work or exercise outside.
Lead	See text on p. 64.

From U.S. Environmental Protection Agency: *EPA criteria air pollutants,* Washington, DC, 2016, Author.

WHAT'S NEW?

CDC Update: Primary Prevention of Lead Exposures for Children

In 2012, the CDC updated recommendations on children's blood lead levels. The shift is to focus on primary prevention of lead exposure to reduce or eliminate dangerous and toxic sources in children's environments. At least 4 million households have children living in them where they are being exposed to high levels of lead. Experts now use a reference level of 5 micrograms per deciliter to identify children with blood lead levels that are much higher than most children's levels. (This new level is based on the U.S. population of children ages 1 to 5 years who are in the highest percentile [2.5% of children] when tested for lead.)

The CDC will update the reference value every 4 years using the most recent National Health and Nutrition Examination Survey (NHANES) based on the 97.5th percentage of blood lead distribution in children.

Still the same is the recommendation when medical treatment is advised for children with high blood lead levels. Chelation therapy is recommended when a child has a blood lead test result greater than or equal to 45 micrograms per deciliter.

Prevent Childhood Lead Poisoning

Exposure to lead can seriously harm a child's health.

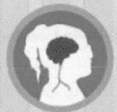
Damage to the brain and nervous system

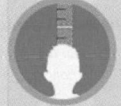
Slowed growth and development

Learning and behavior problems

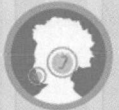
Hearing and speech problems

This can cause:

- Lower IQ
- Decreased ability to pay attention
- Underperformance at school

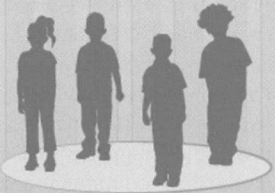

Lead can be found throughout a child's environment.

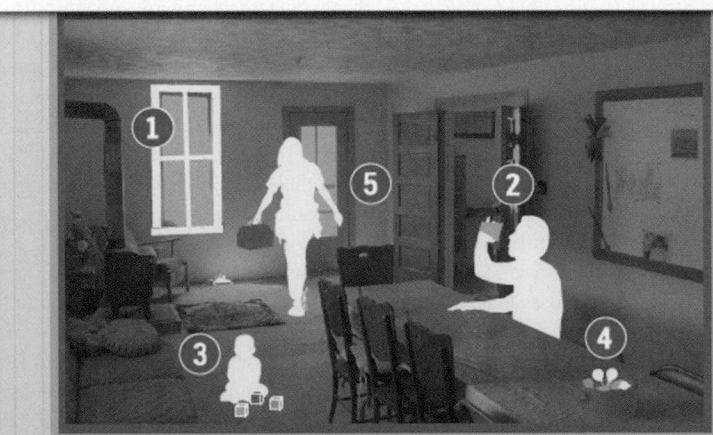

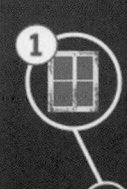
1 Homes built before 1978 (when lead-based paints were banned) probably contain lead-based paint.

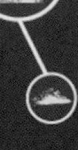
When the paint peels and cracks, it makes lead dust. Children can be poisoned when they swallow or breathe in lead dust.

2 Certain water pipes may contain lead.

3 Lead can be found in some products such as toys and toy jewelry.

4 Lead is sometimes in candies imported from other countries or traditional home remedies.

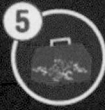
5 Certain jobs and hobbies involve working with lead-based products, like stain glass work, and may cause parents to bring lead into the home.

Data from Centers for Disease Control and Prevention (CDC): *Lead*, Atlanta, GA, 2017, Centers for Disease Control and Prevention, U. S. Department of Health and Human Services, updated February 9, 2017; Centers for Disease Control and Prevention (CDC): *Lead: what do parent's need to know to protect their children?* Atlanta, GA, Author, updated March 15, 2016.

and peeling leaded paint constitutes a major source of current childhood exposure.[42,43] The chipped paint can disintegrate at friction surfaces to form Pb dust.[43] Another source of contamination is Pb dust dispersed along roadways from previous leaded gasoline emissions.[43] When Pb was removed from gasoline, blood lead levels (BLLs) dropped significantly.[44] Previous emissions of leaded fuel created large dispersions of lead dust in the environment. Particulate lead (2 to 10 μm) does not degrade and persists in the environment, making it a notable source of human exposure.[45] Other airborne sources include smelters and piston-engine airplanes.[46] Drinking water exposed to Pb occurs from outdated fixtures, plumbing without corrosion control, and solders.[43] Because well water is not subject to EPA regulation it may not be tested for Pb.[43] Although the average blood levels of Pb in children in the United States have dropped since the 1970s, there are at-risk populations with higher than average BLLs.[43] Children living at or below the poverty line who live in older housing are at greatest risk.[42] Importantly, the Centers for Disease Control and Prevention (CDC) reports "no safe blood lead level in children has been identified."[42] Millions of children are being exposed to lead in their homes, increasing their risks for damage to the brain and nervous system, slowed growth and development, learning and behavior problems (e.g., reduced IQ, attention-deficit/hyperactivity disorder [ADHD], juvenile delinquency, and criminal behavior), and hearing and speech problems.[42] Common sources of Pb are included in Table 2.6.

Lead exposure also remains an important safety and health concern worldwide. Problematic is lead exposure to the fetus during pregnancy because the developing nervous system is especially vulnerable. Compared to adults, developing fetuses and young children absorb lead more easily; the higher intestinal absorption and more permeable blood-brain barrier of children create a high susceptibility to brain damage.[1] Occupational exposure is a common cause of lead poisoning in adults. Approximately 95% of all elevated blood lead levels (BLLs) reported among adults in the United States are work related.[47,48] Industries with the highest number of lead-exposed workers are battery manufacturing, lead and zinc mining, ammunition, and construction and manufacturing. The most common nonoccupational exposures of lead are shooting firearms, remodeling buildings, renovating, painting, possessing retained bullets in the body (gunshot wounds, especially retained bullet in joints), and lead casting.[48]

The organ systems most affected by lead include the nervous, hematopoietic, reproductive, gastrointestinal, cardiovascular, and musculoskeletal systems as well as the kidneys. Exposure occurs through inhalation, ingestion, and uncommonly skin contact. Lead is taken in through direct contact with the mouth, nose, and eyes (i.e., mucous membranes); and through cuts in the skin. Tetraethyl lead, still used in aviation fuel, can pass through skin; but inorganic lead, found in the most common sources of paint, food, and consumer products, is only minimally absorbable through skin.[49,50] Absorption of inorganic lead is primarily from ingestion and inhalation.[49] Most of the absorbed lead (80% to 85%) is incorporated into bone and teeth where it competes with calcium; the half-life in bone is 20 to 30 years.[1] Lead can move from bone to the bloodstream years after the initial exposure.[50] Children store about 70% of absorbed lead in their bones and teeth; thus, other tissues in children are more greatly affected compared to adults.[51] Lead can be reintroduced continuously to the blood from bone remodeling.[51] Other tissues can store lead, including the brain, spleen, kidneys, liver, and lungs; however, not at the levels found in blood, bone, and teeth.[52]

◆PATHOPHYSIOLOGY. The pathogenic effects of lead are multifactorial and complex. The key event underlying effects of Pb exposure in humans is alteration of cellular ion status (disruption of divalent cations, altered ion transport mechanisms, and disruption of protein function from displacement of metal enzyme cofactors) (Fig. 2.20).

An important ion status disruption is calcium (Ca^{++}) homeostasis. Ca^{++} is a crucial cell signal carrier and regulates critical cellular functions.[53] Pb exposure alters the intracellular concentration of Ca^{++} in many cell types, including bone, brain, and red and white blood cells. The change in intracellular Ca^{++} concentrations is probably from alterations in ion transport mechanisms and, importantly, the inhibition of transport proteins such as Na^+-K^+ ATPase and Ca^{++} channels. Pb interferes with these proteins by displacing or competing with normal metal cofactors (e.g., lead binds to calcium-activated proteins with higher affinity than calcium) or through proteins important in Ca^{++}-dependent cell signaling (protein kinase C or calmodulin).[53] Pb disrupts other divalent metals, including zinc and magnesium, leading to alterations in neurotransmitter function, inhibiting heme synthesis, and, from impaired mitochondrial function, decreasing cellular energy. Lead is toxic to multiple enzyme systems. Pb causes abnormal conformational changes in the protein structure resulting in altered protein functions. Antagonism of normal metal ion functions by Pb leads to oxidative stress.[53] Pb-induced oxidative stress is possibly the result of a mutipathway process. Pb-induced oxidative stress results from binding to and subsequently inhibition of the function of delta aminolevulinic acid dehydratase (ALAD) because of competition

TABLE 2.6	COMMON SOURCES OF LEAD
EXPOSURE	**SOURCE**
Environmental	Lead paint, soil, or dust near roadways or lead-painted homes; plastic window blinds; plumbing materials (from pipes or solder); pottery glazes and ceramic ware; lead-core candle wicks; leaded gasoline; water (pipes)
Occupational	Lead mining and refining, plumbing and pipe fitting, auto repair, glass manufacturing, battery manufacturing and recycling, printing shop, construction work, plastic manufacturing, gas station attendant, firing-range attendant
Hobbies	Glazed pottery making, target shooting at firing ranges, lead soldering, preparing fishing sinkers, stained-glass making, painting, car or boat repair
Other	Gasoline sniffing, costume jewelry, cosmetics, contaminated herbal products

Data from Sanborn MD et al: *CMAJ* 166(10):1287–1292, 2002.

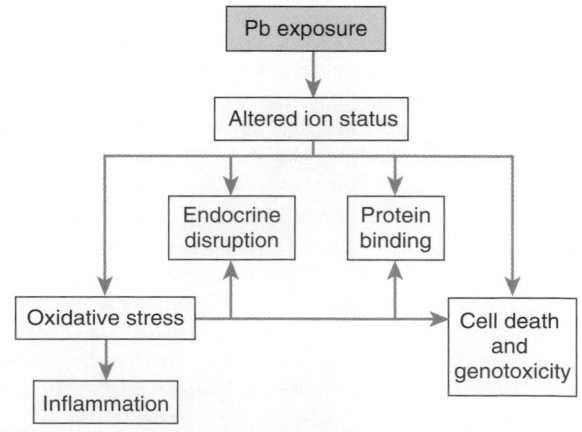

FIGURE 2.20 Key Pathophysiologic Events of Lead Exposure. See text for a discussion of these events and health effects. (Data from Lassiter MG et al: *Toxicology* 330:19–40, 2015.)

TABLE 2.7   SUMMARY OF TOXIC EFFECTS OF CADMIUM AND ARSENIC

METALS	KEY CONCEPTS
Arsenic	Arsenic salts were the poison of choice during the Renaissance in Italy
	Deliberate poisoning by arsenic is rare today; however, its exposure is an important health concern in many areas worldwide
	Arsenic is found naturally in soils and water and used in products (wood preservers, herbicides, agricultural products)
	It can be released from mines and smelting industries and may be present in some Chinese and Indian herbal medicines
	Inorganic arsenic may be present in ground water with large concentrations found in Bangladesh, Chile, and China
	Most toxic forms are the trivalent compounds of arsenic trioxide, sodium arsenite, and arsenic trichloride
	Arsenic trioxide is used as a therapy for acute promyelocytic leukemia; ingestion of large quantities of arsenic causes acute gastrointestinal, cardiovascular, and CNS toxicities that often are fatal
	These effects are partially attributed to replacement of phosphates in ATP and interference of mitochondrial oxidative phosphorylation and the function of some proteins
	Chronic exposure causes skin lesions (hyperpigmentation, hyperkeratosis) and the development of cancers (lung, bladder, skin)
	The mechanism for arsenic carcinogenesis has not been fully defined
	Arsenic present in drinking water has been correlated with nonmalignant respiratory disease
Cadmium	Compared to the other metals discussed, cadmium is a more modern problem
	Pollution in the environment and occupationally is from mining, electroplating, and production of nickel-cadmium batteries, which are often disposed in household waste
	Food is an important source of cadmium because cadmium can contaminate soil and plants directly or from fertilizers and irrigation water
	The most probable mechanism of toxicity is the generation of ROS
	The main toxic effects of excess cadmium are obstructive lung disease and renal tubular damage
	It also can cause skeletal abnormalities associated with calcium loss
	In Japan, cadmium-containing water used to irrigate rice fields caused a disease in postmenopausal women known as "Itai-Itai" (ouch-ouch), which is a combination of osteoporosis and osteomalacia associated with renal disease
	Cadmium is associated with higher risk of lung cancer in populations living near zinc smelters

ATP, adenosine triphosphate; *CNS,* central nervous system; *ROS,* reactive oxygen species.
Data from Kumar V, Abbas A, Aster J: *Robbins & Cotran pathologic basis of disease,* ed 9, Philadelphia, 2015, Saunders.

of Pb ions with normal zinc ions leading to the accumulation of delta-aminolevulinic acid (δ-ALA) in blood and urine. With accumulation of δ-ALA, it undergoes conformational protein change and autooxidation resulting in the generation of ROS.[53] Other sources of Pb-induced oxidative stress are membrane lipid oxidation, NADPH oxidation, and antioxidant depletion.[53] Both abnormalities of cellular ion status and oxidative stress can result in altered inflammation, endocrine disruption, cell death (apoptosis), protein binding, and genotoxicity.[53] These *key* events from Pb exposure affect the nervous system, immune system, and reproductive system and have developmental effects, for example, delayed puberty onset, as well as cancer. A causal relationship is determined for Pb and cardiovascular effects and an association between Pb and renal dysfunction.[53]

◆CLINICAL MANIFESTATIONS. Lead affects all body systems and especially the nervous, cardiovascular, reproductive, endocrine, musculoskeletal, and immune systems, as well as the kidneys and teeth. The recent National Toxicology Program (NTP) has provided the *NTP Monograph: Health Effects of Low-Level Lead* (see Table E 2.1 on Evolve).[54]

◆EVALUATION, PREVENTION, AND TREATMENT. Diagnosis involves the medical history and clinical signs and determination of routes of exposure. The main method of evaluation is laboratory analysis of the blood lead level (BLL). According to the CDC, experts now use a reference level of 5 micrograms per deciliter to identify children with blood lead levels that are much higher than most children's levels.[47]

The most important strategy for lowering exposures to lead is prevention. Prevention methods include individual and family prevention, preventive medicine, and public health. There is an urgent need to focus on preventive strategies, especially for fetal development and the developing child. The key for adults is prevention of exposures at the workplace and home. The main methods of treatment are removal of the source of exposure and, for those with high blood levels, chelation

therapy. Additionally, treatment may include correcting deficiencies of iron, calcium, and zinc; irrigating the bowel; removing strategic bullets or shrapnel; and administering medications for control of seizures.

Cadmium and arsenic. Table 2.7 summarizes toxic effects of cadmium and arsenic.

Mercury. Mercury (quicksilver) is a heavy, silvery white metal that is liquid at room temperature and evaporates easily.[55] Mercury is a global threat to human and environmental health. In nature, mercury is found in the form of cinnabar, a deep red mineral used in the past as a pigment. Cinnabar deposits have been mined for centuries. Mercury also occurs in deposits of other metals, such as lead and zinc, and it is found in small amounts in different rocks including coal and limestone where no cinnabar is found. Mercury can be released into the air, water, and soil through industrial processes including mining, metal and cement production, fuel extraction, and combustions of fossil fuels.[55] Causes from human activity, called anthropogenic, are responsible for about 30% of annual emissions of mercury to air, another 10% from natural geological sources, and the rest (60%) from re-emissions or earlier released mercury that has increased over decades and centuries in surface soil and water.[55] The major sources of anthropogenic mercury emissions to air are artisanal and small-scale gold mining (ASGM) and coal burning. The next major sources are the production of ferrous and nonferrous metals and cement production. Importantly, investigators report that emissions from industrial sectors have increased since 2005.[56] Types of aquatic releases of mercury include industrial sites (power plants, factories), old mines, landfills, and waste disposal locations. Artisanal and small-scale gold mining is significant for aquatic releases. It is estimated that more than 90% of mercury in marine animals is from anthropogenic emissions.[55] Climate change, with thawing of enormous areas of frozen lands, may release even more long-stored mercury and organic matter into lakes, rivers, and oceans.[55]

Mercury is still commonplace in daily life. Consumables used around the world contain mercury, including electrical and electronic devices, switches (including thermostats) and relays, measuring and control equipment, energy-efficient fluorescent light bulbs, batteries, mascara, skin-lightening creams and other cosmetics, and dental amalgams.[55,56] Mercury is found in food products obtained from fish, terrestrial mammals, and other products, such as rice. It is still widely used in healthcare equipment, where much of it is used for measuring in blood pressure devices and thermometers, although their use is declining.[55,56] There are safe and cost-effective replacements for mercury for many healthcare applications and for pharmaceuticals; goals have been set to phase out some mercury-containing devices altogether. Since 2001, no vaccine contains thimerosal (a preservative in multidose vials of vaccines containing ethyl mercury) except inactivated influenza vaccines.

There are three forms of mercury: metallic mercury (elemental mercury), inorganic mercury compounds (mostly mercuric chloride), and organic mercury. A major source of mercury is contaminated fish (mostly methylmercury). Inorganic mercury is converted to organic mercury, such as methylmercury, by bacteria. Methylmercury enters the food chain and, in carnivorous fish (especially swordfish and shark), it may be concentrated to exorbitant levels higher than the surrounding water.[1] Acute exposures from release of methylmercury from industrial sources caused the disaster at Minamata Bay and the Agano River in Japan and led to widespread mortality and morbidity. Known as *Minamata disease,* the disorders included deafness, blindness, intellectual disability, cerebral palsy, and central nervous system (CNS) defects in children exposed in utero. For unclear mechanisms, the developing brain is extremely sensitive to methylmercury.[1] Mercury is found in many species of fish, including grouper, tuna, seabass, marlin, halibut, tilefish, swordfish, shark, and king mackerel.[56] The U.S. Food and Drug Administration (FDA) has recommended that women planning to become pregnant, pregnant women, nursing mothers, and young children avoid eating fish with a high mercury content (>1 part per million [ppm]), such as shark, swordfish, tile fish, and king mackerel. Fish that is lower in methylmercury include shrimp, canned light tuna, salmon, pollock, and catfish.[57] Like Pb, mercury binds with high affinity to sulfhydryl groups in some proteins, leading to tissue damage in the CNS and kidney.[1] Lipid solubility of methylmercury and metallic mercury increases their accumulation in the brain, altering neuromotor, cognitive, and behavioral functions.[1] An antioxidant, intracellular glutathione acting as a sulfhydryl donor, is the main protective mechanism from mercury-induced CNS and kidney damage.

Ethanol

Alcohol *(ethanol)* is the number one mood-altering drug used in the United States. It is estimated there are more than 10 million chronic alcoholics in the United States. Alcohol contributes to more than 100,000 deaths annually with 50% of these deaths from drunk-driving accidents, alcohol-related homicides, and suicides.[1] A blood alcohol concentration of 80 mg/dL is the legal definition of drunk driving in the United States. This level of alcohol in an average person may be reached after consumption of three drinks (three 12-ounce bottles of beer, 15 ounces of wine, and 4 to 5 ounces of distilled liquor). The effects of alcohol vary by age, gender, and percentage body fat; the rate of metabolism affects the blood alcohol level. Importantly, alcohol-related problems include family violence and workplace disabilities. Because alcohol is not only a psychoactive drug but also a food, it is considered part of the basic food supply in many societies.

A large intake of alcohol has enormous effects on nutritional status. Liver and nutritional disorders are the most serious consequences of alcohol abuse. Major nutritional deficiencies include magnesium, vitamin B$_6$, thiamine, and phosphorus. Chronic intake of alcohol and vitamin deficiencies may adversely affect the brain and peripheral nerves (e.g., Wernicke encephalopathy, peripheral neuropathy, Korsakoff psychosis). Folic acid deficiency is a common problem in chronic alcoholic populations. Ethanol alters folic acid (folate) homeostasis by decreasing intestinal absorption of folate, increases liver retention of folate, and increases the loss of folate through urinary and fecal excretion.[33] Folic acid deficiency becomes especially serious in pregnant women who consume alcohol and may contribute to fetal alcohol syndrome.

Most of the alcohol in blood is metabolized to *acetaldehyde* in the liver by three enzyme systems: alcohol dehydrogenase (ADH), the microsomal ethanol-oxidizing system (MEOS; CYP2E1), and catalase (Fig. 2.21). The major pathway involves ADH, an enzyme located in the cytosol of hepatocytes. The microsomal ethanol-oxidizing system (MEOS) depends on cytochrome P-450 (CYP2E1), an enzyme needed for cellular oxidation. Activation of CYP2E1 requires a high ethanol concentration and thus is thought to be important in the accelerated ethanol metabolism (i.e., tolerance) noted in persons with chronic alcoholism. Acetaldehyde has many toxic tissue effects and is responsible for some of the acute effects of alcohol and for development of oral cancers.[58] A recent study showed that head and neck cancer risk may be influenced by alcohol-metabolizing genes (*ADH1B* and *ALDH2*) and oral hygiene.[59,60] Polymorphisms on *ADH1B* and *ALDH2* had significant indirect effects on hepatocellular carcinoma risk.[61]

After ingestion, alcohol is absorbed, unaltered, into the stomach and small intestine from which it is transported to the liver. Fatty foods and milk slow absorption. Alcohol then is distributed to all tissues and fluids of the body in direct proportion to the blood concentration. Individuals differ in their capability to metabolize alcohol. The major effects of acute alcoholism involve the central nervous system (CNS; see below). Genetic differences in metabolism of liver alcohol, including aldehyde dehydrogenases, have been identified. People with chronic alcoholism develop certain levels of tolerance because of enzyme induction, leading to an increased rate of metabolism (e.g., P-450).

Numerous studies have validated the so-called *j-* or *u-shaped* inverse association between alcohol and cardiovascular mortality, such as from myocardial infarction and ischemic stroke. These studies have found that light to moderate (nonbinge) drinkers tend to have lower mortality than nondrinkers, and heavy drinkers have higher mortality.[62] For both men and women, former drinkers and regular heavy drinkers had higher mortality.[62] Light to moderate drinkers in the United States may have reduced mortality, but this may be confounded by medical care and social relationships, especially among women.[62,63] These relationships need further study. The suggested mechanisms for cardioprotection for light to moderate drinkers include increase in levels of high density lipoprotein–cholesterol (HDL-C; recent randomized studies and failure of HDL-C to modify cardiovascular disease have become controversial), decrease in levels of low-density lipoprotein (LDL), prevention of clot formation, reduction in platelet aggregation, decrease in blood pressure, increase in coronary vessel vasodilation, increase in coronary blood flow, decrease in coronary inflammation, decrease in atherosclerosis, a limit in ischemia-reperfusion injury (I/R injury), and a decrease in diabetic vessel pathology.[64] The American Heart Association recommends no more than two drinks per day for men and one drink per day for women (12 oz of beer, 4 oz of wine, 1.5 oz of 80-proof spirits, or 1 oz of 100-proof spirits).

Acute alcoholism (drunkenness) affects the CNS (Box 2.2). Alcohol intoxication causes CNS depression. Depending on the amount consumed, depression is associated with sedation, drowsiness, loss of motor coordination, delirium, altered behavior, and loss of consciousness. Toxic amounts (300 to 400 mg/dL) result in a lethal coma or possibly respiratory arrest because of medullary center depression. Studies are underway to determine the extent of the relationship between alcohol level and

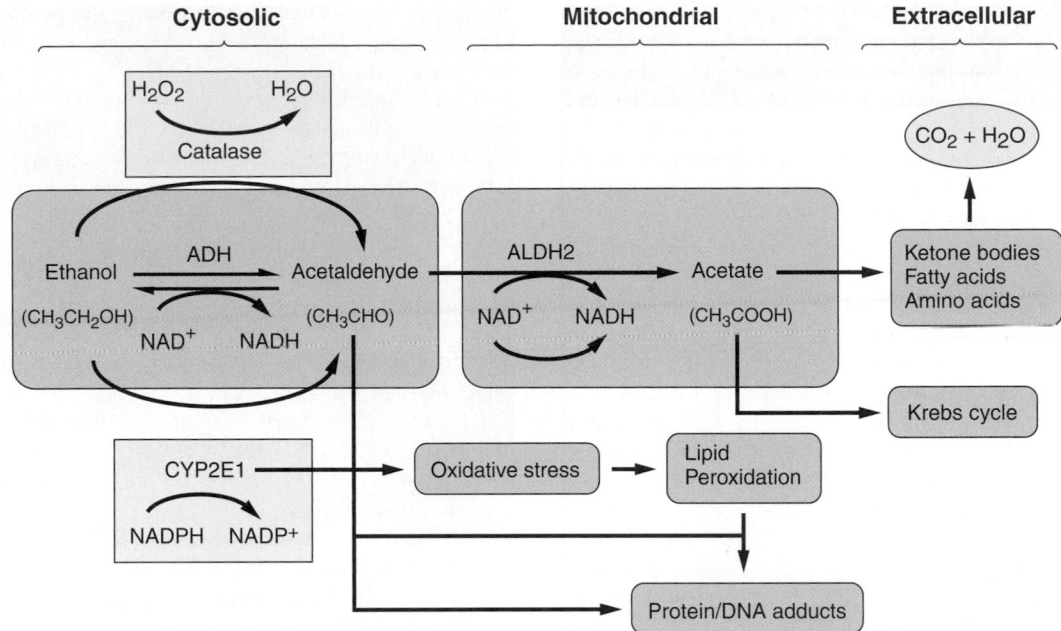

FIGURE 2.21 Ethanol Metabolism Pathway. Ethanol is metabolized into acetaldehyde through the cytosolic enzyme alcohol dehydrogenase (ADH), the microsomal enzyme cytochrome P-450 2E1 (CYP2E1), and the peroxisomal enzyme catalase. The ADH enzyme reaction is the main ethanol metabolic pathway involving an intermediate carrier of electrons, namely, nicotinamide adenine dinucleotide (NAD^+), which is reduced by two electrons to form NADH. Acetaldehyde is metabolized mainly by aldehyde dehydrogenase 2 (ALDH2) in the mitochondria to acetate and NADH before being cleared into the systemic circulation. (Adapted from Zhang Y, Ren J: *Pharmacol Ther* 132[1]:86–92, 2011.)

BOX 2.2   ALCOHOL: GLOBAL BURDEN, ADOLESCENT ONSET, CHRONIC OR BINGE DRINKING

Alcohol is widely consumed worldwide, and in the United States 50% of the adult population (18 years and older) consumes alcohol regularly. Alcohol continues to be the drug of choice among teens and young adults with one-third of twelfth graders and 40% of college students reporting "binge drinking" (four standard alcohol drinks on one occasion in females and five in males). Alcohol abuse is the leading cause of liver-related morbidity and mortality. Chronic and binge drinking causes alcoholic liver disease (ALD) with a spectrum from hepatic steatosis (fatty change) to steatohepatitis (fatty change and inflammation) and cirrhosis. These alterations can eventually lead to hepatocellular carcinoma. The pathogenesis of ALD is not fully characterized, and recent studies reveal a major role of mitochondrial involvement. Animal studies have shown that alcohol causes mitochondrial DNA damage, lipid accumulation, and oxidative stress. Understanding the role of the mitochondria may help identify therapeutic targets.

Investigation of adolescent drinking behaviors, especially binge drinking, is providing evidence of neurocognitive changes, including changes in both gray and white matter. These studies are examining risk-taking behaviors that begin in adolescence and coincide with vulnerable and significant neurodevelopmental changes.

Data from Adams PF et al: *Vital Health Stat* 10(255), 2012; available from www.cdc.gov/nchs/data/series/sr_10/sr10_255.pdf; Hicks BM et al: *Addiction* 107:540–548, 2012; Johnston LD et al: *Monitoring the future national results on adolescent drug use: overview of key findings,* Bethesda, MD, 2009, National Institute on Drug Abuse; Lisdahl KM et al: *Front Psychiatry* 4:53, 2013; Mathews S et al: *Am J Physiol Gastrointest Liver Physiol* 306(10):G819–G823, 2014; Nassir F, Ibdah JA: *World J Gastroenterol* 20(9):2136–2142, 2014; White HR et al: *Alcohol Clin Exp Res* 35:295–303, 2010.

snoring and obstructive sleep apnea (cessation of breathing). Acute alcoholism may induce reversible hepatic and gastric changes.[1] Acetaldehyde has many toxic effects from alcohol oxidation, including the acute effects of alcohol and the development of oral cancers.[1]

Chronic alcoholism causes structural alterations in practically all organs and tissues in the body because most tissues contain enzymes capable of ethanol oxidation or nonoxidative metabolism. The most significant activity occurs in the liver, and alcohol is the leading cause of liver-related morbidity and mortality. Hepatic changes initiated by acetaldehyde include inflammation, deposition of fat, enlargement of the liver, interruption of microtubular transport of proteins and their secretion, increase in intracellular water, decrease in fatty acid oxidation in the mitochondria, increase in membrane rigidity, and development of acute liver necrosis. Chronic or binge alcohol consumption causes alcoholic liver disease (ALD) with a range of alterations from simple fatty liver (steatosis), to steatohepatitis (fatty with inflammation), to cirrhosis. Cirrhosis is associated with portal hypertension and increased risk for hepatocellular carcinoma. A newer hypothesis for the development of ALD is adipose tissue dysfunction, including cell death, inflammation, and insulin resistance.[65] Inflammation plays a crucial role in ALD, and ethanol is implicated in the onset of a variety of immune defects, including the production of cytokines involved in the inflammatory responses.[66] Reactive oxygen and nitrogen species (ROS/RNS) and dysregulated redox signaling pathways are associated with alcohol consumption and provide insight into the molecular basis of hepatic cell dysfunction, destruction, and remodeled tissue or fibrosis.[65,67] Alcohol can induce epigenetic variations in the developmental pathways of many types of immune cells that promote increased inflammation.[68] Chronic alcoholism is a major risk factor for cancers of the oral cavity, larynx, and esophagus. The risk is even greater with concurrent smoking or use of smokeless tobacco.[1] Chronic alcoholism can lead to massive bleeding from gastritis, gastric ulcer, and esophageal varices (associated

BOX 2.3   CONDITIONS AND TYPES OF FETAL ALCOHOL SPECTRUM DISORDERS (FASDS)

FASD conditions include
  Abnormal facial features (e.g., smooth philtrum and others)
  Small head size
  Shorter-than-average height
  Low body weight
  Poor coordination
  Hyperactive behavior
  Difficulty with attention
  Poor memory
  Difficulty in school (especially math)
  Learning disabilities
  Speech and language delays
  Intellectual disability or low IQ
  Poor reasoning and judgment skills
  Sleep and sucking problems as a baby
  Vision or hearing problems
  Problems with the heart, kidneys, or bones
Types of FASDs
  Fetal Alcohol Syndrome (FAS). This is the most involved end of the
    FASD spectrum. Individuals with FAS may have abnormal facial
    features, growth problems, and CNS problems; can have problems
    with learning, memory, attention span, communication, vision, or
    hearing; and may have a hard time in school and trouble getting
    along with others.
  Alcohol-Related Neurodevelopmental Disorder (ARND). Individuals with
    ARND may have intellectual disabilities and problems with behavior
    and learning; might do poorly in school and have difficulties with
    math, memory, attention, and judgment, and poor impulse control.
  Alcohol-Related Birth Defects (ARBDs). People with ARBDs may have
    problems with the heart, kidneys, or bones, or with hearing; and
    may have a mix of these problems.

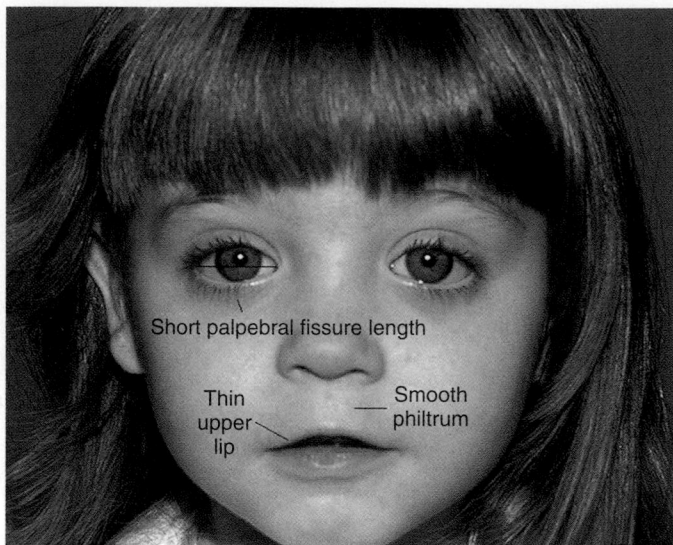

FIGURE 2.22 Diagnostic Facial Features of FAS. Three diagnostic facial features of FAS: (1) short palpebral fissure lengths, (2) smooth philtrum, and (3) thin upper lip. (© 2017 Susan Astley, PhD, University of Washington.)

with cirrhosis). Several effects can occur in the cardiovascular system, including dilated congestive cardiomyopathy and hypertension. Excessive alcohol increases the risk of acute and chronic pancreatitis.

The term **fetal alcohol spectrum disorders (FASDs)** is a range of health effects or disorders of prenatal alcohol exposure, with **fetal alcohol syndrome (FAS)** at the more severe end of the spectrum (Box 2.3). The diagnosis of FAS requires documentation of all three facial abnormalities (smooth philtrum, thin vermilion border, and small palpebral fissures [Fig. 2.22]), documentation of growth deficits, and CNS abnormality.

When the mother drinks so does her baby because of an unimpeded bidirectional movement of alcohol between the fetus and the mother. Alcohol crosses the placenta, reaching the fetus rapidly.[69] There is no known safe amount of alcohol for the mother to drink before she gets pregnant, when she gets pregnant, or during pregnancy.[70] Increased prepregnancy binge drinking rates may estimate alcohol use during very early gestation.[71] The fetus may completely depend on maternal hepatic detoxification because the activity of alcohol dehydrogenase (ADH) in the fetal liver is less than 10% of that of the adult liver. Additionally, the amniotic fluid may act as a reservoir for alcohol, prolonging fetal exposure.[69] Ethanol affects virtually all organ systems and particularly the adult and developing brain. A number of mechanisms have been proposed for ethanol-induced brain damage and include promotion of neuroinflammation, interference of cell

signaling by neurotrophic factors, oxidative stress, changes in retinoid acid signaling, thiamine deficiency, ER stress and unfolded or misfolded proteins, and alterations in autophagy.[72] Acetaldehyde can alter fetal development by disrupting differentiation and growth; DNA and protein synthesis; modification of carbohydrates, proteins, and fats; and the flow of nutrients across the placenta.[69,73] Additionally, alcohol may cause fetal disturbances, even preconceptual effects, epigenetically.[74,75] Recent data identify strong influences of alcohol on methylation and acetylation.[76]

Autopsies of children with FAS have revealed widespread severe damage, including failure of certain brain regions to develop, malformations of brain tissue, and failure of certain cells to migrate to their necessary location during development. Imaging studies reveal that in addition to an overall reduction in brain size, the corpus callosum is reduced in size or missing, the cerebellum is significantly reduced in size, and the basal ganglia and caudate nucleus are significantly reduced.

Social or Street Drugs

The social or "recreational" use of psychoactive drugs is widespread in many parts of the world. Most popular and dangerous are the drugs methamphetamine ("meth"), marijuana, cocaine, and heroin. Illicit use of drugs is a prevalent risk behavior among adolescents. Table 2.9 summarizes the effects of these drugs.

Unintentional and Intentional Injuries

About 199,800 people die from injury (not included here is medical errors) each year, and millions of people are injured and survive.[77] Significant are the numbers of people who face life-long mental, physical, and financial problems. In 2014, 2.5 million people were hospitalized because of injuries and 26.9 million people were treated in an emergency department.[77] Unintentional injury data include motor vehicle crashes as a leading cause of death in the United States with about 35,647 deaths in 2014 alone.[77] Opioid overdoses have quadrupled since 1999, with more than 14,800 deaths from prescription opioid overdoses in 2014. About 48,545 people comprised all poisoning deaths. Older adult falls accounted for 2.7 million people treated in emergency departments. In 2012, about 325,000 children were treated in emergency departments

TABLE 2.8   SOCIAL OR STREET DRUGS AND THEIR EFFECTS

TYPE OF DRUG	DESCRIPTION AND EFFECTS
Marijuana (pot)	*Active substance:* Δ9-Tetrahydrocannabinol (THC), found in resin of *Cannabis sativa* plant With smoking (e.g., "joints"), about 5% to 10% is absorbed through lungs; with heavy use the following adverse effects have been reported: alterations of sensory perception; impairment of cognitive and psychomotor judgments (e.g., inability to judge time, speed, distance); increases in heart rate and blood pressure; increases in susceptibility to laryngitis, pharyngitis, bronchitis; causes cough and hoarseness; may contribute to lung cancer (dosages levels not determined); contains large number of carcinogens; data from animal studies only indicate reproductive changes include reduced fertility, decreased sperm motility, and decreased levels of circulatory testosterone; fetal abnormalities include low birth weight; increased frequency of infectious illness is thought to be the result of depressed cell-mediated and humoral immunity; beneficial effects include decreased nausea secondary to cancer chemotherapy and decreased pain in certain chronic conditions
Methamphetamine (meth)	An amine derivation of amphetamine ($C_{10}H_{15}N$) used as crystalline hydrochloride CNS stimulant; in large doses causes irritability, aggressive (violent) behavior, anxiety, excitement, auditory hallucinations, and paranoia (delusions and psychosis); mood changes are common and abuser can swiftly change from friendly to hostile; paranoiac swings can result in suspiciousness, hyperactive behavior, and dramatic mood swings Appeals to abusers because body's metabolism is increased and produces euphoria, alertness, and perception of increased energy Stages: *Low intensity:* User is not psychologically addicted and uses methamphetamine by swallowing or snorting *Binge and high intensity:* User has psychologic addiction and smokes or injects to achieve a faster, stronger high *Tweaking:* Most dangerous stage; user is continually under the influence, not sleeping for 3–15 days, extremely irritated, and paranoid
Cocaine and crack	Extracted from leaves of cocoa plant and sold as a water-soluble powder (cocaine hydrochloride) liberally diluted with talcum powder or other white powders; extraction of pure alkaloid from cocaine hydrochloride is "free-base" called *crack* because it "cracks" when heated Crack is more potent than cocaine; cocaine is widely used as an anesthetic, usually in procedures involving oral cavity; it is a potent CNS stimulant, blocking reuptake of neurotransmitters norepinephrine, dopamine, and serotonin; also increases synthesis of norepinephrine and dopamine; dopamine induces sense of euphoria, and norepinephrine causes adrenergic potentiation, including hypertension, tachycardia, and vasoconstriction; cocaine can therefore cause severe coronary artery narrowing and ischemia; reason cocaine increases thrombus formation is unclear; other cardiovascular effects include dysrhythmias, sudden death, dilated cardiomyopathy, rupture of descending aorta (i.e., secondary to hypertension); effects on fetus include premature labor, retarded fetal development, stillbirth, hyperirritability
Heroin	Opiate closely related to morphine, methadone, and codeine Highly addictive, and withdrawal causes intense fear ("I'll die without it"); sold "cut" with similar-looking white powder; dissolved in water it is often highly contaminated; feeling of tranquility and sedation lasts only a few hours and thus encourages repeated intravenous or subcutaneous injections; acts on the receptors enkephalins, endorphins, and dynorphins, which are widely distributed throughout body with high affinity to CNS; effects can include infectious complications, especially *Staphylococcus aureus*, granulomas of lung, septic embolism, and pulmonary edema—in addition, viral infections from casual exchange of needles and HIV; sudden death is related to overdosage secondary to respiratory depression, decreased cardiac output, and severe pulmonary edema
Fentanyl	Synthetic opioid analgesic similar to morphine but is 50 to 100 times more potent. The synthetic opioid fentanyl and its analogs have risen across the United States in a variety of forms. Currently, it is documented in connection with a growing number of overdoses and overdose deaths.

CNS, Central nervous system; *HIV,* human immunodeficiency virus.
From Kumar V, Abbas A, Aster J: *Robbins & Cotran pathologic basis of disease,* ed 9, Philadelphia, 2015, Saunders.; Nahas G et al: *N Engl J Med* 343(7):514, 2000.

for sports- and recreation-related injuries, including a diagnosis of concussion or traumatic brain injury.[77] All deaths from firearms were about 33,636 people. According to the CDC, unintentional injury ranks fourth in the United States, a change from 2012 where it ranked fifth. Death and injury from medical care itself is presented in Box 2.4.

According to the CDC, the 10 leading causes of death in 2013 were diseases of the heart, malignant neoplasms, chronic lower respiratory tract diseases, unintentional injuries (accidents), cerebrovascular diseases, Alzheimer disease, diabetes mellitus, influenza and pneumonia, nephritis, nephrotic syndrome and nephrosis, and intentional self-harm (suicide).[78] The more common terms used to describe and classify unintentional and intentional injuries and brief descriptions of important features of these are discussed in Table 2.9.

Asphyxial Injuries

Asphyxial injuries are caused by a failure of cells to receive or use oxygen. Deprivation of oxygen may be partial *(hypoxia)* or total *(anoxia)*. Asphyxial injuries can be grouped into four general categories: suffocation, strangulation, chemical asphyxiants, and drowning.

Suffocation. Suffocation, or oxygen failing to reach the blood, can result from a lack of oxygen in the environment (entrapment in an enclosed space or filling the environment with a suffocating gas) or a blockage of the external airways. Classic examples of these types of asphyxial injuries are a child who is trapped in an abandoned refrigerator or a person who commits suicide by putting a plastic bag over the head. A reduction in the ambient oxygen level to 16% (normal is 21%) is

BOX 2.4   DEATH AND INJURY FROM MEDICAL CARE

Recently, much attention has been given to death and injury from medical care itself. A main concern is the lack of a comprehensive, nationwide system for estimating premature deaths and unintentional injury associated with preventable harm to people. A focus on preventable lethal events is absolutely necessary for safety and to assist educators, clinicians, administrators, and boards of trustees to guarantee a culture of safety for individuals. Studies on U.S. death rates from medical error since 1999 are presented in the following table:

DATES REVIEWED	SOURCE OF INFORMATION	PATIENT ADMISSIONS	ADVERSE EVENT RATE (%)	LETHAL ADVERSE EVENT RATES (%)	% OF EVENTS DEEMED PREVENTABLE	NO. OF DEATHS DUE TO PREVENTABLE ADVERSE EVENT	% OF ADMISSIONS WITH A PREVENTABLE LETHAL ADVERSE EVENT*	EXTRAPOLATION TO 2013 U.S. ADMISSIONS[†]
2000–02	Medicare patients	37,000,000	3.1	0.7	NR	389,576[‡]	0.71	251,454
2008	Medicare patients	838	13.5	1.4	44	12	0.62	219,579
2004	3 tertiary care hospitals	795	33.2	1.1	100	9	1.13	400,201
2002–07	10 hospitals in North Carolina	2341	18.1	0.6	63	14	0.38	134,581
2000–08	–	–	–	–	–	–	0.71	251,454

NOTE: Medical error is a common cause of death in the United States. A December 2015 report from an expert panel convened by the National Patient Safety Foundation identified these strategies for accelerating improvements in safety:

- Ensure that leaders establish and sustain a safety culture.
- Create centralized and coordinated oversight of safety.
- Create a common set of safety metrics that reflect meaningful outcomes.
- Increase funding for research in safety and implementation science.
- Address safety across the entire care continuum.
- Support the healthcare workforce.
- Partner with individuals and families for the safest care.
- Ensure that technology is safe and optimized to improve safety.

*All were considered preventable.

[†]Total number of U.S. hospital admissions in 2013 was 35,416,020.

[‡]Total number of people who died from a preventable lethal adverse event calculated as a point estimate of death rate among hospitalized patients reported in the literature extrapolated to the reported number of patients hospitalized in 2013.

NR, Not reported.

Data from Abbasi J: *J Am Med Assoc* 316(7):698–700, 2016; Makary MA, Daniel M: *BMJ* 353:i2139, 2016.

TABLE 2.9   UNINTENTIONAL AND INTENTIONAL INJURIES

TYPE OF INJURY	DESCRIPTION
FIGURE A. Blunt-force injuries.	Mechanical injury to body resulting in tearing, shearing, or crushing; most common type of injury seen in healthcare settings; caused by blows or impacts; motor vehicle accidents and falls most common cause (Fig. A) *Contusion (bruise):* Bleeding into skin or underlying tissues; initial color will be red-purple, then blue-black, then yellow-brown or green; duration of bruise depends on extent, location, and degree of vascularization; bruising of soft tissue may be confined to deeper structures; *hematoma* is collection of blood in soft tissue; *subdural hematoma* is blood between inner surface of dura mater and surface of brain; can result from blows, falls, or sudden acceleration/deceleration of head as occurs in *shaken baby syndrome; epidural hematoma* is collection of blood between inner surface of skull and dura; is most often associated with a skull fracture *Laceration:* Tear or rip resulting when tensile strength of skin or tissue is exceeded; is ragged and irregular with abraded edges; an extreme example is *avulsion,* where a wide area of tissue is pulled away; lacerations of internal organs are common in blunt-force injuries; lacerations of liver, spleen, kidneys, and bowel occur from blows to abdomen; thoracic aorta may be lacerated in sudden deceleration accidents; severe blows or impacts to chest may rupture heart with lacerations of atria or ventricles *Fracture:* Blunt-force blows or impacts can cause bone to break or shatter

TABLE 2.9 UNINTENTIONAL AND INTENTIONAL INJURIES—cont'd

TYPE OF INJURY	DESCRIPTION

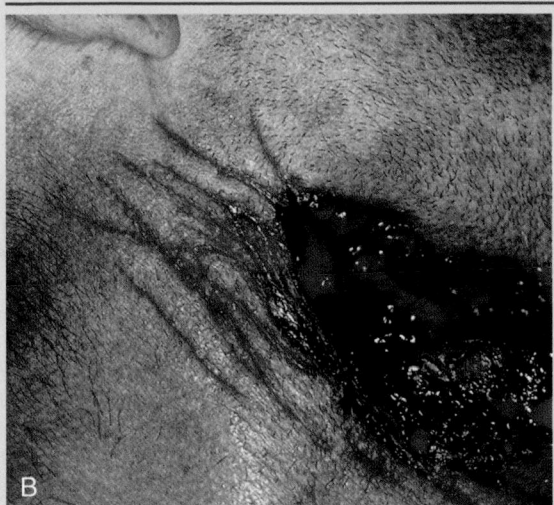

FIGURE B. Sharp-force injuries.

Cutting and piercing injuries accounted for 2609 deaths in 2014; men have a higher rate (1.37/100,000) than women (0.44/100,000)

Incised wound: Wound that is *longer* than it is *deep;* wound can be straight or jagged with sharp, distinct edges without abrasion; usually produces significant external bleeding with little internal hemorrhage; these wounds are noted in sharp-force injury suicides; in addition to a deep, lethal cut, there will be superficial incisions in same area called *hesitation marks* (Fig. B)

Stab wound: Penetrating sharp-force injury that is *deeper* than it is *long;* if a sharp instrument is used, depths of wound are clean and distinct but can be abraded if object is inserted deeply and wider portion (e.g., hilt of a knife) impacts skin; depending on size and location of wound, external bleeding may be surprisingly small; after an initial spurt of blood, even if a major vessel or heart is struck, wound may be almost completely closed by tissue pressure, thus allowing only a trickle of visible blood despite copious internal bleeding

Puncture wound: Instruments or objects with sharp points but without sharp edges produce puncture wounds; classic example is wound of foot after stepping on a nail; wounds are prone to infection, have abrasion of edges, and can be very deep

Chopping wound: Heavy, edged instruments (axes, hatchets, propeller blades) produce wounds with a combination of sharp- and blunt-force characteristics

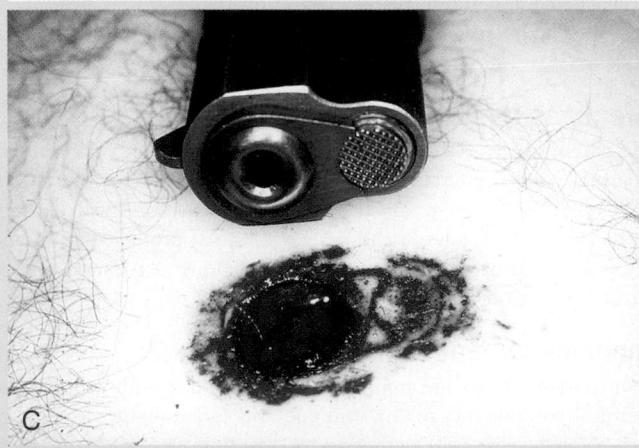

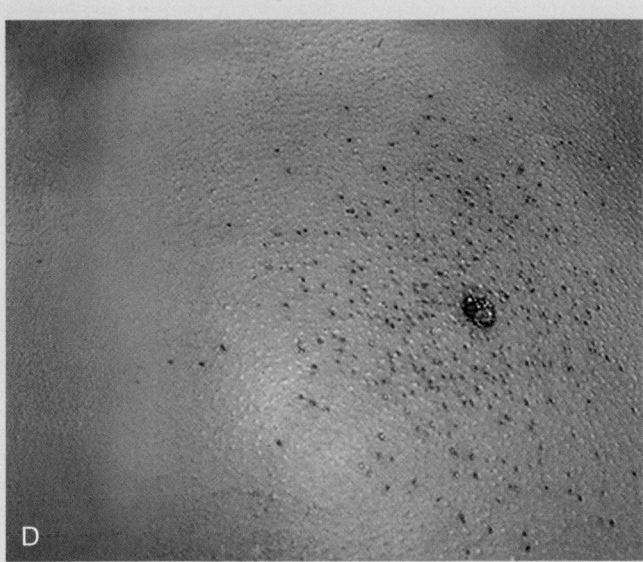

FIGURES C and D. Firearms.

All firearm deaths accounted for 33,599 deaths in the United States in 2014; men more likely to die than women (18.16 vs. 2.73/100,000)

Entrance wound: All wounds share some common features; overall appearance is most affected by range of fire

Contact range entrance wound: Distinctive type of wound when gun is held so muzzle rests on or presses into skin surface; there is searing of edges of wound from flame and soot or smoke on edges of wound in addition to hole; hard contact wounds of head cause severe tearing and disruption of tissue (because of thin layer of skin and muscle overlying bone); wound is gaping and jagged, known as *blow back;* can produce a patterned abrasion that mirrors weapon used (Fig. C)

Intermediate (distance) range entrance wound: Surrounded by gunpowder tattooing or stippling; *tattooing* results from fragments of burning or unburned pieces of gunpowder exiting barrel and forcefully striking skin; *stippling* results when gunpowder abrades but does not penetrate skin (Fig. D)

Indeterminate range entrance wound: Occurs when flame, soot, or gunpowder does not reach skin surface but bullet does; *indeterminate* is used rather than *distant* because appearance may be same regardless of distance; for example, if an individual is shot at close range through multiple layers of clothing the wound may look the same as if the shooting occurred at a distance

Exit wound: Has the same appearance regardless of range of fire; most important factors are speed of projectile and degree of deformation; size cannot be used to determine if hole is an exit or entrance wound; usually has clean edges that can often be reapproximated to cover defect; skin is one of toughest structures for a bullet to penetrate; thus, it is not uncommon for a bullet to pass entirely through body but stop just beneath skin on "exit" side

Wounding potential of bullets: Most damage done by a bullet is a result of amount of energy transferred to tissue impacted; speed of bullet has much greater effect than increased size; some bullets are designed to expand or fragment when striking an object, for example, *hollow-point* ammunition; lethality of a wound depends on what structures are damaged; wounds of brain may not be lethal; however, they are usually immediately incapacitating and lead to significant long-term disability; a person with a "lethal" injury (wound of heart or aorta) also may not be immediately incapacitated

immediately dangerous. If the level is less than 5%, death can ensue within a matter of minutes. The diagnosis of these types of asphyxial injuries depends on the history of the injury, because there will be no specific physical findings.

Diagnosis and treatment in choking asphyxiation (obstruction of the internal airways) depend on locating and removing the obstructing material. Injury or disease also may cause swelling of the soft tissues of the airway, leading to partial or complete obstruction and subsequent asphyxiation. Suffocation also may result from compression of the chest or abdomen (mechanical or compressional asphyxia), preventing normal respiratory movements. Usual signs and symptoms include florid facial congestion and petechiae (pinpoint hemorrhages) of the eyes and face.

Strangulation. Strangulation is caused by compression and closure of the blood vessels and air passages resulting from external pressure on the neck. This causes cerebral hypoxia or anoxia secondary to the alteration or cessation of blood flow to and from the brain. It is important to remember that the amount of force needed to close the jugular veins (2 kg [4.5 lb]) or carotid arteries (5 kg [11 lb]) is significantly less than that required to crush the trachea (15 kg [33 lb]). It is the alteration of cerebral blood flow in most types of strangulation that causes injury or death—not the lack of airflow. With complete blockage of the carotid arteries, unconsciousness can occur within 10 to 15 seconds.

A noose is placed around the neck, and the weight of the body is used to cause constriction of the noose and compression of the neck in hanging strangulations. The body does not need to be completely suspended to produce severe injury or death. Depending on the type of ligature used, there usually is a distinct mark on the neck, an inverted V with the base of the V pointing toward the point of suspension.

In ligature strangulation, the mark on the neck is horizontal, without the inverted V pattern seen in hangings. Petechiae may be more common because intermittent opening and closure of the blood vessels may occur as a result of the victim's struggles. Internal injuries of the neck are rare.

Variable amounts of external trauma on the neck with contusions and abrasions are noted in manual strangulation caused either by the assailant or by the victim clawing at one's own neck in an attempt to remove the assailant's hands. Internal damage can be quite severe, with bruising of deep structures and even fractures of the hyoid bone and tracheal and cricoid cartilages. Petechiae are common.

Chemical asphyxiants. Chemical asphyxiants either prevent the delivery of oxygen to the tissues or block its use. Carbon monoxide (CO) is the most common chemical asphyxiant. Cyanide acts as an asphyxiant by combining with the ferric iron atom in cytochrome oxidase, thereby blocking the intracellular use of oxygen. A victim of cyanide poisoning has the same cherry-red appearance as a carbon monoxide intoxication victim because cyanide blocks the use of circulating oxyhemoglobin. An odor of bitter almonds also may be detected. (The ability to smell cyanide is a genetic trait that is absent in a significant portion of the general population.) Hydrogen sulfide (sewer gas) is a chemical asphyxiant in which victims of hydrogen cyanide poisoning may have brown-tinged blood in addition to the nonspecific signs of asphyxiation.

Drowning. Drowning is an alteration of oxygen delivery to tissues resulting from the breathing in of fluid, usually water. Each year there are thousands of drowning deaths in the United States. The major mechanism of injury is hypoxemia (low blood oxygen levels). Even in freshwater drownings, where large amounts of water can pass through the alveolar-capillary interface, there is no evidence that increases in blood volume cause significant electrolyte disturbances or hemolysis, or that the amount of fluid loading is beyond the compensatory capabilities of the kidneys and heart. Airway obstruction is the more important pathologic abnormality, underscored by the fact that in up to 15% of drownings,

little or no water enters the lungs because of vagal nerve–mediated laryngospasms. This phenomenon is called dry-lung drowning.

No matter what mechanism is involved, cerebral hypoxia leads to unconsciousness in a matter of minutes. Whether this progresses to death depends on a number of factors, including the age and health of the individual. One of the most important factors is the temperature of the water. Irreversible injury develops much more rapidly in warm water than it does in cold water. Submersion times of up to 1 hour with subsequent survival have been reported in children retrieved from very cold water. Complete submersion is not necessary for a person to drown. An incapacitated or helpless individual (such as a person with epilepsy or alcoholism, or an infant) may drown in only a few inches of water.

It is important to remember that there are no specific or diagnostic findings to *prove* that a person recovered from the water is actually a drowning victim. In cases in which water has entered the lung, there may be large amounts of foam coming from the nose and mouth, although this also can be seen in certain types of drug overdoses. A body recovered from water with signs of prolonged immersion could just as easily be a victim of some other type of injury who has been put in the water to obscure the actual cause of death. When working with a living victim recovered from water, it is essential to keep in mind that an underlying condition may have led to the person's becoming incapacitated and submersed—a condition that also may need to be treated or addressed while correcting hypoxemia and dealing with its sequelae.

Infectious Injury

The pathogenicity (virulence) of microorganisms lies in their ability to survive and proliferate in the human body, where they injure cells and tissues. The disease-producing potential of a microorganism depends on its ability to (1) invade and destroy cells, (2) produce toxins, and (3) produce damaging hypersensitivity reactions (see Chapter 9 for further discussion).

Immunologic and Inflammatory Injury

Cellular membranes are injured by direct contact with cellular and chemical components of the immune and inflammatory responses, such as phagocytic cells (lymphocytes, macrophages) and substances such as histamine, antibodies, lymphokines, complement, and proteases. Complement is responsible for many of the membrane alterations that occur during immunologic injury. Membrane alterations are associated with rapid leakage of potassium (K^+) out of the cell and rapid influx of water. Antibodies can interfere with membrane function by binding to and occupying receptor molecules on the plasma membrane. This type of injury is found in certain forms of diabetes mellitus and in myasthenia gravis. Antibodies also can block or destroy cellular junctions, interfering with intercellular communication.

Injurious Genetic/Epigenetic Factors

Genetic disorders may be the result of genetic factors that alter the cell's nucleus and the plasma membrane's structure, shape, receptors, or transport mechanisms. For example, enzymatic genetic defects can lead to abnormalities in membrane transport. Genetic disorders can cause structural alterations of the red blood cell (e.g., sickle cell anemia). Certain human diseases, for example, cancer, can occur because of misregulation of gene expression linked to alterations of epigenetic patterning (see Chapters 6, 12, and 13).

Injurious Nutritional Imbalances

Essential nutrients—micronutrients (vitamins, minerals, trace elements, phytochemicals, and antioxidants) and macronutrients (proteins, carbohydrates, fats)—are required for cells to function normally. If these nutrients are not consumed and transported to the body's cells, or if excessive amounts of nutrients are consumed and transported, pathophysiologic cellular effects develop (*What's New? Phytochemicals and Antiinflammation*).

WHAT'S NEW?

Phytochemicals and Antiinflammation

An increasing number of studies indicate that a diet rich in antiinflammatory phytochemicals may have beneficial effects in reducing the risk of development of chronic disease. The specific mechanisms by which these beneficial effects are mediated are not well understood and include such topics as use of antiinflammatory medications, modulation of gene expression, and implementation of chemopreventive and cardioprotection strategies. One area being investigated is that certain phytochemicals inhibit pattern recognition receptors (PRRs), including Toll-like receptors (TLRs) and nucleotide-binding oligomerization domain proteins (NODs), which detect invading pathogens by recognizing pathogen-associated molecular patterns (PAMPs) and activate innate immune responses for host defense. It is now documented that these PRRs also can be activated by a variety of endogenous molecules derived from tissue injury and elicit sterile (e.g., induced by cell death or injury) inflammation to initiate wound-healing processes. Newer and emerging evidence suggests that PRRs can detect metabolic changes and bridge immune responses to maintain metabolic homeostasis. Dysregulation of this system of response can lead to PRRs vulnerable to chronic inflammation, which in turn can promote the development and progression of chronic disease. Examples of phytochemicals being investigated include curcumin, helenalin, cinnamaldehyde, sulforaphane (e.g., mustard, broccoli), flavonoids (e.g., blueberries), silymarin, parthenolide, allicin (garlic), indole-3-carbinol (cruciferous vegetables), lycopene (tomato), and resveratrol.

Data from Aggarwal BB, Shishodia S: *Biochem Pharmacol* 71(10):1397–1421, 2006; Khuda-Bukhsh AR, Das S, Saha SK: *Nutr Cancer* 66(2):194–205, 2014; Maru GB et al: *World J Biol Chem* 7(1):88–99, 2016; Wang PY et al: *J Diabetes Investig* 7(1):56–69, 2016; Zhao L, Lee JY, Hwang DH: *Nutr Rev* 69(9):310–320, 2011.

(Proteins, which consist of chains of amino acids, are the major structural units of the cell and participate in many enzymatic and hormonal functions. Protein deficiency causes a reduction in the intestinal mucosal mass, decreasing the absorptive function. The integrity of the pancreas is also affected, resulting in diminished exocrine secretion. With starvation or malnutrition, the lowered levels of plasma proteins, particularly albumin, cause fluid to move into the interstitium (edema). Protein-calorie malnutrition (PCM) is the predominant worldwide type of malnutrition. Malnourished children are very susceptible to disease and often die of infectious diseases. Even with adequate protein intake, cellular injury can occur if amino acid transport mechanisms fail or are defective. In Fanconi syndrome, for example, renal tubular cells may contain accumulated protein droplets that have been absorbed but cannot be transported.

Glucose is the major carbohydrate obtained from the breakdown of starch. Hyperglycemia (excessive glucose in the blood) caused by excessive carbohydrate intake may lead to obesity. Deficiencies of glucose result from starvation or from lack of use, as in diabetes. In both conditions the body compensates by metabolizing fat (lipids).

In lipid deficiency, or hypolipidemia, the body compensates by mobilizing fatty acids from adipose tissue. This causes an increase in the production and circulation of ketone bodies, which are acidic byproducts of lipid metabolism. The excretion of ketone bodies results in loss of water and electrolytes and causes dehydration and thirst.

Severe increases in the concentration of ketone bodies cause ketoacidosis, coma, and death. Hyperlipidemia, or an increase in the levels of lipoproteins in the blood, results in deposits of fat in the heart, liver, and muscle.

Vitamins are not sources of energy but are necessary for maintaining normal cellular functions. Adequate vitamin intake is necessary because most vitamins are not synthesized by the body. Research from the 1990s resulted in the identification of 13 vitamins as being essential for humans. These include eight B vitamins (thiamine, niacin, riboflavin, folate, vitamin B_6, vitamin B_{12}, biotin, and pantothenic acid), vitamin C or ascorbic acid, and the fat-soluble vitamins A, D, E, and K. (Minerals are discussed in Chapter 3.) Vitamins are involved in numerous reactions, including metabolism of visual pigments (vitamin A), calcium and phosphate metabolism (vitamin D), prothrombin synthesis (vitamin K), and antioxidation reactions (vitamins E and C). Pyridoxine (vitamin B_6) affects amino acid transfer reactions; flavin adenine dinucleotide (FAD), flavin mononucleotide (FMN), and nicotinamide adenine dinucleotide (NAD) help transfer electrons in various reactions.

Injurious Physical Agents

Injurious physical agents include temperature extremes, atmospheric pressure changes, radiation, illumination, mechanical factors, noise, and prolonged vibration. Physical injury can result from excessive exposure to many environmental agents, as well as to agents used for the diagnosis and treatment of illness.

Climate Change

Climate is changing beyond the range of the recent geological era because levels of carbon dioxide and other greenhouse gases (e.g., methane) in the Earth's atmosphere are exceeding levels recorded in the past millions of years.[79] Strongly correlated with warming of the Earth are the greenhouse gases, particularly CO_2, produced by the combustion of hydrocarbons in automobiles, air travel, marine transportation, railways, and energy plants (coal, natural gas, and oil).[80] Climate change affects social and environmental determinants of health including clean air, safe drinking water, sufficient food, and secure shelter.[81] Climate change will seriously impact human health by increasing several diseases including (1) cardiovascular, cerebrovascular, and respiratory diseases from air pollution and heat waves; (2) gastroenteritis and infectious disease epidemics caused by water and food contamination from flooding, disruption of clean water supplies, and sewage treatment; (3) vector-borne communicable diseases, including dengue, malaria, hantavirus, and cholera;[82] and (4) malnutrition from disruption of crops.[1]

Temperature Extremes

Chilling or freezing of cells causes hypothermic injury. Hypothermia has proved to be strongly injurious to a variety of cells. *Accidental hypothermia* is an unintentional drop in core body temperature below 35° C (95° F). At these temperatures, the compensatory mechanisms that conserve temperature start to fail. Primary accidental hypothermia is the physiologic result of a previously healthy person to the changes that occur with cold. The mortality rate is higher in those who develop secondary hypothermia as a consequence of a serious systemic disorder, for example, endocrine disorders. Primary accidental hypothermia is a worldwide problem with most cases evident in the winter months. Surprisingly, however, it commonly occurs in warmer regions. The highest risks are to the elderly and neonates. The elderly have diminished thermal perception and regulation and are susceptible because of increased likelihood of immobility, impaired nutritional status, the presence of coexisting diseases, and the impact of economic factors. Neonates have high rates of heat loss because of their increased surface-to-mass ratio and lack of shivering and other behavioral responses.

Individuals at increased risks for hypothermia include those with occupations or hobbies that have extensive cold weather exposure, such as people in the military, hunters, sailors, skiers, swimmers, and climbers. Prolonged exposure to low ambient temperature is a common risk factor found in homeless persons. Some causes of secondary hypothermia include hypothyroidism, hypoglycemia, adrenal insufficiency, metabolic alterations associated with uremia, neurologic injury, extensive burns, acute myocardial infarction (can be reversed with resuscitation), skin diseases, and hepatic failure.[83]

Submersion in cold water can induce a high incidence of cardiac dysrhythmias in healthy volunteers.[84] Immersion in cold water is a common cause of death in children and in adults.[85] Deaths caused by cold water have historically been ascribed to hypothermia; however, reports of two newer antagonistic responses are emerging—they are called the *cold shock response* and the *diving response* (Box 2.5).

Hypothermic injury has long been attributed to disturbances of cellular ion balance or homeostasis, especially of sodium balance (i.e., increased intracellular sodium levels). Hypothermia increases the level of intracellular Ca^{++} by slowing Na^+-K^+-ATPase pump activity, leading to Na^+ accumulation intracellularly.[86] In the last decade, however, the role for ROS has gained importance.[87] Hypothermic perfusion of the heart increased superoxide (O_2^-) concentration (see Table 2.3); in turn, O_2^- reacted with nitric oxide (NO) to form another radical peroxynitrite anion ($ONOO^-$).[86] In some cell types, such as hepatocytes and liver endothelial cells, hypothermia can cause pronounced cell injury mediated by ROS. During the body's exposure to cold, injury is inhibited by hypoxia and by a number of antioxidants, especially iron chelators.

Indirect forms of injury occur because of changes in small blood vessels (the microcirculation). Slow chilling can cause vasoconstriction followed by paralysis of vasomotor control, resulting in vasodilation and increased membrane permeability causing cellular and tissue swelling. With an abrupt drop in temperature, vasoconstriction and increased viscosity of the blood cause ischemic injury—infarction and necrosis (cellular death)—in affected tissues. With continued exposure to freezing temperatures, vasodilation produces severe swelling that causes degenerative changes in the myelin sheath that surrounds peripheral nerves, resulting in sensory and motor disturbances. Thrombosis also can occur and may lead to gangrene of the affected part. These conditions often are called *frostbite*.

Therapeutically, hypothermia is widely used to protect cells and tissues against injurious processes. Therapeutic hypothermia (TH) has been used clinically to preserve the heart during surgery and to preserve organs before transplantation.[88] TH in animals to protect the heart against acute infarction has had positive results; however, studies in humans are limited.

Hyperthermia is an uncontrolled increase in body temperature that exceeds the body's ability to lose heat. **Hyperthermic injury** (injury caused by excessive heat) is common and varies depending on the nature, intensity, and extent of the injury. Three types of hyperthermic injury include heat cramps, heat exhaustion (illness), and heat stroke.

Heat cramps (cramping of voluntary muscles) are usually a result of vigorous exercise that causes a loss of salt and water as a consequence of sweat. Treatment is salt replacement.

Heat exhaustion occurs when sufficient salt and water loss results in hemoconcentration. Hypotension occurs secondary to fluid loss (hypovolemia), and the individual feels weak, is nauseated, and can suddenly collapse. Collapsing results from a failure of the cardiovascular system to compensate for hypovolemia. Heat exhaustion is probably the most common heat-related injury.

Heat stroke is a life-threatening condition associated with high environmental temperatures and humidity. Core body temperature rises as a result of thermoregulatory failures. Clinically, a rectal temperature of 41°C (106°F) is considered a life-threatening sign. Generalized peripheral vasodilation and decreased circulating blood volume are significant. At risk are older adults, athletes, military recruits, and people with cardiovascular disorders.

Malignant hyperthermia occurs in individuals with an inherited disorder (e.g., ryanodine receptor intracellular calcium release channel) of skeletal muscle sarcoplasmic reticulum in response to inhalational anesthetics or to succinylcholine.[89] This rare condition is often fatal. The condition includes elevated temperature, increased muscle metabolism, muscle rigidity, rhabdomyolysis, acidosis, and cardiovascular alterations.

Drug-induced hyperthermia has become increasingly common because of the increase in abuse of psychotropic drugs and illicit drugs. Examples of drugs include amphetamines, cocaine, phencyclidine (PCP), and methylenedioxymethamphetamine (MDMA; ecstasy). Lysergic acid diethylamide (LSD), salicylates, lithium, anticholinergics, and sympathomimetics also have been implicated.

Neuroleptic malignant syndrome is hyperthermia caused by the administration of neuroleptic drugs (antipsychotics, phenothiazines, haloperidol, prochlorperazine, metoclopramide) or the withdrawal of dopaminergic drugs and is characterized by lead-pipe muscle rigidity, autonomic dysregulation, hyperthermia, and extrapyramidal side effects.[90]

Burns are caused by local heat injury. A *full-thickness burn* is an open wound involving skin layers—epidermis, dermis, and subcutaneous layers—and causing extensive loss of fluids and plasma proteins. Cellular regeneration is not possible; therefore, skin from a donor or from the host must be grafted to the site. *Partial-thickness burns* result in reddening of the area as a result of dilation of small blood vessels and increased permeability of cellular membranes, with loss of protein-rich fluid, resulting in the typical "burn blister." In surface epithelial cells, membrane permeability increases, causing both cytoplasmic and nuclear swelling. Temperature-sensitive enzymes within certain cells respond to heat by increasing cellular metabolism, with detrimental effects. Intense heat

---

BOX 2.5   COLD WATER IMMERSION AND COLD SHOCK RESPONSE AND THE DIVING RESPONSE

Submersion and breath-holding in cold water can activate two antagonistic responses called the *cold-shock response* and the *diving response*. The cold-shock response triggers tachycardia from activation of the sympathetic nervous system. Sympathetic activation affects the sinoatrial (SA) and atrioventricular (AV) nodes of the heart and the myocardium. The release of breath-holding may be involved, with many dysrhythmias occurring within 10 seconds of stopping breath-holding. Paradoxically, the diving response promotes a parasympathetically mediated brachycardia. The simultaneous activation of both the sympathetic and the parasympathetic branches of the autonomic nervous system is sometimes called "autonomic conflict."

Certain individuals may have vulnerable risk factors including ischemic heart disease, myocardial hypertrophy, acquired (drug-induced) long QT syndrome (LQTS), QT interval mismatch to heart rate, atherosclerosis, and conduction pathologies (e.g., LQTS). There is a strong association between sudden cardiac arrest and swimming in children with LQTS. Certain drugs also may prolong QT interval (e.g., antihistamines, antibiotics, class Ia antiarrhythmics, gastrointestinal prokinetics, and antipsychotics). The actual number of immersion-related deaths because of "autonomic conflict" is unknown and may be undiagnosed because of drowning.

Data from Bowes H et al: *Eur J Appl Physiol* 116(4):759–767, 2016; Patton JF et al: *Brain Res Brain Res Rev* 49:399–404, 2010; Shattock MJ, Tipton MJ: *J Physiol* 590(Pt 14):3219–3230, 2012; Tipton MJ et al: *Aviat Space Environ Med* 81:399–404, 2010.

also damages the vascular endothelium and causes coagulation of the blood vessels.

Epidemiologic investigators have reported a positive relationship between overheating in infants (that is, overdressing infants in the winter) and the prevalence of sudden infant deaths. Sudden infant death syndrome (SIDS), or cot death, is the sudden and unexpected death of an infant less than 1 year of age, with onset of the lethal episode apparently occurring during sleep, that remains unexplained after a thorough investigation.[91] One hypothesis for SIDS is an insufficient cardiorespiratory response to multiple environmental stressors (such as prone sleeping, overwrapping, and infection) during a critical developmental phase in a vulnerable infant.[92] Investigators using neonatal rats did not find a three-way interaction between infection, hyperthermia, and hypoxia but did find independently that heat stress decreased minute ventilation during normal levels of oxygen and increased the hypoxic ventilator response.[92] They also found that administration of lipopolysaccharide (LPS, found normally in the outer membrane of gram-negative bacteria) decreased hypoxia-induced tachycardia.[92] Overall, these investigators found that neonatal cardiorespiratory responses are adversely affected by dual interactions (heat stress and LPS or infection) of environmental stress factors.[92] Recent recommendations to reduce the risk of all sleep-related infant deaths include positioning the infant supine, using a firm sleep surface, breast-feeding, implementing room-sharing without bed-sharing, performing routine immunizations, considering use of a pacifier, and avoiding soft bedding, overheating, and exposure to tobacco smoke, alcohol, and illicit drugs.[93]

Changes in Atmospheric Pressure

Sudden increases or decreases in atmospheric pressure cause blast injury, which can be transmitted by either air (air blast) or water (immersion blast). With sudden increases in pressure, tissue injury is caused by compressive waves of air impinging on the body, followed by a sudden wave of decreased pressure. The pressure changes may collapse the thorax, rupture internal solid organs, and cause widespread hemorrhage. In increased pressure caused by immersion blast, water pressure is applied suddenly to all sides of the body, forcing the body up out of the water. The positive pressure compresses the abdomen and ruptures hollow internal organs, such as the spleen, kidneys, and liver.

Decompression sickness. Decompression sickness (DCS) (diver disease, the bends, or caisson disease) is a condition arising with sudden decreases in pressure; carbon dioxide and nitrogen that are normally dissolved in the blood come out of solution and form tiny bubbles called *gas emboli*. Deep-sea divers, scuba divers, and underwater construction workers who return to the surface too quickly develop decompression sickness. Oxygen is quickly redissolved, but nitrogen bubbles may persist and obstruct blood vessels. Ischemia resulting from gas emboli causes cellular hypoxia, particularly in the muscles, joints, and tendons. Emboli and interstitial gas accumulate around the joints and skeletal muscles, causing the individual to bend in pain. Tissues of the heart and brain also may be affected by emboli, causing necrosis. Dehydration increases the risk of decompression sickness because immersion of the body in water increases venous return to the heart.[94] As a counter-regulatory measure, the cardiac atria secrete atrial natriuretic peptide (ANP), causing diuresis (the Gauer-Henry reflex). At the same time, with a decreased secretion of antidiuretic hormone (ADH) from the hypothalamus, the kidneys excrete water. The result is a reduction of blood volume. During ascent, fluid is lost in expired air. The total volume deficiency changes the rheological (flow of matter) dynamics in blood and promotes the onset of decompression sickness.[94,95] The gases can be promptly redissolved in blood by raising the atmospheric pressure, which is accomplished by placing the individual in a decompression chamber and increasing the pressure until it approximates pressure at the depth to

which the diver had descended. This redissolves the gas bubbles in the blood. Pressure is then decreased gradually until it equals the pressure at the surface of the water. This slows the release of gas bubbles out of solution.

Nitrogen concentrations can have a crippling anesthetic effect on the brain. This narcosis has been referred to as "rapture of the deep," where both physical and cognitive abilities may be seriously impaired.[96] Thus, when diving to great depths, both the volume of nitrogen and the volume of oxygen must be decreased. This is accomplished by the addition of an "inert" gas (one that has no metabolic activity within the body). It has been suggested that problems associated with deep, long-duration dives could be avoided by replacing the nitrogen in a diver's gas supply with helium, an inert gas and nature's second lightest gas.[97] Helium's great advantage is that it does not lead to nitrogen narcosis—it is less soluble in blood and fat than nitrogen.

Decompression sickness can happen with very rapid ascent to high altitude in an aircraft that is not properly pressurized.[98] Although decompression sickness is not a concern when people ascend slowly (e.g., on foot) to a low atmospheric pressure environment, such as altitudes higher than 10,000 feet, there is a significant decrease in available oxygen because of decreased partial pressure of the inspired gases. The hypoxemia that occurs may result in pathologic conditions unique to the hypoxic environment at high altitude.

High altitude illness: HAPE, HACE, AMS. High altitude illness, in the form of high altitude pulmonary edema (HAPE) or high altitude cerebral edema (HACE), is potentially fatal. Both conditions, in addition to a less serious, more common form, are known as *acute mountain sickness* (AMS). Several factors, including rate of ascent to altitude, final altitude reached, altitude at which a person sleeps, and individual physiologic differences, are believed to influence development of these conditions.[99] Additional risk factors include certain preexisting cardiopulmonary conditions, residence at low altitude, prior history of high altitude illness, and level of exertion at altitude.[100]

Acute mountain sickness (AMS) is defined as the presence of a combination of nonspecific symptoms that appear within a few hours after ascent to altitude, and may include headache, loss of appetite, nausea, vomiting, weakness, lassitude, dizziness, and difficulty sleeping.[100,101] Symptoms are usually most noticeable during the first few days at altitude, but may reappear on further ascent to a higher altitude. AMS is usually a relatively benign, self-limited condition and does not include abnormal neurologic symptoms or signs. An increase in severity of symptoms or signs of neurologic dysfunction, such as ataxia or altered consciousness, indicates transition to high altitude cerebral edema (HACE).[102] HACE is a clinical diagnosis defined as the onset of ataxia, altered consciousness (including confusion, impaired mentation, stupor, and coma), and severe lassitude. Severe headache, nausea, and vomiting are frequently present. In both AMS and HACE, headache is most likely initially produced by hypoxemia-induced cerebral vasodilation and a significant increase in blood flow. In addition, recent magnetic resonance imaging (MRI) studies suggest that in persons ascending to high altitudes and suffering moderate to severe AMS, some degree of cerebral edema occurs. However, in milder forms of AMS (a subjective distinction), brain edema is present in some MRI studies, but not in all.[100] The cerebral edema may be either cytotoxic or vasogenic in nature (see Chapter 17).

As potentially lethal as HACE can be, HAPE is actually thought to account for most deaths from high altitude illness.[101] High altitude pulmonary edema (HAPE) is a noncardiogenic pulmonary edema associated with pulmonary hypertension and elevated capillary pressure. The incidence of HAPE also is related to the rate of ascent, the ultimate altitude reached, and the individual's susceptibility. Victims of HAPE have a relatively exaggerated pulmonary hypertensive response on ascent to altitude as a result of augmented hypoxic pulmonary vasoconstriction. Heightened sympathetic nervous system activity, vascular endothelial dysfunction, and hypoxemia resulting from a suboptimal ventilatory response to hypoxia are responsible for the pulmonary vasoconstriction and subsequent pulmonary hypertension. Recent evidence suggests HAPE-prone individuals are characterized by a genetic defect in the transepithelial sodium and water transport mechanism that may impair alveolar fluid clearance.[103] Persons with congenital or acquired pulmonary circulation abnormalities are more susceptible to HAPE, supporting the suggestion that edema results from overperfusion in a restricted pulmonary vascular bed. Another proposed explanation for elevated pulmonary capillary pressure is uneven hypoxic pulmonary vasoconstriction.[102] It is now generally accepted that HAPE is initiated as a noninflammatory unidirectional dysfunction of the alveolar-capillary barrier that is essentially a form of hydrostatic pulmonary edema (i.e., there is an increase in pulmonary capillary pressure, but no elevation in left atrial pressure).

Ionizing Radiation

Ionizing radiation (IR) is any form of radiation capable of removing orbital electrons from atoms, resulting in the production of negatively charged free electrons and positively charged ionized atoms. Ionizing radiation is emitted by x-rays, γ-rays, and alpha and beta particles (which are emitted from atomic nuclei in the process of radioactive decay) and from subatomic particles such as neutrons, deuterons, protons, and pions. Ionizing radiation of three types (x-radiation, gamma radiation, and neutrons) was classified as a carcinogen in 2004.

An important source of exposure to ionizing radiation is the environment. This source includes emission from radioactive material inside the body, cosmic rays from outer space, and radiation emitted from such substances as soil and building materials. Environmental radioactivity is emitted primarily by uranium, thorium, and potassium. Other sources are from medical procedures (e.g., x-rays, computed tomography [CT] scans) used for medical diagnosis and treatment, uranium and thorium mines, nuclear weapons, and nuclear reactors that generate electricity. Medical radiation now comprises about 48% to 50% of the per capita radiation doses compared with 15% in the 1980s; since 1980 medical radiation exposure has increased 600% in the U.S. population (Fig. 2.23). Table 2.10 includes types of ionizing radiation and their magnitude of tissue penetration. (Box 2.6 defines the radiation units.)

TABLE 2.10	TYPES OF IONIZING RADIATION AND THEIR TISSUE PENETRATION
TYPE	**TISSUE PENETRATION**
x-rays	High
Gamma (γ) rays	High
Beta (β) particles	Low
Alpha (α) particles	Very low
Protons	Intermediate between α and β
Neutrons	High

Data from Damjanov I, Linder J, editors: *Anderson's pathology,* ed 10, St Louis, 1996, Mosby.

BOX 2.6   DEFINITIONS OF RADIATION UNITS

Curie (Ci) is the disintegration per second of a radionuclide (radioisotope). It represents the amount of radiation emitted by a source.

Gray (Gy) is a unit that expresses the energy absorbed by the target tissue per unit mass. One gray equals the absorption of 104 erg/g of tissue. A *centigray (cGy)* is the absorption of 100 erg/g of tissue and is equivalent to the older terminology of 100 rad (radiation absorbed dose). cGy has replaced the term *rad* in medical practice.

Sievert (Sv) is a unit of equivalent dose that depends on the biologic rather than the physical effects of radiation and it replaced the older term *rem.* Equivalent dose controls for the variation of damage produced for the same absorbed dose from different types of radiation. It is a uniform measure of biologic dose. The effective dose of x-rays in radiographs and computed tomography is usually expressed in milliSieverts (mSv). For x-radiation, 1 mSv = 1 mGy.

Data from Kumar V, Abbas A, Aster J: *Robbins & Cotran pathologic basis of disease,* ed 9, Philadelphia, 2015, Saunders.

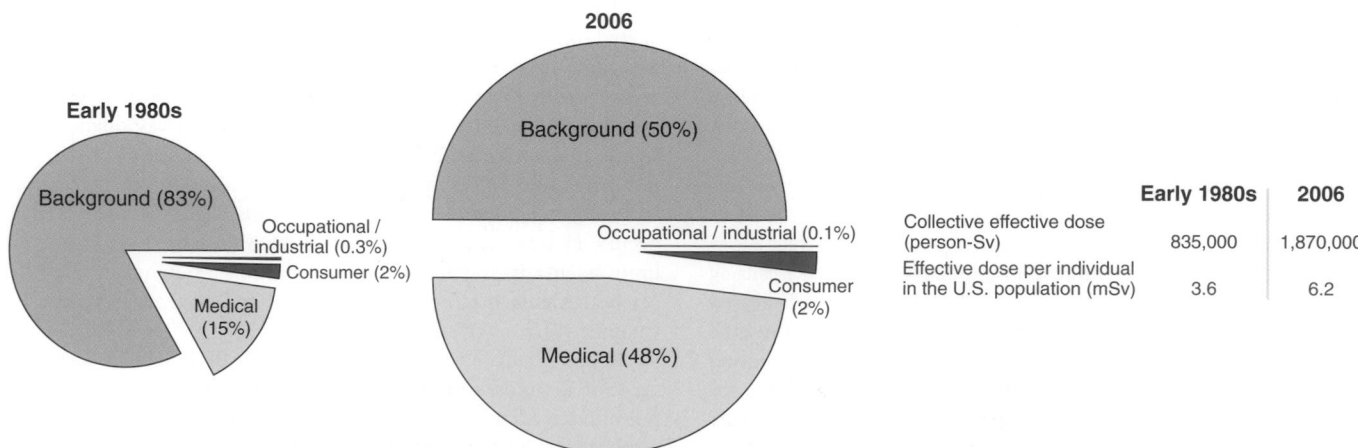

	Early 1980s	2006
Collective effective dose (person-Sv)	835,000	1,870,000
Effective dose per individual in the U.S. population (mSv)	3.6	6.2

FIGURE 2.23 Ionizing Radiation Exposure of the Population of the United States. (From National Council on Radiation Protection & Measurements. (2015). *Ionizing radiation exposure of the population of the United States, NCRP report 160,* Bethesda, MD.)

The main determinants of the biologic effects of ionizing radiation depend on several factors and include the following:

1. *Rate of delivery.* Because the effect of radiant energy is cumulative, divided doses may allow cells to repair between exposures, called *fractionated doses.*
2. *Field size.* Doses of radiation delivered to shielded smaller fields are safer than smaller doses delivered to larger fields, which may be lethal.[1]
3. *Cell proliferation.* Rapidly dividing cells are more vulnerable to injury because ionizing radiation damages DNA. Vulnerable tissues have a high rate of cell division and include *gonads, bone marrow, lymphoid tissue,* and the *mucosa of the gastrointestinal tract.* Injury is manifested early after exposure.
4. *Oxygen effects and hypoxia.* A main mechanism of damage to DNA by ionizing radiation is from generation of reactive oxygen species from reactions with free radicals by radiolysis of water. Tissue with low oxygenation (hypoxia) is less sensitive to radiation, for example, the center of rapidly growing tumors.

5. *Vascular damage.* Endothelial cell damage is an important effect of radiotherapy and can result in narrowing or occlusion of blood vessels, leading to impaired healing, fibrosis, and chronic ischemic atrophy. These changes can appear months or years after exposure.

Late effects in tissues with a low rate of cell proliferation (brain, kidney, liver, muscle, subcutaneous tissue) may include cell death, atrophy, and fibrosis. These effects are associated with vascular damage from the release of proinflammatory mediators in irradiated tissue.[1]

Cellular damage from IR in the absence of effective repair involves two types of damage: (1) early or late tissue reactions (previously called *deterministic*) and (2) stochastic or random effects. High doses of radiation cause substantial cell killing and result in detectable tissue reactions. These reactions occur early (days) or late (months to years) after irradiation (Fig. 2.24).

The International Commission on Radiological Protection (ICRP) emphasizes that protection should be optimized for whole body exposures and for specific tissues, particularly the lens of the eye, the heart, and the cerebrovascular system. The threshold in absorbed doses for the

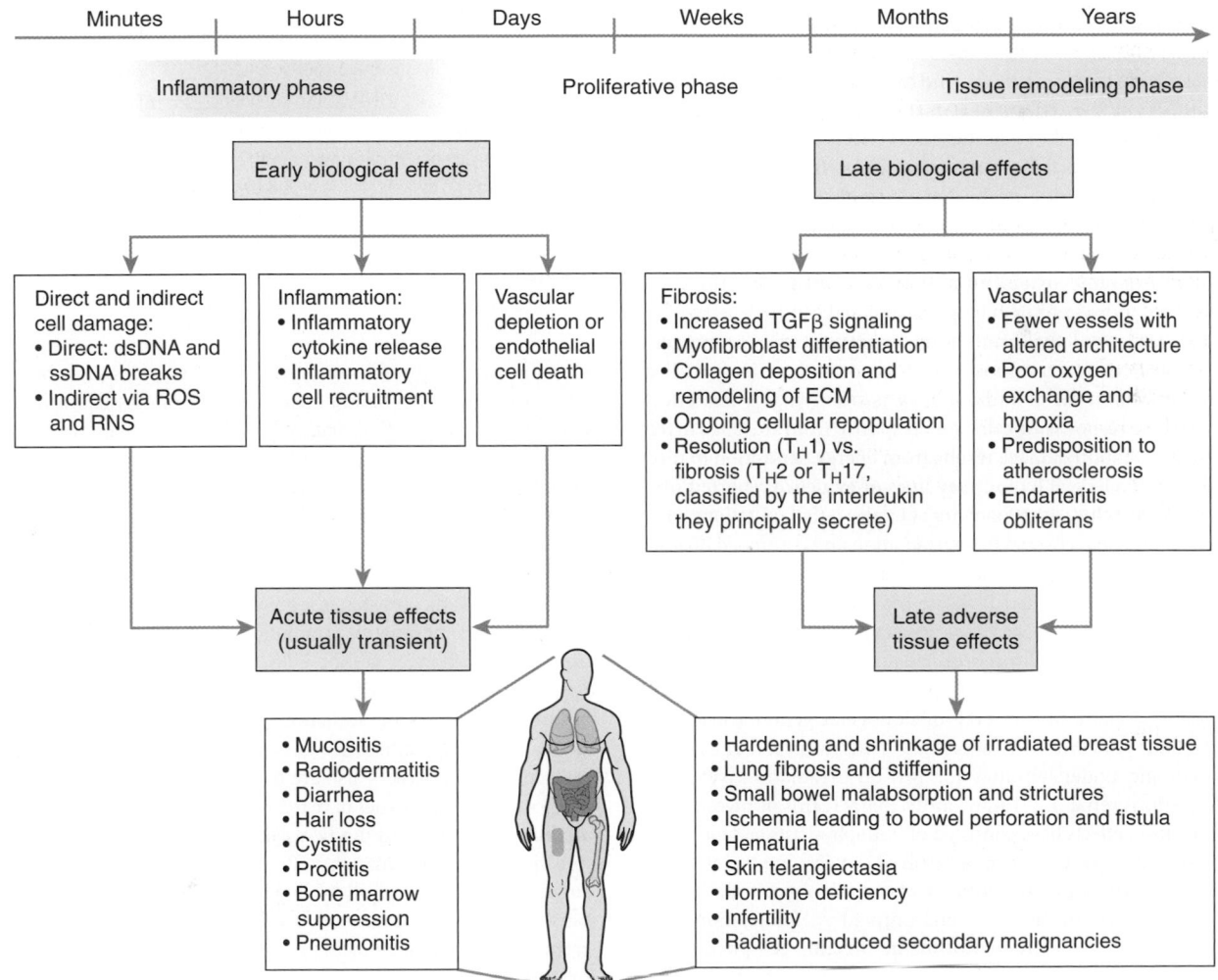

FIGURE 2.24 Early and Late Tissue Effects of Radiation. Early biologic events cause acute effects that are normally transient and resolve within 3 months of completing therapy. These events can lead to biologic effects over time, for example, fibrosis, vascular changes, and secondary malignancies. Severity is increased for these biologic effects with higher radiation dose per fraction. *dsDNA,* Double-stranded DNA; *ECM,* extracellular matrix; *ROS,* reactive oxygen species; *RNS,* reactive nitrogen species; *ssDNA,* single-stranded DNA; *TGFβ,* transforming growth factor-beta; *TH,* T helper cell. (From ICRP: *Ann ICRP* 41[1/2], 2012.)

lens of the eye is now lower and is considered to be 0.5 gray (Gy). The absorbed dose threshold for circulatory disease may be as low as 0.5 Gy to the brain or heart.[104] The emerging science on low-dose radiation and tissue effects is very complicated; for example, for exposures less than 0.5 Gy, the balance of inflammatory markers may shift toward anti-inflammatory effects.[105] *Stochastic effects* are produced at random, without a threshold dose level, and the main effects include carcinogenesis and genetic mutation. The severity of the outcome is *not* related to dose but rather the entire tissue and stress response (see below).[106,107] More simply, ionizing radiation causes damage that initiates DNA repair mechanisms, alterations in gene expression, and various stress responses.

Historically, radiation dose–related cancer risks at low doses were estimated from data of the atomic-bomb survivors and of individuals treated with moderate- to high-dose radiation.[107] The effects of low doses were mathematically extrapolated from high doses. After review from national and international expert committees and publications from 2005 to 2008, the available biologic and biophysical data support a linear no-threshold risk model for cancer.[107] Additionally, this understanding combined with an uncertain dose and a dose rate effectiveness factor for extrapolation from high doses is considered a conservative estimate for radiation protection for low doses and low dose rates.[107] Complicating these standards, however, has been the emerging data from radiobiology suggesting a much more complex understanding regarding low dose and low dose rates because of a complex interplay of various stress response pathways and nontargeted effects (NTEs) of low-dose radiation (e.g., effects in nonirradiated cells near and distant from irradiated cells).[108,109] The **nontargeted effects** of ionizing radiation include bystander effects and genomic instability. **Bystander effects**, or effects on cells not directly in the radiated field, are affected by the radiation and show high levels of mutations, chromosomal aberrations, and membrane signaling changes leading to what some call "horizontal transmission." **Genomic instability** is where generations of cells derived from an irradiated progenitor cell appear normal but time-lethal (i.e., irreversible) and nonlethal mutations appear in distant progeny, sometimes called "vertical transmission."[110] Importantly, a new paradigm shift of the effects of IR or radiobiology is occurring. These effects represent a tissue response or cell stress response from IR. The current theory that all radiation damage results from energy deposition in those cells' DNA was challenged by four key lines of evidence reported from 1986 to 1996 and includes the following: (1) new lethal mutations could occur in cells that had recovered from irradiation and continued dividing for several generations,[111] (2) a delayed appearance of new chromosome aberrations was demonstrated in bone marrow stem cell lines from irradiated stem cells,[112] (3) a very low-dose exposure of alpha radiation resulted in more cells with chromosome damage than would have been predicted mathematically,[113] and (4) the cell medium from irradiated cells was found to cause similar levels of clonogenic genomic instability and cell death as cells *directly* irradiated.[114] Thus, from newer evidence are radiobiologic understandings for low-dose radiation, yet many biologic questions remain.[110] Importantly, many teams of investigators studying radiation effects have consisted of both physicists *and* biologists. Additionally, much research is now involved concerning the effects of radiation on epigenetics, the entire tissue and organismic "stress" response, and the role of the microenvironment.[115,116] Radiation alters the components of the microenvironment, affecting cell phenotypes, tissue composition, and the physical interactions and signaling between cells.[109,117,118] These alterations can contribute to carcinogenesis and therapy resistance.

Ionizing radiation (IR; x-radiation and γ-rays) causes a large spectrum of genetic changes including gene mutations, mini–satellite mutations (altered numbers of tandem repeats of DNA sequences), micronucleus formation (sign of chromosome damage or loss), chromosomal

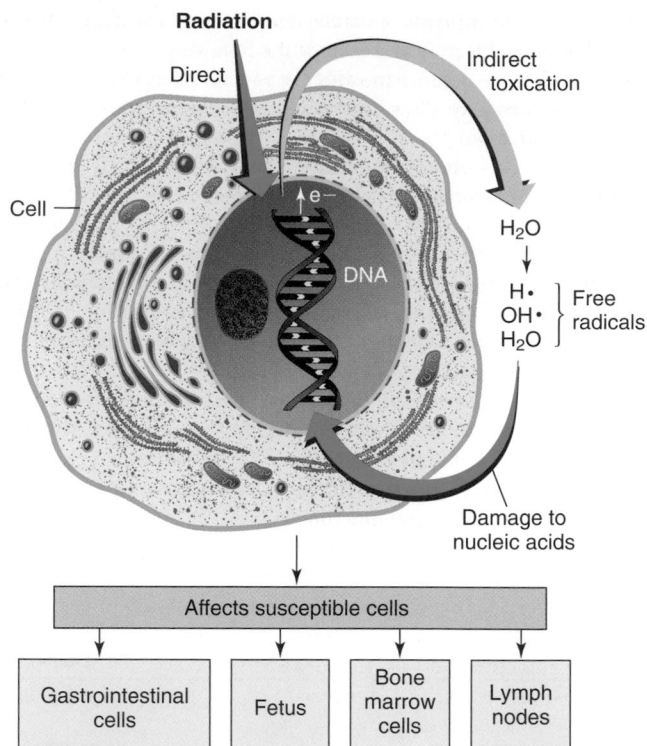

FIGURE 2.25 Cellular Damage Caused by Ionizing Radiation. Radiation can damage macromolecules in two ways: (1) directly, in which the micromolecules are ionized and (2) indirectly, in which water is ionized and produces free radicals that in turn damage macromolecules. Cells that are particularly susceptible to damage are those of the gastrointestinal tract, bone marrow, lymph nodes, fetus, and ovarian follicles.

aberrations (structural or number), ploidy changes (number of sets of chromosomes), DNA strand breaks, and chromosomal instability. DNA may be damaged *directly* or *indirectly* by interaction with reactive products (i.e., free electrons, hydroxyl radicals, hydrogen free radicals) from the degradation of water (Fig. 2.25).

All phases of the cell cycle can be affected by ionizing radiation. Sensitivity of the cell appears to be greatest in G_2, that gap of the cell just before mitosis; irradiation during this phase retards the onset of cell division. Radio-resistance is greatest in the latter part of the S phase. At the time of therapeutic irradiation those cells in the most sensitive parts of the cell cycle will be killed. Those cells in the radio-resistant part of the cell cycle will continue to proliferate and repopulate the tumor—requiring more radiation for a therapeutic effect or cell killing. Irradiation during mitosis induces chromosomal aberrations. Membrane molecules and enzymes also are damaged by radiation.

Not all cells and tissues have the same sensitivity to radiation, although all cells can be affected. Radiosensitivity depends partly on the rate of mitosis and cellular maturity. Because fetal cells both are immature and are undergoing rapid cycling, the fetus is at great risk for injury caused by ionizing radiation. Particularly vulnerable are embryonic germ cells, which are precursors of ova and sperm. Throughout life, cells of the bone marrow, intestinal mucosa, testicular seminiferous epithelium, and ovarian follicles are susceptible to injury because they are always undergoing mitosis, which ensures the presence of vulnerable, immature daughter cells. Exposure to x-radiation and γ-radiation is most strongly correlated with leukemia and cancers of the thyroid, breast, and lung; these correlates have been reported at absorbed low levels, less than 0.2 Gy. The risk of developing these cancers may to some extent depend on age at exposure. The Life Span Study, which had a wide range in age at exposure and a wide dose range (from less than 0.005 Gy to 2–4 Gy), was evidence of a linear dose response for all solid tumors, with significant radiation-associated excess risks observed in most, but not all, types of solid tumors. In utero radiation exposure in the Japanese A-bomb survivors was associated with an increased adult-onset risk of solid tumors.[119] The studies of diagnostic x-rays in utero and the risk of pediatric leukemia and other cancers are characterized by uncertainties, especially a lack of dose measurement data.[107] Ultrasound replaced abdominal x-rays and measurements of the pelvis several decades ago in pregnant women; however, there recently have been reports of increasing levels of radiologic imaging in pregnant women.[120] At the time of the radiologic examination, all women of childbearing potential should be asked if they could be pregnant.[121] If any doubt exists, the results of a pregnancy test should be obtained before proceeding. Many organizations have specific papers on safety and imaging pregnant women, including the American College of Radiology, the American Congress of Obstetricians and Gynecologists, and internationally, for example, the Health & Safety Executive from Great Britain and the International Commission on Radiological Protection Publication (ICRP). Radiation exposure to children may increase the incidence of lymphomas, leukemias, melanomas, breast cancers, and others. The increased frequency of pediatric CT exams in the United States is mainly because of the increased use of fast helical CT, which reduces the need for sedation.[122]

Radiation-induced cancers are found in the "cancer-prone" ages (usually 50 to 80 years of age), independent of age at exposure; therefore, the latency period between radiation exposure and the potential appearance of a cancer decreases significantly with increasing age at exposure.[123] From these effects, more recent analyses of cancer incidence among atomic-bomb (A-bomb) survivors suggest that the lifetime risk of radiation-induced cancer is not so different for exposure at age 5 years vs. exposure at age 55 years.[119,124] Notable research is being done on radiation-induced secondary cancers.

Illumination and Luminance: Light Is Electromagnetic Radiation

Light is electromagnetic radiation, and the portion of the electromagnetic spectrum that interacts with the eye is called **optical radiation** and includes wavelengths from ultraviolet light (100–400 nm), to visible light (400–760 nm), to infrared light (760–10,000+ nm). All radiations like light carry energy, with the shorter wavelengths being the most energetic.[125] Consequently, the smaller the emitting surface the more concentrated the flux in the viewing direction and the higher the luminance.[125] The optical system images everything on the retina, a highly specialized sense organ, and most relevant for retinal illumination is the luminance of the viewed objects. The mechanisms of light-induced damage include (1) heat or thermal damage, called *photothermal* damage; (2) *photochemical* damage, of which sources of damage include blue light, ultraviolet light, and laser beams thought to result mainly from oxidative stress by forming ROS and endoplasmic stress (Fig. 2.26); and (3) *photomechanical* damage, which results from mechanical compression or tensile forces generated by rapid introduction of energy. Thermal damage occurs from absorption of heat and irreversible thermal damage typically occurs after the ambient temperature in the retina is raised by at least 10°C (50°F).[126] The depth of penetration of the radiant energy depends on the incident wavelength and the primary absorbers—melanin and hemoglobin or oxyhemoglobin.[125] Photochemical damage occurs at short visible wavelengths; and for exposure longer than ≈1 ns, it is thought to be the result of light absorption to the chromophore, the most sensitive molecule that absorbs the radiation (light leads to the production of ROS and oxidative stress; the retina is very sensitive

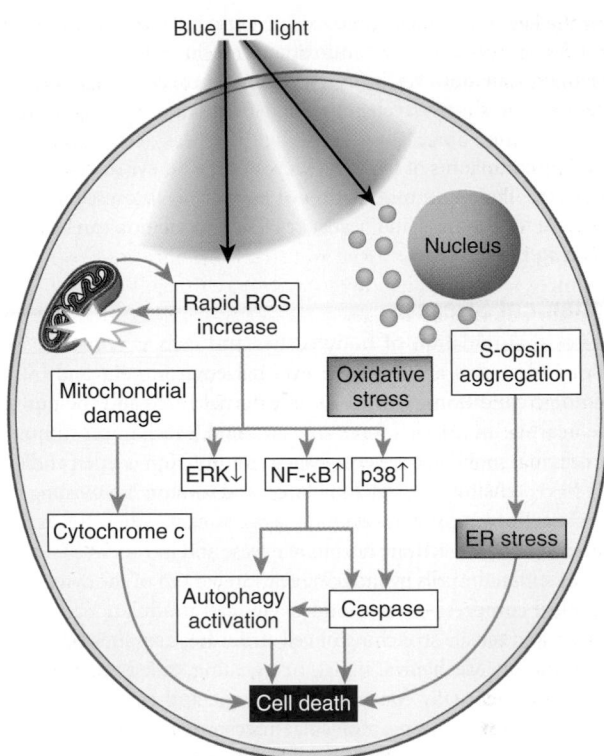

FIGURE 2.26 Photochemical Damage From Blue Light. From an in vitro experiment, blue light induces ROS production and S-opsin (light-sensitive protein) aggregation. The ROS increase is rapid and leads to oxidative damage, cell signaling pathway mitogen-activated protein kinase (MAPK) activation, or the nuclear translocation of NF-κβ. Activated MAPK and NF-κβ induce caspase activation and result in apoptotic cell death. NF-κβ activates autophagy and excessive autophagy leads to cell death. S-opsin aggregation causes endoplasmic (ER) stress. Blue LED light-induced retinal photochemical damage and cell death may be associated with both oxidative stress and ER stress. *ERK,* Extracellular signal-regulated kinases; *NF-kB,* a transcription factor. (Data from Kuse Y et al: *Sci Rep* 4:5223, 2014.)

to oxidative stress).[125] Investigators showed blue light-emitting dioide (LED) light damaged most severely compared to white and green LED light, and *N*-acetylcysteine (NAC), an antioxidant, was photoreceptor specific and protected against the cellular damage.[127] Photomechanical damage occurs with light pulses shorter than ≈1 ns and when the light energy is deposited faster than mechanical relaxation can occur. Tissue is disrupted by shear forces or cavitation (i.e., production of a cavity). The most common clinical application of photomechanical damage in ophthalmology is the use of radiation from the Nd:Yag laser. The laser is typically used to create an iridotomy (puncture-type openings through the iris without removal of iris tissue) in individuals with closed-angle glaucoma or cause retraction of an opacified posterior lens capsule in individuals after cataract surgery. Pulsed lasers are rarely used in vitreoretinal surgery because of the potential for collateral retinal damage, particularly full-thickness retinal defects and hemorrhage.[125,128]

Ocular exposures are accidental and intended (for example, in ophthalmic applications). Adherence to standards for ocular safety is a main concern for protection of the eye from laser exposures and light exposures from ophthalmic instruments. Additionally, to improve the energy performances of artificial light sources and to protect the environment, new light sources are available, such as compact fluorescent lamps or light-emitting diodes (LEDs). The potential risks of these new light sources need safety evaluation to determine health risks, especially hazards to the eye.

Focused light rays can increase oxidative stress, which can be prevented by a wide array of retinal antioxidant mechanisms.[129] Antioxidant mechanisms can, however, be overwhelmed by excessive light exposure, particularly of short-wavelength, high-frequency blue light, and of ultraviolet light. Since fluorescent lighting was introduced to the workplace, complaints of headaches, eyestrain, and eye discomfort have increased.[130] The rapid modulation of light from fluorescent lamps is responsible for eyestrain and headaches. The modulation can be reduced by wearing tinted glasses.

Mechanical Stresses

Mechanical stimulation of body tissues and cells is constant. These stresses and strains are from the external environment and internal physiologic conditions. Gravity as an external force and the pumping of the heart as an internal force are continual. Mechanical stimuli can cause cells to respond in a variety of ways; compression is a perpendicular-acting force, tension is a stretching force, and torsion is a twisting force. Fluid shear forces or layers rubbing against each other, for example, endothelial cells, can activate hormone release and intracellular signaling, as well as stiffen the cells by inducing rearrangement of the cytoskeleton. Mechanical compression of chondrocytes can modulate proteoglycan synthesis, and tensile stretching of cell structures can alter cell motility and orientation. Mechanical signals or signaling, called mechanotransduction, are eventually converted to biologic and chemical responses in the cell. Understanding molecular mechanisms driving cell shape changes is an important topic in cell and tissue structure. Specifically, mechanical forces are sensed by specialized protein complexes at integrin and cadherin adhesions and transformed into biochemical signals that modulate cell shape and function in both development and disease.[131] Mechanical forces at adhesion sites affect gene transcription and protein processes, such as cell proliferation, stemness, and differentiation (Fig. 2.27).[131] Investigators are identifying how adhesion pathways and mechanotransduction affect tissue development and homeostasis.

Acutely mechanical forces elicit adaptive responses (to rapidly alter function) chronically; however, the responses may induce tissue remodeling to accommodate load-bearing capabilities.[132] When the mechanical forces exceed unknown thresholds, injury results.[132] Injury can initiate more reparative responses, transient or continuous dysfunction, or progressive degenerative changes that incorporate nearby and surrounding tissue. Cellularly, the structural responses to deformation and strain (e.g., biomechanical) are causing investigators to focus on the cell membrane. Disruption of cell membranes, or *mechanoporation,* is central to the biologic progression. Investigators are defining mechanoporation

as important for traumatic brain injury because it is a primary source of intraaxonal calcium after contusion. Understanding this physiology is crucial because brain injury is not just an event but rather a process of disruption, and a recoverable state of axon injury persists for hours.[133] Mechanical injury can progress to cell death involving both cell necrosis and delayed apoptosis.[132] The heterogeneous distribution of atherosclerosis in the vasculature is possibly related to biomechanical factors and disturbed hemodynamic flow; that is, certain arteries (e.g., coronary and carotid arteries) and locations (e.g., bifurcations) are more susceptible to plaque formation than others.[134,135] Biomechanical forces probably are not systemic and vary with location. Mechanical stimuli include *shear forces* because of blood flow, strain from pressure distention of the vessel walls, and strain from tethering to a surrounding tissue area (e.g., the heart).[135]

The major focus of occupational biomechanics is the response of tissue to mechanical stress, especially the prevention of overexertion disorders of the lower back and upper extremities. Many mechanical stresses can cause overt injuries (e.g., a head injury when a worker is struck in the head with a dropped object). Most stresses, however, are subtle and can cause *accumulative* injuries and disorders. Table 2.11 summarizes common types of occupational mechanical stresses and associated types of injury. More realistic mechanical models of living cells will contribute greatly to the study of mechanotransduction in humans.

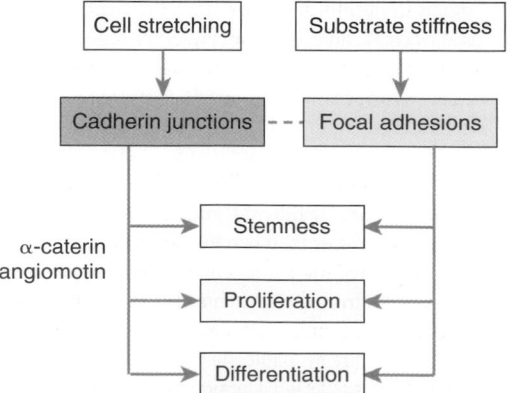

FIGURE 2.27 Mechanotransduction Regulates Gene Transcription. (Adapted from Han MK, de Rooij J: *Trends Cell Biol,* 2016.)

TABLE 2.11	COMMON TYPES OF OCCUPATIONAL MECHANICAL STRESSES AND ASSOCIATED TYPES OF INJURY
MECHANICAL STRESSES	**TYPE OF INJURY**
Forceful exertions (e.g., lifting, pushing, pulling of heavy loads)	Low back pain
Awkward trunk postures (e.g., flexion, lateral bending, axial twisting, prolonged sitting)	Low back pain
Whole body vibration (e.g., vibrating seat or platform)	Low back pain; bone deformities; alterations in nerve conduction (carpal tunnel syndrome)
Repetitive or prolonged exposure (e.g., to any of the above)	Low back pain; numbness and tingling of wrists and hands
Extreme-reaching low temperatures (e.g., exposure to cold air, tools, materials)	Trauma disorders of upper arms (synovitis, Raynaud phenomenon, bursitis, tendinitis)
Vibration (segmental and whole body)	Carpal tunnel syndrome, rotator cuff syndrome, tendinitis, or Raynaud phenomenon
Forceful exertions (e.g., friction, balance, posture, pace, use of heavy objects)	Ulnar deviation of the wrist
Repetitive functions (e.g., walking, climbing stairs, carrying, shoveling, pushing, lifting objects, using computers)	Localized and/or whole body fatigue (shortness of breath, general weakness, hypoxic injury)

Noise

Noise is sound that has the potential for inflicting harm to the body. The most common pathophysiologic effect of noise is hearing impairment. Noise trauma can be caused by acute loud noise, as well as by the cumulative effects of various intensities, frequencies, and durations of noise. Common irritating noise is caused by numerous sources, including lawn care machinery; wood and metal working with electrical equipment; gun target practice; hunting; snowmobiles; outboard motors; chain saws; and high-decibel, low-frequency speakers. According to the National Institutes of Health, more than 10 million Americans suffer some permanent noise-associated hearing loss, and 20 million are exposed to hazardous noise in work environments.[136] The largest increase in hearing loss from noise occurs in people 45 to 64 years old. Noise pollution is now considered a public health threat. Some evidence exists that noise in hospitals is associated with negative outcomes in patients, both psychologically and physiologically.[137]

Two types of hearing loss are associated with noise: (1) acoustic trauma, or instantaneous damage caused by a single sharply rising wave of sound (e.g., gunfire); and (2) noise-induced hearing loss (NIHL), the more common type, which is the result of prolonged exposure to intense sound (e.g., noise associated with the workplace and leisure-time activities). Acoustic trauma can rupture the eardrum, displace the ossicles of the middle ear, and damage the organ of Corti in the inner ear.

If the offending noise has not been too loud or the exposure to it has not been too long, hearing will return to its original level, a type of hearing loss called a *temporary threshold shift* (TTS). If the noise is louder than a certain value or the exposure time is long, the hearing threshold never returns to its original value, causing a *permanent threshold shift* (PTS). Structural changes associated with TTS, although not fully established, include intracellular changes in the sensory cells (hair cells) and swelling of the auditory nerve endings. With PTS, cochlear blood flow may be impaired and hair cells are damaged with each exposure. Noise-induced hearing loss is gradual and painless. Investigators report that cyclooxygenase-2 (Cox-2) is involved in the pathogenesis of NIHL.[138] Symptoms of noise-induced hearing loss include loudness recruitment and tinnitus. In loudness recruitment, soft sounds are not heard but loud sounds are heard normally. Tinnitus is a constant high-pitched ringing that annoys the individual and contributes to loss of sleep. The Occupational Safety and Health Administration (OSHA) requires industries to protect workers when the exposure is more than an 8-hour period and averages 85 decibels.

MANIFESTATIONS OF CELLULAR INJURY

Cellular Manifestations: Accumulations

An important manifestation of cell injury is the resultant metabolic disturbances of intracellular accumulation of abnormal amounts of various substances. Cellular accumulations, also known as infiltrations, occur as a result of not only sublethal injury sustained by cells but also normal (but inefficient) cell function. Two categories of substances can cause accumulations: (1) *a normal cellular substance* (such as water, protein, lipid, and carbohydrate excesses); or (2) an *abnormal substance*, either endogenous (such as a product of abnormal metabolism or synthesis) or exogenous (e.g., infectious agents or a mineral). These products can accumulate transiently or permanently and can be toxic or harmless. Most accumulations are attributed to four types of mechanisms, all abnormal (Fig. 2.28). Abnormal accumulations of these substances can occur in the cytoplasm (frequently in the lysosomes) or in the nucleus if (1) there is insufficient removal of the normal substance because of altered packaging and transport (for example, fatty change in the liver called *steatosis*); (2) an abnormal substance,

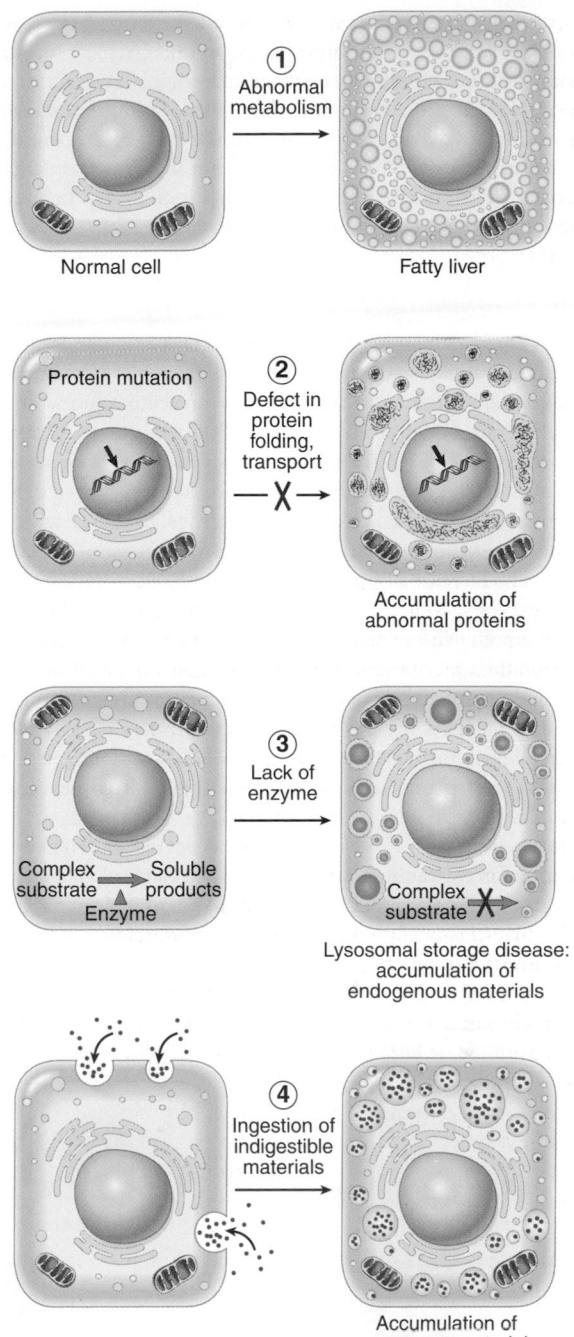

FIGURE 2.28 Mechanisms of Intracellular Accumulations. (From Kumar V et al: Cellular responses to stress and toxic insults: adaptation, injury, and death. In Kumar V, Abbas A, Aster J: *Robbins & Cotran pathologic basis of disease*, ed 9, St Louis, 2015, Saunders.)

often the result of a mutated gene, accumulates because of defects in protein folding, transport, or abnormal degradation; (3) an endogenous substance (normal or abnormal) is not effectively catabolized, usually because of lack of a vital lysosomal enzyme called *storage diseases;* or (4) harmful exogenous materials, such as heavy metals, mineral dusts, or microorganisms, accumulate because of inhalation, ingestion, or infection.

In all storage diseases the cells attempt to digest, or catabolize, the "stored" substances. As a result, excessive amounts of metabolites (products of catabolism) accumulate in the cells and are expelled into the extracellular matrix, where they are taken up by phagocytic cells called *macrophages*. Some of these scavenger cells circulate throughout the body, whereas others remain fixed in certain tissues, such as the liver or spleen. As more and more macrophages and other phagocytes migrate to tissues that are producing excessive metabolites, the affected tissues begin to swell. This is the mechanism that causes enlargement of the liver (hepatomegaly) or the spleen (splenomegaly). Enlargement of one of these organs is a clinical manifestation of many of the storage diseases.

Water

Cellular swelling, the most common degenerative change, is caused by the shift of extracellular water into the cells. In hypoxic injury, movement of fluid and ions into the cell is associated with acute failure of metabolism and loss of ATP production. Normally, the pump that transports sodium ions (Na^+) out of the cell is maintained by the presence of ATP and adenosinetriphosphatase (ATPase), the active transport enzyme. In metabolic failure caused by hypoxia, reduced levels of ATP and ATPase permit sodium to accumulate in the cell, whereas potassium (K^+) diffuses outward. The increase of intracellular sodium concentration increases osmotic pressure, which draws more water into the cell. The cisternae of the ER become distended, rupture, and coalesce to form large vacuoles that isolate the water from the cytoplasm, a process called *vacuolation*. Progressive vacuolation results in cytoplasmic swelling called **oncosis** (which has replaced the old term *hydropic [water] degeneration*) or **vacuolar degeneration** (Fig. 2.29). If cellular swelling affects all cells in an organ, the organ increases in weight and becomes distended and pale.

Cellular swelling is reversible and is considered to be sublethal. It is, in fact, an early manifestation of almost all types of cellular injury, including severe or lethal cell injury. It is also associated with high fever, hypokalemia (abnormally low concentrations of potassium in the blood), and certain infections.

Lipids and Carbohydrates

Certain metabolic disorders result in the abnormal intracellular accumulation of carbohydrates and lipids. The accumulations are caused by inherited disorders with insufficient enzymes or ineffective forms of enzymes. Carbohydrate excess disorders are called **mucopolysaccharidoses (MPSs)**, and accumulations of both carbohydrates and lipids are called **mucolipidoses (MLs)**. MPSs and MLs are classified as **lysosomal storage diseases** because they involve increased storage of carbohydrates or lipids, or both, in lysosomes. Substrate accumulation leads to lysosomal distortion with significant pathologic consequences. These substances may accumulate throughout the body but are found primarily in the cells of the spleen, liver, and central nervous system (CNS). Several of the most prevalent disorders include Tay-Sachs disease, Fabry disease, Gaucher disease, Niemann-Pick disease, the mucopolysaccharidoses, and Pompe disease. Accumulations in cells of the CNS can cause neurologic dysfunction and intellectual disability. The mucopolysaccharidoses are progressive disorders that usually involve multiple organs, including the liver, spleen, heart, and blood vessels. The accumulated mucopolysaccharides are found in reticuloendothelial cells, endothelial cells, intimal smooth muscle cells, and fibroblasts throughout the body. These carbohydrate accumulations can cause corneal clouding, joint stiffness, and intellectual disability.

Although lipids sometimes accumulate in heart, muscle, and kidney cells, the most common site of intracellular lipid accumulation, or **fatty change (steatosis)**, is liver cells. Because hepatic metabolism and secretion of lipids are crucial to proper body function, imbalances and deficiencies in these processes lead to major pathologic changes. The most common cause of fatty change in the liver in developed countries is alcohol abuse. Other causes of fatty change include diabetes mellitus, protein malnutrition, toxins, anoxia, and obesity. As lipids fill the cells, vacuolation pushes the nucleus and other organelles aside. Grossly, the liver looks yellowish and greasy.

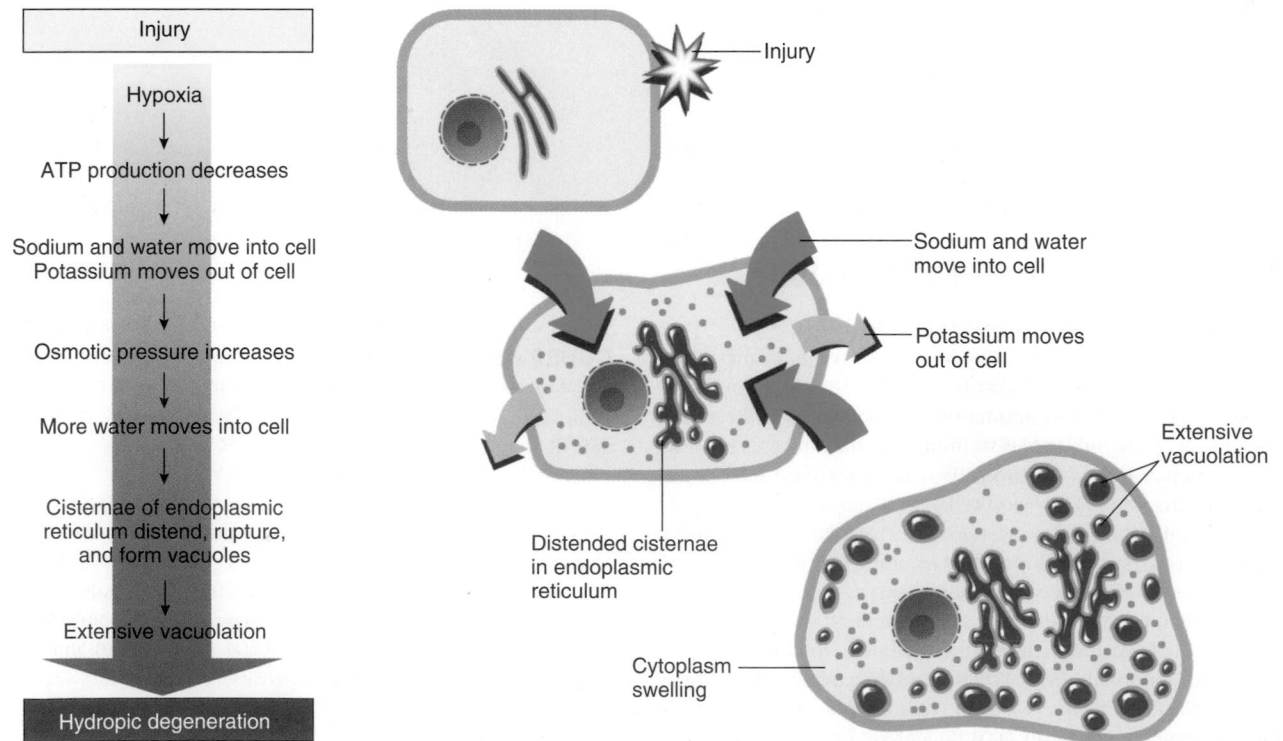

FIGURE 2.29 The Process of Oncosis (Formerly Known as *Hydropic Degeneration*). *ATP*, Adenosine triphosphate.

Lipid accumulation in liver cells occurs after cellular injury sets one or more of the following mechanisms in motion:

1. Increased movement of free fatty acids into the liver (starvation, for example, increases breakdown of triglycerides in adipose tissue, releasing fatty acids that subsequently enter liver cells)
2. Failure of the metabolic process that converts fatty acids to phospholipids, resulting in the preferential conversion of the fatty acids to triglycerides
3. Increased synthesis of triglycerides from fatty acids (increases in amounts of the enzyme α-glycerophosphatase, which can accelerate triglyceride synthesis)
4. Decreased synthesis of apoproteins (lipid-acceptor proteins)
5. Failure of lipids to bind with apoproteins and form lipoproteins
6. Failure of mechanisms that transport lipoproteins out of the cell
7. Direct damage to the endoplasmic reticulum by free radicals released by alcohol's toxic effects

Cholesterol and cholesterol esters can accumulate and are noted in many pathologic states. These states include atherosclerosis, in which atherosclerotic plaques, smooth muscle cells, and macrophages within the intimal layer of the aorta and large arteries are filled with lipid-rich vacuoles of cholesterol and cholesterol esters. Other states include cholesterol-rich deposits in the gallbladder and Niemann-Pick disease (type C), which involve genetic mutations of an enzyme affecting cholesterol transport.

Glycogen

Glycogen storage is important as a readily available energy source in the cytoplasm of normal cells. Intracellular accumulations of glycogen are seen in genetic disorders called *glycogen storage diseases* and in disorders of glucose and glycogen metabolism. Like water and lipid accumulation, glycogen accumulation results in excessive vacuolation of the cytoplasm. The most common cause of glycogen accumulation is diabetes mellitus, a disorder of glucose metabolism.

Proteins

Proteins provide cellular structure and constitute most of the cell's dry weight. The proteins are synthesized on ribosomes in the cytoplasm from the essential amino acids lysine, threonine, leucine, isoleucine, methionine, tryptophan, valine, phenylalanine, and histidine. The accumulation of protein probably damages cells in two ways. First, metabolites (enzymes) produced when the cell attempts to digest some proteins can damage cellular organelles when released from lysosomes. Second, excessive amounts of protein in the cytoplasm push against cellular organelles, disrupting organelle function and intracellular communication.

Excess protein accumulates primarily in the epithelial cells of the renal convoluted tubule of the nephron unit and in the antibody-forming plasma cells (B lymphocytes) of the immune system. Several types of renal disorders cause excessive excretion of protein molecules in the urine (proteinuria). Normally, little or no protein is present in the urine, and its presence in significant amounts indicates cellular injury and altered cellular function in the glomerular membrane.

Accumulations of protein in B lymphocytes can occur during active synthesis of antibodies in the immune response. The excess aggregates of protein are called *Russell bodies*. Russell bodies have been identified in multiple myeloma (plasma cell tumor) (see Chapter 30).

Mutations in protein can slow protein folding, resulting in the accumulation of partially folded intermediates. An example is α_1-antitrypsin deficiency, which can cause emphysema. Certain types of cell injury are associated with the accumulation of cytoskeletal proteins. For example, the *neurofibrillary tangle* found in the brain in Alzheimer disease contains cytoskeletal protein fibrils.

Pigments

Pigment accumulations may be normal or abnormal, endogenous (produced within the body) or exogenous (produced outside the body). Endogenous pigments are derived, for example, from amino acids (e.g., tyrosine, tryptophan). They include melanin and the blood proteins—porphyrins, hemoglobin, and hemosiderin (ferritin). Lipid-rich pigments such as lipofuscin (the aging pigment or spots) give a yellow-brown color to cells undergoing slow, regressive, and often atrophic changes. The most common exogenous pigment is carbon (coal dust), a pervasive air pollutant in urban areas. Inhaled carbon interacts with lung macrophages and is transported by lymphatic vessels to regional lymph nodes. This accumulation blackens lung tissues and involved lymph nodes. Other exogenous pigments include mineral dusts containing silica and iron particles, lead, silver salts, and dyes for tattoos.

Melanin. Melanin accumulates in epithelial cells (keratinocytes) of the skin and retina. It is an extremely important pigment because it protects the skin against long exposure to sunlight and is considered an essential factor in the prevention of skin cancer. Ultraviolet light (e.g., sunlight) stimulates the synthesis of melanin, which probably absorbs ultraviolet rays during subsequent exposure. Melanin also may protect the skin by trapping the injurious free radicals produced by the action of ultraviolet light on skin.

Melanin is a brown-black pigment derived from the amino acid tyrosine. It is synthesized by epidermal cells called *melanocytes* and is stored in membrane-bound cytoplasmic vesicles called *melanosomes*. Melanosomes are particularly abundant in projections of melanocytic cytoplasm, called *dendrites*, from which they are transmitted to neighboring keratinocytes, where melanin accumulation occurs. (Keratinocytes, which constitute 95% of epidermal cells, are discussed with other skin components in Chapter 47.) The dendritic melanocytes form bridges between neighboring keratinocytes and inject melanosomes into the keratinocytes by an unknown mechanism.

Melanin also can accumulate in melanophores (melanin-containing pigment cells), macrophages, or other phagocytic cells in the dermis. Presumably these cells acquire the melanin from nearby melanocytes or from pigment that has been extruded from dying epidermal cells. This is the mechanism that causes freckles.

Although rare, melanin accumulation occurs in the skin of individuals with Addison disease (adrenocortical insufficiency resulting from disorders of the adrenal cortex; see Chapter 22). The increased melanogenesis (melanin production) seen in Addison disease is caused by the loss of feedback control of adrenocorticotropic hormone (ACTH). Decreased hormonal secretion from the adrenal gland causes increased release of ACTH from the pituitary gland. In Addison disease the increase in melanin production occurs presumably because a segment of the ACTH molecule contains the melanin-stimulating hormone (MSH).

An increase in melanin concentration also occurs in the benign form of "pigmented moles" called *nevi*. Malignant melanoma is a cancerous skin tumor that contains melanin and invades normal tissue early and widely and often leads to death.

A decrease in melanin production occurs in the inherited disorder of melanin metabolism called *albinism*. Albinism is often diffuse, involving all the skin, the eyes, and the hair. Albinism is also related to phenylalanine metabolism. In classic forms of this disease, the person with albinism is unable to convert tyrosine to dopa (3,4-dihydroxyphenylalanine), an intermediary in melanin biosynthesis. Melanin-producing cells are present in normal numbers, but they are unable to make melanin. Individuals with albinism are very sensitive to sunlight and quickly become sunburned. They are also at high risk for skin cancer.

Hemoproteins. Hemoproteins are among the most essential of the normal endogenous pigments. They include hemoglobin and the oxidative enzymes—the cytochromes. Knowledge of iron uptake, metabolism, excretion, and storage is central to an understanding of disorders involving these pigments (see Chapter 28). Hemoprotein accumulations in cells are caused by excessive storage of iron, which is transferred to the cells from the bloodstream. Iron enters the blood from three primary sources: (1) tissue stores, (2) the intestinal mucosa, and (3) macrophages that remove and destroy dead or defective red blood cells. The amount of iron in blood plasma also depends on the metabolism of the major iron-transport protein, *transferrin*.

Iron is stored in tissue cells in two forms: as ferritin and, when greater levels of iron are present, as hemosiderin. Hemosiderin is a yellow-brown pigment derived from hemoglobin. With pathologic states, excesses of iron cause hemosiderin to accumulate within cells. Accumulation of hemosiderin often occurs in areas of bruising and hemorrhage and in the lungs and spleen after congestion caused by heart failure. With a local hemorrhage, the skin first appears red-blue and then lysis of the escaped red blood cells occurs, causing the hemoglobin to be transformed to hemosiderin. The color changes noted in bruising reflect this transformation.

Hemosiderosis is a condition in which excess iron is stored as hemosiderin in the cells of many organs and tissues. This condition is common in individuals who have received repeated blood transfusions or prolonged parenteral administration of iron. Hemosiderosis is also associated with increased absorption of dietary iron, conditions in which iron storage and transport are impaired, and hemolytic anemia. Excessive alcohol ingestion also can lead to hemosiderosis. Normally, absorption of excessive dietary iron is prevented by an iron absorption process in the intestines. Failure of this process can lead to total-body iron

accumulations in the range of 60 to 80 grams (g), compared with normal iron stores of 4.5 to 5 g. Excessive accumulations of iron, such as occur in hemochromatosis (a genetic disorder of iron metabolism and the most severe example of iron overload), are associated with liver and pancreatic cell damage.

Bilirubin is a normal yellow-to-green pigment of bile derived from the porphyrin structure of hemoglobin. Excesses of bilirubin within cells and tissues cause jaundice (icterus), or yellowing of the skin. Jaundice occurs when the bilirubin level exceeds 1.5 to 2 mg/dL of plasma, compared with the normal values of 0.4 to 1 mg/dL. Hyperbilirubinemia occurs with (1) diseases that cause destruction of red blood cells (erythrocytes), such as in hemolytic jaundice; (2) diseases affecting the metabolism and excretion of bilirubin in the liver; and (3) diseases that cause obstruction of the common bile duct, such as gallstones or pancreatic tumors.

Certain drugs, specifically chlorpromazine and other phenothiazine derivatives, estrogenic hormones, and halothane (an anesthetic), can cause the obstruction of normal bile flow through the liver.

Because unconjugated bilirubin is lipid soluble, it can injure the lipid components of the plasma membrane. Albumin, a plasma protein, provides significant protection by binding unconjugated bilirubin in plasma. Unconjugated bilirubin causes two cellular effects: uncoupling of oxidative phosphorylation and loss of cellular proteins. These two effects could cause structural injury to the various membranes of the cell.

Calcium

Calcium salts accumulate in both injured and dead tissues (Fig. 2.30). An important mechanism of cellular calcification is the influx of

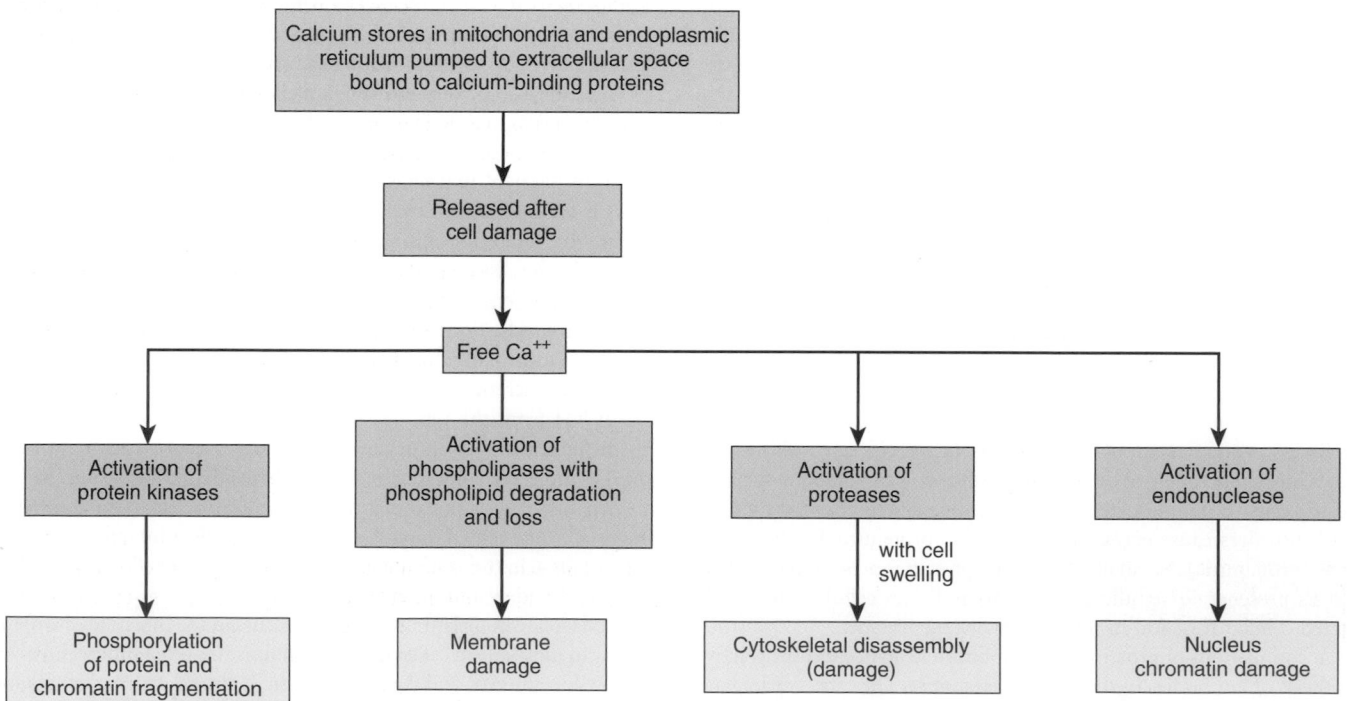

FIGURE 2.30 Free Cytosolic Calcium: A Destructive Agent. Calcium is normally removed from the cytosol by adenosine triphosphate (ATP)–dependent calcium pumps. In normal cells, calcium is bound to buffering proteins, such as calbindin or paralbumin, and is contained in the endoplasmic reticulum and the mitochondria. If there is abnormal permeability of calcium ion channels, direct damage to membranes, or depletion of ATP (i.e., hypoxic injury), calcium level increases in the cytosol. If the free calcium cannot be buffered or pumped out of cells, uncontrolled enzyme activation takes place, causing further damage. Uncontrolled entry of calcium into the cytosol is an important final pathway in many causes of cell death.

extracellular calcium in injured mitochondria. Another mechanism that causes calcium accumulation in alveoli (gas-exchange airways of the lungs), gastric epithelium, and renal tubules is the excretion of acid at these sites, leading to the local production of hydroxyl ions. Hydroxyl ions result in precipitation of calcium hydroxide ($Ca[OH]_2$) and hydroxyapatite ($3Ca_3[PO_4]_2Ca[OH]_2$), a mixed salt. Damage occurs when calcium salts clump and harden, interfering with normal cellular structure and function.

Pathologic calcification can be dystrophic or metastatic. **Dystrophic calcification** occurs in dying and dead tissues in areas of necrosis (types of necrosis: coagulative, caseous, liquefactive, fat). It is present in chronic tuberculosis of the lungs and lymph nodes, in arteries with advanced atherosclerosis (narrowing as a result of plaque accumulation), and often in injured heart valves (Fig. 2.31). Calcification of the heart valves interferes with opening and closing of the valves, causing heart murmurs. Calcification of the coronary arteries predisposes them to severe narrowing and thrombosis, which can lead to myocardial infarction. Another site of dystrophic calcification is the center of tumors. Over time, the center is deprived of oxygen supply, dies, and becomes calcified. The calcium salts appear as gritty, clumped granules that can become hard

as stone. When several layers clump together, they resemble grains of sand and are called **psammoma bodies**.

The exact pathogenic mechanisms responsible for dystrophic calcification are unknown. A popular hypothesis is that with progressive deterioration of dead cells, the exposed denatured (changed) proteins preferentially bind with phosphate ions. The phosphate ions then react with calcium ions to form deposits of phosphate carbonate precipitates and, sometimes, crystalline formations of calcium phosphate. Dystrophic calcification develops slowly and is an explicit marker for the site of dead cells.

Metastatic calcification consists of mineral deposits that occur in undamaged normal tissues as the result of hypercalcemia (excess of calcium in the blood). Conditions that cause hypercalcemia include hyperparathyroidism, toxic levels of vitamin D, hyperthyroidism, idiopathic hypercalcemia of infancy, and Addison disease (adrenocortical insufficiency). Additionally, hypercalcemia is linked with systemic sarcoidosis, milk-alkali syndrome, and the increased bone demineralization that results from bone tumors, leukemia, and disseminated cancers. Hypercalcemia also can occur in some instances of advanced renal failure with phosphate retention, resulting in hyperparathyroidism. As phosphate levels increase, the activity of the parathyroid gland increases, causing higher levels of circulating calcium.

Urate

In humans, uric acid (**urate**) is the major end product of purine catabolism because of the absence of the enzyme urate oxidase. Serum urate concentration is, in general, stable: approximately 5 mg/dL in postpubertal males and 4.1 mg/dL in postpubertal females. Disturbances in maintaining serum urate levels result in hyperuricemia and deposition of sodium urate crystals in the tissues, leading to painful disorders collectively called *gout*. These disorders include acute arthritis, chronic gouty arthritis, tophus (firm nodular subcutaneous deposits of urate crystals surrounded by fibrosis), and nephritis (inflammation of the nephron). Chronic hyperuricemia results in the deposition of urate in tissues, cell injury, and inflammation. Because urate crystals are not degraded by lysosomal enzymes, they persist in dead cells.

Systemic Manifestations

Systemic manifestations of cellular injury include a general sense of fatigue and malaise, a loss of well-being, and an alteration in appetite. Fever is frequently present because of biochemicals produced during the inflammatory response. Table 2.12 summarizes the most significant systemic manifestations of cellular injury.

CELLULAR DEATH

In response to significant external stimuli, cell injury becomes irreversible and cells are forced to die. Cell death has historically been classified as necrosis and apoptosis. **Necrosis** is characterized by rapid loss of the plasma membrane structure, organelle swelling, mitochondrial dysfunction, and the lack of typical features of apoptosis.[139] Apoptosis is known as a regulated or programmed cell process characterized by the "dropping off" of cellular fragments called *apoptotic bodies*. Until recently, only necrosis was considered passive or accidental, occurring after severe and sudden injury. It is the main outcome in several common injuries including ischemia, toxin exposure, certain infections, and trauma. It is now understood that under certain conditions, such as activation of death proteases, necrosis also can be driven by *regulated* or *programmed* molecular pathways.[140] Hence, the new term used is **programmed necrosis**, or **necroptosis**. Historically, programmed cell death only referred to apoptosis; now necrotic cell death is known to depend on genetically defined signaling pathways that have been studied in the

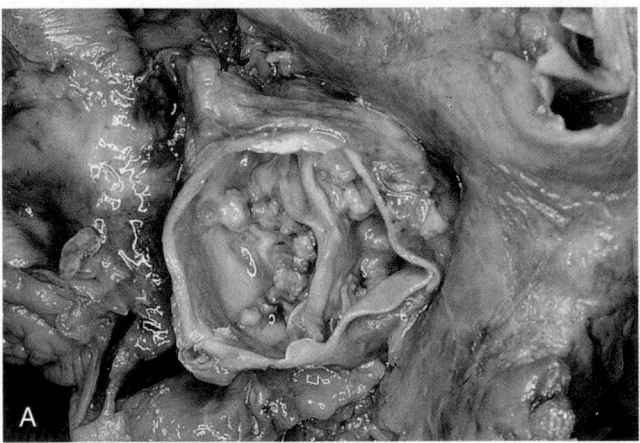

A

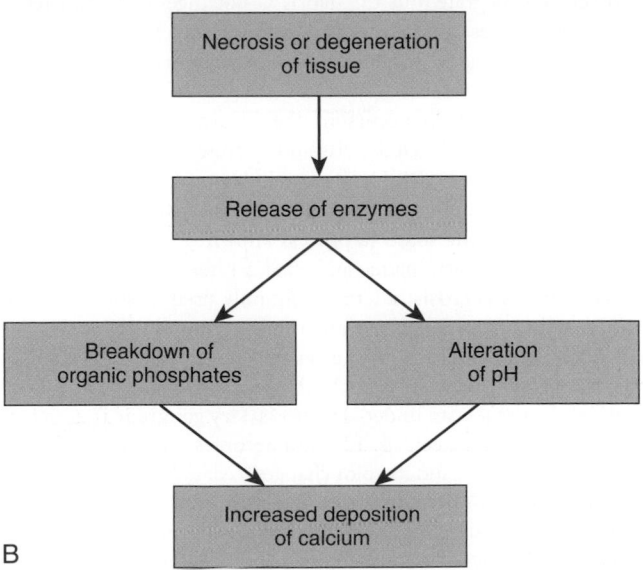

B

FIGURE 2.31 Aortic Valve Calcification. A, Calcified aortic valve. This change is an example of dystrophic calcification. **B,** Algorithm showing the dystrophic mechanism of calcification. (**A** from Damjanov I: *Pathology for the health professions,* ed 4, St Louis, 2012, Elsevier/Saunders.)

TABLE 2.12   SYSTEMIC MANIFESTATIONS OF CELLULAR INJURY

MANIFESTATION	CAUSE
Fever	Release of endogenous pyrogens (interleukin-1, tumor necrosis factor-alpha [TNF-α], prostaglandins) from bacteria or macrophages; acute inflammatory response
Increased heart rate	Increase in oxidative metabolic processes resulting from fever
Increase in number of leukocytes (leukocytosis)	Increase in total number of white blood cells because of infection; normal is 5000–10,000/mm³ (increase is directly related to the severity of the infection)
Pain	Various mechanisms, such as release of bradykinins, obstruction, pressure
Presence of cellular enzymes in extracellular fluid	Release of enzymes from cells of tissue*
Lactate dehydrogenase (LDH) (LDH isoenzymes)	Release from red blood cells, liver, kidney, skeletal muscle
Creatine kinase (CK) (CK isoenzymes)	Release from skeletal muscle, brain, heart
Aspartate aminotransferase (AST)	Release from heart, liver, skeletal muscle, kidney, pancreas
Alanine aminotransferase (ALT)	Release from liver, kidney, heart
Alkaline phosphatase (ALP)	Release from liver, bone
Amylase	Release from pancreas
Aldolase	Release from skeletal muscle, heart
Troponins	Release from heart

*The rapidity of enzyme transfer is a function of the weight of the enzyme and the concentration gradient across the cellular membrane. The specific metabolic and excretory rates of the enzymes determine how long levels of enzymes remain elevated.

pathophysiology of diseases only recently. Fig. 2.32 illustrates the structural changes in cell injury resulting in necrosis or apoptosis. Table 2.13 compares the unique features of necrosis and apoptosis. Other forms of cell loss include autophagy.

Necrosis

Cellular death eventually leads to cellular dissolution, or necrosis. Necrosis is the sum of cellular changes after local cell death and the process of cellular self-digestion, known as *autodigestion* or *autolysis*. Cells die long before any necrotic changes are noted by light microscopy. The structural signs that indicate irreversible injury and progression to necrosis are dense clumping and progressive disruption of genetic material and disruption of the plasma and organelle membranes. Because membrane integrity is lost, necrotic cell contents leak out and may cause the signaling of inflammation in surrounding tissue. In later stages of necrosis, most organelles are disrupted, and karyolysis (nuclear dissolution and lysis of chromatin from the action of hydrolytic enzymes) is underway. In some cells, the nucleus shrinks and becomes a small, dense mass of genetic material (pyknosis). The pyknotic nucleus eventually dissolves (by karyolysis) as a result of the action of hydrolytic lysosomal enzymes on DNA.

External cellular injury that can cause necrosis involves damage to mitochondria with the formation of mitochondrial permeability transition pores in the outer membrane. These channels (pores) allow the spreading of the proton potential, resulting in failure of ATP generation and death of the cell. Emerging evidence shows that programmed necrosis is associated with development, tissue damage during acute pancreatitis, and retinal detachment; and provides an innate immune response to viral infection, thus challenging the historic view of necrosis as passive cell death occurring in a disorganized or unregulated manner.[141,142]

Different types of necroses tend to occur in different organs or tissues and sometimes can indicate the mechanism or cause of cellular injury. The four major types of necroses are coagulative, liquefactive, caseous, and fatty. Another type, gangrenous necrosis, is *not* a distinctive type of cell death but refers to larger areas of tissue death.

Coagulative necrosis, which occurs primarily in the kidneys, heart, and adrenal glands, commonly results from hypoxia caused by severe ischemia or hypoxia caused by chemical injury, especially ingestion of mercuric chloride (Fig. 2.33, A). Coagulation is caused by protein denaturation, which causes the protein albumin to change from a gelatinous, transparent state to a firm, opaque state, similar to that of a cooked egg white. The necrotic tissues appear firm and slightly swollen. The area of coagulative necrosis is called an infarct.

Liquefactive necrosis commonly results from ischemic injury to neurons and glial cells in the brain (Fig. 2.33, B). Dead brain tissue is readily affected by liquefactive necrosis because brain cells are rich in the digestive hydrolytic enzymes and lipids, and the brain contains little connective tissue. As the cells are digested by their own hydrolases, the tissue becomes soft, liquefies, and is walled off from healthy tissue, forming cysts.

Liquefactive necrosis can also result from bacterial infection, particularly by staphylococci, streptococci, and *Escherichia coli*. In this case the hydrolases are released from the lysosomes of neutrophils (phagocytes attracted to the infected area to kill the bacteria). Liquefaction of bacterial cells and neighboring tissue cells by neutrophilic hydrolases results in the accumulation of pus.

Caseous necrosis, which commonly results from tuberculous pulmonary infection, particularly *Mycobacterium tuberculosis*, is a combination of coagulative and liquefactive necrosis (Fig. 2.33, C). The dead cells disintegrate, but the debris is not digested completely by hydrolases. Tissues appear soft and granular and resemble clumped cheese, hence its name. A granulomatous inflammatory wall encloses areas of caseous necrosis.

Fat necrosis, which occurs in the breast, pancreas, and other abdominal structures, is cellular dissolution caused by powerful enzymes called *lipases* (Fig. 2.33, D). Lipases break down triglycerides, releasing free fatty acids, which then combine with calcium, magnesium, and sodium ions, creating soaps (a process known as *saponification*). The necrotic tissue appears opaque and chalk white.

Gangrenous necrosis, a term commonly used in surgical clinical practice, refers to death of tissue and results from severe hypoxic injury, commonly occurring because of arteriosclerosis, or blockage, of major arteries, especially in the lower leg. With hypoxia and subsequent bacterial invasion, the tissues can undergo necrosis. Dry gangrene is usually the result of coagulative necrosis. The skin becomes very dry and shrinks, resulting in wrinkles, and its color changes to dark brown or black (Fig. 2.34). Wet gangrene develops when neutrophils invade the site, causing liquefactive necrosis. This usually occurs in internal organs, causing the site to become cold, swollen, and black. A foul odor is present, produced by pus, and if systemic symptoms become severe, death can ensue.

Gas gangrene, a special type of gangrene, is caused by infection of injured tissue by one of many species of *Clostridium*. These anaerobic

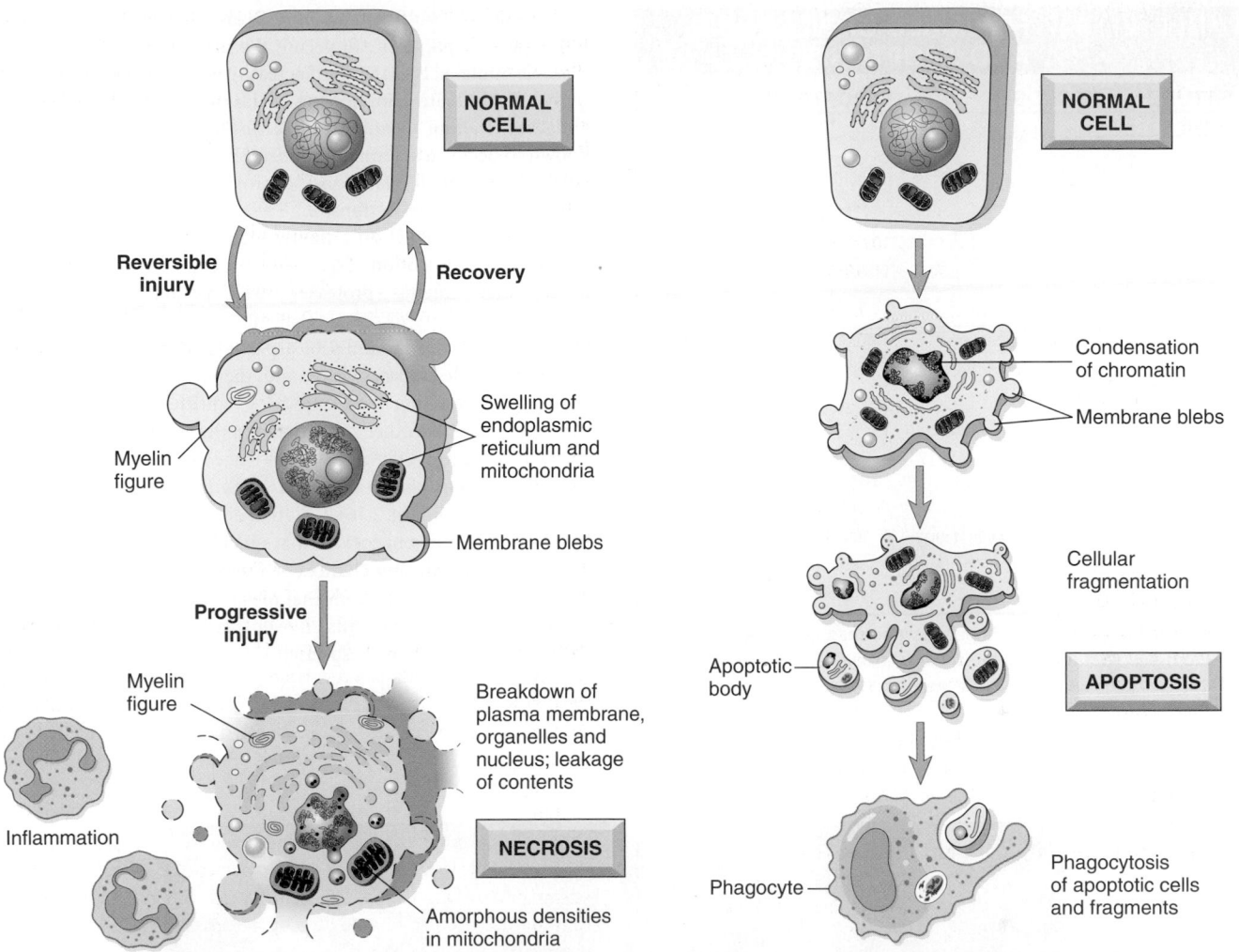

FIGURE 2.32 Schematic Illustration of the Morphologic Changes in Cell Injury Culminating in Necrosis or Apoptosis. Myelin figures come from degenerating cellular membranes and are noted within the cytoplasm or extracellularly. (From Kumar V et al: Cellular responses to stress and toxic insults: adaptation, injury, and death. In Kumar V, Abbas A, Aster J: *Robbins & Cotran pathologic basis of disease*, ed 9, St Louis, 2015, Saunders.)

bacteria produce hydrolytic enzymes and toxins that destroy connective tissue and cellular membranes and cause bubbles of gas to form in muscle cells. Gas gangrene can be fatal if enzymes lyse the membranes of red blood cells, destroying their oxygen-carrying capacity. Death is the result of shock. The condition is treated with antitoxins and supplemental oxygen delivered in a hyperbaric (pressurized) chamber.

Apoptosis

Apoptosis ("dropping off") is an important distinct type of cell death that differs from necrosis in several ways (see Fig. 2.32 and Table 2.13). Apoptosis is an active process of cellular self-destruction—called *programmed cell death (type I)*—in both normal and pathologic tissue changes. It depends on a tightly regulated cellular program for its initiation and execution.[143] The average adult may create 10 billion new cells every day and destroy the same number.[144] Normal physiologic death by apoptosis occurs during embryogenesis; involution of hormone-dependent tissue after hormone withdrawal, such as involution of the lactating breast after weaning; cell loss in proliferating cell populations, such as immature lymphocytes in the bone marrow or thymus that do not express appropriate receptors; and elimination of possibly harmful lymphocytes that may be self-reactive and cause death of cells after

they perform useful functions (e.g., neutrophils after an acute inflammatory reaction). Death by apoptosis causes loss of cells in many pathologic states including the following:

- *Severe cell injury.* When cell injury exceeds repair mechanisms, the cell triggers apoptosis. DNA damage can result either directly or indirectly from production of free radicals.
- *Accumulation of misfolded proteins.* This may result from genetic mutations or free radicals. Excessive accumulation of misfolded proteins in the ER leads to a condition known as endoplasmic reticulum stress (ER stress) (see Chapter 1). ER stress results in apoptotic cell death. This mechanism has been linked to several degenerative diseases of the CNS and other organs (Fig. 2.35).
- *Infections (particularly viral).* Apoptosis may be the result of the virus directly or indirectly by the host immune response. Cytotoxic T lymphocytes respond to viral infections by inducing apoptosis and, therefore, eliminating the infectious cells. This process can cause tissue damage and it is the same for cell death in tumors and rejection of tissue transplants.
- *Obstruction in tissue ducts.* In organs with duct obstruction, including the pancreas, kidney, and parotid gland, apoptosis causes pathologic atrophy.

TABLE 2.13   FEATURES OF NECROSIS AND APOPTOSIS

FEATURE	NECROSIS	APOPTOSIS
Cell size	Enlarged (swelling)	Reduced (shrinkage)
Nucleus	Pyknosis → karyorrhexis → karyolysis	Fragmentation into nucleosome-size fragments
Plasma membrane	Disrupted	Intact; altered structure, especially orientation of lipids
Cellular contents	Enzymatic digestion; may leak out of cell	Intact; may be released in apoptotic bodies
Adjacent inflammation	Frequent	No
Physiologic or pathologic role	Invariably pathologic (culmination of irreversible cell injury)	Often physiologic, means of eliminating unwanted cells; may be pathologic after some forms of cell injury, especially DNA damage

From Kumar V et al: Cellular responses to stress and toxic insults: adaptation, injury, and death. In Kumar V, Abbas A, Fausto N: *Robbins & Cotran pathologic basis of disease,* ed 8, St Louis, 2010, Saunders.

Excessive or insufficient apoptosis is known as *dysregulated apoptosis.* A low rate of apoptosis can permit the survival of abnormal cells, for example, mutated cells that can increase cancer risk. Defective apoptosis may not eliminate lymphocytes that react against host tissue (self-antigens), leading to autoimmune disorders. Increased apoptosis is known to occur in several neurodegenerative diseases, ischemic injury (such as myocardial infarction and stroke), and death of virus-infected cells in many viral infections.

Apoptosis depends on a tightly regulated cellular program for its initiation and execution. This death program involves enzymes that divide other proteins—proteases, which are activated by proteolytic activity in response to signals that induce apoptosis. These proteases are called caspases, a family of aspartic acid–specific proteases. The activated suicide caspases cleave and, thereby, activate other members of the family, resulting in an amplifying "suicide" cascade. The activated caspases then cleave other key proteins in the cell, killing the cell quickly and neatly. The two different pathways that converge on caspase activation are called the *mitochondrial (intrinsic) pathway* and the *death receptor (extrinsic) pathway* (Fig. 2.36). Cells that die by apoptosis release chemical factors that recruit phagocytes that quickly engulf the remains of the dead cell, thus reducing chances of inflammation. With necrosis, cell death is not tidy because cells that die as a result of acute injury swell, burst, and spill their contents all over their neighbors, causing a likely damaging inflammatory response.

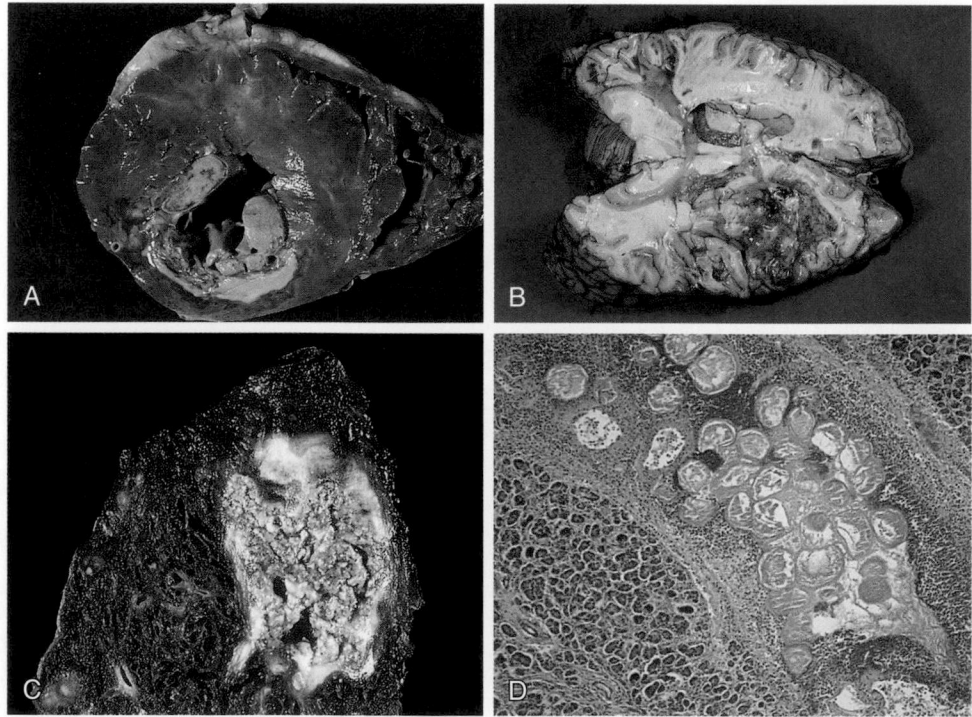

FIGURE 2.33 Types of Necrosis. **A,** Coagulative necrosis of myocardium of posterior wall of left ventricle of heart. A large anemic *(white)* infarct is readily apparent; note also the necrosis of papillary muscle. **B,** Liquefactive necrosis of the brain. The area of infarction is softened as a result of liquefactive necrosis. **C,** Caseous necrosis. Tuberculosis of the lung, with a large area of caseous necrosis containing yellow-white and cheesy debris. **D,** Fat necrosis of pancreas. Interlobular adipocytes are necrotic; these are surrounded by acute inflammatory cells. (**A** and **D** from Damjanov I, Linder J, editors: *Anderson's pathology,* ed 10, St Louis, 1996, Mosby. **B** from Damjanov I: *Pathology for the health professions,* ed 5, St Louis, 2016, Saunders. **C** from Kumar V, Abbas A, Aster J: *Robbins & Cotran pathologic basis of disease,* ed 9, Philadelphia, 2015, Saunders.)

Autophagy

The term **autophagy** is Greek, meaning "eating of self" (Fig. 2.37). Autophagy, as a "recycling factory," is a self-destructive process and a survival mechanism. It degrades cytoplasmic components and organelles in lysosomes (a catabolic function) and salvages key metabolites to promote metabolic and nutrient homeostasis (an anabolic function).[145] Autophagy with its central role in cell homeostasis is considered important in diverse processes such as development, cell proliferation, remodeling, aging, cancer, heart disease, neurodegeneration diseases, antigen presentation, inflammation, infection, metabolic diseases, and cell death. Autophagy is very complex and tissue dependent.[146] When cells are starved or nutrient deprived, the autophagic process institutes

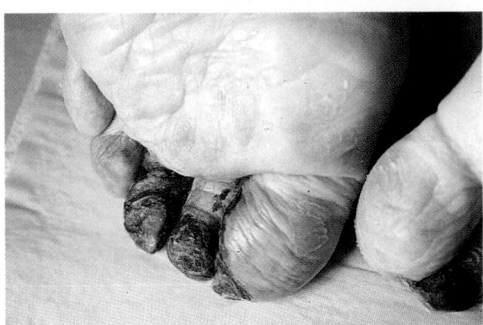

FIGURE 2.34 Gangrene of Toes. Dry gangrene. (From Damjanov I: *Pathology for the health professions,* ed 4, Philadelphia, 2012, Saunders.)

cannibalization and recycles the digested contents.[147,148] Autophagy can maintain cellular metabolism under starvation conditions and remove damaged organelles and misfolded proteins under stress conditions, improving the survival of cells.

With metabolic stress, autophagy provides ATP and other macromolecules as energy sources to enable cell survival; if, however, the stress is excessive, cells may progress to autophagic programmed cell death, which is distinct from apoptosis[149-151] (Fig. 2.38).

Autophagic cell death (**type II programmed cell death**) is characterized by double- or multiple-membrane cytoplasmic vesicles engulfing bulk cytoplasm/cytoplasmic organelles, such as mitochondria and ER. However, in **type I programmed cell death** apoptosis is largely the result of caspase activation and destruction of the cellular components.

Autophagy has been highlighted in cancer. In some contexts, autophagy suppresses tumor development; in most contexts, autophagy facilitates tumor development.[152] Cancers can use autophagy to survive microenvironmental stresses and to increase growth and aggressiveness. The mechanisms of autophagy that promote cancer include suppressing induction of the p53 tumor suppressor protein and maintaining the function of mitochondria.[152] Research efforts are also directed to inhibit autophagy to improve cancer therapy.

Autophagy has been widely characterized in cardiomyocytes, cardiac fibroblasts, endothelial cells, vascular smooth muscle cells, and macrophages.[153] Optimal autophagic activity may be critical to the maintenance of cardiovascular homeostasis and function, and excessive or insufficient levels of autophagic flux can each contribute to cardiac disease.[153]

As a critical garbage collecting and garbage recycling process in healthy cells, the process of autophagy decelerates and may become less discriminating as the cell ages. Consequently, harmful agents accumulate

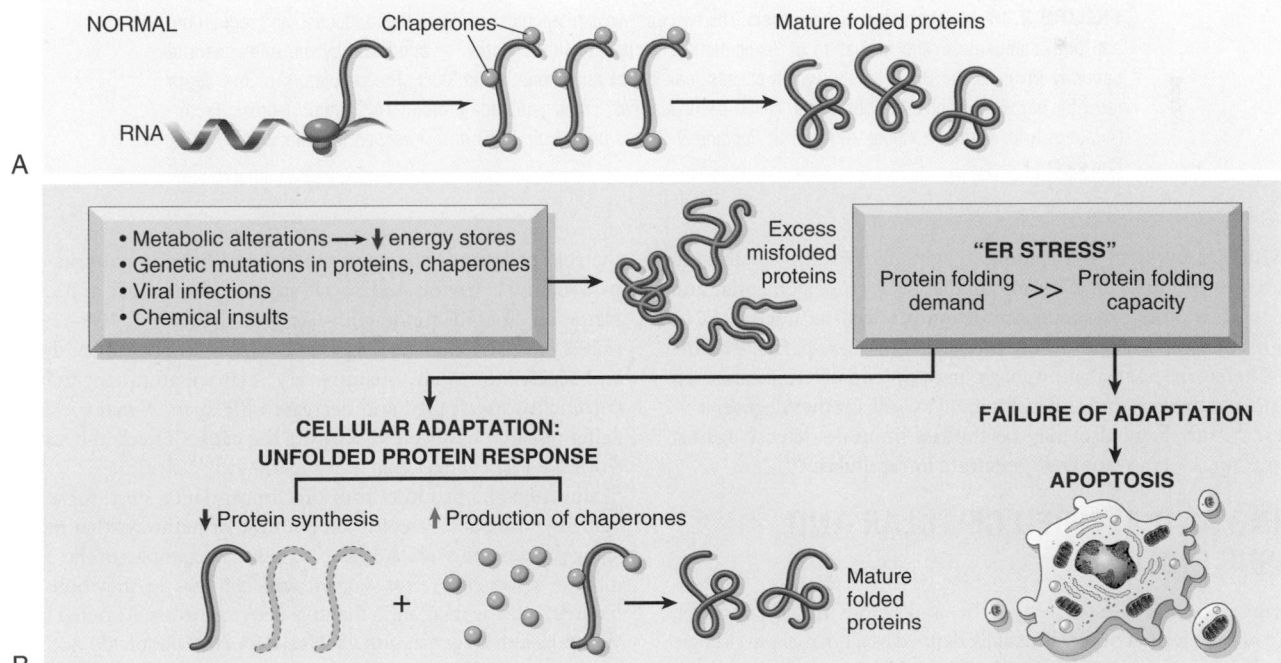

FIGURE 2.35 The Unfolded Protein Response, Endoplasmic Reticulum (ER) Stress, and Apoptosis. **A,** In normal or healthy cells the newly made proteins are folded with help from chaperones and then incorporated into the cell or secreted. **B,** Various stressors can cause ER stress whereby the cell is challenged to cope with the increased load of misfolded proteins. The accumulation of the protein load initiates the *unfolded protein response* in the ER; if restoration of the protein fails, the cell dies by apoptosis. An example of a disease caused by misfolding of proteins is Alzheimer disease. (From Kumar V, Abbas A, Aster J: *Robbins & Cotran pathologic basis of disease,* ed 9, Philadelphia, 2015, Saunders.)

MITOCHONDRIAL (INTRINSIC) PATHWAY   DEATH RECEPTOR (EXTRINSIC) PATHWAY

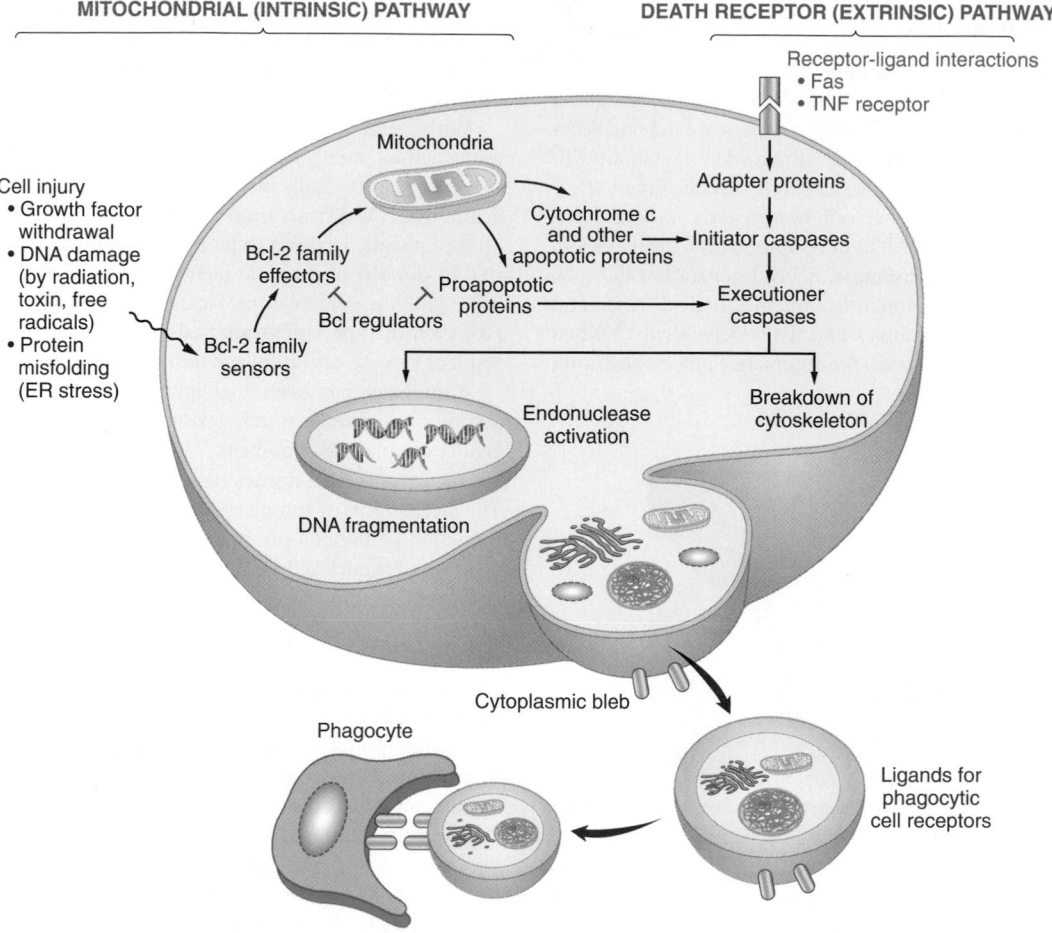

FIGURE 2.36 Mechanisms of Apoptosis. The two pathways of apoptosis differ in their induction and regulation, and both culminate in the activation of "executioner" caspases. The induction of apoptosis by the mitochondrial pathway involves the Bcl-2 family, which causes leakage of mitochondrial proteins. The regulators of the death receptor pathway involve the proteases, called caspases. *Fas,* Transmembrane protein; *TNF,* tumor necrosis factor. (Adapted from Kumar V, Abbas A, Aster J: *Robbins & Cotran pathologic basis of disease,* ed 9, Philadelphia, 2015, Saunders.)

in cells, damaging them and leading to aging. For example, failure to clear protein products in neurons of the CNS cause dementia, and failure to clear ROS-producing mitochondria lead to nuclear DNA mutations and cancer. Thus, these processes may even partially define aging. Therefore, normal autophagy may potentially rejuvenate an organism and prevent cancer development as well as other degenerative diseases.[154] Autophagy also may be the last immune defense against infectious microorganisms that penetrate intracellularly.[155]

AGING AND ALTERED CELLULAR AND TISSUE BIOLOGY

The terms aging and life span tend to be used synonymously; however, they are not equivalent. *Aging* is usually defined as a normal physiologic process that is universal and inevitable, whereas *life span* is the time from birth to death and has been used to study the aging process.[156] **Aging** is the progressive loss of tissues and organs over time.[157] Aging also is a risk factor for a wide variety of chronic diseases. Investigators are focused on genetic, epigenetic, inflammatory, oxidative stress, and metabolic origins of aging. Of interest is the study of genetic signatures in humans with exceptional longevity and the identification of epigenetic mechanisms that modulate gene expression. Other areas being investigated include

the role of intrauterine environment and lifelong patterns of health; personality, behavior, and social support; hormonal and circulating factors, such as insulin/insulin-like growth factor 1 (IGF-1) signaling; mitochondrial dysfunction; and the contributions of cellular dysfunction and senescence to an inflammatory microenvironment that leads to chronic disease, frailty, and decreased life span. A major challenge of aging research has been to separate the causes of cell and tissue aging from the vast changes that accompany it.[158,159]

Investigators propose from preclinical data a need for a "unifying aging hypothesis" as a common pathway or pathways that regulate the aging process and associated disease risks.[160] Examples of these pathways include senescence, proteostasis, and changes in metabolism. Yet, a recurring theme in aging is that it is heterogeneous. As noted in a recent World Health Organization (WHO) report,[161] people do not age at the same rate with the same prevalence of age-related diseases.[160] A recent study in immune factors in identical twins found increasing differences between identical twins, with increasing age suggesting marked influence of nonheritable factors or environmental factors.[162]

Senescence is a process of permanent proliferative arrest on cells in response to various stressors and may be an important contributor to aging and age-related disease.[163] Senescent cells accumulate in various tissues over time and may contribute to tissue dysfunction. Investigators

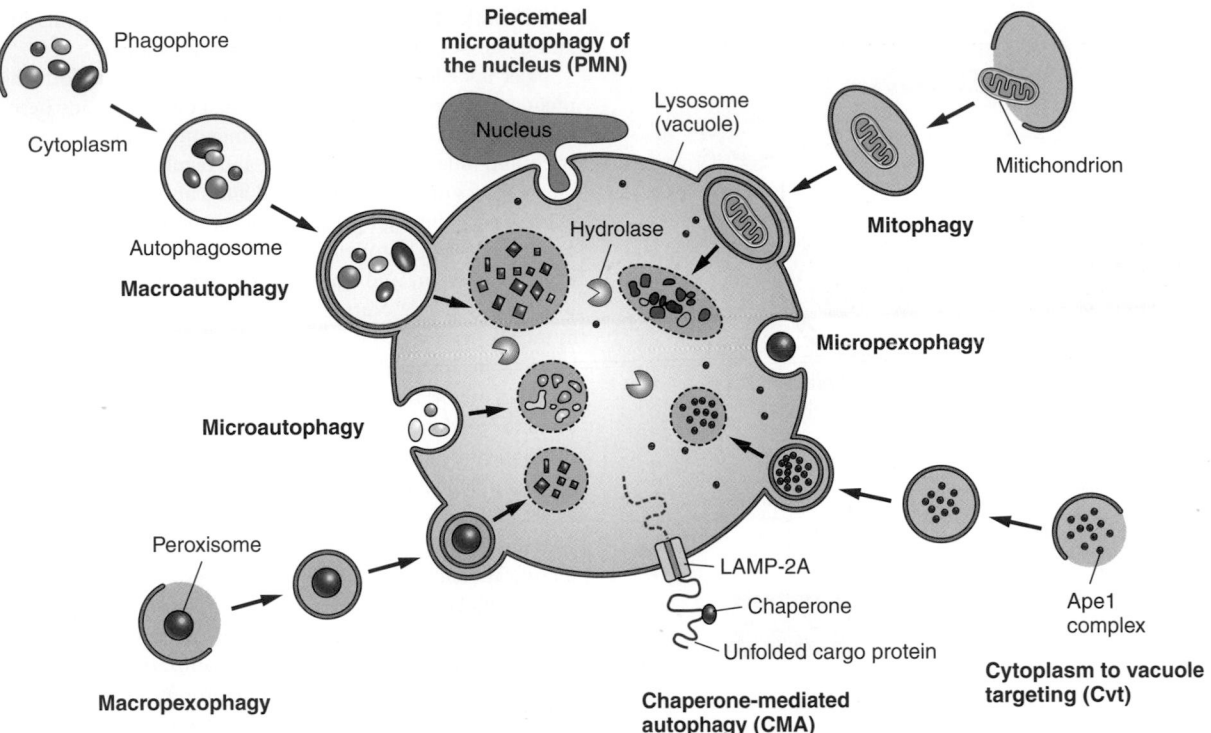

FIGURE 2.37 Autophagy. Three primary modes of autophagy include macrophagy, microphagy, and chaperone-mediated autophagy. Macrophagy is the formation of an autophagosome, a vacuole of nonlysosomal origin; microphagy involves direct uptake of cytosol, inclusions (e.g., glycogen), and organelles (e.g., ribosomes, peroxisomes at the lysosome vacuole); and chaperone-mediated autophagy (CMA) is a translocation process facilitated by certain proteins that are transported across the lysosomal membrane and degraded. Depending on the cargoes, autophagy can be selective or nonselective. During nonselective autophagy, a part of the cytoplasm is confiscated into a double-membrane autophagosome; it then fuses with the lysosome/vacuole. Specific degradation of peroxisomes can be achieved by either macroautophagy (macropexophagy) or microautophagy (micropexophagy). Piecemeal microautophagy of the nucleus causes degradation of a portion of the nucleus. Mitophagy, or degradation of the mitochondria, also occurs. (From Yen WL, Klionsky DJ: *Pathophysiology [Bethesda]* 23[5]:248–262, 2008.)

removed senescent cells in aging mice, increasing their healthy life span and reducing many age-related disease-associated abnormalities[163,164] (see Fig. E 2.1 on Evolve.)

The biologic understanding of senescence in humans is limited, but it seems significant because of two factors: (1) senescence causes a loss of tissue–repair capacity because of cell cycle arrest in progenitor cells and (2) it produces proinflammatory and matrix-degrading molecules in what is known as the *senescence-associated secretory phenotype (SASP).*[163] One of the hallmarks of aging is the accumulation of damaged macromolecules from telomere erosion, DNA damage, epigenetic stress, ROS accumulation, ER stress, and other factors. Aged cells that chronically accumulate damage eventually reach a threshold of cellular stress prompting their permanent withdrawal from the cell cycle.[163] Cellular senescence is a potent anticancer mechanism because senescent cells are permanently arrested and cleared by immune cells recruited because of proinflammatory, chemotactic factors secreted as part of the SASP.[163] Other beneficial functions of senescence include wound healing (limits tissue fibrosis) and embryogenesis.[163]

Aging is associated with increased levels of circulating cytokines and proinflammatory markers.[165] The changes in the immune system with aging, known as *inflammaging,* include immunosenescence and increased secretion of cytokines by adipose tissue and represent the major causes of chronic inflammation.[165] High levels of interleukin 6 (IL-6), IL-1, tumor necrosis factor-alpha, and C-reactive protein (CRP)

are associated in older individuals with increased risk of morbidity and mortality.[165] Studies have indicated TNF-α and IL-6 levels as markers of frailty. Low-grade inflammation underlies sarcopenia, and proinflammatory cytokines from many mechanisms, including platelet activation and endothelial activation, may play a major role in cardiovascular events. Dysregulation of the inflammatory pathways affects the CNS and is associated with many neurodegenerative diseases (e.g., Alzheimer disease, Parkinson disease, amyotrophic lateral sclerosis, and multiple sclerosis).[166] Besides immunosenescence, adipose tissue, through macrophages, produces IL-6, TNF-α, and adipokines. A large amount of visceral tissue or a high-fat diet is correlated with an increase in CRP and IL-6 in obese individuals, and in some who are not obese.[165] Another mechanism of inflammaging is the role of mitochondria and activation of the Nlrp3 inflammasome.[167] The Nlrp3 inflammasome is a mutiprotein complex and, in response to cellular danger, can activate procaspase-1, resulting in the processing and secretion of the proinflammatory cytokines IL-1β and IL-18. Most activators of the Nlrp3 inflammasome generate mitochondrial ROS.[167] Another mechanism that can increase inflammation is increasing activation of the coagulation system with age. Coagulation is part of the inflammatory response with shared components and strong interactions. The increased hypercoagulable state documented in aging may account for the higher incidence of arterial and venous thrombosis in elderly individuals. The microbiota plays a fundamental role on the induction and function of the immune system.[168] Adaptive

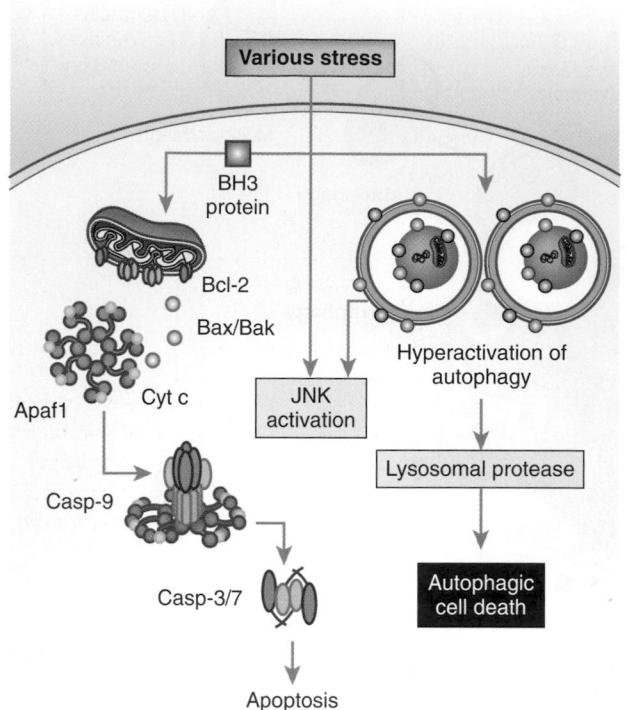

FIGURE 2.38 Molecular Mechanism of Apoptosis and Autophagic Cell Death. Critical for apoptosis to occur is an increase in the outer mitochondrial membrane. The process is regulated by proapoptotic members of the Bcl-2 family (Bax and Bak) leading to the release of cytochrome c into the cytoplasm. Cytochrome c then associates with apoptotic protease activating factor-1 (Apaf1), which activates the caspase cascade to execute apoptotic cell death. When apoptosis is blocked, certain apoptotic stimuli activate autophagy and c-Jun N-terminal kinase (JNK), resulting in the induction of autophagic cell death. Autophagy also mediates programmed cell death as well as other physiologic and pathologic processes. (From Shigeomi S et al: *Int J Mol Sci* 15:3145–3153, 2014.)

immunity declines with age, but innate immunity may result in mild hyperactivity.[169]

The microbiota plays a fundamental role in the induction and function of the immune system.[168] In high-income countries, overuse of antibiotics, changes in diet, and the elimination of helpful partners, such as nematodes, may have caused a microbiota that lacks the resilience and diversity to keep a balanced immune system.[168] These changes also are proposed to account for the dramatic increase in autoimmune and inflammatory disorders in certain parts of the world.

Life span can be experimentally changed in animals.[159,170] Extending life span, however, is not equivalent to delaying aging![159] For example, treatment of an acute infection can prevent death but the fundamental *rate* of aging continues. Critical is extending *health span* with an increase in life span—some experiments increased the proportion of time spent in a frail state.[70] Although the passage of time cannot be stopped (*chronological aging*), it may be possible to delay the concurrent decline in health or *biologic aging*.

Restoration of youthfulness to aged cells and tissues has created so-called *rejuvenating interventions*. Experiments to test whether cells and tissues from an old animal can be restored to a younger self include the approach called *heterochronic* (i.e., young-to-old or old-to-young) transplantations and heterochronic parabiosis, when the systemic circulations of two animals are joined. The systemic environment may become more youthful with restoration of protein components in the blood and tissues, especially chemokines and cytokines.[171]

Diet is believed to have a major influence on both the development and the prevention of age-related diseases. Plant-derived dietary phytochemicals and macro- and micronutrients modulate oxidative stress and inflammatory signaling and regulate metabolic pathways and bioenergetics that can be translated into stable epigenetic patterns of gene expression.[172] Emerging data reveal complex interactions between food components and histone modifications, DNA methylation, non–coding RNA expression, and chromatin remodeling factors that influence inflammaging.[172,173] Nutrients involved in one-carbon metabolism, such as folate, vitamin B_{12}, vitamin B_6, riboflavin, methionine, choline, and betaine, are involved in DNA methylation by regulating levels of the universal methyl donor *S*-adenosylmethionine and the methyltransferase inhibitor *S*-adenosylhomocysteine. Other nutrients and bioactive food components, such as retinoic acid, resveratrol, curcumin, sulforaphane, and tea polyphenols, can modulate epigenetic patterns by altering the levels of *S*-adenosylmethionine and *S*-adenosylhomocysteine or by directing the enzymes that catalyze DNA methylation and histone modifications.[173] Pharmacologic interventions may restore youthfulness at cellular and biochemical levels. The enzyme mammalian target of rapamycin (mTOR) senses cellular nutrient levels, thus regulating rates of protein synthesis and energy utilization.[159] Administration of the drug rapamycin, an mTOR inhibitor, can extend the life span of mice.[174] Some examples of other drugs targeting molecular pathways of aging include metformin, resveratrol, and anticalcitonin gene–regulated peptide (CGRP).

Normal Life Span and Life Expectancy

The maximal life span of humans is between 80 and 100 years and does not vary significantly among populations. In primitive societies, few individuals reach the maximal life span. However, in societies with improved sanitation, housing, nutrition, and health care, many individuals attain the maximal life span. Life expectancy is the average number of years of life remaining at a given age.

Life Expectancy Differences Across America

Although maximal life span has not changed significantly over time, improved public health strategies and health advances in the United States during the last century added about 30 years to life expectancy between 1900 and 2000. This increase in life expectancy has not affected all Americans. In each successive age group from 65 years and older, women outnumber men; thus, women have a greater life expectancy than men. These historic advances in life expectancy resulted in a larger older adult population and, for some, inherent problems of disability, disease, and socioeconomic hardship.

Although U.S. spending on health care far exceeds that of other developed countries, life expectancy and key measures of health lag behind other high-income countries[175] (Table 2.14). U.S. life expectancy for the first time in more than 20 years has declined. The National Center for Health Statistics finds Americans (on average) with a life expectancy of 78.8 years, a decline from 78.9 in 2014. The decline in life expectancy is attributed to rising fatalities from heart disease and stroke; diabetes; drug overdoses; accidents, including unintentional injuries; and other conditions.[176]

In the United States, chronic health conditions associated with modifiable risk factors, such as smoking, nutrition, weight, and physical activity, represent 6 of the 10 costliest medical conditions.[177] These preventable conditions lead to diseases and injuries and cause soaring medical and labor costs that saddle U.S. employers and bankrupt families. All of these conditions are highly amendable to population-based preventive strategies, which have been slow to develop; 20% of adults

TABLE 2.14	U.S. HEALTH RANKINGS FOR LIFE EXPECTANCY, INFANT MORTALITY, AND MATERNAL MORTALITY		
	U.S. RANKING (U.S./TOTAL OTHER COUNTRIES)		
SOURCE	LIFE EXPECTANCY	INFANT MORTALITY	MATERNAL MORTALITY
UN	28/146 (2005–2010 data)	32/146 (2005–2010 data)	n/a
OECD	26/34	30/34 (2008 data)	25/34 (2007 data)
CIA	50/221 (2011 estimated data; in 2010 data, U.S. ranked 49th)	47/222 (2011 estimated data)	52/176 (2011 estimated data)

CIA, Central Intelligence Agency; *n/a,* not available; *OECD,* Organisation for Economic Co-operation and Development; *UN,* United Nations.
Data from Central Intelligence Agency. (2011). *World factbook.* Washington, DC: National Academies Press; Organization for Economic Cooperation and Development. (2009). *Doing better for children.* Paris: OECD Publishing; National Research Council. (2011). *Explaining divergent levels of longevity in high-income countries.* Washington, DC: The National Academies Press.

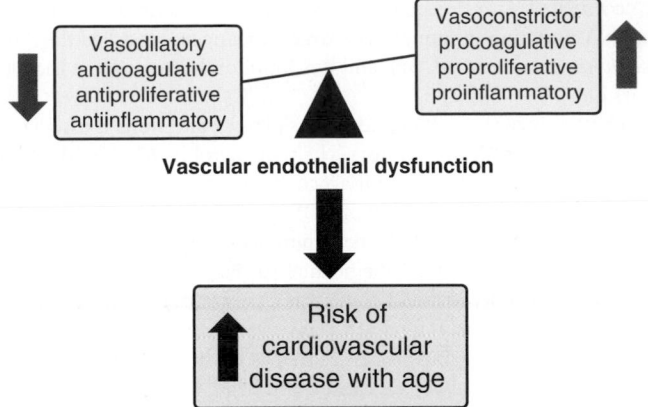

FIGURE 2.39 Vascular Endothelial Function and Increased Risk of Cardiovascular Diseases. Endothelial dysfunction is characterized by a shift from a vasodilatory, anticoagulative, antiproliferative, and antiinflammatory state to a proliferative and proinflammatory state, leading to an increased risk of cardiovascular disease with aging. (Adapted from Seals DR, Jablonski KL, Donato AJ: *Clin Sci* 120:357–375, 2011.)

still smoke and 50% of adults and 20% of children are overweight or obese.[178] It is estimated that one-third of American adults will develop diabetes by 2050 (up from one-tenth today).[179] The current generation of children and young adults in the United States could become the first generation to have shorter life spans, multiple medical conditions, and fewer healthy years of life than those of their parents.[180]

Aging: Degenerative Extracellular Changes

Extracellular factors that affect the aging process include the binding of collagen; the increase in free radicals' effects on cells; the structural alterations of fascia, tendons, ligaments, bones, and joints; and the development of peripheral vascular disease, particularly arteriosclerosis.

Aging affects the extracellular matrix with increased cross-linking, decreased synthesis, and increased degradation of collagen. These changes, together with the disappearance of elastin and changes in proteoglycans and plasma proteins, cause disorders that result in dehydration and wrinkling of the skin. Other age-related defects in the extracellular matrix include skeletal muscle alterations (e.g., atrophy, decreased tone, loss of contractility), cataracts, diverticula, hernias, and rupture of intervertebral disks.

Free radicals of oxygen that result from oxidative stress (e.g., respiratory chain, phagocytosis, prostaglandin synthesis) are known to damage tissues during the aging process. These oxygen products are extremely reactive and can damage nucleic acids, destroy polysaccharides, oxidize proteins, peroxidize unsaturated fatty acids, and kill and lyse cells. Oxidant effects on target cells can lead to malignant transformation, presumably through DNA damage. That progressive and cumulative damage from oxygen radicals may lead to harmful alterations in cellular function is consistent with those alterations of aging. This hypothesis is founded on the wear-and-tear theory of aging, which states that damages accumulate with time, decreasing the organism's ability to maintain a steady state. Because these oxygen-reactive species not only

can permanently damage cells but also may lead to cell death, there is new support for their role in the aging process.

Of much interest is the relationship between aging and the disappearance or alteration of extracellular substances important for blood vessel integrity. Advancing age is an important risk factor for the development of cardiovascular diseases. Vascular oxidative stress increases with age without a compensatory increase in antioxidant defenses.[181] Vascular endothelial dysfunction is characterized by a shift from a vasodilatory, anticoagulative, antiproliferative, and antiinflammatory state to a proinflammatory, proproliferative, and procoagulative state with consequent increased risk for cardiovascular events and diseases (Fig. 2.39).

Oxidative stress plays an important role in initial atherosclerotic lesion formation: its progression and destabilization.[182] With aging, lipid, calcium, and plasma proteins are deposited in vessel walls. These depositions cause basement membrane thickening and alterations in smooth muscle functioning, resulting in arteriosclerosis (a progressive disease that causes serious problems in the aged, including stroke, myocardial infarction, renal disease, and peripheral vascular disease).

Cellular Aging

Cellular changes characteristic of aging include atrophy, decreased function, and loss of cells, possibly by apoptosis. Loss of cellular function from any of these causes initiates the compensatory mechanisms of hypertrophy and hyperplasia of remaining cells, which can lead to metaplasia, dysplasia, and neoplasia. All these changes can alter receptor placement and function, nutrient pathways, cellular product secretion, and neuroendocrine control mechanisms. In the aged cell, DNA, RNA, cellular proteins, and membranes are most susceptible to injurious stimuli. DNA is particularly vulnerable to such injuries as breaks, deletions, and additions. Although it can repair itself with time, the aged cell's capacity for DNA repair is decreased. Lack of DNA repair increases the cell's susceptibility to mutations that may be lethal or may promote the development of neoplasia.

Mitochondria are the organelles responsible for the generation of most of the energy used by eukaryotic cells. Mitochondrial DNA (mtDNA) encodes some of the proteins of the electron-transfer chain, the system necessary for the conversion of adenosine diphosphate (ADP) to ATP. Mutations in mtDNA can deprive the cell of ATP, and mutations are correlated with the aging process. The most common age-related mtDNA mutation in humans is a large rearrangement called the *4977 deletion,* or *common deletion,* and it is found in humans more than 40 years old.

The production of ROS under physiologic conditions is associated with activity of the respiratory chain in aerobic ATP production. Therefore, increased mitochondrial activity by itself can be an "oxidative stress" to cells. The production of ROS is markedly increased in many pathologic conditions in which the respiratory chain is impaired. Because mtDNA, which is essential for normal oxidative phosphorylation, is located in proximity to the ROS-generating respiratory chain, it is more oxidatively damaged than is nuclear DNA. Cumulative damage of mtDNA is implicated in the aging process as well as in the progression of such common diseases as diabetes, cancer, and heart failure.

Tissue and Systemic Aging

It is probably safe to say that every physiologic process can be shown to function less efficiently with increasing age. The most characteristic tissue change with age is a progressive stiffness or rigidity that affects many systems, including the arterial, pulmonary, and musculoskeletal systems. A consequence of blood vessel and organ stiffness is a progressive increase in peripheral resistance to blood flow. The movement of intracellular and extracellular substances also usually decreases with age as does the diffusion capacity of the lung. Blood flow through organs decreases; for example, renal plasma flow decreases.

Changes in the endocrine and immune systems include thymus atrophy. Although this occurs at puberty, it causes a decreased immune response to T-dependent antigens (foreign proteins), increased formation of autoantibodies and immune complexes (antibodies bound to antigen), and an overall decrease in the immunologic tolerance for the host's own cells, which further diminishes the effectiveness of the immune system later in life. The reproductive system loses ova in women, and spermatogenesis in men is decreased. Responsiveness to hormones decreases in the breast and endometrium.

The stomach experiences decreases in the rate of emptying and secretion of hormones and hydrochloric acid. Muscular atrophy diminishes mobility by decreasing motor tone and contractility. **Sarcopenia**, the loss of muscle mass and strength, can occur into old age. The skin of the aged individual is affected by atrophy and wrinkling of the epidermis and by alterations in underlying dermis, fat, and muscle.

Total body changes include a decrease in height; a reduction in circumference of the neck, thighs, and arms; widening of the pelvis; and lengthening of the nose and ears. Several of these changes are the result of tissue atrophy and decreased bone mass caused by osteoporosis and osteoarthritis. Some body composition changes include an increase in body weight, which begins in middle age (men gain until 50 years of age and women until 70 years), and an increase in fat mass followed by a decrease in stature, weight, fat-free mass (FFM), and body cell mass at older ages. FFM includes all minerals, proteins, and water plus all other constituents except lipids. As the amount of fat increases, the percentage of total body water decreases. Increased body fat and centralized fat distribution (abdominal) are associated with non–insulin-dependent diabetes and heart disease. Total body potassium concentration also decreases because of decreased cellular mass. An increased sodium/potassium ratio suggests that the decreased cellular mass is accompanied by an increased extracellular compartment.

Although some of these alterations are probably inherent in aging, others represent consequences of aging. Advanced age increases susceptibility to disease, and death occurs after an injury or insult because of diminished cellular, tissue, and organic function. To determine that an individual "died of old age" would be a monumental if not impossible task.

Frailty

Frailty is a state of increased vulnerability to poor resolution of homeostasis following a stress, which increases the risk of adverse outcomes including falls, delirium, disability, long-term care, and death.[183] Worldwide, population aging is accelerating and the most problematic expression of population aging is frailty. As a consequence of frailty, a minor stress event, such as the introduction of a new drug, a minor infection, or minor surgery, can cause a sudden, often serious, health status change.

The pathophysiology of frailty includes many interrelated physiologic systems (Fig. 2.40). Complex and multiple aging mechanisms are influenced by genetic/epigenetic and environmental factors that regulate the differential expression of genes in cells and may be especially important in aging.[183] For study of the development of frailty, the best-studied systems are the brain and the endocrine, immune, and skeletal muscle systems. Frailty also has been associated with loss of physiologic reserve in the respiratory, cardiovascular, renal, hematopoietic and clotting systems, and nutritional status as important mediating factors.[183] Several physiologic gender differences may explain differing levels of frailty: (1) higher baseline levels of muscle mass for men may

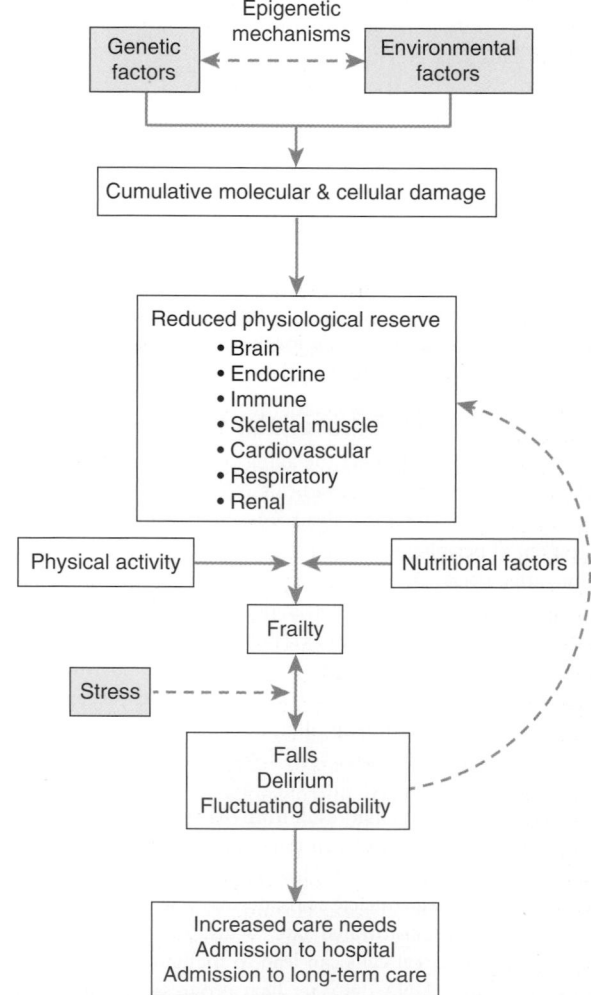

FIGURE 2.40 Frailty. Frailty is a disorder of multiple interrelated physiologic systems. A gradual decline progresses with aging, but in frailty this decline becomes accelerated. Homeostatic mechanisms begin to fail, and vulnerability becomes disproportionate to changes in health status after a relatively minor stressor event. (From Clegg A et al: *Lancet* 381[9868]:752–762, 2013.)

be protective against frailty, (2) testosterone and growth hormone can provide advantages in muscle mass maintenance, (3) cortisol is more dysregulated in older women than in older men, (4) alterations in immune function and immune responsiveness to sex steroids make men more vulnerable to sepsis and infection and women vulnerable to chronic inflammatory conditions and muscle mass loss, and (5) lower levels of activity and caloric intake may influence greater susceptibility to frailty in women.

SOMATIC DEATH

Somatic death is death of the entire person. Unlike the changes that follow cellular death in a live body, postmortem change is diffuse and does not involve components of the inflammatory response. Within minutes of death, manifestations of postmortem change appear, eliminating any difficulty in determining that death has occurred. The most notable manifestations are complete cessation of respiration and circulation. The surface of the skin usually becomes pale and yellowish; however, the lifelike color of the cheeks and lips may persist after death from causes such as carbon monoxide poisoning, drowning, and chloroform poisoning.

Body temperature falls gradually immediately after death and then more rapidly (approximately 1.0° to 1.5° F (−16.9° to −17°C)/hour) until, after 24 hours, body temperature equals that of the environment. After death caused by certain infective diseases, body temperature may continue to rise for a short time. Postmortem reduction of body temperature is called algor mortis.

Blood pressure within the retinal vessels decreases, causing muscle tension to decrease and the pupils to become dilated. The face, nose, and chin begin to look "sharp" or "peaked" as blood and fluids drain from these areas. Gravity causes blood to settle in the most dependent, or lowest, tissues, which develop a purple discoloration called livor mortis. Incisions at this time usually fail to cause bleeding. The skin loses its elasticity and transparency.

Within 6 hours after death, acidic compounds accumulate within the muscles because of the breakdown of carbohydrate and the depletion of ATP. This interferes with ATP-dependent detachment of myosin from actin (contractile proteins), and muscle stiffening, or rigor mortis, develops. The smaller muscles are usually affected first, particularly the muscles of the jaw. Within 12 to 14 hours, rigor mortis usually affects the entire body. Rigor mortis gradually diminishes and the body becomes flaccid in 12 to 14 hours.

Signs of putrefaction—state of decay with foul-smelling odor—are generally obvious about 24 to 48 hours after death. Putrefactive changes vary depending on the temperature of the environment. The most visible is greenish discoloration of the skin, particularly on the abdomen. The discoloration is thought to be related to the diffusion of hemolyzed blood into the tissues and the production of sulfhemoglobin. Slippage or loosening of the skin from underlying tissues occurs at the same time. After this, swelling or bloating of the body and liquefactive changes occur, sometimes causing opening of the body cavities. At a microscopic level, putrefactive changes are associated with the release of enzymes and lytic dissolution called postmortem autolysis.

■ SUMMARY REVIEW

Cellular Adaptation

1. Injury to cells and their surrounding environment, called the *extracellular matrix*, leads to tissue and organ injury. Cellular adaptation is an alteration that enables the cell to maintain a steady state despite adverse conditions.
2. Atrophy is a decrease in cellular size and can affect any organ, but is most common in skeletal muscle, the heart, secondary sex organs, and the brain. The mechanisms probably include decreased protein synthesis, increased protein catabolism, or both.
3. Physiologic atrophy occurs with early development; for example, the thymus gland involutes and atrophies. Pathologic atrophy occurs as a result of decreases in workload, use, pressure, blood supply, nutrition, hormonal stimulation, and nervous stimulation.
4. Aging causes brain cells and endocrine-dependent organs, such as the gonads, to become atrophic.
5. Hypertrophy is an increase in the size of cells caused by increased work demands or hormonal stimulation. Hypertrophy can be physiologic or pathologic. Amounts of protein in the plasma membrane, endoplasmic reticulum, microfilaments, and mitochondria are increased.
6. Hyperplasia is an increase in the number of cells caused by an increased rate of cellular division. Compensatory hyperplasia enables certain organs to regenerate. Hormonal hyperplasia is stimulated by hormones to replace lost tissue or support new growth, such as during pregnancy.
7. Pathologic hyperplasia is the abnormal proliferation of normal cells in response to excessive hormonal stimulation or the effects of growth factors on target cells.
8. Dysplasia, or atypical hyperplasia, is an abnormal change in the size, shape, and organization of mature tissue cells. Importantly, the term dysplasia is not cancer and may not progress to cancer. Dysplasias

that do not involve the entire thickness of the epithelium may be completely reversible.

9. Metaplasia is the reversible replacement of one mature cell type by another, sometimes less differentiated, cell type. It is found in association with tissue damage, repair, and regeneration. Metaplasia develops from a reprogramming of stem cells existing in most epithelia or of undifferentiated mesenchymal cells in connective tissue.

Cellular Injury

1. Injury to cells and to the extracellular matrix (ECM) leads to injury of tissues and organs, ultimately determining the structural patterns of disease. Injured cells may recover (reversible injury) or die (irreversible injury).
2. Cellular injury is caused by a lack of oxygen (hypoxia), free radicals, caustic or toxic chemicals, infectious agents, unintentional and intentional injury, inflammatory and immune responses, genetic factors, insufficient nutrients, or physical trauma from many causes. Injurious stimuli cause cell stress.
3. Cell injury can be acute or chronic, and it can be reversible or irreversible. It can involve necrosis, apoptosis, autophagy, accumulation, or pathologic calcification.
4. Four biochemical themes are important to cell injury: (a) depletion of ATP, (b) decreased levels of oxygen and increased levels of oxygen-derived free radicals, (c) increased concentration of intracellular calcium and loss of calcium steady state, and (d) defects in membrane permeability.
5. The sequence of events leading to cell death is commonly decreased ATP production, failure of active transport mechanisms (the Na^+-K^+ pump), cellular swelling, detachment of ribosomes from the endoplasmic reticulum, cessation of protein synthesis, mitochondrial swelling as a result of calcium accumulation, vacuolation, leakage

of digestive enzymes from lysosomes, autodigestion of intracellular structures, lysis of the plasma membrane, and death.

6. The initial insult in hypoxic injury is usually ischemia—the cessation of blood flow into vessels that supply the cell with oxygen and nutrients. Hypoxia can induce inflammation, and inflamed lesions can become hypoxic.

7. Restoration of oxygen after ischemic injury can result in reperfusion (reoxygenation) injury. Reperfusion injury results from the generation of highly reactive oxygen intermediates or radicals.

8. Inherent reactive oxygen species (ROS) from aerobic metabolism play a crucial biologic role, not just in various diseases but also from cellular communication and cell function. ROS reversibly modulates many intracellular signaling pathways. ROS can affect protein functions through several mechanisms, including regulation of protein expression, posttranslational modifications, and alteration of protein stability.

9. Reduction-oxidation- (redox) dependent regulation and the roles of ROS include both normal physiologic and pathologic roles. These expanding roles include proliferation and differentiation, immune function, stem cell self-renewal, tumor progression, autoimmunity, stem cell exhaustion, senescence, and longevity.

10. Cell injury produced by free radicals, particularly ROS, is an important mechanism of cell damage in many conditions including chemical and radiation injury, ischemia-reperfusion injury, microbial killing by phagocytes, and cellular aging.

11. A significant mechanism of membrane damage is injury caused by free radicals, including oxidative stress. Oxidative stress can activate several intracellular signaling pathways because ROS can modulate enzymes and transcription factors. Free radicals are difficult to control and initiate chain reactions.

12. Free radicals can cause (a) lipid peroxidation or the destruction of unsaturated fatty acids, (b) alterations of proteins, protein loss, and protein misfolding, and (c) mutations in DNA.

13. Mitochondria contain their own DNA, called *mitochondrial DNA* (mtDNA), and can encode proteins involved in energy production. mtDNA encodes enzymes involved in oxidative phosphorylation, and mutations affecting these genes exert their damaging effects on organs most dependent on oxidative phosphorylation, such as the CNS, skeletal muscle, cardiac muscle, liver, and kidneys. Emerging is the role mitochondria has in mediating environmental changes and genomic responses.

14. Humans are exposed to thousands of chemicals that have inadequate toxicologic data. Toxicity pathways or cellular response pathways result in adverse health effects when disturbed. Components of these pathways include oxidative stress, heat shock response, DNA damage response, hypoxia, ER stress, mental stress, inflammation, and osmotic stress.

15. The initial insult in chemical and toxic injury is damage or destruction of the plasma membrane. Two general mechanisms include direct toxicity and conversion to toxic intermediates or metabolites. Examples of chemical agents that cause cellular injury include air pollutants, insecticides, herbicides, alcohol, lead, carbon monoxide, ethanol, mercury, opioids (heroin, morphine, prescription drugs for pain), and social or street drugs.

16. Under investigation are the beneficial effects of chemical compounds called *phytochemicals*. Examples of these products include certain fruits and plants, chamomile, silymarin, carrot, ginger root, milk thistle seed, rosemary leaf, turmeric, and others.

17. The world's largest single environmental health risk is air pollution. From WHO data, every year 4.3 million deaths occur from exposure to indoor air pollution and 3.7 million deaths to outdoor air pollution. Air pollution is contamination of the environment by any chemical, physical, or biologic agent that modifies natural characteristics of the atmosphere.

18. By reducing air pollution levels, countries can lower the burden of diseases from stroke, heart disease, lung cancer, and chronic and acute respiratory diseases, including asthma. Prompt and sustained health benefits can come from improved air quality.

19. Heavy metals commonly associated with harmful effects in humans include lead, mercury, arsenic, and cadmium. Studies of the involvement of metals in pathophysiology include DNA repair mechanisms, tumor suppressor functions, and interference with signal transduction pathways.

20. Unintentional and intentional injuries are an important health problem in the United States. Injuries include motor vehicle crashes, opioid overdoses, poisonings, sports and recreation-related injuries, firearms, falls, blunt force (tearing, shearing, crushing of tissues), asphyxia (suffocation, strangulation, chemical asphyxiants, drowning), and others including injury from medical care itself.

21. Injury from microorganisms lies in their ability to survive and proliferate in the human body. Injury depends on the microorganisms' ability to invade and destroy cells, produce toxins, and produce damaging hypersensitivity reactions.

22. Activation of inflammation and immunity, which occurs after cellular injury or infection, involves powerful biochemicals and proteins capable of damaging normal (uninjured and uninfected) cells.

23. Genetic disorders injure cells by altering the nucleus and the plasma membrane's structure, shape, receptors, or transport mechanisms.

24. Deprivation of essential nutrients (proteins, carbohydrates, lipids, vitamins) can cause cellular injury by altering cellular structure and function, particularly of transport mechanisms, chromosomes, the nucleus, and DNA. Excessive amounts of other nutrients, for example carbohydrates, can lead to obesity, changes with insulin utilization, and diabetes.

25. Injurious physical agents include temperature extremes and climate change, changes in atmospheric pressure, ionizing radiation, illumination, mechanical stresses (e.g., repetitive body movements), and noise.

Manifestations of Cellular Injury

1. Manifestations of cellular injury include accumulations of water, lipids, carbohydrates, glycogen, proteins, pigments, hemosiderin, bilirubin, calcium, and urate.

2. Accumulations harm cells by "crowding" the organelles and by causing excessive (and sometimes harmful) metabolites to be produced during their catabolism. The metabolites are released into the cytoplasm or expelled into the extracellular matrix.

3. Cellular swelling, the accumulation of excessive water in the cell, is caused by the failure of transport mechanisms and is a sign of many types of cellular injury.

4. Accumulations of organic substances—lipids, carbohydrates, glycogen, proteins, and pigments—are caused by disorders in which (a) cellular uptake of the substance exceeds the cell's capacity to catabolize (digest) or use it or (b) cellular anabolism (synthesis) of the substance exceeds the cell's capacity to use or secrete it.

5. Dystrophic calcification (accumulation of calcium salts) is always a sign of pathologic change because it occurs only in injured or dead cells. Free calcium in the cytosol can cause activation of protein kinases, activation of phospholipases and membrane damage, and damage

SUMMARY REVIEW—cont'd

or disassembly of the cytoskeleton. Metastatic calcification, however, can occur in uninjured cells in individuals with hypercalcemia.

6. Disturbances in urate metabolism can result in hyperuricemia and deposition of sodium urate crystals in tissue, leading to a painful disorder called *gout*.

7. Systemic manifestations of cellular injury include fever, leukocytosis, increased heart rate, pain, and serum elevations of enzymes in the plasma.

Cellular Death

1. Cell death has historically been classified as necrosis and apoptosis. Necrosis is characterized by rapid loss of the plasma membrane structure, organelle swelling, mitochondrial dysfunction, and the lack of typical features of apoptosis. Apoptosis is known as regulated or programmed cell process by the "dropping off" of cellular fragments called *apoptotic bodies*. Under certain conditions, necrosis is driven by regulated or programmed molecular pathways, hence the new term programmed necrosis or necroptosis. Other forms of cell loss include autophagy.

2. The four major types of necrosis are coagulative, liquefactive, caseous, and fat. Different types of necrosis occur in different tissues.

3. Gangrenous necrosis, or gangrene, is tissue necrosis caused by hypoxia and subsequent bacterial invasion.

4. Autophagy is a recycling factory, a self-destructive process, and a survival mechanism. It degrades cytoplasmic components and organelles in lysosomes and salvages key metabolites to promote metabolic and nutrient homeostasis. Autophagy has a central role in cell homeostasis. It is important in diverse processes and conditions such as development, cell proliferation, remodeling, aging, cancer, heart disease, neurodegenerative diseases, inflammation, infection, metabolic diseases, and cell death.

Aging

1. Aging is the progressive loss of tissues and organs over time. It is difficult to determine the physiologic (normal) from the pathologic changes of aging. One of the hallmarks of aging is the accumulation of damaged macromolecules.

2. Investigators are focused on genetic, epigenetic, inflammatory, oxidative stress, cell renewal by adult stem cells, and metabolic and endocrine origins of aging.

3. Senescence is a process of permanent proliferative arrest on cells in response to various stressors and may be an important contributor to aging and age-related diseases.

4. Aging is associated with increased levels of circulating cytokines and proinflammatory markers. There are changes in the immune system with aging known as *inflammaging*. The microbiota plays a fundamental role in the induction and function of the immune system. Diet is believed to have a major influence on both the development and the prevention of age-related diseases.

5. Humans have an inherent maximal life span (80 to 100 years) that is dictated by currently unknown intrinsic mechanisms.

6. Although the maximal life span has not changed significantly over time, the average life span, or life expectancy, has decreased for the first time in 20 years in the United States.

7. Frailty is a common clinical syndrome in older adults, leaving a person vulnerable to falls, functional decline, disability, disease, and death. The syndrome is complex, involving oxidative stress, dysregulation of inflammatory cytokines and hormones, malnutrition, physical inactivity, and muscle changes. Women have a higher risk of frailty than men.

Somatic Death

1. Somatic death is death of the entire organism. Postmortem change is diffuse and does not involve the inflammatory response.

2. Manifestations of somatic death include cessation of respiration and circulation, gradual lowering of body temperature, dilation of pupils, loss of elasticity and transparency in the skin, stiffening of muscles (rigor mortis), and discoloration of the skin (livor mortis). Signs of putrefaction are obvious about 24 to 48 hours after death.

KEY TERMS

KEY TERMS—cont'd

Lead (Pb), 64
Life expectancy, 94
Ligature strangulation, 74
Lipid peroxidation, 56
Lipofuscin, 48
Liquefactive necrosis, 88
Livor mortis, 97
Lysosomal storage disease, 84
Macronutrients, 74
Malignant hyperthermia, 76
Manual strangulation, 74
Maximal life span, 94
Mechanotransduction, 82
Melanin, 85
Mercury, 67
Mesenchymal cells, 49
Metaplasia, 49
Metastatic calcification, 87
Micronutrients, 74
Mitochondrial DNA (mtDNA), 56
Mucolipidosis (ML), 84
Mucopolysaccharidosis (MPS), 84

Necrosis, 87
Neuroleptic malignant syndrome, 76
Noise, 83
Nontargeted effect, 80
Nucleophile, 59
Oncosis (vacuolar) degeneration, 84
Optical radiation, 81
Oxidative stress, 54
Pathologic atrophy, 47
Pathologic hyperplasia, 49
Pathologic hypertrophy, 48
Physiologic atrophy, 47
Physiologic hypertrophy, 48
Postmortem autolysis, 97
Postmortem change, 97
Primary accidental hypothermia, 75
Programmed necrosis (necroptosis), 87
Psammoma body, 87
Pyknosis, 88
Reactive oxygen species (ROS), 54
Redox signaling, 54
Reperfusion (reoxygenation) injury, 52

Reversible injury, 49
Rigor mortis, 97
Sarcopenia, 96
Secondary hypothermia, 75
Senescence, 92
Shear force, 82
Somatic death, 97
Strain, 82
Strangulation, 74
Sudden infant death syndrome (SIDS), 77
Suffocation, 71
Tension, 82
Tethering, 82
Thimerosal, 68
Torsion, 82
Toxicophores, 59
Type I programmed cell death, 91
Type II programmed cell death, 91
Urate, 87
Vacuolation, 51
Wet gangrene, 88
Xenobiotics, 59

REFERENCES

1. Kumar V, Abbas A, Aster J, editors: *Robbins & Cotran pathologic basis of disease*, ed 9, Philadelphia, 2015, Saunders.
2. Matkovich SJ, et al: Cardiac disease status dictates functional mRNA targeting profiles of individual microRNAs. *Circ Cardiovasc Genet* 8(6):774–784, 2015.
3. Ucar A, et al: The miRNA-212/132 family regulates both cardiac hypertrophy and cardiomyocyte autophagy. *Nat Commun* 3:1078, 2012.
4. Thum T: Noncoding RNAs and myocardial fibrosis. *Nat Rev Cardiol* 11(11):655–663, 2014.
5. Alberts B, et al: *Molecular biology of the cell*, ed 6, New York, 2015, Garland Science.
6. Hausenloy DJ, Yellon DM: Ischaemic conditioning and reperfusion injury. *Nat Rev Cardiol* 13(4):193–209, 2016.
7. Valko M, et al: Free radicals and antioxidants in normal physiological functions and human disease. *Int J Biochem Cell Biol* 39(1):44–84, 2007.
8. Murphy E, Steenbergen C: Mechanisms underlying acute protection from cardiac ischemia—reperfusion injury. *Physiol Rev* 88(2):581–609, 2008.
9. Murphy E, Steenbergen C: What makes the mitochondria a killer? Can we condition them to be less destructive? *Biochim Biophys Acta* 1813:1302–1308, 2011.
10. Ong SB, et al: The mitochondrial permeability transition pore and its role in myocardial ischemia reperfusion injury. *J Mol Cell Cardiol* 78:23–34, 2015.
11. Holmström KM, Finkel T: Cellular mechanisms and physiological consequences of redox-dependent signaling. *Nat Rev Mol Cell Biol* 15(6):411–421, 2014.
12. Shadel GS, Horvath TL: Mitochondrial ROS signaling in organismal homeostasis. *Cell* 163:560–569, 2015.
13. Konior A, et al: NADPH oxidases in vascular pathology. *Antioxid Redox Signal* 20(17):2794–2814, 2014.
14. Touyz RM, Briones AM: Reactive oxygen species and vascular biology: implications in human hypertension. *Hypertens Res* 34:5–14, 2011.
15. Tse G, et al: Reactive oxygen species, endoplasmic reticulum stress and mitochondrial dysfunction: the link with cardiac arrhythmogenesis. *Front Physiol* 7:313, 2016.
16. Kvietys PR, Granger DN: Role of reactive oxygen and nitrogen species in the vascular responses to inflammation. *Free Radic Biol Med* 52:556–592, 2012.
17. Sovari AA: Cellular and molecular mechanisms of arrhythmia by oxidative stress. *Cardiol Res Pract* 2016:9656078, 2016.
18. Wu F, Tian FJ, Lin Y: Oxidative stress in placenta: health and diseases. *Biomed Res Int* 2015:293271, 2015.
19. Cerdeira AS, Karumanchi SA: Angiogenic factors in preeclampsia and related disorders. *Cold Spring Harb Perspect Med* 2(11):2012.
20. Pereira RD, et al: Angiogenesis in the placenta: the role of reactive oxygen species signaling. *Biomed Res Int* 2015:814543, 2015.
21. Bai J, Cederbaum AI: Mitochondrial catalase and oxidative injury. *Biol Signals Recept* 10(3–4):189–199, 2001.
22. Guo C, et al: Oxidative stress, mitochondrial damage and neurodegenerative diseases. *Neural Regen Res* 8(21):2003–2014, 2013.
23. Young KJ, Bennett JP: The mitochondrial secret(ase) of Alzheimer's disease. *J Alzheimers Dis* 20(Suppl 2):S381–S400, 2010.
24. Ray PD, et al: Reactive oxygen species (ROS) homeostasis and redox regulation in cellular signaling. *Cell Signal* 24:981–990, 2012.
25. Lee J, Giordano S, Zhang J: Autophagy, mitochondria and oxidative stress: cross-talk and redox signaling. *Biochem J* 441(2):523–540, 2012.
26. Huang R, et al: Modeling the TOX21 10K chemical profiles for in vivo toxicity prediction and mechanism characterization. *Nat Commun* 7:10426, 2016, doi:10.1038/ncomms10425.
27. Seeff LB, et al: Herbal products and the liver: a review of adverse effects and mechanisms. *Gastroenterology* 148:517–532.e3, 2015.
28. Gu X, Manautou JE: Molecular mechanisms underlying chemical liver injury. *Expert Rev Mol Med* 14:e4, 2013.
29. Hanzlik RP, et al: The reactive metabolite target protein database (TPDB)—a web-accessible resource. *BMC Bioinformatics* 8:95, 2007.
30. National Institutes of Health and Prevention (NIH): *America's addiction to opioids: heroin and prescription drugs*, Washington, DC, 2014, Author.
31. United Nations Office on Drugs and Crime (UNODC): *World drug report*, 2012. Available at: http://www.unodc.org/unodc/en/data-and-analysis/WDR-2012.html.
32. Substance Abuse and Mental Health Services Administration: Results from the 2012 National Survey on Drug Use and Health: summary of national findings, *NSDUH Series H-46, HHS Publication No. (SMA) 13-4795*, Rockville, MD, 2013, Author.
33. Murray KF, et al: Drug-associated hepatotoxicity and acute liver failure. *J Pediatr Gastroenterol Nutr* 47(5):395–405, 2008.
34. Madrigal-Santillan E, et al: Review of natural products with hepatoprotective effects. *World J Gastroenterol* 20(40):14787–14804, 2014.
35. Singh D, et al: Drug-induced liver toxicity and prevention by herbal antioxidants: an overview. *Front Physiol* 6:363, 2015.
36. World Health Organization (WHO): *Air pollution*, Geneva, 2016, Author. Available at: http://www.who.int/topics/air_pollution/en/.
37. Brook RD, et al: Particulate matter air pollution and cardiovascular disease: an update to the scientific statement from the American Heart Association. *Circulation* 121(21):2331–2378, 2010.
38. Hoek G, et al: Long-term air pollution exposure and cardio-respiratory mortality: a review. *Environ Health* 12(1):43, 2013.
39. Pope CA, et al: Fine-particulate air pollution and life expectancy in the United States. *N Engl J Med* 360:376–386, 2009.
40. U.S. Environmental Protection Agency (EPA): *EPA criteria air pollutants*, Washington, DC, 2016, Author. Available at: https://www.epa.gov/criteria-air-pollutants.
41. Occupational Safety and Health Administration (OSHA): *Lead*, Washington, DC, 2012, U.S. Department of Labor.

42. Centers for Disease Control and Prevention (CDC): *Lead*, Atlanta, GA, 2016, U.S. Department of Health & Human Services, Centers for Disease Control and Prevention. Available at: www.cdc.gov/lead/.

43. Neal AP, Guilarte TR: Mechanisms of lead and manganese neurotoxicity. *Toxicol Res* 2:99–114, 2013.

44. Nichani WI, et al: Blood lead levels in children after phase-out of leaded gasoline in Bombay, India. *Sci Total Environ* 363:95, 2006.

45. Luo XS, et al: Distribution, availability, and sources of trace metals in different particle size fractions of urban soils in Hong Kong: implications for assessing the risk to human health. *Environ Pollut* 159:1317, 2011.

46. United States Environmental Protection Agency (US EPA): *Final revisions to the National Quality Air Standards for lead, lead fact sheet*, Washington, DC, 2008, Author. Available at: www.epa.gov/air/lead/pdfs/20081015pbfactsheet.pdf.

47. Centers for Disease Control and Prevention (CDC): *Adult blood level epidemiology and surveillance (ABLES)*. Available at: www.cdc.gov/lead.

48. National Institute for Occupational Safety and Health (NIOSH): *Adult blood lead epidemiology & surveillance (ABLES)*, Atlanta, GA, 2012, U.S. Department of Health and Human Services, CDC, NIOSH. Available at: www.sdc.gov/niosh/topics/ables/ables.

49. Merrill JC, Morton JJP, Soileau SD: Metals. In Hayes AW, editor: *Principles and methods of toxicology*, ed 5, Milton Park, UK, 2007, Taylor & Francis UK, CRC Press.

50. Patrick L: Lead toxicity, a review of the literature. Part I: exposure, evaluation, and treatment. *Altern Med Rev* 11(1):2–22, 2006.

51. Barbosa F, Jr, et al: A critical review of biomarkers used for monitoring human exposure to lead: advantages, limitations, and future needs. *Environ Health Perspect* 113(12):1669–1674, 2005.

52. Dart RC, Hurlbut KM, Boyer-Hassen LV: Lead. In Dart RC, editor: *Medical toxicology*, ed 3, Philadelphia, 2004, Lippincott Williams & Wilkins.

53. Lassiter MG, et al: Cross–species coherence in effects and modes of action in support of causality determinations in the U. S. Environmental Protection Agency's Integrated Science Assessment for lead. *Toxicology* 330:19–40, 2015.

54. National Institute of Environmental Health Sciences: *National toxicology program: NTP monograph: health effects of low-level lead national toxicology program*, North Carolina, 2012.

55. United Nations Environmental Programme (UNEP): *MERCURY: time to act*, Nairobi, Kenya, 2013, Author.

56. United Nations Environmental Programme (UNEP): *Global mercury assessment 2013: sources, emissions, releases and environmental transport*, Geneva, Switzerland, 2013, UNEP Chemicals Branch.

57. U.S. Food and Drug Administration (US FDA): *Food safety for moms-to-be: before you're pregnant—methylmercury*, Washington, DC, 2016, US FDA, U.S. Department of Health and Human Services.

58. Heard KJ: Acetylcysteine for acetaminophen poisoning. *N Engl J Med* 359(3):285–292, 2008.

59. Kagemoto K, et al: ADH1B and ALDH2 are associated with metachronous SCC after endoscopic submucosal dissection of esophageal squamous cell carcinoma. *Cancer Med* 5(7):1397–1404, 2016.

60. Tsai ST, et al: The interplay between alcohol consumption, oral hygiene, ALDH2, and ADH1B in the risk of head and neck cancer. *Int J Cancer* 135(10):2424–2436, 2014.

61. Liu J, et al: Alcohol drinking mediates the association between polymorphisms of ADH1B and ALDH2 and hepatitis B-related hepatocellular carcinoma. *Cancer Epidemiol Biomarkers Prev* 2016 Jan 2016. [Epub ahead of print].

62. Rostron B: Alcohol consumption and mortality risks in the USA. *Alcohol Alcohol* 47(3):334–339, 2012.

63. Connor J: The life and times of the j-shaped curve. *Alcohol Alcohol* 41:583–584, 2006.

64. Krenz M, Korthius RJ: Moderate ethanol ingestion and cardiovascular protection: from epidemiologic associations to cellular mechanisms. *J Mol Cell Cardiol* 52(1):93–104, 2013.

65. Wang ZG, et al: Adipose tissue-liver axis in alcoholic liver disease. *World J Gastrointest Pathophysiol* 7(1):17–26, 2016.

66. Neuman MG, et al: Markers of inflammation and fibrosis in alcoholic hepatitis and viral hepatitis. *Int J Hepatol* 2012:231210, 2012.

67. Zhu H, et al: Oxidative stress and redox signaling mechanisms of alcoholic liver disease: updated experimental and clinical evidence. *J Dig Dis* 13(3):133–142, 2012.

68. Curtis BJ, et al: Epigenetic targets for reversing immune defects caused by alcohol exposure. *Alcohol Res* 35(1):97–113, 2013.

69. Vaux KK, Chambers C: *Fetal alcohol syndrome*, 2009. Available at: emedicine.medscape.com/article/974016-overview.

70. Centers for Disease Control and Prevention (CDC): *Fetal alcohol spectrum disorders (FASDs)*, Washington, DC, 2015, CDC, U.S. Department of Health & Human Services.

71. Grant TM, et al: Alcohol use before and during pregnancy in western Washington, 1989–2004: implications for the prevention of fetal alcohol spectrum disorders. *Am J Obstet Gynecol* 200(3):278, 2009.

72. Yang F, Luo J: Endoplasmic reticulum stress and ethanol neurotoxicity. *Biomolecules* 5(4):2538–2553, 2015.

73. Gutierrez C, et al: An experimental study on the effects of ethanol and folic acid deficiency, alone or in combination, on pregnant Swiss mice. *Pathology* 39(5):495–503, 2007.

74. Haycock PC: Fetal alcohol spectrum disorders: the epigenetic perspective. *Biol Reprod* 81(4):607–617, 2009.

75. Mason S, Zhou FC: Editorial: Genetics and epigenetics of fetal alcohol spectrum disorders. *Front Genet* 6:146, 2015.

76. Resendiz M, et al: Alcohol metabolism and epigenetic methylation and acetylation. In Patel V, editor: *Molecular aspects of alcohol and nutrition*, ed 1, St Louis, 2015, Elsevier.

77. Centers for Disease Control and Prevention (CDC): *WISQUARS database*, updated 24 June 2015. Available at: www.cdc.gov/ncipc/wisqars.

78. Heron M: Deaths: leading causes for 2013. *Natl Vital Stat Rep* 65(2):1–95, 2016.

79. The National Academies Press: *Abrupt impacts of climate change: anticipating surprises*, Washington, DC, 2013, National Academies of Science.

80. Environmental Protection Agency (EPA): *Overview of greenhouse gases*, Washington, DC, 2016, Author.

81. World Health Organization (WHO): *Climate change and health*, Geneva, Switzerland, 2015, Author.

82. Wu X, et al: Impact of climate change on human infectious diseases: empirical evidence and human adaptation. *Environ Int* 86:14–23, 2016.

83. Danzi D: Hypothermia and frostbite. In Longo DL, et al, editors: *Harrison's principles of internal medicine*, ed 18, New York, 2012, McGraw-Hill.

84. Shattock MJ, Tipton MJ: "Autonomic conflict:" a different way to die during cold water immersion? *J Physiol* 590(Pt 14):3219–3230, 2012.

85. Bierens JJ, Knape JT, Gelissen HP: Drowning. *Curr Opin Crit Care* 8:578–586, 2002.

86. Camara AK, et al: Hypothermia augments reactive oxygen species detected in the guinea pig isolated perfused heart. *Am J Physiol Heart Circ Physiol* 286(4):H1289–H1299, 2004.

87. Rauen U, de Groot H: Mammalian cell injury induced by hypothermia—the emerging role for reactive oxygen species. *Biol Chem* 383(3–4):477–488, 2002.

88. Schwartz BG, et al: Therapeutic hypothermia for acute myocardial infarction and cardiac arrest. *Am J Cardiol* 110(3):461–466, 2012.

89. Lanner JT: Ryanodine receptor physiology and its role in disease. In Islam MS, editor: *Calcium signaling, advances in experimental medicine and biology*, New York, 2012, Springer.

90. Dinarello CA, Porat R: Fever and hypothermia. In Longo DL, et al, editors: *Harrison's principles of internal medicine*, ed 18, New York, 2012, McGraw-Hill.

91. International Society for the Study and Prevention of Infant Death (ISPID): *What is SIDS?* New York, 2015, Author.

92. McDonald FB, et al: Cardiorespiratory control and cytokine profile in response to heat stress, hypoxia, and lipopolysaccharide (LPS) exposure during early neonatal period. *Physiol Rep* 4(2):12688, 2016.

93. Task Force on Sudden Infant Death Syndrome, Moon RY: SIDS and other sleep-related infant deaths: expansion of recommendations for a safe infant sleeping environment. *Pediatrics* 128(5):1030–1039, 2011.

94. Eichhorn L, Leyk D: Diving medicine in clinical practice. *Dtsch Arztebl Int* 112(9):147–158, 2015.

95. Fahlman A, Dromsky DM: Dehydration effects on the risk of severe decompression sickness in a swine model. *Aviat Space Environ Med* 77:102–106, 2006.

96. Lynch JH, Bove AA: Diving medicine: a review of current evidence. *J Spec Oper Med* 9:72–79, 2009.

97. NOAA: *NOAA diving manual: diving for science and technology*, ed 4, Palm Beach Gardens, FL, 2010, Best Publishing.

98. Webb JT, Pilmanis AA: Fifty years of decompression sickness research at Brooks AFB, TX: 1960-2010. *Aviat Space Environ Med* 82(Suppl):A1–A25, 2011.

99. Luks AM, et al: Wilderness Medical Society practice guidelines for the prevention and treatment of acute altitude illness: 2014 update. *Wilderness Environ Med* 25(4 Suppl):S4–S14, 2014.

100. Johnson NJ, Luks AM: High-altitude medicine. *Med Clin North Am* 100(2):357–369, 2016.

101. Bärtsch P, Swenson ER: Clinical practice: acute high-altitude illnesses. *N Engl J Med* 368(24):2294–2302, 2013.

102. Luks AM: Physiology in medicine: a physiologic approach to prevention and treatment of acute high-altitude illness. *J Appl Physiol* 118(5):509–519, 2015.

103. Scherrer U, et al: New insights in the pathogenesis of high-altitude pulmonary edema. *Prog Cardiovasc Dis* 52:485–492, 2010.

104. International Commission for Radiological Protection (ICRP): ICRP statement on tissue reactions and early and late effects of radiation in normal tissues and organs—threshold doses for tissue reactions in a radiation protection context, ICRP Publication No. 118. *Ann ICRP* 41(1/2):2012.

105. Little MP, Lipshultz SE: Low dose radiation and circulatory diseases: a brief narrative review. *Cardiooncology* 1:4, 2015, doi:10.1186/s40959-015-0007-6.

106. Hall E, Giaccia AJ: Milestones in the radiation sciences. In Hall E, Giaccia AJ, editors: *Radiobiology for the radiologist*, ed 6, Philadelphia, 2006, Lippincott Williams & Wilkins.

107. Linet S, et al: Cancer risks associated with external radiation from diagnostic imaging procedures. *CA Cancer J Clin* 62:75–100, 2012.

108. Dauer LT, et al: Review and evaluation of updated research on the health effects associated with low-doses of ionizing radiation. *Radiat Prot Dosimetry* 140:103–136, 2010.

109. Barcellos-Hoff MH, Nguyen DH: Radiation carcinogenesis in context: how do irradiated tissues become tumors? *Health Phys* 97(5):446–457, 2009.

110. Mothersill C, Seymour C: Are epigenetic mechanisms involved in radiation-induced bystander effects? *Front Genet* 3:74, 2012.

111. Seymour CB, Mothersill C, Alper T: High yields of lethal mutations in somatic mammalian cells that survive ionizing radiation. *Int J Radiat Biol Relat Stud Phys Chem Med* 50:167–179, 1986.

112. Kadhim MA, et al: Transmission of chromosomal instability after plutonium alpha-particle irradiation. *Nature* 355:738–740, 1992.

113. Nagasawa H, Little JB: Induction of sister chromatid exchanges by extremely low doses of alpha-particles. *Cancer Res* 52:6394–6396, 1992.

114. Mothersill C, Seymour C: Medium from irradiated human epithelial cells but not human fibroblasts reduces the clonogenic survival of unirradiated cells. *Int J Radiat Biol* 71:421–427, 1997.

115. Barker HE, et al: The tumor microenvironment after radiotherapy: mechanisms of resistance and recurrence. *Nat Rev Cancer* 15:409–425, 2015.

116. Rüegg C, et al: Radiation-induced modifications of the tumor microenvironment promote metastasis. *Bull Cancer* 98(6):47–57, 2011.

117. Leroi N, et al: Impacts of ionizing radiation on the different compartments of the tumor microenvironment. *Front Pharmacol* 7:78, 2016.

118. Park C, Wright EG: Radiation and the microenvironment—tumorigenesis and therapy. *Nat Rev Cancer* 5:867–875, 2005.

119. Preston DL, et al: Solid cancer incidence in atomic bomb survivors: 1958–1998. *Radiat Res* 168:1–64, 2007.

120. Lazarus E, et al: Utilization of imaging in pregnant patients: 10 year review of 5270 examinations in 3285 patients—1997–2006. *Radiology* 251(2):517–524, 2009.

121. UpToDate: Diagnostic imaging procedures during pregnancy. In Post TW, editor: *UpToDate*, Waltham, MA, 2016.

122. Brenner DJ, et al: Estimated risks of radiation-induced fatal cancer from pediatric CT. *AJR Am J Roentgenol* 176:289–296, 2001.

123. Brenner DJ, Shuryak I, Einstein AJ: Impact of reduced patient life expectancy on potential cancer risks. *Radiology* 261(1):193–198, 2011.

124. Shuryak I, Sachs RK, Brenner DJ: Cancer risks after radiation exposure in middle age. *J Natl Cancer Inst* 102(12):1628–1636, 2012.

125. Behar-Cohen F, et al: Light-emitting diodes (LED) for domestic lighting: any risks for the eye? *Prog Retin Eye Res* 30:239–257, 2011.

126. Youssef PN, Sheibani N, Albert DM: Retinal light toxicity. *Eye (Lond)* 25(1):1–14, 2011.

127. Kuse Y, et al: Damage of photoreceptor-derived cells in culture induced by light emitting diode-derived blue light. *Sci Rep* 4:5223, 2014.

128. Organisciak DT, Vaughan DK: Retinal light damage: mechanisms and protection. *Prog Retin Eye Res* 29(2):113–134, 2011.

129. Siu TL, Morley JW, Coroneo MT: Toxicology of the retina: advances in understanding the defence mechanisms and pathogenesis of drug- and light-induced retinopathy. *Clin Experiment Ophthalmol* 36(2):176–185, 2008.

130. Environmental Working Group (EWG): *Health/toxics: mercury*, 2008. Available at: www.ewg.org/mercury.

131. Han MKL, de Rooij J: Converging and unique mechanisms of mechanotransduction at adhesion sites. *Trends Cell Biol* 2016 Mar 29. [Epub ahead of print].

132. Barbee KA: Mechanical cell injury. *Ann N Y Acad Sci* 1066:67–84, 2005.

133. Williams PR, et al: A recoverable state of axon injury persists for hours after spinal cord contusion in vivo. *Nat Commun* 5:5683, 2014.

134. Krenning G, et al: Endothelial plasticity: shifting phenotypes through force feedback. *Stem Cells Int* 2016:9762959, 2016.

135. Van Epps JS, Vorp DA: Mechanopathobiology of atherogenesis: a review. *J Surg Res* 142(1):202–217, 2007.

136. National Institute on Deafness and Other Communication Disorders (NIDCD): *Statistics about hearing disorders, ear infections, and deafness*, Washington, DC, 2005, National Institutes of Health. Available at: www.nidcd.nih.gov/health/statistics/nearing.asp.

137. Ryherd E, West J, Ljungkvist L: Characterizing noise and perceived work environments in a neurological intensive care unit. *J Acoust Soc Am* 123:747–756, 2008.

138. Sun Y, et al: Inhibition of cyclooxygenase-2 by NS398 attenuates noise-induced hearing loss in mice. *Sci Rep* 6:22573, 2016.

139. Cho YS, et al: Physiological consequences of programmed necrosis, an alternative form of cell demise. *Mol Cells* 29(4):327–332, 2010.

140. Linkermann A, Green DR: Necroptosis. *N Engl J Med* 370(5):455–465, 2014.

141. Moquin D, Chan F: The molecular regulation of programmed necrotic cell injury. *Trends Biochem Sci* 35(8):434–441, 2010.

142. Wang Z, et al: The mitochondrial phosphatase PGAM5 functions at the convergence point of multiple necrotic death pathways. *Cell* 148:228–243, 2012.

143. Glick D, Barth S, MacLeod KF: Autophagy: cellular and molecular mechanisms. *J Pathol* 221(1):3–12, 2010.

144. Wyllie AH, Kerr JFR, Currie AR: Cell death: the significance of apoptosis. *Int Rev Cytol* 68:251–306, 1980.

145. Kaur J, Debnath J: Autophagy at the crossroads of catabolism and anabolism. *Nat Rev Mol Cell Biol* 16:461–472, 2015.

146. Mizushima N, Komatsu M: Autophagy: renovation of cells and tissues. *Cell* 147(4):728–741, 2011.

147. Mizushima N: Autophagy: process and function. *Genes Dev* 21(22):2861–2873, 2007, review.

148. Rabinowitz JD, White E: Autophagy and metabolism. *Science* 330(6009):1344–1348, 2010.

149. Rikiishi H: Novel insights into the interplay between apoptosis and autophagy. *Int J Cell Biol* 2012:317645, 2012.

150. Kepp O, et al: Cell death assays for drug discovery. *Nat Rev Drug Discov* 10(3):221–237, 2012.

151. Shigeomi S, et al: Autophagic cell death and cancer. *Int J Mol Sci* 15:3145–3153, 2014.

152. White E: The role for autophagy in cancer. *J Clin Invest* 125(1):42–46, 2015.

153. Lavandero S, et al: Autophagy in cardiovascular biology. *J Clin Invest* 125(1):55–64, 2015.

154. Johnson HA: Is aging physiological or pathological? In Johnson HA, editor: *Relation between normal aging and disease*, New York, 1985, Raven.

155. Hayflick L: Biological aging is no longer an unsolved problem. *Ann N Y Acad Sci* 1100:1–13, 2007, review.

156. Tissenbaum HA: Genetics, life span, health span, and the aging process in *Caenorhabditis elegans*. *J Gerontol A Biol Sci Med Sci* 67A(5):503–510, 2012.

157. Flatt TA: A new definition of aging? *Front Genet* 3:148, 2012.

158. Kaeberlein M, Rabinovitch PS, Martin GM: Healthy aging: the ultimate preventative medicine. *Science* 350(6265):1191–1193, 2015.

159. Rando TA, Chang HY: Aging rejuvenation, and epigenetic reprogramming: resetting the aging clock. *Cell* 148:46–57, 2012.

160. Editorial: Aging: toward avoiding the inevitable. *Nat Med* 21(12):1373, 2015.

161. World Health Organization (WHO): *World report on ageing and health*, Geneva Switzerland, 2015, Author.

162. Brodin P, et al: Variation in the human immune system is largely driven by non-heritable influences. *Cell* 160(1–2):37–47, 2015.

163. Childs BG, et al: Cellular senescence in aging and age-related disease: from mechanisms to therapy. *Nat Med* 21(12):1424–1435, 2015.

164. Baker DJ, et al: Naturally occurring p16(Ink4a)-positive cells shorten healthy lifespan. *Nature* 530:184–189, 2016.

165. Michaud M, et al: Proinflammatory cytokines, aging, and age-related diseases. *J Am Med Dir Assoc* 14(12):877–882, 2013.

166. Glass CK, et al: Mechanisms underlying inflammation in neurodegeneration. *Cell* 140(6):918–934, 2010.

167. Franceschi C, Campisi J: Chronic inflammation (inflammaging) and its potential contribution to age-associated diseases. *J Gerontol A Biol Sci Med Sci* 69(S1):S4–S9, 2014.

168. Belkaid Y, Hand TW: Role of the microbiota in immunity and inflammation. *Cell* 157(1):121–141, 2014.

169. Shaw AC, et al: Aging of the innate immune system. *Curr Opin Immunol* 22:507–513, 2010.

170. Bansal A, et al: Uncoupling lifespan and healthspan in *Caenorhabditis elegans* longevity mutants. *Proc Natl Acad Sci USA* 112(3):E277–E286, 2015.

171. Villeda SA, et al: Age-related changes in the systemic milieu regulate adult neurogenesis. *Nature* 477:90–94, 2011.

172. Szarc vel Szic K, et al: From inflammaging to healthy aging by dietary lifestyle choices: is epigenetics the key to personalized nutrition? *Clin Epigenetics* 7(1):33, 2015.

173. Park LK, Friso S, Choi SW: Nutritional influences on epigenetics and age-related disease. *Proc Nutr Soc* 71(1):75–83, 2012.

174. Harrison DE, et al: Rapamycin fed late in life extends lifespan in genetically heterogeneous mice. *Nature* 460:392–395, 2009.

175. Darzi A, et al: *The five bad habits of healthcare. How new thinking about behaviour could reduce health spending*, Geneva, Switzerland, 2011, World Economic Forum and Imperial College Vlaev.

176. Centers for Disease Control and Prevention (CDC): *Deaths and mortality*, Atlanta GA, 2017, Centers for Disease Control and Prevention, National Center for Health Statistics.

177. Institute of Medicine (IOM): *For the public's health: investing in a healthier future*, Washington, DC, 2012, The National Academies Press.

178. Cory SA, et al: Prevalence of selected risk behaviors and chronic diseases and conditions—steps communities, United States, 2006–2007. *MMWR Surveill Summ* 59(8):1–37, 2010.

179. Boyle J, et al: Projection of the year 2050 burden of diabetes in the US population: dynamic modeling of incidence, mortality, and prediabetes prevalence. *Popul Health Metr* 8(1):29, 2010.

180. Olshansky SJ, et al: A potential decline in life expectancy in the United States in the 21st century. *N Engl J Med* 352(11):1138–1145, 2005.

181. Seals DR, Jablonski KL, Donato AJ: Aging and vascular endothelial function in humans. *Clin Sci* 120:357–375, 2011.

182. Higashi Y, et al: IGF-1, oxidative stress, and atheroprotection. *Trends Endocrinol Metab* 21(4):245–254, 2011.

183. Clegg A, et al: Frailty in elderly people. *Lancet* 381(9868):752–762, 2013.

The Cellular Environment: Fluids and Electrolytes, Acids and Bases

Sue E. Huether

evolve WEBSITE

http://evolve.elsevier.com/McCance/
- Content Updates
- Chapter Summary Review
- Review Questions
- Case Studies
- Animations

CHAPTER OUTLINE

The cells of the body live in a fluid environment that requires electrolyte and acid-base concentrations maintained within a very narrow range. A balance is maintained by an integration of renal, hormonal, and neural functions. Changes in electrolyte concentration affect the electrical activity of nerve and muscle cells and cause shifts of fluid from one compartment to another. Fluid fluctuations also affect blood volume and therefore blood pressure. Alterations in acid-base balance disrupt the cellular function of enzyme systems and can cause cell injury. Disturbances in fluid and electrolyte or acid-base balance are common and can be life threatening. Understanding how alterations occur and the body's ability to compensate or correct the disturbance is important for comprehending many pathophysiologic conditions.

DISTRIBUTION OF BODY FLUIDS

Body fluids are distributed among functional compartments, or spaces, and provide a transport medium for cellular and tissue function. Water moves freely among body compartments and is distributed by osmotic and hydrostatic forces. Two-thirds of the body's water is **intracellular fluid (ICF)** and one-third is in the **extracellular fluid (ECF)** compartments. The two main ECF compartments are the **interstitial fluid** and the **intravascular fluid**, the latter being the blood plasma. Other ECF compartments include the lymph and the transcellular fluids. The major transcellular fluids are summarized in Table 3.1. Other transcellular fluids include pleural, synovial, peritoneal, pericardial, and intraocular fluids (Table 3.1).

TABLE 3.1	APPROXIMATE CONCENTRATIONS OF ELECTROLYTES IN TRANSCELLULAR FLUIDS			
FLUID	**Na^+ (mEq/L)**	**K^+ (mEq/L)**	**Cl^- (mEq/L)**	**HCO_3^- (mEq/L)**
Saliva	33	20	34	40
Gastric juice*	60	9	84	0
Bile	149	5	101	45
Pancreatic juice	141	5	77	92
Ileal fluid	129	11	116	29
Cecal fluid	80	21	48	22
Cerebrospinal fluid	141	3	127	23
Sweat	45	5	58	0

*The Cl^- concentration exceeds the Na^+, K^+ concentration by 15 mEq/L in gastric juice. This largely represents the secretions of hydrochloric acid by parietal cells.

TABLE 3.2	DISTRIBUTION OF BODY WATER	
	% OF BODY WEIGHT	**VOLUME (L)**
Intracellular fluid (ICF)	40	28
Extracellular fluid (ECF)	20	14
Interstitial	(15)	(11)
Intravascular	(5)	(3)
Total body water (TBW)	60	42

TABLE 3.3	TOTAL BODY WATER (%) IN RELATION TO BODY WEIGHT				
BODY BUILD	**ADULT MALE**	**ADULT FEMALE**	**CHILD (1–10 yr)**	**INFANT (1 mo to 1 yr)**	**NEWBORN (up to 1 mo)**
Normal	60	50	65	70	70–80
Lean	70	60	50–60	80	
Obese	50	42	50	60	

NOTE: Total body water is a percentage of body weight.

The sum of fluids within all compartments constitutes the total body water (TBW) (Table 3.2). The volume of TBW is usually expressed as a percentage of body weight in kilograms. The total volume of body water for a 70-kg person is about 42 liters (Table 3.3). The rest of the body weight is composed of fat and fat-free solids, particularly bone.

Although daily fluid intake may fluctuate widely, the body regulates water volume within a relatively narrow range. The primary sources of body water are drinking of fluids, ingestion of water in food, and derivation of water from oxidative metabolism. Normally, the largest amounts of water are lost through renal excretion. Lesser amounts are eliminated through the stool and through vaporization from the skin and lungs (insensible water loss) (Table 3.4).

Although the amount of fluid within the various compartments is relatively constant, exchange of solutes (e.g., salts) and water occurs

TABLE 3.4	NORMAL WATER GAINS AND LOSSES (70-kg MAN)			
	DAILY INTAKE (mL)		**DAILY OUTPUT (mL)**
Drinking ≈60%	1400–1800	Urine ≈60%	1400–1800
Water in food ≈30%	700–1000	Stool ≈2%	100
Water of oxidation ≈10%	300–400	Skin ≈10%	300–500
		Lungs ≈28%	600–800
TOTAL	2400–3200	**TOTAL**	2400–3200

between compartments to maintain their unique compositions. The percentage of TBW varies with the amount of body fat and age. Because fat is water repelling (hydrophobic), very little water is contained in adipose cells. Individuals with more body fat have proportionately less TBW and tend to be more susceptible to fluid imbalances that cause dehydration.

AGING AND DISTRIBUTION OF BODY FLUIDS

The distribution and amount of TBW change with age (see Table 3.3). In newborn infants, TBW is about 70% to 80% of body weight because infants store less fat. In the immediate postnatal period, a physiologic loss of body water occurs, equivalent to about 5% of body weight as the infant adjusts to a new environment. Infants are particularly susceptible to significant changes in TBW because of their high metabolic rate and potential for evaporative fluid loss attributable to their greater body surface area in proportion to total body size. Loss of fluids from diarrhea can represent a significant proportion of body weight in infants. Renal mechanisms that regulate fluid and electrolyte conservation may not be mature enough to counter the losses, so dehydration can develop rapidly.

During childhood, TBW slowly decreases to 60% to 65% of body weight. At adolescence the percentage of TBW approaches adult proportions, and gender differences begin to appear. Males eventually have a greater percentage of body water as a function of increasing muscle mass. Females have more body fat and less muscle as a function of estrogens and therefore have less body water.

With increasing age the percentage of TBW declines further still. The decrease is caused in part by an increased amount of fat and a decreased amount of muscle and by a reduced ability to regulate sodium and water balance. With older age, the kidneys become less efficient at conserving sodium and therefore have difficulty concentrating the urine. Insensible water loss through the skin may increase and thirst perception may be impaired. The normal reduction of TBW in older adults becomes clinically important when the body is under stress, such as development of fever or dehydration; loss of body fluids at such times can be severe and life threatening.

Water Movement Between ICF and ECF

The movement of water between ICF and ECF compartments is primarily a function of osmotic forces. (Osmosis and other mechanisms of passive transport are discussed in Chapter 1.) Water moves freely by diffusion through the lipid bilayer cell membrane and through aquaporins, a family of water channel proteins that provide permeability to water.[1] The osmolality (number of osmoles of solute per kilogram of fluid [Osm/kg]) of TBW is normally at equilibrium. Sodium is responsible for the osmotic balance of the ECF space. Potassium maintains the osmotic balance of the ICF space. The osmotic force of ICF proteins and other nondiffusible substances is balanced by the active transport of ions out of the cell. Water crosses cell membranes freely so the osmolality of TBW is normally at equilibrium. Normally the ICF is not subject to rapid changes in osmolality but when ECF osmolality changes, water moves from one compartment to another until osmotic equilibrium is reestablished.

Water Movement Between Plasma and Interstitial Fluid

The distribution of water and the movement of nutrients and waste products between the plasma in the tissue capillaries and interstitial spaces occur as a result of changes in hydrostatic pressure and osmotic forces at the arterial and venous ends of the capillary (see Fig. 1.33). Water, sodium, and glucose move readily across the capillary membrane. The plasma proteins maintain the effective osmolality (concentration of solutes per kilogram of solution), do not cross the capillary membrane, and generate plasma oncotic pressure. Albumin is the plasma protein that is primarily responsible for the plasma oncotic pressure because it has the highest concentration. Osmotic forces within the capillary are balanced by the hydrostatic pressure, which is primarily determined by blood pressure and blood volume.

As plasma flows from the arterial to the venous end of the capillary, four forces determine if fluid moves out of the capillary and into the interstitial space (filtration) or if fluid moves back into the capillary from the interstitial space (reabsorption):

1. **Capillary hydrostatic pressure (blood pressure)** facilitates the outward movement of water from the capillary to the interstitial space.
2. **Capillary (plasma) oncotic pressure** osmotically attracts water from the interstitial space back into the capillary.
3. **Interstitial hydrostatic pressure** facilitates the inward movement of water from the interstitial space into the capillary.
4. **Interstitial oncotic pressure** osmotically attracts water from the capillary into the interstitial space.

The movement of fluid back and forth across the capillary wall is called **net filtration** and is best described by the **Starling hypothesis**:

$$\textit{Net filtration} = (\text{Forces favoring filtration})\\ - (\text{Forces opposing filtration})$$

$$\textit{Forces favoring filtration} = \text{Capillary hydrostatic}\\ \text{pressure and interstitial oncotic pressure}$$

$$\textit{Forces opposing filtration} = \text{Capillary oncotic pressure}\\ \text{and interstitial hydrostatic pressure}$$

Normally the interstitial forces are negligible because only a very small percentage of plasma proteins crosses the capillary membrane and interstitial fluid moves into cells or is drawn back into the plasma. Thus the major forces for filtration are within the capillary.

As the plasma flows from the arterial to the venous end of the capillary, the force of hydrostatic pressure facilitates the movement of water across the capillary membrane. Oncotic pressure remains fairly constant because plasma proteins normally do not cross the capillary membrane. At the arterial end of the capillary, hydrostatic pressure is greater than capillary oncotic pressure and water filters into the interstitial space. Because of oncotic forces, some water moves back into the capillary, but the net effect is loss of water from the capillary. This loss of water from the plasma decreases the hydrostatic pressure within the capillary; thus, at the venous end of the capillary, oncotic pressure exceeds hydrostatic pressure. Fluids then are attracted back into the circulation, balancing the movement of fluids between the plasma and the interstitial space. The overall effect is filtration at the arterial end and reabsorption at the venous end (Fig. 3.1). Interstitial hydrostatic pressure promotes the movement of interstitial fluid along with small amounts of protein into lymphatic vessels, which is then returned to the circulation.

An important factor in capillary filtration of fluid is the integrity of the capillary membrane. Changes in membrane permeability may permit the escape of plasma proteins into the interstitial space. The normal relationship defined by the Starling hypothesis is altered with the osmotic movement of water into the interstitial space, causing tissue edema.

ALTERATIONS IN WATER MOVEMENT

Edema

Edema is the excessive accumulation of fluid within the interstitial spaces. It is often a problem of fluid distribution and does not necessarily indicate a fluid excess. In some conditions, sequestered fluids can cause both edema and intravascular dehydration. The pathophysiologic process of edema is related to an increase in the forces favoring fluid filtration from the capillaries or lymphatic channels into the tissues. The four most common mechanisms are:

1. Increased capillary hydrostatic pressure
2. Decreased capillary oncotic pressure
3. Increased capillary membrane permeability
4. Lymphatic obstruction (Fig. 3.2)

◆**PATHOPHYSIOLOGY.** Increased capillary hydrostatic pressure can result from venous obstruction or sodium and water retention. Venous obstruction causes hydrostatic pressure to increase behind the obstruction, pushing fluid from the capillaries into the interstitial spaces. Venous blood clots, hepatic obstruction, right heart failure, tight clothing around the extremities, and prolonged standing are common causes of venous obstruction. Right congestive heart failure, renal failure, and cirrhosis of the liver are conditions associated with excessive sodium and water retention, which in turn cause volume overload, increased venous pressure, and edema. The volume of interstitial fluid exceeds the capacity of the lymphatics to return fluid to the vascular system.

Decreased plasma oncotic pressure results from *losses or diminished production of plasma albumin.* Decreased oncotic attraction of fluid within the capillary causes fluid to move into the interstitial space, resulting in edema. Decreased synthesis of plasma protein and decreased oncotic pressure may occur with liver disease or protein malnutrition. Losses of plasma proteins occur with glomerular diseases of the kidney (nephrotic syndrome), hemorrhage, and serous drainage from open wounds or burns.

Increased capillary permeability is usually associated with *inflammation and the immune response.* (Immunity is discussed in Chapters 7, 8, and 9; inflammation is discussed in Chapters 7 and 9.) These responses are often the result of trauma such as burns or crushing injuries, neoplastic disease, allergic reactions, and infection. Excess amounts of fluid escape from the plasma to the interstitial space and produce edema. This type of edema is often very severe because of loss of proteins from the vascular space, which decreases capillary oncotic pressure and increases interstitial oncotic pressure with both processes facilitating fluid movement into the interstitial space.

Lymphatic obstruction occurs when the *lymphatic channels are blocked* because of infection or tumor. Proteins and fluids are not reabsorbed and accumulate in the interstitial space, causing **lymphedema**. Lymphedema of the arm or leg also can occur after surgical removal of axillary or femoral lymph nodes, respectively, for treatment of cancer.[2]

◆**CLINICAL MANIFESTATIONS.** Edema may be localized or generalized. *Localized edema* is usually limited to the site of tissue injury, as in a sprained joint. Local edema can also occur within particular organs,

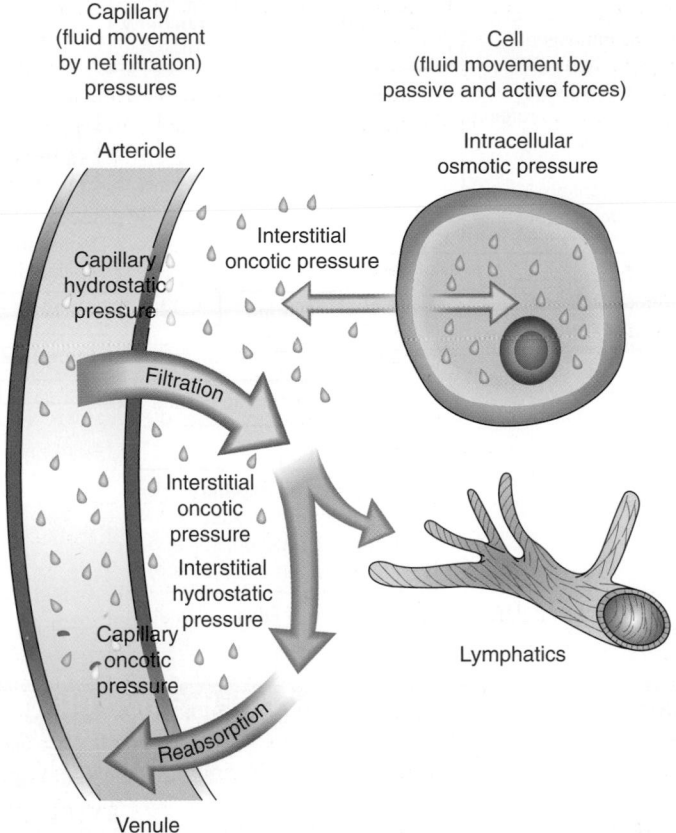

Arterial Capillary Pressures		Venous Capillary Pressures	
Capillary hydrostatic pressure	35 mmHg	Capillary hydrostatic pressure	18 mmHg
Interstitial fluid hydrostatic pressure	2 mmHg	Interstitial fluid hydrostatic pressure	1 mmHg
Net hydrostatic pressure	**33 mmHg**	**Net hydrostatic pressure**	**17 mmHg**
Capillary oncotic pressure	24 mmHg	Capillary oncotic pressure	25 mmHg
Interstitial fluid oncotic pressure	0 mmHg	Interstitial fluid oncotic pressure	0 mmHg
Net oncotic pressure	**24 mmHg**	**Net oncotic pressure**	**25 mmHg**
Net filtration pressure	**+9 mmHg**	**Net filtration pressure**	**−8 mmHg**

FIGURE 3.1 Capillary Filtration Forces. Water, electrolytes, and small molecules exchange freely between the vascular compartment and the interstitial space at the site of capillaries and small venules. The rate and amount of exchange are driven by the physical forces of hydrostatic and oncotic pressures and the permeability and surface area of the capillary membranes. The two opposing hydrostatic pressures are capillary hydrostatic pressure and interstitial hydrostatic pressure. The two opposing oncotic pressures are capillary oncotic pressure and interstitial oncotic pressure. The *forces that favor filtration* from the capillary are capillary hydrostatic pressure and interstitial oncotic pressure, and the *forces that oppose filtration* are capillary oncotic pressure and interstitial hydrostatic pressure. The sum is known as *net filtration pressure*. In the example of normal exchange illustrated here, a small amount of fluid moves to the lymph vessels, which accounts for the net filtration difference between the arterial and venous ends of the capillary.

causing, for example, cerebral edema in the brain, pulmonary edema in the lungs, pleural effusion (fluid accumulation in the pleural space), laryngeal edema, and ascites (accumulation of fluid in the abdomen). Edema of specific organs, such as the brain, lung, or larynx, can be life threatening. *Generalized edema* is manifested by a more uniform distribution of fluid in interstitial spaces throughout the body. *Dependent edema*, in which fluid accumulates in gravity-dependent areas of the body,

might appear in the feet and legs when standing and in the sacral area and buttocks when supine. Dependent edema can be identified by using the fingers to press away edematous fluid in tissues overlying bony prominences. A pit will be left in the skin; hence the term *pitting edema* (Fig. 3.3).

Edema is usually associated with swelling and puffiness, tight-fitting clothes and shoes, and limited movement of the affected area. Weight

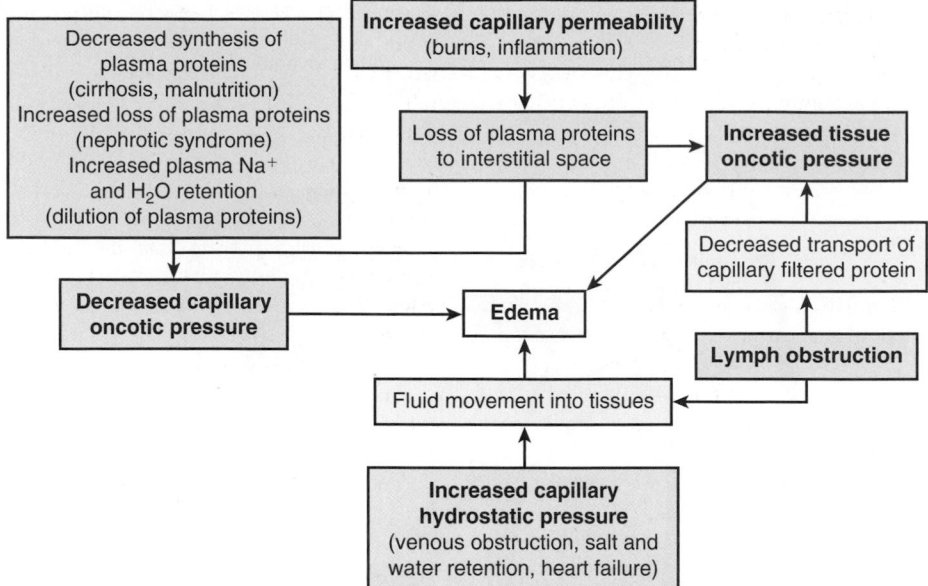

FIGURE 3.2 Mechanisms of Edema Formation.

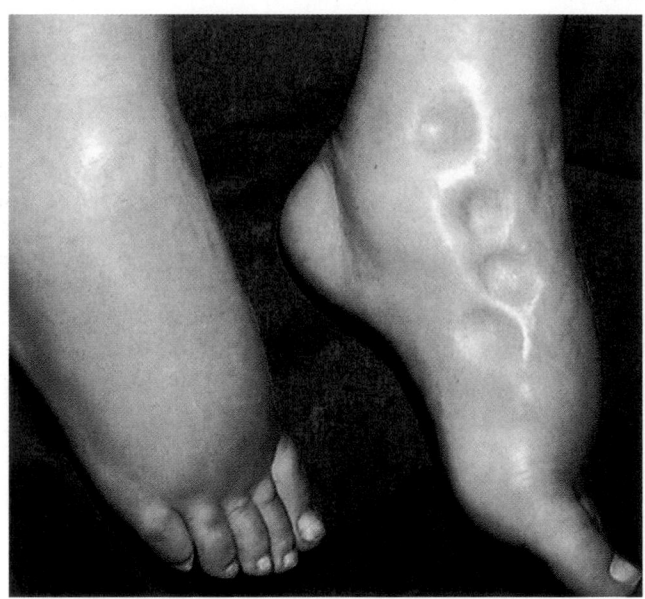

FIGURE 3.3 Pitting Edema. (From Bloom A, Ireland J: *Color atlas of diabetes,* ed 2, St Louis, 1992, Mosby.)

TABLE 3.5	**DISTRIBUTION OF ELECTROLYTES IN BODY COMPARTMENTS**	
	EXTRACELLULAR FLUID (mEq/L)	**INTRACELLULAR FLUID (mEq/L)**
Cations		
Sodium	142	10
Potassium	5	156
Calcium	5	4
Magnesium	2	26
TOTAL	154	196
Anions		
Bicarbonate	24	12
Chloride	104	4
Phosphate	2	40–95
Proteins	16	54
Other anions	8	31–86
TOTAL	154	196 (average)

gain can be significant. The accumulation of fluid increases the distance required for nutrients, oxygen, and wastes to move between capillaries and cells in the tissues. Increased tissue pressure also may diminish capillary blood flow, leading to ischemia. Therefore, wounds heal more slowly and risk of pressure ulcers increase. As edematous fluid accumulates, it is trapped in a "third space" (i.e., the interstitial space) and dehydration can develop as a result of this sequestering of fluid. Such sequestration occurs with severe burns, in which large amounts of vascular fluid are lost to the interstitial spaces, reducing plasma volume and causing shock.

◆**EVALUATION AND TREATMENT.** Specific conditions causing edema require diagnosis. Edema may be treated symptomatically until the underlying disorder is corrected. Supportive measures include elevating edematous limbs, wearing compression stockings or devices, avoiding prolonged standing, restricting salt intake, and taking diuretics.

SODIUM, CHLORIDE, AND WATER BALANCE

The kidneys and hormones have a central role in maintaining sodium and water balance. Because water follows the osmotic gradients established by changes in salt concentration, sodium balance and water balance are intimately related. Sodium is regulated by the renal effects of aldosterone from the adrenal cortex and natriuretic peptides from the heart. Water balance is primarily regulated by the renal response to antidiuretic hormone (ADH; also known as *arginine-vasopressin*) from the posterior pituitary.

Sodium and Chloride Balance

Sodium accounts for 90% of the ECF cations (positively charged ions). The distribution of electrolytes in body compartments is summarized in Table 3.5 and the concentration of electrolytes is summarized in Table 3.1. As the most abundant ECF cation, along with its constituent anions (negatively charged ions) chloride and bicarbonate, sodium regulates extracellular osmotic forces and therefore regulates water balance and ECF volume. Sodium is important in other body functions, including maintenance of neuromuscular irritability for conduction of nerve impulses (in conjunction with potassium and calcium), regulation of acid-base balance (through sodium bicarbonate and sodium phosphate), participation in cellular chemical reactions, and transport of substances across the cellular membrane (see Chapter 1).

The kidney, in conjunction with neural and hormonal mediators, maintains normal serum sodium concentration within a narrow range (135 to 145 mEq/L) primarily through renal tubular reabsorption. Generally, sodium intake matches sodium excretion. The average dietary intake of sodium ranges from 5 to 6 g/day; the minimal daily requirement of sodium is 500 mg. Sweating depletes sodium and water volume and increases the body's sodium requirement.

Hormonal regulation of sodium balance is mediated by **aldosterone**, a mineralocorticoid (steroid) synthesized and secreted from the adrenal cortex as the end product of the renin-angiotensin-aldosterone system (Fig. 3.4). When circulating blood pressure and renal blood flow, or serum sodium concentrations, are reduced, **renin**, an enzyme secreted by the juxtaglomerular cells of the kidney, is released. Renin stimulates the formation of **angiotensin I**, an inactive polypeptide. Angiotensin-converting enzyme (ACE) in pulmonary vessels converts angiotensin I to angiotensin II. **Angiotensin II** causes vasoconstriction, which elevates systemic blood pressure, and stimulates the secretion of aldosterone. Vasoconstriction elevates the systemic blood pressure and restores renal perfusion (blood flow), and aldosterone promotes sodium and water reabsorption by the proximal tubules of the kidneys, thus conserving sodium, blood volume, and blood pressure. Aldosterone also stimulates secretion (and therefore excretion) of potassium by the distal tubule of the kidney, reducing potassium concentrations in the ECF. The restoration of sodium levels, blood volume, and renal perfusion then inhibits further release of renin.

Natriuretic peptides are hormones that include atrial natriuretic peptide (ANP) produced by myoendocrine atrial cells, brain natriuretic peptide (BNP—named brain since it was first discovered in porcine brain) produced by myoendocrine ventricular cells, and urodilatin (renal natriuretic peptide, an ANP analog) synthesized within the kidney. ANP and BNP are released when there is an increase in transmural atrial pressure caused by increased intraatrial volume as may occur with heart failure.[3] ANP and BNP increase sodium and water excretion by the kidneys, which lowers blood volume and pressure (Fig. 3.5). Urodilatin is released from distal tubular kidney cells when there is increased arterial pressure and increased renal blood flow. These hormones are natural antagonists to the renin-angiotensin-aldosterone system. The restoration of lower atrial pressure then inhibits further release of ANP and BNP.

Chloride is the major anion in the ECF and provides electroneutrality, particularly in relation to sodium. Chloride transport is generally passive and follows the active transport of sodium so that increases or decreases in chloride concentration are proportional to changes in sodium concentration. Chloride concentration tends to vary inversely with changes in the concentration of bicarbonate (HCO_3^-), the other major ECF anion.

Water Balance

Water balance is regulated by interactions between sensory organs (carotid and aortic artery volume/pressure receptors and hypothalamic osmoreceptors), **antidiuretic hormone (ADH)** (also known as **arginine-vasopressin**), and the kidney. ADH is secreted when plasma osmolality increases or circulating blood volume decreases and blood pressure drops (Fig. 3.6). Increased plasma osmolality occurs with a water deficit or sodium excess in relation to total body water. The increased osmolality stimulates hypothalamic **osmoreceptors**. In addition to causing thirst and water drinking, the stimulated osmoreceptors signal the posterior pituitary to release ADH. The action of ADH is to increase the permeability of distal renal tubular cells to water, increasing water reabsorption and promoting the restoration of plasma volume and blood pressure. Urine concentration increases, and the reabsorbed water decreases plasma osmolality, returning it toward normal. Like most hormones, ADH is regulated by a feedback mechanism. The restoration of plasma osmolality, blood volume, and blood pressure then inhibits ADH secretion.

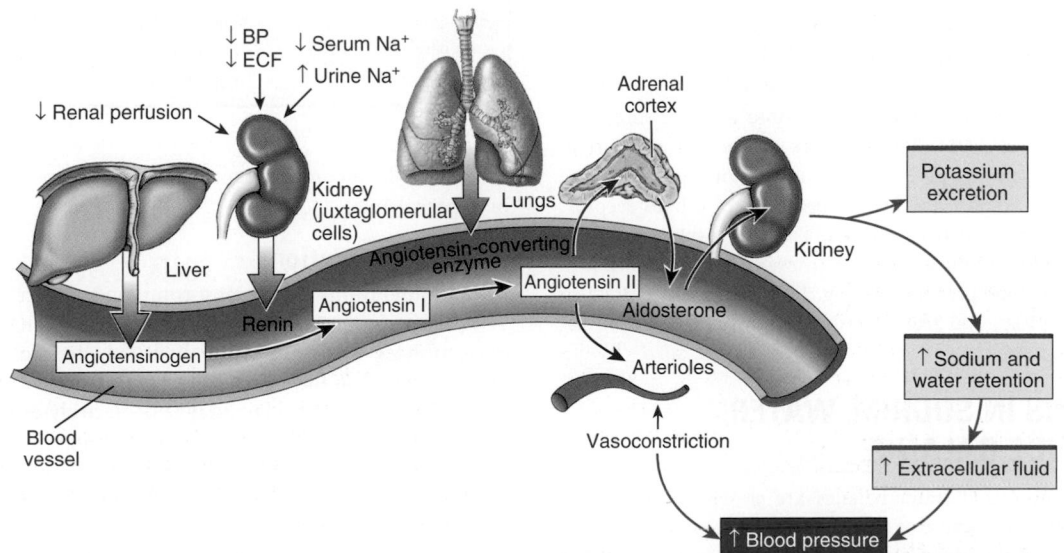

FIGURE 3.4 The Renin-Angiotensin-Aldosterone System. *BP,* Blood pressure; *ECF,* extracellular fluid; *Na⁺,* sodium ion. (Modified from Herlihy B, Maebius N: *The human body in health and disease,* ed 4, Philadelphia, 2011, Saunders. Borrowed from Lewis et al: *Medical-surgical nursing: assessment and management of clinical problems,* ed 9, St Louis, 2014, Mosby.)

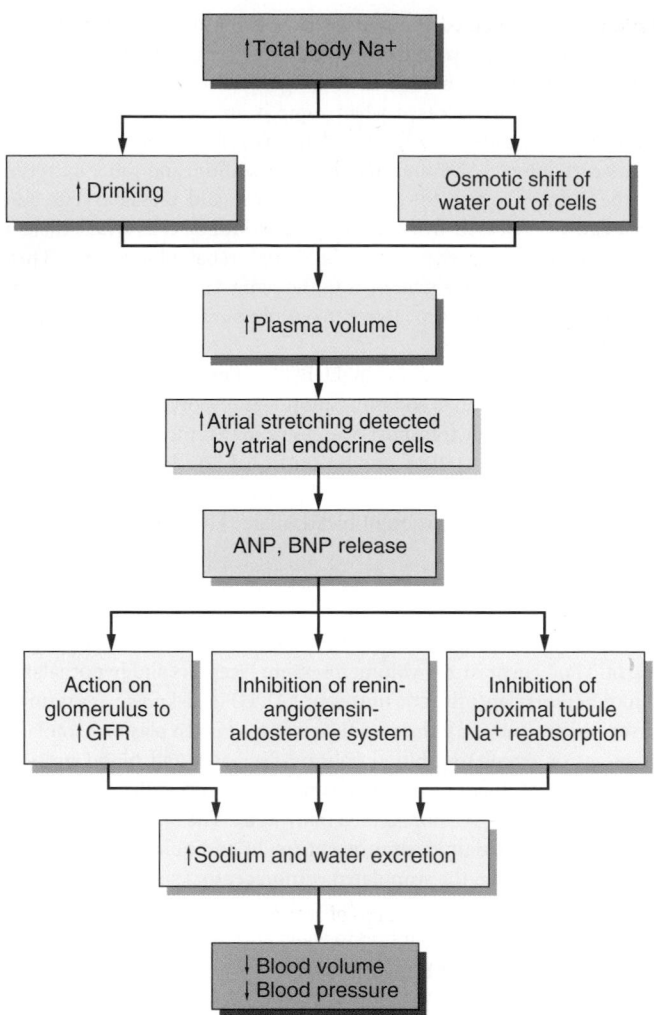

FIGURE 3.5 The Natriuretic Peptide System. *ANP*, atrial natriuretic peptide; *BNP*, brain natriuretic peptide; *GFR*, glomerular filtration rate.

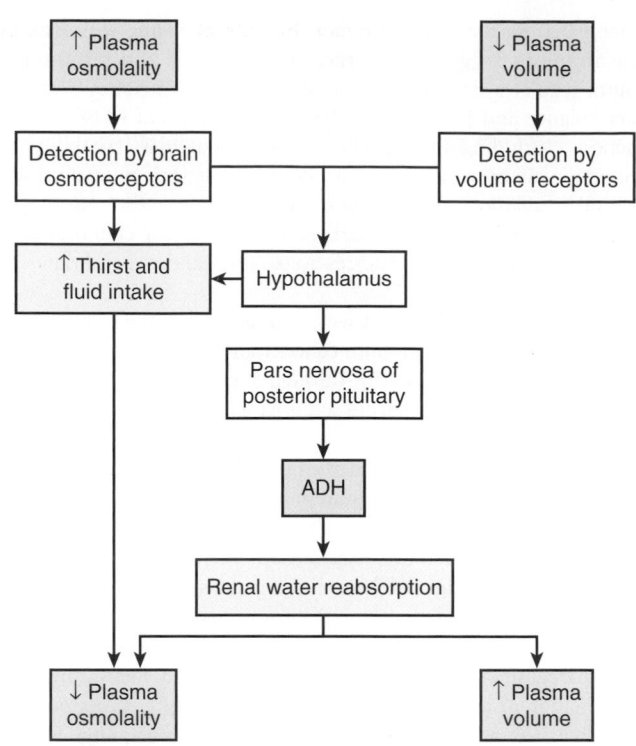

FIGURE 3.6 The Antidiuretic Hormone *(ADH)* System.

TABLE 3.6	WATER AND SOLUTE IMBALANCES
TONICITY	**MECHANISM**
Isotonic (isoosmolar) imbalance	Gain or loss of extracellular fluid (ECF) resulting in a concentration equivalent to a 0.9% sodium chloride (salt) solution (normal saline); no shrinking or swelling of cells
Hypertonic (hyperosmolar) imbalance	Imbalance that results in an ECF concentration >0.9% salt solution; that is, water loss or solute gain; cells shrink in a hypertonic fluid
Hypotonic (hypoosmolar) imbalance	Imbalance that results in an ECF <0.9% salt solution; that is, water gain or solute loss; cells swell in a hypotonic fluid

With fluid loss (dehydration) (e.g., from vomiting, diarrhea, or excessive sweating) and a decrease in blood volume and blood pressure, baroreceptors (volume/pressure sensitive receptors) (stretch receptors that are sensitive to changes in arterial volume and pressure) also stimulate the release of ADH. Baroreceptors are located in the right and left atria and large veins, and in the aorta, pulmonary arteries, and carotid sinus. When arterial and atrial pressure drops, baroreceptors signal the hypothalamus to release ADH. The reabsorption of water mediated by the renal response to ADH promotes the restoration of plasma volume and blood pressure (see Fig. 3.6). Higher concentrations of ADH stimulate peripheral arterial vasoconstriction, thus increasing arterial blood pressure.

ALTERATIONS IN SODIUM, WATER, AND CHLORIDE BALANCE

Alterations in sodium and water balance are closely related. Water imbalances may develop because of changes in osmotic gradients caused by gain or loss of salt. Likewise, sodium imbalances occur with gains or losses of body water volume. Alterations are generally classified as changes in tonicity, the change in concentration of electrolytes in relation to water: isotonic, hypertonic, or hypotonic (Table 3.6 and Fig. 3.7). Changes in tonicity also alter the volume of water in the intracellular

and extracellular compartments, resulting in hypovolemia, euvolemia, or hypervolemia.

Isotonic Alterations

Isotonic alterations are the most common and occur when changes in TBW are accompanied by proportional changes in the concentration of electrolytes. *Isotonic fluid loss* causes dehydration and hypovolemia. For example, if an individual loses pure plasma or ECF, fluid volume is depleted but the number and type of electrolytes (e.g., sodium) and the osmolality remain within a normal range (280 to 294 mOsm). Causes include hemorrhage, severe wound drainage, and excessive diaphoresis (sweating). There is loss of extracellular volume with weight loss, dryness of skin and mucous membranes, decreased urine output, increased hematocrit value, and symptoms of hypovolemia. Indicators of hypovolemia include a rapid heart rate and flattened neck veins, and can present with a normal or decreased blood pressure. In severe states, hypovolemic shock (severe hypotension) can occur. Isotonic fluids containing electrolytes and glucose are given orally, intravenously (i.e.,

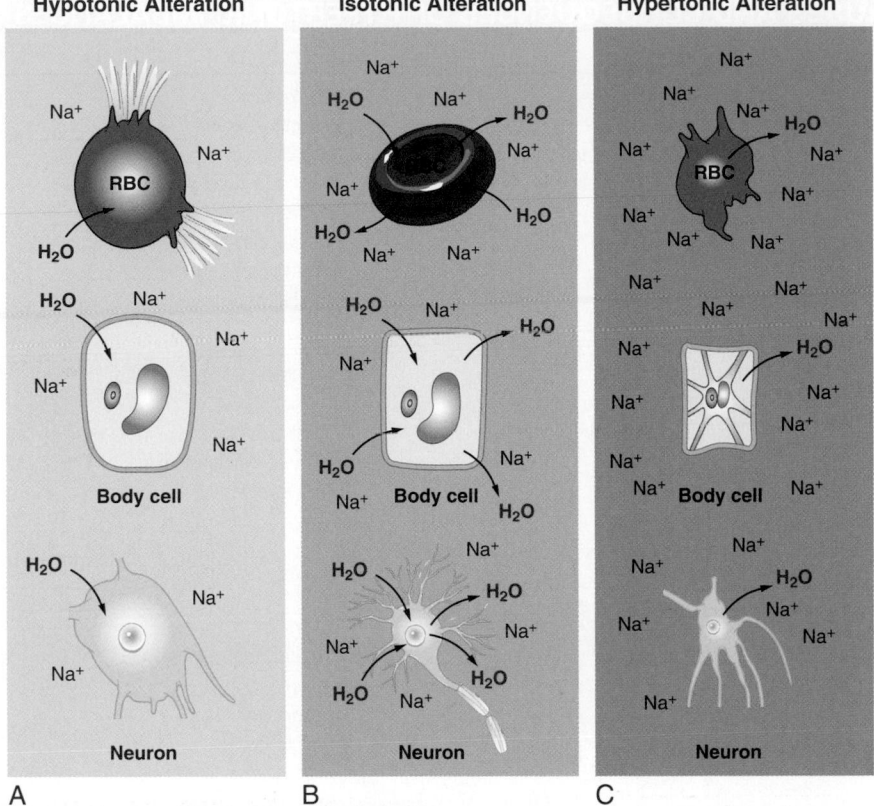

FIGURE 3.7 Effects of Alterations in Extracellular Sodium Concentration in RBCs, Body Cells, and Neurons. **A,** *Hypotonic Alteration:* Decrease in ECF sodium ion *(Na⁺)* concentration (hyponatremia) results in ICF osmotic attraction of water with swelling and potential busting of cells. **B,** *Isotonic Alteration:* Normal concentration of sodium in the ECF and no change in shifts of fluid in or out of cells. **C,** *Hypertonic Alteration:* An increase in ECF sodium concentration (hypernatremia) results in osmotic attraction of water out of cells with cell shrinkage. *RBC,* Red blood cell.

0.9% saline solution or 5% dextrose in 0.225% saline solution, not commonly used), or, in some cases, subcutaneously (hypodermoclysis).

Isotonic fluid excesses result in hypervolemia. Causes include excessive administration of intravenous fluids, hypersecretion of aldosterone, the effects of drugs such as cortisone, or failure of the kidneys. As plasma volume expands, hypervolemia develops with weight gain. The diluting effect of excess plasma volume leads to decreased hematocrit and decreased plasma protein concentration. The neck veins may distend, and the blood pressure increases. Increased capillary hydrostatic pressure leads to edema formation. If the plasma volume is great enough, pulmonary edema and heart failure develop. Diuretics are commonly used for treatment.

Hypertonic Alterations

Hypertonic fluid alterations develop when the osmolality of the ECF is elevated higher than normal (greater than 294 mOsm). The most common causes are an increased concentration of ECF sodium (hypernatremia) or a deficit of ECF free water, or both. In both instances the hypertonicity of the ECF attracts water from the intracellular space, causing ICF dehydration. A primary increase in the amount of ECF sodium causes an osmotic attraction of water and symptoms of *hypervolemia*. In contrast, a hypertonic state caused primarily by free water loss leads to *hypovolemia* (Table 3.7).

Hypernatremia

◆**PATHOPHYSIOLOGY.** Hypernatremia occurs when serum sodium levels exceed 145 mEq/L. Increased levels of serum sodium cause hypertonicity. Hypernatremia can be hypovolemic, euvolemic, or hypervolemic depending on the accompanying ECF water volume. Risk factors include advanced age, impaired mental state, fever, diarrhea, and vomiting. Other factors include uncontrolled diabetes mellitus, tube feedings, and use of diuretics.

Hypovolemic hypernatremia occurs where there is loss of body sodium accompanied by a relatively greater loss of body water. Causes include use of loop diuretics, osmotic diuresis (i.e., from hyperglycemia related to uncontrolled diabetes mellitus or use of mannitol), gastrointestinal losses, or failure of the kidneys to concentrate urine.

Euvolemic hypernatremia is the most common and occurs when there is a *loss of free water* with a near normal body sodium concentration. Causes include inadequate water intake; excessive sweating (sweat is hypotonic); fever with hyperventilation and increased water loss from lungs; burns; vomiting; diarrhea; and central or nephrogenic diabetes insipidus (lack of ADH or inadequate renal response to ADH). Infants with severe diarrhea are vulnerable and have increased risk because they cannot communicate thirst. Insufficient water intake occurs particularly in individuals who are comatose, confused, immobilized, or receiving gastric feedings. Dehydration refers to water deficit but also is commonly used to indicate both sodium and water loss (isotonic or isoosmolar dehydration).[4]

Hypervolemic hypernatremia is rare and occurs when there is increased total body water and a greater increase in total body sodium level, resulting in hypervolemia. Causes include infusion of hypertonic saline solutions (e.g., because sodium replacement for treatment of salt depletion can occur with renal impairment, heart failure, or

TABLE 3.7   CAUSES AND CONSEQUENCES OF HYPERTONIC IMBALANCES

CAUSATIVE FACTOR	MECHANISM	ECF EFFECTS	ICF EFFECTS

Increased sodium (hypernatremia)	Excessive hypertonic salt solutions
	  Intravenous hypertonic sodium
	  Saline-induced abortions
	  Select infant formulas
	Hyperaldosteronism
	Cushing syndrome
		Hypervolemia
		  Weight gain
		  Bounding pulse
		  Increased blood pressure
		  Edema
		  Venous distention
		Neuromuscular symptoms
		  Muscle weakness
		  Seizures
			Intracellular dehydration
			  Thirst
			  Fever
			  Decreased urine output
			  Shrinkage of brain cells
			    Confusion
			    Coma
			    Cerebral hemorrhage

Water deficit	Water deprivation
	  Confusion or coma
	  Inability to communicate
	  Loss of thirst
	Water loss
	  Watery diarrhea
	  Diabetes insipidus
	  Excessive diuresis
	  Excessive diaphoresis
		Hypovolemia
		  Weight loss
		  Weak pulses
		  Postural hypotension
		  Tachycardia
			Intracellular dehydration
			  See above

Other factors	Hyperglycemia	Initial dilutional hyponatremia
		  Polyuria
		  Polydipsia
		  Weight loss
		  Hypovolemia
		  Late hypernatremia
			Intracellular dehydration
			  See above

ECF, Extracellular fluid; *ICF,* intracellular fluid.

gastrointestinal [GI] losses) or oversecretion of adrenocorticotropic hormone (ACTH) or aldosterone (e.g., Cushing syndrome, adrenal hyperplasia), and near–salt water drowning.[5] High amounts of dietary sodium rarely cause hypernatremia in a healthy individual because the sodium is eliminated by the kidneys. Symptoms include weight gain, bounding pulse, and increased blood pressure.

Because chloride follows sodium, **hyperchloremia** (elevation of serum chloride concentration greater than 105 mEq/L) often accompanies hypernatremia, as well as plasma bicarbonate deficits, as in hyperchloremic metabolic acidosis. There are no specific symptoms for chloride excess, and treatment is related to management of the underlying disorder.

◆**CLINICAL MANIFESTATIONS.** When there is excessive sodium in the extracellular space, water is osmotically attracted to the hypertonic extracellular space from the intracellular space, and intracellular dehydration ensues. Central nervous system signs are the most serious and are related to shrinking of brain cells and alterations in membrane potentials. Signs include weakness, lethargy, muscle twitching, and hyperreflexia (hyperactive reflexes). Confusion, coma, and seizures can occur. Hypernatremia with marked water deficit is manifested by signs and symptoms of both intracellular and extracellular dehydration with volume depletion (Box 3.1).

◆**EVALUATION AND TREATMENT.** Serum sodium levels are greater than 145 mEq/L and urine specific gravity will be greater than 1.030. Hematocrit and plasma protein levels will be elevated with water loss. The history, physical examination, and laboratory values provide information about underlying disorders and events. The treatment of hypernatremia and water deficit is to give oral fluids or an isotonic salt-free fluid (5% dextrose in water) until the serum sodium level returns to normal. Fluid replacement must be given slowly to prevent cerebral edema, and

BOX 3.1   SIGNS AND SYMPTOMS OF DEHYDRATION

Increased serum sodium concentration
Thirst
Headache
Weight loss
Oliguria and concentrated urine
Hard stools
Decreased skin turgor
Dry mucous membranes
Decreased sweating and tears
Elevated temperature
Soft eyeballs

Sunken fontanels in infants
Prolonged capillary refill time
Tachycardia
Weak pulses
Low blood pressure
Postural hypotension
Hypovolemic shock
Lethargy
Weakness
Confusion
Coma

serum sodium levels need to be closely monitored. Hypervolemia and hypovolemia require treatment of the underlying clinical condition. Diuretics may be used to enhance sodium excretion.

Hypotonic Alterations

Hypotonic fluid alterations occur when the osmolality of the ECF is less than normal (less than 280 mOsm). The most common causes are sodium deficit (hyponatremia) or free water excess (water intoxication). Both causes lead to an intracellular overhydration (cellular edema) and cell swelling when water moves into the cell, where the osmotic pressure is greater (see Fig. 3.7, *A*). Cerebral and pulmonary edema occur in conjunction with these fluid shifts.[6] With hyponatremia, the plasma

TABLE 3.8	CAUSES AND CONSEQUENCES OF HYPOTONIC IMBALANCES		
CAUSATIVE FACTOR	**MECHANISM**	**ECF EFFECTS**	**ICF EFFECTS**

Decreased sodium (hyponatremia)	Inadequate intake
	Hypoaldosteronism
	Excessive diuretic therapy
	  Furosemide
	  Ethacrynic acid
	  Thiazides
		Extracellular volume contraction and hypovolemia (but may not if there is water excess)	Increased intracellular water; edema
			Brain cell swelling, irritability, depression, confusion
			Systemic cellular edema, including weakness, anorexia, nausea, and diarrhea

Water excess	Excessive pure water intake
	Excessive administration of hypotonic intravenous solutions
	Drinking water to replace isotonic fluid losses
	Tap water enemas
	  Psychogenic polydipsia
	  Renal water retention
	  Syndrome of inappropriate secretion of antidiuretic hormone (SIADH)
		Extracellular volume expands with hypervolemia (but may not if fluid is trapped in intracellular space)	Edema (see above)

Other factors	Isotonic dehydration treated with intravenous D_5W; glucose in D_5W solution is metabolized to water, contributing to hyponatremia Nephrotic syndrome Cirrhosis Cardiac failure	Hypervolemia or hypovolemia	Edema (see above)

D_5W, Dextrose 5% in water; *ECF*, extracellular fluid; *ICF*, intracellular fluid.

volume then decreases, leading to symptoms of hypovolemia. With free water excess, the ECF volume is elevated, causing symptoms of hypervolemia (Table 3.8).

Hyponatremia

◆**PATHOPHYSIOLOGY.** Hyponatremia develops when the serum sodium concentration decreases to less than 135 mEq/L. It is the most common electrolyte disorder in hospitalized individuals and increases morbidity and mortality.[7] Hyponatremia occurs when there is loss of sodium, inadequate intake of sodium, or dilution of sodium by water excess. Hyponatremia can be classified as hypovolemic, euvolemic, or hypervolemic when there are changes in blood volume or as hypotonic, isotonic, or hypertonic when there are changes in effective osmolality. Sodium depletion usually causes hypoosmolality with movement of water into cells (see Fig. 3.7, A).

Hypovolemic hyponatremia occurs with a loss of total body fluid, and there is a greater loss of body sodium (*hypotonic hyponatremia*) than body water. The extracellular volume is decreased. Causes include prolonged vomiting, severe diarrhea, inadequate secretion of aldosterone (e.g., adrenal insufficiency), and renal losses from diuretics. ADH will be released to facilitate repletion of blood volume.

Euvolemic hyponatremia occurs when there is loss of sodium without a significant loss of water (pure sodium deficit and a hypotonic hyponatremia). Causes can include syndrome of inappropriate antidiuretic hormone (SIADH [see Chapter 22]), which enhances water retention), hypothyroidism, pneumonia, and glucocorticoid deficiency. Inadequate intake of dietary sodium is rare but possible in individuals consuming low-sodium diets, particularly with use of diuretics.

Dilutional hypotonic hyponatremia (water intoxication) occurs when there is intake of large amounts of free water or replacement of fluid loss with intravenous 5% dextrose in water, which dilutes sodium. The glucose is metabolized to carbon dioxide and water, leaving a hypotonic solution with a diluting effect. Excessive sweating stimulates

thirst and intake of large amounts of free water (as can occur in endurance athletes), which dilutes sodium concentration. Some individuals with psychogenic disorders develop water intoxication from compulsive water drinking. Other causes can include tap water enemas, near–fresh water drowning, use of selective-serotonin reuptake inhibitors (SSRIs), and SIADH. When the body is functioning normally, it is almost impossible to produce an excess of TBW because water balance is regulated by the kidneys.

Hypervolemic hyponatremia occurs when both TBW and sodium levels are increased, but TBW exceeds the increase in sodium levels, producing a *hypotonic hyponatremia*. Causes include congestive heart failure, cirrhosis of the liver, and nephrotic syndrome. Edema is present.

Hypertonic hyponatremia develops with the shift of water from the ICF to the ECF, as occurs with hyperglycemia, hyperlipidemia, and hyperproteinemia. The osmotic fluid shift to the ECF in turn dilutes the concentration of sodium (pseudohyponatremia) and other electrolytes.

◆**CLINICAL MANIFESTATIONS.** Most individuals are asymptomatic. When serum sodium concentration decreases to less than 120 mEq/L, cellular swelling and deficits of intracellular sodium alter the ability of cells to depolarize and repolarize normally. Nausea and vomiting are more common with less severe hyponatremia (i.e., decreases between 125 and 130 mEq/L). Neurologic symptoms occur with severe hyponatremia (i.e., decreases less than 125 mEq/L) and include lethargy, headache, confusion, apprehension, seizures, and coma.[8] Hypovolemic hyponatremia with pure sodium loss is accompanied by loss of ECF with symptoms of hypotension, tachycardia, and decreased urine output. Hypervolemic hyponatremia is accompanied by weight gain, edema, ascites, and jugular vein distention. Cerebral edema can be a life-threatening complication of hyponatremia caused by increased shifts of fluid to the intracellular space and increased intracranial pressure.

◆**EVALUATION AND TREATMENT.** Evaluation of hyponatremia includes the history, physical examination, and laboratory tests for urine and serum. In hyponatremic states, serum sodium concentration falls to less than 135 mEq/L. With pure sodium deficits, the hematocrit and plasma protein levels may be elevated. Urine specific gravity is less than 1.010 when renal function is normal because sodium is maximally conserved. Evaluation of urine sodium concentration and urine osmolality assists with differential diagnosis. High urine sodium level (normal is 40 to 220 mEq/L in 24 hours) and high urine osmolality are associated with cerebral salt wasting syndrome and adrenal insufficiency. Low urine sodium level (30 mEq/L in 24 hours) and high urine osmolality are associated with extrarenal losses, such as vomiting and diarrhea or severe burns, heart failure, or cirrhosis. Serum osmolality is usually decreased, but secondary conditions of hyperlipidemia, hyperglycemia, or hyperproteinemia can increase serum osmolality.

Treatment of hyponatremia is related to the contributing disorder and severity and acuity of sodium loss. Losses of sodium and water volume are calculated from the clinical evaluation, and appropriate solutions then are selected for replacement. Restriction of water intake is required in most cases of dilutional hyponatremia because body sodium levels may be normal or increased even though serum concentrations are low. Hypertonic saline solutions are used cautiously with severe hyponatremia or the presence of symptoms such as seizures. Rapid correction of chronic hyponatremia can lead to osmotic demyelination syndrome with axonal damage in the brain resulting in neurologic disability or death. Arginine-vasopressin (ADH) receptor antagonists (vaptans) are a class of drugs used for the treatment of hypervolemic and euvolemic hyponatremia, particularly with SIADH.[9] Serum sodium concentration must be monitored.

Hypochloremia

Hypochloremia, a low level of serum chloride (less than 97 mEq/L), usually occurs with hyponatremia or an elevated bicarbonate concentration, as in metabolic alkalosis. Sodium deficit related to restricted intake, use of diuretics, and vomiting is accompanied by chloride deficiency. Cystic fibrosis is a genetic disease characterized by hypochloremia (see Chapters 37 and 43). In all cases, treatment of the underlying cause is required.

ALTERATIONS IN POTASSIUM, CALCIUM, PHOSPHATE, AND MAGNESIUM BALANCE

Potassium

Potassium (K^+) is the major intracellular electrolyte and is found in most body fluids (see Table 3.5.). The ICF concentration of K^+ is about 150 to 160 mEq/L; the ECF concentration is about 3.5 to 5.0 mEq/L. Total body potassium content is about 4000 mEq, with most of it located in the cells. Daily dietary intake of potassium is 40 to 150 mEq/day, with an average of 1.5 mEq/kg body weight.

Potassium balance is highly regulated because of its role in neuromuscular function. About 90% of dietary potassium is absorbed in the gastrointestinal tract. The increased serum K^+ level stimulates insulin, aldosterone, and epinephrine (β-adrenergic stimulation) secretion, which activates K^+ transport into liver and muscle cells. Aldosterone also promotes renal excretion of K^+ by the distal tubules, accounting for 90% to 95% of K^+ excretion (see *What's New? Potassium Intake, Hypertension, and Stroke*).

The difference in the K^+ intracellular to extracellular concentration is maintained by a sodium-potassium active transport system (Na^+-K^+ ATPase pump). The ratio of ICF K^+ concentration to ECF K^+ concentration is the major determinant of the resting membrane potential, which is necessary for the transmission and conduction of nerve impulses, maintenance of normal cardiac rhythms, and contraction of skeletal and smooth muscles (see Fig. 1.34). The constant diffusion of positively

WHAT'S NEW

Potassium Intake, Hypertension, and Stroke

Enriched dietary intake of potassium is associated with a lower risk of hypertension and stroke. Although the American diet often exceeds recommendations for sodium intake, diets are typically deficient in potassium intake. There is increased risk of high blood pressure, cardiovascular disease, and mortality when the plasma ratio of sodium concentration to potassium concentration is high. Potassium attenuates the effects of high dietary salt intake with reduction in blood pressure, stroke rates, and cardiovascular disease risk. The exact mechanism of how potassium affects blood pressure is unknown but is thought to be related to renal handling of sodium, endothelial cell function, decreased vascular resistance, and reduced oxidative stress. A large prospective study of older women showed they were found to have lower risk of ischemic but not hemorrhagic stroke associated with higher intakes of potassium, especially in women without hypertension. Lower risk of mortality was found in all women with higher intakes of potassium. Increased dietary intake of potassium is recommended for most individuals without impaired renal handling of potassium.

Data from Binia A et al: *J Hypertens* 33(8):1509–1520, 2015; Seth A et al: *Stroke* 45(10):2874–2880, 2014; Vinceti et al: *J Am Heart Assoc* 5(10), 2016.

charged K^+ out of the cell (i.e., down its concentration gradient) makes the interior of cells electronegative in relation to the ECF. Changes in the ratio of ICF to ECF potassium concentration are responsible for many of the symptoms associated with K^+ imbalance.

As the predominant ICF ion, K^+ exerts a major influence on the regulation of ICF osmolality and fluid balance, as well as on intracellular electrical neutrality in relation to hydrogen (H^+) and Na^+ levels. Potassium also is necessary for a variety of metabolic functions and is required for glycogen deposition in liver and skeletal muscle cells.

Insulin contributes to the regulation of plasma potassium levels by stimulating the Na^+-K^+ ATPase pump, thereby promoting the movement of K^+ into liver and muscle cells simultaneously with glucose transport. The intracellular movement of K^+ prevents an acute hyperkalemia related to food intake. Insulin also can be used to treat hyperkalemia. However, dangerously low levels of plasma K^+ can result from the administration of insulin when K^+ levels are depressed. Potassium balance is especially significant in the treatment of conditions requiring insulin administration, such as type 1 diabetes mellitus.

Insulin deficiency, aldosterone deficiency, acidosis, and strenuous exercise facilitate the shift of K^+ out of cells. α-Adrenergics impair K^+ entry into cells. Glucagon blocks entry of K^+ into cells, and glucocorticoids promote K^+ excretion. Potassium also will move out of cells along with water when there is increased ECF osmolarity. If cells lyse, they release their intracellular K^+ into the ECF, which can cause an acute rise in plasma K^+ levels. Elevated plasma K^+ concentration causes adrenal secretion of aldosterone and renal excretion of K^+. Alkalosis facilitates the shift of K^+ into cells in exchange for H^+.

The kidney provides the most efficient regulation of K^+ level balance over time. The amount of K^+ excreted varies in proportion to the dietary intake (40 to 150 mEq/day). Potassium is freely filtered by the renal glomerulus, and 90% is reabsorbed by the proximal tubule and loop of Henle. Principal cells in the collecting duct secrete K^+, and intercalated cells in the collecting duct reabsorb K^+. Dietary K^+ intake, aldosterone level, and distal tubule urine flow determine the amount of K^+ excreted from the body. Unlike sodium, the renal mechanism for conserving K^+ is weak, even when total body K^+ stores are depleted. The gut also may sense the amount of K^+ ingested and stimulate renal K^+ excretion.[10] However, a low K^+ intake also suppresses renal K^+ excretion.

The concentration of K^+ in the distal tubular cells is determined primarily by the plasma concentration in the peritubular capillaries. When plasma K^+ concentration increases because of increased dietary intake or shifts from the ICF to the ECF occur, K^+ is secreted into the urine by principal cells in the collecting ducts. Decreased levels of plasma K^+ result in decreased collecting duct secretion and reabsorption by intercalated cells, although K^+ losses of approximately 5 to 15 mEq/day will continue.

Changes in distal tubule flow rate and distal tubule sodium delivery also influence the concentration gradient for K^+ secretion. When the flow rate and sodium delivery are high, as occurs with the administration of diuretics, the concentration of K^+ in the distal tubular urine is lower, favoring the secretion of K^+ into the tubule. Potassium secretion decreases when distal tubule flow rate and sodium delivery are low. However, aldosterone stimulates K^+ secretion by the distal tubule and serves to preserve K^+ secretion and K^+ balance during dehydration and extracellular volume depletion, when tubular delivery of Na^+ and flow rate are reduced.

Changes in pH and thus in hydrogen ion concentration also affect K^+ balance.[11] Hydrogen ions move from the ECF to the ICF during states of acidosis. When hydrogen is moving into the cell, K^+ shifts out of the cell to the ECF to maintain a balance of cations across the cell membrane. This occurs in part because of a decrease in Na^+-K^+ ATPase pump activity. The decreased ICF K^+ level in the distal tubular cells results in decreased secretion of K^+ into the urine, contributing to hyperkalemia (hyperkalemic acidosis), although the total body K^+ level may not change. In contrast, intracellular fluid levels of hydrogen are diminished during states of alkalosis. Alkalosis causes K^+ to shift into the cell, so the distal tubular cells increase their secretion of K^+ into the urine, contributing to hypokalemia (hypokalemic alkalosis). The management of alterations associated with acid-base imbalances requires that the acid-base imbalances must be treated before or concurrently with treatment of changes in K^+ concentration.

In summary, renal regulation of potassium includes:

1. The concentration gradient for K^+ at the distal tubule and collecting duct
2. The distal tubule flow rate and distal tubule sodium delivery
3. The action of aldosterone
4. Changes in pH (causing acidosis or alkalosis)

Potassium loss occurs through normal body functions, but without causing hypokalemia. Average daily losses of K^+ are as follows:

Location	Daily Loss (mEq/L)
Stool	5–10
Sweat	0–20
Urine	40–120

Potassium adaptation is the ability of the body to adapt to increased levels of K^+ intake over time. A sudden increase in K^+ level may be fatal, but if the intake is slowly increased by amounts greater than 120 mEq/day, the kidney can increase the urinary excretion of K^+ and maintain K^+ concentration balance.

Hypokalemia

◆**PATHOPHYSIOLOGY.** Potassium deficiency, or **hypokalemia**, develops when the serum K^+ concentration decreases to less than 3.5 mEq/L. Because intracellular and total body stores of K^+ are difficult to measure, changes in K^+ balance are described by the plasma concentration, although changes in total body K^+ level are not always reflected in the plasma K^+ concentration. Generally, lowered serum K^+ level indicates a loss of total body K^+. Because K^+ is lost from the ECF, the

change in the concentration gradient favors movement of K^+ from the cell to the ECF. The ICF/ECF concentration ratio is maintained, but the amount of total body K^+ is depleted.

Factors contributing to the development of hypokalemia include reduced intake of potassium, increased entry of K^+ into cells, and increased losses of body K^+. Dietary deficiency of K^+ is a rare cause but may occur in elderly individuals with both low protein intake (meat) and inadequate intake of fruits and vegetables, and in individuals with alcoholism or anorexia nervosa. Reduced K^+ intake generally becomes a problem when combined with other causes of K^+ depletion.

ECF hypokalemia can develop without losses of total body K^+ when K^+ is redistributed between the ECF and ICF. Alkalosis, particularly respiratory alkalosis, is the most common clinical cause of these shifts. In alkalosis, ECF hydrogen moves out of the cell to correct the alkalosis, which causes K^+ to move into the cell to maintain an ionic balance. Insulin also promotes cellular uptake of K^+ and can cause an ECF potassium deficit, particularly with the intake of high carbohydrate loads. Severe, even fatal, hypokalemia may occur if insulin is administered without also providing K^+ supplements.

Treatment of pernicious anemia with vitamin B_{12} or folate also may precipitate hypokalemia if the formation of new red blood cells causes enough K^+ uptake to effect an extracellular decrease in K^+ concentration. Familial hypokalemic periodic paralysis is a rare genetically transmitted disease that causes K^+ to shift into the intracellular space.

Hypokalemia also can occur when K^+ shifts from the ICF to the ECF, as occurs in conjunction with renal losses. For example, in diabetic ketoacidosis, the increased hydrogen ion concentration in the ECF causes H^+ to shift into the cell in exchange for K^+ at the same time diuresis is occurring. A normal level of K^+ is maintained in the plasma, but K^+ continues to be lost in the urine, causing a deficit in the amount of total body potassium. Total body K^+ depletion becomes evident when insulin treatment and rehydration therapy are initiated.

Losses of K^+ from body stores are most commonly caused by gastrointestinal and renal disorders. Diarrhea (from any cause), intestinal drainage tubes or fistulae, and laxative abuse also may result in hypokalemia. Normally, only 5 to 10 mEq of potassium and about 100 mL of water are excreted in the stool each day. With diarrhea, fluid and electrolyte losses can be voluminous, with several liters of fluid and 100 to 200 mEq of K^+ lost per day. Vomiting or applying continuous nasogastric suction frequently is associated with K^+ depletion, partly because of the K^+ lost from the gastric fluid but principally because of renal compensation for volume depletion and the metabolic alkalosis (elevated bicarbonate levels) that occurs from sodium, chloride, and hydrogen ion losses. The loss of fluid and sodium stimulates the secretion of aldosterone and ADH, which in turn causes renal loss of K^+. The elevated flow of bicarbonate at the distal tubule contributes to renal excretion of K^+ because of increased tubular lumen electronegativity.

Renal losses of K^+ are related to increased secretion of K^+ by the distal tubule. Use of diuretics, excessive aldosterone secretion, increased distal tubular flow rate, and low plasma magnesium concentration all may contribute to urinary losses of K^+. Many diuretics, including thiazides, furosemide, ethacrynic acid, and osmotic diuretics, inhibit the reabsorption of sodium chloride, causing the diuretic effect. The distal tubular flow rate then increases, promoting K^+ excretion. If sodium loss is severe, the compensating aldosterone secretion (which causes secondary hyperaldosteronism) may further deplete K^+ stores. Primary hyperaldosteronism with excessive secretion of aldosterone from an adrenal adenoma also causes K^+ wasting. Many kidney diseases result in a reduced ability to conserve sodium. The disordered sodium reabsorption produces a diuretic effect, and the increased distal tubule flow rate favors the secretion of K^+. Magnesium deficiency and concomitant hypokalemia increase distal potassium excretion sustaining hypokalemia.[12]

Several antibiotics, including amphotericin B, gentamicin, and carbenicillin, are known to cause hypokalemia.

◆**CLINICAL MANIFESTATIONS.** Mild losses of K⁺ are usually asymptomatic. A wide range of dysfunctions may result from severe hypokalemia (<2.5 mEq/L).[13] Neuromuscular excitability is decreased, causing skeletal muscle weakness, smooth muscle atony, and cardiac dysrhythmias. As Chapter 1 describes, the resting membrane potential (E_m) is determined by the *ratio* of extracellular to intracellular K⁺ ion concentration. Because the concentration of K⁺ in the ECF is small, only small changes in ECF potassium level are required to influence the resting membrane potential and affect neuromuscular excitability (the difference between resting membrane and threshold potentials) (Fig. 3.8, *A*). When extracellular K⁺ levels decrease rapidly, intracellular K⁺ diffuses more readily out of the cell and the resting membrane potential becomes more negative (i.e., from −90 to −100 millivolts). If the threshold potential (E_t) remains stable, the difference between resting membrane potential and threshold potential increases and the cell membrane becomes **hyperpolarized**, requiring a stronger stimulus (decreased excitability) to initiate depolarization and an action potential (Fig. 3.8, *B* [low K⁺]).

The *cardiac effects of hypokalemia* are related to decreased membrane excitability (see Fig. 3.8, *B*). Because K⁺ contributes to the repolarization phase of the action potential, hypokalemia delays ventricular repolarization and the frequency of action potentials. The membrane potential remains partially depolarized with slowed conduction and abnormal pacemaker activity. A variety of dysrhythmias may occur, including sinus bradycardia, atrioventricular block, and paroxysmal atrial tachycardia. The characteristic changes in the electrocardiogram reflect delayed repolarization. For instance, flattening of the T wave, ST-segment depression, and the presence of a U wave (Fig. 3.9). In severe states of hypokalemia, P waves peak and the QRS complex is prolonged. Hypokalemia also increases the risk of digitalis toxicity by slowing the sodium-potassium pump, which augments the action of digitalis in cardiac muscle by excessively increasing intracellular calcium and sodium concentrations.

Plasma calcium concentration also contributes to changes in neuromuscular excitability associated with hypokalemia. Increases in ECF calcium concentration tend to make the threshold potential (E_t) less negative and decrease membrane excitability, potentiating hyperpolarization, decreased excitability, and the neuromuscular effects of hypokalemia (Fig. 3.8, *C*).

Carbohydrate metabolism is affected because hypokalemia depresses insulin secretion and alters hepatic and skeletal muscle glycogen synthesis. Renal function is impaired, with a decreased ability to concentrate urine. Polyuria (increased urine) and polydipsia (increased thirst) are associated with decreased responsiveness to ADH. Chronic potassium deficits lasting more than 1 month may damage renal tissue, with resulting interstitial fibrosis and tubular atrophy.

The onset of symptoms is related to the *rate of potassium depletion*. Because the body can accommodate slow losses of K⁺, the decrease in ECF concentration may be slow enough to allow K⁺ to shift from the intracellular space. The extracellular to intracellular K⁺ concentration gradient then is restored toward normal, with less severe neuromuscular changes. With acute losses of K⁺, changes in neuromuscular excitability are more profound. Skeletal muscle weakness initially occurs in the larger muscles of the legs and arms and ultimately affects the diaphragm and depresses ventilation. Paralysis and respiratory arrest then can occur. Gastrointestinal manifestations include constipation, anorexia, nausea, vomiting, paralytic ileus, and intestinal distention. Table 3.9 contains a summary of K⁺ alterations.

◆**EVALUATION AND TREATMENT.** The diagnosis of hypokalemia is based on serum K⁺ levels; however, it is important to examine the medical history and identify disorders associated with K⁺ loss or shifts

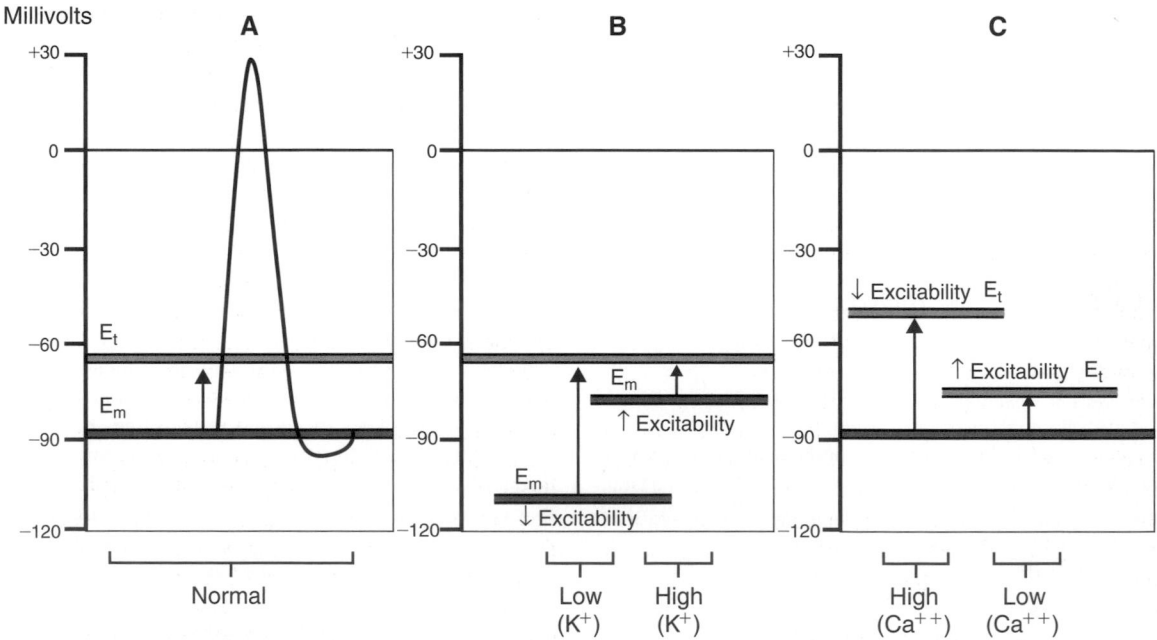

FIGURE 3.8 Effects of Potassium (K⁺) and Calcium (Ca⁺⁺) Ions on Membrane Excitability. **A,** Normal membrane excitability: Potassium affects the resting membrane potential *(E_m)*, and calcium affects the threshold potential *(E_t)*. **B,** Effects of potassium ion (K⁺) changes on membrane potential. **C,** Effect of calcium ion (Ca⁺⁺) on threshold potential. **NOTE:** *Hyperpolarization* can be caused by either hypokalemia (E_m more negative) or hypercalcemia (E_t less negative)—the distance between E_m and E_t is increased (decreased excitability); and *hypopolarization* can be caused by either hyperkalemia (E_m less negative) or hypocalcemia (E_t more negative)—the distance between E_m and E_t is decreased (increased excitability).

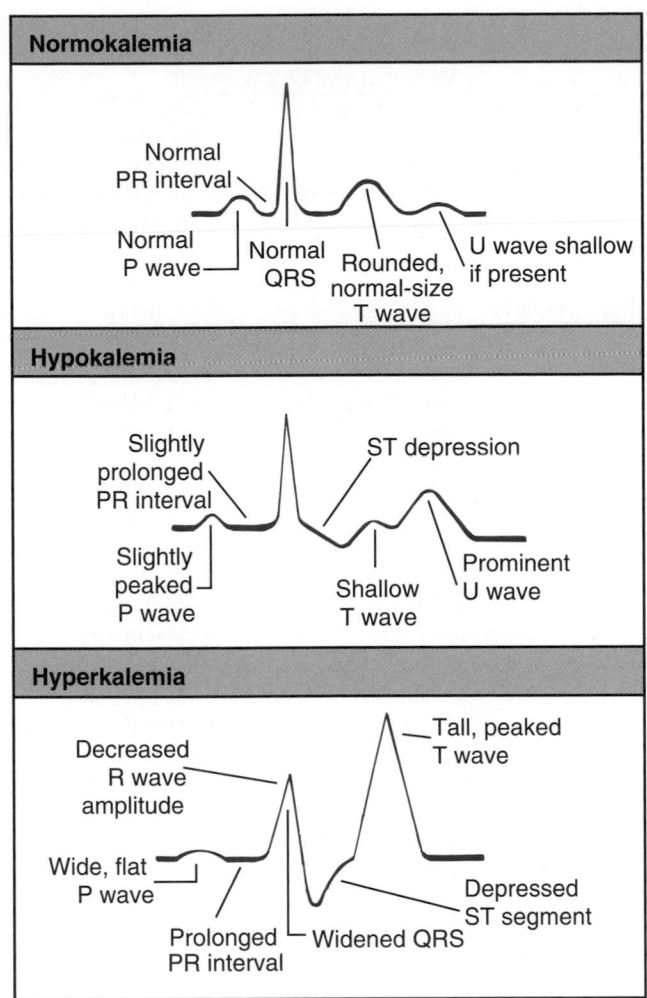

FIGURE 3.9 Electrocardiogram (ECG) Changes With Potassium Imbalance.

of extracellular K^+ to the intracellular space. An electrocardiogram will identify conduction abnormalities or arrhythmias. Treatment involves an estimation of total body K^+ losses and correction of acid-base imbalances. Further losses of K^+ should be prevented, and the individual should be encouraged to eat foods rich in K^+. Potassium replacement is instituted cautiously to prevent hyperkalemia. The maximal rate of oral replacement is 40 to 80 mEq/day if renal function is normal. A maximal safe rate of intravenous (IV) replacement is 20 mEq/hr for adults (usually through a central IV line with cardiac monitoring); 10 mEq/hr is replaced if a peripheral IV is used. Potassium replacement is never given IV push. Because K^+ is irritating to blood vessels, a maximal concentration of 40 mEq/1000 mL should be used. The dosage can range from 10 mEq/hour to 40 mEq/hour depending on the severity of deficiency. The 24-hour dosage should not exceed 200 mEq of potassium. Serum K^+ values can be monitored until normokalemia is achieved. Hypokalemia concurrent with hypomagnesemia is refractory to treatment until magnesium levels are corrected.

Hyperkalemia

◆**PATHOPHYSIOLOGY.** An elevation of ECF potassium concentration *greater than 5.0 mEq/L* constitutes **hyperkalemia**. Because of efficient renal excretion, excesses of total body potassium are relatively rare. Acute increases in serum K^+ concentration are handled quickly through an increase in cellular uptake and renal excretion of body K^+ excesses.

Excesses of serum K^+ may be caused by *excessive intake, a shift of potassium from the ICF to the ECF, or decreased renal excretion.*[14] If renal function is normal, slow, long-term increases in K^+ intake are usually well tolerated through K^+ adaptation, although acute K^+ loading can exceed renal excretion rates. Use of stored whole blood, administration of intravenous boluses of penicillin G, or replacement of K^+ can precipitate hyperkalemia, particularly if renal function is impaired. Dietary excesses of K^+ are uncommon, but accidental ingestion of K^+ salt substitutes can cause toxicity.

Potassium shifts from the ICF to the ECF occur with a *change in cell membrane permeability* (e.g., from cell hypoxia, acidosis, or insulin deficiency). Burns, massive crush injuries, and extensive surgeries can cause cell trauma and loss of ICF potassium to the ECF. If renal function is sustained, K^+ will be excreted. As cell repair begins, hypokalemia develops if the excreted K^+ is not replaced.

Hypoxia can lead to hyperkalemia by diminishing the efficiency of cell membrane active transport, resulting in the escape of K^+ to the ECF. In states of *acidosis*, hydrogen ions shift into the cells in exchange for ICF potassium; hyperkalemia and acidosis therefore often occur together. Because insulin promotes cellular entry of K^+, *insulin deficits*, which occur with conditions such as diabetic ketoacidosis, are accompanied by hyperkalemia. *Digitalis overdose* may cause hyperkalemia by inhibiting the Na^+-K^+ ATPase pump. This pump normally maintains intracellular K^+ concentration and moves sodium and calcium to the ECF (see Chapter 1).

Decreased renal excretion of potassium is commonly associated with hyperkalemia. Renal failure that results in oliguria (urine output <30 mL/hr) is accompanied by elevations of serum K^+ concentration. The severity of hyperkalemia is related to the severity of renal dysfunction, the amount of K^+ intake, and the degree of acidosis from the renal failure. In acute renal failure K^+ levels rise more rapidly with more serious consequences than the slower rises associated with chronic renal failure. *Hypoaldosteronism* also can cause decreases in the urinary excretion of K^+. For example, Addison disease results in decreased production and secretion of aldosterone and thus contributes to hyperkalemia. Drugs that decrease renal potassium excretion (i.e., ACE inhibitors, angiotensin receptor blockers, potassium-sparing diuretics, and aldosterone antagonists) also may contribute to hyperkalemia. Frequently, however, these drugs are used in combination with diuretics that cause K^+ wasting in an attempt to balance renal K^+ gains and losses.

◆**CLINICAL MANIFESTATIONS.** Symptoms of hyperkalemia vary, but common characteristics are muscle weakness or paralysis and dysrhythmias with changes in the electrocardiogram. During mild attacks, increased neuromuscular irritability may be manifested as tingling of lips and fingers, restlessness, intestinal cramping, and diarrhea. Severe hyperkalemia causes muscle weakness, loss of muscle tone, and paralysis. In mild states of hyperkalemia, the more rapid repolarization is reflected in the electrocardiogram as narrow and taller T waves with a shortened QT interval. Severe hyperkalemia (serum levels ≥6 mEq/L) depresses the ST segment, prolongs the PR interval, and widens the QRS complex (loss of atrial activity) (see Fig. 3.9). Delayed conduction and bradydysrhythmias are common in hyperkalemia, with alterations in cardiac conduction causing ventricular fibrillation or cardiac arrest.

As with hypokalemia, changes in the ratio of intracellular to extracellular K^+ concentration contribute to the symptoms of hyperkalemia. If extracellular K^+ concentration increases without a significant change in intracellular K^+ concentration, the resting membrane potential becomes more positive (i.e., changes from −90 to −80 millivolts) and the cell membrane is **hypopolarized** (the inside of the cell becomes less negative or partially depolarized [increased excitability]) (see Fig. 3.8, *B*). (Electrical properties of cells are discussed in Chapter 1.) With relatively mild elevations in extracellular K^+ concentration, the cell more rapidly

TABLE 3.9   POTASSIUM ALTERATIONS

CAUSES	HYPOKALEMIA <3.5 mEq/L	HYPERKALEMIA >5.0 mEq/L
Intake	Decreased intake: starvation or anorexia nervosa, inadequate replacement	Excess dietary or intravenous intake
Loss	Increased renal loss: renal tubular failure, K^+-losing diuretics, hyperaldosteronism, vomiting, diarrhea, use of selected antibiotics	Decreased renal loss: renal failure, K^+-sparing diuretics, hypoaldosteronism
Cellular shifts	Shift from ECF to ICF: metabolic alkalosis, insulin administration	Shift from ICF to ECF: metabolic acidosis, cell injury
ORGAN SYSTEM MANIFESTATIONS		
Cardiovascular	Postural hypotension Dysrhythmias ECG changes (flattened T waves, U waves, ST depression, peaked P wave, prolonged QT interval) Weak, irregular pulse rate Ventricular fibrillation Cardiac arrest	Dysrhythmias ECG changes (peaked T waves, prolonged PR interval, absent P wave with widened QRS complex) Bradycardia Heart block Cardiac arrest
Nervous	Lethargy Fatigue Confusion Paresthesias Decreased tendon reflexes	Anxiety Tingling Numbness
Gastrointestinal	Nausea and vomiting Decreased motility Distention Decreased bowel sounds Ileus	Nausea and vomiting Diarrhea Colicky pain
Kidney	Inability to concentrate urine Water loss Thirst Kidney damage	Oliguria Kidney damage
Skeletal and smooth muscle	Weakness Flaccid paralysis Respiratory arrest Constipation Bladder dysfunction	Early: hyperactive muscles and reflexes Late: weakness and flaccid paralysis

K⁺, potassium; *ECF*, extracellular fluid; *ICF*, intracellular fluid; *ECG*, electrocardiogram.

repolarizes and becomes more irritable (peaked T waves). An action potential then is initiated more rapidly because the distance between the resting membrane potential and the threshold potential has been shortened. With more severe hyperkalemia, the resting membrane potential approaches or exceeds the threshold potential (wide QRS merging with T wave). In this case the cell is not able to repolarize and therefore does not respond to excitation stimuli. The most serious consequence is cardiac standstill.

Like the effects of hypokalemia, the neuromuscular effects of hyperkalemia are related to the rate of increase in the ECF potassium concentration and the presence of other contributing factors, such as acidosis and calcium balance. Long-term increases in ECF potassium concentration result in shifts of K^+ into the cell because the tendency is to maintain a normal ratio of intracellular/extracellular potassium concentrations. Acute elevations of extracellular K^+ concentration affect neuromuscular irritability because this ratio is disrupted.

Because calcium influences the threshold potential, changes in extracellular fluid calcium concentration can augment or override the effects of hyperkalemia. With hypocalcemia the threshold potential becomes more negative, enhancing the neuromuscular effects of hyperkalemia. Hypercalcemia causes the threshold potential to become less negative, counteracting the effects of hyperkalemia on resting membrane potential (see Fig. 3.8, *C*). See Table 3.9 for a summary of potassium alteration.

◆ EVALUATION AND TREATMENT. Hyperkalemia should be investigated when there is a history of renal disease, massive trauma, insulin deficiency, Addison disease, use of potassium salt substitutes, or metabolic acidosis. The acuity of the onset of symptoms may be related to the underlying cause. An electrocardiogram will identify conduction abnormalities or arrhythmias.

Management of hyperkalemia is related to treating the contributing causes and correcting the potassium excess. Normalizing the extracellular potassium concentration can be achieved with a variety of methods; the treatment chosen is related to the cause and severity of the problem. Calcium gluconate can be administered to restore normal neuromuscular irritability when serum potassium levels are dangerously high. Administration of glucose, which readily stimulates insulin secretion, or administration of glucose and insulin for those with diabetes, facilitates cellular entry of potassium. Cation exchange resins can be effective for chronic hyperkalemia, and newer potassium binders are available. Buffered solutions correct metabolic acidosis and lower serum potassium level. Dialysis effectively removes potassium when renal failure has occurred.[15]

Calcium and Phosphate

The total body content of calcium is about 1200 g. Most calcium (99%) is located in bone as hydroxyapatite (an inorganic compound that contributes to bone rigidity), and the remainder is in the plasma and body cells. The total fraction of calcium circulating in the blood is small (9.0 to 10.5 mg/dL) and about 50% is bound to plasma proteins, primarily albumin. About 40% is in the free or ionized form (5.5 to 5.6 mg/dL). Ionized calcium has the most important physiologic functions.

Calcium (Ca^{++}) is a necessary ion for many fundamental metabolic processes. It is the major cation associated with the structure of bones and teeth. It serves as an enzymatic cofactor for blood clotting and is required for hormone secretion and the function of cell receptors. Plasma membrane stability, permeability, and repair are directly related to calcium ions, as is the transmission of nerve impulses and the contraction of muscles. Intracellular calcium is located primarily in the mitochondria.

Phosphate (HPO_4^-) is found primarily in bone (85%), with smaller amounts found within the intracellular and extracellular spaces. In the plasma, phosphate exists in phospholipids and phosphate esters and as inorganic phosphate, which is the ionized form. The normal serum levels of inorganic phosphate range from 2.5 to 4.5 mg/dL and may be as high as 6.0 to 7.0 mg/dL in infants and young children. Intracellular phosphate has many metabolic forms, including the high-energy structures creatine phosphate and adenosine triphosphate (ATP). Phosphate acts as an intracellular and extracellular anion buffer in the regulation of acid-base balance; in the form of ATP it provides energy for muscle contraction.

Calcium and phosphate concentrations are rigidly controlled. They are related by the product of calcium (Ca^{++}) and phosphate (HPO_4^-) concentrations, which is a constant (K) [$Ca^{++} \times HPO_4^- = K$]. Thus, if the concentration of one ion increases or decreases, that of the other increases or decreases.

Calcium and phosphate balance is regulated by three hormones: parathyroid hormone (PTH), vitamin D, and calcitonin. Acting together, these substances determine the amount of dietary calcium and phosphate absorbed from the intestine, the deposition and absorption of calcium and phosphate from bone, and the renal reabsorption and excretion of calcium and phosphate by the kidney.

The parathyroid glands secrete PTH in response to low levels of serum calcium. (The specific actions of PTH in relation to calcium and phosphate are described in Chapter 21.) Parathyroid hormone controls levels of ionized calcium and phosphate in the blood and other extracellular fluids. The renal regulation of calcium and phosphate balance requires PTH. PTH stimulates reabsorption of calcium along the distal tubule of the nephron and inhibits phosphate reabsorption by the proximal tubule of the nephron. The net result is an increase in serum calcium concentration and increased urinary excretion of phosphate. Fig. 3.10 summarizes hormonal regulation of calcium.

Another compound important to calcium and phosphate regulation is vitamin D. Vitamin D (cholecalciferol) is a fat-soluble steroid ingested in food or synthesized in the skin in the presence of ultraviolet light. Several steps of activation are required before vitamin D can act on target tissues. The first step occurs in the liver; final activation is in the kidney. The renal activation of vitamin D begins when the serum calcium level decreases and stimulates secretion of PTH. PTH then acts to increase calcium reabsorption and enhance renal excretion of phosphate, producing decreased phosphate levels. The combination of low calcium level

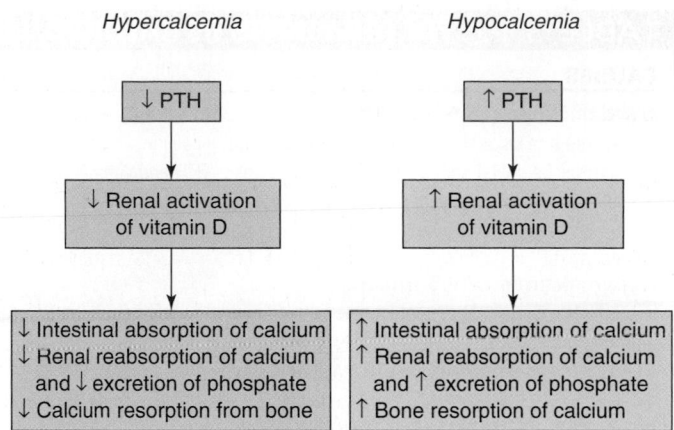

FIGURE 3.10 Hormonal Regulation of Calcium Balance. *PTH,* Parathyroid hormone.

and increased PTH secretion causes the renal activation of vitamin D. The activated vitamin D (vitamin D_3—calcitriol) then circulates as a hormone in the plasma and acts to increase absorption of calcium and phosphate in the small intestine, enhance bone calcification, and increase renal tubular reabsorption of calcium and increase excretion of phosphate. When renal failure occurs, vitamin D is not activated; serum calcium levels decrease; and phosphate levels increase.

As calcium levels increase, an opposite adaptation occurs, leading to suppression of PTH secretion, decreased renal vitamin D activation, decreased intestinal calcium absorption, and increased renal phosphate reabsorption. Calcitonin (produced by C cells of the thyroid gland) primarily decreases calcium levels by inhibiting osteoclastic activity in bone.

The fractions of serum calcium that are freely ionized or bound to plasma proteins are influenced by pH. In states of acidosis, levels of ionized calcium increase. When alkalosis develops, with an increase in pH, the amount of protein-bound calcium increases and the physiologically active, ionized calcium level decreases. The decreased concentration of ionized calcium may be great enough to cause symptoms of hypocalcemia, such as tetany.

Hypocalcemia

◆**PATHOPHYSIOLOGY.** Hypocalcemia occurs when serum total calcium concentrations are less than 9.0 mg/dL and ionized levels are less than 5.5 mg/dL. In general, deficits in calcium are related to inadequate intestinal absorption, decreases in levels of PTH and vitamin D, or deposition of ionized calcium into bone or soft tissue.

Nutritional deficiencies of calcium can occur in the instance of inadequate sources of dairy products or green, leafy vegetables and eating disorders. Excessive amounts of dietary phosphorus also bind with calcium, so neither mineral is absorbed when such an excess occurs. Removal of the parathyroid glands (e.g., during total thyroidectomy) with the resulting loss of PTH also causes hypocalcemia. Vitamin D deficiency, which can result from inadequate intake or avoidance of sunlight, causes decreased intestinal absorption of calcium. Malabsorption of fat, including fat-soluble vitamin D, also may contribute to calcium deficiency. Neoplastic bone metastases tend to inhibit bone resorption and increase calcium deposition into bone, thereby decreasing serum calcium levels.

Blood transfusions are also a common cause of hypocalcemia because the citrate solution used in storing whole blood binds with calcium and makes it unavailable to the tissues. Pancreatitis causes release of lipases into soft tissue spaces, so the free fatty acids that are formed

TABLE 3.10   ALTERATIONS IN CALCIUM, PHOSPHATE, AND MAGNESIUM LEVELS

CAUSES	MANIFESTATIONS
Hypocalcemia (<8.5 mg/dL) Inadequate intestinal absorption, deposition of ionized calcium into bone or soft tissue, blood administration, or decreases in PTH and vitamin D levels; nutritional deficiencies occur with inadequate sources of dairy products or green, leafy vegetables; alkalosis, elevated calcitonin level	Increased neuromuscular excitability; tingling, muscle spasms (particularly in hands, feet, and facial muscles), intestinal cramping, hyperactive bowel sounds; osteoporosis and fractures; severe cases show convulsions and tetany; prolonged QT interval, cardiac arrest
Hypercalcemia (>10.5 mg/dL) Hyperparathyroidism; bone metastases with calcium resorption from breast, prostate, renal, and cervical cancer; sarcoidosis; excess vitamin D; many tumors that produce PTH; calcium-containing antacids	Many nonspecific; fatigue, weakness, lethargy, anorexia, nausea, constipation; impaired renal function, kidney stones; dysrhythmias, bradycardia, cardiac arrest; bone pain, osteoporosis, fractures
Hypophosphatemia (<2.0 mg/dL) Intestinal malabsorption related to vitamin D deficiency, use of magnesium- and aluminum-containing antacids, long-term alcohol abuse, and malabsorption syndromes; respiratory alkalosis; increased renal excretion of phosphate associated with hyperparathyroidism	Conditions related to reduced capacity for oxygen transport by red blood cells and disturbed energy metabolism; leukocyte and platelet dysfunction; deranged nerve and muscle function; in severe cases, irritability, confusion, numbness, coma, convulsions; possibly respiratory failure (because of muscle weakness), cardiomyopathies, bone resorption (leading to rickets or osteomalacia)
Hyperphosphatemia (>4.7 mg/dL) Acute or chronic renal failure with significant loss of glomerular filtration; treatment of metastatic tumors with chemotherapy that releases large amounts of phosphate into serum; long-term use of laxatives or enemas containing phosphates; hypoparathyroidism	Symptoms primarily related to low serum calcium levels (caused by high phosphate levels) similar to symptoms of hypocalcemia; when prolonged, calcification of soft tissues in lungs, kidneys, joints
Hypomagnesemia (<1.5 mEq/L) Malnutrition, malabsorption syndromes, alcoholism, urinary losses (renal tubular dysfunction, loop diuretics)	Behavioral changes, irritability, increased reflexes, muscle cramps, ataxia, nystagmus, tetany, convulsions, tachycardia, hypotension
Hypermagnesemia (>3.0 mEq/L) Usually renal insufficiency or failure; also excessive intake of magnesium-containing antacids, adrenal insufficiency	Lethargy, drowsiness; loss of deep tendon reflexes; nausea and vomiting; muscle weakness; hypotension; bradycardia; respiratory distress; heart block, cardiac arrest

PTH, Parathyroid hormone.

bind calcium, causing a decrease in the concentration of ionized calcium. Metabolic or respiratory alkalosis causes symptoms of hypocalcemia because the change in pH enhances protein binding of ionized calcium. Hypoalbuminemia lowers total serum calcium levels by decreasing the amount of bound calcium in the plasma.

CLINICAL MANIFESTATIONS. The clinical manifestations of hypocalcemia are caused primarily by an increase in neuromuscular excitability. Calcium deficits cause partial depolarization of nerves and muscle as the threshold potential becomes more negative and approaches the resting membrane potential (hypopolarization) (see Fig. 3.8, *C*). Therefore, a smaller stimulus is required for initiating the action potential. The symptoms are related to neuromuscular irritability and include paresthesias around the mouth and in the digits, carpopedal spasm (muscle spasms in the hands and feet), hyperreflexia, and seizures.

Two clinical signs are Chvostek sign and Trousseau sign. *Chvostek sign* is elicited by tapping on the facial nerve just below the temple. A positive sign is a twitch of the nose or lip. *Trousseau sign* is contraction of the hand and fingers when the arterial blood flow in the arm is occluded for 5 minutes with the use of a blood pressure cuff.

Severe symptoms include convulsions and *tetany,* a continuous severe muscle spasm that can cause laryngospasm and death. The characteristic electrocardiogram (ECG) change is a prolonged QT interval, indicating prolonged ventricular depolarization and decreased cardiac contractility. Intestinal cramping and hyperactive bowel sounds also may be present because hypocalcemia affects the smooth muscles of the gastrointestinal

tract. Table 3.10 contains a summary of the manifestations of calcium level alterations.

EVALUATION AND TREATMENT. The health history may signify underlying pathologic conditions that require further evaluation and treatment. Severe symptoms of hypocalcemia require emergency treatment with intravenous 10% calcium gluconate. Oral calcium replacement should be initiated, and serum calcium levels should be monitored. Decreasing phosphate intake facilitates long-term management of hypocalcemia.[16]

Hypercalcemia

PATHOPHYSIOLOGY. Hypercalcemia with total serum calcium concentrations exceeding 10.5 mg/dL can be caused by a number of diseases.[17] The most common among these are hyperparathyroidism (which can be associated with thyrotoxicosis); bone metastases with calcium resorption from breast, prostate, or cervical cancer, or hematologic malignancy; sarcoidosis; and excess vitamin D. Many tumors produce PTH and elevate the serum calcium levels. Sarcoidosis appears to increase vitamin D levels. Prolonged immobilization can also lead to hypercalcemia from enhanced bone resorption and decreased calcium deposition into bone. Acidosis decreases serum binding of calcium to albumin, increasing ionized calcium levels.

CLINICAL MANIFESTATIONS. Many symptoms of hypercalcemia are nonspecific. Because serum calcium levels are increased, a greater amount of calcium is also contained inside the cells. The threshold potential becomes more positive (hyperpolarized) (e.g., moves from

−60 to −50 millivolts) and the cell membrane becomes refractory to depolarization (decreased excitability) because there is a greater difference between threshold potential and resting membrane potential (see Fig. 3.8, *C*). Thus many of the symptoms are related to loss of cell membrane excitability. (Membrane potentials and membrane excitability are discussed in Chapter 1.) Fatigue, weakness, lethargy, anorexia, nausea, and constipation are common.

Mental status changes and confusion may occur. Impaired renal function frequently develops, and kidney stones form as precipitates of calcium salts. A shortened QT segment and depressed widened T waves also may be observed on the ECG, with bradycardia and varying degrees of heart block. Table 3.10 contains a summary of the manifestations of alterations in calcium levels.

◆**EVALUATION AND TREATMENT.** With elevated serum calcium levels, often a reciprocal decrease in serum phosphate values occurs. Specific diagnostic procedures to identify the contributing pathologic condition are required.

Treatment is related to the severity of symptoms and the underlying disease. When renal function is normal, oral phosphate administration is effective. When acute illness and high calcium levels are present, treatment options include intravenous administration of large amounts of normal saline to enhance renal excretion of calcium, administration of bisphosphonates in the absence of renal failure, and administration of calcitonin. Denosumab is given for hypercalcemia related to malignancies.[18] Ultimately, the underlying pathologic condition must be treated.

Hypophosphatemia

◆**PATHOPHYSIOLOGY.** Hypophosphatemia is a serum phosphate level less than 2.0 mg/dL and is usually an indication of phosphate deficiency. In some conditions, total body phosphate concentration is normal but serum concentrations are low. The most common causes are intestinal malabsorption and increased renal excretion of phosphate. Inadequate absorption is associated with vitamin D deficiency, use of magnesium- and aluminum-containing antacids (which bind with phosphorus), long-term alcohol abuse, malabsorption syndromes, and refeeding syndromes after starvation. Respiratory alkalosis can cause severe hypophosphatemia because of cellular use of phosphorus for accelerated glycolysis (ATP) formation. Increased renal excretion of phosphorus is associated with hyperparathyroidism.

◆**CLINICAL MANIFESTATIONS.** The consequences of phosphate deficiency are not clinically evident until hypophosphatemia is severe. There is reduced capacity for oxygen transport by red blood cells and disturbed energy metabolism. Transport and release of oxygen are associated with 2,3-diphosphoglycerate (2,3-DPG) and ATP levels. When phosphate is depleted, 2,3-DPG and ATP levels become low and diminish release of oxygen to the tissues, leading to hypoxia with bradycardia and varying degrees of heart block.

Leukocyte and platelet dysfunctions also are associated with hypophosphatemia. There is a greater risk of infection and blood-clotting impairment, with potential for hemorrhage. Nerve and muscle function can be affected because of derangement in energy metabolism. Muscle weakness may become serious enough to cause respiratory failure, and cardiomyopathies also can develop. Irritability, confusion, numbness, coma, and convulsions develop with severe phosphate losses. In response to low phosphate levels, bone resorption occurs and may lead to rickets or osteomalacia. (Table 3.10 contains a summary of the manifestations of phosphate level alterations.)

◆**EVALUATION AND TREATMENT.** To correct the condition, the underlying cause must be identified and treated. The rate and amount of replacement are determined by the cause and presenting symptoms.[19] (Table 3.10 contains a summary of the manifestations of alterations in phosphate levels.)

Hyperphosphatemia

◆**PATHOPHYSIOLOGY.** Hyperphosphatemia, or an elevated serum phosphate level of more than 4.7 mg/dL, develops with exogenous or endogenous addition of phosphorus to the ECF or with significant loss of glomerular filtration and chronic kidney disease. Because most phosphate is located in cells, the cell destruction associated with treatment of metastatic tumors with chemotherapy can release large amounts of phosphate into the ECF. Long-term use of phosphate-containing enemas or laxatives also may lead to hyperphosphatemia. Hypoparathyroidism can cause elevated phosphate levels by increasing renal tubular reabsorption of phosphate.

High levels of serum phosphate also lower serum calcium levels, and increased amounts of phosphate and calcium are deposited in bone and soft tissues. Serum calcium levels may become low enough to cause symptoms of hypocalcemia, including tetany.

◆**CLINICAL MANIFESTATIONS.** Symptoms of hyperphosphatemia are related primarily to low serum calcium levels and thus are comparable to symptoms of hypocalcemia. With prolonged hyperphosphatemia, calcification of soft tissues occurs in the lungs, kidneys, and joints. (Table 3.10 contains a summary of the manifestations of alterations in phosphate concentration.)

◆**EVALUATION AND TREATMENT.** To correct hyperphosphatemia, the underlying pathologic condition must be identified and treated. Aluminum hydroxide may be administered because it binds phosphate in the gastrointestinal tract and is then eliminated; however, aluminum can be toxic, causing encephalopathy and osteomalacia. Non-aluminum, non–calcium phosphate binders (lanthanum carbonate or sevelamer), and iron-based binders are being evaluated, but cost and toxicity are concerns.[20] Dialysis is required for management of renal failure.

Magnesium

Magnesium (Mg^{++}) is a major intracellular cation, second to potassium. About 40% to 60% is stored in muscle and bone with 30% in the cells. A small amount (1%) is in the serum. Plasma concentration is 1.5 to 3.0 mg/dL with about one-third bound to plasma proteins and the rest in ionized form. Regulation of magnesium metabolism is balanced by the small intestine and kidney. Low serum levels cause renal conservation of magnesium. Magnesium is a cofactor in intracellular enzymatic reactions, protein synthesis, nucleic acid stability, and neuromuscular excitability. Calcium and magnesium often interact in reactions at the intracellular level with magnesium being an antagonist of calcium.[21]

Hypomagnesemia occurs when serum magnesium concentration is less than 1.5 mEq/L and clinical symptoms are present.[22] Malnutrition, malabsorption syndromes, alcoholism, renal tubular dysfunction, metabolic acidosis, use of loop and thiazide diuretics, and prolonged use of proton pump inhibitors can cause magnesium losses. Hypomagnesemia is associated with insulin resistance, diabetes mellitus, left ventricular hypertrophy, systemic inflammation, hypoalbuminemia, and osteoporosis. Because magnesium inhibits potassium channels, loss of magnesium results in movement of potassium out of the cell, with renal excretion resulting in hypokalemia. Signs and symptoms of hypomagnesemia are similar to those of hypocalcemia. Depression, confusion, irritability, increased reflexes, muscle weakness, ataxia, nystagmus, tetany, convulsions, and tachydysrhythmias may be observed. Treatment is intramuscular or intravenous administration of magnesium sulfate. Magnesium supplementation may be beneficial in the treatment of preeclampsia, migraine, depression, coronary artery disease, and asthma.[21] Magnesium improves myocardial metabolism and cell function; improves vascular smooth muscle tone (reduces peripheral vascular resistance and afterload); reduces cardiac dysrhythmias; and improves lipid and glucose metabolism. Magnesium also reduces vulnerability to oxygen-derived free radicals and systemic inflammation, improves human endothelial function, and inhibits platelet function, including platelet aggregation and adhesion.

Hypermagnesemia, in which magnesium concentration is greater than 3.0 mEq/L, is rare and usually is caused by renal failure. Magnesium-containing antacids (e.g., Gaviscon, Gelusil) can potentiate excess magnesium levels. Excess magnesium concentration depresses skeletal muscle contraction and nerve function. Signs and symptoms include nausea and vomiting, muscle weakness, hypotension, bradycardia, and respiratory depression. Treatment is avoidance of magnesium-containing substances and removal of magnesium by dialysis.[23] (Table 3.10 contains a summary of the manifestations of magnesium level alterations.)

ACID-BASE BALANCE

Acid-base balance and hydrogen ion concentration must be regulated within a narrow range for the body to function normally. Slight changes in amounts of hydrogen and pH changes can significantly alter biologic processes in cells and tissues. Hydrogen ion is necessary to maintain membrane integrity and the speed of enzymatic reactions. Most pathologic conditions disturb acid-base balance, and the degree of severity may be more harmful than the disease process.

Hydrogen Ion and pH

The hydrogen ion concentration, $[H^+]$, is commonly expressed as the pH, the negative logarithm of hydrogen ions in solution. The symbol **pH** represents the acidity or alkalinity of a solution. The logarithmic value means that as the pH changes 1 unit (e.g., from 7.0 to 6.0), the $[H^+]$ changes 10-fold (i.e., from 0.0000001 to 0.000001). The relationship is commonly expressed as follows:

$$pH = \log\frac{1}{[H^+]} \text{ or } pH = -\log_{10}[H^+]$$

As the $[H^+]$ increases, the pH decreases; likewise, as the $[H^+]$ decreases, the pH increases. The greater the $[H^+]$, the more acidic the solution and the lower the pH. The lower the $[H^+]$, the more basic the solution and the higher the pH. In biologic fluids, a pH of less than 7.4 is defined as acidic and a pH greater than 7.4 is defined as basic.

Different body fluids have different pH values as follows:

Body Fluid	pH
Gastric juices	1.0–3.0
Urine	5.0–6.0
Arterial blood	7.38–7.42
Venous blood	7.32–7.36
Cerebrospinal fluid	7.28–7.32
Pancreatic fluid and bile	7.8–8.0
Small intestinal fluid	6.5–7.5

Body acids are formed as end products of cellular metabolism. The average person generates 50 to 100 mEq/day of acid from the metabolism of proteins, carbohydrates, and fats and from loss of alkaline fluids in the stools. To maintain a normal pH, an equal amount of acid therefore must be neutralized or excreted. The lungs, kidneys, and bone are the major organs involved in the regulation of acid-base balance. The systems are interrelated and work together to regulate short- or long-term changes in acid-base status. Body acids exist in two forms: **volatile** (respiratory acids—eliminated as carbon dioxide [CO_2] gas) and **nonvolatile** (metabolic acids—eliminated by the kidney or metabolized by the liver). The volatile acid is carbonic acid (H_2CO_3), which is formed from the hydration of carbon dioxide:

Regulated by lung   Regulated by kidney

$$CO_2 + H_2O \leftrightarrow H_2CO_3 \leftrightarrow HCO_3^- + H^+$$

Carbonic acid is a weak acid, and in the presence of carbonic anhydrase, it readily dissociates into carbon dioxide and water. CO_2 is produced as an end product of oxidative metabolism. The more oxygen that is consumed, the more CO_2 is produced. The carbon dioxide is then eliminated by pulmonary ventilation. Sulfuric, phosphoric, and other metabolic acids (lactic acid, pyruvic acid, and keto acids [such as acetoacetic acid and β-hydroxybutyric acid, associated with diabetes mellitus]) are nonvolatile strong acids produced from the incomplete metabolism of proteins, carbohydrates, and fats. (Strong acids are those that readily give up their hydrogen; weak acids do not.) Nonvolatile acids are eliminated by the renal tubules in conjunction with the regulation of the concentration of bicarbonate (HCO_3^-). Thus the lungs and kidneys, with the help of body buffer systems, are the prime regulators of acid-base balance.

Buffer Systems

Buffering occurs in response to changes in acid-base status. **Buffers** can absorb excessive H^+ (acid) or hydroxyl ion (OH^-) (base) to minimize fluctuations in pH. The buffer systems are located in both the ICF and the ECF compartments, and they function at different rates. Buffer systems exist as buffer pairs, consisting of a weak acid and its conjugate base (Table 3.11). The most important plasma buffer systems are bicarbonate–carbonic acid and hemoglobin. Phosphate and protein are the most important intracellular buffers and provide a first line of defense. Ammonia and phosphate can attach hydrogen ion and are important renal buffers.

An important factor for effective buffering is a function known as the *pK value*, which represents the pH at which a buffer pair is half dissociated. Buffer pairs can associate and dissociate (see Table 3.11).

The pK provides a rate constant for the chemical reaction. A buffer system is most effective when the pK for the buffer is close to the pH of the fluid in which the buffer is acting. There is an equal concentration of acid and its conjugate base when pK equals pH. For the bicarbonate–carbonic acid buffer system, the pK is 6.1. This value is not as high as the pK for other buffer systems (see Table 3.11), but this buffer system is still very effective because carbon dioxide is rapidly removed from the blood by the lungs.

The pK value is also a term in the equation used to determine pH. The relationships among pH, pK, and the ratio of bicarbonate to carbonic acid can be expressed as follows by the *Henderson-Hasselbalch equation*:

$$pH = pK + \log\frac{[HCO_3^-]}{[H_2CO_3]}$$

The pH then can be determined when specific values are included in the equation:

$$pH = pK + \log\frac{[HCO_3^-]}{[H_2CO_3]}$$
$$= 6.1 + \log\frac{24}{1.2}$$
$$= 6.1 + \log\frac{20}{1}$$
$$= 6.1 + 1.3$$
$$= 7.40$$

Carbonic Acid–Bicarbonate Buffering

The **carbonic acid–bicarbonate buffer** pair operates in both the lung and the kidney. The greater the carbon dioxide partial pressure (P_{CO_2}),

TABLE 3.11   BUFFER SYSTEMS

BUFFER PAIRS	BUFFER SYSTEM	pK VALUES	REACTION	RATE
HCO_3^-/H_2CO_3	Bicarbonate	6.1	$H^+ + HCO_3^- \rightleftharpoons H_2O + CO_2$	Instantaneous
Hb^-/HHb	Hemoglobin	7.3	$HHb \rightleftharpoons H^+ + Hb^-$	Instantaneous
$HPO_4^=/H_2PO_4^-$	Phosphate	6.8	$HPO_4^- + H^+ \rightleftharpoons H_2PO_4^-$	Instantaneous
Pr^-/HPr	Plasma proteins	6.7	$HPr \rightleftharpoons H^+ + Pr^-$	Instantaneous

ORGANS	MECHANISM	RATE
Lungs	Regulates retention or elimination of CO_2 and therefore H_2CO_3 concentration	Minutes to hours
Ionic shifts	Exchange of intracellular potassium and sodium for hydrogen	2–4 hours
Kidneys	Bicarbonate reabsorption and regeneration, ammonia formation, phosphate buffering	Hours to days
Bone	Exchanges of calcium and phosphate, release of carbonate	Hours to days

H^+, Hydrogen ion; HCO_3^-, bicarbonate; H_2CO_3, carbonic acid; Hb^-, hemoglobin; HHb, hydrogenated hemoglobin; $H_2PO_4^-$, monobasic phosphate; $HPO_4^=$, dibasic phosphate; HPr, hydrogenated protein; Pr^-, protein.

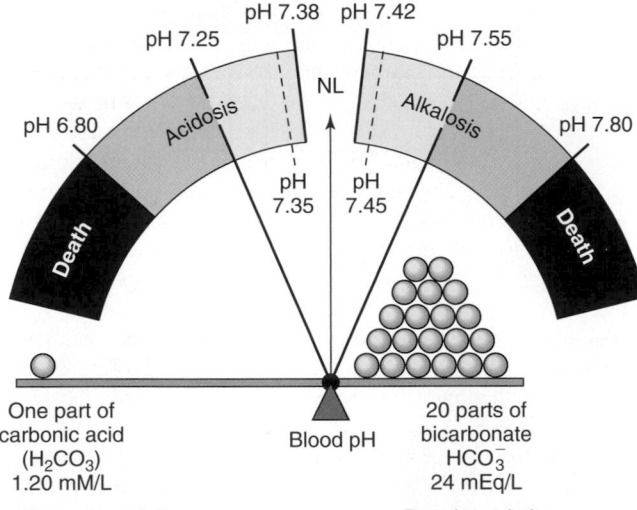

FIGURE 3.11 Ratio of Carbonic Acid and Bicarbonate Concentration in Maintaining pH Within Normal Limits. An increase in H_2CO_3 or decrease in HCO_3^- concentration causes acidosis. A decrease in H_2CO_3 or increase in HCO_3^- concentration causes alkalosis. *NL,* Normal. (From Monahan FD et al: *Medical-surgical nursing: health and illness perspectives,* ed 8, St Louis, 2007, Mosby.)

the more carbonic acid is formed. The relationship that exists between carbonic acid concentration ([H_2CO_3]) and carbon dioxide partial pressure (Pco_2) can be expressed as follows:

$$[H_2CO_3] = 0.03 \times P_{CO2}(mmHg)$$

The 0.03 represents the solubility coefficient for carbon dioxide in water. The Pco_2 of arterial blood ($Paco_2$) is normally about 40 mmHg. Therefore, the amount of H_2CO_3 is equal to about 1.2 mmol/L (0.03 × 40). As the amount of carbon dioxide increases or decreases, the amount of H_2CO_3 changes in the same direction.

The relationship between the levels of bicarbonate and carbonic acid is usually expressed as a ratio. When the pH is 7.40, this ratio is 20:1 (bicarbonate/carbonic acid) (Fig. 3.11). The ratio is defined by the amount of bicarbonate and carbon dioxide (carbonic acid) in the arterial blood. Bicarbonate concentration ([HCO_3^-]) is normally about 24 mEq/L. Therefore, the 20:1 ratio can be developed as follows:

$$\frac{[HCO_3^-] = 24 \text{ mEq/L}}{[H_2CO_3] = (0.03 \times 40 \text{ mmHg})} = \frac{24}{1.2} = \frac{20}{1}$$

When the values for [HCO_3^-] and $Paco_2$ ([H_2CO_3]) increase or decrease proportionately, the 20:1 ratio is maintained.

The lungs can decrease the amount of carbonic acid by exhaling CO_2 and leaving water. The kidneys can reabsorb bicarbonate or regenerate new bicarbonate from CO_2 and water. The renal mechanism does not act as rapidly as the lungs, but the two systems are very effective together because acid concentration can be rapidly adjusted by the lungs and bicarbonate is easily reabsorbed or regenerated by the kidneys. The pH equation can be symbolically expressed as follows:

$$pH = \frac{Base}{Acid} \text{ or } pH = \frac{Renal \text{ regulation (slow)}}{Pulmonary \text{ regulation (fast)}}$$

$$or$$

$$pH = \frac{Metabolic \text{ acid-base function}}{Respiratory \text{ acid-base function}}$$

Changes in either the numerator or the denominator will change the pH. For example, if the amount of bicarbonate is decreased, the pH also decreases, causing a state of acidosis. The pH can be returned to a normal range if the value of the denominator or the amount of carbonic acid also decreases. When a disease process causes an alteration in the bicarbonate/carbonic acid ratio, the kidneys or lungs (i.e., the organ not responsible for causing the alteration) respond to restore the ratio and maintain a normal pH. Renal and respiratory adjustments to *primary* changes in pH are known as **compensation**. With compensation, a 20:1 ratio may be achieved, but the actual values for HCO_3^- and H_2CO_3 concentrations are not normal. The respiratory system compensates for changes in pH by increasing or decreasing ventilation, a rapid response occurring within minutes to hours. The renal system compensates by producing more acidic or more alkaline urine, which may take hours to days. **Correction** occurs when the values for both components of the buffer pair ratio (bicarbonate and carbonic acid) return to normal (Fig. 3.12).

Protein Buffering

Both intracellular and extracellular proteins have negative charges and can serve as buffers for H^+, but because most proteins are inside cells, they are primarily an intracellular buffer system. Hemoglobin (Hb) is an excellent intracellular blood buffer because of its ability to bind with H^+ (forming HHb) and carbon dioxide (forming $HHbCO_2$). Hemoglobin bound to H^+ becomes a weak acid. Less oxygen-saturated hemoglobin (venous blood) is a better buffer than hemoglobin saturated with oxygen (arterial blood). The pH control system is illustrated in Fig. 3.13.

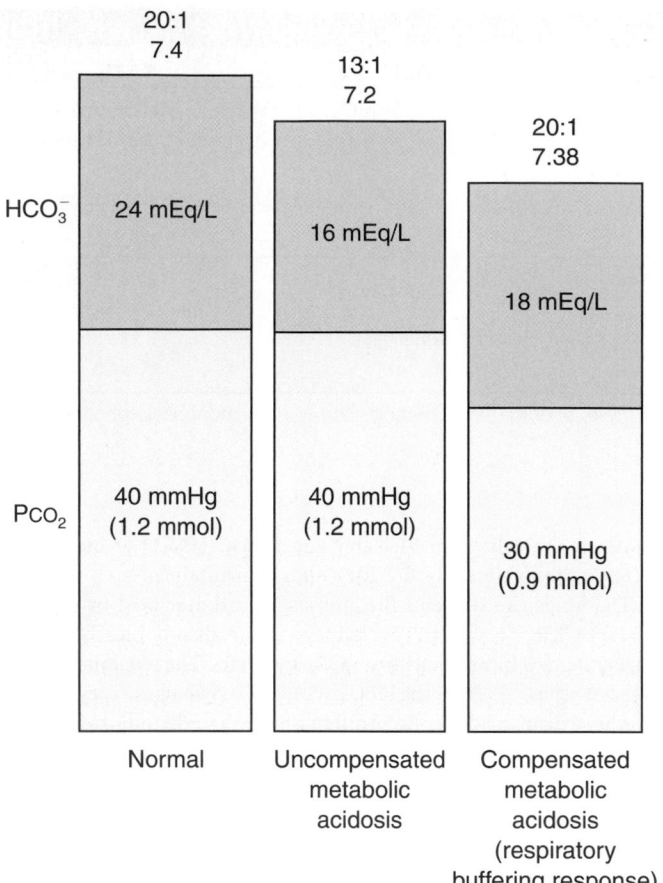

FIGURE 3.12 Compensated Maintenance of $[HCO_3^-]/Pco_2$ (H_2CO_3) Ratio in Metabolic Acidosis.

Respiratory and Renal Buffering

The respiratory system regulates acid-base balance by controlling the rate of ventilation when there is metabolic acidosis or alkalosis. Central chemoreceptors sense increases or decreases in pH and $Paco_2$ When acidemia exists, the respiratory rate increases (eliminating CO_2 and reducing carbonic acid concentration) (see Fig. 3.13). When alkalemia occurs, the respiratory rate decreases (retaining CO_2 and increasing carbonic acid concentration).

The distal tubule of the kidney regulates acid-base balance by secreting hydrogen into the urine and regenerating bicarbonate with a maximum urine acidity of a pH of about 4.4 to 4.7. Buffers in the tubular fluid combine with hydrogen ions, allowing more H^+ to be secreted before the limiting pH value is reached. Dibasic phosphate $(HPO_4^=)$ and ammonia (NH_3) are two important renal buffers because they can attach hydrogen ions and be secreted into the urine. Dibasic phosphate is filtered at the glomerulus. About 75% is reabsorbed, and the remainder is available for buffering H^+. Secreted H^+ combines with $HPO_4^=$ to form monobasic phosphate $(H_2PO_4^-)$. The remaining negative charge on the molecule makes it lipid insoluble, preventing it from diffusing back across the tubular cells and into the blood. Thus the $H_2PO_4^-$ containing the secreted H^+ is excreted in the urine (Fig. 3.14).

Ammonia (NH_3) is an important renal buffer; it is not ionized (does not carry a charge), and therefore it is lipid soluble and can cross the tubular cell membrane. The presence of NH_3 in the tubular cells creates a concentration gradient, and it diffuses into the renal tubular fluid, where it combines with hydrogen to form ammonium ion (NH_4^+), which is eliminated in the urine (see Fig. 3.14). NH_4^+ is lipid insoluble and does not readily diffuse back into the tubular cells. The renal buffering

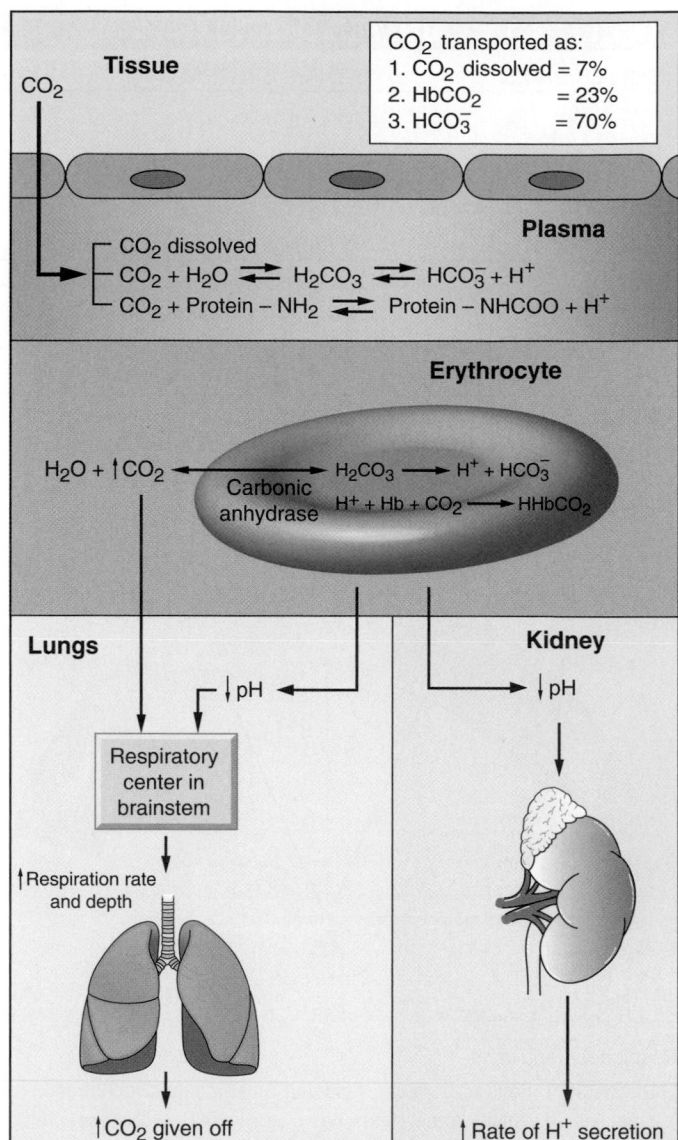

FIGURE 3.13 Integration of pH Control Mechanisms. CO_2 is produced in tissue cells and diffuses to plasma, where it is transported as dissolved CO_2, or it combines with water to form carbonic acid (H_2CO_3), or it combines with protein from which hydrogen has been released. Most of the CO_2 diffuses into the red blood cells and combines with water to form H_2CO_3. The H_2CO_3 dissociates to form hydrogen ion (H^+) and bicarbonate (HCO_3^-). Hydrogen ion combines with hemoglobin that has released its oxygen to form HHb, which buffers the hydrogen ion and makes venous blood slightly more acidic than arterial blood. The increase in H^+ concentration coupled with elevated CO_2 levels results in $HHbCO_2$ and an increase in the respiratory rate (eliminates CO_2) and secretion of H^+ by the kidneys.

of hydrogen ions requires the use of CO_2 and H_2O to form H_2CO_3. The enzyme carbonic anhydrase catalyzes the formation of $H^+ + HCO_3^-$. The hydrogen is secreted from the tubular cell and buffered in the lumen by phosphate and ammonia. The bicarbonate is reabsorbed. The end effect is the addition of new bicarbonate, which contributes to the alkalinity of the plasma, because the hydrogen ion is excreted from the body (see Fig. 3.14).

Other Buffers

A cellular ion exchange mechanism is also an important buffering system. The best example is the shift of potassium in exchange for hydrogen

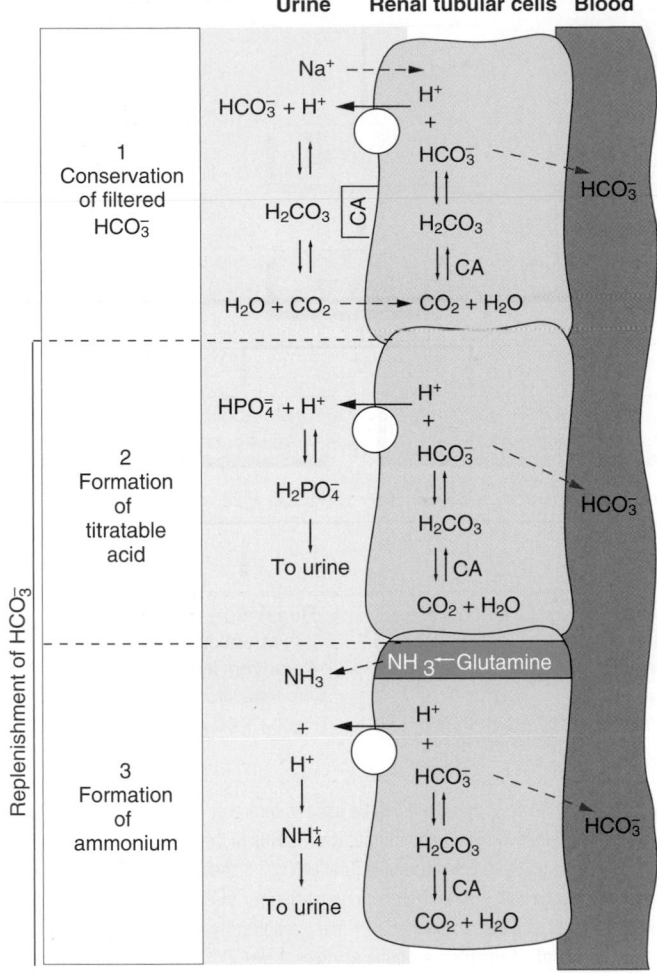

FIGURE 3.14 Renal Excretion of Acid. **1,** *Conservation of Filtered Bicarbonate.* Filtered bicarbonate (HCO_3^-) combines with secreted hydrogen ion (H^+) in the presence of carbon anhydrase (CA) to form carbonic acid (H_2CO_3), which then dissociates to water (H_2O) and carbon dioxide (CO_2); both diffuse into the renal tubular cell. The CO_2 and H_2O combine to form H_2CO_3 in the presence of CA, and the resulting bicarbonate ion (HCO_3^-) is reabsorbed into the blood. **2,** *Formation of Titratable Acid.* Hydrogen ion (H^+) is secreted and combines with dibasic phosphate ($HPO_4^=$) to form monobasic phosphate ($H_2PO_4^-$). The secreted hydrogen ion (H^+) is formed from the dissociation of H_2CO_3, and the remaining HCO_3^- is reabsorbed into the blood. **3,** *Formation of Ammonium.* Ammonia (NH_3) is produced from glutamine in the renal tubular cell and diffuses to the urine where it combines with H^+ to form ammonium ion (NH_4^+). Once NH_4^+ has been formed it cannot return to the renal tubular cell (diffusional trapping) and the bicarbonate remaining in the renal tubular cell is reabsorbed into the blood. **NOTE**: The white circles with the arrows on top represent a renal tubular cell active transport pump.

during states of acidosis or alkalosis. During acidosis, potassium tends to leave the intracellular space in exchange for hydrogen. The reverse occurs during alkalosis. Although the ionic shifts facilitate buffering, the changes in intracellular or extracellular potassium concentrations may have serious consequences (e.g., hyperkalemia or hypokalemia).

Acid-Base Imbalances

Pathophysiologic changes in the concentration of hydrogen ion or base in the blood lead to acid-base imbalances. Acidemia is a state in which the pH of arterial blood is less than 7.35. A systemic increase in hydrogen ion concentration or a loss of base is termed acidosis. Alkalemia is a

TABLE 3.12	CAUSES OF METABOLIC ACIDOSIS	
INCREASED NON–CARBONIC ACIDS (ELEVATED ANION GAP)	**BICARBONATE LOSS (NORMAL ANION GAP)**
Increased H^+ load—overproduction of acid	Diarrhea
Ketoacidosis (e.g., diabetes mellitus,	Ureterosigmoidoscopy
alcoholic ketoacidosis, starvation)	Early renal failure
Lactic acidosis (e.g., shock)	Proximal renal tubule acidosis
Ingestions (e.g., ammonium chloride,	
ethylene glycol, methanol, salicylates,	
paraldehyde)	
Decreased H^+ excretion	
Advanced renal failure	
Distal renal tubule acidosis	

state in which the pH of arterial blood is greater than 7.45. A systemic decrease in hydrogen ion concentration or an excess of base is termed alkalosis. Acid-base imbalances may have a metabolic or respiratory etiology or may be of mixed etiology. Acid-base imbalances are assessed using a measurement of arterial blood gases that includes the reporting of pH, $Paco_2$, and HCO_3^- concentration. The medical history is important to determining the cause of the disorder.[24] Fig. 3.15 summarizes the relationships among pH, $Paco_2$, and bicarbonate concentration during different primary acid-base alterations and the associated renal and respiratory compensatory changes. The ratio of the concentration of HCO_3^- and Pco_2 is altered.

Metabolic Acidosis

◆PATHOPHYSIOLOGY. In metabolic acidosis, the concentration of non–carbonic acids increases or bicarbonate (base) is lost from the extracellular fluid or cannot be regenerated by the kidney (Table 3.12). This can occur quickly, as in from poor perfusion or hypoxemia, or more slowly, as in renal failure (failure to excrete acid), starvation states, or diabetic ketoacidosis (excess production of keto acids from lack of insulin) (see Chapter 22). There is a decrease in the 20:1 ratio of HCO_3^- and H_2CO_3.

The buffer systems compensate for the excess acid and attempt to maintain the arterial pH within a normal range. Hydrogen ions will move to the intracellular space, and potassium will move to the extracellular space to maintain an ionic balance. Buffering by bicarbonate lowers the serum value of hydrogen ions and increases the pH. The respiratory system compensates for a metabolic acidosis as the reduced pH stimulates hyperventilation, lowering the $Paco_2$ and the amount of H_2CO_3 circulating in the blood. The kidneys excrete the excess acid as NH_4^+ and titratable acid ($H_2PO_4^-$). When acidosis is severe, buffers become depleted and cannot compensate for the increasing H^+ load and the pH continues to decrease. The ratio of bicarbonate to carbonic acid decreases to less than 20:1 (Fig. 3.16). In states of metabolic acidosis, potassium is redistributed from the intracellular to the extracellular space, and is reabsorbed at the apical membrane of the renal collecting tubule. There is also an increase in the levels of ionized calcium because acidosis decreases the amount of calcium bound to albumin.

The evaluation of the anion gap can be helpful when used cautiously to distinguish different types of metabolic acidosis.[25] Normally, the concentrations of cations and anions in the plasma are equivalent. Some anions, such as protein, sulfates, phosphates, and organic acids, however, are not measured in the common laboratory evaluations of the blood. Therefore the normal anion gap represents these unmeasured negative ions (sulfate, phosphate, lactate, keto acids, albumin). A

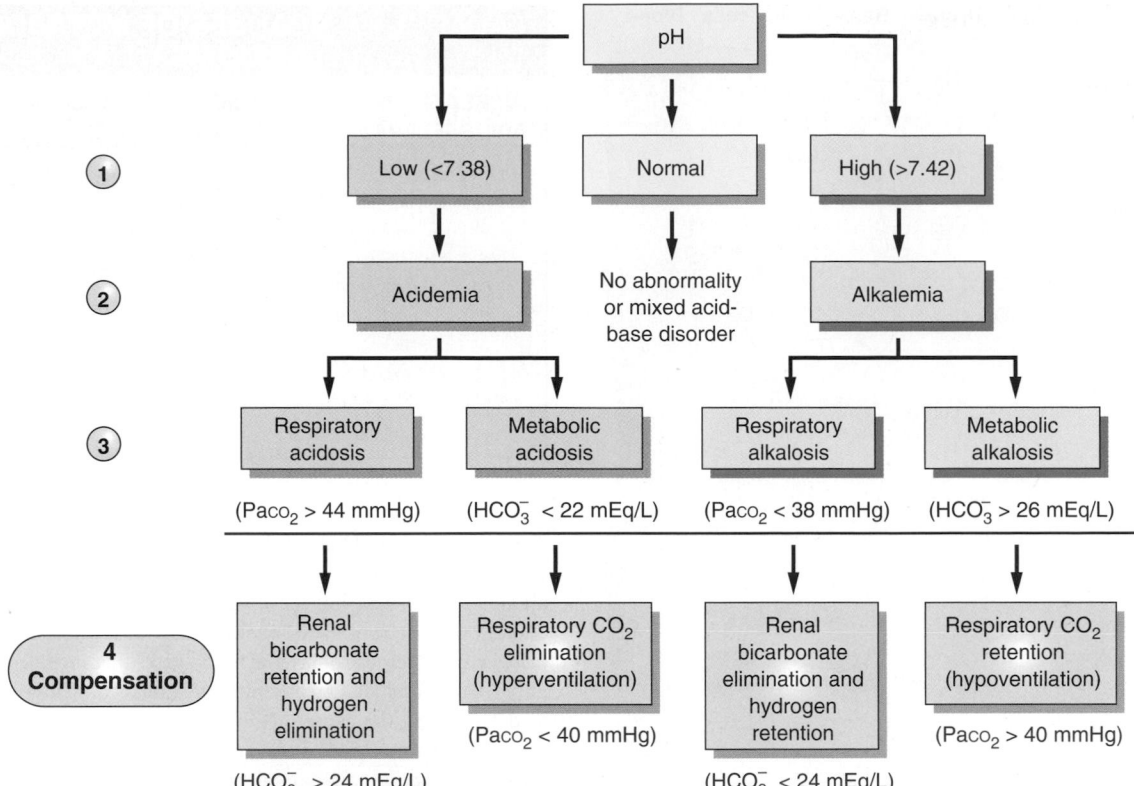

FIGURE 3.15 **Primary and Compensatory Acid-Base Changes.** A systematic approach can be used to interpret the cause of an acid-base imbalance. **1,** Is the pH low or high? **2,** If the pH is low there is acidemia; if the pH is high there is alkalemia. **3,** If the pH is low (acidemia), is the cause respiratory (high $PaCO_2$) or metabolic (low HCO_3^-)? If the pH is high (alkalemia), is the cause respiratory (low $PaCO_2$) or metabolic (high HCO_3^-)? **4,** Is there compensation for the primary acid-base disorder? *(a)* HCO_3^- will be ≥24 mEq/L if there is renal compensation for a primary respiratory acidosis; *(b)* $PaCO_2$ will be <40 mmHg if there is respiratory compensation of a primary metabolic acidosis; *(c)* HCO_3^- will be ≤24 mEq/L if there is renal compensation for primary respiratory alkalosis; *(d)* $PaCO_2$ will be >40 mmHg if there is respiratory compensation for primary metabolic alkalosis. **NOTE:** Examine the pH first. Then examine the changes in HCO_3^- and $PaCO_2$. HCO_3^- concentration will be elevated when there is primary metabolic alkalosis or renal compensation for primary respiratory acidosis. HCO_3^- concentration will be decreased when there is primary metabolic acidosis or renal compensation for primary respiratory alkalosis. $PaCO_2$ will be elevated when there is primary respiratory acidosis or respiratory compensation for primary metabolic alkalosis. $PaCO_2$ will be decreased when there is primary respiratory alkalosis or respiratory compensation for metabolic acidosis.

convenient measure of the anion gap is the difference between the sum of Na^+ and K^+ concentrations and the sum of HCO_3^- and Cl^- concentrations, or about 10 to 12 mEq/L:

$$\text{Anion gap} = [Na^+ (140) + K^+ (4.0)] - [HCO_3^- (24) + Cl^- (110)] = 10 - 12 \text{ mEq/L}$$

In metabolic acidosis a **normal anion gap** is characteristic of conditions related to bicarbonate loss with retention of chloride to maintain an ionic balance. This is called **hyperchloremic metabolic acidosis** and it occurs with renal failure or prolonged diarrhea with bicarbonate loss. An elevated anion gap is characteristic of acidosis associated with accumulation of anions other than chloride (see Table 3.12).

◆**CLINICAL MANIFESTATIONS.** Metabolic acidosis is manifested by changes in the neurologic, respiratory, gastrointestinal, and cardiovascular systems. Headache and lethargy are early symptoms, which progress to confusion and coma with severe acidosis. Deep, rapid respirations (Kussmaul respirations) are indicative of respiratory compensation. Anorexia, nausea, vomiting, diarrhea, and abdominal discomfort are common. Severe acidosis can compromise ventricular contraction and produce life-threatening dysrhythmias.

◆**EVALUATION AND TREATMENT.** The diagnosis of metabolic acidosis is established from the health history, clinical symptoms, and laboratory findings. Arterial blood pH is below 7.35, and bicarbonate concentration is less than 22 mEq/L. The anion gap can isolate the specific cause. The oxyhemoglobin curve is shifted to the right (see Fig. 35.16), reducing hemoglobin affinity for oxygen.

The underlying condition must be diagnosed to establish effective treatment with a buffering solution. During severe acidosis (pH ≤7.1), base administration is required to elevate the pH to a safe level, particularly if there is renal failure. Accompanying sodium and water deficits must also be corrected.[26]

Metabolic Alkalosis

◆**PATHOPHYSIOLOGY.** Metabolic alkalosis occurs when bicarbonate concentration is increased, usually caused by excessive loss of metabolic acids. There is an increase in the 20:1 ratio of HCO_3^- and H_2CO_3. Conditions that can result in metabolic alkalosis are hydrogen and chloride depletion (i.e., prolonged vomiting, gastric suctioning), excessive bicarbonate intake, hyperaldosteronism with hypokalemia, and diuretic therapy.[27]

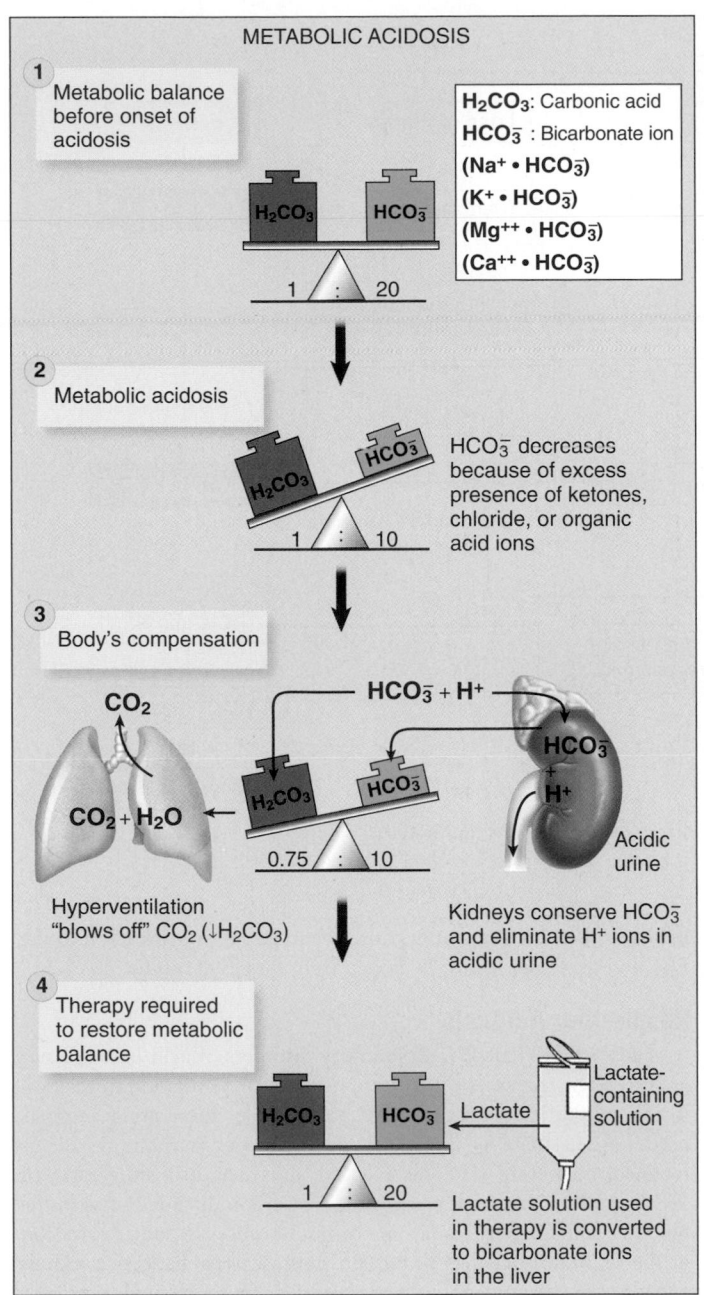

METABOLIC ACIDOSIS

1 Metabolic balance before onset of acidosis

H_2CO_3: Carbonic acid
HCO_3^- : Bicarbonate ion
$(Na^+ \cdot HCO_3^-)$
$(K^+ \cdot HCO_3^-)$
$(Mg^{++} \cdot HCO_3^-)$
$(Ca^{++} \cdot HCO_3^-)$

H_2CO_3 HCO_3^- 1 : 20

2 Metabolic acidosis

H_2CO_3 HCO_3^- 1 : 10

HCO_3^- decreases because of excess presence of ketones, chloride, or organic acid ions

3 Body's compensation

CO_2
$CO_2 + H_2O$
$HCO_3^- + H^+$
H_2CO_3 HCO_3^- 0.75 : 10
$HCO_3^- + H^+$
Acidic urine

Hyperventilation "blows off" CO_2 ($\downarrow H_2CO_3$)

Kidneys conserve HCO_3^- and eliminate H^+ ions in acidic urine

4 Therapy required to restore metabolic balance

H_2CO_3 HCO_3^- 1 : 20
Lactate
Lactate-containing solution

Lactate solution used in therapy is converted to bicarbonate ions in the liver

FIGURE 3.16 Metabolic Acidosis With Compensation and Correction. See text for abbreviations. (From Patton KT, Thibodeau GA: *Anatomy & physiology*, ed 9, St Louis, 2016, Mosby.)

METABOLIC ALKALOSIS

1 Metabolic balance before onset of alkalosis

H_2CO_3: Carbonic acid
HCO_3^- : Bicarbonate ion
$(Na^+ \cdot HCO_3^-)$
$(K^+ \cdot HCO_3^-)$
$(Mg^{++} \cdot HCO_3^-)$
$(Ca^{++} \cdot HCO_3^-)$

H_2CO_3 HCO_3^- 1 : 20

2 Metabolic alkalosis

H_2CO_3 HCO_3^- 1 : 40

HCO_3^- increases because of loss of chloride ions or excess ingestion of sodium bicarbonate

3 Body's compensation

$CO_2 + H_2O$
CO_2
CO_2
$H^+ + HCO_3^-$
H_2CO_3 HCO_3^- 1.25 : 30
$H^+ + HCO_3^-$
Alkaline urine

Hypoventilation retains CO_2 ($\uparrow H_2CO_3$)

Kidneys conserve H^+ ions and eliminate HCO_3^- in alkaline urine

4 Therapy required to restore metabolic balance

H_2CO_3 HCO_3^- Cl^- 1 : 20
Chloride-containing solution

HCO_3^- ions replaced by Cl^- ions

FIGURE 3.17 Metabolic Alkalosis With Compensation and Correction. See text for abbreviations. (From Patton KT, Thibodeau GA: *Anatomy & physiology*, ed 9, St Louis, 2016, Mosby.)

Respiratory compensation for metabolic alkalosis occurs when the elevated pH inhibits the respiratory center. The rate and depth of ventilation are decreased, causing retention of carbon dioxide. The ratio of HCO_3^- concentration to H_2CO_3 concentration is reduced toward normal. Respiratory compensation is not very efficient, however, and chronic or severe metabolic alkalosis requires therapeutic intervention (Fig. 3.17).

Hypochloremic metabolic alkalosis occurs when acid loss is caused by vomiting or gastric suctioning with depletion of ECF sodium, chloride, and potassium. Renal compensation is not very effective because the volume depletion and loss of electrolytes stimulate a paradoxical response by the kidneys. The kidneys increase bicarbonate reabsorption to maintain an anionic balance because the ECF chloride concentration is decreased. The resulting excretion of H^+ and reabsorption of bicarbonate prevent correction of the alkalosis (Fig. 3.18). The kidneys also increase sodium reabsorption. When potassium concentration is depleted, hydrogen ion moves to the intracellular space and is excreted to maintain an electrochemical balance.

With alkalemia, hydrogen ions are redistributed from the intracellular to the extracellular space and potassium moves to the intracellular space to preserve electroneutrality. With hyperaldosteronism, the excess aldosterone causes sodium retention and loss of hydrogen and potassium ions. Mild volume expansion ensues, and bicarbonate is retained along with the sodium, thereby causing alkalosis. Diuretics, such as thiazides,

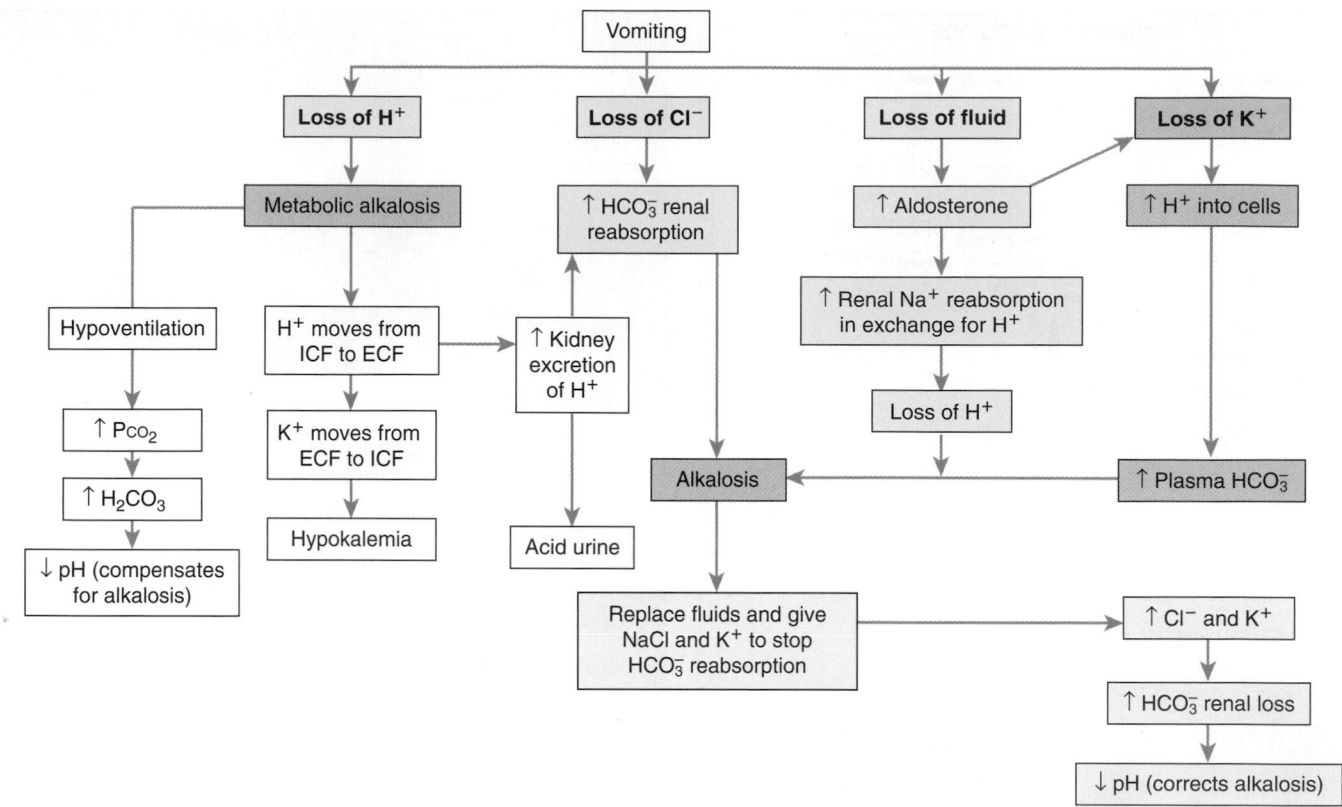

FIGURE 3.18 Hypochloremic Metabolic Alkalosis. See text for abbreviations.

ethacrynic acid, and furosemide, produce mild alkalosis by enhancing sodium, potassium, and chloride excretion more than bicarbonate excretion.

◆**CLINICAL MANIFESTATIONS.** Because of the many causes of metabolic alkalosis, the symptoms vary. Some common symptoms, such as weakness, muscle cramps, and hyperactive reflexes, are related to volume depletion and electrolyte losses. Because alkalosis increases binding of Ca^{++} to plasma proteins (albumin), ionized calcium concentration decreases, causing excitable cells to become hypopolarized, which initiates an action potential more easily. Paresthesias (especially numbness/tingling of the fingertips and perioral area), tetany, and seizures may develop (see Hypocalcemia).

Respirations are slow and shallow to increase carbon dioxide retention. Confusion and convulsions occur with severe alkalosis. Atrial tachycardia is a potential problem. The oxyhemoglobin curve is shifted to the left (see Fig. 35.16), decreasing the dissociation of oxyhemoglobin and increasing the risk of dysrhythmias.

◆**EVALUATION AND TREATMENT.** The health history provides significant clues to the diagnosis of metabolic alkalosis. The arterial pH is greater than 7.45, and bicarbonate levels exceed 26 mEq/L. With respiratory compensation, the $Paco_2$ rises above 40 mmHg. With hypochloremic metabolic alkalosis, serum chloride values are below normal. Serum potassium levels are usually depleted because hydrogen is released from the cells in exchange for potassium to help regulate the pH level. The potassium is then secreted from renal distal tubule cells into the urine.

With hypochloremic alkalosis or contraction alkalosis with volume depletion, a sodium chloride solution is required for *correction*. The renal stimulus to increase ECF volume by retaining Na^+ is diminished, and HCO_3^- can be excreted as $NaHCO_3$ in the urine. The administration of potassium corrects alkalosis caused by hyperaldosteronism or

hypokalemia. The potassium causes hydrogen to move back into the ECF and decreases loss of hydrogen from the distal tubule.

Respiratory Acidosis

◆**PATHOPHYSIOLOGY.** Respiratory disorders of acid-base balance are caused by increases or decreases of alveolar ventilation in relation to the metabolic production of carbon dioxide. Respiratory acidosis occurs when there is alveolar hypoventilation. Carbon dioxide is retained, increasing $[H^+]$ (as H_2CO_3), thus decreasing the ratio of HCO_3^- to Pco_2, and producing acidosis. Carbon dioxide excess in the blood is called hypercapnia. The common causes include depression of the respiratory center (brainstem trauma, oversedation), paralysis of the respiratory muscles, disorders of the chest wall (kyphoscoliosis, pickwickian syndrome, flail chest), and disorders of the lung parenchyma (e.g., pneumonitis, pulmonary edema, and chronic obstructive lung disease).

Respiratory acidosis may be acute or chronic.[28] Airway obstruction is the most common cause of acute respiratory acidosis. Acute compensation for respiratory acidosis is not effective because the renal buffer mechanism takes time to function. Further, the protein buffers provide marginal compensation, and HCO_3^- is not a good buffer for CO_2. Acute uncompensated respiratory acidosis is characterized by decreased arterial pH, elevated $Paco_2$, and normal or slightly increased bicarbonate concentration.

Chronic respiratory acidosis is commonly associated with chronic obstructive pulmonary disease and deformities of the chest wall or neuromuscular disorders. Renal compensation is effective and is established over several days. The acidosis produced from CO_2 retention stimulates the kidney to secrete hydrogen ions and regenerate bicarbonate. Serum bicarbonate and $Paco_2$ levels are elevated, and pH is restored toward normal (Fig. 3.19).

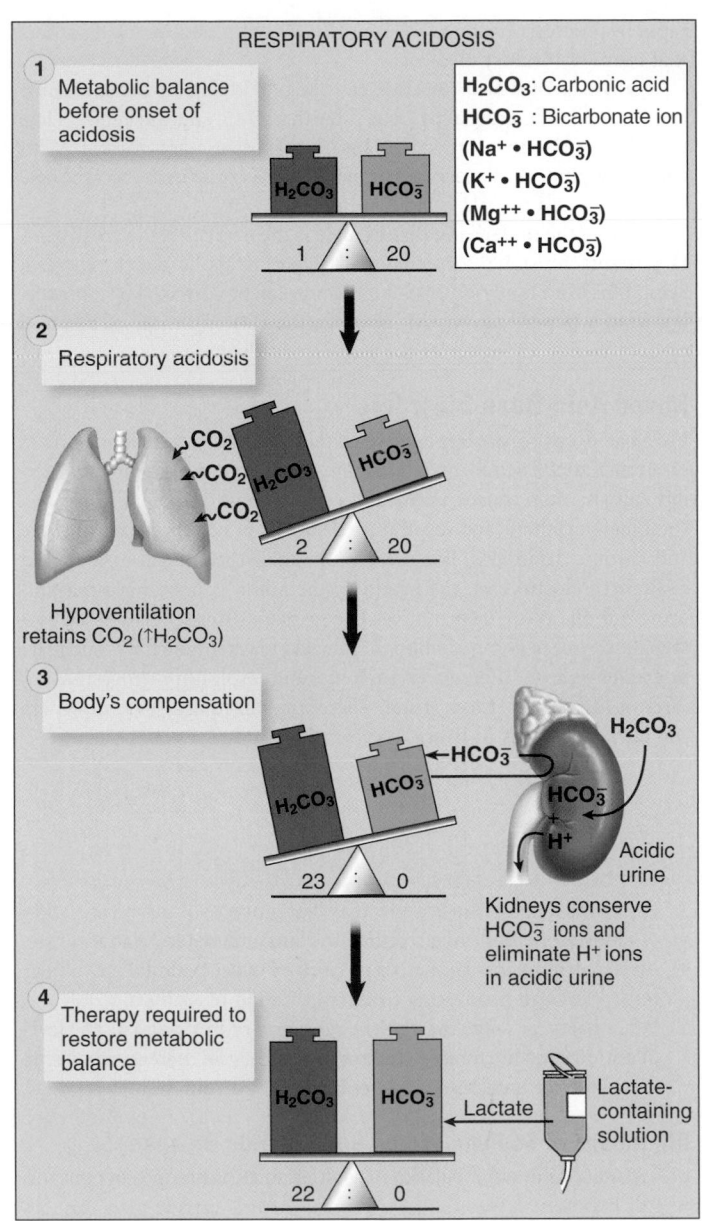

FIGURE 3.19 Respiratory Acidosis With Compensation and Correction. See text for abbreviations. (From Patton KT, Thibodeau GA: *Anatomy & physiology*, ed 9, St Louis, 2016, Mosby.)

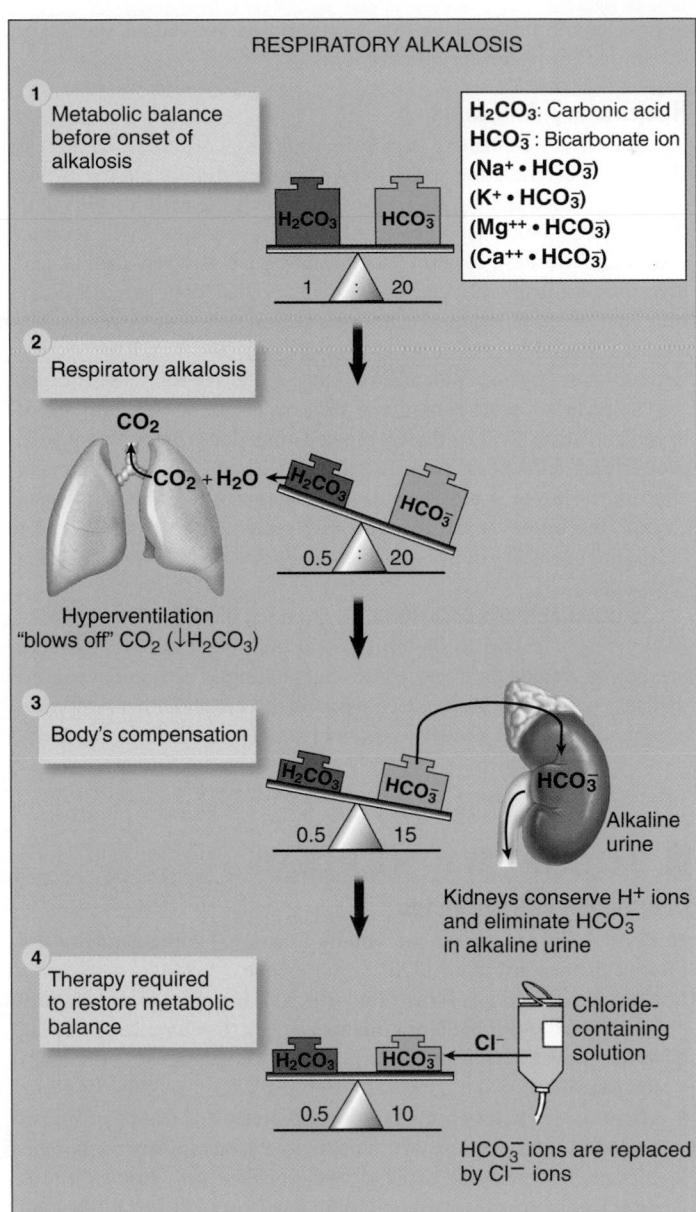

FIGURE 3.20 Respiratory Alkalosis With Compensation and Correction. See text for abbreviations. (From Patton KT, Thibodeau GA: *Anatomy & physiology*, ed 9, St Louis, 2016, Mosby.)

◆**CLINICAL MANIFESTATIONS.** The symptoms of respiratory acidosis are related to acuity of onset and severity of $Paco_2$ retention. Initial symptoms include headache, restlessness, blurred vision, and apprehension. Lethargy, muscle twitching, tremors, convulsions, and coma follow. Chronic acidosis causes myocardial depression, arrhythmias, and hypotension. Neurologic symptoms are caused by a decrease in the pH of cerebrospinal fluid and vasodilation because CO_2 readily crosses the blood-brain barrier. The respiratory rate is rapid at first and gradually becomes depressed because over time, the respiratory center adapts to increasing levels of CO_2. Cyanosis does not occur unless there is an accompanying hypoxemia, and the skin may instead be pink from vasodilation caused by the elevated CO_2 level.

◆**EVALUATION AND TREATMENT.** The primary diagnostic indicators are an arterial pH less than 7.35 and hypercapnia. Acute respiratory acidosis must be distinguished from chronic acidosis; the health history and clinical laboratory data are therefore helpful.

In many cases, restoration of adequate alveolar ventilation removes excess CO_2. If alveolar ventilation cannot be maintained spontaneously because of drug overdose or neuromuscular disorders, mechanical ventilation is required. When the hypercapnia is caused by alterations in gas diffusion at the alveolar-capillary membrane, ventilation may not be effective. The values of arterial pH, Pco_2, Po_2, and HCO_3^- must be carefully monitored. Rapid reduction of $Paco_2$ can cause respiratory alkalosis with seizures and death.

The underlying diseases are treated to achieve maximal ventilation. In the presence of hypoxemia and hypercapnia, oxygen can function as a respiratory depressant when the respiratory center is no longer stimulated by the lower pH and elevated $Paco_2$ value. Therefore, when oxygen is administered in this situation, the individual should be monitored for respiratory depression.

Respiratory Alkalosis

◆**PATHOPHYSIOLOGY.** **Respiratory alkalosis** occurs when there is alveolar hyperventilation and decreased concentration of plasma carbon dioxide (termed **hypocapnia**), thus increasing the ratio of HCO_3^- to Pco_2 (H_2CO_3). Stimulation of ventilation is precipitated by hypoxemia (i.e., high altitudes); hypermetabolic states such as fever, anemia, and thyrotoxicosis; early salicylate intoxication; or anxiety or panic disorder. Improper use of mechanical ventilators can cause iatrogenic respiratory alkalosis. Secondary respiratory alkalosis may develop from hyperventilation stimulated by metabolic acidosis, causing a mixed acid-base disorder.

The onset of acute respiratory alkalosis occurs within minutes of hyperventilation. Cellular buffers provide immediate compensation (i.e., protein and shifts of H^+ from ICF to ECF). The H^+ shifts are not very effective, however, if the $Paco_2$ level is significantly decreased. When chronic respiratory alkalosis is present, renal compensation restores pH toward normal by decreasing H^+ excretion and bicarbonate absorption (Fig. 3.20).

◆**CLINICAL MANIFESTATIONS.** Respiratory alkalosis, like metabolic alkalosis, is irritating to the central and peripheral nervous systems. Symptoms include dizziness, confusion, tingling of extremities (paresthesias), convulsions, and coma. Carpopedal spasm and other symptoms of hypocalcemia are similar to those of metabolic alkalosis. Deep and rapid respirations (tachypnea) are primary symptoms of the disorders that cause respiratory alkalosis.

◆**EVALUATION AND TREATMENT.** The underlying disturbance must be identified. The arterial pH is greater than 7.45, and the $Paco_2$ is less than 38 mmHg. In acute states, bicarbonate levels are normal. With chronic respiratory alkalosis, a compensatory decrease in the bicarbonate level occurs and the pH is closer to normal.

Treating the underlying disturbance is the most effective treatment. Hypoxemia must be corrected and hypermetabolic states reversed. Symptoms from hysterical hyperventilation can be corrected by rebreathing from a paper bag, which increases the concentration of inspired carbon dioxide and reverses the respiratory alkalosis.

Mixed Acid-Base Disorders

Mixed acid-base disorders are two or more primary acid-base disorders occurring at the same time. They are more common in hospitalized individuals, often those in critical care with comorbid conditions (i.e., combined metabolic and respiratory disorders or combinations of acute and chronic disorders). For these individuals the clinical history and analysis of electrolytes, medications, the anion gap, and plasma and urine osmolality are informative. The primary disorder is assessed and then the degree of compensation is evaluated to determine if it is adequate or greater or lesser than expected. Renal and respiratory compensation rarely returns the pH to normal. Therefore, mixed acid-base disorders can have alterations in $Paco_2$ and bicarbonate and a normal pH.[29,30]

■ SUMMARY REVIEW

Distribution of Body Fluids
1. Body fluids are distributed among functional compartments and are classified as ICF or ECF.
2. The sum of all fluids is the TBW, which varies with age and amount of body fat and is higher in infants because they have less body fat.
3. Water moves between the ICF and ECF compartments principally by osmosis.
4. Water moves between the plasma and interstitial fluid by osmosis and hydrostatic pressure, which occur across the capillary membrane.
5. Movement across the capillary wall is called *net filtration* and is described according to the Starling law (forces favoring filtration minus forces opposing filtration).

Alterations in Water Movement
1. Edema is a problem of fluid distribution that results in accumulation of fluid within the interstitial spaces.
2. Edema is caused by venous or lymphatic obstruction (increases hydrostatic pressure), plasma protein losses (decreases plasma oncotic pressure), increased capillary permeability, and increased vascular volume.
3. The pathophysiologic process that leads to edema is related to an increase in forces favoring fluid filtration from the capillaries into the tissues.
4. Edema may be localized or generalized and usually is associated with swelling and puffiness, tighter-fitting clothes and shoes, limited movement of the affected area, and, in severe cases, weight gain.

Sodium, Chloride, and Water Balance
1. Sodium balance and water balance are intimately related; chloride levels are generally proportional to changes in sodium levels.
2. Sodium balance is regulated by aldosterone, which increases reabsorption of sodium by the distal tubule of the kidney.
3. Renin and angiotensin are enzymes that promote or inhibit secretion of aldosterone and thus regulate sodium and water balance.
4. Atrial natriuretic hormone is also involved in decreasing renal tubular resorption and promoting urinary excretion of sodium.
5. Water balance is regulated by the sensation of thirst and by the level of antidiuretic hormone, which is initiated by an increase in plasma osmolality or a decrease in circulating blood volume.

Alterations in Sodium, Water, and Chloride Balance
1. Alterations in water balance may be classified as isotonic, hypertonic, or hypotonic.
2. Isotonic alterations occur when changes in TBW are accompanied by proportional changes in concentrations of electrolytes.
3. Hypertonic alterations develop when the osmolality of the ECF is elevated above normal, usually because of an increased concentration of ECF sodium or a deficit of ECF water.
4. Hypernatremia (sodium levels >145 mEq/L) may be caused by an acute increase in sodium level or a loss of water.
5. Water deficit, or hypertonic dehydration, can be caused by lack of access to water, pure water losses, hyperventilation, arid climates, or increased renal clearance.
6. Hyperchloremia is caused by an excess of sodium or a deficit of bicarbonate.
7. Hypotonic alterations occur when the osmolality of the ECF is less than normal.
8. Hyponatremia occurs when the serum sodium concentration decreases to less than 135 mEq/L, and may be caused by inadequate intake of sodium or dilution of the body's sodium level.
9. Water excess is rare but can be caused by compulsive water drinking, decreased urine formation, or the syndrome of inappropriate secretion of ADH.
10. Hyponatremia usually causes movement of water into cells.

■ SUMMARY REVIEW—cont'd

11. Hypochloremia is usually the result of hyponatremia or elevated bicarbonate concentrations.

Alterations in Potassium, Calcium, Phosphate, and Magnesium Balance

1. Potassium is the predominant ICF ion; it functions to regulate ICF osmolality, maintain the resting membrane potential, and deposit glycogen in liver and skeletal muscle cells.
2. Potassium balance is regulated by the kidney, by aldosterone and insulin secretion, and by changes in pH.
3. A mechanism known as *potassium adaptation* allows the body to accommodate slowly to increased levels of potassium intake.
4. Hypokalemia (serum potassium concentration <3.5 mEq/L) indicates loss of total body potassium, although ECF hypokalemia can develop without losses of total body potassium, and plasma K$^+$ levels may be normal or elevated when the amount of total body potassium is depleted.
5. Hypokalemia may be caused by reduced potassium intake, increased ICF to ECF potassium concentration, loss of potassium from body stores, increased aldosterone secretion (e.g., caused by hypernatremia), and increased renal excretion.
6. Hyperkalemia (potassium levels >5.0 mEq/L) may be caused by increased potassium intake, a shift from ICF to ECF potassium, or decreased renal excretion.
7. Calcium is a necessary ion in the structure of bones and teeth, in blood clotting, in hormone secretion and the function of cell receptors, and in membrane stability.
8. Phosphate acts as a buffer in acid-base regulation and provides energy for muscle contraction.
9. Calcium and phosphate concentrations are rigidly controlled by PTH, vitamin D, and calcitonin.
10. Hypocalcemia (total serum calcium concentration <9.0 mg/dL) is related to inadequate intestinal absorption, deposition of ionized calcium into bone or soft tissue, blood administration, or decreased PTH and vitamin D levels.
11. Hypercalcemia (serum calcium concentration >10.5 mg/dL) can be caused by a number of diseases, including hyperparathyroidism, bone metastases, sarcoidosis, and excess vitamin D.
12. Hypophosphatemia is a serum phosphate level less than 2.0 mg/dL and is usually caused by intestinal malabsorption and increased renal excretion of phosphate.
13. Hyperphosphatemia is a serum phosphate level more than 4.7 mg/dL and develops with acute or chronic renal failure with significant loss of glomerular filtration.
14. Magnesium is a major intracellular cation and is principally regulated by PTH.
15. Magnesium functions in enzymatic reactions and often interacts with calcium at the cellular level.
16. Hypomagnesemia (serum magnesium concentrations <1.5 mEq/L) may be caused by malabsorption syndromes.
17. Hypermagnesemia (serum magnesium concentrations >3.0 mEq/L) is rare and is usually caused by renal failure.

Acid-Base Balance

1. Hydrogen ions, which maintain membrane integrity and the speed of enzymatic reactions, must be concentrated within a narrow range if the body is to function normally.
2. Hydrogen ion concentration is expressed as pH, which represents the negative logarithm of hydrogen ions in solution.
3. Different body fluids have different pH values.
4. The renal and respiratory systems, together with the body's buffer systems, are the principal regulators of acid-base balance.
5. Buffers are substances that can absorb excessive acid or base to minimize fluctuations in pH.
6. Buffers exist as acid-base pairs; the principal plasma buffers are bicarbonate, protein (hemoglobin), and phosphate.
7. Buffer pairs can associate and dissociate; the pK value is the pH at which a buffer pair is half dissociated.
8. The lungs and kidneys act to compensate for changes in pH by increasing or decreasing ventilation and by producing more acidic or more alkaline urine.
9. Correction is a process different from compensation; correction occurs when the values for both components of the buffer pair are returned to normal.
10. Acid-base imbalances are caused by changes in the concentration of H$^+$ in the blood; an increase causes acidosis, and a decrease causes alkalosis.
11. An abnormal increase or decrease in bicarbonate concentration causes metabolic acidosis or metabolic alkalosis; changes in the rate of alveolar ventilation produce respiratory acidosis or respiratory alkalosis.
12. Metabolic acidosis is caused by an increase in the concentrations of non–carbonic acids or by loss of bicarbonate from the extracellular fluid.
13. Metabolic alkalosis occurs with an increase in bicarbonate concentration usually caused by loss of metabolic acids from conditions such as vomiting, gastrointestinal suctioning, excessive bicarbonate intake, hyperaldosteronism, and diuretic therapy.
14. Respiratory acidosis occurs with a decrease of alveolar ventilation and an increase in levels of carbon dioxide, or hypercapnia.
15. Respiratory alkalosis occurs with alveolar hyperventilation and excessive reduction of carbon dioxide concentration, or hypocapnia.

■ KEY TERMS

KEY TERMS—cont'd

Hypernatremia, 111
Hyperphosphatemia, 121
Hyperpolarized, 116
Hypertonic fluid alterations, 111
Hypertonic hyponatremia, 113
Hypervolemic hypernatremia, 111
Hypervolemic hyponatremia, 113
Hypocalcemia, 119
Hypocapnia, 130
Hypochloremia, 114
Hypochloremic metabolic alkalosis, 127
Hypokalemia, 115
Hypomagnesemia, 121
Hyponatremia, 113
Hypophosphatemia, 121
Hypopolarized, 117
Hypotonic fluid alterations, 112
Hypotonic hyponatremia, 113
Hypovolemic hyponatremia, 113

Hypovolemic hypernatremia, 111
Inadequate intake of dietary sodium, 113
Increased capillary hydrostatic pressure, 106
Increased capillary permeability, 106
Intercalated cell, 114
Interstitial fluid, 104
Interstitial hydrostatic pressure, 106
Interstitial oncotic pressure, 106
Intracellular fluid (ICF), 104
Intravascular fluid, 104
Isotonic alteration, 110
Lymphatic obstruction, 106
Lymphedema, 106
Magnesium (Mg^{++}), 121
Metabolic acidosis, 125
Metabolic alkalosis, 126
Mixed acid-base disorders, 130
Natriuretic peptide, 109
Net filtration, 106

Nonvolatile, 122
Normal anion gap, 126
Osmoreceptor, 109
Parathyroid hormone (PTH), 119
pH, 122
Phosphate ($HPO_4^=$), 119
Potassium adaptation, 115
Principal cell, 114
Pure sodium deficit, 113
Renin, 109
Respiratory acidosis, 128
Respiratory alkalosis, 130
Sodium, 108
Starling hypothesis, 106
Total body water (TBW), 105
Vitamin D, 119
Volatile, 122

REFERENCES

1. Day RE, et al: Human aquaporins: regulators of transcellular water flow. *Biochim Biophys Acta* 1840(5):1492–1506, 2014.
2. Hespe GE, et al: Pathophysiology of lymphedema-Is there a chance for medication treatment? *J Surg Oncol* 115(1):96–98, 2017.
3. Song W, Wang H, Wu Q: Atrial natriuretic peptide in cardiovascular biology and disease (NPPA). *Gene* 569(1):1–6, 2015.
4. Cheuvront SN, et al: Physiologic basis for understanding quantitative dehydration assessment. *Am J Clin Nutr* 97(3):455–462, 2013.
5. Liamis G, Filippatos TD, Elisaf MS: Evaluation and treatment of hypernatremia: a practical guide for physicians. *Postgrad Med* 128(3):299–306, 2016.
6. Sterns RH, Silver SM: Complications and management of hyponatremia. *Curr Opin Nephrol Hypertens* 25(2):114–119, 2016.
7. Buffington MA, Abreo K: Hyponatremia: a review. *J Intensive Care Med* 31(4):223–236, 2016.
8. Espay AJ: Neurologic complications of electrolyte disturbances and acid-base balance. *Handb Clin Neurol* 119:365–382, 2014.
9. Filippatos TD, Liamis G, Elisaf MS: Ten pitfalls in the proper management of patients with hyponatremia. *Postgrad Med* 128(5):516–522, 2016.
10. Youn JH: Gut sensing of potassium intake and its role in potassium homeostasis. *Semin Nephrol* 33(3):248–256, 2013.

11. Lee Hamm L, Hering-Smith KS, Nakhoul NL: Acid-base and potassium homeostasis. *Semin Nephrol* 33(3):257–264, 2013.
12. Medford-Davis L, Rafique Z: Derangements of potassium. *Emerg Med Clin North Am* 32(2):329–347, 2014.
13. Theisen-Toupal J: Hypokalemia and hyperkalemia. *Hosp Med Clin* 4(1):34–50, 2015.
14. Viera AJ, Wouk N: Potassium disorders: hypokalemia and hyperkalemia. *Am Fam Physician* 92(6):487–495, 2015.
15. Sterns RH, Grieff M, Bernstein PL: Treatment of hyperkalemia: something old, something new. *Kidney Int* 89(3):546–554, 2016.
16. Fong J, Khan A: Hypocalcemia: updates in diagnosis and management for primary care. *Can Fam Physician* 58(2):158–162, 2012.
17. Žofková I: Hypercalcemia. Pathophysiological aspects. *Physiol Res* 65(1):1–10, 2016.
18. Thosani S, Hu MI: Denosumab: a new agent in the management of hypercalcemia of malignancy. *Future Oncol* 11(21):2865–2871, 2015.
19. Felsenfeld AJ, Levine BS: Approach to treatment of hypophosphatemia. *Am J Kidney Dis* 60(4):655–661, 2012.
20. Negri AL, Ureña Torres PA: Iron-based phosphate binders: do they offer advantages over currently available phosphate binders? *Clin Kidney J* 8(2):161–167, 2015.

21. de Baaij JH, Hoenderop JG, Bindels RJ: Magnesium in man: implications for health and disease. *Physiol Rev* 95(1):1–46, 2015.
22. Pham PC, et al: Hypomagnesemia: a clinical perspective. *Int J Nephrol Renovasc Dis* 7:219–230, 2014.
23. Chang WT, Radin B, McCurdy MT: Calcium, magnesium, and phosphate abnormalities in the emergency department. *Emerg Med Clin North Am* 32(2):349–366, 2014.
24. Gooch MD: Identifying acid-base and electrolyte imbalances. *Nurse Pract* 40(8):37–42, 2015.
25. Berend K, de Vries AP, Gans RO: Physiological approach to assessment of acid-base disturbances. *N Engl J Med* 372(2):195, 2015.
26. Kraut JA, Kurtz I: Treatment of acute non-anion gap metabolic acidosis. *Clin Kidney J* 8(1):93–99, 2015.
27. Soifer JT, Kim HT: Approach to metabolic alkalosis. *Emerg Med Clin North Am* 32(2):453–463, 2014.
28. Bruno CM, Valenti M: Acid-base disorders in patients with chronic obstructive pulmonary disease: a pathophysiological review. *J Biomed Biotechnol* 2012:915150, 2012.
29. Adrogué HJ: Mixed acid-base disturbances. *J Nephrol* 19(Suppl 9):S97–S103, 2006.
30. Dzierba AL, Abraham P: A practical approach to understanding acid-base abnormalities in critical illness. *J Pharm Pract* 24(1):17–26, 2011.

Genes and Genetic Diseases

Lynn B. Jorde

evolve WEBSITE

http://evolve.elsevier.com/McCance/
- Content Updates
- Chapter Summary Review
- Review Questions
- Case Studies
- Animations

CHAPTER OUTLINE

In the nineteenth century, microscopic studies of cells led scientists to suspect that the nucleus of the cell contained the important mechanisms of inheritance. Scientists found that chromatin, the substance that gives the nucleus a granular appearance, is observable in nondividing cells. Just before the cell divides, the chromatin condenses to form microscopically observable, threadlike structures called *chromosomes*. (Cell division and chromosomes are discussed in Chapter 1.) With the rediscovery of Gregor Mendel's important breeding experiments at the turn of the twentieth century, it soon became apparent that the chromosomes contained genes, the basic units of inheritance. Genes are composed of sequences of deoxyribonucleic acid (DNA), a primary constituent of chromosomes; the other primary constituent consists of proteins, such as histones, that cause the DNA to coil into a highly compressed structure (Fig. 1.2, Chapter 1). By serving as the blueprints of proteins

in the body, genes ultimately influence all aspects of body structure and function. Humans have approximately 20,000 to 25,000 genes. An error in one of these genes can lead to a recognizable genetic disease.

To date, more than 23,000 human genetic traits have been identified and cataloged.[1] About one-third of pediatric inpatients are children with genetic diseases.[2,3] In addition, many common diseases that affect primarily adults, such as hypertension, coronary heart disease, diabetes, and cancer, are now known to have important genetic components. (These diseases are also affected by environmental factors. The interaction between genetic and environmental components is discussed in Chapter 5.)

Great progress is being made in the diagnosis of genetic diseases and the understanding of genetic mechanisms underlying them. Genetic testing is used increasingly to guide drug choice and dosage, and gene therapy—the direct alteration of genes in cells—is now carried out effectively for some diseases. Genetics is now one of the most rapidly advancing fields of medicine (Boxes 4.1 and 4.2).

DNA, RNA, AND PROTEINS: HEREDITY AT THE MOLECULAR LEVEL
DNA
Composition and Structure

Genes are composed of DNA, and the most important constituent of DNA is four types of nitrogenous bases (Fig. 4.1). The four bases, adenine, cytosine, guanine, and thymine, are commonly represented by their first letters: A, C, G, and T, respectively.

In the early 1950s, James Watson and Francis Crick determined the physical structure of DNA. They proposed the now-famous **double-helix model**, in which DNA can be envisioned as a twisted ladder with chemical bonds as its rungs (see Fig. 4.1). Projecting from each side of the ladder, at regular intervals, are the nitrogenous bases. The base projecting from one side is bound to the base projecting from the other by a weak hydrogen bond. Therefore, the nitrogenous bases form the rungs of the ladder; adenine pairs with thymine, and guanine pairs with cytosine. Each DNA subunit—consisting of one deoxyribose molecule, one phosphate group, and one base (Fig. 4.2)—is called a **nucleotide**.

BOX 4.1   GENETIC TESTING

The genetic causes of several thousand different diseases have now been identified, and the pace of discovery is accelerating. Consequently, it is now possible to perform genetic tests to help determine whether an individual carries specific disease-causing mutations. Chromosome disorders, such as trisomy 21, are routinely detected using karyotypes or other, more automated approaches. Nearly 5000 diseases can now be diagnosed by testing for specific mutations (www.ncbi.nlm.nih.gov/sites/GeneTests/). In addition, genetic tests have been developed to help predict susceptibility for a number of common, genetically complex diseases. Genetic testing can be applied in a variety of contexts, including the following:

1. *Carrier screening.* Genetic tests can identify heterozygous carriers for many recessive diseases, such as cystic fibrosis, sickle cell disease, and Tay-Sachs disease. It is becoming increasingly common for couples to undergo carrier screening to help make reproductive decisions, especially in populations in which specific diseases are relatively common (e.g., Tay-Sachs disease in the Ashkenazi Jewish population, β-thalassemia in Mediterranean populations). As a result, the prevalence of some of these diseases has declined dramatically in the past two decades.
2. *Prenatal diagnosis.* Several forms of prenatal genetic diagnosis are available, including the following:
   a. *Amniocentesis.* This procedure, which is usually carried out at about 16 weeks' gestation, involves the withdrawal of a small amount of amniotic fluid from the uterus. This fluid contains fetal cells, which can be cultured and karyotyped to detect chromosome abnormalities. In addition, genetic testing for single-gene disorders can be undertaken using DNA from these cells. Neural tube defects (spina bifida and anencephaly) can be detected as an elevation of α-fetoprotein level in amniotic fluid. The risk of fetal loss as a result of this procedure is now estimated to be about 1/500 higher than the background loss rate.
   b. *Chorionic villus sampling (CVS).* Carried out at 10 to 12 weeks' gestation, CVS is performed by extracting a small amount of villous tissue directly from the chorion. This procedure does not require in vitro culturing of cells for chromosome analysis because sufficient numbers of dividing cells are directly available in the extracted tissue. Chorionic villus sampling involves a slightly higher fetal loss rate (approximately 1%) than that of amniocentesis.
   c. *Preimplantation genetic diagnosis (PGD).* This relatively new procedure is carried out on early embryos (typically 8 to 12 cells) created by in vitro fertilization. One or two cells are removed from the embryo (which causes no damage), and these cells can be tested for chromosome abnormalities or single-gene disorders. If a genetic disorder is found in the cell, the embryo is not implanted in the mother's uterus and another embryo is chosen.
   d. *Analysis of fetal DNA in maternal circulation.* By approximately 6 to 8 weeks' gestation, fetal cells, as well as cell-free fetal DNA, can be found in the mother's bloodstream and can be tested for disease-causing mutations. This approach is developing rapidly and has the advantages of early diagnosis and minimal risk to the mother and fetus. Recently, whole-genome fetal DNA sequences have been obtained from a small sample of maternal blood. In addition to these diagnostic procedures, prenatal screening is now routinely carried out by measuring various analytes in maternal serum samples to assess the risk of conditions, such as trisomies 21, 13, and 18, and neural tube defects. Newborn screening also is commonly performed for a variety of genetic conditions such as PKU and galactosemia. A positive screening result is an indication for a subsequent diagnostic test (e.g., amniocentesis for a positive prenatal screening result or DNA sequencing for a positive newborn screening result).
3. *Presymptomatic diagnosis.* Many hereditary diseases, such as familial breast or colon cancer, can be tested genetically before an individual develops the disease. For some of these conditions, measures can be taken either to diagnose the disease early (e.g., colonoscopy or mammography) or to minimize the risk of developing the disease.
4. *Testing for drug efficacy or sensitivity.* A number of genes are now known to be associated with sensitivity to specific therapeutic drugs, and people are sometimes tested for variants in these genes to help guide drug treatment. For example, abacavir, an antiviral drug used in treating human immunodeficiency virus (HIV) infection, can cause severe adverse reactions in those who have a specific HLA-B variant (HLA-B*57:01, seen in about 7% of persons of European ancestry). The Food and Drug Administrtion now recommends testing for this variant before administering abacavir. For other drugs, such as warfarin, genetic testing for variants in specific genes (*CYP2C9* and *VKORC1*) may help to guide drug dosage.

Although genetic testing can be very informative, it also has limitations. Genetic testing usually reveals the presence or absence of a disease-causing mutation, but many genetic diseases have incomplete penetrance. For example, a woman who carries a mutation in the *BRCA1* or *BRCA2* genes has a lifetime breast cancer risk of approximately 70% to 80% (but not 100%). In addition, the absence of a disease-causing mutation does not guarantee that the disease in question will not occur (e.g., a woman who does not have a *BRCA1* or *BRCA2* mutation still has nearly the same risk of developing breast cancer as do other women because these genes account for only a few percent of all cases of breast cancer). Individuals and families should be advised of these and other limitations of genetic testing.

Data from Katsanis SH, Katsanis N: *Nat Rev Genet* 14:415–426, 2013.

BOX 4.2   GENE THERAPY

Gene therapy, in which the harmful effects of a disease-causing mutation are corrected by altering the person's DNA, has been a long-sought goal in human genetics. Hundreds of individuals are currently enrolled in dozens of clinical trials of gene therapy. Many technical challenges have arisen, but gene therapy is now beginning to yield positive therapeutic results.

In somatic cell gene therapy, the DNA of a specific set of an individual's somatic cells is altered. (It is also possible to perform germline therapy, which affects all cells, including reproductive cells; however, for technical and ethical reasons, this is not being pursued in humans.) Most commonly, somatic cell therapy is used for conditions in which a mutation has caused the absence of a gene product in a cell (e.g., adenosine deaminase in T cells, which leads to immunodeficiency). A "vector" is used to carry a normal copy of the mutated gene into the individual's cells. These vectors are usually viruses, such as retroviruses, lentiviruses, or adenoviruses, which have been genetically modified so that they contain the normal human gene and cannot make copies of themselves (otherwise they could cause a viral infection). Once inside the individual's cells, the normal human gene begins to encode the missing gene product.

This approach faces a number of technical hurdles, including immune responses against the vector and difficulties in producing sufficient quantities of the desired gene product. In one case, an immune response against an adenoviral vector proved fatal. Another challenge is that commonly used retroviral vectors integrate randomly into the genome. In several people with severe combined immunodeficiency, a modified retrovirus was inserted near an oncogene, activating it and causing leukemia. This issue has been addressed by designing alternative vectors and by implementing new developments in targeted genome modification using the CRISPR/Cas genome editing system.

Gene therapy has now been successful in treating a number of inherited conditions, including two forms of severe combined immunodeficiency (SCID), Wiskott-Aldrich syndrome, Leber congenital amaurosis, β-thalassemia, hemophilia B, and X-linked adrenoleukodystrophy. In some cases, symptoms have been completely reversed through gene therapy. When hematopoietic stem cells are altered, the beneficial effects of gene therapy can be permanent. In addition to the treatment of hereditary diseases, gene therapy is being used to alter cells of the immune system to combat specific tumor cells, improving the treatment of various types of cancer. It is hoped that further research will lead to safe, efficient, and cost-effective treatment of many human diseases through gene therapy.

Data from Naldini L: *Nature* 526:351–360, 2015.

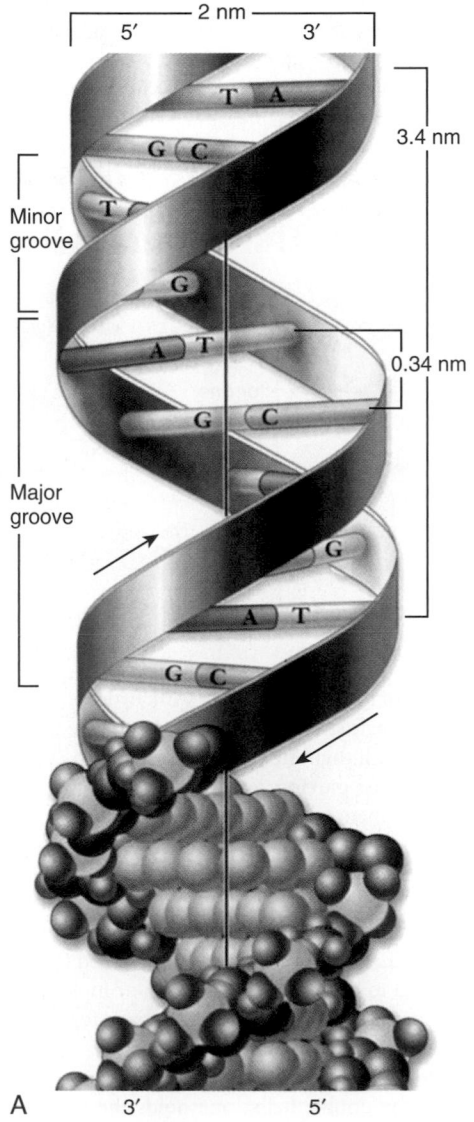

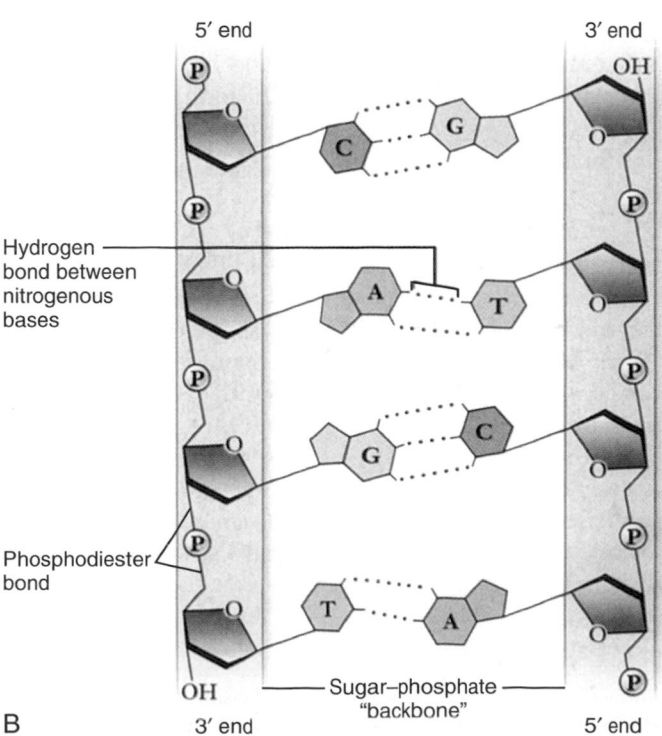

FIGURE 4.1 Structure of DNA. **A,** Double helix. Shown with the phosphodiester backbone as a ribbon on top and a space-filling model on the bottom. The bases protrude into the interior of the helix where they hold it together by base pairing. The backbone forms two grooves, the larger major groove and the smaller minor groove. **B,** Base pairing holds strands together. The hydrogen (H)-bonds that form between A and T and between G and C are shown with dashed lines. These produce AT and GC base pairs that hold the two strands together. This always pairs a purine with a pyrimidine, keeping the diameter of the double helix constant. *A,* Adenine; *C,* cytosine; *G,* guanine; *T,* thymine. (From Raven PH et al: *Biology,* ed 8, New York, 2008, McGraw-Hill.)

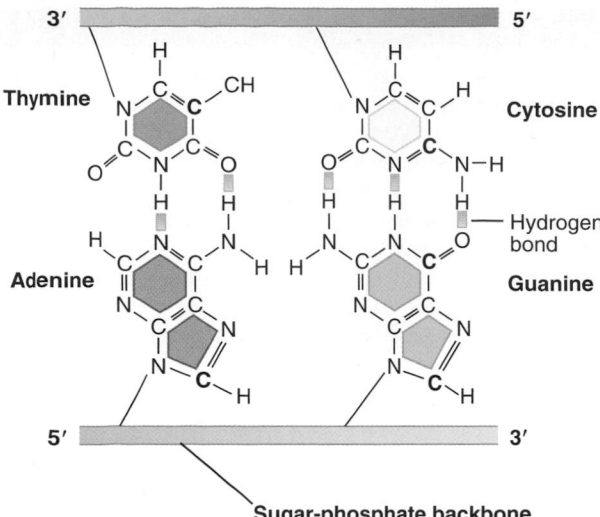

FIGURE 4.2 Chemical Structure of Nucleotides. Chemical structure of the four bases, which shows hydrogen bonds between base pairs. Three hydrogen bonds are formed between cytosine–guanine pairs, and two bonds are formed between adenine–thymine pairs. (From Jorde LB et al: *Medical genetics,* ed 5, Philadelphia, 2016, Elsevier.)

DNA as the Genetic Code

To serve as the basis of genetic inheritance, DNA must be able to provide a code for all the body's proteins. **Proteins** are composed of one or more **polypeptides** (intermediate protein compounds), which are in turn composed of sequences of **amino acids** (organic acids containing NH_2). The body contains 20 different types of amino acids, and the amino acid sequences that make up polypeptides must in some way be specified by the DNA molecule.

Because there are 20 possible amino acids and only 4 bases, each single nucleotide cannot specify an amino acid. Similarly, the amino acids cannot be specified by couplets of bases (e.g., adenine-guanine, thymine-guanine, guanine-cytosine) because there are only 4×4, or 16, possible couplets. If series of 3 bases are translated into amino acids, however, there are $4 \times 4 \times 4$, or 64, possible combinations—more than enough to specify each different amino acid. By manufacturing synthetic nucleotide sequences and allowing them to direct the formation of amino acids in the laboratory, it was proved that amino acids were specified by these triplets of bases, or **codons**.

Of the 64 possible codons, 3 signal the end of a gene and are known as **stop**, or **nonsense**, **codons**. The remaining 61 all specify amino acids, which means that most amino acids can be specified by more than 1 codon. The genetic code is thus said to be redundant, although each codon can specify only one amino acid.

Another significant feature of the genetic code is that it is nearly universal: with the exception of ciliated protozoa and some plants, all organisms use precisely the same DNA codes to specify proteins. Within cells, a general exception to this rule occurs in mitochondria—cytoplasmic organelles that are the sites of cellular respiration (see Chapter 1). The mitochondria have their own extranuclear DNA. Several codons of **mitochondrial DNA (mtDNA)** encode different amino acids than do the same nuclear DNA codons.

Replication

In addition to having the ability to specify amino acid sequences, DNA must be able to replicate itself accurately during cell division so that the genetic code can be preserved in subsequent cell generations. DNA

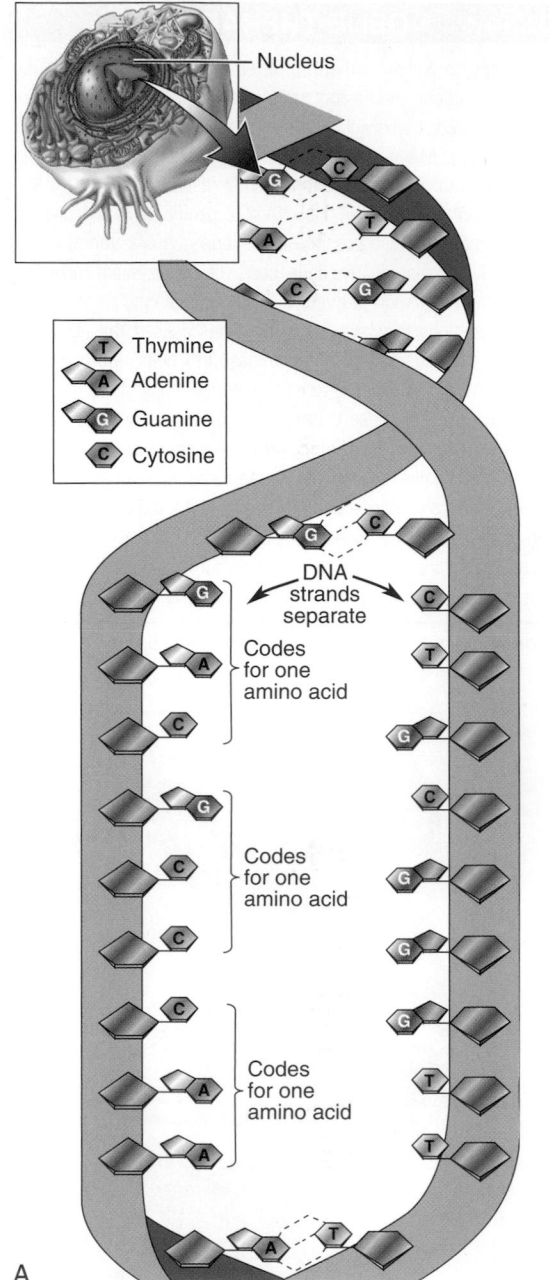

A

FIGURE 4.3 Replication and Action of DNA. **A,** Replication of DNA.

replication consists of the breaking of the weak hydrogen bonds between the bases, leaving a single strand with each base unpaired. The consistent pairing of adenine with thymine and of guanine with cytosine, known as **complementary base pairing**, is the key to accurate replication. The principle of complementary base pairing dictates that the unpaired base will attract a free nucleotide only if the nucleotide has the proper complementary base. Thus a portion of a single strand with a sequence of bases labeled ATTGCT will bond with a series of free nucleotides with the bases TAACGA. When replication is complete, a new double-stranded molecule identical to the original is formed (Fig. 4.3, *A*). The single strand is said to be a **template (guide)**, or molecule on which a complementary molecule is built, and is the basis for synthesizing the new double strand.

Several different proteins are involved in DNA replication. One protein unwinds the double helix, one holds the strands apart, and

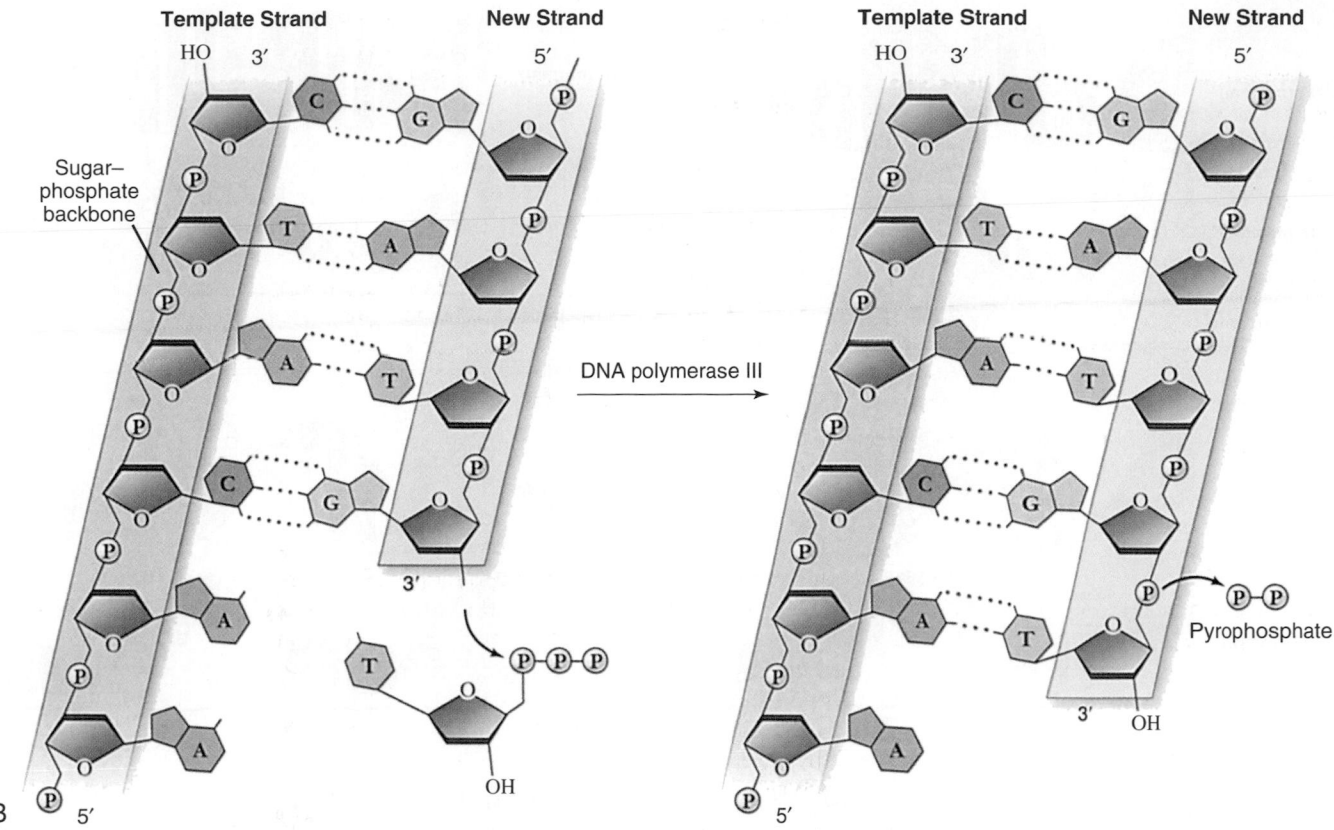

FIGURE 4.3, cont'd B, Action of DNA polymerase. DNA polymerases add nucleotides to the 3′ end of a growing chain. The nucleotide added depends on the base that is in the template strand. Each new base must be complementary to the base in the template strand. With the addition of each new nucleotide, triphosphate, two of its phosphates are cleaved off as pyrophosphate. *A,* Adenine; *T,* thymine; *G,* guanine; *C,* cytosine. (**A** from Herlihy B: *The human body in health and illness,* ed 5, St Louis, 2015, Saunders; **B** adapted from Raven PH et al: *Biology,* ed 8, New York, 2008, McGraw-Hill.)

others perform different distinct functions. The most important of these proteins is the enzyme known as **DNA polymerase**. This enzyme travels along the single DNA strand, adding the correct nucleotides to the free end of the new strand (see Fig. 4.3, *B*). Besides adding the new nucleotides, the DNA polymerase performs a proofreading procedure. After the new nucleotide has been added to the chain, the DNA polymerase checks to make sure that its base is actually complementary to the template base. If it is not, the incorrect nucleotide is excised and replaced with a correct one. This procedure, one of the mechanisms of DNA repair, substantially enhances the accuracy of DNA replication.

Mutation

A **mutation** is any inherited alteration of genetic material. Microscopically observable alterations of chromosome number or structure are examples of mutations. Some mutations are much too small to be observed under a microscope. An example is the **base pair substitution**, in which one base pair is replaced by another. Because of the redundancy of the genetic code, a base pair substitution sometimes has no consequence (i.e., it does not alter the amino acid sequence). When the substitution alters a single amino acid, it is termed a **missense mutation** (Fig. 4.4, *A*). When the substitution produces any of the three stop or nonsense codons, it is termed a **nonsense mutation** (Fig. 4.4, *B*). Missense and nonsense mutations can have profound consequences, and they cause many of the serious genetic diseases discussed later.

A second major type of mutation is the **frameshift mutation**. This alteration involves the insertion or deletion of one or more base pairs

to the DNA molecule. As Fig. 4.5 shows, these mutations can change the entire "reading frame" of the DNA sequence because codons consist of groups of three base pairs. A frameshift mutation thus can greatly alter the resulting amino acid sequence and typically results in a premature stop codon.

A large number of agents, known collectively as **mutagens**, can increase the frequency of mutations. Radiation, such as that produced by x-rays and nuclear fallout, is an important mutagen and is known to cause cell damage (see Chapters 12 and 13). Radiation can fragment the DNA molecule and it can cause chemical reactions that can alter a DNA base. A variety of chemicals also can induce mutations, often because they are chemically similar to DNA bases. Other chemicals mimic the effects of ionizing radiation, and still others interfere with the process of base pairing. Hundreds of chemicals (some of which are human-generated and some of which occur naturally) are now known to be mutagenic in humans or laboratory animals, such as nitrogen mustard, vinyl chloride, alkylating agents, formaldehyde, and sodium nitrite. Some of these chemicals, however, are much more potent mutagens than others. Nitrogen mustard, for example, is extremely mutagenic, whereas sodium nitrate is a weak mutagen.

Measurement of the mutation rate in humans is difficult, in part because mutations are very rare events. Current estimates are that the **mutation rate** in humans is about 10^{-4} to 10^{-7} per gene per generation. This rate appears to vary from one gene to another, with greater mutation rates for larger genes. At the nucleotide level, the human mutation rate is approximately 10^{-8} per nucleotide per generation. Certain DNA

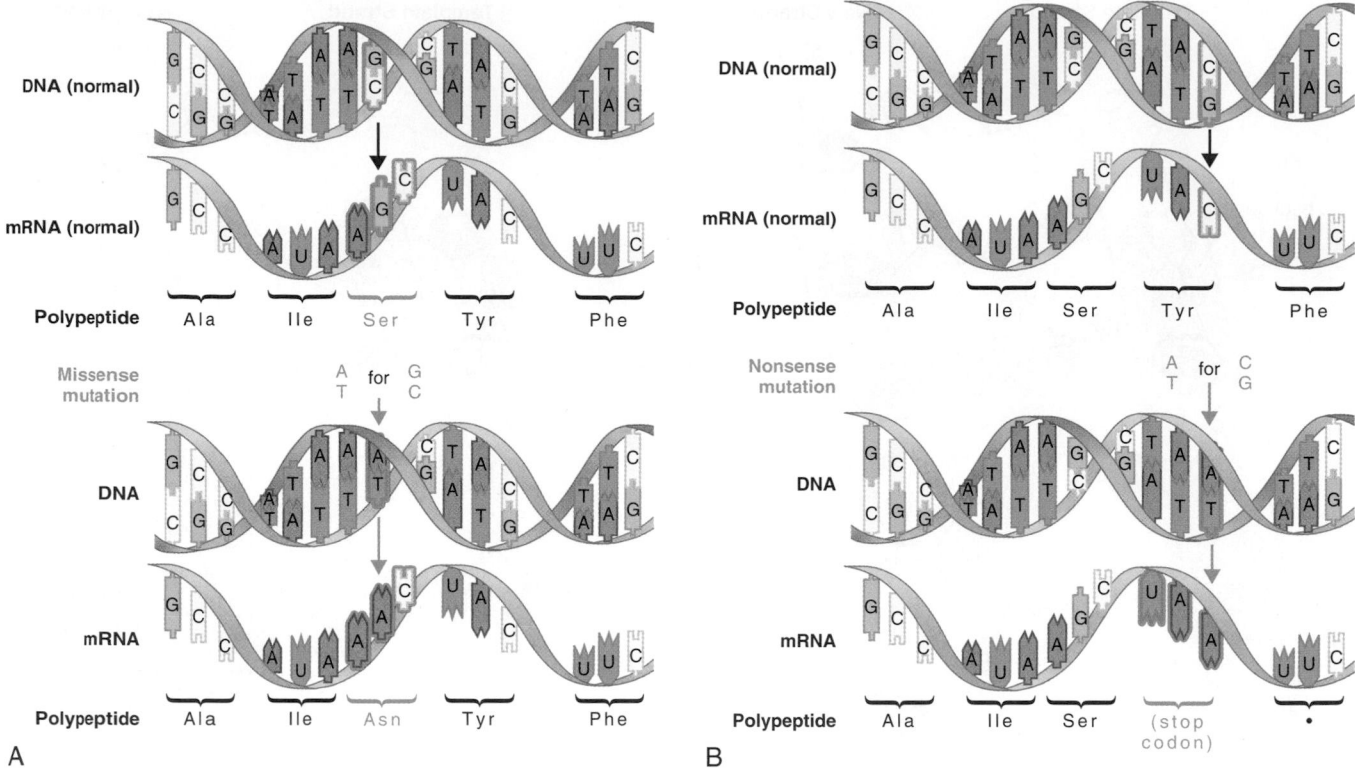

FIGURE 4.4 Base Pair Substitution. Missense mutations **(A)** produce a single amino acid change, whereas nonsense mutations **(B)** produce a stop codon in the mRNA. Stop codons terminate translation of the polypeptide. (From Jorde LB et al: *Medical genetics,* ed 5, Philadelphia, 2016, Elsevier.)

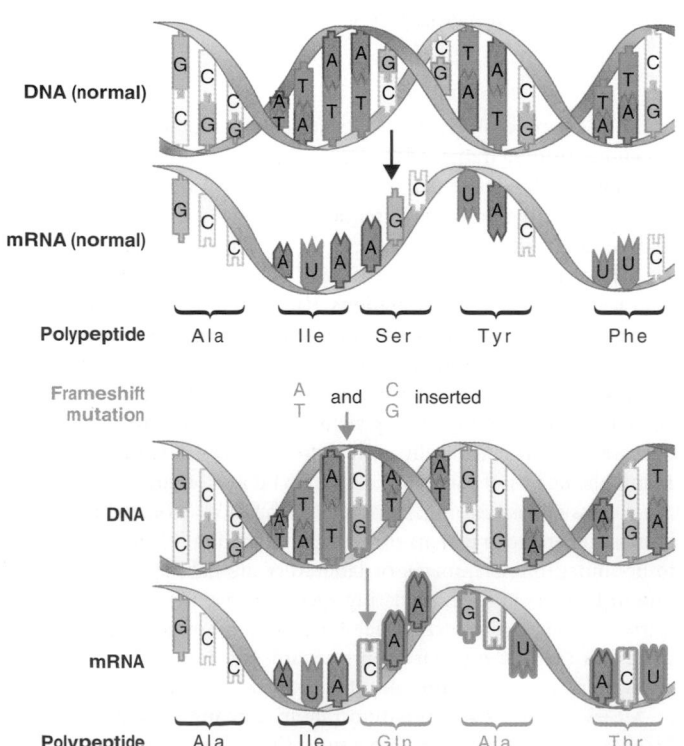

FIGURE 4.5 Frameshift Mutations. Frameshift mutations result from the addition or deletion of a number of bases that is not a multiple of 3. This mutation alters all of the codons downstream from the site of insertion or deletion. (From Jorde LB et al: *Medical genetics,* ed 5, Philadelphia, 2016, Elsevier.)

sequences have particularly high mutation rates and are known as **mutational hot spots.** In particular, sequences consisting of a cytosine base followed by a guanine base *(CG)* are highly susceptible to mutation and are known to account for a disproportionately large percentage of disease-causing mutations.[4]

From Genes to Proteins

Whereas DNA is formed and replicated in the cell nucleus, protein synthesis takes place in the cytoplasm. The transport of the DNA code from nucleus to cytoplasm and the subsequent protein formation involve two basic processes: transcription and translation. Both of these processes are mediated by **ribonucleic acid (RNA),** a type of nucleic acid that is chemically very similar to DNA. RNA differs from DNA in that uracil rather than thymine is one of the four nitrogenous bases. The other bases of RNA, as in DNA, are adenine, cytosine, and guanine. Uracil is structurally very similar to thymine, so it also can pair with adenine. Whereas DNA usually occurs as a double strand, RNA usually occurs as a single strand.

Transcription

Transcription is the process by which RNA is synthesized from a DNA template. The result is the formation of **messenger RNA (mRNA)** from the base sequence specified by the DNA molecule. Transcription of a gene begins when an enzyme called **RNA polymerase** binds to a **promoter site** on the DNA. A promoter site is a sequence of DNA that specifies the beginning of a gene. In addition to RNA polymerase, proteins called **transcription factors** bind to DNA sequences called **transcription factor binding sites** near genes to regulate the timing of transcription, as well as the specific tissues in which genes are actively transcribed (e.g., clotting

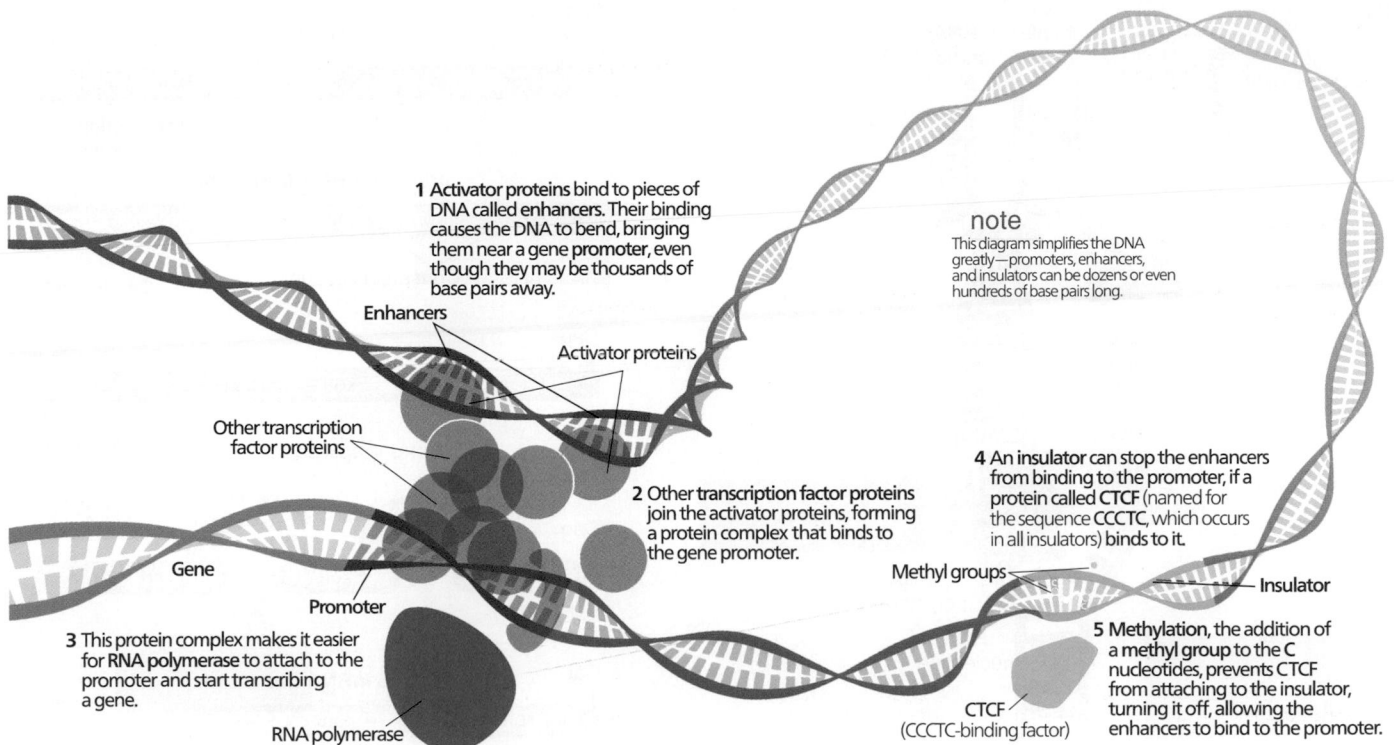

1 Activator proteins bind to pieces of DNA called **enhancers**. Their binding causes the DNA to bend, bringing them near a gene **promoter**, even though they may be thousands of base pairs away.

Enhancers

Activator proteins

note
This diagram simplifies the DNA greatly—promoters, enhancers, and insulators can be dozens or even hundreds of base pairs long.

Other transcription factor proteins

2 Other transcription factor proteins join the activator proteins, forming a protein complex that binds to the gene promoter.

4 An insulator can stop the enhancers from binding to the promoter, if a protein called **CTCF** (named for the sequence **CCCTC**, which occurs in all insulators) binds to it.

Gene

Methyl groups

Insulator

Promoter

3 This protein complex makes it easier for RNA polymerase to attach to the promoter and start transcribing a gene.

RNA polymerase

CTCF (CCCTC-binding factor)

5 Methylation, the addition of a methyl group to the C nucleotides, prevents CTCF from attaching to the insulator, turning it off, allowing the enhancers to bind to the promoter.

FIGURE 4.6 Transcription Factors and Simplified Schematic of Gene Expression. Transcription factors are proteins and bind to specific sites on DNA. They read and interpret the genetic blueprint of the DNA, thereby controlling transcription or the flow of genetic information from DNA to mRNA. Transcription factors are essential for gene expression (e.g., proteins that function as receptors, enzymes, or biomarkers). Not only do transcription factors act downstream from biological stimuli but they can be downstream of signaling cascades promoted by various environmental stimuli (hormones, temperature). Transcription factors can alter gene expression to promote pathophysiology. (From Song K: Transcription Factors. *Wikimedia Commons*. Dec 20, 2012. https://commons.wikimedia.org/wiki/File:Transcription_Factors.svg.)

factor VIII primarily in hepatocytes) (Fig. 4.6). Transcription factors can either activate or repress the expression of genes. In addition, transcription is sometimes up-regulated by the binding of nearby DNA sequences called **enhancers**. The RNA polymerase pulls a portion of the DNA strands apart from one another, allowing unattached DNA bases to be exposed. One of the DNA strands then provides the template for the sequence of mRNA nucleotides.

The sequence of bases in the mRNA is thus complementary to that of the template strand, and with the exception of the presence of uracil instead of thymine, the mRNA sequence is identical to that of the other DNA strand. Transcription continues until a DNA sequence called a **termination sequence** is reached. Then the RNA polymerase detaches from the DNA, and the transcribed mRNA is freed to move out of the nucleus and into the cytoplasm. Fig. 4.7 summarizes the process of transcription.

RNA Splicing

After the mRNA first has been transcribed from the DNA template, it reflects exactly the base sequence of the DNA. In eukaryotes an important step takes place before this RNA leaves the nucleus. Many of the RNA sequences are removed, and the remaining sequences are spliced together to form the functional mRNA that will migrate to the cytoplasm (Fig. 4.8). The excised sequences are called **introns**, and the sequences that are left to code for proteins are called **exons**. The functions of most introns remain poorly understood.

Translation

Translation is the process by which RNA directs the synthesis of a polypeptide (Fig. 4.9). However, mRNA cannot code directly for amino acids. Instead, it interacts with **transfer RNA (tRNA)**, a cloverleaf-shaped strand of about 80 nucleotides. The tRNA molecule has a site for the attachment of an amino acid. At the opposite side of the cloverleaf is a sequence of three nucleotides called the **anticodon**. The anticodon undergoes complementary base pairing with an appropriate codon in the mRNA. The mRNA thus specifies the sequence of amino acids by acting through the tRNA. As each codon is processed, an amino acid is translated by the interaction of mRNA and tRNA, which is aided by cytoplasmic structures called **ribosomes**. Bonds are formed between adjacent amino acids to make a growing polypeptide. When the ribosome arrives at a termination signal on the mRNA sequence, translation and polypeptide formation cease. The mRNA, ribosome, and polypeptide separate from one another, and the polypeptide is released into the cytoplasm to perform its required function.

Noncoding RNA. The progression from DNA to RNA to proteins, as described here, is a core concept in genetics and molecular biology. However, several forms of RNA are never translated into amino acid sequences but have key functions. **MicroRNAs (miRNAs)** are small RNA sequences, 17 to 27 nucleotides in length, that bind to specific mRNA sequences and down-regulate their expression. More than 1000 miRNAs have been identified, and some of them play important roles

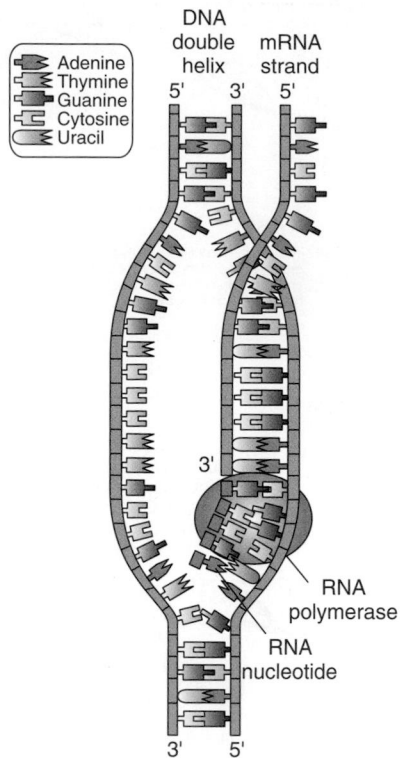

FIGURE 4.7 General Scheme of RNA Transcription. In transcription of messenger RNA *(mRNA),* a DNA molecule "unzips" in the region of the gene to be transcribed. RNA nucleotides already present in the nucleus temporarily attach themselves to exposed DNA bases along one strand of the unzipped DNA molecule according to the principle of complementary pairing. As the RNA nucleotides attach to the exposed DNA, they bind to each other and form a chainlike RNA strand called a *messenger RNA (mRNA)* molecule. Notice that the new mRNA strand is an exact copy of the base sequence on the opposite side of the DNA molecule. As in all metabolic processes, the formation of mRNA is controlled by an enzyme—in this case, the enzyme is called *RNA polymerase.* (From Ignatavicius DD, Workman LD: *Medical-surgical nursing,* ed 6, St Louis, 2010, Saunders.)

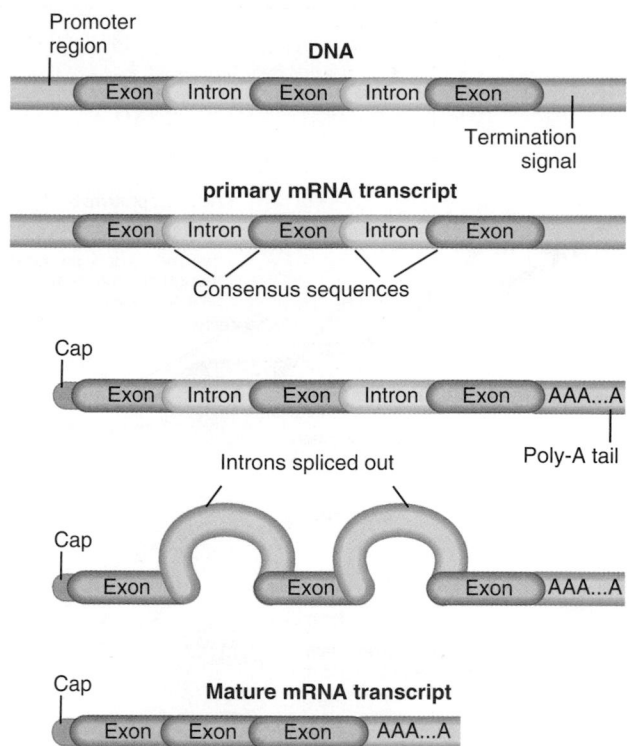

FIGURE 4.8 RNA Splicing. Gene splicing. Introns are precisely removed from the primary mRNA transcript to produce a mature mRNA transcript. Consensus sequences mark the sites at which splicing occurs. (From Jorde LB et al: *Medical genetics,* ed 5, Philadelphia, 2016, Elsevier.)

in regulating genes involved in cancer. Each miRNA can bind to multiple mRNA targets and therefore can regulate many different genes. In contrast, small interfering RNAs (siRNAs), another type of short RNA sequence, have single, specific binding targets and are used in cancer therapy and some forms of gene therapy (see Box 4.2). Another non-translated RNA, classified as having a length greater than 200 nucleotides, is termed long noncoding RNA (lncRNA). The genome contains at least 10,000 lncRNAs and, like miRNA and siRNA, some lncRNAs are involved in gene regulation.

CHROMOSOMES

Human cells can be categorized into two types: germline cells (sperm and egg cells, or gametes, and their precursor cells) and somatic cells (which include all other cells). Mutations in germline cells can be transmitted to the next generation, whereas mutations in somatic cells are not. Each somatic cell has 46 chromosomes in its nucleus. These are diploid cells, meaning that the chromosomes occur in pairs. Thus each cell contains 23 pairs of chromosomes. One member of each pair comes from an individual's mother, and one comes from the father. New somatic cells are formed through mitosis and cytokinesis, through which the cell nucleus and cytoplasm are replicated. (The division process that creates new

copies of somatic cells is described in Chapter 1.) Gametes are haploid cells: they have only 1 member of each chromosome pair, giving them a total of 23 chromosomes. The process by which these haploid cells are formed from diploid cells is called meiosis (Fig. 4.10).

In 22 of the 23 chromosome pairs, the 2 members of each pair are virtually identical in microscopic appearance and DNA sequence and are thus said to be homologous to each other. These 22 chromosome pairs are homologous in both males and females and are termed autosomes. The remaining pair of chromosomes, the sex chromosomes, consists of two homologous X chromosomes in females and a nonhomologous pair, X and Y, in males.

Fig. 4.11, *A,* illustrates a metaphase spread, which is a photograph of the chromosomes as they appear in the nucleus of a somatic cell during metaphase. (Chromosomes are easiest to visualize during this stage of mitosis.) A karyogram (also termed a karyotype) is an ordered display of chromosomes. In Fig. 4.11, *B,* the chromosomes are arranged according to size, with the homologous chromosomes paired. The 22 autosomes are numbered according to length, with chromosome 1 as the longest and chromosome 22 as the shortest. Some natural variation in relative chromosome length can be expected from person to person, however, so it is not always possible to distinguish each chromosome by its length. Therefore, the position of the centromere is also used to classify the chromosomes (Fig. 4.12).

The chromosomes in Fig. 4.11, *A,* were stained with a substance that binds preferentially to certain areas of chromosomes. The resulting distinctive chromosome bands are evident in various patterns in the different chromosomes so that each chromosome can be distinguished easily. One of the most commonly used stains is Giemsa stain. By using banding techniques, chromosomes can be unambiguously numbered,

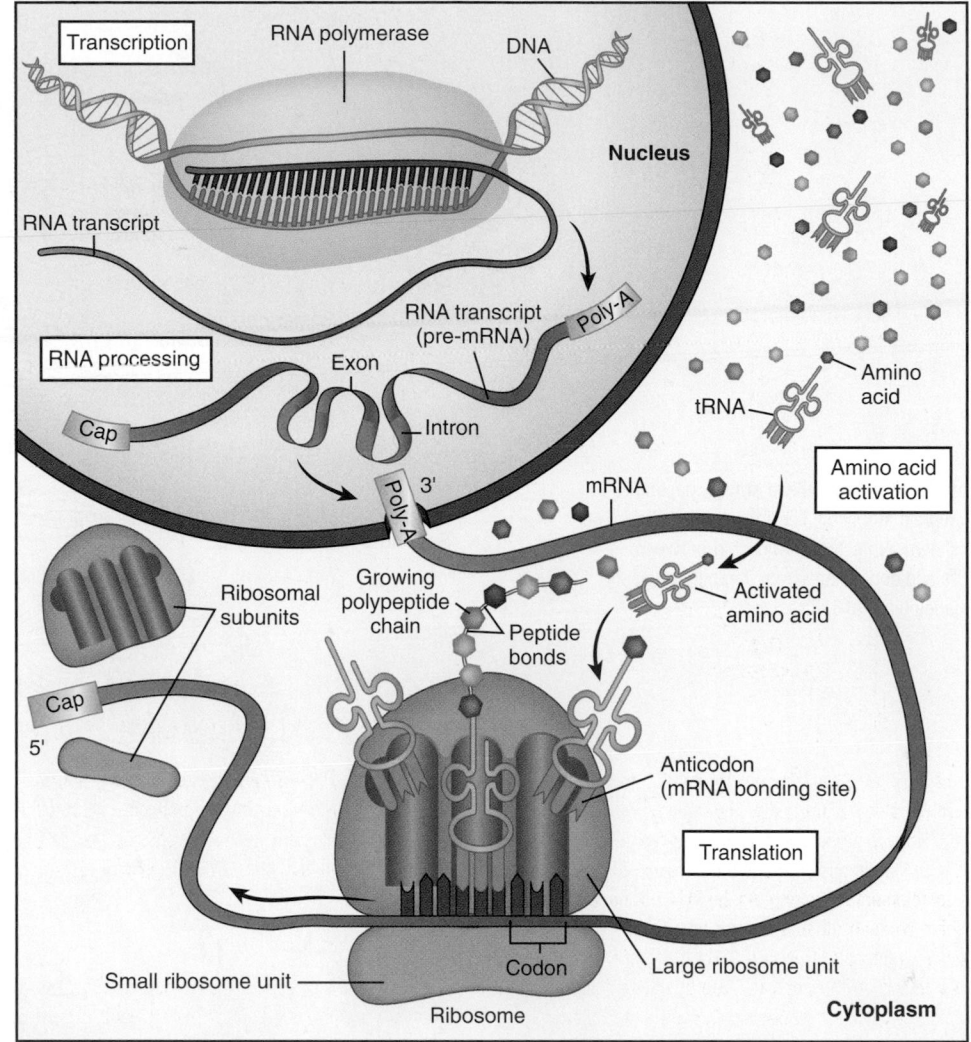

FIGURE 4.9 Protein Synthesis. The site of transcription is the nucleus, and the site of translation is the cytoplasm. See the text for details.

and individual variation in chromosome composition can be studied. Missing or duplicated portions of chromosomes, which often result in serious diseases, also can be readily identified.

Chromosome Aberrations and Associated Diseases

Chromosome abnormalities are the leading known cause of intellectual disability and spontaneous pregnancy loss. A major chromosome aberration occurs in more than half of conceptions. Most of these fetuses do not survive to term; in fact, about 50% of all recovered first-trimester spontaneous abortuses have major chromosomal aberrations.[5] About 1 in 150 live births has a major diagnosable chromosome abnormality.[6]

Polyploidy

Cells that have a multiple of the normal number of chromosomes are said to be **euploid cells** (Greek *eu,* "good" or "true"; *ploid,* "number"). Because normal gametes are haploid and most normal somatic cells are diploid, they are both euploid forms. When a euploid cell has more than the diploid number of chromosomes, it is said to be a **polyploid cell.** Several types of body tissues, including some liver, bronchial, and epithelial tissues, are normally polyploid. A zygote having three copies of each chromosome, rather than the usual two, has a form of polyploidy

called **triploidy.** **Tetraploidy,** a condition in which euploid cells have 92 chromosomes, also has been observed. Nearly all triploid and tetraploid conceptions are spontaneously aborted or stillborn, and the small proportion that survive to term die shortly after birth. Triploidy and tetraploidy are relatively common conditions at conception, accounting for approximately 10% of all known miscarriages.[5]

Aneuploidy

Aneuploid cells are defined as those that do not contain a multiple of 23 chromosomes. An aneuploid cell containing three copies of one chromosome is said to be trisomic (a condition termed **trisomy**). **Monosomy,** the presence of only one copy of a given chromosome in a diploid cell, is the other common form of aneuploidy. Among the autosomes, monosomy of any chromosome is lethal, but newborns with trisomy of chromosomes 13, 18, or 21 can survive. This difference illustrates an important principle: loss of chromosome material has more serious consequences than duplication of chromosome material.

Aneuploidy of the sex chromosomes is usually less serious than that of the autosomes. For the Y chromosome, this is true because very little genetic material is located on this chromosome. For the X chromosome, inactivation of extra chromosomes largely diminishes their effect. A zygote bearing *no* X chromosome, however, will not survive.

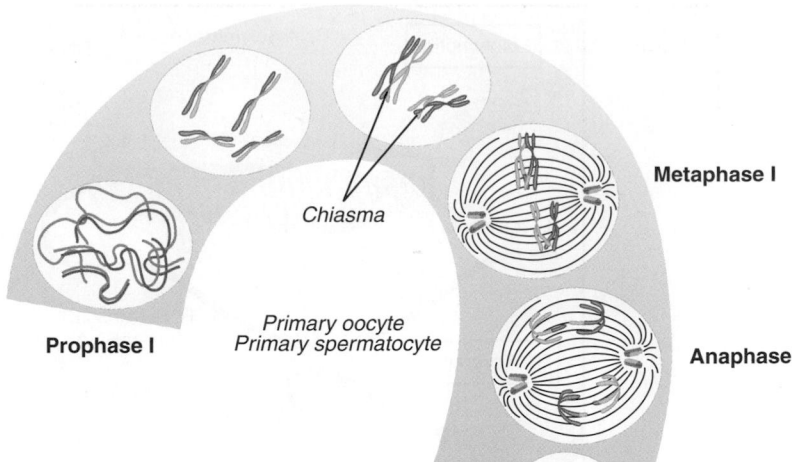

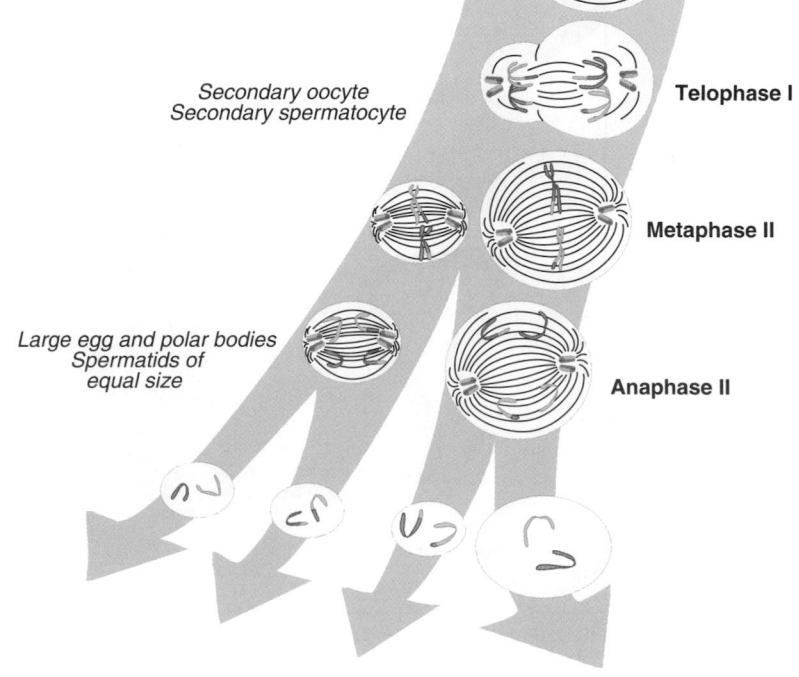

FIGURE 4.10 Stages of Meiosis. From these stages, haploid gametes are formed from a diploid stem cell. For brevity, prophase II and telophase II are not shown. Note the relationship between meiosis and spermatogenesis and oogenesis. (From Jorde LB et al: *Medical genetics,* ed 5, Philadelphia, 2016, Elsevier.)

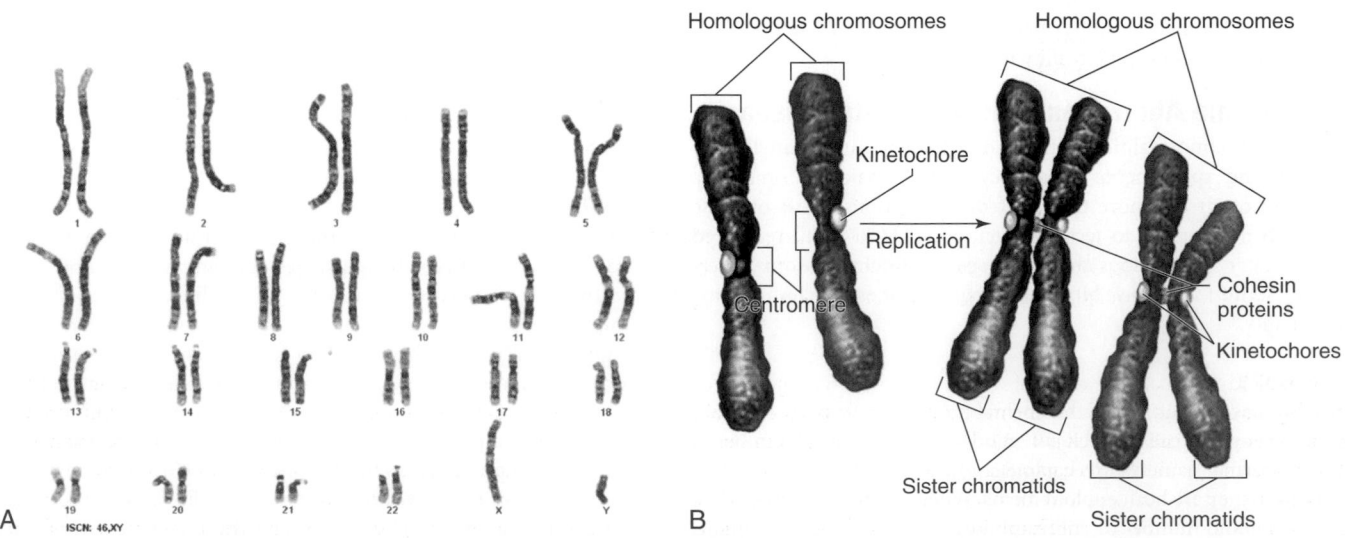

FIGURE 4.11 Karyogram of Chromosomes. **A,** Metaphase Spread; human karyogram. **B,** Homologous chromosomes and sister chromatids. (**A** courtesy the Clinical Cytogenetics Section, Laboratory of Pathology, National Cancer Institute, National Institutes of Health, Bethesda, MD. **B** from Raven PH et al: *Biology,* ed 8, New York, 2008, McGraw-Hill.)

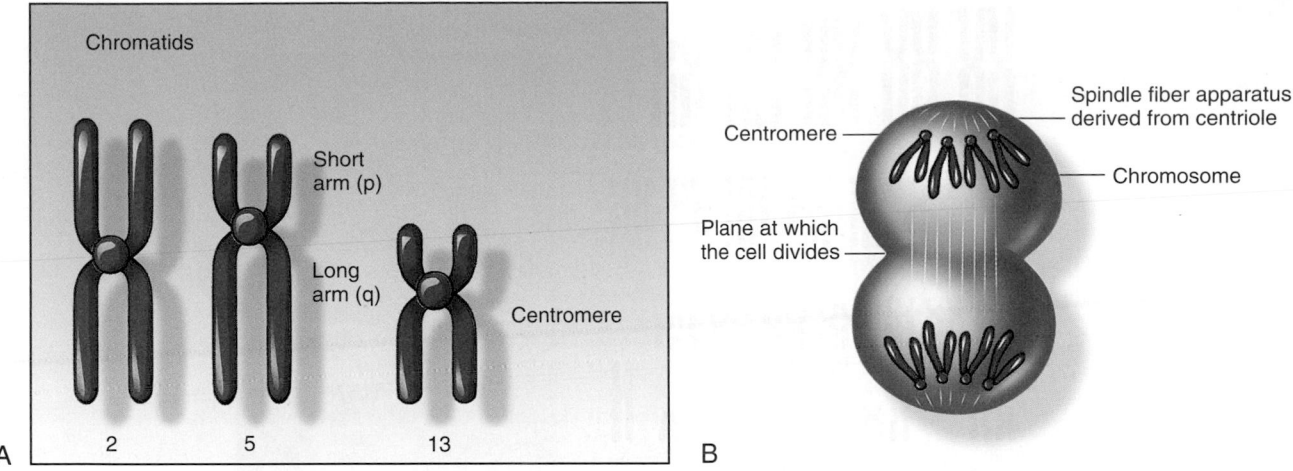

FIGURE 4.12 Structure of Chromosomes. **A,** Human chromosomes 2, 5, and 13. Each is replicated and consists of two chromatids. Chromosome 2 is a metacentric chromosome because the centromere is close to the middle; chromosome 5 is submetacentric because the centromere is set off from the middle; chromosome 13 is acrocentric because the centromere is at or very near the end. **B,** During mitosis, the centromere divides and chromosomes move to opposite poles of the cell. At the time of centromere division, the chromatids are designated chromosomes.

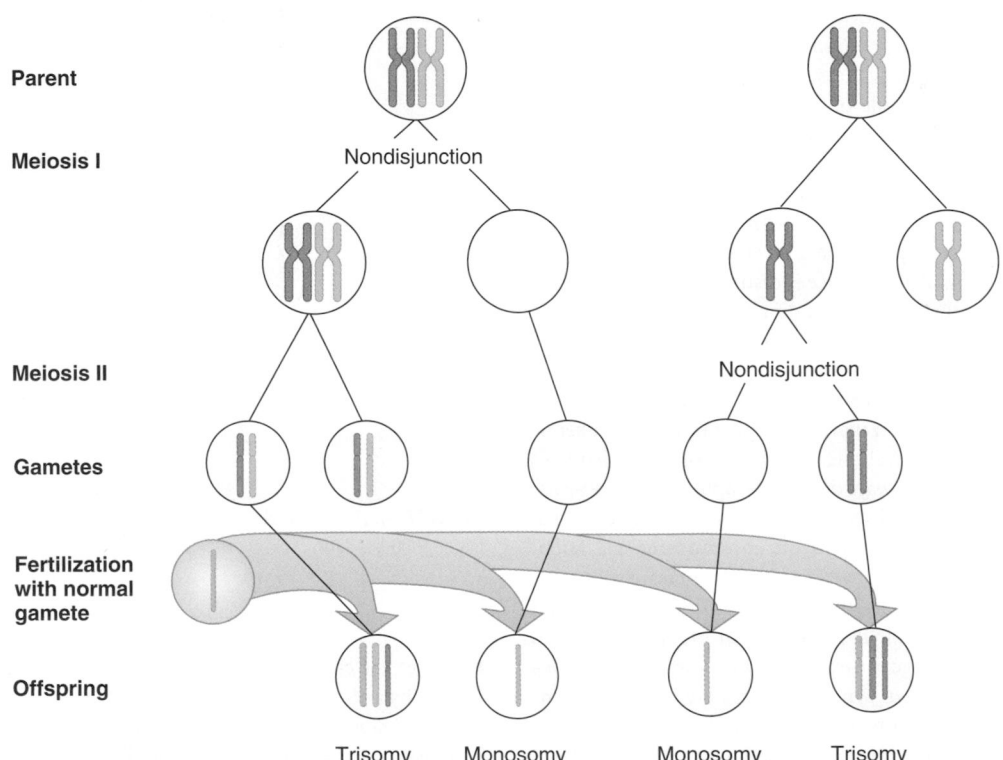

FIGURE 4.13 Nondisjunction Causes Aneuploidy When Chromosomes or Sister Chromatids Fail to Divide Properly. (From Jorde LB et al: *Medical genetics,* ed 5, Philadelphia, 2016, Elsevier.)

Aneuploidy is usually the result of **nondisjunction,** an error in which homologous chromosomes or sister chromatids fail to separate normally during meiosis or mitosis (Fig. 4.13). Nondisjunction during either stage of meiosis produces some gametes that have two copies of a given chromosome and others that have no copies of the chromosome. When such gametes unite with normal haploid gametes, the resulting zygote is monosomic or trisomic for that chromosome.

Autosomal Aneuploidy. Trisomy can occur for any chromosome at conception, but the only forms seen with an appreciable frequency in live births are trisomies of the thirteenth, eighteenth, or twenty-first chromosome. Fetuses with most other chromosomal trisomies do not survive to term. Trisomy 16, for example, is the most commonly known trisomy among abortuses, but it is not seen in live births.[5]

Partial trisomy, in which only an extra portion of a chromosome is present in each cell, also can occur. The consequences of partial trisomies are not as severe as those of complete trisomies. Trisomies also may occur in only some cells of the body. Individuals thus affected are said to be **chromosomal mosaics,** meaning that the body has two

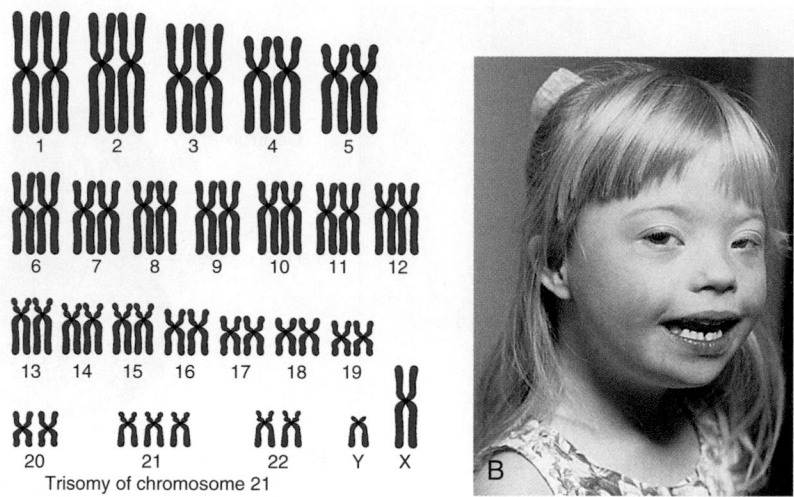

FIGURE 4.14 Down Syndrome. **A,** The karyotype of Down syndrome consists of 47 chromosomes and shows trisomy 21. **B,** A child with Down syndrome. (**A** from Damjanov I: *Pathology for the health professions*, ed 4, Philadelphia, 2012, Saunders; **B** courtesy Olney A, MacDonald M, University of Nebraska Medical Center, Omaha, NE.)

or more different cell lines, each of which has a different karyotype. Mosaics are usually formed by early mitotic nondisjunction occurring in one embryonic cell but not in others.

The most well-known example of aneuploidy in an autosome is trisomy of the twenty-first chromosome, which causes Down syndrome (named after J. Langdon Down, who first described the disease in 1866). Down syndrome was formerly called *mongolism*, but this inappropriate term is no longer used. Down syndrome is seen in 1 in 800 live births.[5] Individuals with this disease typically have intelligence quotients (IQs) between 25 and 70. The facial appearance is distinctive (Fig. 4.14), with a low nasal bridge, epicanthal folds, protruding tongue, and flat, low-set ears. Poor muscle tone (hypotonia) and short stature are both characteristic. Congenital heart defects affect about one-third to one-half of live-born children with Down syndrome; a reduced ability to fight respiratory tract infections and an increased susceptibility to leukemia also contribute to reduced survival rate. By 40 years of age, individuals with Down syndrome virtually always develop symptoms that are nearly identical to those of Alzheimer disease because one of the genes that can cause Alzheimer disease is located on chromosome 21. About three-fourths of fetuses known to have Down syndrome are spontaneously aborted or stillborn. About 10% to 20% of infants born with Down syndrome die during their first 10 years of life. For those who survive beyond 10 years, average life expectancy is now about 60 years.

Approximately 97% of Down syndrome cases are caused by nondisjunction during the formation of one of the parent's gametes or during early embryonic development. The remaining 3% result from translocations (discussed later). In 90% to 95% of cases, the nondisjunction occurs in the formation of the mother's egg cell. Paternal nondisjunction is responsible for the remaining cases. Among individuals with Down syndrome, about 1% to 3% are known to be mosaics. Because mosaics have a large number of normal cells, the effects of the trisomic cells are attenuated and symptoms are sometimes less severe.

The risk of having a child with Down syndrome increases greatly with maternal age. As Fig. 4.15 demonstrates, women younger than 30 years have a risk ranging from about 1 in 1000 births to 1 in 2000 births. The risk begins to rise substantially after 35 years of age, and it reaches 3% to 5% for women older than 45 years of age. This dramatic increase in risk is a consequence of the age of maternal egg cells, which are held in an arrested state of prophase I from the time they are formed

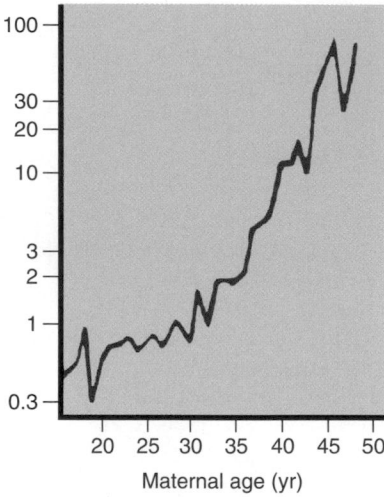

FIGURE 4.15 Down Syndrome Risk Increases With Maternal Age. Rate is per 1000 live births related to maternal age.

in the female embryo until they are shed in ovulation. Thus an egg cell formed by a 45-year-old woman is itself 45 years old. This long suspended state may allow for the accumulation of errors leading to nondisjunction. The risk of Down syndrome, as well as that of other trisomies, does not appear to increase with paternal age.[7]

Sex Chromosome Aneuploidy. Among live births, about 1 in 400 males and 1 in 650 females have a form of sex chromosome aneuploidy.[8] Because these conditions are generally less severe than autosomal aneuploidies, all forms except complete absence of an X chromosome allow at least some individuals to survive.

One of the most common sex chromosome aneuploidies, affecting about 1 in 1000 newborn females, is trisomy X. Instead of two X chromosomes, these females have three X chromosomes in each cell. Most of them have no overt physical abnormalities, although sterility, menstrual irregularity, or cognitive deficits are sometimes seen. A very small proportion of females have four or even five X chromosomes, and their mental function is more severely compromised. Another sex

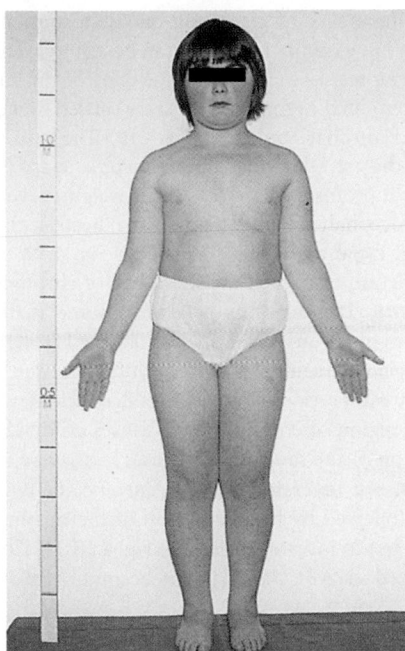

FIGURE 4.16 Turner Syndrome. A sex chromosome is missing, and the person's chromosomes are 45,X. Characteristic signs are short stature, female genitalia abnormality, webbed neck, shieldlike chest with underdeveloped breasts and widely spaced nipples, and imperfectly developed ovaries. (From Patton KT, Thibodeau GA: *Anatomy & physiology*, ed 8, St Louis, 2013, Mosby.)

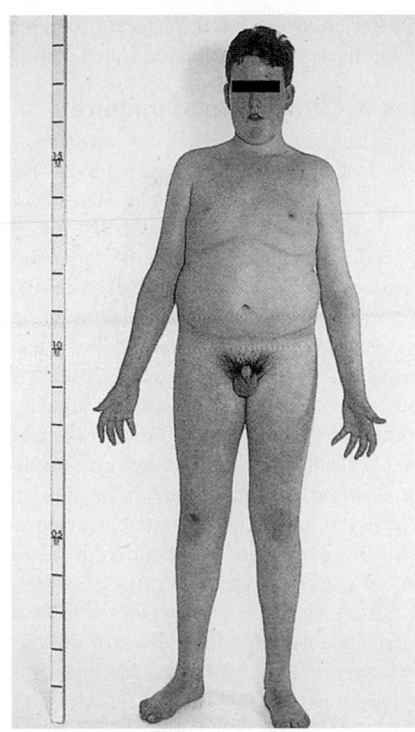

FIGURE 4.17 Klinefelter Syndrome. This young man exhibits many characteristics of Klinefelter syndrome: small testes, some development of the breasts, sparse body hair, and long limbs. This syndrome results from the presence of two or more X chromosomes with one Y chromosome (genotypes XXY or XXXY, for example). (Courtesy Nancy S. Wexler, PhD, Columbia University. Picked up from Patton KT, Thibodeau GA: *Anatomy & physiology*, ed 9, St Louis, 2016, Mosby.)

chromosome aneuploidy is the presence of a single X chromosome and no homologous X or Y chromosome, resulting in a total of 45 chromosomes. The karyotype is designated 45,X, and it causes a set of symptoms known as Turner syndrome (Fig. 4.16). Because they have no Y chromosome, persons with Turner syndrome are always female. They are usually sterile, however, and have gonadal streaks rather than ovaries. These streaks of connective tissue are susceptible to cancer in mosaic fetuses who have some cells containing a Y chromosome. Other features of the disorder include short stature, webbing of the neck in about half of cases, widely spaced nipples, coarctation (narrowing) of the aorta (in 15% to 20% of cases), edema of the feet in newborns, and sparse body hair. Their IQs are typically in the normal range, although they often have some impairment of spatial and mathematical reasoning ability. About three-fourths of recognized 45,X conceptions inherit their X chromosome from the mother. Thus most cases are caused by a loss of the paternally transmitted X chromosome.

The frequency of Turner syndrome is low compared with that of other sex chromosome aneuploidies: only about 1 in 2500 newborn females is affected.[9] The 45,X karyotype is more common among conceptions, however, and about 15% to 20% of spontaneous abortions with chromosome abnormalities have this karyotype, making it one of the most common single-chromosome aberrations. Thus the condition is highly lethal during gestation: less than 1% of 45,X conceptions survive to term. Most fetuses that survive to term are mosaics, with combinations of 45,X cells and XX, XXX, or XY cells. It is likely that the presence of some normal cells in mosaic fetuses enhances fetal survival.

Teenagers with Turner syndrome are typically treated with estrogen to promote the development of secondary sexual characteristics. The dose is then continued at a reduced level to maintain these characteristics and to help avoid osteoporosis. Human growth hormone is sometimes administered to increase stature.

Individuals with at least two X chromosomes and a Y chromosome in each cell (47,XXY karyotype) have a disorder known as Klinefelter syndrome (Fig. 4.17). Because of the presence of a Y chromosome, these individuals have a male appearance, but they are usually sterile, and about half develop female-like breasts (a condition called *gynecomastia*). The testes are small, body hair is sparse, the voice is often somewhat high pitched, stature is elevated, and a moderate degree of mental impairment may be present. Klinefelter syndrome is found in about 1 in 1000 male births. About two-thirds of the cases are caused by nondisjunction of the X chromosomes in the mother, and the frequency of the disorder rises with maternal age. Individuals with the 48,XXXY and 49,XXXXY karyotypes also are considered to have Klinefelter syndrome, and the degree of physical and mental impairment increases with each additional X chromosome. Regardless of the number of X chromosomes, however, these individuals have a male appearance. The presence of a single Y chromosome, which causes the undifferentiated gonads to become testes, always produces a male. Mosaicism is sometimes seen in Klinefelter syndrome and results in less severe disease; the most prevalent combination is XXY and XY cells.

About 1 in 1000 males has an extra Y chromosome, producing the 47,XYY karyotype. Individuals with this karyotype tend to be taller than average, and they have a 10- to 15-point reduction in average IQ. This condition, which causes few serious physical problems, achieved notoriety when it was found that its incidence was significantly elevated in prison populations. This discovery led to the suggestion that this chromosome might predispose affected individuals to violent, criminal behavior. Several dozen studies have addressed this issue, and they have shown that 47,XYY males are not inclined to commit violent crimes.

However, even after adjusting for the effects of decreased IQ, some evidence exists for an increased incidence of behavioral disorders.

Abnormalities of Chromosome Structure

In addition to the loss or gain of whole chromosomes, parts of chromosomes can be lost or duplicated as gametes are formed, and the arrangement of genes on chromosomes can be altered. Unlike aneuploidy and polyploidy, these changes sometimes do not have serious consequences for an individual's health. Some of them can even remain entirely unnoticed, especially when very small pieces of chromosomes are involved. Nevertheless, abnormalities of chromosome structure also can produce serious disease in individuals or their offspring.

During meiosis and mitosis, chromosomes usually maintain their structural integrity very well, but chromosome breakage occasionally does occur. Mechanisms exist to "heal" these breaks, and generally the break is repaired perfectly with no damage resulting to the daughter cell. Sometimes, however, the breaks remain, or they heal in a fashion that alters the structure of the chromosome. Chromosome breakage occurs spontaneously, but it also can be caused by ionizing radiation, some viral infections, and certain chemicals.

Deletions. Broken chromosomes and loss of DNA cause deletions (Fig. 4.18, *A*). Usually a gamete with a deletion unites with a normal gamete to form a zygote. The zygote thus has one chromosome with the normal complement of genes and one with some missing genes. Because a fairly large number of genes can be lost in a deletion, serious consequences can result even though one copy of the chromosome is normal. An often-cited example of a disease caused by a chromosomal deletion is the cri du chat syndrome (Fig. 4.19). The term, which literally means "cry of the cat," describes the characteristic cry of the affected child. Other symptoms include low birth weight, severe intellectual disability, microcephaly (smaller than normal head size), heart defects, and the typical facial appearance shown in Fig. 4.19. The disease is caused by a deletion of part of the short arm of chromosome 5.

Duplications. Duplications of chromosome material are, like deletions, a form of chromosome aberration (see Fig. 4.18, *B*). Because a deficiency of genetic material is more harmful than an excess, duplications usually have less serious consequences than deletions. For example, a deletion of a region of chromosome 5 causes cri du chat syndrome, but a duplication of the same region causes less severe disease.

Inversions. An inversion is the occurrence of two breaks on a chromosome, followed by the reinsertion of the missing fragment at its original site but in inverted order (see Fig. 4.18, *C*). Thus a chromosome symbolized as ABCDEFG might become ABEDCFG after an inversion.

Unlike deletions and duplications, inversions result in no loss or gain of genetic material. They are thus said to be a "balanced" alteration of chromosome structure, and they often have no apparent physical effect. Genes are sometimes influenced by neighboring DNA sequences, however, and this position effect, a change in a gene's expression caused by its position, does sometimes result in disease in persons with inversions.

The serious problems caused by inversions usually occur in the offspring of individuals who carry the inversion. Because chromosomes must align in perfect order during prophase I, a chromosome with an inversion must form a loop to align with its normal homolog. Crossing

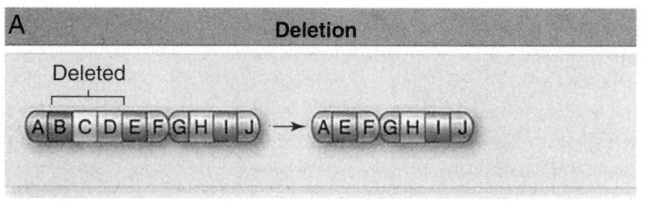

A   Deletion

Deleted

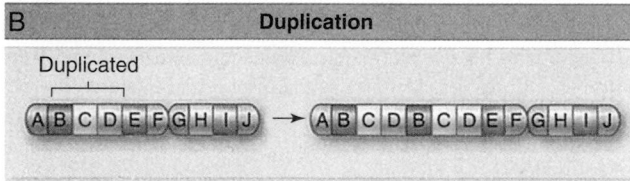

B   Duplication

Duplicated

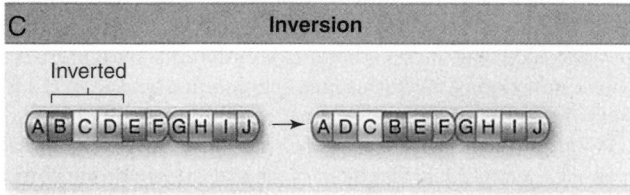

C   Inversion

Inverted

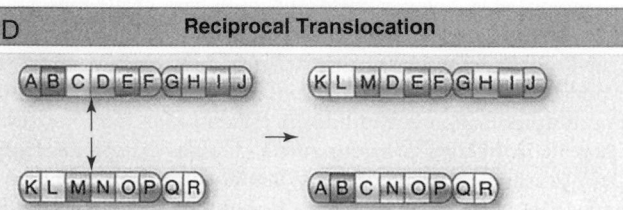

D   Reciprocal Translocation

FIGURE 4.18 Chromosome Structural Alterations. Larger-scale changes in chromosomes are also possible. Material can be deleted **(A)**, duplicated **(B)**, and inverted **(C)**. Translocations occur when one chromosome is broken and becomes part of another chromosome. This often occurs where both chromosomes are broken and exchange material, an event called a *reciprocal translocation* **(D)**. (From Raven PH et al: *Biology*, ed 8, New York, 2008, McGraw-Hill.)

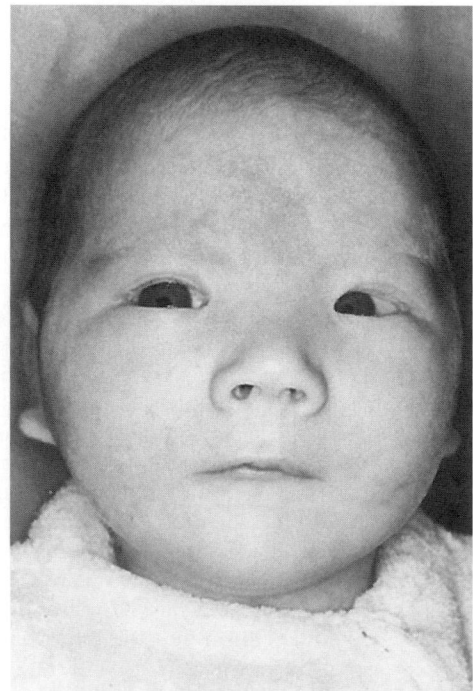

FIGURE 4.19 Infant With Cri Du Chat Syndrome. This syndrome is caused by deletion of part of the short arm of chromosome 5. (From Nussbaum RL, McInnes RR, Willard HF: *Thompson & Thompson genetics in medicine*, ed 7, Philadelphia, 2007, Saunders.)

over within this loop can result in duplications or deletions in the chromosomes of daughter cells. Thus the offspring of individuals who carry inversions often have chromosome deletions or duplications.

Translocations. The interchanging of genetic material between nonhomologous chromosomes is called translocation, and the most clinically significant type of translocation is termed a Robertsonian translocation. In this translocation the long arms of two nonhomologous chromosomes fuse at the centromere, forming a single chromosome (Fig. 4.20). Robertsonian translocations are confined to chromosomes 13, 14, 15, 21, and 22 because the short arms of these chromosomes are very small and contain no essential genetic material. When a Robertsonian translocation takes place, the short arms are usually lost during subsequent cell divisions. Because the carriers of Robertsonian translocations (about 1 in 500 individuals) lose no important genetic material, they are normal, although they have only 45 chromosomes in each cell. Their offspring, however, may have serious deletions or duplications (see Fig. 4.20). For example, a common Robertsonian translocation involves the fusion of the long arms of chromosomes 21 and 14. An offspring who inherits a gamete carrying the fused chromosome receives an extra copy of the long arm of chromosome 21 and thus develops Down syndrome. Robertsonian translocations are responsible for approximately 3% to 5% of Down syndrome cases. Parents who carry a Robertsonian translocation involving chromosome 21 have an increased risk for producing multiple offspring with Down syndrome.

A reciprocal translocation occurs when breaks take place in two different chromosomes and the material is exchanged (see Fig. 4.18, *D*). As with Robertsonian translocations, the carrier of a reciprocal translocation is usually normal because the individual has a normal complement of genetic material. However, the carrier's gametes can be normal, can carry the translocation, or can have duplications and deletions.

Fragile Sites. A number of areas on chromosomes develop microscopically observable breaks and gaps when the cells are cultured in a folate-deficient medium. Most of these fragile sites have no apparent relationship to disease. However, one fragile site, located on the long arm of the X chromosome, is associated with a disorder of considerable importance, both clinically and genetically. This disorder is known as *fragile X syndrome,* and it is associated with substantial cognitive impairment. With a relatively high population prevalence (affecting approximately 1 in 4000 males and 1 in 8000 females), fragile X syndrome is the second most common genetic cause of intellectual disability (after Down syndrome).[10]

Fragile X syndrome is usually caused by an elevated number (more than about 200) of repeated DNA sequences in the first exon of the fragile X gene. These "repeats" consist of CGG sequences that are duplicated many times. Most individuals have fewer than 50 of these repeats, but those who have 50 to 200 are more likely to produce affected offspring because DNA replication becomes unstable.[10] An increase in the number of these repeated sequences in successive generations can lead to expression of fragile X syndrome. More than 20 other genetic diseases also are caused by this mechanism.[11]

ELEMENTS OF FORMAL GENETICS

Many traits can be attributed primarily to single genes and are often called *mendelian traits* (after Gregor Mendel). Each gene occupies a position along a chromosome known as a locus. The genes at a particular locus can take different forms (i.e., they can be composed of different nucleotide sequences) called alleles. For example, most people have a type of hemoglobin known as *hemoglobin A.* A few individuals have an alternative form of hemoglobin, termed *hemoglobin S,* which differs from hemoglobin A by a single amino acid substitution in the β-globin

component of the hemoglobin molecule. The β-globin locus thus has two different alleles, one that encodes hemoglobin A and another that encodes hemoglobin S. A locus containing two or more alleles that each occur with an appreciable frequency in a population is said to be polymorphic or a polymorphism.

Because humans are diploid organisms, each chromosome is represented twice, with one member of the chromosome pair contributed by the father and one by the mother. At a given locus an individual has one allele whose origin is paternal and one whose origin is maternal. When the two alleles are identical, the individual is homozygous at that locus. When the alleles are not identical, the individual is heterozygous at the locus.

Phenotype and Genotype

The composition of genes at a given locus is known as the genotype. The outward appearance of an individual, which is the result of both genotype and environment, is the phenotype (see also Chapter 6, Epigenetics). For example, an infant who is born with an inability to metabolize the amino acid phenylalanine has the single-gene disorder known as *phenylketonuria (PKU)* and thus has the PKU genotype. If the condition is left untreated, abnormal metabolites of phenylalanine will begin to accumulate in the infant's brain and irreversible intellectual disability will occur. Intellectual disability is thus one aspect of the PKU phenotype. By imposing dietary restrictions to limit the intake of food containing phenylalanine, however, cognitive impairment can be prevented. Although the child still has the PKU genotype, a modification of the environment (in this case the child's diet) produces an outwardly normal phenotype.

Dominance and Recessiveness

In many loci the effects of one allele mask those of another when the two are found together in a heterozygote. The allele whose effects are observable is said to be dominant. The allele whose effects are hidden is said to be recessive (from the Latin root for "hiding"). Traditionally, for loci having two alleles, the dominant allele is denoted by an uppercase letter and the recessive allele is denoted by a lowercase letter. When one allele is dominant over another, the heterozygote genotype *Aa* has the same phenotype as the dominant homozygote *AA.* For the recessive allele to be expressed, it must exist in the homozygote form, *aa.*

When the heterozygote is distinguishable from both homozygotes, the locus is said to exhibit codominance. For example, in the MN blood group, both alleles, *M* and *N,* of the heterozygote are detectable and therefore codominant. Another example is the ABO blood group, in which heterozygotes having the *A* and *B* alleles express both of them as A and B antigens on their red cells (forming blood group AB).

A carrier is an individual who has a disease-causing allele but is phenotypically normal. Most recessive disease-causing alleles occur in heterozygotes who carry one copy of the allele but do not express the disease. Because many recessive alleles are lethal in the homozygous state, they are eliminated from the population when they occur in homozygotes. By "hiding" in carriers, however, most recessive alleles survive to be passed on to the next generation.

TRANSMISSION OF GENETIC DISEASES

An important aspect of a genetic disease is the pattern in which it is inherited through the generations of a family, or its mode of inheritance. Once the mode of inheritance is known, much can be learned about the disease-causing gene itself, and more reliable genetic counseling can be given to members of families in which the disease is present.

Modes of inheritance were systematically studied by Mendel, who formulated two basic laws of inheritance. His principle of segregation

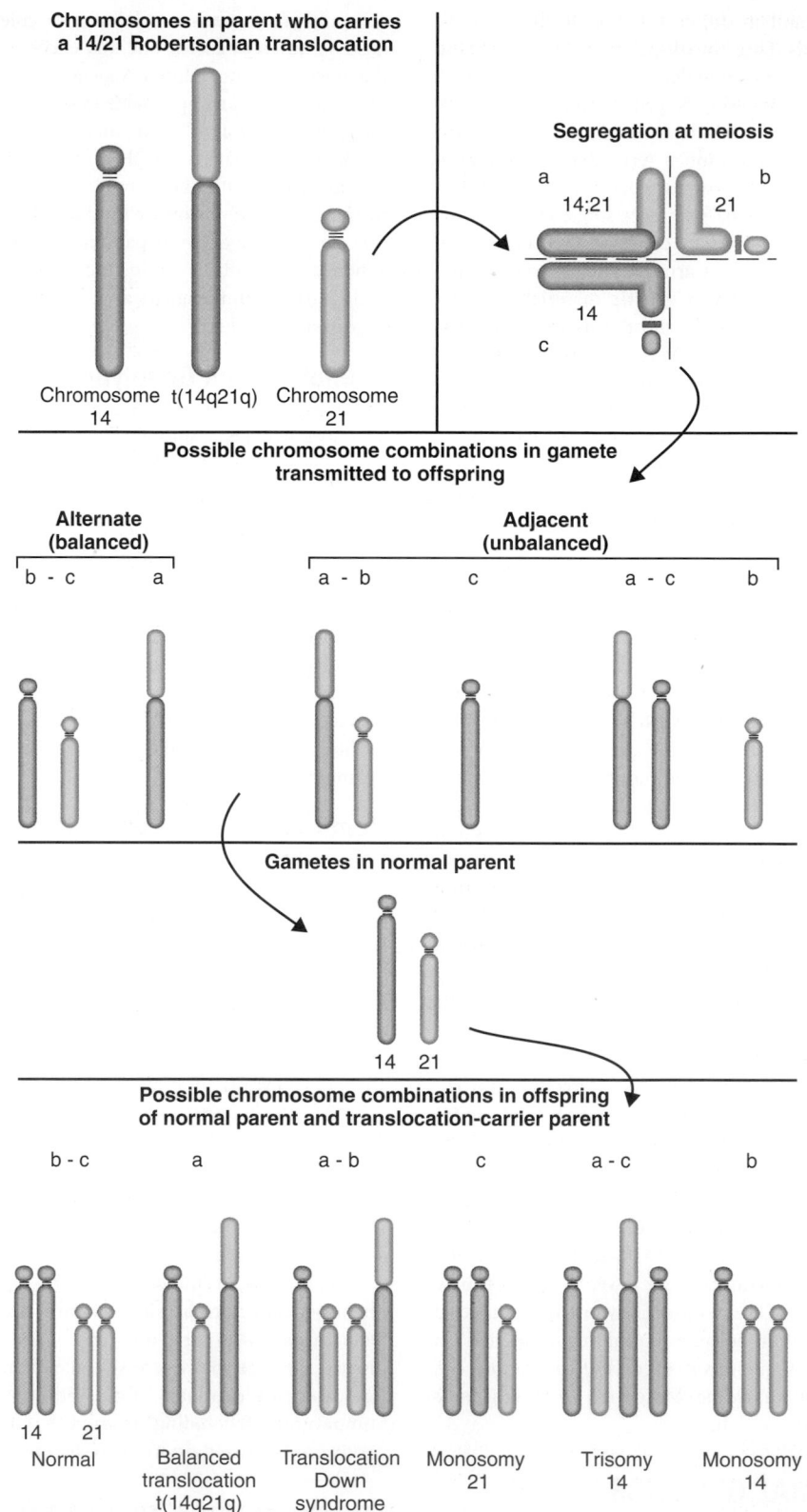

FIGURE 4.20 Possible Segregation Patterns for the Gametes Formed by a Carrier of a Robertsonian Translocation. Alternate segregation (quadrant a alone, or quadrant b with quadrant c) produces either a normal chromosome constitution or a translocation carrier with a normal phenotype. Adjacent segregation (quadrant a with b, quadrant c alone, quadrant a with c, or quadrant b alone) produces unbalanced gametes and results in conceptions with translocation Down syndrome, monosomy 21, trisomy 14, or monosomy 14, respectively. For example, monosomy 14 is produced when the parent who carries the translocation transmits a copy of chromosome 21 but does not transmit a copy of chromosome 14 (as in the lower right corner). (From Jorde LB et al: *Medical genetics,* ed 5, Philadelphia, 2016, Elsevier.)

states that homologous genes separate from one another during reproduction and that each reproductive cell carries only one of the homologous genes. Mendel's second law, the **principle of independent assortment**, states that the hereditary transmission of one gene has no effect on the transmission of another. Mendel discovered these laws in the mid-nineteenth century by performing breeding experiments with garden peas. He had no knowledge of chromosomes. Early in the twentieth century geneticists found that the behavior of chromosomes does essentially correspond to Mendel's laws, which now form the basis for the **chromosome theory of inheritance**.

The known single-gene diseases can be classified into four major modes of inheritance: autosomal dominant, autosomal recessive, X-linked dominant, and X-linked recessive. The first two types involve genes known to occur on the 22 pairs of autosomes. The last two types occur on the X chromosome; only a few disease-causing genes, primarily affecting male fertility, are found on the Y chromosome. The number of diseases assigned to each category is growing rapidly. Current catalogs of single-gene traits, which include disease-producing and nonclinical traits (e.g., attached earlobes), list nearly 22,000 known autosomal traits and nearly 1200 X-linked traits.[1]

An important tool in the analysis of modes of inheritance is the **pedigree** chart. It summarizes family relationships and shows which members of a family are affected by a genetic disease (Fig. 4.21). Generally, the pedigree begins with one individual in the family, the **proband**, also termed the **propositus** (male) or **proposita** (female). This individual is usually the first person in the family diagnosed or seen in a clinic.

Autosomal Dominant Inheritance
Characteristics of Pedigrees

Diseases caused by autosomal dominant genes are relatively rare. The most common occur in fewer than 1 in 500 individuals, so it is uncommon for 2 individuals both affected by the same autosomal dominant disease to produce offspring together. Fig. 4.22, *A*, illustrates this unusual pattern. More often, affected offspring are produced by the union of a normal parent with an affected heterozygous parent. The diagram (Punnett square) in Fig. 4.22, *B*, illustrates this mating. The affected parent can pass either a disease gene or a normal gene to the children. Each event has a probability of 0.5; thus, on average, half of the children will be heterozygous and will the disease, and half will be normal.

Fig. 4.23, *A*, is a typical pedigree showing the transmission of an autosomal dominant allele. The allele shown here causes achondroplasia (Fig. 4.23, *B*). Several important characteristics of this pedigree support the conclusion that the trait is caused by an autosomal dominant allele:
1. The two sexes exhibit the trait in approximately equal proportions, and males and females are equally likely to transmit the trait to their offspring.
2. There is no skipping of generations. If an individual has achondroplasia, one parent must also have it. If neither parent has the trait, none of the children has it (with the exception of new mutations, as discussed later).
3. Affected heterozygous individuals transmit the trait to approximately half of their children, but because gamete transmission is subject to chance fluctuations, it is possible that all or none of the children of an affected parent may have the trait. When large numbers of matings of this type are studied, however, the proportion of affected children will closely approach one-half.

Recurrence Risks

Parents at risk for producing children with a genetic disease nearly always ask the question, "What is the *chance* that the child will have this disease?" The probability that a family member will have a genetic

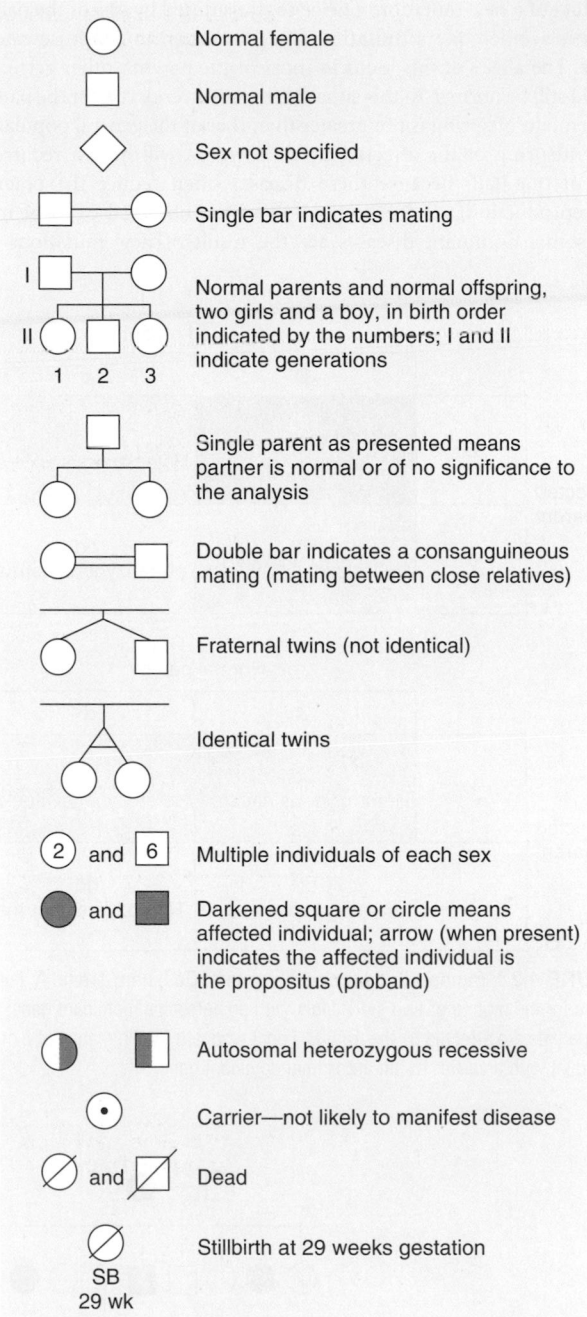

FIGURE 4.21 Symbols Commonly Used in Pedigrees.

disease is termed the **recurrence risk**. When one parent is affected by an autosomal dominant disease (and is a heterozygote) and the other is unaffected, the recurrence risks for each child are one-half.

An important principle is that each birth is an independent event, much like a coin toss. Thus, even though parents may already have had a child with the disease, their recurrence risk remains one-half. If they have had several children, all affected (or all unaffected) by the disease, the law of independence dictates that the probability that their next child will have the disease is still one-half. Parents' misunderstanding of this principle is a common problem encountered in genetic counseling.

If a child has been born with an autosomal dominant disease and there is no history of the disease in the family, the child is probably the product of a new mutation. The gene transmitted by one of the parents has thus undergone a mutation from a normal to a disease-causing allele. The alleles at this locus in most of the parent's other germ cells would still be normal. In this situation the recurrence risk for the parent's subsequent offspring is not greater than that of the general population. The offspring of the affected child, however, will have a recurrence risk of one-half. Because these diseases often reduce the potential for reproduction, a large proportion of the observed cases of many autosomal dominant diseases are the result of new mutations. For

example, approximately seven-eighths of all cases of achondroplasia are caused by new mutations.

Occasionally, two or more offspring will present symptoms of an autosomal dominant disease when there is no family history of the disease. Because mutation is a rare event, it is unlikely that this disease would be a result of multiple mutations in the same family. The mechanism most likely to be responsible is termed **germline mosaicism**. During the embryonic development of one of the parents, a mutation occurred that affected all or part of the germline but few or none of the somatic cells of the embryo. Thus the parent carries the mutation in the germline but does not actually express the disease. As a result, the unaffected parent can transmit the mutation to multiple offspring. This phenomenon, although relatively rare, can have significant effects on recurrence risks.[12]

Penetrance and Expressivity

An important variation seen in some genetic diseases is incomplete penetrance. The **penetrance** of a trait is the percentage of individuals with a specific genotype who also exhibit the expected phenotype. Incomplete penetrance means that individuals who have a disease-causing allele may not exhibit the disease phenotype at all, even though the allele and the associated disease may be transmitted to the next generation. A pedigree illustrating the transmission of an autosomal dominant allele with incomplete penetrance is given in Fig. 4.24. Retinoblastoma, the most common malignant eye tumor affecting children, typically exhibits incomplete penetrance. About 10% of the individuals who are **obligate carriers** of the allele (i.e., those who have an affected parent and affected children and therefore must themselves carry the allele) do not have the disease. The penetrance of the disease-causing genotype is then said to be 90%.

The gene responsible for retinoblastoma encodes a **tumor-suppressor gene**, the normal function of which is to regulate the cell cycle so that cells do not divide in an uncontrollable manner. When a mutation alters the protein, its tumor-suppressing capacity is lost and a tumor can form[13,14] (see Chapter 12).

Huntington disease is another well-known autosomal dominant condition, and its main features are progressive dementia and increasingly

Affected parent

	D	d
D	DD Homozygous affected (usually rare)	Dd Heterozygous affected
d	Dd Heterozygous affected	dd Homozygous normal

A

Normal parent

	d	d
D	Dd Heterozygous affected	Dd Heterozygous affected
d	dd Homozygous normal	dd Homozygous normal

B

(Affected parent on left axis for both)

FIGURE 4.22 Punnett Square and Autosomal Dominant Traits. **A,** Punnett square for the mating of two individuals with an autosomal dominant gene. Here both parents are affected by the trait. **B,** Punnett square for the mating of a normal individual with a carrier for an autosomal dominant gene.

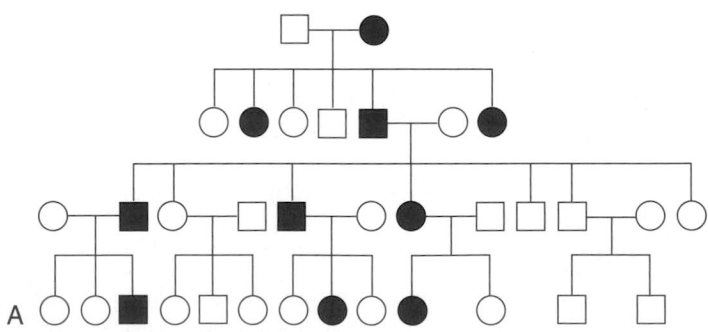

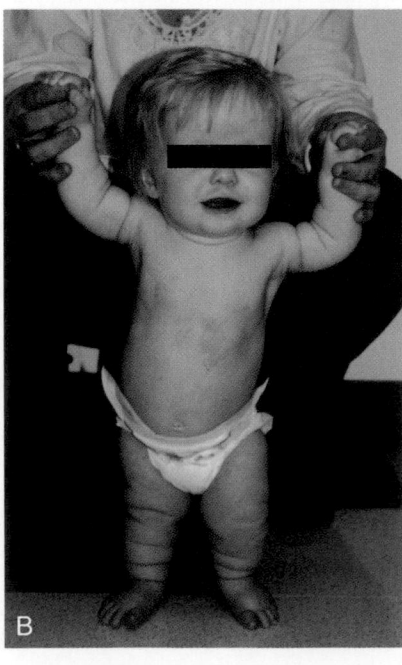

FIGURE 4.23 Achondroplasia. **A,** Pedigree showing the transmission of an autosomal dominant disease. **B,** Achondroplasia. This girl has short limbs relative to trunk length. She also has a prominent forehead, a low nasal bridge, and redundant skin folds in the arms and legs. (**B** from Jorde LB et al: *Medical genetics*, ed 5, Philadelphia, 2016, Elsevier.)

uncontrollable movements of the limbs (discussed further in Chapter 17). The latter is known as chorea (Greek *khoreia,* "dance"; the disease is sometimes called *Huntington chorea*).

One of the key features of this disease is that symptoms are not usually seen until age 40 years or later, a pattern known as **age-dependent penetrance.** Thus people who develop the disease often have had children before they are aware that they have the disease-causing allele. If the disease was present at birth, nearly all those affected would die before reaching reproductive age, and the occurrence of the allele in the population would be much lower. Individuals whose parent has the disease have a 50% chance of developing it during middle age. Individuals are thus confronted with a torturous question: "Should I have children, knowing that there is a 50-50 chance that I may have this disease gene and pass it to half my children?" Age-dependent penetrance characterizes a number of important genetic diseases, including familial breast cancer, familial colon cancer, hemochromatosis, and polycystic kidney disease.

Most genetic diseases exhibit variable expressivity. **Expressivity** is the extent of variation in phenotype associated with a particular genotype. If the expressivity of a disease is variable, the penetrance may be complete but the severity of the disease can vary greatly. A well-known example of variable expressivity in an autosomal dominant disease is type 1 neurofibromatosis, or von Recklinghausen disease. Like the retinoblastoma gene, the neurofibromatosis gene normally encodes a tumor suppressor.[15] The expression of this condition can vary from a few harmless café-au-lait spots ("coffee with milk," describing the light brown color) on the skin to malignant tumors, scoliosis, seizures, gliomas,

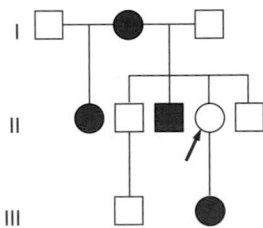

FIGURE 4.24 Pedigree for Retinoblastoma Showing Incomplete Penetrance. The female with the marked arrow in line II must be heterozygous, but the trait is not expressed.

hypertension, learning disabilities, and neuromas (Fig. 4.25). A parent with mild expression of the disease—so mild that the individual is not aware of it—can transmit the gene to a child, who can then exhibit severe expression of the disease. Several factors can cause variation in expressivity. Genes at other loci can sometimes modify the expression of a disease-causing gene (these are termed *modifier genes*). Environmental factors also can influence the expression of a disease-causing gene. Finally, different types of mutations at a locus can cause variation in severity. For example, a base substitution resulting in a single amino acid change (a missense mutation) usually produces a mild form of the clotting disorder hemophilia A. A nonsense mutation (which produces a stop codon and thus premature termination of translation) usually produces a more severe form of hemophilia A.

Autosomal Recessive Inheritance
Characteristics of Pedigrees

Like autosomal dominant diseases, those caused by autosomal recessive alleles are rare in populations, although the frequency of carriers for recessive diseases can be high. The most common lethal recessive disease in white children, cystic fibrosis, occurs in about 1 in 2500 births. Approximately 1 in 25 whites carries 1 copy of an allele that can cause cystic fibrosis (see Chapter 35). Because an individual must be homozygous for a recessive allele to express the disease, the carriers are phenotypically normal. Because most recessive alleles are maintained in normal carriers, they are able to survive in the population from one generation to the next. As with many autosomal dominant diseases, many autosomal recessive diseases are characterized by delayed age of onset, incomplete penetrance, and variable expressivity.

Fig. 4.26 shows a pedigree for cystic fibrosis. The cystic fibrosis gene encodes a protein product that forms chloride channels in the membranes of specialized epithelial cells.[16] Defective transport of chloride ions leads to a salt imbalance that results in secretions of abnormally thick, dehydrated mucus. Some of the digestive organs, particularly the pancreas, become obstructed, causing malnutrition, and the lungs become clogged with mucus, making them highly susceptible to bacterial infections (especially *Pseudomonas*). Death from lung disease or heart failure occurs on average by about 40 years of age. In the pedigree shown, the two affected individuals are the offspring of the marriage of two first cousins.

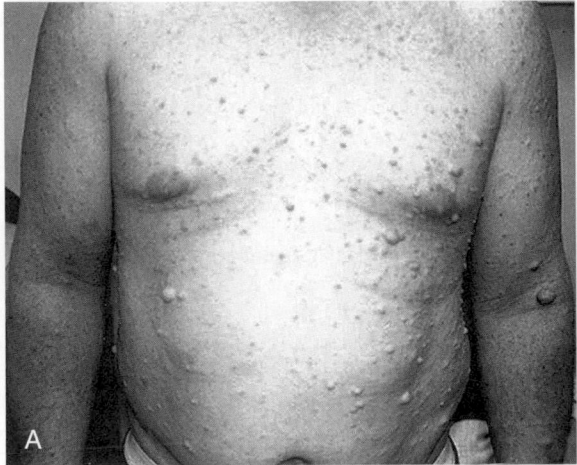
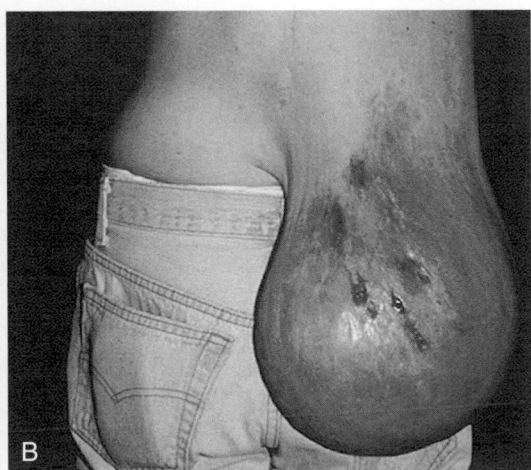

FIGURE 4.25 Neurofibromatosis. **A,** Young adult with multiple dermal neurofibromas of the trunk. **B,** Individual has a large plexiform neurofibroma hanging from lower right back, causing considerable inconvenience and discomfort (substantially improved by surgical removal of tumor). (**A** from Jorde LB et al: *Medical genetics,* ed 3, St Louis, 2003, Mosby. **B** courtesy Dr. D. Viskochil, University of Utah Health Sciences Center, Salt Lake City, UT.)

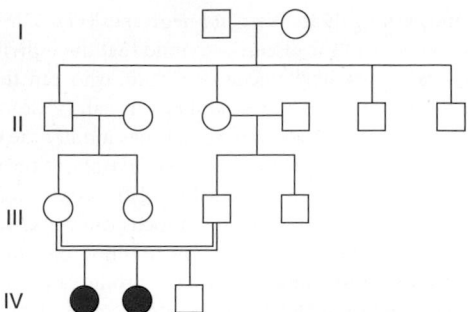

FIGURE 4.26 Pedigree for Cystic Fibrosis.

	D	d
D	DD Homozygous normal	Dd Heterozygous carrier
d	Dd Heterozygous carrier	dd Homozygous affected

FIGURE 4.27 Punnett Square for the Mating of Heterozygous Carriers. This is typical of most cases of recessive disease.

Marriage between related individuals, termed consanguinity (from the Latin root meaning "with blood"), is often a factor in producing children with recessive diseases because related individuals are more likely to share the same recessive disease-causing alleles. Consanguinity is seen most often in rare recessive diseases because carriers of common recessive diseases (such as cystic fibrosis) have a fairly high probability of encountering one another just by chance.

Important criteria for discerning autosomal recessive inheritance include the following:

1. Males and females are affected in equal proportions.
2. Consanguinity is sometimes present.
3. The disease is seen in siblings but usually not in their parents.
4. On average, one-fourth of the offspring of carrier parents will be affected.

Recurrence Risks

In most cases of recessive disease, both parents of affected individuals are heterozygous carriers. On average, one-fourth of their offspring will be normal homozygotes, one-half will be phenotypically normal carrier heterozygotes, and one-fourth will be homozygotes with the disease (Fig. 4.27). Thus the recurrence risk for the offspring of carrier parents is 25%. In any given family, chance fluctuations are likely, but a study of a large number of families would yield figures close to these proportions.

If two parents have a recessive disease, they each must be homozygous for the disease. Therefore, when two parents are affected by a recessive disease, all their children also must be affected. This observation helps to distinguish recessive from dominant inheritance, because two parents both affected by a dominant disease are nearly always both heterozygotes, and thus one-fourth of their children will be unaffected.

Because carrier parents usually are unaware that they both carry the same recessive gene, they often produce an affected child before realization of their condition. Carrier detection tests can identify heterozygotes by direct examination of the disease locus for a mutation.

Such testing is especially valuable for siblings of known carriers, who may themselves be carriers. Genetic testing is now available for nearly 5000 diseases.

Consanguinity

Consanguinity and inbreeding are related concepts. *Consanguinity* refers to the mating of two related individuals, and the offsprings of such matings are said to be *inbred*. Consanguinity is often an important characteristic of pedigrees for recessive diseases because relatives share a certain proportion of alleles received from a common ancestor. The proportion of shared alleles depends on the closeness of their biologic relationship. For example, siblings share one-half of their DNA, on average, because of their descent from the same parents. With each decreasing degree of relationship, this proportion is reduced by one-half. Uncles share one-fourth of their DNA with nephews and nieces; first cousins share one-eighth; first cousins once removed (offspring of one's own first cousins) share one-sixteenth; second cousins share one-thirty-second; and so on. The frequency of recessive disorders increases significantly in the offspring of consanguineous unions. Most empirical studies show that the proportion of offspring of marriages of first cousins who are affected by genetic diseases is approximately double that of the general population.[17] Marriages between first cousins are prohibited in most states of the United States. (*First cousins* are the offspring of two siblings and thus share a set of grandparents.) Marriages between closer relatives are prohibited throughout the United States.

X-Linked Inheritance

Not all genetic diseases are caused by genes located on the 22 autosomes. Some conditions are instead caused by genes located on the sex chromosomes, and that mode of inheritance is referred to as sex-linked. The Y chromosome contains only a few dozen genes, so most sex-linked traits are located on the X chromosome and are said to be X-linked. With the exception of fragile X syndrome (discussed earlier), which is considered to be X-linked dominant with incomplete penetrance, X-linked dominant diseases are relatively rare. Only the more common X-linked recessive diseases are discussed here.

Females receive two X chromosomes, one from the father and one from the mother, so they can be homozygous for a disease allele at a given locus, homozygous for the normal allele at the locus, or heterozygous. Males, having only one X chromosome, are said to be hemizygous for genes on this chromosome. A male who inherits a recessive disease allele on the X chromosome will be affected by the disease because the Y chromosome does not carry a normal allele to counteract the effects of the disease-causing allele. Consequently, males are more frequently affected by X-linked recessive diseases, with the difference becoming more pronounced as the disease becomes rarer.

X Inactivation

In the late 1950s, Mary Lyon proposed that one X chromosome in the somatic cells of females is permanently inactivated, a process termed X inactivation.[18] This explains why most gene products coded by the X chromosome are present in roughly equal amounts in males and females, even though males have only one X chromosome and females have two X chromosomes. This phenomenon is called dosage compensation. The inactivated X chromosomes are observable in many interphase cells as highly condensed chromatin bodies, termed Barr bodies (after Barr and Bertram, who discovered them in the late 1940s). Normal females have one Barr body in each somatic cell, whereas normal males have no Barr bodies.

The process of inactivation occurs very early in embryonic development—approximately 7 to 14 days after fertilization. In each somatic cell, one of the two X chromosomes is inactivated. In some cells the X chromosome contributed by the father is inactivated; in others the maternally contributed X chromosome is inactivated. Because the inactivation process is random, the maternal X chromosome is inactivated in approximately half the cells and the paternal X chromosome is inactivated in approximately half the cells. Once the X chromosome has been inactivated in a cell, all the descendants of that cell have the same chromosome inactivated. Thus inactivation is said to be *random* but *fixed*.

Some individuals do not have the normal number of X chromosomes in their somatic cells. For example, males with Klinefelter syndrome typically have two X chromosomes and one Y chromosome and they have one Barr body in each cell. Females whose cell nuclei have three X chromosomes have two Barr bodies in each cell, and females whose cell nuclei have four X chromosomes have three Barr bodies in each cell. Females with Turner syndrome have only one X chromosome and no Barr bodies. Thus the number of Barr bodies is always one less than the number of X chromosomes in the cell. All but one X chromosome are always inactivated.

People with abnormal numbers of X chromosomes, such as those with Turner syndrome or Klinefelter syndrome, are not physically normal. This situation presents a puzzle because they presumably have only one active X chromosome, the same as individuals with normal numbers of chromosomes. However, the distal portions of the short and long arms of the X chromosome, as well as other regions on the chromosome, are not inactivated. In total, about 15% of the genes on the human X chromosome escape inactivation. Thus X inactivation is also said to be *incomplete*.

Although the mechanism underlying X inactivation is still incompletely understood, the gene responsible for initiating X inactivation, *XIST*, has been located.[19] This gene encodes a lncRNA that coats the copy of the X chromosome on which it is expressed, which then inactivates most of the genes on the chromosome. Methylation of X chromosome DNA, a process in which DNA is inactivated when cytosine bases are enzymatically converted to 5-methylcytosine, occurs on the inactivated X chromosome. Inactive X chromosomes can be at least partially reactivated in vitro by administering 5-azacytidine, a demethylating agent.

Sex Determination

The process of sexual differentiation, in which the embryonic gonads become either testes or ovaries, begins during the sixth week of gestation. A key principle of sex determination in mammals is that one copy of the Y chromosome is sufficient to initiate the process of gonadal differentiation that produces a male fetus (Fig. 4.28, *A*). The number of X chromosomes does not alter this process. For example, an individual with two X chromosomes and one Y chromosome in each cell is still phenotypically a male. Thus it is logical that the Y chromosome must contain a gene that begins the process of male gonadal development.

This gene, termed *SRY* (for "sex-determining region on the Y"), has been located on the short arm of the Y chromosome.[20,21] The *SRY* gene lies immediately proximal to the distal tip of the Y chromosome, known as the **pseudoautosomal** region (see Fig. 4.28, *B*). This portion of the Y chromosome is so named because it pairs with the distal tip of the short arm of the X chromosome during meiosis and exchanges genetic material with it (crossover), just as autosomes do. The DNA sequences of these regions on the X and Y chromosomes are highly similar. The remainder of the X and Y chromosomes, however, do not exchange material and are not similar in DNA sequence. An important piece of evidence that supports *SRY* as the male-determining gene is that female mouse embryos injected with this gene develop as phenotypic males.

Although the *SRY* gene is located on the Y chromosome, the other genes that contribute to male differentiation are located on other

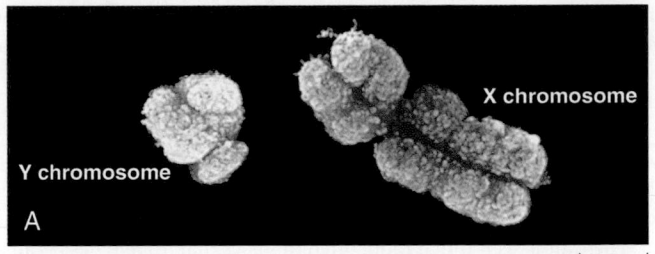

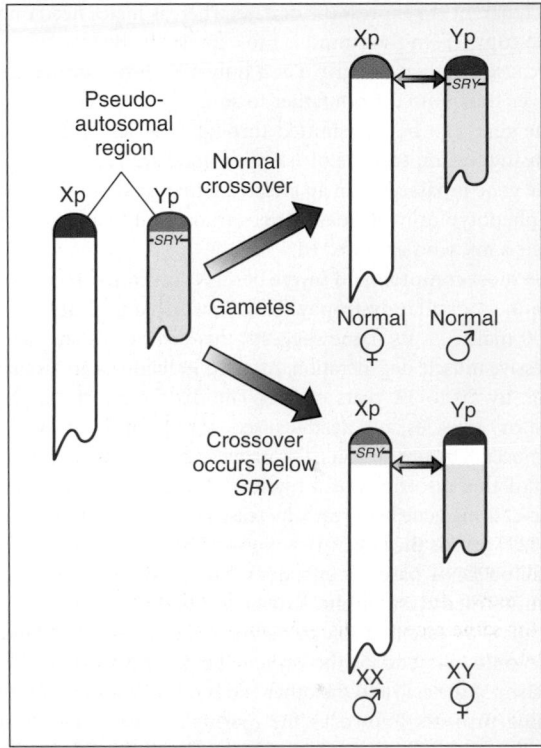

FIGURE 4.28 The Distal Short Arms of the X and Y Chromosomes Exchange Material During Meiosis in the Male. A, X and Y chromosomes. **B,** The region of the Y chromosome in which this crossover occurs is called the *pseudoautosomal region.* (Xp and Yp refer to the short arms of each chromosome.) The *SRY* gene, which triggers the process leading to male gonadal differentiation, is located just outside the pseudoautosomal region. Occasionally, the crossover occurs on the centromeric side of the *SRY* gene, causing it to lie on an X chromosome instead of a Y chromosome. An offspring receiving this X chromosome will be an XX male, and an offspring receiving the Y chromosome will be an XY female. (**A** from Raven PH et al: *Biology,* ed 8, New York, 2008, McGraw-Hill. **B** from Jorde LB et al: *Medical genetics,* ed 5, Philadelphia, 2016, Elsevier.)

chromosomes. Thus *SRY* appears to act as a trigger that initiates the action of genes on other chromosomes (e.g., those that control Sertoli cell differentiation or secretion of müllerian-inhibiting substance). This concept is supported by the fact that the *SRY* gene is similar in sequence to other genes that are known to regulate the transcription of DNA (i.e., they turn other genes on and off).

Occasionally the crossover between X and Y occurs closer to the centromere than it should, placing the *SRY* gene on the X chromosome after crossover (see Fig. 4.28, *B*). This event can result in offspring with an apparently normal XX karyotype but a male phenotype. Such XX males are seen in about 1 in 20,000 live births and closely resemble males with Klinefelter syndrome, although their stature is normal. Conversely, it is possible to inherit a Y chromosome that has lost the *SRY* gene (because of either a crossover error or a deletion of the gene). This situation produces an XY female. Such females have gonadal streaks rather than ovaries and have poorly developed secondary sex characteristics.

Characteristics of Pedigrees

Pedigrees for X-linked recessive conditions show the following distinctive features:

1. The trait is seen much more often in males than in females because females must inherit two copies of the recessive allele (one from each parent) to express the disease, whereas males need only inherit one copy (from their mother) to express the disease.
2. Because a father can give a son only a Y chromosome, the trait is never transmitted from father to son.
3. The gene can be transmitted through a series of carrier females, causing the appearance of "skipped generations."
4. The gene is passed from an affected father to all his daughters, who, as phenotypically normal carriers, transmit it to approximately half their sons, who are affected.

The most common and severe of all X-linked recessive disorders is Duchenne muscular dystrophy (DMD), which affects approximately 1 in 3500 males. As its name suggests, this disorder is characterized by progressive muscle degeneration. Affected individuals are usually unable to walk by 10 to 12 years of age. The disease affects the heart and respiratory muscles, and death caused by respiratory or cardiac failure usually occurs before 20 years. For many years, the underlying pathologic origin of this disorder was a mystery. However, identification of the disease-causing gene has greatly increased our understanding of DMD.[21] The *DMD* gene is the largest gene known in the human, spanning about 2.5 million DNA bases. It encodes a previously undiscovered muscle protein, termed **dystrophin**. Extensive study of dystrophin indicates that it plays an essential role in maintaining the structural integrity of muscle cells: one end of the protein binds to actin filaments in the cytoplasm of the cell, and the other end binds to a group of membrane-spanning proteins known as the *dystrophin-associated glycoproteins*. When dystrophin is absent, as in individuals with DMD, the muscle cell cannot survive, and muscle deterioration ensues.

Most cases of Duchenne muscular dystrophy are caused by deletions of portions of the *DMD* gene. They usually involve frameshift deletions in which all the amino acids following the deletion are altered and a premature stop codon occurs. An "in frame" deletion (in which a multiple of three bases is deleted, and the amino acids following the deletion are not altered) produces a milder form of muscular dystrophy, the Becker type. These two types of muscular dystrophy are examples of a disease in which different types of mutations at the same locus produce variable expression of the disease.

Recurrence Risks

The most common mating type involving X-linked recessive genes is the combination of a carrier female and a normal male. On average, the carrier mothers will transmit the disease-causing allele to half their sons and half their daughters. As Fig. 4.29, *A*, shows, half the daughters in such a mating will be carriers, whereas half will be normal. Half the sons will be normal, on average, whereas half will have the disease.

The other common mating type is an affected father and a normal mother (see Fig. 4.29, *B*). In this situation all the sons must be normal because the father can transmit only his Y chromosome to them. Because all the daughters must receive the father's X chromosome, they will all be heterozygous carriers. None of the children will express the disease.

The final mating pattern, less common than the other two, involves an affected father and a carrier mother (see Fig. 4.29, *C*). With this pattern, on average, half the daughters will be heterozygous carriers

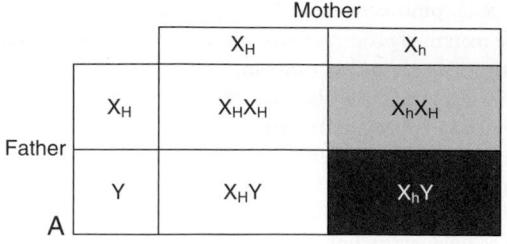

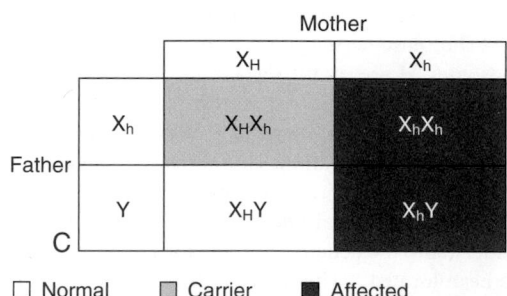

□ Normal   ▨ Carrier   ■ Affected

FIGURE 4.29 Punnett Square and X-Linked Recessive Traits. **A,** Punnett square for the mating of a normal male (X_HY) and a female carrier of an X-linked recessive gene (X_HX_h). **B,** Punnett square for the mating of a normal female (X_HX_H) with a male affected by an X-linked recessive disease (X_hY). **C,** Punnett square for the mating of a female who carries an X-linked recessive gene (X_HX_h) with a male who is affected with the disease caused by the gene (X_hY).

and half will be homozygous for the disease allele and thus affected. Half the sons will be normal, and half will be affected. Some X-linked recessive diseases, such as DMD, are fatal or incapacitating before the affected individual reaches reproductive age, and therefore affected fathers are rare or nonexistent.

Sex-Limited and Sex-Influenced Traits

Confusion sometimes exists regarding the difference between traits that are sex-linked and those that are sex-limited or sex-influenced. A **sex-limited trait** is one that can occur in only one of the sexes, often because of anatomic differences. Inherited uterine and testicular defects are two obvious examples.

A **sex-influenced trait** is one that occurs much more often in one sex than in the other. A good example of a sex-influenced trait is male-pattern baldness, which occurs in both males and females but is much more common in males. Another example is breast cancer, which is approximately 70 times more common in females than males.

Evaluation of Pedigrees

With complications such as incomplete or age-dependent penetrance, variable expressivity, and sex-influenced traits, it is not always possible simply to look at a disease pedigree and determine the mode of inheritance. Sophisticated statistical approaches have evolved to deal with such complications. Incorporated into computer programs, these statistical techniques assess the probability of observing a certain pedigree if a particular mode of inheritance (e.g., autosomal dominant with incomplete penetrance) is in effect.

LINKAGE ANALYSIS AND GENE IDENTIFICATION

Locating the positions of genes on chromosomes has been one of the most important endeavors in human genetics. It is often an important first step in identifying a disease-causing gene and can be used to predict the likelihood that certain individuals will develop a genetic disease.

Mendel's second law, the principle of independent assortment, states that an individual's genes will be transmitted to the next generation independently of one another. This law is only partly true, however, because genes located close together on the same chromosome *do* tend to be transmitted together to the offspring. Thus Mendel's principle of independent assortment holds true for most pairs of genes but not those that occupy the same region of a chromosome. Such loci demonstrate linkage and are said to be linked.

During the first meiotic stage, the arms of homologous chromosome pairs intertwine and sometimes exchange portions of their DNA (Fig. 4.30) in a process known as crossing over. During crossing over, new combinations of alleles can be formed. For example, two loci on a chromosome have alleles *A* and *a* and alleles *B* and *b*. Alleles *A* and *B* are located together on one chromosome arm, and alleles *a* and *b* are located on the other arm. The genotype of this individual is denoted as *AB/ab*.

As Fig. 4.30, *A*, shows, the allele pairs *AB* and *ab* would be transmitted together when no crossing over occurs. However, when crossing over does occur (see Fig. 4.30, *B*), all four possible pairs of alleles can be transmitted to the offspring: *AB, aB, Ab,* and *ab*. The process of forming such new arrangements of alleles is called recombination. Crossing

over does not necessarily lead to recombination, however, because double crossing over between two loci can result in no actual recombination of the alleles at the loci (see Fig. 4.30, *C*).

The rate of crossing over can be used to infer the distance between two loci on a chromosome because the probability of crossovers occurring between two loci increases as the loci become more distant. For example, if an individual with genotype *AB/ab* produces recombinant offspring gametes (composition of *Ab* and *aB*) 2% of the time, it is said that the two loci are two map units apart. One map unit equals a 1% recombination rate between two loci. When loci on the same chromosome are 50 or more map units apart, they are considered unlinked because their recombination frequency is just as great as it would be if they were on different chromosomes (where the probability of being transmitted together must equal one-half). Recombination frequencies provide a good estimate of actual physical distance between loci: on average, each map unit is equal to approximately 1 million DNA base pairs.

An important early goal of the Human Genome Project was to establish a "map" of markers (polymorphic loci with known chromosome locations that could be assayed easily in laboratories) spanning the entire genome. In pedigrees in which a mendelian disease is being transmitted, the recombination rate between the disease-causing gene and each marker locus is assessed. When a marker locus shows little or no recombination with the disease locus, we know that the disease locus must be located near the position of the marker, and an approximate location for the disease locus has been established. This principle was used to establish the chromosome locations of most of the diseases shown in Fig. 4.31.

Once a close linkage has been established between a disease locus and a marker, it can be predicted whether a relative of an affected individual will develop the disease. If, for example, the recombination rate between a disease locus and a marker polymorphism is less than 1%, family members can simply have the marker locus assayed to determine, with 99% or greater certainty, whether each member carries the disease-causing allele.

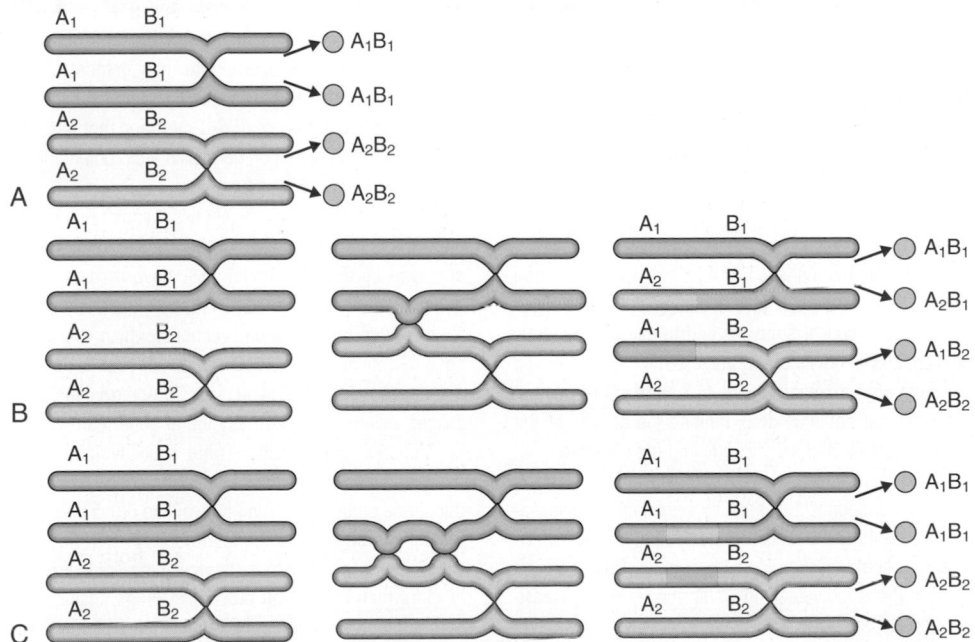

FIGURE 4.30 The Genetic Results of Crossing Over. A, No crossing over: A_1 and B_1 remain together after meiosis. **B,** Crossing over between A and B results in a recombination: A_1 and B_2 are inherited together on one chromosome, and A_2 and B_1 are inherited together on another chromosome. **C,** A double crossover between A and B results in no recombination of alleles.

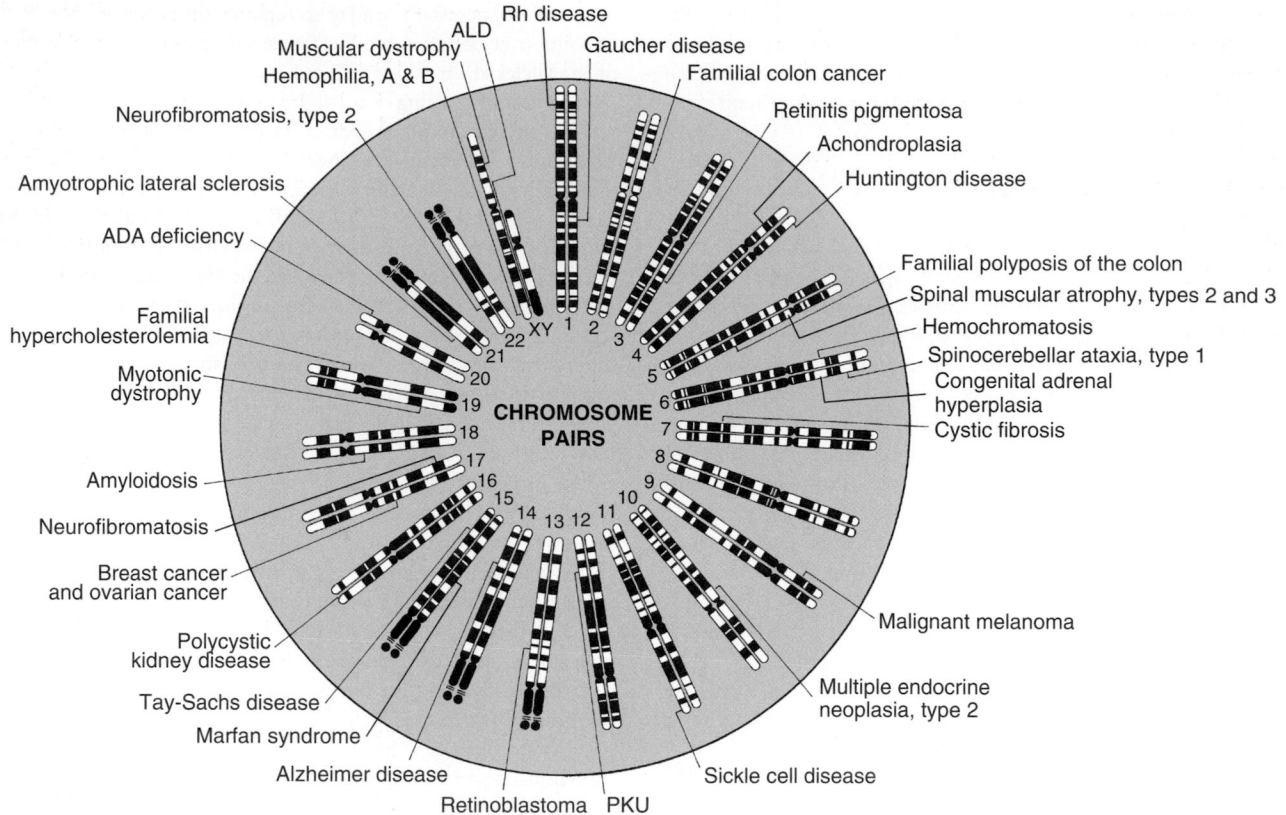

FIGURE 4.31 Example of Diseases: A Gene Map. *ADA,* Adenosine deaminase; *ALD,* adrenoleukodystrophy; *PKU,* phenylketonuria.

BOX 4.3   GENETICS AND PRECISION MEDICINE

Precision medicine, also known as *personalized* medicine, is a healthcare model in which each person's unique genetic and environmental risk factors are taken into account in the diagnosis and management of disease. Because genes contribute to susceptibility to nearly all human diseases, and because each individual is genetically unique, it follows that genetics is an important component of precision medicine. As the technology to interrogate the genome becomes more advanced and more affordable, genetics will play an increasingly prominent role in precision medicine.

Genetic analysis, including genetic testing (see Box 4.2), has become integral to the diagnosis of many diseases. For example, genetic testing of tumor samples is done frequently to help diagnose cancer subtypes and to guide therapeutic treatment. Tumor cells from people with breast cancer are tested for overexpression of the *HER2* gene, which is seen in approximately 20% to 30% of primary breast tumors. Trastuzumab, a monoclonal antibody drug, inhibits the activity of the cell surface receptor encoded by *HER2* and significantly improves survival.

As the price of whole-genome DNA sequencing continues to decline, it is becoming increasingly common to diagnosis disease by searching for disease-causing variants in the person's entire DNA sequence (or in the **exome,** which is the 1.5% of the genome that contains protein-coding exons). This approach can be particularly powerful in those individuals in whom the cause of disease is unknown. Currently, "diagnostic odysseys," which can continue for years and can cost hundreds of thousands of dollars, can sometimes be resolved quickly and accurately through whole-genome sequencing. The challenges encountered

in whole-genome sequencing include the interpretation of "variants of unknown significance" and the appropriate management of incidental genetic findings (e.g., a person referred because of an undiagnosed neurologic disorder who is found to have a *BRCA1* or *BRCA2* mutation that has a high probability of causing breast or ovarian cancer or, perhaps more problematically, a mutation that causes familial Alzheimer disease).

Perhaps the area in which genetics is contributing most significantly to precision medicine is in the guidance of therapeutic drug prescription. Of the 1200 drugs approved by the FDA, about 15% have recommendations on their labels for genetic testing to guide administration and dosage. Genetic testing can help to avoid severe adverse drug reactions, which are estimated to cause 2 million hospitalizations and 100,000 deaths per year in the United States. For example, a variant in the *TPMT* gene, seen in homozygous form in 1 in 300 Europeans, causes severe and potentially lethal bone marrow suppression upon exposure to thiopurine drugs used to treat acute lymphocytic leukemia. Consequently, genetic testing to avoid this reaction is done routinely in the administration of thiopurine drugs. In addition to avoiding drugs harmful to the individual, genetic testing can be used to formulate drug dosage more precisely. Variants in the *CYP2D6* gene (which encodes a cytochrome P-450 enzyme) influence the metabolism of more than 25% of all prescribed drugs, including tricyclic antidepressants, beta-adrenergic receptor blockers, and neuroleptics. Testing of *CYP2D6,* as well as other genes involved in drug metabolism, can reduce trial-and-error in estimating appropriate drug dosage levels.

Data from Relling MV, Evans WE: *Nature* 526:343–350, 2015; Topol EJ: *Cell* 157:241–253, 2014; Wilke RA et al: *Nat Rev Drug Discov* 6:904–916, 2007.

For most genetic diseases, it is now possible to test directly for the disease-causing mutation, often by sequencing the germline DNA in family members. In some cases, however, the actual disease-causing mutation cannot be identified, but linked marker loci can be assayed to provide an indirect genetic test. Genetic tests are now used routinely to confirm diagnosis of a genetic disease, to identify carriers of recessive diseases, and to presymptomatically identify individuals who are at risk for inheriting a disease with delayed age of onset, such as autosomal dominant breast or colon cancer, Huntington disease, and many others. In some cases, testing can help provide preventive treatment, such as prophylactic oophorectomy in women who have inherited a dominant allele that can cause breast or ovarian cancer.

As the cost of sequencing whole human genomes has declined, it is now common to search for a disease-causing mutation in an individual or a family by evaluating their entire germline DNA sequence (genome).[22] Their sequences are compared with those of unaffected individuals, and statistical methods are used to determine which, if any, of their DNA variants cause disease. Linkage results, as discussed previously, can help to define a specific chromosome region that contains a disease-causing variant in a family. Currently, the genetic causes of about 4700 mendelian conditions have been determined,[1] enabling genetic testing, more accurate diagnosis, and in some cases more effective treatment of disease (Box 4.3).

SUMMARY REVIEW

DNA, RNA, and Proteins: Heredity at the Molecular Level

1. Genes, the basic units of inheritance, are composed of DNA and are located on the chromosomes.
2. The most important constituent of DNA is the four types of nitrogenous bases, labeled A, C, G, and T. The physical structure of DNA is a double helix.
3. The DNA bases code for amino acids, which in turn make up proteins. The amino acids are specified by triplet codons of nitrogenous bases.
4. DNA replication is based on complementary base pairing, in which a single strand of DNA serves as the template for attracting bases that form a new strand of DNA.
5. DNA polymerase is the primary enzyme involved in replication. It adds bases to the new DNA strand and performs "proofreading" functions.
6. A mutation is an inherited alteration of genetic material (i.e., DNA).
7. Substances that cause mutations are called *mutagens*.
8. The mutation rate in humans varies from locus to locus and ranges from 10^{-4} to 10^{-7} per gene per generation.
9. Transcription and translation, the two basic processes in which proteins are specified by DNA, both involve RNA. RNA is chemically similar to DNA, but it is single stranded and has uracil rather than thymine as one of its four nitrogenous bases.
10. Transcription is the process by which DNA specifies a sequence of mRNA.
11. Much of the RNA sequence is spliced from the mRNA before the mRNA leaves the nucleus. The excised sequences are called *introns*, and those that remain to code for proteins are called *exons*.
12. MicroRNAs (miRNAs) are small RNA sequences, 17 to 27 nucleotides in length, that bind to specific mRNA sequences and down-regulate their expression. Another nontranslated RNA, classified as having a length greater than 200 nucleotides, is termed *long noncoding RNA* (lncRNA). The genome contains at least 10,000 lncRNAs, and, like miRNA, some lncRNAs are involved in gene regulation.
13. Transcription factors bind to DNA sequences called *transcription factor binding sites* near genes to regulate the timing of transcription, as well as the specific tissues in which genes are actively transcribed.
14. Translation is the process by which RNA directs the synthesis of polypeptides. This process takes place in the ribosomes.
15. During translation, mRNA interacts with tRNA, a molecule that has an attachment site for a specific amino acid.

Chromosomes

1. Human cells consist of diploid somatic cells (body cells) and haploid gametes (sperm and egg cells).
2. Humans have 23 pairs of chromosomes: 22 of these pairs are autosomes. The remaining pair consists of the sex chromosomes. Females have two homologous X chromosomes as their sex chromosomes; males have an X and a Y chromosome.
3. A karyotype is an ordered display of chromosomes arranged according to length and the location of the centromere.
4. Various types of stains can be used to make chromosome bands more visible.
5. About 1 in 150 live births has a major diagnosable chromosome abnormality. Chromosome abnormalities are the leading known cause of intellectual disability and miscarriage.
6. Polyploidy is a condition in which a euploid cell has some multiple of the normal number of chromosomes. Humans have been observed to have triploidy (three copies of each chromosome) and tetraploidy (four copies of each chromosome); both conditions are lethal.
7. Somatic cells that do not have a multiple of 23 chromosomes are aneuploid. Aneuploidy is usually the result of nondisjunction.
8. Trisomy is a type of aneuploidy in which one chromosome is present in three copies in somatic cells. A partial trisomy is one in which only part of a chromosome is present in three copies.
9. Monosomy is a type of aneuploidy in which one chromosome is present in only one copy in somatic cells.
10. In general, monosomies cause more severe physical defects than do trisomies, illustrating the principle that the loss of chromosome material has more severe consequences than the duplication of chromosome material.
11. Down syndrome, a trisomy of chromosome 21, is the most well-known disease caused by a chromosome aberration. It affects 1 in 800 live births and is much more likely to occur in the offspring of women older than 35 years of age.
12. Most aneuploidies of the sex chromosomes have less severe consequences than those of the autosomes.
13. The most commonly observed sex chromosome aneuploidies are the 47,XXX karyotype; 45,X karyotype (Turner syndrome); 47,XXY karyotype (Klinefelter syndrome); and 47,XYY karyotype.
14. Abnormalities of chromosome structure include deletions, duplications, inversions, and translocations.

Elements of Formal Genetics

1. Mendelian traits are caused by single genes, each of which occupies a position, or locus, on a chromosome.
2. Alleles are different forms of genes located at the same locus on the chromosome.
3. At any given locus in a somatic cell, an individual has two genes, one from each parent. An individual may be homozygous or heterozygous for a locus.

■ SUMMARY REVIEW—cont'd

4. An individual's genotype is the person's genetic makeup, and the phenotype reflects the interaction of genotype and environment.

5. At a heterozygous locus, a dominant gene's effects mask those of a recessive gene. The recessive gene is expressed only when it is present in two copies.

Transmission of Genetic Diseases

1. Genetic diseases caused by single genes usually follow autosomal dominant, autosomal recessive, or X-linked recessive modes of inheritance.

2. Pedigree charts are an important tool in the analysis of modes of inheritance.

3. Recurrence risks specify the probability that future offspring will inherit a genetic disease. For single-gene diseases, recurrence risks remain the same for each offspring, regardless of the number of affected or unaffected offspring.

4. The recurrence risk for autosomal dominant diseases is usually 50%.

5. Germline mosaicism can alter recurrence risks for genetic diseases because unaffected parents can produce multiple affected offspring. This situation occurs because the germline of one parent is affected by a mutation but the parent's somatic cells are unaffected.

6. Skipped generations are not seen in classic autosomal dominant pedigrees.

7. Males and females are equally likely to exhibit autosomal dominant diseases and to pass them on to their offspring.

8. A gene that is not always expressed phenotypically is said to have incomplete penetrance.

9. Penetrance may be age-dependent, as in Huntington disease and familial breast cancer.

10. Variable expressivity is a characteristic of many genetic diseases.

11. Most commonly, parents of children with autosomal recessive diseases are both heterozygous carriers of the disease gene. In this case, the recurrence risk for autosomal recessive diseases is 25%.

12. Males and females are equally likely to be affected by autosomal recessive diseases.

13. Consanguinity is sometimes present in families with autosomal recessive diseases, and it becomes more prevalent with rarer recessive diseases.

14. Carrier detection tests for an increasing number of autosomal recessive diseases are available.

15. The frequency of genetic diseases approximately doubles in the offspring of first-cousin matings.

16. In each normal female somatic cell, one of the two X chromosomes is inactivated early in embryogenesis.

17. X inactivation is random, fixed, and incomplete (i.e., only part of the chromosome is actually inactivated). It may involve methylation.

18. Gender is determined embryonically by the presence of the *SRY* gene on the Y chromosome. Embryos that have a Y chromosome (and thus the *SRY* gene) become males, whereas those lacking the Y chromosome become females. When the Y chromosome lacks the *SRY* gene, an XY female can be produced. Similarly, an X chromosome that contains the *SRY* gene can produce an XX male.

19. X-linked genes are those that are located on the X chromosome. Nearly all known X-linked diseases are caused by X-linked recessive genes.

20. Males are hemizygous for genes on the X chromosome.

21. X-linked recessive diseases are seen much more often in males than in females because males need only one copy of the gene to express the disease.

22. Fathers cannot pass X-linked genes to their sons.

23. Skipped generations are often seen in X-linked recessive disease pedigrees because the gene can be transmitted through carrier females.

24. Recurrence risks for X-linked recessive diseases depend on the carrier and affected status of the mother and father.

25. A sex-limited trait is one that occurs in only one of the sexes.

26. A sex-influenced trait is one that occurs more often in one sex than in the other.

Linkage Analysis and Gene Identification

1. During meiosis I, crossing over occurs and can cause recombinations of alleles located on the same chromosome.

2. The frequency of recombinations can be used to infer the map distance between loci on the same chromosome.

3. A marker locus, when closely linked to a disease-gene locus, can be used to predict whether an individual will develop a genetic disease.

4. The complete human genome sequence will facilitate gene identification, diagnosis, and disease treatment.

■ KEY TERMS

KEY TERMS—cont'd

REFERENCES

1. *Mendelian inheritance in man*. Available at www.omim.org.
2. Bell CJ, et al: Carrier testing for severe childhood recessive diseases by next generation sequencing. *Sci Transl Med* 3(65):65ra4, 2011.
3. McCandless SE, Brunger JW, Cassidy SB: The burden of genetic disease on inpatient care in a children's hospital. *Am J Hum Genet* 74:121–127, 2004.
4. Segurel L, Wyman MJ, Przeworski M: Determinants of mutation rate variation in the human germline. *Annu Rev Genomics Hum Genet* 15:47–70, 2014.
5. Nagaoka SI, Hassold TJ, Hunt PA: Human aneuploidy: mechanisms and new insights into an age-old problem. *Nat Rev Genet* 13:493–504, 2012.
6. Curry CJ: Autosomal trisomies. In Rimoin DL, editor: *Emery and Rimoin's principles and practice of medical genetics*, ed 6, Philadelphia, 2013, Elsevier.
7. Hunter AGW: Down syndrome. In Cassidy SB, Allanson JE, editors: *Management of genetic syndromes*, Hoboken, NJ, 2010, Wiley-Liss, pp 309–336.

8. Jorde LB, et al: *Medical genetics*, ed 5, Philadelphia, 2016, Elsevier.
9. Gravholt CH: Sex chromosome abnormalities. In Rimoin DL, Pyeritz RE, Korf BR, editors: *Emery and Rimoin's principles and practice of medical genetics*, ed 6, Philadelphia, 2013, Elsevier.
10. Rooms L, Kooy RF: Advances in understanding fragile X syndrome and related disorders. *Curr Opin Pediatr* 23:601–606, 2011.
11. Nelson DL, Orr HT, Warren ST: The unstable repeats—three evolving faces of neurological disease. *Neuron* 77:825–843, 2013.
12. Biesecker LG, Spinner NB: A genomic view of mosaicism and human disease. *Nat Rev Genet* 14:307–320, 2013.
13. McDermott U, Downing JR, Stratton MR: Genomics and the continuum of cancer care. *N Engl J Med* 364:340–350, 2011.
14. Vogelstein B, et al: Cancer genome landscapes. *Science* 339:1546–1558, 2013.
15. Pasmant E, et al: Neurofibromatosis type 1: from genotype to phenotype. *J Med Genet* 49:483–489, 2012.

16. Cutting GR: Cystic fibrosis genetics: from molecular understanding to clinical application. *Nat Rev Genet* 16:45–56, 2015.
17. Jorde LB: Inbreeding in human populations. In Dulbecco R, editor: *Encyclopedia of human biology*, (vol 5), New York, 1997, Academic Press.
18. Lyon MF: Sex chromatin and gene action in the mammalian X-chromosome. *Am J Hum Genet* 14:135–148, 1962.
19. Lee JT, Bartolomei MS: X-inactivation, imprinting, and long noncoding RNAs in health and disease. *Cell* 152:1308–1323, 2013.
20. Larney C, Bailey TL, Koopman P: Switching on sex: transcriptional regulation of the testis-determining gene Sry. *Development* 141:2195–2205, 2014.
21. Wein N, Alfano L, Flanigan KM: Genetics and emerging treatments for Duchenne and Becker muscular dystrophy. *Pediatr Clin North Am* 62:723–742, 2015.
22. Biesecker LG, Green RC: Diagnostic clinical genome and exome sequencing. *N Engl J Med* 370:2418–2425, 2014.

Genes, Environment-Lifestyle, and Common Diseases

Lynn B. Jorde

evolve WEBSITE

http://evolve.elsevier.com/McCance/
- Content Updates
- Chapter Summary Review
- Review Questions
- Case Studies
- Animations

CHAPTER OUTLINE

Chapter 4 focuses on diseases that are caused by single genes or by abnormalities of single chromosomes. Much progress has been made in identifying specific mutations that cause these diseases, leading to better risk estimates and, in some cases, more effective treatment of the disease. However, these conditions form only a small portion of the total burden of human genetic disease. Most congenital malformations are not caused by single genes or chromosome defects. Many common adult diseases, such as cancer, heart disease, and diabetes, have genetic components, but again they are usually not caused by single genes or by chromosomal abnormalities. These diseases, whose treatment collectively occupies the attention of most healthcare practitioners, are the result of a complex interplay of multiple genetic and environmental factors.

FACTORS INFLUENCING INCIDENCE OF DISEASE IN POPULATIONS

Concepts of Incidence and Prevalence

How common is a given disease, such as diabetes, in a population? Well-established measures are used to answer this question.[1] The incidence rate is the number of new cases of a disease reported during a specific period (typically 1 year) divided by the number of individuals in the population. The denominator is often expressed as *person-years*. The incidence rate can be contrasted with the prevalence rate, which is the proportion of the population affected by a disease at a specific point in time. Prevalence is thus determined by both the incidence rate and the length of the survival period in affected individuals. For example, the prevalence rate of acquired immunodeficiency syndrome (AIDS) is larger than the yearly incidence rate because most people with AIDS survive for at least several years after diagnosis.

Many diseases vary in prevalence from one population to another. Cystic fibrosis is relatively common among Europeans, occurring about once in every 2500 births. In contrast, it is quite rare in Asians, occurring only once in every 90,000 births. Similarly, sickle cell disease affects approximately 1 in 600 American blacks, but it is seen much less frequently in whites. Both of these diseases are single-gene disorders, and they vary among populations because disease-causing mutations are more or less common in different populations. (This is in turn the result of differences in the evolutionary history of these populations.) Nongenetic (environmental) factors have little influence on the current prevalence of these diseases.

The picture often becomes more complex with the common diseases of adulthood. For example, colon cancer was until recently relatively rare in Japan, but it is the second most common cancer in the United

States. Stomach cancer, on the other hand, is common in Japan but relatively rare in the United States. These statistics, in themselves, cannot distinguish environmental from genetic influences in the two populations. However, because large numbers of Japanese emigrated first to Hawaii and then to the U.S. mainland, we can observe what happens to the rates of stomach and colon cancer among the migrants. It is important that the Japanese émigrés maintained a genetic identity, marrying largely among themselves. Among first-generation Japanese in Hawaii, the frequency of colon cancer rose several-fold—not yet as high as in the U.S. mainland but higher than that in Japan. Among second-generation Japanese on the U.S. mainland, colon cancer rates rose to 5%, equal to the U.S. average. At the same time, stomach cancer has become relatively rare among Japanese-Americans.

These observations strongly indicate an important role for environmental factors in the etiology of cancers of the colon and stomach. In each case, diet is a likely culprit—a high-fat, low-fiber diet in the United States is thought to increase the risk of colon cancer, whereas techniques used to preserve and season the fish commonly eaten in Japan are thought to increase the risk of stomach cancer. It is interesting that the incidence of colon cancer in Japan has increased dramatically during the past several decades as the Japanese population has adopted a more "Western" diet. These results do not, however, rule out the potential contribution of genetic factors in common cancers. Genes also play a role in the etiology of colon and other cancers.

Analysis of Risk Factors

The comparison just discussed is one example of the analysis of risk factors (in this case, diet) and their influence on the prevalence of disease in populations. A common measure of the effect of a specific risk factor is the **relative risk**. This quantity is expressed as a ratio:

$$\frac{\text{Increased rate of the disease among individuals exposed to a risk factor}}{\text{Incidence rate of the disease among individuals } not \text{ exposed to a risk factor}}$$

A classic example of a relative risk analysis was carried out in a sample of more than 40,000 British physicians to determine the relationship between cigarette smoking and lung cancer. This study compared the incidence of death from lung cancer in physicians who smoked with those who did not. The incidence of death from lung cancer was 1.66 (per 1000 person-years) in heavy smokers (more than 25 cigarettes daily), but it was only 0.07 in the nonsmokers. The ratio of these two incidence rates is 1.66/0.07, which yields a relative risk of 23.7 deaths. Thus, it is concluded that the risk of dying from lung cancer increased by about 24-fold in heavy smokers compared with nonsmokers. Many other studies have obtained similar risk figures.

Although cigarette smoking clearly increases one's risk of developing lung cancer (as well as heart disease, as will be seen later), it is equally clear that *most* smokers do not develop lung cancer. Other lifestyle factors are likely to contribute to one's risk of developing this disease (e.g., exposure to cancer-causing substances in the air, such as asbestos fibers). In addition, differences in genetic background may be involved. Smokers who have variants in genes that are involved in the metabolism of components of tobacco smoke (such as *CYP1A1* and *GSTM1*) are at significantly increased risk of developing lung cancer.

Many factors can influence the risk of acquiring a common disease such as cancer, diabetes, or high blood pressure. These include age, gender, diet, amount of exercise, and family history of the disease. Usually, complex interactions occur among these genetic and nongenetic factors. The effects of each factor can be quantified in terms of relative risks.

The following discussion demonstrates how genetic and environmental factors contribute to the risk of developing common diseases.

PRINCIPLES OF MULTIFACTORIAL INHERITANCE

Basic Model

Traits in which variation is thought to be caused by the combined effects of multiple genes are **polygenic** ("many genes"). When environmental factors are also believed to cause variation in the trait, which is usually the case, the term **multifactorial trait** is used.[2] Many **quantitative traits** (those, such as blood pressure, that are measured on a continuous numeric scale) are multifactorial. Because they are caused by the additive effects of many genetic and environmental factors, these traits tend to follow a normal, or bell-shaped, distribution in populations.

An example illustrates this concept. To begin with the simplest case, suppose (unrealistically) that height is determined by a single gene with two alleles, *A* and *a*. Allele *A* tends to make people tall, whereas allele *a* tends to make them short. If there is no dominance at this locus, then the three possible genotypes (*AA, Aa, aa*) will produce three phenotypes: tall, intermediate, and short, respectively. Assume that the gene frequencies of *A* and *a* are each 0.50. When looking at a population of individuals, the height distribution depicted in Fig. 5.1, *A*, will be observed.

Now suppose, a bit more realistically, that height is determined by two loci instead of one. The second locus also has two alleles, *B* (tall) and *b* (short), and they affect height in exactly the same way as alleles *A* and *a*. There are now nine possible genotypes in our population: *aabb, aaBb, aaBB, Aabb, AaBb, AaBB, AAbb, AABb,* and *AABB*. An individual may have zero, one, two, three, or four "tall" alleles, so now five distinct phenotypes are possible (see Fig. 5.1, *B*). Although the height distribution in this fictional population is still not normal compared with an actual population, it approaches a normal distribution more closely than in the single-gene case just described.

From extension of this example, *many* genes and environmental factors influence height, each having a small effect. Then many phenotypes are possible, each differing slightly from the others, and the height distribution of the population approaches the bell-shaped curve shown in Fig. 5.1, *C*.

It should be emphasized that the individual genes underlying a multifactorial trait such as height follow the mendelian principles of segregation and independent assortment, just like any other gene. The only difference is that many of them *act together* to influence the trait. More than 200 genes have now been shown to be associated with variation in human height.

Blood pressure is another example of a multifactorial trait. A correlation exists between parents' blood pressures (systolic and diastolic) and those of their children. The evidence is good that this correlation is partially caused by genes, but blood pressure is also influenced by environmental factors, such as diet, exercise, and stress. Two goals of genetic research are the identification and measurement of the relative roles of genes and environment in the causation of multifactorial diseases.

Threshold Model

A number of diseases do not follow the bell-shaped distribution. Instead, they appear to be either present or absent in individuals, yet they do not follow the inheritance patterns expected of single-gene diseases. A commonly used explanation for such diseases is that there is an underlying **liability distribution** for the disease in a population (Fig. 5.2). Those individuals who are on the "low" end of the distribution have little chance of developing the disease in question (i.e., they have few of the

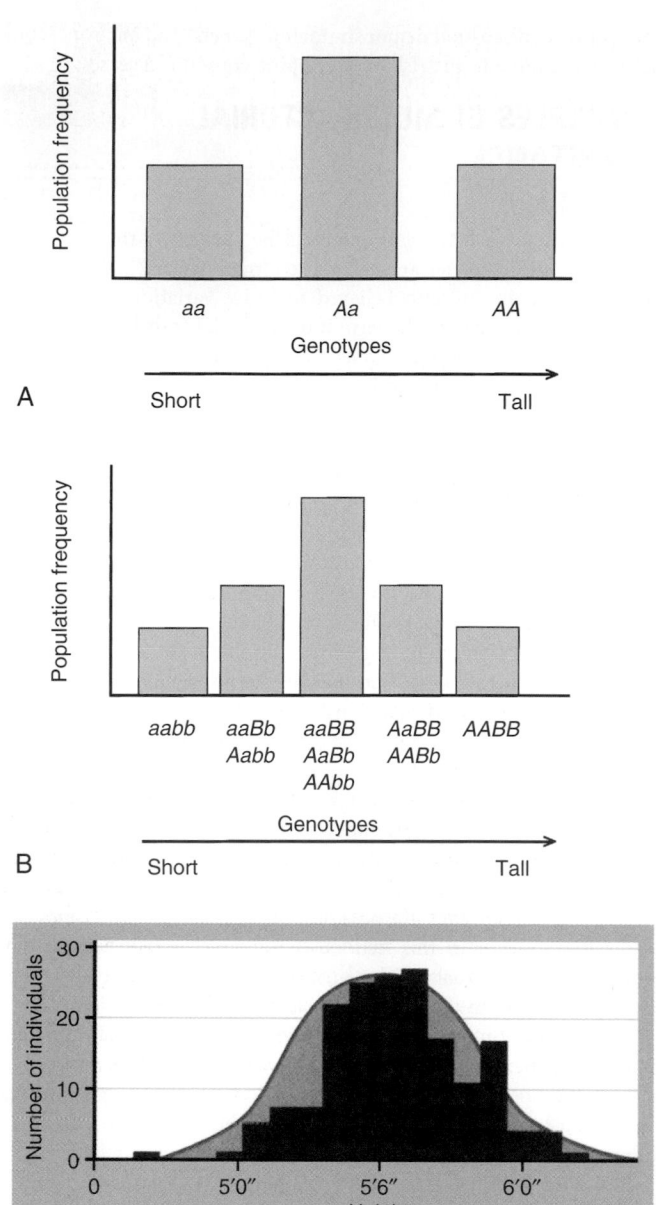

C

FIGURE 5.1 Distribution of Height. A, Distribution of height in a population, assuming that height is controlled by a single locus with genotypes *AA, Aa,* and *aa*. **B,** Distribution of height, assuming that height is controlled by two loci. Five distinct genotypes are shown instead of three, and the distribution begins to look more like the normal distribution. **C,** Height is portrayed, realistically, as a trait with a continuous statistical distribution. Because many genes contribute to height and tend to segregate independently of one another, the cumulative contribution of different combinations of alleles to height forms a continuous distribution of possible heights, in which the extremes are much rarer than the intermediate values. Variation also can be caused by environmental factors such as nutrition. (**A** and **B** adapted from Jorde LB et al: *Medical genetics,* ed 5, Philadelphia, 2016, Elsevier; **C** from Raven PH et al: *Biology,* ed 8, New York, 2008, McGraw-Hill.)

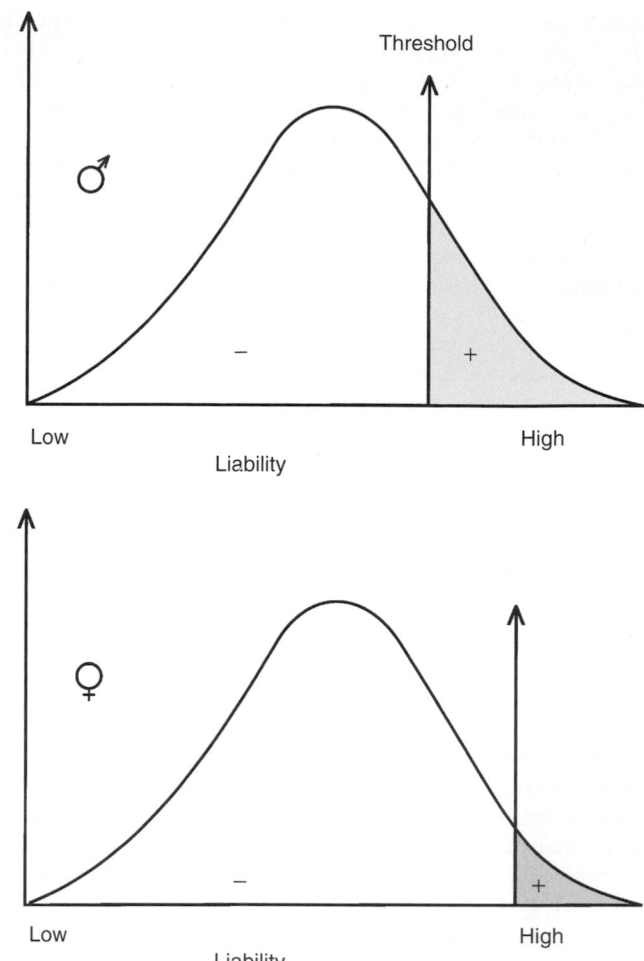

FIGURE 5.2 A Liability Distribution in a Population for a Multifactorial Disease. To be affected with the disease, an individual must exceed the threshold on the liability distribution. This figure shows two thresholds, a lower one for males and a higher one for females (as in pyloric stenosis; see text). (From Jorde LB et al: *Medical genetics,* ed 5, Philadelphia, 2016, Elsevier.)

disease is expressed. Below the threshold, an individual appears normal; above it, he or she is affected by the disease.

A disease that is thought to correspond to this threshold model is *pyloric stenosis*, a disorder that presents shortly after birth and is caused by a narrowing or obstruction of the pylorus, the area between the stomach and intestine. Chronic vomiting, constipation, weight loss, and imbalance of electrolyte levels result from the condition, but it sometimes resolves spontaneously or can be corrected by surgery. The prevalence of pyloric stenosis is about 3 per 1000 live births in whites. It is much more common in males than females, affecting 1 of 200 males and 1 of 1000 females. It is thought that this difference in prevalence reflects two thresholds in the liability distribution—a lower one in males and a higher one in females (see Fig. 5.2). A lower male threshold implies that fewer disease-causing factors are required to generate the disorder in males.

The liability threshold concept may explain the pattern of recurrence risks for pyloric stenosis seen in Table 5.1. Note that males, having a lower threshold, always have a higher risk than females. However, the sibling recurrence risk also depends on the sex of the proband (i.e., the first affected individual diagnosed in a family). It is higher when the proband is female than when the proband is male. This reflects the

alleles or environmental factors that would cause the disease). Individuals who are closer to the "high" end of the distribution have more of the disease-causing genes and environmental factors and are more likely to develop the disease. For diseases that are either present or absent, it is thought that a **threshold of liability** must be crossed before the

TABLE 5.1	RECURRENCE RISKS (%) FOR PYLORIC STENOSIS, SUBDIVIDED BY GENDERS OF AFFECTED PROBANDS AND RELATIVES			
	MALE PROBANDS		**FEMALE PROBANDS**	
RELATIVES	**LONDON**	**BELFAST**	**LONDON**	**BELFAST**
Brothers	3.8	9.6	9.2	12.5
Sisters	2.7	3.0	3.8	3.8

NOTE: The risks differ somewhat between the two populations. Data from Carter CO: *Br Med Bull* 32(1):21–26, 1976.

TABLE 5.2	RECURRENCE RISKS (%) FOR FIRST-, SECOND-, AND THIRD-DEGREE RELATIVES			
	RISK			
DEGREE	**FIRST DEGREE**	**SECOND DEGREE**	**THIRD DEGREE**	**GENERAL POPULATION**
Cleft lip/palate	4	0.7	0.3	0.1
Clubfoot	2.5	0.5	0.2	0.1
Congenital hip dislocation	5	0.6	0.4	0.2

concept that females, having a higher liability threshold, must be exposed to more disease-causing factors than males to develop the disease. Thus a family with an affected female must have more genetic and environmental risk factors, producing a higher recurrence risk for pyloric stenosis in future offspring. It would be expected that the highest risk category would be *male* relatives of *female* probands; Table 5.1 shows that this is the case.

A similar pattern has been observed in studies of *autism spectrum disorder*, a behavioral disorder in which the male to female ratio is approximately 4 : 1. As expected for a multifactorial disorder, the recurrence risk for siblings of male probands (10%) is lower than that of siblings of female probands (12%).[3] When the sex ratio for a disease is reversed (i.e., more affected females than males), one would expect a higher recurrence risk when the proband is male.

A number of other congenital malformations are thought to correspond to this model. They include isolated *cleft lip and/or cleft palate (CL/P), neural tube defects (anencephaly, spina bifida), clubfoot (talipes),* and some forms of congenital heart disease. In this context, "isolated" means that this is the only observed disease feature (i.e., the feature is not part of a larger constellation of findings, as in CL/P secondary to trisomy 13). In addition, many common adult diseases, such as *hypertension, coronary heart disease, stroke, diabetes mellitus* (types 1 and 2), and *some cancers,* are caused by complex genetic and environmental factors and can thus be considered multifactorial diseases.

Recurrence Risks and Transmission Patterns

Whereas sibling recurrence risks can be given with confidence for single-gene diseases (e.g., 50% for typical autosomal dominant diseases, 25% for autosomal recessive diseases), the situation is more complicated for multifactorial diseases. This is because the number of genes contributing to the disease is usually not known, the precise allelic constitution of the parents is not known, and the extent of environmental effects can vary substantially. For most multifactorial diseases, empirical risks (i.e., risks based on direct observation of data) have been derived. To estimate empirical risks, a large series of families is examined in which one child has developed the disease (the proband). Then the siblings of each proband are surveyed to calculate the percentage of siblings who also have developed the disease. For example, in the United States about 3% of siblings of individuals with neural tube defects also have neural tube defects (Box 5.1). Thus the recurrence risk for parents who have had one child with a neural tube defect is 3% in the United States. For conditions such as CL/P that are not lethal or severely debilitating, recurrence risks also can be estimated for the offspring of affected parents. Because each multifactorial disease has different numbers and types of risk factors, empirical recurrence risks vary for each disease.

In contrast to most single-gene diseases, recurrence risks for multifactorial diseases can change substantially from one population to another because gene frequencies as well as environmental factors can differ among populations (note the differences between the London and Belfast populations in Table 5.1).

It is sometimes difficult to distinguish polygenic or multifactorial diseases from single-gene diseases that have reduced penetrance or variable expression. Large data sets and good epidemiologic data are necessary to make the distinction. Several criteria are commonly used to define multifactorial inheritance.

First, *the recurrence risk becomes higher if more than one family member is affected.* For example, the sibling recurrence risk for a *ventricular septal defect* (VSD, a type of congenital heart defect) is 3% if one sibling has been affected by a VSD but increases to approximately 10% if two siblings have been diagnosed with VSDs.[4] The same trend is seen for other multifactorial diseases like neural tube defects and autism. In contrast, the recurrence risk for single-gene diseases remains the same regardless of the number of affected siblings. It should be emphasized that this increase does not mean that the family's risk has actually *changed.* Rather, it means that there is more information about the family's true risk; because they have had two affected children, they are probably located higher on the liability distribution than a family with only one affected child. In other words, they have more risk factors (genetic or environmental) and are more likely to produce an affected child.

Second, *if the expression of the disease in the proband is more severe, the recurrence risk is higher.* This is again consistent with the liability model because a more severe expression indicates that the affected individual is at the extreme tail end of the liability distribution (see Fig. 5.2). His or her relatives are thus at a higher risk for inheriting disease genes. For example, the occurrence of a bilateral (both sides) CL/P confers a higher recurrence risk on family members than does the occurrence of a unilateral (one side) cleft.

Third, *the recurrence risk is higher if the proband is of the less commonly affected sex* (see the preceding discussion of pyloric stenosis). This is because an affected individual of the less susceptible sex is usually at a more extreme position on the liability distribution.

Fourth, *the recurrence risk for the disease usually decreases rapidly in more remotely related relatives* (Table 5.2). Whereas the recurrence risk for single-gene diseases decreases by 50% with each degree of relationship (e.g., an autosomal dominant disease has a 50% recurrence risk for siblings, 25% for uncle-nephew relationships, 12.5% for first cousins), it decreases much more quickly for multifactorial diseases. This reflects the fact that many genes and environmental factors must combine to produce a trait. All the necessary risk factors are unlikely to be present in less closely related family members.

Finally, *if the prevalence of the disease in a population is f, the risk for offspring and siblings of probands is approximately* $\sqrt{f}$. This does not hold true for single-gene traits because their recurrence risks are largely

BOX 5.1   NEURAL TUBE DEFECTS

Neural tube defects (NTDs), which include *anencephaly*, *spina bifida*, and *encephalocele* (as well as several other less common forms), are one of the most important classes of birth defects, and they are seen in 0.5 to 2 of 1000 pregnancies. The prevalence of NTDs among different populations varies considerably, with an especially high rate among some northern Chinese populations (as high as 6 or more per 1000 births). The prevalence of NTDs has been decreasing in many parts of the United States and Europe during the past three decades, partly because of dietary changes.

Normally the neural tube closes at about the fourth week of gestation. A defect in closure, or a subsequent reopening of the neural tube, results in a neural tube defect. Spina bifida (Fig. 5.3, A) is the most commonly observed NTD and consists of a protrusion of spinal tissue through the vertebral column (the tissue usually includes meninges, spinal cord, and nerve roots). About 75% of individuals with spina bifida have secondary hydrocephalus, which sometimes in turn produces intellectual disability. Paralysis or muscle weakness, lack of sphincter control, and clubfeet are often observed. A study conducted in British Columbia showed that survival rates for people with spina bifida have improved dramatically over the past several decades. Less than 30% of people born between 1952 and 1969 survived to 10 years of age, whereas 65% of those born between 1970 and 1986 survived to this age. Anencephaly (see Fig. 5.3, *B*) is characterized by partial or complete absence of the cranial vault and calvarium and partial or complete absence of the cerebral hemispheres. At least two-thirds of newborns with anencephaly are stillborn; term deliveries do not survive more than a few hours or days.

NTDs are thought to arise from a combination of genetic and environmental factors. In most populations surveyed thus far, empirical recurrence risks for siblings of affected people range from 2% to 5%. Consistent with a multifactorial model, the recurrence risk increases with additional affected siblings. Studies conducted in Great Britain showed that the sibling recurrence risk was approximately 5% when one sibling was affected and 10% when two were affected. A Hungarian study showed that the overall prevalence of NTDs was 1 in 300 births and that the sibling recurrence risks were 3%, 12%, and 25% after one, two, and three affected offspring, respectively. Recurrence risks tend to be slightly lower in populations with lower NTD prevalence rates, as predicted by the multifactorial model. Recurrence risk data support the idea that the major forms of NTDs are caused by similar factors. An anencephalic conception increases the recurrence risk for subsequent spina bifida conceptions, and vice versa.

NTDs can usually be diagnosed prenatally, sometimes by ultrasound and usually by an elevation in α-fetoprotein (AFP) level in the maternal serum or amniotic fluid (see Chapter 20). A spina bifida lesion can be either open or closed (i.e., covered with a layer of skin). Fetuses with open spina bifida are more likely to be detected by AFP assays.

A major epidemiologic finding is that mothers who supplement their diet with folic acid at the time of conception are less likely to produce children with NTDs. This result has been replicated in several different populations and thus appears to be well confirmed. It has been estimated that as many as 50% to 70% of NTDs can be avoided simply by dietary folic acid supplementation. (Traditional prenatal vitamin supplements have little effect because administration does not usually begin until well after the time that the neural tube closes.) It is now recommended that all women of reproductive age supplement their diet with 0.4 mg of folic acid each day; many foods in the United States are supplemented with folic acid. Consequently, average folate levels in U.S. females have doubled, and the incidence of neural tube defects has declined by 30% to 50% in the past decade.

Because mothers would be likely to ingest similar amounts of folic acid from one pregnancy to the next, folic acid deficiency could well account for at least part of the elevated sibling recurrence risk for NTDs. This is an important example of a *nongenetic* factor that contributes to familial clustering of a disease. It is likely that there is genetic variation in response to folic acid, which helps to explain why most mothers with folic acid deficiency do not bear children with NTDs and why some who ingest adequate amounts of folic acid nonetheless bear children with NTDs. To address this issue, researchers are testing for associations between NTDs and variants in several genes whose products (e.g., methylene tetrahydrofolate reductase) are involved in folic acid metabolism.

Data from Copp AJ, Stanier P, Greene NDE: *Lancet Neurol* 12:799–810, 2013; Daly LE et al: *JAMA* 274(21):1698–1702, 1995.

---

independent of population prevalence. It is not an absolute rule for multifactorial traits either, but many such diseases tend to conform to this prediction. Examination of the risks given in Table 5.2 shows that the first three diseases follow the prediction fairly well. However, the observed sibling risk for the fourth disease, infantile autism, is substantially higher than that predicted by $\sqrt{f}$.

NATURE AND NURTURE: DISENTANGLING THE EFFECTS OF GENES AND ENVIRONMENT

Family members share genes and a common environment. Family resemblance in traits such as blood pressure reflects both genes (nature) and environment (nurture). For centuries people have debated the relative importance of these two types of factors. It is a mistake, of course, to view them as mutually exclusive. Few traits are influenced only by genes or only by environmental factors. Most are influenced by both. It is useful to try to determine the *relative* influence of genetic and environmental factors (Fig. 5.4). This can lead to a better understanding of disease etiology. It can also help in planning public health strategies. A disease in which the genetic influence is relatively small, such as lung cancer, may be prevented most effectively through emphasis on lifestyle changes (avoidance of tobacco). When a disease has a relatively larger genetic component, as in breast cancer, examination of family history should be emphasized in addition to lifestyle modification. Here, two

research strategies are reviewed that often are used to estimate the relative influence of genes and environment: twin studies and adoption studies.

Twin Studies

Twins occur with a frequency of about 1 in 100 births in white populations. They are a bit more common in blacks and a bit less common among Asians. **Monozygotic (MZ, identical) twins** originate when the developing embryo divides to form two separate but identical embryos. Because they are genetically identical, MZ twins are an example of natural clones. **Dizygotic (DZ, fraternal) twins** are the result of a double ovulation followed by the fertilization of each egg by a different sperm. Thus dizygotic twins are genetically no more similar than siblings. Because two different sperm cells are required to fertilize the two eggs, it is possible for each DZ twin to have a different father. Whereas MZ twinning rates are constant across populations, DZ twinning rates vary somewhat. DZ twinning increases with maternal age until about 40 years, after which it declines.

Because MZ twins are genetically identical, any differences between them should be caused only by environmental effects.[5] MZ twins should thus resemble one another very closely for traits that are strongly influenced by genes. DZ twins provide a convenient comparison because their environmental differences should be similar to those of MZ twins, but their genetic differences are as great as those between siblings. Twin studies thus usually consist of comparisons between MZ and DZ twins.[6]

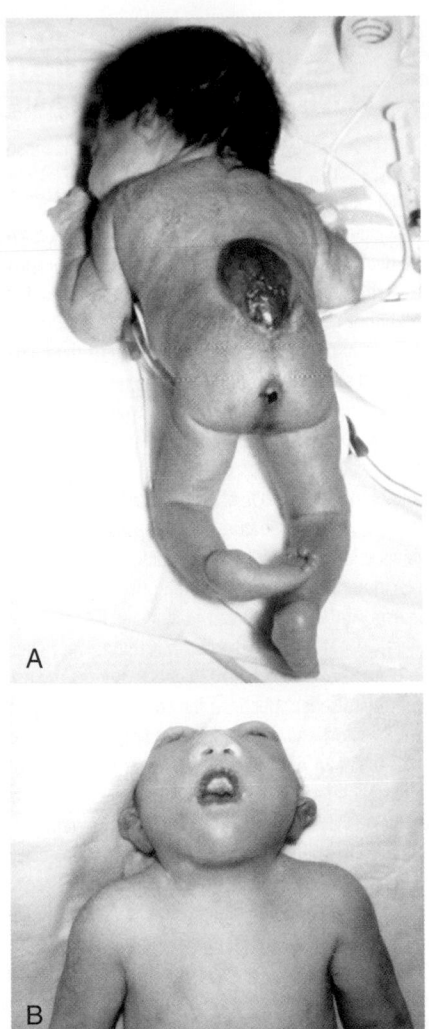

A

B

FIGURE 5.3 Spina Bifida and Anencephaly. **A,** Spina bifida in a newborn. **B,** Anencephaly, showing the absence of the cranial vault. (From Jones KL: *Smith's recognizable patterns of human malformation,* ed 6, Philadelphia, Saunders, 2006, p. 705.)

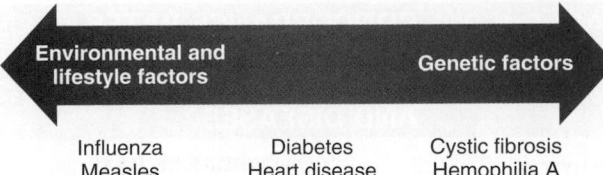

Environmental and lifestyle factors		Genetic factors
Influenza	Diabetes	Cystic fibrosis
Measles	Heart disease	Hemophilia A

FIGURE 5.4 Continuum of Genetic Diseases. Some diseases (e.g., cystic fibrosis) are strongly determined by genes, whereas others (e.g., infectious diseases) are strongly determined by environmental factors. (Adapted from Jorde LB et al: *Medical genetics,* ed 5, Philadelphia, 2016, Elsevier.)

If both members of a twin pair share a trait (e.g., a cleft lip), they are said to be **concordant**. If they do not share the trait, they are **discordant**. For a trait determined totally by genes, MZ twins should always be concordant, whereas DZ twins should be concordant less often, because they, like full siblings, share only 50% of their DNA. Concordance rates may differ between opposite-sex DZ twin pairs and same-sex DZ pairs for some traits, such as those that have different frequencies in males and females. For such traits, only same-sex DZ twin pairs should be used when comparing MZ and DZ concordance rates, because MZ twins are necessarily of the same sex.

Table 5.3 gives concordance rates for a number of traits. Note that the concordance rates for contagious diseases such as measles are quite similar in MZ and DZ twins. This is expected because a contagious disease is unlikely to be influenced markedly by genes. On the other hand, the concordance rates are quite dissimilar for *schizophrenia* and *bipolar affective disorder,* suggesting a sizable genetic component for these diseases. The MZ correlations for dermatoglyphics (fingerprints), which are determined almost entirely by genes, are close to 1.0.

At one time, twins were thought to provide a perfect "natural laboratory" in which to determine the relative influences of genetics and environment, but several difficulties arose. One of the most important is the assumption that the environments of MZ and DZ twins are equally similar. As one would expect, MZ twins are often treated more similarly than DZ twins. A greater similarity in environment can make MZ twins more concordant for a trait, inflating the apparent influence of genes. In addition, MZ twins may be more likely to seek the same type of environment, further reinforcing environmental similarity. On the other hand, it has been suggested that MZ twins tend to develop personality differences in an attempt to assert their individuality.

Adoption Studies

Studies of adopted children also are used to estimate the genetic contribution to a multifactorial trait. Children born to parents who have a disease but are then subsequently adopted by parents lacking the disease can be studied to find out whether these children develop the disease. In some cases such children develop the disease more often than a comparative control population (i.e., adopted children who were born to parents who do *not* have the disease). This provides some evidence that genes may be involved in the causation of the disease, because the adopted children do not share an environment with their affected natural parents. For example, about 8% to 10% of adopted children of a schizophrenic parent develop *schizophrenia,* whereas only 1% of adopted children of unaffected parents develop schizophrenia.

As with twin studies, several precautions must be exercised in interpreting the results of adoption studies. First, prenatal environmental influences could have long-lasting effects on an adopted child. Second, children are sometimes adopted after they are several years old, ensuring that some environmental influence would have been imparted by the natural parents. Finally, adoption agencies sometimes try to match the adoptive parents with the natural parents in terms of background, socioeconomic status, and other factors. All of these factors could exaggerate the apparent influence of biologic inheritance.

These reservations, as well as those summarized for twin studies, underscore the need for caution in basing conclusions on twin and adoption studies. These approaches do not provide definitive measures of the role of genes in multifactorial disease, nor can they identify specific genes responsible for disease. Instead, they serve a useful purpose in providing a preliminary indication of the extent to which a multifactorial disease may be caused by genetic factors. Sophisticated molecular techniques are being used to identify the specific genes that underlie predisposition to multifactorial diseases.

This discussion should make clear that most common diseases are not the result of either genetics *or* environment. Instead, genetic and nongenetic factors usually interact to influence one's likelihood of developing a common disease. In some cases a genetic predisposition may interact with an environmental factor to increase the risk of disease acquisition to a much higher level than would either factor acting alone. A good example of a **gene-environment interaction** is given by α_1-antitrypsin deficiency, a genetic condition that causes pulmonary emphysema and is greatly exacerbated by cigarette smoking (Box 5.2).

TABLE 5.3	CONCORDANCE RATES IN MZ AND DZ TWINS FOR SELECTED TRAITS AND DISEASES		
TRAIT OR DISEASE	**CONCORDANCE RATE**		
	MZ TWINS	**DZ TWINS**	**HERITABILITY**
Affective disorder (bipolar)	0.79	0.24	>1*
Affective disorder (unipolar)	0.54	0.19	0.7
Alcoholism	>0.6	<0.3	0.6
Autism	0.92	0	>1
Blood pressure (diastolic)†	0.58	0.27	0.62
Blood pressure (systolic)†	0.55	0.25	0.6
Body fat percentage†	0.73	0.22	>1
Body mass index†	0.95	0.53	0.84
Cleft lip/palate	0.38	0.08	0.6
Clubfoot	0.32	0.03	0.58
Dermatoglyphics (finger ridge count)†	0.95	0.49	0.92
Diabetes mellitus	0.45–0.96	0.03–0.37	>1
Diabetes mellitus (type 1)	0.55	–	–
Diabetes mellitus (type 2)	0.9	–	–
Epilepsy (idiopathic)	0.69	0.14	>1
Height†	0.94	0.44	1
Intelligence quotient (IQ)†	0.76	0.51	0.5
Measles	0.95	0.87	0.16
Multiple sclerosis	0.28	0.03	0.5
Myocardial infarction (males)	0.39	0.26	0.26
Myocardial infarction (females)	0.44	0.14	0.6
Schizophrenia	0.47	0.12	0.7
Spina bifida	0.72	0.33	0.78

NOTE: Heritability, which is defined as the proportion of the variation in a trait that is due to genetic factors, can be measured as $2(C_{MZ} - C_{DZ})$, where C_{MZ} and C_{DZ} are the concordance rates for MZ twins and DZ twins, respectively. These figures were compiled from a large variety of sources and represent primarily European and U.S. populations.
*Several heritability estimates exceed 1. Because it is impossible for >100% of the variance of a trait to be genetically determined, these values indicate that other factors, such as shared environmental factors, must be operating.
†Because these are quantitative traits, correlation coefficients are given rather than concordance rates.
DZ, Dizygotic; *MZ*, monozygotic.

BOX 5.2 α_1-ANTITRYPSIN DEFICIENCY: THE INTERACTION OF GENES AND ENVIRONMENT-LIFESTYLE

α_1-Antitrypsin (AAT) deficiency is one of the most common autosomal recessive disorders among whites, affecting approximately 1 in 2500 members of this ethnic group. AAT, synthesized primarily in the liver, is a serine protease inhibitor. It does bind trypsin, as its name suggests. However, AAT binds much more strongly to neutrophil elastase, a protease that is produced by neutrophils (a type of leukocyte) in response to infections and irritants. It carries out its binding and inhibitory role primarily in the lower respiratory tract, where it prevents elastase from digesting the alveolar septi of the lung.

Individuals with less than 10% to 15% of the normal level of AAT activity will experience significant lung damage and typically develop emphysema during their 30s, 40s, or 50s. In addition, at least 10% develop liver cirrhosis as a result of the accumulation of variant AAT molecules in the liver; AAT deficiency accounts for nearly 20% of all nonalcoholic liver cirrhosis cases in the United States. An important feature of this disease is that cigarette smokers with AAT deficiency develop emphysema much earlier than do nonsmokers. This is because cigarette smoke irritates lung tissue, increasing secretion of neutrophil elastase. At the same time it inactivates AAT, so there is also less inhibition of elastase. One study showed that the median age of survival of nonsmokers with AAT deficiency was 62 years, whereas it was only 40 years for smokers with this disease. Because the combination of cigarette smoking (an environmental factor) and the AAT mutation (a genetic factor) produces more severe disease than either factor alone, it is an example of a gene-environment interaction.

Typically, AAT deficiency is tested first by a straightforward assay for reduced serum AAT concentration. Because a variety of conditions can reduce serum AAT level, additional testing, through a type of protein electrophoresis or DNA testing, is carried out to confirm a diagnosis of AAT deficiency. Direct DNA testing became feasible with the identification of *SERPINA1*, the gene that encodes AAT. More than 100 *SERPINA1* mutations have been identified, but only 2 missense variants, labeled the *S* and *Z* alleles, are common and clinically significant. Approximately 95% of cases of AAT deficiency are either *ZZ* homozygotes or *SZ* compound heterozygotes. The latter genotype generally produces less severe disease symptoms. Two large studies have indicated that the risk of developing emphysema among *ZZ* homozygotes is 70% for nonsmokers and 90% for smokers.

Data from Abboud RT et al: *Appl Clin Genet* 4:55–65, 2011; Stockley RA, Turner AM: *Trends Mol Med* 20:105–115, 2014.

GENETICS OF COMMON DISEASES

Some common multifactorial disorders, the congenital malformations, are by definition present at birth. Others, including heart disease, cancer, diabetes, and most psychiatric disorders, are seen primarily in adolescents and adults. Because these disorders are complex, unraveling their genetics is a daunting task. Nonetheless, significant progress is being made.

Congenital Malformations

Congenital diseases are present at birth. Approximately 2% of newborns present with a congenital malformation; most of these are multifactorial in etiology. Table 5.4 lists some more common congenital malformations. Sibling recurrence risks for most of these disorders range from 1% to 5%.

Some congenital malformations, such as CL/P and pyloric stenosis, are relatively easy to repair and thus are not considered to be serious problems. Others, such as neural tube defects, usually have more severe consequences. Although some cases of congenital malformations occur in the absence of any other problems, it is quite common for them to be associated with other disorders. For example, hydrocephaly and

TABLE 5.4	PREVALENCE RATES OF COMMON CONGENITAL MALFORMATIONS IN WHITES

DISORDER	PREVALENCE PER 1000 BIRTHS (APPROXIMATE)
Cleft lip/palate	1
Clubfoot	1
Congenital heart defects	4–8
Hydrocephaly	0.5–2.5
Isolated cleft palate	0.4
Neural tube defects	1–3
Pyloric stenosis	3

TABLE 5.5	PREVALENCE OF COMMON ADULT DISEASES IN THE UNITED STATES

DISEASE	NUMBER AFFECTED (APPROXIMATE)
Alcoholism	14 million
Alzheimer disease	4 million
Arthritis	43 million
Asthma	17 million
Cancer	8 million
Cardiovascular disease (all forms)	
Coronary artery disease	13 million
Congestive heart failure	5 million
Congenital defects	1 million
Hypertension	50 million
Stroke	5 million
Depression and bipolar disorder	17 million
Diabetes (type 1)	1 million
Diabetes (type 2)	15 million
Epilepsy	2.5 million
Multiple sclerosis	350,000
Obesity*	60 million
Parkinson disease	500,000
Psoriasis	3–5 million
Schizophrenia	2 million

*Body mass index >30.
Data from National Center for Chronic Disease Prevention and Health Promotion; American Heart Association (*2002 Heart and Stroke Statistical Update);* National Institute on Alcohol Abuse and Alcoholism; Office of the U.S. Surgeon General; American Academy of Allergy, Asthma and Immunology; Cown WM, Kandel ER: *JAMA* 285:594–600, 2001; Flegal et al: *JAMA* 288:1723–1727, 2002.

clubfoot are often seen secondary to spina bifida, CL/P is often seen in babies with trisomy 13, and congenital heart defects are seen in children with many other disorders, including Down syndrome.

Environmental factors also cause some congenital malformations. An example is thalidomide, a sedative used during pregnancy in the early 1960s. When ingested during early pregnancy this drug often caused phocomelia (severely shortened limbs) in babies. Maternal exposure to retinoic acid, which is used to treat acne, can cause congenital defects of the heart, ear, and central nervous system. Maternal rubella infection can cause congenital heart defects.

Multifactorial Disorders in the Adult Population

Until quite recently, very little was known about specific genes responsible for common adult diseases. With the more powerful laboratory and analytic techniques now available, this situation is changing. This section reviews recent progress in understanding the genetics of the major common adult diseases. Table 5.5 gives approximate prevalence figures for these disorders in the United States.

Coronary Heart Disease

It is well known that coronary heart disease (CHD) is the leading killer of Americans, accounting for approximately 25% of all deaths in the United States. It is caused by *atherosclerosis* (narrowing as a result of the formation of lipid-laden lesions) of the coronary arteries. This narrowing impedes blood flow to the heart and can eventually result in a *myocardial infarction* (destruction of heart tissue caused by an inadequate supply of oxygen). When atherosclerosis occurs in arteries supplying blood to the brain, a *stroke* can result. Many risk factors for heart disease have been identified, including obesity, cigarette smoking, hypertension, elevated cholesterol level, and positive family history (usually defined as having one or more affected first-degree relatives). Many studies have examined the role of family history in CHD, and they show that an individual with a positive family history is two to seven times more likely to have heart disease than is an individual with no family history (this would be the relative risk of heart disease as a result of a positive family history). Generally, these studies also show that the risk increases if (1) there are more affected relatives; (2) the affected relative or relatives are female (the less commonly affected sex) rather than male; and (3) the age of onset in the affected relative is early (before 55 years). For example, one study showed that men between the ages of 20 and 39 years had a relative risk of 3 for CHD if they had one affected first-degree relative. The relative risk increased to 13 if two first-degree relatives were affected with CHD before 55 years of age.[7]

What part do genes play in the familial clustering of heart disease? Because of the key role of lipids in atherosclerosis, many studies are focusing on the genetic determination of various lipoproteins.[8] An important advance in this area has been the identification of several genes that encode the processing of low-density lipoproteins and that, when mutated, can cause *familial hypercholesterolemia* (Box 5.3). Many other genes involved in lipid variation, coagulation, and hypertension have been identified, including several genes encoding apolipoproteins (the protein components of lipoproteins) (Table 5.6).[9] Functional analysis of these genes is leading to an increased understanding, and eventually more effective treatment, of CHD.

Environmental factors, many of which are easily modified, are also important causes of CHD. Abundant epidemiologic evidence shows that cigarette smoking and obesity increase the risk of CHD, whereas exercise and a diet low in saturated fats decrease the risk. Indeed, the approximate 50% decline in CHD prevalence in the United States during the past 40 years is usually attributed to a decrease in the proportion of adults who smoke cigarettes, a decreased consumption of saturated fats, and an increased emphasis on exercise and a generally healthier lifestyle.

BOX 5.3   FAMILIAL HYPERCHOLESTEROLEMIA

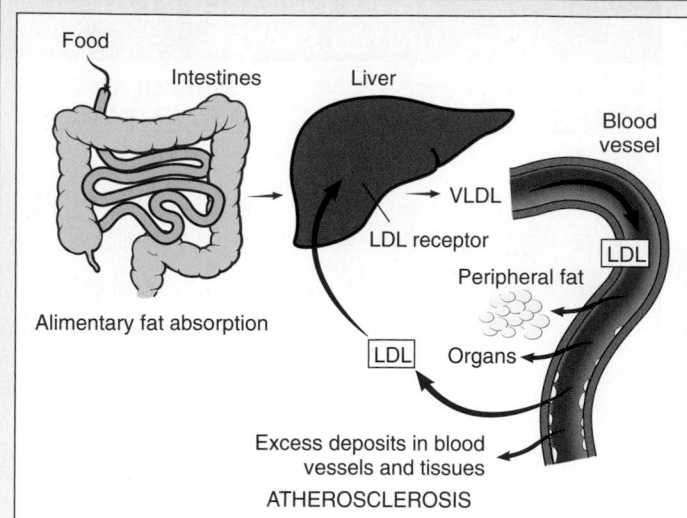

surface but incapable of normal binding to LDL. Class 4 mutations, which are comparatively rare, produce receptors that are normal except that they do not migrate specifically to coated pits and thus cannot carry LDL into the cell. The final group of mutations, class 5, produces an LDL receptor that cannot dissociate from the LDL particle after entry into the cell. The receptor cannot return to the cell surface and is degraded. Each class of mutations reduces the number of effective LDL receptors, resulting in decreased LDL uptake and hence elevated levels of circulating cholesterol. The number of effective receptors is reduced by about half in FH heterozygotes, and homozygotes have virtually no functional LDL receptors.

Understanding the defects that lead to FH has helped to develop effective therapies for the disorder. Dietary reduction of cholesterol (primarily through the reduced intake of saturated fats) has only modest effects on cholesterol levels in FH heterozygotes. Because cholesterol is reabsorbed into the gut and then recycled through the liver (where most cholesterol synthesis takes place), serum cholesterol levels can be reduced by the administration of bile acid–absorbing resins, such as cholestyramine. The absorbed cholesterol is then excreted. It is interesting that reduced recirculation from the gut causes the liver cells to form additional LDL receptors, lowering circulating cholesterol levels. However, the decrease in the concentration of intracellular cholesterol also stimulates cholesterol synthesis by liver cells, so the overall reduction in plasma LDL level is only about 15% to 20%. This treatment is much more effective when combined with agents that reduce cholesterol synthesis by inhibiting 3-hydroxy-3-methylglutaryl coenzyme A (HMG-CoA) reductase (the "statin" class of drugs). Decreased synthesis leads to further production of LDL receptors. When these therapies are used in combination, serum cholesterol levels in FH heterozygotes can be reduced to approximately normal levels.

The picture is less encouraging for FH homozygotes. The therapies just discussed can enhance cholesterol elimination and reduce its synthesis, but they are largely ineffective because homozygotes have few or no LDL receptors. Liver transplants, which provide hepatocytes that have normal LDL receptors, have been successful in some cases, but this option is often limited by a lack of donors. Plasma exchange, carried out every 1 to 2 weeks, in combination with drug therapy, can reduce cholesterol levels by about 50%. However, this therapy is difficult to continue for long periods. Somatic cell gene therapy, in which hepatocytes carrying normal LDL receptor genes are introduced into the portal circulation, is now being tested. It may eventually prove to be an effective treatment for FH homozygotes.

FH also can be caused by inherited mutations in the gene that encodes apolipoprotein B. In addition, a small number of FH cases are caused by mutations in the gene that encodes PCSK9 (proprotein convertase subtilisin/kexin type 9), an enzyme that plays a key role in degrading LDL receptors. Gain-of-function mutations in the *PCSK9* gene reduce the number of LDL receptors, causing FH. Loss-of-function mutations in this gene can increase the number of LDL receptors, resulting in exceptionally low circulating LDL levels. These findings have led to the development of drugs that inhibit PCSK9 activity, thus lowering LDL cholesterol levels. These drugs, which have been approved for clinical use, can reduce LDL cholesterol levels by approximately 50% in the general population of persons with hypercholesterolemia and produce significant effects even in those who are using statin drugs.

The FH story illustrates how medical research has made important contributions both to our understanding of basic cell biology and to our advances in clinical therapy. The process of receptor-mediated endocytosis, elucidated largely by research on the LDL receptor defects, is of fundamental significance for cellular processes throughout the body. Equally important is that this research, by clarifying how cholesterol synthesis and uptake can be modified, has led to significant improvements in therapy for this important cause of heart disease. The discovery of rare mutations in PCSK9 has led to PCSK9 inhibitor drugs that may benefit millions of persons with high cholesterol levels.

Autosomal dominant familial hypercholesterolemia (FH) is an important cause of heart disease, accounting for approximately 5% of myocardial infarctions in individuals less than 60 years of age. FH is one of the most common autosomal dominant disorders: in most populations surveyed to date, about 1 in 500 people is a heterozygote. Plasma cholesterol levels are approximately twice as high as normal (i.e., about 300 to 400 mg/dL), resulting in substantially accelerated atherosclerosis and distinctive cholesterol deposits in skin and tendons (*xanthomas* [Fig. 5.5]). Data compiled from five studies showed that approximately 75% of men with FH developed coronary disease, and 50% had a fatal myocardial infarction by 60 years. The corresponding percentages for women were lower (45% and 15%) because women generally develop heart disease at a later age than men.

Consistent with Hardy-Weinberg predictions, about 1 in 1 million births is homozygous for the FH gene. Homozygotes are much more severely affected, with cholesterol levels ranging from 600 to 1200 mg/dL. Most experience myocardial infarctions before 20 years of age, and a myocardial infarction at 18 months of age has been reported. If untreated, most FH homozygotes die before 30 years of age.

All cells require cholesterol as a component of their plasma membrane. They can either synthesize their own cholesterol or, preferably, obtain it from the extracellular environment, where it is carried primarily by low-density lipoprotein (LDL). In a process known as *endocytosis,* LDL-bound cholesterol is taken into the cell via LDL receptors on the cell's surface (Fig. 5.6). FH is most commonly caused by a reduction in the number of functional LDL receptors on cell surfaces. Lacking the normal number of LDL receptors, cellular cholesterol uptake is reduced and circulating cholesterol levels increase.

Much of what we know about endocytosis has been learned through the study of LDL receptors. The process of endocytosis and the processing of LDL in the cell are described in detail in Fig. 5.6 (endocytosis is discussed in Chapter 1). These processes result in a fine-tuned regulation of cholesterol levels within cells, and they influence the level of circulating cholesterol as well.

The identification of the LDL receptor gene in 1984 was critical in understanding exactly how LDL receptor defects cause FH. More than 1000 different mutations, including missense and nonsense substitutions as well as insertions and deletions, have been identified in the LDL receptor gene. These can be grouped into five broad classes according to their effects on the activity of the receptor. Class 1 mutations result in no detectable protein product. Thus, heterozygotes would produce only half the normal number of LDL receptors. Class 2 mutations in the LDL receptor gene result in production of the LDL receptor, but it is altered such that it cannot leave the endoplasmic reticulum. It is eventually degraded. Class 3 mutations produce an LDL receptor that is capable of migrating to the cell

VLDL, very-low-density lipoprotein.
Data from Brautbar A et al: *Curr Atheroscler Rep* 17:491, 2015; Roberts R: *Trends Cardiovasc Med* 64(23):2525–2540, 2014; Varret MM et al: *Clin Genet* 73(1):1–13, 2008.

Hypertension

Systemic hypertension, which has a worldwide prevalence of approximately 25% to 30%, is a key risk factor for heart disease, stroke, and kidney disease. Studies of blood pressure correlations within families indicate that about 20% to 40% of the variation in both systolic and diastolic blood pressure is caused by genetic factors. The fact that this figure is substantially less than 100% indicates that environmental factors also must be important causes of blood pressure variation. The most important environmental risk factors for hypertension are increased sodium intake, decreased physical activity, psychosocial stress, and obesity (but, as discussed later, the latter factor is itself influenced by both genes and environment).

Blood pressure regulation is a highly complex process that is influenced by many physiologic systems, including various aspects of kidney function, cellular ion transport, and heart function.[10] Because of this complexity, much research is now focused on specific components that may influence blood pressure variation, such as the renin-angiotensin system (involved in sodium reabsorption and vasoconstriction), vasodilators such as nitric oxide and the kallikrein-kinin system, and ion-transport systems such as adducin and sodium-lithium countertransport (Fig. 5.7). These individual factors are more likely to be under the control of smaller numbers of genes than is blood pressure itself, simplifying the task of identifying these genes and their role in blood pressure regulation. For example, linkage and association studies have implicated several genes involved in the renin-angiotensin system (e.g., the genes that encode angiotensinogen, angiotensin-converting enzyme, angiotensin receptors) in the causation of hypertension.

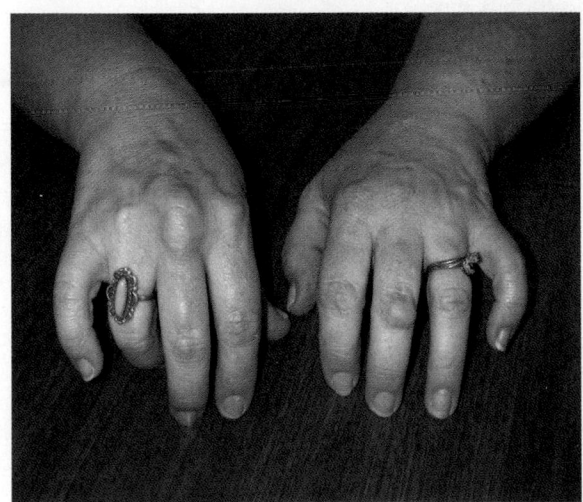

FIGURE 5.5 Xanthoma. Fatty deposits, referred to as xanthomas as seen here on the knuckles, are often noted in individuals with familial hypercholesterolemia. (From Jorde LB et al: *Medical genetics,* ed 5, Philadelphia, 2016, Elsevier.)

Cancer

Cancer is the second leading cause of death in the United States. It is well established that many major types of cancer (e.g., breast, colon, prostate, ovarian) cluster strongly in families. This is caused by both inherited genes and shared environmental factors. Although numerous cancer-causing genes are being isolated,[11] environmental factors also play an important role in causing cancer. In particular, tobacco use is estimated to account for one-third of all cancer cases in the United States, making it the most important known cause of cancer.[12] Typically,

TABLE 5.6	LIPOPROTEIN GENES KNOWN TO CONTRIBUTE TO CORONARY ARTERY DISEASE RISK	
GENE	**CHROMOSOME LOCATION**	**FUNCTION OF PROTEIN PRODUCT**
Apolipoprotein A-I	11q	HDL component; LCAT cofactor
Apolipoprotein A-IV	11q	Component of chylomicrons and HDL; may influence HDL metabolism
Apolipoprotein C-III	11q	Allelic variation associated with hypertriglyceridemia
Apolipoprotein B	2p	Ligand for LDL receptor; involved in formation of VLDL, LDL, IDL, and chylomicrons
Apolipoprotein D	2p	HDL component
Apolipoprotein C-I	19q	LCAT activation
Apolipoprotein C-II	19q	Lipoprotein lipase activation
Apolipoprotein E	19q	Ligand for LDL receptor
Apolipoprotein A-II	1p	HDL component
LDL receptor	19p	Uptake of circulating LDL particles
Lipoprotein(a)	6q	Cholesterol transport
Lipoprotein lipase	8p	Hydrolysis of lipoprotein lipids
Hepatic triglyceride lipase	15q	Hydrolysis of lipoprotein lipids
LCAT	16q	Cholesterol esterification
Cholesterol ester transfer protein	16q	Facilitates transfer of cholesterol esters and phospholipids between lipoproteins

HDL, High-density lipoprotein; *IDL,* intermediate-density lipoprotein; *LCAT,* lecithin cholesterol acyltransferase; *LDL,* low-density lipoprotein; *VLDL,* very-low-density lipoprotein.
Adapted in part from King RA, Rotter JI, editors: *The genetic basis of common diseases,* ed 2, New York, 2002, Oxford University Press.

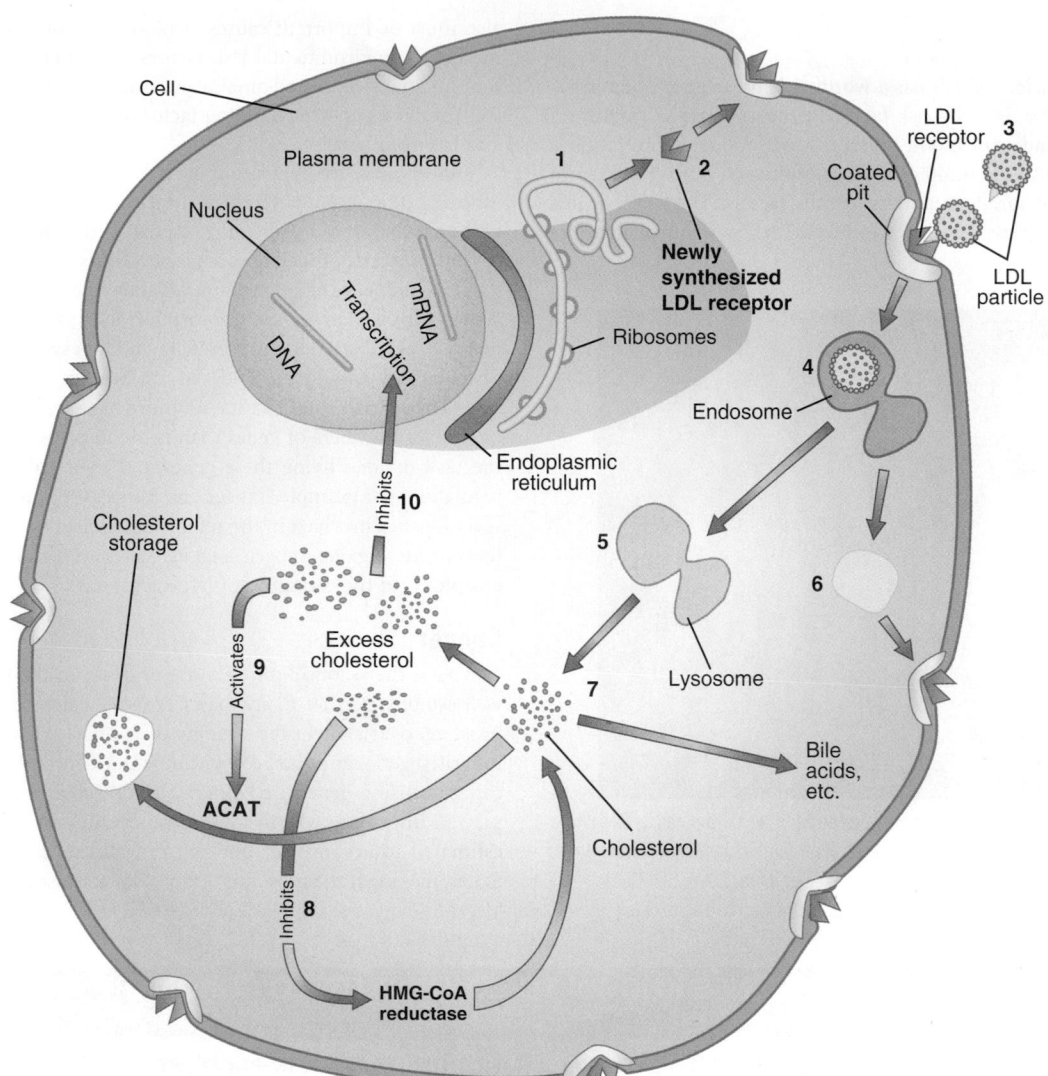

FIGURE 5.6 Process of Receptor-Mediated Endocytosis. Numbers in parentheses correspond to numbers shown in the figure. **1,** The low-density lipoprotein *(LDL)* receptors, which are glycoproteins, are synthesized in the endoplasmic reticulum of the cell. **2,** From here, they pass through the Golgi apparatus to the cell surface, where part of the receptor protrudes outside the cell. **3,** The circulating LDL particle is bound by the LDL receptor and localized in cell surface depressions called *coated pits* (so named because they are coated with a protein called *clathrin*). **4,** The coated pit invaginates, bringing the LDL particle inside the cell. **5,** Once inside the cell, the LDL particle is separated from the receptor, taken into a lysosome, and broken down into its constituents by lysosomal enzymes. **6,** The LDL receptor is recirculated to the cell surface to bind another LDL particle (each LDL receptor goes through this cycle approximately once every 10 minutes even if it is not occupied by an LDL particle). **7,** Free cholesterol is released from the lysosome for incorporation into cell membranes or metabolism into bile acids or steroids. Excess cholesterol can be stored in the cell as a cholesterol ester or removed from the cell by associating with high-density lipoprotein (HDL). **8,** As cholesterol levels in the cell rise, cellular cholesterol synthesis is reduced by inhibition of the rate-limiting enzyme 3-hydroxy-3-methylglutaryl coenzyme A *(HMG-CoA)* reductase. **9,** Rising cholesterol levels also increase the activity of acyl coenzyme A (acyl CoA):cholesterol acyltransferase *(ACAT)*, an enzyme that modifies cholesterol for storage as cholesterol esters. **10,** In addition, the number of LDL receptors is decreased by lowering the transcription rate of the LDL receptor gene itself. This decreases cholesterol uptake. (From Jorde LB et al: *Medical genetics,* ed 5, Philadelphia, 2016, Elsevier.)

these environmental factors cause cancer by creating somatic mutations (see Chapter 4) in specific cell types. Thus, cancer can be caused both by inherited genetic variants and by noninherited somatic mutations acquired during an individual's lifetime.

Breast Cancer. Breast cancer is the most common cancer among women, affecting approximately 12% of American women who live to 85 years or older. Formerly the leading cause of cancer death among women, it has been surpassed by lung cancer. Breast cancer aggregates strongly in families; for example, if a woman has one affected first-degree relative, her risk of developing breast cancer doubles. This risk increases further if the age of onset in the affected relative is early and if the cancer is bilateral (tumors in both breasts).

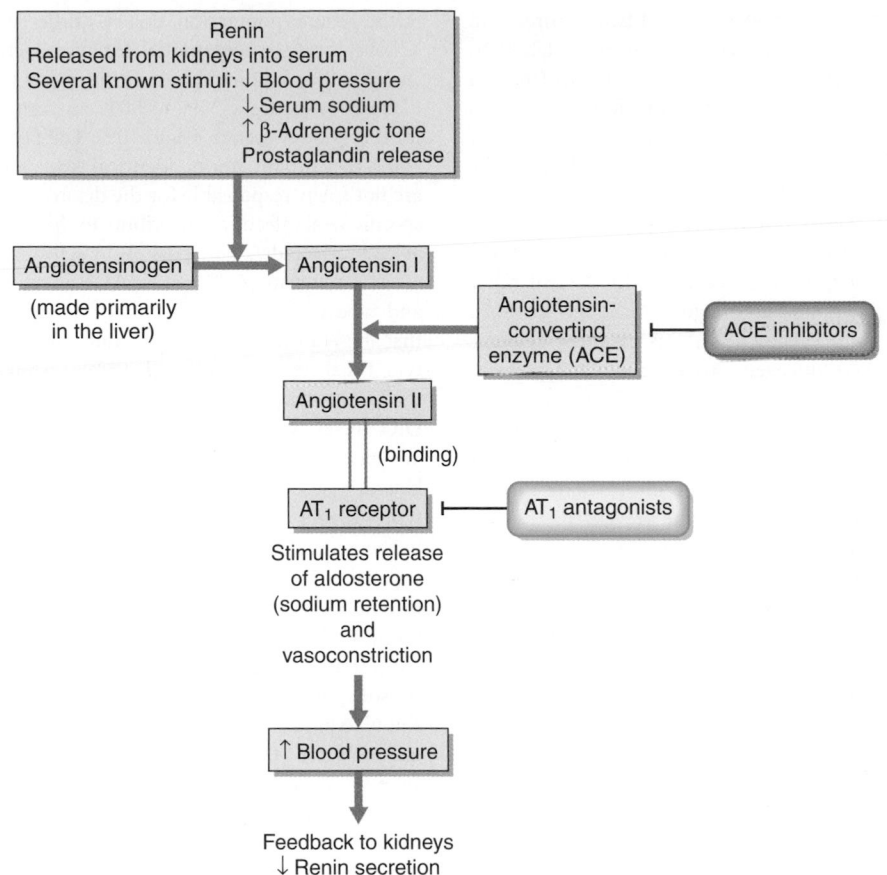

FIGURE 5.7 Renin-Angiotensin-Aldosterone System. (Modified from King RA, Rotter JI, Motulsky AG, editors: *The genetic basis of common diseases,* New York, 1992, Oxford University Press.)

An autosomal dominant form of breast cancer accounts for approximately 5% to 10% of breast cancer cases in the United States. Genes responsible for this form of breast cancer have been identified on chromosomes 17 *(BRCA1)* and 13 *(BRCA2),* and these genes can be tested for inherited cancer-causing mutations.[13] Women who inherit a mutation in *BRCA1* or *BRCA2* experience a 50% to 80% lifetime risk of developing breast cancer.[14] *BRCA1* mutations also increase the risk of ovarian cancer among women (20% to 50% lifetime risk), and they confer a modestly increased risk of prostate and colon cancers. *BRCA2* mutations also confer an increased risk of ovarian cancer (10% to 20% lifetime prevalence). Approximately 6% of males who inherit a *BRCA2* mutation will develop breast cancer, representing a 100-fold increase over the risk in the general male population. Evaluation of the *BRCA1* and *BRCA2* gene products, which are both involved in deoxyribonucleic acid (DNA) repair, is yielding valuable evidence on the etiology of breast cancer in general.

Although *BRCA1* and *BRCA2* mutations are the most common known causes of inherited breast cancer, this disease also can be caused by inherited mutations in several other genes (e.g., *CHK2, ATM, PALB2,* and *TP53).* Germline mutations in a tumor-suppressor gene called *PTEN* are responsible for Cowden disease, which is characterized by multiple benign tumors and an increased susceptibility to breast cancer. Despite the significance of these genes, it should be emphasized that more than 90% of breast cancer cases are not inherited as mendelian diseases.

Colorectal Cancer. Colorectal cancer is second only to lung cancer in the number of cancer deaths occurring annually in the United States, with approximately 134,000 new cases (and 49,000 deaths) estimated in 2016.[15] Approximately 1 in 21 Americans will develop colorectal

cancer. Like breast cancer, it clusters in families (in fact, familial clustering of this form of cancer was reported in the medical literature as early as 1881). The risk of colorectal cancer in people with one affected first-degree relative is two to three times higher than that in the general population.

This familial aggregation is caused in part by subsets of colorectal cancer cases that are inherited as single-gene traits. For example, *familial adenomatous polyposis* occurs in approximately 1 in 8000 whites. The gene responsible for this disorder, *APC,* encodes a tumor suppressor.[16] Importantly, somatic mutations of *APC* are found in at least 85% of all colon tumors. Thus although inherited *APC* mutations cause rare familial adenomatous polyposis, somatic mutations are involved in the great majority of all common colorectal cancers.

Hereditary nonpolyposis colorectal cancer, which may account for as many as 5% of colorectal cancer cases, is caused by mutations in any of six genes.[17] Research has shown that all of these genes are involved in the vital process of DNA repair. When this function is compromised, cancer-causing mutations can persist in cells, leading eventually to growth of a tumor.

Other colorectal cancer cases are likely to be caused by a complex interaction of multiple genes. In addition, environmental factors, such as a high-fat, low-fiber diet, are thought to increase the risk of colorectal cancer.

Prostate Cancer. Prostate cancer is the second most commonly diagnosed cancer in men (after skin cancer), with approximately 220,000 new cases annually in the United States. Prostate cancer is second only to lung cancer as a cause of cancer death in men, causing more than 27,000 deaths each year. Having an affected first-degree relative increases the risk of developing prostate cancer by a factor of two to three, and the heritability of prostate cancer is estimated to be approximately 40%.

The relatively late age of onset of most prostate cancer cases (median age 72 years) makes genetic analysis especially difficult. However, loss of heterozygosity (see Chapter 12) has been observed in a number of genomic regions in prostate tumor cells, possibly indicating the presence of genetic alterations in these regions. In addition, genome-wide association studies have identified several dozen polymorphisms associated with prostate cancer risk. Several of these are located in chromosome 8q24, which contains polymorphisms associated with several other cancers as well (colon, pancreas, and esophagus). Although the 8q24 region contains no protein-coding genes, it contains enhancer elements that affect expression of the *MYC* oncogene, located about 250 kilobytes (kb) from 8q24.

Nongenetic risk factors for prostate cancer may include a high-fat diet. Because prostate cancer usually progresses slowly and because it can be detected by digital examination and by the prostate-specific antigen (PSA) test, fatal metastasis can usually be prevented.

Cancer Gene Identification. Recently developed techniques, including large-scale DNA sequencing, have identified hundreds of genes that are mutated in various cancers. Some of these genes contribute directly to a growth advantage in tumors and are considered primary causes of cancer. Approximately 150 such driver genes have been described.[11] A much larger number of genes undergo somatic mutations during tumorigenesis, but these genes do not directly confer a growth advantage to cells; these are termed passenger genes. The gene responsible for retinoblastoma (see Chapter 4), which normally acts as a "brake" on cell division, is an example of a well-known driver gene. The *APC* gene, discussed previously, is another example.

Although many types of cancer, such as retinoblastoma or familial adenomatous polyposis, are relatively rare, study of the causative genes has provided many important insights into the nature of carcinogenesis in general. This can lead to more effective treatment and prevention of all cancers.

Diabetes Mellitus. Like the other disorders discussed in this chapter, the etiology of diabetes mellitus is complex and not fully understood. Nevertheless, progress is being made in understanding the genetic basis of this disorder, which is a leading cause of blindness, heart disease, and kidney failure.[18,19] An important advance has been the recognition that diabetes is actually a heterogeneous group of disorders, all characterized by elevated blood glucose level. The focus here is on the two major types of diabetes: type 1 (insulin-dependent diabetes mellitus [IDDM]) and type 2 (non–insulin-dependent diabetes mellitus [NIDDM]).

Type 1 Diabetes. Type 1 diabetes, which is characterized by T-cell infiltration of the pancreas and destruction of the insulin-producing beta cells, usually (though not always) presents before age 40. Individuals with type 1 diabetes must receive exogenous insulin to survive. In addition to T-cell infiltration of the pancreas, autoantibodies are formed against pancreatic cells; the latter can be observed long before clinical symptoms occur. These findings, along with a strong association between type 1 diabetes and the presence of several major histocompatibility complex (MHC) class II alleles, indicate that this is an autoimmune disease. Over the past few decades, the incidence of type 1 diabetes has increased substantially.

Siblings of individuals with type 1 diabetes face a substantial elevation in risk: approximately 6%, as opposed to a risk of about 0.3% to 0.5% in the general population. The recurrence risk is also elevated when there is a diabetic parent, although this risk varies with the sex of the affected parent. The risk for offspring of diabetic mothers is only 1% to 3%, whereas it is 4% to 6% for the offspring of diabetic fathers (because type 1 diabetes affects males and females in roughly equal proportions

in the general population, this risk difference is inconsistent with the sex-specific threshold model for multifactorial traits). Twin studies show that the empirical risks for identical twins of people with type 1 diabetes range from 30% to 50%. In contrast, the concordance rates for dizygotic twins are 5% to 10%. The fact that type 1 diabetes is not 100% concordant among identical twins indicates that genetic factors are not solely responsible for the disorder. There is good evidence that specific viral infections contribute to the causation of type 1 diabetes in at least some individuals, possibly by activating an autoimmune response.

The association of specific MHC class II alleles (see Chapter 22) and type 1 diabetes has been studied extensively, and it is estimated that these alleles account for about 40% of the familial clustering of type 1 diabetes. Approximately 95% of whites with type 1 diabetes have the human leukocyte antigen (HLA) (part of the MHC), DR3, and/or DR4 alleles, whereas only about 50% of the general white population has either of these alleles. If an affected proband and a sibling are heterozygous for the DR3 and DR4 alleles, the sibling's risk of developing type 1 diabetes is nearly 20% (i.e., about 40 times higher than the risk in the general population). In addition, the presence of aspartic acid at position 57 of the HLA DQ chain is strongly associated with resistance to type 1 diabetes. In fact, those who do not have this amino acid at position 57 (and instead are homozygous for a different amino acid) are 100 times more likely to develop type 1 diabetes. The aspartic acid substitution alters the shape of the HLA class II molecule and thus its ability to bind and present peptides to T cells. Altered T-cell recognition may help protect individuals with the aspartic acid substitution from an autoimmune episode.

The insulin gene, which is located on the short arm of chromosome 11, is another logical candidate for type 1 diabetes susceptibility. Polymorphisms within and near this gene have been tested for association with type 1 diabetes. It is estimated that inherited genetic variation in the insulin region accounts for approximately 10% of the familial clustering of type 1 diabetes.

Many additional genes have been shown to be associated with susceptibility to type 1 diabetes. The most significant of these are cytotoxic lymphocyte associated-4 (*CTLA4*), which encodes a protein involved in the regulation of T-cell proliferation, and *PTPN22*, which encodes a lymphoid-specific tyrosine phosphatase that negatively regulates T-cell activation. It is interesting that variation in the latter gene has been associated with several other autoimmune diseases, including systemic lupus erythematosus (SLE), rheumatoid arthritis, and autoimmune thyroid disease.

Type 2 Diabetes. Type 2 diabetes accounts for more than 90% of all diabetes cases and affects 10% to 20% of the adult populations of many developed countries. A number of features distinguish it from type 1 diabetes. There is nearly always some endogenous insulin production in people with type 2 diabetes, and the disease can often be treated successfully with dietary modification and/or oral drugs. People with type 2 diabetes suffer from insulin resistance (i.e., their cells have difficulty in using insulin). This disease typically occurs among people older than age 40 and, in contrast to type 1 diabetes, is seen more commonly among the obese. The incidence of type 2 diabetes is rising dramatically among adolescents and young adults in developed countries, however, and is strongly correlated with an increased incidence of obesity. Neither MHC associations nor autoantibodies are commonly seen in this form of diabetes. Monozygotic twin concordance rates are substantially higher than those seen in type 1 diabetes, ranging from 70% to 90% (because of age dependence, the concordance rate increases if older subjects are studied). The empirical recurrence risks for first-degree relatives of type 2 diabetes cases are higher than those for type 1, generally ranging from 15% to 40%. The differences between type 1 and type 2 diabetes are summarized in Table 5.7.

TABLE 5.7   COMPARISON OF MAJOR FEATURES OF TYPES 1 AND 2 DIABETES

FEATURE	TYPE 1 DIABETES	TYPE 2 DIABETES
Age of onset	Usually <40 yr	Usually >40 yr (except maturity-onset diabetes of the young [MODY])
Insulin production	None	Partial
Insulin resistance	No	Yes
Autoimmunity	Yes	No
Obesity	Not common	Common
Monozygotic (MZ) twin concordance	0.55	0.90
Sibling recurrence risk	1–6%	10–15%

Hundreds of studies have been undertaken to identify genes that may contribute to type 2 diabetes susceptibility, and nearly 100 genes are now known to be associated with risk of this disease. An important risk factor is *TCF7L2*, which encodes a transcription factor involved in the secretion of insulin. A variant of *TCF7L2* is associated with a 50% increased risk of developing type 2 diabetes. A significant association has also been observed between type 2 diabetes and a common allele of the gene that encodes peroxisome proliferator–activated receptor-gamma (PPAR-γ), a nuclear receptor that is involved in adipocyte differentiation and glucose metabolism. This receptor is the target of thiazolidinediones (TZDs), a class of drugs commonly used to increase insulin sensitivity in those with type 2 diabetes. Although the disease-associated allele confers only a 25% increase in the risk of developing type 2 diabetes, it is found in more than 75% of individuals of European descent and thus helps to account for a significant proportion of type 2 diabetes cases. Variation in *KCNJ11*, which encodes a potassium channel necessary for glucose-stimulated insulin secretion, confers an additional 20% increase in type 2 diabetes susceptibility. The associations between diabetes susceptibility and each of these genes have been widely replicated in multiple populations.

The two most important risk factors for type 2 diabetes are positive family history and obesity; the latter increases insulin resistance. The disease tends to rise in prevalence when populations adopt a diet and exercise pattern typical of U.S. and European populations. Increases have been seen, for example, among Japanese immigrants to the United States and among some native populations of the South Pacific, Australia, and the Americas. Several studies, conducted on male and female subjects, have shown that regular exercise can substantially lower one's risk of developing type 2 diabetes, even among individuals with a family history of the disease. This is partly because exercise reduces obesity. However, even in the absence of weight loss, exercise increases insulin sensitivity and improves glucose tolerance.

Because of the dramatic increase in obesity in the United States and other developed countries, the prevalence of type 2 diabetes is also rising rapidly, and the average age of onset is decreasing. A small proportion of type 2 diabetes cases occurs early in life, often before 25 years of age, and typically exhibits autosomal dominant inheritance (unlike most type 2 diabetes cases). This subset is termed *maturity-onset diabetes of the young* (MODY). Studies of MODY pedigrees have shown that about half of cases of the disease are caused by mutations in the glucokinase gene. Glucokinase converts glucose to glucose-6-phosphate in the pancreas. In addition to the glucokinase gene, five other genes, all of which are involved in pancreatic development or regulation of insulin levels, have now been shown to be causes of MODY.

Obesity

Obesity is most commonly defined as a body mass index (BMI) greater than 30. (BMI is defined as W/H^2, in which W is weight in kilograms and H is height in meters.) Using this criterion, more than one-third of American adults are obese, and an additional one-third are overweight (BMI greater than 25 but less than 30). The proportion of obese adults and children continues to increase rapidly. Although obesity itself is not a "disease," it is an important risk factor for several common diseases, including heart disease, stroke, type 2 diabetes, and cancers of the prostate, breast, and colon.

As one might expect, there is a strong correlation between obesity in parents and their children. This could easily be ascribed to common environmental effects: parents and children usually share similar dietary and exercise habits. However, there is good evidence for genetic components as well. Four adoption studies each showed that the body weights of adopted individuals correlated significantly with their natural parents' body weights but not with those of their adoptive parents. Twin studies also provide evidence for a genetic effect on body weight, with most studies yielding heritability estimates between 0.60 and 0.80.

Research, aided substantially by mouse models, has shown that many genes each play a role in human obesity. Important among these are the genes that encode leptin (Greek, "thin") and its receptor. The leptin hormone is secreted by adipocytes (fat storage cells) and binds to receptors in the hypothalamus, the site of the body's appetite control center. Cloning of the human leptin gene and its receptor led to optimistic predictions that leptin could be a key to weight loss in humans (without the perceived unpleasantness of dieting and exercise). Although mutations in the human leptin gene and its receptor have been identified in a few humans with severe obesity (BMI >40), they both appear to be extremely rare. Clinical trials using recombinant leptin have demonstrated moderate weight loss in a subset of obese individuals. In addition, leptin participates in important interactions with other components of appetite control, such as neuropeptide Y and α-melanocyte-stimulating hormone and its receptor, the melanocortin-4 receptor (MC4R). Mutations in the gene that encodes MC4R have been found in 3% to 5% of severely obese individuals. Homozygosity for a DNA variant in the *FTO* gene (which is seen in 16% of whites) has been associated with 40% and 70% increases in the risks of overweight and obesity, respectively. Recent evidence shows that the *FTO* variant is part of an enhancer that binds to the *IRX* gene, which is located 2 million base pairs away from *FTO* and is involved in regulation of fat mass. Identification of these human genes is leading to a better understanding of natural weight control in the human, and it could eventually lead to effective treatments for some cases of obesity.

Alzheimer Disease

Alzheimer disease (AD), which is responsible for 60% to 70% of cases of progressive cognitive impairment among older adults, affects approximately 5% to 10% of the population older than 65 years of age and 40% of the population older than 85 years of age. Because of the aging of the population, the number of Americans with AD is predicted to increase substantially during the coming decade. AD is characterized by progressive dementia and memory loss and by the formation of amyloid plaques and neurofibrillary tangles in the brain, particularly in the cerebral cortex and hippocampus. The plaques and tangles lead to progressive neuronal loss, and death usually occurs within 7 to 10 years after the first appearance of symptoms.

The risk of developing AD doubles in individuals who have an affected first-degree relative. Although most cases do not appear to be caused by single loci, approximately 10% follow an autosomal dominant mode of transmission. About 3% to 5% of AD cases occur before age 65 and are considered early onset; these are much more likely to be inherited in autosomal dominant fashion.[20]

AD is a genetically heterogeneous disorder. Approximately half of early-onset cases can be attributed to mutations in any of three genes, all of which affect amyloid-β deposition.[20]

Two of the genes, presenilin 1 (PS1) and presenilin 2 (PS2), are very similar to one another, and their protein products are involved in cleavage of the amyloid-β precursor protein (APP). When APP is not cleaved normally, a long form of it accumulates excessively and is deposited in the brain. This is thought to be a primary cause of AD. Mutations in PS1 typically result in early-onset AD, with the first occurrence of symptoms in the fifth decade of life.

A small number of cases of early-onset AD are caused by mutations of the gene that encodes APP itself, which is located on chromosome 21. These mutations disrupt normal cleavage sites in APP, again leading to the accumulation of the longer protein product. It is interesting that this gene is present in three copies in trisomy 21 individuals, in which the extra gene copy leads to amyloid deposition and the occurrence of AD in those with Down syndrome (see Chapter 4). High-throughput DNA sequencing (techniques allowing the sequencing of massive amounts of DNA at once) studies have revealed an allele in APP that is protective against Alzheimer disease and may help to prevent cognitive decline.

An important risk factor for the more common late-onset form of AD is allelic variation in the apolipoprotein E (APOE) locus, which has three major alleles: ε2, ε3, and ε4. Studies conducted in diverse populations have shown that persons who have one copy of the ε4 allele are at least 2 to 5 times more likely to develop AD, whereas those with two copies of this allele are at least 5 to 10 times more likely to develop AD. The risk varies somewhat by population, with higher ε4-associated risks in Europeans and Japanese and relatively lower risks in Hispanics and blacks. Despite the strong association between ε4 and AD, approximately half of individuals who develop late-onset AD do not have a copy of the ε4 allele, and many who are homozygous for ε4 remain free of AD even at advanced age. The apolipoprotein E protein product is not involved in cleavage of APP but instead appears to be associated with clearance of amyloid from the brain.

Alcoholism

At some point, alcoholism is diagnosed in approximately 10% of adult males and 3% to 5% of adult females in the United States. The national cost of alcoholism, in terms of lost productivity and direct medical costs, is approximately $250 billion per year. More than 100 studies have shown that this disease clusters in families.[21] The risk of developing alcoholism among individuals with one affected parent is three to five times higher than for those with unaffected parents.

Most twin studies have yielded concordance rates for DZ twins less than 30% and concordance rates for MZ twins in excess of 60%. Adoption studies have shown that the offspring of an alcoholic parent, even when raised by nonalcoholic parents, have a fourfold increased risk of developing the disorder. To control for possible prenatal effects in an alcoholic mother, some studies have included only the offspring of alcoholic fathers. The results have remained the same. One study showed that the offspring of nonalcoholic parents, when reared by alcoholics, did *not* have an increased risk of developing alcoholism. These data argue that there may be genetic variants that predispose some people to alcoholism.

It has long been known that an individual's physiologic response to alcohol can be influenced by variation in the key enzymes responsible for alcohol metabolism: alcohol dehydrogenases (ADHs), which convert ethanol to acetaldehyde; and aldehyde dehydrogenases (ALDHs), which convert acetaldehyde to acetate. In particular, an allele of the ALDH2 gene (ALDH2*2) results in excessive accumulation of acetaldehyde and thus in facial flushing, nausea, palpitations, and lightheadedness. Because of these unpleasant effects, individuals who have the ALDH2*2 allele are much less likely to become alcoholics. This "protective" allele is common in some Asian populations but is rare in other populations.

A number of other genes are associated with susceptibility to alcohol addiction, including genes that encode components of gamma-aminobutyric acid (GABA) receptors. This finding is biologically plausible, because the GABA neurotransmitter system inhibits excitatory signals in neurons, exerting a calming effect. Alcohol has been shown to increase GABA release, and allelic variation in GABA receptor genes may modulate this effect.

It should be underscored that genes may increase one's *susceptibility* to alcoholism. Obviously this is a disease that requires an environmental component, regardless of genetic constitution.

Psychiatric Disorders

The major psychiatric diseases, schizophrenia and affective disorder, have been the subjects of numerous genetic studies.[22] Twin, adoption, and family studies have shown that both disorders aggregate in families.

Schizophrenia. *Schizophrenia* is a severe emotional disorder characterized by delusions, hallucinations, retreat from reality, and bizarre, withdrawn, or inappropriate behavior. (Contrary to popular belief, schizophrenia is not a "split personality" disorder.) The lifetime recurrence risk for schizophrenia among the offspring of one affected parent is approximately 8% to 10%, which is about 10 times higher than the risk in the general population.[23] As one might expect, the empirical risks increase when more relatives are affected. For example, an individual with an affected sibling and an affected parent has a risk approaching 20% and an individual with two affected parents has a risk of nearly 50%. The risks decrease when the affected family member is a second- or third-degree relative. Details are given in Table 5.8. On inspection of Table 5.8, it may seem puzzling that the proportion of schizophrenic probands who have a schizophrenic parent is only about 5%, which is substantially lower than the risk for other first-degree relatives (e.g., siblings, affected parents and their offspring). This can

TABLE 5.8	RECURRENCE RISKS FOR RELATIVES OF SCHIZOPHRENIC PROBANDS
RELATIONSHIP TO PROBAND	**RECURRENCE RISK (%)**
Monozygotic twin	44.3
Dizygotic twin	12.1
Offspring	9.4
Sibling	7.3
Niece/nephew	2.7
Grandchild	2.8
First cousin	1.6
Spouse	1

NOTE: Figures are based on multiple studies of Western European populations.
Data from McGue M, Gottesman II, Rao DC: *Behav Genet* 16(1):75–87, 1986.

be explained by the fact that people with schizophrenia are less likely to marry and produce children than are other individuals. Thus substantial selection against schizophrenia occurs in the population.

Twin and adoption studies also indicate that genetic factors are likely to be involved in schizophrenia. Data pooled from five different twin studies show a 47% concordance rate for MZ twins, compared with a concordance rate of only 12% for DZ twins. When the offspring of a schizophrenic parent are adopted by normal parents, their risk of developing the disease is about 10%, which is approximately the same as the risk when raised by a schizophrenic biologic parent. Large-scale genetic studies have revealed more than 100 loci that are associated with risk of schizophrenia. Many of these genes encode components of the dopaminergic and glutamatergic neuronal signaling pathways. These findings are biologically plausible because the major therapeutic drugs used to treat schizophrenia block dopamine receptors.

Bipolar Disorder. *Bipolar disorder,* also known as *manic-depressive disorder,* is a form of psychosis with extreme mood swings and emotional instability. The incidence of the disorder in the general population is approximately 0.5%, but it rises to 5% to 10% among those with an affected first-degree relative. Twin and family studies show that approximately 60% of the risk for bipolar disorder is attributable to genetic factors, whereas about 30% of the risk for unipolar disorder (major depression) is because of genetic factors.[24]

As with schizophrenia, many large-scale studies have been undertaken to identify genes associated with susceptibility to bipolar disorder. Some of these loci were identified because their products are involved in neurotransmitter systems that are targets of drugs used to treat the disease (e.g., the serotonin, dopamine, and noradrenaline systems). Some of the best-replicated genetic studies implicate genes that encode voltage-gated calcium channels. Ion-channel modulating drugs are frequently used as mood stabilizers, lending the genetic results functional plausibility. Many of the genes associated with bipolar disorder also are associated with schizophrenia.

Genetic studies of psychiatric disorders are especially challenging because these disorders are undoubtedly heterogeneous, reflecting the influence of numerous genetic and environmental factors. Also, definition of the phenotype is not always straightforward and it may change through time, significantly complicating genetic analysis.

Other Complex Disorders

The disorders discussed in this chapter represent some of the most common multifactorial disorders and those for which significant progress has been made in identifying genes. Many other multifactorial disorders are being studied as well, and in some cases specific susceptibility genes have been identified. These include, for example, Parkinson disease, hearing loss, multiple sclerosis, amyotrophic lateral sclerosis, epilepsy, asthma, inflammatory bowel disease, and some forms of blindness.

Some General Principles and Conclusions

Some general principles can be deduced from the results obtained thus far on the genetics of complex disorders. First, the more strongly inherited forms of complex disorders generally have an earlier age of onset (e.g., breast cancer, AD, heart disease). Often these represent subsets of cases in which there is single-gene inheritance. Second, when laterality is a component, the bilateral forms are more likely to cluster strongly in families (e.g., breast cancer, CL/P). Third, although the sex-specific threshold model fits some of the complex disorders (e.g., pyloric stenosis, CL/P, autism, heart disease), it fails to fit others (e.g., type 1 diabetes).

A tendency exists, particularly among the lay public, to assume that the presence of a genetic component means that the course of a disease cannot be altered. *This is incorrect.* Most of the diseases discussed in this chapter have both genetic and environmental components. Thus lifestyle modification (e.g., diet, exercise, stress reduction) often can reduce risk significantly. Such modification may be especially important for individuals with a family history of a disease because they are likely to develop the disease earlier in life. Those with a family history of heart disease, for example, can often add many years of productive living with relatively minor lifestyle alterations. By targeting those who can benefit most from intervention, genetics helps to serve the goal of preventive medicine.

In addition, it should be stressed that the identification of a specific genetic lesion can lead to more effective prevention and treatment of the disease. Identification of mutations that cause autosomal dominant breast cancer may enable early screening and prevention of metastasis. Pinpointing a gene responsible for a neurotransmitter defect in a behavioral disorder such as schizophrenia could lead to the development of more effective drug treatments. In some cases, such as those with familial hypercholesterolemia, targeted drug therapy or gene therapy may prove to be useful in treating the disease. It is important for healthcare practitioners to help individuals understand these facts.

Although the genetics of common disorders is complex and often confusing, the community health effect of these diseases, together with the evidence for hereditary factors in their etiology, demands that genetic studies be pursued. Substantial progress is already being made. The next decade will undoubtedly witness many further advances in the understanding and treatment of these disorders.

■ SUMMARY REVIEW

Factors Influencing Incidence of Disease in Populations

1. The incidence rate is the number of new cases of a disease reported during a specific period (typically 1 year) divided by the number of individuals in the population.
2. The prevalence rate is the proportion of the population affected by a disease at a specific point in time. This rate, and the incidence rate, can be used to compare population variations in disease frequency.
3. Relative risk is a common measure of the effect of a specific risk factor. It is expressed as a ratio of the incidence rate of the disease among individuals exposed to a risk factor divided by the incidence of the disease among individuals *not* exposed to a risk factor.
4. Many factors can influence the risk of acquiring a common disease, such as cancer, diabetes, or hypertension. The factors can include age, gender, diet, exercise, and family history of the disease.

Principles of Multifactorial Inheritance

1. Traits in which variation is thought to be caused by the combined effects of multiple genes are polygenic.
2. The term *multifactorial* is used when environmental factors also are believed to cause variation in the trait.
3. Many quantitative traits (e.g., blood pressure) are multifactorial.
4. Because traits are caused by the additive effects of many genetic and environmental factors, they tend to follow a normal or bell-shaped distribution in populations.
5. Those diseases, however, that do not follow a bell-shaped distribution appear to be either present or absent in individuals. They do not follow the inheritance patterns of single-gene disease. Instead, such diseases may follow an underlying liability distribution. It is thought that a threshold of liability must be crossed before the disease is expressed.

SUMMARY REVIEW—cont'd

6. Examples of diseases that correspond to the liability model include pyloric stenosis, neural tube defects, CL/P, and some forms of congenital heart disease.

7. Many of the common adult diseases, such as hypertension, coronary heart disease, stroke, diabetes mellitus (types 1 and 2), and some cancers, are caused by complex genetic and environmental factors and are thus multifactorial diseases.

8. For most multifactorial diseases, empirical risks (risks based on direct observation of data) have been derived.

9. In contrast to most single-gene diseases, recurrence risks for multifactorial diseases can change significantly from one population to another because gene frequencies, as well as environmental factors, can differ among populations.

10. Several criteria are used to define multifactorial inheritance: (a) the recurrence risk becomes higher if more than one family member is affected; (b) if the expression of the disease in a proband is more severe, the recurrence risk is higher; (c) the recurrence risk is higher if the proband is of the less commonly affected sex; (d) the recurrence risk for the disease usually decreases rapidly in more remotely related relatives; and (e) if the prevalence of the disease in a population is f, the risk for offspring and siblings of probands is approximately $\sqrt{f}$.

Nature and Nurture: Disentangling the Effects of Genes and Environment

1. Family members share genes and a common environment; therefore, resemblance in traits, such as high blood pressure, reflects both genetic and environmental factors (nature and nurture, respectively).

2. Few traits are influenced *only* by genes or *only* by environment. Most are influenced by both.

3. When a disease has a relatively larger genetic component, as in breast cancer, examination of family history should be emphasized in addition to lifestyle modification.

4. Two research strategies often are used to estimate the relative influence of genes and environment-lifestyle: twin studies and adoption studies.

5. Monozygotic twins originate when the developing embryo divides to form two separate but identical embryos.

6. Dizygotic twins are the result of a double ovulation followed by the fertilization of each egg by a different sperm.

7. If both members of a twin pair share a trait, they are said to be *concordant*. If they do not share the same trait, they are *discordant*.

8. Studies of adopted children also are used to estimate the genetic contribution to a multifactorial trait.

9. A genetic predisposition may interact with an environmental-lifestyle factor to increase the risk of disease; this is called a *gene-environment interaction*.

Genetics of Common Diseases

1. Congenital diseases are those present at birth. Most of these diseases are multifactorial in etiology.

2. Multifactorial diseases in adults include coronary heart disease, hypertension, breast cancer, colon cancer, diabetes mellitus, obesity, AD, alcoholism, schizophrenia, and bipolar affective disorder.

3. It is incorrect to assume that the presence of a genetic component means that the course of a disease cannot be altered—most diseases have *both* genetic and environmental aspects.

KEY TERMS

Concordant, 165
Congenital disease, 166
Discordant, 165
Dizygotic (DZ, fraternal) twin, 164
Driver genes, 172
Empirical risk, 163

Gene-environment interaction, 165
Incidence rate, 160
Liability distribution, 161
Monozygotic (MZ, identical) twin, 164
Multifactorial trait, 161
Passenger genes, 172

Phocomelia, 167
Polygenic, 161
Prevalence rate, 160
Quantitative trait, 161
Relative risk, 161
Threshold of liability, 162

REFERENCES

1. Rothman KJ, Greenland S, Lash TL: *Modern epidemiology*, ed 3, New York, 2012, Lippincott.

2. Duarte CW, et al: Multifactorial inheritance and complex diseases. In Rimoin DL, et al, editors: *Emery and Rimoin's principles and practice of medical genetics*, ed 6, Philadelphia, 2012, Elsevier.

3. Risch N, et al: Familial recurrence of autism spectrum disorder: evaluating genetic and environmental contributions. *Am J Psychiatry* 171:1206–1213, 2014.

4. Clarke A: *Harper's practical genetic counseling*, ed 8, London, 2017, Hodder Arnold.

5. van Dongen J, et al: The continuing value of twin studies in the omics era. *Nat Rev Genet* 13:640–653, 2012.

6. Kaprio J, Silventoinen K: Advanced methods in twin studies. *Methods Mol Biol* 713:143–152, 2011.

7. Hunt SC, Williams RR, Barlow GK: A comparison of positive family history definitions for defining risk of future disease. *J Chronic Dis* 39(10):809–821, 1986.

8. Roberts R: A genetic basis for coronary artery disease. *Trends Cardiovasc Med* 25:171–178, 2015.

9. O'Donnell CJ, Nabel EG: Genomics of cardiovascular disease. *N Engl J Med* 365(22): 2098–2109, 2011.

10. Munroe PB, Barnes MR, Caulfield MJ: Advances in blood pressure genomics. *Circ Res* 112:1365–1379, 2013.

11. Vogelstein B, et al: Cancer genome landscapes. *Science* 339:1546–1558, 2013.

12. Peto J: Cancer epidemiology in the last century and the next decade. *Nature* 411(6835):390–395, 2001.

13. Easton DF, et al: Gene-panel sequencing and the prediction of breast-cancer risk. *N Engl J Med* 372:2243–2257, 2015.

14. Couch FJ, Nathanson KL, Offit K: Two decades after BRCA: setting paradigms in personalized cancer care and prevention. *Science* 343(6178): 1466–1470, 2014.

15. American Cancer Society (ACS): *Cancer facts & figures 2016*, Atlanta, GA, 2016, Author.

16. Jasperson KW, et al: Hereditary and familial colon cancer. *Gastroenterology* 138:2044–2058, 2010.

17. Raskov H, et al: Colorectal carcinogenesis—update and perspectives. *World J Gastroenterol* 20(48): 18151–18164, 2014.

18. Mohlke KL, Boehnke M: Recent advances in understanding the genetic architecture of type 2 diabetes. *Hum Mol Genet* 24:R85–R92, 2015.

19. Stankov K, Benc D, Draskovic D: Genetic and epigenetic factors in etiology of diabetes mellitus type 1. *Pediatrics* 132:1112–1122, 2013.

20. Karch CM, Goate AM: Alzheimer's disease risk genes and mechanisms of disease pathogenesis. *Biol Psychiatry* 77:43–51, 2015.

21. Enoch MA: Genetic influences on the development of alcoholism. *Curr Psychiatry Rep* 15:412, 2013.

22. Doherty JL, Owen MJ: Genomic insights into the overlap between psychiatric disorders: implications for research and clinical practice. *Genome Med* 6:29, 2014.

23. Gejman PV, et al: Genetics of schizophrenia: new findings and challenges. *Annu Rev Genom Hum Genet* 12(1):121–144, 2011.

24. Geschwind DH, Flint J: Genetics and genomics of psychiatric disease. *Science* 349(6255):1489–1494, 2015.

Epigenetics and Disease

Diane P. Genereux

e**volve** WEBSITE

http://evolve.elsevier.com/McCance/
- Content Updates
- Chapter Summary Review
- Review Questions
- Case Studies
- Animations

CHAPTER OUTLINE

Humans exhibit an impressive diversity of physical and behavioral traits. Much of this diversity is attributable to genetic variation. Another substantial contributor is epigenetic ("upon genetic") modification. The specific definition of epigenetic remains a topic of discussion among biologists.[1,2] Under one definition, the term is reserved for modifications that are not encoded in nucleotide sequence but are nevertheless transmitted when a somatic cell divides (mitotic inheritance), when gametes are produced (germline inheritance), or both.[3] In this chapter, the term epigenetic is used to refer to processes that modulate how a given set of genomic information gives rise to phenotype. Under this definition, epigenetic mechanisms include chemical modifications to DNA and associated histones, the production of small regulatory RNA molecules, and, more generally, gene regulation by epigenetic processes at the level of either transcription or translation.

Epigenetic modification is essential to fundamental processes of human development, including the differentiation of embryonic stem cells into specific cell types, and the inactivation of one of the two X chromosomes in each cell of a genetic female. Some genes are said to be *imprinted,* meaning that they are inherited from the mother and the father in predictable and distinct epigenetic states. At imprinted loci, it is always either the allele from the mother or the allele from the father that is expressed in the offspring.[4-6]

A variety of diseases can result from abnormal epigenetic states. For example, metabolic disease can occur when there is abnormal expression from both alleles at a locus that is typically imprinted; exposure to environmental stressors can markedly increase the risk of abnormal epigenetic states and is strongly associated with some cancers. Because of their increasingly clear role in a wide range of pathologies, such epigenetic perturbations are currently a focus of both preventative efforts and pharmaceutical interventions.

OVERVIEW OF EPIGENETIC MECHANISMS

Epigenetic marks include DNA methylation and hydroxymethylation, chemical modifications that alter the charges of the histone proteins around which DNA is wound for compaction within the nucleus, and RNA-based mechanisms (Fig. 6.1).

DNA Methylation

DNA methylation occurs through the attachment of a methyl group to the carbon-5 position of a cytosine. In the somatic cells of adults, DNA methylation occurs principally at cytosines that are followed by a guanine base (sometimes known as cytosines in "CpG dinucleotides"); in human embryonic stem cells, methylation also can occur at cytosines outside of the CpG context.[7]

DNA methylation plays a prominent role in human health and disease. For example, in each cell of a normal human female, one of the two X chromosomes has dense methylation at most regions. Dense methylation is a key feature of heterochromatin, a structure consisting of DNA tightly wound around histones into a condensed state and not actively transcribed. The heterochromatization of the so-called "inactive X" accounts for the cytologic observations that each cell from a human female has a region of densely stained DNA. This region was later confirmed to be the highly condensed inactive X chromosome.[8,9]

Most regions of the other X chromosome in a cell from a human female, the so-called *active X chromosome,* are largely devoid of DNA

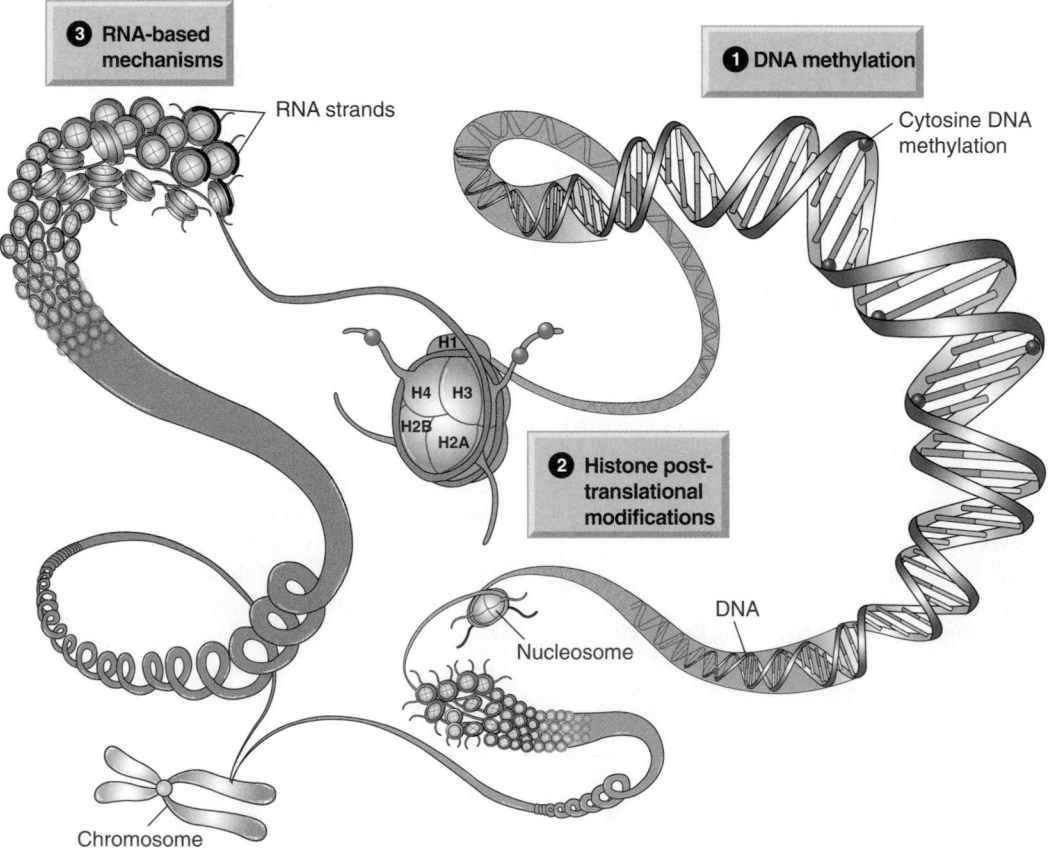

FIGURE 6.1 Three Major Types of Epigenetic Processes. Investigators are studying the following epigenetic mechanisms: **(1)** DNA methylation, **(2)** histone modifications, and **(3)** RNA based-mechanisms. See text for discussion.

methylation. The active X chromosome is said to be a transcriptionally active *euchromatic* state. Epigenetic inactivation of one of the two X chromosomes occurs in each cell of a human female during gastrulation, a phase of early embryonic development. The determination of which chromosome is to be silenced, either the copy from the father or the copy from the mother, occurs at random and independently in each cell; the silent state of that chromosome and the active state of the other are inherited by descendant cells. If a woman's two X chromosomes carry different alleles at a given locus, random X inactivation in early development can lead to somatic mosaicism, wherein differences between the alleles active in two cells can confer two very different traits. Visually notable examples include the patchy coloration of calico cats and *anhidrotic ectodermal dysplasia,* the patchy presence and absence of sweat glands in the skin of human females with one X chromosome bearing a normal allele and one X chromosome bearing a mutant allele. It is important to note that somatic mosaicism because of random inactivation can arise for any X-encoded trait. As a result, females who inherit one normal allele and one disease allele at an X-encoded gene tend to have less severe disease phenotypes than do males whose lone X chromosome bears a disease allele. This pattern is reflected in the typically lower severity in females as compared to males for color blindness, fragile X syndrome, and other phenotypes that arise from mutations on the X chromosome.

Aberrant DNA methylation, either the presence of dense methylation where it is typically absent or the absence of methylation where it is typically present, is associated with misregulation of tumor-suppressor genes and oncogenes. Specific alterations to DNA methylation states are a common feature of several human cancers, including those of the colon[10] and breast;[11] the details of these alterations can be useful in assessing disease prognosis[12] (see Figs. 6.1 and 6.4; also see Chapter 12).

DNA Hydroxymethylation

DNA hydroxymethylation is most common in cells that are undergoing epigenetic transition. DNA hydroxymethylation differs from DNA methylation in that it is a hydroxymethyl group, rather than methyl group, that is affixed to the C5 of cytosine. Discovery of this alternate DNA modification has helped to resolve long-standing uncertainties as to how genomic regions dense in DNA methylation undergo methylation loss, as observed, for example, in early embryonic development.[13]

In 2011, Wossidlo and colleagues[14] found that genome-wide declines in DNA methylation in early murine zygotes occur in concert with genome-wide increases in DNA hydroxymethylation. They also found that this loss of methylation, as well as the parallel gain in hydroxymethylation, were obliterated in zygotes deficient in the Tet3 enzyme. These two findings helped to establish that Tet enzymes can convert DNA methylation into hydroxymethylation. The name *Tet* derives from the term "ten-eleven translocation," a reference to the discovery of these enzymes through their association with a chromosomal translocation between chromosomes 10 and 11 that is commonly observed in some forms of leukemia.[15] Though the specific functional impacts of hydroxymethylation remain an area of active investigation, one recent proposal is that it is associated with the activation of lineage-specific enhancers and so could play a role in specifying cell lineages.[16]

Histone Modifications

Histones are the positively charged proteins around which negatively charged DNA molecules are wound, facilitating compaction of DNA into the cellular nuclei. When all of the DNA that comprises the human genome is wound around histones, it is only 1/40,000 as long as it would be in its uncondensed state. A set of histones and the segment of DNA wound around them are, together, known as individual nucleosomes. The total chromatin in a cell, a combination of DNA and its associated histones and RNA molecules, is made up of individual nucleosome units.

When a given segment of DNA is bound tightly to its associated histones it is said to be heterochromatic, such that, as noted previously in describing the inactive X chromosome, it is not accessible by transcription factors and so cannot be used to guide the production of mRNA. By contrast, if a given segment of DNA is only loosely bound to associated histones it is said to be euchromatic, such that, as noted previously in describing the active X chromosome, transcription factors are able to access it and use it as a template for production of mRNA. Whether a given segment of DNA is heterochromatic or euchromatic depends largely on chemical modifications to histone tails, parts of the histone-protein complex that extend away from the main part of the nucleosome.

Researchers are only beginning to understand the full diversity and complexity of these histone modifications.[17] The two modifications best studied are histone acetylation and histone methylation. Histone acetylation tends to diminish the positive charge of histones, reducing the strength of their binding to negatively charged DNA and, ultimately, making DNA more accessible for transcription. Histone methylation can either increase or decrease the strength of bonding between DNA and histones, depending on the specific parts of the histones to which the methyl groups are added.

Whether individual segments of the genome are in heterochromatic or euchromatic states play a critical role in determining the developmental potential of a given cell—that is, its capacity to give rise to a diverse set of differentiated cell types. For example, chromatin states differ substantially between embryonic stem cells, which are poised to give rise to all of the different cell types that comprise an individual, and terminally differentiated cells, which are committed to a specific developmental path. The fraction of DNA that is in the heterochromatic state typically increases as cells differentiate, in parallel to the reduction in the number of genes that are active as a cell lineage transitions from pluripotency, when they have the capacity to give rise to a large number of descendant cell types, to terminal differentiation, and when they are able to produce only a cell of a single specified type.[18] Mutations in genes that encode histone-modifying proteins have been implicated in various pathologic states, including congenital heart disease,[19] highlighting histone modification as critical to normal development.

In contrast to the vast majority of other cell types, including oocytes, sperm cells express not histones but protamines, which are evolutionarily derived from histones.[20] Protamines enable sperm DNA to achieve compaction even greater than for the histone-bound DNA in somatic cells. This tight compaction improves the hydrodynamic features of sperm cells, facilitating their movement.

Noncoding RNAs

Noncoding RNAs (ncRNAs) play an important role in regulating a wide variety of cellular processes, including RNA splicing and DNA replication. Of particular relevance to gene regulation are microRNAs (miRNAs), which are encoded by DNA sequences approximately 22 nucleotides long and typically reside within the introns of genes or in noncoding intergenic regions. In contrast to DNA methylation and histone modification, both of which principally impact gene expression at the level of transcription, miRNAs typically modulate the stability and translational efficiency of messenger RNAs (mRNAs) encoded at other loci. Interaction between miRNAs and the mRNAs they target for degradation is typically mediated by regions of partial sequence complementarity. As a result, miRNAs can at once be specific enough so that they do not bind to *all* of the mRNAs in a cell and general enough to regulate a large set of different mRNA sequences. miRNAs can also modulate translation by impairing ribosomal function. miRNAs regulate diverse signaling pathways; those that stimulate cancer development and progression are called oncomirs. For example, miRNAs have been linked to carcinogenesis because they alter the activity of oncogenes and tumor-suppressor genes (see Chapter 12). Like other classes of genomic elements, the sequences that encode miRNAs can be transcriptionally silenced by DNA methylation. Insofar as the expression of miRNAs can modulate the formation and growth of tumors, epigenetic modification of the sequences that encode them is a key area for exploration of strategies for characterizing and perhaps even treating cancer.[21]

EPIGENETICS AND HUMAN DEVELOPMENT

Each of the cells in the early embryo has the potential to give rise to a somatic cell of any type. These embryonic stem cells are therefore said to be totipotent ("possessing all powers"). A key process in early development is the differential epigenetic modification of specific DNA nucleotide sequences in these embryonic stem cells, ultimately leading to the differential gene-expression profiles that characterize differentiated somatic cell types. Early modifications ensure that specific genes are expressed only in the cells and tissue types in which their gene products typically function (e.g., factor VIII expression primarily in hepatocytes, and dopamine-receptor expression in neurons).

Epigenetic modifications early in development processes also highlight a fundamental feature of genetic as compared to epigenetic information: all of the cells in a given individual contain almost exactly the same genetic information. It is the epigenetic information eventually placed "on top of" these sequences that enables them to achieve the diverse functions of differentiated somatic cells. A small percentage of genes, termed housekeeping genes, are necessary for the function and maintenance of all cells. These genes escape epigenetic silencing and remain transcriptionally active in all or nearly all cells. Housekeeping genes include those encoding histones, DNA and RNA polymerases, and ribosomal RNA genes.

How do embryonic stem cells achieve epigenetic states typical of totipotency, whereby they can give rise to all of the diverse cell types that comprise a fully developed organism? One explanation is that early embryogenesis, which occurs during the 10 or so days just after fertilization, is characterized by rapid fluctuation in genome-wide DNA methylation densities. Fertilization triggers a global loss of DNA methylation at most loci in both the oocyte-contributed and the sperm-contributed genomes. This loss of methylation is accomplished in part by suppression of the DNA methyltransferases, the enzymes that add methyl groups to DNA. Methylation is not directly copied by the DNA replication process. Instead, immediately following replication, the methyltransferases read the pattern of methylation on the parent DNA strand and use that information to determine which daughter-strand cytosines should be methylated. As embryonic cell division proceeds in the absence of DNA methyltransferases, cell division continues, eventually yielding cells that have nearly all of their loci in unmethylated, transcriptionally active states. Around the time of implantation in the uterus, the DNA methyltransferases become active again, permitting establishment of the cell lineage–specific marks required for the establishment of organ systems.

GENOMIC IMPRINTING

A baby inherits two copies of each autosomal gene: one from its mother and one from its father. For a large subset of these genes, expression is biallelic, meaning that both the maternally and the paternally inherited copies contribute to offspring phenotype. As noted earlier, for another, smaller subset of these genes, expression is stochastically monoallelic,[22]

meaning that the maternal copy is randomly chosen for inactivation in some somatic cells and the paternal copy is randomly chosen for inactivation in other somatic cells. For a third and smaller subset of autosomes (about 1%), either the maternal copy or the paternal copy is imprinted, meaning that either the copy inherited through the sperm or the copy inherited through the egg is inactivated and remains in this inactive state in all of the somatic cells of the individual.

The subset of genes that are subject to imprinting is highly enriched for loci relevant to organismal growth. The genetic conflict hypothesis[22] was developed as a potential explanation for this pattern. The logic of this hypothesis is as follows. Although both the mother and the father benefit genetically from the birth and survival of offspring, their interests are not entirely aligned. Because mothers make a large physiologic investment in each child, it is in their evolutionary best interest to limit the flow of energetic resources to any given offspring so as to maintain their physiologic capacity to bear subsequent children. By contrast, except in cases of lifelong monogamy, it is in the best interest of the fathers for their child to extract maximum resources from its mother, since the fathers' reproductive success is tied to the survival of their own child but not to the mother's ability to bear additional offspring in the future. Therefore, imprinted genes expressed from the maternal genome are predicted to limit offspring size, whereas imprinted genes expressed from the paternal genome are predicted to result in larger offspring. Available data are broadly consistent with these predictions.

One hallmark of imprinting-associated disease is that the phenotype of affected individuals is critically dependent on whether the mutation is inherited from the mother or from the father. Some examples are included in the following.

Prader-Willi and Angelman Syndromes

A well-known disease example of imprinting is associated with a deletion of about 4 million base pairs of the long arm of chromosome 15. When this deletion is inherited from the father, the child manifests Prader-Willi syndrome, with features that include short stature, hypotonia, small hands and feet, obesity, mild to moderate intellectual disability, and hypogonadism[23,24] (Fig. 6.2, A). The same deletion, when inherited from the mother, causes Angelman syndrome, which is characterized by severe intellectual disability, seizures, and an ataxic gait (Fig. 6.2, B).[25] These diseases are each observed in about 1 of every 15,000 live births; chromosome deletions are responsible for about 70% of cases of both diseases. The deletions that cause Prader-Willi and Angelman syndromes are indistinguishable at the DNA sequence level and affect the same group of genes.

It was unclear for several decades how the same deletion could produce such disparate results in different individuals. Further analysis showed that the 4 million base-pairs deletion (the critical region) contains several genes that are normally transcribed only on the copy of chromosome 15 that is inherited from the father.[26] These genes are imprinted on the copy of chromosome 15 inherited from the mother, meaning that they are transcriptionally silenced. Similarly, other genes in the critical region are transcriptionally active only on the chromosome copy inherited from the mother and are inactive, or imprinted, on the chromosome inherited from the father (Fig. 6.3). If the single active copy of one of these genes is lost because of a chromosome deletion, then no gene product is produced, resulting in disease.

Molecular analysis has revealed a great deal about genes in this critical region of chromosome 15.[26] The gene responsible for Angelman syndrome encodes a ligase involved in protein degradation during brain development, an observation that may help to explain the intellectual disability and ataxia observed in this disorder. In the brain, this gene is active only on the chromosome copy inherited from the mother. Consequently, a maternally-transmitted deletion removes the single active copy of this gene. Several genes in the critical region are associated with Prader-Willi syndrome and they are transcribed only on the chromosome transmitted by the father. A paternally-transmitted deletion removes the only active copies of these genes producing the features of Prader-Willi syndrome.

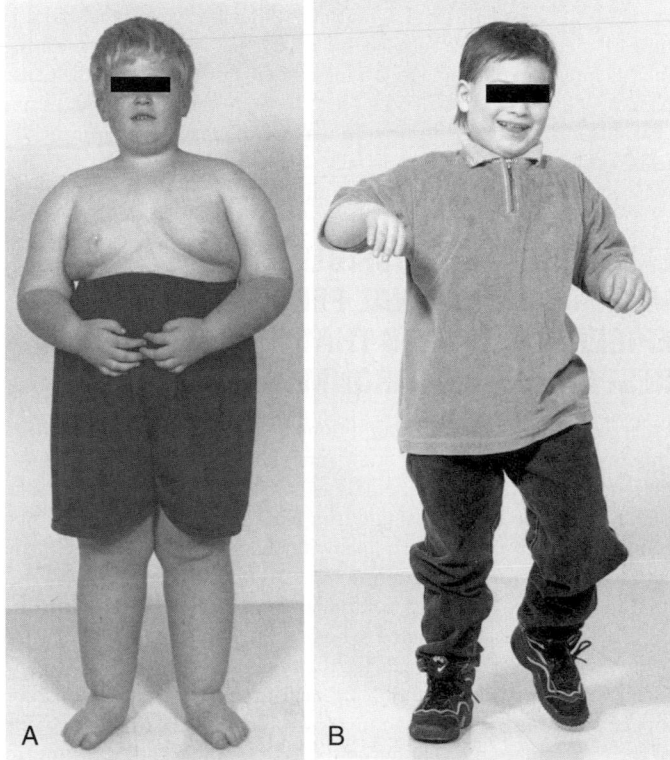

FIGURE 6.2 Prader-Willi and Angelman Syndromes. **A,** A child with Prader-Willi syndrome (truncal obesity, small hands and feet, inverted V-shaped upper lip). **B,** A child with Angelman syndrome (characteristic posture, ataxic gait, bouts of uncontrolled laughter). (From Jorde LB, Carey JC, Bamshad MJ: *Medical genetics,* ed 4, Philadelphia, 2010, Mosby.)

Beckwith-Wiedemann Syndrome

Another well-known example of imprinting is Beckwith-Wiedemann syndrome, an overgrowth condition accompanied by an elevated risk of cancer. Beckwith-Wiedemann syndrome is usually identifiable at birth because of the large size for gestational age, neonatal hypoglycemia, a large tongue, creases on the earlobe, and omphalocele (birth defect of infant's intestines).[27] Children with Beckwith-Wiedemann syndrome have an increased risk of developing Wilms tumor or hepatoblastoma. Both of these tumor types can be treated effectively if they are detected early; thus, screening at regular intervals is an important part of management. Some children with Beckwith-Wiedemann syndrome also develop asymmetrical overgrowth of a limb or one side of the face or trunk (hemihyperplasia).

As with Angelman syndrome, a minority of Beckwith-Wiedemann syndrome cases (about 20% to 30%) are caused by the inheritance of two copies of chromosome 11 from the father and no copy of the chromosome from the mother, in a process known as uniparental disomy. Several genes on the short arm of chromosome 11 are imprinted on either the paternally- or the maternally-transmitted chromosome. These genes are found in two separate, differentially methylated regions (DMRs). In DMR1, the gene that encodes insulin-like growth factor 2 *(IGF2)* is inactive on the maternally-transmitted chromosome but active on the paternally-transmitted chromosome, such that a normal individual has only one active copy of *IGF2.* When two copies of the paternal chromosome are inherited (i.e., paternal uniparental disomy) or there is loss of imprinting on the maternal copy of *IGF2,* an active *IGF2* gene is present in double dose. These changes produce increased levels of *IGF2* during fetal development, contributing to the overgrowth features of Beckwith-Wiedemann syndrome. Thus, in contrast to Prader-Willi and Angelman syndromes, which are produced by a missing gene product, Beckwith-Wiedemann syndrome is caused, in part, by overexpression of a gene product.

Russell-Silver Syndrome

Russell-Silver syndrome is characterized by growth retardation; proportionate short stature; leg length discrepancy; and a small, triangular-shaped face. About one-third of Russell-Silver syndrome cases are caused

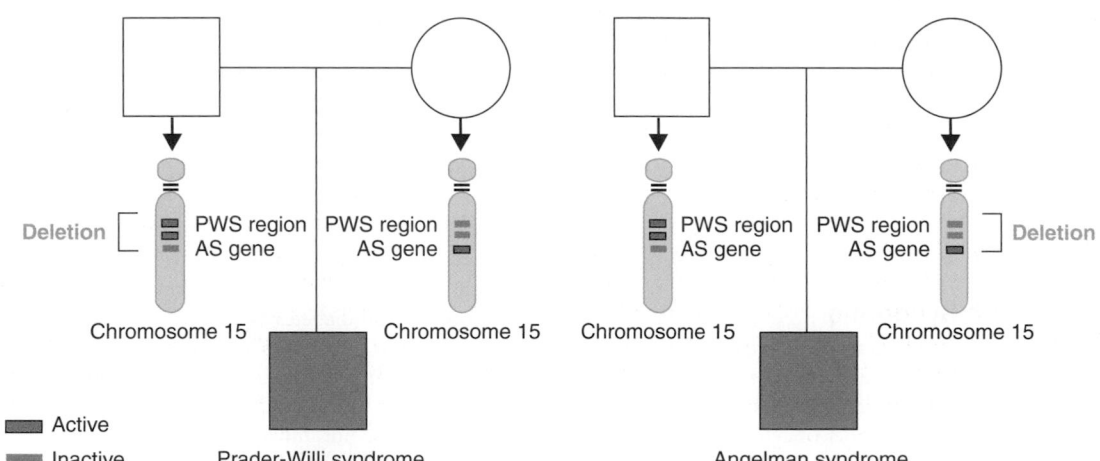

Active
Inactive

Prader-Willi syndrome

Angelman syndrome

FIGURE 6.3 Prader-Willi Syndrome (PWS) and Angelman Syndrome (AS) Pedigrees. These pedigrees illustrate the inheritance patterns of Prader-Willi syndrome, which can be caused by a 4 million base pair deletion of chromosome 15q when inherited from the father. In contrast, Angelman syndrome can be caused by the same deletion but only when it is inherited from the mother. The reason for this difference is that different genes in this region are normally imprinted (inactivated) in the copies of 15q transmitted by the mother and the father in Prader-Willi and Angelman syndromes, respectively. (From Jorde LB, Carey JC, Bamshad MJ: *Medical genetics,* ed 4, Philadelphia, 2010, Mosby.)

by imprinting abnormalities of chromosome 11p15.5 that lead to down-regulation of *IGF2* and therefore diminished growth. Another 10% of cases of Russell-Silver syndrome are caused by maternal uniparental disomy. Thus, while it is upregulation, or extra copies, of active *IGF2* that causes overgrowth in Beckwith-Wiedemann syndrome, it is downregulation of *IGF2* that causes the diminished growth seen in Russell-Silver syndrome.

EPIGENETICS IN COGNITIVE DEVELOPMENT AND MENTAL HEALTH

Several lines of evidence suggest a role for epigenetic abnormalities in disorders of cognitive development.

Epigenetics and Ethanol Exposure in Utero

The impact of ethanol exposure *in utero* on skeletal and neural development was first reported in 1973,[28] and led to broad awareness of fetal alcohol syndrome. It was not until recently, however, that population-based and molecular-level studies began to clarify the epigenetic signals that are associated with these developmental abnormalities. Initially, researchers found that alcohol exposure in utero can impact the DNA methylation states of various genomic elements but without specific emphasis on loci directly relevant to skeletal and neural development.[29] Later experiments revealed that treating cultured neural stem cells with ethanol impairs their ability to differentiate to functional neurons; this impairment seems to be correlated with aberrant, dense methylation at loci that are active in normal neuronal tissue.[30] One possible explanation for these effects is that ethanol exposure in utero modulates fetal expression of the DNA methyltransferases.[31]

Epigenetics and Mental Health

Several emerging lines of evidence suggest an association between altered epigenetic states and mental health. A recent study found that children who grow up under conditions of poverty have atypical methylation at a serotonin receptor, suggesting DNA methylation as a mechanistic link between early-life socioeconomic stress to an increased propensity to depression.[32] Similarly, in individuals with posttraumatic stress disorder (PTSD), alterations in gene expression in key neural pathways are associated with atypical methylation in a large set of genes.[33] Among individuals with PTSD, specific changes in methylation are associated with suicidal ideation and behavior.[34] Autism-spectrum disorder also is associated with altered DNA methylation at some loci.[35] In these cases, as in the connection of epigenetic abnormality to depression and PTSD, it is not clear whether epigenetic alteration plays a mechanistic role in the etiology of cognitive syndromes, or whether information on this link is useful principally for suggesting biomarkers potentially useful for diagnosis.

Fragile X Syndrome: A Genetic/Epigenetic Syndrome

Fragile X syndrome can be described as a genetic and epigenetic disease, insofar as abnormalities of both sorts are observed at the fragile X locus, *FMR1*, in affected individuals. The most common *genetic* abnormality at *FMR1* involves expansion in the number of cytosine-guanine (CG) dinucleotide repeats in the gene promoter. Females who have CG repeats in excess of the ⊕35 that are typical at this locus are at risk for fragile X–associated primary ovarian insufficiency, characterized by an elevated risk of early menopause.[36] Males with moderate expansions are at risk of fragile X tremor ataxia syndrome (FXTAS), characterized by a late-onset intention tremor.[37] Both of these conditions seem to arise through accumulation of excess levels of *FMR1* mRNAs in nuclear inclusion bodies.[38,39] Individuals with 200 repeats are at risk of fragile

X syndrome, characterized by reduced IQ and a set of behavioral abnormalities.

Remarkably, while possession of a large CG repeat in the *FMR1* promoter dramatically increases the probability that an individual will have fragile X syndrome, the disease can be at once present in males who have the large repeat and absent in their brothers who have inherited an allele of very similar size.[40]

This can be explained at least in part by the observation that acquisition of methylation-based silencing at *FMR1* is stochastic, meaning that the presence of a large repeat increases the probability of the dense promoter methylation that could lead to gene silencing, but does not guarantee it. It remains to be seen whether dietary or environmental features can modulate the probability that dense methylation at *FMR1* will accrue in individuals with the full-mutation allele.

EXPLORING THE POSSIBLE MULTIGENERATIONAL PERSISTENCE OF EPIGENETIC STATES THAT ARISE IN RESPONSE TO ENVIRONMENTAL FACTORS

Emerging data suggest that conditions encountered in utero, during childhood, and even during adolescence or later can have long-term impacts on epigenetic states. Some data have been interpreted to indicate that epigenetic changes arising during an individual's lifetime can be transmitted through the germline, with the potential to impact gene expression in future generations.

Some reports of transgenerational inheritance of environment-induced epigenetics have failed to be replicated in subsequent work by other researchers. For example, Iqbal and colleagues[41] sought to follow up on an earlier report[42] that the epigenetic impacts of endocrine disruptors can be transmitted, by an unknown mechanism, to the germline of the grandchildren of the mice exposed. Although they did confirm the capacity of endocrine disruptors to induce epigenetic changes in tissues and gametes directly exposed, they found no evidence that any differences can persist to the germline of exposed animals' grandchildren. Further investigation will be required to explain the disparity between these conflicting findings. A few examples of such apparent connections between environment and inheritance of epigenetic states are discussed below; all of the examples remain under active investigation.

Epigenetics and Nutrition

During the winter of 1943, millions of people in urban areas of the Netherlands suffered starvation conditions as a result of a Nazi blockage that prevented shipments of food from agricultural area. When researchers sought to investigate how exposure to famine during this Dutch Hunger Winter had impacted individuals born in a historically prosperous country, they found that individuals who had been in utero during this interval of severe nutritional deprivation were more likely to suffer from obesity and diabetes as adults than were other individuals from the Netherlands. There also seemed to be a transgenerational impact, in that the children of individuals who were in utero during the Dutch Hunger Winter were found to be significantly smaller than were the children of those not impacted by the blockade. Other datasets reveal elevated risk of cardiovascular and metabolic disease for offspring of individuals exposed during early development to fluctuations in food availability.[43]

The specific molecular mechanisms that may mediate these apparent relationships between nutritional deprivation and disease risk on one or more generations are largely unknown. From some animal models, it seems that the *IGF2* gene is a possible target of epigenetic modifications arising through nutritional deprivation. Exposure in utero and through lactation to some chemicals (including bisphenol-A, a constituent of plastics sometimes used in food preparation and storage) seems to lead to epigenetic modifications similar to those that arise through nutritional deprivation in early life.[44]

Epigenetics and Maternal Care

There is increasing evidence that parenting style can impact epigenetic states, and that this information can be transmitted from one generation to the next. Mice and other rodents can exhibit two alternate styles of nursing behavior. One style is characterized by frequent arched-back nursing, with a high level of licking and grooming behavior. An alternate style is characterized by infrequent arched-back nursing and less licking and grooming behavior. In one study,[45] pups of mothers that engaged in frequent arched-backed nursing were found to have significantly lower methylation levels and higher transcription activity of a glucocorticoid receptor–encoding locus. Because the glucocorticoid receptor is involved in a pathway that intensifies fearfulness and response to stress, these findings suggest that alteration to methylation states could help explain the finding that exposure to stress early in life can modulate behavior in adulthood. These findings also highlight the concept that epigenetic processes can help store information about the environment, and that the relevant epigenetic modifications can modulate behavior later in life.

EPIGENETIC CHANGE OVER THE LIFE SPAN

Twin Studies Reveal Epigenetic Changes over Time

Identical (monozygotic) twins, whose DNA sequences are essentially the same, offer a unique opportunity to isolate and examine the trajectory of epigenetic change over the life span. A recent study found that, as twins age, they exhibit increasingly substantial differences in methylation patterns of the DNA sequences of their somatic cells; these changes are often reflected in increasing numbers of phenotypic differences. Twins with significant lifestyle differences (e.g., smoking vs. nonsmoking) tend to accumulate larger numbers of differences in their methylation patterns. These results, along with findings generated in animal studies, suggest that changes in epigenetic states may be an important part of the aging process.[46]

Epigenetics and Aging

The occurrence of epigenetic change over the life span, as suggested by studies in twins, is echoed by broader studies in both human and nonhuman systems. In yeast, a shift in histone modification, as well as an overall decline in histone abundance, is a marker of replicative aging and is associated with dysregulation of gene expression.[47] Chemical labeling techniques have revealed that the genome-wide abundance of hydroxymethylcytosine increases with time in the brains of adult mice.[48] In view of these and similar findings, some authors have proposed that senescence, itself, can be characterized as an epigenomic phenomenon.[49] From this perspective, while accrual of adverse exposures over the life span is to some degree unavoidable, understanding environmental impacts on epigenetic states could lead to a new paradigm for life span extension.

This apparent relationship between epigenetics and aging could help to explain the long-standing observation that metformin, a drug used to treat insulin resistance, also is effective in slowing senescence in yeast.[50] Studies in human populations suggest that long-term use of metformin may even extend mean life span in diabetic people beyond that expected for untreated, nondiabetic individuals.[51] Initially, these effects, which echo the increase in life span occurring under caloric restriction in primate models,[52] were thought to operate directly through the impact of metformin on metabolism. However, metformin has recently been found specifically to alter the expression of *SIRT1*, the gene encoding sirtuin, a protein that modulates the metabolic response to energy limitation. Therefore, it is possible that a drug that has long been used to treat insulin resistance may modulate epigenetic pathways, with possible opportunities for life span extension in humans.[49]

MOLECULAR AND COMPUTATIONAL TOOLS FOR EXPLORING EPIGENETIC STATES

Epigenetic information is not encoded DNA sequence. Therefore, specialized methods must be used to detect and quantify it.

Detecting DNA Methylation in Populations of Molecules: Methyl-Sensitive Restriction Enzymes

Many restriction enzymes are sensitive to methylation, and so they cleave DNA only at unmethylated cytosines. Clues to the overall level of methylation in DNA isolated from a given individual can, therefore, be gathered by treating DNA with a methyl-sensitive enzyme, and then comparing banding patterns for enzyme-treated and nonenzyme-treated samples.[53]

Detecting DNA Methylation in Single Molecules: Bisulfite Conversion

Sometimes it is of interest to gather information about methylation on individual molecules. For example, among males who inherit a full-mutation fragile X allele, there is a strong correlation between the severity of the syndrome and the number of cells in which the fragile X allele is densely methylated.[40] To collect information on the methylation states of individual molecules, DNA can be subjected to bisulfite conversion before sequencing. Bisulfite treatment does not alter most nucleotides, including methylated cytosines, but deaminates unmethylated cytosines to uracil.[54] Because uracil complements adenine, not guanine, in double-stranded DNA, methylated and unmethylated cytosines can be distinguished in conventional sequence data, provided that the original sequence of that region is known and can be used to distinguish between true thymines and converted, unmethylated cytosines. Either subcloning followed by Sanger sequencing or single-molecule sequencing technologies can then be applied to ascertain the detailed methylation patterns of individual molecules.

Detecting DNA Hydroxymethylation: Fluorescence Resonance Energy Transfer

Following Wossidlo and colleagues'[14] discovery that loss of DNA methylation and the gain of DNA hydroxymethylation during early development, there has been considerable interest in exploring the specific functional impacts and mechanisms of this transition. However, efforts in this area have been hampered by lack of a method to detect relative levels of DNA methylation and DNA hydroxymethylation within individual molecules. Recently, Song and colleagues[55] introduced a promising solution. Under their new method, DNAs are first treated with two different fluorophores. Of these, one binds methyl groups and the other binds hydroxymethyl groups. When samples are examined using fluorescence assays, the methylation and hydroxymethylation can be distinguished visually. This new method will undoubtedly enable critical insight into the basic biology of epigenetic transitions and, perhaps, into the mechanisms of epigenetic disease.

Identifying Histone-Modification States: Chromatin Immunoprecipitation

The identity of DNA-bound proteins can provide important clues as to the activity states of individual regions. The goal of chromatin immunoprecipitation (ChIP) is to ascertain the sequences bound by specific proteins of interest. Broadly, this is achieved in seven steps:

1. **Cross-link** DNA-bound proteins to the specific genomic regions to which they are attached. At this step, binding is not specific, meaning that all proteins, regardless of identity, are cross-linked to DNA.
2. **Shear** DNA, lysing DNA regions that are not protein bound. Proteins prevent sheering of the DNA to which they are bound.
3. **Select** for proteins of interest, using a protein-specific antibody.
4. **Capture** protein-DNA complexes by using a secondary antibody that can bind to the first, and by washing away any remaining unbound DNA fragments.
5. **Remove** protein-DNA cross-links and wash away proteins.
6. **Sequence** DNA fragments to profile the portion of genome that was bound by the protein of interest.
7. **Repeat** to characterize DNAs bound to any other proteins of interest.

Detecting DNA Accessibility States: DNase Hypersensitivity Testing

DNase enzymes cleave uncondensed, transcriptionally active euchromatic DNA, but not condensed, transcriptionally silent heterochromatic DNA. Genomic regions that are euchromatic in a given cell type therefore can be identified through DNase treatment of bulk DNA samples. This approach can be readily applied at the genome scale,[56] opening opportunities to compare transcriptionally active states across cells under various differentiation states and culture conditions.

Detecting DNA Accessibility States in Single Molecules: Assay for Transposase-Accessible Chromatin

Like DNase hypersensitivity testing, the recently introduced assay for transposase-accessible chromatin (ATAC-seq) is focused on identifying genomic regions whose "open," euchromatic states suggest that they could be transcriptionally active.[57] However, in contrast to DNase assays under which transcriptionally active states are identified by their overall sensitivity to DNase enzyme cleavage, ATAC-seq uses a transpose for which cleavage of accessible sites is followed immediately by specific ligation of a linker that bears barcodes that differ among cells. Genomic regions that have been ligated to adapters can then be isolated, amplified, and sequenced. In contrast to earlier approaches, which collect population-level summaries of active and inactive states of individual genomic locations, the use of single-cell barcodes in ATAC-seq enables comparison of epigenomes across individual cells in a sample.[58] Using single-cell ATAC-seq, one group found that there is an unexpectedly high level of variation among the epigenetic states of individual intestinal lymphoid cells, and that this variation is shaped by the microbiome.[59]

Publicly Available Resources Enable Exploration of Epigenetic States at Genome Scale

One of the great advances of the genomics era is the emergence of public, online data repositories for researchers to share their findings, enabling insights that might not be accessible from the work of any single research group. Such publicly available datasets have provided unprecedented opportunities to compare epigenomic profiles over developmental time and between tissues in disparate functional states.

The Encyclopedia of DNA Elements (ENCODE), a project supported by the National Human Genome Research Institute (NHGRI), is providing great insights as a catalog of the epigenomic signatures of cells grown in culture.[60] The Roadmap Epigenomics Project, a cooperative venture of epigenomic biologists worldwide sponsored by the U.S. National Institutes of Health, is expanding this goal to provide information on freshly sampled cells and tissues.[61]

Although it is possible for users to browse data using a visual interface, the most efficient way to leverage these publicly available resources is to use a command-line approach to download, process, and analyze available datasets. In just the past 3 years, data available through ROADMAP have provided insight into the genomic architecture underlying disorders of gonadal development,[62] juvenile arthritis,[63] and attention-deficit/hyperactivity disorder (HDAD).[64]

EPIGENETICS AND CANCER
DNA Methylation and Cancer

Some of the most extensive evidence for the association of epigenetic modification with human disease comes from studies of cancer[65,66] (Fig. 6.4). Tumor cells often exhibit decreased methylation genome-wide, relative to normal cells of the same type, which can increase the activity of oncogenes (see Chapter 12). Genome-wide loss of methylation tends to continue as tumors progress from benign neoplasms to malignancy. In addition, the promoter regions of tumor-suppressor genes are often hypermethylated, decreasing their rate of transcription and thus their ability to inhibit tumor formation. Hypermethylation of the promoter region of the *RB1* gene is often seen in retinoblastoma,[67] and hypermethylation of the *MLH1* locus is associated with colorectal cancer.[68] It is important to note that the observation of perturbed DNA methylation states in tumors is not, itself, an indication that perturbation in DNA methylation state is the proximate cause of cancer.[69] However, as described in the following, the finding that many tumors have epigenetic abnormalities hints at exciting new opportunities for minimally invasive cancer screening and diagnosis.

Global Epigenomic Alterations and Cancer

A major feature of one form of inherited colon cancer (hereditary nonpolyposis colorectal cancer [HNPCC]) is the methylation of the promoter region of a gene, *MLH1*, whose protein product repairs damaged DNA. Inactivation of *MLH1*, a DNA mismatch repair enzyme, is associated with accrual of DNA damage, another common feature of colon tumors (see Fig. 42.28). Abnormal methylation of tumor-suppressor genes also is common in the progression of Barrett's esophagus,[70] a condition in which the esophagus is lined with cells that have features typically associated with the lower intestinal tract.

Epigenetic Screening for Cancer

As noted previously, specific epigenetic abnormalities are often a defining feature of a tumor, but cannot necessarily be inferred to be the cause of disease. Regardless of the nature of the connection between epigenetic abnormality and any particular cancer, the ability to screen for abnormal epigenetic states raises the possibility that epigenetic screening approaches could complement or even replace existing early-detection methods. In some cases, epigenetic screening can be implemented using bodily fluids, such as urine or sputum, eliminating the need for the more invasive, costly, and risky strategies that are currently standard. For example, screening for epigenetic misregulation of miRNAs has shown promise as a tool for detecting and characterizing cancers of the colon,[71] breast,[72] and prostate.[73] Other epigenetics-based screening approaches have shown promise for detecting and characterizing cancers of the bladder,[74] lung,[75,76] and prostate.[77]

Screening for epigenetic abnormality to detect cancer may be especially powerful in conjunction with emerging methods for detecting tumors in blood and sputum samples.[76,78] These "liquid-biopsy" methods are minimally invasive and so could be useful not only for characterizing abnormalities after diagnosis but also for performing routine, simultaneous screening for multiple types of cancers, even in individuals without

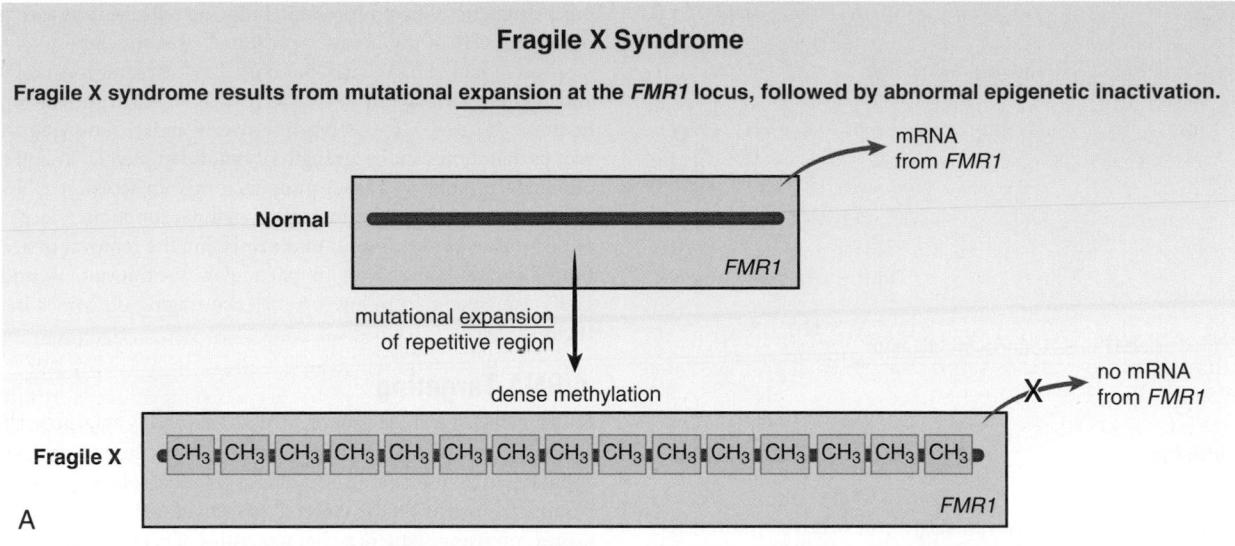

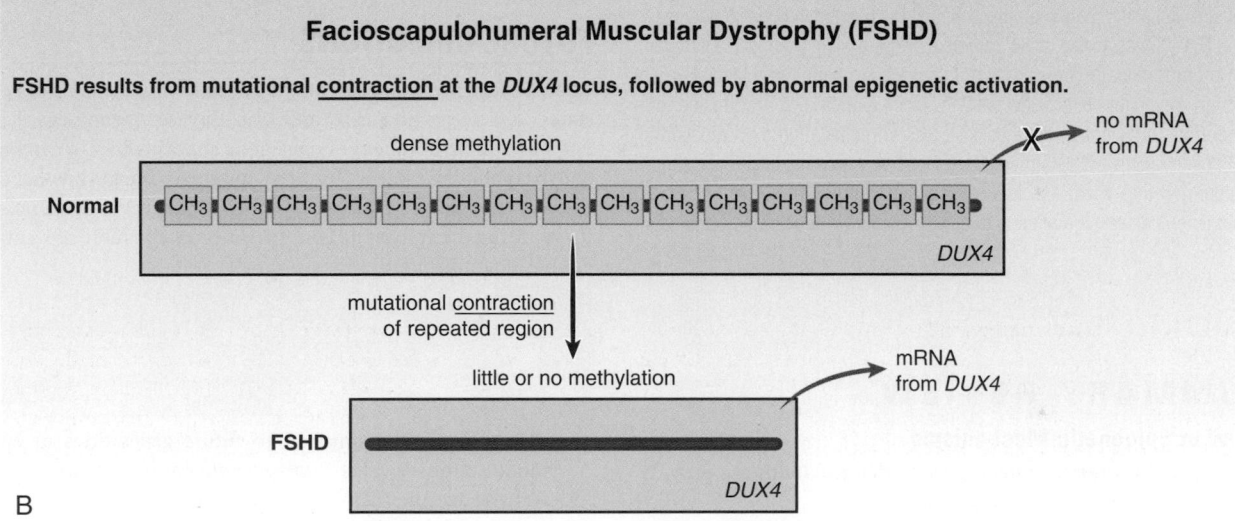

FIGURE 6.4 Comparing the Molecular Mechanisms of Fragile X and FSHD. **A,** *FMR1* in normal, expanded permutation, and full-mutation states. **B,** *DUX4* in normal and contracted states.

signs of disease, and for detecting the emergence of drug-resistance mutations in individuals undergoing chemotherapy.

Misregulation of miRNAs in Cancer

Hypermethylation also is seen in microRNA genes, which encode small (22 base pair) RNA molecules that bind to the ends of mRNAs, degrading them and preventing their translation. More than 1000 microRNA sequences have been identified in humans, and hypermethylation of specific subgroups of micoRNAs is associated with tumorigenesis.

EMERGING STRATEGIES FOR THE TREATMENT OF EPIGENETIC DISEASE

Epigenetic modifications are potentially reversible: DNA can be demethylated, histones can be modified to change the transcriptional state of nearby DNA, and miRNA-encoding loci can be up- or down-regulated. This raises the prospect for treating epigenetic disease with pharmaceutical agents that directly reverse the changes associated with the disease phenotype. In recent years, interventions involving all three types of epigenetic modulators (DNA methylation, histone modification, and miRNAs) have shown considerable promise for the treatment of disease.

DNA Demethylating Agents

5-Azacytidine has been used as a therapeutic drug in the treatment of leukemia and myelodysplastic syndrome.[79] A cytosine analog, 5-azacytidine, is incorporated into DNA opposite its complementary nucleotide, guanine. Chemical differences between 5-azacytidine and conventional cytosine (Fig. 6.5) cause it to achieve irreversible binding to the DNA methyltransferases. As a result, the administration of 5-azacytidine tends to reduce the density of DNA methylation,[80] offering prospects for reversing the aberrant accumulation of methylation at tumor-suppressor loci. Though associated with various side effects, including digestive disturbance, treatment with 5-azacytidine has shown promise in the treatment of diseases, including pancreatic cancer[81] and myelodysplastic syndromes.[82]

Histone Deacetylase Inhibitors

The activity of the histone deacetylases (HDACs) increases chromatin compaction, decreasing transcriptional activity. In many cases, excessive activity of HDACs results in transcriptional inactivation of tumor-suppressor genes, leading ultimately to the development of tumors. Treatment with HDAC inhibitors, either alone or in combination with

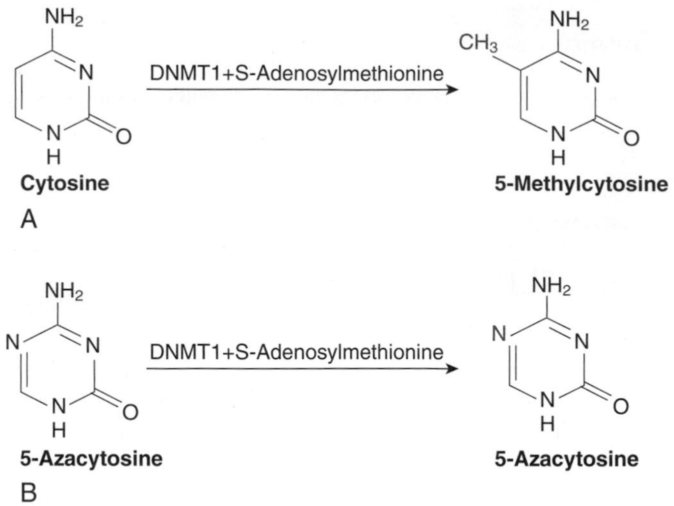

FIGURE 6.5 **5-Azacytosine as Demethylating Agent. A,** Unmethylated cytosines in DNA are typically subject to the addition of methyl groups by DNMT1, a DNA methyltransferase, using methyl groups supplied by the methyl donor *S*-adenosylmethionine. **B,** In 5-Azacytosine, the 5′ carbon of cytosine is replaced with a nitrogen. This chemical difference is sufficient both to block the addition of a methyl group and to confer irreversible binding to DNMT1. Incorporation of 5-azacytosine into DNA is therefore sufficient to drive passive loss of methylation from replicating DNA, and thus to reactivate hypermethylated loci. 5-Azacytosine, bound to a sugar, can be integrated into DNA, and has been administered with some success in treating epigenetic diseases that arise through hypermethylation of individual loci.

other drugs, has shown promise in reducing cell-division rates in culture cells of cancers of the breast,[83] prostate,[84] and pancreas.[85]

Most recently, HDACs have been used to treat some forms of leukemia and lymphoma that are characterized by transcriptional repression. In those diseases, HDACs become overly active, removing the acetyl groups that diminish the strength of bonds between DNA and histones, ultimately preventing transcription factors from accessing DNA regions whose activity is required for proper cellular function. A large number of drugs have proven useful in diminishing the removal of acetylation from histones. One drug in particular, abexinostat, is undergoing safety assessment to follow up on encouraging outcomes in a Phase II clinical trial.[86]

miRNA Targeting

A major challenge in developing drugs that modify epigenetic alterations is to target only the genes responsible for a specific cancer. Therapeutic approaches that use microRNAs offer a potential solution to this problem because treatment can be targeted to individual loci that have aberrant expression using sequence characteristics of relevant RNA molecules.

FUTURE DIRECTIONS

Robust experimental observations are clarifying the roles of epigenetic states in determining cell fates and disease phenotypes. The well-documented involvement of epigenetic abnormalities in carcinogenesis and the mounting evidence for these epigenetic changes in other common diseases (discussed in other chapters) will likely elucidate possibilities for reversing the epigenetic abnormalities and possibly preventing their establishment in utero.

▮ S U M M A R Y   R E V I E W

Overview of Epigenetic Mechanisms

1. Differences between the phenotypes of identical twins can provide novel insights into epigenetic phenomena.
2. To be both effective and safe, pharmaceutical strategies for treating epigenetic abnormalities must be targeted to affected genomic regions.
3. Epigenetics modification alters gene expression without changes to DNA sequence.
4. Investigators are studying three major types of epigenetic processes: (a) DNA methylation, which results from attachment of a methyl group to a cytosine; in the somatic cells, all or nearly all methylation occurs at cytosines that are followed by guanines ("CpG dinucleotides"); (b) histone modification, through the addition of various chemical groups including methylation and acetylation; and (c) noncoding RNAs (ncRNAs or miRNAs), short nucleotides derived from introns of protein coding genes or transcribed as independent genes from regions of the genome whose functions, if any, remain poorly understood. MicroRNAs regulate diverse signaling pathways.
5. DNA methylation is, at present, the best-studied epigenetic process. When a gene becomes heavily methylated, the DNA is less likely to be transcribed into mRNA.
6. Methylation, along with histone hypoacetylation and condensation of chromatin, inhibits the binding of proteins that promote transcription, such that the gene becomes transcriptionally inactive.
7. Environmental factors, such as diet gene exposure to certain chemicals, may cause epigenetic modifications.

8. The heritable transmission to future generations of epigenetic modifications is called *transgenerational inheritance.*
9. As twins age, they demonstrate increasing differences in methylation patterns of their DNA sequences, causing increasing numbers of phenotypic differences.
10. In studies of twins with significant lifestyle differences (e.g., smoking vs. nonsmoking) large numbers of differences in their methylation patterns are observed to accrue over time.

Genomic Imprinting

1. For some human genes, a given gene is transcriptionally active on only one copy of a chromosome (e.g., the copy inherited from the father). On the other copy of the chromosome (the one inherited from the mother), the gene is transcriptionally inactive. This process of gene silencing, in which genes are silenced depending on which parent transmits them, is known as *imprinting;* the transcriptionally silenced genes are said to be "imprinted."
2. When an allele is imprinted, it typically has dense DNA methylation; the nonimprinted allele is typically not methylated.
3. A well-known disease example of imprinting is associated with a deletion of about 4 million base pairs (Mb) of the long arm of chromosome 15. When this deletion is inherited from the father, the child manifests Prader-Willi syndrome.
4. The same 4-Mb deletion, when inherited from the mother, causes Angelman syndrome.
5. Another well-known example of imprinting is Beckwith-Wiedemann syndrome, an overgrowth condition accompanied by an increased predisposition to cancer.

SUMMARY REVIEW—cont'd

6. Whereas upregulation, or extra copies, of active *IGF2* causes overgrowth in Beckwith-Wiedemann syndrome, downregulation of *IGF2* causes the diminished growth seen in Russell-Silver syndrome.

Epigenetics in Cognitive Development and Mental Health

1. Consumption of alcohol during pregnancy has long been associated with the cognitive abnormalities of fetal alcohol syndrome. Recent findings suggest that alcohol may affect these changes through altered methylation of genes involved in neuronal differentiation.
2. Individuals with autism and with PTSD have altered DNA methylation profiles; current work is investigating the potential functional relevance of these alterations.
3. Fragile X syndrome results from a complex interaction of genetic and epigenetic abnormalities.
4. Fetal alcohol syndrome, which results from ethanol exposure in utero, may be mediated by the repressive impact of ethanol on the DNA methyltransferases.
5. Both abnormal gain of methylation, as in the case of fragile X syndrome, and abnormal loss of methylation, as in the case of FSHD, can produce disease phenotypes.

Exploring the Possible Multigenerational Persistence of Epigenetic States That Arise in Response to Environmental Factors

1. Events encountered in utero, in childhood, and in adolescence can result in specific epigenetic changes that yield a wide range of phenotypic abnormalities, including metabolic syndromes.

Epigenetic Change over the Life Span

1. Identical twins diverge in their epigenetic states over time at rates potentially modulated by environmental factors, such as tobacco use.
2. Metformin, a drug useful in treating insulin resistance, also may prolong life through epigenetic mechanisms.

Molecular and Computational Tools for Exploring Epigenetic States

1. Bisulfite conversion induces chemical changes in the binding properties of cytosine and methylcytosine, such that they can be distinguished in sequence data.

2. Assay for transposase-accessible chromatin (ATAC-seq) uses a transposase to introduce DNA cell-specific barcodes into euchromatic DNA regions, permitting comparison of chromatin states across cells.

Epigenetics and Cancer

1. The best evidence for epigenetic effects on disease risk comes from studies of human cancer.
2. Methylation densities decline as tumors progress, which can increase the activity of oncogenes, causing tumors to progress from benign neoplasms to malignancy. Additionally, the promoter regions of tumor-suppressor genes are often hypermethylated. These elevated methylation levels decrease their rate of transcription at these critical genes, thus reducing the ability to inhibit tumor formation.
3. Hypermethylation also is seen in microRNA genes and is associated with tumorigenesis.
4. 5-Azacytidine, a demethylating agent, has been used as a therapeutic drug in the treatment of leukemia and myelodysplastic syndrome.

Emerging Strategies for the Treatment of Epigenetic Disease

1. In diseases associated with aberrant, dense methylation of individual loci, treatment with 5-azacytidine, a cytosine analog that is refractory to the addition of methyl groups, can lead to clinically beneficial reduction in methylation densities.
2. miRNAs can be used to regulate the expression of loci whose altered epigenetic states are associated with disease.
3. Histone–deacetylase inhibitors have shown promise in treating cancers of the breast, prostate, and pancreas.

Future Directions

1. Robust experimental observations are defining the roles of epigenetic states in shaping cell fates.
2. The well-documented involvement of epigenetic abnormalities in carcinogenesis and the mounting evidence for these epigenetic changes in other common diseases (discussed throughout the text) will likely elucidate new therapies with the possibilities of reversing the epigenetic abnormalities.

KEY TERMS

Angelman syndrome, 180
Assay for transposase-accessible chromatin (ATAC-seq), 184
Beckwith-Wiedemann syndrome, 181
Biallelic, 180
Bisulfite conversion, 183
Chromatin immunoprecipitation (ChIP), 183
DNA hydroxymethylation, 179
DNA methylation, 178
DNA methyltransferase, 180
Embryonic stem cell, 180
Encyclopedia of DNA Elements (ENCODE), 184
Epigenetic, 182

Euchromatin (euchromatic), 179
Fragile X syndrome, 182
Genetic conflict hypothesis, 180
Heterochromatin (heterochromatic), 178, 179
Histone, 179
Histone modification, 179
Housekeeping gene, 180
Imprinted, 180
MicroRNA (miRNA), 179
Monoallelic, 180
Noncoding RNA (ncRNA), 179
Nucleosome, 179
Oncogene, 179

Oncomir, 180
Prader-Willi syndrome, 180
Protamines, 179
Roadmap Epigenomics Project, 184
Russell-Silver syndrome, 181
Somatic mosaicism, 179
Totipotent, 180
Transcription factor, 179
Tumor-suppressor gene, 179
Uniparental disomy, 181
X inactivation, 179

REFERENCES

1. Bird A: Perceptions of epigenetics. *Nature* 447(7143):396–398, 2007.
2. Deans C, Maggert KA: What do you mean, "epigenetic"? *Genetics* 199(4):887–896, 2015.
3. Miska EA, Ferguson-Smith AC: Transgenerational inheritance: models and mechanisms of non–DNA sequence–based inheritance. *Science* 354(6308):59–63, 2016.
4. Barlow DP, et al: The mouse insulin-like growth factor type 2 receptor is imprinted and closely linked to the Tme locus. *Nature* 349:84–87, 1991.
5. Bartolomei MS, Zemel S, Tilghman SM: Parental imprinting of the mouse H19 gene. *Nature* 351:153–155, 1991.
6. DeChiara TM, Robertson EJ, Efstratiadis A: Parental imprinting of the mouse insulin-like growth factor II gene. *Cell* 64:849–859, 1991.
7. Lister R, Pelizzola M, Dowen RH, et al: Human DNA methylomes at base resolution show widespread epigenomic differences. *Nature* 462(7271):315–322, 2009.
8. Lyon MF: Gene action in the X-chromosome of the mouse (*Mus musculus* L.). *Nature* 190(4773):372–373, 1961.
9. Ohno S, Kaplan WD, Kinosita R: Formation of the sex chromatin by a single X-chromosome in liver cells of *Rattus norvegicus*. *Exp Cell Res* 18:415–418, 1959.
10. Cui J, et al: Epigenetic silencing of TPM2 contributes to colorectal cancer progression upon RhoA activation. *Tumour Biol* 37(9):12477–12483, 2016.
11. Tang Q, et al: DNA methylation array analysis identifies breast cancer associated-RPTOR, MGRN1 and RAPSN hypomethylation in peripheral blood DNA. *Oncotarget* 7(39):64191–64202, 2016.
12. Zhang M, et al: DNA methylation patterns can estimate nonequivalent outcomes of breast cancer with the same receptor subtypes. *PLoS ONE* 10(11):e0142279, 2015.
13. Smith ZD, Meissner A: DNA methylation: roles in mammalian development. *Nat Rev Genet* 14(3):204–220, 2013.
14. Wossidlo M, et al: 5-Hydroxymethylcytosine in the mammalian zygote is linked with epigenetic reprogramming. *Nat Commun* 2:241, 2011.
15. Lorsbach RB, et al: TET1, a member of a novel protein family, is fused to MLL in acute myeloid leukemia containing the t(10;11)(q22;q23). *Leukemia* 17:637–641, 2003.
16. Szyf M: The elusive role of 5′-hydroxymethylcytosine. *Epigenomics* 8(11):1539–1551, 2016.
17. Biswas M, et al: Role of histone tails in structural stability of the nucleosome. *PLoS Comput Biol* 7(12):e1002279, 2011.
18. Meshorer E, Misteli T: Chromatin in pluripotent embryonic stem cells and differentiation. *Nat Rev Mol Cell Biol* 7(7):540–546, 2006.
19. Yuan S, Zaidi S, Brueckner M: Congenital heart disease: emerging themes linking genetics and development. *Curr Opin Genet Dev* 23(3):352–359, 2013.
20. Balhorn R: The protamine family of sperm nuclear proteins. *Genome Biol* 8(9):227, 2007.
21. Schliesser MG, et al: Prognostic relevance of miRNA-155 methylation in anaplastic glioma. *Oncotarget* 7(50):82028–82045, 2016.
22. Deng Q, et al: Single-cell RNA-seq reveals dynamic, random monoallelic gene expression in mammalian cells. *Science* 343(6167):193–196, 2014.

23. Cassidy SB, Dykens E, Williams CA: Prader-Willi and Angelman syndromes: sister imprinted disorders. *Am J Med Genet* 97(2):136–146, 2000.
24. Cassidy SB, et al: Prader-Willi syndrome. *Genet Med: Offic J Am Coll Med Genet* 14(1):10–26, 2012.
25. Williams CA, et al: Angelman syndrome 2005: updated consensus for diagnostic criteria. *Am J Med Genet A* 140(5):413–418, 2006.
26. Horsthemke B, Wagstaff J: Mechanisms of imprinting of the Prader-Willi/Angelman region. *Am J Med Genet A* 146A(16):2041–2052, 2008.
27. Elliott M, et al: Clinical features and natural history of Beckwith-Wiedemann syndrome: presentation of 74 new cases. *Clin Genet* 46(2):168–174, 1994.
28. Jones KL, Smith DW: Recognition of the fetal alcohol syndrome in early infancy. *Lancet* 302(7836):999–1001, 1973.
29. Kaminen-Ahola N, Ahola A: *Postnatal growth restriction and gene expression changes in a mouse model of fetal alcohol syndrome, research part A*, Wiley Online Library, 2010. Available at http://onlinelibrary.wiley.com/doi/10.1002/bdra.20729/full.
30. Zhou FC, et al: Alcohol alters DNA methylation patterns and inhibits neural stem cell differentiation. *Alcohol Clin Exp Res* 35(4):735–746, 2011.
31. Mukhopadhyay P, et al: Alcohol modulates expression of DNA methyltransferases and methyl CpG-/CpG domain-binding proteins in murine embryonic fibroblasts. *Reprod Toxicol* 37:40–48, 2013.
32. Swartz JR, Hariri AR, Williamson DE: An epigenetic mechanism links socioeconomic status to changes in depression-related brain function in high risk adolescents. *Mol Psychiatry* 22(2):209–214, 2016.
33. Bam M, et al: Dysregulated immune system networks in war veterans with PTSD is an outcome of altered miRNA expression and DNA methylation. *Sci Rep* 6(Aug):31209, 2016.
34. Sadeh N, et al: Epigenetic variation at SKA2 predicts suicide phenotypes and internalizing psychopathology. *Depress Anxiety* 33(4):308–315, 2016.
35. Loke YJ, Hannan AJ, Craig JM: The role of epigenetic change in autism spectrum disorders. *Front Neurol* 6:107, 2015.
36. Lieb-Lundell CC: Three faces of fragile X. *Phys Ther* 96(11):1782–1790, 2016.
37. Tassone F, Hagerman PJ: The molecular biology of FXTAS. In Tassone F, Berry-Kravis EM, editors: *The fragile X-associated tremor ataxia syndrome (FXTAS)*, New York, 2010, Springer, pp 77–93.
38. Lu C, et al: Fragile X premutation RNA is sufficient to cause primary ovarian insufficiency in mice. *Hum Mol Genet* 21(23):5039–5047, 2012.
39. Tassone F, et al: Intranuclear inclusions in neural cells with premutation alleles in fragile X associated tremor/ataxia syndrome. *J Med Genet* 41(4):e43, 2004.
40. Stöger R, et al: Epigenetic variation illustrated by DNA methylation patterns of the fragile-X gene FMR1. *Hum Mol Genet* 6(11):1791–1801, 1997.
41. Iqbal K, et al: Deleterious effects of endocrine disruptors are corrected in the mammalian germline by epigenome reprogramming. *Genome Biol* 16:59, 2015.
42. Anway MD, et al: Transgenerational effect of the endocrine disruptor Vinclozolin on male spermatogenesis. *J Androl* 27(6):868–879, 2006.

43. Bygren LO: Intergenerational health responses to adverse and enriched environments. *Annu Rev Public Health* 34:49–60, 2013.
44. van Esterik JCJ, et al: Programming of metabolic effects in C57BL/6JxFVB mice by exposure to bisphenol A during gestation and lactation. *Toxicology* 321:40–52, 2014.
45. Szyf M, et al: Maternal programming of steroid receptor expression and phenotype through DNA methylation in the rat. *Front Neuroendocrinol* 26(3-4):139–162, 2005.
46. Fraga MF: Genetic and epigenetic regulation of aging. *Curr Opin Immunol* 21(4):446–453, 2009.
47. Dang W, et al: Histone H4 lysine 16 acetylation regulates cellular lifespan. *Nature* 459(7248):802–807, 2009.
48. Song C-X, et al: Selective chemical labeling reveals the genome-wide distribution of 5-hydroxymethylcytosine. *Nat Biotechnol* 29(1):68–72, 2011.
49. Pal S, Tyler JK: Epigenetics and aging. *Sci Adv* 2(7):e1600584, 2016.
50. Cabreiro F, et al: Metformin retards aging in C. elegans by altering microbial folate and methionine metabolism. *Cell* 153(1):228–239, 2013.
51. Anisimov VN: Metformin: do we finally have an anti-aging drug? *Cell Cycle* 12(22):3483–3489, 2013.
52. Colman RJ, et al: Caloric restriction reduces age-related and all-cause mortality in rhesus monkeys. *Nat Commun* 5:3557, 2014.
53. Bird AP, Southern EM: Use of restriction enzymes to study eukaryotic DNA methylation: I. The methylation pattern in ribosomal DNA from *Xenopus laevis. J Mol Biol* 118(1):27–47, 1978.
54. Frommer M, et al: A genomic sequencing protocol that yields a positive display of 5-methylcytosine residues in individual DNA strands. *Proc Natl Acad Sci USA* 89(5):1827–1831, 1992.
55. Song C-X, et al: Simultaneous single-molecule epigenetic imaging of DNA methylation and hydroxymethylation. *Proc Natl Acad Sci USA* 113(16):4338–4343, 2016.
56. Crawford GE, et al: Genome-wide mapping of DNase hypersensitive sites using massively parallel signature sequencing (MPSS). *Genome Res* 16(1):123–131, 2006.
57. Buenrostro JD, et al: ATAC-seq: a method for assaying chromatin accessibility genome-wide. *Curr Protoc Mol Biol* 109:21–29, 2015.
58. Buenrostro JD, et al: Single-cell chromatin accessibility reveals principles of regulatory variation. *Nature* 523(7561):486–490, 2015.
59. Gury-BenAri M, et al: The spectrum and regulatory landscape of intestinal innate lymphoid cells are shaped by the microbiome. *Cell* 166(5):1231–1246, 2016.
60. Siggens L, Ekwall K: Epigenetics, chromatin and genome organization: recent advances from the ENCODE project. *J Intern Med* 276(3):201–214, 2014.
61. Romanoski CE, et al: Epigenomics: roadmap for regulation. *Nature* 518(7539):314–316, 2015.
62. Ohnesorg T, et al: Using ROADMAP data to identify enhancers associated with disorders of sex development. *Sex Dev* 10(2):59–65, 2016.
63. Hu Z, et al: Complexity and specificity of the neutrophil transcriptomes in juvenile idiopathic arthritis. *Sci Rep* 6:27453, 2016.
64. Tong JHS, et al: Separating the wheat from the chaff: systematic identification of functionally relevant noncoding variants in ADHD. *Mol Psychiatry* 21(11):1589–1598, 2016.

65. Neidhart M: DNA methylation and cancer. In Neidhart M, editor: *DNA methylation and complex human disease*, St Louis, 2016, Elsevier, pp 103–134.

66. Øster B, et al: Non-CpG island promoter hypomethylation and miR-149 regulate the expression of SRPX2 in colorectal cancer. *Int J Cancer* 132(10):2303–2315, 2013.

67. Giacinti C, Giordano A: RB and cell cycle progression. *Oncogene* 25(38):5220–5227, 2006.

68. Hitchins MP: Constitutional epimutation as a mechanism for cancer causality and heritability? *Nat Rev Cancer* 15(10):625–634, 2015.

69. Sproul D, Meehan RR: Genomic insights into cancer-associated aberrant CpG island hypermethylation. *Brief Funct Genomics* 12(3):174–190, 2013.

70. Zhai R, et al: Genome-wide DNA methylation profiling of cell-free serum DNA in esophageal adenocarcinoma and Barrett esophagus. *Neoplasia* 14(1):29–33, 2012.

71. Tao K, et al: Prognostic value of miR-221-3p, miR-342-3p and miR-491-5p expression in colon cancer. *Am J Transl Res* 6(4):391–401, 2014.

72. Wang B, et al: miRNA expression in breast cancer varies with lymph node metastasis and other clinicopathologic features. *IUBMB Life* 66(5):371–377, 2014.

73. Ren Q, et al: Epithelial and stromal expression of miRNAs during prostate cancer progression. *Am J Transl Res* 6(4):329–339, 2014.

74. Mikhailenko DS, Kushlinskii NE: The somatic mutations and aberrant methylation as potential genetic markers of urinary bladder cancer. *Klin Lab Diagn* 61(2):78–83, 2016, (Article in Russian.).

75. Hsu H-S, et al: Characterization of a multiple epigenetic marker panel for lung cancer detection and risk assessment in plasma. *Cancer* 110(9):2019–2026, 2007.

76. Hulbert A, et al: Early detection of lung cancer using DNA promoter hypermethylation in plasma and sputum. *Clin Cancer Res* 2016 October 11. [Epub ahead of print].

77. Zhang SQ, Zhang GQ, Zhang L: Correlation between methylation of the E-cadherin gene and malignancy of prostate cancer. *Genet Mol Res* 15(2):2016.

78. Qin Z, et al: Cell-free circulating tumor DNA in cancer. *Chin J Cancer* 35:36, 2016.

79. Di Costanzo A, et al: Epigenetic drugs against cancer: an evolving landscape. *Arch Toxicol* 88(9):1651–1668, 2014.

80. Christman JK, Schneiderman N, Acs G: Formation of highly stable complexes between 5-azacytosine-substituted DNA and specific non-histone nuclear proteins. Implications for 5-azacytidine-mediated effects on DNA methylation and gene expression. *J Biol Chem* 260(7):4059–4068, 1985.

81. Zhang JS, et al: Keratin 23 (K23), a novel acidic keratin, is highly induced by histone deacetylase inhibitors during differentiation of pancreatic cancer cells. *Genes Chromosomes Cancer* 30(2):123–135, 2001.

82. Jabbour E, et al: Prognostic factors associated with disease progression and overall survival in patients with myelodysplastic syndromes treated with decitabine. *Clin Lymphoma Myeloma Leuk* 13(2):131–138, 2013.

83. Wilson-Edell KA, et al: mTORC1/C2 and pan-HDAC inhibitors synergistically impair breast cancer growth by convergent AKT and polysome inhibiting mechanisms. *Breast Cancer Res Treat* 144(2):287–298, 2014.

84. Ruscetti M, et al: HDAC inhibition impedes epithelial-mesenchymal plasticity and suppresses metastatic, castration-resistant prostate cancer. *Oncogene* 35(29):3781–3795, 2016.

85. Feng W, et al: Combination of HDAC inhibitor TSA and silibinin induces cell cycle arrest and apoptosis by targeting survivin and cyclinB1/Cdk1 in pancreatic cancer cells. *Biomed Pharmacother* 74:257–264, 2015.

86. Ribrag V, et al: Safety and efficacy of abexinostat, a pan-histone deacetylase inhibitor, in non-Hodgkin lymphoma and chronic lymphocytic leukemia: results of a phase 2 study. *Haematologica* 2017 Jan 25. [Epub ahead of print].

CHAPTER

7

Innate Immunity: Inflammation and Wound Healing

Neal S. Rote

evolve WEBSITE

http://evolve.elsevier.com/McCance/
- Content Updates
- Chapter Summary Review
- Review Questions
- Case Studies
- Animations

CHAPTER OUTLINE

People are exposed daily to an environment containing a large variety of toxic substances and potentially infectious and disease-causing microorganisms. Without an efficient system of protection most individuals would succumb to these hazards early in life. That system consists of multiple complementary and interdependent layers. An outer layer of specialized epithelium, including the skin and mucosal surfaces, is relatively resistant to most environmental hazards and resists infection with disease-causing microorganisms.[1] If the epithelial barrier is damaged, a highly efficient local and systemic response (inflammation) is mobilized to limit the extent of damage, protect against infection,

and initiate repair of the damaged tissue. The natural epithelial barrier and inflammation confer innate resistance and protection, commonly referred to as innate immunity, also known as natural or native immunity. Inflammation associated with infection usually initiates an adaptive process that results in a long-term and very effective immunity to the infecting microorganism, referred to as adaptive immunity, also known as acquired or specific immunity. Adaptive immunity is relatively slow to develop but has memory and more rapidly targets and eradicates a second infection with a particular disease-causing microorganism.

The information presented in this chapter introduces the components and processes of innate immunity and sets the stage for Chapter 8, which discusses adaptive immunity. Although inflammation and adaptive immunity provide protection, either genetic or acquired aberrations in these processes can lead to disease. Diminution of innate or adaptive immunity may lead to critically decreased resistance to infection. Excessive inflammation or adaptive immunity may lead to damage to normal tissue or organs. Both may result in severe and potentially fatal disease, examples of which are discussed in Chapter 9. Many microorganisms that cause disease have developed methods of bypassing our protective systems. These are discussed in Chapter 10. Each chapter is designed to render an overview and is not intended to be all-inclusive. Protective mechanisms consist of a very large number of soluble factors and cells and would require many more pages to discuss in adequate detail. Different classes or groups of molecules and cells will be discussed, but only a few examples will be described in detail. Some components directly participate in the protective response, whereas others are designed to limit the extent of the response.

HUMAN DEFENSE MECHANISMS

Innate immunity includes two lines of defense: natural barriers and inflammation (Table 7.1). Natural barriers are physical, mechanical, and biochemical barriers at the body's surfaces and are in place at birth to prevent damage by substances in the environment and thwart infection by pathogenic microorganisms. If the surface barriers are breached, the second line of defense, the inflammatory response, is activated to protect the body from further injury, prevent infection of the injured tissue, and promote healing. The inflammatory response is a rapid activation of biochemical and cellular processes that is relatively nonspecific, with similar responses being initiated against a wide variety of causes of tissue damage.

FIRST LINE OF DEFENSE: PHYSICAL, MECHANICAL, AND BIOCHEMICAL BARRIERS AND NORMAL MICROBIOME

Physical and Mechanical Barriers

The physical barriers that protect against damage and infection are composed of tightly associated epithelial cells including those of the skin and of the membranous sheets lining the gastrointestinal, genito-urinary, and respiratory tracts (Fig. 7.1). The mucosal epithelial cells are highly interconnected junctions that prohibit the passage of microorganisms into the underlying tissue. The normal turnover of the cells in these sites as well as mechanisms for "washing" the surfaces may mechanically remove many infectious microorganisms and prevent their residence on the epithelial surfaces. For instance, the routine sloughing off and replacement of dead skin cells also removes adherent bacteria. Mechanical cleansing of the surfaces includes vomiting and urination. Goblet cells of the upper respiratory tract produce mucus that coats the epithelial surface and traps microorganisms that are removed by hairlike cilia that mechanically move the mucus upward to be expelled by coughing or sneezing. Additionally, the low temperature on the skin and low pH of the skin and stomach generally inhibit microorganisms, most of which prefer temperatures near 37°C (98.6°F) and a pH near neutral for more efficient growth.

Biochemical Barriers

Epithelial surfaces also provide biochemical barriers by synthesizing and secreting substances meant to trap or destroy microorganisms (epithelial-derived chemicals).[2] Mucus, perspiration (or sweat), saliva, tears, and earwax are all examples of biochemical secretions that can trap and kill potential disease-causing microorganisms. Sebaceous glands in the skin secrete antibacterial and antifungal fatty acids and lactic

TABLE 7.1 OVERVIEW OF HUMAN DEFENSES

CHARACTERISTICS	INNATE IMMUNITY		ADAPTIVE (ACQUIRED) IMMUNITY
	BARRIERS	INFLAMMATORY RESPONSE	
Level of defense	First line of defense against infection and tissue injury	Second line of defense; occurs as a response to tissue injury or infection	Third line of defense; initiated when innate immune system signals the cells of adaptive immunity
Timing of defense	Constant	Immediate response	Delay between primary exposure to antigen and maximum response; immediate against secondary exposure to antigen
Specificity	Broadly specific	Broadly specific	Response is very specific toward "antigen"
Cells	Epithelial cells	Mast cells, granulocytes (neutrophils, eosinophils, basophils), monocytes/macrophages, natural killer (NK) cells, platelets, endothelial cells	T lymphocytes, B lymphocytes, macrophages, dendritic cells
Memory	No memory involved	No memory involved	Specific immunologic memory by T and B lymphocytes
Peptides	Defensins, cathelicidins, collectins, lactoferrin, bacterial toxins	Complement, clotting factors, kinins	Antibodies, complement
Protection	Protection includes anatomic barriers (i.e., skin and mucous membranes), cells and secretory molecules or cytokines (e.g., lysozymes, low pH of stomach and urine), and ciliary activity	Protection includes vascular responses, cellular components (e.g., mast cells, neutrophils, macrophages), secretory molecules or cytokines, and activation of plasma protein systems	Protection includes activated T and B lymphocytes, cytokines, and antibodies

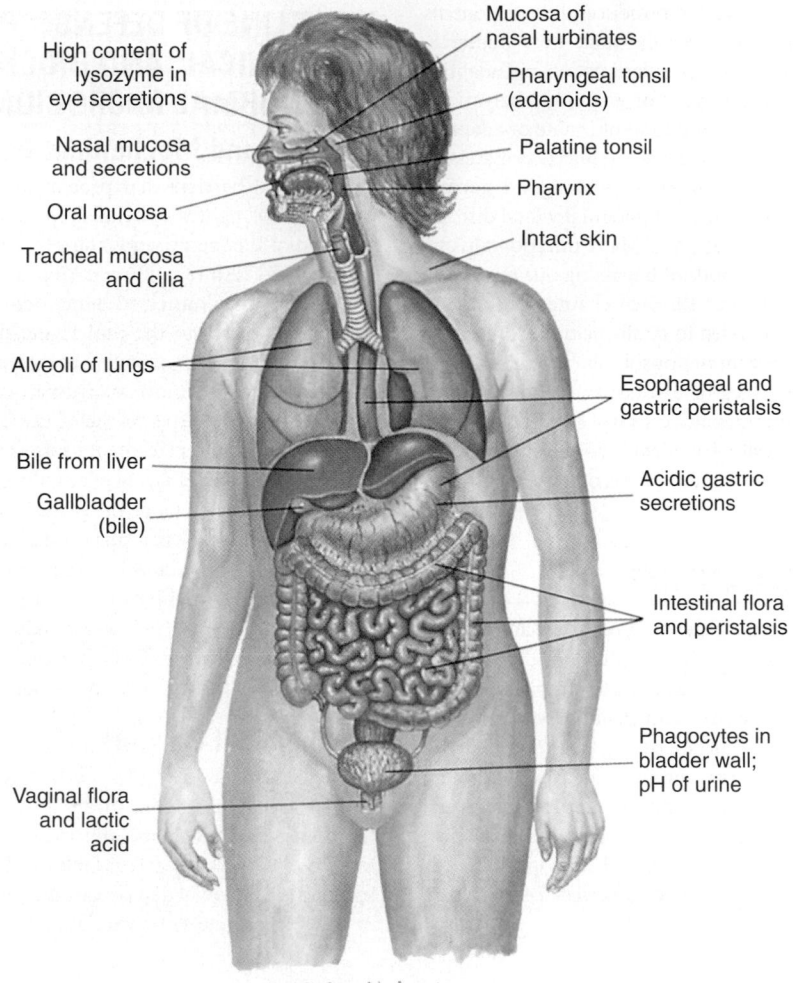

High content of
lysozyme in
eye secretions

Nasal mucosa
and secretions

Oral mucosa

Tracheal mucosa
and cilia

Alveoli of lungs

Bile from liver

Gallbladder
(bile)

Vaginal flora
and lactic
acid

Mucosa of
nasal turbinates

Pharyngeal tonsil
(adenoids)

Palatine tonsil

Pharynx

Intact skin

Esophageal and
gastric peristalsis

Acidic gastric
secretions

Intestinal flora
and peristalsis

Phagocytes in
bladder wall;
pH of urine

G.J.Wassilchenko

FIGURE 7.1 The Closed Barrier. The digestive, respiratory, and genitourinary tracts and the skin form closed barriers between the internal organs and the environment. (From Grimes DE: *Infectious diseases*, St Louis, 1991, Mosby.)

acid. Perspiration, tears, and saliva contain an enzyme (lysozyme) that attacks the cell walls of gram-positive bacteria. These glandular secretions result in an acidic skin surface (pH 3 to 5), which is an inhospitable environment for most bacteria.

Epithelial cells secrete a complex array of proteins that destroy potential pathogens. Small-molecular-weight **antimicrobial peptides** are generally positively charged polypeptides of approximately 15 to 95 amino acids and can be divided into two classes—cathelicidins and defensins—based on their three-dimensional chemical structures. Both classes are in very high local concentrations and are toxic to several bacteria, fungi, and viruses. **Cathelicidins** have a linear α-helical shape, and only one is currently known to function in humans. In contrast, about 50 different defensins have been identified thus far. All are triple-stranded β-sheet structures. **Defensin** molecules contain 3 intrachain disulfide bonds and can be further subdivided into α (at least 6 identified in humans) and β types (at least 10 identified, but perhaps up to 40 different molecules), depending on how the cysteine residues are connected during formation of the disulfide linkages.[3] The α-defensins often require activation by proteolytic enzymes, whereas the β-defensins are synthesized in active forms. Bacteria have cholesterol-free cell membranes, which may allow cathelicidins to insert into and disrupt their membranes. Given the similarity in their chemical charges, defensins may kill bacteria in the same way. These same chemicals also may

contribute to other means of protection because they are also produced by monocytes, macrophages, and neutrophils, which are components of the inflammatory response. Cathelicidin is stored in neutrophils, mast cells, and a variety of epithelial cells. The α-defensins are particularly rich in the granules of neutrophils and may contribute to the killing of bacteria by those cells. They are also found in Paneth cells lining the small intestine, where they protect against a variety of disease-causing microorganisms. The β-defensins are found in epithelial cells lining the respiratory, urinary, and intestinal tracts, as well as in the skin. In addition to antibacterial properties, β-defensins may also help protect epithelial surfaces from human immunodeficiency virus (HIV) infection. Both classes of antimicrobial peptides also can activate cells of innate and adaptive immunity.

The lung also produces and secretes a family of glycoproteins, **collectins**, which includes surfactant proteins A through D and mannose-binding lectin.[4] Collectins react with different affinities to carbohydrates and lipids on the surfaces of a wide array of pathogenic microorganisms. Collectin binding facilitates recognition of the microorganism by macrophages, enhancing macrophage attachment, phagocytosis, and killing. **Mannose-binding lectin (MBL)** recognizes a sugar commonly found on the surface of microbes and is a powerful activator of a plasma protein system (complement) resulting in damage to bacteria or increased recognition by macrophages.

Other *epithelial antimicrobials* include resistin-like molecule β, bactericidal/permeability-inducing protein, and antimicrobial lectins. **Resistin-like molecule β** is found in the intestinal goblet cells, where it appears to protect against helminth infections. **Bactericidal/permeability-inducing (BPI) protein** is stored in neutrophils and intestinal epithelium. BPI protein specifically reacts with lipopolysaccharide on the surface of gram-negative bacteria, resulting in bacterial lysis. **Antimicrobial lectins** are carbohydrates that are found in intestinal epithelium and have activity against gram-positive bacteria.

Normal Microbiome

The body's surfaces are colonized with a spectrum of microorganisms, the **normal microbiome**. Each surface, including the skin and the mucous membranes of the eyes, upper and lower gastrointestinal tracts, urethra, and vagina, is colonized by a combination of bacteria and fungi that is unique to the particular location and individual (Fig. 7.2).[5] The microorganisms in the microbiome do not normally cause disease, although several are opportunistic in that they can cause disease if the integrity of the body surface is compromised or the individual's immune or inflammatory systems are defective. The relationship of the microbiome with humans has been referred to as *commensal* (to the benefit of one organism without affecting the other); however, the relationship may be more *mutualistic* (to the benefit of both organisms). Using the colon for an example, at birth the lower gut is relatively sterile but colonization with bacteria begins quickly, with the number, diversity,

and concentration increasing progressively during the first year of life. To the benefit of humans, many of these microorganisms help digest fatty acids, large polysaccharides, and other dietary substances; produce biotin and vitamin K; and assist in the absorption of ions, such as calcium, iron, and magnesium.

These bacteria contribute to the human body's innate protection against pathogenic microorganisms in the colon. They compete with pathogens for nutrients and block attachment to the epithelium. Members of the normal microbiome also produce chemicals (ammonia, phenols, indoles, and other toxic materials) and toxic proteins *(bacteriocins)* that inhibit colonization by pathogenic microorganisms. Prolonged treatment with broad-spectrum antibiotics can alter the normal intestinal microbiome, decreasing its protective activity, and lead to an overgrowth of opportunistic pathogenic microorganisms, such as the yeast *Candida albicans* or the bacteria *Clostridium difficile* (overgrowth can cause pseudomembranous colitis, an infection of the colon). Additionally, the normal microbiome of the gut helps train the adaptive immune system by inducing the growth of gut-associated lymphoid tissue (where cells of the adaptive immune system reside) and the development of both local and systemic adaptive immune systems.[6]

The bacterium *Lactobacillus* is a major constituent of the normal vaginal microbiome in healthy women: at least 22 different species of *Lactobacillus* have been identified in the vaginal microbiome, with 4 of those being predominantly represented.[7] This microorganism produces a variety of chemicals (e.g., hydrogen peroxide, lactic acid, bacteriocins)

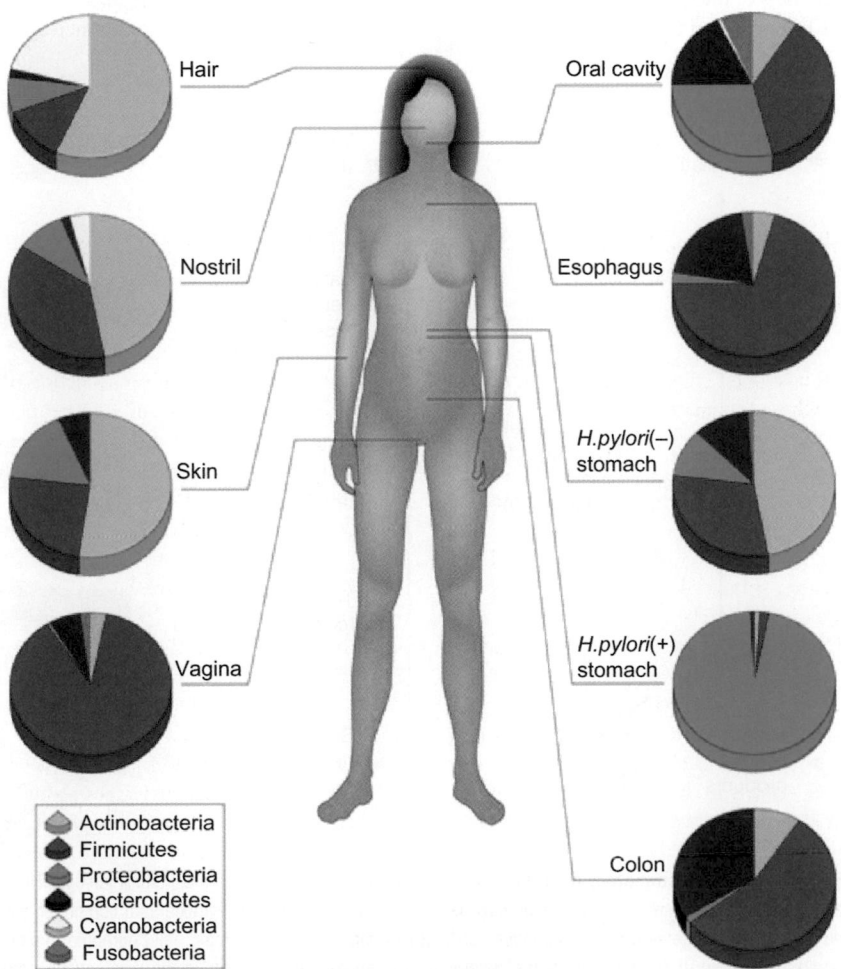

FIGURE 7.2 The Human Microbiome. Typical phylum-level composition of the human microbiota that vary at each site. (From Cho I, Blaser MJ: *Nat Rev Genet* 13:260–270, 2012.)

that help prevent infections of the vagina and urinary tract by other bacteria and yeast. Prolonged antibiotic treatment can diminish colonization with *Lactobacillus* and increase the risk for urologic or vaginal infections, such as vaginosis.

Opportunistic microorganisms are normally controlled by the innate and adaptive immune systems and contribute to the human body's defenses. For example, *Pseudomonas aeruginosa* is a member of the normal microbiome of the skin and produces a toxin that protects against infections with staphylococcal and other bacteria. However, severe burns compromise the integrity of the skin and may lead to life-threatening systemic pseudomonal infections.

SECOND LINE OF DEFENSE: INFLAMMATION

Whereas the physical and chemical barriers of the innate immune system are relatively static, inflammation is programmed to respond to cellular or tissue damage, whether the damaged tissue is septic (contaminated with microorganisms) or sterile. The inflammatory response is a rapid initiation and interactive system of humoral (soluble in the blood) and cellular systems designed to limit the extent of tissue damage, destroy contaminating infectious microorganisms, initiate the adaptive immune response, and begin the healing process (Fig. 7.3). The inflammatory response (1) occurs in tissues with a blood supply (vascularized); (2) is activated rapidly (within seconds) after damage occurs; (3) depends on the activity of both *cellular and chemical components,* including plasma proteins; and (4) is *nonspecific,* meaning that it takes place in approximately the same way regardless of the type of stimulus or whether exposure to the same stimulus has occurred in the past.

Vascular Response

Virtually any injury to vascularized tissue will activate inflammation. Injury may result from a variety of causes including infection or necrosis (e.g., trauma, oxygen deprivation [ischemia], nutrient deprivation, genetic or immune defects, chemical injury, foreign bodies, temperature extremes, ionizing radiation). The classic symptoms of acute inflammation include *redness* (erythema), *heat, swelling* (edema), and *pain.* This tetrad represents the "cardinal signs of inflammation" and was identified in the first century by a Roman writer, Celsus. A fifth sign was added later: *loss of function.* Microscopically, inflammatory changes can be seen at the vascular level (Fig. 7.4). The three characteristic changes in the microcirculation (arterioles, capillaries, and venules) near the site of an injury include the following:

1. Vasodilation (increased size of the blood vessels) causes slower blood velocity and increases blood flow to the injured site.
2. Increased vascular permeability (the blood vessels become porous from contraction of endothelial cells) and leakage of fluid out of the vessel (exudation) cause swelling (edema) at the site of injury; as plasma moves outward, blood in the microcirculation becomes more viscous and flows more slowly, and the increased blood flow and increasing concentration of red cells at the site of inflammation cause locally increased redness (erythema) and warmth.
3. White blood cells adhere to the inner walls of vessels, and they migrate through enlarged junctions between the endothelial cells lining the vessels into the surrounding tissue (diapedesis).

The effects of inflammation are visible within seconds. First, arterioles near the site of infection or injury constrict briefly. Vasodilation then causes slower blood velocity and increases local blood flow to the injured

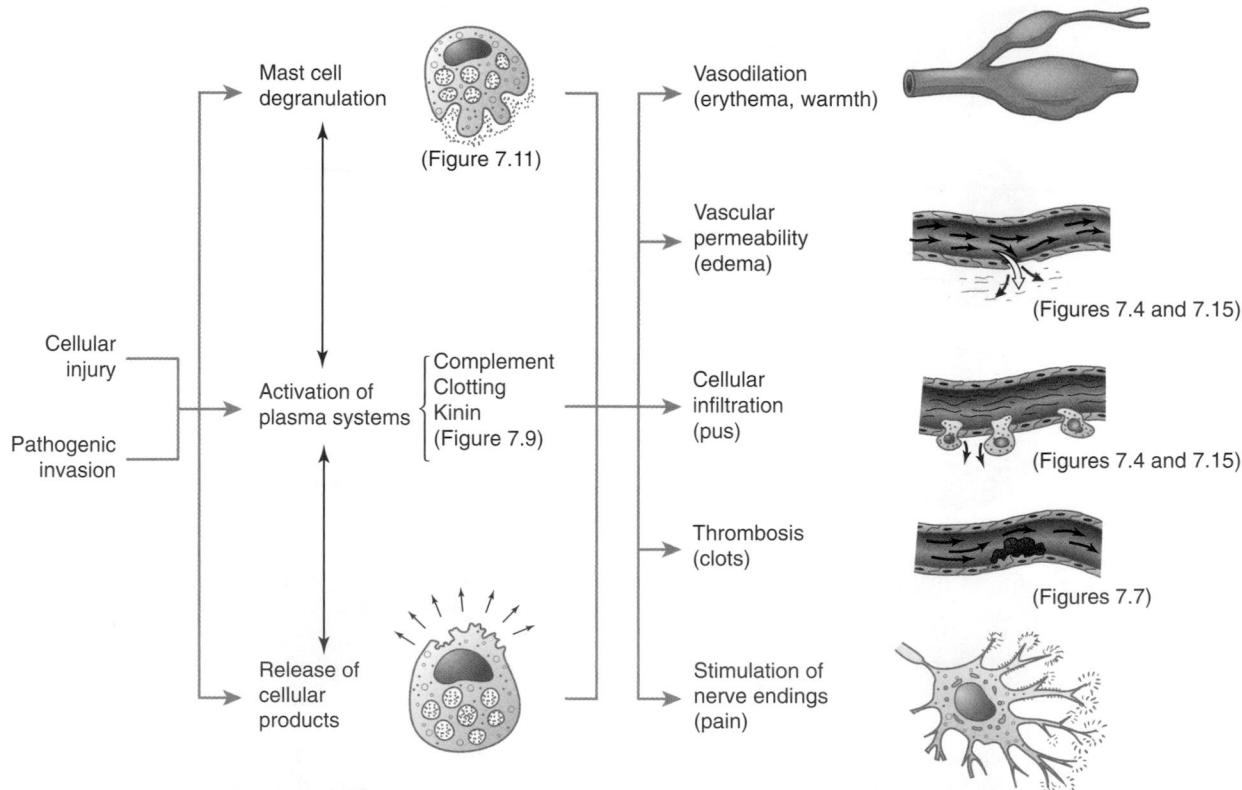

FIGURE 7.3 Acute Inflammatory Response. Inflammation is usually initiated by cellular injury, which results in mast cell degranulation, the activation of three plasma systems, and the release of subcellular components from the damaged cells. These systems are interdependent, so that induction of one (e.g., mast cell degranulation) can result in activation of the other two. The result is the development of microscopic changes in the inflamed site, as well as characteristic clinical manifestations. The figure numbers refer to those in which more detailed information may be found on that portion of the response.

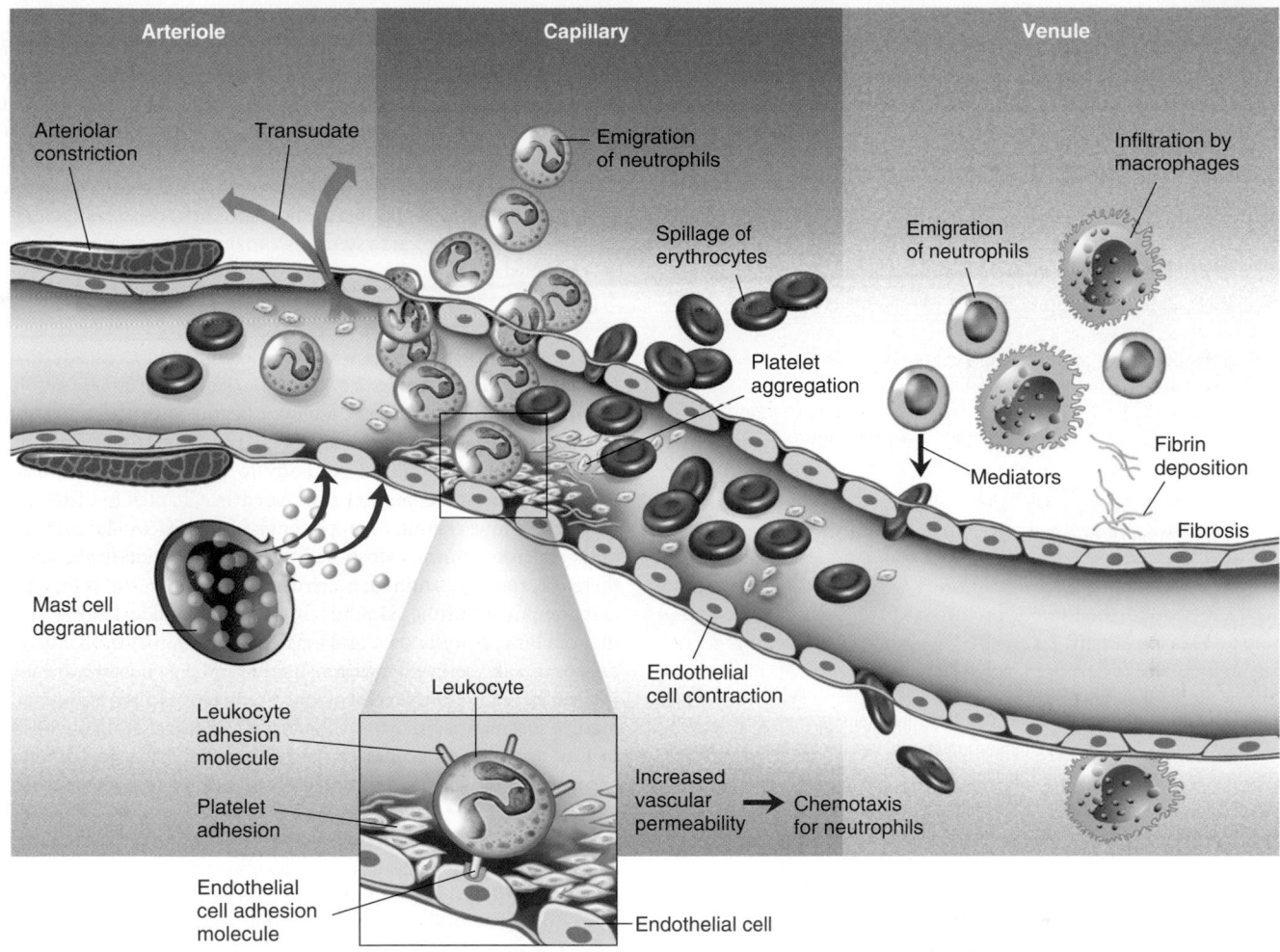

FIGURE 7.4 Sequence of Events in the Acute Inflammatory Response. See text for details.

site. The increased flow and capillary permeability result in leakage of plasma from the vessels, causing edema in the surrounding tissue. As plasma moves outward, blood remaining in the microcirculation flows more slowly and becomes more viscous. The increased blood flow and increasing concentration of red cells at the site of inflammation cause locally increased warmth and redness. Leukocytes adhere to vessel walls. At the same time, biochemical mediators (e.g., histamine, bradykinins, leukotrienes, prostaglandins) stimulate the endothelial cells that line capillaries and venules to retract, creating spaces at junctions between the cells, allowing leukocytes and plasma to enter the surrounding tissue (intercellular junctions are described in Chapter 1).

Each of the characteristic changes associated with inflammation is the direct result of the activities and interactions of a host of chemicals and cellular components found in the blood and tissues. The vascular changes deliver leukocytes (particularly neutrophils), plasma proteins, and other biochemical mediators to the site of injury where they act in concert.

Benefits of inflammation include:

1. Prevention of infection and further damage by contaminating microorganisms through the influx of fluid to dilute toxins produced by bacteria and released from dying cells, the influx and activation of plasma protein systems that help destroy and contain bacteria (e.g., complement system, clotting system), and the influx of cells (e.g., neutrophils, macrophages) that "eat" and destroy cellular debris and infectious agents.

2. Limitation and control of the inflammatory process through the influx of plasma protein systems (e.g., clotting system), plasma enzymes, and cells (e.g., eosinophils) that prevent the inflammatory response from spreading to areas of healthy tissue.

3. Interaction with components of the adaptive immune system to elicit a more specific response to contaminating pathogen(s) through the influx of macrophages and lymphocytes.

4. Preparation of the area of injury for healing through removal of bacterial products, dead cells, and other products of inflammation (e.g., by way of channels through the epithelium or drainage by lymphatic vessels) and initiation of mechanisms of healing and repair.

Extravascular fluid and debris that accumulate at an inflamed site are drained by lymphatic vessels. This process also facilitates the development of adaptive immunity because microbial antigens in lymphatic fluid pass through the lymph nodes, where they activate both B and T lymphocytes. (This process is discussed in Chapter 8, and the lymphatic system is described in Chapter 28.) The lymphatic vessels may, themselves, become secondarily inflamed. Lymphangitis of the lymph vessels and lymphadenitis of the nodes, which become hyperplastic, enlarge and frequently become painful.

Inflammation and repair can be divided into several phases (Fig. 7.5). The characteristics of the early (i.e., acute) inflammatory response differ from those of the later (i.e., chronic) response, and each phase involves different biochemical mediators and cells that function together. The acute inflammatory response is of short duration; that is, it continues

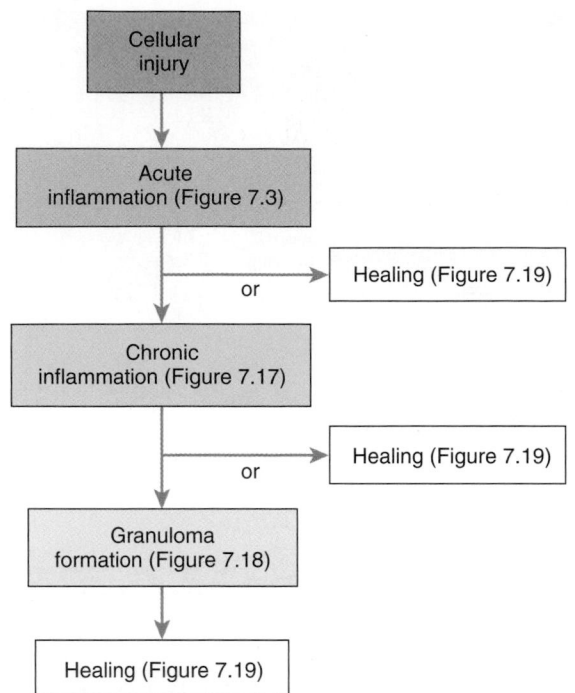

FIGURE 7.5 Inflammatory Phases. Cellular injury leads to acute inflammation and may result in resolution and healing of the injured site or may progress into chronic inflammation. Chronic inflammation in turn may result in healing or progress to development of a granuloma. The final step of the inflammatory process is usually healing and reconstruction of the damaged tissue. The figure numbers refer to those in which more detailed information on that portion of the process may be found.

only until the immediate threat to the host is eliminated. This usually takes 8 to 10 days from onset to healing. (Mechanisms of cellular injury are described in Chapter 2.)

Plasma Protein Systems

Three key **plasma protein systems** are essential to an effective inflammatory response. These are the complement system, the clotting system, and the kinin system (Figs. 7.6, 7.7, and 7.8, respectively). Although each system has a unique role in inflammation, they also have many similarities. Each system consists of multiple proteins in the blood. To prevent activation in unnecessary situations, each protein is normally in an inactive form. Several of the proteins are enzymes that circulate in inactive forms as **proenzymes**. Each system contains a few proteins that can be activated early in inflammation. Activation of the first component of a system results in sequential activation of other components, leading to a biologic function that helps protect the individual. This sequential activation is referred to as a *cascade*. Thus, we refer to the complement cascade, the clotting cascade, or the kinin cascade. In some cases, activation of a protein may require that it be enzymatically cut into two pieces or fragments of different size. Usually the larger fragment continues the cascade by activating the next component, and the smaller fragment frequently has potent biologic activities to promote inflammation.

Complement System

The **complement system** consists of several plasma proteins (sometimes called *complement components*) that together constitute about 10% of the total circulating serum protein. Activation of the complement system produces several factors that can destroy pathogens directly and can activate or collaborate with other components of the innate and adaptive

immune responses. Factors produced during activation of the complement system are among the body's most potent defenders, particularly against bacterial infection.[8]

Activation of the complement system can be accomplished in three different pathways, all of which converge at the third component (C3) of the pathway:

1. **Classical pathway**: activated by proteins of the adaptive immune system (antibodies) bound to their specific targets (antigen)
2. **Lectin pathway**: activated by mannose-containing bacterial carbohydrates
3. **Alternative pathway**: activated by gram-negative bacterial and fungal cell wall polysaccharides

The principal routes by which the **complement cascade** may be activated are shown in Fig. 7.6.

Activation of the *classical pathway* begins with the activation of complement protein C1 and is preceded by formation of a complex between an antigen and an antibody to form an **antigen-antibody complex (immune complex)** (discussed in Chapter 8). The antigen may be a unique chemical component of the surface of a bacterium or other microorganism. Most pathogens express multiple antigens; therefore, multiple antibodies are usually bound in the complex. The first component of the classical complement cascade, C1, has six sites that can bind to antibodies, and efficient activation of the complement cascade usually requires concurrent binding of C1 to at least two antibody molecules. The complex formed by antigen-antibody-complement binding is shown in Fig. 7.6. C1 is a macromolecular complex consisting of C1q and two molecules each of C1r and C1s. A conformational change in C1 results in an enzymatically active molecule whose substrates are C4 and C2. The resultant complex formed by the interaction of C1, C4, and C2 uses C3 as a substrate, resulting in the production of C3a and C3b. A complex that has C3 as a substrate is generally referred to as a **C3 convertase**. The addition of C3b to the complex changes the substrate specificity to C5, resulting in the conversion of C5 to C5a and C5b. A complex that has C5 as a substrate is generally called a **C5 convertase**. Thus activation of C1 initiates the sequential enzymatic activation of all other components of the classical pathway, ultimately resulting in the activation of C5. The classical pathway also can be activated to a lesser degree by biologic molecules other than antibody, including heparin (a charged molecule that prevents clotting), deoxyribonucleic acid (DNA) or ribonucleic acid (RNA), and C-reactive protein, which is increased in the blood during inflammation.

Even under normal conditions small amounts of circulating C3 are spontaneously broken down into C3b and C3a by a number of naturally occurring enzymes in the blood. The rate of C3 spontaneous activation is generally very low, and C3b is readily inactivated by complement regulator proteins in the blood (e.g., factor H and factor I). However, materials produced by some infectious microorganisms (e.g., lipopolysaccharides [endotoxins] on the bacterial surface, yeast cell wall carbohydrates [zymosans]) can bind the naturally produced C3b and protect it from inactivation. This will initiate activation of the *alternative complement pathway*. The C3b bound to bacterial products can react with another normally occurring component, factor B. The complex of C3b and factor B is recognized by an enzyme, factor D, which activates factor B, producing factor Bb. The resultant C3b/Bb complex is very unstable unless it binds to properdin (P). The C3b/Bb/P complex is a C3 convertase that produces further C3b, resulting in a C3b/Bb/P/C3b complex that is a C5 convertase, which activates C5.

The *lectin pathway* is similar to the classical pathway but is antibody independent. It is activated by a plasma protein called *mannose-binding lectin (MBL)*. MBL is similar to C1q and binds to bacterial polysaccharides containing the carbohydrate mannose and activates complement through two MBL-associated serine proteases (MASP-1 and MASP-2) that

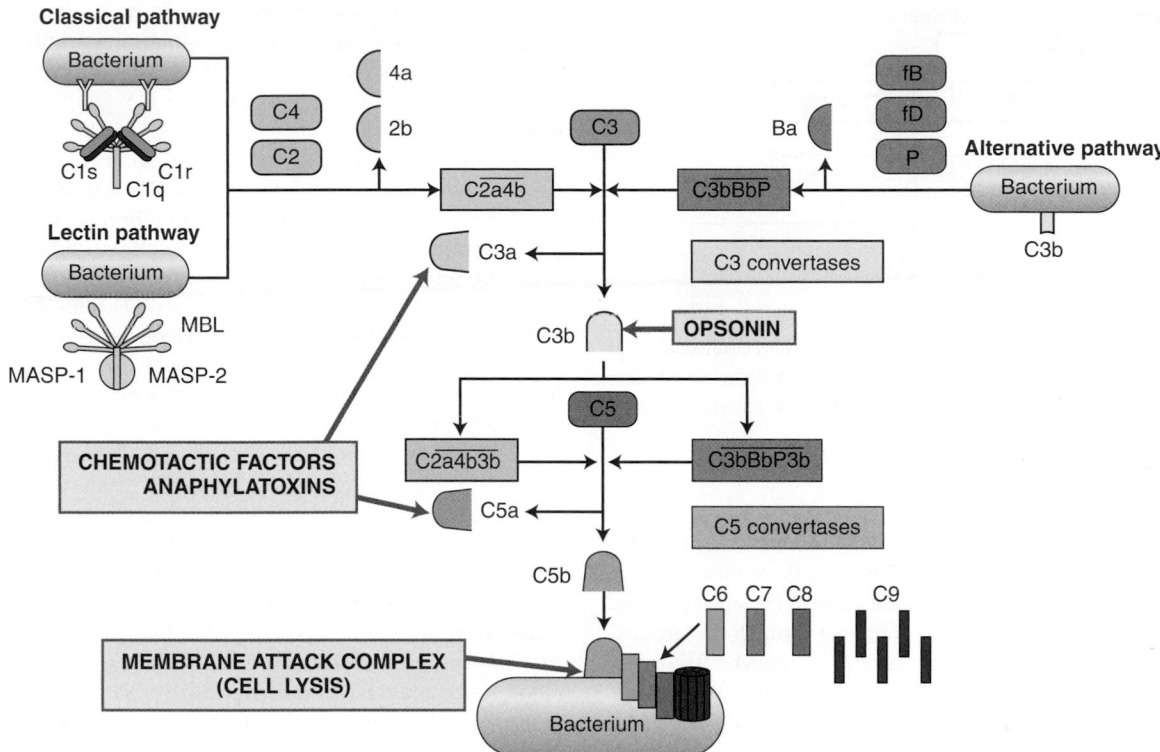

FIGURE 7.6 Pathways of Complement Cascade Activation. The complement system is activated by three pathways: the classical pathway, the lectin pathway, and the alternative pathway. During activation, many complement components are cleaved into fragments (2b, 4a, Ba, C3a, and C5a). The smaller fragments frequently have potent biologic activities and may serve as chemotactic factors and anaphylatoxins. The larger activated fragments are usually converted into active enzymes (indicated by the bar above the names) and form complexes with additional components in the cascade. The classical pathway is usually activated by antigen-antibody complexes through component C1, which consists of C1q and two C1r and C1s molecules. As indicated, the C1q must simultaneously bind to two antibody molecules (indicated by Y-shaped structures). The lectin pathway is activated by mannose-binding lectin *(MBL)*, which binds to two mannose-rich pathogen-associated molecular patterns on the surface of a bacterium. MBL contains two associated enzymes, MASP-1 and MASP-2, and functions in a manner similar to C1. C1 and MBL each activate complement components C4 and C2. The alternative pathway is activated by many agents, such as bacterial polysaccharides, which bind and stabilize C3b, which is produced by normal breakdown of C3 in the blood. The C3b forms the site of binding of factor B *(fB)*, which is activated by factor D *(fD)* into Bb and the small fragment Ba. Properdin *(P)* helps stabilize the complex. Each pathway produces C3 and C5 convertases, which are enzymatically active complexes that activate C3 and C5, respectively. C3b produced by the C3 convertase can function as an opsonin. C5b initiates assemblage of the membrane attack complex (MAC), which results in multiple C9 molecules forming a pore in the bacterial membrane.

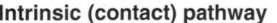

Intrinsic (contact) pathway

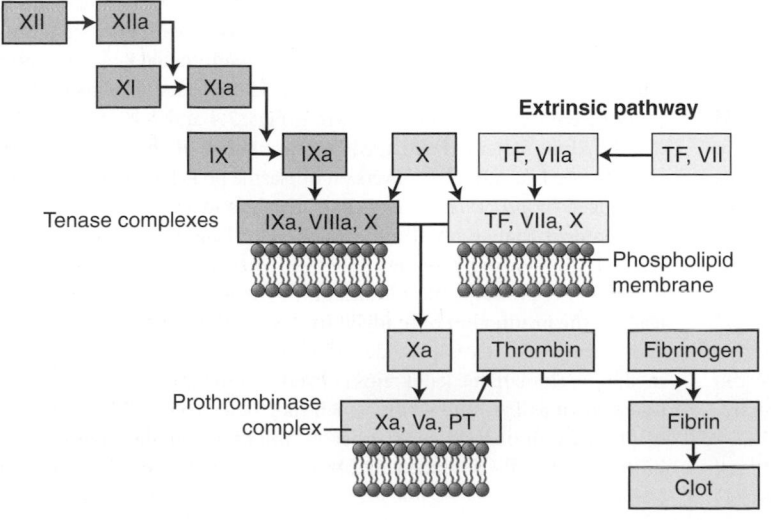

FIGURE 7.7 Coagulation Cascade. Clotting is activated through two pathways: the intrinsic (contact) pathway and the extrinsic pathway. The intrinsic pathway is initiated by the activation of Hageman factor *(XII)* into XIIa (activated factors are enzymes and are indicated by a lowercase *a*). The sequential activation of other intrinsic pathway components results in formation of a complex of IXa, VIIIa, and X. The extrinsic pathway is activated by exposure of tissue factor *(TF)* during tissue damage. TF complexes with factor VII, which is activated *(VIIa)* and forms a complex with factor X *(TF, VIIa, X)*. Both the intrinsic and the extrinsic pathway complexes are dependent on calcium, form on phospholipid membranes that are rich in phosphatidylserine, and have "tenase" activity (can activate factor X into Xa). Factor X begins a common pathway in which Xa complexes with Va and prothrombin *(PT)*, with calcium and phospholipid membranes, to form an active prothrombinase (activates prothrombin into thrombin). Thrombin is an enzyme that cuts high-molecular-weight fibrinogen into fibrin molecules. Fibrin polymerizes to form a clot.

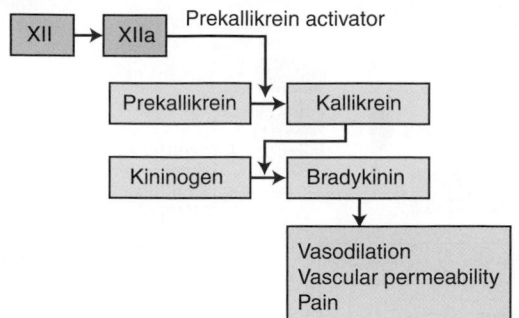

FIGURE 7.8 **Plasma Kinin Cascade.** The kinin pathway is activated by factor XIIa from the clotting system, which functions as an enzyme (prekallikrein activator) to convert prekallikrein into kallikrein. Enzymatically active kallikrein converts kininogen into bradykinin.

substitute for C1r and C1s and activate C4 and C2 to create a C3 convertase.[9] Thus, infectious agents that do not activate the alternative pathway may be susceptible to complement through the lectin pathway.

After activation of C5, the cascade continues through the terminal components C6, C7, C8, and C9. Components C5b through C9 assemble to form complexes (*membrane attack complex, or MAC*) capable of creating pores in cell membranes and permitting the influx of water and ions and may ultimately result in cell lysis.

The most important result of complement activation is the production of fragments during the activation of C4, C2, C3, and C5. The fragments C4a, C2b, C3a, and C5a are soluble and of low-molecular-weight that contribute in other ways to the inflammatory response. C2b affects smooth muscle, causing vasodilation and increased vascular permeability. C3a and C5a, and to a limited extent C4a, are anaphylatoxins; that is, they induce rapid mast cell degranulation (release of granular contents) and the release of histamine (see Fig. 7.12), causing vasodilation and increased capillary permeability.[10] C5a is the major chemotactic factor for neutrophils. C3a is approximately 100 times less potent in chemotactic and anaphylatoxic activity. A chemotactic factor is a biochemical substance that attracts leukocytes to the site of inflammation.

The dual functions of a chemotactic factor and an anaphylatoxin are not needed simultaneously or to the same degree. Anaphylatoxic activity is necessary early in inflammation and occurs close to the inflammatory site to induce local mast cell degranulation and to increase the number of soluble mediators available to enhance vascular permeability and vasodilation. Chemotactic activity, on the other hand, is required for a much longer period and occurs distal to the inflammatory site to attract leukocytes from the circulation. Thus it is beneficial to an effective inflammatory response to limit the range of anaphylatoxic activity while allowing widespread chemotactic activity. A plasma enzyme, a carboxypeptidase, removes a terminal arginine on both C3a and C5a peptides, thereby producing "C3a desArg" and "C5a desArg," respectively, which are inactive as anaphylatoxins but retain chemotactic activity. Thus chemotactic activity is retained, while not inducing distal mast cell degranulation that would result in considerable enlargement of the inflammatory response to the detriment of surrounding healthy tissue.

C3b adheres to the surface of a pathogenic microorganism and serves as an efficient opsonin. Opsonins are molecules that "tag" microorganisms for destruction by cells of the inflammatory system (primarily neutrophils and macrophages). C3b on the cell surface also can be broken down by several enzymes in the blood into inactive fragments (e.g., iC3b), which retain opsonic activity.

In summary, the complement cascade can be activated by at least three different means, and its products have four functions: (1)

anaphylatoxic activity resulting in mast cell degranulation (C3a, C3b), (2) leukocyte chemotaxis (C5a), (3) opsonization (C3b), and (4) cell lysis (C5b-C9, MAC).

Clotting System

The clotting (coagulation) system is a group of plasma proteins that, when activated sequentially, forms a blood clot at an injured or inflamed site. A blood clot is a meshwork of protein (fibrin) strands that contains platelets (the primary cellular initiator of clotting) and traps other cells, such as erythrocytes, phagocytes, and microorganisms. This (1) prevents the spread of infection to adjacent tissues, (2) traps microorganisms and foreign bodies at the site of inflammation for removal by infiltrating cells (e.g., neutrophils and macrophages), (3) forms a clot that stops bleeding, and (4) provides a framework for future repair and healing. The main substance in this fibrinous mesh is an insoluble protein called *fibrin* that is the end product of the coagulation cascade.

The clotting system can be activated by many substances that are released during tissue injury and infection, including collagen, proteinases, kallikrein, and plasmin, as well as by bacterial products such as endotoxins. Like the complement cascade, the coagulation cascade can be activated through different convergent pathways (see Fig. 7.7). The tissue factor (extrinsic) pathway is activated by tissue factor (TF) (also called *tissue thromboplastin*) that is released by damaged endothelial cells in blood vessels and reacts with activated factor VII (VIIa).[11] The intrinsic (contact) pathway is activated when the vessel wall is damaged and Hageman factor (factor XII) in plasma contacts negatively charged subendothelial substances. The pathways converge at factor X. Activation of factor X begins a common pathway leading to activation of fibrin that polymerizes to form a fibrin clot. The coagulation system is discussed in more detail and illustrated again in Chapter 28.

As with the complement system, activation of the clotting system produces protein fragments that enhance the inflammatory response. Two low-molecular-weight fibrinopeptides, A and B, are released from fibrinogen when fibrin is produced. Both fibrinopeptides (especially fibrinopeptide B) are chemotactic for neutrophils and increase vascular permeability of endothelial cells by enhancing the effects of bradykinin (formed from the kinin system).

Kinin System

The third plasma protein system, the kinin system, augments inflammation in several ways. The primary product from the kinin system is bradykinin, which causes dilation of blood vessels, acts with prostaglandins to stimulate nerve endings and induce pain, causes smooth muscle cell contraction, increases vascular permeability, and may increase leukocyte chemotaxis (see Fig. 7.3). Bradykinin induces smooth muscle contraction more slowly than histamine and, along with prostaglandins of the E series, is probably responsible for endothelial cell retraction and increased vascular permeability in the later phases of inflammation (endothelial cell retraction is shown in Figs. 7.4 and 7.16).

The kinin system is activated by stimulation of the plasma kinin cascade (see Fig. 7.8). The conversion of plasma prekallikrein to kallikrein is induced by *prekallikrein activator,* which is identical to factor XIIa (the product that results from activation of Hageman factor—factor XII) of the clotting cascade. Kallikrein then converts kininogen to bradykinin. Although the plasma kinin cascade is one pathway that leads to the production of bradykinin, tissue kallikreins in saliva, sweat, tears, urine, and feces provide other sources for this inflammatory mediator. These tissue kallikreins convert serum kininogens to kallidin, also known as *Lys-bradykinin,* which may be converted to bradykinin by plasma aminopeptidase. In order to limit the extent of inflammation, kinins are rapidly degraded by kininase enzymes present in plasma and tissues.

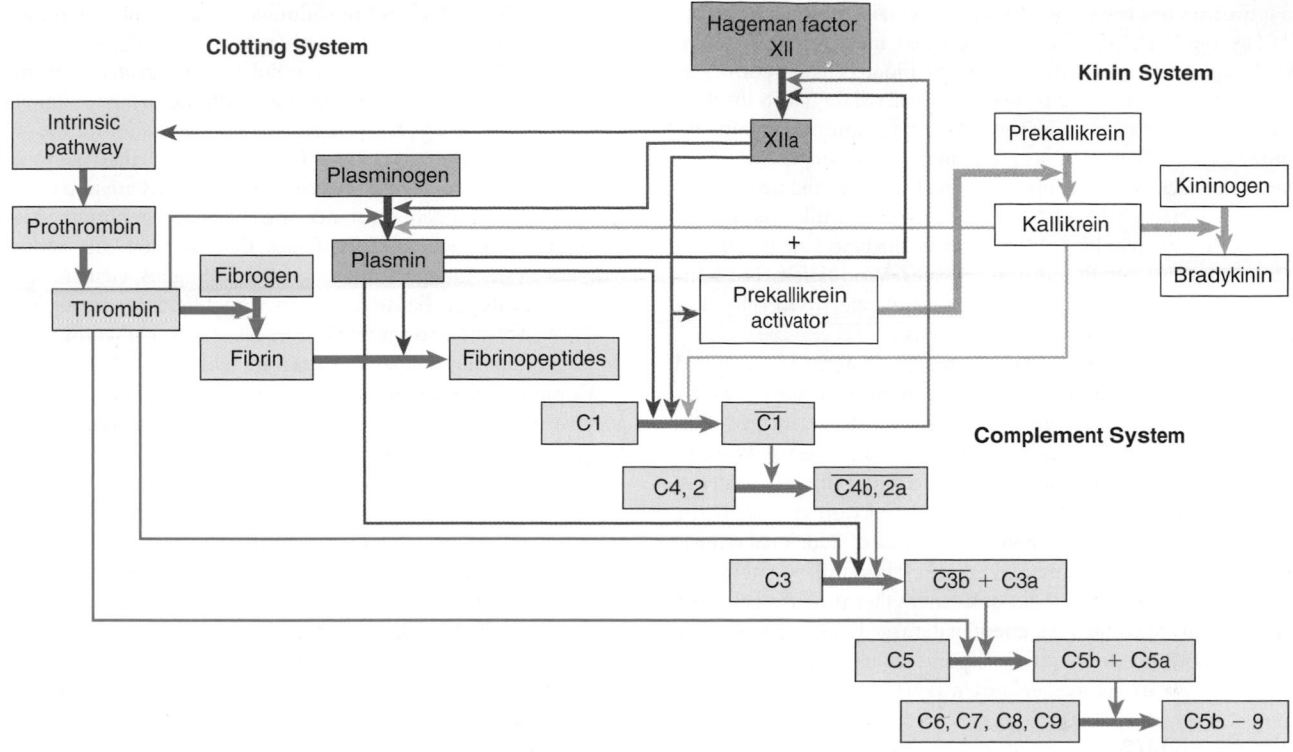

FIGURE 7.9 Interactions between the Complement, Clotting, and Kinin Systems. *Thick colored arrows* denote the activation of factors within a system. *Thin colored arrows* denote the interaction between systems.

Control and Interactions of Plasma Protein Systems

The three plasma protein systems are highly interactive so that activation of one system results in the production of a large number of very potent, biologically active substances that further activate the other systems (Fig. 7.9). Very tight control of these processes is essential for two reasons:

1. The inflammatory process is critical for an individual's survival; thus, efficient activation must be guaranteed regardless of the cause of tissue injury.
2. The biochemical mediators generated during these processes are so potent and potentially detrimental to the individual, and their actions must be strictly confined to injured or infected tissues.

Multiple mechanisms are available to either *activate* or *inactivate (regulate)* these plasma protein systems. For instance, the plasma that enters the tissues during inflammation (edema) contains enzymes that destroy mediators of inflammation. **Carboxypeptidase** inactivates the anaphylatoxic activities of C3a and C5a, and kininases degrade kinins. **Histaminase** degrades histamine and kallikrein and down-regulates the inflammatory response.

The formation of clots also activates a **fibrinolytic system** that is designed to limit the size of the clot and remove the clot after bleeding has ceased. Thrombin activates **plasminogen** in the blood to form the enzyme plasmin. The primary activity of **plasmin** is to degrade fibrin polymers in clots. However, plasmin also can activate the complement cascade through components C1, C3, and C5 and the kinin cascade by activating factor XII and producing prekallikrein activator. Activation of Hageman factor has four effects that impact all three of the plasma protein systems:

1. Activation of the clotting cascade through factor XI
2. Control of clotting through conversion of plasminogen proactivator to plasminogen activator, resulting in the generation of plasmin

3. Activation of the kinin system by activated Hageman factor (prekallikrein activator)
4. Activation of C1 in the complement cascade

The activity of plasmin itself is also regulated because it is synthesized as a proenzyme, plasminogen. Plasminogen is converted to plasmin by several factors, including plasminogen activator generated from the kallikrein system, thrombin generated from the clotting system, bacterial factors such as streptokinase produced by hemolytic streptococci, plasminogen activators produced by endothelial cells, and several cellular enzymes released during tissue destruction.

Another example of a common regulator is **C1-esterase inhibitor (C1-inh).**[12] C1-inh inhibits complement activation through reactivity with C1 (classical pathway), MASP-2 (lectin pathway), and C3b (alternative pathway). It is also a major inhibitor of clotting and kinin pathway components (e.g., kallikrein, XIIa). A genetic defect in C1-inh (C1-inh deficiency) results in **hereditary angioedema**, which is a self-limiting edema of cutaneous and mucosal layers resulting from stress, illness, or relative minor or unapparent trauma. The disease is characterized by hyperactivation of all three plasma protein systems, although excessive production of bradykinin appears to be the principal cause of increased vascular permeability.

Cellular Mediators of Inflammation

Inflammation is a process in vascular tissue; thus, the cellular components are found in the blood and in the tissue surrounding the blood vessels. The vessels are lined with endothelial cells, which under normal conditions actively maintain normal blood flow. During inflammation the vascular endothelium becomes a principal coordinator of blood clotting and the passage of cells and fluid into the tissue. The tissue close to the vessels contains mast cells, which are probably the most important activators of inflammation, and dendritic cells, which connect the innate and adaptive immune responses. The blood contains a complex mixture of cells (see Fig. 7.4). Blood cells are divided into erythrocytes (red blood cells), platelets, and leukocytes (white blood cells). Erythrocytes carry oxygen to the tissues, and platelets are small cell fragments involved in blood clotting. Leukocytes are subdivided into **granulocytes** (containing many enzyme-filled cytoplasmic granules), monocytes, and lymphocytes. Granulocytes are the most common leukocytes and are classified by the type of stains needed to visualize their granules (basophils, eosinophils, and neutrophils). Monocytes in the blood are precursors of macrophages that are found in the tissues. Various forms of lymphocytes participate in the innate (e.g., natural killer [NK] cells) and the adaptive immune response (B and T cells).

Cells of both innate and acquired immune systems are recruited and activated by biochemical mediators produced at the site of cellular damage. These molecules originate from destroyed or damaged cells, contaminating microbes, activation of the plasma protein systems, or secretions by other cells of the innate or acquired immune systems. Activation may result in the cell gaining a function critical to the inflammatory response or induction of the release of additional cellular products that increase inflammation, or both. These inflammatory cells and protein systems, along with the substances they produce, act at the site of tissue injury to confine the extent of damage, kill microorganisms, and remove the debris of "battle" in preparation for healing: tissue regeneration or repair (processes known as *resolution*).

Cellular Receptors

Cells of both innate and adaptive immunity must recognize and respond to their environment, whether to products of damaged cells or to potential pathogenic microorganisms. Each cell has receptors on the cell surface that specifically bind soluble substances (ligands) produced during tissue damage or infection. The binding of a ligand to its receptor results in activation of intracellular signaling pathways and activation of the cell. As will be discussed in Chapter 8, B and T lymphocytes of the adaptive immune system have evolved surface receptors (i.e., the T-cell receptor, or TCR, and the B-cell receptor, or BCR) that bind a large spectrum of antigens. Cells involved in innate resistance have evolved a different set of receptors that recognize a much more limited array of specific molecules. These are referred to as **pattern recognition receptors (PRRs)**, and they recognize molecular "patterns" on infectious agents or their products (**pathogen-associated molecular patterns, or PAMPs**), or products of cellular damage (necrosis or apoptosis; **damage-associated molecular patterns, or DAMPs**).[13] PRRs are generally found on cells at the interface of the host and environment (i.e., skin, respiratory tract, gastrointestinal tract, genitourinary tract), where they monitor for products of cellular damage and potentially infectious microorganisms. Although most PRRs are on the cell surface, some are secreted or intracellular.[14] An example of a secreted PRR is mannose-binding lectin of the lectin pathway of complement activation. Cellular PRRs include Toll-like receptors, complement receptors (CRs), scavenger receptors, glucan receptors, and mannose receptors.

In humans, at least 11 different **Toll-like receptors (TLRs)** have been described, 10 of which are functional.[15] They are expressed on the surface of many cells that have direct and early contact with potential pathogenic microorganisms. These include mucosal epithelial cells, mast cells, neutrophils, macrophages, dendritic cells, and some subpopulations of lymphocytes. (Dendritic cells are found in the skin, mucosa, and lymphoid tissues, where they have developed from Langerhans cells and function as highly specialized initiators of the adaptive immune response.) TLRs recognize a large variety of PAMPs located on the microorganism's cell wall or surface (e.g., bacterial lipopolysaccharide [LPS], peptidoglycans, lipoproteins, yeast zymosan, viral coat proteins), other surface structures (e.g., bacterial flagellin), or microbial nucleic

acid (e.g., bacterial DNA, viral double-stranded RNA). Some TLRs recognize host factors that are produced by "stressed" or damaged cells (e.g., breakdown products of extracellular matrix proteins, chromatin). Interactions between PAMPs and TLRs, with the collaboration of other cellular receptors (e.g., CD14), can result in activation of the cell and the release of soluble products (e.g., cytokines) that increase local resistance to the pathogenic microorganism. TLRs are also one of the bridges between innate resistance and the adaptive immune response through the induction of cytokines that increase the response of lymphocytes to foreign antigens on the pathogens. Genetic polymorphisms in TLRs may explain some observed differences among individuals' resistance and susceptibility to infections. Information on each of the TLRs found in humans is shown in Table 7.2.

Complement receptors are found on many cells of the innate and adaptive immune responses (e.g., granulocytes, monocytes/macrophages, lymphocytes, mast cells, erythrocytes, platelets), as well as some epithelial cells. They recognize several fragments produced through activation of the complement system.[16] Under a variety of normal and disease-related conditions, immune complexes of antibody, antigen, and complement form in the blood and are removed by cells expressing surface complement receptor-1 (CR1), which binds to C4b, C3b, and C3b breakdown products (e.g., iC3b). CR2 is found on B lymphocytes, as well as dendritic cells and some epithelial cells, and recognizes C3b breakdown products (particularly iC3b). CR2 appears to facilitate B-cell function and antibody production. Both CR3 and CR4 are integrins that primarily recognize C3b breakdown products (particularly iC3b). CR3 (integrin αMβ2, also called CD11b/CD18) facilitates phagocytosis by neutrophils and monocytes/macrophages. CR4 (αXββ2, also called CD11c/CD18) is found primarily on platelets. (**Integrins** are cell surface receptors that have a role in cell adhesion and attachment and mediate intracellular signaling within the extracellular matrix [see Fig. 1.17].)

Scavenger receptors are primarily expressed on macrophages and facilitate recognition and phagocytosis of bacterial pathogens, as well as damaged cells and altered soluble lipoproteins associated with vascular damage (e.g., high-density lipoprotein [HDL], acetylated low-density lipoprotein [LDL], oxidized LDL).[17] More than eight receptors have been identified. Some scavenger receptors (e.g., SR-PSOX) recognize the cell membrane phospholipid phosphatidylserine (PS). PS is normally sequestered on the cytoplasmic surface of the cell membrane, but it is externalized under a very limited variety of conditions, including erythrocyte senescence and cellular apoptosis. Thus, macrophages, through this receptor, can identify and remove old red blood cells and cells undergoing apoptosis. Another important scavenger receptor is CD14, which recognizes the complex of LPS and LPS-binding protein. LPS-binding protein is up-regulated during inflammation by the cytokines interleukin-6 (IL-6) and IL-1 and helps remove bacterial LPS (endotoxin) from the circulation.

NOD-like receptors (NLRs) are cytoplasmic receptors that recognize products of microbes and damaged cells.[18] At least 22 NLRs have been identified in humans. NOD-1 and NOD-2 are cytoplasmic and recognize fragments of peptidoglycans from intracellular bacteria and initiate production of proinflammatory mediators, such as tumor necrosis factor (TNF) and IL-6. Some NLRs associate with intracellular multiprotein complexes called **inflammasomes**. Inflammasomes primarily bind cellular stress–related molecules, a type of DAMP, and through the activation of caspases-1 control the activation and secretion of inflammatory cytokines, such as IL-1β.[19]

Cellular Products

To elicit an effective inflammatory (or adaptive immune) response, intercellular communication and cooperation are necessary. **Cytokines** constitute a large family of small-molecular-weight soluble

TABLE 7.2	CELLULAR SOURCE AND MICROBIAL TARGET FOR EACH TOLL-LIKE RECEPTOR (TLR)	
RECEPTOR	**CELLULAR EXPRESSION PATTERN**	**PAMP RECOGNITION**
TLR1	Cell surface (ubiquitous): neutrophils, monocytes/macrophages, dendritic cells, T cells, B cells, NK cells	Fungal, bacterial, viral; forms heterodimer with TLR2 (TLR2 recognition)
TLR2	Cell surface: neutrophils, monocytes/macrophages, dendritic cells	Fungal (yeast zymosan), bacterial (gram-positive bacterial peptidoglycan, lipoproteins), viral (lipoproteins)
TLR3	Intracellular: monocytes/macrophages, dendritic cells, T cells, NK cells, epithelial cells	Double-stranded RNA produced by many viruses
TLR4	Cell surface: granulocytes, monocytes/macrophages, dendritic cells, T cells, B cells, epithelial cells	Bacterial (primarily gram-negative bacterial LPS, lipoteichoic acids), viral (RSV F protein, hepatitis C)
TLR5	Cell surface: granulocytes, monocytes/macrophages, dendritic cells, NK cells, epithelial cells	Bacterial (flagellin); forms heterodimer with TLR4
TLR6	Cell surface: monocytes/macrophages, dendritic cells, B cells, NK cells	Fungal, bacterial, viral; forms heterodimer with TLR2 (TLR2 recognition)
TLR7	Intracellular: monocytes/macrophages, dendritic cells, B cells	Natural ligand uncertain; may bind viral single-strand RNA
TLR8	Cell surface: monocytes/macrophages, dendritic cells, NK cells	Natural ligand uncertain; may bind fungal PAMPs or viral single-stranded RNA
TLR9	Intracellular: monocytes/macrophages, dendritic cells, B cells	Bacterial (unmethylated DNA [CpG dinucleotides])
TLR10	Cell surface: monocytes/macrophages, dendritic cells, B cells	Natural ligand uncertain; may form heterodimers with TLR2
TLR11	TLR11 gene does not code a full-length protein in humans	No known immune response

DNA, Deoxyribonucleic acid; *LPS,* lipopolysaccharide; *NK,* natural killer; *PAMPs,* pathogen-associated molecular patterns; *RNA,* ribonucleic acid; *RSV,* respiratory syncytial virus.

intercellular-signaling molecules that are secreted, bind to specific cell membrane receptors, and regulate innate or adaptive immunity (Fig. 7.10). Cytokines may be either *proinflammatory* or *antiinflammatory* in nature, depending on whether they tend to induce or inhibit the inflammatory response. These molecules usually diffuse over short distances, but some effects occur over long distances, such as the systemic induction of fever by some cytokines (i.e., endogenous pyrogens) that are produced at an inflammatory site. Binding of cytokines to a target cell often induces synthesis of additional cellular products. For example, binding of the cytokine TNF-α to a cell may result in synthesis and release of IL-1.

The actions of chemokines and cytokines are *pleiotropic,* indicating that the same molecule may have a large variety of different biologic activities depending on the particular target cell to which it binds. In addition, the same molecule may be produced by a large spectrum of cells, many of which are not part of inflammation or the immune system. These molecules may be *synergistic,* so that their combined activity exceeds the sum of their individual activities, or have *antagonistic* properties that cause them to inhibit each other. (A partial list cytokines that are particularly relevant to the acquired immune response is provided in Chapter 8, Table 8.4.)

A large number of cytokines have been described and are classified into several families. The terms lymphokines and monokines refer respectively to cytokines secreted from lymphocytes or monocytes, although cytokines are secreted by many different types of cells. Chemokines are members of a special family of cytokines that are chemotactic and primarily attract leukocytes to sites of inflammation. Chemokines are synthesized by many cell types, including macrophages, fibroblasts, and endothelial cells, in response to proinflammatory cytokines, such as TNF-α. To date, more than 50 different human chemokines have been described. Examples include those that primarily attract macrophages (e.g., monocyte/macrophage chemotactic proteins [MCP-1, MCP-2, and MCP-3], macrophage inflammatory proteins [MIP-1α and MIP-1β]) or neutrophils (e.g., IL-8).

Cytokines. The majority of important cytokines are classified as interleukins or interferons. Other critical cytokines, however, are not classified as either. Many of these same cytokines are produced by cells of the acquired immune system in response to specific antigens and are discussed further in Chapter 8.

The interleukins (ILs) are biochemical messengers produced predominantly by macrophages and lymphocytes in response to stimulation of PRRs or by other cytokines. More than 30 interleukins have been identified. Their effects include the following:

1. Alteration of adhesion molecule expression on many types of cells
2. Attraction of leukocytes to a site of inflammation (chemotaxis)
3. Induction of proliferation and maturation of leukocytes in the bone marrow
4. General enhancement or suppression of inflammation
5. Mediation of development of the acquired immune response

Two major proinflammatory interleukins are IL-1 and IL-6, which cooperate closely with another cytokine, tumor necrosis factor-alpha (TNF-α). Interleukin-1 (IL-1) is produced in two forms (IL-1α and IL-1β) mainly by macrophages. IL-1 activates monocytes, other macrophages, and lymphocytes, thereby enhancing both innate and acquired immunity, and acts as a growth factor for many cells.[20] It has several effects on neutrophils, including induction of proliferation (resulting in an increase in the number of circulating neutrophils), attraction to an inflammatory site (chemotaxis), and an increase in cellular respiration and lysosomal enzyme activity (both effects resulting in increased cellular killing of bacteria). IL-1 is an endogenous pyrogen (i.e., fever-causing cytokine) that reacts with receptors on cells of the hypothalamus and affects the body's thermostat, resulting in fever.

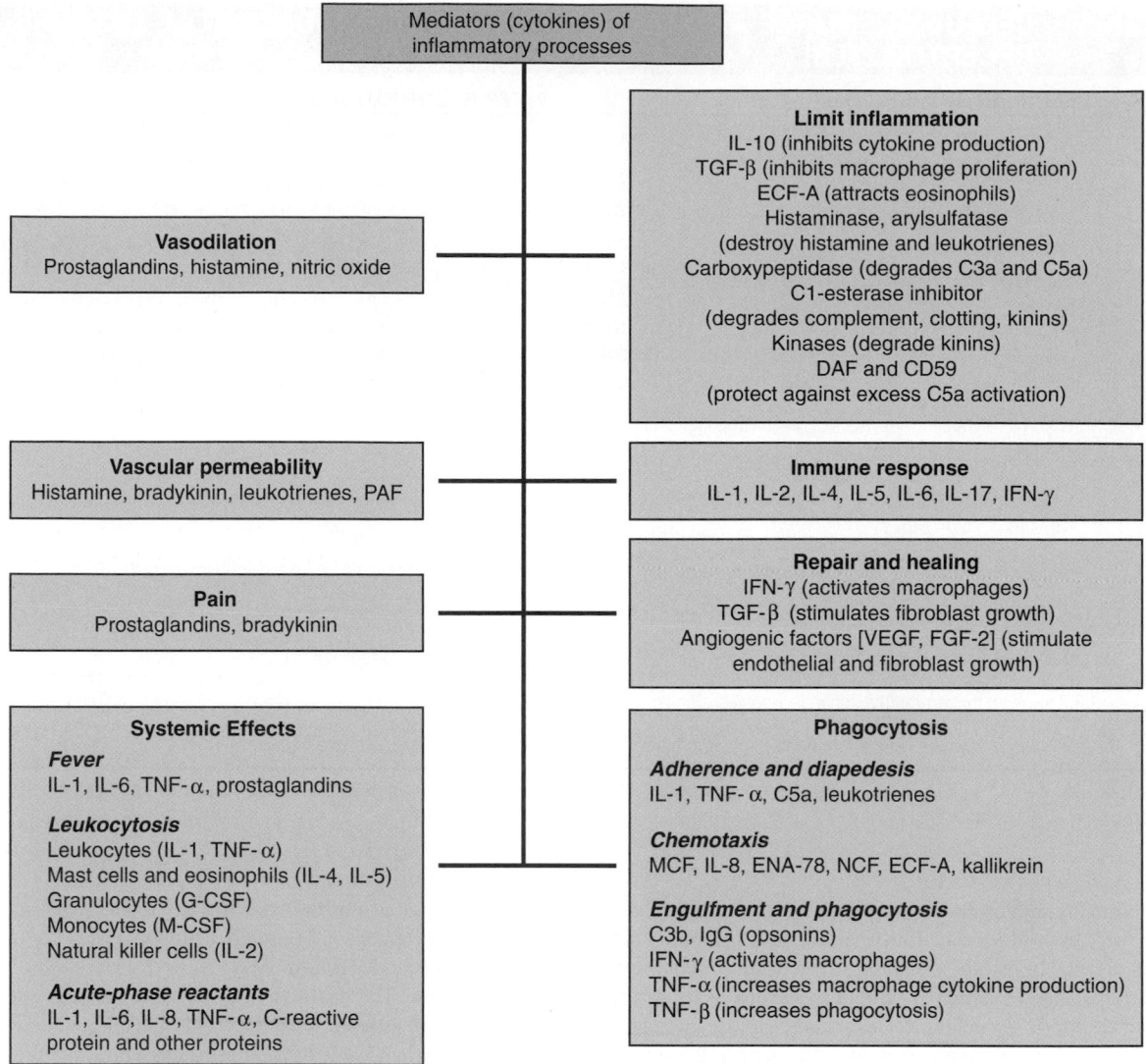

Mediators (cytokines) of inflammatory processes

Vasodilation
Prostaglandins, histamine, nitric oxide

Vascular permeability
Histamine, bradykinin, leukotrienes, PAF

Pain
Prostaglandins, bradykinin

Systemic Effects

Fever
IL-1, IL-6, TNF-α, prostaglandins

Leukocytosis
Leukocytes (IL-1, TNF-α)
Mast cells and eosinophils (IL-4, IL-5)
Granulocytes (G-CSF)
Monocytes (M-CSF)
Natural killer cells (IL-2)

Acute-phase reactants
IL-1, IL-6, IL-8, TNF-α, C-reactive protein and other proteins

Limit inflammation
IL-10 (inhibits cytokine production)
TGF-β (inhibits macrophage proliferation)
ECF-A (attracts eosinophils)
Histaminase, arylsulfatase
(destroy histamine and leukotrienes)
Carboxypeptidase (degrades C3a and C5a)
C1-esterase inhibitor
(degrades complement, clotting, kinins)
Kinases (degrade kinins)
DAF and CD59
(protect against excess C5a activation)

Immune response
IL-1, IL-2, IL-4, IL-5, IL-6, IL-17, IFN-γ

Repair and healing
IFN-γ (activates macrophages)
TGF-β (stimulates fibroblast growth)
Angiogenic factors [VEGF, FGF-2] (stimulate endothelial and fibroblast growth)

Phagocytosis

Adherence and diapedesis
IL-1, TNF-α, C5a, leukotrienes

Chemotaxis
MCF, IL-8, ENA-78, NCF, ECF-A, kallikrein

Engulfment and phagocytosis
C3b, IgG (opsonins)
IFN-γ (activates macrophages)
TNF-α (increases macrophage cytokine production)
TNF-β (increases phagocytosis)

FIGURE 7.10 Principal Mediators of Inflammation. *C3b,* Large fragment produced from complement component C3; *C5a,* small fragment produced from complement component C5; *ECF-A,* eosinophil chemotactic factor of anaphylaxis; *ENA,* epithelial-dermoid neutrophil attractant; *FGF,* fibroblast growth factor; *G-CSF,* granulocyte colony–stimulating factor; *IFN,* interferon; *IgG,* immunoglobulin G (predominant class of antibody in the blood); *IL,* interleukin; *MCF,* monocyte chemotactic factor; *M-CSF,* monocyte colony–stimulating factor; *NCF,* neutrophil chemotactic factor; *PAF,* platelet-activating factor; *TGF,* T-cell growth factor; *TNF,* tumor necrosis factor; *VEGF,* vascular endothelial growth factor.

Interleukin-6 (IL-6) is produced by macrophages, lymphocytes, fibroblasts, and other cells. IL-6 directly induces hepatocytes (liver cells) to produce many of the proteins needed in inflammation (acute-phase reactants, discussed later in this chapter).[21] IL-6 also stimulates growth and differentiation of blood cells in the bone marrow and the growth of fibroblasts (required for wound healing).

Although not classified as an interleukin, **tumor necrosis factor-alpha (TNF-α)** is secreted by macrophages and other cells (e.g., mast cells) in response to recognition of PAMPs by TLRs.[22] Macrophages secrete TNF-α in response to recognition of PAMPs by TLRs. TNF-α is initially synthesized as a membrane-anchored protein, which is cleaved into a soluble form by a membrane-associated protease, TNF-converting enzyme (TACE). Soluble TNF-α induces a multitude of proinflammatory effects, including enhancement of endothelial cell adhesion molecule expression and induction of chemokine production by both endothelial cells and

macrophages. When secreted in large amounts, TNF-α has systemic effects as well:

1. Induces fever by acting as an endogenous pyrogen
2. Causes increased synthesis of proinflammatory serum proteins by the liver
3. Causes muscle wasting (cachexia) and intravascular thrombosis as a consequence of prolonged production in cases of severe infection or cancer
4. Probably responsible for fatalities from shock caused by gram-negative bacterial infections

Some cytokines are antiinflammatory and diminish the inflammatory response. The most important are IL-10 and transforming growth factor-beta (TGF-β). **Interleukin-10 (IL-10)** is primarily produced by lymphocytes and suppresses the growth of other lymphocytes and the production of proinflammatory cytokines by macrophages, leading to the downregulation of both inflammation and the adaptive immune response. **Transforming growth factors**, including **transforming growth factor-beta (TGF-β)**, are produced by many types of cells in response to inflammation and induce cell division and differentiation of other cell types, such as immature blood cells.

Interferons (IFNs) are members of a family of low-molecular-weight proteins that primarily protect against viral infections and modulate the inflammatory response. (Mechanisms of viral infection are described in Chapter 10.) Type I interferons (primarily IFN-α, IFN-β) are produced and released by virally infected cells in response to viral double-stranded RNA and other viral PAMPs.[23] Type I IFNs do not kill viruses directly but instead are secreted from virally infected cells, attach to a receptor on neighboring cells, and, if the neighboring cells are uninfected, stimulate the production of a variety of antiviral proteins that will interfere with transcription of viral nucleic acids or with viral replication. Interferons are species specific, meaning that human interferon is effective only in humans; however, these cytokines are not virus specific, meaning that they are effective against almost all viruses.

Type II interferon (IFN-γ) is produced primarily by lymphocytes; it activates macrophages, resulting in increased capacity to kill infectious agents (including viruses and bacteria), and it enhances the development of acquired immune responses against viruses.

Chemokines. Chemokines are members of a family of low-molecular-weight (8 to 10 kDa) peptides that function primarily to induce leukocyte chemotaxis.[24] This response can be elicited either by soluble chemokines or by chemokines that are bound to extracellular glycosaminoglycan carbohydrates. Chemokines can be synthesized by multiple cell types, including macrophages, fibroblasts, and endothelial cells, in response to proinflammatory cytokines. Macrophages can be stimulated to produce chemokines by recognition of either infectious microorganisms or a β-defensin (both through TLR4). To date, more than 40 different human chemokines have been described, the vast majority of which are classified as either CC-chemokines (β-chemokines) or CXC-chemokines (α-chemokines), depending on the arrangement of cysteine amino acids in the protein. This amino acid arrangement also determines which target cell(s) will respond to a given chemokine. CC-chemokines affect mainly monocytes, lymphocytes, and eosinophils, whereas CXC-chemokines generally affect neutrophils. Examples of CC-chemokines include RANTES (regulated on activation, normal T expressed and secreted), monocyte/macrophage chemotactic proteins (MCP-1, MCP-2, and MCP-3), and macrophage inflammatory proteins (MIP-1α and MIP-1β). CXC-chemokines include IL-8 and epithelial-dermoid neutrophil attractant (ENA-78).

Mast Cells and Basophils

The mast cell is probably the most important cellular activator of the inflammatory response. **Mast cells**, first described by Paul Ehrlich[25] in 1877, are cellular bags of granules located in the loose connective tissues close to blood vessels near the body's outer surfaces (i.e., in the skin and lining the gastrointestinal and respiratory tracts) (Fig. 7.11). **Basophils** are found in the blood and probably function in the same way as tissue mast cells. A great number of stimuli activate mast cells to release potent soluble inducers of inflammation. These are released by (1) *degranulation* (the release of the contents of mast cell granules) and (2) *synthesis* (the new production and release of mediators in response to a stimulus). Typical causes of mast cell activation include (1) physical injury (e.g., heat, mechanical trauma, ultraviolet light, and x-rays), (2) chemical agents (e.g., toxins, snake and bee venoms, proteolytic enzymes, and antimicrobial peptides), (3) immunologic means (e.g., anaphylatoxins released during activation of complement components or particular types of antibody [e.g., immunoglobulin E (IgE)] produced by cells of the adaptive immune response [see Chapter 8]),

and (4) activation of TLRs by bacteria and viruses. Soluble and extremely potent chemicals from the mast cell are responsible for its effects on inflammation. Mast cells are also involved in initiating many allergic responses (discussed in Chapter 9).

Degranulation. In response to a stimulus, biochemical mediators in the mast cell granules, including histamine, chemotactic factors (e.g., neutrophil chemotactic factor, eosinophil chemotactic factor of anaphylaxis or ECF-A), and cytokines (e.g., TNF-α, IL-4), are released within seconds and exert their effects immediately (see Fig. 7.11).

Histamine is a small-molecular-weight molecule with potent effects on many other cells, particularly those that control the circulation. Histamine, along with serotonin (found in many cells, but not human mast cells), is called a *vasoactive amine*. Histamine causes temporary, rapid constriction of smooth muscle and dilation of the postcapillary venules, both of which result in increased blood flow into the microcirculation. Histamine also causes increased vascular permeability resulting from retraction of endothelial cells lining the capillaries and increased adherence of leukocytes to the endothelium (see Fig. 7.4). The pharmacologic effects of histamine are partially determined by histamine receptors on the person's target cells. Two main histamine receptors are the H1 and H2 receptors (Fig. 7.12), and two other receptors, H3 and H4, have been described.[26] Binding of histamine to the *H1 receptor* is essentially proinflammatory; that is, it promotes inflammation. On the other hand, binding to the *H2 receptor* is generally antiinflammatory because it results in suppression of leukocyte function. The H1 receptor is present on smooth muscle cells, especially those of the bronchi, and causes bronchial smooth muscle to contract (bronchoconstriction) when stimulated. Both types of receptors are distributed among many different cells and are often present on the same cells and may act in an antagonistic fashion. For instance, neutrophils express both types of receptors, with stimulation of H1 receptors resulting in the augmentation of neutrophil chemotaxis, and H2 stimulation resulting in its inhibition. The H2 receptor is especially abundant on parietal cells of the stomach mucosa and induces the secretion of gastric acid as part of the normal physiology of the stomach. The role of H1 and H2 receptors is discussed further in Chapter 9.

Mast cell granules also contain chemotactic factors, two of which are **neutrophil chemotactic factor (NCF)** and **eosinophil chemotactic factor of anaphylaxis (ECF-A)**. **Chemotaxis** is directional movement of cells along a chemical gradient formed by a chemotactic factor (see Fig. 7.4). Neutrophils (attracted by NCF) are the predominant leukocytes at work during the early phases of acute inflammation, and eosinophils (attracted by ECF-A) have several functions in the inflammatory process; both of these important inflammatory cells are discussed in more detail later in this chapter.

Synthesis of Mediators. Activated mast cells initiate synthesis of other mediators of inflammation, including those derived from plasma membrane lipids (leukotrienes, prostaglandins, platelet-activating factor),[27] cytokines (TNF-α, various interleukins), and factors that stimulate cell growth and angiogenesis. **Leukotrienes** (also known as **slow-reacting substances of anaphylaxis [SRS-A]**) are products of arachidonic acid, which is released from mast cell membranes by an intracellular phospholipase that acts on membrane phospholipids (Fig. 7.13). Leukotrienes are acidic, sulfur-containing lipids produced by *lipoxygenase* that produce effects similar to those of histamine: smooth muscle contraction, increased vascular permeability, and perhaps neutrophil and eosinophil chemotaxis. Leukotrienes appear to be important in the later stages of the inflammatory response because they stimulate slower and more prolonged responses than do histamines.

Prostaglandins are long-chain unsaturated fatty acids produced from arachidonic acid by the action of the enzyme *cyclooxygenase (COX)* and are classified into groups (E, D, A, F, and B) according to their

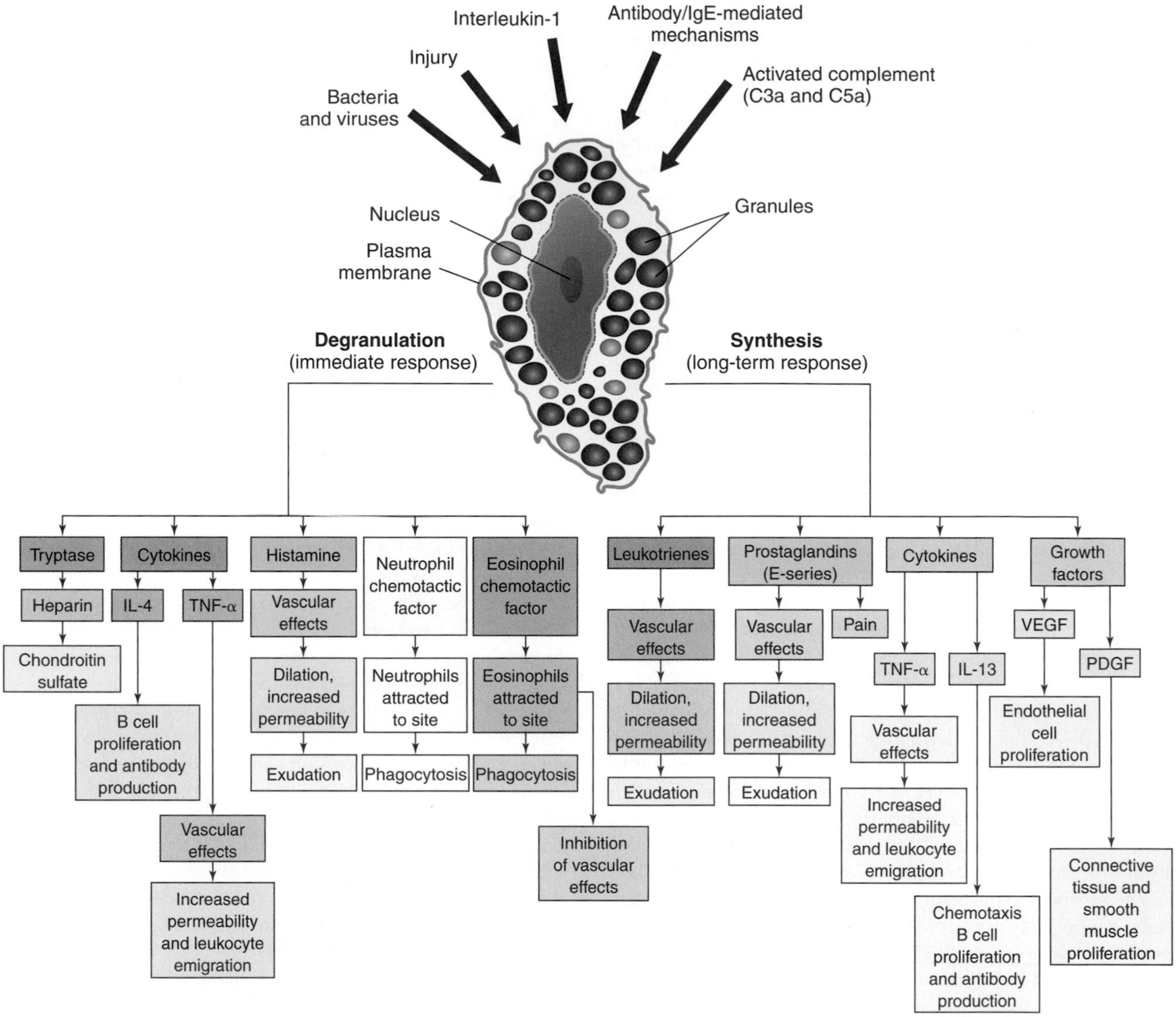

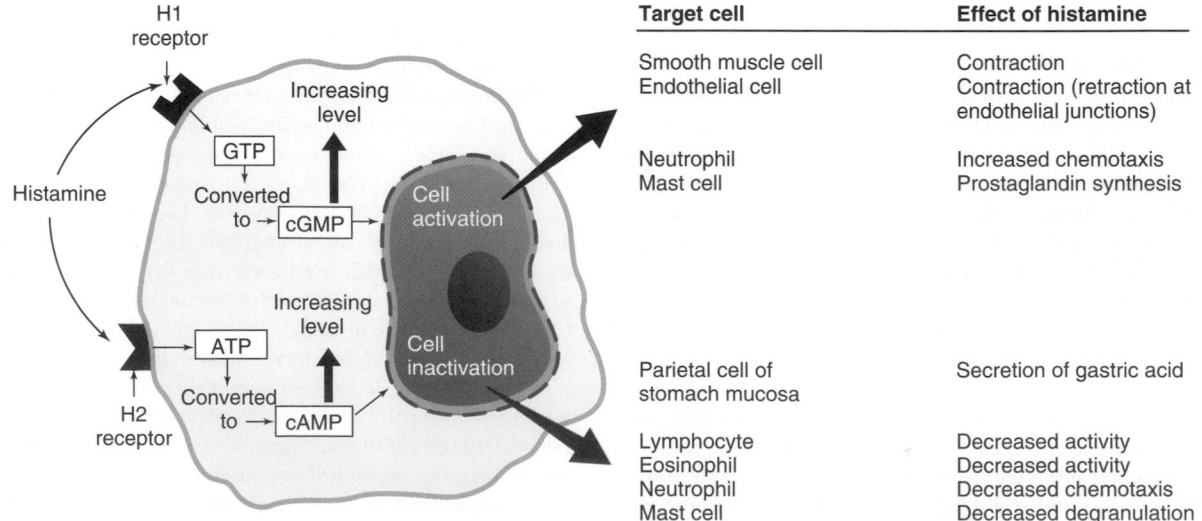

FIGURE 7.11 Effects of Degranulation *(left)* and Synthesis *(right)* by Mast Cells. The depiction of a tissue mast cell shows darkly stained granules in the cytoplasm. *IGE,* Immunoglobulin E; *IL-4,* interleukin-4; *IL-13,* interleukin-13; *PDGF,* platelet-derived growth factor; *TNF-α,* tumor necrosis factor-alpha; *VEGF,* vascular endothelial growth factor.

Target cell	Effect of histamine
Smooth muscle cell	Contraction
Endothelial cell	Contraction (retraction at endothelial junctions)
Neutrophil	Increased chemotaxis
Mast cell	Prostaglandin synthesis
Parietal cell of stomach mucosa	Secretion of gastric acid
Lymphocyte	Decreased activity
Eosinophil	Decreased activity
Neutrophil	Decreased chemotaxis
Mast cell	Decreased degranulation

FIGURE 7.12 Effects of Histamine through H1 and H2 Receptors. Effects depend on (1) density and affinity of H1 or H2 receptors on the target cell, and (2) the identity of the target cell. *ATP,* Adenosine triphosphate; *cAMP,* cyclic adenosine monophosphate; *cGMP,* cyclic guanosine monophosphate; *GTP,* guanosine triphosphate.

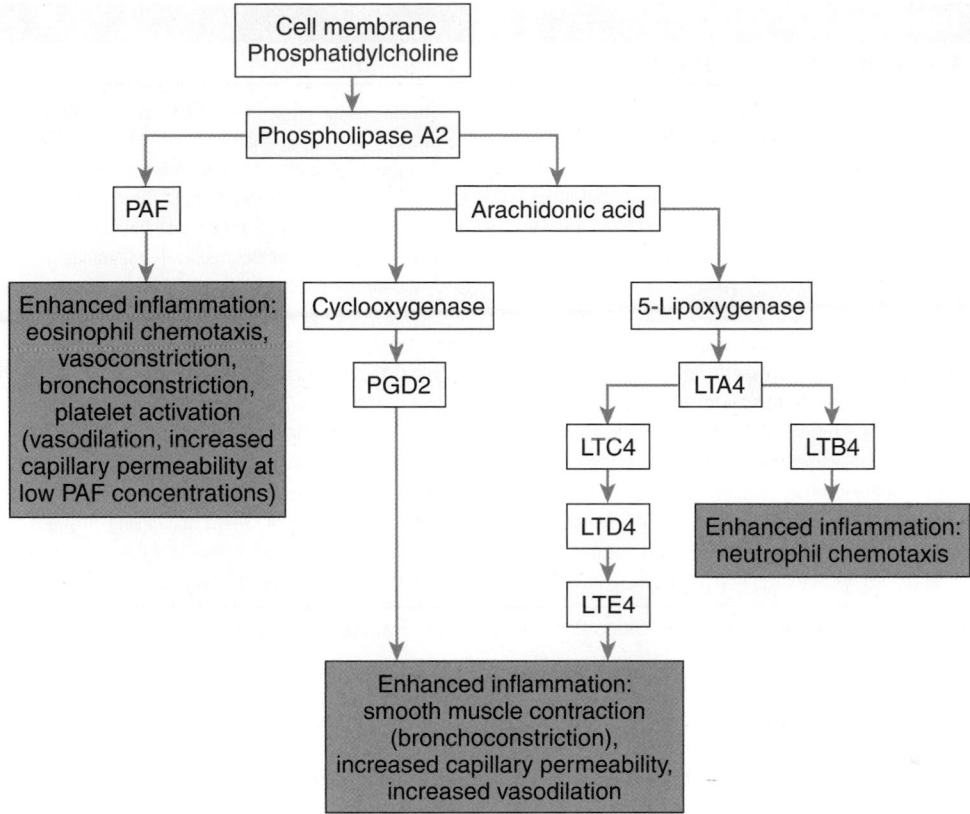

FIGURE 7.13 Production of Lipid Vasoactive Substances by Mast Cells. *LTA4, LTC4, LTD4, LTE4, LTB4,* Various leukotriene molecules; *PAF,* platelet-activating factor; *PGD2,* prostaglandin D$_2$.

structure. Prostaglandins E$_1$ and E$_2$ cause increased vascular permeability and smooth muscle contraction, apparently acting directly on postcapillary venules. They can inhibit some aspects of inflammation by suppressing both the release of histamine from mast cells and the release of lysosomal enzymes (enzymes responsible for killing and digesting microorganisms) from neutrophils. Enhancement or suppression of the inflammatory response may be related to the concentration of prostaglandins. Cyclooxygenase exists in two different forms: COX-1 is found in most tissues and COX-2 is associated with inflammation. Aspirin and other nonsteroidal antiinflammatory drugs (NSAIDs) inhibit both COX-1 and COX-2, blocking synthesis of prostaglandins of the E series, but inhibition of COX-1 causes complications, such as gastrointestinal toxicity. Selective COX-2 inhibitors are now available. Dietary free fatty acids also promote antiinflammatory effects (see *Nutrition & Disease:* Essential Fatty Acids and Inflammation).

Platelet-activating factor (PAF) is produced by removal of a fatty acid from the plasma membrane phospholipid phosphatidylcholine by phospholipase A$_2$. Although mast cells are a major source of PAF, this molecule also can be produced during inflammation by neutrophils, monocytes, endothelial cells, and platelets. The biologic activity of PAF is virtually identical to that of leukotrienes: causing endothelial cell retraction to increase vascular permeability, leukocyte adhesion to endothelial cells, and platelet activation.

Endothelium

The blood vessel walls consist of a layer of endothelial cells that adhere to an underlying matrix of connective tissue that contains a variety of proteins, including collagen, fibronectin, and laminins. Circulating cells and platelets and components of plasma protein systems continually contact endothelial cells, which contribute to regulation of normal blood flow by preventing spontaneous activation of platelets and members of the clotting system.[28] Nitric oxide (NO) produced from arginine and prostacyclin (PGI$_2$) from arachidonic acid maintain blood flow and pressure and inhibit platelet activation. PGI$_2$ and NO are synergistic. NO is released continually to relax vascular smooth muscle and suppress the effects of low levels of cytokines, thus maintaining vascular tone. PGI$_2$ production varies a great deal and is increased when additional regulation is needed.

Damage to the endothelial cell lining of the vessel exposes the subendothelial connective tissue matrix, which is prothrombogenic and initiates platelet activation and formation of clots (the contact activation [intrinsic] clotting pathway). Proinflammatory mediators (e.g., histamine, prostacyclin, and many others) affect the endothelium, resulting in adherence of leukocytes to the vessel surface, invasion of leukocytes into the tissue, and efflux of plasma from the vessel.

Platelets

Platelets (thrombocytes) are anucleate cytoplasmic fragments formed from megakaryocytes. They circulate in the bloodstream until vascular injury occurs, resulting in platelet activation. Platelets can be activated by many products of both the innate and the adaptive immune responses, including collagen, thrombin, thromboxane, PAF, and antigen-antibody complexes.[29] Activated platelets (1) relocate plasma membrane phosphatidylserine to the cell surface, which provides a foundation for interaction with components of the coagulation cascade to stop bleeding; (2) degranulate to release biochemical mediators such as serotonin (a vasoactive amine with histamine-like vasoactive effects); and (3) synthesize thromboxane A$_2$ (TXA$_2$) from prostaglandin H$_2$. Platelets contain alpha (α) granules and dense granules. *Alpha granules* generally contain polypeptides that affect inflammation, including coagulation proteins (e.g., fibrinogen, factor V), soluble adhesion molecules (e.g., von Willebrand factor, vitronectin), growth factors that promote wound healing (e.g., platelet-derived growth factor, epidermal growth factor), protease inhibitors (e.g., plasminogen activator inhibitor-1, α_2-antiplasmin), and membrane adhesion molecules (e.g., P-selectin, αIIbβ3).[30] *Dense granules* contain several small molecules, including adenosine diphosphate (ADP), serotonin, calcium, and magnesium. TXA$_2$ is a potent vasoconstrictor and inducer of platelet aggregation. Prolonged use of low-dose aspirin preferentially suppresses production of TXA$_2$ without interfering with the production of antiinflammatory PGI$_2$ by endothelium. (Platelet function is described in detail in Chapter 28.)

Phagocytes

The primary role of most granulocytes (neutrophils, eosinophils, basophils) and monocytes/macrophages is **phagocytosis**, the process by which a cell ingests and disposes of damaged cells and foreign material, including microorganisms.

Neutrophil. The **neutrophil**, or **polymorphonuclear neutrophil (PMN)**, is a member of the granulocytic series of white blood cells and is named for the characteristic staining pattern of its granules, as well as its multilobed nucleus. Neutrophils are the predominant **phagocytes** in the early inflammatory site, arriving within 6 to 12 hours after the initial injury, where they ingest (phagocytose) bacteria, dead cells, and cellular debris. Several inflammatory mediators (e.g., some bacterial proteins, complement fragments C3a and C5a, and mast cell neutrophil chemotactic factor) specifically attract neutrophils from the circulation and activate them. Macrophages and lymphocytes, on the other hand, enter the site later, usually after 24 hours, and gradually replace the neutrophils.

Because the neutrophil is a mature cell incapable of division and sensitive to the acidic environment it is short-lived at the inflammatory site and becomes a component of the purulent exudate, or *pus,* which is removed from the body through the epithelium or through the lymphatic system. (The lymphatic system is described in Chapter 28.) The primary roles of the neutrophil are removal of debris in sterile lesions, such as burns, and phagocytosis of bacteria in nonsterile lesions.

Eosinophil. Another population of granulocytes is the **eosinophil**. Although eosinophils are only mildly phagocytic, they have two specific functions: (1) to serve as the body's primary defense against parasites and (2) to help regulate vascular mediators released from mast cells. Their role in resistance to parasites occurs in collaboration with specific antibodies produced by the adaptive immune system and will be discussed in Chapter 8.

Regulation of mast cell–derived inflammatory mediators is critical for control of inflammation. The acute inflammatory response is needed only in a circumscribed area and for a limited time. Therefore, control mechanisms are necessary to prevent biochemical mediators from evoking more inflammation than necessary. Mast cells' ECF-A attracts eosinophils to the site of inflammation. Eosinophil lysosomal granules contain enzymes that degrade vasoactive molecules, thereby controlling the vascular effects of inflammation.[31] Histaminase degrades histamine, and arylsulfatase B degrades leukotrienes.

Basophil. The **basophil** is the least prevalent granulocyte in the blood. It is very similar to mast cells in the content of its granules and, in addition, is an important source of the cytokine IL-4, which is a key regulator of the adaptive immune response.[32] Although often associated with allergies and asthma, its primary role is yet unknown.

Dendritic Cells. **Dendritic cells** provide one of the major links between the innate and acquired immune responses. They are the primary phagocytic cells located in the peripheral organs and skin, where molecules released from infectious agents are encountered, recognized through PRRs, and internalized through phagocytosis. Dendritic cells then migrate through the lymphatic vessels to lymphoid tissue, such as lymph nodes, and interact with T lymphocytes to generate an acquired immune response.[33] Through the production of a family of cytokines, they guide development of a subset of T cells (helper cells) that coordinate the development of functional B and T cells (discussed in Chapter 8).

Monocyte and Macrophage. **Monocytes** are the largest normal blood cells (14 to 20 μm in diameter) and have a nucleus that is often indented, or horseshoe shaped. Monocytes are produced in the bone marrow, enter the circulation, and migrate to the inflammatory site where they develop into macrophages. Monocytes also appear to be the precursors of macrophages that are found in tissues (tissue macrophages, discussed in Chapter 8), including Kupffer cells in the liver, alveolar macrophages in the lungs, and microglia in the brain. **Macrophages** are generally larger (20 to 40 μm) and are more active as

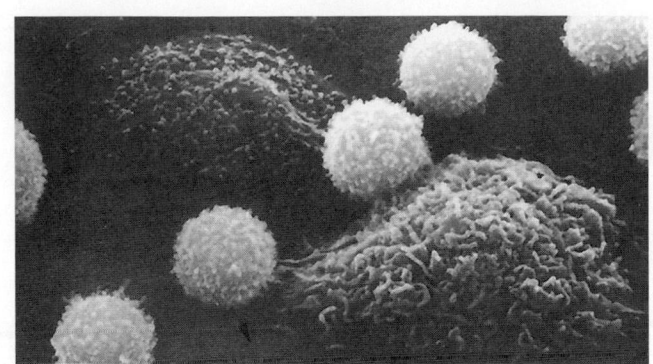

FIGURE 7.14 Scanning Electron Micrograph of Lymphocytes and Macrophages. The lymphocytes are small and spherical; the macrophages are larger and more irregular in shape. (From Raven PH, Johnson GB: *Biology*, St Louis, 1992, Mosby.)

phagocytes than their monocytic precursors. Macrophages, particularly those residing in the tissues, are often important cellular initiators of the inflammatory response (Fig. 7.14).

Monocyte-derived macrophages from the circulation may appear at the inflammatory site as soon as 24 hours after the initial neutrophil infiltration, but usually arrive 3 to 7 days later. Neutrophils and monocytes/macrophages are cooperative but differ chiefly in the following ways:

1. *Speed:* Neutrophils arrive at the injury site first, whereas macrophages move more sluggishly.
2. *Active life span:* Macrophages survive and divide in the acidic inflammatory site, whereas neutrophils cannot.
3. *Chemotactic factors:* Neutrophils and macrophages are not attracted by the same factors, such as macrophage chemotactic factor, which is released by neutrophils.
4. *Content of their lysosomes, or digestive vacuoles:* Neutrophils produce large amounts of reactive oxygen species, myeloperoxidase, and antimicrobial proteins compared to macrophages.
5. *Role in the immune response:* Macrophages, but not neutrophils, are involved in activation of the adaptive immune system.
6. *Role in wound repair:* Macrophages are the primary cells that infiltrate tissue in wounds, remove cells and cellular debris, promote angiogenesis, and produce cytokines and growth factors that suppress further inflammation and initiate healing by promoting epithelial cell division, activating fibroblasts, and promoting synthesis of extracellular matrix and collagen.

Phagocytosis. The two most important phagocytes are neutrophils and macrophages. Both cells are circulating in the blood and must first leave the circulation and migrate to the site of inflammation before initiating phagocytosis (Fig. 7.15). Under normal conditions, the circulation in the capillaries and venules is rapidly moving with red blood cells in the main stream and neutrophils and other leukocytes tending to flow more slowly along the vessel's periphery. Many of the biochemical products produced early at inflammatory sites (e.g., histamine, TNF-α, bradykinin, leukotrienes, prostaglandins) diffuse to the vessels and affect both leukocytes and endothelial cells.

Both cell populations respond by expressing new cell adhesion molecules (CAMs) on their surfaces. CAMs are a family of transmembrane proteins that provide adhesion between cells or between a cell and components of extracellular matrix (e.g., fibronectin, collagen, fibrinogen). The most important CAMs related to vascular inflammation are selectins and integrins. Selectins are CAMs that bind carbohydrate ligands on transmembrane glycoproteins: E-selectins are found on endothelial cells, L-selectins on leukocytes, and P-selectins on platelets

and endothelial cells. Integrins are proteins consisting of alpha (α) and beta (β) chains that primarily provide cell-to-cell adhesion by binding to ligands on another cell. Their affinity for a ligand is dependent on conformational changes of the integrin molecule. The reciprocal change in adhesion molecules on leukocytes (from low-affinity integrins to high-affinity integrins), as well as platelets, promotes their interaction with the endothelial cells.[34] The initial change of surface molecules increases the adhesion, or stickiness, between leukocytes and endothelial cells, causing the leukocytes to adhere more avidly to the walls of the capillaries and postcapillary venules in a process called margination, or pavementing (see Fig. 7.15). Adhesion molecules, such as platelet endothelial cell adhesion molecules (PCAMs), that are expressed later lead to diapedesis or emigration of the cells through the endothelial junctions that have retracted in response to the same mediators.[35] The leukocytes digest the basement membrane and migrate into the surrounding tissues.

Additionally, endothelial cells release NO, a gas that under normal conditions maintains vascular tone. Inflammation induces additional endothelial nitric oxide synthase, increasing the amount of NO production. Effects of NO on inflammation include vasodilation by inducing relaxation of vascular smooth muscle, a response that is local and short-lived, and suppression of mast cell function as well as platelet adhesion and aggregation.

Once inside the connective tissue in the perivascular space, leukocytes migrate to the inflammatory site by means of chemotaxis. They detect chemotactic factors in the environment through chemoreceptors at multiple locations on their plasma membranes and migrate in the direction of highest concentration (see Fig. 7.15). The primary chemotactic factors include many bacterial products, complement fragments C3a and C5a, kallikrein, plasminogen activator, products of fibrin degradation (fibrinopeptides), and chemokines, such as IL-8. Eosinophils and neutrophils also respond to chemotactic factors released from mast cells (ECF-A, neutrophil chemotactic factor [NCF]). Monocytes are attracted toward a factor (monocyte chemotactic factor) that has been released by neutrophils already at the site of injury. And although histamine is not itself chemotactic, it may facilitate the chemotactic effects of other factors.

Once the phagocytic cell enters the inflammatory site, the process of phagocytosis involves four steps: (1) *opsonization* (*recognition* of the target and *adherence* of the phagocyte to it); (2) *engulfment* (ingestion or endocytosis) and *formation of phagosome*; (3) *fusion of the phagosome* with lysosomal granules within the phagocyte to form a phagolysosome; and (4) *destruction* of the target (see Fig. 7.15, *C*) (lysosomes are described in Chapter 1). Throughout the process, both the ingested material and the digestive enzymes are isolated within membrane-bound vesicles. Isolation protects the phagocyte itself from the harmful effects of a microorganism, as well as its own enzymes.

Most phagocytes can trap and engulf bacteria using cellular PRRs and PAMPs normally expressed on the bacterial surface (see Fig. 7.15, *B*). However, that process is slow and inefficient. Opsonization, usually by antibody or complement component C3b, greatly enhances both recognition and adherence. Phagocytosis of a red blood cell is illustrated in Fig. 7.16. Opsonins function as "glue" between the phagocyte and the target cell because receptors on the phagocyte are specific for sites on the opsonin (Fc receptors for antibody, C3b receptors for C3b). This enables the phagocyte to bind an opsonized target very tightly to its surface. Antibody forms a stronger attachment, but the signal through the C3b receptor activates the phagocytic process to a greater extent.

Although the inflammatory response is considered to be nonspecific, opsonins and other recognition molecules add a degree of specificity to efficient phagocytosis. Antibodies on the surface of bacteria are directed against antigens that are highly specific to that particular microorganism.

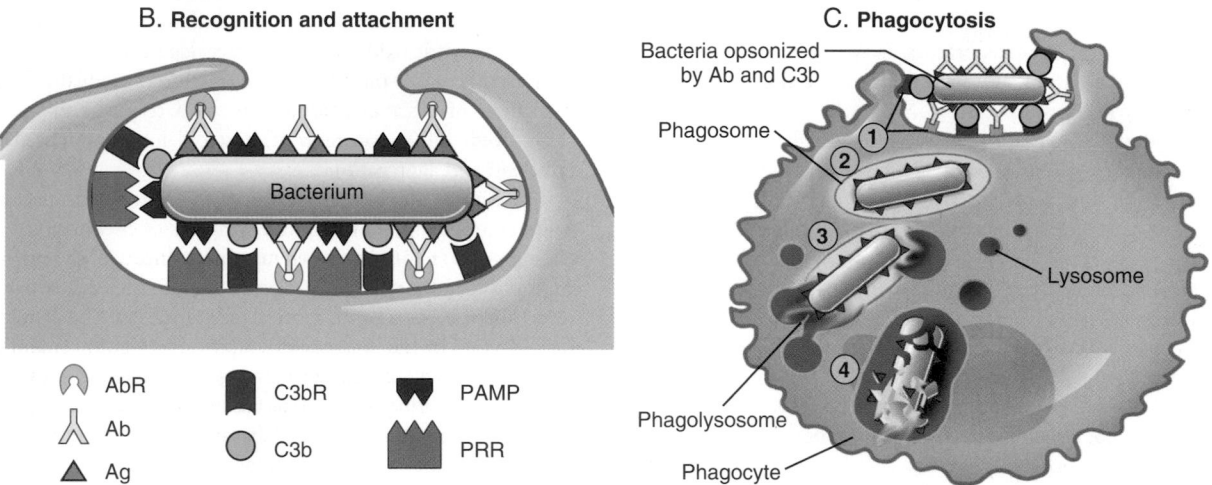

FIGURE 7.15 Process of Phagocytosis. The process that results in phagocytosis is characterized by three interrelated steps: adherence and diapedesis, tissue invasion by chemotaxis, and phagocytosis. **A, Tissue damage.** *Adherence, margination, and diapedesis:* The primary phagocyte in the blood is the neutrophil, which usually moves freely within the vessel **(1)**. At sites of inflammation, the neutrophil progressively develops increased adherence to the endothelium, leading to accumulation along the vessel wall (margination or pavementing) **(2)**. At sites of endothelial cell retraction, the neutrophil exits the blood by means of diapedesis **(3)**. *Chemotaxis:* In the tissues, the neutrophil detects chemotactic factor gradients through surface receptors **(1)** and migrates toward higher concentrations of the factors **(2)**. The high concentration of chemotactic factors at the site of inflammation immobilizes the neutrophil **(3)**. **B, Recognition and attachment.** *Specific receptors and ligands for recognition and attachment.* **C, Phagocytosis.** **(1)** Opsonized microorganisms are recognized and bind to the surface of a phagocyte through specific receptors. **(2)** The microorganism is engulfed (ingested) into a phagocytic vacuole, or phagosome. **(3)** Lysosomes fuse with the phagosome, resulting in the formation of a phagolysosome. During this process the microorganism is exposed to products of the lysosomes, including a variety of enzymes and products of the hexose-monophosphate shunt (e.g., H_2O_2, O_2^-). **(4)** The microorganism is killed and digested. *Ab,* Antibody; *AbR,* antibody receptor; *Ag,* antigen; *C3b,* complement component C3b; *C3bR,* complement C3b receptor; *PAMP,* pathogen-associated molecular pattern; *PRR,* pattern recognition receptor.

Certain bacterial and fungal polysaccharide coatings activate the alternative and lectin pathways of complement activation resulting in C3b deposition.

Engulfment (endocytosis) is carried out by small pseudopods that extend from the plasma membrane and surround the adherent microorganism, forming an intracellular phagocytic vacuole, or **phagosome** (see Figs. 7.15 and 7.16). The membrane that surrounds the phagosome consists of inverted plasma membrane. Lysosomes converge on and fuse with the phagosome, creating a **phagolysosome**. The **primary lysosomal granules** *(azurophilic granules)* contain a variety of bactericidal molecules, including myeloperoxidase, lysozyme, defensins, acid hydrolases, elastase, and others. Most phagocytes also contain **secondary granules** *(specific granules)* with molecules that are bactericidal and involved in remodeling the surrounding tissue, including lysozyme, collagenase, lactoferrin, and other proteases. Destruction of the bacterium takes place within the phagolysosome and is accomplished by both oxygen-dependent and oxygen-independent mechanisms.

Oxygen-dependent killing mechanisms result from the production of toxic oxygen species. Phagocytosis is accompanied by a burst of oxygen uptake by the phagocyte, termed the "respiratory burst," which results

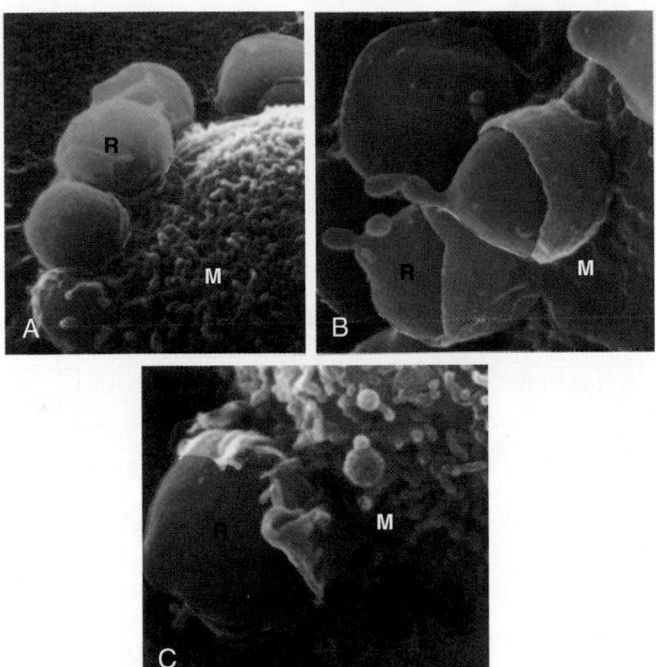

FIGURE 7.16 **Steps in Phagocytosis.** This scanning electron micrograph shows the progressive steps in phagocytosis. **A,** Red blood cells *(R)* attach to the surface of a macrophage *(M)*. **B,** Part of the macrophage *(M)* membrane starts to enclose the red cell *(R)*. **C,** The red blood cells are almost totally engulfed by the macrophage. (From King DW, Fenoglio CM, Lefwitch JH: *General pathology: principles and dynamics,* Philadelphia, 1983, Lea & Febiger.)

from a shift in much of the cell's glucose metabolism to the hexose-monophosphate shunt. The nicotinamide adenine dinucleotide phosphate (NADPH) that is produced because of this shift is used by a membrane-associated enzyme, NADPH oxidase, to generate superoxide, a reactive oxygen intermediate that is converted to hydrogen peroxide and other reactive oxygen species. Many of the reactive oxygen species are directly toxic to the microorganism. Hydrogen peroxide also can collaborate with the lysosomal enzyme *myeloperoxidase* and halide anions (Cl^- and Br^-) to form acids, such as hypochlorous (HClO) and hypobromous (HBrO) acids. These acids probably kill bacteria and fungi by adding Cl^- or Br^- to the surface of these cells.

Oxygen-independent mechanisms of microbial killing include (1) the acidic pH (3.5 to 4.0) of the phagolysosome caused by lactic acid production; (2) cationic proteins, such as defensins and cathelicidins, that bind to and damage cell membranes; (3) enzymatic attack of the microorganism's cell wall by lysozyme and other enzymes; and (4) inhibition of bacterial growth by lactoferrin that binds iron.

When a phagocyte dies at an inflammatory site, it frequently lyses (breaks open) and releases its cytoplasmic contents into the tissue. Although released lysosomal products may contribute to inflammation by increasing vascular permeability, attracting additional monocytes, and activating the complement and kinin systems, they also may increase the tissue destruction associated with inflammation. For instance, the contents of neutrophil primary granules (e.g., lysozyme, hydrolases, neutral proteases) and secondary granules (e.g., lysozyme, collagenase, gelatinase) can digest the connective tissue matrix. The destructive effects of many enzymes and reactive oxygen molecules released by dying phagocytes are minimized by natural inhibitors found in the blood, such as superoxide dismutase (breaks down superoxide), catalase (breaks down hydrogen peroxide), and the antiproteinases α_1-antitrypsin and α_2-macroglobulin (both produced by the liver). An inherited deficiency

of α_1-antitrypsin often results in chronic lung damage and emphysema as a result of inflammation. (The pulmonary effects of α_1-antitrypsin deficiency are described in Chapter 36.)

Macrophage Activation. Several bacteria are resistant to killing by granulocytes and can even survive inside macrophages. Microorganisms such as *Mycobacterium tuberculosis* (tuberculosis), *Mycobacterium leprae* (leprosy), *Salmonella typhi* (typhoid fever), *Brucella abortus* (brucellosis), and *Listeria monocytogenes* (listeriosis) can remain dormant or even multiply inside the phagolysosomes of macrophages.

The bactericidal activity of macrophages can be markedly increased by activation. Macrophage activation results in two subpopulations of cells. *M1 macrophages* are activated through TLRs by substances found in sites of inflammation (e.g., microbial products, endotoxin, or interferon-γ [IFN-γ]) and produce NO and cytokines, release lysosomal granules, and have greater bacterial killing capacity. *M2 macrophages* are activated by cytokines produced by subsets of T lymphocytes of the adaptive immune system (e.g., IL-4, IL-13) and are primarily involved in healing and repair. Activated macrophages have increased (1) phagocytic activity, (2) size, (3) ruffling of the plasma membrane to increase surface area, (4) glucose metabolism, and (5) number of lysosomes.[36] Activated macrophages also secrete factors that stimulate the growth, differentiation, and activation of other inflammatory cells as well as control the initiation of healing processes. These include granulocyte colony–stimulating factor (G-CSF), IFN-γ, IL-1β, angiogenic factor, fibroblast activating factor, and growth factors that promote regeneration of damaged tissues. Macrophages are also the primary cells that infiltrate wounds to remove cellular debris and initiate the regenerative process. In some cases, inadequate macrophage activation results from defects in the adaptive immune responses and deficits in the production of appropriate cytokines. For example, a form of leprosy called *lepromatous leprosy* is characterized by the survival of phagocytosed *M. leprae* bacteria in macrophage phagolysosomes. In individuals with lepromatous leprosy, cells of the adaptive immune system have failed to secrete the cytokines necessary to transform macrophages into highly efficient killing cells.

Natural Killer Cells and Lymphocytes

The main function of natural killer (NK) cells is recognition and elimination of cells infected with viruses, although they are also somewhat effective at elimination of other abnormal cells, specifically cancer cells. NK cells seem to be more efficient in this role when they encounter abnormal cells within the circulatory system as opposed to within tissues. Along with TLRs, NK cells have additional inhibitory and activating receptors that allow differentiation between infected or tumor cells and normal cells. If the NK cell binds to a target cell through activating receptors, it produces several cytokines and toxic molecules that can kill the target. NK cells and lymphocytes, which are the principal cells of the adaptive immune response, will be discussed in much more detail in Chapter 8.

LOCAL MANIFESTATIONS OF INFLAMMATION

The cells and plasma protein systems described previously interact to produce all the characteristics of inflammation, whether local or systemic, as well as determine the duration of inflammation, either acute or chronic. Local inflammation accompanies all types of cellular and tissue injury, whether infected or sterile, from fractures or strains of the musculoskeletal system to burn injuries (see Chapters 2 and 49), and is responsible for initiating healing.

All the *local* manifestations of acute inflammation (i.e., swelling, pain, heat, and redness) result from vascular changes and the subsequent leakage of circulating components into the tissue. Heat and redness are the result of vasodilation and increased blood flow through the injured site. Swelling occurs as exudate (fluid and cells) accumulates. Swelling is usually accompanied by pain caused by pressure exerted by exudate accumulation, as well as the presence of soluble biochemical mediators such as prostaglandins and bradykinin.[37] Loss of function at the cellular, tissue, or organ level is associated with these manifestations.

Exudate varies in composition, depending on the stage of the inflammatory response and, to some extent, the injurious stimulus. In early or mild inflammation, the exudate is watery (serous) with very few plasma proteins or leukocytes. An example of serous exudate is the fluid in a blister. In more severe or advanced inflammation, the exudate may be thick and clotted (fibrinous exudate), such as in the lungs of individuals with pneumonia. If a large number of leukocytes accumulate, as in persistent bacterial infections, the exudate consists of pus and is called a purulent (suppurative) exudate. Purulent exudate is characteristic of walled-off lesions (cysts or abscesses). If bleeding occurs, the exudate is filled with erythrocytes and is described as a hemorrhagic exudate.

Although the local manifestations of inflammation can affect all vascularized tissues, lesions vary depending on the organ or tissue involved. The lesion resulting from widespread cellular death (necrosis), for example, differs in myocardial (heart muscle), brain, and hepatic (liver) tissues. Cellular death resulting from myocardial infarction (deprivation of oxygen caused by cessation of blood flow) causes a response that proceeds to replacement of the dead tissue with a fibrinous scar. The same injury to brain tissue is more likely to result in the formation of an abscess filled with necrotic tissue (types of necrosis are described in Chapter 2). Destruction of liver tissue stimulates the regrowth, or regeneration, of liver cells.

SYSTEMIC MANIFESTATIONS OF ACUTE INFLAMMATION

The three primary *systemic* changes associated with the acute inflammatory response are fever, leukocytosis (a transient increase in the levels of circulating leukocytes), and plasma protein synthesis (increased levels of circulating plasma proteins).

Fever

Fever is an early systemic response, which is partially induced by specific cytokines, for example, IL-1 released from neutrophils and macrophages. These fever-causing cytokines are known as endogenous pyrogens to differentiate them from pathogen-produced *exogenous pyrogens*. Pyrogens act directly on the hypothalamus, the portion of the brain that controls the body's thermostat. The release of endogenous pyrogens by inflammatory cells occurs after phagocytosis, after exposure to bacterial endotoxins, or after exposure to antigen-antibody complexes. (Mechanisms of temperature regulation are discussed in Chapter 16.)

A febrile response can be beneficial because the microorganisms that cause some conditions (e.g., those that cause syphilis or gonococcal urethritis) are highly sensitive to small increases in body temperature. On the other hand, fever may have some harmful side effects because it may enhance the person's susceptibility to the effects of endotoxins associated with gram-negative bacterial infections (bacterial toxins are described in Chapter 10).

Leukocytosis

Leukocytosis is an increase in the number of circulating white blood cells (greater than $11,000/mL^3$ in adults). During many infections, leukocytosis may be accompanied by a *left shift* in the ratio of immature to mature neutrophils, so that the more immature forms of neutrophils, such as band cells, metamyelocytes, and occasionally myelocytes, are

TABLE 7.3	CIRCULATING LEVELS OF ACUTE-PHASE REACTANTS DURING INFLAMMATION	
FUNCTION	**INCREASED**	**DECREASED**
Coagulation components	Fibrinogen Prothrombin Factor VIII Plasminogen	None
Protease inhibitors	α_1-Antitrypsin α_1-Antichymotrypsin	Inter-α-antitrypsin
Transport proteins	Haptoglobin Hemopexin Ceruloplasmin Ferritin	Transferrin
Complement components	C1s, C2, C3, C4, C5, C9, factor B, C1 inhibitor	Properdin
Miscellaneous proteins	α_1-Acid glycoprotein Fibronectin Serum amyloid A (SAA) C-reactive protein (CRP)	Albumin Prealbumin α_1-Lipoprotein β-Lipoprotein

present in relatively greater than normal proportions. (Chapter 28 discusses the development and maturation of blood cells.) Production of immature leukocytes increases primarily from proliferation and release of granulocyte and monocyte precursors in the bone marrow, which is stimulated by several products of inflammation, including complement product C3a and G-CSF.

Plasma Protein Synthesis

The synthesis of many plasma proteins, mostly products of the liver, is increased during inflammation. These proteins, which can be either proinflammatory or antiinflammatory in nature, are referred to as acute-phase reactants (Table 7.3). Acute-phase reactants reach maximal circulating levels within 10 to 40 hours of initial infection. IL-1 is indirectly responsible for the synthesis of acute-phase reactants through the induction of IL-6, which directly stimulates liver cells to synthesize most of the acute-phase reactants.

Common laboratory tests for inflammation measure levels of acute-phase reactants. For example, an increase in blood levels of acute-phase reactants, primarily fibrinogen, is associated with an increased adhesion among erythrocytes and a corresponding increase in the sedimentation rate. The alteration in plasma proteins probably leads to an enhanced erythrocyte rouleaux formation (stacking of erythrocytes, as in a stack of coins) and thereby an increased rate of sedimentation. Although increased erythrocyte sedimentation is a nonspecific reaction, it is considered a good indicator of an acute inflammatory response. Other symptoms of acute inflammation include somnolence (drowsiness), malaise (generalized feeling of discomfort or illness), anorexia (lack of desire to eat), and muscle aching.

CHRONIC INFLAMMATION

Superficially, the difference between acute and chronic inflammation is purely one of duration, in that chronic inflammation lasts 2 weeks or longer regardless of cause. Characteristic histologic and mechanistic differences also may be present (Fig. 7.17). Chronic inflammation is sometimes preceded by an unsuccessful acute inflammatory response.

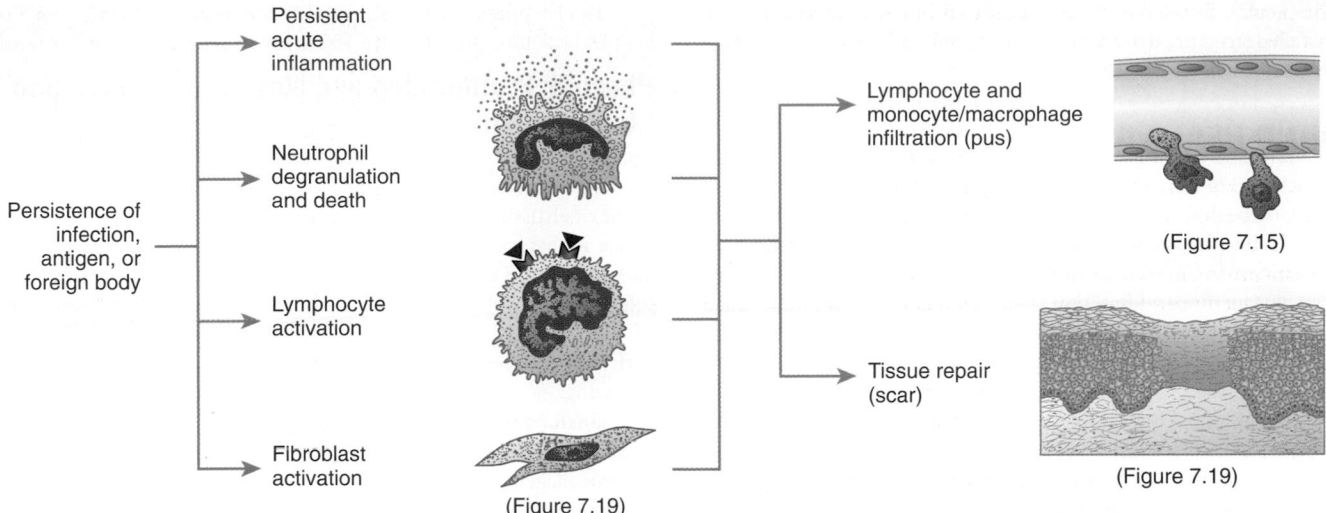

(Figure 7.15)

(Figure 7.19)

(Figure 7.19)

FIGURE 7.17 The Chronic Inflammatory Response. Inflammation usually becomes chronic because of the persistence of an infection, an antibody, or a foreign body in the wound. Chronic inflammation is characterized by the persistence of many of the processes of acute inflammation. In addition, the presence of large amounts of neutrophil degranulation and death, the activation of lymphocytes, and the concurrent activation of fibroblasts result in the release of mediators that induce the infiltration of more lymphocytes and monocytes/macrophages and the beginning of wound healing and tissue repair.

For example, if bacterial contamination or foreign objects (e.g., dirt, wood splinters, glass) persist in a traumatic wound, an acute response may be prolonged beyond 2 weeks. Pus formation, suppuration (purulent discharge), and incomplete wound healing may characterize this type of chronic inflammation.

Chronic inflammation can occur also as a distinct process without much previous acute inflammation. Some microorganisms (e.g., mycobacteria that cause tuberculosis) have cell walls with a very high lipid and wax content, making them relatively insensitive to degradation by phagocytes and therefore relatively resistant to clearance in an acute inflammatory response. Other microorganisms, such as those that cause leprosy, syphilis, and brucellosis, can survive within the macrophage and thereby also avoid clearance by the acute inflammatory response. Other microorganisms produce toxins that damage tissue and cause persistent inflammation even after the microorganism is killed. Finally, chemicals, particulate matter, or physical irritants (e.g., inhaled dusts, wood splinters, and suture material) also can cause a prolonged inflammatory response.

Chronic inflammation is characterized by a dense infiltration of lymphocytes and macrophages. If macrophages are unable to limit the tissue damage or infection, the body attempts to wall off and isolate the infected area, thus forming a granuloma (Fig. 7.18). Granulomas may form if neutrophils and macrophages are unable to destroy microorganisms during the acute inflammatory response. For example, infections caused by some bacteria (*Listeria* sp., *Brucella* sp.), fungi (histoplasmosis, coccidioidomycosis), and parasites (leishmaniasis, schistosomiasis, toxoplasmosis) can result in granuloma formation. Large antigen-antibody complexes such as those present in rheumatoid arthritis also can result in the formation of these structures. TNF-α primarily drives granuloma formation. Some macrophages differentiate into large epithelioid cells, cells that are incapable of phagocytosing large bacteria but are capable of taking up debris and other small particles. Other macrophages fuse into multinucleated giant cells, which are active phagocytes that can engulf very large particles—larger than those that can be engulfed by a single macrophage. These two types of specialized cells form the center of the granuloma, which is surrounded by a wall

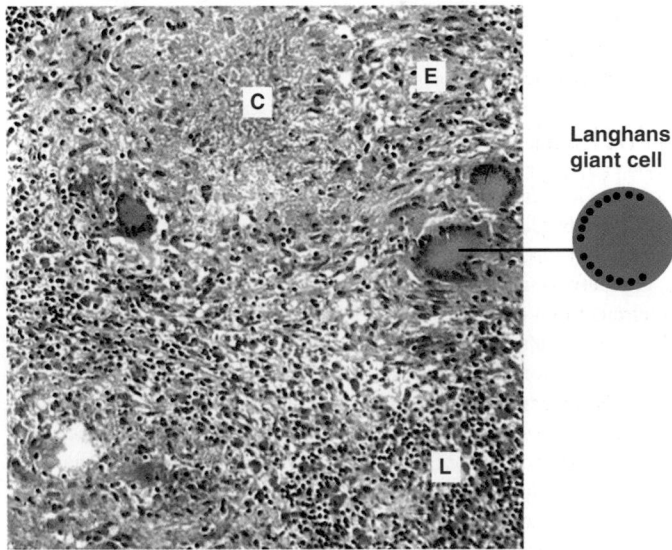

Langhans giant cell

FIGURE 7.18 Tuberculous Granuloma. A central area of amorphous caseous necrosis *(C)* is surrounded by a zone of lymphocytes *(L)* and enlarged epithelioid cells *(E)*. Activated macrophages frequently fuse to form multinucleated cells (Langhans giant cells). In tuberculoid granulomas the nuclei of the giant cells move to the cellular margins in a horseshoe-like formation.

of lymphocytes. The granuloma itself is also often encapsulated by fibrous deposits of collagen and may become cartilaginous or possibly calcified by deposits of calcium carbonate and calcium phosphate.

The classic granuloma associated with tuberculosis is characterized by a wall of epithelioid cells surrounding a cheeselike proteinaceous center derived from dead and decaying tissue (caseous necrosis, see Chapter 2) and mycobacteria. Decay of cells within the granuloma results in the release of acids and the enzymatic contents of lysosomes from dead phagocytes. In this inhospitable environment, the cellular debris is broken down and a clear fluid may remain (liquefaction necrosis, see Chapter 2). Eventually this fluid diffuses out and leaves a hollow, thick-walled structure that has replaced normal tissue and reduces organ function.

WOUND HEALING

The conclusion of inflammation is healing and repair. The most favorable outcome of healing is tissue **regeneration** (replacement of damaged tissue with healthy tissue, such as occurs in the epithelia of the skin and intestines, and in some organs, such as liver) with complete return to normal structure and function (Fig. 7.19). This restoration is called **resolution**, may take up to 2 years, and local production of IL-10 appears to play a critical role. Resolution may not be possible if extensive damage is present, the tissue is not capable of regeneration, infection results in abscess or granuloma formation, or fibrin persists in the lesion. In those cases, repair takes place instead of resolution. **Repair** is the replacement of destroyed tissue with scar tissue. **Scar tissue** is composed primarily of collagen that fills in the lesion and restores strength but cannot carry out the physiologic functions of destroyed tissue, resulting in loss of function.

Wound healing involves processes that (1) fill in, (2) seal, and (3) shrink the wound. These characteristics of healing vary in importance and duration among different types of wounds. A clean incision, such as a paper cut or a sutured surgical wound, heals primarily through the process of collagen synthesis. Because this type of wound has minimal tissue loss and close apposition of the wound edges, very little sealing (**epithelialization**) and shrinkage (**contraction**) are required. Wounds that heal under conditions of minimal tissue loss are said to heal by **primary intention** (see Fig. 7.19).

Other wounds do not heal as easily. Healing of an open wound, such as a stage IV pressure injury (bedsore), requires a great deal of tissue replacement so that epithelialization, scar formation, and contraction take longer and healing occurs through **secondary intention** (see Fig. 7.19). Healing by either primary or secondary intention may occur at different rates for different types of tissue injury.

Epidermal wounds that heal by secondary intention and unsutured internal lesions are not completely restored by healing. At best, repaired tissue regains 80% of its original tensile strength. Only epithelial, hepatic (liver), and bone marrow cells are capable of the complete mitotic regeneration of the normal tissue known as *compensatory hyperplasia*. In fibrous connective tissue, such as joints and ligaments, normal healing results in replacement of the original tissue with new tissue that does not have exactly the same structure or function as that of the original. Some tissues heal without replacement of cells. For example, damage resulting from myocardial infarction heals with a scar composed of fibrous tissue rather than with cardiac muscle. Wound healing occurs in three overlapping phases: inflammation, proliferation and new tissue formation, and remodeling and maturation.[37a]

Phase I: Inflammation

The early phase of wound healing, the transition from acute inflammation to healing, begins almost immediately. The **inflammatory phase** includes coagulation and the infiltration of cells that participate in wound healing, including platelets, neutrophils, and macrophages.[38] The fibrin mesh of the blood clot acts as a scaffold for cells that participate in healing. Platelets contribute to clot formation and, as they degranulate, release growth factors that initiate proliferation of undamaged cells. Neutrophils and macrophages clear the wound of debris (fibrin from dissolved clots, microorganisms, erythrocytes, and dead tissue cells). This cleanup of the lesion, which also involves dissolution of fibrin clots (or scabs) by fibrinolytic enzymes, is called **débridement**. After débridement the remaining debris is drained away by blood vessels and lymphatics, and

the vascular dilation and permeability associated with inflammation are reversed, thus preparing the lesion for either regeneration or repair.

Phase II: Proliferation and New Tissue Formation (Reconstruction)

The proliferative phase begins 3 to 4 days after the injury and continues for as long as 2 weeks. The wound is sealed and the fibrin clot is replaced by normal tissue or scar tissue during this phase. The **proliferative phase** is characterized by macrophage invasion of the dissolving clot and recruitment and proliferation of fibroblasts (connective tissue cells), followed by fibroblast collagen synthesis, epithelialization, contraction of the wound, and cellular differentiation.[39] Macrophages secrete a variety of biochemical mediators that promote healing, including the following:

1. **Transforming growth factor-beta (TGF-β)** stimulates fibroblasts entering the lesion to synthesize and secrete the collagen precursor procollagen.
2. **Angiogenesis factors**, such as vascular endothelial growth factor (VEGF) and fibroblast growth factor-2 (FGF-2), stimulate vascular endothelial cells to form capillary buds that grow into the lesion; decreased pH and decreased wound oxygen tension also promote angiogenesis.
3. **Matrix metalloproteinases (MMPs)** degrade and remodel extracellular matrix proteins (e.g., collagen and fibrin) at the site of injury.[40]

Granulation tissue grows into the wound from surrounding healthy connective tissue and consists of invasive cells, new lymphatic vessels, and new capillaries derived from capillaries in the surrounding tissue, giving the granulation tissue a red, granular appearance. Capillary buds sprout from vascular endothelial cells around the wound and extend into the débrided areas. Loops form when the young capillaries join (*anastomose*). The loops are more fragile and permeable than mature vessels, resulting in leakage of erythrocytes and neutrophils. The erythrocytes are phagocytosed by macrophages, and the neutrophils assist in further débridement of the inflammatory lesion. Many of the new capillaries differentiate into larger vessels as repair continues, promoting influx of nutrients and removal of metabolic wastes. New lymphatic vessels also grow into the granulation tissue by a similar process.

The healing wound must be protected during this process. Epithelialization is the process by which epithelial cells grow into the wound from surrounding healthy tissue. Epithelial cells migrate under the clot or scab using MMPs to unravel collagen. Migrating epithelial cells contact similar cells from all sides of the wound and seal it. The epithelial cells remain active, undergoing differentiation to give rise to the various epidermal layers. Epithelialization of a skin wound can be hastened if the wound is kept moist, preventing the fibrin clot from becoming a scab.

Fibroblasts are important cells during healing because they secrete collagen and other connective tissue proteins. Fibroblasts are stimulated by macrophage-derived TGF-β to proliferate, enter the lesion, and deposit connective tissue proteins in débrided areas about 6 days after the fibroblasts have entered the lesion. **Collagen** is the most abundant protein in the body. It contains high concentrations of the amino acids glycine, proline, and lysine, many of which are enzymatically modified. Modification of proline and lysine requires several cofactors that are absolutely necessary for proper collagen polymerization and function. These include iron, ascorbic acid (vitamin C), and molecular oxygen (O_2); absence of any of these results in impaired wound healing.

Immature collagen (i.e., procollagen) is secreted by fibroblasts as a complex of three polypeptide chains cross-linked by intermolecular bonds. Procollagen is converted to mature collagen by the proteolytic removal of small polypeptide sequences at both ends of the trimer. As healing progresses, collagen molecules are cross-linked by intramolecular

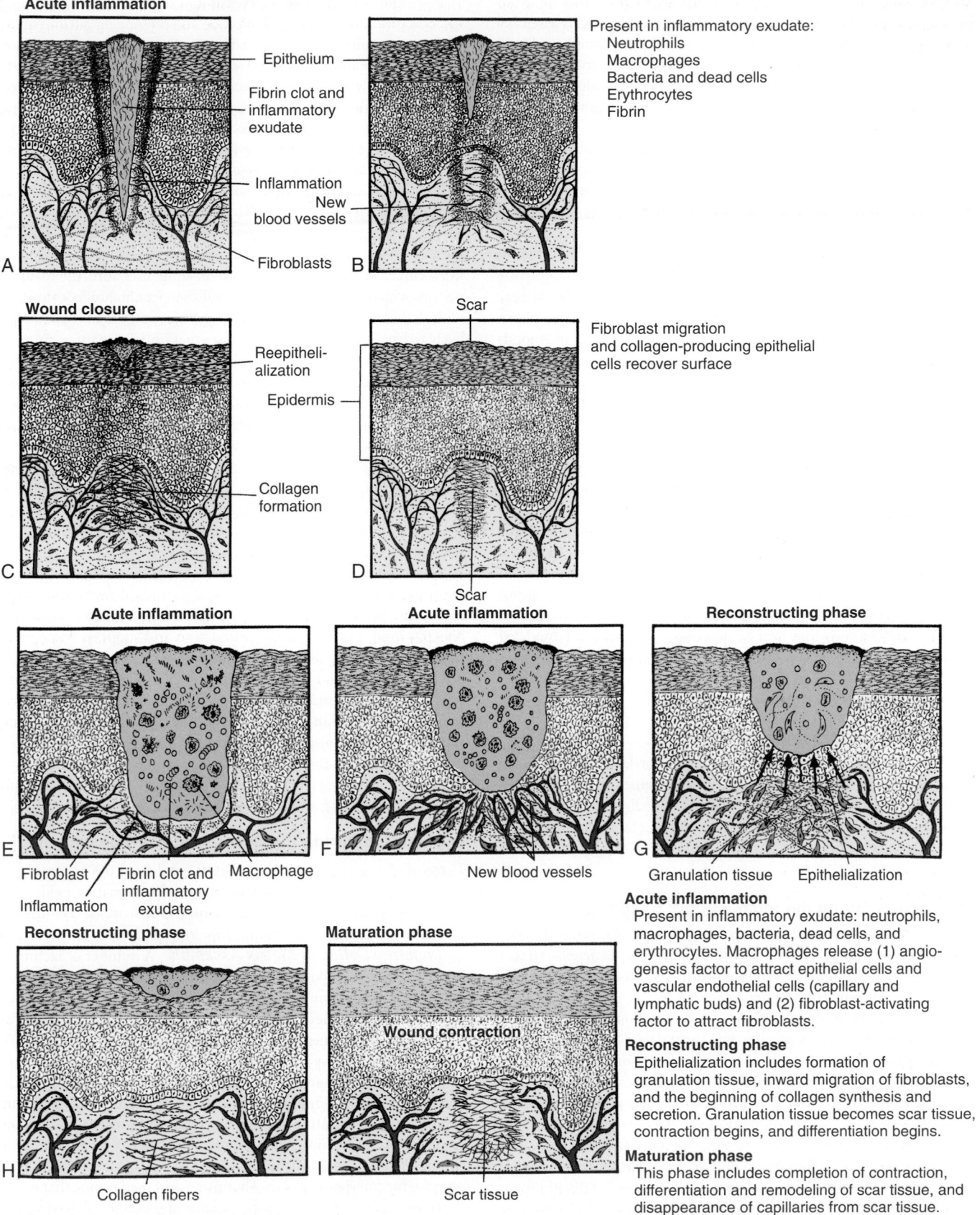

Acute inflammation

A — Epithelium
— Fibrin clot and inflammatory exudate
— Inflammation
New blood vessels
— Fibroblasts

B — Present in inflammatory exudate:
Neutrophils
Macrophages
Bacteria and dead cells
Erythrocytes
Fibrin

Wound closure

C — Reepitheli-alization
Epidermis
— Collagen formation

Scar
D — Fibroblast migration and collagen-producing epithelial cells recover surface
Scar

Acute inflammation

E — Fibroblast / Fibrin clot and inflammatory exudate / Macrophage
Inflammation

Acute inflammation

F — New blood vessels

Reconstructing phase

G — Granulation tissue   Epithelialization

Acute inflammation
Present in inflammatory exudate: neutrophils, macrophages, bacteria, dead cells, and erythrocytes. Macrophages release (1) angio-genesis factor to attract epithelial cells and vascular endothelial cells (capillary and lymphatic buds) and (2) fibroblast-activating factor to attract fibroblasts.

Reconstructing phase
Epithelialization includes formation of granulation tissue, inward migration of fibroblasts, and the beginning of collagen synthesis and secretion. Granulation tissue becomes scar tissue, contraction begins, and differentiation begins.

Maturation phase
This phase includes completion of contraction, differentiation and remodeling of scar tissue, and disappearance of capillaries from scar tissue.

Reconstructing phase

H — Collagen fibers

Maturation phase

Wound contraction

I — Scar tissue

FIGURE 7.19 Wound Repair by Primary or Secondary Intention. **A–D,** Healing by primary intention. **E–I,** Healing by secondary intention.

covalent bonds to form collagen fibrils that are further cross-linked to form collagen fibers. The process of complete collagen matrix assembly takes several months because collagen is initially deposited randomly but then is remodeled by repeated dissolution (by MMPs) and reassembly. During this remodeling period, collagen fibers orient along the lines of mechanical stress; further cross-linking adds strength to the final collagen matrix.

Wound contraction is the final process of the reconstruction of new tissue. It is necessary for closure of all wounds, but especially those that heal by secondary intention. Contraction is noticeable 6 to 12 days after injury and may amount to inward movement of the wound edge by approximately 0.5 mm/day in normal healing. In granulation tissue, TGF-β induces some fibroblasts to transition into myofibroblasts, specialized cells responsible for wound contraction.[41] Myofibroblasts have features of both smooth muscle cells and fibroblasts. They appear microscopically similar to fibroblasts but differ in that their cytoplasm contains bundles of parallel fibers similar to those found in smooth muscle cells. Wound contraction occurs as extensions from the plasma membrane of myofibroblasts establish connections between neighboring cells, contract their fibers, and exert tension on the neighboring cells while anchoring themselves to the wound bed.

Phase III: Remodeling and Maturation

Tissue remodeling and maturation begins several weeks after injury and is normally complete within 2 years. During this phase, there is continuation of cellular differentiation, scar formation, and scar remodeling. The fibroblast is the major cell of tissue remodeling with the deposition of collagen into an organized matrix. Tissue regeneration and wound contraction continue in the remodeling and maturation phase—a phase for recovering normal tissue structure that can persist for years. For wounds that heal by scarring, scar tissue is remodeled and capillaries disappear, leaving the scar avascular. Within 2 to 3 weeks after maturation has begun, the scar tissue has gained about two-thirds of its eventual maximal strength.

Dysfunctional Wound Healing

Dysfunctional wound healing and impaired epithelialization may occur during any phase of the healing process. The causes of dysfunctional wound healing include ischemia; excessive bleeding; excessive fibrin deposition; a predisposing disorder, such as diabetes mellitus; obesity; wound infection; inadequate nutrients; numerous drugs; and tobacco smoke.

Dysfunction during the Inflammatory Response

Oxygen-deprived (ischemic) is susceptible to cellular death and infection, which prolongs inflammation and delays healing. *Ischemia* reduces energy production and impairs collagen synthesis and the tensile strength of regenerating connective tissue.

Healing may be prolonged if bleeding is not stopped during acute inflammation. *Hemorrhage* in a damaged area delays healing for several reasons. Initially the excess blood cells that accumulate at the site of injury must be cleared—a process that requires additional time. Formation of a clot increases the amount of space that granulation tissue must fill and serves as a mechanical barrier to oxygen diffusion. *Hypovolemia*—decreased blood volume—hinders inflammation. The physiologic response to hypovolemia is vessel constriction rather than the dilation required to deliver inflammatory cells to the site of injury. The great amount of fibrin that is deposited during hemorrhage also must eventually be reabsorbed in order to prevent its organization into *fibrous adhesions.* Adhesions formed in the pleural, pericardial, or abdominal cavities, can bind organs together by fibrous bands and distort or strangulate the affected organ.

Accumulated blood also serves as an excellent culture medium for bacteria, promoting continued infection and prolonging inflammation by increasing purulent exudate formation. Prolonged infection can promote *excess scar formation* or even prevent healing completely. Continued infection of a wound, termed *wound sepsis,* can be clinically treated in several ways. Most important is the débridement of necrotic tissue and foreign bodies. This removal is accomplished either through surgery or through the use of absorbent dressings. Wound irrigation and antibiotic therapy also may assist in combating continued infection.

Optimal nutrition is important during all phases of healing because metabolic needs are increased. The most essential nutrients for healing are glucose, oxygen, and amino acids. Leukocytes need glucose to produce the adenosine triphosphate (5′-ATP) needed for chemotaxis, phagocytosis, intercellular killing, and initiation of healing; therefore, the wounds of persons with diabetes who receive insufficient insulin heal poorly. Persons with diabetes also are at risk for ischemic wounds because they are likely to have both small-vessel diseases that impair the microcirculation and altered (glycosylated) hemoglobin, which has an increased affinity for oxygen and thus does not readily release oxygen in tissues. Oxygen delivery is also compromised by hypoxemic states because ischemic tissue is susceptible to infection. *Hypoproteinemia* prolongs inflammation because the associated decrease in available amino acids is an impediment to fibroblast proliferation and collagen synthesis. Other nutrients, including iron, zinc, manganese, copper, and vitamins A and C, also are required as cofactors for collagen synthesis. Malnutrition increases risk for wound infection, delays healing, and reduces wound tensile strength.

Medications, including antineoplastic (anticancer) agents, nonsteroidal antiinflammatory drugs (NSAIDs), and steroids, delay wound healing. Antineoplastic agents slow cell division and inhibit angiogenesis. Although NSAIDs inhibit prostaglandin production and suppress acute inflammation and relieve pain, they also can delay wound healing, particularly bone formation, and may contribute to the formation of excessive scarring. Antiinflammatory steroids prevent macrophages from migrating to the site of injury and inhibit release of collagenase and plasminogen activator. Steroids also inhibit fibroblast migration into the wound during the proliferative phase and delay epithelialization. Toxic agents in tobacco smoke (i.e., nicotine, carbon monoxide, and hydrogen cyanide) delay wound healing and increase the risk for wound infection.

Dysfunction during the Reconstructive Phase of Healing

Three of the essential processes that occur during the reconstructive phase are assembly and remodeling of the collagen matrix, epithelialization of the wound bed, and contraction of the wound. Dysfunctional wound healing can result from the impairment of any of these processes.

Impaired Collagen Matrix Assembly. A number of factors may interfere with the production of collagen in healing tissues, most being nutritional. Scurvy, for example, is a condition caused by a deficiency in ascorbic acid, one of the cofactors required for the amino acid modification that is necessary for proper collagen matrix assembly. The complication of scurvy is a poorly formed collagen matrix and, therefore, greatly impaired wound healing. Other nutrients, including iron, copper, and calcium, play additional roles in the enzymatic reactions required for collagen modification and assembly. Usually, however, such minute amounts of these substances are required that deficiencies are not clinically significant. Nutritionally, appropriate protein intake is also essential for collagen synthesis. The amino acid methionine that is found in proteins is converted to cysteine, the role of which in collagen synthesis is twofold: (1) it functions as an important cofactor in the enzymatic reactions required for collagen synthesis; and (2) it contains sulfur, which contributes to formation of the strong covalent bonds in cross-linked collagen fibrils.

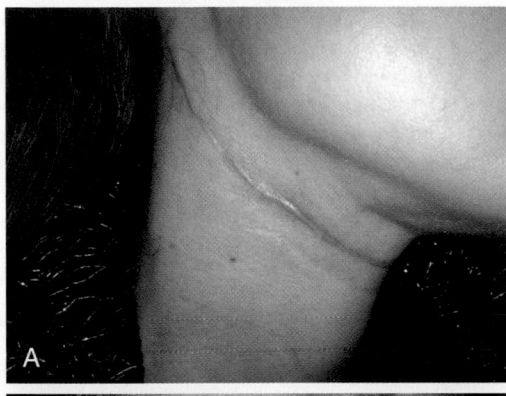

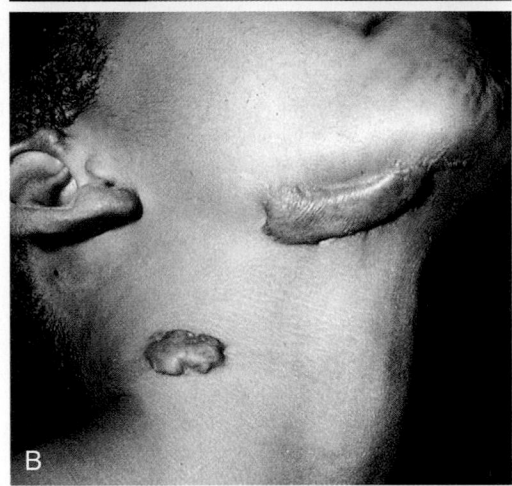

FIGURE 7.20 Hypertrophic Scar and Keloid Scar Formation. Hypertrophic scar (**A**) and keloid scar (**B**) caused by excessive synthesis of collagen at suture sites. (**A** from Flint PW et al: *Cummings otolaryngology: head & neck surgery,* ed 6, Philadelphia, 2015, Mosby; **B** from Damjanov I, Linder J: *Anderson's pathology,* ed 10, St Louis, 1996, Mosby.)

Dysfunctional collagen synthesis may involve excessive production of collagen, causing surface "overhealing," leading to a hypertrophic scar or keloid. A hypertrophic scar is raised but remains within the original boundaries of the wound and tends to regress over time (Fig. 7.20, *A*). A keloid is a raised scar that extends beyond the original boundaries of the wound, invades surrounding tissue, and is likely to recur after surgical removal (Fig. 7.20, *B*). A familial tendency to keloid formation has been observed, with a greater incidence in blacks than whites.

Similar to a keloid, a hypertrophic scar is also raised but differs in that it remains within the original boundaries of the wound. Hypertrophic scars tend to regress over time, whereas keloids do not. Both keloids and hypertrophic scars are caused by an imbalance between collagen synthesis and collagen degradation in which synthesis is increased relative to degradation. Although the precise mechanism of this imbalance is unknown, recent evidence suggests that keloid fibroblasts have lower rates of apoptosis and an inability to respond to normal suppressive feedback.

Impaired Epithelialization. The process of epithelialization is suppressed by antiinflammatory steroids, hypoxemia, and nutritional deficiencies. Antiinflammatory steroids inhibit phagocyte production of the biochemical mediators required for epithelialization, hypoxemia deprives cells of the energy required for the process, and dietary zinc is necessary for the MMP activity that is crucial to cellular migration.

Wound care techniques also may greatly influence epithelial cell migration. External wounds that are draining or healing by secondary intention often are clinically débrided and protected with dressings. The ideal dressing is one that absorbs some drainage without being incorporated into the clot or granulation tissue. Because epithelial cells must migrate across the wound during healing, dressings that débride healthy epithelial cells along with necrotic tissue prolong epithelialization. Many solutions that traditionally have been used to clean or irrigate wounds are now known to be deleterious to the fragile new cells in the wound bed. Normal saline is the most innocuous solution that can be used to cleanse or irrigate a wound that is healing primarily by epithelialization. Solutions such as povidone-iodine and hydrogen peroxide are desiccating (drying) and, as such, inhibit rather than promote epithelial cell migration.

Impaired Contraction. Excessive wound contraction may result in a deformity or contracture. Burn wounds are especially susceptible to the development of contractures. Internal contractures may occur as well, and are common in cirrhosis of the liver. Internally, scar tissue that becomes contracted constricts blood flow that may contribute to the development of portal hypertension and esophageal varices. Other types of internal contraction deformity include duodenal strictures caused by dysfunctional healing of an ulcer and esophageal strictures caused by chemical burns.

Proper positioning and range-of-motion exercises, as well as surgery, are among the physical means used to overcome the excessive myofibroblast-derived tension that results in contractures. Clinical use of pharmacologic methods for control of wound contracture is still largely experimental, but includes control of myofibroblast contraction by the administration of smooth muscle cell inhibitors such as colchicine and inhibition of proper collagen matrix assembly with drugs that prevent either collagen cross-linking or MMP activity. These latter treatments are based on the knowledge that myofibroblast binding to collagen can "lock" contracted cells into position.

Wound Disruption

Finally, a potential complication in the healing of wounds that are sutured closed is dehiscence, in which the wound pulls apart at the suture line. The greatest incidence of dehiscence occurs 5 to 12 days after suturing, paradoxically at the time when collagen synthesis is at its peak. Approximately 50% of dehiscence occurrences are associated with wound sepsis, although dehiscence also may occur when sutures break as a result of excessive strain. Obesity increases the risk of suture breakage because adipose tissue is difficult to suture. Wound dehiscence usually is heralded by an increase in serous drainage from the wound. In addition, patients may report a feeling that "something gave way." Prompt surgical attention is required.

PEDIATRICS: INNATE IMMUNITY IN THE NEWBORN CHILD

Neonates commonly have transiently depressed inflammatory and immune function since they are being born from a sterile environment. For example, neutrophils and perhaps monocytes may not be capable of efficient chemotaxis. Insufficient response to chemotactic factors appears to be caused by lack of fluidity in the phagocyte's plasma membrane so that pseudopod formation and migration are impaired. Neonates are prone to infections associated with chemotactic defects, including cutaneous abscesses caused by staphylococci and cutaneous candidiasis. Further, neutrophils in neonates who were stressed by in utero infection or respiratory insufficiency have diminished oxidative and bacterial responses. (Acquired phagocytic defects, which may be induced by a variety of infections, metabolic disorders, nutrition deficiencies, or drugs, are described in Chapter 9.)

Neonates also are partially deficient in complement, especially components of the alternative pathway. They tend to have a relative deficiency of factor B and to develop severe, overwhelming sepsis and meningitis when infected with bacteria against which there is no transferred maternal antibody. Low levels of mannose-binding lectin increase the risk for neonatal hospital-acquired sepsis. Neonates also may be deficient in some of the collectins and collectin-like proteins. This is especially true of preterm neonates. Some preterm infants with respiratory distress syndrome are deficient in at least one collectin, which provides innate defense against respiratory tract infections.

AGING: INNATE IMMUNITY IN THE OLDER ADULT POPULATION

The older adult population is also at risk for impaired inflammation and wound healing. In some cases, impaired healing is not directly associated with aging in general but can instead be linked to a chronic illness, such as cardiovascular disease or diabetes mellitus.[42] Aging also alters the tissue microenvironment and macrophage function with changes in wound healing neoangiogenesis and fibrosis.[43] In addition, many older adults require medications such as antiinflammatory steroids that can interfere with the healing process.

Older adults have increased susceptibility to bacterial infections of the lungs, urinary tract, and skin. Because of impaired sensation or mobility and physiologic changes in the skin, older adults are at increased risk for sustaining various wounds. With aging, subcutaneous fat is lost, diminishing a layer of protection. Collagen fibers become thicker and a certain percentage of elastin is lost, further contributing to loss of protection. The regenerative capability of the skin is maintained with aging, but the epidermis undergoes age-associated changes that include atrophy of the underlying capillaries. The consequent decrease of perfusion makes older adults more susceptible than younger people to the adverse effects of hypoxia in the wound bed. In addition, aging fibroblasts may have a slower rate of proliferation, and therefore wound healing is attenuated.

Immunosenescence affects both innate and adaptive immune systems, limiting responses to both infections and vaccines. Several cellular components of innate resistance are deficient in number (e.g., alveolar macrophages) or have diminished activity (e.g., neutrophil chemotaxis, degranulation, and phagocytosis). One explanation for this diminished inflammatory cellular activity is an age-related decrease in expression and function of several, if not all, TLRs. Alterations in T cells and NK cells also occur. The levels of proinflammatory cytokines (e.g., IL-6, TNF-α, and IL-1β) are elevated with aging and can contribute to systemic disease.[44,45]

SUMMARY REVIEW

Human Defense Mechanisms

1. There are three layers of human defense: barriers; innate immunity, which includes the inflammatory response; and adaptive (acquired) immunity.

First Line of Defense: Physical, Mechanical, and Biochemical Barriers and Normal Microbiome

1. Physical and mechanical barriers are the first lines of defense that prevent damage to the individual and prevent invasion by pathogens; these include the skin and mucous membranes.
2. Antibacterial peptides in mucous secretions, perspiration, saliva, tears, and other secretions provide a biochemical barrier against pathogenic microorganisms.
3. The normal bacterial flora provides protection by releasing chemicals that prevent colonization by pathogens.

Second Line of Defense: Inflammation

1. Inflammation is a rapid and nonspecific protective response to cellular injury from any cause. It can occur only in vascularized tissue.
2. The macroscopic hallmarks of inflammation are redness, swelling, heat, pain, and loss of function of the inflamed tissues.
3. The microscopic hallmark of inflammation is an accumulation of fluid and cells at the inflammatory site.
4. Inflammation is mediated by three key plasma protein systems: the complement system, the clotting system, and the kinin system. The components of all three systems are a series of inactive proteins that are activated sequentially.
5. The complement system can be activated by antigen-antibody reactions (through the classical pathway) or by other products, especially bacterial polysaccharides (through the lectin pathway or the alternative pathway), resulting in the production of biologically active fragments and the destruction of cells.
6. The most biologically potent products of the complement system are C3b (opsonin), C3a (anaphylatoxin), and C5a (anaphylatoxin, chemotactic factor).
7. The clotting system stops bleeding, localizes microorganisms, and provides a meshwork for repair and healing.
8. Bradykinin is the most important product of the kinin system and causes vascular permeability, smooth muscle contraction, and pain.
9. Many different types of cells are involved in the inflammatory process including mast cells, endothelial cells, platelets, phagocytes (neutrophils, eosinophils, monocytes and macrophages, dendritic cells), natural killer (NK) cells, and lymphocytes.
10. Most cells express plasma membrane pattern recognition receptors (PRRs) that recognize molecules produced by infectious microorganisms (pathogen-associated molecular patterns, or PAMPs), or products of cellular damage (damage-associated molecular patterns, or DAMPs).
11. The cells of the innate immune system secrete many biochemical mediators (cytokines) that are responsible for activating other cells; these cytokines include interleukins, chemokines, interferons, and other molecules.
12. The most important proinflammatory cytokines are IL-1, IL-6, and tumor necrosis factor-alpha (TNF-α).
13. Interferons are produced by cells that are infected by viruses. Once released from infected cells, interferons can stimulate neighboring healthy cells to produce substances that prevent viral infection.
14. Chemokines are synthesized by a number of different cells and induce leukocyte chemotaxis.
15. The most important activator of the inflammatory response is the mast cell, which initiates inflammation by releasing biochemical mediators (histamine, chemotactic factors) from preformed cytoplasmic granules and synthesizing other mediators (prostaglandins, leukotrienes) in response to a stimulus.

SUMMARY REVIEW—cont'd

16. Histamine is the major vasoactive amine released from mast cells. It causes dilation of capillaries and retraction of endothelial cells lining the capillaries, which increases vascular permeability.

17. The endothelial cells lining the circulatory system (vascular endothelium) normally regulate circulating components of the inflammatory system and maintain normal blood flow by preventing spontaneous activation of platelets and members of the clotting system.

18. During inflammation the endothelium expresses receptors that help leukocytes leave the vessel and retract to allow fluid to pass into the tissues.

19. Platelets interact with the coagulation cascade to stop bleeding and release a number of mediators that promote and control inflammation.

20. The polymorphonuclear neutrophil (PMN), the predominant phagocytic cell in the early inflammatory response, exits the circulation by diapedesis through the retracted endothelial cell junctions and moves to the inflammatory site by chemotaxis.

21. Eosinophils release products that control the inflammatory response and are the principal cell that kills parasitic organisms.

22. The macrophage, the predominant phagocytic cell in the late inflammatory response, is highly phagocytic, is responsive to cytokines, and promotes wound healing.

23. Dendritic cells connect the innate and acquired immune systems by collecting antigens at the site of inflammation and transporting them to sites, such as the lymph nodes, where immunocompetent B and T cells reside.

24. Phagocytosis is a multistep cellular process for the elimination of pathogens and foreign debris. The steps include recognition and attachment, engulfment, formation of a phagosome and phagolysosome, and destruction of pathogens or foreign debris. Phagocytic cells engulf microorganisms and enclose them in phagocytic vacuoles (phagolysosomes), within which toxic products (especially metabolites of oxygen) and degradative lysosomal enzymes kill and digest the microorganisms.

25. Opsonins, such as antibody and complement component C3b, coat microorganisms and make them more susceptible to phagocytosis by binding them more tightly to the phagocyte.

Local Manifestations of Inflammation

1. Local manifestations of inflammation are the result of the vascular changes associated with the inflammatory process, including vasodilation and increased capillary permeability. The symptoms include redness, heat, swelling, and pain.

Systemic Manifestations of Acute Inflammation

1. The principal systemic effects of inflammation are fever and increases in levels of circulating leukocytes (leukocytosis) and plasma proteins (acute-phase reactants).

Chronic Inflammation

1. Chronic inflammation can be a continuation of acute inflammation that lasts 2 weeks or longer. It also can occur as a distinct process without much preceding acute inflammation.

2. Chronic inflammation is characterized by a dense infiltration of lymphocytes and macrophages. The body may wall off and isolate the infection to protect against tissue damage by formation of a granuloma.

Wound Healing

1. Resolution (regeneration) is the return of tissue to nearly normal structure and function. Repair is healing by scar tissue formation.

2. Damaged tissue proceeds to resolution (restoration of the original tissue structure and function) if little tissue has been lost or injured tissue is capable of regeneration. This is called healing by primary intention.

3. Tissues that sustained extensive damage or those incapable of regeneration heal by the process of repair, resulting in the formation of a scar. This is called healing by secondary intention.

4. Resolution and repair occur in two separate phases: the reconstructive phase in which the wound begins to heal and the maturation phase in which the healed wound is remodeled.

5. Dysfunctional wound healing can be related to ischemia, excessive bleeding, excessive fibrin deposition, a predisposing disorder (such as diabetes mellitus), wound infection, inadequate nutrients, numerous drugs, or altered collagen synthesis.

6. Dehiscence is a disruption in which the wound pulls apart at the suture line.

7. A contracture is a deformity caused by the excessive shortening of collagen in scar tissue.

Pediatrics: Innate Immunity in the Newborn Child

1. Neonates often have transiently depressed inflammatory function, particularly neutrophil chemotaxis and alternative complement pathway activity.

Aging: Innate Immunity in the Older Adult Population

1. Older adults are at risk for impaired wound healing, usually because of chronic illnesses.

2. Alterations in both the innate and the adaptive immune systems occur with aging and affect responses to inflammation, infection, and vaccination.

KEY TERMS

α₁-Antitrypsin, 209
α₂-Macroglobulin, 209
Abscess, 210
Acquired immunity, 190
Acute-phase reactant, 210
Adaptive immunity, 190
Adhesion, 214
Adhesion molecule, 202
Alternative pathway, 196

Anaphylatoxin, 198
Angiogenesis factor, 212
Antigen-antibody complex (immune complex), 196
Antimicrobial lectin, 193
Antimicrobial peptide, 192
Bactericidal/permeability-inducing (BPI) protein, 193
Basophil, 203, 206
Bradykinin, 198

C1-esterase inhibitor (C1-inh), 199
C3 convertase, 196
C5 convertase, 196
C3b receptor, 207
Carboxypeptidase, 198, 199
Cathelicidin, 192
Cell adhesion molecule (CAM), 207
Cell lysis, 198
Chemokine, 201, 203

■ KEY TERMS—cont'd

REFERENCES

1. Ramanan D, Cadwell K: Intrinsic defense mechanisms of the intestinal epithelium. *Cell Host Microbe* 19(4):434–441, 2016.
2. Rivera A, et al: Innate cell communication kick-starts pathogen-specific immunity. *Nat Immunol* 17(4):356–363, 2016.
3. Suarez-Carmona M, et al: Defensins: "simple" antimicrobial peptides or broad-spectrum molecules? *Cytokine Growth Factor Rev* 26(3):361–370, 2015.
4. Jaillon S, et al: Fluid phase recognition molecules in neutrophil-dependent immune responses. *Semin Immunol* 28(2):109–118, 2016.
5. Lloyd-Price J, Abu-Ali G, Huttenhower C: The healthy human microbiome. *Genome Med* 8(1):51, 2016.
6. Shen SJ, Wong CHY: Bugging inflammation: role of the gut microbiota. *Clin Transl Immunology* 5(4):e72, 2016.
7. Nunn KL, Forney LJ: Unraveling the dynamics of the human vaginal microbiome. *Yale J Biol Med* 89(3):331–337, 2016.
8. Ricklin D, Reis ES, Lambris JD: Complement in disease: a defence system turning offensive. *Nat Rev Nephrol* 12(7):383–401, 2016.
9. Beltrame MH, et al: MBL-associated serine proteases (MASPs) and infectious diseases. *Mol Immunol* 67(1):85–100, 2015.

10. Karpman D, et al: Complement interactions with blood cells, endothelial cells and microvesicles in thrombotic and inflammatory conditions. *Adv Exp Med Biol* 865:19–42, 2015.
11. Witkowski M, Landmesser U, Rauch U: Tissue factor as a link between inflammation and coagulation. *Trends Cardiovasc Med* 26(4):297–303, 2016.
12. Bork K: A decade of change: recent developments in pharmacotherapy of hereditary angioedema (HAE). *Clin Rev Allergy Immunol* 51(2):183–192, 2016.
13. Mullen LM, Chamberlain G, Sacre S: Pattern recognition receptors as potential therapeutic targets in inflammatory rheumatic disease. *Arthritis Res Ther* 17:122, 2015.
14. Cao X: Self-regulation and cross-regulation of pattern-recognition receptor signaling in health and disease. *Nat Rev Immunol* 16(1):35–50, 2016.
15. Joosten LAB, et al: Toll-like receptors and chronic inflammation in rheumatic diseases: new developments. *Nat Rev Rheumatol* 12(6):344–357, 2016.
16. Mathern DR, Heeger PS: Molecules great and small: the complement system. *Clin J Am Soc Nephrol* 10(9):1636–1650, 2015.
17. Penberthy KK, Ravichandran KS: Apoptotic cell recognition receptors and scavenger receptors. *Immunol Rev* 269(1):44–59, 2016.

18. Kim YK, Shin J-S, Nahm MH: NOD-like receptors in infection, immunity, and disease. *Yonsei Med J* 57(1):5–14, 2016.
19. Patel S: Inflammasomes, the cardinal pathology mediators are activated by pathogens, allergens and mutagens: A critical review with focus on NLRP3. *Biomed Pharmacother* 92:819–825, 2017.
20. Schett G, Dayer JM, Manger B: Interleukin-1 function and role in rheumatic disease. *Nat Rev Rheumatol* 12(1):14–24, 2016.
21. Schmidt-Arras D, Rose-John S: IL-6 pathway in the liver: from physiopathology to therapy. *J Hepatol* 64(6):1403–1415, 2016.
22. Kalliolias GD, Ivashkiv LB: TNF biology, pathogenic mechanisms and emerging therapeutic strategies. *Nat Rev Rheumatol* 12(1):49–62, 2016.
23. Teijaro JR: Type I interferons in viral control and immune regulation. *Curr Opin Virol* 16:31–40, 2016.
24. Proudfoot AEI, Uguccioni M: Modulation of chemokine responses: synergy and cooperativity. *Front Immunol* 7:183, 2016.
25. Ehrlich P: Dietbage zur Kenntnis der Anilinsfarb und Ihrer Verwendung nin ungen der Mikroskopichen technik. *Arch Mikr Anat* 13:263, 1877.
26. Tichenor MS, et al: Functional profiling of 2-aminopyrimidine histamine H4 receptor modulators. *J Med Chem* 58(18):7119–7127, 2015.

27. Dennis EA, Norris PC: Eicosanoid storm in infection and inflammation. *Nat Rev Immunol* 15(8):511–523, 2015.

28. Daiber A, et al: Targeting vascular (endothelial) dysfunction. *Br J Pharmacol* 2016 May 17. [Epub ahead of print].

29. Kapur R, et al: Nouvelle cuisine: platelets served with inflammation. *J Immunol* 194(12):5579–5587, 2015.

30. Kral JB, et al: Platelet interaction with innate immune cells. *Transfus Med Hemother* 43(2):78–88, 2016.

31. Long H, et al: A player and coordinator: the versatile roles of eosinophils in the immune system. *Transfus Med Hemother* 43(2):96–108, 2016.

32. Otsuka A, Nonomura Y, Kabashima K: Roles of basophils and mast cells in cutaneous inflammation. *Semin Immunopathol* 38(5):563–570, 2016.

33. Macri C, et al: Targeting dendritic cells: a promising strategy to improve vaccine effectiveness. *Clin Transl Immunology* 5(3):e66, 2016.

34. Sergé A: The molecular architecture of cell adhesion: dynamic remodeling revealed by videonanoscopy. *Front Cell Dev Biol* 4:36, 2016.

35. Hordijk PL: Recent insights into endothelial control of leukocyte extravasation. *Cell Mol Life Sci* 73(8):1591–1608, 2016.

36. Weiss G, Schaible UE: Macrophage defense mechanisms against intracellular bacteria. *Immunol Rev* 264(1):182–203, 2015.

37. Luo J, et al: Molecular and cellular mechanisms that initiate pain and itch. *Cell Mol Life Sci* 72(17):3201–3223, 2015.

37a. Childs DR, Murthy AS: Overview of wound healing and management. *Surg Clin North Am* 97(1):189–207, 2017.

38. Sugimoto MA, et al: Resolution of inflammation: what controls its onset? *Front Immunol* 7:160, 2016.

39. Landén NX, Li D, Ståhle M: Transition from inflammation to proliferation: a critical step during wound healing. *Cell Mol Life Sci* 73(20):3861–3885, 2016.

40. Dufour A: Degradomics of matrix metalloproteinases in inflammatory diseases. *Front Biosci (Schol Ed)* 7:150–167, 2015.

41. Rittlé L: Cellular mechanisms of skin repair in humans and other mammals. *J Cell Commun Signal* 10(2):103–120, 2016.

42. Eming SA, Martin P, Tomic-Canic M: Wound repair and regeneration: mechanisms, signaling, and translation. *Sci Transl Med* 6(265):265sr6, 2014.

43. Goh J, Ladiges WC: Exercise enhances wound healing and prevents cancer progression during aging by targeting macrophage polarity. *Mech Ageing Dev* 139:41–48, 2014.

44. Linton PJ, Thoman ML: Immunosenescence in monocytes, macrophages, and dendritic cells: lessons learned from the lung and heart. *Immunol Lett* 162(1 Pt B):290–297, 2014.

45. Pera A, et al: Immunosenescence: implications for response to infection and vaccination in older people. *Maturitas* 82(1):50–55, 2015.

Adaptive Immunity

Neal S. Rote, Kathryn L. McCance

e**volve** WEBSITE

http://evolve.elsevier.com/McCance/
- Content Updates
- Chapter Summary Review
- Review Questions
- Case Studies
- Animations

CHAPTER OUTLINE

The third line of defense in the human body is adaptive (acquired) immunity, often called the immune response or immunity, and consists of lymphocytes (Fig. 8.1) and serum proteins called *antibodies*. Once constitutive protective mechanisms at external barriers (first line of defense) have been compromised and inflammation (see Chapter 7) has been activated (second line of defense), the adaptive immune response is called into action. Thus inflammation is the "first responder" that contains the initial injury and slows spread of infection, whereas adaptive immunity is the "secondary responder" that augments the initial defenses against infection and provides long-term security against reinfection. Innate immunity, especially inflammation, and adaptive immunity are highly interactive and complementary. Components of innate resistance are necessary for the development of the adaptive immune response. Conversely, products of the adaptive immune response activate components of the innate immune system. Thus both systems are essential for complete protection against infectious disease.

Inflammation and adaptive immunity differ in several key ways. First, adaptive immunity develops more slowly than inflammation. The components of inflammation preexist in the blood and tissues and are activated immediately after and as a result of tissue damage. Adaptive immunity is *inducible*. The effectors of the immune response, lymphocytes and antibodies, do not preexist but must be produced in response to infection. Second, each inflammatory response is similar (although not identical) regardless of differences in the cause of tissue damage or whether the inflammatory site is sterile or contaminated with microorganisms. The adaptive immune response is exquisitely *specific*. The lymphocytes and antibodies induced in response to a particular infectious agent are extremely specific to that agent. A different infectious agent will induce a different battery of lymphocytes and antibodies. Third, the residual mediators of inflammation must be removed quickly to limit damage to surrounding healthy tissue and allow healing. The effectors of the adaptive immune response are *long-lived* and systemic, providing long-term protection against a specific infectious agent. Fourth, activation of the inflammatory response to recurrent tissue damage or repeated infection with the same microorganism is generally identical. The adaptive immune response has *memory*. If reinfected with the same microorganism, protective lymphocytes and antibody are produced rapidly, thus providing permanent long-term protection. Thus the adaptive immune response is distinguished by being inducible, specific, and long-lived, and by having memory.

The collaborative and beneficial nature of inflammation and adaptive immunity can, on occasion, fail. Chapter 9 discusses these medically relevant aberrations in both inflammation and immunity, including allergies, diseases that involve unwanted immunologic destruction of healthy tissue, and diseases that are caused by a deficiency in the normal immune or inflammatory responses. Chapter 10 presents an overview of infection and Chapter 11 discusses the connection between stress

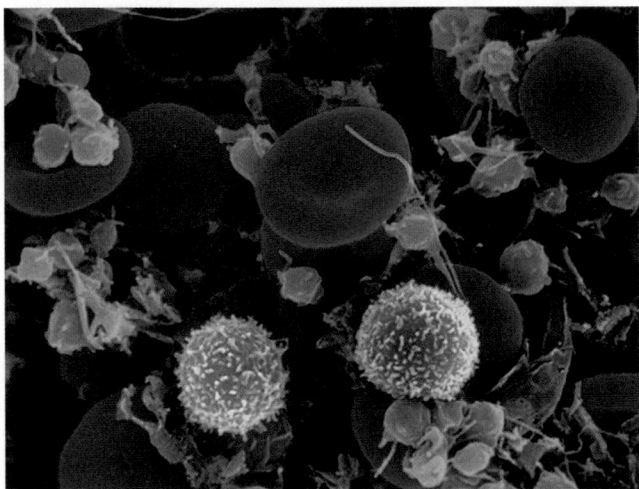

FIGURE 8.1 Scanning Electron Micrograph Showing Lymphocytes *(Yellow)*, Red Blood Cells, and Platelets. (Copyright Dennis Kunkel Microscopy, Inc.)

and disease and the interrelatedness of the immune, nervous, and endocrine systems.

GENERAL CHARACTERISTICS OF ADAPTIVE IMMUNITY

The adaptive immune system has its own vocabulary (Fig. 8.2). The immune system of the normal adult is continually challenged by a spectrum of substances that it may recognize as foreign, or "nonself." These substances, called *foreign antigens,* are often associated with pathogens such as viruses, bacteria, fungi, or parasites, although they are also found on noninfectious environmental agents such as pollens, foods, and bee venom, and still others are associated with clinically derived drugs, vaccines, transfusions, and transplanted tissues (Table 8.1). The products (i.e., effectors) of the adaptive immune response include antibodies (sometimes called **immunoglobulins**) and lymphocytes that are specific for particular antigens.

Specificity and memory are primary characteristics that differentiate the immune response from other protective mechanisms. This chapter first discusses the nature of that specificity by defining the various types of antigens recognized by the immune system, the ways in which they are recognized by antibodies and lymphocytes, and the specific intercellular recognition molecules that are necessary for effective immune responses. After the recognition molecules are defined, the development of the immune response is discussed. An immune response can be divided into two phases (see Fig. 8.2). In the fetus, well before being exposed to any infectious microorganisms, lymphocytes undergo extensive differentiation and proliferation. These events occur in the primary lymphoid organs (thymus and bone marrow). Some lymphoid stem cells in humans enter the thymus and differentiate into **T lymphocytes** (**T cells**, T indicating thymus derived) and others enter specific regions in the bone marrow and differentiate into **B lymphocytes** (**B cells**, B indicating bone marrow derived). Each type of cell develops origin-specific cell surface proteins that identify them as T or B cells. Both B and T cells also develop cell surface antigen receptors. The receptors are remarkable because an individual B or T cell is programmed to

ANTIGEN SOURCE	PROTECTION: COMBAT ACTIVE DISEASE	PROTECTION: VACCINATION	DIAGNOSIS	THERAPY
Infectious agents	Neutralize or destroy pathogenic microorganisms (e.g., antibody response against viral infections)	Induce safe and protective immune response (e.g., recommended childhood vaccines)	Measure circulating antigen from infectious agent or antibody (e.g., diagnosis of hepatitis B infection)	Passive treatment with antibody to treat or prevent infection (e.g., administration of antibody against hepatitis A)
Cancers	Prevent tumor growth or spread (e.g., immune surveillance to prevent early cancers)	Prevent cancer growth or spread (e.g., vaccination with cancer antigens)	Measure circulating antigen (e.g., circulating PSA for diagnosis of prostate cancer)	Immunotherapy (e.g., treatment of cancer with antibodies against cancer antigens)
Environmental substances	Prevent entrance into body (e.g., secretory IgA limits systemic exposure to potential allergens)	No clear example	Measure circulating antigen or antibody (e.g., diagnosis of allergy by measuring circulating IgE)	Immunotherapy (e.g., administration of antigen for desensitization of individuals with severe allergies)
Self-antigens	Immune system tolerance to self-antigens, which may be altered by an infectious agent leading to autoimmune disease (see Chapter 9)	Some cases of vaccination alter tolerance to self-antigens leading to autoimmune disease	Measure circulating antibody against self-antigen for diagnosis of autoimmune disease (see Chapter 9)	No clear example

TABLE 8.1 CLINICAL USE OF ANTIGEN OR ANTIBODY

IgA, Immunoglobulin A; *PSA,* prostate-specific antigen.

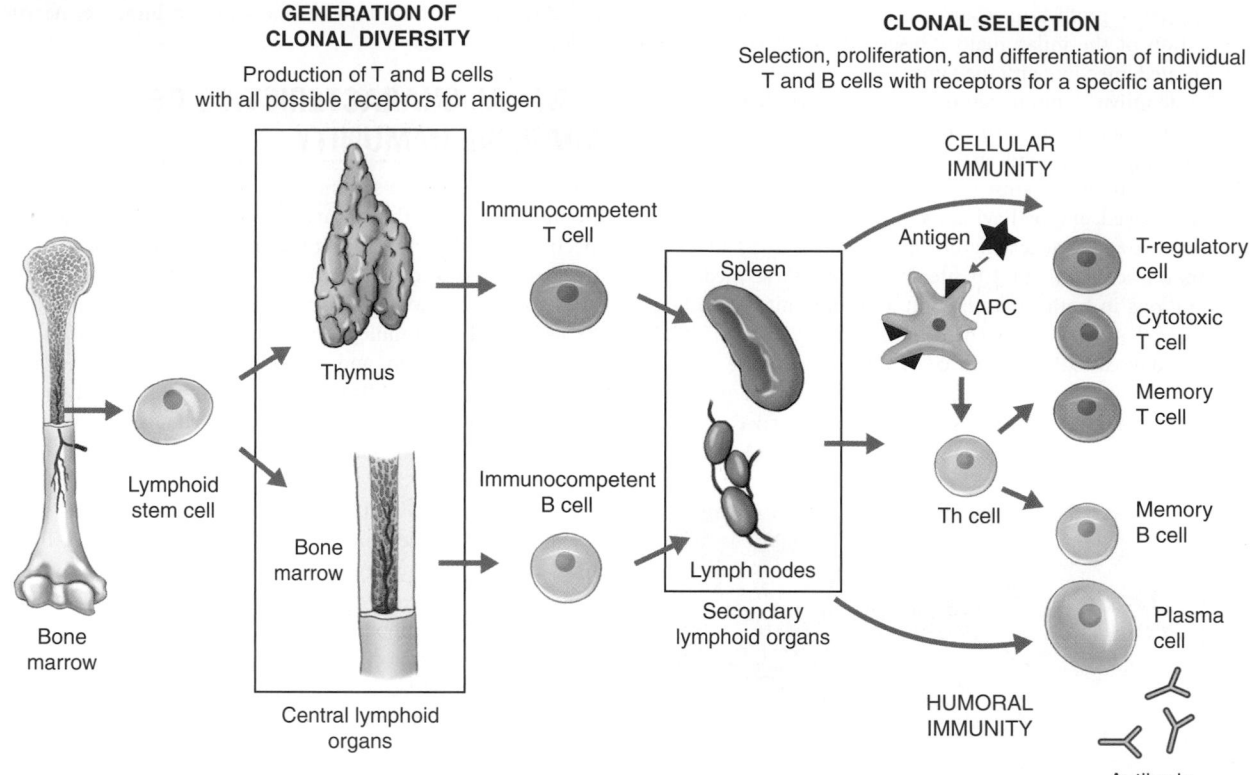

**GENERATION OF
CLONAL DIVERSITY**

Production of T and B cells
with all possible receptors for antigen

CLONAL SELECTION

Selection, proliferation, and differentiation of individual
T and B cells with receptors for a specific antigen

CELLULAR
IMMUNITY

Bone
marrow

Lymphoid
stem cell

Thymus

Bone
marrow

Central lymphoid
organs

Immunocompetent
T cell

Immunocompetent
B cell

Spleen

Lymph nodes

Secondary
lymphoid organs

Antigen

APC

Th cell

T-regulatory
cell

Cytotoxic
T cell

Memory
T cell

Memory
B cell

Plasma
cell

HUMORAL
IMMUNITY

Antibody

FIGURE 8.2 Overview of Immune Response. The immune response can be separated into two phases: the *generation of clonal diversity* and *clonal selection.* During the generation of clonal diversity, lymphoid stem cells from the bone marrow migrate to the central lymphoid organs (the thymus or regions of the bone marrow), where they undergo a series of cellular division and differentiation stages resulting in either immunocompetent T cells from the thymus or immunocompetent B cells from the bone marrow. (This process is outlined in more detail in Figs. 8.9 and 8.12.) These cells are still naïve in that they have never encountered foreign antigen. The immunocompetent cells enter the circulation and migrate to the secondary lymphoid organs (e.g., spleen and lymph nodes), where they take up residence in B- and T-cell–rich areas. The clonal selection phase is initiated by exposure to foreign antigen. The antigen is usually processed by antigen-presenting cells (APCs) for presentation to helper T cells (Th cells) (more detail in Fig. 8.16). The intercellular cooperation among APCs, Th cells, and immunocompetent T and B cells results in a second stage of cellular proliferation and differentiation (more details in Figs. 8.18 and 8.21). Because antigen has "selected" those T and B cells with compatible antigen receptors, only a small population of T and B cells undergoes this process at one time. The result is an active cellular immunity or humoral immunity, or both. Cellular immunity is mediated by a population of "effector" T cells that can kill targets (cytotoxic T cells) or regulate the immune response (T-regulatory cells), as well as a population of memory cells (memory T cells) that can respond more quickly to a second challenge with the same antigen. Humoral immunity is mediated by a population of soluble proteins (antibodies) produced by plasma cells and by a population of memory B cells that can produce more antibody rapidly to a second challenge with the same antigen.

recognize only one specific antigen before having encountered that antigen. It is estimated that each person has produced a population of B and T cells with an extensive diversity of antigen receptors capable of recognizing at least 10^8 different antigens. This process is called **generation of clonal diversity** (see Fig. 8.2).

Lymphocytes leave the primary lymphoid organs as immunocompetent but naïve B and T cells. They are **immunocompetent** in that they have the capacity to respond to antigen, but naïve in that they have not yet encountered antigen. These cells enter the blood and lymphatic vessels and migrate to the secondary lymphoid organs (e.g., lymph nodes, spleen) of the systemic immune system (Fig. 8.3). Some take up residence in B-cell– and T-cell–rich areas of those organs and others reenter the circulation. Approximately 60% to 70% of circulating lymphocytes are immunocompetent T cells, and 10% to 20% are immunocompetent B cells.

The second phase, called **clonal selection**, is initiated by exposure to foreign antigen usually related to infection (see Fig. 8.2). Antigen reacts with, or selects, clones of B and T cells with surface receptors against that specific antigen and initiates a process of further differentiation and proliferation into mature effector cells. The process requires the cooperation among a variety of cells in the secondary lymphoid organs; most antigens need to be processed (antigen processing) by phagocytic cells, primarily dendritic cells, that also present the processed antigen on their surfaces and present **(antigen presentation)** the antigen to lymphocytes. These cells are generally called antigen-processing or **antigen-presenting cells (APCs)**. Thus begins a symphony of cellular interactions that define clonal selection, involving APCs and several subsets of B and T cells, intercellular adhesion through antigen receptors and specific intercellular adhesion molecules, the production and response to multiple cytokines, and eventual differentiation of immunocompetent

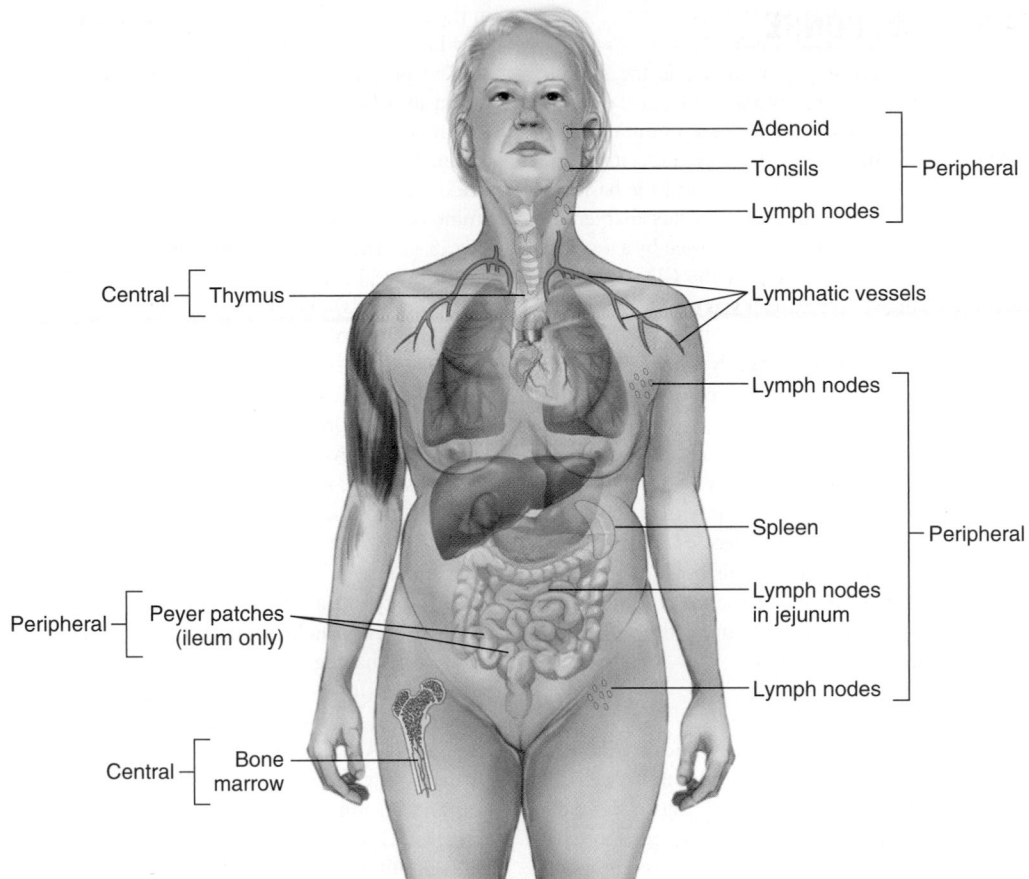

FIGURE 8.3 Lymphoid Tissues: Sites of B-Cell and T-Cell Differentiation. Immature lymphocytes migrate through central (primary) lymphoid tissues: the bone marrow (central lymphoid tissue for B lymphocytes) and the thymus (central lymphoid tissue for T lymphocytes). Mature lymphocytes later reside in the T- and B-lymphocyte–rich areas of the peripheral (secondary) lymphoid tissues.

B and T cells into highly specialized effector cells. B cells develop into plasma cells that become factories for the production of antibody. T cells develop into several subsets that identify and kill a target cell (T-cytotoxic cell [Tc cell]), regulate the immune response by helping the clonal selection process (T-helper cell [Th cell]), or suppress or limit the immune response (T-regulatory cell [Treg cell]). Both B and T cells also differentiate into very long-lived memory cells that exist for decades or, in some cases, the life of the individual. Memory cells "remember" the initial antigen and are rapidly activated if a second exposure occurs to the same microorganism.

Humoral and Cell-Mediated Immunity

The immune response has two arms: antibody and T cells, both of which protect against infection. Antibody circulates in the blood and in secretions and defends against extracellular microbes found in those fluids and microbial toxins. This interaction can result in direct inactivation of the microorganism or activation of a variety of inflammatory mediators (e.g., complement, phagocytes) that will destroy the pathogen. Antibody is primarily responsible for protection against many bacteria and viruses. This arm of the immune response is termed the humoral immune response, or humoral immunity.

Effector T cells are found in the blood and in tissues and organs and defend against intracellular pathogens (e.g., some viruses) and cancer cells. T cells may produce cytokines that stimulate the protective response of other leukocytes. Others develop into Tc cells that attack and kill cellular targets directly. This arm of the immune response is termed the cellular immune response, or cellular immunity. The humoral and cellular immune responses are interdependent at many levels. In the end, the success of an acquired immune response depends on the functions of both the humoral and the cellular responses, as well as the appropriate interactions between them.

Active vs. Passive Immunity

Adaptive immunity can be either active or passive, depending on whether the antibodies or T cells are produced by the individual in response to antigen or are administered directly. Active immunity (active acquired immunity) is produced by an individual either after natural exposure to an antigen or after immunization, whereas passive immunity (passive acquired immunity) does not involve the host's immune response at all. Rather, passive immunity occurs when preformed antibodies or T lymphocytes are transferred from a donor to the recipient. This can occur naturally, as in the passage of maternal antibodies across the placenta to the fetus, or artificially, as in a clinic using immunotherapy for a specific disease. Unvaccinated individuals who are exposed to particular infectious agents (e.g., hepatitis A virus, rabies virus) often will be given immunoglobulins that are prepared from individuals who already have antibodies against that particular pathogen (see Table 8.1). Whereas active acquired immunity is long-lived, passive immunity is only temporary because the donor's antibodies or T cells are eventually destroyed.

RECOGNITION AND RESPONSE

The foundation of any successful immune response is the specific recognition of antigen by antibody or receptors on the surface of B or T cells, followed by a set of complex intercellular communications among a variety of APCs and lymphocytes. To fully understand the immune response, it is necessary to initially understand the basis for that recognition. Many of the molecules discussed in this chapter are part of a nomenclature that uses the prefix "CD" followed by a number (e.g., CD1 or CD2) (Table 8.2). The definition of the CD (cluster of differentiation) format has changed over time. It was originally used to describe proteins found on the surface of lymphocytes. Currently, CD is the accepted format for labeling a very large family of proteins found on the surface of many cells. Many have alternative names related to their function, which may be used in this chapter. The list of identified molecules is constantly increasing (the number of molecules with a CD designation is probably in excess of 370). In a similar fashion, the list of known cytokines is continually growing, with more than 70 having been identified so far. A large number of CD molecules and cytokines contribute to the acquired immune response. This book attempts to focus on a small number of highly important examples to illustrate the immensely complicated, but highly effective, interactions that take place to produce a protective immune response.

Antigens and Immunogens

Initially, we need to understand the molecules against which an immune response is directed. Although the terms antigen and immunogen are commonly used as synonyms, there are clinically important differences between the two. Antigen is a commonly used term to describe a molecule that can *react with* binding sites on antibodies or antigen receptors on B and T cells. Most, but not all, antigens are also immunogens. An antigen that is immunogenic will *induce* an immune response, resulting in the production of antibodies or functional T cells. Thus a substance may be antigenic yet not be immunogenic.

The precise portion of the antigen that is configured for recognition and binding is called its antigenic determinant, or epitope. The matching portion on the antibody or the lymphocyte receptor is sometimes referred to as the *antigen-binding site*, or paratope. The size of an antigenic determinant is relatively small, perhaps just a few amino acids or carbohydrate residues on the surface of a large molecule (Fig. 8.4). Antigenic determinants may be linear or conformational. For instance, linear antigenic determinants consist of amino acids (or other chemicals) that are adjacent in the molecule's primary structure; thus they are stable when the molecule is denatured. Conformational antigenic determinants consist of amino acids that are only adjacent when the molecule is folded appropriately. When the molecule is denatured or processed, that antigenic determinant is destroyed. Therefore macromolecules (e.g., proteins, polysaccharides, nucleic acids) usually contain multiple and diverse antigenic determinants, and the immune response against the macromolecule will usually consist of a mixture of specific antibodies against several of these determinants.

Certain criteria influence the degree to which an antigen is immunogenic. These include (1) being foreign to the host, (2) being appropriate in size, (3) having an adequate chemical complexity, and (4) being present in a sufficient quantity.

Foremost among the criteria for immunogenicity is the antigen's foreignness. A self-antigen is part of the individual's makeup that fulfills all these criteria *except* foreignness and does not normally elicit an immune response. Thus most individuals are *tolerant* to their own antigens. The immune system has an exquisite ability to distinguish self (self-antigens) from nonself (foreign antigens). Tolerance was once thought to be a state of nonresponsiveness in which the immune system passively allowed self-antigens to persist, but tolerance is now known

TABLE 8.2	SELECT CD MOLECULES AND THEIR FUNCTIONS	
CD MOLECULES	**PRIMARY LOCATION**	**FUNCTIONS**
CD1	APCs	Presents lipid antigens
CD2	All T cells, NK cells	T-cell marker; adhesion molecule that binds to CD58 (LFA-3) and provides a costimulatory signal
CD3	All T cells	Associated with TCR and provides intracellular signaling
CD4	Th cells	Binds to MHC class II as co-receptor with the TCR
CD8	Tc cells	Binds to MHC class I as co-receptor with the TCR
CD19	B cells	Complexes with CD21 to form a co-receptor for B cells
CD20	B cells	Major regulator of B-cell function
CD21	B cells	Receptor for complement that complexes with CD19 to form a co-receptor for B cells
CD25	Activated T cells	α chain of IL-2 receptor
CD28	T cells	Adhesion molecule that binds to CD80 to provide costimulatory signal for Tc cells
CD40	B cells, macrophages	Adhesion molecule that binds to CD154 to provide costimulatory signal for B cells
CD45	All lymphocytes	Has multiple types; augments antigen signal
CD58 (LFA-3)	Most cells	Adhesion molecule that binds to CD2 to provide a costimulatory signal
CD80 (B7-1)	APCs	Adhesion molecule that binds to CD28 to provide a costimulatory signal
CD154 (CD40L)	Th2 cells	Adhesion molecule that binds to CD40 to provide a costimulatory signal

APCs, Antigen-presenting cells; *IL,* interleukin; *MHC,* major histocompatibility complex; *NK,* natural killer; *Tc,* cytotoxic; *TCR,* T-cell receptor; *Th,* T-helper.

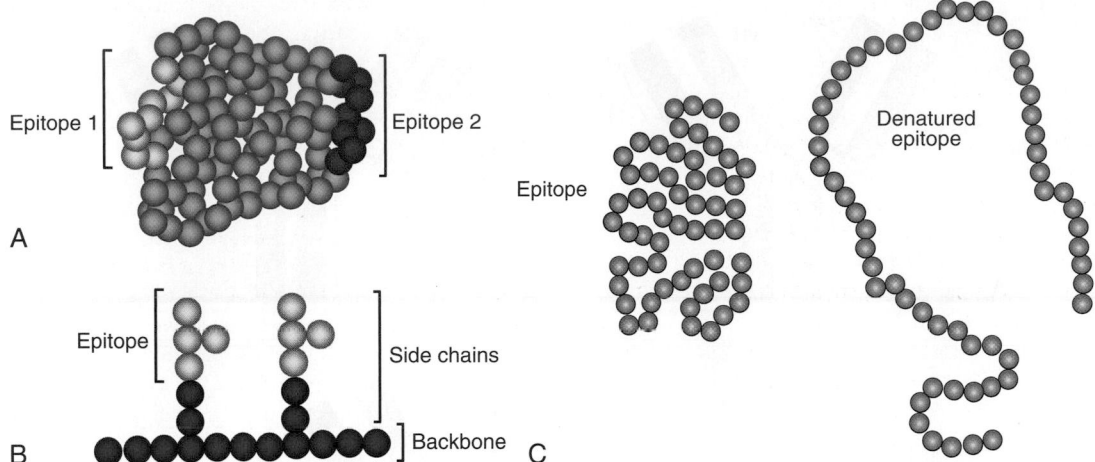

FIGURE 8.4 Antigenic Determinants (Epitopes). Shown are generic examples of linear epitopes on protein **(A)** and polysaccharide **(B)** molecules and conformational epitopes on protein **(C).** In **A,** an antigenic protein may have multiple different epitopes (epitopes 1 and 2) that react with different antibodies. Each sphere represents an amino acid, with the yellow spheres representing epitope 1 and the red spheres representing epitope 2. Individual epitopes may consist of eight or nine amino acids. In **B,** a polysaccharide is constructed of a backbone with branched side chains. Each sphere represents an individual carbohydrate, with the yellow spheres representing the carbohydrates that form the epitope. In this example, two identical epitopes are shown that would bind two identical antibodies. In **C,** an epitope consists of amino acids from different portions of the primary sequence that are placed near each other during folding of the molecule. When the molecule is denatured, the epitope is destroyed.

to have a variety of mechanisms. In some cases, a state of central tolerance exists, in which lymphocytes with receptors against self-antigens have been eliminated during generation of clonal diversity. In other cases, tolerance is peripheral tolerance that is mediated by Treg cells (see Fig. 8.2). Rather than merely tolerating some self-antigens, the immune system actively prevents or limits their recognition by lymphocytes and antibodies. Some pathogens have developed a survival advantage by their capacity to mimic self-antigens and avoid inducing an immune response.

Molecular size also contributes to an antigen's immunogenicity. In general, large molecules (those bigger than 10,000 daltons), such as proteins, polysaccharides, and nucleic acids, are most immunogenic. Low-molecular-weight molecules, such as amino acids, monosaccharides, fatty acids, and the purine and pyrimidine bases, tend to be unable to induce an immune response. Many small molecules can function as haptens: antigens that are too small to be immunogenic by themselves but become immunogenic after binding with larger molecules that function as carriers for the hapten. For example, the antigens of penicillin (a β-lactam antibiotic of about 243 daltons) and poison ivy (which contains urushiol, an oily sap of about 1500 daltons) are haptens, but they initiate allergic responses only after binding to large-molecular-weight proteins in the allergic individual's blood or skin. Antigens that induce an allergic response are also called allergens. Allergic conditions are discussed in Chapter 9.

Chemical complexity affects immunogenicity. The best immunogens contain a diversity of chemically different components. For instance, a large synthetic protein consisting only of the amino acid alanine would not be very immunogenic despite its size and foreignness. However, if other amino acids, such as tyrosine, tryptophan, or phenylalanine, were inserted into the structure, the degree of immunogenicity would increase greatly.

Finally, antigens that are present in extremely small or large quantities may be unable to elicit an immune response and therefore by definition are also nonimmunogenic. In many cases, exposure to high or low extremes of antigen quantities may induce a state of tolerance rather than immunity.

Even if an antigen fulfills all these criteria, the quality and intensity of the immune response may still be affected by a variety of additional factors. For example, the route and vehicle of antigenic entry or administration are critical to the immunogenicity of some antigens. This has important clinical implications. The most common routes for clinical administration of antigen, such as vaccines, are intravenous, intraperitoneal, subcutaneous, intranasal, and oral. Each route preferentially stimulates a different set of lymphocyte-containing (lymphoid) tissues and therefore results in the induction of different types of cell-mediated or humoral immune responses. For some vaccines, the route may affect the protectiveness of the immune response so that the individual is protected if immunized by one route, but may remain susceptible to infection if administered through a different route. Immunogenicity of an antigen also may be altered by being delivered along with substances that stimulate the immune response; these substances are known as *adjuvants.* Finally, the genetic makeup of a host can play a critical role in the immune system's ability to respond to many antigens; some individuals appear to be unable to respond to immunization with a particular antigen, whereas they respond well to other antigens. For instance, a small percentage of the population may fail to produce a measurable immune response to a common vaccine, despite multiple injections, whereas they will respond well to a different vaccine. Many other factors can modulate the immune response. These include the individual's age, nutritional status, and reproductive status, as well as the exposure to traumatic injury, the presence of concurrent disease, or the use of immunosuppressive medications. These are discussed further in Chapter 9.

Molecules That Recognize Antigen

Antigen is directly recognized by three molecules: circulating antibody and antigen receptors on the surface of B lymphocytes (**B-cell receptor,** or **BCR**) and T lymphocytes (**T-cell receptor,** or **TCR**) (Fig. 8.5).

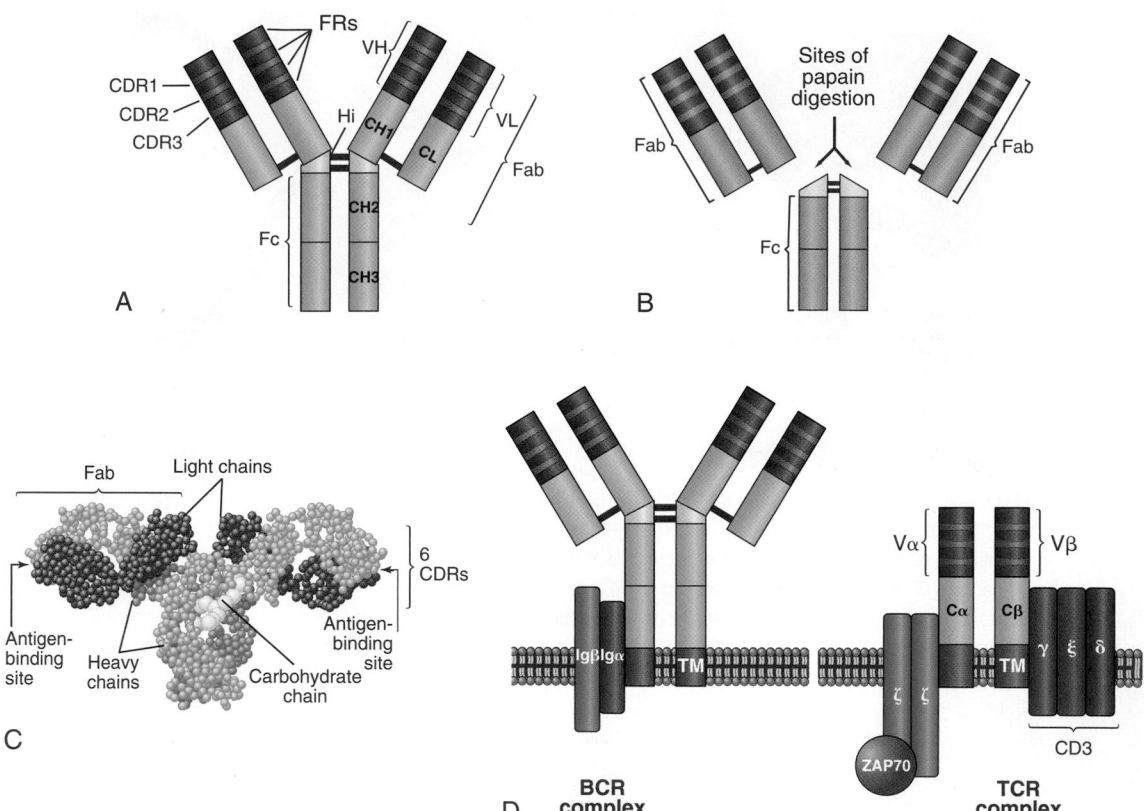

FIGURE 8.5 Antigen-Binding Molecules. Antigen-binding molecules include soluble antibody **(A, B, C)** and cell surface receptors **(D)**. **A,** The typical antibody molecule consists of two identical heavy chains and two identical light chains connected by interchain disulfide bonds (– between chains in the figure). Each heavy chain is divided into three regions with relatively constant amino acid sequences *(CH1, CH2,* and *CH3)* and a region with a variable amino acid sequence *(VH)*. Each light chain is divided into a constant region *(CL)* and a variable region *(VL)*. The hinge region *(Hi)* provides flexibility in some classes of antibody. Within each variable region are three highly variable complementary-determining regions *(CDR1, CDR2, CDR3)* separated by relatively constant framework regions *(FRs)*. **B,** Fragmentation of the antibody molecule by limited digestion with the enzyme papain has identified three important portions of the molecule: a fragment crystallizable (Fc) and two identical fragment antigen binding (Fab) fragments. Both Fab fragments bind antigen. As the antibody folds **(C),** the CDRs are placed in proximity to form the antigen-binding site. **D,** The antigen receptor on the surface of B cells *(BCR complex)* is a monomeric antibody with a structure similar to that of circulating antibody, with an additional hydrophobic transmembrane region *(TM)* that anchors the molecule to the cell surface. The active BCR complex contains molecules *(Igα* and *Igβ)* that are responsible for intracellular signaling after the receptor has bound antigen. The T-cell receptor *(TCR)* consists of an α chain and a β chain joined by a disulfide bond. Each chain consists of a constant region *(Cα* and *Cβ)* and a variable region *(Vα* and *Vβ)*. Each variable region contains CDRs and FRs in a structure similar to that of antibody. The active TCR is associated with several molecules that are responsible for intracellular signaling. These include CD3, which is a complex of γ (gamma), ε (epsilon), and δ (delta) subunits, and a complex of two ζ (zeta) molecules. The ζ molecules are attached to a cytoplasmic protein kinase (ZAP70) that is critical to intracellular signaling. (**C** adapted from Patton KT, Thibodeau GA: *Anatomy & physiology,* ed 9, St Louis, 2016, Mosby.)

Antibody

An understanding of antibodies and how they react with antigen will provide a foundation for more complex topics, such as the B-cell and T-cell receptors for antigen. An **antibody**, or immunoglobulin, is a serum glycoprotein produced by plasma cells in response to a challenge by an immunogen. The term *immunoglobulin* is used as a generic description of a general group of antibodies, whereas the term *antibody* commonly denotes one particular set of immunoglobulins known to have specificity for a specific antigen.

Classes. There are five molecular classes of immunoglobulins (IgG, IgA, IgM, IgE, and IgD) that are characterized by differences in antigenicity, structure, and function. Within two of the immunoglobulin classes are several distinct subclasses including four subclasses of IgG and two subclasses of IgA (Table 8.3).

IgG is the most abundant class of immunoglobulins, constituting 80% to 85% of those circulating in the body and accounting for most of the protective activity against infections (see Table 8.3). Maternal IgG is transported across the placenta during pregnancy and protects the newborn child during the first 6 months of life. Four subclasses of IgG have been described: IgG1, IgG2, IgG3, and IgG4.

IgA can be divided into two subclasses, IgA1 and IgA2. IgA1 molecules are found predominantly in the blood, whereas IgA2 is the predominant class of antibody found in normal body secretions (**secretory IgA [sIgA]**).

TABLE 8.3 PROPERTIES OF IMMUNOGLOBULINS

	IgG	IgM	IgA	sIgA	IgD	IgE

Physiochemical Properties of Immunoglobulins

	IgG	IgM	IgA	sIgA	IgD	IgE
Subclasses	IgG1, IgG2, IgG3, IgG4	IgM	IgA1, IgA2	IgA1, IgA2	IgD	IgE
Heavy chain	γ_1, γ_2, γ_3, γ_4	μ	α_1, α_2	α_1, α_2	Δ	ϵ
MW	146,000	970,000	160,000	385,000	184,000	190,000
Serum levels*	850, 290, 95, 50	135	290, 50	5	3	0.03

Biologic Properties of Immunoglobulins

	IgG	IgM	IgA	sIgA	IgD	IgE
Complement activation	Yes IgG3 > IgG1 > IgG2	Yes	No	No	No	No
Fc binds to phagocytes	Yes IgG1, IgG3	No	No	No	No	No
Fc binds to mast cells	Yes IgG4	No	No	No	No	Yes
Fc binds to platelets	Yes	No	No	No	No	No
Placental transfer	Yes IgG1 = IgG3 > IgG4 > IgG2	No	No	No	No	No

Biologic Function

	IgG	IgM	IgA	sIgA	IgD	IgE
Biologic Function	Toxin neutralization, complement activation, opsonization, long-term immunity	Initial antibody produced, agglutination, complement fixation, B-cell receptor	Neutralization	In secretions, toxin and bacterial neutralization	B-cell receptor	Protection against infections with worms, allergies

*Average adult levels (mg/dL) arranged by subclass.
Fc, Fragment crystallizable; *MW*, molecular weight in daltons.

sIgA molecules are dimers anchored together through a J chain and "secretory piece." This secretory piece is attached to the IgA dimer inside mucosal epithelial cells and protects these immunoglobulins against degradation by enzymes also found in the secretions.

IgM is the largest of the immunoglobulins and usually exists as a pentamer (a molecule consisting of five identical smaller molecules) that is stabilized by a J (joining) chain. It is the first antibody produced during the initial, or primary, response to antigen. IgM is usually synthesized early in neonatal life, but may be increased as a response to infection in utero.

Information on the role of IgD is limited. This class of immunoglobulins is found in very low concentrations in the blood. IgD functions as an antigen receptor on the surface of early B lymphocytes.

IgE is normally at low concentrations in the circulation. It functions as a mediator of many common allergic responses (see Chapter 9) and in the defense against parasitic infections.

Molecular Structure. Structural analysis of immunoglobulins began with Porter's early studies on the effects of the enzyme papain to digest IgG.[1] IgG was cleaved into three fragments, two of which were identical. The two identical fragments retained the ability to bind antigen, and each was termed an antigen-binding fragment (Fab).[2] The third fragment crystallized when separated from the Fab portions and was termed the crystalline fragment (Fc) (see Fig. 8.5).

The Fab portions contain identical recognition sites (receptors) for antigenic determinants and confer the molecule's specificity toward a particular antigen. The Fc portion is responsible for most of the biologic functions of antibodies that have bound antigen, including activation of the complement cascade and opsonization by binding to Fc receptors on the surface of the cells of the innate immune system.

The basic structure of an antibody molecule consists of four polypeptide chains—two identical light (L) chains and two identical heavy (H) chains (see Fig. 8.5). The class of antibody is determined by which heavy chain is used: gamma (IgG), mu (IgM), alpha (IgA), epsilon (IgE), or delta (IgD). The light chains of an antibody molecule are of either the kappa (κ) or the lambda (λ) type. The light and heavy chains are held together by two major forces: noncovalent bonds and disulfide linkages. A set of disulfide bridges between the heavy chains occurs in the hinge region and in some instances lends a degree of molecular flexibility at that site so that the Fab regions can move. An individual plasma cell produces only one type of H chain and one type of L chain at a time; for instance, one plasma cell may produce only IgGκ, whereas other plasma cells will be producing other antibody classes with either κ or λ light chains.

Light and heavy chains are further subdivided into constant (C) and variable (V) regions. The constant regions have relatively stable amino acid sequences within a particular immunoglobulin class or subclass or a particular light chain type. Thus the amino acid sequence of the constant region of one IgG1 heavy chain should be almost identical with the sequence of the same region of another IgG1 heavy chain, even if they react with different antigens. This holds true for light chains also; all λ chains possess highly similar constant regions that differ from those in κ chains. The amino acid sequences of the variable regions in heavy and light chains, however, differ greatly and determine the antigen-binding specificity of the molecule. Therefore two IgG1 molecules against different antigens may have similar constant regions but have many differences in the amino acid sequence of their variable regions. The diversity of amino acid sequences in the variable region is localized into three regions of the variable region. These three areas were once called *hypervariable regions*, but are now called complementary-determining regions (CDRs). The four regions separating the CDRs have relatively stable amino acid sequences and are called framework regions (FRs).

Antigen Binding

The antigen-binding site is formed by folding an antibody molecule so that the CDRs of the variable regions of both the heavy (V_H) and the light (V_L) chains are moved into close proximity, resulting in a binding site that is lined by the three CDRs of the heavy chain and the three CDRs of the light chain (see Fig. 8.5). Most proteins will naturally fold and take on secondary or tertiary structures. The FRs control the accuracy of folding in the variable regions of antibodies so that the CDRs in both variable regions are placed into accurate positions to bind antigen.[3] The specificity of an antibody toward a particular antigen is determined by the chemical nature of the particular amino acids in the six CDRs and the shape of the binding site. The antigen that will bind most strongly must have complementary chemistry and topography with the binding site formed by the antibody.[4] The antigen fits into this binding site with the specificity of a key into a lock and is held there by noncovalent chemical interactions (Fig. 8.6). In some cases the substitution of a single critical amino acid in a CDR may have a significant effect on the shape of the binding site and the specificity of the antibody molecule.

Because the heavy and light chains are identical within the same antibody molecule, the two binding sites are also identical and have specificity for the same antigen. The number of functional antigen-binding sites is called the antibody's valence. Most antibody classes (i.e., IgG, IgE, IgD, and circulating IgA) have a valence of 2, but secretory IgA has a valence of 4. IgM, being a pentamer, has a theoretical valence of 10, but can simultaneously use only about 5 binding sites because a large antigenic molecule binding to 1 site blocks antigen binding to other sites.

B-Cell Receptor Complex

The B-cell receptor (BCR) is a complex of antibody bound to the cell surface and other molecules involved in intracellular signaling (see Fig. 8.5). Its role is to recognize antigen and communicate that information

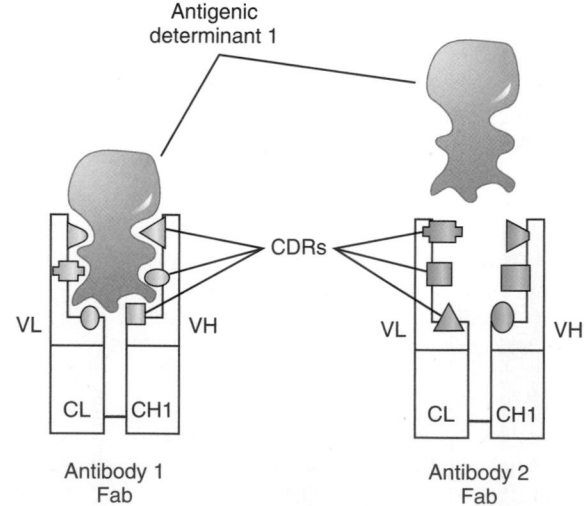

FIGURE 8.6 Antigen-Antibody Binding. The specificity required for antibody binding with an antigen is determined by the shape and chemistry of the six complementary-determining regions *(CDRs)* in the combining site on the variable region of the antibody. This figure indicates two different antibodies (Fab portions of antibody 1 and antibody 2) that have different sets of CDRs and therefore different specificities. As indicated, the antigenic determinant that reacts well with antibody 1 is unable to react with antibody 2 because of differences in the antibody combining site. *CH,* Constant region of the heavy chain; *CL,* constant region of the light chain; *Fab,* antigen-binding fragment; *V,* variable; *VH,* variable heavy chain; *VL,* variable light chain.

to the cell's nucleus. Therefore the BCR complex consists of antigen-recognition molecules and accessory molecules involved in intracellular signaling (Igα and Igβ). BCRs on the surface of immunocompetent B cells are membrane-associated IgM (mIgM) with or without IgD (mIgD) immunoglobulins. The immunoglobulin portion of the BCR is produced from the same genes used by plasma cells for soluble antibodies and has the same antigen specificity as circulating antibodies produced from the same cell after clonal selection. As a BCR, however, mIgM is a monomer rather than the pentamer, and both mIgM and mIgD express an extra hydrophobic transmembrane region that anchors to the hydrophobic regions of the plasma membrane.

The BCR signaling complex consists of two Igα and Igβ heterodimers that are closely associated with the BCR and contain tyrosine kinase signaling activity. The antibody portion of the BCR complex is responsible for recognition and binding to an antigen, but by itself cannot provide the intracellular signals required to activate the B cell and complete its maturation into antibody-producing plasma cells. That message is conveyed by the Igα and Igβ heterodimers.

T-Cell Receptor Complex

T lymphocytes use a similar but distinct array of proteins in their recognition and response to antigens. The T-cell receptor (TCR) complex is composed of an antibody-like transmembrane protein (TCR) and a group of accessory proteins (collectively referred to as CD3) that are involved in intracellular signaling (see Fig. 8.5). The most common TCR resembles an antibody Fab region and consists of two protein chains, α and β chains, each of which has a variable and constant region and is encoded from genes located independently of the antibody heavy and light chains. Similar to the BCR, the TCR is responsible for recognition and binding to the antigen, whereas the accessory proteins are responsible for the intracellular signaling necessary for activation and differentiation of the T cell. Each of the individual components of the TCR complex is important, and several severe defects in the T-cell immune response have been related to mutations in individual components of the complex (see Chapter 9).

Molecules That Present Antigen

For an effective immune response, most antigens must be processed by APCs and presented on the cell surface by specialized molecules, molecules of the major histocompatibility complex (MHC) (Fig. 8.7). MHC molecules in humans also are called *human leukocyte antigens* (HLAs) (discussed in greater detail in Chapter 9 related to their role in transplantation). Some types of antigen are processed only by highly specialized cells: APCs. Other types of antigen can be processed and presented by almost any type of cell. Several sets of cell surface molecules have the responsibility for appropriately presenting antigen. These molecules are described next.

Major Histocompatibility Complex

MHC molecules are glycoproteins found on the surface of all human cells except red blood cells. They are divided into two general classes, class I and class II, based on their molecular structure, distribution among cell populations, and function in antigen presentation. MHC class I molecules are heterodimers composed of a large alpha (α) chain and a smaller chain called *β₂-microglobulin*. MHC class II molecules are also heterodimers composed of α and β chains. The α and β chains of the MHC molecules are encoded from different genetic loci in a large complex of genes on the short arm of human chromosome 6 (β_2-microglobulin is found on chromosome 15). The MHC also contains other genes that control the quality and quantity of an immune response, which are commonly referred to as *class III MHC genes*. The general properties of each of the MHC classes are summarized in Fig. 8.7.

The primary MHC class I genes consist of three closely linked loci labeled A, B, and C. The primary MHC class II genes are located within an area called the *D region*, which actually consists of three separate and independent loci: DR, DP, and DQ.

MHC loci are the most genetically diverse (polymorphic) of any human genetic loci. Within the human population, the number of possible different alleles (i.e., forms of the gene) expressed by each locus is astounding: approximately 700 at the A locus, 1000 at the B locus, 350 at the C locus, 600 at the DR locus (α and β), 125 at the DQ locus (α and β), and 150 at the DP locus (α and β). These numbers are based on the polymorphism of observed DNA sequences and may not reflect differences in function. Clearly, not every allele is expressed in the same individual. Humans have two copies of each MHC locus (one inherited from each parent) that are codominant so that molecules encoded by each parent's genes are expressed on the cell surface. Within an individual, each locus will be expressing only one allele. For instance, each person will have only two different A proteins (one from each parent).

Transplantation. The diversity of MHC molecules is clinically relevant during organ transplantation. Cells in transplanted tissue or organs from one individual will have a different set of MHC surface antigens than those of the recipient; therefore the recipient can mount an immune response against the foreign MHC antigens, resulting in rejection of the transplanted tissue. As a result of studies of transplantation, the human MHC molecule is also referred to as human leukocyte antigen (HLA), and the different MHC genetic loci are commonly called HLA-A, HLA-B, HLA-C, HLA-DR, HLA-DQ, and HLA-DP. To minimize the chance of tissue rejection, the donor and recipient are often *tissue typed* beforehand to identify differences in HLA antigens. The more similar two individuals are in their HLA tissue type, the more likely a transplant from one to the other will be successful. Because of the large number of different alleles, it is highly unlikely that a perfect "match" can be found in the general population between a potential donor and the recipient.

The specific combination of alleles at the six major HLA loci on one chromosome (A, B, C, DR, DQ, and DP) is termed a haplotype. Each individual has two HLA haplotypes, one from the paternal chromosome 6 and another from the maternal chromosome. Because the different HLA loci within the MHC are in such close proximity to one another, haplotypes are not *usually* disrupted by recombination and are thus inherited intact. One HLA haplotype from each parent is passed to each of the offspring, meaning that children usually share one haplotype with each parent (Fig. 8.8). Odds dictate that children of the same parents will share one haplotype with half of their siblings and either no haplotypes or both haplotypes with a quarter of their siblings. Thus the chance of finding a match among siblings is much higher (25%) than that from the general population. Identical twins, originating from the same egg and sperm, will have a complete set of identical genes, including HLA molecules.

It should be noted, however, that although HLA alleles are the primary contributor to rejection of a transplant, a number of other antigens also have a role in determining tissue compatibility. Some of these are encoded on other chromosomes and are inherited independently of HLA antigens. This means that although two people have the same HLA makeup, a graft or transplant still may be rejected because of differences between other antigens. It is preferable to obtain a graft or transplant from a closely related individual, such as a sibling, because the chance of sharing both the same HLA antigens and other undetermined antigenic differences encoded outside the MHC is much greater.

CD1

Another set of antigen-presenting molecules are members of the CD1 group. CD1 molecules have very low genetic polymorphism and a

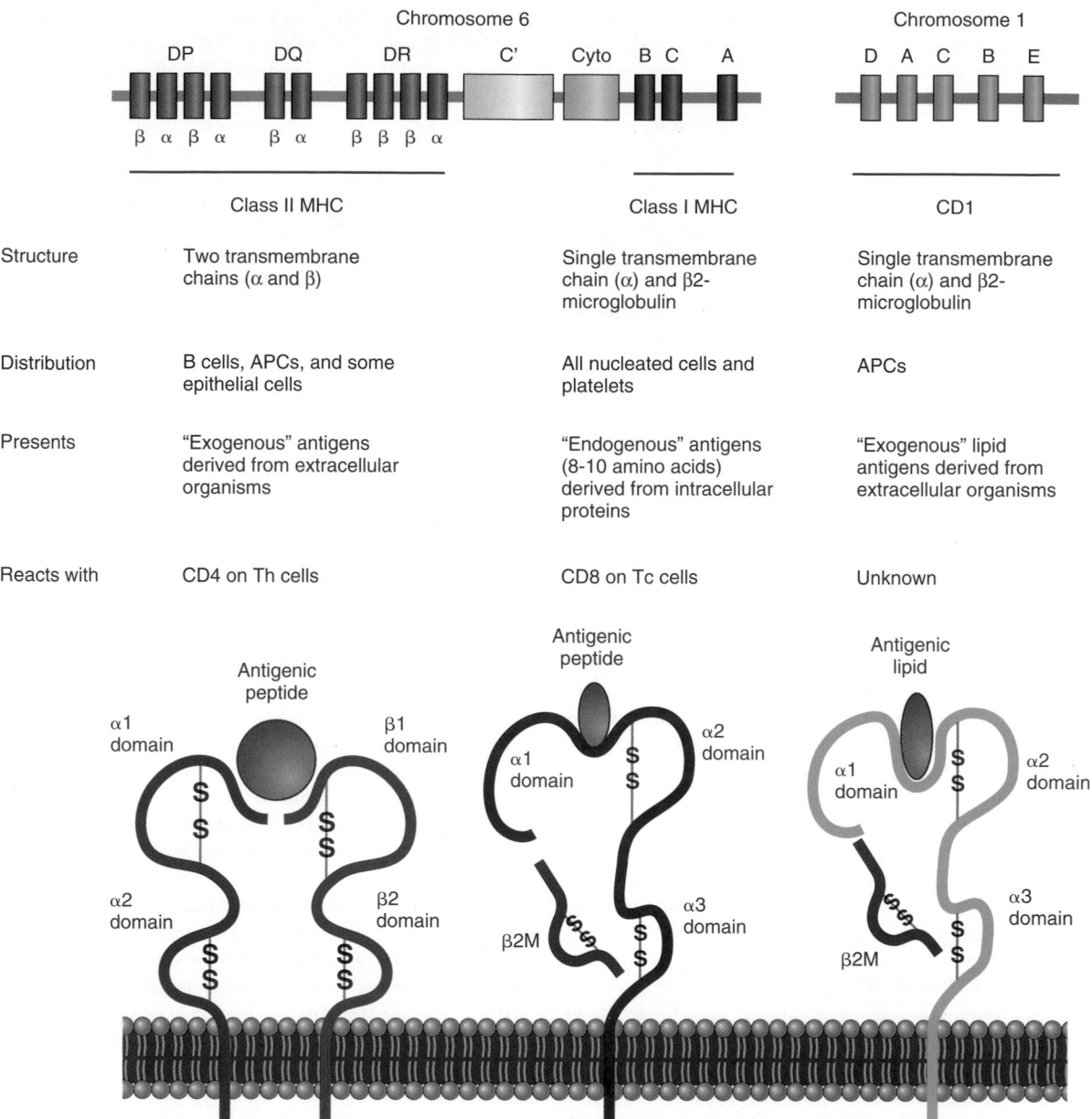

	Class II MHC	Class I MHC	CD1
Structure	Two transmembrane chains (α and β)	Single transmembrane chain (α) and β2-microglobulin	Single transmembrane chain (α) and β2-microglobulin
Distribution	B cells, APCs, and some epithelial cells	All nucleated cells and platelets	APCs
Presents	"Exogenous" antigens derived from extracellular organisms	"Endogenous" antigens (8-10 amino acids) derived from intracellular proteins	"Exogenous" lipid antigens derived from extracellular organisms
Reacts with	CD4 on Th cells	CD8 on Tc cells	Unknown

FIGURE 8.7 **Genetics and Structure of Antigen-Presenting Molecules.** Three sets of molecules are primarily responsible for antigen presentation: MHC class I, MHC class II, and CD1. The major histocompatibility complex (MHC) molecules are encoded from the MHC region on chromosome 6, which contains information for class I and class II molecules, as well as for several other molecules that participate in the innate or immune responses. These include several complement proteins *(C')* and cytokines *(Cyto),* which are referred to as *MHC class III molecules.* Three principal class I molecules, HLA-A, HLA-B, and HLA-C, are presented here, but this region contains information for the α chains of several other molecules, including HLA-E, HLA-F, and HLA-G. The MHC class I products complex with β₂-microglobulin, which is encoded by a gene on chromosome 15. The MHC class I molecules present small peptide antigens in a pocket formed by the α1 and α2 domains of the α chain. The conformation of the molecule is stabilized by β₂-microglobulin *(β2M)* as well as by intrachain disulfide bonds (-S-S-). The α and β chains of class II molecules are also encoded in this region: HLA-DR, HLA-DP, and HLA-DQ. In some cases, multiple genes for α and β chains are available. The MHC class II molecules present peptide antigens in a pocket formed by the α1 domain of the α chain and the β1 domain of the β chain. The genes for CD1 molecules are encoded on chromosome 1, which contains genes for five α chains (CD1A-E), and the α chains complex with β₂-microglobulin to present lipid antigens in a pocket formed by the α1 and α2 domains. All three sets of antigen-presenting molecules are anchored to the plasma membrane by hydrophobic regions on the ends of the α and chains. *APCs,* antigen-presenting cells; *Tc,* T cytotoxic; *Th,* T-helper.

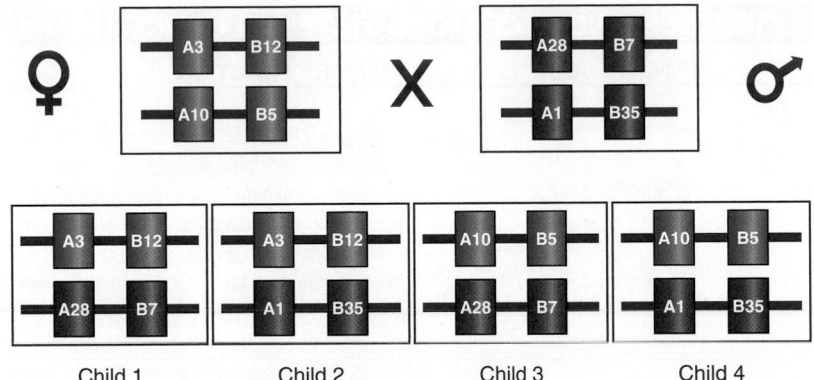

FIGURE 8.8 Inheritance of Human Leukocyte Antigen. Human leukocyte antigen (HLA) alleles are inherited in a codominant fashion so that both maternal and paternal antigens are expressed. Specific HLA alleles are commonly given numbers to indicate different antigens. In this example, the mother has linked genes for HLA-A3 and HLA-B12 on one chromosome 6 and genes for HLA-A10 and HLA-B5 on the second chromosome 6. The father has HLA-A28 and HLA-B7 on one chromosome and HLA-A1 and HLA-B35 on the second chromosome. On one particular chromosome, the HLA antigens are firmly linked, with crossovers occurring in only 1% of individuals. The children from this pairing may have one of four possible combinations of maternal and paternal HLA.

BOX 8.1	IMPORTANT ADHESION MOLECULE PAIRINGS	
Th-cell CD4	⇔	MHC class II on APC
Tc-cell CD8	⇔	MHC class I on APC
Tc-cell CD2	⇔	CD58 (LFA-3) on APC
Tc-cell CD28	⇔	CD80 (B7-1) on APC
Tc-cell LFA-1	⇔	ICAM-1 on APC
Th-cell CD40L (CD154)	⇔	CD40 on B cell
Th-cell CD40L (CD154)	⇔	CD40 on APC

APC, Antigen-presenting cell; *ICAM,* intercellular adhesion molecule; *LFA,* lymphocyte function associated antigen; *MHC,* major histocompatibility complex; *Tc,* T-cytotoxic; *Th,* T-helper.

structure similar to that of MHC class I, and they are found primarily on APCs and cells in the thymus.[5] Unlike MHC molecules that present proteins, the CD1 molecules appear to specialize in presenting lipid antigens contained in lipoproteins, glycolipids, and other molecules. These antigens are commonly important factors in infections with bacteria of the *Mycobacterium* spp. (e.g., *Mycobacterium tuberculosis* that causes tuberculosis and *Mycobacterium leprae* that causes leprosy), which have a very large amount of lipid in their cell membranes.

Molecules That Hold Cells Together

The efficient development of an immune response requires several antigen-independent interactions between cells. The interactions between specific cellular receptors and their ligands result in intracellular signaling events that are independent of the TCR or BCR complexes but are necessary complements to the antigen-specific signal. Several of these molecules are listed in Box 8.1.

Cytokines and Their Receptors

As discussed in Chapter 7, cytokines are low-molecular-weight proteins or glycoproteins that function as chemical signals between cells. A large number of cytokines are secreted by APCs and lymphocytes and provide both positive and negative regulation of the immune response. The effects of particular cytokines depend on binding to specific cellular receptors, which are linked to intracellular signaling pathways. The lymphocyte may respond in many ways. One of the most common

responses is an increase in the production of proteins, many of which are other cytokines or cytokine receptors. Many cytokines also cause a lymphocyte to proliferate and differentiate. The participation of cytokines is essential to the development of an adequate immune response, and in general the precise combination of cytokines influences the ultimate response of a given cell. Specific deficiencies in the immune response that result from genetic mutations that lead to defective cytokine production or defective cytokine receptors are discussed in Chapter 9. Table 8.4 provides information about key cytokines and receptors that are known to influence the immune response.

GENERATION OF CLONAL DIVERSITY

The immune response occurs in two phases: generation of clonal diversity and clonal selection (Table 8.5 and see Fig. 8.2).[6,7] During generation of clonal diversity, a large population of T cells and B cells is produced before birth. These lymphocytes have the capacity to recognize almost any foreign antigen found in the environment. This process occurs mostly in specialized lymphoid organs (the primary [central] lymphoid organs): the thymus for T cells and the bone marrow for B cells. The result is differentiation of lymphoid stem cells into B and T lymphocytes. Lymphoid stem cells are precursor cells formed in the liver (in the fetus) or in the bone marrow (of a child or adult) that do not have antigen-specific receptors (BCR and TCR) or other B-cell–specific and T-cell–specific surface proteins. After maturation in the central lymphoid organs, these stem cells develop into immunocompetent cells with antigen-specific receptors without encountering foreign antigen. Although each B or T cell expresses receptors against a single specific antigen, the total population of immunocompetent cells may have receptors that can react with more than 10^8 different antigenic determinants. Thus before the individual is exposed to any foreign antigen, millions of different T- and B-cell antigen receptors must be constructed to recognize *any* potential antigenic determinant. Immunocompetent lymphocytes are released to the circulation and many reside in secondary (peripheral) lymphoid organs (e.g., spleen, lymph nodes, adenoids, tonsils, Peyer patches).

Although generation of clonal diversity primarily occurs in the fetus, it probably continues to a low degree throughout most of adult life. The endless array of possible antibodies and TCRs certainly cannot be constructed from the amount of deoxyribonucleic acid (DNA) that is

TABLE 8.4   KEY CYTOKINES AND RECEPTORS THAT INFLUENCE THE IMMUNE RESPONSE

CYTOKINE	PRIMARY SOURCE	PRIMARY FUNCTION
Interleukin (IL)		
IL-1	APCs	Stimulates proliferation and differentiation of T cells; induces acute-phase proteins in inflammatory response; endogenous pyrogen
IL-2	Th1 cells, NK cells	Stimulates proliferation and differentiation of T cells and NK cells
IL-4	Th2 cells, mast cells	Induces B-cell proliferation and differentiation; up-regulates MHC class II expression; induces class-switch to IgE
IL-5	Th2 cells, mast cells	Induces eosinophil proliferation and differentiation; induces B-cell proliferation and differentiation
IL-6	Th2 cells, APCs	Induces B-cell proliferation and differentiation into plasma cells; induces acute-phase proteins in inflammatory response
IL-7	Thymic epithelial cells, bone marrow stromal cells	Major cytokine for induction of B- and T-cell proliferation and differentiation in central lymphoid organs
IL-8	Macrophages	Chemotactic factor for neutrophils
IL-10	Th cells, B cells	Inhibits cytokine production; activator of B cells
IL-12	B cells, APCs	Induces NK-cell proliferation; increases production of IFN-γ
IL-13	Th2 cells	IL-4–like properties; decreases inflammatory responses
IL-17	Th17 cells	Increases inflammation; increased influx of neutrophils and macrophages; increased epithelial cell chemokine production
IL-22	Th17 cells	Increases inflammation; increased epithelial cell production of antimicrobial peptides
Interferon (IFN)		
IFN-α, IFN-β	Macrophages, some virally infected cells	Antiviral; increases expression of MHC class I; activates NK cells
IFN-γ	Th1 cells, NK cells, Tc cells	Increases expression of MHC class II; activates macrophages and NK cells
Tumor Necrosis Factor (TNF)		
TNF-α (cachectin)	Macrophages	IL-1–like properties; induces cellular proliferation
TNF-β (lymphotoxin)	Tc cells	Kills some cells; increases phagocytosis by macrophages and neutrophils
Transforming Growth Factor (TGF)		
TGF-β	Lymphocytes, macrophages, fibroblasts	Chemotactic for macrophages; increases macrophage IL-1 production; stimulates wound healing

CYTOKINE RECEPTORS	LIGAND	ADDITIONAL INFORMATION
Class I receptor dimers (α and β chains)	IL-3, IL-5, IL-6, IL-11, IL-12, IL-13	IL-3 and IL-5 share a common α chain; IL-6 and IL-11 share a common β chain
Trimers (α, β, and γ chains)	IL-2, IL-4, IL-7, IL-9, IL-15	All share a common γ chain
Class II receptors	IFN-α, -β, and -γ	Two chains
TNF receptors	TNF-α, TNF-β, CD40, Fas	Single chain
Immunoglobulin-like receptors	IL-1	Single chain with immunoglobulin-like characteristics

APCs, Antigen-presenting cells; *Fas,* death receptor; *MHC,* major histocompatibility complex; *NK,* natural killer; *Tc,* T-cytotoxic; *Th,* T-helper.

in the nucleus of a human lymphocyte. The enormous repertoire of specificities with appropriate conservation of DNA is made possible by rearrangement of smaller regions of existing DNA during T- and B-cell development in the primary lymphoid organs. Loci in the DNA that encode parts of the variable regions of immunoglobulins and TCRs are rearranged, a process known as somatic recombination, in a unique way to generate receptors that collectively can recognize and bind to any possible antigen.

B-Cell Maturation
Central Lymphoid Organ

Lymphoid stem cells destined to become B cells percolate through specialized regions of the bone marrow, where they are exposed to hormones and cytokines that induce proliferation and differentiation into immunocompetent B cells (Fig. 8.9).[8] They interact with stromal cells through a variety of intercellular adhesion molecules (e.g., stem cell factor [a cytokine bound to the membrane of stromal cells and sometimes known as steel factor]). As the stem cell begins to mature, it progressively develops a variety of necessary surface markers, one of the earliest being the interleukin-7 (IL-7) receptor. IL-7, produced by the stromal cells, is critical in driving the further differentiation and proliferation of the B cell.[9] The next stage in development is formation of the B-cell receptor.

Production of the B-Cell Receptor (BCR)

The BCR is a complex of antibody that is anchored to the plasma membrane and other molecules involved in intracellular signaling. Its role is to recognize an antigen and communicate that information to the cell nucleus. BCRs on immunocompetent B cells are membrane-associated IgM (mIgM) with or without concurrent mIgD that have identical specificities for antigen.

TABLE 8.5   GENERATION OF CLONAL DIVERSITY VS. CLONAL SELECTION

	GENERATION OF CLONAL DIVERSITY	CLONAL SELECTION
Purpose?	To produce large numbers of T and B lymphocytes with the maximum diversity of antigen receptors	Select, expand, and differentiate clones of T and B cells against a specific antigen
When does it occur?	Primarily in the fetus	Primarily after birth and throughout life
Where does it occur?	Central lymphoid organs: thymus for T cells, bone marrow for B cells	Peripheral lymphoid organs, including lymph nodes, spleen, and other lymphoid tissues
Is foreign antigen involved?	No	Yes; antigen determines which clones of cells will be selected
What hormones/cytokines are involved?	Thymic hormones, IL-7, others	Many cytokines produced by Th cells and APCs
Is tolerance induced?	Central tolerance induced as autoreactive cells are deleted	Peripheral tolerance induced as autoreactive cells are regulated
Final product?	Immunocompetent T and B cells that can react with antigen but have not seen antigen, and migrate to the secondary lymphoid organs	Plasma cells that produce antibody, effector T cells that help (Th), kill targets (Tc), or regulate immune responses (Treg); memory B and T cells

APCs, Antigen-presenting cells; *IL,* interleukin; *Tc,* T-cytotoxic; *Th,* T-helper; *Treg,* regulatory T cells.

The enormous repertoire of specificities is related to the sum of diversities of CDRs in the heavy and light chain variable regions. The CDRs are encoded by multiple sets of genes that undergo somatic recombination. The process of recombination is simplest for the antibody light chains (Fig. 8.10). The segments of DNA that encode either kappa (κ) (chromosome 2) or lambda (λ) (chromosome 22) light chain are clustered in *V, J,* and *C* genes. Diversity is accomplished by random rearrangement of *V* and *J* gene regions encoding the V region. The *V* genes encode the first two CDRs and intervening FR regions of the V region. The *J* genes (joining genes) encode the third CDR (CDR3) and FR4. To create the V region of the light chain, one *V* gene and one *J* gene are randomly selected and rearranged so that the *V* and *J* are moved to adjacent positions, and the intervening DNA is excised and spliced, resulting in a *VJ* region that encodes the V region of the light chain. Somatic recombination is controlled by enzymes encoded by *recombination activating genes (RAG-1, RAG-2)* that cut and remove intervening DNA between the selected *V* and *J* gene regions and splice the *VJ* together.[10]

Some *V* gene regions are defective; however, estimates of functional gene regions range from 40 to 70. About 5 *J* gene regions appear to be available. Thus recombination of a light chain may result in as many as 350 *VJ* possible recombinants. Within a particular differentiating B cell, a precise order of light chain rearrangement exists so that a successful *VJ* rearrangement prevents any attempts to any rearrangement of light chain genes on other chromosomes, and each B cell only produces one light chain. The primary mRNA transcript contains information for the *VJ* region, an intervening intron, and the *C* region gene. Processing of the mRNA (RNA splicing) removes the intron, resulting in a mRNA with contiguous *VJC* regions that is transcribed into an intact light chain.

The gene for the heavy chain on chromosome 14 undergoes similar somatic recombination. Unlike the light chain organization of *V, J,* and *C* gene regions, the heavy chain loci consist of approximately 50 *V,* 30 *D,* and 6 *J* gene regions and 9 *C* regions, with the gene for the mu (μ) constant region being closest to the *VDJ* region, and the delta (δ) constant region gene being next in sequence (see Fig. 8.10). Somatic rearrangement of the *V* region genes is a two-step process with rearrangement to a contiguous *DJ* followed by formation of *VDJ.* During both rearrangements, intervening sequences of DNA are excised and repaired. The *V* gene region encodes the CDR1 and CDR2 regions and

intervening *FR* regions. The genetic information for the CDR3 is a composite of a small amount of DNA from the *V* gene region, the entire *D* region, and a portion of the *J* gene region. Somatic recombination may result in more than 13,500 different heavy chain variable regions.

The primary mRNA contains five exons: *VDJ,* μ constant region (*Cμ*), a μ transmembrane region (*TMμ*), δ constant region (*Cδ*), and a *TMμ* region (Fig. 8.11). There are no stop signals between the *Cμ* and *Cδ* so that both will be transcribed in the same mRNA.[11] A stop signal is present after the information for *Cδ* so that other constant regions will not be transcribed. During RNA splicing all introns will be excised and all mRNA molecules will retain the same *VDJ* region. All cells will produce a population of mRNA containing the *Cμ* and its *TM* region. Through alternative splicing, many cells also will produce concurrently a second group of mRNA containing the *Cδ* and its *TM* region. Within a single developing immunocompetent B cell, alternatively spliced mRNA may be translated into μ and δ heavy chains that have identical V regions and have *TM* regions for anchoring to the cell membrane. The light chains are assembled with two μ chains to form monomeric IgM or with two δ chains to form IgD antibody. Initially, the developing B cell rearranges and expresses heavy chain that is followed by the rearrangement of either the κ or the λ light chain so that only one type is produced. The hydrophobic *TM* regions will result in insertion into the plasma membrane and simultaneous expression of mIgM and mIgD with identical CDRs and antigen specificities. A very rough calculation of the diversity resulting from this process would be the diversity of the H chain (13,500) × the diversity of the κ light chain (350) + the H chain diversity (13,500) × the λ light chain (350) = 9.45×10^6 combinations of H and L chain CDRs.

The BCR signaling complex is further constructed by the addition of two Igα and Igβ heterodimers that are closely associated with the BCR and contain tyrosine kinase signaling activity. The antibody portion of the BCR complex is responsible for recognition and binding to an antigen but, by itself, cannot provide the intracellular signals required to activate the B cell and complete its later maturation into plasma cells. That message is conveyed by the Igα and Igβ heterodimers.

Changes in Characteristic Surface Markers

B-cell differentiation is also characterized by the development of a variety of important surface molecules. These include CD21 (a complement

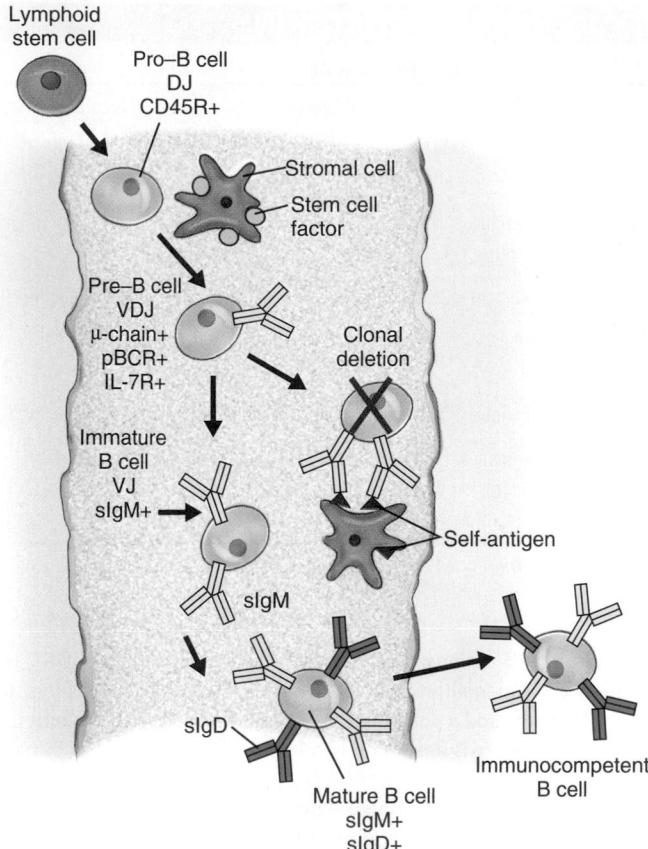

FIGURE 8.9 B-Cell Development in the Bone Marrow. During the generation of clonal diversity, lymphoid stem cells enter portions of the bone marrow that serve as the central lymph organ for B-cell development. Interactions with a series of bone marrow stromal cells guide the proliferation and differentiation process through direct cell-to-cell contact and the production of cytokines and hormones by the stromal cells, but without the presence of foreign antigen. A simplified scheme for that process is presented here. The differentiation process of B cells is characterized by the upregulation of many important surface molecules (only some of which are shown) and the random development of a huge number of different B-cell receptors. The early B cell (pro–B cell) binds to a membrane-bound cytokine (stem cell factor) on the stromal cell and initiates expression of the surface molecule CD45R and begins to rearrange the *DJ* regions of the antibody heavy-chain gene. As the cell progresses to the pre–B-cell stage, it concludes DNA rearrangement of the heavy chain *(VDJ)* and begins expressing cytoplasmic mu (μ) heavy chain. The μ chain is incorporated into a pre–B-cell receptor *(pBCR)* using a surrogate protein in place of the light chain. The cell also up-regulates the IL-7 receptor *(IL-7R)*, which interacts with IL-7 produced by the stromal cells to drive the remaining steps in differentiation. Some pBCRs have specificities toward self-antigen. Many of these encounter self-antigen expressed on the stromal cells and undergo negative selection (clonal deletion). The surviving cells (immature B cells) rearrange the light-chain DNA *(VJ)* and express a BCR consisting of light chain and the μ heavy chain (membrane-bound IgM [mIgM]). In the mature B cell, changes in processing of the heavy-chain precursor RNA result in coexpression of mIgM and mIgD (see Fig. 8.11 for more details).

receptor) and CD40 (adhesion molecule required for later interactions with Th cells).

Central Tolerance

Because assembly of the *VJ* and *VDJ* regions is random, B-cell receptors will be produced that react with self-antigens *(autoreactive B cells)*. Further development and release of these autoreactive cells into the

circulation would result in a catastrophic immune attack against the individual's own tissues. One stage at which immune tolerance (suppression or limitation of immune responses against self-antigens) occurs is the deletion of autoreactive B cells in the bone marrow, which is referred to as central tolerance (induction of tolerance within the central lymphoid organs). During the very earliest stages of formation of the BCR in the bone marrow, a large number of autoreactive B cells undergo apoptosis *(clonal deletion)* if exposed to self-antigen. This process of *negative selection* induces the death of more than 90% of developing B cells. Some autoreactive clones persist and must be controlled by other means in the lymphoid organs (peripheral tolerance).

T-Cell Maturation
Central Lymphoid Organ

The process of T-cell generation of clonal diversity is similar to that for B cells. The primary lymphoid organ for T-cell development is the thymus, which is an organ located near the heart. Lymphoid stem cells migrate to the thymus and enter the subcapsular region. As the cells journey through the thymic cortex to the medulla, they are instructed by interactions with various thymic cells (epithelial cells, macrophages, and dendritic cells), thymic hormones (e.g., thymosin, thymopoietin, thymostimulin, and others produced by the thymic epithelium), and the cytokine IL-7 to undergo proliferation and progressive development of the characteristics of immunocompetent T cells (Fig. 8.12). Changes include development of the T-cell receptor complex and expression of characteristic surface molecules. The final immunocompetent T cells are released into the blood vessels and lymphatic vessels to establish residence in the secondary lymphoid organs to await antigen.

Production of the T-Cell Receptor

Within the thymic cortex, the cells begin rearranging the variable region genes necessary for forming a functional T-cell receptor. The basic process of TCR rearrangement is essentially identical with formation of the BCR and, although the structure of the TCR closely resembles a Fab portion of antibody, the TCR uses different genes than are used for antibody (see Fig. 8.5). The most common TCR contains α and β chains, each of which has a variable region and a constant region.

The variable regions of the TCR α and β chains also undergo somatic recombination: the α chain gene (chromosome 14) rearranges V and J regions and the β chain gene (chromosome 7) rearranges V, D, and J regions. Somatic recombination of the α chain proceeds as described for the antibody light chain using a set of at least 70 V region genes and at least 50 J region genes (see Fig. 8.10). Thus potentially 3500 different α chains may be generated. Rearrangement of the β chain occurs similarly as described for antibody heavy chain rearrangement. A major difference, however, is the option of using two separate C gene regions ($C\beta_1$ and $C\beta_2$) each of which is adjacent to its own set of D and J gene regions. Somatic rearrangement of the β chain gene segments uses at least 60 V gene regions and 2 $C\beta$ regions (each containing at least 1 D and 6 or 7 J gene regions). As many as 720 different β chains may be produced. As with the generation of antibody diversity, the primary mRNA for α and β chains contains V region and C region exons with an intervening intron that is removed by RNA processing. Assembly of the α and β chains results in TCR diversity that potentially represents 2.5×10^6 (3500 α chains × 720 β chains) antigenic specificities.

For both α and β chains, the V region genes encode the amino acid sequences that include CDR1 and CDR2 and their appropriate FR regions. The J regions contain information for CDR3 and FR4. The TCR β chain D regions encode a short amino acid sequence found in the CDR3 and greatly increase the diversity of the β chain CDR3.

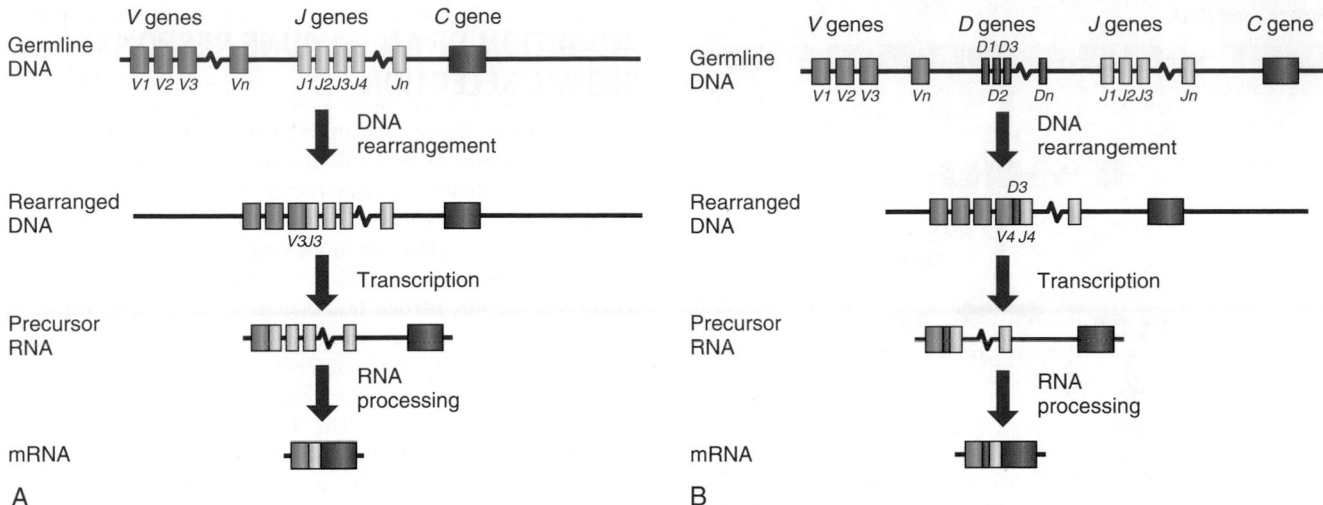

FIGURE 8.10 DNA Rearrangement of Genes for Antigen-Binding Molecules. During the generation of clonal diversity, a tremendous number of different antigen-binding molecules are produced. These include the B-cell receptor (BCR), which consists of a membrane-bound antibody molecule, and the T-cell receptor (TCR). The process by which receptor diversity is created is identical for all antigen-binding molecules and is summarized in this figure. Maximum diversity with minimum use of DNA is accomplished by random rearrangement of sets of genes that encode different portions of the variable regions. **A,** The variable regions of the light chain of antibody and the α chain of the TCR independently rearrange two sets of genes: V region genes and J region genes. The light chain uses its own set of genes, and the α chain uses a completely different set. In either case is the exact number of V or J region genes known; therefore in this figure they are numbered from *1* to an unknown value *(n)*. In a particular cell's DNA, one V gene is randomly selected and moved to a position immediately adjacent to a randomly selected J gene. In this example, *V3* and *J3* were selected. The DNA between the selected genes is enzymatically removed and the DNA repaired, so that the rearranged DNA in this example is missing the portion found in the germline DNA between *V3* and *J3*. This product is transcribed into a precursor ribonucleic acid (RNA) that contains information for the rearranged *VJ* pair, a span containing other unselected *J* regions, and information for the appropriate constant region *(C gene)* of the molecule. The RNA between the *VJ* and the *C* regions is not translated; therefore it is removed by RNA processing to produce a messenger RNA *(mRNA)* that is translated. **B,** The variable region of the antibody heavy chain and the TCR β chain result from a similar DNA rearrangement, with the added diversity contributed by a group of *D* region genes. The joining of *D* and *J* occurs first, with the removal of intervening DNA. In this example, *D3* and *J4* were chosen. This is followed by rearrangement of the *V* gene (e.g., *V4*) and formation of a *VDJ* region in the rearranged DNA. The precursor RNA contains information for the *VDJ*, the intervening portion of DNA, and the appropriate constant region. After RNA processing, an mRNA is formed for the intact antibody heavy chain or the TCR β chain. Once the DNA is rearranged and spliced in a given B or T cell, all of the antigen receptors produced by that cell employ the same *V, D,* and *J* segments and have the same specificity.

As with somatic rearrangement of antibody light and heavy gene regions, the level of diversity, especially for the CDR3 regions, may be increased further by other factors. Imprecise joining increases the diversity of the CDR3 regions. For example, the sites of VJ and VDJ joining may shift slightly, resulting in an amino acid being inserted or deleted from the protein.

Although the αβ TCR is the preferred antigen receptor, some T cells (about 5% of the total T-cell population) use alternative genes: gamma (γ) (chromosome 7) and delta (δ) (chromosome 14, in the middle of α chain genes). T cells with γδ TCRs appear to migrate to unique areas of the body (the epithelial areas in the skin, reproductive tract, intestine, respiratory tract) and have different and less well understood functions than the T cells with αβ TCRs.

A functional TCR requires intracellular signaling molecules. Insertion of the TCR into the plasma membrane is associated with expression and association with TCR accessory molecules (collectively called *CD3*) that provide signaling to the nucleus after the binding of antigen to the TCR. CD3 is a marker for T cells that successfully form a TCR complex and are immunocompetent.

Changes in Characteristic Surface Markers

Differentiation of T cells in the thymus also results in changes in a variety of important surface molecules. Much of T-cell development is controlled by hormones and cytokines in the thymus, and an early step in maturation is expression of the receptor for interleukin-7 (IL-7R), which is a major cytokine that drives the differentiation process.[12] Transit through the thymic cortex initiates expression of the molecule CD2 on the cell surface. CD2 is expressed on virtually every subpopulation of cells that have undergone development in the thymus and is thus a T-cell marker.

The developing T cell also begins making two other important surface proteins, CD4 and CD8, which are concurrently expressed on the developing cell's surface at this stage.[13] CD4+, CD8+ cells are often called "double-positive" cells. After entering the medulla of the thymus, the double-positive cells become "single-positive." That is, some of the cells suppress production of the CD8 molecule and remain only CD4+, whereas others suppress CD4 production and remain CD8+. The phenotypic change to single-positive cells is driven by exposure of CD4+,

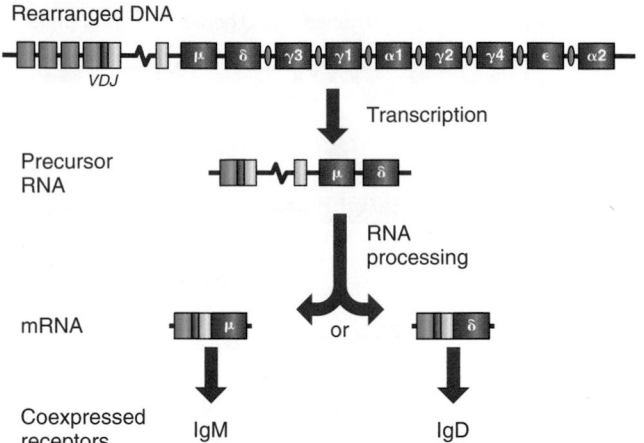

FIGURE 8.11 Coexpression of IgM and IgD B-Cell Receptors. Most mature immunocompetent B cells express both membrane-bound IgM and IgD as the B-cell receptor. In the germline DNA, the heavy-chain gene complex consists of a series of V, D, J, and constant region genes. In humans, each class and subclass of antibody has a unique constant region gene arranged in the indicated order. Switch regions occur preceding every constant region gene, except mu (μ) (IgM) and delta (δ) (IgD). After successful DNA rearrangement of the VDJ regions, a ribonucleic acid (RNA) molecule is transcribed that contains the information from the VDJ, intervening DNA, the μ constant region, and the δ constant region. Precursor RNA molecules are alternatively processed to produce messenger RNAs (mRNAs) containing either μ or δ. Initially, RNA processing favors the μ chain and production of membrane-bound IgM (see Fig. 8.10), but as the B cell matures, both mRNA molecules are produced. IgD, immunoglobulin D; IgM, immunoglobulin M.

CD8+ cells to MHC antigen expressed on cells of thymus. The CD4 and CD8 molecules react specifically with MHC class II molecules or MHC class I molecules, respectively. For instance, if a double-positive cell initially comes into contact with MHC class II molecules on the thymic cells, the T cell will suppress expression of CD8 and become CD4 single-positive. However, if initial reactivity occurs between the CD8 and MHC class I molecules, the cells will become CD8 single-positive. Thus this *positive selection* process results in two groups of immunocompetent cells with different functional characteristics: CD4 cells develop into T-helper cells (Th cells) in the clonal selection process, whereas CD8 cells become mediators of cell-mediated immunity and kill other cells directly (e.g., Tc cells). Approximately 60% of immunocompetent T cells in the circulation express CD4 and 40% express CD8.

Central Tolerance

During the random rearrangement of VJ and VDJ genes to produce the T-cell receptor, some combinations result in specificities that recognize self-antigens. If some of these *autoreactive* T cells were allowed to progress further in development and leave the thymus, a severe immunologic reaction against the individual's own tissues could result. One stage at which tolerance for self-antigens is maintained is the deletion of autoreactive T cells in the thymus, which is referred to as central tolerance.

A large spectrum of self-antigens is expressed on the surface of thymic macrophages, dendritic cells, and especially epithelial cells.[14] If a developing T-cell's TCR binds strongly with a self-antigen, it will undergo apoptosis *(clonal deletion)*. Although this process of *negative selection* induces more than 95% of T cells to undergo apoptosis in the thymus, a limited number of autoreactive clones persist and must be controlled by other means in the peripheral lymphoid organs (peripheral tolerance, discussed in the section titled Antigens and Immunogens).

INDUCTION OF AN IMMUNE RESPONSE: CLONAL SELECTION

Antigens initiate the second phase of the immune response, clonal selection. The process proceeds through three finely tuned sets of intercellular collaborations that result in the production of effector cells (Th cells, plasma cells, Tc cells) and memory cells that provide long-term specific protection against infectious microorganisms. Step 1 is antigen processing and presentation. This is the "selection" component of clonal selection in that the particular antigen is selective for maturing those B and T cells with related TCR and BCR specificities. Step 2 is induction of a population of Th cells. Immunocompetent CD4+ T cells respond to presented antigen and proliferate and differentiate into populations of effector Th cells (e.g., Th1, Th2, Th17 cells). Step 3 is induction of immunocompetent B cells into plasma cells and immunocompetent CD8+ T cells into Tc cells. This step requires the presence of antigen presentation and effector Th cells. Steps 2 and 3 are dependent on highly regulated interactions among cells: APCs and immunocompetent Th cells in step 2 and APCs, effector Th cells, and immunocompetent B or CD8+ T cells in step 3. Successful intercellular collaborations depend on three complementary signaling events: antigen-specific recognition through the TCR complex, intercellular adhesion between specific cell surface receptors/ligands, and secretion of and response to specific groups of cytokines. Without all of these signaling events, a protective immune response would not be produced.

Clonal selection usually begins at birth and proceeds throughout the life of the individual as new antigens are encountered, although it can begin as early as the eighth week of gestation in humans if foreign antigens are encountered in utero. Most commonly, foreign antigens encountered in utero are related to fetal infection during the last third of gestation.

Secondary Lymphoid Organs

Most aspects of clonal selection begin in the secondary lymphoid organs: the spleen, lymph nodes, adenoids, tonsils, Peyer patches (intestines), and the appendix (see Fig. 8.3). Immunocompetent lymphocytes enter the secondary lymphoid organs through the blood and enter specialized small veins, called high endothelial venules (HEVs), where they bind to the endothelium through a family of adhesion molecules. The lymphocytes migrate from the vessels into the lymphoid tissues, which contain B- and T-cell–rich areas. B lymphocytes that encounter antigen in the secondary lymph organs usually undergo a process of differentiation and proliferation that results in the formation of specialized germinal centers in these organs (Fig. 8.13).[15]

Antigen Processing and Presentation

Most antigens do not react directly with T or B cells, but require processing and presentation in the appropriate fashion. This is the duty of APCs. Most cells have the capacity to present antigen to some degree, but dendritic cells, macrophages, and B lymphocytes are so efficient at antigen presentation that they are considered "professional" APCs. Each is responsible for the presentation of antigens of different types and from different sources. B cells can process soluble antigens and present them to Th cells that facilitate development of the humoral immune response. Macrophages are effective APCs for the development of immune responses against antigenic components of infectious agents (e.g., bacteria). Contamination of tissue by infectious microbes usually initiates an inflammatory response and the infiltration of macrophages into the site. Macrophages also are very effective in presenting antigen to memory Th cells in order to initiate a rapid response to antigens that have been previously encountered by the immune system.

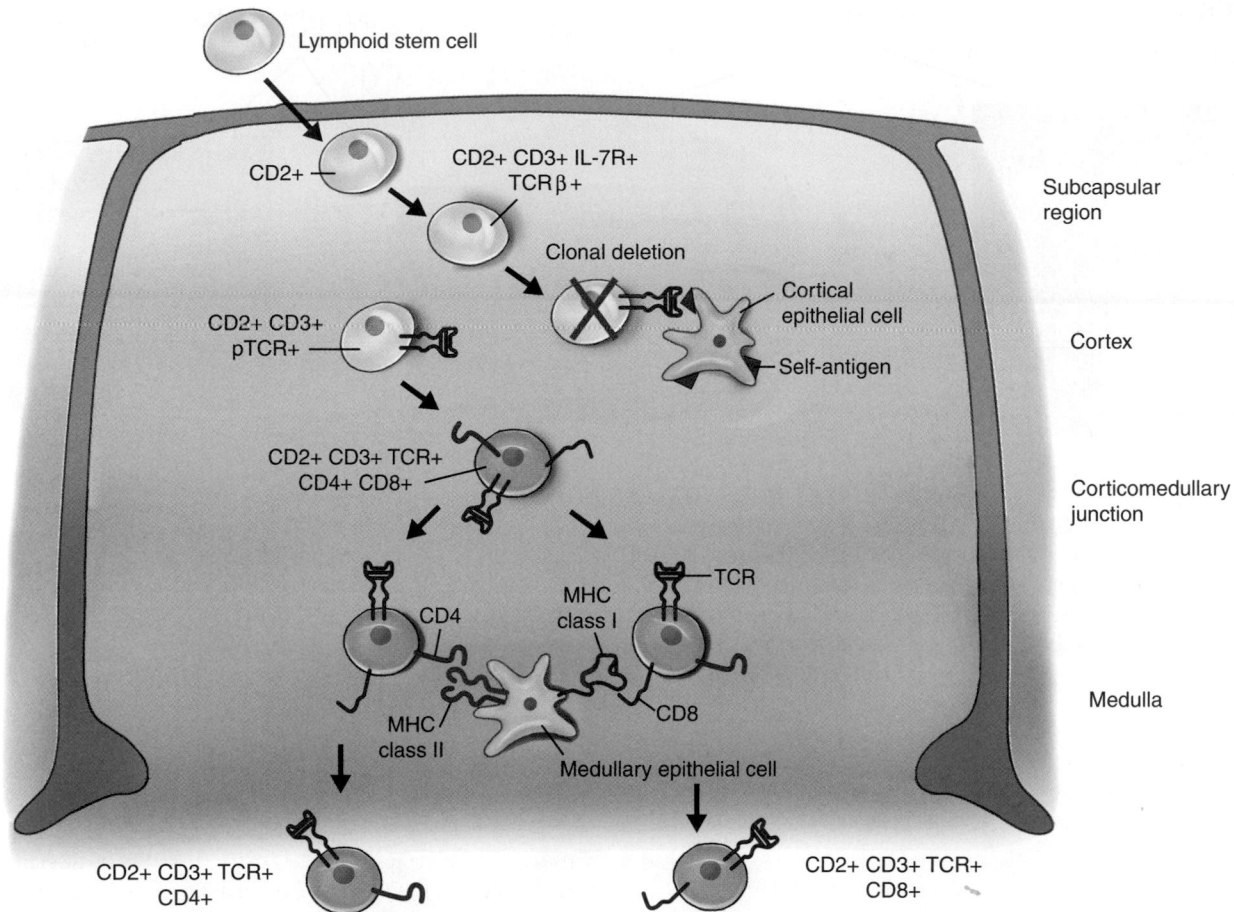

FIGURE 8.12 T-Cell Development in the Thymus. During the generation of clonal diversity in the fetus, lymphoid stem cells undergo several stages of cellular division and differentiation in a central lymphoid organ (the thymus) under the control of hormones but without the influence of foreign antigen. A simplified scheme for that process is presented here. The differentiation process is characterized by the upregulation of many important surface molecules (only some of which are shown) and the random development of a huge number of different T-cell receptors against all possible antigens that the adult may encounter. The lymphoid stem cell enters the subcapsular region of the thymus, where it begins to undergo differentiation. One of the first surface changes is the appearance of the molecule CD2, which is a marker for all T cells. In the cortex of the thymus, the developing cell encounters epithelial cells that guide most of the early differentiation process. The pre–T cell begins expressing the surface receptor for the cytokine IL-7, which is produced by the epithelial cell along with other thymic hormones to drive the T-cell differentiation process. At this stage the T cell begins constructing the T-cell receptor (TCR) by first rearranging and expressing the TCR β chain (more detail is provided in Fig. 8.10) and expressing CD3 molecules. Although the TCR α chain has not yet been produced, the β chain is expressed on the surface as a pre-TCR (pTCR) using a protein that acts as a surrogate for the α chain. Because of the randomness of the process, some pTCRs are produced with specificities toward self-antigens. Many of these undergo negative selection and are deleted (clonal deletion) by apoptosis induced through interactions with self-antigens presented by the epithelial cells. Survivors of negative selection move toward the thymic cortex and begin expressing the TCR α chain, the normal TCR, and both CD4 and CD8 on their surfaces. These CD4+, CD8+ "double-positive" cells encounter medullary epithelial cells that express both MHC class I and MHC class II molecules. The phenotype of the developing T cell is positively selected so that interaction between CD4 and MHC class II selects for retention of CD4 expression, whereas interaction between CD8 and MHC class I favors the CD8 phenotype. Thus two populations of "single-positive" immunocompetent T cells leave the thymus: one cell is CD4+, CD8– (destined to be a helper T [Th] cell) and the other is CD4–, CD8+ (destined to be a cytotoxic T [Tc] cell).

The dendritic cells are perhaps the most effective in presenting antigen to naïve immunocompetent Th cells.[16] Dendritic cells develop from bone marrow precursor cells, either of myeloid or of lymphoid lineage (at least two populations of dendritic cells have been described). They migrate to the peripheral tissues (e.g., skin, intestinal tract) and to the secondary lymphoid organs. Immature dendritic cells at a site of inflammation function as phagocytes, and the process of phagocytosis can initiate differentiation and directed migration of dendritic cells to the secondary lymphoid organs, particularly the lymph nodes (Fig. 8.14). Thus dendritic cells can carry processed antigen from a site of inflammation to the T-cell–rich areas of the lymph nodes.

Additionally, infectious microbes or fragments of the microbe may be drained by lymphatic vessels to lymph nodes. The lymph nodes are extremely rich in dendritic cells and macrophages. Pathogens entering

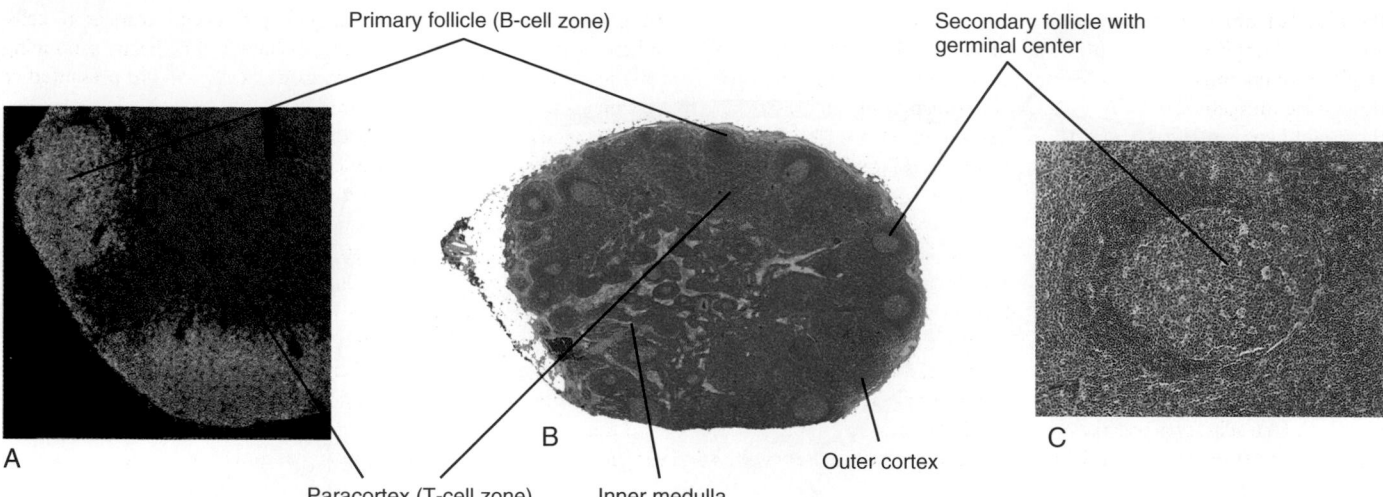

Primary follicle (B-cell zone)

Secondary follicle with germinal center

A

B

C

Paracortex (T-cell zone)   Inner medulla   Outer cortex

FIGURE 8.13 Histology of a Secondary Lymphoid Organ. A, The lymph node contains areas (primary follicles) that are rich in immunocompetent B cells (stained green), and T cells (stained red) in the paracortex. **B,** A lymph node is organized into an outer cortex and an inner medulla. **C,** In response to antigen, B cells undergo proliferation, resulting in the formation of secondary follicles with germinal centers. (Modified from Kumar V, Abbas A, Fausto N: *Robbins & Cotran pathologic basis of disease,* ed 8, Philadelphia, 2010, Saunders.)

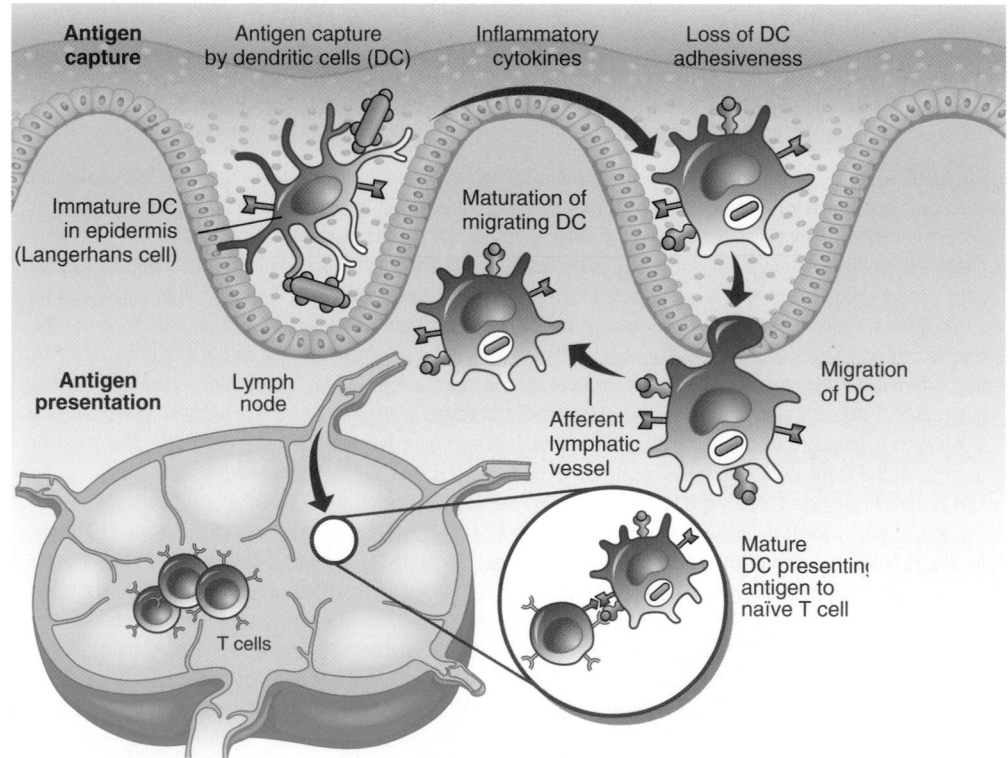

Antigen capture   Antigen capture by dendritic cells (DC)   Inflammatory cytokines   Loss of DC adhesiveness

Immature DC in epidermis (Langerhans cell)

Maturation of migrating DC

Migration of DC

Antigen presentation   Lymph node

Afferent lymphatic vessel

Mature DC presenting antigen to naïve T cell

T cells

FIGURE 8.14 The Role of the Dendritic Cell in Capturing Antigen. Immature dendritic cells in the tissues encounter and phagocytose antigen, which results in the production of inflammatory cytokines and a loss of adhesive interactions with neighboring cells. The maturing dendritic cell migrates through the lymphatic vessels to a regional lymph node, where it presents the antigen to immunocompetent T cells to initiate the clonal selection process. (Redrawn from Kumar V, Abbas A, Fausto N: *Robbins & Cotran pathologic basis of disease,* ed 8, Philadelphia, 2010, Saunders.)

the bloodstream may be removed by phagocytic cells in the spleen and other lymphoid tissues. In either case, the phagocytic cells that engulf foreign microbes or their fragments are also responsible for processing antigens from the pathogen and displaying or presenting those antigens on the phagocyte's surface to neighboring lymphocytes in order to initiate the adaptive immune response against that specific pathogen.

Pathways of Antigen Processing and Presentation

In general, the immune system responds to two types of antigens: exogenous and endogenous. Using infection as a model, *exogenous antigens* are carried on microorganisms that are trapped and killed by phagocytic cells; therefore they come from outside the cell. *Endogenous antigens* are synthesized within a cell. These include viral antigens because viruses infect cells and use the normal cellular protein-synthesizing machinery to translate the viral genes into viral proteins. Endogenous

antigens also may include those uniquely produced by cancerous cells. When many cells undergo malignant change, they begin producing unique proteins that are specific to cancer cells and are presented as foreign antigens on the cell surface.

Exogenous and endogenous antigens are preferentially presented by different classes of MHC molecules: class I MHC molecules generally present endogenous antigens, and class II molecules prefer exogenous antigens (Fig. 8.15). Because class I MHC molecules are expressed on all cells, except red blood cells, any change in that cell attributable to viral infection or malignancy may result in foreign antigen being presented by MHC class I. Class II MHC molecules are coexpressed with MHC class I molecules on a more limited number of cells that have APC function, including macrophages, dendritic cells, B lymphocytes, activated T lymphocytes, and some endothelial cells.

Thus the term **antigen processing** relates to the process by which exogenous and endogenous antigens are linked with the appropriate

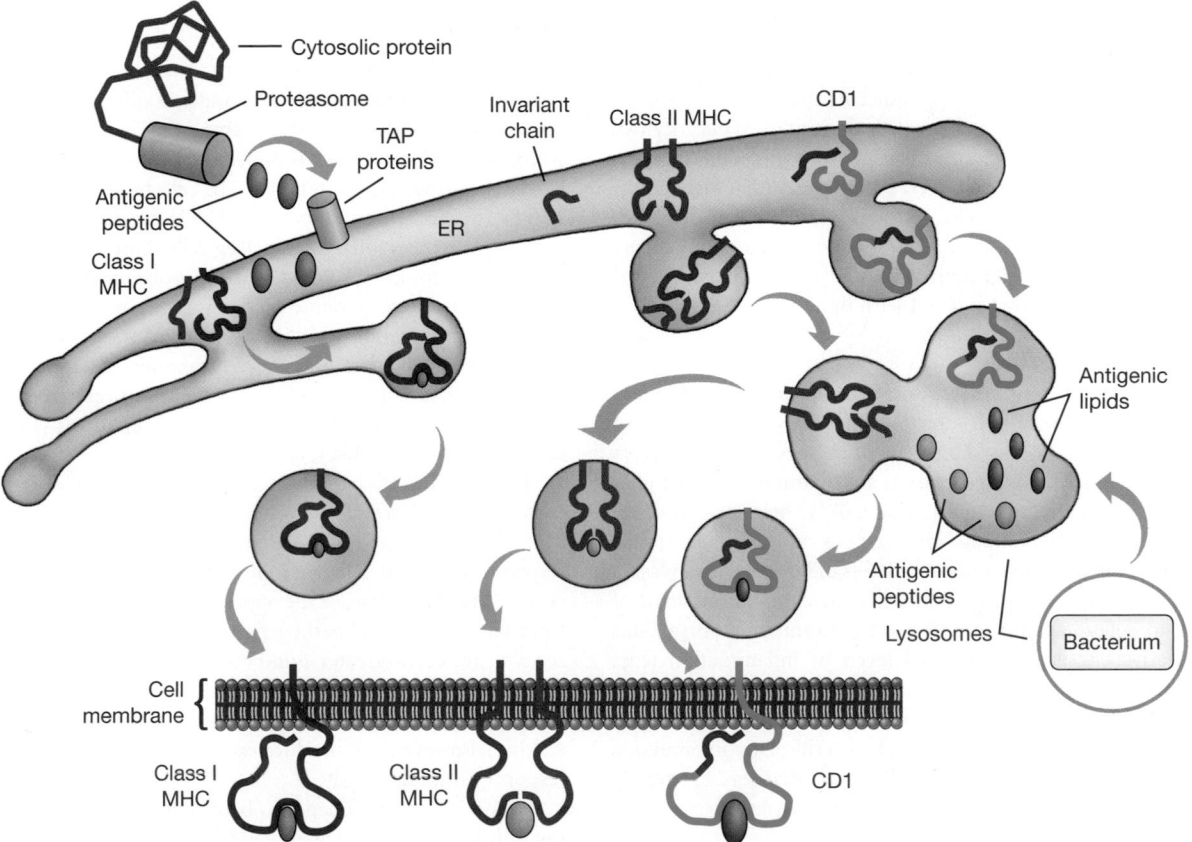

FIGURE 8.15 Antigen Processing and Presentation. Antigen processing and presentation are required for initiation of most immune responses. Foreign antigen may be either endogenous (cytosolic protein) or exogenous (e.g., bacterium). Endogenous antigenic determinants (antigenic peptides) are produced by cellular proteasomes and transported by transporter associated with antigen processing (TAP) proteins into the endoplasmic reticulum (ER) where the major histocompatibility complex (MHC) and CD1 molecules are being assembled. In the ER, antigenic peptides bind to the α chains of the MHC class I molecule, and the complex is transported to the cell surface. In the ER, the α and β chains of the MHC class II molecules are also being assembled, but the antigen-binding site is blocked by a small molecule (invariant chain) to prevent interactions with endogenous antigenic peptides. The MHC class II–invariant chain complex is transported to lysosomes, where exogenous antigenic fragments have been generated as a result of phagocytosis. In the lysosomes, the invariant chain is digested and replaced by exogenous antigenic peptides, after which the MHC class II–antigen complex is inserted into the cell membrane. CD1 is also assembled in the ER, but its antigen-binding site is specific for lipid antigenic determinants and does not bind endogenous antigenic peptides. The CD1 molecule is transported to the lysosomes and may encounter and bind antigenic lipids produced by phagocytic digestion of engulfed bacteria. The CD1-antigen complex is transported to the cell membrane and presents lipid antigens.

MHC molecules. Endogenous antigens are usually components of proteins synthesized in the cytosol.[17] They are degraded into small peptides in the cytosol by proteasomes and transported by TAP (transporter associated with antigen processing) proteins (TAP-1 and TAP-2) into the endoplasmic reticulum, where MHC class I and class II molecules are assembled.[18] The class I MHC molecules have open antigen-binding sites so that antigen, the class I MHC α chain, and a β2-microglobulin molecule form a stable complex that is transported through the Golgi apparatus to the plasma membrane. The antigenic peptides presented by class I MHC molecules are usually very small, 8 to 10 amino acids in length.

MHC class II molecules are also assembled in the endoplasmic reticulum but do not bind with endogenous antigen because the antigen-binding site is blocked by a small protein called invariant chain.[19] Exogenous antigens are internalized by phagocytosis and small antigenic molecules produced by digestion in the lysosomes. The MHC class II complexes of the class II α and β chains, with invariant chain, are transported to the lysosomes where the invariant chain is digested and replaced by antigenic molecules that are usually slightly larger (in excess of 12 amino acids in length) than those presented by MHC class I molecules.[20]

CD1 is a third antigen-presenting molecule that presents a variety of lipid-containing antigens that are usually derived from phagocytosis and digestion of infectious microorganisms with very high lipid content in their cell membranes. Therefore CD1 complexes with antigen in the lysosomes, in a fashion similar to MHC class II. The "pocket" that holds antigen for presentation by CD1 is generally more narrow and deeper than that described for MHC molecules, and it is lined with many hydrophobic amino acids that interact with lipid.

T-Helper Lymphocytes

Formation of a robust immune response depends on generation of a spectrum of highly specialized effector cells, Th cells. A group of immunocompetent CD4+ cells (Th precursor cells) responds to antigen presentation by undergoing proliferation and maturation into a phenotypically diverse population of cells that will (1) help immunocompetent CD8+ T cells differentiate into Tc cells and T-memory cells (Th1 cells), (2) help immunocompetent B cells differentiate into plasma cells and B-memory cells (Th2 cells), (3) increase the capacity of phagocytes to defend against infection with chronic microorganisms that are relatively resistant to normal levels of inflammation (e.g., organisms that cause tuberculosis or leprosy) (Th17 cells), and (4) limit the immune response to control excessive damage to normal tissue (Treg cells). These subpopulations of Th cells are critical to most immune responses, and a variety of major Th-cell defects that lead to severely diminished immune responses are discussed in Chapter 9.

APC-Th Cooperation

Cells that are destined to become Th cells emerge from the thymus with characteristic cell surface markers. They have a functional αβ TCR complex and express the surface molecule CD4 and lack CD8. These are generally referred to as *precursor Th cells*, or sometimes Thp cells (Fig. 8.16). Three critical and concurrent signals between APCs and Thp cells are necessary to initiate the Th-cell differentiation process. The first is an antigen-specific signal. The APC presents antigen held by the polymorphic regions (α1 and β1) of the α and β chains of MHC class II molecules.[20] The antigen also binds to the TCR complex on the Th cell. The strength of the intercellular antigen binding is increased by CD4 on the Th cell, which binds to a nonpolymorphic (a region of amino acids shared by all MHC class II molecules) sequence of the β2 region of the MHC class II molecule. As a result of collaborative binding of the TCR to the MHC class II/antigen complex, the cytoplasmic

portions of CD3 (the TCR signaling complex) and the CD4 molecule interact and initiate a series of enzymatic interactions that send a signal to the nucleus.

A second costimulatory signal results from the interactions of a variety of adhesion molecules. The antigenic signal alone is inadequate and may even inactivate the Th cell if costimulatory signals are not present.[21] The most critical interaction is between B7 on the APC and CD28 on the Th cell, which activates the enzymatic activity of the cytoplasmic portion of CD28 and initiation of additional intracellular signaling pathways.

The third signal occurs through Th-cell cytokine receptors. In the early stages of Th-cell differentiation, IL-1 secreted by the APC provides this signal through the IL-1 receptor on the Th cell (see Fig. 8.16). Initially, the Th cell responds by producing the cytokine IL-2 and upregulation of IL-2 receptors. IL-2 is secreted and acts in an autocrine (self-stimulating) fashion to induce further maturation and proliferation of the Th cell. Without IL-2 production, the Th cell cannot efficiently mature into a functional helper cell.

Th Subsets

At this point and depending on the predominant cytokines in the immediate environment, Th cells undergo differentiation into one of several subsets: Th1, Th2, Th17, or Treg cells. These subsets have different primary functions: Th1 cells preferentially provide help in developing Tc cells (cell-mediated immunity), Th2 cells provide help for developing B cells (humoral immunity), Th17 cells are cytokine-secreting cells that activate macrophages, and Treg cells limit the immune response (these functions are discussed in the sections on cellular interactions). The Th subsets are cytokine-secreting (lymphokine-secreting) T cells but differ considerably in the spectrum of molecules they produce, their cytokine receptors, and intercellular adhesion molecules. Th1 cells produce IL-2, tumor necrosis factor-beta (TNF-β), and interferon-gamma (IFN-γ);[22] Th2 cells produce IL-4, IL-5, IL-6, and IL-13,[23] and Th17 cells produce IL-17, IL-21, and IL-22.[24]

Th1 and Th2 cells have different cytokine receptors and may suppress each other (Th1 cell IFN-γ will inhibit development of Th2 cells and Th2 cell IL-4 will inhibit development of Th1 cells) so that the immune response may favor either antibody formation with suppression of a cell-mediated response, or the opposite.[25] For example, antigens derived from viral or bacterial pathogens and those derived from cancer cells seem to induce a greater number of Th1 cells relative to Th2 cells, whereas antigens derived from multicellular parasites and allergens may result in production of more Th2 cells. Many antigens (e.g., tetanus vaccine), however, will produce excellent humoral- and cell-mediated responses simultaneously.

How a Th cell is guided into becoming a Th1, Th2, or Th17 cell is not fully known. Some evidence indicates that different subpopulations of APCs influence the choice by secreting different profiles of cytokines that may favor one route of differentiation over another (see Fig. 8.16).

B-Cell Clonal Selection: The Humoral Immune Response

When an immunocompetent B cell encounters an antigen for the first time, only those cells with specific BCRs complementary to that antigen's determinant sites are stimulated to proliferate and differentiate (clonal selection), resulting in multiple copies of that particular B cell. The differentiated B cell becomes a plasma cell and can be found in the blood, secondary lymphoid organs (primarily spleen and lymph nodes), and some inflammatory sites. Each plasma cell is a factory for antibody production and is dedicated to the secretion of a single class or subclass of antibody with one variable region and therefore specificity against one antigenic determinant.

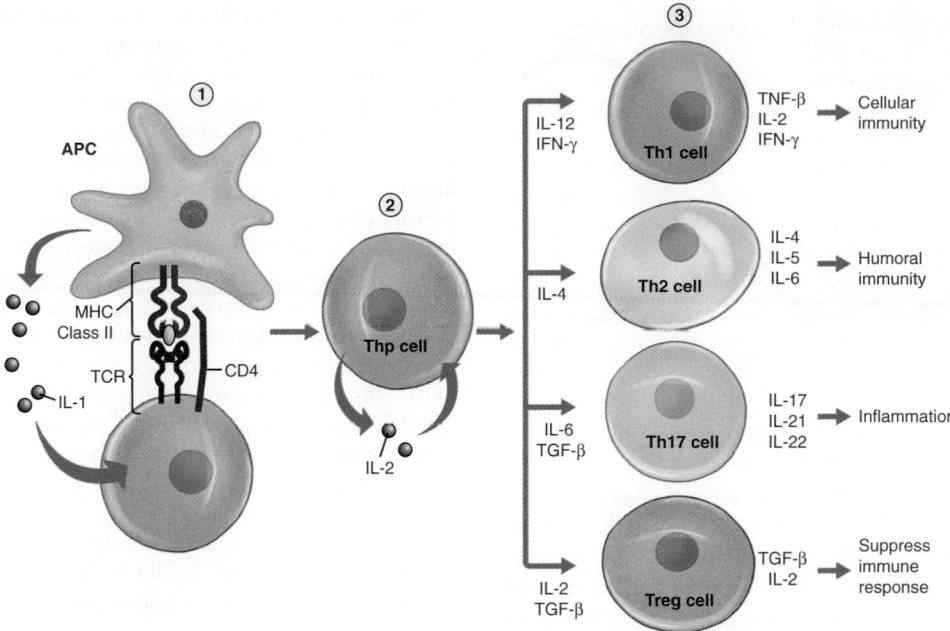

FIGURE 8.16 Development of T-Cell Subsets. The most important step in clonal selection is the production of populations of T helper (Th) cells (Th1, Th2, and Th17) and regulatory T (Treg) cells that are necessary for the development of cellular and humoral immune responses. In this model, APCs (probably multiple populations) may influence whether a precursor Th cell (Thp cell) will differentiate into a Th1, Th2, Th17, or Treg cell. Differentiation of the Thp cell is initiated by three signaling events. **(1)** The antigen signal is produced by the interaction of the T-cell receptor *(TCR)* and CD4 with antigen presented by MHC class II molecules. A set of costimulatory signals is produced from interactions between adhesion molecules (e.g., CD80 and CD28) (not shown). A third signal is produced by the interactions of cytokines (particularly interleukin-1 [IL-1]) with appropriate cytokine receptors (IL-1R) on the Thp cell. **(2)** The Thp cell up-regulates IL-2 production and expression of the IL-2 receptor (IL-2R), which act in an autocrine fashion to accelerate Thp-cell differentiation and proliferation. **(3)** Commitment to a particular phenotype results from the relative concentrations of other cytokines. IL-12 and IFN-γ produced by some populations of APCs favor differentiation into the Th1-cell phenotype; IL-4, which is produced by a variety of cells, favors differentiation into the Th2-cell phenotype; IL-6 and TGF-β (T-cell growth factor) facilitate differentiation into Th17 cells; IL-2 and TGF-β induce differentiation into Treg cells. The Th1 cell is characterized by the production of cytokines that assist in the differentiation of cytotoxic T (Tc) cells, leading to cellular immunity, whereas the Th2 cell produces cytokines that favor B-cell differentiation and humoral immunity. Th1 and Th2 cells affect each other through the production of inhibitory cytokines: IFN-γ will inhibit the development of Th2 cells, and IL-4 will inhibit the development of Th1 cells. Th17 cells produce cytokines that affect phagocytes and increase inflammation. Treg cells produce immunosuppressive cytokines that prevent the immune response from being excessive. *APC,* Antigen-presenting cell; *IFN,* interferon; *MHC,* major histocompatibility complex; *TGF,* transforming growth factor; *TNF-β,* tumor necrosis factor-beta.

Primary and Secondary Immune Responses

The immune response to antigenic challenge has classically been divided into two phases—the primary and secondary responses. These phases occur for development of both humoral and cellular immunity but can be most easily demonstrated by serologic tests that measure plasma concentrations of antibody over time (Fig. 8.17). On initial or primary exposure to most antigens, there is a latent period, or lag phase. After approximately 5 to 7 days, IgM antibody specific for that antigen can be detected in the circulation followed by the production of IgG against the same antigen. The quantity of IgG produced may be about equal to or less than the amount of IgM production. The amount of antibody in a serum sample is frequently referred to as the *titer*; a higher titer indicates more antibodies. This is the primary immune response. The lag phase is a result of the time necessary for clonal selection, including processing and presentation of antigens, induction of Th cells, interactions between immunocompetent B cells and Th cells, and maturation and proliferation of the B cells into plasma cells and memory cells. If no further exposure to the antigen occurs, the circulating antibody is catabolized (broken down) and measurable quantities fall. The individual's immune system, however, has been primed.

A second challenge by the same antigen results in the secondary (anamnestic) immune response, which is characterized by a very rapid production of a larger amount of antibody than that produced by the primary response. The rapidity of the secondary immune response is the result of the presence of memory cells that require little further differentiation into plasma cells. IgM may be transiently produced in the secondary response, and the quantity may be about the same as that produced in the primary response. IgG production is increased considerably, making it the predominant antibody class of the secondary response. It is often present in concentrations severalfold larger than those of IgM, and levels of circulating IgG specific for that antigen may remain elevated for an extended period of time. Natural infection (e.g., the virus rubella) may result in measurable levels of protective IgG for the life of the individual. Some vaccines (e.g., polio) also may produce extremely long-lived protection, although most vaccines require boosters at specified intervals.

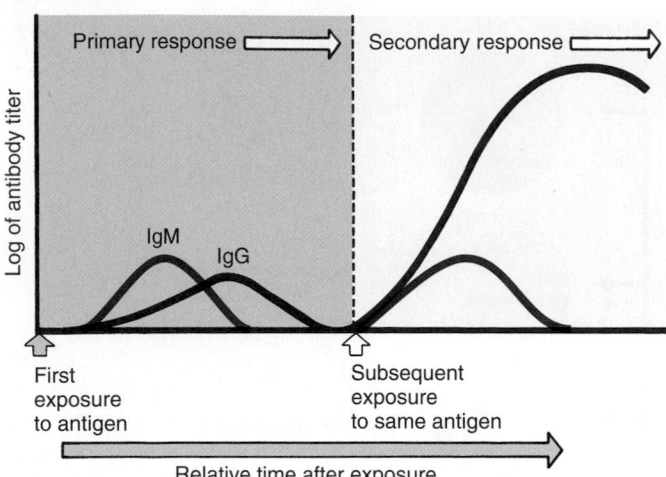

FIGURE 8.17 Primary and Secondary Immune Responses. Antigen responses are dominated by two classes of immunoglobulins, IgM and IgG. IgM predominates on initial exposure to the antigen in the primary response, with IgG appearing later. After the host's immune system is primed, another challenge by the same antigen induces the secondary response in which some IgM and larger amounts of IgG are produced.

The existence of a prolonged and protective secondary immune response explains how vaccinations provide protection against certain pathogenic microorganisms. Edward Jenner, an English physician of the late eighteenth century, performed the first well-documented vaccine trial.[26,27] Although some of the stories about Jenner's experiments are fanciful, it is known that Jenner recognized that milkmaids were protected from the deadly smallpox virus if they had previously developed cowpox, a bovine equivalent of smallpox that causes only mild disease in humans. Jenner took material from a cowpox pustule on the hand of an infected milkmaid and injected it into the arm of an 8-year-old boy. After the boy's initial inflammatory reaction to the injection subsided, Jenner injected the boy again, this time with material from a smallpox pustule. Fortunately, the experiment was a success because Jenner is reported to have injected smallpox virus into the boy at least 20 times without the child becoming ill. In Jenner's experiment, the antigens on the cowpox virus and the smallpox virus were sufficiently similar that the cowpox antigen functioned as an altered or attenuated smallpox antigen. The antibodies and lymphocytes that recognized and destroyed cowpox also were able to recognize the smallpox virus, thereby protecting the immunized child against smallpox. In 1798, Jenner used the term *vaccination* (*vacca* = cow) to describe his technique.

Cellular Interactions

A further sequence of cellular interactions is required to produce an effective antibody response (Fig. 8.18). The immunocompetent B cell is also an APC and expresses surface mIgM and mIgD BCRs. Unlike the T-cell receptor that can only "see" processed and presented antigen,

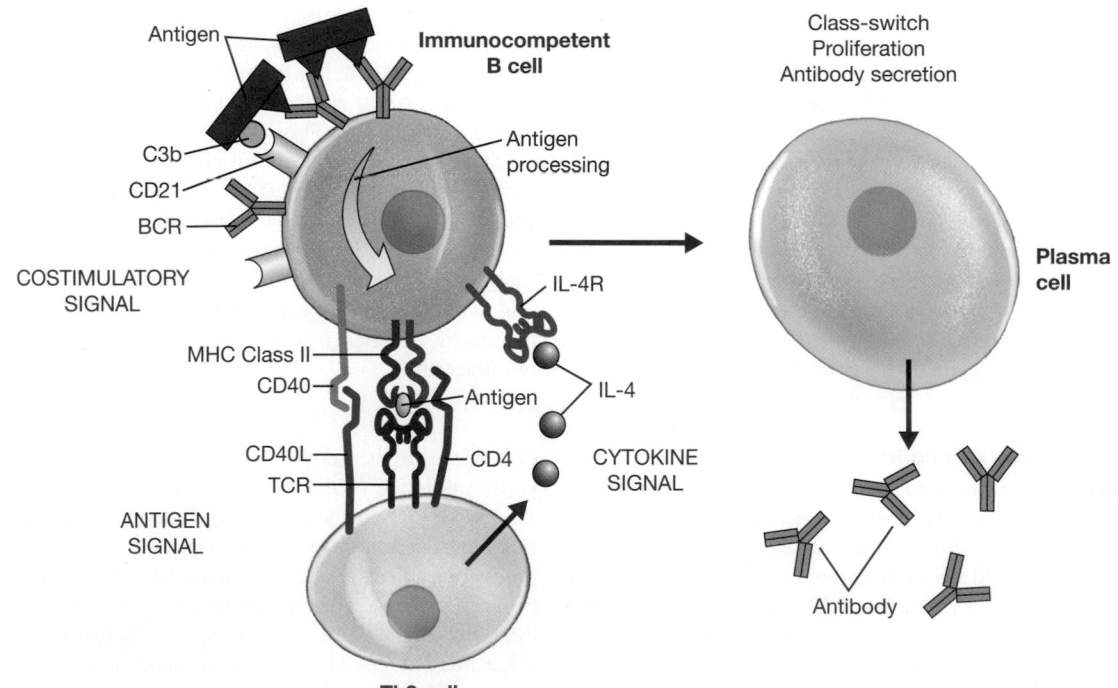

FIGURE 8.18 B-Cell Clonal Selection. Immunocompetent B cells undergo proliferation and differentiation into antibody-secreting plasma cells. Three signals are necessary. The antigen signal is provided by the B cell itself. A B cell can recognize soluble antigen directly through the B-cell receptor and co-receptors, such as complement receptors *(CD21),* which usually involve accessory molecules such as CD19 (not shown). Antigen is internalized and processed for presentation by major histocompatibility complex (MHC) class II molecules, which interact with the T-cell receptor *(TCR)* and CD4 on Th2 cells. Costimulatory signals are provided through adhesion molecules, particularly CD40 and CD40L (CD154). The cytokine signal is provided by Th2 cytokines (particularly interleukin *[IL]-4*) binding to appropriate cytokine receptors *(IL-4R)* on the B cell. Additional cytokines influence switch to particular classes or subclasses of antibody.

the BCR can react with soluble antigen that has not been processed.[28] B cells also express surface CD21, which is a receptor for **opsonins** produced by the complement system. Circulating antigen released from the surface of a microbial pathogen will have activated the complement system through the alternative or lectin pathways. Thus complement receptors on the B cell, such as CD21 and CD19, act as co-receptors to bind antigen. Antigen binding through the BCR complex and CD21 activates the B cell to internalize, process, and present a complex of antigenic molecules and MHC class II molecules to neighboring Th2 cells. The Th2 cell binds to the presented antigen through its TCR and CD4. The intercellular bridge created through antigen induces the Th2 cell to up-regulate additional surface receptors and secrete cytokines. Interactions between CD40 on the B-cell surface and the CD40 ligand (CD40L, also called *CD154*) on the Th2 cell, as well as between B7 on the B cell and CD28 on the Th cell, provide necessary costimulatory signals. The cytokine signal is provided by Th2-cell cytokines (particularly IL-4) binding to the appropriate cytokine receptors (e.g., IL-4R) on the B cell and initiating B-cell proliferation and maturation into a plasma cell.

Class-Switch

A major component of maturation is antibody **class-switch**, the process that results in the change in antibody production from one class to another during the primary immune response.[11] The immunocompetent B cell produces mIgM and mIgD before clonal selection. After encountering antigen, however, each B cell has the option of changing the class of antibody to a secreted form of one of the four IgG subclasses, one of the two IgA subclasses, or IgE, or continuing to produce IgM but changing to a secreted form, usually a pentamer. This process is called class- or **isotype-switch**. During this process the variable region of the antibody heavy chain is conserved, and the light chain remains unchanged from that used in the BCR; therefore the antigenic specificity of new classes of antibody also remains unchanged.

The mechanism of class-switch involves another round of somatic recombination, during which the *VDJ* region encoding the heavy chain's variable region is moved to another site on the DNA that is adjacent to the gene for a different constant region. This step is under the control of activation-induced cytidine deaminase (AICD) (Fig. 8.19). The intervening DNA is cut and mended with removal of the DNA that was between the *VDJ* site and the new constant region. Specific recognition sites (switch regions) precede each constant region gene, and the particular constant region chosen for class-switch appears to be, at least partially, under the control of specific Th2 cytokines. For instance, IL-4 and IL-13 appear to preferentially stimulate switch to IgE secretion, and transforming growth factor-beta (TGF-β) and IL-5 appear to play major roles in class-switch to IgA secretion.[29] Thus during clonal selection a B cell may produce a population of plasma cells that are capable of producing many different classes and subclasses of antibodies against the same antigen.

A few antigens can bypass the need for Th cells and can directly stimulate B-cell maturation and proliferation. These are called *T cell–independent antigens* (Fig. 8.20). They are mostly bacterial products that are large and are likely to have repeating antigenic determinants (multiple identical antigenic determinant sites) that bind and cross-link several B-cell receptors. The accumulated intracellular signal is adequate to induce differentiation to a plasma cell but is not adequate to induce class-switch. The CD40-CD40L interaction is a necessary component of the signal that leads to class-switch. T cell–independent antigens usually induce a relatively pure IgM primary and secondary immune response.

During the differentiation of B cells into plasma cells, the CDR portions of the antibody variable region are prone to somatic point mutations that lead to changes in single amino acids. Some of these

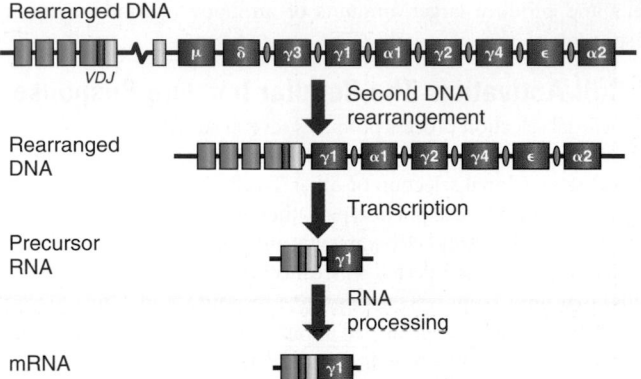

FIGURE 8.19 Genetics of Class-Switch. During clonal selection, most B cells switch from expression of surface IgM and IgD to a different class or subclass of antibody. A first set of DNA rearrangements during the generation of clonal diversity resulted in formation of the *VDJ* region. The class-switch process involves a second DNA rearrangement during which the *VDJ* region is moved to a switch region *(orange ovals)* immediately preceding the new class/subclass of antibody. In this example, the B cell undergoes class-switch to a γ1 heavy chain and secretion of an IgG1 antibody. The intervening DNA between the *VDJ* and the selected switch region is excised, and the DNA is repaired (DNA after second rearrangement) and transcribed into a precursor ribonucleic acid (RNA). The RNA is processed to a messenger RNA (mRNA) with information for the new heavy chain.

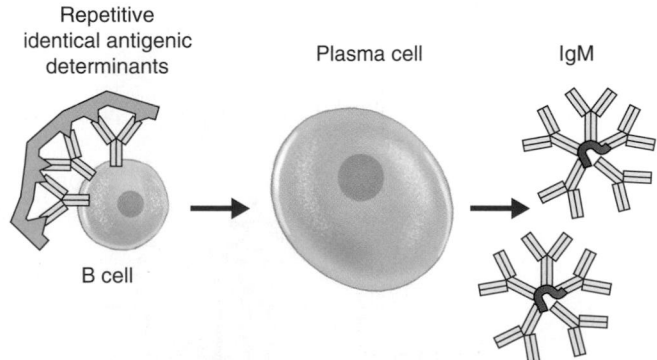

FIGURE 8.20 Activation of a B Cell by a T-Cell–Independent Antigen. Molecules containing repeating identical antigenic determinants may interact simultaneously with several receptors on the surface of the B cell and induce the proliferation and production of immunoglobulins, mainly IgM.

changes produce better antibodies that bind more strongly (higher affinity) to the antigen. The presence of antigen creates a positive selective pressure toward the developing B cells that express the higher-affinity antibody, which results in a process called *affinity maturation* and an improved quality of circulating antibody over time. Plasma cells may migrate to special regions of the spleen, lymph nodes, and mucosal-associated lymphoid tissues that support the plasma cell's long-term survival and function so that an adequate level of protective antibody may be available in the circulation for decades after vaccination or resolution of infection.

B Memory Cells

During the clonal selection process, B cells differentiate into antibody-producing plasma cells and into a set of long-lived memory cells. Memory cells remain inactive until subsequent exposure to the same antigen. Upon reexposure, these memory cells do not require much further differentiation and will therefore differentiate rapidly into new plasma cells and produce larger amounts of antibody (secondary immune response).

T-Cell Activation: The Cellular Immune Response

The clonal selection process produces several subsets of effector T cells (different phenotypes of Th cells have been discussed in the section on Th subsets). Clonal selection of other T-cell phenotypes is dependent on help by the Th1 cell phenotype. Other effector cells include Tc cells that attack and destroy cells expressing antigens of intracellular (endogenous) origins (virus-infected cells, cancer cells), T-regulatory cells (Treg cells) that limit (suppress) the immune response, and T-memory cells that provide a rapid cell-mediated immune reaction to repeated exposure to the same antigen (secondary immune response).

Cellular Interactions

During the clonal selection phase of the cell-mediated immune response, immunocompetent CD8+ T cells in the peripheral lymphoid organs must recognize antigen that has been processed and presented by MHC class I molecules (Fig. 8.21). The antigen is usually an endogenous antigen expressed on the surface of cells infected with a virus or cells that have become malignant. The antigen-driven signal for Tc-cell clonal selection is recognition of the presented antigen by the TCR combined with CD8 binding to a constant region of the MHC class I molecule α chain. The presence of the CD8 molecule confines antigen recognition to MHC class I molecules; therefore CD8+ T cells are *class I restricted*. The co-recognition of the MHC-antigen complex by the TCR and CD8

brings the CD8 cytoplasmic region into proximity with the CD3 components of the TCR complex, which initiates a series of enzymatic interactions among other molecules associated with the cytoplasmic portions of CD3 and CD4, as was described for Th-cell activation.[30] These molecules activate a signaling pathway from the TCR to the T-cell nucleus.

Interactions of costimulatory adhesion molecules and cytokines are also necessary for proliferation and maturation of Tc cells. The costimulatory signals for Tc-cell maturation are virtually the same as has been described for Th-cell maturation: B7 on the cell-presenting antigen and CD28 on the T cell, CD48 on the antigen-presenting cell and CD2 on the T cell, and a variety of other adhesion molecules. Development of Tc cells also requires cytokines, especially IL-2, produced by the Th1 cell. As with B cells, some of the Tc cells that become activated in response to antigen presentation will not become effectors that destroy infected targets, but instead develop into a population of T-memory cells.[31] These cells have the capacity to rapidly respond to further exposure to the same antigen.

Superantigens

Several pathogenic viruses and bacteria manipulate the normal interaction between APCs and Th1 cells to the detriment of the individual and the benefit of the microbe. A group of microbial molecules called **superantigens (SAgs)** binds to a portion of the TCR outside its normal antigen-specific binding site (usually to the V region of the β chain) and to MHC class II molecules outside their antigen-presentation sites

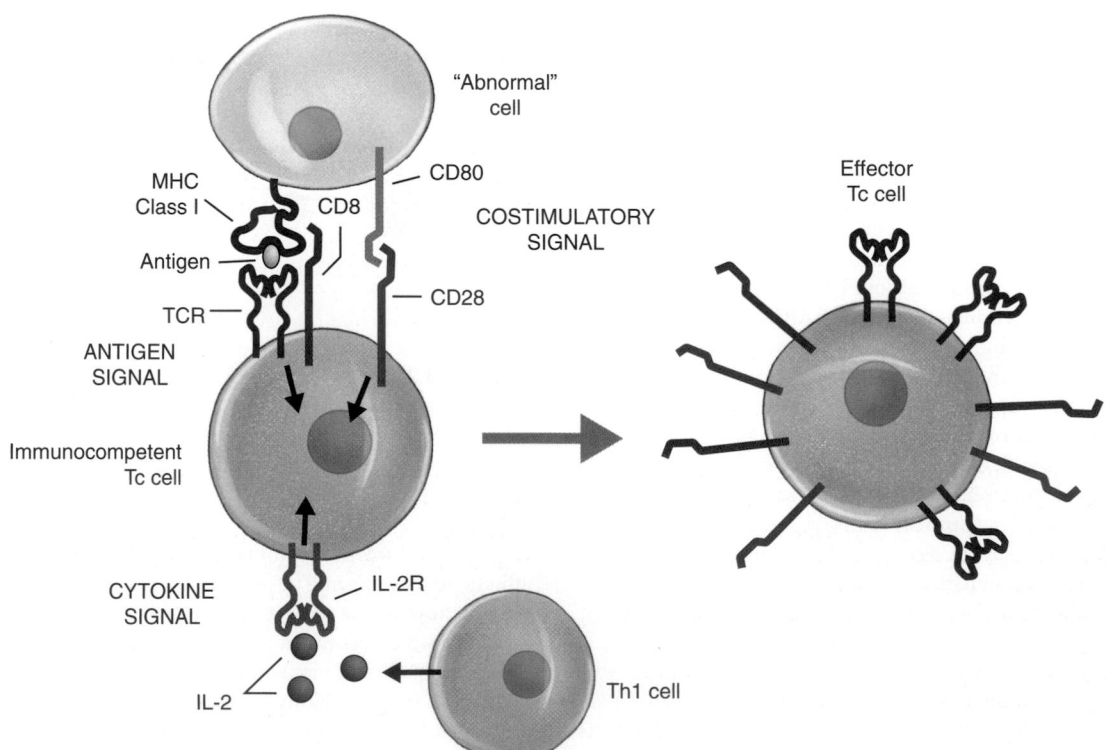

FIGURE 8.21 Tc-Cell Clonal Selection. The development of effector T-cytotoxic *(Tc)* cells during clonal selection results from three cooperative signaling events provided by antigen, costimulatory adhesion molecules, and cytokines. The immunocompetent Tc cell "sees" antigen presented by major histocompatibility complex (MHC) class I molecules on the surface of a virally infected or cancerous "abnormal" cell. The antigen–MHC class I complex is recognized simultaneously by the T-cell receptor (TCR), which binds to antigen, and CD8, which binds to the MHC class I molecule. The proximity of signaling molecules associated with the cytoplasmic portions of CD8 and the TCR results in intracellular signaling. A separate signal results from the interaction of several groups of adhesion molecules (e.g., CD80 and CD28 in this example). The third signal is provided by the interaction of cytokine, particularly IL-2 from type 1 T-helper (Th1) cells, and the appropriate receptor.

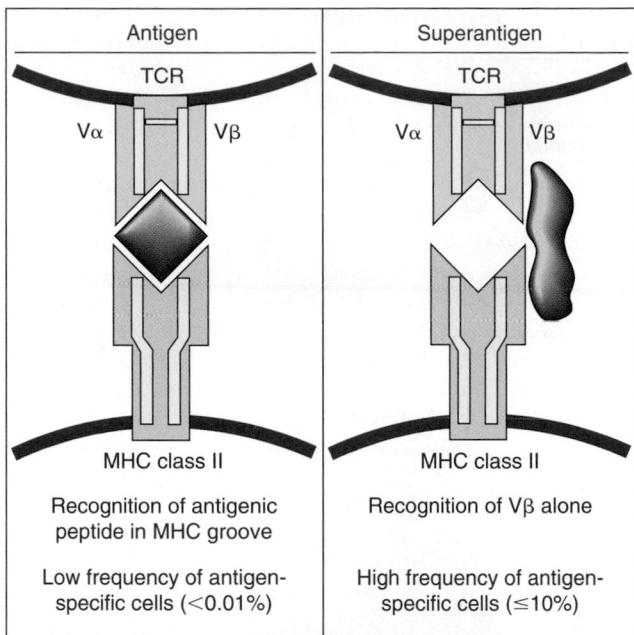

Antigen	Superantigen
TCR	TCR
Vα Vβ	Vα Vβ
MHC class II	MHC class II
Recognition of antigenic peptide in MHC groove	Recognition of Vβ alone
Low frequency of antigen-specific cells (<0.01%)	High frequency of antigen-specific cells (≤10%)

FIGURE 8.22 Superantigens. The T-cell receptor (TCR) and a major histocompatibility complex (MHC) class II molecule normally simultaneously interact with a processed antigen to induce T-cell differentiation. Superantigens, such as some bacterial toxins, bind directly to the TCR and the MHC class II molecules. Superantigens activate Th cells independently of TCR antigen specificity. *V*, Variable; *Vα*, variable region of the α chain; *Vβ*, variable region of the β chain.

(either to the α or to the β chain, depending on the particular SAg) (Fig. 8.22). These molecules are not digested and processed by an APC to be presented to an immune cell. Binding results in adherence of the TCR and MHC class II molecules, independent of antigen recognition, and provides a signal for Th-cell activation and proliferation. Other SAgs may bind to costimulatory molecules, such as CD28, and induce similar polyclonal Th-cell activation.

The normal antigen-specific recognition between Th cells and APCs results in activation of relatively few cells (fewer than 0.1% of Th cells): only those cells with specific TCRs against that antigen. SAgs induce polyclonal Th-cell activation (up to 25% of Th cells) regardless of the antigen specificity of the TCRs. SAg-activated T cells overproduce cytokines, especially IFN-γ, which is an activator of phenotype macrophage 1 (M1) macrophages. Extensive M1 macrophage activation leads to secretion of IL-1, IL-6, and TNF-α, which are primary mediators of systemic inflammatory responses. The overproduction of inflammatory cytokines results in symptoms of a systemic inflammatory reaction, including fever, low blood pressure, and, potentially, fatal shock. Some examples of SAgs are the bacterial toxins produced by *Staphylococcus aureus* and *Streptococcus pyogenes* (including the superantigens that cause toxic shock syndrome and food poisoning).[32]

EFFECTOR MECHANISMS
Antibody Function
Protection Against Infection

The chief function of circulating antibodies is to protect against infection. Protection can be afforded by antibody in several ways, either directly or indirectly (Fig. 8.23). Directly, antibody can cause neutralization (inactivating or blocking the binding of an antigen to a receptor), agglutination (clumping insoluble particles that are in suspension), or precipitation (making a soluble antigen into an insoluble precipitate) of

infectious agents or their toxic products. Indirectly, antibodies activate several components of innate immunity, including complement and phagocytes.

Direct Effects. Many pathogens initiate infection by attaching to specific receptors on cells. Viruses that cause the common cold or influenza must attach to specific receptors on respiratory epithelial cells. Some bacteria, such as *Neisseria gonorrhoeae* that causes gonorrhea, must attach to specific sites on urogenital epithelial cells. Antibodies may protect against infection by covering sites on the microorganism that are needed for attachment. Neutralization, or prevention of attachment to the host cell, thereby prevents infection of the host. Many viral infections can be prevented by vaccination with inactivated or attenuated (weakened) viruses designed to induce neutralizing antibody production at the site of the entrance of the virus into the body. Vaccination against influenza using an inhaled vaccine particularly induces protective IgA in the respiratory tract. Viruses found in the bloodstream also may be agglutinated by antibody, rendering them unable to infect cells.

Some bacteria secrete toxins that harm individuals. For instance, specific bacterial toxins cause the symptoms of tetanus or diphtheria. Most toxins are proteins that bind to surface molecules on cells and damage those cells. Protective antibodies produced against the toxin (referred to as *antitoxins*) can bind to the toxins, prevent their interaction with cells, and neutralize their biologic effects. Additionally, antibody may precipitate soluble toxins and prevent binding to cells. Detection of the presence of an antibody response against a specific toxin can aid in the diagnosis of diseases. Group A streptococcal bacteria produce a toxin, streptolysin O, that destroys cells, particularly erythrocytes and leukocytes. The infected individual produces an antibody that can neutralize this toxin (antistreptolysin O) and can be detected in laboratory tests as a useful diagnostic tool for infections with group A streptococci.

Vaccines that induce protective antibody against toxins are commonly used. To prevent harming the recipient of immunization, bacterial toxins are chemically inactivated to destroy their harmful properties but still retain immunogenicity. These are referred to as *toxoids*. Examples of bacterial pathogens for which immunization with toxoids can provide immunologic protection include those that cause diphtheria and tetanus (others are discussed in Chapter 10).

Indirect effects. Indirectly, through the Fc portion, antibodies activate components of innate immunity, including complement and phagocytes (see Fig. 8.23). Through the classical pathway, complement component C1 will be activated by binding simultaneously to the Fc regions of two adjacent antibodies bound to a microbe, resulting in activation of the entire cascade (see Chapter 7). Phagocytic cells express receptors that bind the Fc portion of antibody and components of the complement cascade (e.g., C3b); thus antibody and complement are opsonins that facilitate phagocytosis of bacteria. Additionally, activation of the complement cascade may damage or destroy some infectious microbes. IgM is the best complement-activating antibody, and IgG is the best opsonin.

Because bacteria are coated with several proteins and carbohydrates, each of which has multiple antigenic determinants, a normal antibody response usually consists of a mixed population of classes, specificities, and capacity to provide the functions previously listed. Some of these antibodies are more protective than others. It is now a common procedure to clone the "best" antibodies (monoclonal antibodies) for use in diagnostic tests and for therapy (see Box E 8.1 on Evolve).

Secretory Immune Response

Immunocompetent lymphocytes migrate among secondary lymphoid organs and tissues as part of the systemic immune system. A distinct set of lymphoid tissues makes up another, partially independent, immune

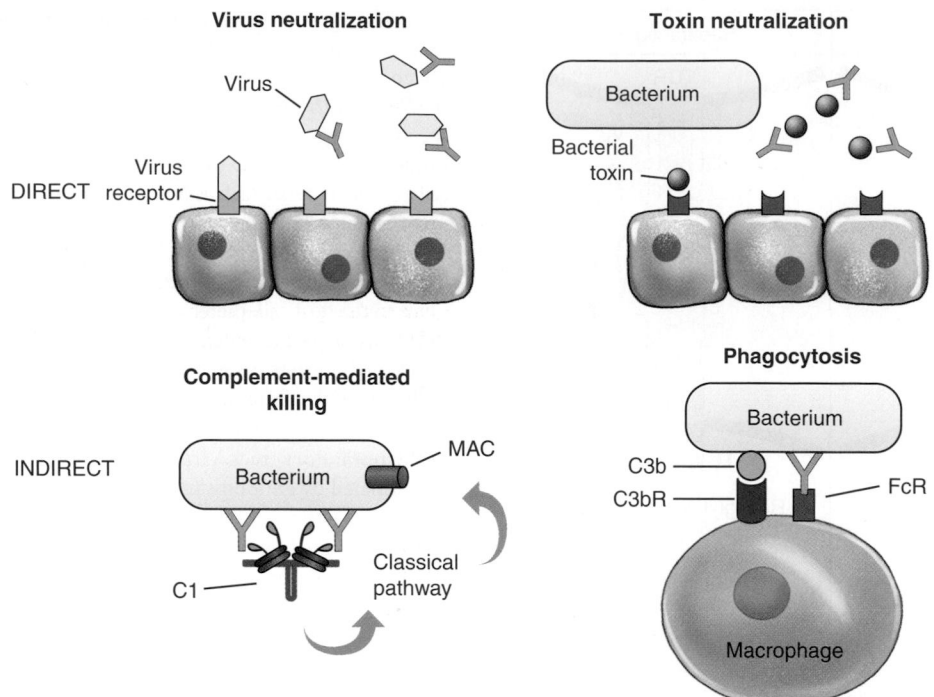

FIGURE 8.23 Direct and Indirect Functions of Antibody. Protective activities of antibodies can be direct (through the action of antibody alone) or indirect (requiring activation of other components of the innate immune response, usually through the Fc region). Direct means include neutralization of viruses or bacterial toxins before they bind to receptors on the surface of the host's cells. Indirect means include activation of the classical complement pathway through C1, resulting in formation of the membrane attack complex (MAC), or by increased phagocytosis of bacteria opsonized with antibody and complement components bound to appropriate surface receptors (FcR and C3bR).

system that protects the external surfaces of the body through lacrimal and salivary glands and a network of lymphoid tissues residing in the breast, bronchi, intestines, and genitourinary tract. This system is called the secretory (mucosal) immune system (Fig. 8.24). Immunocompetent lymphocytes of the systemic immune system travel through the spleen and lymph nodes where they undergo clonal selection and mature into plasma cells. Lymphocytes destined for the secretory immune system undergo a different pattern of migration to mucosal areas where they undergo clonal selection and maturation. Plasma cells in those sites secrete antibodies (secretory immunoglobulins) into bodily secretions, such as tears, sweat, saliva, mucus, and breast milk, to prevent pathogenic microorganism from infecting the body's surfaces and possibly penetrating to cause systemic disease.

IgA is the dominant secretory immunoglobulin, although IgM and IgG also are present in secretions. The primary role of IgA is to prevent the attachment and invasion of pathogens through mucosal membranes, such as those of the gastrointestinal, pulmonary, and genitourinary tracts.[33] Dimeric IgA antibodies containing the J chain are produced by plasma cells of the mucosa. Mucosal epithelium expresses a cell surface immunoglobulin receptor that binds and internalizes IgA. The IgA, along with the epithelial receptor (secretory piece), is secreted as secretory IgA (sIgA).

The lymphoid tissues of the secretory immune system are connected; thus many foreign antigens in a mother's gastrointestinal tract (e.g., poliovirus) induce secretion of specific antibodies into the breast milk (colostral antibodies). Colostral antibodies may protect the nursing newborn against infectious disease agents that enter through the gastrointestinal tract. Although colostral antibodies provide the newborn with passive immunity against gastrointestinal infections, they do not provide systemic immunity because transport across the newborn's gut

into the bloodstream shuts down after the first 24 hours of life. Maternal antibodies that pass across the placenta into the fetus before birth provide passive systemic immunity.

Local protection is a distinct advantage to combat infectious microorganisms that are inhaled, swallowed, or otherwise come into contact with external body surfaces. Once they have taken up residence in the external layers of the body, harmful microorganisms can cause local disease or possibly penetrate the barriers described in Chapter 7 to cause systemic disease. Alternatively, the microorganisms may reside in the mucosal membranes without causing disease, and may be shed and cause infection in other individuals. For instance, in the 1950s two different vaccines were developed to prevent infection with poliovirus, which enters through the gastrointestinal tract. The Sabin vaccine was administered orally as an attenuated (i.e., inactivated so as to render the virus relatively harmless) live virus. This route caused a transient, limited infection and induced effective systemic and secretory immunity, preventing both the disease and the establishment of a carrier state. The Salk vaccine, on the other hand, consisted of killed viruses that were administered by injection into the skin. It induced adequate systemic protection but did not generally prevent an intestinal carrier state. Thus recipients of the Salk vaccine were protected from disease but could still shed the virus and infect others.

The mechanisms and functions of antigen-antibody binding are the same in the secretory immune system as they are in the systemic immune systems; that is, binding neutralizes or opsonizes the antigen, preventing it from harming the host. The major differences between the two systems include (1) the order of utilization—the secretory immune response is incorporated as part of the body's first-line defense, whereas the systemic response is the body's final defense to prevent spread of infection to internal organs; (2) the lymphocytes of each system follow different

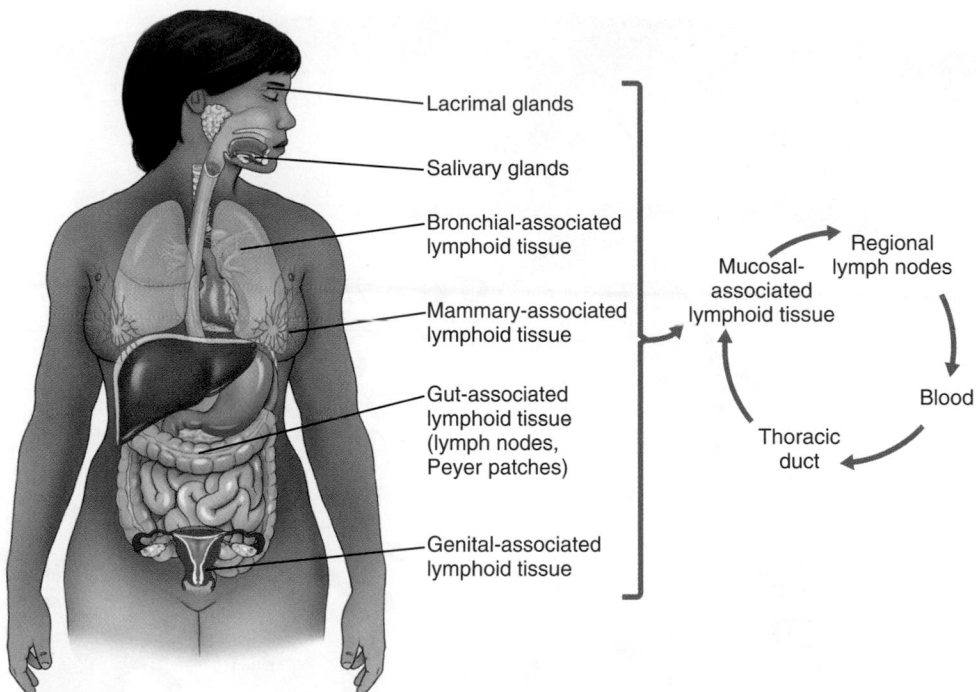

FIGURE 8.24 Secretory Immune System. Lymphocytes from the mucosal-associated lymphoid tissues circulate throughout the body in a pattern separate from other lymphocytes. For example, lymphocytes from the gut-associated lymphoid tissue circulate through the regional lymph nodes, the thoracic duct, and the blood and return to other mucosal-associated lymphoid tissues rather than to lymphoid tissue of the systemic immune system.

paths of migration and pass through different secondary lymphoid tissues; and (3) the secretory response occurs locally and externally (in body secretions), whereas the systemic response occurs systemically and internally (in blood and tissues).

IgE

IgE is a special class of antibody that is designed to help protect the individual from infection with large parasitic worms (helminths).[34] However, when IgE is produced against relatively innocuous environmental antigens, it is also the primary cause of common allergies (e.g., hay fever, dust allergies, bee stings). The role of IgE in allergies is discussed in Chapter 9.

Large multicellular parasites usually invade mucosal tissues (Fig. 8.25). In response to parasitic antigens, a variety of different antibody classes are produced with many B cells class-switching to IgE-secreting plasma cells under the direction of Th2 cells primarily producing IL-4 and IL-13. IgG, IgM, and IgA bind to the surface of parasites, activate complement, generate chemotactic factors for neutrophils and macrophages, and serve as opsonins for those phagocytic cells. The influx of neutrophils and macrophages progressively leads to development of a granulomatous response around the parasite. Unique to parasitic infections, the eosinophil is a primary cell in the granuloma and the only cell that can adequately damage the parasite because of the special contents of its granules: major basic protein (binds to heparin sulfate proteoglycans), eosinophil cationic protein (a member of the RNase A family), eosinophil peroxidase, and eosinophil neurotoxin. The influx of eosinophils results from IgE-triggered mast cell degranulation.

Mast cells in the tissues have very high affinity Fc receptors for IgE. IgE antibody against antigens of the parasite are rapidly bound to the mast cell surface. Soluble parasite molecules with multiple antigenic determinants diffuse to neighboring mast cells and bind to multiple IgE-Fc receptors and initiate mast cell degranulation (see Chapter 7).

Eosinophil chemotactic factor of anaphylaxis (ECF-A) is released from mast cell granules and attracts eosinophils to the site of infection, as well as up-regulates surface receptors for IgG and complement component C3b. Eosinophil attachment to the parasite through these opsonins results in degranulation, releasing a variety of very toxic proteins at the eosinophil/parasite interface. These can cause extensive and lethal damage to the parasite if an adequate number of eosinophils are involved.

T-Lymphocyte Function
Killing Abnormal Cells

T-Cytotoxic Lymphocytes. T-cytotoxic lymphocytes (Tc cells) are responsible for the cell-mediated destruction of tumor cells or cells infected with viruses. In a fashion similar to intercellular recognition during the clonal selection process, the Tc cell must directly adhere to the target cell through TCR/CD8 recognition of antigen presented by MHC class I molecules (Fig. 8.26). Because of the broad cellular distribution of MHC class I molecules, Tc cells can recognize antigen on the surface of almost any type of cell that has been infected by a virus or has become cancerous. Unlike clonal selection, the roles of costimulatory signals through adhesion molecules and cytokines are of less importance here.

After attachment to a target cell, killing can occur by at least two different mechanisms that induce apoptosis: through the actions of perforin and granzyme or by direct receptor interactions. Perforins and granzymes are contained in Tc-cell lysosomal granules, which are released onto the surface of the target cell. Perforin acts in a fashion similar to C9 of the complement cascade and penetrates, polymerizes, and forms pores in the target cell's plasma membrane. The granzymes enter the target cell through the perforin-lined pores and activate cellular enzymes (caspases) that initiate apoptosis and death of the target. Additionally, target cell apoptosis can be induced directly through the stimulation

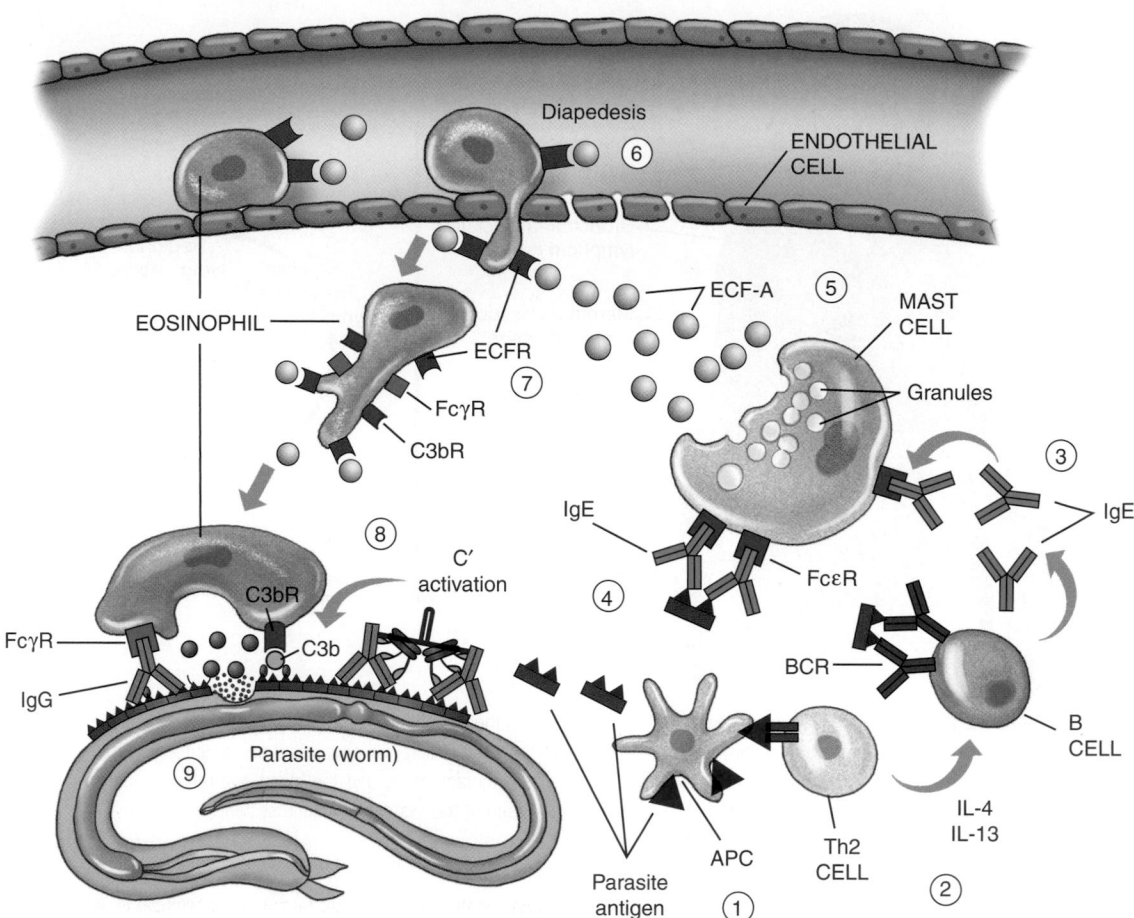

FIGURE 8.25 IgE Function. Soluble antigens from a parasitic infection are processed by local antigen-presenting cells *(APCs)* and presented to Th2 cells **(1),** which respond by producing cytokines that favor class-switch to IgE production **(2).** B cells bind soluble parasite antigen, and some switch to producing IgG, whereas others switch to IgE. The secreted IgE molecules bind to IgE-specific receptors *(FcεR)* on the mast cell surface **(3).** Additional soluble parasite antigen cross-links IgE-FcεR complexes on the mast cell surface **(4),** leading to mast cell degranulation and release of many proinflammatory products, including eosinophil chemotactic factor of anaphylaxis *(ECF-A)* **(5).** Eosinophils have receptors for ECF-A *(ECFR)* and are stimulated to increase adherence to the vessel walls and initiate diapedesis **(6)** and invasion of the surrounding tissue. The eosinophil also responds by increasing the density of surface receptors for IgG (FcγR) and complement component C3b *(C3bR)* **(7).** IgG had previously attached to the antigens on the parasite's surface and activated the complement cascade *(C' activation)* in a failed attempt to damage the parasite. The eosinophil attaches to the parasite's surface through Fc and C3b receptors **(8).** Once bound to the parasite, the eosinophil releases its lysosomal enzymes onto the parasite, damaging its outer membrane **(9).** *Th2,* Type 2 T-helper cell.

of specific receptors on the cell surface. For instance, Tc cells express a surface molecule called *Fas ligand,* which is very similar to TNF-α and reacts with a protein called *Fas* (CD95) on the target cell surface. Activation of Fas signals the target cell to undergo apoptosis.

Other Cells That Kill Abnormal Cells. Various other cells kill targets in a fashion similar to Tc lymphocytes. Prominent among these cells are natural killer (NK) cells (see Chapter 7). NK cells are a special group of lymphoid cells that are similar to Tc cells.[35] NK cells are not selected in the thymus and lack antigen-specific receptors. Instead, they express a variety of cell surface activation receptors (similar to pattern recognition receptors, see Chapter 7) that identify protein changes on the surface of cells infected with viruses or that have become cancerous. After attachment, the NK cell kills its target in a manner similar to that of Tc cells. NK cells also have receptors for MHC class I. However, NK cells lack CD8 so that binding to MHC class I molecules results in an inactivation signal in the NK cell.

NK cells complement the target cell specificity of Tc cells; Tc cells kill targets that express MHC class I, and NK cells kill targets that do not express MHC class I (see Fig. 8.26). In some instances, a virus infected or cancerous cell will "protect" itself by down-regulating MHC class I molecule expression. Without surface MHC class I molecules a cell becomes resistant to Tc-cell recognition and killing. However, suppression of MHC class I results in vulnerability to NK cells. Thus Tc cells kill abnormal cells that continue to express MHC class I, whereas NK cells kill abnormal cells that have suppressed MHC class I expression.

NK cells, as well as some macrophages, can specifically kill targets through the use of antibodies. NK cells express Fc receptors for IgG (CD16, a marker for NK cells). If antigens on the cell are infected with virus or a cancerous cell binds IgG, the NK cell can attach through the Fc receptors and activate its normal killing mechanisms. This is referred to as **antibody-dependent cell-mediated cytotoxicity (ADCC)** (see Fig. 8.26).

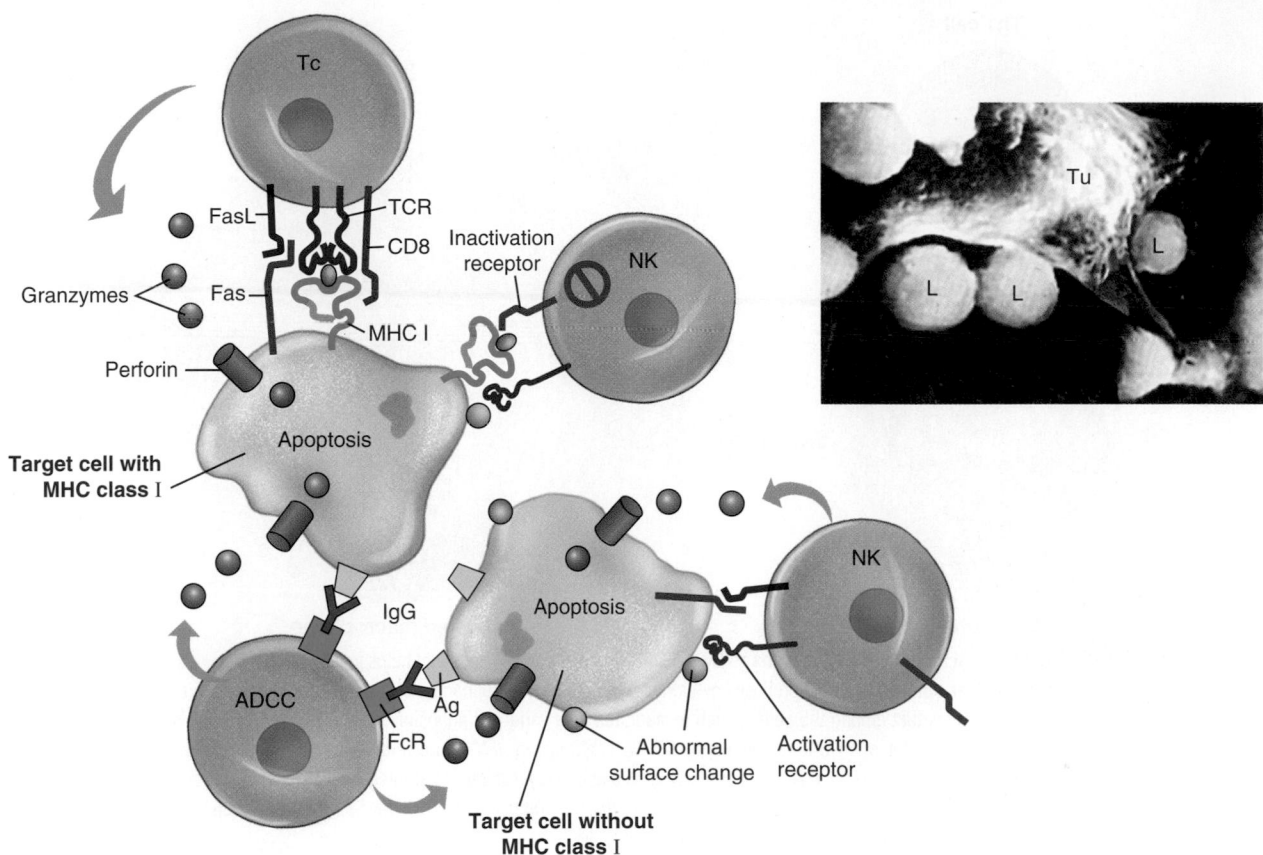

FIGURE 8.26 Cell Killing Mechanisms. Several cells have the capacity to kill abnormal (e.g., virally infected, cancerous) target cells. T-cytotoxic *(Tc)* cells recognized endogenous antigen presented by major histocompatibility complex *(MHC)* class I molecules *(cell on upper left).* The intercellular interaction is enhanced through a variety of costimulatory adhesion molecules (not shown). The Tc cell mobilizes multiple killing mechanisms that induce apoptosis of the target cell, including the secretion of perforin that creates pores for the entrance of granzymes into the target cell and stimulation of Fas molecules on the target cell surface by Fas ligand *(FasL)* on the Tc cell. Natural killer *(NK)* cells *(cells on right)* use the same mechanisms to kill target cells through activation receptors that recognize "abnormal surface changes." NK cells specifically kill targets that have down-regulated expression of surface MHC class I molecules. Targets expressing MHC class I molecules inactivate NK cells through a variety of inactivation receptors *(cell on upper right).* Several cells, including macrophages and NK cells, can kill by antibody-dependent cell-mediated cytotoxicity *(ADCC).* IgG antibody binds to foreign antigen on the target cell. Cells involved in ADCC *(cell on lower left)* bind IgG through Fc receptors *(FcRs)* and initiate killing. The insert is a scanning electron microscopic view of Tc cells *(L)* attacking a much larger tumor cell *(Tu).* (Insert from Abbas A, Lichtman A: *Cellular and molecular immunology,* ed 5, Philadelphia, 2003, Saunders.)

Another population of NK-like cells has been identified, NK-T cells. NK-T cells are produced in the thymus and more closely resemble Tc cells. However, they express TCRs that have very limited variability and recognize antigens presented by CD1.

T Cells That Activate Macrophages

Th1, Th2, and Th17 cells produce cytokines that amplify inflammation. Th1 cells secrete cytokines that activate M1 macrophages to increase phagocytosis and microbial killing[36] (see Fig. 8.27 and described in Chapter 7). The most important Th1-cell cytokine for M1 macrophage activation is interferon-γ (IFN-γ). IFN-γ–induced macrophage activation is also achieved by NK cells and CD8+ Tc cells. Additional signals (e.g., the CXC chemokine macrophage migration inhibitory factor) retain macrophages at inflammatory sites and increase intercellular adhesion between the Th1 cell (CD40L) and the macrophage (CD40). Th2 cells secrete cytokines (e.g., IL-4, IL-13) that activate M2 macrophages for healing and repair of damaged tissue (described in Chapter 7). Th17

cells secrete a set of cytokines (e.g., IL-17, IL-21, IL-22) that recruit phagocytic cells, particularly neutrophils and macrophages, to a site of inflammation.[37] Th17 cell cytokines also may activate cells, particularly epithelial cells, to produce antimicrobial proteins in defense against certain bacterial and fungal pathogens. IL-17 cytokines induce epithelial cell chemokines and neutrophil infiltration, and IL-22 affects production of antimicrobial protein by epithelial cells. Thus Th17 cells control many aspects of inflammation, including chronic inflammation.

T-Regulatory Lymphocytes

T-regulatory (Treg) cells are a diverse group of T cells that control the immune response, usually suppressing the response and maintaining tolerance against self-antigens. This process occurs in the secondary lymphoid organs and other tissues; therefore it is referred to as *peripheral tolerance*,[38] in contrast to the process of central tolerance described earlier. This population of Treg cells that differentiates from the Th-cell population expresses CD4 and binds to antigens presented by MHC

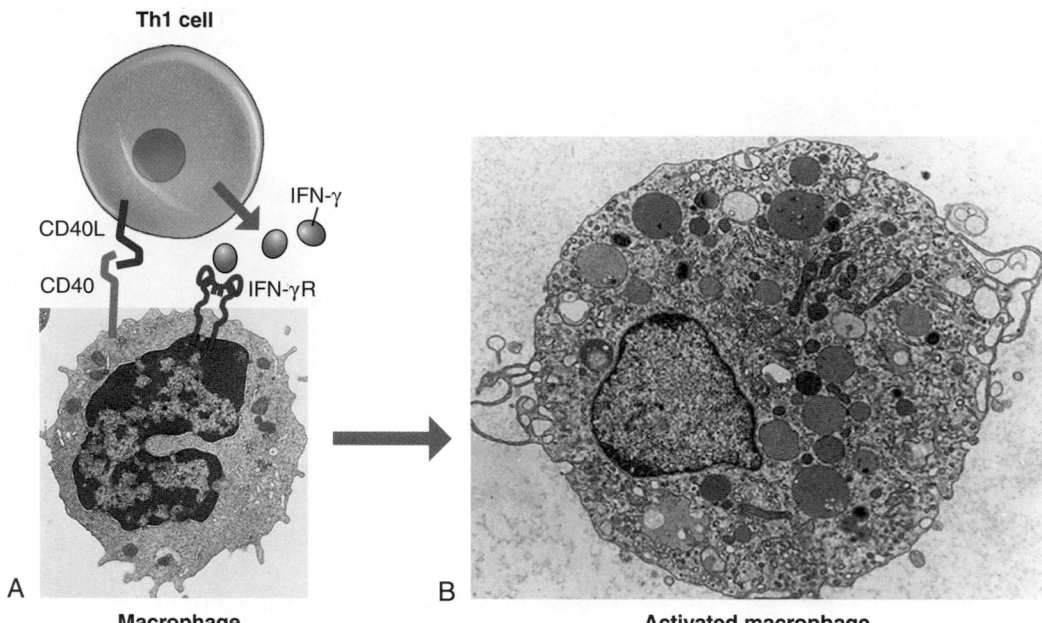

Th1 cell

CD40L

CD40

IFN-γ

IFN-γR

A
Macrophage

B
Activated macrophage

FIGURE 8.27 Activation of a Macrophage by a T Cell. A population of T cells that helps immune and inflammatory responses (T-helper cells or Th1 cells) produces cytokines that activate macrophages. Optimal macrophage activation also requires close contact among the cells, which is mediated by a variety of adhesion molecules expressed on the surface of each cell (CD40L and CD40 shown here). *CD40L*, CD40 ligand; *IFN-γ*, interferon-gamma; *IFN-γR*, receptor for interferon-gamma. (Micrograph in **A** courtesy Dr. Noel Weidner, Department of Pathology, University of California, San Diego. **B** from Fawcett DW: *Bloom and Fawcett: a textbook of histology*, ed 12, New York, 1994, Chapman & Hall. With kind permission of Springer Science and Business Media.)

class II molecules (see Fig. 8.16). Unlike other Th cells, however, Treg cells express consistently high levels of CD25 (the α chain of the IL-2 receptor) and are frequently designated CD4+, CD25+ Treg cells. Differentiation from the Th precursor cell is controlled primarily by TGF-β and IL-2. Treg cells produce very high levels of the immunosuppressive cytokines TGF-β and IL-10, which generally decrease Th1 and Th2 activity by suppressing antigen recognition and Th-cell proliferation.

B-regulatory (Breg) cells contain a population of B cells that functions in a similar fashion to Treg cells. Breg cells control peripheral tolerance through the production of immunosuppressive cytokines (IL-10, IL-35, TGF-β) that suppress proliferation of autoreactive Th cells.[39]

FETAL AND NEONATAL IMMUNE FUNCTION

The normal human infant is immunologically immature at birth. Although cell-mediated immunologic capabilities begin developing early in gestation and probably are completely functional at birth, phagocytic activity, antibody production, and complement activity are clearly deficient. In the last trimester, the fetus appears capable of producing a primary immune response (almost entirely IgM) to in utero infections (e.g., cytomegalovirus, rubella virus, and *Toxoplasma gondii*) but is unable to produce a significant IgG response. Although some IgA can be detected, the capacity to produce IgA is underdeveloped.

To protect the child against infectious agents both in utero and during the first few postnatal months, a system of active transport facilitates the passage of maternal antibodies into the fetal circulation (Fig. 8.28). In the placenta, maternal and fetal blood is separated by a layer of specialized multinucleate cells termed *syncytiotrophoblasts*. Immunoglobulins are too large to diffuse across this cellular layer so the trophoblastic cells actively transport immunoglobulins from the maternal to the fetal circulation. Active transport of maternal IgG is

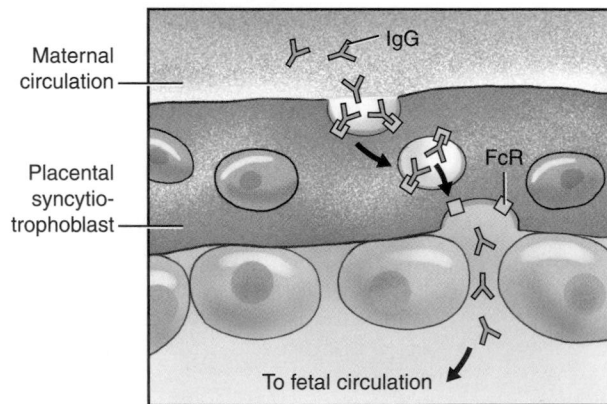

Maternal circulation

IgG

Placental syncytio-trophoblast

FcR

To fetal circulation

FIGURE 8.28 Transport of IgG Across the Syncytiotrophoblast. The human placenta is covered with a specialized multinucleated cell, the syncytiotrophoblast. Transport of maternal IgG across the syncytiotrophoblast and into the fetal circulation is an active process. Maternal IgG binds to Fc receptors on the surface of the syncytiotrophoblast and is internalized by the process of endocytosis. Receptors on the syncytiotrophoblast are specific for the Fc portion of IgG and do not bind other classes of immunoglobulins. Interaction of IgG with Fc receptors protects the antibody from lysosomal digestion during transport of the vacuole across the cell (i.e., transcytosis). On the fetal side of the syncytiotrophoblast, IgG is released by exocytosis (see Chapter 1).

mediated by surface receptors that are specific for the Fc portion of free IgG but not for IgM, IgE, or IgA. Active transport sometimes results in higher antibody titers in umbilical cord blood than in maternal blood. (Active transport mechanisms are discussed in Chapter 1.)

At birth, total IgG levels in the umbilical cord are near adult levels (Fig. 8.29). When the source of maternal antibodies is severed at birth,

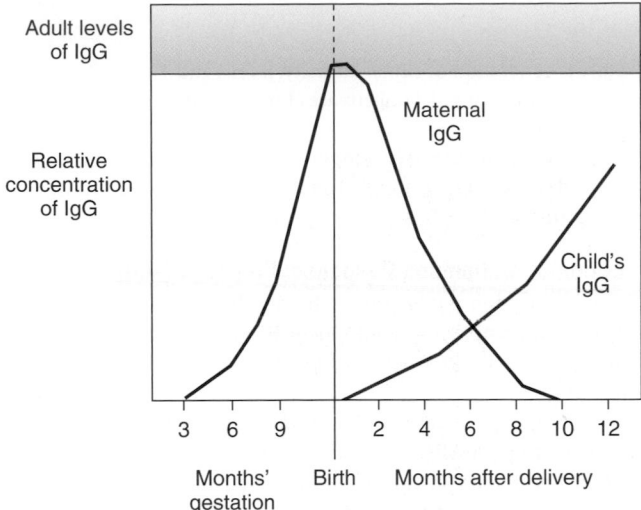

FIGURE 8.29 Antibody Levels in Umbilical Cord Blood and in Neonatal Circulation. Early in gestation, maternal IgG begins crossing the placenta and enters the fetal circulation. At birth, the fetal circulation may contain nearly adult levels of IgG, which is almost exclusively from the maternal source. The fetal immune system has the capacity to produce IgM and small amounts of IgA before birth (not shown). After delivery, maternal IgG is rapidly catabolized and neonatal IgG production increases.

antibody titers in the newborn begin to drop as maternal antibody is catabolized. Thus antibody titers drop rapidly as the neonate's production of IgG is beginning to rise. The rate of catabolism is usually more rapid than the rate of production so that the total immunoglobulin levels reach a minimum at 5 to 6 months in the normal child, occasionally causing transient hypogammaglobulinemia (insufficient quantities of circulating immunoglobulins). Many normal infants experience recurrent mild respiratory tract infections at this age.

AGING AND IMMUNE FUNCTION

Immune function decreases with age as a result of changes in both lymphocyte function and relative lymphocyte populations. Individuals older than 60 years of age generally exhibit decreased T-cell activity as demonstrated by laboratory assays of T-cell function, as well as in vivo reductions in cell-mediated responses to infections. The thymus, where T cells begin their development, reaches its maximum size at sexual maturity and then undergoes involution until the thymus is only 15% of its maximum size by middle age.[40] Decrease in thymic activity is accompanied by decreased production of thymic hormones, and the capacity to mediate T-cell differentiation decreases with this atrophy. Although the total number of circulating T cells does not decrease with age, there is a shift in the populations of T-cell subtypes.

B-cell function is also altered with age as shown by decreases in specific antibody production in response to antigenic challenge, with concomitant increases in circulating immune complexes and in circulating autoantibodies (antibodies against self-antigens). A decrease in the number of circulating memory B cells is also observed.

SUMMARY REVIEW

General Characteristics of Adaptive Immunity

1. The third line of defense is adaptive immunity, often called the immune response. It consists of lymphocytes and serum proteins called antibodies. The adaptive immune response develops more slowly than inflammation and is exquisitely specific in response to a particular infectious agent.

2. Compared with the innate inflammatory response, the adaptive immune response is slower, is specific (rather than nonspecific or general), and has "memory" that makes it much longer lived.

3. The adaptive immune response is most often initiated by cells of the innate system. These cells process and present portions of invading pathogens (i.e., antigens) to lymphocytes in peripheral lymphoid tissue.

4. The adaptive immune response is mediated by two different types of lymphocytes—B lymphocytes and T lymphocytes. Each has distinct functions. B cells are responsible for humoral immunity that is mediated by circulating antibodies, whereas T cells are responsible for cell-mediated immunity, in which they kill targets directly or stimulate the activity of other leukocytes.

5. Both T cells and B cells are programmed to recognize only one specific antigen before having encountered that antigen. B and T cells have an extensive diversity of antigen receptors capable of recognizing different antigens. This process is called clonal diversity. Clonal selection is initiated by exposure to foreign antigen usually related to infection.

6. Most antigens need to be processed (antigen processing) by phagocytic cells, primarily dendritic cells. These cells also present processed antigen on their surfaces and present (antigen presentation) the antigen to lymphocytes. These antigen-presenting cells (APCs) define clonal selection involving APCs and subsets of B and T cells. B cells develop into plasma cells and become factories for the production of antibody.

7. T cells develop into subsets that identify and kill a target cell (T-cytotoxic [Tc cell]), regulate the immune response (T-helper cell [Th cell]), or suppress or limit the immune response (T-regulatory [Treg cell]). Both B and T cells also differentiate into very long-lived memory cells.

8. Antibodies and T cells both protect against infection. Antibody is primarily responsible for protection against many bacteria and viruses. This arm of the immune response is termed the humoral immune response, or humoral immunity.

9. Effector T cells are found in the blood and in tissues and organs and defend against intracellular pathogens (e.g., some viruses) and cancer cells. This arm of the immune response is termed the cellular immune response, or cellular immunity.

10. Active immunity (active acquired immunity) is produced by an individual either after natural exposure to an antigen or after immunization, whereas passive immunity (passive acquired immunity) does not involve the host's immune response at all. Rather, passive immunity occurs when preformed antibodies or T lymphocytes are transferred from a donor to the recipient.

11. Passive immunity can occur naturally, as in the passage of maternal antibodies across the placenta to the fetus, or artificially, as in a clinic using immunotherapy for a specific disease.

Recognition and Response

1. Antigens are the molecules that can react with components of the adaptive immune system, including antibodies and lymphocyte

■ SUMMARY REVIEW—cont'd

surface receptors. Immunogens are antigens that can initiate the adaptive immune response. To be immunogenic, an antigen must be of the correct type, size, and complexity and be present in sufficient quantities. Haptens are small-molecular-weight antigens that are not themselves immunogenic.

2. Both B and T lymphocytes bind antigen through cognate receptor complexes on their surfaces. These receptor complexes (i.e., the BCR and TCR complexes, respectively) work in conjunction with accessory proteins to produce lymphocyte activation.

3. The antigen-binding molecule of the BCR is antibody. Antibodies are composed of four polypeptide chains—two identical heavy chains and two identical light chains—held together by disulfide bonds. Each heavy chain has a variable region and a large constant region. Each light chain has a variable region and a short constant region. The class of antibody is determined by which constant regions make up their heavy chains, giving each class a slightly different molecular structure. The classes include IgG (the most prevalent), IgA (mostly in secretions), IgE (the most rare), IgD, and IgM (the first and largest immunoglobulin produced). The parts of antibody that bind antigen are called the Fab, and the part that reacts with cells and molecules of the innate system is called the Fc. Antigen binds to hypervariable regions (complementary-determining regions, or CDRs) of both the heavy and the light chains.

4. For most antigens to elicit an immune response, they must be presented to lymphocytes by molecules on the surface of antigen-presenting cells. Endogenous protein antigens are presented by class I molecules of MHC. Exogenous protein antigens are presented by class II MHC molecules. Lipid antigens are presented by CD1.

5. The MHC is a cluster of genes found on human chromosome 6. The products of these genes are also called *HLA antigens*. The MHC genes are highly polymorphic, having many different possible alleles. An individual will carry only two alleles at each locus, one from each parent. The particular combination of alleles given individuals carry define their MHC haplotype.

6. For an immune response to develop, a variety of cells must interact through surface adhesion molecules.

7. During their interactions, cells must communicate with each other through soluble cytokines. In addition to their roles in the innate immune response, cytokines have multiple functions in the adaptive immune response including both positive and negative regulation of B-cell and T-cell maturation. In general, it is the precise combination of cytokines influencing a given cell that ultimately determines that cell's response.

Generation of Clonal Diversity

1. The generation of clonal diversity occurs in the primary lymphoid organs (thymus for T cells, bone marrow for B cells) in the fetus.

2. An individual's population of T cells and B cells has the collective ability to respond to virtually any antigen. This ability results from genetic rearrangement of various genes to form the variable regions for the TCR and BCR. Rearrangement of *V* and *J* genes results in the variable regions of the TCR α chain and the BCR light chain, and rearrangement of *V, D,* and *J* genes results in the variable regions of the TCR β chain and the BCR heavy chain.

3. Differentiation of B cells and T cells in the primary lymphoid organs results in expression of several characteristic surface markers, such as CD4 on helper T cells, CD8 on cytotoxic T cells, and CD21 and CD40 on B cells.

4. During generation of clonal diversity, B cells and T cells that produce receptors against self-antigens are eliminated by a process of central tolerance.

5. Cells leaving the primary lymphoid organs are immunocompetent (capable of reacting to antigen) and enter the circulation and secondary lymphoid organs.

Induction of an Immune Response: Clonal Selection

1. Clonal selection is the process by which antigen selects lymphocytes with complementary TCRs or BCRs and induces an immune response with the production of specific antibody or cytotoxic T cells, or both.

2. For lymphocyte activation, most antigens must be processed and presented by an APC in the context of the appropriate molecule, either MHC class I, MHC class II, or CD1 molecules.

3. Most immune responses require T-helper cells (Th cells). Precursor Th cells interact with APCs through the TCR-CD4 complex, a variety of adhesion molecules, and cytokines, especially IL-1, and develop into either Th1 or Th2 subsets. Th1 cells are responsible for helping to activate macrophages and cytotoxic T cells, whereas Th2 cells are responsible for helping to activate B cells.

4. Another set of Th cells, Th17 cells, provides help in developing inflammation, particularly attraction of neutrophils and macrophages and induction of chemokine and antimicrobial protein production by epithelial cells.

5. B-cell activation results from recognition of soluble antigen by the BCR, processing of the antigen, and presentation by MHC class II antigens to Th2 cells. Interactions between the B cells and Th2 cells through adhesion molecules (e.g., CD40 and CD40L) are also required. Depending on the particular combination of cytokines produced by the Th2 cell, the B cells can undergo class-switch from making IgM antibody to making and secreting either IgA, IgE, or IgG.

6. The humoral immune response is divided into two phases, primary and secondary. These differ in the relative amounts of IgG produced—the secondary response having a much higher proportion of IgG relative to IgM. The two responses also differ in the speed with which each occurs after antigen challenge—the secondary response being much more rapid than the primary response because of the presence of memory cells in the secondary phase.

7. B cells become activated upon recognition of a particular antigen to proliferate and differentiate either into plasma cells that function as factories for the synthesis of large amounts of antibody that is specific for the recognized antigen or into memory B cells.

8. T-cell activation results from recognition by the TCR and CD8 of antigen presented by MHC class I. Appropriate intercellular adhesion molecules and cytokines, such as IL-2 from Th1 cells, are also necessary for efficient differentiation. T cells become cytotoxic T lymphocyte (CTLs) or memory T cells.

9. Superantigens are molecules produced by infectious agents that can bind to the TCR of the Th cell outside the normal antigen-binding site and to class II MHC on the APCs, resulting in activation of a large number of Th cells and excessive production of proinflammatory cytokines that may cause shock and death of the patient. Examples of these antigens, called *superantigens,* include the bacterial toxins that can cause toxic shock syndrome and food poisoning.

Effector Mechanisms

1. The antibodies that are produced by B cells affect antigens by several different mechanisms that can be categorized as either direct or indirect. Direct mechanisms are mediated by the antigen-binding

SUMMARY REVIEW—cont'd

portions of antibodies (the Fab portions containing the variable regions). This binding results in neutralization of the biologic activity of antigens and possibly removal of the antigen by agglutination or precipitation. Indirect mechanisms depend on both the Fab and the non–antigen-binding portion of antibodies (the Fc portions containing the constant regions), which interact with components of innate immunity.

2. Antibodies of the systemic immune system function throughout the body, whereas antibodies of the secretory (mucosal) immune system—primarily immunoglobulins of the IgA class—are associated with bodily secretions and function to prevent pathogenic infection on epithelial surfaces.

3. T-cytotoxic cells (Tc cells) adhere directly to antigen presented by MHC class I on target cells (virus-infected cells or cancer cells) through the TCR, CD8, and a variety of adhesion proteins. This contact results in killing of the target by apoptosis through the release of perforin and granzymes and/or direct stimulation of apoptotic receptors on the target (e.g., Fas).

4. NK cells kill targets in a fashion similar to that of Tc cells. However, NK cells recognize target cells that do not express MHC class I.

5. Th1, Th2, and Th17 cells produce cytokines that amplify inflammation. Th1 cells secrete cytokines that activate M1 macrophages to increase phagocytosis and microbial killing. The most important Th1 cell cytokine for M1 macrophage activation is interferon-γ (IFN-γ). Th2 cells secrete cytokines (e.g., IL-4, IL-13) that activate M2 macrophages for healing and repair of damaged tissue (described in Chapter 7). Th17 cells secrete a set of cytokines (e.g., IL-17, IL-21, IL-22) that recruit phagocytic cells, particularly neutrophils and macrophages, to a site of inflammation.

6. T-regulatory (Treg) cells are a diverse group of T cells that control the immune response, usually suppressing the response and maintaining tolerance against self-antigens. This process occurs in the secondary lymphoid organs and other tissues; therefore it is referred to as peripheral tolerance.

7. B-regulatory (Breg) cells contain a population of B cells that functions in a similar fashion to Treg cells. Breg cells control peripheral tolerance through the production of immunosuppressive cytokines (IL-10, IL-35, TGF-β) that suppress proliferation of autoreactive Th cells.

Fetal and Neonatal Immune Function

1. The human neonate has a poorly developed immune response, particularly in the production of IgG. The fetus and neonate are protected in utero and during the first few postnatal months by maternal antibody that was actively transported across the placenta.

2. The maternal antibodies are slowly catabolized after birth until they disappear altogether by about 10 months of age. At birth, total IgG levels in the umbilical cord are near adult levels. The neonate begins producing IgG at birth, and the child's antibodies reach protective levels after about 6 months of age.

Aging and Immune Function

1. T-cell activity is deficient in older adults, and a shift in the balance of T-cell subsets is observed. These changes may result in increased susceptibility to infection.

2. Antibody production to specific antigens is inferior, although older adults tend to have increased levels of circulating autoantibodies.

KEY TERMS

Active immunity (active acquired immunity), 223
Adaptive (acquired) immunity, 220
Agglutination, 245
Allergen, 225
Antibody, 226
Antibody-dependent cell-mediated cytotoxicity (ADCC), 248
Antibody titer, 250
Antigen, 224
Antigen-binding fragment (Fab), 228
Antigen presentation, 222
Antigen-presenting cell (APC), 222
Antigen processing, 239
Antigenic determinant, 224
Attenuated virus, 245
B lymphocyte (B cell), 221
B-cell receptor (BCR), 225
B-cell receptor (BCR) complex, 228
Bone marrow, 231
Carrier, 225
CD3, 229
CD4, 235
CD8, 235
CD (cluster of differentiation), 224
Cellular immunity, 223
Central tolerance, 234
Class-switch, 243
Clonal selection, 222

Complementary-determining region (CDR), 228
Crystalline fragment (Fc), 228
Epitope, 224
Framework region (FR), 228
Generation of clonal diversity, 222
Haplotype, 229
Hapten, 225
High endothelial venule (HEV), 236
Hinge region, 228
Human leukocyte antigen (HLA), 229
Humoral immunity, 223
Immune tolerance, 234
Immunity, 220
Immunocompetent, 222
Immunogen, 224
Immunogenic, 224
Immunoglobulin, 221
Invariant chain, 240
Isotype-switch, 243
Lymphocyte, 220
Lymphoid stem cell, 231
Major histocompatibility complex (MHC), 229
Memory cell, 223
MHC class I gene, 229
MHC class II gene, 229
Neutralization, 245
Opsonin, 243
Opsonization, 228

Paratope, 224
Passive immunity (passive acquired immunity), 223
Peripheral tolerance, 234
Plasma cell, 240
Precipitation, 245
Primary (central) lymphoid organ, 231
Primary immune response, 241
Secondary (anamnestic) immune response, 241
Secondary (peripheral) lymphoid organ, 231
Secretory (mucosal) immune system, 246
Secretory immunoglobulin A (sIgA), 226
Self-antigen, 224
Somatic recombination, 232
Superantigen (SAg), 244
Systemic immune system, 245
T-cell receptor (TCR), 225
T-cell receptor (TCR) complex, 229
T-cytotoxic cell (Tc cell), 223
Th1 cell, 240
Th2 cell, 240
Th17 cell, 240
T-helper cell (Th cell), 223
T lymphocyte (T cell), 221
T-memory cell (Th1 cell), 240
T-regulatory (Treg) cell, 223
Thymus, 231
Valence, 228

REFERENCES

1. Porter RR: The hydrolysis of rabbit γ-globulin and antibodies with crystalline papain. *Biochem J* 73:119–126, 1959.
2. Schroeder HW, Jr, Cavacini L: Structure and function of immunoglobulins. *J Allergy Clin Immunol* 125(2 Suppl 2):S41–S52, 2010.
3. Janda A, et al: Ig constant region effects on variable region structure and function. *Front Microbiol* 7:22, 2016.
4. Zhang X, et al: Functional assessment and structural basis of antibody binding to human papillomavirus capsid. *Rev Med Virol* 26(2):115–128, 2016.
5. Van Rhijn I, et al: Lipid and small-molecule display by CD1 and MR1. *Nat Rev Immunol* 15(10):643–654, 2016.
6. Burnet FM: *The clonal selection theory of acquired immunity*, London, 1959, Cambridge University Press.
7. Jerne NK: The natural-selection theory of antibody formation. *Proc Natl Acad Sci USA* 41:849–857, 1955.
8. Mercier FE, Ragu C, Scadden DT: The bone marrow at the crossroads of blood and immunity. *Nat Rev Immunol* 12(1):49–60, 2012.
9. Perry JS, Hsieh CS: Development of T-cell tolerance utilizes both cell-autonomous and cooperative presentation of self-antigen. *Immunol Rev* 271(1):141–155, 2016.
10. Lovely GA, Sen R: Evolving adaptive immunity. *Genes Dev* 30(8):873–875, 2016.
11. Senger K, et al: Antibody isotype switching in vertebrates. *Results Probl Cell Differ* 57:295–324, 2015.
12. Seo W, Taniuchi I: Transcriptional regulation of early T-cell development in the thymus. *Eur J Immunol* 46(3):531–538, 2016.
13. Xiong Y, Bosselut R: CD4-CD8 differentiation in the thymus: connecting circuits and building memories. *Curr Opin Immunol* 24(2):139–145, 2012.
14. Guerder S, et al: Differential processing of self-antigens by subsets of thymic stromal cells. *Curr Opin Immunol* 24(1):99–104, 2012.
15. Shlomchik MJ, Weisel F: Germinal center selection and the development of memory B and plasma cells. *Immunol Rev* 247(1):52–63, 2012.
16. Benvenuti F: The dendritic cell synapse: a life dedicated to T cell activation. *Front Immunol* 7:70, 2016.
17. Stern LJ, Santambrogio L: The melting pot of the MHC II peptidome. *Curr Opin Immunol* 40:70–77, 2016.
18. Krüger E, Kloetzel P-M: Immunoproteasomes at the interface of innate and adaptive immune responses: two faces of one enzyme. *Curr Opin Immunol* 24(1):77–83, 2012.
19. Schröder B: The multifaceted roles of the invariant chain CD74 – more than just a chaperone. *Biochim Biophys Acta* 1863(6 Pt A):1269–1281, 2016.
20. Fooksman DR: Organizing MHC class II presentation. *Front Immunol* 5:58, 2014.
21. Gascoigne NR, et al: Co-receptors and recognition of self at the immunological synapse. *Curr Top Microbiol Immunol* 340(1):171–189, 2010.
22. Oestreich KJ, Weinmann AS: Transcriptional mechanisms that regulate T helper 1 cell differentiation. *Curr Opin Immunol* 24(2):191–195, 2012.
23. Paul WE, Zhu J: How are T$_H$2-type immune responses initiated and amplified? *Nat Rev Immunol* 10(4):225–235, 2010.
24. Rutz S, Ouyang W: Regulation of interleukin-10 and interleukin-22 expression in T helper cells. *Curr Opin Immunol* 23(5):605–612, 2011.
25. Starbeck-Miller GR, Harty JT: The role of IL-12 and type I interferon in governing the magnitude of CD8 T cell responses. *Adv Exp Med Biol* 850:31–41, 2015.
26. Eyler JM: Smallpox in history: the birth, death, and impact of a dread disease. *J Lab Clin Med* 142(4):216–220, 2003.
27. Jenner E: *An inquiry into the causes and effects of the variolae vaccinae: a disease discovered in some of the western counties of England, particularly Gloucestershire, and known by the name of the cow pox*, London, 1798, Sampson Low.
28. Avalos AM, Ploegh HL: Early BCR events and antigen capture, processing, and loading on MHC class II on B cells. *Front Immunol* 5:92, 2014.
29. Tong P, Wesemann DR: Molecular mechanisms of IgE class switch recombination. *Curr Top Microbiol Immunol* 388:21–37, 2015.
30. Conley JM, Gallagher MP, Berg LJ: T cells and gene regulation: the switching on and turning up of genes after T cell receptor stimulation in CD8 T cells. *Front Immunol* 7:76, 2016.
31. Di Rosa F, Gebhardt T: Bone marrow T cells and the integrated functions of recirculating and tissue-resident memory T cells. *Front Immunol* 7:51, 2016.
32. Proft T, Fraser JD: Streptococcal superantigens: biological properties and potential role in disease. In Ferretti JJ, Stevens DL, Fischetti VA, editors: *Streptococcus pyogenes: basic biology to clinical manifestations*, Oklahoma City, OK, 2016, University of Oklahoma Health Sciences Center. Available at:: http://www.ncbi.nlm.nih.gov/books/NBK333435/.
33. Geuking MB, McCoy KD, Macpherson AJ: The function of secretory IgA in the context of the intestinal continuum of adaptive immune response in host-microbial mutualism. *Semin Immunol* 24(1):36–42, 2012.
34. Fitzsimmons CM, Falcone FH, Dunne DW: Helminth allergens, parasite-specific IgE, and its protective role in human immunity. *Front Immunol* 5:61, 2014.
35. Michel T, et al: Human CD56bright NK cells: an update. *J Immunol* 196(7):2923–2931, 2016.
36. Schultze JL, Schmidt SV: Molecular features of macrophage activation. *Semin Immunol* 27(6):416–423, 2015.
37. Burkett PR, Meyer zu Horste G, Kuchroo VK: Pouring fuel on the fire: Th17 cells, the environment, and autoimmunity. *J Clin Invest* 125(6):2211–2219, 2015.
38. Campbell DJ: Control of regulatory T cell migration, function, and homeostasis. *J Immunol* 95(6):2507–2513, 2015.
39. Rosser EC, Mauri C: Regulatory B cells: origin, phenotype, and function. *Immunity* 42(4):607–612, 2015.
40. Chaudhry MS, et al: Thymus: the next (re) generation. *Immunol Rev* 271(1):56–71, 2016.

Alterations in Immunity and Inflammation

Neal S. Rote, Kathryn L. McCance

evolve WEBSITE

http://evolve.elsevier.com/McCance/
- Content Updates
- Chapter Summary Review
- Review Questions
- Case Studies
- Animations

CHAPTER OUTLINE

The immune system is a finely tuned network that protects the host against foreign antigens, particularly infectious agents. Sometimes this network breaks down, causing the immune system to react inappropriately. Inappropriate immune responses may be (1) exaggerated against environmental antigens (allergy); (2) misdirected against the host's own cells (autoimmunity); (3) directed against beneficial foreign tissues, such as transfusions or transplants (alloimmunity); or (4) be insufficient to protect the host (immune deficiency). All of these can be serious or life threatening. Exaggerated immune responses (allergy) are the most common, but usually the least life threatening.

HYPERSENSITIVITY: ALLERGY, AUTOIMMUNITY, AND ALLOIMMUNITY

Hypersensitivity is an altered immunologic response to an antigen that results in disease or damage to the host. *Hypersensitivity reactions* can be classified in two ways: by the source of the antigen that the immune system is attacking (allergy, autoimmunity, alloimmunity; Table 9.1) and by the mechanism that causes disease (types I, II, III, and IV; see Table 9.3). Allergy originally denoted both facets of the immune response: immunity, which is beneficial, and hypersensitivity, which is harmful. Allergy has now come to mean the deleterious effects of

hypersensitivity to environmental antigens, and immunity means the protective responses to antigens expressed by disease-causing agents.

Autoimmunity is a disturbance in the immunologic tolerance of self-antigens. The immune system normally does not strongly recognize the individual's own antigens. Healthy individuals of all ages, but particularly older adults, may produce low quantities of antibodies against their own antigens *(autoantibodies)*, without development of overt autoimmune disease. Therefore, the presence of low quantities of autoantibodies does not necessarily indicate a disease state. Autoimmune diseases occur when the immune system reacts against self-antigens to such a degree that the person's own tissues are damaged by autoantibodies or autoreactive T cells. Many clinical disorders are associated with autoimmunity and are collectively referred to as autoimmune diseases (Table 9.2).

Alloimmunity (also termed *isoimmunity*) occurs when the immune system of one individual produces a reaction against tissues of another individual. Alloimmunity can be observed during immunologic reactions against transfusions, transplanted tissue, or the fetus during pregnancy.

The mechanism that initiates the onset of hypersensitivity, whether it consists of allergy, autoimmunity, or alloimmunity, is not completely understood. It is generally accepted that genetic, infectious, and possibly

TABLE 9.1   RELATIVE INCIDENCES AND EXAMPLES OF HYPERSENSITIVITY REACTIONS*

TARGET ANTIGEN	MECHANISM			
	TYPE I (IMMUNOGLOBULIN E–[IgE] MEDIATED)	TYPE II (TISSUE SPECIFIC)	TYPE III (IMMUNE COMPLEX)	TYPE IV (CELL-MEDIATED)
Allergy	++++	+	+	++
Environmental antigens	Hay fever	Hemolysis in drug allergies	Gluten (wheat) allergy	Poison ivy allergy
Autoimmunity	±	++	+++	+
Self-antigens	May contribute to some type III reactions	Autoimmune thrombocytopenia	Systemic lupus erythematosus	Hashimoto thyroiditis
Alloimmunity	±	++	+	++
Another person's antigens	May contribute to some type III reactions	Hemolytic disease of the newborn	Anaphylaxis to IgA in IV gamma-globulin	Graft rejection

*The frequency of each reaction is indicated in a range from rare (±) to very common (++++). An example of each reaction is given.

environmental factors contribute to hypersensitivity. Most diseases caused by hypersensitivity develop because of the interactions of at least three variables: (1) an original "insult," which alters immunologic homeostasis (a steady state of tolerance to self-antigens or lack of immune reaction against environmental antigens); (2) the individual's genetic makeup, which determines the degree of the resultant immune response from the effects of the insult; and (3) an immunologic process that causes the symptoms of the disease.

Mechanisms of Hypersensitivity

Diseases caused by hypersensitivity reactions can be characterized also by the particular immune mechanism that results in the disease (see Table 9.1). These mechanisms are apparent in most hypersensitivity reactions and have been divided into four distinct types: type I (immunoglobulin E [IgE]–mediated) hypersensitivity reactions, type II (tissue-specific) hypersensitivity reactions, type III (immune complex–mediated) hypersensitivity reactions, and type IV (cell-mediated) hypersensitivity reactions (Table 9.3).[1] This classification is artificial and seldom is a particular disease associated with only a single mechanism. The four mechanisms are interrelated, and in most hypersensitivity reactions, several mechanisms can be at work simultaneously or sequentially. Some of the mechanisms are secondary to the disease and not directly involved in the pathologic process, whereas others are the primary cause of tissue destruction.

Hypersensitivity reactions require *sensitization* against a particular antigen that results in primary and secondary immune responses. An individual is sensitized when an adequate amount of antibodies or T cells is available to cause a noticeable reaction on reexposure to the antigen. Some individuals become sensitized quite rapidly (after an apparent single exposure to the antigen), whereas others require multiple exposures that may occur over years. After sensitization has been achieved, hypersensitivity reactions can be immediate or delayed, depending on the time between reexposure to the antigen and the onset of clinical symptoms. Reactions that occur within minutes to a few hours are termed immediate hypersensitivity reactions. Delayed hypersensitivity reactions may take several hours to appear and are at maximum severity days after reexposure to the antigen.

The most rapid and severe immediate hypersensitivity reaction is anaphylaxis. Anaphylaxis occurs within minutes of reexposure to the antigen and can be either systemic (generalized) or cutaneous (localized).[2] Symptoms of systemic anaphylaxis include itching, erythema, headaches, vomiting, abdominal cramps, diarrhea, and breathing difficulties. The most severe reactions may include contraction of bronchial smooth muscle, laryngeal edema, and vascular collapse and decreased blood pressure that can lead to shock and death. Examples of systemic anaphylaxis are allergic reactions to bee stings, peanuts, eggs, and shellfish. Cutaneous anaphylaxis results in local symptoms, such as pain, swelling, and redness, which occur at the site of exposure to an antigen (e.g., a painful local reaction to an injected vaccine or drug).

Type I: IgE-Mediated Hypersensitivity Reactions

Type I (IgE-mediated) hypersensitivity reactions are mediated by antigen-specific IgE and the products of tissue mast cells[3] (Fig. 9.1). Most common allergies (e.g., pollen allergies) are type I reactions. In addition, most type I reactions occur against environmental antigens and are therefore allergic. Because of this strong association, many healthcare professionals use the term *allergy* to indicate only IgE-mediated reactions. However, IgE can contribute to a few autoimmune and alloimmune diseases, and many common allergies (e.g., poison ivy) are not mediated by IgE.

In some individuals, exposure to an environmental antigen causes primarily IgE production. Repeated exposure to the antigen usually is required to elicit enough IgE so that the person becomes "sensitized." IgE has a relatively short life span in the blood because it rapidly binds to very-high-affinity Fc receptors on the plasma membranes of mast cells (see Fig. 9.1). The subclass IgG4 also has specific receptors on the mast cell and may contribute to the type I mechanism. Antibody that binds to mast cells is termed cytotropic antibody (able to bind to cell surfaces) or reagin (skin-sensitizing antibody). Unlike Fc receptors on phagocytes, which bind IgG that has reacted with antigen, the Fc receptors on mast cells bind with IgE that has not previously interacted with antigen.

If further exposure of a sensitized individual to the antigen occurs, one molecule of antigen may bind simultaneously to two molecules of IgE-Fc receptor complexes on the mast cell's surface (cross-link) resulting in activation of intracellular signaling pathways and mast cell degranulation (see Fig. 9.1, *B*, and Chapter 7). The antigen that triggers cross-linking must have at least two antigenic determinants on the same molecule. Sometimes an IgE-mediated response is beneficial to the host, as is the case of some immune reactions against parasites. (This mechanism is described in Chapter 8 and illustrated in Fig. 8.25.) The products of mast cell degranulation can modulate almost all aspects of an acute inflammatory response. (The effects of biochemical mediators released by mast cells are illustrated in Fig. 7.11).

The most potent mediator is histamine, which affects several key target cells. Acting through the H1 receptors, histamine contracts bronchial smooth muscles, causing bronchial constriction; increases vascular permeability, causing edema; and causes vasodilation, increasing

TABLE 9.2 DISORDERS ASSOCIATED WITH AUTOIMMUNITY

SYSTEM DISEASE	ORGAN OR TISSUE	PROBABLE SELF-ANTIGEN
Endocrine System		
Hyperthyroidism (Graves disease)	Thyroid gland	Receptors for thyroid-stimulating hormone on plasma membrane of thyroid cells
Autoimmune thyroiditis	Thyroid gland	Thyroglobulin; microsomes
Primary myxedema	Thyroid gland	Microsomes
Insulin-dependent diabetes	Pancreas	Islet cells, insulin, and insulin receptors on pancreatic cells
Addison disease	Adrenal gland	Surface antigens on steroid-producing cells; microsomes of adrenal cortex
Premature gonadal failure	Ovary	Interstitial cells; corpus luteum
Male infertility	Testis	Surface antigens on spermatozoa
Orchitis	Testis	Germinal epithelium
Female infertility	Ovary	Zona pellucida
Idiopathic hypoparathyroidism	Parathyroid gland	Surface antigens on chief cells (epithelial cells of gland)
Partial pituitary deficiency	Pituitary gland	Prolactin-producing cells; growth hormone–producing cells
Skin		
Pemphigus vulgaris	Skin	Intercellular substances in stratified squamous epithelium
Bullous pemphigoid	Skin	Basement membrane
Dermatitis herpetiformis	Skin	Basement membrane (immunoglobulin A [IgA])
Vitiligo	Skin	Surface antigens on melanocytes (melanin-producing cells)
Neuromuscular Tissue		
Polymyositis (dermatomyositis)	Muscle	Nuclear materials; myosin
Multiple sclerosis	Neural tissue	Unknown
Myasthenia gravis	Neuromuscular junction	Acetylcholine receptors; striations of skeletal and cardiac muscle
Polyneuritis	Nerve cell	Peripheral myelin
Rheumatic fever	Heart	Cardiac tissue (subsarcolemmal membrane); cross reaction with group A streptococcal antigen
Cardiomyopathy	Heart	Cardiac muscle
Postvaccinal or postinfectious encephalitis	Central nervous system	Central nervous system myelin or basic protein
Gastrointestinal System		
Celiac disease (gluten-sensitive enteropathy)	Intestine	Gluten
Ulcerative colitis	Colon	Mucosal cells
Crohn disease	Ileum	Unknown
Pernicious anemia	Stomach	Surface antigens of parietal cells; intrinsic factor
Atrophic gastritis	Stomach	Parietal cells
Primary biliary cirrhosis	Liver	Mitochondria; cells of bile duct
Chronic active hepatitis	Liver	Surface antigens, nuclei, microsomes, mitochondria or hepatocytes; smooth muscle
Eye		
Sjögren syndrome	Lacrimal gland	Antigens of lacrimal gland, salivary gland, thyroid, and nuclei of cells; immunoglobulin G (IgG)
Uveitis	Uveal structures	Antigens of the iris, ciliary body, and choroid

Continued

TABLE 9.2   DISORDERS ASSOCIATED WITH AUTOIMMUNITY—cont'd

SYSTEM DISEASE	ORGAN OR TISSUE	PROBABLE SELF-ANTIGEN
Connective Tissue		
Ankylosing spondylitis	Joints	Sacroiliac and spinal apophyseal joint
Rheumatoid arthritis	Joints	IgG; collagen
Systemic lupus erythematosus	Multiple sites	Numerous antigens in nuclei, organelles, and extracellular matrix
Mixed connective tissue disease	Multiple sites	Ribonucleoprotein and numerous other nucleoproteins
Polyarteritis nodosa (necrotizing vasculitis)	Arterioles (small arteries)	Unknown
Scleroderma (progressive systemic sclerosis)	Multiple organs	Nuclear antigens; IgG
Felty syndrome	Joints	IgG
Antiphospholipid antibody syndrome	Platelets, endothelial cells, trophoblast of placenta	Membrane phospholipids, especially phosphatidylserine
Renal System		
Immune complex glomerulonephritis	Kidney	Numerous immune complexes
Goodpasture syndrome	Kidney	Glomerular basement membrane
Hematologic System		
Idiopathic neutropenia	Neutrophil	Surface antigens on polymorphonuclear neutrophils
Idiopathic lymphopenia	Lymphocytes	Surface antigens on lymphocytes
Autoimmune hemolytic anemia	Erythrocytes	Surface antigens on erythrocytes
Autoimmune thrombocytopenic purpura	Platelets	Surface antigens on platelets
Respiratory System		
Goodpasture syndrome	Lung	Septal membrane of alveolus

TABLE 9.3   IMMUNOLOGIC MECHANISMS OF TISSUE DESTRUCTION

TYPE	NAME	RATE OF DEVELOPMENT	CLASS OF ANTIBODY INVOLVED	PRINCIPAL EFFECTOR CELLS INVOLVED	COMPLEMENT PARTICIPATION	EXAMPLES OF DISORDERS
I	IgE-mediated reaction	Immediate	IgE	Mast cells	No	Seasonal allergic rhinitis
II	Tissue-specific reaction	Immediate	IgG, IgM	Macrophages in tissues	Frequently	Autoimmune thrombocytopenic purpura, Graves disease, autoimmune hemolytic anemia
III	Immune complex–mediated reaction	Immediate	IgG, IgM	Neutrophils	Yes	Systemic lupus erythematosus
IV	Cell-mediated reaction	Delayed	None	Lymphocytes, macrophages	No	Contact sensitivity to poison ivy and metals (jewelry)

Ig, Immunoglobulin.

blood flow into the affected area (see Figs. 7.3 and 7.12). The interaction of histamine with H2 receptors results in increased gastric acid secretion and a decrease of histamine released from mast cells and basophils. The action of histamine through H2 receptors suggests an important negative-feedback mechanism that stops degranulation. That is, the released histamine inhibits release of additional histamine by interacting with H2 receptors on the mast cells. Histamine also may affect control of the immune response through H2 receptors on most cells of the immune system. Another important activity of histamine is enhancement of the chemotactic activity of other factors, such as eosinophil chemotactic factor of anaphylaxis (ECF-A), which attracts eosinophils into sites of allergic inflammatory reactions and prevents them from migrating out of the inflammatory site. (The role of the eosinophil in inflammation is discussed in Chapter 7.) Blocking histamine receptors with antihistamines can control some type I responses.

Mast cells also initiate synthesis of bioactive lipid-derived mediators, such as leukotrienes, platelet-activating factor (PAF), and prostaglandins. Each is released much more slowly than histamine and can mediate similar, yet more prolonged, clinical symptoms, such as recruiting inflammatory cells (e.g., neutrophils, eosinophils), promoting vascular permeability and edema, inducing bronchoconstriction or rhinitis, and inducing further release of histamine from mast cells.[4] Therapy includes the use of competitive inhibitors of receptors for lipid mediators. Montelukast (a leukotriene receptor inhibitor), rupatadine (a PAF receptor inhibitor), and others are in clinical use.

Type II: Tissue-Specific Hypersensitivity Reactions

Type II (tissue-specific) hypersensitivity reactions are generally characterized by a specific cell or tissue being the target of an immune response. In addition to major histocompatibility locus antigens (i.e.,

human leukocyte antigens [HLAs]; discussed in Chapter 8), most cells have other antigens on their surfaces. Some of these other antigens are called tissue-specific antigens because they are expressed on the plasma membranes of only certain cells in specific tissues. Platelets, for example, have groups of antigens that are found on no other cells of the body. The symptoms of many type II diseases are determined by which tissue or organ expresses the particular antigen. Environmental antigens (e.g., drugs or their metabolites) may bind to the plasma membranes of specific

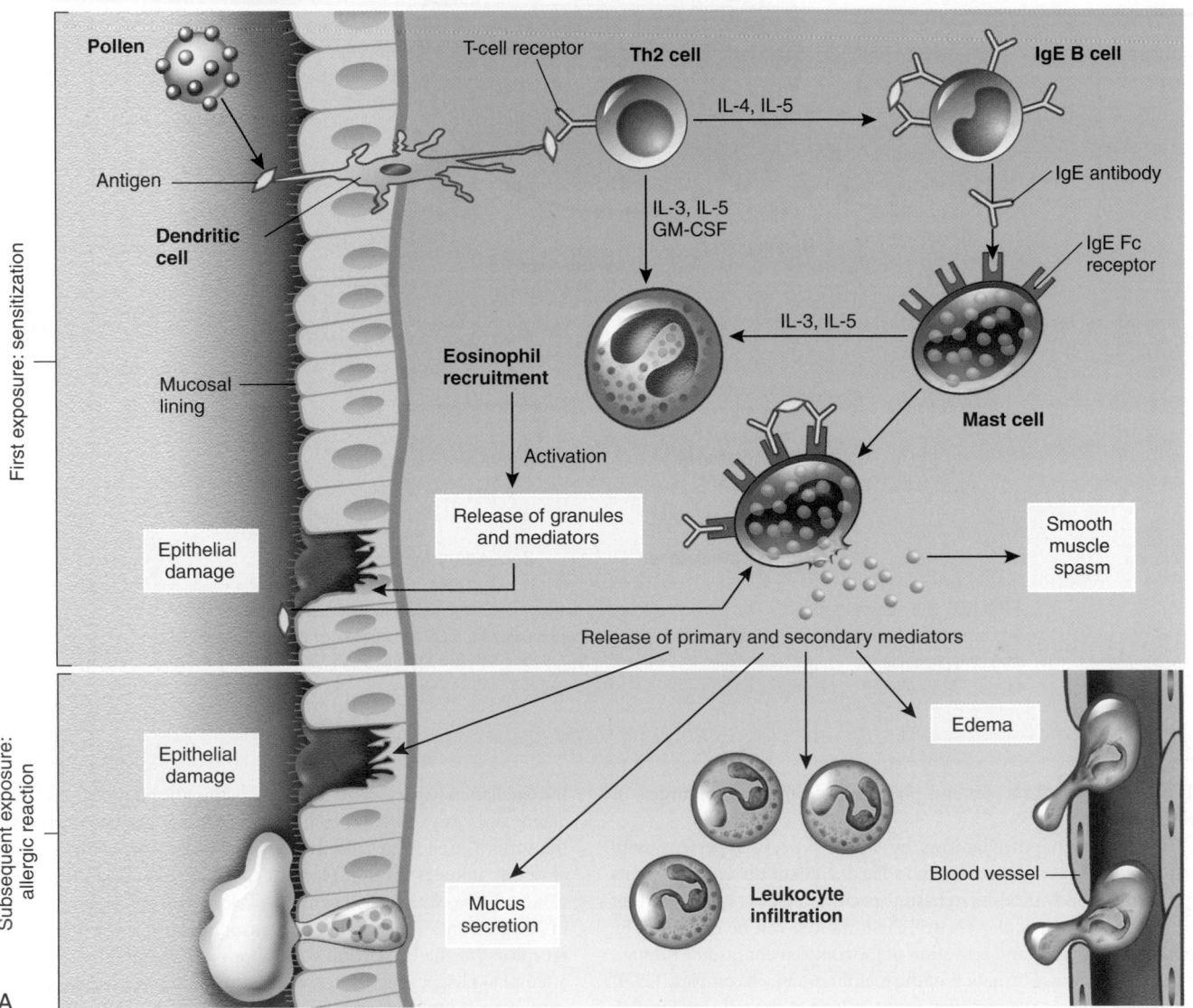

FIGURE 9.1 Mechanism of Type I IgE–Mediated Reactions. A, Th2 cells are activated by antigen-presenting dendritic cells to produce cytokines, including IL-3, IL-4, IL-5, and granulocyte-macrophage colony-stimulating factor (GM-CSF). IL-3, IL-5, and GM-CSF attract and promote the survival of eosinophils. Other cytokines (e.g., IL-4) induce B cells to class-switch to IgE-producing plasma cells. The IgE coats the surface of the mast cell by binding with IgE-specific Fc receptors on the mast cell's plasma membrane (sensitization). Further exposure to the same allergen cross-links the surface-bound IgE and activates signals from the cytoplasmic portion of the IgE Fc receptors. These signals initiate two parallel and interdependent processes: mast cell degranulation and discharge of preformed mediators (e.g., histamine, eosinophil-chemotactic factor of anaphylaxis) and production of newly formed mediators such as arachidonic metabolites (leukotrienes, prostaglandins). Many local type I hypersensitivity reactions have two well-defined phases. The initial phase is characterized by vasodilation, vascular leakage, and, depending on the location, smooth muscle spasm or glandular secretions. These changes usually become evident within 5 to 30 minutes after exposure to the antigen. The late phase occurs 2 to 8 hours later without additional exposure to the antigen. The late phase has more intense infiltration of tissues with eosinophils, neutrophils, basophils, monocytes, and Th cells and tissue destruction in the form of mucosal epithelial cell damage.   *Continued*

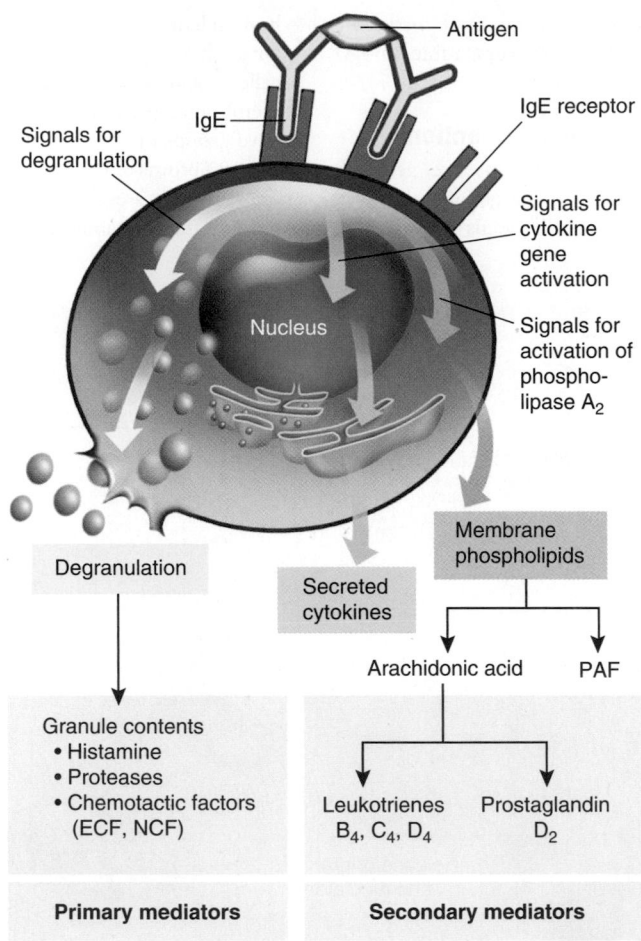

FIGURE 9.1, cont'd B, Activation of mast cells leading to degranulation of preformed mediators (primary mediators) and synthesis of newly formed (de novo) mediators (secondary mediators). *ECF,* Eosinophilic chemotactic factor; *Fc,* fragment crystallizable; *Ig,* immunoglobulin; *IL,* interleukin; *NCF,* neutrophil chemotactic factor; *PAF,* platelet-activating factor; *Th,* T-helper.

cells (especially erythrocytes and platelets) and function as targets of type II reactions.

The five general mechanisms by which type II hypersensitivity reactions can affect cells are shown in Fig. 9.2. All of these mechanisms begin with antibody binding to tissue-specific antigens or antigens that have attached to particular tissues. First, the cell can be destroyed by antibody (IgG or IgM) and activation of the complement cascade through the classical pathway. Formation of the membrane attack complex (C5-9) damages the membrane and may result in lysis of the cell (see Fig. 9.2, *A*). For example, erythrocytes are destroyed by complement-mediated lysis in individuals with autoimmune hemolytic anemia (see Chapter 29) or as a result of an alloimmune reaction to ABO-mismatched transfused blood cells.

Second, antibody may cause cell destruction through phagocytosis by macrophages. IgG and also C3b of the complement system are opsonins that bind to receptors on the macrophage (see Fig. 9.2, *B*). Phagocytosis of the target cell follows. (Phagocytosis is illustrated in Figs. 7.15 and 7.16.) For example, antibodies against platelet-specific antigens or against red blood cell antigens of the Rh system coat those cells at low density, resulting in their preferential removal by phagocytosis in the spleen, rather than by complement-mediated lysis.

Third, antibody and complement may attract neutrophils. Either antigen expressed normally on the vessel walls or soluble antigen in the circulation (e.g., released from cells within the body or from infectious agents or by way of drugs or medications) that has been deposited on the surface of endothelial cells may bind antibody (see Fig. 9.2, *C*). The antibody initiates the complement cascade, resulting in the release of C3a and C5a, which are chemotactic for neutrophils, and deposition of complement component C3b. Neutrophils bind to the tissues through receptors for the Fc portion of antibody (Fc receptor) or for C3b and attempt to phagocytose the tissue. Because the tissue is large, phagocytosis cannot be completed; even so, neutrophils release their granules onto the healthy tissue. The components of neutrophil granules, as well as the several toxic oxygen products produced by these cells, will damage the tissue.

The fourth mechanism is antibody-dependent cell-mediated cytotoxicity (ADCC) (see Fig. 9.2, *D*). This mechanism involves a subpopulation of cytotoxic cells that are not antigen specific (natural killer [NK] cells). Antibody on the target cell is recognized by Fc receptors on the NK cells, which release toxic substances that destroy the target cell.

The fifth mechanism does not destroy the target cell, but rather causes it to malfunction. In this mechanism of type II injury, the antibody is usually directed against antigenic determinants associated with specific cell surface receptors, and the symptoms of the disease are a result of a direct effect of antibody binding alone (see Fig. 9.2, *E*). The antibody reacts with the receptors on the target cell surface and modulates the

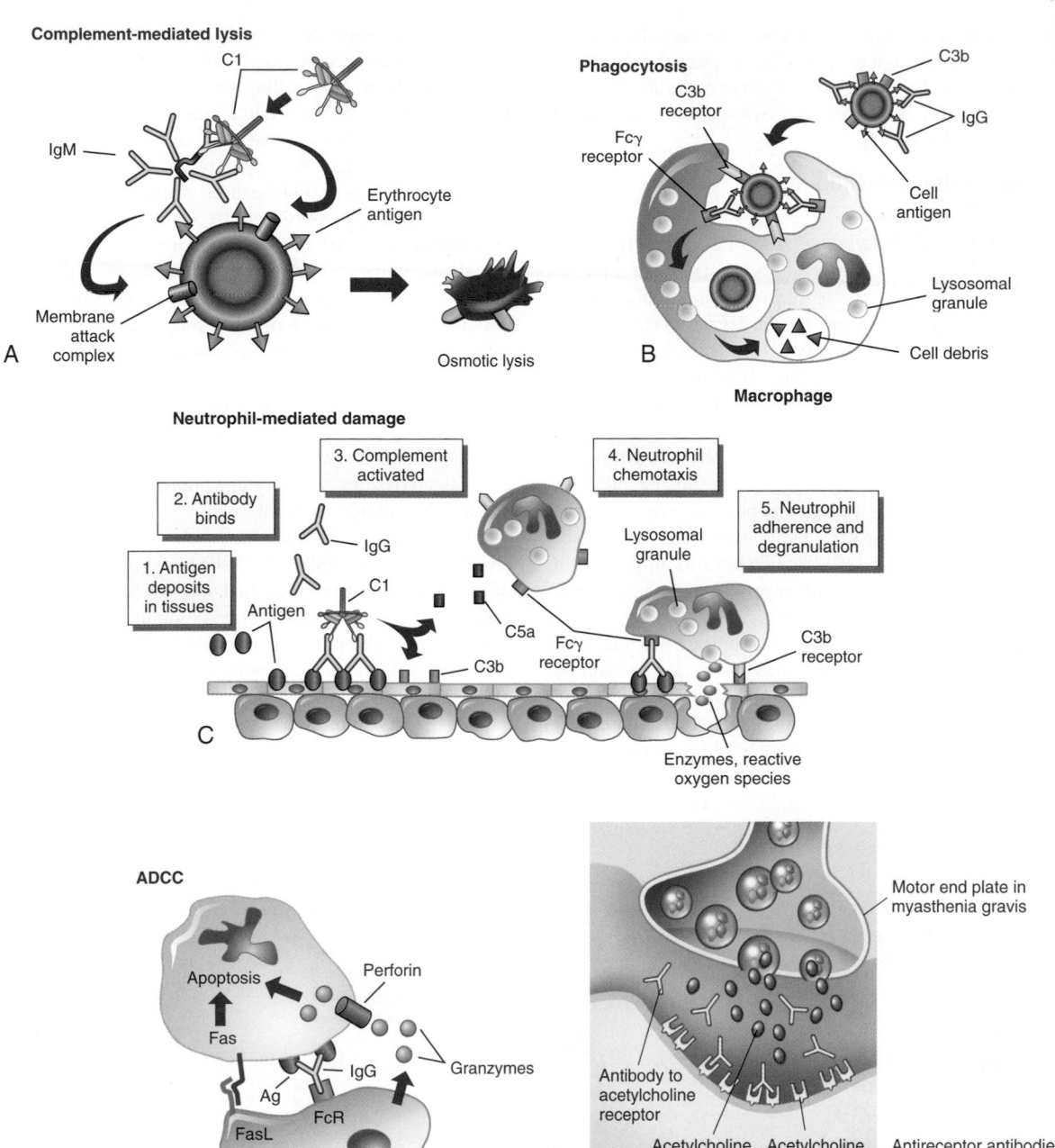

FIGURE 9.2 Mechanisms of Type II, Tissue-Specific, Reactions. Antigens on the target cell bind with antibody and are destroyed or prevented from functioning by **A,** complement-mediated lysis (an erythrocyte target is illustrated here); **B,** clearance (phagocytosis) by macrophages in the tissue; **C,** neutrophil-mediated immune destruction; **D,** antibody-dependent cell-mediated cytotoxicity (ADCC) (apoptosis of target cells is induced by granzymes and perforin produced by natural killer [NK] cells and interactions of Fas ligand [FasL] on the surface of NK cells with Fas on the surface of target cells); or **E,** modulation or blocking the normal function of receptors by antireceptor antibody. This example of mechanism **E** depicts myasthenia gravis in which acetylcholine receptor antibodies block acetylcholine from attaching to its receptors on the motor end plates of skeletal muscle, thereby impairing neuromuscular transmission and causing muscle weakness. *C1,* Complement component C1; *C3b,* complement fragment produced from C3, which acts as an opsonin; *C5a,* complement fragment produced from C5, which acts as a chemotactic factor for neutrophils; *Fcγ receptor,* cellular receptor for the Fc portion of IgG; *FcR,* Fc receptor.

function of the receptor by preventing interactions with their normal ligands, replacing the ligand and inappropriately stimulating the receptor, or destroying the receptor. For example, in the hyperthyroidism (excessive thyroid activity) of Graves disease, autoantibody binds to and activates receptors for thyroid-stimulating hormone (TSH) (a pituitary hormone that controls the production of the hormone *thyroxine* by the thyroid). In this way the antibody stimulates the thyroid cells to produce thyroxine. Under normal conditions, the increasing levels of thyroxine in the blood would signal the pituitary to decrease TSH production, which would result in less stimulation of the TSH receptor in the thyroid and a concomitant decrease in thyroxine production. Because the level of anti-TSH receptor antibody is not controlled by the pituitary, increasing amounts of thyroxine in the blood have no effect on antibody levels, and thyroxine production continues to increase despite decreasing amounts of TSH (see Chapter 22).

Type III: Immune Complex–Mediated Hypersensitivity Reactions

Mechanisms of Type III Hypersensitivity. Most type III (immune complex–mediated) hypersensitivity reactions are caused by antigen-antibody (immune) complexes that are formed in the circulation and deposited later in vessel walls or extravascular tissues (Fig. 9.3). The primary difference between type II and type III mechanisms is that in type II hypersensitivity antibody binds to the antigen on the cell surface, whereas in type III the antibody binds to soluble antigen that was released into the blood or body fluids, and the complex is then deposited in the tissues. Type III reactions are not organ specific, and symptoms have little to do with the particular antigenic target of the antibody. The harmful effects of immune complex deposition are caused by complement activation, particularly through the generation of chemotactic factors for neutrophils. The neutrophils bind to antibody and C3b contained in the complexes and attempt to ingest the immune complexes.

They are often unsuccessful because the complexes are bound to large areas of tissue. During the attempted phagocytosis, large quantities of lysosomal enzymes are released into the inflammatory site instead of into phagolysosomes. The attraction of neutrophils and the subsequent release of lysosomal enzymes cause most of the resulting tissue damage.

Immune complexes can be of various sizes, depending on the relative amounts of antigen and antibody. Fairly large immune complexes are cleared rapidly from the circulation by tissue macrophages, whereas very small complexes eventually are filtered from blood through the kidneys, without any pathologic consequences. Intermediate-sized immune complexes (formed at a ratio of antigen to antibody that has a slight excess of antigen) are likely to be deposited in certain target tissues, where they have severe pathologic consequences, such as inflammation in the kidneys (glomerulonephritis), the vessels (vasculitis), or the joints (arthritis or degenerative joint disease).

Immune Complex Disease. The nature of the immune complexes may change during the progression of the disease, with resultant changes in the severity of the symptoms. Immune complex formation is dynamic because variations in the ratio of antigen to antibody, the class and subclass of antibody, and the quantity and quality of circulating antigen occur. Thus complexes formed early in a disease process may differ from those formed later, and several types of immune complexes may be present simultaneously. With the tremendous potential heterogeneity of immune complexes, it is not surprising that immune complex diseases are characterized by a variety of symptoms and periods of remission or exacerbation of symptoms.

Because many immune complexes activate complement very effectively, complement levels in the blood may decrease during active disease. At times the individual's blood may become hypocomplementemic (i.e., contains below normal amounts of complement activity). During type I, II, or IV hypersensitivity reactions, complement levels are unaffected, or some components of the complement cascade, such as C3, may even be increased.

Two prototypic models of type III hypersensitivity help explain the variety of diseases in this category. Serum sickness is a model of systemic type III hypersensitivities, and the Arthus reaction is a model of localized or cutaneous reactions.

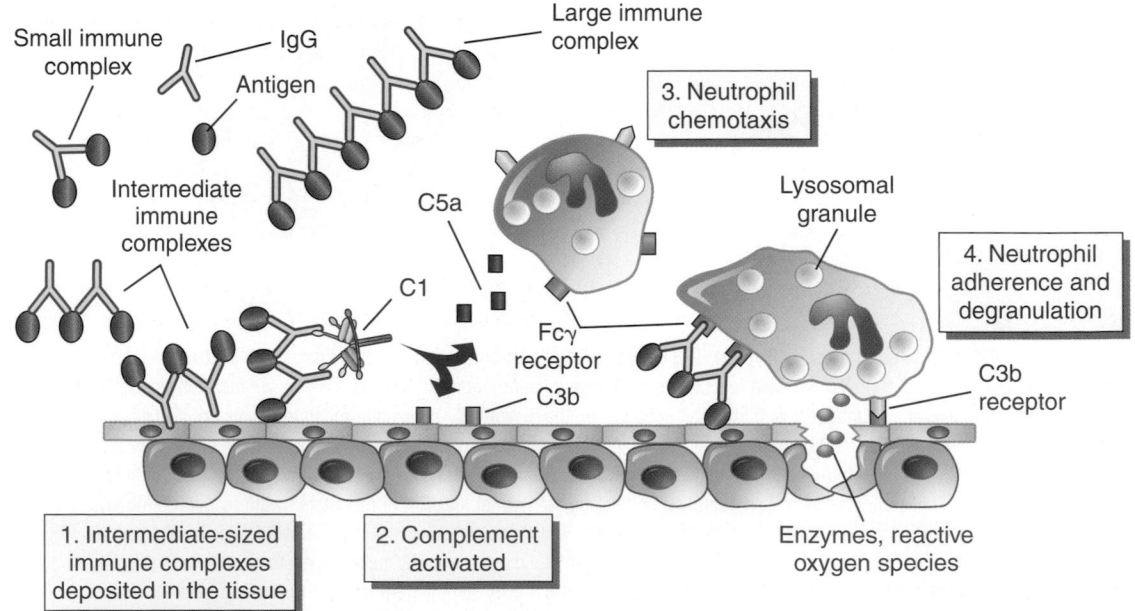

FIGURE 9.3 Mechanism of Type III, Immune Complex–Mediated, Reactions. Immune complexes form in the blood from circulating antigen and antibody. Both small and large immune complexes are removed successfully from the circulation and do not cause tissue damage. Intermediate-sized complexes are deposited in certain target tissues in which the circulation is slow or filtration of the blood occurs. The complexes activate the complement cascade through C1 and generate fragments including C5a and C3b. C5a is chemotactic for neutrophils, which migrate into the inflamed area and attach to the IgG and C3b in the immune complexes. The neutrophils attempt unsuccessfully to phagocytose the tissue and in the process release a variety of degradative enzymes that destroy the healthy tissues. Fcγ receptor is the cellular receptor for the Fc portion of IgG.

Serum Sickness. The systemic prototype of immune complex–mediated disease is called serum sickness because it was initially described as being caused by the therapeutic administration of foreign serum, such as horse serum that contained antibody against tetanus toxin.[5] Foreign serum generally is not administered to individuals today, although serum sickness reactions can be caused by the repeated intravenous administration of other antigens, such as drugs, and the characteristics of serum sickness are observed in systemic type III autoimmune diseases. Serum sickness–type reactions are caused by the formation of immune complexes in the blood and their subsequent generalized deposition in target tissues. Typically, affected tissues are the blood vessels, joints, and kidneys. Other symptoms include fever, enlarged lymph nodes, rash, and pain at sites of inflammation.

A form of serum sickness is Raynaud phenomenon, a condition caused by the temperature-dependent deposition of immune complexes in the capillary beds of the peripheral circulation. Certain immune complexes precipitate at temperatures below normal body temperature, particularly in the tips of the fingers, toes, and nose, and are called cryoglobulins. The precipitates block the circulation and cause localized pallor and numbness, followed by cyanosis (a bluish tinge resulting from oxygen deprivation) and eventually gangrene if the circulation is not restored.

Arthus Reaction. An Arthus reaction is the prototypic example of a localized immune complex–mediated inflammatory response.[6] It is caused by repeated local exposure to an antigen that reacts with preformed antibody and forms immune complexes in the walls of the local blood vessels. Symptoms of an Arthus reaction begin within 1 hour of exposure and peak 6 to 12 hours later. The lesions are characterized by a typical inflammatory reaction, with increased vascular permeability, an accumulation of neutrophils, edema, hemorrhage, clotting, and tissue damage.

Type IV: Cell-Mediated Hypersensitivity Reactions

Whereas types I, II, and III hypersensitivity reactions are mediated by antibody, type IV (cell-mediated) hypersensitivity reactions are mediated by T lymphocytes and do not involve antibody (Fig. 9.4). Type IV mechanisms occur through either cytotoxic T lymphocytes (Tc cells) or lymphokine-producing Th1 and Th17 cells. Tc cells attack and destroy cellular targets directly. Th1 and Th17 cells produce cytokines that recruit and activate phagocytic cells, especially macrophages. Destruction of the tissue is usually caused by direct killing by toxins from Tc cells or by the release of soluble factors, such as lysosomal enzymes and toxic reactive oxygen species (ROS), from activated macrophages.

Clinical examples of type IV hypersensitivity reactions include graft rejection and allergic reactions resulting from contact with such substances as poison ivy and metals. A type IV component also may be present in many autoimmune diseases. For example, T cells against type II collagen (a protein present in joint tissues) contribute to the destruction of joints in rheumatoid arthritis; T cells against a thyroid cell surface antigen contribute to the destruction of the thyroid in autoimmune thyroiditis (Hashimoto disease); and T cells against an antigen on the surface of pancreatic beta cells (the cell that normally produces insulin) are responsible for beta-cell destruction in insulin-dependent (type 1) diabetes mellitus.

A type IV hypersensitivity reaction in the skin was thoroughly described first by Ehrlich in 1891 and led to the development of a diagnostic skin test for tuberculosis.[7] The reaction follows an intradermal injection of tuberculin antigen into a suitably sensitized individual and is called a *delayed hypersensitivity skin test* because of its slow onset—24 to 72 hours to reach maximum intensity. The reaction site is infiltrated with T lymphocytes and macrophages, resulting in a clear hard center (induration) and a reddish surrounding area (erythema).

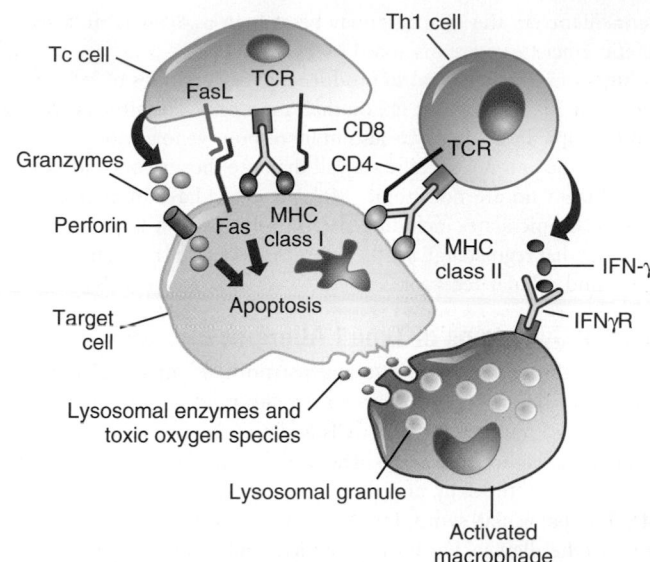

FIGURE 9.4 Mechanism of Type IV, Cell-Mediated, Reactions. Antigens from target cells stimulate T cells to differentiate into cytotoxic T cells (Tc cells), which have direct cytotoxic activity, and helper T cells (Th1 cells) involved in delayed hypersensitivity. The Th1 cells produce lymphokines (especially interferon-gamma *[IFN-γ]*) that activate the macrophage through specific receptors (e.g., IFN-γ receptor *[IFNγR]*). The macrophages can attach to targets and release enzymes and reactive oxygen species that are responsible for most of the tissue destruction.

Antigenic Targets of Hypersensitivity Reactions
Allergy

Allergy is a hypersensitivity response against an environmental antigen (allergen). Allergies are the most common hypersensitivity reactions. The most common allergies are type I hypersensitivities, although any of the other three mechanisms of hypersensitivity may cause allergic responses depending on the particular allergen.

Typical allergens that induce type I hypersensitivity include pollens (e.g., ragweed), molds and fungi (e.g., *Penicillium notatum*), foods (e.g., milk, eggs, shellfish), animals (e.g., cat dander, dog dander), cigarette smoke, components of house dust (e.g., fecal pellets of house mites), and almost anything else encountered in the environment. Allergens that primarily elicit type IV allergic hypersensitivities include plant resins (e.g., poison ivy, poison oak), metals (e.g., nickel, chromium), acetylates, and chemicals in rubber, cosmetics, detergents, and topical antibiotics (e.g., neomycin). Type II and type III allergic hypersensitivities are relatively rare but may include antibiotics (e.g., penicillin, sulfonamides) and soluble antigens produced by infectious agents (e.g., hepatitis B).

Usually a sensitization process involving multiple exposures to the allergen occurs before adequate amounts of antibody or T cells are available to elicit a hypersensitivity response. In some instances, exposure to a particular allergen may not be apparent in the case of allergens that are drugs, additives, or preservatives in food. For example, an individual may become sensitized by drinking milk that contains trace amounts of penicillin used for treating cows for mastitis. Thus the first therapeutic exposure to penicillin may cause an unexpected hypersensitivity reaction. Additionally, penicillin shares a β-lactam structure with cephalosporin, so that one antibiotic may be sensitive against another.

Genetic Predisposition. Certain individuals are genetically predisposed to develop allergies, particularly type I allergies, and are called atopic. In families in which one parent has an allergy, allergies develop in about 40% of the offspring. If both parents have allergies, the incidence in the offspring may be as high as 80%. (Principles of genetic inheritance are discussed in Chapter 4.)

Atopic individuals tend to produce higher quantities of IgE and to have more Fc receptors for IgE on their mast cells. The airways and the skin of atopic individuals are also more responsive to a wide variety of both specific and nonspecific stimuli than are the airways and skin of individuals who are not atopic. Multiple genes have been associated with the atopic state, including polymorphisms in a large variety of cytokines that regulate IgE synthesis (e.g., interleukin [IL]-4, IL-5, IL-12, IL-13) and cellular receptors.

Clinical Symptoms of Type I Allergies

The clinical manifestations of type I reactions are attributable mostly to the biologic effects of histamine. Tissues most commonly affected contain large numbers of mast cells and are sensitive to the effects of histamine released from them. These tissues are found in the gastrointestinal tract, the skin, and the respiratory tract (Fig. 9.5 and Table 9.4). The particular symptoms frequently reflect the main portal of entry for the allergen. For instance, pollens and other airborne allergens usually cause respiratory symptoms.

Effects of allergens on the mucosa of the eyes, nose, and respiratory tract include conjunctivitis (inflammation of the membranes lining the eyelids), rhinitis (inflammation of the mucous membranes of the nose), and asthma (constriction of the bronchi). Symptoms are caused by vasodilation, hypersecretion of mucus, edema, and swelling of the respiratory mucosa. Because the mucous membranes lining the respiratory tract (accessory sinuses, nasopharynx, and upper and lower respiratory tracts) are continuous, they are all adversely affected. The degree to which each is affected determines the symptoms of the disease.

Urticaria, or hives, is a dermal (skin) manifestation of type I allergic reactions (see Fig. 9.5). The underlying mechanism is the localized release of histamine and increased vascular permeability, resulting in limited areas of edema. Urticaria is characterized by white fluid-filled blisters (wheals) surrounded by areas of redness (flares). The wheal and flare reaction is usually accompanied by itching. Not all urticarial symptoms are caused by allergic (immunologic) reactions. Some, termed *nonimmunologic urticaria,* result from exposure to cold temperatures, emotional stress, medications, systemic diseases, hyperthyroidism, or malignancies (e.g., lymphomas).

Gastrointestinal allergies are caused primarily by allergens that enter through the mouth—usually foods or medicines. When food is the allergen, the active immunogen may be a product of food breakdown by digestive enzymes. Symptoms usually occur rapidly (frequently within minutes) and include vomiting, diarrhea, or abdominal pain and may be severe enough to result in malabsorption or protein-losing enteropathy, if the reactions are prolonged or recurrent. Systemic symptoms may range from urticaria to life-threatening anaphylactic reactions. The most common food allergies are milk, chocolate, eggs, soy, wheat, tree nuts, peanuts, shellfish, and fish.[8] The incidence of food allergies in children is estimated at 2% to 10% and has been increasing. Most children (about 75%) outgrow food allergies, but most individuals with peanut allergy (about 80%) will remain sensitive through adulthood with the potential of severe reactions.

If possible, avoidance of the allergen is the best method to limit allergic responses. Approximately 30% of laboratory animal handlers have allergies to animal dander and must use face masks or other devices to avoid contact.

Although some type I allergic responses can be controlled by blocking histamine receptors with antihistamines, the primary mechanism of

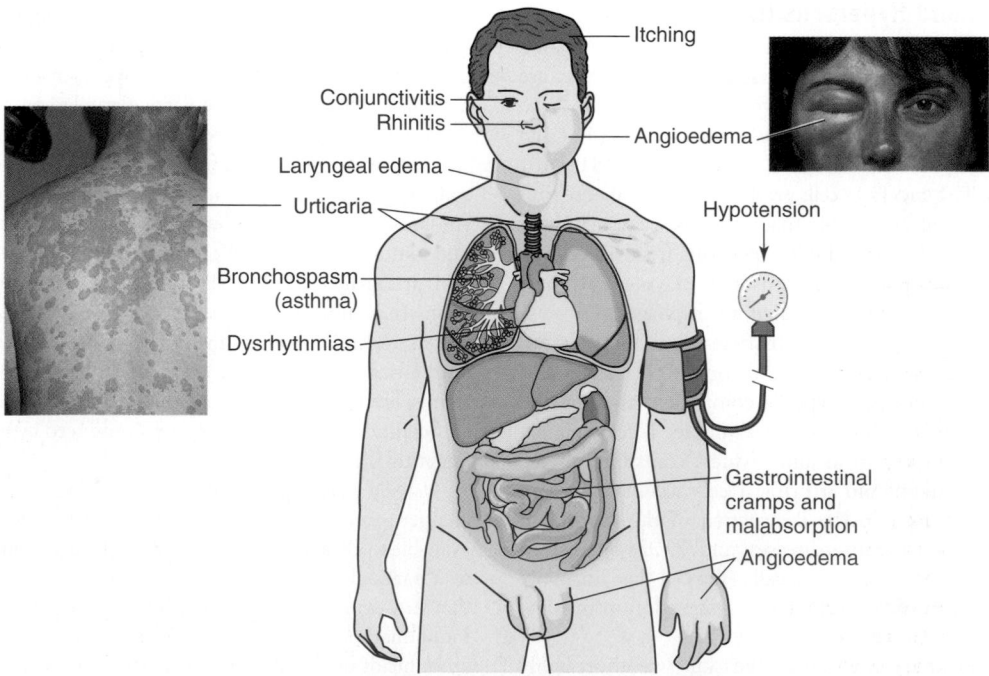

FIGURE 9.5 Type I Hypersensitivity Reactions. Manifestations of allergic reactions as a result of type I hypersensitivity include itching, angioedema (swelling caused by exudation), edema of the larynx, urticaria (hives), bronchospasm (constriction of airways in the lungs), hypotension (low blood pressure), and dysrhythmias (irregular heartbeat) because of anaphylactic shock, and gastrointestinal cramping caused by inflammation of the gastrointestinal mucosa. Photographic inserts show a diffuse allergic-like eye and skin reaction on an individual. The skin lesions have raised edges and develop within minutes or hours, with resolution occurring after about 12 hours. (Inserts from Male D et al: *Immunology,* ed 8, St Louis, 2013, Mosby.)

TABLE 9.4	CAUSES OF CLINICAL MANIFESTATIONS OF ALLERGY	
TYPICAL ALLERGEN	MECHANISM OF HYPERSENSITIVITY	CLINICAL MANIFESTATION
Ingestants		
Foods	Type I	Gastrointestinal allergy
Drugs	Types I, II, III	Urticaria, immediate drug reaction, hemolytic anemia, serum sickness
Inhalants		
Pollens, dust, molds	Type I	Allergic rhinitis, bronchial asthma
Aspergillus fumigatus	Types I, III	Allergic bronchopulmonary aspergillosis
Thermophilic actinomycetes*	Types III, IV	Extrinsic allergic alveolitis
Injectants		
Drugs	Types I, II, III	Immediate drug reaction, hemolytic anemia, serum sickness
Bee venom	Type I	Anaphylaxis
Vaccines	Type III	Localized Arthus reaction
Serum	Types I, III	Anaphylaxis, serum sickness
Contactants		
Poison ivy, metals	Type IV	Contact dermatitis

*An order of fungi that is stimulated by warmth to grow and proliferate.
Modified from Bellanti JA: *Immunology III*, Philadelphia, 1985, Saunders.

control is the autonomic nervous system. The autonomic nervous system includes biochemical mediators (e.g., epinephrine, acetylcholine) that, like the mediators of the inflammatory response, have profound effects on cells. These mediators bind to appropriate receptors on mast cells and the target cells of inflammation (e.g., smooth muscle), thereby controlling (1) the release of inflammatory mediators from mast cells and (2) the degree to which target cells respond to inflammatory mediators (see Chapter 7).

Allergic Disease: Bee Sting Allergy

An example of a life-threatening allergy is an anaphylactic reaction to a bee sting. Bee venoms contain a mixture of enzymes and other proteins that may serve as allergens. About 1% of children may have an anaphylactic reaction to bee venom. Within minutes they may develop excessive swelling (edema) at the bee sting site, followed by generalized hives, itching, and swelling in areas distal from the sting (e.g., eyes, lips), and other systemic symptoms including flushing, sweating, dizziness, and headache. The most severe symptoms may include gastrointestinal (e.g., stomach cramps, vomiting), respiratory (e.g., tightness in the throat, wheezing, difficulties breathing), and vascular (e.g., low blood pressure, shock) reactions. Severe respiratory and vascular reactions may lead to death.

If a child has had a previous anaphylactic reaction to bee stings, the chance of having another is about 60%. During the reaction the administration of antihistamines has little effect because histamine has already bound H1 receptors and initiated severe bronchial smooth muscle contraction. Most individuals carry self-injectable epinephrine. Autonomic nervous system mediators, such as epinephrine, bind to specific receptors on smooth muscle and reverse the effects of histamine and result in muscle relaxation. Similar anaphylactic reactions have been described against peanuts and other nuts, shellfish, fish, milk, eggs, and some medications.

Tests of IgE-Mediated Allergy

Allergic reactions can be life threatening; therefore, it is essential that severely allergic individuals be made aware of the specific allergen against which they are sensitized and instructed to avoid contact with that material. Several tests are available, including food challenges, skin tests with allergens, and laboratory tests for measurements of total IgE and allergen-specific IgE in the blood.[9]

Reactivity to a particular food allergen may be tested by controlled administration of small doses of the suspected allergen in order to evoke a mild allergic response. This approach can be dangerous if the individual has a history of anaphylactic responses. A safer approach is injection of an allergen into (intradermal) or onto (epicutaneous or prick test) the skin. If the individual is allergic to a particular allergen, a local wheal and flare reaction may occur within a few minutes at the site of injection. The diameter of the flare reaction is usually indicative of the individual's degree of sensitivity to that allergen. In the most severely allergic individuals, even the extremely small amounts of allergen used for the skin test may evoke a systemic anaphylaxis. Skin test is also contraindicated if the individual is using medications that may affect the test or has diffuse dermatitis, which would make the reaction difficult to interpret.

A variety of laboratory tests can detect IgE antibodies in serum. These assays have various commercial acronyms, depending on whether they are radioimmunoassays (RIAs; reactivity detected by measuring a radioactive reagent) or enzyme immunoassays (EIAs or ELISA [enzyme-linked immunosorbent assay]; reactivity detected by measuring a color change caused by an enzyme-labeled reagent). One set of assays measures circulating levels of total IgE, with atopic individuals usually having elevated levels. Other assays are capable of measuring circulating levels of specific IgE antibodies against selected allergens. The amount of IgE against a specific allergen correlates well with the degree of skin test reactivity and the severity of clinical symptoms related to the same allergen, although the laboratory text is less sensitive.

Desensitization. Clinical desensitization to allergens can be achieved in some individuals. Minute quantities of the allergen are injected in increasing doses over a prolonged period. The procedure may reduce the severity of the allergic reaction in the treated individual and works best for routine respiratory tract allergens and biting insect allergies (80% to 90% rate of desensitization over 5 years of treatment). However, this form of therapy is associated with a risk of systemic anaphylaxis, which can be severe and life threatening. Food allergies have been very difficult to suppress, but some promising trials are underway to evaluate desensitization by oral or sublingual administration of increasing amounts of allergen.[10]

The mechanisms by which desensitization occurs may be several, one of which is the production of large amounts of so-called blocking antibodies, usually circulating IgG. A blocking antibody presumably competes in the tissues or in the circulation for binding with antigenic determinants on the allergen so that the allergen is "neutralized" and is unable to bind with IgE on mast cells. Sublingual desensitization (another approach that works best with some food allergies) produces sIgA and circulating IgG that may prevent the allergen from accessing mast cells. Desensitization injections also may stimulate the generation of clones of T-regulatory lymphocytes, which inhibit hypersensitivity by suppressing the production of IgE or modifying the Th1/Th2 interactions in favor of production of antiinflammatory cytokines.

Other approaches to suppressing type I allergic responses have been tested, with some preliminary success. An example is injection of anti-IgE antibody directed against the Fc portion of the IgE in order to decrease binding of IgE to mast cells.

Type IV Allergic Hypersensitivities. The allergens that induce a type IV allergic reaction are mostly haptens that react with normal self-proteins in the skin. When presented in this fashion, these antigens are recognized by pattern recognition receptors (PRRs) on antigen-presenting cells in the skin and induce a cell-mediated response. (Pattern recognition receptors are discussed in Chapter 7.) The primary result is an allergic contact dermatitis that is confined to the area of contact with the allergen. The best-known example is poison ivy (Fig. 9.6). The antigen in that instance is a plant catechol, *urushiol*, that reacts with normal skin proteins and evokes a cell-mediated immune response.

As noted, type I hypersensitivity reactions may result in a skin reaction (e.g., hives formed during an allergic reaction to a particular food). The distribution of the lesions may suggest whether the reaction is caused by immediate (type I) or delayed (type IV) hypersensitivity mechanisms. Immediate hypersensitivity reactions, termed atopic dermatitis, are usually characterized by widely distributed lesions, whereas contact dermatitis (delayed hypersensitivity) consists of lesions only at the site of contact with the allergen, such as a metal allergy to jewelry (see Fig. 9.6).[11]

Types II and III Allergic Hypersensitivities. Type II allergic hypersensitivities are usually against allergic haptens that bind to the surface of cells and elicit an IgG or IgM response. For instance, allergic reactions against many drugs (e.g., penicillin, sulfonamides) occur after the drug binds to proteins on the plasma membranes of a person's cells and becomes immunogenic. The immune system attacks the allergen on the cell membrane and destroys the cell as well. In allergic reactions to penicillin, the immunogenic antigen is a metabolite of penicillin catabolism that binds to the plasma membranes of erythrocytes or platelets and induces an antibody response that destroys the cells (type

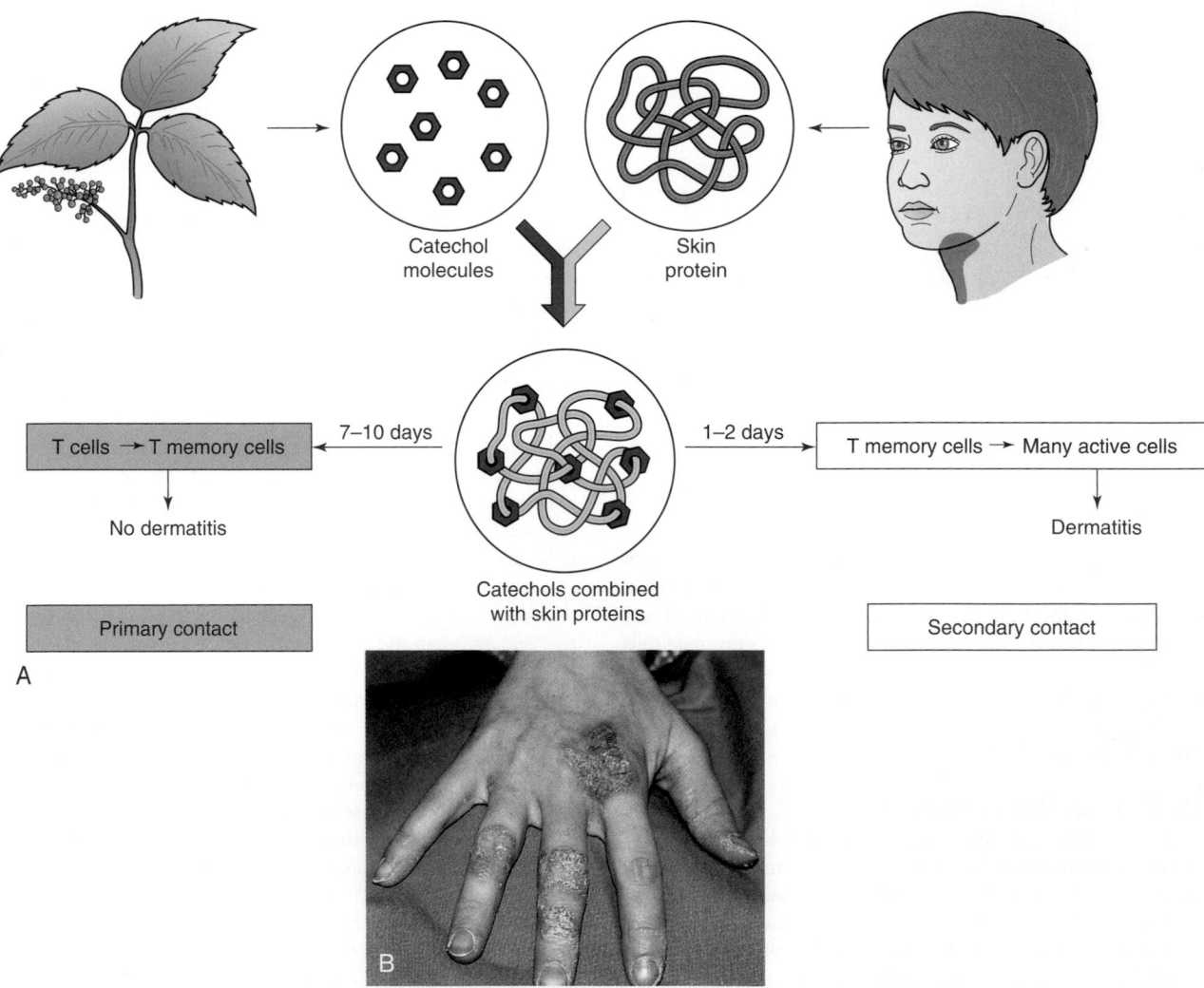

FIGURE 9.6 Development of Allergic Contact Dermatitis, a Delayed Hypersensitivity Reaction. **A,** Shown here is the development of allergy to catechols from poison ivy. No dermatitis results from the primary contact because the antigens (catechols) are sensitizing the immune response and producing memory T cells. Secondary contact, however, quickly activates a type IV, cell-mediated reaction that causes dermatitis. **B,** This contact dermatitis was caused by a delayed hypersensitivity reaction that led to vesicles and scaling at the sites of contact. (From Damjanov I, Linder J: *Anderson's pathology,* ed 10, St Louis, 1996, Mosby.)

II hypersensitivity), causing anemia or thrombocytopenia. Type II allergic reactions also can occur against antigens of infectious diseases. For instance, encephalitis secondary to a rubella infection may result from damage to cells of the nervous system by an immune response against rubella virus antigen on the cell's plasma membrane.

Type III allergic reactions occur after the formation of immune complexes containing soluble allergens. For instance, Arthus reactions may be observed after injection, ingestion, or inhalation of allergens. Skin reactions can follow subcutaneous or intradermal inoculation with drugs, fungal extracts, or antigens used in skin tests. Gastrointestinal reactions, such as gluten-sensitive enteropathy (celiac disease), follow ingestion of antigen, usually gluten from wheat products (see Chapter 42). Allergic alveolitis is a type III acute hemorrhagic inflammation of the air sacs (alveoli) of the lungs resulting from inhalation of fungal antigens, usually particles from moldy hay (farmer's lung) or pigeon feces (pigeon breeder's disease) (see Chapter 36). Circulating drugs (e.g., penicillin) or antigens produced from infectious diseases (e.g., hepatitis B, streptococcal infection) may form circulating immune complexes that are deposited in the circulation (vasculitis) or the kidneys (glomerulonephritis).

Autoimmunity

Autoimmune diseases originate from the coincidence of an initiating event in a genetically predisposed individual leading to an autoimmune mechanism that affects specific target tissues or cells. Some autoimmune diseases can be familial and attributed to the presence of a very small number of susceptibility genes. Affected family members may not all develop the same disease, but have different disorders characterized by a variety of hypersensitivity reactions, including autoimmune and allergic. For instance, the HLA antigen B27 (HLA is discussed further under Transplantation and Transfusion) is a risk factor for developing **ankylosing spondylitis (AS)**, an autoimmune inflammatory disease of the spine. Ninety-five percent of individuals diagnosed with AS express HLA-B27, whereas only 4% to 8% of the general population expresses this antigen (Table 9.5). Although most autoimmune diseases appear as isolated events without a positive family history, susceptibility for developing such diseases appears to be linked to a combination of multiple genes.

Genetic Factors. Genetic factors that contribute to autoimmunity are easier to identify than the original insult that initiates the disease. It is fairly well established that autoimmune diseases can be familial. Affected family members may not all develop the same disease, but several members may have different disorders characterized by a variety of hypersensitivity reactions, including autoimmune and allergic reactions.

Associations with particular autoimmune diseases have been identified for a variety of major histocompatibility complex (MHC) alleles (see Chapter 8) or non-MHC genes. The specific HLA alleles of susceptible and resistant individuals have been analyzed for almost every known disease and, almost universally, individuals with certain diseases are more likely than the general population to have a specific HLA allele or set of alleles.[12] Some associations are strong; others are more tenuous (see Table 9.5). The reason some HLA alleles are associated with inappropriate immune function is unclear, but it may directly involve the ability of particular HLA molecules to present antigen or the use of particular HLAs as receptors for disease-causing microorganisms. These genes may determine an individual's susceptibility to specific infectious agents or the capacity of that individual to mount an immune response against specific antigens. Therefore, an individual of a specific HLA type may have an inappropriate or exaggerated immune responses against a microorganism resulting in a hypersensitivity reaction.

TABLE 9.5	EXAMPLES OF ASSOCIATIONS BETWEEN SPECIFIC HLA ALLELES AND DISEASE	
DISEASE	**HLA ALLELE**	**RR**
Acute anterior uveitis	B27	14
Addison disease	DR3	6
Ankylosing spondylitis	B27	90
Behçet syndrome	B51	4
Celiac disease	DR3	11
Chronic active hepatitis	DR3	13
Dermatitis herpetiformis	DR3	16
Diabetes (type 1)	DR3	5
	DR4	6
	DR3/DR4	20
Goodpasture syndrome	DR2	16
Graves disease	DR3	4
Hashimoto disease	DR11	3
Multiple sclerosis	DR2	4
Myasthenia gravis	DR3	3
Pemphigus vulgaris	DR4	13
Postgonococcal arthritis	B27	14
Reiter syndrome	B27	37
Rheumatoid arthritis	DR4	4
Sjögren syndrome	DR3	9
Systemic lupus erythematosus	DR3	6

HLA, Human leukocyte antigen; *RR*, the approximate relative risk, which is the frequency of a disease in individuals with the particular HLA allele compared with individuals without that allele.

A large variety of non-MHC genes also have been identified as risk factors for the development of specific autoimmune diseases. Most of these genes encode for inflammatory cytokines or costimulatory molecules found on the cell surface.

Breakdown of Tolerance. Individuals are usually tolerant to their own antigens. Tolerance is a state of immunologic control so that the individuals do not make a detrimental immune response against their own cells and tissues. *Central tolerance* develops in humans during the embryonic period as autoreactive lymphocytes are either eliminated or suppressed in the primary lymphoid organs during differentiation and proliferation of immature T or B lymphocytes (see Figs. 8.9 and 8.12). Clones of cells with antigen receptors for self-antigens are deleted. *Peripheral tolerance* is maintained in the secondary lymphoid organs through the action of T-regulatory lymphocytes or antigen-presenting dendritic cells. The key term in the definition of tolerance is *detrimental immune response* because autoimmune antibodies frequently are present at low, but measurable, levels in the blood of most individuals. They may perform a useful function, such as removing low levels of cellular debris from the blood, and are quantitatively and qualitatively regulated to avoid autoimmune disease. Autoimmune disease results more commonly from a breakdown of this peripheral tolerance rather than a defect in central tolerance.

An initiating event results in a breakdown of tolerance to an individual's own antigens. A great deal of research has progressively identified genetic risk or predisposing factors in autoimmune diseases, but, in the vast majority of autoimmune diseases, the nature of the initiating event and the mechanism by which it breaks tolerance are unclear. Several potential mechanisms have been suggested.

Sequestered Antigen. The induction of central tolerance requires that the self-antigen be present in the fetus and exposed to the developing fetal immune system. Some self-antigens may not normally encounter the immune system in either fetal or adult life, but are sequestered or hidden from the immune system in immunologically privileged sites, so named because foreign tissues can be transplanted into these sites with less chance of immunologic rejection. For example, several sites (e.g., anterior chamber of the eye, the brain) are separated from the circulation by barriers (blood-ocular and blood-brain barriers) that offer protection against many immune cells and lead to relatively poor lymphatic drainage. Lymphocytes that enter these sites encounter tissue that expresses Fas ligand (FasL) and tumor necrosis factor (TNF)–related apoptosis-inducing ligand (TRAIL). These molecules induce the lymphocytes to undergo apoptosis, thus protecting the tissue. Self-antigens in these sites are protected by sequestration and an active protective mechanism. However, if the barriers are damaged, antigenic sensitization can occur, and the resultant antibodies and lymphocytes can enter the site and cause additional damage to the tissue. For instance, physical trauma to one eye may result in release of sequestered antigen into the blood or lymphatics, resulting in immunologic injury to the other eye (sympathetic uveitis).[13]

Infectious Disease. A long-standing hypothesis is that foreign antigens from infectious microorganisms can initiate autoimmune disease through a process of molecular mimicry. Some antigens of infectious agents so closely resemble (mimic) a particular self-antigen that antibodies or T cells produced to protect against the infection also recognize the self-antigen as foreign (cross-reactive antibody or T cell). The relationship between many autoimmune diseases and predisposing infections, such as the link between enterovirus infection and type 1 diabetes, and the link between a variety of infectious microorganisms and autoimmune thyroid disease are being investigated.[14,15]

The only clearly defined example so far is acute rheumatic fever that may occur after a group A streptococcal sore throat.[16] In some individuals with group A streptococcal sore throat or infection of the skin or mucosa, the M protein and group A carbohydrate in the bacterial capsule mimic (antigenic mimicry) normal antigens in the heart valves and induce antibodies that also react with proteins (e.g., cardiac myosin and others) in the heart valve, damaging the valve, and allowing the influx of CD4+ cells with specificities towards normal valvular antigens. Only a small number of individuals whose heart proteins have similar antigens to the bacterial capsular antigens are normally affected. Thus acute rheumatic fever is initiated by a type II autoimmune hypersensitivity that may be augmented by a type IV hypersensitivity.

Additionally, some streptococcal infections also release soluble bacterial antigens into the blood that form circulating immune complexes with antibacterial antigens. The complexes may deposit in the kidneys and initiate an immune complex–mediated glomerulonephritis (inflammation of the kidney). Thus soluble streptococcal antigens may, by a type III hypersensitivity mechanism, elicit a poststreptococcal glomerulonephritis. Because the circulating antigens are bacterial and thus environmental, this complication may be defined as a type III allergic reaction.

Neoantigen. In certain situations, a neoantigen that induces an allergic reaction may also lead to autoimmunity. Many neoantigens (new antigens) are haptens that become immunogenic after binding to self-proteins. The immune reaction against the neoantigen may lead to an immunologic reaction against normal antigenic determinants on the protein. Other new antigenic determinants may result from posttranslational modifications of a normal protein so that one or more amino acids are chemically altered (e.g., addition or removal of amino acid side groups, phosphorylation) without affecting the protein's function. Many experimental autoimmune diseases (e.g., experimental autoimmune thyroiditis) can be initiated by immunization with molecules containing neoantigenic determinants.

Neoantigens may result from genetic or epigenetic modifications or posttranslational modification, particularly in response to lifestyle (e.g., smoking, diet, consumption of alcohol or coffee, exposure to organic solvents). These conditions are under investigation, but to date only associations rather than clear causative relationships have been found.[17]

Forbidden Clone. During differentiation and proliferation of lymphoid stem cells into immature T and B lymphocytes (see Figs. 8.9 and 8.12), some lymphocytes produce receptors that react with self-antigens. Many autoreactive lymphocytes interact with self-antigens and other costimulatory molecules on the surface of thymic epithelial cells and are induced to undergo clonal deletion by a process of apoptosis. Thus lymphocytes reactive against self-antigen are prevented, or "forbidden," from maturing. Autoimmunity may result from the survival of a forbidden clone and its proliferation later in life.

Defective Peripheral Tolerance. Tolerance to some self-antigens is controlled in the secondary lymphoid organs. This process is controlled by a variety of cells, including antigen-presenting dendritic cells and members of a family of T-regulatory lymphocytes (Treg cells) that normally suppress immune responses against self. Defects in particular regulatory cells may result in expansion of clones of autoreactive cells and the development of autoimmune disease. Systemic lupus erythematosus, which is characterized by the production of a large array of autoantibodies, may be caused by a general breakdown in the regulatory network.

Silent Imitators of Autoimmune Disease. The mechanism for imitation of autoimmune diseases may already be within all humans. Two very interesting potential mechanisms are being explored (see *What's New? Silent Initiators of Autoimmune Disease: Microchimerism and Endogenous Retroviruses*).

Alloimmunity

Alloimmunity occurs when an individual's immune system reacts against antigens on the tissues of other members of the same species. Genetic diversity is the norm in humans. Diversity also is observed among self-antigens, so that two individuals may have different antigens on their tissues and, therefore, make an immune response against each other's tissues. Some self-antigens, such as the ABO blood group, have limited diversity with very few different antigens being expressed in the population, whereas others, such as the HLA system, have tremendous diversity.

Two clinically relevant examples of this reactivity are (1) several transient neonatal diseases (in which the maternal immune system becomes sensitized against antigens expressed by the fetus) and (2) transplant rejection and transfusion reactions (in which the immune system of a recipient of an organ transplant or blood transfusion reacts against antigens on the donor cells).

Transient Neonatal Alloimmunity. Because the fetus is a hybrid between the mother and father, it expresses paternal antigens that are not found in the mother. Occasionally these fetal antigens cross the placenta and elicit an immune response in the mother (e.g., production of alloantibodies against the fetal antigens). The maternal alloantibody

WHAT'S NEW?

Silent Initiators of Autoimmune Disease: Microchimerism and Endogenous Retroviruses

Two normally silent conditions have been studied in relationship to the onset of autoimmune diseases. Both microchimerism and endogenous retroviruses are conditions that have unknown roles in normal physiology, but may be triggers for autoimmune diseases.

A rapidly growing body of evidence suggests that humans are in a state of microchimerism (Mc): possessing a small number of cells originating from another individual.[1] The placenta routinely allows bidirectional passage of both maternal and fetal cells beginning as early as 6 months' gestation. Most gravid women (having been pregnant) have detectable fetal cells (fetal Mc) in their blood and many organs (e.g., white blood cells, hepatocytes, kidney tubular epithelium, neurons and glia, cardiomyocytes, endothelial cells, intestinal epithelium, and islet beta cells), which apparently originated as fetal stem cells that differentiated in the maternal tissues. Microchimerism persists for decades after pregnancy.

The fetal cells appear to be regulated by T-cell cytokines: TGF-β and IL-10.[2] If regulation is diminished, the fetal cells may initiate a chronic inflammatory reaction leading to tissue damage and potential autoimmune reactions. Many autoimmune diseases are associated with increased numbers of male cells in the diseased organs (e.g., scleroderma, dermatomyositis, Sjögren syndrome, thyroiditis, primary biliary cirrhosis, hyper- and hypothyroidism, and systemic lupus erythematosus), suggesting that Mc may contribute to the etiology of these diseases.[1] The role of microchimerism in autoimmune thyroid disease is enveloped in contradictory data. Levels of fetal cells are elevated in the blood in women with autoimmune thyroid diseases: Graves and Hashimoto disease,[3] whereas others have reported fewer fetal cells associated with these diseases.[4] Thus it cannot yet be determined whether the foreign cells are initiators of autoimmune damage. Thus these observations remain intriguing but of unknown significance.

Another silent potential trigger of autoimmune disease is activation of human endogenous retroviruses (HERVs). Infectious retroviruses, such as HIV, are well-known. What most do not know is that 8% of the human genome is of retroviral

origin. It appears that 30 to 40 million years ago, humans were infected by simple retroviruses that inserted themselves into the genome of gametes, thus becoming inheritable.[5] The endogenous retroviral inserts contained regions of control of expression, the *gag* gene that encoded matrix and capsid proteins (Gag proteins), the *pol* region that encoded retroviral enzymes, and the *env* gene for envelope (Env) proteins. Most HERV genes are inactivated. The genome contains approximately 10,000 retroviral sequences, but only about 50 functional open reading frames so that several Gag, Pol, and Env proteins can be expressed. These genes are usually silent until activated for unknown reasons.

Several HERV genes are activated and expressed in tissues undergoing autoimmune processes. They have been described in tissue related to rheumatoid arthritis (RA), systemic lupus erythematosus (SLE), multiple sclerosis, systemic sclerosis, and Sjögren syndrome. An unresolved hypothesis is that some HERV proteins mimic normal proteins, inducing autoantibodies that attack normal proteins, and triggering autoimmune inflammation.[6] Gag proteins are expressed by HERV K-10 and the Fc region of IgG1, which also is the target for rheumatoid factor, a pathologic autoantibody associated with RA. Several HERVs, especially HRES-1 Gag protein, are activated during SLE. HRES-1 Gag has homology with at least nine autoantigens that are common targets in SLE. Two HERV loci (HERV-Fc1 on the X chromosome and HERV-K13 on chromosome 19) appear to synergize and increase the risk for Mc.[7]

References:
1. Nelson JL: *Trends Immunol* 33(8):421–427, 2012.
2. Stevens AM: *Best Pract Res Clin Obstet Gynaecol* 31(2):121–130, 2016.
3. Boddy AM et al: *Bioessays* 37(10):1106–1118, 2015.
4. Cirello V et al: *Eur J Endocrinol* 173(1):111–118, 2015.
5. Weiss RA: *APMIS* 124(1–2):4–10, 2016.
6. Trela M, Nelson PN, Rylance PB: *APMIS* 124(1–2):88–104, 2016.
7. Nexø BA et al: *BMC Neurology* 16:57, 2016.

may be transported across the placenta into the fetal circulation, bind to the fetal cells, and produce alloimmune disease in the fetus and neonate. The mother's immune system produces the antibody, but because the cells do not express the target antigen, the mother has no symptoms of the disease.

Neonatal alloimmune disease may be secondary to maternal autoimmune diseases in which the mother produces an IgG autoantibody specific for maternal self-antigens that are found on fetal cells as well. Therefore, symptoms of the same autoimmune disease may affect mother and child, even though the autoantibody is being produced only by the mother's immune system. This form of disease usually occurs only in association with type II (tissue-specific) hypersensitivity reactions. It does not occur in association with IgE-mediated (type I) reactions, immune complex–mediated (type III) reactions, or cell-mediated (type IV) reactions because the immunologic factors (IgE, immune complexes, T cells) that cause these reactions do not readily cross the placenta and enter the fetal circulation in sufficient quantity.

Symptoms of the alloimmune disease may be present in utero or immediately after birth and may be fatal to the fetus or neonate. At birth, maternal circulating antibody can no longer enter the child, and if symptoms are successfully treated, the disease will disappear as the maternal antibody is catabolized.[18] Examples of maternal immunologic hypersensitivity diseases in which the child can be affected include the following antibody-mediated diseases:

1. Graves disease—an autoimmune disease in which maternal antibody against the receptor for TSH causes neonatal hyperthyroidism

2. Myasthenia gravis—an autoimmune disease in which maternal antibody binds with receptors for neural transmitters on muscle cells (acetylcholine receptors), causing neonatal muscular weakness (see Chapter 18)

3. Immune thrombocytopenic purpura—a disease in which both autoimmune and alloimmune variants in maternal antiplatelet antibody destroy platelets in the fetus and neonate (see Chapter 30)

4. Alloimmune neutropenia—a disease in which maternal antibody against neutrophils destroys neutrophils in the neonate

5. Systemic lupus erythematosus—an autoimmune disease in which diverse maternal autoantibodies induce anomalies (e.g., congenital heart defects) in the fetus or cause pregnancy loss

6. Rh and ABO alloimmunization (e.g., erythroblastosis fetalis)—a disease in which maternal antibody against erythrocyte antigens induces anemia in the child (see Chapter 31)

Autoimmune and Alloimmune Diseases

Many examples of autoimmune or alloimmune diseases have been described. Several basic principles are exemplified by two examples: systemic lupus erythematosus (an autoimmune disease) and tissue rejection (i.e., transplant rejection or transfusion reaction) (an alloimmune phenomenon). Most of the classic autoimmune diseases, including disorders of the endocrine system (autoimmune thyroiditis and Graves disease), hematologic system (the hemolytic and pernicious anemias), nervous system (myasthenia gravis), and connective tissue in joints (rheumatoid arthritis), are discussed in Unit II of this book.

Systemic Lupus Erythematosus

Systemic lupus erythematosus (SLE) is a chronic, multisystem, inflammatory disease and is one of the most common, complex, and serious of the autoimmune disorders. SLE is characterized by multiple immune disorders that result in the production of a large variety of autoantibodies against nucleic acids, erythrocytes, coagulation proteins, phospholipids, lymphocytes, platelets, and many other self-components.[19] The most characteristic autoantibodies produced in SLE are against nucleic acids (e.g., single-stranded deoxyribonucleic acid [DNA], double-stranded DNA), histones, ribonucleoproteins, and other nuclear materials.

Deposition of circulating immune complexes containing antibody against DNA produces tissue damage in individuals with SLE. DNA and DNA-containing immune complexes have a high affinity for glomerular basement membranes and therefore may be selectively deposited in the glomerulus (Fig. 9.7). (Kidney structures are described in Chapter 38.) The presence of DNA in the circulation increases from cellular damage in response to trauma, drugs, or infections and is usually removed in the liver. Removal of circulating DNA is slowed in the presence of immune complexes, thereby increasing the potential for deposition in the kidney. (The liver's role in removing waste products from the blood is discussed in Chapter 41.) Deposition of immune complexes composed of DNA and antibody also causes inflammatory lesions in the renal tubular basement membranes, brain (choroid plexus), heart, spleen, lung, gastrointestinal tract, skin (see Fig. 9.7), and peritoneum.

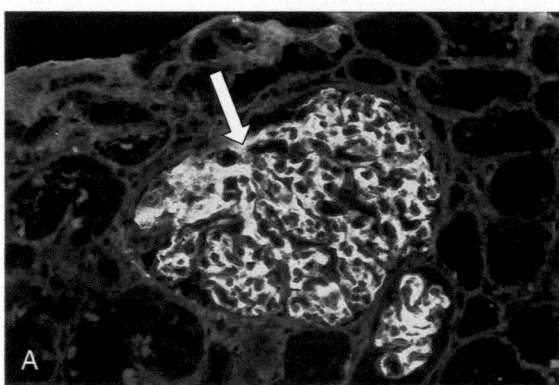
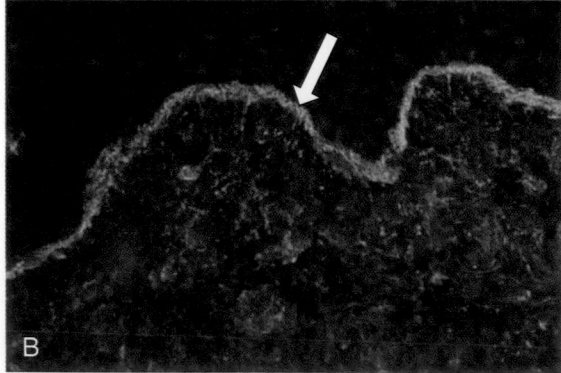

FIGURE 9.7 Deposition of IgG in the Kidney and Skin of Individuals With Lupus. These photographs of tissue were obtained from individuals with lupus and stained with fluorescent anti-IgG. **A,** Section from a kidney showing a glomerulus with deposits of IgG (*arrow,* indicating bright areas of staining). **B,** Section of the skin showing deposition of IgG along the dermal-epidermal junction (*arrow,* indicating bright green staining). (**A** courtesy Dr. Helmut Rennke, Department of Pathology, Brigham and Women's Hospital, Boston; **B** courtesy Dr. Richard Sontheimer, Department of Dermatology, University of Texas Southwestern Medical School, Dallas.)

SLE, as with most autoimmune diseases, occurs more often in women (approximately a 10:1 predominance of females), especially in the 20- to 40-year-old age group. Blacks are affected more often than whites (about an eightfold increased risk). A genetic predisposition for the disease has been implicated on the basis of increased incidence in twins and the existence of autoimmune disease in the families of individuals with SLE.

A transient lupus-like syndrome that is indistinguishable both clinically and in the laboratory from spontaneously occurring SLE can develop from the prolonged use of medications, particularly hydralazine (an antihypertensive agent) and procainamide (an antidysrhythmic drug). In genetically susceptible individuals, certain environmental agents, such as ultraviolet light, and several infectious agents may trigger lupus-like immune reactions.

Clinical manifestations of SLE include arthralgias or arthritis (90% of individuals), vasculitis and rash (70% to 80% of individuals), renal disease (40% to 50% of individuals), hematologic abnormalities (50% of individuals, with anemia being the most common complication), and cardiovascular diseases (30% to 50% of individuals). A recent study of male and female individuals with SLE reported gender-based differences in the incidence of SLE-related symptoms.[20] Females more commonly developed alopecia, photosensitivity, oral ulcers, malar rash, lupus anticoagulant, arthritis, and serositis with pleurisy, whereas males more commonly developed thrombocytopenia, anti-dsDNA, and renal involvement.

As with most autoimmune diseases, the disease process develops slowly (up to 10 years from occurrence of the first autoantibody until diagnosis)[21] and is characterized by frequent remissions and exacerbations. Because the signs and symptoms affect almost every body system and tend to be intermittent, SLE is extremely difficult to diagnose. This has led to the development of a list of 11 common clinical findings,[22] which has been modified slightly to increase sensitivity of the diagnosis.[23] The serial or simultaneous presence of at least four of them indicates that the individual has SLE:[24]

1. Facial rash confined to the cheeks (malar rash)
2. Discoid rash (raised patches, scaling)
3. Photosensitivity (development of skin rash developed as a result of exposure to sunlight)
4. Oral or nasopharyngeal ulcers
5. Nonerosive arthritis of at least two peripheral joints
6. Serositis (pleurisy, pericarditis)
7. Renal disorder (persistent proteinuria of >0.5 g/day or >3 g/day on dipstick or cellular casts)
8. Neurologic disorders (seizures or psychosis in the absence of known causes)
9. Hematologic disorders (hemolytic anemia, leukopenia, lymphopenia, or thrombocytopenia)
10. Immunologic disorders (antibodies against double-stranded DNA [dsDNA] or Smith [Sm] antigen, false-positive serologic test for syphilis, or antiphospholipid antibodies [anticardiolipin antibody or lupus anticoagulant])
11. Presence of antinuclear antibody (ANA)

Laboratory diagnosis is usually based on a positive ANA screening test; about 98% of persons with SLE are positive, but a substantial number of false-positives occur in healthy individuals and those with other diseases. Because SLE is a progressive and slowly developing disease, some laboratory tests, including the ANA, may be positive years before the onset of clinical symptoms.[25] Detection of a positive ANA is usually followed by one or more specific tests (e.g., antibodies against Sm, dsDNA) that are complicated by low sensitivity (only a portion of individuals with SLE will be positive, although the number of false-positives is low).

There is no cure for SLE or most other autoimmune diseases. In the 1950s, the expected survival rate at 5 years after diagnosis was only 50%. Because of improved diagnosis and treatment of SLE the 2004 expected survival rate 20 years after diagnosis was 78%.[26] Fatalities resulting from SLE are usually related to cardiovascular disease with infection and other organ failure almost as common. The goals of treatment are to control symptoms and prevent further damage by suppressing the autoimmune response. Mild forms of SLE are treated with nonsteroidal antiinflammatory drugs, such as aspirin, ibuprofen, or naproxen, to reduce inflammation and relieve pain. Low-dose corticosteroids, such as prednisone, are often prescribed with higher doses used for more serious active disease. Antimalarial medications (e.g., hydroxychloroquine) are preferred treatments for individuals with stable disease. Immunosuppressive drugs (e.g., methotrexate, azathioprine, or cyclophosphamide) are used to treat individuals with severe symptoms involving internal organs who have not responded to high-dose corticosteroids. Ultraviolet light can worsen symptoms (known as flares), and protection from sun exposure is helpful. Prolonged use of certain drugs can cause transient SLE-like symptoms, and the medication history is important for diagnostic evaluation.

Other therapeutic approaches have been attempted for SLE and other autoimmune diseases. Several decades ago preparations of intravenous immune globulin (IVIg), which was routinely used to replenish antibodies in persons with antibody deficiencies, were administered to children with autoimmune thrombocytopenia (an autoimmune disease in which platelets were destroyed by an autoantibody). IVIg therapy resulted in a rebound of platelet levels and temporary resolution of the thrombocytopenia. IVIg is currently being used for a variety of autoimmune diseases, including SLE. A monoclonal antibody, belimumab, inhibits a factor that activates B cells and has been used in some individuals with SLE. Other reagents have specifically targeted and suppressed B and T cells that are participating in autoimmune responses.[27] This approach has been somewhat successful in SLE, rheumatoid arthritis, and other autoimmune diseases. Improved outcomes may be available in the future with the continued advances in medical research and the use of stem cell treatments.

Transfusion Reactions

Red blood cells (erythrocytes) express several important surface antigens, known collectively as the blood group antigens, that can be targets of alloimmune reactions. More than 80 different red cell antigens are grouped into several dozen blood group systems. The most important of these, because they provoke the strongest humoral alloimmune response, are the ABO and Rh systems.

ABO System. Human blood transfusions were carried out as early as 1818, but they were often unsuccessful. Sometimes after a transfusion, the recipient's red blood cells would clump together, thereby blocking the capillaries and causing death in some instances. In 1901 Karl Landsteiner reported that this reaction was related to the ABO antigens located on the surface of erythrocytes.

The ABO blood group consists of two major carbohydrate antigens, labeled A and B (Fig. 9.8), that are expressed on virtually all cells. These are codominant so that both A and B can be simultaneously expressed, resulting in an individual having any one of four different blood types. The erythrocytes of persons with blood type A express the type A carbohydrate antigen (i.e., carry the A antigen), those with blood type B express the B antigen, those with blood type AB express both A and B antigens on the same cell, and those of blood type O express neither

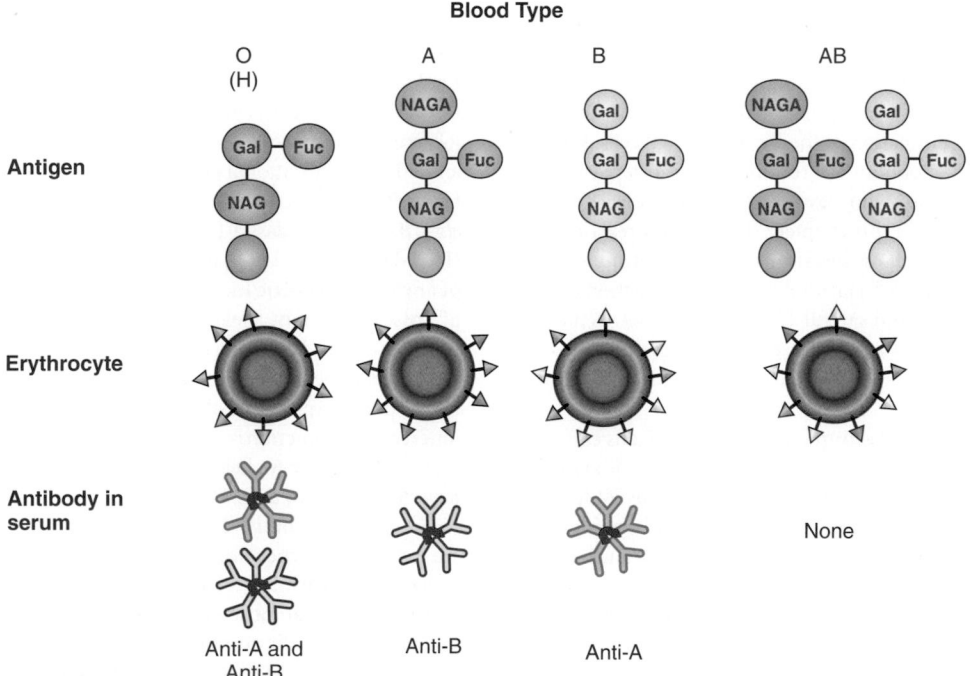

FIGURE 9.8 ABO Blood Types. This figure shows the antigens and antibodies associated with the ABO blood groups. The surfaces of erythrocytes of individuals with blood group O have the core H antigenic carbohydrate. Their sera contain IgM antibodies against both A and B carbohydrates. In individuals of the blood group A, some of the H antigens have been modified into A antigens by the addition of *N*-acetylgalactosamine *(NAGA)*. The sera of these individuals have IgM antibodies against the B antigen. In individuals with blood group B, some of the H antigens have been modified into B antigens by the addition of galactose *(Gal)*. These individuals have IgM antibodies against the A antigen in their sera. In individuals of the blood group AB, some of the H antigens have been modified into both the A and the B antigens. These individuals do not have antibody to either A or B antigens. *Fuc,* Fucose.

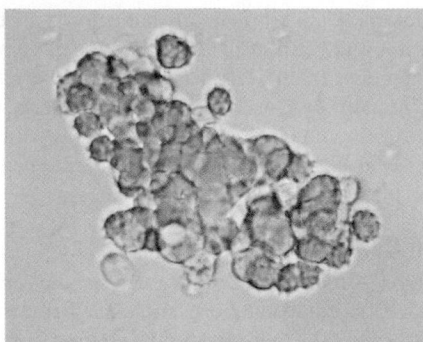

FIGURE 9.9 Mismatched Transfused Blood Cells. Agglutination of erythrocytes caused by anti-A blood-typing serum. (Copyright Ed Reschke.)

the A nor the B antigen. A person with type A blood also has circulating antibodies to the B carbohydrate antigen. If this person receives blood containing B antigens (i.e., blood from a type AB or B individual), a severe transfusion reaction occurs and the transfused erythrocytes are destroyed by agglutination (Fig. 9.9) or complement-mediated lysis. Similarly, a type B individual (whose blood contains anti-A antibodies) cannot receive blood from a type A or type AB donor. Type O individuals, who have neither A nor B antigen but have both anti-A and anti-B antibodies, cannot accept blood from any of the other three types. These naturally occurring antibodies, called isohemagglutinins, are IgM and are induced early in life by similar antigens expressed on naturally occurring bacteria in the intestinal tract.[28]

Because individuals with type O blood lack both types of antigens, they are considered universal donors, meaning that anyone can accept their red blood cells. Similarly, type AB individuals are considered universal recipients because they lack both anti-A and anti-B antibodies and can be transfused with any ABO blood type. When large volumes of *whole blood* (i.e., cells plus plasma) are transfused, however, antibodies in the *donor's* blood can bind to antigenic determinants on the *recipient's* erythrocytes, causing agglutination of the recipient's own cells. Preparations of pooled immunoglobulins are routinely administered intravenously (IVIg) to treat those who have immune deficiencies lacking antibodies (discussed later in this chapter). Transfusion reactions can occur if the IVIg contains excess levels of isohemagglutinins against the recipient's A or B antigens.[29] Harmful transfusion reactions can be prevented only by complete and careful ABO matching between donor and recipient.[30] Because ABO antigens are also expressed on all other cells, except platelets, ABO typing and matching also must be performed before organ transplantation.

Rh System. The Rh blood group is a group of antigens expressed only on red blood cells. This group is the most polymorphic system of red cell antigens, consisting of at least 50 separate antigens. At least five major antigens and a large number of rare variants have been identified and are expressed primarily on erythrocytes. The major antigens are contained on two proteins encoded from two closely linked genes, *RHD* and *RHCE*. The RhD protein expresses the dominant antigen, which determines whether an individual is Rh-positive or Rh-negative. Individuals who express the D antigen on the RhD protein are Rh-positive, whereas individuals who do not express the D antigen are Rh-negative. The letter *d* is used to indicate lack of D. Rh-positive individuals can have either a *DD* or a *Dd* genotype, whereas Rh-negative individuals have the *dd* genotype. About 15% of North American whites are Rh-negative, whereas the Rh-negative genotype is much less common among members of other ethnic groups. Rh-negative individuals can make anti-D if exposed to Rh-positive erythrocytes, but because the letter *d* is used to indicate the lack of the D antigen and does not represent a

different antigen, Rh-positive individuals do not produce an antibody against *d*. The second protein, RhCE, expresses two different antigens, C and E, each of which has two different alleles (*C* or *c*, *E* or *e*). Therefore, four potential haplotypes of C and E antigens are commonly observed: *CE*, *Ce*, *cE*, and *ce*.

A disease called hemolytic disease of the newborn was most commonly caused by IgG anti-D alloantibody produced by Rh-negative mothers against erythrocytes of their Rh-positive fetuses (see Chapter 31).[31] The mother's antibody crossed the placenta and destroyed the red blood cells of the fetus. The occurrence of this particular form of the disease has decreased dramatically because of the use of prophylactic IgG anti-D immunoglobulin (e.g., Rh$_o$[D] immunoglobulin).[32] By mechanisms that are still not completely understood, administration of anti-D antibody within a few days of exposure to RhD-positive erythrocytes completely prevents sensitization against the D antigen. Because hemolytic disease of the newborn related to the D antigen has been controlled, alloantibodies against the other Rh antigens (usually C, c, or E) have become more important. In general, these alloantibodies are associated with a less severe hemolytic disease.

A form of autoimmune hemolytic anemia is often caused by autoantibodies against Rh antigens, especially the e antigen.[33] This variant is caused by IgG antibodies that react with erythrocytes at normal body temperature (thus called *warm autoimmune hemolytic anemia*) and increase phagocytic destruction of the red blood cell. This characteristic differentiates the warm variant from another form of autoimmune hemolytic anemia, which is caused by IgM autoantibodies that react optimally with erythrocytes in the cooler portions of the body (e.g., fingers, toes) and is referred to as *cold autoimmune hemolytic anemia*.

Graft Rejection

Molecules of the major histocompatibility complex (MHC) were discussed in Chapter 8 as antigen-presenting molecules. MHC molecules also are a major target of transplant rejection. As a result of studies of transplantation, the human MHC molecules are also referred to as human leukocyte antigens (HLAs), and the different MHC genetic loci are commonly called HLA-A, HLA-B, HLA-C, HLA-DR, HLA-DQ, and HLA-DP. Additional genes for complement components (e.g., C4, factor B) also are contained in the MHC region and are referred to as *class III loci*. The class I (HLA-A, -B, and -C) and class II MHC loci (HLA-DR, -DQ, and -DP) are the most genetically diverse (polymorphic) of any human genetic loci. Within the human population, the number of possible different alleles (i.e., forms of the gene) expressed by each locus is astounding. For example, more than 300 different HLA-A molecules are expressed in the population. These numbers are based on the polymorphism of observed DNA sequences and may not reflect differences in function.

Clearly, not every allele is expressed in the same individual. Humans have two copies of each MHC locus (one inherited from each parent) that are codominant so that molecules encoded by each parent's genes are expressed on the surface of every cell, except erythrocytes. Within an individual, each locus will express only one allele. For instance, each person will have at most two different HLA-A proteins (one from each parent). The specific combination of alleles at the six major HLA loci on one chromosome (A, B, C, DR, DQ, and DP) is termed a *haplotype*. Each individual has two HLA haplotypes, one from the paternal chromosome 6 and another from the maternal chromosome. Odds dictate that children will share one haplotype with half their siblings and either no haplotypes or both haplotypes with a quarter of their siblings. Thus the chance of finding a match among siblings is 25%. Because of the tremendous number of possible alleles expressed throughout the population, the probability of matching any two unrelated individuals is extremely small.

Not all HLA loci are equally important; matching at the HLA-DR locus appears to be the most critical for graft acceptance, and matching at HLA-A and HLA-B of slightly lesser importance. (These loci also are discussed in Chapter 8.)

Transplant rejection may be classified as hyperacute, acute, or chronic, depending on the amount of time that elapses between transplantation and rejection. **Hyperacute rejection** is immediate and rare. When the circulation is reestablished to the grafted area, the graft may immediately turn white (the so-called *white graft*) instead of a normal pink. Hyperacute rejection usually occurs in recipients with preexisting antibody (type II reaction) to HLA antigens on vascular endothelium in the graft. The antibodies may have resulted from rejection of a previous graft or from prior blood transfusions that contained platelets and white blood cells with foreign HLA. Additionally, about half of women who have had multiple pregnancies have circulating antibodies against their husband's HLA antigens. As the circulation to the graft is established, antibodies bind to the vascular endothelial cells in the grafted tissue and activate the inflammatory response, including the coagulation cascade, which results in stasis of blood flow into the tissue (see Fig. E 9.1 on Evolve). (Coagulation is described in Chapters 7 and 28.) Biopsies of the graft often show deposits of antibody (IgG and IgM), complement, and neutrophils. This condition is rare because of effective pretransplantation cross-matching during which a recipient is tested for antibodies against the HLA antigens of the potential donor.

Acute rejection is primarily a cell-mediated immune response that occurs within days to months after transplantation. This type of rejection occurs when the recipient develops an immune response against unmatched HLAs after transplantation. Sensitization is usually initiated by the recipient's lymphocytes interacting with the donor's dendritic cells within the transplanted tissue, resulting in induction of recipient Th1 and Tc cells against the donor's antigens. The Th1 cells release cytokines that activate infiltrating macrophages, and the Tc cells directly attack the endothelial cells in the transplanted tissue. A biopsy of the rejected organ usually shows an infiltration of lymphocytes and macrophages characteristic of a type IV reaction. Immunosuppressive drugs may delay or lessen the intensity of acute rejection.

Another form of acute rejection, *acute antibody-mediated rejection,* has recently been recognized and accounts for about 10% of acute rejections. This form of rejection is mediated by antibody and complement. The predominant antibodies are against HLA antigens or, on occasion, autoantigens in the graft (e.g., vimentin, angiotensin receptor), but, unlike those antibodies that cause hyperacute rejection, are not present at the time of transplantation. Sensitization takes 2 weeks or longer and results in the accumulation of antibody, complement, neutrophils, and thrombi in the vasculature of the graft (a type II hypersensitivity reaction).

Chronic rejection may occur after a period of months or years of normal function. It is characterized by slow, progressive organ failure. Chronic rejection usually results from a weak cell-mediated immunologic (type IV) reaction against minor histocompatibility antigens on the grafted tissue. However, antibodies against HLA and other antigens also may cause chronic rejection through activation of complement or antibody-dependent cellular cytotoxicity (ADCC) with NK cells.

DEFICIENCIES IN IMMUNITY

Disorders resulting from immune deficiency are the clinical sequelae (results) of impaired function of one or more components of the immune or inflammatory response (e.g., B cells, T cells, phagocytes, complement) (Table 9.6). An **immune deficiency** is the failure of these mechanisms of self-defense to function at their normal capacity, resulting in increased susceptibility to infections. A **primary (congenital) immune** deficiency is caused generally by a genetic anomaly, whereas a **secondary (acquired) immune deficiency** is caused by another illness, such as cancer or viral infection, or by normal physiologic changes, such as aging. Acquired forms of immune deficiency are far more common than the congenital forms.

Initial Clinical Presentation

The clinical hallmark of immune deficiency is a tendency to develop unusual or recurrent, severe infections. The most severe primary immune deficiencies develop in young children 2 years old and younger. Frequent infections are normal in preschool and school-age children, who normally have 6 to 12 infections per year, of which 3 or 4 are ear infections, and adults may have 2 to 4 infections per year. Most of these are not severe and are limited to viral infections of the upper respiratory tract, recurrent streptococcal pharyngitis, or mild otitis media.

Potential immune deficiencies are considered if the individual has had severe, documented bouts of pneumonia, severe otitis media, sinusitis, bronchitis, septicemia, or meningitis or infections with rare opportunistic microorganisms that normally are not pathogenic or usually confined to one site (e.g., *Pneumocystis jirovecii,* disseminated *Candida* infection, cytomegalovirus [CMV]). Infections are generally recurrent with only short intervals of relative health, and multiple simultaneous infections are common. Individuals with primary immune deficiencies often have eight or more purulent ear infections, two or more serious sinus infections, and two or more pneumonias, recurrent abscesses or infections in unusual sites, or persistent fungal infections (particularly thrush in a child at least 1 year old) within a year. Invasive fungal infections are rare in healthy individuals and strongly indicate a defective immune system. Recurrent internal infections, such as meningitis, osteomyelitis, or sepsis, are common. Prolonged antibiotic use is commonly ineffective by oral or injected routes and may necessitate intravenous administration. Children frequently present with failure to thrive because of chronic diarrhea and other chronic symptoms. A familial history of immune deficiency may be found in some types of primary deficiency.

Routine care of individuals with immune deficiencies must be tempered with the knowledge that the immune system may be totally ineffective. It is unsafe to administer conventional immunizing agents or blood products to many of these individuals because of the risk of causing an uncontrolled infection. Infection is a particular problem when attenuated vaccines that contain live but weakened microorganisms are used (e.g., live polio vaccine; vaccines against measles, mumps, and rubella).

The type of recurrent infections that manifest may indicate the type of immune defect. Deficiencies in T-cell immune responses associated with recurrent infections are caused by certain viruses (e.g., varicella, vaccinia, herpes, cytomegalovirus), fungi and yeasts (e.g., *Candida, Histoplasma*), or certain atypical microorganisms (e.g., *P. jirovecii*). B-cell deficiencies and phagocyte deficiencies, however, are suggested if the individual has documented, recurrent infections with microorganisms that require opsonization (e.g., encapsulated bacteria) or viruses against which humoral immunity is normally effective (e.g., rubella). Some complement deficiencies resemble defects in antibody or phagocyte function, but others are characterized by disseminated infections with bacteria of the genus *Neisseria* (*Neisseria meningitidis* and *Neisseria gonorrhoeae*).

Much of the current understanding of the development of the immune system and the interactions of the cells in the immune response was developed by studying congenital and acquired immune deficiencies or, as they have been called, "experiments of nature." Many immune deficiencies result from selective alteration or removal of one component of the immune system. The importance of that component can be

TABLE 9.6   CLASSES OF PRIMARY IMMUNE DEFICIENCIES

CLASSIFICATION	EXAMPLE	MUTATION	IMMUNE DEFICIENCY
Combined Deficiencies Without Nonimmunological Abnormalities			
SCID: No WBC stem cells	Reticular dysgenesis	Unknown	Complete lack of white blood cells
SCID: Enzyme defects	Adenosine deaminase (ADA) deficiency	*ADA*	Complete, few, or no T, B, or NK cells
	Purine nucleoside phosphorylase (PNP) deficiency	*PNP*	Few T or NK cells
SCID: Cytokine receptor defects	X-linked	*IL-2Rγ*	Partial or no maturation of Th and NK cells (T−, B+, NK−)
	Autosomal	*JAK3*	Absence of T and NK cells (T−, B+, NK−)
	Janus kinase 3 deficiency	*IL-7Rα*	Absence of T cells (T−, B+, NK+)
	IL-7 receptor deficiency		
SCID: Antigen presentation defects	Bare lymphocyte syndrome MHC class I deficiency	*TAP1* or *TAP2*	Abnormal cytotoxic T-cell activity
	Bare lymphocyte syndrome MHC class II deficiency	Multiple	Abnormal helper T-cell activity
SCID: TCR/BCR defects	RAG-1 or RAG-2 deficiency	*RAG-1/RAG-2*	Lack of maturation of T or B cells; normal NK cells
SCID: TCR defects	CD45 deficiency	CD45	Partial to incomplete T-cell maturation, normal B and NK cells
	CD3 deficiency	CD3 γ, δ, or ε chains	
	ZAP-70 deficiency	*ZAP-70*	
Combined Deficiencies With Nonimmunological Abnormalities			
Cytoskeletal defect	Wiskott-Aldrich syndrome (WAS)	*WASP*	Altered T and B cells; decreased IgM; thrombocytopenia, eczema
DNA repair defect	Ataxia-telangiectasia (AT)	*ATM*	Altered T and B cells; absent IgA; ataxia, telangiectasia
Defective primary lymphoid organ for T-cell development	DiGeorge syndrome	Development of 3rd and 4th pharyngeal pouches	Little or no T-cell maturation; small or absent thymus, hypoparathyroidism (diminished Ca levels, tetany), facial defects
Predominantly Antibody Deficiencies			
B-cell receptor signaling	Bruton/X-linked agammaglobulinemia	*Btk*	Little or no B-cell maturation or antibody
	Autosomal agammaglobulinemia	IgM μ chain	
Class-switch: hyper-IgM	X-linked hyper-IgM syndrome	CD40 ligand	Little or no class-switch to IgG or IgA, with overproduction of IgM
	Autosomal hyper-IgM syndrome	CD40	
	AICD deficiency	*AICD*	
Class-switch: selective	IgG subclass deficiency	Unknown	Defective switch to an IgG subclass
	Selective IgA deficiency	Unknown	Defective switch to IgA
	Common variable immune deficiency	Multiple	Defective switch to ≥1 antibody class
Immune Dysregulation			
Decreased cellular killing	Perforin deficiency	Perforin *(PRF1)*	Decreased or absent Tc and NK cells
Bacterial killing defect	Chédiak-Higashi syndrome	*CHS1*	Defective lysosomal granules
Phagocyte Defects			
Neutropenia	Severe congenital neutropenia	Elastase, neutrophil-expressed *(ELAINE)*	Severe deficiency in neutrophils
	Cyclic neutropenia	Elastase *(ELA2)*	Mild periodic neutropenia
Bacterial killing	Chronic granulomatous disease	NADPH oxidase	Defective production of H_2O_2
	Myeloperoxidase deficiency	Myeloperoxidase *(MPO)*	Mild killing defect
Diapedesis defect	Leukocyte adhesion deficiency-1 (LAD-1)	CD18	Defective invasion
	Leukocyte adhesion deficiency-2 (LAD-2)	Glycosylation pathway	Defective invasion
Innate Immunity Defects			
Macrophage response defect	Chronic mucocutaneous candidiasis	Mutations in Th17 or macrophage IL-17 receptor	Little or no response to *Candida*

TABLE 9.6 CLASSES OF PRIMARY IMMUNE DEFICIENCIES—cont'd

CLASSIFICATION	EXAMPLE	MUTATION	IMMUNE DEFICIENCY
Autoinflammatory Disorders			
Control of inflammasome	Familial Mediterranean fever	*MEFV*	Excess IL-1β production
Complement Defects			
Classical pathway	C1q, r, s; C4; or C2 deficiency	C1q, r, or s; C4; or C2	Defective classical pathway, intact alternative pathway
Lectin pathway	Mannose-binding lectin (MBL) deficiency	*MBL*	Defective lectin pathway
Alternative pathway	Properdin, factor D or B deficiency	Properdin, factor D or B	Defective alternative pathway
	Factor H, factor I deficiency	Factor H, factor I	Secondary C3 deficiency
C3	C3 deficiency	C3	Entire complement cascade blocked
Terminal pathway	C5, C6, C7, C8, or C9 deficiency	C5, C6, C7, C8, or C9	Membrane attack complex blocked, normal opsonization and chemotaxis

AICD, Activation-induced cytidine deaminase; *ATM,* ataxia-telangiectasia mutated serine/threonine kinase; *Btk,* Bruton tyrosine kinase; *CHS1,* Chédiak-Higashi syndrome 1 (also known as *LYST,* lysosomal trafficking regulator); *IL-2Rγ,* interleukin-2 receptor gamma chain; *IL-7Rα,* interleukin-7 receptor alpha chain; *MEFV,* Mediterranean fever gene; *MHC,* major histocompatibility complex; *NADPH,* nicotinamide adenine dinucleotide phosphate; *NK,* natural killer cell; *RAG,* recombination activating gene; *SCID,* severe combined immune deficiency; *TAP,* transporter associated with antigen processing; *TCR/BCR,* T-cell receptor/B-cell receptor; *WASP,* Wiskott-Aldrich syndrome protein; *WBC,* white blood cell; *ZAP,* zeta-chain associated protein.

understood by observing the effect of its removal on the remainder of the immune response.

Primary Immune Deficiencies

Most primary immune deficiencies are the result of single gene defects (Fig. 9.10). Generally, the mutations are sporadic and not inherited: a family history exists in only about 25% of individuals. The sporadic mutations occur before birth, but the onset of symptoms may be early in neonatal life or later, depending on the particular syndrome. In approximately 60% of the cases, symptoms of immune deficiency appear within the first 2 years of life, whereas other immune deficiencies are progressive, with the onset of symptoms appearing in the second or third decade of life. The most common symptoms include sinusitis (68% of individuals), pneumonia (51%), ear infections (51%), diarrhea (30%), and bronchitis (55%), with the incidence varying depending on the specific syndrome.

Individually, primary immune deficiencies are very rare. For instance, only 30 to 50 new cases of severe combined immune deficiency are diagnosed in the United States yearly. However, more than 200 different genetic defects resulting in immune deficiencies have been identified, and the number is growing rapidly. Together, primary immune deficiencies are more common than cystic fibrosis, hemophilia, childhood leukemia, or many other well-known diseases. Many are subtle with minor deficiencies, but several lead to recurrent life-threatening infections. An estimated 50,000 cases of clinically significant primary immune deficiency have been reported in the United States. The gender distribution depends on the specific disease, but in general those diagnosed within the first 2 years of life have a male preponderance (5:1) because many are X-linked, whereas those diagnosed later are evenly distributed. The three most commonly diagnosed deficiencies are common variable immune deficiency (34% of individuals with primary immune deficiencies), selective IgA deficiency (24%), and IgG subclass deficiency (17%).

Primary immune deficiencies have recently been reclassified into nine groups, based on which principal component of the immune or inflammatory systems is defective.[34] On occasion a particular immune deficiency may be listed under two categories because the predominant mechanism may not be fully understood. To provide a better understanding of the diversity and severity of primary immune deficiencies, only a very few selected examples will be discussed.

Combined Deficiencies without Nonimmunologic Abnormalities

A great deal of knowledge about the evolution of bone marrow stem cells into functional lymphocytes came from studying children with deficiencies of more than one type of lymphocyte (combined immune deficiencies). The most severe group of immune deficiencies is severe combined immune deficiency (SCID). The most severe form of SCID is reticular dysgenesis (failure of blood cells to develop), in which a common stem cell for all white blood cells is absent; therefore, T cells, B cells, and phagocytic cells never develop (see Fig. 9.10). Most children with reticular dysgenesis die in utero or very soon after birth. Most typically, a defect occurs after stem cells become committed to developing into lymphocytes (lymphoid stem cells); therefore, most individuals with SCID have normal numbers of granulocytes.

Most individuals with SCID have few detectable lymphocytes in the circulation and secondary lymphoid organs (spleen, lymph nodes). The thymus is usually underdeveloped because of the absence of T cells. Immunoglobulin levels, especially IgM and IgA, are absent or greatly reduced.

At least 20 different forms of SCID have been identified. Depending on the specific genetic mutation, the defect may involve T cells, B cells, and NK cells or may suppress the function of one cell type more severely with relatively minor effects on the others. SCID often results in few or absent T and B lymphocytes in the circulation and secondary lymphoid organs (spleen, lymph nodes). The thymus is usually hypoplastic (underdeveloped) because of the absence of T cells. Immunoglobulin levels, especially of IgM and IgA, are absent or greatly reduced, although IgG levels may be almost normal in the first months of life because of the presence of maternal antibodies. In the most severe defects, death occurs at about 1 year of life.

All three cells are adversely affected (T–, B–, NK–) in SCID; it develops from an autosomal recessive enzymatic defect in adenosine deaminase (ADA) deficiency, resulting in the accumulation of toxic purine metabolites to which rapidly dividing cells, such as lymphocytes, are

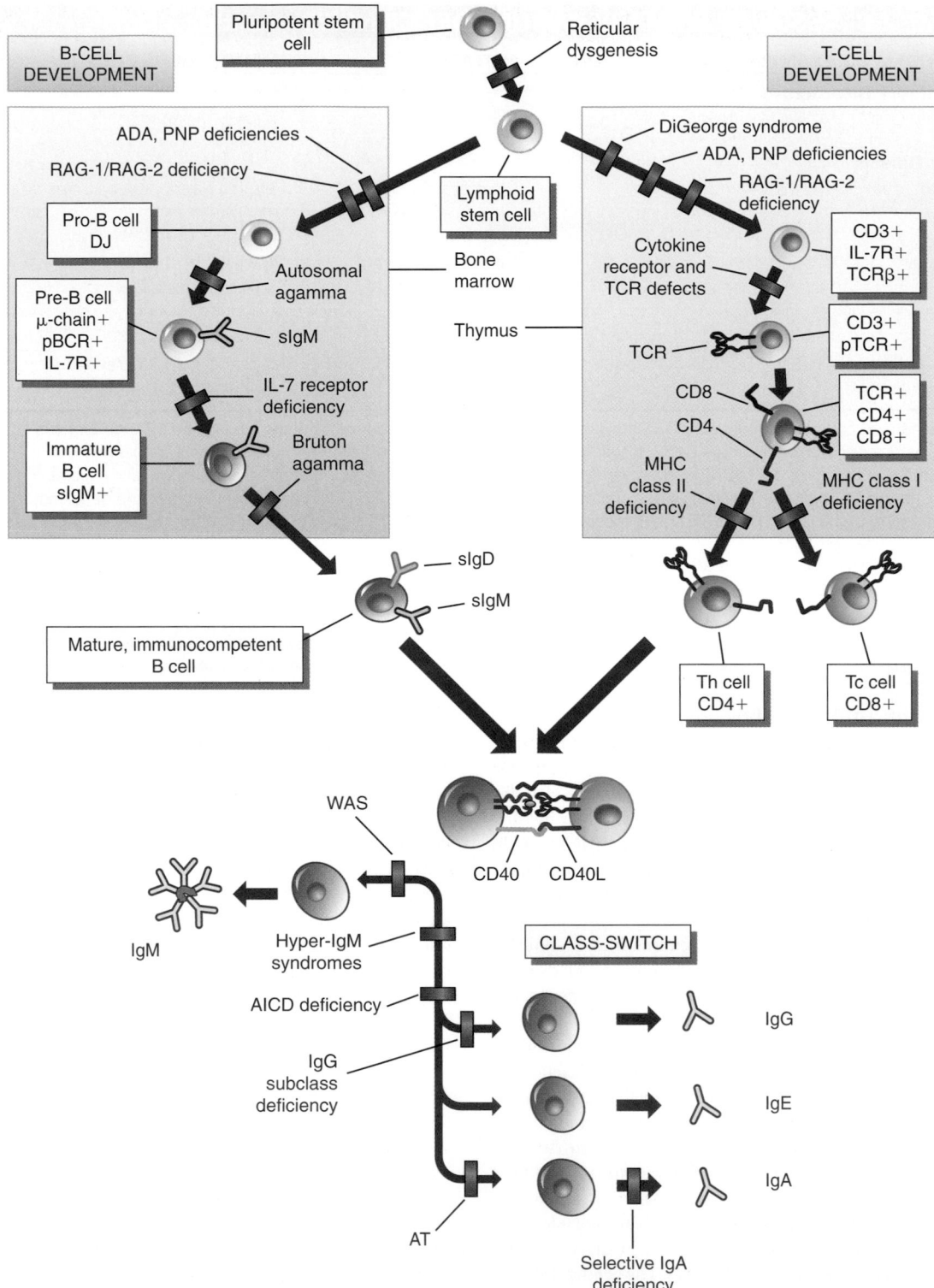

FIGURE 9.10 Lymphocyte Development Defects. This diagram shows defects in lymphocyte development that may account for congenital (primary) immune deficiencies. See the text and refer to Figs. 8.9 and 8.12 for more detailed information. Pluripotent stem cell indicates the common stem cells for lymphocytic, granulocytic, and monocytic lineages. Cytokine receptor defects include X-linked severe combined immunodeficiency (SCID) (IL-2 receptor defect), JAK3 defects, and IL-7 receptor defects. T-cell receptor (TCR) defects include defects in CD3, CD45, and ZAP-70. Neither common variable immune deficiency nor chronic mucocutaneous candidiasis is included in this figure because the cause of these defects remains unknown. See Table 9.6 for further information on each defect. *ADA,* Adenosine deaminase deficiency; *agamma,* agammaglobulinemia; *AICD deficiency,* activation-induced cytidine deaminase deficiency; *AT,* ataxia-telangiectasia; *MHC,* major histocompatibility complex; *PNP,* purine nucleoside phosphorylase deficiency; *RAG,* recombination-activating enzyme; *sIgM* and *sIgD,* surface IgM and IgD, respectively; *WAS,* Wiskott-Aldrich syndrome.

especially sensitive (see Fig. 9.10). ADA deficiency accounts for about 16% of all persons with SCID. The development of T cells, B cells, and NK cells is arrested very early, and very few lymphocytic cells are found in the blood. Mutation of another purine metabolism enzyme, purine nucleoside phosphorylase (purine nucleoside phosphorylase [PNP] deficiency), is less severe than ADA deficiency (see Fig. 9.10). T cells and NK cells appear to be more susceptible to mutations in PNP so that B-cell function can be relatively normal (T−, B+, NK−).

X-linked SCID results from a common defect in most of the important cytokine receptors needed for lymphocyte maturation (e.g., IL-2, IL-4, IL-7, and others). T cells and NK cells are preferentially affected (T−, B+, NK−), but the defect often results in the production of immature B cells that cannot respond well to antigen because of the lack of Th cells. The most common (44% of those with SCID) is an X-linked SCID resulting from a defect in the IL-2 receptor gamma (γ)-chain (IL-2Rγ). This protein is a component of several receptors for cytokines, including IL-2, IL-4, IL-7, IL-9, IL-15, and IL-21. A similar, but autosomal, deficiency occurs with a mutation in JAK3 (JAK3 deficiency), which is an enzyme (a tyrosine kinase) that associates with IL-2Rγ in normal cells and communicates information from the receptor to the nucleus. Thus cells with defects in JAK3 cannot respond to cytokines that bind to these receptors on the cell surface. Another autosomal form of SCID results from mutations in the α chain of the IL-7 receptor (IL-7 receptor deficiency). IL-7 is necessary for the maturation of T cells within the thymus, so that this deficiency has relatively normal levels of B cells and NK cells (T−, B+, NK+).

Even if nearly adequate numbers of B and T cells are produced, their cooperation may be defective. The bare lymphocyte syndrome is a group of immune deficiencies characterized by an inability of lymphocytes and macrophages to produce major histocompatibility complex (MHC) class I or class II molecules. Without MHC molecules, antigen presentation and intercellular cooperation cannot occur effectively (see Fig. 9.10). MHC class I deficiency results from mutations in the genes for the transporters associated with antigen processing (TAP1 or TAP2), which control the transport of antigenic protein fragments across the endoplasmic reticulum and the formation of MHC class I/antigen complexes for transportation to the cell surface (see Fig. 8.15). Because MHC class I molecules preferentially present antigen to CD8+ Tc cells, the resultant deficiency is of CD8+ cytotoxic cells, with normal levels of CD4+ helper cells and normal antibody production. MHC class II deficiency is more severe. A variety of mutations prevent normal production of MHC class II molecules, which present antigen to CD4+ helper cells. Because of defective recruitment of T-helper cells, normal antibody responses are greatly suppressed. Children with this deficiency develop life-threatening infections and usually die before age 5 years.

T and B lymphocytes possess receptors for antigen, whereas NK cells do not. Those receptors result from a process of genetic rearrangement of V and J genes to form the variable regions of the L chain (B-cell receptor [BCR]) and the α chain (T-cell receptor [TCR]) and the V, D, and J genes to form the variable regions of the H chain (BCR) and the β chain (TCR). Successful genetic rearrangement is controlled by two recombination activating enzymes (RAG-1 and RAG-2). RAG-1 or RAG-2 deficiencies are autosomal recessive and result in arrested lymphocyte development from blocked recombination of variable regions of B-cell and T-cell receptors (see Fig. 9.10), whereas NK cells are not affected (T−, B−, NK+).

Forms of partial SCID, with the defect being primarily of T cells, arise from mutations in several components of the TCR complex (see Fig. 9.10). The TCR is a complex organization of proteins that react with antigen (α and β chains) and then provide an intracellular signal to the nucleus (γ, δ, and ε chains [collectively called CD3] and the associated molecules CD45 and ZAP-70). Examples of these deficiencies include mutations in CD3, CD45, or ZAP-70. The T-cell defect in each can range from mild to severe in nature, with normal B lymphocytes and NK cells (T−, B+, NK+). Although B cells are normal, antibody production may be depressed because of the lack of Th cells.

Combined Deficiencies with Nonimmunologic Abnormalities

Some combined immune deficiencies are associated with other characteristic defects, some of which appear to be unrelated to the immune system yet may be life threatening by themselves. These associated symptoms can be useful diagnostically and can clarify the pathophysiology of the disease. Wiskott-Aldrich syndrome (WAS, an X-linked recessive disorder) results from sporadic mutations in the WAS protein (WASP), which is involved in intracellular signaling and regulation of the cell's actin cytoskeleton (see Fig. 9.10). Defects in the cytoskeleton lead to the classic symptoms of thrombocytopenia (with resultant bleeding disorders), scaly eczema, and recurrent infections. IgA and IgG levels are usually normal, but antibody responses against antigens that elicit primarily an IgM response, such as polysaccharides from bacterial capsules (e.g., *Pseudomonas aeruginosa, Streptococcus pneumoniae [S. pneumoniae], Haemophilus influenzae [H. influenzae]*) are deficient. Persons with WAS also have a very high risk of lymphoid malignancies (leukemias and lymphomas).

Ataxia-telangiectasia (AT) is an autosomal recessive disorder resulting from a large variety of sporadic mutations in the *ATM* gene, which encodes a protein involved in repair of double-stranded breaks in DNA. Affected infants often develop ataxia (unsteady gait), which usually becomes apparent when the child is learning to walk. The neurologic defect may eventually lead to confinement in a wheelchair. Telangiectasia (dilation of capillaries) can occur in the eyes and skin, especially on the ears, neck, and extremities. Both B cells and T cells are variably affected and unrepaired double-stranded DNA breaks are commonly observed in the regions encoding the T-cell and B-cell receptors. About 70% of those with AT are IgA deficient, occasionally accompanied by deficiencies in IgG (see Fig. 9.10). Individuals with AT are at high risk for developing leukemias and lymphomas.

DiGeorge syndrome (congenital thymic aplasia or hypoplasia and diminished parathyroid gland development) is caused by the lack or partial lack of the thymus, resulting in greatly decreased T-cell numbers and function and life-threatening viral, fungal, and intracellular bacterial infections.[35] The defect is usually attributed to deletions on chromosome 22 (some deletions also have been identified on chromosome 10),[36] about 25% of which are inherited. The deleted region encodes information for formation of organs that originate from the third and fourth pharyngeal pouches during the twelfth week of gestation. Defective development of the third and fourth pharyngeal pouches during embryogenesis results in the thymic defects, lack of the parathyroid gland (causing an inability to regulate calcium concentration), major structural defects in the heart and the aorta (resulting in inadequate blood flow and inadequate oxygenation of the tissues), and abnormal facial characteristics (e.g., underdeveloped chin, low-set ears, shortened structure of the upper lip) (see Fig. E 9.2 on Evolve). Low blood calcium levels cause the development of tetany or involuntary rigid muscular contraction.

Predominantly Antibody Deficiencies

Predominantly antibody deficiencies result from defects in B-cell maturation or function and are the most common immune deficiencies. T-cell immune responses are not affected in pure B-lymphocyte deficiencies. These deficiencies are widely characterized by lower levels of circulating immunoglobulins (hypogammaglobulinemia) or occasionally totally or nearly absent immunoglobulins (agammaglobulinemia). Recurrent infections range from life threatening to mild, depending on the severity of the deficiency. Characteristic infections include encapsulated bacteria (e.g., *S. pneumoniae, H. influenzae*) that may cause pneumonia or sepsis and other microorganisms that cause infections of the sinuses, ears, and gastrointestinal tract.

One of the most severe B-lymphocyte deficiencies is Bruton agammaglobulinemia. This condition results from mutations in the gene for Bruton tyrosine kinase *(Btk)*—an enzyme involved in intracellular signaling from several B-cell receptors, including the IgM B-cell antigen receptor, the IL-5 receptor, and the IL-6 receptor. Ineffective signaling results in the arrest of the development in the bone marrow of early cells in the B-cell lineage into mature B cells[37] (see Fig. 9.10). Somewhat less than a third of the mutations are sporadic. Few or no circulating mature B cells are present, although T-cell number and function are normal. At 6 months of life, the approximate normal serum concentrations of immunoglobulins are the following: IgG, 400 mg/dL; IgM, 40 mg/dL; and IgA, 30 mg/dL. In 6-month-old children with Bruton agammaglobulinemia, serum IgG levels are much less than 100 mg/dL, and IgM and IgA are almost absent.

An autosomal recessive form of agammaglobulinemia (autosomal agammaglobulinemia) results from other mutations in the B-cell receptor. The most common is a mutation of the mu (μ) chain of the IgM portion of the receptor. This mutation prevents intracellular signaling after antigen binds to the receptor, leading to blocked maturation, the absence of antibody production, and very severe infections.

Common variable immune deficiency is the most commonly diagnosed immune deficiency. As the name implies, the presentation is very heterogeneous. It is characterized by hypogammaglobulinemia, but the particular class of antibody that is decreased varies. Most individuals have low amounts of IgG, which may or may not be accompanied by decreased levels of IgA or IgM, or both, with normal numbers of B cells. Some may have accompanying T-cell defects. Multiple genetic defects in terminal differentiation account for this condition, although the specific defects have not been identified in most people. The age of onset of symptoms, such as recurrent bacterial respiratory tract infections, is generally later than most primary immune deficiencies (late 20s). Secondary complications include arthritis (infectious and noninfectious), gastrointestinal symptoms (malabsorption, chronic diarrhea), autoimmune disease (anemia, thrombocytopenia, endocrine diseases), and cancer (of the lymphoid system, skin, and gastrointestinal tract).

Some defects may involve a particular class of antibody, such as selective IgA deficiency, in which only IgA is suppressed. Because many affected individuals are asymptomatic, the true incidence is uncertain, although clinically relevant symptoms may occur in 1 in 700 to 1 in 400 individuals. Individuals with selective IgA deficiency are able to produce other classes of immunoglobulins but fail to produce IgA (see Fig. 9.10). Many will have B cells that have undergone class-switch to IgA but, for unknown reasons, cannot undergo the terminal steps of differentiation to IgA-secreting plasma cells.

Affected individuals may have a history of recurring sinus, pulmonary, and gastrointestinal infections, particularly chronic intestinal candidiasis (infection with *C. albicans*). Complications of IgA deficiency include severe allergic disease and autoimmune diseases. Selective IgA deficiency is two or three times more common in atopic individuals than in others. Secretory IgA normally may prevent the uptake of allergens from the environment, so that IgA deficiency may lead to a more intense challenge to the immune system by prolonged exposure to environmental antigens.

One of the most severe complications of IgA deficiency is an anaphylactic reaction that can follow administration of blood products that contain IgA. Serious anaphylactic reactions can occur in individuals totally lacking IgA because the immune system recognizes donor IgA as a foreign antigen. Initial sensitization can occur in fetal life through exposure to maternal IgA that leaks across the placenta or later through the ingestion of maternal IgA in breast milk or bovine IgA in cow's milk. Sensitization also can occur with initial administration of blood products containing IgA. The individual's primed immune system then acts against donor IgA on subsequent exposure.

Several defects in antibody class-switch have been identified (see Fig. 9.10). A defect in a DNA editing enzyme (activation-induced cytidine deaminase deficiency; AICD deficiency) also inhibits class-switch. During class-switch and movement of the H chain genetic information for the variable region to a different constant region gene, the double-stranded DNA must be cut and mended. This enzyme is responsible for cutting and mending the DNA; thus IgM may be overproduced and levels of IgG and IgA diminished.

Deficiencies in certain subclasses of antibody (IgG subclass deficiency), particularly IgG2, may result from a defect in switch to a particular subclass constant region (see Fig. 9.10). The level of IgG2 subclass is often increased in response to polysaccharide antigens such as those on the surface of encapsulated bacteria. Low levels of IgG2 may be responsible for recurrent risk for pneumonias caused by these bacteria. Whether IgG subclass deficiencies are unique immune deficiency conditions is unclear because many are apparently early indications of the development of common variable immune deficiency or are secondary to selective IgA deficiency.

X-linked or autosomal recessive hyper-IgM syndrome results from a mutation in the CD40 ligand (CD40L deficiency) or, less commonly, the CD40 receptor (CD40 deficiency), respectively.[38] The CD40/CD40L interaction provides an important signal between T-helper (Th) cells and B cells during the initiation of class-switch (see Fig. 8.18). A critical ligand-receptor interaction occurs between the receptor CD40 on the B cell and its ligand (CD154 or CD40L) on the Th cell. A mutation in CD40L or CD40 results in defective class-switch, decreased or absent production of IgG and IgA, poor development of memory B cells, and overproduction of IgM, resulting in increased infections with opportunistic bacteria. T-cell immunity is not affected. This particular immune deficiency is co-listed as a combined immune deficiency because of the potential of mutations that affect either the Th cell or the B cell.

Immune Dysregulation

The classification of immune dysregulation presents causes of immune deficiencies and includes conditions in which the regulation of components of the immune system is predominant.

Perforin deficiency results from a mutation in perforin, which is an important component of cellular killing by cytotoxic T cells and NK cells (see Fig. 8.26), resulting in decreased or absent Tc and NK cells. Several other deficiencies result from mutations in secretory vesicle function, including fusion with the cell membrane and other aspects of the process. Mutations in interleukin IL-10 or its receptor IL-10R suppress the production or response to IL-10 (an immunosuppressive cytokine), resulting in excessive inflammation and an increased risk for early-onset inflammatory bowel disease, or recurrent respiratory disease.[39]

Chédiak-Higashi syndrome results from a defect in the movement of cytoplasmic granules and is caused by an autosomal recessive mutation in the lysosomal trafficking regulator gene *(CHS1)*. The CHS1 protein helps control movement of granules to cellular membranes in preparation for degranulation. As a result of these mutations, the granules remain in the cytoplasm and form large aggregates that are readily apparent microscopically. Leukocytes from individuals with Chédiak-Higashi syndrome have decreased chemotaxis, granular fusion, and bacterial killing. Platelet granules also may be affected, resulting in prolonged bleeding, and partial albinism can occur because of defects in melanocyte granules. Affected children develop recurrent infections of the skin, respiratory tract, and mucous membranes, especially with gram-positive bacteria.

Phagocyte Defects: Numbers, Function, or Both

Phagocyte defects range from inadequate numbers of phagocytes (e.g., severe congenital neutropenia) to defects in phagocyte function that can result in recurrent infections (Fig. 9.11). Because phagocytosis is generally aided by bacterial opsonization with IgG or C3b, infection occurs with the same group of microorganisms (encapsulated bacteria) that are associated with antibody and complement deficiencies.

Inadequate numbers of phagocytes, particularly neutrophils (severe congenital neutropenias), result in a variety of recurrent and severe bacterial infections beginning early in life. Approximately 50% of these individuals have mutations in the gene for elastase, neutrophil-expressed (ELANE). Other mutations have been identified (e.g., WAS gene) in the other 50%. A milder form, cyclic neutropenia, is autosomal dominant with almost 100% of affected individuals having a mutation in the ELA2 gene. Changes in neutrophil levels are cyclic and may remain at or near normal for 2 to 3 weeks, followed by periods of neutropenia lasting a few days to weeks. During the neutropenia, the individual has increased susceptibility to recurrent bacterial infections.

Chronic granulomatous disease (CGD) is group of disorders resulting from severe X-linked (about 70% of the individuals) or autosomal defects in the respiratory burst necessary for the myeloperoxidase–hydrogen peroxide system, a major means of bacterial destruction using the enzyme myeloperoxidase, halides (e.g., chloride ion), and hydrogen peroxide (H_2O_2).[40] Neutrophils and other phagocytes switch much of their glucose metabolism to the hexose-monophosphate shunt during phagocytosis. A byproduct of this pathway is the conversion of molecular oxygen by nicotinamide adenine dinucleotide phosphate (NADPH) oxidase into highly reactive oxygen derivatives, including hydrogen peroxide. Mutations in NADPH oxidase or other components of the NADPH oxidase complex result in deficient production of hydrogen peroxide and other oxygen products. Thus affected individuals have adequate myeloperoxidase in the primary granules and halide but lack the necessary hydrogen peroxide, resulting in recurrent severe pneumonias; tumor-like granulomata in lungs, skin, and bones; and other infections with some opportunistic microorganisms, such as *Staphylococcus aureus*, *Serratia marcescens*, and *Aspergillus* spp. The symptoms usually appear in the first 2 years of life.

Recurrent infections occur with rather innocuous catalase-positive microorganisms, whereas infections with more virulent catalase-negative microorganisms (e.g., *S. pneumoniae*) are rare. Most microorganisms produce their own hydrogen peroxide as a byproduct, which accumulates in the phagocytic vacuole and can be used by the phagocyte's myeloperoxidase to kill the microorganism. Some microorganisms also produce the enzyme catalase, which breaks down hydrogen peroxide. Thus catalase-negative microorganisms donate hydrogen peroxide to the phagocyte's myeloperoxidase, leading to their own death. Catalase-positive

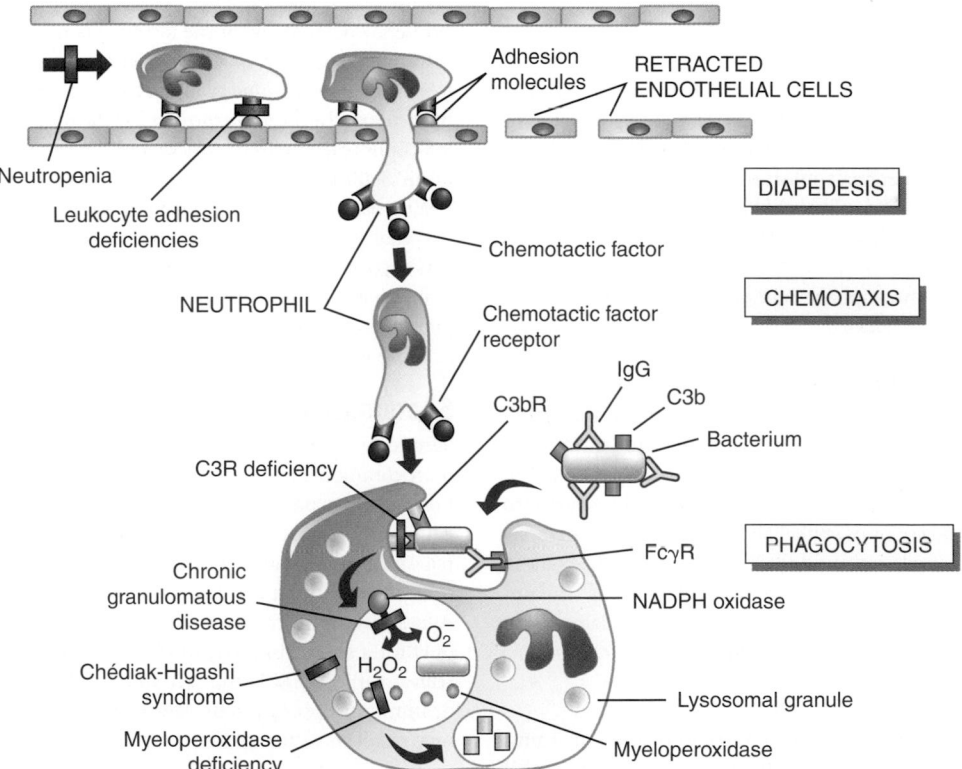

FIGURE 9.11 Phagocytic Defects. Several genetic defects in the process leading up to and including phagocytosis result in increased susceptibility to bacterial infections. See the text and refer to Fig. 7.15 for more detailed information. The phagocyte leaves the bloodstream and enters the tissue through interactions between leukocyte and endothelial adhesion molecules and the process of diapedesis. The cell is attracted to the inflammatory site by chemotaxis, where it encounters opsonized bacteria, and attaches to and engulfs the microorganism. Inside the phagocyte the bacteria are killed and broken down by the combination of lysosomal granule constituents and reactive oxygen products of the hexose-monophosphate shunt and nicotinamide adenine dinucleotide phosphate (NADPH) oxidase. *C3R*, C3 receptor, which includes the C3b receptor *(C3bR)*; *FcγR*, receptor for the Fc portion of IgG; *H₂O₂*, hydrogen peroxide; *O₂⁻*, reactive oxygen.

microorganisms, however, destroy the bacterial hydrogen peroxide and survive to cause infection.

A deficiency in another component of the myeloperoxidase–hydrogen peroxide system, myeloperoxidase deficiency, is a relatively mild disorder characterized by a complete or partial deficiency in myeloperoxidase. Individuals do not have severe recurrent infections because most infectious bacteria are sensitive to direct killing by many of the toxic oxygen molecules produced by NADPH oxidase. The exception is the person with concurrent diabetes, who may have recurrent disseminated candidiasis.

Other phagocytic deficiencies include defects in various leukocyte adhesion molecules (leukocyte adhesion deficiency) that prevent adherence to the vascular endothelium and diapedesis. Leukocyte adhesion deficiency, type 1 (LAD-1) results from an autosomal recessive mutation in CD18, which is a β_2-integrin chain that is shared by several different receptors. Leukocyte adhesion deficiency, type 2 (LAD-2) results from a defect in adding the monosaccharide fucose to carbohydrates on the phagocyte surface. Surface carbohydrates with fucose are ligands for selectins on the endothelium and leukocytes. These and other defects in leukocyte adhesion molecules usually result in increased levels of neutrophils in the blood (leukocytosis, because they cannot leave the circulation) and in increased recurrent bacterial and fungal infections.

Additional deficiencies diminish the leukocyte's capacity to respond to cytokines. Defects in the interferon-γ receptor result in increased susceptibility to infection with pathogenic intracellular bacteria, such as *Mycobacteria* and *Salmonella*.

Defects in Innate Immunity

Some immune deficiencies are characterized by a defect in the capacity to produce a protective innate response against microorganisms. The inherited form of chronic mucocutaneous candidiasis presents with mild to extremely severe recurrent infections of the skin, nails, and mucous membranes with *Candida albicans*. In this condition, the response of macrophages to Th17 lymphocytes is defective because of mutations in IL-17 produced by Th17 lymphocytes or the IL-17 receptor on macrophages.[41] Thus the macrophage cannot be adequately activated to defend against *Candida albicans*.

Autoinflammatory Disorders

Autoinflammatory disorders are characterized by abnormally high levels of inflammation secondary to mutations in control of inflammasome activation or in defects in cellular receptors of cytokines designed to decrease inflammation. These disorders are frequently related to diminished control of infections of epithelial surfaces. Familial Mediterranean fever is an autosomal recessive disorder in eastern Mediterranean populations that results in uncontrolled release of IL-1β by inflammasomes in granulocytes and monocytes.[42] Affected individuals present with skin rashes, usually of the lower extremities, and fever.

Complement Deficiencies

Complement activation is a necessary component of protection against many infectious agents, particularly bacteria. IgG and complement components, such as C3b, are opsonins and facilitate phagocytosis by neutrophils and macrophages. Thus complement deficiencies often resemble antibody deficiencies. Recurrent life-threatening infections at an early age with encapsulated bacteria (e.g., *Haemophilus influenzae* and *Streptococcus pneumoniae*) that are very sensitive to opsonin-assisted phagocytosis may occur.

Activation of C3 is central to the complement cascade. All three pathways of complement activation (i.e., classical, alternative, and lectin pathways) result in activation of C3 into C3b and C3a; C3b is a major opsonin and also is the activator of the terminal components of the cascade (C6 through C9). C3 deficiency is the most severe complement deficiency (Fig. 9.12). Factor I and factor H are major regulators of the complement cascade and control the level of spontaneous activation of C3. Factor I deficiency and factor H deficiency can be severe because they lead to increased spontaneous destruction of C3 and a secondary C3 deficiency.

Deficiencies of lesser severity have been described in each of the pathways of complement activation. Defects in the classical pathway (i.e., C1, C2, C4) result in increased risk for recurrent infections, sometimes severe, with encapsulated bacteria at an early age.[43] Defects in the early components of the classical pathway also result in a SLE-like syndrome that may be complicated by kidney disease (glomerulonephritis), suggesting a role of these components in removal of naturally occurring immune complexes from the circulation.[44] C2 deficiency, more so than C1 or C4 deficiencies, also has an increased risk for recurrent respiratory tract infections with encapsulated bacteria. Mannose-binding lectin (MBL) deficiency is the primary defect of the lectin pathway of complement activation.[45] The defect results in increased risk of infection with microorganisms that have polysaccharide capsules rich in mannose, particularly the yeast *Saccharomyces cerevisiae*, and encapsulated bacteria such as *Neisseria meningitides* and *S. pneumonia*. Properdin deficiency is the most common defect in the alternative pathway, is associated with recurrent infections with *Neisseria meningitides*, and is X-linked, whereas all other complement deficiencies are autosomal recessive. Symptoms generally appear in the second decade of life.

Deficiencies of any of the terminal components of the complement cascade (C5, C6, C7, or C8 deficiencies) are associated with increased infections with only one group of bacteria—those of the genus *Neisseria*, particularly *Neisseria meningitides*. *Neisseria* usually causes localized infections (meningitis or gonorrhea), but terminal pathway defects result in an 8000-fold increased risk for systemic infections with atypical strains of these microorganisms. C9 deficiency is the most common terminal pathway defect, appears primarily in Japanese populations, and is generally asymptomatic. The other deficiencies of the terminal pathway are extremely rare, but are characterized by more aggressive infections. The risk for systemic infections with *Neisseria* is also increased in those with deficiencies of C2, factor D, factor B, and properdin.

Secondary Immune Deficiencies

Secondary, or acquired, immune and inflammatory deficiencies are far more common than primary deficiencies. These deficiencies are complications of other physiologic or pathophysiologic conditions (Table 9.7). Although secondary deficiencies are common, many are not clinically relevant. In many cases, the degree of the immune deficiency is relatively minor and without any apparent increased susceptibility to infection. Alternatively, the immune system may be substantially suppressed, but only for a short duration, thus minimizing the incidence of clinically relevant infections. Some secondary immune deficiencies (e.g., AIDS or immunosuppression by cancer), however, are extremely severe and may result in recurrent life-threatening infections.

Normal Physiologic Conditions

The competence of an individual's immune system varies throughout life. Pregnancy itself is considered by many to be an immunocompromised condition. Pregnant women may have decreased reactivity or altered results in several tests of the immune system, including skin tests against various antigens, circulating numbers of T lymphocytes, and other very general tests. Pregnancy itself, however, is not associated with a marked change in infections, suggesting that the mother's immune system is not severely altered.

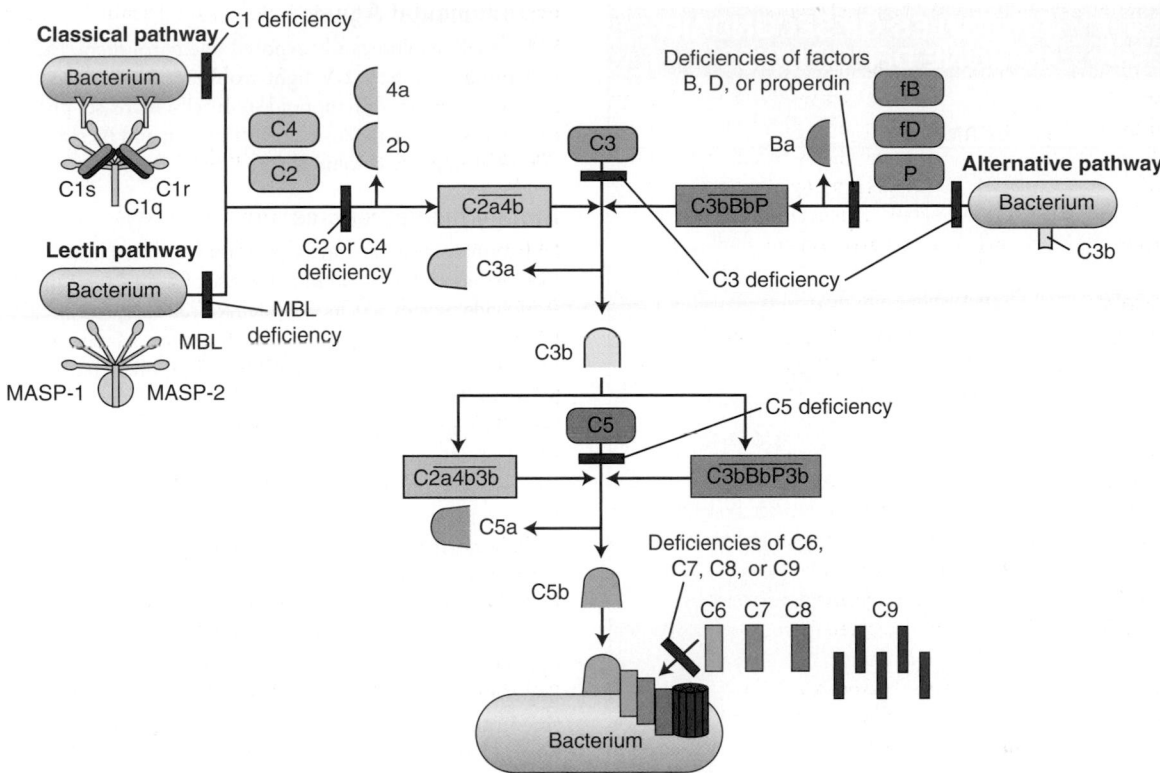

FIGURE 9.12 Complement Defects. The complement cascade is initiated through three pathways: the classical pathway, the lectin pathway, and the alternative pathway. Each of the three pathways produces a C3 convertase, which activates C3 leading to the formation of a C5 convertase. The activation of C5 initiates formation of the membrane attack complex. For more details, see the text and Fig. 7.6. The most severe defect is a C3 deficiency because it blocks all three pathways. *MASP*, MBL-associated serine protease; *MBL*, mannose-binding lectin.

The newborn child is immunologically immature. Although T-cell immune responses may be normal or near normal, other components of the immune system (especially antibody production) are just beginning to mature. Beginning at about 32 weeks of pregnancy, the placenta transports maternal antibodies into the fetal blood to protect the child during the first months of life (see Fig. 8.29). After the delivery, the level of the mother's antibodies slowly decreases in the newborn so that maternal antibodies no longer protect the child by about 6 months of life. By 6 to 8 months, the newborn should be efficiently protected by antibodies produced by its own B cells. In some infants, the development of antibody production is delayed, and a transient low level of antibody may persist for several months (**transient hypogammaglobulinemia of infancy**), during which the child has increased susceptibility to infections. Premature infants are particularly immunologically immature and are at increased risk for neonatal infections. The blood of infants born before 32 weeks' gestation is generally devoid of maternal antibody. However, if the infant is born prematurely, the degree of immunologic immaturity is greater and places the child at a significant risk of developing infections.

Aging is also associated with a progressive depression in immune responses. Older adults generally have more severe bacterial and fungal infections, greater difficulty resolving those infections, and lower responses to vaccination. Several meaningful changes occur during aging, although variations in the degree of change and a corresponding increased susceptibility to infection can be considerable among individuals. The thymus involutes over time, resulting in decreased production of fresh T cells. A concurrent depletion of T-memory cells results in depressed responses to both new and "recall" antigens. A shift toward Th2 cells also may occur with a resultant decrease in Th1 cytokines.

Total numbers of B cells may decrease. Numbers of NK cells may remain normal, although their activity is decreased. Similarly, neutrophil numbers may remain normal, with decreased phagocytosis and killing.

Psychologic Stress

The relationship between emotional stress and depressed immune function has become an area of intense clinical and research interest. For many decades anecdotal reports have suggested that increased incidences of infection and malignancy are associated with periods of both intense stress (e.g., the loss of a loved one, divorce) and relatively minor stress (e.g., final examination periods at colleges and universities). In addition, early studies showed that immune function, as demonstrated by delayed hypersensitivity skin test results, could be depressed through posthypnotic suggestion.

The mechanisms of the relationship between emotional stress and the immune system are now beginning to be understood. Many lymphoid organs are innervated and can be affected by nerve stimulation. In addition, lymphocytes have receptors for many hormones (e.g., sex hormones, neurotransmitters, and neuropeptides) and can respond to changing levels of these chemicals with increased or decreased function. For instance, stress-induced catecholamines affect the expression of adhesion molecules and the movement of lymphocytes among lymphoid organs. (Further discussion of the effects of stress on susceptibility to disease is the subject of Chapter 11.)

Physical Trauma

Trauma that compromises the epithelial barrier also predisposes an individual to infection. Burn victims are susceptible to severe bacterial infections. Thermal burns appear to be associated with suppressed

TABLE 9.7 EXAMPLES OF SECONDARY IMMUNE DEFICIENCIES

CAUSE OF DEFICIENCY	EXAMPLES
Normal physiologic conditions	Pregnancy Premature infants Infancy Aging
Psychologic stresses	Emotional trauma Eating disorders
Dietary insufficiencies	Protein-calorie malnutrition Protein loss syndromes (e.g., nephrotic syndrome, protein-losing enteropathy) Vitamin deficiencies
Malignancies	Hematologic malignancies (e.g., Hodgkin disease, acute or chronic leukemia, myeloma) Solid tumors (e.g., sarcomas, carcinomas)
Chronic diseases	Diabetes Cystic fibrosis Alcoholic cirrhosis Sickle cell disease Aplastic anemia Autoimmune diseases (e.g., systemic lupus erythematosus)
Chromosome abnormalities	Trisomy 21 (Down syndrome)
Environmental agents	Ultraviolet light Ionizing radiation Chronic hypoxia
Physical trauma	Burns
Medical treatments	Stress from surgery Anesthesia Immunosuppressive treatments (e.g., corticosteroids, antilymphocyte antibodies) Splenectomy Anticonvulsive medications Cancer treatment (e.g., cytotoxic drugs, ionizing radiation) Hematopoietic stem cell transplants
Infections	Congenital infections (e.g., rubella, cytomegalovirus, hepatitis B) Acquired infections (e.g., AIDS)
Lifestyle	Alcohol abuse

Environmental Agents

Individuals are constantly exposed to environmental agents that affect the immune system. UV light from sun exposure or tanning salons induces apoptosis of lymphoid stem cells, increases production of Treg cells that suppress defenses against cancer, and increases production of antiinflammatory cytokines.

Dietary Insufficiencies

Nutritional status can have a profound effect on immune function, and malnutrition is the predominant cause of secondary immune deficiencies worldwide. Severe deficits in protein or calorie (protein-calorie malnutrition) intake lead to immune deficiencies. Marasmus (deficiency in calories) and kwashiorkor (deficiency in protein, but adequate calories) have similar outcomes. T-cell–rich areas of primary (thymus) and secondary lymphoid tissue are greatly affected, resulting in impaired T-cell function. Antibody levels are normal but neutrophil function (chemotaxis, phagocytosis, bacterial killing), complement levels, and NK activity are impaired, resulting in infections with microorganisms that are normally destroyed by opsonization and phagocytosis.

Deficient zinc intake can profoundly depress both T- and B-cell function. Zinc is required as a cofactor for at least 70 different enzymes, some of which are found in lymphocytes and are necessary for their function. Secondary zinc deficiencies may be associated with malabsorption syndrome (failure to absorb zinc), chronic renal disease (loss of zinc in the urine), chronic diarrhea (loss of zinc through the gut), or burns or severe psoriasis (loss of zinc through the skin). Deficiencies of other enzyme cofactors, such as vitamins (e.g., pyridoxine, pantothenic acid, folic acid, and vitamins A, C, E, and B_{12}), also may result in severe depressions of B- and T-cell function, phagocytosis, and complement activity.

Chronic Diseases

Chronic diseases of the cardiovascular, gastrointestinal, and renal systems are commonly complicated by a secondary immune suppression. Nephrotic syndrome from inflammation of the kidneys results in loss of protein through the kidneys, proteinuria (increased protein in the urine), and resultant hypoproteinemia (diminished protein in the blood). The loss of IgG may increase susceptibility of infection. Protein-losing enteropathy results from conditions that damage the surface of the gastrointestinal tract (e.g., inflammatory bowel diseases, such as Crohn disease, ulcerative colitis, celiac disease, gastrointestinal [GI] infections, cancer of the GI tract). Although circulating levels of immunoglobulin are diminished because of loss through the GI tract and catabolism, increased susceptibility to infections is rare.

Metabolic Diseases or Genetic Syndromes

Diabetes results in altered glucose metabolism and suppresses many aspects of the immune and inflammatory responses, including phagocytosis and chemotaxis, and lymphocyte proliferation. The effects of trisomy 21 are less severe, but primarily include diminished neutrophil function. People with cystic fibrosis have decreased airway clearance of bacteria, thus increasing the probability of major respiratory tract infections.

Malignancies

Many malignancies are complicated by a wasting syndrome (cachexia) in the later stages, which can suppress the immune system secondary to the resultant malnutrition. The effect is commonly nonspecific, resulting in a generalized deficiency of the immune response and a greatly increased susceptibility to developing life-threatening infections. In fact, many people with malignancies die from infection rather than from direct effects of the tumor.

neutrophil function (especially chemotaxis), complement levels, cell-mediated immunity, and primary humoral responses, although secondary humoral responses are normal. The mechanism of this immunosuppression may be twofold. Blood from burned individuals contains nonspecific immunosuppressive factors (all immune responses are suppressed, regardless of the antigen involved). In addition, burn victims also have increased regulatory T-cell function, which may increase antigen-specific suppression.

Other malignancies (e.g., lymphomas, leukemias, plasmacytomas) present with an early and more specific immune depression. Non-Hodgkin lymphoma may result in an antibody deficiency in the most advanced stages of the disease. Hodgkin lymphoma, however, may suppress the immune system even before the onset of symptoms, with worsening of the suppression as the disease progresses. Individuals usually present with depletion of T cells with normal production of T-cell–independent antibodies. In general, leukemia is characterized by normal T- and B-cell responses until progression to terminal stages. Chronic lymphocytic leukemia commonly suppresses B-cell differentiation but does not affect T-cell function. Depressed production of antibodies results in increased susceptibility to fatal infection. Plasmacytomas (malignancies of plasma cells) result in greatly diminished antibodies because the malignant cells are displacing normal plasma cells and increased catabolism of immunoglobulins results in increased susceptibility to infections against which antibody is protective. T-cell immunity remains intact.

Medical Treatments

Medical treatments themselves may produce suppression of immune responses. Surgery and administration of anesthesia can suppress T- and B-cell function. Transient, severe lymphopenia (loss of circulating lymphocytes) is a common postoperative condition that can last as long as a month. Surgery to remove the spleen (splenectomy) can result in a depressed IgM response against encapsulated bacteria (especially *S. pneumoniae, H. influenzae, Staphylococcus aureus,* Group A streptococci, and *Neisseria meningitidis*) and decreased levels of opsonins.

Corticosteroids are intentionally used to suppress the immune system and control hypersensitivity diseases (especially autoimmune disease) or prevent rejection of transplants. They predominantly inhibit T-cell function, prevent lymphocyte proliferation, inhibit production of critical cytokines, and suppress monocyte/macrophage functions; but they do not affect neutrophils. Because of their nonspecific activity, however, immune responses against infectious agents also can be suppressed, increasing an individual's susceptibility to infection.

Many drugs and other treatments that are used to fight cancer (e.g., cytotoxic cancer chemotherapeutic agents, irradiation) are not specific for cancer cells, but are designed to attack cells in susceptible stages in their cell cycles or rapidly proliferating cells, which includes cells of the immune system as well as malignant cells. Cytotoxic agents may affect all lymphocyte subsets or may only affect a specific stage of the immune response. For instance, azathioprine and methotrexate affect response after antigenic challenge, whereas cyclophosphamide affects response before and after exposure to antigen. Cyclosporine A preferably affects CD4+ cells. The immunosuppressive effects of chemotherapeutic drugs are exacerbated by concurrent treatment with ionizing radiation (x-rays), which also affects rapidly dividing cells. T cells, particularly CD4+ cells, are most sensitive. Phagocytes, which have a much slower proliferation rate, are relatively resistant to the effects of irradiation. Depending on the dose of irradiation administered, the entire immune system may be depleted.

The list of medications that affect the immune response is ever increasing and includes analgesics, antithyroid medications, anticonvulsants, antihistamines, antimicrobial agents, antilymphocyte antibodies, and tranquilizers.

Infections

Many infectious microorganisms successfully invade the human body using mechanisms for fighting off specific immune/inflammatory responses against themselves (discussed in Chapter 10). However, some infectious agents more broadly suppress the immune response. HIV is one of the few microorganisms that directly attacks the central processes involved in the development of an immune response (discussed in detail in Chapter 10). It infects and destroys the T-helper cell, which is necessary to provide help for the maturation of both plasma cells and T-cytotoxic cells. Therefore, HIV suppresses the immune response against itself and secondarily creates a generalized immune deficiency by suppressing the development of immune responses against other pathogens and opportunistic microorganisms.

Several other viruses (e.g., measles; hepatitis B; and herpes viruses, such as Epstein-Barr virus [EBV], cytomegalovirus [CMV], and herpes simplex viruses) may suppress various components of the immune response. CMV, herpes virus, and hepatitis B virus in particular can establish congenital infections through transmission from an infected mother to the child in utero or at birth when the child's immune system is immature. These children may have suppressed immune responses, although the degree of the deficiency is not usually severe. However, as the child's immune system develops, the viral antigens may be partially seen as "self" so that a chronic infection is established.

Measles virus can infect both B and T cells and macrophages. Infection may result in lymphopenia and a suppressed T-cell response that are generally transient. Acute infections with herpes viruses may transiently suppress the immune system. EBV infects B cells and may cause infectious mononucleosis, although most EBV infections are asymptomatic. The virus enters a stage of latency in memory B cells. In some cases, EBV may suppress both CD4+ and CD8+ T cells and NK cells. Immunosuppression is generally transient and not severe. CMV infects mucosal epithelium and can infect macrophages where antigen processing and presentation may be impaired.

Other infections may lead to a relatively broad suppression of immune responses. *Mycobacterium leprae* causes two forms of leprosy: tuberculoid leprosy, in which an active T-cell immunity contains and kills the infecting bacteria; and lepromatous leprosy, in which the infected individual's T-cell immunity is severely depressed but high levels of antibody are produced. The T-cell deficit is characterized by suppressed T-cell IL-2 production and antigen-specific T-cell responses. Some fungal infections may suppress the immune response. In disseminated *Candida albicans* infections, T-cell responses and neutrophil chemotaxis are suppressed to various degrees. Similar immunosuppression may be observed in individuals with disseminated histoplasmosis (infections with *Histoplasma capsulatum*). The most severe form of acute malaria (caused by the parasite *Plasmodium falciparum*) suppresses specific antibody responses against protein and polysaccharide antigens by dysregulation of CD4+ T-cell function and decreased IL-2 production.

Evaluation and Care of Those with Immune Deficiency

Routine care of individuals with immune deficiencies must be tempered with the knowledge that the immune system may be totally ineffective. Administration of conventional immunizing agents or blood products to these individuals may be unsafe because of the risk that the immunizing agent will cause an uncontrolled infection. Attenuated vaccines contain live but weakened microorganisms (e.g., live polio vaccine; vaccines against measles, mumps, and rubella) that can cause disseminated infection. Although the vaccine virus is attenuated enough to be destroyed by a normal immune system, it can survive, multiply, and cause severe disease in an immune-deficient recipient. Additionally, even healthy recipients of vaccines containing live microorganisms can shed those microorganisms for a short time, increasing the risk of infection to family members or other close associates who are immune deficient. Even simple procedures, such as penetrating the skin for routine blood tests, may lead to fatal septicemia (bacterial infection of the blood) in the immune-deficient person.

Individuals with immune deficiencies are also at risk for graft-versus-host disease (GVHD). Mature T cells in a transplanted graft (e.g., transfused blood) are capable of a destructive cell-mediated reaction against unmatched histocompatibility antigens on the tissues in the graft recipient. Symptoms of an acute graft-versus-host reaction usually appear within 10 to 30 days after the transplant. The primary targets for GVHD are the skin (e.g., rash, loss or increase of pigment, thickening of skin), liver (e.g., damage to bile duct, hepatomegaly), mouth (e.g., dry mouth, ulcers, infections), eyes (e.g., burning, irritation, dryness), and gastrointestinal tract (e.g., severe diarrhea) and may lead to death from infections.

GVHD is not a problem when the recipient is immunocompetent, that is, has an immune system that can control the donor's lymphocytes. If, however, the recipient's immune system is deficient, the grafted T cells remain unchecked and attack the recipient's tissues. Most GVHD is prevented by treating whole blood with irradiation to kill white blood cells before transfusion.

The most common presenting symptom of immune deficiencies is recurrent severe infections. Significant information concerning the nature of the specific immune deficiency can be obtained by noting the types of infection, as well as certain characteristics of the affected individual, including gender, age of disease onset, the presence of any associated anomalies, family history, and risk factors associated with secondary immune deficiencies.[46] Humoral deficiencies are generally characterized by recurrent sinopulmonary infections with encapsulated bacteria, gastrointestinal malabsorption, and poor growth. T-cell defects generally present with failure to thrive, chronic diarrhea, persistent thrush, and opportunistic infections (e.g., *Mycobacterium, Pneumocystis, Candida,* and certain viruses). Phagocytic defects are usually associated with recurrent abscesses, oral ulcers, and infections with specific bacteria (e.g., catalase-positive bacteria). Complement defects may be linked to SLE-like disease and recurrent and disseminated infections with *Neisseria* spp.

A variety of laboratory tests are available to evaluate specific immune deficiencies (Table 9.8). The choice of which particular tests to perform is determined on the characteristics described previously. A basic screening test is a complete blood count (CBC) with a differential. The CBC provides information on the numbers of red cells, white cells, and platelets, and the differential indicates the quantities of lymphocytes,

granulocytes, and monocytes in the blood. Quantitative determination of immunoglobulins (IgG, IgM, IgA) is a screening test for antibody production, and an assay for total complement (total hemolytic complement, CH_{50}) is useful if a complement defect is suspected.

Many PIDs result from single gene mutations.[41] Diagnosis can frequently be confirmed by appropriate genetic analysis. If the nature of the immune deficiency remains uncertain after the screening tests, additional relatively common tests can be performed. For instance, subpopulations of lymphocytes (T or B) can be quantified using characteristic surface markers, such as surface immunoglobulin for B cells and CD3 for T cells. T-cell populations can be further subdivided using additional surface markers, such as CD4 (T-helper cells) or CD8 (T-cytotoxic cells). For antibodies, routine assays are available to quantify subclasses of IgG, such as IgG2.

An additional level of testing would include determination of immune responses against specific antigens. Determination of isohemagglutinins is informative about antigen-specific IgM production. Antibody responses to vaccines (e.g., tetanus, pertussis, measles, diphtheria, hepatitis B) are usually indicative of IgG responses. T-cell immunity against specific antigens can be measured by skin tests against antigens to which the individual had been exposed: "recall antigens." These include antigens from vaccines (e.g., mumps, tetanus) or from microorganisms with which the person had a previous active infection (e.g., *Candida*). An adequate T-cell immunity results in a positive delayed hypersensitivity skin test reaction.

If the tests do not identify the immune deficiency, more esoteric tests are offered by reference laboratories or research laboratories. These include quantification of individual complement components, in vitro proliferation (mitogenic response) of T or B cells to antigens or nonspecific mitogens, and a variety of tests of phagocyte function (e.g., nitroblue tetrazolium test [NBT] for hexose-monophosphate shunt activity, specific tests for phagocytosis, chemotaxis, or bacterial killing).

Replacement Therapies for Immune Deficiencies

Diagnosis of primary immune deficiencies (PIDs) and administration of appropriate therapy remain a problem. Most individuals with such deficiencies are initially seen by primary care physicians, particularly family practice physicians or pediatricians. Most primary immune deficiencies are rare, affecting about 1 in 1200 individuals in the United

TABLE 9.8	LABORATORY EVALUATION OF IMMUNODEFICIENCIES	
FUNCTION TESTED	**LABORATORY TEST**	**INTERPRETATION OF TEST**
Tests of Humoral Immune Function		
Antibody production	Total immunoglobulin levels	Presence of antibody-producing B cells
	Levels of isohemagglutinins	Capacity to produce specific IgM antibodies
	Levels of antibodies against vaccines—especially diphtheria and tetanus toxoids	Capacity to produce specific IgG antibodies
B-cell numbers	Numbers of lymphocytes with surface immunoglobulin	Presence of circulating B cells
Tests of Cellular Immune Function		
Delayed hypersensitivity	Skin test reaction against previously encountered antigens—especially *Candida albicans* or tetanus toxoid	Presence of antigen-responsive T cells and skin test cellular interactions (e.g., lymphokine activity and macrophage function)
T-cell numbers	Numbers of T cells forming rosettes with sheep erythrocytes or expressing membrane CD3 or CD11 antigen	Presence of circulating T cells
T-cell proliferation in vitro	Proliferative response to nonspecific mitogens (e.g., phytohemagglutinin)	Capacity of all T cells to divide in response to nonspecific stimulation (mitogens)
	Proliferative response to antigens (e.g., tetanus toxoid)	Capacity of antigen-reactive T cells to respond to antigen

States. The most common primary immune deficiency disease is common variable immune deficiency (about 1 in 2400 individuals). The variable presentations of this disorder lead to difficult diagnosis. The average time span from onset of the immune deficiency to diagnosis has been estimated to be longer than 12 years. The most common PIDs handled by primary care physicians are selective IgA deficiency and chronic granulomatous disease.[47]

Gamma-Globulin Therapy

Many immune deficiencies can be successfully treated by replacing the missing component of the immune system. Individuals with B-cell deficiencies that cause hypogammaglobulinemia or agammaglobulinemia are usually treated by administration of immune gamma-globulin by intramuscular or intravenous (IVIg) routes. Administration by subcutaneous injection has been recently approved and is replacing intramuscular injections. Ig contains antibody-rich fractions prepared from plasma pooled from large numbers of donors. Administration of gamma-globulin replaces the individual's antibodies temporarily; these antibodies have a half-life of 3 to 4 weeks. Thus individuals must be treated repeatedly to maintain a protective level of antibodies in the blood. Gamma-globulin therapy has become routine for common variable immune deficiency, hyper-IgM syndromes, SCID, and X-linked agammaglobulinemia (Bruton).

The schedule and dosage of gamma-globulin vary among individuals and are primarily determined by body weight, the degree of gamma-globulinemia, and the incidence of infections in the individual. Commercial gamma-globulin preparations usually contain small amounts of IgM and IgA. Individuals with selective IgA deficiency occasionally develop allergic reactions to IgA in gamma-globulin preparations.

Individuals who need larger amounts of IgM or IgA can be given fresh frozen plasma in monthly IV infusions. Complications associated with plasma therapy include the potential transmission of blood-borne viruses for which no assay is yet available. The plasma is irradiated to destroy immunocompetent T cells to avoid GVHD in individuals with accompanying T-cell deficiencies. Administration of fresh frozen plasma is successful in individuals with WAS (IgM deficient), AT (IgA deficient), or complement component deficiencies.

Transplantation and Transfusion

Several primary immune deficiencies originate from defects in lymphoid stem cells that interfere with their development in the primary lymphoid organs. Some of these (e.g., SCID, WAS, leukocyte adhesion defect) have benefited from replacement of stem cells through transplantation of bone marrow, umbilical cord cells, or other cell populations that are rich in stem cells.

The source of donor cells, particularly bone marrow, may contain a mixed population of stem cells and more mature T lymphocytes. In order to avoid GVHD, the preferred donor would be matched with the recipient for HLA antigens. Several other diseases involving depletion of the bone marrow (i.e., aplastic anemia, leukemia requiring eradication of tumor cells in the marrow) also are treated by bone marrow transplantation. At least 75% of bone marrow transplants between individuals who are matched for HLA are accepted. In immunocompetent recipients, most rejections of HLA-matched transplants occur because of recognition of minor histocompatibility antigens by individuals who have received multiple blood transfusions and are, as a result, sensitized against those antigens, which are not evaluated in tissue typing. For stem cell transplants, differences in minor histocompatibility antigens may lead to GVHD. Because HLA antigens are inherited in a codominant fashion, the preferred donor would be a relative, especially a sibling. Although the donor is not tested for minor histocompatibility antigens, the use of a close relative also would minimize differences at those loci.

Chronic GVHD appears in 30% to 50% of transplants between HLA-matched siblings and in 60% to 70% of transplants between unrelated donors. Symptoms may appear about 4 to 7 months after the transplant, but may begin much earlier or later. Depletion of T cells from bone marrow before transplantation significantly lowers the incidence of both acute and chronic GVHD. One method of doing this is to infuse the graft with monoclonal antibody against plasma membrane antigens found only on mature T cells. Another method is to use fetal tissue as the graft. For example, fetal liver, which contains stem cells but not immunocompetent lymphocytes, is sometimes grafted in place of bone marrow if an HLA-matched donor cannot be found.

Steroids are commonly used to suppress GVHD in recipients of bone marrow transplants performed to treat certain malignancies or primary immune deficiencies. In cases where steroids are ineffective, promising new data support the use of mesenchymal stem cells (MSCs). Stem cells are relatively undifferentiated cells and can be obtained from a variety of sources (e.g., embryos, bone marrow, adult tissues). MSCs are present in all adult tissues. These particular stem cells undergo differentiation into other cell types and, more importantly, have potent immunosuppressive properties. Several recent clinical trials have demonstrated complete suppression of GVHD in a large number of recipients of MSCs.

Reconstitution of thymic function can benefit individuals lacking a thymus or thymic function (e.g., DiGeorge syndrome, ataxia-telangiectasia, or chronic mucocutaneous candidiasis). The procedure involves transplantation of fetal thymic tissue, which lacks immunocompetent T cells, or thymic epithelial cells (the cells that produce the thymic hormones) from which mature T cells have been removed. In some individuals transplantation increases the number of circulating mature T cells, but in most cases improvement is only temporary.

Enzymatic defects that cause SCID (e.g., adenosine deaminase deficiency) have been treated successfully with transfusions of glycerol frozen-packed erythrocytes. The donor erythrocytes contain the needed enzyme and can, at least temporarily, provide sufficient enzyme for normal lymphocyte function. An alternative method is administration of purified adenosine deaminase that has been stabilized with polyethylene glycol (PEG).

Treatment with Soluble Immune Modulators

The administration of soluble materials that affect lymphocyte function can restore T-cell function, especially in individuals with WAS or chronic mucocutaneous candidiasis. Successful for some individuals is the use of transfer factor, a low-molecular-weight nucleoprotein prepared from lymphocyte lysates, which can confer specific reactivity against certain antigens. Thymosin, a thymic hormone, also has been used, although with limited success. Cytokine therapy also has been effective in some cases of chronic granulomatous disease.

Gene Therapy

The first successful therapeutic replacement of defective genes was performed in two girls with SCID caused by an ADA deficiency.[48] The normal gene for ADA was cloned and inserted into a retroviral vector.[49] The gene for ADA replaced some retroviral genes, resulting in a virus that carried the normal human gene but was thought not to cause disease. The virus was used to infect bone marrow stem cells from these children. The retrovirus inserted the normal ADA gene into the individuals' genetic material. The genetically altered stem cells were infused into the children, resulting in partial reconstitution of their immune systems, although multiple treatments were needed and the need for infusion of packed erythrocytes was still required. However, retroviral-mediated gene therapy for other diseases, such as X-linked SCID, chronic granulomatous disease (CGD), and Wiskott-Aldrich Syndrome (WAS), but not to treat ADA deficiency, resulted in the induction of leukemia.[50] Current gene therapy using alternative modified viral vectors has alleviated those complications.[51] New gene therapy trials using newly developed vectors have been performed for ADA deficiency, X-linked SCID, CGD, and WAS. The outcomes have significantly improved for ADA deficiency (100% survival) with most individuals gaining protective immunity and no complications related to viral vector.[52] Gene therapy has become standard care for individuals without well-matched sibling donors for stem cell transplant.

SUMMARY REVIEW

Hypersensitivity: Allergy, Autoimmunity, and Alloimmunity

1. Inappropriate immune responses are misdirected responses against the host's own tissues (autoimmunity); directed responses against beneficial foreign tissues, such as transfusions or transplants (alloimmunity); exaggerated responses against environmental antigens (allergy); or insufficient responses to protect the host (immune deficiency).

2. Allergy, autoimmunity, and alloimmunity are collectively known as hypersensitivity reactions.

3. Mechanisms of hypersensitivity are classified as type I (IgE-mediated) reactions, type II (tissue-specific) reactions, type III (immune complex–mediated) reactions, and type IV (cell-mediated) reactions.

4. Hypersensitivity reactions can be immediate (developing within minutes to a few hours) or delayed (developing within several hours or days).

5. Anaphylaxis, the most rapid immediate hypersensitivity reaction, is an explosive reaction that occurs within minutes of reexposure to the antigen and can lead to cardiovascular shock.

6. Allergens are antigens that cause allergic responses.

7. Type I (IgE-mediated) hypersensitivity reactions are mediated through the binding of IgE to Fc receptors on mast cells and cross-linking of IgE by antigens that bind to the Fab portions of IgE. Cross-linking causes mast cell degranulation and the release of histamine (the most potent mediator) and other inflammatory substances.

8. Histamine, acting through the H1 receptor, contracts bronchial smooth muscles, causing bronchial constriction; increases vascular permeability, causing edema; and causes vasodilation, increasing blood flow into the affected area. Histamine with H2 receptors results in increased gastric acid secretion and a decrease of histamine released from mast cells and basophils.

9. Histamine enhances the chemotaxis of eosinophils into sites of type I allergic reactions.

10. Atopic individuals tend to produce higher quantities of IgE and to have more Fc receptors for IgE on their mast cells.

11. Type II (tissue-specific) hypersensitivity reactions are caused by five possible mechanisms: complement-mediated lysis, opsonization and phagocytosis, neutrophil-mediated tissue damage, antibody-dependent cell-mediated cytotoxicity, and modulation of cellular function.

12. Type III (immune complex–mediated) hypersensitivity reactions are caused by the formation of immune complexes that are deposited in target tissues, where they activate the complement cascade, generating chemotactic fragments that attract neutrophils into the inflammatory site. Neutrophils release lysosomal enzymes that result in tissue damage.

13. Intermediate-sized immune complexes are the most likely to have severe pathologic consequences.

14. Immune complex disease can be a systemic reaction, such as serum sickness, or a localized response, such as the Arthus reaction.

15. Type IV (cell-mediated) hypersensitivity reactions are caused by either cytotoxic T lymphocytes (Tc cells) or lymphokine-producing Th1 cells.

16. Typical allergens include pollen, molds and fungi, certain foods (milk, eggs, fish, peanuts), animals, certain drugs, cigarette smoke, and house dust.

17. Clinical manifestations of allergic reactions usually are confined to the areas of initial intake or contact with the allergen. Ingested allergens induce gastrointestinal symptoms, airborne allergens induce respiratory tract or skin manifestations, and contact allergens induce allergic responses at the site of contact.

18. Autoimmune diseases originate from the coincidence of an initiating event in a genetically predisposed individual leading to an autoimmune mechanism that affects specific target tissues or cells. Central tolerance develops during the embryonic period. Peripheral tolerance is maintained in secondary lymphoid organs by regulatory T lymphocytes or antigen-presenting dendritic cells.

19. Autoimmune disease can be caused by the exposure of a previously sequestered antigen, the development of a neoantigen, the complications of infectious disease, the emergence of a forbidden clone of lymphocytes, or the consequence of ineffective peripheral tolerance. The mechanism for imitation of autoimmune diseases may already be within humans.

20. Alloimmunity is the immune system's reaction against antigens on the tissues of other members of the same species.

21. Alloimmune disorders include transient neonatal disease, in which the maternal immune system becomes sensitized against antigens expressed by the fetus; transplant rejection; and transfusion reactions, in which the immune system of the recipient of an organ transplant or blood transfusion reacts against foreign antigens on the donor's cells.

22. SLE is a chronic, multisystem, inflammatory disease and is one of the most serious of the autoimmune disorders. SLE is characterized by the production of a large variety of autoantibodies.

23. Hyperacute graft rejection (preexisting antibody) is immediate and rare, acute rejection is cell mediated and occurs days to months after transplantation, and chronic rejection is caused by inflammatory damage to endothelial cells as a result of a weak cell-mediated reaction.

24. Red blood cell antigens may be the targets of autoimmune or alloimmune reactions. The most important of these, because they provoke the strongest humoral immune response, are the ABO and Rh systems.

Deficiencies in Immunity

1. Disorders resulting from immune deficiency are the clinical sequelae of impaired function of components of the immune or inflammatory response, phagocytes, or complement.

2. Immune deficiency is the failure of mechanisms of self-defense to function in their normal capacity.

3. Immune deficiencies are either congenital (primary) or acquired (secondary). Primary immune deficiencies are caused by genetic defects that disrupt lymphocyte development, whereas secondary immune deficiencies are secondary to disease or other physiologic alterations.

SUMMARY REVIEW—cont'd

4. The clinical hallmark of immune deficiency is a propensity to unusual or recurrent severe infections. The type of infection usually reflects the immune system defect.

5. The most common infections in individuals with defects of the cell-mediated immune response are fungal and viral, whereas infections in individuals with defects of the humoral immune response or complement function are primarily bacterial.

6. Defects in B-cell function are diverse, ranging from a complete lack of the human bursal equivalent function, the lymphoid organs required for B-cell maturation (as in Bruton agammaglobulinemia), to deficiencies in a single class of immunoglobulins (e.g., selective IgA deficiency).

7. DiGeorge syndrome (congenital thymic aplasia or hypoplasia) is characterized by complete or partial lack of the thymus (resulting in depressed T-cell immunity) and the parathyroid glands (resulting in hypocalcemia) and the presence of cardiac anomalies.

8. SCID is a total lack of T-cell function and a severe (either partial or total) lack of B-cell function. SCID can result from mutations in critical enzymes (ADA deficiency, PNP deficiency), in cytokine receptors (X-linked SCID, JAK3 deficiency, IL-7 receptor deficiency), or in antigen receptors (RAG-1/RAG-2 deficiencies, CD45 deficiency, CD3 deficiency, ZAP-70 deficiency). Other combined defects may result from deficiencies in antigen-presenting molecules (bare lymphocyte syndrome), cytoskeletal proteins (WAS), or DNA repair (ataxia-telangiectasia).

9. Almost any portion of the complement cascade may be defective. The most severe defect is C3 deficiency, which results in recurrent life-threatening bacterial infections. Defects in proteins of the membrane attack complex usually result in unusual disseminated infections with bacteria of the *Neisseria* spp.

10. Defects in phagocyte function, which include insufficient numbers of phagocytes or defects of chemotaxis, phagocytosis, or killing, can result in recurrent life-threatening infections such as septicemia and disseminated pyogenic lesions.

11. Autoinflammatory disorders are characterized by abnormally high levels of inflammation secondary to mutations in control of inflammasome activation or in defects in cellular receptors of cytokines designed to decrease inflammation. These disorders are frequently related to diminished control of infections of epithelial surfaces. Autoinflammatory disorders are characterized by abnormally high levels of inflammation secondary to mutations in control of inflammasome activation or in defects in cellular receptors of cytokines designed to decrease inflammation. These disorders are frequently related to diminished control of infections of epithelial surfaces.

12. Acquired immunodeficiencies are caused by superimposed conditions, such as aging, malnutrition, infections, malignancies, physical or psychologic trauma, environmental factors, some medical treatments, or other diseases.

13. Deficiencies in immunity usually are treated by replacement therapy. Deficient antibody production is treated by replacement of missing immunoglobulins with commercial gamma-globulin preparations. Lymphocyte deficiencies are treated with the replacement of host lymphocytes with transplants of bone marrow, fetal liver, or fetal thymus from a donor.

KEY TERMS

ABO blood group, 271
Activation-induced cytidine deaminase deficiency (AICD deficiency), 278
Acute rejection, 273
Adenosine deaminase (ADA) deficiency, 275
Agammaglobulinemia, 277
Allergen, 263
Allergy, 255
Alloimmune disease, 269
Alloimmunity, 255
Anaphylaxis, 256
Ankylosing spondylitis (AS), 267
Antibody-dependent cell-mediated cytotoxicity (ADCC), 260
Arthus reaction, 263
Ataxia-telangiectasia (AT), 277
Atopic, 263
Atopic dermatitis, 266
Autoimmune disease, 255
Autoimmunity, 255
Autosomal agammaglobulinemia, 278
Autosomal recessive hyper-IgM syndrome, 278
Bare lymphocyte syndrome, 277
Blocking antibody, 265
Blood group antigen, 271
B-lymphocyte deficiency, 278
Bruton agammaglobulinemia, 278
CD40 deficiency, 278
CD40L deficiency, 278
C1 deficiency, 280
C2 deficiency, 280
C3 deficiency, 280
C4 deficiency, 280

C9 deficiency, 280
Chédiak-Higashi syndrome, 278
Chronic granulomatous disease (CGD), 279
Chronic mucocutaneous candidiasis, 280
Chronic rejection, 273
Common variable immune deficiency, 278
Complement deficiency, 280
Complete blood count (CBC), 284
Contact dermatitis, 266
Cross-reactive antibody (T cell), 268
Cryoglobulin, 263
Cyclic neutropenia, 279
Cytotropic antibody, 256
Defective class-switch, 278
Delayed hypersensitivity reaction, 256
Desensitization, 265
DiGeorge syndrome, 277
Factor H deficiency, 280
Factor I deficiency, 280
Familial Mediterranean fever, 280
Graft-versus-host disease (GVHD), 284
Hemolytic disease of the newborn, 272
Human leukocyte antigen (HLA), 272
Hyperacute rejection, 273
Hypersensitivity, 255
Hypocomplementemic, 262
Hypogammaglobulinemia, 277
IgG subclass deficiency, 278
IL-7 receptor deficiency, 277
Immediate hypersensitivity reaction, 256
Immune deficiency, 273
Immunologic homeostasis, 256
Immunologically privileged site, 268

Isohemagglutinin, 272
JAK3 deficiency, 277
Leukocyte adhesion deficiency, type 1 (LAD-1), 280
Leukocyte adhesion deficiency, type 2 (LAD-1), 280
Major histocompatibility complex (MHC), 272
Mannose-binding lectin (MBL) deficiency, 280
Mesenchymal stem cell (MSC), 285
MHC class I deficiency, 277
MHC class II deficiency, 277
Microchimerism, 269
Molecular mimicry, 268
Myeloperoxidase deficiency, 280
Neoantigen, 268
Perforin deficiency, 278
Phagocyte defects, 279
Predominantly antibody deficiency, 277
Primary (congenital) immune deficiency, 273
Properdin deficiency, 280
Purine nucleoside phosphorylase (PNP) deficiency, 277
RAG-1 deficiency, 277
RAG-2 deficiency, 277
Raynaud phenomenon, 263
Reagin, 256
Reticular dysgenesis, 275
Rh blood group, 272
Secondary (acquired) immune deficiency, 273
Selective IgA deficiency, 278
Serum sickness, 263
Severe combined immune deficiency (SCID), 275
Severe congenital neutropenia, 279
Systemic lupus erythematosus (SLE), 270
Tissue-specific antigen, 259

288   **UNIT III** Mechanisms of Self-Defense

▋KEY TERMS—cont'd

Transient hypogammaglobulinemia of infancy, 281

Type I (immunoglobulin E [IgE]–mediated) hypersensitivity reaction, 256

Type II (tissue-specific) hypersensitivity reaction, 259

Type III (immune complex–mediated) hypersensitivity reaction, 262

Type IV (cell-mediated) hypersensitivity reaction, 263

Universal donor, 272

Universal recipient, 272

Urticaria (hives), 264

Wheal and flare reaction, 264

Wiskott-Aldrich syndrome (WAS), 277

X-linked hyper-IgM syndrome, 278

X-linked SCID, 277

REFERENCES

1. Gell PGH, Coombs RRA, Lachman PT: *Clinical aspects of immunology*, Oxford, England, 1975, Blackwell Scientific.
2. Portier P, Richet C: De l'action anaphylactique de certains venins. *Comptes Rendus Societie Biologie (Paris)* 54:170, 1902.
3. Oettgen HC: Fifty years later: emerging functions of IgE antibodies in host defense, immune regulation, and allergic diseases. *J Allergy Clin Immunol* 137(6):1631–1645, 2016.
4. Schauberger E, et al: Lipid mediators of allergic disease: pathways, treatments, and emerging therapeutic targets. *Curr Allergy Asthma Rep* 16(7):48, 2016.
5. Pirquet C, Schick B: *Serum sickness*, Leipzig, Germany, 1905, Franz Denticke.
6. Arthus M, Breton M: Lésions cutanées produites par les injections de sérum. *Compt Rendus Soc Biol* 55:817, 1903.
7. Koch R: Fortsetzung der mitteilungen, uber ein heilmittel gegen tuberkulose. *Deutsche Med Wochenschr* 17:100–102, 1891.
8. Iweala OI, Burks AW: Food allergy: our evolving understanding of its pathogenesis, prevention, and treatment. *Curr Allergy Asthma Rep* 16(5):37, 2016.
9. Platts-Mills TAE, et al: IgE in the diagnosis and treatment of allergic disease. *J Allergy Clin Immunol* 137(6):1662–1670, 2016.
10. Commins SP, et al: Peanut allergy: new developments and clinical implications. *Curr Allergy Asthma Rep* 16(5):35, 2016.
11. McKee AS, Fontenot A: Interplay of innate and adaptive immunity in metal-induced hypersensitivity. *Curr Opin Immunol* 42:25–30, 2016.
12. Pociot F, Lernmark A: Genetic risk factors for type 1 diabetes. *Lancet* 387(10035):2331–2339, 2016.
13. Song J, et al: Ocular diseases: immunological and molecular mechanisms. *Int J Ophthalmol* 9(5):780–788, 2016.
14. Benvenga S, Guarneri F: Molecular mimicry and autoimmune thyroid disease. *Rev Endocr Metab Disord* 17(4):485–498, 2016.
15. Rewers M, Ludvigsson J: Environmental risk factors for type 1 diabetes. *Lancet* 387(10035):2340–2348, 2016.
16. Cunningham MW: Post-streptococcal autoimmune sequelae: rheumatic fever and beyond. In Ferretti JJ, Stevens DL, Fischetti VA, editors: *Streptococcus pyogenes: basic biology to clinical manifestations*, Oklahoma City, OK, 2016, University of Oklahoma Health Sciences Center. [Internet publication.].
17. Anaya J-M, et al: The autoimmune ecology. *Front Immunol* 7:139, 2016.
18. Lewin S, Bussel JB: Review of fetal and neonatal immune cytopenias. *Clin Adv Hematol Oncol* 13(1):35–43, 2015.
19. Bengtsson AA, Rönnblom L: Systemic lupus erythematosus: still a challenge for physicians. *J Intern Med* 281(1):40–43, 2016.
20. Boodhoo KD, Liu S, Zuo X: Impact of sex disparities on the clinical manifestations in patients with systemic lupus erythematosus: a systemic review and meta-analysis. *Medicine (Baltimore)* 95(29):e4272, 2016.
21. Arbuckle MR, et al: Development of autoantibodies before the clinical onset of systemic lupus erythematosus. *N Engl J Med* 349(16):1526–1533, 2003.
22. Hochberg MC: Updating the American College of Rheumatology revised criteria for the classification of systemic lupus erythematosus. *Arthritis Rheum* 40(9):1725, 1997.
23. Petri M, et al: Deviation and validation of the Systemic Lupus International Collaborating Clinics classification for systemic lupus erythematosus. *Arthritis Rheum* 64(8):2677–2686, 2012.
24. American College of Rheumatology: *Systemic lupus erythematosus*, 2012. Available at www.rheumatology.org/practice/clinical/patients/diseases_and_conditions/lupus.asp.
25. Kirtakidou M, et al: Systemic lupus erythematosus. *Ann Int Med* 159(1):ITC4-1–ITC4-16, 2013.
26. Fors Nieves CE, Izmirly PM: Mortality in systemic lupus erythematosus: an update review. *Curr Rheumatol Rep* 18(4):21, 2016.
27. Durcan L, Petri M: Immunomodulators in SLE: clinical evidence and immunological actions. *J Autoimmun* 74(1):73–84, 2016.
28. Branch DR: Anti-A and anti-B: what are they and where do they come from? *Transfusion* 55(Suppl 2):S74–S79, 2015.
29. Flegel WA: Pathogenesis and mechanisms of antibody-mediated hemolysis. *Transfusion* 55(Suppl 2):S47–S58, 2015.
30. Menendez JB, Edwards B: Early identification of acute hemolytic transfusion reactions: realistic implications for best practice in patient monitoring. *Medsurg Nurs* 25(2):88–90, 2016.
31. de Haas M, et al: Haemolytic disease of the fetus and newborn. *Vox Sang* 109(2):99–113, 2015.
32. Aitken SL, Tichy EM: Rh(O)D immune globulin products for prevention of alloimmunization during pregnancy. *Am J Health Syst Pharm* 72(4):267–276, 2015.
33. Quist E, Koepsell S: Autoimmune hemolytic anemia and red blood cell autoantibodies. *Arch Pathol Lab Med* 139(11):1455–1458, 2015.
34. Al-Herz W, et al: Primary immunodeficiency diseases: an update on the classification from the International Union of Immunological Societies Expert Committee for Primary Immunodeficiency. *Front Immunol* 5:162, 2014.
35. DiGeorge AM: Congenital absence of the thymus and its immunologic consequences. In Bergsma D, McKusick FA, editors: *Immunologic deficiency diseases in man, National Foundation—March of Dimes original article series*, Baltimore, MD, 1968, Williams & Wilkins.
36. Demczuk S, Aurias A: DiGeorge syndrome and related syndromes associated with 22q11.2 deletions. *Ann Genet* 38:59, 1995.
37. Bruton OC: Agammaglobulinemia. *Pediatrics* 9(6):722–728, 1952.
38. Leven EA, et al: Hyper IgM syndrome: a report from the USIDNET registry. *J Clin Immunol* 36:490–501, 2016.
39. Lehman HK: Autoimmunity and immune dysregulation in primary immune deficiency disorders. *Curr Allergy Asthma Rep* 15:53, 2015.
40. Roos D: Chronic granulomatous disease. *Br Med Bull* 118(1):50–63, 2016.
41. Casanova J-L: Severe infectious diseases of childhood as monogenic inborn errors of immunity. *Proc Natl Acad Sci USA* 112(51):E7128–E7137, 2015.
42. Gurung P, Kanneganti T-D: Autoinflammatory skin disorders: the inflammasomme in focus. *Trends Mol Med* 22(7):545–564, 2016.
43. Truedsson L: Classical pathway deficiencies – a short analytical review. *Mol Immunol* 68(1):14–19, 2015.
44. Macedo ACL, Isaac L: Systemic lupus erythematosus and deficiencies of early components of the complement classical pathway. *Front Immunol* 7:55, 2016.
45. Beltrame MH, et al: MBL-associated serine proteases (MASPs) and infectious diseases. *Mol Immunol* 67(1):85–100, 2015.
46. Lehman H, Hernandez-Trujillo V, Ballow M: Diagnosing primary immunodeficiency: a practical approach for the non-immunologist. *Curr Med Res Opin* 31(4):697–706, 2015.
47. Orange JS, et al: Family physician perspectives on primary immunodeficiency diseases. *Front Med* 3:12, 2016.
48. Blaese RM: Development of gene therapy for immunodeficiency: adenosine deaminase deficiency. *Pediatr Res* 33(Suppl 1):S49–S53, 1993.
49. Onodera M, et al: Gene therapy for severe combined immunodeficiency caused by adenosine deaminase deficiency: improved retroviral vectors for clinical trials. *Acta Haematol* 101(2):89–96, 1999.
50. Fischer A, Hacein-Bey-Abina S, Cavazzana-Calvo M: Gene therapy for primary adaptive immune deficiencies. *J Allergy Clin Immunol* 127(6):1356–1359, 2011.
51. Kumar SRP, et al: Clinical development of gene therapy: results and lessons from recent successes. *Mol Ther Methods Clin Dev* 2016:3, 2016.
52. Kuo CY, Kohn DB: Gene therapy for the treatment of primary immune deficiencies. *Curr Allergy Asthma Rep* 16(5):39, 2016.

CHAPTER OUTLINE

For most of human history infection was the primary disease-related cause of death including bubonuc/pneumonic plague, Spanish influenza and smallpox. Modern public health initiatives, vaccination programs, and the use of antibiotics have greatly progressed prevention and treatment of infectious diseases. As a result of these initiatives, naturally occurring smallpox has been eradicated from the globe (the last reported case was in 1975 in Somalia), measles is almost eradicated in the Western Hemisphere, and many diseases, such as tuberculosis and polio, are on the decline. In the United States in 2014, influenza/pneumonia was the eighth and septicemia was the eleventh ranked cause of death in adults, and bacterial sepsis was the seventh leading cause of neonatal deaths.[1] However, infectious disease remains a significant threat to life in many parts of the world, particularly in low income countries where prevention is less effective. In these countries 5 of the top 10 causes of death are attributable to infection: lower respiratory tract infections (#1), HIV/AIDS (#2), diarrheal diseases (#3), malaria (#6), and tuberculosis (#8).

Infectious disease remains a significant cause of morbidity and mortality because of the emergence of previously unknown infections, the reemergence and spread of old infections that were thought to be under control, and the development of infectious agents that are resistant to multiple antibiotics. The causes for these occurrences are numerous and include the following:
- Vast and rapid urbanization in many areas of the world, resulting in a breakdown in public health programs and a more rapid spread of infection
- Poverty and social inequality
- War and famine
- Global travel, allowing more rapid spread of disease from isolated areas to virtually any point around the world in a few hours
- Human encroachment into wilderness areas, resulting in contact with previously sequestered infectious agents
- Practice of prescribing antibiotics excessively or not taking antibiotics for a complete course of therapy; or, even when appropriately used, over administration of antibiotics facilitates the emergence of antibiotic-resistant microorganisms
- Denial of a problem by governments, allowing infections to spread in an uncontrolled way
- Diminished use of effective insecticides
- Increased global warming, allowing insect vectors to spread into and breed in areas that were previously too cool for them

EMERGING INFECTIONS

The emergence of previously unknown infections is not a new event in human history. However, the current rate may be unprecedented. Within 1 generation, more than 40 previously unknown infections have arisen. Some of these infections were harbored in animals and spread to humans with significant clinical impacts (e.g., severe acute respiratory syndrome [SARS-coronavirus] from bats, Middle East respiratory syndrome [MERS] from dromedary camels).[3] These are referred to as zoonotic infections. Zika virus also is an example of a recently emerging infection that has spread globally (see *What's New? Zika Virus*). Several have extremely high mortality rates of more than 50%, including SARS (in those older than 65 years), Ebola virus, Marburg virus, "mad cow" disease, Nipah virus (up to 75%), and acquired immunodeficiency syndrome (AIDS) (almost 100% in untreated persons). However, most either spread very slowly (e.g., AIDS) or initially appear in relatively isolated areas and are effectively controlled by quarantine (e.g., Ebola virus). Although none of these infections has developed into worldwide scourges, the potential of reversion to more rapidly spreading variants is a concern of public health agencies. In 2015 the World Health Organization (WHO) developed a list of emerging viral diseases that need urgent attention based on the probability of causing severe epidemics and the lack of medical countermeasures.[4] These included MERS, SARS-coronavirus, Nipah virus, and hemorrhagic fevers associated with Ebola, Marburg virus, Lassa fever, Rift Valley fever, and Crimean Congo hemorrhagic fever.

At least 20 previously known infections have reemerged including a new strains of cholera, malaria, yellow fever, dengue fever, diptheria, plague, and Marburg virus. The incidence of tuberculosis has risen by almost 33% between the mid-1980s and early 1990s. Although the United States is relatively free of most of these diseases, the effects of global warming and relaxed control of vectors may result in resurgence. West Nile virus, spread by mosquitoes, has spread throughout the continental United States, Canada, and Mexico.[5]

Many common infections previously controlled by antibiotics or vaccination have reemerged because of antibiotic resistance or secondary to decreased compliance with recommended vaccinations. Examples of these infections include *Streptococcus pneumoniae, Staphylococcus aureus,* tuberculosis, diarrheal diseases, malaria, meningitis, respiratory tract infections, sexually transmitted infections (STIs), and human immunodeficiency virus (HIV). Additionally, noncompliance with recommended vaccinations has led to outbreaks of diseases that were once under control (e.g., measles and pertussis).

Added to this collage of microbiologic dangers is the rising risk of bioterrorism. Agents such as smallpox, anthrax, and plague are continuing threats to public health and safety.

MICROORGANISMS AND HUMANS: A DYNAMIC RELATIONSHIP

For many microorganisms the human body is a hospitable site in which to grow and flourish because of sufficient nutrients and appropriate

WHAT'S NEW?

Zika Virus

The spread of Zika virus (ZIKV) is the most recent example of an infection emerging from a limited geographical region and rapidly becoming a global health risk of yet unknown impact. Extensive discussions of ZIKV can be found at numerous websites, particularly at those of the World Health Organization (WHO) and the Centers for Disease Control and Prevention (CDC). ZIKV was discovered in rhesus monkeys in 1947 in the Zika forest of Uganda and in 1948 in local mosquitoes. ZIKV is a member of the Flavivirus family, which includes West Nile virus, dengue virus, yellow fever virus, and tick-borne encephalitis virus. The principal vectors are *Aedes aegypti* and occasionally *A. albopictus.* One or both of these mosquitoes are distributed throughout most of the United States.[1]

The first human cases were found in Uganda and neighboring Tanzania in 1952 and in Nigeria in 1953. ZIKV was progressively detected in western Africa and southern Asia, but human infection was rare. In 2007 the first major outbreak occurred. On the island of Yap in Micronesia about 5000 individuals (73% of the population) were infected.[2] Symptoms were relatively mild, and most individuals were asymptomatic. In 2008 the first case in the United States was reported. The number of sexually transmitted cases has progressively increased. ZIKV has been found in semen, sperm, and vaginal fluid and can be transmitted during virtually any kind of sexual activity.[3] Semen contains infectious virus for up to 6 months after the onset of symptoms and is transmissible at any stage (i.e., before, during, and well after symptoms) or from an individual with a subclinical infection.

ZIKV can be transmitted from mother to child during pregnancy or delivery. Transmission through breast-feeding has not been reported. ZIKV appears to be neurotropic (specifically infects neural tissue). Major fetal complications include miscarriage, fetal death, microcephaly, and ocular disorders. In asymptomatic pregnant women, the risk of microcephaly is relatively low (approximately 1%). In symptomatic women, the incidence is higher (some estimate as high as 29%). Congenital microcephaly presents as a significantly smaller head because of diminished cerebral cortex development and frequently results in early neonatal death.[4]

Adult complications are relatively few but also neurologic, primarily a postinfection Guillain-Barré syndrome (GBS) that occurs in about 2 of 10,000 individuals.[5] GBS is a suspected autoimmune disorder of peripheral nerves leading to peripheral symptoms (e.g., weakness, tingling in the arms or legs, difficulty breathing, complete paralysis, and potentially death because of respiratory failure).

The CDC has been closely monitoring ZIKV infections within the United States and U.S. territories. As of September 6 2017, the CDC has reported 231 symptomatic cases in the United States and 554 cases in U.S. territories.[6]

Very few alternatives are available to limit the spread of ZIKV and attempts to eradicate the vector by destruction of breeding sites are the most effective approach. Prevention includes limiting travel to sites where ZIKV is endemic preventing access of mosquitoes to homes, using insect repellents on exposed skin, and wearing clothing that covers most of the body surfaces in ZIKV-infected areas.

References

1. Wikan N, Smith DR: Zika virus: history of a newly emerging arbovirus. *Lancet Infect Dis* 16(7):e119–e126, 2016.
2. Petersen LR, et al: Zika virus. *N Engl J Med* 374(16):1552–1563, 2016.
3. Moreira J, et al: Sexually acquired Zika virus: a systemic review. *Clin Microbiol Infect* 23(5):296–305, 2017.
4. Chibueze EC, et al: Zika virus infection in pregnancy: a systematic review of disease course and complications. *Reprod Health* 28;14(1):28, 2017.
5. Lessler J, et al: Review summary: assessing the global threat from Zika virus. *Science* 353(6300):663, 2016.
6. Centers for Disease Control and Prevention (CDC): *2017 Case counts in the US*, July 20, 2017. https://www.cdc.gov/zika/reporting/2017-case-counts .html.

conditions of temperature and humidity. Frequently, a symbiotic relationship exists, in which both humans and microorganisms benefit (Box 10.1). These microorganisms make up the *normal microbiome*—the resident microorganisms found in different parts of the body, including the skin, mouth, gastrointestinal tract, respiratory tract, and genital tract (see Chapter 7). For instance, the normal bacterial microbiome of the human gut is provided with nutrients from ingested food, produces enzymes that facilitate the digestion and use of many of the more complex molecules found in the human diet, produces antibacterial factors (e.g., bacteriocins, colicins) that prevent colonization by pathogenic microorganisms, and produces usable metabolites (e.g., vitamin K, B vitamins). This beneficial homeostasis is normally maintained through the physical integrity of the gut and other mechanisms that sequester these microorganisms on the mucosal surface.

MICROORGANISMS AND INFECTIONS

Clinical Infectious Disease

Microorganisms are generally classified based on different morphologic characteristics and life cycles. However, groups of disease-causing microorganisms share many properties related to clinical disease, processes of infection, and evasion of human protective systems. The clinical process of infection occurs in the following four distinct stages:

- *Incubation period*—the period from initial exposure to the infectious agent and the onset of the first symptoms, during which the microorganisms have entered the individual, undergone initial colonization, and begun multiplying, but are at insufficient numbers to cause symptoms; this period may last from several hours to years
- *Prodromal stage*—the occurrence of initial symptoms, which are often very mild and include a feeling of discomfort and tiredness
- *Invasion period*—the pathogen is multiplying rapidly, invading farther and affecting the tissues at the site of initial colonization as well as other areas; the immune and inflammatory responses have been triggered; symptoms may be specifically related to the pathogen or to the inflammatory response
- *Convalescence*—in most instances, the individual's immune and inflammatory systems successfully remove the infectious agent and symptoms decline; alternatively, the disease may be fatal or may enter a latency phase with resolution of symptoms until reactivation at a later time

Clinical manifestations of infectious disease vary depending on the pathogen, the organ system affected, and the intensity of the inflammatory response. The disease may be clinical (measurable infection-related symptoms) or subclinical (no apparent symptoms although the individual is infected). Effects of infection may be acute or chronic, secondary to the immune and inflammatory responses, or a direct consequence of toxins or injury to infected cells. The initial symptoms are typically fatigue, malaise, weakness, and loss of concentration. Generalized aching and loss of appetite are common complaints. However, the hallmark of most infectious diseases is fever.

Fever is not failure of the body to regulate temperature; rather, body temperature is being regulated to a higher level than normal. The hypothalamus functions as a central thermostat and regulates temperature (see Chapter 16). Pyrogens are agents that can produce fever. Those derived from outside the host are termed exogenous pyrogens and those produced by the individual's inflammatory response are termed endogenous pyrogens. Exogenous pyrogens indirectly affect the hypothalamus through the release of endogenous pyrogens by cells of the host. A number of cytokines have been identified as endogenous pyrogens: interleukin-1 and interleukin-6 (IL-1 and IL-6), interferon (IFN), tumor necrosis factor (TNF), and others (see Fig. 16.8). These cytokines raise the thermoregulatory set point through stimulation of prostaglandin synthesis in both thermoregulatory (brain) and non-thermoregulatory (peripheral) tissue. Fever is considered a beneficial adaptive host-defense response in infection (e.g., killing of temperature-sensitive microorganisms).

Several factors influence the capacity of a microorganism to cause disease:

- *Communicability:* the ability to spread from one individual to others and cause disease (measles and pertussis spread very easily; HIV is of lower communicability)
- *Immunogenicity:* the ability to induce an immune response
- *Infectivity:* the ability to invade and multiply in the host
- *Mechanism of action:* how the microorganism damages tissue
- *Pathogenicity:* the ability to produce disease—success depends on communicability, infectivity, extent of tissue damage, and virulence
- *Portal of entry:* the route by which a microorganism infects the host (e.g., direct contact, inhalation, ingestion, or bites of an animal or insect)
- *Toxigenicity:* the ability to produce soluble toxins or endotoxins, factors that greatly influence the degree of virulence
- *Virulence:* the capacity to cause severe disease, for example, measles virus is of low virulence; rabies virus is highly virulent

Infectious diseases also are classified by their prevalence and spread within the community:

- *Endemic:* diseases with relatively high but constant rates of infection in a particular population
- *Epidemic:* the number of new infections in a particular population greatly exceeds the number usually observed
- *Pandemic:* an epidemic that spreads over a large area, such as a continent or worldwide (see Table E 10.1 on Evolve)

As a consequence of the relative severity of clinical infection and the ability to successfully treat the infection, some infections are considered relatively minor inconveniencies, such as the common cold, and others have a major impact because of severe morbidity and mortality. In the United States, the Centers for Disease Control and Prevention (CDC) have developed a National Notifiable Diseases Surveillance System.[6] An evolving list of notifiable infectious diseases is maintained to monitor, control, and prevent the spread of disease. STIs are among the most common reportable diseases in 2015: *Chlamydia* (>1.5 million cases), gonorrhea (about 400,000 cases), HIV (>33,000 cases), and syphilis (>23,000 cases).

Process of Infection

The process of infection includes colonization, invasion, multiplication, and dissemination of pathogenic microorganisms. Many potentially pathogenic microorganisms reside within the normal microbiome without causing severe disease. The symbiotic relationship with the normal flora is maintained by physical barriers (e.g., skin and lining of respiratory and intestinal tracts), the complexity of the microbiome, and inflammatory and immune systems. Microorganisms that may cause infection if the protective barriers or defensive systems are weakened are referred to as *opportunistic microorganisms*. Physical damage to the intestinal tract during trauma or surgery releases intestinal bacteria into the bloodstream, potentially leading to sepsis, shock, and death. Cuts in the skin may allow normally contained bacteria (e.g., *S. aureus*) to cause local infections (e.g., abscesses, boils) and invade further and infect various organs. Alterations in the microbiome by antibiotics may allow local overgrowth of opportunistic microorganisms (e.g., *Clostridium difficile, Candida albicans*). Immune deficiencies may allow invasive systemic infections (e.g., systemic fungal infections) (see Chapter 9).

Unlike opportunistic infectious agents, *true pathogens* have devised means to circumvent the individual's defenses (discussed in Chapters 7 and 8) and cause infection. Infection with these agents is usually dependent on adequate numbers of microorganisms rather than compromise of the host's defenses. The estimated minimum number of microorganisms needed to cause infection (minimum infective dose) varies greatly with the particular pathogen: *Vibrio cholerae* (10^3 to 10^8 microorganisms), norovirus and rotavirus (10–100), *Giardia lamblia* parasitic diarrhea (10), and *Mycobacterium tuberculosis* (<10).

Pathogenic microorganisms usually exist in reservoirs (a natural habitat where the microorganism can multiply), such as the environment (e.g., contaminated water, soil), vertebrate animals, or another human who is infected. An individual may obtain an infectious microorganism from a reservoir either directly or indirectly.

Direct transmission may occur through direct contact with infections of another individual, such as the skin lesions of impetigo *(S. aureus, Streptococcus pyogenes)*, fungal skin infections (athlete's foot), scabies (mites), lice (head or body lice), oral herpes, and STIs (see Chapter 27).

Vertical transmission is the spread of microorganisms from mother to child across the placenta (e.g., *T. pallidum, Listeria monocytogenes*, cytomegalovirus [CMV], *Toxoplasma gondii*), ascending the birth canal from vaginal colonization or during delivery (e.g., group B *Streptococcus, Escherichia coli, C. trachomatis, N. gonorrhoeae*, hepatitis B virus, HIV, *C. albicans*), or through the breast milk (e.g., *S. aureus*, HIV). Spread of microorganisms from one person to another is *horizontal transmission*.

Indirect transmission occurs from contact with contaminated materials, which can range from towels to food or through a vector. Transmission by indirect physical contact may occur with materials that the infected individual came in contact (e.g., towels, sheets, clothing, toys, bandages) and is a common route of transmission for *S. aureus*. Iatrogenic transmission occurs inadvertently as a result of medical procedures, such as contaminated transfusions, transplants, implants, and catheters. Many infectious microorganisms are transmitted on the surface of objects that penetrate the skin or from dirt that contaminates wounds, such as spores of *Clostridium perfringens* (gas gangrene) and *C. tetani* (tetanus).

Respiratory transmission may occur by means of several mechanisms. Coughing or sneezing generally creates a mist that can be inhaled from the air for considerable time. This mechanism readily transmits many viral diseases, including the common cold, influenza, mumps, and measles. Infected individuals also may produce airborne droplets that settle on environmental surfaces. Several viral and bacterial diseases may be spread in this manner, including pertussis, influenza, pneumonia, legionnaires disease, and rubella. Other microorganisms may be airborne by circulating air that carries microorganisms picked up from the soil, dried droppings, or other sites. Most pathogenic fungi (e.g., *Histoplasma capsulatum, Coccidioides immitis, Blastomyces dermatitidis*) grow as saprophytes in the environment and are transmitted by inhalation of spores and initially present as pulmonary infections but may spread to other sites in the body.

Many ingested substances (food, water) may be contaminated by minuscule amounts of human feces *(fecal-oral transmission)* that transmits *Salmonella* (salmonella food poisoning), cholera, hepatitis A virus,

poliovirus, rotavirus, norovirus, *Giardia lamblia,* and many others that cause minor or major gastrointestinal diseases.

Zoonotic infections may be directly transmitted from animals, such as transmission of the rabies virus through bites. Most zoonotic infections are transmitted indirectly by means of *vector-borne transmission* (primarily insects). Mechanical vectors (e.g., housefly) passively transfer parasitic, bacterial, fungal, or viral microorganisms on the outside of their body from contaminated material to an individual. Biologic vectors (e.g., insects [*arthropods*]) feed off the blood of infected individuals. The infectious agent usually undergoes part of its life cycle within the arthropod, including multiplication, and is transmitted through bites or stings. Biologic vectors are responsible for some of the most severe blood-borne diseases. Important arthropods include mosquitoes (spreads malaria [*Plasmodium* spp.], arboviruses [arthropod-borne viruses], dengue hemorrhagic fever), tsetse fly (spreads trypanosomes such as *Trypanosoma cruzi*, which causes Chagas disease in South America, and *T. brucei*, which causes sleeping sickness in Africa), fleas (plague [*Yersinia pestis*], typhus [*Rickettsia prowazekii*], leishmaniasis [protozoan parasite *Leishmania* spp.]), and deer tick (Lyme disease [*Borrelia burgdorferi*]).

During transmission successful pathogens usually undergo initial adherence to tissue at the site of entrance to the body. Several produce localized infections without tissue invasion (e.g., *V. cholera* in the intestinal tract), whereas others require spread from the initial site of colonization. Colonization begins when the microorganism stabilizes adherence to tissue through specific surface receptors. Adherence helps protect the microorganism from removal by mechanical, nonspecific forces, such as coughing of respiratory mucus. Adherence occurs between ligands/receptors on the microorganism and on the surface of cells, the specificity of which results in localization of an infectious agent to particular sites (tissue tropism), such as the confinement of common cold viruses to the respiratory tract.

Although discussions of infectious diseases generally focus on single microorganisms that can be isolated and identified, they frequently exist in the body as part of complex multicellular masses called biofilms.[7] Biofilms consist of mixed species of microorganisms, including bacteria and fungi, immersed in a highly organized extracellular matrix produced by the microorganisms. Growth in biofilms offers survival advantages of protection by trapping components of the host's defenses and antibiotics.[8] The closely organized structure allows for exchange of genetic information for antibiotic resistance and other defense mechanisms. Biofilms form on implanted medical devises (e.g., catheters, pacemakers, implanted heart valves, prosthetic joints, dentures) and are associated with chronic infections (e.g., persistent nasopharyngeal colonization with staphylococci; otitis media; diabetes-associated foot ulcers; infected burns; vaginitis; osteomyelitis; pneumonia secondary to cystic fibrosis; diseases of the oral cavity related to dental plaque, such as dental caries and periodontitis).

Invasion follows colonization. Successful infectious agents have developed mechanisms to penetrate the tissues and evade the host's nonspecific and specific defenses (inflammation and immunity). The process of invasion is closely linked to tissue damage. Extracellular pathogens generally invade by means of direct extension into the surrounding tissue and access to the lymphatics and bloodstream, from which they spread to internal organs. This form of invasion requires a variety of virulence factors, including adhesion molecules and toxins, which may directly lead to tissue damage. Obligate intracellular pathogens, such as intracellular bacteria, parasites, and viruses, spread directly from cell to cell or by release of infectious microorganisms into extracellular fluid or blood from which they infect another cell. Some intracellular microorganisms may enter a latency phase within infected cells without spread or cellular damage until reactivation of the microbe occurs (e.g., herpes simplex virus, CMV, tuberculosis).

TABLE 10.1   CLASSES OF MICROORGANISMS INFECTIOUS TO HUMANS

CLASS	SIZE	SITE OF REPRODUCTION	EXAMPLE
Bacteria	0.8–15 mcg	Skin Mucous membranes Extracellular Intracellular	Staphylococcal wound infection Cholera Streptococcal pneumonia Mycobacterium tuberculosis
Chlamydiae Rickettsiae Mycoplasma	200–1000 nm 300–1200 nm 125–350 nm	Intracellular Intracellular Extracellular	Urethritis Rocky Mountain spotted fever Atypical pneumonia
Fungi	2–200 mcg	Skin Mucous membranes Extracellular Intracellular	Tinea pedis (athlete's foot) Candida (e.g., thrush) Sporotrichosis Histoplasmosis
Protozoa	1–50 mm	Mucosal Extracellular	Giardiasis Sleeping sickness
Helminths	3 mm–10 m	Intracellular Extracellular	Trichinosis Filariasis
Virus	20–300 nm	Intracellular	Poliomyelitis

The presence of infectious microorganisms in the blood is generally referred to as bacteremia (bacteria in blood), viremia (viruses in blood), or fungemia (fungi in blood) and is usually related to transport and spread to other organs. Septicemia is multiplication of microorganisms (particularly bacteria) in the blood.

Classes of Infectious Microorganisms

Infectious disease can be caused by microorganisms that range in size from 20 nm (poliovirus) to 10 m (tapeworm). Classes of pathogenic microorganisms and their characteristics are summarized in Table 10.1 and discussed in detail in the following sections.

Infectious Bacteria

Bacteria are prokaryotic unicellular microorganisms with no nuclei, mitochondria, or membrane-bound organelles. They are generally divided into several groups:

- *True bacteria* divide by binary fission and may have a variety of morphologies, including cocci (spherical), bacilli (rod shaped), vibrios (comma-shaped rods), or spirilla (twisted, rod shaped). Most disease-causing bacteria fall into this classification.
- *Filamentous bacteria* may have branching, mycelium-like structures that resemble fungi. Examples include *Mycobacterium tuberculosis* and *Mycobacterium leprae* that respectively cause tuberculosis and leprosy.
- *Spirochetes* are flexible spiral filaments that are motile and most are anaerobic. Pertinent examples include *Borrelia recurrentis* (relapsing fever), *Treponema pallidum* (syphilis), and *Borrelia burgdorferi* (Lyme disease).
- *Mycoplasma* lack a rigid cell wall and are small and pleomorphic. They are the smallest and simplest members of the bacteria. *Mycoplasma pneumoniae* causes atypical pneumonia, and *Mycoplasma genitalium* is a suspected cause of urethritis and pelvic inflammatory disease.
- *Rickettsia* are strict intracellular parasites that can be rod-shaped, spherical, or pleomorphic. They are typically spread by insect vectors and cause Rocky Mountain spotted fever *(Rickettsia rickettsii)* and typhus *(R. prowazekii)*.

- *Chlamydia* are also strict intracellular parasites, but with more complex intracellular life cycles. The primary chlamydial pathogen is *Chlamydia trachomatis*, which causes the most common bacterial STI (pelvic inflammatory disease) and eye infections (conjunctivitis).

Bacteria also can be categorized as gram negative or gram positive. Gram-negative bacteria do not retain crystal violet dye in the Gram-staining process whereas gram-positive bacteria do retain crystal violet dye. Gram-negative bacteria also have a lipopolysaccharide (LPS) coat in the outer membrane, which consists of lipid A, a core polysaccharide, and O antigen. The LPS coat also is known as endotoxin (Fig. 10.1). Common bacterial pathogens are listed in Table 10.2.

Mechanisms of Bacterial Invasion and Tissue

Bacterial Invasion. Many bacteria have specialized surface structures that contribute to the structural integrity of biofilms and provide adherence to cells and tissue during invasion. Pili (also called fimbriae) are thin, rodlike projections from the bacterial surface[9] (Fig. 10.2). Pathogenic strains of *E. coli* involved in urinary tract infections have a variety of different specific pili-associated adhesion molecules (i.e., adhesins), including mannose-binding protein that binds with glycoproteins specifically expressed on the bladder epithelium.

Flagella (used for bacterial motion) also express adhesins. *Vibrio cholerae* expresses adhesins for fibronectin, a common component of mucosal cell surfaces. Adhesion to connective tissue components, such as fibronectin (*S. pyogenes* [group A streptococci], *S. aureus*, *T. pallidum*), collagen, laminin, and vitronectin are common sites of bacterial adherence.

Several microorganisms use complement-related receptors for initial attachment. *Neisseria* spp. adhere to urinary tract epithelial cell membrane–associated cofactor protein (CD46), which is a complement-regulatory protein that protects cells by inactivating C3b and C4b. Others use different components of the CR3-C3b/C3bi receptor-ligand system on the surface of monocytes/macrophages for adherence including *Bordetella pertussis*, *Legionella pneumophila* (legionnaires disease), and *M. tuberculosis*.

Toxins and Bacterial Products. Bacterial pathogens produce a variety of toxic molecules that may kill the individual's cells, disrupt the tissue, and protect against inflammation. Exotoxins are proteins

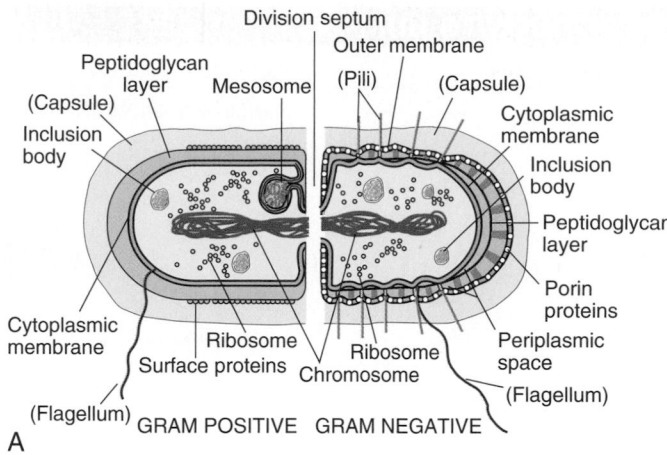

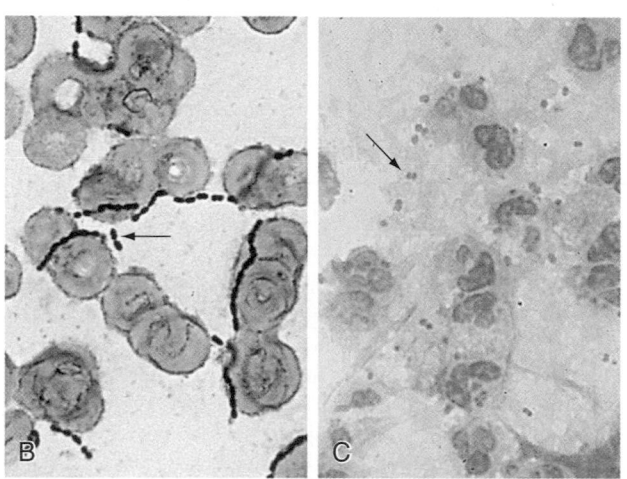

FIGURE 10.1 Gram-Positive and Gram-Negative Bacteria. **A,** The structure of the bacterial cell wall determines its staining characteristics with Gram stain. Gram-positive bacteria have a thick layer of peptidoglycan *(left)*. Gram-negative bacteria have a thin peptidoglycan layer and an outer membrane of lipopolysaccharide (LPS) *(right)*. **B,** Example of a gram-positive (darkly stained microorganisms, *arrow*) group A *Streptococcus*. This microorganism consists of cocci that frequently form chains. **C,** Example of a gram-negative (pink microorganisms, *arrow*) *Neisseria meningitidis* in cerebrospinal fluid. *Neisseria* form complexes of two cocci (diplococci). (**A** from Murray PR et al: *Medical microbiology,* ed 7, Philadelphia, 2013, Saunders; **B, C** from Murray PR et al: *Medical microbiology,* ed 4, St Louis, 2002, Mosby.)

released during microbial growth and they may have specific or broad effects on connective tissue and cells. Exotoxins are classified by their mode of action. Type I toxins bind to the cell surface and alter cell function, type II toxins cause membrane damage, and type III toxins enter the cell.

Type I toxins include superantigens and heat-stable enterotoxins (i.e., toxins that target the intestinal tract). Superantigens (SAgs) (discussed in Chapter 8) are molecules that react with major histocompatibility complex (MHC) class II proteins on the surface of antigen-presenting cells and the T-cell receptor (TCR), independent of the specificity of the TCR. SAgs activate many more cells than a specific antigen would and lead to overproduction of proinflammatory cytokines, such as IL-1, IL-6, and TNF-α. SAgs are responsible for several diseases, including food poisoning (heat-stable enterotoxins of *S. aureus* and *C. perfringens*), toxic shock syndrome (toxic shock syndrome toxin [TSST] of *S. aureus*), and scarlet fever (erythrogenic toxin of *S. pyogenes*). *E. coli* secretes small-molecular-weight heat-stable enterotoxins that bind to membrane-bound guanylate cyclase, resulting in increased levels of cyclic guanosine monophosphate (cGMP) and loss of cellular electrolytes and water.

Type II toxins are membrane-damaging molecules of several subtypes. Cholesterol-dependent toxins are cytolytic. They bind to the cell surface and assemble to construct an extremely large pore, similar to C9 of the complement system and perforin produced by T-cytotoxic cells[10] (see Chapters 7 and 8). Cholesterol is required for formation of the pore. The pore leads to rapid exchange of calcium and water and cell death. *S. pneumoniae* secretes the cholesterol-dependent toxin pneumolysin, which can facilitate colonization of the lungs as well as protect the bacteria from macrophages. Type II toxins also include a subtype called *RTX cytotoxins,* which contain repeats in protein sequence. An example is α-hemolysin from *E. coli.* The α-hemolysin is a virulence factor that predominantly causes urinary tract infection and lysis of erythrocytes as a source of nutrients, but also protects *E. coli* by lysis of macrophages and lymphocytes. A third subtype of type II toxins includes enzymatically active toxins. *C. perfringens,* found in soil and as a wound contaminant, is the cause of gas gangrene. The major virulence factor is an α-toxin with phospholipase activity that results in hemolysis, as well as hydrolysis of membrane phospholipids of other cells.

Type III toxins are generally A-B toxins and the most common bacterial toxin. *A-B toxins* are referred to as *binary toxins* because two different components are required for activity: separately secreted A (active) and B (binding) components. The B components are activated by proteases

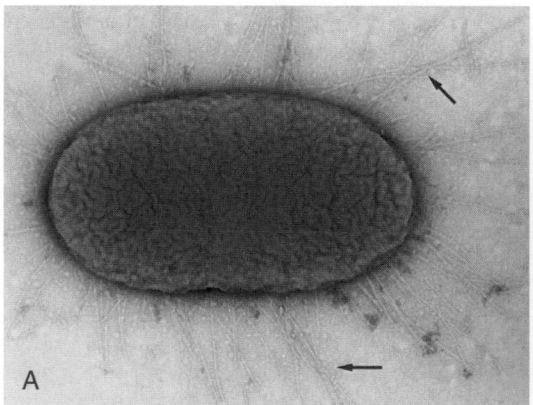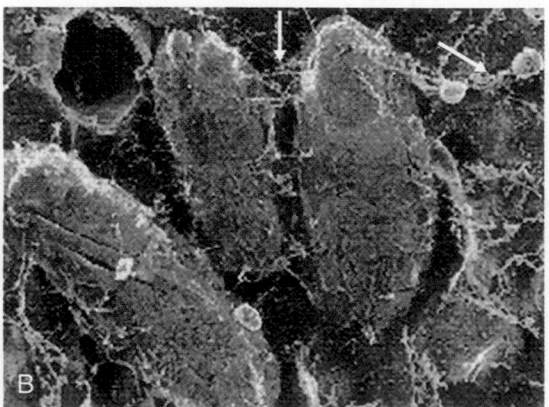

FIGURE 10.2 Attachment of *Escherichia coli* through Pili. **A,** Transmission electron micrograph showing pili *(arrows)* of pathogenic *E. coli.* **B,** Scanning electron micrograph of *E. coli (orange)* attached by pili *(arrows)* to bladder epithelium *(blue).* (**A** courtesy Eric Buckles and Paula J. Fernandes; **B** modified from Wein A et al: *Campbell-Walsh urology,* ed 9, Philadelphia, 2007, Saunders.)

TABLE 10.2 COMMON BACTERIAL INFECTIONS

MICROORGANISM	GRAM STAIN	RESPIRATORY PATHWAY	INTRACELLULAR OR EXTRACELLULAR
Respiratory Tract Infections			
Upper Respiratory Tract Infections			
Corynebacterium diphtheriae (diphtheria)	Gram +	Facultative anaerobic	Extracellular
Haemophilus influenzae	Gram −	Facultative anaerobic	Extracellular
Streptococcus pyogenes (group A)	Gram +	Facultative anaerobic	Extracellular
Otitis Media			
Haemophilus influenzae	Gram −	Facultative anaerobic	Extracellular
Moraxella catarrhalis	Gram −	Aerobic	Extracellular
Streptococcus pneumoniae	Gram +	Facultative anaerobic	Extracellular
Lower Respiratory Tract Infections			
Bacillus anthracis (pulmonary anthrax)	Gram +	Facultative anaerobic	Extracellular
Bordetella pertussis (whooping cough)	Gram −	Aerobic	Extracellular
Chlamydia pneumoniae	Not stainable	Aerobic	Obligate intracellular
Escherichia coli	Gram −	Facultative anaerobic	Extracellular
Haemophilus influenzae	Gram −	Facultative anaerobic	Extracellular
Klebsiella pneumoniae	Gram −	Facultative anaerobic	Extracellular
Legionella pneumophila	Gram −	Aerobic	Facultative intracellular
Mycobacterium tuberculosis	Weak gram +	Aerobic	Extracellular
Mycoplasma pneumoniae	Not stainable	Aerobic	Extracellular
Neisseria meningitidis (develops into meningitis)	Gram −	Aerobic	Extracellular
Pseudomonas aeruginosa	Gram −	Aerobic	Extracellular
Streptococcus agalactiae (group B; develops into meningitis)	Gram +	Facultative anaerobic	Extracellular
Streptococcus pneumoniae	Gram +	Facultative anaerobic	Extracellular
Yersinia pestis (plague)	Gram −	Facultative anaerobic	Extracellular
Gastrointestinal Tract Infections			
Inflammatory Gastrointestinal Tract Infections			
Bacillus anthracis (gastrointestinal anthrax)	Gram +	Facultative anaerobic	Extracellular
Clostridium difficile	Gram +	Anaerobic	Extracellular
Escherichia coli 0157:H7	Gram −	Facultative anaerobic	Extracellular
Vibrio cholerae	Gram −	Facultative anaerobic	Extracellular
Vibrio parahaemolyticus	Gram −	Facultative anaerobic	Extracellular
Invasive Gastrointestinal Tract Infections			
Brucella abortus (brucellosis, undulant fever leading to sepsis, heart infection)	Gram −	Aerobic	Intracellular
Campylobacter jejuni	Gram −	Microaerophilic	Extracellular
Francisella tularensis	Gram −	Strict anaerobic	Facultative intracellular
Helicobacter pylori (gastritis and peptic ulcers)	Gram −	Microaerophilic	Extracellular
Listeria monocytogenes (leading to sepsis and meningitis)	Gram +	Aerobic	Intracellular
Salmonella typhi (typhoid fever)	Gram −	Anaerobic	Extracellular
Shigella sonnei	Gram −	Facultative anaerobic	Extracellular
Food Poisoning			
Bacillus cereus	Gram +	Facultative anaerobic	Extracellular
Clostridium botulinum	Gram +	Anaerobic	Extracellular
Clostridium perfringens	Gram +	Anaerobic	Extracellular
Staphylococcus aureus	Gram +	Facultative anaerobic	Extracellular
Sexually Transmitted Infections			
Chlamydia trachomatis (pelvic inflammatory disease)	Not stainable	Aerobic	Intracellular
Neisseria gonorrhoeae (urethritis)	Gram −	Aerobic	Facultative intracellular
Treponema pallidum (spirochete; syphilis)	Gram −	Aerobic	Extracellular
Skin and Wound Infections			
Bacillus anthracis (cutaneous anthrax)	Gram +	Facultative anaerobic	Extracellular
Borrelia burgdorferi (Lyme disease; spirochete)	Gram −	Aerobic	Extracellular

Continued

TABLE 10.2   COMMON BACTERIAL INFECTIONS—cont'd

MICROORGANISM	GRAM STAIN	RESPIRATORY PATHWAY	INTRACELLULAR OR EXTRACELLULAR
Clostridium tetani (tetanus)	Gram +	Anaerobic	Extracellular
Clostridium perfringens (gas gangrene)	Gram +	Anaerobic	Extracellular
Mycobacterium leprae (leprosy)	Gram + (weakly)	Aerobic	Extracellular
Pseudomonas aeruginosa	Gram −	Aerobic	Extracellular
Rickettsia prowazekii (rickettsia; typhus)	Gram −	Aerobic	Obligate intracellular
Staphylococcus aureus	Gram +	Facultative anaerobic	Extracellular
Streptococcus pyogenes (group A)	Gram +	Facultative anaerobic	Extracellular
Eye Infections			
Chlamydia trachomatis (conjunctivitis)	Not stainable	Aerobic	Obligate intracellular
Haemophilus aegyptius (pink eye)	Gram −	Facultative anaerobic	Extracellular
Zoonotic Infections			
Bacillus anthracis (anthrax)	Gram +	Facultative anaerobic	Extracellular
Brucella abortus (brucellosis, also called undulant fever)	Gram −	Aerobic	Intracellular
Borrelia burgdorferi (spirochete; Lyme disease)	Gram −	Aerobic	Extracellular
Listeria monocytogenes	Gram +	Aerobic	Intracellular
Rickettsia rickettsii (rickettsia; Rocky Mountain spotted fever)	Gram −	Aerobic	Obligate intracellular
Rickettsia prowazekii (rickettsia; typhus)	Gram −	Aerobic	Obligate intracellular
Yersinia pestis (plague)	Gram −	Facultative anaerobic	Extracellular
Nosocomial Infections			
Enterococcus faecalis	Gram +	Facultative anaerobic	Extracellular
Enterococcus faecium	Gram +	Facultative anaerobic	Extracellular
Escherichia coli (cystitis)	Gram −	Facultative anaerobic	Extracellular
Pseudomonas aeruginosa	Gram −	Obligate anaerobic	Extracellular
Staphylococcus aureus	Gram +	Facultative anaerobic	Extracellular
Staphylococcus epidermidis	Gram +	Facultative anaerobic	Extracellular

either in the extracellular fluid or on the surface membrane of the target cell. Multiple activated B components organize on the cell membrane to form a complex with which A components bind for transportation into the cell. Overgrowth of *C. difficile* in the colon is a common complication of prolonged antibiotic therapy that kills much of the commensal microbiome. *C. difficile* secretes membrane-disrupting toxins A (an enterotoxin) and B (a cytotoxin) that damage the mucosa and result in watery diarrhea and potentially life-threatening pseudomembranous colitis.[11] *Clostridium botulinum* produces the most potent toxin known, botulinum toxin, which is a paralytic neurotoxin that blocks the release of acetylcholine at nerve-muscle synapses and results in flaccid paralysis and death. Examples of A-B toxins include botulinum, tetanospasmin, *Corynebacterium diptheriae* (diptheria cytotoxin), *P. aeruginosa* (exotoxin A), and *Bacillus anthracis* (anthrax toxin).

A subset of A-B toxins is AB$_5$ toxins, examples of which are *B. pertussis* (pertussis toxin), *S. dysenteriae* (Shiga toxin), and *V. cholerae* (cholera heat-labile enterotoxin). AB$_5$ toxins form a complex of an A component noncovalently bound in a ring of five B components. During endocytosis, the A component is activated and alters cellular function usually by inactivating signaling pathways, increasing intracellular cyclic adenosine monophosphate (cAMP), or other means. The A component of anthrax A-B toxin is a zinc-metalloproteinase that prevents intracellular signaling. Diphtheria is a respiratory tract infection with systemic complications caused by an A-B toxin that inhibits messenger RNA (mRNA) translation and causes low blood pressure, necrosis in the heart and liver, degeneration of myelin sheaths, and death. The AB$_5$ cholera toxin leads to increased adenylate cyclase activity, which affects chloride channels, causing an efflux of chloride, water, and other salts into the intestinal lumen. Shiga toxin, another AB$_5$ toxin, binds to carbohydrates on the cell surface of the endothelium of the intestine, kidney, and brain. Shiga toxin is secreted by several pathogens, including *E. coli* O157:H7, a contaminant of food or water. Ingestion of Shiga toxin may initially cause bloody diarrhea followed by hemolytic uremic syndrome (hemolytic anemia, acute kidney failure, thrombocytopenia), which is especially severe and fatal in children.[12]

Another type of toxin is endotoxin. Unlike secreted exotoxins, endotoxin (also called lipopolysaccharide [LPS]) is contained in the cell walls of gram-negative bacteria and is released during lysis (or destruction) of the bacteria (see Fig. 10.1). The innermost part of LPS, *lipid A*, is made of polysaccharides and fatty acids and is responsible for the substance's toxic effects. Endotoxin also may be released during bacterial growth or during treatment with antibiotics. Therefore antibiotics cannot prevent the effects of the endotoxin.

The release of a sufficient amount of endotoxin can lead to fatal endotoxic shock (septic shock), which is one of the leading causes of death in intensive care units. Bacteria that produce endotoxins are called *pyrogenic bacteria* because they stimulate the release of inflammatory mediators that produce fever and cause the local and systemic effects of inflammation (Fig. 10.3). Once in the blood, endotoxins cause the release of vasoactive peptides and cytokines that affect blood vessels, producing vasodilation, which reduces blood pressure; causes decreased oxygen delivery; and produces subsequent cardiovascular shock (see Chapter 49). Endotoxin can activate the coagulation cascade, leading to the syndrome of disseminated (or diffuse) intravascular coagulation

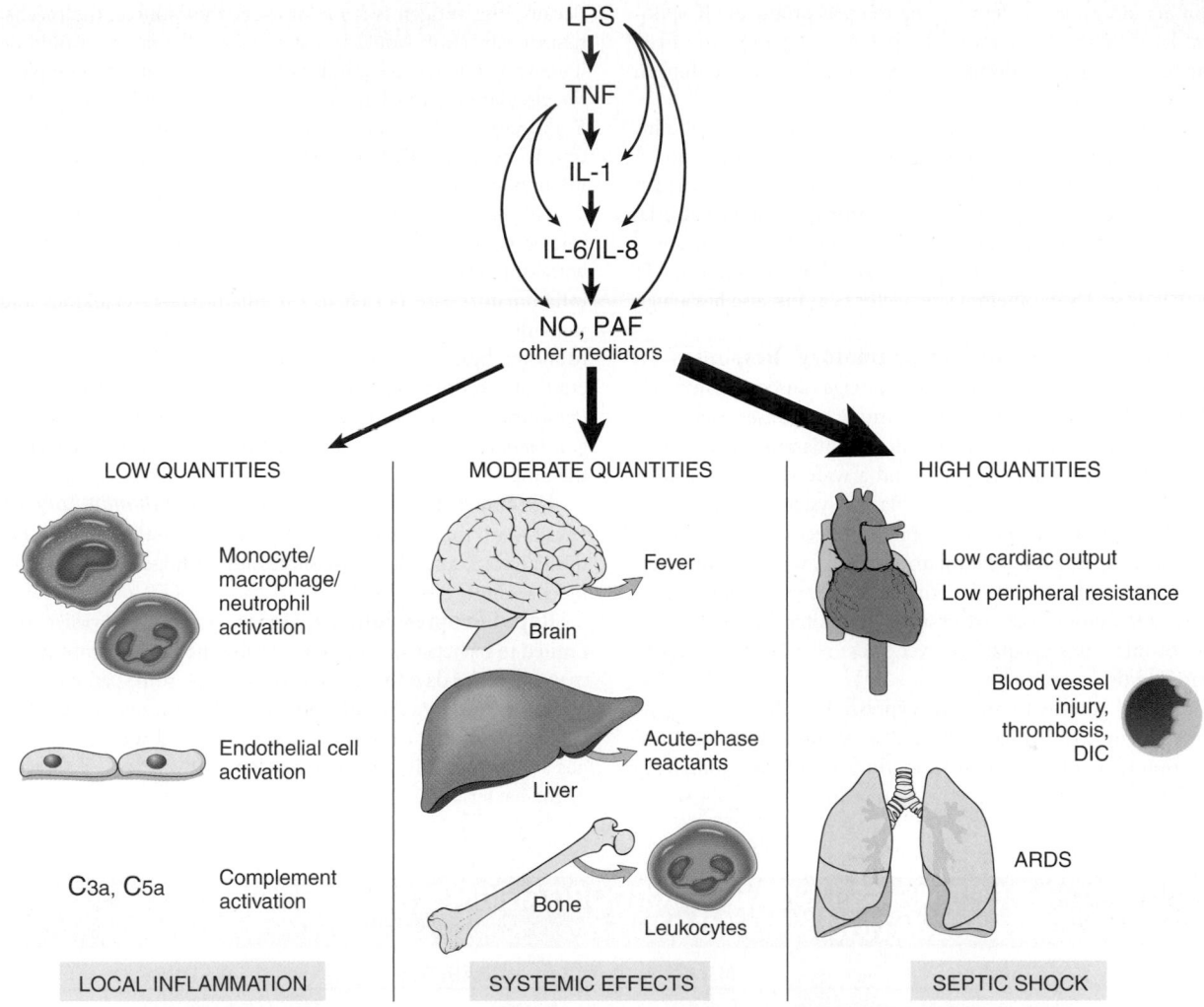

LPS

TNF

IL-1

IL-6/IL-8

NO, PAF
other mediators

LOW QUANTITIES

Monocyte/
macrophage/
neutrophil
activation

Endothelial cell
activation

C3a, C5a — Complement
activation

LOCAL INFLAMMATION

MODERATE QUANTITIES

Fever

Brain

Acute-phase
reactants

Liver

Bone

Leukocytes

SYSTEMIC EFFECTS

HIGH QUANTITIES

Low cardiac output

Low peripheral resistance

Blood vessel
injury,
thrombosis,
DIC

ARDS

SEPTIC SHOCK

FIGURE 10.3 The Many Activities of Lipopolysaccharide (LPS). Bacterial endotoxin *(LPS)* activates almost every aspect of inflammation. The release of LPS from gram-negative bacteria triggers successive waves of cytokine production, including tumor necrosis factor *(TNF)*, interleukin-1 *(IL-1)*, interleukin-6 *(IL-6)*, and interleukin-8 *(IL-8)*, and secondary mediators of inflammation, such as nitric oxide *(NO)* and platelet-activating factor *(PAF)*. At low levels of LPS the effect is local. Moderate levels of LPS cause more systemic inflammatory responses. High levels of LPS may lead to septic shock and death. *ARDS*, Acute respiratory distress syndrome; *DIC*, disseminated intravascular coagulation. (From Kumar V, Abbas A, Fausto N: *Robbins & Cotran pathologic basis of disease*, ed 7, Philadelphia, 2005, Saunders; Modified from Abbas AK et al: *Cellular and molecular immunology*, ed 4, Philadelphia, 2000, WB Saunders.)

(see Chapter 29). Additionally, endotoxin induces the release of TNF-α by macrophages. TNF is a potent proinflammatory cytokine, also called *cachectin* because of its role in promoting cachexia (wasting syndrome) in individuals with cancer. (Cachexia is discussed in Chapter 12; cytokines are discussed in Chapters 7 and 8.)

In addition to toxins, bacteria can also release enzymes that promote infection. The enzymes are not specific for any particular cell or cell receptor, but facilitate spread of the microorganism and are sometimes called *invasins*. A secondary effect may be considerable damage to the tissues and organs.

The site of infection contains a broad spectrum of proteases, lipases, deoxyribonucleases (DNases), and other enzymes secreted by microorganisms. The secretion of most toxic enzymes is common to broad groups of pathogens, whereas others discussed here are more limited to particular strains. Some proteases contribute to the defense against the immune and inflammatory systems by digesting components of the plasma systems (complement, clotting, fibrinolysis), immunoglobulins, cytokines,

and antimicrobial peptides. Most also will weaken the surrounding connective tissue to allow invasion. Connective tissue is vulnerable to digestion by proteases that break down hyaluronic acid, collagen, fibrin, elastin, laminin, and glycosaminoglycans. Hyaluronidase is frequently produced by streptococci, staphylococci, and clostridia to break down hyaluronic acid polymers in the matrix. Collagenase is a product of several clostridia, breaking down the intercellular matrix in muscle during gangrene. Neuraminidase is especially useful for intestinal pathogens, such as *V. cholerae* and *S. dysenteriae,* degrading the sialic acid that strengthens the intestinal epithelial junctions. Kinases, such as streptokinase and staphylokinase, activate plasminogen to digest large clots that interfere with bacterial spread.

Many enzymes also will digest membranes of tissue cells leading to lysis and release of nutrients that are useful to the microorganisms. Some hemolysins (those that lyse erythrocytes) or leukocidins (those that lyse phagocytes) are pore-forming toxins, but others are enzymes (e.g., lecithinases or phospholipases) that digest lipids in the membrane, resulting in hemolysis or cell death. *C. perfringens* produces phospholipases and lecithinases that remove the polar head groups from cell membrane phospholipids or destroy phosphatidylcholine (lecithin) in the membranes of most cells.

Several enzymes perform a secondary role in invasion as adhesins to matrix components.[13] *Yersinia pestis* (plague) expresses a plasminogen activator protease that can activate plasminogen to plasmin, which can dissolve clots and activate collagenase. When expressed on the bacterial surface, it binds strongly to laminin in the matrix and facilitates invasion. *S. agalactiae* (group B *Streptococcus*) produces a serine protease, a C5a peptidase, that degrades the chemotactic factor C5a, but also has a high binding affinity for fibronectin.

Destructive Immune and Inflammatory Responses to Bacterial Infection. Much of the tissue damage caused by infections is secondary to the inflammatory and immune responses. Infectious microorganisms routinely initiate an immune and inflammatory response, including infiltrates of phagocytic cells and a wide variety of T cells, production of antibody, and activation of plasma systems (complement, clotting) (see Chapters 7, 8, and 9). Some are specific to antigens (T cells, antibodies) expressed by the microorganism, whereas others are not antigen-specific (phagoytes). Cytokines and chemokines secreted by inflammatory and immune cells are designed to inhibit the proliferation and spread of infectious agents; however, most also are damaging to the surrounding tissue.

Antibodies will react with antigens expressed by the microorganism. Overproduction of antigen released as soluble molecules will lead to reaction with antibody and formation of immune complexes in the circulation or in tissue and activation of inflammatory systems.

Because the antigen is from an exogenous source, the mechanism of tissue destruction would be classified as allergic and would be type II if expressed on the cell surface or type III if immune complexes are in the circulation (see Chapter 9). For example, individuals infected with *S. pyogenes* or *T. palladium* are at risk for developing symptoms of type III hypersensitivity reactions including kidney disease and vascular inflammation.

The typical immune and inflammatory reaction against intracellular microorganisms or persistent infections involves a cell-mediated response with infiltration of T cells and macrophages, as well as neutrophils. The inflammatory site is rich in proinflammatory cytokines and as the individual's response increases so do the destructive effects on surrounding healthy tissue. Many of these infections are very difficult to eradicate, leading to progressively increasing production of cytokines. Persistent infections (e.g., *M. tuberculosis*) may lead to formation of *granulomas,* which cause further destruction of the infected organ (e.g., the lung).

Bacterial Evasion of Immune and Inflammatory Systems. Evasion of the individual's immune and inflammatory systems is multifaceted, and the most successful pathogens incorporate several mechanisms (Table 10.3).

Rapid Progression. Rapid progression is an evasive mechanism limited to bacteria and viruses. Because the primary immune response may take 3 to 5 days to reach protective levels, some pathogens proliferate at rates that surpass the development of the immune system. An example is *V. cholerae,* that causes severe vomiting and watery diarrhea, which has a 60% mortality rate and develops within 2 to 3 days of ingestion of the bacteria.

TABLE 10.3	MECHANISMS USED BY MICROORGANISMS TO DEFEND AGAINST INFLAMMATION AND IMMUNITY			
STRATEGY	BACTERIA	FUNGI	PARASITES	VIRUSES
Rapid division	Initial proliferation in protective environment	NA	NA	Rapid proliferation of viruses with small genomes
Protection against phagocytosis and intracellular destruction	Intracellular bacteria block granule fusion, survive in phagolysosomes, enter and multiply in cytoplasm. Capsules with antiphagocytic and anticomplement activities, toxins to kill phagocytes (e.g., α-toxin and leukocidin).	Multiplication in phagosomes, inhibition of lysosomal enzymes. Polysaccharide capsule, toxins that inhibit phagocytosis.	Resistance to lysosomal enzymes, block granule fusion, enter and multiply in cytoplasm. Glycocalyx, toxins that inhibit phagocytosis.	Obligative intracellular life cycle, latency (e.g., herpes simplex virus in dorsal root ganglia)
Blocking antigen recognition	Adsorption of fibronectin or IgG (e.g., protein A), sialic acid capsule. Large diversity of surface molecules, phase changes in pili or membrane proteins, strain-to-strain serotype differences.	Changes in surface antigens	Adsorption of IgG by Fc receptor. Changing morphologic forms during life cycle, antigen switching.	Enveloped viruses with plasma membrane. Viral enzymes that produce translational errors, antigen shift and drift, diversity of serotypes.
Blocking the immune response	Proteases for IgA and IgG, degrade complement, defensins, and cathelicidins. Shedding of surface antigens. Proteases degrade complement (e.g., C3b, C5a), capsules that prevent complement deposition, inhibitors of complement components and convertases. Induction of anergy, direct suppression of Th cell development.	Stimulation of antiinflammatory cytokines, inhibition of proinflammatory cytokines.	IgG and IgA proteases. Shedding of surface antigens. Degrade or inactivate C3b, C3a, and C5a; break down C3 convertase. Release of soluble antigens that induce "tolerance," polyclonal B-cell activation, induction of antiinflammatory cytokines, cytotoxic molecules.	Secretion of viral proteins to neutralize antibody, molecules to neutralize cytokines. Cellular complement inhibitors in envelope. Infect and kill immune cells, inhibit Tc and natural killer (NK) recognition of major histocompatibility complex (MHC), inhibit antigen presentation.

IgA, Immunoglobulin A; *IgG,* immunoglobulin G; *NA,* not applicable; *Th,* T helper cell.

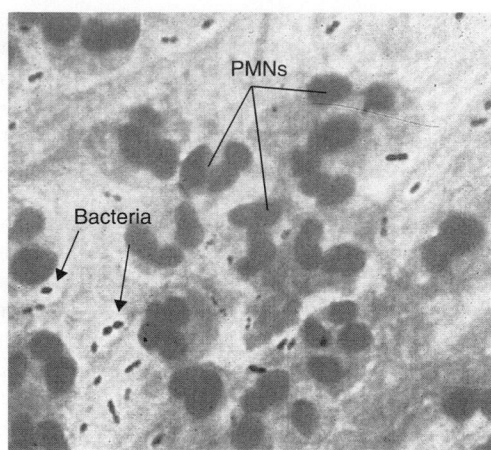

FIGURE 10.4 Bacterial Capsule. Gram stain of a sputum sample from an individual with pneumococcal pneumonia (×1000 magnification). The sputum is rich in polymorphonuclear *(PMN)* cells and slightly elongated, gram-negative cocci *(Streptococcus pneumoniae).* Clear areas *(arrows)* around the bacteria indicate capsules. (Modified from Mandell G, Bennett J, Dolin R: *Principles and practice of infectious diseases,* ed 7, Philadelphia, 2010, Churchill Livingstone.)

Bacterial Protection Against Phagocytosis and Intracellular Destruction. Antiphagocytic capsules are expressed by most bacterial pathogens involved in pneumonia and meningitis (Fig. 10.4). Capsules are mostly polysaccharide, although proteins also may be capsular components. Examples include the thick polysaccharide covering of the pneumococcus *(S. pneumoniae),* the waxy capsule surrounding the tubercle bacillus *(M. tuberculosis),* the polysaccharide "slime" capsule of *P. aeruginosa,* and the M protein of *S. pyogenes.*

Some bacterial toxins and extracellular enzymes kill phagocytic cells (e.g., *P. aeruginosa* exotoxin A). Staphylococcal hemolysins and toxins from *B. anthracis* and *B. pertussis* decrease phagocytic and chemotactic activities and may be toxic to the cell. Streptococcal products, such as streptolysin O, bind to cholesterol in the membrane of the phagolysosome and initiate destruction through the cytoplasmic release of lysosomal enzymes.

Normally a macrophage would efficiently kill bacteria, but mechanisms for intracellular survival have evolved to the benefit of the infectious agent. *Intracellular bacteria* can survive and even multiply in macrophages *(Brucella, Listeria, M. leprae, M. tuberculosis)* or in other cells. Bacterial killing results from fusion of lysosomal granules with the phagosome to produce a phagolysosome and activation of oxygen-dependent and oxygen-independent mechanisms. *M. tuberculosis* produces toxins that prevent phagosome-lysosome fusion so that the environment in the phagosome remains relatively nontoxic.

A second means of avoiding killing is neutralization of the toxic environment of the phagolysosome. Production of catalase and superoxide dismutase *(N. gonorrhoeae, Brucella abortus)* destroys toxic oxygen products produced by the hexose-monophosphate shunt.

A third means of avoiding killing is escape from the phagosome. Lysins (e.g., hemolysin of *Shigella,* listeriolysin O and phospholipase C of *L. monocytogenes,* phospholipase A of *Rickettsia* spp.) are secreted enzymes that break down the phagosome membrane, releasing the bacteria into the cytoplasm where they multiply.[14]

Blocking Recognition of Bacterial Antigens. Pathogens that coat themselves with human proteins may "fool" the immune system by masking antigens. Some bacterial surface proteins (e.g., protein G of *S. pyogenes*) bind the Fc portion of antibody, thus forming a protective coat of "self" protein. Binding through the Fc holds the antibody in an orientation that does not allow complement activation or phagocytosis.

T. pallidum coats itself with fibronectin. Capsules may contain sialic acid (e.g., *E. coli* K-12), which closely resembles the sialic acid on the surface of most human cells, or hyaluronic acid (e.g., group A streptococci), which is the basic substance in normal connective tissue.

Antigenic variation allows the pathogen to alter surface antigens that are the targets of protective immune responses. Thus as the individual develops protective levels of antibodies, the pathogen responds by changing antigens and becoming resistant. The three primary mechanisms of antigenic variation are *mutation* (a change or error in gene structure that results in variant expression of antigen); *recombination* (the exchange of DNA fragments between cells resulting in a new DNA sequence and variance of antigen expression); and *gene switching* (the switching of genes on and off resulting in variation of antigen expression).

Neisseria use pili to adhere to epithelium, and antibody against these antigens can abrogate adherence. *Neisseria* undergoes *phase shifts* during which pilar antigens are changed by progressive silencing of 1 set of 10 or 11 available pili genes and activation of others that express different antigens. Many bacteria have a large number of different antigenic types (serotypes) across the species. At least 80 different strains of group A streptococci express different serotypes of the capsular M protein. *S. pneumoniae* has at least 100 different serotypes based on capsular polysaccharides. Some gram-negative bacteria can revert to "rough" forms in which serotype-specific carbohydrates are deleted, thus becoming resistant to antibody and activation of complement.

Blocking the Immune Response to Bacteria. Bacteria may spontaneously release surface molecules that bind to and neutralize antibody. These include endotoxin from gram-negative bacteria and capsular antigens from *S. pneumoniae* and *N. meningitidis.* The secretion of large amounts of soluble antigen may lead to formation of immune complexes.

Bacteria may break down molecules of the immune or inflammatory system. An IgA protease produced by meningitis-causing microorganisms and other related bacteria *(N. gonorrhoeae, N. meningitidis, H. influenzae, S. pneumoniae)* cleaves IgA at the hinge region into ineffective Fc and Fab'$_2$ regions. *Salmonella* membrane protease degrades nonspecific antimicrobial molecules like defensins and cathelicidins.

Complement is a major component of the defense against bacterial infection through production of opsonin (C3b) and chemotactic factors (C3a, C5a) for neutrophils. Teichoic acid in the gram-positive cell wall provides resistance against complement-mediated lysis. Bacterial regulatory proteins (e.g., *Borrelia* complement-regulator-acquiring protein, *Neisseria* porins, and members of the *Streptococcus* M protein family) affect complement activation, including destabilization of the C3 convertase complex or degradation of the opsonin C3b.[15] *Pseudomonas* produces elastase (breaks down C3 of the complement system) and a 56-kDa protease (breaks down the chemotactic factor C5a).

Some bacterial pathogens can broadly suppress immune responses against their own antigens, as well as other antigens unrelated to the infectious agent. Chronic bacterial infections, like leprosy *(M. leprae)* and tuberculosis *(M. tuberculosis),* induce anergy (suppressed response to multiple antigens) in infected hosts. *Helicobacter pylori* releases LPS that binds to dendritic cells and blocks development of T-helper 1 (Th1) cells, produces toxins that block the T-cell IL-2 receptor signaling pathway, thus inhibiting maturation of Th cells, and induces a Th17 response that impairs inflammatory responses.[16]

One of the most common bacterial infections is *Staphylococcus aureus* and it is described in Box 10.2.

Infectious Fungi

Fungi are eukaryotic microorganisms with thick, rigid cell walls and the capacity to form a variety of complex structures (Fig. 10.5). Fungi

BOX 10.2   EXAMPLE OF BACTERIAL PATHOGENESIS: *STAPHYLOCOCCUS AUREUS*

Infection with *S. aureus* is an example of how mechanisms of bacterial pathogenesis come together. *S. aureus* is a commensal microorganism that resides on the skin and nasal passages (30% of individuals are nasal carriers), but also is an opportunistic pathogen. Minor skin infections may result if the integrity of the skin is compromised by cuts or abrasions or if hair follicles are infected. Most infections are relatively mild and localized as red and swollen eruptions on the skin containing pus or other drainage (see Figure). If not treated appropriately, more severe abscesses (pus-filled nodules in skin tissue), boils (pus-filled nodular infection of hair follicle), carbuncles (cluster of boils), or cellulitis (red and diffuse infection of inner layers of skin, dermis, and subcutaneous fat) may develop.

Invasive disease results from more extensive skin damage (e.g., eczema, trauma, surgical wounds, or injection sites for intravenous drug abuse). Extensive biofilms can develop on inert materials (e.g., intravenous catheters, indwelling medical devices, or prosthetic joints). *S. aureus* can spread to the circulation (bacteremia, septicemia) and infect the heart valves (endocarditis), bones (osteomyelitis), and joints (infectious arthritis), and form abscesses in internal organs.

Chronic medical conditions requiring hospitalization (e.g., diabetes, cancer, vascular disease, pulmonary disease, or surgery) weaken the immune system and increase the risk for invasive *S. aureus* infection. For instance, *S. aureus* is a major cause of diabetic foot ulcers resulting in limb amputation or death.[1] *S.* aureus also has become a major cause of hospital-acquired (nosocomial) infections. Healthcare providers and visitors to hospitals can easily become carriers by direct skin-to-skin contact or contact with items or surfaces (e.g., clothing, towels, or bandages) contaminated by another individual's infection. Untreated *S. aureus* bacteremia has an 80% fatality rate. Because of the prevalence of multiple antibiotic resistance (see Emerging Infections), even appropriate treatment has a 15% to 50% fatality rate depending on the individual's age and health.

An unusually large number of virulence factors contribute to invasive infection by *S. aureus*. Invasion is initiated by adherence to extracellular matrix (e.g., laminin, fibrin, fibronectin) and endothelium. Two fibronectin-binding proteins bridge between fibronectin and cellular $\alpha5\beta1$ integrin, triggering bacterial uptake by endocytosis in endothelium, epithelial cells, and other cells. *S. aureus* can proliferate within cells and destroy infected cells. Adherence to fibronectin also facilitates the formation of biofilms.[2] Spread to bone and joints, enhanced by attachment to collagen, occurs in osteomyelitis and septic arthritis–causing strains. Staphylococci also produce a polysaccharide capsule that mediates attachment to prosthetic devices, as well as protects against phagocytosis.

S. aureus is very susceptible to antibody and complement-mediated neutrophil phagocytosis, but has developed a variety of effective defenses. IgG antibody is neutralized by cell surface staphylococcal protein A (SPA) and secreted staphylococcal binder of immunoglobulin. Both bind IgG at the Fc region. This IgG orientation prevents binding to surface antigens, prevents activation of complement, and masks the bacterium with human proteins. Additional masking with self-protein is provided by bacterial coagulase that activates coagulation to produce a coat of fibrin, which also inhibits phagocytosis. *S. aureus* inhibits the complement cascade at several key points. The thick peptidoglycan layer and a thin capsule prevent complement from binding with the bacterial membrane. Secreted complement inhibitor proteins and enzymes (e.g., staphylokinase) inhibit or break down most protective components of the complement cascade.

Neutrophil phagocytic and bactericidal functions are directly inhibited by *S. aureus*. The primary mechanism of bacterial killing by neutrophils involves recognition of bacterial products by Toll-like receptor-2 (TLR2) and activation of oxygen-dependent killing. *S. aureus* produces chemokine receptor blockers (e.g., staphopain A), chemotaxis inhibitors that prevent neutrophil binding to endothelium and extravascularization (e.g., chemotaxis inhibitory protein, superantigen-like protein), metalloprotease inhibitors to prevent migration through tissue, phagocytosis inhibitors, and lysins that kill neutrophils. Bacterial protection includes blocking of TLR2 recognition of staphylococcal lipoproteins and peptidoglycan, several enzymatic inhibitors of oxygen-dependent killing in phagosomes (e.g., catalase, superoxide dismutase, hydrogen peroxide reductase, and glutathione peroxidase), and inhibitors of lysosomal granule proteases (e.g., elastase). Bacterial production of adenosine, an antiinflammatory molecule, inhibits the neutrophil respiratory burst, degranulation, and platelet-activated coagulation. *S. aureus* also produces a cell-bound pigment (carotenoid) that "quenches" singlet oxygen within the phagocyte.

S. aureus modifies B- and T-cell responses. A variety of superantigens interfere with normal T-cell function, including diminished proliferation of antigen-specific T-helper cells. Adenosine secretion modulates T-cell activation, decreases expression of antigen-presenting major histocompatibility molecules in macrophages and dendritic cells, and suppresses the production of IL-12 that normally drives differentiation of Th1 cells.

Secretion of exotoxins contributes to the pathophysiology of *S. aureus* infection. Many toxins are the result of uptake of new extrachromosomal genetic information from the environment, conjugation with other bacteria, or infection of bacteria with phages (viruses that infect bacteria).[3] Thus different strains of *S. aureus* express different toxin profiles. More than 20 type I toxins (superantigens, heat-stable enterotoxins) have been associated with *S. aureus* infections. Staphylococcal enterotoxins are the most common cause of food poisoning with vomiting and diarrhea. The staphylococcal toxic-shock syndrome toxin-1 (TSST-1)

FIGURE *Staphylococcus aureus* Infections. Different strains of *S. aureus* (gram-positive cocci in sputum from an individual with pneumonia [center photograph]) cause a variety of infections. The particular infection may depend on the toxin produced: exfoliative toxin (scalded skin syndrome), enterotoxins A–G (food poisoning), or toxic shock syndrome toxin-1 *(TSST-1).* (Toxic shock syndrome, carbuncle, impetigo, and wound infection photos from Cohen J, Powderly WG: *Infectious diseases,* ed 3, St Louis, 2010, Mosby; Folliculitis photo from Goldman L, Ausiello D: *Cecil medicine,* ed 24, Philadelphia, 2012, Saunders; Center photo and photos of food poisoning and endocarditis from Kumar V et al: *Robbins & Cotran pathologic basis of disease,* ed 8, Philadelphia, 2010, Saunders; Furuncle photo from Long S et al: *Principles and practice of pediatric infectious diseases,* ed 4, Philadelphia, 2012, Saunders; Scalded skin syndrome and pneumonia photos from Mandell G et al: *Principles and practice of infectious diseases,* ed 7, Philadelphia, 2010, Churchill Livingstone.)

BOX 10.2   **EXAMPLE OF BACTERIAL PATHOGENESIS: *STAPHYLOCOCCUS AUREUS*—cont'd**

causes the most common form of that potentially fatal disease. Exfoliative toxins are responsible for scalded skin syndrome in newborns.[4] These toxins are enzymes that digest the intercellular desmosomes that maintain the integrity of skin, causing separation of the epidermis. The skin peels off as would burned skin.

A battery of membrane-damaging toxins (hemolysins) mediates destruction of cells from outside (to protect against phagocytosis or open cellular barriers for invasion) or from inside (escape from phagocytic cells). *S. aureus* α-hemolysin (i.e., alpha-toxin) is a type II toxin that produces large pores in cell membranes, resulting in lysis of erythrocytes, breakdown of epithelial barriers, escape from a phagosome, and lysis of the macrophage plasma membrane, causing escape into the surrounding environment. Leukocidins are lytic toxins that bind to receptors on the cell surface and lyse most phagocytes. Although not yet fully understood, these leukocidins are expressed mostly by strains that cause necrotizing skin infections.

S. aureus additionally secretes a variety of enzymes that nonspecifically aid invasion and defend against the immune and inflammatory response. These include lipases, proteases (e.g., a neutral protease, collagenase), nucleases (e.g.,

DNase), catalases, coagulases (e.g., staphylocoagulase and von Willebrand factor that activate prothrombin and deposit small amounts of fibrin on the bacteria, preventing phagocytosis and contributing to formation of abscesses and biofilms), and staphylokinase (activates plasminogen to allow escape from fibrin clots).

References

1. Dunyach-Remy C, et al: Staphylococcus aureus toxins and diabetic foot ulcers: role in pathogenesis and interest in diagnosis. *Toxins (Basel)* 8(7):1–20, 2016.
2. Foster TJ: The remarkably multifunctional fibronectin binding proteins of Staphylococcus aureus. *Eur J Clin Microbiol Infect Dis* 35(12):1923–1931, 2016.
3. Kong C, Neoh H-M, Nathan S: Targeting Staphylococcus aureus toxins: a potential form of anti-virulence therapy. *Toxins (Basel)* 8(3):1–20, 2016.
4. Mishra AK, Yadav P, Mishra A: A systemic review on Staphylococcal scalded skin syndrome (SSSS): a rare and critical disease of neonates. *Open Microbiol J* 20(1):150–159, 2016.

TABLE 10.4   **COMMON PATHOGENIC FUNGI**

PRIMARY SITE OF INFECTION	FUNGUS	DISEASE (PRIMARY)	SYMPTOMS
Cutaneous (no tissue invasion, inflammatory response)	Dermatophytes	Tinea pedis (athlete's foot)	Scaling, fissures, itching
	Trichophyton mentagrophytes	Tinea cruris (jock itch)	Rash, itching
	Trichophyton rubrum	Tinea corporis (ringworm)	Lesion, raised border, scaling
	Candida albicans	Cutaneous candidiasis	Lesions in most areas of skin, mucous membranes, thrush, vaginal infection
Subcutaneous (tissue invasion)	*Sporothrix schenckii*	Sporotrichosis	Ulcers or abscesses on skin and other organ systems
Systemic (dimorphic; causes disease in healthy individuals)	*Stachybotrys chartarum* or "black mold"	Black mold disease	Rash, headaches, nausea, pains
	Coccidioides immitis	Coccidioidomycosis	Valley fever, flulike symptoms
	Histoplasma capsulatum	Histoplasmosis	Lung, flulike symptoms, disseminates to multiple organs, eye
	Blastomyces dermatitidis	Blastomycosis	Flulike symptoms, chest pains
Systemic (opportunistic)	*Aspergillus fumigatus*, *Aspergillus flavus*	Aspergillosis	Invasive to lungs and other organs
	Pneumocystis jiroveci	Pneumocystis pneumonia (PCP)	Pneumonia
	Cryptococcus neoformans	Cryptococcosis	Pneumonia-like illness, skin lesions, disseminates to brain, meningitis
	Candida albicans	Systemic candidiasis	Sepsis, endocarditis, meningitis

may grow as a mold with branched filaments or as a meshwork mycelium structure (e.g., *Aspergillus* spp., causing aspergillosis), yeast with ovoid or spherical shapes (*Candida albicans*, which causes candidiasis), or dimorphic with a yeastlike appearance in tissue and mycelium in culture (e.g., *Histoplasma capsulatum*, which causes histoplasmosis, a respiratory disease). Molds are aerobic and yeasts are facultative anaerobes. The cell wall is composed of polysaccharides that differ from the peptidoglycans of bacteria and are resistant to bacterial cell wall inhibitors, such as penicillin and cephalosporin. In contrast to bacteria, the cytosol of fungi contains organelles: mitochondria, Golgi apparatus, microtubules, microvesicles, endoplasmic reticulum, and nuclei. Many of the antifungal drugs (e.g., amphotericin B, ketoconazole, fluconazole) used to treat deep or systemic infections are toxic to the host because the

fungal cell composition is similar to that of the human cell. Common pathologic fungi are summarized in Table 10.4.

Infection with a fungus is called mycosis. Many pathogenic fungi (e.g., *H. capsulatum*, *Coccidioides immitis*, *Blastomyces dermatitidis*) grow as saprophytes in the environment and are transmitted by inhalation or contamination of wounds. Other medically relevant fungi either exist as human commensals or cause relatively mild infections (superficial mycoses) of the skin, nails, hair, and mucous membranes of the mouth and vagina. These include dermatophytes (e.g., tineas) and yeasts (e.g., *Candida*, *Aspergillus*, *Cryptococcus*).

Human-to-human transmission is the primary means of transmission of dermatophytes, for instance, *Tinea pedis* (athlete's foot), *T. capitis* (ringworm of scalp), and *T. unguium* (fungal infection of nails). Systemic

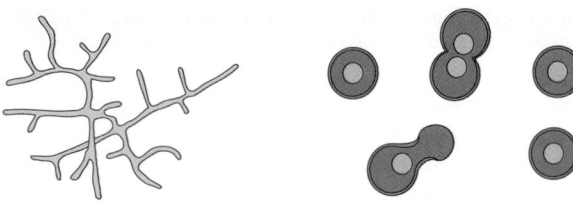

MOLDS
Filamentous fungi grow as multinucleate, branching hyphae, forming a mycelium (i.e., ringworm)

YEASTS
Yeasts grow as ovoid or spherical; single cells multiply by budding and division (i.e., *Histoplasma*)

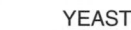

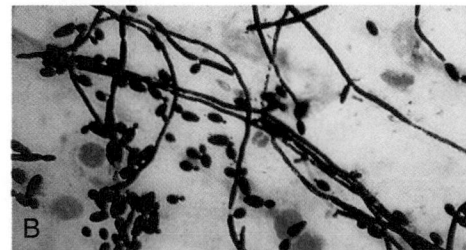

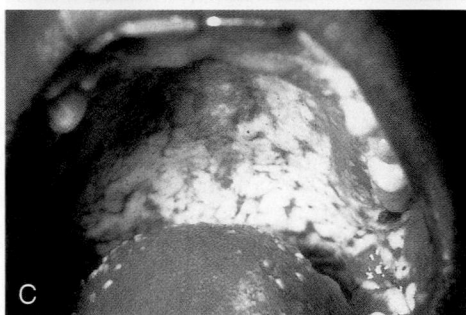

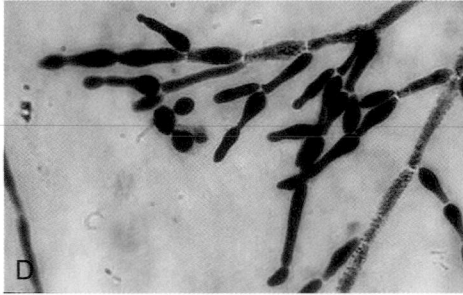

FIGURE 10.5 *Candida albicans* Morphology and Disease. **A,** Fungi may be either mold or yeast forms, or dimorphic. **B,** Photograph showing *Candida albicans* with both the mycelial and the yeast forms. **C,** Oral candidiasis (i.e., thrush). **D,** Gram stain of sputum showing that clinical isolates of *C. albicans* present as chains of elongated budding yeasts (×1000). (**A, B** from Goering R et al: *Mims' medical microbiology*, ed 5, London, 2013, Saunders; **C** from McPherson R, Pincus M: *Henry's clinical diagnosis and management by laboratory methods*, ed 22, Philadelphia, 2012, Saunders; **D** courtesy Dr. Stephen Raffanti.)

mycosis generally results from inhalation of spores present in a contaminated environment and initially presents as a pulmonary infection. Infection that disseminates to other organs can be life threatening. Systemic mycosis caused by opportunistic fungi is usually secondary to immunosuppression caused by genetic defects, infections such as HIV, cancer, and drugs used to prevent transplant rejection.

Fungi are diagnosed by microscopic observation of specimens treated with potassium hydroxide and stained to enhance visualization of spheres

and filaments. Specimens also can be cultured. Skin tests are available for species of *Aspergillus*.

Mechanisms of Fungal Invasion and Tissue Destruction. Specific adherence to the epithelium is provided by several polysaccharides on the fungal surface. Glucan, mannan, glycoprotein, and chitin molecules adhere with host receptors, including Toll-like receptors (TLRs), mannose receptors, and cadherins. A cell wall adhesion molecule, agglutinin-like sequence 3 (ALS3), on several fungi (e.g., *C. albicans*) promotes adherence to epithelial cells as well as silicone, thus facilitating infection of implants and other medical devices.

Pneumocystis jiroveci infection is a major concern in individuals with AIDS. As with many fungi, *Pneumocystis* has two life-cycle forms: a cyst form and a trophic form. The cyst form is dormant, more globular with a thick wall, and when ruptured releases multiple spores. The trophic form (trophozoite) is the infectious and proliferative form. Two surface proteins, glycoprotein A (gpA) and major surface glycoprotein (MSG), mediate attachment of the trophozoite to alveolar epithelial cells leading to the development of pneumonia.

Fungal Toxins and Products. Pathogenic fungi do not commonly produce toxins as virulence factors. The only identified peptide toxin related to virulence is a cytolytic toxin (candidalysin) that is crucial for *C. albicans* infection of mucosa.[17] A sulfur-containing mycotoxin that induces apoptosis of many cells of the inflammatory and immune system is produced by *A. fumigatus*. Several toxins secreted by molds in the environment cause disease without fungal infection. Mycotoxins are produced by molds that grown on nuts, beans, and grains. Ingestion of these toxins affects muscle coordination, causes tremors, and may be fatal. Other fungal toxins may cause cancer; aflatoxins produced by some *Aspergillus* are especially carcinogenic.

By mechanisms similar to those described for bacteria, fungal infections damage tissue directly by secretion of enzymes and indirectly by initiation of an inflammatory response. Secreted enzymes, such as proteases, phospholipases, and elastases, damage cells and intercellular matrix, leading to breakdown of tissue and cellular necrosis.

Destructive Immune and Inflammatory Responses to Fungal Infection. The typical immune and inflammatory reaction against fungal infections involves a cell-mediated response with infiltration of T cells, macrophages, and neutrophils. Fungal infections can be very difficult for these systems to eradicate, leading to progressively increasing production of proinflammatory cytokines. Hyperinflammatory responses enhance virulence of *A. fumigatus* by increasing adhesion and invasiveness. Thus as the host's response increases so do the destructive effects on surrounding healthy tissue. In cases of persistent infection, granulomas form and compromise the normal function of the infected tissue.

Pulmonary exposure to spores or soluble antigens also may elicit an IgE response and allergic pneumonitis (inflammation of the lungs). Examples include allergic bronchopulmonary aspergillosis and allergic fungal sinusitis, both of which are type I allergic reactions (see Chapter 9). Excessive degranulation of mast cells may even cause anaphylactic shock.

Fungal Evasion of Immune and Inflammatory Systems. The host defense against fungal infection includes the fungistatic properties of neutrophils and macrophages. T lymphocytes are crucial in limiting the extent of infection and producing cytokines to further activate macrophages.

Resistance to the individual's protective mechanisms is a complex process that requires the expression of multiple genes at different stages and different sites of infection. Pathologic fungi are generally dimorphic (e.g., *H. capsulatum, B. dermatitidis, C. immitis*) and readily adapt to the host environment, responding to temperature variations, low oxygen levels, more alkaline pH, and other conditions in the host tissue by undergoing changes in morphology and switching from avirulent mold forms to virulent yeast forms. Similar conditions also trigger yeasts (e.g., *C. albicans*) to switch from the yeast form to its more virulent hyphal form. As with parasites, rapid progression is not a major factor in immune evasion by fungi.

Fungal Protection Against Phagocytosis and Intracellular Destruction.
Encapsulated yeast cells (e.g., *Cryptococcus neoformans*) are more resistant to phagocytosis than unencapsulated yeast. A capsule is antiphagocytic by masking surface PAMPs (pathogen associated molecular patterns) and inhibiting recognition by PRRs (pattern recognition receptors) on phagocytes and epithelial cells (see Chapter 7).

Aspergillus fumigatus and many other fungi produce toxic metabolites (e.g., gliotoxin) that inhibit macrophage and neutrophil phagocytosis. Molecules like gliotoxin may suppress inflammation, including suppression of mast cell activation, degranulation, and secretion of leukotrienes and cytokines.

Even if successfully ingested by phagocytic cells, fungi have developed complex processes for intracellular survival. Pathologic fungi are generally dimorphic (e.g., *H. capsulatum, B. dermatitidis, C. immitis*) and readily adapt to the host environment, responding to temperature variations, low oxygen levels, more alkaline pH, and other conditions in the host tissue by undergoing changes in morphology and switching from avirulent mold forms to virulent yeast forms. The yeast form of *Histoplasma* replicates in phagosomes and phagolysosomes. Some yeasts also produce proteins that inhibit the activity of lysosomal proteases. The macrophage may be destroyed as a result of membrane modification by the fungus or, in the case of *Histoplasma*, may harbor the fungus in granulomas. Breakdown of the granulomas over time results in release of viable fungi and recurrence of the infection.

Blocking Recognition of Fungal Antigens. Altered antigen expression affords protection against the developing immune responses, although this defense strategy is used only by selected fungal pathogens. *Pneumocystis* contains approximately 80 different gpA and MSG genes, only 1 of which is expressed at a time. Modulation of these antigens provides resistance against immune destruction.

Blocking the Immune Response. Several yeasts stimulate the production of immunosuppressive cytokines, resulting in down-regulation of the individual's immune response. The yeast *C. neoformans* suppresses inflammation by inhibiting production of the proinflammatory cytokines TNF-α and IL-12 and inducing production of the antiinflammatory cytokine IL-10. The overall result is suppression of macrophage function and protection against killing.

Candida albicans is a common cause of infection reviewed in Box 10.3.

Infectious Parasites and Protozoans
Parasitic organisms establish symbiosis with another species in which the parasite benefits at the expense of the other species. Parasites range from unicellular protozoa to large worms. Parasitic worms (helminths) include intestinal and tissue nematodes (roundworms such as hookworms, pinworms, and ascariasis) and flatworms such as flukes (e.g.,

---

BOX 10.3 EXAMPLE OF FUNGAL PATHOGENESIS: *CANDIDA ALBICANS*

C. albicans is the most common cause of fungal infections in humans. It is an opportunistic microorganism that is a commensal in the normal microbiome of many healthy individuals, residing in the skin, gastrointestinal tract, mouth (in 30% to 55% of healthy individuals), and vagina (in 20% of healthy women), and is normally under the control of local defense mechanisms, including members of the bacterial microbiome that produce antifungal agents. In healthy individuals, infection remains localized to the dermis (e.g., diaper rash, thrush, mild vaginal yeast infection). In those whose normal microbiome has been disturbed by antibiotic therapy (e.g., resulting in diminished levels of *Lactobacillus* in the vaginal microbiome) *Candida* overgrowth may occur, resulting in more severe vaginitis or oropharyngeal infection.

In immunocompromised individuals, particularly those with diminished levels of neutrophils (neutropenia), disseminated infection may occur. *Candida* is the most common fungal infection in people with cancer (particularly acute leukemia and other hematologic cancers), transplantation (bone marrow and solid organ), and HIV/AIDS.

Invasive candidiasis may result from biofilms on materials that provide direct entrance into the blood (e.g., indwelling catheters, intravenous lines, peritoneal dialysis) and medical implants or other devices (e.g., pacemakers, prosthetic joints, dentures). More than 5 million central venous catheters are placed yearly. Most recipients are immunosuppressed secondary to their illness or therapy, and more than 50% develop biofilms resulting in about 100,000 deaths.[1] The strength of the biofilm results partially from strong intercellular adherence mediated by hyphal cells.

Like most pathogenic yeasts, *Candida* is dimorphic and undergoes morphologic changes from unicellular yeast to filamentous hyphal forms under conditions found in the environment (e.g., alkaline pH, elevated temperature, and changes in serum factors) or inside phagolysosomes (e.g., low pH, hydrolytic enzymes, antimicrobial peptides, and the presence of reactive oxygen species).

Candida expresses diverse surface adhesion molecules that permit adherence to materials in implants, epithelium, extracellular matrix, and formation of the biofilm and tissue invasion. *Candida* can colonize a variety of sites in the individual, apparently the result of adhesins that have broad specificity.[2]

The biofilm also contains a very complex extracellular matrix with fungal enzymes and other components that provide extensive resistance to the immune response, antibiotics, and environmental changes that could damage the fungus. Individuals must be treated with very high doses of antifungal antibiotics with potential toxicity to the kidneys and liver. Antibiotic resistance increases, however, as *Candida* up-regulates expression of efflux pumps that are the primary means of antibiotic resistance (see the section on Antimicrobials).

Adaptation to the environment also results in altered profiles of surface antigens and surface carbohydrates that are identified as pathogen-associated molecular patterns (PAMPs) and a resultant increased resistance to destruction by innate and acquired immunity. Immune suppression may occur secondary to induction of the cytokine granulocyte-monocyte colony-stimulating factor (GM-CSF) that suppresses monocyte/macrophage function, including antigen presentation and production of components of the complement cascade. Decreased production of C3 results in less opsonization (C3b) and production of chemotactic activity (C3a) for phagocytes.

Disseminated candidiasis may involve several internal organs, including abscesses in the kidney, brain, liver, and heart, and is characterized by persistent or recurrent fever, gram-negative shocklike symptoms (hypotension, tachycardia), disseminated intravascular coagulation (DIC), and death. The mortality rates of sepsis or disseminated candidiasis are in the range of 30% to 40%. *Candida* secretes several enzymes that function as virulence factors and contribute to spread and tissue destruction.

References
1. Nobile CJ, Johnson AD: Candida albicans biofilms and human disease. *Annu Rev Microbiol* 69:71–92, 2015.
2. Cota E, Hoyer LL: The Candida albicans agglutinin-like sequence family of adhesins: functional insights gained from structural analysis. *Future Microbiol* 10(10):1635–1648, 2015.

TABLE 10.5   PARASITES THAT ARE IMPORTANT IN HUMANS

CATEGORY	SUBGROUP	SPECIES	DISEASE	ORGANS AFFECTED/SYMPTOMS
Protozoa	Amoeboid	*Entamoeba histolytica*	Amebiasis	Dysentery, liver abscess
	Flagellate	*Giardia lamblia*	Giardiasis*	Diarrhea
		Leishmania donovani, L. tropica	Leishmaniasis	Sores on skin, progression to liver, spleen
		Trichomonas vaginalis	Trichomoniasis	Inflammation of reproductive organs
		Trypanosoma cruzi, T. brucei	Chagas disease: African sleeping sickness	Generalized, blood, lymph nodes, progressing to cardiac and central nervous system (CNS)
	Ciliate	*Balantidium coli*	Balantidiasis	Small intestines, invasion of colon, diarrhea
	Sporozoa (nonmotile)	*Cryptosporidium parvum, C. hominis*	Cryptosporidiosis*	Intestine, diarrhea
		Plasmodium spp.	Malaria	Blood, liver
		Toxoplasma gondii	Toxoplasmosis*	Intestine, eyes, blood, heart, liver
Helminths	Flukes (trematodes)	*Fasciola hepatica*	Fasciolosis	Liver destruction
		Paragonimus westermani	Lung fluke disease	Granuloma in lung, spinal cord
		Schistosoma mansoni	Schistosomiasis	Blood, diarrhea, bladder, generalized symptoms
	Tapeworms (cestodes)	*Taenia solium*	Pork tapeworm	Encysts in muscle, brain, liver
	Roundworms (nematodes)	*Ascaris lumbricoides*	Ascariasis	Intestinal obstruction, bile duct obstruction
		Necator americanus (hookworm)	Hookworm disease	Intestinal parasite
		Trichuris trichiura (whipworm)	Trichuriasis	Diarrhea
		Trichinella spiralis	Trichinosis*	Intestine, diarrhea, muscle, CNS, death
		Wuchereria bancrofti	Filariasis, elephantiasis	Lymphatics
		Enterobius vermicularis (pinworm)	Pinworm infection	Intestines
		Strongyloides stercoralis (threadworm)	Strongyloidiasis	Intestinal parasite, skin infection
		Onchocerca volvulus	Onchocerciasis	Blindness, dermatitis

*Most common in the United States.

liver fluke, lung fluke, blood fluke) and tapeworms. A protozoan is a eukaryotic, unicellular microorganism with a nucleus and cytoplasm. Pathogenic protozoa primarily include sporozoa (e.g., *Plasmodium*, which causes malaria, and *Cryptosporidium*, which causes diarrhea), amoebae (e.g., *Entamoeba histolytica*, which causes amoebic dysentery), and flagellates (e.g., *Giardia lamblia*, which causes diarrhea, *Trypanosoma*, which causes sleeping sickness, and *Leishmania*, which causes skin ulcers and a visceral form that infects the spleen and liver). The most common parasitic infections in the United States include *Toxoplasma gondii* (a lifelong infection that may cause of blindness and miscarriage) and *Trichomonas vaginalis* (a common STI). Parasites are common causes of infections worldwide, with a significant effect on mortality and morbidity in developing countries. Important parasites of humans are listed in Table 10.5.

Mechanisms of Parasite Invasion and Tissue Destruction

Parasite Invasion. Parasite invasion of tissue can be broadly characterized as by extracellular or intracellular mechanisms. There is considerable variation within both mechanisms because of complex life cycles, means of transmission, and unique adaptations among parasites. A common component of invasion is adherence to and breakdown of connective tissue and basement membranes.

Helminths may infect the gastrointestinal tract or enter through the skin. An example is *Schistosoma mansoni*, a blood fluke infection where the aquatic larval form attaches to and penetrates the skin using a family of proteases that degrade elastin and other skin components. After entering the circulatory system, the parasite may burrow into other organs.

Extracellular parasites enter through the gastrointestinal tract (e.g., *Entamoeba histolytica, Giardia lamblia*), the vagina as STIs (*Trichomonas vaginalis*), or through the skin in bites (*Trypanosoma brucei*). After

attachment to the lining of the gastrointestinal tract or vagina, extracellular parasites undergo evolution to more invasive forms.

Most intracellular protozoan parasites can only reproduce within host cells and are therefore obligatory intracellular parasites. These include *Leishmania* spp. (leishmaniasis causing ulcers of skin and internal organs), *Toxoplasma gondii* (toxoplasmosis with possible latent infection of the brain and eye), *Cryptosporidium parvum* (cryptosporidiosis causing watery diarrhea), and *Plasmodium* spp. (malaria). Infections are obtained by ingestion of contaminated food or water or through bites from insect vectors. Invasion is mediated by adhesion to lectins on cells near the site of infection and invasion of the tissue using a host of proteases and other enzymes. Very soon these protozoa invade cells (i.e., fibroblasts, mesenchymal cells) or undergo phagocytosis (i.e., macrophages) where reproduction occurs resulting in progressive cell lysis and spread to neighboring cells.

Toxins and Parasite Products. Toxins are not as prevalent in the pathogenesis of parasitic diseases as in bacterial diseases. *C. parvum* produces hemolysin H4, which is very similar to *E. coli* O157:H7 and disrupts cell membranes. *E. histolytica* produces a small-molecular weight pore-forming toxin (amoebapore) that inserts pores into the membrane of intestinal cells resulting in increased calcium influx, efflux of water, and diarrhea. Endotoxin is normally associated with gram-negative bacteria, but similar molecules are produced by African trypanosomes and *Plasmodium falciparum* (most severe form of malaria).

Most of the tissue damage caused by parasites is secondary to the release of enzymes such as proteases and phospholipases. These enzymes help invasion by destroying surrounding extracellular matrix and tissue.

Destructive Immune and Inflammatory Responses to Parasite Infection. Because of their size, tissue damage caused by large multicellular parasites is generally a direct result of parasitic accumulation in the tissue or secondary to the individual's immune and inflammatory responses. Large infestations may lead to physical loss of function in a tissue or organ. For instance, a large number of intestinal parasites (e.g., the roundworm *Ascaris lumbricoides,* tapeworms, and *Giardia* spp.) compete for and prevent uptake of nutrients, leading to various forms of malabsorption, blocked uptake of fats, or anemia from malabsorption of B$_{12}$, or from large amounts of blood loss. Some roundworms (e.g., *Wuchereria bancrofti* and *Brugia malayi*) block the lymphatics and cause accumulation of large amounts of lymph in tissues (i.e., elephantiasis). The larvae of tapeworms (e.g., *Taenia solium*) encyst in and prevent normal function of organs (e.g., muscle, liver, eye), which is particularly dangerous in the human brain.

Parasitic infections may also damage tissue through exacerbated inflammation or initiation of immune hypersensitivity reactions. *C. parvum* induces considerable release of proinflammatory cytokines from epithelial cells, inducing influx of inflammatory cells and increased tissue destruction. Ascaris larvae migrate to bronchi causing pulmonary inflammation. IgE-mediated anaphylactic responses have been observed associated with infections with helminths and African trypanosomes. Helminth parasites (e.g., schistosomiasis) may deposit eggs in organs (e.g., the liver) leading to a chronic cell-mediated response and persistent production of proinflammatory cytokines with formation of granulomas. Rapid progression is not used as a protective mechanism for parasites.

Parasite Protection Against Phagocytosis and Intracellular Destruction.
Several parasites (*Leishmania* spp.) are obligative intracellular organisms of monocytes and macrophages. *Leishmania* uses components of the complement system for entrance into macrophages. Once in the macrophage, several mechanisms are used to facilitate survival of parasites. *T. gondii* produces toxins that prevent phagosome-lysosome fusion so that the environment in the phagosome remains relatively nontoxic. *E. histolytica* (amoebiasis) releases phospholipase and pore-forming proteins that disrupt the phagocyte's plasma membrane. *T. cruzi* (Chagas disease, sleeping sickness) escapes from the phagosome and grows in the macrophage cytoplasm. *Leishmania* reproduces within phagocytic cells and inhibits respiratory burst and chemotaxis.

Blocking Recognition of Parasitic Antigens. Pathogens that coat themselves with human proteins may be disguised and "fool" the immune system. For instance, schistosomes and trypanosomes mask their antigens by absorbing IgG by the Fc portion of the molecule.

Much more commonly, those pathogens that undergo part of their life cycle in humans, or may assume multiple morphologic forms during infection, also will undergo antigenic changes related to the stage in the life cycle or morphology. Some protozoa have developed very complex alterations in surface antigens using gene switching. For example, African trypanosomes, carried by tsetse flies, can vary the structure of their antigenic coat (variant surface glycoproteins) using gene switching thus allowing them to be protected from immune defenses. Newly produced antibodies will not recognize the variant antigen coat allowing the trypanosome to survive.

Parasite Blocking of the Immune Response. Parasites use an array of mechanisms to block protective immune responses including: (1) secretion of enzymes that degrade immunoglobulins (schistosomes); (2) inactivation of complement (e.g. *Echinococcus* spp., *Leishmania* spp. and trypansomes); (3) prevention of antigen processing by macrophages (*Leishmania*); (4) inhibition of complement mediated phagocyte chemotaxis (*E. hisolytica*); and (5) inhibition of T-cell function (schistosomes). These responses may be pathogen specific or non-specific.

Malaria, a plasmodium parasite, has been very successful at mounting immune defenses and is a significant cause of morbidity and mortality throughout the world. Details related to malaria are presented in Box 10.4.

Infectious Viruses

Viruses are extremely simple microorganisms and do not possess any of the metabolic organelles found in prokaryotes (e.g., bacteria) or eukaryotes (e.g., human cells). The basic viral structure (virion) consists of nucleic acid protected by a protein shell, the capsid. The capsid may take many characteristic shapes: helical, icosahedral, or large pleomorphic (Fig. 10.6). Some viruses also have the capsid surrounded by a protective envelope, which consists of the plasma membrane from the previously infected cell.

Viruses are classified by the format of nucleic acid in the virion, which may be RNA or DNA and either single-stranded (ss) or double-stranded (ds), and by whether the virus uses the enzyme reverse transcriptase (RT) for replication. Thus seven classifications are used: dsDNA (e.g., herpesvirus, smallpox virus), ssDNA (parvovirus), dsRNA (rotavirus), ssRNA +sense (+sense functions as mRNA) (e.g., hepatitis A and C viruses, SARS virus, poliovirus, rhinovirus), ssRNA −sense (e.g., Ebola virus, Marburg virus, influenza virus, hantavirus, Lassa virus, and viruses that cause measles, mumps, and rabies), ssRNA +sense with RT (e.g., HIV), and dsDNA with RT (e.g., hepatitis B virus).

Viral diseases are the most common afflictions of humans. Examples of human diseases caused by specific viruses are listed in Table 10.6.

Mechanisms of Invasion and Tissue Destruction

Viral Invasion. Viral pathogens directly destroy or damage cells as part of their replication in infected cells. Viruses are obligatory

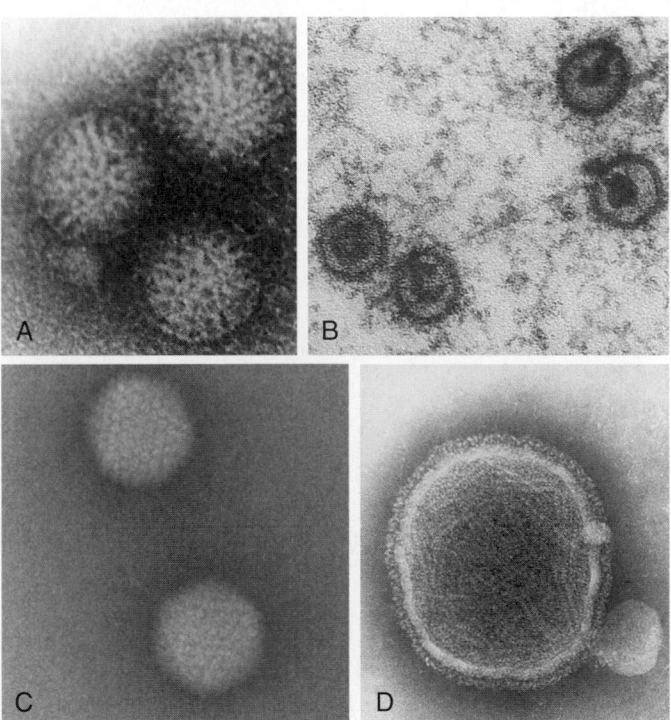

FIGURE 10.6 Electron Micrographs of Representative Viral Structures. A, Rotavirus: particles with a double shell and a characteristic "wheel-and-spoke" appearance. **B,** Epstein-Barr virus: icosahedral enveloped DNA virus. **C,** Adenovirus: particles with characteristic icosahedral structures. **D,** Paramyxovirus: spherical enveloped RNA virus. RNA is seen spilling out of the disrupted virus. (**A** from Long S, Pickering L, Prober C: *Principles and practice of pediatric infectious diseases,* ed 3, Philadelphia, 2005, Saunders; **B** and **D** photos courtesy Science Source; © Photo Researchers, Inc., New York, NY; **C** from Mandell GL, Bennett JE, Dolin R: *Mandell, Douglas, and Bennett's principles and practice of infectious diseases,* ed 7, Philadelphia, 2010, Churchill Livingstone.)

BOX 10.4 PARASITIC PATHOGENESIS: *PLASMODIUM* AND *MALARIA*

Malaria is one of the most common debilitating infections worldwide. The WHO estimated that in 2015 there were 214 million new cases of malaria worldwide and more than 400,000 malaria-related deaths, more than 90% occurring in Africa, and most of whom were children.[1] Malaria is caused by five species of *Plasmodium* parasites that infect humans (*P. falciparum, P. vivax, P. ovale, P. malariae, P. knowlesi* [a simian parasite that causes human malaria primarily in Malaysia]), although two species account for the most cases and deaths.[2] *Plasmodium falciparum* is the most prevalent in Africa and accounts for most fatalities. Infection results in severe chills, high fever, sweating, headache, muscle pains, vomiting, severe anemia, and pulmonary edema. Neurologic complications may result from infected red blood cells (RBCs) adhering to endothelium in capillaries of the brain causing hypoxia and degradation of neural tissue.[3] The most severely affected individuals may develop cardiovascular collapse, shock, coma, and death. *P. vivax* is the primary cause of malaria outside of Africa. Symptoms are severe flulike in nature and with less morbidity and mortality than observed with *P. falciparum*. All forms of malaria are characterized by paroxysm (cyclic chills followed by fever). Cycles range from every 2 days for *P. vivax* to 36 hours for *P. falciparum*.

The life cycle of *Plasmodium* requires two hosts: mosquito and human. The parasite undergoes a sexual reproductive cycle in the salivary gland of the female *Anopheles* mosquito and is transmitted to humans during a blood meal. The infectious form (sporozoite) enters the tissue and migrates to the bloodstream. The sporozoite has the capacity to traverse through cells in the tissue, mediated by a variety of parasitic proteins that bind to specific substance on the cell surface and facilitate entry.[4]

The parasite enters hepatocytes using sporozoite proteins that bind to sulfated molecules on endothelial cells and Kupffer cells. Protection against malaria may occur by means of stage-specific immune responses against different phases of the life cycle: invasive stage, hepatic stage, pre-erythrocyte stage, erythrocyte stage, and sexual stages. Phagocytic cells, like Kupffer cells, are the primary means of protection against the prehepatic invasive stage and hepatic stage. Traversal of phagocytic cells results in modulation of the cell's cytokine profile, causing downregulation of proinflammatory cytokines (e.g., IL-6, TNF-α) and upregulation of antiinflammatory cytokines (e.g., IL-10), blocked production of reactive oxygen species, and reduced expression of class I MHC to suppress antigen presentation.[5] The parasite in the blood avoids destruction by phagocytes in the spleen by expressing adhesion proteins that cause adherence and sequestration along the walls of the small vessels.

Sequestration in the liver begins an asymptomatic stage during which several rounds of multiplication occur. *P. vivax* and *P. ovale* can remain dormant in the liver for years, protected from the immune system by intracellular residence. In the hepatocytes, the parasites transform to the merozoite form, thousands of which are released into the blood during hepatocyte rupture and infect erythrocytes.

The blood-borne phase and infection of erythrocytes begin the symptomatic stage of the disease (see Figure). *P. falciparum* uses a variety of parasite surface proteins (e.g., merozoite surface protein-1 [MSP-1]) for adhesion to erythrocyte membrane glycophorins and entrance into the cell.[6] *P. vivax* seems to use the erythrocyte Duffy antigen for adhesion. Thus individuals who are negative for the Duffy blood group antigen are naturally resistant to *P. vivax* malaria.

Symptoms of malaria occur after an approximate 2-week period from the initial mosquito bite and are the result of asexual multiplication in the erythrocytes and cell lysis upon the release of daughter parasites that reinfect other erythrocytes. During this erythrocytic cycle, the merozoites mature into male and female gametocytes within the erythrocyte, which after another blood meal can establish another cycle of further sexual multiplication in the mosquito vector. The erythrocytic cycle will resolve, but many relapses will occur upon new cycles of merozoite release from infected hepatocytes.

During the erythrocytic cycle, the infected individual produces protective antibodies against antigens expressed on the surface of infected erythrocytes. *Plasmodium* expresses several families of antigens on the erythrocyte's surface and uses antigen variation through gene switching diversity to mitigate the effects of antibody.

Other antigen-directed responses contribute to protection of the parasite. Antibodies against *P. falciparum* asparagine-rich protein enhance merozoite invasion of erythrocytes, which is further facilitated by the addition of complement. The *Pf*EMP1 antigen also can protect the infected erythrocyte by epitope masking. The antigen contains Fc binding sites where IgM antibody, regardless of specificity, is bound by its Fc region, thus masking the *Pf*EMP1 epitopes. Parasites also can bind complement regulator factor, factor H, which protects the parasite from damage by activated complement factors.

Malarial infection also may induce immune suppression by inhibiting macrophage and dendritic cell phagocytosis, as well as inducing apoptosis of antigen-presenting cells. Phagocytic cell function is diminished by a malarial pigment (hemozoin), which is taken up and reduces the ability to phagocytize merozoites or infected erythrocytes. Numbers of CD4 and CD8 T-cells are diminished by apoptosis combined with induction of immunosuppressive Treg cells.

Malarial parasites have developed broad drug resistance including against chloroquine, the previous mainstay of the preventive and therapeutic arsenal of antimalarial drugs. Drug resistance appears to result from increased activity of drug transporters that eliminate the drugs from the parasitic microorganism.

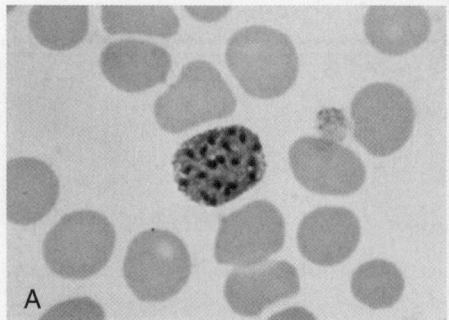
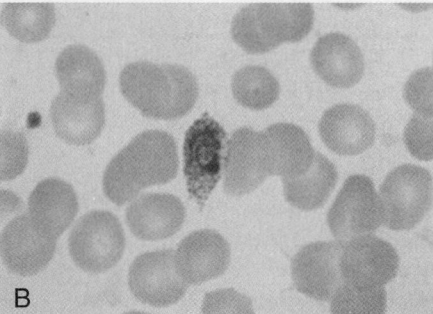
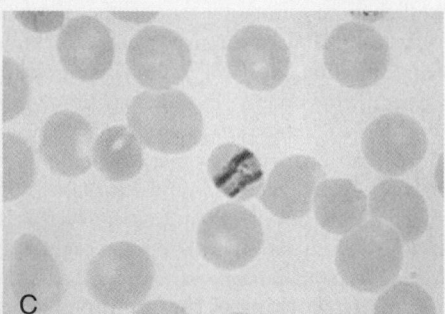

FIGURE Malaria Giemsa-stained smears. **A,** *Plasmodium vivax* schizont. **B,** *Plasmodium ovale* trophozoite. **C,** Characteristic band from trophozoite of *Plasmodium malariae* containing intracellular pigment hemozoin. (From Kliegman R et al: *Nelson textbook of pediatrics*, ed 19, St Louis, 2011, Saunders.)

References

1. World Health Organization (WHO): Eliminating malaria, Geneva, Switzerland, 2016, Author, pp 1–24. http://apps.who.int/iris/bitstream/10665/205565/1/WHO_HTM_GMP_2016.3_eng.pdf.
2. Cowman AF, et al: Malaria: biology and disease. *Cell* 167(3):610–624, 2016.
3. Wah ST, et al: Molecular basis of human cerebral malaria development. *Trop Med Health* 44(33):1–7, 2016.
4. Yang ASP, Boddey JA: Molecular mechanisms of host cell traversal by malaria sporozoites. *Int J Parasitol* 47(2-3):129–136, 2017.
5. Gomes PS, et al: Immune escape strategies of malaria parasites. *Front Microbiol* 7(1617):1–7, 2016.
6. Satchwell TJ: Erythrocyte invasion receptors for Plasmodium falciparum: new and old. *Transfus Med* 26(2):77–88, 2016.

TABLE 10.6 HUMAN DISEASES CAUSED BY SPECIFIC VIRUSES

BALTIMORE CLASSIFICATION	FAMILY	VIRUS	ENVELOPE	MAIN ROUTE OF TRANSMISSION	DISEASE
dsDNA	Adenoviruses	Adenovirus	No	Droplet contact	Acute febrile pharyngitis
	Herpesviruses	HSV-1	Yes	Direct contact with saliva or lesions	Lesions in mouth, pharynx, conjunctivitis
		HSV-2	Yes	Sexually, contact with lesions during birth	Sores on labia, meningitis in children
		HSV-8	Yes	Saliva and genital body fluids	Kaposi sarcoma
		Epstein-Barr virus (EBV), HSV-4	Yes	Saliva	Mononucleosis, Burkitt lymphoma
		Cytomegalovirus (CMV), HSV-5	Yes	Body fluids, mother's milk, transplacental	Mononucleosis, congenital infection
		Varicella-zoster virus (VZV)	Yes	Droplet contact	Chickenpox, shingles
ssDNA	Papovaviruses	Papillomavirus	No	Direct contact	Warts, cervical carcinoma
dsRNA	Reoviruses	Rotavirus	No	Fecal-oral	Severe diarrhea
ssRNA+	Picornaviruses	Coxsackievirus	No	Fecal-oral, droplet contact	Nonspecific febrile illness, conjunctivitis, meningitis
		Hepatitis A virus	No	Fecal-oral	Acute hepatitis
		Poliovirus	No	Fecal-oral	Poliomyelitis
		Rhinovirus	No	Droplet contact	Common cold
	Flaviviruses	Hepatitis C virus	Yes	Blood, sexually	Acute or chronic hepatitis, hepatocellular carcinoma
		Yellow fever virus	Yes	Mosquito vector	Yellow fever
		Dengue virus	Yes	Mosquito vector	Dengue fever
		West Nile virus	Yes	Mosquito vector	Meningitis, encephalitis
	Togaviruses	Rubella virus	Yes	Droplet contact, transplacental	Acute or congenital rubella
	Coronaviruses	SARS	Yes	Droplets in aerosol or direct contact	Severe respiratory disease
	Caliciviruses	Norovirus	No	Fecal-oral	Gastroenteritis
ssRNA−	Orthomyxoviruses	Influenza virus	Yes	Droplet contact	Influenza
	Paramyxoviruses	Measles virus	Yes	Droplet contact	Measles
		Mumps virus	Yes	Droplet contact	Mumps
		Parainfluenza virus	Yes	Droplet contact	Croup, pneumonia, common cold
		Respiratory syncytial virus (RSV)	Yes	Droplet contact, hand-to-mouth	Pneumonia, influenza-like syndrome
	Rhabdoviruses	Rabies virus	Yes	Animal bite, droplet contact	Rabies
	Bunyaviruses	Hantavirus	Yes	Aerosolized animal fecal material	Viral hemorrhagic fever
	Filoviruses	Ebola virus	Yes	Direct contact with body fluids	Viral hemorrhagic fever
		Marburg virus	Yes	Direct contact with body fluids	Viral hemorrhagic fever
	Arenavirus	Lassa virus	Yes	Aerosolized animal fecal material	Viral hemorrhagic fever
ssRNA+ with RT	Retroviruses	HIV	Yes	Sexually, blood products	AIDS
dsDNA with RT	Hepadnaviruses	Hepatitis B virus	Yes	All body fluids	Acute or chronic hepatitis, hepatocellular carcinoma

AIDS, Acquired immunodeficiency syndrome; *DNA,* deoxyribonucleic acid; *ds,* double-stranded; *HIV,* human immunodeficiency virus; *HSV,* herpes simplex virus; *RNA,* ribonucleic acid; *RT,* reverse transcriptase; *SARS,* severe acute respiratory syndrome; *ss,* single-stranded.

intracellular microorganisms; thus transmission is frequently from one infected cell to an uninfected cell. The viral life cycle involves several steps: *attachment* to the target cell (determines host range and tropism), *penetration* (by endocytosis or membrane fusion), *uncoating* (release of viral nucleic acid from the viral capsid by viral or host enzymes), replication (synthesis of viral proteins and mRNA), *assembly* (formation of new virions), and *release* (by lysis or budding).

Attachment involves specific interactions between surface proteins on the virus and receptors on the cell to be infected. The specificity of the virus for these receptors and the distribution of receptors throughout the individual's tissues dictate the range of host cells that a particular virus can infect. An example is epstein-Barr virus (EBV, which causes mononucleosis) binds to complement receptor 2 (CR2) on B lymphocytes. Once bound, the virion penetrates the plasma membrane by envelope fusion with cellular membranes or receptor-mediated endocytosis (Fig. 10.7).

Most RNA viruses directly produce mRNA, which is translated into viral proteins, and genomic RNA, which is eventually packaged into

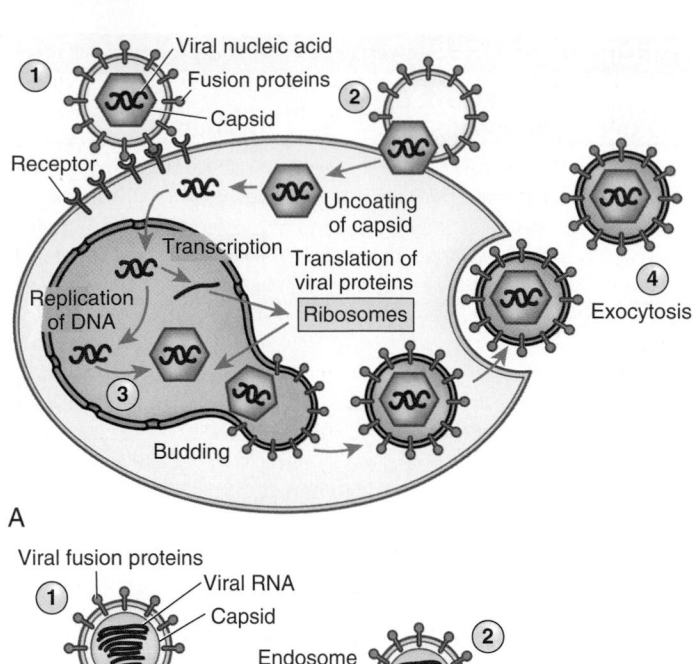

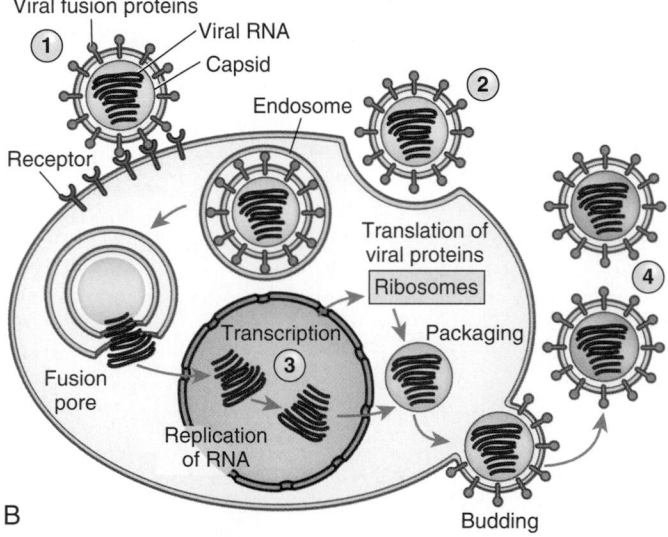

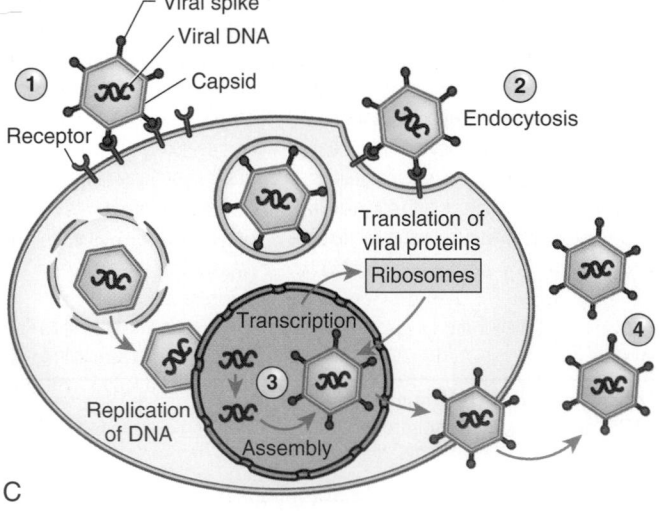

FIGURE 10.7 Stages of Viral Entrance during Infection of a Cell. The viral life cycle includes **1,** attachment; **2,** uncoating; **3,** replication; and **4,** release. Viral entrance into a cell is by one of three mechanisms. **A,** Some enveloped viruses (e.g., HIV) express fusion proteins that **(1)** bind to receptors on the target cell and **(2)** mediate membrane fusion and release of the viral nucleocapsid directly into the cytoplasm. **(3)** Within the cytoplasm the virus uncoats the protective nucleocapsid and releases viral nucleic acid and **(4)** release by exocytosis. **B,** Other enveloped viruses (e.g., influenza virus) **(1)** bind to receptors that trigger **(2)** receptor-mediated endocytosis of the virion particle. **(3)** The endosome fuses with lysosomes. The relative acidic conditions in the endosome trigger membrane fusion, formation of fusion pores, breakdown of the capsid, and **(4)** release of viral nucleic acid into the cytoplasm. **C,** Viral particles without an envelope (e.g., poliovirus) **(1)** express viral spikes that bind to the cell membrane and **(2)** initiate receptor-mediated endocytosis of the viral particle. **(3)** The acidic conditions in the endosome cause capsid breakdown and formation of pores in the endosomal membrane through which viral nucleic acid enters the cytoplasm and **(4)** release of virus.

new viruses. DNA viruses are transcribed in the nucleus into mRNA before protein translation in the cytoplasm. Some viruses can enter a period of latency during which production of a new virus ceases with concurrent resolution of disease symptoms. One particular family of viruses, retroviruses (e.g., HIV), carries the enzyme *reverse transcriptase* that creates a double-stranded DNA provirus that integrates into the host cell's chromosomal DNA, and may be transmitted to the daughter cells during mitosis. By this process, viral genes can become part of the genetic information of the cell and its progeny. Insertion into the DNA is random. If viral DNA is inserted at a nonessential site the cell may be unaffected, if into an essential gene the cell may undergo death, and if insertion modifies genes related to normal growth the cell may be transformed (become cancerous). Episomal latency is associated with viral genes outside the cell DNA *(episome),* in a linear or circular conformation, either in the cytoplasm or in the nucleus. Episomal latency is characteristic of herpesviruses (e.g., HSV-1 and 2, EBV). Latency must be actively maintained by *latency-associated transcript (LAT)* genes that inhibit apoptosis. The infected cell will remain functional, and the virus will remain dormant until activated. HSV1 (herpes simplex) is latent as a circular double-stranded DNA in the nuclei of peripheral neurons and may be reactivated to a lytic cycle in response to stress, sunlight, diet, or other events.[20] Reactivation results in shedding of virions from nerves into the mucosa of the mouth or genitals.

At the end of the replicate phase, new virus particles are released from the cell for transmission of the viral infection to neighboring uninfected cells. The method of release depends on the particular virus. Enveloped viruses are released through *budding,* in which shed viral particles are enveloped in the plasma membrane from the surface of the infected cell. Viral envelope proteins are inserted into the membrane and cluster at sites of budding. Translation of viral-specific mRNA produces capsid and matrix proteins that assemble and incorporate viral nucleic acid. Budding is not immediately destructive to the cell, whereas nonenveloped viruses are commonly released in large numbers concurrent with the destruction of the cell. Some viruses induce a progressive apoptosis during which virions are packaged in apoptotic vesicles. The vesicles are portions of the plasma membrane released from the dying cell. Vesicles will break down and release virions into the surrounding environment. Apoptotic vesicles also may undergo phagocytosis by macrophages and establish infections (e.g., HIV) in the macrophage. Other viruses are released by exocytosis, during which the cell may not be destroyed. New viral particles in the cytoplasm are packaged in vesicles, transported to the cell surface, and released. This process is generally used by nonenvelope viruses.

Toxins and Viral Products. Generally, viruses rarely produce toxins or other destructive products that cause tissue damage. The products of viral genes are directed toward adherence to target cells, providing components of the reproductive cycle, and evasion of immune and inflammatory responses. Some products that are important to the viral life cycle may therefore indirectly lead to cellular destruction. An exception to the rarity of viral toxins is the rotavirus nonstructural protein (NSP4). NSP4 is an enterotoxin that affects intracellular calcium levels in intestinal cells resulting in water efflux and diarrhea, particularly in infants and children.

Destructive Immune and Inflammatory Responses to Viral Infection.
Most of the symptoms of viral infection (e.g., fever, aches, nausea) are generally mild, caused by the individual's own inflammatory response to infection, and usually resolve in a relatively short time. More severe local cellular effects may result from destruction of infected cells by lymphocytes. The dermal and ocular lesions of HSV infection result from T-cell mediated cytotoxicity of infected epithelial cells. A Th2 cell response is primarily responsible for severe respiratory syncytial virus related lesions in the lower respiratory tract (see Chapter 8). Many viruses induce excessive production of proinflammatory cytokines (e.g., IL-1, IL-2, IL-6, and many more), mediators (e.g., prostaglandins, histamines), and reactive oxygen species, all of which contribute to tissue damage.

Hepatitis viruses provoke immune and inflammatory responses that may damage infected and noninfected hepatic cells. Hepatitis A (HAV) and hepatitis B (HBV) viruses may cause acute liver damage, whereas hepatitis C (HCV) virus infection is usually subclinical with no apparent liver damage. The degree of T cell infiltration of the liver is related to the degree of liver pathology. CD8-positive T-cytotoxic cells attack and destroy virus-infected liver cells (see Chapter 8). HBV and HCV activate Th17 cells that contribute to inflammation of the liver. Individuals with high amounts of circulating viral antigen (e.g., hepatitis B) are at risk for developing symptoms of type III hypersensitivity reactions including kidney disease and vascular inflammation (see Chapter 9).

Viral Evasion of Immune and Inflammatory Systems
Rapid Progression of Viruses. Some viruses, particularly those with small genomes, rapidly proliferate after the initial infection and produce a large number of virions more quickly than the immune system can develop. By the development of an effective adaptive immune response in 4 or 5 days, the virus has spread and caused severe clinical disease.

Viral Protection Against Phagocytosis and Intracellular Destruction.
Viruses are the prime examples of intercellular survival. As obligatory intracellular pathogens, viruses hide and proliferate within cells and away from normal inflammatory or immune responses. Viral particles that spread through the blood to infect other cells encounter antibodies, which in most cases cure the infection. Thus most viral infections are self-limiting.

Interferons are particularly effective against many viral infections, and viral survival mechanisms have evolved to mitigate these effects.

A great many viruses have developed methods of blocking every step of type I interferon cascade, thus preventing production of IFN1 by infected cells and induction of antiviral substances in neighboring cells.

Viruses encounter intracellular PRRs designed to bind viral substances and initiate protective innate responses (discussed in Chapter 7). Successful viral pathogens have developed mechanisms to either block TLR recognition of viral substances or prevent TLR signaling.

Blocking Recognition of Viral Antigens. Enveloped viruses are excellent examples of how this mechanism may succeed. The viral capsid is completely surrounded by a cellular plasma membrane that is highly similar to that of an uninfected cell. Only a few critical differences

exist. In order to infect another cell, the virion expresses membrane-associated viral envelope proteins that are critical for the intercellular fusion process. These proteins are virus-specific and targets for protective immune responses. Other viruses, such as the HCV, coat themselves with normal proteins from the infected host, such as lipoproteins, that mask the viral epitopes from circulating antibody.

Some viruses (e.g., HIV) increase antigenic diversity by incorporating frequent functional translational errors. Viral enzymes can create small errors in reading mRNA leading to minor changes in the viral proteins. These changes are not at functionally critical sites but may provide resistance to specific and nonspecific defense mechanisms. In a manner similar to bacteria, other viruses have multiple stable antigenic serotypes. A person who recovers from an infection with one serotype may not have protective immunity against other serotypes of the same virus. At least 100 different serotypes of rhinovirus can cause the "common cold," which explains why individuals can catch many colds throughout their lives.

Blocking the Immune Response to Viral Infection. HIV and other viruses have developed the capacity to infect and kill immune cells, thus protecting themselves but also leading to a broad immunosuppression against other antigens. This process is discussed more thoroughly in the section on AIDS.

Some viruses have developed mechanisms for interfering with antigen processing and presentation by major histocompatibility complex (MHC) class I molecules. Endogenous antigens, such as viral antigens, are normally degraded by proteasomes, transported into the endoplasmic reticulum, and complexed with MHC class I molecules for expression on the cell surface and presentation to appropriate cells of the immune response (see Chapter 8). Many of the herpesviruses and retroviruses prevent steps in this process. For instance, EBV inhibits degradation by the proteasomes. HSV can prevent binding of the antigenic peptide to MHC class I. Inhibition of antigen presentation by MHC class I prevents the generation of effective T-cell immune responses.

CMV has developed a unique modification of affecting MHC processing. Natural killer (NK) cells are the principal defenders against tumor cells or virally infected cells that are not recognized by T-cytotoxic cells because of downregulated MHC expression. NK cell function is suppressed, however, if the infected cell expresses class I MHC molecules. CMV is capable of preventing antigen presentation by MHC class I and stimulates the expression of a MHC-like molecule that cannot present antigen but suppresses NK cells. Thus CMV-infected cells are protected from both T-cytotoxic cells and NK cell killing.

Some viruses also have the capacity to produce molecules that mimic cytokines or their ligands and neutralize the effects of cytokines, such as IL-1 and TNF-α. Cells infected with vaccinia virus (the less virulent vaccine relative of smallpox virus) produce a protein that can bind to IL-1. These molecules are frequently called *cytokine decoys*.

Viruses are sensitive to complement activation. Protection can be provided by incorporation of complement inhibitors into the envelope (e.g., HIV and vaccinia). CMV induces complement inhibitors on the surface of infected cells. HSV expresses a cell surface protein (glycoprotein C-1) that binds and inhibits C3b, as well as blocks formation of the membrane attack complex.

Influenza viruses causes significant seasonal epidemics throughout the world. Box 10.5 reviews the pathogenesis of influenza.

HUMAN IMMUNODEFICIENCY VIRUS AND ACQUIRED IMMUNODEFICIENCY SYNDROME
Acquired Immunodeficiency Syndrome
The most notable form of secondary or acquired immune deficiency is caused by the human immunodeficiency virus (HIV). HIV causes

BOX 10.5   THE PATHOGENESIS OF INFLUENZA

Influenza is an ssRNA (−strand) virus with a segmented genome. It is transmitted through aerosols or body fluids and is highly infectious. The virions attach to and enter respiratory epithelial cells. Symptoms begin 1 to 4 days after infection and may include chills, fever, sore throat, muscle aches, severe headaches, coughing, weakness, and generalized discomfort. Nausea and vomiting may occur in children. Infection may lead to viral pneumonia or secondary bacterial pneumonia, both of which can be fatal, particularly in young children and older adults. The normal rate of infectivity is about 5% to 15%, with a mortality rate of about 0.1%, and in most cases recovery occurs in 1 to 2 weeks.

The influenza virion is enveloped and expresses two surface proteins that are essential to virulence: hemagglutinin (HA) and neuraminidase (NA). The HA is a glycoprotein that binds to the carbohydrate sialic acid which is richly expressed on the surface of respiratory epithelium. The HA molecule is cut by a human protease, thus signaling a process of endocytosis that internalizes the virus into an endosomal vacuole.[1] The endosomal vacuole is acidic (about pH 5), which initiates HA-dependent fusion between the viral envelope and endosomal membrane.[2] The viral core disassembles and releases viral RNA (vRNA) and core proteins into the cytoplasm. The virion carries an RNA-dependent RNA polymerase that transcribes the vRNA into +strand ssRNA copies that are used to produce more vRNA. Viral proteins are translated and new HA and NA molecules are inserted into the plasma membrane and cluster. Copies of vRNA and capsid proteins are assembled underneath the HA and NA clusters and begin the budding process. HAs on the budding virus remain attached to surface glycans; new virions must be released by the action of the neuraminidase (NA) that cuts the sialic acid. Thus HA is essential for entrance and NA is essential for release of new virions. The infected cell usually dies during this process.

Antibodies against the HA and NA antigens are responsible for protection against influenza infection. Infections are seasonal and protection gained from the previous year's infection is partial and does not totally protect against influenza in the following year because the HA and NA antigens undergo yearly change. Usually antigenic variation is relatively minor (**antigenic drift**) and results from mutations. Yearly revaccination is necessary to produce immunity against changes resulting from antigenic drift. Two major groups of influenza virus, influenza A and influenza B, infect humans and both undergo drift. Influenza A and influenza B contain 8 RNA segments that encode at least 10 proteins. Influenza A infects birds and some mammals. Influenza B infects mostly humans and seals and undergoes antigenic drift much more slowly than influenza A.

Several major variants of HA (18 forms, numbered 1–18) and NA (11 forms, numbered 1–11) have been identified for influenza A. One particular viral strain will express a single HA and a single NA. The particular HA and NA variant being expressed becomes part of the nomenclature of the particular yearly viral strains (e.g. strain H3N2), important for the development of yearly vaccines.

Influenza A periodically undergoes major antigenic changes (**antigenic shifts**) (see Figure). Shifts occur in animals coinfected by a human and an avian strain of influenza. Because the genome is segmented, the segments can undergo recombination during which the human virus obtains a new HA or NA antigen. When such changes occur, previous protective antibodies may not be effective, resulting in a major pandemic and more severe disease.

As with most vaccines, not everyone is protected. Research is in progress to induce protective antibody responses against common surface antigens shared by genetically diverse influenza viruses thus providing a long lasting protection.

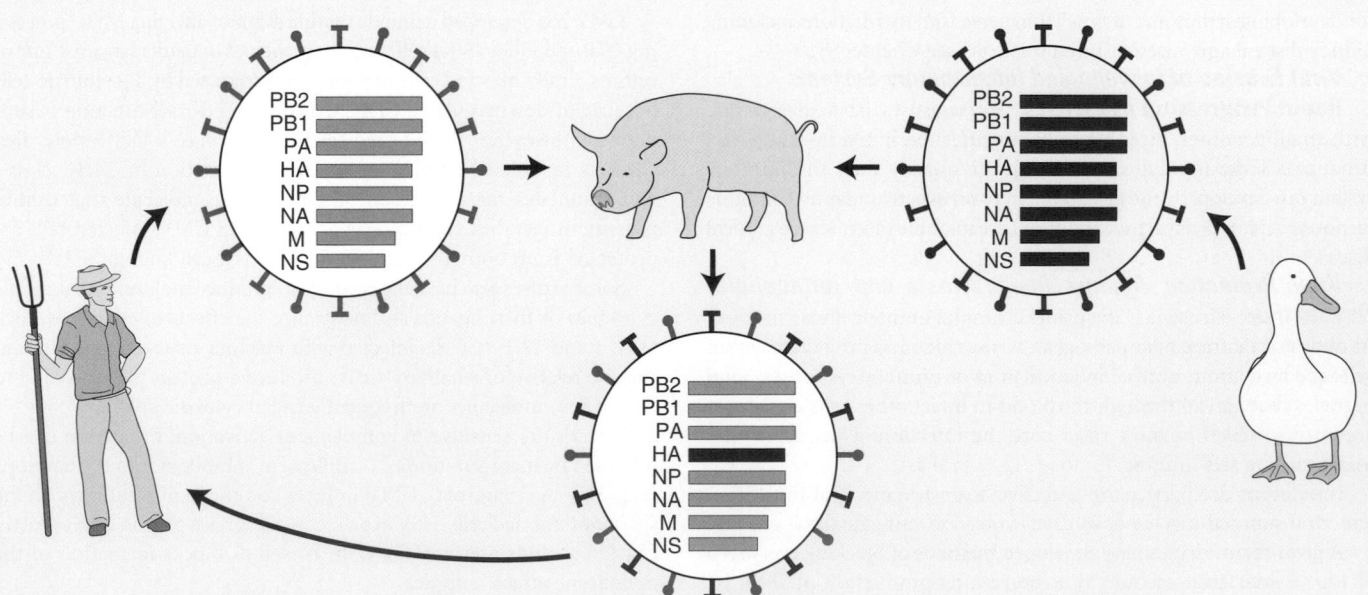

FIGURE Antigenic Shifts in Influenza Virus. One theory proposes that antigenic shifts occur when a human influenza virus *(blue)* and an avian influenza virus *(red)* coinfect a species that is permissive for both. The eight ssRNA strands are coexpressed in the same infected cell, resulting in mixing of the strands so that a hybrid virus can be produced. The hybrid virus indicated here contains all the genetic information of the original virus that infected humans, but contains a new hemagglutinin *(HA)*-containing strand from the avian virus. This virus expresses a new HA antigen and will be less susceptible to residual immunity that normally provides partial protection against yearly influenza infections. *M,* Matrix (M1) and membrane protein (M2); *NA,* neuramidase; *NP,* nucleoprotein; *NS,* nucleotide sequences; *PA,* polymerase acidic protein; *PB1,* polymerase basic protein 1; *PB2,* polymerase basic protein 2.

BOX 10.5   THE PATHOGENESIS OF INFLUENZA—cont'd

Pharmacologic therapy may lessen the severity of symptoms. Competitive neuraminidase inhibitors, such as oseltamivir (Tamiflu), bind to NA and inhibit enzymatic activity, thus preventing spread of the virions between cells. If the NA mutates, the drugs may lose inhibitory capacity, which may explain observations of the rapid development of drug resistance.

Several variables affect the pathophysiology of influenza infections. Less aggressive strains primarily infect epithelium lining the upper respiratory tract. The proliferation of virus within infected cells results in tissue damage far in excess to what is seen with cold viruses. More aggressive strains can infect cells that are deeper in the lungs and produce even more tissue damage. The differences are related somewhat to the particular HA antigen expressed on the virus. The HA normally binds to α2-6 sialylated glycans in the upper respiratory tract. The highly pathogenic H5N1 influenza virus binds to upper respiratory tract cells and also to α2-3 sialylated glycans on pneumocytes (cells lining the alveoli of the lungs) leading to severe pneumonia.

Influenza has several virulence factors that contribute to the pathophysiology. All influenza strains can inhibit the innate antiviral interferon response. The influenza ssRNA is recognized by intracellular pattern recognition receptors (PRRs), such as Toll-like receptor-7 (TLR7) which induce the production of antiviral type I interferons (IFNs).

The primary difference between strains of low or high pathogenicity is the intensity of cytokine and chemokine production. Tissue damage typically attracts macrophages that induce apoptosis of epithelial cells, thus increasing the amount of damage. The more pathogenic viruses induce more tissue damage and a level of cytokine and chemokine production that is referred to as a *cytokine storm*. Pulmonary damage is greatly exacerbated, resulting in diffuse alveolar damage, hyaline membrane formation, and fibrin deposition, all of which may lead to respiratory failure. Systemic cytokine levels are greatly elevated, resulting in multiorgan dysfunction. The unexpectedly large number of deaths in the 20 to 39 age group during the 1918 influenza pandemic appeared to be related to an excessive number of neutrophils attracted to the lungs and to an intense cytokine storm reflecting their healthy and highly responsive immune systems.

References

1. Greber UF: Virus and host mechanics support membrane penetration and cell entry. *J Virol* 90(8):3802–3805, 2016.
2. Jakubová L, Holly J, Varečková E: The role of fusion activity of influenza A viruses in their biological properties. *Acta Virol* 60(2):121–135, 2016.

acquired immunodeficiency syndrome (AIDS). HIV is a retrovirus that infects and depletes a portion of the immune system (CD4+ Th cells), making individuals extremely susceptible to life-threatening infections and malignancies (Fig. 10.8).

When AIDS was recognized as a major health epidemic in sub-Saharan Africa and in the United States in the early 1980s, an AIDS diagnosis was considered a death sentence, with a near 100% mortality rate within 2 years of the diagnosis of AIDS. With the advent of aggressive treatment with antiretroviral drugs in the mid-1990s and widespread public health campaigns, HIV/AIDS has become a chronic and manageable illness with many infected individuals having a near normal life span. Currently, about half of the 18 million individuals living with HIV/AIDS in Africa are being administered antiretroviral drugs.[21] As yet, however, antiviral medications are not fully available at an affordable price in many parts of the world where HIV/AIDS remains the major cause of morbidity and mortality.

The transmission of HIV in Africa is predominantly heterosexual, whereas the distribution of individuals with HIV/AIDS in the United States reflects the primary means of transmission within the original cohort. Although isolated cases of what was later identified as AIDS occurred in the United States as early as 1959, the appearance of the AIDS epidemic has been linked to several gay males who had contracted HIV infection during visits to the Caribbean, probably Haiti.[22] Initial reports of outbreaks in the United States were of gay men who developed *Pneumocystis carinii* pneumonia[23] and aggressive Kaposi sarcoma,[24] both of which were uncommon and mostly observed in immune-deficient individuals. The epidemic then spread to intravenous drug abusers and heterosexuals. In 2014 (the latest available statistics) 44,073 men and women were newly diagnosed with HIV infection with gay or bisexual men representing 67% of all individuals and 83% newly diagnosed men.[25] Women represented 19% of newly diagnosed individuals with 87% of women contracting HIV through heterosexual encounters. As a result of aggressive antiretroviral therapy and public education, the transmission to women had declined by about 40% over the previous decade. About 6% of all individuals newly diagnosed with HIV were associated with

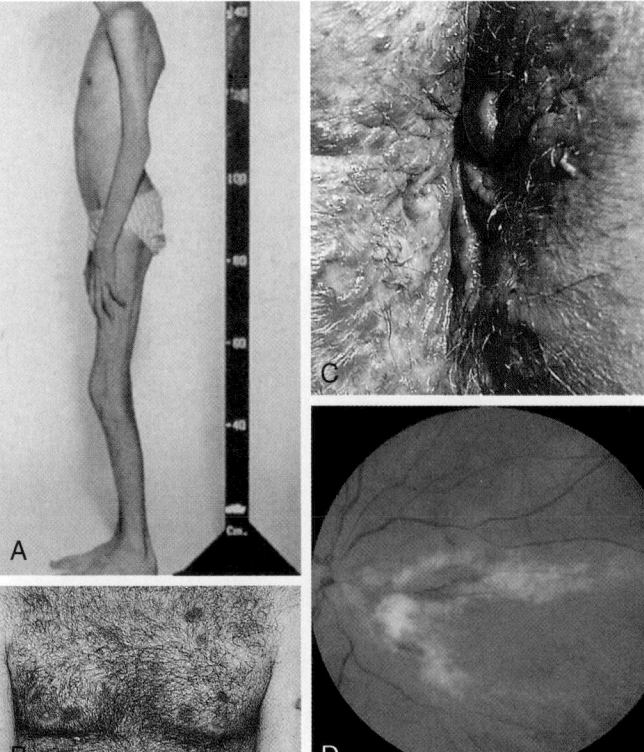

FIGURE 10.8 Clinical Symptoms of AIDS. **A,** Severe weight loss and anorexia. **B,** Biopsy-proven Kaposi sarcoma lesions. **C,** Perianal vesicular and ulcerative lesions of herpes simplex infection. **D,** Deterioration of vision from cytomegalovirus retinitis leading to areas of infection; unless treated, the progressive impairment will lead to blindness. (**A** and **D** from Taylor PK: *Diagnostic picture tests in sexually transmitted diseases,* London, 1995, Mosby; **B** and **C** from Morse SA, Holmes KK, Ballard RC, editors: *Atlas of sexually transmitted diseases and AIDS,* ed 4, London, 2011, Saunders.)

intravenous drug abuse. In 2015, 18,303 people were diagnosed with AIDS, and since the early 1980s, 1,216,917 people have been diagnosed with AIDS. In 2014, 6721 deaths were attributed directly to HIV infection. An estimated 650,000 individuals with a diagnosis of AIDS have died since the early 1980s.

Transmission of HIV

HIV is a blood-borne pathogen present in body fluids with the typical routes of transmission: blood or blood products, intravenous drug abuse, heterosexual and homosexual activity, and maternal-child transmission before or during birth. The CDC estimates that 91% of new HIV infections in the United States result from sexual activity with those who are undiagnosed or diagnosed but not treated for HIV infection.

As with all blood-borne infections, healthcare providers are at increased risk of contracting the infection from an individual's blood. Since the strict implementation of universal precautions and the use of post-exposure prophylaxis with antiretroviral drugs, infection of healthcare providers is extremely rare.

Pathogenesis of HIV

HIV-1 was initially isolated by researchers at the Pasteur Institute as the lymphadenopathy/AIDS virus (LAV), a discovery for which they received the 2008 Nobel Prize in Medicine.[26] A second major and less virulent variant, HIV-2, was identified later and is found mostly in western Africa. HIV is a member of the retrovirus family, which carries genetic information in the form of two identical copies of single-stranded RNA (Fig. 10.9 see the genetic map of HIV-1, Fig. E 10.1 on Evolve). The RNA copies are packaged in the viral particle within a capsid constructed of viral capsid protein p24. The capsid also contains two viral enzymes: reverse transcriptase and integrase. Retroviral particles are contained in a plasma membrane envelope originating during release

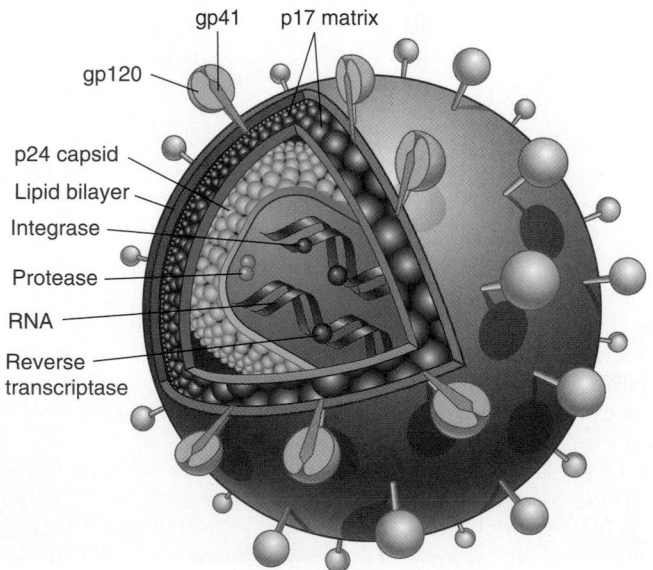

FIGURE 10.9 HIV-1: Structure. The HIV-1 virion consists of a core of two identical strands of viral RNA molecules, three viral enzymes (integrase [IN], protease [PR], and reverse transcriptase [RT]) and a capsid. The capsid is further encased in a matrix consisting primarily of a viral protein. The outer surface is an envelope consisting of the plasma membrane of the cell from which the virus budded (lipid bilayer) and two viral glycoproteins: a transmembrane gp41 and a noncovalently attached surface protein, gp120. (Modified from Kumar V et al: *Robbins & Cotran pathologic basis of disease,* ed 9, Philadelphia, 2015, Saunders.)

from the infected cell. The membrane contains two viral proteins (gp41 and gp120), referred to as envelope proteins. Between the envelope and capsid are viral matrix proteins underlying the envelope and another viral enzyme, a protease.

As with all other viruses, the life cycle must begin with attachment and entrance into its cellular target. HIV is primarily tropic for CD4+ T-helper cells, although macrophages and dendritic cells also express CD4 and can be infected. Attachment occurs between the viral envelope proteins and CD4 (Fig. 10.10). The envelope protein gp41 is anchored in the plasma membrane and is referred to as the TM (transmembrane) protein. The N-terminal portion of TM consists of very hydrophobic amino acids. The TM associates with a gp120 envelope protein, called the SU (surface protein), which contains binding sites for CD4. When the SU protein attaches to CD4, it undergoes a conformational change that allows further recognition of cell surface chemokine receptors, primarily CCR5, and exposure of the TM hydrophobic tail, which interacts with the lipid region of the T cell and initiates a process of fusion between the viral envelope and the cellular membrane. The fusion event releases the viral capsid into the cellular cytoplasm, where it undergoes uncoating (shedding of capsid proteins) and release of viral RNA and enzymes.

The third step in the life cycle, integration, is controlled by **reverse transcriptase**, which converts single-stranded viral RNA into double-stranded DNA. The viral **integrase** inserts viral DNA into the infected cell's DNA, where it may remain dormant. If replication is activated, the *gag* gene encodes a large precursor protein that undergoes post-translational modification by the viral protease to generate smaller matrix (e.g., p17) and capsid proteins (e.g., p24). The *env* gene encodes a large gp160 glycoprotein that is processed by a cellular protease (furin) into the TM and SU proteins. The capsid and nuclear components of the virus undergo assembly in the cytoplasm, and the Env proteins are inserted into the plasma membrane. The assembled particle buds from the cell surface as an infectious virion.

The major immunologic finding in AIDS is the striking decrease in the number of CD4+ Th cells. Several mechanisms of Th cell killing are used.[27] The replication and release of new virions triggers apoptotic cell death of the infected cell. The release of death ligands (e.g., Fas ligand [FasL], TNF) initiates apoptosis in neighboring uninfected Th cells. The infected Th cell also becomes a target for killing by CD8+ T-cytotoxic cells.

Clinical Manifestations of HIV

With the advent of antiretroviral drugs, the early identification of HIV infection is essential. The CDC has issued a new system for staging HIV infection at diagnosis and during monitoring of therapeutic effectiveness and managing the disease.[28] The stages are adapted for every age group and based primarily on diagnostic laboratory tests. Stage 0 disease covers the first 180 days after infection, and stages 1 to 3 are based primarily on the CD4 cell counts to monitor disease progression.

The lymphoid areas of the mucosal surfaces are the primary sites of initial infection, particularly if the mucosa has been damaged. Dendritic cells and mucosal T cells probably spread the infection to other peripheral lymphoid organs (especially follicular dendritic cells in the lymph nodes). Production of new virus particles proceeds rapidly with increasing viremia. HIV RNA may be detected in the plasma by 10 days after an acute infection and HIV p24 antigen detected about 4 to 10 days after viral RNA (Fig. 10.11). Indication of an individual's immune response quickly follows. HIV-specific IgM antibody is detected about 3 to 5 days after p24 antigen and levels of IgG begin rising soon afterwards and remain elevated throughout the disease process. As with most immune responses against viral diseases, the IgM levels are usually

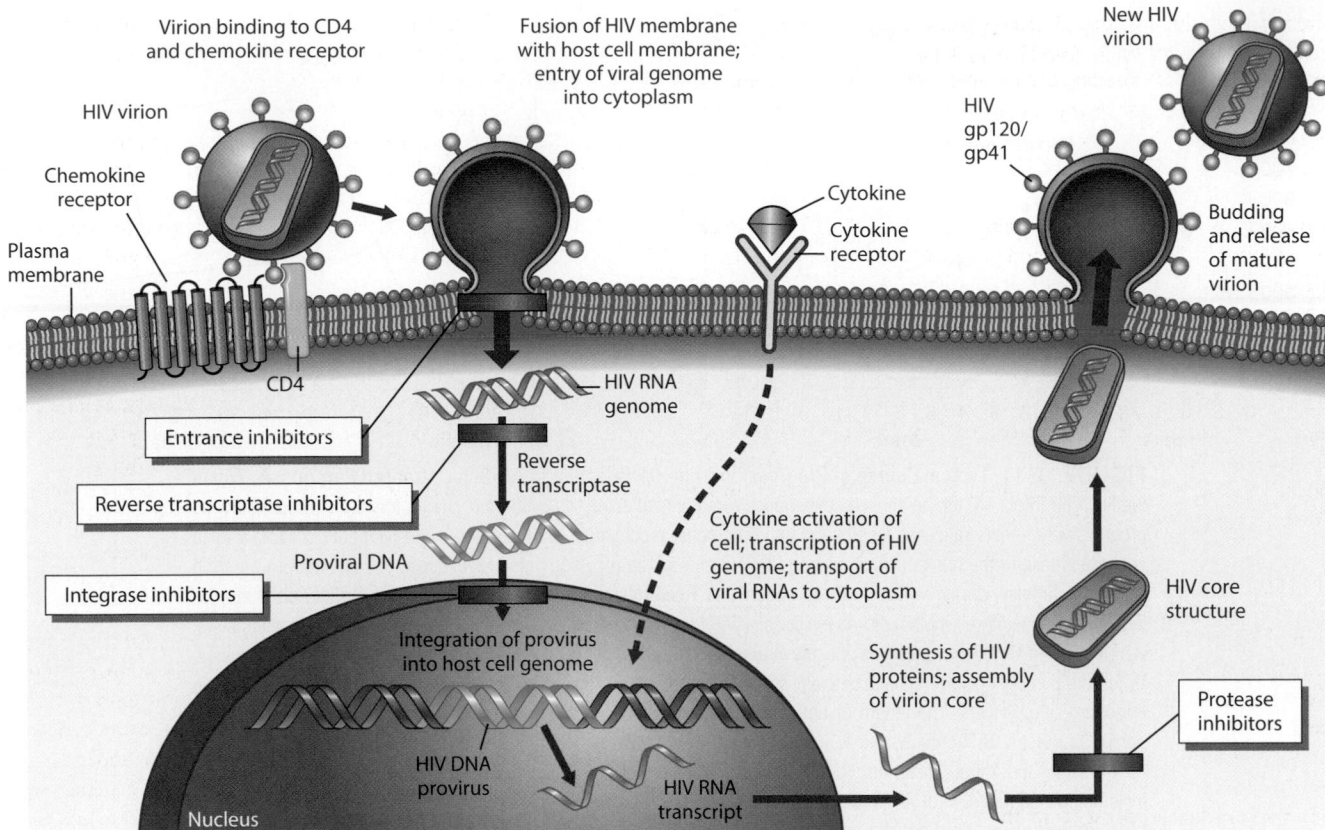

FIGURE 10.10 Life Cycle and Possible Sites of Therapeutic Intervention of HIV-1. The HIV-1 life cycle is susceptible to blockage at several sites. Some agents could block the attachment and entrance of the virus (entrance inhibitors). Reverse transcriptase inhibitors (e.g., azidothymidine [AZT]) prevent the reverse transcription of viral RNA into DNA. Drugs also may be able to inhibit the viral integrase (integrase inhibitors) and prevent insertion of the provirus into the host's chromosomes. Protease inhibitors specifically inhibit the viral protease and prevent the processing of the gp160 into viral capsid and matrix proteins. (Modified from Kumar V et al: *Robbins & Cotran pathologic basis of disease,* ed 9, Philadelphia, 2015, Saunders.)

transient. The appearance of viral RNA in the plasma is indicative of viremia and the appearance of infectious virus in the body fluids, an indication that infected individuals can transmit HIV to other individuals.

From 40% to 90% of individuals in stage 0 will experience symptoms of acute viral syndrome. Symptoms may include fever, fatigue, headache, lymphadenopathy, pharyngitis, myalgia (muscle pain), arthralgia (joint pain), and a skin rash that can be extensive. Without knowledge of exposure to HIV, the infected individual may suspect a self-limiting influenza or infectious mononucleosis condition. By 180 days, the initial burst of viremia and acute viral syndrome will have resolved. The infected individual will be asymptomatic, yet infectious HIV is present in body fluids and the process of HIV-mediated destruction of CD4 cells has just begun.

Stages 1 through 3 are determined by diminishing CD4 T-cell counts, adjusted for normal age-related levels. In the first year of life, the normal CD4 T-cell count is the highest and decreases with age. For instance, stage 1 disease is classified after 180 days of infection and the CD4 T-cell counts are still normal: ≥1500 cells/μL at <1 year, ≥1000 cells/μL at 1 through 5 years, and ≥500 cells/μL at 6 years to adult. Stage 2 is characterized by diminished numbers of CD4 T cells: 750 to 1499 cells/μL at <1 year, 500 to 999 cells/μL at 1 through 5 years, and 200 to 499 cells/μL at 6 years to adult. Stage 3 is defined as AIDS, determined by

CD4 T-cell counts of <750, <500, or <200 cells/μL for the respective age groups, or the development of AIDS-related opportunistic infections, regardless of the CD4 T-cell count (Box 10.6).

Treatment and Prevention of HIV

The current regimen of **highly active antiretroviral therapy (HAART)** for treatment of HIV infection is a combination of drugs that attack different portions of the viral replication pathway.[29] Since the FDA approval of zidovudine (AZT), more than 25 antiretroviral agents representing 6 different classes have been approved to treat HIV/AIDS and several others are in various stages of testing.

Classes of antiretroviral agents include inhibitors of the enzyme reverse transcriptase (nucleoside/nucleotide reverse transcriptase inhibitors [NRTIs] and non-nucleoside reverse transcriptase inhibitors [NNRTIs]), inhibitors of the viral protease (protease inhibitors [PIs]), entry and intercellular fusion inhibitors that prevent attachment of the virus to the target cell or prevent fusion between HIV and the cell membrane, and inhibitors of the viral integrase enzyme (integrase strand transfer inhibitors [INSTIs]).[29] A sixth group of drugs are pharmacokinetic enhancers, such as cobicistat (COBI), that are administered with some PIs and INSTIs. Enhancers affect intestinal transport proteins and liver enzyme that would normally break down some antiretroviral drugs, thus allowing smaller doses to be used. Many other drugs are in clinical testing,

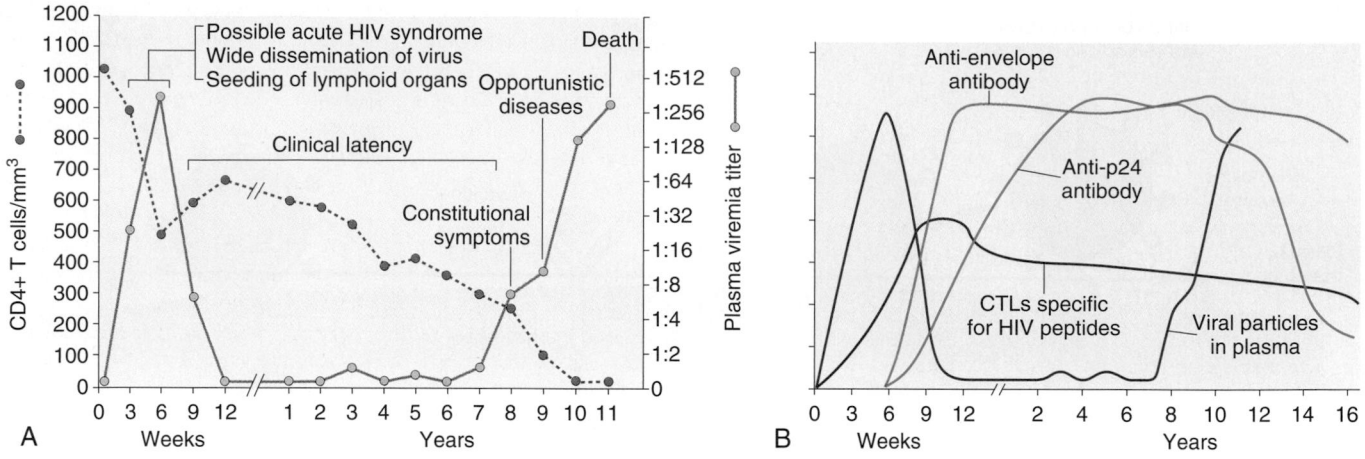

FIGURE 10.11 Typical Course of Progression from HIV Infection to AIDS in Untreated Persons. **A,** Within weeks after infection, the person may experience symptoms of acute HIV syndrome. During this early period the virus progressively infects mucosal T cells and dendritic cells, propagates, and spreads to the lymphoid organs, with a sharp decrease in the number of circulating CD4+ Th cells. The resulting immune response usually induces a period of clinical latency, during which viral replication and T-cell destruction continue in the lymph nodes, although the individual is generally asymptomatic. As the disease progresses, the person may develop HIV-related disease (constitutional symptoms)—a variety of symptoms of acute viral infection that do not involve opportunistic infections or malignancies. When the number of CD4+ cells is critically suppressed, the person becomes susceptible to a variety of opportunistic infections and cancers. The length of time for progression from HIV infection to AIDS may vary considerably from person to person. **B,** Antibody and Tc cell (cytotoxic T lymphocytes [CTLs]) levels change during the progression to AIDS. During the initial phase, antibodies against HIV-1 are not yet detectable (window period), but viral products, including p24 antigen, viral RNA, and infectious virus, may be detectable in the blood a few weeks after infection. Most antibodies produced against envelope proteins in the early phase are absorbed onto viral particles in the blood and are not detectable by most routine assays. During the latent phase of infection, antibody levels against p24 and other viral proteins, as well as HIV-specific CTLs, generally increase and then remain constant until the development of AIDS. As the immune system becomes severely depressed and excess viral antigen is released into the blood, measurable antibody levels decrease. Disease progression usually ends in the death of the untreated individual. (**A** redrawn from Fauci AS, Lane HC: Human immunodeficiency virus disease: AIDS and related conditions. In Fauci AS et al, editors: *Harrison's principles of internal medicine,* ed 14, New York, 1997, McGraw-Hill; **B** from Kumar V, Abbas A, Fausto N: *Robbins & Cotran pathologic basis of disease,* ed 8, Philadelphia, 2010, Saunders.)

including Gag maturation inhibitors (prevent enzymatic activation of Gag precursor protein), gp120 inhibitors (prevent conformational changes necessary for attachment and entry process), and broadly neutralizing antibodies (bind to proteins on viral envelope and prevent attachment).

The recommended first-line treatment is a combination of two NRTIs and a third drug from another class (see Fig. 10.10). Many drug combinations are available in a single pill, facilitating compliance. The specific regimen and drugs may vary based on a variety of an individual's characteristics. Other drugs (e.g., entry inhibitors) are reserved for those who develop resistance to first-line drugs.

The goals of therapy are reduction of viral load in fluids, reduced HIV-associated morbidity, prolonged survival, and prevention of HIV transmission. The plasma viral load is frequently suppressed below detectable levels within weeks. With treatment beginning at the time of diagnosis, transmission has decreased by about 90%. Retroviral preventive treatment of uninfected partners of those who are HIV infected has diminished transmission by 96%. Without treatment, the progression from acute infection to AIDS takes 9 to 10 years, with death occurring within 2 to 3 years. Death from AIDS-related diseases has been reduced significantly since the introduction of HAART; those who

respond well to HAART may survive for several decades. Continued suppression of HIV/AIDS progression absolutely requires daily and continuous use of medications.

However, many people do not respond to HAART therapy; those who do respond are not "cured," and resistant variants to these drugs have been identified. Individuals who initiate antiretroviral therapy will still have a shortened life expectancy secondary to HIV-associated persistent immune activation. Continued systemic inflammation secondary to persistent HIV infection and toxicity of available drugs increase the risk for developing chronic and potentially fatal morbidities. Complications include dyslipidemia (imbalance of blood lipids), insulin resistance, lipodystrophy (changes in body composition, either loss or accumulation of fat), decreased bone density and increase in incidence of fractures, diabetes, renal disease, and liver disease. The risk of cardiovascular disease is increased twofold.[30]

Antiretroviral drug therapy does not cure HIV/AIDS because the HIV genome incorporates into the DNA of the infected cells that may act as reservoirs and release viral particles if therapy is stopped. The primary reservoir is probably long-lived CD4+ memory T cells, although contribution to the reservoir may include other infected cells, such as macrophages, dendritic cells, astrocytes, microglia, and hematopoietic

STAGE 3 AIDS-DEFINING OPPORTUNISTIC INFECTIONS AND NEOPLASMS FOUND IN INDIVIDUALS WITH HIV INFECTION

Protozoal and Helminthic Infections

Cryptosporidiosis, chronic intestinal (>1 month's duration)

Isosporiasis, chronic intestinal (>1 month's duration)

Toxoplasmosis of brain, onset at age >1 month

Fungal Infections

Candidiasis (esophageal, bronchi, tracheal, or pulmonary)

Coccidioidomycosis, disseminated or extrapulmonary

Cryptococcosis, extrapulmonary

Histoplasmosis, disseminated or extrapulmonary

Pneumocystis jiroveci (previously known as *"Pneumocystis carinii"*) pneumonia

Bacterial Infections

Bacterial infections, multiple or recurrent*

Mycobacterium avium complex or *Mycobacterium kansasii,* disseminated or extrapulmonary

Mycobacterium tuberculosis of any site, pulmonary,* disseminated, or extrapulmonary

Mycobacterium, other species or unidentified species, disseminated or extrapulmonary

Pneumonia, recurrent*

Salmonella septicemia, recurrent

Viral Infections

Cytomegalovirus disease (other than liver, spleen, or nodes), onset at age >1 month

Cytomegalovirus retinitis (with loss of vision)

Herpes simplex: chronic ulcers (>1 month's duration) or bronchitis, pneumonitis, or esophagitis (onset at age >1 month)

Progressive multifocal leukoencephalopathy

Varicella-zoster virus (localized or disseminated)

Neoplasms

Cervical cancer, invasive[†]

Kaposi sarcoma

Lymphoma, Burkitt (or equivalent term)

Lymphoma, immunoblastic (or equivalent term)

Lymphoma, primary, of brain

HIV-Associated Disorders[‡]

Encephalopathy attributed to HIV

Wasting syndrome attributed to HIV

Adapted from Selik RM et al: 2014, *MMWR Morb Mortal Wkly Rep* 63(RR-03):1–10, 2014.

*Only among children aged <6 years.

[†]Only among adults, adolescents, and children aged ≥6 years.

[‡]Suggested diagnostic criteria for these illnesses, which might be particularly important for HIV encephalopathy and HIV wasting syndrome, are described in the following references: Data from 1993 revised classification system for HIV infection and expanded surveillance case definition for AIDS among adolescents and adults, *MMWR Recomm Rep* 41(RR-17):1–19, 1992; 1994 revised classification system for human immunodeficiency virus infection in children less than 13 years of age, *MMWR Recomm Rep* 43(RR-12), 1994.

progenitors.[31] HIV also may persist in regions where the antiviral drugs are not as effective, such as the central nervous system (CNS). HIV penetrates the CNS early in the infection and persists despite successful treatment with antiretroviral drugs. Neural infection leads to viral encephalitis and apoptosis of neurons. The incidence of HIV-associated dementia was about 20% in untreated individuals, but antiretroviral therapy has reduced that number to about 5% and decreased the severity. Dementia is now rarely seen.

Ultimately, the best hope for preventing the spread of HIV infection is development of an effective vaccine. Most common antiviral vaccines (e.g., rubella, mumps, influenza) induce protective antibodies that block the initial infection. Only one vaccine (rabies) is used after the infection has occurred. That approach is successful because the rabies virus proliferates and spreads very slowly. Whether an HIV vaccine would be effective in either preventing or treating HIV infection is problematic, and the results of recent vaccine trials have for the moment dampened enthusiasm. Characteristics of HIV have been difficult to overcome. HIV-1 commonly undergoes random mutations that result in an extreme and changing antigenic diversity.[32] During transmission, bodily fluids may contain a variety of viral antigenic types so that effective vaccines may need to induce protection against a broad spectrum of HIV surface antigens.

Pediatric HIV

Neonates become HIV infected from their mothers by the passage of the virus across the placenta during pregnancy, by contact with infected maternal blood at childbirth, or through the milk during breast-feeding. The transmission rate in the United States was about 13%, but has been reduced to 1% with the use of prenatal antiviral therapy beginning early in pregnancy, the implementation of neonatal prophylaxis, and the avoidance of breast-feeding.

Without prenatal treatment, symptoms of HIV infection usually develop within 6 months of neonatal life, 20% get opportunistic infections within the first year, and life expectancy is generally less than 3 years. Because of aggressive clinical intervention, there are currently fewer than 50 cases of pediatric HIV infection diagnosed yearly in the United States.

The presence of passive maternal antibody limits the use of HIV antibody testing in infants in the high-risk category up to 18 months of age. The current recommended diagnostic procedure is testing initially for HIV nucleic acid: viral RNA in plasma, or DNA within cells. Determination of whether the child is infected is based on repeated negative test results.[27] Two negative nucleic acid test results at 2 and 4 weeks after birth is considered a "presumptive" uninfected state. A "definitive" uninfected is defined as two nucleic acid test results at 1 and 4 months. Combined HAART is initiated immediately in infants and leads to reduced viral latency, a 76% reduction in AIDS-related mortality, and many children reaching the adolescent period with functional immune systems.

Complications in children undergoing HAART are related to metabolic disorders, including insulin resistance and dyslipidemia.[27] Because of the metabolic complications of HAART and the ongoing HIV-associated inflammation, half of HIV-infected children are at increased risk of coronary disease. Most HIV-infected children who reach adulthood will have indications of coronary artery abnormalities. A third or less of children will present with low bone density, but with no increase in fractures.

A particularly vulnerable site of HIV infection in infants and children is the CNS. HIV encephalopathy is more common in the advanced stages. Because survival of children with HIV has been prolonged with effective treatment, the incidence of progressive encephalopathy has increased. For diagnosis of HIV-related neurologic effects, at least one of the following progressive findings needs to be present for at least 2 months, in the absence of a concurrent illness other than HIV that could explain the following findings:

- Failure to attain or loss of developmental milestones, or loss of intellectual ability, verified by standard developmental scale or neuropsychologic tests
- Impaired brain growth or acquired microcephaly demonstrated by head circumference measurements or brain atrophy demonstrated by computed tomography (CT) or magnetic resonance imaging (MRI) with serial imaging required in children less than 2 years of age
- Acquired symmetrical motor deficits manifested by affecting a child 1 month of age or older

The onset of progressive encephalopathy may be a prognostic indicator of a poor outcome.

Other insults may accompany HIV in a young child and affect growth and development, such as drug exposure, prematurity, chronic illness, and a chaotic social atmosphere. The pathogenesis of HIV encephalopathy in children is poorly understood, but the presence of inflammatory mediators may be a contributing factor.

COUNTERMEASURES AGAINST PATHOGENS

An extremely effective means of countering infectious microorganisms is rigorous use of environmental infection control measures, including control of insect vector populations, establishment of modern sanitation facilities, provision of clean water and uncontaminated food supplies, and other measures. Additionally, prophylactic or therapeutic procedures have been developed to prevent pathogens from initiating disease (vaccines) or to subdue the pathogen once the disease process has started (antimicrobials). Vaccine development has focused successfully on preventing the most severe and common infections (Table 10.7). With the initial success of antibiotic therapy there was no perceived need for vaccination against many common and non–life-threatening infections. The increasing problem of antibiotic-resistant pathogens, however, forced a reappraisal of that strategy, and a greater emphasis is being placed on the development of new vaccines.

Infection Control Measures

Although effective means of safeguarding populations from exposure to infectious disease are well known, lack of implementation or breakdowns in application of these initiatives have led to the reemergence of some infectious diseases. These diseases include cholera, dengue fever and West Nile virus.

Sewage removal and other public health initiatives are now the expected norm in developed countries. The quality of water and food, as well as disposal of human and animal waste, remains poor in many developing countries. Rapid urbanization as well as other problems (e.g., poverty, overcrowding, mass relocation of people because of war, rapid destruction of forests) has put pressure on already inadequate systems. A 1991 outbreak of cholera in Peru resulted in an estimated 1100 deaths in Peru and more than 4000 deaths in Latin America, and was attributed to problems with infrastructure, including inadequate sanitation.

Additionally, previously successful programs designed to control the breeding of insect vectors have been reversed. Despite an international emphasis on draining standing water that provides breeding grounds for mosquitoes, large unmanaged areas still abound. A very successful international mosquito eradication program resulted in decreasing incidence of mosquito-borne diseases. Some regions were declared "free" of mosquito-borne diseases. However, lack of access to pesticides, and

TABLE 10.7   REDUCTION IN VACCINE-PREVENTABLE DISEASES IN THE UNITED STATES

DISEASE	BASELINE 20th CENTURY ANNUAL CASES*	2015 CASES[†]	% REDUCTION
Diphtheria	175,885	0	100.0
Measles	503,282	188	99.9
Mumps	152,209	1329	95.1
Pertussis	147,271	20,762	85.9
Smallpox	48,164	0	100.0
Polio	16,316	0	100.0
Rubella	47,745	5	99.9
Tetanus	1314	29	97.8
Haemophilus influenzae type b, invasive	20,000	4138	79.9

*Average number of reported cases over multiple years before initiation of vaccine (Centers for Disease Control and Prevention: *MMWR Morb Mortal Wkly Rep* 48[12]:243–248, 1999; *Morb Mortal Wkly Rep* 57[11]:289–291, 2008).
[†]CDC: *MMWR Morb Mortal Wkly Rep* 65(46):1306–1321, 2016. http://dx.doi.org/10.15585/mmwr.mm6546a9.
From National Institute of Allergy and Infectious Disease, National Institutes of Health: *Vaccine, vaccine benefits.* Updated May 11, 2010. http://www.niaid.nih.gov/topics/vaccines/understanding/pages/vaccinebenefits.aspx.

failure or delay in initiating fumigation and larvacide programs for mosquitoes has resulted in rebound of mosquito-related diseases in previously disease-free regions in some parts of the world. The consequence is increasingly severe outbreaks of viral disease. An example is outbreaks of dengue virus and West Nile virus in areas of India in the last several years. This problem is exacerbated by the development of insecticide-resistant mosquitoes.

Antimicrobials

Antibiotics are natural products of fungi, bacteria, and related microorganisms and kill or inhibit the growth of other microorganisms. They are basically microbial defense mechanisms by which one microorganism can defend itself against another. The goal of antibiotic therapy is elimination of the pathogenic microorganism. Some antibacterial antibiotics are bactericidal (kill the organism), whereas others are bacteriostatic (inhibit growth until the organism is destroyed by the individual's own protective mechanisms). The mechanisms of action of most antibiotics are (1) inhibition of the function or production of the cell wall, (2) prevention of protein synthesis, (3) blockage of DNA replication, or (4) interference with folic acid metabolism. Because viruses use the biochemical pathways of the host's cells, there has been far less success in developing specific antiviral antibiotics.

Antibiotic resistance observed clinically is of major importance and has become a problem worldwide. As the use of penicillin became widespread, Alexander Fleming, the discoverer of penicillin, frequently warned about the development of penicillin resistance, and the first bacterial penicillinase (enzyme that destroyed penicillin; β-lactamase) was described in 1940 by Fleming's collaborators. At least 1000 variations of β-lactamase have since been discovered. Being natural products of microorganisms that exist in nature, resistance mechanisms also developed in nature. Genes related to antibiotic resistance have been characterized from samples of permafrost that were dated at 30,000 years ago from the oral microbiome of 2000-year-old skeletons, from the gut microbiome of a Peruvian mummy dated near 1000 AD, and from several other samples that greatly predate the era of therapeutic antibiotics.[33] As might be expected, environment antibiotic resistance has increased greatly since the use of antibiotics in agriculture.

The CDC publishes a list of antibiotic resistance threats ranked as urgent, serious, and concerning available at: https://www.cdc.gov/drugresistance/biggest_threats.html and https://www.cdc.gov/drugresistance/threat-report-2013/index.html.[34] They estimated that more than 2 million antibiotic-resistant illnesses occur in the United States yearly, resulting in more than 23,000 deaths. The trend is progressing toward more infectious agents being resistant to multiple antibiotics, such as the classification of extensively drug-resistant TB that is resistant to all of the first- and second-line drugs and the cases of some vancomycin-resistant infections that are resistant to almost all antibiotics (see *What's New?* Totally Antibiotic-Resistant Infections Are Here!).

Antibiotic resistance may result from a variety of inherited processes that can coexist in different combinations in the same microorganism. Resistance genes can be spread within the bacterial community by *horizontal gene transfer*. Genetic information can be transferred by means of transformation (uptake of short DNA fragments from the environment), by transduction (transfer of DNA by means of viruses that infect bacteria, bacteriophages), or by conjugation (transfer of DNA, usually in the form of circular *plasmids*, through pili connecting the bacteria). A single plasmid may contain a large amount of genetic information for multiple types of antibiotic resistance.

Enzymatic inactivation of antibiotics is one of the most common forms of resistance. The β-lactam antibiotics contain a β-lactam ring central to their structures and are bactericidal by inhibiting formation of the bacterial cell wall. The initial class of β-lactam antibiotics (e.g., penicillin, cephalosporins) blocked synthesis of the gram-positive cell wall, whereas newer broad-spectrum β-lactam antibiotics (e.g., carboxypenicillins) also affect gram-negative cell wall synthesis. Resistance is conferred by enzymatic (β-lactamase) destruction of the antibiotic. Another class of antibiotics, aminoglycosides (e.g., streptomycin, neomycin, gentamicin), is bactericidal primarily to gram-negative aerobic bacteria and against tuberculosis by binding to sites on ribosomal RNA (rRNA) and inhibiting protein synthesis. Resistance is conferred by

WHAT'S NEW?

Totally Antibiotic-Resistant Infections Are Here!

The apparently unstoppable evolution by which bacteria add and horizontally transfer plasmids containing new antibiotic resistance genes has increased the fear of encountering microorganisms with total resistance to all available antibiotics (pan-antibiotic resistance).

Two antibiotics have been used as drugs-of-last-resort to treat infections with gram-negative microorganisms. Carbapenem is a β-lactam antibiotic similar to penicillin but with greater resistance to standard β-lactamases. Colistins (polymyxin E) are polypeptide antibiotics used to treat many gram-negative infections. Resistance genes have been recently described. In 2008, the enzyme New Delhi metallo-β-lactamase (NDM)-1 gene (*bla*$_{NDM-1}$) conferred resistance to multiple carbapenems and in 2015 the colistin resistance 1 gene (*mcr-1*) was reported in China. Both resistance genes have spread globally. The presence of either NDM-1 or *mcr-1* resistance gene on a plasmid with other resistance genes may confer a state of pan-antibiotic resistance. Several reports of this scenario have been published recently. In Germany, 2 individuals infected with *Serratia marcescens* with the *NDM-1* gene in addition to other resistance genes were resistant to 32 different antibiotics representing 8 different groups of antimicrobials.[1] In India, an individual with an aggressive eye infection (keratitis) with *Pseudomonas aeruginosa* was resistant to multiple antibiotics representing eight groups of antimicrobials.[2] The danger of increased incidences of pan-antibiotic resistance has increased even further when a German group discovered bacteria with *mcr-1* and *NDM-1* genes on the same plasmid.[3]

Pan-antibiotic resistant infections have now been identified in the United States. The first report of an infection with a microorganism expressing *mcr-1* came from Pennsylvania. The individual presented with a urinary tract infection with *E. coli* that expressed *mcr-1*.[4] A similar case from New Jersey involved an elderly man with a urinary tract infection with *E. coli* that contained both *mcr-1* and an *NDM* gene. The infection was resistant to both colistin and carbapenems.[5] In both reports, the infection remained treatable only because the bacterial plasmid did not carry the entire repertoire of available resistance genes.

The most recent report, however, confirms the presence of pan-antibiotic resistant microorganisms in the United States. An elderly female presented in Nevada with a wound infected with *Klebsiella pneumoniae* resistant to all 26 available antibiotics and died of septic shock 2 months after being admitted to the hospital.[6] She had a history of multiple hospital admissions in India (where bacteria expressing the *NDM-1* resistance gene are prevalent) related to a broken femur and osteomyelitis.

Although a major effort is being taken to prevent pan-antibiotic resistant infections from entering the United States and spreading from individual to individual, encountering these microorganisms more often should be expected. These highly dangerous infections will not be limited to bacteria. A case of pan-antibiotic resistant, opportunistic yeast, *Trichosporon dermatis*, was recently reported in the Netherlands.[7] The persistent infection was resistant to all conventional therapy and the individual died from multiorgan failure.

References

1. Gruber TM, et al: Pathogenicity of pan-drug-resistant *Serratia marcescens* harbouring *bla*$_{NDM-1}$. *J Antimicrob Chemother* 70(4):1026–1030, 2015.
2. Fernandes M, et al: Extensively and pan-drug resistant *Pseudomonas aeruginosa* keratitis: clinical features, risk factors, and outcome. *Graefes Arch Clin Exp Ophthalmol* 254(2):315–322, 2016.
3. Falgenhauer L, et al: Colistin resistance gene *mcr-1* in extended-spectrum β-lactamase-producing and carapenemase-producing Gram-negative bacteria in Germany. *Lancet Infect Dis* 16(3):282–283, 2016.
4. McGann P, et al: *Escherichia coli* harboring *mcr-1* and *bla*$_{CTX-M}$ on a novel IncF plasmid: first report of *mcr-1* in the United States. *Antimicrob Agents Chemother* 60(7):4420–4421, 2016.
5. Mediavilla JR, et al: Colistin- and carbapenem-resistant *Escherichia coli* harboring *mcr-1* and *bla*$_{NDM-5}$, causing a complicated urinary tract infection in a patient from the United States. *MBio* 7(4):2016.
6. Chen L, et al: Notes from the field: pan-resistant New Delhi metallo-beta-lactmase-producing *Klebsiella pneumoniae*-Washoe County, Nevada. *MMWR Morb Mortal Wkly Rep* 66(1):33–2017.
7. dos Santos CO, et al: Emerging pan-resistance in *Trichosporon* species: a case report. *BMC Infect Dis* 16:279, 2016.

aminoglycoside-modifying enzymes (AMEs), which acetylate and inactivate aminoglycoside.

Another major form of antibiotic resistance is caused by multi–drug-resistance transporters (MDRs). MDRs are members of a diverse and widely expressed family of transmembrane proteins that are designed to protect the cell by diminishing the rate of intracellular accumulation of antimicrobials by preventing entrance or, more commonly, increasing active efflux of the antibiotic. At least six different bacterial MDR families have been identified, with their genes also primarily carried on plasmids that can be transferred to other bacteria.[35] Expression of MDRs is not limited to bacteria; C. albicans uses multiple MDRs as efflux pumps for antibiotics. Individual MDRs are capable of transporting and simultaneously protecting microorganisms from several antibiotics (e.g., kanamycin, erythromycin, doxycycline).

Other methods of antibiotic resistance are less common, but still important in understanding the combination of protective mechanisms leading to multidrug resistance.[36] Antibiotics gain entrance to bacteria by passing through the cell wall. Resistance may result from sequestration or decreased uptake of the antibiotic. Thickened cell walls or biofilms trap antibiotics in the extracellular matrix to prevent access to bacteria. Decreased uptake also may result from modification of the cell wall; P. aeruginosa undergoes minor changes in cell wall chemistry and becomes resistant to the uptake of β-lactam antibiotics. Additional mechanisms protect the molecular target of particular antibiotics. The target may be altered by mutation or other means.

Genetic amplification and overproduction of the target molecule result in excessive numbers of targets and reduced antibiotic sensitivity (e.g., increased resistance to sulfonamides in some streptococci). Target bypass is a resistance mechanism resulting from switch from an antibiotic-sensitive metabolic to one that is more antibiotic resistant. Some bacteria have gained resistance to sulfonamide by converting from use of environmental para-aminobenzoic acid for conversion to folic acid, which is an antibiotic-sensitive step in nucleic acid synthesis, to the direct use of environmental folic acid. The target molecule also can be protected by novel bacterial proteins that block the antibiotic binding site. Multi–antibiotic resistance results from the simultaneous application of a combination of mechanisms. Methicillin-resistant Staphylococcus aureus (MRSA) caused an international healthcare crisis. Outside of the United States, MRSA accounts for 80% of S. aureus infections. MRSA produces a β-lactamase. Normally β-lactamase–resistant broad-spectrum antibiotics (e.g., methicillin) can be substituted. However, MRSA also carries an extra-chromosomal gene mecA for resistance to methicillin. The mecA gene encodes a penicillin-binding protein (PBP2a) with a lower affinity for β-lactams and, therefore, less sensitivity to inhibition by antibiotics. Resistance to aminoglycoside antibiotics is accomplished by expression of AMEs, production of excess para-aminobenzoic acid, and spontaneous mutation of rRNA with a lower affinity for antibiotics. Resistance to the glycopeptide antibiotic vancomycin is controlled by the gene vanA, which results in alterations in peptidoglycans and loss of the vancomycin-binding site. Antibiotic sequestration also occurs in the thick peptidoglycan layer and within biofilms. MRSA expresses four different classes of multi–drug-resistance transporters.[37] Fusidic acid, one of few drugs for MRSA, binds to the ribosome and prevents protein synthesis. Resistance results from small proteins that bind to the target and prevent interactions with the antibiotic.[38]

Multiple antibiotic resistance has appeared and can be related to overuse of antibiotics and not completing an antibiotic regimen. Overuse of antibiotics leads to the destruction of the normal microbiome, allowing the selective overgrowth of antibiotic-resistant strains or pathogens that had previously been kept under control. For example, treatment with clindamycin can compromise the normal intestinal microbiome allowing the overgrowth of C. difficile and the development of

pseudomembranous colitis. Lack of compliance in completing a therapeutic antibiotic regimen allows the selective resurgence of microorganisms that are more relatively resistant to the antibiotic.

With the development of multiple antibiotic–resistant strains, creativity in addressing this challenge must be rekindled. New antibiotics may solve a portion of the problem or may exacerbate it further as pathogens develop resistance to new antibiotics as well. Available antibiotics that prove to be no longer effective must be replaced with alternative forms of therapy, including the increased development and use of vaccines.

In that context, an old treatment has been revisited: the administration of lytic bacteriophages. Bacteriophages are viruses that specifically infect bacteria and, in the case of lytic phages, result in bacterial death and lysis. The advantages of bacteriophage therapy are numerous: cocktails of complementary phages can be used, phages can progressively infiltrate a biofilm that traps antibiotics, and phages can be genetically engineered to express enzymes that weaken the biofilm. Bacterial resistance to phages may occur related to alteration of phage receptors on the bacteria. However, this therapeutic agent clearly needs to be explored further and studies are in progress to test the effect of bacteriophage therapy on P. aeruginosa chronic lung infections.[39]

Active Immunization: Vaccines

Contracting and surviving an infectious disease is the most effective means of developing lifelong immunity against a particular pathogen. However, some infections cause a great deal of morbidity and mortality. The purpose of vaccination is to induce active immunologic protection before exposure to the risks of debilitating or fatal infection. For each vaccine an initial immunization protocol is developed to produce large numbers of memory cells and a sustained protective secondary immune response in the greatest number of individuals. Even under optimized protocols, vaccines are not completely protective. For every vaccine a small percentage of recipients do not produce a protective immune response, referred to as primary vaccine failure. Failure to induce an immune response occurs in about 10% of recipients of measles (rubeola), mumps, rubella, and hepatitis B vaccines, and inactivated influenza vaccine may only protect 30% to 40% of adults 65 or older.[40] A recently approved, high-dose injectable vaccine with four times the amount of influenza antigen is now recommended for increased protection of adults 65 or older.

In general, vaccine-induced protection does not persist as long as infection-induced immunity; thus booster injections may be necessary to maintain protection throughout life. Secondary vaccine failure results if appropriate booster immunizations are not administered. Many adults vaccinated against diseases that are more severe in childhood will not get routine boosters. Although not developing debilitating illness, they may become asymptomatic carriers and infect unvaccinated children. The CDC maintains the most current immunization schedules for people of all ages.

Mass vaccination programs have led to major changes in the health of the world's population.[41] For example global eradication of smallpox by 1979. In 1994 polio was declared officially eradicated in all the Americas. The goal of the WHO is to eradicate polio worldwide by 2022.

Rubella and congenital rubella syndrome were declared eliminated in the Americas in 2015, and in 2016 measles was eradicated. Although eliminated in the Americas, measles and rubella have not been eliminated elsewhere and infected visitors from other countries may transmit the infection to individuals who have not been vaccinated. A certain percentage of the population (usually about 85%, with a range of 75% to 99% depending on the particular microorganism) should be immunized in order to achieve protection of the total population, referred to as herd immunity. The principles of calculating herd immunity are based on several parameters: the number of susceptible individuals who may become infected in an unvaccinated population from an initial case, the time interval over which the infection may spread, and the effectiveness of the vaccine.

An individual infected with measles can infect 12 to 18 other individuals over about 2 weeks. If the desired level of herd immunity is not achieved, outbreaks of infection can occur. The WHO declared that measles was eradicated in the United States in 2000, and many parents became either complacent or resistant to immunization. This resulted in at least 23 outbreaks of measles in 2014 triggered by exposure to infected visitors to the United States or travel by U.S. citizens to areas where measles was still endemic. Most of the infected individuals had no history of immunization and the required level of herd immunity had not been maintained.[42] The incidence of pertussis (whooping cough) in the United States has also reflected resistance to vaccination. In 2004, 32 pertussis outbreaks were published; analysis of 8 of these found that 59% to 93% of infected individuals were intentionally not vaccinated. Immunization programs in several European countries have been disrupted by anti–vaccine groups. As a result, the incidence of pertussis increased by 10 to 100 times compared with neighboring countries that maintained a high incidence of immunization.

Resistance to routine vaccination has arisen for many reasons, particularly potential vaccine dangers. As with any medicine, complications can arise, including pain and redness at the injection site, fever, allergic reactions to vaccine ingredients, infection associated with attenuated viruses in immunodeficient individuals, and others. Additionally, some individuals in the United States and Europe became concerned that vaccines, particularly those containing the preservative thimerosal, induced autism in children. Thimerosal is a mercury-containing compound that has been used as a preservative since the 1930s. Multiple studies concluded that neither vaccines nor thimerosal was associated with the onset of autism.[43,44] The debate related to thimerosal and many other environmental chemicals to autism is still under investigation.[45,46] Although no cases of mercury toxicity have been reported secondary to vaccination, thimerosal was removed from all vaccines by 2001 with the exception of inactivated influenza vaccines.

Development of a successful vaccine depends on many factors. These include characterizing the desired protective immune response (e.g., antibody, T cell), identifying the appropriate antigen to induce that response (i.e., immune responses against some antigens on an infectious agent are ineffective or even increase the risk for infection), determining the most effective route of administration (e.g., injected, oral, inhaled), optimizing the number and timing of vaccine doses to induce protective immunity in a large proportion of the at-risk population, and deciding the most effective, yet safe, form in which to administer the vaccine. For instance, most vaccines against viral infections (e.g., measles, mumps, rubella, *Varicella zoster* [chickenpox], yellow fever) contain live viruses that are weakened (**attenuated**) to continue expressing the appropriate antigens but are unable to establish more than a limited and easily controlled infection. The limited proliferative capacity of attenuated live viruses appears to afford better long-term protection than using purified viral antigen. Exceptions are the vaccines against hepatitis B, which uses a recombinant viral protein, and hepatitis A, which is an inactivated (killed) virus.

Even attenuated viruses can, however, establish life-threatening infections in vaccine recipients whose immune system is congenitally deficient or suppressed (see Chapter 9). Two different vaccines were developed against polio. The Sabin vaccine is an attenuated virus that is administered orally (oral polio vaccine [OPV]). It provides systemic protection and induces a secretory immune response to prevent growth of the poliovirus in the intestinal tract. The live attenuated vaccine causes polio in some children who have unsuspected immune deficiencies (about 1 case in 2.4 million doses). The Salk vaccine is a completely

inactivated virus administered by injection (inactivated polio vaccine [IPV]). It induces protective systemic immunity but does not provide adequate secretory immunity. Therefore even if the individual is protected from systemic infection the "wild-type" poliovirus can transiently infect the intestinal mucosa, be shed, and spread to others. For example, when polio was epidemic, the live oral vaccine was preferred; however, about eight cases of paralytic polio per year in the United States result from the vaccine strain proliferating in individuals with inadequate immune systems. As a result, the CDC currently recommends vaccination with the killed virus.

Some common bacterial vaccines are killed microorganisms or extracts of bacterial antigens. *S. pneumoniae* (pneumococcus) is a major cause of pneumonia, particularly in the young and adults with compromised lung function secondary to smoking, asthma, and other lung diseases. Of the more than 90 known strains of this microorganism, only a few cause the most severe illnesses. The current vaccines against pneumococcal pneumonia consist of a mixture of capsular polysaccharides. The conjugated vaccine is recommended for young children in whom the pure polysaccharide vaccine is not very immunogenic. A similar vaccine is available for *H. influenzae* type B (Hib), which is a cause of pneumonia and meningitis in children.

Some bacterial diseases are caused by potent bacterial toxins that act locally or systemically. These include diphtheria, cholera, and tetanus. Vaccination against the toxins is achieved using **toxoids**—purified toxins that have been chemically detoxified without loss of immunogenicity. Pertussis (whooping cough) vaccine was changed from a killed whole cell vaccine to an acellular vaccine that contained the pertussis toxin and additional bacterial antigens.

With so many available vaccines there has been an effort to mix vaccines in order to minimize the number of required injections. An example is DPT, now usually contains diphtheria (D) and tetanus (T) toxoids and acellular pertussis vaccine (aP). More recent mixtures include DTaP mixed with inactivated poliovirus, hepatitis B vaccine, or *H. influenzae* antigen or a mixture of these.

Passive Immunotherapy

Passive immunotherapy is a form of countermeasure against pathogens in which preformed antibodies are given to the individual. This form of therapy has been used for decades. Horse serum that contained antibodies was used to treat diphtheria, pneumococcal pneumonia, tetanus, and other diseases in the early twentieth century. However, because of foreign proteins in the serum, many individuals developed an immune reaction against the horse proteins and an immune complex–mediated serum sickness. Passive immunotherapy with human immunoglobulin has been approved for several infections, including hepatitis B and hepatitis A. Treatment of potential rabies infection after a bite combines passive and active immunization. The rabies virus proliferates very slowly. Individuals who have been bitten receive a one-time injection with human rabies immune globulin to further slow viral proliferation, followed by multiple injections with a killed viral vaccine to induce greater protective immunity.

A recent example of passive immunotherapy is the 2014 to 2016 outbreak of Ebola virus in West Africa, the largest outbreak of Ebola infection ever observed: 28,616 cases with 11,310 fatalities (a 40% mortality rate). No vaccine was available. An experimental mixture of monoclonal antibodies against the virus rapidly increased circulating antibody titers and diminished viral load by more than eightfold.[47]

In the past, vaccines and therapeutic antibodies were developed for only the deadliest pathogens. With the increase in antibiotic-resistant microorganisms, the development and widespread use of new vaccines and passively administered antibodies against these microorganisms must be considered.

SUMMARY REVIEW

Emerging Infections

1. Emergence of previously unknown infections, reemergence of old infections thought to be controlled, and the development of infections resistant to multiple antibiotics or vaccination are significant causes of death and morbidity.

Microorganisms and Humans: A Dynamic Relationship

1. The human body is a hospitable site for microorganisms to grow and flourish. These microorganisms make up the *normal microbiome* of the body.
2. The beneficial homeostasis between humans and microorganisms is maintained through the physical integrity of the gut and other mechanisms that sequester these microorganisms on the mucosal surface.
3. The symbiotic relationship with the normal microbiome can be altered by injury, compromising protective barriers including the skin and mucous membranes.

Microorganisms and Infections

1. Clinical infectious disease occurs in four distinct stages: (1) incubation period, (2) prodromal state, (3) invasion period, and (4) convalescence.
2. The hallmark of most infectious diseases is fever. Body temperature is regulated at a higher than normal level.
3. Several factors influence the capacity of a pathogen to cause disease, including communicability, immunogenicity, infectivity, mechanisms of action, pathogenicity, entry portal, toxigenicity, and virulence.
4. Infectious diseases also are classified by their prevalence and spread as endemic, epidemic, and pandemic.
5. The process of infection includes colonization, invasion, multiplication, and dissemination.
6. When an individual's immune system is deficient, the person can become infected with opportunistic infections.
7. True pathogens in adequate numbers can circumvent an individual's defenses and directly cause infection.
8. Infectious microorganisms usually exist in reservoirs (e.g., contaminated soil, contaminated water or food, breast milk), animals, or another human.
9. Direct transmission of pathogens can occur by direct physical contact, ingestion or inhalation, or placental transfer.
10. *Indirect transmission* occurs from contact with contaminated materials, which can range from towels to food or through a vector.
11. As part of colonization, the microorganism stabilizes the adherence to tissue through surface receptors and can then invade surrounding tissue.
12. Because tissue is warm and nutrient rich, most microorganisms undergo *rapid* multiplication. Viral pathogens replicate within infected cells, and some bacteria are intracellular pathogens and replicate in macrophages and other cells.
13. Successful spreading requires a variety of virulence factors, including adhesion molecules, toxins, and the ability to evade immunity.
14. Mixed species of microorganisms can come together and form slimy biofilms and anchor themselves to various surfaces and resist immune defenses.
15. Stable colonization of bacteria requires adhesion. Many bacteria attach through pili (fimbriae), surface glycoproteins, or complement-related receptors.
16. Invasion results in direct confrontation with an individual's defense mechanisms, including complement, antibodies, and phagocytes (neutrophils, macrophages). Evasion of these defenses can result in bacteremia or viremia or fungemia and sepsis.

17. Bacteria can protect against phagocytosis by producing toxins that destroy phagocytic cells and extracellular enzymes that digest complement, clotting factors, immunoglobulins, cytokines, and antimicrobial peptides and promote extracellular spreading.
18. Classes of infectious microorganisms include bacterial, fungal, parasitic, protozoal, and viral.
19. Bacteria are divided into several groups—"true bacteria," filamentous, spirochetes, mycoplasma, rickettsia, and chlamydia—and can be categorized as gram negative or gram positive.
20. Many bacteria have specialized surface structures such as pili and flagella that promote adhesion and tissue invasion.
21. Bacteria can produce a variety of toxic molecules that may kill the individual's cells, disrupt tissue, and protect the individual against inflammation.
22. Exotoxins are released by bacteria during bacterial growth and can damage cell membranes, activate second messengers, and inhibit protein synthesis.
23. Endotoxins are contained in the cell walls of gram-negative bacteria and released during lysis of the bacteria. Bacteria that produce endotoxins are called *pyrogenic bacteria* because they activate inflammation and produce fever. They also can activate the coagulation cascade and release cachectin (TNF).
24. Inflammatory and immune responses to infection can cause tissue damage through excessive production of inflammatory cytokines, excessive activation of antibodies, and infiltration of T cells, macrophages, and neutrophils.
25. Other self-protective mechanisms for bacteria and other pathogens include degradation of immune molecules, neutralization of immune molecules, complement evasion, immune suppression, and escape from the phagosome.
26. Some bacteria (and viruses) proliferate more rapidly than the development of immune defenses causing severe clinical disease.
27. Some bacteria (like viruses) evade immune defenses by surviving inside immune cells.
28. Some bacteria can coat the Fc portion of an individual's antibody, preventing complement activation or phagocytosis.
29. Antigenic variation allows pathogens to alter surface molecules that express antigens that are the targets of protective immune responses. The pathogen thus becomes resistant.
30. Some bacteria can release molecules that bind to and neutralize antibody or form immune complexes that deposit in tissue, causing damage.
31. Some bacteria can degrade immunoglobulins or components of the complement system.
32. Some bacteria can suppress immune responses that block T cells or impair the signals in the inflammatory response or interfere with antigen processing and presentation.
33. *S. aureus* has numerous virulence factors that promote invasive infection. It has become a major cause of hospital-acquired (nosocomial) infections and antibiotic resistance.
34. Fungal infection is called *mycosis*. Most pathologic fungi are from the environment and transmitted by human-to-human contact, inhalation, or contamination of wounds.
35. Fungi have polysaccharide surface molecules that promote adhesion to epithelial tissue.
36. Fungi can produce toxins that promote infection, evade immune responses, or cause cancer (aflatoxins).
37. Some fungi secrete enzymes that damage tissue and initiate pathogenic inflammatory responses including hypersensitivity reactions.
38. Some fungi can survive in phagocytes and resist lysosomal destruction.

▍SUMMARY REVIEW—cont'd

39. *C. albicans* is the most common cause of fungal infections in humans. It resides in the skin, gastrointestinal tract, mouth, and vagina. Local defense mechanisms, including members of the bacterial microbiome, produce antifungal agents. The infection remains localized in individuals with an intact immune system.

40. Parasitic organisms establish a symbiosis with another species, whereby the parasite benefits. They range from unicellular protozoa to large worms.

41. Parasites adhere to and break down connective tissue and basement membranes allowing penetration and entry to the circulatory system.

42. Some parasites only reproduce within host cells (obligatory intracellular parasites).

43. Some parasites evade immune defenses by secreting cytotoxic molecules or by antigenic variation.

44. Malaria is one of the most common infections worldwide. It is transmitted through the bite of an infected *Anopheles* mosquito. The parasite *(Plasmodium)* enters the bloodstream, survives in the liver, and invades parenchymal cells. After several rounds of division, the liver cell ruptures and thousands of parasites enter the blood, infecting red blood cells.

45. Viruses are intracellular microorganisms. The viral life cycle is completely intracellular and involves several stages: attachment, penetration, uncoating, replication, assembly, and release of new virions.

46. Viruses are classified by the format of nucleic acid in the virion, (RNA or DNA and either single-stranded [ss] or double-stranded [ds]), and by whether the virus uses the enzyme reverse transcriptase (RT) for replication.

47. Successful viruses use a variety of mechanisms for bypassing immune rejection, including rapid division, intracellular survival, coating with self-proteins, antigenic variation, neutralization, complement evasion, and immune suppression.

48. Viruses inside the infected cell have several harmful effects, including inhibition of DNA, RNA, or protein synthesis; disruption of lysosomal membranes, resulting in lytic enzyme release; promotion of cell apoptosis; fusion of adjacent cells (i.e., giant cells); transformation into a neoplastic cell; and alteration of antigenic properties (i.e., decreasing immune effectiveness).

49. An example of viral infection is influenza, an ssRNA virus transmitted through aerosol and body fluids, and there are several variant forms. Influenza viruses undergo antigen shifts allowing them to evade protection from vaccines.

Human Immunodeficiency Virus and Acquired Immunodeficiency Syndrome

1. AIDS is a viral disease caused by HIV.

2. HIV infects and depletes a portion of the immune system (Th cells), making individuals susceptible to life-threatening infections and malignancies.

3. HIV/AIDS remains a major cause of death worldwide.

4. Aggressive antiretroviral therapy and public health campaigns have stabilized the number of new cases and deaths in the United States from HIV/AIDS and other parts of the world where there is access to therapy.

5. HIV is a blood-borne pathogen present in body fluids with typical routes of transmission: blood or blood products, intravenous drug abuse, heterosexual and homosexual activity, and maternal-child transmission before or during birth.

6. The primary surface receptor on HIV is the envelope glycoprotein gp120, which binds to the CD4 molecule found mostly on the surface of T-helper cells. Several other important co-receptors have been identified.

7. HIV is a member of the *retrovirus* family, which carries genetic information in the form of RNA. An enzyme, reverse transcriptase (RT), converts RNA into a double-stranded DNA. Another enzyme, an *integrase,* inserts the new DNA into the infected cell's genetic material. On activation, translation of the viral information may be initiated, forming new virions, resulting in lysis and death of the infected cell, and shedding infectious HIV particles.

8. The major immunologic finding in AIDS is the striking decrease in the number of CD4+ Th cells.

9. The presence of circulating antibody against HIV indicates infection by the virus, although many individuals are asymptomatic.

10. The current treatment for HIV infection is a combination of drugs called highly active antiretroviral therapy (HAART) that attacks different portions of the viral replication pathway.

11. Mother-to-child transmission has been reduced to 1% with prenatal treatment of HIV infection.

12. Neonates become HIV infected by placental transmission or through breast-feeding.

13. Children with HIV are at increased risk of coronary artery disease.

Countermeasures Against Pathogens

1. Effective means of countering infectious microorganisms are rigorous use of environmental infection control measures, including control of insect vector populations, establishment of modern sanitation facilities, and provision of clean water and uncontaminated food supplies. Prophylactic or interventive procedures include vaccines and antimicrobials.

2. Passive immunotherapy has been effective using previously formed human immunoglobulin for diseases such as hepatitides A and B, rabies, and ebola.

3. With antibiotic-resistant pathogens, a greater emphasis is placed on the development of new vaccines.

▍KEY TERMS

Acquired immunodeficiency syndrome (AIDS), 311
Aminoglycoside-modifying enzymes (AMEs), 318
Antibiotic resistance, 316
Antigenic drift, 310
Antigenic shift, 310
Antigenic variation, 299
Attenuated, 319
Bacteremia, 293

Bactericidal, 316
Bacteriophages, 318
Bacteriostatic, 316
β-Lactamase, 317
Biofilms, 292
Capsule, 299
Dimorphic, 301
Endogenous pyrogen, 291

Endotoxic shock (septic shock), 296
Endotoxin, 296
Exogenous pyrogen, 291
Exotoxin, 293
Fever, 291
Fungemia, 293
Gene switching, 305
Highly active antiretroviral therapy (HAART), 313

KEY TERMS—cont'd

Human immunodeficiency virus (HIV), 290
IgA protease, 299
Integrase, 312
Lipopolysaccharide (LPS), 296
Methicillin-resistant *Staphylococcus aureus*
    (MRSA), 318
Mold, 301

Multi–drug-resistance transporters (MDRs), 318
Mycosis, 301
Obligatory intracellular parasites, 304
Passive immunotherapy, 319
Pili (fimbriae), 293
Reverse transcriptase, 312
Sepsis, 289

Septicemia, 293
Tissue tropism, 292
Toxoid, 319
Viremia, 293
Yeast, 301
Zoonotic infection, 290

REFERENCES

1. Kochanek KD, et al: Deaths: final data for 2014. *National Vital Stat Rep* 65(4):1–122, 2016.
2. World Health Organization (WHO): *The top 10 causes of death, fact sheet #310*. Updated May 2014. http://www.who.int/mediacentre/factsheets/fs310/en/index.html.
3. Guan Y, Drosten C: Editorial overview: emerging viruses: interspecies transmission. *Curr Opin Virol* 16:v–vi, 2016.
4. World Health Organization (WHO): *Report of the workshop on prioritization of pathogens, 8-9 December 2015*, Geneva, 2015, Author. http://www.who.int/csr/research-and-development/meeting-report-prioritization.pdf.
5. National Institute of Allergy and Infectious Diseases: *West Nile virus*. https://www.niaid.nih.gov/diseases-conditions/west-nile-virus.
6. Centers for Disease Control and Prevention (CDC): *National notifiable diseases surveillance system fact sheet*. https://www.cdc.gov/nndss/document/NNDSS-Fact-Sheet.pdf.
7. Flemming H-C, et al: Biofilms: an emergent form of bacterial life. *Nat Rev Microbiol* 14(9):563–575, 2016.
8. Liu W, et al: Interspecific bacteria interactions are reflected in multispecies biofilm spatial organization. *Front Microbiol* 7(1366):1–8, 2016.
9. Moorthy S, Keklak J, Klein EA: Perspective: adhesion mediated signal transduction in bacterial pathogens. *Pathogens* 5(23):1–8, 2016.
10. Dal Peraro M, van der Goot FG: Pore-forming toxins: ancient, but never really out of fashion. *Nat Rev Microbiol* 14(2):77–92, 2016.
11. Di Bella S, et al: *Clostridium difficile* toxins A and B: insights into pathogenic properties and extraintestinal effects. *Toxins (Basel)* 8(5):1–25, 2016.
12. Chan YS, Ng TB: Shiga toxins: from structure and mechanism to applications. *Appl Microbiol Biotechnol* 100(4):1597–1610, 2016.
13. Jarocki VM, Tacchi JL, Djordjevic SP: Non-proteolytic functions of microbial proteases increase pathological complexity. *Proteomics* 15(5-6):1075–1088, 2015.
14. Pizarro-Cerdá J, et al: Manipulation of host membranes by bacterial pathogens *Listeria, Francisella, Shigella* and *Yersinia*. *Semin Cell Dev Biol* 60:155–167, 2016.
15. Doorduijn DJ, et al: Complement resistance mechanisms of *Klebsiella pneumoniae*. *Immunobiology* 221(10):1102–1109, 2016.
16. Larussa T, et al: *Helicobacter pylori* and T helper cells: mechanisms of immune escape and tolerance. *J Immunol Res* 2015:981328, 2015.
17. Moyes DL, et al: Candidalysin is a fungal peptide toxin critical for mucosal infection. *Nature* 532:64–68, 2016.
18. Reference deleted in pages.
19. Reference deleted in pages.
20. Cliffe AR, Wilson AC: Restarting lytic gene transcription at the onset of herpes simplex virus reactivation. *J Virol* 91(2):2017.
21. Kagaayi J, Serwadda D: The history of the HIV/AIDS epidemic in Africa. *Curr HIV/AIDS Rep* 13(4):187–193, 2016.
22. Worobey M, et al: 1970s and 'Patient 0' HIV-1 genomes illuminate early HIV/AIDS history in North America. *Nature* 539(7627):98–101, 2016.
23. Centers for Disease Control and Prevention (CDC): *Pneumocystis* pneumonia – Los Angeles. *MMWR Morb Mortal Wkly Rep* 30(21):250–252, 1981.
24. Centers for Disease Control and Prevention (CDC): Kaposi's sarcoma and *Pneumocystis* pneumonia among homosexual men – New York City and California. *MMWR Morb Mortal Wkly Rep* 30(25):305–308, 1981.
25. Centers for Disease Control and Prevention (CDC): *HIV in the United States: at a glance*. Updated Oct 22, 2016. https://www.cdc.gov/hiv/statistics/overview/ataglance.html.
26. Barre-Sinoussi F, et al: Isolation of a T-lymphotropic retrovirus from a patient at risk for acquired immune deficiency syndrome (AIDS). *Science* 220(4599):868–871, 1983.
27. Smith C, McFarland EJ: Update on pediatric human immunodeficiency virus infection. *Adv Pediatr* 63(1):147–171, 2016.
28. Selik RM, et al: Revised surveillance case definition for HIV infection–United States, 2014. *MMWR Morb Mortal Wkly Rep* 63(RR03):1–10, 2014.
29. Cihlar T, Fordyce M: Current status and prospects of HIV treatment. *Curr Opin Virol* 18:50–56, 2016.
30. Kaplan-Lewis E, Aberg JA, Lee M: Arterosclerotic cardiovascular disease and anti-retroviral therapy. *Curr HIV/AIDS Rep* 13(5):297–308, 2016.
31. Churchill MJ, et al: HIV reservoirs: what, where and how to target them. *Nat Rev Microbiol* 14(1):55–60, 2016.
32. Haynes BF, et al: HIV-host interactions: implications for vaccine design. *Cell Host Microbe* 19(3):292–303, 2016.
33. Perry J, Waglechner N, Wright G: The prehistory of antibiotic resistance. *Cold Spring Harb Perspect Med* 6(6):1–8, 2016.
34. Centers for Disease Control and Prevention (CDC): *Antibiotic resistance threats in the United States, 2013*, Atlanta, GA, 2013, Author, pp 1–113. https://www.cdc.gov/drugresistance/pdf/ar-threats-2013-508.pdf.
35. Mousa JJ, Bruner SD: Structural and mechanistic diversity of multidrug transporters. *Nat Prod Rep* 33(11):1255–1267, 2016.
36. Yilmaz Ç, Özcengiz G: Antibiotics: pharmacokinetics, toxicity, resistance and multidrug efflux. *Biochem Pharmacol* 133:43–62, 2017.
37. Jang S: Multidrug efflux pumps in *Staphylococcus aureus* and their clinical implications. *J Microbiol* 54(1):1–8, 2016.
38. Tomlinson JH, et al: A target-protection mechanism of antibiotic resistance at atomic resolution: insights into FusB-type fusidic acid resistance. *Sci Rep* 6:19524, 2016.
39. Darch SE, Kragh KN, Abbott EA, et al: Phage inhibit pathogen dissemination by targeting bacterial migrants in a chronic infection model. *M Bio* 4;8(2):e00240, 2017.
40. Poland GA, et al: Vaccinology in the third millennium: scientific and social challenges. *Curr Opin Virol* 17:116–125, 2016.
41. Hussein IH, et al: Vaccines through centuries: major cornerstones of global health. *Front Public Health* 3:269, 2015.
42. Phadke VK, et al: Association between vaccine refusal and vaccine-preventable diseases in the United States: a review of measles and pertussis. *JAMA* 315(11):1149–1158, 2016.
43. DeStefano F, Price CS, Weintraub ES: Increasing exposure to antibody-stimulating proteins and polysaccharides in vaccines is not associated with risk of autism. *J Pediatr* 163(2):561–567, 2013.
44. Taylor LE, Swerdfeger AL, Eslick GD: Vaccines are not associated with autism: an evidence-based meta-analysis of case-control and cohort studies. *Vaccine* 32(29):3623–3629, 2014.
45. Geier DA, et al: Thimerosal: clinical, epidemiologic and biochemical studies. *Clin Chim Acta* 444(1):212–220, 2015.
46. Kalkbrenner AE, Schmidt RJ, Penlesky AC: Environmental chemical exposures and autism spectrum disorders: a review of the epidemiological evidence. *Curr Probl Pediatr Adolesc Health Care* 44(10):277–318, 2014.
47. Zeitlin L, et al: Antibody therapeutics for Ebola virus disease. *Curr Opin Virol* 17(1):45–49, 2016.

Stress and Disease

Lorey K. Takahashi, Kathryn L. McCance, Margaret F. Clayton

evolve WEBSITE

http://evolve.elsevier.com/McCance/

- Content Updates
- Chapter Summary Review
- Review Questions
- Case Studies
- Animations

CHAPTER OUTLINE

To observe the obvious, modern society is full of stress. As a culture, Westerners are champions of the work ethic, a Protestant philosophy originating in the sixteenth century that views idleness as taboo. Stressful experiences include daily hassles, major life events (e.g., loss of loved one, life-threatening illness, loss of job), social isolation, early-life social deprivation, abuse, trauma, work-related stress, work-life balance, low-socioeconomic status (SES), and many other events. For example, the pressure to remain in contact despite illness, travel, vacation, and other events that used to provide socially acceptable temporary absences is now customary in the American, and indeed global, culture. When added to other well-identified stressors, such as financial problems, the individual may suffer and develop symptoms that reflect the so-called *stress-related disorders.*

When thinking about stress, one must consider the factors producing a perception of stress, which begin when the brain perceives a stimulus as stressful and then, in turn, promote adaptational and survival-related physiologic responses. However, when the psychologic perception of environmental demand exceeds the adaptive capacity of the individual to cope, stress may lead to negative affective and health-related disease states.[1,2] Another way to think about stress involves the short- or long-term consequences of stress. Today, most researchers consider acute stress to be immunoenhancing (protective) whereas chronic, unremitting stress is thought to be immunosuppressive (destructive).[1,2] A variety of adverse life circumstances affects the pool of circulating leukocytes, involves transcription with increased expression of genes that promote inflammation, and decreased expression of genes that promote antiviral responses.[3] Chronic inflammation contributes to many diseases and drives contemporary morbidity and mortality.

HISTORICAL BACKGROUND AND GENERAL CONCEPTS

Walter B. Cannon used the term *stress* to encompass both physiologic and psychologic ideas as early as 1914.[4] He applied the engineering concept of stress and strain in a physiologic context and believed that emotional stimuli also were capable of causing stress. In 1946 Hans Selye popularized these same findings, viewing stress as a biologic phenomenon.[5] Originally, Selye inadvertently discovered the biologic syndrome of stress while he was attempting to discover a new sex hormone by injecting crude ovarian extracts into rats.[5] He repeatedly found that three structural changes occurred: (1) enlargement of the cortex of the adrenal gland, (2) atrophy of the thymus gland and other lymphoid structures, and (3) development of bleeding ulcers in the stomach and duodenal lining. Selye soon discovered that these manifestations were not specific to injected ovarian extracts but also occurred after he exposed the rats to other noxious stimuli, such as cold, surgical injury, and restraint. He called these stimuli *stressors.* Selye concluded that this triad or syndrome of manifestations represented a nonspecific response to noxious stimuli, naming it the **general adaptation syndrome (GAS).** He identified the three following successive stages of the GAS: (1) the alarm stage or

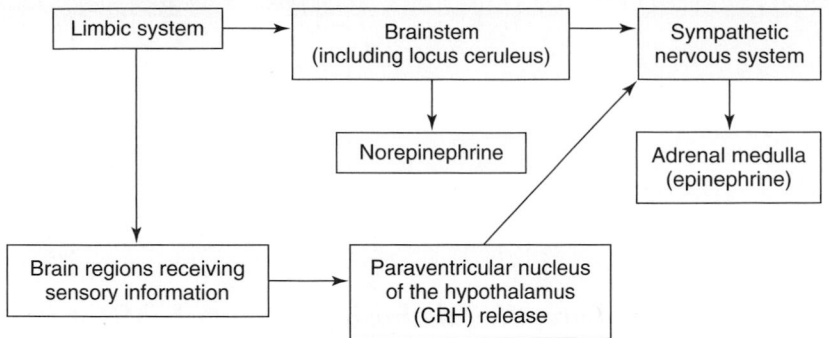

FIGURE 11.1 Neural Recognition and Response to Real or Predicted Stressors. *CRH*, Corticotrophin-releasing hormone.

reaction, in which the central nervous system (CNS) is aroused and the body's defenses are mobilized (e.g., "fight or flight") (Fig. 11.1); (2) the stage of resistance or adaptation, during which mobilization contributes to "fight or flight"; and (3) the stage of exhaustion, where continuous stress causes the progressive breakdown of compensatory mechanisms (acquired adaptations) and homeostasis. Exhaustion marks the onset of certain diseases (diseases of adaptation).

Initially one becomes alarmed by a stressor that activates the hypothalamus and sympathetic nervous system (see Figs. 11.1 and 11.2). The resistance or adaptation phase begins with the actions of the hormones cortisol, norepinephrine, and epinephrine. Exhaustion (also known as allostatic overload; discussed later) occurs if stress continues and adaptation is not successful, ultimately causing impairment of the immune response, heart failure, and kidney failure, leading to death.

From a physiologic perspective, what is emerging across the disciplines involved—molecular biology, immunology, neurology, endocrinology, and behavioral science—is a more holistic and complex model that involves biochemical relationships of the CNS, autonomic nervous system (ANS), the hypothalamic-pituitary-adrenal (HPA) axis (Fig. 11.3), and the immune system that causes the stress responses identified by Selye.

CONCEPTS OF STRESS, HOMEOSTASIS, AND ALLOSTASIS

Selye believed that stressors cause a general or nonspecific response. However, research in the past 50 years has shown the remarkable sensitivity of the central nervous system and endocrine system to psychologic influences (emotion is included as a psychologic factor that modulates social stress). Thus, although Selye's identification of the GAS is regarded as tremendously important and the cornerstone of stress research, the idea that stress is a purely physiologic response is vastly oversimplified. In the mid-1950s, studies showed that activation of the adrenal cortex occurred in humans in response to psychologic stressors,[6] in monkeys with conditioned emotional responses,[7] and in humans subjected to a stressful interview technique.[8] In the early 1960s, researchers found that plasma cortisol levels increased in groups of subjects exposed to war movies and decreased while they viewed Disney nature films.[9,10] Mason later demonstrated that the initiation of the GAS depended on psychologic factors surrounding the stressors.[11] He also showed that various factors, such as degrees of discomfort or unpleasantness or the suddenness of the stress, could account for the presence or absence of physiologic stress responses.[11]

Although the term *stress* was used by many disciplines and with numerous disagreements over its definition, in recent years, stress was defined as a *transactional* or *interactional concept*. Transactionally, stress

is viewed as the state of affairs arising when a person relates to (i.e., interacts or transacts with) situations in certain ways. People are not disturbed by situations per se but by the ways they appraise and react to situations. In general, a person experiences stress when a demand *exceeds* a person's coping abilities, resulting in reactions such as disturbances of cognition, emotion, and behavior that can adversely affect well-being. Moreover, psychologic stressors can elicit reactive or anticipatory stress responses. The reactive response is a physiologic response derived from psychologic stressors. For example, the stress of an examination may produce an increased heart rate and dry mouth in the unprepared student. The anticipatory response occurs when physiologic responses develop in anticipation of disruption of the optimal steady-state, also known as homeostasis. These anticipatory responses can be generated either by species-specific innate programs, such as reacting to the presence of predators and unfamiliar situations, or by experience-dependent memory programs created by conditioning.[12] Anticipatory responses are learned responses under fine control by regions located in the brain regions most frequently associated with learning and memory and include the hippocampus, amygdala, and prefrontal cortex. In order for these regions to elicit a stress response, the paraventricular nucleus (PVN) of the hypothalamus must be stimulated. These brain structures interact with the PVN through intermediary neurons, some of which are primarily used for the reactive response.

In a conditional response one learns that specific stimuli (i.e., objects or situational context) are associated with danger, and as such anticipation of subsequent encounters with the stimulus produces a physiologic stress response. For example, a child abused by a parent may experience a physiologic stress response in anticipation of further abuse when the parent enters the room. Under some circumstances these memory programs may become so strong that psychologic disorders, such as phobias, develop. In a similar fashion, some persons develop posttraumatic stress disorder (PTSD) in response to the memory, as opposed to the anticipation of traumatic events. PTSD is characterized by flashback memories, sleep disturbances, depression, and other symptoms. These symptoms have the potential to greatly compromise normal activities, such as employment, personal relationships, and quality of life. Today, evidence implicates stress as a precipitating factor across a range of diseases and health conditions. The term allostasis, as opposed to *homeostasis*, is currently used in stress research as a better way to understand how stress influences the development of disease. Unlike having a set point and physiologic equilibrium in Selye's homeostasis view of physiologic stress systems, the allostasis view proposes that physiologic systems are dynamic and capable of changing set-points after exposure to stress. This change in physiologic set point (e.g., chronic stress–induced elevation in cortisol secretion) may be the

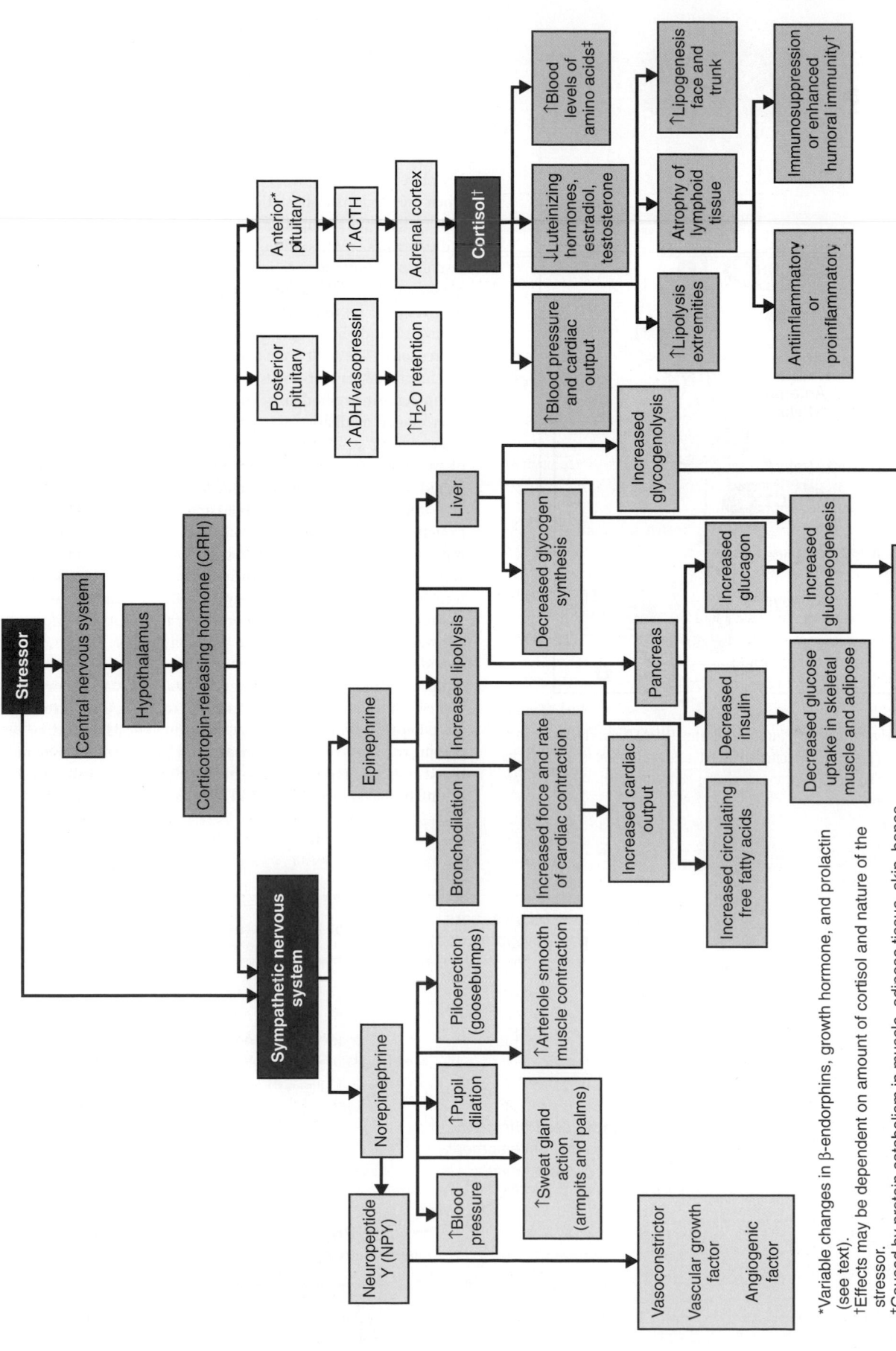

FIGURE 11.2 The Stress Response.

*Variable changes in β-endorphins, growth hormone, and prolactin (see text).

†Effects may be dependent on amount of cortisol and nature of the stressor.

‡Caused by protein catabolism in muscle, adipose tissue, skin, bones, and lymphoid tissue.

ADH, Antidiuretic hormone; *ACTH,* adrenocorticotropic hormone.

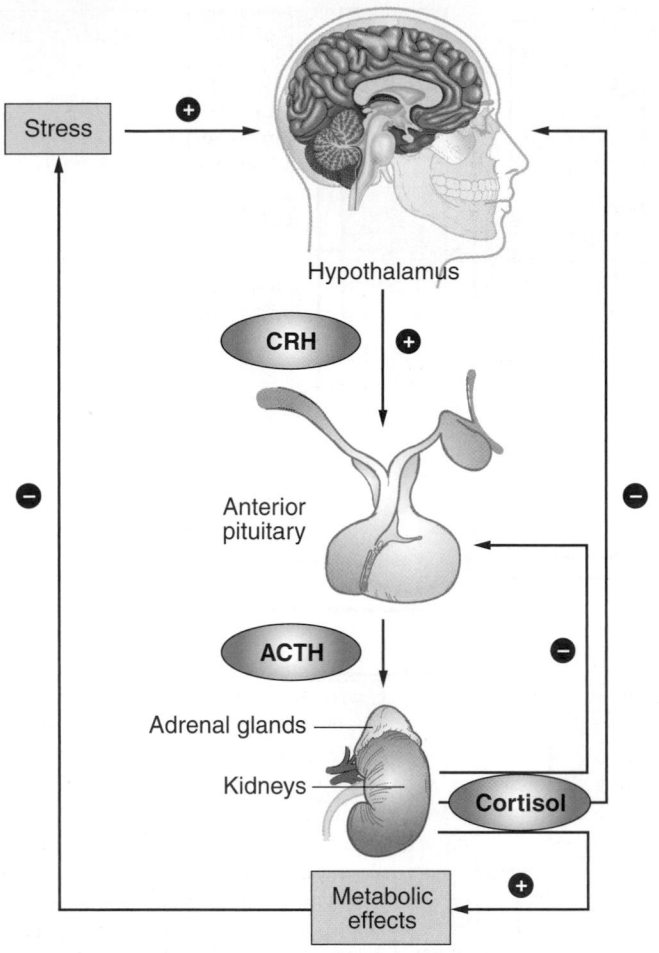

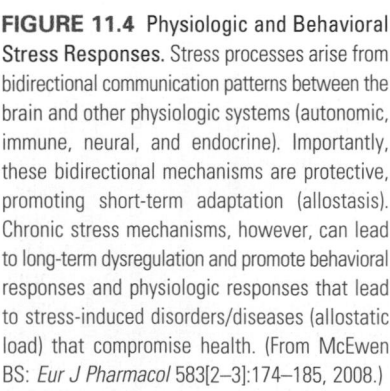

FIGURE 11.3 Hypothalamic-Pituitary-Adrenal (HPA) Axis. The response to stress begins in the brain. The hypothalamus is the control center in the brain for many hormones including corticotropin-releasing hormone (CRH). *ACTH,* Adreno-corticotropic hormone.

culprit underlying pathophysiologic conditions. Allostatic load (Fig. 11.4) is the individualized cumulative effects of stressors that exist in people's lives and influence their physiologic responses. Allostatic load may result from a vulnerable physiologic/genetic makeup, lifestyle (including damaging health behaviors), daily stressful encounters, and extraordinary events (such as disasters).[2,13] Over time this load exacts a toll on people's bodies (i.e., "wear and tear"). Because the brain is a key player in deciding what is stressful, it is influential in determining when they feel toxic allostatic overload. Under conditions of allostatic overload, the parasympathetic system may decrease its restraint of the sympathetic system, resulting in increased or prolonged inflammatory responses.[2,14] Furthermore, in response to acute and chronic stress some regions of the brain (the hippocampus, amygdala, and prefrontal cortex) may respond by undergoing structural remodeling, which can alter behavioral and physiologic responses (such as cognitive impairment or depression).[2] The adult brain and the developing brain possess structural and functional plasticity in response to stress, including neuronal replacement, dendritic remodeling, and synapse turnover.[15] Many intra- and intercellular mediators and processes are involved in changing the brain during stress and recovery from stress experiences. Examples of molecules that are necessary or permissive for brain remodeling include brain-derived neurotrophic factor (BDNF), tissue plasminogen activator (tPA), corticotropin releasing hormone (CRH), the secreted protein Lipocalin-2, and endocannabinoids (eCBs).[16] Stress causes an imbalance of neural circuitry that serves cognition, decision-making, and anxiety and mood that can disrupt behavioral states.[16] The imbalance can then affect systemic physiology through neuroendocrine, autonomic, immune, and metabolic mediators.[16] Key mediators and biomarkers of allostatic overload (exaggerated pathophysiologic responses to stress) include the glucocorticoid cortisol, catecholamines (released from sympathetic nervous system activation), and proinflammatory cytokines. A prevalent example is sleep deprivation resulting from excessive stress. Sleep deprivation has significant damaging effects, including elevated evening cortisol level; elevated insulin and blood glucose levels; increased blood pressure; reduced parasympathetic activity; increased levels of proinflammatory cytokines; and increased concentrations of the gut

FIGURE 11.4 Physiologic and Behavioral Stress Responses. Stress processes arise from bidirectional communication patterns between the brain and other physiologic systems (autonomic, immune, neural, and endocrine). Importantly, these bidirectional mechanisms are protective, promoting short-term adaptation (allostasis). Chronic stress mechanisms, however, can lead to long-term dysregulation and promote behavioral responses and physiologic responses that lead to stress-induced disorders/diseases (allostatic load) that compromise health. (From McEwen BS: *Eur J Pharmacol* 583[2–3]:174–185, 2008.)

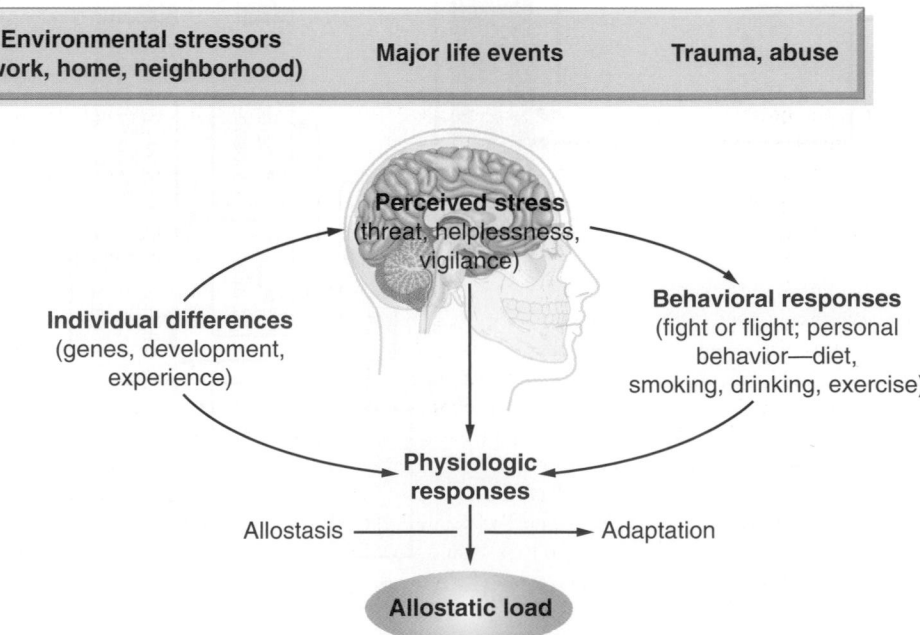

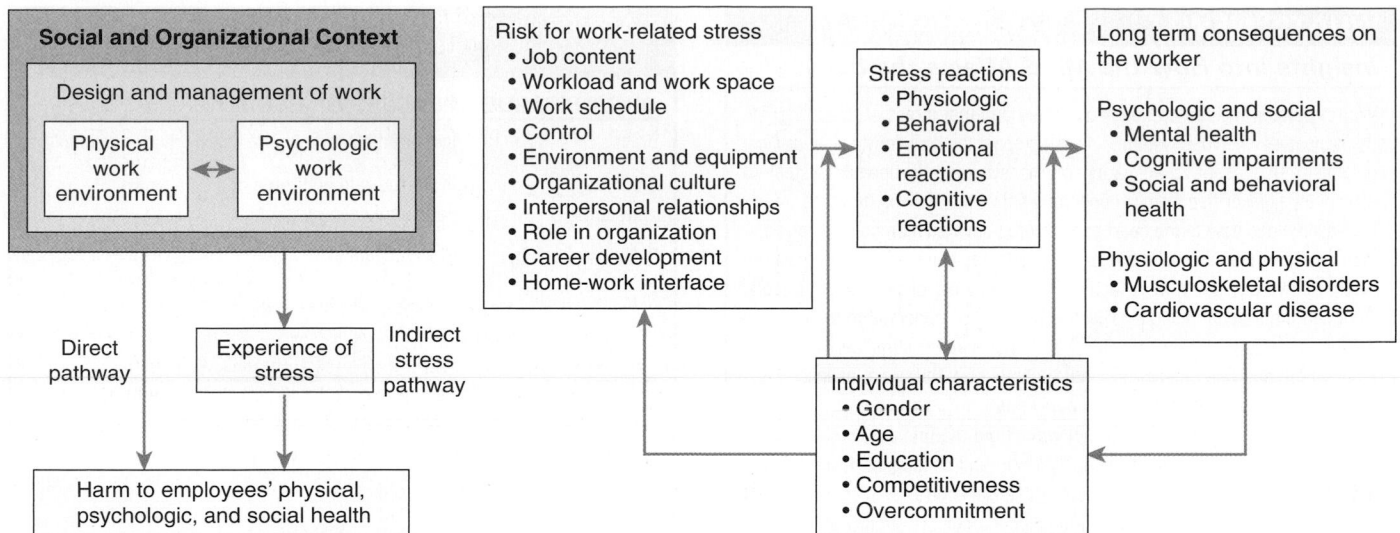

FIGURE 11.5 Psychosocial Work Environment and Work-Related Stress (Data from Leka S, Jain A: *Health impact of psychosocial hazards at work: An overview*, Geneva, 2010, Institute of Work, Health & Organizations, University of Nottingham, World Health Organization.)

hormone ghrelin, which stimulates appetite. Altogether, these physiologic alterations induced by the cumulative effects of insomnia can lead to increased caloric intake, depressed mood, cognitive problems, and a host of other potential health issues.[17]

As studies point increasingly to the important role that stress plays in certain disease processes, research has begun to focus on the mechanisms and interactions among social, psychologic, biologic, and behavioral risk factors responsible for these mind-body interactions. Molecular biologists, immunologists, neurologists, clinicians, and behavioral scientists are now exploring the role of the other half of the mind-body (dualistic) model—that is, the mind. What is emerging is a more holistic and complex model of health and disease states. This model involves the biochemical relationships of the central and autonomic nervous systems, the endocrine system, and their relationships to stress-elicited coping behaviors that can modify the integrity of the immune system. Discoveries of these complex links have led to the creation of the field of psychoneuroimmunology.

Psychoneuroimmunologic Mediators of Stress

Psychoneuroimmunology (PNI) is the study of how the consciousness *(psycho)*, the brain and spinal cord *(neuro)*, and the body's defenses against infection and abnormal cell division *(immunology)* interact. Psychoneuroimmunology assumes that all immune-mediated diseases result from interrelationships among psychosocial, emotional, genetic, and behavioral factors with the neurologic, endocrine, and immune systems.[18-20] The immune system is integrated with other physiologic processes and is sensitive to changes in CNS and endocrine functioning that accompany psychologic states. **Stressors** (e.g., infection, noise, decreased oxygen supply, pain, malnutrition, heat, cold, trauma, prolonged exertion, radiation, responses to life events [including anxiety, depression, anger, fear, loss, and excitement], obesity, old age, drugs, disease, surgery, and medical treatment) can elicit the stress response through the action of the nervous and endocrine systems.

The field of PNI has generated a large body of research, some of which has led to strenuous scientific debate. For example, mouse models suggest a strong link between stress and breast cancer progression, yet this effect is not consistently found in humans,[21,22] especially with respect to the causal role of personality in cancer mortality and morbidity.[21] Current understanding in the PNI field is that hormones released by stress influence many metabolic systems and corresponding physiologic events. Furthermore, data now suggest that psychosocial stressors or interventions modulate the immune system to impact health outcomes.[2,14,17,23-37] Studies support the link between psychosocial stressors and health outcomes for infectious disease and wound healing.[38-43] A meta-analysis of 10 studies conducted among persons living in England found that any level of psychologic distress is associated with increased mortality and increased risk of death from cardiovascular disease, external causes, and cancer (albeit only at higher levels of distress); 68,000 persons were used in this study and personal factors, such as age, smoking, and alcohol use, were adjusted accordingly.[44] Investigators studied workplace stressors and health outcomes.[45] Using meta-analysis of 228 studies they found that job insecurity increases the odds of reporting poor health by about 50%, high job demands raise the odds of having a diagnosed illness by 35%, and long work hours increase mortality by almost 20%.[45] Work-related stress can cause both behavioral and psychosocial problems. The World Health Organization (WHO) report focuses on the stress and health outcomes from work.[46] Fig. 11.5 summarizes psychosocial hazards that may affect both psychologic and physical health directly or indirectly through the experience of stress and risks for work-related stress.

STRESS RESPONSE

The perception of stress initiates a series of events in the central and peripheral nervous systems (see Fig. 11.1). In the brain, stress elicits an anticipatory response that activates the limbic system; the brain area responsible for motivation, emotions, and cognition. The limbic system also indirectly elicits both an endocrine stress response by stimulating neural pathways responsible for receiving sensory information and the release of norepinephrine from the locus ceruleus (LC). Norepinephrine release promotes arousal, increased vigilance, and anxiety, as well as other protective emotional responses. The fast-acting sympathetic adrenal medullary system in the periphery releases the catecholamines norepinephrine and epinephrine and the slower-acting HPA system culminates in the secretion of cortisol. The activation of these two stress systems redirects adaptive energy to the CNS and peripheral body sites to cope with stress (see *What's New?* Insights into How the Mind Affects the Body).

WHAT'S NEW?

Insights into How the Mind Affects the Body

Walter Cannon recognized nearly a century ago that stress or threat triggers the sympathetic nervous system to rapidly prepare the body for the *fight-or-flight* response. This adaptive activation of the sympathetic nervous system to effectively fight or flee from a dangerous situation involves, to name a few, increased blood flow to the heart and viscera, elevated metabolism, and pupil dilation. Catecholamine secretion from the adrenal medulla into the circulatory system plays a major role in facilitating this myriad of physiologic effects. Although the adrenal medulla is well-known to be connected to sympathetic neurons that project from the thoracic spinal cord to stimulate release of epinephrine and norepinephrine, until recently how the brain influences this adrenal-medullary system has been a mystery.

Using a technique to trace the pathways from the primate cerebral cortex that are linked to the adrenal medulla, Dunn and colleagues found cortical motor areas of the frontal lobe and somatosensory cortex also are involved in facilitating visceromotor and skeletomotor output. This cortical pathway coordinates the body's motor system required to cope with stress with increased metabolism through adrenal medulla catecholamine secretion. Another pathway from the medial prefrontal cortex plays a role in regulating cognitive and emotional processing. Cognitive control over a stressful situation determines the degree or intensity of adrenal medulla secretion of catecholamines. Failure to assess or cope with a stressful situation may then lead to uncontrolled emotional states, heightened activation of the sympathetic nervous system, and the onset disorders, such as posttraumatic stress disorder or chronic psychosomatic illness. In summary, this study identifies key cortical brain regions involved in coordinating motor, cognitive, and emotional functions with adrenal medulla catecholamine secretion. This research offers insights into the mind-body connection underlying health and psychosomatic illness.

Data from Dunn RP et al: *Proc Natl Acad Sci U S A* 113(35):9922–9927, 2016.

TABLE 11.1	PHYSIOLOGIC EFFECTS OF CATECHOLAMINES*
ORGAN/TISSUE	**PROCESS OR RESULT**
Brain	Increased blood flow; increased glucose metabolism
Cardiovascular system	Increased rate and force of contraction Peripheral vasoconstriction
Pulmonary system	Bronchodilation
Skeletal muscle	Increased glycogenolysis Increased contraction Increased dilation of muscle vasculature Decreased glucose uptake and utilization (decreases insulin release)
Liver	Increased glucose production Increased glycogenolysis
Adipose tissue	Increased lipolysis Decreased glucose uptake
Skin	Decreased blood flow
Gastrointestinal and genitourinary tracts	Decreased protein synthesis Decreased smooth muscle contraction Increased renin release Increased gastrointestinal sphincter tone
Lymphoid tissue	Acute and chronic stress inhibits several components of innate immunity, particularly decreasing number of natural killer cells
Macrophages	Inhibit and stimulate macrophage activity Depend on availability of type 1/proinflammatory cytokines, presence or absence of antigenic stressors, and peripheral corticotropin-releasing hormone (CRH)

*Some of these responses require glucocorticoids (e.g., cortisol) for maximal activity (see text for explanation).
Data from Elenkov IJ, Chrousos GP: *Ann N Y Acad Sci* 966:290–303, 2002; Granner DK: Hormones of the adrenal medulla. In Murray RK et al, editors: *Harper's biochemistry*, ed 25, New York, 2000, McGraw Hill.

Sympathetic Nervous System
Catecholamines

Stress activates the sympathetic nervous system (SNS) to stimulate the release of catecholamines (epinephrine and norepinephrine) from the adrenal medulla into the bloodstream and nerve endings that innervate peripheral organs and tissues. The adrenal medulla is an extension of the SNS because preganglionic fibers from the splanchnic nerve terminate in the medulla to innervate chromaffin cells that produce catecholamines. These adrenergic effector molecules have multiple effects on gene expression and cellular function in the nervous, endocrine, cardiovascular, gastrointestinal, respiratory, reproductive, and immune systems. Each adrenergic system regulates cellular functions through distinct receptors (α_1, α_2, β_1, β_2, β_3) coupled to G-protein–mediated signal transduction pathways. For example, acute fight-or-flight responses increase heart rate by activating β_1-adrenergic receptors in the heart muscle; blood from superficial tissues is redistributed to long muscles by activating vascular α_1- and β_2-adrenergic receptors; respiratory rate is increased by activating bronchial α_1- and β_2-adrenergic receptors; energy is mobilized by activating β_2- and β_3-adrenergic receptors in adipose tissue and the liver; and immune cells, such as natural killer (NK) cells, are mobilized into circulation by activating β_2-adrenergic receptors on leukocytes.[47] The physiologic effects of the catecholamines on organs and tissues are summarized in Table 11.1 and Fig. 11.2.

Epinephrine is rapidly transported to and acts on several organs, but it is metabolized quickly, making it short-acting. Metabolically, epinephrine causes transient hyperglycemia (high blood glucose level),

decreases glucose uptake in the muscles and other organs, and decreases insulin release from the pancreas. This is accomplished by activating enzymes whose actions promote glucose formation (gluconeogenesis) and glycogen breakdown (glycogenolysis) in the liver, while inhibiting glycogen formation. This prevents glucose from being taken up by peripheral tissue and preserves it for the CNS. Further, very little adrenal norepinephrine reaches distal tissue; thus the effects caused by norepinephrine during the stress response are primarily elicited from the SNS.[48,49]

Epinephrine has a greater influence on cardiac action and is the principal catecholamine involved in metabolic regulation. Epinephrine enhances myocardial contractility (inotropic effect), increases heart rate (chronotropic effect), and increases venous return to the heart, all of which increase cardiac output and blood pressure. Epinephrine dilates blood vessels of skeletal muscle, allowing for greater oxygenation. Epinephrine in the liver and skeletal muscles is rapidly metabolized and dilates blood vessels supplying skeletal muscles, allowing for more oxygenation. Epinephrine also mobilizes free fatty acids and cholesterol by stimulating lipolysis, freeing triglycerides and fatty acids from fat

TABLE 11.2	PHYSIOLOGIC ACTIONS OF α- AND β-ADRENERGIC RECEPTORS	
RECEPTOR	**PHYSIOLOGIC ACTIONS**
α_1	Increased glycogenolysis; smooth muscle contraction (blood vessels, genitourinary tract)
α_2	Smooth muscle relaxation (gastrointestinal tract); smooth muscle contraction (some vascular beds); inhibition of lipolysis, renin release, platelet aggregation, and insulin secretion
β_1	Stimulation of lipolysis; myocardial contraction (increased rate, increased force of contraction)
β_2	Increased hepatic gluconeogenesis; increased hepatic glycogenolysis; increased muscle glycogenolysis; increased release of insulin, glucagon, and renin; smooth muscle relaxation (bronchi, blood vessels, genitourinary tract, gastrointestinal tract)

stores, and by inhibiting the degradation of circulating cholesterol to bile acids. The metabolic actions of epinephrine aid the metabolic actions of cortisol, which are similar.

Table 11.2 summarizes the actions of the two subclasses of adrenergic receptors. Epinephrine binds to and activates both α- and β-adrenergic receptors. Norepinephrine at physiologic concentrations binds primarily to α-adrenergic receptors.[50]

Catecholamines can modify the numbers of cells of the immune system circulating in the blood.[51] Injection of epinephrine into healthy human subjects is associated with a transient increase of the number of lymphocytes (e.g., T cells and natural killer [NK] cells) in the peripheral blood. Specifically, the levels of T cytotoxic and especially NK cells increase,[51] whereas little change occurs in the levels of B lymphocytes. Qualitatively, lymphocyte responsiveness of T and B lymphocytes is reduced. Similar quantitative and qualitative changes are found 5 to 6 minutes after exposure to a psychologic or physical stressor.[52] However, the effects of acute elevation of catecholamine levels on the alteration of lymphocyte function are short-lived, lasting only about 2 hours.[53]

Catecholamines also increase proinflammatory cytokine production, for example, causing increased heart rate and blood pressure. Glucocorticoids are known to inhibit this proinflammatory production; however, inhibition depends on dose and cell or tissue type.[31] More simply, glucocorticoids can also promote inflammation depending on dose and cell type.[14] The possibility that chronic and dysfunctional HPA axis stimulation (as may occur during chronic inflammation) increases inflammation in the brain and other tissue may contribute to other diseases, including osteoporosis, metabolic disease (diabetes, obesity), and cardiovascular disease.[32] Additionally, these interactions are nonlinear and are very complex (Fig. 11.6).

Parasympathetic System

The parasympathetic system balances the sympathetic nervous system and, thus, it influences adaptation or maladaptation to stressful events. The parasympathetic system also has antiinflammatory effects and opposes the sympathetic (catecholamine) responses, for example, by slowing the heart rate.[14] Researchers evaluate the relative balance of the parasympathetic and sympathetic nervous systems using a technique known as heart rate variability (the measurement of R wave variability from heartbeat to heartbeat).

Neuroendocrine Regulation
Hypothalamic-Pituitary-Adrenal System

In sequence, the PVN of the hypothalamus secretes corticotropin-releasing hormone (CRH), which binds to specific receptors on anterior pituitary cells that, in turn, produce adrenocorticotropic hormone (ACTH). ACTH is then transported through the blood to the adrenal glands located on the top of the kidneys. After binding to specific receptors on the adrenal glands, the glucocorticoid hormones (primarily cortisol; from the adrenal cortex) are released. Cortisol (hydrocortisone is a synthetically produced but chemically identical version of cortisol) initiates a series of metabolic changes (see the following section Glucocorticoids: Cortisol); however, these hormones overall are thought to enhance immunity during acute stress and suppress immunity during chronic stress because of prolonged exposure and increased concentration.[1] Cortisol also sends a negative feedback signal to the pituitary and hypothalamus to terminate the HPA stress response.[23] Cortisol reaches *all* tissues, including the brain; easily penetrates cell membranes; and reacts with numerous intracellular glucocorticoid receptors. Because they spare almost no tissue or organ and influence a large proportion of the human genome, they exert significant diverse biologic actions.[23]

Glucocorticoids: Cortisol

Cortisol circulates in the plasma, both protein-bound and free. The main plasma-binding protein is called transcortin or corticosteroid-binding globulin. The unbound, or free, fraction is approximately 8% of the total plasma cortisol and is biologically active.[50] Cortisol mobilizes substances needed for cellular metabolism. One of the primary effects of cortisol is the stimulation of gluconeogenesis, or the formation of glucose from noncarbohydrate sources, such as amino acids or free fatty acids in the liver. In addition, cortisol enhances the elevation of blood glucose level promoted by other hormones, such as epinephrine, glucagon, and growth hormone. This action by cortisol is said to be *permissive* for the actions of other hormones. Cortisol also inhibits the uptake and oxidation of glucose by many body cells. The overall action of cortisol increases blood glucose concentration, thereby enabling the body to combat the stressor. The physiologic effects of cortisol are summarized in Table 11.3.

Cortisol also affects protein metabolism. It has an anabolic effect; that is, it increases the rate of synthesis of proteins and ribonucleic acid (RNA) in the liver. The anabolic effect of cortisol, however, is countered by its catabolic effect on protein stores in other tissues. Protein catabolism acts to increase levels of circulating amino acids, and chronic exposure to excess cortisol can severely deplete protein stores in muscle, bone, connective tissue, and skin. Further, cortisol acts to reduce protein synthesis in nonhepatic tissues, a loss for which dietary protein cannot compensate. Some evidence suggests that cortisol depresses transport of amino acids into muscle cells while enhancing their uptake into the liver. Finally, cortisol promotes gastric secretion in the stomach and intestines, potentially causing gastric ulcers. This could account for the gastrointestinal ulceration observed by Selye. In contrast, norepinephrine reduces gastric secretion.

Chronic Stress–Induced Effects of Glucocorticoids. Chronic secretion of glucocorticoids, along with catecholamines and the immune system, contributes to the development of the metabolic syndrome and the pathogenesis of obesity (Box 11.1). Elevated secretion of cortisol, norepinephrine (NE), epinephrine, and interleukin-6 (IL-6) promotes insulin release and decreases levels of growth and sex hormones. Over time, visceral fat increases accompanied by the loss of muscle mass (sarcopenia) and bone mass (osteoporosis).[54] The increase in adipose tissue is accompanied by the secretion of IL-6 and other cytokines. As a result, a low-grade, systemic inflammatory state emerges that induces

Staying on the Good Side of the Stress Spectrum

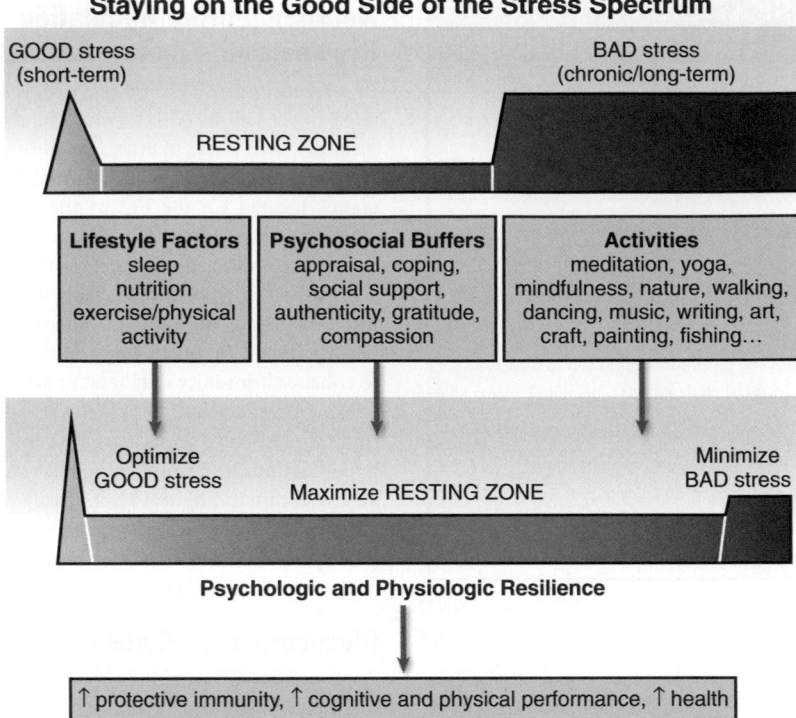

FIGURE 11.6 Stress Interactions Are Nonlinear and Complex. GOOD stress is shown on the left of the spectrum and involves a rapid biologic response to the stressor, followed by a rapid shutdown of the response upon cessation of the stressor. These responses support physiologic conditions that are likely to enhance protective immunity, cognitive and physical performance, and overall health. BAD stress, represented on the right of the spectrum, involves exposure to chronic or long-term biologic changes that are likely to result in dysregulation or suppression of immune function, a decrease in cognitive and physical performance, and an increased likelihood of disease. Short- and/or long-term stress is generally superimposed on a psychophysiologic RESTING ZONE of low/no stress that also represents a state of health maintenance/restoration. To maintain health, one needs to optimize GOOD stress, maximize the RESTING ZONE, and minimize BAD stress. Achieving psychologic and physiologic resilience involves a multipronged approach. Sleep of a quality and duration that helps one feel rested in the morning, a moderate and healthy diet, and consistent and moderate exercise or physical activity are three *Lifestyle Factors* that are likely to enable one to stay on the "good" side of the stress spectrum. Effective appraisal and coping mechanisms, genuine gratitude, social support, and compassion toward others and oneself are likely to provide *Psychosocial Buffers* against bad stress and enable one to stay on the "good" side of the stress spectrum. Additionally, depending on individual preferences, *Activities,* such as, meditation, yoga, being in nature, exercise/physical activity, music, art, craft, dance, fishing, painting, also may reduce BAD stress, extend The RESTING ZONE, and optimize GOOD stress. Such personal activities are likely to involve different strokes for different folks and need not always be meditative or reflective in nature. (Adapted from Dhabhar FS, McEwen BS: Bidirectional effects of stress on immune function: possible explanations for salubrious as well as harmful effects. In Ader R, editor: *Psychoneuroimmunology IV,* San Diego, 2007, Elsevier.)

insulin resistance and the onset of type 2 diabetes mellitus, tumor growth, atherosclerosis, and neurodegeneration.[55,56]

Epidemiologic evidence suggests that prenatal stress or elevations in levels of glucocorticoids may increase the subsequent risk of disease in offspring.[57] One study reported that high maternal cortisol concentration during pregnancy was associated with low birth weight.[58] This cortisol-induced low birth weight increases the offspring's risk of disease in later life, for example, obesity; cardiovascular conditions, such as hypertension; and behavioral disorders attributed to altered brain structure.[35,58,59] Thus abnormal glucocorticoid elevation in utero dramatically affects human pathophysiology and, consequently, longevity.[2,23,60]

The inhibitory effects of chronic glucocorticoid secretion on the growth axis are caused, in part, by elevated CRH secretion, which increases somatostatin, the inhibitor of growth hormone (GH) from the pituitary. Evidence linking the role of the HPA system to growth is found in

studies showing that children who experienced abuse may have decreased levels of GH and short stature, which is reversed when removed from the abusive, stressful environment and in children with Cushing syndrome where chronic exposure to glucocorticoids leads to arrested growth.[61]

The brain is a target of glucocorticoids and neurotransmitters that alters physiologic, behavioral, cognitive, and immune functions. When exposed to chronic stress, specific brain regions that have glucocorticoid (GC), catecholamine, and excitatory amino acid receptors may undergo dendritic retraction or expansion, cell death, or inhibition of neurogenesis to alter the brain functions.

GCs are involved in stress and circadian regulation and produce actions through the GC receptor (GR). GR can function as a nuclear transcription factor.[62] Just like the nuclear genome, the mitochondria contain a small genome, the mitochondrial DNA (mtDNA), that encodes 13 polypeptides. Recent work has found that in the brain and other

TABLE 11.3 PHYSIOLOGIC AND ACUTE EFFECTS OF CORTISOL

FUNCTIONS AFFECTED	PHYSIOLOGIC EFFECTS
Carbohydrate and lipid metabolism	Diminishes peripheral uptake and utilization of glucose; promotes gluconeogenesis in liver metabolism cells; enhances gluconeogenic response to other hormones; promotes lipolysis in adipose tissue
Protein metabolism	Increases protein synthesis in liver and decreases protein synthesis (including immunoglobulin synthesis) in muscle, lymphoid tissue, adipose tissue, skin, and bone; increases plasma level of amino acids; stimulates deamination in liver
Antiinflammatory effects (systemic effects)	High levels of cortisol used in drug therapy suppress inflammatory response; inhibit proinflammatory activity of many growth factors and cytokines; however, over time some individuals may develop tolerance to glucocorticoids, causing an increased susceptibility to both inflammatory and autoimmune disease
Proinflammatory effects (possible local effects)	Cortisol levels released during stress response may increase proinflammatory effects
Lipid metabolism	Lipolysis in extremities and lipogenesis in face and trunk
Immune effects	*Treatment* levels of glucocorticoids are immunosuppressive; thus they are valuable agents used in numerous diseases; the T-cell or innate immunity system is particularly affected by these larger doses of glucocorticoids with suppression of Th1 function or innate immunity; *stress* can cause a different pattern of immune response; these nontherapeutic levels can suppress innate (Th1) and increase adaptive (Th2) immunity—the so-called *Th1 to Th2 shift;* several factors influence this complex physiology and include long-term adaptations, reproductive hormones (i.e., overall, androgens suppress and estrogens stimulate immune responses), defects of hypothalamic-pituitary-adrenal axis, histamine-generated responses, and acute vs. chronic stress; thus stress seems to cause a Th2 shift *systemically* whereas *locally,* under certain conditions, it can induce proinflammatory activities and by these mechanisms may influence onset or course of infections and autoimmune/inflammatory, allergic, and neoplastic diseases
Digestive function	Promotes gastric secretion
Urinary function	Enhances excretion of calcium
Connective tissue function	Decreases proliferation of fibroblasts in connective tissue (thus delaying healing)
Muscle function	Maintains normal contractility and maximal work output for skeletal and cardiac muscle
Bone function	Decreases bone formation
Vascular system/myocardial function	Maintains normal blood pressure; permits increased responsiveness of arterioles to constrictive action of adrenergic stimulation; optimizes myocardial performance
Central nervous system function	Somehow modulates perceptual and emotional functioning; essential for normal arousal and initiation of daytime activity
Possible synergism with estrogen in pregnancy?	Suppresses maternal immune system to prevent rejection of fetus?

systems, GR is translocated from the cytosol to the mitochondria and that stress and corticosteroids have a direct influence on mtDNA transcription and mitochondrial physiology.[62] Investigators also found that both acute and chronic stress and GC were linked with changes in the function of brain mitochondria.[62]

The hippocampus has GRs that support the HPA negative feedback systems. Activation of hippocampal GRs by moderate stress also may lead to temporary hippocampal dendritic shrinkage and loss of spines. However, chronic stress may lead to cell death and inhibit neurogenesis. The loss of hippocampal neurons compromises the HPA negative feedback system and promotes the chronic increase in glucocorticoid secretion. This elevated, prolonged stress-induced increase in glucocorticoids is linked to cognitive deficits and major depression.[16] Furthermore, chronic stress-induced elevations to glucocorticoids may be a risk factor for Alzheimer disease.[63] Middle-aged women exposed to heightened stress are at increased risk of developing Alzheimer disease.[64] An animal study showed that stress and glucocorticoid secretion impaired memory and increased Tau kinases and hyperphosphorylated Tau in the hippocampus and prefrontal cortex.[65] This study provides insight into how the cumulative effects of stress and glucocorticoid exposure

over time may progress to Alzheimer disease through the onset of Tau, which mediates the pathogenic actions of amyloid β.

Another brain region influenced by stress is the amygdala, a major site linked to fear and anxiety. Here, chronic stress expands the dendritic field and the synthesis of CRH neurons. The increase in amygdala CRH neurons is associated with increased fear and autonomic and HPA functioning found in anxiety disorders, such as posttraumatic stress disorder.[16]

The prefrontal cortex modulates higher order cognitive functions, such as abstract thinking, executive decision-making processing, and goal-directed behavior. Exposure to chronic stress causes dendritic shrinkage in the medial prefrontal cortex, which may lead to cognitive rigidity or inflexible thinking. However, another region, the orbitofrontal cortex, shows neurons with an expanded dendritic field that may lead to increased fear vigilance. These alterations in the prefrontal cortex disrupt the balance between the fear-generating amygdala and cognitive control or coping with stress.[16,66] People exposed to high levels of stress have high levels of HPA hormones and catecholamines, impairments in working memory, and the ability to switch to flexible goal-directed behavior. Of relevance to mental disorders, stress may exacerbate the

BOX 11.1   GLUCOCORTICOIDS, INSULIN, INFLAMMATION, AND OBESITY

The signs and symptoms of Cushing syndrome (e.g., excess glucocorticoids [GCs]) include truncal obesity, relatively thin extremities, a "moon face," and a "buffalo [neck] hump." In such individuals the possibility of associated hypertension is high as well as increased risk of infection and metabolic syndrome or frank type 2 diabetes. In addition, the likelihood of an elevated ratio of intraabdominal subcutaneous fat mass to nonabdominal fat mass is high because the glucocorticoids mediate the redistribution of stored calories into the abdominal region. The specific increase in abdominal fat stores is a consequence of elevated levels of glucocorticoids combined with increased insulin action. However, the increased levels of glucocorticoids need not be present in the circulation, but can be generated locally in fat by conversion of inactive cortisone to active cortisol through the action of the isoenzyme 11β-hydroxysteroid dehydrogenase (11β-HSD) type-1. This conversion is referred to as "pre-receptor" metabolism of cortisol. The active steroid is secreted directly to the liver through the portal vein. In vitro insulin

synthesis and secretion from the pancreas are inhibited by the glucocorticoids. However, increasing levels of glucocorticoids in vivo are associated with increasing insulin secretion possibly because of an antiinsulin effect on the liver, which appears to be vulnerable to the negative effects of glucocorticoids on insulin action. Hepatic insulin resistance is strongly associated with abdominal obesity.

Recent data reveal that the plasma concentration of inflammatory mediators, such as tumor necrosis factor-alpha (TNF-α) and interleukin-6 (IL-6), is increased in the insulin-resistant states of obesity and type 2 diabetes. Two mechanisms might be involved in the pathogenesis of inflammation: (1) glucose and macronutrient intake (i.e., which can be mediated through chronic stress) causes oxidative stress; and (2) the increased concentrations of TNF-α and IL-6 associated with obesity and type 2 diabetes might interfere with insulin signal transduction. This interference might promote inflammation. Chronic overnutrition (obesity) might thus be a proinflammatory state with oxidative stress.

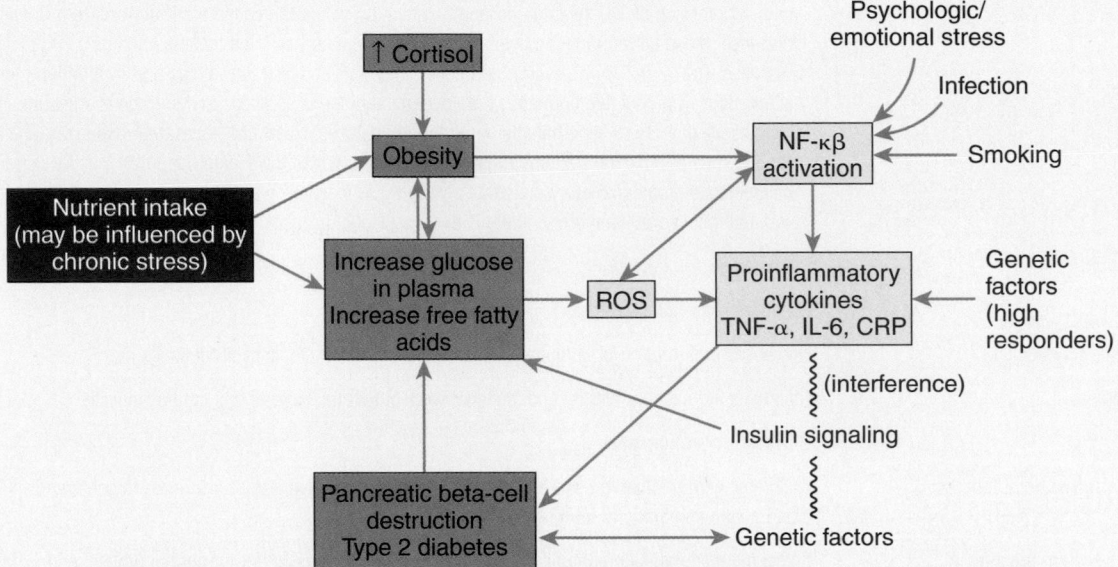

FIGURE Stress, Inflammation, Obesity, and Type 2 Diabetes. The induction of reactive oxygen species (ROS) generation and inflammation through the proinflammatory transcription factor, NF-κβ, activate most proinflammatory genes. Macronutrient intake, obesity, free fatty acids, infection, smoking, psychologic stress, and genetic factors increase the production of ROS. Interference with insulin signaling (insulin resistance) leads to hyperglycemia and proinflammatory changes. Proinflammatory changes increase the levels of TNF-α and IL-6, and also lead to the inhibition of insulin signaling and insulin resistance. Inflammation in pancreatic beta cells leads to beta-cell dysfunction, which in combination with insulin resistance leads to type 2 diabetes. *CRP*, C-reactive protein.

onset of schizophrenia. In addition, stress may facilitate the conversion from euthymia to bipolar disorder.

In summary, the stress-induced alterations in the brain associated with emotional and cognitive disorders may develop because of an inability of the brain to readily induce synaptic changes that promote recovery and resilience. Effective clinical treatments may be unlocking these inflexible neuronal functions and brain circuits and returning the brain to a functional state capable of generating adaptive cognitive and behavioral programs.

Glucocorticoids, Stress, and the Immune System. Glucocorticoids or cortisol secretion during stress exerts beneficial effects by inhibiting initial inflammatory effects, for example, vasodilation and increased capillary permeability.[32] Cortisol also promotes resolution and repair. These actions are mainly accomplished by facilitating the effects of GR, namely, the transcription of genetic material (through

DNA binding) within leukocytes.[32] Because GR is so widely expressed, glucocorticoids influence virtually all immune cells. However, whether cortisol-induced effects are adaptive or destructive may depend on the intensity, type, and duration of the stressor; the tissue involved; and the subsequent concentration and length of cortisol exposure. Finally, glucocorticoids are shown to induce T-cell apoptosis.[32]

Cortisol acts to suppress the activity of Th1 cells, which leads to a decrease in innate immunity and the proinflammatory response. Cortisol also stimulates the activity of Th2 cells, which increases adaptive immunity and the antiinflammatory response. Epinephrine and norepinephrine have a similar effect: a decrease in Th1 activity and an increase in Th2 activity.

Initially, immune responses are regulated by cells of *innate immunity* called *antigen-presenting cells (APCs)*, such as monocytes/macrophages, dendritic cells, and other phagocytic cells, and by Th1 and Th2 lymphocytes (cells involved in *adaptive immunity*). These cells secrete chemical messengers, called cytokines, that regulate innate and adaptive immune responses. Cytokines, such as interferons, interleukins, and tumor necrosis factors, can stimulate or inhibit various components of the immune system. Antigen-presenting cells also release cytokines that induce T cells to differentiate into Th1 cells. Th1 cells and APC cytokines work together to stimulate the activity of cytotoxic T cells, natural killer cells, and activated macrophages—the major components of innate immunity. These cytokines also stimulate the synthesis of nitric oxide and other inflammatory mediators that increase chronic delayed-type inflammatory responses. Because of this effect, these cytokines are sometimes referred to as proinflammatory cytokines.

The cytokines secreted by the Th2 cells act to inhibit Th1 cells and can promote adaptive immunity by stimulating the growth and activation of mast cells and eosinophils, as well as the differentiation of B-cell immunoglobulins. Thus these cytokines are sometimes referred to as antiinflammatory cytokines[67] (Fig. 11.7). Moreover, cytokines can act synergistically, antagonistically, or reciprocally. However, the roles of

cytokines are highly complex and much remains unknown. Regardless, the decrease in Th1 activity and the increase in Th2 activity are sometimes called a Th1 to Th2 shift. Individuals experiencing a Th1 to Th2 shift are more likely to experience allergic responses, infections, and temporary worsening of autoimmune conditions such as arthritis.

The preceding description of the effect of stress hormones on the Th1-Th2 balance may not be accurate for certain local responses.[67,68] That is, the release of catecholamines (epinephrine and norepinephrine) can cause certain epithelial cells of the lung to release cytokines that promote recruitment of leukocytes, potentially enhancing inflammation and worsening lung function. This paradoxical stress-induced potentiation of inflammation in the lungs may explain why "acute respiratory distress syndrome" often develops in individuals with major infections associated with profound activity of the stress response.[69]

For years, stress hormones, especially glucocorticoids (cortisol), have been used therapeutically as powerful antiinflammatory/immunosuppressive agents. The synthetic forms of glucocorticoid hormones (exogenous types of antiinflammatory glucocorticoids

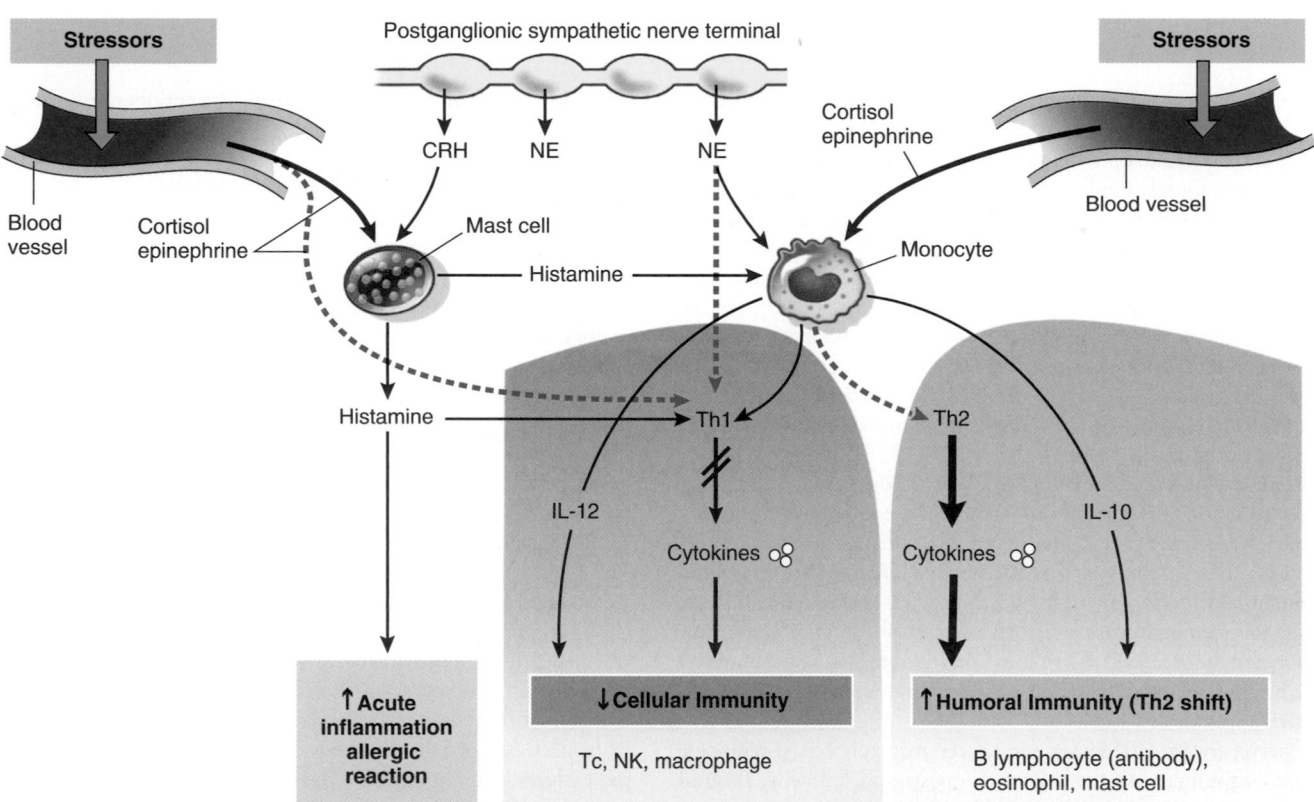

FIGURE 11.7 Effect of Corticotropin-Releasing Hormone (CRH)—Mast Cell—Histamine Axis, Cortisol, and Catecholamines on the Th1/Th2 Balance—Innate and Adaptive Immunity. Adaptive immunity provides protection against multicellular parasites, extracellular bacteria, some viruses, soluble toxins, and allergens. Innate immunity provides protection against intracellular bacteria, fungi, protozoa, and several viruses. Type 1 cytokines or proinflammatory cytokines include IL-12, interferon-gamma (IFN-γ), and tumor necrosis factor-alpha (TNF-α). Type 2 cytokines or antiinflammatory cytokines include IL-10 and IL-4. Solid lines *(black)* represent stimulation, whereas dashed lines *(blue)* represent inhibition (i.e., Th1 and Th2 are mutually inhibitory, IL-12 and IFN-γ inhibit Th2, and vice versa; IL-4 and IL-10 inhibit Th1 responses). Stress and CRH modulate inflammatory/immune and allergic responses by stimulating cortisol (glucocorticoid), catecholamines, and peripheral (immune) CRH secretion and by changing the production of regulatory cytokines and histamines. *CRH* (peripheral, immune), *CRH,* Corticotropin-releasing hormone; *IL,* interleukin; *NE,* norepinephrine; *NK,* natural killer cell; *Tc,* cytotoxic T cell; *Th,* helper T cell. *Dashed lines,* decreased (inhibited); *solid lines,* increased (stimulation). (Redrawn from Elenkov IJ, Chrousos GP: *Trends Endocrinol Metab* 10[9]:359–368, 1999.)

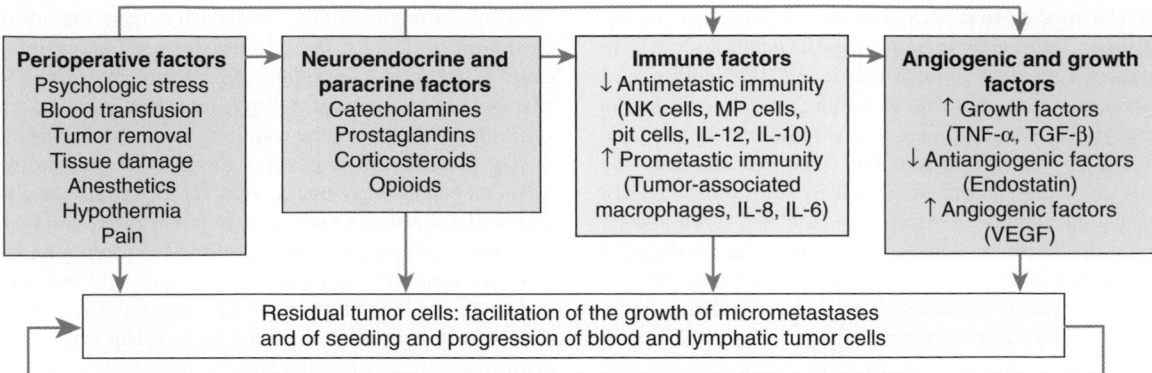

FIGURE 11.8 The Perioperative Period and the Excision of the Primary Tumor Can Promote the Development of Metastases. The perioperative timeframe is critical in determining long-term cancer outcomes. Various aspects of surgery, with the consequent paracrine and neuroendocrine responses and immunologic changes, can directly and indirectly affect malignant tissue. The cancer outcome is affected by surgery-related anxiety and stress, nutritional status, anesthetics and analgesics, hypothermia, blood transfusion, tissue damage, and levels of sex hormones. *IL*, Interleukin; *MP*, mononuclear phagocyte cells; *NK*, natural killer cells; *TGF*, transforming growth factor; *VEGF*, vascular endothelial growth factor. (Data from Horowitz M et al: *Nat Rev Clin Oncol* 12:213–226, 2015.)

administered for a pharmaceutical reaction) are poorly metabolized when compared to endogenous glucocorticoids, leading to a longer half-life and no circadian rhythm for these compounds. Moreover, these synthetic compounds bind to different targets, so each has a unique effect.[14] Therapeutic levels of glucocorticoids inhibit the accumulation of leukocytes at the site of inflammation and inhibit the release of substances involved in the inflammatory response (i.e., kinins, plasminogen-activating factor, prostaglandins, and histamine) from the leukocytes. Glucocorticoids inhibit fibroblast proliferation and function at the site of an inflammatory response. This inhibition accounts for the poor wound healing, increased susceptibility to infection, and decreased inflammatory response that often are noted in individuals with chronic glucocorticoid excess.

Paradoxically, elevated levels of glucocorticoids and catecholamines (epinephrine and norepinephrine)—both endogenous and exogenously administered—may decrease innate immunity and increase autoimmune responses. These effects, which can accentuate inflammation in general and potentially increase neuronal death (e.g., in stroke victims),[14] may explain the seemingly contradictory stress response of immunosuppression and the increased risk of infection (decreased innate immunity) with a heightened antibody response and autoimmune disease (increased adaptive immunity).

A perioperative risk factor for cancer recurrence is psychologic distress, beginning with the cancer diagnosis and following surgical and adjuvant treatment, when individuals experience stress, anxiety, and depression.[70,71] Psychologic stress was reported to down-regulate cellular immune factors, including natural killer (NK) and cytotoxic T lymphocyte (CTL) activity, macrophage motility, and phagocytosis.[72-75] Stress hormones, catecholamines, opioids, and glucocorticoids were relatedly shown in animal experiments to causally promote metastatic progression.[76,77] Importantly, from animal experiments a single exposure to stress or stress hormones during a critical period of tumor progression could increase cancer mortality.[76] Surgery, itself, profoundly suppresses cell-mediated immunity.[78] Surgery, and associated neuroendocrine and paracrine responses, increased secretion of cortisol, leading to immune suppression and decreases in the number and function of NK, Th1, and CTL cells.[79,80] These responses begin before surgery, are increased following surgery, and dissipate during the first few postoperative days

or weeks.[80,81] Immunosuppression during the perioperative period can increase long-term cancer recurrence rates (Fig. 11.8).[77,82]

Corticotropin-Releasing Hormone (CRH)

CRH influences the immune system indirectly by the activation of cortisol (glucocorticoids) and catecholamines. CRH is secreted by the hypothalamus and also peripherally at inflammatory sites (called peripheral [immune] CRH).[26,67] Peripheral (immune) CRH is proinflammatory, causing an increase in vasodilation and vascular permeability.[83] Therefore it appears that mast cells are the target of peripheral CRH. Mast cells release histamine, a well-known mediator of acute inflammation and allergic reactions (see Fig. 11.7). Recent evidence suggests that immune cells have histamine receptors and that histamine may have an effect similar to that of catecholamines. This finding suggests that histamine induces acute inflammation and allergic reactions while suppressing Th1 activity (decreasing innate immunity) and promoting Th2 activity (increasing adaptive immunity).[69,83,84] A number of stress factors initiate CRH production, including high levels of interleukin-1 (IL-1) and IL-6. Increased CRH secretion facilitates cortisol secretion, which in turn inhibits further cytokine release by macrophages and monocytes. The observation that IL-1 can elicit changes in the nervous and endocrine systems by stimulating CRH production in the hypothalamus is part of a growing body of evidence demonstrating immune-induced regulation of the CNS. The release of the immune inflammatory mediators IL-6, tumor necrosis factor-alpha (TNF-α), and interferon is triggered by bacterial or viral infections, cancer, and tissue injury that in turn initiate a stress response through the HPA pathway. Enhanced systemic production of these cytokines also induces other CNS and behavior changes during the acute phase of an infectious episode, acting either directly in a distant, systemic "endocrine" way or indirectly through the mediation of neuropeptides. These effects include pyrogenesis (fever), induction of slow-wave sleep, and anorexia, which together are adaptive responses to infection and possibly cancer. Slow-wave sleep is associated with enhanced release of growth hormone (GH) and a reduction in levels of cortisol, which is beneficial for tissue repair and enhanced immune response.

In summary, stress can activate an excessive immune response and, through cortisol and catecholamines, suppress the Th1 response, causing a Th1 to Th2 shift. Locally, stress can exert proinflammatory or anti-inflammatory effects depending on the chemicals that are released in the local environment and the way that cells of the local environment respond to those chemicals. Moreover, different types of stressors may have variable effects on the immune response. Thus *systemic responses to stress* may cause a decrease in innate immunity and an enhancement in adaptive immunity, whereas *local responses to stress,* under certain conditions, may induce proinflammatory activities that influence the onset and cause of infectious, autoimmune/inflammatory, allergic, and neoplastic diseases.

Other Hormones

The immune system is integrated with other physiologic processes and is sensitive to changes in CNS and endocrine functioning, such as those that accompany psychologic states. For example, neuropeptide Y (NPY), a sympathetic neurotransmitter and growth factor for many cells, is a stress-mediator implicated in atherosclerosis and tissue remodeling.[51] Other hormones that influence the stress response are listed in Table 11.4. Neuropeptides and hormones have a significant effect on the immune response. This effect on immune function depends on the

TABLE 11.4	OTHER HORMONES THAT INFLUENCE THE STRESS RESPONSE	
HORMONE	**SOURCE**	**ACTION**
β-Endorphins (endogenous opiates)	Pituitary and hypothalamus	Activates endorphin (opiate) receptors on peripheral sensory nerves, leading to pain relief or analgesia Hemorrhage increases levels to inhibit blood pressure or delay compensatory changes that would increase blood pressure[1]
Growth hormone (GH, somatotropin)	Anterior pituitary gland	Affects protein, lipid, and carbohydrate metabolism Counters effects of insulin Involved in tissue repair May participate in growth and function of immune system[2] Levels increase after a variety of stressful stimuli (cardiac catheterization, electroshock therapy, gastroscopy, surgery, fever, physical exercise) Increased levels associated with psychologic stimuli (taking examinations, viewing violent or sexually arousing films, certain psychologic performance tests) Prolonged stress (chronic stress) suppresses growth hormone
Prolactin	Anterior pituitary gland; numerous extrapituitary tissue sites	Increases in response to many stressful stimuli (including procedures such as gastroscopy, proctoscopy, pelvic examination, and surgery)[3] Requires more intense stimuli than those leading to increases in catecholamine or cortisol levels Levels show little change after exercise
Oxytocin	Hypothalamus	Promotes bonding and social attachment In animals it is associated with reduced hypothalamic-pituitary-adrenal (HPA) activation levels and reduced anxiety[4]
Testosterone	Leydig cells in testes	Regulates male secondary sex characteristics and libido Levels decrease after stressful stimuli (anesthesia, surgery, marathon running, mountain climbing)[5] Decreased by psychologic stimuli; however, some data indicate that psychologic stress associated with competition (e.g., pistol shooting) increases both testosterone and cortisol levels, especially in athletes older than 45 years[6] Markedly reduced in individuals with respiratory failure, burns, and congestive heart failure[7] Decreased levels occur during aging and are associated with a lower cortisol responsiveness to stress-induced inflammation[8]
Estrogen	Ovaries	Works in concert with oxytocin, exerting a calming effect during stressful situations[9]
Melatonin	Produced by pineal gland	Increases during stress response; release is suppressed by light and increased in the dark; receptors have been identified on lymphoid cells, possibly higher density of receptors on T cells than B cells; suppression of lymphocyte function by trauma was reversed by melatonin[10]
Somatostatin (SOM)	Produced by sensory nerve terminals found in and released from lymphoid cells and hypothalamus	Natural killer (NK) function and immunoglobulin synthesis are decreased by SOM; growth hormone secretion decreased by SOM
Vasoactive intestinal peptide (VIP)	Found in neurons of central nervous system (CNS) and in peripheral nerves	VIP increases during stress; VIP-containing nerves are located in both primary and secondary lymphoid tissues, around blood vessels, and in gastrointestinal tract; VIP receptors are on both T and B cells; VIP may influence lymphocyte maturation; cytokine production by T cells is modified by VIP; B cells and antibody production are influenced by VIP

Continued

TABLE 11.4 OTHER HORMONES THAT INFLUENCE THE STRESS RESPONSE—cont'd

HORMONE	SOURCE	ACTION
Calcitonin gene–related peptide (CGRP)	Found in spinal cord motor neurons and in sensory neurons near dendritic cells of skin and in primary and secondary lymphoid tissues	CGRP receptors are present on T and B lymphocytes; thus it is likely that CGRP can modulate immune function; CGRP may enhance acute inflammatory response because it is a vasodilator; maturation of immune B lymphocytes is inhibited by CGRP; IL-1 is inhibited by CGRP, which is important for activation of T cells; it has been shown to interfere with lymphocyte activation
Neuropeptide Y (NPY)	Present in neurons of CNS and in neurons throughout body; co-localized in nerve terminals in lymphatic tissues with norepinephrine	Lymphocytes have receptors for NPY and thus may modulate their function;[11] several lines of evidence suggest that NPY is a neurotransmitter and neurohormone involved in stress response; increased levels of NPY occur in plasma in response to severe or prolonged stress; it may be responsible for stress-induced regional vasoconstriction (splanchnic, coronary, and cerebral); it may also increase platelet aggregation[2]
Substance P (SP)	Produced by a neuropeptide classified as tachykinin (increases heart rate subsequent to lowering blood pressure) found in brain, as well as nerves innervating secondary lymphoid tissues	SP increases in response to stress; receptors for SP are found on membranes of both T and B cells, mononuclear phagocytic cells, and mast cells; proinflammatory activity induces release of histamine from mast cells during stress response; causes smooth muscle contraction, causes macrophages and T cells to release cytokines, and increases antibody production

References

1. Amico JA et al: *J Neuroendocrinol* 16(4):319–324, 2004.
2. Rabin BS: The nervous system—immune system connection. In *Stress, immune function, and health: the connection*, New York, 1999, Wiley-Liss.
3. Rohleder N et al: *J Neuroimmunol* 126(1–2):69–77, 2002.
4. Marucha PT, Kiecolt-Glaser JK, Favagehi M: *Psychosom Med* 60(3):362–365, 1998.
5. Chesnokova V, Melmed S: *Endocrinology* 143(5):1571–1574, 2002.
6. Guezennec CY et al: *Int J Sports Med* 16(6):368–372, 1995.
7. Bauer-Wu SM: *Clin J Oncol Nurs* 6(3):167–170, 2002.
8. Bauer-Wu SM: *Clin J Oncol Nurs* 6(4):243–246, 2002.
9. Repka-Ramirez MS, Baraniuk JN: *Clin Allergy Immunol* 17:1–17, 2002.
10. Maestroni GJ: *Adv Exp Med Biol* 460:396, 1999.
11. Petito JM, Huang Z, McCarthy DB: *J Neuroimmunol* 54:81, 1994.

type of factor secreted, with some factors enhancing activity, some suppressing activity, and some both enhancing and suppressing activity, depending on the concentration and length of exposure, the target cell, and the specific immune function studied.

Hormones of the Female Reproductive System. The HPA axis exerts powerful, multilevel effects on the female reproductive system. Stress generally inhibits the female reproductive system (Fig. 11.9), primarily through the HPA axis by (1) CRH suppression of hypothalamic gonadotropin-releasing hormone (GnRH) secretion and CRH stimulation of β-endorphin release; (2) cortisol-inhibited secretion of luteinizing hormone (LH), estradiol, progesterone, and possibly testosterone;[85,86] and (3) cortisol-induced target tissue resistance by estradiol.[87,88] The locus ceruleus–norepinephrine (LC/NE) system provides positive input to the reproductive system, which is frequently altered by the stress-activated HPA axis. Sexual stimulation and GnRH neuron activation, however, may cause the gonadal axis to be resistant to suppression by the HPA axis. Table 11.5 presents potential pathologic effects of central and peripheral CRH in women.

Estrogen stimulates the HPA axis, and HPA responsiveness is greater in women than in men.[88] Estrogen directly stimulates the CRH gene promoter and the central NE system, which may explain the effects of estradiol fluctuations on adult women's slight hypercortisolism, increases in affective anxiety and eating disorders, mood cycles, and vulnerability to autoimmune and inflammatory disease. Estradiol down-regulates glucocorticoid receptor binding in the anterior pituitary, hypothalamus, and hippocampus, which tends to *increase* HPA activity by interfering with glucocorticoid-negative feedback, whereas progesterone opposes these effects.[89] Thus alterations in estradiol levels during normal menses, perimenopause (including increases as well as decreases), and menopause modify the regulatory feedback loop, and adaptations over time develop as a new equilibrium is established in the relationship (see Fig. 11.9). Over time, these changes increase the incidence of mood alterations, eating disorders, anxiety, depression, weight alterations, and inflammatory and immune disorders.

Endorphins and Enkephalins. Endorphins and enkephalins (endogenous opiates) are released into the blood as part of the response to stressful stimuli. These proteins found in the brain have pain-relieving capabilities. Stressful stimuli include traumatic injury and an acute, intense stress situation, such as first-time parachute jumping. In inflamed tissue, immune cell–derived endorphins activate endorphin receptors on peripheral sensory nerves, leading to pain relief or analgesia.[90] Hemorrhage increases β-endorphin levels, which inhibits blood pressure increases or delays compensatory changes that increase blood pressure.[91] Thus endogenous opiates modulate blood pressure instability and neuroendocrine and cytokine responses to blood losses.[92,93]

In conditions or activities when endogenous opiate activity increases, people not only experience insensitivity to pain but also report increased feelings of excitement, positive well-being, or euphoria. In addition, cells of the immune system synthesize and release opioids when lymphoid cells are activated.[94] T and B lymphocytes and mononuclear phagocytic cells have receptors for opioids. Endorphins may play a role in the excitement and exhilaration produced by dancing, contact sports, and

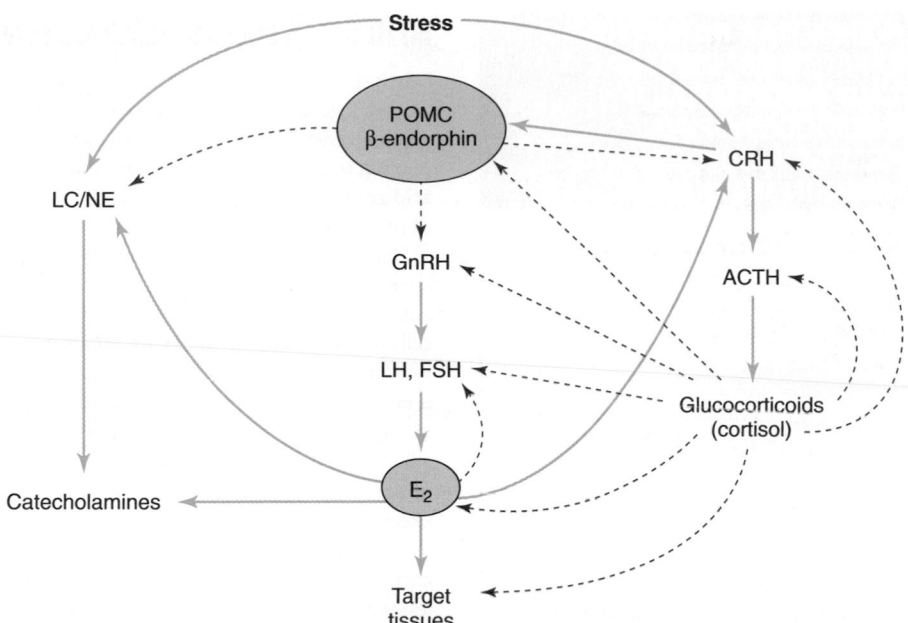

FIGURE 11.9 Stress and the Female Reproductive System. Interactions of the reproductive system with the hypothalamic-pituitary-adrenal (HPA) axis and locus ceruleus–norepinephrine system (LC/NE). Corticotropic cells of the pituitary gland express proopiomelanocortin (POMC) peptides. Stress generally inhibits the female reproductive system primarily through the HPA by (1) suppressing hypothalamic gonadotropin-releasing hormone (GnRH) secretion by corticotropin-releasing hormone (CRH) and CRH-induced β-endorphins; (2) inhibiting GnRH, pituitary luteinizing hormone (LH), and ovarian estradiol (E2) secretion by cortisol; and (3) enhancing cortisol-induced target tissue resistance to estradiol. The LC/NE system provides positive input to the reproductive system, which can be overridden by the stress-activated HPA. Estradiol can cause the reproductive system to stimulate the stress system by stimulating CRH secretion and inhibiting reuptake and catabolism of catecholamines. *ACTH,* Adrenocorticotropic hormone; *FSH,* follicle-stimulating hormone. Dashed lines refer to inhibitory pathways. Solid lines refer to direct stimulatory pathways. (Adapted from Chrousos GP et al: *Ann Intern Med* 129[3]:229–240, 1998.)

combat. Little direct evidence, however, links the endorphin system to most of these activities.

Prolactin. Prolactin is released from the anterior pituitary gland as well as numerous extrapituitary tissue sites. It is necessary for lactation and breast development. Prolactin receptors are present in many different tissues, including the liver, kidney, intestine, and adrenals. Prolactin is also produced by lymphoid cells.[95] Prolactin is necessary for lactation and breast development. Plasma prolactin levels also increase after exposure to a variety of stressful stimuli, including gastroscopy, proctoscopy, pelvic examination, and surgery; after taking examinations; and after receiving various sexual stimuli, for example, stimulation of the nipple or areola in women. Unlike GH, prolactin levels show little change after exercise. However, similar to GH, prolactin secretion appears to require more intense stimuli than those leading to increases in catecholamine or cortisol levels. Immune cells also are influenced by prolactin. Prolactin acts as a second messenger for IL-2 and has a positive influence on B-cell activation and differentiation. Several classes of lymphocytes have receptors for prolactin, suggesting a direct effect of prolactin on immune function.

Oxytocin. Oxytocin, a peptide hormone and neurotransmitter produced in the hypothalamus, is well-known to be secreted by the posterior pituitary in females to induce parturition and lactation. In the brain, oxytocin acts on brain circuits, including the amygdala, HPA, and sympathetic nervous systems, to modulate or buffer fear and anxiety and attenuate the HPA stress response.[96] Animal studies further indicate that oxytocin stimulates prosocial behavior, such as maternal or parental

care and mother-infant bonding. In humans, oxytocin facilitates interpersonal gaze; social support; maternal care;[97,98] and, when secreted during orgasm in both sexes, the prosocial hormone may promote bonding and social attachment. Some but not all studies further suggest oxytocin may have a role in promoting trust.[98] In summary, oxytocin is increasingly recognized as a prosocial hormone that strengthens social relationships, social support, and protection and also attenuates psychosocial stressful events.

Testosterone. Testosterone, a hormone secreted by Leydig cells, regulates male secondary sex characteristics and libido. Testosterone levels decrease after stressful stimuli. This decrease in testosterone level occurs after stimuli such as ether or anesthetic administration, surgery, marathon running, and mountain climbing. The mechanism causing decreased levels of testosterone is thought to be exerted by cortisol and β-endorphin.

Psychologic stimuli also lead to a decrease in testosterone levels. Men engaged in rigorous combat training and those engaged in the first several weeks of officer candidate school experience significant drops in testosterone levels.[99,100] However, other data have shown that the psychologic stress associated with some types of competition (e.g., pistol shooting) *increases* both testosterone and cortisol levels, especially in athletes older than 45 years.[101] Moreover, individuals with acute illness, such as respiratory failure, burns, and congestive heart failure, show a marked reduction in plasma testosterone level.[102]

The direct immunologic effects of sex hormones contribute to the sexual dimorphism seen in the incidence of autoimmune disease[103] and

TABLE 11.5	POTENTIAL PATHOLOGIC EFFECTS OF CENTRAL AND PERIPHERAL CORTICOTROPIN-RELEASING HORMONE (CRH) IN WOMEN
CHANGES	**ALTERATIONS**
Central CRH	
Increased secretion	Hypercortisolism
	Melancholic depression
	Eating disorders
	Chronic active alcoholism
	Chronic active exercise
	Consequences: osteoporosis, visceral obesity, infertility
	Tau protein misfolding-Alzheimer disease?*
Decreased secretion	Atypical depression
	Seasonal affective disorder
	Chronic fatigue and fibromyalgia syndromes
	Rheumatoid arthritis
	Postpartum blues, depression, and autoimmunity
	Premenstrual tension syndrome
	Menopausal depression
Peripheral CRH	
Increased secretion of immune CRH	Inflammatory disorders
Increased secretion of placental CRH	Premature labor
Decreased secretion of placental CRH	Delayed labor
Decreased secretion of ovarian CRH	Ovarian dysfunction
	Anovulation
	Defective corpus luteum function
Increased secretion of ovarian CRH	Early menopause
Decreased secretion of endometrial CRH	Infertility
	Early spontaneous abortion

*New line of investigation: Filipcik P et al: *Cell Mol Neurobiol* 32(5):837–845, 2012.
Data from Chrousos GP et al: *Ann Intern Med* 129(3):229–240; Kalantaridou SN et al: *J Reprod Immunol* 62(1–2):61–68, 2004.

the greater susceptibility to sepsis and mortality in males following injury.[104] Estrogens generally are associated with a depression of T-cell–dependent immune function and an enhancement of B-cell functions, and androgens suppress both T- and B-cell responses.[102] In injury, however, males produce greater amounts of proinflammatory cytokines, a profile that is associated with poor outcome.[105] Additionally, androgens appear to induce a greater degree of immune cell apoptosis following injury, a mechanism that may elicit a greater immunosuppression in injured males vs. females.[106] (A list of other hormones, including melatonin, substance P, neuropeptide Y, calcitonin gene–related peptide, somatostatin, and vasoactive intestinal peptide, is contained in Table 11.4.)

STRESS, ILLNESS, AND COPING

Cortisol secretion during stress may be beneficial for several reasons. Gluconeogenesis prompted by cortisol ensures an adequate source of glucose (energy) for body tissues, and nerve cells in particular. The pooling of amino acids from catabolized proteins may ensure amino acid availability for protein synthesis in certain cells. The redistribution of protein to sites where replacement is critical, such as muscle or cells of damaged tissue, would be beneficial. Short-term, cortisol-induced alterations in immune cell distribution (e.g., traffic) patterns may be adaptive, with a decrease in peripheral blood cell numbers as effector cells locate to sites of injury or inflammation. In addition, decreased immune cell activity by cortisol is beneficial in some situations because it prevents immune-mediated tissue damage by prolonged cell exposure to high levels of certain cytokines. Whether cortisol-induced effects are adaptive or destructive may depend on the intensity, type, and duration of the stressor, and the subsequent concentration and length of cortisol exposure that target cells of the individual experience.

Extreme physiologic stressors, such as severe burn injury, represent a predictable stimulus for the stress responses described previously. A less severe and defined event or situation, however, can be a stressor for one person and not for another. Many stressors, such as fasting or temperature changes, do not necessarily cause a physiologic stress response if psychologic factors are minimized. Stress itself is not an independent entity but a system of interdependent processes that are moderated by the nature, intensity, and duration of the stressor and the perception, appraisal, and coping efficacy of the affected individual, all of which in turn mediate the psychologic and physiologic response to stress. Further, adjustment to repetitive stressors is based on a person's appraisal of a situation.[107] Illustrating the influence of an individualized stress appraisal on physiologic processes, a meta-analysis of the relationships between stressors and immunity found that a higher *perception* of stress was associated with reduced T-cytotoxic (Tc) cell cytotoxicity although not with levels of circulating Th or Tc lymphocytes.[108] Appraisals of highly threatening stressors also are coupled to intense cognition rumination and greater inflammatory stress responses.[109,110] Of relevance to the importance of mental well-being in the context of overall health, a recent study reported that after adjusting for age, sex, follow-up year, all psychiatric and physical conditions, and socioeconomic factors, individuals who perceived higher levels of stress were at increased risk of requiring hospitalization or rehospitalization.[111]

Psychosocial distress may be predictive of psychologic and physical health outcomes. In psychologic distress, the individual feels a general state of unpleasant arousal after exposure to life events that manifest as physiologic, emotional, cognitive, and behavioral changes. Periods of depression and emotional upheaval often are associated with adverse life events and place the affected individual at risk for immunologic deficits, increasing the risk of ill health.[112] An older meta-analysis of studies demonstrates the longstanding relationship between depression and reduction in lymphocyte proliferation and NK cell activity.[113] Multiple moderating factors may be important in immune modulation in depressed individuals, including comorbidities such as alcoholism. Adverse life events having the most negative effect on immunity are characterized as uncontrollable, undesirable, and overtaxing the individual's ability to cope.

Low socioeconomic status (SES), as indicated in terms of income, education, or occupation, is found to be associated with higher rates of mortality and morbidity. People of lower SES may be confronted with situations characterized by uncontrollable exposure to psychosocial stress or allostatic overload that increase the risk for disease by continuously activating the sympathetic and HPA systems.[114] Indeed, low SES individuals exhibit higher basal levels of cortisol and catecholamines than those with higher income and education.[115] This association between SES and physiologic measures was independent of race, age, gender, and body mass.

Evidence also points to the emerging connection between early stressful life events and a range of chronic illnesses in later life. Childhood adversity (e.g., abuse, neglect, a dysfunctional family lifestyle, low SES) increases the risk of developing cardiovascular disease, type 2 diabetes, cancer, and a number of somatic disorders. Exposure to stress-induced dysregulation of the immune system in vulnerable children may be a major factor responsible for the subsequent onset of chronic diseases and premature death[116] (see *What's New? How Childhood Poverty Compromises Adaptive Body and Brain Functions* located on the Evolve site).

It should be further noted that the developing HPA axis is hypothesized to be influenced by parental rearing styles. Inconsistent parental discipline and monitoring are related to a flatter diurnal cortisol slope (e.g., lower morning and elevated evening cortisol secretion), problem behavior of children characterized by aggression and defiance,[117] and decreased physical and mental health.[1] This altered diurnal cortisol secretion pattern is reported to be a reflection of chronic exposure to stress occurring in young children.[118]

Animal studies reported that stress contributes to the initiation, growth, and metastasis of certain tumors.[119] In humans, stress affects important processes in cancer including antiviral responses, deoxyribonucleic acid (DNA) repair, and aspects of cellular aging.[119] The role of epigenetics and stress is an emerging field with strong implications for the intersection between stress and disease. A very recent study suggests that breast cancer bone metastases may be influenced by chronic stress by increasing the levels of Receptor Activator of Nuclear Factor κB Ligand (RANKL) that are expressed by osteoblasts, a known chemoattractant for RANK-expressing breast cancer cells.[120] However, the overall evidence is mixed from prospective studies linking stress with cancer incidence and progression. Although stress may influence the progression and recurrence of cancer, critical prospective studies have not always been supportive.[121] Studies examining impairments in antiviral immunity and chronic activation of hormonal responses (e.g., HIV-related tumors, hepatocellular carcinoma, and cervical cancer) may be more successful for defining the stress-related mechanisms.[119] Previous and current evidence show a relationship between immune stimulation and heart disease.[122] The relationship between stress and cardiovascular health may be mediated by stress-induced changes in immune function, which may potentiate proinflammatory processes and permit alterations leading to heart disease.[123] A new study of heart disease and inflammation demonstrates that monocytes and splenic macrophages invade atherosclerotic plaques after an initial myocardial infarction (heart attack), rendering them unstable and as such contribute to secondary heart attacks.[124]

In the past decade, evidence has accumulated linking severe psychosocial stress resulting from negative life events to a chronic syndrome with mental and physical consequences. Posttraumatic stress disorder (PTSD) has been described in many populations.[125-127] A cascade model has been proposed to describe the pathogenesis and clinical course illustrating the clinical, epidemiologic, neurobiologic, and psychosocial components of PTSD.[128] The study of PTSD has contributed to the knowledge concerning mechanisms involved in the chronic stress and disease relationship. Recently an appreciation of the association of chronic stress with high levels of cortisol production and paradoxical biounavailability (i.e., bound to plasma protein and therefore not bioavailable) of cortisol has been gained.[129]

Another well-documented finding is that exposure to major stressful life events, such as interpersonal loss (e.g., death of spouse, job termination) or the advent of serious health-threatening issues (e.g., cancer

diagnosis, cardiovascular disease), increases the risk of major depressive disorder.[130] Furthermore, studies suggest that stressors dramatically disrupt the person's life plans and goals and not only promote major depression but also increase the likelihood of developing diverse health problems that may be mediated and exacerbated at least, in part, by inflammation, such as asthma, rheumatoid arthritis, chronic pain, certain cancers,[1,131-133] and cardiovascular disease, the leading cause of death in major depression.[134]

This complex interplay connecting stress, depression, and inflammation may be understood in the context that stress is known to up-regulate proinflammatory cytokines.[133,135] One mechanism involving proinflammatory cytokines on major depression is the effects of TNF-α, IL-2, and IL-6 in breaking down tryptophan, the essential amino acid of serotonin synthesis.[136-138] IL-6 and TNF-α also may deplete serotonin levels by metabolizing to 5-hydroxyindoleacetic acid. Over time, stress-induced proinflammatory cytokines reduce serotonin synthesis or increase serotonin degradation that together contribute to alterations in mood, emotion, and motivational states and the eventual onset of major depression.

Another contributing factor that increases the risk of stress-induced inflammation and depression is oxidative stress, which potentially damages or shortens the telomeres and accelerates cellular aging.[139,140] Telomeres are DNA-protein complexes that cap the chromosomal DNA ends to protect the chromosome from damage. Although telomere shortening is part of the normal aging process, chronic stress accelerates telomere shortening and over time increases the risk of a number of age-related diseases, including cancer, cardiovascular disease, diabetes, obesity, Alzheimer disease, and early death.[141,142] Toxic exposure to glucocorticoids and catecholamines that promote oxidation, inflammation, and telomere shortening also is linked to depression, bipolar, and possibly anxiety disorders, especially when exposed to childhood maltreatment or trauma.[143-145]

The influence of repetitive but episodic stress on cancer survivors demonstrates a connection between events such as mammography and activation of the HPA axis. Early research with breast cancer survivors by Cordova and colleagues[146] demonstrated a link between sympathetic activity and HPA axis activation, noting that some women reported symptoms of PTSD (heart palpitations, panic, shakiness, nausea) during thoughts of recurrence triggered by events such as finding themselves near the hospital where they received initial treatment.[146] HPA axis activation also influences organs and tissues that enable bidirectional communication processes (feedback loops) between neuroendocrine and immune processes.[147] For example, among breast cancer survivors 3 to 5 years post diagnosis, elevated baseline cortisol levels and blunted cortisol reactivity were reported in response to the anticipation of a real, regularly scheduled mammogram, and alterations in cortisol level and heart rate variability were reported in women simulating the threat of cancer with a controlled laboratory stressor.[148,149] Further, Ma and colleagues[148] reported that the threat of cancer recurrence (using a simulated mammography event as a stressor to elicit thoughts of cancer recurrence) elicited greater alterations in heart rate variability when compared with another simulated controlled stressor. These studies suggest activation of the autonomic nervous system to events, such as mammography, that occur repeatedly throughout breast cancer survivorship, although the timing of onset of these autonomic activation responses to a stressor is unclear. Similar ANS activation may occur in association with events particular to the management of many other types of chronic illnesses as well as interactions with the healthcare system (see *What's New? Attenuating the Effects of Stress on Cancer*).

These additional stresses may affect the course of illness as well as interfere with the efficacy of the medical intervention. Identifying

Attenuating the Effects of Stress on Cancer

Chronic exposure to psychosocial stress can compromise health by increasing inflammation and promoting the development of diseases including cancer. Preclinical research demonstrates that prolonged stress-induced activation of the sympathetic nervous system (SNS) increases the progression of tumors by recruiting inflammatory cells to tumors and forming blood vessels that provide routes for tumor cell transport. In addition, the lymphatic system, which is innervated by the SNS and involved in immune function, also may influence cancer progression by providing a means for tumor cells to disperse through the lymphatic vasculature and a source of chemokines that promote the invasion of tumor cells.

Of interest, a preclinical study by Le and colleagues recently showed the effects of stress on tumor lymphatic vasculature and tumor breast cancer cell progression. In this study, investigators using an animal model of chronic stress reported an increase in intratumoral lymphatic vessel density (LVD), as well as increased dilation of lymphatic vessels that drain metastatic tumor cells into the lymphatic circulation. The investigators then examined whether blocking the stress-induced effects of norepinephrine on β-adrenoceptors, which are present on both tumor and inflammatory cells, will attenuate the increase in intratumoral LVD. Mice treated with the beta-blocker propranolol, a drug used clinically to treat hypertension, reduced stress-induced intratumoral LVD and tumor cell dissemination. The potential benefits of using propranolol treatment to limit LVD were then investigated in 956 people who had breast cancer. Analysis revealed that beta-blocker treatment significantly reduced the risk of lymph node metastasis. Thus inhibition of SNS signaling through the norepinephrine β-adrenoceptor attenuates in animal models the effects of chronic stress on intratumoral LVD and metastasis in people with breast cancer. The researchers conclude the results offer a promising treatment strategy to reduce the adverse effects of stress-induced SNS signaling on lymphatic vascular remodeling and the progression of cancer.

Data from Cole SW et al: *Nat Rev Cancer* 15:563–572, 2015; Le CP et al: *Nat Comm* 7:10634, 2016.

and reducing stress in the clinical setting have particular applicability in both disease prevention and illness management. In addition to medical procedures, patient-provider communication also provides an important area for future research. Recent studies of cancer communication and patient-provider interaction have demonstrated a link between communication events and emotional outcomes, such as uncertainty and mood state in breast cancer survivors.[150,151] Although a logical extension, it remains to be seen if these emotional outcomes affect physiologically based health outcomes caused by activation of the HPA axis and subsequent immune processes.

As indicated previously, coping can be considered as adaptive or maladaptive. Adaptive coping strategies, especially those that are problem focused and those that encourage seeking social support, are beneficial during stressful experiences. The extent to which an individual responds to distress, using effective positive coping strategies, determines the degree of successful moderation of the stress challenge. Conversely, ineffective negative coping attempts may exacerbate the effects of distress on health, thus augmenting the potential for illness. Mediating factors that may influence stress susceptibility or resilience include age, socioeconomic status, gender, social support status, personality and lifestyle, self-esteem, genetics, life events, past experiences, and current health status.[152] Evidence suggests that effective intervention may result in greater stress resilience and improved psychologic and physiologic

outcomes. In a study of nursing home residents randomly assigned to control or social support intervention groups, improved psychologic measures and immune function (NK cell activity) were observed in the experimental group at 6 weeks.[153] In another study, women with recurrent metastatic breast cancer were given either routine follow-up (routine care) or weekly support group sessions. Survival in the support treatment group was an average of 19 months longer than in the routine care group, suggesting a mediating influence of additional support for these women.[26,154] The importance of social support for seriously ill individuals has focused attention on the health and well-being of family members who function as caregivers. Significant stress manifested as depression, anxiety, and fatigue has been noted in family caregivers of those with cancer, Alzheimer disease, and burn trauma.[155] A recent study reported that a substantial percentage of spousal or common law caregivers may be at risk of clinical depression or suffer from psychologic health, especially in caregivers without a sense of control, social support, and low socioeconomic income.[156] Individuals and caretakers exhibited suppression of various measures of immune function, with improved function associated with better perceived social support.[157-159] Gender-based coping differences may be attributed, in part, to the hormonal milieu of the individual, with females more likely to offer social support, a behavior with an oxytocin/estrogen association.[94]

Interventions to prevent or manage stress-related psychologic or physical problems include both short- and long-term coping strategies. Stress management consists of educational components specific to the individual's problems and relaxation techniques, which may include meditation, imagery, massage, and biofeedback. These approaches may be used on an individual or a support group basis. Incorporation of these approaches into clinical training facilitates their use in the clinical arena. Research should focus on the efficacy of such approaches with various populations (*What's New?* Stress and Resilience).

AGING AND STRESS: STRESS-AGE SYNDROME

A set of neurohormonal and immune alterations, as well as tissue and cellular changes, sometimes develops with aging. These changes, which recently have been defined as stress-age syndrome, include the following:[152,160]

- Alterations in the excitability of structures of the limbic system and hypothalamus
- Increase of the blood concentrations of catecholamines, antidiuretic hormone (ADH), ACTH, and cortisol
- Decrease of the concentrations of testosterone, thyroxine, and others
- Alterations of opioid peptide concentration
- Alterations in immunodepression and patterns of chronic inflammation
- Alterations in levels of lipoproteins
- Hypercoagulation of the blood
- Free radical damage of cells

Some of the alterations are adaptational, whereas others are potentially damaging. These stress-related alterations of aging can influence the course of developing stress reactions and lower adaptive reserve and coping.[152]

In summary, it is clear that the mind and body are connected through a multitude of complex physical and emotional interactions. Understanding the complexity of these interactions is a challenge for many researchers. Areas of promise include investigating relationships between the potential for illness with respect to stressors, as well as developing effective stress management techniques and approaches that can be easily and cost-effectively employed.

WHAT'S NEW?

Stress and Resilience

People encounter many stressful experiences in modern society. In some people, stress may induce maladaptive coping behavior accompanied by pathophysiologic disorders, whereas other people are able to overcome adversity and keep in check adaptive psychologic and physiologic functioning. This latter group of individuals is considered to be resilient to the negative, toxic effects of stress and recent studies are investigating the basis of resilience.

A hypothesized neuroprotective factor underlying resilience is neuropeptide Y (NPY), a neurotransmitter that modulates stress. Higher plasma NPY levels were found in Special Forces soldiers than in non–Special Forces people and predicted better psychologic performance under stressful training situations. Another factor contributing to resilience may be testosterone. Secretion of testosterone is elevated in dominant male animals and in men who won an athletic competition. The hormone is associated with feelings of success and positive mood. In contrast, low blood levels of testosterone are found in men with posttraumatic stress disorder (PTSD) and major depressive disorder. Of further interest, testosterone may have resilient effects in men compared to women who are more likely to develop PTSD and depression. Other protective hormones may include dehydroepiandrosterone (DHEA) and DHEA sulfate ester (DHEAS). These hormones, secreted by the adrenal cortex, are some of the most abundant steroid hormones and suggested to modulate fat, mineral metabolism, and sexual functioning along with antiglucocorticoid, antiinflammatory, and antioxidant effects. Studies show that soldiers undergoing underwater navigation stress tests performed physically and cognitively better when DHEA levels are elevated or when the DHEA-to-cortisol ratio in blood is high. DHEA and DHEAS may serve to buffer the potential deleterious effects of stress and lead to superior performance effects. Another example of

the potential basis of resilience is the serotonin transporter promoter polymorphism (5HTTLPR). Carriers of the "short" (S) variant, which is less transcriptionally efficient than the "long" (L) variant, are vulnerable to major depression and anxiety. In contrast, people with the L allele are better able to cope and recover from stress. An L genetic variation in 5HTTLPR appears to promote emotional resilience.

Studies also demonstrate that people with high cognitive control that is associated with increased prefrontal cortex activity exhibit more appropriate emotional responses compared to people diagnosed with PTSD. Volunteers with high trait resilience show insula and amygdala activation only to aversive pictures compared to low-trait resilience participants. Resilient people appear better able to appropriately appraise and adjust the level of emotional resources required to meet the demands of stressful situations. Programs are currently offered to train and prepare people (e.g., firefighters, soldiers) who are likely to encounter dangerous situations by developing stress management skills, such as relaxation training. This type of training involves developing skills to manage the thoughts and perception that one will recover from stressful life events. Mindfulness-based stress reduction (MBSR) is another resilience program associated with higher levels of physical and mental health and is used as a potential treatment for PTSD, anxiety and depression disorders, and chronic pain. MBSR focuses awareness on present mental processes, such as sensations, thoughts, and feelings, in order to reduce negative emotions and improve health and coping. Overall, cognitive-based training programs play a proactive role in promoting the development of skills to become resilient to the long-term negative effects of stress disorders.

Data from Horn SR et al: *Exp Neurol* 284(Pt B):119–132, 2016; Osorio C et al: *Behav Med* 2016 Apr 21 [Epub ahead of print]; Russo SJ et al: *Nat Neurosci* 15:1475–1484, 2012.

■ SUMMARY REVIEW

Historical Background and General Concepts

1. Modern society is full of stress.

2. In general, a person experiences stress when a demand exceeds a person's coping abilities.

3. Hans Selye identified three structural changes in rats subjected repeatedly to noxious stimuli (stressors): enlargement of the cortex of the adrenal gland, atrophy of the thymus gland and other lymphoid tissues, and ulceration of the gastrointestinal tract.

4. Selye believed that the three changes were caused by a nonspecific physiologic response to any long-term stressor. He called this response the general adaptation syndrome (GAS).

5. The GAS occurs in three stages: the alarm stage, the stage of resistance or adaptation, and the stage of exhaustion. Diseases of adaptation develop if the stage of resistance or adaptation does not restore homeostasis.

6. Selye identified three components of physiologic stress: the stressor, the physiologic or chemical disturbance produced by the stressor, and the body's adaptational response to the stressor.

7. It is now known that, while important, the physiologic view of stress as outlined in the GAS is an oversimplified model of stress responses.

8. The stress response is currently viewed as the product of the interaction of the mind and body and how the cumulative effects of stress or allostatic overload may lead to disease and mental disorders. Allostatic overload refers to how long-term functional changes in the stress-related hypothalamic-pituitary-adrenal (HPA) axis and

the sympathetic nervous system (SNS) may compromise the immune system and health of the individual.

Concepts of Stress, Homeostasis, and Allostasis

1. Psychologic stress may cause or exacerbate (worsen) several disease states. Stress is related to the severity of symptoms and the outcomes of diseases and conditions. Research is focused on the mechanisms responsible for these mind-body interactions.

2. Stress has been defined as the state of affairs arising when a person relates to (i.e., interacts or transacts with) situations in a certain way. The way a person appraises and reacts to situations has a profound impact on stress.

3. The nonspecific physiologic response consists of interaction among the sympathetic branch of the autonomic nervous system (ANS) and other neural signals that activate the endocrine system, known as the hypothalamic-pituitary-adrenal (HPA) axis.

4. The nonspecific physiologic response is a common residual response and can be elicited with diverse agents such as cold, heat, x-rays, adrenaline, insulin, tubercle bacilli, and muscular exercise. Although the reactions of these stages are nonspecific, evidence supports the coexistence of highly specific, adaptive reactions to any of these agents.

5. As with a physically mediated stress response, psychologic stressors can elicit a reactive stress response; that is, a physiologic response can be derived from psychologic stressors.

■ S U M M A R Y   R E V I E W — cont'd

6. Another type of psychologic-mediated stress response is the anticipatory response.

7. In a conditioned response, the organism learns that specific stimuli are associated with danger and anticipation of subsequent encounters with that particular stimulus produces a physiologic stress response (e.g., PTSD).

8. Psychoneuroimmunology (PNI) is the study of the interaction of consciousness *(psycho)*, the brain and spinal cord *(neuro),* and the body's defense against external infection and abnormal cell division *(immunology).*

9. Psychoneuroimmunology assumes that all immune-related disease is multifactorial. The immune system is integrated with other physiologic processes and is sensitive to changes in CNS and endocrine functioning, such as those that accompany psychologic states.

10. CRH is released centrally from the brain and peripherally at inflammatory sites.

Stress Response

1. The stress response is initiated by the CNS and endocrine system. Where the stress response begins depends on whether the stressor is perceived or real.

2. Perceived stressors elicit an anticipatory response that usually begins in the limbic system of the brain. The limbic system elicits an endocrine stress response indirectly by stimulating neural pathways responsible for receiving sensory information and elicits a central response directly by stimulating the LC to release LC/NE.

3. Real stressors elicit a reactive response that can begin either in the limbic system or in the brain in response to specific sensory information. This information is then relayed to the paraventricular nucleus (PVN). The PVN stimulates the LC and both central and endocrine stress responses.

4. The neuroendocrine response to stress consists of sympathetic stimulation of the adrenal medulla to secrete catecholamines (norepinephrine and epinephrine) and stressor-induced stimulation of the hypothalamus to secrete CRH, which in turn stimulates the pituitary to secrete ACTH, which then stimulates the adrenal cortex to secrete steroid hormones, particularly cortisol.

5. In general, the catecholamines prepare the body to act, and cortisol mobilizes energy stores (e.g., glucose) and other substances needed to fuel the action.

6. Epinephrine exerts its chief effects on the cardiovascular system. Epinephrine increases cardiac output and increases blood flow to the heart, brain, and skeletal muscles by dilating vessels that supply these organs. It also dilates the airways, thereby increasing delivery of oxygen to the bloodstream.

7. Norepinephrine's chief effects complement those of epinephrine. Norepinephrine constricts blood vessels of the viscera and skin; this has the effect of shifting blood flow to the vessels dilated by epinephrine. Norepinephrine also increases mental alertness.

8. CRH influences the immune system indirectly by the activation of glucocorticoids (cortisol) and catecholamines. Peripheral CRH is proinflammatory, causing vasodilation and vascular permeability. It appears that the mast cells are the target of peripheral CRH.

9. Cortisol's chief effects involve metabolic processes. By inhibiting the use of metabolic substances while promoting their formation, cortisol mobilizes glucose, amino acids, lipids, and fatty acids and delivers them to the bloodstream.

10. Glucocorticoids or cortisol secretion during stress exerts beneficial effects by inhibiting inflammation and promoting resolution and repair. Paradoxically, elevated levels of glucocorticoids and catecholamines (epinephrine and norepinephrine), administered both endogenously and exogenously, can decrease innate immunity and increase autoimmune (adaptive) responses. These immunosuppressive effects can accentuate inflammation in general and potentially increase neuronal death (e.g., in stroke victims). In addition, chronic exposure to stress alters adaptive functions throughout the body and brain to increase the risk of developing a host of diseases including obesity, the metabolic syndrome, cardiovascular disease, and cognitive impairments, such as Alzheimer disease, and mental disorders, such as major depression, schizophrenia, and posttraumatic stress disorder.

11. The nervous, endocrine, and immune systems communicate through the common use of signal molecules and their receptors, which in turn regulate the behavior of cells in each system during stress challenge.

12. There are direct and indirect pathways of influence among the nervous, endocrine, and immune systems. Neuropeptides have direct effects on immune cells, as well as indirect influences through neuromediated endocrine modulation of immune function. Endocrine products (cortisol) also influence nerve cell behavior. Immune cell products affect both nerve and endocrine cell function, reflecting an adaptive role for the immune system as a "signal" organ to alert other systems of threatening stimuli.

13. Other hormones are affected by the stress response and include increased circulating levels of β-endorphins, growth hormone, prolactin, and oxytocin and a decrease in antidiuretic hormone level with extreme stress. Concentrations of luteinizing hormone, estradiol, progesterone, and possibly testosterone decrease during the stress response.

Stress, Illness, and Coping

1. Stress is a system of interdependent processes that are moderated by the nature, intensity, and duration of the stressor and the coping efficacy of the affected individual, all of which in turn mediate the psychologic and physiologic response to stress.

2. Many studies have linked psychologic distress with altered immune function, and evidence strengthens the association of stress with potential for illness in humans, especially in vulnerable young children who are unable to control the adverse effects of stress, such as poor housing and negative parental rearing conditions.

3. Adaptive coping strategies, especially those that are problem focused and those that encourage seeking social support, are beneficial during stressful experiences.

Aging and Stress: Stress-Age Syndrome

1. With aging, sometimes a set of neurohormonal and immune alterations develop; these changes have been defined as stress-age syndrome.

2. These stress-related alterations of aging can influence the course of developing stress reactions and lower adaptive reserve and coping.

KEY TERMS

Adrenocorticotropic hormone (ACTH), 329
Allostasis, 324
Allostatic load, 326
Allostatic overload, 326
Anticipatory response, 324
Catecholamine, 328
Conditional response, 324
Coping, 338
Corticosteroid-binding globulin, 329
Corticotropin-releasing hormone (CRH), 329

Cortisol, 329
Cytokine, 333
General adaptation syndrome (GAS), 323
Homeostasis, 324
Hypothalamic-pituitary-adrenal (HPA) axis, 324
Inflammation, 323
Neuropeptide Y (NPY), 335
Peripheral (immune) CRH, 334
Posttraumatic stress disorder (PTSD), 324
Psychologic distress, 338

Psychoneuroimmunology (PNI), 327
Reactive response, 324
Stress, 324
Stressor, 327
Stress response, 324
Sympathetic nervous system (SNS), 328
Th1 to Th2 shift, 333
Transcortin, 329

REFERENCES

1. Chrousos GP: Stress and disorders of the stress system. *Nat Rev Endocrinol* 5:374–381, 2009.
2. McEwen BS: Central effects of stress hormones in health and disease: understanding the protective and damaging effects of stress and stress mediators. *Eur J Pharmacol* 583(2-3):174–185, 2008.
3. Powell ND, et al: Social stress up-regulates inflammatory gene expression in the leukocyte transcriptome via β-adrenergic induction of myelopoiesis. *Proc Natl Acad Sci USA* 110(41): 16574–16579, 2013.
4. Cannon WB, Bringer CAL, Fritz R: Experimental hyperthyroidism. *Am J Physiol* 36:363, 1914.
5. Selye H: The general adaptation syndrome and the diseases of adaptation. *J Clin Endocrinol* 6:117–230, 1946.
6. Hill SR, et al: Studies on adrenocortical and psychological responses to stress in man. *Arch Intern Med* 97:269, 1956.
7. Mason JW, Brady JV: Plasma 17-hydroxycorticosteroid changes related to reserpine effects on emotional behaviors. *Science* 124:983, 1956.
8. Hetzel BS, et al: Changes in urinary 17-hydroxycorticosteroid excretion during stressful life experiences in man. *J Clin Endocrinol Metab* 15(9):1057–1068, 1955.
9. Handlon JH, et al: Psychological factors lowering plasma 17-hydroxycorticosteroid concentration. *Psychosom Med* 24:535–541, 1962.
10. Wadeson RW, et al: Plasma and urinary 17-OHCS responses to motion pictures. *Arch Gen Psychiatry* 14:146–156, 1963.
11. Mason JW: Organization of psychoendocrine mechanisms: a review and reconsideration of research. In Greenfield NS, Steinbach RA, editors: *Handbook of psychophysiology*, New York, 1972, Holt, Rinehart, & Winston.
12. Herman JP, et al: Central mechanisms of stress integration: hierarchical circuitry controlling hypothalamo-pituitary-adrenocortical responsiveness. *Front Neuroendocrinol* 24(3): 151–158, 2003.
13. Seeman T, et al: Socio-economic differentials in peripheral biology: cumulative allostatic load. *Ann N Y Acad Sci* 1186:223–239, 2010.
14. Sorrells SF, et al: The stressed CNS: when glucocorticoids aggravate inflammation (review). *Neuron* 64(1):33–39, 2009.
15. McEwen BS, Gray JD, Nasca C: Redefining neuroendocrinology: stress, sex and cognitive and emotional regulation. *J Endocrinol* 226(2): T67–T83, 2015.
16. McEwen BS, et al: Mechanisms of stress in the brain. *Nat Neurosci* 18(10):1353–1363, 2015.
17. McEwen BS: Sleep deprivation as neurobiologic and physiologic stressor, allostasis and allostatic load. *Metabolism* 55:S20–S23, 2006.

18. Kiecolt-Glaser JK, et al: Psychoneuroimmunology: psychological influences on immune function and health. *J Consult Clin Psychol* 70(3):537–547, 2002.
19. Bauer-Wu SM: Psychoneuroimmunology. Part I: Physiology. *Clin J Oncol Nurs* 6(3):167–170, 2002.
20. Bauer-Wu SM: Psychoneuroimmunology. Part II: Mind-body interventions. *Clin J Oncol Nurs* 6(4):243–246, 2002.
21. Ranchor AV, Sanderman R, Coyne JC: Invited commentary: personality as a causal factor in cancer risk and mortality—time to retire a hypothesis? *Am J Epidemiol* 172(4):386–388, 2010.
22. Sloan EK, et al: The sympathetic nervous system induces a metastatic switch in primary breast cancer. *Cancer Res* 70(18):7042–7052, 2010.
23. Chrousos GP, Kino T: Glucocorticoid signaling in the cell: expanding clinical complications to complex human behavioral and somatic disorders. *Ann N Y Acad Sci* 1179:153–166, 2009.
24. Liu LY, et al: School examinations enhance airway inflammation to antigen challenge. *Am J Respir Crit Care Med* 165(8):1062–1067, 2002.
25. Cacioppo JT, et al: Autonomic, neuroendocrine, and immune responses to psychological stress: the reactivity hypothesis. *Ann N Y Acad Sci* 840:664–673, 1998.
26. Calcagni E, Elenkov I: Stress system activity, innate and T helper cytokines, and susceptibility to immune-related diseases (review). *Ann N Y Acad Sci* 1069:62–76, 2006.
27. Maier SF, Watkins LR: Cytokines for psychologists: implications of bidirectional immune-to-brain communication for understanding behavior, mood, and cognition. *Psychol Rev* 105(1):83–107, 1998.
28. Charmandari E, Tsigos C, Chrousos G: Endocrinology of the stress response (review). *Annu Rev Physiol* 67:259–284, 2005.
29. Carrillo-Vico A, et al: A review of the multiple actions of melatonin on the immune system (review). *Endocrine* 27(2):189–200, 2005.
30. Bruunsgard H, Pedersen BK: Age-related inflammatory cytokines and disease. *Immunol Allergy Clin North Am* 23(1):15–39, 2003.
31. MacPherson A, Dinkel K, Sapolsky R: Glucocorticoids worsen excitoxin-induced expression of proinflammatory cytokines in hippocampal cultures. *Exp Neural* 194(2):376–383, 2005.
32. Coutinho AE, Chapman KE: The anti-inflammatory and immunosuppressive effects of glucocorticoids, recent developments and mechanistic insights. *Mol Cell Endocrinol* 335(1):2–13, 2010.
33. Thayer JF, Lane RD: A model of neurovascular integration in emotion regulation and dysregulation. *J Affect Disord* 61:201–216, 2000.
34. Alevizaki M, et al: High anticipatory stress plasma cortisol levels and sensitivity to glucocorticoids

predict severity of coronary artery disease in subjects undergoing coronary angiography. *Metabolism* 56:222–226, 2007.
35. Kajantie E, et al: Body size at birth predicts hypothalamic-pituitary-adrenal axis response to psychosocial stress at 60 to 70 years. *J Clin Endocrinol Metab* 92(11):4094–4100, 2007.
36. Elenkov IJ, et al: Cytokine dysregulation, inflammation, and well-being. *Neuroimmunomodulation* 12(5):255–269, 2005.
37. Kox M, et al: Voluntary activation of the sympathetic nervous system and attenuation of the innate immune response in humans. *Proc Natl Acad Sci USA* 111(20):7379–7384, 2014.
38. Cohen S, et al: Types of stressors that increase susceptibility to the common cold in healthy adults. *Health Psychol* 17(3):214–223, 1998.
39. McCain NL, et al: A randomized clinical trial of alternative stress management interventions in persons with HIV infection. *J Consult Clin Psychol* 76(3):431–441, 2008.
40. Glaser R, et al: Chronic stress modulates the immune response to a pneumococcal pneumonia vaccine. *Psychosom Med* 62(6):804–807, 2000.
41. Marucha PT, Kiecolt-Glaser JK, Favagehi M: Mucosal wound healing is impaired by examination stress. *Psychosom Med* 60(3):362–365, 1998.
42. Pacak K, et al: Heterogeneous neurochemical responses to different stressors: a test of Selye's doctrine of nonspecificity. *Am J Physiol* 275(4 Pt 2):R1247–R1255, 1998.
43. Repka-Ramirez MS, Baraniuk JN: Histamine in health and disease. *Clin Allergy Immunol* 17:1–25, 2002.
44. Russ TC, et al: Association between psychological distress and mortality: individual participant pooled analysis of 10 prospective cohort studies. *BMJ* 345:e4933, 2012.
45. Goh J, Pfeffer J, Zenios SA: Workplace stressors & health outcomes: health policy for the workplace. *Behav Sci Policy* 1(1):43–52, 2015.
46. Leka S, Jain A: *Health impact of psychosocial hazards at work: An overview*, Geneva, 2010, Institute of Work, Health & Organizations, University of Nottingham, World Health Organization.
47. Sapolsky RM, editor: *Why zebras don't get ulcers: a guide to stress, stress-related diseases, and coping*, New York, 1994, Freeman.
48. Dimsdale JE, Ziegler MG: What do plasma and urinary measures of catecholamines tell us about human response to stressors? *Circulation* 83(4 Suppl):II36–II42, 1991.
49. Herd JA: Cardiovascular response to stress. *Physiol Rev* 71(1):305–330, 1991.
50. Sapolsky RM, Romero LM, Munck AU: How do glucocorticoids influence stress responses? Integrating permissive, suppressive, stimulatory,

and preparative actions. *Endocr Rev* 21(1):55–89, 2000.

51. Rabin BS: The nervous system—immune system connection. In Rabin BS, editor: *Stress, immune function, and health: the connection*, New York, 1999, Wiley-Liss.

52. Moyna NM, et al: The effects of incremental submaximal exercise on circulating leukocytes in physically active and sedentary males and females. *Eur J Appl Physiol Occup Physiol* 74(3):211–218, 1996.

53. Kapcala LP, et al: The protective role of the hypothalamic-pituitary-adrenal axis against lethality produced by immune, infections, and inflammatory stress. *Ann N Y Acad Sci* 771: 419–437, 1995.

54. Kyrou I, Tsigos C: Chronic stress, visceral obesity and gonadal dysfunction. *Hormones* 7:287–293, 2008.

55. Kyrou I, Tsigos C: Stress hormones: physiological stress and regulation of metabolism. *Curr Opin Pharmacol* 9:787–793, 2009.

56. Odengaard JI, Chawla A: Leukocyte set points in metabolic disease. *F1000 Biol Rep* 4:13, 2012.

57. Seckl JR, Holmes MC: Mechanisms of disease: glucocorticoids, their placental metabolism and fetal 'programming' of adult pathophysiology. *Nat Clin Pract Endocrinol Metab* 3:479–488, 2007.

58. Reynolds RM: Glucocorticoid excess and the developmental origins of disease: two decades of testing the hypothesis—2012 Curt Richter Award winner. *Psychoneuroendocrinology* 38:1–11, 2013.

59. Painter RC, Roseboom TJ, de Rooij SR: Long-term effects of prenatal stress and glucocorticoid exposure. *Birth Defects Res C Embryo Today* 96(4):315–324, 2012.

60. Monaghan P: Organismal stress, telomeres and life histories. *J Exp Biol* 217(Pt 1):57–66, 2014.

61. Nicolaides NC, et al: Stress, the stress system and the role of glucocorticoids. *Neuroimmunomodulation* 22:6–19, 2015.

62. Hunter RG, et al: Stress and glucocorticoids regulate rat hippocampal mitochondrial DNA gene expression via the glucocorticoid receptor. *Proc Natl Acad Sci USA* 113(32):9099–9104, 2016.

63. Wilson RS, et al: Proneness to psychological distress is associated with risk of Alzheimer's disease. *Neurology* 61:1479–1485, 2003.

64. Johansson L, et al: Common psychosocial stressors in middle-aged women related to longstanding distress and increased risk of Alzheimer's disease: a 38-year longitudinal population study. *BMJ Open* 3:e003142, 2013.

65. Sotiropoulos I, et al: Stress acts cumulatively to precipitate Alzheimer's disease-like Tau pathology and cognitive deficits. *J Neurosci* 31:7840–7847, 2011.

66. Arnsten AFT: Stress weakens prefrontal networks: molecular insults to higher cognition. *Nat Neurosci* 18:1376–1385, 2015.

67. Elenkov IJ, Chrousos GP: Stress hormones, proinflammatory and antiinflammatory cytokines, and autoimmunity. *Ann N Y Acad Sci* 966: 290–303, 2002.

68. Elenkov IJ: Glucocorticoids and the Th1/Th2 balance. *Ann N Y Acad Sci* 1024:138–146, 2004. review.

69. Meduri GU, Chrousos GP: Duration of glucocorticoid treatment and outcome in sepsis: is the right drug used the wrong way? *Chest* 114(2): 355–360, 1998.

70. Seok JH, et al: Psychological and neuroendocrinological characteristics associated with depressive symptoms in breast cancer patients at the initial cancer diagnosis. *Gen Hosp Psychiatry* 32(5):503–508, 2010.

71. Thornton LM, Andersen BL, Blakely WP: The pain, depression, and fatigue symptom cluster in advanced breast cancer: covariance with the hypothalamic-pituitary-adrenal axis and the sympathetic nervous system. *Health Psychol* 29(3):333–337, 2010.

72. Ben-Eliyahu S, et al: Suppression of NK cell activity and of resistance to metastasis by stress: a role for adrenal catecholamines and beta-adrenoceptors. *Neuroimmunomodulation* 8(3):154–164, 2000.

73. Li Q, et al: Effect of electric foot shock and psychological stress on activities of murine splenic natural killer and lymphokine-activated killer cells, cytotoxic T lymphocytes, natural killer receptors and mRNA transcripts for granzymes and perforin. *Stress* 8(2):107–116, 2005.

74. Palermo-Neto J, et al: Effects of physical and psychological stressors on behavior, macrophage activity, and Ehrlich tumor growth. *Brain Behav Immun* 17(1):43–54, 2003.

75. Stefanski V: Social stress in laboratory rats: behavior, immune function, and tumor metastasis. *Physiol Behav* 73(3):385–391, 2001.

76. Inbar S, et al: Do stress responses promote leukemia progression? An animal study suggesting a role for epinephrine and prostaglandin-E2 through reduced NK activity. *PLoS ONE* 6(4): e19246, 2011.

77. Neeman E, Ben-Eliyahu S: The perioperative period and promotion of cancer metastasis: new outlooks on mediating mechanisms and immune involvement. *Brain Behav Immun* 30(Suppl): S32–S40, 2013.

78. Shakhar G, Ben-Eliyahu S: Potential prophylactic measures against postoperative immunosuppression: could they reduce recurrence rates in oncological patients? *Ann Surg Oncol* 10(8):972–992, 2003.

79. Bartal I, et al: Immune perturbations in patients along the perioperative period: alterations in cell surface markers and leukocyte subtypes before and after surgery. *Brain Behav Immun* 24(3): 376–386, 2010.

80. Greenfeld K, et al: Immune suppression while awaiting surgery and following it: dissociations between plasma cytokine levels, their induced production, and NK cell cytotoxicity. *Brain Behav Immun* 21(4):503–513, 2007.

81. Faist E, Schinkel C, Zimmer S: Update on the mechanisms of immune suppression of injury and immune modulation. *World J Surg* 20(4):454–459, 1996.

82. Horowitz M, et al: Exploiting the critical perioperative period to improve long-term cancer outcomes. *Nat Rev Clin Oncol* 12:213–226, 2015.

83. Chrousos GP, Elenkov IJ: Interactions of the endocrine and immune systems. In DeGroot LG, Jameson JL, editors: *Endocrinology*, ed 4, Philadelphia, 2001, Saunders.

84. Rocklin RE, editor: *Histamine and H2 antagonists in inflammation and immunodeficiency*, New York, 1990, Marcel Dekker.

85. Chrousos GP, Gold PW: The concepts of stress and stress system disorders: overview of physical and behavioral homeostasis. *JAMA* 267(9): 1244–1252, 1992.

86. Chrousos GP, et al: Interactions between the hypothalamic-pituitary-adrenal axis and the female reproductive system. *Ann Intern Med* 129(3):229–240, 1998.

87. Kalantaridou SN, et al: Stress and the female reproductive system. Review. *J Reprod Immunol* 62(1-2):61–68, 2004.

88. Gallucci WT, et al: Sex differences in sensitivity of the hypothalamic-pituitary-adrenal axis. *Health Psychol* 12(5):420–425, 1993.

89. Peiffer A, Lapointe B, Barden H: Hormonal regulation of type II glucocorticoid receptor messenger ribonucleic acid in rat brain. *Endocrinology* 129(4):2166–2174, 1991.

90. Machelska H, et al: Opioid control of inflammatory pain regulated by intercellular adhesion molecule-1. *J Neurosci* 22(13): 5588–5596, 2002.

91. Molina PE: Stress-specific opioid modulation of haemodynamic counter-regulation. *Clin Exp Pharmacol Physiol* 29(3):248–253, 2002.

92. Jochem J, Josko J, Gwozdz B: Endogenous opioid peptides system in haemorrhagic shock—central cardiovascular regulation. *Med Sci Monit* 7(3): 545–549, 2001.

93. Molina PE: Opiate modulation of hemodynamic, hormonal, and cytokine responses to hemorrhage. *Shock* 15(6):471–478, 2001.

94. Cabot PJ, et al: Immune cell-derived beta-endorphin: production, release, and control of inflammatory pain in rats. *J Clin Invest* 100(1): 142–148, 1997.

95. Van De Weerdt C, et al: Far upstream sequences regulate the human prolactin promoter transcription. *Neuroendocrinology* 71(2):124–137, 2000.

96. Cardoso C, Kingdon D, Ellenbogen MA: A meta-analytic review of the impact of intranasal oxytocin administration on cortisol concentrations during laboratory tasks: moderation by method and mental health. *Psychneuroendocrinology* 49:161–170, 2014.

97. Meyer-Lindenberg A, et al: Oxytocin and vasopressin in the human brain: social neuropeptides for translational medicine. *Nat Rev Neurosci* 12:524–538, 2011.

98. Nave G, Camerer C, McCullough M: Does oxytocin increase trust in humans? A critical review of research. *Perspect Psychol Sci* 10(6): 772–789, 2015.

99. Aakvaag A, et al: Testosterone and testosterone-binding globulin (TeBG) in young men during prolonged stress. *Int J Androl* 1:22, 1978.

100. Kreuz LE, Rose RM, Jennings JR: Suppression of plasma testosterone levels and psychological stress: a longitudinal study of young men in Officer Candidate School. *Arch Gen Psychiatry* 26(5): 479–482, 1972.

101. Guezennec CY, et al: Effect of competition stress on tests used to assess testosterone administration in athletes. *Int J Sports Med* 16(6):368–372, 1995.

102. Rose RM: Psychoendocrinology. In Wilson JD, Foster DW, editors: *Williams textbook of endocrinology*, ed 7, Philadelphia, 1985, Saunders.

103. Da Silva JA: Sex hormones and glucocorticoids: interactions with the immune system. *Ann N Y Acad Sci* 876: 102–117, 1999.

104. Offner PJ, Moore EE, Biffl WL: Male gender is a risk factor for major infections after surgery. *Arch Surg* 134(9):935–938, 1999.

105. Angele MK, et al: Sex steroids regulate pro- and anti-inflammatory cytokine release by macrophages after trauma-hemorrhage. *Am J Physiol* 277(1 Pt 1):C35–C42, 1999.

106. Angele MK, et al: Gender dimorphism in trauma-hemorrhage–induced thymocyte apoptosis. *Shock* 12(4):316–322, 1999.

107. McEwen BS: Protective and damaging effects of stress mediators. *N Engl J Med* 338(3):171–179, 1998.

108. Segerstrom SC, Miller GE: Psychological stress and the human immune system: a meta-analytic study of 30 years of inquiry. *Psychol Bull* 130(4): 601–630, 2004.

109. Watkins E: Appraisals and strategies associated with rumination and worry. *Pers Individ Differ* 37:679–694, 2004.

110. Wirtz PH, et al: Variations in anticipatory cognitive stress appraisal and differential proinflammatory cytokine expression in response to acute stress. *Brain Behav Immun* 21:851–859, 2007.

111. Prior A, et al: Perceived stress, multimorbidity, and risk for hospitalizations for ambulatory care–sensitive conditions: a population-based cohort study. *Med Care* 55(2):131–139, 2016.

112. Rozlog LA, et al: Stress and immunity: implications for viral disease and wound healing. *J Periodontol* 70(7):786–792, 1999.

113. Irwin M: Immune correlates of depression. *Adv Exp Med Biol* 461:1–24, 1999.

114. Adler NE, editor: *Socioeconomic status and health in industrial nations: social, psychological, and biological pathways*, New York, 1999, New York Academy of Sciences.

115. Cohen S, et al: Socioeconomic status is associated with stress hormones. *Psychosom Med* 68:414–420, 2006.

116. Miller GE, et al: Psychological stress in childhood and susceptibility to the chronic diseases of aging: moving toward a model of behavioral and biological mechanisms. *Psychol Bull* 137:959–997, 2011.

117. Lahey BB, et al: Is parental knowledge of their offspring's whereabouts and peer associations spuriously associated with offspring delinquency? *J Abnorm Child Psychol* 36:807–823, 2008.

118. Fries E, et al: A new view on hypocortisolism. *Psychoneuroendocrinology* 30:1010–1016, 2005.

119. Antoni MH, et al: The influence of bio-behavioral factors on tumor biology: pathways and mechanisms. *Nat Rev Cancer* 6(3):240–248, 2006.

120. Campbell JP, et al: Stimulation of host bone marrow stromal cells by sympathetic nerves promotes breast cancer bone metastasis in mice. *PLoS Biol* 10(7):e1001363, 2012.

121. Vedhara K, Irwin M, editors: *Human pyschoimmunology*, Oxford, England, 2005, Oxford University Press.

122. Sharma R, Coats AJ, Anker SD: The role of inflammatory mediators in chronic heart failure: cytokines, nitric oxide, and endothelin-1. *Int J Cardiol* 72(2):175–186, 2000.

123. Sher L: Effects of psychological factors on the development of cardiovascular pathology: role of the immune system and infection. *Med Hypotheses* 53(2):112–113, 1999.

124. Dutta P, et al: Myocardial infarction accelerates atherosclerosis. *Nature* 487(7407):325–329, 2012.

125. Bremner JD, et al: Neural correlates of memories of childhood sexual abuse in women with and without posttraumatic stress disorder. *Am J Psychiatry* 156(11):1787–1795, 1999.

126. Clohessy S, Ehlers A: PTSD symptoms, response to intrusive memories and coping in ambulance service workers. *Br J Clin Psychol* 38(Pt 3):251–265, 1999.

127. Donnelly CL, Amaya-Jackson L, March JS: Psychopharmacology of pediatric posttraumatic stress disorder. *J Child Adolesc Psychopharmacol* 9(3):203–220, 1999.

128. Heim C, Ehlert U, Hellhammer DH: The potential role of hypocortisolism in the pathophysiology of stress-related bodily disorders. *Psychoneuroendocrinology* 25(1):1–35, 2000.

129. Alarcon RD, Glover SG, Deering CG: The cascade model: an alternative to comorbidity in the pathogenesis of posttraumatic stress disorder. *Psychiatry* 62(2):114–124, 1999.

130. Kendler KS, Karkowski LM, Prescott CA: Causal relationship between stressful life events and the onset of major depression. *Am J Psychiatry* 156:837–848, 1999.

131. Bower JE, Crosswell AD, Slavich GM: Childhood adversity and cumulative life stress: risk factors for cancer-related fatigue. *Clin Psychol Sci* 2:108–115, 2014.

132. Cohen S, Janicki-Deverts D, Miller GE: Psychological stress and disease. *JAMA* 298:1685–1687, 2007.

133. Slavich GM, Irwin MR: From stress to inflammation and major depressive disorder: a social signal transduction theory of depression. *Psychol Bull* 140:774–815, 2014.

134. Assies J, et al: Effects of oxidative stress on fatty acid- and one-carbon-metabolism in psychiatric and cardiovascular disease comorbidity. *Acta Psychiatr Scand* 130:163–180, 2014.

135. Hodes GE, et al: Neuroimmune mechanisms of depression. *Nat Neurosci* 18:1386–1393, 2015.

136. Dantzer R, et al: From inflammation to sickness and depression: when the immune system subjugates the brain. *Nat Rev Neurosci* 9:46–57, 2008.

137. Schwarcz R, et al: Kynurenines in the mammalian brain: when physiology meets pathology. *Nat Rev Neurosci* 13:465–477, 2012.

138. Leonard B, Maes M: Mechanistic explanations how cell-mediated immune activation, inflammation and oxidative and nitrosative stress pathways and their sequels and concomitants play a role in the pathophysiology of unipolar depression. *Neurosci Biobehav Rev* 36:764–785, 2012.

139. Wolkowitz OM, et al: Depression gets old fast: do stress and depression accelerate cell aging? *Depress Anxiety* 27:327–338, 2010.

140. Epel ES: Psychological and metabolic stress: a recipe for accelerated cellular aging? *Hormones* 8:7–22, 2009.

141. Blackburn EH, Epel ES: Too toxic to ignore. *Nature* 490:169–171, 2012.

142. Rizvi S, et al: Telomere length variations in aging and age-related diseases. *Curr Aging Sci* 7:161–167, 2014.

143. Danese A, McEwen BS: Adverse childhood experiences, allostasis, allostatic load, and age-related disease. *Physiol Behav* 106:29–39, 2012.

144. Lindqvist D, et al: Psychiatric disorders and leukocyte telomere length: underlying mechanisms linking mental illness with cellular aging. *Neurosci Biobehav Rev* 55:333–364, 2015.

145. Verhoeven JE, et al: Major depressive disorder and accelerated cellular aging: results from a large psychiatric cohort study. *Mol Psychiatry* 19:895–901, 2014.

146. Cordova MJ, et al: Frequency and correlates of posttraumatic-stress-disorder-like symptoms after treatment for breast cancer. *J Consult Clin Psychol* 63(6):981–986, 1995.

147. Reiche EMV, Nunes SOV, Morimoto HK: Stress, depression, the immune system, and cancer (review). *Lancet Oncol* 5(10):617–625, 2004.

148. Ma Z, Faber A, Dube L: Exploring women's psychoneuroendocrine responses to cancer threat: insights from a computer-based guided imagery task. *Can J Nurs Res* 39(1):98–115, 2007.

149. Porter LS, et al: Cortisol levels and responses to mammography screening in breast cancer survivors: a pilot study. *Psychosom Med* 65(5):842–848, 2003.

150. Clayton MF, Dudley WN, Musters A: Communication with breast cancer survivors. *Health Commun* 23(3):207–221, 2008.

151. Clayton MF, Mishel MH, Belyea M: Testing a model of symptoms, communication, uncertainty, and well-being, in older breast cancer survivors. *Res Nurs Health* 29(1):18–39, 2006.

152. Frolkis VV: Stress-age syndrome. *Mech Ageing Dev* 69(1-2):93–107, 1993.

153. Kiecolt-Glaser J, et al: Psychosocial enhancement of immunocompetence in a geriatric population. *Health Psychol* 4(1):25–41, 1985.

154. Spiegel D: Psychosocial intervention in cancer. *J Natl Cancer Inst* 85(15):1198–1205, 1993.

155. Pinquart M, Sörensen S: Differences between caregivers and noncaregivers in psychological health and physical health: a meta-analysis. *Psychol Aging* 18(2):250–267, 2003.

156. Cameron JI, et al: One-year outcomes in caregivers of critically ill patients. *N Engl J Med* 374(19):1831–1841, 2016.

157. Baron RS, et al: Social support and immune function among spouses of cancer patients. *J Pers Soc Psychol* 59(2):344–352, 1990.

158. Kiecolt-Glaser J, et al: Chronic stress and immune function in family caregivers of Alzheimer's disease victims. *Psychosom Med* 45(5):523, 1987.

159. Shelby J, et al: Severe burn injury: effects on psychologic and immunologic function in noninjured close relatives. *J Burn Care Rehabil* 13(1):58–63, 1992.

160. Mazzeo RS: Aging, immune function, and exercise: hormonal regulation. *Int J Sports Med* 21(Suppl 1):S10–S13, 2000. Review.

CHAPTER

12

Cancer Biology

Neal S. Rote

evolve WEBSITE

http://evolve.elsevier.com/McCance/
- Content Updates
- Chapter Summary Review
- Review Questions
- Case Studies
- Animations

CHAPTER OUTLINE

Cancer is a leading cause of suffering and death in the developed world. Over the past 35 years intensive research has led to a significantly enhanced understanding of this complex and frightening disease. It is now understood that cancer is a collection of more than 100 different diseases, each caused by a specific and often unique age-related accumulation of genetic and epigenetic alterations. Environment, heredity, and behavior interact to modify the risk of developing cancer and the response to treatment. Improvements in treatment strategies and supportive care, coupled with new, often individualized therapies based on advances of the basic pathophysiology of malignancy, have contributed to an increasing number of effective options for these diverse, often lethal, disorders collectively called *cancer*.

CANCER CHARACTERISTICS AND TERMINOLOGY

Any discussion of cancer must start with a definition of what it is and what it is not. Although most readers may have an intuitive understanding of this disorder, composing an exact definition that encompasses this broad category is more challenging.

The term *cancer* derives from the Greek word for crab, *karkinoma*, which the physician Hippocrates used to describe the appendage-like projections extending from tumors. The word tumor originally referred to any swelling that was caused by inflammation, but is now generally reserved for describing a new growth, or neoplasm, resulting from an

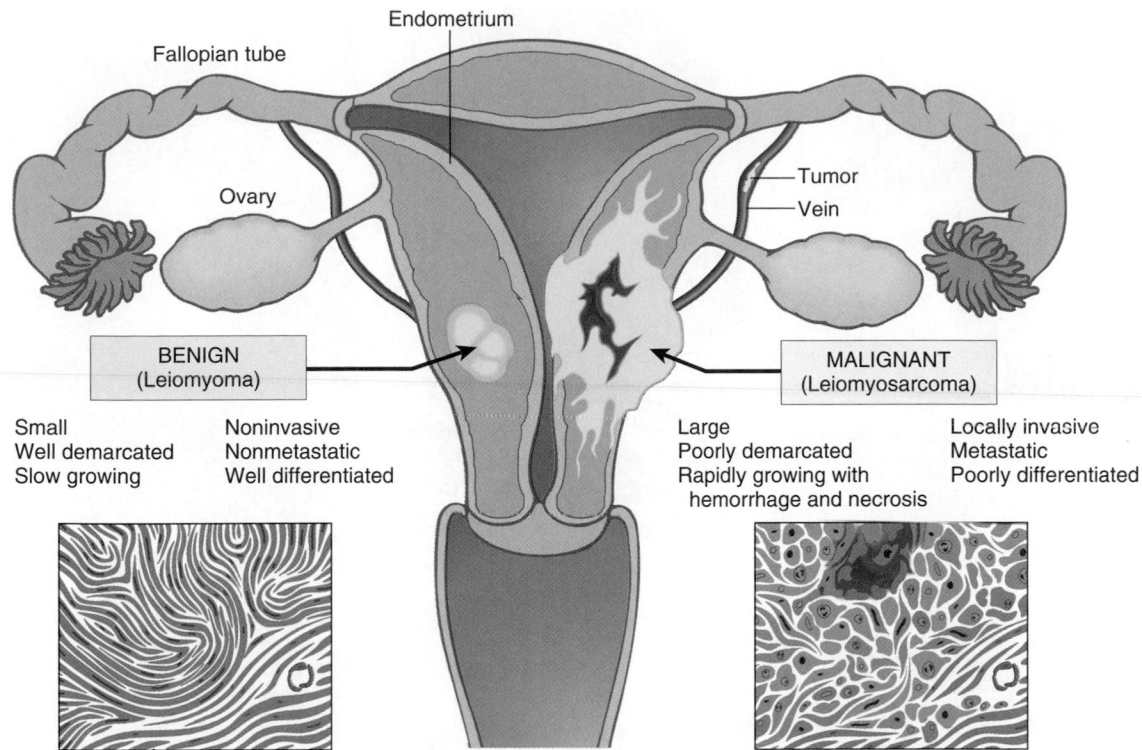

FIGURE 12.1 Comparison Between a Benign Tumor and a Malignant Tumor of the Same Origin. (From Kumar V et al: *Robbins and Cotran pathologic basis of disease*, ed 9, Philadelphia, 2015, Saunders.)

abnormal growth following uncontrolled proliferation and serving no physiologic purpose. Not all tumors or neoplasms, however, are cancer. The term cancer refers to a *malignant* tumor and is not used to refer to *benign* growths, such as lipomas or hypertrophy of an organ. The National Cancer Institute (NCI) of the National Institutes of Health (NIH) defines cancer as "diseases in which abnormal cells divide without control and are able to invade other tissues."[1] The definitions of benign vs. malignant are presented in the following text and shown in Fig. 12.1.

Tumor Classification and Nomenclature

Proper identification of a cancer is important for many reasons. Different cancers will have different causes, different rates and patterns of progression, and different responses to treatment. The classification starts with knowing the tissue and organ of origin, the extent of distribution to other sites, and the microscopic appearance of the lesion. Increasingly, it also includes a detailed description of the critical genetic changes in the cancer.

Benign tumors, which are not referred to as cancers, are usually encapsulated with connective tissue and contain fairly well-differentiated cells and well-organized stroma (see Fig. 12.1). They retain recognizable normal tissue structure and do not invade beyond their capsule, nor do they spread to regional lymph nodes or distant locations. Mitotic cells are very rarely present during microscopic analysis. Benign tumors are generally named according to the tissues from which they arise with the suffix "-oma," which indicates a tumor or mass. For example, a benign tumor of the smooth muscle of the uterus is a *leiomyoma,* and a benign tumor of fat cells is a *lipoma.* Benign tumors of the colon or stomach usually present as colonic or gastric polyps, and those of melanocytes present as dark-colored nevi (e.g., birthmark, mole). It is important to understand that benign tumors can become extremely

large and, depending on their location in the body, can cause morbidity or be life-threatening by compressing normal tissue, preventing blood flow to the region (ischemia), or causing necrotic death of normal tissue. For example, a benign meningioma at the base of the skull may cause symptoms by compressing adjacent normal brain tissue. Benign tumors of endocrine organs may lead to overproduction of hormones.

Some tumors initially described as benign can progress to cancer and then are referred to as malignant tumors, which are distinguished from benign tumors by more rapid growth rates and specific microscopic alterations, including loss of differentiation and absence of normal tissue organization (Fig. 12.2). One of the microscopic hallmarks of cancer cells is anaplasia, the loss of cellular differentiation. Malignant cells are also pleomorphic, with marked variability of size and shape. They often have large darkly stained nuclei, and mitotic cells are common. Malignant tumors may have a substantial amount of stroma, but it is disorganized, with loss of normal tissue structure. Malignant tumors lack a capsule and grow to invade nearby blood vessels, lymphatics, and surrounding structures. The most important and deadliest characteristic of malignant tumors is their ability to spread far beyond the tissue of origin, a process known as metastasis.

Unlike benign tumors, which are named related to the tissue of origin, cancers are generally named according to the cell type from which they originate. Cancers arising in epithelial tissue are called carcinomas, and if they arise from or form ductal or glandular structures are named adenocarcinomas. Hence, a malignant tumor arising from breast glandular tissue is a mammary adenocarcinoma, whereas an example of a benign breast tumor is a fibroadenoma. Cancers arising from mesenchymal tissue (including connective tissue, muscle, and bone) usually have the suffix sarcoma. For example, malignant cancers of skeletal muscle are known as *rhabdomyosarcomas.* Cancers of lymphatic

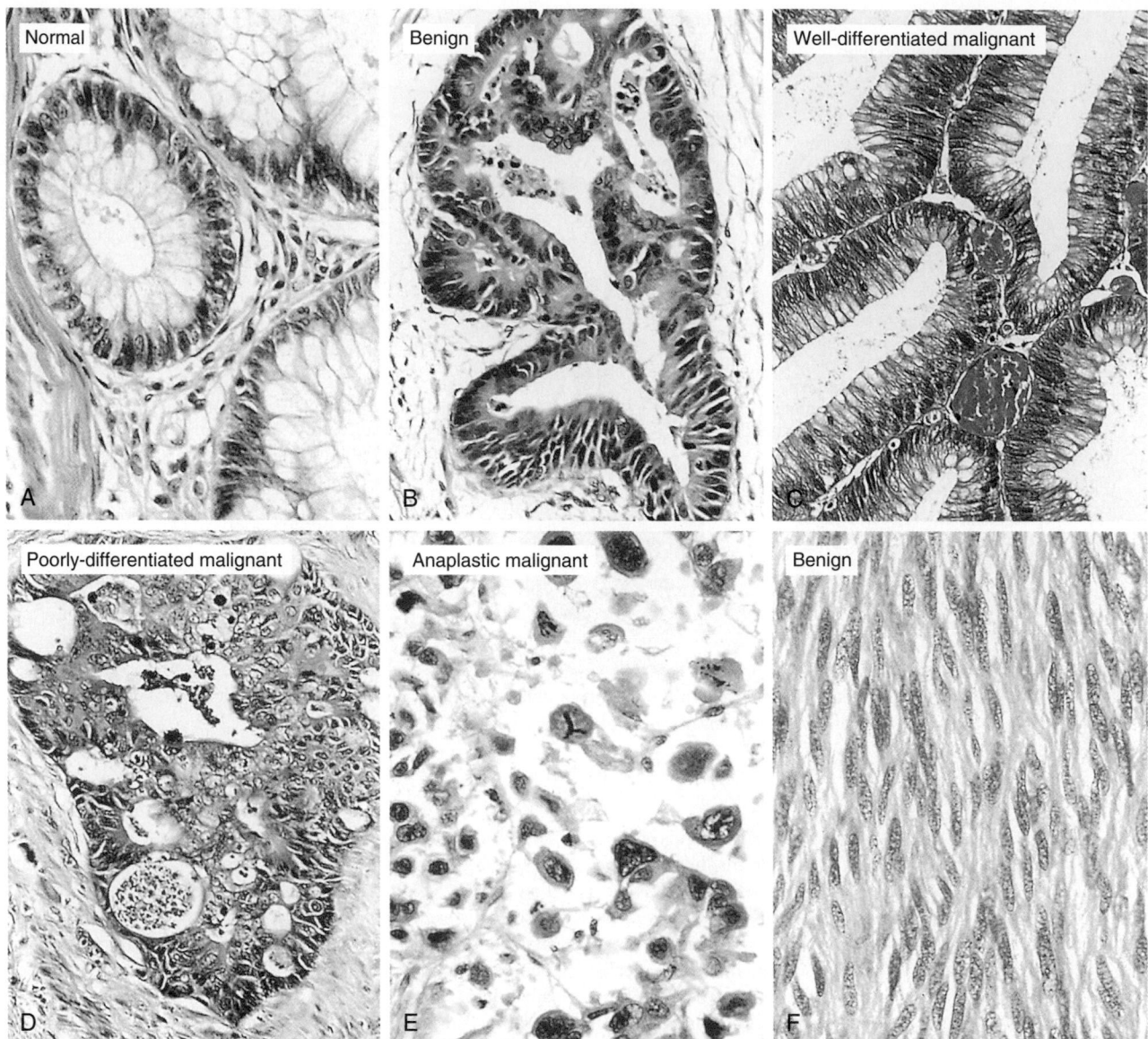

FIGURE 12.2 Loss of Cellular and Tissue Differentiation During the Development of Cancer. The cells of a benign neoplasm **(B)** resemble those of the normal colonic epithelium **(A),** in that they are columnar and have an orderly arrangement. Loss of some degree of differentiation is evident in that the neoplastic cells do not show much mucin vacuolization. Cells of the well-differentiated malignant neoplasm **(C)** of the colon have a haphazard arrangement and although gland lumina are formed, they are architecturally abnormal and irregular. Nuclei vary in shape and size, especially when compared with those illustrated in **A.** Cells in the poorly differentiated malignant neoplasm **(D)** have an even more haphazard arrangement, with very poor formation of gland lumina. Nuclei show greater variation in shape and size compared with the well-differentiated malignant neoplasm in **C.** Cells in anaplastic malignant neoplasms **(E)** bear no relation to the normal epithelium, with no recognizable gland formation. Tremendous variation is found in the size of cells and their nuclei, with very intense staining (hyperchromatic nuclei). Not knowing the site of origin would make it impossible to classify this tumor by microscopic appearance alone. Well-differentiated tumors often resemble their cell of origin, as shown in the example of a benign tumor of smooth muscles **(F).** (From Stevens A, Lowe J: *Pathology*, ed 2, London, 2000, Mosby.)

tissue are called lymphomas, whereas cancers of blood-forming cells are called leukemias. However, many cancers, such as Hodgkin disease and Ewing sarcoma, are named for historical reasons that do not follow this nomenclature convention.

Carcinoma in situ (often abbreviated CIS) refers to preinvasive epithelial tumors of glandular or squamous cell origin. Cancers develop incrementally, as they accumulate specific genetic mutations. Careful surveillance for cancer often detects abnormal growths in epithelial tissues that have atypical cells and an increased proliferation rate compared with normal surrounding tissues. These early stage cancers are localized to the epithelium and have not penetrated the local basement membrane or invaded the surrounding stroma. Based on these characteristics, they

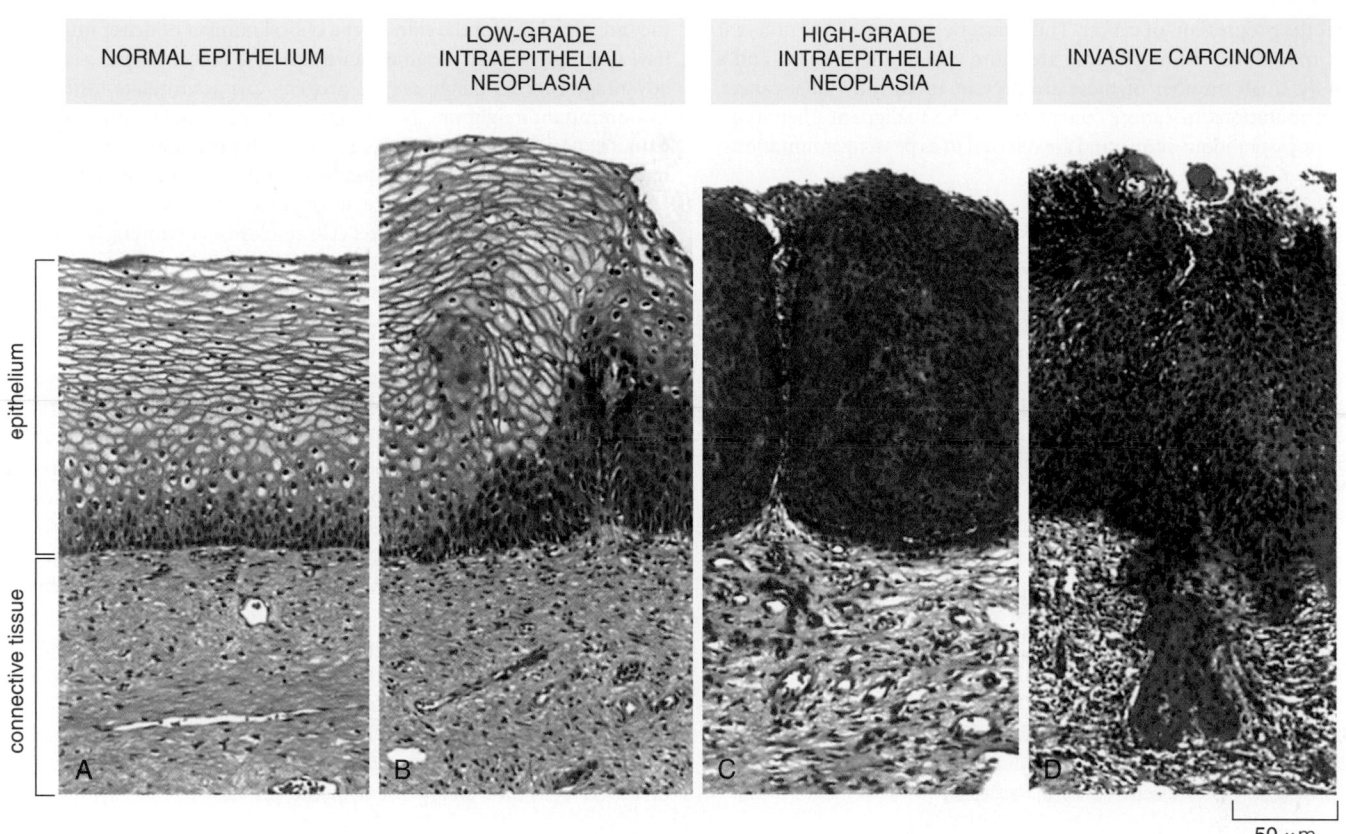

| NORMAL EPITHELIUM | LOW-GRADE INTRAEPITHELIAL NEOPLASIA | HIGH-GRADE INTRAEPITHELIAL NEOPLASIA | INVASIVE CARCINOMA |

50 μm

FIGURE 12.3 Progression from Normal to Neoplasm in the Uterine Cervix. A sequence of cellular and tissue changes progressing from low-grade to high-grade intraepithelial neoplasms (also called *carcinoma in situ*) and then to invasive cancer is seen often in the development of cancer. In this example of the early stages of cervical neoplastic changes, the presence of anaplastic cells and the loss of normal tissue architecture signify the development of cancer. The high rate of cell division and the presence of local mutagens and inflammatory mediators all contribute to the accumulation of genetic abnormalities that lead to cancer. (From Alberts B et al: *Molecular biology of the cell*, ed 5, New York, 2002, Garland.)

are not malignant but are often called CIS. CIS occurs in a number of sites, including the cervix, skin, oral cavity, esophagus, and bronchus. In glandular epithelium, in situ lesions occur in the stomach, endometrium, breast, and large bowel. In the breast, ductal carcinoma in situ (DCIS) fills the mammary ducts but has not progressed to local tissue invasion. CIS lesions can have one of the following three fates: (1) they can remain stable for a long time, (2) they can progress to invasive and metastatic cancers, or (3) they can regress and disappear. CIS can vary from low-grade to high-grade dysplasia, with the high-grade lesions having the highest likelihood of becoming invasive cancers. The time that such preinvasive lesions remain in situ before becoming invasive is unknown. Some carcinomas of the cervix appear as preinvasive lesions in situ for several years before they progress to invasive carcinoma and metastatic tumors (Fig. 12.3). Knowing how to best treat low-grade CIS lesions is challenging because the proportion that progress to cancer vs. the proportion that will never cause clinical problems is usually not known. Although most persons prefer removal of any CIS as opposed to "watchful waiting," this topic continues to be a source of great debate.

THE BIOLOGY OF CANCER CELLS

In two seminal publications, Drs. Douglas Hanahan and Robert Weinberg[2,3] described what they considered the hallmarks of cancer. Both articles stimulated considerable discussion and, especially, debate.

The original publication contained six hallmarks, but with time and new research findings, increased to eight hallmarks and two traits that enable cancer progression. Their analysis remains the leading overview of why a cell is malignant. The following discussion is organized in the context of those 10 hallmarks/enablers (Fig. 12.4). Two fundamental concepts are the foundation for understanding the biology of cancer. Cancer is a complex genetic disease, and the microenvironment of a tumor is a heterogeneous mixture of cells, both cancerous and benign.

Cancer is a disease of cumulative genetic changes during aging. The fraction of individuals who develop cancer increases dramatically with age. Genetic changes may occur by both mutational and epigenetic mechanisms. Mutation generally means an alteration in the DNA sequence affecting expression or function of a gene (Fig. 12.5). Mutations include small-scale changes in DNA, such as point mutations; the alteration of one or a few nucleotide base pairs (see Chapter 4). This type of mutation can have profound effects on the activity of resultant proteins. Chromosome translocations are large changes in chromosome structure in which a piece of one chromosome is translocated to another chromosome. Gene amplification is the result of repeated duplication of a region of a chromosome, so that instead of the normal two copies of a gene, tens or even hundreds of copies are present. Gene expression also may be altered indirectly by epigenetic effects including DNA methylation, histone acetylation, or altered expression of non–coding RNA (see Chapter 6).[4] Some mutations, referred to as driver mutations, "drive" the progression of cancer. There may be as many as 140 different driver mutations, although some are more critical than others, and a relatively small number of these are present in an individual cancer. Not all mutations in cancer contribute to the malignant phenotype. Some are just random events, and are referred to as passenger mutations;

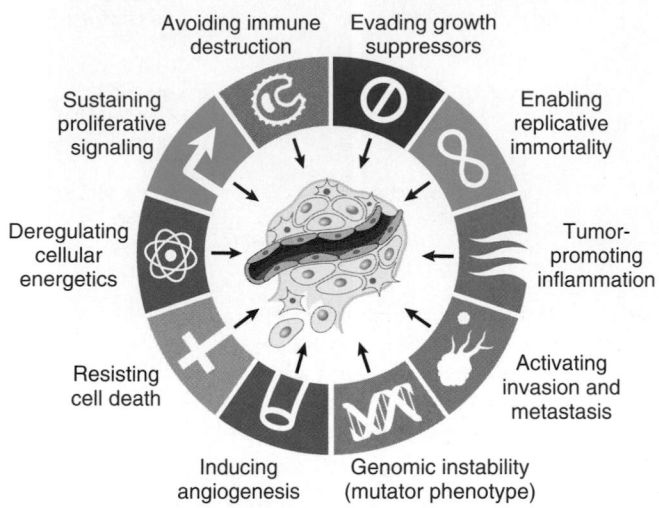

FIGURE 12.4 Hallmarks of Cancer. (Adapted from Hanahan D, Weinberg RA: *Cell* 144(5):646–674, 2011. Found in Kumar V et al: *Robbins and Cotran pathologic basis of disease*, ed 9, Philadelphia, 2015, Saunders.)

they are just along for the ride. After a critical number of driver mutations have occurred, the cell becomes cancerous. The cancer cell has a selective advantage over its neighbors; its progeny can accumulate faster than its nonmutant neighbors. This is referred to as clonal proliferation or clonal expansion (Fig. 12.6). As a clone with mutations proliferates, it may become an early stage tumor, for example, a carcinoma in situ or a benign colonic polyp. The increasingly rapid cell division and impaired DNA repair mechanisms of cancer cells result in a continuing accumulation of mutations throughout the progression to the most aggressive metastatic lesion. Thus malignant transformation, the process by which a normal cell becomes a cancer cell, is directed by progressive accumulation of genetic changes that alter the basic nature of the cell and drive it to malignancy. The process of tumor development is a form of Darwinian evolution; cells with a heritable change that confers a survival advantage out-compete their neighbors. Each cancer cell may develop its own set of mutations resulting in a genomically *heterogeneous* mixture of cancer cells with subsets that have accumulated more and more mutations that increase the cell's malignant potential.[5] The degree of intratumor mutational heterogeneity may vary considerably among tumors. For instance, melanomas have a rather high degree of genetic homogeneity, whereas pancreatic cancers are more heterogeneous and appear to arise from independent mutational events in the pancreas. Thus many cancer cells that do not accumulate a critical set of mutations lose the competition and die during this process.

The processes occurring during the development of cancer are, in many ways, analogous to wound healing. The initial proliferation of cancer cells and enlargement of the tumor elicit the synthesis of

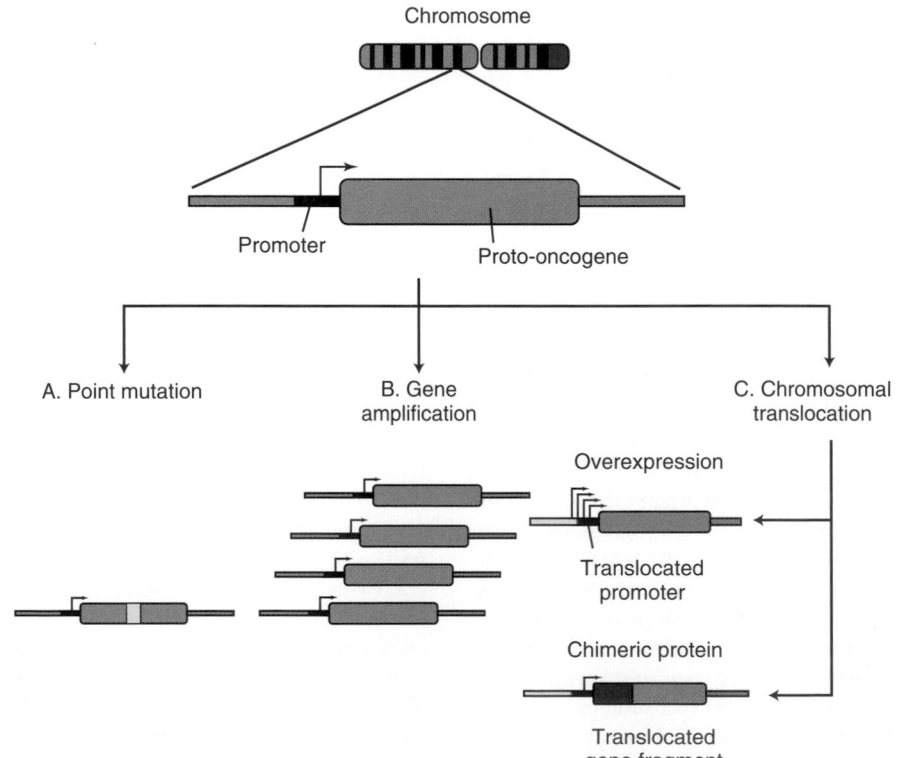

FIGURE 12.5 Oncogene Activation Mechanisms. Cellular genes may become cancerous oncogenes as a result of **(A)** point mutations that alter one or a few nucleotide base pairs, causing the production of a protein that is activated as a result of the altered sequence (e.g., *ras*); **(B)** amplification of the cellular gene, resulting in higher levels of protein expression (e.g., N-myc in neuroblastoma); or **(C)** chromosomal translocations that either lead to the juxtaposition of a strong promoter, causing increased protein expression (c-myc in Burkitt lymphoma), or produce a novel fusion protein that is derived from gene fragments normally present on different chromosomes (BCR-ABL in chronic myeloid leukemia). (From Haber DA: *Molecular genetics of cancer*. In *ACP medicine*, Danbury, CT, 2004, WebMD.)

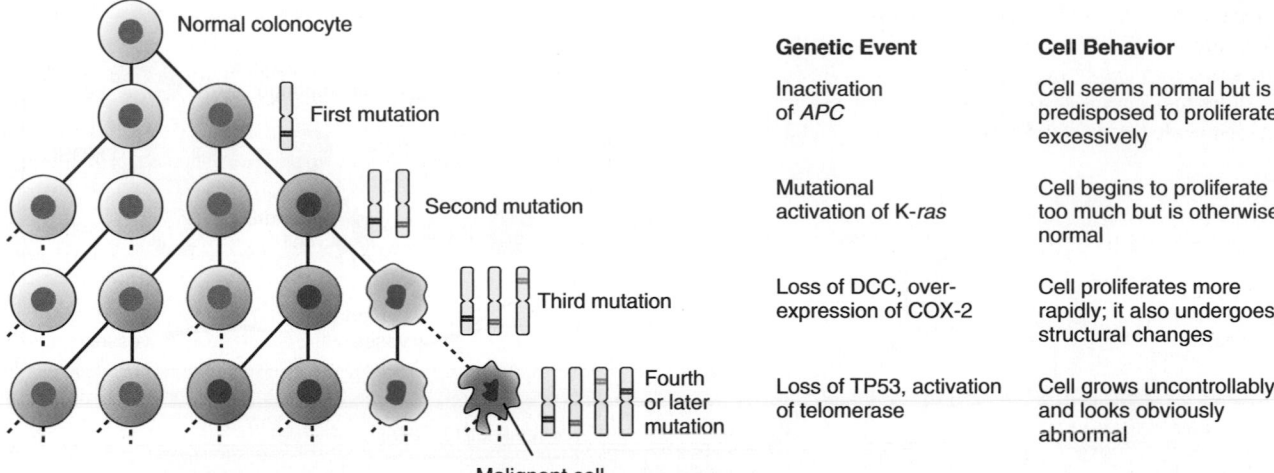

Genetic Event	Cell Behavior
Inactivation of *APC*	Cell seems normal but is predisposed to proliferate excessively
Mutational activation of K-*ras*	Cell begins to proliferate too much but is otherwise normal
Loss of DCC, over-expression of COX-2	Cell proliferates more rapidly; it also undergoes structural changes
Loss of TP53, activation of telomerase	Cell grows uncontrollably and looks obviously abnormal

FIGURE 12.6 Clonal Proliferation Model of Neoplastic Progression in the Colon. During clonal proliferation, progressively altered populations of colon cells (colonocytes) arise over time. As genetic and epigenetic changes occur, different subclones (indicated by different color cells) coexist for a time. Clones that grow the fastest out-compete other clones, producing even more malignant, and abnormal-appearing, growths. The sequential accumulation of mutations has been well studied in the progression from a normal colon cell to a benign intestinal polyp to a malignant colon cancer. One of the earliest mutations in colon cancer is loss of the tumor-suppressor gene *APC.* Additional mutations (often in the oncogene *RAS*), activation of COX-2, and loss of the tumor suppressors *DCC* and TP53 occur as the lesion progresses from a benign polyp to an invasive carcinoma. *APC,* Adenomatous polyposis coli; *COX-2,* cyclooxygenase-2; *DCC,* deleted in colon cancer; TP53, *p53* gene. (Modified from Mendelsohn I et al: *The molecular basis of cancer,* ed 2, Philadelphia, 2001, Saunders; and Kumar V et al: *Basic pathology,* ed 6, Philadelphia, 1997, Saunders.)

proinflammatory mediators by the cancer cells and adjacent nonmalignant cells. As with wound healing, mediators recruit inflammatory/immune cells (primarily T lymphocytes and macrophages, but also B cells and neutrophils) and cells normally associated with tissue repair (fibroblasts, adipocytes, mesenchymal stem cells, endothelial cells, and pericytes). These cells form the stroma (tumor microenvironment) that surrounds and infiltrates the tumor[6] (Fig. 12.7). In some conditions, stromal cells may make up 90% of the tumor mass. Extensive paracrine signaling among the stromal and cancer cells affects both populations; cancer cells increase proliferation and become more heterogeneous during tumor growth, and several populations of stromal cells undergo evolution to phenotypes that promote cancer progression and metastatic potential. Cancer heterogeneity arises from ongoing proliferation and mutation. Tumor-associated endothelial cells, fibroblasts, and inflammatory cells develop different and distinct gene expression profiles with unique cell surface molecules and patterns of secreted molecules. During this process there is generally a great deal of cancer cell death, but the surviving cells are more aggressive and many take on a metastatic phenotype. Because continuing somatic mutations may be random, cancer cells in different regions of the tumor may be genetically diverse. Additionally, a population of cancer stem cells may arise, the origin of which is still unclear. Many of the hallmarks of cancer are consequences of cancer-stromal interactions (discussed later).

Several of the hallmarks/enablers are primarily genomic alterations that initiate and maintain development of cancer. These will be discussed first and include sustained proliferative signaling, evading growth suppression, genomic instability, and replicative immortality (see Fig. 12.4). Other hallmarks/enablers are cellular adaptations secondary to genomic change and include inducing angiogenesis and reprogramming energy metabolism. A third group, tumor resistance to destruction by the host's protective mechanisms, includes resisting apoptotic cell death, promoting tumor inflammation, and avoiding immune destruction.

The last hallmark is the culmination of the previous nine: activating invasion and metastasis.

Genomic Hallmarks
Sustained Proliferative Signaling

The first and foremost hallmark of cancer is uncontrolled cellular proliferation. Normal cells generally only enter proliferative phases in response to growth factors that bind to specific receptors (receptor tyrosine kinases [RTKs]) on the cell surface. The cytoplasmic components of the receptors are associated with signaling molecules that undergo activation and in turn activate intracellular signaling pathways leading to induction/activation of regulatory factors affecting DNA synthesis, entrance into the cell cycle, and changes in expression of other genes related to cell metabolism for optimal growth (Fig. 12.8). One example is initiation of cell proliferation by epidermal growth factor (EGF). EGF binds and cross-links two EGF receptors (EGFRs) on the cell surface.[7] The cytoplasmic portions of the receptors are tyrosine kinases that attach phosphorus to tyrosine in neighboring proteins, including each other (autophosphorylation). Phosphorylation allows the receptor to attach to bridging protein, which links the EGF receptors to plasma membrane–associated inactive RAS. RAS is an acronym for "rat sarcoma," where it was found originally. Inactive RAS is associated with guanine diphosphate (GDP). Association between the EGF receptor and inactive RAS modifies the binding of GDP, which is replaced with guanine triphosphate (GTP). GTP activates RAS, which is a GTPase that converts GTP to GDP, during which it can activate signaling pathways such as the mitogen-activated protein kinase pathway (MAPK pathway) and the phosphatidylinosityl-3-kinase pathway (PI3K pathway). These signaling pathways phosphorylate other cytoplasmic proteins and affect activity and nuclear localization of transcription factors, such as MYC (myelocytomatosis viral oncogene homolog), that govern the

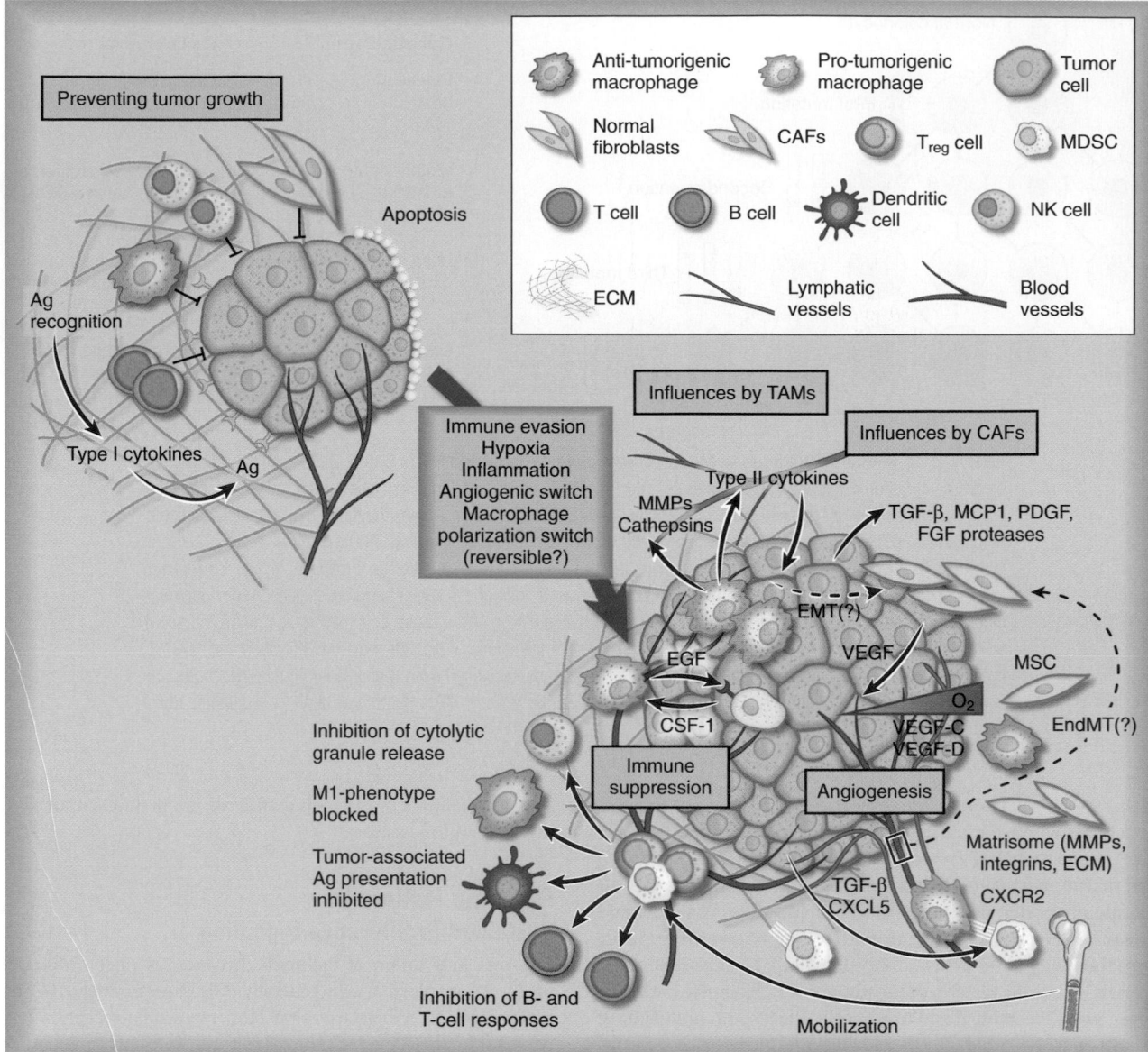

FIGURE 12.7 Cancers Live in a Complex Microenvironment. Cancer cells express tumor-specific antigens that ideally can be recognized by cells of the immune system and inflammatory systems (natural killer cells, antitumor M1 macrophages, T-cytotoxic cells) and destroyed by apoptosis or undergo growth suppression by type I cytokines. However, successful cancers produce a variety of cytokines and chemokines that are chemoattractants for stromal cells that infiltrate the tumor and undergo change to pro-tumor phenotypes. These include tumor-associated M2 macrophages (TAMs), cancer-associated fibroblasts (CAFs), mesenchymal stem cells (MSCs), and immune suppressor cells of T-cell origin (T-regulatory cells) and myeloid origin (myeloid-derived suppressor cells). Through multiple receptor-mediated interactions between other stromal cells and the cancer cells, the stromal cells, as well as the cancer cells, collectively produce a battery of additional cytokines (e.g., TGF-β, type II cytokines), chemokines (e.g., CXCL5), growth factors (e.g., VEGF, EGF, CSF-1, FGF, PDGF), and proteases (e.g., MMPs) and secrete components of the extracellular matrix (ECM). The stromal reaction promotes tumor progression, including new blood vessel growth (angiogenesis), tumor cell proliferation and differentiation, suppression of immune rejection and tumor cell apoptosis, invasion, and commitment to metastasis. *CAF,* Cancer-associated fibroblast; *CSF-1,* colony-stimulating factor-1; *CXCL5,* C-X-C motif chemokine 5; *ECM,* extracellular matrix; *EGF,* epidermal growth factor; *FGF,* fibroblast growth factor; *MSC,* mesenchymal stem cell; *MMP,* matrix metalloproteinase; *NK,* natural killer cell; *PDGF,* platelet-derived growth factor; *TAM,* tumor-associated macrophage; *TGF-β,* tumor growth factor-beta; *T_reg,* T-regulatory cell; *VEGF,* vascular endothelial cell growth factor. (Modified from Quail DF, Joyce JA: Microenvironmental regulation of tumor progression and metastasis, *Nat Med* 19[11]:1423–1437, 2013.)

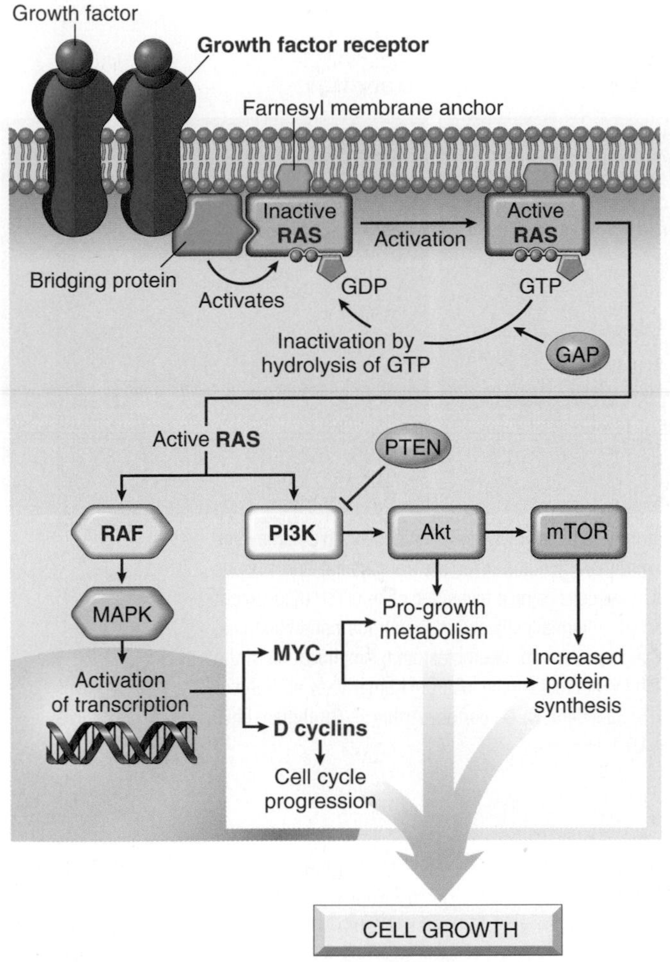

FIGURE 12.8 Growth Factor Signaling Pathways in Cancer. Growth factor receptors, RAS, PI3K, MYC, and D cyclins are oncoproteins that are activated by mutations in various cancers. GAPs apply brakes to RAS activation, and PTEN serves the same function for PI3K. *GAP*, GTPase-activating protein; *GDP*, guanosine diphosphate; *GTP*, guanosine triphosphate; *MAPK*, mitogen-activated protein kinase; *PI3K*, phosphatidylinositide-3-kinase; *PTEN*, phosphatase and tensin homolog. (From Kumar V et al: Robbins and Cotran pathologic basis of disease, ed 9, Philadelphia, 2015, Saunders.)

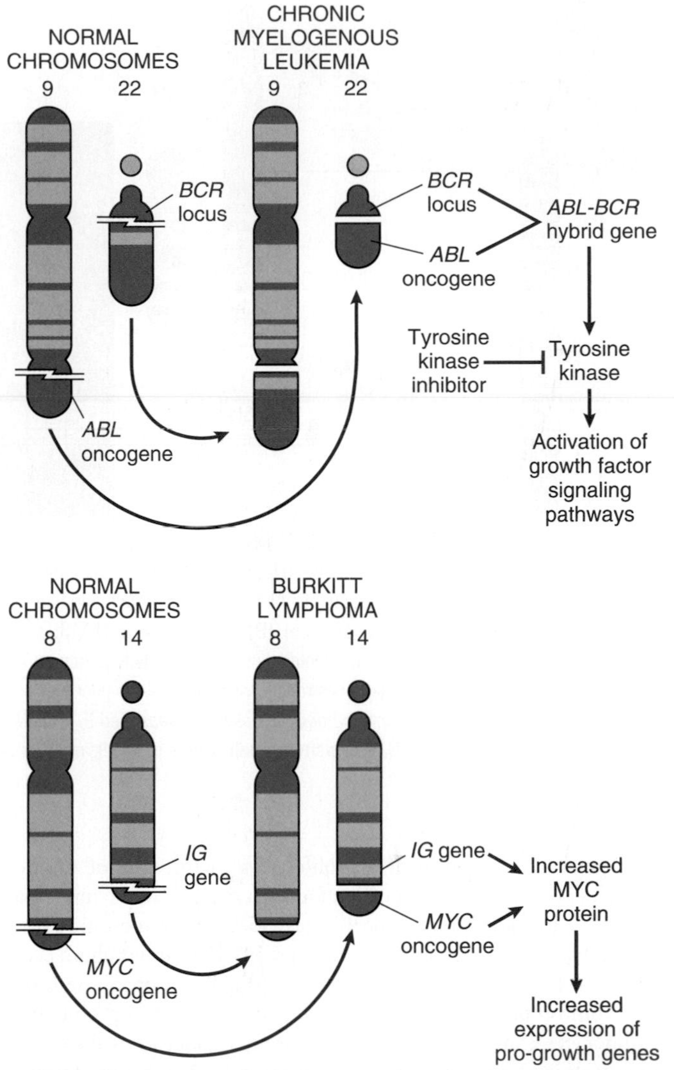

FIGURE 12.9 Examples of Chromosomal Translocations and Associated Oncogenes. See text for further explanation. (From Kumar V et al: *Robbins and Cotran pathologic basis of disease,* ed 9, Philadelphia, 2015, Saunders.)

transcription of cell cycle regulators, such as cyclins, and entrance into cellular proliferation. Proliferation can be discontinued through this pathway by decreased levels of growth factors in the environment or inactivation of signaling pathway components.

The genes that encode components of receptor-mediated pathways designed to regulate normal cellular proliferation are collectively called **proto-oncogenes**. Cancerous cells characteristically express mutated or overexpressed proto-oncogenes, which are referred to as **oncogenes**. Oncogenes are independent of normal regulatory mechanisms; thus the cell is driven into a state of unregulated constitutive expression of proliferation signals and uncontrolled cell growth. Oncogenes can affect any portion of the growth factor pathways, such as described for EGF. For instance, most growth factors originate from neighboring cells, but some cancers acquire the ability to secrete growth factors that stimulate their own growth, a process known as **autocrine stimulation**. As described later in this chapter, noncancerous stromal cells within a tumor are frequently modified to benefit the cancer. In some instances, stromal cells produce excessive growth factors that drive the proliferation of cancer cells. Other cancers increase the expression of RTKs; for example, in breast cancer production of the **human epidermal growth factor receptor 2 (HER2)**, also known as the *epidermal growth factor receptor gene [ERBB-2]*) is up-regulated and is hyperresponsive to low levels of EGF. Some breast and lung cancers are effectively treated by inhibitors of HER2 and other EGF receptors that block this pathway.

Oncogenes may lead to constitutive activation of the signal cascade from the cell surface receptor to the nucleus. Up to a third of all cancers have an activating mutation in the *RAS* gene resulting in a continuous cell growth signal even when growth factors are missing (see Fig. 12.8). Other mutations in the EGF receptor pathway include excessive proliferation signaling by hyperactivation of the PI3 kinase.

Several types of genetic events can activate oncogenes. A point mutation that is frequently observed in lung cancer results in continuous activation of the EGF **receptor tyrosine kinase**. A point mutation in the *RAS* gene converts it from a regulated proto-oncogene to an unregulated oncogene. Activating point mutations in *RAS* are found in many cancers, especially pancreatic and colorectal cancer. Specialized tests, such as direct DNA sequencing, can detect such point mutations in clinical samples.

Translocations can activate oncogenes in one of two distinct mechanisms (Fig. 12.9). First, a translocation can cause excess and

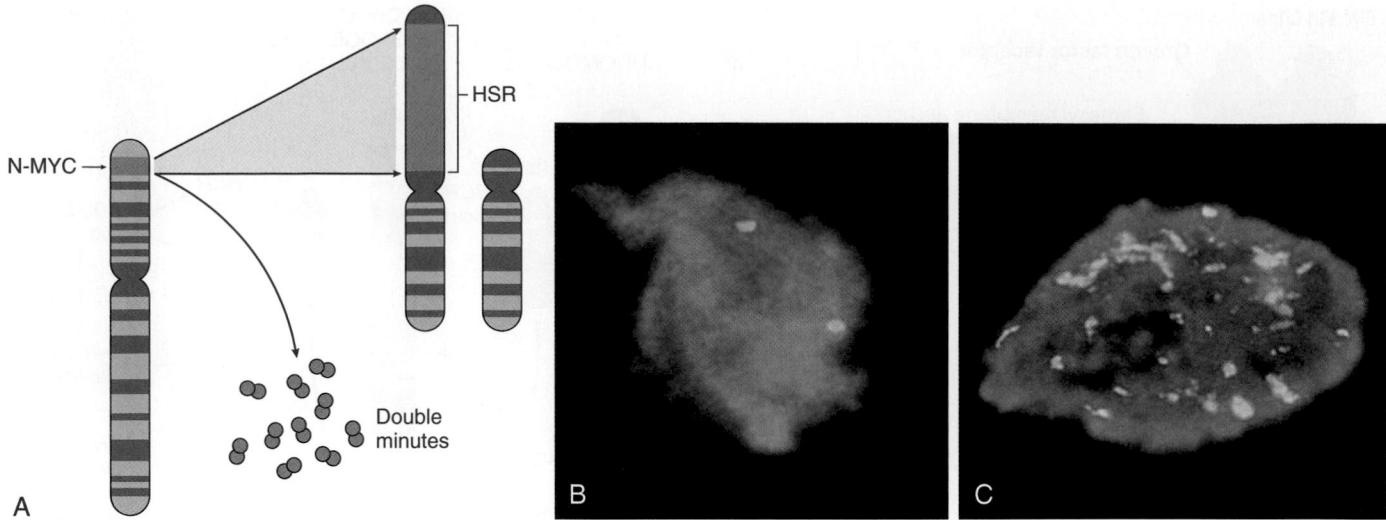

FIGURE 12.10 N-Myc Gene Amplification in Neuroblastoma. **(A)** The N-Myc gene is present on chromosome 2, becomes amplified, and is seen either as extra chromosomal double minutes or as a chromosomal homologous staining region. The N-Myc gene is detected in human neuroblastoma cells using a technique called FISH (fluorescent in situ hybridization). **(B)** A single pair of N-Myc genes is detected in normal cells and in low-grade neuroblastoma. **(C)** Multiple, amplified copies of the N-Myc gene are detected in some cases of neuroblastoma. Amplification of the N-Myc gene is strongly associated with a poor prognosis in childhood neuroblastoma. (**A** from Kumar V, et al: *Robbins and Cotran pathologic basis of disease,* ed 9, Philadelphia, 2015, Saunders; **B, C** courtesy Arthur R. Brothman, PhD, FACMG, University of Utah School of Medicine, Salt Lake City, UT.)

inappropriate production of a proliferation factor. One of the best examples is the t(8;14) translocation found in many Burkitt lymphomas; t(8;14) designates a chromosome that has a piece of chromosome 8 fused to a piece of chromosome 14 (see Chapter 30). Burkitt lymphoma is an aggressive cancer of B lymphocytes. The Myc proto-oncogene found on chromosome 8 is normally activated at low levels in proliferating lymphocytes and is inactivated in mature lymphocytes. If the t(8;14) translocation occurs (reciprocal translocation[t] or exchange of genetic material between chromosomes designated t[8, for chromosome 8, and 14, for chromosome 14]) the *Myc* gene is aberrantly placed under the control of a B-cell immunoglobulin gene *(IG)* present on chromosome 14. The *IG* gene is very active in maturing B lymphocytes. The t(8;14) translocation alters the control of *MYC;* its normal low-level expression is switched to high levels, as directed by an *IG* gene promoter. Hyperproduction of MYC protein drives proliferation and blocks differentiation.

Second, chromosome translocations can lead to production of novel proteins with growth-promoting properties. In chronic myeloid leukemia (CML) a specific chromosome translocation is almost always present. This translocation, t(9;22), was first identified in association with CML in Philadelphia in 1960 and is often referred to as the Philadelphia chromosome. Translocation fuses two chromosomes in the middle of two different genes: *Bcr* (break point cluster region gene) on chromosome 9 and *Abl* (Abelson gene) on chromosome 22. The result is production of a BCR-ABL fusion protein containing the first half of BCR and the second half of ABL (a nonreceptor tyrosine kinase). BCR-ABL is an unregulated protein tyrosine kinase that promotes growth of myeloid cells. Imatinib, a drug that specifically targets this tyrosine kinase, represents the first successful chemotherapy targeted against the product of a specific oncogenic mutation. Imatinib and related tyrosine kinase inhibitors (TKIs) are highly effective in the treatment of CML and, because of their specificity, lack the toxic side effects noted with non-specific anticancer drugs. However, imatinib is not effective in cancers that do not have the t(9;22) translocation or related mutations. In

modern personalized cancer therapy, knowledge of the specific genetic alteration can dictate the optimal drugs for the individual.

Oncogenes also may be activated by gene amplification (Fig. 12.10). Gene amplification results in increased expression of an oncogene, or in some cases drug resistance genes. The N-Myc oncogene, a member of the Myc family, is amplified in 25% of childhood neuroblastomas and confers a poor prognosis. The HER2 gene *(ERBB2)* is amplified in 20% of breast cancers.

Evading Growth Suppressors

Uncontrolled cancer cell proliferation also is related to inactivation of tumor-suppressor genes. Tumor-suppressor genes normally regulate the cell cycle, inhibit proliferation resulting from growth signals, stop cell division when cells are damaged, and prevent mutations. Hence, they also have been referred to as *anti-oncogenes*. Whereas oncogenes are *activated* in cancers, tumor suppressors must be *inactivated* to allow cancer to occur (Table 12.1 and Fig. 12.11). A single genetic event can activate an oncogene because it can act in a dominant manner in the cell. However, each individual has two copies of each tumor-suppressor gene, one from each parent. Both copies must be inactivated; therefore two mutations are necessary.

A prototypical tumor-suppressor gene is the retinoblastoma *(RB)* gene. Normal cells receive diverse "antigrowth" signals from their normal environment. Contact with other cells, with basement membranes, and with some soluble factors normally signal cells to stop proliferating. Tumor-suppressor genes, such as *RB*, monitor antigrowth cellular signals and block activation of the growth/division phase in the cell cycle; thus mutations in *RB* lead to persistent cell growth. Antiproliferative activity of *RB* depends on the degree of protein phosphorylation. Low levels of phosphorylation (hypophosphorylation) result in *RB* binding to and inhibiting transcription factors that regulate genes controlling passage through the cell cycle. Growth factor–regulated kinases increase phosphorylation (hyperphosphorylation) and inactivation of *RB*. A variety

TABLE 12.1	COMPARISON OF CANCER GENE TYPES	
GENE TYPE	**NORMAL FUNCTION**	**MUTATION EFFECT**
Caretaker	DNA and chromosome stability	Chromosome instability and increased rates of mutation
Dominant oncogenes*	Encode proteins that promote growth (e.g., growth factors)	Overexpression or amplification causes gain of function
Tumor suppressors (recessive oncogenes)	Encode proteins that inhibit proliferation and prevent or repair mutations	Requires loss of function of both alleles to increase cancer risk

*Nonmutant state referred to as proto-oncogene.

TABLE 12.2	SOME FAMILIAL CANCER SYNDROMES CAUSED BY LOSS OF TUMOR-SUPPRESSOR GENE FUNCTION
SYNDROME	**GENE**
Retinoblastoma	*RB1*
Li-Fraumeni syndrome	*p53* (TP53)
Familial melanoma	*p16^INK4a* (CDKN2A)
Neurofibromatosis	*Neurofibromin (NF1)*
Familial adenomatous polyps	*APC*
Breast cancer	*BRCA1*

of genetic mutations in cancers also inactivate *RB*, resulting in unregulated and continuous cellular proliferation. *RB* is mutated in childhood retinoblastoma, and in many lung, breast, and bone cancers as well. The *RB* gene resides on chromosome 13, in a region referred to as q14 (13q14). Most individuals with *RB* mutations have a subtle mutation, such as a point mutation, in one allele. The *RB* gene in the other chromosome may be inactivated through loss of the 13q14 region or epigenetic mechanisms.

Another classic tumor-suppressor gene is the p53 tumor-suppressor gene (TP53). The protein p53 has been called the *guardian of the genome*. TP53 monitors intracellular signals related to stress and activates caretaker genes—genes that are responsible for the maintenance of genomic integrity (Fig. 12.12). Many types of cellular stress (e.g., anoxia, oncogene expression, nuclear damage) produce intracellular signals (e.g., levels of nucleotides and glucose, degree of oxygenation, DNA damage, and other indicators of cellular abnormalities) detectable by p53. Normally p53 is in an inactive complex with inhibitor molecules. Stress activates kinases that phosphorylate p53 into an active suppressor of cell division and activator of caretaker genes. Caretaker genes encode proteins that are involved in repairing damaged DNA, such as with errors in DNA replication, mutations caused by ultraviolet or ionizing radiation, and mutations caused by chemicals and drugs. The p53 protein also controls initiation of cellular senescence or apoptosis, and suppresses cell division until DNA repair is complete or other effects of stress are corrected. If not corrected, the cell enters senescence or apoptosis, thus preventing further DNA damage and mutations. Loss of function of TP53 or caretaker genes leads to increased mutation rates and cancer.

Because inactivation of tumor-suppressor genes requires at least two mutations (one in each allele), a single mutation in the germline cells (sperm or egg) results in the transmission of cancer-causing genes from one generation to the next, producing families with a high risk for specific cancers. These inherited mutations that predispose to cancer are almost invariably in tumor-suppressor genes because only a single additional mutation is needed to inactivate completely the tumor-suppressor gene (Table 12.2).

An example of increased risk for cancer that can be inherited is the familial form of retinoblastoma. A mutation in one *RB* allele is inherited so that only one additional mutation in the normal allele will lead to cancer. Approximately half of children with retinoblastoma have the inheritable form and most will develop tumors in both eyes (bilateral retinoblastoma). Also, Li-Fraumeni syndrome is a very rare inheritable loss-of-function mutation in TP53 in one allele resulting in a 25-fold increase of developing malignancy at early age (<50 years of age). These malignancies may include breast cancer, brain tumors, acute leukemia,

soft tissue sarcomas, bone sarcoma, and adrenal cortical carcinoma. Other familial cancers with inheritable mutations in tumor-suppressor genes include Wilms tumor, a childhood cancer of the kidney (*WT1* gene); neurofibromatosis (*NF1* gene); and familial polyposis coli or adenomas of the colon (*APC* gene). Characterization of cancer-causing genes and other genetic factors helps identify individuals prone to developing cancer and contributes to the understanding of sporadic cancers. Individuals known to carry mutations in tumor-suppressor genes are offered targeted cancer screening to facilitate early cancer detection and therapy.

Genomic Instability

Genomic instability refers to an increased tendency of alterations—mutability—in the genome during the life cycle of cells. Inherited and acquired mutations in caretaker genes that protect the integrity of the genome and DNA repair increase the level of genomic instability and risk for developing cancer.[8] Acquired mutations in "guardians of the genome," such as TP53, that detect DNA damage and activate repair mechanisms result in an increasing accumulation of mutations. Xeroderma pigmentosum is a defect in the repair of DNA pyrimidine dimers created by ultraviolet (UV) light that increases the risk for skin cancers. Hereditary nonpolyposis colorectal cancer results from an inherited defect in repairing DNA base pair mismatches that occur occasionally during DNA replication. Affected individuals have an increased rate of small insertions and deletions in DNA, leading to a high rate of colon and other cancers. Some inherited mutations threaten the integrity of entire chromosomes. Bloom syndrome, caused by mutations in a DNA helicase, presents with an increased risk of several forms of cancer, and those with Fanconi aplastic anemia, caused by loss of function for repairing DNA double-strand breaks, have a particularly increased risk of acute myelogenous leukemia. These examples are autosomal recessive disorders in which affected individuals demonstrate marked chromosomal instability.

Genomic instability also may result from increased epigenetic silencing or modulation of gene function (Chapters 4 and 6). Many cancers have increased methylation of DNA in the promoter region of tumor-suppressor genes. They also have associated changes in the modification of histones in the chromatin, often correlated with methylation of DNA. These changes alter the promoter regions of genes, leading to their silencing or altered gene expression.

Changes in gene regulation can affect not just single genes, but also entire intracellular signaling networks. Gene expression networks can be regulated by changes in microRNAs (miRNAs, or miRs) and other non–coding RNAs (ncRNAs). miRs regulate diverse signaling pathways; the miRs that stimulate cancer development and progression are termed

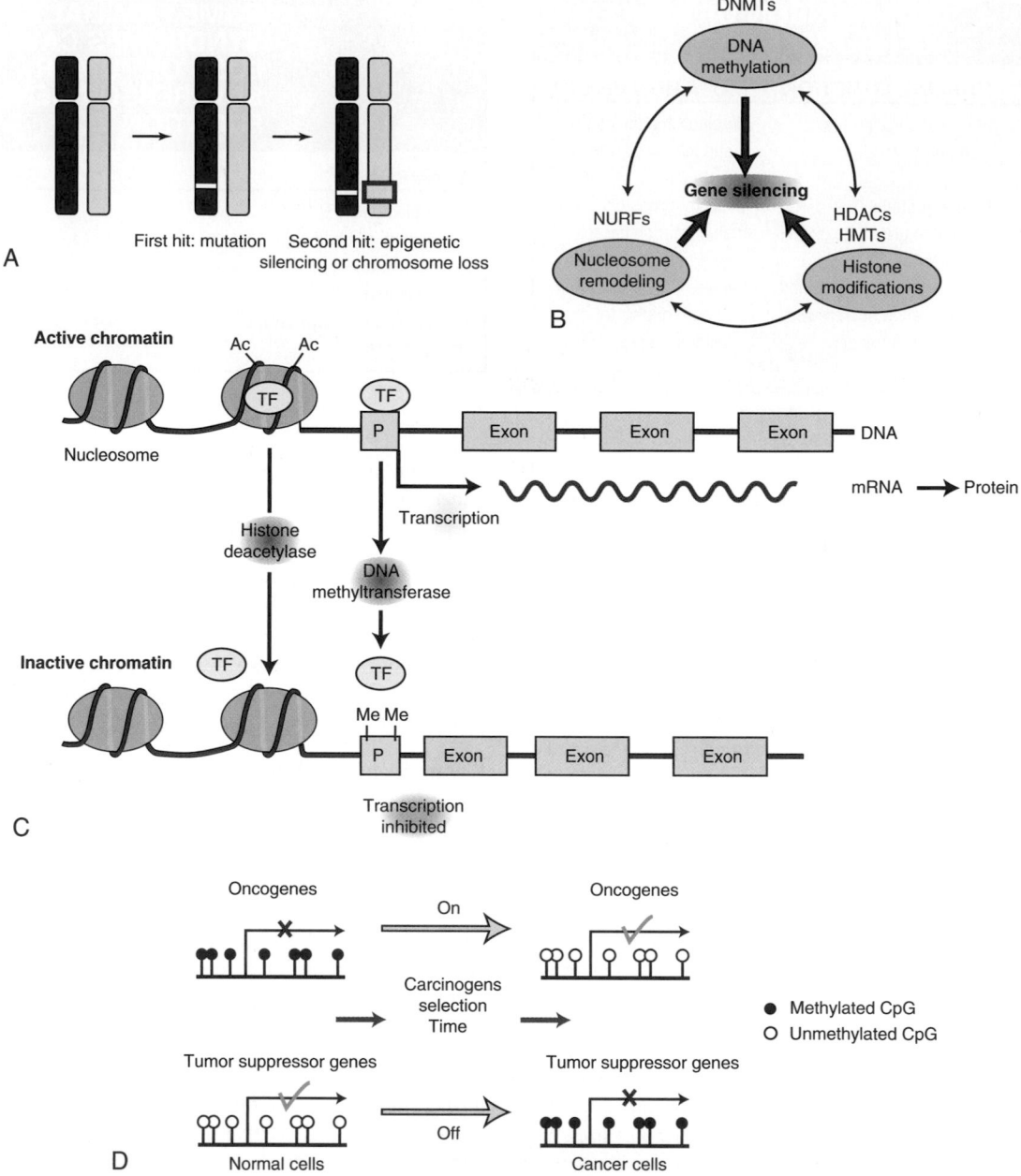

FIGURE 12.11 Silencing Tumor-Suppressor Genes by Epigenetic Alterations. Tumor-suppressor genes can be turned off by a variety of mechanisms. **A,** In this example, the first hit is a point mutation in a tumor-suppressor gene *(white box),* followed by either epigenetic silencing or chromosome loss of the second allele *(red box).* **B,** Genes can normally be silenced by a variety of interacting processes including DNA methylation, histone modifications, nucleosome remodeling, and microRNAs (not shown). A number of cellular enzymes contribute to these modifications, including DNA methyltransferases *(DNMTs),* histone deacetylases *(HDACs),* histone methyltransferases *(HMTs),* and complex nucleosomal remodeling factors *(NURFs).* Gene silencing is essential for normal development and differentiation. **C,** Histone modification and promoter methylation regulate gene expression. Genes are transcribed when chromatin is modified by addition of acetyl *(Ac)* groups to specific lysine groups in histones. Gene expression can be turned off when specific acetyl groups are removed by HDACs or when the CpG-rich promoter regions of genes are modified by direct DNA methylation (by DNA methyltransferase). In addition, small endogenous RNA molecules (microRNAs or miRNA) can bind to mRNA and reduce gene expression. **D,** Changes in promoter methylation turn cancer genes off and on. Oncogenes can be turned on by promoter hypomethylation, and tumor-suppressor genes can be turned off by promoter hypermethylation. Each of these changes can produce selective growth and survival advantage for the cancer cell. (**B** adapted from Jones PA, Baylin SB: *Cell* 128:683–692, 2007; **C** from Gluckman PD et al: *N Engl J Med* 359[1]:66, 2008; **D** from Shames DS, Minna JF, Gazdar AF: *Curr Mol Med* 7:85–102, 2007.)

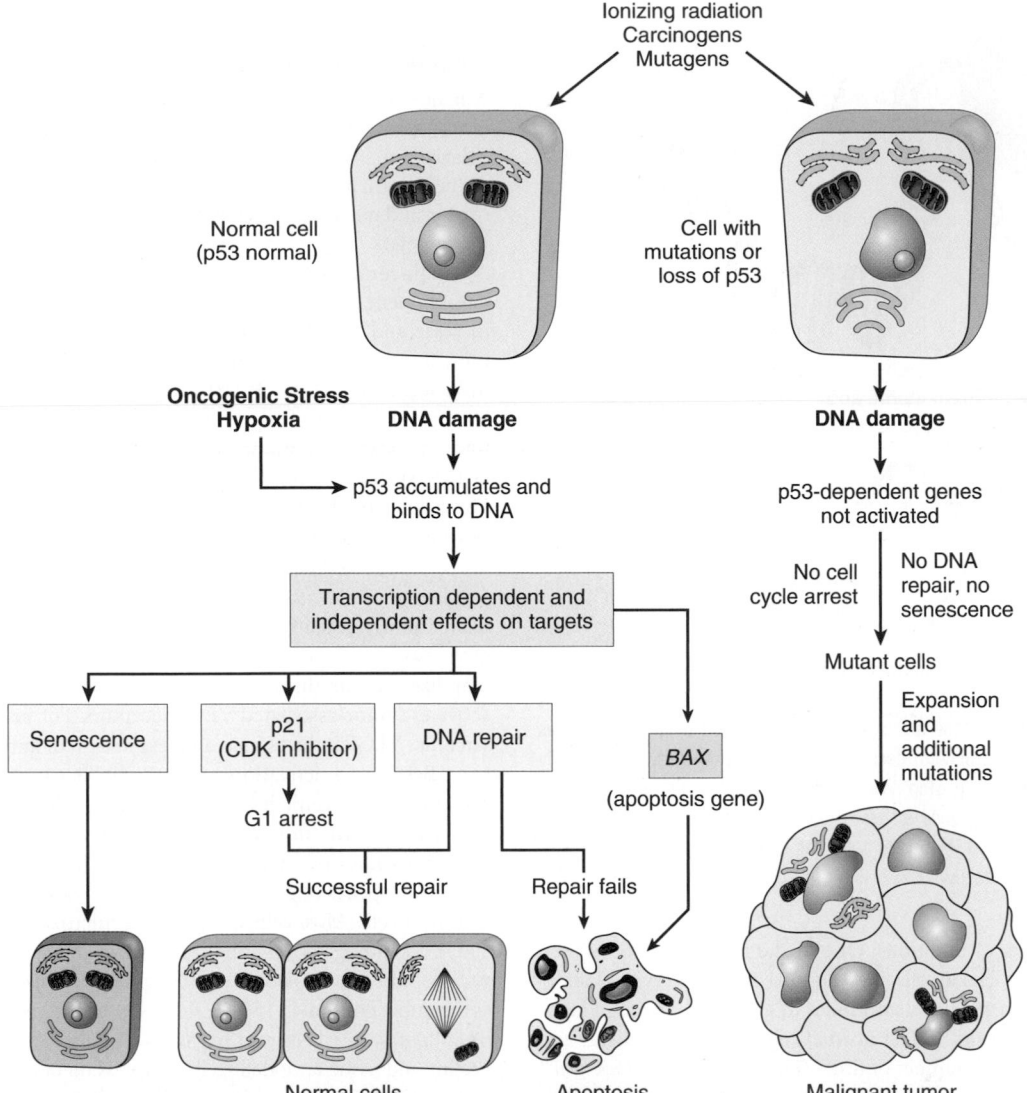

FIGURE 12.12 The Role of p53 in Maintaining the Integrity of the Genome. Activation of normal p53 by DNA-damaging agents or by hypoxia leads to cell cycle arrest in G_1 by up-regulation of the cell cycle inhibitor p21 and induction of DNA repair transcriptional up-regulation of the cyclin-dependent kinase inhibitor *CDKN1A* (encoding the cyclin-dependent kinase inhibitor p21) and the *GADD45* genes. Successful repair of DNA allows cells to proceed with the cell cycle. If DNA repair fails, *p53* triggers either apoptosis or senescence. In cells with loss or mutation of the *p53* gene, DNA damage does not induce cell cycle arrest or DNA repair, and genetically damaged cells proliferate, giving rise eventually to malignant neoplasms. (From Kumar V et al: *Robbins and Cotran pathologic basis of disease,* ed 9, Philadelphia, 2015, Saunders.)

oncomirs. miRs decrease the stability and expression of other genes by pairing with mRNA.

Mutations in *BRCA1* and *BRCA2* (breast cancer 1 and 2, early onset genes, respectively) are currently of clinical importance. Both are tumor-suppressors and caretaker genes that repair double-stranded DNA breaks. Inherited mutations in either gene greatly increase the risk for a variety of tumors, especially breast cancer in both women and men, and ovarian or prostate cancers.[9] Approximately 12% of women generally will develop breast cancer within their lifetime, whereas about 60% of women with a high-risk *BRCA1* mutation and 45% with a *BRCA2* mutation will develop cancer by age 70.[10] Ovarian cancer occurs in approximately 1.4% of the general population, but about 39% of women with an inherited mutation in *BRCA1* and about 15% with a

mutation in *BRCA2* will develop ovarian cancer by age 70. At-risk women are currently offered prophylactic surgery to reduce the risk of cancer.

In addition to specific gene mutations and abnormal epigenetic silencing, chromosome instability also appears to be increased in malignant cells, resulting in a high rate of chromosome loss, as well as loss of heterozygosity and chromosome amplification. The underlying mechanism of this instability is not clear but may be caused by malfunctions in the cellular machinery that regulates chromosome segregation at mitosis.

Enabling Replication Immortality

A hallmark of cancer cells is their immortality, in that they seem to have an unlimited life span and will continue to divide for years under

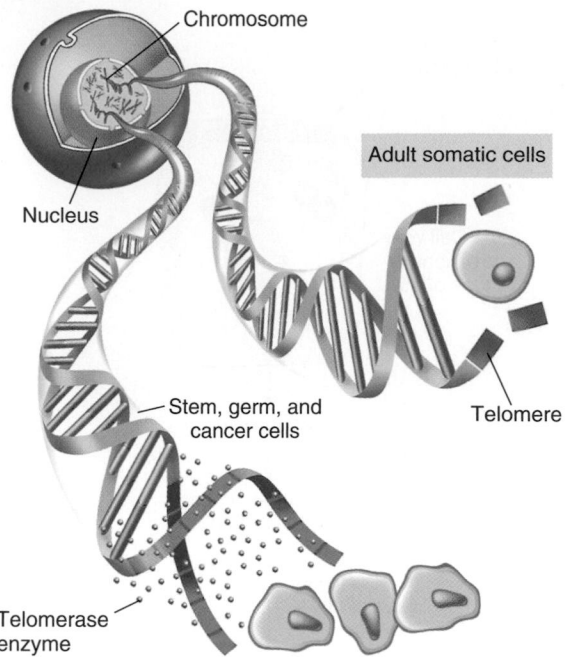

FIGURE 12.13 Control of Immortality: Telomeres and Telomerase. Normal adult somatic cells cannot divide indefinitely because the ends of their chromosomes are capped by telomeres. In the absence of the telomerase enzyme, telomeres become progressively shorter with each division until, when they are critically short, they signal to the cell to stop dividing. In germ cells, adult stem cells, and cancer cells the telomerase gene is "switched on," producing an enzyme that rebuilds the telomeres. Thus, like germ cells, the cancer cell becomes immortal and able to divide indefinitely without losing its telomeres.

appropriate laboratory conditions. One of the most commonly used laboratory cell lines, HeLa cells, was derived from a cervical cancer specimen obtained in 1951 that continues to grow and divide in laboratories around the world.[11] Most normal cells are not immortal and can divide only a limited number of times (known as the *Hayflick limit*) before they either enter senescence (cease dividing) or enter crisis (apoptosis) and die. One major block to unlimited cell division (i.e., immortality) is the size of a specialized structure called the telomere. Telomeres are protective ends, or caps, of repeating hexanucleotides (six nucleotide units) on each chromosome and are placed and maintained by a specialized enzyme called telomerase (Fig. 12.13). As one might expect, telomerase is usually active only in germ cells (in ovaries and testes) and in stem cells. All other cells of the body lack telomerase activity. Therefore when non–germ cells begin to proliferate abnormally their telomere caps shorten with each cell division. Short telomeres normally signal the cell to cease cell division. If the telomeres become critically small, the chromosomes become unstable and fragment, and the cells die.

Cancer cells are very heterogeneous and many cells die as the cancer develops. When they reach a critical age, most cancer cells activate telomerase to restore and maintain their telomeres, thereby allowing continuous division.[12] The trigger for reexpression of telomerase activity remains unclear, but seems to require expression of specific oncogenes, such as *RAS* or *Myc*, and loss of function of certain tumor-suppressor molecules, such as p53 and RB. Telomerase activity is restored in about 90% of cancers. The remaining cancers appear to recruit or originate from stem cells, becoming cancer stem cells that maintain levels of telomerase activity characteristically found in somatic stem cells. Because telomerase is specifically activated in cancer cells, and potentially in cancer stem cells, it is an attractive therapeutic target.

Cellular Adaptations
Inducing Angiogenesis

A major component of wound healing is the process of establishing new blood vessels within the tissue undergoing repair (called neovascularization or angiogenesis). Access to a blood supply also is obligatory to the growth and spread of cancer. Without a blood supply to deliver oxygen and nutrients, growth of a tumor is limited to about a millimeter in diameter.

Angiogenic factors and angiogenic inhibitors normally control development of new vessels. In cancerous tumors several mechanisms increase and maintain secretion of angiogenic factors by the cancer cells, as well as prevent release of angiogenic inhibitors. Hypoxia-inducible factor-1α (HIF-1α), an oxygen-sensitive transcription factor, is a major regulator of angiogenesis in normal tissue; HIF-1α is stabilized under hypoxic conditions and induces expression of pro-angiogenic factors, such as vascular endothelial growth factor (VEGF) and basic fibroblast growth factor (bFGF).[13] Inactivation of tumor-suppressor genes (e.g., *p53*) or increased expression of oncogenes (e.g., HER2) leads to increased expression of HIF-1α–regulated angiogenic factors and increased vascularization. Increased expression of HIF-1α also is related to increased resistance to chemotherapy, increased tumor cell glycolysis, increased metastasis, and a poor prognosis. These effects may likely occur through an autocrine mechanism by which VEGF activates tumor-associated VEGF receptors. For instance, in soft tissue sarcomas VEGF induces increased expression of anti-apoptotic proteins (e.g., Bcl-2) and activation of intracellular survival signal pathways. The use of angiogenic inhibitors targeting VEGF signaling can inhibit angiogenesis and diminish tumor growth.

Other routes of angiogenic factor induction include mutations in cancer oncogenes (e.g., *RAS*, Myc) that increase transcription of VEGF by cancer cells. Most cells in the tumor microenvironment also secrete VEGF, including tumor-infiltrating monocytes, endothelial cells, adipocytes, and cancer-associated fibroblasts. Angiogenesis inhibitors, such as thrombospondin-1 (TSP-1), normally bind to cellular surface receptors on inflammatory cells and negatively regulate angiogenesis in wound healing and tissue remodeling. The expression of angiogenesis inhibitors is under the control of p53, which is suppressed in cancer cells, thus diminishing the control of stromal inflammatory cell secretion of angiogenic factors.

Cancer cells and stromal cells may increase production of matrix metalloproteinases (e.g., MMP-9)[14] (Fig. 12.14). MMPs are zinc-dependent proteases that digest the surrounding extracellular matrix (ECM). The ECM contains stored latent (inactive) forms of some angiogenic factors (e.g., bFGF, transforming growth factor-beta [TGF-β]). MMPs activate the stored forms into functional angiogenic factors.

The vessels formed within tumors differ from those in healthy tissue. They originate from endothelial sprouting from existing capillaries and irregular branching, rather than regular branching seen in healthy tissue. The interendothelial cell contact is less tight so the vessels are more porous and prone to hemorrhage, as well as allowing passage of tumor cells into the vascular system.

Reprograming Energy Metabolism

Cancer cells live in a distinct environment from normal cells and have different nutritional requirements from nonproliferating cells. The successful cancer cell divides rapidly, with the consequent requirement for the building blocks to construct new cells. Nonmalignant cells in the presence of adequate oxygen normally generate adenosine triphosphate (ATP) by mitochondrial oxidative phosphorylation (OXPHOS), generating 36 ATP molecules from each glucose molecule that is broken down to water and carbon dioxide. In the absence of sufficient oxygen

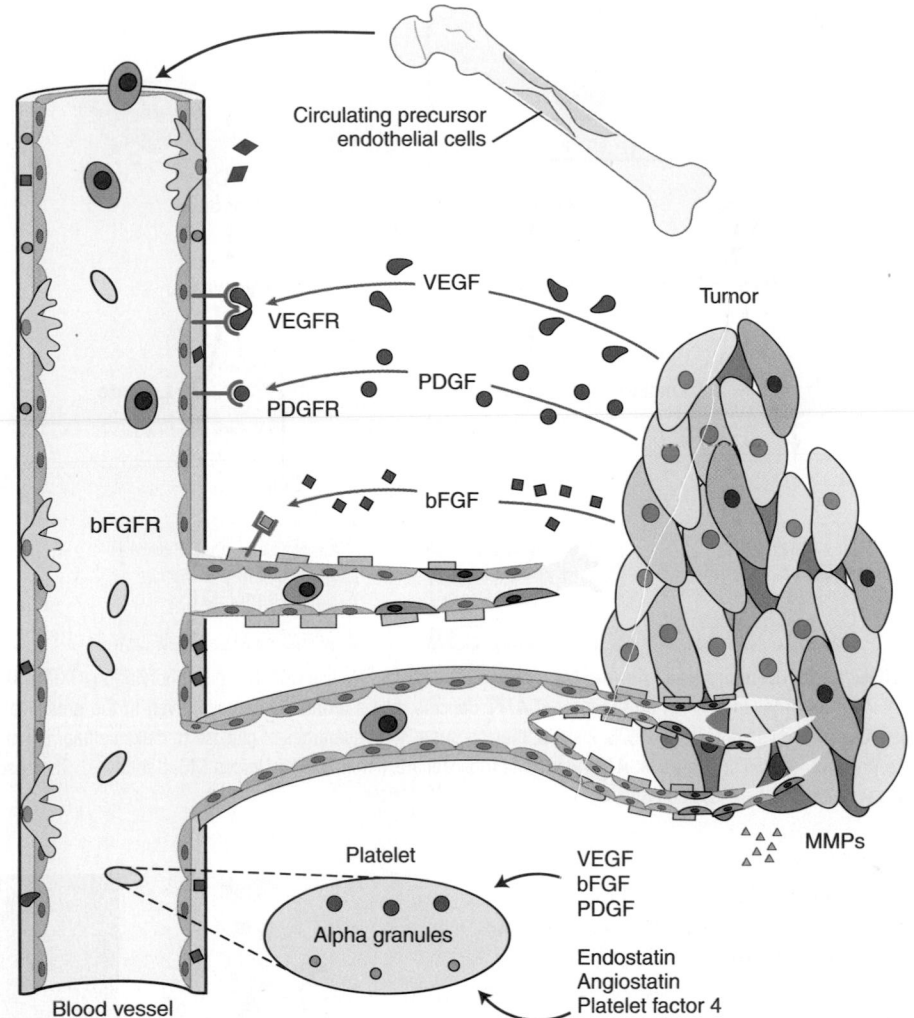

FIGURE 12.14 Tumor-Induced Angiogenesis. Malignant tumors secrete angiogenic factors and tissue-remodeling matrix metalloproteinases *(MMPs)* that actively induce formation of new blood vessels. New blood vessels are formed from both local endothelial cells and circulating precursor cells recruited from the bone marrow. Circulating platelets can also release regulatory proteins into the tumor. *bFGF* and *bFGFR,* Basic fibroblast growth factor and its receptor, respectively; *PDGF* and *PDGFR,* platelet-derived growth factor and its receptor, respectively; *VEGF* and *VEGFR,* vascular endothelial growth factor and its receptor, respectively. (Adapted from Folkman J: *Nat Rev Drug Discov* 6[4]: 273–286, 2007.)

(hypoxia) normal cells perform glycolysis (anaerobic glycolysis), generating only two ATP molecules per molecule of glucose, with lactic acid and pyruvate as byproducts.

Even in the presence of adequate oxygen, cancer cells may not use OXPHOS, but are reprogrammed to glycolysis (Warburg effect) (Fig. 12.15). Thus the Warburg effect is the use of glycolysis under normal oxygen conditions, hence the name aerobic glycolysis.[15] Although aerobic glycolysis was postulated to arise from cancer-specific mitochondrial dysfunction, it is now apparent that this is instead a highly regulated and beneficial adaptation for cancer cells. The shift from OXPHOS to glycolysis allows lactate and other products of glycolysis to be used for the more efficient production of lipids, nucleosides, amino acids, and other molecular building blocks needed for rapid cell growth.

A new model, the reverse Warburg effect, may play a role in certain cancers. Cancer cells may continue using OXPHOS to generate large amounts of ATP. However, they also may manipulate the cancer-associated fibroblasts (CAFs), perhaps by inducing oxidative stress, to undergo aerobic glycolysis and secrete metabolites (e.g., lactate, pyruvate)

that the cancer cells can use in the citric acid cycle (Krebs cycle) to feed OXPHOS and produce ATP. A secondary consequence would be induction of autophagy in the CAFs, resulting in consumption of the CAFs and release of materials needed by the cancer cell in the synthesis of new organelles.

Promoters of aerobic glycolysis are activated by oncogenes and mutated tumor-suppressor molecules. Up-regulation of GLUT1 (glucose transporter 1) under the control of oncogenes (e.g., *RAS, Myc*) and mutant tumor suppressors (e.g., TP53) increases transport of glucose into the cytoplasm. These and other oncogenes or mutant tumor-suppressor genes inhibit OXPHOS and promote the aerobic glycolytic pathway and related metabolic pathways that support the rapid growth of cancers.

Clinically the high glucose utilization of a cancer can be exploited for its detection. ^{18}F-Fluorodeoxyglucose (FDG) is incorporated into cells in the same way as glucose, with two key differences. Because it is missing a key hydroxyl group it cannot be broken down by glycolysis and, thus, FDG accumulates in cells. Because it is tagged with ^{18}F, it can

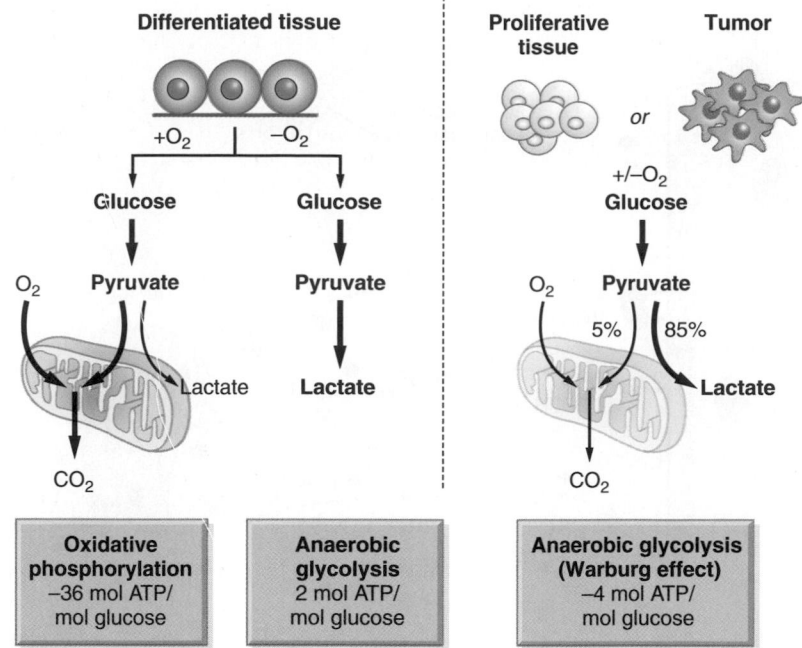

FIGURE 12.15 Cancers Have Altered Metabolism. Normal tissues use oxidative phosphorylation (OXPHOS) to turn glucose into CO_2 and energy (in the form of ATP). Cancers take a different approach; even in the presence of oxygen, usually they do not use OXPHOS. Instead, they consume large quantities of glucose to make cellular building blocks, supporting rapid proliferation. *ATP,* Adenosine triphosphate. (From Van der Heiden MG, Cantley LC, Thompson CB: *Science* 324:1029–1033, 2009.)

be imaged by a positron emission tomography (PET) scan. Small metastatic tumor masses that are consuming huge amounts of glucose can readily be detected with this imaging method (Fig. 12.16).

Resistance to Destruction
Resisting Apoptotic Cell Death

Programmed cell death (apoptosis) is a mechanism by which individual cells can self-destruct under conditions of tissue remodeling or as a protection against aberrant cell growth that may lead to malignancy. Two pathways may trigger apoptosis (Fig. 12.17). The intrinsic pathway (mitochondrial pathway) monitors cellular stress. Cellular stress may include DNA damage, genomic instability, aberrant proliferation, loss of adhesion to extracellular matrix or to adjacent cells, and other causes and characteristics of abnormal cellular physiology. The extrinsic pathway is activated through a plasma membrane receptor complex linked to intracellular activators of apoptosis (known as the *death receptor*).

The balance between proapoptotic (e.g., Bcl-2–associated X protein [BAX] and Bcl-2–homologous antagonist/killer [BAK]) and antiapoptotic (e.g., BCL2 [B-cell lymphoma 2]) members of the Bcl-2 family regulates apoptosis. Both groups regulate mitochondrial release of proapoptotic molecules (e.g., cytochrome *c*). As mentioned previously, expression of the tumor-suppressor gene TP53 is affected by intracellular stress, particularly DNA damage. If DNA damage is irreparable, p53 is activated by phosphorylation and induces transcription of proapoptotic factors.

The extrinsic pathway is relatively dormant until the death receptor is activated. The principal apoptotic receptor is called Fas/CD95 (the CD95 nomenclature is an alternative for Fas) (see Fig. 12.17). Fas is a receptor for Fas ligand (FasL) and similar molecules, such as tumor necrosis factor (TNF). Cytotoxic T lymphocytes and NK cells express surface and soluble FasL and can produce TNF, thus inducing apoptosis

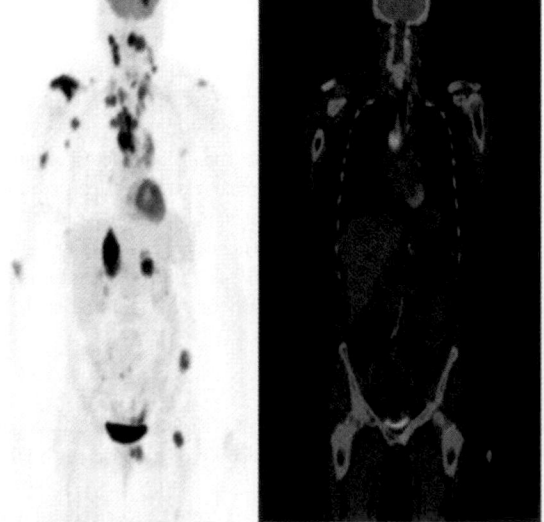

FIGURE 12.16 Intense Glucose Requirement Aids in Diagnosis of Metastatic Non–Small Cell Lung Cancer. This 54-year-old woman had a non–small cell lung cancer (NSCLC) resected from the left upper lobe. Five years later, these studies were obtained. The positron emission tomography (PET) scan using 18-fluorodeoxyglucose (FDG) shows metastatic lesions in the brain, right shoulder, and mediastinal and cervical lymph nodes, as well as in the liver, left pelvis, and proximal femur. *PET whole-body image (left):* Representative coronal image from the whole-body FDG-PET/CT–fused image of the same patient *(right).* The fused image consists of the computed tomography (CT) image with the metabolic information superimposed in color. The pattern of spread is most likely from the primary tumor to the large mediastinal lymph nodes, followed by lymphatic spread to cervical nodes. Blood-borne dissemination produced the bone, brain, and liver metastases. Normally, only the heart, brain, and bladder show a strong signal in PET scans. (Images courtesy John Hoffman, MD, Huntsman Cancer Institute, Salt Lake City, UT.)

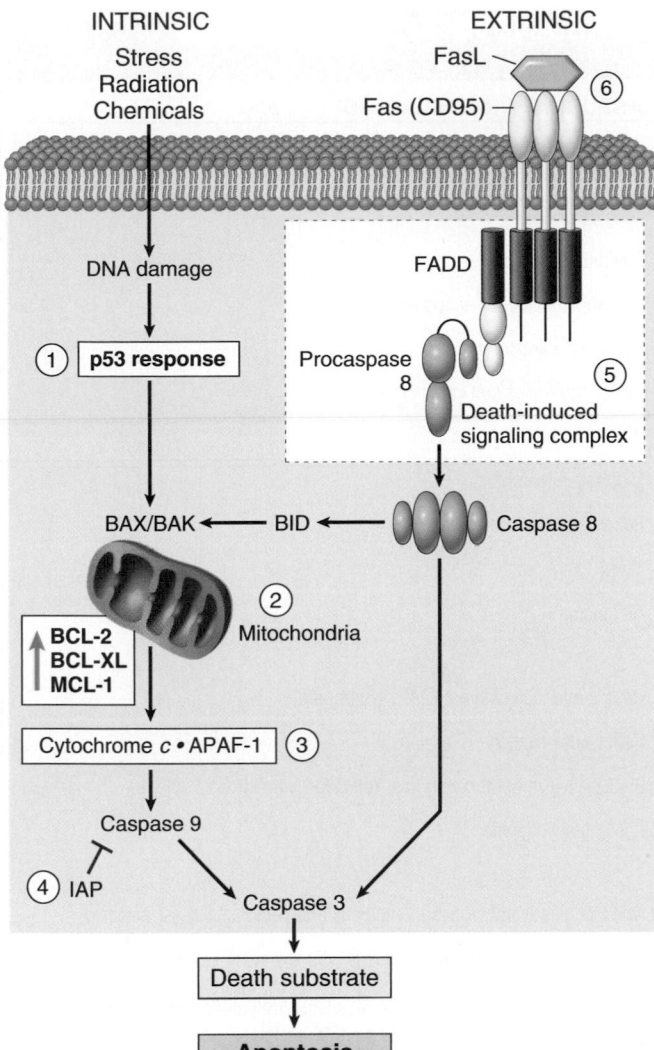

FIGURE 12.17 Extrinsic and Intrinsic Pathways of Apoptosis and Mechanisms Used by Tumor Cells to Evade Cell Death. (1) Loss of p53 leading to reduced function of proapoptotic factors, such as BAX. **(2)** Reduced egress of cytochrome *c* from mitochondria as a result of up-regulation of antiapoptotic factors, such as BCL-2. **(3)** Loss of apoptotic peptidase-activating factor 1 *(APAF-1).* **(4)** Up-regulation of inhibitors of apoptosis *(IAP).* **(5)** Reduced CD95 levels. **(6)** Inactivation of death domain signaling complex *(FADD).* (From Kumar V et al: *Robbins and Cotran pathologic basis of disease,* ed 9, Philadelphia, 2015, Saunders.)

in target cells. The Fas receptor is linked to a complex of intracellular proteins (FADD, the Fas-associated death domain signaling complex) that triggers apoptosis.

Both pathways activate a series of intracellular effector enzymatic molecules (caspases). Proapoptotic molecules released by mitochondria in the intrinsic pathway activate caspase 9, which in turn activates caspase 3. Caspase 3 cuts DNA and other substrates, leading to cell death. Activation of the extrinsic pathway activates caspase 8, which can directly activate caspase 3.

Apoptotic pathways are dysregulated in most cancers. Most commonly, loss-of-function mutations to the TP53 gene suppress activation of apoptosis during DNA damage. The balance between pro- and anti-apoptotic molecules also can be affected by overexpression of anti-apoptotic molecules or diminished expression of anti-apoptotic molecules

resulting from mutations. Overexpression of Bcl-2 occurs in the vast majority of follicular B-cell lymphomas. Excess expression of other anti-apoptotic members of the Bcl-2 family also may provide increased resistance to chemotherapeutic drugs, many of which act through induction of apoptosis. Other mechanisms of providing resistance to apoptosis include downregulation of caspases or production of caspase inhibitors. Whichever mechanism, or combination of mechanisms, is used successful cancers suppress apoptotic pathways and increase resistance to cell death.

Tumor-Promoting Inflammation

Historically, an immune/inflammatory response to cancer was considered a detrimental condition that successful tumors evolved methods of evading. It is now realized that the relationship between a cancer and the inflammatory system is much more complex. The inflammatory response may contribute to the onset of cancer and be manipulated throughout the process to benefit tumor progression and spread.

Chronic inflammation has been recognized for close to 150 years as being an important factor in the development of cancer. Chronic inflammations may result from many causes, for example, solar irradiation, asbestos exposure (mesothelioma), pancreatitis, and infection (Table 12.3). Additionally, some organs appear to be more susceptible to the oncogenic effects of chronic inflammation (e.g., the gastrointestinal [GI] tract, prostate, thyroid gland). Individuals who have suffered with ulcerative colitis for 10 years or more have up to a 30-fold increase in the risk of developing colon cancer. Chronic viral hepatitis caused by hepatitis B virus (HBV) or hepatitis C virus (HCV) infection markedly increases the risk of liver cancer.

A specific example is the association between gastric inflammation induced by infection with the bacterium *Helicobacter pylori (H. pylori)* and the risk for gastric cancer. *H. pylori* is a bacterium that infects more than half of the world's population. Chronic infection with *H. pylori* is an important cause of peptic ulcer disease and is strongly associated with gastric carcinoma, a leading cause of cancer deaths worldwide. It also is associated with a less common cancer, gastric mucosa–associated lymphoid tissue (MALT) lymphomas. *H. pylori* infection is often acquired in childhood and disproportionately affects lower socioeconomic classes. Although most infections are asymptomatic, prolonged chronic inflammation can lead to increased gastric acid secretion, atrophic gastritis, and duodenal ulcers, or benign cellular proliferation that can in a small fraction of individuals progress to dysplastic changes and finally gastric adenocarcinoma. *H. pylori* infection can both directly and indirectly produce genetic and epigenetic changes in cells of infected stomachs, including mutations in TP53 and alterations in the methylation of specific genes. Eradication of *H. pylori* from infected individuals before the development of dysplasia may prevent the development of cancer. However, there is no expert consensus on the value of population screening and treatment strategies. The MALT lymphomas associated with chronic *H. pylori* infections may depend on chronic inflammation and antigenic stimulation associated with infections, and therefore treatment with antibiotics may be useful even in cases of early lymphoma.

Once cells with malignant phenotypes have developed, additional complex interactions occur between the tumor and the surrounding stroma and cells of the immune and inflammatory systems. Cancers disrupt the environment, initiate or enhance inflammation, and in turn recruit local and distant cells (macrophages, lymphocytes, and other cellular components of inflammation). The acute inflammatory response is initially designed to eliminate infection, but evolves to initiate and direct the healing process (see Chapter 7). Successful tumors appear capable of manipulating cells of the inflammatory response from a rejection response toward the phenotypes associated with wound healing

TABLE 12.3   CHRONIC INFLAMMATORY CONDITIONS AND INFECTIOUS AGENTS ASSOCIATED WITH NEOPLASMS

INFLAMMATORY CONDITIONS	ASSOCIATED NEOPLASM(S)
Inflammatory Conditions	
Asbestosis, silicosis	Mesothelioma, lung carcinoma
Bronchitis	Lung carcinoma
Cystitis, bladder inflammation	Bladder carcinoma
Gingivitis, lichen planus	Oral squamous cell carcinoma
Inflammatory bowel disease, Crohn disease, chronic ulcerative colitis	Colorectal carcinoma
Lichen sclerosus	Vulvar squamous cell carcinoma
Chronic pancreatitis, hereditary pancreatitis	Pancreatic carcinoma
Reflux esophagitis, Barrett esophagus	Esophageal carcinoma
Sialadenitis	Salivary gland carcinoma
Sjögren syndrome, Hashimoto thyroiditis	MALT lymphoma
Skin inflammation	Melanoma
Infectious Agent (Nonviral)	
Helicobacter pylori	Gastric adenocarcinoma, MALT lymphoma
Chronic bacterial cholecystitis	Gallbladder cancer
Schistosomiasis	Bladder, liver, rectal carcinoma; follicular lymphoma of spleen
Liver flukes	Cholangiocarcinoma
Infectious Agent (Viral)	
Human immunodeficiency virus type 1 (HIV-1)	Non-Hodgkin lymphoma, squamous cell carcinomas, Kaposi sarcoma
Hepatitis B and hepatitis C	Hepatocellular carcinoma
Epstein-Barr virus	B-cell non-Hodgkin lymphoma, Burkitt lymphoma, nasopharyngeal carcinoma
Kaposi sarcoma-associated herpesvirus (KSHV/HHV8)	Kaposi sarcoma
Human Papilloma Virus (HPV)-16, -18, -31, others	Cervical, anogenital warts
Human T-cell lymphotropic virus 1 (HTLV-1)	Adult T-cell leukemia/lymphoma

MALT, mucosa-associated lymphoid tissue.
Modified from Kuper H et al: *J Intern Med* 248(3):171–183, 2000.

and tissue regeneration; a process that includes induction in the damaged tissue of cellular proliferation, neovascularization, and local immune suppression. These activities benefit cancer progression, as well as increase resistance to chemotherapeutic agents.

One of the key cells that promote tumor survival is the tumor-associated macrophage, or TAM. Tumors commonly produce cytokines and chemokines that are chemotactic factors for monocytes/macrophages (e.g., colony-stimulating factor-1 [CSF1; also known as *macrophage colony stimulating factor* or M-CSF], the chemokine ligand 2 [CCL2; also known as *monocyte chemotactic protein-1* or MCP-1]). Levels of CCL2 in human breast cancer and cancers of the esophagus are related to the degree of macrophage infiltration and progression of the tumor. Most tumors have large numbers of TAMs, whose presence frequently correlates with a worse prognosis. Thus monocytes are attracted from the blood and into the tumor, where they mature into macrophages. Monocytes have the capacity to differentiate into several macrophage phenotypes, depending upon the conditions in the microenvironment. The classic proinflammatory macrophage (M1) is the primary macrophage in the acute inflammatory response and is responsible for removal

and destruction of infectious agents. During healing, however, a different phenotype (M2) produces antiinflammatory mediators to suppress ongoing inflammation and induce cellular proliferation, angiogenesis, and wound healing. TAMs appear to phenotypically mimic the M2 phenotype.

TAMs have diminished cytotoxic response, and develop the capacity to block T-cytotoxic cell and NK-cell functions and produce cytokines that are advantageous for tumor growth and spread. TAMs secrete cellular growth factors (e.g., TGF-β and fibroblast growth factor-2 [FGF-2]) that favor tumor cell proliferation, angiogenesis, and tissue remodeling, similar to their activities in wound healing. They also secrete angiogenesis factors (e.g., VEGF) that induce neovascularization and matrix metalloproteinases (MMPs) that degrade intercellular matrix. The overall effect is increased tumor growth, invasion of the blood vessels, increased oxygen to the tumor, and invasion through the degraded matrix into the local tissue.

Cancer-associated fibroblasts (CAFs) synthesize the extracellular matrix that surrounds and permeates the tumor. Cytokines and growth factors stored in the matrix as well as growth factors, metalloproteases, proteoglycans, and other molecules secreted by CAFs contribute greatly to cancer progression, local spread, and metastasis.[16]

Evading Immune Destruction

Many cancers express cell surface antigens that are not generally found on normal cells from the same tissue. Tumor-associated antigens include products of oncogenes, antigens from oncogenic viruses, oncofetal antigens (expressed in embryonic tissues and tumors), and altered glycoproteins and glycolipids. Viral and tumor antigens are processed by the tumor cell and presented on the cell surface by MHC class I molecules and are targets of CD8+ T-cytotoxic cells (Tcyto) (see Chapter 8). NK cells recognize altered cell surface glycoproteins and glycolipids. Thus cancer cells should be recognized as foreign and destroyed by the immune system. In the laboratory, T lymphocytes and NK cells recognize and kill cancer cells. This observation gave rise to two concepts—*immune surveillance* and *immunotherapy*. The immune surveillance hypothesis predicts that most developing malignancies are suppressed by an efficient immune response against tumor-associated antigens. The rationale for immunotherapy predicts that the immune system could be used to target tumor-associated antigens and destroy tumors clinically. Immunotherapy could be either active, by immunization with tumor antigens to elicit or enhance the immune response against a particular cancer, or passive, by injecting the individual with cancer with antibodies or lymphocytes directed against the tumor antigens. However, the interactions between cancer and the immune system are more complex than originally envisioned and both hypotheses remain controversial.

What is the role of the immune system in protecting against cancer? The most clearly documented effective immune response is prophylactic and directed against oncogenic viruses. Several viruses have been associated with human cancer; human papillomavirus (HPV), Epstein-Barr virus (EBV; also known as HHV4), Kaposi sarcoma herpesvirus (KSHV; also known as HHV8), and hepatitis B and C viruses (HBV, HCV) are associated with about 15% of all human cancers worldwide.[17] Cancer of the cervix and hepatocellular carcinoma account for approximately 80% of virus-linked cancer cases.

Virtually all cervical cancer is caused by infection with specific types of HPV, which infects basal skin cells and commonly causes warts. There are more than 120 HPV types, but only about 40 can infect human mucosal tissue, and only a few (HPV-16, -18, -31, and -45) are associated with the highest risk for developing cervical, anogenital, and penile cancer. Most HPV infection is handled effectively and rapidly by the immune system and does not cause cancer. Cancer is more common in people with prolonged infection with HPV (a decade or more), during which the viral DNA becomes integrated into the genomic DNA of the infected basal cell of the cervix and directs the persistent production of viral oncogenes. Early oncogenic HPV infection is readily detected by the Papanicolaou (Pap) test, an examination of cervical epithelial scrapings. Early detection of atypical cells in a Pap test alerts healthcare providers to the possibility of cervical carcinoma in situ, which can be effectively treated. The Pap test is probably the most effective cancer-screening test developed to date. For women age 30 to 65 years old, additional testing for HPV infection of cervical cells (HPV test) should be added. Vaccines protecting against the common oncogenic HPV types (HPV-16 and HPV-18 [types that cause 70% of cervical cancers] and HPV-6 and HPV-11 [types that cause 90% of genital warts]) were approved for clinical use beginning in 2006; if these vaccines are administered to young women and men before an initial HPV infection, this is likely to prevent many cases of cervical cancer.

Chronic hepatitis B infections are common in parts of Asia and Sub-Saharan Africa and confer up to a 200-fold increased risk of developing liver cancer. Chronic hepatitis C infections have become increasingly recognized in Western countries. Up to 80% of liver cancer cases worldwide are associated with chronic hepatitis caused either by HBV or by HCV. The initial infection with hepatitis B or C is not associated with cancer; instead, it is acquisition of a chronic viral hepatitis that markedly increases cancer risk. In both cases, it appears that a lifetime of chronic liver inflammation predisposes to the development of hepatocellular carcinoma. Widespread use of the HBV vaccine is expected to significantly decrease the incidence of chronic hepatitis B and hence hepatocellular carcinoma. Unfortunately, a vaccine for HCV is not yet available.

For most other human tumor viruses, immunoprophylaxis is not yet available. EBV and HHV8 are members of the Herpesviridae family. More than 90% of adults have been infected with EBV, usually as children and without symptoms. EBV infection during adolescence may cause infectious mononucleosis. The virus infects B lymphocytes and stimulates their limited proliferation and usually becomes latent throughout the individual's life. If the individual is immunosuppressed because of HIV infection or because of drugs given for an organ transplant, persistent EBV infection can lead to the development of B-cell lymphomas. EBV infection also is associated with Burkitt lymphoma in areas of endemic malaria and with nasopharyngeal carcinoma, a cancer endemic in Chinese populations in Southeast Asia. HHV8 is linked to the development of Kaposi sarcoma, a cancer that was once seen primarily in older men but now occurs in a markedly more virulent form in immunosuppressed individuals, especially those with acquired immunodeficiency syndrome (AIDS). HHV8 also has been linked to several rare lymphomas. Human T-cell lymphotropic virus type 1 (HTLV-1) is an oncogenic retrovirus linked to the development of adult T-cell leukemia and lymphoma (ATLL). HTLV is transmitted vertically (that is, inherited by children from infected parents) and horizontally (e.g., by breast-feeding, sexual intercourse, blood transfusions, and exposure to infected needles). Infection with HTLV may be asymptomatic, and only a small fraction of infected individuals develop ATLL, often many years after acquiring the virus.

Thus immunization has proven beneficial in preventing viral-induced cancers. The immune surveillance hypothesis, however, would predict that components of the immune system, especially T cells, monitor the body and destroy most nascent tumors, even those not caused by viruses. If the immune surveillance hypothesis is correct, compromise of the immune system by immunosuppressive drugs or development of genetic or acquired immune deficiencies would result in increased incidences of all types of cancer. However, defective immune responses generally only increase the risk for lymphoid cancers, many of which are associated with viral infections. For instance, individuals taking chronic powerful immunosuppressive drugs, such as those given for kidney, heart, or liver transplant, have a much higher risk of developing viral-associated cancers, with a 10-fold increased risk of non-Hodgkin lymphoma (caused by EBV) and up to a 1000-fold increased risk of Kaposi sarcoma (caused by HHV8). The same immunosuppressed individuals, however, have only a slight increase in the risk of common cancers such as lung and colon cancer (and this could well be because of increased inflammation at those sites), and no increase in the risk of breast or prostate cancer.

However, many tumors have an abundance of tumor-infiltrating lymphocytes (TILs). Although the immune cells frequently found in tumors were once thought to be futile attempts at an antitumor response, instead it appears that cancers actively recruit an immune and stromal response to assist in remodeling of tissues, formation of new blood vessels, and promotion of metastasis. NK cells are generally in low amounts in tumors. The predominant TILs are T-regulatory (Treg) cells. Treg cells are CD4+ cells that differentiate under the control of specific cytokines, primarily TGF-β. The role of Treg cells during wound healing is to control or limit the immune response to protect the host's own tissues against autoimmune reactions. Their role in tumors is manipulated to prevent a destructive antitumor immune response and provide cytokines that facilitate tumor cell proliferation and spread.[18] Treg cells and TAMs, as well as other stromal cells, produce very high levels of TGF-β and interleukin-10 (IL-10). IL-10 is an immunosuppressive cytokine, which generally decreases T-helper cell 1 (Th1) and Th2 activity, suppresses antigen recognition and cell proliferation by Th cells, and suppresses the capacity of CD8+ T-cytotoxic (Tcyto) cells to recognize, proliferate, and kill tumor cells. The goal of current immunotherapy regimens is to reverse this relationship and facilitate T-cell–mediated cancer cell death (discussed later in this chapter).

The release of immunosuppressive factors into the tumor microenvironment also increases resistance of the tumor to chemotherapy and radiotherapy. Increased levels of Treg cells in blood and lymph nodes and infiltrating the tumor correlate with poor outcomes in breast and GI tumors. In advanced non–small cell lung cancer an elevated ratio of Treg to Tcyto cells is related to a poor response to platinum-based chemotherapy. Immunosuppressive cytokines additionally lower the cancer cell's sensitivity to immune-mediated death (Fig. 12.18). With increasing heterogeneity of cells within the tumor, subpopulations of antigen-negative cancer cell variants may selectively outgrow more immune-sensitive cells. Variants may suppress the production of particular antigens or suppress levels of antigen-presenting MHC class I.

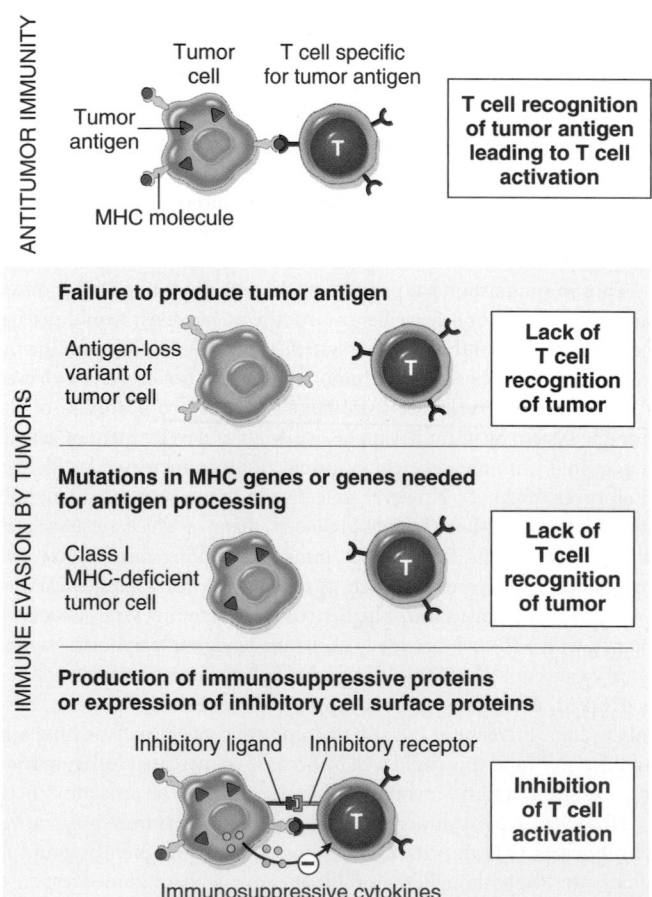

FIGURE 12.18 Mechanisms by Which Tumor Cells Evade the Immune System. Tumors may evade the immune response by losing expression of antigens or major histocompatibility complex *(MHC)* molecules or by producing immunosuppressive cytokines or ligands for inhibitory receptors on T cells. (From Kumar V et al: *Robbins and Cotran pathologic basis of disease,* ed 9, Philadelphia, 2015, Saunders.)

Other cytokines appear to increase the cancer cells' resistance to apoptosis. For example, the Th2 cytokine IL-4 increases the resistance of thyroid cancer to chemotherapy; IL-6 produced by Th cells, adipocytes, and fibroblasts activates survival pathways in breast cancer leading to resistance to radiotherapy; and adipocytes enhance the transcription of the anti-apoptotic factor Bcl-2 in leukemia cells.

Activating Invasion and Metastasis

Metastasis is the spread of cancer cells from the site of the original tumor to distant tissues and organs through the body. Metastasis is a defining characteristic of cancer and is the major cause of death from cancer. Cancer that has not metastasized can often be cured by a combination of surgery, chemotherapy, and radiation. These same therapies are frequently ineffective against cancer that has metastasized. For example, in appropriately treated women with localized low-stage breast cancer, the 5-year survival rate is often greater than 90%. Tragically, less than 30% of women with metastatic breast cancer are still alive 5 years after diagnosis. A growing body of basic and clinical research is defining the biologic principles of metastasis, with the hope that this improved understanding will lead to novel diagnostic approaches and better therapies to prevent and treat metastatic cancers.

How do cancer cells develop the ability to metastasize? Metastasis is a highly inefficient process. Cancer cells must surmount multiple physical and physiologic barriers in order to spread, survive, and proliferate in distant locations, and the destination must be receptive to the growth of the cancer. Changes in the tumor microenvironment initiate the metastatic process and may include stromal cell adaptation to increase tumor mass and intratumor hypoxia. As this diversity increases within the changing tumor microenvironment, some cancer cells evolve with multiple new abilities that can facilitate metastasis. The model for transition to metastatic cancer cells is called *epithelial-mesenchymal transition.*

Epithelial-mesenchymal transition (EMT) has been most extensively described for carcinomas, which originate from highly differentiated and polarized epithelial cells that form structured sheets stabilized by multiple adherences to neighboring cells and to a basement membrane (an extracellular meshwork of collagens and other connective tissue proteins) along the cell's basal surface.[19] Although the degree of malignant transformation resulting in a primary carcinoma may be adequate for local expansion of the tumor, neoplastic cells usually retain some epithelial-like characteristics that prevent dissociation from the extracellular matrix and preclude successful metastasis to distal sites. A greater degree of cellular "dedifferentiation" is necessary to produce the phenotype that can separate from the primary tumor and flourish in a potentially hostile secondary site. This results from a programmed transition of the still partially epithelial-like carcinoma to a more undifferentiated mesenchymal-like phenotype (Fig. 12.19). A similar process occurs with tumors of endothelial origin (endothelial-mesenchymal transition).

EMT is a process that occurs normally in embryonic development, as well as wound healing and tissue repair. Generally, cells that have transitioned into a mesenchymal-like phenotype have suppressed expression of adhesion molecules with a loss of polarity, increased migratory capacity, and elevated resistance to apoptosis, and have demonstrated the potential to redifferentiate into other cell types. The transition to a mesenchymal-like phenotype is, in most cases, driven by cytokines and chemokines produced within the tumor microenvironment. IL-8 is an effective driver of carcinoma cells into EMT.

Invasion, or local spread, is a prerequisite for metastasis. In its earliest stages local invasion may occur by direct tumor extension. Eventually, however, cells migrate away from the primary tumor and invade the surrounding tissues (see Fig. 12.19). Invasion is a multistep process

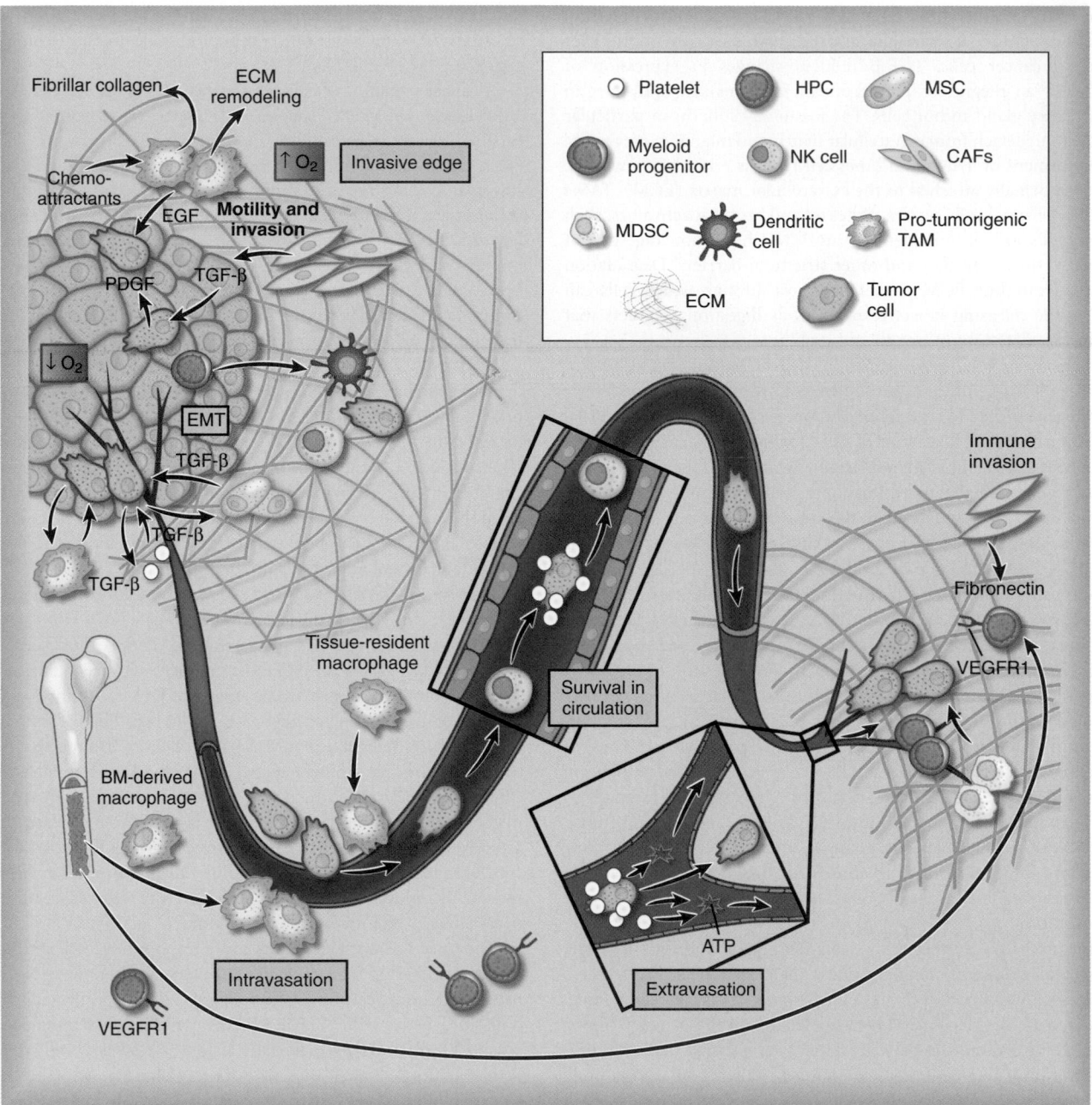

FIGURE 12.19 Epithelial-Mesenchymal Transition and Metastasis. The microenvironment supports metastatic dissemination and colonization at secondary sites. Stromal cells (e.g., mesenchymal stem cells *[MSCs]*), possibly facilitated by a relative decrease in oxygen levels in the tumor, contribute to the epithelial-to-mesenchymal transition *(EMT)* through which tumor cells develop a metastatic phenotype characterized by suppression of adhesion molecules and reduced adherence to adjacent cells and extracellular matrix, increased local invasion, and access to the blood and lymphatic circulations. One major mediator of this process is TGF-β, which is secreted by the tumor stroma. Intravascularization of tumor cells into the circulation is facilitated by protumorigenic TAMs, and CAFs tend to cluster at the leading edge of the invading cancer cells and secrete matrix metalloproteinases that promote digestion and remodeling of the surrounding ECM. Survival in the circulation is promoted by association with platelets and clotting factors that shield the cancer cells from cytotoxic immune cells (T-cytotoxic cells and NK cells) that are also suppressed by myeloid-derived suppressor cells *(MDSCs)*. Potential metastatic sites are prepared by induction of fibronectin, which provides a site for the influx of hematopoietic progenitor cells *(HPCs)* that have receptors for VEGF. HPCs appear essential for establishment of a metastatic site. At a metastatic site, cancer cells will adhere to local vascular endothelium, undergo extravascularization facilitated by the effects of ATP on the endothelium, and undergo mesenchymal-to-epithelial transition *(MET)*. The premetastatic niche may have been prepared by molecular signaling from the cancer and initiation of a favorable microenvironment. *CAF,* Cancer-associated fibroblast; *ECM,* extracellular matrix; *NK,* natural killer cell; *PDGF,* platelet-derived growth factor; *TAM,* tumor-associated macrophage; *TGF-β,* tumor growth factor-beta; *Treg,* T-regulatory cell; *VEGF,* vascular endothelial cell growth factor. (Modified from Quail DF, Joyce JA: *Nat Med* 19[11]:1423–1437, 2013.)

within EMT that includes diminished cell-to-cell adhesion, digestion of the surrounding extracellular matrix, and increased motility of individual cancer cells. TGF-β induces changes in expression of E-cadherin (an integral component of tight junctions) and of β_4-integrin in mammary gland tumor cells. The loss of E-cadherin in particular allows cells to detach from extracellular matrix and migrate more readily.

Recruitment of TAMs and other cell types is critical for invasion. Cells are normally attached to the extracellular matrix (ECM). TAMs and other stromal cells secrete proteases and protease activators, such as the MMPs and plasminogen activators, which promote digestion of connective tissue capsules and other structural barriers. Degradation of the surrounding ECM creates pathways through which cells can move, while releasing bioactive peptides as digestion products that further stimulate tumor growth and mobility.

Normal cells, when separated from their ECM, undergo anoikis, a form of apoptosis. Tumor cells adapted to a hypoxic environment have already been selected for resistance to apoptosis, often by loss of normal cell death pathways. The process of EMT frequently increases resistance to apoptosis. For example, neuroblastomas with loss of the proapoptotic caspase 8 genes are able to avoid apoptosis after loss of integrins, and are more able to metastasize than the same cells with normal levels of caspase 8. Accordingly, individuals whose neuroblastomas have low levels of caspase 8 have a poor prognosis.

To transition from local to distant metastasis, the cancer cells must also be able to invade local blood and lymphatic vessels, a task facilitated by stimulation of neoangiogenesis and lymphangiogenesis by factors such as VEGF. After release from the ECM and digestion of basement membranes, mobile cancer cells gain access to the circulation, perhaps facilitated by the leaky newly made vessels and attraction of the cells because of chemoattractants coming from these new vessels. Once in the circulation, metastatic cells must be able to withstand the physiologic stresses of travel in the blood and lymphatic circulation, including high shear rates and exposure to immune cells. One mechanism is for tumor cells to bind to blood platelets, giving them a protective coat of non-malignant blood cells that both shields the tumor cells and creates a small tumor embolus, or cancer clot, that can promote cancer cell survival in distant locations.

Cancer cells spread through vascular and lymphatic pathways. The neovascularization of a cancer offers malignant cells direct access into the venous blood and draining lymphatic vessels. The venous and lymphatic drainage networks associated with the primary tumor frequently determine the pattern of metastasis. Single cells, clumps, and even tumor fragments can disseminate by these routes. Anatomic patterns of lymphatic and venous blood flow help determine how colon cancers spread to the liver, liver cancers spread through the portal vein to the lungs, lung cancers spread through the systemic circulation to the brain, and breast cancer spreads through the lymphatics to axillary lymph nodes (Fig. 12.20). Cancers often spread first to regional lymph nodes through the lymphatics and then to distant organs through the bloodstream.

There also is a major yet poorly understood selectivity of different cancers for different sites. Metastatic breast cancer often spreads through the bloodstream to bones but rarely to kidney or spleen, whereas lymphomas often spread to the spleen but uncommonly spread to bone. In a key study, different types of cancer cells were injected into the carotid artery of mice.[20] In spite of identical blood flow–mediated distribution of the cancer cells, each cell type produced cancers in very different parts of the brain. This tissue selectivity is likely caused by specific interactions between the cancer cells and specific receptors on the small blood vessels in different organs. Experimental metastasis studies in mice are beginning to reveal additional molecular reasons for this tissue specificity. Examples include interaction between α3β1

integrins binding to laminin-5 receptors in the lung, and the chemokine receptor CXCR4 on breast cancer cells promoting homing to lung tissues expressing the ligand CXCL12.

A cancer's ability to establish a metastatic lesion in a new location requires that the cancer survive in the specific environment and be capable of forming complex and heterogeneous tumors. In some cases, these tumor-initiating cells are very rare. Human cancers transplanted into special immune-deficient mice will grow and can metastasize. Experiments have been performed to determine how few cancer cells are capable of establishing a tumor; only 1 in 10,000 human colon cancer cells are able to re-form a complex and heterogeneous colon cancer in mice; however, in human melanomas 1 in 4 cells can initiate a complex tumor in the appropriate mouse model. Thus the number of potentially metastatic cells may vary greatly with the particular cancer.

The degree of dedifferentiation may be variable, but most cells undergoing EMT acquire stem cell traits that facilitate initial growth in a new microenvironment. The EMT is not a stable transition; after taking residence in the metastatic site, the tumor tends to regain some characteristics of the primary tumor, thus reverting to some extent to its epithelial origins. Because metastasis requires successful completion of each and every step, there may be many opportunities to interrupt this potentially lethal pathway.

However, metastasis does not universally result in proliferation at a new site. Some cancer cells survive at a new site but do not proliferate to form a clinically relevant metastatic site. These cancer cells appear to exist in a state of *dormancy*. Cellular dormancy is cellular quiescence—a stable, nonproliferative state that is reversible. Cells may remain quiescent for years before initiating proliferation. About two-thirds of breast cancer deaths occur after a 5-year disease-free interval. In other conditions, solitary tumor cells can be detected in the blood years after a complete clinical remission in individuals, and many people with detectable micrometastases will not develop clinically obvious metastases. Cancer cell dormancy may be extremely common, even without a history of clinical cancer. Studies of deceased individuals without any history of cancer suggest that most individuals have dormant cancer cells that never adjusted to form a malignant tumor.

The causes of dormancy and, more importantly, escape from dormancy and development of malignant cancer are unknown. Dormancy may result from features of the cell or the environmental niche, or both. Individuals with clinical cancers may shed disseminated tumor cells very early from premetastatic lesions. These early cells may have developed inadequately to a metastatic phenotype and thus cannot recruit cells into a supportive stroma or initiated angiogenesis. Another consideration is the niche itself. It is not clear whether a developing cancer secretes factors that enter the bloodstream and prepare potential metastatic niches. If so, early disseminated cancer cells may encounter nonsupportive niches that foster dormancy. A clear understanding of dormancy is needed because existing cancer therapies do not address this condition.

CLINICAL MANIFESTATIONS OF CANCER

Paraneoplastic Syndromes

Paraneoplastic syndromes are symptom complexes that are triggered by a cancer but are not caused by direct local effects of the tumor mass. They are most commonly caused by biologic substances released from the tumor (e.g., hormones) or by an immune response triggered by the tumor. For example, a small fraction of carcinoid tumors release hormones, including serotonin, into the bloodstream that cause flushing, diarrhea, wheezing, and rapid heartbeat. A number of cancers trigger an antibody response that attacks the nervous system, causing a variety

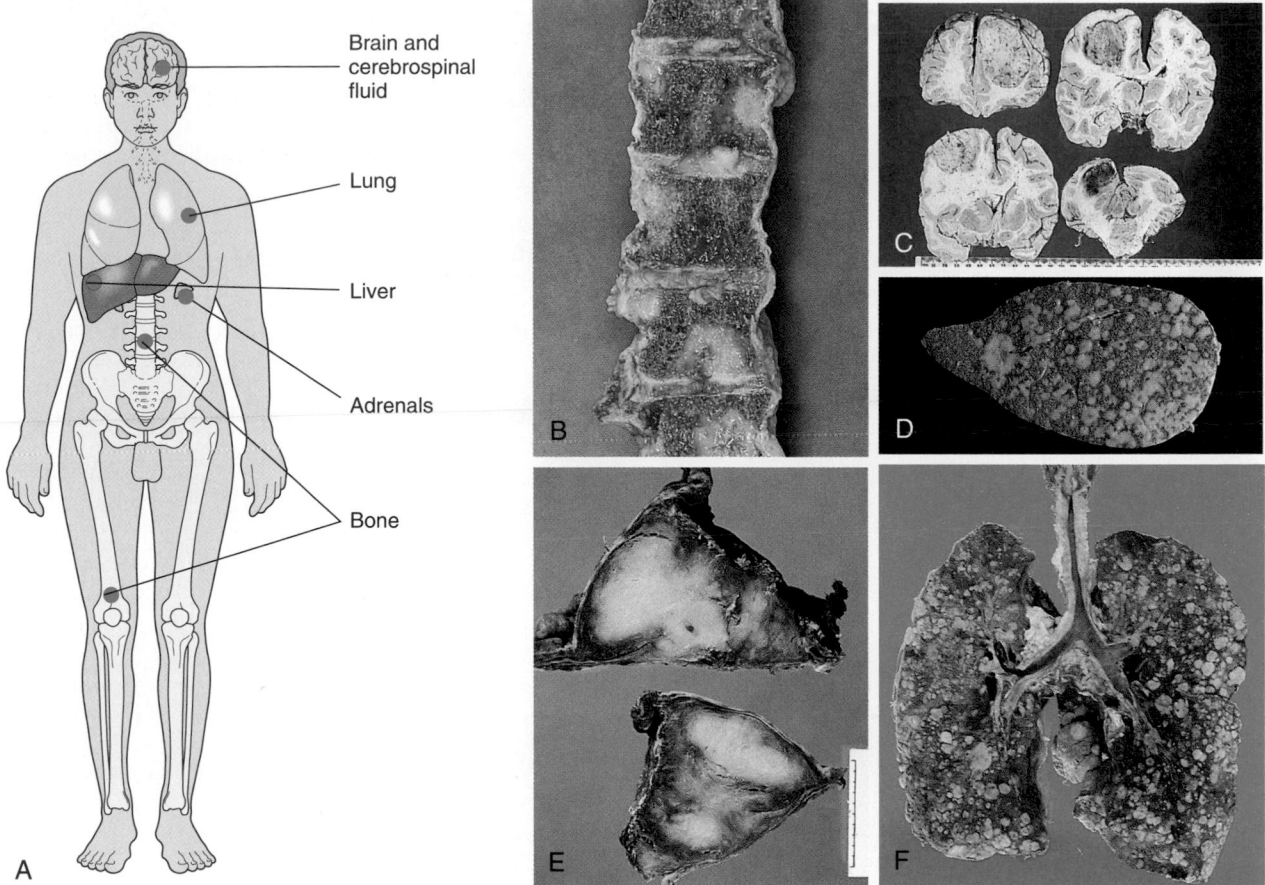

FIGURE 12.20 Patterns of Metastatic Spread. **A,** Sites of hematogenous metastasis. Blood-borne tumor metastasis leads to growth of secondary tumors in several main sites. The macroscopic appearance of bone metastasis is shown in **B,** where lesions are seen in vertebrae. **C,** Numerous metastases from a neoplasm of the stomach are seen in the brain. **D,** The liver is the most common site for metastases from tumors in the gastrointestinal tract that arose from a colonic neoplasm. **E,** Metastatic tumor has replaced both adrenal glands, as is commonly seen with spread from lung and breast tumors. **F,** The lung is the most common site for blood-borne metastases from tumors outside the spinal tract, particularly mesenchymal tumors.

of neurologic disorders that can precede other symptoms of cancer by months.

Although infrequent, paraneoplastic syndromes are significant because they may be the earliest symptom of an unknown cancer and, in affected individuals, can be serious, often irreversible, and sometimes life-threatening. Table 12.4 presents the classifications of paraneoplastic syndromes. Other clinical manifestations of cancer are summarized in Box 12.1 and Table 12.5.

Molecular Mechanisms of Cachexia

Cachexia is a multiorgan syndrome that has been discussed as a type of energy balance disorder where energy intake is decreased and energy expenditure is increased (Fig. 12.21). Energy intake and expenditure depends on the tumor type and its growth phase. Because individuals who are being administered total parenteral nutrition still lose weight, increased resting energy expenditure may be the cause of the wasting syndrome. Investigators are studying the role of both mitochondria and sarcoplasmic reticulum (SR) in muscle function and its relationship to cachexia. Hypotheses related to these functions include increased production of peroxisome proliferator–activated receptor-γ co-activator-1α (PGC1α), which can activate a mitochondrial protein (mitofusin-2

[MFN2]) that interacts with muscle SR and controls interorganelle calcium (Ca^{++}) signaling. Therefore one hypothesis is the overexpression of PGC1α can activate MFN2 expression, leading to Ca^{++} deregulation, which is closely associated with muscle wasting. Muscle weakness and fatigue is related to loss of myofibrillar proteins in muscle cells. Abnormalities in protein and amino acid metabolism are noted in cachectic muscle (Fig. 12.22).

Contributing further to muscle wasting are an increase in apoptosis and an impaired capacity for regeneration. Many signaling pathways are involved in protein turnover leading to the wasting process and are activated by inflammatory mediators including cytokines, myostatin, and tumor-derived factors. In addition to muscle wasting, miRNAs may be involved in stimulating the breakdown of adipose tissue. In cancer cachexia, skeletal muscle loss includes major loss of white adipose tissue (WAT). The WAT loss is thought to be caused by (1) increased lipolysis, (2) decreased activity of lipoprotein lipase (LPL), and (3) decreased new or de novo lipogenesis in adipose tissue. New data show that WAT cells undergo a "browning" process during cancer cachexia where they change to beige cells called *BAT-like cells*. Browning is associated with increased thermogenesis. Tumor-derived compounds, such as IL-6 (which also may be released by immune cells) and

TABLE 12.4   PARANEOPLASTIC SYNDROMES

CLINICAL SYNDROMES	MAJOR FORMS OF UNDERLYING CANCER	CAUSAL MECHANISM
Endocrinopathies		
Cushing syndrome	Small cell carcinoma of lung Pancreatic carcinoma Neural tumors	ACTH or ACTH-like substance
Syndrome of inappropriate antidiuretic hormone (SIADH) secretion	Small cell carcinoma of lung; intracranial neoplasms	Antidiuretic hormone or atrial natriuretic hormones
Hypercalcemia	Squamous cell carcinoma of lung Breast carcinoma Renal carcinoma Adult T-cell leukemia/lymphoma Ovarian carcinoma	Parathyroid hormone–related protein (PTHRP), TGF-α, TNF, IL-1
Hypoglycemia	Fibrosarcoma Other mesenchymal sarcomas Hepatocellular carcinoma	Insulin or insulin-like substance
Carcinoid syndrome	Bronchial adenoma (carcinoid) Pancreatic carcinoma Gastric carcinoma	Serotonin, bradykinin
Polycythemia	Renal carcinoma Cerebellar hemangioma Hepatocellular carcinoma	Erythropoietin
Nerve and Muscle Syndrome		
Myasthenia	Bronchogenic carcinoma	Immunologic
Disorders of central and peripheral nervous systems	Breast carcinoma	
Dermatologic Disorders		
Acanthosis nigricans	Gastric carcinoma Lung carcinoma Uterine carcinoma	Immunologic; secretion of epidermal growth factor
Dermatomyositis	Bronchogenic, breast carcinoma	Immunologic
Osseous, Articular, and Soft Tissue Changes		
Hypertrophic osteoarthropathy and clubbing of the fingers	Bronchogenic carcinoma	Unknown
Vascular and Hematologic Changes		
Venous thrombosis (Trousseau phenomenon)	Pancreatic carcinoma Bronchogenic carcinoma Other cancers	Tumor products (mucins that activate clotting)
Nonbacterial thrombotic endocarditis	Advanced cancers	Hypercoagulability
Anemia	Thymic neoplasms	Unknown
Others		
Nephrotic syndrome	Various cancers	Tumor antigens, immune complexes

ACTH, Adrenocorticotropic hormone; *IL*, interleukin; *TGF*, transforming growth factor; *TNF*, tumor necrosis factor.
From Kumar V, Abbas AK, Fausto N: *Pathologic basis of disease*, ed 7, Philadelphia, 2005, Saunders.

parathyroid hormone–related protein (PTHRP), may be the drivers of thermogenesis.

An unusual and frustrating component of cancer care is the person's early satiety, or a sense of being full after only a few mouthfuls of food. Brain mediators are involved in the regulation of food intake and include appetite, satiation, taste, and smell of food. Therefore the brain is an important organ in anorexia and consequently altered energy balance. Profoundly altered are both orexigenic (appetite-stimulating) and anorexigenic (appetite-suppressing) brain pathways. (Cytokines are discussed in detail in Chapters 7 and 8.)

BOX 12.1 COMMON SIDE EFFECTS OF CANCER AND CANCER THERAPY

Anemia: Commonly associated with malignancy, with 20% of persons diagnosed with cancer having hemoglobin concentrations less than 9 g/dL (normal value = 15 g/dL). Mechanisms of anemia include chronic bleeding (resulting in iron deficiency), severe malnutrition, cytotoxic chemotherapy, and malignancy in blood-forming organs. Chronic bleeding and iron deficiency can accompany colorectal or genitourinary malignancy. Iron also is malabsorbed in individuals with gastric, pancreatic, or upper intestinal cancer.

Bone Density Loss: Osteoporosis, or less severe osteopenia, may occur secondary to hormone treatment, such as used for breast cancer and prostate cancer, or in individuals treated with steroids.

Cachexia: A syndrome that includes many symptoms including anorexia, early satiety (filling), weight loss, anemia, asthenia (marked weakness), taste alterations, and altered protein, lipid, and carbohydrate metabolism. It is the most severe form of malnutrition associated with cancer and results in wasting, emaciation, and decreased quality of life. Cytokines and metabolites from the tumor may contribute to cachexia.

Cardiac and Pulmonary Damage: Chemotherapy and localized radiation can damage the heart and lungs, resulting in increased risk for heart failure and decreased pulmonary function.

Fatigue: Severe fatigue is the most frequently reported and persistent symptom of cancer and cancer treatment, particularly chemotherapy. Suggested causes include sleep disturbances, chronic inflammation, anemia, depression, level of activity, nutritional status, and other environmental and physical factors.

Gastrointestinal Tract (GI): Rapidly proliferating cells of the GI tract are particularly sensitive to radiation and chemotherapy, leading to oral ulcers (stomatitis), malabsorption, and diarrhea, as well as increased risk for infection from the individual's own microbiome.

Hair Loss (Alopecia) and Skin: Some chemotherapy generally affects hair follicles, whereas radiation is more localized. It is usually temporary, although hair may regrow with a different texture initially. Decreased renewal rates of the epidermal layers in the skin may lead to skin breakdown and dryness, altering the normal barrier protection against infection. Radiation therapy may cause skin erythema (redness) and contribute to breakdown.

Infection: The most significant cause of complications and death in people with malignant disease is infection. Immune suppression, lymphopenia, and granulocytopenia may result from the underlying cancer or secondary to treatment increasing the risk of serious microbial (bacterial and fungal) infections. (Factors that predispose individuals with cancer to infection are summarized in Table 12.5.) The prevalence of hospital-acquired (nosocomial) infections increases because of indwelling medical devices, inadequate wound care, and the introduction of microorganisms from visitors and other individuals.

Infertility: Male or female infertility may be secondary to the cancer, surgical treatment, or treatment with chemotherapy or radiation. Many infertility clinics will freeze sperm, eggs, or embryos before initiation of therapy.

Leukopenia and Thrombocytopenia: Causes can include many chemotherapeutic drugs and radiation therapy because they are toxic to the bone marrow, often causing granulocytopenia and thrombocytopenia. Thrombocytopenia is a major cause of hemorrhage in people with cancer and is often treated with platelet transfusions.

Lymphedema: Accumulation of fluid in the tissues results from damage to the lymphatic system from lymphoid cancer or metastatic disease, surgery, or radiation treatment.

Pain: Pain may occur during the early stages of malignant disease but intensifies with disease progression. Direct pressure, obstruction, invasion of a sensitive structure, stretching of visceral surfaces, tissue destruction, infection, and inflammation all can cause pain. Chronic pain may result from nerve damage secondary to surgery, chemotherapy, or radiation.

TABLE 12.5 FACTORS PREDISPOSING INDIVIDUALS WITH CANCER TO INFECTION

FACTOR	BASIS
Age	Many common malignancies occur mostly in older age. Immunologic functions decline with age. General debility reduces immunocompetence. Immobility predisposes to infection. Far-advanced cancer often results in immobility and general debility that worsen with age. Elderly persons are predisposed to nutritional inadequacies. Malnutrition impairs immunocompetence.
Tumor	Nutritional derangements can result. Sites and circumstances favorable to growth of microorganisms (obstruction, serous or blood effusion, ulceration) can be created. Far-advanced disease predisposes individuals to debility and immobility. Humoral or cellular immune defects may result. Metastasis to bone marrow may cause leukopenia or other defects in immunity.
Leukemias	Inadequate granulocyte production can occur (e.g., neutropenia, impaired phagocytosis). Thrombocytopenia (bleeding) can occur. Late effect: chronic lung disease from *Pneumocystis carinii* pneumonia can develop during therapy.
Lymphomas and other mononuclear phagocyte malignancies	Humoral and cellular immune defects (anergy, altered immunoglobulin production) result. Late effect: splenectomy in children can cause increased susceptibility to infection.
Surgical treatment	Invasive procedure interrupts first lines of defense. Radical nature of surgery (removal of large blocks of tissue in lengthy procedures) causes hemorrhage, decreased tissue perfusion, creation of dead spaces, and tissue necrosis. Procedure may be "dirty" surgery (bowel, infected, or contaminated areas). Surgery patients are often older and at poor risk. Long preoperative hospitalization often precedes surgery. Patients may have received previous adrenocorticosteroid therapy. Patients may have infections at sites remote from the operative area. Nutritional derangements (especially important in head and neck surgery) may result. Lymph node dissection may predispose patient to local infection and impair containment to area. Gynecologic surgery may result in fistulae. Lung surgery may cause bronchopleural fistulae. Debility and immobility may result.

Data from Donovan MI, Girton SF: *Cancer care nursing,* ed 2, New York, 1984, Appleton-Century-Crofts; Murphy GP et al: *Clinical oncology,* ed 2, New York, 1994, American Cancer Society.

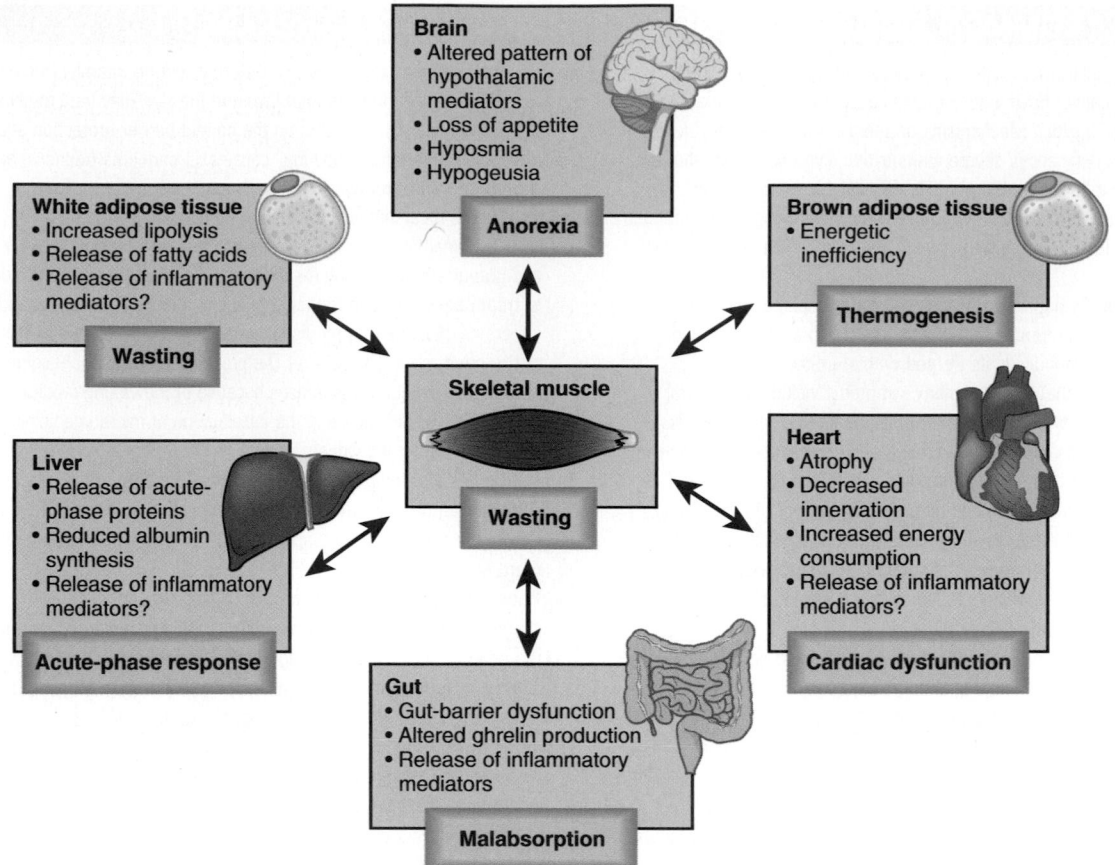

FIGURE 12.21 Cachexia: A Multiorgan Syndrome. Loss of skeletal muscle and adipose tissue are major contributors to cachexia. But many other organs have a role in the cachexia syndrome and the wasting that takes place in muscle may be dependent on alterations in these other organs or tissues. Changes in hypothalamic function and activation of brown adipose tissue, as well as alterations in liver and heart function, also are involved in the syndrome. Recent studies support a role for gut microbiota in cancer cachexia and the possibility of a gut–microbiota–skeletal muscle relationship. Recent data suggest that the conversion of white adipose tissue to brown adipose tissue is triggered by both humoral inflammatory mediators, such as interleukin-6 (IL-6), and tumor-derived compounds, such as parathyroid hormone–related protein (PTHRP). (From Bindels LB, Delzenne NM: *Int J Biochem Cell Biol* 45:2186–2190, 2013; Bindels LB et al: *PLoS One* 7[6]:e37971, 2012.)

TABLE 12.6	OBTAINING TISSUE—THE BIOPSY	
PROCEDURE	**PURPOSE**	**EXAMPLE**
Excisional biopsy	Complete removal, usually with a margin of normal tissue	Full resection (e.g., mastectomy, partial colectomy)
Incisional biopsy	Removal of a portion of a lesion	Lymph node biopsy, muscle mass biopsy
Core needle biopsy	Often performed with direct vision, or guided with ultrasound or computed tomography (CT)	Needle biopsy of prostate or liver mass
Fine-needle aspiration	Obtains dissociated cells for cytologic study but does not preserve tissue structure	Thyroid, breast mass
Exfoliative cytology	Cells shed from the surface, for example, from cervix, sputum (lung), or urine	Brushings from lung or colon endoscopy

DIAGNOSIS AND STAGING OF CANCER

Histologic Staging

Cancer can be discovered in many ways: after screening tests, from routine examinations, and after investigation of symptoms. The symptoms a cancer produces are as diverse as the types of cancer. The location of the cancer can determine symptoms by physical pressure, obstruction, and loss of normal function or a cancer can cause problems far away from its source by pressing on nerves or secreting bioactive compounds.

Whatever the initial complaint, once the diagnosis is suspected and a tumor has been identified, it is essential that tumor tissue be obtained to establish a definitive diagnosis and correctly classify the disease. Various methods of obtaining tissue are described in Table 12.6.

If the diagnosis of cancer is established, it is critical to determine if the cancer has spread, known as the stage of the cancer. Cancer staging initially involves determining the size of the tumor, the degree to which it has locally invaded, and the extent to which it has spread (metastasized) (Fig. 12.23). Specific molecular tests are increasingly used in staging as well. Diverse schemes are used for staging different tumors. In general, a four-stage system is used, with carcinoma in situ regarded as a special case. Cancer confined to the organ of origin is stage 1; cancer that is locally invasive is stage 2; cancer that has spread to regional structures, such as lymph nodes, is stage 3; and cancer that has spread to distant sites, such as a liver cancer spreading to lung or a prostate cancer spreading to bone, is stage 4. One common scheme for standardizing staging is the World Health Organization's TNM system: *T* indicates tumor spread, *N* indicates node involvement, and *M* indicates the presence of distant metastasis. The prognosis generally worsens with increasing tumor size, lymph node involvement, and metastasis. Staging also may alter the choice of therapy, with more aggressive therapy being delivered to more invasive disease.

Tumor Markers

During surveillance or diagnosis of cancer as well as following therapy, specific biochemical markers of tumors have proven to be helpful. These **tumor markers** are substances produced by both benign and malignant cells that are either present in or on tumor cells or found in blood, spinal fluid, or urine. Some tumor markers have been known for many decades. Tumor markers include hormones, enzymes, genes, antigens, and antibodies. If the tumor marker itself has biologic activity, then it can cause symptoms, such as those described in Table 12.7. For example, the adrenal medulla normally secretes the catecholamine epinephrine (adrenaline). Benign tumors of the adrenal medulla (pheochromocytoma) can produce catecholamines (e.g., adrenaline) in vast excess, leading to rapid pulse rate, high blood pressure, diaphoresis (i.e., sweating), and tremors. Detection of elevated blood or urine levels of catecholamines helps to confirm the diagnosis, and treatment of the disease relieves the symptoms. Tumor markers can be used in three ways: (1) to screen and identify individuals at high risk for cancer; (2) to help diagnose the specific type of tumor in individuals with clinical manifestations relating to their tumor, as in adrenal tumors or enlarged liver or prostate; and (3) to follow the clinical course of a tumor.

To date, no tumor marker has proven satisfactory to screen populations of healthy individuals for cancer. Testing large populations will always detect a few normal individuals with test results at the high end of the normal distribution (the "false positives"), which can lead to expensive and invasive additional tests, and unnecessary concern. Similarly, some individuals with disease will have test results in the

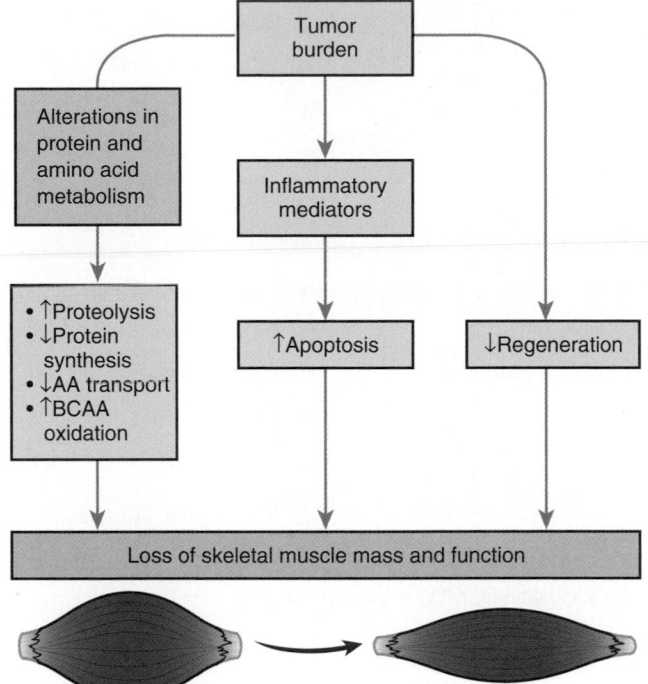

FIGURE 12.22 Wasting of Skeletal Muscle. Inflammation plays a major role in muscle wasting and is linked to alterations in protein and amino acid metabolism, activation of muscle cell apoptosis, and decreased regeneration. *AA*, amino acids; *BCAA*, branched-chain amino acids. (Adapted from Argilés JM et al: *Nat Rev Cancer* 14[11]:754–762, 2014.)

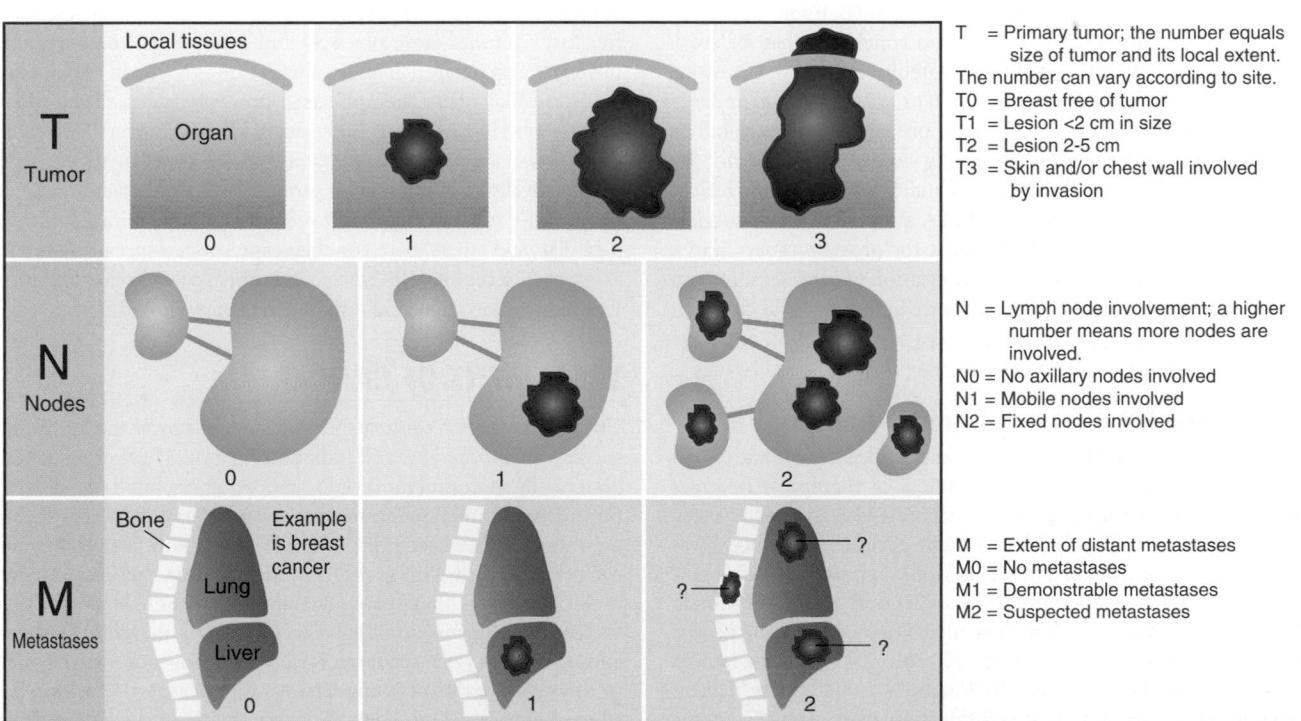

FIGURE 12.23 Tumor Staging by the TNM System. Example of staging for breast cancer.

TABLE 12.7 EXAMPLES OF TUMOR MARKERS IN BODY FLUIDS

MARKER NAME	NATURE	TYPE OF TUMOR
Adrenocorticotropic hormone (ACTH)	Peptide hormone	Pituitary adenomas
Alpha fetoprotein (AFP)	70-kDa protein	Hepatic, germ cell
Beta-2-microglobulin (β2M)	11-kDa protein	Multiple myeloma, CLL
Beta-human chorionic gonadotropin (β-hCG)	Glycopeptide hormone β-chain	Germ cell, choriocarcinoma
CA15-3/CA27-29	Large MW glycoproteins	Breast
CA-125	Large MW glycoprotein	Ovary
CA19-9	201-kDa glycoprotein	Pancreas, gallbladder, bile duct, gastric
Calcitonin	3.4-kDa polypeptide hormone	Thyroid
Carcinoembryonic antigen (CEA)	200-kDa glycoprotein	GI, pancreas, lung, breast, etc.
Catecholamines	Epinephrine and precursors	Pheochromocytoma (adrenal medulla)
CD20	33–36-kDa glycosylated phosphoprotein	Non-Hodgkin lymphoma
Chromogranin A (CgA)	48-kDa protein	Neuroendocrine
Homovanillic acid/vanillylmandelic acid (HVA/VMA)	Catecholamine metabolites	Neuroblastoma
Prostate-specific antigen (PSA)	33-kDa glycoprotein	Prostate
Urinary Bence-Jones protein	Ig light chain	Multiple myeloma

CLL, Chronic lymphocytic leukemia; *GI,* gastrointestinal; *Ig,* immunoglobulin; *kDa,* kilodalton(s); *MW,* molecular weight.

normal range ("false negatives"). More importantly, some nonmalignant conditions also can produce tumor markers. The presence of an elevated tumor marker therefore may suggest a specific diagnosis, but it is not used alone as a definitive diagnostic test. For instance, prostate tumors secrete *prostate specific antigen (PSA)* into the blood. However, enthusiasm has waned for routine testing for PSA levels. Most men (approximately 75%) with elevated levels of PSA do not have cancer upon biopsy.[21] A taskforce to study the use of PSA detection concluded that for every 1000 men (ages 55 to 69) screened repeatedly, only 0 to 1 prostate cancer-related deaths would be avoided, 100 to 120 men would undergo unnecessary biopsies with some complications, and 110 men would be diagnosed with prostate cancer (frequently slow growing and not life threatening) and 50 of these would have major complications related to treatment. However, falling levels of PSA after radiation or surgical therapy may indicate successful treatment for prostate cancer, and a later rise may indicate a recurrence. Identification of ideal sensitive and specific tumor markers that are elevated early in the course of common cancers remains a high priority because the early detection of cancer often improves the treatment outcome.

Immunohistochemical and Genetic Analysis

Because knowledge about the cellular and molecular alterations in individual cancers can influence the choices of therapy, it becomes increasingly important for clinicians to accurately classify each cancer. The classification, and hence the treatment decisions, of cancers was originally based on gross and light microscopic appearance, and is now commonly accompanied by immunohistochemical analysis of protein expression. Increasingly, this is supplemented by a more extensive genetic analysis of the tumors. The range of genetic analysis is expanding rapidly. A single gene may be examined (for example, to determine if there is a characteristic chromosomal translocation diagnostic of chronic myelogenous leukemia [CML]) or a panel of genes and proteins may be examined (e.g., in breast cancer) to determine if the tumor expresses estrogen receptor, progesterone receptor, and the epidermal growth factor (EGF) receptor HER2 or if there are mutations in specific genes that modify response to therapy. In a research setting and increasingly in clinical settings, global gene expression and mutation analysis can be measured using polymerase chain reaction (PCR), microarray, or advanced DNA sequencing technology. These analyses can be used to classify tumors more precisely and may predict the most effective therapy.[22] This detailed analysis of each tumor is a form of personalized medicine that offers therapy based on a very detailed knowledge of the characteristics of each individual's specific cancer. This enhanced molecular characterization subdivides cancers into therapeutically and prognostically relevant smaller groups. As an example, breast cancers can now be subclassified into over four types (luminal A, luminal B, basal-like, and others) based on their expression of specific markers, such as estrogen receptor, HER2/Neu, and other specific genes and proteins. Each subtype has a different response to therapy and a different prognosis.

TREATMENT OF CANCER

Until late in the last century the mainstays of cancer therapy have been surgery, chemotherapy, and radiation therapy. These approaches have been highly successful for certain types of cancer, but have many limitations. Immunotherapy has been the Holy Grail of cancer therapists, but successes have been few. Cancer therapy is now in a process of rapid evolution. Armed with a clearer understanding that cancer is in fact multiple diseases that share general hallmarks/enablers and that the specific mechanisms underlying each hallmark may vary considerably among cancers (e.g., the large variety of oncogenes that may be used to differentiate cancers), modern cancer therapy is reaching a stage where complete genetic analysis of an individual cancer may determine the appropriate combination of therapies. Thus effective therapy may include a combination of reagents targeting several hallmarks and under constant modification to target the evolving cancer cells.

Classic Approaches
Surgery

Surgery plays many roles in the care of individuals with cancer. The multiple approaches to obtaining tissue for diagnosis have been discussed. Surgery is often the definitive treatment of cancers that do not spread beyond the limits of surgical excision. If melanoma can be diagnosed when localized to the skin, surgical removal can result in a cure rate of 98%.[23] Cancers detected early in the prostate, testis, or thyroid have cure rates of 99%, 95%, and 98%, respectively.

Surgery also is indicated for the relief of symptoms, for instance, those caused by tumor mass obstruction. In selected high-risk diseases, surgery plays a role in the prevention of cancer. For example, individuals with familial adenomatous polyposis because of germline mutations of the *APC* gene have close to a 100% lifetime risk of colon cancer, so a prophylactic colectomy is indicated. Similarly, women with *BRCA1/2* mutations have a markedly increased risk of breast and ovarian cancer, and often choose prophylactic mastectomy or bilateral salpingo-oophorectomy (removal of ovaries and fallopian tubes), or both.

Key principles apply specifically to cancer surgery, including obtaining adequate surgical margins during a resection to prevent local recurrences and obtaining adequate tissue specimens during biopsies so that the pathologist can be confident of the diagnosis. Additionally, the surgeon provides critical staging information by inspection, sampling, and removal of local and regional lymph nodes during procedures.

Radiation Therapy

Radiation therapy is used to kill cancer cells while minimizing damage to normal structures. Ionizing radiation damages cells by imparting enough energy to cause molecular damage, especially to DNA. The damage may be lethal, in which the cell is killed by radiation; potentially lethal, in which the cell is so severely affected by radiation that modifications in its environment will cause it to die; or sublethal, in which the cell can subsequently repair itself. Areas with rapidly renewing cells are more radiosensitive. Effective cell killing by radiation also requires good local delivery of oxygen, something not always present in large cancers. Radiation produces slow changes in most cancers and irreversible changes in normal tissues as well. Because of these irreversible changes, each tissue has a maximum lifetime dose of radiation it can tolerate. Radiation is well suited to treat localized disease in areas that are hard to reach surgically, for example, in the brain and pelvis. A number of radiation delivery methods are available, with external beam being the most common. Radiation sources, such as small ^{125}I-labeled capsules (also called *seeds*), can also be temporarily placed into body cavities, a delivery method termed brachytherapy. Brachytherapy is useful in the treatment of cervical, prostate, and head and neck cancers.

Chemotherapy

The era of modern chemotherapy began with the observation in World War II that mustard gas exposure caused suppression of the bone marrow. Related compounds, such as nitrogen mustard and cyclophosphamide, were then tested and produced clinical responses in hematologic malignancies, including lymphomas. Also in the late 1940s, based on the remarkable clinical observation that the vitamin folic acid could *increase* leukemia growth, antifolate drugs were developed (leading ultimately to methotrexate) that produced remissions in previously untreatable leukemia.

All chemotherapeutic agents attack pathways that exist in rapidly dividing normal cells, but cancer cells utilize more and are severely affected. Antimetabolites, such as methotrexate and L-asparaginase, block normal growth pathways in all cells, but leukemia and other cancer cells are exquisitely sensitive to folic acid and asparagine deprivation, whereas nonmalignant cells are far less sensitive. Similarly, some cancer cells are highly sensitive to DNA-damaging agents, such as cyclophosphamide and anthracyclines, because of the oncogenic mutations that accelerate the cell cycle and DNA synthesis. Cellular checkpoints prevent normal cells treated with microtubule-directed drugs, such as vincristine and the taxanes, from undergoing mitosis, whereas cancer cells treated with these agents lack normal checkpoints, continue through mitosis, and undergo mitotic catastrophe.

Single chemotherapeutic agents often shrink cancers, but these drugs given alone rarely, if ever, provide a cure. Hence, chemotherapy drugs are usually given in combinations designed to attack a cancer from many different weaknesses at the same time and to limit the dose and therefore the toxicity of any single agent. Cancers contain a very large number of cells, and commonly a small fraction of those cells may be resistant to a particular drug. However, those cells are likely to be sensitive to the second or third drug in a chemotherapy cocktail. Scheduling of drug administration is also very important, with many studies showing cancers are more likely to develop drug resistance if there are significant delays between planned courses of chemotherapy.

Induction chemotherapy seeks to cause shrinkage or disappearance of tumors, but success depends greatly on the type of tumor, the stage, and the individual's age at diagnosis. In Hodgkin lymphoma, for example, chemotherapy alone can be used in some cases to cure the disease. If used as part of a drug cocktail, treated individuals have a 5-year cure rate of 86%.[23] In other settings, chemotherapy may shrink the tumor and improve symptoms without ultimately providing a cure. Adjuvant chemotherapy is given after surgical excision of a cancer with the goal of eliminating micrometastases. Neoadjuvant chemotherapy is given before localized (surgical or radiation) treatment of a cancer. As with induction chemotherapy, the effectiveness of neoadjuvant therapy can be determined by measuring the size of the tumor. Neoadjuvant therapy can shrink a cancer so that surgery may spare more normal tissue. For example, in the bone cancer osteogenic sarcoma, neoadjuvant therapy often converts a large tumor mass into a much smaller mass, allowing the surgeon to perform a limb-sparing excision rather than an amputation.

Some leukemia is very effectively treated with chemotherapy. Acute lymphoblastic leukemia (ALL) is most common in children and adolescents. Primarily using chemotherapy, the 5-year cure rate is about 90%.[23] Acute myelogenous leukemia (AML) and chronic lymphoblastic leukemia (CLL) occur in children, but more often in adults. Chemotherapy of AML may lead to 5-year cure rates of 65%, but it is not as effective in adults (about 40% in adults younger than 60 years, but only about 10% in adults older than 60 years). CLL occurs more in the elderly (median age of 71 at diagnosis), and chemotherapy results in a 82% 5-year cure rate.[23]

A major complication of chemotherapy is death of rapidly dividing cells that are not cancer, such as those of the bone marrow. Hematopoietic growth factors also have been used to counter the effects of chemotherapy on bone marrow cells, for example, erythropoietin to increase numbers of red blood cells, IL-11 to increase platelet levels, and colony-stimulating factors to increase granulocytes (G-CSF) or both granulocytes and monocytes (GM-CSF).

Immunotherapy

The expression of unique antigens on cancer cells that can be targeted by T cells has driven the quest for effective therapies to initiate an immune response, boost a currently inadequate immune response, or convert a tumor-protective immune response to a destructive one.[24] Since the 1950s this quest has been characterized by promises and frustrations.

Tumor cell vaccines were one of the first attempts at immunotherapy for cancer. Vaccines have been extremely effective in protecting individuals against infective agents. Killed whole tumor cell vaccines prepared from an individual's own cancer (autologous) or from cancers from other individuals (allogeneic) were attempted. Several allogeneic cancer cell vaccines using protein extracts or peptides continue to be tested, but so far none have been shown to be effective enough to be licensed.[25]

WHAT'S NEW?

Engineering T Cells for Better Anticancer Killing

The specificity and function of T-cytotoxic cells (Tc cells) is controlled by three signals: (1) the T-cell receptor (TCR) that binds antigen and is associated with a complex of transmembrane signaling molecules (CD3) (see Chapter 7); (2) the transmembrane co-receptor CD8 that binds to class I major histocompatibility complex (MHC) that is presenting antigen, resulting in proximity of CD3 with the intracellular portion of CD8 leading to activation of a signaling molecule; and (3) transmembrane accessory molecules, such as CD28, that bind to ligands on the target cell surface and provide an additional activation signal (Fig. A). Cancers have developed multiple mechanisms for escaping the cytotoxic effects of Tc cells, among which are suppression of antigen presentation, reduction of CD3 expression, and inhibition of the CD28 signal by expression of soluble CTLA-4, which competes for binding to the CD28 ligand. Thus recognition of cancer-associated antigens by the Tc cell may be completely suppressed.

A variety of approaches have been designed to bypass suppression of the TCR. Initial attempts included cloning Tc cells expressing high-affinity TCRs for tumor antigen. However, suppression of antigen presentation by the tumor prevented recognition by these Tc cells. This has led to a unique approach of engineering T cells with chimeric antigen receptors (CAR T cells). Early success with these novel cells has led to further sophisticated approaches to constructing more complex CARs.

The process involves collection of circulating white blood cells from the blood of an individual with cancer using leukapheresis. The lymphocytes are enriched, induced to proliferate, and transfected by a virus containing the genetically engineered CAR. The CAR T cells are cloned in bulk, verified for expression of the CAR, and cryopreserved. When used, the cells are thawed and infused into the individual with cancer.

The CAR receptors are V_H and V_L regions cloned from monoclonal antibodies and inserted in tandem into the *CAR* gene. Because tumors suppress MHC presented antigen, the CAR receptors are designed against other surface molecules that do not require presentation. The *CAR* gene also contains information for hydrophobic transmembrane regions, followed by genetic information for costimulatory signals. Initially the costimulatory signals included the cytoplasmic portions of CD28 and CD3, but more recently developed CARs include multiple costimulatory signaling peptides. Thus binding of the receptor to a cancer-related molecule activates linked intracellular signaling peptides, such as CD3, CD28, and others, contained sequentially in the *CAR* gene.

Targets for CAR T cells have included CD19, CD20, and CD22 on hematologic cancers and HER2, EGFR, and others on solid tumors. The most notable success has been treatment of CD19-positive B-cell malignancies. CD19 is expressed on cancer cells at a very high level related to normal B cells. Infusion of CAR T cells has led to remissions of greater than 80% of people with ALL and about 50% of those with CLL. Success against solid tumors has been less spectacular.

The next generation of CAR T cells is in development. These include the addition of more costimulatory signals, simultaneous expression of two CAR molecules on the T cell (both targeted to the same cancer-related molecule, but one CAR providing a strong TCR-like signal and the second providing a costimulatory signal), CARs directed to apoptosis-inducing molecules or cytokine receptors, and the use of engineered allogeneic T cells. The use of allogeneic T cells would accelerate treatment by circumventing the current 2- to 3-week process of preparing CAR T cells from the individual's own cells.

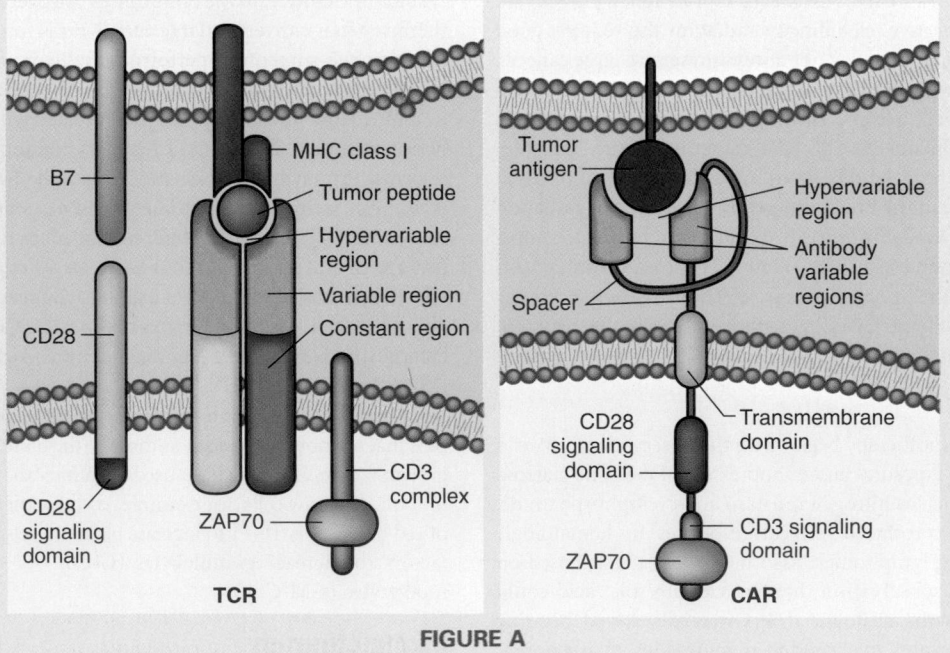

FIGURE A

ALL, acute lymphocytic leukemia; *CLL,* chronic lymphocytic leukemia.
Data from Fesnak AD, June CH, Levine BL: *Nat Rev Cancer* 16(9):566–581, 2016; Lim WA, June CH: *Cell* 168(4):724–740, 2017; Sadelain M: *Curr Opin Immunol* 41:68–76, 2016.

One innovative approach using sipuleucel-T has been approved by the Food and Drug Administration (FDA) for the treatment of metastatic prostate cancer that is resistant to conventional therapy. One therapy is sipuleucel-T using dendritic cells obtained from an individual with prostate cancer and incubated with a protein resulting from the fusion of prostatic acid phosphatase (a cancer antigen found in 95% of prostate cancers) and granulocyte-macrophage colony–stimulating factor (GM-CSF, an immune cell–stimulating cytokine). The dendritic cells process and present the antigen and are infused back into the individual. In clinical trials, treatment with sipuleucel-T extended the lives of individuals by 4.1 months. These results may not seem spectacular, but were meaningful in this group with very advanced and terminal disease. Other similar vaccine approaches against B-cell lymphoma and melanoma have shown promising results.

Passive immunotherapy using lymphocytes against cancer cell antigens has been attempted, with limited success, since the early 1970s. In recent years, passive administration of tumor-targeting lymphocytes (adoptive cell therapy, ACT) treated ex vivo with cytokines seems promising. The use of cytokines or adoptive cell therapy assumes the individual with cancer has remaining cancer-specific Tc cells and NK, which may not be true. Cytokines have been injected into individuals with cancer to enhance T-cell function. The cytokines IL-2 and Interferon-alfa (trade name for interferon-alpha, IFN-α) increase proliferation and cytotoxic activity of Tc and NK cells and have been approved by the FDA to treat metastatic kidney cancer and melanoma. Lymphocytes that have infiltrated the tumor (TILs) are more likely to contain active tumor-specific Tc and NK cells. TILs can be obtained from excised tumor tissue and further activated in the laboratory. Treatment of TILs with IL-2 before reinjection has been successful in some individuals. This approach is being improved by engineering T-cell receptors (TCRs) to increase the effectiveness of cancer-specific killing (see *What's New? Engineering T Cells for Better Anticancer Killing*).

A family of monoclonal antibodies are currently approved for use against cancer. One group is designed to directly bind to and damage cancer cells. Dinutuximab is a monoclonal antibody against ganglioside GD2. It reacts with CD2-expressing tumor cells, such as malignant melanoma, neuroblastoma, osteosarcoma, and small cell carcinomas of the lung, and induces complement-mediated cytotoxicity or provides a site for NK cells and others with Fc receptors to bind and initiate antibody-dependent cellular cytotoxicity (ADCC) (see Chapter 7). Bispecific monoclonal antibodies have been created that, unlike other antibodies, are engineered to express two different antigen binding sites on the same molecule. One example is an antibody in which one binding site is specific for CD19 and the other is against CD3; thus the antibody bridges CD19-positive ALL cells and CD3-positive T cells, facilitating T-cell killing of these leukemia cells.

A group of highly effective monoclonal antibodies are called **immune checkpoint inhibitors**. Immune checkpoints are where signals from costimulatory molecules may suppress or allow T-cell–mediated cytotoxicity, thus protecting normal cells. These antibodies are directed against the costimulatory molecules involved in repressing T-cell immune responses (see Chapter 8). Ipilimumab was the first immune checkpoint inhibitor approved by the FDA for treatment of advanced melanoma. This monoclonal antibody blocks the costimulatory molecule cytotoxic T-lymphocyte–associated protein-4 (CTLA-4) on the surface of Tc cells so they retain tumor-killing capacity. Two other approved drugs block protein cell death protein-1 (PD-1) on the surface of Tc cells (nivolumab) and the respective ligand (PD-L1 and PD-L2) on the surface of tumor cells (pembrolizumab). These have been approved for treatment of advanced melanoma, urothelial carcinoma, non–small cell lung cancer, and renal cell carcinoma.

TARGETED DISRUPTION OF CANCER

As discussed previously, cancers appear to share a variety of hallmarks that contribute to the malignant phenotype. Recent molecular and genetic analyses of groups of cancer can classify an individual's cancer by the spectrum of mutations underlying the cancer phenotype. Targeted cancer therapy is designed to address unique growth characteristics of a specific class of tumor and directly interfere with that process. Tumor growth and progression are dependent on a variety of mutations leading to expression of oncogenes, inactivation of tumor-suppressor molecules, and interactions with inflammatory cells in the tumor microenvironment that foster angiogenesis, resistance to apoptosis and immune-mediated cancer cell death, altered tumor cell metabolism, and metastasis. A more efficacious therapeutic approach, therefore, may be a combination of drugs highly targeted to cancer hallmarks.[26] More than 25 drugs are listed at the National Cancer Institute as cancer-targeting agents that inactivate oncogenes, block angiogenesis, and affect cancer cell metabolism. For instance, imatinib mesylate is a competitive inhibitor of tyrosine kinases, primarily the BCR-ABL tyrosine kinase. It is highly effective in treating CML and ALL that expresses the Philadelphia chromosome but ineffective in virtually all other cancers.

Some monoclonal antibodies have been effective in delivering targeted cancer therapy. Monoclonal antibodies against the CD20 antigen (rituximab) expressed on some non-Hodgkin lymphomas and those against CD52 (alemtuzumab) on CLL can induce apoptosis of the cancer cell. Monoclonal antibodies against the epidermal growth factor (EGF) receptor on colon cancers and head and neck cancers and also the HER2 EGF receptor on breast cancer have been relatively successful. Bevacizumab inhibits tumor angiogenesis by targeting the interaction between VEGF secreted by tumor cells and the VEGF receptor.

Monoclonal antibodies also have been used as targeted carriers (immunoconjugates) of radioactive molecules or toxins. Examples include ^{90}Y-ibritumomab, a monoclonal antibody that targets CD20 on non-Hodgkin lymphoma cells to deliver yttrium-90; and ado-trastuzumab emtansine that delivers the drug DM1 (inhibits cell proliferation) to HER2-positive breast cancer cells. These drugs are so tightly targeted they have much less toxicity than conventional chemotherapies that have targets in virtually all cells.

SUMMARY REVIEW

Cancer Terminology and Characteristics

1. Benign tumors are usually encapsulated and contain fairly well-differentiated cells and well-organized stroma, and they do not spread to distant locations.
2. Malignant tumors, compared with benign tumors, have more rapid growth rates, specific microscopic alterations (anaplasia, loss of differentiation), absence of normal tissue organization, and no capsule.

They invade blood vessels and lymphatics and have distant metastases.
3. Carcinomas arise from epithelial tissue, and leukemias are cancers of blood-forming cells. Carcinoma in situ (CIS) refers to preinvasive epithelial tumors of glandular or squamous cell origin. These early-stage cancers are localized to the epithelium and have not penetrated the local basement membrane or invaded the surrounding stroma.

▌S U M M A R Y   R E V I E W—cont'd

The Biology of Cancer Cells

1. Genetic changes are the basis of cancer. These changes include small and large DNA mutations that alter genes, chromosomes, and non–coding RNAs, as well as epigenetic changes because of altered chemical modifications of DNA and histones.

2. Mutations include point mutations that alter a few nucleotide base pairs, which has a profound effect on the activity of resultant proteins. Other genetic alterations include chromosome translocations, gene amplification, DNA methylation, histone acetylation, or altered expression of non–coding RNA.

3. Some mutations, referred to as driver mutations, drive the progression of cancer and some are just random events, referred to as passenger mutations, and are just along for the ride.

4. Each cancer cell may develop its own set of mutations resulting in a genomically heterogenous mixture of cancer cells with subsets that have accumulated more and more mutations increasing the cell's malignant potential.

5. The processes occurring during the development of cancer are in many ways analogous to wound healing. The initial proliferation of cancer cells and enlargement of the tumor elicit the synthesis of proinflammatory mediators by the cancer cells and adjacent nonmalignant cells.

6. As with wound healing, mediators recruit inflammatory/immune cells and cells normally associated with tissue repair. These cells form the stroma that surrounds and infiltrates the tumor.

7. Extensive paracrine signaling among the stromal and cancer cells affects both populations; cancer cells increase proliferation and become more heterogenous during tumor growth and stromal cells undergo evolution to phenotypes that promote cancer progression and metastatic potential.

8. Cancer heterogeneity arises from ongoing proliferation and mutation.

9. Many of the hallmarks of cancer are consequences of cancer-stromal interactions.

10. Several of the hallmarks/enablers are mostly genomic alterations that initiate and maintain development of cancer. These hallmarks include sustained proliferative signaling, evading growth suppression, genomic instability, and replicative immortality.

11. Other hallmarks/enablers are cellular adaptations secondary to genomic change and include inducing angiogenesis and reprogramming energy metabolism. A third group of hallmarks/enablers are the host's protective mechanisms including apoptotic cell death, promoting tumor inflammation, and avoiding immune destruction. The last hallmark is the culmination of the previous nine: activating invasion and metastasis.

12. Cancerous cells characteristically express mutated or overexpressed proto-oncogenes, referred to as oncogenes, which are independent of normal regulatory mechanisms and signal uncontrolled proliferation.

13. Some oncogenes, such as *RAS*, result from point mutations.

14. Oncogenes can result from genetic translocations. The Philadelphia chromosome in chronic myeloid leukemia (CML) results from a translocation that creates a novel protein fusion of the *BCR* and *ABL* genes and expression of an unregulated promoter of cell growth.

15. Tumor-suppressor genes must be inactivated in cancer cells by mutations to each allele, one from each parent.

16. A common mutation in cancer cells is inactivation of the tumor-suppressor gene tumor protein p53 (TP53), which controls expression of many genes that repair DNA damage, suppression of cellular proliferation during genomic repair, and initiation of apoptosis. Inactivation of p53 results in increased mutation rates and cancer.

17. In rare families, an initial inheritable mutation in a tumor-suppressor gene, such as TP53, the retinoblastoma gene *(RB)*, or the breast cancer genes *(BRCA1* and *BRCA2)*, may lead to a greatly increased risk for developing particular cancers.

18. Caretaker genes are responsible for maintaining genomic integrity. Inherited mutations can disrupt caretaker genes and cause genomic instability.

19. Abnormal gene silencing is emerging as a major factor in cancer progression. Gene expression can be regulated in a heritable manner (i.e., passed from a parent to a child or from a single cell to its progeny) by an "epigenetic" mechanism called silencing.

20. Changes in gene regulation can affect not just single genes, but entire networks of signaling. Gene expression networks can be regulated by changes in microRNAs (miRNAs or miRs) and other non–coding RNAs (ncRNAs).

21. Cancer cells are immortal.

22. When they reach a critical age, cancer cells activate telomerase to restore and maintain their telomeres, thereby allowing cancer cells to divide repeatedly or become immortal.

23. Like many normal adult tissues, cancers can contain rare stem cells that provide a source of immortal cells. To fully eradicate a cancer, it may be necessary to target the cancer stem cell.

24. Most of the genetic and epigenetic alterations that cause cancer occur within the somatic tissues during the lifetime of the individual.

25. Access to the vascular system is essential for tumor growth.

26. Stromal cells and cancer cells can secrete multiple factors, such as vascular endothelial growth factor (VEGF), that stimulate new blood vessel growth (called neovascularization or angiogenesis).

27. The successful cancer cell divides rapidly, with the consequent requirement for the building blocks of new cells; cancer cell division often occurs in a hypoxic and acidic environment. Many cancer genes also encourage aerobic glycolysis and promote high glucose utilization of a cancer.

29. In cancer, defects in the intrinsic or extrinsic pathways, or both, provide resistance to apoptotic cell death.

30. Overexpression of BCL-2 blocks apoptosis in most follicular B-cell lymphomas.

31. Some conditions of chronic inflammation increase the risk of developing cancer. A prime example is the association between gastric cancer and infection with *Helicobacter pylori*. Additionally, some organs appear to be more susceptible to the oncogenic effects of chronic inflammation.

32. One of the key cells that promote tumor survival is the tumor-associated macrophage, or TAM. The classic proinflammatory macrophage (M1) is the primary macrophage in the acute inflammatory response. During tissue healing, the M2 macrophage phenotype produces antiinflammatory mediators to suppress ongoing inflammation and induce cellular proliferation, angiogenesis, and wound healing. TAMs appear to mimic the M2 phenotype.

33. Cancer-associated fibroblasts (CAFs) synthesize the extracellular matrix that surrounds and permeates the tumor. Molecules secreted by CAFs contribute greatly to cancer progression, local spread, and metastasis.

34. The most clearly documented effective immune response is prophylactic and directed against oncogenic viruses. Viruses are

∎ SUMMARY REVIEW—cont'd

associated with about 15% of all human cancers worldwide. Cancer of the cervix and hepatocellular carcinoma account for approximately 80% of virus-linked cancer cases.

35. Antibodies induced by vaccines against oncogenic viruses, such as human papillomavirus (HPV) and hepatitis B virus (HBV), are expected to protect against initial infection and development of cervical and liver tumors, respectively.

36. Unique antigens and other markers on tumor cells can be recognized by T cells and NK cells of the immune system, leading to destruction of the tumor cell.

37. Cancer cells can evade rejection by the immune system by production of immunosuppressive factors, induction of immunosuppressive T-regulator cells, evolution of tumor-antigen negative variants, or suppressed expression of antigen-presenting MHC class I molecules.

38. Metastasis is the major cause of death from cancer.

39. Metastasis is a complex process that requires cells to have many new abilities, including the ability to invade, survive, and proliferate in a new environment.

40. Invasion consists of loss of cell-to-cell contact, degradation of the extracellular matrix (ECM), and migration of tumor cells to the vascular or lymphatic systems. Stromal cells, particularly TAMs, are essential to this process.

41. Carcinomas undergo a process of epithelial-mesenchymal transition (EMT) during which many epithelial-like characteristics are lost (e.g., polarity, adhesion to basement membrane), resulting in increased migratory capacity, increased resistance to apoptosis, and a dedifferentiated stem cell–like state that favors growth in foreign microenvironments and establishment of metastatic disease.

42. Some cancers appear to selectively move or home to particular metastatic sites, which may be a result of expression of particular receptors for ligands expressed by cells at the site.

Clinical Manifestations of Cancer

1. Paraneoplastic syndromes are rare symptom complexes, often caused by biologically active substances released from a tumor or by an immune response triggered by a tumor, that manifest as symptoms not directly caused by the local effects of the cancer.

2. Clinical manifestations of cancer include pain, cachexia, anemia, leukopenia, thrombocytopenia, and infection.

3. Pain is generally associated with the late stages of cancer. It can be caused by pressure, obstruction, invasion of a structure sensitive to pain, stretching, tissue destruction, and inflammation.

4. Fatigue is the most frequently reported symptom of cancer and cancer treatment.

5. Cachexia is a multiorgan syndrome with many clinical manifestations including anorexia; muscle wasting; thermogenesis; altered heart and liver function; gut malabsorption; early satiety; taste alterations; and altered protein, lipid, and carbohydrate metabolism. Two factors are most significant: muscle loss and inflammation. Muscle wasting involves many protein signaling pathways and inflammatory mediators. Profoundly altered are both appetite-stimulating and appetite-suppressing brain pathways.

6. Anemia associated with cancer usually occurs because of malnutrition, chronic bleeding and resultant iron deficiency, chemotherapy, radiation, and malignancies in the blood-forming organs.

7. Leukopenia is usually a result of chemotherapy (which is toxic to bone marrow) or radiation (which kills circulating leukocytes).

8. Thrombocytopenia is usually the result of chemotherapy or malignancy in the bone marrow.

9. Infection may be caused by leukopenia, immunosuppression, or debility associated with advanced disease. It is the most significant cause of complications and death.

10. The gastrointestinal tract relies on rapidly growing cells to provide an absorptive surface for nutrients. Both chemotherapy and radiation therapy may cause decreased cell turnover, thereby leading to oral ulcers (stomatitis), malabsorption, and diarrhea.

11. Alopecia (hair loss) results from chemotherapy effects on hair follicles. Alopecia is usually temporary, although hair may initially regrow with a different texture. Not all chemotherapeutic agents cause alopecia. Decreased renewal rates of the epidermal layers in the skin may lead to skin breakdown and dryness, altering the normal barrier protection against infection.

Diagnosis, Characterization, and Treatment of Cancer

1. The diagnosis of cancer requires examination of tumor tissue by a pathologist. Cancer classification is established by a variety of tests.

2. Tumor staging involves the size of the tumor, the degree to which it has locally invaded, and the extent to which it has spread. A standard scheme for staging is the T (tumor spread), N (node involvement), and M (metastasis) system.

3. The classification, and hence the treatment decisions, of cancers was originally based on gross and light microscopic appearance, and is now commonly accompanied by immunohistochemical analysis of protein expression. Increasingly, this is supplemented by a more extensive molecular analysis of the tumors.

4. Tumor markers are substances (i.e., hormones, enzymes, genes, antigens, antibodies) found in cancer cells and in blood, spinal fluid, or urine. They are used to screen and identify individuals at high risk for cancer, to help diagnose specific types of tumors, and to follow the clinical course of cancer.

5. Cancer therapy is now in a process of rapid evolution. Although cancer is treated routinely with surgery, radiation therapy, chemotherapy, and combinations of these modalities, they have many limitations.

6. Surgical therapy is used for nonmetastatic disease and as a palliative measure to alleviate symptoms.

7. Ionizing radiation causes cell damage; therefore the goal of radiation therapy is to damage the tumor without causing excessive toxicity or damage to nondiseased structures.

8. The theoretic basis of chemotherapy is the vulnerability of tumor cells in various stages of the cell cycle.

9. Modern chemotherapy uses combinations of drugs with different targets and different toxicities.

10. Immunotherapy attempts to modify the immune system from a cancer-protective state to a destructive condition.

11. Future treatment of tumors will, most likely, use a careful histologic and genetic analysis of individual cancers that prescribes a combination of tumor-targeting drugs to simultaneously disrupt multiple hallmarks of that particular cancer.

12. Prevention of cancer has become increasingly urgent with researchers studying lifestyle changes to lower the risks of cancers including diet, exercise, cessation of smoking, air pollution, occupational hazards, synthetic chemicals, sunlight and ionizing radiation, and many other factors. These factors are discussed in Chapter 13.

KEY TERMS

Adenocarcinoma, 347
Adjuvant chemotherapy, 373
Aerobic glycolysis, 359
Anaplasia, 347
Angiogenesis, 358
Angiogenic factor, 358
Angiogenic inhibitor, 358
Anoikis, 366
Anorexigenic brain pathway, 368
Apoptosis, 360
Autocrine stimulation, 353
Benign tumor, 347
Brachytherapy, 373
Cachexia, 367
Cancer, 347
Cancer-associated fibroblast (CAF), 359
Cancer heterogeneity, 351
Cancer staging, 370
Carcinoma, 347
Carcinoma in situ (CIS), 348
Caretaker gene, 355
Cellular dormancy, 366
Chromosome instability, 357
Chromosome translocation, 349
Clonal expansion, 350
Clonal proliferation, 350
DNA methylation, 349
Driver mutations, 349
E-cadherin, 366
Epigenetic, 349

Epigenetic silencing, 355
Epithelial-mesenchymal transition (EMT), 364
Gene amplification, 349
Genomic instability, 355
Human epidermal growth factor receptor 2 (HER2), 353
Human T-cell lymphotropic virus type 1 (HTLV-1), 363
Hypoxia-inducible factor-1α (HIF-1α), 358
Immortal, 358
Immune checkpoint inhibitor, 375
Immune surveillance hypothesis, 363
Immunotherapy, 363
Induction chemotherapy, 373
Leukemia, 348
Lymphoma, 348
Malignant transformation, 350
Malignant tumor, 347
Mammary adenocarcinoma, 347
Matrix metalloproteinase (MMP), 358
Metastasis, 347
MicroRNA (miRNA, miR), 355
Mitogen-activated protein kinase pathway (MAPK pathway), 351
MYC protein, 354
Neoadjuvant chemotherapy, 373
Neoplasm, 346
Neovascularization, 358
Non–coding RNA, 349
Oncogene, 353

Oncomir, 357
Orexigenic brain pathway, 368
p53 tumor-suppressor gene (TP53), 355
Paraneoplastic syndrome, 366
Passenger mutations, 350
Personalized medicine, 372
Philadelphia chromosome, 354
Phosphatidylinosityl-3-kinase pathway (PI3K pathway), 351
Pleomorphic, 347
Point mutation, 349
Proto-oncogene, 353
RAS, 351
Receptor tyrosine kinase, 353
Retinoblastoma (RB) gene, 354
Reverse Warburg effect, 359
Sarcoma, 347
Stage of the cancer, 370
Stroma, 351
Telomerase, 358
Telomere, 358
Thrombospondin-1 (TSP-1), 358
Tumor, 346
Tumor-associated antigen, 363
Tumor-associated macrophage (TAM), 362
Tumor-infiltrating lymphocyte (TIL), 363
Tumor marker, 371
Tumor-suppressor gene, 354
Warburg effect, 359
White adipose tissue (WAT), 367

REFERENCES

1. National Cancer Institute (NCI): *Fact sheet: what is cancer?* 2015. Available at: http://www.cancer.gov/about-cancer/understanding/what-is-cancer.
2. Hanahan D, Weinberg RA: Hallmarks of cancer. *Cell* 100(1):57–70, 2000.
3. Hanahan D, Weinberg RA: Hallmarks of cancer: the next generation. *Cell* 144(5):646–674, 2011.
4. Bradner JE, Hnisz D, Young RA: Transcriptional addition in cancer. *Cell* 168(4):629–643, 2017.
5. McGranahan N, Swanton C: Clonal heterogeneity and tumor evolution: past, present, and the future. *Cell* 168(4):613–628, 2017.
6. Hanahan D, Coussens LM: Accessories to the crime: functions of cells recruited to the tumor microenvironment. *Cancer Cell* 21(3):309–322, 2012.
7. Hsu JL, Hung M-C: The role of HER2, EGFR, and other receptor tyrosine kinases in breast cancer. *Cancer Metastasis Rev* 35(4):575–588, 2016.
8. Tubbs A, Nussenzweig A: Endogenous DNA damage as a source of genomic instability in cancer. *Cell* 168(4):644–656, 2017.
9. Nielsen FC, van Overeem Hansen T, Sørensen CS: Hereditary breast and ovarian cancer: new genes in confined pathways. *Nat Rev Cancer* 16(9):599–612, 2016.
10. National Cancer Institute (NCI): *Fact sheet: BRCA1 and BRCA2: cancer risk and genetic testing*, 2015. Available at: http://www.cancer.gov/about-cancer/causes-prevention/genetics/brca-fact-sheet.
11. Lucey BP, et al: HeLa cells, and cell culture contamination. *Arch Pathol Lab Med* 133(9):1463–1467, 2009.
12. Arndt GM, MacKenzie KL: New prospects for targeting telomerase beyond the telomere. *Nat Rev Cancer* 16(8):508–524, 2016.
13. Nakazawa MS, Keith B, Simon MC: Oxygen availability and metabolic adaptations. *Nat Rev Cancer* 16(10):663–673, 2016.
14. Jackson HW, et al: TIMPs: versatile extracellular regulators in cancer. *Nat Rev Cancer* 17(1):38–53, 2017.
15. Vander Heiden MG, DeBerardinis RJ: Understanding the intersections between metabolism and cancer biology. *Cell* 168(4):657–669, 2017.
16. Kalluri R: The biology and function of fibroblasts in cancer. *Nat Rev Cancer* 16(9):583–598, 2016.
17. Smith AJ, Smith LA: Viral carcinogenesis. *Prog Mol Biol Transl Sci* 144:121–168, 2016. doi:101016/bs.pmbts.2016.09.007.
18. Munn DH, Bronte V: Immune suppressive mechanisms in the tumor microenvironment. *Curr Opin Immunol* 39(1):1–6, 2016.
19. Lambert AW, Pattabiraman DR, Weinberg RA: Emerging biological principles of metastasis. *Cell* 168(4):870–891, 2017.
20. Fidler IJ, et al: The biology of melanoma brain metastasis. *Cancer Metastasis Rev* 18(3):387–400, 1999.
21. National Cancer Institute (NCI): *Fact sheet: prostate-specific antigen (PSA) test*, 2012. Available at: www.cancer.gov/types/prostate/psa-fact-sheet.
22. Hyman DM, Taylor BS, Baselga J: Implementing genome-driven oncology. *Cell* 168(4):584–599, 2017.
23. Miller KD, et al: Cancer treatment and survivorship: statistics, 2016. *CA Cancer J Clin* 66(4):271–289, 2016.
24. Schumacher TN, Hacohen N: Neoantigens encoded in the cancer genome. *Curr Opin Immunol* 41(4):98–103, 2016.
25. Romero P, et al: The Human Vaccines Project: a roadmap for cancer vaccine development. *Sci Transl Med* 8(334):1–7, 2016.
26. Hanahan D: Rethinking the war on cancer. *Lancet* 383(9916):558–563, 2014.

Cancer Epidemiology

Kathryn L. McCance

CHAPTER OUTLINE

Although cancer arises from a complicated and an interacting web of multiple etiologies, avoiding high-risk behaviors and exposure to individual carcinogens, or cancer-causing substances, will prevent many types of cancer (Fig. 13.1). In fact, estimates as high as 80% to 90% for smoking-related cancers, such as lung and oropharyngeal cancer, and as high as 60% for other common lifestyle cancers, such as colorectal and bladder cancer, are preventable.[1] Lifestyle behaviors, dietary and environmental factors (such as exposure to ultraviolet radiation and infections), and occupational exposure contribute to cancer cases and deaths. In this context, any of the following factors can contribute to the development of cancer[2-4]:

Lifestyle choices, such as smoking, alcohol use, nutritional intake
Lack of physical exercise and overweight/obesity
Infections, sexual practices
Environmental conditions, air pollution, sunlight, natural and medical
  radiation, workplace exposures, and involuntary or unknown
  exposures
Prescribed and illicit medications
Socioeconomic factors that affect exposures and susceptibility
Carcinogenic substances present in air, water, and soil

Estimates of environmental factors and their attributable risk for cancer vary. The International Agency for Research on Cancer (IARC) is part of the World Health Organization (WHO). A major goal for the IARC is to identify causes of cancer. The IARC has evaluated more than 900 candidate carcinogens and placed them into the following groups: Group 1: Carcinogenic to humans, Group 2A: Probably carcinogenic to humans, Group 3: Unclassifiable as to carcinogenicity in humans, and Group 4: Probably not carcinogenic to humans. Because it is difficult to test candidate carcinogens, most are listed as probable, possible, or unknown risk. About 100 chemicals, occupations, physical agents, biologic agents, and other agents are classified as carcinogenic to humans.[2] Simplified tables with a list of classifications by cancer sites with sufficient or limited evidence in humans are contained in Table 13.1.

GENETICS, EPIGENETICS, AND TISSUE

Cancers are caused by environmental-lifestyle and genetic factors. Cancer is *driven* by genetic alterations and changes in epigenetic regulation[5-7] (see Chapter 12). Critical cancer genes include oncogenes and tumor-suppressor genes. These genes become altered by a combination of genetic and epigenetic alterations to drive cancer progression.[8] Critical

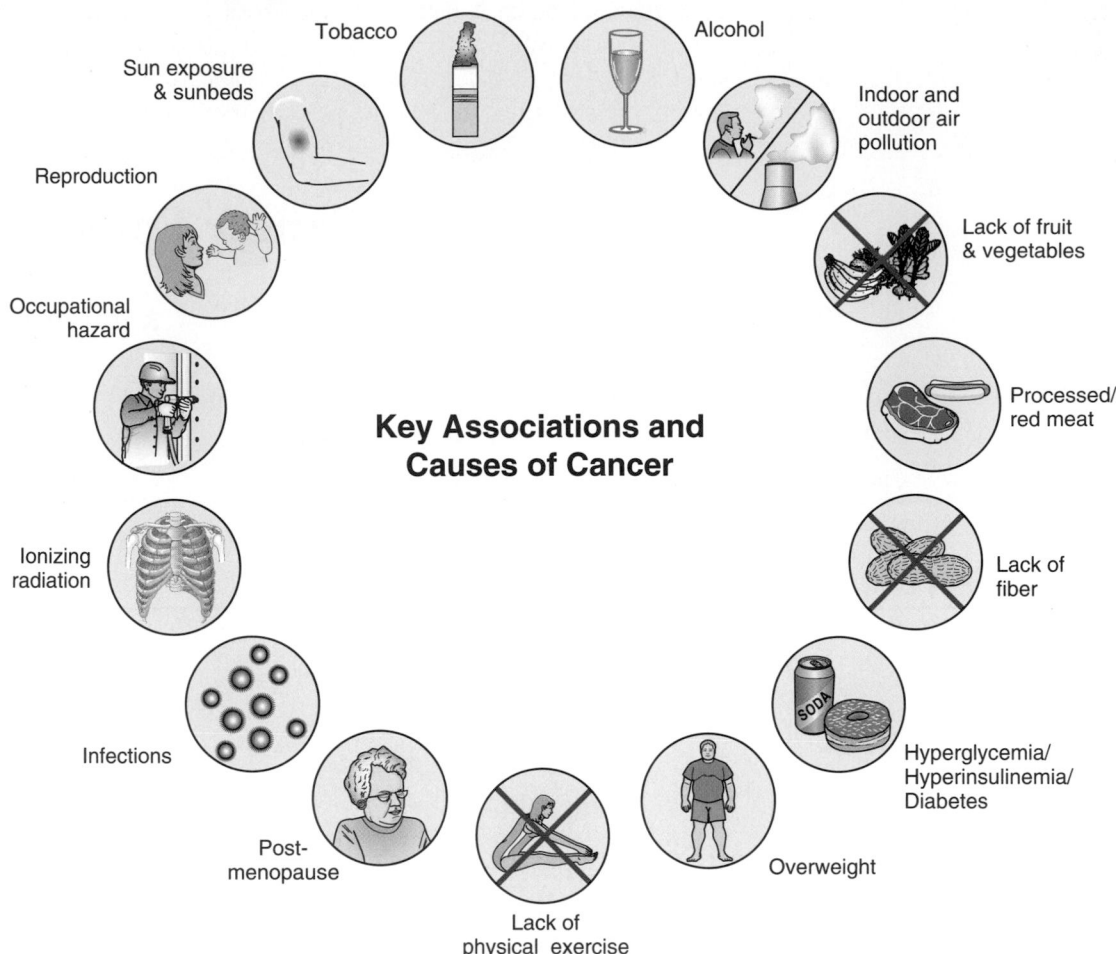

FIGURE 13.1 Key Associations and Causes of Cancer. Tobacco, diet and alcohol, obesity, lack of physical activity, air pollution, hormones, infections, ionizing radiation, occupational hazards, reproductive factors, and ultraviolet light are key associations and causes of cancer. Although diet is key and known to affect cancer risk, determining specific dietary factors has been very difficult and is emerging.

genes for cancer regulate when cells grow, divide, differentiate, or die. A subclass of tumor-suppressor genes helps maintain genome integrity.[8] Although driver and passenger genetic alterations are key, a wealth of data now indicate the importance of epigenetic processes, especially those with resultant gene silencing (not broken, but mute) of key regulatory genes (see Chapters 6 and 12). Different combinations of mutations and epigenetic changes are found in different types of cancers.[8] Neoplastic cells undergo dynamic and reversible transitions between multiple phenotypic states, including epithelial-mesenchymal plasticity in cancer (see Chapter 12). This plasticity is enabled by changes in epigenetic regulation.[7,9] Interacting factors that influence cancer risk include detoxifying enzymes, DNA repair genes, immune/inflammation systems, and the cell's immediate environment. The biologic environment surrounding cells includes metabolic and hormonal factors, for example, excess estrogen production, inflammation, and disordered glucose and lipid metabolism. The cell's biologic environment is modified by metabolic requirements, physical activity, infections, nutrition, occupational carcinogens, air pollution, and many other environmental factors. Investigators are challenged to connect the complex web between genotype, phenotype, and environment-lifestyle factors to understand a person's chances of developing cancer (see *What's New?* New Models to Understand Intrinsic and Extrinsic Cancer Risk).

Cancer development and progression involve the tissue microenvironment or stroma (see Chapter 12). The microenvironment participates in a complex signaling process that facilitates tumor promotion and metastasis because stromal tissue has various immune cells that can promote inflammation. Extensive clinical and experimental evidence shows that infiltrating immune cells cause chronic inflammation and, therefore, create a permissive tumor-progressing environment. Chronic inflammation also can *precede* and presumably initiate malignant change, as for example in inflammation-induced colon cancer.[10] It is well documented that chronic inflammation induced by bacteria, viruses, autoimmune processes, and toxins promotes common types of cancer, including colon, liver, and lung cancer. Inflammation can be caused by numerous environmental factors, for example, inhaling tobacco smoke, asbestos fibers, or fine particles in the air from diesel engine exhaust and industrial sources. These sources are major factors in lung and other respiratory tract cancers.[11,12] Cancer development in the presence of chronic inflammation involves the continuous presence of cytokines, chemokines, reactive oxygen species (ROS), oncogenes, cyclooxgenase-2 (COX-2), 5-lipoxygenase (5-LOX), and matrix metalloproteinases (MMPs), as well as the activation of essential transcription factors, such as nuclear factor κB (NF-κB).

INCIDENCE AND MORTALITY TRENDS

Cancer is reported to become a major cause of morbidity and mortality in the coming decades in all regions of the world. According to a report

Text continued on p. 385

TABLE 13.1 LIST OF CLASSIFICATIONS BY CANCER SITES WITH SUFFICIENT OR LIMITED EVIDENCE IN HUMANS

CANCER SITE	CARCINOGENIC AGENTS WITH SUFFICIENT EVIDENCE IN HUMANS	AGENTS WITH LIMITED EVIDENCE IN HUMANS
Lip, Oral Cavity, and Pharynx		
Lip		Solar radiation
Oral cavity	Alcoholic beverages Betel quid with tobacco Betel quid without tobacco Human papillomavirus type 16 Tobacco, smokeless Tobacco smoking	
Salivary gland	X-radiation, γ-radiation	Radioiodines, including iodine-131
Tonsil	Human papillomavirus type 16	
Pharynx	Alcoholic beverages Betel quid with tobacco Human papillomavirus type 16 Tobacco smoking	Asbestos (all forms) Mate drinking, hot Printing presses Tobacco smoke, secondhand
Nasopharynx	Epstein-Barr virus Formaldehyde Salted fish, Chinese-style Wood dust	
Digestive tract, upper	Acetaldehyde associated with consumption of alcoholic beverages	
Digestive Organs		
Esophagus	Acetaldehyde associated with consumption of alcoholic beverages Alcoholic beverages Betel quid with tobacco Betel quid without tobacco Tobacco, smokeless Tobacco smoking X-radiation, γ-radiation	Dry cleaning Mate drinking, hot Pickled vegetables (traditional Asian) Rubber production industry Tetrachloroethylene
Stomach	*Helicobacter pylori* Rubber production industry Tobacco smoking X-radiation, γ-radiation	Asbestos (all forms) Epstein-Barr virus Lead compounds, inorganic Nitrate or nitrite (ingested) under conditions that result in endogenous nitrosation Pickled vegetables (traditional Asian) Salted fish (Chinese style)
Colon and rectum	Alcoholic beverages Tobacco smoking X-radiation, γ-radiation	Asbestos (all forms) *Schistosoma japonicum*
Anus	Human immunodeficiency virus type 1 Human papillomavirus type 16	Human papillomavirus types 18, 33
Liver and bile duct	Aflatoxins Alcoholic beverages *Clonorchis sinensis* Estrogen-progestogen contraceptives Hepatitis B virus Hepatitis C virus *Opisthorchis viverrini* Plutonium thorium-232 and its decay products Tobacco smoking (in smokers and in smokers' children) Vinyl chloride	Androgenic (anabolic) steroids Arsenic and inorganic arsenic compounds Betel quid without tobacco Human immunodeficiency virus type 1 Polychlorinated biphenyls *Schistosoma japonicum* Trichloroethylene X-radiation, γ-radiation

Continued

TABLE 13.1   LIST OF CLASSIFICATIONS BY CANCER SITES WITH SUFFICIENT OR LIMITED EVIDENCE IN HUMANS—cont'd

CANCER SITE	CARCINOGENIC AGENTS WITH SUFFICIENT EVIDENCE IN HUMANS	AGENTS WITH LIMITED EVIDENCE IN HUMANS
Gallbladder	Thorium-232 and its decay products	
Pancreas	Tobacco, smokeless Tobacco smoking	Alcoholic beverages Thorium-232 and its decay products X-radiation, γ-radiation
Digestive tract, unspecified		Radioiodines, including iodine-131
Respiratory Organs		
Nasal cavity and paranasal sinus	Isopropyl alcohol production Leather dust Nickel compounds Radium-226 and its decay products Radium-228 and its decay products Tobacco smoking Wood dust	Carpentry and joinery Chromium (VI) compounds Formaldehyde Textile manufacturing
Larynx	Acid mists, strong inorganic Alcoholic beverages Asbestos (all forms) Tobacco smoking	Human papillomavirus type 16 Mate drinking, hot Rubber production industry Sulfur mustard Tobacco smoke, secondhand
Lung	Aluminum production Arsenic and inorganic arsenic compounds Beryllium and beryllium products Bis(chloromethyl) ether; chloromethyl methyl ether (technical grade) Cadmium and cadmium compounds Chromium (VI) compounds Coal, indoor emissions from household combustion Coal gasification Coal-tar pitch Coke production Hematite mining (underground) Iron and steel founding MOPP (vincristine-prednisone-nitrogen mustard-procarbazine mixture) Nickel compounds Painting Plutonium Radon-222 and its decay products Rubber production industry Silica dust, crystalline Soot Sulfur mustard Tobacco smoke, secondhand Tobacco smoking X-radiation, γ-radiation	Acid mists, strong inorganic Art glass, glass containers, and pressed ware (manufacture of) Biomass fuel (primarily wood), indoor emissions from household combustion of Bitumens, oxidized, and their emissions during roofing Bitumens, hard, and their emissions during mastic asphalt work Carbon electrode manufacture α-Chlorinated toluenes and benzyl chloride (combined exposure) Cobalt metal with tungsten carbide Creosotes Engine exhaust, diesel Frying, emissions from high-temperature Insecticides, nonarsenical (occupational exposures in spraying and application) Printing processes 2,3,7,8-Tetrachlorodibenzo-*para*-dioxin Welding fumes
Bone, Skin, and Mesothelium, Endothelium, and Soft Tissue		
Bone	Plutonium radium-224 and its decay products Radium-226 and its decay products Radium-228 and its decay products X-radiation, γ-radiation	Radioiodines, including iodine-131
Skin (melanoma)	Solar radiation Ultraviolet-emitting tanning devices	

TABLE 13.1	**LIST OF CLASSIFICATIONS BY CANCER SITES WITH SUFFICIENT OR LIMITED EVIDENCE IN HUMANS—cont'd**	
CANCER SITE	**CARCINOGENIC AGENTS WITH SUFFICIENT EVIDENCE IN HUMANS**	**AGENTS WITH LIMITED EVIDENCE IN HUMANS**
Skin (other malignant neoplasms)	Arsenic and inorganic arsenic compounds Azathioprine Coal-tar distillation Coal-tar pitch Cyclosporine Methoxsalen plus ultraviolet A Mineral oils, untreated or mildly treated Shale oils Solar radiation Soot X-radiation, γ-radiation	Creosotes Human immunodeficiency virus type 1 Human papillomavirus types 5 and 8 (in individuals with epidermodysplasia verruciformis) Nitrogen mustard Petroleum refining (occupational exposures) Ultraviolet-emitting tanning devices Merkel cell polyomavirus (MCV)
Mesothelium (pleura and peritoneum)	Asbestos (all forms) Erionite Painting	
Endothelium (Kaposi sarcoma)	Human immunodeficiency virus type 1 Kaposi sarcoma herpesvirus	
Soft tissue		Polychlorobiphenols or their sodium salts (combined exposures) Radioiodines, including iodine-131 2,3,7,8-Tetrachlorodibenzo-*para*-dioxin
Breast and Female Genital Organs		
Breast	Alcoholic beverages Diethylstilbestrol Estrogen-progestogen contraceptives Estrogen-progestogen menopausal therapy X-radiation, γ-radiation	Estrogen menopausal therapy Ethylene oxide Shift work that involves circadian disruption Tobacco smoking
Vulva	Human papillomavirus 16	Human immunodeficiency virus type 1
Vagina	Diethylstilbestrol (exposure in utero) Human papillomavirus 16	Human immunodeficiency virus type 1
Uterine cervix	Diethylstilbestrol (exposure in utero) Estrogen-progestogen contraceptives Human immunodeficiency virus type 1 Human papillomavirus types 16, 18, 31, 33, 35, 39, 45, 51, 52, 56, 58, 59 Tobacco smoking	Human papillomavirus types 26, 53, 66, 67, 68, 70, 73, 82 Tetrachloroethylene
Endometrium	Estrogen menopausal therapy Estrogen-progestogen menopausal therapy Tamoxifen	Diethylstilbestrol
Ovary	Asbestos (all forms) Estrogen menopausal therapy Tobacco smoking	Talc-based body powder (perineal use) X-radiation, γ-radiation
Male Genital Organs		
Penis	Human papillomavirus type 16	Human immunodeficiency virus type 1 Human papillomavirus type 18
Prostate		Androgenic (anabolic) steroids Arsenic and inorganic arsenic compounds Cadmium and cadmium compounds Rubber production industry Thorium-232 and its decay products X-radiation, γ-radiation
Testis		Diethylstilbestrol exposure in utero

Continued

TABLE 13.1	LIST OF CLASSIFICATIONS BY CANCER SITES WITH SUFFICIENT OR LIMITED EVIDENCE IN HUMANS—cont'd	
CANCER SITE	**CARCINOGENIC AGENTS WITH SUFFICIENT EVIDENCE IN HUMANS**	**AGENTS WITH LIMITED EVIDENCE IN HUMANS**
Urinary Tract		
Kidney	Tobacco smoking X-radiation, γ-radiation	Arsenic and inorganic arsenic compounds Cadmium and cadmium compounds Printing processes
Renal pelvis and ureter	Aristolochic acids, plants containing phenacetin Phenacetin, analgesic mixtures containing Tobacco smoking	Aristolochic acids
Urinary bladder	Aluminum production 4-Aminobiphenyl Arsenic and inorganic arsenic compounds Auramine production Benzidine Chlornaphazine Cyclophosphamide Magenta production 2-Naphthylamine Painting Rubber production industry *Schistosoma haematobium* Tobacco smoking *ortho*-Toluidine X-radiation, γ-radiation	4-Chloro-*ortho*-toluidine Coal-tar pitch Coffee Dry cleaning Engine exhaust, diesel Hairdressers and barbers (occupational exposure) Printing processes Soot Textile manufacturing
Eye, Brain, and Central Nervous System		
Eye	Human immunodeficiency virus type 1 Ultraviolet-emitting tanning devices Welding	Solar radiation
Brain and central nervous system	X-radiation, γ-radiation	Radiofrequency electromagnetic fields (including from wireless phones)
Endocrine Glands		
Thyroid	Radioiodines, including iodine-131 X-radiation, γ-radiation	
Lymphoid, Hematopoietic, and Related Tissue		
Leukemia and/or lymphoma	Azathioprine Benzene Busulfan 1,3-Butadiene Chlorambucil Cyclophosphamide Cyclosporine Epstein-Barr virus Etoposide with cisplatin and bleomycin Fission products, including strontium-90 Formaldehyde *Helicobacter pylori* Hepatitis C virus Human immunodeficiency virus type 1 Human T-cell lymphotropic virus type 1 Kaposi sarcoma herpesvirus Melphalan	Bis(chloroethyl)nitrosourea (BBCNU) Chloramphenicol Ethylene oxide Etoposide Hepatitis B virus Magnetic fields, extremely low frequency (childhood leukemia) Mitoxantrone Nitrogen mustard Painting (childhood leukemia from maternal exposure) Petroleum refining (occupational exposures) Polychlorophenols or their sodium salts (combined exposures) Radioiodines, including iodine-131 Radon-222 and its decay products Styrene Teniposide

TABLE 13.1	LIST OF CLASSIFICATIONS BY CANCER SITES WITH SUFFICIENT OR LIMITED EVIDENCE IN HUMANS—cont'd	
CANCER SITE	**CARCINOGENIC AGENTS WITH SUFFICIENT EVIDENCE IN HUMANS**	**AGENTS WITH LIMITED EVIDENCE IN HUMANS**
	MOPP (vincristine-prednisone-nitrogen mustard-procarbazine mixture)	Tetrachloroethylene
	Phosphorus-32	Trichloroethylene
	Rubber production industry	2,3,7,8-Tetrachlorodibenzo-*para*-dioxin
	Semustine (methyl-CCNU)	Tobacco smoking (childhood leukemia in smokers' children)
	Thiotepa	Malaria (caused by infection with *Plasmodium falciparum* in holoendemic areas)
	Thorium-23 and its decay products	
	Tobacco smoking	
	Treosulfan	
	X-radiation, γ-radiation	
Multiple or Unspecific Sites		
Multiple sites (unspecified)	Cyclosporine	Chlorophenoxy herbicides
	Fission products, including strontium-90	Plutonium
	X-radiation, γ-radiation (exposure in utero)	
All cancer sites (combined)	2,3,7,8-Tetrachlorodibenzo-*para*-dioxin	

NOTE: This table does not include factors not covered in the IARC Monographs, notably genetic traits, reproductive status, and some nutritional factors.
Adapted from Cogliano VJ et al: *J Natl Cancer Inst* 103:1–13, 2011. http://jnci.oxfordjournals.org/content/early/2011/12/11/jnci.djr483.short?rss=1.

by GLOBACAN, an estimated 14.1 million new cancer cases and 8.2 million cancer deaths were reported and 32.6 million people were found to be living with cancer (diagnosed in the past 5 years) worldwide in 2012.[13] The age-standardized rate for all cancers (excluding nonmelanoma skin cancer) for men and women combined was 182 per 100,000 in 2012; the rate was higher for men (205 per 100,000) than women (165 per 100,000). The highest cancer rate for men and women together was found in Denmark with 338 people per 100,000 being diagnosed in 2012. The age-standardized rate was at least 300 per 100,000 for 9 countries (Denmark, France, Australia, Belgium, Norway, United States, Ireland, Republic of Korea, and The Netherlands). The countries in the top 10 come from Europe, Oceania, Northern America, and Asia.[13]

In the 2016 annual report to the nation, the National Cancer Institute, the American Cancer Society, the Centers for Disease Control and Prevention, and the North American Association of Central Cancer registries collaborated to provide updates on cancer incidence, death rates, and trends in these rates for the United States from 2003 to 2012.[14] The overall incidence rates (new cases per 100,000 persons in the United States) decreased for men and stayed about the same for women. During this period, 7 of the 17 more common cancers in men showed decreases in incidence, including colorectal, lung and bronchus, prostate, stomach, larynx, bladder, and brain cancers. Six of the more common cancers in women showed decreases in incidence, including cancers of the colorectum, cervix, lung and bronchus, bladder, ovary, and stomach. Importantly, the decline in the incidence of lung cancer corresponded with a decrease in tobacco use. During this same period, cancer incidence increased among people ages 0 to 19 years. The annual report's highlight included a special section on liver cancer. In all racial and ethnic populations, men had about a threefold higher liver cancer incidence rate than women. In 2012, the most recent year for which data are available, 28,012 people were diagnosed with liver cancer in the United States (excluding Nevada). Of this total, 20,207 were men and 7805 were women.[14] Liver cancer incidence rates were higher among people born between 1945 and 1965 than among those born in other periods because of higher rates of hepatitis C virus (HCV) infection. Among persons born in this cohort, HCV infection was highest among nonHispanic whites, nonHispanic blacks, and Hispanics. Cirrhosis or scarring of the liver also is a precursor to liver cancer. Risk factors for cirrhosis include a history of liver disease, a history of heavy alcohol use, and some rare genetic disorders. In the United States, alcohol overuse contributes to about 8% to 16% of liver cancer deaths.[14]

Researchers found continued declines in cancer death rates or mortality rates for men, women, and children. Deaths caused by liver cancer, however, increased at the highest rate of all reported cancer sites, and liver cancer incidence rates increased sharply. The mortality rates for men from liver cancer were more than double the rate of those from women, with 15,563 deaths among men and 7409 deaths among women.

IN UTERO AND EARLY LIFE CONDITIONS

From studies of the etiology of certain cancers, it is widely accepted that a long latency period precedes the onset of adult cancers. Accumulating data suggest early life events influence later susceptibility to certain chronic diseases (Fig. 13.2).[15] Developmental plasticity is the degree to which an organism's development is contingent on its environment. Specifically, the developmental origins' hypothesis postulates that nutrition and other environmental factors affect cellular pathways during gestation, enabling a single genotype to produce a broad range of adult phenotypes.[16] *Plasticity* refers to the ability of genes to organize physiologically or structurally in response to environmental conditions during fetal development. The hypothesis also postulates that persistent epigenetic adaptations that occur early in development in response to maternal and paternal nutrition and the environment are associated with increased susceptibility to cancer and other adult-onset chronic diseases.[17,18] Throughout in utero development, the placenta plays a major role in controlling growth and development.[19] Because the placenta is a regulator of the intrauterine environment and can be influenced

WHAT'S NEW?

New Models to Understand Intrinsic and Extrinsic Cancer Risk

Vigorous debate has surrounded two possibly opposing explanations of why cancers are distributed unevenly among organs. Some organs are more likely to develop malignant tumors than others, and children and adults develop very different types of cancers. These biases in cancer formation, adult versus child and organ specificity, are explained, in part, by organ-specific susceptibilities to carcinogens or inherited oncogenic mutations. The specific contributions, however, to these or other factors are unknown. The understanding of these factors that lead to cancer development is crucial for prevention and treatment. Thus investigators have proposed recent hypotheses. The "bad luck" hypothesis states that many cancers arise following the generation of mutations that occur by chance in highly-replicative stem cell populations, rather than following exposure to environmental factors. The implication of this hypothesis is that these cancers are not preventable. This hypothesis has undergone a great deal of scrutiny and is strongly contested. Importantly, recent mathematical modeling estimated that 70% to 90% of the causal factors driving the most common cancers are extrinsic or environmental factors.

The controversy from these studies has occurred because of the use of different mathematical approaches to correlate selected human cancer incidence data with various metrics of stem cell proliferation data. Investigators, therefore, approached the problem using experimental in vivo studies with defined populations of both neonatal and adult mice. These investigators found that tumor incidence is determined by the lifelong generative capacity of mutated cells, supporting the hypothesis that *stem cells dictate organ cancer risk.* Damage-induced activation of stem cell function significantly increases cancer risk. Therefore a combination of stem cell mutagenesis and environmental (extrinsic) factors that damage tissue and increase the proliferation of these cells creates the "perfect storm" and ultimately determines organ cancer risk. Tissue damage and inflammation are well-recognized determinants of cancer risk. The risk of an organ developing cancer following the introduction of oncogenic mutations into a stem cell population is significantly associated with their lifelong generative capacity and this holds true regardless of the developmental stage, supporting the finding that the mutation of stem cells dictates cancer risk. Chronic tissue injury plays a critical role in tumor development and progression because it can reactivate generative and tumorigenic capacity in stem cells. In this model, damaging the liver reactivated a neonatal-like stem cell program promoting their proliferation and liver repair. The reactivation increases their susceptibility to transformation providing direct evidence that *cell generative capacity* can be a major determinant of organ cancer risk (see Figures A and B).

1. Normal stem cells

Stem cells can be asleep

When needed, for example to repair damage, they replicate to make more stem cells or other cells the body needs.

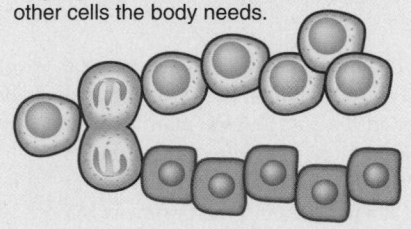

2. DNA mistakes in stem cells

Sometimes stem cells acquire random mistakes in their DNA as they replicate

Things in the environment can increase DNA mistakes

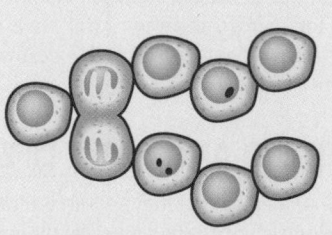
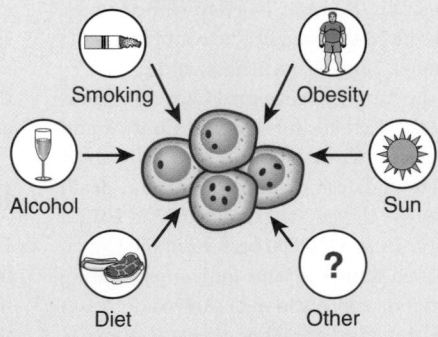

Smoking   Obesity

Alcohol   Sun

Diet   Other   ?

3. What happens to stem cells with DNA mistakes?

If stem cells with DNA mistakes are sleeping, no cancer develops

But if stem cells with DNA mistakes are replicating, cancer can develop

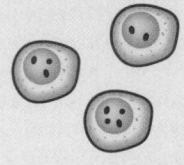
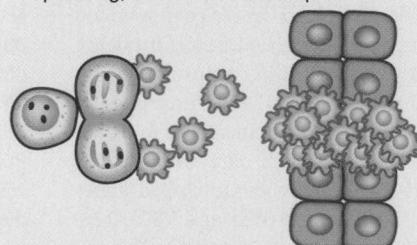

FIGURE A New research has demonstrated how cancers can start in stem cells.

WHAT'S NEW?

New Models to Understand Intrinsic and Extrinsic Cancer Risk—cont'd

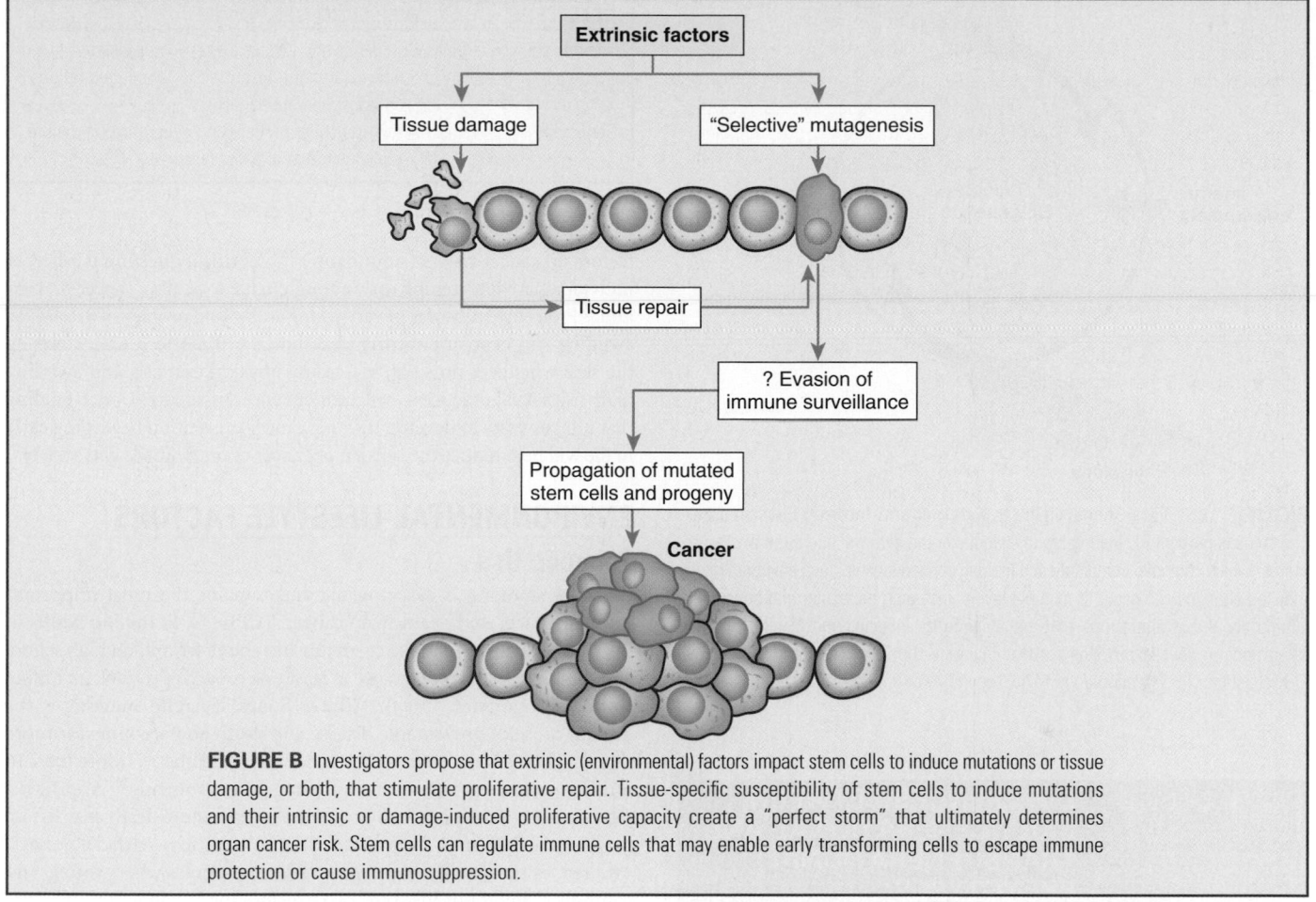

FIGURE B Investigators propose that extrinsic (environmental) factors impact stem cells to induce mutations or tissue damage, or both, that stimulate proliferative repair. Tissue-specific susceptibility of stem cells to induce mutations and their intrinsic or damage-induced proliferative capacity create a "perfect storm" that ultimately determines organ cancer risk. Stem cells can regulate immune cells that may enable early transforming cells to escape immune protection or cause immunosuppression.

Data from Ashford NA et al: *Science* 347:727, 2015; Gotay C, Dummer T, Spinelli J: *Science* 347:728, 2015; Howlader N et al: *SEER cancer statistics review*, 1975-2009, Bethesda, MD, 2012, National Cancer Institute; O'Callaghan M: Science 347:729, 2015; Potter JD, Prentice RL: *Science* 347:727, 2015; Song M, Giovannucci EL: *Science* 347:728–729, 2015; Wild C et al: *Science* 347:728, 2015; Wu S et al: *Nature* 529:43–47, 2016; Zhu L et al: *Cell* 166(5):1132–1146, 2016.

by exposures throughout pregnancy,[19,20] research is being done with DNA methylation linking environmental cues to placental pathologies and adult life. The Dutch Famine Birth Cohort is a well-known study of the effects of prenatal undernutrition in humans. Undernutrition was linked to increased heart disease, metabolic disorders, and a possible link with breast cancer decades later.[21] Early versus late undernutrition in pregnancy indicated that the first trimester of pregnancy is particularly vulnerable to disease outcome in adulthood.[22] A striking experiment in mice demonstrated how extra vitamin doses during pregnancy in the mother's diet changed the fur color of her pups.[23] This was the first study to show maternal nutrition and subsequent phenotype changes. The nutrients (B_{12}, folic acid, choline, and betaine) silenced the gene that rendered mice fat and yellow but did not alter its DNA sequence. Silencing, or switching the gene off, linked prenatal diet to such diseases as diabetes, obesity, and cancer. More research is needed to understand nutrition in pregnancy and child vulnerabilities later in life (Fig. 13.3).

Perhaps one of the best examples of early life events and future cancer is the chemical exposure to diethylstilbestrol (DES), a synthetic estrogen. This medication was prescribed between 1938 and 1971 to attempt to prevent multiple pregnancy-related problems, such as miscarriage, premature birth, and abnormal bleeding.[24] By the 1950s it became clear that DES interfered with the *development* of the reproductive system in the fetus and it did not prevent miscarriage. Recent data suggest that the DES-associated increase in clear cell adenocarcinoma is elevated throughout a woman's reproductive years.[25] Other studies have revealed that daughters of women who took DES during pregnancy may have a slightly increased risk of breast cancer before age 40 (i.e., 1.9 times the risk compared with unexposed women at age 40).[26] For every 1000 DES-exposed women ages 45 to 49 it is estimated that 4 will be diagnosed with breast cancer.

Research from animal studies has demonstrated a relationship between DES exposure and an increased rate of a rare type of testicular cancer (rete testis) and prostate cancer.[27,28] In terms of in utero exposures, testicular cancer has been linked to exposure to abnormal levels of estrogen,[29] and testicular cancer is a risk factor for men with undescended testicles, a factor in some studies correlated with DES exposure. However, studies in humans determining the risk of testicular or prostate cancer and DES exposure are unclear and continuing. Investigators from a

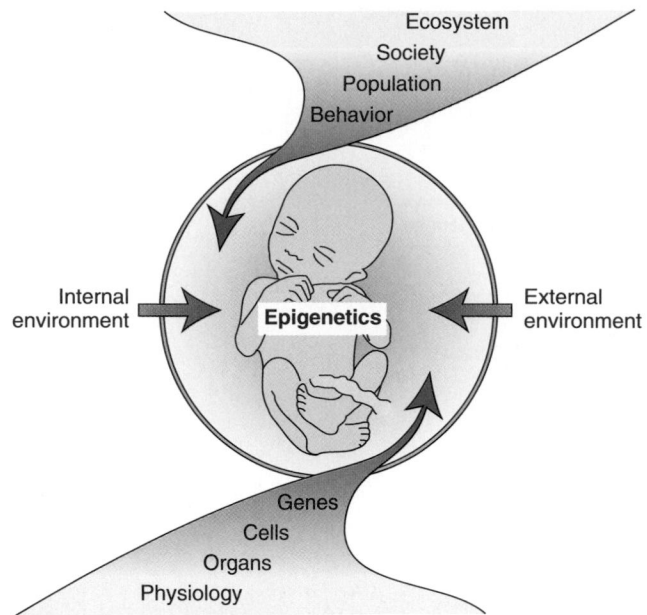

FIGURE 13.2 Fetal Vulnerability to External and Internal Environments. The fetus is particularly vulnerable to changes in the external and internal environments, which can have immediate and lifelong consequences. Such environmentally induced changes can occur at multiple levels, including molecular and behavioral. Ultimately these alterations may be epigenetic, inducing mitotically heritable alterations in gene expression without changing the DNA. (Adapted from Crews E, McLachlan JA: *Endocrinology* 147[6 Suppl]:S4–S10, 2006.)

TABLE 13.2	DIFFERENCES BETWEEN MULTIGENERATIONAL AND TRANSGENERATIONAL PHENOTYPES	
PHENOTYPE	**EXPOSURE**	**DEFINITION**
Multigenerational	Direct	Simultaneous exposure of multiple generations to an environmental factor
Transgenerational	Initial germline exposure (ancestral)	Transgenerational phenotype is transmitted to future generations through germline inheritance

recent study reported early life exposure to endocrine disrupting chemicals (EDCs), including DES, can increase the incidence, multiplicity, and overall size of uterine fibroids in the Eker rat model.[30]

In summary, epidemiologic and animal studies reveal that small changes in the developmental environment can alter phenotypic changes, resulting in individual responses in adulthood. Continuing evidence indicates that epigenetic mechanisms are responsible for tissue-specific gene expression during cellular differentiation and that these mechanisms modulate developmental phenotypic changes. The phenotypic effects of epigenetic modifications during development may need long latency periods, such as in cancer, thus manifesting later in life. In addition, epigenetic effects may help explain transgenerational effects (Tables 13.2 and 13.3).

Lifestyle habits are modifiable, and changing them can translate to reduced cancer risk and prevention of cancer. Examples of environmental

TABLE 13.3	SOMATIC VS. GERM CELL INHERITANCE
CELL TYPE	**BIOLOGIC RESPONSE**
Somatic cells	Critical for adult-onset disease in exposed individual; not transmitted to future generations as transgenerational effect
Germ cells	Allow transmission between generations; promote transgenerational phenotype

factors on cancer risk are abundant.[1,31,32] A critical question is whether individuals are intervening early enough in life to achieve cancer prevention.[33] Protective measures in very young and young people—for example, avoiding sun exposure during peak hours (10 AM to 3 PM), covering the skin whenever possible, increasing physical exercise, and avoiding high-risk sexual practices—will reduce cancer incidence. Understanding that it takes years to develop tumors, cancer prevention beginning early in life will help reduce the burden of cancer on individuals and society.[33]

ENVIRONMENTAL-LIFESTYLE FACTORS

Tobacco Use

Cigarette smoking is carcinogenic and remains the most important cause of cancer and death from cancer.[34] Close to 40 million adults in the United States still smoke cigarettes and about 4.7 million high school and middle school students use at least one tobacco product, including electronic cigarettes.[35] In the United States, cigarette smoking is the leading cause of preventable disease and death and accounts for more than 480,000 deaths each year, or 1 of every 5 deaths.[35,36] More than 16 million Americans live with a smoking-related disease.[36] Worldwide, tobacco use is a major preventable cause of premature death and disease in which 5.4 million people die each year from tobacco-related illnesses.[37] The risk is greatest in those who begin to smoke when young and continue throughout life, but tobacco smoking is pandemic, affecting all ages. Current cigarette smoking was higher among persons aged 18 to 24 years, 25 to 44 years, and 45 to 64 years than among those 65 years and older.[38] The eradication of tobacco use can only be achieved by preventing children and adolescents from starting tobacco use. Men are more likely to smoke (16.7%) than women (13.6%).[38] According to race and ethnicity, smoking occurs more often in nonHispanic American Indians/Alaska Natives (29.2%), nonHispanic whites (18.2%), nonHispanic blacks (17.5%), nonHispanic multiple race individuals (27.9%), and nonHispanic Asians (9.5%). Cigarettes remained the most commonly used tobacco product, and young adults aged 18 to 24 years reported the highest prevalence of use of emerging tobacco products, including water pipes/hookahs and e-cigarettes.[39] Globally, tobacco use is greatest in developing countries, where 84% of 1.3 billion current smokers live.[40] Asia is now considered the largest tobacco producer and consumer in the world.[41]

Smoking affects nearly every organ of the body[42,43] (Fig. 13.4). Since the first Surgeon General's report on smoking and health in 1964, more than 20 million Americans have died as a result of smoking.[43] Most of these deaths were adults with a history of smoking, but about 2.5 million were nonsmokers who died from lung cancer and heart disease from secondhand smoke[43] (see Fig. 13.4). Secondhand smoke, also called environmental tobacco smoke (ETS), is the combination of sidestream smoke (burning end of a cigarette, cigar, or pipe) and mainstream smoke (exhaled by the smoker). More than 7000 chemicals have been identified in mainstream tobacco smoke. Nonsmokers who live with smokers are at greatest risk for lung cancer as well as numerous

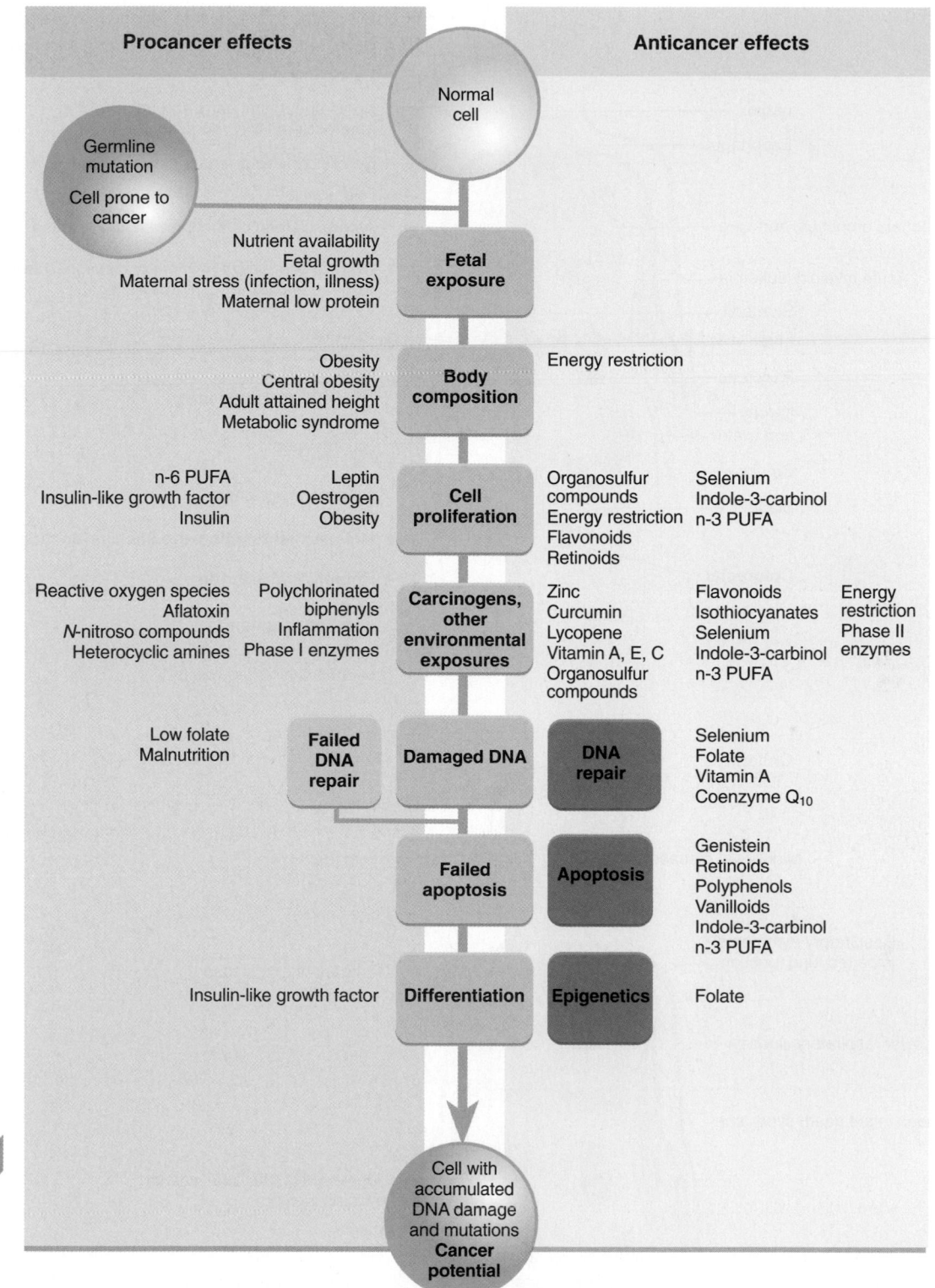

FIGURE 13.3 Pro- and Anticancer Effects. *PUFA,* Polyunsaturated fatty acids. (From World Cancer Research Fund/American Institute for Cancer Research: *Food, nutrition, physical activity, and the prevention of cancer: a global perspective,* Washington, DC, 2007, AICR.)

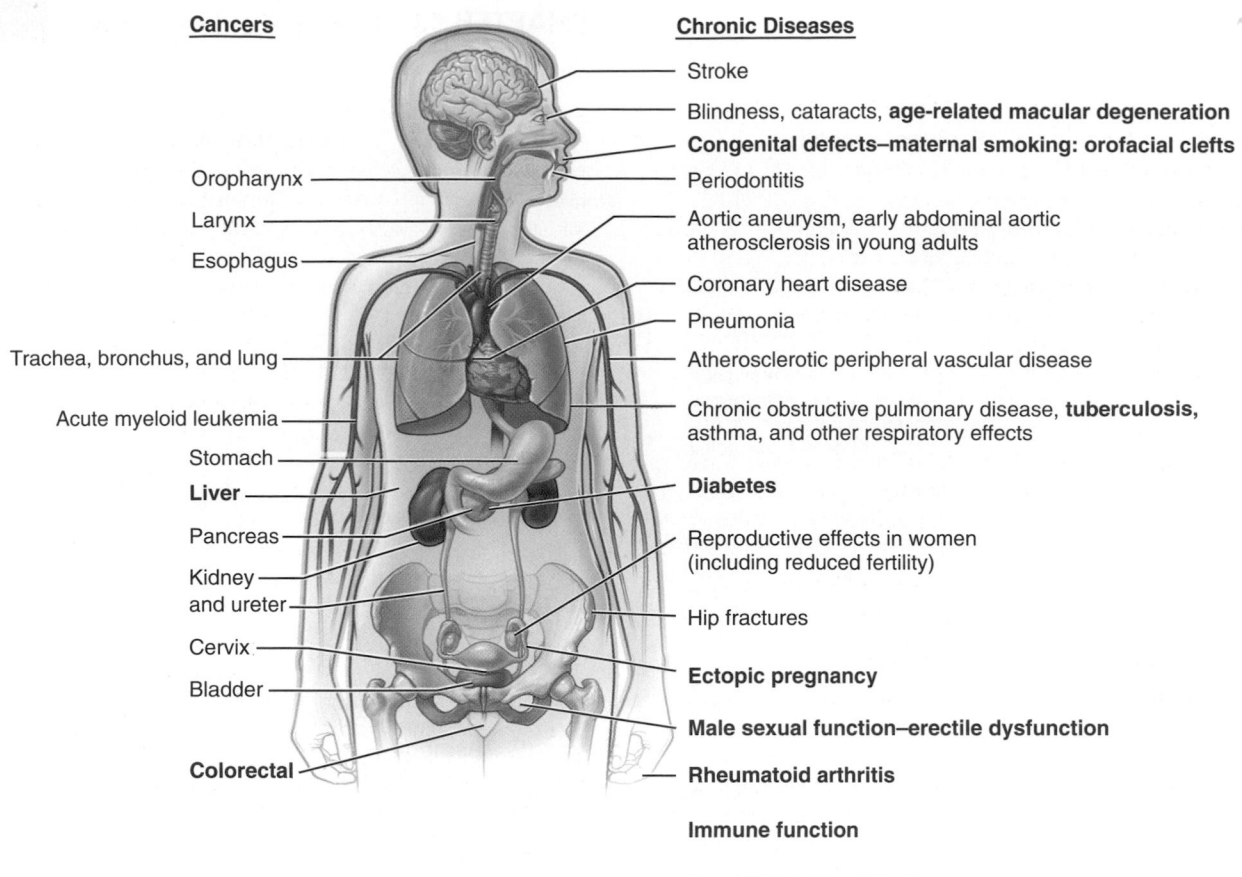

Cancers

Oropharynx

Larynx

Esophagus

Trachea, bronchus, and lung

Acute myeloid leukemia

Stomach

Liver

Pancreas

Kidney and ureter

Cervix

Bladder

Colorectal

Chronic Diseases

Stroke

Blindness, cataracts, **age-related macular degeneration**

Congenital defects–maternal smoking: orofacial clefts

Periodontitis

Aortic aneurysm, early abdominal aortic atherosclerosis in young adults

Coronary heart disease

Pneumonia

Atherosclerotic peripheral vascular disease

Chronic obstructive pulmonary disease, **tuberculosis, asthma, and other respiratory effects**

Diabetes

Reproductive effects in women (including reduced fertility)

Hip fractures

Ectopic pregnancy

Male sexual function–erectile dysfunction

Rheumatoid arthritis

Immune function

Overall diminished health

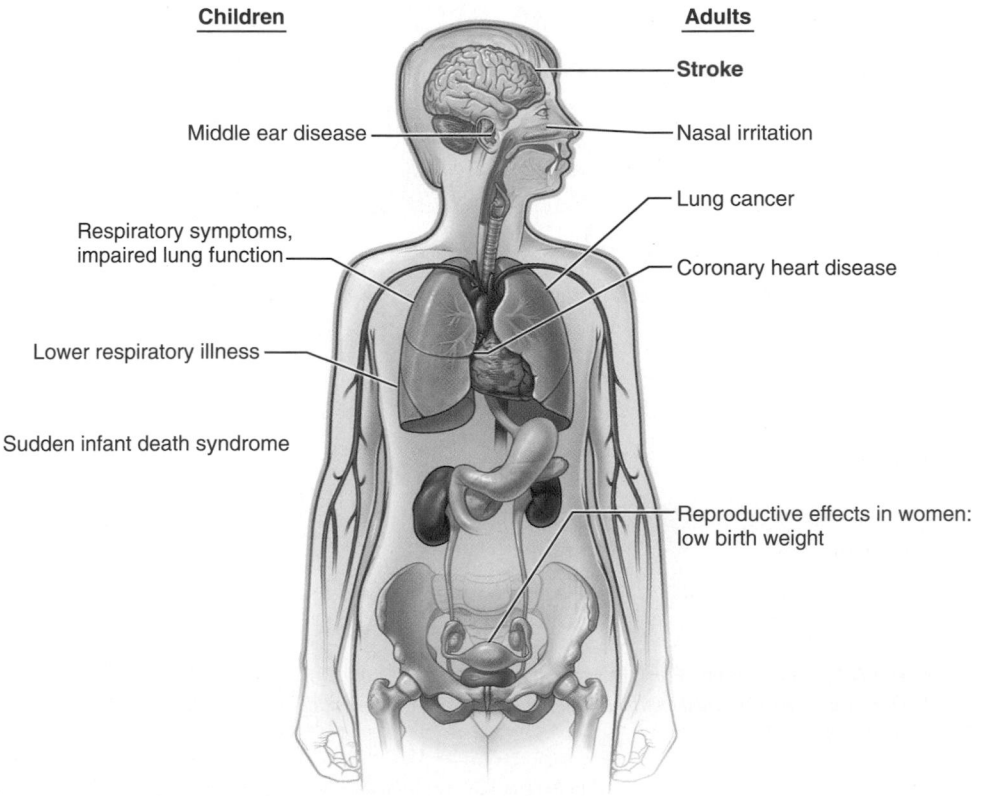

Children

Middle ear disease

Respiratory symptoms, impaired lung function

Lower respiratory illness

Sudden infant death syndrome

Adults

Stroke

Nasal irritation

Lung cancer

Coronary heart disease

Reproductive effects in women: low birth weight

FIGURE 13.4 Health Consequences Linked to Smoking. **NOTE:** The conditions in red are new diseases that have causally been linked to smoking. See text for discussion. Stroke is a new disease causally linked to secondhand smoke. (From U.S. Department of Health and Human Services [USDHHS]: *The health consequences of smoking—50 years of progress: a report of the Surgeon General,* Atlanta, 2014, U.S. Department of Health and Human Services, Centers for Disease Control and Prevention, National Center for Chronic Disease Prevention and Health Promotion, Office on Smoking and Health.)

noncancerous conditions.[44] Additionally, another 100,000 fatalities were babies who died of sudden infant death syndrome (SIDS) or complications from low birth weight or other conditions as a result of parental smoking, particularly from the mother.[43]

Smoking tobacco is linked to cancers of the lung, upper aerodigestive tract (oral cavity, pharynx, larynx, nasal cavity, paranasal sinuses, esophagus), stomach, lower urinary tract (renal pelvis, penis, and bladder), kidney, pancreas, cervix, and uterus, as well as myeloid leukemia (see Fig. 13.4). The new list of disease risks includes liver cancer and colorectal cancer. Secondhand smoke is a cause of stroke; it increases the risk of death in people with cancer and cancer survivors as well as those with age-related macular degeneration, tuberculosis, ectopic pregnancy, and diabetes mellitus; increases inflammation; impairs immunity; and is a cause of rheumatoid arthritis. Smoking causes even more deaths from vascular, respiratory, and other diseases than from cancer. The epidemic of smoking ranks among the greatest health catastrophes of the century and has caused an enormous avoidable public health tragedy.[44]

Cigars have the same toxic and carcinogenic compounds found in cigarettes; they are not a safe alternative to cigarettes.[45,46] Cigars have a much higher concentration of nicotine (100 to 200 mg or higher [444 mg]) than cigarettes (about 8 mg), and cigarettes deliver about 1 to 2 mg of nicotine to the smoker.[47] Full-size cigars can have as much nicotine as an entire pack of cigarettes.[47] Regular cigar smoking is associated with increased risk for cancers of the lung, esophagus, larynx, and oral cavity (lip, tongue, mouth, throat). Cigar smoking is linked to gum disease and tooth loss. Heavy cigar smoking increases the risk for lung diseases, including emphysema and chronic bronchitis.[48] Heavy cigar smokers and those who inhale deeply may be at increased risk for developing coronary heart disease.[46]

Hookahs are water pipes used to smoke specialized tobacco that comes in different flavors, including apple, mint, cherry, chocolate, coconut, licorice, cappuccino, and watermelon.[49] Hookah smoking has many of the same health risks as cigarette smoking, but is often assumed by users to be less harmful.[49] Other names for Hookahs include *narghile, argileh, shisha, hubble-bubble,* and *goza.* Hookah pipes vary in size, shape, and style and typical smoking is done in groups with the same mouthpiece passed from person to person. Hookah use is increasing worldwide, including Britain, France, Russia, the Middle East, and the United States, and in young people and college students.[49] Data from Monitoring the Future survey found that, among high school seniors in the United States, about 1 in 5 boys (17%) and 1 in 6 girls (15%) had used a hookah in the past year.[50] Compared to smoking a cigarette where it involves about 20 puffs, an hour-long hookah smoking session involves 200 puffs. The smoke inhaled during a typical hookah session is about 90,000 milliliters (mL), compared with 500 to 600 mL inhaled when a cigarette is smoked.[49] Hookah smokers may be at risk for some of the same diseases as cigarette smokers, including oral cancer, lung cancer, stomach cancer, esophageal cancer, reduced lung function, and decreased fertility. Secondhand smoke from hookahs is a health risk for nonsmokers.

Pipe smokers have an increased risk of dying from cancers of the lung, throat, esophagus, larynx, pancreas, and colorectum.[51] Smoking *bidi,* a small amount of tobacco wrapped in the leaf of another plant (used in South Asia), delivers higher amounts of nicotine per gram of tobacco and comparable or greater amounts of tar compared with cigarettes.[52] Bidi smokers have the same risks of cancers and higher risks of heart attacks and chronic bronchitis than those found in nonsmokers.[51] *Kreteks,* or clove cigarettes, are a tobacco product with the same health risks as cigarettes.

Electronic cigarettes (e-cigarettes) are a type of electronic nicotine delivery system (ENDS). ENDS include e-pens, e-pipes, e-hookahs, and e-cigars. Over 3 million high school and middle school students were current users of e-cigarettes in 2015.[53] As a small battery-operated device, e-cigarettes look like a cigarette. When a smoker puffs on the e-cigarette, the system delivers a vapor (aerosol) of nicotine, flavorings, and other chemicals.[51] The vapor is inhaled just like smoke from a regular cigarette and absorbed into the lungs. Colorful "vape pens" or "e-hookahs" are marketed to appeal to youth with flavors like candy and fruit.[51] These products contain liquid nicotine, flavorings, propylene glycol, glycerin, and other ingredients.[53] Since 2016, the Food and Drug Administration (FDA) regulates the manufacture, import, packaging, labeling, advertising, promotion, sale, and distribution of ENDS.[53] Beginning in 2018, all newly regulated covered tobacco products must have the following statement "WARNING: This product contains nicotine. Nicotine is an addictive chemical."[53]

A recent genetics study found the total mutation burden is elevated in smokers versus nonsmokers with lung adenocarcinoma, larynx, liver, and kidney cancers.[54] United Kingdom researchers reported for the first time that starting smoking results in epigenetic changes or DNA methylation associated with the development of cancer.[55] Investigators are studying the genetic and epigenetic effects of secondhand smoke and smoking (both maternal and paternal) during pregnancy on prenatal exposure and subsequent chronic diseases. Fig. 13.5 illustrates a working model of carcinogenesis by cigarette smoke. Measures that prevent young adults from starting smoking would substantially avoid future disease burden. A strong public health approach is one that *prevents* young people from *starting* smoking and helps others *stop* smoking.

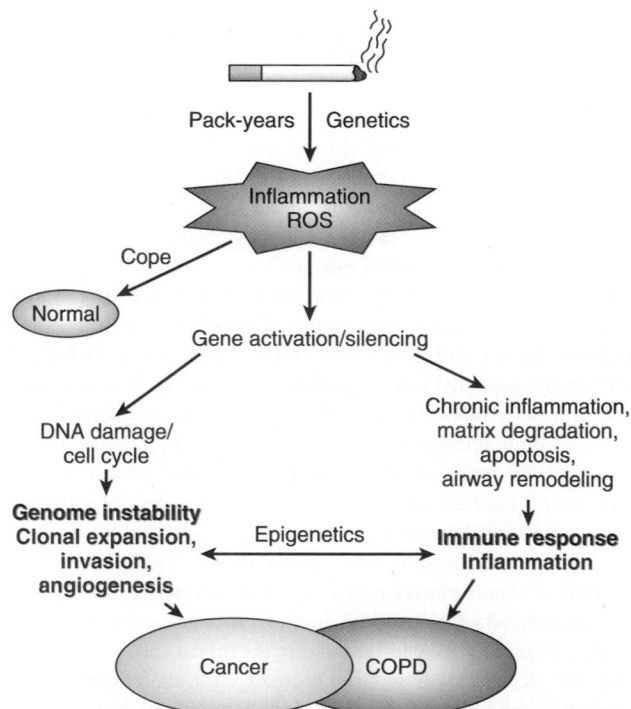

FIGURE 13.5 Working Model of Carcinogenesis by Cigarette Smoke. The major inducer of both lung cancer and chronic obstructive pulmonary disease *(COPD)* is cigarette smoke. Nonsmokers may develop these diseases caused by other environmental or genetic/epigenetic factors. Cigarette smoke induces an inflammatory response and causes an increase in reactive oxygen species *(ROS)*, causing oxidative stress. Oxidative stress is a risk factor for many diseases because it can alter many cellular proteins. A combination of immune-inflammatory signals and epigenetic events may increase the risk for individuals with COPD developing lung cancer. (From Adcock IM et al: *Respiration* 81[4]:265–284, 2011.)

Diet

Understanding dietary factors that increase the risk for cancer can be difficult. The ways in which diet affects one's likelihood of developing cancer are complicated by the variety of foods consumed, the many constituents of foods, the metabolic consequences of eating, and the temporal changes in the patterns of food use. Cancer risks in older adults may depend as much on diet in early life as on current eating practices. In addition, studies in humans targeting diet and disease associations face a variety of challenges including measurements of specific nutrients, food types, and dietary patterns.

A summary of convincing and probable judgments related to food (diet and nutrition), physical activity, and weight risk factors and the prevention of cancer is presented in Fig. 13.6. Dietary components can act directly as mutagens or interfere with mutagen elimination. Abundant evidence exists that nutritional factors in many processes are related to cancer development (Fig. 13.7).

Research is ongoing to understand the complexity of genomics, epigenomics, transcription factors (transcriptomics), proteomics, and metabolic factors (metabolomics) and the way that modifying any one, or more, influences cancer risk. Nutrigenomics is the study of the effects of nutrition on the phenotypic variability of individuals based on genomic differences (see Fig. 13.7).

Nutrition, Obesity, Alcohol Consumption, and Physical Activity: Impacts on Cancer

What people eat, how much they weigh, and how much they move influence their risks of developing cancer. Mounting evidence is clear—everyday *choices* impact their chances of getting or preventing cancer. Ongoing tedious and comprehensive investigative work is linking diet, body weight, and exercise to risk of specific cancers.

Nutrition

Data from epidemiologic and clinical research independent of aging are revealing that lifestyle and nutrition are associated with development or progression, or both, of major human cancers.[56,57] These cancers include some of the most common including breast, prostate, colorectal tumors, and other diet-related cancers.[56]

The Mediterranean diet (MD) has been reported to reduce mortality rates for chronic illnesses, including cardiovascular diseases, neurodegenerative diseases, and cancer.[56] Two meta-analyses of conformity with the MD were associated with a significant reduction in the risk of overall cancer mortality/incidence, as well as the incidence of several cancer types (colorectal, aerodigestive tract, breast, stomach, pancreas, prostate, liver, and head and neck).[58,59] Overall risk of cancer mortality was evaluated in 11 cohort studies; 6 of these cohorts did not show a significant correlation between adherence to an MD and cancer risk. Pooling all 11 cohort studies, however, a meta-analysis yielded a 13% risk reduction of overall cancer mortality when comparing the highest to the lowest adherence to the MD.[59] Box 13.1 presents research outcomes of components of the Mediterranean diet. Recent data of two intervention studies, the MedDiet study and the DiMeSa project, are reviewed assessing the effects of the Mediterranean diet or its components on both plasma and urine biomarkers (see Box 13.1).

Many bioactive dietary components have been implicated as promoting or protective factors in cancer development.[59] Examples of food components reported to have cancer-preventive potential include polyphenols, selenium, methyl group donors, retinoids, isothiocyanates, allyl compounds, and mono- and poly-unsaturated fatty acids.[57] Although important cellular processes affected by nutrition include the cell cycle, the balance between cell proliferation and cell death (e.g., apoptosis); cell differentiation; oxidative stress and genes, including oncogenes and

tumor-suppressor genes; DNA damage and repair; cell signaling; cellular microenvironment that influences gene expression; hormonal regulation; carcinogen metabolism; and inflammation and immunity (Fig. 13.8), the epigenome is being implicated as a major target for nutrition-induced changes of gene expression and function (Fig. 13.9, *A*).[56,60] Emerging evidence is revealing epigenetic processes act in synergy with genetic changes during carcinogenesis and tumor progression.[61-63]

B vitamins, coenzymes in one-carbon metabolism (vitamins B_2, B_6, B_{12}), also are modulators of DNA methylation.[64] To date there are limited human studies of the effects of methyl donor supply on methylation of specific genomic sequences.[65] However, a study[66] found that periconceptional maternal supplementation with 400 micrograms (mcg) of folic acid per day was associated with increased methylation in offspring aged 17 months. Higher methylation levels were observed as being small for gestational age (SGA) compared to appropriate for gestational age (AGA) infants with maternal folic acid supplementation.[67] In the Waterland study, methylation effects were found to be similar in all tissues examined, suggesting that the mechanism may alter markings in stem cells early in embryogenesis before tissue differentiation, and persist into adult life.[23] Choline deficiency in pregnancy results in hypermethylation of genomic DNA and of the *IGF2* gene.[68] Several studies have reported that severe folate deficiency (which increases risk of hepatocellular cancer) induces hypomethylation of the *p53* tumor-suppressor gene.[69] Women with folate deficiency were 3.6 times more likely to display LINE-1 (interspersed genetic elements) hypomethylation than women with no folate deficiency. A dietary pattern characterized by low fruit consumption and folate deficiency is associated with LINE-1 hypomethylation and with cancer risk.[70] In vitro studies have shown that several bioactive food components, including tea polyphenols and bioflavonoids, inhibit DNA methyltransferase-1 (DNMT-1)–mediated DNA methylation in a dose-dependent manner[71] (Fig. 13.9, *B*). Acetylation and deacetylation are mediated by enzyme histones (see Fig. 6.1), histone acetyl transferase (HAT), and histone deacetylation (HDAC). There is evidence for the epigenetic effects of organosulfur compounds from garlic and of isothiocyanates from cruciferous vegetables.[72,73] The chemopreventive effects of garlic may be attributed to the antiinflammatory properties of its sulfur-containing components, for example, diallyl disulfide (DADS).[73] Interest in resveratrol, a polyphenolic compound with antiinflammatory, antioxidant, and anticancer activities, is growing because of its demonstrable role from in vitro and animal studies as cardioprotective, neuroprotective, chemopreventive, and antiaging properties.[74] In an animal model, investigators gave resveratrol immediately after onset of sepsis and found it inhibited endoplasmic stress activated nuclear factor-κB in the kidney.[75] Examples of food sources of resveratrol include grapes, peanuts, mulberry, and cocoa. The epigenetic functions of resveratrol include DNA methyltransferase (DNMT) and histone deacetylase (HDAC) inhibition, and mRNA regulation.[76] Butyrate produced in the colon by bacterial fermentation of nonstarch polysaccharide (fiber), diallyl disulfide from garlic and other allium vegetables, and sulforaphane from cruciferous vegetables can act as histone deacetylase inhibitors to maintain DNA stability or modify transcription.[77]

MicroRNA (miRNA) expression in response to diet may be involved in several cancers.[77] Several dietary factors, including macronutrients (fat, protein, and alcohol) and micronutrients (folate and vitamin E), alter the expression of many miRNAs in animals and humans[65] (see Chapter 12). Investigators indicate for the first time that select dietary agents impact stem cell regulatory networks, somewhat, by modulating steady-state levels of miRNAs.[78]

Bioactive components have a profound effect on differentiation, and a major area of investigation is on the differentiation of cancer stem cells. Cancer stem cells have been isolated and identified in

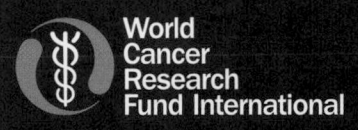
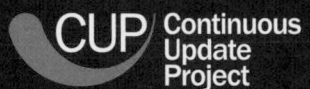
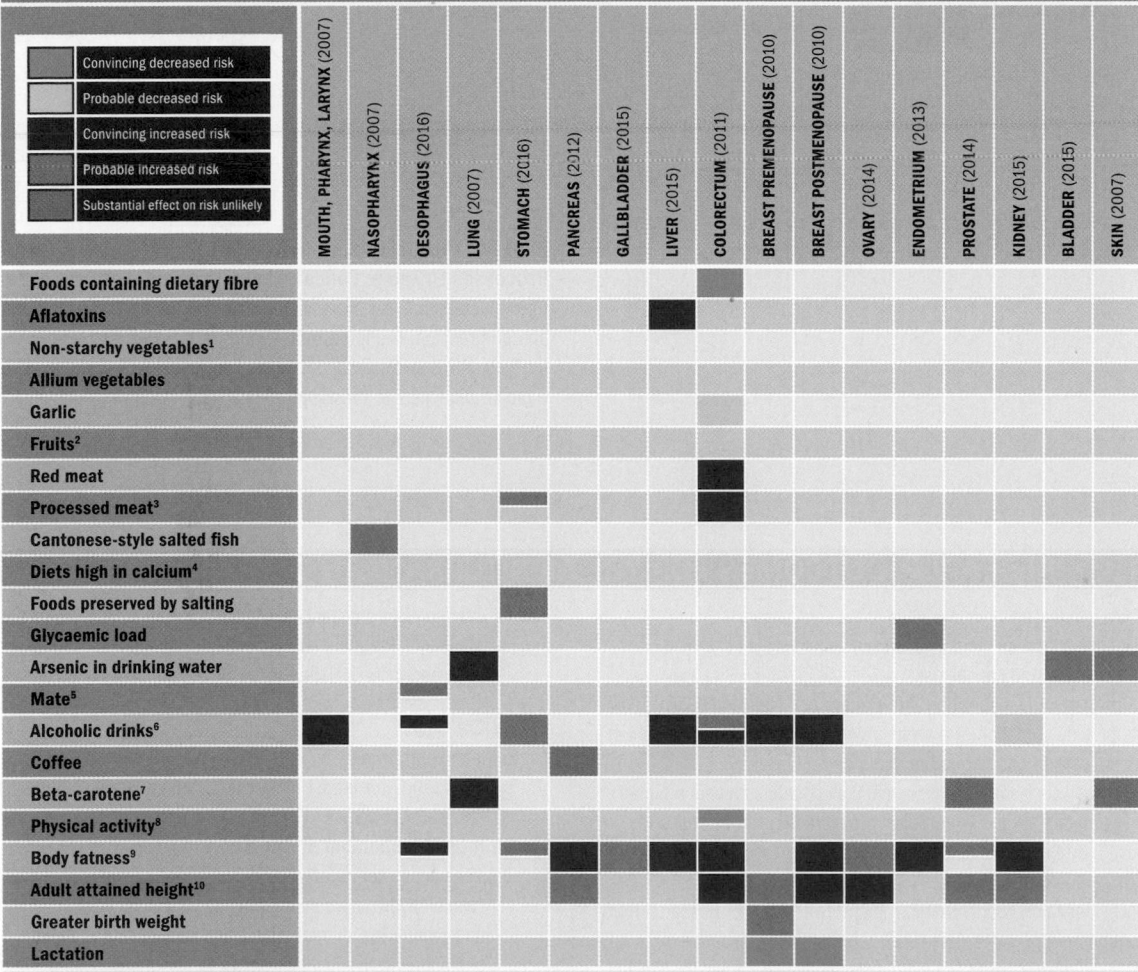

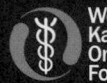
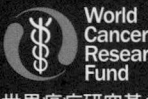

FIGURE 13.6 Summary of Strong Evidence on Diet, Nutrition, Physical Activity, and Prevention of Cancer. Evidence is presented as part of the Continuous Update Project (CUP), an ongoing program to analyze global research on how diet, nutrition, physical activity, and weight affect cancer risk and survival. Scientific research from around the world is collated and added to a database continuously reviewed by experts at the Imperial College London. The CUP database now contains 9037 publications on breast, colorectal, pancreatic, endometrial, ovarian, prostate, liver, gallbladder, kidney, bladder, and stomach cancers, as well as breast cancer survivors. (From Continuous Update Project [CUP]: London, April 2016, WCRF International.)

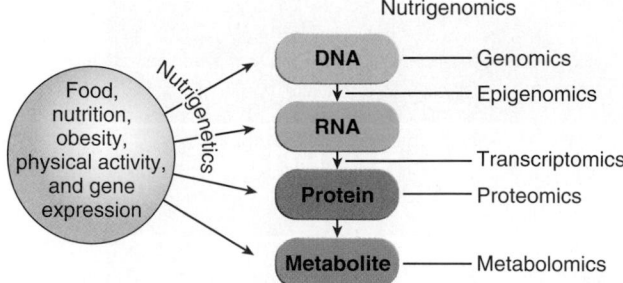

FIGURE 13.7 Basis for the Study of Food, Nutrition, Obesity, Physical Activity, and the Cancer Process. The genetic message in the DNA code is translated to RNA, and then into protein synthesis, and so determines metabolic processes. Research methods, called *"-omics,"* address these different stages. (Adapted from World Cancer Research Fund/American Institute for Cancer Research: *Food, nutrition, physical activity, and the prevention of cancer: a global perspective,* Washington, DC, 2007, AICR.)

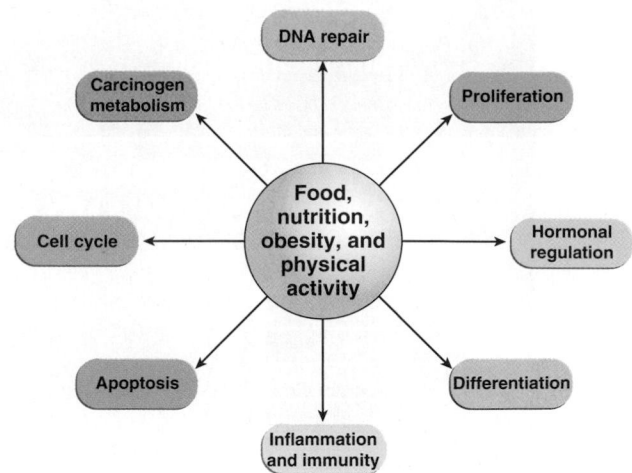

FIGURE 13.8 Food, Nutrition, Obesity, Physical Activity, and Cellular Processes Linked to Cancer. Food, nutrition, and physical activity can influence fundamental processes shown here, which may promote or inhibit cancer development and progression. (Adapted from World Cancer Research Fund/American Institute for Cancer Research: *Food, nutrition, physical activity, and the prevention of cancer: a global perspective,* Washington, DC, 2007, AICR.)

BOX 13.1 RESEARCH OUTCOMES FOR THE MEDITERRANEAN DIET AND CANCER

Fruits and Vegetables
Prospective cohort studies yield inconsistent results regarding fruit and vegetable intake and cancer risk.

European Prospective Investigation into Cancer and Nutrition (EPIC) cohorts provide evidence of a weak inverse association between high consumers of fruit and vegetable users and lower risk.

Recent meta-analysis from 16 prospective cohort studies reveal a higher consumption of fruit and vegetables correlated with a decrease in all-cause mortality, albeit, not with a significant reduction in cancer-related death.

World Cancer Research Fund/American Institute for Cancer Research from the Continuous Update Project (CUP) reports strong evidence of *probable decrease cancer risk* from nonstarchy vegetables for cancers (mouth, pharynx, larynx, esophagus) and for fruits *probable decreased cancer risk* for cancers (mouth, pharynx, larynx, esophagus, and lung). Data for fruits include evidence on foods containing carotenoids for mouth, pharynx, larynx and lung; foods containing beta-carotene for esophagus; foods containing vitamin C for esophagus.

Biologic Mechanism of Action: Antioxidant, antiinflammatory, antimutagenic, or antiproliferative.

Fish
Recent meta-analyses show inconsistent and inconclusive results.

Biologic Mechanism of Action: Antiinflammatory affects *n*-3 fatty acids.

Whole Grain
Whole grains and dietary fiber were inversely associated with risk of developing colorectal cancer in meta-analyses.

Intervention and observational studies showed dietary fiber is associated with reduced risk of insulin resistance.

Biologic Mechanism of Action: Enlargement of the bulk of stool leading to decreased transit time and decreasing impact of potential carcinogenic substances. Metabolizing of fiber to short-chain fatty acids by intestinal bacteria may prevent dedifferentiation of colonic cells and increase apoptosis.

Olive Oil
Epidemiologic studies on effects of olive oil showed decreased risks or odds ratios for breast cancer and cancers of the digestive system and respiratory tract.

Biologic Mechanism of Action: Extra-virgin olive oil is rich both in monounsaturated fatty acids and in polyphenolic compounds (e.g., tyrosol, hydroxytyrosol, oleuropein). Phenolic content of extra-virgin and virgin olive oil may affect oncogenes. It may exert chemopreventive effects, including direct antioxidant effects, cancer cell signaling, and cell cycle progression.

Alcohol and Red Wine in Moderate Amounts
Some observational studies showed light amounts of alcohol (<30 g of ethanol/day for men; <20 g of ethanol/day for women) with a focus on red wine to be associated with a reduced risk of cardiovascular disease.

Alcoholic beverages, however, ≥30 g of ethanol/day, are associated with increased risks of different cancers (e.g., pharynx, larynx, esophagus, colorectal, breast, and liver).

The effects of light alcohol drinking on cancer development and progression are controversial.

Biologic Mechanism of Action: Metabolism of alcohol converts ethanol to a highly reactive, toxic chemical called *acetaldehyde*. To prevent excessive increases in acetaldehyde, human cells contain three aldehyde dehydrogenase (ALDH) enzymes (ALDH1A1, ALDH2, and ALDH1B1) that can metabolize acetaldehyde into acetate. Inherited deficiency of the ALDH2 enzyme is present in approximately 36% of ethnic Japanese, Chinese, and Koreans. The deficiency is linked to facial flushing and, more recently, to squamous cell

---

BOX 13.1   RESEARCH OUTCOMES FOR THE MEDITERRANEAN DIET AND CANCER—cont'd

esophageal cancer. The ALDH enzymes can be overwhelmed by high quantities of alcohol, causing acetaldehyde to increase. This can lead to DNA mutations that can eventually lead to cancer.

Red and Processed Meat

Red and processed meats (sometimes poultry) are regarded to be unfavorable compounds. Meta-analyses link high consumption of meat or processed meat, or both, with an increased risk of cancer mortality. Meta-analyses of 21 observational studies showed high consumption of red/processed meat is associated with increased risk of colorectal adenomas.

Biologic Mechanism of Action: The exact mechanism is unknown but may be related to chemicals found in meat (heme, N-nitroso, iron?). Cooking meat at high temperatures, such as grilling or barbequing, can create chemical carcinogens.

Dairy Products

Controversial and contradictory results are reported with consumption of milk and dairy products and risk of cancer.

Two Experimental Intervention Studies: The MedDiet Study and the DiMeSa Project for the Mediterranean Diet
From the MedDiet Study Two Important Findings:

1. Both hydroxyl and methoxy estrogen derivatives account for the majority of endogenous estrogens in human urine. Urinary estrogen profiles are considered closer to intratissue estrogen content than respective plasma values (parent estrogens [E2, E1, E3] represent a limited fraction [5% to 8%] of total endogenous estrogens).

2. The traditional Mediterranean diet may reduce the risk of developing breast cancer through its effects on estrogen metabolism, whereby hydroxylation of E2, a process that leads to the formation of genotoxic metabolites, was strongly decreased in the intervention group (e.g., controlled Mediterranean diet) and unchanged in the control group.

From the DiMeSa Project: Primary Prevention

Only preliminary data are currently available.

The randomized intervention is a clinical trial to test the assessment of the health impact of extra-virgin olive oil (EVO) on two cohorts of study subjects: healthy postmenopausal women and those with breast cancer. Two different EVOs were used: one at lower (BL) and one at higher (CS) polyphenols and oleocanthal.

Preliminary data reveal consumption of BL EVO resulted in significant changes of various biomarkers in plasma in both healthy subjects and breast cancer subjects. These biomarkers included reduction of glycemia, insulinemia, and total cholesterol.

Consumption of CS EVO changes included a significant increase of high density lipoprotein (HDL) cholesterol, a reduction of low density lipoprotein (LDL) cholesterol, and a reduction of plasma levels of estradiol.

Under current analysis are results of gene expression, microRNA profiling, and patterns of urinary sex steroids.

Limitations of Research

Mediterranean diet (MD) is a complex food pattern.
Methodologic issues are needed to identify adherence to MD.

Data from Andrici J, Hu SX, Eslick GD: *Cancer Epidemiol* 40:31–38, 2016; Arts IC, Hollman PC: *Am J Clin Nutr* 81(1 Suppl):317S–325S, 2005; Aune D et al: *BMJ* 343:d6617, 2011; Bagnardi V et al: *Ann Oncol* 24(2):301–308, 2013; Benetou V et al: *Cancer Epidemiol Biomarkers Prev* 17(2):387–392, 2008; Boffetta P et al: *J Natl Cancer Inst* 102(8):529–537, 2010; Brooks PJ et al: *PLoS Med* 6(3):e50, 2009; Carruba G, et al: *Immun Ageing* 13:13, 2016; Corona G, Spencer JP, Dessi MA: *Toxicol Ind Health* 25(4–5):285–293, 2009; Haas P et al: *Int J Food Sci Nutr* 60(s6):1–13, 2009; Han YJ et al: *Eur J Clin Nutr* 67(2):147–154, 2013; Jin M et al: *Ann Oncol* 24(3):807–816, 2013; O'Sullivan TA et al: *Am J Public Health* 103(9):e31–e42, 2013; Schwingshackl L, Hoffmann G: *Ann Intern Med* 161(6):455–456, 2014; Schwingshackl L, Hoffmann G: *Lipids Health Dis* 13:154, 2014; Sotiroudis TG, Kyrtopoulos SA: *Eur J Nutr* 47(Suppl 2):69–72, 2008; Williams MT, Hord NG: *Nutr Clin Pract* 20(4):451–459, 2005; World Cancer Research Fund (WCFR)/American Institute for Cancer Research (AICR): *Food, nutrition, physical activity, and the prevention of cancer: a global perspective,* Washington, DC, 2007, AICR; WCRF/AICR Continuous Update Project: *Diet, Nutrition, Physical Activity and Esophageal Cancer,* 2016; Xu X et al: *Int J Cancer* 132(2):437–448, 2013; Zheng J-S et al: *BJM* 346:f3705, 2013.

---

hematopoietic and epithelial cancers, including cancers of the brain, breast, ovary, prostate, colon, and stomach.[77,79] Although still mysterious biologically, stem cells are found among most adult tissues, where they maintain and regenerate tissues. Stem cells are capable of both self-renewal and differentiation to generate functional tissue.[80] The balance between self-renewal and differentiation is critical to understand not only normal development but also disruption of normal development, which can lead to cancer.[80] Musashi (named after samurai Miyamoto Musashi), a family of RNA-binding proteins discovered originally in *Drosophila*, has arisen as a key signal that allows and protects the stem cell state across organisms.[80] Emerging evidence shows that RNA-binding proteins (RBPs) play important roles in the regulation of self-renewal by assisting metabolism of coding and non–coding RNAs in normal tissue and cancers.[81] The ways in which all of these processes are influenced by bioactive components need much study. Evidence from both drug and bioactive food constituents shows modifications in cancer stem cell self-renewal capabilities; for example, retinoic acid may promote differentiation of breast cancer stem cells.[82] Adequate consumption of specific food compounds, including vitamins A and D, genistein, green tea, epigallocatechin gallate (EGCG), sulforaphane, theanine, curcumin,

choline, and possibly many others, may suppress cancer stem renewal.[79,83] Uncontrolled self-renewal process may be initiated by abnormal developmental signals that come from the extracellular microenvironment known as "niches." The loss of regulation in self-renewal signals, including Wnt, Notch, and hedgehog pathways, is a characteristic of cancer stem cells.[79] Various food bioactive components can modulate the signaling pathway.

A variety of food constituents may influence DNA repair[77] (Fig. 13.10). Investigators demonstrate that certain miRNAs have a role in the interplay among the DNA damage response and bioactive compounds, including epigallocatechin-3-gallate, curcumin, resveratrol, and n3-polyunsaturated fatty acids.[84] In vivo studies have demonstrated that healthy adults consuming kiwi fruits, cooked carrots, or supplemental coenzyme Q_{10} improved their DNA repair.[77]

Humans are constantly exposed to a variety of compounds termed **xenobiotics** (Greek *xenos,* "foreign"; *bios,* "life") that include toxic, mutagenic, and carcinogenic chemicals. Many of these chemicals are found in the human diet. Most xenobiotics are transported in the blood by lipoproteins and penetrate lipid membranes. These chemicals can react with cellular macromolecules, such as proteins and DNA, or can

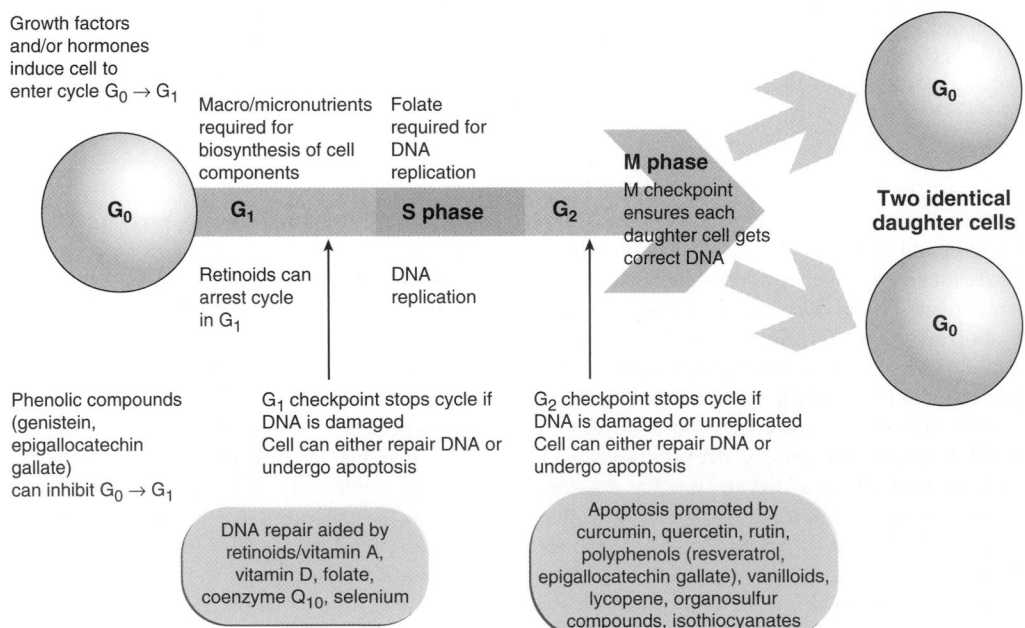

FIGURE 13.9 Dietary Components as Epigenetic-Regulating Agents and DNA Methylation and Cancer. **A,** Epigenetics and gene transcriptional regulation together create a microenvironment for cancer development with alterations in cell proliferation, differentiation, metabolism, DNA repair, and movement. The main epigenetic modifications regulated by dietary components include DNA methylation, histone modifications (acetylation/deacetylation, methylation/demethylation), and microRNAs. DNA methylation and histone modifications can alter chromatin structure and microRNAs can degrade mRNA and affect the translation process. Data are needed on these processes, as well as the potential synergistic effects of dietary components, to revert chemotherapy resistance, side effects from chemotherapy, and increase chemotherapy sensitivity. **B,** Certain dietary factors (see Table 13.5) may supply methyl groups ($+CH_3$) that can be donated through *S*-adenosylmethionine *(SAM)* to many acceptors in the cell (DNA, proteins, lipids, and metabolites). Donation and removal (demethylation) are affected by numerous enzymes, including DNA methyltransferase *(DNMT)*. Increased DNMT activity occurs in many tumor cells. Hypermethylation can inhibit or silence tumor-suppressor genes (see Chapter 12), and DNA methylation inhibitors as anticancer agents can block DNMT activity, thus reactivating tumor-suppressor genes. DNA hypomethylation can reactivate and mutate genes, including cancer-causing oncogenes. *CpG,* Cytosine guanine nucleotide; *HATs,* histone acetyltransferases; *HDACs,* histone deacetylases; *HMTs,* histone methyltransferases; *SAH, S*-adenosylhomocysteine. (**A** adapted from Chang L, Yu Y: *BioMedicine* 6910:9–16, 2016.)

FIGURE 13.10 Cell Cycle and Nutrition Regulation. Nutrition may influence the regulation of the normal cell cycle, which ensures correct DNA replication. G_0 represents the resting phase, G_1 the growth and preparation of the chromosome for replication, S the synthesis of DNA, G_2 the preparation of the cell for division, and M mitosis. (Adapted from World Cancer Research Fund/American Institute for Cancer Research: *Food, nutrition, physical activity, and the prevention of cancer: a global perspective,* Washington, DC, 2007, AICR.)

react directly with cell structures to cause cell damage.[85] The body has two main defense systems for counteracting these effects: (1) detoxification enzymes and (2) antioxidant systems (see Chapter 2). Enzymes that activate xenobiotics are called phase I activation enzymes and are represented by the multigene cytochrome P-450 family, aldehyde oxidase, xanthine oxidases, and peroxidases. Phase II detoxification enzymes then protect further against a large array of reactive intermediates and nonactivated xenobiotics.[77] These enzymes are located predominantly in the liver and provide clearance of compounds through the portal circulation, thereby preventing the potentially carcinogenic agent(s) from entering the body through the gastrointestinal tract and portal circulation. They also occur in the skin epithelia and can be induced in other extrahepatic tissue, such as the lung. They represent a potential target to influence carcinogen metabolism. Isothiocyanates from cruciferous vegetables induce the expression of phase II detoxification enzymes. Food and nutrition modify carcinogen metabolism and may modify carcinogenesis. Some examples include selenium, allyl sulfur, sulforaphane, and isoflavonoids. The enzyme CYP3A4 is involved in the metabolism of many drugs and is sensitive to foods.[77] For example, interactions have been reported for grapefruit juice, red wine, garlic, and drugs.

Glutathione-S-transferases (GSTs) are enzyme housekeepers involved in the metabolism of environmental carcinogens and reactive oxygen species. Individuals who lack these enzymes may be at higher risk for cancers because of decreased capacity to dispose of activated carcinogens. For example, the fungi that produce aflatoxins can grow on certain crops, such as peanuts and some cereal (e.g., grains). Aflatoxins are carcinogens activated by phase I enzymes in the liver that can produce DNA adducts. Individuals lacking these enzymes are at higher risk of colon cancer. Diets high in isothiocyanates (from cruciferous vegetables) may decrease this risk.[86]

Individuals who consume diets high in red meat and processed meat have an increased risk of developing colorectal cancer.[77,87,88] Processed meats include those preserved by preservatives or by smoking, curing, or salting. The IARC has classified processed meat as a carcinogen and red meat as a probable carcinogen.[89] The European Prospective Investigation into Cancer and Nutrition (EPIC) study, which included 478,040 people from 10 countries, reports that the most convincing data are from meats, including sausages, bratwursts, frankfurters, and hot dogs, all of which have nitrites, nitrates, or other preservatives. Potential mechanisms of how processed meat/red meat may increase cancer include the concepts that (1) red meat contains the heme form of iron, which may cause alterations of the lining of the colon; (2) red meat stimulates the production of N-nitroso compounds, which can increase nitrogenous residues in the colon and cause DNA damage; and (3) cooking meat at high temperatures (e.g., grilling) produces two cancer promoters: heterocyclic amines (HCAs) and polycyclic aromatic hydrocarbons (PAHs). Certain single-nucleotide polymorphisms (SNPs) in the N-acetyltransferase gene alter the activity of the enzyme involved in the activation of heterocyclic amines from cooking meat at high temperatures and may increase the risk of colon cancer.[77] Other foods that alter the metabolism of carcinogens and induce GSTs include cruciferous vegetables, especially brussels sprouts and red cabbage. Red cabbage leads to changes in meat-derived mutagens in urine.[77] Flavonoids found in plants may alter carcinogen metabolism.

Chronic inflammation and immune function may help explain patterns of cancer around the world. Chronic inflammation assists cancer initiation, progression, and dissemination.[90] People who are undernourished or live in poverty may have impaired immune status, which can be a factor in cancers caused by infectious agents, for example, cancers of the liver and cervix.[77] Undernutrition can include deficiencies in vitamin A, riboflavin, vitamin B_{12}, folic acid,

vitamin C, selenium, and zinc, and these nutrient deficiencies may be related to chronic inflammation and immune alterations.[77] The cytokine interleukin-6 (IL-6) can act as either a proinflammatory or an antiinflammatory cytokine; consequently, it can enhance both innate and adaptive immunity as well as stimulate or suppress tumor growth (see Chapter 12).

In summary, epidemiologic and laboratory evidence suggests that diet has important consequences for cancer development and perhaps its rate of progression. Diet affects many pathways to cancer including cell cycle control, differentiation, DNA repair, gene silencing, inflammation, apoptosis, and carcinogen metabolism. Many of these processes are likely influenced, if not regulated, by DNA methylation, an epigenetic mechanism that affects gene function. As illustrated in Fig. 13.2, it is possible that many environmental factors interact with the genome to produce altered epigenetic markers that change the expression of cancer-causing genes, tumor-suppressor genes, and oncogenes. Future research is needed to define robust biomarkers of cancer risk.

Obesity

Obesity in most developed countries (and in urban areas of many developing countries) has been increasing rapidly over the past 20 years. Obesity in the United States is an epidemic and constitutes a startling setback to major improvements in other areas of health during the past century.[91] Childhood obesity also is increasing and disproportionately affects children from low-income families.[92] Numerous health conditions are linked to obesity and physical inactivity. The substantial suffering and long-term human and societal costs of obesity underlie the urgency to accelerate progress in obesity prevention.[91] This will require a comprehensive approach including the involvement of knowledgeable healthcare personnel, the provision of appropriate education from schools, the access to healthy food and beverage choices, and the promotion of physical activity.

Studies have significantly improved the understanding of the relationship between overweight/obesity, energy balance and cancer risk, cancer recurrence, and survival (see Fig. E 13.1 on Evolve). Being overweight or obese, measured using the body mass index (BMI), is linked to an increased risk of developing 11 cancers: liver, advanced prostate, ovarian, gallbladder, kidney, colorectal, esophageal (adenocarcinoma), postmenopausal breast, pancreatic, endometrial, and stomach (cardia) (Fig. 13.11).

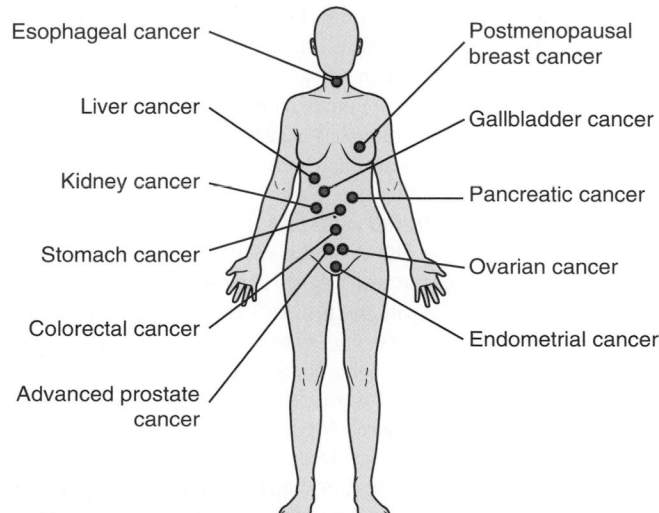

FIGURE 13.11 Overweight and Obesity and Increased Risk for 11 Cancers. (From World Cancer Research Fund [WCRF]: *International weight & cancer continuous update project*, London, 2016, WCRF International.)

TABLE 13.4	WORLD HEALTH ORGANIZATION CLASSIFICATION OF BODY MASS INDEX	
BMI (kg/mm²)*	WHO CLASSIFICATION	OTHER DESCRIPTIONS
<18.5	Underweight	Thin
18.5–24.9	Normal range	"Healthy," "normal," or "acceptable" weight
25–29.9	Grade 1 overweight	Overweight
30–39.9	Grade 2 overweight	Obese
≥40	Grade 3 overweight	Morbidly overweight

*The cutoffs are somewhat arbitrary, although they are derived from epidemiologic studies of body mass index (BMI) and overall mortality. It is important to understand that within each category of BMI there can be substantial individual variation in total and visceral adiposity and in related metabolic factors. These variations are also true for the normal range BMI.

The IARC identified additional cancers with sufficient evidence that the absence of body fatness lowers cancer risk for thyroid and multiple myeloma.[93] Importantly, obesity is recognized as a poor prognostic factor for several cancers.[94,95]

The only globally accepted criteria for overweightness and obesity are based on BMI. Widely accepted standards based on BMI criteria for overweightness and obesity are recommended by the WHO[96,97] and supported by other panels and federal agencies (WHO classifications are shown in Table 13.4).

Worldwide estimates suggest that 2 billion adults are overweight (BMI ≥25 to 29.9 kg/m²) and 500 million are obese (BMI ≥30 kg/m²).[98] The prevalence of overweight and obesity was highest in the WHO regions of the Americas (61% for overweight in both sexes, and 27% for obesity) and lowest in the WHO region for South East Asia (22% overweight in both sexes and 5% for obesity).[98] More than 50% of women in the WHO region of the Americas and European and Eastern Mediterranean regions were overweight. In all three of these regions, nearly half of overweight women were obese (25% in Europe, 24% in the Eastern Mediterranean, 30% in the Americas). In all WHO regions, women were more likely to be obese than men. In the WHO African, Eastern Mediterranean, and South East Asia regions, women had approximately double the obesity prevalence of men.[98] In 2014, 41 million children less than 5 years of age in the world were overweight, approximately 10 million more than two decades earlier.[98] Globally, the prevalence of overweight children has increased between 1990 and 2014 from 4.8% to 6.1%. This disturbing rise is occurring across all income groups and in all regions.[98]

Mechanisms Associated with Energy Balance and Obesity.

The Institute of Medicine (IOM) and National Cancer Policy Forum convened to discuss mechanisms of obesity and cancer, cancer recurrence and mortality, research needs, and future directions.[99] A simple model based on energy balance and energy expenditure was utilized. Energy balance measures intake-absorbable energy against the energy demands of the body. Energy expenditure is comprised of (1) the resting metabolic rate (RMR), the energy required for normal body functions, which constitutes the majority of energy needs; (2) the thermic effect of food, or the amount of energy needed to digest and metabolize food; and (3) physical activity, a moderate and modifiable part of energy expenditure. This model does not include body composition (i.e., lean tissue, adipose tissue) or the dynamic state of body composition. Because lean mass determines resting metabolic rate, it is unknown whether obesity

WHAT'S NEW?

Insulin, Insulin Receptor, Insulin-Like Growth Factors, and Cancer

Investigators are studying the growth-promoting effect of insulin, the insulin receptor (IR), insulin-related growth factors (insulin-like growth factor 1 [IGF-1] and IGF-2), hyperinsulinemia, insulin resistance, hyperglycemia, and diabetes as factors that interfere with the host and the malignant cell responses. These factors are all important for the obese individual and cancer because insulin resistance and hyperinsulinemia are metabolic abnormalities of most obese individuals. Known for years is that cancer cells require insulin for optimal in vitro growth. Recent data indicate that (1) insulin stimulates growth mainly through its own IR and not the IGF-1 receptor and (2) the IR is overexpressed in many cancer cells and the A isoform is more predominant than the B isoform. The IR-A isoform has a major mitogenic effect that can cause proliferation. Altogether, these factors promote a growth advantage to malignant cells when exposed to insulin. IR overexpression has been found in neoplastic cells but not in stromal adipocytes and inflammatory cells. Increased IR content has been found in breast, colon, lung, ovary, and thyroid carcinomas

All conditions of hyperinsulinemia, both endogenous (prediabetes, metabolic syndrome, obesity, type 2 diabetes before pancreas exhaustion, and polycystic ovary syndrome) and exogenous (the requirement for exogenous insulin [type 1 diabetes]), will increase the risk of cancer. Cancer-related mortality is increased in individuals exposed to hyperinsulinemia; however, other factors related to different diseases also may contribute. Hyperinsulinemia is often associated with hyperglycemia. Cancer cells have an abnormal metabolism and, compared to normal cells, mainly rely on aerobic glycolysis for energy needed for accelerated growth (Warburg effect). To satisfy this increased energy requirement cancer cells need more sugar ("sugar fuels cancer").

Currently, it is difficult to determine from human data if the diabetic state and which specific mechanism of diabetes may affect fructose absorption in humans. Dietary fructose intake has increased dramatically and recent studies suggest that glucose homeostasis and fructose absorption interact. Using mouse studies, investigators found fructose derived from sucrose facilitated lung metastasis from breast tumors through inflammation. Given the potential importance of fructose metabolism worldwide, more investigation into this subject is needed.

Data from Dotimas JR et al: *eLife* 5:e18313, 2016; Jiang Y et al: *Cancer Res* 76(1):24–29, 2016; Vigneri R, Goldfine ID, Frittitta L: *J Endocrinol Invest* 39(12):1365–1376, 2016.

itself drives cancer progression or whether components of energy balance (i.e., too much consumed or too little expended) have a greater impact, and therefore it is uncertain which factors hold more promise for cancer control and prevention.[100]

The mechanisms of obesity-associated cancer risks are unclear and may vary by type of tumor and distribution of body fat. Emerging, however, are three main factors related to obesity and cancer: (1) the insulin–insulin-like growth factor axis (see *What's New: Insulin, Insulin Receptor, Insulin-like Growth Factors, and Cancer*), (2) sex hormones, and (3) adipokines or adipocyte-derived cytokines.[101] These three factors are linked to metabolic dysregulation of adipose tissue and endocrine and paracrine altered signaling of adipose tissue in obesity.[101,102] The factors strongly implicated include insulin, insulin-like growth factor 1 (IGF-1) more than IGF-2, leptin, adiponectin, and IL-6. Metabolic changes in adipose tissue from obesity result in several alterations and include insulin resistance, hyperglycemia, dyslipidemia, hypoxia, and chronic inflammation.[101,103]

Emerging is a newer focus also on the consequences of local adipose inflammation.[104,105] Obesity-associated lipolysis releases saturated fatty acids that induce activation of macrophages and stimulate NF-κB signaling. This signaling activates transcription of proinflammatory genes, including *cyclooxygenase-2,* IL-6, IL-1β, and tumor necrosis factor-alpha (TNF-α); altogether, the elevated levels of proinflammatory mediators cause both local and systemic effects.[104] With breast cancer, for example, the increased transcription of the *CYP19* gene encodes aromatase, an enzyme for estrogen synthesis.[104] Animal studies of pancreatic ductal adenocarcinoma reveal obesity is a *pro-desmoplastic* (insult leading to ECM alterations including dense, fibrosis changes) condition.[105] Obesity leads to adipocyte dysfunction and immune cell recruitment, leading to cytokine production, inflammation, and, ultimately, fibrosis and reduced response to chemotherapy.[105] Because tumor growth is regulated by interactions between tumor cells and their tissue microenvironment or stromal compartments that are rich in adipose tissue, adipocytes function as endocrine cells and critically shape the tumor microenvironment. Dysfunctional adipose tissue can create altered signaling pathways that involve proinflammatory mediators, macrophages, and cancer-associated fibroblasts. All of these cells are tumor-promoting cell types and, with insulin resistance and hypoxia, can trigger compensatory angiogenesis and an energy reservoir for the embedded cancer cells.[101] The cancer-associated adipocytes (CAAs) undergo both structural and functional alterations during cancer progression that altogether create an environment toward increased cancer invasiveness and aggression[101] (Fig. 13.12).

Adipose tissue can have greater effects on the physiology of other tissue (see Chapter 23). The metabolic function of adipose tissue is derived in part because it can secrete many proteins, collectively called **adipokines**.[106] The adipokine leptin enhances the production of inflammatory factors and TNF-α.[100] These inflammatory factors also are modulated by sex hormones (e.g., estradiol and testosterone) and growth factors, especially vascular endothelial growth factor (VEGF). Importantly, increased adiposity is correlated with *lower* levels of adiponectin that normally induce apoptosis, thus increasing cell proliferation.[100] Lower levels of adiponectin also give rise to insulin resistance and to compensatory hyperinsulinemia. Adipokines have both proinflammatory and antiinflammatory activities and their balance can contribute to the initiation and progression of obesity-induced metabolic changes that can affect other organs (including the brain, heart, vasculature, liver, and muscle) and increase the risk of cancer, cardiovascular disease, and metabolic disturbances.[106]

Studies have linked levels of circulating free hormones (e.g., estradiol) and hormonally driven cancers as an important mechanism (Chapters 22, 25, and 26 contain discussions on hormones and cancer risk). Obesity can increase aromatase expression, resulting in increased estradiol levels, which can promote the growth of estrogen-dependent cancers (e.g., breast and endometrial cancers).

Cancers have altered metabolism. Normal tissues use oxidative phosphorylation (OXPHOS) to convert glucose into CO_2 and energy (i.e., ATP). Even with adequate oxygen, cancer cells may not use OXPHOS, but are reprogrammed to glycolysis or the *Warburg effect* (see Chapter 12).

Recent studies reveal a link between glucose availability and protein acetylation, an epigenetic change.[107] Importantly, in the context of constant glucose levels, metabolite levels seem to oscillate in a circadian way within cells and tissues.[107] Food metabolism and circadian cycles are linked, and impairment of clock regulation (e.g., disrupted night sleep and light; shift work) results in dysregulated metabolism.[108] **Circadian rhythms** pervade mammalian biology (Fig. 13.13). They manifest and permeate temporal organization in behavioral, physiologic, cellular, and neuronal processes.[109,110] This ancient timekeeper interacts with multiple cell systems, including signaling mechanisms, and the cell cycle, thus impacting disease. Evidence is emerging that circadian mechanisms are linked to cell proliferation and its control at the DNA

(epigenetic), RNA, and protein levels. Circadian disruption accelerates malignant growth.[110,111] In addition to nutrient levels oscillating metabolically, circadian rhythms appear to affect detoxification cycles.[108,110] Mutations in internal clock genes alter glucose and lipid metabolism and affect the function of the kidney.[112]

The survivorship literature is growing and data suggest that increasing BMI is related to less favorable outcomes for recurrence, survival, and comorbidities (e.g., cardiovascular disease, diabetes, wound healing).[100] Researchers have documented the development of obesity and diabetes mellitus in aging survivors of childhood cancer, as well as other endocrine disturbances.[113]

Alcohol Consumption

Alcohol is classified by the International Agency for Cancer Research (IACR) as a human carcinogen. Alcohol plays a contributory role in several common cancers. Overall, there are convincing data that alcohol increases the risk of cancer of the mouth, pharynx, larynx, esophagus, liver, and pre- and postmenopausal breast cancer in women and colorectal cancer in men (possibly also in women) (Table 13.5).[114,115] The evidence does not show any "safe limit" of intake, and the effect is from ethanol regardless of the type of drink.[77] Modifiable causes of premature death (before the age of 70) in middle-aged persons in Western Europe included smoking, poor diet, overweight and obesity, hypertension, physical inactivity, and excessive alcohol consumption.[116]

Several factors contribute to alcohol-induced cancer development, including acetaldehyde, oxidative stress, and nutritional deficiencies, especially folate, a B vitamin (see Chapter 2). Variations in several genes modulate the risk of alcohol-induced carcinogenesis. New data suggest that the *ADH1B* gene *ARG47His* variant was associated with a decreased risk of esophageal cancer.[117] Increasing evidence suggests aberrant patterns of DNA methylation are part of the alcohol-induced mechanisms of carcinogenesis.[118] The molecular actions of ethanol are believed to include site-specific changes to histone modifications and alterations of one-carbon metabolism causing methylation changes.[107] MicroRNA expression has been linked to alcohol consumption in a case-controlled study of head and neck cancer (i.e., head and neck squamous cell carcinoma [HNSCC]).[119] The risk may be modified by alcohol dehydrogenase genes.[120] Alcohol interacts with smoke, increasing the risk of malignant tumors including lung cancer, possibly by acting as a solvent for the carcinogenic chemicals in smoke products.

Physical Activity

Studies suggest that regular exercise decreases the risk of breast cancer, colon cancer, and endometrial cancer, independent of weight changes. The World Cancer Research Fund summarized the effects as *convincing* for cancers of the colorectal and *probable* for postmenopausal breast cancer and endometrial cancer[77,121] (Table 13.6). Annual deaths attributable to physical inactivity are reported between 3.2 and 5.3 million deaths per year.[122,123] Investigators confirm irrefutable evidence of the effectiveness of regular physical activity in the primary and secondary prevention of several chronic diseases, including cardiovascular disease, hypertension, diabetes, cancer, obesity, depression, osteoporosis, and premature death.[124]

Several biologic mechanisms suggest physical activity may protect against cancers of the breast and endometrium, by decreasing insulin and IGF levels, decreasing obesity, altering inflammatory mediators, decreasing oncogenes, decreasing levels of circulating sex hormones and metabolic hormones, improving immune function, and enhancing cytochrome P-450 activity, thus modifying carcinogen activation. A new mechanism from exercise is the release of **myokines** or proteins from contracting muscles and their antitumor effects (see *What's New? Exercise and Anticancer Effects of Myokines*).

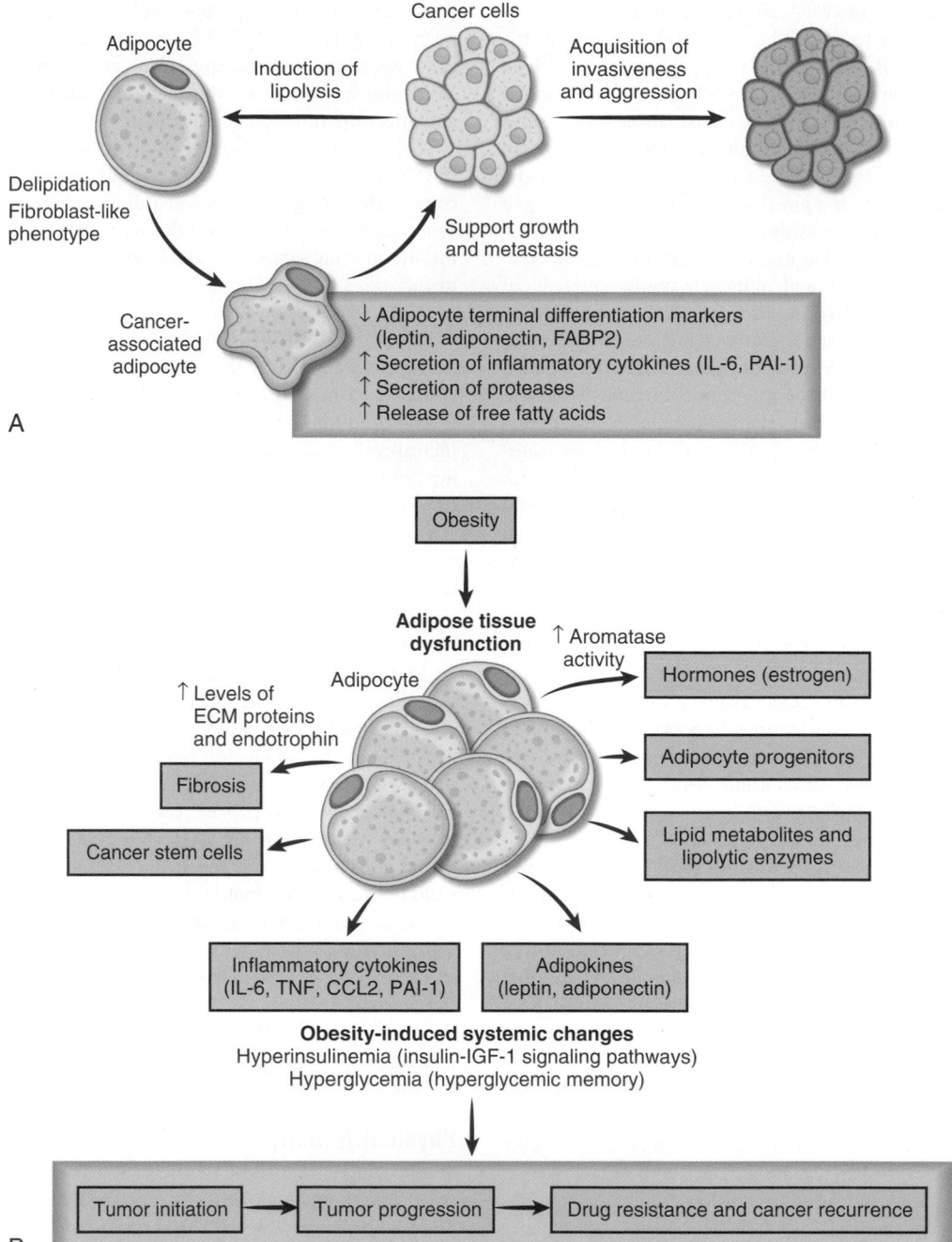

FIGURE 13.12 Structural and Functional Changes in Adipocytes and Interaction with the Microenvironment Contribute to Cancer Progression and Metastases: A Working Model. **A,** Signaling interactions occur between cancer cells and cancer-associated adipocytes. This interaction within the tumor microenvironment creates a place or *niche* permissive for cancer growth. Cancer cells stimulate the breakdown of lipids in adipocytes, leading to *delipidation* and the emergence of a fibroblast-like phenotype in adipocytes. The continuing alterations are associated with functional changes in the cells and include increased secretion of inflammatory mediators (cytokines) and proteases, and increased release of free fatty acids. All of these changes can support tumor growth and invasiveness. **B,** Obesity leads to excessive levels of proinflammatory cytokines, sex hormones, lipid metabolites, and altered adipokines. The altered adipose tissue becomes a source of various extracellular matrix proteins, cancer stem cells, and cancer-associated adipokines. Collectively these alterations contribute to tumor initiation, growth, and recurrence. The systemic metabolic changes of obesity—hyperinsulinemia and hyperglycemia—can further contribute to a tumor-permissive environment. *CCL2,* chemokine ligand 2; *ECM,* extracellular matrix; *FABP2,* fatty acid-binding protein 2; *IGF,* insulin-like growth factor; *IL,* interleukin; *TNF,* tumor necrosis factor. (Adapted from Park J et al: *Nat Rev Endocrinol* 10[8]:455–465, 2014.)

TABLE 13.5   ALCOHOLIC DRINKS AND RISK OF CANCER*

	DECREASES RISK		INCREASES RISK	
	EXPOSURE	CANCER SITE	EXPOSURE	CANCER SITE
Convincing			Alcoholic drinks	Mouth, pharynx and larynx, esophagus Colorectum (men)† Breast (pre- and postmenopause)
Probable			Alcoholic drinks	Liver‡ Colorectum (women)†
Limited—suggestive				
Substantial effect on risk unlikely	Alcoholic drinks (adverse effect): kidney§			

*In the judgment of the World Cancer Research Fund/American Institute for Cancer Research Panel, the factors listed modify the risk of cancer. Judgments are graded according to the strength of the evidence.
†The judgments for men and women are different because there are fewer data for women. Increased risk is only apparent above a threshold of 30 g/day of ethanol for both genders.
‡Cirrhosis is an essential precursor of liver cancer caused by alcohol. The International Agency for Research on Cancer has graded alcohol as a class 1 carcinogen for liver cancer. Alcohol alone only causes cirrhosis in the presence of other factors.
§The evidence was sufficient to judge that alcoholic drinks are unlikely to have an adverse effect on the risk of kidney cancer; it was inadequate to draw a conclusion regarding the protective effect.
Adapted from World Cancer Research Fund/American Institute for Cancer Research (WCRF/AICR): *Second expert report: food, nutrition, physical activity, and the prevention of cancer: a global perspective*, London, 2007, Author.

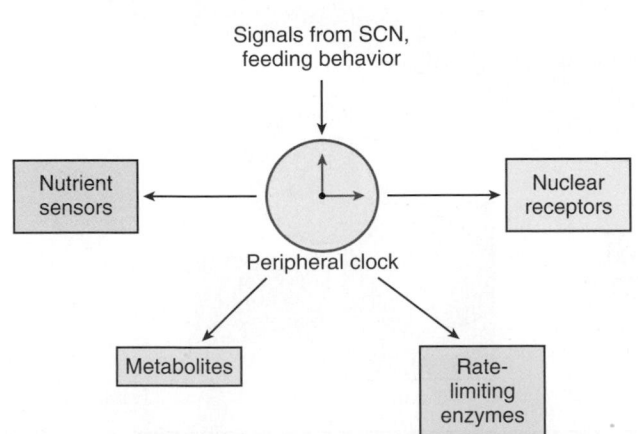

FIGURE 13.13 Regulation of Metabolism by the Circadian Clock. Peripheral clocks, such as that in the liver, are regulated by the master clock present in the suprachiasmatic nucleus *(SCN)*. The liver clock can regulate multiple metabolic pathways by various mechanisms. These mechanisms include regulation of rate-limiting steps, control of metabolite levels, interaction of nutrient sensors, and modulation of nuclear sensors. (Adapted from Sahar S, Sassone-Corsi P: *Trends Endocrinol Metab* 23[1]:1–8, 2011.)

TABLE 13.6   PHYSICAL ACTIVITY AND RISK OF CANCER*,†

	DECREASES RISK	INCREASES RISK
Convincing	Colon‡	
Probable	Breast (postmenopausal)	
	Endometrium	
Limited—suggestive	Lung	
	Pancreas	
	Breast (premenopausal)	
Substantial effect on risk unlikely	None identified	

*In the judgment of the World Cancer Research Fund/American Institute for Cancer Research Panel, physical activity† modifies the risk of the cancers. Judgments are graded according to the strength of the evidence.
†Physical activity of all types: occupational, household, transport, and recreational.
‡Much of the evidence grouped colon cancer and rectal cancer together categorized as "colorectal cancer." The Panel judges that the evidence is stronger for colon cancer than for rectal cancer.
Adapted from World Cancer Research Fund/American Institute for Cancer Research (WCRF/AICR): *Second expert report: food, nutrition, physical activity, and the prevention of cancer: a global perspective*, London, 2007, Author.

WHAT'S NEW?

Exercise and Anticancer Effects of Myokines

A newer, exercise-induced anticancer mechanism in contracting muscle fibers (from exercise) releases proteins called *myokines* into the bloodstream, which have beneficial effects, such as increasing insulin sensitivity on many systems. Additionally, myokines can induce apoptosis in breast cancer and colon cancer cells. Other investigators found antitumorigenic effects of another myokine, IL-6, from working muscles and epinephrine from the adrenal glands that result in increased mobilization of NK cells that migrate into tumors and destroy tumor cells.

Continued

Exercise and Anticancer Effects of Myokines—cont'd

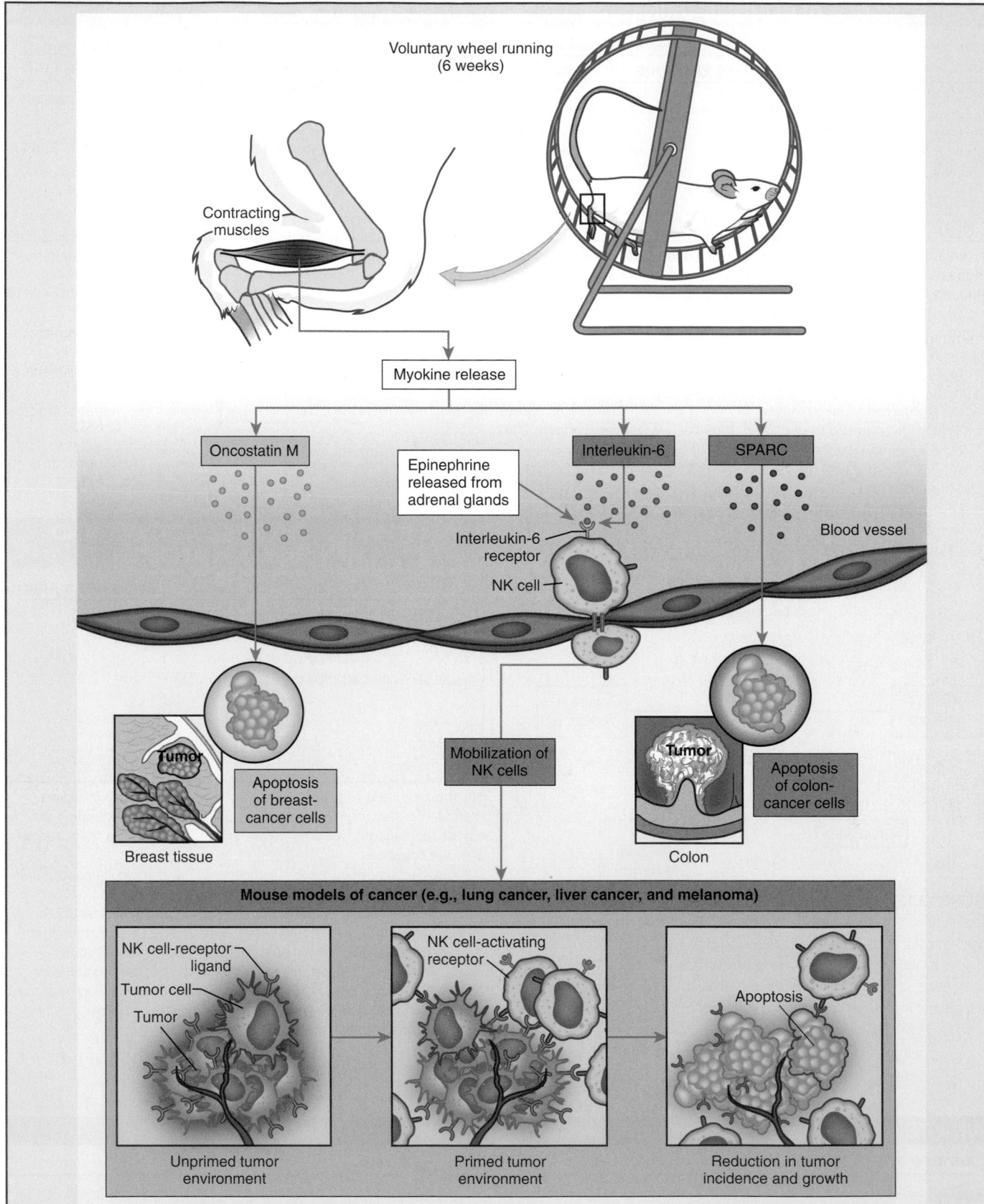

Anticancer Effects of Exercise-Induced Myokines. Exercise and contracting muscle fibers release myokines into the bloodstream, which can induce apoptosis in breast and colon cancer cells. In mouse models, investigators Pedersen and colleagues show antitumor effects from myokine IL-6, which is elevated after exercise. IL-6 and epinephrine released from the adrenal gland move to the bloodstream and result in increased mobilization of natural killer (NK) lymphocytes, which migrate into tumors and destroy tumor cells.

Adapted from Lucia A, Ramirez M: *NEJM* 375(9):892–894, 2016; Pedersen L et al: *Cell Metab* 23:554–562, 2016.

A randomized trial found that, after 12 months of moderate-intensity exercise, postmenopausal women had significantly decreased levels of serum estrogens.[125] A new study from national and international researchers, including those from the National Cancer Institute (NCI), National Institutes of Health (NIH), and American Cancer Society (ACS), of the relationship between physical activity and cancer has shown that greater levels of leisure-time physical activity were associated with a lower risk of developing 13 different types of cancer. The risk of developing 7 cancer types was 20% (or more) lower among the most active participants (90th percentile of activity) as compared with the least active participants (10th percentile of activity). Leisure-time physical activity was associated with a lower risk of colon, breast, endometrial, esophageal (adenocarcinoma), liver, kidney, and cancer of the gastric cardia and myeloid leukemia.[126] This study also showed physical activity reduced risks of heart disease and risk of death from all causes.

Many questions are unanswered regarding frequency, intensity, and duration of exercise. The World Health Organization (WHO) recommends at least 600 metabolic equivalent (MET) minutes of total activity per week for benefits; this is about 150 minutes/week of brisk walking or 75 minutes/week of running.[127] A recent review and dose-response meta-analysis, however, found 3000 to 4000 MET minutes/week is strongly associated with a lower risk of breast cancer, colon cancer, diabetes, ischemic heart disease, and ischemic stroke.[128] Several reports suggest that physical activity after a cancer diagnosis is associated with better cancer-specific sequelae and improved overall survival time with early-stage breast, prostate, and colorectal cancers.[100] Further research is needed on cancer outcomes and physical activity.

Air Pollution

Research reviews done by the U.S. Environmental Protection Agency, WHO, and others show that long-term exposure to ambient air pollution increases mortality and morbidity and shortens life expectancy from cardiovascular, respiratory disease, and lung cancer[129] (Table 13.7). The 2015 Global Burden of Diseases, Injuries, and Risk Factors Study identified air pollution as a leading cause of global disease burden, particularly in low-income and middle-income countries.[129] Long-term exposure to fine particle air pollution ($PM_{2.5}$) caused 4.2 million deaths and 103.1 million lost years of healthy life in 2015, making it the 5th ranked global risk factor in 2015 or 7.6% of total global mortality[129] (Fig. 13.14). An additional 254,000 deaths were linked to exposure to ozone.[129] The risk factor rank for deaths for the top 10 countries attributable to ambient particulate matter pollution include China (1), India (2), Russia (3), Pakistan (4), Bangladesh (5), United States of America (6), Indonesia (7), Japan (8), Brazil (9), and Nigeria (10).[129] Household air pollution from solid fuel use was responsible for 2.8 million deaths and 85.6 million disability-adjusted life-years, or DALYs, in 2015.[129]

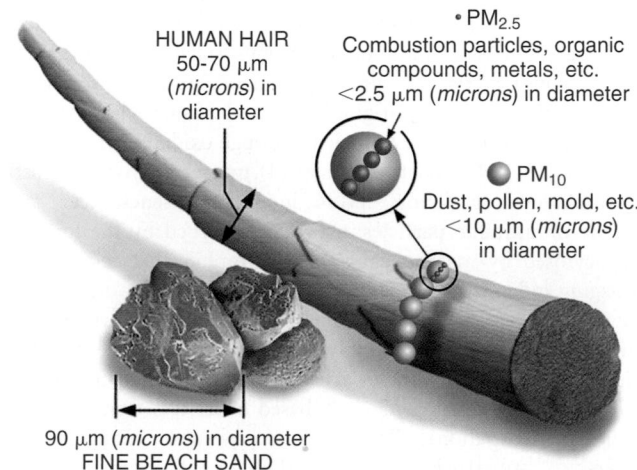

FIGURE 13.14 Particle Sizes and Pollution. (From Environmental Protection Agency: *Particulate matter updated March 18, 2013*, Washington, DC, 2013, Author.)

TABLE 13.7 **GLOBAL DEATHS, DISABILITY-ADJUSTED LIFE-YEARS, AND AGE-STANDARDIZED RATES ATTRIBUTABLE TO AMBIENT PARTICULATE MATTER POLLUTION IN 2015**

	DEATHS, IN THOUSANDS (95% UI)	AGE-STANDARDIZED DEATHS PER 100,000 PEOPLE (95% UI)	DALYS, IN THOUSANDS (95% UI)	AGE-STANDARDIZED DALYS PER 100,000 PEOPLE (95% UI)
All Causes	4241.1 (3698.0-4776.7)	66.0 (57.2-74.8)	103,066.2 (90,829.6-115,072.6)	1490.9 (1312.4-1665.6)
Disease				
Lower respiratory infection	675.0 (491.9-889.0)	10.1 (7.4-13.4)	28,359.9 (21,141.8-35,796.9)	390.9 (290.9-494.3)
Lung cancer	283.3 (178.4-398.7)	4.4 (2.7-6.1)	6209.1 (3934.9-8689.3)	90.9 (57.5-127.3)
Ischemic heart disease	1521.1 (1231.7-1821.2)	23.6 (18.9-28.5)	32,406.0 (27,078.2-37,427.4)	470.7 (394.6-543.0)
Cerebrovascular disease	898.1 (717.6-1083.6)	14.0 (11.0-17.1)	19,242.8 (16,095.9-22,679.7)	281.2 (234.4-331.4)
Chronic obstructive pulmonary disease	863.6 (538.5-1212.8)	14.0 (8.7-19.6)	16,848.2 (10,517.4-23,590.0)	257.2 (160.3-360.6)
Sex				
Male	2455.4 (2140.2-2752.9)	83.9 (72.5-94.7)	62,894.7 (55,545.7-70,098.2)	1888.8 (1659.4-2113.6)
Female	1785.7 (1546.2-2049.2)	50.8 (44-0-58.4)	40,171.5 (35,205.5-45,382.8)	1127.4 (986.6-1275.4)
Age				
Children <5 years	202.6 (152.7-254.6)	30.1 (22.7-37.8)	17,431.1 (13,139.7-21,906.3)	2585.9 (1949.1-3249.5)
Elderly >70 years	2228.3 (1842.0-2653.9)	562.7 (465.1-670.8)	25,073.0 (20,775.2-29,511.1)	6302.2 (5226.3-7419.8)

DALYS, Disability-adjusted life years; *UI*, unit interval.
Data from Cohen AJ et al: *Lancet*, 2017. (Epub ahead of print.)

Outdoor air pollution is a complex mixture of many known carcinogens and has been studied for over 50 years on its relationship to lung cancer.[130] High levels of particulate-based smog can cause dramatic increases in daily mortality.[131,132] The Harvard Six Cities Study published in 1993 revealed that air pollution was positively associated with death from lung cancer and cardiopulmonary disease.[133] **Particulate matter**, also known as *particle pollution,* is a mixture of extremely small particles and liquid droplets. Particle pollution is made up of a complex mix of acids (such as nitrates and sulfates), organic chemicals, metals, and soil or dust particles. The International Agency for Research on Cancer (IARC) concluded that exposure to outdoor air pollution and to particulate matter (PM) in outdoor air is carcinogenic to humans (IARC Group 1) and causes lung cancer.[134,135] Specifically, focused reviews of lung cancer risk are with prominent components of PM in outdoor air ($PM_{2.5}$ particles with aerodynamic diameter ≤ 2.5 µm, or fine particles and PM_{10} [≤ 10 µm, or inhalable particles]) (see Fig. 13.14). The major components of PM are transition metals, ions (sulfate, nitrate), radicals of carbonaceous material, organic compound, minerals, reactive gases, and other materials of biologic origin.[136] The mechanisms of adverse cellular effects of PM include (1) cytotoxicity through oxidative stress, (2) ROS generation, (3) DNA oxidative damage, (4), mutagenicity, (5) stimulation of proinflammatory factors, and (6) induction of senescence.[136,137]

Fine or ultrafine particles are easily absorbed by the lungs and phagocytosed by macrophages and neutrophils that release tissue-damaging inflammatory mediators. *Acute* exposure to diesel exhaust that contains fine particles is linked to lung, throat, and eye irritations; asthma attacks; and myocardial ischemia.[138] From three decades of epidemiologic research, diesel exhaust was classified as a carcinogen in humans by the IARC in 2012, based on results from two recent studies of occupational diesel exhaust exposures among nonmetal miners[139,140] and truck drivers[141,142] (Fig. 13.15). Importantly, from the WHO, diesel exhaust is carcinogenic and causes lung cancer.[143] Perhaps similar to cigarette smoking where it took time to understand that it causes cancer of numerous other sites (see Fig. 13.4), diesel exhaust will be studied for its role to other cancer sites including urinary bladder, larynx, and colon.[144] Critical questions are urgent, including how much of the carcinogenicity of air pollution is related to diesel exhaust and its specific role in cardiovascular disease.[142] The central hypothesis, based on rat studies, for the mechanisms related to particle-induced lung carcinogenesis is that insoluble particles cause pulmonary inflammation (e.g., cytokine release, ROS) which leads to oxidative stress and oxidation of DNA, proliferative response, and tissue remodeling progressing toward fibrosis and tumor development.

Living close to certain industries is a recognized cancer risk factor.[145] Overall, fine particle pollution also is linked to other health problems and includes (1) premature death in people with heart or lung disease, (2) nonfatal heart attacks, (3) irregular heartbeat, (4) aggravated asthma, (5) decreased lung function, and (6) respiratory symptoms including irritation of the airways, coughing, and shortness of breath. Additionally, other effects of particle pollution include reduced visibility (haze); environmental damage in lakes and streams, coastal waters, and river basins; depletion of nutrients in soil; and damage to forests and food crops.[146]

Indoor pollution generally is considered worse than outdoor pollution, partly because of cigarette smoke (Fig. 13.16). Environmental tobacco smoke (ETS; passive smoking) can cause the formation of reactive oxygen free radicals and thus DNA damage. The IARC has classified ETS as a human carcinogen. In China, some regions report very high levels of lung cancer in women who spend much of their time indoors. Exposures from heating and cooking combustion sources (e.g., oil vapors, volatile toxicants) are identified as risk factors for lung cancer.[147,148] In addition, domestic coal use and ETS increase the risk of lung cancer in women and men.[149]

Another significant indoor air pollutant is radon gas. **Radon** is a natural radioactive gas derived from the radioactive decay of uranium that is ubiquitous in rock and soil; it can become trapped in houses and gives rise to radioactive decay products known to be carcinogenic to humans. The most hazardous houses can be identified by testing and then can be modified to prevent further radon contamination. Exposure levels are greater from underground mines than from houses. Most of the lung cancers associated with radon are bronchogenic; however, small cell carcinoma does occur with greater frequency in underground miners. Radon increases the risk of lung cancer in underground miners whether they smoke or not.

Ionizing Radiation

Much of the knowledge of the effects of ionizing radiation (IR) on human cancer has stemmed from observations of the Hiroshima and Nagasaki atomic bomb (A-bomb) exposures, particularly the Life Span Study. These data provide estimates of human cancer risk over the dose range from 20 to 250 centigray (cGy) for low linear energy transfer (LET) radiation, such as x-rays or γ-rays. Other evidence is derived from groups exposed for medical reasons, underground miners exposed to radon gas, and other occupational exposures (Table 13.8). The atomic bomb exposures in Japan caused acute leukemias in adults and children and increased frequencies of thyroid and breast carcinomas. Lung, stomach, colon, esophageal, and urinary tract cancers and multiple myeloma have been added to the list. At Nagasaki and Hiroshima, leukemia incidence in individuals 15 years or younger reached its peak 6 to 7 years after the explosions and has steadily declined since 1952. People 45 years and older at the time of exposure had a latent period of 20 years before developing acute leukemia.

Age at the time of radiation exposure is one of the important factors in radiation-induced cancer. Recently, standard models and evaluations of age of exposure to radiation and radiation-induced cancer risks have been questioned.[150-153] Epidemiologic data from Japanese atomic bomb survivors and from children exposed to radiation for medical intervention suggest that excess relative risks (ERRs) for radiation-induced cancers at a given age are exceptionally higher for individuals exposed during childhood than for those exposed at older ages.[154] These data also are published by the International Commission on Radiological Protection

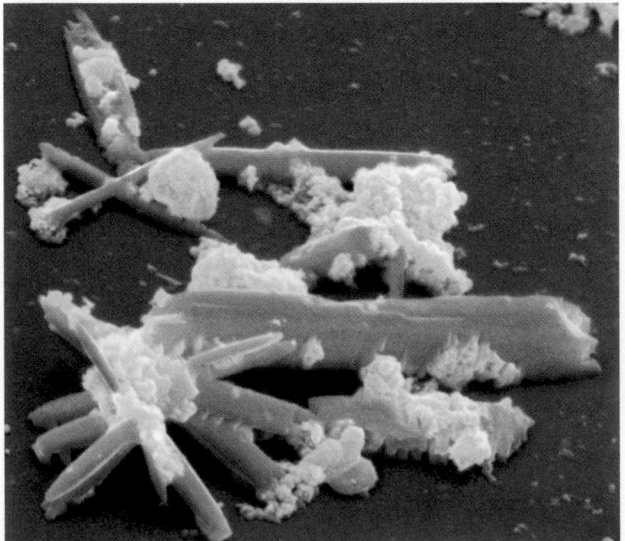

FIGURE 13.15 Exhaust Particulate Matter. Diesel exhaust is carcinogenic and causes lung cancer. (From Science Photo Laboratory.)

WHAT'S IN THE
AIR INDOORS?

Particulate matter is a mixture of very small solids and liquid droplets that float in the air. Some particles come from a specific source (such as a burning candle), while others form as a result of complicated chemical reactions.

Most Americans spend about **90%** of their time indoors.[1]

While much is known about the health effects of exposure to particulate matter outdoors, the effects of indoor exposure are less well-understood. However, indoor exposure to particulate matter is gaining attention as a potential source of adverse health effects.

The National Academies of Sciences, Engineering, and Medicine recently convened a workshop to examine the issues.

WHAT ARE SOME SOURCES OF PARTICULATE MATTER INDOORS?

outdoor sources that enter indoors through heating, ventilation, and air conditioning systems; open doors and windows; and leakage through walls and roofs[1]

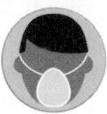

airborne allergens and bacteria in outdoor air and that come from people and their pets and plants indoors[2]

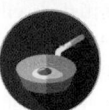

emissions from food as it's cooking[3]

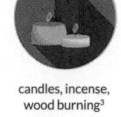

candles, incense, wood burning[3]

cleaning activities like dusting, vacuuming, and ironing[3]

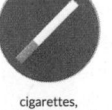

cigarettes, e-cigarettes, and other smoking materials[4]

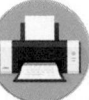

desktop laser printers and 3-D printers[1]

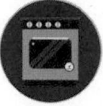

gas and electric ranges and stoves[1]

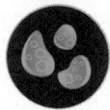

mold that grows on indoor surfaces[2]

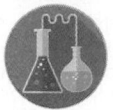

chemical reactions between elements in the air and materials inside of buildings[5]

HOW BIG IS PARTICULATE MATTER, AND WHY IS THE SIZE A CONSIDERATION?

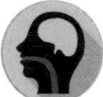

PARTICULATE MATTER IS TYPICALLY CLASSIFIED INTO THREE SIZE CATEGORIES:

- Coarse particles are 2.5 to 10 micrometers in diameter (a strand of human hair is 60-120 micrometers wide[6]).
- Fine particles are 2.5 micrometers in diameter or smaller.
- Ultrafine particles are 100 nanometers (0.1 micrometers) or smaller.

Fine and ultrafine particles may be small enough to pass through the throat and nose and enter deeper into the body.[7]

WHAT ARE THE POTENTIAL HEALTH EFFECTS?

A body of epidemiologic research has shown associations between short-term and long-term exposures to particulate matter and a broad array of respiratory and cardiovascular effects.[8] Results from scientific studies are converging to indicate that exposures both to fine and ultrafine particles may produce such adverse effects.[8] The size and shape of inhaled particles influence where and how much mass will be deposited in various regions of the respiratory system.[9]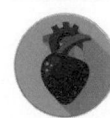

WHAT ARE SOME WAYS OF ALTERING THE LEVELS OF PARTICULATE MATTER INDOORS?

The source of indoor particulate matter may be affected by:
- limiting indoor smoking [3,10]
- using a correctly installed range hood when cooking[3,10]
- avoiding burning candles and incense [3]
- performing regular surface cleaning [10]

Ventilation may reduce the levels of particulate matter generated indoors, but it increases the amount of outdoor-generated particulate matter that comes inside.[10]

Filtration may lower the concentrations of particulate matter in indoor air.[3,10]

To download the free workshop summary, visit **nationalacademies.org/IndoorPM.**

1. Brent Stephens, Illinois Institute of Technology
2. Sergey Grinshpun, University of Cincinnati College of Medicine
3. Brett Singer, Lawrence Berkeley National Laboratory
4. Barbara Turpin, UNC Gillings School of Global Public Health
5. Charles Weschler, Rutgers University
6. William Hallmann, Rutgers University
7. Mark Weisskopf, Harvard T.H. Chan School of Public Health
8. National Research Council (NRC). 2010. *Review of the Department of Defense Enhanced Particulate Matter Surveillance Program Report*
9. NRC. 2004. *Research Priorities for Airborne Particulate Matter: IV. Continuing Research Progress*
10. William Fisk, Lawrence Berkeley National Laboratory

The National Academies of
SCIENCES · ENGINEERING · MEDICINE

FIGURE 13.16 What's in the Air Indoors. (From Science Photo Library.)

TABLE 13.8	CANCER ASSOCIATED WITH EXPOSURE TO IONIZING RADIATION							
CANCER TYPE	AB	AS	PM	TC	TH	RP	UM	RD
Leukemia	X	X			X			X
Thyroid	X			X				
Breast	X		X					
Lung	X	X			X		X	
Bone						X		
Stomach	X	X						
Esophagus	X	X						
Lymphoma	X	X						X
Brain			X				X	
Liver				X				
Skin				X			X	X

AB, Atomic bomb survivors; *AS,* ankylosing spondylitis patients; *PM,* postpartum mastitis patients; *TC,* tinea capitis patients; *TH,* individuals receiving thorotrast; *RP,* radium dial painters; *UM,* underground miners; *RD,* radiologists.
Data from Jones JA, Casey RC, Karouia F: Ionizing radiation as a carcinogen. In McQueen E, editor: *CA comprehensive toxicology,* ed 2, St Louis, 2010, Elsevier.

(ICRP) and the National Academy of Sciences Committee on the Biological Effects of Ionizing Radiation (BEIR Committee).[155] What is at question is the ERRs of radiation exposure in adulthood and radiation-induced cancer risk. Recent analyses of Japanese bomb survivors suggest that the ERR for cancer induction decreases with increasing age at exposure only until exposure ages of 30 to 40 years; with radiation exposure at older ages, the ERR does not decrease further and for many individual cancer sites (liver, colon, lung, stomach, and bladder) the ERR may actually increase in all solid cancers combined.[151,153,154,156] These new data present a challenge to the conceptual understanding of the mechanisms of cancer induction.[153] Biologic models of cancer development all predict that ERRs should decrease continuously with increasing age of radiation exposure. Recent models, however, of radiation carcinogenesis show IR acts not only as an initiator of premalignant cell clones but also as a promoter of preexisting premalignant cell alterations.[151,153,156] Promotion is used here to mean the process by which an initiated cell clonally expands. Therefore promotional processes from radiation can result in increasing excess lifetime cancer risks with increasing age at exposure. From these new data, investigators propose that radiation-induced cancer risks after exposure in middle age may be almost twice as high as previously estimated.[153]

Human exposure to IR includes emissions from the environment (e.g., radon), x-rays, computed tomography (CT) scans, radioisotopes, and other radioactive sources (Fig. 13.17). Health risks involve not only neoplastic diseases but also cardiovascular disease and stroke following high doses in therapeutic medicine and lower doses in A-bomb survivors (BEIR VII).[155,157] Late effects of radiation in A-bomb survivors show persistent elevations in the levels of inflammatory markers, implying immunologic damage may be the cause of later cardiovascular effects.[158] Investigators for the first time using a model of umbilical vein endothelial

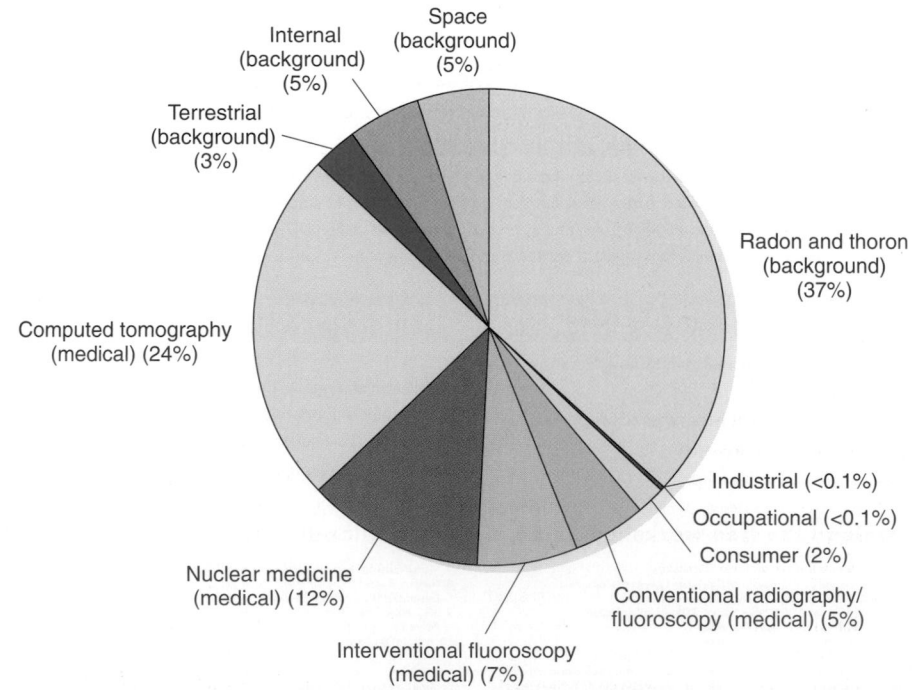

FIGURE 13.17 Pie Chart Showing Sources of Exposure to Ionizing Radiation. Percent contribution of various sources of exposure to the total collective effective dose (1,870,000 person-Sv) and the total effective dose per individual in the U.S. population (6.2 mSv) for 2006. Percent values have been rounded to the nearest 1%, except those <1%. *Sv,* Sievert. (From NCRP: *2009 Ionizing radiation exposure of the population of the United States,* NCRP Report No. 160, Bethesda, MD, Author.)

BOX 13.2 **POTENTIAL RADIOPROTECTIVE EFFECTS OF NANOFORMULATION OF CURCUMIN, GREEN TEA, AND GRAPE SEED EXTRACTS**

Investigators using an irradiated THP-1 macrophage model treated irradiated macrophages with a nanoformulation of curcumin (DNC). The curcumin suppressed IR-induced oxidative damage, inflammation, and foam cell formation in macrophages through multiple mechanisms. Another group of investigators studied the radioprotective effects of green tea extract (GTE) and grape seed extract (GSE) on radiation-induced immune suppression in rats. The level of proinflammatory cytokines significantly decreased by the GTE and GSE mixture. These results indicate the possible role of these compounds as radioprotectors that may be used as an adjuvant during radiotherapy. These findings need more research.

IR, Ionizing radiation; *THP-1,* is a human monocytic leukemia cell line. Data from El-Desouky W, Hanafi A, Abbas MM: *Int J Radiat Biol* 94(4):433-439, 2017; Soltani B et al: *Int J Radiat Biol* 93(3):303-314, 2017.

cells showed that low doses (0.05 Gy) of x-rays induce DNA damage and apoptosis in endothelial cells. These data will need continued research.[159] Cardiac and blood vessel damage may manifest years after completion of radiation therapy (Box 13.2).[160]

Exposure to ionizing radiation induces apoptosis and senescence. Less is known about senescence. In vitro studies suggest endothelial cell senescence can lead to endothelial dysfunction by altering vasodilation and hemostasis, induction of oxidative stress and inflammation, and inhibition of angiogenesis.[161] The underlying biology of radiation-induced cardiovascular disease is poorly described; however, investigators report the role of the 5-lipooxygenase/leukotriene pathway as a possible therapeutic target.[162] Chronic inflammation is increasingly implicated in radiation-induced late tissue injury.[163] Other risks from IR include somatic mutations and tissue alterations that may contribute to other diseases (e.g., respiratory diseases, birth defects, and eye maladies) and, from animal studies, inherited mutations that may affect the incidence of diseases in future generations. Exposure to relatively low doses of ionizing radiation may be harmful to the lens of the eye and increase risk of cataract formation.[164-166] Conclusions from low dose cohorts suggest an elevated risk of posterior subcapsular cataract (PSC) as well as cortical cataracts.[166] The human embryo and fetus are particularly sensitive to ionizing radiation; the health consequences of exposure even at doses too low to immediately affect the mother can be severe.[167] The consequences include growth retardation, malformations, impaired brain function, and cancer.[167] An important summary point in BEIR VII[155] is the concern from medical exposure, for example, CT. The National Council on Radiation Protection and Measurements reported in 2006 that Americans were exposed to more than 7 times as much IR from medical procedures compared to their exposure in the 1980s[168] (Fig. 13.18). The increase in imaging is likely driven by several factors, including improvements in the technology, that have led to increased clinical applications, patient demand, physician demand, defensive medical practices, and medical uncertainty.[169,170] A major concern is the cumulative exposure doses of repetitive tests and the inappropriate utilization of these imaging techniques.

Evidence, usually epidemiologic, shows cancer associated with exposure to IR (see Table 13.8). Evidence includes animal models and in vitro studies as well as exposed groups including atomic/nuclear survivors, survivors of industrial accidents and the Techa River basin

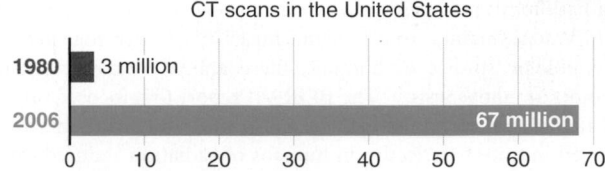

CT scans in the United States

1980	■	3 million
2006		67 million

0 10 20 30 40 50 60 70

MEDIAN EFFECTIVE RADIATION DOSE FOR EACH TYPE OF CT STUDY			
ANATOMIC AREA, STUDY TYPE	MEDIAN (mSv)	RANGE (mSv)	DOSE EQUIVALENT (NO. OF CHEST X-RAYS)
Head and Neck			
Routine head	2	0.3-6	30
Routine neck	4	0.7-9	55
Suspected stroke	14	4-56	199
Chest			
Chest, no contrast	8	2-24	117
Chest, with contrast	8	2-19	119
Suspected pulmonary embolus	10	2-30	137
Coronary angiogram	22	7-39	309
Abdomen-Pelvis			
Routine abdomen-pelvis, no contrast	15	3-43	220
Routine abdomen-pelvis, with contrast	16	4-45	234
Multiphase abdomen pelvis	31	6-90	442
Suspected aneurysm or dissection	24	4-68	347

FIGURE 13.18 CT Scans in the United States. National Council Radiation Protection estimates that 67 million CT scans (compared to 3 million in 1980), 18 million nuclear medicine procedures, and 17 million interventional fluoroscopy procedures were performed in the United States in 2006. (From NCRP: *2009 Ionizing radiation exposure of the population of the United States,* NCRP Report No. 160, Bethesda, MD, Author.)

in Siberia, and medical diagnostic/therapeutic data. The studies of exposed groups are large enough to allow epidemiologists to derive detail concerning the dose and quality, age at exposure, and other factors on cancer incidence in a large variety of organs.[171] From data collected over several decades, exposed cohorts reveal that IR is a potent carcinogen.[171] Additionally, reports of occupational exposures may have increased the incidence of certain types of cancer, for example, underground miners and lung cancer.[172] Certain medical conditions, especially those with a genetic basis, predispose individuals to ionizing radiation–induced injury.[171] The most well-known condition is ataxia-telangiectasia (AT), a rare (1 in 300,000 people) condition in which individuals have a strong sensitivity to IR. Individuals with *BRCA1/BRCA2* pathway mutations have increased radiosensitivity caused by insufficient DNA repair and cell cycle control mechanisms.[173]

Investigations conducted jointly by the U.S. Air Force and NASA from 1963 to 1969 studied the relative biologic effectiveness (RBE) of different types of radiation exposures on rhesus monkeys and mice.[171] Long-term follow-up studies of the exposed animals showed an induction of solid tumors and leukemia, and the extent of life shortening depended on dose and not on proton energy level.[174] The general characteristics of radiation carcinogenesis were determined from studies done after World War II, mainly from rats and mice.[171] However, together with epidemiologic studies of humans, these animal studies elucidated radiation carcinogenesis.[175] The BEIR VII report that focused on low-level radiation determined that the radiation-induced life shortening observed in mice is reflective in humans of radiation-induced cancer mortality.[176] These studies are important because they show that IR is universally carcinogenic to animals and humans and that there are wide differences in radiation responses according to species, organ, and radiation distribution.[171]

The universal nature of radiation as a carcinogen relates to its ability to penetrate cells and deposit energy in tissues at random. By the 1980s, using in vitro models, the *general* characteristics of IR-induced carcinogenesis were well established.[177] The past two decades have focused on *specific* cellular and molecular mechanisms that relate to the induction of cancer, including dose-response relationships for chromosome aberrations, cell transformation, gene expression (genetic and epigenetic), alternative targets, mutagenesis in somatic cells, and the biologic effects that occur in nonirradiated cells (i.e., **nontargeted effects [NTEs]**) and effects on the microenvironment.[171] Through much of the twentieth century, radiobiology was thought to be a relatively simple science and was dominated by physicists. Now, with biologists entering the field, it has become apparent that radiobiology is not so simple and involves much more understanding beyond a DNA-centric model, including alternative targets, such as membranes, repair, and rescue within a biologic system.[178] Because models and underlying assumptions are incomplete, investigators are working hard to understand induced repair, adaptive responses, hormesis, low-dose hypersensitivity, nontargeted effects, microenvironment, immune landscape, signaling, exosomes, and long-term persistence of radiation damage and clonal heterogeneity.[178,179]

Oncogenes and Tumor-Suppressor Genes

Part of the biologic response of radiation-induced cancer is oncogene activation. Although evidence suggests that interindividual differences in radiation responses may be attributed to certain genes, IR can activate oncogenes, resulting in uncontrolled cell growth[171] (see Chapter 12). Tumor-suppressor genes also are sensitive to IR. Several tumor-suppressor genes have been identified that are deactivated by IR that promotes carcinogenesis.[171] Recent research has shown that cells can detect and respond epigenetically, altering gene expression after low doses of radiation.[171] Gene expression can change as a function of radiation dose and radiation type.[171]

Chromosomal Aberrations

IR is a mutagen and carcinogen; it can penetrate cells and tissues and deposit energy in tissues at random in the form of ionizations (e.g., removal of an electron from the target atom). Importantly, arising from IR is the localized release of large amounts of energy that can break a chemical bond (electron volts [eV] is the energy per ionizing event). Damage from IR can occur either *directly* from biologic macromolecules (e.g., DNA) or *indirectly*, in the medium from which organelles are suspended in mostly water, and *irreversibly* from ionizations that can attack by water-based free radicals (e.g., H•, OH•) [radiolysis]).[180] Electromagnetic radiations, such as x-rays and γ-rays, damage by reactive species produced by ionizations elsewhere in the cell and thus have indirect action. The biologic effects of indirect action include cell killing (days), mutation (generation), and carcinogenesis (years). IR affects many cell processes, including gene expression, mitochondrial function disruption, cell cycle arrest, and cell death. IR is a potent DNA-damaging agent, causing cross-linking, nucleotide base damage, and single- and double-strand breaks (SSBs and DSBs, respectively) (Fig. 13.19). Damage to DNA and disrupted cellular regulation processes can lead to carcinogenesis.[181-183] The **double-strand break (DSB)** is considered the important lesion in the induction of both chromosomal abnormalities and gene mutations (Fig. 13.20). Persistent disturbance by oxidative metabolism can cause DSBs long after exposure to radiation.[184] The misrepair of DSBs could lead to substantial chromosomal instability.[185] The nonhomologous end-joining (NHEJ) pathway plays a dominant role in repair of DSBs.[186] Another pathway is by homologous recombination (HR); for example, *BRCA1* and *BRCA2* are tumor-suppressor genes and one of their functions is DNA repair by HR.[187,188] These two mechanisms of DSB repair act at different phases of the cell cycle. Irradiated human cells unable to execute the NHEJ pathway are supersensitive to the introduction of large-scale mutations and chromosomal aberrations.[180]

Cell Transformation

Cell transformation describes the total changes associated with loss of normal homeostatic control.[171] The majority of studies on cell transformation in vitro have been quantitative, using rodent-derived models. Few human-derived assays have been conducted. Overall, the exposure to high-LET radiation results in a higher transformation frequency than exposure to low-LET radiation.[171] There is no tendency, however, for the response per unit dose to decrease at low doses or low dose rates, and a number of studies have shown an enhanced effect.[171]

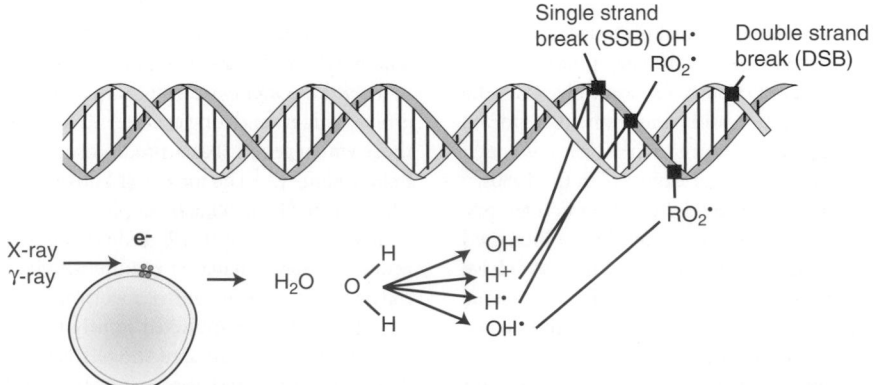

FIGURE 13.19 Free Radicals. Free radicals formed by water nearby and around DNA cause indirect effects. These effects have a short life of single free radicals. Oxygen can modify the reaction, enabling longer lifetimes of oxidative free radicals.

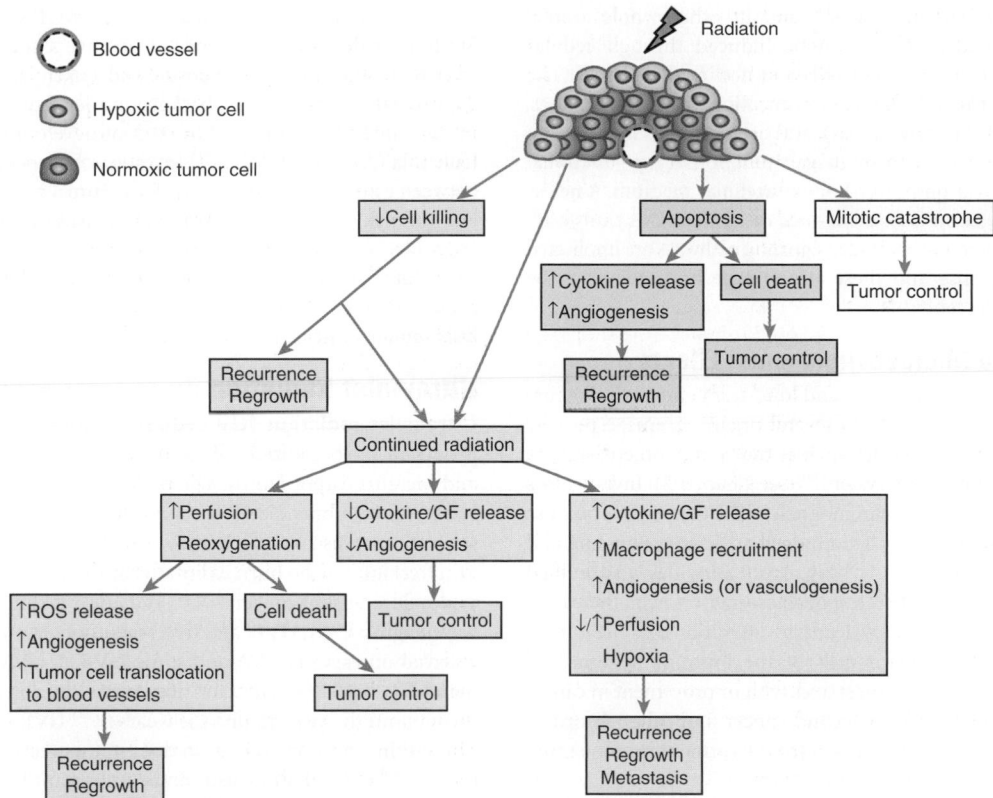

FIGURE 13.20 Simplified Model of the Effects of Radiation on Tumor Microenvironment. Tumor cells that are not hypoxic cells (i.e., called *normoxic*) are more sensitive to radiation and hence more susceptible to cell death (apoptosis) and mitotic catastrophe or destruction. In some cases, however, proapoptotic mechanisms can cause the release of cytokines that promote tumor regrowth and recurrence. Hypoxic cells are resistant to radiation therapy and more likely lead to tumor recurrence. Continuous radiation (especially fractionated) can lead to reoxygenation, which can improve radiation-induced cell killing or promote release of reactive oxygen species (ROS) and angiogenesis and/ or induce tumor cell movement to blood vessels; both mechanisms can result in tumor regrowth and recurrence. Decreased cytokine production and destruction of blood vessels from continued administration of high doses of radiation can increase tumor cell killing. In certain situations, however, irradiation is associated with the production of an aggressive phenotype of the remaining cells that survive radiation therapy. This failure is caused by the release of protective cytokines and/or growth factors *(GFs)*, the recruitment of macrophages, altered perfusion of blood, and hypoxia that increase angiogenesis or blood vessel growth, resulting in tumor regrowth and recurrence and/or metastasis. Importantly, the effects of radiation on tumor microenvironment depend on many factors. (Adapted from Fokas E, McKenna WG, Muschel RJ: *Cancer Metastasis Rev* 31[3–4]:823–842, 2012.)

Nontargeted Effects

A long-held assumption is that cellular alterations—mutations and malignant transformation—occur only in cells directly radiated. There is clear evidence indicating that cells not directly traversed by a radiation particle, but in the vicinity of a cell that has been exposed to or received signals from irradiated cells, can participate in the damage response.[189] The **DNA damage response (DDR)** is a coordinated series of events that allows DNA damage detection, signaling that includes cell cycle checkpoint activation, and repair.[190,191] Emerging and important data indicate that the DDR should be considered not only at the DNA level but also in the chromatin of cell nuclei where DNA envelopes histone proteins.[192] Additionally, the importance of the plasticity of the microenvironment is becoming integrated into the radiation response.

It is now known that cells not directly exposed to radiation, but instead the progeny of cells that were irradiated many cell divisions previously, may express a high level of gene mutations, cell lethality, and chromosomal aberration. Altogether these effects are called **genomic**

instability. Genomic instability can initiate cancer, increase cancer progression, and affect the prognosis.[193] Therapeutic targeting of genomic instability and antitumor responses includes lifestyle, diet, and nutrition to inhibit proliferative signaling, decrease oncogenic metabolism, and block inflammation.[193] Multiple, complex genetic pathways, such as DNA damage repair, oxidative stress, and cell cycle control, may contribute to the development of radiation- and chemotherapy-related second primary cancers, supporting a polygenic model for sensitivity to treatment-related cancers.[194] The directly irradiated cells also can lead to genetic effects in so-called *bystander cells* or *innocent cells* (called **bystander effects**) even though they themselves received no direct radiation exposure.[189] The bystander and genomic instability effects also have been termed *nontargeted effects (NTEs)*.

The vast majority of bystander effects have been described in cell culture systems. However, investigators, using an in vivo mouse model, found an unexpected enhancement of medulloblastoma in the cerebellum of radiosensitive *Patched-1* (*Ptch*) heterozygous mice after radiation exposure to their bodies.[195] The bystander effect has been demonstrated in three-dimensional human tissues[196] and in other whole animal organisms.[197,198] Bystander effects can be induced through cellular communication between irradiated cells and nonirradiated cells. The signals that mediate this cellular communication include cytokines, ROS and nitric oxide (oxidative stress), and even microRNAs that can be transferred between cells through gap junctions (gap junctional intercellular communication [GJIC]) or extracellular medium. A newer process under investigation is *exosome-mediated microRNA transfer*.[199] Numerous intercellular and intracellular signaling pathways are implicated in the bystander response and these effects have been shown to be transmitted to their descendants.

Acute, Latent, and Microenvironmental Effects

IR causes acute and persistent short- and long-term effects.[200-202] Acute exposure to IR can cause damage to several organ systems, especially those with highly proliferative cells, such as the hematopoietic system, the skin, and the gastrointestinal system[203] (see Chapter 2). Investigators have postulated that radiation's carcinogenic potential persists because of nontargeted radiation effects that alter cell and tissue signaling and change the microenvironment.[204,205] Fig. 13.20 provides a simplified model of the effects of radiation on tumor microenvironment. Increasing evidence shows that radiotherapy leads to alterations in the tumor microenvironment, especially for cells of the immune system.[206-208] Radiotherapy is a treatment for cancer and, with improvement in cancer survival, the long-term risks of a second cancer and other disorders (e.g., atherosclerotic risk factors, stroke) from treatment become more important.[209,210]

Radiation-induced cancer in humans has latent periods, usually 5 to 10 years, but can be decades.[171,211] British investigators reported the following results: for solid cancers, radiation-related excess risk starts to appear about 5 years after exposure in therapeutically irradiated groups; and for leukemia, it starts to appear within 5 years of exposure.[212] Using U.S. Surveillance Epidemiology and End Results (SEER) data, the estimated excess of second cancers that could be related to radiotherapy is about 8%; data from the United Kingdom, which included diagnostic procedures and excluded therapeutic irradiation, yielded an estimation of 15%.[209,212]

Low Dose and Dose Rate

New studies on low doses of radiation have resulted in three paradigm shifts: (1) bystander effects have been observed in which nonhit cells may respond as well as hit cells; (2) radiation-induced changes in gene expression at very low radiation doses alter response pathways, some of which appear to involve adaptive or protective responses; and (3) early changes in the initiation phase of radiation-induced cancer were thought to be induced by gene mutation and chromosomal aberrations only; however, it is now understood that genomic instability that leads to the loss of genetic control may have a role in the development of cancer.[186] Constant debate involves risk estimates for human exposure at low-dose, low-LET ionizing radiation (0 to 100 mSv or less than 0.1 Gy). Much uncertainty exists about the risks of leukemia and lymphoma after repeated or protracted low-dose radiation typical of exposures from occupational, environmental, and diagnostic settings.[213] The first and most striking late effect of radiation exposure from the Life Span Study (Hiroshima and Nagasaki atomic bomb survivors) was a marked increase in leukemia risks. Although the leukemia excess risks generally declined with attained age or time since exposure, the radiation-associated excess leukemia risk, especially for acute myeloid leukemia, persisted through the follow-up period to 55 years after the bombings. There was a weak suggestion of a radiation dose response for nonHodgkin lymphoma among men and no indication of an effect for women. There was no evidence of radiation-associated excess risks for either Hodgkin

lymphoma or multiple myeloma.[214] The INWORKS International Cohort Study provides strong evidence of positive associations between protracted low-dose radiation exposure and leukemia.[213] Investigators report an association between the background level of terrestrial γ-radiation in the United Kingdom and the risk of developing acute lymphocytic leukemia (ALL) in children.[215] Investigators report a linear correlation between estimated bone marrow dose from a head CT scan in children and the risk of developing ALL.[216] The risks of low doses of radiation are controversial and the uncertainties associated with the best estimates are great.[217] Theoretical models to understand low-dose radiation are presented in Box 13.3. The risk of neoplastic transformation in bystander cells remains unclear.

Ultraviolet Radiation

Ultraviolet radiation (UV radiation) comes from sunlight and is produced in specialized lights, including tanning lamps, black lights, and mercury-vapor lamps. The most preventable cause of skin cancer is exposure to ultraviolet (UV) light either from the sun or from artificial sources, such as tanning beds.[218] Individuals who tan poorly, whose skin freckles, or who burn easily after sun exposure are most susceptible to developing skin cancer.[219] UV radiation is divided into three major wavelengths: UVA, UVB, and UVC radiation. Most of the UV radiation received on earth is UVA and some UVB.[220] UVA radiation is weaker than UVB, but UVA penetrates deeper into the skin and is more constant throughout the year despite the weather.[220] UVB affects the outer layer of the skin, and UVC radiation does not increase health risks as much as UVB.[220] UV radiation also can be important to health and produces vitamin D that helps in the absorption of calcium and phosphorus from food, both of which are important for bone development. Food sources of vitamin D include some types of fish, foods with added vitamin D, juices, dairy products, and egg yolks.[221] More importantly, continued time in the sun will increase skin cancer risk.[221] Prolonged human exposure to solar UV radiation can result in acute and chronic health effects on the skin, eye, and immune system.[222] Organ transplant recipients receiving immunosuppressive drugs have an increased risk of skin cancer, particularly squamous cell carcinoma (SCC). Arsenic exposure increases the risk of cutaneous SCC.[219]

There are three main types of skin cancer: (1) cancer that forms in melanocytes (pigment cells) derived from the neural crest, called melanoma; (2) cancer in the lower part of the epidermis or outer layer of the skin, called basal cell carcinoma (BCC); and (3) cancer in the flat cells that form the surface of the skin, called squamous cell carcinoma (SCC) (see Chapter 47). Solid evidence shows sun and UV radiation exposure are associated with an increased risk of BCC and SCC.[219] Melanoma, the most lethal form of skin cancer, can occur on any skin surface and also may arise from mucosal surfaces or other sites from which neural crest cells migrate, including the uveal (intraocular) tract; however, in men it is often found on the skin on the head, the neck, between the shoulders, and on the hips. In women it is more commonly found on the skin on the lower legs, between the shoulders, and on the hips. Although rare in people with dark skin, melanoma is usually found under the fingernails, under the toenails, on the palms of the hands, or on the soles of the feet.[223] Based on fair evidence, *intermittent acute sun exposure* leading to sunburn is associated with an increased risk of melanoma.[219] Melanomas on sun-exposed skin are heterogeneous tumors and can be classified on the basis of their cumulative levels of exposure to UV radiation. Basal cell carcinoma commonly occurs on the head and neck. Squamous cell carcinoma is found more commonly in men who work outdoors, but can occur in anyone. SCC occurs on sun-exposed areas of the skin including the nose, ears, lower lip, and dorsa of the hand. SCCs are composed of keratinizing cells and are more aggressive than BCC, but the development into invasive SCC is low.[224]

BOX 13.3 THEORETIC MODELS TO UNDERSTAND LOW-DOSE RADIATION

Several models include the linear no-threshold (LNT) relationship, in which any dose, including very low doses, has the potential to cause mutations (see **A**). Another model, the linear-quadratic relationship, proposes there is a risk mathematical term that is directly proportional to the dose (linear term) and another term proportional to the square of the dose (quadratic term) (see **B**). The threshold model proposes a threshold dose below which radiation may not cause cancer in humans (see **C**). Proponents of this model argue that such thresholds are

derived, for example, from the ability to repair damage caused by lower doses of radiation. There is some evidence that low doses may actually produce a higher level of risk per unit of dose, which is called the *supralinear hypothesis* (see **D**). **E**, Stochastic or random probability is a major model for understanding low-dose radiation. Currently, the shape of the response curve for the low-dose region is really unknown.

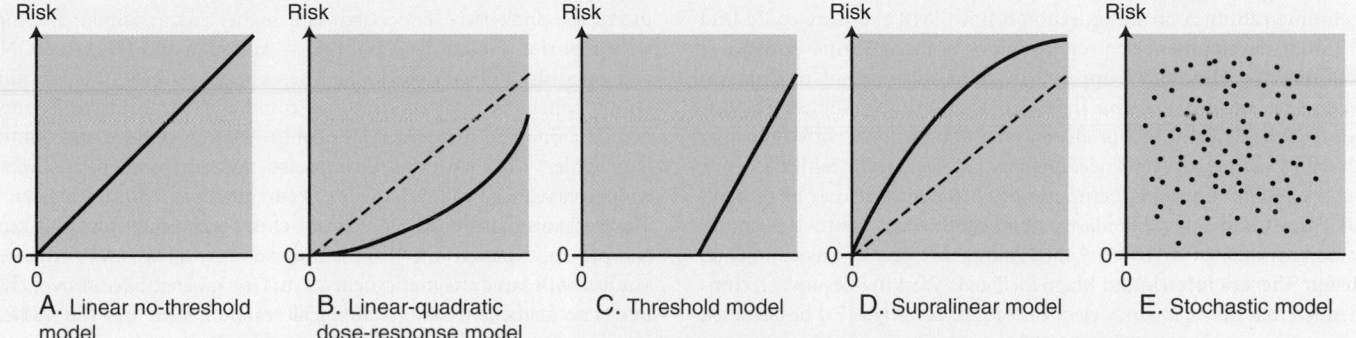

A. Linear no-threshold model

B. Linear-quadratic dose-response model

C. Threshold model

D. Supralinear model

E. Stochastic model

Theoretic Models for Estimating Risk of Low-Dose Ionizing Radiation. Collective population dose is expressed as a person-rem (roentgen equivalent, man). Estimating a collective dose then enables an application of a "constant risk factor" to obtain a statistical estimate of the number of additional cancers (above background radiation) from that exposure. These computations apply to low doses–low dose rates only **(A)**. Many propose the best fit is the linear no-threshold (LNT) model **(B)**. The most common alternative to the LNT model is the linear-quadratic model. The quadratic term is the square of the dose. The linear term is equal to zero **(C)**. The threshold model is a threshold below which there is *no* increase in cancer risk. Proponents of this model argue that because some toxic chemicals/materials exhibit such thresholds, radiation must also have a threshold. Their arguments are related to repair of the radiation damage caused by lower doses of radiation **(D)**. Some evidence exists that low levels of radiation produce a higher level of risk per unit dose, which is called the *supralinear model*. The stochastic model is where effects are random and the events cannot be predicted **(E)**. (Adapted from Makhijani A, Smith B, Thorne MC: Takoma Park, MD, 2006, Institute for Energy and Environmental Research.)

Data from Hoel DG: *Ann N Y Acad Sci* 1076:309-331, 2006; Preston DL et al: *Radiat Res* 160:381–407, 2003.

The pathogenesis of nonmelanoma skin cancers involves specific gene mutations, DNA methylation and histone modifications, oxidative stress, inflammation, and reduced immune surveillance. For a more complete discussion about these skin cancers, see Chapter 47.

Skin cancer is the most common malignancy diagnosed in the United States. The actual number of nonmelanoma skin cancers is difficult to estimate because they are not reported to cancer registries. In 2016 an estimated 76,380 cases of melanoma will be diagnosed and 10,100 will die from the disease. Although melanoma accounts for about 1% of all skin cancer cases, it is responsible for substantial morbidity and the vast majority of deaths.[225] Because mortality rates have not risen as rapidly, however, controversy exists as to whether the incidence increase is a true increase in clinically significant melanoma or is a result of overdiagnosis.[226] The U.S. Preventive Services Task Force (USPSTF) concludes that the current evidence is insufficient for early detection of skin cancer and the balance of benefit and harms of visual skin examination by a clinician to screen for skin cancer in asymptomatic adults cannot be determined.[227] A major harm is overdiagnosis and overtreatment (see Chapter 47).

Death rates varied by race and ethnicity with white men and women more likely to die of melanoma than any other group.[228] Risk factors vary for different types of skin cancer but, in general, the risk factors include a lighter natural skin color; a family history of skin cancer; a personal history of skin cancer; exposure to the sun through work and

play; a history of sunburns, especially early in life; a history of indoor tanning; skin that burns, freckles, reddens easily, or becomes painful in the sun; blue or green eyes; blonde or red hair; and certain types of moles and a large number of moles.[228] Higher coffee intake was associated with a modest decrease in risk of melanoma in a large U.S. cohort study.[229]

Electromagnetic Radiation

Electromagnetic radiation (EM or EMR) is energy in the form of transverse magnetic and electric waves. Health risks associated with EM are very controversial and have been a concern since at least the 1950s. The early concerns were with radar and other radio and microwave sources.[230] The biologic effects of nonionizing radiation have been difficult to establish, particularly the effects of long-term low-level exposures. A recent emphasis has arisen from the potential effects of low-intensity fields; intermediate radiofrequency (RF); and higher-frequency radiation from devices, such as phones, broadcast antennas, Wi-Fi, security monitors, and others.[230] Exposure to electric and magnetic fields is widespread. Electric fields are shielded or weakened by walls and other objects; however, magnetic fields are not.[231] Electromagnetic fields (EMFs) are, for example, generated by RF sources coupled with the body and result in induced electric and magnetic fields with associated currents inside tissue.[232] The most common sources of **radiofrequency electromagnetic radiation (RF-EMR)** are wireless telecommunication devices and equipment, including cell phones and smart meters, and portable wireless devices, such as laptop computers and tablets.[231] Other common sources also include radio and television signals, radar, satellite stations, magnetic resonance imaging (MRI) devices, microwave ovens, cordless phones, television and computer screens, and wireless local area networks (Wi-Fi).[231] From household appliances that require electricity, magnetic fields are highest near the source and decrease rapidly with distance.

The major debate for more than five decades has focused on the association of exposure to EMR and resultant health consequences, including cancer. A critical question is how EMR exposure could lead to tumor development or progression, or both. Scientific evidence is accumulating although hampered by the availability of methods to accurately measure exposure, the lack of a clear dose-response relationship, and the difficulty in reproducing effects. In addition, with competing priorities such as convenience, financial interest, and health necessity, a consensus of the risk/benefit ratio of EMR exposure may be difficult to achieve, and safety standards significantly vary, up to 1000 times among countries.[233,234] In 1998, the National Institute of Environmental Health Sciences Electric and Magnetic Fields Working Group[235] recommended that low-frequency electromagnetic fields (EMFs) be classified as possible carcinogens. The possibility of a causal effect between low levels of low-frequency EMF and cancer led to the classification of EMF by the World Health Organizations International Agency for Research on Cancer (IARC) as a possible cause of cancer.[236,237]

The National Institute of Environmental Health Sciences is conducting a large-scale study on rodents exposed to radiofrequency energy (cell phone type). Preliminary results were released in May 2016 and the findings were reviewed by expert peer reviewers selected by the National Toxicology Program (NTP) and the National Institutes of Health (NIH).[238] These studies are the largest and most complex ever conducted by the NTP. For the studies, rats and mice were exposed to frequencies and modulations currently used in cellular communication in the United States. They were exposed for 10-minute on and 10-minute off increments, totaling more than 9 hours a day from birth through 2 years of age. NTP found low incidences of glioma in the brains and schwannomas of the heart of male rats but not in female rats. Studies in mice are continuing. These studies are very important but are limited in that (1) they are done in rats and not humans, (2) the rats were exposed to large amounts of radiation that may not be the same exposures as humans, (3) some of the rats that developed tumors lived longer than control group rats, and (4) the full analysis of the data is ongoing. Replication of these studies is required.

Overall, there is limited evidence that magnetic fields cause childhood leukemia[231] (see Chapter 14). Studies of magnetic field exposure from power lines and electric blankets in adults reveal little evidence of an association with leukemia, brain tumors, or breast cancer.[231]

Most exposure to EMF from occupational sources comes from near-field sources; the highest exposure to the general population comes from transmitters close to the body, such as hand-held devices like mobile telephones.[232] Epidemiologic evidence for an association between EMF and cancer has been derived from case-control, cohort, and time-trend studies. The most extensively studied exposure is from use of wireless telephones (mobile and cordless); other exposures include occupational settings and sources from the general environment[232] (also see Chapter 14). The pooled analyses from the INTERPHONE study included 2708 glioma cases and 2972 controls.[239] The odds ratios (ORs) in terms of time spent on the phone showed that the highest time spent on the phone (>1640 hours of use) was related to glioma risk (OR 1.40; 95% confidence interval [CI] 1.03–1.89). There was a suggestion of increased risk of tumors on the same side of the head as the phone use (ipsilateral exposure) in the temporal lobe, where radiofrequency

(RF) EMF exposure is highest.[232] The OR for glioma increased with increasing RF dose for exposure 7 years or more before diagnosis, and there was no association with estimated dose for exposure less than 7 years before diagnosis.[232] A Swedish investigative group performed a pooled analysis of two similar studies between the relationship of glioma, acoustic neuroma, and meningioma manifestation and mobile and cordless phone use.[240] Study participants who used a mobile phone for more than 1 year had an OR for glioma of 1.3 (95% CI 1.1–1.6). The OR increased with increasing time since first use and with total call time, 3.2 (2.0–5.1) for more than 2000 hours of use.[232] Ipsilateral use of the phone was associated with higher risk.[232] Similar findings were reported for cordless phones.[232] Although the INTERPHONE and Swedish studies were judged susceptible to bias, the Working Group concluded that the findings could not be dismissed because of bias alone and a causal relationship between phones and glioma is possible.[232] The Working Group also reviewed numerous studies' endpoints relevant to mechanisms of carcinogenicity from RF-EMF.[232] The mechanisms included genotoxicity, effects on immune function, gene and protein expression, cell signaling, oxidative stress, and apoptosis. Studies with large magnetic fields, 1 mT or greater, have shown that magnetic fields can change chemical reaction rates and free radical concentrations.[230] ROS, such as superoxide O_2^-, and nitrogen radicals, such as NO, are both signaling molecules and can attack bacteria and other microorganisms. NO is released by neutrophils and is involved in the activation of macrophages. Additionally, a very large number of molecules are affected by magnetic fields from a free radical mechanism for phosphorylation in many biologic signaling systems and promotion of different biologic processes.[241] Investigators reported that reductions of the Earth's magnetic field inhibited growth of fibrosarcoma HT1080 cells.[242] A working hypothesis is that weak magnetic fields change the rate of recombination for radical pairs that are generated by the metabolic activity in cells and this changes the concentration of radicals, such as O_2^- and H_2O_2. The overall effects include generation of antioxidants and activation of the immune system; however, long-term exposure to elevated magnetic fields may lead to increased radical concentrations, which are associated with aging, cancers, and Alzheimer disease.[230] Oxidative stress can activate many transcription factors leading to the expression of genes, including those for growth factors, inflammatory cytokines, chemokines, cell cycle regulators, and antiinflammatory molecules.[243] Although research results are inconsistent, an additional mechanism from exposure to magnetic fields may be decreased production of melatonin.

Concern is for children in whom the effects may be compounded because of increased vulnerability to radiation and their longer use of cell phones into adulthood. In response to the NTP study discussed earlier, the American Academy of Pediatrics issued specific recommendations to reduce wireless cell phone exposure (Box 13.4). Ongoing unbiased research is desperately needed. Chapter 14 discusses cancer in children.

Infection, Sexual and Reproductive Behavior, Human Papillomaviruses

Infections with certain viruses, bacteria, and parasites are an important contributor to cancer worldwide. Of the 14 million new cancer cases in 2012, 2.2 million (15.4%) were attributable to carcinogenic infections[244] (Table 13.9). Infection and cancer rates vary widely between countries and level of socioeconomic development; the higher the development, the lower the attributable fraction (AF) for infection. However, some highly developed countries continue to show a large burden of infection-attributable cancer because of the long interval between infection and cancer development.[244] In less-developed countries, infections account for about one in four cancers. The AFs for infection varied from less

BOX 13.4	CELL PHONE RADIATION AND CHILDREN'S HEALTH: WHAT PARENTS NEED TO KNOW

Use text messaging when possible and use cell phones in speaker mode or with the use of hands-free kits

When talking on the cell phone, try holding it an inch or more away from the head

Make only short or essential calls on cell phones

Avoid carrying the phone against the body like in a pocket, sock, or bra; cell phone manufacturers cannot guarantee that the amount of radiation absorbed will be at a safe level

Do not talk on the phone or text while driving; this increases the risk of automobile crashes

Exercise caution when using a phone or texting while walking for performing other activities; "distracted walking" injuries also are on the rise

If planning to watch a movie on the device, download it first, then switch to airplane mode while watching it to avoid unnecessary radiation exposure

Keep an eye on signal strength (i.e., number of bars); the weaker the cell signal, the harder the phone has to work and the more radiation it gives off; it is better to wait until there is a stronger signal before using the device

Avoid making calls in cars, elevators, trains, and buses; the cell phone works harder to get a signal through metal so the power level increases

Remember that cell phones are not toys or teething items

Data from American Academy of Pediatrics June 13, 2016. http://www.healthychildren.org.

than 5% in the United States, Canada, Australia, New Zealand, and some countries in western and northern Europe to more than 50% in some countries in sub-Saharan Africa.[244] The most significant infections worldwide together accounting for 92% of all infection-attributable cancers were *Helicobacter pylori* (*H. pylori* [770,000 cases]), human papillomavirus (640,000), hepatitis B virus (HBV [420,000]), hepatitis C virus (HCV [170,000]), and Epstein-Barr virus (EBV [120,000]). *H. pylori* was the most significant infectious cause of cancer in countries with high and very high development. Liver cancers attributable to HBV and HCV varied greatly with indices of the human development index (HDI). HBV was more significant than HCV as a cause of liver cancer in low-HDI and medium-HDI countries, and the opposite was true in countries with high and very high HDI because of early spread of HCV in some countries with very high HDI and the decreasing prevalence of HBV with increasing HDI.[244]

HPV caused more than half of the total infection-attributable cancers in women worldwide.[244] In low-HDI countries, HPV accounted for half of infection-attributable cancers in both sexes combined. Increased rates of cervical cancer resulted from poor screening and treatment of precancerous lesions combined with high prevalence of HPV and HIV infections.[245] It has been estimated that *H. pylori* accounts for about 75% of all stomach cancers.[246] Epstein-Barr virus (EBV) is associated with a subset of Hodgkin lymphoma, a subset of diffuse large B-cell lymphoma (DLBCL); Burkitt lymphoma; EBV-associated malignant B-cell lymphoma; age-related EBV-positive B-lymphoproliferative diseases (LPDs) that pathologically range from reactive hyperplasia to monomorphous lymphoma; EBV-associated T-/NK-cell LPDs; nasopharyngeal carcinoma; and gastric adenocarcinoma.[247] Human herpesvirus type 8 (HHV-8) accounted for about 2% of infection-attributable cancers

| TABLE 13.9 | NUMBER OF NEW CANCER CASES IN 2012 ATTRIBUTABLE TO INFECTION, BY INFECTIOUS AGENT |

	NUMBER OF NEW CASES*	PROPORTION OF NEW CASES ATTRIBUTABLE TO EACH INFECTIOUS AGENT (%)	NUMBER OF NEW CASES ATTRIBUTABLE TO INFECTION BY SEX			NUMBER OF NEW CASES ATTRIBUTABLE TO INFECTION BY AGE GROUP		
			MALES	FEMALES	<50 YEARS	50–69 YEARS	+70 YEARS
Helicobacter pylori	770,000	35.4	500,000	270,000	91,000	340,000	330,000
Human papillomavirus	640,000	29.5	66,000	570,000	270,000	280,000	90,000
Hepatitis B virus	420,000	19.2	300,000	120,000	84,000	190,000	140,000
Hepatitis C virus	170,000	7.8	110,000	55,000	26,000	76,000	66,000
Epstein-Barr virus	120,000	5.5	80,000	40,000	61,000	44,000	14,000
Human herpesvirus type B	44,000	2.0	29,000	15,000	32,000	7600	4500
Schistosoma haematobium	7000	0.3	4900	2200	1300	3700	2100
Human T-cell lymphotropic virus, type 1	3000	0.1	1700	1200	630	1200	1200
Opisthorchis viverrini or *Clonorchis sinensis*	1300	0.1	820	470	130	670	490
All infectious agents	2,200,000	100.0	1,100,000	1,100,000	570,000	950,000	650,000

*Numbers are rounded to two significant digits.
Data from Plummer M et al: *Lancet Global Health* 4:e609–e616, 2016.

worldwide and is associated with Kaposi sarcoma, a major public health concern in Africa. Human T-cell lymphotropic virus type 1 (HTLV-1) is associated with adult T-cell leukemia-lymphoma (ATL).

Human papillomavirus (HPV) is the most common sexually transmitted virus in the United States. HPV is extremely common worldwide.[248] About 14 million people become infected with HPV each year and about 79 million Americans are currently infected with HPV.[249] Most sexually active women and men will be infected at some point in their lives and some are infected repeatedly.[248] HPVs are a group of more than 200 related viruses of which at least 13 are cancer causing.[248] HPV is mainly transmitted through sexual contact and most people are infected with HPV shortly after the onset of sexual activity. *High-risk,* or oncogenic, *HPVs* (types 16 and 18) cause about 70% of cervical cancers and precancerous cervical lesions.[248] HPV has been linked with cancers of the anus, vulva, vagina, and penis. *Low-risk HPVs* do not cause cancer but can cause skin warts, called *condylomata acuminata.* Most high-risk HPV infections occur without any symptoms, may cause cytologic abnormalities or abnormal cell changes that disappear within 1 to 2 years, and do not cause cancer.[250] Persistence of infection with high-risk HPV is a prerequisite for the development of cervical intraepithelial neoplasia (CIN) (see Fig. 25.19), lesions, and invasive cervical cancers.[251] HPV can cause anal cancer, with about 85% of all cases caused by HPV-16.[250] HPV types 16 and 18 also have been found to be responsible for almost half of vaginal, vulvar, and penile cancers.[252] Investigators from prospective cohort studies have confirmed that infection with HPV-16 precedes by several years the diagnosis of oropharyngeal cancer (OPC).[253] HPV infections have been found to cause cancer of the oropharynx (most commonly base of the tongue, tonsils, and pharynx).[250] More than half of the oropharyngeal cancers diagnosed in the United States are linked to HPV-16.[254] The incidence of HPV-associated oropharyngeal cancer has increased during the past 20 years, especially among men, and it has been estimated that by 2020 HPV will cause more oropharyngeal cancers than cervical cancers in the United States.[255] Persistent chronic inflammation-related HPV infection might drive oropharyngeal carcinogenesis, and myeloid-derived suppressor cells (MDSCs [e.g., VEGF, GM-CSF, IL-1]) may play a role in this development because they facilitate tumor-induced immune suppression.[256] Factors that may increase the risk of developing cancer following a high-risk HPV infection include smoking, decreased immunity, having many children (for increased risk of cervical cancer), long-term oral contraceptive use (for increased risk of cervical cancer), poor oral hygiene (for increased risk of oropharyngeal cancer), and chronic inflammation.[257]

HPVs infect epithelial cells that cover the inside and outside surfaces of the body, including the skin, throat, genital tract, and anus. HPV types can easily be spread through direct sexual contact.[250] Vertical transmission also is possible in utero and during vaginal birth (see Chapter 27). Once an HPV virus enters an epithelial cell, the virus begins to make proteins that can interfere with normal functions in the cell, enabling the cell to grow in an uncontrolled manner, and to avoid apoptosis.[250] These infected cells are often recognized by the immune system and eliminated. Sometimes, however, infected cells are not destroyed and a persistent infection results. As the persistently infected cells continue to grow, they may develop mutations that promote even more cell growth, leading to the formation of a high-grade lesion and, ultimately, a tumor.[250] Investigators believe that it can take between 10 and 20 years from the time of an initial HPV infection until tumor formation. However, even high-grade lesions do not always lead to cancer[250] (see *What's New?* HPV Vaccine in Chapter 27).

Other Viruses and Microorganisms

A discussion of the relationship between viruses, bacteria, and cancer is contained in Chapter 12 and appropriate chapters in Part Two.

Other microorganisms involved in carcinogenesis include parasites such as *Opisthorchis viverrini* and *Schistosoma haematobium.* Their specific roles in carcinogenesis are thought to be related to cofactors or carcinogens, or both. Some viruses, bacteria, and parasites can cause chronic inflammation.

CHEMICALS AND OCCUPATIONAL HAZARDS AS CARCINOGENS

An estimated 100,000 synthetic chemicals are used in the United States;[258] however, a full set of basic toxicity information is available for only about 7% of these chemicals.[259] Another 1000 chemicals are added each year.[260] The list of chemicals has, therefore, expanded greatly, and other cancer risks related to the workplace now include ergonomic (e.g., sedentary), organizational (e.g., shift work), and biologic factors (e.g., infectious agents, endocrine disruptors). Exposure to chemicals occurs every day—they are present in air, soil, food, water, household products, toys, personal care products, workplaces, and homes. The number of known carcinogens in experimental animals is large. It is suspected that most of these chemical carcinogens are potentially carcinogenic in humans but documentation is lacking. An extensive list of potential occupational carcinogens is published by NIOSH and is available at https://www.cdc.gov/niosh/topics/cancer/npotocca.html. Table 13.1 provides a summary of a limited number of chemicals according to sufficient or limited evidence by IARC in humans by cancer site. A simplified overview of Occupational Safety and Health (OSH)-relevant carcinogenic factors is presented in Table 13.10.

Chemical carcinogenesis involves genotoxic mechanisms and nongenotoxic mechanisms (Fig. 13.21). The nongenotoxic mechanisms include inflammation, immunosuppression, oxidative stress (ROS), receptor activation, and epigenetic silencing.[261-263] According to the director of the National Institute of Environmental Health Sciences, "…exposure to gene-altering substances, particularly in the womb and shortly after birth, can lead to increased susceptibility to disease. There is a huge potential impact from these exposures, partly because the changes may be inherited across generations."[264]

Millions of U.S. workers are exposed to substances tested as carcinogens in animal studies or possibly found to be carcinogenic in human studies.[265] Shift work that involves circadian disruption and sedentary work have recently been identified as possible contributing factors to the development of work-related cancer.[266] Additionally, emerging from animal studies is that specific nonionizing radiation may be linked to human cancer risks.[238] Work-related stress may indirectly lead to cancers because coping strategies can include smoking, alcohol use, drug intake, and excessive and high-risk diets.[266] Newer risks identified are from nanomaterials, for example, carbon nanotubes, and from endocrine-disrupting compounds (EDCs).[266-268] In February 2013, WHO and the United Nations Environment Programme (UNEP) published a report on EDCs.[269] The authors reported emerging evidence of a link between exposure to EDCs and an increase in certain cancers, such as breast, endometrial, ovarian, testicular, prostate, and thyroid cancer. These cancers have been increasing over the past 40 to 50 years.[269] Occupational exposure to pesticides and to some polychlorinated biphenyls (PCBs) and exposure to arsenic are being studied as causes of prostate cancer. Additionally, concern was for workplace risks to reproduction because many substances also are reprotoxicants.[266] Research projects are needed to identify high-risk vulnerable groups (for example, pregnant women, young workers, and those exposed to high levels of carcinogens) for contracting occupational cancer. Model solutions need development to reduce exposure for such groups. In the service sector, awareness is low and workers have little training on how to protect themselves, they may have limited access to preventive services, and

TABLE 13.10   OVERVIEW OF OSH-RELEVANT CARCINOGENIC FACTORS

GROUP	EXAMPLE	GROUP	EXAMPLE
Chemicals		**Emerging Factors**	
Gases	Vinyl chloride	Air pollution and fine particulate matter	Emissions from motor vehicles, industrial processes, power generation, and other sources polluting the ambient air
	Formaldehyde		
Liquids, volatile	Trichloroethylene		
	Tetrachloroethylene		
	Methylchloride	Endocrine-disrupting compounds	Certain pesticides
	Styrene		Certain flame retardants
	Benzene		
	Xylene	**Biologic Factors**	
Liquids, nonvolatile	Metalworking fluids	Bacteria	*Helicobacter pylori*
	Mineral oils	Viruses	Hepatitis B
	Hair dyes		Hepatitis C
Solids, dust	Silica	Mycotoxin-producing fungi	Bulk handling of agricultural foodstuffs (nuts, grain, maize, coffee), animal-feed production, brewing/malting, waste management, composting, food production, working with indoor molds, horticulture
	Wood dust		
	Talc containing asbestiform fibers		
Solids, fibers	Asbestos		
	Man-made mineral fibers, for example, ceramic fibers		
Solids	Lead		
	Nickel compounds	*Aspergillus flavus, A. parasiticus*	Aflatoxin (A1)
	Chromium VI compounds	*Penicillium griseofulvum*	Griseofulvin (IARC group 2B)
	Arsenic	*A. ochraceus, A. carbonarius, P. verrucosum*	Ochratoxin A (group 2B)
	Beryllium		
	Cadmium	*A. versicolor, Emericella nidulans, Chaetomium spp., A. flavus, A. parasiticus*	Sterigmatocystin (group 2B)
	Carbon black		
	Bitumen		
Fumes, smoke	Welding fumes	*Fusarium spp.*	Fumonisin B1 (group 2B)
	Diesel emissions		
	Coal tar fumes	**Physical Factors**	
	Bitumen fumes	Ionizing radiation	Radon
	Fire, combustion emissions		X-rays
	PAHs	Ultraviolet radiation (UVR)	Solar radiation
	Tobacco smoke		Artificial UVR
Mixtures	Solvents	Ergonomics	Sedentary work
Pesticides		**Other**	
Halogenated organic compounds	DDT	Work organization	Shift work that involves circadian disruption
	Ethylene dibromide		Static work
Others	Amitrole		Prolonged sitting and standing
Pharmaceuticals		Lifestyle factors	Stress-related obesity, smoking, drinking, drug consumption
Antineoplastic drugs	MOPP (Mustargen, oncovin, procarbazine, and prednisone, a combination chemotherapy regimen used to treat Hodgkin disease) and other combined chemotherapy, including alkylating agents	**Combinations of Various Factors**	
		Chemicals and radiation	Methoxsalen and UVA radiation
			Some chemicals, called *promoters*, can increase the cancer-causing ability of UVR. Conversely, UVR can act as a promoter and increase the cancer-causing ability of some chemicals, particularly coal tar and pitch.
Anesthetics	There is evidence from in vitro experiments that isoflurane increases cancer cells' potential to grow and migrate		
		Work organization and chemicals	Shift work and solvents

DDT, Dichlorodiphenyltrichloroethane; *IARC*, International Agency for Research on Cancer; *PAHs*, polycyclic aromatic hydrocarbons; *UVA*, ultraviolet A.

Data from European Agency for Safety and Health at Work: *Exposure to carcinogens and work-related cancer: a review of assessment methods European Risk Observatory Report*, Luxembourg, 2014, European Agency for Safety and Health at Work Eu-OSHA. http://europa.eu.

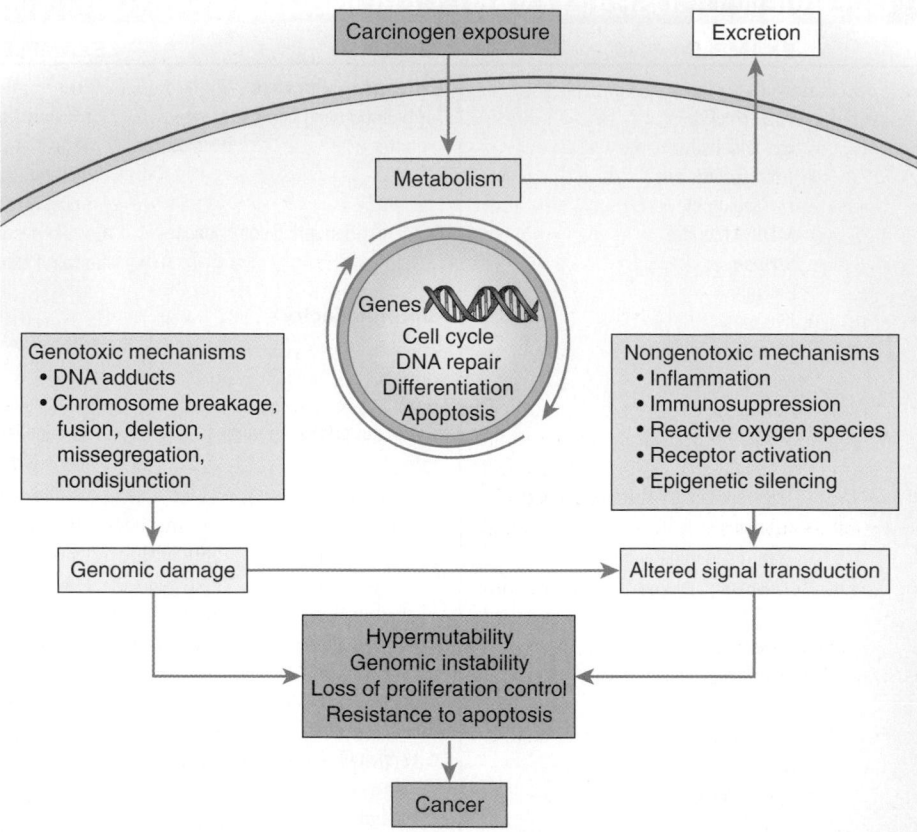

FIGURE 13.21 Mechanisms of Chemical Carcinogenesis. Cellular internalization of chemical carcinogens results in metabolic products that are either excreted or retained by the cell. Within the cell, carcinogens or their metabolic products can directly or indirectly affect the regulation and expression of genes involved in cell cycle control, DNA repair, cell differentiation, or apoptosis. Some chemical carcinogens act by *genotoxic* mechanisms, such as DNA adducts, chromosomal breakage, fusion, deletion, missegregation, and nondisjunction. Other carcinogens act by *nongenotoxic* mechanisms, such as induction of inflammation, immunosuppression, formation of reactive oxygen species (oxidative stress), activation of receptors, and epigenetic mechanisms, such as silencing. Both genotoxic and nongenotoxic mechanisms can alter signal-transduction pathways that result in many features of cancer cells. (Adapted from Luch A: *Nat Rev Cancer* 5:113–125, 2005.)

they are infrequently consulted on workplace measures.[266] It has been estimated that 3% to 6% of all cancers worldwide are caused by workplace exposures to carcinogens.

A substantial percentage of cancers of the upper respiratory passages (lung, bladder, and peritoneum) is attributed to occupational factors; however, fewer studies of nonsmokers exist.[270,271] Textile industry workers are exposed to a number of chemicals (dyes, solvents, fiber dusts, others) continuously with known carcinogenic properties.[272] Exposure to different kinds of chemicals and physical factors in the textile industry induce occupational cancer, including lung, bladder, colorectal, and breast cancer, as a long-term effect among textile industry workers.[272] One notable occupational factor is asbestos, which increases the risk of asbestosis, lung cancer, and mesothelioma. Asbestos was used in homes and buildings built before the 1970s to insulate ceiling tiles, flooring, and pipe covers. Asbestos also has been used for decades in thousands of commercial products, including fireproofing materials, automotive brakes, textile products, cement, and wallboard materials. In Western Europe, the epidemic of mesothelioma in building workers and other workers born after 1940 did not become apparent until the 1990s because of long latency. No exposure to asbestos is without risk and a large number of countries still use, export, and import asbestos-containing products (see Table 13.1). Many residential and commercial settings still contain asbestos.[273]

Carcinoma of the bladder has been linked with the manufacture of dyes, rubber, paint, and aromatic amines, especially β-naphthylamine and benzidine. Benzol inhalation is linked to leukemia in shoemakers and in workers in the rubber cement, explosives, and dyeing industries. Other notable occupational hazards include heavy metals (e.g., high-nickel alloy, chromium VI compounds, inorganic arsenic), silica, polycyclic aromatic hydrocarbons, sulfuric acid, and chloromethyl ether. Occupational exposure to diesel exhaust, especially to underground miners, has been linked to eye and nose irritation, headaches, nausea, and asthma. NIOSH and the EPA have classified diesel exhaust as a possible carcinogen.[274] The IARC classifies diesel engine exhaust as carcinogenic to humans and is based on sufficient evidence that it is linked to an increased risk of lung cancer. Disentangling data related to lung cancer, air pollution, and occupational risks is complex, especially in combination with active and passive smoking and the interplay of environmental factors and genetic polymorphisms at multiple loci.

SUMMARY REVIEW

Genes, Epigenetics, and Tissue

1. Cancers are caused by environmental-lifestyle and genetic factors. Environmental factors and lifestyle behaviors contribute to a very large number of cancer cases. Biologically, cancer is driven by genetic alterations and changes in epigenetic regulation. Different combinations of mutations and epigenetic changes are found in different types of cancer. Avoiding high-risk behaviors and exposures to individual carcinogens, or cancer-causing substances, will prevent many types of cancer.
2. Investigators are connecting the intricate web between genotype, phenotype, high-risk lifestyle behaviors, the environment, and carcinogenesis.
3. Interacting factors that influence cancer risk include detoxifying enzymes, DNA repair genes, immune/inflammation systems, and the cell's immediate environment. The cell's biologic environment is modified by metabolic requirements, physical activity, infections, nutrition, carcinogens, air pollution, and many other environmental factors.
4. Cancer development and progression involve the tissue microenvironment or stroma.
5. The microenvironment participates in a complex signaling process that facilitates tumor promotion and metastases because stromal tissue has immune cells. Chronic inflammation from infiltrating immune cells can be caused by numerous environmental factors, for example, inhaling tobacco smoke.
6. Cancer development in the presence of chronic inflammation involves the continuous presence of cytokines, ROS, COX-2, 5-LOX, MMPs, and essential transcription factors (e.g., NF-κB).

Incidence and Mortality Trends

1. Cancer is reported to become a major cause of morbidity and mortality in the coming decades in all regions of the world.
2. Data for the United States from 2003 to 2012 showed incidence of 7 of the 17 more common cancers in men decreased and overall incidence stayed close to the same for women. The decline in lung cancer corresponded to a decrease in tobacco use. Cancer incidence, however, increased among people ages 0 to 19 years. In all racial and ethnic populations, men had about a threefold higher liver cancer incidence than women.
3. Death rates continued to decrease for men, women, and children. Deaths caused by liver cancer, however, increased at the highest rate of all reported cancer sites.

In Utero and Early Life Conditions

1. Accumulating data suggest early life events influence later susceptibility to certain chronic conditions, including cancer.
2. Developmental plasticity is the degree to which an organism's development is contingent on its environment. An emerging hypothesis is that persistent epigenetic adaptations that occur early in development in response to parental nutrition and the environment are associated with increased susceptibility to cancer and other adult-onset chronic diseases.
3. Epidemiologic and animal studies reveal that small changes in the developmental environment can alter phenotypic changes, resulting in individual responses in adulthood.

Environmental-Lifestyle Factors
Tobacco Use

1. Cigarette smoking is carcinogenic and the most important cause of cancer and death from cancer. The risk is greatest in those who begin to smoke when young and continue throughout life.
2. Worldwide, tobacco use is a major preventable cause of premature death and disease where 5.4 million people die each year from tobacco-related illnesses. More than 16 million Americans live with a smoking-related disease.
3. Smoking affects nearly every organ of the body. Since the first Surgeon's General report on smoking and health in 1964, more than 20 million Americans have died as a result of smoking. Smoking causes even more deaths from vascular, respiratory, and other diseases than from cancer.
4. Smoking tobacco is linked to cancers of the lung, upper aerodigestive tract (oral cavity, pharynx, larynx, nasal cavity, paranasal sinuses, esophagus), stomach, lower urinary tract (renal pelvis, penis, bladder), kidney, pancreas, cervix, and uterus, as well as myeloid leukemia. The new list of disease risks includes liver cancer and colorectal cancer.
5. Secondhand smoke or environmental tobacco smoke (both sidestream smoke [burning end of cigarette, cigar, or pipe] and mainstream smoke exhaled by the smoker) is a cause of stroke; it increases the risk of death in people with cancer and cancer survivors, as well as those with age-related macular degeneration, tuberculosis, ectopic pregnancy, and diabetes mellitus; it increases inflammation and impairs immunity; and it is a cause of rheumatoid arthritis.
6. Nonsmokers who live with smokers are at greatest risk for lung cancer, as well as other noncancerous conditions. Parental smoking is linked to babies who died of sudden infant death syndrome or complications from low birth weight or other conditions. In utero effects from maternal or paternal smoking and subsequent disease are being investigated.
7. Regular cigar smoking is associated with increased risk for cancers of the lung, esophagus, larynx, and oral cavity (lip, tongue, mouth, throat). Heavy cigar smoking increases the risk for lung diseases, including emphysema and chronic bronchitis. Cigar smoking is linked to gum disease and tooth loss. Pipe smokers have an increased risk of dying from cancers of the lung, throat, esophagus, larynx, pancreas, and colorectum. Compared to nonsmokers, bidi smokers have the same risks of cancer and higher risks of heart attacks and chronic bronchitis. Kreteks are a tobacco product.
8. An e-cigarette delivers a vapor (aerosol) of nicotine, flavorings, and other chemicals when puffed. The vapor is inhaled just like smoke from a regular cigarette and absorbed into the lungs. Colorful "vape pens" or "e-hookahs" are marketed to appeal to youth with flavors like candy and fruit. The electronic nicotine delivery system (ENDS) is designed to deliver nicotine, which is addictive. Many questions have been raised as to the safety of e-cigarettes because ENDS cartridges are *not* labeled with their ingredients.

Nutrition, Obesity, Alcohol Consumption, and Physical Activity

1. Abundant evidence exists that dietary factors are related to cancer development. Emerging is the interaction of dietary factors with genomics, epigenomics, transcription factors (transcriptomics), proteomics, and metabolic factors (metabolomics) and how they influence cancer risk. Nutrigenomics is the study of the effects of nutrition on the phenotypic variability of individuals based on genomic differences.
2. What people eat, how much they weigh, and how much they move influence their risks of developing cancer and other chronic diseases. Everyday choices impact their chances of getting or preventing cancer. Lifestyle and nutrition are associated with development or progression, or both, of major human cancers, including some of the most common (e.g., breast, prostate, colorectal, and others).

3. Researchers are studying types of diet that either prevent or reduce mortality rates for cancer and other chronic diseases. Much attention is the research on the Mediterranean diet.

4. Examples of food components reported to have cancer-preventive potential include polyphenols, selenium, methyl group donors, retinoids, isothiocyanates, allyl compounds, and mono- and polyunsaturated fatty acids. Several dietary factors alter the expression of many miRNAs in animals and humans.

5. Various food components can influence DNA repair.

6. Sources of carcinogenic substances include compounds produced in the cooking of fat, meat, or protein, and naturally occurring carcinogens associated with plant food substances, such as alkaloids or mold byproducts.

7. Dietary components can act directly as mutagens or interfere with the elimination of mutagens.

8. Dietary factors may affect the cell cycle, differentiation, DNA damage and repair, stem cell renewal, hormonal axes, the balance of cellular proliferation and cell death, the microenvironment, cell signaling, inflammation, and immunity.

9. Xenobiotics that include toxic, mutagenic, and carcinogenic chemicals are found in the human diet.

10. Food and nutrition modify carcinogen metabolism and include the examples selenium, allyl sulfur, sulforaphane, and isoflavonoids.

11. Diets high in red meat and processed meat are linked to an increased risk of developing colorectal cancer. Several mechanisms are proposed for effects of meat and cancer, for example, *N*-nitroso compounds can increase nitrogenous residues in the colon and cause DNA damage.

12. Undernutrition can be a factor in cancers caused by infectious agents, for example, cancers of the liver and cervix.

13. Future research is needed to define robust biomarkers of cancer risk.

14. Obesity has been increasing in most developed countries and in urban areas of developing countries. Obesity in the United States is an epidemic.

15. Childhood obesity has been increasing. There is considerable concern for children with early onset of obesity.

16. The substantial suffering and long-term human and societal costs of obesity underlie the urgency to accelerate progress in obesity prevention.

17. Studies have significantly improved the understanding of the relationship between overweight/obesity, energy balance and cancer risk, cancer recurrence, and survival.

18. Consensus now exists that obesity is a risk factor for developing the following cancers: liver, advanced prostate, ovarian, gallbladder, kidney, colorectal, esophageal (adenocarcinoma), postmenopausal breast, pancreatic, endometrial, and stomach (cardia) (see Fig. 13.13). The IARC identified additional cancers with sufficient evidence that the absence of body fatness lowers cancer risk for thyroid and multiple myeloma.

19. Obesity is recognized as a poor prognostic factor for several cancers.

20. The mechanisms of obesity-associated cancer risks are unclear and may vary by type of tumor and distribution of body fat. Three main factors related to obesity and cancer are the insulin–insulin-like growth factor axis, sex hormones, and adipokines.

21. Metabolic changes in adipose tissue from obesity result in several alterations and include insulin resistance, hyperglycemia, dyslipidemia, hypoxia, and chronic inflammation.

22. Obesity leads to adipocyte dysfunction and immune cell recruitment leading to cytokine production, inflammation, and, ultimately,

fibrosis and reduced response to chemotherapy. Adipocytes function as endocrine cells and critically shape the tumor microenvironment.

23. Obesity can increase aromatase expression, resulting in increased estradiol levels, which can promote the growth of estrogen-dependent cancers.

24. Cancers have altered metabolism. Tumors consume large quantities of glucose to make cellular building blocks, called the *Warburg effect*.

25. Food metabolism and circadian cycles are linked, and impairment of inner clock regulation results in dysregulated metabolism.

26. Overall, there are strong data supporting alcohol as a cause of cancers of the mouth, pharynx, larynx, esophagus, and liver; colorectal cancer in men; and postmenopausal breast cancer.

27. Factors contributing to alcohol-induced cancer development include acetaldehyde, oxidative stress, and nutritional deficiencies, especially folate, a B vitamin.

28. Variations in several genes modulate the risk of alcohol-induced carcinogenesis, and increasing evidence suggests aberrant patterns of DNA methylation also contribute.

29. Physical activity reduces the risk for breast cancer, colon cancer, and endometrial cancer, independent of weight changes.

30. Biologic mechanisms for the protective effects of exercise include decreasing insulin and IGF levels, decreasing obesity, increasing free-radical scavenger systems, changing inflammatory mediators, decreasing oncogenes, decreasing the levels of circulating sex hormones and metabolic hormones, improving immune function, and enhancing cytochrome P-450 function, thus modifying carcinogen activation and increasing gut motility.

31. Several reports suggest that implementing a physical activity program after a cancer diagnosis is associated with better cancer-specific outcomes and overall survival with early-stage breast, prostate, and colorectal cancers.

32. Many unanswered questions remain regarding the frequency, intensity, and duration of exercise required for optimal health benefits.

Air Pollution

1. Ambient air pollution increases mortality and morbidity and shortens life expectancy from cardiovascular, respiratory disease, and lung cancer.

2. Air pollution is a leading cause of global disease burden. Long-term exposure to fine particle air pollution ($PM_{2.5}$) caused 4.2 million deaths and 103.1 million lost years of healthy life in 2015. An additional 254,000 deaths were linked to exposure to ozone.

3. The IARC concluded that exposure to outdoor air pollution and to particulate matter (PM) in outdoor air is carcinogenic to humans and causes lung cancer. Fine or ultrafine particles are easily absorbed by the lungs and phagocytosed by macrophages and neutrophils that release tissue-damaging inflammatory mediators.

4. The mechanisms of adverse cellular effects of PM include (1) cytotoxicity through oxidative stress, (2) ROS generation, (3) DNA oxidative damage, (4) mutagenicity, (5) stimulation of proinflammatory factors, and (6) induction of cell senescence.

5. The indoor air pollution environmental tobacco smoke (ETS; passive smoking) can cause the formation of reactive oxygen free radicals and thus DNA damage. The IARC has classified ETS as a human carcinogen.

6. In 2012 diesel exhaust was classified as a carcinogen in humans by the IARC.

SUMMARY REVIEW—cont'd

7. The central hypothesis for cancer pathogenesis is that insoluble particles cause pulmonary inflammation (e.g., cytokine release, ROS) which leads to oxidative stress and oxidation of DNA, proliferative response, and tissue remodeling progressing toward fibrosis and tumor development.

Ionizing Radiation, Ultraviolet Radiation, and Electromagnetic Radiation

1. Much of the knowledge of the effects of ionizing radiation (IR) on human cancer has stemmed from observations of the Hiroshima and Nagasaki atomic bomb exposures, particularly the Life Span Study. Other evidence is derived from groups exposed for medical reasons, underground miners exposed to radon gas, and other occupational exposures.

2. The atomic bomb exposures in Japan caused acute leukemias in adults and children and increased frequencies of thyroid and breast carcinomas. Lung, stomach, colon, esophageal, and urinary tract cancers and multiple myeloma have been added to the list.

3. Recent models of radiation carcinogenesis show ionizing radiation (IR) acts not only as an initiator of premalignant cell clones but also as a promoter of preexisting premalignant cell alterations.

4. Health risks from IR involve cancers, cardiovascular diseases, respiratory diseases, birth defects, and eye maladies.

5. In 2009 the National Council on Radiation Protection and Measurements reported Americans were exposed to more than 7 times as much IR from medical procedures compared to IR exposure in the 1980s.

6. Ionizing radiation is a mutagen and carcinogen and can penetrate cells and tissues and deposit energy in tissues at random in the form of ionizations.

7. The past two decades have focused on cellular and molecular mechanisms that relate to the induction of cancer, including dose-response relationships for chromosome aberrations and for cell transformation; gene expression (genetic and epigenetic); alternative targets, such as membranes; mutagenesis in somatic cells; the biologic effects that occur in nonirradiated cells (i.e., nontargeted effects); and effects on the microenvironment.

8. Exposure to ionizing radiation induces apoptosis and senescence. Emerging data are identifying these effects in endothelial cells and the biology of radiation-induced cardiovascular disease.

9. Because models and underlying assumptions of IR and cell damage are incomplete, investigators are working hard to understand induced repair, adaptive responses, hormesis, low-dose hypersensitivity, nontargeted effects, signaling, exosomes, and long-term persistence of radiation damage and clonal heterogeneity.

10. A long-held assumption is that cellular alterations—mutations and malignant transformation—occur only in cells directly radiated. It is now known that radiation may induce a type of genomic instability to the progeny of the directly irradiated cells over many cell generations and can affect so-called *innocent bystander cells*.

11. Epigenetic events after radiation include alterations in pathways affecting cell adhesion, extracellular matrix interactions, and cell-to-cell communication.

12. The principal source of UV radiation is sunlight. Solid evidence shows sun and ultraviolet (UV) radiation causes basal cell carcinoma and squamous cell carcinoma. Fair evidence showing intermittent acute sun exposure leading to sunburn is associated with an increased risk of melanoma. The most preventable cause of skin cancer is exposure to UV light from the sun or from artificial sources, such as tanning beds.

13. The degree of damage in skin depends on the intensity and wavelength content—ultraviolet A (UVA) or ultraviolet B (UVB).

14. The pathogenesis of nonmelanoma skin cancers involves specific gene mutations, DNA methylation and histone modifications, oxidative stress, inflammation, and reduced immune surveillance. The relationship between sun exposure and the risk of melanoma remains complex.

15. ROS can induce a number of transcription factors (e.g., activator protein 1 [AP-1] and NF-κB) and increase the levels of regulating genes that induce inflammation. Inflammation is a critical component of tumor progression.

16. The incidence of melanoma in the United States has been increasing annually. Because mortality rates have not risen as rapidly, however, controversy exists as to whether the incidence increase is a true increase in clinically significant melanoma or is a result of overdiagnosis.

17. Health risks associated with electromagnetic radiation (EMR) are controversial. Exposure to electric and magnetic fields is widespread. EMRs are a type of nonionizing and low-frequency radiation.

18. EMRs generated by radiofrequency sources couple with the body and result in induced electric and magnetic fields with associated currents inside tissue.

19. Microwaves, radar, mobile and cell phones, mobile phone base stations, appliances, power frequency radiation associated with electricity and radio waves, fluorescent lights, computers, and other electric equipment create EMRs of varying strength.

20. Data measuring the relationships between EMR exposure and cancer are limited because of inadequate methods to accurately measure exposure, lack of clear dose-response relationships and reproduction of effects, financial interests, and other priorities such as convenience.

21. Most exposure to EMFs from occupational sources comes from near-field sources; the highest exposure to the general population comes from transmitters close to the body, such as hand-held devices like mobile telephones.

22. The WHO International Agency for Research on Cancer Monograph Working Group reported that the INTERPHONE and Swedish studies were judged susceptible to bias, the findings could not be dismissed because of bias alone, and a causal relationship between phones and glioma is possible. The National Institute of Environmental Health Sciences is doing a large-scale study on rodents exposed to radiofrequency energy (cell phone type). Early preliminary data have been reported.

23. The outcome of the Working Group was to classify RF-EMF as "possibly carcinogenic to humans" (Group 2B). The mechanisms included genotoxicity, effects on immune function, gene and protein expression, cell signaling, oxidative stress, apoptosis, and, possibly, the blood-brain barrier.

24. There are no studies of adults who have used cell phones as children or adolescents. Concern is for children in whom the effects may be compounded because of increased vulnerability to radiation and their longer use of cell phones into adulthood.

Infection

1. Infections with certain viruses, bacteria, and parasites are an important contributor to cancer worldwide. Of the 14 million new cancer cases in 2012, 2.2 million (15.4%) were attributable to carcinogenic infections.

2. Infection and cancer rates vary widely between countries and level of socioeconomic development.

SUMMARY REVIEW—cont'd

3. The top notable infections and new cancer cases include *Helicobacter pylori (H. pylori),* human papillomavirus (HPV), hepatitis B virus (HBV), hepatitis C virus (HCV), and Epstein-Barr virus (EBV).

4. Hepatitis B and hepatitis C can infect the liver and together account for the large majority of liver cancer diagnoses. HPV caused more than half of the total infection-attributable cancers in women worldwide. HPV is the most common viral infection of the reproductive tract. Most sexually active women and men will be infected at some point in their lives and some may be repeatedly infected. *H. pylori* accounts for an estimated 75% of all stomach cancers. EBV is associated with a subset of Hodgkin lymphoma and Burkitt lymphoma, and other types of cancer.

5. HPVs are a group of more than 200 related viruses of which 13 are cancer causing. High-risk or oncogenic HPVs (types 16 and 18) cause about 70% of cervical cancers and precancerous cervical lesions. HPV has been linked with cancers of the anus, vulva, vagina, and penis. Prospective studies have confirmed that infection with HPV-16 precedes by several years the diagnosis of oropharyngeal cancer (OPC).

6. Factors that may increase the risk of developing cancer following a high-risk HPV infection include smoking, decreased immunity, having many children (for increased risk of cervical cancer), long-term oral contraceptive use (for increased risk of cervical cancer), poor oral hygiene (for increased risk of oropharyngeal cancer), and chronic inflammation.

Chemicals and Occupational Hazards as Carcinogens

1. An estimated 100,000 synthetic chemicals are used in the United States. Of those, only about 7% have been tested for their health effects and another 1000 are added each year.

2. Chemicals are present in air, soil, food, water, personal care products, toys, household products, medications, workplaces, and homes. The list of chemicals has expanded and added to other cancer risks related to the workplace, including ergonomic, organizational, and biologic factors.

3. An extensive list of potential occupational carcinogens is published by the NIOSH, and known and probable carcinogenic agents are updated by the International Agency for Research on Cancer (IARC).

4. Chemical carcinogenesis involves genotoxic and nongenotoxic mechanisms. The nongenotoxic mechanisms include inflammation, immunosuppression, oxidative stress (ROS), receptor activation, and epigenetic silencing.

5. Work-related stress may indirectly lead to cancer because coping strategies include smoking, alcohol, drug intake, and excessive high-risk diets.

6. A substantial percentage of cancers of the upper respiratory passages, lung, bladder, and peritoneum are attributed to occupational factors; however, fewer studies of nonsmokers exist.

7. Disentangling data related to lung cancer, air pollution, and occupational factors is complex, especially in combination with active and passive smoking, environmental factors, and multiple interacting genes.

KEY TERMS

Adipokine, 399
Asbestos, 416
Basal cell carcinoma (BCC), 410
Bystander effect, 409
Circadian rhythm, 399
Developmental plasticity, 385
DNA damage response (DDR), 409
Double-strand break (DSB), 408
Electromagnetic radiation (EM or EMR), 411
Electronic cigarettes (e-cigarettes), 391

Energy balance, 398
Environmental tobacco smoke (ETS), 388
Genomic instability, 409
Individual carcinogen, 379
Insulin-like growth factor-1 [IGF-1], 398
Melanoma, 410
Myokine, 399
Nontargeted effect (NTE), 408
Nutrigenomics, 392
Particulate matter, 404

Phase I activation enzyme, 397
Phase II detoxification enzyme, 397
Radiofrequency electromagnetic radiation (RF-EMR), 411
Radon, 404
Squamous cell carcinoma (SCC), 410
Ultraviolet radiation (UV radiation), 410
Xenobiotics, 395

REFERENCES

1. Colditz GA, Sutcliffe S: The preventability of cancer; stacking the deck. *JAMA Oncol* 2(9): 1131–1133, 2016.

2. Cogliano VJ, et al: Preventable exposures associated with cancers. *J Natl Cancer Inst* 103:1–13, 2011.

3. Institute of Medicine (IOM): *Rebuilding the unity of health and the environment: a new vision of environmental health for the 21st century. Workshop summary,* Washington, DC, 2001, National Academies Press.

4. National Toxicology Program: *Report on carcinogens,* ed 12, Washington, DC, 2011, U.S. Department of Health and Human Services.

5. Esteller M: Epigenetics in cancer. *N Engl J Med* 358:1148–1159, 2008.

6. Jones PA, Baylin SB: The epigenomics of cancer. *Cell* 128:683–692, 2007.

7. Tam WL, Weinberg RA: The epigenetics of epithelial-mesenchymal plasticity in cancer. *Nat Med* 19(11):1438–1449, 2013.

8. Alberts B, et al: *Molecular biology of the cell,* ed 6, Garland Science. New York, 2015, Taylor & Francis Group.

9. Lambert AW, Pattabiraman DR, Weinberg RA: Emerging biological principles of metastasis. *Cell* 168(4):670–691, 2017.

10. O'Hagan HM, et al: Oxidative damage targets complexes containing DNA methyltransferases, SIRT1, and polycomb members to promoter CpG islands. *Cancer Cell* 20(5):606–619, 2011.

11. International Agency for Research on Cancer (IARC): *Special report: policy—a review of human carcinogens—part C: metals, arsenic, dusts, and fibres,* 2012. Available at http://monographs .iarc.fr/ENG/Monographs/vol100C/index.php.

12. Straif K, et al: A review of human carcinogens—part C: metals, arsenic, dusts, and fibres. *Lancet Oncol* 10(5):453–454, 2009.

13. Ferlay J, et al: *GLOBOCAN 2012 v1.1, Cancer incidence and mortality worldwide: IARC CancerBase No. 11 [Internet],* Lyon, France, 2014, Author. Available at http://globocan.iarc.fr.

14. National Cancer Institute (NCI): *Annual report to the nation on the status of cancer, 1975-2012,* Bethesda, MD, 2016, National Institutes of Health, National Cancer Institute.

15. Gluckman PD, et al: Effect of in utero and early-life conditions on adult health and disease. *N Engl J Med* 359(1):61–73, 2008.

16. Bateson P, et al: Developmental plasticity and human health. *Nature* 430:419–421, 2004.

17. Lee HS: Impact of maternal diet on the epigenome during in utero life and the developmental programming of diseases in childhood and adulthood. *Nutrients* 7(11): 9492–9507, 2015.

18. Waterland RA, Jirtle RJ: Early nutrition, epigenetic changes at transposons and imprinted genes, and enhanced susceptibility to adult chronic disease. *Nutrition* 20:63–68, 2004.

19. Koukoura O, et al: DNA methylation in the human placenta and fetal growth. *Mol Med Rep* 5:883–889, 2012.

20. Marsit CJ: Placental epigenetics in children's environmental health. *Semin Reprod Med* 34(1): 36–41, 2016.

21. Painter RC, et al: Early onset of coronary artery disease after prenatal exposure to the Dutch famine. *Am J Clin Nutr* 84:322–327, 2006.

22. Jang H, Serra C: Nutrition, epigenetics, and diseases. *Clin Nutr Res* 3(1):1–8, 2014.

23. Waterland RA, Jirtle RL: Transposable elements: targets for early nutritional effects on epigenetic gene regulation. *Mol Cell Biol* 23:5293–5300, 2003.

24. Rubin MM: Antenatal exposure to DES: lessons learned…future concerns. *Obstet Gynecol Surv* 62(8):548–555, 2007.

25. Triosi R, Potischman N, Hoover RN: Exploring the underlying hormonal mechanisms of prenatal risk factors for breast cancer: a review and commentary. *Cancer Epidemiol Biomarkers Prev* 16(9):1700–1712, 2007.

26. Palmer JR, et al: Prenatal diethylstilbestrol exposure and risk of breast cancer. *Cancer Epidemiol Biomarkers Prev* 15(8):1509–1514, 2006.

27. McLachlan JA: Commentary: prenatal exposure to diethylstilbestrol (DES): a continuing story. *Int J Epidemiol* 35(4):868–870, 2006.

28. Newbold RR, et al: Proliferative lesions and reproductive tract tumors in male descendants of mice exposed developmentally to diethylstilbestrol. *Carcinogenesis* 21:1355–1363, 2000.

29. Petridou E, et al: Baldness and other correlates of sex hormones in relation to testicular cancer. *Int J Cancer* 71(6):982–985, 1997.

30. Yang Q, Diamond MP, Al-Hendy A: Early life adverse environmental exposures increase the risk of uterine fibroid development: role of epigenetic regulation. *Front Pharmacol* 7:40, 2016.

31. Song M, Giovannucci E: Preventable incidence and mortality of carcinoma associated with lifestyle factors among whites in the United States. *JAMA Oncol* 2(9):1154–1161, 2016.

32. Wu S, et al: Substantial contribution of extrinsic risk factors to cancer development. *Nature* 529: 43–47, 2016.

33. Colditz GA, Wolin KY, Gehlert S: Applying what we know to accelerate cancer prevention. *Sci Transl Med* 4(127):127rv4, 2012.

34. National Cancer Institute (NCI): *Tobacco*, Washington, DC, 2015, U.S. Department of Health and Human Services, National Institutes of Health, National Cancer Institute.

35. Center for Disease Control and Prevention (CDC): *At a glance 2016 tobacco use: extinguishing the epidemic*, Atlanta GA, 2017, Office on Smoking and Health, National Center for Chronic Disease Prevention and Health promotion.

36. U.S. Department of Health and Human Services (USDHHS): *The health consequences of smoking—50 years of progress: a report of the Surgeon General*, Atlanta, 2014, U.S. Department of Health and Human Services, Centers for Disease Control and Prevention, National Center for Chronic Disease Prevention and Health Promotion, Office on Smoking and Health.

37. Centers for Disease Control and Prevention (CDC): *Global tobacco control*, Atlanta, GA, 2017, Office on Smoking and Health, Centers for Disease Control and Prevention, National Center for Chronic Disease Prevention and Health Promotion, U.S. Department of Health & Human Services.

38. Centers for Disease Control and Prevention (CDC): *Current cigarette smoking among adults in the United States*, Atlanta, GA, 2017, Centers for Disease Control and Prevention, National Center

for Chronic Disease Prevention and Health Promotion, U.S. Department of Health & Human Services.

39. Hu SS, et al: Tobacco product use among adults—United States, 2013-2014. *MMWR Morb Mortal Wkly Rep* 65(27):685–691, 2016.

40. World Health Organization (WHO): *WHO report on the global tobacco epidemic, 2011. Warning about the dangers of tobacco, executive summary*, Geneva, Switzerland, 2011, Author.

41. Zeng W, et al: Burden of total and cause-specific mortality related to tobacco smoking among adults aged ≥45 years in Asia: a pooled analysis of 21 cohorts. *PLoS Med* 11(4):e1001631, 2014.

42. Lushniak BD: A historic moment: the 50th anniversary of the first Surgeon General's Report on smoking and health. *Public Health Rep* 129(1):5–6, 2014.

43. Office of the Surgeon General: *The health consequences of smoking—50 years of progress. A report of the Surgeon General executive summary*, Rockville, MD, 2014, U.S. Department of Health and Human Services.

44. Centers for Disease Control and Prevention (CDC): *Smoking and secondhand smoke*. Available at www.cdc.gov/cancer/lung.

45. Campaign for Tobacco-Free Kids: *The rise of cigars and cigar-smoking harms*, Washington, DC, 2016, Author. Available at http:// www.tobaccofreekids.org/who_we_are.

46. National Cancer Institute (NCI): *Cigars: health effects and trends. Smoking and Tobacco Control Monograph No. 9*, Bethesda, MD, 1998, National Institutes of Health, National Cancer Institute.

47. American Cancer Society (ACS): *Is any type of smoking safe?* Atlanta, GA, 2015, Author.

48. Centers for Disease Control and Prevention (CDC): *Cigars*, Atlanta, GA, 2016, U.S. Department of Health & Human Services Office on Smoking and Health, National Center for Chronic Disease Prevention and Health Promotion.

49. Centers for Disease Control and Prevention (CDC): *Smoking and tobacco use: hookahs*, Atlanta, GA, 2016, U.S. Department of Health & Human Services, Centers for Disease Control and Prevention, National Center for Chronic Disease Prevention and Health Promotion Office on Smoking and Health.

50. U.S. Department of Health and Human Services (USDHHS): *Preventing tobacco use among youth and young adults: a report of the Surgeon General*, Atlanta, GA, 2012, U.S. Department of Health and Human Services, Centers for Disease Control and Prevention, Office on Smoking and Health.

51. American Cancer Society (ACS): *Is any type of smoking safe?* Atlanta, GA, 2016, Author. Available at: http://www.cancer.org/cancer/cancercauses/ tobaccocancer/is-any-type-of-smoking-safe? Revised Sept 14, 2016.

52. American Cancer Society (ACS): *What about exotic forms of smoking tobacco, such as clove cigarettes, bidis, and hookahs?* Atlanta, GA, 2011, Author.

53. U.S. Food and Drug Administration (FDA): *Vaporizers, e-cigarettes, and other electronic nicotine delivery systems (ENDS)*, updated April 18, 2017, Silver Spring MD, 2017, Author.

54. Alexandrov LB, et al: Mutational signatures associated with tobacco smoking in human cancer. *Science* 354(6312):618–622, 2016.

55. Ma YT, et al: Smoking initiation is followed by the early acquisition of epigenetic change in cervical epithelium: a longitudinal study. *BMJ* 104(9):1500–1504, 2011.

56. Carruba G, et al: Nutrition, aging and cancer: lessons from dietary intervention studies. *Immun Ageing* 13:13, 2016.

57. World Cancer Research Fund/American Institute for Cancer Research (WCRF/AICR): *Food, nutrition, physical activity, and the prevention of cancer: a global perspective*, Washington, DC, 2007, American Institute for Cancer Research.

58. Schwingshackl L, Hoffmann G: Adherence to Mediterranean diet and risk of cancer: a systematic review and meta-analysis of observational studies. *Int J Cancer* 135(8): 1884–1897, 2014.

59. Schwingshackl L, Hoffmann G: Adherence to Mediterranean diet and risk of cancer: an updated systemic review and meta-analysis of observational studies. *Cancer Med* 4(12): 1933–1947, 2015.

60. Daniel M, Tollefsbol TO: Epigenetic linkage of aging, cancer and nutrition. *J Exp Biol* 218(Pt 1):59–70, 2015.

61. Ballestar E, Esteller M: Epigenetic gene regulation in cancer. *Adv Genet* 61:247–267, 2008.

62. Feinberg AP, Koldsbskiy MA, Göndör A: Epigenetic modulators, modifiers and mediators in cancer aetiology and progression. *Nat Rev Genet* 17:284–299, 2016.

63. Kanwal R, Gupta S: Epigenetic modifications in cancer. *Clin Genet* 81:303–311, 2012.

64. Choi S-W, Corrocher R, Friso S: Nutrients and DNA methylation. In Choi S-W, Frisco S, editors: *Nutrients and epigenetics*, Boca Raton, FL, 2009, CRC Press Taylor & Francis Group, pp 105–126.

65. Mathers JC, Strathdee G, Relton CL: Induction of epigenetic alterations by dietary and other environmental factors. *Adv Genet* 71:3–39, 2010.

66. Steegers-Theunissen RP, et al: Periconceptional maternal folic acid use of 4000 microg per day is related to increased methylation of the IGF2 gene in the very young child. *PLoS ONE* 4(11):e7845, 2009.

67. Qian YY, et al: Effects of maternal folic acid supplementation on gene methylation and being small for gestational age. *J Hum Nutr Diet* 29(5): 643–651, 2016.

68. Kovacheva VP, et al: Gestational choline deficiency causes global and Igf2 gene DNA hypermethylation by up-regulation of Dnmt1 expression. *J Biol Chem* 282(43):31777–31788, 2007.

69. Kim YI, et al: Folate deficiency in rats induces DNA strand breaks and hypomethylation within the p53 tumor suppressor gene. *Am J Clin Nutr* 65(1):46–52, 1997.

70. Agodi A, et al: Low fruit consumption and folate deficiency are associated with LINE-1 hypomethylation in women of a cancer-free population. *Genes Nutr* 10(5):480, 2015.

71. Lee WJ, Shim JY, Zhu BT: Mechanisms for the inhibition of DNA methyltransferases by tea catechins and bioflavonoids. *Mol Pharmacol* 68(4):1018–1030, 2005.

72. Delage B, Dashwood RH: Dietary manipulation of histone structure and function. *Annu Rev Nutr* 28:347–366, 2008.

73. Saud SM, et al: Diallyl disulfide (DADS), a constituent of garlic, inactivates NF-κB and prevents colitis-induced colorectal cancer by inhibiting GSK-3β. *Cancer Prev Res (Phila)* 9(7):607–615, 2016.

74. Shindikar A, et al: Curcumin and resveratrol as promising natural remedies with nanomedicine approach for the effective treatment of triple negative breast cancer. *J Oncol* 2016:9750785, 2016.

75. Wang N, et al: Resveratrol protects against early polymicrobial sepsis-induced acute kidney injury through inhibiting endoplasmic reticulum stress-activated NF-κB pathway. *Oncotarget* 2017 Apr 5. [Epub ahead of print].

76. Daniel M, Tollefsbol TO: Epigenetic linkage of aging, cancer and nutrition. *J Exp Biol* 218(Pt 1):59–70, 2015.

77. World Cancer Research Fund/American Institute for Cancer Research (WCRF/AICR): *Second expert report: food, nutrition, physical activity, and the prevention of cancer: a global perspective*, London, 2007, Author.

78. Shah MS, et al: Comparative effects of diet and carcinogen on microRNA expression in the stem cell niche of the mouse colonic crypt. *Biochim Biophys Acta* 1862(1):121–134, 2016.

79. Kim YS, et al: Cancer stem cells: potential target for bioactive food components. *J Nutr Biochem* 23:691–698, 2012.

80. Fox RG, et al: Musashi signaling in stem cells and cancer. *Annu Rev Cell Dev Biol* 31:249–267, 2015.

81. Hattori A, Buac K, Ito T: Regulation of stem cell self-renewal and oncogenesis by RNA-binding proteins. *Adv Exp Med Biol* 907:153–188, 2016.

82. Ginestier C, et al: Retinoid signaling regulates breast cancer stem cell differentiation. *Cell Cycle* 8:3297–3302, 2009.

83. Kasdagly M, et al: Colon carcinogenesis: influence of Western diet-induced obesity and targeting stem cells using dietary bioactive compounds. *Nutrition* 30(11-12):1242–1256, 2014.

84. Carotenuto F, et al: How diet intervention via modulation of DNA damage response through microRNAs may have an effect on cancer prevention in aging, an in Silico Study. *Int J Mol Sci* 17(5):2016.

85. Omiecinski CJ, et al: Xenobiotic metabolism, disposition, and regulation by receptors: from biochemical phenomenon to predictors of major toxicities. *Toxicol Sci* 120(Suppl 1):S49–S75, 2011.

86. Yang G, et al: Isothiocyanate exposure, glutathione S-transferase polymorphisms, and colon cancer risk. *Am J Nutr* 91(3):704–711, 2010.

87. World Cancer Research Fund/American Institute for Cancer Research (WCRF/AICR): *Continuous update project report. Food, nutrition, physical activity, and the prevention of colorectal cancer*, London, 2011, Author.

88. Vieira AR, et al: Foods and beverages and colorectal cancer risk: a systematic review and meta-analysis of cohort studies, an update of the evidence of the WCRF-AICR Continuous Update Project. *Ann Oncol* 2017 Apr 12. [Epub ahead of print].

89. Bouvard V, et al: Carcinogenicity of consumption of red and processed meat. *Lancet Oncol* 16(16):1599–1600, 2016.

90. Lowe D, Storkus WJ: Chronic inflammation and immunologic-based constraints in malignant disease. *Immunotherapy* 3(10):1265–1274, 2011.

91. Glickman D, et al: *Accelerating progress in obesity prevention: solving the weight of the nation*, Washington, DC, 2012, The National Academies Press.

92. Centers for Disease Control and Prevention (CDC): *Childhood obesity*, Atlanta GA, 2017, Facts Division of Nutrition, Physical Activity, and Obesity, National Center for Chronic Disease Prevention and Health Promotion.

93. Lauby-Secretan B, et al: Body fatness and cancer—viewpoint of the IARC Working Group. *NEJM* 375:794–798, 2016.

94. Calle EE, et al: Overweight, obesity, and mortality from cancer in a prospective studies cohort of U.S. adults. *N Engl J Med* 348(17):1625–1638, 2003.

95. Cao Y, Ma J: Body mass index, prostate cancer-specific mortality, and biochemical recurrence: a systematic review and meta-analysis. *Cancer Prev Res (Phila)* 4:486–501, 2011.

96. World Health Organization (WHO): *Global strategy on diet, physical activity, and health (online)*, Geneva, 2004, Author. Available at www.who.int/dietphysicalactivity/strategy/eb11344/en/.

97. Centers for Disease Control and Prevention (CDC): *About adult BMI*, Atlanta GA, 2015, Division of Nutrition, Physical Activity, and Obesity, National Center for Chronic Disease Prevention and Health Promotion.

98. World Health Organization (WHO): *Managing child and adolescent overweight and obesity: early nutrition-focused intervention for lifelong benefit*, Geneva, 2016, Author. Available at http://www.who.int/nutrition/topics/seminar_23Aug2016/en/.

99. Institute of Medicine (IOM): *The role of obesity in cancer survival and recurrence: workshop summary*, Washington, DC, 2012, The National Academies Press.

100. Demark-Wahnefried W, et al: The role of obesity in cancer survival and recurrence. *Cancer Epidemiol Biomarkers Prev* 21(8):1244–1259, 2012.

101. Park J, et al: Obesity and cancer—mechanisms underlying tumor progression and recurrence. *Nat Rev Endocrinol* 10(8):455–465, 2014.

102. Park J, et al: Paracrine and endocrine effects of adipose tissue on cancer development and progression. *Endocr Rev* 32(4):550–570, 2011.

103. Pérez-Hernández AI, et al: Mechanisms linking excess adiposity and carcinogenesis promotion. *Front Endocrinol (Lausanne)* 5:65, 2014.

104. Howe LR, et al: Molecular pathways: adipose inflammation as a mediator of obesity-associated cancer. *Clin Cancer Res* 19(22):6074–6083, 2013.

105. Incio J, et al: Obesity-induced inflammation and desmoplasia promote pancreatic cancer progression and resistance to chemotherapy. *Cancer Discov* 6(8):852–869, 2016.

106. Ouchi N, et al: Adipokines in inflammation and metabolic disease. *Nat Rev Immunol* 11:85–97, 2011.

107. Wellen KE, Thompson CB: A two-way street: reciprocal regulation of metabolism and signaling. *Nat Rev Mol Cell Biol* 13:270–276, 2012.

108. Asher G, Schibler U: Crosstalk between components of circadian and metabolic cycles in mammals. *Cell Metab* 13:125–137, 2011.

109. Altman BJ: Cancer clocks out for lunch: disruption of circadian rhythm and metabolic oscillation in cancer. *Front Cell Dev Biol* 4:62, 2016.

110. Reddy AB, O'Neill JS: Health clocks, healthy body, healthy mind. *Trends Cell Biol* 20(1):36–44, 2010.

111. Papagiannakopoulos T, et al: Circadian rhythm disruption promotes lung tumorigenesis. *Cell Metab* 24(2):324–331, 2016.

112. Sahar S, Sassone-Corsi P: Regulation of metabolism: the circadian clock dictates the time. *Trends Endocrinol Metab* 23(1):1–8, 2011.

113. Mostoufi-Moab S, et al: Endocrine abnormalities in aging survivors of childhood cancer: a report from the Childhood Cancer Survivor Study. *J Clin Oncol* 34(27):3240–3247, 2016.

114. American Cancer Society (ACS): *Alcohol and cancer*, Atlanta, GA, 2016, Author.

115. World Cancer Research Fund/American Institute for Cancer Research (WCRF/AICR): *Recommendations for cancer prevention*, Washington, DC, 2016, American Institute for Cancer Research.

116. Muller DC, et al: Modifiable causes of premature death in middle-age in Western Europe: results from the EPIC cohort study. *BMC Med* 14:87, 2016.

117. Mao N, et al: Association between alcohol dehydrogenase-2 gene polymorphism and esophageal cancer risk: a meta-analysis. *World J Surg Oncol* 14(1):191, 2016.

118. Varela-Ray M, et al: Alcohol, DNA methylation, and cancer. *Alcohol Res* 35(1):25–35, 2013.

119. Avissar M, et al: Micro RNA expression in head and neck cancer associates with alcohol consumption and survival. *Carcinogenesis* 30:2059–2063, 2009.

120. Chang JS, Strif K, Guha N: The role of alcohol dehydrogenase genes in head and neck cancers: a systematic review and meta-analysis of ADH1B and ADH1C. *Mutagenesis* 27(3):275–286, 2012.

121. American Institute for Cancer Research (AICR): *Being physically active decreases risk of these cancers: postmenopausal breast, colorectal, endometrial, continuous update project (CUP)*, Washington, DC, 2015, Author.

122. Lee IM, et al: Annual deaths attributable to physical inactivity: whither the missing 2 million? *Lancet* 381(9871):992–993, 2013.

123. World Health Organization (WHO): *Noncommunicable diseases*, Geneva, 2016, WHO Media Centre.

124. Warburton DER, Nicol CW, Bredin SSD: Health benefits of physical activity: the evidence. *CMAJ* 174(6):801–809, 2006.

125. McTiernan A, et al: Effect of exercise on serum estrogens in postmenopausal women: a 12-month randomized clinical trial. *Cancer Res* 64(8):2923–2928, 2004.

126. Moore SC, et al: Leisure-time physical activity and risk of 26 types of cancer in 1.44 million adults. *JAMA Int Med* 176(6):816–825, 2016.

127. World Health Organization (WHO): *Global Physical Activity Questionnaire (GPAQ) analysis guide: surveillance and population-based prevention*, Geneva, 2008, Author. Available at: http://www.who.int/chp/steps/resources/GPAQ_Analysis_Guide.pdf.

128. Kyu HH, et al: Physical activity and risk of breast cancer, colon cancer, diabetes, ischemic heart disease, and ischemic stroke events: systematic review and dose-response meta-analysis for the Global Burden of Disease Study 2013. *BMJ* 9:354, 2016.

129. Cohen AJ, et al: Estimates and 25-year trends of the global burden of disease attributable to ambient air pollution: an analysis of data from the Global Burden of Diseases Study 2015. *Lancet* 2017 April 10. [Epub ahead of print].

130. Hamra GB, et al: Outdoor particulate matter exposure and lung cancer: a systematic review and meta-analysis. *Environ Health Perspect* 122(9):906–911, 2014.

131. Schwartz J: Air pollution and daily mortality: a review and metaanalysis. *Environ Res* 64(1):36–52, 1994.

132. Schwartz J, Dockery DW, Neas LM: Is daily mortality associated specifically with fine particles? *J Air Waste Manag Assoc* 46:927–939, 1996.

133. Dockery DW, et al: An association between air pollution and mortality in six U.S. cities. *N Engl J Med* 329:1753–1759, 1993.

134. International Agency for Research on Cancer (IARC): *Outdoor air pollution, IARC Monogr Eval Carcinog Risks Hum Volume 109*, Lyon, France, 2013.

135. Loomis D, et al: The carcinogenicity of outdoor air pollution. *Lancet Oncol* 14:1262–1263, 2013.

136. Valavanidis A, Fiotakis K, Vlachogianni T: Airborne particulate matter and human health: toxicological assessment and importance of size and composition of particles for oxidative damage and carcinogenic mechanisms. *J Environ Sci Health C Environ Carcinog Ecotoxicol Rev* 26(4): 339–362, 2008.

137. Rivas-Santiago CE, et al: Air pollution particulate matter alters antimycobacterial respiratory epithelium innate immunity. *Infect Immun* 83:2507–2517, 2015.

138. Puett RC, et al: Chronic fine and course particulate exposure, mortality, and coronary heart disease in the Nurses' Health Study. *Environ Health Perspect* 117(11):1697–1701, 2009.

139. Attfield MD, et al: The Diesel Exhaust in Miners Study: a cohort mortality study with emphasis on lung cancer. *J Natl Cancer Inst* 104:869–883, 2012.

140. Silverman DT, et al: The Diesel Exhaust in Miners Study: a nested case-control study of lung cancer and diesel exhaust. *J Natl Cancer Inst* 104:855–868, 2012.

141. Garshick E, et al: Lung cancer and elemental carbon exposure in trucking industry workers. *Environ Health Perspect* 120:1301–1306, 2012.

142. Silverman DT: Diesel exhaust causes lung cancer-now what? *Occup Environ Med* 74(4): 233–234, 2017.

143. Gulland A: Diesel engine exhaust causes lung cancer, says WHO. *BMJ* 344:e4174, 2012.

144. International Agency for Research on Cancer (IARC): *Diesel and gasoline engine exhausts and some nitroarenes Vol 105, IARC monographs on the evaluation of the carcinogenic risks to humans,* Lyon, France, 2013.

145. Boffetta P, et al: Mortality among workers employed in the titanium dioxide production industry in Europe. *Cancer Causes Control* 15(7): 697–706, 2004.

146. Environmental Protection Agency (EPA): *Particulate matter updated March 18, 2013,* Washington DC, 2013, Author.

147. Boffetta P: Involuntary smoking and lung cancer. *Scand J Work Environ Health* 28(Suppl 2):30–40, 2002.

148. Hecht SS, et al: Elevated levels of volatile organic carcinogen and toxicant biomarkers in Chinese women who regularly cook at home. *Cancer Epidemiol Biomarkers Prev* 19(5):1185–1192, 2010.

149. Zhao Y, et al: Air pollution and lung cancer risks in China—meta-analysis. *Sci Total Environ* 366(2-3):500–513, 2006.

150. Heidenreich WF, et al: Promoting action of radiation in the atomic bomb survivor carcinogenesis data? *Radiat Res* 168(6):750–756, 2007.

151. Little MP: Heterogeneity of variation of relative risk by age at exposure in the Japanese atomic bomb survivors. *Radiat Environ Biophys* 48(3): 253–262, 2009.

152. Shuryak I, et al: A new view of radiation-induced cancer: integrating short- and long-processes. Part l: approach. *Radiat Environ Biophys* 48(3): 263–274, 2009.

153. Shuryak I, Sachs RK, Brenner DJ: Cancer risks after radiation exposure in middle age. *J Natl Cancer Inst* 102(21):1606–1609, 2010.

154. Preston DL, et al: Solid cancer incidence in atomic bomb survivors: 1958-1998. *Radiat Res* 168(1): 1–64, 2007.

155. Committee on the Biological Effects of Ionizing Radiation: *Health risks from exposure to low levels of ionizing radiation, BEIR VII Phase 2,* Washington, DC, 2006, National Academies Press.

156. Walsh L: Heterogeneity of variation of relative risk by age at exposure in Japanese atomic bomb survivors. *Radiat Environ Biophys* 48(3):345–347, 2009.

157. Preston DL, et al: Studies of mortality of atomic bomb survivors. Report 13: solid cancer and noncancer disease mortality: 1950-1997. *Radiat Res* 160:381–407, 2003.

158. Hoel DG: Ionizing radiation and cardiovascular disease. *Ann N Y Acad Sci* 1076:309–317, 2006.

159. Rombouts C, et al: Differential response to acute low dose radiation in primary and immortalized endothelial cells. *Int J Radiat Biol* 89(10):841–850, 2013.

160. Yusuf SW, Sami S, Daher IN: Radiation-induced heart disease: a clinical update. *Cardiol Res Pract* 2011:317659, 2011.

161. Wang Y, Boerma M, Zhou D: Ionizing radiation-induced endothelial cell senescence and cardiovascular diseases. *Radiat Res* 186(2): 153–161, 2016.

162. Halle M, Christersdottir T, Back M: Chronic adventitial inflammation, vasa vasorum expansion, and 5-lipoxygenase up-regulation in irradiated arteries from cancer survivors. *FASEB J* 30(11):3845–3852, 2016.

163. Mathias D, et al: Low-dose irradiation affects expression of inflammatory markers in the heart of ApoE mice. *PLoS ONE* 10(3):e0119661, 2015.

164. International Commission on Radiological Protection (ICRP): ICRP statement on tissue reactions. *Ann ICRP* 41:1–322, 2012.

165. Klieman NJ: Radiation cataract. *Ann ICRP* 41(3-4):80–97, 2012.

166. Rao SB: Biological bases for the revision of doses limits to the eye lens. *J Med Phys* 41(4):211–213, 2016.

167. Centers for Disease Control and Prevention (CDC): *Radiation and pregnancy: a fact sheet for clinicians,* Atlanta, GA, 2014, Centers for Disease Control and Prevention, National Center for Environmental Health (NCEH)/Agency for Toxic Substances and Disease Registry (ATSDR), National Center for Injury Prevention and Control (NCIPC).

168. National Council on Radiation Protection & Measurements (NCRP): *Report no.160, ionizing radiation exposure of the population of the United States,* Bethesda, MD, 2015, Author.

169. Smith-Bendman R, et al: Use of diagnostic imaging studies and associated radiation exposure for patients enrolled in large integrated health care system, 1996-2010. *JAMA* 307(22):2400–2409, 2012.

170. Studdert DM, et al: Defensive medicine among high-risk specialist physicians in a volatile malpractice environment. *JAMA* 293(21): 2609–2617, 2005.

171. Jones JA, Casey RC, Karouia F: Ionizing radiation as a carcinogen. In McQueen CA, editor: *Comprehensive toxicology,* ed 2, St Louis, 2010, Elsevier.

172. Lubin JH, et al: Lung cancer in radon-exposed miners and estimation of risk from indoor exposure. *J Natl Cancer Inst* 87(11):817–827, 1995.

173. Ernestos B, et al: Increased chromosomal radiosensitivity in women carrying BRCA1/ BRCA2 mutations assessed with the G2 assay. *Int J Radiat Oncol Biol Phys* 76(4):1199–1205, 2010.

174. Dalrymple GV, et al: A review of the USAF/NASA proton bioeffects project: rationale and acute effects. *Radiat Res* 126(2):117–119, 1991.

175. United Nations Scientific Committee on the Effects of Atomic Radiation (UNSCEAR): *Report to the general assembly, with scientific annexes,* New York, 1993, Author.

176. Committee on the Biological Effects of Ionizing Radiation: *Health risks from exposure to low levels of ionizing radiation, BEIR VII Phase 2,* Washington, DC, 2006, The National Academies Press.

177. Little JB: Radiation carcinogenesis. *Carcinogenesis* 21(3):397–404, 2000.

178. Mothersill C, Seymour C: Changing paradigms in radiobiology. *Mutat Res* 750(2):85–95, 2012.

179. Barcellos-Hoff MH, et al: Systems biology perspectives on the carcinogenic potential of radiation. *J Radiat Res* 55:i145–i154, 2014.

180. Little JB: Cellular radiation effects and the bystander response. *Mutat Res* 597:113–118, 2006.

181. Barcellos-Hoff MH: Integrative radiation carcinogenesis: interactions between cell and tissue responses to DNA damage. *Semin Cancer Biol* 15:138 148, 2005.

182. Kovalchuk O, Baulch JE: Epigenetic changes and nontargeted radiation effects—is there a link? *Environ Mol Mutagen* 49(1):16–25, 2008.

183. Sowa M, et al: Effects of ionizing radiation on cellular structures, induced instability and carcinogenesis. *EXS* 96:293–301, 2006.

184. Azzam EI, Jay-Gerin JP, Pain D: Ionizing radiation-induced metabolic oxidative stress and prolonged cell injury. *Cancer Lett* 327:48–60, 2012.

185. Jeggo PA, Lobrich M: Contribution of DNA repair and cell cycle checkpoint arrest to the maintenance of genomic stability. *DNA Repair (Amst)* 5:1192–1198, 2006.

186. National Council on Radiation Protection and Measurement (NCRP): *Commentary no. 24 health effects of low doses of radiation: perspectives on integrating radiation biology and epidemiology,* Bethesda, MD, 2015, National Council on Radiation Protection and Measurements.

187. Pellegrini L, et al: Insights into DNA recombination from the structure of a RAD51-BRCA2 complex. *Nature* 420:287–293, 2002.

188. Tutt A, Ashworth A: The relationship between the roles of BRCA genes in DNA repair and cancer predisposition. *Trends Mol Med* 8:571–576, 2002.

189. Hei TK, et al: Radiation induced non-targeted response: mechanism and potential clinical implications. *Curr Mol Pharmacol* 4:96–105, 2011.

190. Ciccia A, Elledge SJ: The DNA damage response: making it safe to play with knives. *Mol Cell* 40: 179–204, 2010.

191. Giglia-Mari G, Zotter A, Vermeulen W: DNA damage response. *Cold Spring Harb Perspect Biol* 3(1):2011.

192. Soria G, Polo SE, Almouzni G: Prime, repair, restore: the active role of chromatin in the DNA response. *Mol Cell* 46(6):722–734, 2012.

193. Ferguson LR, et al: Genomic instability in human cancer: molecular insights and opportunities for therapeutic attack and prevention through diet and nutrition. *Semin Cancer Biol* 35:S5–S24, 2015.

194. National Cancer Institute (NCI): *Second primary cancers,* National Cancer Institute Division of Cancer Epidemiology & Genetics. Available at http://dceg.cancer.gov/research/what-we-study/second-cancers.

195. Mancuso M, et al: Oncogenic bystander radiation effects in patched heterozygous mouse cerebellum. *Proc Natl Acad Sci USA* 105:12445–12450, 2008.

196. Belyako OV, et al: Biological effects in unirradiated human tissue induced by radiation damage up to 1 mm away. *Proc Natl Acad Sci USA* 102:14203–14208, 2005.

197. Bertucci A, et al: Microbeam irradiation of the C. elegans nematode. *J Radiat Res* 50:A49–A54, 2009.

198. Chai Y, Hei TK: Radiation induced bystander effect *in vivo. Acta Med Nagasaki* 53:S65–S69, 2008.

199. Xu S, et al: Exosome-mediated microRNA transfer plays a role in radiation-induced bystander effect. *RNA Biol* 12(12):1355–1363, 2015.

200. Mancuso M, et al: Oncogenic bystander radiation effects in patched heterozygous mouse cerebellum. *Proc Natl Acad Sci USA* 105(34):12445–12450, 2008.

201. Nguyen DH, et al: Radiation acts on the microenvironment to affect breast carcinogenesis by distinct mechanisms that decrease cancer latency and affect tumor type. *Cancer Cell* 19:640–651, 2011.

202. Ojima M, et al: Persistence of DNA double-strand breaks in normal human cells induced by radiation-induced bystander effect. *Radiat Res* 175:90–96, 2011.

203. Chute JP: To survive radiation injury, remember you're aPCs. *Nat Med* 18(7):1013–1014, 2012.

204. Barcellos-Hoff MH, Nguyen DH: Radiation carcinogenesis in context: How do irradiated tissues become tumors? *Health Phys* 97(5):446–457, 2009.

205. Wright EG: Manifestations and mechanisms of non-targeted effects of ionizing radiation. *Mutat Res* 687(1–2):28–33, 2010.

206. Gupta A, et al: Radiotherapy promotes tumor-specific effector CD8+ T cells via dendritic cell activation. *J Immunol* 189(2):558–566, 2012.

207. Sharma A, et al: Radiotherapy of human sarcoma promotes an intratumoral immune effector signature. *Clin Cancer Res* 19(17):4843–4853, 2013.

208. Surace L, et al: Complement is a central mediator of radiotherapy-induced tumor-specific immunity and clinical response. *Immunity* 42(4):767–777, 2015.

209. Barrington de Gonzalez A, et al: Proportion of second cancers attributable to radiotherapy treatment in adults: a prospective cohort study in the US SEER cancer registries. *Lancet Oncol* 12(4):353–360, 2011.

210. Fullerton HJ, et al: Recurrent stroke in childhood cancer survivors. *Neurology* 85(12):1056–1064, 2015.

211. Nakashima M, et al: Foci formation of P53-binding protein 1 in thyroid tumors: activation of genomic instability during thyroid carcinogenesis. *Int J Cancer* 122(5):1082–1088, 2008.

212. Parkin DM, Darby SC: Cancers in 2010 attributable to ionising radiation exposure in the UK. *Br J Cancer* 105:S57–S65, 2011.

213. Leuraud K, et al: Ionising radiation and risk of death from leukaemia and lymphoma in radiation-monitored workers (INWORKS): an international cohort study. *Lancet Haematol* 12(7):e276–e281, 2015.

214. Hsu WL, et al: The incidence of leukemia, lymphoma and multiple myeloma among atomic bomb survivors: 1950-2001. *Radiat Res* 179(3):361–382, 2013.

215. Kendall GM, et al: A record-based case-control study of natural background radiation and the incidence of childhood leukaemia and other cancers in Great Britain during 1980-2006. *Leukemia* 27(1):3–9, 2013.

216. Pearce MS, et al: Radiation exposure from CT scans in childhood and subsequent risk of leukaemia and brain tumors: a retrospective cohort study. *Lancet* 380:499–505, 2012.

217. Brenner DJ: We don't know enough about low-dose radiation risk, *Nature News*, 2011.

218. Centers for Disease Control and Prevention (CDC): *Basic information about skin cancer*, Atlanta, GA, 2017, Division of Cancer Prevention and Control, Author.

219. National Cancer Institute: (NCI): *Skin cancer prevention (PDQ)–health professional version*, Bethesda, MD, 2016, National Institutes of Health, National Cancer Institute.

220. Centers for Disease Control and Prevention (CDC): *Radiation and your health*, Atlanta, GA, 2017, Author. Available at: www.cdc.gov/nceh/radiation/.

221. Centers for Disease Control and Prevention (CDC): *Are there benefits to spending time outdoors?* Atlanta, GA, 2016, Division of Cancer Prevention and Control, Author.

222. World Health Organization (WHO): *Health effects of UV radiation*, Geneva, 2016, Author.

223. National Cancer Institute (NCI): *Types of skin cancer*, Washington, DC, 2011, National Institutes of Health. Available at: www.cancer.gov/cancertopics/wyntk/skin/page4.

224. National Cancer Institute (NCI): *Cellular classification of skin cancer*, Washington, DC, 2013, National Institutes of Health.

225. American Cancer Society (ACS): *Cancer facts & figures 2016*, Atlanta, GA, 2016, Author.

226. Welch HG, Black WC: Overdiagnosis in cancer. *J Natl Cancer Inst* 102:605–613, 2010.

227. U.S. Preventive Services Task Force (USPSTF): Screening for skin cancer: US Preventive Services Task Force recommendation statement. *JAMA* 316(4):429–435, 2016.

228. Centers for Disease Control and Prevention (CDC): *Skin cancer rates by race and ethnicity*, Atlanta, GA, 2016, Author.

229. Loftfield E, et al: Coffee drinking and cutaneous melanoma risk in the NIH-AARP diet and health study. *J Natl Cancer Inst* 107(2):2015.

230. Barnes F, Greenebaum B: Some effects of weak magnetic fields on biological systems: RF fields can change radical concentrations and cancer cell growth rates. *IEEE Power Electronics Magazine* 3(1):60–68, 2016.

231. National Cancer Institute (NCI): *Electromagnetic fields and cancer*, Washington, DC, 2016, National Institutes of Health.

232. Baan R, et al: Carcinogenicity of radiofrequency electromagnetic fields. *Lancet Oncol* 12(7):624–626, 2011.

233. Belyaev IY: Dependence of non-thermal biological effects of microwaves on physical and biological variables: implications for reproducibility and safety standards. *Eur J Oncol Library* 5:187–219, 2010.

234. Genuis SJ: Fielding a current idea: exploring the public health impact of electromagnetic radiation. *Public Health* 122(2):113–124, 2008.

235. National Institute of Environmental Health Sciences (NIEHS) Working Group Report: *Assessment of health effects from exposure to power-line frequency electric and magnetic fields*, Washington, DC, 1998, U.S. Government Printing Office.

236. International Agency for Research on Cancer (IARC): *IARC classifies radiofrequency electromagnetic fields as possibly carcinogenic to humans, IARC communications international agency for research on cancer*, Lyon, France, 2011, World Health Organization.

237. International Agency for Research on Cancer (IARC): *Non-ionizing radiation, Part 2: Radiofrequency electromagnetic fields, IARC monographs on the evaluation of carcinogenic risks to humans*, Lyon, France, 2013, World Health Organization. Available at http://monographs.iarc.fr/ENG/Monographs/vol102/index.php.

238. Wyde M: *Report of partial findings from the National Toxicology Program carcinogenesis studies of cell phone radiofrequency radiation in Hsd: Sprague Dawley (SD) rats (whole body exposure) bioRxiv the preprint server for biology*, Cold Spring Harbor, NY, 2016, Cold Spring Harbor Laboratory. Available at http://dx.doi.org/10.1101/055699.

239. INTERPHONE Study Group: Brain tumour risk in relation to mobile telephone use: results of the INTERPHONE International Case-control Study. *Int J Epidemiol* 39:675–694, 2010.

240. Hardell L, Carlberg M, Mild K: Pooled analysis of case-control studies on malignant brain tumours and the use of mobile and cordless phones including living and deceased subjects. *Int J Oncol* 38:1465–1474, 2011.

241. Buchachenko A, Kuznetsov D: Magnetic control of enzymatic phosphorylation. *J Phys Chem Biophys* 4(2):9, 2014.

242. Martino C, et al: Reduction of the Earth's magnetic field inhibits growth rates of model cancer cell lines. *Bioelectro Magn* 31(8):649–655, 2010.

243. Reuter S, et al: Oxidative stress, inflammation, and cancer: How are they linked? *Free Radic Biol Med* 49(11):1603–1616, 2010.

244. Plummer M, et al: Global burden of cancers attributable to infections in 2012: a synthetic analysis. *Lancet Glob Health* 4:e609–e616, 2016.

245. Crosbie EJ, et al: Human papillomavirus and cervical cancer. *Lancet* 382:889–899, 2013.

246. Dart H, Wolin KY, Colditz GA: Commentary: eight ways to prevent cancer: a framework for effective prevention messages for the public. *Cancer Causes Control* 23(4):601–608, 2012.

247. Ko Y-H: EBV and human cancer. *Exp Mol Med* 47:e130, 2015.

248. World Health Organization (WHO): *Human papillomavirus and cervical cancer*, Geneva, 2016, Author.

249. Centers for Disease Control and Prevention (CDC): *Human papillomavirus (HPV)*, Atlanta, 2016, Division of STD Prevention; National Center for HIV/AIDS, Viral Hepatitis, STD, and TB Prevention, Centers for Disease Control and Prevention.

250. National Cancer Institute (NCI): *HPV and cancer*, Washington, DC, 2015, Author.

251. Bosch FX, de Sanjose S: Human papillomavirus and cervical cancer—burden and assessment of causality. *J Natl Cancer Inst Monogr* 31:3–13, 2003.

252. Watson M, et al: Using population-based cancer registry data to assess the burden of human papillomavirus-associated cancers in the United States: overview of methods. *Cancer* 113(Suppl 10):2841–2854, 2008.

253. Agalliu I, et al: Associations of oral α-, β-, and γ-human papillomavirus types with risk of incident head and neck cancer. *JAMA Oncol* 2016 Jan 21. [Epub ahead of print].

254. Jayaprakash V, et al: Human papillomavirus types 16 and 18 in epithelial dysplasia of oral cavity and oropharynx: a meta-analysis, 1985-2010. *Oral Oncol* 47(11):1048–1054, 2011.

255. Chaturvedi AK, et al: Human papillomavirus and rising oropharyngeal cancer incidence in the United States. *J Clin Oncol* 29(32):4294–4301, 2011.

256. Liu X, et al: Chronic inflammation-related HPV: a driving force speeds oropharyngeal carcinogenesis. *PLoS ONE* 10(7):e0133681, 2015.

257. Schiffman M, et al: Human papillomavirus and cervical cancer. *Lancet* 370(9590):890–907, 2007.

258. Agency for Toxic Substances and Disease Registry (ATSDR): *Chemicals, cancer, and you*, Atlanta, GA, 2016, Author, Division of Health Assessment and Consultation, U.S. Department of Health and Human Services. Available at: www.atsdr.cdc.gov/…/Chemicals,%20Cancer,%20and%20You%20FS.pdf.

259. Gray J: *State of the evidence 2008: the connection between breast cancer and the environment*, San Francisco, 2008, Breast Cancer Fund.

260. Agency for Toxic Substances and Disease Registry (ATSDR): *Chemicals, cancer, and you*, Agency for Toxic Substances and Disease Registry Division. Available at www.atsdr.cdc.gov/emes/public/docs/Chemicals,%20Cancer,%20and%20You%20FS.pdf.

261. Kakehashi A, et al: Oxidative stress in the carcinogenicity of chemical carcinogens. *Cancers (Basel)* 5(4):1332–1354, 2013.

262. Klaunig JE, et al: Oxidative stress and oxidative damage in chemical carcinogenesis. *Toxicol Appl Pharmacol* 254(2):86–99, 2011.

263. Luch A: Nature and nurture—lessons from chemical carcinogenesis. *Nat Rev Cancer* 5:113–125, 2005.

264. Hileman B: *Chemicals can turn genes on and off; new tests needed, scientists say, Environmental Health News*, Charlottesville, VA, 2009, National Institute of Environmental Health Sciences.

265. National Institute for Occupational Safety and Health (NIOSH): *Hazard evaluations, and field studies*, Atlanta, GA, 2015, Occupational Cancer National Institute for Occupational Safety and Health Division of Surveillance, CDC.

266. European Agency for Safety and Health at Work: *Exposure to carcinogens and work-related cancer: a review of assessment methods European Risk Observatory Report*, Luxembourg, 2014, European Agency for Safety and Health at Work Eu-OSHA. Available at http://europa.eu.

267. Centers for Disease Control and Prevention (CDC): *Chemicals, cancer, and you*, Atlanta, GA, 2013, Agency for Toxic Substances and Disease Registry, Division of Health Assessment and Consultation Centers for Disease Control.

268. Clapp RW, Jacobs MM, Loechler EL: *Environmental and occupational causes of cancer: new evidence, 2005-2007*, Lowell, MA, 2007, Lowell Center for Sustainable Production.

269. Bergman A, et al: *State of the science of endocrine disrupting chemicals*, 2012. Available at http://www.who.int/ceh/publications/endocrine/en/index.html.

270. Malhotra J, et al: Risk factors for lung cancer worldwide. *Eur Respir J* 48(3):889–902, 2016.

271. Neuberger JS, Field RW: Occupation and lung cancer in nonsmokers. *Rev Environ Health* 18(4): 251–267, 2003, review.

272. Singh Z, Chadha P: Textile industry and occupational cancer. *J Occup Med Toxicol* 11:39, 2016.

273. National Institute for Occupational Safety and Health (NIOSH): *Asbestos*, Atlanta, GA, 2013, Centers for Disease Control and Prevention, National Institute for Occupational Safety and Health Respiratory Health Division, CDC.

274. National Institute for Occupational Safety and Health (NIOSH): *Mining topic: diesel exhaust*, Atlanta, GA, 2015, National Institute for Occupational Safety and Health. Updated Feb 19, 2015.

Cancer in Children

Lauri A. Linder

CHAPTER OUTLINE

Cancer in children and adolescents is rare, but it is still the leading cause of death from disease in this patient population. The 5-year survival rates among children and adolescents with cancer have improved from 59% in the 1970s to nearly 85% today.[1,2] Factors leading to improved cure rates in children and adolescents with cancer include the use of combination chemotherapy; the development of targeted therapies, including immunotherapy; and the participation in clinical trials.

INCIDENCE AND TYPES OF CANCER

More than 15,500 children and adolescents (from birth to 19 years of age) in the United States will be diagnosed with cancer each year. Just less than 2000 deaths from cancer occur in this age group each year. Deaths from cancer in this age group most commonly result from central nervous tumors, followed by leukemias.[1,3]

The types of malignancies in children and adolescents are vastly different from those that affect adults. The most common types of cancer among adults include prostate, breast, lung, and colon. Many adult cancers have associated lifestyle factors and many cancers may be prevented (see Chapter 13).

Among children up to 14 years of age, leukemias and brain tumors account for 61% of childhood cancers; solid tumors, such as neuroblastoma and soft tissue or bone sarcomas, are less common.[3] Lymphomas (including Hodgkin and nonHodgkin subtypes) are the most common

type of cancer among adolescents (15 to 19 years of age). Leukemia, thyroid carcinoma, brain tumors, and germ cell tumors also are among the most common adolescent cancers.[1,4] Although very few environmental factors have been linked to pediatric and adolescent malignancies, more data are emerging that the developing child may be affected by parental exposures before conception, exposures in utero, and the contents of breast milk. These exposures may result in epigenetic changes, creating an increased vulnerability to the development of childhood cancer.[5,6]

Most childhood and adolescent cancers originate from the meso-dermal germ layer that gives rise to connective tissue, bone, cartilage, muscle, blood, blood vessels, gonads, kidney, and the lymphatic system. Thus the more common childhood cancers are leukemias, sarcomas, and embryonal tumors. Embryonal tumors originate during intrauterine life. These tumors contain abnormal cells that appear to be immature embryonic tissue, unable to mature or differentiate into fully developed functional cells. Embryonal tumors are diagnosed early in life (usually before 5 years of age). Embryonal tumors often contain the term blast cell in their name, which refers to the immature nature of the cells. Examples of embryonal tumors include retinoblastoma, neuroblastoma, and Wilms tumor (nephroblastoma).

Leukemia is the most common malignancy in children, with most cases occurring in children between 2 and 5 years of age. The most common type of leukemia is acute lymphoblastic leukemia (ALL), which represents approximately 75% of all childhood and 67% of all adolescent leukemia cases.[1] Although the presenting signs of the various types of leukemia may be similar, the treatment and response to treatment of childhood leukemias vary greatly (see Chapter 31).

Central nervous system (CNS) tumors are the most common types of solid tumors in children and account for 21% of all childhood cancers and 10% of adolescent cancers[1] (see Chapter 20). Not all brain tumors are diagnosed malignant by histologic studies; however, even a benign tumor can have devastating effects, depending on the anatomic location. The treatment for brain tumors in children often presents difficulties because therapies, such as radiation, may have debilitating effects on the developing brain, particularly in children younger than 3 years of age.

Lymphomas, including Hodgkin and non-Hodgkin subtypes, are malignancies that occur in children, adolescents, and adults. The subtypes of lymphoma and subsequent treatment often differ across the life span.

Many pediatric solid tumors usually develop in children and adolescents, but in very rare instances, may occur in adults. Examples of these tumors include neuroblastoma, Wilms tumor, rhabdomyosarcoma, retinoblastoma, osteosarcoma, and Ewing sarcoma. Likewise, solid tumors that occur more frequently in adults, such as hepatocellular carcinoma, can occur in children and adolescents.

Childhood and adolescent cancers are often associated with specific peak times of physical growth and may occur as a consequence of altered cellular regulatory mechanisms at a given time in the child's or adolescent's development. Embryonal tumors most often develop before the age of 5 years, acute lymphoblastic leukemia occurs most often in younger children, and bone tumors occur most often in adolescents. In general, childhood and adolescent cancers are extremely fast growing, with 80% having distant spread (metastases) at diagnosis. Overall, cancer is 10% to 25% more common in white than in black children. Boys are more likely to develop cancer than girls.

ETIOLOGY

The causes of cancer in children are largely unknown. A few environmental factors are known to predispose a child to cancer, but causal factors have not been established for most childhood cancers. A number of host factors, many of which are genetic risk factors or congenital conditions, have been implicated in the development of childhood cancer (Table 14.1). The interaction of many factors most likely produces cancer, a concept referred to as multiple causation or **multifactorial etiology**. According to this premise, cancer develops because of the predisposing characteristics of the person and the interaction with environmental factors.

A **multiple causation model** is useful when the results of epidemiologic studies are interpreted. For example, laboratory and epidemiologic studies may indicate that exposure to a certain chemical or ionizing radiation can cause leukemia, but not all children exposed to that chemical will develop leukemia. Additional studies will be needed to determine what other factors must interact with chemical exposure to cause the disease.

Genetic Factors

Oncogenes and tumor-suppressor genes are associated with the development of childhood cancer (Table 14.2; also see Chapter 12). **Proto-oncogenes** code for proteins that help regulate normal cell growth and differentiation. If mutated, proto-oncogenes become oncogenes that help to turn normal cells into cancer cells. Changes produced by specific oncogenes cause the cell cycle to become dysregulated. An example of an oncogene identified in pediatric cancer is *MYCN*, which is involved in neuroblastoma and glioblastoma. Tumor-suppressor genes are protective genes that normally suppress cancer cell proliferation but have lost

TABLE 14.1	CONGENITAL FACTORS ASSOCIATED WITH CHILDHOOD CANCER
SYNDROME	**ASSOCIATED CHILDHOOD CANCER**
Chromosomal Alterations	
Down syndrome	Acute leukemia
13q syndrome	Retinoblastoma
Chromosomal Instability	
Ataxia-telangiectasia	Lymphoma
Bloom syndrome	Acute leukemia, lymphoma, Wilms tumor
Fanconi anemia	Nonlymphocytic leukemia, myelodysplastic syndrome, hepatic tumors
Hereditary Syndromes	
Beckwith-Wiedemann syndrome	Wilms tumor, sarcoma, brain tumors, neuroblastoma, hepatoblastoma
Neurofibromatosis type 1	Brain tumors, sarcomas, neuroblastomas, Wilms tumor, nonlymphocytic leukemia
Neurofibromatosis type 2	Meningioma (malignant or benign), acoustic neuroma/schwannoma, gliomas, ependymomas
Tuberous sclerosis	Glial tumors
Li-Fraumeni syndrome	Sarcoma, adrenocortical carcinoma
von Hippel-Lindau disease	Cerebellar hemangioblastoma, retinal angioma, renal cell carcinoma, pheochromocytomas
Ataxia-telangiectasia	Leukemia, lymphoma, brain tumors
Gorlin syndrome	Medulloblastoma, skin tumors
Immune Deficiency Disorders	
Congenital	
Agammaglobulinemia	Lymphoma, leukemia, brain tumors
Immunoglobulin A (IgA) deficiency	Lymphoma, leukemia, brain tumors
Wiskott-Aldrich syndrome	Leukemia, lymphoma
Acquired	
Aplastic anemia	Leukemia
Organ transplantation	Leukemia, lymphoma
Congenital Malformation Syndromes	
Aniridia, hemihypertrophy, hamartoma, genitourinary anomalies	Wilms tumor
Cryptorchidism	Testicular tumor
Gonadal dysgenesis	Gonadoblastoma
Family Susceptibility	
Twin or sibling with leukemia	Leukemia

TABLE 14.2   SELECTED ONCOGENES AND TUMOR-SUPPRESSOR GENES ASSOCIATED WITH CHILDHOOD CANCER

GENE	ASSOCIATED PEDIATRIC TUMOR
Oncogenes	
BCR-ABL	Acute lymphoblastic leukemia
MYCN	Neuroblastoma
MYB	Neural tumors, leukemia, lymphoma, rhabdomyosarcoma, Wilms tumor, neuroblastoma
EGFR/ErbB	Glioblastomas
NRAS	Neuroblastoma, leukemia, rhabdomyosarcoma
KRAS	Leukemia
ATM	Lymphoma, leukemia
Tumor-Suppressor Genes	
RB1	Retinoblastoma, sarcoma
WT1, WT2	Wilms tumor, leukemia
WTC	Wilms tumor
NF-1	Sarcoma, primitive neuroectodermal tumor, juvenile chronic myelocytic leukemia
NF-2	Brain tumors, melanoma, meningiomas
CDKN2A	Melanoma, Ewing sarcoma
PTEN	Glioma, melanoma
INK4A/ARF	Leukemia, glioma
TP53	Sarcoma, leukemia, brain tumors, lymphoma
DCC	Ewing sarcoma, rhabdomyosarcoma, neuroblastoma
ARF	Glioma, T-cell ALL
CDC2L1	Non-Hodgkin lymphoma, neuroblastoma

Data from OMIM Online Mendelian inheritance in man: *An online catalog of human genes and genetic disorders.* Available at http://www.omim.org.

their suppressor function. When both copies of a tumor-suppressor gene acquire mutations, normal cell function is lost and cancer can develop. Some childhood and adolescent cancers identified with tumor-suppressor genes include osteosarcoma, leukemia, rhabdomyosarcoma, retinoblastoma, and Wilms tumor.[7]

Other genetic factors involve chromosomal aberrations, including both germline and acquired abnormalities. These chromosomal abnormalities include aneuploidy, amplifications, deletions, and translocations. Some chromosomal disorders and congenital malformations are associated with the development of pediatric cancer; however, the mechanisms associated with cancer development are not fully understood. Trisomy 21 (Down syndrome) is the most common genetic defect linked to the development of acute leukemia. Children with Down syndrome have a 10- to 20-fold increased risk of developing acute lymphoblastic and myelogenous leukemias and a higher risk for developing acute megakaryocytic leukemia. The risk is highest between 1 and 4 years of age.[8] The risk of leukemia also is increased for children with congenital malformations involving the circulatory system.[9]

Wilms tumor may occur in combination with other congenital anomalies, including aniridia or congenital absence of the iris of the eye, ambiguous genitalia, and intellectual disability (WAGR syndrome). WAGR syndrome is caused by a mutation on the short arm of chromosome 11. This region includes the Wilms tumor gene *(WT1)* as well as the *PAX6* gene that is associated with ocular development. Wilms tumor also is associated with neurofibromatosis and Beckwith-Wiedemann syndrome.[10] Most cases of Wilms tumor, however, do not occur in children with underlying congenital syndromes.

Population-based studies indicate that children with congenital malformations involving the nervous system are at increased risk for cancer, including cancer in the central nervous system.[9] Additionally, the siblings of children with congenital malformations involving the central nervous system, eye, ear, face, or neck are at an increased risk for cancer compared with the siblings of unaffected children.[11]

Retinoblastoma, a malignant embryonal tumor of the eye, results from deletions in the long arm of chromosome 13, which is the locus for the *RB1* gene, a tumor-suppressor gene. Deletions may occur as germline or acquired mutations. Germline deletions are associated with familial retinoblastoma, whereas acquired deletions are associated with sporadic cases (see Chapter 20).

Translocations, or the exchange of chromosomal material between nonhomologous chromosomes, also are associated with childhood and adolescent cancers. A well-known chromosomal translocation is the Philadelphia chromosome, which involves chromosomes 9 and 22. The Philadelphia chromosome results in the production of the BCR-Abl fusion protein, which accelerates cell division and inhibits DNA repair. It is commonly found in chronic myelogenous leukemia and some cases of acute lymphoblastic leukemias.[12] Chromosomal translocations also are commonly observed in sarcomas.

Several single-gene disorders have been associated with the subsequent development of childhood and adolescent cancers. Fanconi anemia and Bloom syndrome are autosomal recessive conditions that are risk factors for the development of cancer. Fanconi anemia results in altered DNA repair, and the majority of affected individuals develop acute myelogenous leukemia. Bloom syndrome results in chromosomal fragility leading to increased mutations. It is associated with a spectrum of cancers including leukemias, lymphomas, and carcinomas.

Li-Fraumeni syndrome (LFS) is an autosomal dominant disorder involving mutations in the tumor protein p53 *(TP53)* gene, a tumor-suppressor gene on the short arm of chromosome 17. For individuals carrying a TP53 mutation, the risk of developing cancer as a child or adult is significantly higher than that seen in the unaffected population. Children and adults in these families are at risk for soft tissue sarcoma, breast cancer, leukemia, osteosarcoma, melanoma, and cancer of the colon, pancreas, adrenal cortex, and brain. Individuals with LFS also are at increased risk for developing multiple primary cancers.[13]

An increased familial risk has been observed in some pediatric cancers. Although the majority of pediatric cancers are not genetically transmitted as single-gene disorders, shared genetic and environmental risk factors may contribute to an increased familial risk. A child who has a sibling with leukemia has a risk for the development of leukemia that is 2 to 4 times greater than that for children with healthy siblings. The occurrence of leukemia in monozygous twins is estimated as being as high as 25%. Although susceptibility gene loci have been identified for ALL, they explain only a relatively small portion of the familial risk for recurrence of ALL among siblings. Additional currently unidentified genetic loci are likely to contribute to the additional familial risk.[14] The heritability of adult cancers across the life span also is increased among both monozygotic and dizygotic twins.[15]

Cancers in children and adolescents are associated with fewer genetic mutations compared with adult cancers; however, efforts to understand

WHAT'S NEW?

Cancer Predisposition Genes and Pediatric Cancer

Genetic technologies are providing insights into the prevalence of genetic mutations that may predispose children and adolescents to cancer. A recent study used genome sequencing techniques to identify the presence of germline mutations in 565 genes associated with cancer development in 1120 children and adolescents with cancer and 966 individuals who did not have cancer. The investigators found that 8.5% of individuals with cancer had a mutation associated with cancer development compared with only 1.1% of the individuals who did not have cancer. Mutations most frequently occurred in the *TP53* gene, a gene involved in regulating cell division and preventing tumor formation. Other frequently affected genes were *APC* and *BRCA2*. The majority of children and adolescents with mutations in cancer predisposition genes did not have a family history of cancer.

The results of this study will guide additional epidemiologic studies, as well as studies investigating mechanisms of cancer development in children and adolescents. Identifying the presence of these predisposition mutations also may help guide treatment, as well as genetic testing and counseling of other family members.

the scope of predisposing mutations in pediatric cancer are ongoing. A recent study identified a greater frequency of germline mutations in cancer predisposition genes among children and adolescents with cancer compared with individuals who do not have cancer. More than one-half of the children and adolescents with germline mutations did not have a family history of cancer[16] (see *What's New? Cancer Predisposition Genes and Pediatric Cancer*).

Mutations in individual genes also may result in epigenetic modifications that, in turn, increase an individual's vulnerability to cancer. For example, mutations in genes encoding histone proteins can decrease the expression of other genes without changing the sequence of these genes. This subsequent decreased gene expression can alter cell differentiation, leading to cancer development. Such epigenetic changes are being investigated in relation to the development of diffuse intrinsic pontine glioma (DIPG), an incurable brain tumor, as well as sarcomas.[17,18]

Environmental Factors

Although many adult cancers are associated with exposure to environmental agents, few childhood tumors share a similar strong association. Because of the lengthy latency period required between exposure and development of cancer, early exposure to carcinogens is presumed not to result in cancer until the child is an adult. To date, exposures to high-dose and high-dose rate ionizing radiation have been established as risk factors for childhood leukemia.[19] Multiple other possible environmental risk factors for childhood cancer have been explored. Results of these studies have been mixed, and no definitive causal pathway for childhood cancer has been determined.

Prenatal Exposure

Prenatal exposure to some drugs, however, has been linked to childhood cancers. The most well-described drug is diethylstilbestrol (DES), which was prescribed by physicians to prevent spontaneous miscarriage (in women with previous miscarriage). In 1971 DES was identified as a transplacental chemical carcinogen because a small percentage of the daughters of the women who took DES developed adenocarcinomas of the vagina and cervix. Since then, other studies have attempted to identify drugs taken by pregnant women that may cause cancer in their offspring, but no other drugs have been found. Prior research suggested an association between antenatal x-ray exposure and childhood cancer,

but studies have not been replicated or supported in recent literature. In 2006 the Office of the U.S. Surgeon General suggested evidence of a causal relationship between childhood leukemia, lymphoma, and brain tumors and prenatal or postnatal environmental tobacco smoke exposure.

Results of recent meta-analyses have suggested associations between parental exposure to pesticides and other potential environmental toxins before or during pregnancy and subsequent development of childhood cancer.[6] Recent studies suggest that the risk of leukemia and lymphoma is increased when the mother was exposed to pesticides in the prenatal period, and the risk of brain tumors is associated with paternal exposure (occupational or household use) either before or after birth.[20,21] Results of a European population-based study, however, did not suggest an association between parental occupational pesticide exposure and the development of childhood brain tumors.[22] In contrast, however, a meta-analysis of 1426 cases of neuroblastoma failed to show an association between paternal occupational exposure to pesticide and development of disease.[23] An Italian case-control study suggested that maternal exposure to hair dyes and occupational chemical exposure was associated with an increased risk of neuroblastoma.[24]

Childhood Exposure

Childhood exposure to ionizing radiation, drugs, and viruses has been associated with the risk of developing cancer.[25] Although high doses of ionizing radiation are established risk factors for the development of childhood cancer, evidence is emerging about the role of lower doses as well as additional variables that may further convey an increased risk. Retrospective studies have demonstrated significant positive correlations between radiation-induced malignancies from radiotherapy (cancer treatment) and from radiation exposure from diagnostic imaging and the development of childhood cancer.[26-28] A case-control study of more than 1000 children in Finland with leukemia who were less than 15 years of age did not demonstrate an overall association of childhood leukemia with background gamma radiation.[29] This study did, however, demonstrate an increased risk of leukemia in relation to increasing radiation dose among children between 2 and 7 years of age. Additionally, this study also identified a positive association between leukemia with high hyperdiploid features and radiation dose. A similar increased risk was not identified for leukemia with other genetic features. Few studies have followed children for a long enough period of time to determine whether the risk of cancer remains increased in adulthood, although current studies with more rigorous methodology are assessing this risk[30-32] (see *What's New? CT Scans in Childhood Appear to Increase Cancer Risk*).

In addition to the drug and environmental agents that are known to cause cancer in adults and therefore also are risks for exposure during childhood, a few drugs may particularly increase cancer risk during childhood (Table 14.3). Exposures during childhood to unspecified residential pesticides and insecticides have been associated with childhood leukemia.[33]

The relationship between childhood cancer and exposure to radon[34-36] and electromagnetic fields has been the focus of many epidemiologic studies, yet no conclusive evidence has been observed. In 2007 a task group of scientific experts convened by the World Health Organization (WHO) reported that it could not confirm the existence of any health consequences from exposure to low-level magnetic fields.[37] A review of studies from 1997 to 2013 indicated that magnetic field exposure may be associated with an increased incidence of childhood leukemia.[38]

The strongest association between viruses and the development of cancer in children has been the relationship between exposure to Epstein-Barr virus (EBV) and development of Burkitt lymphoma, nasopharyngeal carcinoma, and Hodgkin disease. Children with acquired

TABLE 14.3   DRUGS THAT MAY INCREASE RISK OF CHILDHOOD CANCER

DRUG CLASS	USES	CANCER RISK
Anabolic androgenic steroids	Stimulate bone growth and appetite Induce puberty Increase muscle mass and physical strength	Hepatocellular carcinoma Brain tumors
Cytotoxic chemotherapy	Used in cancer treatment	Leukemia
Immunosuppressive agents	Prevent organ rejection following transplantation surgery	Lymphoma

WHAT'S NEW?

CT Scans in Childhood Appear to Increase Cancer Risk

A growing number of international studies are providing evidence of an increased risk of childhood cancer following computed tomography (CT) scans. The findings from a recent study of 176,587 children suggest that those who had 2 or 3 CT scans of the head before age 22 years were 3 times as likely to develop brain cancer as those in the general population, and the risk of developing leukemia was 3 times as great in those who received 5 to 10 CT scans. A follow-up study involving this same cohort of children addressed underlying unreported conditions that could have introduced bias. Results indicated a lower estimated relative risk for both leukemia and brain tumors than initially reported. The study results did, however, continue to demonstrate an increased risk of childhood cancer following CT exposure and that a significant dose-response risk was present. Although CT scans are important diagnostic imaging studies for children, the results of the study emphasize that children receive scans only when necessary using the lowest dose of radiation possible.

Data from Mathews JD et al: *BMJ* 346:f2360, 2013; Pearce MS et al: *Lancet* 380(9840):499-505, 2012.

immunodeficiency syndrome (AIDS) have an increased risk of developing non-Hodgkin lymphoma and Kaposi sarcoma. However, with the use of highly active antiretroviral therapy (HAART) in the developed world, the incidence of AIDS-related malignancies has declined dramatically[39] Current evidence, however, indicates that the rate of non-AIDS–related malignancies is increasing among children and adolescents receiving

HAART. Hypothesized mechanisms include oxidative stress and premature aging resulting from shortened telomeres as an adverse effect of HAART.[39,40]

PROGNOSIS

Nearly 85% of children and adolescents diagnosed with cancer are cured. Mortality rates have declined from 6.5 per 100,000 in 1969 to 2.3 per 100,000 in 2013, largely because of advances in treatment and increased participation in clinical trials.[1,2]

Some of the factors leading to improved cure rates in pediatric oncology include the use of combination chemotherapy and multimodal treatment for childhood solid tumors. Additionally, development of research centers for comprehensive childhood cancer treatment, cooperation among treatment institutions, and development of cooperative study groups enable the most efficient advancement of treatment regimens. Currently, clinical trials are being conducted by the Children's Oncology Group (COG) at more than 180 hospitals across the United States and are funded by the National Cancer Institute through CureSearch for Children's Cancer. Clinical trials are continually focusing on more effective, targeted therapies with fewer side effects. Side effects of treatment are better managed as a result of improvements in nursing and supportive care, recognition of the psychologic effects of cancer treatment, and continued follow-up care to track trends in the late effects of cancer treatment. Young children are particularly prone to long-term sequelae of cancer therapy. Supportive care guidelines to manage acute side effects of cancer treatment, as well as long-term follow-up guidelines,[41] are available to guide the care of individuals who are survivors of childhood and adolescent cancers.

SUMMARY REVIEW

Incidence and Types of Cancer

1. Cancer in children and adolescents is rare, but it is still the leading cause of death from disease in this population.
2. Leukemias and brain tumors account for 61% of cancer in children from birth to 14 years of age, with neuroblastoma and soft tissue or bone sarcomas less common.
3. The most common cancers among the adolescent and young adult populations (15 to 39 years of age) are Hodgkin lymphoma, leukemia, germ cell tumors (particularly testicular), central nervous system (CNS) tumors, non-Hodgkin lymphoma, thyroid cancer, melanoma, sarcomas, and breast, cervical, liver, and colorectal cancers.

Etiology

1. The interaction of many factors most likely produces cancer in children and adolescents, a concept referred to as multiple causation or multifactorial etiology.
2. Oncogenes and tumor-suppressor genes have been associated with childhood and adolescent malignancies.

3. Chromosomal aberrations or single-gene defects including aneuploidy, amplifications, deletions, translocations, and fragility are associated with the development of childhood cancer.
4. Wilms tumor and retinoblastoma are pediatric malignancies that are linked in a familial manner.
5. Childhood exposure to ionizing radiation, drugs, or viruses has been associated with the risk of developing cancer.

Prognosis

1. Nearly 85% of children and adolescents diagnosed with cancer are cured.
2. Mortality rates have declined significantly in the past 45 years largely because of advances in treatment and increased participation in clinical trials.
3. Young children are particularly prone to long-term sequelae of cancer therapy. The development of more effective, targeted therapies with fewer side effects is imperative.

KEY TERMS

Blast cell, 426
Embryonal tumors, 426

Mesodermal germ layer, 426
Multifactorial etiology, 427

Multiple causation model, 427
Proto-oncogenes, 427

REFERENCES

1. American Cancer Society (ACS): *Cancer facts and figures 2017*, Atlanta, 2017, Author.
2. Howlader N, et al, editors: *SEER cancer statistics review, 1975-2013*, Bethesda, MD, 2016, National Cancer Institute. Available at http://seer.cancer.gov/csr/1975_2013/. based on Nov 2015 SEER data submission.
3. Siegel RL, Miller KD, Jemal A: Cancer statistics, 2016. *CA Cancer J Clin* 66(1):7–30, 2016.
4. National Cancer Institute (NCI): *Adolescents and young adults with cancer*. Available at http://www.cancer.gov/cancertopics/aya/types.
5. Ghantous A, et al: Characterizing the epigenome as a key component of the fetal exposome in evaluating in utero exposures and childhood cancer risk. *Mutagenesis* 30(6):733–742, 2015.
6. Turner MC, Wigle DT, Krewski D: Residential pesticides and childhood leukemia: a systematic review and meta-analysis. *Environ Health Perspect* 118(1):33–41, 2010.
7. Plon SE, Malkin D: Childhood cancer and heredity. In Pizzo PA, Poplack DG, editors: *Principles and practice of pediatric oncology*, ed 6, Philadelphia, 2011, Lippincott Williams & Wilkins, pp 17–37.
8. Margolin JF, et al: Acute lymphoblastic leukemia. In Pizzo PA, Poplack DG, editors: *Principles and practice of pediatric oncology*, ed 6, Philadelphia, 2011, Lippincott Williams & Wilkins, pp 518–565.
9. Sun Y, Overvad K, Olsen J: Cancer risks in children with congenital malformations in the nervous and circulatory system—a population-based cohort study. *Cancer Epidemiol* 38(4):393–400, 2014.
10. Fernandez C, et al: Renal tumors. In Pizzo PA, Poplack DG, editors: *Principles and practice of pediatric oncology*, ed 6, Philadelphia, 2011, Lippincott Williams & Wilkins, pp 861–885.
11. Sun Y, et al: Cancer risk in siblings of children with congenital malformations. *Cancer Epidemiol* 44(1):59–64, 2016.
12. Alvarnez JC, et al: Acute lymphoblastic leukemia. *J Natl Comp Canc Netw* 10(7):858–914, 2012.
13. Mai PL, et al: Risks of first and subsequent cancers among TP53 mutation carriers in the National Cancer Institute Li-Fraumeni syndrome cohort. *Cancer* 122(23):3673–3681, 2016.
14. Kharazmi E, et al: Familial risks for childhood acute lymphoblastic leukaemia in Sweden and Finland: far exceeding the effects of known germline variants. *Br J Haematol* 159(5):585–588, 2012.
15. Mucci LA, et al: Familial risk and heritability of cancer among twins in Nordic countries. *JAMA* 315(1):68–76, 2016.

16. Zhang J, et al: Germline mutations in predisposition genes in pediatric cancer. *N Engl J Med* 373(24):2336–2346, 2015.
17. Lewis PW, Allis CD: Poisoning the "histone code" in pediatric gliomagenesis. *Cell Cycle* 12(20):3241–3242, 2013.
18. Lu C, et al: Histone H3K36 mutations promote sarcomagenesis through altered histone methylation landscape. *Science* 352(6287):844–849, 2016.
19. Hsu WL, et al: The incidence of leukemia, lymphoma, and multiple myeloma among atomic bomb survivors: 1950-2001. *Radiat Res* 179(3):361–382, 2013.
20. Van Maele-Fabry G, Hoet P, Lison D: Parental occupational exposure to pesticides as risk factor for brain tumors in children and young adults: a systematic review and meta-analysis. *Environ Int* 56:19–31, 2013.
21. Vinson F, et al: Exposure to pesticides and risk of childhood cancer: a meta-analysis of recent epidemiological studies. *Occup Environ Med* 68(9):694–702, 2011.
22. Febvey O, et al: Risk of central nervous system tumors in children related to parental occupational pesticide exposures in three European case-control studies. *J Occup Environ Med* 58(10):1046–1052, 2016.
23. Moore A, Enquobahrie DA: Paternal occupational exposure to pesticides and risk of neuroblastoma among children: a meta-analysis. *Cancer Causes Control* 22(11):1529–1536, 2011.
24. Parodi S, et al: Risk of neuroblastoma, maternal characteristics and perinatal exposures: the SETIL study. *Cancer Epidemiol* 38(6):686–694, 2014.
25. Linet MS, et al: International long-term trends and recent patterns in the incidence of leukemias and lymphomas among children and adolescents ages 0–19 years. *Int J Cancer* 138(8):1862–1874, 2016.
26. Berrington de Gonzalez A, et al: Relationship between paediatric CT scans and subsequent risk of leukaemia and brain tumours: assessment of the impact of underlying conditions. *Br J Cancer* 114:388–394, 2016.
27. Buka I, et al: Trends in childhood cancer incidence: review of environmental linkages. *Pediatr Clin North Am* 54(1):177–203, 2007.
28. Pearce MS, et al: Radiation exposure from CT scans in childhood and subsequent risk of leukemia and brain tumors: a retrospective cohort study. *Lancet* 380:499–505, 2012.

29. Nikkilä A, et al: Background radiation and childhood cancer: a nationwide register-based case-control study. *Int J Cancer* 139(9):1975–1982, 2016.
30. Krille L, et al: Risk of cancer incidence before the age of 15 years after exposure to ionising radiation from computed tomography: results from a German cohort study. *Radiat Environ Biophys* 54(1):1–12, 2015.
31. Linet MS, et al: Cancer risks associated with external radiation from diagnostic imaging procedures. *CA Cancer J Clin* 62:75–100, 2012.
32. Miglioretti DL, et al: Pediatric computed tomography and associated radiation exposure and estimated cancer risk. *JAMA Pediatr* 167(8):700–707, 2013.
33. Chen M, et al: Residential exposure to pesticide during childhood and childhood cancers: a meta-analysis. *Pediatrics* 136(4):721–729, 2015.
34. Del Risco Kollerud R, Blaasaas KG, Claussen B: Risk of leukaemia or cancer in the central nervous system among children living in an area with high indoor radon concentrations: results from a cohort study in Norway. *Br J Cancer* 111(7):1413–1420, 2014.
35. Hauri D, et al: Domestic radon exposure and risk of childhood cancer: a prospective census-based cohort study. *Environ Health Perspect* 121(10):1239–1244, 2013.
36. Peckham EC, et al: Residential radon exposure and incidence of childhood lymphoma in Texas, 1995-2011. *Int J Environ Res Public Health* 12(10):12110–12126, 2015.
37. Repacholi M: Concern that "EMF" magnetic fields from power lines causes cancer. *Sci Total Environ* 426:454–458, 2012.
38. Zhao L, et al: Magnetic fields exposure and childhood leukemia risk: a meta-analysis based on 11,699 cases and 13,194 controls. *Leuk Res* 38(3):269–274, 2014.
39. Chiappini E, et al: Pediatric human immunodeficiency virus infection and cancer in the highly active antiretroviral treatment (HAART) era. *Cancer Lett* 347(1):38–45, 2014.
40. Torres RA, Lewis W: Aging and HIV/AIDS: pathogenic role of therapeutic side effects. *Lab Invest* 94(2):120–128, 2014.
41. Children's Oncology Group: *Long-term follow-up guidelines for survivors of childhood, adolescent, and young adult cancers (version 4.0)*, 2013. Available at http://www.survivorshipguidelines.org/pdf/LTFUResourceGuide.pdf.

Pathophysiologic Alterations: Organs and Systems

CHAPTER

15

Structure and Function of the Neurologic System

Russell J. Butterfield

CHAPTER OUTLINE

The nervous system is a remarkable structure responsible for the body's ability both to interact with the environment and to regulate and control activities involving internal organs, muscles, and glands. It is a network composed of complex structures that transmit electrical and chemical signals between the brain and the body's many organs and tissues.

OVERVIEW AND ORGANIZATION OF THE NERVOUS SYSTEM

Although the components of the nervous system are considered individually to facilitate a better understanding of their function, it is important to recognize that these distinct parts of the nervous system function as a unified whole. Most broadly, the nervous system is divided into the central nervous system and the peripheral nervous system. The central nervous system (CNS) consists of the brain and spinal cord, enclosed within the protective cranial vault and vertebrae, respectively. The peripheral nervous system (PNS) is composed of the cranial nerves, which project from the brain and pass through foramina (openings) in the skull, and the spinal nerves, which project from the spinal cord and pass through intervertebral foramina. PNS pathways can be divided into ascending, afferent pathways that carry sensory information toward the CNS, and descending, efferent pathways that innervate effector organs, such as skeletal, cardiac, and smooth muscle, as well as glands. Most peripheral nerves carry a combination of both afferent and efferent pathways. Cranial nerves are viewed most correctly as modified spinal nerves. Cranial nerves control motor and sensory function similarly to spinal nerves, but also can have specialized sensory tasks, such as smell, taste, sight, and hearing (see Peripheral Nervous System).

Functionally, the PNS can be divided into the somatic nervous system and the autonomic nervous system. The somatic nervous system consists of motor and sensory pathways regulating voluntary motor control of skeletal muscle. The autonomic nervous system (ANS) also consists of motor and sensory components and is involved with regulation of the body's internal environment (viscera) through involuntary control of organ systems. The ANS is further divided into sympathetic and parasympathetic divisions. Although most aspects of the ANS are involuntary, some aspects can be controlled through mental practice with or without biofeedback techniques.

CELLS OF THE NERVOUS SYSTEM

Two basic types of cells comprise nervous tissue: neurons and supporting neuroglia. The neuron is an electrically excitable cell and transmits electrical or chemical information between other neurons or to an effector organ. Neuroglial cells provide structural support, protection, and nutrition for the neurons, and facilitate neurotransmission.[1] Neuroglial cells include astrocytes, microglia, and oligodendrocytes in the CNS; and Schwann (neurilemma) and satellite cells in the PNS.

Neurons

Working alone or in units, neurons detect environmental changes and initiate body responses to maintain a dynamic steady state. Neuronal structure varies markedly so that each neuron is adapted to perform specialized functions. Although they may vary somewhat in function, neurons (Fig. 15.1) have three common components: a cell body (soma), dendrites (thin branching fibers of the cell), and the axons. Cell bodies for most neurons, even those extending axons into peripheral nerves, are located within the CNS. Dense collections of cell bodies in the CNS are called nuclei. In the PNS, cell bodies can be found in groups called ganglia, or plexuses (group of relay nerves). The dendrites are extensions that carry nerve impulses *toward* the cell body. The dendritic zone is the receptive portion of a neuron that receives a stimulus and either propagates or diminishes conduction. Axons are long projections that carry nerve impulses *away* from the cell body. The axon hillock is a cone-shaped process where the axon leaves the cell body. The first part of the axon hillock has the lowest threshold for stimulation so action potentials often begin there. The principle of *divergence* refers to the ability of axonal branches to influence many different neurons. *Convergence* applies when branches of various numbers of neurons "converge" on and influence a single neuron.

The cellular constituents of a typical neuron include microtubules (transport substances within the cell), neurofibrils (thin supportive fibers that extend throughout the neuron), microfilaments (proteins thought to be involved in transport of cellular products), and Nissl substances/bodies (endoplasmic reticulum and ribosomes) that are involved in protein synthesis. Although most neurons are nondividing cells, some neurons continue to divide after birth; for example, olfactory neurons in the nose continue to divide throughout life.

A typical neuron has only one axon, which may be tightly wrapped with a segmented layer of lipid material called myelin, an insulating substance. In the brain and spinal cord, myelin is formed by oligodendrocytes. Regions of the brain and spinal cord with a high level of myelination constitute the white matter, whereas regions lacking significant myelination (typically primarily composed of cell bodies) are gray matter. In the PNS, the myelin sheath of motor and sensory axons is formed by Schwann cells. Myelin sheaths are interrupted at regular intervals by the nodes of Ranvier. Axons can branch at the nodes of Ranvier.

Nutrient exchange is not possible through the myelin sheath, although it can occur at the nodes of Ranvier where the axon is not insulated. Myelin acts as an insulator that allows an action potential to leap between the nodes of Ranvier rather than flow along the entire length of the membrane, yielding increased velocity of conduction. This mechanism is referred to as saltatory conduction. Disorders of the myelin sheath (demyelinating diseases), such as multiple sclerosis, Guillain-Barré syndrome, and Charcot-Marie-Tooth disease, demonstrate the important role myelin plays in nerve conduction (see Chapter 18). Conduction velocities depend not only on the myelin coating but also on the diameter of the axon. Larger axons transmit impulses at a faster rate.

Neurons are structurally classified on the basis of the number of processes (projections) extending from the cell body. There are four basic types of cell configuration: (1) unipolar, (2) pseudounipolar, (3) bipolar, and (4) multipolar (Fig. 15.2). Unipolar neurons have one process that branches shortly after leaving the cell body. One example is found in the retina. Pseudounipolar neurons (some authors call them *unipolar*) also have one process. The dendritic portion of each of these neurons extends away from the CNS, and the axon portion projects into the CNS. The configuration is typical of sensory neurons in both cranial and spinal nerves. Bipolar neurons have two distinct processes arising from the cell body. This type of neuron connects to rod and cone cells of the retina. Multipolar neurons are the most common and have multiple processes capable of extensive branching. A motor neuron is typically multipolar.

Functionally, there are three types of neurons (with their direction of transmission and typical configuration noted in parentheses): (1) sensory (afferent, mostly pseudounipolar), (2) associational (interneurons, multipolar), and (3) motor (efferent, multipolar). Sensory neurons carry impulses from peripheral sensory receptors to the CNS (Box 15.1). Association neurons (interneurons) transmit impulses from neuron to neuron and are located solely within the CNS. Motor neurons transmit impulses away from the CNS to an effector organ (i.e., skeletal muscle or organs). In skeletal muscle, the end processes of an axon form a specialized structure called a neuromuscular junction.

Neuroglia and Schwann Cells

Neuroglia ("nerve glue") are the general classification of non-neuronal cells that support the neurons of the CNS. Conduction velocities depend not only on the myelin coating and nodes of Ranvier, but also on the diameter of the axon. Larger axons transmit impulses at a faster rate. Oligodendroglia (oligodendrocytes) form myelin sheaths within the brain and spinal cord. Regions of the brain and spinal cord with a high level of myelination constitute the white matter, whereas regions lacking significant myelination (typically primarily composed of cell bodies)

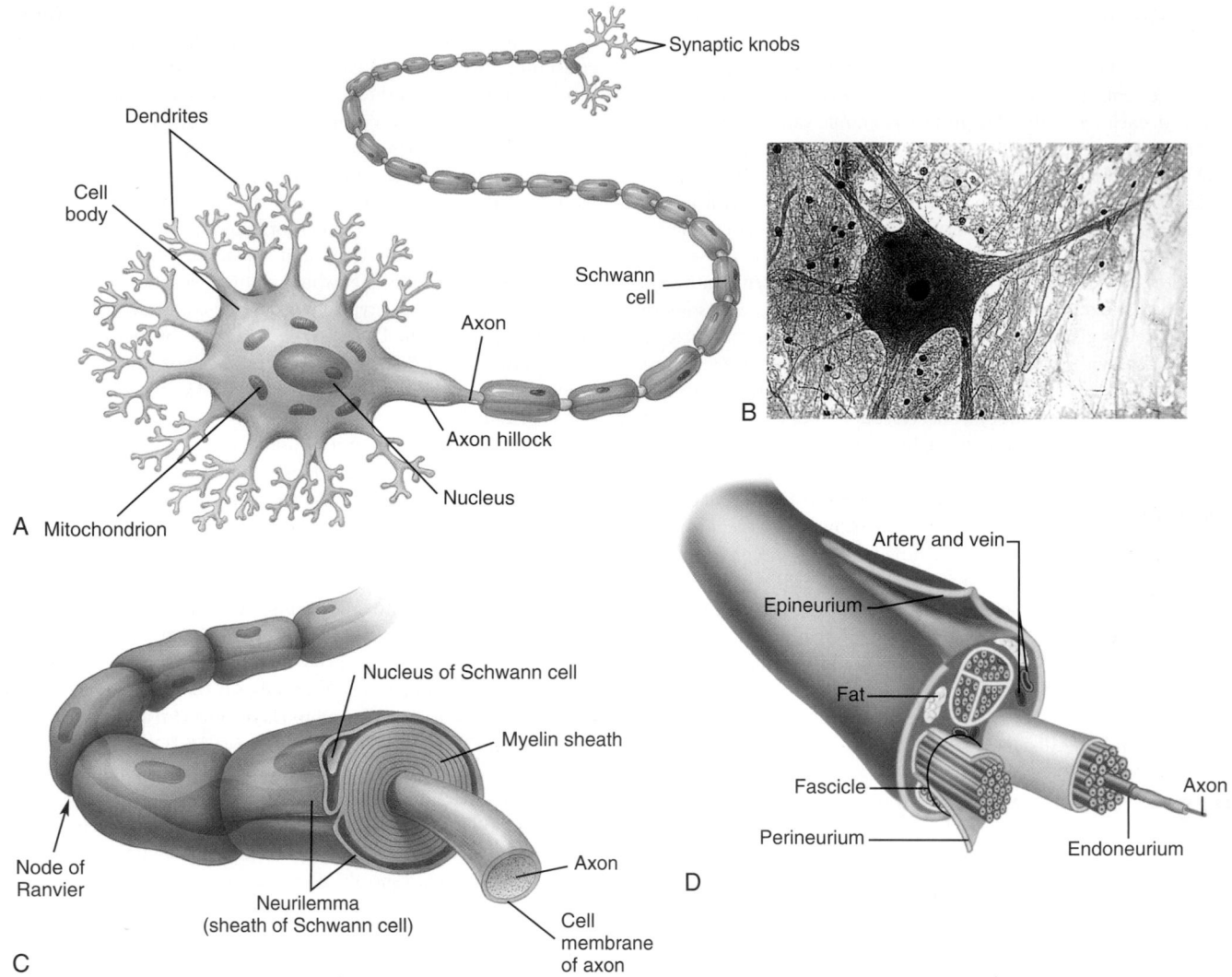

FIGURE 15.1 Structure of a Typical Neuron. A, Multiple dendrites carry nerve impulses to the cell body, and a single long axon carries nerve impulses away from the cell body. Long axons are encased at intervals by a myelin sheath. **B,** Photomicrograph of a neuron. **C,** A segment of myelinated fiber in cross section, showing myelin sheath composed of several layers of myelin, which insulate the axon. **D,** Axons bundled into fascicles. (**A** and **C** from Thibodeau GA, Patton KT: *Structure and function of the human body,* ed 12, St Louis, 2004, Mosby; **B** copyright Edward Reschke; **D** from Patton KT, Thibodeau GA: *Anatomy & physiology,* ed 8, St Louis, 2013, Mosby.)

BOX 15.1	**MAJOR TYPES OF SENSORY RECEPTORS**

Nociceptors (pain)

Mechanoreceptors (touch, pressure, and mechanical deformation or encapsulated endings)

Photochemical (light on the retina)

Chemoreceptors (flavors, odors, oxygen levels, osmolarity of body fluids, and carbon dioxide levels in the blood)

Thermoreceptors (heat and cold)

Proprioception (sensing location of body parts)

Audition and balance (sound and positional movement)

are gray matter. Schwann cells form the myelin sheath around axons in the peripheral nervous system and direct axonal regrowth and functional recovery of injured neurons (see *What's New?* Schwann Cells). Nonmyelinating Schwann cells provide metabolic support. Characteristics of neuroglia and Schwann cells are summarized in Fig. 15.3 and Table 15.1.

Nerve Injury and Regeneration

Mature neurons do not divide, and injury in the CNS causes permanent loss of damaged neurons. Peripheral nerves can repair themselves through local, anterograde, and retrograde changes. This is known as the axonal reaction. *Local changes* occur when the axon is severed. The cut ends retract and the axolemma covers the cut ends, diminishing the escape of axoplasm. Macrophages and Schwann cells begin to phagocytize damaged tissue. The cell body undergoes chromatolysis with swelling, loss of Nissl

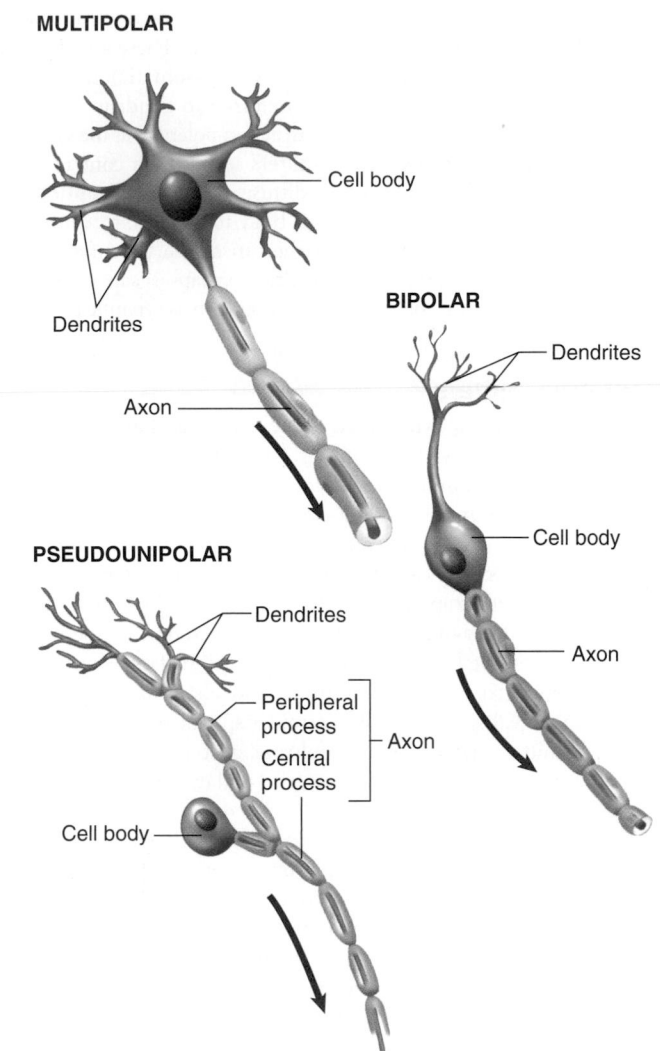

MULTIPOLAR

Cell body

Dendrites

Axon

BIPOLAR

Dendrites

Cell body

Axon

PSEUDOUNIPOLAR

Dendrites

Peripheral process

Central process

Axon

Cell body

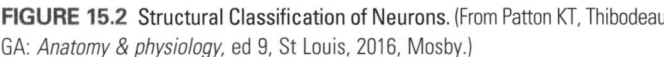

FIGURE 15.2 Structural Classification of Neurons. (From Patton KT, Thibodeau GA: *Anatomy & physiology*, ed 9, St Louis, 2016, Mosby.)

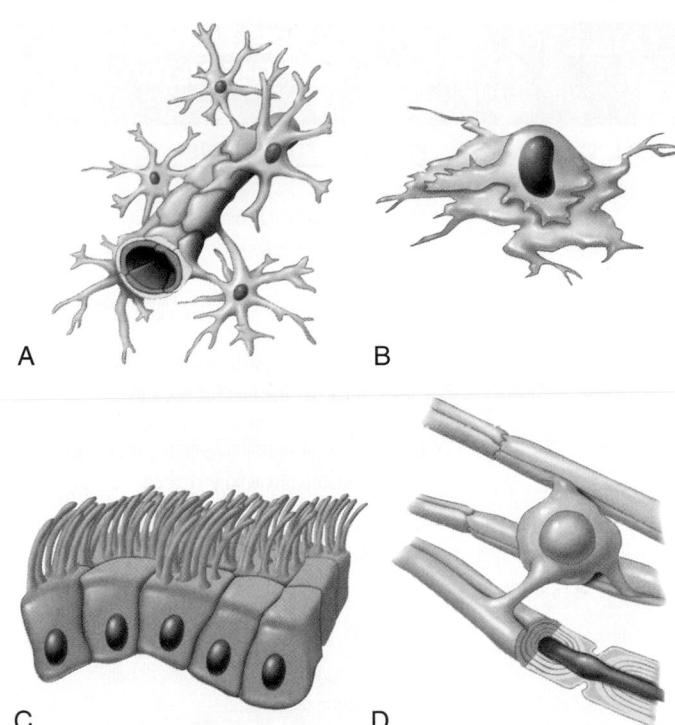

A

B

C

D

FIGURE 15.3 Types of Neuroglial Cells. **A,** Astrocyte attached to brain capillary. **B,** Microglial cell. **C,** Ependymal cells that form sheets to line fluid cavities in brain. **D,** Oligodendrocyte wrapped around CNS nerve fiber forming myelin. (From Patton KT et al: *Essentials of anatomy & physiology*, St Louis, 2012, Mosby.)

bodies, and lateral migration of the nucleus. Antegrade *(Wallerian) degeneration* occurs in the distal axon: (1) a characteristic swelling appears in the axon terminal, and it degenerates and loses contact with the postsynaptic membrane within 7 days; (2) macrophages and Schwann cells phagocytize the remnants of the axon terminal; and (3) Schwann cells proliferate, forming a column or tube of Schwann cells enclosed by the original basal lamina of the endoneurium. *Retrograde changes* occur at the proximal end of the injured axon and are similar to antegrade changes but only back to the next node of Ranvier. Approximately 7 to 14 days after the injury, new terminal sprouts project from the proximal segment guided by Schwann cells and enter the sustaining substrate of the Schwann cell column or tubes for axonal regrowth. Fig. 15.4 contains a more detailed representation of these events. This process is very slow (about 1 mm per day) and is limited to myelinated fibers in the PNS. The regeneration of axonal constituents in the CNS is limited by an increased incidence of glial scar formation (gliosis) and the different nature of myelin formed by the oligodendrocyte.

Nerve regeneration depends on many factors, such as the location of the injury, the type of injury, the presence of inflammatory responses, and the process of scarring. The closer the injury is to the cell body of

WHAT'S NEW?
Schwann Cells

Schwann cells (SCs) are peripheral neuroglial cells derived from the neural crest. They are the most common cell type in the peripheral nervous system. There are several subtypes in addition to the myelin-forming cells. These include non–myelin-forming autonomic nervous system cells, perisynaptic cells, and perineuronal satellite cells of the dorsal root ganglia and of the autonomic ganglia. SCs are important for maintenance of normal nervous system function, repair of neural injury, immune modulation, and upregulation of pain. Myelin-forming SCs form spirals of compact myelin lamellae in both small and large neurons. Increasing layers of lamellae increase the speed of salutatory conduction. These cells also can recognize antigen and be the target of autoimmune responses as occur with Guillain-Barré syndrome. Most neural cells in the peripheral nervous system are unmyelinated, and SCs in these nerves, as well as the dorsal root and sympathetic and parasympathetic ganglia, provide an axonal sheath but do not form myelin. With peripheral nerve injury, perineuronal satellite cells can up-regulate nerve growth factor and other molecules important to peripheral chronic pain syndromes. At the neuromuscular junction (NMJ), nonmyelinating SCs function to facilitate neurotransmission and repair damage. Transplant of SCs and use of exogenous neurotrophic factors are in the preclinical stage of evaluation.

Data from Armati PJ, Mathey EK: *J Neurol Sci* 333(1–2):68–72, 2013; Armati PJ, Mathey EK: *J Peripher Nerv Syst* 19(1):14–23, 2014; Jones S, Eisenberg HM, Jia X: *Int J Mol Sci* 17(9), 2016; Monk KR, Feltri ML, Taveggia C: *Glia* 63(8):1376–1393, 2015; Namgung U: *Cells Tissues Organs* 200(1):6–12, 2014.

TABLE 15.1	SUPPORT CELLS (GLIAL CELLS) OF THE NERVOUS SYSTEM
CELL TYPE	**PRIMARY FUNCTIONS**
Astrocytes	Form specialized contacts between neuronal surfaces and blood vessels
	Provide rapid transport for nutrients and metabolites
	Believed to form an essential component of the blood-brain barrier
	Appear to be the scar-forming cells of the CNS, which may be the foci for seizures
	Participate in CNS immune function
	Appear to work with neurons in processing information and memory storage
Oligodendroglia (oligodendrocytes)	Formation of myelin sheath and neurilemma in the CNS
Schwann cells	Formation of myelin sheath and neurilemma in the PNS
Microglia	Responsible for clearing cellular debris (phagocytic properties)
Ependymal cells	Serve as a lining for ventricles and choroid plexuses involved in production of CSF

CNS, Central nervous system; *CSF,* cerebrospinal fluid; *PNS,* peripheral nervous system.

the nerve, the greater the chances that the nerve cell will die and not regenerate. A crushing injury allows recovery more fully than does a cut injury. Crushed nerves sometimes recover fully, whereas cut nerves often form connective tissue scars that block or slow regenerating axonal branches. Peripheral nerves injured close to the spinal cord recover poorly and slowly because of the long distance between the cell body and the peripheral termination of the axon.[2]

NERVE IMPULSE

Neurons generate and conduct electrical impulses by selectively changing the conductance across their plasma membrane and influencing other nearby neurons by the release of chemical signals (neurotransmitters). An unexcited neuron maintains a resting membrane potential. When the membrane potential is raised sufficiently, an action potential is generated and propagated to other parts of the neuron (see Fig. 1.39). The action potential occurs only when the stimulus is strong enough; if it is too weak the membrane remains unexcited. This property is sometimes termed the *all-or-none response*.

Synapses

Neurons are not physically continuous with one another but form points of contact with adjacent neurons with a specialized structure called a synapse. The synapse is composed of a small bulbous end of the presynaptic neuron (synaptic knob) that is separated from the postsynaptic neuron by a synaptic cleft. Impulses are transmitted across the synapse by chemical (Fig. 15.5 and see Fig. 15.16) and electrical conduction; only chemical conduction is discussed here. Chapter 1 contains information on electrical conduction. The neurons that conduct a nerve impulse are named according to whether they relay impulses *toward* (presynaptic neurons) or *away* from the synapse (postsynaptic

neurons). Four basic types of connections occur in regions of contact between the presynaptic and postsynaptic neurons. These are between axons (axo-axonic), from axon to cell body (axo-somatic), from axon to dendrite (axo-dendritic), and from dendrite to dendrite (dendro-dendritic). In response to the arrival of an action potential at the synaptic knob, vesicles containing neurotransmitters release their contents into the synaptic cleft. Neurotransmitters diffuse across the synaptic cleft (the space between the neurons) and bind to specific receptors on postsynaptic neurons, where they trigger an action potential in the postsynaptic neuron (see Fig. 15.5). Brain synapses can change in strength and number throughout life; this is known as synaptic plasticity or neuroplasticity.

Neurotransmitters

Neurotransmitters are synthesized in the neuron and localized in the presynaptic terminal (synaptic bouton). Neurotransmitters are released into the synaptic cleft in response to the arrival of an electrical impulse and bind to a receptor site (binding site) on the postsynaptic membrane of an adjacent neuron or other effector. Here, binding of the neurotransmitter to its receptor causes a change in conductance of postsynaptic membrane allowing propagation of the impulse (see Fig. 15.5). Efficient termination of the signal requires rapid degeneration of the neurotransmitter in the cleft or on the postsynaptic cell surface. Neurons can synthesize more than one neurotransmitter, and postsynaptic membranes can contain more than one type of transmitter-specific receptor. Common neurotransmitters include norepinephrine, acetylcholine, dopamine, histamine, and serotonin. These have varied and overlapping functions[3] that are summarized in Table 15.2.

Because the neurotransmitter is normally stored on the presynaptic side of the synaptic cleft and the receptor sites are on the postsynaptic side, chemical synapses operate in one direction. Therefore action potentials are transmitted along a multineuronal pathway in one direction. The binding of the neurotransmitter at the receptor site changes the permeability of the postsynaptic membrane and, consequently, its membrane potential. Two possible scenarios can follow: (1) the postsynaptic neuron may be excited (depolarized; excitatory postsynaptic potentials [EPSPs]), or (2) the postsynaptic membrane may be inhibited (hyperpolarized; inhibitory postsynaptic potentials [IPSPs]).[4] (Chapter 1 contains a review of electrical impulses and membrane potentials.)

Usually, a single postsynaptic potential cannot induce a neuron's action potential and the propagation of the nerve impulse. Whether an action potential occurs depends on the number and frequency of excitatory and inhibitory potentials the postsynaptic neuron receives, a concept known as summation. Temporal summation refers to the effects of successive, rapid impulses received from a single neuron on the same synapse. Spatial summation is the combined effects of impulses from a number of neurons on a single synapse at the same time. Facilitation refers to the effect of multiple EPSPs on the plasma membrane potential. The plasma membrane is facilitated when summation brings the membrane closer to the threshold potential and decreases the stimulus required to induce an action potential. The effect of a neurotransmitter on the membrane potential depends on the balance of these effects. The mechanisms of convergence (many neurons firing and converging on one neuron), divergence (one neuron firing and diverging on many neurons), summation, and facilitation allow for the integrative processes of the nervous system.

Two points could be helpful in understanding the complexity of brain physiology. First, the aforementioned neuromodulators appear to function to raise or lower the membrane potentials of neurons. These chemicals facilitate or inhibit the effect of neurotransmitters. Second, reciprocal synapses between dendrites—that is, one dendrite being able to depolarize or hyperpolarize the membrane potential of

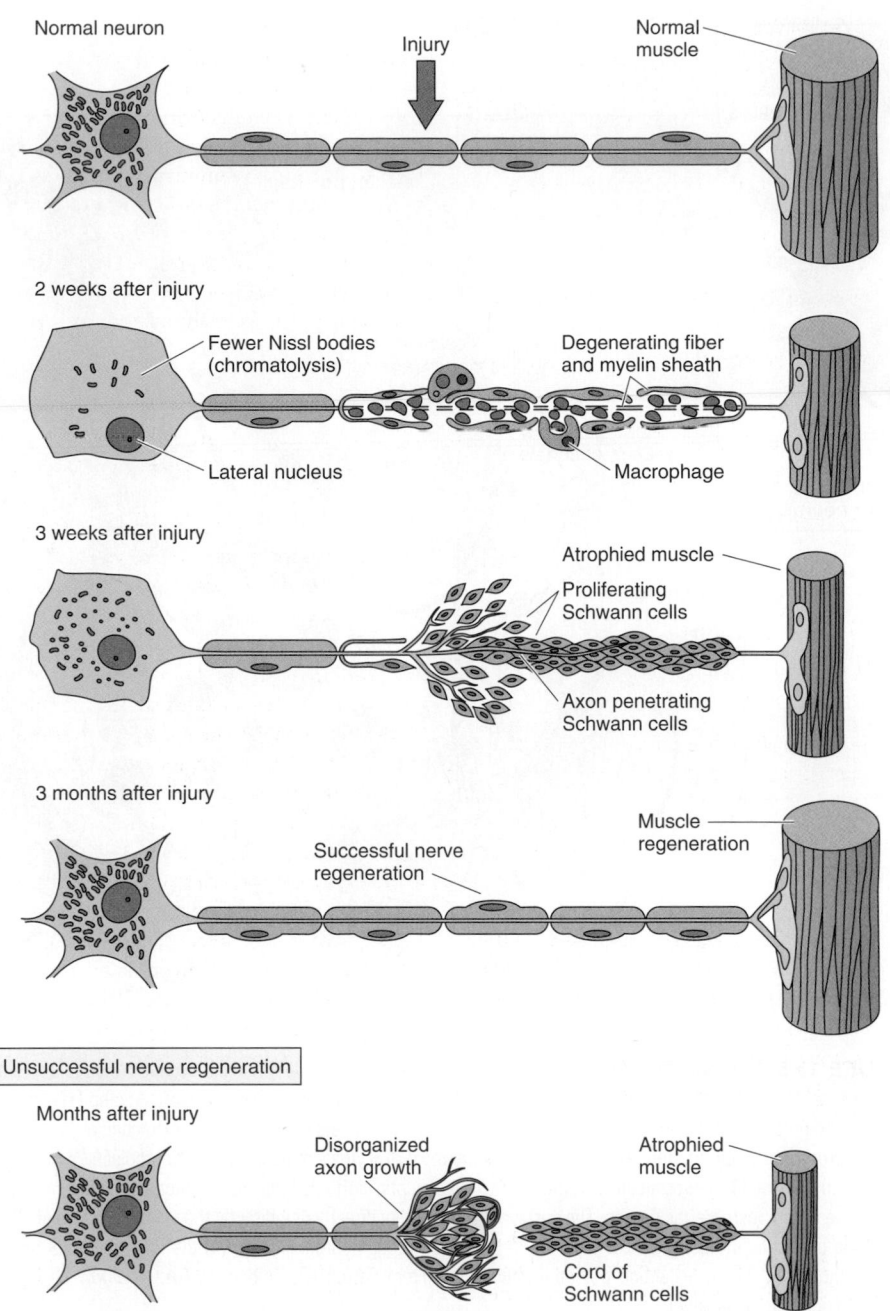

FIGURE 15.4 Peripheral Nerve Regeneration Following Injury. Schwann cells detach from the axons, proliferate, and, with recruited macrophages, help to clear cellular and myelin debris. At the same time, expression of growth factors by Schwann cells creates a favorable environment for nerve regrowth toward the target organ. A damaged motor axon can regrow to its distal connection only if the neurilemma remains intact (to form a guiding tunnel) and if scar tissue does not block its pathway. (From Gartner LP: *Textbook of histology*, ed 4, Philadelphia, 2017, Elsevier.)

another dendrite through the use of neurotransmitters—demonstrate that the interactions between neurons are far more complicated than postulated by simple on-off models of brain function.

CENTRAL NERVOUS SYSTEM

The **central nervous system (CNS)** is composed of the brain and the spinal cord. The neuron is the basic structure of the CNS.

Brain

The **brain** is a functionally integrated circuit of millions of neurons with different structures, molecular composition, networks, and connections. It weighs only 3 pounds but receives 15% to 20% of the total cardiac output. The brain enables a person to reason, function intellectually, express personality and mood, and perceive and interact with the environment.

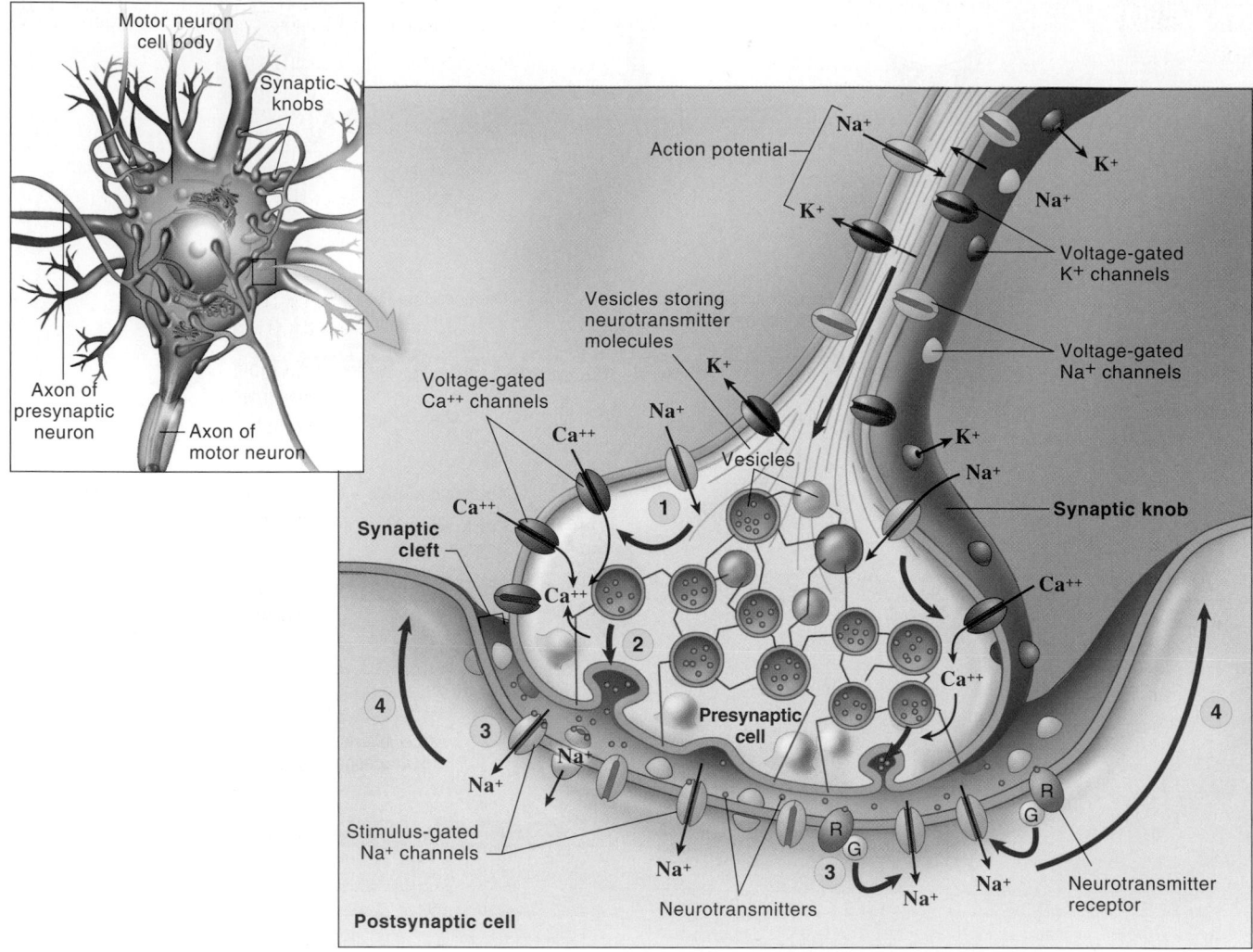

FIGURE 15.5 **Neuronal Transmission and Synaptic Cleft.** Details illustrate the synaptic knob (axon terminal) of a presynaptic neuron, the plasma membrane of a postsynaptic neuron, and a synaptic cleft. At step **(1)**—the arrival of an action potential at the synaptic knob—voltage-gated Ca^{++} channels open and allow extracellular Ca^{++} to diffuse into the presynaptic cell. At step **(2)** the Ca^{++} triggers the rapid exocytosis of neurotransmitter molecules from vesicles in the knob. At step **(3)** neurotransmitter diffuses into the synaptic cleft and binds to receptor molecules in the plasma membrane of the postsynaptic neuron. The postsynaptic receptors directly or indirectly trigger the opening of stimulus-gated ion channels, initiating a local potential in the postsynaptic neuron. At step **(4)** the local potential may move toward the axon, where an action potential may begin. (From Patton KT, Thibodeau GA: *Anatomy & physiology,* ed 8, St Louis, 2013, Mosby.)

The three major structural divisions of the brain are (1) the forebrain (prosencephalon), which includes the telencephalon and diencephalon; (2) the midbrain (mesencephalon), which connects the pons to the diencephalon and includes the corpora quadrigemina, tegmentum, and cerebral peduncles; and (3) the hindbrain (rhombencephalon), which includes the cerebellum, pons, and medulla (Table 15.3 and Fig. 15.6). The midbrain, medulla, and pons comprise the **brainstem**, which connects the hemispheres of the brain, cerebellum, and spinal cord. A collection of nuclei within the brainstem collectively constitute the **reticular formation**. The reticular formation is a large network of diffuse nuclei that connect the brainstem to the cortex and control vital reflexes, such as cardiovascular function and respiration. It is essential for maintaining wakefulness and attention and, therefore, is referred to as the **reticular activating system** (Fig. 15.7).

Divisions of the brain are associated with specific functions, but it is important to recognize that most brain functions require integration of multiple different inputs from different parts of the brain. However, for clinical considerations, functional specificity is useful for localizing pathologic conditions in various nervous system regions. Korbinian Brodmann, a German neuroanatomist, was among the first to define structural and functional aspects of brain anatomy. Brodmann's areas are still used to correlate functional activities to many regions of the cerebral cortex.[5] Fig. 15.8, *C,* illustrates these regions and describes some of the areas. The mapping of **brain networks** (interconnected areas of the brain) using functional MRI (fMRI) and other advanced imaging techniques is helping to discover new insights into the function of these complex and interconnected pathways[6,7] (Box 15.2).

TABLE 15.2   SUBSTANCES THAT ARE NEUROTRANSMITTERS OR NEUROMODULATORS

SUBSTANCE	LOCATION	EFFECT	CLINICAL EXAMPLE
Acetylcholine	Many parts of the brain, spinal cord, neuromuscular junction of skeletal muscle, and many ANS synapses	Excitatory or inhibitory	Alzheimer disease (a type of dementia) is associated with a decrease in the number of acetylcholine-secreting neurons. Muscle weakness caused by myasthenia gravis results from an autoimmune response to acetylcholine receptors on the postsynaptic terminal.
Monoamines			
Norepinephrine	Many areas of the brain and spinal cord; also in some ANS synapses	Excitatory or inhibitory	CNS: Sleep-wake cycles and mood. Cocaine and amphetamines* result in overstimulation of postsynaptic neurons. PNS: Sympathetic nerve transmission.
Serotonin	Many areas of the brain and spinal cord	Generally inhibitory	Is involved with mood, anxiety, and sleep induction. Levels of serotonin are elevated in schizophrenia (delusions, hallucinations, withdrawal).
Dopamine	Some areas of the brain and ANS synapses	Generally excitatory	Parkinson disease (depression of voluntary motor control) results from destruction of dopamine-secreting neurons. Drugs used to increase dopamine can induce vomiting and hallucinations.
Histamine	Posterior hypothalamus	Excitatory (H1 and H2 receptors) and inhibitory (H3 receptors)	There is no clear indication of histamine-associated pathologic conditions. Histamine is involved with arousal and attention and links to other brain transmitter systems.
Amino Acids			
Gamma-aminobutyric acid (GABA)	Most neurons of the CNS have GABA receptors	Majority of postsynaptic inhibition in the brain	Drugs that increase GABA function have been used to treat epilepsy by inhibiting excessive discharge of neurons.
Glycine	Spinal cord	Most postsynaptic inhibition in the spinal cord	Glycine receptors are inhibited by strychnine.
Glutamate and aspartate	Widespread in brain and spinal cord	Excitatory	Drugs that block glutamate or aspartate, such as riluzole, are used to treat amyotrophic lateral sclerosis. These drugs might prevent overexcitation from seizures and neural degeneration.
Neuropeptides			
Endorphins and enkephalins	Widely distributed in the CNS and PNS	Generally inhibitory	Morphine and heroin bind to endorphin and enkephalin receptors on presynaptic neurons and reduce pain by blocking the release of neurotransmitter.
Substance P	Spinal cord, brain, and sensory neurons associated with pain, GI tract	Generally excitatory	Substance P is a neurotransmitter involved in pain transmission pathways. Blocking release of substance P by morphine reduces pain.
Vasoactive intestinal peptide	Gastrointestinal tract	Generally excitatory	Stimulates secretion, vasodilation, and smooth muscle relaxation (vasodilation, sphincter relaxation).

*Increase the release and block the reuptake of norepinephrine.
ANS, Autonomic nervous system; *CNS,* central nervous system; *GI,* gastrointestinal; *PNS,* peripheral nervous system.
From Mtui E, Gruener G, Dockery P: *Fitzgerald's clinical neuroanatomy and neuroscience,* ed 7, Philadelphia, 2016, Elsevier.

Forebrain

Telencephalon. The telencephalon (cerebral hemispheres) consists of the cerebral cortex (the largest portion of the brain) and the basal ganglia (composed of several *nuclei*). The surface of the cerebral cortex is covered with convolutions called *gyri* (see Fig. 15.8, *A*) that greatly increase the cortical surface area and the number of neurons. Grooves between adjacent gyri are termed sulci; deeper grooves are fissures. The cerebral cortex contains an outer layer of cell bodies of neurons (gray matter). Gray matter is organized into columns perpendicular to the surface that receive, integrate, store, and transmit information. White matter lies beneath the cerebral cortex and is composed of myelinated nerve fibers (axons).

The two cerebral hemispheres are separated by a deep groove known as the longitudinal fissure. The surface of each hemisphere is divided into lobes named after the region of the skull under which each lobe lies. The posterior margin of the frontal lobe is the central sulcus (fissure of Rolando) and it borders inferiorly on the lateral sulcus (sylvian fissure, lateral fissure) (see Fig. 15.8, *A*). The prefrontal area is responsible for goal-oriented behavior (i.e., ability to concentrate), short-term or recall memory, and the elaboration of thought and inhibition on the limbic (emotional) areas of the CNS. The premotor area (Brodmann area 6) (see Fig. 15.8, *C*) is involved in programming motor movements. This area also contains the cell bodies that form part of the basal ganglia system (extrapyramidal system,

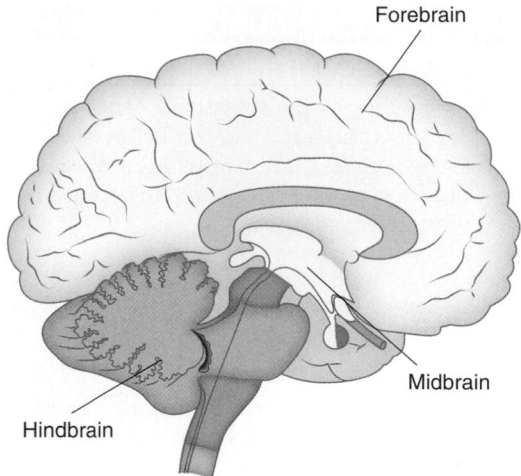

FIGURE 15.6 Structural Divisions of the Brain. (From Standring S: *Gray's anatomy: the anatomical basis of clinical practice,* ed 40, Philadelphia, 2008, Elsevier.)

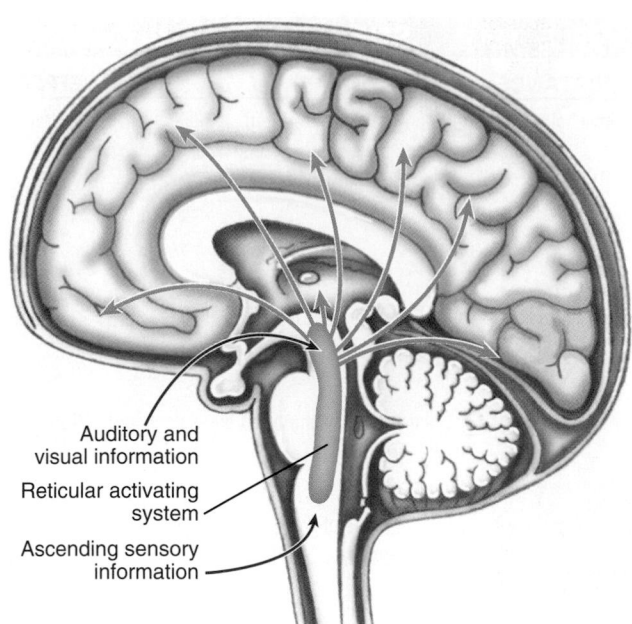

FIGURE 15.7 Reticular Activating System. The reticular activating system consists of nuclei in the brainstem reticular formation plus fibers (axons) that conduct to the nuclei from below and fibers that conduct from the nuclei to widespread areas of the cerebral cortex. Functioning of the reticular activating system is essential for maintaining consciousness.

TABLE 15.3	DIVISIONS OF THE CENTRAL NERVOUS SYSTEM	
PRIMARY VESICLES	**SECONDARY VESICLES**	**ASSOCIATED STRUCTURES**
Forebrain (prosencephalon)	Telencephalon	Cerebral hemispheres
		Cerebral cortex
		Rhinencephalon (olfaction)
		Basal ganglia
	Diencephalon	Epithalamus
		Thalamus
		Hypothalamus
		Subthalamus
Midbrain (mesencephalon)	Mesencephalon	Tectum (corpora quadrigemina)
		Tegmentum
		Red nucleus
		Substantia nigra
		Cerebral peduncles
Hindbrain (rhombencephalon)	Metencephalon	Cerebellum
		Pons
	Myelencephalon	Medulla oblongata
Spinal cord	Spinal cord	Spinal cord

efferent pathways outside the pyramids of the medulla oblongata). The frontal eye fields (the lower portion of Brodmann area 8), which are involved in controlling eye movements, are located in the middle frontal gyrus.

The **primary motor area (Brodmann area 4)** is located along the **precentral gyrus** forming the **primary voluntary motor area**, which has a somatotopic organization that often is referred to as a *homunculus* (little man) (Fig. 15.9). Electrical stimulation of specific areas of this cortex causes specific muscles of the body to move. For example, stimulation of Brodmann area 4 in the medial longitudinal fissure affects the lower limb and foot, whereas stimulation of the superior lateral

surface of the precentral gyrus affects the torso and arm, the middle third of the hand, and the lower third of the face and mouth/throat. The axons traveling from the cell bodies in and on either side of this gyrus project fibers (axons) that form the **pyramidal system**. This system includes the **corticobulbar tract** that synapses in the brainstem and provides voluntary control of muscles in the head and neck, and the **corticospinal (pyramidal) tracts** that descend into the spinal cord and provide voluntary control of muscles throughout the body. Cerebral impulses control function on the opposite side of the body, a phenomenon called *contralateral control* (Fig. 15.10, *A*). **Broca area** in the inferior frontal lobe (Brodmann areas 44, 45) is an important center for speech and language processing. This area, rostral to the inferior edge of the premotor area (Brodmann area 6) on the inferior frontal gyrus, is usually most important in the left hemisphere. Injury to this area results in difficulty forming or inability to form words (expressive aphasia or dysphasia) (see Chapter 17).

The **parietal lobe** lies within the borders of the central, parietooccipital, and lateral sulci. This lobe contains the major area for somatic sensory input, located along the **postcentral gyrus** (Brodmann areas 3, 1, 2) (see Fig. 15.8), which is adjacent to the primary motor area in the **precentral gyrus**. Communication between the motor and sensory areas (and among other regions in the cortex) is provided by **association fibers**. Much of this region is involved in sensory association (storage, analysis, and interpretation of stimuli). Fig. 15.9 shows the distribution of functions associated with both the primary motor area and the primary sensory area of the cerebral cortex (note the somatotopic organization of both primary motor and primary sensory areas).

The **occipital lobe** lies caudal to the parietooccipital sulci and superior to the cerebellum. The primary visual cortex (Brodmann area 17) is located in this region and receives input from the retinas. Much of the remainder of this lobe is involved in visual association (Brodmann areas 18, 19). The **temporal lobe** lies inferior to the lateral fissure and

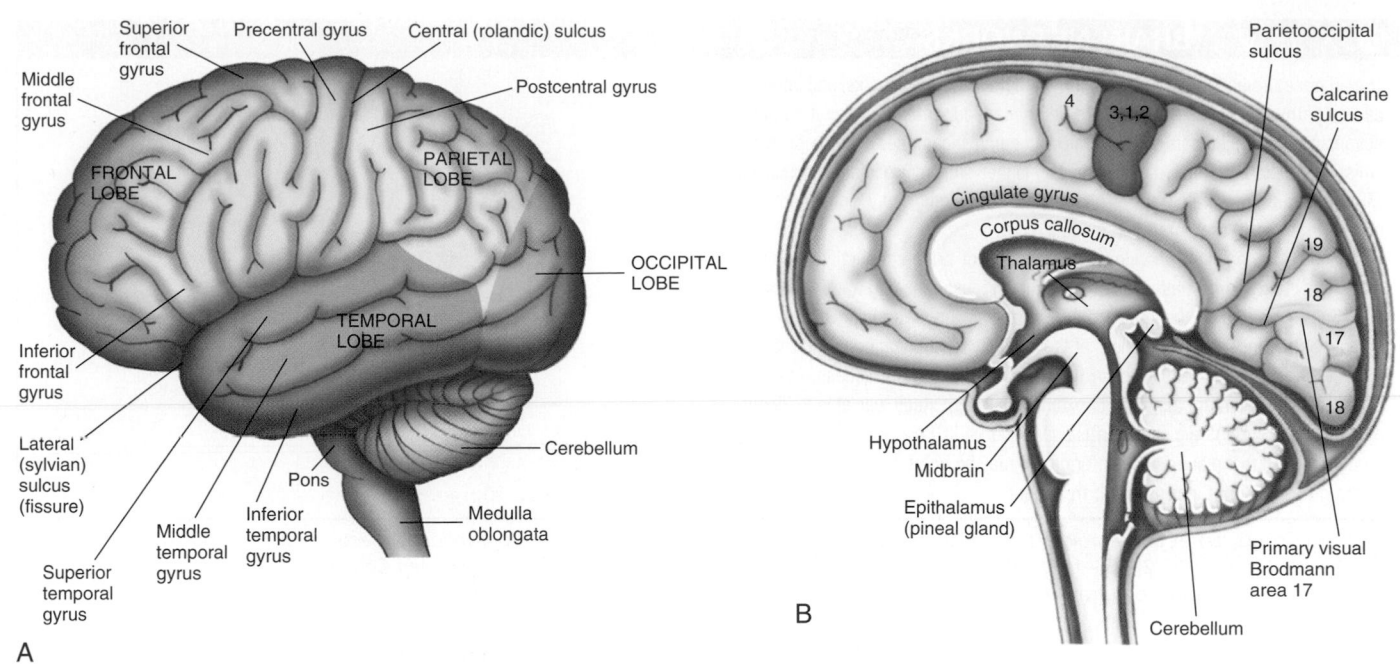

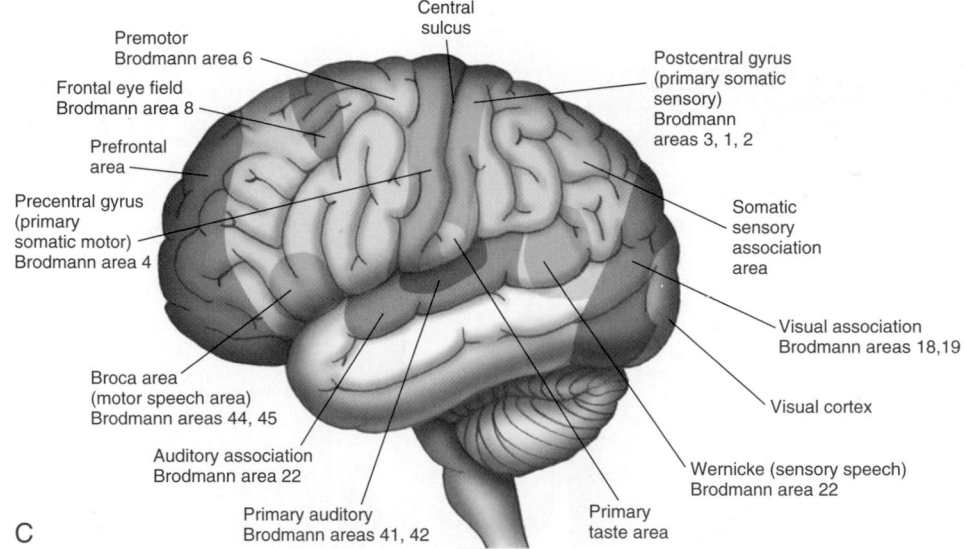

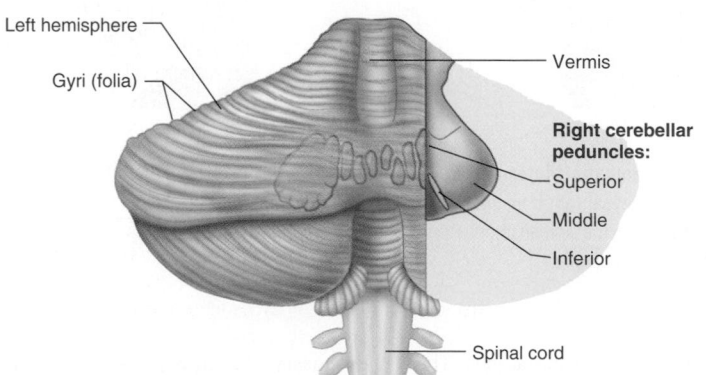

FIGURE 15.8 Cerebral Hemispheres. A, Left hemisphere of cerebrum *(lateral view).* **B,** Functional areas of the cerebral cortex *(midsagittal view).* **C,** Functional areas of the cerebral cortex *(lateral view).* **D,** Cerebellum *(posterior view);* coordination of voluntary movement, balance, and posture. (From Patton KT, Thibodeau GA: *Anthony's textbook of anatomy and physiology,* ed 20, St Louis, 2013, Mosby.)

BOX 15.2   BRAIN NETWORKS

The architecture and integrated function of neural nodes, networks, and interconnected pathways within the brain are being mapped with high resolution in the advancing field of human connectomics. Imaging techniques include positron-emission tomography, trace diffusion tensor magnetic resonance imaging, functional MRI, magnetoencephalography, and electroencephalography combined with mathematical and computational models.

The figure at the right provides an illustration of brain connectivity showing interconnecting cortical pathways using diffusion tensor imaging tracking technology. Such mapping of the brain contributes to an understanding of the commonalities and individual differences of the normally functioning brain and changes associated with aging and disease (i.e., degenerative brain disease, epilepsy, schizophrenia, and brain tumors). For example, a recent study was able to identify dysfunctional cholinergic and perfusion networks in Parkinson disease using functional MRI techniques. Such information may be helpful in identifying areas of brain function that improve with treatment.

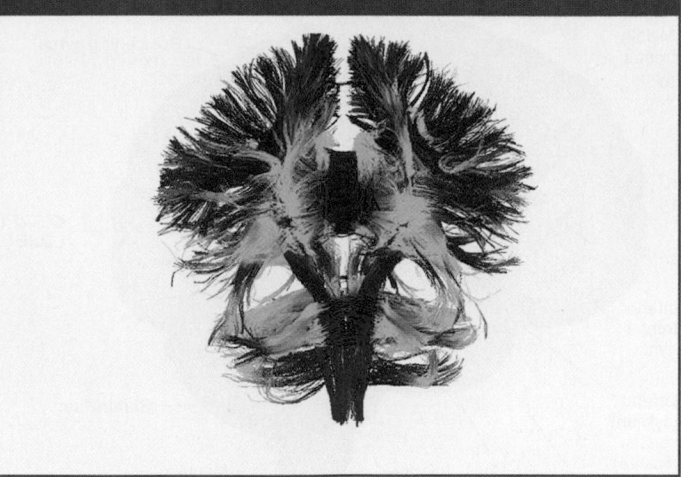

Data from Colloby SJ et al: *Neurology* 87(2):178–185, 2016; Fornito A, Bullmore ET: *Eur Neuropsychopharmacol* 25(5):733–748, 2015; Pollock JD et al: *Trends Neurosci* 37(2):106–123, 2014; Sporns O: *Neuroimage* 80:53–61, 2013; also see the *Human Connectome Project* at http://humanconnectomeproject.org. Image from Filippi M et al: *Lancet Neurol* 12[12]:1189–1199, 2013.

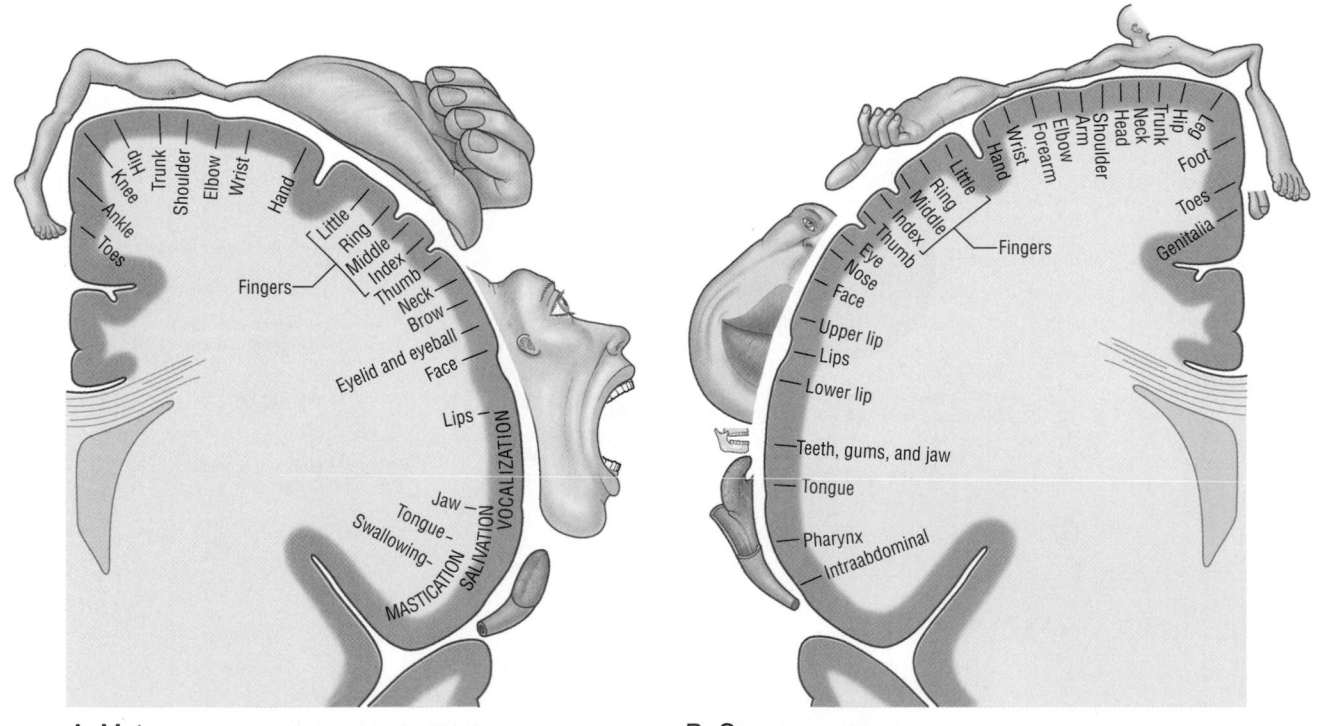

A Motor   B Sensory

FIGURE 15.9 Primary Somatic Motor and Sensory Areas of the Cortex. **A,** The motor homunculus shows proportional somatotopic representation in the main motor area. **B,** The sensory homunculus shows proportional somatotopic representation in the somaesthetic cortex. (From Standring S et al, editors: *Gray's anatomy,* ed 40, Edinburgh, 2008, Churchill Livingstone.)

is composed of the superior, middle, and inferior temporal gyri. The primary auditory cortex (Brodmann area 41) and its related association area (Brodmann area 42) lie deep within the lateral sulcus on the superior temporal gyrus. **Wernicke area** (posterior portion of Brodmann area 22), along with adjacent portions of the parietal lobe, constitutes a *sensory speech area*. This area is responsible for reception and interpretation of speech, and dysfunction may result in receptive aphasia or

dysphasia. The temporal lobe also is involved in memory consolidation and smell.

The **insula (insular lobe)** lies hidden in the lateral sulci between the temporal and frontal lobes of each hemisphere. The insula processes sensory and emotional information and routes the information to other areas of the brain. Lying directly beneath the longitudinal fissure, the **corpus callosum (transverse commissural fibers)** is a bundle of

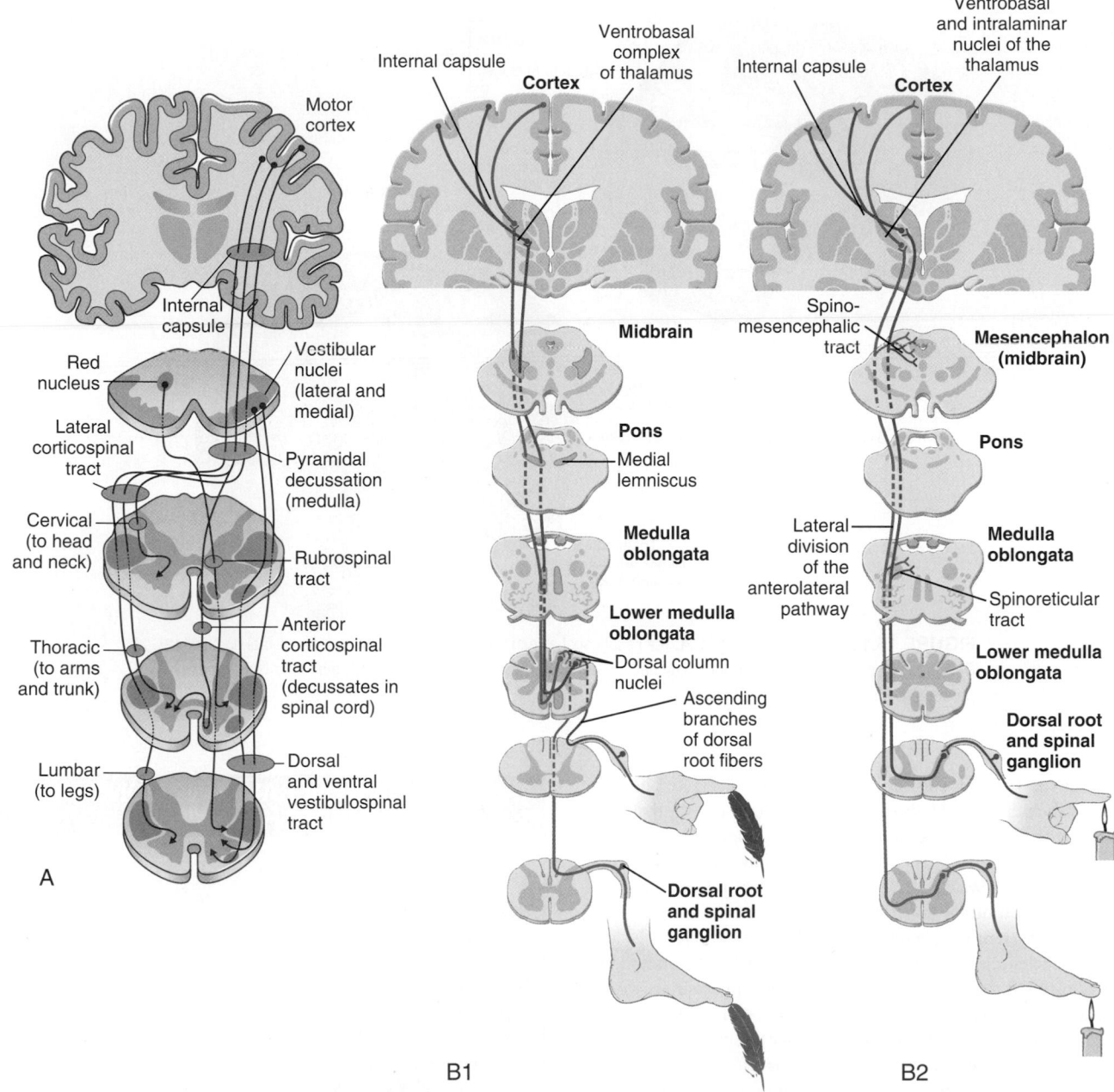

FIGURE 15.10 Examples of Somatic Motor and Sensory Pathways. **A,** Motor pathways. The pyramidal pathway through the lateral corticospinal tract and the extrapyramidal pathways through the rubrospinal, reticulospinal, and vestibulospinal tracts. **B,** Sensory pathways. **B1,** The dorsal column-medial lemniscal pathway for transmitting critical types of tactile signals: touch/proprioception. Note the later corticospinal tract decussation is in the lower medulla. The corticobulbar tract is not shown. **B2,** Anterior and lateral divisions of the anterolateral sensory pathway: pain/temperature. Note the decussation is in the spinal cord. (**A** from Compston A et al: *McAlpines's multiple sclerosis,* ed 4, London, 2006, Churchill Livingstone; **B** from Hall JE: *Guyton and Hall textbook of medical physiology,* ed 13, Philadelphia, 2016, Saunders.)

myelinated fibers that connects the two cerebral hemispheres. The corpus callosum conveys contralateral projection of axons and is essential in coordinating activities between hemispheres (see Fig. 15.8, *B*).

Deep inside the cerebrum are numerous white matter tracts and gray matter nuclei and the major **cerebral nuclei** of the basal ganglia (basal nuclei) system. The **basal ganglia system** is a group of nuclei that includes the caudate nucleus, putamen, and globus pallidus. The putamen and globus pallidus together are called the *lentiform nuclei.*

The caudate nucleus and putamen together are called the *striatum*[5] (Fig. 15.11). Other structures in the basal ganglia include the substantia nigra, the nucleus accumbens (not shown), and the subthalamic nucleus (not shown). The nuclei of the basal ganglia are important for coordination of voluntary movement and cognitive and emotional functions.

The **internal capsule** is a white matter tract in which afferent (sensory) and efferent (motor) pathways are conveyed to and from the cerebral cortex by passing through the center of the cerebral hemispheres and

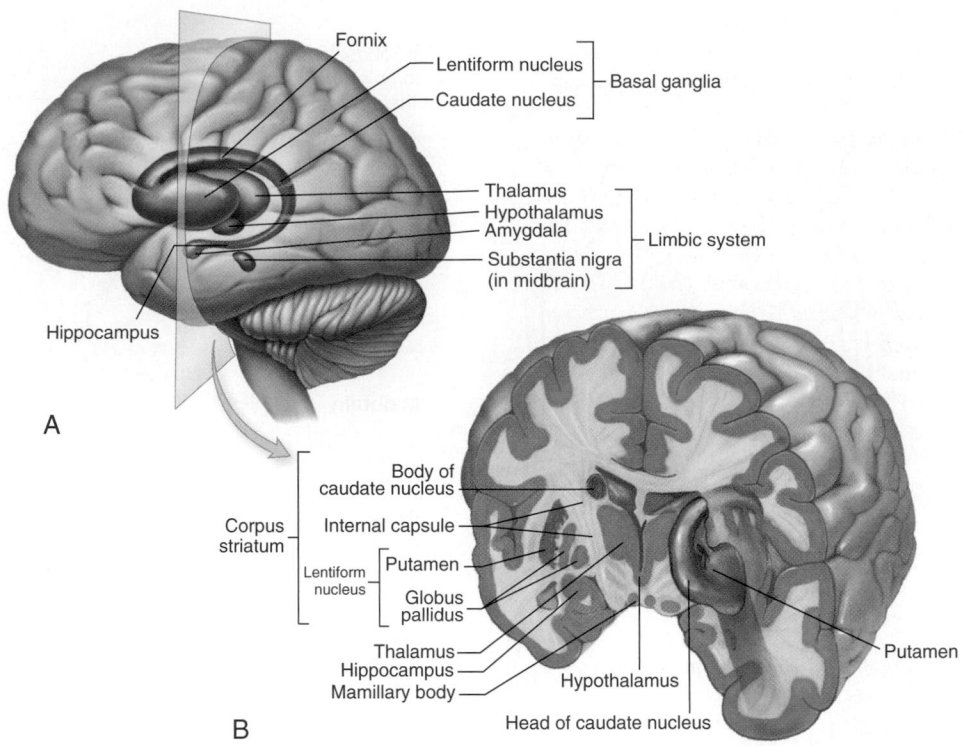

Fornix
Lentiform nucleus ⎤
Caudate nucleus ⎦ Basal ganglia

Thalamus
Hypothalamus
Amygdala ⎤ Limbic system
Substantia nigra ⎦
(in midbrain)

Hippocampus

A

Body of
caudate nucleus
Corpus striatum
Internal capsule
Lentiform nucleus ⎰ Putamen
Globus pallidus
Thalamus
Hippocampus
Mamillary body
Hypothalamus
Head of caudate nucleus
Putamen

B

FIGURE 15.11 The Basal Ganglia. **A,** The basal ganglia seen through the cortex of the left cerebral hemisphere. **B,** The basal ganglia seen in a frontal (coronal) section of the brain. (From Patton KT, Thibodeau GA: *Anatomy & physiology*, ed 9, St Louis, 2016, Mosby.)

between the caudate and lentiform nuclei (see Fig. 15.11, *B*). The basal ganglia and their direct and indirect interconnections with the thalamus, premotor cortex, red nucleus, reticular formation, and spinal cord are part of the extrapyramidal system. The extrapyramidal system is a part of the motor control system that causes involuntary reflexes and has a stabilizing effect on motor control.

The limbic system is a group of interconnected structures located between the telencephalon and diencephalon and surrounding the corpus callosum. It is composed of the amygdala, hippocampus, fornix, hypothalamus, and related autonomic nuclei (see Fig. 15.11). The limbic system mediates emotion and long-term memory through connections in the prefrontal cortex (limbic cortex). Its principal effects are involved in primitive behavioral responses, visceral reaction to emotion, motivation, mood, feeding behaviors, biologic rhythms, and the sense of smell.

Diencephalon. The diencephalon (interbrain), surrounded by the cerebrum and sitting on top of the brainstem, has four divisions: epithalamus, thalamus, hypothalamus, and subthalamus (see Table 15.3 and Fig. 15.8, *B*). The epithalamus forms the roof of the third ventricle and composes the most superior portion of the diencephalon. The diencephalon controls vital functions and visceral activities and is closely associated with those of the limbic system.

The largest component of the diencephalon is the thalamus. It borders and surrounds the third ventricle and is a major integrating center for afferent (sensory) impulses to the cerebral cortex. Various sensations are perceived at this level, but cortical processing is required for interpretation. The thalamus also serves as a relay center for information from the basal ganglia and cerebellum to the appropriate motor area.

The hypothalamus forms the ventral part of the diencephalon and functions to maintain a constant internal environment and implement behavioral patterns. Integrative centers control autonomic nervous system (ANS) function, regulate body temperature and endocrine

BOX 15.3	**GENERAL FUNCTIONS OF THE HYPOTHALAMUS**

Visceral and somatic responses
Affectual responses
Hormone synthesis
Sympathetic and parasympathetic activity
Temperature regulation
Feeding responses
Physical expression of emotions
Sexual behavior
Pleasure-punishment centers
Level of arousal or wakefulness

function, and adjust emotional expression. (Temperature regulation is discussed in Chapter 16.) The hypothalamus exerts its influence through the endocrine system, as well as neural pathways (Box 15.3). The subthalamus flanks the hypothalamus laterally and serves as an important basal ganglia center for motor activities.

Midbrain (Mesencephalon)

The midbrain (mesencephalon) (see Table 15.3) connects the forebrain with the hindbrain and is composed of the tectum (corpora quadrigemina [forms roof of midbrain]), the tegmentum, and the cerebral peduncles. The tectum includes the two pairs of superior colliculi and two pairs of inferior colliculi. The superior colliculi are involved with voluntary and involuntary visual motor movements (e.g., the ability of the eyes to *track* moving objects in the visual field). The inferior colliculi accomplish similar motor activities but involve movements affecting the auditory system (e.g., positioning the head to improve hearing). The inferior colliculus also is a major relay center along the auditory pathway. The **tegmentum** (floor of the midbrain) is composed of the red nucleus and substantia nigra. The **red nucleus** receives ascending sensory information from the cerebellum and projects a minor motor pathway, the rubrospinal tract, to the cervical spinal cord. The **substantia nigra** synthesizes **dopamine.** Dysfunction of dopaminergic neurons in the substantia nigra is associated with Parkinson disease and schizophrenia. The **cerebral peduncles** of the anterior midbrain are made up of efferent fibers of the corticospinal, corticobulbar, and corticopontocerebellar tracts (tracts that link the cortex to the brainstem).

Other notable structures of this region are the nuclei of the third and fourth cranial nerves. The **cerebral aqueduct (aqueduct of Sylvius),** which carries cerebrospinal fluid (CSF) between the third and fourth ventricles, also traverses this structure. Obstruction of this aqueduct is a common cause of hydrocephalus.

Hindbrain

Metencephalon. The major structures of the **metencephalon** are the cerebellum and the pons. The **cerebellum** (see Fig. 15.8, *A* and *B*) is composed of two lobes of gray and white matter, and its cortical surface is convoluted like the surface of the cerebrum. The lobes are divided by a central fissure and connected by a midline structure, the vermis.

The cerebellum is responsible for reflexive, involuntary fine-tuning of motor control and for maintaining balance and posture through extensive neural connections with the medulla (through the inferior cerebellar peduncle) and with the midbrain (through the superior cerebellar peduncle). The two hemispheres are connected to the pons by the middle cerebellar peduncles. These connections allow extensive sampling of visual, vestibular, and proprioceptive data from other regions of the CNS and periphery. The cerebellum has ipsilateral (same side) control of the body, in contrast to the cerebral cortex, which has contralateral (opposite side) control of the body.

The **pons** (bridge) is easily recognized by its bulging appearance below the midbrain and above the medulla. Primarily it transmits information from the cerebellum to the brainstem between the two cerebellar hemispheres. The nuclei of the fifth through eighth cranial nerves are located in the pons.

Myelencephalon. The **myelencephalon (medulla oblongata)** forms the lowest portion of the brainstem. Reflex activities, such as heart rate, respiration, blood pressure, coughing, sneezing, swallowing, and vomiting, are controlled in this area. The nuclei of cranial nerves IX through XII are located in this region (see Table 15.6 for details).

A major portion of the descending motor pathways (i.e., corticospinal tracts) cross to the other side, or decussates at the inferior medulla (see Fig. 15.10, *A*). These pathways, together with other areas of decussation in the CNS, are the basis for the phenomenon of contralateral control. Sleep-wake rhythms also are processed by neural influences from lower brain centers and are associated with a complex group of diffuse structures and functions including the reticular activating system (see Fig. 15.7).

Spinal Cord

The **spinal cord** lies within the vertebral canal and is surrounded and protected by the vertebral column. One of the primary functions of the spinal cord is to transmit long motor and sensory tracts that originate in the brain and synapse with cell bodies in gray matter of the spinal cord before exiting to the body. Additional significant functions include somatic and autonomic reflexes, motor pattern control centers, and sensory and motor modulation. The spinal cord originates in the medulla oblongata (Fig. 15.12) and ends at the **conus medullaris,** a cone shaped

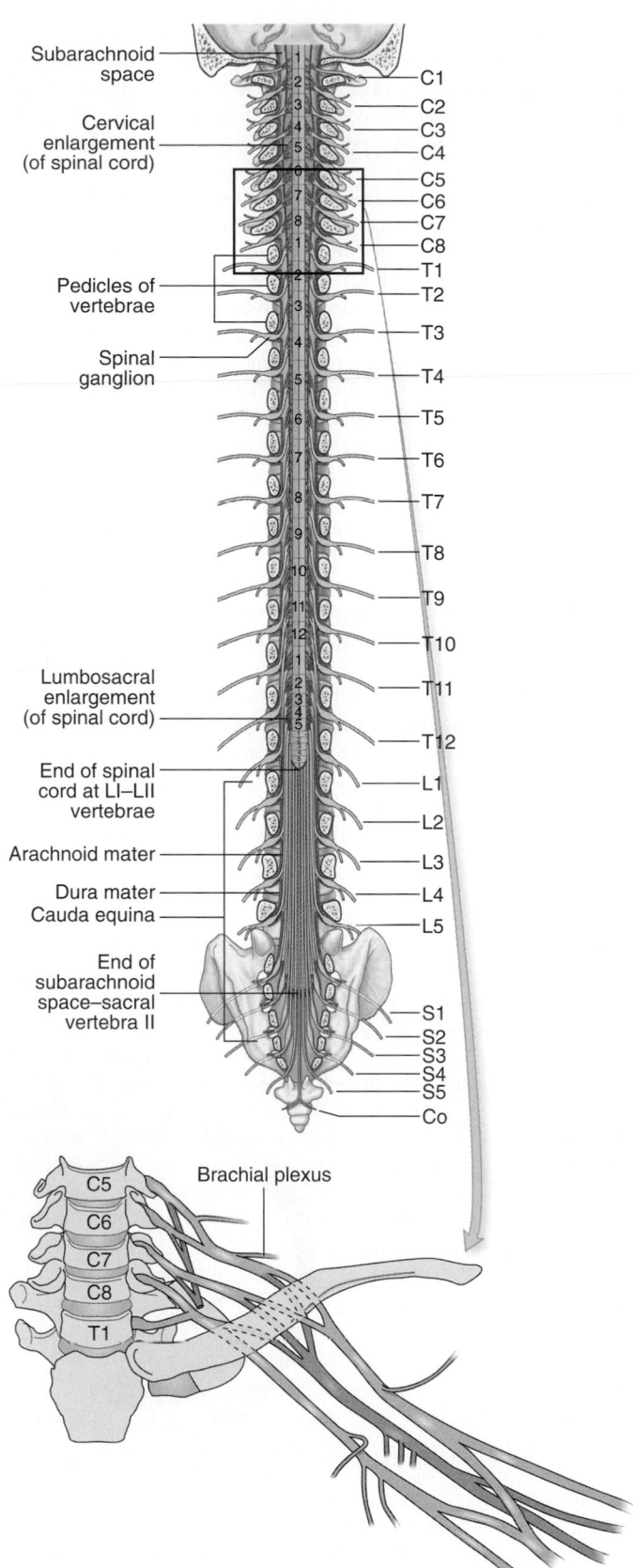

FIGURE 15.12 Vertebral Canal, Spinal Cord, and Spinal Nerves. Enlarged segment of the brachial plexus is shown. (From Drake R, et al: *Gray's anatomy for students,* ed 3, London, 2015, Churchill Livingstone. *Inset,* from Chung KC, et al: *Practical management of pediatric and adult brachial plexus palsies,* London, 2012, Saunders.)

structure at the level of the first or second lumbar vertebra in adults (Fig. 15.13). Spinal nerves extend from the conus medullaris and form a nerve bundle called the cauda equina. A thin filament, the filum terminale, extends from the conus medullaris and anchors it to the coccyx. The coverings of the spinal cord mirror those of the brain and are illustrated in Fig. 15.13.

Grossly, the spinal cord is divided into sections (8 cervical, 12 thoracic, 5 lumbar, 5 sacral, and 1 coccygeal) that correspond to paired nerves (see Fig. 15.12). A cross section of the spinal cord (see Figs. 15.13 and 15.14) is characterized by a butterfly-shaped inner core of gray matter (containing nerve cell bodies) surrounded by white matter tracts. The central canal extends through the spinal cord from its origin in the fourth ventricle. The gray matter of the spinal cord is divided into three regions and displays specific functional characteristics. These regions include the posterior horn (dorsal horn), composed primarily of interneurons and axons from sensory neurons whose cell bodies lie in the dorsal root ganglion. At the tip of the posterior horn is the substantia gelatinosa, a structure involved in pain transmission (see Chapter 16). The lateral horn contains cell bodies involved with the ANS. The anterior horn (ventral horn) contains the nerve cell bodies for efferent (motor) pathways that leave the spinal cord by way of spinal nerves. The terms *anterior* and *posterior* are preferred by many authors for describing human spinal cord anatomy, whereas *dorsal* and *ventral* are the common zoologic (veterinary) terms.

Surrounding the gray matter is white matter that forms ascending and descending pathways called spinal tracts and short ascending and descending integrative pathways. Spinal tracts are named to denote their beginning and ending points. For example, the spinothalamic tract carries nerve impulses from the spinal cord to the thalamus in the diencephalon. Numerous spinal tracts are grouped into columns

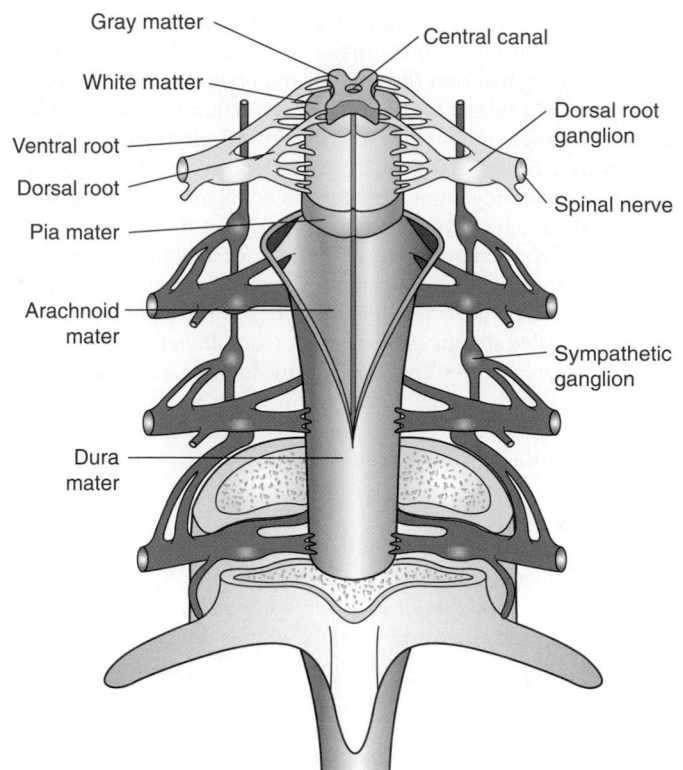

FIGURE 15.13 Coverings of the Spinal Cord. The dura mater is shown in purple. Note how it extends to cover the spinal nerve roots and nerves. The arachnoid mater is highlighted in pink and the pia mater in orange. (From Patton KT, Thibodeau GA: *Structure and function of the body,* ed 15, St Louis, 2016, Mosby.)

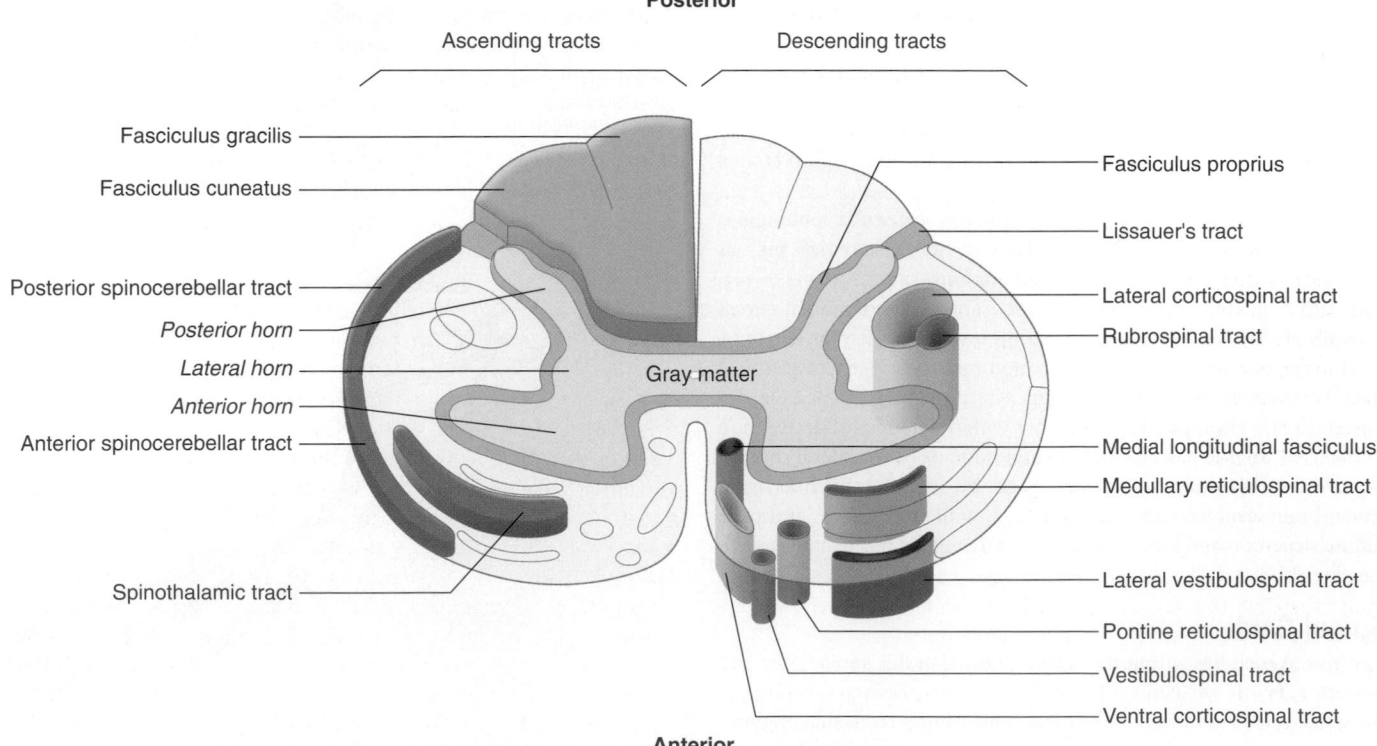

FIGURE 15.14 Ascending and Descending Tracts of the Spinal Cord. Ascending (*sensory*) tracts are emphasized on the left side and descending (*motor*) tracts are emphasized on the right side. The locations of Lissauer's tract and the fasciculus proprius (which contain both ascending and descending fibers) are also shown. (From Crossman AR, Neary D: *Neuroanatomy: an illustrated colour text,* ed 4, London, 2015, Churchill Livingstone.)

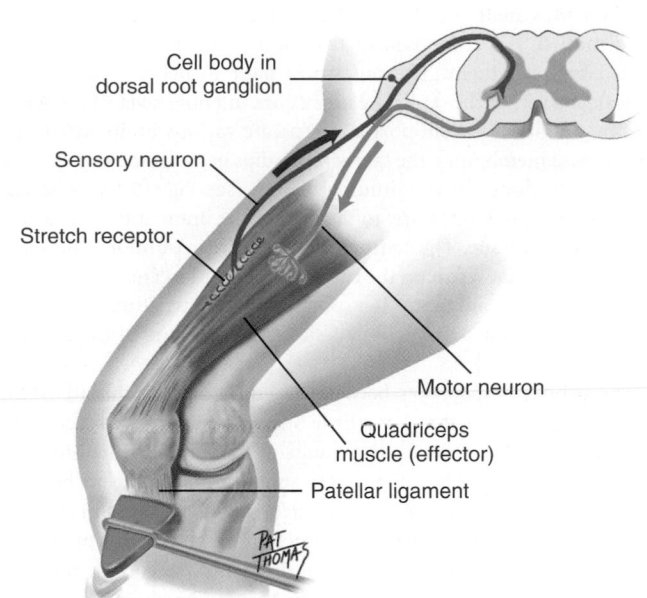

FIGURE 15.15 Cross Section of Spinal Cord Showing Simple Reflex Arc. (From Jarvis C: *Physical examination & health assessment*, ed 7, St Louis, 2016, Mosby.)

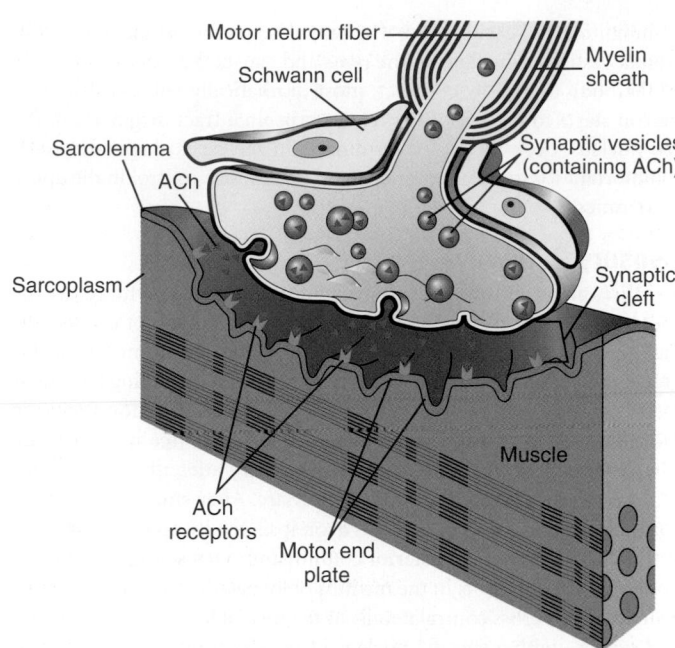

FIGURE 15.16 Normal Neuromuscular Junction. This figure shows how the distal end of a motor neuron fiber forms a synapse with an adjacent muscle fiber. Acetylcholine *(ACh)* is released from the neuron's synaptic vesicles and diffuses across the synaptic cleft, where it stimulates receptors in the motor end-plate region of the sarcolemma. (From Damjanov I: *Pathology for the health professions*, ed 4, St Louis, 2012, Saunders.)

according to their location within the white matter. These include the **anterior column**, **lateral column**, and **posterior column** (the fasciculus gracilis and fasciculus cuneatus). Ascending tracts are found in all columns. Descending tracts are found only in the lateral and anterior columns. Fig. 15.14 identifies the location and principal activities of the major spinal tracts and the horns of the gray matter.

Neural circuits in the spinal cord, when activated, display specific sets of motor responses. **Reflex arcs** form basic units that respond to stimuli and provide protective circuitry for motor output. Structures mandatory for a reflex arc (monosynaptic reflex) are a receptor, an **afferent (sensory) neuron**, an **efferent (motor) neuron**, and an effector muscle or gland. A simple reflex arc (e.g., knee jerk reflex) contains only two neurons. In most cases, simple reflex arcs are modulated by interneurons that provide a link between sensory and motor neurons (Fig. 15.15 illustrates a reflex arc). The motor effects of reflex arcs generally occur before the event is perceived in the brain's higher centers. Much internal environmental regulation is mediated by reflex activity involving the ANS (e.g., cardiac muscle and smooth muscle contraction/relaxation and glandular responses).

Afferent pathways transmit information from peripheral receptors with eventual termination in the cerebral or cerebellar cortex, or both. Efferent pathways primarily relay information from the cerebrum to the brainstem or spinal cord (see Fig. 15.10, *A*). **Upper motor neurons** (i.e., corticospinal and corticobulbar tracts) are completely contained within the CNS (see Fig. 17.32). Their primary roles are controlling fine motor movement and influencing/modifying spinal reflex arcs and circuits. Generally, upper motor neurons form synapses with interneurons, which then form synapses with lower motor neurons that project into the periphery. **Lower motor neurons** directly influence muscles. Their cell bodies lie in the gray matter of the brainstem and anterior horn of the spinal cord, but their processes extend out of the CNS and into the PNS (see Fig. 15.10, *A* and Fig. 17.33). Destruction of upper motor neurons usually results in initial paralysis followed within days or weeks by partial recovery, whereas destruction of the lower motor neurons

often leads to permanent paralysis, unless peripheral nerve damage is followed by nerve regeneration and recovery.

Muscle activity (i.e., stimulation and contraction) is regulated by nerve impulses. Motor neurons innervate one or more muscle cells, forming a **motor unit** which consists of a single motor neuron and all of the skeletal muscle fibers it stimulates. The junction between the axon of the motor neuron and the plasma membrane of the muscle cell is called the **neuromuscular (myoneural) junction** (Fig. 15.16). Injury to motor neurons is discussed in Chapter 18.

Motor Pathways (Tracts)

Clinically relevant motor pathways are the corticospinal and corticobulbar (bulbar refers to brainstem) pyramidal tracts; and the extrapyramidal reticulospinal, vestibulospinal, and rubrospinal tracts. The corticospinal (see Fig. 15.10, *A*) and corticobulbar tracts (cortex to medulla) (see Fig. 17.31) consist of a two-neuron chain. The cell bodies (upper motor neurons) originate in and around the precentral gyrus; pass through the corona radiata of the cerebrum, the internal capsule, and the middle three-fifths of the basis pedunculi, pons, and pyramid; and decussate (cross contralaterally) in the medulla oblongata and form the lateral corticospinal tract of the spinal cord (see Fig. 15.14). The lateral corticospinal tract axons descend in the spinal cord and leave the white matter tract to synapse with specific interneurons or motor neurons in the anterior horn of the spinal cord. The lateral corticospinal tract has the same somatotopic organization as the body. The corticobulbar tract axons synapse on motor cranial nuclei within the brainstem that control muscles of the face, head, and neck. Lower motor neurons project from the anterior horn of the spinal cord through nerves to specific muscles.

The **extrapyramidal tracts** are involved in precise motor movements (see Fig. 15.14). The reticulospinal tract modulates motor movement by inhibiting and exciting spinal activity. The vestibulospinal tract arises from a vestibular nucleus in the pons and causes the extensor muscles of the body to rapidly contract, most dramatically witnessed when a person starts to fall backward. The rubrospinal tract originates in the red nucleus, decussates, and terminates in the cervical spinal cord. It is important for muscle movement and fine muscle control in the upper extremities.

Sensory Pathways

The three clinically important spinal afferent (sensory) pathways are the posterior column, anterior spinothalamic, and lateral spinothalamic (see Fig. 15.14; also see Figs. 16.2 and 16.3). The posterior column (fasciculus gracilis and fasciculus cuneatus) carries fine-touch (including two-point discrimination), vibration, and proprioceptive information (epicritic information). The posterior column is formed by a three-neuron chain. The first neurons of the chain are the primary afferent neuron. They are also the sensory neuron of the reflex arc. After entering the spinal cord, the primary neuron sends its axon ipsilaterally up the spinal cord in a specific part of the posterior column and synapses in one of three posterior column nuclei in the medulla oblongata. The axons of second-order neurons cross contralaterally at the medial lemniscus and ascend and synapse with a specific nucleus of the thalamus. The third-order neurons originate in the thalamus and continue the tract into the internal capsule, corona radiata, and postcentral gyrus (Brodmann areas 3, 1, 2) (see Fig. 15.8, C).

The anterior and lateral spinothalamic tracts are responsible for vague touch and for pain and temperature perception, respectively (see Fig. 15.10, B2). These modalities are referred to as protopathic. These tracts also form a three-neuron chain. However, their primary afferent neurons synapse in the posterior horn of the spinal cord, not just at the level they enter the intervertebral foramen but in a number of spinal segments above and below their point of entry. This is an example of divergence. The axons of the second-order neurons in the posterior horn cross to the contralateral side in the spinal cord in the lateral column, and ascend to the same thalamic nucleus as the posterior column pathway and continue on with the posterior column pathway to the postcentral gyrus.

Protective Structures
Cranium

The cranial vault functions to enclose and protect the brain and its associated structures. The bony cranium is composed of eight bones (frontal, two parietal, two temporal, ethmoid, sphenoid, and occipital). The galea aponeurotica is a thick, fibrous band of tissue overlying the cranium between the frontal and occipital muscles. This structure affords added protection to the bony structure of the skull. The subgaleal space has venous connections with the dural sinuses, and with increased intracranial pressure, blood can be shunted to this space, thus reducing pressure in the intracranial cavity. The subgaleal space is also a common site for placement of wound drains after intracranial surgery.

The floor of the cranial vault is irregular and contains many foramina (openings) that act as exit sites for cranial nerves, blood vessels, and the spinal cord. The cranial floor is divided into three fossae (depressions). The frontal lobes lie in the anterior fossa; the temporal lobes and base of the diencephalon lie in the middle fossa (temporal fossa); and the cerebellum lies in the posterior fossa. These terms are commonly used anatomic landmarks to describe the location of intracranial lesions.

Meninges

Surrounding the brain and spinal cord are three protective membranes: the dura mater, the arachnoid, and the pia mater. Collectively they are called the meninges (Fig. 15.17, C). The dura mater (meaning literally "hard mother") is composed of two layers, with the venous sinuses formed between them. The outermost layer forms the periosteum (endosteal layer) of the skull. The inner dura (meningeal layer) provides rigid membranes that support and separate various brain structures. One of these membranes, the falx cerebri, dips between the two cerebral hemispheres along the longitudinal fissure (see Fig. 15.17). The falx cerebri is anchored anteriorly to the base of the brain at the crista galli of the ethmoid bone. The tentorium cerebelli, a common landmark, is a membrane that separates the cerebellum from the cerebral structures above. The arachnoid mater is a spongy, weblike structure just underneath the dura mater that loosely follows the contours of the cerebral structures.

The subdural space lies between the dura and arachnoid. Many small bridging veins that have little structural support traverse the subdural space. Their disruption results in a subdural hematoma (see Chapter 18 and Figs. 18.5 and 18.6). The subarachnoid space lies between the arachnoid and the pia mater and cerebrospinal fluid (CSF) (see Fig. 15.17). Unlike the dura mater and arachnoid, the delicate pia mater closely adheres to the surface of the brain and spinal cord. It provides support for blood vessels serving brain tissue. The choroid plexuses arise from the pia membrane and function to produce cerebrospinal fluid (CSF). The spinal cord is anchored to the vertebrae by extensions of the meninges called denticulate ligaments. The meninges continue beyond the end of the spinal cord (at vertebrae levels L1 and L2) to the lower portion of the sacrum. CSF, contained within the subarachnoid space, also circulates down to the large lumbar cistern, which extends from the second lumbar vertebra to the second sacral vertebra. Cisterns are expanded areas of the subarachnoid space. The cerebellomedullary cistern (cisterna magna) and the pontine cistern are two other important cisterns.

The meninges form potential and real spaces important to understanding functional and pathologic mechanisms. For example, between the dura mater and skull lies a potential space termed the epidural space (see Fig. 15.17). The arterial supply to the meninges consists of blood vessels that lie within grooves in the skull. A skull fracture can severe one of these vessels and produce an epidural hematoma.

Cerebrospinal Fluid and the Ventricular System

Cerebrospinal fluid (CSF) is a clear, colorless fluid similar to blood plasma and interstitial fluid. The intracranial and spinal cord structures float in CSF and are thereby partially protected from jolts and blows. The buoyant properties of the CSF also prevent the brain from tugging on meninges, nerve roots, and blood vessels. (Constituents of CSF are listed in Table 15.4.) Between 125 and 150 mL of CSF is circulating within the ventricles (small cavities) and subarachnoid space at any given time. Approximately 600 mL of CSF is produced daily.

The choroid plexuses in the lateral, third, and fourth ventricles produce the major portion of CSF. (Ventricles are illustrated in Fig. 15.17.) These plexuses are characterized by a rich network of blood vessels, supplied by the pia mater, that lie close to the ependymal cells of the ventricles. The tight junctions of the choroid blood vessel provide a limiting barrier between the CSF and blood that functions similarly to the blood-brain barrier (see Blood-Brain Barrier).

The CSF exerts pressure within the brain and spinal cord. When a person is supine, CSF pressure is approximately 80 to 180 mm of water pressure but can double when the person moves to an upright position. CSF flow results from the pressure gradient between the arterial system and the CSF-filled cavities. Beginning in the lateral ventricles, the CSF flows through the interventricular foramen (foramen of Monro) into the third ventricle and then passes through the cerebral aqueduct (aqueduct of Sylvius) into the fourth ventricle. From the fourth ventricle, the

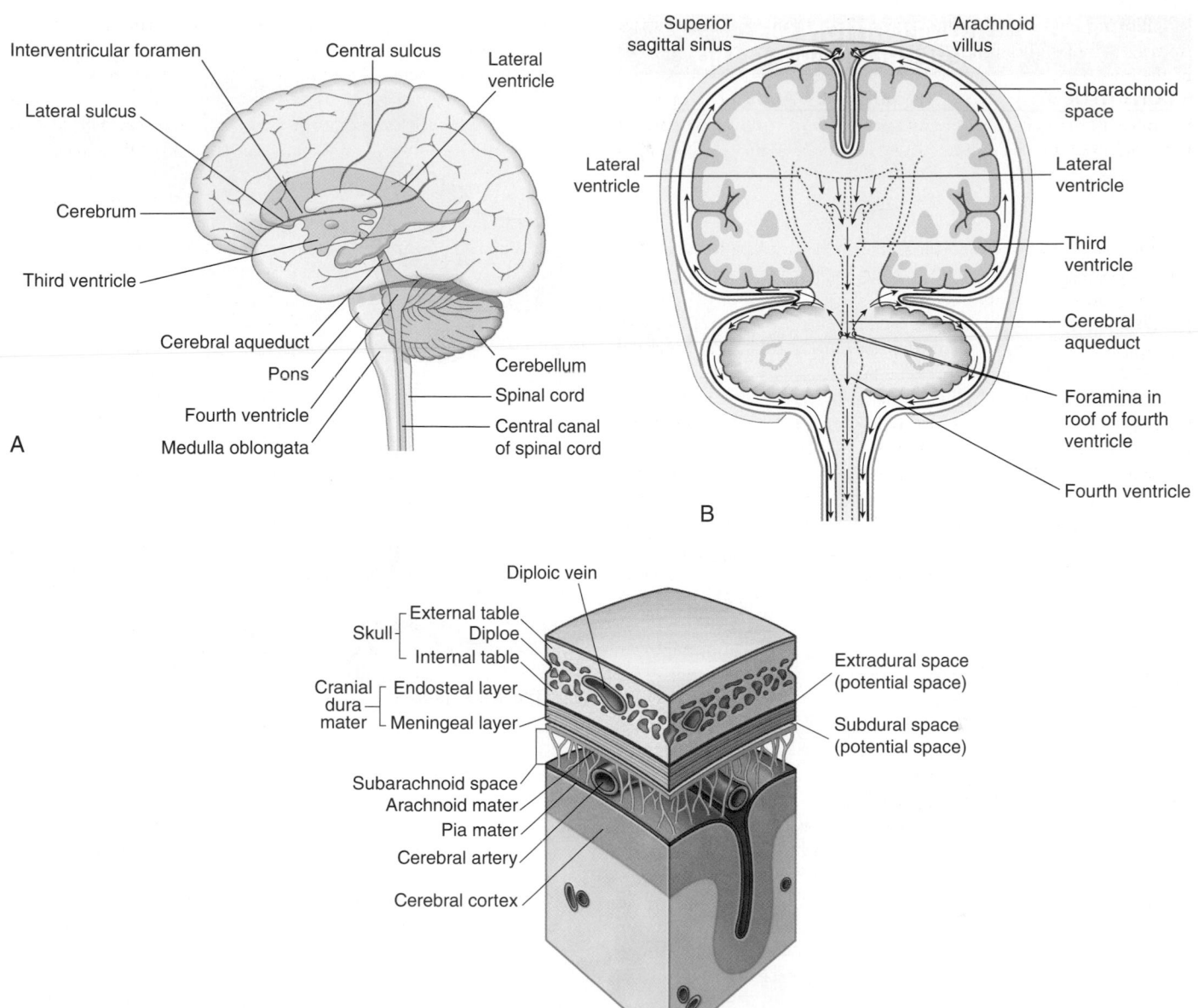

FIGURE 15.17 Flow of Cerebrospinal Fluid and Meninges of the Brain **A,** Ventricles highlighted in blue within a translucent brain in a left lateral view. **B,** Flow of cerebrospinal fluid. The fluid produced by filtration of blood by the choroid plexus of each ventricle flows inferiorly through the lateral ventricles, interventricular foramen, third ventricle, cerebral aqueduct, fourth ventricle, and subarachnoid space to the blood. **C,** Meninges of the brain. (**A, B** from Waugh A, Grant A: *Ross and Wilson anatomy and physiology in health and illness,* ed 12, London, 2012, Churchill Livingstone; **C** from Drake R et al: *Gray's anatomy for students,* ed 3, London, 2015, Churchill Livingstone.)

CSF may pass through either the paired lateral apertures (foramina of Luschka) or the median aperture (foramen of Magendie) before communicating with the subarachnoid spaces of the brain and spinal cord. CSF is produced continually but does not accumulate. Instead, it is reabsorbed into the venous circulation through a pressure gradient between the arachnoid villi and the cerebral venous sinuses. The arachnoid villi protrude from the arachnoid space, through the dura mater, and lie within the blood flow of the venous sinuses. The villi function as one-way valves directing CSF outflow into the blood but preventing blood flow into the subarachnoid space. Thus CSF is formed from the blood and, after circulating throughout the CNS, it returns to the blood.

Vertebral Column

The **vertebral column** (Fig. 15.18) is composed of 33 vertebrae: 7 cervical, 12 thoracic, 5 lumbar, 5 fused sacral, and 4 fused coccygeal. Between each vertebra (except the fused sacral and coccygeal vertebrae) is an **intervertebral disk** (Fig. 15.19). At the center of the intervertebral disk is the **nucleus pulposus,** a pulpy mass of elastic fibers. The intervertebral disk functions to absorb shocks, preventing damage to the vertebrae. The intervertebral disk is also a common source of back problems. If too much stress is applied to the vertebral column, the disk contents may rupture and protrude into the spinal canal, causing compression of the spinal cord or nerve roots. The disks also can degenerate.

TABLE 15.4	COMPOSITION OF CEREBROSPINAL FLUID
CONSTITUENT	**NORMAL VALUE**
Na^+	148 mM
K^+	2.9 mM
Cl^-	125 mM
HCO_3^-	22.9 mM
Glucose (fasting)	50–75 mg/dL (60% of serum glucose)
pH	7.3
Protein	15–45 mg/dL
Albumin	80%
Gamma-globulin	6–10%
Cells	
White (lymphocytes)	0–6/mm³
Red (red blood cell [RBC])	0/mm³

Cl⁻, Chloride; *HCO₃⁻*, bicarbonate; *K⁺*, potassium; *Na⁺*, sodium.

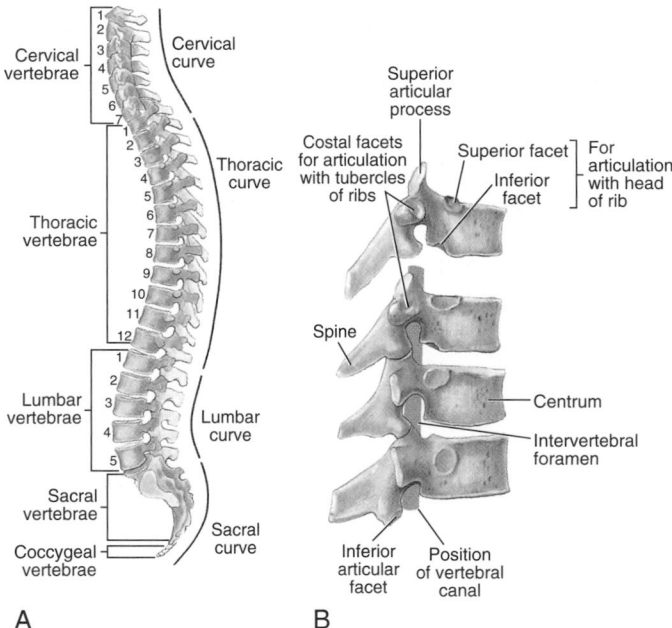

FIGURE 15.18 Vertebral Column. **A,** The normal curves and regions of the vertebral column. The vertebrae in each region are numbered. **B,** Lateral view of several vertebrae showing how they articulate. (From Solomon E: *Introduction to human anatomy and physiology,* ed 4, St Louis, 2010, Mosby.)

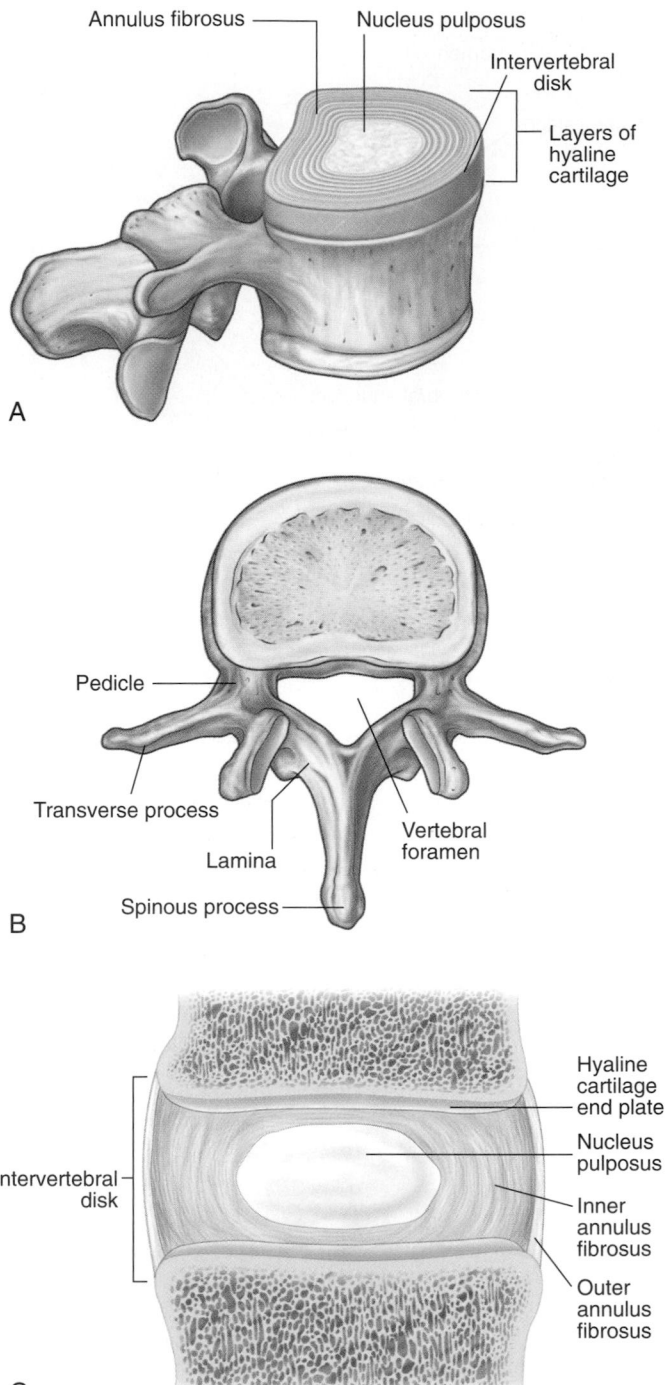

FIGURE 15.19 Intervertebral Disk. **A,** Sagittal view. **B,** Superior view. **C,** Magnified illustration. (**A** and **B** from Drake R, Vogl AW, Mitchell AWM: *Gray's anatomy for students,* ed 3, London, 2015, Churchill Livingston; **C** from Lawry GV, et al: *Fam's musculoskeletal examination and joint injection techniques,* ed 2, Philadelphia, 2010, Mosby.)

Blood Supply of the Central Nervous System
Blood Supply to the Brain

The brain receives approximately 20% of the cardiac output, or 800 to 1000 mL of blood flow per minute. Carbon dioxide serves as a primary regulator for blood flow within the CNS. It is a potent vasodilator in the CNS, and its effects ensure an adequate blood supply.

The brain derives its arterial supply from two systems: the internal carotid arteries (anterior circulation) and the vertebral arteries (posterior circulation) (Fig. 15.20). The internal carotid arteries supply a proportionately greater amount of blood flow. They originate at the common carotid arteries, enter the cranium through the base of the skull, and pass through the cavernous sinus. After entering the skull, these arteries divide into the anterior and middle cerebral arteries (Fig. 15.21). The vertebral arteries originate at the subclavian arteries and pass through the transverse foramina of the cervical vertebrae, entering the

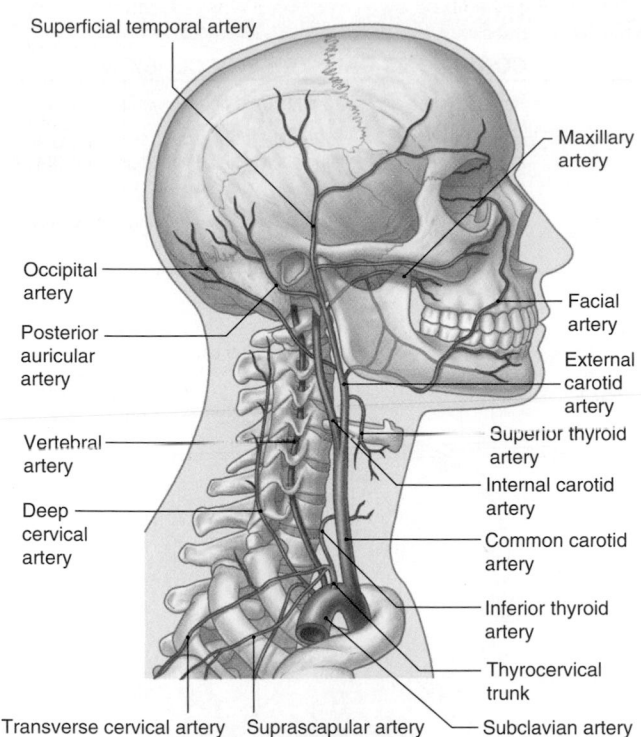

Superficial temporal artery

Maxillary artery

Occipital artery

Posterior auricular artery

Facial artery

External carotid artery

Superior thyroid artery

Vertebral artery

Internal carotid artery

Deep cervical artery

Common carotid artery

Inferior thyroid artery

Thyrocervical trunk

Transverse cervical artery   Suprascapular artery   Subclavian artery

FIGURE 15.20 Major Arteries of the Head and Neck. The internal carotid artery branches are not shown; it branches to the ophthalmic, anterior choroidal, anterior cerebral, middle cerebral, and posterior communicating arteries. (From Moses KP et al: *Atlas of clinical gross anatomy*, ed 2, Philadelphia, 2013, Saunders.)

cranium through the foramen magnum. They join at the junction of the pons and medulla oblongata to form the basilar artery. The basilar artery divides at the level of the midbrain to form paired posterior cerebral arteries.

Three major paired arteries perfuse the cerebellum and brainstem: the posterior inferior cerebellar artery, the anterior inferior cerebellar artery, and the superior cerebellar arteries. They originate from the basilar artery. The basilar artery also gives rise to small pontine arteries. The large arteries on the surface of the brain and their branches are called **superficial arteries (conducting arteries).** Small branches that project into the brain are termed **projecting arteries (nutrient arteries).**

The **circle of Willis** (see Fig. 15.21) provides an alternative route for blood flow when one of the contributing arteries is obstructed (collateral blood flow). The circle of Willis is formed by the posterior cerebral arteries, posterior communicating arteries, internal carotid arteries, anterior cerebral arteries, and anterior communicating artery. The anterior cerebral, middle cerebral, and posterior cerebral arteries leave the arterial circle and extend to various brain structures. (Table 15.5 and Fig. 15.22 illustrate structures served, functional relationships, and pathologic considerations related to occlusion of cerebral arteries.)

Cerebral venous drainage does not parallel its arterial supply, whereas the venous drainage of the brainstem and cerebellum does parallel the arterial supply of the structures. The cerebral veins are classified as superficial veins and deep cerebral veins. The veins drain into venous plexuses and dural sinuses (formed between the dural layers) and eventually join the internal jugular veins at the base of the skull (Fig. 15.23). Adequacy of venous outflow can have a significant effect on intracranial pressure. For example, in individuals with head injury, turning or letting the head fall to the side partially occludes venous

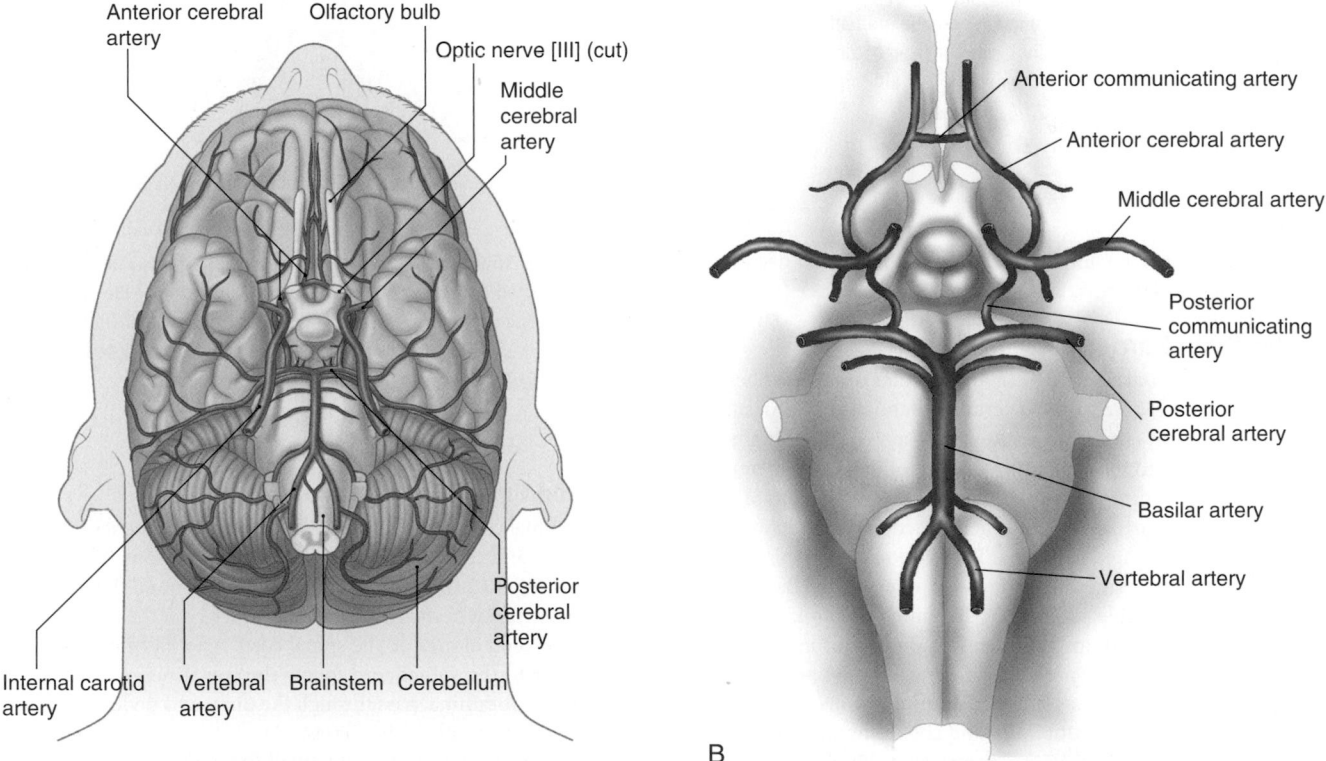

Anterior cerebral artery

Olfactory bulb

Optic nerve [III] (cut)

Middle cerebral artery

Anterior communicating artery

Anterior cerebral artery

Middle cerebral artery

Posterior communicating artery

Posterior cerebral artery

Basilar artery

Vertebral artery

Internal carotid artery   Vertebral artery   Brainstem   Cerebellum

Posterior cerebral artery

A

B

FIGURE 15.21 Arteries at the Base of the Brain. The arteries that compose the circle of Willis are the two anterior cerebral arteries, joined to each other by the anterior communicating artery and two short segments of the internal carotids, off of which the posterior communicating arteries connect to the posterior cerebral arteries. (**A** from Moses KP et al: *Atlas of clinical gross anatomy*, ed 2, Philadelphia, 2013, Saunders; **B** from Hagen-Ansert S: *Textbook of diagnostic sonography*, ed 7, St Louis, 2012, Mosby.)

TABLE 15.5   ARTERIAL SYSTEMS SUPPLYING THE BRAIN

ARTERIAL ORIGIN	STRUCTURES SERVED	CONDITIONS CAUSED BY OCCLUSION
Anterior cerebral artery	Basal ganglia; corpus callosum; medial surface of cerebral hemispheres; superior surface of frontal and parietal lobes	Hemiplegia on contralateral side of body, greater in lower extremities than in upper extremities
Middle cerebral artery	Frontal lobe; parietal lobe; temporal lobe (primarily cortical surfaces)	Aphasia in dominant hemisphere and contralateral hemiplegia (see Chapter 17)
Posterior cerebral artery	Part of diencephalon and temporal lobe; occipital lobe	Visual loss; sensory loss; contralateral hemiplegia if cerebral peduncle affected

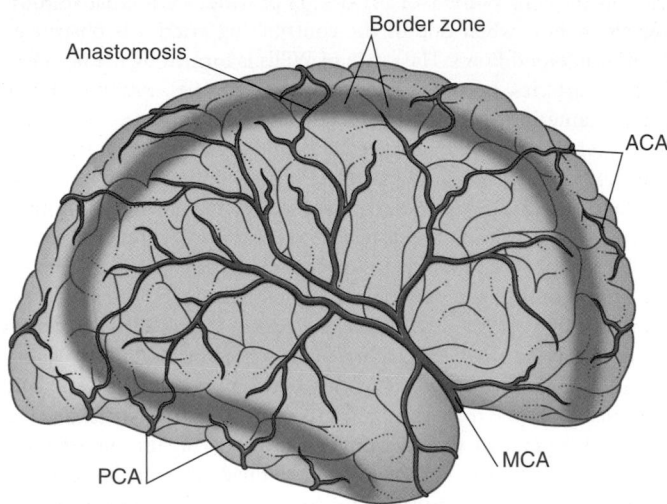

FIGURE 15.22 Areas of the Brain Affected by Occlusion of the Anterior, Middle, and Posterior Cerebral Artery Branches. *ACA*, Gray area affected by occlusion of branches of anterior cerebral artery; *MCA*, pink area affected by occlusion of branches of middle cerebral artery; *PCA*, orange area affected by occlusion of branches of posterior cerebral artery. Occlusions can occur in the cortical or deep areas of the border zone. (From Fitzgerald MJT et al: *Clinical neuroanatomy and neuroscience,* ed 6, Philadelphia, 2012, Saunders.)

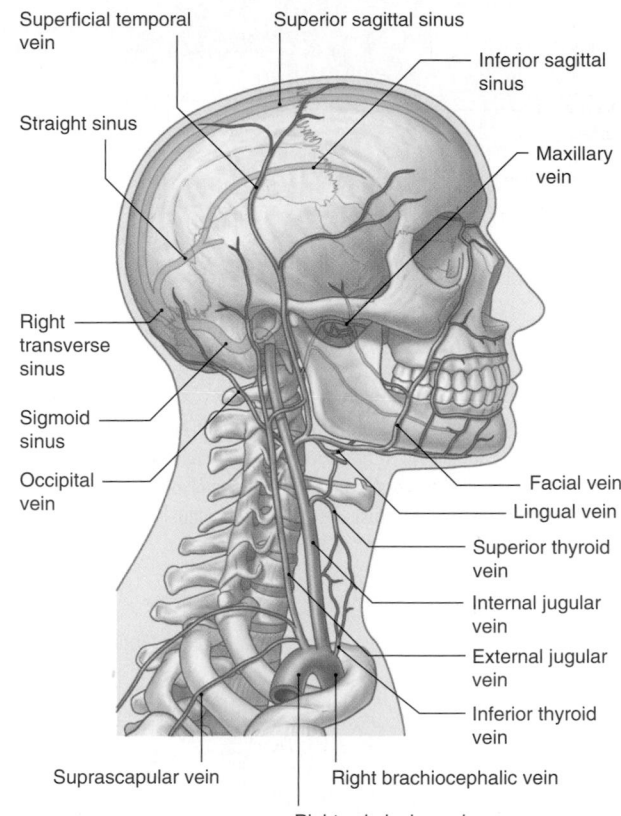

FIGURE 15.23 Veins of the Head and Neck. Deep veins and dural sinuses are projected on the skull. Note two superficial veins in the face are tributaries that send blood through emissary veins in the skull foramen into deep veins inside the skull terminating in the internal jugular vein. (From Moses KP et al: *Atlas of clinical gross anatomy,* ed 2, Philadelphia, 2012, Saunders.)

return and can increase intracranial pressure because of decreased flow through the jugular veins.

Blood-Brain Barrier

The **blood-brain barrier (BBB)** (neurovascular unit) describes cellular structures that selectively inhibit certain potentially harmful substances in the blood from entering the interstitial spaces of the brain or CSF, allowing neurons to function normally. Endothelial cells in brain capillaries with their intracellular tight junctions are the site of the BBB (Fig. 15.24). Supporting cells and their functional interactions include astrocytes, pericytes, and microglia. The exact nature of this mechanism is controversial but permeability is high for water, carbon dioxide, oxygen, and most lipid-soluble substances, including alcohol; moderate for electrolytes, such as sodium, chloride, and potassium; and almost totally impermeable to plasma proteins and most non–lipid-soluble large organic molecules. This has substantial implications for drug therapy because certain types of antibiotics and chemotherapeutic drugs show a greater propensity than others for crossing the blood-brain barrier. Dysfunction or increased permeability of the BBB as occurs in hypoxia can contribute to neuroinflammation, cerebral edema, and neurodegeneration. The epithelium of the choroid plexus and the arachnoid membrane also provide barrier functions.[8]

Blood Supply to the Spinal Cord

The spinal cord derives its blood supply from branches off the vertebral arteries and from branches from various regions of the descending aorta (Fig. 15.25). The **anterior spinal arteries** and the paired **posterior spinal arteries** branch off the vertebral artery at the base of the cranium and descend alongside the spinal cord. Arterial branches from vessels exterior to the spinal cord follow the spinal nerve through the intervertebral foramina, pass through the dura, and divide into the anterior and posterior radicular arteries.

The radicular arteries eventually reconnect to the spinal arteries. Branches from the radicular and spinal arteries form plexuses whose branches penetrate the spinal cord, supplying the deeper tissues. Venous drainage parallels the arterial supply closely and drains into venous sinuses located between the dura and periosteum of the vertebrae.

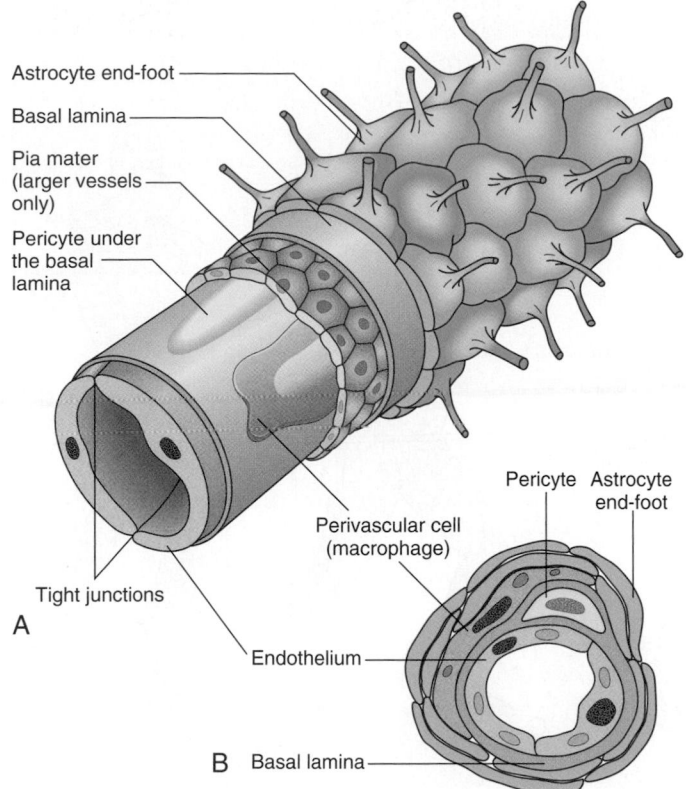

A

B

FIGURE 15.24 Blood-Brain Barrier. **A,** Cellular structure of brain capillary. Endothelial cell membranes with tight junctions create a physical barrier between capillary blood and the brain, restricting movement of bacteria or neurotoxic substances. The pia mater is present only in larger vessels. **B,** Cross section. (From Standring S: *Gray's anatomy,* ed 41, London, 2016, Elsevier.)

PERIPHERAL NERVOUS SYSTEM

The **peripheral nervous system (PNS)** includes the nerves outside the central nervous system. The **somatic nervous system** is the part of the PNS that controls voluntary muscle movement (efferent nerves) and sensory information (afferent nerves). The cranial and spinal nerves, including their branches and ganglia, constitute the PNS. A peripheral nerve is composed of individual axons/dendrites, with most wrapped in a myelin sheath. These individual fibers are arranged in bundles called *fascicles* (see Fig. 15.1 and Fig. 15.26, *B*). The coverings provide structural support, a blood supply, and interstitial compartments necessary for the delivery of essential electrolytes to support nerve impulse conduction.

The 31 pairs of **spinal nerves** derive their names from the vertebral level from which they exit. There are 8 cervical, 12 thoracic, 5 lumbar, 5 sacral pairs of spinal nerves, and 1 coccygeal. The first cervical nerve exits above the first cervical vertebra, and the rest of the spinal nerves exit below their corresponding vertebrae. From the thoracic region (and inferiorly), nerves correspond to the vertebral level above their exit (see Fig. 15.12).

Spinal nerves contain both sensory and motor neurons and are called **mixed nerves.** They arise as rootlets lateral to the anterior and posterior horn cells of the spinal cord. These two spinal nerve roots converge in the region of the intervertebral foramen to form the spinal nerve trunk (see Fig. 15.13). Shortly after converging, the spinal nerve divides into anterior and posterior rami (branches). The anterior rami (except the thoracic) initially form plexuses (networks of nerve fibers), which then branch into the peripheral nerves. Instead of forming plexuses, the thoracic nerves pass through the intercostal spaces and innervate regions of the thorax.

The main spinal nerve plexuses innervate the skin and the underlying muscles of the limbs. The **brachial plexus,** for example, is formed by

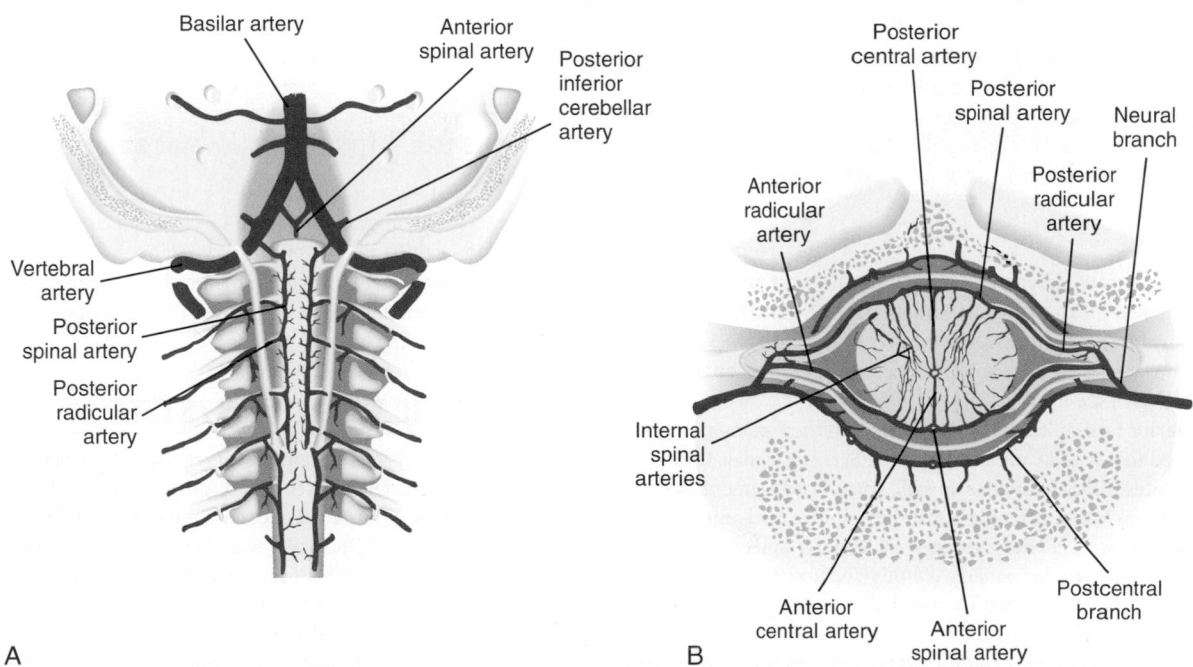

A

B

FIGURE 15.25 Arteries of the Spinal Cord. **A,** Arteries of cervical cord exposed *(posterior view).* **B,** Arteries of spinal cord shown in horizontal section. (From Rudy EB, editor: *Advanced neurological and neurosurgical nursing,* St Louis, 1984, Mosby.)

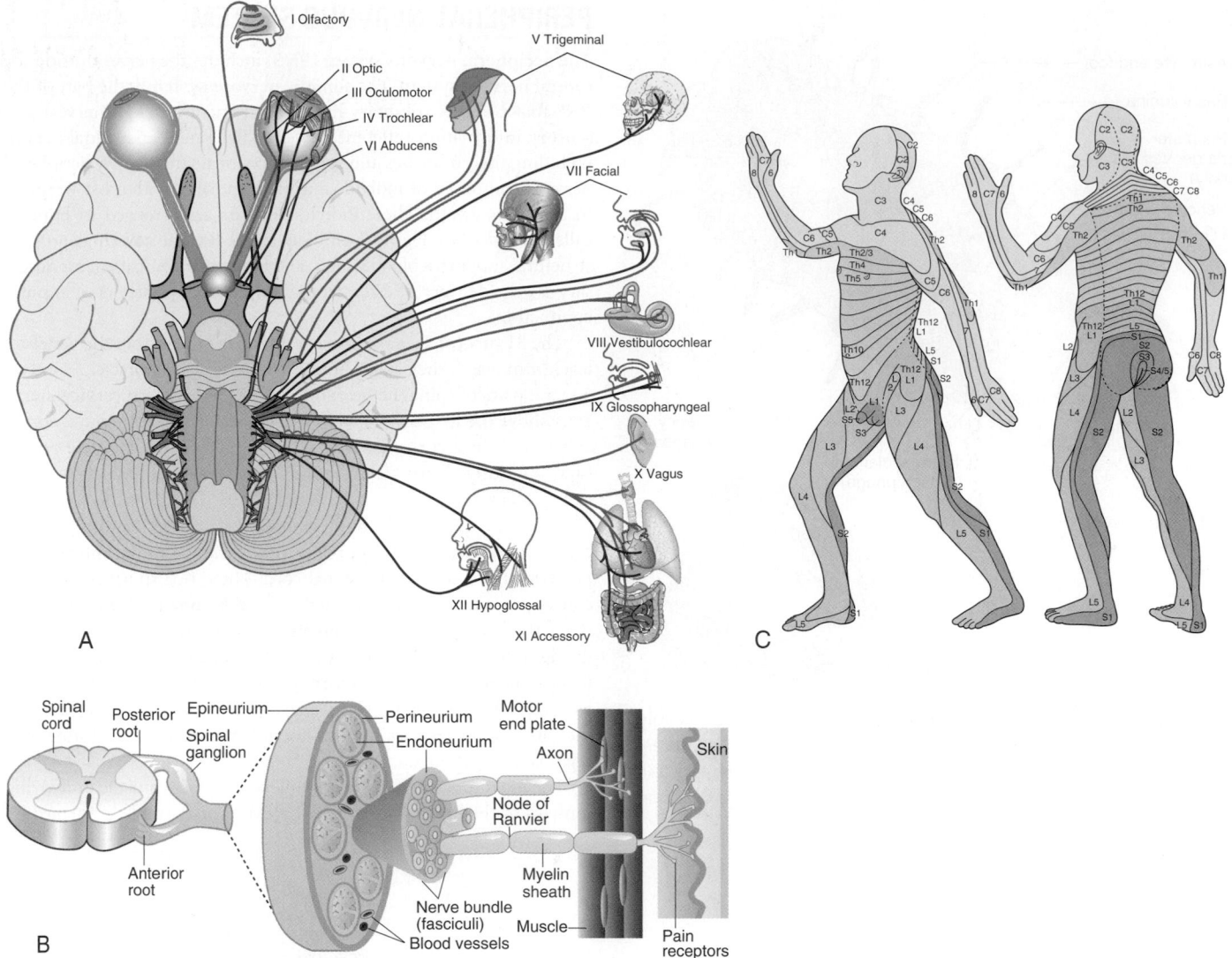

FIGURE 15.26 Cranial and Peripheral Nerves and Skin Dermatomes. **A,** Ventral surface of the brain showing origin of the cranial nerves. The red lines indicate motor function, and the blue lines indicate sensory function. **B,** Peripheral nerve trunk and coverings. **C,** Dermatome map, anterolateral view *(left)* and posterolateral view *(right).* (**A** from Applegate E: *The anatomy and physiology learning system,* ed 4, St Louis, 2011, Saunders; **C** from Salvo SG: *Mosby's pathology for massage therapists,* ed 3, St Louis, 2014, Mosby.)

the last four cervical nerves (C5–C8) and the first thoracic nerve (T1). The brachial plexus innervates the nerves of the arm, wrist, and hand. The lumbar plexus (L2–L4) and sacral plexus (L5–S5) contain nerves that innervate the anterior and posterior portions of the lower body, respectively (see Fig. 15.12).

The posterior rami of each spinal nerve, with their many processes, are distributed to a specific area in the body. Sensory signals thus arise from specific sites associated with a specific spinal cord segment. Specific areas of cutaneous (skin) innervation at these spinal cord segments are called dermatomes. The dermatomes of various spinal nerves are distributed in a fairly regular pattern, although adjacent regions between dermatomes can be innervated by more than one spinal nerve (see Fig. 15.26, *C*).

Like spinal nerves, cranial nerves are categorized as peripheral nerves. Most of these are mixed nerves (like the spinal nerves), although some are purely sensory or purely motor. For example, some cranial nerves carry only special sensory information (e.g., vision, hearing, and taste).

Cranial nerves project to nuclei in the brain and brainstem. Fig. 15.26, *A,* illustrates their location, and Table 15.6 describes structural and functional characteristics.

AUTONOMIC NERVOUS SYSTEM

The autonomic nervous system (ANS) regulates the involuntary function of internal organs. The structure and function of the ANS are complex and still not well understood. Components of the ANS are located in both the CNS and the PNS; however, the ANS is considered part of the efferent division of the PNS, even though visceral afferent neurons are an important part of this system. Many neurons of the ANS travel in spinal nerves and in certain cranial nerves. The widespread activity of this system indicates that its components are distributed over the entire body. The peripheral autonomic nerves carry mainly efferent fibers. The motor component of the ANS is a two-neuron system consisting of preganglionic (myelinated) neurons and postganglionic

TABLE 15.6   THE CRANIAL NERVES

NUMBER AND NAME	ORIGIN AND COURSE	FUNCTION	HOW TESTED
I. Olfactory	Fibers arise from nasal olfactory epithelium and form synapses with olfactory bulbs that transmit impulses to temporal lobe	Purely sensory; carries impulses for sense of smell	Person is asked to sniff aromatic substances, such as oil of cloves and vanilla, and to identify them
II. Optic	Fibers arise from retina of eye to form optic nerve, which passes through sphenoid bone; two optic nerves then form optic chiasma (with partial crossover of fibers) and eventually end in occipital cortex	Purely sensory; carries impulses for vision	Vision and visual field tested with an eye chart and by testing point at which person first sees an object (finger) moving into visual field; inside of eye is viewed with ophthalmoscope to observe blood vessels of eye interior
III. Oculomotor	Fibers emerge from midbrain and exit from skull and extend to eye	Contains motor fibers to inferior oblique and to superior, inferior, and medial rectus extraocular muscles that direct eyeball; levator muscles of eyelid; smooth muscles of iris and ciliary body; and proprioception (sensory) to brain from extraocular muscles	Pupils examined for size, shape, and equality; pupillary reflex tested with a penlight (pupils should constrict when illuminated); ability to follow moving objects
IV. Trochlear	Fibers emerge from posterior midbrain and exit from skull to run to eye	Proprioceptor and motor fibers for superior oblique muscle of eye (extraocular muscle)	Tested in common with cranial nerve III relative to ability to follow moving objects
V. Trigeminal	Fibers emerge from pons and form three divisions that exit from skull and run to face and cranial dura mater	Both motor and sensory for face; conducts sensory impulses from mouth, nose, surface of eye, and dura mater; also contains motor fibers that stimulate chewing muscles	Sensations of pain, touch, and temperature tested with safety pin and hot and cold objects; corneal reflex tested with a wisp of cotton; motor branch tested by asking subject to clench teeth, open mouth against resistance, and move jaw from side to side
VI. Abducens	Fibers leave inferior pons and exit from skull and extend to eye	Contains motor fibers to lateral rectus muscle and proprioceptor fibers from same muscle to brain	Tested in common with cranial nerve III relative to ability to move each eye laterally
VII. Facial	Fibers leave pons and travel through temporal bone and extend to face	Mixed: (1) supplies motor fibers to muscles of facial expression and to lacrimal and salivary glands, and (2) carries sensory fibers from taste buds of anterior part of tongue	Anterior two-thirds of tongue tested for ability to taste sweet (sugar), salty, sour (vinegar), and bitter (quinine) substances; symmetry of face checked; subject asked to close eyes, smile, whistle, and so on; tearing tested with ammonia fumes
VIII. Vestibulocochlear (acoustic)	Fibers run from inner ear (hearing and equilibrium receptors in temporal bone) to enter brainstem just below pons	Purely sensory; vestibular branch transmits impulses for sense of equilibrium; cochlear branch transmits impulses for sense of hearing	Hearing checked by air and bone conduction by use of a tuning fork; vestibular tests: Bárány and caloric tests
IX. Glossopharyngeal	Fibers emerge from midbrain and leave skull and extend to pharynx, salivary glands, and tongue	Mixed: (1) motor fibers serve pharynx (throat) and salivary glands, and (2) sensory fibers carry impulses from pharynx, posterior tongue (taste buds), and pressure receptors of carotid artery	Gag and swallow reflexes checked; subject asked to speak and cough; posterior one-third of tongue may be tested for taste
X. Vagus	Fibers emerge from medulla, pass through skull, and descend through neck region into thorax and abdominal region	Fibers carry sensory and motor impulses for pharynx; a large part of this nerve is parasympathetic motor fibers, which supply smooth muscles of abdominal organs; receives sensory impulses from viscera	Same as for cranial nerve IX (IX and X are tested in common) because they both serve muscles of the throat
XI. Spinal accessory	Fibers arise from medulla and superior spinal cord and extend to muscles of neck and back	Provides sensory and motor fibers for sternocleidomastoid and trapezius muscles and muscles of soft palate, pharynx, and larynx	Sternocleidomastoid and trapezius muscles checked for strength by asking subject to rotate head and shrug shoulders against resistance
XII. Hypoglossal	Fibers arise from medulla and exit from skull and extend to tongue	Carries motor fibers to muscles of tongue and sensory impulses from tongue to brain	Subject asked to stick out tongue, and any position abnormalities are noted

(unmyelinated) neurons. This arrangement contrasts with the somatic nervous system, in which a single motor neuron travels from the CNS to the innervated structure. Visceral afferent neurons have their cell bodies in some sensory and cranial ganglia and their fiber processes traveling in peripheral nerves.

The CNS has autonomic areas in the intermediolateral horns of the spinal cord, the cardiovascular and respiratory centers in the reticular formation, and both sympathetic and parasympathetic areas in the hypothalamus. CNS pathways interconnect all these areas.

The ANS coordinates and maintains a steady-state among visceral (internal) organs, such as regulation of cardiac muscle, smooth muscle, and the glands of the body. This system is considered an involuntary system because one generally cannot *will* these functions to happen. The ANS is separated structurally and functionally into two divisions: (1) the sympathetic nervous system and (2) the parasympathetic nervous system (Fig. 15.27).

Anatomy of the Sympathetic Nervous System

The sympathetic nervous system mobilizes energy stores in times of need (e.g., in the fight-or-flight response) (see Chapter 11 and Fig. 11.2). The sympathetic division receives its innervation from cell bodies located from the first thoracic (T1) through the second lumbar (L2) regions of the spinal cord and is therefore called the thoracolumbar division. The preganglionic axons of the sympathetic division form synapses shortly after leaving the spinal cord in the sympathetic (paravertebral) ganglia. Preganglionic axons travel one of several different pathways: (1) directly synapsing with postganglionic neurons in the sympathetic chain ganglion at their level, (2) traveling up or down the sympathetic chain ganglion before forming synapses with a higher or lower postganglionic neuron (divergence), or (3) passing through the sympathetic chain ganglion postganglionic neurons within collateral ganglia (see Fig. 15.27). Some preganglionic axons form pathways called splanchnic nerves, which lead to collateral ganglia on the front of the aorta. The collateral ganglia are named according to the branches of the aorta nearest them, namely, the celiac, superior mesenteric, and inferior mesenteric. These postganglionic neurons leave the collateral ganglia and innervate the viscera below the diaphragm.

Preganglionic sympathetic neurons that innervate the adrenal medulla also travel in the splanchnic nerves and do not synapse before reaching the gland. The secretory cells in the adrenal medulla are considered modified postganglionic neurons. Because preganglionic sympathetic fibers are all myelinated, travel to the adrenal medulla is quick and innervation causes the rapid release of epinephrine and norepinephrine, which mediate the fight-or-flight response (see Chapter 11).

Anatomy of the Parasympathetic Nervous System

The parasympathetic nervous system functions to conserve and restore energy. The nerve cell bodies of this division are located in the cranial nerve nuclei and in the sacral region of the spinal cord, and therefore constitute the craniosacral division. Unlike the sympathetic division, the preganglionic fibers in the parasympathetic division travel to ganglia close to the organs they innervate before forming synapses with the relatively short postganglionic neurons (see Fig. 15.27). Parasympathetic nerves arising from nuclei in the brainstem travel to the viscera of the head, thorax, and abdomen within cranial nerves—including the oculomotor (III), facial (VII), glossopharyngeal (IX), and vagus (X) nerves.

Preganglionic parasympathetic nerves that originate from the sacral region of the spinal cord run either separately or together with spinal nerves. The preganglionic axons join to form the pelvic nerve, which innervates the viscera of the pelvic cavity. These preganglionic axons synapse with postganglionic neurons in terminal ganglia located close to the organs they innervate.

Neurotransmitters and Neuroreceptors

Sympathetic preganglionic fibers and parasympathetic preganglionic and postganglionic fibers release acetylcholine—the same neurotransmitter released by somatic efferent neurons (Fig. 15.28). These fibers are characterized by cholinergic transmission. Most postganglionic sympathetic fibers release norepinephrine (adrenaline) and thus are considered to function by adrenergic transmission. A few postganglionic sympathetic fibers, such as those that innervate the sweat glands, release acetylcholine.

The action of catecholamines (epinephrine, norepinephrine, dopamine) varies with the type of neuroreceptor stimulated. It should be remembered that catecholamines also are released by the adrenal medulla that physiologically and biochemically resembles the sympathetic nervous system. Two types of adrenergic receptors exist: α and β. Cells of the effector organs may have only one or both types of adrenergic receptors. The α-adrenergic receptors have been further subdivided according to the action produced: α_1-adrenergic activity is associated mostly with excitation or stimulation; α_2-adrenergic activity is associated with relaxation or inhibition. Most of the α-adrenergic receptors on effector organs belong to the α_1-adrenergic class. The β-adrenergic receptors are classified as β_1-adrenergic receptors (which facilitate increased heart rate and contractility and cause the release of renin from the kidney), and β_2-adrenergic receptors (which facilitate all of the remaining effects attributed to β-adrenergic receptors).

Norepinephrine stimulates all α-adrenergic and β_1-adrenergic receptors and only certain β_2-adrenergic receptors. The most significant response from norepinephrine, however, is stimulation of the α_1-adrenergic receptors that cause vasoconstriction. Epinephrine strongly stimulates all four types of receptors and induces general vasodilation because of the predominance of β-adrenergic receptors in muscle vasculature. (Table 15.7 summarizes the effects of neuroreceptors on their effector organs.)

Dopamine is a precursor of norepinephrine and epinephrine and is a brain neurotransmitter synthesized in the substantia nigra and the ventral tegmental areas of the brain. There are five types of dopamine receptors distributed throughout the brain, D_1, D_2, D_3, D_4, and D_5. They have varying functions including pleasure, motivation, cognition, attention, memory, learning, fine motor control, sleep regulation, hormonal regulation, sympathetic regulation, penile erection, and immune function.[9]

Functions of the Autonomic Nervous System

Many body organs are innervated by the sympathetic and parasympathetic nervous systems. The two divisions frequently cause opposite responses; for example, sympathetic stimulation of the gastrointestinal (GI) tract causes decreased peristalsis, whereas parasympathetic stimulation of the GI tract increases peristalsis. In general, sympathetic stimulation promotes responses that are concerned with the protection of the individual. For example, sympathetic activity increases blood glucose levels and temperature and raises blood pressure. In emergency situations a generalized and widespread discharge of the sympathetic system occurs and is known as the "fight or flight" reflex or acute stress response (see Chapter 11). This is accomplished by an increased firing frequency of sympathetic fibers and by activation of sympathetic fibers normally silent (fibers to the sweat glands, pilomotor muscles, and the adrenal medulla, as well as vasodilator fibers to muscle). Regulation of vasomotor tone is considered the single most important function of the sympathetic nervous system. (Fig. 15.29 illustrates some of the most important functions of the sympathetic nervous system; also see Fig. 11.2.)

Increased parasympathetic activity promotes rest and tranquility and is characterized by reduced heart rate and enhanced visceral functions leading to digestion. Stimulation of the vagus nerve in the GI tract

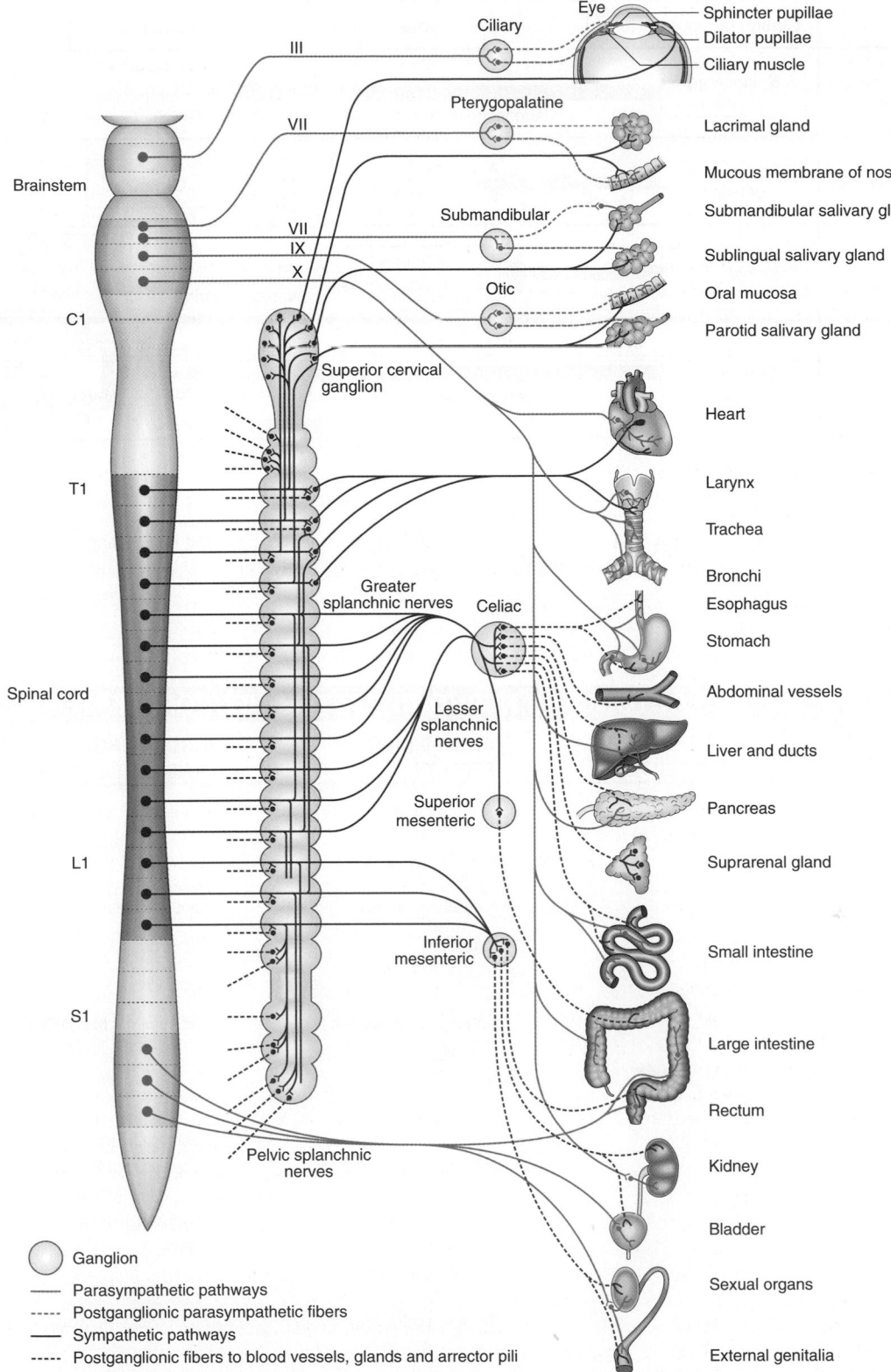

FIGURE 15.27 **Sympathetic and Parasympathetic Divisions of the Autonomic Nervous System.** Parasympathetic neuron cell bodies are located in the brainstem and sacral spinal cord ("craniosacral" division). Cell bodies of sympathetic neurons are located in the thoracic and upper lumbar cord segments ("thoracolumbar" division). The axons of these neurons synapse with postganglionic neurons, which innervate smooth muscle, cardiac muscle, and glands of the body. The postganglionic neuron cell bodies may be located in distinct autonomic ganglia (represented with circles), or in or very near the wall of the innervated visceral organ. Note that sympathetic fibers provide the only innervation to peripheral effectors (sweat glands, arrector pili muscles, adipose tissue, and blood vessels). (From Cramer D et al: *Basic and clinical anatomy of the spine, spinal cord and ANS,* ed 2, St Louis, 2005, Elsevier Mosby.)

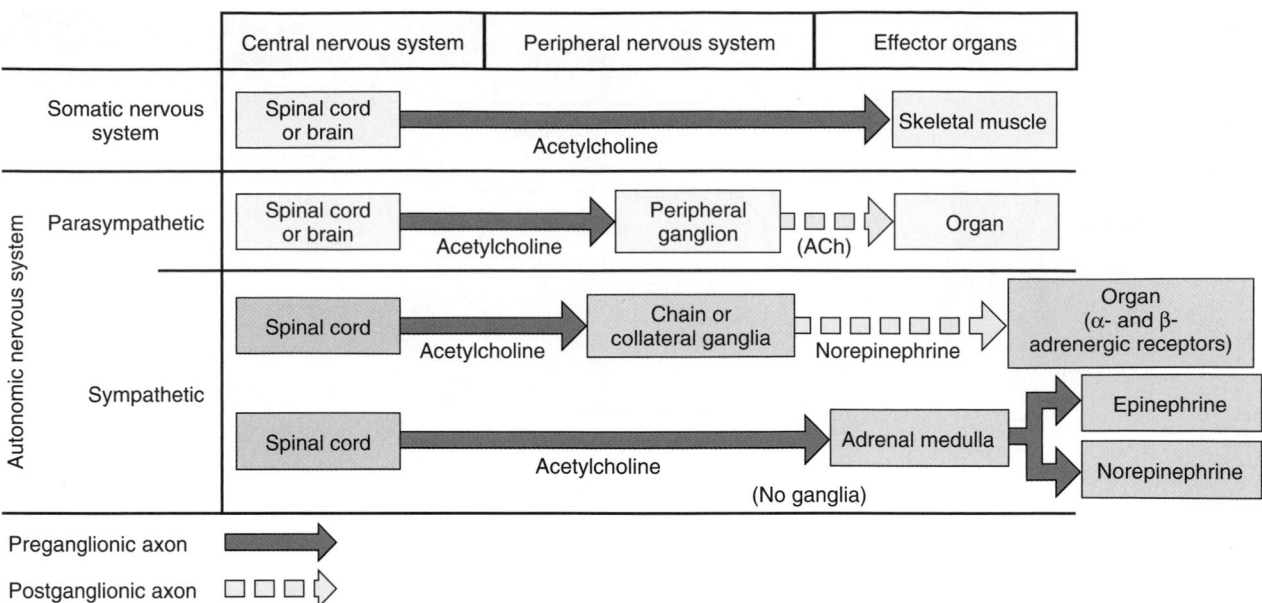

FIGURE 15.28 Autonomic Nervous System and Type of Neurotransmitters Secreted by Preganglionic and Postganglionic Fibers. Note that all preganglionic fibers are cholinergic (acetylcholine [ACh]). A somatic nerve is used for comparison.

TABLE 15.7	ACTIONS OF AUTONOMIC NERVOUS SYSTEM NEURORECEPTORS		
EFFECTOR ORGAN OR TISSUE	**ADRENERGIC RECEPTORS**	**ADRENERGIC EFFECTS**	**CHOLINERGIC EFFECTS (NICOTINE AND MUSCARINIC* RECEPTORS)**
Eye			
Iris			
Radial muscle	α_1	Dilation	–
Sphincter muscle	–	–	Constriction
Ciliary muscle	β_2	Relaxation for far vision	Contraction for near vision
Lacrimal glands	α_1	Secretion	Secretion
Nasopharyngeal glands	–	–	Secretion
Salivary glands	α_1	Secretion of potassium and water	Secretion of potassium and water
	β	Secretion of amylase	–
Heart			
Sinoatrial (SA) node	β_1, β_2	Increase heart rate	Decrease heart rate; vagus arrest
Atrial	β_1, β_2	Increase contractility and conduction velocity	Decrease contractility; shorten action potential duration
Atrioventricular (AV) junction	β_1, β_2	Increase automaticity and propagation velocity	Decrease automaticity and propagation velocity
Purkinje system	β_1, β_2	Increase automaticity and propagation velocity	–
Ventricles	β_1, β_2	Increase contractility	Slight decrease in contraction
Arterioles			
Coronary	$\alpha_1, \alpha_2, \beta_2$	Constriction, dilation	Dilation
Skin and mucosa	α_1, α_2	Constriction	Dilation
Skeletal muscle	α, β_2	Dilation, constriction	Dilation
Cerebral	α_1	Constriction (slight)	Dilation
Pulmonary	α_1, β	Constriction, dilation	Dilation
Mesenteric	α_1	Constriction	Dilation
Renal	$\alpha_1, \beta_1, \beta_2$	Constriction, dilation	Dilation
Salivary glands	α_1, α_2	Constriction	Dilation
Veins, systemic	$\alpha_1, \alpha_2, \beta_2$	Constriction, dilation	–

TABLE 15.7	ACTIONS OF AUTONOMIC NERVOUS SYSTEM NEURORECEPTORS—cont'd		
EFFECTOR ORGAN OR TISSUE	**ADRENERGIC RECEPTORS**	**ADRENERGIC EFFECTS**	**CHOLINERGIC EFFECTS (NICOTINE AND MUSCARINIC* RECEPTORS)**
Lung			
Bronchial muscle	α_2	Relaxation	Contraction
Bronchial glands	α_1, β_2	Decrease secretion; increase secretion	Stimulation
Stomach			
Motility	α_1, α_2, β_1, β_2	Decrease (usually)	Increase
Sphincters	α_1	Contraction (usually)	Relaxation (usually)
Secretion	α_2	Inhibition	Stimulation
Liver	α_1, β_2	Glycogenolysis and gluconeogenesis	–
Gallbladder and ducts	β_2	Relaxation	Contraction
Pancreas			
Acini	α	Decrease secretion	Secretion
Islet cells	α_2, β_2	Decrease secretion; increase secretion	–
Intestine			
Motility and tone	α_1, α_2, β_1, β_2	Decrease	Increase
Sphincters	α_1	Contraction	Relaxation (usually)
Secretion	α_2	Inhibition	Stimulation
Adrenal medulla	–	Secretion of epinephrine and norepinephrine (nicotinic effect)	
Kidney			
Renin secretion	α_1, β_1	Decrease; increase	–
Ureter			
Motility and tone	β_1	Increase	Increase (?)
Urinary bladder			
Detrusor	β_2	Relaxation	Contraction
Trigone and sphincter	α_1	Contraction	Relaxation
Sex organs, male	α_1	Ejaculation	Erection
Skin			
Pilomotor muscles	α_1	Contraction	–
Sweat glands	α_1	Localized secretion	–
Fat cells	α_2, β_1, β_2, β_3	Inhibition of lipolysis; stimulation of lipolysis	–
Pineal gland	β	Melatonin synthesis	–

*Muscarinic receptors respond to circulating muscarinic antagonists.
Modified from Brunton LL et al, editors: *Goodman & Gilman's the pharmacological basis of therapeutics*, ed 12, New York, 2010, McGraw-Hill; Yagiela JA et al: *Pharmacology and therapeutics for dentistry*, ed 6, St Louis, 2011, Mosby.

increases peristalsis and secretion, as well as relaxation of sphincters. Activation of parasympathetic fibers traveling with cranial nerves III, VII, and IX causes pupillary constriction, tear secretion, and increased salivary secretion. Stimulation of the sacral division of the parasympathetic system contracts the urinary bladder and facilitates the process of genital erection.

The parasympathetic system lacks the generalized and widespread response of the sympathetic system. Specific parasympathetic fibers are activated to regulate particular functions. Although the actions of the parasympathetic and sympathetic systems usually are antagonistic, there are exceptions. Changes in the shape of the lens (for near vision) require only oculomotor parasympathetic activity. Most of the blood vessels

involved in the control of blood pressure are innervated by sympathetic nerves. Peripheral vascular resistance is increased and decreased by the relative activity of the sympathetic division without a counteracting parasympathetic component. To decrease blood pressure, therefore, it is more important to block the continuous (tonic) discharge of the sympathetic system than to promote parasympathetic activity.

AGING AND THE NERVOUS SYSTEM

The CNS mechanisms involved in the aging process are extremely complex, and many questions concerning the neurologic effects of aging have yet to be answered. Some of the identified mechanisms associated

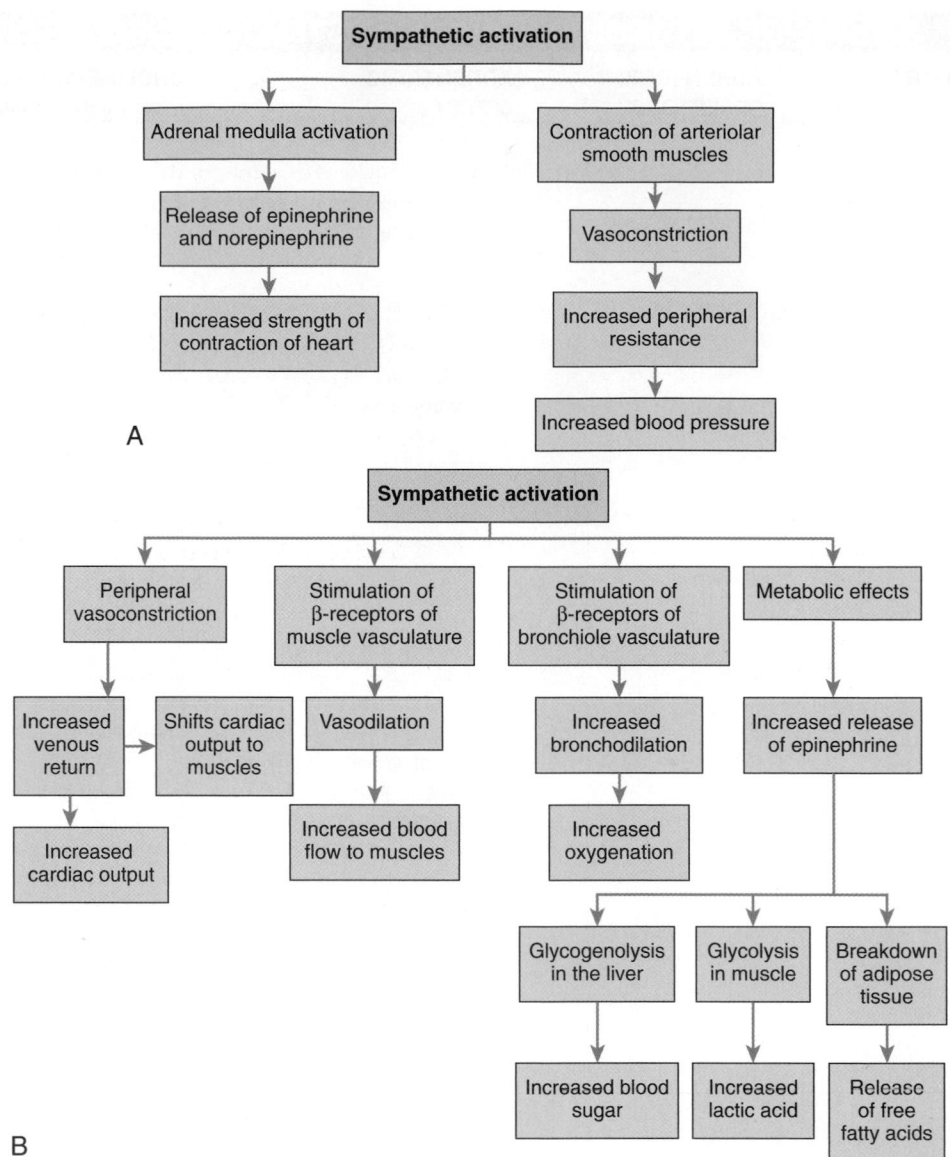

FIGURE 15.29 Important Functions of the Sympathetic Nervous System. **A,** Regulation of vasomotor tone. **B,** Regulation of strenuous muscular exercise (fight-or-flight response). (See also Chapter 11 and Fig. 11.2 for more detail of the stress response.)

with aging are pathologic, but the distinction between these mechanisms and those that are a part of the normal aging process remains somewhat ambiguous. Box 15.4 contains information on the structural, cellular, cerebrovascular, and functional changes that occur in the nervous system with aging.

TESTS OF NERVOUS SYSTEM STRUCTURE AND FUNCTION

Skull and Spine Roentgenograms

Roentgenograms (x-ray films) of the skull or spine from multiple angles (views) are used primarily to localize bony defects, bone density, erosion, or calcified structures. The pineal gland in older people becomes calcified and is useful as an internal brain landmark. Probably the most commonly used radiologic studies are x-ray films.

Computed Tomography

Computed tomography (CT) creates two-dimensional reconstructions from multiple radiologic images (x-rays) using computer-assisted analysis. It is capable of demonstrating fine distinctions in shape, size, and densities of a variety of tissues based on differential absorption of x-rays. CT imaging is a noninvasive procedure used in evaluating cranial and spinal structures, as well as hemorrhages, tumors, and distortions in the brain caused by pressure differences. A variety of contrast media also are commonly used in conjunction with this procedure to aid in enhanced delineation of selected structures. Spiral or helical CT uses a multidetector scanner mounted on a rotating gantry to provide several axial images of a large continuous anatomic area in a matter of seconds. Helical CT angiography uses contrast media for detection of aneurysms or ruptured aneurysms.

BOX 15.4   AGING AND THE NERVOUS SYSTEM

Structural Changes with Aging

Decreased brain weight and size, particularly frontal regions

Fibrosis and thickening of the meninges

Narrowing of gyri and widening of sulci

Increase in size of ventricles

Cellular Changes with Aging

Decrease in the number of neurons, not consistently related to changes in mental function

Decreased amount of myelin

Lipofuscin deposition (a pigment resulting from cellular autodigestion)

Decreased number of dendritic processes and synaptic connections

Activation of microglial function, increased neuroinflammation and loss of protective brain mechanisms

Formation of intracellular neurofibrillary tangles; significant accumulation in hippocampus and cortex associated with Alzheimer dementia

Imbalance in the amount and distribution of neurotransmitters

Atrophy of epithelial cells and thickening of the basement membrane in the choroid plexus can increase or decrease CSF production

Declines in melatonin level can alter circadian rhythms and brain energy metabolism

Cerebrovascular Changes with aging

Arterial atherosclerosis (may cause infarcts and scars)

Increased permeability of the blood-brain barrier (escape of toxins into the brain)

Decreased vascular density

Functional Changes with Aging

Decreased tendon reflexes

Skeletal muscle atrophy

Progressive deficit in taste and smell

Decreased vibratory sense

Decrease in accommodation and color vision

Decrease in neuromuscular control with change in gait and posture

Sleep disturbances

Memory impairments

Cognitive alterations associated with chronic disease

Functional changes and nervous system aging have significant individual variation; the plasticity of the brain and variations in genetics, diet, exercise, environment, and chronic disease significantly affect brain changes and sensory-motor and cognitive abilities in older adults.

Data from Kennedy KM, Ra N: Normal aging of the brain. In Toga AW, editor: *Brain mapping: an encyclopedic reference*, London, 2015, Academic Press, pp. 603–617; Khan ZU et al: *Prog Mol Biol Transl Sci* 122:1–29, 2014; Magnusson KR, Brim BL: The aging brain. In *Reference module in biomedical sciences*, St Louis, 2014, Elsevier, pp. 76–80; Mather M: *Annu Ref Psychol* 67:213-238, 2016; Nissen JC: *Int J Mol Sci* 18(3), 2017.

Magnetic Resonance Imaging

Magnetic resonance imaging (MRI) uses a static magnetic field, instead of x-rays, to orient physiologic atomic particles. Disruption of this orientation by excitation of the particles using serial radiofrequency pulsations provides the image data. The specific tissue reaction is computer-analyzed to give an image with much better spatial resolution than that provided by CT. The MRI also provides reconstruction of images in three views at right angles (i.e., axial, sagittal, coronal). MRI is reported to have none of the adverse effects associated with radiation examinations. Magnetic resonance spectroscopy (MRS) can be completed at the same time as a standard MRI by analyzing the chemical composition of proton (hydrogen) or phosphorous-based molecules and is useful for differentiating the chemical composition and function of various regions of the brain. Functional MRI (fMRI) detects changes in blood oxygenation and flow and can be used to produce maps showing the parts of the brain that are functioning during a mental process. Diffusion tensor imaging (DTI) is an MRI technique that quantifies the size and direction of white matter tracts by measuring asymmetries in the magnitude and direction of the diffusion of water molecules. Color coding and fiber tracking (tractography) add detail.

Magnetic Resonance Angiography

Magnetic resonance angiography (MRA) uses special imaging techniques to visualize blood vessels in great detail. MRA can be used in conjunction with cerebral angiography to detect and localize pathologic lesions of the circulatory system of the brain, particularly the arterial system. In some cases contrast agents are used.

Positron-Emission Tomography Scan

The positron-emission tomography (PET) scan uses CT imaging to detect the emission of positive electrons from trace amounts of radioactive substances injected into the bloodstream or administered as inhaled gases. With radioactive decay, radioactive substances emit a positron. As they are distributed in tissues, they display characteristic patterns that indicate physiologic and metabolic processes, for example, glucose and oxygen uptake, cerebral blood flow, neural and neurotransmitter function, and the effects of drugs. As a research tool, PET is being used to visualize the specific brain sites that are involved in the processing of information in the brain.

Single Photon Emission Computed Tomography

Single photon emission computed tomography (SPECT) uses radiotracers that have longer half-lives than PET. Images are created by CT after radionuclide substances (technetium [^{99m}Tc]) have been introduced into the bloodstream. For example, visualization of tissue uptake of the radioactive agent provides an indication of blood-brain barrier integrity (increased uptake of the agent indicates disruption). This scanning technique also can identify abnormalities in blood flow dynamics and cellular metabolic function. The brain scan is particularly helpful in detecting abnormal vascularity resulting from neoplasms, abscesses, and vascular lesions.

Cerebral Angiography

Cerebral angiography is a radiologic technique that demonstrates cerebrovascular blood flow. This technique commonly is performed by the introduction of a small catheter into the femoral artery. The catheter is then passed to the level of the cerebral circulation and through the aorta, and a contrast dye is injected. Serial x-ray films are then taken. These films demonstrate flow of the dye through the cerebral vasculature and provide information on patency, location, size, and flow pattern of the vessels. Another technique used in cerebral angiography is the retrograde (reverse flow) injection of the dye through catheterization of a brachial, axillary, subclavian, or femoral vein.

Echoencephalography (Ultrasound)

Echoencephalography, or ultrasound, is a safe, noninvasive procedure using sound waves that are deflected at differing rates, depending on the density of the tissue. Information is processed and displayed on an oscilloscope screen. It is useful primarily in the detection of structural characteristics of intracranial space–occupying mass lesions and the determination of ventricular dimensions, especially in newborns where open fontanelles provide good acoustic windows.

Electroencephalography

The electroencephalograph (EEG) is a recording of electrical impulses arising from the cortical surface of the brain that are detected by scalp electrodes. The recording of brain wave patterns is analyzed for alterations or localization (or both) of specific electrical activity. This test is especially useful in detecting and localizing foci that initiate seizure activity. It is also an important technique in assessment of encephalopathy (altered mental status). Complete absence of electrical activity is seen in individuals who are legally "brain dead."

Magnetoencephalography

Magnetoencephalography (MEG) is a specialized imaging technique used to measure magnetic fields induced by electrical activity in the brain. Electrical activity in the brain, such as that detected by EEG, induces an orthogonally oriented magnetic field. MEG uses multiple sensors that allow vectoring and ultimately localization of the origin of the electrical activity that generated the field. Use of MEG has the advantage over EEG in that the induced magnetic field is not significantly dispersed by passing through the skull and soft tissues of the scalp. Co-registration of MEG and MRI data allow precise localization of the electrical focus for seizure onset.

Evoked Potentials

Evoked potentials (EPs) are a method of detecting electrical brain activity that results from a stimulus—primarily auditory, visual, or peripheral sensory. Electrical activity is computer formatted to display changes in trends. The primary uses of EPs include perioperative detection of sensory pathway integrity and disease- or drug-related sensory dysfunction.

Cerebrospinal Fluid Analysis

CSF generally is obtained from the lumbar or cisternal subarachnoid space by means of a hollow needle that allows passive flow. The lumbar puncture is performed most often at the L3–L4 interspace (below the level of the spinal cord at L1–L2). Cisternal puncture is performed by the insertion of a needle into the cerebellomedullary cistern using an approach from the back of the neck in the region of the foramen magnum. CSF pressure is commonly measured during these procedures. The CSF can be analyzed also for gross characteristics and constituents (color, blood cells, electrolytes, and protein) and cultured for microorganisms (Table 15.8).

TABLE 15.8 CEREBROSPINAL FLUID ANALYSIS

PARAMETERS	NORMAL	ABNORMAL	POSSIBLE CAUSE
Pressure (initial readings)	12–18 cm H_2O (9–14 mmHg)	<6 cm H_2O	Faulty needle placement Dehydration Spinal block along subarachnoid space Block of foramen magnum
		>20 cm H_2O	Muscle tension Abdominal compression Brain tumor Subdural hematoma Brain abscess Brain cyst Cerebral edema (any cause) Hydrocephalus
Color (turbidity)	Clear, colorless	Cloudy	Increased cell count Increased microorganisms (meningitis)
		Yellow	Xanthochromic (caused by red blood cell [RBC] pigments) High protein content
		Smoky	Presence of RBCs
Red blood cells	None	Blood-tinged	Traumatic tap
		Grossly bloody	Traumatic tap Subarachnoid hemorrhage
White blood cells	0–6/mm³	>10/mm³ (cell counts range from <100/mm³ to many thousands depending on causative factor; all are abnormal findings)	Occurs in many conditions: Bacterial infections of meninges Viral infections of meninges Neurosyphilis Tuberculous meningitis Metastatic neoplastic lesions Parasitic infections Acute demyelinating diseases Following introduction of air or blood into subarachnoid space

TABLE 15.8	CEREBROSPINAL FLUID ANALYSIS—cont'd		
PARAMETERS	**NORMAL**	**ABNORMAL**	**POSSIBLE CAUSE**
Protein*	15–45 mg/dL (1% of serum protein)	<10 mg/dL	Little clinical significance

		>60 mg/dL	Occurs in many conditions:
			    Complete spinal block
			    Guillain-Barré syndrome
			    Carcinomatosis of meninges
			    Tumors close to pial or ependymal surfaces or in cerebellopontine angle
			    Acute and chronic meningitis
			    Meningeal hemorrhage
			    Demyelinating disorders
			    Degenerative diseases

Glucose (CSF/serum ratio)	0.6 (approximately 60% of blood glucose level: 50–55 mg/dL)	<0.4: <40 mg/dL >0.6: >60 mg/dL	Acute bacterial meningitis Tuberculous meningitis Meningeal carcinomatosis Acute viral meningitis Glucose transporter deficiency
		>100 mg/dL	Diabetes
Chloride	700–750 mg/dL 116–130 mEq/L	<625 mg/dL <110 mEq/L >800 mg/dL	Hypochloremia Tuberculous meningitis Not of neurologic significance; correlates with blood levels of chloride

*NOTE: If CSF contains blood, this will raise the protein level.
Data from Larson D, Hayden J, Nair H, editors: *Clinical chemistry: fundamental and laboratory techniques,* St Louis, 2017, Elsevier; Marx JA, editor in chief: *Rosen's emergency medicine,* Philadelphia, 2010, Saunders.

SUMMARY REVIEW

Overview and Organization of the Nervous System

1. The divisions of the nervous system have been categorized as either structural (CNS and PNS) or functional (somatic nervous system and ANS).
2. The CNS is contained within the brain and spinal cord.
3. The PNS is composed of cranial and spinal nerves that carry impulses toward the CNS (afferent) and away from the CNS (efferent) to target organs or skeletal muscle.
4. The somatic nervous system consists of motor and sensory pathways regulating voluntary motor control of skeletal muscle.
5. The ANS consists of motor and sensory involuntary control of organ systems.

Cells of the Nervous System

1. The neuron and neuroglial cells make up nervous tissue. The neuron is specialized to transmit and receive electrical and chemical impulses, and the neuroglial cell provides supportive functions.
2. The neuron is composed of a cell body, one or more dendrites, and an axon. A myelin sheath around selected axons forms an insulation that allows quicker nerve impulse conduction, referred to as *saltatory conduction.*
3. Neurons have four basic types of cell configuration: (a) unipolar, (b) pseudounipolar, (c) bipolar, and (d) multipolar. The three function types of neurons are sensory, associational, and motor.
4. Neuroglial cells ("nerve glue") support the CNS and comprise approximately half of the total brain and spinal cord volume.
5. Nerve injury in peripheral neurons triggers a sequence of events known as the *axonal reaction* and includes local, antegrade, and

retrograde changes in the injured neuron that can lead to recovery of function. CNS neuron injury usually leads to permanent loss of function.

Nerve Impulse

1. The region between adjacent neurons is the synapse, and the region between the neuron and muscle is the myoneural junction.
2. Neurotransmitters are responsible for chemical conduction across the synapse and myoneural junction. The nerve impulse is predominantly regulated by a balance of IPSPs and EPSPs, temporal and spatial summation, and convergence and divergence.

Central Nervous System

1. The brain is contained within the cranial vault and is divided into three distinct regions: (a) forebrain, (b) midbrain, and (c) hindbrain.
2. The forebrain comprises the two cerebral hemispheres (telencephalon) and includes the cerebral cortex and basal ganglia and is associated with conscious perception of internal and external stimuli, cognition and memory processes, and voluntary control of skeletal muscles. The posterior portion of the forebrain is termed the *diencephalon* (thalamus, hypothalamus, epithalamus, and subthalamus), which relays sensory information, controls autonomic functions, and links to the limbic system for memory and emotion. The center for voluntary control of skeletal muscle movements is located along the precentral gyrus in the frontal lobe, whereas the center for sensory perception is along the postcentral gyrus in the parietal lobe. The Broca area (anterior to the postcentral gyrus)

■ SUMMARY REVIEW—cont'd

and the Wernicke area (superior posterior temporal lobe) are major speech and language centers.

3. The midbrain connects the forebrain and hindbrain and is primarily a relay center for some motor and sensory tracts, as well as a center for auditory and visual reflexes, temperature control, sleep-wake cycles, arousal, and attention.

4. The hindbrain consists of the metencephalon (cerebellum and pons) and the myelencephalon (medulla oblongata). The metencephalon allows sampling and comparison of sensory data from the periphery and motor impulses from the cerebral hemispheres for the purpose of coordination and refinement of skeletal muscle movement. The medulla controls activities such as heart rate, blood pressure, and reflex activities, such as swallowing, coughing, and vomiting. The reticular formation maintains wakefulness and attention.

5. The midbrain, medulla, and pons comprise the brainstem, which connects the hemispheres of the brain, cerebellum, and spinal cord.

6. The spinal cord contains the majority of nerve fibers connecting the brain with the periphery and is divided into cervical, thoracic, lumbar, and sacral regions. The gray matter (cell bodies) of the spinal cord is divided into regions: the anterior (contains the lower motor neurons), posterior (sensory neurons), and lateral horns (autonomic neurons). The white matter is divided into posterior, lateral, and anterior columns. Ascending (sensory) tracts are found in all columns. Descending (motor) tracts are found only in the lateral and anterior columns. Reflex arcs are completed in the spinal cord and influenced by the higher centers in the brain.

7. The major motor tracts are the corticobulbar, lateral corticospinal, and anterior corticospinal and carry motor neurons of the pyramidal tract. The reticulospinal, vestibulospinal, and rubrospinal tracts are extrapyramidal tracts that modulate fine motor movement.

8. The major sensory pathways are the posterior column, spinothalamic, and spinocerebellar tracts.

9. The CNS is protected by the scalp, bony cranium, meninges, vertebral column, and CSF. The CSF is formed from blood components in the choroid plexuses of the ventricles and is reabsorbed in the arachnoid villi (located in the dural venous sinuses) after circulating through the brain and spinal cord.

10. The paired carotid and vertebral arteries supply blood to the brain and connect to form the circle of Willis. The major branches projecting from the circle of Willis are the anterior, middle, and posterior cerebral arteries. Drainage of blood from the brain is accomplished through the venous sinuses and jugular veins.

11. Blood supply to the spinal cord originates from the vertebral arteries and branches arising from the aorta.

12. The blood-brain barrier is composed of endothelial cells in brain capillaries and associated supporting cells. The barrier prevents harmful substances from entering the brain.

Peripheral Nervous System

1. The PNS functions to relay information from the CNS to muscle and effector organs through cranial and spinal nerve tracts arranged in fascicles (multiple fascicles bound together form the peripheral nerve).

2. The 31 pairs of spinal nerves contain sensory and motor neurons.

Autonomic Nervous System

1. The ANS is responsible for the maintenance of a steady state in the internal environment. Two opposing systems constitute the ANS: (a) the sympathetic nervous system responds to stress by mobilizing energy stores and prepares the body to defend itself, and (b) the parasympathetic nervous system conserves energy and the body's resources.

Aging and the Nervous System

1. Major structural changes with aging include a decrease in number of neurons and a decrease in brain weight and size.

2. Decreased amounts of myelin, deposition of lipofuscin, and the presence of neuritic (amyloid) plaques, multiple neurofibrillary tangles, and Lewy bodies are common cellular changes with aging.

3. Cerebral atherosclerosis, decreased vascular density, and increased permeability of the blood-brain barrier occur with aging.

4. Functional changes with aging include diminished sensory functions, sleep disturbances, and memory impairments.

Tests of Nervous System Structure and Function

1. Tests of nervous system structure and function include x-ray films, CT, MRI and MRA, PET, SPECT, cerebral angiography, echoencephalography, electroencephalography, magnetoencephalography, EPs, and analysis of CSF.

■ KEY TERMS

Acetylcholine, 458
α-Adrenergic receptor, 458
β-Adrenergic receptor, 458
Adrenergic transmission, 458
Afferent pathway, 435
Afferent (sensory) neuron, 449
Anterior column, 449
Anterior fossa, 450
Anterior horn (ventral horn), 448
Anterior spinal artery, 454
Anterior spinothalamic tract, 450
Arachnoid mater, 450
Association fiber, 442
Association neuron (interneuron), 435
Autonomic nervous system (ANS), 456
Axon, 435
Axonal reaction, 436
Axon hillock, 435
Basal ganglia system, 445

Bipolar neuron, 435
Blood-brain barrier (BBB), 454
Brachial plexus, 455
Brain, 439
Brain network, 440
Brainstem, 440
Broca area, 442
Cauda equina, 448
Celiac branch of aorta, 458
Central canal, 448
Central nervous system (CNS), 439
Central sulcus (fissure of Rolando), 441
Cerebellomedullary cistern (cisterna magna), 450
Cerebellum, 447
Cerebral angiography, 463
Cerebral aqueduct (aqueduct of Sylvius), 447
Cerebral cortex, 441
Cerebral nuclei, 445

Cerebral peduncle, 447
Cerebrospinal fluid (CSF), 450
Cholinergic transmission, 458
Choroid plexus, 450
Circle of Willis, 453
Collateral ganglia, 458
Computed tomography (CT), 462
Conus medullaris, 447
Convergence, 438
Corpus callosum (transverse commissural fiber), 444
Corticobulbar tract, 442
Corticospinal (pyramidal) tract, 442
Cranial nerve, 456
Craniosacral division, 458
Dendrite, 435
Dendritic zone, 435
Denticulate ligament, 450
Dermatome, 456

KEY TERMS—cont'd

Diencephalon (interbrain), 446
Diffusion tensor imaging (DTI), 463
Divergence, 438
Dopamine, 447
Dorsal root ganglion, 448
Dura mater, 450
Echoencephalography (ultrasound), 463
Effector organ, 435
Efferent (motor) neuron, 449
Efferent pathway, 435
Electroencephalograph (EEG), 464
Epidural space, 450
Epithalamus, 446
Evoked potential (EP), 464
Excitatory postsynaptic potential (EPSP), 438
Extrapyramidal tract, 449
Facilitation, 438
Falx cerebri, 450
Filum terminale, 448
Fissure, 441
Frontal lobe, 441
Functional MRI (fMRI), 463
Galea aponeurotica, 450
Ganglia, 435
Gray matter, 441
Helical CT angiography, 462
Hypothalamus, 446
Inferior colliculi, 446
Inferior mesenteric branch of aorta, 458
Inhibitory postsynaptic potential (IPSP), 438
Inner dura (meningeal layer), 450
Insula (insular lobe), 444
Internal capsule, 445
Intervertebral disk, 451
Lateral column, 449
Lateral horn, 448
Lateral spinothalamic tract, 450
Lateral sulcus (sylvian fissure, lateral fissure), 441
Limbic system, 446
Longitudinal fissure, 441
Lower motor neuron, 449
Lumbar cistern, 450
Lumbar plexus, 456
Magnetic resonance angiography (MRA), 463
Magnetic resonance imaging (MRI), 463
Magnetic resonance spectroscopy (MRS), 463
Magnetoencephalography (MEG), 464
Meninges, 450
Metencephalon, 447
Microfilament, 435
Microtubule, 435

Midbrain (mesencephalon), 446
Middle fossa (temporal fossa), 450
Mixed nerve, 455
Motor neuron, 435
Motor unit, 449
Multipolar neuron, 435
Myelencephalon (medulla oblongata), 447
Myelin, 435
Myelin sheath, 435
Neurofibril, 435
Neuroglia, 435
Neuroglial cell, 435
Neuromuscular junction, 435
Neuromuscular (myoneural) junction, 449
Neuron, 435
Neuroplasticity, 438
Neurotransmitter, 438
Nissl substance/bodies, 435
Nodes of Ranvier, 435
Nonmyelinating Schwann cells, 436
Nuclei, 435
Nucleus pulposus, 451
Occipital lobe, 442
Oligodendroglia, 435
Parasympathetic nervous system, 458
Parietal lobe, 442
Pelvic nerve, 458
Periosteum (endosteal layer), 450
Peripheral nervous system (PNS), 455
Pia mater, 450
Pons, 447
Positron-emission tomography (PET) scan, 463
Postcentral gyrus, 442
Posterior column, 449
Posterior fossa, 450
Posterior horn (dorsal horn), 448
Posterior spinal artery, 454
Postganglionic (unmyelinated) neurons, 456
Postsynaptic neuron, 438
Precentral gyrus, 442
Prefrontal area, 441
Preganglionic (myelinated) neuron, 456
Premotor area, 441
Presynaptic neuron, 438
Primary motor area (Brodmann area 4), 442
Primary voluntary motor area, 442
Projecting artery (nutrient artery), 453
Protopathic, 450
Pseudounipolar neuron, 435

Pyramidal system, 442
Red nucleus, 447
Reflex arc, 449
Reticular activating system, 440
Reticular formation, 440
Roentgenogram (x-ray film), 462
Sacral plexus, 456
Saltatory conduction, 435
Satellite cell, 435
Schwann (neurilemma) cell, 435, 436
Sensory neuron, 435
Single photon emission computed tomography (SPECT), 463
Somatic nervous system, 455
Spatial summation, 438
Spinal cord, 447
Spinal nerve, 455
Spinal tract, 448
Spinothalamic tract, 448
Spiral (helical) CT, 462
Splanchnic nerve, 458
Subarachnoid space, 450
Subdural space, 450
Substantia gelatinosa, 448
Substantia nigra, 447
Subthalamus, 446
Sulci, 441
Summation, 438
Superficial artery (conducting artery), 453
Superior colliculi, 446
Superior mesenteric branch of aorta, 458
Sympathetic (paravertebral) ganglia, 458
Sympathetic nervous system, 458
Synapse, 438
Synaptic cleft, 438
Tectum, 446
Tegmentum, 447
Telencephalon (cerebral hemisphere), 441
Temporal lobe, 442
Temporal summation, 438
Tentorium cerebelli, 450
Thalamus, 446
Thoracolumbar division, 458
Ultrasound, 463
Unipolar neuron, 435
Upper motor neuron, 449
Ventricle, 450
Vertebral column, 451
Wernicke area, 444
White matter, 441

REFERENCES

1. Gundersen V, Storm-Mathisen J, Bergersen LH: Neuroglial transmission. *Physiol Rev* 95(3):695–726, 2015.
2. Jones S, Eisenberg HM, Jia X: Advances and future applications of augmented peripheral nerve regeneration. *Int J Mol Sci* 17(9):2016.
3. Mustafa AK, Gazi SK: Neurotransmitters: overview. In Aminoff MJ, Daroff RB, editors: *Reference module in biomedical sciences, encyclopedia of the neurological sciences*, ed 2, St Louis, 2014, Elsevier, pp 565–572.
4. Kolb B, Whishaw IQ: *An introduction to brain and behavior.* New York, 2011, Worth.
5. Vanderah T, Gould D: *Nolte's the human brain: an introduction to its functional anatomy*, ed 7, St Louis, 2015, Mosby.
6. Craddock RC, Tungaraza RL, Milham MP: Connectomics and new approaches for analyzing human brain functional connectivity. *Gigascience* 4:13, 2015.
7. Fornito A, Bullmore ET: Connectomics: a new paradigm for understanding brain disease. *Eur Neuropsychopharmacol* 25(5):733–748, 2015.
8. Serlin Y, et al: Anatomy and physiology of the blood-brain barrier. *Semin Cell Dev Biol* 38:2–6, 2015.
9. Beaulieu JM, Espinoza S, Gainetdinov RR: Dopamine receptors—IUPHAR review 13. *Br J Pharmacol* 172(1):1–23, 2015.

Pain, Temperature Regulation, Sleep, and Sensory Function

Sue E. Huether, George W. Rodway

WEBSITE

http://evolve.elsevier.com/McCance/
- Content Updates
- Chapter Summary Review
- Review Questions
- Case Studies
- Animations

CHAPTER OUTLINE

Alterations in sensory function may involve dysfunctions of the general or the special senses. Dysfunctions of the general senses include chronic pain and abnormal temperature regulation. Somatosensory alterations include tactile, proprioceptive, and vestibular dysfunction.

Pain is a unique sensory experience that, although universally described as unpleasant, is nonetheless essential to an individual's survival. Pain provides protection by signaling the presence of disease or injury. Unlike pain, which need not be a part of everyday life, temperature is carefully monitored and regulated within clearly defined normal limits. Like pain, however, variations in temperature can signal disease. Fever is a common manifestation of dysfunction and is often the first symptom observed in an infectious or inflammatory condition.

Sleep is a normal, cyclic process that restores the body's energy and maintains normal functioning. Sleep is so essential to physiologic and psychologic function that sleep deprivation causes a wide range of clinical manifestations. Prolonged deprivation or disruption of sleep ultimately leads to serious dysfunction.

The special senses of vision, hearing, touch, smell, and taste are the means by which individuals perceive stimuli that are essential for interacting with the environment. Special sensory receptors are connected to specific areas of the brain through the afferent pathways of the peripheral and central nervous system (CNS). Each of the special senses thus involves a connected system of organs and tissues that receives stimuli and sends sensory messages to areas of the CNS, where they are processed and guide behavior. Dysfunctions of the special senses include visual, auditory, olfactory, and gustatory (taste).

PAIN

Pain is one of the body's most important adaptive and protective mechanisms. It is a complex experience composed of dynamic interactions among physical, cognitive, spiritual, emotional, and environmental factors and cannot be characterized as only a response to injury. The International Association for the Study of Pain (IASP) and accepted by the American Pain Society and the World Health Organization define pain as "an unpleasant sensory and emotional experience associated with actual or potential tissue damage or described in terms of such damage."[1] McCaffery defined pain as "whatever the experiencing person says it is, existing whenever he says it does."[2] Waddell defines pain as "a symptom, not a clinical sign, diagnosis or disease."[3]

Theories of Pain

The theories of pain include the specificity theory, pattern theory, gate control theory, and neuromatrix theory.[4] Specificity theory proposes that pain and touch are carried on distinct pathways that project to distinct brain centers. Injury activates only specific pain receptors and fibers that project to the brain. *Intensity of pain* is directly related to the amount of associated tissue injury (i.e., pricking one's finger with a needle would cause minimal pain, whereas cutting one's hand with a knife would produce more pain). The theory is useful when applied to specific injuries and the acute pain associated with them. It does not account for chronic pain or cognitive and emotional elements that contribute to more complex types of pain.[5]

Pattern theory proposes that any somatic sense organs respond to a dynamic range of stimulus intensities. Different sense organs have different levels of responsiveness to stimuli with different spatial and temporal profiles of firing. The patterns of impulse intensity are encoded in the central nervous system (CNS). The pattern theory is limited because it does not account for all types of pain experiences.[4]

Gate control theory (GCT) integrates and builds upon features of the other theories to explain the complex multidimensional aspects of pain perception and pain modulation. Pain transmission is modulated by a balance of impulses conducted to the spinal cord where cells in the substantia gelatinosa function as a "gate." The spinal gate regulates pain transmission to higher centers in the CNS. Large myelinated A-delta fibers and small unmyelinated C fibers respond to a broad range of painful stimuli (mechanical, thermal, and chemical). These fibers terminate on interneurons in the substantia gelatinosa (laminae in the dorsal horn of the spinal cord) and "open" the spinal gate to transmit the perception of pain. Closure or partial closure of the spinal gates can occur from nonnociceptive stimulation (i.e., from touch sensors in the skin) carried on large A-beta fibers decreasing pain perception. This is why rubbing a painful area may alleviate some of the discomfort. Other efferent CNS pathways descend to the spinal cord and may close, partially close, or open the gate modulating the pain experience. The gate control theory, bolstered by progress in understanding neuronal pathways in the peripheral and central nervous systems, has greatly advanced the understanding of pain. As good as the GCT has been, however, there are observations about phantom pain in paraplegics and other pain syndromes that "do not fit the theory."[6]

Neuromatrix theory is an advancement of the gate control theory and proposes that the brain produces patterns of nerve impulses drawn from various inputs, including genetic, sensory-discriminative, affective-motivational, and evaluative-cognitive experiences.[7] The qualities individuals normally feel from the body, including pain, also can be felt in the absence of inputs from the body (as noted with phantom limb pain). In other words, stimuli may trigger the patterns but do not produce them. Neuromatrix patterns are normally activated by sensory inputs from the periphery, but may originate independently in the brain with no external input. The pain experience involves an extensive network of brain regions and networks that may shift and evolve over time.[8] The neuromatrix theory illustrates the plasticity (adaptable change in structure and function) of the brain.[9] It does not supplant the understanding of the gate theory and what has been learned about peripheral inflammation, spinal modulation, and midbrain descending control of pain. The neuromatrix theory expands on the gate control theory by explicating a body-self that provides a holistic, integrated, dynamic consideration of pain. However, there are many different kinds of pain, and no single theory is adequate to explain the complex dynamics of the pain experience. Continuing research is advancing the understanding of the neural mechanisms of pain.

Neuroanatomy of Pain

The integrated function of three components of the nervous system mediates the sensation, perception, and response to pain:

1. The afferent pathways, which begin in the peripheral nervous system (PNS), travel to the spinal gate in the dorsal horn and then ascend to higher centers in the CNS
2. The interpretive centers located in the brainstem, midbrain, diencephalon (thalamus, hypothalamus, epithalamus, and subthalamus), and cerebral cortex
3. The efferent pathways that descend from the CNS to the dorsal horn of the spinal cord

The processing of potentially harmful (noxious) stimuli through a normally functioning nervous system is called nociception. Nociceptors are free nerve endings in the afferent peripheral nervous system that selectively respond to different chemical, mechanical, and thermal stimuli. When stimulated, they cause nociceptive pain. Nociceptors are unevenly distributed throughout the body, so the relative sensitivity to pain differs according to their location (Table 16.1). For example, fingertips have more nociceptors than the skin of the back, and all skin has many more

TABLE 16.1	STIMULI THAT ACTIVATE NOCICEPTORS (PAIN RECEPTORS)
LOCATION OF RECEPTOR	**PROVOKING STIMULI**
Skin	Pricking, cutting, crushing, burning, freezing, inflammation
Gastrointestinal tract	Engorged or inflamed mucosa, distention or spasm of smooth muscle, traction on mesenteric attachment
Skeletal muscle	Ischemia, injuries of connective tissue sheaths, necrosis, hemorrhage, prolonged contraction, injection of irritating solutions
Bone	Periosteal injury, inflammation, fractures, tumors
Joints	Synovial membrane inflammation
Arteries	Piercing, inflammation
Head	Traction, inflammation, or displacement of arteries, meningeal structures, and sinuses; prolonged muscle contraction
Heart	Ischemia and inflammation

nociceptors than the internal organs. Unlike sensory neurons of the special senses of vision, gustation, and olfaction (discussed later), which are required to detect only one type of sensory stimulus (e.g., light for the sense of vision), primary nociceptive afferents have the remarkable ability to detect a wide range of stimuli. To do this, nociceptors are equipped with an array of transduction channels that can sense different forms of noxious stimulation and at different intensities. In addition to the previously well-studied voltage-gated potassium, sodium, and calcium channels, there are multiple types of transmembrane receptors (called *transient receptor potential [TRP] channels*), which reside on "naked nerve endings" and respond to a variety of physical, chemical, and thermal stimuli.[10]

Nociceptors *(primary order neurons)* are categorized according to the stimulus to which they respond and by the properties of the axons associated with them. **A-delta (Aδ) fibers** are lightly myelinated, medium-sized fibers that are stimulated by severe mechanical deformation *(mechanonociceptors)* or by mechanical deformation and/or extremes of temperature *(mechanothermal nociceptors)*. Aδ fibers rapidly transmit sharp, well-localized "fast" pain sensations. These fibers are responsible for causing reflex withdrawal of the affected body part from the stimulus before a pain sensation is perceived. The smaller **unmyelinated C fibers** are polymodal and are stimulated by mechanical, thermal, and chemical nociceptors. The unmyelinated C fibers slowly transmit dull, aching, or burning sensations that are poorly localized and longer lasting. **A-beta (Aβ) fibers** are large myelinated fibers that transmit touch and vibration sensations. They do not normally transmit pain but play a role in pain modulation.[11] Nociception involves four phases: transduction (stimulation of nociceptors in the periphery), transmission (axonal conduction), perception (cortical processing of stimuli), and modulation (descending pathways and neurotransmitters that inhibit or amplify pain).

Pain transduction begins when tissue is damaged by exposure to chemical (acids or chemicals of inflammation, such as bradykinin, histamine, leukotrienes, prostaglandins, interleukin [IL]-1, IL-6, IL-7, IL-17), mechanical (pressure or stretch), or thermal (extreme temperatures) noxious stimuli and is translated into electrophysiological activity. This causes activation of nociceptors.

Pain transmission is the conduction of pain impulses along the Aδ and C fibers (primary order neurons) into the dorsal horn of the spinal cord (Fig. 16.1). Here they form synapses with excitatory or inhibitory interneurons (second-order neurons) that may branch into ascending or descending collaterals for one or two cord segments in neuronal projections called the *dorsolateral tract*. Eventually all of the primary afferents terminate on interneurons in the *marginal layer* (laminae I) or *substantia gelatinosa* (laminae II) of the spinal cord (Fig. 16.2). The impulses then synapse with projection neurons (third order neurons), cross the midline of the spinal cord, and ascend to the brain through two lateral spinothalamic tracts. The neospinothalamic tract (anterior spinal thalamic tract) carries fast impulses for acute sharp pain. The paleospinothalamic tract (lateral spinothalamic tract) carries slow impulses for dull or chronic pain. The fast sharp pain is perceived first, followed by dull, throbbing pain. These tracts connect to the reticular formation, hypothalamus, thalamus (the major relay station of sensory information), and limbic system. The impulses are then projected to the somatosensory cortex for interpretation of location and intensity of pain, and to other areas of the brain for an integrated response to pain (Fig. 16.3).[12]

Pain perception is the conscious awareness of pain that occurs primarily in the reticular and limbic systems and the cerebral cortex. Three systems interact to produce the perception of pain and it changes with age (Table 16.2). The **sensory-discriminative system** is mediated

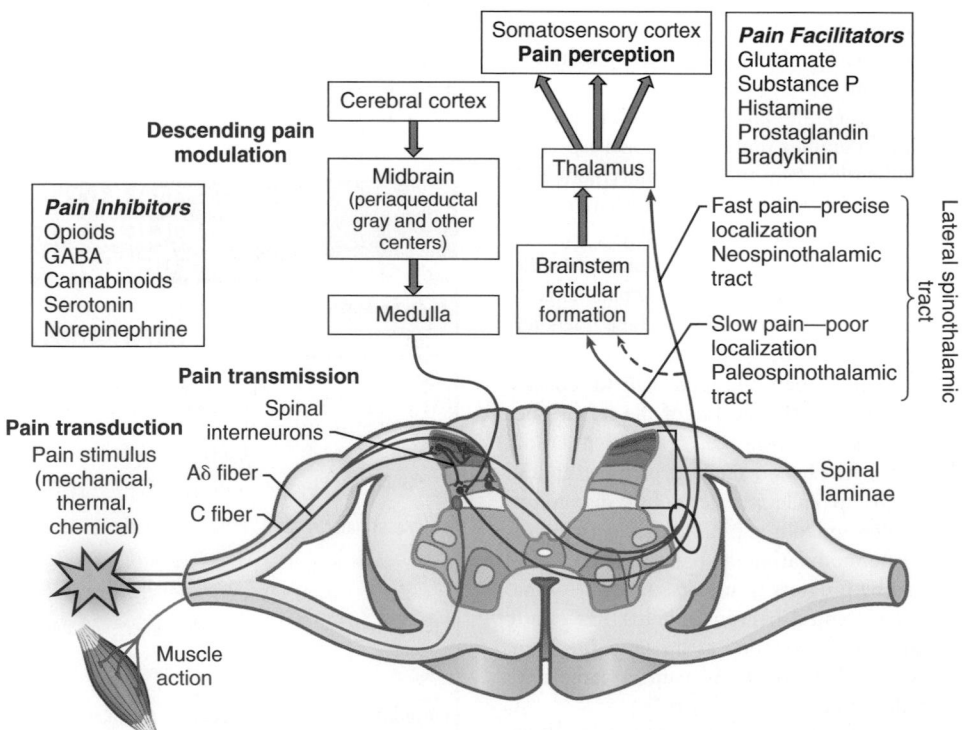

FIGURE 16.1 Transmission of Pain Sensations. The Aδ and C fibers synapse in the laminae of the dorsal horn, cross over to the contralateral spinothalamic tract, and then ascend to synapse in the midbrain through the neospinothalamic (lateral spinothalamic tract) and paleospinothalamic tracts (anterior spinothalamic tracts). Impulses are then conducted to the sensory cortex. Descending pain inhibition is initiated in the cerebral cortex or from the midbrain and medulla. *GABA,* Gamma-aminobutyric acid.

by the somatosensory cortex and is responsible for identifying the presence, character, location, and intensity of pain. The affective-motivational system determines an individual's conditioned avoidance behaviors and emotional responses to pain. It is mediated through the reticular formation, limbic system, and brainstem with projections to the prefrontal cortex. The cognitive-evaluative system overlies the individual's learned behavior concerning the experience of pain and can modulate perception of pain. It is mediated through the cerebral cortex. Pain threshold and tolerance are subjective phenomena that influence an individual's perception of pain. They can be influenced by genetics, gender, cultural perceptions, expectations, role socialization, physical and mental health, and age.

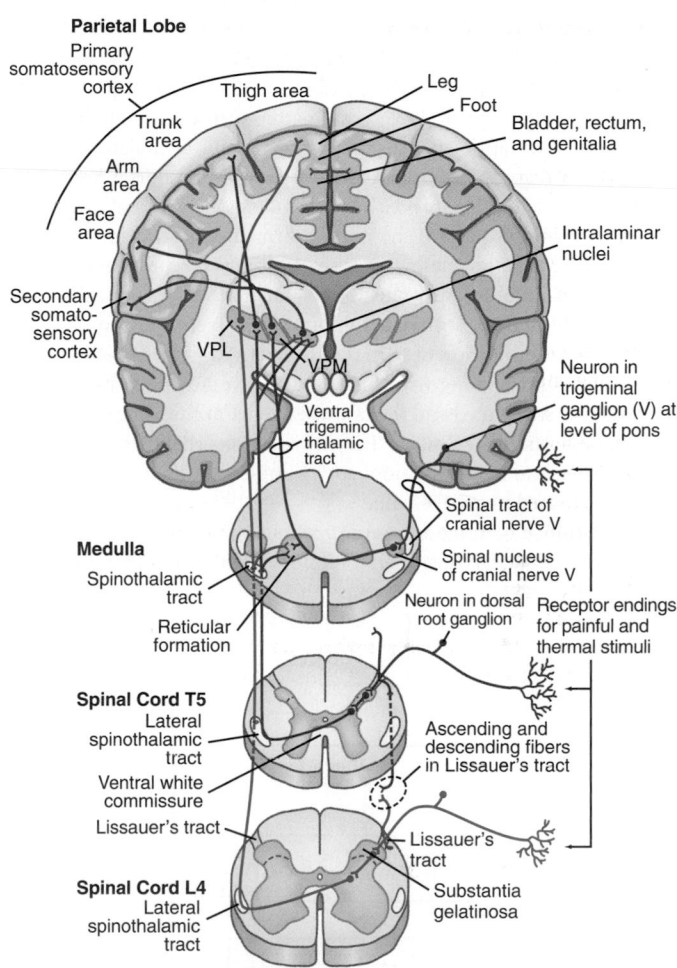

FIGURE 16.2 Nociception Pathways. Aδ and C fibers comprise the primary, first-order sensory afferents coming into the gate at the dorsal horn of the spinal cord. Second-order neurons cross the cord ("decussate") and ascend to the thalamus as part of the spinothalamic tract. Third-order afferents project to higher brain centers of the limbic system, the frontal cortex, and the primary sensory cortex of the postcentral gyrus of the parietal lobe.

FIGURE 16.3 Central Nervous System Pathways That Mediate the Sensations of Pain and Temperature. *VPL*, Ventral posterior lateral thalamic nuclei; *VPM*, ventral posterior medial thalamic nuclei.

TABLE 16.2	**PAIN PERCEPTION IN INFANTS, CHILDREN, AND OLDER PERSONS**		
	INFANTS	**CHILDREN**	**OLDER PERSONS**
Pain threshold	Painful neonatal experiences increase pain sensitivity (lower threshold); pain may be increased with future procedures	Lower or same as adults	Individual responses may vary but pain threshold may be lower
Physiologic symptoms	Increased heart rate, blood pressure, and respiratory rate; flushing or pallor, sweating, and decreased oxygen saturation	Same as infants; nausea and vomiting	Same as infants and children; nausea and vomiting; may be decreased in individuals with cognitive impairment
Behavioral responses	Changes in facial expression, crying, and body movements, with lowered brows drawn together; vertical bulge and furrows in forehead between brows; broadened nasal root; tightly closed eyes; angular, square-shaped mouth, chin quiver; withdrawal of affected limbs, rigidity, flailing	Individual responses vary	Individual responses vary and may be influenced by presence of painful chronic diseases and decline in renal, intestinal, hepatic, cardiovascular, and neurologic function; individuals with cognitive impairment may demonstrate changes in behavior (e.g., combative or withdrawn, increased confusion)

Data from Maxwell LG et al: *Clin Perinatol* 40(3):457-469, 2013; Molton IR, Terrill AL: *Am Psychol* 69(2):197-207, 2014; Tracy B, Sean Morrison R: *Clin Ther* 35(11):1659-1668, 2013; Walker SM: *Paediatr Anaesth* 24(1):39-48, 2014.

Pain Modulation

Pain modulation involves many different mechanisms that increase or decrease the transmission of pain signals throughout the nervous system. Depending on the mechanism, modulation can occur before, during, or after pain is perceived.[13]

Pathways of Modulation

Descending inhibitory or facilitatory pathways, nuclei, and neurotransmitters inhibit or facilitate pain. Afferent stimulation of particularly the periaqueductal gray (PAG; gray matter surrounding the cerebral aqueduct) and raphe nucleus in the midbrain stimulates efferent pathways, which inhibit afferent pain signals at the dorsal horn. The rostroventromedial medulla (RVM) stimulates efferent pathways that facilitate or inhibit pain in the dorsal horn through the dorsal lateral funiculus.[14] Inhibitory pathways activate opioid receptors and inhibit release of excitatory neurotransmitters, facilitate release of inhibitory neurotransmitters, or stimulate inhibitory interneurons (Fig. 16.4).

Segmental inhibition of pain occurs when Aβ fibers (which synapse in the dorsal horn along with their nociceptive Aδ and C fiber counterparts) are stimulated and the impulses arrive at the same spinal level as impulses from Aδ or C fibers. They stimulate an inhibitory interneuron and decrease pain transmission. An example is rubbing an area that has been injured to relieve pain.[13]

Conditioned pain modulation (previously known as *diffuse noxious inhibitory control [DNIC]*) is an inhibitory pain system that involves a spinal-medullary-spinal pathway. Pain is relieved when two noxious stimuli occur at the same time from different sites (pain inhibiting pain). This also is known as *heterosegmental pain inhibition* (simultaneous pain stimulation and pain inhibition) and is the basis for pain relief with acupuncture, deep massage, or intense cold or heat.[15]

Expectancy-related cortical activation (placebo effect [positive expectations] or nocebo effect [adverse expectations]) can exert control over analgesic systems to attenuate or intensify pain. In other words, cognitive expectations can cause real, measurable physiologic effects that share some of the same descending pain pathways as the pain modulatory systems.[16]

Neurotransmitters of Pain Modulation

A wide variety of neurotransmitters act to modulate control over transmission of pain impulses in the periphery, spinal cord, and brain (Box 16.1).[17,18] The peripheral triggering mechanisms that initiate release of excitatory neurotransmitters include tissue injury and inflammation (prostaglandins, histamine, bradykinin, tumor necrosis factor-alpha [TNF-α], nitric oxide) and chronic inflammatory lesions (lymphokines). Activity within nociceptors or damage to them causes release of peptides and neurotransmitters, such as tachykinins (e.g., substance P and neurokinins), calcitonin gene–related peptide (CGRP), and adenosine triphosphate (ATP). Glutamate, aspartate, substance P, and calcitonin are common excitatory neurotransmitters in the brain and spinal cord. These substances reduce the activation threshold, leading to increased responsiveness of nociceptors

Inhibitory neurotransmitters in the spinal cord include gamma-aminobutyric acid (GABA) and glycine. Norepinephrine and 5-hydroxytryptamine (serotonin) contribute to pain inhibition in the medulla and pons but can excite peripheral nerves.[18,19]

Endogenous opioids are a family of morphine-like neuropeptides that inhibit transmission of pain impulses in the spinal cord, brain, and periphery. Their receptors also play a role in various central nervous,

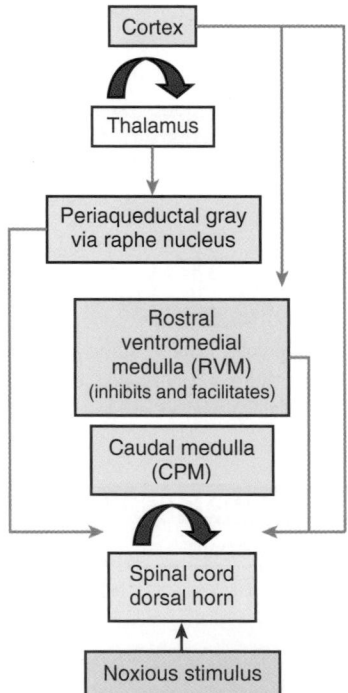

FIGURE 16.4 Diagram Representing the Central Mechanisms of Pain Modulation. A noxious peripheral stimulus activates both segmental and top-down (corticofugal and bulbospinal heterosegmental) modulatory mechanisms, which either accentuate or inhibit afferent pain transmission to the brain. The most important and widespread source of top-down (corticofugal) modulation arises from the cortex. Both thalamic and prethalamic nociceptive relays are under the influence of this top-down control. The dorsal horn of the spine is also under the influence of the caudal medulla through conditioned pain modulation (CPM). (Modified from Villanueva L, Fields HL: *The pain system in normal and pathological states: a primer for clinicians,* Seattle, 2004, IASP Press.)

BOX 16.1   MEDIATORS THAT ACTIVATE NOCICEPTORS

Excitatory Mediators (Inflammatory)
Bradykinin
Leukotrienes
Prostaglandins
Serotonin
Substance P
Interleukins 1, 6, 7, 17
Tumor necrosis factor-alpha
Nitric oxide
ATP
Neurokinins
Calcitonin gene–related peptide

Excitatory Transmitters
Glutamate (fast pain)
NMDA
AMPA
Tachykinins
Neurokinin A

Neurokinin B
Substance P
Calcitonin gene–related peptides
Somatostatins
Bombesins
Cholecystokinins

Inhibitory Mediators
Gamma-aminobutyric acid (GABA)
Glycine
Descending pain modulators
　　Norepinephrine–α₂-receptors
　　Serotonin (5-hydroxytryptamine)
Opioids (μ, δ, κ receptors)
Endorphins ⎫ Released from PAG
Enkephalins ⎬ and NRM and
Dynorphins ⎭ other areas of
　　　　　　　the brain

AMPA, α-Amino-3-hydroxy-5-methyl-4-isoxazole-propionate; *ATP,* adenosine triphosphate; *NMDA, N*-methyl-D-aspartate; *NRM,* nucleus raphes magnus; *PAG,* periaqueductal gray.

gastrointestinal, immune, and other organ system disorders. There are four types of opioid neuropeptides: (1) *enkephalins,* (2) *endorphins,* (3) *dynorphins,* and (4) *endomorphins.* These neurohormones act as neurotransmitters by binding to one or more G-protein-coupled opioid receptors. There are three specific types of neuron opioid receptors: mu (μ), kappa (κ), and delta (δ). A fourth receptor subtype is nociception-opioid peptide (NOP), and its ligand is nociceptin/orphanin FQ.

Each receptor type binds differently with the various types of opioids. They inhibit ion channels in the dorsal horn, preventing the release of excitatory neurotransmitters, such as substance P and glutamate, or other areas of the brain such as the PAG or rostral ventromedial nuclei in the brainstem (Fig. 16.5). In the midbrain they influence descending inhibitory pathways.[20] In peripheral inflamed tissue, opioids are produced and released from leukocytes and activate opioid receptors on sensory nerve terminals.[21] Because leukocyte opioids do not cross the blood-brain barrier, they do not have central nervous system side effects, such as respiratory depression, somnolence, or addiction. Opioid receptors are widely distributed throughout the body and are responsible for general sensations of well-being and modulation of many physiologic processes, including control of respiratory and cardiovascular functions, stress and immune responses, gastrointestinal function, reproduction, and neuroendocrine control.[22,23]

Enkephalins are the most prevalent of the natural opioids and bind to δ opioid receptors. They are concentrated in the hypothalamus, the PAG matter, the nucleus raphe magnus of the medulla, and the dorsal horns of the spinal cord.

Endorphins (endogenous morphine) are produced in the brain. The best studied endorphin, β-endorphin, binds to μ receptors in the hypothalamus and pituitary gland and is purported to produce the greatest sense of exhilaration as well as substantial natural pain relief.

Dynorphins are the most potent of the endogenous opioids binding strongly with κ receptors to impede pain signals in the brain. They play a role in mood disorders and drug addiction and paradoxically in stimulating chronic pain.[24] Endomorphins-1 and -2 bind with μ receptors throughout the brain, brainstem, and gastrointestinal tract and have analgesic and antiinflammatory effects.[25,26]

Nociceptin/orphanin FQ produces antiopioid hyperalgesic effects in supraspinal pain pathways, while exerting analgesic properties in spinal pain pathways. It does not interact with opioid receptors. The nociceptin receptor (κ-type 3 opioid receptor) is widely distributed throughout the peripheral and central nervous system; is associated with inflammation, immune regulation, feeding behavior, and mood elevation; and blunts addictive behavior.[27]

In addition to analgesic effects, endogenous opioids are involved in a variety of other functions throughout the body, including modulation of stress and anxiety, feeding behavior, cough suppression, immune and inflammatory responses, and alcohol intake.[28] Endogenous opioids of one type or another are found to bind to almost all tissues in the body and thus affect numerous biologic functions.[29]

Pain Threshold and Pain Tolerance

Pain threshold is the point at which a stimulus is perceived as pain, and it does not vary significantly among people or in the same person over time. Intense pain at one location, however, may cause an increase in the threshold in another location. For example, a person with severe pain in one knee is more likely to experience chronic back pain that is less intense. This phenomenon is called perceptual dominance. Because of perceptual dominance, pain at one site may mask other painful areas.

Pain tolerance is the duration of time or the intensity of pain that an individual will endure before initiating overt pain responses and is generally decreased with repeated exposure to pain. Pain tolerance is influenced by the person's cultural perceptions, expectations, role behaviors, physical and mental health, gender, age, fatigue, anger, boredom, apprehension, and sleep deprivation (see Table 16.2). Tolerance

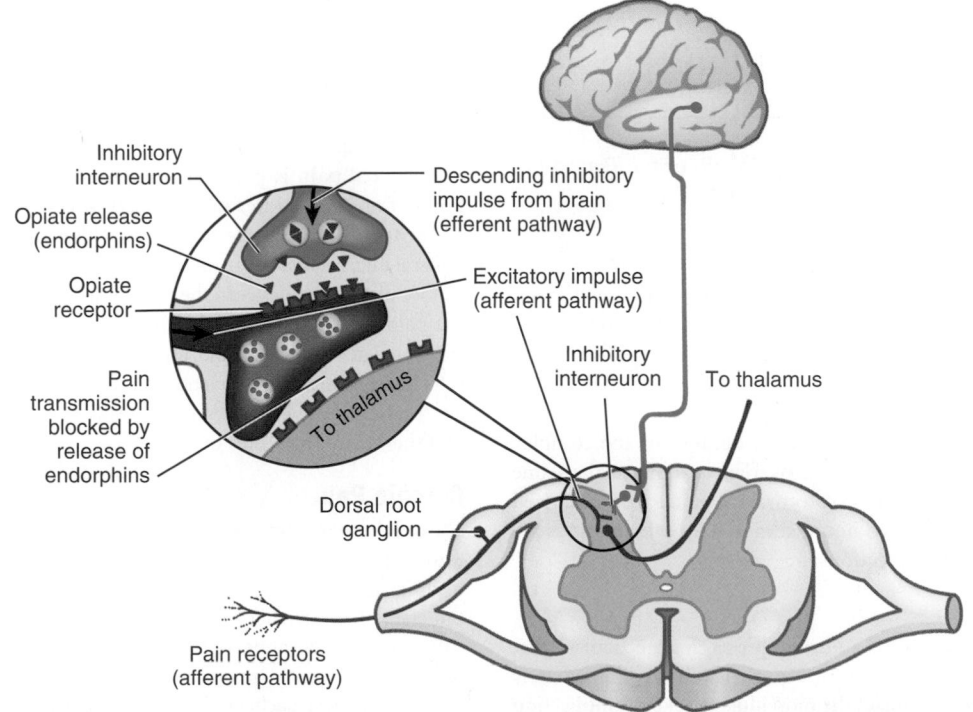

FIGURE 16.5 Descending Pathway and Endorphin Response. In this figure, a descending inhibitory impulse is transmitted from the brain to an inhibitory interneuron in the dorsal horn, stimulating the release of endorphin. The endorphin activates a mu opioid receptor and results in inhibition of pain transmission to ascending pathways.

BOX 16.2 CATEGORIES OF PAIN

I.   Neurophysiologic Pain
A. Nociceptive pain
   1. Somatic (e.g., fracture, thermal, or traumatic injury)
   2. Visceral (e.g., bowel obstruction, endometriosis, gastritis)
   3. Referred (e.g., ureteral distention localizes to testicle, angina localizes to arm, neck, or back)
B. Neuropathic (nonnociceptive)
   1. Central pain (lesion/dysfunction in brain or spinal cord)
   2. Peripheral pain (lesion/dysfunction in peripheral nervous system [PNS])

II.   Neurogenic Pain
A. Neuralgia (pain in the distribution of a nerve)
B. Constant
   1. Sympathetically independent
   2. Sympathetically dependent

III.   Temporal Pain (Time Related)
A. Acute pain
B. Chronic

IV.   Regional Pain
A. Abdominal pain
B. Chest pain
C. Headache
D. Low back pain
E. Orofacial pain
F. Pelvic pain
G. Joint pain

V.   Etiologic Pain
A. Cancer pain
B. Dental pain
C. Inflammatory pain (e.g., infection, trauma)
D. Ischemic pain
E. Vascular pain
F. Postoperative pain

Adapted from Derasari MD: Taxonomy of pain syndromes: classification of chronic pain syndromes. In Raj PP, editor: *Practical management of pain*, ed 3, St Louis, 2000, Mosby.

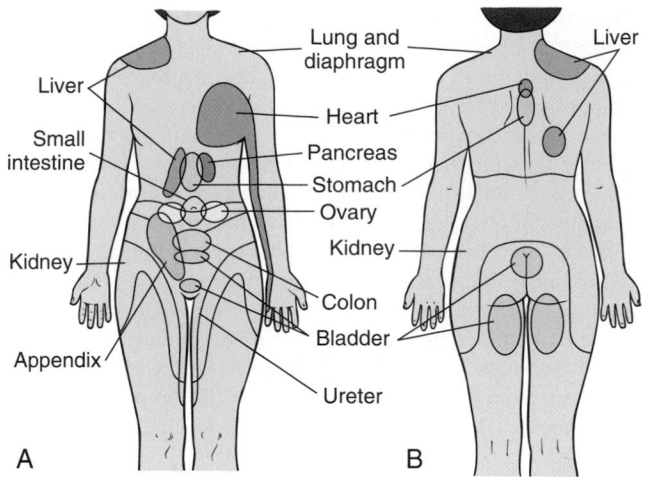

FIGURE 16.6 Sites of Referred Pain. **A,** Front. **B,** Back.

may be increased by alcohol consumption, persistent use of pain medication, hypnosis, warmth, distracting activities, and strong beliefs or faith.[30]

Clinical Descriptions of Pain

Pain can be described in a variety of ways. Because of the complex nature of pain, however, many terms overlap and more than one description is often used. The broad categories of pain are summarized in Box 16.2. Some of the most common clinical pain presentations are summarized in the following sections.

Acute Pain

Acute pain (nociceptive pain) is a normal protective mechanism that alerts the individual to a condition or experience that is immediately harmful to the body and mobilizes the individual to take prompt action to relieve it. Acute pain is transient, usually lasting seconds to days, and sometimes up to 3 months.[31] It begins suddenly and is relieved after the chemical mediators that stimulate pain receptors are removed.

Stimulation of the autonomic nervous system results in physical manifestations including increased heart rate, hypertension, diaphoresis, and dilated pupils. Anxiety related to the pain experience, including its cause, treatment, and prognosis, is common and there is expectation of limited duration.

Acute pain arises from cutaneous and deep somatic tissue, or from visceral organs, and can be classified as (1) somatic, (2) visceral, or (3) referred. Somatic pain arises from muscle, bone, joints, and skin. It is either sharp and well localized (especially fast pain carried by Aδ fibers) or dull, aching, throbbing, and poorly localized as seen in polymodal C fiber transmissions.

Visceral pain is transmitted by C fibers and refers to pain in internal organs and the lining of body cavities with an aching, gnawing, throbbing, or intermittent cramping quality. It is transmitted by sympathetic afferents and tends to be poorly localized, because of the lesser number of nociceptors in the visceral structures. Visceral pain is associated with nausea and vomiting, hypotension, restlessness, and, in some cases, shock. It often radiates (spreads away from the actual site of the pain) or is referred.

Referred pain is pain felt in an area removed or distant from its point of origin. The area of referred pain is supplied by the same spinal segment as the actual site of pain. Impulses from many cutaneous and visceral neurons converge on the same ascending neuron, and the brain cannot distinguish between the two. Because the skin has more receptors, the painful sensation is experienced at the referred site instead of the site of origin.[32] For example, an inflamed gallbladder or pancreas may refer pain to the shoulder and scapular regions. Referred pain can be acute or chronic. Fig. 16.6 illustrates common areas of referred pain and their associated sites of origin.

Chronic Pain

Chronic or persistent pain is usually defined as lasting for more than 3 to 6 months and is pain lasting well beyond the expected normal healing time. Chronic or persistent pain serves no purpose, is poorly understood, is often accompanied by anxiety and depression, and causes suffering. It often appears to be out of proportion to any observable tissue injury. It may be ongoing (e.g., low back pain) or intermittent (e.g., migraine headaches). Changes in the peripheral and central nervous systems that cause dysregulation of nociception and pain modulation processes (peripheral and central sensitization) are thought to lead to chronic pain (see Neuropathic Pain, described later in this section).

TABLE 16.3	COMPARISON OF ACUTE AND CHRONIC PAIN	
CHARACTERISTIC	**ACUTE PAIN**	**CHRONIC PAIN**
Experience	An event	A situation; state of existence
Source	External agent or internal disease usually known	Unknown; if known, treatment is prolonged or ineffective
Onset	Usually sudden	May be sudden or develop insidiously
Duration	Transient (up to 6 months)	Prolonged and persistent (months to years)
Pain identification	Painful and nonpainful areas generally well identified	Painful and nonpainful areas less easily differentiated; change in sensations becomes more difficult to evaluate
Clinical signs	Increased pulse rate, elevated blood pressure, increased respiratory rate, diaphoresis, dilated pupils	Response patterns vary; fewer overt signs (adaptation)
Significance	Significant (informs person something is wrong)	Person looks for significance
Pattern	Self-limiting or readily corrected	Continuous or intermittent; intensity may vary or remain constant
Course	Suffering usually decreases over time	Suffering usually increases over time
Actions	Leads to actions to relieve pain	Leads to actions to modify pain experience
Prognosis	Likelihood of eventual complete relief	Complete relief usually not possible

Data from Black RG: *Surg Clin North Am* 55(4):999, 1975.

Neuroimaging studies (functional, structural, and neurochemical imaging) have demonstrated brain changes (neuroplasticity) in individuals with chronic pain which can lead to the maintenance of pain even in the absence of the original nociceptive input. These negative manifestations of chronic pain are thought to be caused by, in part, the stress of coping with continuous pain and may be reversible when pain is controlled.[33,34] Because it is not yet possible to predict when acute pain will develop into chronic pain, early treatment of acute pain is encouraged.

Neuropathic pain is chronic pain initiated or caused by a primary lesion or dysfunction in the nervous system and leads to long-term changes in pain pathway structures (neuroplasticity) and abnormal processing of sensory information.[35] There is amplification of pain without stimulation by injury or inflammation. Neuropathic pain is often described as burning, shooting, shocklike, or tingling. It is characterized by hyperalgesia, increased sensitivity to a normally painful stimulus (touch, pressure, pinprick, cold, and heat), or allodynia, the induction of pain by normally nonpainful stimuli.[36] Neuropathic pain is classified as either peripheral or central and is associated with central and peripheral sensitization.[37]

Peripheral neuropathic pain is caused by peripheral nerve lesions and an increase in the sensitivity and excitability of primary sensory neurons and cells in the dorsal root ganglion (peripheral sensitization). Examples include nerve entrapment, diabetic neuropathy, or chronic pancreatitis. Central neuropathic pain is caused by a lesion or neuroplastic changes in the brain or spinal cord. A progressive repeated stimulation of group C neurons (wind-up) in the dorsal horn leads to increased sensitivity of central pain signaling neurons (central sensitization). This results in pathologic changes in the CNS that cause chronic pain. Examples include brain or spinal cord trauma, tumors, vascular lesions, multiple sclerosis, Parkinson disease, postherpetic neuralgia, and phantom limb pain.

The following mechanisms have been implicated in the cause of neuropathic pain:[35,38]

- Changes in sensitivity of neurons—lower threshold with peripheral and central sensitization
- Spontaneous impulses from regenerating peripheral nerves

- Alterations in the dorsal root ganglion in response to peripheral nerve injury and neurotransmitters—reorganization of nociceptive neurons (deafferentation pain)
- Loss of GABAergic pain inhibition in the spinal cord
- Activation of microglia and upregulation of nociceptive chemokines and their receptors
- Structural and functional alterations in brain processing neural networks

Comparison of acute and chronic pain is summarized in Table 16.3. Common chronic pain conditions are listed in Table 16.4.

An Overview of Chronic Pain Syndromes. Specific spinal pain (i.e., intervertebral disk degeneration) and nonspecific spinal pain (i.e., low back pain not attributable to a specific pathologic source) are global, common, chronic, and disabling pain conditions (see Chapter 18). The prevalence of nonspecific low back pain is about 23% with 11% to 12% of those affected being disabled.[39,40] Prevalence estimates and definition of risk factors vary among studies depending on the definition of low back pain used. Acute back pain is relatively rare, and many individuals of all ages have chronic recurrent back pain. Common causes include muscle tension and spasm (i.e., fibromyalgia; degeneration, including disk hernia, lumbar stenosis, and osteoarthritis; and fractures, mostly in those with osteoporosis).[41] Both cortical and spinal alterations in pain processing are associated with low back pain.[42] Treatment is individualized and often ineffective, and the personal and societal burden is great.[43,44]

Myofascial pain syndrome (MPS) is a regional pain syndrome associated with injury to muscle, fascia, and tendons and includes myositis, fibrositis, myofibrositis, myalgia (see Chapter 45 for fibromyalgia), and muscle strain. These conditions involve myofascial trigger points within a taut band of skeletal muscle. The pain may be the result of low-threshold mechanosensitive afferents projecting to sensitized dorsal horn neurons and the development of peripheral and central sensitization.[45] Neuroaxonal degeneration with alterations in neuromuscular transmission (i.e., extra leakage of acetylcholine at the neuromuscular junction induces persistent contraction) may occur.[46] Compression of the trigger point causes referred pain, motor dysfunction, and autonomic responses. During the early stages of the disorder the

TABLE 16.4   COMMON CHRONIC PAIN CONDITIONS

CONDITION	DESCRIPTION
Persistent low back pain	Most common chronic pain condition Results from poor muscle tone, inactivity, muscle strain, or sudden, vigorous exercise
Myofascial pain syndromes	Second most common chronic pain condition Pain results from muscle spasm, tenderness, and stiffness Examples include myositis, fibrositis, myofibrositis, myalgia, and muscle strain—conditions that involve injury to the muscle and fascia As disorder progresses, pain becomes increasingly generalized
Chronic postoperative pain	Chronic pain that can occur with disruption or cutting of sensory nerves
Cancer pain	Can be pain attributed to advance of disease, associated with treatment, or attributed to coexisting disease entities
Deafferentation pain	Painful condition resulting from damage to a peripheral nerve Common types include severe burning pain triggered by various stimuli, such as cold, light touch, or sound, and reflex sympathetic dystrophies (occur after peripheral nerve injury and are characterized by continuous, severe, burning pain associated with vasomotor changes and muscle wasting)
Hyperesthesias	Increased sensitivity and decreased pain threshold to tactile and painful stimuli Pain is diffuse, modified by fatigue and emotion, and mixed with other sensations May result from chronic irritations of central nervous system areas
Hemiagnosia	Loss of ability to identify source of pain on one side of the body Painful stimuli on that side produce discomfort, anxiety, moaning, agitation, and distress but no attempt to withdraw from the stimulus Associated with stroke
Phantom limb pain	Pain experienced in amputated limb after stump has completely healed; may be immediate or occur months later Influenced by emotions or sympathetic stimulation Trigger points—small hypersensitive regions in muscle or connective tissues that, when stimulated, produce pain in a specific area
Complex regional pain syndrome	Chronic pain usually associated with limb injury, surgery, or fractures Characterized by autonomic and neuroinflammatory features and pain out of proportion to expected pain

pain is localized, but as the disorder progresses it becomes deep, aching, and more generalized. These, like many other chronic conditions, begin as a result of poor muscle tone, inactivity, muscle or tendon strain, or sudden vigorous exercise and can evolve into a chronic pain state.[47]

Chronic postoperative pain occurs in some individuals and includes nerve injury, complex regional pain syndrome, phantom limb pain, chronic donor site pain, postthoracotomy pain syndrome, postmastectomy pain syndrome, joint arthroplasty pain, and postsurgical abdominal and pelvic pain. Plastic changes in the peripheral nervous system (PNS) and CNS contribute to allodynia and hypersensitivity. Multimodal approaches to analgesia are needed for pain management including adequate management of preoperative pain and postoperative management of acute pain.[48,49]

Cancer pain is often chronic and the cause is unknown. Cancers generate and secrete mediators that sensitize and activate primary afferent nociceptors in the area of the tumor, resulting in neurochemical reorganization of the spinal cord, which contributes to spontaneous activity and enhanced pain responsiveness. Cancer pain is greater than inflammatory pain and has decreased expression of the μ-opioid receptor on dorsal root ganglia. Tumors also can secrete neurotrophic factors that contribute to enhanced responsiveness to pain.[50] Increasing pressure of a growing tumor on nerve endings, tissue destruction, distention of visceral surfaces, obstruction of ducts and intestine, chemotherapy, radiation therapy, and surgical procedures also cause pain.[51] Therapeutic approaches to the management of cancer pain have advanced significantly in recent years, particularly in palliative care and hospice programs.

Frequent assessment of pain, management of breakthrough pain, and implementation of individualized interdisciplinary therapeutic strategies (including pharmacotherapeutic, anesthetic, neurosurgical, psychologic, and rehabilitative techniques along with frequent evaluations) are essential to optimal cancer pain management.[52-54]

Central poststroke pain is a form of central pain associated with stroke which occurs along the spinothalamocortical pathway and produces hypersensitivity on one-half of the body. There may be hyperexcitation in the damaged sensory pathways, damage to the central inhibitory pathways, or a combination of the two. The pain can be persistent or intermittent; burning or aching (more common); or stabbing, widespread, or focused. Allodynia may occur. The symptoms usually develop weeks or months after the stroke and can be difficult to differentiate from other causes of pain.[55,56]

Phantom limb pain is pain that an individual feels in an amputated limb, usually distally (hands and feet) after the stump has completely healed (1 to 3 months after amputation). Nonpainful phantom limb sensations occur in almost all amputees, but the sensations usually fade with time. This is distinguished from the syndrome of phantom limb pain, a chronic pain occurring in 60% to 80% of amputees.[57] It is more likely to appear in individuals who experienced pain in the limb before amputation. Theories about the cause of phantom limb pain include regeneration or hyperactivity of injured or cut peripheral nerves, scar tissue or neuroma formation in the cut peripheral nerves, spinal cord deafferentation (loss of sensory fibers), nerve injury causing sensitization of dorsal horn neurons mediated by release of glutamate and neurokinins, and alterations in the thalamus and cortex. It has been proposed that CNS integration, including reorganization and plastic changes of the somatosensory cortex, results in the perception of pain from receptors associated with the amputated limb even though the limb itself is no longer present. The absence of inhibitory effects of sensory input from the missing peripheral body part may cause increased autonomous activity of dorsal horn neurons with pain transmission. The cause is likely multifactorial, contributing to the difficulty of prevention or effective treatment.[58]

Complex regional pain syndrome (CRPS) is chronic neuropathic pain usually associated with limb injury. Two forms are described: complex regional pain syndrome-I (CRPS-I) (previously termed *reflex sympathetic dystrophy syndrome*) associated with injury but no apparent nerve injury; and complex regional pain syndrome II (CRPS-II) (previously termed *causalgia*) with evidence of nerve injury. The symptoms of both forms are similar.[59] CRPS is distinguished from other chronic pain disorders by signs of autonomic and inflammatory changes in the pain region of the injured nerve. There are *autonomic symptoms*: changes in skin color, temperature, and sweating and alterations in hair and nail growth for the affected limb; *motor symptoms*: tremor or weakness may be present; and *sensory symptoms*: hypersensitivity and allodynia.[60] CRPS is further distinguished as "warm CRPS," associated with a warm, red, and edematous extremity; and "cold CRPS," associated with a cold, dusky, and sweaty extremity. Acute CRPS is more often associated with a warm CRPS presentation, whereas chronic CRPS is more often characterized by a cold CRPS presentation. Peripheral and central sensitization contribute to the pain syndrome, but the mechanisms are unknown. A combination of injury and the presence of inflammatory cytokines and neuropeptides may lead to peripheral nociceptive sensitization and physiologic change in pain transmission and in autonomic and motor systems.[61]

PEDIATRICS AND PERCEPTION OF PAIN

Infants and children have the anatomic and functional ability to perceive pain. Pain pathways and cortical and subcortical centers for pain perception, as well as neurochemicals associated with pain transmission and modulation, are functional in preterm and newborn infants. The nociceptor system is functional in fetuses by 15 to 20 weeks' gestation, and painful fetal procedures require adequate analgesia.[62,63] Repetitive, painful experiences and prolonged exposure to analgesic drugs in preterm infants may permanently alter developing synaptic and neuronal pain processing networks, causing irreversible hypersensitivity to pain with subsequent injury. Alterations occur in both the excitatory and inhibitory pathways in the spinal cord and descending inhibitory processing from the brainstem. Repeated painful procedures require increased amounts of analgesia.[64] Preterm infants experiencing the stress of repeated painful procedures also have delayed postnatal growth and poor early neurodevelopment with long-term consequence in both cognitive and motor functions.[65,66] More research is needed to guide selection of analgesic and anesthetic agents and nonpharmacologic therapies for infant pain management in relation to effects on long-term neurodevelopment.[67-69]

Facial expression, crying, body movements, and lack of consolability are the most consistent expressions of pain in infants. The painful facial expression includes lowered brows drawn together; presence of a vertical bulge and furrows in the forehead between the brows; broadened nasal root; tightly closed, scourged eye fissures; angular, tongue cupping, squarish mouth; and chin quiver (Fig. 16.7). There may be finger clenching, writhing, back arching, and head banging. Physiologic responses include increases in heart rate, blood pressure, and respiratory rate, although these measures lack sensitivity and specificity. There may be flushing or pallor, sweating, and decreased oxygen saturation. Toddlers also express

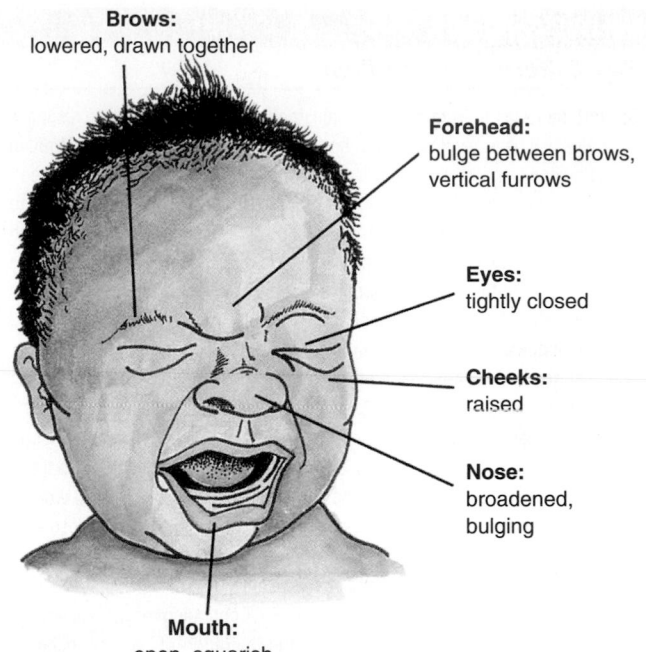

Brows: lowered, drawn together

Forehead: bulge between brows, vertical furrows

Eyes: tightly closed

Cheeks: raised

Nose: broadened, bulging

Mouth: open, squarish

FIGURE 16.7 Painful Facial Expression of Infants. (From Hockenberry MJ: *Wong's nursing care of infants and children*, ed 7, St Louis, 2003, Mosby.)

pain with crying, facial expression, and body language (tensed body, guarding, and hands holding body).[70] Older children, between ages 5 and 18 years, tend to have a lower pain threshold than do adults. Children, like adults, have highly individual responses to pain. Any behavioral and physiologic indicators of pain must be carefully and accurately assessed[71,72] and adequately treated for children of all ages.[73,74]

AGING AND PERCEPTION OF PAIN

Studies on pain perception in the older adult population have yielded conflicting evidence. Some studies show an increase in pain threshold with aging; others show no change.[75-77] The varied results are probably a function of independent variation in the sensory-discriminative, motivational-affective, and cognitive-evaluative components of the pain experience. In general, studies confirm that an increase in the pain threshold occurs in some older adults. This change may be caused by peripheral neuropathies and changes in the thickness of the skin or cognitive impairment. (Neuropathies are discussed in Chapter 18.) A decrease in pain tolerance is also evident in some older adults and may be related to decreased descending inhibitory modulation, decreased synthesis of neurotransmitters, or decreased opioid receptor density.[78] Women appear to be more sensitive to pain than are men[79] (see *What's New? Sex Differences and Pain*). Pain in the older adult is also influenced by cognitive function and liver and renal function, including alterations in metabolism of drugs and metabolites and age-associated brain changes. Pain must be accurately assessed in relation to its effect on cognitive function, coexisting disease, drug interactions, other reactions to treatment, and an individual's ability to express pain and maintain safety.[80,81] Poorly managed pain can result in depression, inactivity, and failure to maintain activities of daily living.[82]

TEMPERATURE REGULATION

Human thermoregulation is achieved through precise balancing of heat production, heat conservation, and heat loss. The normal range

WHAT'S NEW?
Sex Differences and Pain

Sex differences in the experience of pain, modulation of pain, and the response to analgesics have been studied in both animal and human research. Women report higher pain levels or have less tolerance for pain stimuli, such as heat, cold, pressure, and electrical stimulation. The differences may be related to mechanisms of excitatory and inhibitory control. Sex differences also exist in the prevalence of painful chronic diseases; for example, women are more affected by interstitial cystitis, fibromyalgia, and rheumatoid arthritis, and men are more affected by cluster headache. Pain symptoms differ for men and women for diseases such as coronary artery disease, irritable bowel syndrome, appendicitis, and cancer. Sex hormones are known to have an effect on the mechanisms and outcomes of opiate analgesia, and in rodents, morphine analgesia is more effective in males than in females. Pain sensitivities in women also vary across the phases of the menstrual cycle. Recent human and animal studies suggests that κ-opioid receptor analgesia is greater in women than in men and may reflect a difference in endogenous pain circuits mediated by different opiate receptor subtypes and influenced by effects of estrogen and progesterone. Sex differences with respect to pain also are influenced by role socialization, cognitive factors, and culture. Continuing research is needed to further understand sex differences in the operation of pain mechanisms and the development of more specific pain management strategies.

Data from Kvachadze I, Tsagareli MG, Dumbadze Z: *Georgian Med News* (238):102-108, 2015; Loyd DR, Murphy AZ: *Exp Neurol* 259:57-63, 2014; Palmeira CC, Ashmawi HA, Pieretti S et al: *Ann 1st Super Sanita* 52(2):184-189, 2016; Posso Ide P: *Rev Bras Anestesiol* 61(6):814-828, 2011; Racine M et al: *Pain* 153(3):602-618, 2012.

of body temperature is 36.2° to 37.7°C (97.2° to 99.9°F) overall, but a person's individual body parts will vary in temperature. The extremities are generally cooler than the trunk, and the temperature at the core of the body (as measured by rectal temperature) is generally 0.5°C (0.9°F) higher than the surface temperature (as measured by oral temperature). Internal temperature varies in response to activity, environmental temperature, and daily fluctuations (circadian rhythm). Oral temperatures fluctuate within 0.2° to 0.5°C (0.36° to 0.9°F) during a 24-hour period. Women tend to have wider fluctuations that follow the menstrual cycle, with a sharp rise in temperature just before ovulation. The daily fluctuating temperature is similar in both sexes.[83] Maintenance of body temperature within the normal range is necessary for life.

Control of Temperature

Temperature regulation (thermoregulation) is mediated primarily by the preoptic anterior area of the hypothalamus. Peripheral thermoreceptors in the skin and abdominal organs (unmyelinated C fibers and thinly myelinated Aδ fibers) and central thermoreceptors in the spinal cord and trigeminal ganglia provide the hypothalamus with information about skin and core temperatures. These peripheral thermoreceptors have heat-sensitive ion channels (TRP cation channels) which are activated at variable temperatures and provide thermotransduction of energy into a neural signal to the hypothalamus.[84] If these temperatures are low or high, the hypothalamus responds by triggering heat production, heat conservation, or heat loss mechanisms.

Body heat is produced by the chemical reactions of metabolism and skeletal muscle tone and contraction. The heat-producing mechanism (chemical or nonshivering thermogenesis) begins with hypothalamic thyrotropin-stimulating hormone-releasing hormone (TSH-RH); it stimulates the anterior pituitary to release thyroid-stimulating hormone

(TSH), which acts on the thyroid gland and stimulates the release of thyroxine. Thyroxine then acts on the adrenal medulla, causing the release of epinephrine into the bloodstream. Epinephrine causes vasoconstriction, stimulates glycolysis, and increases metabolic rate, thus increasing body heat. Norepinephrine and thyroxine activate brown fat thermogenesis, where energy is released as heat instead of as adenosine triphosphate (ATP). Heat is distributed by the circulatory system.

The hypothalamus also triggers heat conservation by stimulating the sympathetic nervous system, which stimulates the adrenal cortex and results in increased skeletal muscle tone, initiating the shivering response, and producing vasoconstriction. By constricting peripheral blood vessels, centrally warmed blood is shunted away from the periphery to the core of the body where heat can be retained. This involuntary mechanism takes advantage of the insulating layers of the skin and subcutaneous fat to protect core temperature. The hypothalamus relays information to the cerebral cortex about cold, and voluntary responses result. Individuals typically bundle up, keep moving, or curl up in a ball. These types of voluntary physical activities respectively provide insulation, increase skeletal muscle activity, and decrease the amount of skin surface available for heat loss through radiation, convection, and conduction.

The hypothalamus responds to warmer core and peripheral temperatures by reversing the same mechanisms. The TSH-RH pathway is shut down. The sympathetic pathway is prompted to produce cutaneous vasodilation, decreased muscle tone, and increased sweat production. Hypothalamic stimulation of the cerebral cortex provokes voluntary behavior to reduce heat production and promote heat loss. Table 16.5 summarizes further information about heat production and loss.

Mechanisms of Heat Production

Chemical Reactions of Metabolism. The *chemical reactions* that occur during the ingestion and metabolism of food and those required to maintain the body at rest (basal metabolism) require energy and produce heat. These processes occur in the body core (primarily the liver) and are in part responsible for the maintenance of core temperature.

Skeletal Muscle Contraction. Skeletal muscles produce heat through two mechanisms: (1) gradual increase in muscle tone and (2) production of rapid muscle oscillations (*shivering*—which does not occur in neonates). Both increasing muscle tone and shivering are controlled by the posterior hypothalamus and occur in response to cold. As peripheral temperature drops, muscle tone increases and shivering begins. Shivering is a fairly effective method for increasing heat production because no work is performed and all the energy produced is retained as heat.[85]

Chemical Thermogenesis. Chemical thermogenesis, also called *nonshivering thermogenesis* or *adrenergic thermogenesis,* results from the release of epinephrine and norepinephrine. Epinephrine and norepinephrine produce a rapid, transient increase in heat production by raising the body's basal metabolic rate. Chemical thermogenesis seems to be different from hormone-triggered increases in the basal metabolic rate. Chemical thermogenesis produces a quick, brief rise in basal metabolic rate, whereas the hormone thyroxine triggers a slow, prolonged rise. Chemical thermogenesis occurs in brown and beige adipose tissue (see Chapter 23 for adipose tissue as an endocrine organ). Brown adipose tissue is rich with mitochondria and blood vessels and is essential for nonshivering thermogenesis. Beige (bright) adipocytes are found within subcutaneous white adipose tissue.[85] White adipocytes store energy, and brown and beige adipocytes produce heat. Beige adipocytes demonstrate transdifferentiation to white adipocytes, and such plasticity allows direct conversion of one cell type into the other. With chronic cold exposure white-to-beige conversion increases thermogenesis.[86]

TABLE 16.5 MECHANISMS OF HEAT PRODUCTION AND HEAT LOSS

CONDITION	DESCRIPTION
Heat Production	
Chemical reactions of metabolism	Occurs during ingestion and metabolism of food and while maintaining body at rest (basal metabolism); occurs in body core (e.g., liver)
Skeletal muscle contraction	Gradual increase in muscle tone or rapid muscle oscillations (shivering); controlled by posterior hypothalamus
Chemical (nonshivering) thermogenesis	Epinephrine and norepinephrine are released and produce rapid, transient increase in heat production by raising basal metabolic rate; quick, brief effect that counters heat lost through conduction and convection; occurs in brown and beige adipose tissue (thermogenic adipocytes), which decreases markedly in older adults; thyroid hormone increases metabolism and heat production
Heat Loss	
Radiation	Heat loss through electromagnetic waves emanating from surfaces with temperature higher than surrounding air
Conduction	Heat loss by direct molecule-to-molecule transfer from one surface to another, so that warmer surface loses heat to cooler surface
Convection	Transfer of heat through currents of gases or liquids; exchanges warmer air at body's surface with cooler air in surrounding space
Vasodilation	Diverts core-warmed blood to surface of body, with heat transferred by conduction to skin surface and from there to surrounding environment; occurs in response to autonomic stimulation under control of hypothalamus
Evaporation	Body water evaporates from surface of skin and linings of mucous membranes; major source of heat reduction connected with increased sweating in warmer surroundings
Decreased muscle tone	Exhausted feeling caused by moderately reduced muscle tone and curtailed voluntary muscle activity
Increased respiration	Air is exchanged with environment through normal process; minimal effect
Voluntary mechanisms	"Stretching out" and "slowing down" in response to high body temperatures; increasing body surface area available for heat loss; dressing in light-colored, loose-fitting garments
Adaptation to warmer climates	Gradual process beginning with lassitude, weakness, and faintness; proceeding through increased sweating, lowered sodium content, decreased heart rate, and increased stroke volume and extracellular fluid volume; and terminating in improved warm weather functioning and decreased symptoms of heat intolerance (work output, endurance, and coordination increase; subjective feelings of discomfort decrease)

Mechanisms of Heat Loss

Heat loss is achieved through many mechanisms: (1) radiation, (2) conduction, (3) convection, (4) vasodilation, (5) decreased muscle tone, (6) evaporation, (7) increased pulmonary ventilation, (8) voluntary measures, and (9) adaptation to warmer climates.

Radiation. Radiation refers to heat loss through electromagnetic waves. These waves emanate from surfaces with temperatures higher than the surrounding air temperature. Thus, if the temperature of the skin is higher than that of the air, the skin and therefore the body lose heat to the air.

Conduction. Conduction refers to heat loss by direct molecule-to-molecule transfer from one surface to another. Through conduction, the warmer surface loses heat to the cooler surface. Thus the skin loses heat through direct contact with cooler air, water, or another surface. In the same manner, the core of the body loses heat to the cooler body surface.

Convection. Convection is the transfer of heat through currents of gases or liquids. It greatly aids heat loss through conduction by exchanging warmer air at the surface of the body with cooler air in the surrounding space. Convection occurs passively as warmer air at the surface of the body rises away from the body and is replaced by cooler air, but the process may be aided by fans or wind. (The combined effect of conduction and convection by wind is conventionally measured as the *windchill factor*.)

Vasodilation. Peripheral vasodilation increases heat loss by diverting core-warmed blood to the surface of the body. As the core-warmed blood passes through the periphery, heat is transferred by conduction to the skin surface and from the skin to the surrounding environment. Because heat loss through conduction depends on the surrounding temperature, it is minimal to nonexistent if the surrounding air or water is warmer than the body surface.

Vasodilation occurs in response to autonomic stimulation under the control of the hypothalamus. It is useful in instances of moderate temperature elevation. As core temperature increases, vasodilation increases until maximal dilation is achieved. At that point the body must use additional heat loss mechanisms.

Decreased Muscle Tone. To decrease heat production, muscle tone may be moderately reduced and voluntary muscle activity curtailed. These mechanisms explain in part the "washed-out" feeling associated with high temperatures and warm weather. Decreased muscle tone and reduced activity have a limited effect on decreasing heat production, however, because muscle tone and heat production cannot be reduced below basal body requirements.

Evaporation. Evaporation of body water from the surface of the skin and the linings of the mucous membranes is a major source of heat reduction. Insensible water loss (in the absence of perceptible sweating) accounts for a loss of about 600 mL of water per day. Heat is lost as surface fluid is converted to gas, so that heat loss by evaporation is increased if more fluids are available at the body surface. To speed this process, fluids are actively secreted through the sweat glands. As much as 2.2 L of fluid per hour may be lost by sweating. Electrolytes are lost with the water. Therefore loss of large volumes through sweating may result in decreased plasma volume, decreased blood pressure, weakness, and fainting. (Alterations in fluid balance are discussed in Chapter 3.)

Like other heat reduction mechanisms, stimulation of sweating occurs in response to sympathetic neural activity and depends on a favorable temperature difference between the body and the environment. In addition, heat loss through evaporation is affected by the relative humidity of the air. If the humidity is low, sweat evaporates quickly, but if the humidity is high, sweat does not evaporate and instead remains on the skin or drips off it.

Increased Pulmonary Ventilation. Exchanging air with the environment through the normal pulmonary ventilation provides some heat loss, although it is minimal in humans. As air is inhaled, the air draws heat from the upper respiratory tract. The air is further warmed in the alveoli by blood in the microcirculation. This warmed air then is exhaled into the environment. This normal process occurs faster at higher body temperatures through an increase in ventilatory rates. Thus hyperventilation is associated with hyperthermia. (Normal pulmonary function is discussed in Chapter 35.)

Voluntary Mechanisms. In response to high body temperatures, people physically "stretch out," thereby increasing the body surface area available for heat loss. They also "slow down" or "take it easy," thereby decreasing skeletal muscle work, and they "dress for warm weather" with light-colored, loose-fitting garments to reflect heat and promote convection, conduction, and evaporation.

Heat Adaptation. The body of an individual who moves from a cooler to a much warmer climate undergoes a period of adjustment, a process that takes several days to weeks. At first the individual experiences feelings of lassitude, weakness, and faintness with even moderate activity. Body temperatures rise with any work. Within several days, however, the individual experiences an earlier onset of sweating, the volume of sweat is increased, the sodium content is lowered, and skin blood flow increases. Heart rate is decreased and stroke volume increased so that cardiac output remains unchanged. Extracellular fluid volume increases, as does plasma volume. These physiologic adaptations result in improved warm weather functioning and decreased symptoms of heat intolerance. People's work output, endurance, and coordination increase, and their subjective feelings of discomfort decrease.[87,88]

Mechanisms of Heat Conservation

Vasoconstriction. By constricting peripheral blood vessels, centrally warmed blood is shunted away from the periphery (where radiation, conduction, and convection would allow heat loss) to the core of the body, where heat can be retained. This mechanism takes advantage of the insulating layers of the skin and subcutaneous fat to protect core temperature.

Voluntary Mechanisms. In response to lower body temperatures, individuals typically "bundle up," "keep moving," or "curl up in a ball." Bundling up involves dressing with several layers of clothes that allow air to be trapped between the skin and the clothing, thus providing an additional layer of insulation. Keeping moving, stamping feet, clapping hands, jogging, and other types of physical activity increase skeletal muscle activity and thus promote heat production. Curling up in a ball decreases the amount of skin surface available for heat loss through radiation, convection, and conduction.

PEDIATRICS AND TEMPERATURE REGULATION

Infants and older adults require special attention to maintenance of body temperature. Term infants produce body heat primarily through the metabolism of brown fat, but it may not be adequately developed for cold stress.[89] They also are unable to efficiently conserve heat because of the infant's small body size, greater ratio of body surface area to body weight with heat loss through conduction and convection, and decreased ability to shiver. Infants have a thin layer of subcutaneous fat and thus are not as well insulated as adults.[90] Therefore it is important to keep infants warm with hats, clothing, and blankets. Children also have a greater ratio of body surface area to body weight, fewer sweat glands, lower sweating rate, higher peripheral blood flow in the heat, and a greater extent of vasoconstriction in the cold than adults. They can acclimatize to changes in environmental temperatures, but do so at a lower rate than that seen in adults.[91]

AGING AND TEMPERATURE REGULATION

Older adults have lower body temperatures than younger people. They have poor responses to environmental temperature extremes as a result of slowed blood circulation, structural and functional changes in the skin, an overall decrease in heat-producing activities, and the presence of disease (e.g., congestive heart failure, chronic lung disease, diabetes mellitus, or peripheral vascular disease). Cold stress in older adults also decreases coronary perfusion.[92] Other factors affecting thermal regulation in the older adult population include decreased shivering response (delayed onset and decreased effectiveness), slowed metabolic rate, sedentary lifestyle, decreased vasoconstrictor and vasodilator responses, diminished or absent sweating, decreased amount of brown fat, desynchronization of circadian rhythm, undernutrition, and decreased perception of heat and cold.[93,94]

Pathogenesis of Fever

Fever (febrile response or pyrexia) is a temporary resetting of the hypothalamic thermostat to a higher level in response to pyrogenic cytokines (previously known as endogenous pyrogens) and exogenous pyrogens.[95] The pathophysiologic mechanism of fever begins with the introduction of exogenous pyrogens or endotoxins produced by pathogens. The most frequently encountered exogenous pyrogens are the lipopolysaccharide complexes in the cell wall of gram-positive bacteria and viruses released with rupture of the cell wall when the microbe dies. Pyrogenic cytokines, including tumor TNF-α, IL-1, IL-6, and interferon-γ, are produced by phagocytic cells as they destroy microorganisms within the host. The final common step for fever generation by pyrogens is the production of prostaglandin E_2 (PGE_2) in both the periphery and the brain. PGE_2 acts on warm sensitive neurons in the preoptic area of the hypothalamus. An integrated behavioral, endocrine, and autonomic nervous system response is then initiated. Centers in the hypothalamus and brainstem signal an increase in heat production and heat conservation to raise the set point for body temperature regulation (Fig. 16.8). Peripheral vasoconstriction occurs with shunting of blood from the skin to the body core. Epinephrine release increases metabolic rate, and muscle tone increases. Decreased release of vasopressin reduces the volume of body fluid to be heated. Shivering also may occur. The individual dresses more warmly, decreases body surface area by curling up, and may go to bed in an effort to get warm. Body temperature is maintained at the new level until the fever "breaks."

The "acute phase response" is a reaction that occurs when pyrogenic and other cytokines are released in response to infection and inflammation. In addition to fever, other symptoms occur including anorexia, fatigue, malaise, somnolence, and loss of concentration. At the cellular level, inflammatory pyrogenic cytokines promote muscle catabolism and hyperglycemia (gluconeogenesis, glycogenolysis, and insulin resistance) by stimulating release of adrenocorticotropic hormone and glucocorticoids to support glucose-consuming cells. The hepatic acute phase response involves increasing or decreasing protein synthesis. C-reactive protein, mannose-binding protein, complement factors,

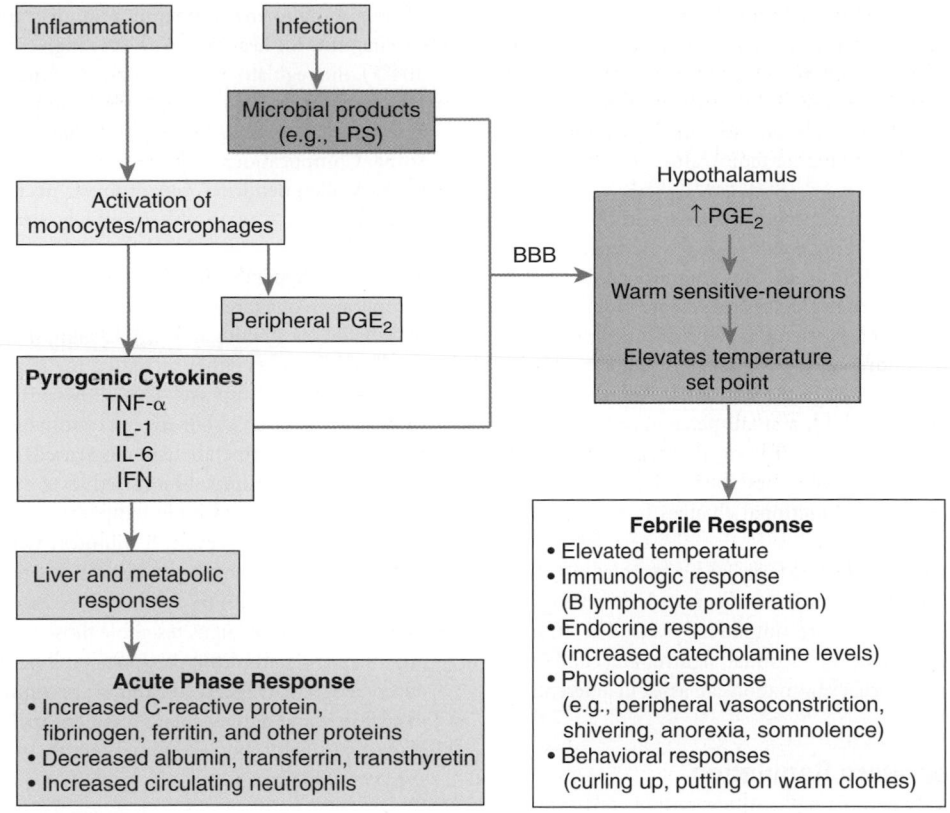

FIGURE 16.8 Pathogenesis of Fever and Acute Phase Response. Inflammation and infection initiate the release of pyrogenic cytokines and exogenous pyrogens. Exogenous pyrogens lead to production of PGE$_2$ in the periphery and the brain, and pyrogenic cytokines stimulate PGE$_2$ release in the brain. PGE$_2$ acts on warm-sensitive neurons in the hypothalamus, setting a higher temperature set point and initiating an integrated febrile response. Concurrently, pyrogenic cytokines initiate the acute phase response. *BBB,* blood-brain barrier; *IFN,* interferon; *IL-1, IL-6,* interleukin-1, interleukin-6; *LPS,* lipopolysaccharide; *PGE$_2$,* prostaglandin E$_2$; *TNF-α,* tumor necrosis factor-alpha. (Adapted from Bennett JE et al: *Mandell, Douglas, and Bennett's principles and practice of infectious disease,* ed 8, Philadelphia, 2015, Saunders.)

ferritin, ceruloplasmin, serum amyloid A, fibrinogen, and haptoglobin are increased. Albumin, transferrin (binds iron), retinol-binding proteins, and transthyretin (transports thyroid hormone) are reduced. The erythrocyte sedimentation rate (ESR) increases as the increase in fibrinogen and other plasma proteins decrease rouleaux formation, allowing the red blood cells to fall faster. Acute phase proteins and the ESR can serve as biomarkers for the inflammatory response.[96] The general functions of increased acute phase proteins are to opsonize and trap microorganisms and their products, activate complement, neutralize enzymes, and modulate the host's immune response (see Chapter 7).

During fever, arginine vasopressin (AVP), α-melanocyte-stimulating hormone (α-MSH), and corticotropin-releasing factor are released from the brain, and systemic antiinflammatory cytokines (i.e., IL-1 receptor agonist and IL-10) can act as endogenous cryogens or antipyretics to help diminish and control the febrile response.[97,98] This antipyretic effect constitutes a negative-feedback loop. The antipyretic effect may help explain fluctuations in the febrile response. When the fever breaks, the set point is returned to normal. The hypothalamus responds by signaling a decrease in heat production and an increase in heat reduction mechanisms. The result is decreased muscle tone, peripheral vasodilation, flushed skin, and sweating. The individual feels very warm, replaces warm clothing with cooler clothes, throws off the covers, and stretches out. Once the body has returned to a normal temperature, the individual feels more comfortable and the hypothalamus adjusts thermoregulatory mechanisms to maintain the new temperature.

Benefits of Fever

Moderate fever aids responses to infectious processes through several mechanisms.[99] A raised body temperature kills many microorganisms and has adverse effects on the growth and replication of others. Higher body temperatures decrease serum levels of iron, zinc, and copper, all of which are needed for bacterial replication. The body switches from burning glucose to a metabolism based on lipolysis and proteolysis, thereby depriving bacteria of a food source. Increased temperature also causes lysosomal breakdown and autodestruction of cells, thus preventing viral replication in infected cells. Acute-phase proteins produced by the liver during inflammation bind cations necessary for bacterial reproduction. Heat increases lymphocytic transformation and motility of polymorphonuclear neutrophils, thus facilitating the immune response. Phagocytosis is enhanced, and production of antiviral interferon may be augmented.[100]

Because fever is a beneficial response to infection, suppressing fever with antipyrogenic medications should be reviewed carefully.[101] Such treatment should be used only if the fever is high enough to produce serious side effects, such as nerve damage or convulsion, although more studies are needed to guide practice.[102]

Infection and fever responses in older adults and in children may vary from those in the adult. Older individuals may have decreased or no fever response to infection. The absence of fever responses to infection and therefore the beneficial aspects of fever production may explain the increase in morbidity and mortality rates seen in very old individuals.[103] In contrast, children develop higher temperatures than do adults for relatively minor infections.

Febrile seizures may occur with temperatures greater than 38°C (100.4°F), although most children do not develop febrile seizures until temperatures are much higher. Febrile seizures are more predominant in boys before age 5 years, and genetic factors contribute to susceptibility.[104] Febrile seizures are generally brief and self-limiting, lasting less than 5 minutes in 40% of children and less than 20 minutes in 75% of children (see Chapter 20). Although in most instances there appear to be no long-term effects on the child, a small percentage of children (1% to 2%) may develop epilepsy.[105] Prolonged febrile seizures are associated with the development of temporal lobe epilepsy in children and are probably associated with functional changes in neurons and neural networks.[106]

Fever of unknown origin (FUO) is a fever with a body temperature greater than 38.3°C (101°F) that remains undiagnosed after 3 days of hospital investigation or two or more outpatient visits. The clinical categories of FUO include classic, nosocomial, neutropenic, and HIV associated. The history and clinical examination can assist in differentiating possible causes.[107,108]

Disorders of Temperature Regulation

Internal body temperature is maintained within a narrow range. Alterations in the regulation of heat production or heat loss can be life-threatening.

Hyperthermia

Hyperthermia is elevation of the body temperature without an increase in the hypothalamic set point. Hyperthermia can produce nerve damage, coagulation of cell proteins, and death. At 41°C (105.8°F), nerve damage produces convulsions in the adult. Death results at 43°C (109.4°F). Hyperthermia may be therapeutic, accidental, or associated with stroke or head trauma. Prevention of hyperthermia in stroke and head trauma assists in limiting brain injury.[109] **Therapeutic hyperthermia** is a form of local, regional, or whole-body induced hyperthermia used to destroy pathologic microorganisms or tumor cells by facilitating the host's natural immune process or tumor blood flow.[110]

The forms of **accidental hyperthermia** are summarized as follows:[111]

1. **Heat cramps**—severe, spasmodic cramps in the abdomen and extremities that follow prolonged sweating and associated sodium loss. They usually occur in those not accustomed to heat or those performing strenuous work in very warm climates. Fever, rapid pulse rate, and increased blood pressure accompany the cramps. Treatment involves administration of dilute salt solutions through oral or parenteral routes.

2. **Heat exhaustion**—results from prolonged high core or environmental temperatures, which cause profound vasodilation and profuse sweating, leading to dehydration, decreased plasma volumes, hypotension, decreased cardiac output, and tachycardia. Symptoms include weakness, dizziness, confusion, nausea, and fainting. The symptoms of heat exhaustion cause the individual to stop work, lie down, and rest. Ceasing activity decreases muscle work, causing decreased heat production. Lying down redistributes vascular volume. The individual should be encouraged to drink cool fluids to replace fluid lost through sweating.

3. **Heat stroke**—a potentially lethal result of an overstressed thermoregulatory center. Heat stroke can be caused by exertion, by overexposure to environmental heat, or from impaired physiologic mechanisms for heat loss. With very high core temperatures (>40°C; 104°F), the regulatory center ceases to function and the body's heat loss mechanisms fail. Symptoms include high core temperature, absence of sweating, rapid pulse rate, confusion, agitation, and coma. Complications include cerebral edema, degeneration of the CNS, swollen dendrites, renal tubular necrosis, and hepatic failure with delirium, coma, and eventually death if treatment is not undertaken.[112]

4. **Malignant hyperthermia**—a potentially lethal hypermetabolic complication of a rare inherited muscle disorder that may be triggered by inhaled anesthetics and depolarizing muscle relaxants.[113,114] The syndrome involves either increased myoplasmic calcium release or decreased calcium uptake. This allows intracellular calcium levels to rise, producing sustained, uncoordinated muscle contractions; muscle cell hypermetabolism; increased muscle work; increased oxygen consumption; and a raised level of lactic acid production. Acidosis develops and body temperature rises (body temperature may rise 1°C [1.8°F] every 5 minutes) with resulting tachycardia and cardiac dysrhythmias, hypotension, decreased cardiac output, and cardiac arrest. The syndrome is caused by a defect in the ryanodine receptor. Signs resemble those of coma: unconsciousness, absent reflexes, fixed pupils, apnea, and occasionally a flat electroencephalogram. Oliguria and anuria are common. It is most common in children and adolescents. Treatment includes withdrawal of the provoking agents, body cooling therapy, and drugs that antagonize the ryanodine receptor.[114]

Hypothermia

Hypothermia (core body temperature less than 35°C [95°F]) produces depression of the central nervous and respiratory systems, vasoconstriction, alterations in microcirculation and coagulation, and ischemic tissue damage. In a controlled situation, such as a surgical procedure, most tissues can tolerate temperatures as low as 33°C (91.4°F). In severe hypothermia (less than 28°C [82.4°F]), ice crystals forming on the inside of the cell cause cells to rupture and die. Tissue hypothermia slows the rate of chemical reactions (tissue metabolism), increases the viscosity of the blood, slows blood flow through the microcirculation, impairs platelet function and blood coagulation, stimulates profound vasoconstriction, suppresses myocardial contractility, and induces arrhythmias. Hypothermia may be accidental or therapeutic. In accidental hypothermia, high-energy phosphates (e.g., ATP) are depleted, and in therapeutic hypothermia, ATP storage is preserved.[115]

Accidental Hypothermia. Accidental hypothermia is generally the result of sudden immersion in cold water or prolonged exposure to cold environments. At particular risk for accidental hypothermia are infants and older adults, because thermoregulatory mechanisms are immature or altered in these two groups. Also at risk are individuals with conditions that diminish the ability to generate heat. Such conditions include hypothyroidism, hypopituitarism, decreased liver function, malnutrition, Parkinson disease, and rheumatoid arthritis. Other risk factors include chronic increased vasodilation and decreased thermoregulatory control caused by cerebral injuries, ketoacidosis, uremia, and drug overdoses. In acute hypothermia, peripheral vasoconstriction shunts blood away from the cooler skin to the core in an effort to decrease heat loss, which produces peripheral tissue ischemia. Intermittent reperfusion of the extremities (the Lewis phenomenon) helps preserve peripheral oxygenation. Intermittent peripheral perfusion continues until core temperatures drop dramatically.

The hypothalamic center stimulates **shivering** in an effort to increase heat production. Severe shivering occurs at core temperatures of 35°C (95°F) and continues until core temperature (measure by esophageal probe) drops to about 30° to 32°C (86° to 89.6°F). Prolonged shivering can lead to exhaustion of liver glycogen stores. Thinking becomes sluggish and coordination is decreased at 34°C (93.2°F). As hypothermia deepens, paradoxical undressing may occur as hypothalamic control of vasoconstriction is lost and vasodilation occurs with loss of core heat to the periphery. The hypothermic individual therefore feels suddenly warm and begins to remove clothing.[116]

At 30°C (86°F), the individual becomes stuporous, heart rate and respiratory rate decline, and cardiac output is diminished. Cerebral blood flow is decreased. Metabolic rate declines, further decreasing core temperature. Sinus node depression occurs with slowing of conduction through the atrioventricular node. In severe hypothermia (core temperature of 26° to 28°C [78.8° to 82.4°F]), pulse and respirations may be undetectable and require resuscitation. Acidosis is moderate to severe. Coagulopathy, ventricular fibrillation, and asystole are common.[117] Surface cooling may cause frostbite and fat necrosis.

If hypothermia is mild, passive rewarming may be sufficient. If core temperature is greater than 30°C (86°F), active rewarming also may be required. Active rewarming uses warm-water baths, warm blankets, heating pads, and warm oral fluids when the individual is fully alert. Core rewarming may be accomplished through administration of warm intravenous (IV) solutions, warm gastric lavage, warm peritoneal lavage, inhalation of warmed gases, and, in extreme cases, exchange transfusions, warming blood in a pump oxygenator circuit, and mediastinal lavage.[118]

Rewarming generally should proceed no faster than a few degrees per hour. Short-term complications of rewarming include acidosis, rewarming shock, and dysrhythmias. Long-term complications include congestive heart failure, hepatic and renal failure, abnormal erythropoiesis, myocardial infarction, pancreatitis, and neurologic dysfunctions.[119]

Therapeutic Hypothermia. Therapeutic hypothermia is used to slow metabolism and preserve ischemic tissue after brain trauma or during brain surgery, after cardiac arrest, and in neonatal hypoxic encephalopathy.[120] Hypothermia protects the brain by reduction in metabolic rate, ATP consumption, oxidative stress, and the critical threshold for oxygen delivery; modulation of excitotoxic neurotransmitters and calcium antagonism; preservation of protein synthesis and the blood-brain barrier; decreased edema formation; and modulation of the inflammatory response.[121-123]

Trauma and Temperature Regulation

Major body trauma has varying effects on temperature regulation, depending on the body systems involved. Five types of traumatic injury that usually affect temperature regulation are: (1) CNS trauma (discussed in Chapter 18), (2) accidental injury, (3) hemorrhagic shock, (4) major surgery, and (5) thermal burns.

Central Nervous System Trauma. CNS trauma that causes CNS damage, inflammation, increased intracranial pressures, or intracranial bleeding typically produces a temperature greater than 39°C (102.2°F). This temperature, often referred to as *neurogenic or central fever,* appears with or without relative bradycardia and is not caused by infection. The temperature is sustained, does not induce sweating, and is highly resistant to antipyretic therapy.[124,125]

Accidental Injuries. Mild accidental injuries may produce a slight elevation in core temperature. Moderate to severe injuries result in peripheral vasoconstriction with decreased surface and core temperatures. Core temperature is thought to be inversely related to the severity of the injury and may be a result of decreased oxygen transport to the tissues. In severe injuries, shivering is absent and some alteration in thermoregulation is evident.[126]

Hemorrhagic Shock. Loss of blood volume in hemorrhage triggers peripheral vasoconstriction and hypoxia, contributing to hypothermia.

Risk for subsequent decreases in core temperature occurs when hemorrhagic shock is treated with unwarmed, volume-expanding solutions and surgery. Volume expansion with warmed solutions is recommended to prevent the deleterious effects of hypothermia on cardiac output, cardiac rhythm, and the immune system.

Major Surgery. Major surgery often induces significant hypothermia through exposure of body cavities to the relatively cool operating room environment, irrigation of body cavities with room temperature solutions, infusion of room temperature intravenous solutions, use of drugs that impair thermoregulatory mechanisms, and inhalation of unwarmed anesthetic agents. Anesthesia induces hypothermia, reduces platelet function, and impairs the coagulation cascade, contributing to transfusion requirements and postoperative complications. Use of warmed irrigating and intravenous solutions and perioperative forced air and skin warming procedures reduce intraoperative hypothermia and postoperative complications.[127]

Thermal Burns. Large burn injuries produce significant hypothermia because of the loss of the skin barrier to fluid evaporation and the loss of control of the microcirculation in the skin. Severe burns also compromise the normal insulation of the skin and subcutaneous tissues. (Burns are discussed in Chapter 49.)

SLEEP

Sleep is an active, multiphase process that provides restorative functions and promotes memory consolidation. Complex neural circuits in the hypothalamus, thalamus, brainstem, and cortex interacting with hormones and neurotransmitters control the timing of the sleep-wake cycle and coordinate this cycle with circadian rhythms (24-hour rhythm cycles).[128] Normal sleep has two independent phases that can be documented by electroencephalogram (EEG): rapid eye movement (REM) sleep and non-REM (NREM) slow wave sleep. NREM and REM sleep alternate, with each cycle lasting for approximately 90 to 100 minutes. NREM sleep is further divided into three stages (N1, N2, N3) from light to deep sleep followed by REM sleep. Four to six cycles of REM and NREM sleep occur each night in an adult. The first cycle of the night begins with stage N1. The individual then progresses through stages N2, N3, and REM sleep. A new cycle, beginning with stage N2, follows each REM sleep. With each successive cycle, the amount of time spent in stage N3 sleep decreases and the amount of time spent in REM sleep increases (Fig. 16.9). The individual who is awakened begins the next cycle with stage N1.

A complex interaction of neural networks and neurotransmitters promote wakefulness and sleep. The hypothalamus, brainstem, and basal forebrain are involved in promoting wakefulness. The neurotransmitters include brainstem and basal forebrain serotonin, norepinephrine, dopamine acetylcholine (ACh), and glutamine. Hypothalamic wakefulness is associated with orexin and histamine. The production of these neurotransmitters decreases during sleep. Neurons in the preoptic area and basal forebrain induce sleep. The primary neurotransmitters are GABA and galanin. Other sleep promoters, particularly for NREM sleep, are melanin-concentrating hormone and adenosine, prostaglandin D2, nitric oxide, and cytokines. ACh, GABA, and glutamate also promote REM sleep.[129] The phases of sleep are based on changes in the EEG pattern (Fig. 16.10):

Awake—Wakefulness with eyes closed and predominated by alpha waves (8 to 25 Hz)
NREM sleep (75% to 80% of sleep time):
    N1—Light sleep, with alpha waves (6 to 8 Hz) interspersed with low-frequency theta waves; slow eye movements; cycle lasts 10 to 12 minutes (3% to 8% of sleep time)

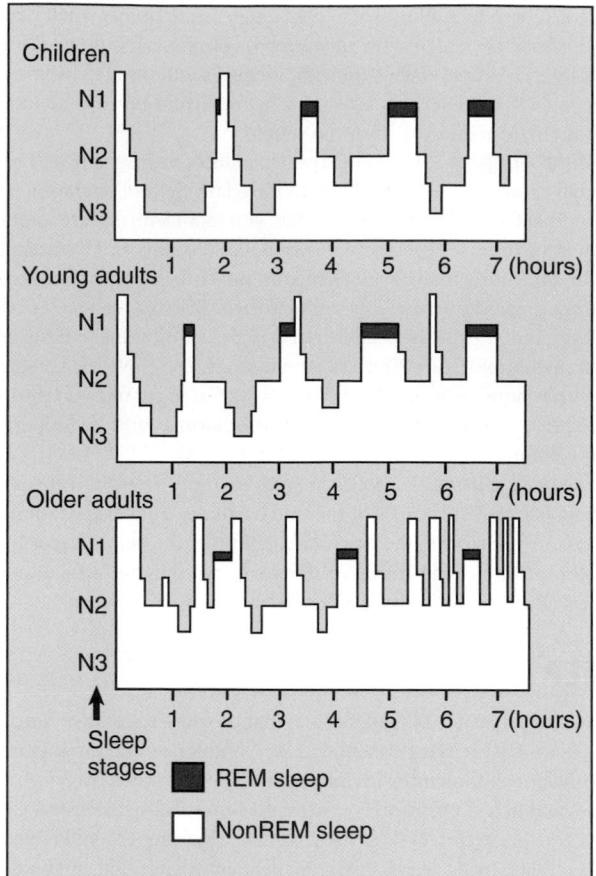

FIGURE 16.9 Normal Sleep Cycles. Rapid eye movement *(REM)* sleep occurs cyclically throughout the night at intervals of approximately 90 minutes in all age groups. REM sleep shows little variation in the different age groups, whereas stage N3 sleep decreases with age. In addition, older adults awaken frequently and show a marked increase in total time awake.

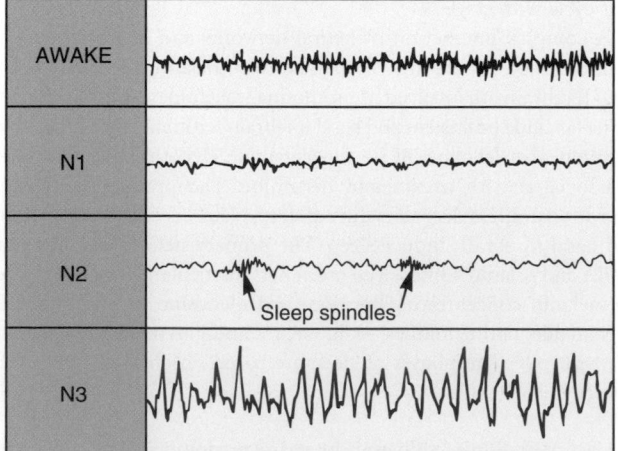

FIGURE 16.10 Electroencephalogram (EEG) Stages of Wakefulness and NREM Sleep. *Awake,* Low-voltage fast activity; *stage N1,* falling asleep; *stage N2,* light sleep with sleep spindles; *stage N3,* slow delta waves. Rapid eye movement (REM) sleep looks similar to awake and stage N1 sleep. Sleep spindles are bursts of brain activity associated with onset of sleep.

N2—Further slowing of the EEG (4 to 7 Hz) with the presence of sleep spindles and slow eye movements; cycle lasts 30 to 60 minutes (45% to 55% of sleep time)

N3—Low-frequency (1 to 3 Hz) high-amplitude delta waves with occasional sleep spindles—also known as *slow-wave sleep*; no slow eye movements (13% to 23% of sleep time)

REM sleep—time of most dreaming (20% to 25% of sleep time)

Non–Rapid Eye Movement Sleep

Non-REM (NREM) slow wave sleep is initiated when inhibitory signals are released from the hypothalamus. Sympathetic tone is decreased and parasympathetic activity is increased during NREM sleep, creating a state of reduced activity. The basal metabolic rate falls by 10% to 15%; temperature decreases 0.5° to 1.0°C (0.9° to 1.8°F); heart rate, respiration, blood pressure, and muscle tone decrease; and knee jerk reflexes are absent. Pupils are constricted. During stages N1 and N2, cerebral blood flow to the brainstem and cerebellum is decreased. During stage N3, cerebral blood flow to the cortex is decreased.[130] Growth hormone is released during stage N3, and levels of corticosteroids and catecholamines are depressed.

Rapid Eye Movement Sleep

Rapid eye movement (REM) sleep is initiated by *REM-on* and *REM-off* neurons in the pons and mesencephalon. *REM-on* cells use the transmitter gamma-aminobutyric acid (GABA), glycine, acetylcholine, and glutamate. *REM-off* cells use the transmitters norepinephrine, epinephrine, serotonin, histamine, and GABA.[131] REM sleep occurs about every 90 minutes beginning 1 to 2 hours after NREM sleep begins. This sleep is known as *paradoxical sleep* because the EEG pattern is similar to that of the normal awake pattern and the brain is very active with dreaming. REM and NREM sleep alternate throughout the night, with lengthening intervals of REM sleep and fewer intervals of deeper stages of NREM sleep toward morning. The changes associated with REM sleep include increased parasympathetic activity and variable sympathetic activity associated with rapid eye movement; antigravity muscle relaxation or atonia (requires GABA and glycine inhibition of motor neurons); loss of temperature regulation; altered heart rate, blood pressure, and respiration; penile erection in men and clitoral engorgement in women; release of steroids; and many memorable dreams. Respiratory control appears largely independent of metabolic requirements and oxygen variation. Loss of normal voluntary muscle control in the tongue and upper pharynx may produce some respiratory obstruction. Cerebral blood flow and brain oxygen consumption increase.[131]

PEDIATRICS AND SLEEP PATTERNS

Sleep patterns of children change as they age. Newborns sleep about 16 to 18 hours per day on an irregular schedule related to culture and parental and family influences. About 53% of that time is spent in active sleep (REM sleep), 23% in quiet sleep (NREM sleep), and the remainder in an indeterminate phase. The infant sleep cycle is approximately 50 to 60 minutes long, with 20 minutes of NREM sleep and 10 to 45 minutes of REM sleep, in contrast to the adult sleep cycle. Newborns enter REM sleep immediately on falling asleep[132] and have well developed sleep-wake cycling.[133] At about 1 year of age, an infant spends approximately 45% of total sleep time in quiet sleep and 41% in REM sleep. Total sleep time decreases slightly from birth to 1 year. In the young child, the sleep cycle length is 45 to 60 minutes, in contrast to 90 to 100 minutes in the adult. The child assumes the adult sleep pattern at some point during the first 3 to 5 years of life and sleeps 9 to 10 hours per night.[134] Sleep for infants and children is important for growth and neurocognitive development. Sudden infant death syndrome (SIDS) is presented in Chapter 37. Sleep disorders are common in children and include insomnia and dyssomnias.[135] Obstructive sleep apnea syndrome (OSAS) in children is related to anatomic obstruction, collapse of airways, and adenotonsillar inflammation.[136] Sleep deprivation in adolescents is associated with obesity, depression, anxiety disorders, poor academic performance, and safety issues.[137]

AGING AND SLEEP PATTERNS

The sleep pattern of the older adult differs from that of the younger adult or child and is variable among individuals. Total sleep time is decreased, and the older individual takes longer to initiate and maintain sleep. Older adults tend to go to sleep earlier in the evening and awaken more frequently during the night and earlier in the morning. REM and NREM sleep decreases and the amount of time awake at night increases. Decreased NREM sleep is more common in men over 70 years of age. Changes in the older adult's sleep pattern may be associated with loss of orexin synthesis or sensitivity, changes in lifestyle, presence of chronic disease, lack of daily routine, desynchronization of circadian rhythm, and use of medications.[138] Growth hormone and cortisol levels are diminished in the older adult and decrease slow wave sleep.[139] The alteration in sleep pattern typically appears about 10 years later in women than in men. Older adults are less able than younger individuals to tolerate sleep deprivation, and good sleep quality in middle age promotes better cognitive function and memory in older age.[140,141]

Sleep Disorders

The classification of sleep disorders is complex. A system has been established by the American Academy of Sleep Medicine and includes four classifications:[142] (1) dyssomnias (disorders of initiating and maintaining sleep and disorders of excessive sleepiness), (2) parasomnias (disorders that primarily do not cause a complaint of insomnia or excessive sleepiness), (3) sleep disorders associated with medical/psychiatric disorders, and (4) proposed sleep disorders. The most common, dyssomnias and parasomnias, are reviewed here.

Common Dyssomnias

The dyssomnias are sleep disorders related to difficulty in initiating or maintaining sleep or the presence of excessive sleepiness. The most common dyssomnias include insomnia, restless legs syndrome, obstructive sleep apnea syndrome, circadian rhythm disorder, and hypersomnia.

Insomnia is the inability to fall or stay asleep; it is accompanied by fatigue during wakefulness and may be mild, moderate, or severe. It may be transient, lasting a few days or months (primary insomnia), and related to travel across time zones or caused by acute stress.[143] Chronic insomnia can be idiopathic, start at an early age, and be associated with drug or alcohol abuse, chronic pain disorders, chronic depression, the use of certain drugs (amphetamines, steroids, central adrenergic blockers, bronchodilating agents, and caffeine), obesity, aging, genetics, and environmental factors that result in hyperarousal, reduced cortical GABA, increased arousals during REM sleep, and dysregulation of sleep-wake cycles.[144]

Restless legs syndrome (RLS) is a sensorimotor disorder associated with unpleasant sensations (prickling, tingling, crawling) and a compelling urge to move the legs for relief that occurs at rest and is worse in the evening or at night. Sensations also may be experienced in the arms. The syndrome can lead to insomnia and affect quality of life. The age of onset is 30 to 40 years and is more common in women and individuals with iron deficiency. RLS has a familial tendency and may be related to diurnal variation in iron transport across the blood-brain barrier

and a loss of dopamine in the substantia nigra. Iron is a cofactor in dopamine production. Treatment options include alpha-2-delta drugs, such as gabapentin; dopamine agonists; and iron administration.[145]

Obstructive sleep apnea syndrome (OSAS) is a disorder of breathing during sleep related to repetitive upper airway collapse (obstruction) that is associated with reduced blood oxygen saturation and hypercapnia. OSAS is the most commonly diagnosed sleep disorder. An estimated 1% to 5% of children, 9% of women, and 24% of men younger than 65 years of age in the United States have diagnosable sleep-disordered breathing. The incidence increases in those older than 65 years. Major risk factors include obesity, male sex, older age, and postmenopausal status (not on hormone therapy) in women.[146] The typical classification of the severity of this disease uses the Apnea Hypopnea Index (AHI).[147] This index represents how many apnea (total airway closure) or hypopnea (partial airway closure) episodes occur per night—the number of which is then divided by the night's total sleep time to give an average number of apnea or hypopnea episodes per hour. The AHI severity scale is as follows:

- *Normal:* 0 to 5 abnormal sleep episodes per hour
- *Mild:* 5 to 15 abnormal sleep episodes per hour
- *Moderate:* 15 to 29 abnormal sleep episodes per hour
- *Severe:* more than 30 abnormal sleep episodes per hour

OSAS is increasingly prevalent in the rapidly expanding older adult population.[148] Premenstrual women may be protected from sleep-disordered breathing because the female hormone progesterone is a respiratory stimulant. The longer pharyngeal airway in males also may contribute to increased risk for OSAS. Women have different symptoms than men such as insomnia, restless legs, depression, nightmares, palpitations, and hallucinations. Men are more likely to report snoring and apneic episodes. Obese individuals often have a short, thick neck; pharyngeal airway collapse; impaired respiratory mechanics; and depressed respiratory control, particularly during sleep.[149] Obesity hypoventilation syndrome (obesity, daytime hypoventilation, and sleep-disordered breathing not related to other causes) may be related to leptin resistance because leptin is also a respiratory stimulant.[150] It is important to note that the current obesity pandemic has not spared the pediatric population, and there has been an increased prevalence of OSAS among obese children.[151]

OSAS results from partial or total upper airway collapse related to pharyngeal anatomy or decreased pharyngeal dilator muscle tone. There is obstruction to airflow recurring during sleep with excessive loud snoring, gasping, and multiple apneic episodes that last 10 seconds or longer. The periodic breathing eventually produces arousal, which interrupts the sleep cycle, reducing total sleep time, and sleep stage fragmentation with REM deprivation. Associated conditions include decreased sensitivity to carbon dioxide and oxygen tensions, upper airway obstruction, a small airway, and decreased pharyngeal dilator muscle activation.[152] The level of negative intrathoracic pressure is the most likely stimulus for arousal, possibly mediated by mechanoreceptors in the upper airway. Sleep apnea produces hypercapnia and low oxygen saturation and eventually leads to polycythemia, pulmonary hypertension, systemic hypertension, stroke, right-sided congestive heart failure, dysrhythmias, liver congestion, cyanosis, and peripheral edema. There also is increasing recognition that OSAS may accelerate the loss of kidney function.[153] The mechanisms responsible for renal damage from OSAS are not completely clear, but activation of the renin-angiotensin system has been proposed as a contributor.[154]

Laboratory polysomnography and home sleep testing are used to diagnose OSAS in addition to history and physical examination. Treatments include use of continuous positive airway pressure (treatment of choice), dental devices, surgery of the upper airway and jaw in selected individuals, and management of obesity.[155] Adenotonsillar hypertrophy is the major cause of obstructive sleep apnea in children, and obesity increases risk. Adenotonsillectomy is the treatment of choice.

Hypersomnia is excessive daytime sleepiness and is commonly associated with voluntary sleep deprivation. There may also be an underlying sleep disorder such as OSAS or narcolepsy. Individuals may fall asleep while driving, working, or even conversing, resulting in significant concerns for safety.[156] Treatment is symptomatic with reinforcement of good sleeping habits.[157]

Narcolepsy is hypersomnolence characterized as Type 1, with excessive daytime sleepiness, cataplexy (brief spells of involuntary muscle weakness or paralysis), and hypocretin-1 deficiency; and Type 2, absence of cataplexy and normal levels of hypocretin-1. The disorder is a REM sleep disorder, with hypothalamic hypocretin (orexin) deficiency and immune-mediated T-cell destruction of hypocretin-secreting cells. There is a genetic association with HLA DQB1*06:02 allele, infections, and vaccination (H1N1 Pandemrix vaccine).[131,158] Older adults with narcolepsy are far more likely to have associated sleep disorders, such as OSAS and RLS.[159]

Circadian rhythm sleep disorders are common disorders of the sleep-wake schedule and occur with rapid time-zone changes (jet-lag syndrome) and in about 5% to 10% of shift workers.[160] There is an alteration in sleep schedule with an advance (advanced sleep-wake phase disorder), a delay (delayed sleep-wake phase disorder) of 3 hours or more in sleep time, changes in sleep patterns from day to day (non-24-hour sleep-wake rhythm disorder [N24SWD], a problem occurring in totally blind individuals), and irregular sleep-wake rhythm disorder (ISWRD).[161] These changes in the timing of established sleep schedules have been shown to desynchronize circadian rhythm. Affected shift workers exhibit a decrease in vigilance, accuracy, and work performance, as well as increased accident proneness. Individuals may experience short sleep episodes called *microsleeps* without being aware of decreased vigilance. For similar reasons, people suffering from jet-lag syndrome require several days to adapt to a new time zone. Travel across time zones requires 2 days to adjust the sleep-wake schedule, 5 days to adjust the body temperature cycle, and 8 days to adjust cortisol level secretion. There is a need to phase delay sleep when traveling from east to west, and to phase advance sleep when traveling from west to east. Bright light exposure and administration of exogenous melatonin provide some success in retiming or resetting the body clock before or after time-zone shifts.[162]

Sleep deprivation can result in neuropsychologic effects, including:[163-165]
1. A marked impact on performance through decreases in cognitive functions and specific effects on brain regions that support cognitive function (vigilance, attention, learning, memory, decision making)
2. Decreased speed of mental processing
3. Declines in attention and vigilance with distinct intraindividual variability
4. Abnormal activation in the prefrontal cortex, parietal lobes, thalamus, and temporal lobes as shown by functional neuroimaging
5. Task performance decreases as sleep debt accumulates in a manner that is "dose dependent"

Sleep disturbance and resultant sleep deprivation also are associated with increased risk for heart disease, stroke, obesity, diabetes, infection, and depression.[137,166-168] Sleep of poor quality and quantity also is now recognized as an important biomarker for cerebral pathologies other than just sleep disturbance-related large and small vessel stroke. There has been increasing recognition that insidious and progressive neurodegenerative diseases are now associated with sleep disorders.[169]

Common Parasomnias

Parasomnias are complex behaviors related to awakening from REM sleep or partial arousal from NREM sleep and disorders of sleep stage transitions. Three types of parasomnias include *arousal disorders* such as confusional arousals, sleepwalking (somnambulism), night terrors (dream anxiety attacks), rearranging furniture, eating food, violent behavior, bruxism (teeth grinding), and sleep enuresis; *sleep-wake transition disorders* such as rhythmic movements (head banging), sleep talking, and nocturnal leg cramps; and *disorders associated with REM sleep* such as sleep paralysis and nightmares, sleep apnea, and SIDS (see Chapter 37). Parasomnias are more common in children and may be familial.[170]

REM sleep behavior disorder is loss of normal skeletal muscle atonia during REM sleep and may cause injury from the acting-out of dreams. It is caused by alterations to the brainstem circuits that mediate REM sleep atonia and is more common in older adult men. It is an early symptom (i.e., 5 years) associated with Parkinson disease and other neurodegenerative diseases.[171]

SOMATOSENSORY FUNCTION AND THE SPECIAL SENSES

The somatosensory system includes the peripheral receptors and central nervous system pathways that detect internal and external information, which is then processed and interpreted by the brain. This system includes touch, proprioception and vestibular function, and the special senses—sight, hearing, smell, and taste.

Touch

Touch is not a uniform sensory experience. The sensation of touch involves the fusion of several qualities, including modality, intensity, location, and duration of the sensory stimulus. Receptors sensitive to touch are present in the skin. Meissner and pacinian corpuscles are rapidly adapting receptors, whereas Merkel disks and Ruffini endings are slowly adapting touch receptors. Touch receptors are most numerous in the skin of the fingers and lips and are more scarce in the skin of the trunk. Specific sensory input is carried to the higher levels of the CNS by the dorsal column of the spinal cord and the anterior spinothalamic tract.

Much of the development of the cutaneous senses takes place before birth, but structural growth of the cutaneous senses continues into early adulthood at a reduced rate. Then a gradual decline occurs.[172] Studies have documented loss in tactile sensitivity with advancing age.[173,174] This occurs simultaneously with an increase in the size of pacinian corpuscles and a decrease in the number of corpuscles.

Abnormal tactile perception may be caused by alterations at any level of the nervous system, from the receptor to the cerebral cortex. Any factor that interrupts or impairs reception, transmission, perception, or interpretation of touch also alters tactile sensation. Trauma, tumor, infection, metabolic changes, vascular changes, and degenerative diseases thus may cause tactile dysfunction, which may involve heightened or diminished tactile perceptions.

In addition, most tactile sensations evoke affective responses that determine whether the sensation is unpleasant, pleasant, or neutral. Cerebral and hypothalamic centers influence this response. Sedative drugs and prefrontal injury, which interrupt connections between the prefrontal cortex and subcortical centers, diminish the interpretation of tactile sensations.

Proprioception

Perception and awareness of the position and movement of the body and its parts depend on impulses from the inner ear and from receptors in joints and ligaments. The role of muscle, tendon, and cutaneous receptors is indefinite. Sensory data are transmitted to higher centers, primarily through the dorsal columns and the spinocerebellar tracts, with some data passing through the medial lemnisci and thalamic radiations to the cortex. These stimuli are necessary for the coordination of movements, the grading of muscular contraction, and the maintenance of equilibrium and postural control.

A progressive loss of proprioception has been reported in older adults with increased risk for falls and injury.[175] Proprioceptive dysfunction may be caused by alterations at any level of the nervous system. As with tactile dysfunction, any factor that interrupts or impairs the reception, transmission, perception, or interpretation of proprioceptive stimuli also alters proprioception. Two common causes of proprioceptive dysfunction are vestibular dysfunction and neuropathy.

Specific vestibular dysfunctions are vestibular nystagmus and vertigo. Vestibular nystagmus is the constant, involuntary movement of the eyeball caused by ear disturbances. This condition occurs when the semicircular canal system is overstimulated. Vestibular vertigo (dizziness) is the sensation of spinning that occurs with inflammation of the semicircular canals or displacement of otoliths in the utricle and saccule of the semicircular canal system (benign positional vertigo). The individual may feel either that he or she is moving in space or that the world is revolving. Vertigo often causes loss of balance and may be accompanied by nausea. Vertigo and nystagmus may occur in a variety of conditions, including labyrinthitis, vestibular neuritis, acute toxic labyrinthitis, benign paroxysmal positional vertigo (displacement of otoliths in the utricle and saccule of the semicircular canal system), migrainous vertigo, and Ménière disease.[176]

Ménière disease (endolymphatic hydrops) is an idiopathic episodic vestibular disorder resulting from neuroepithelial damage related to abnormalities in the quantity, composition, and pressure of the endolymph in the middle ear.[177] The individual with Ménière disease experiences vertigo, hearing loss, tinnitus (ringing or buzzing sounds), and aural fullness and may have proprioceptive dysfunction and headache. Standing or walking may be impossible because of loss of balance. Ménière syndrome, or secondary endolymphatic hydrops, is secondary to other conditions that alter the production or absorption of endolymph.

Peripheral neuropathies also can cause proprioceptive dysfunctions.[178] Neuropathies may be caused by a variety of conditions and commonly are associated with renal disease and diabetes mellitus. Although the exact sequence of events is unknown, neuropathies are thought to be caused by a metabolic disturbance of the neuron itself. The result is a diminished or absent sense of body position or position of body parts. Gait changes often occur. (Neuropathies are further discussed in Chapter 18.)

Vision

The eyes are complex sense organs responsible for vision. Within a protective casing, each eye has receptors, a lens system for focusing light on the receptors, and a system of nerves for conducting impulses from the receptors to the brain. Visual dysfunction may be caused by abnormal ocular movements or alterations in visual acuity, refraction, color vision, or accommodation. Visual dysfunction also may be the secondary effect of another neurologic disorder.

The External Eye

Protective external eye structures include the eyelids (palpebrae), conjunctivae, and lacrimal apparatus (Fig. 16.11). The eyelids are used to control the amount of light reaching the eyes, and the conjunctivae line the eyelids. Tears released from the lacrimal apparatus bathe the surface of the eye and prevent friction, maintain hydration, and wash out foreign bodies and other irritants.

Infection and inflammatory responses are the most common conditions affecting the supporting structures of the eyes. Blepharitis is an

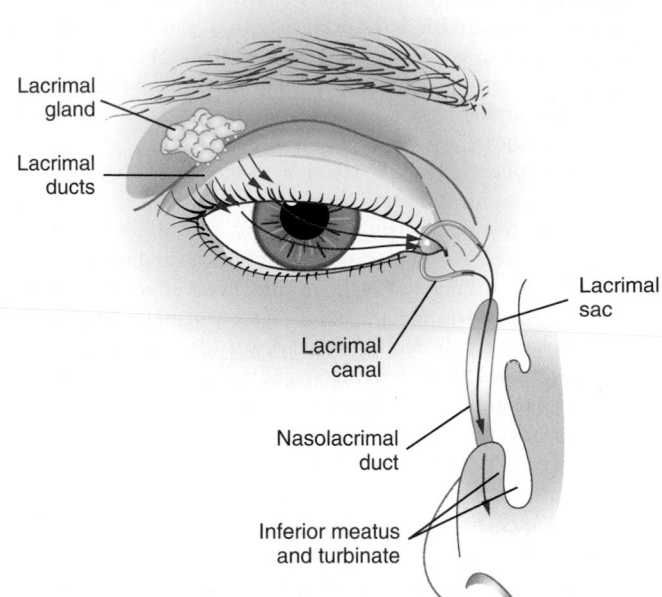

FIGURE 16.11 Lacrimal Apparatus. Fluid produced by lacrimal glands (tears) streams across the eye surface, enters the canals, and then passes through the nasolacrimal duct to enter the nose. (From Applegate E: *The anatomy and physiology learning system,* ed 4, St Louis, 2011, Saunders.)

inflammation of the eyelids caused by *Staphylococcus* or seborrheic dermatitis. Redness, edema, tearing, and itching are common symptoms. An external hordeolum (anterior blepharitis [stye]) is an infection of the sebaceous glands of the eyelids, and an internal hordeolum is an infection of the eyelid margin. A chalazion (posterior blepharitis) is a noninfectious lipogranuloma of the meibomian (oil-secreting) gland and may be associated with an internal hordeolum. These conditions present with redness, swelling, and tenderness and are treated symptomatically.[179] Entropion is a common eyelid malposition in which the lid margin turns inward against the eyeball. In ectropion, the eyelid turns outward away from the eye. Trichiasis is abnormally positioned eyelashes that grow back toward the eye. There are both surgical and nonsurgical treatments to reposition the lid margin.[180]

Conjunctivitis

Conjunctivitis ("red eye") is an inflammation of the conjunctiva (mucous membrane covering the front part of the eyeball). Conjunctivitis may be caused by bacteria, viruses, allergies, or chemical irritations. The inflammatory response produces photophobia, visual blurring, redness, edema, pain, and lacrimation. Treatment is related to cause.[181]

Acute bacterial conjunctivitis (pinkeye) is highly contagious and often is caused by gram-positive organisms (*Staphylococcus, Haemophilus, Streptococcus pneumoniae,* and *Moraxella catarrhalis*), although other bacteria may be involved. The onset is acute, characterized by mucopurulent drainage from one or both eyes. In children younger than 6 years, *Haemophilus* infection often leads to otitis media (conjunctivitis-otitis syndrome). Preventing spread of the organism with meticulous handwashing and use of separate towels is important. The disease often is self-limiting and resolves spontaneously in 10 to 14 days. Antibiotic eyedrops usually are effective.

Viral conjunctivitis is caused by an adenovirus. Again, it is contagious with symptoms of watering, redness, and photophobia. Some strains of virus cause conjunctivitis and pharyngitis (pharyngoconjunctival fever), and others cause keratoconjunctivitis. Both diseases are contagious, with watering, redness, and photophobia. Treatment is symptomatic.

Allergic conjunctivitis is associated with a variety of antigens, including pollens. Ocular itching is associated with photophobia, burning, and gritty sensations in the eye. Treatment is symptomatic and may include antihistamines, low-dose corticosteroids, mast cell stabilizers, and vasoconstrictors.

Chronic conjunctivitis is the result of any persistent conjunctivitis. The cause requires identification for effective treatment.

Trachoma (chlamydial conjunctivitis) is caused by *Chlamydia trachomatis*. It often is associated with poor hygiene and is the leading cause of preventable blindness in the world. The severity of the disease varies, but it can involve inflammation with scarring of the conjunctiva and eyelids causing distorted lashes to abrade the cornea, leading to corneal scarring and blindness. Chlamydial organisms are sensitive to local or systemic antibiotics. The World Health Organization aims to eliminate trachoma as a public health problem by 2020 using the SAFE Strategy: Surgery for inturned lashes, Antibiotics, Facial cleanliness, and Environmental improvement.[182]

Keratitis. **Keratitis** is an inflammation of the cornea that can be noninfectious or caused by bacteria, viruses, fungus, or amoebae. Bacterial infections often cause corneal ulceration and require intensive antibiotic treatment. *Staphylococcus aureus* is the most common bacterial infection. Type 1 herpes simplex virus can involve the cornea and conjunctiva. Predisposing factors include contact lens use, trauma, and penetrating keratoplasty (corneal grafting). *Acanthamoeba* is associated with contact lens use and is a severe sight-threatening corneal infection.[183] Common symptoms include photophobia, pain, and lacrimation. Severe ulcerations with residual scarring require corneal transplantation.

The Eye

The wall of the eye is formed of three layers: sclera, choroid, and retina (Fig. 16.12). The **sclera** is the thick, white, outermost layer. It becomes transparent at the **cornea**, the portion of the sclera in the central anterior region that allows light to enter the eye. The **choroid** is the deeply pigmented middle layer that prevents light from scattering inside the eye. The **iris**, part of the choroid, has a round opening, the **pupil**, through which light passes. Smooth muscle fibers control the size of the pupil so that in close vision and bright light the pupil constricts and in distant vision and dim light the pupil dilates.

The **retina** is the innermost layer of the eye and contains millions of rods and cones, special photoreceptors that convert light energy into nerve impulses. **Rods** mediate peripheral and dim light vision and are densest at the periphery. **Cones**, densest in the center of the retina, are color and detail receptors. The photoreceptive rods and cones are distributed over the entire retina, except where the optic nerve leaves the eyeball. Lack of rods and cones in this area form the **optic disc**, or blind spot. Lateral to each optic disc is the **macula**, a yellow disc that absorbs ultraviolet light. The **fovea centralis** is a tiny central area of the macula that contains only cones and provides the greatest visual acuity (see Fig. 16.12).

The **optic nerve** (second cranial nerve) is composed of retinal cell axons. As shown in Fig. 16.13, nerve impulses pass through the optic nerves after leaving the retinas. At the optic chiasm the fibers from the inner (nasal) halves of the retinas cross to the opposite side, where they join fibers from the outer (temporal) halves of the retinas to form the optic tracts. The fibers of the optic tracts synapse in the dorsal lateral geniculate nucleus, and from there the geniculocalcarine fibers pass by way of the optic radiation (or geniculocalcarine tract) to the primary visual cortex in the occipital lobe of the brain. Some fibers terminate in the suprachiasmatic nucleus (located above the optic chiasm) and are involved in regulating the sleep-wake cycle.

Light entering the eye is focused on the retina by the **lens**—a flexible, biconvex, crystal-like structure. In youth the lens is transparent and has the consistency of hardened jelly. The flexibility of the lens allows a change in curvature with contraction of the ciliary muscles. This is called **accommodation**, and it allows the eye to focus on objects at different distances. Anterior to the lens are the iris and the aqueous chamber, which is filled with **aqueous humor**. The aqueous humor helps to maintain the pressure inside the eye and provides nutrients to the lens and cornea. Aqueous humor is free-flowing fluid, secreted by the ciliary processes and reabsorbed into the canal of Schlemm. If drainage is blocked, pressure within the eye increases (as it does with glaucoma). Posterior to the lens is the vitreous chamber, which is filled with a gel-like substance called **vitreous humor**. Vitreous humor helps prevent the eyeball from collapsing inward.

The central retinal artery provides blood to the inner retinal surface. Nutrients and oxygen are supplied to the outer surface of the retina by the choroid, a vascular layer that lies between the retina and sclera. Six extrinsic eye muscles, attached to the outer surface of each eye, allow gross eye movements and permit the eyes to follow a moving object (Fig. 16.14).

AGING AND VISION

Changes in the visual and motor components of the eye caused by aging begin at an early age, particularly in the lens of the eye. Changes caused by aging are summarized in Table 16.6. Structural changes combined with chronic diseases, including dementias and diabetes mellitus, result in a decline in visual acuity and extraocular motor muscle function.[184]

Visual Dysfunction

Alterations in Ocular Movements. Abnormal ocular movements occur as a result of oculomotor, trochlear, or abducens cranial nerve dysfunction (see Table 15.6). The three types of eye movement disorders are (1) strabismus, (2) nystagmus, and (3) paralysis of individual extraocular muscles.

Strabismus is the deviation of one eye from the other when a person is looking at an object; it results in failure of the two eyes to simultaneously focus on the same image and therefore loss of binocular vision. The deviation may be upward, downward, inward, or outward, resulting from a weak or hypertonic muscle in one of the eyes. Strabismus may be caused by a neuromuscular disorder of the eye muscle, diseases involving the cerebral hemispheres, or thyroid disease.[185]

The primary symptom of strabismus is **diplopia** (double vision). Strabismus in children requires early intervention to prevent the development of amblyopia (reduced vision in the affected eye without ocular pathology and with full optical correction). Surgery may be helpful to both children and adults with strabismus.[186]

Nystagmus is an involuntary unilateral or bilateral rhythmic movement of the eyes and can occur in infants (congenital) or adults (acquired). It may be present at rest, or it may occur with eye movement. The two major forms of nystagmus are pendular nystagmus and jerk nystagmus. **Pendular nystagmus** is characterized by a regular alternating forward and backward movement of the eyes in which both phases of the movement are equal in length. In **jerk nystagmus** one phase of the eye movement is faster than the other. Nystagmus may be caused by an imbalance in the normally coordinated reflex activity of the inner ear, vestibular nuclei (connecting the vestibular nerve with vestibulospinal tracts), cerebellum, medial longitudinal fascicle (connecting the mesencephalon with the upper portion of the spinal cord), or nuclei of the oculomotor, trochlear, and abducens cranial nerves (see Table 15.6). Drugs, retinal disease, and diseases involving the cervical cord also may

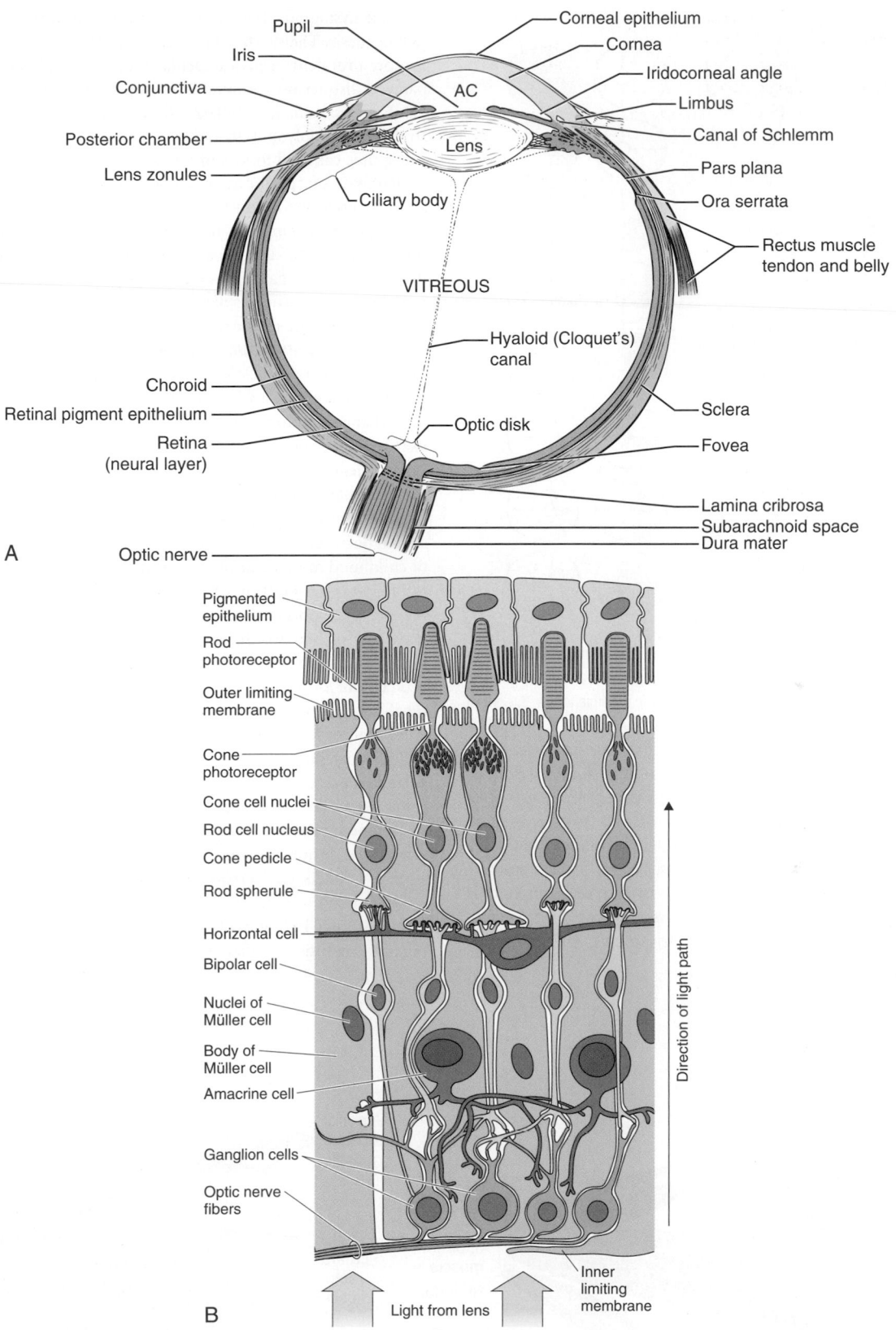

FIGURE 16.12 Structure of the Eyeball and Cell Layers of the Retina. A, The right eye is viewed from above (horizontal section). **B,** The various layers and cells of the retina. *AC,* Anterior chamber. (**A** from Forrester JV et al: *The eye: basic sciences in practice,* ed 4, St Louis 2016, Elsevier; **B** from Gartner LP: *Textbook of histology,* ed 4, Philadelphia, 2017, Elsevier.)

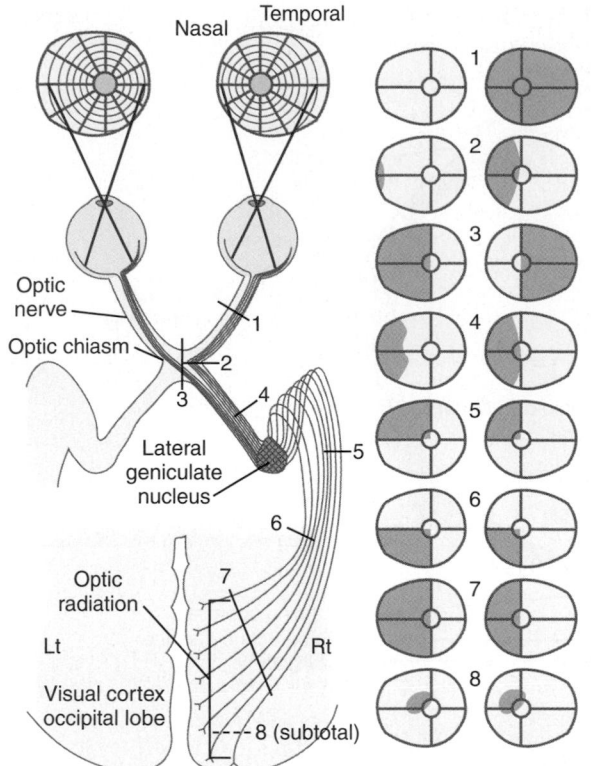

FIGURE 16.13 Visual Fields and Defects That Accompany Damage to the Right Visual Pathways. **1,** Optic nerve: blindness. **2,** Lateral optic chiasm: grossly incongruous, incomplete (contralateral) homonymous hemianopsia. **3,** Central optic chiasm: bitemporal hemianopsia. **4,** Optic tract: incongruous, incomplete homonymous hemianopsia. **5,** Temporal loop of the optic radiation: congruous partial or complete (contralateral) homonymous superior quadrantanopia. **6,** Parietal *(superior)* projection of the optic radiation: congruous partial or complete homonymous inferior quadrantanopia. **7,** Complete parietooccipital interruption of the optic radiation: complete congruous homonymous hemianopsia with psychophysical shift of the foveal point, often sparing central vision and resulting in "macular sparing." **8,** Incomplete (subtotal) damage to the visual cortex: congruous homonymous scotomas, usually encroaching at least acutely on central vision. (From Goldman C, editor: *Goldman's Cecil medicine,* ed 24, vol 2, Philadelphia, 2012, Saunders.)

produce nystagmus. Infantile nystagmus syndrome has an unknown pathogenesis. The syndrome develops in the first 6 months of age and is more prevalent in males. Ocular motor control and anterior visual pathway disturbances are under investigation. One disease-causing gene has been identified, X-linked *FRMD7.* There may be an associated strabismus, amblyopia, torticollis, or visual impairment.[187] Untreated nystagmus can lead to loss of visual acuity.[188]

Paralysis of specific extraocular muscles may cause a variety of abnormalities, including limited abduction, abnormal closure of the eyelid, ptosis (drooping of the eyelid), and diplopia. The abnormalities occur as a result of unopposed muscle activity. Trauma or pressure in the area of the cranial nerves may cause paralysis of specific extraocular muscles. Diseases such as diabetes mellitus and myasthenia gravis also may affect specific extraocular muscles.

Alterations in Visual Acuity. Visual acuity is the ability to see objects in sharp detail. With advancing age the eye's lens becomes less flexible and less adjustable, and visual acuity declines. Visual acuity also may change or diminish for many other reasons. Specific causes of visual acuity changes include: (1) amblyopia, (2) scotoma, (3) cataracts, (4) papilledema, (5) dark adaptation, (6) glaucoma, (7) retinal detachment, and (8) macular degeneration.

Amblyopia (lazy eye) is a reduction or dimness of vision related to altered development of the visual cortex and is the most common cause of childhood monocular blindness. It does not result from a change in refraction (i.e., deviation of light rays) or from any visible changes in the eye. Amblyopia is associated with strabismus, anisometropia (refractive error in one eye differs from that of the other eye), ametropia (severe refractive error in both eyes), stimulus deprivation (congenital cataracts or orbital lesions); with diseases such as diabetes mellitus, renal failure, and malaria; and with toxic substances, such as alcohol and tobacco. Early detection is required to restore vision. Treatment includes patching the unaffected eye for extended times to ensure a period of use of the affected eye, or administering atropine eyedrops (blurring vision). Research related to brain plasticity with bilateral treatment approaches, including visual perceptual learning and video gaming, is promising for visual restoration in both children and adults.[189,190] Refractive errors are treated with corrective lenses.

A scotoma is a circumscribed defect of the central field of vision. It can be caused by lesions of the central retina or a sequela to demyelinating optic neuritis, an inflammatory lesion of the optic nerve frequently

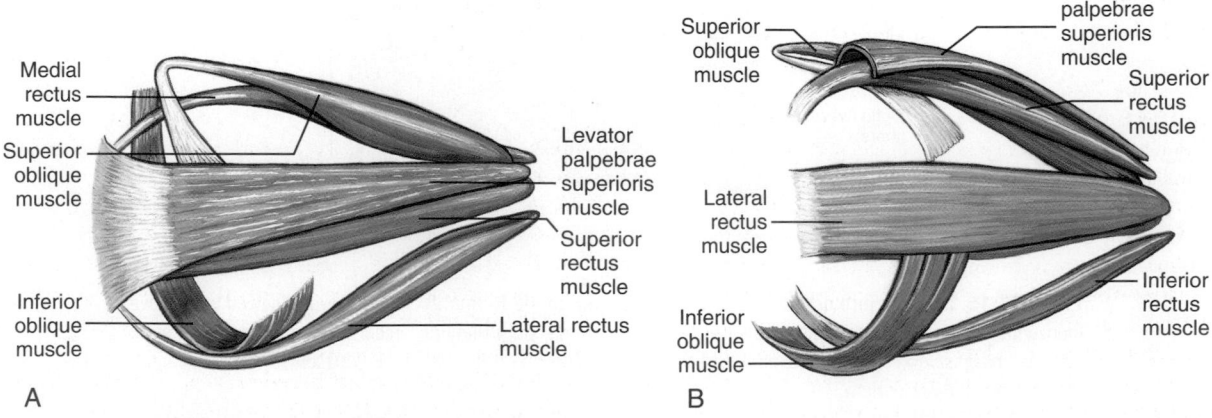

A   B

FIGURE 16.14 Extrinsic Muscles of the Right Eye. **A,** Superior view. **B,** Inferior view. (From Dutton JJ: *Atlas of clinical and surgical orbital anatomy,* ed 2, Philadelphia, 2011, Saunders.)

TABLE 16.6   CHANGES IN THE EYE CAUSED BY AGING

STRUCTURE	CHANGE	CONSEQUENCE
Cornea	Thicker and less curved; decreased sensitivity to touch	Increase in astigmatism
	Formation of a gray ring at the edge of cornea (arcus senilis)	Not detrimental to vision
Anterior chamber	Decrease in size and volume caused by thickening of lens	Occasionally exerts pressure on Schlemm canal and may lead to increased intraocular pressure and glaucoma
Lens	Increase in thickness and opacity (yellowing)	Decrease in refraction with increased light scattering and decreased color vision (green and blue); delayed dark adaptation; cataracts
	Loss of elasticity	Loss of accommodation (presbyopia: loss of focus for near objects)
Ciliary muscles	Reduction in pupil diameter; atrophy of radial dilation muscles	Persistent constriction (senile miosis); decrease in critical flicker frequency*
Retina	Reduction in number of rods at periphery; loss of rods and associated nerve cells	Increase in the minimum amount of light necessary to see an object
Macula	Atrophy (age-related macular degeneration)	Loss of vision
Vitreous	Liquefaction of vitreous and decrease in gel volume	Posterior vitreous detachment causing "floaters;" risk for retinal detachment

*The rate at which consecutive visual stimuli can be presented and still be perceived as separate.

associated with optico-spinal multiple sclerosis (see Chapter 18). Age-related macular degeneration is associated with scotoma. Less common causes include the compression of one optic nerve by a retroorbital tumor, neuromyelitis optica (autoantibody-related inflammation of the optic nerve and spinal cord), pernicious anemia, and toxic or metabolic causes such as methyl alcohol poisoning and use of tobacco. The precise mechanisms for these conditions causing a scotoma are uncertain, but the result is always a serious impairment in visual acuity.[191]

A cataract is a cloudy or opaque area in the ocular lens and leads to visual loss when located on the visual axis. The incidence of cataracts increases with age as the lens enlarges. Cataracts develop because of alterations of metabolism and transport of nutrients within the lens. Although the most common form of cataract is degenerative, cataracts also may occur congenitally or as a result of infection, radiation, trauma, drugs, or diabetes mellitus. Cataracts cause decreased visual acuity, blurred vision, glare, and decreased color perception. Cataracts are treated by removal of the entire lens and replacement with an intraocular artificial lens.[192]

Dark adaptation also affects visual acuity. Low illumination causes impaired visual acuity, particularly in older adults. The average 80-year-old person needs more than twice as much light as a 20-year-old person to see equally well. Changes in the quantity and quality of rhodopsin, a substance found in the rods and responsible for low-light vision, are thought to be responsible for reduced dark adaptation in older adults.[193] Vitamin A deficiencies can cause the same phenomenon in individuals of any age.

Glaucomas are the second leading cause of blindness and are characterized by intraocular pressures greater than 12 to 20 mmHg, with death of retinal ganglion cells and optic nerve axons. Family history is a risk factor, and several glaucoma-associated genes have been identified.[194] The types of glaucoma are summarized in Table 16.7 and Fig. 16.15. Most forms of glaucoma are associated with resistance to aqueous humor outflow. Primary open-angle glaucoma is the most common and is associated with alterations in the trabecular meshwork. Chronic increased intraocular pressure causes death of retinal ganglions and optic nerve degeneration with loss of peripheral vision, followed by central vision impairment and blindness. Extremely high pressures can cause blindness within days or hours. Loss of visual acuity results from pressure on the optic nerve, which is believed to block the flow of cytoplasm from neuronal bodies in the retina to peripheral optic nerve

TABLE 16.7   TYPES OF GLAUCOMA

TYPE	MECHANISM OF INCREASED PRESSURE
Open-angle	Obstruction of outflow of aqueous humor at trabecular meshwork or Schlemm canal; myopia may be a risk factor
Normal or low-tension	Form of open-angle glaucoma with symptomless damage to the optic nerve and gradual vision loss when intraocular pressure is within normal range (12-20 mmHg)
Narrow-angle (angle-closure)	Forward displacement of iris toward cornea with narrowing of iridocorneal angle and obstruction to outflow of aqueous humor from anterior chamber
Acute angle-closure	Acute closure of iridocorneal angle with a sudden rise in intraocular pressure, producing pain, redness, and visual disturbances
Chronic angle-closure	Progressive, permanent closure of anterior chamber angle
Secondary	Open- or closed-angle obstruction caused by, for example, uveitis, hemorrhage, rupture of lens or tumors
Congenital glaucoma	Malformation of trabecular meshwork and excess extracellular matrix in outer meshwork

fibers entering the brain. Lack of nutrients, ischemia, oxidative stress associated with mitochondrial failure, inflammatory cytokines, excessive apoptosis, and altered immune mechanisms may lead to death of the involved neurons.[195] Initially there are no symptoms. With increasing pressure acute pain may result, and there is loss of peripheral vision and progression to blindness. Early detection and treatment prevent optic neuropathy and visual impairment. Screening programs assist in identifying this silent disease. Glaucoma often is treated with pharmaceutical eyedrops to reduce secretion or increase absorption of aqueous humor. Surgery may be needed to open the spaces of the trabeculae and reduce intraocular pressure. Neuroprotective therapies are being evaluated.[196]

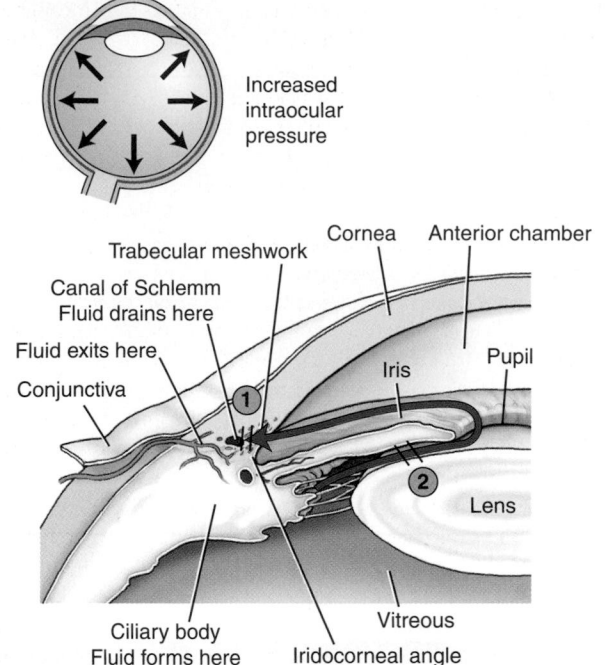

FIGURE 16.15 Glaucoma. **1,** Open-angle glaucoma. The obstruction to aqueous flow lies in the trabecular meshwork. **2,** Closed-angle glaucoma. The iris presses against the lens, blocking aqueous flow into the anterior chamber and raising intraocular pressure.

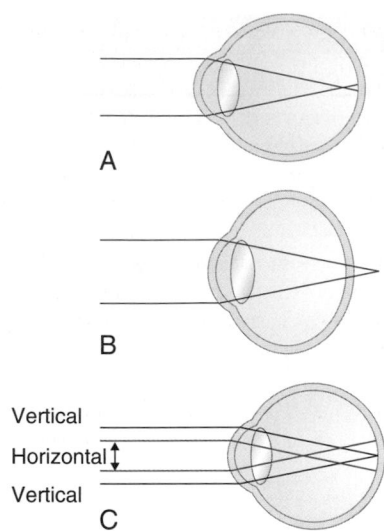

FIGURE 16.16 Alterations in Refraction. **A,** Myopic eye. Parallel rays of light are brought to a focus in front of the retina. **B,** Hyperopic eye. Parallel rays of light come to a focus behind the retina in the nonaccommodative eye. **C,** Simple myopic astigmatism. The vertical bundle of rays is focused on the retina; the horizontal rays are focused in front of the retina and the image is blurred. (From Stein HA, Stein RM, Freeman MI: *The ophthalmic assistant: a text for allied and associated ophthalmic personnel,* ed 9, Philadelphia, 2013, Saunders.)

Retinal detachment is a common cause of visual impairment and blindness. Risk factors include retinal holes and vitreoretinal traction. Fluid (exudate, hemorrhage, or liquid vitreous) separates the photoreceptors from the retinal pigment epithelium. The separation deprives the outer retina of oxygen and nutrients because the diffusion distance is increased. Communication is also disrupted between the pigment epithelium and photoreceptors. **Rhegmatogenous retinal detachment** (full thickness retinal breaks caused by vitreoretinal traction) is the most common form of retinal detachment. Causes include intracapsular cataract extraction, severe myopia, age-related lattice degeneration, vitreoretinal traction, and trauma. Contraction of fibrous membranes can cause tractional separation of the retinal layers as occurs in proliferative diabetic retinopathy. Treatment involves immediate surgical retinal reattachment.[197]

Age-related macular degeneration (AMD) is a severe and irreversible loss of vision and a major cause of central blindness in older individuals. Risk factors include older age, hypertension, cigarette smoking, diabetes mellitus, previous cataract surgery, and family history of AMD. The degeneration usually occurs after the age of 60 years.

There are two forms: atrophic (dry, nonexudative–geographic atrophic) and neovascular (wet, exudative). The atrophic form is more common and is slowly progressive with inflammation and accumulation of lipofuscin (a lysosomal pigmented residue) and drusen (waste products from photoreceptors) in the retina. Symptoms include limited night vision and difficulty reading. The neovascular form includes accumulation of drusen and lipofuscin, abnormal choroidal blood vessel growth, leakage of blood or serum, retinal detachment, fibrovascular scarring, loss of photoreceptors, and more severe and rapid loss of central vision. Treatment for wet AMD includes antivascular endothelial growth factor (anti-VEGF) injections; new treatments are under investigation.[198] Two carotenoids, lutein and zeaxanthin, are antioxidants that selectively accumulate in the macula. Supplements of lutein and zeaxanthin may enhance vision in early dry AMD.[199]

Alterations in Accommodation. Accommodation is the process whereby the thickness of the lens changes with contraction of the ciliary muscles. Accommodation is needed for clear vision and is mediated through the oculomotor nerve (cranial nerve III). Pressure, inflammation, and disease of the oculomotor nerve may alter accommodation. Symptoms include diplopia, blurred vision, and headache. Loss of accommodation in adults beginning at ages 45 to 50 years is termed **presbyopia,** a condition in which the ocular lens becomes larger, firmer, and less elastic in response to ciliary muscle contraction. The major symptom is reduced near vision, causing the individual to hold reading material at arm's length. Correction of presbyopia is accomplished through reading glasses or bifocal lenses, accommodative intraocular lenses, or surgical treatment.[200]

Alterations in Refraction. Alterations in refraction are the most common visual problem. Errors in refraction are caused by irregularities of the corneal curvature, the focusing power of the lens, and the length of the eye. The major symptoms of refraction alterations are blurred vision and headache. Three types of refraction alterations are myopia, hyperopia, and astigmatism (Fig. 16.16).

In **myopia** (nearsightedness), the axis of the eyeball is lengthened and light rays are focused in front of the retina when a person is looking at a distant object, resulting in blurred vision. The cause is unknown. A concave lens is needed for correction. Myopia requires frequent changes of eyeglasses while the eyeball is lengthening in childhood. Myopia is a risk factor for retinal detachment, cataract formation, and glaucoma.

In **hyperopia** (farsightedness), the axis of the eyeball is too short and light rays are focused behind the retina when a person is looking at a near object. **Astigmatism** is caused by an unequal curvature of the cornea. In astigmatism, light rays are bent unevenly and do not come to a single focus on the retina. Astigmatism may coexist with myopia, hyperopia, or presbyopia. Hyperopia is corrected with a convex lens or laser refractive surgery.

Alterations in Color Vision. Normal sensitivity to color diminishes with age because of the progressive yellowing of the lens that occurs with aging. All colors become less intense, although color discrimination for blue and green is most greatly affected. Color vision deteriorates more rapidly for individuals with diabetes mellitus than for the general population. The deterioration is thought to be an accelerated version of senile color vision deterioration.

Abnormal color vision also may be caused by color blindness, an inherited trait. Color blindness is generally an X-linked recessive characteristic affecting 6% to 8% of the male population and 0.5% of the female population. Although many forms of color blindness exist, most commonly the affected individual cannot distinguish red from green.[201] In the most severe form individuals see only shades of gray, black, and white.

Neurologic Disorders Causing Visual Dysfunction. Various neurologic disorders may cause visual dysfunction.[202] Vision may be disrupted at many points along the visual pathway, causing a variety of defects in fields of vision. Visual changes do not always cause defects or blindness in the entire visual field; hemianopia is the term that describes defective vision in half of a visual field. (Fig. 16.13 illustrates the many areas along the visual pathway that may be damaged and the associated visual changes.) Because of the anatomy of the optic nerves, injury to the optic nerve causes ipsilateral (same side) blindness but a normal contralateral (opposite side) visual field. Injury to the optic chiasm (the X-shaped crossing of the optic nerves), often caused by atherosclerotic ischemia or external compression from trauma or aneurysm, can cause a variety of defects, depending on the location of injury. These defects vary because at the optic chiasm, nerve fibers from the medial half of each retina separate from the lateral half and enter the opposite optic tract.

Because of the normal structure of the visual pathways, destruction of one optic tract causes homonymous hemianopsia (complete loss of vision in the inner half of one eye and the outer half of the other). Thus, if an injury to the left optic tract occurs, the individual is blind in the right eye's medial (inner) field and the left eye's lateral (outer) field. If the compression of the optic tract is asymmetric, an incongruous (or uneven) homonymous defect results. Injury to one optic radiation (an ocular pathway in the internal capsule, temporal lobe, or occipital lobe) also causes a homonymous (same field) defect. A major injury in the optic radiation causes homonymous hemianopsia. A lesser injury may cause an upper quadrant homonymous defect. Generally the defects are the same size in both eyes. When the homonymous hemianopsia is caused by an occipital lobe lesion, the area of hemianopsia is split. Although visual acuity may remain unimpaired, reading is difficult because of the inability to group words.

Papilledema is edema of the optic nerve at its point of entrance into the eyeball. Papilledema is caused by increased intracranial pressure (e.g., brain tumors, intracranial hemorrhage, hydrocephalus). The subarachnoid space of the brain is continuous with the optic nerve sheath. As cerebrospinal fluid (CSF) pressure increases, the pressure is transmitted to the optic nerve, and the optic nerve sheath compresses the nerve and impedes axoplasmic transport. This leads to accumulation of axoplasmic substances at the level of the lamina cribrosa (a meshlike structure in the sclera where the retinal nerves exit the eye and form the optic nerve), resulting in the characteristic swelling of the optic disc. Obliteration of the physiologic cup (a bright area normally located in the center of the optic disc) follows. Later the optic disc becomes raised above the level of the surrounding retina, and the margins become blurred and indistinct. With severe swelling, hemorrhage and patches of white exudate (caused by nerve infarcts) surround the disc margins. The edematous nerves compress the small retinal veins, causing venous stasis and engorgement. Headache is common, and there may be no visual changes, blurred vision, or constriction of visual fields.

Hearing

The external auditory canal is surrounded by the bones of the cranium. The opening (meatus) of the canal is just above the mastoid process (Fig. 16.17). The air-filled sinuses, called mastoid air cells, are located

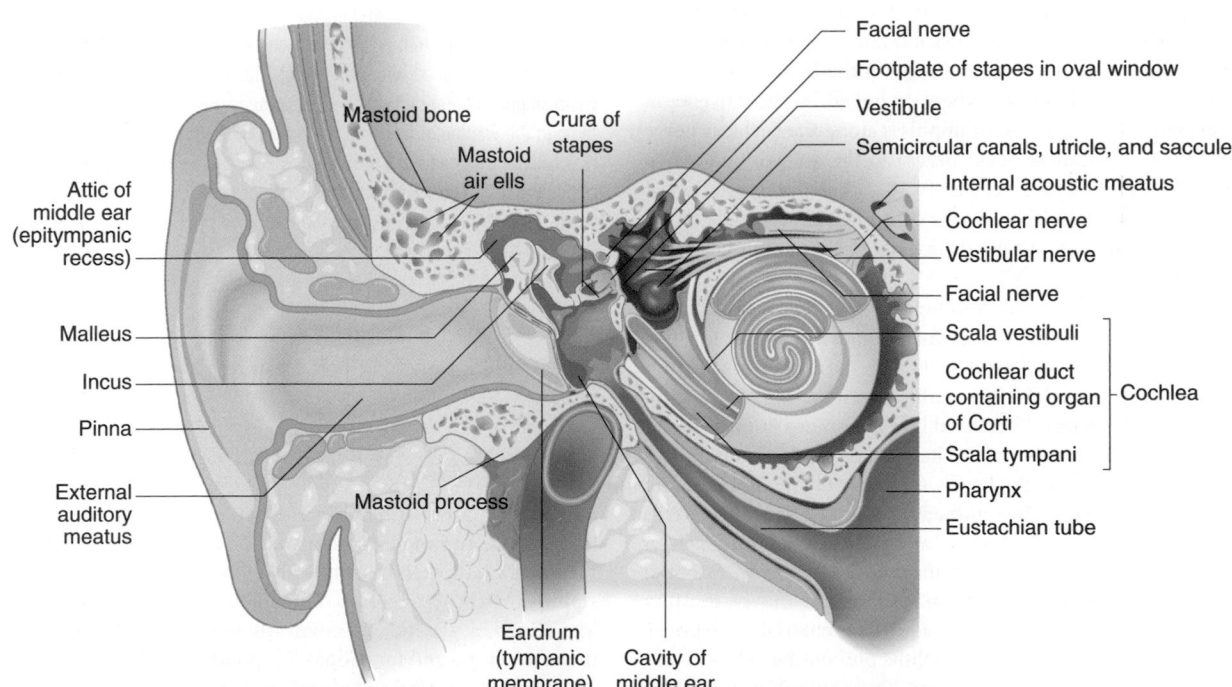

FIGURE 16.17 The Ear. External, middle, and inner ear structures. (From Glynn M, Drake WM: *Hutchison's clinical methods: an integrated approach to clinical practice*, ed 23, London, 2012, Elsevier.)

in the mastoid process and promote conductivity of sound between the external and the middle ear. Mastoid air cells communicate with the middle ear cavity through the entrance to the mastoid antrum.

The Ear

The ear is divided into three areas: (1) the external ear, involved only with hearing; (2) the middle ear, involved only with hearing; and (3) the inner ear, involved with both hearing and equilibrium. The external ear is composed of the pinna (auricle), which is the visible portion of the ear, and the external auditory canal, a tube that leads to the middle ear (see Fig. 16.17). Sound waves entering the external auditory canal hit the tympanic membrane (eardrum) and cause it to vibrate. The tympanic membrane separates the external ear from the middle ear.

The middle ear is composed of the tympanic cavity, a small chamber in the temporal bone. Three ossicles (small bones known as the malleus [hammer], incus [anvil], and stapes [stirrup]) transmit the vibration of the tympanic membrane to the inner ear. When the tympanic membrane moves, the malleus moves with it and transfers the vibration to the incus, which passes it on to the stapes. The stapes presses against the oval window, a small membrane of the inner ear. The movement of the oval window sets the fluids of the inner ear in motion (Fig. 16.18).

The eustachian (pharyngotympanic) tube connects the middle ear with the thorax. Normally flat and closed, the eustachian tube opens briefly when a person swallows or yawns, and it equalizes the pressure in the middle ear with atmospheric pressure. Equalized pressure permits the tympanic membrane to vibrate freely. Through the eustachian tube the mucosa of the middle ear is contiguous with the mucosal lining of the throat.

The inner ear is a system of osseous labyrinths (bony, mazelike chambers) filled with a fluid called perilymph. The bony labyrinth is divided into the cochlea, the vestibule, and the semicircular canals (see Fig. 16.18). Suspended in the perilymph is the endolymph-filled membranous labyrinth that basically follows the shape of the bony labyrinth.

Within the cochlea is the organ of Corti, which contains hair cells (hearing receptors). Sound waves that reach the cochlea through vibrations of the tympanic membrane, ossicles, and oval window set the cochlear fluids into motion. Receptor cells on the basilar membrane are stimulated when their hairs are bent or pulled by the movement. Once stimulated, hair cells transmit impulses along the cochlear nerve (a division of the vestibulocochlear nerve) to the auditory cortex of the temporal lobe in the brain (see Fig. 16.18), where interpretation of the sound occurs. Directional hearing is controlled by the angle of the sound source to both ears and by the axonal delay in conduction in groups of neurons.

The semicircular canals and vestibule of the inner ear contain equilibrium receptors. In the semicircular canals the dynamic equilibrium receptors respond to changes in direction of movement. Within each semicircular canal is the crista ampullaris, a receptor region composed of a tuft of hair cells covered by a gelatinous cupula. When the head is rotated, the endolymph in the canal lags behind and moves in the direction opposite to the head's movement. The hair cells are stimulated, and impulses are transmitted through the vestibular nerve (a division of the vestibulocochlear nerve) to the cerebellum.

The vestibule in the inner ear contains maculae, receptors essential to the body's sense of static equilibrium. As the head moves, otoliths (small pieces of calcium salts) move in a gel-like material in response to changes in the pull of gravity. The otoliths pull on the gel, which in turn pulls on the hair cells in the maculae. Nerve impulses in the hair cells are triggered and transmitted to the brain (see Fig. 16.18). Thus the ear not only permits the hearing of a large range of sounds but also

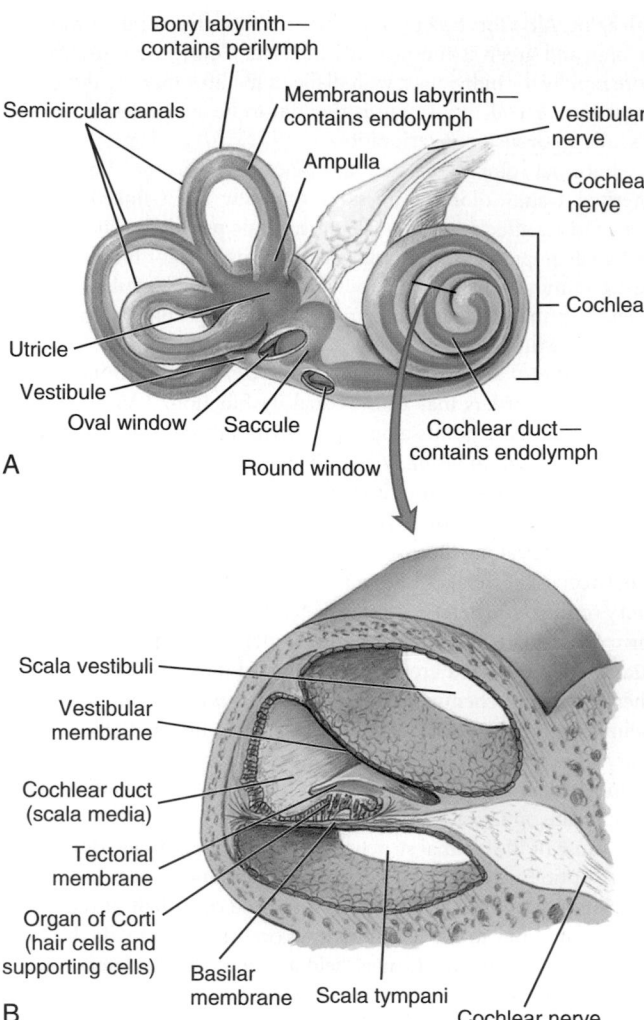

FIGURE 16.18 The Inner Ear. A, The bony labyrinth *(tan)* is the hard outer wall of the entire inner ear and includes semicircular canals, vestibule, and cochlea. Within the bony labyrinth is the membranous labyrinth *(purple),* which is surrounded by perilymph and filled with endolymph. Each ampulla in the vestibule contains a crista ampullaris that detects changes in head position and sends sensory impulses through the vestibular nerve to the brain. **B,** Section of the membranous cochlea. Hair cells in the organ of Corti detect sound and send the information through the cochlear nerve. The vestibular and cochlear nerves join to form the eighth cranial nerve. (From Applegate E: *The anatomy and physiology learning system,* ed 4, St Louis, 2011, Saunders.)

assists with maintaining balance through the sensitive equilibrium receptors.

AGING AND HEARING

Presbycusis is loss of hearing in older age.[203] Auditory changes caused by aging are common, incremental, and with considerable individual variation. Changes in hearing with aging are summarized in Table 16.8. Approximately 30% to 40% of people older than 65 years have hearing loss caused by genetic and environmental factors. Changes may occur in the structural and functional components of the peripheral or central auditory system. Accumulative damage to the middle ear and inner ear, particularly of hair cells (sensory presbycusis) and the cochlea (neural presbycusis), is caused by damaging factors such as noise, inflammation,

TABLE 16.8	CHANGES IN HEARING CAUSED BY AGING

CHANGES IN STRUCTURE	CHANGES IN FUNCTION
Cochlear hair cell degeneration	Inability to hear high-frequency sounds (presbycusis, sensorineural loss); interferes with understanding speech; hearing may be lost in both ears at different times
Loss of auditory neurons in spiral ganglia of organ of Corti	Inability to hear high-frequency sounds (presbycusis, sensorineural loss); interferes with understanding speech; hearing may be lost in both ears at different times
Degeneration of basilar (cochlear) conductive membrane of cochlea	Inability to hear at all frequencies, but more pronounced at higher frequencies (cochlear conductive loss)
Decreased vascularity of cochlea	Equal loss of hearing at all frequencies (strial loss); inability to disseminate localization of sound
Loss of cortical auditory neurons	Equal loss of hearing at all frequencies (strial loss); inability to disseminate localization of sound

toxins, oxidative stress, and vascular damage (i.e., atherosclerosis and diabetes mellitus).

Ototoxic drugs include antibiotics, such as streptomycin, neomycin, gentamicin, and vancomycin; diuretics, such as ethacrynic acid and furosemide; chemicals, such as salicylate, quinine, carbon monoxide, nitrogen mustard, arsenic, mercury, gold, tobacco, and alcohol; and cancer drugs (i.e., cisplatin). Because of increased concentrations of antibiotics in the endolymph, these drugs generally cause damage to the cells of the cochlea or the hair cells of the organ of Corti. Diuretics affect hearing primarily by altering the sodium-potassium balance, causing extracellular fluid accumulation and changes in the microstructure of secretory cells. Quinine, mercury, and lead affect the neural pathways of hearing, including the spinal ganglia, the eighth cranial nerve, and the cochlear nucleus.

Loss of hearing for sounds in the high-frequency range is most common and interferes with understanding speech, particularly high-frequency consonant sounds (e.g., s, sh, f). Hearing may be lost in both ears but not at the same time. The ability to discriminate localization of sound varies with high and low frequencies and diminishes with age. In the low-frequency range, sound localization is a function of the timing of sound arrival between the two ears; localization of high-frequency sounds is a function of sound intensity. Because older adults tend to lose high-frequency hearing first, they may have difficulty localizing high-frequency sounds and understanding speech. Cognitive impairment and poor quality of life are associated with presbycusis.[204]

Auditory Dysfunction

Between 5% and 10% of the general population have a hearing impairment. The major categories of auditory dysfunction are conductive hearing loss, sensorineural hearing loss, mixed hearing loss, and functional hearing loss.

Conductive Hearing Loss. Conductive hearing loss occurs when a change in the outer or middle ear impairs sound from being conducted from the outer to the inner ear. Conductive hearing loss occurs when there is interference in air conduction. Conditions that commonly cause a conductive hearing loss include impacted cerumen, foreign bodies lodged in the ear canal, benign tumors of the middle ear, carcinoma of the external auditory canal or middle ear, eustachian tube dysfunction, otitis media, acute viral otitis media, chronic suppurative otitis media, cholesteatoma, and otosclerosis (impaired mobility of the stapes footplate in the presence of dense sclerotic bone).

Symptoms of conductive hearing loss include diminished hearing and soft speaking voice. The voice is soft because often the individual hears his or her voice, conducted by bone, as loud. In addition, although the cause is unknown, the individual often hears better in a noisy environment than in a quiet one (a condition called *paracusia willisiana*). Treatment of the underlying cause generally improves hearing, and a hearing aid can improve quality of life.[205]

Sensorineural Hearing Loss. A sensorineural hearing loss is caused by impairment of the organ of Corti or its central connections. The hearing loss may be gradual or sudden. Conditions that commonly cause sensorineural hearing loss include congenital and hereditary factors, noise exposure, aging, Ménière disease, ototoxicity (see drugs associated with presbycusis above), and systemic disease (syphilis, Paget disease, collagen diseases, diabetes mellitus). Congenital and neonatal sensorineural hearing loss may be caused by maternal rubella, cytomegalovirus, ototoxic drugs, prematurity, traumatic delivery, erythroblastosis fetalis, and congenital hereditary malfunction.[206] Diagnosis often is made when delayed speech development is noted. Treatment includes hearing aids and cochlear implant. Gene therapy and allotransplantation of stem cells are under investigation.[207]

Mixed Hearing Loss. A mixed hearing loss is caused by a combination of conductive and sensorineural losses.

Functional Hearing Loss. A functional hearing loss occurs for no organic reason. The individual does not respond to voice and appears not to hear. Functional hearing loss is thought to be caused by emotional or psychologic factors. It occurs only rarely.

Ear Infections

Otitis Externa. Otitis externa is inflammation of the external ear canal with or without infection and may include parts of the outer ear. It is commonly acute rather than chronic. Regular swimming is a risk factor. Alterations in the normal acidic environment, lack of cerumen, and trauma to skin epithelium can lead to bacterial and, less commonly, fungal infections with inflammation. The most frequently found microorganisms are *Pseudomonas, Escherichia coli,* and *Staphylococcus aureus*. Infection usually follows prolonged exposure to moisture (swimmer's ear). The earliest symptoms are inflammation with swelling, tenderness, and itching with clear drainage progressing to purulent drainage and obstruction of the canal. Treatment includes topical antibiotics and steroids.[208]

Otitis Media. Otitis media is an infection of the middle ear and is the most common infection of infants and children. Otitis media is the leading cause of healthcare visits and drug prescriptions throughout the world, with 50% occurring in the under 5-year age group.[209] Most children have one episode by 3 years of age. The most common pathogens are *Haemophilus influenzae, Moraxella catarrhalis, Streptococcus pneumonia,* and *Staphylococcus aureus*. Respiratory viruses also may have an etiologic role.[210] Predisposing factors include allergy, sinusitis, submucous cleft palate, adenoidal hypertrophy, and immune deficiency. Breast-feeding is a protective factor.

Acute otitis media (AOM) is associated with ear pain, fever, irritability, inflamed tympanic membrane, and fluid in the middle ear. The tympanic membrane progresses from erythema to opaqueness with bulging as fluid accumulates. An increasing prevalence of AOM is caused by methicillin-resistant microorganisms. Otitis media with effusion (OME) is the presence of fluid in the middle ear without symptoms of acute infection. Treatment includes antimicrobial therapy for AOM, particularly in children 2 years and younger. Reduction in the incidence of AOM has accompanied the widespread use of bacterial and viral vaccines in young children, including pneumococcal conjugate and influenza vaccines.[211]

Chronic otitis media (COM) is persistent or recurring infection of the middle ear. Chronic suppurative OM (CSOM) is associated with ear drum perforation and purulent discharge. Conductive hearing loss occurs when the effusion prevents the middle ear ossicles from effectively relaying sound vibrations from the ear drum to the oval window of the inner ear. Sensorineural hearing loss occurs when inflammatory mediators penetrate into the inner ear through the round window with loss of hair cells in the cochlea. Placement of tympanostomy tubes is considered when bilateral effusion persists for 3 months and for significant hearing loss. Mastoidectomy combined with tympanostomy ventilation tubes may be required when there is cholesteatoma (skin growth into the middle ear associated with perforation of the eardrum). Complications include mastoiditis, brain abscess, meningitis, and chronic otitis media with hearing loss. Speech, language, and cognitive disabilities may be affected by persistent middle ear effusions. Eosinophilic COM is associated with bronchial asthma and with sensitization to bacterial or fungal ear infection.[212]

Olfaction and Taste

Olfaction (smell) dysfunction and taste (gustation) dysfunction may occur separately or jointly. The strong relationship between smell and taste creates the sensation of flavor. If either sensation is impaired, the perception of flavor is altered. (Olfactory structures are illustrated in Fig. 16.19.)

Olfaction is a function of cranial nerve I (olfactory) and part of cranial nerve V (trigeminal). The receptor cells for smell are located in the olfactory epithelium. Seven primary classes of olfactory stimulants have been identified: (1) camphoraceous, (2) musky, (3) floral, (4) peppermint, (5) ethereal, (6) pungent, and (7) putrid. Olfaction is important for detection of hazards in the environment, generating feelings of pleasure, promoting adequate nutrition, influencing sexuality, and maintenance of mood.[213]

Olfactory dysfunctions include hyposmia, anosmia, hallucinations, and parosmia. Hyposmia is the impaired sense of smell, and anosmia is the complete loss of smell. Both conditions are associated with aging, neurodegenerative and nasal/sinus disorders, and head trauma. When hyposmia or anosmia occurs bilaterally, it is usually the result of rhinitis (inflammation of nasal mucosa), sinusitis, nasal polyps, or excessive smoking. Unilateral hyposmia or anosmia may indicate compression of one olfactory bulb (a bulblike portion of the olfactory nerves) or nerve tract (olfactory nerve pathway), possibly by tumor or head trauma. Olfactory hallucinations arise from hyperactivity in cortical neurons and involve smelling odors that are not really present. They are associated with temporal lobe seizures and rarely with schizophrenia. Parosmia, an abnormal or perverted sense of smell, may occur with severe depression and in Parkinson and Alzheimer disease.[214]

Taste is a function of multiple nerves in the tongue, soft palate, uvula, pharynx, and upper esophagus, including cranial nerves VII (facial) and IX (glossopharyngeal). Taste buds (fungiform, foliate, and circumvallate) sensitive to each of the primary sensations are located in specific areas of the tongue and are continuously renewing.[215]

The primary sensations of taste are sour, salty, sweet, bitter, and umami (savoriness). Taste buds sensitive to each of the primary sensations are located on the circumvallate, fungiform, and foliate papillae in specific areas of the tongue. Taste receptors also are found on airway smooth muscle (bitter) and in the gastrointestinal tract (bitter and sweet). Their function is not for taste. In the lung they stimulate bronchodilation, and in the gastrointestinal tract they may participate in metabolic and digestive regulation.[216,217]

Alterations in taste can be caused by injury, medications, oral infections, or aging. A change in taste also may be attributable to impairment of smell associated with injury near the hippocampus.

Hypogeusia is a decrease in taste sensation, and ageusia is the absence of taste. Ageusia affecting the entire tongue may follow head injury. Hypogeusia and ageusia occur with viral respiratory and oral infections. Autoimmune disease (i.e., systemic lupus erythematosus) and cancer chemotherapy alter taste sensitivity. Damage to the glossopharyngeal nerve (cranial nerve IX, which innervates the posterior one third of the tongue) causes the loss of the ability to detect bitterness. This loss occurs because the receptors for bitter are located on the base of the tongue. Damage to the facial nerve (cranial nerve VII, which innervates the anterior two-thirds of the tongue) causes loss of the ability to detect sour, sweet, and salty tastes. Only bitter tastes can be detected. These losses occur because sour, sweet, and salt receptors are located on the anterior portion of the tongue.[218]

AGING AND OLFACTION AND TASTE

Sensitivity to odors declines steadily with aging.[219] A study of odor identification indicates an increasing ability from childhood to adolescence and then a decline after 60 years of age. The sense of smell begins to degenerate with loss of olfactory sensory neurons and loss of cells from the olfactory bulbs. The mechanism of loss is unknown. Loss of olfactory sensitivity and odor identification may diminish appetite and food selection and thus may lead to malnutrition. Safety also may be compromised by an inability to smell spoiled food or hazardous gases.[220]

Parageusia is a perversion of taste in which substances possess an unpleasant flavor. Parageusia occasionally develops for no apparent reason in older adults, leading to anorexia and malnutrition. The decline in taste sensation is more gradual than that of smell and is associated with loss of olfaction. Higher concentrations of flavors are required, and older adults have difficulty differentiating combinations of flavors. Taste changes with aging are associated with decline in the number of fungiform papillae on the tongue, and changes in taste receptor function.[218] Taste also may be affected by decreased salivary gland secretion. Amylase, contained in saliva, facilitates perception of sweet flavors.

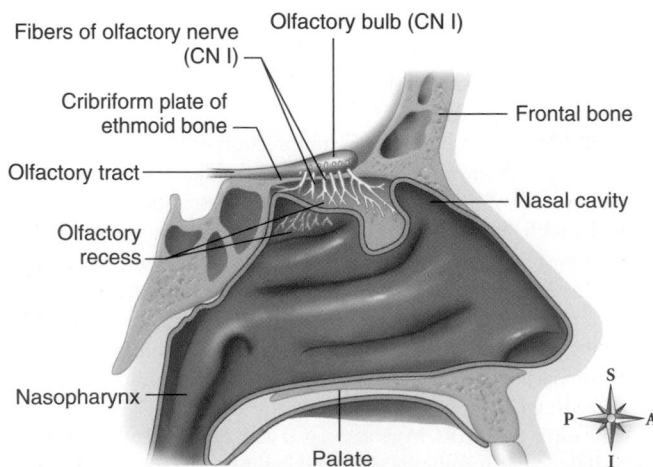

FIGURE 16.19 Olfaction. Midsagittal section of the nasal area shows the locations of major olfactory sensory structures. (From Patton KT, Thibodeau GA, Douglas MM: *Essentials of anatomy & physiology*, St Louis, 2012, Mosby.)

SUMMARY REVIEW

Pain

1. Pain is a protective and a complex phenomenon composed of sensory experiences (time, space, intensity) and emotion, cognition, and motivation.

2. The portions of the nervous system responsible for the sensation and perception of pain may be divided into three areas: (a) the afferent pathways; (b) the interpretive centers in the brainstem, midbrain, and diencephalon; and (c) the descending pathways from the brain to the dorsal horn of the spinal cord.

3. Nociceptors are pain receptors that detect a wide range of stimuli and respond to chemical, mechanical, and thermal stimulation.

4. The afferent system is composed of nociceptors, Aδ and C fibers (first-order neurons); the dorsal horn of the spinal column (second-order neurons); and afferent neurons in the spinothalamic tract (third-order neurons).

5. Myelinated Aδ receptor transmission is fast and conveys mechanical and thermal, sharp, localized pain. Unmyelinated polymodal C fiber transmission is slower and conveys diffuse burning and aching sensations. These primary-order neurons terminate on second-order neurons.

6. Three classes of second-order neurons modulate pain transmission: projection cells, excitatory interneurons, and inhibitory interneurons. The second-order neurons are located in the spinal cord laminae and function as a pain gate to regulate pain transmission.

7. Second-order neurons cross over the cord and ascend primarily in the lateral spinothalamic tract to projection centers including the thalamus, reticular formation, and PAG matter.

8. Third-order neurons carry information to the sensory cortex and reticular and limbic systems for pain processing and interpretation.

9. Efferent pathways from the PAG are responsible for modulation or inhibition of afferent pain signals. The thalamus, cortex, and postcentral gyrus perceive, describe, and localize pain. The reticular formation and limbic system control the emotional and affective response to pain.

10. Pain threshold is the point at which pain is perceived. Pain threshold does not vary significantly among people or within the same person over time.

11. Pain tolerance is the duration of time or the intensity of pain that an individual will endure before initiating overt pain response. Tolerance varies widely among individuals and in the same individual over time.

12. Descending inhibitory or facilitatory pathways, nuclei, and neurotransmitters inhibit or facilitate pain. Segmental inhibition is the peripheral stimulation of nociceptors by touch, vibration, or pressure resulting in closure of the spinal cord pain gate. The higher brain centers also can influence painful stimuli (heterosegmental control of nociception) as well as inhibition from the caudal medulla (diffuse noxious inhibitory controls). Thus pain can be modulated with stimulation from the periphery or by descending impulses from the brain.

13. Cognitive expectation can attenuate or intensify pain, and this is known as the placebo and nocebo effects.

14. Pain neurotransmitters can be classified as inflammatory, excitatory, and inhibitory modulators of pain. Inflammatory neurotransmitters are usually excitatory. Gamma-aminobutyric acid (GABA) and glycine are inhibitors of pain.

15. Endogenous opioids are a family of morphine-like neuropeptides that inhibit transmission of pain by acting on specific opioid receptors (mu [μ], kappa [κ], and delta [δ]).

16. Classifications of pain include nociceptive pain (with a known physiologic cause), nonnociceptive pain (neuropathic pain), acute pain (signal to the person of a harmful stimulus), and chronic pain (persistence of pain of unknown cause or unusual response to therapy).

17. Acute pain may be (a) somatic (superficial), (b) visceral (internal), or (c) referred (present in an area distant from its origin).

18. Somatic pain arises from connective tissue, muscle, bone, and skin and is sharp and localized.

19. Visceral pain is from internal organs and is transmitted by sympathetic afferents and is poorly localized.

20. Referred pain usually arises from the viscera and terminates in an area of the spinal cord that is conjoined with fibers originating in the skin and other areas and thereby produces the perception of pain at the referred site.

21. Physiologic responses to acute pain include increased heart rate, respiratory rate, and blood pressure; pallor or flushing; dilated pupils; and diaphoresis. Blood glucose level is elevated; gastric secretion and motility are decreased; and blood flow to the viscera and skin is decreased.

22. Chronic pain generally lasts at least 3 months and may be persistent, for example, low back pain, myofascial pain syndromes, chronic postoperative pain, and chronic pain associated with cancer.

23. Neuropathic pain is usually chronic, results from nerve trauma or disease, and leads to abnormal peripheral and central pain processing. Types of neuropathic pain include deafferentation pain, sympathetically maintained pain, central poststroke pain, phantom limb pain, and complex regional pain syndrome.

24. Newborns and young children have the anatomic and functional ability to perceive pain. Repeated pain experienced by infants may have prolonged effects on brain neurodevelopment and motor and cognitive function.

25. Older individuals may or may not have an increased pain threshold. In all age groups, women appear to be more sensitive to pain than are men.

26. Pain in older adults is influenced by liver and renal function, including alterations in the metabolism of drugs and metabolites.

Temperature Regulation

1. Temperature regulation (thermoregulation) is achieved through precise balancing of heat production, heat conservation, and heat loss. Body temperature is maintained around 37°C (98.6°F).

2. Temperature regulation is mediated by the hypothalamus. Peripheral thermoreceptors in the skin and central thermoreceptors in the hypothalamus, spinal cord, and abdominal organs provide the hypothalamus with information about skin and core temperatures.

3. Heat is produced through chemical reactions of metabolism, skeletal muscle contraction (shivering), and brown fat (nonshivering) thermogenesis.

4. Heat is lost through radiation, conduction, convection, vasodilation, decreased muscle tone, evaporation of sweat, increased ventilation, and voluntary mechanisms.

5. Heat conservation is accomplished through vasoconstriction and voluntary mechanisms.

6. Infants and older adults require special attention to maintenance of body temperature. Because of their greater body surface area to mass ratio and decreased subcutaneous fat, infants do not conserve heat well. Older individuals have poor responses to environmental temperature extremes as a result of slowed blood circulation,

■ SUMMARY REVIEW—cont'd

structural and functional changes in skin, and an overall decrease in heat-producing activities.

7. Fever is triggered by the release of pyrogens from leukocytes and other cells involved in the immune response (endogenous pyrogens) and bacteria (exogenous pyrogens). Fever is both a symptom of a disease and a normal immunologic mechanism.

8. Fever involves resetting the hypothalamic thermostat to a higher level. When a fever breaks, the set point is returned to normal.

9. Fever production aids responses to infectious processes. Higher temperatures kill many microorganisms and decrease serum levels of iron, zinc, and copper that are needed for bacterial replication.

10. Endogenous cryogens diminish and control the febrile response.

11. Hyperthermia (marked warming of core temperature) can produce nerve damage, coagulation of cell proteins, and death. Therapeutic hyperthermia is used in the treatment of infection to treat cancer. Forms of accidental hyperthermia include heat cramps, heat exhaustion, heat stroke, and malignant hyperthermia. Heat stroke and malignant hyperthermia are potentially lethal developments.

12. Hypothermia (marked cooling of core temperature) slows the rate of chemical reaction (tissue metabolism), increases the viscosity of the blood, slows blood flow through the microcirculation, facilitates blood coagulation, and stimulates profound vasoconstriction. Hypothermia may be accidental or therapeutic and used to reduce metabolic needs and for neuroprotection.

13. Temperature regulation can be disrupted by central nervous system trauma, bodily injury, hemorrhagic shock, major surgery, and thermal burns.

Sleep

1. Sleep may be divided into REM and NREM stages, each of which has its own series of stages. While asleep, an individual progresses through the three stages of NREM (slow-wave) sleep and REM sleep in a predictable cycle. Restorative, reparative, and growth processes occur during NREM sleep.

2. NREM sleep is initiated when inhibitory signals are released from the hypothalamus. There is decreased sympathetic tone, temperature, blood pressure, and muscle tone. Parasympathetic activity increases.

3. REM sleep is mediated in the pons and mesencephalon and is associated with increased parasympathetic activity and variable sympathetic activity associated with rapid eye movement, atonia, loss of temperature regulation, and changes in heart rate, blood pressure, and respiration.

4. The sleep patterns of the newborn and young child vary from those of the adult in total sleep time, cycle length, and percentage of time spent in each sleep cycle. Older adults experience a total decrease in sleep time.

5. Sleep deprivation can cause profound changes in personality and functioning.

6. Sleep disorders include: (a) dyssomnias; (b) parasomnias; (c) sleep disorders associated with mental, neurologic, or other medical disorders; and (d) proposed sleep disorders.

7. Common dyssomnias include insomnia, RLS, OSAS, hypersomnia, narcolepsy, and circadian rhythm disorder.

8. Common parasomnias include arousal disorders, sleep-wake transition disorder, and disorders associated with REM sleep.

Somatosensory Function and the Special Senses

1. The sensation of touch involves the fusion of several qualities, including modality, intensity, location, and duration of the sensory stimulus.

2. Receptors sensitive to touch are present in the skin; these include Meissner and pacinian corpuscles and Merkel disks and Ruffini endings. The sensory response is conducted to the brain through the dorsal column and anterior spinothalamic tract.

3. Abnormal tactile perception may be caused by alterations at any level of the nervous system, from the receptor to the cerebral cortex.

4. Proprioception is the perception of the position and location of the body and its parts. Proprioceptors are located in the inner ear, joints, and ligaments. Proprioceptive stimuli are necessary for balance, coordinated movement, and grading of muscular contraction.

5. Disorders of proprioception can be caused by alterations at any level of the nervous system. Two common causes of proprioceptive dysfunction are vestibular dysfunction and peripheral neuropathy.

Vision

1. The eyelids, conjunctivae, and lacrimal apparatus protect the eye. Infections are the most common disorders; they include blepharitis, conjunctivitis, chalazion, and hordeolum.

2. Conjunctivitis can be acute or chronic, bacterial, viral, or allergic. Redness, edema, pain, and lacrimation are common symptoms. Trachoma (chlamydial conjunctivitis) is the leading cause of blindness in the world and is associated with poor sanitary conditions.

3. Keratitis is a bacterial or viral infection of the cornea that can lead to corneal ulceration. Photophobia, pain, and tearing are common symptoms.

4. The wall of the eye has three layers: sclera, choroid, and retina. The retina contains millions of photoreceptors known as rods and cones that receive light through the lens and then convey signals to the optic nerve and subsequently to the visual cortex of the brain.

5. The eye is filled with vitreous and aqueous humor, which prevent it from collapsing.

6. Structural eye changes caused by aging or chronic disease result in decreased visual acuity.

7. The major alterations in ocular movement include strabismus, nystagmus, and paralysis of the extraocular muscles.

8. Alterations in visual acuity can be caused by amblyopia, scotoma, cataracts, papilledema, macular degeneration, retinal detachment, and glaucoma.

9. Alterations in accommodation develop with increased intraocular pressure, inflammation, and disease of the oculomotor nerve. Presbyopia is loss of accommodation caused by loss of lens elasticity with aging.

10. Alterations in refraction, including myopia, hyperopia, and astigmatism, are the most common visual disorders.

11. Alterations in color vision occur with disorders of the cornea and the inherited trait of color blindness.

12. Trauma or disease of the optic nerve pathways, or optic radiations, can cause blindness in the visual fields. Homonymous hemianopsia is caused by damage of one optic tract.

Hearing

1. The ear is composed of external, middle, and inner structures. The external structures are the pinna, auditory canal, and tympanic membrane. The tympanic cavity (containing three bones: malleus, incus, and stapes), oval window, eustachian tube, and fluid compose the middle ear and transmit sound vibrations to the inner ear.

2. The inner ear includes the bony and membranous labyrinths that transmit sound waves through the cochlea to the division of the eighth cranial nerve (i.e., vestibulocochlear). The semicircular canals

SUMMARY REVIEW—cont'd

and vestibule help maintain balance through the equilibrium receptors.

3. Approximately one-third of all people older than 65 years have hearing loss.

4. Hearing loss can be classified as conductive, sensorineural, mixed, or functional.

5. Conductive hearing loss occurs when sound waves cannot be conducted through the middle ear.

6. Sensorineural hearing loss develops with impairment of the organ of Corti or its central connections. Presbycusis is age-related hearing loss and is the most common form of sensorineural hearing loss.

7. A combination of conductive and sensorineural loss is a mixed hearing loss.

8. Loss of hearing with no known organic cause is a functional hearing loss.

9. Otitis externa is an infection of the outer ear. Otitis media, an infection of the middle ear, is common in children and can be acute or chronic.

10. Acute otitis media is an infection of the middle ear associated with ear pain, fever, an inflamed tympanic membrane, and fluid in the middle ear.

11. Chronic otitis media is persistent or recurrent middle ear infection.

Olfaction and Taste

1. The perception of flavor is altered if olfaction or taste dysfunctions occur. Sensitivity to odor and taste decreases with aging.

2. Hyposmia is a decrease in the sense of smell, and anosmia is the complete loss of smell. Inflammation of the nasal mucosa and trauma or tumors of the olfactory nerve lead to a diminished sense of smell.

3. Hypogeusia is a decrease in taste sensation, and ageusia is the absence of taste. Loss of taste buds or trauma to the facial or glossopharyngeal nerves decreases taste sensation.

4. Parageusia is a perversion of taste in which substances possess an unpleasant flavor.

KEY TERMS

A-beta (Aβ) fiber, 470
Accidental hyperthermia, 482
Accommodation, 488
Acute bacterial conjunctivitis (pinkeye), 487
Acute otitis media (AOM), 495
Acute pain (nociceptive pain), 474
Acute phase response, 480
A-delta (Aδ) fiber, 470
Affective-motivational system, 471
Age-related macular degeneration (AMD), 492
Ageusia, 496
Allergic conjunctivitis, 488
Allodynia, 475
Amblyopia, 490
Anosmia, 496
Antipyretic, 481
Aqueous humor, 488
Astigmatism, 492
Blepharitis, 487
Cancer pain, 476
Cataract, 491
Central neuropathic pain, 475
Central poststroke pain, 476
Central sensitization, 475
Chalazion, 487
Choroid, 488
Chronic conjunctivitis, 488
Chronic otitis media (COM), 496
Chronic or persistent pain, 474
Chronic postoperative pain, 476
Circadian rhythm sleep disorder, 486
Cochlea, 494
Cognitive-evaluative system, 471
Color blindness, 493
Complex regional pain syndrome (CRPS), 477
Conditioned pain modulation, 472
Conduction, 479
Conductive hearing loss, 495
Cone, 488
Conjunctivitis, 487
Convection, 479
Cornea, 488
Crista ampullaris, 494
Dark adaptation, 491
Descending facilitatory pathways, 472
Descending inhibitory pathways, 472

Diplopia, 488
Dynorphin, 473
Dyssomnia, 485
Ectropion, 487
Endogenous cryogen, 481
Endogenous opioid, 472
Endomorphin, 473
Endorphin, 473
Enkephalin, 473
Entropion, 487
Equilibrium receptor, 494
Eustachian (pharyngotympanic) tube, 494
Excitatory neurotransmitter, 472
Exogenous pyrogen, 480
Expectancy-related cortical activation, 472
External auditory canal, 493
Febrile seizures, 482
Fever, 480
Fever of unknown origin (FUO), 482
Fovea centralis, 488
Functional hearing loss, 495
Gate control theory (GCT), 469
Glaucoma, 491
Hair cell, 494
Heat cramp, 482
Heat exhaustion, 482
Heat stroke, 482
Hemianopia, 493
Homonymous hemianopsia, 493
Hordeolum (anterior blepharitis [stye]), 487
Hyperalgesia, 475
Hyperopia, 492
Hypersomnia, 486
Hyperthermia, 482
Hypogeusia, 496
Hyposmia, 496
Hypothermia, 482
Incus (anvil), 494
Infantile nystagmus syndrome, 490
Inhibitory neurotransmitter, 472
Insomnia, 485
Iris, 488
Jerk nystagmus, 488
Keratitis, 488
Lens, 488
Macula, 488

Malignant hyperthermia, 482
Malleus (hammer), 494
Mastoid air cell, 493
Mastoid process, 493
Ménière disease (endolymphatic hydrops), 487
Ménière syndrome, 487
Mixed hearing loss, 495
Myofascial pain syndrome (MPS), 475
Myopia, 492
Narcolepsy, 486
Neuromatrix theory, 469
Neuropathic pain, 475
Nocebo effect, 472
Nociceptin/orphanin FQ, 473
Nociception, 469
Nociceptive pain, 469
Nociceptor, 469
Nonnociceptive stimulation, 469
Non-REM (NREM) slow wave sleep, 484
Nonspecific spinal pain, 475
Nystagmus, 488
Obesity hypoventilation syndrome, 485
Obstructive sleep apnea syndrome (OSAS), 485
Olfaction, 496
Olfactory hallucination, 496
Optic chiasm, 493
Optic disc, 488
Optic nerve, 488
Organ of Corti, 494
Otitis externa, 495
Otitis media, 495
Otoliths, 494
Oval window, 494
Pain modulation, 472
Pain perception, 470
Pain threshold, 473
Pain tolerance, 473
Pain transduction, 470
Pain transmission, 470
Papilledema, 493
Parageusia, 496
Parosmia, 496
Pattern theory, 469
Pendular nystagmus, 488
Perceptual dominance, 473

KEY TERMS—cont'd

Perilymph, 494
Peripheral neuropathic pain, 475
Peripheral sensitization, 475
Phantom limb pain, 476
Pinna, 494
Placebo effect, 472
Presbycusis, 494
Presbyopia, 492
Pupil, 488
Pyrogenic cytokines, 480
Radiation, 479
Rapid eye movement (REM) sleep, 484
Referred pain, 474
Restless legs syndrome (RLS), 485
Retina, 488

Retinal detachment, 492
Rhegmatogenous retinal detachment, 492
Rods, 488
Sclera, 488
Scotoma, 490
Segmental inhibition of pain, 472
Semicircular canal, 494
Sensorineural hearing loss, 495
Sensory-discriminative system, 470
Shivering, 482
Sleep, 483
Somatic pain, 474
Specific spinal pain, 475
Specificity theory, 469
Stapes (stirrup), 494

Strabismus, 488
Taste, 496
Therapeutic hyperthermia, 482
Thermoregulation, 478
Trachoma, 488
Trichiasis, 487
Tympanic cavity, 494
Tympanic membrane, 494
Unmyelinated C fiber, 470
Vertigo, 487
Vestibular nystagmus, 487
Vestibule, 494
Viral conjunctivitis, 487
Visceral pain, 474
Vitreous humor, 488

REFERENCES

1. International Association for the Study of Pain: *IASP taxonomy*. Available at http://www.iasp-pain.org/AM/Template.cfm?Section=Pain_Definitions&;Template=/CM/HTMLDisplay.cfm&ContentID=1728.
2. McCaffery M: *Nursing practice theories related to cognition, bodily pain and nonenvironment interactions*, Los Angeles, Calif, 1968, University of California at Los Angeles Students' Store.
3. Waddell G: *The back pain revolution*, ed 2, London, 2004, Churchill Livingstone.
4. Moayedi M, Davis KD: Theories of pain: from specificity to gate control. *J Neurophysiol* 109(1):5–12, 2013.
5. Melzack R, Wall PD: Pain mechanisms: a new theory. *Science* 150:971, 1965.
6. Mendell LM: Constructing and deconstructing the gate theory of pain. *Pain* 155(2):210–216, 2014.
7. Melzak R: Toward a new concept of pain for the new millennium. In Waldman SD, editor: *Interventional pain management*, ed 2, Philadelphia, 2001, Saunders.
8. Iannetti GD, Mouraux A: From the neuromatrix to the pain matrix (and back). *Exp Brain Res* 205(1):1–12, 2010.
9. Melzack R: Evolution of the neuromatrix theory of pain. *Pain Pract* 5(2):85–94, 2005.
10. Mickle AD, Shepherd AJ, Mohapatra DP: Sensory TRP channels: the key transducers of nociception and pain. *Prog Mol Biol Transl Sci* 131:73–118, 2015.
11. Todd AJ: Neuronal circuitry for pain processing in the dorsal horn. *Nat Rev Neurosci* 11(12):823–836, 2010.
12. Bourne S, Machado AG, Nagel SJ: Basic anatomy and physiology of pain pathways. *Neurosurg Clin N Am* 25(4):629–638, 2014.
13. Marchand S: The physiology of pain mechanisms: from the periphery to the brain. *Rheum Dis Clin North Am* 34:285–309, 2008.
14. Ossipov MH, Morimura K, Porreca F: Descending pain modulation and chronification of pain. *Curr Opin Support Palliat Care* 8(2):143–151, 2014.
15. Baeumler PI, et al: Acupuncture-induced changes of pressure pain threshold are mediated by segmental inhibition—a randomized controlled trial. *Pain* 156(11):2245–5225, 2015.
16. Colloca L, Grillon C: Understanding placebo and nocebo responses for pain management. *Curr Pain Headache Rep* 18(6):419, 2014.
17. Fields HL, et al: Central nervous system mechanism of pain modulation. In McMahon S, Koltzenburg M, editors: *Wall and Melzack's*

textbook of pain, ed 5, Edinburgh, Scotland, 2005, Churchill Livingstone.
18. Ossipov MH, Dussor GO, Porreca F: Central modulation of pain. *J Clin Invest* 120(11):3779–3787, 2010.
19. Guo D, Hu J: Spinal presynaptic inhibition in pain control. *Neuroscience* 283:95–106, 2014.
20. Lau BK, Vaughan CW: Descending modulation of pain: the GABA disinhibition hypothesis of analgesia. *Curr Opin Neurobiol* 29C:159–164, 2014.
21. Ninkovic J, Roy S: Role of the mu-opioid receptor in opioid modulation of immune function. *Amino Acids* 45(1):9–24, 2013.
22. Bodnar RJ: Endogenous opiates and behavior: 2009. *Peptides* 31(12):2325–2359, 2010.
23. Busch-Dienstfertig M, Stein C: Opioid receptors and opioid peptide-producing leukocytes in inflammatory pain—basic and therapeutic aspects. *Brain Behav Immun* 24(5):683–694, 2010.
24. Podvin S, Yaksh T, Hook V: The emerging role of spinal dynorphin in chronic pain: a therapeutic perspective. *Annu Rev Pharmacol Toxicol* 56:511–533, 2016.
25. Lazarus LH, Okada Y: Engineering endomorphin drugs: state of the art. *Expert Opin Ther Pat* 22(1):1–14, 2014.
26. Perlikowska R, Janecka A: Bioavailability of endomorphins and the blood-brain barrier—a review. *Med Chem* 10(1):2–17, 2014.
27. Toll L, et al: Nociceptin/orphanin FQ receptor structure, signaling, ligands, functions, and interactions with opioid systems. *Pharmacol Rev* 68(2):419–457, 2016.
28. Bodnar RJ: Endogenous opiates and behavior. *Peptides* 31(12):2325–2359, 2009.
29. Sauriyal DS, Jaggi AS, Singh N: Extending pharmacological spectrum of opioids beyond analgesia: multifunctional aspects in different pathophysiological states. *Neuropeptides* 45(3):175–188, 2011.
30. Defrin R, Eli I, Pud D: Interactions among sex, ethnicity, religion, and gender role expectations of pain. *Gend Med* 8(3):172–183, 2011.
31. American Pain Society: *Principles of analgesic use in the treatment of acute pain and cancer pain*, ed 6, Glenview, IL, 2008, Author.
32. Naftel JP: Viscerosensory pathways. In Haines DE, editor: *Fundamental neuroscience for basic and clinical applications*, ed 4, Philadelphia, 2013, Saunders, pp 260–266.
33. May A: Chronic pain may change the structure of the brain. *Pain* 137:7–15, 2008.

34. Schmidt-Wilcke T: Neuroimaging of chronic pain. *Best Pract Res Clin Rheumatol* 29(1):29–41, 2015.
35. Gilron I, Baron R, Jensen T: Neuropathic pain: principles of diagnosis and treatment. *Mayo Clin Proc* 90(4):532–545, 2015.
36. Jensen TS, Finnerup NB: Allodynia and hyperalgesia in neuropathic pain: clinical manifestations and mechanisms. *Lancet Neurol* 13(9):924–935, 2014.
37. Pozek JP, et al: The acute to chronic pain transition: can chronic pain be prevented? *Med Clin North Am* 100(1):17–30, 2016.
38. Vranken JH: Elucidation of pathophysiology and treatment of neuropathic pain. *Cent Nerv Syst Agents Med Chem* 12(4):304–314, 2012.
39. Balagué F, et al: Non-specific low back pain. *Lancet* 379(9814):482–491, 2012.
40. Hoy D, et al: The epidemiology of low back pain. *Best Pract Res Clin Rheumatol* 24(6):769–781, 2010.
41. Braun J, et al: Assessment of spinal pain. *Best Pract Res Clin Rheumatol* 28(6):875–887, 2014.
42. Izzo R, et al: Spinal pain. *Eur J Radiol* 84(5):746–756, 2015.
43. Hooten WM, Cohen SP: Evaluation and treatment of low back pain: a clinically focused review for primary care specialists. *Mayo Clin Proc* 90(12):1699–1718, 2015.
44. Webster LR, Markman J: Medical management of chronic low back pain: efficacy and outcomes. *Neuromodulation* 17(Suppl 2):18–23, 2014.
45. Shah JP, Gilliams EA: Uncovering the biochemical milieu of myofascial trigger points using in vivo microdialysis: an application of muscle pain concepts to myofascial pain syndrome. *J Body Mov Ther* 12(4):371–384, 2008.
46. Zhuang X, Tan S, Huang Q: Understanding of myofascial trigger points. *Chin Med J* 127(24):4271–4277, 2014.
47. Roldan CJ, Hu N: Myofascial pain syndromes in the emergency department: what are we missing? *J Emerg Med* 49(6):1004–1010, 2015.
48. Lovich-Sapola J, Smith CE, Brandt CP: Postoperative pain control. *Surg Clin North Am* 95(2):301–318, 2015.
49. Reddi D, Curran N: Chronic pain after surgery: pathophysiology, risk factors and prevention. *Postgrad Med J* 90(1062):222–227, 2014.
50. Schmidt BL: The neurobiology of cancer pain. *Neuroscientist* 20(5):546–562, 2014.
51. Smith TJ, Saiki CB: Cancer pain management. *Mayo Clin Proc* 90(10):1428–1439, 2015.

52. Davies AN: Breakthrough cancer pain. *Curr Pain Headache Rep* 18(6):420, 2014.

53. Kahan B: Cancer pain and current theory for pain control. *Phys Med Rehabil Clin North Am* 25(2):439–456, 2014.

54. Moeschler SM, et al: Interventional modalities to treat cancer-related pain. *Hosp Pract (1995)* 42(5):14–23, 2014.

55. Kim JS: Pharmacological management of central post-stroke pain: a practical guide. *CNS Drugs* 28(9):787–797, 2014.

56. Singer J, et al: Central poststroke pain: a systematic review. *Int J Stroke* 12(4):343–355, 2017.

57. Pirowska A, et al: Phantom phenomena and body scheme after limb amputation: a literature review. *Neurol Neurochir Pol* 48(1):52–59, 2014.

58. Nikolaisen L, Springer JS, Haroutiunian S: Phantom limb pain. In Benzon HT, et al, editors: *Practical management of pain*, ed 5, St Louis, 2014, Mosby, pp 369–377.

59. Bruehl S: Complex regional pain syndrome. *BMJ* 351:h2730, 2015.

60. International Association for the Study of Pain: *Classification of chronic pain*, ed 2 (revised). Available at http://www.iasppain.org/files/Content/ContentFolders/Publications2/Classificationof ChronicPain/Part_II-A.pdf.

61. Birklein F, Schlereth T: Complex regional pain syndrome-significant progress in understanding. *Pain* 156(Suppl 1):S94–S103, 2015.

62. Derbyshire SW: Fetal pain: do we know enough to do the right thing? *Reprod Health Matters* 16(Suppl 31):117–126, 2008.

63. Sekulic S, et al: Appearance of fetal pain could be associated with maturation of the mesodiencephalic structures. *J Pain Res* 9:1031–1038, 2016.

64. Beggs S: Long-term consequences of neonatal injury. *Can J Psychiatry* 60(4):176–180, 2015.

65. Ranger M, Grunau RE: Early repetitive pain in preterm infants in relation to the developing brain. *Pain Manag* 4(1):57–67, 2014.

66. Valeri BO, Holsti L, Linhares MB: Neonatal pain and developmental outcomes in children born preterm: a systematic review. *Clin J Pain* 31(4):355–362, 2015.

67. Allegaert K, van den Anker JN: Neonatal pain management: still in search for the Holy Grail. *Int J Clin Pharmacol Ther* 54(7):514–523, 2016.

68. Davidson AJ, et al: Anesthesia and the developing brain: a way forward for clinical research. *Paediatr Anaesth* 25(5):447–452, 2015.

69. McPherson C, Grunau RE: Neonatal pain control and neurologic effects of anesthetics and sedatives in preterm infants. *Clin Perinatol* 41(1):209–227, 2014.

70. Krauss BS, et al: Current concepts in management of pain in children in the emergency department. *Lancet* 387(10013):83–92, 2016.

71. Arif-Rahu M, Fisher D, Matsuda Y: Biobehavioral measures for pain in the pediatric patient. *Pain Manag Nurs* 13(3):157–168, 2012.

72. Hatfield LA, Ely EA: Measurement of acute pain in infants: a review of behavioral and physiological variables. *Biol Res Nurs* 17(1):100–111, 2015.

73. Pillai Riddell RR, et al: Non-pharmacological management of infant and young child procedural pain. *Cochrane Database Syst Rev* (12):CD006275, 2015.

74. Tobias JD: Acute pain management in infants and children-Part 1: pain pathways, pain assessment, and outpatient pain management. *Pediatr Ann* 43(7):e163–e168, 2014.

75. Yezierski RP: The effects of age on pain sensitivity: preclinical studies. *Pain Med* 13(Suppl 2):S27–S36, 2012.

76. Gagliese L, et al: Age-related patterns in adaptation to cancer pain: a mixed-method study. *Pain Med* 10(6):1050–1061, 2009.

77. Gibson SJ, Farrell M: A review of age differences in the neurophysiology of nociception and the perceptual experience of pain. *Clin J Pain* 20(4):227–239, 2004.

78. Rastogi R, Meek BD: Management of chronic pain in elderly, frail patients: finding a suitable, personalized method of control. *Clin Interv Aging* 8:37–46, 2013.

79. Bartley EJ, Fillingim RB: Sex differences in pain: a brief review of clinical and experimental findings. *Br J Anaesth* 111(1):52–58, 2013.

80. Molton IR, Terrill AL: Overview of persistent pain in older adults. *Am Psychol* 69(2):197–207, 2014.

81. Tracy B, Sean Morrison R: Pain management in older adults. *Clin Ther* 35(11):1659–1668, 2013.

82. Chai E, Horton JR: Managing pain in the elderly population: pearls and pitfalls. *Curr Pain Headache Rep* 14(6):409–417, 2010.

83. Mortola JP: Gender and the circadian pattern of body temperature in normoxia and hypoxia. *Respir Physiol Neurobiol* 2016. [Epub ahead of print.].

84. Zhang X: Molecular sensors and modulators of thermoreception. *Channels (Austin)* 9(2):73–81, 2015.

85. Tansey EA, Johnson CD: Recent advances in thermoregulation. *Adv Physiol Educ* 39(3):139–148, 2015.

86. Contreras C, et al: The brain and brown fat. *Ann Med* 47(2):150–168, 2015.

87. Taylor NA: Human heat adaptation. *Compr Physiol* 4(1):325–365, 2014.

88. Yamazaki F: Effectiveness of exercise-heat acclimation for preventing heat illness in the workplace. *J UOEH* 35(3):183–192, 2013.

89. Hillman NH, Kallapur SG, Jobe AH: Physiology of transition from intrauterine to extrauterine life. *Clin Perinatol* 39(4):769–783, 2012.

90. Lyon AJ, Freer Y: Goals and options in keeping preterm babies warm. *Arch Dis Child Fetal Neonatal Ed* 96(1):F71–F74, 2011.

91. Gomes LH, Carneiro-Júnior MA, Marins JC: Thermoregulatory responses of children exercising in a hot environment. *Rev Paul Pediatr* 31(1):104–110, 2013.

92. Gao Z, et al: Altered coronary vascular control during cold stress in healthy older adults. *Am J Physiol Heart Circ Physiol* 302(1):H312–H318, 2012.

93. Blatteis CM: Age-dependent changes in temperature regulation—a mini review. *Gerontology* 58(4):289–295, 2012.

94. Greaney JL, Alexander LM, Kenney WL: Sympathetic control of reflex cutaneous vasoconstriction in human aging. *J Appl Physiol (1985)* 119(7):771–782, 2015.

95. Roth J, Blatteis CM: Mechanisms of fever production and lysis: lessons from experimental LPS fever. *Compr Physiol* 4(4):1563–1604, 2014.

96. Markanday A: Acute phase reactants in infections: evidence-based review and a guide for clinicians. *Open Forum Infect Dis* 2(3):ofv098, 2015.

97. Roth J: Endogenous antipyretics. *Clin Chim Acta* 371(1-2):13–24, 2006.

98. Shido O, Sugimoto N: Possible human endogenous cryogens. *Curr Protein Pept Sci* 12(4):288–292, 2011.

99. Evans SS, Repasky EA, Fisher DT: Fever and the thermal regulation of immunity: the immune system feels the heat. *Nat Rev Immunol* 15(6):335–349, 2015.

100. Harden LM, et al: Fever and sickness behavior: friend or foe? *Brain Behav Immun* 50:322–333, 2015.

101. Carey JV: Literature review: should antipyretic therapies routinely be administered to patients with [corrected] fever? *J Clin Nurs* 19:2377–2393, 2010.

102. Niven DJ, Laupland KB: Pharmacotherapy of fever control among hospitalized adult patients. *Expert Opin Pharmacother* 14(6):735–745, 2013.

103. Matheï C, et al: Infections in residents of nursing homes. *Infect Dis Clin North Am* 21(3):761–772, 2007.

104. Camfield P, Camfield C: Febrile seizures and genetic epilepsy with febrile seizures plus (GEFS+). *Epileptic Disord* 17(2):124–133, 2015.

105. Patterson JL, et al: Febrile seizures. *Pediatr Ann* 42(12):249–254, 2013.

106. Gupta A: Febrile seizures. *Continuum (Minneap Minn)* 22(1Epilepsy):51–59, 2016.

107. Cunha BA, Lortholary O, Cunha CB: Fever of unknown origin: a clinical approach. *Am J Med* 128(10):1138.e1–1138.e15, 2015.

108. Hayakawa K, Ramasamy B, Chandrasekar PH: Fever of unknown origin: an evidence-based review. *Am J Med Sci* 344(4):307–316, 2012.

109. Wang H, et al: Brain temperature and its fundamental properties: a review for clinical neuroscientists. *Front Neurosci* 8:307, 2014.

110. Mallory M, et al: Therapeutic hyperthermia: the old, the new, and the upcoming. *Crit Rev Oncol Hematol* 97:56–64, 2016.

111. Gomez CR: Disorders of body temperature. *Handb Clin Neurol* 120:947–957, 2014.

112. Leon LR, Bouchama A: Heat stroke. *Compr Physiol* 5(2):611–647, 2015.

113. Bandschapp O, Girard T: Malignant hyperthermia. *Swiss Med Wkly* 142:w13652, 2012.

114. Rosenberg H, et al: Malignant hyperthermia: a review. *Orphanet J Rare Dis* 10:93, 2015.

115. Søreide K: Clinical and translational aspects of hypothermia in major trauma patients: from pathophysiology to prevention, prognosis and potential preservation. *Injury* 45(4):647–654, 2014.

116. Jurkovich GJ: Environmental cold-induced injury. *Surg Clin North Am* 87(1):247–267, 2007.

117. Zafren K: Out-of-hospital evaluation and treatment of accidental hypothermia. *Emerg Med Clin North Am* 35(2):261–279, 2017.

118. Lantry J, Dezman Z, Hirshon JM: Pathophysiology, management and complications of hypothermia. *Br J Hosp Med (Lond)* 73(1):31–37, 2012.

119. Rischall ML, Rowland-Fisher A: Evidence-based management of accidental hypothermia in the emergency department. *Emerg Med Pract* 18(1):1–18, 2016.

120. Lampe JW, Becker LB: State of the art in therapeutic hypothermia. *Annu Rev Med* 62:79–93, 2011.

121. Alshimemeri A: Therapeutic hypothermia after cardiac arrest. *Ann Card Anaesth* 17(4):285–291, 2014.

122. Andresen M, et al: Therapeutic hypothermia for acute brain injuries. *Scand J Trauma Resusc Emerg Med* 23:42, 2015.

123. Merchant N, Azzopardi D: Early predictors of outcome in infants treated with hypothermia for hypoxic-ischaemic encephalopathy. *Dev Med Child Neurol* 57(Suppl 3):8–16, 2015.

124. Agrawal A, Timothy J, Thapa A: Neurogenic fever. *Singapore Med J* 48(6):492–494, 2007.

125. Hocker SE, et al: Indicators of central fever in the neurologic intensive care unit. *JAMA Neurol* 70(12):1499–1504, 2013.

126. Block J, et al: Evidence-based thermoregulation for adult trauma patients. *Crit Care Nurs Q* 35(1): 50–63, 2012.

127. Campbell G, et al: Warming of intravenous and irrigation fluids for preventing inadvertent perioperative hypothermia. *Cochrane Database Syst Rev* (4):CD009891, 2015.

128. Albrecht U: Timing to perfection: the biology of central and peripheral circadian clocks. *Neuron* 74(2):246–260, 2012.

129. Monti JM: The neurotransmitters of sleep and wake, a physiological reviews series. *Sleep Med Rev* 17(4):313–315, 2013.

130. Brown RE, et al: Control of sleep and wakefulness. *Physiol Rev* 92(3):1087–1187, 2012.

131. Fraigne JJ, et al: REM sleep at its core—circuits, neurotransmitters, and pathophysiology. *Front Neurol* 6:123, 2015.

132. Danker-Hopfe H: Growth and development of children with a special focus on sleep. *Prog Biophys Mol Biol* 107(3):333–338, 2011.

133. Korotchikova I, et al: Sleep-wake cycle of the healthy term newborn infant in the immediate postnatal period. *Clin Neurophysiol* 127(4): 2095–2101, 2016.

134. Leo G: Parasomnias. *World Med J* 102(1):32–35, 2003.

135. Bharti B, Mehta A, Malhi P: Sleep problems in children: a guide for primary care physicians. *Indian J Pediatr* 80(6):492–498, 2013.

136. Wilhelm CP, et al: The nose, upper airway, and obstructive sleep apnea. *Ann Allergy Asthma Immunol* 115(2):96–102, 2015.

137. Owens J, Adolescent Sleep Working Group, Committee on Adolescence: Insufficient sleep in adolescents and young adults: an update on causes and consequences. *Pediatrics* 134(3):e921–e932, 2014.

138. Pace-Schott EF, Spencer RM: Sleep-dependent memory consolidation in healthy aging and mild cognitive impairment. *Curr Top Behav Neurosci* 25:307–330, 2015.

139. Copinschi G, Caufriez A: Sleep and hormonal changes in aging. *Endocrinol Metab Clin North Am* 42(2):371–389, 2013.

140. Mander BA, Winer JR, Walker MP: Sleep and human aging. *Neuron* 94(1):19–36, 2017.

141. Scullin MK, Bliwise DL: Sleep, cognition, and normal aging: integrating a half century of multidisciplinary research. *Perspect Psychol Sci* 10(1):97–137, 2015.

142. American Academy of Sleep Medicine, Diagnostic Classification Steering Committee: *International classification of sleep disorders, revised: diagnostic and coding manual*, Westchester, IL, 2005, Author.

143. Ellis JG, et al: Acute insomnia: current conceptualizations and future directions. *Sleep Med Rev* 16(1):5–14, 2012.

144. Levenson JC, Kay DB, Buysse DJ: The pathophysiology of insomnia. *Chest* 147(4): 1179–1192, 2015.

145. Garcia-Borreguero D, Cano-Pumarega I: New concepts in the management of restless legs syndrome. *BMJ* 356:j104, 2017.

146. Wimms A, et al: Obstructive sleep apnea in women: specific issues and interventions. *Biomed Res Int* 2016:1764837, 2016.

147. Ruehland WR, et al: The new AASM criteria for scoring hypopneas: impact on the apnea hypopnea index. *Sleep* 32(2):150–157, 2009.

148. Cherniack EP, Cherniack NS: Obstructive sleep apnea, metabolic syndrome, and age: will geriatricians be caught asleep on the job? *Aging Clin Exp Res* 22(1):1–7, 2010.

149. Isono S: Obesity and obstructive sleep apnoea: mechanisms for increased collapsibility of the passive pharyngeal airway. *Respirology* 17(1): 32–42, 2012.

150. Pierce AM, Brown LK: Obesity hypoventilation syndrome: current theories of pathogenesis. *Curr Opin Pulm Med* 21(6):557–562, 2015.

151. Alonso-Álvarez M, et al: Obstructive sleep apnea in obese community-dwelling children: the NANOS study. *Sleep* 37(5):943–949, 2014.

152. Pham LV, Schwartz AR: The pathogenesis of obstructive sleep apnea. *J Thorac Dis* 7(8): 1358–1372, 2015.

153. Hanly PJ, Ahmed SB: Sleep apnea and the kidney: is sleep apnea a risk factor for chronic kidney disease? *Chest* 146(4):1114–1122, 2014.

154. Ayas NT, et al: New frontiers in obstructive sleep apnea. *Clin Sci* 127(4):209–216, 2014.

155. Malhotra A, Orr JE, Owens RL: On the cutting edge of obstructive sleep apnoea: where next? *Lancet Respir Med* 3(5):397–403, 2015.

156. Hirsch Allen AJ, Bansback N, Ayas NT: The effect of OSA on work disability and work-related injuries. *Chest* 147(5):1422–1428, 2015.

157. Saini P, Rye DB: Hypersomnia: evaluation, treatment, and social and economic aspects. *Sleep Med Clin* 12(1):47–60, 2017.

158. Liblau RS, et al: Hypocretin (orexin) biology and the pathophysiology of narcolepsy with cataplexy. *Lancet Neurol* 14(3):318–328, 2015.

159. Nevsimalova S, et al: Narcolepsy: clinical differences and association with other sleep disorders in different age groups. *J Neurol* 260(3):767–775, 2013.

160. Abbott SM, Reid KJ, Zee PC: Circadian rhythm sleep-wake disorders. *Psychiatr Clin North Am* 38(4):805–823, 2015.

161. Auger RR, et al: Clinical practice guideline for the treatment of intrinsic circadian rhythm sleep-wake disorders: advanced sleep-wake phase disorder (ASWPD), delayed sleep-wake phase disorder (DSWPD), non-24-hour sleep-wake rhythm disorder (N24SWD), and irregular sleep-wake rhythm disorder (ISWRD). An update for 2015: an American Academy of Sleep Medicine clinical practice guideline. *J Clin Sleep Med* 11(10):1199–1236, 2015.

162. Reid KJ, Abbott SM: Jet lag and shift work disorder. *Sleep Med Clin* 10(4):523–535, 2015.

163. Basner M, et al: Sleep deprivation and neurobehavioral dynamics. *Curr Opin Neurobiol* 23(5):854–863, 2013.

164. Goel N, et al: Circadian rhythms, sleep deprivation, and human performance. *Prog Mol Biol Transl Sci* 119:155–190, 2013.

165. Prince TM, Abel T: The impact of sleep loss on hippocampal function. *Learn Mem* 20(10): 558–569, 2013.

166. Irwin MR: Why sleep is important for health: a psychoneuroimmunology perspective. *Annu Rev Psychol* 66:143–172, 2015.

167. Kohansieh M, Makaryus AN: Sleep deficiency and deprivation leading to cardiovascular disease. *Int J Hypertens* 2015:615681.

168. Meerlo P, Havekes R, Steiger A: Chronically restricted or disrupted sleep as a causal factor in the development of depression. *Curr Top Behav Neurosci* 25:459–481, 2015.

169. Anderson KN: An update in sleep neurology: the latest bedtime stories. *J Neurol* 262(2):487–491, 2015.

170. Galbiati A, et al: Behavioural and cognitive-behavioural treatments of parasomnias. *Behav Neurol* 2015:786928.

171. Howell MJ, Schenck CH: Rapid eye movement sleep behavior disorder and neurodegenerative disease. *JAMA Neurol* 72(6):707–712, 2015.

172. Besne I, Descombes C, Breton L: Effect of age and anatomical site on density of sensory innervation in human epidermis. *Arch Dermatol* 138(11): 1445–1450, 2002.

173. Kalisch T, Tegenthoff M, Dinse HR: Repetitive electric stimulation elicits enduring improvement of sensorimotor performance in seniors. *Neural Plast* 2010:690531.

174. Shaffer SW, Harrison AL: Aging of the somatosensory system: a translational perspective. *Phys Ther* 87(2):193–207, 2007.

175. Hughes CM, et al: Upper extremity proprioception in healthy aging and stroke populations, and the effects of therapist- and robot-based rehabilitation therapies on proprioceptive function. *Front Hum Neurosci* 9:120, 2015.

176. Wipperman J: Dizziness and vertigo. *Prim Care* 41(1):115–131, 2014.

177. Espinosa-Sanchez JM, Lopez-Escamez JA: Ménière's disease. *Handb Clin Neurol* 137:257–277, 2016.

178. Buetti B, Luxon LM: Vestibular involvement in peripheral neuropathy: a review. *Int J Audiol* 53(6):353–359, 2014.

179. Pflugfelder SC, Karpecki PM, Perez VL: Treatment of blepharitis: recent clinical trials. *Ocul Surf* 12(4):273–284, 2014.

180. Fea A, et al: Ectropion, entropion, trichiasis. *Minerva Chir* 68(6 Suppl 1):27–35, 2013.

181. Tarff A, Behrens A: Ocular emergencies: red eye. *Med Clin North Am* 101(3):615–639, 2017.

182. Taylor HR, et al: Trachoma. *Lancet* 384(9960): 2142–2152, 2014.

183. Maycock NJ, Jayaswal R: Update on acanthamoeba keratitis: diagnosis, treatment, and outcomes. *Cornea* 35(5):713–720, 2016.

184. Nylén P, et al: Vision, light and aging: a literature overview on older-age workers. *Work* 47(3): 399–412, 2014.

185. Peragallo JH, Pineles SL, Demer JL: Recent advances clarifying the etiologies of strabismus. *J Neuroophthalmol* 35(2):185–193, 2015.

186. Kushner BJ: The efficacy of strabismus surgery in adults: a review for primary care physicians. *Postgrad Med J* 87(1026):269–273, 2011.

187. Richards MD, Wong A: Infantile nystagmus syndrome: clinical characteristics, current theories of pathogenesis, diagnosis, and management. *Can J Ophthalmol* 50(6):400–408, 2015.

188. Thurtell MJ, Leigh RJ: Nystagmus and saccadic intrusions. *Handb Clin Neurol* 102:333–378, 2011.

189. Bonaccorsi J, Berardi N, Sale A: Treatment of amblyopia in the adult: insights from a new rodent model of visual perceptual learning. *Front Neural Circuits* 8:82, 2014.

190. DeSantis D: Amblyopia. *Pediatr Clin North Am* 61(3):505–518, 2014.

191. Brass SD, Zivadinov R, Bakshi R: Acute demyelinating optic neuritis: a review. *Front Biosci* 13:2376–2390, 2008.

192. Pershing S, Kumar A: Phacoemulsification versus extracapsular cataract extraction: where do we stand? *Curr Opin Ophthalmol* 22(1):37–42, 2011.

193. Jackson RG, Owsley C, McGwin G, Jr: Aging and dark adaptation. *Vision Res* 39(23):3975–3982, 1999.

194. Wiggs JL: Glaucoma genes and mechanisms. *Prog Mol Biol Transl Sci* 134:315–342, 2015.

195. Pinazo-Durán MD, et al: Oxidative stress and mitochondrial failure in the pathogenesis of glaucoma neurodegeneration. *Prog Brain Res* 220:127–153, 2015.

196. M K: Present and new treatment strategies in the management of glaucoma. *Open Ophthalmol J* 9:89–100, 2015.

197. Feltgen N, Walter P: Rhegmatogenous retinal detachment—an ophthalmologic emergency. *Dtsch Arztebl Int* 111(1-2):12–21, 2014.

198. Stuart A, et al: Anti-VEGF therapies in the treatment of choroidal neovascularisation secondary to non-age-related macular degeneration: a systematic review. *BMJ Open* 5(4):e007746, 2015.

199. Carneiro Â, Andrade JP: Nutritional and lifestyle interventions for age-related macular degeneration: a review. *Oxid Med Cell Longev* 2017:6469138.

200. Gil-Cazorla R, Shah S, Naroo SA: A review of the surgical options for the correction of presbyopia. *Br J Ophthalmol* 100(1):62–70, 2016.

201. Neitz J, Neitz M: The genetics of normal and defective color vision. *Vision Res* 51(7):633–651, 2011.

202. Swienton DJ, Thomas AG: The visual pathway—functional anatomy and pathology. *Semin Ultrasound CT MR* 35(5):487–503, 2014.

203. Roth TN: Aging of the auditory system. *Handb Clin Neurol* 129:357–373, 2015.

204. Panza F, Solfrizzi V, Logroscino G: Age-related hearing impairment-a risk factor and frailty marker for dementia and AD. *Nat Rev Neurol* 11(3):166–175, 2015.

205. Bainbridge KE, Wallhagen MI: Hearing loss in an aging American population: extent, impact, and management. *Annu Rev Public Health* 35:139–152, 2014.

206. Cohen BE, Durstenfeld A, Roehm PC: Viral causes of hearing loss: a review for hearing health professionals. *Trends Hear* 18, 2014.

207. Yu YQ, et al: Genetic effects on sensorineural hearing loss and evidence-based treatment for sensorineural hearing loss. *Chin Med Sci J* 30(3):179–188, 2015.

208. Wipperman J: Otitis externa. *Prim Care* 41(1):1–9, 2014.

209. Monasta L, et al: Burden of disease caused by otitis media: systematic review and global estimates. *PLoS ONE* 7(4):e36226, 2012.

210. Sáfadi MA, Jarovsky D: Acute otitis media in children: a vaccine-preventable disease? *Braz J Otorhinolaryngol* 83(3):241–242, 2017.

211. Thomas NM, Brook I: Otitis media: an update on current pharmacotherapy and future perspectives. *Expert Opin Pharmacother* 15(8):1069–1083, 2014.

212. Kanazawa H, Yoshida N, Iino Y: New insights into eosinophilic otitis media. *Curr Allergy Asthma Rep* 15(12):76, 2015.

213. Patel RM, Pinto JM: Olfaction: anatomy, physiology, and disease. *Clin Anat* 27(1):54–60, 2014.

214. Ottaviano G, et al: Olfaction deterioration in cognitive disorders in the elderly. *Aging Clin Exp Res* 28(1):37–45, 2016.

215. Roper SD: Taste buds as peripheral chemosensory processors. *Semin Cell Dev Biol* 24(1):71–79, 2013.

216. Calvo SS, Egan JM: The endocrinology of taste receptors. *Nat Rev Endocrinol* 11(4):213–227, 2015.

217. Grassin-Delyle S, Naline E, Devillier P: Taste receptors in asthma. *Curr Opin Allergy Clin Immunol* 15(1):63–69, 2015.

218. Feng P, Huang L, Wang H: Taste bud homeostasis in health, disease, and aging. *Chem Senses* 39(1):3–16, 2014.

219. Attems J, Walker L, Jellinger KA: Olfaction and aging: a mini-review. *Gerontology* 61(6):485–490, 2015.

220. Mobley AS et al: Aging in the olfactory system. *Trends Neurosci* 37(2):77–84, 2014.

Alterations in Cognitive Systems, Cerebral Hemodynamics, and Motor Function

Barbara J. Boss, Sue E. Huether

CHAPTER OUTLINE

A person achieves cognitive and behavioral functional adequacy by integrated processes of cognitive systems, sensory systems, and motor systems. Alterations in any or all of these affect functional adequacy. The purpose of this chapter is to present the concepts and processes of these alterations as an approach to understanding the manifestation of neurologic dysfunction. Some specific diseases are also presented (i.e., Parkinson disease, Huntington disease, and amyotrophic lateral sclerosis) because they fit best here. The manifestations for specific central and peripheral nervous system disorders are presented in Chapter 18. Alterations in sensory function are presented in Chapter 16.

 The neural systems essential to cognitive function are: (1) attentional systems that provide arousal and maintenance of attention over time; (2) memory and language systems by which information is communicated; and (3) affective or emotive systems that mediate mood, emotion, and intention. These core systems are fundamental to the processes of abstract thinking and reasoning. The products of abstraction and reasoning are organized and made operational through the executive attentional networks. The normal functioning of these systems manifests through the motor system in a behavioral array viewed by others as being appropriate to human activity and successful living.

ALTERATIONS IN COGNITIVE SYSTEMS

Full consciousness is a state of awareness both of oneself and of the environment and a set of responses to that environment. The fully conscious individual responds to external stimuli with a wide array of responses. Any decrease in this state of awareness and varied responses is thus a decrease in consciousness.

 Consciousness has two distinct components: arousal (state of awakeness) and awareness (content of thought). Arousal is mediated by the reticular activating system, which regulates aspects of attention and information processing and maintains consciousness (see Fig. 15.7). Cognitive cerebral functions require a functioning reticular activating system. Awareness encompasses all cognitive functions and is mediated by attentional systems, memory systems, language systems, and executive systems.

Alterations in Arousal

Alterations in level of arousal may be caused by structural, metabolic, or psychogenic (functional) disorders.

◆**PATHOPHYSIOLOGY.** Structural alterations in arousal are divided according to original location of the pathologic condition: supratentorial (above the tentorium cerebelli); infratentorial (subtentorial, below the tentorium cerebelli); subdural (below the dura mater [see Figs. 15.17 and 17.18]); extracerebral (outside the brain tissue); and intracerebral (within the brain tissue). Causes include infection, vascular alterations, neoplasms, traumatic injury, congenital alterations, degenerative changes, polygenic traits, and metabolic disorders.

Supratentorial disorders (above the tentorium cerebelli) produce changes in arousal by either diffuse or localized dysfunction. Diffuse dysfunction may be caused by disease processes affecting the cerebral cortex or the underlying subcortical white matter (e.g., encephalitis). Disorders outside the brain but within the cranial vault (extracerebral) also can produce diffuse dysfunction, including neoplasms, closed-head trauma with subsequent bleeding, and subdural empyema (accumulation of pus). Disorders within the brain substance (intracerebral)—bleeding, infarcts, emboli, and tumors—function primarily as masses. Such localized destructive processes directly impair function of the thalamic or hypothalamic activating systems.

Infratentorial disorders (below the tentorium cerebelli) produce a decline in arousal by (1) direct destruction of the reticular activating system (RAS) and its pathways (e.g., accumulations of blood or pus, neoplasms, and demyelinating disorders), or (2) the brainstem (midbrain, pons, medulla) may be destroyed either by direct invasion or by indirect impairment of its blood supply. The most common cause of direct destruction is cerebrovascular disease. Demyelinating diseases, neoplasms, granulomas, abscesses, and head injury also may cause brainstem destruction by tissue compression. This compression may occur because of (1) direct pressure on the pons and midbrain, producing ischemia

and edema of the neurons of the RAS; (2) upward herniation of the cerebellum through the tentorial notch, thus compressing the upper midbrain and diencephalon; or (3) downward herniation of the cerebellum through the foramen magnum, compressing and displacing the medulla oblongata.

Metabolic alterations in arousal produce a decline in arousal by alterations in delivery of energy substrates as occurs with hypoxia, electrolyte disturbances, or hypoglycemia. Metabolic disorders caused by liver or renal failure cause alterations in neuronal excitability because of failure to metabolize or eliminate drugs and toxins. All the systemic diseases that eventually produce nervous system dysfunction are part of this metabolic category.

Psychogenic alterations in arousal (unresponsiveness), although uncommon, may signal general psychiatric disorders (see Chapter 19). Despite apparent unconsciousness, the person actually is physiologically awake and the neurologic examination reflects a normal response.

◆**CLINICAL MANIFESTATIONS AND EVALUATION.** Five patterns of neurologic function are critical to the evaluation process: (1) level of consciousness, (2) pattern of breathing, (3) pupillary reaction, (4) oculomotor responses, and (5) motor responses. Patterns of clinical manifestations help determine the extent of brain dysfunction and serve as indices for identifying increasing or decreasing central nervous system (CNS) function. Distinctions are made between metabolic and structurally induced manifestations (Table 17.1). The types of manifestations suggest the cause of the altered arousal state (Table 17.2).

Level of Consciousness

Level of consciousness is the most critical clinical index of nervous system function with changes indicating either improvement or deterioration of the individual's condition. A person who is alert and oriented to self, others, place, and time is considered to be functioning at the highest level of consciousness, which implies full use of all the person's cognitive capacities. From this normal alert state, levels of

TABLE 17.1 CLINICAL MANIFESTATIONS OF METABOLIC AND STRUCTURAL CAUSES OF ALTERED AROUSAL

MANIFESTATION	METABOLICALLY INDUCED	STRUCTURALLY INDUCED
Blink to threat (cranial nerves II, VII)	Equal	Asymmetric
Discs (cranial nerve II)	Flat, good pulsation	Papilledema
Extraocular movement (cranial nerves III, IV, VI)	Roving eye movements; normal doll's eyes and calorics	Gaze paresis, nerve III palsy, medial longitudinal fasciculus (MLF) syndrome (internuclear ophthalmoplegia)
Pupils (cranial nerves II, III)	Equal and reactive; may be large (e.g., atropine), pinpoint (e.g., opiates), or midposition and fixed (e.g., glutethimide [Doriden])	Asymmetric and/or nonreactive; may be midposition (midbrain injury), pinpoint (pons injury), large (tectal injury)
Corneal reflex (cranial nerves V, VII)	Symmetric response	Asymmetric response
Grimace to pain (cranial nerve VII)	Symmetric response	Asymmetric response
Motor function movement	Symmetric	Asymmetric
Tone	Symmetric	Paratonic, spastic, flaccid, especially if asymmetric
Posture	Symmetric	Decorticate, especially if symmetric; decerebrate, especially if asymmetric
Deep tendon reflexes	Symmetric	Asymmetric
Babinski sign	Absent or symmetric response	Present
Sensation	Symmetric	Asymmetric

TABLE 17.2   DIFFERENTIAL CHARACTERISTICS OF DISORDERS CAUSING ALTERED AROUSAL

MECHANISM	MANIFESTATIONS
Supratentorial mass lesions compressing or displacing diencephalons or brainstem	Initiating signs usually of focal cerebral dysfunction Signs of dysfunction progress rostral to caudal Neurologic signs at any given time point to one anatomic area (e.g., diencephalon, mesencephalon, medulla) Motor signs often asymmetric
Infratentorial mass or destruction, causing coma	History of preceding brainstem dysfunction or sudden onset of coma Localizing brainstem signs precede or accompany onset of coma and always include oculovestibular abnormality Cranial nerve palsies; usually manifest as "bizarre" respiratory patterns that appear at onset
Metabolic coma Exogenous toxins (drugs) Endogenous toxins (organ system failure)	Confusion and stupor commonly precede motor signs Motor signs usually are symmetric Pupillary reactions usually are preserved Asterixis, myoclonus, tremor, and seizures are common Acid-base imbalance with hyperventilation or hypoventilation is common
Psychiatric unresponsiveness	Lids close actively Pupils reactive or dilated (cycloplegics) Oculocephalic reflexes are unpredictable; oculovestibular reflexes are physiologic (nystagmus is present) Motor tone is inconsistent or normal Eupnea or hyperventilation is usual No pathologic reflexes are present Electroencephalogram (EEG) is normal

TABLE 17.3   LEVELS OF ALTERED CONSCIOUSNESS

STATE	DEFINITION
Confusion	Loss of ability to think rapidly and clearly; impaired judgment and decision making
Disorientation	Beginning loss of consciousness; disorientation to time followed by disorientation to place and impaired memory; lost last is recognition of self
Lethargy	Limited spontaneous movement or speech; easy arousal with normal speech or touch; may not be oriented to time, place, or person
Obtundation	Mild to moderate reduction in arousal (awakeness) with limited response to the environment; falls asleep unless stimulated verbally or tactilely; answers questions with minimum response
Stupor	A condition of deep sleep or unresponsiveness from which the person may be aroused or caused to open eyes only by vigorous and repeated stimulation; response is often withdrawal or grabbing at stimulus
Light coma	Associated with purposeful movement on stimulation
Coma	No verbal response to the external environment or to any stimuli; noxious stimuli such as deep pain or suctioning yields motor movement
Deep coma	Associated with unresponsiveness or no response to any stimulus

consciousness diminish in stages from confusion and disorientation (can occur simultaneously) to coma, each of which is clinically defined (Table 17.3).

Pattern of Breathing

Respiratory patterns help evaluate the level of brain dysfunction and coma. Rate, rhythm, and pattern should be evaluated. Breathing patterns can be categorized as hemispheric or brainstem (Table 17.4 and Fig. 17.1).

With normal breathing, a neural center in the forebrain (cerebrum) produces a rhythmic breathing pattern. When consciousness decreases, lower brainstem centers regulate the breathing pattern by responding only to changes in Paco2 levels, called posthyperventilation apnea (PHVA).

Cheyne-Stokes respiration is an abnormal rhythm of ventilation (periodic breathing) with alternating periods of hyperventilation and apnea (crescendo-decrescendo pattern). In the damaged brain, higher levels of Paco2 are required to stimulate ventilation, and increases in Paco2 lead to tachypnea. The Paco2 level then decreases to below normal, and breathing stops (apnea) until the carbon dioxide reaccumulates and again stimulates tachypnea (see Fig. 17.1). In cases of opiate or sedative drug overdose, the respiratory center is depressed and the rate of breathing gradually decreases until respiratory failure occurs.

Central neurogenic hyperventilation is a respiratory pattern of sustained hyperventilation caused by a lesion in the central pons. Apneustic respirations have prolonged inspiratory and expiratory phases caused by injury to the pons or upper medulla. Cluster respirations are characterized by periods or clusters of rapid respirations of near equal depth resulting from trauma or compression to the medulla or from chronic opioid abuse. Ataxic respirations are irregular respirations with prolonged periods of apnea associated with damage to the medulla (see Fig. 17.1).

TABLE 17.4 PATTERNS OF BREATHING

BREATHING PATTERN	DESCRIPTION	LOCATION OF INJURY
Hemispheric Breathing Patterns		
Normal	After a period of hyperventilation that lowers the arterial carbon dioxide pressure ($PaCO_2$), the individual continues to breathe regularly but with a reduced depth.	Response of the nervous system to an external stressor—not associated with injury to the central nervous system (CNS)
Posthyperventilation apnea	Respirations stop after hyperventilation has lowered the $PaCO_2$ level below normal. Rhythmic breathing returns when the $PaCO_2$ level returns to normal. (Usually an intact cerebral cortex will trigger breathing within 10 seconds regardless of $PaCO_2$.)	Associated with diffuse bilateral metabolic or structural disease of the cerebrum
Cheyne-Stokes respirations	Breathing pattern has a smooth increase (crescendo) in the rate and depth of breathing (hyperpnea), which peaks and is followed by a gradual smooth decrease (decrescendo) in the rate and depth of breathing to the point of apnea when the cycle repeats itself. The hyperpneic phase lasts longer than the apneic phase (represents an amplitude change).	Bilateral dysfunction of the deep cerebral or diencephalic structures; seen with supratentorial injury and metabolically induced coma states unrelated to neurologic dysfunction; may see also in congestive heart failure (CHF)
Brainstem Breathing Patterns		
Central reflex hyperpnea (central neurogenic hyperventilation)	A sustained deep rapid but regular pattern (hyperpnea) occurs, with a decreased $PaCO_2$ and a corresponding increase in pH and increased PO_2.	May result from CNS damage or disease that involves the lower midbrain and upper pons; seen after increased intracranial pressure and blunt head trauma
Apneusis	A prolonged inspiratory cramp (a pause at full inspiration) occurs. A common variant of this is a brief end-inspiratory pause of 2 or 3 seconds, often alternating with an end-expiratory pause.	Indicates damage to the respiratory control mechanism located at the pontine level; most commonly associated with pontine infarction but documented with hypoglycemia, anoxia, and meningitis
Cluster breathing	A cluster of breaths has a disordered sequence with irregular pauses between breaths.	Dysfunction in the lower pontine and high medullary areas
Ataxic breathing	Completely irregular breathing occurs, with random shallow and deep breaths and irregular pauses. Often the rate is slow.	Originates from a primary dysfunction of the medulla
Gasping breathing pattern (agonal gasps)	A pattern of deep "all-or-none" breaths is accompanied by a slow respiratory rate.	Indicative of a failing medullary respiratory center

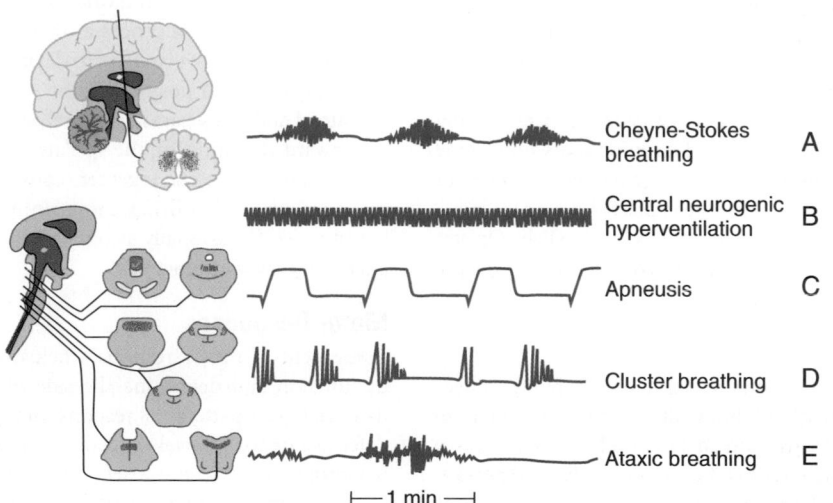

Cheyne-Stokes breathing **A**

Central neurogenic hyperventilation **B**

Apneusis **C**

Cluster breathing **D**

Ataxic breathing **E**

├── 1 min ──┤

FIGURE 17.1 Abnormal Respiratory Patterns with Corresponding Level of Central Nervous System Injuries. A, Cheyne-Stokes respiration is seen with metabolic injury and lesions in the forebrain and diencephalon. **B,** Central neurogenic hyperventilation is most commonly seen with metabolic encephalopathies (lesion of midbrain, pons, or medulla). **C,** Apneustic breathing (inspiratory pauses) is seen in patients with bilateral pontine lesions. **D,** Cluster breathing and ataxic breathing are seen in lesions at the pontine medullary junction. **E,** Ataxic breathing occurs when the medullary ventral respiratory nuclei are injured. (From Urden LD et al: *Critical care nursing: diagnosis and management,* ed 6, St Louis, 2010, Mosby.)

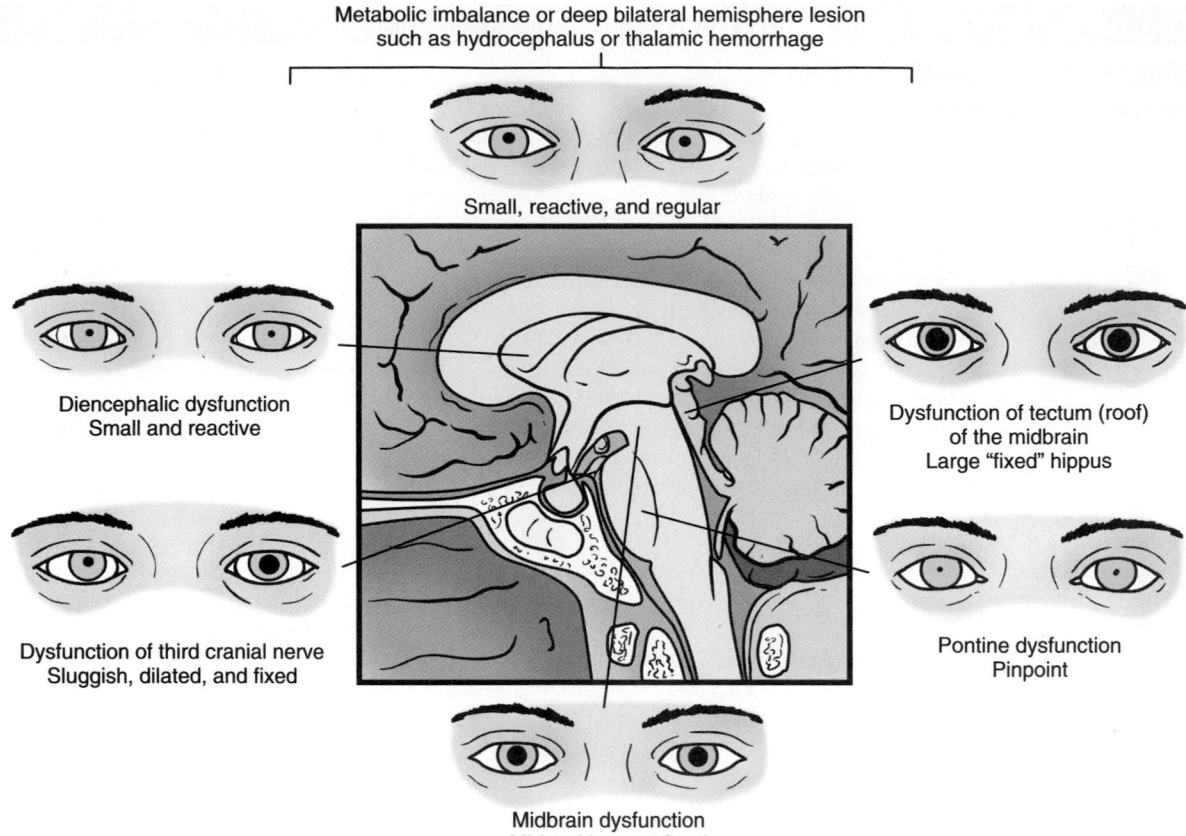

Metabolic imbalance or deep bilateral hemisphere lesion
such as hydrocephalus or thalamic hemorrhage

Small, reactive, and regular

Diencephalic dysfunction
Small and reactive

Dysfunction of tectum (roof)
of the midbrain
Large "fixed" hippus

Dysfunction of third cranial nerve
Sluggish, dilated, and fixed

Pontine dysfunction
Pinpoint

Midbrain dysfunction
Midposition and fixed

FIGURE 17.2 Appearance of Pupils at Different Levels of Consciousness.

Pupillary Changes

Brainstem areas that control arousal are adjacent to areas that control the pupils. Pupillary changes thus are a valuable guide to evaluating the presence and level of brainstem dysfunction (Fig. 17.2). For example, severe ischemia and hypoxia usually produce dilated, fixed pupils. Hypothermia may cause fixed pupils.

Some drugs affect pupils and must be considered in evaluating individuals in comatose states. Large doses of atropine and scopolamine fully dilate and fix pupils. Doses of sedatives (e.g., glutethimide) in sufficient amounts to produce coma cause the pupils to become midposition or moderately dilated, unequal, and commonly fixed to light. Opiates cause pinpoint pupils. Severe barbiturate intoxication may produce fixed pupils.

Oculomotor Responses

Oculomotor responses (resting, spontaneous, and reflexive eye movements) change at various levels of brain dysfunction in comatose individuals (Table 17.5). Persons with metabolically induced coma, except in cases of barbiturate-hypnotic and phenytoin (Dilantin) poisoning, generally retain ocular reflexes, however, even when other signs of brainstem damage, such as central neurogenic hyperventilation, are present.

The presence of brisk oculocephalic reflexes and roving eye movements, as well as the failure to elicit nystagmus with instillation of cold or warm water into the external ear canal, indicates a decrease in consciousness (loss of cortical influence) but an intact brainstem (Figs. 17.3 and 17.4).

Destructive or compressive injury to the brainstem causes specific abnormalities of the oculocephalic and oculovestibular reflexes. For example, a skewed deviation, in which one eye diverges downward and the other looks upward, indicates brainstem dysfunction. Destructive or compressive disease processes that involve an oculomotor nucleus or nerve cause the involved eye to deviate outward, producing a resting dysconjugate lateral position of the eyes (each eye diverges laterally). Unilateral abducens paralysis (paralysis of cranial nerve VI) results in an upward deviation of the ipsilateral eye. With bilateral abducens paralysis, the eyes come together (converge). Reflexive eye movements may be suppressed by drugs, most commonly phenytoin, tricyclics, and barbiturates. Occasionally alcohol, phenothiazines, and diazepam may alter reflex eye movements.

Motor Responses

Assessment of motor responses helps to evaluate the level of brain dysfunction and determine the side of the brain that is maximally damaged. The pattern of response noted may be (1) purposeful (a defensive or withdrawal movement of limbs to noxious stimuli); (2) inappropriate, or not purposeful (generalized motor movement, posturing, grimacing, or groaning); or (3) not present (unresponsive, no motor response). Purposeful movement requires an intact corticospinal system. Nonpurposeful movement is evidence of severe dysfunction of the corticospinal system.

Motor signs indicating loss of cortical inhibition are commonly associated with decreased consciousness and include primitive reflexes and rigidity (paratonia) (Fig. 17.5). Primitive reflexes include grasping, reflex sucking, snout reflex, and palmomental reflex, all of which are

TABLE 17.5	**CHANGES IN OCULOMOTOR RESPONSES**	
STATE	**RESTING AND SPONTANEOUS EYE MOVEMENTS**	**REFLEXIVE EYE MOVEMENTS**
Full consciousness	Eyes at rest, still (cortical gaze centers inhibit spontaneous roving eye movements)	Eyes move as the head turns Oculocephalic responses not elicited or inconsistently elicited (frontal gaze centers inhibit brainstem reflexes that fix gaze straight ahead) Oculovestibular (caloric) stimulation produces nystagmus
Cortical dysfunction or disruption of efferent pathways	Conjugate, horizontal, roving eye movements may well be present (cortical gaze centers no longer inhibit these brainstem-generated roving eye movements)	Gaze fixed straight ahead regardless of head position—positive doll's eyes reaction (normal oculocephalic reflexes are no longer inhibited by frontal gaze centers)
Diffuse anoxic damage to cortex	"Ocular dipping"—slow, dysrhythmic downward movement followed by faster, upward movement	Nystagmus is no longer induced by caloric stimulation (normally a cold-water stimulus produces deviation of the eyes opposite the irrigated ear; a warm-water stimulus deviates the eyes to the same [ipsilateral] side) With an injury that depresses cortical gaze center function, the eyes (and often the entire head) deviate or appear to look toward the side of the injured hemisphere With an injury that irritates (stimulates) the neurons of the cortical gaze center, the eyes (and often the entire head) deviate away from the injured hemisphere (all fibers from the frontal gaze centers decussate and therefore control the function of the contralateral pontine gaze center, which moves the eyes in the ipsilateral direction)
Mesencephalon dysfunction	Roving eye movements cease, and the eyes become immobile and directed ahead (roving eye movements require an intact brainstem) Eyes may turn down and inward	Oculovestibular reflexes become inconsistent and abnormal Loss of Bell phenomenon (upward deviation of eyes on stimulation) (requires intact eye movement pathways from the mesencephalon to pons)
Pontine dysfunction	Loss of spontaneous blinking (requires an intact pons) "Ocular bobbing"—brisk, conjugate, downward movement of eyes with loss of horizontal eye movements	

TABLE 17.6	**ABNORMAL MOTOR RESPONSES WITH DECREASED RESPONSIVENESS**	
MOTOR RESPONSE	**DESCRIPTION OF MOTOR RESPONSES**	**LOCATION OF INJURY**
Decorticate posturing/rigidity: upper extremity flexion, lower extremity extension (Fig. 17.6)	Slowly developing flexion of the arm, wrist, and fingers with abduction in the upper extremity and extension, internal rotation, and plantar flexion of the lower extremity	Hemispheric damage above midbrain releasing medullary and pontine reticulospinal systems
Decerebrate posturing/rigidity: upper and lower extremity extensor responses (Fig. 17.6)	Opisthotonos (hyperextension of the vertebral column) with clenching of the teeth; extension, abduction, and hyperpronation of the arms; and extension of the lower extremities In acute brain injury, shivering and hyperpnea may accompany unelicited recurrent decerebrate spasms	Associated with severe damage involving midbrain or upper pons Acute brain injury may cause limb extension regardless of location
Extensor responses in the upper extremities accompanied by flexion in the lower extremities		Pons
Flaccid state with little or no motor response to stimuli		Lower pons and upper medulla

normal in the newborn but disappear in infancy. Abnormal flexor and extensor responses in the upper and lower extremities are defined in Table 17.6 and illustrated in Fig. 17.6.

Vomiting, yawning, and hiccups are complex reflex-like motor responses that are integrated by neural mechanisms in the lower brainstem. These responses may be produced by compression or diseases involving tissues of the medulla oblongata (e.g., infection, neoplasm, infarct, or other more benign stimuli to the vagal nerve). Most CNS disorders produce nausea and vomiting. Vomiting without nausea indicates direct involvement of the central neural mechanism (or pyloric obstruction). Vomiting often accompanies CNS injuries that (1) involve the vestibular nuclei or its immediate projections, particularly when double vision (diplopia) also is present; (2) impinge directly on the floor of the fourth ventricle; or (3) produce brainstem compression secondary to increased intracranial pressure.

Outcomes of Alterations in Arousal

Outcomes of alterations in arousal fall into two categories: *extent of disability (morbidity)* and *mortality*. Outcomes depend on the cause and extent of brain damage and the duration of coma. Some individuals may recover consciousness and an original level of function, some may have permanent disability, and some may never regain consciousness and experience neurologic death. Two forms of neurologic death—brain death and cerebral death—result from severe pathologic conditions and are associated with irreversible coma. Other possible outcomes are a vegetative state, a minimally conscious state, or locked-in syndrome. The extent of disability has four subcategories: recovery of consciousness, residual cognitive function, psychologic function, and vocational function.

Brain death (total brain death) occurs when brain damage is so extensive that it can never recover (irreversible) and cannot maintain the body's internal homeostasis. State laws define brain death as irreversible cessation of function of the entire brain, including the brainstem and cerebellum. On postmortem examination, the brain is autolyzing (self-digesting) or already autolyzed. Brain death has occurred when there is no evidence of brain function for an extended period.[1] The abnormality of brain function must result from structural or known metabolic disease and must *not* be caused by a depressant drug, alcohol poisoning, or hypothermia. An isoelectric, or flat, electroencephalogram (EEG) (electrocerebral silence) for 6 to 12 hours in a person who is not hypothermic and has not ingested depressant drugs indicates brain death. The clinical criteria used to determine brain death are noted in Box 17.1. A task force for determination of brain death in children recommended the same criteria as for adults but with a longer observation period.[1]

Cerebral death or irreversible coma is death of the cerebral hemispheres exclusive of the brainstem and cerebellum. Brain damage is permanent, and the individual is unable to ever respond behaviorally in any significant way to the environment. The brainstem may continue to maintain internal homeostasis (i.e., body temperature, cardiovascular functions, respirations, and metabolic functions). The survivor of cerebral

FIGURE 17.3 Test for Oculocephalic Reflex Response (Doll's Eyes Phenomenon). **A,** Normal response—eyes turn together to side opposite from turn of head. **B,** Abnormal response—eyes do not turn in conjugate manner. **C,** Absent response—eyes do not turn as head position changes. (**A** and **C** from Rudy EB: *Advanced neurological and neurosurgical nursing*, St Louis, 1984, Mosby.)

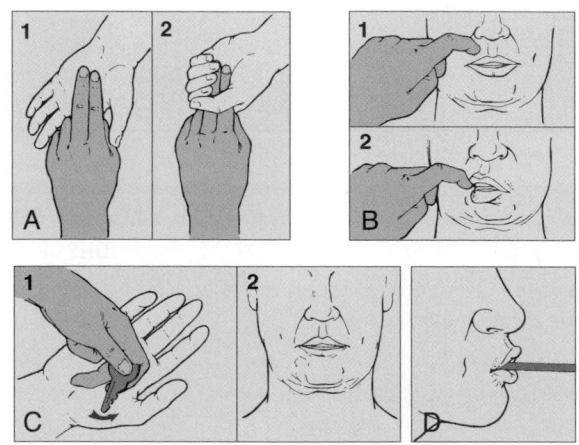

FIGURE 17.5 Pathologic Reflexes. **A,** Grasp reflex. **B,** Snout reflex. **C,** Palmomental reflex. **D,** Suck reflex.

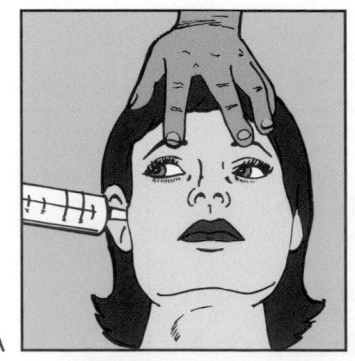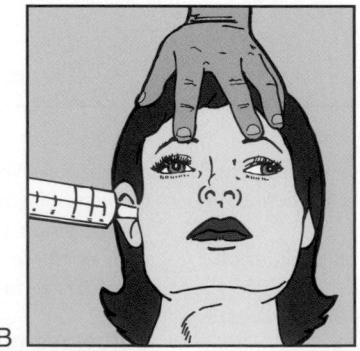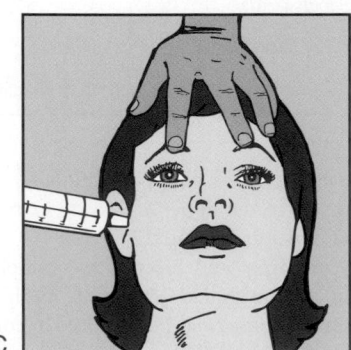

FIGURE 17.4 Test for Oculovestibular Reflex (Caloric Ice-Water Test). **A,** Normal response—conjugate eye movements. **B,** Abnormal response—dysconjugate or asymmetric eye movements. **C,** Absent response—no eye movements.

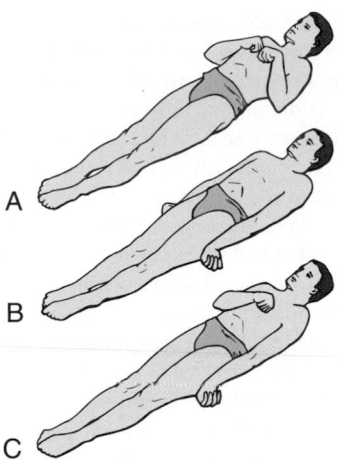

FIGURE 17.6 Decorticate and Decerebrate Responses. A, *Decorticate response (flexor posturing):* bilateral flexion of elbows and wrists with shoulder adduction in upper extremities. Extension, internal rotation of lower extremities (lesions above the midbrain). **B,** *Decerebrate response (extensor posturing):* all four extremities in rigid extension, internal rotation of shoulders with hyperpronation of forearms (midbrain lesions). **C,** *Decorticate response on right side of body and decerebrate response on left side of body:* the most pronounced response differences are in the upper body. (From Rudy EB: *Advanced neurological and neurosurgical nursing,* St Louis, 1984, Mosby.)

BOX 17.1   CRITERIA FOR BRAIN DEATH

1. Completion of all appropriate diagnostic and therapeutic procedures with no possibility of brain function recovery
2. Unresponsive coma (no motor or reflex movements)
3. No spontaneous respiration (apnea)
4. No brainstem functions (ocular responses to head turning or caloric stimulation; dilated, fixed pupils; no gag or corneal reflex [see Figs. 17.3 and 17.4])
5. Isoelectric (flat) EEG (electrocerebral silence)
6. Persistence of these signs for an appropriate observation period

EEG, electroencephalogram.
Summarized from Wijdicks EF et al: *Neurology* 74(23):1911-1918, 2010.

---

death may remain in a coma or emerge into a persistent vegetative state (VS) or a minimally conscious state (MCS). In coma, the eyes are usually closed with no eye opening. The person does not follow commands, speak, or have voluntary movement (Table 17.7).

A **persistent vegetative state (VS),** or **unresponsive wakefulness syndrome,** is complete unawareness of the self or surrounding environment and complete loss of cognitive function. The individual does not speak any comprehensible words or follow commands.[2] Sleep-wake cycles are present, eyes open spontaneously, and blood pressure and breathing are maintained without support. Brainstem reflexes (pupillary, oculocephalic, chewing, swallowing) are intact but cerebral function is lost. There may be random hand, extremity, or head movements. There is bowel and bladder incontinence. Recovery is unlikely if the state persists for 12 months.

In a minimally conscious state (MCS) individuals may follow simple commands; manipulate objects; gesture or give yes/no responses; have intelligible speech; and have movements, such as blinking or smiling, that occur in a meaningful relationship to the eliciting stimulus and are not attributable to reflexive activity.

With **locked-in syndrome (ventral pontine syndrome)** there is complete paralysis of voluntary muscles with the exception of eye movement. Content of thought and level of arousal are intact but the efferent pathways are disrupted (injury at the base of the pons with the reticular formation intact, often caused by basilar artery occlusion).[3] The individual cannot communicate either through speech or through body movement but is fully conscious with intact cognitive function. The upper cranial nerves (I through IV) often are preserved, so that the person possesses vertical eye movement and blinking as a means of communication.

Akinetic mutism (AM) is a neurobehavioral state characterized by a severe loss of motivation to move or inability to voluntarily initiate motor responses, or both. It exemplifies an inability to voluntarily execute motor functions including speech, gestures, and facial expression. Generally, these individuals are alert, orient to external stimuli, and can follow the examiner with their eyes but do not initiate other voluntary activity or movement. This is not attributable to decreased wakefulness, motor weakness, or paralysis. The neuropathology is different when compared with the vegetative state and locked-in syndrome and involves damage to the frontal lobe or bilateral cingulate cortex (a component of the limbic system).[4,5] Combined deficits of vigilance, detection, and working memory accompanied by other deficits of the cognitive systems are common.

TABLE 17.7   COMPARATIVE CLINICAL FEATURES OF ALTERATIONS IN LEVELS OF AROUSAL

DIAGNOSIS	AROUSAL	AWARENESS	COMMUNICATION
Coma	Eyes do not open spontaneously or in response to stimulation	No evidence of perception, communication ability, only reflexes and postural responses	None
Persistent vegetative state	Eyes open spontaneously; no visual tracking; sleep-wake cycle resumes or state of chronic wakefulness; arousal often sluggish	No evidence of cognitive function or purposeful motor activity	None
Akinetic mutism	Eyes open spontaneously; normal sleep-wake cycle; arousal level is normal	Visual tracking present; little or no following of commands	Little or no volitional speech or movement
Minimally conscious state	Eyes open spontaneously; normal to abnormal sleep-wake cycle; arousal level ranges from obtunded to normal	Inconsistent evidence of perception, communication ability, or purposeful motor activity; visual tracking often intact	Inconsistent verbalization and gesturing
Locked-in syndrome	Full arousal; sleep-wake cycle present; quadriplegic	Perceptions and emotions intact	Cannot speak or move muscles except vertical eye movement and blinking

Data from Giacino JT et al: *Neurology* 58(3):349-353, 2002; Owen AM: *Ann N Y Acad Sci* 1125:225–238, 2008.

Alterations in Awareness

Awareness (content of thought) encompasses all cognitive functions, including awareness of self, environment, and affective states (i.e., moods). Awareness is mediated by all of the core networks under the guidance of executive attention networks, including selective attention and memory. Executive attention networks involve abstract reasoning, planning, decision making, judgment, error correction, and self-control. Each attentional function is a network of interconnected brain circuits and not localized to a single brain area.

Selective attention (orienting) refers to the ability to select specific information to be processed from available, competing environmental and internal stimuli and to focus on that stimulus (i.e., to concentrate on a specific task without being distracted).[6] *Selective visual (spatial) attention* is the ability to select objects/events from multiple visual stimuli (location and movement in visual space) and process them to complete a task. *Selective auditory* or *hearing attention* is the ability to select or filter specific sounds and process them to complete a task. Multiple areas of the brain are involved in selective attention, including cortical areas, thalamic nuclei, and the limbic system. Frontal and parietal regions of the right hemisphere contribute to selective attention. The engage component (identifying the target of attention) is mediated by the pulvinar nucleus of the thalamus and regulates cortical synchrony[7] (Fig. 17.7). The disengagement mechanism (shifting attention to a new target and re-engaging on the new target) is mediated by the right parietal lobe. The motor consequences of attention are mediated by the superior colliculi for visual orienting and spatial attention.[8]

Selective attention deficits can be temporary, permanent, or progressive. Disorders associated with selective attention deficits include seizure activity, parietal lobe contusions, subdural hematomas, stroke, gliomas or metastatic tumor, late Alzheimer dementia, frontotemporal dementia, and psychotic disorders. Disorders of selective attention related to visual orienting behavior are produced by disease that involves portions of the midbrain. Disease affecting the superior colliculi manifests as a slowness in orienting attention. Parietal lobe disease may produce *unilateral neglect syndrome,* which is failure to report, respond, or orient to visual, auditory, or tactile stimuli that are presented contralateral to a brain lesion, provided this failure is not explained by primary sensory or motor disorders. For example, an individual with neglect following a right hemisphere lesion may fail to recognize a left limb, read from the left side of a book, ignore the food on the left side of the plate, remain unaware of numerals on the left side of a clock, or have an abnormal rightward shift in head and eye position. The person is able to recognize individual sensory input from the ipsilateral side (the side with the hemispheric lesion) when asked, but ignores (i.e., neglects, extinguishes) the sensory input from the contralateral side when stimulated from both sides. This phenomenon is called *extinction.*[9] The entire complex of sensory inattentiveness, loss of recognition of one's own body parts, and extinction, sometimes referred to as *neglect syndrome,* is common after stroke, generally in the right hemisphere.[10]

Memory is the recording, retention, and retrieval of information. Two types of long-term memory exist: declarative and nondeclarative[11] (Fig. 17.8). Declarative memory involves the learning and remembrance of *episodic memories* (personal history, events, and experiences) and *semantic memories* (facts and information). Declarative memory is mediated by domain-specific cortical areas of the association areas. This includes: (1) areas of the temporal, parietal, and occipital lobes (Fig. 17.9), where long-term memories are thought to be stored; and (2) domain-independent areas of the medial temporal lobe (i.e., hippocampus), the diencephalon (thalamic structures and hypothalamus), and the basal forebrain (located ventral to the striatum and produces acetylcholine) (Fig. 17.10), where it is thought distinct domain-specific features of an experience are related or bound.[11]

Nondeclarative memory (nonconscious), also called *reflexive, procedural, or implicit memory,* is the memory for actions, behaviors (habits), skills, and outcomes.[11] It is not a language memory but a motor memory. Nondeclarative memory involves the construction of the motor pattern so that the action, behavior, or skill becomes increasingly automatic. The striatum of the basal ganglia supports this learning across trials (stimulus-response learning), as well as probabilistic classification learning, which supports outcome prediction. All skills and habits are stored in this memory network.[12] *Cerebellar memory* is involved in working memory (short term memory), in addition to motor coordination and nonmotor functions of cognition, emotion, and learning.[13] *Emotional memory* is mediated by the amygdala (located on the inner surface of the temporal lobe) (see Fig. 17.10) and other neural networks. The amygdala attaches positive (e.g., pleasure) or negative (e.g., fear) dispositions to stimuli in the absence of conscious recollection of the circumstances of the emotional experience.[14]

Amnesia is the loss of memory and can be mild or severe. Two types of amnesia are retrograde amnesia and anterograde amnesia. The person experiencing retrograde amnesia has difficulty retrieving past personal history memories or past factual memories. In anterograde amnesia, new personal or factual memories cannot be formed, but memories of the distant past are retained and retrieved. These are disorders of domain-independent declarative memory networks, and the hippocampus and other temporal lobe structures often are involved. These memory disorders may be temporary (e.g., after a seizure) or permanent (e.g., after severe head injury or in Alzheimer disease). There may be only the memory disorder, or the memory disorder may be associated with other cognitive disorders. Global amnesia is a combination of anterograde and retrograde amnesia and involves the hippocampus. *Transient global amnesia* has a sudden onset and lasts less than 24 hours. The causal mechanisms are not clear, but it can be associated with migraine headache and cerebrovascular ischemia.[15] *Permanent global amnesia* is rare and associated with damage to the hippocampus.[16] *Domain–specific declarative memory loss* can manifest as agnosias (agnosias are in the section on Data Processing Deficits).

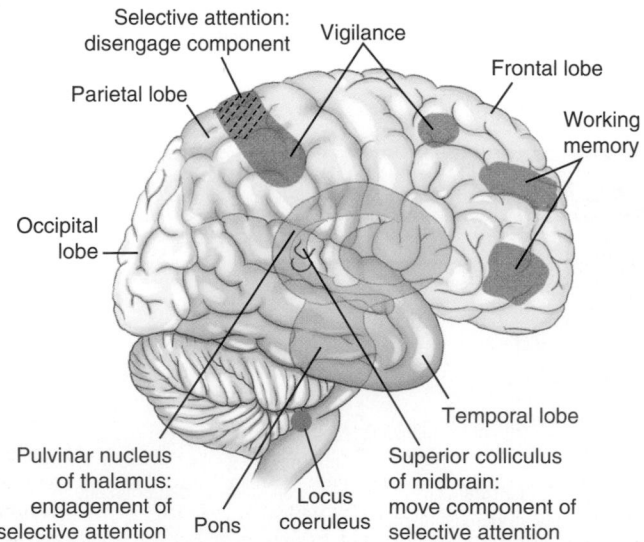

FIGURE 17.7 Right Cortical, Subcortical, and Brainstem Areas of the Brain—Mediating Cognitive Functions. (From Boss BJ, Wilkerson R: Communication: language and pragmatics. In Hoeman SP, editor: *Rehabilitation nursing: prevention, intervention, & outcomes,* ed 4, p 508, St Louis, 2008, Mosby.)

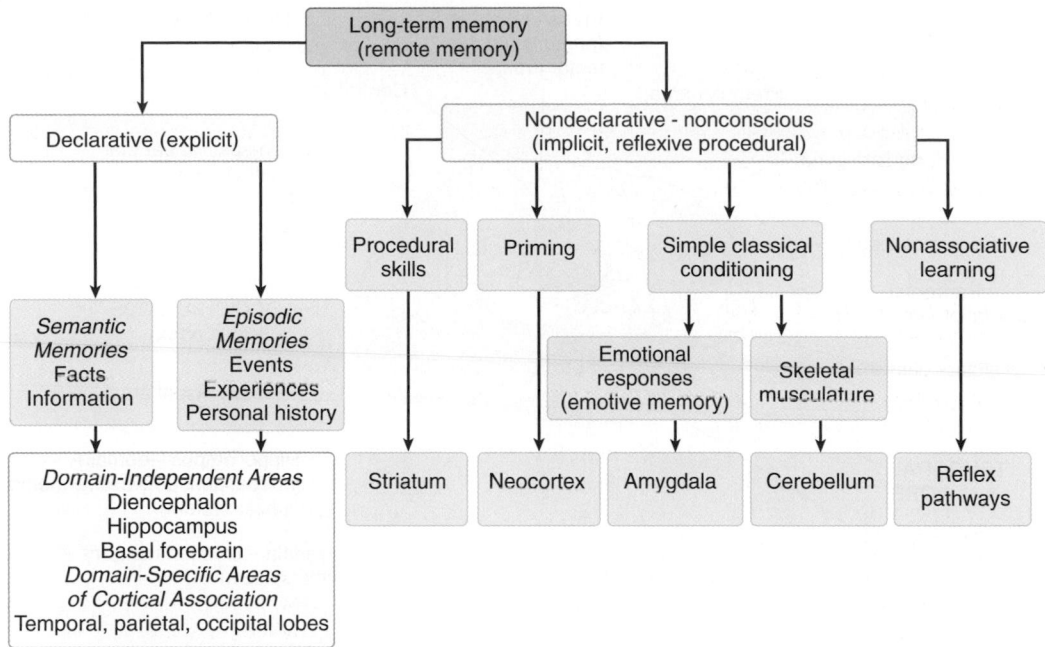

FIGURE 17.8 Types of Memory and Associated Brain Systems. (From Miller RD et al: *Miller's anesthesia,* ed 7, Philadelphia, 2010, Churchill Livingstone.)

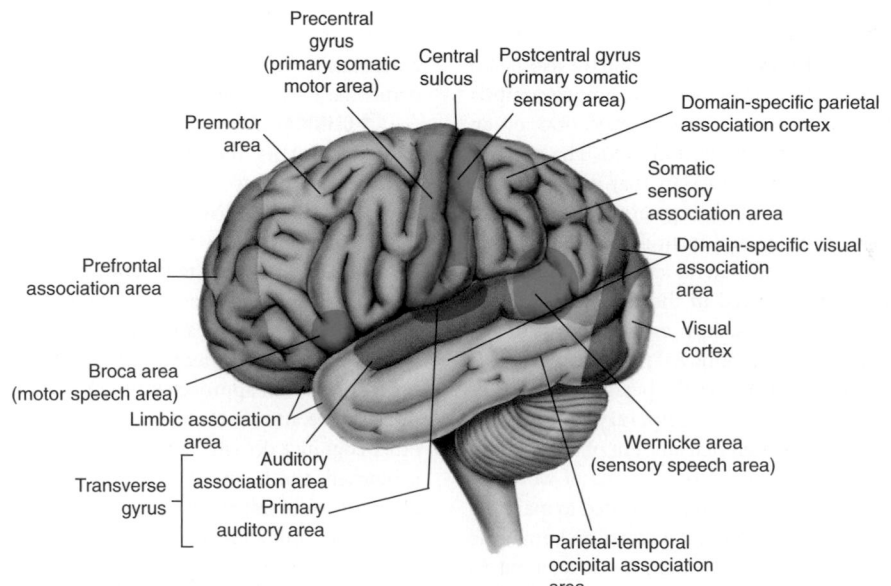

FIGURE 17.9 Cortical Areas of the Left (Dominant) Hemisphere. (Adapted from Patton KT, Thibodeau GA: *The human body in health & disease,* ed 7, St Louis, 2018, Elsevier.)

Image processing is a higher level of memory function and includes the ability to use sensory data and language to form concepts, assign meaning, and make abstractions. Alterations in image processing include an inability to form concepts and generalizations or to reason. Thinking is very concrete. These memory disorders may be temporary (e.g., after a seizure or postconcussive states) or permanent (e.g., after severe head injury, severe stroke, or in Alzheimer disease). There may be only the memory disorder, or the memory disorder may be associated with other cognitive disorders.

The prefrontal areas mediate several cognitive functions, called *executive attention functions* (planning, problem solving, goal setting). The *vigilance system* provides the person with the ability to maintain a sustained state of alertness or concentration for searching and scanning activities and involves the right frontal areas and the locus ceruleus (LC) (located in the rostral pons) (see Fig. 17.7). Through the neurotransmitter norepinephrine from the LC, the speed of the orienting (selective attention) network is increased and the detection function of the anterior cingulate gyrus (see Fig. 17.10) is decreased.

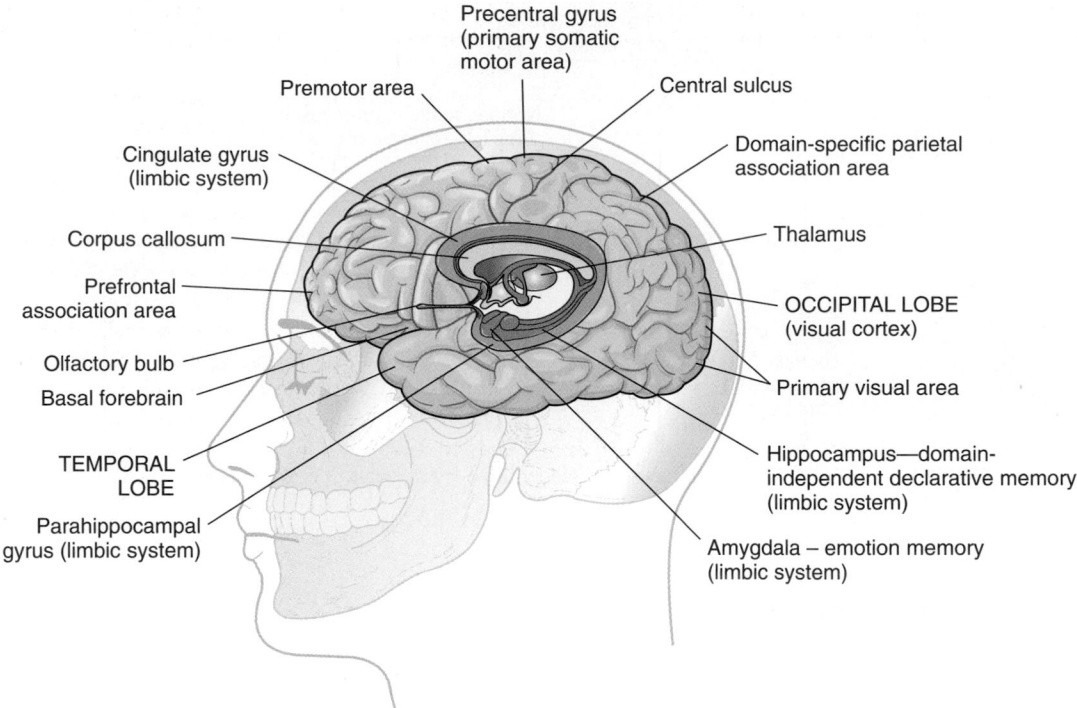

FIGURE 17.10 Midline Cortical and Deep Areas of the Cerebral Hemisphere.

Detection is the recognition of the object's identity and the realization that the object fulfills a desired goal (i.e., target selection among competing, complex contingencies). There is conscious execution of an instruction, ensuring that the instructions are followed. The anterior cingulate cortex inhibits automatic responses so that a less routine response can be given. The basal ganglia and cingulate, as well as other frontal areas, function in color, motion, and form detection.

The anterior cingulate plus the ventrolateral and dorsolateral prefrontal cortex (see Fig. 17.10) are involved in the representations of information in the absence of a stimulus, such as spatial position of visual events in memory when the event is removed from view. Working memory (short-term or recent memory) gives the person control over information processing (see Fig. 17.7). These temporary storage areas permit the brain to maintain or discard a limited amount of information (i.e., to retrieve instructions, such as strings or patterns of words or colors) and other information (i.e., strings of digits) needed to maintain a current stream of thought, resist distraction, and perform an immediate task. When attention is diverted, long-term memory is required to complete the task.[11] Isolated (pure) vigilance deficit, detection deficit, and working memory deficits are uncommon and involve focal lesions of the prefrontal cortex. Whether these losses are temporary or permanent depends on the cause and severity of injury.[17,18]

Executive attention deficits include the inability to maintain sustained attention and a working memory deficit. Sustained attention deficit is an inability to plan, set goals, and recognize when an object meets a goal. A working memory deficit is an inability to focus and remember instructions and information needed to guide behavior and complete a single task. Executive attention deficits may be temporary, progressive, or permanent.

PATHOPHYSIOLOGY. Very generally, the primary pathophysiologic mechanisms that operate in disorders of awareness are (1) direct destruction because of direct ischemia and hypoxia or indirect destruction as a result of compression and (2) the effects of toxins and chemicals or metabolic derangement, including processes related to dementia. The pathophysiologic processes are summarized in Fig. 17.11.

CLINICAL MANIFESTATIONS. Clinical manifestations of selective attention deficits, memory deficits, and executive attention function deficits are presented in Table 17.8.

EVALUATION AND TREATMENT. Immediate medical management is directed at diagnosing the cause and treating reversible factors. Rehabilitative measures for cognitive system deficits generally are either compensatory or restorative in nature and have been greatly facilitated by computer technology and other electronic-assisted devices. Approaches based on behavioral techniques tend to be compensatory, whereas process-oriented approaches, it is hoped, are restorative.

Selective attention and executive attention deficits masquerade as other cognitive deficits. Differential diagnosis of other cognitive deficits is blocked, and learning potential is largely obscured, by the presence of an attention deficit. Therefore diagnosis and treatment of attention deficits are fundamental.

Data Processing Deficits

Data processing deficits are problems associated with recognizing and processing sensory information and include agnosias, aphasias, and acute confusional states.

Agnosia

Agnosia is a defect of pattern recognition—a failure to recognize the form and nature of objects. Agnosia can be tactile, visual, or auditory, but only one sense is generally affected. For example, an individual may be unable to identify a safety pin by touching it with a hand but able to name it when looking at it. Agnosia may be as minimal as a finger agnosia (failure to identify by name the fingers of one's hand) or more extensive, such as a color agnosia.

Agnosia is produced by dysfunction in the primary sensory area or in the interpretive areas of the cerebral cortex (temporo-occipital area) (see Fig. 17.9). The types of agnosia and the associated area that is most commonly involved with each are presented in Table 17.9. Although agnosia most commonly is associated with cerebrovascular accidents, it may arise from any pathologic process that injures these specific areas of the brain.

Aphasia

Aphasia is impairment of comprehension or production of language with impaired written or verbal communication. The terms aphasia and dysphasia are often used interchangeably; the term aphasia is used here.[19] Aphasia results from dysfunction in the left cerebral hemisphere (i.e., Broca area [inferior frontal gyrus] and Wernicke area [superior temporal gyrus]) and the subcortical and cortical connecting networks (see Fig. 15.8, *C*). Aphasias are usually associated with a cerebrovascular accident involving the middle cerebral artery or one of its many branches (see Fig. 15.22). Language disorders, however, may arise from a variety of injuries and diseases including vascular, neoplastic, traumatic,

degenerative, metabolic, or infectious causes. Most language disorders result from acute processes or a chronic residual deficit of the acute process.

Aphasias have been classified anatomically (i.e., Wernicke or Broca area aphasias) or functionally as disorders of fluency (quality and content of speech). Expressive or motor aphasia, also known as *Broca, motor,* or *nonfluent aphasia,* involves loss of ability to produce spoken or written language with slow or difficult speech. Verbal comprehension is usually present. Expressive aphasia is differentiated from *dysarthria,* in which words cannot be articulated clearly as a result of cranial nerve damage or muscle impairment. Receptive aphasia, also known as *Wernicke, sensory,* or *fluent dysphasia,* involves an inability to understand written or spoken language. Speech is fluent, flowing at a normal rate but words and phrases have no meaning. Anomic aphasia is a sensory aphasia distinguished by difficulty finding words and naming a person or object. Circumlocution, or describing an object as a way of trying to name something, is common in anomic aphasia. Auditory comprehension is

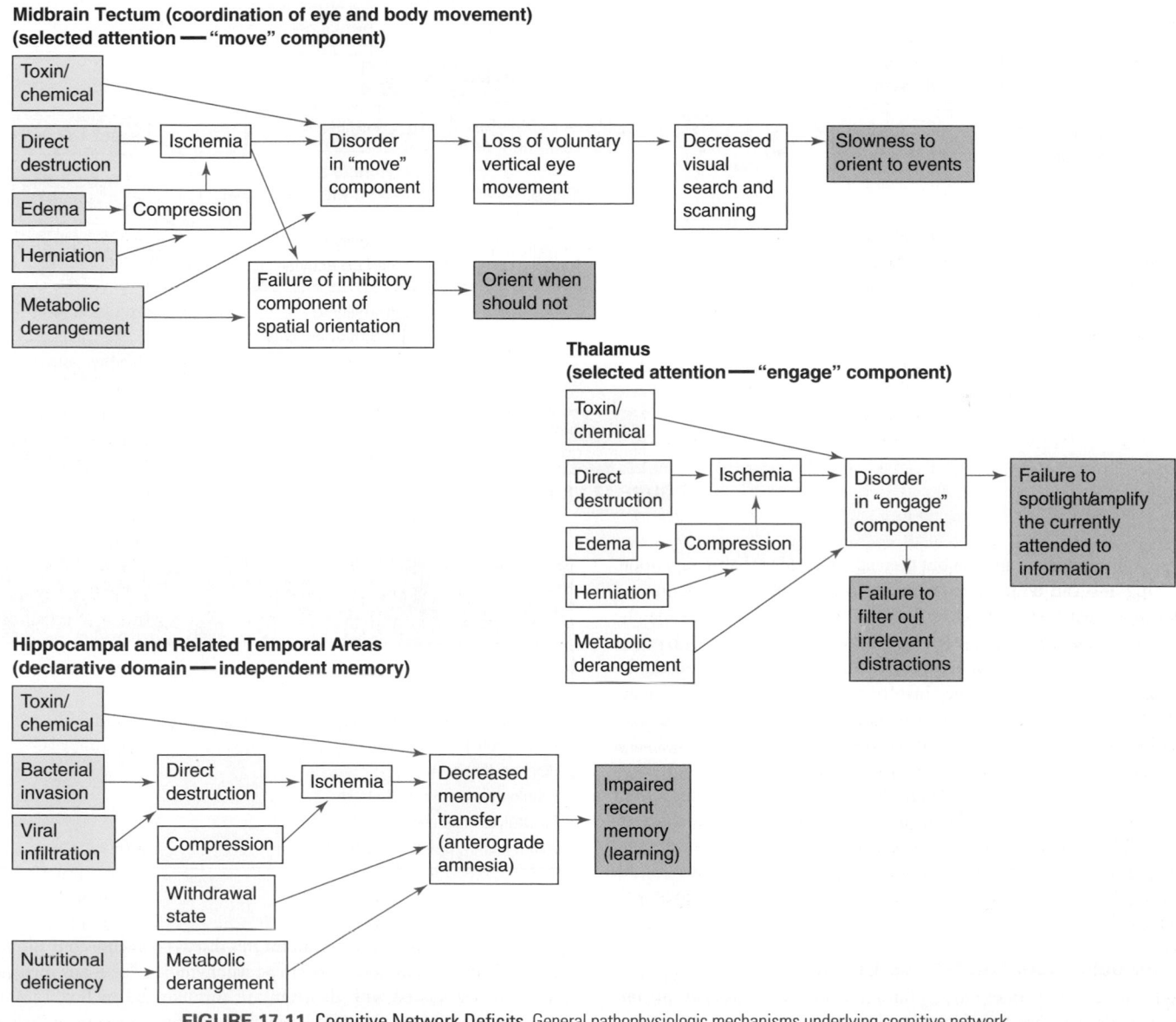

FIGURE 17.11 Cognitive Network Deficits. General pathophysiologic mechanisms underlying cognitive network deficits.   *Continued*

Cortical Association Areas
(selective attention, disengage components, declarative domain—specific memory)
(image formation)

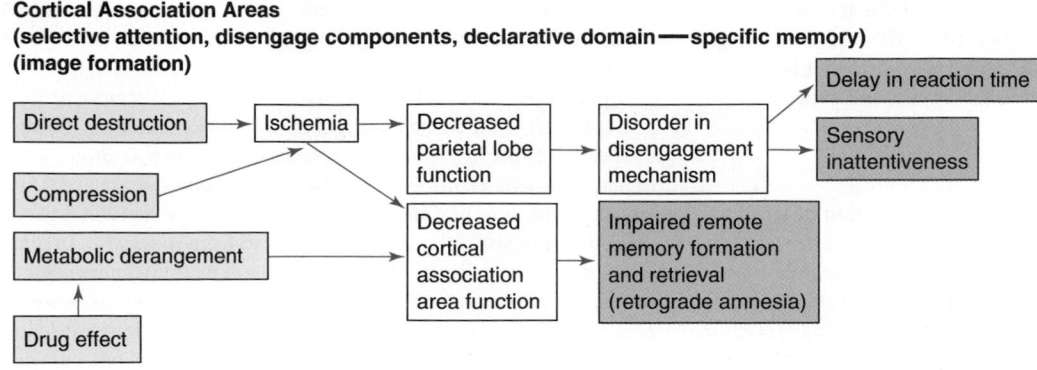

Frontal Areas
(vigilance, detection, working memory)

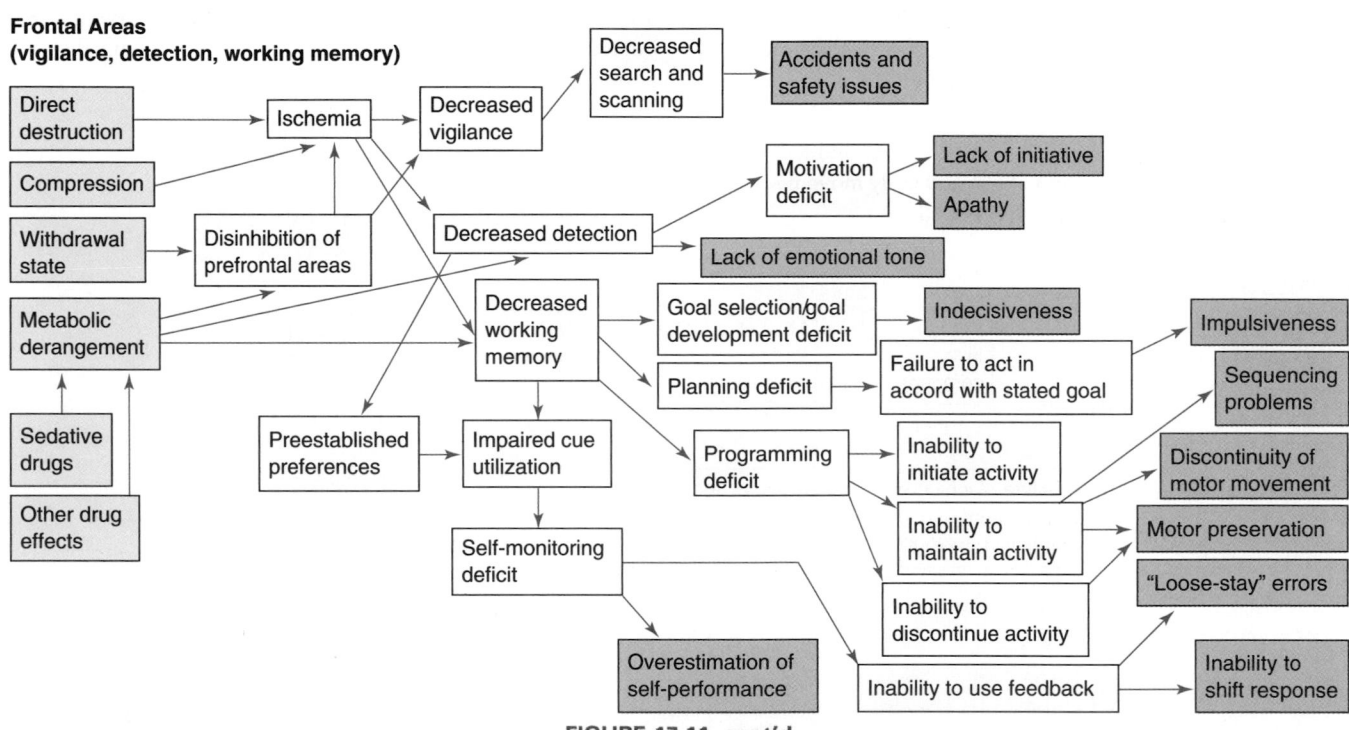

FIGURE 17.11, cont'd

present in conductive aphasia but there is impaired verbatim repetition. Naming also can be impaired. The person recognizes the errors and tries to correct them. Speech is fluent but words and sounds may be transposed. Damage is in the left hemisphere to networks that connect Broca and Wernicke areas. Transcortical aphasias are rare and can be motor, sensory, or mixed. They involve areas of the brain that connect into the language centers. Global aphasia is the most severe aphasia and involves both expressive and receptive aphasia. The individual is nonfluent or mute; cannot read or write; and has impaired comprehension, naming, reading, and writing. Global aphasia is usually associated with a cerebrovascular accident involving the middle cerebral artery. Table 17.10 compares types of aphasia, and Table 17.11 illustrates some of the language disturbances. Pure aphasias are rare and are often mixed, making diagnosis difficult. All types of aphasia usually improve with speech rehabilitation.

Acute Confusional States and Delirium

Acute confusional states (ACSs) (also may be known as *acute organic brain syndromes*) are transient disorders of awareness and may have either a sudden or a gradual onset. Delirium can be considered as a

BOX 17.2	CONDITIONS CAUSING ACUTE CONFUSIONAL STATES OR DELIRIUM

Drug intoxication
Alcohol or drug withdrawal
Metabolic disorders (i.e., hypoglycemia, thyroid storm)
Brain trauma or surgery
Postanesthesia
Febrile illnesses or heat stroke
Electrolyte imbalance, dehydration
Heart, kidney, or liver failure

type of acute confusional state, but for this discussion acute confusional states and delirium are considered to be synonymous. The many medical conditions associated with delirium are summarized in Box 17.2. It most commonly occurs in critical care units, following surgery, or during withdrawal from central nervous system depressants (i.e., alcohol or

TABLE 17.8	CLINICAL MANIFESTATIONS OF COGNITIVE NETWORK DEFICITS	
DEFICIT	**CLINICAL SIGNS**	**SYMPTOMS**
Attention		
Selective attention (orienting)	Inability to focus attention; decreased eye, head, and body movements associated with focusing on the stimuli; decreased search and scanning; faulty orientation to stimuli causing safety problems	Person reports inability to focus attention, failure to perceive objects and other stimuli (history of injuries, falls, and safety problems)
Memory (Long Term, Remote)		
Domain-independent declarative	*Left hemisphere:* disorientation to time, situation, place, name, person (verbal identification); impaired language memory (e.g., names of objects); impaired semantic memory *Right hemisphere:* disorientation to self, person (visual), place (visual); impaired episodic memory (personal history), impaired emotional memory *Either or both hemispheres:* confusion; behavioral change	Person reports disorientation, confusion, "not listening," "not remembering"; reports by others of person being disoriented, not able to remember, not able to learn new information
Domain-specific declarative	*Left hemisphere:* inability to retrieve personal history, past medical history; unaware of recent current events *Right hemisphere:* inability to recognize persons, places, objects, music, etc., from the past	Person reports remote memory problems; others report that person cannot recall formerly known information
Image processing (semantic processing)	Inability to categorize (identify similarities and differences), sort; inability to form concepts; inability to analyze relationships; misinterpretation; inability to interpret proverbs Inability to perform deductive reasoning (convergent reasoning); inability to perform inductive reasoning (divergent reasoning); inability to abstract; concrete reasoning demonstrated; delusions	Reports by others of frequent misinterpretation of data; failure to conceptualize or generalize information Reports by others of predominantly concrete thinking; lack of understanding of everyday situations, healthcare regimens, delusional thinking
Executive Attention Deficits		
Vigilance	Failure to search and scan environment	Person reports accidents, safety issues
Detection	Lack of initiative (anergy); lack of ambition; lack of motivation; flat affect; no awareness of feelings; appears depressed, apathetic, and emotionless; fails to appreciate deficit; disinterested in appearance; lacks concern about childish or crude behavior	Reports by others of laziness or apathy, flat affect or lack of emotional expression, failing to exhibit or be aware of feelings
Mild	Responds to immediate environment but no new ideas; grooming and social graces are lacking	Reports by others of lack of ambition, motivation, or initiative; failure to carry out adult tasks; lack of social graces and new ideas
Severe	Motionless, lack of responding to even internal cues; does not respond to physical needs; does not interact with surroundings Inability to use feedback regarding behavior; failure to recognize omissions and errors in self-care, speech, writing, and arithmetic; impaired cue utilization; overestimation of performance Failure to shift response set; failure to change behavior when conditions change; cue utilization may be impaired	Reports by others of failure to groom or toilet self, unawareness of surroundings and own physical needs Reports by others of not changing behavior when requested; unawareness of limitations; does not recognize and correct errors in dressing, grooming, toileting, eating; fails to recognize speech and arithmetic errors; careless speech Reports by others of failure to use feedback; inability to incorporate feedback (does not correct when feedback is given)
Working memory (recent memory, short-term memory)	Inability to set goals or form goals; indecisiveness Failure to make plans; inability to produce a complete line of reasoning; inability to make up a story; appears impulsive Failure to initiate behavior; failure to maintain behavior; failure to discontinue behavior; slowness to alternate response for the next step; motor perseveration	Reports by others of failure to set goals, indecisiveness Reports by others of failure to plan, impulsiveness, "does not think things through" Reports by others of not knowing where to begin, inability to carry out sequential acts (maintain a behavior), inability to cease a behavior

narcotic agents). Hospitalized older individuals are at greatest risk for delirium.[20]

◆**PATHOPHYSIOLOGY.** Acute confusional states arise from disruption of a widely distributed neural network involving the reticular activating system of the upper brainstem and its projections into the thalamus, basal ganglion, and specific association areas of the cortex and limbic areas (see Figs. 17.7, *B* and 17.10). Delirium is associated with autonomic nervous system hyperactivity and typically develops over 2 to 3 days. Hyperactive delirium (hyperactive confusional state) is associated with right-upper middle-temporal gyrus or left-temporal-occipital junction

TABLE 17.9 TYPES OF AGNOSIA (CONCEPT DISORDERS)

TYPE OF AGNOSIA	DEFINITION	LOCATION OF INJURY
Tactile agnosia (astereognosis)	Inability to recognize objects by touch	Parietal lobe
Spatial agnosia	Incapacity to find one's way around familiar places; disturbance of perception of space (disorders of [1] topographic [extrapersonal] orientation or [2] topographic and geographic memory [construction])	Parietal lobe
Gerstmann syndrome	Loss of spatial orientation of fingers, body, sides, and numbers	Left angular gyrus (parietal lobe)
Finger agnosia (digital agnosia)	Inability to identify the names of one's fingers	
Right-left confusion	Inability to distinguish right from left	
Agraphia	Inability to write	
Acalculia	Inability to perform mathematic calculations	
Visual agnosia		
Object agnosia	Inability to recognize objects and pictures	Temporo-occipital area
Prosopagnosia	Inability to recognize faces	Temporo-occipital lobe, ventromedial region
Color agnosia	Inability to understand colors as qualities of objects; faulty color concepts and inability to evoke color images in the absence of color blindness; specific types: (1) "hue" problem, (2) color anomia (cannot name color)	Inferior occipital cortex in left hemisphere
Body image agnosias (may be spatial)		
Anosognosia	Ignorance or denial of existence of the disease	Right parietal lobe
Autotopagnosia	Loss of ability to identify the body, in whole or in part, or to recognize relationships among various parts	Right parietal lobe
Word blindness (alexia/dyslexia)	Inability to recognize written symbols	Left parietotemporal region
Auditory agnosia (pure word deafness)	Inability to recognize speech sounds	Superior temporal area
Amusia (music deafness)	Loss of capacity to recognize tones and melodies	Right superior temporal area

disruption. Several neurotransmitters are involved, including decreased acetylcholine and/or melatonin; excess in dopamine, norepinephrine, and/or glutamate release; and variable alterations (e.g., either a decreased or increased activity, depending on delirium presentation and cause) in serotonin, histamine, and/or γ-aminobutyric acid.[21] Inflammatory cytokines, including C-reactive protein, interleukins, interferon, and tumor necrosis factor-alpha (TNF-α), may contribute to delirium by altering blood-brain barrier permeability causing oxidative stress, altering cerebral blood flow, and activating microglia, all affecting neurotransmission and subsequent neurobehavioral and cognitive symptoms.[22] Most metabolic disturbances (i.e., hypoglycemia, thyroid disorders, liver or kidney disease) that produce delirium interfere with neuronal metabolism or synaptic transmission. Many drugs and toxins also interfere with neurotransmission function at the synapse. Hypoactive delirium (hypoactive confusional state) is more likely to be associated with right-sided frontal-basal ganglion disruption.

◆**CLINICAL MANIFESTATIONS.** Delirium initially manifests as difficulty in concentrating and focusing attention, restlessness, irritability, insomnia, tremulousness, and poor appetite. Some persons experience seizures. Unpleasant, even terrifying dreams, hallucinations or delusions may occur. In a fully developed delirium state, the individual is completely inattentive and perceptions are grossly altered, with extensive misperception and misinterpretation. The person appears distressed and often perplexed; conversation is incoherent. Frank tremor and high levels of restless movement are common. Violent behavior may be present. The individual cannot sleep, is flushed, and has dilated pupils, a rapid pulse rate (tachycardia), elevated temperature, and profuse sweating (diaphoresis).

Excited delirium syndrome (ExDS), also known as *agitated delirium*, is a type of hyperkinetic delirium that can lead to sudden death. Its symptoms include altered mental status, combativeness, aggressiveness, tolerance to significant pain, rapid breathing, sweating, severe agitation, elevated temperature, noncompliance or poor awareness to direction

from police or medical personnel, inability to become fatigued, unusual or superhuman strength, and inappropriate clothing for the current environment. Hypoglycemia, thyroid storm, certain kinds of seizures, cocaine or methamphetamine intoxication, and/or catecholamine-induced fatal arrhythmias are associated with ExDS.[23]

Hypoactive delirium is associated with underactivity and may occur in individuals who have fevers or metabolic disorders (i.e., chronic liver or kidney failure) or who are under the influence of central nervous system depressants or are postoperative. The individual exhibits decreases in mental function, specifically alertness, attention span, accurate perception, interpretation of the environment, and reaction to the environment. Forgetfulness, confusion, and apathy are prominent, speech may be slow, and the individual dozes frequently. Hypoactive delirium can be mistaken for depression or dementia.[24]

Mixed delirium is a combination of both types of delirium fluctuating from one to the other. Delirium resolves suddenly or gradually in 2 to 3 days, although delirium states occasionally persist for weeks.

◆**EVALUATION AND TREATMENT.** An ACS is an acute medical problem. The initial goal is to establish that the individual is confused, and to identify the cause and contributing factors. Hypokinetic delirium will need to be differentiated from depression or an underlying dementia[25,26] (Table 17.12). A complete history and physical examination, as well as laboratory tests including an electrocardiogram and blood, urine, cerebral spinal fluid (CSF), and imaging studies are needed. Several assessment scales are available to guide evaluation.[27-29]

Once the cause is established, treatment is directed at controlling the primary disorder. Drugs that may be contributing to or causing the condition are discontinued unless the problem is the result of drug withdrawal. Both nonpharmacologic (i.e., orientation to surroundings, pain management, hydration, nutrition, early mobilization, sleep maintenance) and pharmacologic (i.e., antipsychotics) interventions may be implemented.[30,31] Delirium is preventable in some individuals with management of risk factors and early intervention.

TABLE 17.10 MAJOR TYPES OF APHASIA

TYPE	EXPRESSION	VERBAL COMPREHENSION	REPETITION	READING COMPREHENSION	WRITING	LOCATION OF LESION	CAUSE OF LESION
Expressive							
Broca, nonfluent or motor aphasia	Cannot find words, difficulty writing	Relatively intact	Impaired	Variable	Impaired	Left posteroinferior frontal lobe (Broca area)	Occlusion of one or several branches of left middle cerebral artery supplying inferior frontal gyrus
Transcortical motor, nonfluent aphasia	Halting speech	Intact	Intact	Impaired	Impaired	Anterior superior frontal lobe	Occlusion at the border zone between two arterial territories
Receptive							
Wernicke, receptive fluent or sensory aphasia	Meaningless verbal language, inappropriate words or unable to monitor language for correctness so errors are not recognized. Intonation, accent, cadence, rhythm, and articulation normal	Impaired; disturbance in understanding all language	Impaired	Impaired	Impaired	Left posterosuperior temporal lobe (Wernicke area)	Occlusion of inferior division of left middle cerebral artery
Conductive aphasia	Difficulty repeating words, phrases spoken to them; naming is impaired	Intact	Severely impaired	Variable	Variable	Inferior and posterior temporal lobe; parietotemporal junction	Occlusion in distributions of left middle cerebral artery
Anomic aphasia	Hesitancy, difficulty recalling names, objects, or numbers	Intact	Impaired	Variable	Intact except for anomia	Left temporoparietal zones; arcuate fasciculus	Diffuse left hemisphere brain disease
Transcortical sensory, fluent aphasia	Repeats words and phrases spoken to them	Poor	Intact	Impaired	Impaired	Posterior temporal lobe	Occlusion at the border zone between two cerebral arterial territories
Other							
Transcortical mixed motor and sensory, nonfluent	Repeats words and phrases spoken to them	Impaired	Intact	Impaired	Impaired	Left cerebral hemisphere; spares the perisylvian cortex	Occlusion at the border zone between two cerebral arterial territories
Global or nonfluent; summation of motor and sensory aphasia	Mute	Impaired	Impaired	Impaired	Impaired	Large areas of the left cortex and subcortical regions	Occlusion of left middle cerebral artery of left internal carotid artery, tumors, other mass lesions, hemorrhage, embolic occlusion of ascending parietal or posterior temporal branch of middle cerebral artery

TABLE 17.11   EXAMPLES OF APHASIA

DISORDER	EXAMPLE
Wernicke/Fluent/Sensory Aphasia	
Verbal paraphasia	*Question:* What did the car do? *Patient:* The car would spit sweetly down the road. (The car sped swiftly down the road.)
Literal paraphasia	*Request:* Say "persistence is essential to success." *Patient:* Mesastence is instans to success.
Neologism	*Question:* What do you call this? (Pointing to a plant.) *Patient:* It's a logper.
Anomic aphasia (circumlocution example)	*Question:* What do you call this? (Pointing to a plant.) *Patient:* Something that grows. *Patient:* It's … Or *Question:* What did you do this morning? *Patient:* Reading. *Question:* Were you reading a book or newspaper? *Patient:* One of those.
Broca or Motor Aphasia	
Telegraphic style	*Question:* Where is your daughter? *Patient:* New Orleans … home … Monday.

From Boss BJ: *J Neurosurg Nurs* 16(3):151-160, 1984.

TABLE 17.12   COMPARISON OF DELIRIUM AND DEMENTIA

FEATURE	DELIRIUM	DEMENTIA
Age	Usually older	Usually older
Onset	Acute—common during hospitalization	Usually insidious; acute in some cases of strokes/trauma
Associated conditions	Urinary tract infection, thyroid disorders, hypoxia, hypoglycemia, toxicity, fluid-electrolyte imbalance, renal insufficiency, trauma, multiple medications	May have no other conditions Brain trauma
Course	Fluctuating; remits with treatment	Chronic slow decline, usually starts with memory loss
Duration	Hours to weeks	Months to years
Attention	Impaired	Intact early; often impaired late
Sleep-wake cycle	Disrupted	Usually normal or fragmented
Alertness	Impaired	Normal
Orientation	Impaired	Intact early; impaired late
Behavior	Agitated, withdrawn/depressed	Intact early
Speech	Incoherent, rapid/slowed	Word-finding problems
Thoughts	Disorganized, delusions	Impoverished
Perceptions	Hallucinations/illusions	Usually intact early

Adapted from Caplan JP, Rabinowitz T: *Med Clin North Am* 94(6): 1103-1116, ix, 2010.

Dementia

Dementia is an acquired deterioration and a progressive failure of many cerebral functions that includes impairment of intellectual processes with a decrease in orienting, memory, language, judgment, and decision making. Because of declining intellectual ability, the individual may exhibit alterations in behavior, for example, agitation, wandering, and aggression.

Dementias can be classified according to etiologic factors (e.g., trauma, tumors, vascular disorders, infections) and to associated clinical and laboratory signs. Dementing processes also have been grouped as cortical, subcortical, or both. Box 17.3 lists the potentially reversible and irreversible causes of dementia. Alzheimer disease (AD) is the most common cause followed by vascular dementia, then dementia associated with Lewy bodies (i.e., Parkinson disease [see section on Parkinson Disease]), and frontotemporal dementia.[32,33] In people younger than 60 years, frontotemporal dementia (FTD) rivals AD in terms of frequency.[34]

◆**PATHOPHYSIOLOGY.** Mechanisms leading to dementia include neuron degeneration, compression of brain tissue, atherosclerosis of cerebral vessels, and brain trauma. Genetic predisposition (Table 17.13) is associated with the neurodegenerative diseases, including Alzheimer, Huntington (see section on Huntington Disease), and Parkinson diseases (see section on Parkinson Disease). CNS infections, including the human immunodeficiency virus (HIV) and prions in Creutzfeldt-Jakob disease (Table 17.13 and Box 17.4), also lead to nerve cell degeneration and brain atrophy.

◆**CLINICAL MANIFESTATIONS.** Clinical manifestations of the major dementias are presented in Table 17.14.

◆**EVALUATION AND TREATMENT.** Establishing the cause for a dementia may be complicated, but individuals with clinical manifestations of dementia should be evaluated with laboratory and neuropsychologic testing to identify underlying conditions that may be treatable. Unfortunately, no specific cure exists for most progressive dementias. Therapy is directed at maintaining and maximizing use of the remaining capacities, restoring functions if possible, and accommodating to lost abilities. Helping the family to understand the process and to learn ways to assist the individual is essential.

Alzheimer Disease. Alzheimer disease (dementia of Alzheimer type [DAT], senile disease complex) is the leading cause of severe cognitive dysfunction in older adults. The three forms of AD are nonhereditary sporadic or late-onset AD (70% to 90%), early-onset familial AD (FAD), and early-onset AD (very rare). An estimated 5.3 million Americans have AD, and two-thirds of these individuals are women.[35] The greatest risk factors are age and family history. Other proposed risk factors include diabetes, midlife hypertension, hyperlipidemia, midlife obesity, smoking, depression, cognitive inactivity or low educational attainment, female gender, estrogen deficit at the time of menopause, physical inactivity, head trauma, elevated serum homocysteine and cholesterol levels, oxidative stress, and neuroinflammation (Fig. 17.12). Proposed protective factors include lifelong activity, the presence of *apoE2* and antioxidant substances, omega-3 fatty acids, estrogen replacement at the time of surgical menopause, low-calorie diet, and use of nonsteroidal anti-inflammatory agents.[36-39] Statins are being investigated for their role in preventing AD; recent reviews do not support their use.[40]

BOX 17.3   CAUSES OF DEMENTIA

Potentially Reversible Causes of Dementia

Infection
Encephalitis
Meningitis
Neurosyphilis

Normal Pressure Hydrocephalus

Chronic Subdural Hematoma

Nutritional Deficiencies
Vitamin B₁ (thiamine) deficiency
Vitamin B₁₂ (cobalamin) deficiency
Nicotinic acid deficiency (pellagra)

Chronic Drug Intoxication
Alcohol*
Sedatives

Metabolic Disorders
Thyroid abnormalities
Chronic hepatic encephalopathy
Cerebral vasculitis
Sarcoidosis

Some Types of Tumors
Frontal and temporal lobe
Pseudodementia of depression

Medical Side Effects
Anticholinergics
Antihypertensives
Antihistamines

Irreversible Causes of Dementia

Neurodegenerative Disorders
Alzheimer disease*
Dementia with Lewy bodies
Frontotemporal dementia
Pick disease
Huntington disease
Parkinson disease

Vascular Disease
Vascular dementia*
Multi-infarct
Strategic single infarct
Binswanger disease* (diffuse white matter disease)
Amyloid angiopathy

Infection
Creutzfeldt-Jakob disease (CJD)
Postencephalitic dementia
Dementia associated with HIV

*Most common.

BOX 17.4   CREUTZFELDT-JAKOB DISEASE

Creutzfeldt-Jakob disease is a progressive, fatal, dementing neurologic illness caused by an infectious protein known as a *prion*. Prions are composed of misfolded prion proteins and are able to self-replicate and cause spongiform encephalopathy (numerous small vacuoles within the grey matter). The incidence is about 1 in 1.5 million population per year, and 10% of cases are genetic. Most cases are sporadic. Diagnosis is made by clinical evaluation, magnetic resonance imaging, and electroencephalography. Spinal fluid analysis shows the presence of 14-3-3 protein or human prion protein (PrP^{Sc}), and it also may be detected in olfactory epithelium, blood, and/or urine samples. There is progressive dementia and at least two of the four following features: myoclonus, visual or cerebellar disturbance, pyramidal or extrapyramidal signs, and akinetic mutism. The disease is fatal in an average of 8 months, and there is no treatment. Tissue from persons with prion disease must not be transplanted. Animal forms of prion disease include scrapie in sheep; chronic wasting disease in deer, elk, and moose; and bovine spongiform encephalopathy (BSE) in cows. BSE can be transmitted to humans by consumption of infected meat and is known as *new variant Creutzfeldt-Jakob disease.*

Data from Iwasaki Y: Creutzfeldt-Jakob disease, *Neuropathology* 37(2):174-188, 2017; Kim MO, Geschwind MD: *Curr Opin Neurol* 28(3):302-310, 2015; Lee J et al: *J Med Virol* 87(1):175-186, 2015.

◆PATHOPHYSIOLOGY. The exact cause of AD is unknown. Early-onset FAD is autosomal dominant and has been linked to three genes with mutations on chromosome 21 (abnormal amyloid precursor protein 14 [APP14], abnormal presenilin 1 [PSEN1], and abnormal presenilin 2 [PSEN2]). The major genetic risk for late-onset AD is related to apolipoprotein E gene-allele 4 (apoE4) on chromosome 19, which interferes with amyloid beta clearance from the brain and also is processed into neurotoxic fragments found in the plaques and tangles in the brain of people with AD.[41] Studies are ongoing to classify the genetic variations of AD; genome-wide association studies have identified numerous single nucleotide variations for late-onset Alzheimer disease.[42] Epigenetic mechanisms are associated with the pathology of Alzheimer disease, but the mechanisms are yet to be determined.[43]

Sporadic late-onset AD is the most common and does not have a specific genetic association; however, the cellular pathology is the same as that for gene-associated early- and late-onset AD.[44] Pathologic alterations in the brain include accumulation of extracellular neuritic plaques containing a core of abnormally folded amyloid beta and tau proteins, intraneuronal neurofibrillary tangles, and degeneration of basal forebrain cholinergic neurons with loss of acetylcholine. Failure to process and clear amyloid precursor protein results in the accumulation of toxic fragments of amyloid beta protein that leads to formation of diffuse neuritic plaques, disruption of nerve impulse transmission, and death of neurons. Aging and injury may result in changes that contribute to the development and progression of this disease. Misfolded and aggregated proteins trigger immune responses with activation of glial cells and release of cytokines leading to neuroinflammation and oxidative stress; decreased oxygen and glucose transport; molecular changes in vascular smooth muscle and in the blood-brain barrier; and mitochondrial defects that alter cell metabolism and processing of proteins, including amyloid (apolipoprotein-4) (apoE4), that lead to cell death.[45-48]

Amyloid also is deposited in the smooth muscle of cerebral arteries, causing an amyloid angiopathy and disturbance in blood flow[49] (Fig. 17.13). The tau protein, a microtubule-binding protein, in neurons detaches and forms an insoluble filament called a **neurofibrillary tangle**, contributing to neuronal death. Tangles are flame-shaped (Fig. 17.14). Neuritic plaques and neurofibrillary tangles are more concentrated in the cerebral cortex and hippocampus (important for memory). The loss of neurons results in brain atrophy with decreases in weight and volume. The sulci widen and the gyri thin, especially in the frontal and temporal lobes, and the ventricles enlarge to fill the space (Fig. 17.15). Loss of synapses, acetylcholine, and other neurotransmitters contributes to the decline of memory and attention and the loss of other cognitive functions associated with AD.

◆CLINICAL MANIFESTATIONS. AD has a long preclinical and prodromal course, and pathophysiologic changes can occur decades before the appearance of the clinical dementia syndrome. The disease progresses from mild short-term memory deficits to total loss of cognition and executive functions. Initial clinical manifestations are insidious and often attributed to forgetfulness, emotional causes, or other illness. The individual becomes progressively more forgetful over time, particularly in relation to recent events. Memory loss increases as the disorder advances, and the person becomes disoriented, confused, and loses the ability to concentrate. Abstraction, problem solving, and judgment gradually deteriorate with failure in mathematic calculation ability, language, and visuospatial orientation. Dyspraxia may appear. The mental status changes induce behavioral changes, including irritability, agitation, and restlessness. Mood changes also result from the deterioration in cognition. The person may become anxious, depressed, hostile, emotionally labile, and prone to mood swings. Motor changes may occur if the posterior frontal lobes are involved, causing rigidity and

TABLE 17.13   THE MOLECULAR BASIS FOR DEGENERATIVE DEMENTIA

DEMENTIA	MOLECULAR MECHANISM	CAUSAL GENES (CHROMOSOME)	SUSCEPTIBILITY GENES (CHROMOSOME)	PATHOLOGY
Alzheimer disease (familial)	Amyloid beta protein	Early onset: autosomal dominant: <2% carry these mutations APP (21), PSEN1 (14), PSEN2 (1) (most mutations are in PSEN1)	Late onset: risk gene apoE4 (19) CUGBP2 (10p)	Amyloid plaques, neurofibrillary tangles; neuronal and synaptic loss in the brain
Creutzfeldt-Jakob disease (hereditary form)	PrPSC proteins type 1 and 2	Prion (20) (up to 15% of cases carry these dominant mutations)	PRNP codon 129 homozygosity for methionine or valine	Tau inclusions, spongiform changes, gliosis
Dementia with Lewy bodies	Alpha-synuclein	Very rare alpha-synuclein (4) (dominant)	Unknown	Alpha-synuclein inclusions (Lewy bodies)
Behavioral variant frontotemporal dementia	Microtubule-associated protein tau (MAPT) Progranulin (PGRN)	Tau exon and intron mutation (17) (about 10% of familial cases) PGRN (17) (10% of familial cases)	Tau haplotypes (H1 and H2)	Tau inclusions, Pick bodies, neurofibrillary tangles
Huntington disease (autosomal dominant)	Huntingtin protein (polyglutamine)	Autosomal dominant: HD-IT15 (4) (trinucleotide repeat expansion)	None known	Neuronal degeneration, astrogliosis
Parkinson disease Dementia	Autosomal dominant: Alpha-synuclein Leucine-rich repeat kinase 2 Autosomal recessive: Parkin (juvenile onset) DJ-1 protein PTEN-induced putative kinase 1	Autosomal dominant: SNCA-PARK1 (4) LRRK2-PARK8 (12) Autosomal recessive: PARK2 (4) oncogene DJ-1 (PARK7) PINK1 (PARK6)	GBA (glucosidase beta acid) SNCAIP (alpha-synuclein interacting protein) NR4A2 (orphan nuclear receptor) UCH-L1 (PARK5) ubiquitin C-terminal hydrolase Other low-risk genes	Neuronal degeneration, alpha-synuclein inclusions (Lewy bodies), gliosis; neuronal degeneration

APP, Amyloid precursor protein; PRNP, prion protein; PrPSC, prion protein scrapie form; PSEN, presenilin; PTEN, phosphatase and tensin homolog.

TABLE 17.14   CLINICAL DIFFERENTIATION OF THE MAJOR DEGENERATIVE DEMENTIAS

DISEASE	MENTAL STATUS	NEUROBEHAVIOR	NEUROLOGIC EXAMINATION
Alzheimer disease	Memory loss, disorientation to place and time, loss of facial recognition	Initially normal; progressive cognitive, language, abstraction, and judgment impairment	Initially normal
Creutzfeldt-Jakob disease	Variable, frontal/executive, focal cortical, memory	Depression, anxiety, decreased cognitive function, and memory loss	Myoclonus, rigidity, parkinsonism
Dementia with Lewy body (Lewy body dementia)	Initially affects concentration and attention, then memory or cognition loss but unpredictable levels of ability, attention, or alertness; delirium prone	Visual hallucinations, depression, sleep disorder, delusions, transient loss of consciousness	Parkinsonism Changes in walking or movement may present first
Frontotemporal disorders/ degeneration/ dementia	PPA variant Language loss with talking less and speech becoming hesitant, or loss of understanding of language, which may precede memory loss; spares drawing	Behavioral variant FTD Loss of empathy (emotional blunting), apathy, increased inappropriate or decline in personal or social conduct, loss of judgment and reasoning, hyperorality, euphoria, depression	Caused by CBD and PSP variants
Huntington disease		Apathy, loss of interest early; impaired cognition, judgment, and memory occur later	Chorea, bradykinesia, dystonia
Vascular dementia	Frontal/executive, cognitive slowing; memory can be intact	Often but not always sudden, usually within 3 months of a stroke; variable; apathy, falls, focal weakness, delusions, anxiety	Usually motor slowing, spasticity; can be normal or may have symptom improvement with stroke recovery

FTD, frontotemporal dementia; CBD, corticobasal degeneration; PPA, primary progressive aphasia; PSP, progressive supranuclear palsy.
Data from Bott NT et al: Neurodegener Dis Manag 4(6):439-454, 2014; Darrow MD: Prim Care 42(2):195-204, 2015; Hugo J, Ganguli M: Clin Geriatr Med 30(3):421-442, 2014; Nordberg A: Nat Rev Neurol 11(2):69-70, 2015.

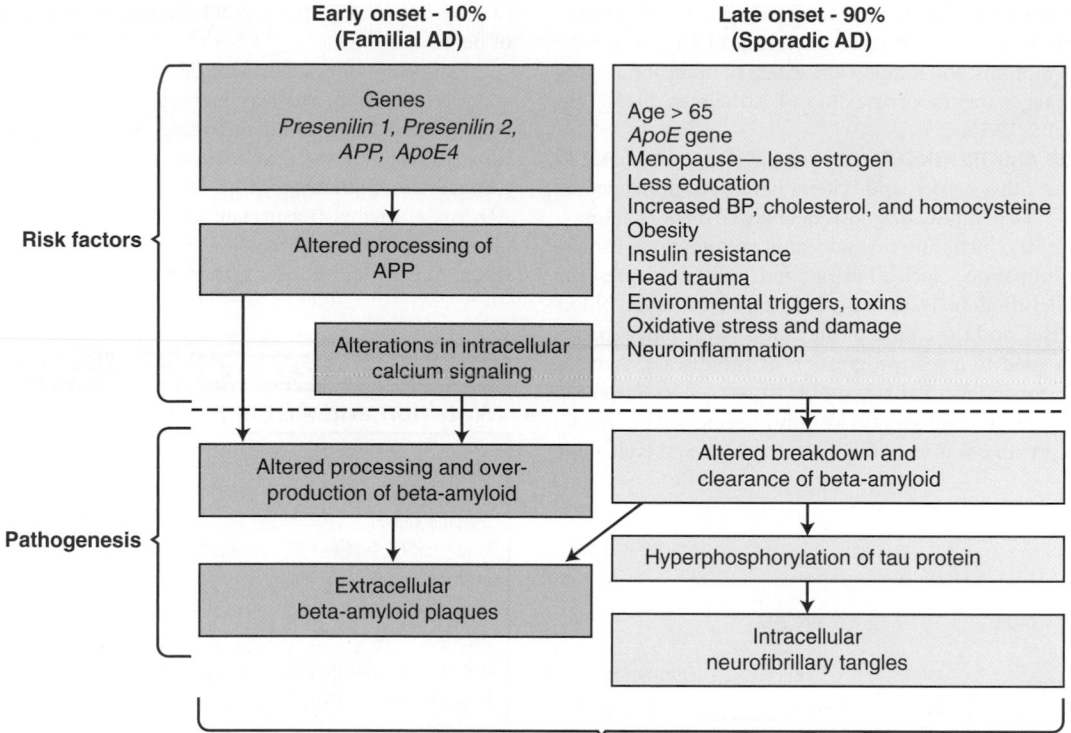

FIGURE 17.12 Proposed Risk Factors and Pathogenesis of Alzheimer Disease (AD). *ApoE,* Apolipoprotein E; *APP,* amyloid precursor protein; *BP,* blood pressure. (Data from Barnes DE, Yaffe K: *Lancet Neurol* 10[9]:819-828, 2011; de la Monte SM: *Drugs* 72[1]:49-66, 2012; Daviglus ML et al: *Arch Neurol* 68[9]:1185-1190, 2011; Hasan MK, Mooney RP: *W V Med J* 107[3]:26-29, 2011.)

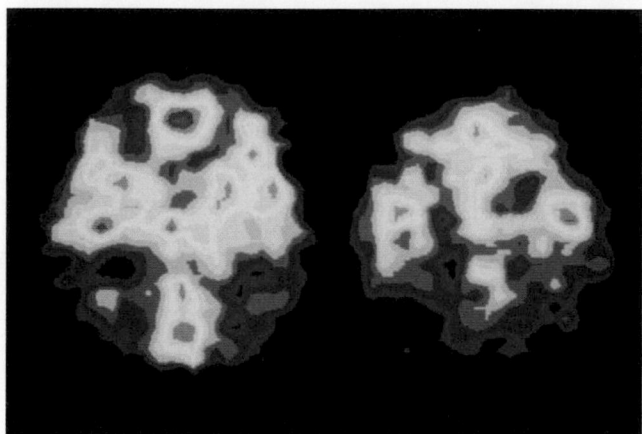

FIGURE 17.13 Altered Cerebral Blood Flow in Alzheimer Disease. Single photon emission computerized tomography scan showing reduction of temporoparietal blood flow *(right)* compared with normal blood flow *(left).* (From Perkin GD et al: *Atlas of clinical neurology,* ed 3, Philadelphia, 2011, Saunders.)

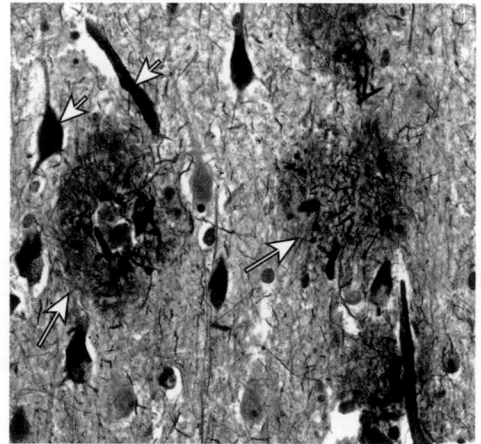

FIGURE 17.14 Major Histopathologic Changes in Alzheimer Disease. Beta-amyloid protein deposits (plaques) in the neutrophil *(long arrows)* and neurofibrillary tangles *(short arrows).* (From Kumar V, Abbas AK, Aster J: *Robbins basic pathology,* ed 9, Philadelphia, 2013, Saunders.)

flexion posturing. Weight loss can be significant (see *Nutrition & Disease*: Diet and Alzheimer Disease). Great variability in age of onset, intensity and sequence of symptoms, and location and extent of brain abnormalities is common. Stages for the progression of Alzheimer disease are summarized in Table 17.15.

◆**EVALUATION AND TREATMENT.** The clinical diagnosis of AD is made by ruling out other causes, and criteria have been developed to assist diagnosis.[50-52] The definitive diagnosis can only be made at autopsy.

The clinical history, including mental status examinations (mini–mental status examination, clock drawing, and geriatric depression scale), cerebrospinal fluid analysis, brain imaging of structure, blood flow and metabolism, and the course of the illness (which may span 5 years or more) is used to assess progression of the disease. Genetic susceptibility tests for *PSEN1*, *PSEN2*, and *APP* are used to screen for early-onset AD.[53] Efforts are underway to identify imaging and biochemical markers to assist with risk assessment, early diagnosis, and evaluation of progression of Alzheimer-type and other neurodegenerative causes of dementia.[54,55]

Treatment is directed at using devices to compensate for the impaired cognitive function, such as memory aids; maintaining unimpaired cognitive functions; and maintaining or improving the general state of hygiene, nutrition, and health. There are no disease-modifying therapies. Cholinesterase inhibitors (ChE-Is) are used in mild cases to moderate AD. An *N*-methyl-D-aspartate (NMDA) receptor antagonist blocks glutamate activity and may slow progression of disease in moderate to severe AD.[56,57] Anti-amyloid drugs are in clinical trials.

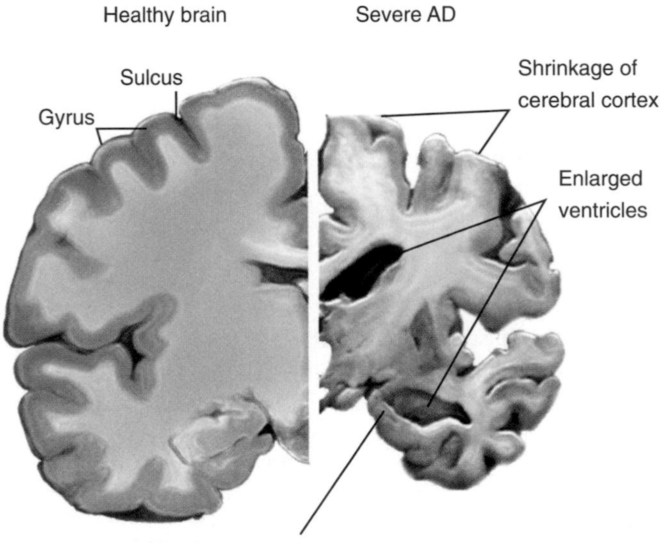

FIGURE 17.15 Comparison of Normal and Alzheimer Brain. The brain decreases in volume and weight, the sulci widen, and the gyri thin, especially in the temporal and frontal lobes. The ventricles enlarge to fill the space. (From National Institute on Aging Scientific Images, *Brain images.* Available at https://www.nia.nih.gov/alzheimers/scientific-images.)

NUTRITION & DISEASE
Nutrition and Alzheimer Disease (AD)

Research is in progress to evaluate the effects of nutrition on delaying the onset and preventing the progression of AD. Nutrition has a role in arresting the pathogenesis of dementia, particularly processes related to oxidative stress, inflammation, and vascular disease. Dietary patterns that include a diet high in fruits, vegetables, other plant-derived products, fish and lower intakes of meat, saturated fats, and added refined sugar have been associated with reduced cognitive decline. Diets and supplements that include docosahexaenoic acid (DHA-an omega-3 fatty acid), the vitamin B family, antioxidant vitamins E and C, and vitamin D have shown some evidence in sustaining healthy neurons. Adherence to a Mediterranean diet also has shown reduced risk for AD. Weight loss is a major concern for older adults with AD and it may precede onset of the classic motor symptoms. Weight loss may be a result of (1) increased incidence of infection, (2) increased energy output because of constant pacing, (3) olfactory and taste changes making food less appealing, (4) inadequate food intake, (5) decreased independence and difficulty in self-feeding, and (6) loss of neural regulation of appetite. Dementia may lead to memory loss, social isolation, depression, and poor food intake with resultant weight loss. Individuals may forget or refuse to eat, fail to communicate the need to eat, throw away or hide food, eat spoiled food or nonfood substances, eat favorite foods to the exclusion of other foods, take a long time to eat, have difficulty in preparing foods, and be unable to feed themselves. Reduced lean body mass has been associated with brain atrophy and declining cognitive performance. Nutritional intervention is an important component of care for individuals with Alzheimer disease.

Data from Barnard ND et al: *Neurobiol Aging* 35(Suppl 2):S74-S78, 2014; Droogsman E, van Asselt D, De Deyn PP: *Z Gerontol Geriatr* 48(4):318-324, 2015; Mohajeri MH, Troesch B, Weber P: *Nutrition* 31(2):261-275, 2015; Singh B et al: *J Alzheimers Dis* 39(2):271-282, 2014; Swaminathan A, Jicha GA: *Front Aging Neurosci* 6:282, 2014; eCollection 2014; van de Rest O et al: *Adv Nutr* 6(2):154-168, 2015.

TABLE 17.15 PROGRESSION OF ALZHEIMER DISEASE

STAGE	MILD COGNITIVE IMPAIRMENT	EARLY STAGE	MIDDLE STAGE	LATE STAGE	END STAGE
Cognitive	Mild memory loss, particularly for recent event (episodic memory) and new information (semantic memory)	Measurable short-term memory loss; difficulty planning; disorientation to location	Significant forgetfulness; easy to get lost; may dress inappropriately; may have hallucinations	Little cognitive ability; language not clear; personality change; does not recognize family members; wandering; repetitive behavior	No significant cognitive function; loss of word speech
Functional	Possibly depression (vs. apathy); mild anxiety	Mild IADL problems	IADL-dependent; some ADL problems	ADL-dependent; incontinent; difficulty eating	Nonambulatory/bedbound; unable to eat

ADL, Activities of daily living; *IADL*, instrumental activities of daily living.
Adapted from National Conference of Gerontological Nurse Practitioners and the National Gerontological Nursing Association, *Counseling Points* 1(1):6, 2008.

Vascular Dementia. Vascular dementia is a progressive disease caused by reduced brain blood flow and accounts for 10% to 15% of cases. The pathology can be variable, including multiple infarcts and hemorrhages that occur in different parts of the brain, and can be related to stroke and small vessel disease. The disease can be difficult to clinically differentiate from AD, and the symptoms can be much more variable. The diseases often coexist. Loss of executive functions, attention deficit, and loss of information processing often occur first. Brain imaging provides the most definitive diagnosis. There is no specific treatment.[32,58]

Frontotemporal Dementia. Frontotemporal dementia (FTD), previously known as *Pick disease,* is a form of dementia and a degenerative disease of the frontal lobes. There is a familial association with an age of onset less than 60 years and an estimated incidence of 15 per 100,000. The majority of cases involve mutations of genes encoding tau protein or progranulin. Three distinct clinical syndromes have been described depending on the site of atrophy: behavioral variant of frontotemporal dementia, progressive nonfluent aphasia, and semantic dementia. Neuroimaging identifies atrophy of the frontal and temporal lobes. The specific mechanism of pathogenesis is unknown, and there is no specific treatment.[59,60]

Seizure Disorders

Seizure disorders represent a manifestation of disease and not a specific disease entity. A seizure is a sudden, transient disruption in brain electrical function caused by abnormal excessive discharges of cortical neurons.[61] Epilepsy is "a disease of the brain with: (1) at least two unprovoked (or reflex) seizures occurring more than 24 hours apart; (2) one unprovoked (or reflex) seizure and a probability of further seizures similar to the general recurrence risk (at least 60%) after two unprovoked seizures, occurring over the next 10 years; (3) diagnosis of an epilepsy syndrome."[62] The term convulsion is sometimes applied to seizures and refers to the tonic-clonic (jerky, contract-relax) movement associated with some seizures. Epilepsy was estimated to have affected about 4.3 million adults and 750,000 children in the United States in 2013.[63] Seizures in children are presented in Chapter 20.

Conditions Associated with Seizure Disorders

Any disorder that alters the neuronal environment may cause seizure activity. Conditions that may produce a seizure are metabolic disorders, congenital malformations, genetic predisposition, perinatal injury, postnatal trauma, myoclonic syndromes, infection, brain tumor, vascular disease, and drug or alcohol abuse. The onset of seizures also may indicate the presence of an ongoing primary neurologic disease. Metabolic and structural causes of recurrent seizures in adults are summarized in Table 17.16. The cause of seizures is often unknown.

The threshold for seizures may be lowered by hypoglycemia; fatigue or lack of sleep; emotional or physical stress; fever; large amounts of water ingestion (hyponatremia); constipation; use of antipsychotic drugs (i.e., chlorpromazine and clozapine), especially when combined with alcohol; or hyperventilation (respiratory alkalosis). Some environmental stimuli, such as blinking lights, a poorly adjusted television screen, loud noises, certain music, certain odors, or merely being startled, have been known to initiate a seizure. Women may have increased seizure activity immediately before or during menses.[64,65]

Types of Seizure

Seizures are classified in different ways: clinical manifestations, site of origin and pattern of spread, EEG correlates, or response to therapy. Types of seizures and clinical manifestation are presented in Table 17.17.

◆**PATHOPHYSIOLOGY.** Epilepsy is considered to be the result of the interaction of complex genetic mutations with environmental effects

TABLE 17.16	STRUCTURAL/METABOLIC CAUSES OF RECURRENT SEIZURES IN ADULTS
AGE AT ONSET	**PROBABLE CAUSE**
Young adults (18-35 yr)	Alcohol or drug withdrawal (e.g., barbiturates, benzodiazepines)
	Brain tumor
	Idiopathic
	Illicit drug use (e.g., cocaine, amphetamines)
	Posttraumatic brain injury
	Perinatal insults
Older adults (>35 yr)	Alcohol or drug withdrawal (e.g., barbiturates, benzodiazepines)
	Brain tumor
	Cerebrovascular disease (e.g., stroke, aneurysm, arteriovenous malformations)
	CNS degenerative diseases (e.g., Alzheimer disease, multiple sclerosis)
	Major depression
	Idiopathic
	Metabolic disorders (e.g., uremia, hepatic failure, electrolyte abnormalities, hypoglycemia)
	Posttraumatic brain injury

CNS, Central nervous system.
Data from Daroff RB et al: *Bradley's neurology in clinical practice,* ed 7, Philadelphia, 2016, Elsevier.

that cause abnormalities in synaptic transmission, an imbalance in the brain's neurotransmitters, or the development of abnormal nerve connections or loss of nerves after injury.[66,67] The International League Against Epilepsy has proposed six groups for categorizing causes of epilepsy: genetic, structural, metabolic, immune, infectious, and unknown. These categories may be interrelated and continue to be revised[68] (Fig. 17.16).

A group of neurons may exhibit a paroxysmal depolarization shift and function as an epileptogenic focus. These neurons are hyperexcitable and are more easily activated by hyperthermia, hypoxia, hypoglycemia, hyponatremia, repeated sensory stimulation, and certain sleep phases. Epileptogenic neurons fire more frequently and with greater amplitude. When the intensity reaches a threshold point, cortical excitation spreads. Excitation of the subcortical, thalamic, and brainstem areas corresponds to the tonic phase (muscle contraction with increased muscle tone) and is associated with loss of consciousness. The clonic phase (alternating contraction and relaxation of muscles) begins when inhibitory neurons in the cortex, anterior thalamus, and basal ganglia react to the cortical excitation. The seizure discharge is interrupted, producing intermittent muscle contractions that gradually decrease and finally cease. The epileptogenic neurons are exhausted.

During seizure activity, oxygen is consumed at a high rate—about 60% greater than normal. Although cerebral blood flow also increases, oxygen is rapidly depleted along with glucose, and lactate accumulates in brain tissue. Continued, severe seizure activity has the potential for progressive brain injury and irreversible damage. In addition, if a seizure focus in the brain is active for a prolonged period, a mirror focus may develop in contralateral normal tissue and cause seizure activity, particularly with focal (i.e., temporal or frontal lobe) epilepsy.[69]

The person is still in a postictal state (a state that follows an epileptic seizure and returns to baseline) when the next seizure begins. Status epilepticus most often results from abrupt discontinuation of antiseizure medications but also may occur in untreated or inadequately treated

TABLE 17.17 TYPES OF SEIZURES AND DESCRIPTION OF SEIZURE EVENT

TYPE	DESCRIPTION OF SEIZURE EVENT
Focal seizures (previously partial seizures)	Seizures originating in one area of the brain; an aura is common *Motor* Tonic: stiffening of body muscles with falling; loss of consciousness; can occur in sleep; more common in infants and children Atonic: sudden, brief loss of muscle tone with falling (drop attacks); usually no loss of consciousness Myoclonic: sudden brief shocklike jerks or twitches of the arms and/or legs; may drop things; no impairment of consciousness; frequently occurs shortly after awakening Tonic-clonic: Abrupt loss of consciousness, body stiffening (tonic) and then shaking (clonic); may begin with sudden cry, sometimes loss of bladder control or biting of tongue; usually lasts about two minutes, followed by a period of confusion, agitation, and fatigue; headaches and soreness are common afterwards Hypermotor: bimanual or bipedal motor activity such as kicking and thrashing, clapping and rubbing of both hands, hugging, sometimes with sexual automatisms and autonomic changes with or without preserved awareness *Nonmotor* Sensory: numbness, tingling or burning sensation, flashing lights, auditory experiences Cognitive: aphasia, hallucination, memory or attention impairment Emotional or affective: fear, agitation, anger, crying, laughing, paranoia Autonomic: blushing, pallor, increased or decreased heart rate, hyper- or hypoventilation nausea
Without loss of awareness	Recall, responsiveness, and consciousness are intact
Impaired awareness (also known as *complex focal seizure*)	Loss of consciousness or awareness; vague or dreamlike state
Awareness unknown	Unable to determine awareness
Focal to bilateral tonic-clonic seizure	Begins in one part of brain (focal seizure) and spreads to both sides of brain followed by generalized tonic-clonic seizure; loss of consciousness
Generalized seizures	Seizures originating in both sides of the brain simultaneously; can include tonic, atonic, clonic, myoclonic, myoclonic-atonic, clonic-tonic-clonic activity (see above descriptions)
Epileptic spasms (formerly known as *infantile spasms*)	Episodes of sudden flexion or extension involving neck, trunk, and extremities; clinical manifestations range from subtle head nods to violent body contractions (jackknife seizures); onset between 3 and 12 months of age; may occur after infancy, may be idiopathic, genetic, result of metabolic disease, or in response to CNS insult; spasms occur in clusters of 5 to 150 times per day; EEG shows large-amplitude, chaotic, and disorganized pattern called "hypsarrhythmia"
Epilepsy syndromes (examples)	Seizure disorder that displays a group of signs and symptoms that occur collectively and characterize or indicate a particular condition; usually associated with genetic or developmental cause
Neonatal seizures	Wide variety of abnormal clinical activity, including rhythmic eye movements, chewing, and swimming movements; common in neonatal seizures; there are five main types of neonatal seizures: (1) subtle seizures (50%), (2) tonic seizures (5%), (3) clonic seizures (25%), (4) myoclonic seizures (20%), (5) nonparoxysmal repetitive behaviors
Lennox-Gastaut syndrome	Epileptic syndrome with onset in early childhood, 1 to 5 years of age; includes various generalized seizures (tonic-clonic, atonic [drop attacks], akinetic, absence, and myoclonic); EEG has characteristic "slow spike and wave" pattern; results in intellectual disability and delayed psychomotor developments
Juvenile myoclonic epilepsy	Generalized epilepsy syndrome with onset in adolescence; multifocal myoclonus; seizures often occur early in morning, aggravated by lack of sleep or after excessive alcohol intake; occasional generalized convulsions; requires long-term medication treatment
Unclassified epileptic seizures	Etiology remains unknown; seizures do not have distinct clinical and EEG features
Simple febrile seizures	Common in children younger than 5 to 6 years of age; brief (less than a few minutes) generalized convulsions associated with high fever; important to exclude meningitis as cause of seizures; usually do not develop epilepsy
Pseudoseizures	Nonepileptic phenomena that look like epileptic seizures; diagnosis often requires video-EEG monitoring to capture spells, and determine that EEG is normal during clinical events; frequently occurs in setting of child abuse
Status Epilepticus	Continuing or recurring seizure activity in which recovery from seizure activity is incomplete; unrelenting seizure activity can last 30 min or more; other forms can evolve into status epilepticus; medical emergency that requires immediate intervention

CNS, Central nervous system; *EEG,* electroencephalogram.

Data from: Fisher RS, et al: Operational classification of seizure types by the International League Against Epilepsy, 2016, available at: http://www.ilae.org/Visitors/Centre/documents/ClassificationSeizureILAE-2016.pdf, accessed June 2, 2017; Scheffer IE, et al: *Epilepsia Open* 1(1-2):37-44, 2016.

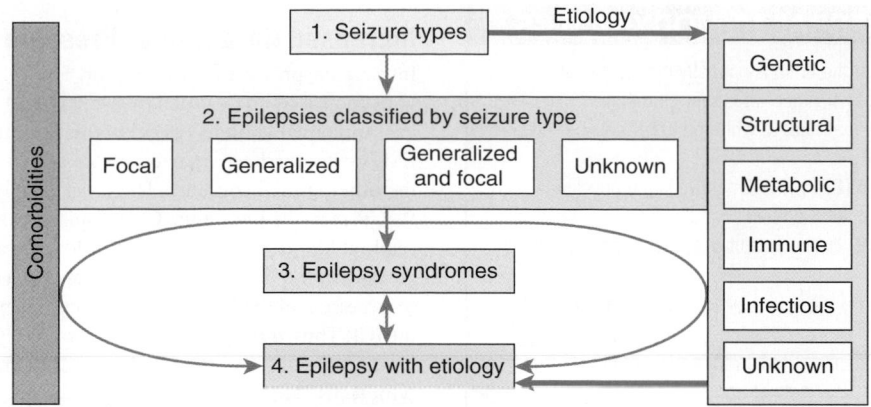

FIGURE 17.16 Framework for Classification of Epilepsy. (From Scheffer IE, et al: *Epilepsia Open* 1(1-2):37-44, 2016.)

TABLE 17.18	**TERMINOLOGY USED TO DESCRIBE PHASES OF A SEIZURE**
TERM	**DEFINITION**
Prodroma	Early clinical manifestations, such as malaise, headache, or a sense of depression, that may occur hours to a few days before the onset of a seizure
Aura	A focal seizure experienced as a peculiar sensation preceding the onset of a generalized seizure or complex partial seizure that may take the form of gustatory, visual, or auditory experience; a feeling of dizziness or numbness; or just "a funny feeling"
Ictus	The episode of the seizure
Tonic phase	A state of muscle contraction in which there is excessive muscle tone
Clonic phase	A state of alternating contraction and relaxation of muscles
Postictal state	The period immediately following the cessation of seizure activity

persons with seizure disorders. The situation is a medical emergency because of the resulting cerebral hypoxia. Intellectual disability, dementia, other brain damage, and even death are serious threats. Aspiration also is a great risk.

CLINICAL MANIFESTATIONS. The phases associated with a seizure are summarized in Table 17.18. Two types of symptoms signal the preictal phase of a generalized tonic-clonic seizure: prodroma, early manifestations occurring hours to days before a seizure and may include anxiety, depression, or inability to think clearly; and a focal seizure or aura that immediately precedes the onset of a generalized tonic-clonic seizure. Both may become familiar to the person experiencing recurrent generalized seizures and may enable the person to prevent injuries during the seizure. The ictus is the episode of the epileptic seizure with tonic-clonic activity. Relaxation of urinary and bowel sphincters may occur, leading to bladder and bowel incontinence. Airway maintenance needs to be ensured. Status epilepticus in adults is a state of continuous tonic-clonic seizures lasting more than 5 minutes, or rapidly recurring seizures before the person has fully regained consciousness from the preceding seizure, or a single seizure lasting more than 30 minutes. It is a condition requiring prompt diagnosis and treatment because of the resulting cerebral hypoxia. Long-term consequences can include neuronal death, neuronal injury, and alteration of neuronal networks.[70] The postictal state follows an epileptic seizure and can include signs of headache, confusion, aphasia, memory loss, and paralysis that may last hours or a day or two. Deep sleep also is common.

EVALUATION AND TREATMENT. Health history is the most critical aspect in diagnosing a seizure disorder and establishing the cause and onset. The health history is supplemented by the physical examination and laboratory tests of blood and urine (blood glucose, serum calcium, blood urea nitrogen, urine sodium, and creatinine clearance measurements) to identify any systemic diseases known to have seizures as a clinical manifestation. Brain imaging and CSF examination are useful for identifying any neurologic diseases associated with seizures. The EEG is useful in assessing the type of seizure and may help determine its focus. Combined EEG and functional magnetic resonance imaging (fMRI) are useful in identifying neural networks involved in epileptic activity. Differentiating a generalized epilepsy from a focal epilepsy is vital to treatment and prognosis.[71,72]

Treatment for a seizure disorder is first to correct or control its cause, if possible. If this is not possible, the major means of management is the judicious administration of antiseizure medications. The therapeutic goal is complete suppression of seizure activity without intolerable side effects of the drug or drug resistance. Dietary treatments (e.g., ketogenic and modified Adkins diet) are effective for some individuals.[73] Surgical interventions can improve seizure control and quality of life in people with drug-resistant epilepsy.[74] Vagus nerve stimulation can reduce seizure frequency in persons with drug-resistant focal seizures.[75]

ALTERATIONS IN CEREBRAL HEMODYNAMICS

An injured brain reacts with structural, chemical, and pathophysiologic changes. Primary brain injury is the original trauma, and secondary brain injury (see Chapter 18) is a consequence of alterations in cerebral blood flow, intracranial pressure, and oxygen delivery. Several relevant features of cerebral hemodynamics relate to cerebral oxygenation (Box 17.5).

Alterations in cerebral blood flow may be related to three injury states: inadequate cerebral perfusion, normal cerebral perfusion but with an elevated intracranial pressure, and excessive cerebral blood volume (CBV). Treatments for these injury states are directed at improving or maintaining cerebral perfusion pressure (CPP), as well as controlling intracranial pressure. Target values for relevant clinical parameters are presented in Table 17.19.

BOX 17.5   CEREBRAL HEMODYNAMICS

Cerebral blood flow (CBF) to the brain is normally maintained at a rate that matches local metabolic needs of the brain. CBF to gray matter is about 3 to 4 times greater than that to white matter because of the increased metabolic activity.

Cerebral perfusion pressure (CPP) (70-90 mmHg) is the pressure required to perfuse the cells of the brain.

Cerebral blood volume (CBV) is the amount of blood in the intracranial vault at a given time.

Cerebral blood oxygenation is measured by oxygen saturation in the internal jugular vein.

Intracranial pressure (ICP) is normally 1 to 15 mmHg, or 60 to 180 cm H_2O.

TABLE 17.19   THERAPEUTIC MANAGEMENT GOALS FOR INDIVIDUALS WITH ALTERED CEREBRAL HEMODYNAMICS

CLINICAL PARAMETER	TARGET VALUE
Central perfusion pressure	>70 mmHg
Intracranial pressure	<20 mmHg
Arterial CO_2 pressure ($PaCO_2$)	35 mmHg
Mean arterial pressure	90 mmHg
Temperature	34-36°C (93.2-96.8°F)
Pulmonary capillary wedge pressure	10-15 mmHg

Increased Intracranial Pressure

Intracranial pressure (ICP) normally is 5 to 15 mmHg, or 60 to 180 mm H_2O. **Increased intracranial pressure (IICP)** may result from an increase in intracranial content (as occurs with tumor growth), edema, excess CSF, or hemorrhage. It necessitates an equal reduction in volume of the other cranial contents. The most readily displaced content is CSF. If ICP remains high after CSF displacement out of the cranial vault, cerebral blood volume and blood flow are altered.

In *stage 1 of intracranial hypertension,* vasoconstriction and external compression of the venous system occur in an attempt to further decrease the ICP. Thus, during the first stage of IICP, ICP may not change because of the effective compensatory mechanisms, and there may be few symptoms (Fig. 17.17). Small increases in volume, however, cause an increase in pressure, and the pressure may take longer to return to baseline. This can be detected with ICP monitoring.

In *stage 2 of intracranial hypertension,* there is continued expansion of intracranial contents. The resulting increase in ICP may exceed the brain's compensatory capacity to adjust. The pressure begins to compromise neuronal oxygenation, and systemic arterial vasoconstriction occurs in an attempt to elevate the systemic blood pressure sufficiently to overcome the IICP. Clinical manifestations at this stage are usually subtle and transient, including episodes of confusion, restlessness, drowsiness, and slight pupillary and breathing changes (see Fig. 17.17).

In *stage 3 of intracranial hypertension,* the ICP begins to approach arterial pressure, the brain tissues begin to experience hypoxia and hypercapnia, and the individual's condition rapidly deteriorates. Clinical manifestations include decreasing levels of arousal or central neurogenic hyperventilation, widened pulse pressure, bradycardia, and pupils that become small and sluggish (see Fig. 17.17).

Dramatic sustained rises in ICP are not seen until all compensatory mechanisms have been exhausted. Then dramatic rises in ICP occur

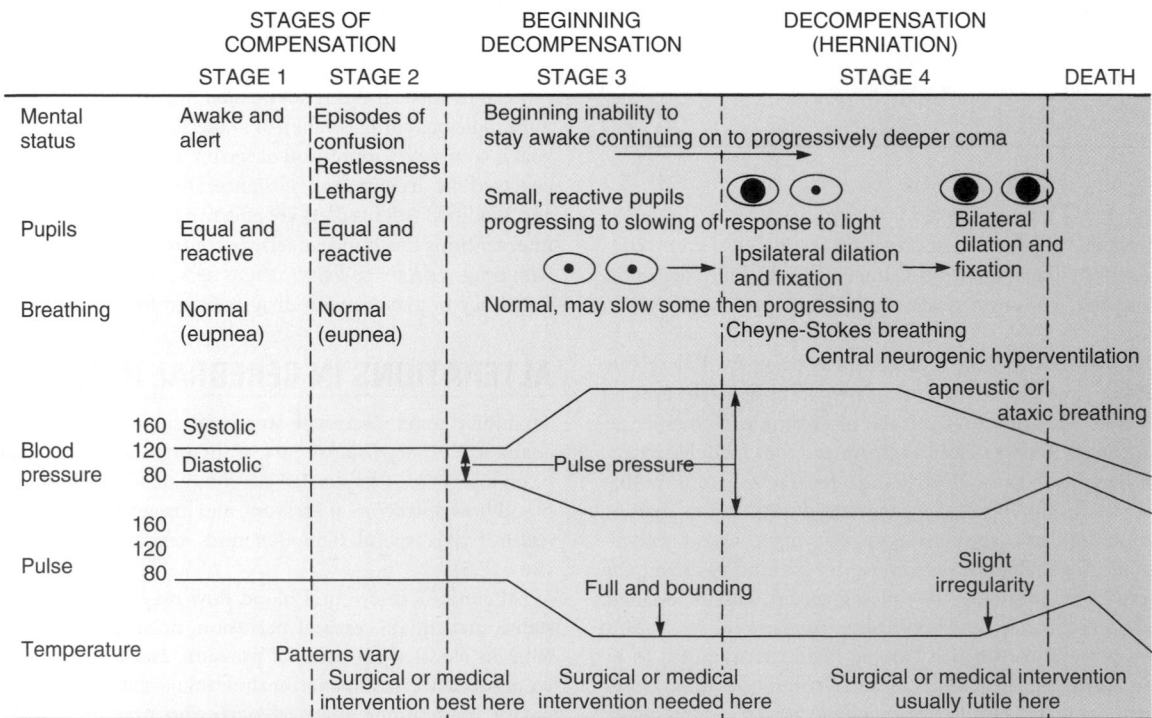

FIGURE 17.17 Clinical Correlates of Compensated and Uncompensated Phases of Intracranial Hypertension.
(From Beare PG, Myers JL: *Principles and practice of adult health nursing,* ed 3, St Louis, 1998, Mosby.)

over a very short period. Autoregulation, the compensatory alteration in the diameter of the intracranial blood vessels designed to maintain a constant blood flow during changes in cerebral perfusion pressure, is lost with progressively increased ICP. Accumulating carbon dioxide may still cause vasodilation locally, but without autoregulation this vasodilation causes the hydrostatic (blood) pressure in the vessels to drop and blood volume to increase. The increasing pressure may obstruct venous outflow. The brain volume is thus further enhanced, and ICP continues to rise. Small increases in volume cause dramatic increases in ICP, and the pressure takes much longer to return to baseline. As the ICP begins to approach systemic blood pressure, cerebral perfusion pressure falls and cerebral perfusion slows dramatically. The brain tissues experience severe hypoxia, hypercapnia, and acidosis, all of which cause cerebrovascular vasodilation.

In *stage 4 of intracranial hypertension,* brain tissue shifts (herniates) from the compartment of greater pressure to a compartment of lesser pressure, and ICP in one compartment of the cranial vault is not evenly distributed throughout the other vault compartments (see Figs. 17.17 and 17.18). With this shift in brain tissue, the herniating brain tissue's blood supply is compromised, causing further ischemia and hypoxia in the herniating tissues. The volume of content within the lower pressure compartment increases, exerting pressure on the brain tissue that normally occupies that compartment and impairing its blood supply. Small hemorrhages often develop in the involved brain tissue. Obstructive hydrocephalus may develop. The herniation process markedly and rapidly increases ICP. Mean systolic arterial pressure soon equals ICP, and cerebral blood flow ceases at this point. The types of herniation syndromes are outlined in Box 17.6.

Cerebral Edema

Cerebral edema is an increase in the fluid content of brain tissue (Figs. 17.19 and 17.20). The result is increased extracellular or intracellular tissue volume. It occurs after brain insult from trauma, infection, toxicity, hemorrhage, tumor, ischemia, infarction, or hypoxia. The harmful effects of cerebral edema are caused by the distortion of blood vessels, the

BOX 17.6   BRAIN HERNIATION SYNDROMES

Supratentorial Herniation

1. *Uncal herniation.* This occurs when the uncus or hippocampal gyrus, or both, shifts from the middle fossa through the tentorial notch into the posterior fossa, compressing the ipsilateral third cranial nerve, the contralateral third cranial nerve, and the mesencephalon. Uncal herniation generally is caused by an expanding mass in the lateral region of the middle fossa. The classic manifestations of uncal herniation are a decreasing level of consciousness, pupils that become sluggish before fixing and dilating (first the ipsilateral, then the contralateral pupil), Cheyne-Stokes respirations (which later shift to central neurogenic hyperventilation), and the appearance of decorticate and then decerebrate posturing.
2. *Central herniation.* This is the straight downward shift of the diencephalon through the tentorial notch. It may be caused by injuries or masses located around the outer perimeter of the frontal, parietal, or occipital lobes; extracerebral injuries around the central apex (top) of the cranium; bilaterally positioned injuries or masses; and unilateral cingulate gyrus herniation. The individual rapidly becomes unconscious; moves from Cheyne-Stokes respirations to apnea; develops small, reactive pupils and then dilated, fixed pupils; and passes from decortication to decerebration.
3. *Cingulate gyrus herniation.* This occurs when the cingulate gyrus shifts under the falx cerebri. Little is known about its clinical manifestations.
4. *Transcalvarial herniation.* The brain shifts through a skull fracture or a surgical opening in the skull. This type of external herniation may occur during a craniectomy—surgery in which a flap of skull is removed, preventing the piece of skull from being replaced.

Infratentorial Herniation

The most common syndrome is *cerebellar tonsillar.* The cerebellar tonsil shifts through the foramen magnum because of increased pressure within the posterior fossa. The clinical manifestations are an arched stiff neck, paresthesias in the shoulder area, decreased consciousness, respiratory abnormalities, and pulse rate variations. Occasionally the force produces an *upward transtentorial* herniation of a cerebellar tonsil or the lower brainstem. There is increased intracranial pressure but no specific set of clinical manifestations associated with infratentorial herniation (see Fig. 17.18).

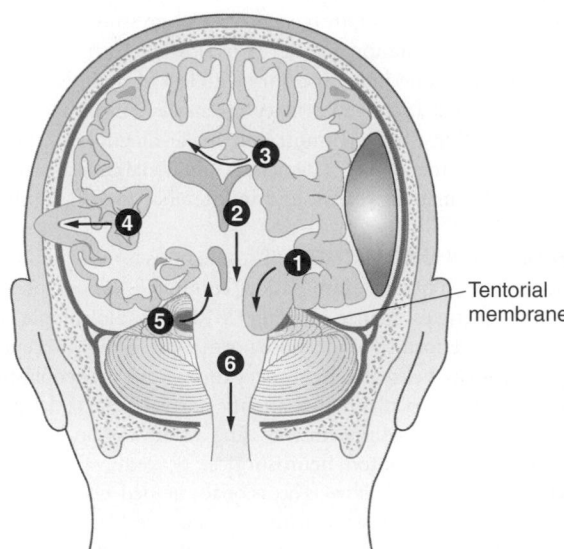

FIGURE 17.18 Brain Herniation. Herniations can occur both above and below the tentorial membrane. *Supratentorial:* **1,** uncal (transtentorial); **2,** central; **3,** cingulate; **4,** transcalvarial (external herniation through an opening in the skull). *Infratentorial:* **5,** upward herniation of cerebellum; **6,** cerebellar tonsil moves down through foramen magnum.

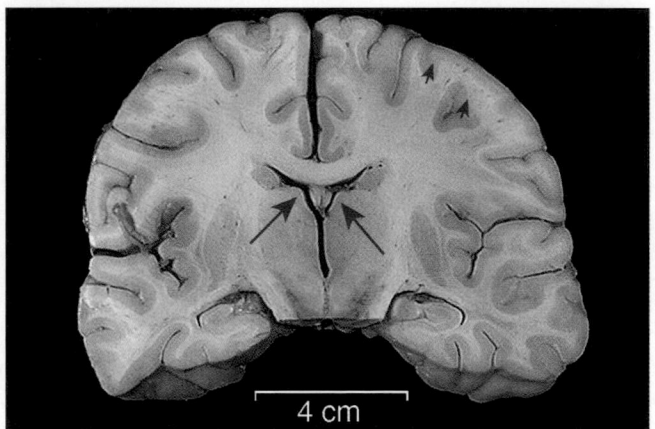

FIGURE 17.19 Brain Edema. This coronal section of cerebrum demonstrates marked compression in the lateral ventricles *(long arrows)* and flattening of gyri *(short arrows)* from extensive bilateral cerebral edema. Edema increases intracranial pressure, leading to herniation. (From Klatt EC: *Robbins and Cotran atlas of pathology,* ed 2, Philadelphia, 2010, Saunders.)

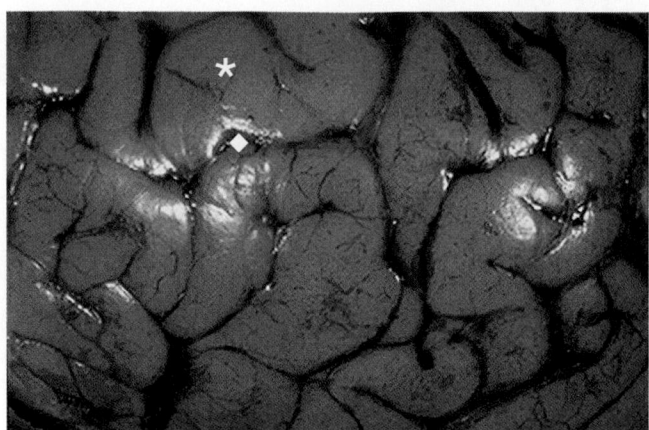

FIGURE 17.20 Cerebral Edema, Gross. The surface of the meninges of the brain with cerebral edema shows widened, flattened gyri (*) with narrowed sulci (◇). (From Klatt EC: *Robbins and Cotran atlas of pathology*, ed 2, Philadelphia, 2010, Saunders.)

displacement of brain tissues, increase in ICP, and the eventual herniation of brain tissue from one brain compartment to another.

Three types of cerebral edema are (1) vasogenic edema, (2) cytotoxic (metabolic) edema, and (3) interstitial edema. Vasogenic edema is clinically the most common form. It is caused by the increased permeability of the capillaries that form the blood-brain barrier. Plasma proteins leak into the extracellular spaces, drawing water to them, and increasing the water content of brain parenchyma, particularly the white matter. Vasogenic edema begins in the area of injury and spreads with fluid accumulating in the white matter of the ipsilateral side because the parallel myelinated fibers separate more easily. Edema promotes more edema because of ischemia from the increasing ICP.

Clinical manifestations of vasogenic edema include focal neurologic deficits, disturbances of consciousness, and a severe increase in ICP. Vasogenic edema resolves by slow diffusion.

In cytotoxic (metabolic) edema, toxic factors directly affect the cellular elements of the brain parenchyma (neuronal, glial, and endothelial cells), causing failure of the active transport systems. The most common cause is ischemia/hypoxia. The blood-brain barrier is not disrupted. The cells lose their potassium and gain larger amounts of sodium because of failure of cell membrane ion pumps. Water follows by osmosis into the cell so that the cells swell (intracellular edema). Cytotoxic edema occurs principally in the gray matter and may increase vasogenic edema because of the loss of endothelial tight junctions.[76]

Interstitial edema is seen most often with noncommunicating hydrocephalus (see following section and Chapter 20). The edema is caused by transependymal movement of CSF from the ventricles into the extracellular spaces of the brain tissues. The brain fluid volume thus is increased predominantly around the ventricles. The hydrostatic pressure within the white matter increases, and the size of the white matter is reduced because of the rapid disappearance of myelin lipids.

Hydrocephalus

The term hydrocephalus refers to various conditions characterized by an excess of fluid within the cerebral ventricles, subarachnoid space, or both (see Figs. 15.17 and 20.11). Hydrocephalus occurs because of interference with CSF flow caused by increased fluid production, obstruction within the ventricular system, or defective reabsorption of the fluid. A tumor of the choroid plexus may, in rare instances, cause overproduction of CSF (Fig. 17.21). Hydrocephalus may develop from infancy through adulthood.

Types of Hydrocephalus

Noncommunicating hydrocephalus (obstructive) *(internal or intraventricular hydrocephalus)* is caused by obstruction within the ventricular system and occurs more often in children. Impaired absorption of CSF from the subarachnoid space occurs when an obstructive process disrupts the flow of CSF through the subarachnoid space. The fluid is prevented from reaching the convex portion of the cerebrum, where the arachnoid granulations are located.

Communicating hydrocephalus (nonobstructive) *(extraventricular)* results from impaired reabsorption of CSF in the absence of obstruction between the ventricles and subarachnoid space. The most common causes of communicating hydrocephalus are subarachnoid hemorrhage, developmental malformation, head injury, neoplasm, inflammation (i.e., meningitis), high venous pressure in the sagittal sinus, and increased CSF secretion by the choroid plexus. It occurs more commonly in adults.

Normal-pressure hydrocephalus (dilation of the ventricles without increased pressure) is a slowly developing form of communicating hydrocephalus that occurs mostly in late middle age. The ventricles are enlarged and the cerebrospinal fluid pressure is minimally elevated. This form of hydrocephalus is idiopathic, occurs secondarily as a complication of head injury or subarachnoid hemorrhage, or is associated with a benign external hydrocephalus (enlarged frontal subarachnoid spaces) in infancy.[77]

Acute hydrocephalus may develop in several hours in persons who have sustained head injuries. Acute hydrocephalus contributes significantly to increased ICP.

PATHOPHYSIOLOGY. The obstruction of CSF flow associated with hydrocephalus produces increased pressure and dilation of the ventricles proximal to the obstruction. The increased pressure and dilation cause atrophy of the cerebral cortex and degeneration of the white matter tracts. Selective preservation of gray matter occurs. When excess CSF fills a defect caused by atrophy, a degenerative disorder, or a surgical excision, this fluid is not under pressure; therefore atrophy and degenerative changes are not induced. This is known as hydrocephalus ex vacuo.

CLINICAL MANIFESTATIONS. Most cases of hydrocephalus develop gradually and insidiously over time. Acute hydrocephalus presents with signs of rapidly developing increased ICP. The person rapidly deteriorates into a deep coma if not promptly treated. Normal-pressure hydrocephalus has a long-term presentation and develops slowly over time. A triad of symptoms, including declining memory with loss of cognitive function; unsteady, broad-based gait; and urinary urgency and incontinence from detrusor overactivity, are common and make diagnosis difficult to differentiate from other causes of dementia. Additional clinical manifestations are apathy, inattentiveness, and indifference to self, family, and the environment.[78,79]

EVALUATION AND TREATMENT. The diagnosis is made on the basis of clinical history, physical examination, computed tomography (CT) scan, and magnetic resonance imaging (MRI). A radioisotopic cisternogram may be performed to diagnose normal-pressure hydrocephalus. Hydrocephalus can be treated by surgery to resect cysts, neoplasms, or hematomas or by ventricular bypass into the normal intracranial channel or into an extracranial compartment using a shunting procedure, one of the three most common neurosurgical procedures. Excision or coagulation of the choroid plexus is occasionally needed when a papilloma is present. In normal-pressure hydrocephalus, reduction in CSF is achieved through diuresis or placement of a ventriculoperitoneal shunt.[80]

ALTERATIONS IN NEUROMOTOR FUNCTION

Movements are complex patterns of activity controlled by the cerebral cortex, the pyramidal system, the extrapyramidal system, and the muscle

Normal   Hydrocephalus

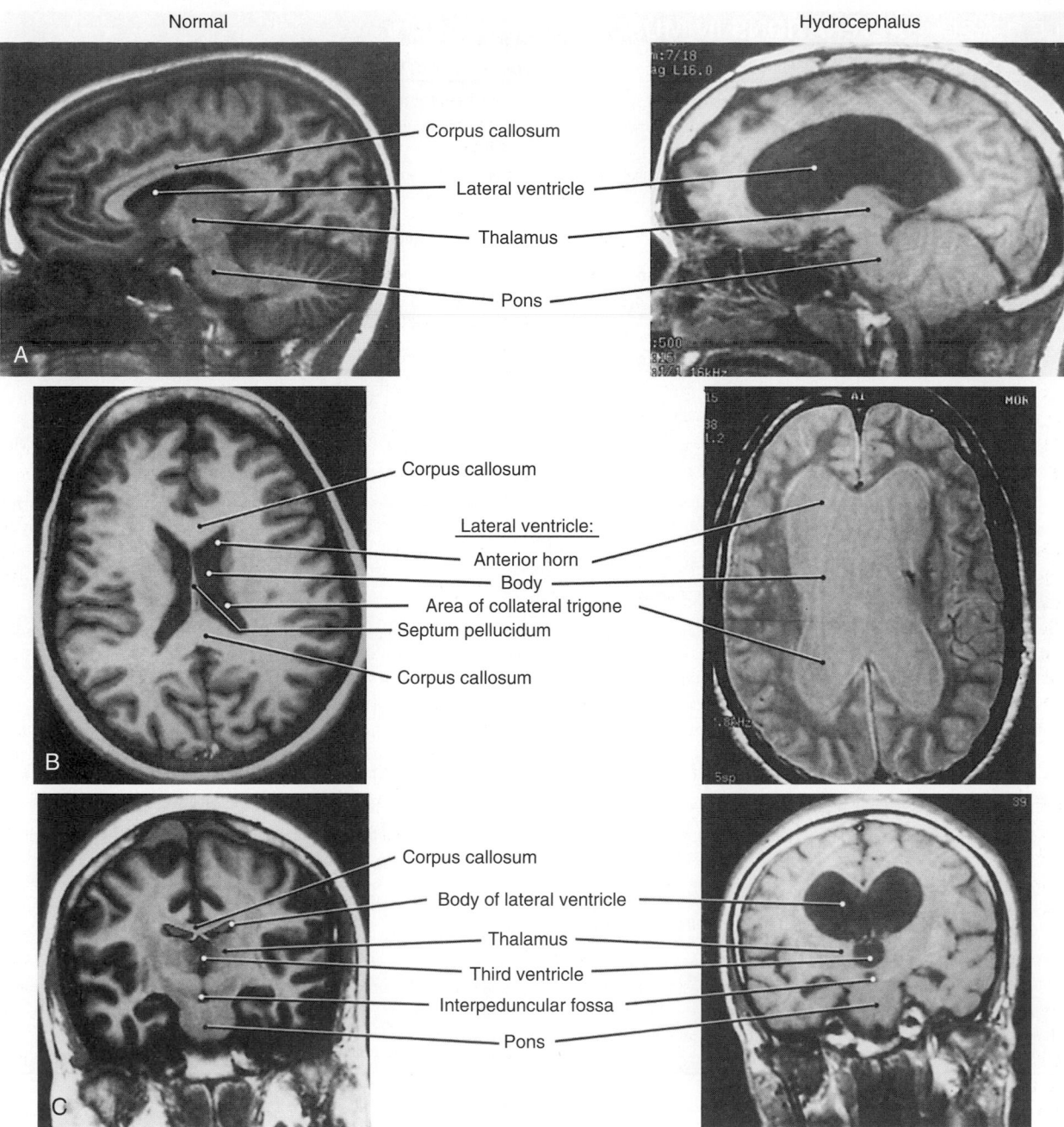

FIGURE 17.21 Comparison of Normal and Hydrocephalic Brains. **A,** Sagittal; **B,** axial; and **C,** coronal planes as seen in magnetic resonance imaging (MRI). (From Haines DE, editor: *Fundamental neuroscience for basic and clinical applications,* ed 4, Philadelphia, 2013, Saunders.)

motor units. Dysfunction in any of these areas can cause motor dysfunction. General motor dysfunctions are associated with changes in muscle tone, movement, and complex motor performance.[81,82]

Alterations in Muscle Tone

Normal muscle tone involves a slight resistance to passive movement. The resistance is smooth, constant, and even throughout the range of motion. The alterations of muscle tone and their characteristics and causes are presented in Table 17.20.

Hypotonia

In **hypotonia (decreased muscle tone),** passive movement of a muscle occurs with little or no resistance. Hypotonia is a symptom of cerebellar

and pure pyramidal tract damage (a rare occurrence). It is thought to be caused by decreased muscle spindle activity secondary to decreased excitability of neurons. Hypotonia contributes to the ataxia and intention tremor in cerebellar damage and manifests with minimal weakness and normal or slightly exaggerated reflexes. A pure pyramidal tract injury produces hypotonia and weakness. Hypotonia, often described as flaccidity (a state in which the muscle may be moved rapidly without resistance), occurs when nerve impulses necessary for muscle tone are lost, such as in spinal cord injury or cerebrovascular accident.

Individuals with hypotonia report that they tire easily (asthenia) or are weak. They may have difficulty rising from a sitting position, sitting down without using arm support, or walking up and down stairs, as well as an inability to stand on their toes. Because of their weakness,

TABLE 17.20   ALTERATIONS IN MUSCLE TONE

ALTERATIONS	CAUSE	CHARACTERISTICS
Hypotonia	Thought to be caused by decreased muscle spindle activity as a result of decreased excitability of neurons Occurs typically when nerve impulses necessary for muscle tone are lost	Passive movement of a muscle mass with little or no resistance Difficult to detect; extremity is floppy and allows excessive movement when displaced Muscles may be rapidly moved without resistance
Flaccidity		Associated with limp, atrophied muscles and paralysis
Hypertonia	Results when the lower motor unit reflex arc continues to function but is not mediated or regulated by higher centers	Increased muscle resistance to passive movement May be associated with paralysis May be accompanied by muscle hypertrophy (see Fig. 17.25)
Spasticity	Exact mechanism unclear; appears to arise from an increased excitability of the alpha motor neurons to any input because of absence of the descending inhibition of the pyramidal systems	A gradual increase in tone causing increased resistance until tone suddenly is reduced, which results in clasp-knife phenomenon Velocity dependent (may be absent with slow speed of displacement) Selective distribution (predominates in flexors of upper extremities and extensors of lower extremities and in pronators compared with supinators)
Paratonia (gegenhalten)	Exact mechanism unclear; associated with frontal lobe injury	Resistance to passive movement, which varies in direct proportion to force applied
Dystonia	Loss of central nervous system (CNS) inhibitory function with sustained muscular contraction	Sustained involuntary twisting and repetitive movements or abnormal posture
Rigidity	Occurs as a result of constant, involuntary contraction of muscle	Muscle resistance to passive movement of a rigid limb that is uniform in both flexion and extension throughout the motion Not velocity dependent Activated by contraction of muscles in contralateral extremities Uniform through range in displacement
Plastic or lead-pipe	Associated with basal ganglion damage	Increased muscular tone relatively independent of degree of force used in passive movement; does not vary throughout the passive movement
Cogwheel	Associated with basal ganglion damage	The uniform resistance may be interrupted by a series of brief jerks resulting in movements much like a ratchet, "cogwheel" phenomenon
Gamma	Loss of excitation of extensor inhibitory areas by the cerebral cortex, decreasing the inhibition of alpha and gamma motor neurons	Characterized by extensor posturing (decerebrate rigidity)
Alpha	Loss of cerebellum input to lateral vestibular nuclei	Impaired relaxation characterized by extensor rigidity of skeletal muscle after the contraction
Myotonia		Impaired relaxation of skeletal muscle after the contraction

accident proneness during locomotion and self-care activities is common. The joints become hyperflexible, so people with hypotonia may be able to assume positions that require extreme joint mobility. The joints may appear loose. The muscle mass atrophies because of decreased input entering the motor unit. Muscle cells gradually are replaced by connective tissue and fat. The muscles are flabby on palpation and are flat in appearance. Fasciculations may be present in some cases.

Hypertonia

In **hypertonia (increased muscle tone)**, passive movement of a muscle occurs with resistance to stretch and is caused by upper motor neuron damage. The four types of hypertonia are spasticity, paratonia (gegenhalten), dystonia, and rigidity.

Spasticity results from hyperexcitability of the stretch reflexes (overactivation of the alpha motor neurons) and is associated with damage to the motor, premotor, and supplementary motor areas, as well as lateral corticospinal tract damage (Fig. 17.22). Spasticity is

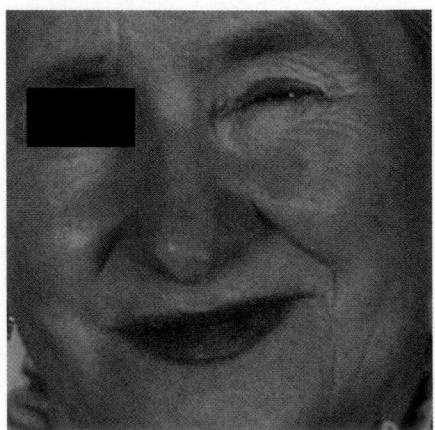

FIGURE 17.22 Left-Sided Hemifacial Spasm. (From Perkin GD: *Mosby's color atlas and text of neurology,* London, 1998, Mosby-Wolfe.)

accompanied by increased deep tendon reflexes (hyperreflexia) and the spread of reflexes (clonus).

Paratonia (gegenhalten) is resistance to passive movement that increases with velocity of movement. Dystonia is increased involuntary muscle contraction, manifested as sustained, involuntary twisting movements. It is caused by slow muscle contraction and may be caused by a failure in appropriate reciprocal inhibition of the muscles (Figs. 17.23 and 17.24). Injury to the putamen or its outflow tracts also is associated with hemidystonia.

Rigidity produced by tonic reflex activity mediated by gamma motor neurons may be continuous or intermittent. The involved muscles are firm and tense; the increase in muscle movement is even and uniform throughout the range of passive movement. Four types of rigidity are described: plastic, or lead-pipe; cogwheel; gamma; and alpha (see Table 17.20).

Individuals with hypertonia may tire easily (asthenia) or be weak. Passive movement and active movement are equally affected, except in paratonia, in which more active than passive movement is possible. As a result of hypertonia and weakness, accident proneness during locomotion and self-care activities is common.

The muscles may atrophy because of decreased use. However, hypertrophy occasionally occurs from overstimulation of muscle fibers. Overstimulation occurs when the motor unit reflex arc remains intact and functioning but is not inhibited by higher centers. The loss of inhibition and the constant state of excitation cause continual muscle contraction, resulting in enlargement of the muscle mass. The muscles are firm on palpation (Fig. 17.25).

Alterations in Muscle Movement

Movement requires a change in the contractile state of muscles. Abnormal movements may occur when a variety of CNS dysfunctions alter muscular innervation. *Dopamine*, a neurotransmitter, has a role in several movement disorders. Some movement disorders (e.g., the akinesias) result from too little dopaminergic activity, whereas others (e.g., chorea, ballism, tardive dyskinesia) result from too much dopaminergic activity. Still others are not related primarily to dopamine function. Movement disorders are not associated necessarily with mass, strength, or tone but are neurologic dysfunctions with either an excess of movement or a lack of voluntary movement. Muscle strength is quantitatively evaluated on a scale of 0 to 4+ or 0 to 5, in which 4+ or 5 is normal and 0 indicates an inability to move against gravity (Table 17.21).

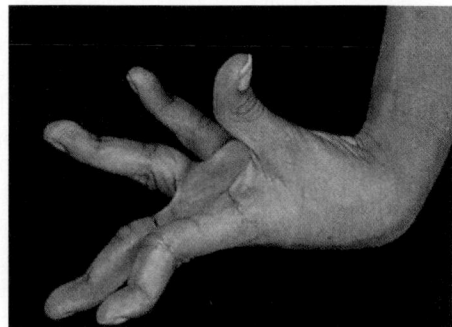
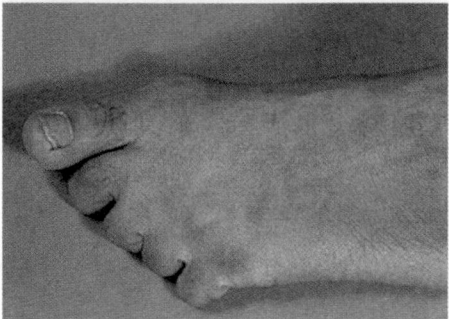

FIGURE 17.23 Dystonic Posturing of the Hand and Foot. (From Perkin GD: *Mosby's color atlas and text of neurology*, London, 1998, Mosby-Wolfe.)

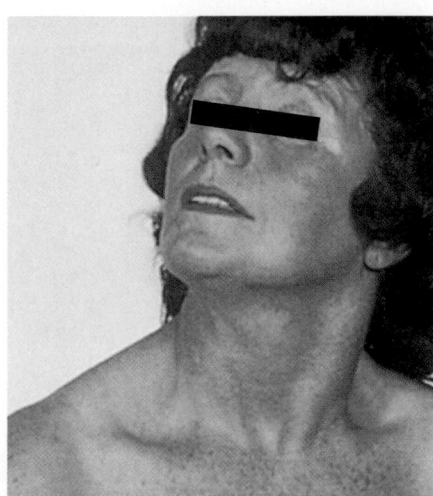

FIGURE 17.24 Spasmodic Torticollis. A characteristic head posture related to spasticity. (From Perkin GD et al: *Atlas of clinical neurology*, ed 3, Philadelphia, 2011, Saunders.)

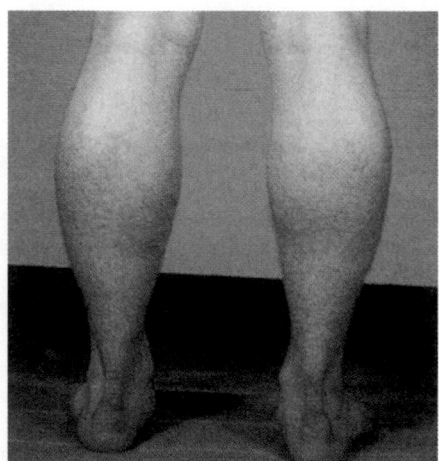

FIGURE 17.25 Pseudohypertrophy of the Calf Muscles. (From Perkin GD et al: *Atlas of clinical neurology*, ed 3, Philadelphia, 2011, Saunders.)

TABLE 17.21	UNITED KINGDOM MEDICAL RESEARCH COUNCIL CLASSIFICATION OF MUSCLE POWER
GRADE	**DEFINITION**
0	Total paralysis—no muscle contraction
1	Flicker of contraction—no joint movement
2	Movement with gravity eliminated
3	Movement against gravity but not resistance
4	Movement against resistance but incomplete
5	Normal power against resistance

Data from Vanhoutte EK et al: *Brain* 135(Pt 5):1639-1649, 2012.

Hyperkinesia

Hyperkinesia is excessive, purposeless movement. Within this category are a number of specific dysfunctions including tremors (Table 17.22). Also included under the general category of hyperkinesias are *dyskinesias* and abnormal involuntary movements. Huntington disease symptoms are the hallmark of hyperkinesia.

Paroxysmal dyskinesias are abnormal, involuntary movements that occur as spasms. The type of dyskinesia varies depending on the specific disorder.

Tardive dyskinesia (slow onset dyskinesia) is the involuntary movement of the face, trunk, and extremities. Although the condition occurs occasionally in individuals with Parkinson disease, it usually occurs as a side effect of prolonged antipsychotic drug therapy.[83] The antipsychotic drugs cause denervation hypersensitivity, thereby mimicking the effect of excessive dopamine. The most common symptom of tardive dyskinesia is rapid, repetitive, stereotypic movements, such as continual chewing with intermittent protrusions of the tongue, lip smacking, and facial grimacing. The symptoms also are called *extrapyramidal symptoms* because the extrapyramidal system controls involuntary reflexes and coordination of movement and posture (see section on Extrapyramidal Motor Syndromes).

Other movement disorders in this category are (1) complex repetitive movements, including automatism (unconscious behavior), stereotypy (ritualistic behavior such as rocking), complex tics such as Tourette syndrome [see *What's New? Tourette Syndrome*], compulsions, perseverations, and mannerisms; (2) excessive reactions to certain stimuli; and (3) paroxysmal excessive activity, including cataplexy and excessive startle reaction.

Hypokinesia is decreased amplitude of movement, bradykinesia is decreased speed of movement, and akinesia is absence of voluntary movement. These are all terms that represent a deficit of voluntary movement. Parkinson disease symptoms are the hallmark of a lack of voluntary movement.

Huntington Disease

Huntington disease (HD), also known as *chorea*, is a relatively rare, hereditary, degenerative hyperkinetic movement disorder diffusely involving the basal ganglia and cerebral cortex. The onset of HD is usually between 25 and 45 years of age, when the trait may already have been passed to the person's children. The disorder has a prevalence rate of approximately 5 to 10 per 100,000 persons, occurs in all races, and rates vary in different regions across the world.[84]

◆**PATHOPHYSIOLOGY.** HD is inherited from one or both parents who have the autosomal dominant trait with high penetrance. The genetic defect of HD is on the short arm of chromosome 4. There is an abnormally long polyglutamine tract in the huntingtin (htt) protein with abnormal folding that is toxic to neurons caused by a cytosine-adenine-guanine (CAG) trinucleotide repeat expansion (40 to 70 repeats instead of 9 to 34). Age of symptom onset is related to the length of the repeat sequences and mechanisms of toxicity. Repeat lengths greater than 60 cause the juvenile form of the disease.[85] Fathers, but not mothers, with high normal alleles do not develop HD but are at risk of transmitting potentially penetrant HD alleles (≥36) to their offspring, who can develop HD.[86]

The principal pathologic feature of HD is severe degeneration of the striatum. The degeneration of the basal ganglia leaves enlarged lateral ventricles (Fig. 17.26) and there is widespread degeneration in late stages of the disease. Expression of the *huntingtin* gene produces tangles of protein that collect in brain cells and chains of glutamine on the abnormal molecules that adhere to each other. The mechanism of neuronal death is unknown. The excitotoxic theory of striatal and cortical degeneration proposes that the mutated huntingtin protein produces excitotoxic pathways mediated by glutamate function that also induce concomitant dysregulation of dopaminergic function. Lysosomal autophagy is disrupted, resulting in accumulation of misfolded proteins. The huntingtin protein also alters cellular organelles, including mitochondrial function, axon transport, and synapses. Apoptotic pathways may be activated and cause neuronal death. Neurotrophic factors also may be depleted, contributing to loss of neurons.[87,88]

WHAT'S NEW?

Tourette Syndrome

There is growing evidence that Tourette syndrome (TS) occurs worldwide and has common features across all races and cultures. The hallmark of TS is the presence of motor tics (sudden, rapid, repetitive nonrhythmic movements) and vocal tics. The tics may be either simple, involving only an individual muscle group (e.g., eye blinking or grunting), or complex, requiring coordinated movement of muscle groups (e.g., head banging or repeating of another person's words). Sensory tics involve unpleasant sensations in the face, head, and neck areas. Probably underdiagnosed, the onset of TS is typically between the ages of 2 and 15 years, with the tics lessening in adulthood. The syndrome has a complex multifactorial etiology with undetermined genetic, environmental, immune, and hormonal factors. The pathophysiology of TS is unclear and currently under study. There is evidence of cortico-striato-thalamocortical dysfunction and, in some cases, altered dopaminergic neurotransmission and abnormalities in brain GABA (loss of inhibition). TS is often diagnosed in association with anxiety, depression, attention-deficit/hyperactivity disorder (ADHD), and obsessive-compulsive disorder. Habit reversal therapy of the urge to move is the most common behavioral therapy, and all behavioral therapy needs further investigation. Pharmacologic treatments target symptoms and can have significant side effects. New drugs are being evaluated to identify the best outcomes. Deep brain stimulation is under investigation.

GABA, gama-aminobutyric acid.
Data from Hallett M: *Brain Dev* 37(7):651-655, 2015; Hirschtritt ME et al: *J Am Med Assoc Psychiatry* 72(4):325-333, 2015; Schrock LE et al: *Mov Disord* 30(4):448-471, 2015; Serajee FJ, Mahbubul Huq AH: *Pediatr Clin North Am* 62(3):687-701, 2015.

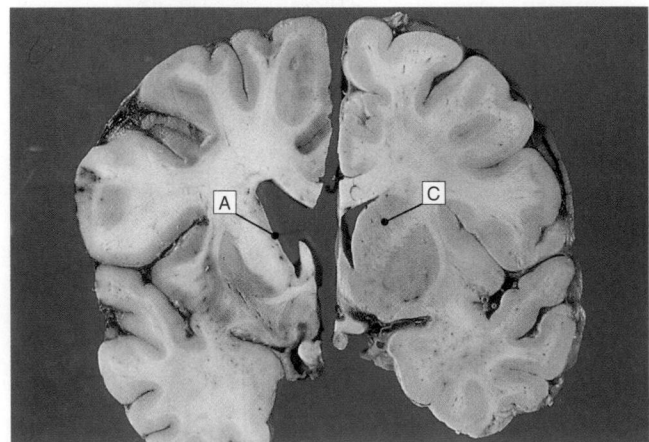

FIGURE 17.26 Huntington Disease. On the right is a normal brain with a normal caudate *(C)*; on the left is a brain from an individual with Huntington disease showing severe atrophy of the caudate *(A)* and an enlarged lateral ventricle. (From Stevens A, Lowe J, Scott I: *Core pathology*, ed 3, London, 2009, Mosby.)

TABLE 17.22	**TYPES OF HYPERKINESIA SYNDROMES**	
TYPE	**CHARACTERISTICS**	**CAUSES**
Chorea*	Nonrepetitive muscular contractions, usually of the extremities of the face; random pattern of irregular, involuntary rapid contractions of groups of muscles; disappears with sleep, decreases with resting; increases with emotional stress and attempted voluntary movement	Associated with excess concentration of or a supersensitivity to dopamine within basal ganglia
Athetosis*	Disorder of distal-muscle postural fixation; slow, twisting, sinuous, irregular movements most obvious in the distal extremities, more rhythmic than choreiform movements and always much slower; movements accompany characteristic hand posture; slowly fluctuating grimaces	Occurs most commonly as a result of injury to the putamen of the basal ganglion; exact pathophysiologic mechanism is not known
Ballism	Disorder of proximal-muscle postural fixation with wild flinging movement of the limbs; movement is severe and stereotyped, usually lateral; does not lessen with sleep; ballism is most common on one side of the body, a condition termed *hemiballism*	Results from injury to the subthalamic nucleus (one of the nuclei that comprise the basal ganglia); thought to be caused by reduced inhibitory influence in the nucleus, a release phenomenon; hemiballism results from injury to the contralateral subthalamic nucleus
Hyperactivity	State of prolonged, generalized, increased activity that is largely involuntary but may be subject to some voluntary control; not highly stereotyped but rather manifests as continual changes in total body posture or in excessive performance of some simple activity, such as pacing under inappropriate circumstances	May be caused by frontal and reticular activating system injury
Wandering	Tendency to wander without regard for environment	"Release" phenomenon; associated with bilateral injury to globus pallidus or putamen
Akathisia	Special type of hyperactivity; mild compulsion to move (usually more localized to legs); severe frenzied motion possible; movements are partly voluntary and may be transiently suppressed; carrying out the movement brings a sense of relief; a frequent complication of antipsychotic drugs	Dopaminergic transmission may be involved
Tremor at rest	Rhythmic, oscillating movement affecting one or more body parts	Caused by regular contraction of opposing groups of muscles
Parkinsonian tremor	Regular, rhythmic, slow flexion-extension contraction; involves principally the metacarpophalangeal and wrist joints; alternating movements between thumb and index finger described as "pill rolling"; disappears during voluntary movement	Loss of inhibitory influence of dopamine in the basal ganglia, causing instability of basal ganglia feedback circuit within the cerebral cortex
Postural Tremor		
Asterixis (tremor of hepatic encephalopathy)	Irregular flapping movement of the hands accentuated by outstretching arms	Caused by transient inhibition of muscles that maintain posture; thought to be related to accumulation of products normally detoxified by the liver
Metabolic	Rapid, rhythmic tremor affecting fingers, lips, and tongue; accentuated by extending the body part; enhanced physiologic tremor	Occurs in conditions associated with disturbed metabolism or toxicity, as in thyrotoxicosis (hyperthyroidism), alcoholism, and chronic use of barbiturates, amphetamines, lithium, amitriptyline (Elavil); exact mechanism responsible unknown
Essential (familial)	Tremor of fingers, hands, and feet; absent at rest but accentuated by extension of body part, prolonged muscular activity, and stress	Not associated with any other neurologic abnormalities; cause unknown
Intentional Tremor		
Cerebellar	Tremor initiated by movement, maximal toward end of movement	Occurs in disease of the dentate nucleus (one of the deep cerebellar nuclei responsible for efferent output) and the superior cerebellar peduncle (a stalklike structure connected to the pons); caused by errors in feedback from the periphery and errors in preprogramming goal-directed movement
Rubral	Rhythmic tremor of limbs that originates proximally by movement	Results from lesions involving the dentatorubrothalamic tract (a spinothalamic tract connecting the red nucleus in the reticular formation and the dentate nucleus in the cerebellum)
Myoclonus	Series of shocklike, nonpatterned contractions of a portion of a muscle, entire muscle, or group of muscles that cause throwing movements of a limb; usually appear at random but frequently triggered by sudden startle; do not disappear during sleep	Associated with an irritable nervous system and spontaneous discharge of neurons; structures associated with myoclonus include the cerebral cortex, cerebellum, reticular formation, and spinal cord

*Choreoathetosis involves chorea and athetosis; precise pathophysiology unknown.

◆**CLINICAL MANIFESTATIONS.** Symptoms of Huntington disease progress slowly and include involuntary fragmentary movements, such as chorea, athetosis, and ballism (see Table 17.22). Chorea, the most common type of abnormal movement, begins in the face and arms, eventually affecting the entire body. There is emotional lability and progressive dysfunction of intellectual and thought processes (dementia) that may precede motor symptoms. Cognitive deficits include loss of working memory and reduced capacity to plan, organize, and sequence. Thinking is slow and apathy is present. Any one of these features may mark the onset of the disease. Restlessness, disinhibition, and irritability are common. Euphoria or depression may be present.

◆**EVALUATION AND TREATMENT.** The diagnosis of HD is based on family history, clinical presentation of the disorder, and genetic testing. Neuroradiologic abnormalities can be demonstrated up to 15 years before clinical symptoms. No known treatment is effective in halting the degeneration or progression of symptoms, and the disease is fatal. Efforts are underway to identify biomarkers for early diagnosis and to monitor disease progression.[89] Symptomatic drug therapies are available.[90]

Hypokinesia

Hypokinesia (decreased movement) is loss of voluntary movement despite preserved consciousness and normal peripheral nerve and muscle function. Types of hypokinesia include akinesia, bradykinesia, and loss of associated movement.

Akinesia and Bradykinesia. Akinesia is a decrease in voluntary and associated movements. It is related to dysfunction of the extrapyramidal system and caused by either a deficiency of dopamine or a defect of the postsynaptic dopamine receptors, which occurs in parkinsonism. Bradykinesia is slowness of voluntary movements. All voluntary movements become slow, labored, and deliberate with difficulty in (1) initiating movements, (2) continuing movements smoothly, and (3) performing synchronous (at the same time) and consecutive tasks. Both akinesia and bradykinesia involve a delay in the time it takes to start to perform a movement.

Loss of Associated Movement. In hypokinesia, the normal, habitually associated movements that provide skill, grace, and balance to voluntary movements are lost. Decreased associated movements accompanying emotional expression cause an expressionless face, a statue-like posture, absence of speech inflection, and absence of spontaneous gestures. Decreased associated movements accompanying locomotion cause reduction in arm and shoulder movements, hip swinging, and rotary motion of the cervical spine.

Parkinson Disease

Parkinson disease (PD) is a complex motor disorder accompanied by systemic nonmotor and neurologic symptoms. Etiologic classification of parkinsonism includes primary parkinsonism and secondary parkinsonism. The onset of primary PD begins after 40 years of age, with the incidence increasing after 60 years. Approximately 60,000 new cases are diagnosed in the United States each year, and an estimated 10 million people worldwide are living with PD. Men are 150% more likely to have PD than women.[91] The familial form represents about 10% of PD; however, the majority of cases are sporadic or idiopathic. Secondary parkinsonism is parkinsonism caused by other neurodegenerative diseases and acquired disorders. Drug-induced parkinsonism is the most common secondary form and is usually reversible (Box 17.7).

◆**PATHOPHYSIOLOGY.** The pathogenesis of primary PD is unknown. Several gene mutations have been identified, the most significant of which are listed in Table 17.13. The hallmark pathologic features of PD are loss of dopaminergic pigmented neurons in the substantia nigra (SN) pars compacta with dopaminergic deficiency in the putamen portion of the striatum (the striatum includes the putamen and caudate

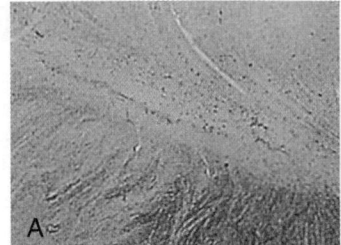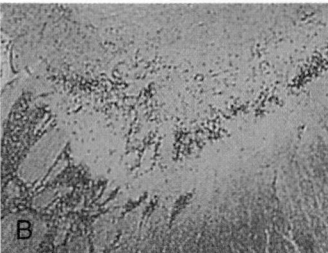

FIGURE 17.27 A, Atrophic substantia nigra. **B,** Compared with normal control. (From Perkin GD et al: *Atlas of clinical neurology,* ed 3, Philadelphia, 2011, Saunders.)

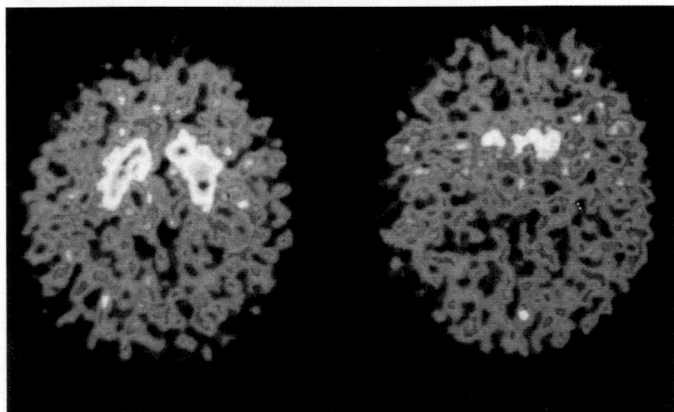

FIGURE 17.28 Reduced Fluorodopa in Parkinson Disease. Positron-emission tomography scan showing reduced fluorodopa uptake in the basal ganglia consistent with neurodegeneration *(right)* compared with a normal control *(left).* (From Perkin GD et al: *Atlas of clinical neurology,* ed 3, Philadelphia, 2011, Saunders.)

nucleus) (Fig. 17.27). Dopamine loss in other brain areas, including the brainstem, thalamus, and cortex, also occurs.[92] The primary pathology is degeneration of the basal ganglia (corpus striatum, globus pallidus, subthalamic nucleus, and substantia nigra) (Fig. 17.28) with formation of Lewy bodies (fibrillar intracellular eosinophilic inclusions with high concentrations of alpha-synuclein, ubiquitin, tau protein, tuberculin, and other proteins) in the substantia nigra and dorsal striatum. There is loss of dopaminergic pigmented neurons in the substantia nigra (SN) pars compacta (see Fig. 17.27) with dopaminergic deficiency in the putamen portion of the striatum (the striatum includes the putamen and caudate nucleus). Dopamine loss occurs in other brain areas, including the brainstem, thalamus, and cortex. Degeneration of the locus coeruleus (LC), which contains noradrenergic neurons, also occurs in PD. Norepinephrine is thought to be neuroprotective, and loss of LC neurons may be associated with a worsening of disease progression and the behavioral symptoms of PD.[93] Molecular events thought to be associated with the neurodegeneration of PD include mitochondrial dysfunction, oxidative stress, abnormal folding and accumulation of alpha-synuclein, abnormal phosphorylation, and dysfunction of the ubiquitin proteasome system (which regulates intracellular protein processing).[94,95] The resulting depletion of dopamine, an inhibitory neurotransmitter, and relative excess of cholinergic (excitatory) activity in the feedback circuit are manifested by hypertonia (tremor and rigidity) and akinesia, producing a syndrome of abnormal movement called parkinsonism (Parkinson syndrome, parkinsonian syndrome, paralysis agitans) (Fig. 17.29). Neuroimaging shows degeneration of dopaminergic neurons preceding the onset of motor symptoms by as long as 3 to 6 years.[91] Dementia may develop over decades with infiltration of Lewy

BOX 17.7   PRIMARY AND SECONDARY CAUSES OF PARKINSONISM

Primary Parkinsonism
Sporadic (idiopathic); most common form
Genetic: autosomal dominant; autosomal recessive
Phenotype may be influenced by gene-environment interactions

Secondary Parkinsonism
Neurodegenerative disorders (sporadic or genetic)
   Disorders associated with alpha-synuclein pathology
      Multiple system atrophies (glial and neuronal inclusions)
         Nigrostriatal degeneration
         Olivopontocerebellar atrophy
         Shy-Drager syndrome
         Motor neuron disease with Parkinson disease (PD) features
      Dementia with Lewy bodies (cortical and brainstem neuronal inclusions)
   Disorders associated with primary tau pathology ("tauopathies")
      Progressive supranuclear palsy
      Corticobasal degeneration
      Frontotemporal dementia
   Disorders associated with primary amyloid pathology ("amyloidopathies")
      Alzheimer disease with parkinsonism
Genetically mediated disorders with occasional parkinsonian features
   Wilson disease
   Hallervorden-Spatz disease
   Chédiak-Higashi syndrome
   SCA-3 spinocerebellar ataxia
   X-linked dystonia-parkinsonism *(DYT3)*
   Fragile X permutation associated with ataxia-tremor-parkinsonism syndrome
   Huntington disease (Westphal variant)
   Prion disease
   Rett syndrome

Miscellaneous acquired conditions
   Vascular parkinsonism: atherosclerosis, amyloid angiopathy
   Normal pressure hydrocephalus
   Catatonia
   Cerebral palsy
Repeated head trauma ("dementia pugilistica" with parkinsonian features)
Infectious and postinfectious diseases
   Postencephalitic PD
   Creutzfeldt-Jakob disease
   Neurosyphilis
Metabolic conditions
   Hypoparathyroidism or pseudohypoparathyroidism with basal ganglia calcifications
   Nonwilsonian hepatolenticular degeneration
Multiple sclerosis
Neoplastic disease
Drugs
   Neuroleptics (typical antipsychotics)
   Selected atypical antipsychotics
   Antiemetics (e.g., prochlorperazine, metoclopramide)
   Dopamine-depleting agents (reserpine, tetrabenazine)
   α-Methyldopa
   Lithium carbonate
   Valproic acid
   Fluoxetine
Toxins
   1-Methyl-1,2,4,6-tetrahydropyridine (MPTP)
   Manganese
   Cyanide
   Methanol
   Carbon monoxide
   Carbon disulfide
   Hexane
   Pesticides (i.e., paraquat, rotenone)

Data from Checkoway H, Nielsen SS, Racette BA: Chapter 12: Environmental exposures and risks for Parkinson's disease. In Aschner M, editor: *Environmental factors in neurodevelopmental and neurodegenerative disorders*, Amsterdam, 2015, Academic Press, pp 253-265; Fahn S, Jankovic J, Hallett M: Atypical parkinsonism, parkinsonism-plus syndromes, and secondary parkinsonian disorders. In Fahn S, Jankovic J, Hallett M, editors: *Principles and practice of movement disorders*, ed 2, Philadelphia, 2011, Saunders, pp 197-240; Singer HS et al, editors: *Movement disorders in childhood*, ed 2, Amsterdam, 2016, Academic Press, pp 301-316.

bodies and plaque formation similar to Alzheimer disease.[96] Loss of cholinergic subcortical input into the cortex is associated with nonmotor symptoms of PD.[97]

CLINICAL MANIFESTATIONS. The classic manifestations of Parkinson disease are resting tremor, rigidity, bradykinesia/akinesia, postural disturbance, dysarthria, and dysphagia. They may develop alone or in combination but, as the disease progresses, all are usually present. There is no true paralysis. Onset of symptoms is insidious, and symptoms appear after a 70% to 80% loss of pigmented nigral neurons and a 60% to 70% loss of striatal dopamine.[98] The symptoms are always bilateral but usually involve one side early in the illness. Because the onset is insidious, the beginning of symptoms is difficult to document. Reflex status, sensory status, and mental status usually are normal early in the disease.

Postural abnormalities (flexed, forward leaning), difficulty walking, and weakness develop as neurodegeneration progresses (Fig. 17.30). Disorders of equilibrium result from postural abnormalities. The person with PD is unable to make the appropriate postural adjustment to tilting or falling and falls like a post when starting to tilt. The short, accelerating steps of the person with PD are an attempt to maintain an upright position while walking. Individuals also are unable to right themselves when changing from a reclining or crouching position to a standing position. Speech may be slurred.

Nonmotor symptoms are common. Sleep disorders and excessive daytime sleepiness are commonly experienced. Sensory disturbances (pain and impaired smell and vision), urinary urgency, difficulty concentrating, depression, apathy, and hallucinations are some of the nonmotor symptoms of Parkinson disease. Loss of smell can be an early nonmotor symptom.[99] Autonomic-neuroendocrine changes also contribute to nonmotor symptoms and include inappropriate diaphoresis, orthostatic hypotension, drooling, gastric retention, constipation, and urinary retention.[100]

Progressive dementia is more common in persons older than 70 years with alterations in executive function (concept formation, planning, abstraction, calculations, and judgment) and memory and visuospatial (complex perceptual discrimination and spatial orientation) deficits.[101]

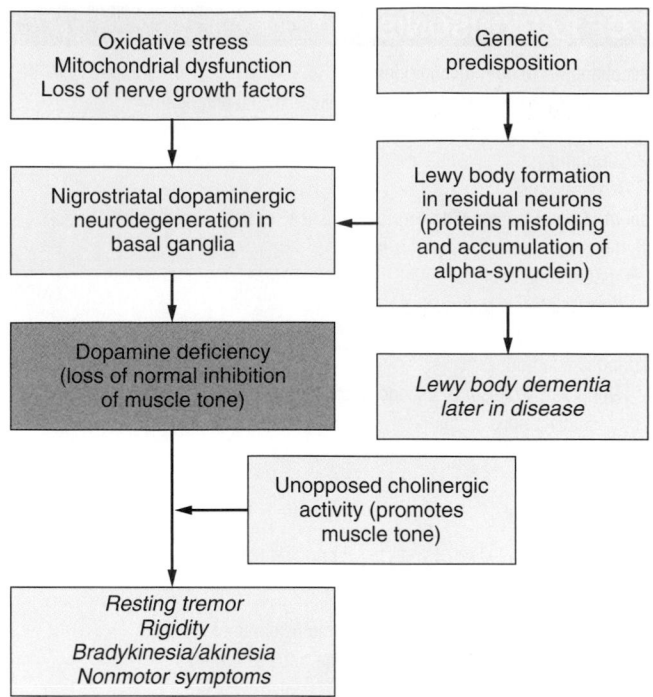

FIGURE 17.29 Pathophysiology of Parkinson Disease.

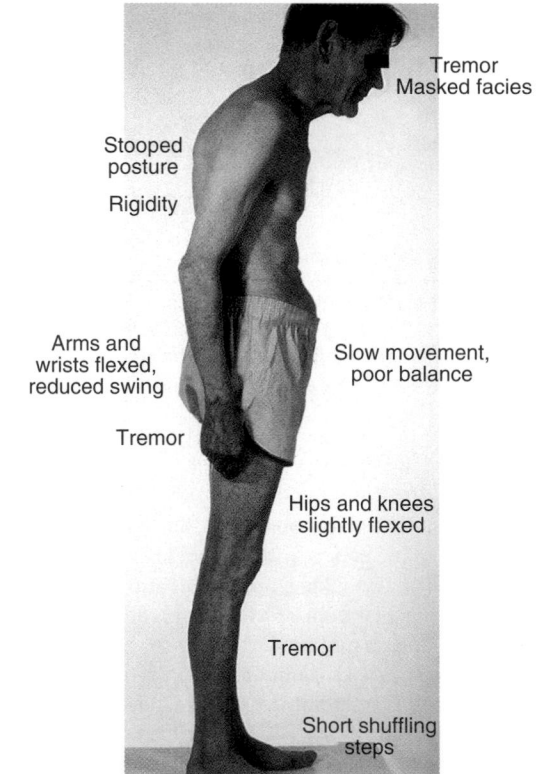

FIGURE 17.30 Stooped Posture of Parkinson Disease. (From Perkin DG et al: *Mosby's color atlas and text of neurology*, ed 2, London, 2002, Mosby.)

Lewy bodies are distributed diffusely in many neurons causing a Lewy body dementia.[33] Mental status may be further compromised by the side effects of the medication taken to control symptoms.

◆**EVALUATION AND TREATMENT.** There is no diagnostic marker for PD.[102] The diagnosis of PD is based on the history and clinical features

of the disease. Causes of secondary parkinsonism are first excluded. Specific gene panels and imaging studies are evolving for early diagnosis.[103] Early nonmotor symptoms of PD can precede motor symptoms, and their identification may assist early diagnosis and guide disease-modifying strategies.[104] Treatment of PD is symptomatic, with drug therapy to protect or restore striatal dopamine levels and decrease akinesia and manage nonmotor symptoms.[105] However, because of troublesome side effects and loss of effectiveness, drug therapy may not be started until the symptoms become incapacitating.[106,107] Recent studies of the gut microbiome in mice indicate that gut dysbiosis is a cause of synucleinopathies and neuroinflammation, with early manifestations of subtle motor and gastrointestinal symptoms, such as constipation. More research is needed to assist with early diagnosis and preventive strategies.[108] Deep brain stimulation (i.e., subthalamic neurostimulation) is replacing surgery to treat persons unresponsive to drug therapy. Implants of stem cells and fetal cells, as well as gene therapy, are strategies for future treatments.[109] Nonmotor symptoms and general immobility are special problems requiring interdisciplinary efforts to improve functional status.[110]

Upper and Lower Motor Neuron Syndromes

Paresis and paralysis are symptoms of upper and lower motor neuron syndromes (Table 17.23). **Paresis (weakness)** is impairment of motor function, that is, partial paralysis with incomplete loss of muscle power. **Paralysis** is loss of motor function so that a muscle group is unable to overcome gravity.

Upper Motor Neuron Syndromes. Upper motor neuron syndromes are the result of damage to descending motor pathways at cortical, brainstem, or spinal cord levels. Upper motor neurons direct the lower motor neurons to produce movements, such as walking or chewing. Upper motor neuron paresis/paralysis also is known as *spastic paresis/paralysis,* and different terms are used to describe the specific disorders (Box 17.8).

Upper motor neuron paresis/paralysis is associated with a pyramidal motor syndrome. The **pyramidal motor syndrome** involves a series of motor dysfunctions resulting from interruption of the pyramidal system (Figs. 17.31 and 17.32). The injury may be in the cerebral cortex, the subcortical white matter, the internal capsule, the brainstem, or the spinal cord. The clinical manifestations reflect overactivity and include excessive movements, such as clonus and spasms, occurring regularly as a result of loss of higher motor control. The clinical manifestations can vary depending on the location of the lesion, suddenness of onset, and age of the individual.

Spinal shock is the temporary loss of all spinal cord functions below the lesion (below the level of the pons). It is characterized by complete flaccid paralysis, absence of reflexes, and marked disturbances of bowel and bladder function. Hypotension can occur from loss of sympathetic

TABLE 17.23 UPPER AND LOWER MOTOR NEURON SIGNS AND SYMPTOMS

UPPER MOTOR NEURON (PYRAMIDAL CELLS [MOTOR CORTEX])	LOWER MOTOR NEURON (VENTRAL HORN [SPINAL CORD], MOTOR NUCLEI [BRAINSTEM])
Muscle groups are affected	Individual muscles may be affected
Mild weakness	Mild weakness
Minimal disuse muscle atrophy	Marked muscle atrophy
No fasciculations	Fasciculations
Increased muscle stretch reflexes (clasp-knife spasticity; resistance to passive flexion that releases abruptly to allow easy flexion)	Decreased muscle stretch reflexes
Clonus may be present	Clonus not present
Hypertonia, spasticity	Hypotonia, flaccidity Hyporeflexia
Pathologic reflexes (Babinski and Hoffmann signs, loss of abdominal reflexes)	No Babinski sign
Often initial impairment of only skilled movements	Asymmetric and may involve one limb only in beginning to become generalized as disease progresses

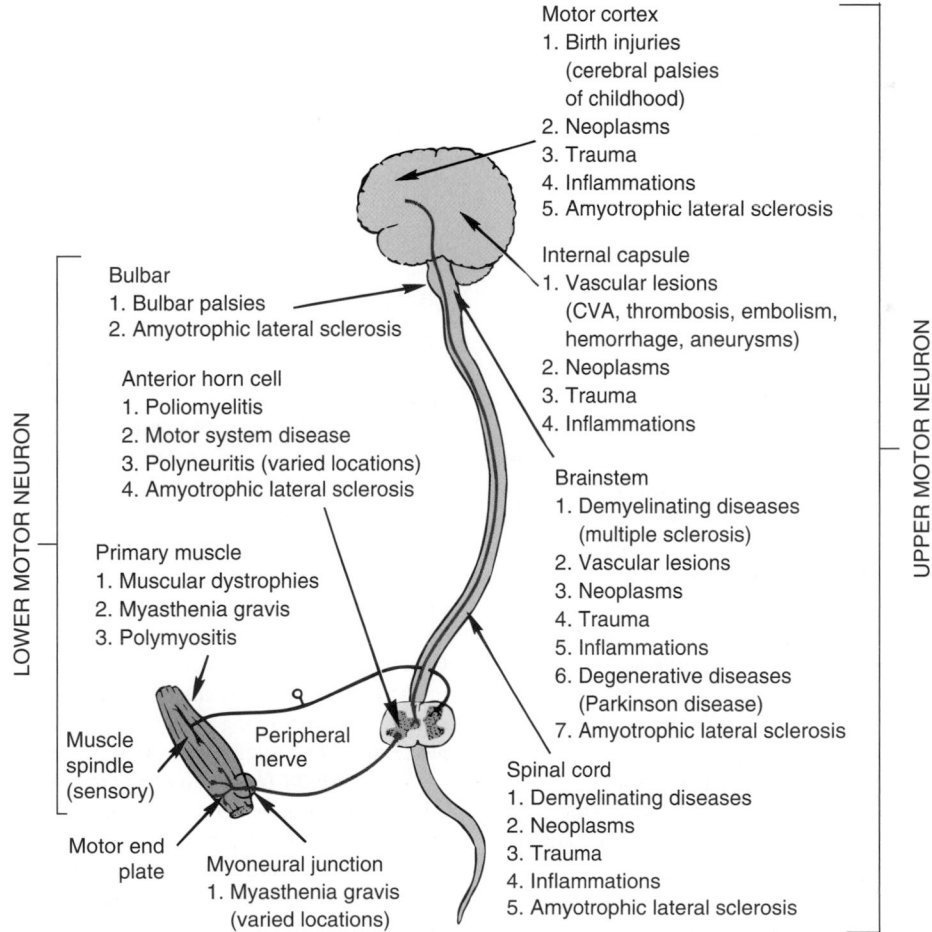

Motor cortex
1. Birth injuries (cerebral palsies of childhood)
2. Neoplasms
3. Trauma
4. Inflammations
5. Amyotrophic lateral sclerosis

Internal capsule
1. Vascular lesions (CVA, thrombosis, embolism, hemorrhage, aneurysms)
2. Neoplasms
3. Trauma
4. Inflammations

Brainstem
1. Demyelinating diseases (multiple sclerosis)
2. Vascular lesions
3. Neoplasms
4. Trauma
5. Inflammations
6. Degenerative diseases (Parkinson disease)
7. Amyotrophic lateral sclerosis

Spinal cord
1. Demyelinating diseases
2. Neoplasms
3. Trauma
4. Inflammations
5. Amyotrophic lateral sclerosis

Bulbar
1. Bulbar palsies
2. Amyotrophic lateral sclerosis

Anterior horn cell
1. Poliomyelitis
2. Motor system disease
3. Polyneuritis (varied locations)
4. Amyotrophic lateral sclerosis

Primary muscle
1. Muscular dystrophies
2. Myasthenia gravis
3. Polymyositis

Muscle spindle (sensory)

Peripheral nerve

Motor end plate

Myoneural junction
1. Myasthenia gravis (varied locations)

LOWER MOTOR NEURON

UPPER MOTOR NEURON

FIGURE 17.31 Disturbances in Motor Function. Disturbances in motor function are classified pathologically along upper and lower motor neuron structures. It should be noted that neoplasms occur at more than one site in an upper motor neuron *(above right)*. A few pathologic conditions, such as amyotrophic lateral sclerosis, involve upper and lower motor neuron structures. Other lesion sites include myoneural junctions and primary muscles, making it possible to classify conditions as neuromuscular and muscular, respectively. *CVA,* Cerebrovascular accident.

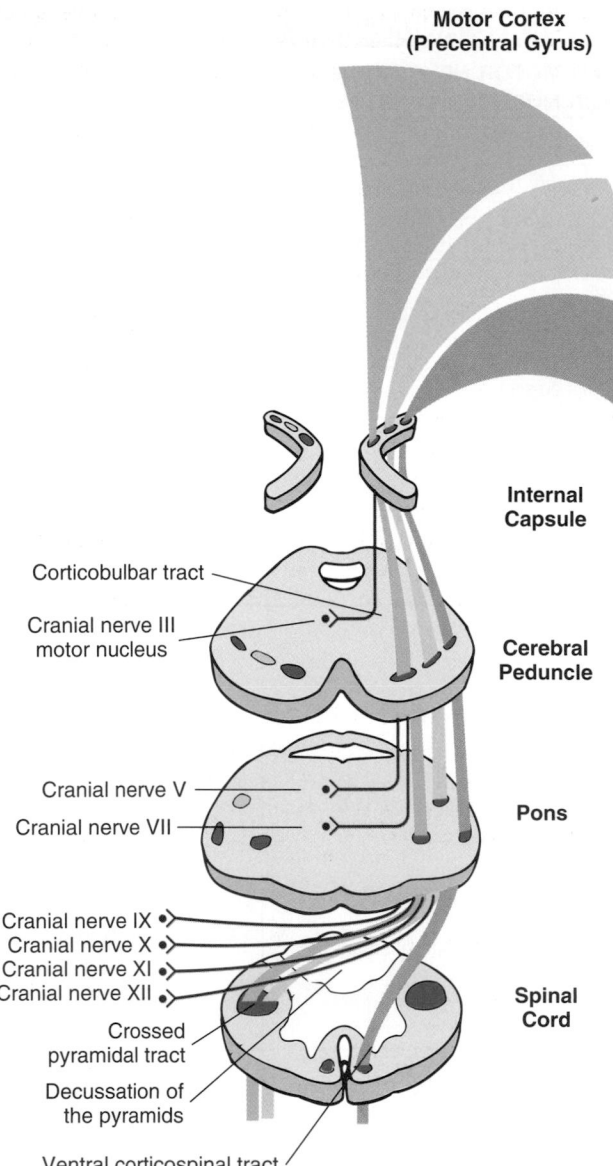

FIGURE 17.32 Structures of the Upper Motor Neuron, or Pyramidal, System. Pyramidal system fibers are shown to originate primarily in the cells in the precentral gyrus of the motor cortex; to converge at the internal capsule; to descend to form the central third of the cerebral peduncle; to descend further through the pons, where small fibers supply cranial nerve motor nuclei along the way; to form pyramids at the medulla, where most of the fibers decussate; and then to continue to descend in the lateral column of the white matter of the spinal cord. A few fibers descend without crossing at the medulla level.

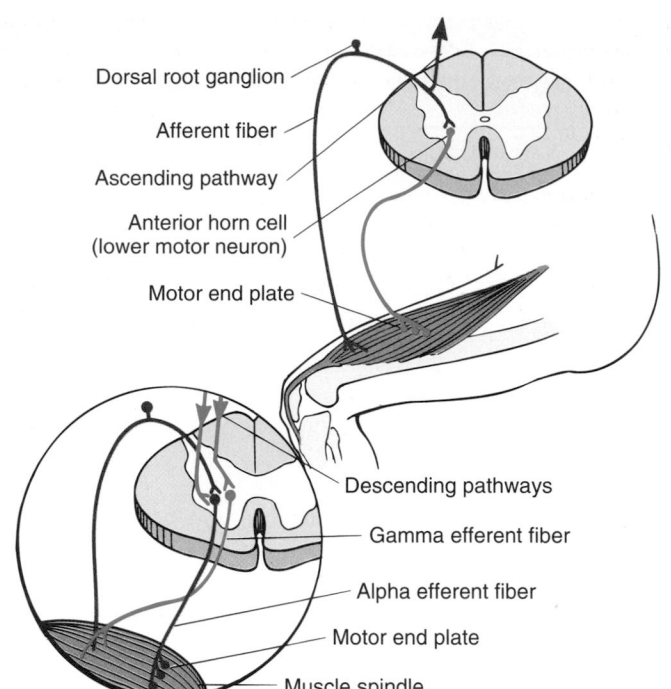

FIGURE 17.33 Component Structure of a Lower Motor Neuron, Including Motor (Efferent) and Sensory (Afferent) Elements. *Top,* Anterior horn cell (in anterior gray column of spinal cord and its axon), terminating in motor end plate as it innervates extrafusal muscle fibers in the quadriceps muscle. *Detailed enlargement:* Sensory and motor elements of the gamma loop system. The gamma efferent fiber is shown innervating the polar, or end, region of the muscle spindle (sensory receptor of skeletal muscle). Contraction of muscle spindle fibers stretches the central portion of the spindle and causes the afferent spindle fiber to transmit the impulse centrally to the cord. Muscle spindle afferent fibers in turn synapse on the anterior horn cell and are transmitted by way of gamma efferent fibers to skeletal (extrafusal) muscle, causing it to contract. Muscle spindle discharge is interrupted by active contraction of extrafusal muscle fibers.

tone at higher levels of spinal cord injury. A major factor in spinal shock is the sudden destruction of the efferent pathways from the motor cortex and brainstem. If destruction occurs more slowly, spinal shock may not develop (see Chapter 18).

If the pyramidal system is interrupted above the level of the pons, the hand and arm muscles are greatly affected. Paralysis rarely involves all the muscles on one side of the body, even when the hemiplegia results from complete damage to the internal capsule. Bilateral movements, such as those of the eye, jaw, and larynx, are affected only slightly, if at all. Predominantly the limbs are influenced. Because of their bilateral control, trunk muscles are much less affected.

Paralysis associated with a pyramidal motor syndrome rarely remains flaccid for a prolonged time. After a few days or weeks, a gradual return of spinal reflexes marks the end of spinal shock. Reflexes then become hyperactive, and muscle tone is increased significantly, particularly in antigravity muscles. Spasticity is common, although rigidity occasionally occurs. Most often, passive range of motion causes the "clasp-knife" phenomenon, probably by activating stretch receptors in the muscle spindles and Golgi tendon organ. (Muscle function is discussed in Chapter 44.) With pyramidal motor syndrome, predominantly the flexors of the arms and the extensors of the legs are affected. The Babinski sign is present (stroking the sole of the foot causes extension of the big toe rather than flexion, and fanning of the other toes).

Lower Motor Neuron Syndromes. Lower (primary, alpha) motor neurons are the large motor neurons in the anterior (ventral) horn of the spinal cord and the motor nuclei of the brainstem. The axons from these nerve cell bodies bring nerve impulses from upper motor neurons to the skeletal muscles through the anterior spinal roots or cranial nerves (Fig. 17.33). **Lower motor neuron syndromes** impair voluntary and involuntary movement. The degree of paralysis or paresis is proportional to the number of lower motor neurons affected. If only some of the motor units that supply a muscle are affected, only partial paralysis or paresis results. If all the motor units are affected, a complete paralysis results. Other clinical manifestations also are proportional to the degree of dysfunction, but the precise manifestations depend on the location of the dysfunction in the motor unit and in the CNS.

Small motor (gamma) neurons, which function to maintain muscle tone and protect the muscle from injury, also are necessary for normal motor movement. They depend on input from the muscle spindle (arriving through an afferent limb rising to the cord). Dysfunction in this motor system (the gamma loop) impairs tone and reduces the tendon reflexes, causing hyporeflexia. The muscles become susceptible to damage from hyperextensibility because the normal protective mechanisms that prevent muscle fiber injury are impaired. The degree of tone loss and the loss of tendon reflexes are proportional to the dysfunction in these reflex motor units.

Generally, the large and small motor neuron systems are equally affected. Therefore the muscle has reduced or absent tone and is accompanied by hyporeflexia or areflexia (loss of tendon reflexes) and flaccid paresis/paralysis.

Denervated muscles (i.e., muscles that have lost their nervous system input) atrophy over weeks to months, mostly from disuse, and demonstrate fasciculations (muscle rippling or quivering under the skin). Occasionally denervated muscles cramp. Fibrillation is isolated contraction of a single muscle fiber because of metabolic changes in denervated muscle and is not clinically visible.

Motor Neuron Diseases

Motor neuron diseases result from progressive degeneration of upper or lower motor neurons in the spinal cord, brainstem, or cortex. Amyotrophic lateral sclerosis (see section on Amyotrophic Lateral Sclerosis) and paralytic poliomyelitis (see Chapter 10) are examples of these diseases.

Several pathologic processes may generate motor neuron diseases that can be sporadic or inherited. A virally induced or postinfectious or postvaccination inflammatory process may injure or destroy anterior horn cells or cranial nerve cell bodies. Most of these inflammatory processes are mild and are followed by rapid cellular recovery (Box 17.9).

In motor neuron disease, muscle strength, muscle tone, and muscle bulk are affected in the muscles innervated by the involved motor neurons. The paresis and paralysis associated with anterior horn cell injury are segmental, but because each muscle is supplied by two or more roots, the segmental character of the weakness may be difficult to recognize. When cranial nerve motor nuclei are affected (these lack nerve roots and have only small rootlets near the point of exit from the brainstem), the distribution of the motor weakness follows that of the peripheral nerve. The weakness may involve distal muscles, proximal muscles, and the muscles of midline structures. Hypotonia and hyporeflexia or areflexia are present.

The atrophy associated with motor neuron disease is segmental when the anterior horn cells of the spinal cord are involved and follows the distribution of the peripheral nerve when the motor nuclei of the cranial nerves are affected. The atrophy may be in distal, proximal, or midline muscles. Fasciculations are particularly associated with primary motor neuron injury, and muscle cramps are common. Mild fatigue is a common complaint. If the pathologic process is limited to the primary motor neuron, no sensory changes are evident.

Because degenerative disorders can cause loss of nerve cells in the anterior horn or motor nuclei, the surviving cells are small and shrunken and filled with lipofuscin. Lost neurons are replaced by astrocytes. The roots or rootlets are thin, and the muscles show denervation and atrophy.

Several brainstem syndromes involve damage to one or more of the cranial nerve nuclei. These are called *cranial nerve palsy* (Table 17.24) and may be caused by vascular occlusion, tumor, aneurysm, tuberculosis, or hemorrhage.

The anterior horn cells and the motor nuclei of the cranial nerves may be affected secondarily in many severe pathologic processes that primarily involve the peripheral nerves. The condition may extend proximally to affect the nerve roots or rootlets and the motor neurons themselves, a process commonly seen, for example, in Guillain-Barré syndrome (see Chapter 18). If sufficient numbers of motor neurons

BOX 17.9   BELL PALSY

The etiology of Bell palsy (facial nerve palsy) remains unknown. There is usually an inflammatory reaction compressing the facial nerve in the fallopian (facial) canal of the middle ear, particularly in the narrowest labyrinthine segment, followed by demyelinating neural change. The most distressing symptoms are unilateral facial weakness and inability to smile or whistle. Bell palsy may be caused by reactivation of herpesviruses in cranial nerve VII (facial) geniculate ganglia or an autoimmune response. The signs usually have an acute onset (within 72 hours). Herpes simplex type 1 has been detected in up to 78% of cases and herpes zoster in 30% of cases. Severe pain with facial palsy and a vesicular rash in the ear or mouth suggest herpes zoster infection. Ramsay Hunt syndrome (herpes zoster oticus) is rare, but complete recovery is less than 50%. Recovery from Bell palsy is usually complete and may not require treatment. Both disorders may be treated with antivirals, corticosteroids, or both, and physiotherapy. Treatment should be individualized according to severity of symptoms.

Data Vakharia K, Vakharia K. *Facial Plast Surg Clin North Am* 24(1):1-10, 2016; Glass GE, Tzafetta K: *Fam Pract* 31(6):631-642, 2014; Eviston TJ et al: *J Neurol Neurosurg Psychiatry* 86(12):1356-1361, 2015.

TABLE 17.24	EXAMPLES OF CRANIAL NERVE PALSIES	
TYPE OF NUCLEAR PALSY	**CAUSES**	**ASSOCIATED CLINICAL MANIFESTATIONS**
Ocular	Upper brainstem tumor	Other cranial nerve signs
	Cerebrovascular disease in the vertebrobasilar system	Contralateral spastic hemiparesis/hemiplegia
		Contralateral hyperreflexia
	Aneurysm	Contralateral extensor plantar
	Intramedullary bleeding	reflex
Facial	Pontine tumor	Paresis/paralysis of both upper
	Cerebrovascular disease in the vertebrobasilar system	and lower facial muscles for both voluntary movement and emotionally induced movement
Vagal	Intramedullary tumor	Ipsilateral loss of pain and temperature sensations of the face
	Cerebrovascular disease in the vertebrobasilar system	Contralateral spastic arm and leg paresis/hemiplegia
		Ipsilateral cerebellar signs
Hypoglossal	Intramedullary tumor	Contralateral loss of position sense and vibration in the arm and leg
	Cerebrovascular disease in the vertebrobasilar system	Contralateral spastic hemiparesis/hemiplegia

are destroyed, permanent loss of motor function results because regeneration of the damaged axons requires a living neuronal cell body.

A group of degenerative disorders principally cause progressive motor cell atrophy. One of these is progressive spinal muscular atrophy, in which the degenerated anterior horn cells of the spinal cord are the affected motor neurons. This disorder occurs in adults and closely resembles the familial progressive muscular atrophies that occur in infants and children and that are considered inherited metabolic disorders (see Chapter 46). If the motor nuclei of the cranial nerves are affected instead of the anterior horn cells, the disorder is labeled progressive bulbar palsy, so named because the myelencephalon (medulla and upper cranial nerves) originally was called the *bulb* and a degenerative process causes a progressively more serious condition. When any lower motor neuron syndrome involves the cranial nerves that arise from the bulb (i.e., cranial nerves IX, X, and XII), the dysfunction is called a bulbar palsy.

The clinical manifestations of bulbar palsy include paresis or paralysis of the jaw, face, pharynx, and tongue musculature. Articulation is affected, especially articulation of the lingual *(r, n, l)*, labial *(b, m, p, f)*, dental *(d, t)*, and palatal *(k, g)* consonants. Modulation is impaired, making the voice rasping or nasal. Pharyngeal reflexes are diminished or lost. Palate and vocal cord movement during phonation is impaired, and chewing and swallowing are affected. The facial muscles are weak, and the face appears to droop. The jaw jerk reflex is decreased. Atrophy eventually becomes apparent, as do fasciculations. All these manifestations become progressively worse, leading to aspiration, malnutrition, possible dehydration, and an inability to communicate verbally.

Amyotrophic Lateral Sclerosis

Amyotrophic lateral sclerosis (ALS) (sporadic motor system disease, sporadic motor neuron disease, motor neuron disease, Lou Gehrig disease) is a worldwide degenerative disorder with loss of lower and upper motor neurons resulting in progressive muscle weakness. *Amyotrophic* (without muscle nutrition or progressive muscle wasting) refers to the predominant lower motor neuron component of the syndrome. *Lateral sclerosis*, scarring of the corticospinal tract in the lateral column of the spinal cord, refers to the upper motor neuron component of the syndrome.

ALS may begin at any time from the fourth decade of life; its peak occurrence is between 60 and 69 years of age with about 3.9 cases per 100,000 population in the United States. The prevalence is higher in males.[111] Most cases of ALS are sporadic. A subset (about 10% to 20%) have a familial form with genetic mutations in C9ORF72 (chromosome 9 open reading frame 72), superoxide dismutase *(SODI)*, and fused in sarcoma *(FUS)* that contribute to the neurotoxicity affecting motor neurons. Mutated TAR RNA-binding protein 43 *(TDP-43)* is a major constituent of the toxic ubiquitinated protein inclusions found in motor neurons and glial cells. More than 40 ALS-associated genes have been identified.[112,113] Gene and environmental interactions are being evaluated as a cause of ALS.[114] Genetic testing is available.

◆**PATHOPHYSIOLOGY.** The cause of ALS is unknown. Apoptotic factors, abnormal synthesis of filament units, defects in axonal transport, glutamate excitotoxicity, oxidative stress, growth factors, mitochondrial dysfunction, and neuroinflammation are under investigation.[115]

The principal pathologic feature of ALS is degeneration and death of upper and lower motor neurons, including the neuromuscular junction. There is a decrease in large motor neurons in the spinal cord, brainstem, and cerebral cortex (premotor and motor areas) with ongoing degeneration in the remaining motor neurons. The nuclei of cranial nerves III, IV, and VI usually are not involved. Death of the motor neuron results in axonal degeneration and secondary demyelination with glial proliferation and sclerosis (scarring) along the corticospinal tract. Inclusion bodies containing the protein *ubiquitin* are found in surviving neurons. However, there also is widespread neural degeneration of nonmotor neurons in the spinal cord and motor cortices, as well as in the premotor, sensory, and temporal cortices.[116] Altered astrocytes and microglial functions are suspected to exist.

Lower motor neuron degeneration denervates motor units. Adjacent, still-viable lower motor neurons attempt to compensate by distal intramuscular sprouting, reinnervation, and enlargement of motor units.

◆**CLINICAL MANIFESTATIONS.** Presentation of symptoms can be variable among individuals because of the numerous genes and multiple systems involved. The initial onset of ALS can be subtle with cramping or weakness that affects a limb, incoordination, slurring of speech, and difficulty swallowing. About 60% of individuals have a spinal form of the disease with focal muscle weakness beginning in the arms and legs and progressing to muscle atrophy, spasticity, and loss of manual dexterity and gait. No associated mental, sensory, or autonomic symptoms are present.[117] Muscle weakness in ALS exhibits the following characteristics:
1. Paresis usually begins in a single muscle group.
2. Corresponding muscle groups are asymmetrically affected in a mottled distribution.
3. Gradual involvement occurs in all striated muscles, except extraocular and heart muscles, and progresses to paralysis with no remissions.
4. Flaccid and spastic paresis may coexist in a single muscle group; flaccid paresis may mask spasticity, which is usually mild.
5. Urethral and anal sphincter weakness is uncommon.

The lower motor neuron syndrome of flaccid paresis consists of weakness of individual muscles, progressing to paralysis, associated with hypotonia and primary muscle atrophy (i.e., atrophy caused by denervation). Hypotonia is manifested by (1) decreased resistance to passive movement, (2) hypoactive or absent deep tendon reflexes, (3) absent abdominal and cremasteric reflexes, and (4) absent Babinski sign. Primary atrophy is manifested by (1) severe, irreversible muscular wasting; (2) fasciculations and fibrillation; (3) metabolically related changes in the skin and appendages; and (4) specific electromyographic (EMG) findings. Metabolic changes include: (1) thinning of the skin, (2) thickening of the nails, (3) loss of body hair, and (4) decreased perspiration.

The upper motor neuron syndrome of spastic paresis consists of weakness of movement patterns, progressing to paralysis, associated with spasticity and, in some cases, atrophy secondary to disuse. Spasticity is manifested by (1) clasp-knife phenomenon, evident with passive movement; (2) hyperactive deep tendon reflexes and clonus with severe spasticity; (3) absent abdominal and cremasteric reflexes; and (4) presence of Babinski sign. The coexistence of frontal dementia and ALS has been demonstrated and may be related to common gene mutations.[118]

◆**EVALUATION AND TREATMENT.** The diagnosis of ALS is based predominantly on medical history and physical examination with no evidence of other neuromuscular disorders. Electromyography and muscle biopsy results verify lower motor neuron degeneration and denervation. Imaging studies and cerebrospinal fluid biomarkers can assist in making the diagnosis. Riluzole (Rilutek), an antiglutamate, is the only drug approved by the Food and Drug Administration for treatment of ALS and prolongs life for months. Supportive and rehabilitation management is directed at relief of symptoms, prevention of complications, maintenance of maximal function, and maintenance of optimal quality of life. Special problems requiring preventive and symptomatic management are communication difficulties caused by dysmasesis and dysphonia, salivation problems with either thick saliva or excessively thin saliva (sialorrhea), and dyspnea caused by diaphragmatic and intercostal weakness. Ventilatory issues become prominent. Psychologic support of the affected individual and the family is extremely important in this disorder. ALS is fatal from respiratory failure usually within 3 years of diagnosis. A small percentage of individuals live 5 to 10 years or longer.[117]

Alterations in Complex Motor Performance

The alterations in complex motor performance include disorders of posture (stance), disorders of gait, and disorders of expression.

Disorders of Posture (Stance)

An inequality of tone in muscle groups because of a loss of normal postural reflexes results in a posturing of limbs. Many reflex systems govern tone and posture, but the most important factor in posture control is the stretch reflex, in which extensor (antigravity) muscles stretching causes increased extensor tone and inhibited flexor tone. Four types of disorders of posture are described: (1) dystonic posture, (2) decerebrate posture, (3) basal ganglion posture, and (4) senile posture. Equilibrium and balance are disrupted when postural disorders are present.

Dystonia is the maintenance of an abnormal posture through muscular contractions. When muscular contractions are sustained for several seconds, they are called dystonic movements; when contractions last for longer periods, they are called dystonic postures, such as in torticollis. Dystonic postures may last for weeks, causing permanent fixed contractures. Dystonia has been associated with basal ganglia abnormality, but the exact pathophysiologic mechanisms are unknown (Box 17.10). One dystonic posture discussed earlier in this chapter is decorticate posture (striatal posture or upper motor neuron dysfunction posture), which may be unilateral or bilateral in occurrence.

Decorticate posture (antigravity posture or hemiplegic posture) is characterized by upper extremities that are flexed at the elbows and held close to the body and by lower extremities that are externally rotated and extended (see Fig. 17.6). Decorticate posture/response is believed to occur when the brainstem is not inhibited by the motor function of the cerebral cortex. Upper motor neuron posture is more commonly described as the arm flexed at the elbow with a wristdrop; the leg inadequately bent at the knee, the hip excessively circumducted, and the presence of a footdrop.

Decerebrate posture refers to increased tone in extensor muscles and trunk muscles, with active tonic neck reflexes. When the head is in a neutral position, all four limbs are rigidly extended (see Fig. 17.6). The decerebrate posture is caused by severe injury to the brain and brainstem, resulting in overstimulation of the postural righting and vestibular reflexes.

Basal ganglion posture refers to a stooped, hyperflexed posture with a narrow-based, short-stepped gait. This posture abnormality results

from the loss of normal postural reflexes and not from defects in proprioceptive, labyrinthine, or visual function. Dysfunctional equilibrium results when the individual loses stability and cannot make the appropriate postural adjustment to tilting or loss of balance, falling instead. Dysfunctional righting is the inability to right oneself when changing from a lying or crouching to a standing position or when rolling from the supine to the lateral or prone position. Dysfunctional postural fixation is the involuntary flexion of the head and neck, causing the person difficulty in maintaining an upright trunk position while standing or walking. Basal ganglion dysfunction, with loss of dopaminergic and cholinergic neurons, accounts for this posture.

Disorders of Gait

Four predominant types of gait associated with neurologic disorders are (1) upper motor neuron dysfunction gait, (2) cerebellar (ataxic) gait, (3) basal ganglion gait, and (4) frontal lobe ataxic gait. As with posture, equilibrium and balance are affected with gait disturbances.[119]

Several upper motor neuron gaits exist. With mild forms, the individual may have footdrop with fatigue and hip and leg pain. A spastic gait, which is associated with unilateral injury, is manifested by a shuffling gait with the leg extended and held stiff, causing a scraping over the floor surface. The leg swings improperly around the body rather than being appropriately lifted and placed. The foot may drag on the ground, and the person tends to fall to the affected side. A scissors gait is associated with bilateral injury and spasticity. The legs are adducted, causing them to touch each other. As the person walks, the legs are still swung around the body but then cross in front of each other because of adduction. Injury to the pyramidal system accounts for these gaits (e.g., stroke, cerebral palsy, multiple sclerosis, spinal cord tumor).

A cerebellar gait is wide-based with the feet apart and often turned outward or inward for greater stability. The pelvis is held stiff and the individual staggers when walking. Cerebellar dysfunction with loss of coordination accounts for this particular gait.

A basal ganglion gait is a wide-based gait in which the person walks with small steps and a decreased arm swing. The head and body are flexed and the arms are semiflexed and abducted, whereas the legs are flexed and rigid in more advanced states. Basal ganglion dysfunction accounts for this gait and is associated with PD.

A frontal lobe ataxic gait also is wide-based with increased body sway and falls, loss of control of truncal motion, gait ignition failure, start hesitation, shuffling, and freezing. The gait is associated with frontal lobe damage or degeneration. The pattern may change as the frontal disease progresses. The slowness of walking, lack of heel-shin or upper limb ataxia, dysarthria, or nystagmus distinguishes the wide stance from cerebellar gait ataxia.[120]

Gait disorders are often accompanied by balance, coordination, and sensory dysfunction that further alter mobility and increase risk for falls. Assessment and intervention strategies are important for prevention of injury.

Disorders of Expression

Disorders of expression involve the motor aspects of communication and include (1) hypermimesis, (2) hypomimesis, and (3) dyspraxias and apraxias. Hypermimesis is a disinhibition phenomenon that most commonly manifests as pathologic laughter or crying. Pathologic laughter is associated with right hemisphere injury, and pathologic crying is associated with left hemisphere injury. The exact pathophysiology is not known. Hypomimesis manifests as aprosody, or the loss of voice modulation (pitch, speed, emphasis, emotion). Receptive aprosody involves an inability to understand emotion in speech and facial expression, whereas expressive aprosody involves the inability to express emotion

---

BOX 17.10 BOTULINUM TOXIN THERAPEUTIC EFFECTIVENESS IN DYSTONIA

Botulinum toxin, both A and B, is effective in relieving cervical dystonia (spasmodic torticollis) symptoms in adults and is the mainstay of modern treatment for focal dystonia and pain. The effectiveness of other drugs (benzodiazepines, gamma-aminobutyric acid [GABA] inhibitors, atypical anticonvulsants, dopaminergic agonists and antagonists), as well as the effect of surgical interventions or physical therapies, is not empirically known. Deep brain stimulation also is an option when other procedures are ineffective.

Data from Fox MD, Alterman RL: *JAMA Neurol* 72(6):713-719, 2015; Jinnah HA, Factor SA: *Neurol Clin* 33(1):77-100, 2015; Skogseid IM: *Acta Neurol Scand Suppl* 198:13-19, 2014.

TABLE 17.25   DYSPRAXIAS AND APRAXIAS

TYPES	DESCRIPTION	LOCATION
Ideomotor apraxia	Impairment in selecting, sequencing, and spatial orientation of movements involved in gestures (spatial and temporal production errors)	Left parietal cortex (angular gyrus) or supramarginal gyrus
Posterior form	Difficulty performing in response to command and imitation; cannot discriminate well between poorly performed and well-performed acts	Left parietal cortex (angular gyrus or supramarginal gyrus) lesion
Anterior form	Performs poorly to command and imitation but comprehends and discriminates pantomime	Lesions anterior to the supramarginal gyrus, which disconnects visual kinesthetic motor engrams from premotor and motor areas
Conduction apraxia	Greater impairment in performance when imitating movements than when pantomiming to command; comprehends pantomime and gesture but cannot perform the movements	Location unknown at this time
Disassociation apraxia	Inability to gesture normally to command and required verbal mediation; has good performance with imitation and actual tools and objects	Callosal abnormalities, but not all locations known
Ideational apraxia	Inability to carry out an ideational plan or a series of acts in the proper sequence	Location unclear at this time
Conceptual apraxia	Cannot recall type of action associated with specific tools, utensils, or objects (content and tool selection errors; may be unable to recall which tool is associated with a specific object or may have impaired mechanical knowledge)	Bilateral frontal and parietal dysfunction

TABLE 17.26   PYRAMIDAL VS. EXTRAPYRAMIDAL MOTOR SYNDROMES

MANIFESTATIONS	PYRAMIDAL MOTOR SYNDROME	EXTRAPYRAMIDAL MOTOR SYNDROME
Unilateral movement	Paralysis of voluntary movement	Little or no paralysis of voluntary movement
Tendon reflexes	Increased tendon reflexes	Normal or slightly increased tendon reflexes
Babinski sign	Present	Absent
Involuntary movements	Absence of involuntary movements	Presence of tremor, chorea, athetosis, or dystonia
Muscle tone	Spasticity in muscles (e.g., clasp-knife phenomenon)	Plastic (equal throughout movement) rigidity or intermittent (generalized but predominantly in flexors of limbs and trunk) rigidity (cogwheel rigidity)
	Hypertonia present in flexors of arms and extensors of legs	Hypotonia, weakness, and gait disturbance in cerebellar disease

in speech and facial expression. Aprosody is associated with right hemisphere damage.

Dyspraxia is the partial inability and apraxia is the complete inability to perform purposeful or skilled motor acts in the absence of paralysis, sensory loss, abnormal posture and tone, abnormal involuntary movement, incoordination, or inattentiveness. These are disorders of learned skilled movements (i.e., arm and hand movement [eating], standing and turning around, blowing out a candle).[121] Dyspraxia and apraxia are associated with left hemisphere vascular disorders, particularly stroke, trauma, tumor, degenerative disorders, infections, and metabolic disorders. Both motor and sensory neural networks play a role in skilled movements[121] (Table 17.25).

True dyspraxias occur when the connecting pathways between the left and right cortical areas are interrupted, causing language-motor and motor representation disconnections between the hemispheres. Dyspraxias may result from any pathologic process that disrupts the cortical areas necessary for the conceptualization and execution of a complex motor act or the communication pathways within the left hemisphere or between the hemispheres.

Extrapyramidal Motor Syndromes

Because the extrapyramidal system encompasses all the motor pathways except the pyramidal system, two types of motor dysfunction comprise the extrapyramidal motor syndromes: (1) the basal ganglia motor syndromes and (2) the cerebellar motor syndromes. Unlike pyramidal motor syndromes, both extrapyramidal motor syndromes result in movement or posture disturbance without significant paralysis, along with other distinctive symptoms (Table 17.26).

Basal ganglia motor syndromes are movement disorders that involve either a paucity or an excess of movements. Stress and nervous tension typically worsen the symptoms, whereas relaxation improves motor performance. Akinesia may occur despite normal strength. Involuntary movements, such as tremor, chorea, ballism, athetosis, and dystonia, also may occur and probably are caused by the loss of the normal modulating effects of the corpus striatum and other parts of the basal ganglia. They can be associated with brain trauma, stroke tumors, infection, metabolic disorders, multiple sclerosis, progressive supranuclear palsy, PD, and medication side effects.

TABLE 17.27	CEREBELLAR MOTOR SYNDROMES
ANATOMIC LOCATION OF DYSFUNCTION	**CHARACTERISTICS**
Rostral vermis (so-called *anterior lobe*)	Ataxia of stance and gait with varying degrees of instability of the trunk and ataxia of legs; anteroposterior body sway; presence of Romberg sign
Caudal vermis (including flocculonodular lobe)	Truncal, postural, and gait ataxia; omnidirectional body sway; Romberg negative; tendency to fall; saccadic slow pursuit, nystagmus; inability to suppress vestibulo-ocular reflex (doll's eyes)
Cerebellar hemisphere (neocerebellar syndrome)	Severe disturbance in ipsilateral limb movements; hypotonia in acute situation; dysmetria (extremity overshooting its target); decomposition of movement; kinetic tremor, past-pointing; deviation of gait; dysarthria
Pancerebellum (combines all other syndromes)	Ataxia of trunk and bilateral limbs; ataxia of gait and stance; dysarthria; oculomotor disturbance

Data from McGee S: *Evidence-based physical diagnosis*, ed 4, St Louis, 2018, Elsevier; Timmann D, Diener HC: Coordination and ataxia. In Goetz GC, editor: *Textbook of clinical neurology*, St Louis, 2007, Saunders.

Basal ganglia motor syndromes also are characterized by alterations in muscle tone and posture. Rigidity, together with the cogwheel phenomenon, is present in all muscle groups but is most prominent in those that maintain flexed position. Postural abnormalities result from the loss of normal postural reflexes. Dysfunctional equilibrium results from the loss of postural stability.

Cerebellar motor syndromes involve the cerebellum and may result in (1) acute loss of muscle tone; (2) difficulty with coordination of voluntary movements (ataxia); (3) minor degrees of muscle weakness, tendency toward fatigue, and impairment of associated movements; and (4) disorders of equilibrium, posture, and gait. They are associated with hereditary ataxias and stroke, brain trauma, multiple sclerosis or tumors; or with systemic disorders (toxin exposure, celiac disease, heat stroke); or they are idiopathic. Cerebellar effects can be ipsilateral (primarily affecting the same side of the body), so damage to the right cerebellum generally causes symptoms on the right side of the body. Predominant symptoms depend on the area and extent of damage within the cerebellum. The four cerebellar syndromes are the rostral vermis, caudal vermis, cerebellar hemisphere, and pancerebellum[122] (Table 17.27).

Diagnosis of a cerebellar motor syndrome is based on the symptoms, but these may vary because of the individual's attempts at compensation. Further, the nervous system often can operate well despite destruction of parts of the cerebellum, although the mechanisms responsible for this retained function are not fully understood.

SUMMARY REVIEW

Alterations in Cognitive Systems

1. Three systems support cognitive function: attentional systems, memory and language systems, and affective or emotive systems.
2. Full consciousness is an awareness of oneself and the environment and includes an ability to respond to external stimuli with a wide variety of responses.
3. Consciousness has two components: arousal (state of awakeness) and awareness (content of thought).
4. Alterations in level of arousal may be caused by structural, metabolic, or psychogenic disorders.
5. Levels of consciousness can diminish in stages from alert and oriented to confusion and coma.
6. An alteration in breathing pattern and level of coma reflects the level of hemispheric and brainstem dysfunction.
7. Pupillary changes reflect changes in level of brainstem function, drug action, and response to hypoxia and ischemia.
8. Abnormal eye movements, including nystagmus and divergent gaze, reflect alterations in brainstem function.
9. Level of brain function manifests by changes in generalized motor responses or the presence of no responses.
10. Loss of cortical inhibition associated with decreased consciousness includes abnormal flexor and extensor movements.
11. Brain death represents irreversible total brain damage including an inability to maintain cardiac, respiratory, and other vital functions. Cerebral death or irreversible coma is death of the cerebral hemispheres exclusive of the brainstem and cerebellum.
12. Arousal returns in the vegetative state and minimally conscious state, but content of thought is absent or markedly reduced, respectively.
13. With locked-in syndrome (ventral pontine syndrome) content of thought and level of arousal are intact but the efferent pathways are disrupted with complete paralysis.
14. Akinetic mutism is a neurobehavioral state characterized by a severe loss of motivation to move or inability to voluntarily initiate motor responses, or both.
15. Alterations in awareness encompass all cognitive functions including awareness, selective attention, and memory.
16. With a deficit in selective attention, mediated by the brainstem, the parietal lobe structures, and the pulvinar nucleus of the thalamus, the individual cannot focus on selective stimuli and thus neglects those stimuli, causing a neglect syndrome.
17. Amnesia can be retrograde (loss of past memories) or anterograde (retention of old memories but an inability to form new ones). Global amnesia is a combination of both.
18. Frontal areas mediate vigilance, detection, and working memory (temporary storage of information). With a vigilance deficit, the person cannot maintain search and scanning activities. With a detection deficit, the person is unmotivated and unable to use feedback.
19. Data processing deficits are problems associated with recognizing and processing sensory information and include agnosias, aphasia, and acute confusional states.

SUMMARY REVIEW—cont'd

20. Agnosias are a defect of recognition and may be tactile, visual, or auditory. They are caused by dysfunction in the primary sensory area or the interpretive areas of the cerebral cortex.
21. Aphasia is an impairment of comprehension (sensory) or production of language (expressive or motor).
22. Expressive aphasia involves loss of ability to produce spoken or written language with slow or difficult speech.
23. Receptive aphasia is a disturbance in understanding all language—verbal and reading comprehension.
24. Anomic aphasia is an inability to name objects, people, or qualities.
25. Transcortical aphasias can be motor, sensory, or mixed.
26. Global aphasia involves anterior and posterior speech areas, with expressive and receptive aphasia.
27. Acute confusional states are characterized chiefly by defects in attention and coherence of thoughts and actions and, in the case of hyperactive delirium, an intense, autonomic nervous system hyperactivity.
28. Dementia is an acquired impairment of intellectual function, memory, and language with alteration in behavior and can be caused by trauma, vascular disease, infection, and progressive neurodegeneration.
29. AD is the most common chronic, irreversible dementia with accumulations of amyloid and tau protein neurofibrillary tangles in the brain. Less common forms include vascular and frontotemporal dementia.
30. Seizures represent abnormal, excessive hypersynchronous discharges of cerebral neurons with transient alterations in brain function. Seizures may be focal or generalized. The categories of seizures include genetic, structural, metabolic, immune, infectious, and unknown.

Alterations in Cerebral Hemodynamics

1. Cerebral oxygenation is a critical management issue.
2. Cerebral perfusion pressure determines cerebral blood flow.
3. An injured brain may experience cerebral oligemia, normal cerebral blood flow but with increased intracranial pressure, or cerebral hyperemia.
4. Increased intracranial pressure may result from edema, excess CSF, hemorrhage, or tumor growth. When intracranial pressure approaches arterial pressure, hypoxia and hypercapnia produce brain damage.
5. Cerebral edema is an increase in the fluid content of the brain resulting from infection, hemorrhage, tumor, ischemia, infarct, or hypoxia.
6. The shifting or herniation of brain tissue from one compartment to another disrupts the blood flow of both compartments and damages brain tissue.
7. Supratentorial herniation involves temporal lobe and hippocampal gyrus shifting from the middle fossa to the posterior fossa; transtentorial herniation with a downward shift of the diencephalon through the tentorial notch; and shifting of the cingulate gyrus herniation under the falx.
8. The most common infratentorial herniation is a shift of the cerebellar tonsils through the foramen magnum.
9. Hydrocephalus comprises a variety of disorders characterized by an excess of fluid within the cranial vault, subarachnoid space, or both. Hydrocephalus occurs because of interference with CSF flow caused by increased fluid production or obstruction within the ventricular system or by defective reabsorption of the fluid.

Alterations in Neuromotor Function

1. Motor dysfunction may be characterized as alterations of motor tone, movement, and complex motor performance.
2. Hypotonia and hypertonia are the main categories of altered muscle tone.
3. Four types of hypertonia exist: spasticity, paratonia (gegenhalten), dystonia, and rigidity.
4. Alteration in muscle movement includes hyperkinesia (excessive movement), hypokinesia (slow movement), and dyskinesias (abnormal voluntary movement).
5. Included in the category of hyperkinesia are chorea, athetosis, ballism, akathisia, tremor, and myoclonus.
6. HD (chorea) is a rare hereditary irreversible disease involving the basal ganglia and frontal cerebral cortex with a depletion of neurons that secrete GABA (an inhibitory neurotransmitter) that causes involuntary, fragmentary movements accompanied by emotional lability and progressive dementia.
7. Types of hypokinesia include akinesia, bradykinesia, and loss of associated movements.
8. PD is a common degenerative disorder of the basal ganglia (corpus striatum) involving degeneration of the dopamine-secreting nigrostriatal pathway resulting in overactivity by the subthalamic nucleus, causing tremor, rigidity, and bradykinesia. Involvement of the limbic system causes emotional lability. Progressive dementia may be associated with an advanced stage of the disease.
9. Two subtypes of paresis and paralysis are described: upper motor neuron and lower motor neuron.
10. An upper motor neuron syndrome is characterized by spastic paresis or paralysis, hypertonia, and hyperreflexia from interruption of the pyramidal system.
11. Interruption of the pyramidal tract below the pons results in spinal shock with complete flaccid paralysis, absence of reflexes, and marked disturbances of bowel and bladder function.
12. Lower motor neuron syndromes manifest with impaired voluntary and involuntary movements and flaccid paralysis.
13. Partial paralysis occurs with only partial loss of alpha motor neurons, and total paralysis is complete loss of alpha motor neurons. Loss of gamma motor neurons impairs muscle tone and decreases deep tendon reflexes.
14. Motor neuron diseases result from progressive degeneration of upper or lower motor neurons in the spinal cord, brainstem, or cortex.
15. Nuclear palsies involve damage to the cranial nerve nuclei.
16. Bulbar palsies involve cranial nerves IX, X, and XII.
17. ALS is a motor neuron disease. The pathogenesis of ALS is not fully known; however, lower and upper motor neuron degeneration occurs as well as degeneration of the nonmotor neurons in the cortices and spinal cord. Clinical manifestations of ALS may include weakness in all muscles that may begin in a single muscle group, slurring of speech, and difficulty swallowing. Flaccid paresis progressing to paralysis is characteristic of the lower motor neuron syndrome.
18. Alterations in complex motor performance include disorders of posture (stance), disorders of gait, and disorders of expression.
19. Disorders of posture include dystonic posture, decerebrate posture, basal ganglion posture, and senile posture.
20. Disorders of gait include upper motor neuron gaits, cerebellar gait, basal ganglion gait, and senile gait.

SUMMARY REVIEW—cont'd

21. Disorders of expression include hypermimesis, hypomimesis, and dyspraxia or apraxia.
22. Dyspraxia is the partial inability and apraxia is the complete inability to perform purposeful or skilled motor acts.
23. Extrapyramidal motor syndromes include basal ganglia and cerebellar motor syndromes.

24. Basal ganglia disorders manifest with alterations in muscle tone and posture, including rigidity, involuntary movements, and loss of postural reflexes.
25. Cerebellar motor syndromes result in loss of muscle tone, difficulty with coordination, and disorders of equilibrium and gait.

KEY TERMS

Acute confusional state (ACS), 516
Acute hydrocephalus, 530
Agnosia, 514
Akinesia, 534, 536
Akinetic mutism (AM), 511
Alzheimer disease (dementia of Alzheimer type [DAT], senile disease complex), 520
Amnesia, 512
Amyotrophic lateral sclerosis (ALS) (sporadic motor system disease, sporadic motor neuron disease, motor neuron disease, Lou Gehrig disease), 542
Aphasia, 515
Apneustic respiration, 506
Apraxia, 544
Arousal, 504
Ataxic respiration, 506
Aura, 527
Autoregulation, 529
Awareness (content of thought), 512
Basal ganglia motor syndrome, 544
Basal ganglion gait, 543
Basal ganglion posture, 543
Bradykinesia, 534, 536
Brain death (total brain death), 510
Bulbar palsy, 542
Central neurogenic hyperventilation, 506
Cerebellar gait, 543
Cerebellar motor syndrome, 545
Cerebral blood flow (CBF), 528
Cerebral blood volume (CBV), 527
Cerebral death (irreversible coma), 510
Cerebral edema, 529
Cerebral perfusion pressure (CPP), 527
Cheyne-Stokes respiration, 506
Clonic phase, 525
Cluster respiration, 506
Communicating hydrocephalus (nonobstructive), 530
Consciousness, 504
Convulsion, 525
Cytotoxic (metabolic) edema, 530
Decerebrate posture, 543
Declarative memory, 512
Decorticate posture (antigravity posture, hemiplegic posture), 543
Delirium, 517

Dementia, 520
Detection, 514
Detection deficit, 514
Diplegia, 538
Dyspraxia, 544
Dystonia, 533, 543
Dystonic movement, 543
Dystonic posture, 543
Epilepsy, 525
Epileptogenic focus, 525
Extrapyramidal motor syndrome, 544
Executive attention deficit, 514
Focal seizure (partial seizure), 526
Frontal lobe ataxic gait, 543
Frontotemporal dementia (FTD) (Pick disease), 525
Generalized seizure, 526
Hemiparesis, 538
Hemiplegia, 538
Herniation syndrome, 529
Hiccups, 509
Huntington disease (HD), 534
Hydrocephalus, 530
Hydrocephalus ex vacuo, 530
Hyperkinesia (excessive movement), 534
Hypermimesis, 543
Hypertonia (increased muscle tone), 532
Hypokinesia (decreased movement), 534, 536
Hypomimesis, 543
Hypotonia (decreased muscle tone), 531
Ictus, 527
Image processing, 513
Intracranial pressure (ICP), 528
Increased intracranial pressure (IICP), 528
Interstitial edema, 530
Irreversible coma, 510
Isolated (pure) vigilance deficit, 514
Level of consciousness, 505
Locked-in syndrome (ventral pontine syndrome), 511
Lower motor neuron syndrome, 540
Memory, 512
Metabolic alterations in arousal, 505
Mirror focus, 525
Neglect syndrome, 512
Neurofibrillary tangle, 521

Noncommunicating hydrocephalus (obstructive), 530
Nondeclarative memory (nonconscious), 512
Normal-pressure hydrocephalus (low-pressure, adult, occult hydrocephalus), 530
Oculomotor response, 508
Paralysis, 538
Paraparesis, 538
Paraplegia, 538
Paratonia (gegenhalten), 533
Paresis (weakness), 538
Parkinson disease (PD), 536
Parkinsonism (Parkinson syndrome, parkinsonian syndrome), 536
Paroxysmal dyskinesia, 534
Persistent vegetative state (VS; unresponsive wakefulness syndrome), 511
Pick disease, 525
Post-hyperventilation apnea (PHVA), 506
Postictal state, 527
Preictal phase, 527
Progressive bulbar palsy, 542
Progressive spinal muscular atrophy, 542
Psychogenic alteration in arousal (unresponsiveness), 505
Pyramidal motor syndrome, 538
Quadriparesis, 538
Quadriplegia, 538
Rigidity, 533
Scissors gait, 543
Seizure, 525
Seizure disorder, 525
Selective attention, 512
Selective attention deficits, 512
Spastic gait, 543
Spasticity, 532
Spinal shock, 538
Status epilepticus, 527
Structural alterations in arousal, 505
Tardive dyskinesia (slow onset dyskinesia), 534
Tonic phase, 525
Upper motor neuron syndromes, 538
Vasogenic edema, 530
Vomiting, 509
Working memory deficit, 514
Yawning, 509

REFERENCES

1. Nakagawa TA, et al: Guidelines for the determination of brain death in infants and children: an update of the 1987 task force recommendations. *Crit Care Med* 39(9): 2139–2155, 2011.
2. Bender A, et al: Persistent vegetative state and minimally conscious state: a systematic review and meta-analysis of diagnostic procedures. *Dtsch Arztebl Int* 112(14):235–242, 2015.
3. Balami JS, Chen RL, Buchan AM: Stroke syndromes and clinical management. *QJM* 106(7):607–615, 2013.
4. Shetty AC, Morris J, O'Mahony P: Akinetic mutism—not coma. *Age Ageing* 38(3):350–351, 2009.
5. Tengvar C, Johansson B, Sorensen J: Frontal lobe and cingulate cortical metabolic dysfunction in acquired akinetic mutism: a PET study of the interval form of carbon monoxide poisoning. *Brain Inj* 18(6):615–625, 2004.
6. Carrasco M: Visual attention: the past 25 years. *Vision Res* 51(13):1484–1525, 2011.
7. Saalmann Y, et al: The pulvinar regulates information transmission between cortical areas based on attention demands. *Science* 337(6095): 753–756, 2012.

8. Krauzlis RJ, Lovejoy LP, Zénon A: Superior colliculus and visual spatial attention. *Annu Rev Neurosci* 36:165–182, 2013.

9. de Haan B, Karnath HO, Driver J: Mechanisms and anatomy of unilateral extinction after brain injury. *Neuropsychologia* 50(6):1045–1053, 2012.

10. Li K, Malhotra PA: Spatial neglect. *Pract Neurol* 15(5):333–339, 2015.

11. Squire LR, Dede AJ: Conscious and unconscious memory systems. *Cold Spring Harb Perspect Biol* 7(3):a021667, 2015.

12. Lisman J, Sternberg EJ: Habit and nonhabit systems for unconscious and conscious behavior: implications for multitasking. *J Cogn Neurosci* 25(2):273–283, 2013.

13. Luis EO, et al: Successful working memory processes and cerebellum in an elderly sample: a neuropsychological and fMRI study. *PLoS ONE* 10(7):e0131536, 2015.

14. Hermans EJ, et al: How the amygdala affects emotional memory by altering brain network properties. *Neurobiol Learn Mem* 112:2–16, 2014.

15. Arena JE, Rabinstein AA: Transient global amnesia. *Mayo Clin Proc* 90(2):264–272, 2015.

16. Szabo K: Hippocampal stroke. *Front Neurol Neurosci* 34:150–156, 2014.

17. Kirova AM, Bays RB, Lagalwar S: Working memory and executive function decline across normal aging, mild cognitive impairment, and Alzheimer's disease. *Biomed Res Int* 2015:748212, 2015.

18. Matthews BR: Memory dysfunction. *Continuum (Minneap Minn)* 21(3Behavioral Neurology and Neuropsychiatry):613–626, 2015.

19. Worrall L, et al: Let's call it "aphasia": rationales for eliminating the term "dysphasia". *Int J Stroke* 11(8):848–851, 2016.

20. Slooter AJ, Van De Leur RR, Zaal IJ: Delirium in critically ill patients. *Handb Clin Neurol* 141:449–466, 2017.

21. Maldonado JR: Neuropathogenesis of delirium: review of current etiologic theories and common pathways. *Am J Geriatr Psychiatry* 21(12):1190–1222, 2013.

22. Piva S, McCreadie VA, Latronico N: Neuroinflammation in sepsis: sepsis associated delirium. *Cardiovasc Hematol Disord Drug Targets* 15(1):10–18, 2015.

23. Vilke GM, et al: Excited delirium syndrome (ExDS): treatment options and considerations. *J Forensic Leg Med* 19(3):117–121, 2012.

24. Peritogiannis V, et al: Recent insights on prevalence and correlations of hypoactive delirium. *Behav Neurol* 2015:416792, 2015.

25. Fong TG, et al: The interface between delirium and dementia in elderly adults. *Lancet Neurol* 14(8):823–832, 2015.

26. Roden M, Simmons BB: Delirium superimposed on dementia and mild cognitive impairment. *Postgrad Med* 126(6):129–137, 2014.

27. Devlin JW, et al: Optimising the recognition of delirium in the intensive care unit. *Best Pract Res Clin Anaesthesiol* 26(3):385–393, 2012.

28. Grover S, Kate N: Assessment scales for delirium: a review. *World J Psychiatry* 2(4):58–70, 2012.

29. Morandi A, et al: Tools to detect delirium superimposed on dementia: a systematic review. *J Am Geriatr Soc* 60(11):2005–2013, 2012. Erratum in *J Am Geriatr Soc* 61(1):174, 2013.

30. Jackson P, Khan A: Delirium in critically ill patients. *Crit Care Clin* 31(3):589–603, 2015.

31. Trogrlić Z, et al: A systematic review of implementation strategies for assessment, prevention, and management of ICU delirium and their effect on clinical outcomes. *Crit Care* 19:157, 2015.

32. O'Brien JT, Thomas A: Vascular dementia. *Lancet* 386(10004):1698–1706, 2015.

33. Walker Z, et al: Lewy body dementias. *Lancet* 386(10004):1683–1697, 2015.

34. Waldö ML: The frontotemporal dementias. *Psychiatr Clin North Am* 38(2):193–209, 2015.

35. Alzheimer's Association: 2015 Alzheimer's disease facts and figures. *Alzheimers Dement* 11(3):332–384, 2015. Available at: http://www.alz.org/facts/downloads/facts_figures_2015.pdf.

36. Beydoun MA, et al: Epidemiologic studies of modifiable factors associated with cognition and dementia: systematic review and meta-analysis. *BMC Public Health* 14:643, 2014.

37. Imtiaz B, et al: Future directions in Alzheimer's disease from risk factors to prevention. *Biochem Pharmacol* 88(4):661–670, 2014.

38. Rocca WA, Grossardt BR, Shuster LT: Oophorectomy, estrogen, and dementia: a 2014 update. *Mol Cell Endocrinol* 389(1-2):7–12, 2014.

39. Solomon A, et al: Advances in the prevention of Alzheimer's disease and dementia. *J Intern Med* 275(3):229–250, 2014.

40. McGuinness B, et al: Statins for the prevention of dementia. *Cochrane Database Syst Rev* (1):CD003160, 2016.

41. Michaelson DM: APOE ε4: the most prevalent yet understudied risk factor for Alzheimer's disease. *Alzheimers Dement* 10(6):861–868, 2014.

42. Kanatsu K, Tomita T: Molecular mechanisms of the genetic risk factors in pathogenesis of Alzheimer disease. *Front Biosci (Landmark Ed)* 22:180–192, 2017.

43. Bennett DA, et al: Epigenomics of Alzheimer's disease. *Transl Res* 165(1):200–220, 2015.

44. Loy CT, et al: Genetics of dementia. *Lancet* 383(9919):828–840, 2014.

45. Bolós M, Perea JR, Avila J: Alzheimer's disease as an inflammatory disease. *Biomol Concepts* 8(1):37–43, 2017.

46. Gonzalez B, et al: Tau spread, apolipoprotein E, inflammation, and more: rapidly evolving basic science in Alzheimer disease. *Neurol Clin* 35(2):175–190, 2017.

47. Heneka MT, et al: Neuroinflammation in Alzheimer's disease. *Lancet Neurol* 14(4):388–405, 2015.

48. Kang S, Lee YH, Lee JE: Metabolism-centric overview of the pathogenesis of Alzheimer's disease. *Yonsei Med J* 58(3):479–488, 2017.

49. Tai LM, et al: The role of APOE in cerebrovascular dysfunction. *Acta Neuropathol* 131(5):709–723, 2016.

50. Alzheimer's Association: *New diagnostic criteria and guidelines for Alzheimer's disease.* Available at: http://www.alz.org/research/diagnostic_criteria/.

51. Cummings JL, et al: International Work Group criteria for the diagnosis of Alzheimer disease. *Med Clin North Am* 97(3):363–368, 2013.

52. Moore A, et al: Canadian Consensus Conference on the Diagnosis and Treatment of Dementia. Fourth Canadian Consensus Conference on the Diagnosis and Treatment of Dementia: recommendations for family physicians. *Can Fam Physician* 60(5):433–438, 2014.

53. Reitz C: Genetic diagnosis and prognosis of Alzheimer's disease: challenges and opportunities. *Expert Rev Mol Diagn* 15(3):339–348, 2015.

54. Kovacs GG: Molecular pathological classification of neurodegenerative diseases: turning towards precision medicine. *Int J Mol Sci* 17(2):2016.

55. Shimojo M, et al: Imaging multimodalities for dissecting Alzheimer's disease: advanced technologies of positron emission tomography and fluorescence imaging. *Front Neurosci* 9:482, 2015.

56. Scheltens P, et al: Alzheimer's disease. *Lancet* 388(10043):505–517, 2016.

57. Waite LM: Treatment for Alzheimer's disease: has anything changed? *Aust Prescr* 38(2):60–63, 2015.

58. Venkat P, Chopp M, Chen J: Models and mechanisms of vascular dementia. *Exp Neurol* 272:97–108, 2015.

59. Bang J, Spina S, Miller BL: Frontotemporal dementia. *Lancet* 386(10004):1672–1682, 2015.

60. Kelley RE, El-Khoury R: Frontotemporal dementia. *Neurol Clin* 34(1):171–181, 2016.

61. Lowenstein DH: Seizures and epilepsy. In Fauci AS, et al, editors: *Harrison's principles of internal medicine*, ed 15, New York, 2008, McGraw-Hill.

62. Fisher RS, et al: ILAE official report: a practical clinical definition of epilepsy. *Epilepsia* 55(4):475–482, 2014.

63. Centers for Disease Control and Prevention (CDC): *Epilepsy fast facts.* Available at: http://www.cdc.gov/epilepsy/basics/fast-facts.htm.

64. Berg AT, et al: Revised terminology and concepts for organization of seizures and epilepsies: report of the ILAE Commission on Classification and Terminology, 2005-2009. *Epilepsia* 51(4):676–685, 2010.

65. Stanuszek A, et al: Seizure-precipitating factors in relation to medical recommendations: especially those limiting physical activity. *J Child Neurol* 30(12):1569–1573, 2015.

66. Casillas-Espinosa PM, et al: Regulators of synaptic transmission: roles in the pathogenesis and treatment of epilepsy. *Epilepsia* 53(Suppl 9):41–58, 2012.

67. Jefferys JG: Are changes in synaptic function that underlie hyperexcitability responsible for seizure activity? *Adv Exp Med Bio* 813:185–194, 2014.

68. Fisher RS, et al: Instruction manual for the ILAE 2017 operational classification of seizure types. *Epilepsia* 58(4):531–542, 2017.

69. Wu Y, Liu D, Song Z: Neuronal networks and energy bursts in epilepsy. *Neuroscience* 287:175–186, 2015.

70. Trinka E, et al: A definition and classification of status epilepticus—report of the ILAE Task Force on Classification of Status Epilepticus. *Epilepsia* 56(10):1515–1523, 2015.

71. Bates K: Epilepsy: current evidence-based paradigms for diagnosis and treatment. *Prim Care* 42(2):217–232, 2015.

72. Tolaymat A, et al: Diagnosis and management of childhood epilepsy. *Curr Probl Pediatr Adolesc Health Care* 45(1):3–17, 2015.

73. Martin K, et al: Ketogenic diet and other dietary treatments for epilepsy. *Cochrane Database Syst Rev* (2):CD001903, 2016.

74. Ryvlin P, Cross JH, Rheims S: Epilepsy surgery in children and adults. *Lancet Neurol* 13(11):1114–1126, 2014.

75. Panebianco M, et al: Vagus nerve stimulation for partial seizures. *Cochrane Database Syst Rev* (4):CD002896, 2015.

76. Stokum JA, et al: Mechanisms of astrocyte-mediated cerebral edema. *Neurochem Res* 40(2):317–328, 2015.

77. Bradley WG, Jr: CSF Flow in the brain in the context of normal pressure hydrocephalus. *AJNR Am J Neuroradiol* 36(5):831–838, 2015.

78. Paidakakos N, Borgarello S, Naddeo M: Indications for endoscopic third ventriculostomy in normal pressure hydrocephalus. *Acta Neurochir Suppl* 113:123–127, 2012.

79. Shprecher D, Schwalb J, Kurlan R: Normal pressure hydrocephalus: diagnosis and treatment. *Curr Neurol Neurosci Rep* 8(5):371–376, 2008.

80. Torsnes L, Blåfjelldal V, Poulsen FR: Treatment and clinical outcome in patients with idiopathic

normal pressure hydrocephalus—a systematic review. *Dan Med J* 61(10):A4911, 2014.

81. Fahn S: Classification of movement disorders. *Mov Disord* 26(6):947–957, 2011.

82. Moore AP: Classification of movement disorders. *Neuroimaging Clin North Am* 20(1):1–6, 2010.

83. Voelker R: Tardive dyskinesia drug approved. *JAMA* 317(19):1942, 2017.

84. Rawlins MD, et al: The prevalence of Huntington's disease. *Neuroepidemiology* 46(2):144–153, 2016.

85. Labbadia J, Morimoto RI: Huntington's disease: underlying molecular mechanisms and emerging concepts. *Trends Biochem Sci* 38(8):378–385, 2013.

86. Ross CA, Tabrizi SJ: Huntington's disease: from molecular pathogenesis to clinical treatment. *Lancet Neurol* 10(1):83–98, 2011.

87. Dayalu P, Albin RL: Huntington disease: pathogenesis and treatment. *Neurol Clin* 33(1): 101–114, 2015.

88. De Souza RA, Leavitt BR: Neurobiology of Huntington's disease. *Curr Top Behav Neurosci* 22:81–100, 2015.

89. Mestre TA, Sampaio C: Huntington disease: linking pathogenesis to the development of experimental therapeutics. *Curr Neurol Neurosci Rep* 17(2):18, 2017.

90. Coppen EM, Roos RA: Current pharmacological approaches to reduce chorea in Huntington's disease. *Drugs* 77(1):29–46, 2017.

91. Parkinson Disease Foundation: Statistics on Parkinson's. 2016. Available at: www.pdf.org/en/parkinson_statistics.

92. Schneider SA, Obeso JA: Clinical and pathological features of Parkinson's disease. *Curr Top Behav Neurosci* 22:205–220, 2015.

93. Espay AJ, LeWitt PA, Kaufmann H: Norepinephrine deficiency in Parkinson's disease: the case for noradrenergic enhancement. *Mov Disord* 29(14):1710–1719, 2014.

94. Abdel-Salam OM: The paths to neurodegeneration in genetic Parkinson's disease. *CNS Neurol Disord Drug Targets* 13(9):1485–1512, 2014.

95. Macchi B, et al: Inflammatory and cell death pathways in brain and peripheral blood in Parkinson's disease. *CNS Neurol Disord Drug Targets* 14(3):313–324, 2015.

96. Hirsch EC, et al: Pathogenesis of Parkinson's disease. *Mov Disord* 28(1):24–30, 2013.

97. Yarnall A, et al: The interplay of cholinergic function, attention, and falls in Parkinson's disease. *Mov Disord* 26(14):2496–2503, 2011.

98. Mullin S, Schapira AH: Pathogenic mechanisms of neurodegeneration in Parkinson disease. *Neurol Clin* 33(1):1–17, 2015.

99. Goldman JG, Postuma R: Premotor and nonmotor features of Parkinson's disease. *Curr Opin Neurol* 27(4):434–441, 2014.

100. Bernal-Pacheco O, et al: Nonmotor manifestations in Parkinson disease. *Neurologist* 18(1):1–16, 2012.

101. Ding W, et al. Neurodegeneration and cognition in Parkinson's disease: a review. *Eur Rev Med Pharmacol Sci* 19(12):2275–2281, 2015.

102. Miller DB, O'Callaghan JP: Biomarkers of Parkinson's disease: present and future. *Metabolism* 64(3 Suppl 1):S40–S46, 2015.

103. Cosottini M, et al: Comparison of 3T and 7T susceptibility-weighted angiography of the substantia nigra in diagnosing Parkinson disease. *AJNR Am J Neuroradiol* 36(3):461–466, 2015.

104. Chao YX, et al: Nonmotor symptoms in sporadic versus familial forms of Parkinson's disease. *Neurodegener Dis Manag* 5(2):147–153, 2015.

105. Rana AQ, et al: Parkinson's disease: a review of non-motor symptoms. *Expert Rev Neurother* 15(5):549–562, 2015.

106. Goetz CG, Pal G: Initial management of Parkinson's disease. *BMJ* 349:g6258, 2014.

107. Johnson KE: Approach to the patient with Parkinson disease. *Prim Care* 42(2):205–215, 2015.

108. Sampson TR, et al: Gut microbiota regulate motor deficits and neuroinflammation in a model of Parkinson's disease. *Cell* 167(6):1469–1480, 2016.

109. Rowland NC, et al: Combining cell transplants or gene therapy with deep brain stimulation for Parkinson's disease. *Mov Disord* 30(2):190–195, 2015.

110. van der Marck MA, Bloem BR: How to organize multispecialty care for patients with Parkinson's disease. *Parkinsonism Relat Disord* 20(Suppl 1):S167–S173, 2014.

111. Mehta P, et al: Prevalence of amyotrophic lateral sclerosis—United States, 2010-2011. *MMWR Surveill Summ* 63(Suppl 7):1–14, 2014.

112. Ludolph AC, Brettschneider J: TDP-43 in amyotrophic lateral sclerosis—is it a prion disease? *Eur J Neurol* 22(5):753–761, 2015.

113. Peters OM, Ghasemi M, Brown RH, Jr: Emerging mechanisms of molecular pathology in ALS. *J Clin Invest* 125(5):1767–1779, 2015.

114. Al-Chalabi A, Hardiman O: The epidemiology of ALS: a conspiracy of genes, environment and time. *Nat Rev Neurol* 9(11):617–628, 2013.

115. Robelin L, Gonzalez De Aguilar JL: Blood biomarkers for amyotrophic lateral sclerosis: myth or reality? *Biomed Res Int* 525097:2014.

116. Wijesekera LC, Leigh PN: Amyotrophic lateral sclerosis. *Orphanet J Rare Dis* 4:3, 2009.

117. Valadi N: Evaluation and management of amyotrophic lateral sclerosis. *Prim Care* 42(2): 177–187, 2015.

118. Lattante S, Ciura S, Rouleau GA, et al: Defining the genetic connection linking amyotrophic lateral sclerosis (ALS) frontotemporal dementia (FTD). *Trends Genet* 31(5):263–273, 2015.

119. Jankovic J: Gait disorders. *Neurol Clin* 33(1): 249–268, 2015.

120. Thompson PD: Frontal lobe ataxia. *Handb Clin Neurol* 103:619–622, 2012.

121. Foundas AL: Apraxia: neural mechanisms and functional recovery. *Handb Clin Neurol* 110: 335–345, 2013.

122. McGee S: *Evidence-based physical diagnosis*, ed 3, Philadelphia, 2012, Saunders.

Disorders of the Central and Peripheral Nervous Systems and the Neuromuscular Junction

Barbara J. Boss, Sue E. Huether

CHAPTER OUTLINE

Alterations in central nervous system (CNS) structure and function are caused by traumatic injury, vascular disorders, tumor growth, infectious and inflammatory processes, metabolic derangements (including those arising from nutritional deficiencies and drugs/chemicals), and degenerative processes. Alterations in peripheral nervous system function involve the nerve roots (radiculopathies), a nerve plexus, the nerves themselves (neuropathies), or the neuromuscular junction.

CENTRAL NERVOUS SYSTEM DISORDERS
Traumatic Brain and Spinal Cord Injury
Traumatic Brain Injury

Traumatic brain injury (TBI) is an alteration in brain function or other evidence of brain pathology caused by an external force. The most common causes are falls for children and older adults followed by unintentional blunt trauma and motor vehicle accidents. Males have the highest incidence in every age group.[1] The incidence of TBI is highest among American Indian/Alaska Natives and blacks and in lower- and median-income families. In recent years, individuals with TBI have shown improved survival outcomes. Advancements have been made in enhanced safety measures (e.g., passive seat restraints, air bags, protective head gear), reduced transport time to hospitals or trauma centers, improved on-scene medical management, imaging of brain injury, prevention and management of secondary brain injury, and a better understanding of long-term consequences of all degrees of brain injury severity.

TBI can be classified as primary and secondary. Primary brain injury is caused by the direct impact or injury and can be focal, affecting one area of the brain, or diffuse (diffuse axonal injury [DAI]), involving more than one area of the brain.[2] Both types of injury can be associated with the same initiating event. Focal brain injury and diffuse axonal injury each account for half of all injuries. Focal brain injury accounts for more than two-thirds of head injury deaths and DAI accounts for less than one-third of deaths. Secondary injury is an indirect consequence of the primary injury and includes systemic responses and a cascade of molecular and chemical events that affect the brain (Fig. 18.1). TBI can be mild, moderate, or severe. The Glasgow Coma Scale (GCS) is commonly used to grade severity of injury (Table 18.1). Other scales also may be used, including the Abbreviated Injury Scale, Injury Severity Score, and the length of posttraumatic amnesia.[3] Most TBIs are mild.

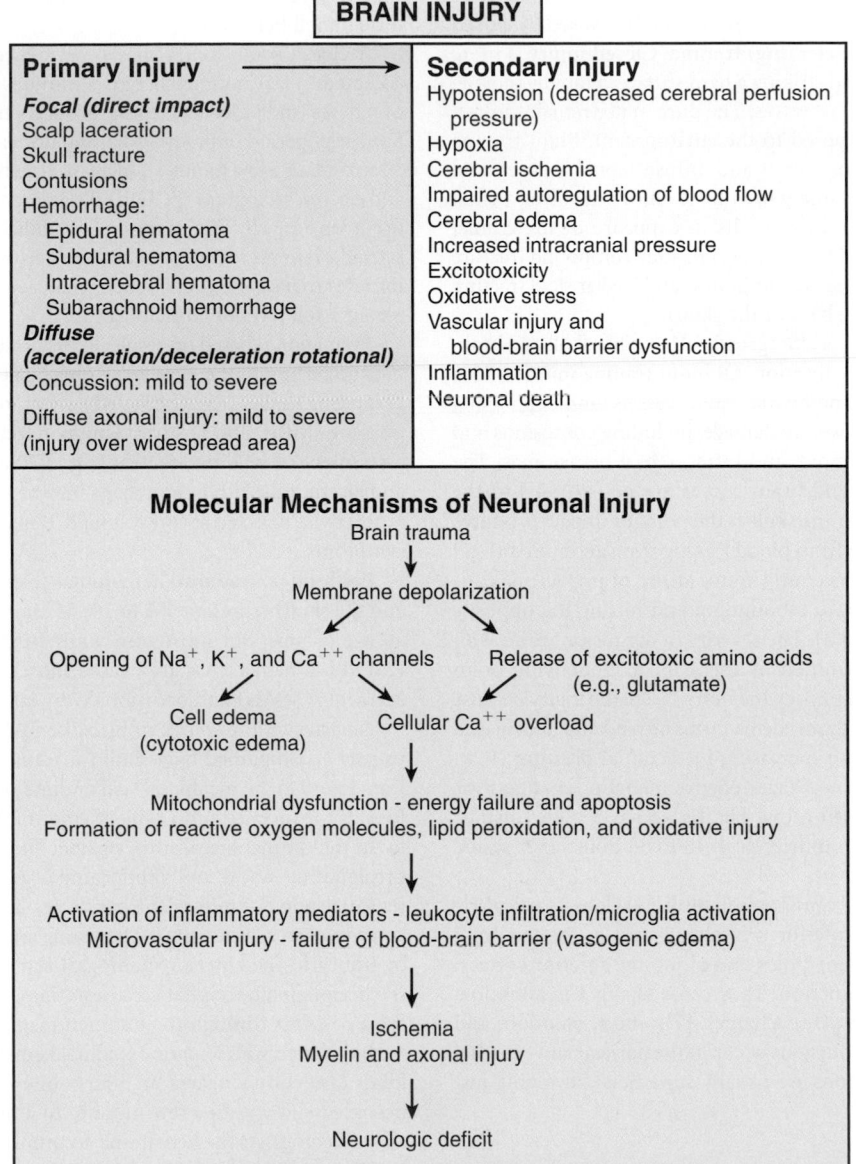

FIGURE 18.1 Pathophysiology of Brain Injury.

TABLE 18.1   GLASGOW COMA SCORE*

SCORE†	BEST EYE RESPONSE SCORE (4)	BEST VERBAL RESPONSE SCORE (5)	BEST MOTOR RESPONSE SCORE (6)
1	No eye opening	No verbal response	No motor response
2	Eye opening to pain	Incomprehensible sounds	Extension to pain
3	Eye opening to verbal command	Inappropriate words	Flexion to pain
4	Eyes open spontaneously	Confused	Withdrawal from pain
5	NA	Oriented	Localizing pain
6	NA	NA	Obeys commands

*The Glasgow Coma Score (GCS) is scored between 3 and 15, with 3 being the worst and 15 the best. It is composed of the sum of three parameters: Best Eye Response, Best Verbal Response, and Best Motor Response. Mild Brain Injury, 13 or higher; Moderate Brain Injury, 9 to 12; Severe Brain Injury, 8 or less.

†It is important to break the scoring report into its components, for example, E3V3M5 = GCS 11. A total score is meaningless without this information. Age affects the GCS. Elderly individuals with traumatic brain injury (TBI) have better GCS scores than younger individuals with TBI with similar TBI severity (i.e., elderly individuals have higher GCS scores than younger individuals with TBI with similar anatomic TBI severity). Data from Teasdale G, Jennett B: *Lancet* 2:81-84, 1974; Salottolo K et al: *J Am Med Assoc Surg* 149(7):727-734, 2014.

Primary Brain Injury

Focal Brain Injury. Focal brain injury can be caused by closed (blunt) trauma or open (penetrating) trauma. Closed injury is more common and involves the head striking a hard surface, a rapidly moving object striking the head, or blast waves. The dura mater remains intact, and brain tissues are not exposed to the environment. Blunt trauma can result in both focal brain injuries and diffuse axonal injuries, and they can occur at the same time. Open head injury involves a skull fracture, and a break in the dura results in exposure of the cranial contents to the environment. Skull fractures include compound fracture or perforated fracture and linear, comminuted, and basilar skull fracture (in the cranial vault or at the base of the skull).

Closed head injuries are specific, grossly observable skull and brain lesions that occur in a precise location. Of blunt trauma injuries, 75% to 90% are mild. Injury to the cranial vault, vessels, and supporting structures can produce more severe damage, including contusions and epidural, subdural, subarachnoid, and intracerebral hematomas. The dura mater remains intact, and brain tissues are not exposed to the environment. Compression of the skull at the point of impact produces contusions or brain bruising from blood leaking from an injured vessel (Fig. 18.2). The injury may be coup (injury at site of impact) or contrecoup (injury from the brain rebounding and hitting the opposite side of skull) or both (Fig. 18.3). The severity of contusion varies with the amount of energy transmitted by the skull to underlying brain tissue. The smaller the area of impact, the more severe the injury because of the concentration of force. Brain edema forms around and in damaged neural tissues, contributing to increasing intracranial pressure (ICP) (see Chapter 17). Multiple hemorrhages, edema, infarction, and necrosis can occur within the contused areas. The tissue has a pulpy quality. The maximal effects of these injuries peak 18 to 36 hours after severe head injury.

Contusions are found most commonly in the frontal lobes, particularly at the poles and along the inferior orbital surfaces; in the temporal lobes, especially at the anterior poles and along the inferior surface; and at the frontotemporal junction. They cause changes in attention, memory, executive functions (see Chapter 17), affect, emotion, and behavior. Less commonly, contusions occur in the parietal and occipital lobes. Focal cerebral contusions are usually superficial, involving just

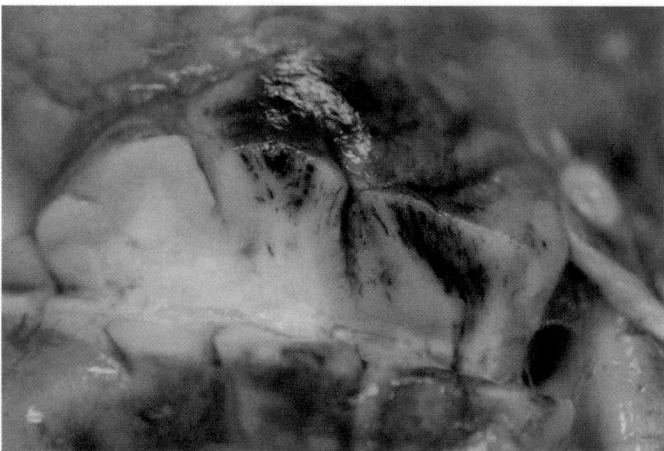

FIGURE 18.2 Cerebral Contusion. Close-up view of a contused brain region with characteristic streaklike, densely arranged hemorrhages in the cortex (cut surface here). Such lesions represent "bruises" on the surface of the brain caused by violent contact between the delicate brain parenchyma and the hard inner surface of the skull. (From Pollak S, Saukko P: Blunt injury, forensic medicine/causes of death, *Encyclopedia of forensic sciences*, London, 2013, Academic Press.)

the gyri. Hemorrhagic contusions may coalesce into a large confluent intracranial hematoma.

A closed brain injury may be evidenced by immediate (generally accepted to last no longer than 5 minutes) loss of consciousness, loss of reflexes (individual falls to the ground), transient cessation of respiration, brief period of bradycardia, and decrease in blood pressure (lasting 30 seconds to a few minutes). Increased cerebrospinal fluid (CSF) pressure and electrocardiogram (ECG) and electroencephalogram (EEG) changes occur on impact. Vital signs may stabilize to normal values in a few seconds; reflexes then return and the person regains consciousness over minutes to days. Residual deficits may persist, and some persons never regain a full level of consciousness.

Evaluation is based on results of the health history, level of consciousness according to the Glasgow Coma Scale (see Table 18.1), outcomes of imaging studies (e.g., computed tomography [CT], magnetic resonance imaging [MRI], and positron emission tomography [PET] scans), and assessment of vital parameters (e.g., ICP and EEG). Large contusions and lacerations with hemorrhage may be surgically excised. Treatment is otherwise directed at controlling ICP, neuroprotection, and managing symptoms.

Epidural (extradural) hematomas (bleeding between the dura mater and the skull) represent 1% to 2% of major head injuries and occur in all age groups, but most commonly in those 20 to 40 years of age. Extradural hematomas are caused most commonly by motor vehicle accidents (MVAs) and occasionally by falls and sporting accidents.

An artery is the source of bleeding in 85% of epidural hematomas, usually accompanied by a skull fracture; 15% of these injuries result from injury to the meningeal vein or dural sinus (Fig. 18.4). The temporal fossa is the most common site of epidural hematoma caused by injury to the middle meningeal artery or vein. The temporal lobe shifts medially, precipitating uncal and hippocampal gyrus herniation through the tentorial notch. Epidural hemorrhages are found occasionally in the subfrontal area, especially in the young and elderly populations, caused by injury to the anterior meningeal artery or a venous sinus; and in the occipital-suboccipital area, resulting in herniation of the posterior fossa contents through the foramen magnum (see Fig. 17.18).

Individuals with temporal epidural hematomas (i.e., over the temporal lobe) lose consciousness at injury; one-third of those affected then become lucid within a few minutes to a few days (if a vein is causing slow bleeding). As the hematoma accumulates, a headache of increasing severity, vomiting, drowsiness, confusion, seizure, and hemiparesis may develop. Because temporal lobe herniation occurs, the level of consciousness is rapidly lost with ipsilateral pupillary dilation and contralateral hemiparesis. A CT scan or MRI is usually needed to diagnose epidural hematoma. The prognosis is good if intervention is initiated before bilateral dilation of the pupils occurs. Epidural hematomas are almost always medical emergencies requiring monitoring and evaluation and surgical evacuation of the hematoma.[4]

Subdural hematomas (bleeding between the dura mater and the brain) arise in 10% to 20% of TBIs. *Acute subdural hematomas* develop rapidly, usually within hours, and are commonly located at the top of the skull (the cerebral convexities). Bilateral hematomas occur in 15% to 20% of persons. The expanding clots directly compress the brain. As the ICP rises the bleeding veins are compressed. Thus bleeding is self-limiting, although cerebral compression and displacement of brain tissue can cause temporal lobe herniation. Symptoms classically begin with headache, drowsiness, restlessness or agitation, slowed cognition, and confusion. These symptoms worsen over time and progress to loss of consciousness, respiratory pattern changes, and pupillary dilation (i.e., the symptoms of temporal lobe herniation). Homonymous hemianopia (defective vision in either the right or the left field [see Fig. 16.13]), dysconjugate gaze, and gaze palsies also may occur.

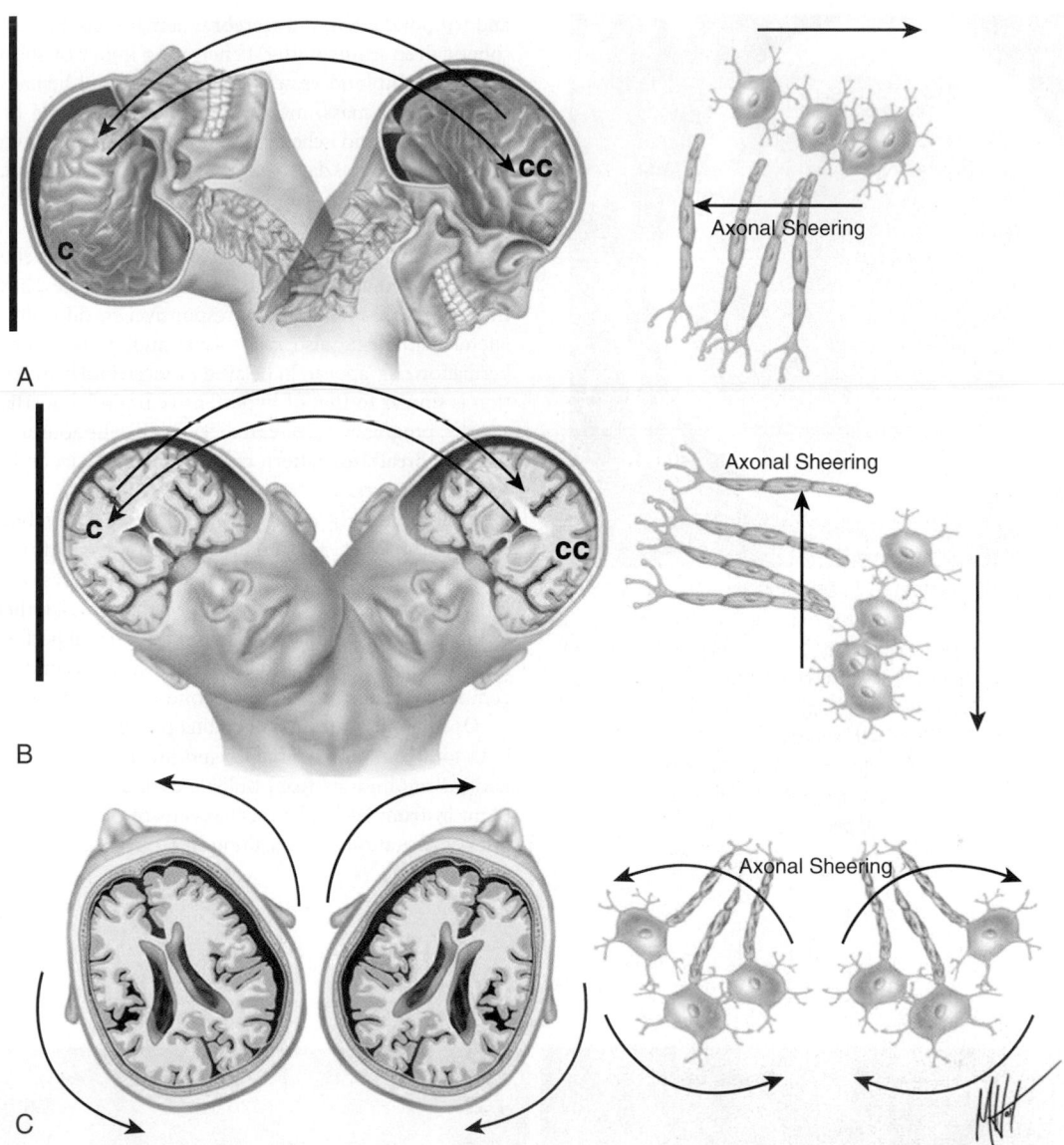

FIGURE 18.3 Coup and Contrecoup Brain Injury Following Blunt Trauma. A, Sagittal force causing coup *(c)* and contrecoup injury *(cc)*. **B,** Lateral force causing coup *(c)* and contrecoup *(cc)* injury. **C,** Axial or rotational injury with shearing of axons, particularly at base of brain. Acceleration/deceleration axonal shearing injury occurs throughout the brain (red and blue directional arrows in all three images). (Borrowed from Pascual JM, Preito R: Surgical management of severe closed head injury in adults. In Quinones-Hinojosa A, editor: *Schmidek and Sweet operative neurosurgical techniques*, ed 6, vol 2, Philadelphia, 2012, Saunders, pp 1513-1538. Originally redrawn from Adams JH: *Brain damage in fatal non-missile head injury in man.* In Braakman R, editor: *Handbook of clinical neurology, head injury*, vol 13, Amsterdam, 1990, Elsevier Science Publishers BV, pp 43-63; Gennarelli TA et al: *Ann Neurol* 12:564-574, 1982.)

Subacute subdural hematomas develop more slowly, often over 48 hours to 2 weeks. Bridging veins (extending from the dura into the surface of the brain) tear, causing both rapidly and subacutely developing subdural hematomas, although torn cortical veins or venous sinuses and contused tissue also may be the source (Fig. 18.5). They occur more commonly in older adults and those who abuse alcohol because they have some degree of brain atrophy with a subsequent increase in the size of the extradural space. These subdural hematomas act like expanding masses, increasing ICP that eventually compresses the bleeding vessels. Brain herniation can result.

Chronic subdural hematomas develop over weeks to months. The existing subdural space contains the liquefied clot from the acute bleed and/or accumulation of blood from a leaking vein. A vascular membrane

forms around the hematoma in approximately 2 weeks (Fig. 18.6). Of those individuals affected by chronic subdural hematomas, 80% have chronic headaches and tenderness over the hematoma on palpation. They may have confusion, memory loss, or coma, difficulty speaking or swallowing, and weakness with difficulty walking, loss of sensation, or seizures. Chronic subdural hematomas require a craniotomy to evacuate the gelatinous blood and to prevent brain herniation. Percutaneous drainage for chronic subdural hematomas has proven successful; however, reaccumulation often occurs. Subarachnoid hemorrhage is presented in the section on Subarachnoid Hemorrhage.

Intracerebral hematomas (bleeding within the brain) occur in 2% to 3% of head injuries, may be single or multiple, and are associated with contusions. Although most are commonly located in the frontal

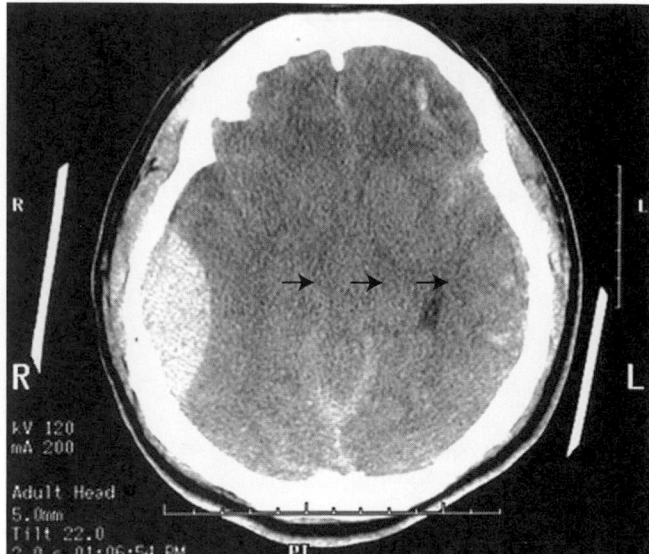

FIGURE 18.4 Epidural Hematoma, CT Image. Note the large right epidural hematoma with a lens-shaped outline as the smooth dura becomes indented against the underlying cortex on the right lateral aspect of the cerebrum. The epidural hematoma is confined within an area bounded by cranial sutures where the dura is firmly adherent to the skull. Note the mass effect with effacement of the lateral ventricles and the shift of midline to the left *(arrows)*. In this case the individual fell from a height and struck the right side of the head, severing the middle meningeal artery. This epidural hematoma collected within hours. *CT,* Computed tomography. (From Klatt EC: *Robbins and Cotran atlas of pathology,* ed 3, Philadelphia, 2015, Saunders.)

and temporal lobes, intracerebral hematomas may occur in the hemispheric deep white matter. Penetrating injury or shearing forces traumatize small blood vessels. The intracerebral hematoma then acts as an expanding mass, increasing ICP, compressing brain tissues, and causing edema and ischemia (Fig. 18.7). Delayed intracerebral hematomas may appear 3 to 10 days after the head injury. Intracerebral hematomas also can occur with nontraumatic brain injury, such as hemorrhagic stroke (see the section on Hemorrhagic Stroke).

Intracerebral hematomas cause a decreasing level of consciousness. Coma or a confusional state from other injuries, however, can make the cause of this increasing unresponsiveness difficult to detect. Contralateral hemiplegia also may occur and, as ICP rises, temporal lobe herniation may appear. In delayed intracerebral hematoma, the presentation is similar to that of hypertensive brain hemorrhage with sudden, rapidly progressive decreased level of consciousness with pupillary dilation; breathing pattern changes; hemiplegia; and bilateral positive Babinski reflexes.

History and physical examination help to establish the diagnosis, and CT scan, MRI, and cerebral angiography confirm it. Evacuation of a singular intracerebral hematoma has only occasionally been helpful, mostly for subcortical white matter hematomas. Otherwise, treatment is directed at reducing ICP to maintain cerebral perfusion pressure and allowing the hematoma to reabsorb slowly. Secondary brain injury is common (see the section on Secondary Brain Injury).

Open brain trauma (trauma that penetrates the dura mater) produces both focal and diffuse injuries and includes compound skull fractures and missile injuries (e.g., bullets, rocks, shell fragments, knives, and blunt instruments). The mechanisms of open brain trauma are crush injury (laceration and crushing of tissue touched by the missile) and

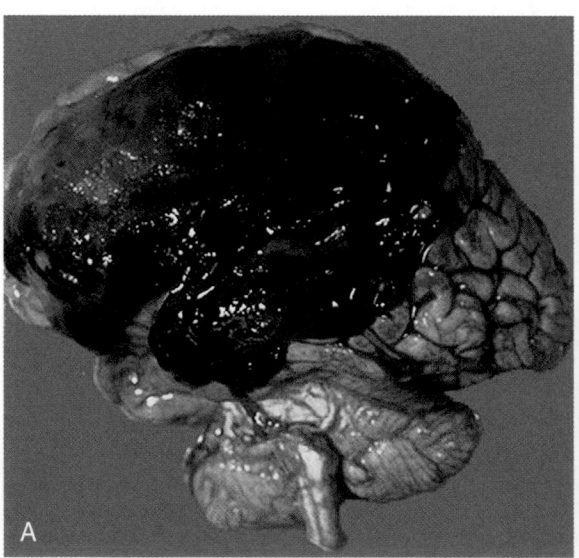
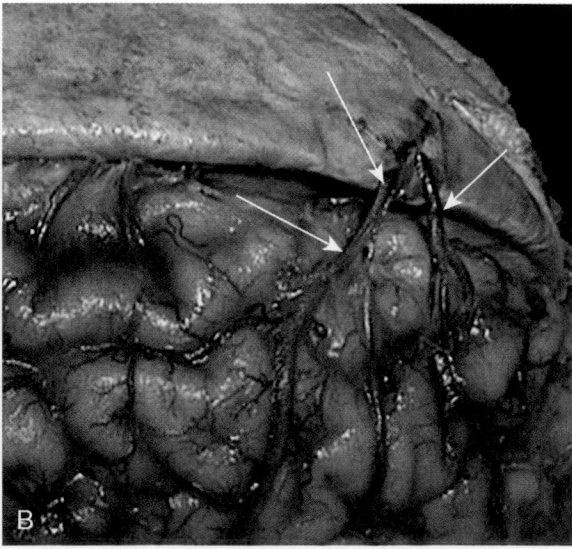

FIGURE 18.5 Subdural Hematoma, Gross, and Bridging Veins, Gross. A large subdural hematoma **(A)** is seen in the frontoparietal region. A subdural hematoma forms after head trauma that severs the bridging veins from dura to brain, shown in the right panel **(B),** where the dura has been folded back to reveal the normal appearance of the bridging veins that extend across to the superior aspect of the cerebral hemispheres. Older adults and the very young are at greater risk because their cerebral veins are more vulnerable to injury. Because the bleeding is venous, blood collects over hours to weeks, with variable onset of symptoms. Because the blood collects beneath the dura, a subdural hematoma can be seen to cross the region of cranial sutures. (From Klatt EC: *Robbins and Cotran atlas of pathology,* ed 3, Philadelphia, 2015, Saunders.)

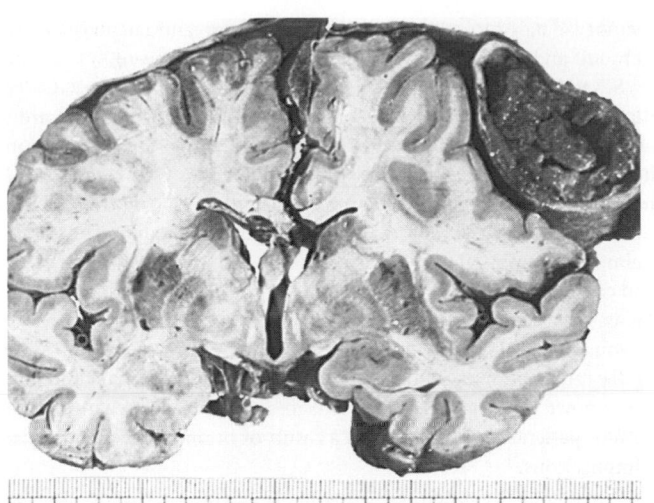

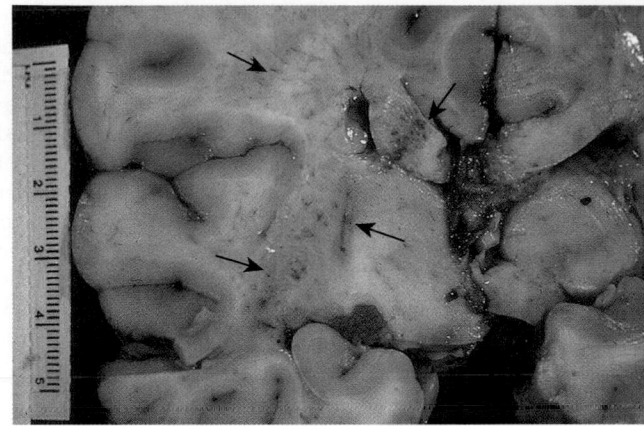

FIGURE 18.8 Diffuse Axonal Injury. Gross photograph demonstrating characteristic hemorrhage lesions within the corpus callosum. (Courtesy Walter Kemp, MD, Department of Pathology, University of Texas Southwestern Medical School, Dallas. From Kumar V, Cotran RS, Robbins SL: *Robbins basic pathology,* ed 7, Philadelphia, 2003, Saunders.)

FIGURE 18.6 Chronic Subdural Hematoma. Compression of underlying brain and lateral ventricle. Note the capsule around the hematoma. (From Kissane JM, editor: *Anderson's pathology,* ed 9, St Louis, 1993, Mosby.)

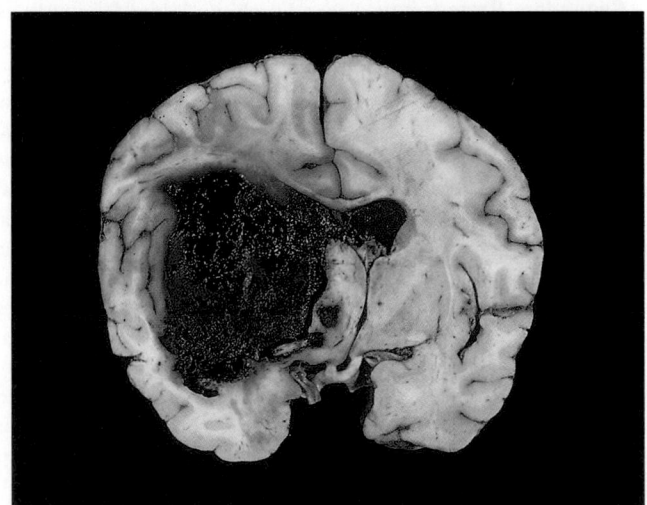

FIGURE 18.7 Acute Intracerebral Hemorrhage. A fresh hematoma has disrupted and expanded the left cerebral hemisphere, causing the midline structures to shift to the right. Uncontrolled hypertension is an important cause of this catastrophic lesion. (From Kumar V, Cotran RS, Robbins SL: *Robbins basic pathology,* ed 7, Philadelphia, 2003, Saunders.)

remove blood clots and debris, thereby reducing ICP. ICP also is managed with dehydrating agents, osmotic diuretics, or a combination of these drugs.

A compound fracture may be diagnosed through physical examination, skull radiographs, or both. Basilar skull fracture is determined on the basis of clinical findings (i.e., involvement of cranial nerves, ecchymosis around the eyes, ears and nose or spinal fluid leaking from the ear or nose.). Skull radiographs often do not demonstrate the fracture, although intracranial air or air in the sinuses on radiograph, CT, or MRI is indirect evidence of a basilar skull fracture, A compound fracture is débrided and bone grafts may be required. Antibiotics are administered after surgery. Bed rest and close observation for meningitis and other complications are prescribed for a basilar skull fracture.

Diffuse Axonal Injury. Diffuse axonal injury (DAI) involves neurons in widespread areas of the brain and occurs with all severities of brain injury. Mechanical effects from high levels of acceleration and deceleration, such as whiplash, and rotational forces, cause stretching and shearing of delicate axonal fibers and white matter tracts that project to the cerebral cortex (see Fig. 18.3). The most severe axonal injuries are located more peripheral to the brainstem, causing extensive cognitive and affective impairments. Axonal damage reduces the speed of information processing and responding and disrupts cognitive function.[5]

Pathophysiologically, axonal damage can be seen only with an electron microscope and involves numerous axons, either alone or in conjunction with actual tissue tears. Advanced imaging techniques using MRI are assisting to define areas and extent of injury. Areas where axons and small blood vessels are torn appear as small hemorrhages (Fig. 18.8), located particularly in the parasagittal white matter near the cerebral cortex, corpus callosum, and brainstem and at the superior cerebellar peduncle.[6] More damaged axons are visible 12 hours to several days after the initial injury. The severity of DAI correlates with the amount of shearing force. DAI is not associated with intracranial hypertension immediately after injury. However, acute brain swelling from increased intravascular blood flow within the brain, loss of cerebrovascular autoregulation, vasodilation, and increased cerebral blood volume is often seen and can result in death. DAI may induce long-term neurodegenerative processes, with progressive axonal pathology that may continue for years after injury and may play a role in the development of chronic traumatic encephalopathy and Alzheimer disease-like pathologic changes.[7]

stretch injury (damage of blood vessels and nerves not directly contacted, occurring as a result of stretching).

A compound skull fracture opens a communication between the cranial contents and the environment and should be investigated whenever there are lacerations of the scalp, tympanic membrane, a sinus, an eye, or mucous membranes. Such fractures may involve the cranial vault or the base of the skull (basilar skull fracture). A basilar skull fracture can involve the temporal, sphenoid, and occipital bones. Severity of brain damage is related to the severity of skull fracture. Infection is a significant complication. Bone fragments or debris from projectiles may contuse brain tissues or lacerate blood vessels.

Most victims lose consciousness with open-head injury. The depth and duration of the coma are related to the location of injury, extent of damage, and amount of bleeding. Open brain injury often requires débridement of the traumatized tissues to prevent infection and to

There is currently a lack of consensus regarding the terminology to grade or define the clinical syndromes associated with TBI, and several categories exist: mild concussion and classic concussion, and mild, moderate, and severe TBI.[8-13] The symptoms associated with grades of concussion or TBI are often the same. Concussion has been described as a set of symptoms with or without neuropathologic damage that may or may not involve loss of consciousness following TBI.[14,15] However with new imaging techniques and discovery of molecular markers associated with mild and moderate TBI, it is likely that DAI occurs in mild, moderate, and severe TBI[16] (see *What's New?* Biomarkers and Concussion). Methods of grading severity of TBI are arbitrary, with the GCS most commonly used along with clinical evaluation of neurologic function. Recommendations are available to direct imaging of TBI.[17] The discussion presented here considers the severity of grades of concussion and TBI as the same.

WHAT'S NEW?

Biomarkers and Concussion

Biomarker research has focused on proteins abundant in cells impacted by TBI. Glial fibrillary acidic protein (GFAP) and ubiquitin C-terminal hydrolase L1 (UCH-L1) have been studied in both animals and humans and show promise for diagnosis of suspected TBI and mild to moderate concussion. Both markers cross the blood-brain barrier after TBI and are detectable in the blood. Subjects were assessed for blunt head trauma with loss of consciousness, amnesia, or disorientation and a Glasgow Coma Scale score of 9 to 15. Both GFAP and UCH-L1 were detectible within 1 hour of injury. GFAP peaks in 20 hours and declines slowly over 72 hours. UCH-L1 rises rapidly and peaks in 8 hours. The markers distinguished mild to moderate concussion with and without a neurosurgical intervention and provided values consistent with CT findings with 97% accuracy. The ultimate goal is to use the biomarkers for diagnosis, for monitoring progression of injury and recovery, and avoid radiation exposing CT scans, particularly in children with TBI.

Data from Kulbe JR, Geddes JW: *Exp Neurol* 275 Pt 3:334-352, 2016; Papa L et al: *JAMA Neurol* 73(5):551-560, 2016; Mannix R et al: *J Neurotrauma* 31(11):1072-1075, 2014.

Mild traumatic brain injury (mild concussion) is characterized by immediate but transitory clinical manifestations without loss of consciousness, or loss of consciousness that is momentary or less than 30 minutes. Most blunt trauma injuries cause mild TBI.[18] The GCS is 13 to 15.[19] Posttraumatic anterograde amnesia also may exist transiently to less than 24 hours.[20] There may be no findings with diagnostic imaging. Persons may experience headaches, nausea and vomiting, confusion, disorientation, attention deficit, dizziness, and impaired ability to concentrate for days after the injury. Diffuse axonal injury, metabolic impairment, alterations in neural activation, and cerebral blood flow perturbations can occur and may contribute to acute symptomatology. Lesions may be detected with advanced MRI imaging. Biomarkers are under investigation to assist with diagnosis of mild TBI.[18]

Moderate traumatic brain injury (moderate cerebral concussion) is any loss of consciousness lasting more than 30 minutes, accompanied by posttraumatic anterograde amnesia lasting 24 hours or more. A GCS between 8 and 13 is classified as moderate TBI. A basal skull fracture may be present with moderate TBI, but there is no brainstem injury. There is transitory decerebration or decortication (see Fig. 17.6) with unconsciousness lasting days or weeks. The person is confused and experiences a long period of posttraumatic amnesia. There often are permanent deficits in selective attention, vigilance, detection, working memory, data processing, vision or perception, and language, as well as mood and affect changes ranging from mild to severe.

Severe traumatic brain injury (severe concussion) is a GCS less than 8 associated with brainstem signs (pupillary reaction, cardiac and respiratory symptoms, posturing) and intracranial contusions, hematomas, or lacerations. Loss of consciousness lasts more than 24 hours. The person experiences immediate autonomic dysfunction that resolves in a few weeks. Increased ICP appears 4 to 6 days after injury. Pulmonary complications occur frequently, with profound sensorimotor and cognitive system deficits. Severely compromised coordinated movements and verbal and written communication, inability to learn and reason, and inability to modulate behavior also are evident. Severe injury causes permanent neurologic deficits (20% of adults) and it has been shown that up to 14% remain in a vegetative state, and 20% to 40% of patients end up dying as a result of brain injury or secondary complications.[21]

The goal of treatment is to maintain cerebral perfusion and oxygenation, promote neuroprotection, and mitigate long-term neurologic deficits. The Corticosteroid Randomisation After Significant Head Injury (CRASH) trial showed corticosteroids increase mortality with acute TBI; consequently these drugs are no longer used. Guidelines are available to direct evaluation and treatment.[18,22]

Secondary Brain Injury. **Secondary brain injury** is an indirect result of primary brain injury (see Fig. 18.1), including trauma and stroke syndromes. Systemic and cerebral processes are contributing factors. Systemic processes include hypotension, hypoxia, anemia, hypoglycemia, hyperglycemia, and hypercapnia or hypocapnia. Cerebral contributions include inflammation, oxidative stress, alterations in the blood-brain barrier, excitotoxicity, cerebral edema, increased intracranial pressure (IICP), decreased cerebral perfusion pressure, cerebral ischemia, and brain herniation. Cellular and molecular brain damage from the effects of primary injury develops hours to days later. Cerebrovascular autoregulation (vasoconstriction or vasodilation in response to increases or decreases in cerebral perfusion pressure) is impaired after brain injury and may be transient or persistent with alterations in CO_2 reactivity (i.e., CO_2 vasodilation). Vasospasm commonly occurs, contributing to brain hypoperfusion, and is caused by chronic depolarization of vascular smooth muscle, release of endothelin (vasoconstrictor), and decreased availability of nitric oxide (vasodilator).

Ischemia contributes to excitotoxicity with release of excitatory neurotransmitters, such as glutamate that escapes from stretched and injured neurons. They cause cellular influx of calcium and stimulate neuronal hyperexcitability by depolarizing the membrane potential (excitotoxicity). A hypermetabolic state, poor perfusion, influx of inflammatory mediators, fluctuations in cellular sodium and potassium ion channels, and mitochondrial failure all contribute to cytotoxic edema, axonal swelling, and neuronal death.[23]

Mitochondrial failure, anaerobic metabolism, lactic acid production, and increased levels of reactive oxygen species (ROS), phospholipases, and other enzymes damage proteins and the phospholipid components of cell and organelle membranes. Cell swelling, vacuolization, and, ultimately, necrotic or programmed cell death (apoptosis) occur.[24] These events lead to failure of the capillary blood-brain barrier and *vasogenic edema*. The influx of sodium and water results in intracellular cytotoxic edema in neurons, astrocytes, and microglia irrespective of the integrity of the vascular endothelial wall. Edema increases ICP, contributing to tissue hypoxia and cerebral ischemia. Inflammation occurs immediately and persists for weeks. Inflammation is critical for wound healing; immune cells, including neutrophils, macrophages, and T-cell lymphocytes, need to infiltrate injured tissue and clear debris, thus promoting formation of scar tissue. However, an overactive response leads to occlusion of the microvasculature with leukocytes and platelets. The release of inflammatory cytokines (e.g., tumor necrosis factor-alpha [TNF-α], interleukins, and interferons), proteases, free radicals, prostaglandins, and complement proteins alters the blood-brain barrier and causes vasoconstriction, brain edema, IICP, reduced cerebral perfusion, and ischemia, aggravating secondary brain injury.[25] Activation of astrocytes and microglia contributes to persistent neuroinflammation, alters the blood-brain barrier, and can cause progressive neurodegeneration that occurs over weeks after traumatic injury.[26]

Intracranial hemorrhage, whether traumatic or related to a stroke syndrome, may contribute to secondary brain injury. The bleeding is often accompanied by IICP, ischemia, oxidative damage, and vasogenic and cytotoxic edema as previously described. In addition, the vascular injury can cause activation of platelets, which contribute to vasoconstriction in large arteries and vasodilation in small arteries with spreading cortical ischemia. Activated platelets also trigger the release of free radicals from granulocytes, enhancing oxidative stress. Vascular injury causes coagulation disorders from release of increased amounts of tissue factor from endothelial cells, which initiates the coagulation cascade and overwhelms the normal factors that control coagulation. Free heme and free iron are released from red blood cells, and both cause the induction of free radicals, lipid peroxidation, and further nerve damage.[27]

The management of secondary brain trauma includes removal of hematomas and management of hypotension, hypoxemia, anemia, ICP, fluid and electrolyte balance, body temperature, ventilation, and nutrition. Numerous agents are under investigation and may be neuroprotective by decreasing excitotoxicity, neuroinflammation, apoptosis, mitochondrial failure, blood-brain barrier disruption, edema, and other mechanisms of secondary injury.[28,29] Progress is difficult because of lack of predictive biomarkers and drugs that can cross the blood-brain barrier. Fluid and nutrition management have emerged as critically important in the care of individuals with severe brain injury.[30] Long-term recovery can be influenced by systemic complications, such as pneumonia, fever, infections, and immobility.

Complications of Traumatic Brain Injury. Many complications are associated with TBI and are related to the severity of injury and the parts of the brain that are affected. Altered states of consciousness can range from confusion to deep coma (see Table 17.3). Cognitive deficits, hydrocephalus, and sensory-motor disorders, including pain, paresis, and loss of coordination, may be present. Three of the most common posttraumatic brain syndromes are summarized next.

Postconcussion syndrome occurs with mild TBI including sports concussion.[31] Symptoms are nonspecific and include headache, dizziness, fatigue, nervousness or anxiety, irritability, insomnia, photophobia, depression, inability to concentrate, and forgetfulness, and may last for weeks to months. Treatment entails reassurance and symptomatic relief in addition to 24 hours of close observation after the concussion in the event bleeding or swelling in the brain occurs. Symptoms requiring further evaluation and treatment include drowsiness or confusion, nausea or vomiting, severe headache, memory deficit, seizures, drainage of CSF from the ear or nose, weakness or loss of feeling in the extremities, asymmetry of the pupils, and double vision. Guidelines for the management of pediatric and adult mild TBI are available.[32-34] Guidelines also have been published for the management of sports-related concussion.[35,36]

Posttraumatic seizures (epilepsy) occur in about 10% of TBIs, with the highest risk among open brain injuries.[37] Seizures can occur early, within days, and up to 2 to 5 years or longer after the trauma. Causal mechanisms are poorly understood, and cellular and molecular changes in the brain associated with injury and repair, such as sprouting of new neurons with hyperexcitability and decreases in GABAergic inhibition, may cause the hyperexcitable state that leads to epileptogenesis. Seizure prevention using drugs, such as phenytoin, is initiated for moderate to severe TBI at the time of injury. Neuromodulation with implantable devices is under evaluation. Clinical trials are ongoing to test drugs that prevent the development of posttraumatic seizures.[38]

Chronic traumatic encephalopathy (CTE) (previously called *dementia pugilistica*) is a progressive dementing disease that develops with repeated brain injury associated with sporting events, blast injuries in soldiers, or work-related head trauma. Tau neurofibrillary tangles are present in the brain. CTE is associated with violent behaviors, loss of control, depression, suicide, memory loss, and cognitive change. Research is in progress to discover the mechanistic link between neurotrauma and CTE. It is diagnosed from history and clinical evaluation, and at autopsy.[39]

Spinal Cord and Vertebral Injury

Approximately 282,000 people were living with spinal cord injury (SCI) in the United States, with approximately 17,000 new cases in 2016. About 80% are males, and the average age is 42 years. Since 2010, the causes include vehicular crashes (38%), falls (30%), violence (14%), and sports (9%). The extent of injury has been 45% incomplete quadriplegia, 14% complete quadriplegia, 21% incomplete paraplegia, and 20% complete paraplegia.[40]

◆PATHOPHYSIOLOGY. Primary spinal cord injury occurs with the initial mechanical trauma and immediate tissue destruction from shearing, compression, or penetration. Injuries to the cord are summarized in Table 18.2. Primary spinal cord injury also can occur if an injured spine is not adequately immobilized immediately following injury. Primary spinal cord injury may occur in the absence of vertebral fracture or dislocation from longitudinal stretching of the cord with or without flexion or extension of the vertebral column, or both. The stretching causes altered axon transport, edema, myelin degeneration, and retrograde or wallerian degeneration (see Chapter 15).

Secondary spinal cord injury is a pathophysiologic cascade of vascular, cellular, and biochemical events that begins within a few minutes after injury and continues for weeks. Edema, ischemia, excitotoxicity (excessive stimulation by excitatory neurotransmitters such as glutamate), inflammation, oxidative damage, and activation of necrotic and apoptotic cell death signal events similar to those previously described for TBI[41,42] (see the Secondary Brain Injury section).

With secondary spinal cord injury, microscopic hemorrhages appear in the central gray matter and pia-arachnoid, increasing in size until the entire gray matter is hemorrhagic and necrotic. Edema in the white matter occurs, impairing the microcirculation of the cord. Hemorrhages and edema are followed by loss of autoregulation and reduced vascular perfusion and development of ischemic areas, which are maximal at the level of injury and two cord segments above and below it. Cellular and subcellular alterations with myelin disruption, axonal degeneration, and tissue necrosis occur. Impaired perfusion is aggravated by systemic responses, including neurogenic or hemorrhagic shock, and dysrhythmias. Cord swelling increases the individual's degree of dysfunction, making it difficult to distinguish functions permanently lost from those temporarily impaired. In the cervical region, cord swelling may be life-threatening. Diaphragm function may be impaired because phrenic nerves exit at C3 to C5. Cardiovascular and respiratory functions mediated by the medulla oblongata can be lost. Efforts are in progress to identify biomarkers that reflect severity of injury and guide treatment.[43]

Circulation in the white matter tracts of the spinal cord returns to normal in about 24 hours, but gray matter circulation remains altered. Phagocytes appear 36 to 48 hours after injury, and microglia proliferate with altered astrocytes promoting inflammation.[44] Red blood cells then begin to disintegrate, and resorption of hemorrhages and edema begins. Degenerating axons are engulfed by macrophages in the first 10 days after injury. The traumatized cord is replaced by acellular collagenous tissue, usually in 3 to 4 weeks. Meninges thicken as part of the scarring process.

Vertebral injuries result from acceleration, deceleration, rotation, or deformation forces at impact. These forces cause vertebral fractures, dislocations, and bone fragments that can cause compression or exert traction (tension) on the tissues, or shear tissues so they slide into one another (Figs. 18.9 through 18.12). Vertebral injuries can be classified as (1) simple fracture—a single break usually affecting transverse or spinous processes; (2) compressed (wedged) vertebral fracture, that is, a vertebral body compressed anteriorly; (3) comminuted (burst) fracture—vertebral body shattered into several fragments; and (4) dislocation.

The vertebrae fracture readily with direct and indirect trauma. When the supporting ligaments are torn, the vertebrae move out of alignment, and dislocations occur. A horizontal force moves the vertebrae straight forward; if the individual is in a flexed position at the time of injury, the vertebrae are then in an angulated position. Flexion and extension injuries may result in dislocations. (Mechanisms of vertebral injury are presented in Table 18.3.) Vertebral injuries in adults occur most often at vertebrae C1-C2 (cervical), C4-C7, and T10 to L2 (thoracic-lumbar) (see Fig. 15.18), the most mobile portions of the vertebral column. The

TABLE 18.2	SPINAL CORD INJURIES
INJURY	**DESCRIPTION**
Cord concussion	Results in a temporary disruption of cord-mediated functions
Cord contusion	Bruising of the neural tissue causing swelling and temporary loss of cord-mediated functions
Cord compression	Pressure on the cord causing ischemia to tissues; must be relieved (decompressed) to prevent permanent damage to the spinal cord
Laceration	Tearing of the neural tissues of the spinal cord; may be reversible if only slight damage is sustained by the neural tissues; may result in permanent loss of cord-mediated functions if spinal tracts are disrupted
Transection	Severing of the spinal cord, causing permanent loss of function
Complete	All tracts in the spinal cord are completely disrupted; all cord-mediated functions below the transection are completely and permanently lost
Incomplete	Some tracts in the spinal cord remain intact, together with functions mediated by these tracts; has the potential for recovery although function is temporarily lost
Preserved sensation only	Some demonstrable sensation below the level of injury
Preserved motor nonfunctional	Preserved motor function without useful purpose; sensory function may or may not be preserved
Preserved motor functional	Preserved voluntary motor function that is functionally useful
Hemorrhage	Bleeding into the neural tissue because of blood vessel damage; usually no major loss of function
Damage or obstruction of spinal blood supply	Causes local ischemia

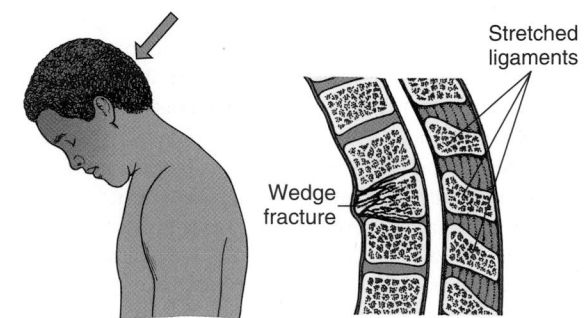

FIGURE 18.10 **Flexion Injury of the Spine.** Hyperflexion produces translation (subluxation) of vertebrae that compromises the central canal and compresses spinal cord parenchyma or vascular structures.

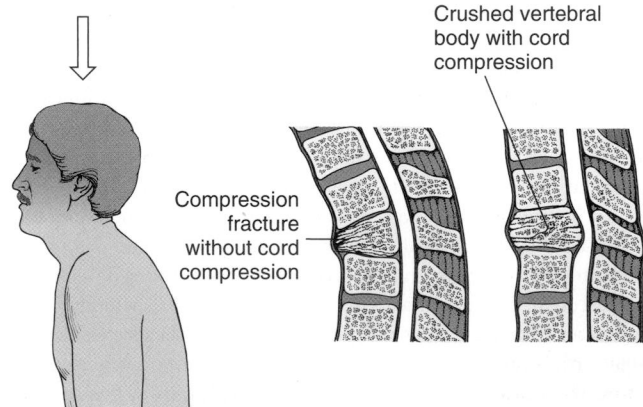

FIGURE 18.11 **Axial Compression Injuries of the Spine.** In axial compression injuries of spine, the spinal cord is contused directly by retropulsion of bone or disk material into the spinal canal.

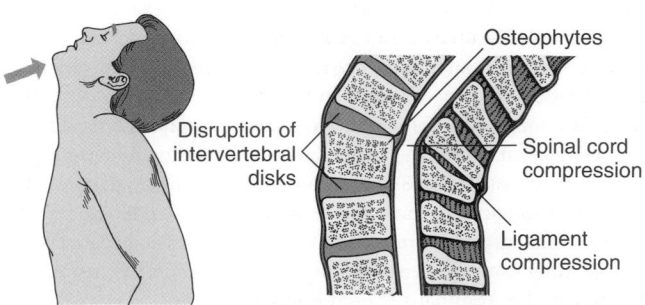

FIGURE 18.9 **Hyperextension Injuries of the Spine.** Hyperextension injuries of the spine can result in fracture or nonfracture injuries with spinal cord damage.

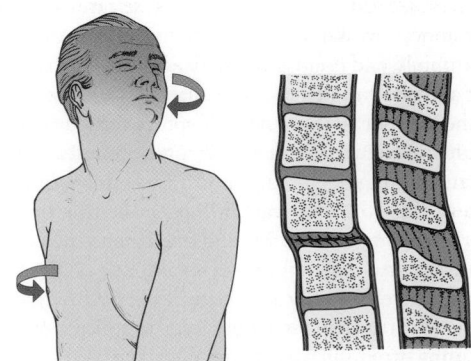

FIGURE 18.12 **Flexion-Rotation Injuries of the Spine.**

TABLE 18.3   MECHANISMS OF VERTEBRAL INJURY

MECHANISMS OF INJURY	VERTEBRAL INJURY	FORCES OF INJURY	LOCATION OF INJURY
Hyperextension	Fracture and dislocation of posterior elements such as spinous processes, transverse processes, laminae, pedicles, or posterior ligaments	Results from forces of acceleration-deceleration and the sudden reduction in the anteroposterior diameter of the spinal cord	Cervical area
Hyperflexion	Fracture or dislocation of the vertebral bodies, disks, or ligaments	Results from sudden and excessive force that propels the neck forward or causes an exaggerated lateral movement of the neck to one side	Cervical area
Vertical compression (axonal loading)	Shattering fractures	Results from a force applied along an axis from the top of the cranium through the vertebral bodies	T12-L2
Rotational forces (flexion-rotation)	Ruptures support ligaments in addition to producing fractures	Adds shearing force to acceleration-deceleration forces	Cervical area

spinal cord occupies most of the vertebral canal in the cervical and lumbar regions, so it also can be easily injured in these locations.

CLINICAL MANIFESTATIONS. Spinal shock develops immediately after injury because of loss of continuous tonic discharge from the brain or brainstem and inhibition of suprasegmental impulses caused by cord hemorrhage, edema, or anatomic transection. All motor, sensory, reflex, and autonomic functions cease below any transected area and may cease below concussive, contused, compressed, or ischemic areas. There is flaccid paralysis, absence of sensation, loss of bladder and rectal control, transient drop in blood pressure, and poor venous circulation. The condition also results in disturbed thermal control because the sympathetic nervous system is damaged. The hypothalamus cannot regulate body heat through vasoconstriction and increased metabolism; therefore the individual assumes the temperature of the air (poikilo-thermia).[45] Spinal shock generally lasts 7 to 20 days, with a range of a few days to 3 months. It terminates with the reappearance of reflex activity, hyperreflexia, spasticity, and reflex emptying of the bladder. Table 18.4 summarizes the clinical manifestations of spinal cord injury.

Neurogenic shock, also called vasogenic shock, occurs with cervical or upper thoracic cord injury above T6 and may be seen in addition to spinal shock. Neurogenic shock is caused by the absence of sympathetic activity through loss of supraspinal control and unopposed parasympathetic tone mediated by the intact vagus nerve and may last up to 5 weeks after injury. Symptoms include vasodilation, hypotension, bradycardia, and hypothermia (failure of body temperature regulation). Neurogenic shock may be complicated by hypovolemic or cardiogenic shock if there is concurrent heart failure or blood loss[46] (see Chapter 33).

Continued loss of motor and sensory function depends on the extent and level of injury. Paralysis of the lower half of the body with both legs involved is termed *paraplegia*. Paralysis involving all four extremities is termed *quadriplegia* (tetraplegia). In complete quadriplegia the level of injury is above C6, and all upper extremity function is lost. In incomplete quadriplegia, function at or above C6 is preserved, leaving the shoulder, upper arm, and some forearm muscle control intact. With acceleration injuries the greatest stress point is C4-C5. With a deceleration force the greatest stress point is at C5-C6. The initial clinical manifestations associated with acute spinal cord injury are (1) rapid loss of voluntary movements in body parts below the level of injury, (2) loss of sensations in the lower extremities and possibly lower trunk (depending on the level of injury), and (3) loss of spinal and autonomic reflexes below the level of injury. The duration of this areflexic state is highly variable. In most persons, reflex activity returns in 1 to 2 weeks. Return of spinal neuron excitability occurs slowly. Depending on the degree of damage, either of the following can occur: (1) motor, sensory, reflex,

and autonomic functions return to normal; or (2) autonomic neural activity in the isolated segment develops. Spasticity is common with hyperreflexia, clonus, and painful muscle spasms. Sometimes after several months, episodes of autonomic hyperreflexia occur.

Autonomic hyperreflexia (dysreflexia) is a syndrome of sudden, life-threatening massive reflex sympathetic discharge associated with spinal cord injury at level T6 or above where descending inhibition is blocked (Fig. 18.13). It may occur after spinal shock resolves and can be a recurrent complication. Characteristics include paroxysmal hypertension (up to 300 mmHg, systolic), a pounding headache, blurred vision, sweating above the level of the lesion with flushing of the skin, nasal congestion, nausea, piloerection caused by pilomotor spasm, and bradycardia (30 to 40 beats/min). The symptoms may develop singly or in combination. The condition can cause serious complications (stroke, seizures, myocardial ischemia, and death) and requires immediate treatment.[47]

In autonomic hyperreflexia, sensory receptors below the level of the cord lesion are stimulated. The intact autonomic nervous system reflexively responds with an arteriolar spasm that increases blood pressure. Baroreceptors in the cerebral vessels, the carotid sinus, and the aorta sense the hypertension and stimulate the parasympathetic system. The heart rate decreases, but the visceral and peripheral vessels do not dilate because efferent impulses cannot pass through the cord.

The most common cause is a distended bladder or rectum; however, any sensory stimulation (i.e., skin or pain receptors) can elicit autonomic hyperreflexia. Emptying of the bladder or bowel usually relieves the syndrome, and the head of the bed should be elevated. Drug therapy, including nifedipine (a calcium channel blocker) and nitrates (e.g., nitroglycerine paste or sublingual nitroglycerine), may be required to lower blood pressure and reduce complications. Bladder, bowel, and skin care management are important preventive strategies. Education of the individual and family regarding triggers and acute management is important, as is wearing a medic alert tag.[48]

EVALUATION AND TREATMENT. Diagnosis of spinal cord injury is made on the basis of physical examination and imaging studies (e.g., MRI). Neurogenic shock must be differentiated from other kinds of shock (i.e., hypovolemic shock). For a suspected or confirmed vertebral fracture or dislocation, regardless of the presence or absence of spinal cord injury, the immediate intervention is immobilization of the spine to prevent further injury. Decompression and surgical fixation should be performed early. High-dose methylprednisolone steroid therapy has been given within 8 hours of the time of injury to decrease secondary cord injury. There are no clinical trials indicating this treatment is effective, and more research is needed.[49] Therapeutic hypothermia (32°C to 34°C; 89.6° to 93.2°F) has shown some encouraging evidence for

TABLE 18.4   CLINICAL MANIFESTATIONS OF SPINAL CORD INJURY

STAGE	MANIFESTATIONS
Spinal Shock Stage	
Complete spinal cord transection	Loss of motor function 　1. Quadriplegia with injuries of cervical spinal cord 　2. Paraplegia with injuries of thoracic spinal cord Muscle flaccidity Loss of all reflexes below level of injury Loss of pain, temperature, touch, pressure, and proprioception below level of injury Pain at site of injury caused by a zone of hyperesthesia above the injury Atonic bladder and bowel Paralytic ileus with distention Loss of vasomotor tone in lower body parts; low and unstable blood pressure Loss of perspiration below level of injury Loss or extreme depression of genital reflexes such as penile erection and bulbocavernosus reflex Dry and pale skin, possible ulceration over bony prominences Respiratory impairment
Partial spinal cord transection	Asymmetric flaccid motor paralysis below level of injury Asymmetric reflex loss Preservation of some sensation below level of injury Vasomotor instability less severe than with complete cord transection Bowel and bladder impairment less severe than that seen with complete cord transection Preservation of ability to perspire in some portions of the body below level of injury *Brown-Séquard syndrome* (associated with penetrating injuries, hyperextension and flexion, locked facets, and compression fractures) 　1. Ipsilateral paralysis or paresis below level of injury 　2. Ipsilateral loss of touch, pressure, vibration, and position senses below level of injury 　3. Contralateral loss of pain and temperature sensations below level of injury *Central cervical cord syndrome* (acute cord compression between bony bars or spurs anteriorly and thickened ligamentum flavum posteriorly associated with hyperextension) 　1. Motor deficits in upper extremities, especially hands; more dense than in lower extremities 　2. Varying degrees of bladder dysfunction *Burning hand syndrome* (variant of central cord syndrome; half of cases have an underlying spine fracture/dislocation present) 　1. Severe burning paresthesias and dysesthesias in the hands and/or feet *Anterior cord syndrome* (compromise of anterior spinal artery by occlusion or pressure effect of disk) 　1. Loss of motor function below level of injury 　2. Loss of pain and temperature sensations below level of injury 　3. Touch, pressure, position, and vibration senses intact *Posterior cord syndrome* (associated with hyperextension injuries with fractures of vertebral arch) 　1. Impaired light touch and proprioception *Conus medullaris syndrome* (compression injury at T12 from disk herniation or burst fracture of body of T12) 　1. Flaccid paralysis of legs 　2. Flaccid paralysis of anal sphincter 　3. Variable sensory deficits *Cauda equina syndrome* (compression of nerve roots below L1 caused by fracture and dislocation of spine or large posterocentral intervertebral disk herniation) 　1. Lower extremity motor deficits 　2. Variable sensorimotor dysfunction 　3. Variable reflex dysfunction 　4. Variable bladder, bowel, and sexual dysfunction *Syndrome of neuropraxia* (seen as post–athletic injury, associated with congenital spinal stenosis) 　1. Dramatic but transient neurologic deficits including quadriplegia *Horner syndrome* (injury to preganglionic sympathetic trunk or postganglionic sympathetic neurons of superior cervical ganglion) 　1. Ipsilateral pupil smaller than contralateral pupil 　2. Sunken ipsilateral eyeball 　3. Ptosis of affected eyeball 　4. Lack of perspiration on ipsilateral side of face

TABLE 18.4	CLINICAL MANIFESTATIONS OF SPINAL CORD INJURY—cont'd
STAGE	**MANIFESTATIONS**
Heightened Reflex Activity Stage	Emergence of Babinski reflexes, possibly progressing to a triple reflex; possible development of still later flexor spasms
	Reappearance of ankle and knee reflexes, which become hyperactive
	Contraction of reflex detrusor muscle, leading to urinary incontinence
	Appearance of reflex defecation
	Mass reflex with flexion spasms, profuse sweating, piloerection, and bladder and occasional bowel emptying may be evoked by an autonomic stimulation of skin or from a full bladder
	Episodes of hypertension
	Defective heat-induced sweating
	Eventual development of extensor reflexes, first in muscles of hip and thigh, later in leg
	Possible paresthesias below level of transaction: dull, burning pain in lower back, abdomen, buttocks, and perineum

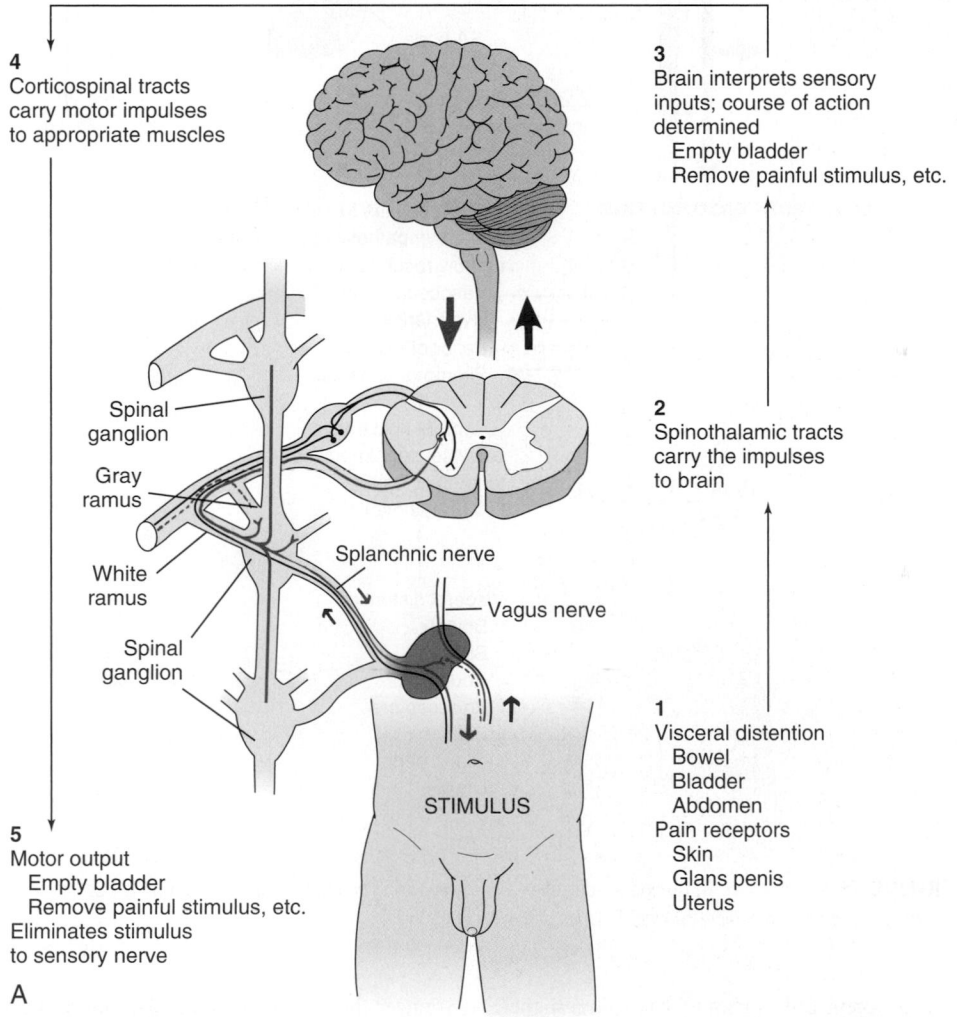

FIGURE 18.13 Autonomic Hyperreflexia. **A,** Normal response pathway.

improved outcomes, particularly for cervical cord injuries, but more research is needed.[50] Clinical trials are in progress to treat acute spinal cord injury, including cell-based therapies, immune modulators, vasculature selective treatments, functional electrical stimulation, and tissue engineering (hydrogels, nanofibers, and gene therapy).[51,52]

Nutrition; lung function; skin integrity, particularly prevention of pressure ulcers; and bladder and bowel management must be addressed. Plans for rehabilitation require early consideration. Impairments are permanent because endogenous repair events fail to restore the damaged axonal circuits.

Degenerative Disorders of the Spine
Low Back Pain

Low back pain (LBP) affects the area between the lower rib cage and gluteal muscles and often radiates into the thighs. The percentage of

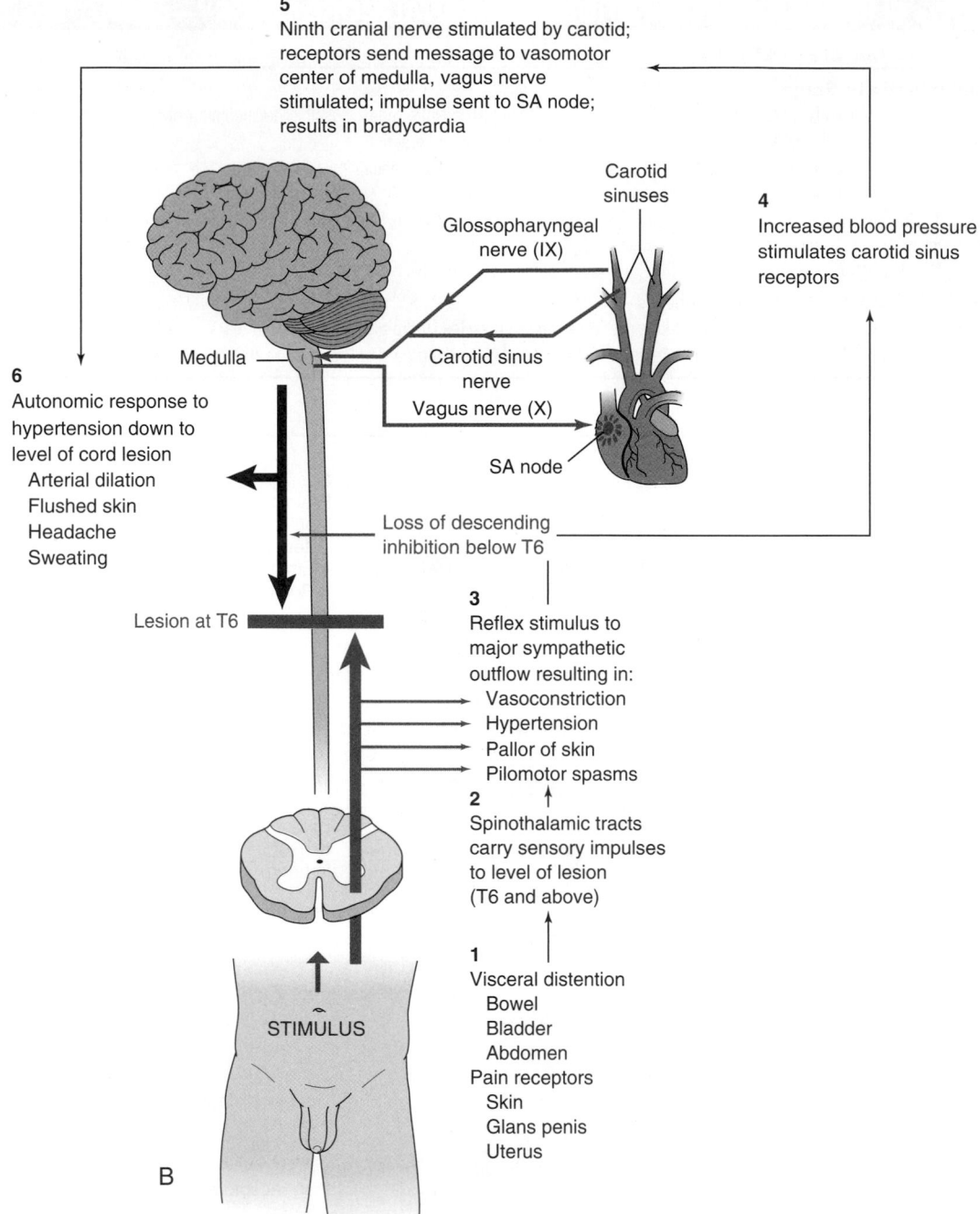

5
Ninth cranial nerve stimulated by carotid; receptors send message to vasomotor center of medulla, vagus nerve stimulated; impulse sent to SA node; results in bradycardia

Carotid sinuses

Glossopharyngeal nerve (IX)

4
Increased blood pressure stimulates carotid sinus receptors

Medulla

Carotid sinus nerve
Vagus nerve (X)

SA node

6
Autonomic response to hypertension down to level of cord lesion
  Arterial dilation
  Flushed skin
  Headache
  Sweating

Loss of descending inhibition below T6

Lesion at T6

3
Reflex stimulus to major sympathetic outflow resulting in:
  Vasoconstriction
  Hypertension
  Pallor of skin
  Pilomotor spasms

2
Spinothalamic tracts carry sensory impulses to level of lesion (T6 and above)

1
Visceral distention
  Bowel
  Bladder
  Abdomen
Pain receptors
  Skin
  Glans penis
  Uterus

STIMULUS

B

FIGURE 18.13, cont'd B, Autonomic dysreflexia pathway. *SA,* Sinoatrial. (Modified from Rudy EB: *Advanced neurological and neurosurgical nursing,* St Louis, 1984, Mosby.)

the population affected with recent LBP is about 29%, with a higher percentage among older individuals, particularly women older than age 60.[53] Most people will experience back pain at some time in their lives. LBP is the primary cause of disability worldwide.[54] The burdens of disability include psychologic, financial, occupational, and social effects on the person and family members.

Risk factors include occupations that require repetitive lifting in the forward bent-and-twisted position, exposure to vibrations caused by vehicles or industrial machinery, obesity, and cigarette smoking.

◆**PATHOPHYSIOLOGY.** Most cases of LBP are idiopathic or nonspecific, and no precise diagnosis is possible.[55] Acute LBP is often associated with muscle or ligament strain and is more common in individuals younger than 50 years of age without a history of cancer. Common causes of chronic LBP include degenerative disk disease and lumbar disk herniation. Genetic causes include isthmic spondylolisthesis (vertebra slides forward or slips in relation to a vertebra below), spinal osteochondrosis, and spinal stenosis associated with achondroplasia.[56] Other causes include tension caused by tumors or disk prolapse, bursitis, synovitis, rising venous and tissue pressures (found in degenerative joint disease), abnormal bone pressures, spinal immobility, inflammation caused by infection (as in osteomyelitis), and pain referred from viscera or the posterior peritoneum. Systemic causes of LBP include bone diseases, such as osteoporosis or osteomalacia, and hyperparathyroidism. Anatomically, low back pain must originate from innervated structures, but deep pain is widely referred and varies. The nucleus pulposus has no intrinsic innervation but, when extruded or herniated through a prolapsed disk, it irritates the spinal nerve dural membranes and causes pain referred to the segmental area.[57] Diskogenic pain also may be related to nerve sprouting and inflammation within the disk.[58]

The interspinous bursae can be a source of pain between L3, L4, L5, and S1, but also may affect L1, L2, and L3 spinous processes. The anterior and posterior longitudinal ligaments of the spine and the interspinous and supraspinous ligaments are abundantly supplied with pain receptors, as is the ligamentum flavum. All of these ligaments are vulnerable to traumatic tears (sprains) and fracture.

◆**CLINICAL MANIFESTATIONS.** About 1% of individuals with acute LBP have sciatica or pain along the distribution of a lumbar nerve root (radicular pain), most commonly involving the sciatic nerve (sciatica). Sciatica is often accompanied by neurosensory and motor deficits, such as tingling, numbness, and weakness in various parts of the leg and foot. Major or progressive motor or sensory deficit, cauda equina syndrome (new-onset bowel or bladder incontinence or urinary retention, loss of anal sphincter tone, saddle anesthesia), history of cancer metastasis to bone, and suspected spinal infection can be associated with chronic LBP.

◆**EVALUATION AND TREATMENT.** Diagnosis of LBP is based on the history and physical examination. Imaging and nerve conduction studies are obtained with severe neurologic deficit or serious underlying disease. Diagnosis and treatment guidelines are available to plan therapy.[59,60] Most individuals with acute LBP benefit from nonspecific short-term treatment, including nonsteroidal antiinflammatory medications, exercises, physical therapy, and education. Individuals with chronic LBP (pain for more than 3 months) can be treated with antiinflammatory and muscle relaxant medications, exercise programs, massage, topical heat, spinal manipulation, acupuncture, cognitive-behavioral therapy, and interdisciplinary care.[61] There is scant evidence for efficacy of opioids for chronic LBP, and there is high risk for addiction.[62] Surgical treatments for identified pathologic conditions include diskectomy and spinal fusions. Radiotherapy is used for treatment of facet-related pain after diagnostic nerve block. Evaluation of treatment outcomes should include pain, function, and quality of life.[63]

Spondylolysis. Spondylolysis is a structural defect (degeneration, fracture, or developmental defect) in the pars interarticularis of the vertebral arch (the joining of the vertebral body to the posterior structures). The lumbar spine at L5 is affected most often. Mechanical pressure may cause an anterior displacement of the deficient vertebra (spondylolisthesis). This defect occurs in the portion of the lamina between the superior and inferior articular facets called the *pars interarticularis.* Heredity plays a significant role, and spondylolysis is associated with an increased incidence of other congenital spinal defects. As a result of torsional and rotational stress, "microfractures" occur at the affected site and eventually cause dissolution of the pars interarticularis. Symptoms include lower back and lower limb pain.

Cervical spondylolysis is facet hypertrophy and disk degeneration with narrowing in the cervical spine predominantly at C5-C6 and C6-C7.[64] It may present as a cervical radiculopathy or a cervical myelopathy. Clinical manifestations of cervical radiculopathy include neck or occipital pain as well as pain in the medial aspects of the scapula, shoulder, or arm. Sensory symptoms, such as tingling or numbness, follow a dermatomal pattern; weakness follows the pattern of innervation of the affected nerve root. Occipital or suboccipital headache is another symptom. Cervical myelopathy can also cause difficulty walking, altered sensation in the feet, and sphincter disturbances (occurs late).

Spondylolisthesis. Spondylolisthesis is an osseous defect of the pars interarticularis allowing a vertebra to slide forward in relation to the vertebra below, commonly occurring at L5-S1. It is more prevalent

in adolescent athletes.[65] Grades 1 and 2 have symptoms of pain in the lower back and buttocks, muscle spasms in the lower back and legs, and tightened hamstrings. Conservative management includes exercise, rest, and back bracing. Vertebral slippage in grades 3 and 4 usually requires surgical decompression, stabilization, or both.

Spinal Stenosis. Spinal stenosis is a narrowing of the spinal canal that causes pressure on the spinal nerves or cord and can be congenital or acquired (more common) and associated with trauma or arthritis. It is categorized by the area of the spine affected: cervical, thoracic, or lumbar. Acquired conditions include a bulging disk, facet hypertrophy, or a thick ossified posterior longitudinal ligament. Symptoms are related to the area of the spine affected and can produce pain; numbness; and tingling in the neck, hands, arms, or legs with weakness and difficulty walking. Surgical decompression is recommended for those with chronic symptoms and those who do not respond to medical management.

Degenerative Disk Disease

Degenerative disk disease (DDD) is common in individuals 30 years of age and older. It is, in part, a process of normal aging as a response to continuous vertical compression of the spine (axial loading). DDD includes a genetic component involving over expression of genes that code the cartilage intermediate layer protein (CILP). The combination of environmental interactions and genetic predisposition increases susceptibility to nontraumatic lumbar disk disease by disrupting normal building and maintenance of cartilage.[58] Causes include biochemical (e.g., inflammatory mediators) and biomechanical alterations (e.g., mechanical loading and compression) of the intervertebral disk tissue. For example, loss of disk proteoglycans and collagen with disk dehydration and loss of hydrostatic pressure alters disk structure and function. The annulus can tear and the disk can herniate, pinching nerves or placing strain on the spine. Fibrocartilage replaces the gelatinous mucoid material of the nucleus pulposus as the disk changes with age. There may be shrinkage of the nucleus pulposus that produces prolapse or folding of the annulus with secondary osteophyte formation at the margins of the adjacent vertebral body. The pathologic findings in DDD include disk protrusion, spondylolysis and/or spondylolisthesis, degeneration of vertebrae, and spinal stenosis. Lumbar disk disease causes one-third of all back pain that affects 70% to 90% of adults at some point in their lives. However, only a small percentage of people with DDD have any functional incapacity because of pain.[66]

Symptoms result from either (1) protrusion of the disk or annulus or (2) narrowing of the spinal canal or intervertebral foramen by osteophytes. A congenital narrow canal or congenitally short pedicles may be present. Posterior disk protrusion in the cervical, thoracic, and lumbar regions leads to spinal cord compression causing *myelopathy* (pathology in the spinal cord). Posterolateral disk protrusions, with or without a contribution from the vertebral body or apophyseal joint osteophytes, lead to nerve root compression causing *radiculopathy* (nerve root damage).

Thoracic disk disease is rarely symptomatic. Lumbosacral disk disease *(lumbar spondylosis)* involves degeneration of the lower two lumbar disks in 90% of persons. There may be (1) lateral disk protrusion (10% of cases), manifesting as pain referred to the anterior thigh and leg; (2) posterolateral disk protrusion; or (3) central disk protrusion, manifesting with pain, lower extremity weakness, impaired sphincter function, and saddle anesthesia. Clinical manifestations of posterolateral protrusions (Fig. 18.14) include pain in the back, the sacroiliac joint, and the medial aspect of the buttock and upper thigh; radicular pain exacerbated by movement and straining (medial calf suggests L5, lateral calf suggests S1 root compression); sensory symptoms that are common and segmental in distribution; focal tenderness on palpation of the back; limited range of motion in the back and scoliosis secondary to paravertebral spasms;

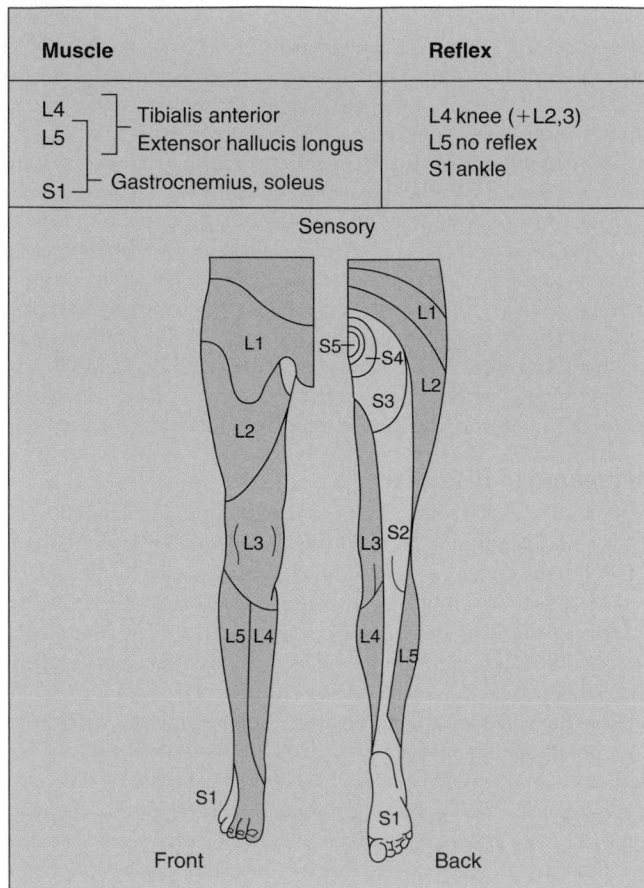

Muscle		Reflex
L4 ⎤⎤ L5 ⎦ S1 ⎦	Tibialis anterior Extensor hallucis longus Gastrocnemius, soleus	L4 knee (+L2,3) L5 no reflex S1 ankle

FIGURE 18.14 Motor, Sensory, and Reflex Changes in Lumbosacral Root Disorders. (From Perkin DG et al: *Atlas of clinical neurology,* ed 3, Philadelphia, 2011, Saunders.)

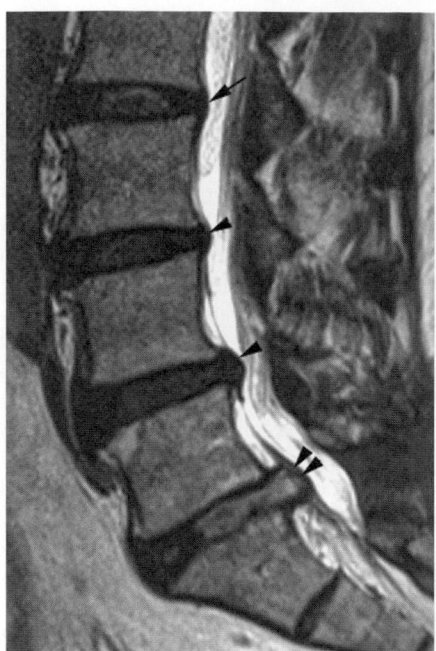

FIGURE 18.15 Disk Bulge, Protrusion, and Herniation. Sagittal T2-weighted image demonstrates examples for all stages of disk pathology. Viewing from rostral to caudal, a disk bulge *(arrow),* a small and more prominent protrusion *(arrowheads),* and a herniation *(double arrowhead)* are seen. (From Daroff RB et al: *Bradley's neurology in clinical practice,* Philadelphia, 2012, Saunders.)

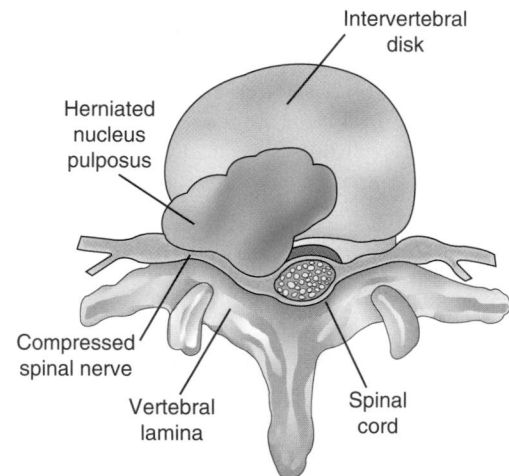

FIGURE 18.16 Herniated Nucleus Pulposus.

restricted straight-leg raising (root at or below L5); positive femoral stretch test (roots of L2, L3, or L4); and focal signs that are determined by the root affected.

Herniated Intervertebral Disk

Herniation of an intervertebral disk is a displacement of the nucleus pulposus or annulus fibrosus beyond the intervertebral disk space[67] (Figs. 18.15 and 18.16). Rupture of an intervertebral disk is usually caused by trauma, degenerative disk disease, or both. Risk factors are weight-bearing sports; light weight lifting; and certain work activities, such as repeated lifting. Men are more affected than women, with the highest incidence in the 30- to 50-year age group. The lumbosacral disks L4-L5 and L5-S1 are most commonly affected. Herniation is typically at higher vertebrae in older persons. Disk herniation occasionally occurs in the cervical area, usually at C5-C6 and C6-C7. Herniations at the thoracic level are extremely rare. The herniation may occur immediately, within a few hours, or months to years after injury.

PATHOPHYSIOLOGY. In a herniated disk, the ligament and posterior capsule of the disk usually are torn, allowing the gelatinous material (the nucleus pulposus) to extrude and compress the nerve root. The vascular supply may be compromised and cause inflammatory changes in the nerve root (radiculitis). Occasionally, the injury tears the entire disk loose, causing the disk capsule and nucleus pulposus to protrude onto the nerve root or compress the spinal cord. Multiple nerve root compression may be found at the L5-S1 level, where the cauda equina may be compressed, causing cauda equina syndrome.

CLINICAL MANIFESTATIONS. The location and size of the herniation into the spinal canal, together with the amount of space in the canal, determine the clinical manifestations associated with the injury (see Fig. 18.14). Compression or inflammation, or both, of a spinal nerve resulting from disk herniation follows a dermatomal distribution called **radiculopathy** (Fig. 18.17). A herniated disk in the lumbosacral area is associated with pain that radiates along the sciatic nerve course over the buttock and into the calf or ankle. The pain occurs with straining, including coughing and sneezing, and usually on straight-leg raising. Other clinical manifestations include limited range of motion of the lumbar spine; tenderness on palpation in the sciatic notch and along the sciatic nerve; impaired pain, temperature, and touch sensation in the L5-S1 or L4-L5 dermatomes of the leg and foot; decreased or absent ankle jerk reflex; and mild weakness of the foot. More rarely, there is development of cauda equina syndrome (saddle anesthesia, decreased

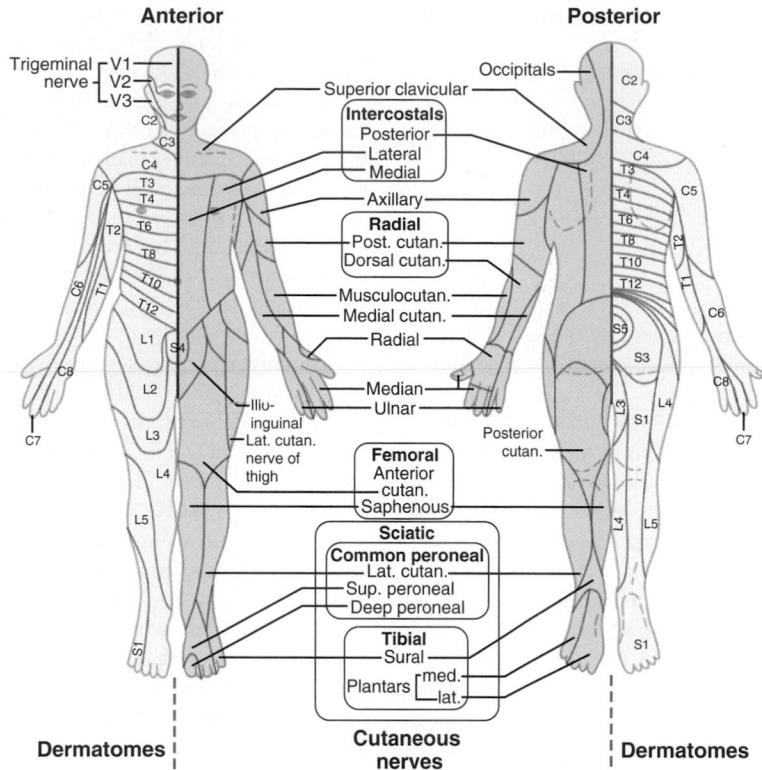

FIGURE 18.17 Sensory Nerve Distribution of Skin Dermatomes. (Redrawn from Patton HD, et al, editors: *Introduction to basic neurology*, Philadelphia, 1976, WB Saunders. Borrowed from Canale ST, Beaty JH: *Campbell's operative orthopaedics*, ed 12, St Louis, 2013, Mosby.)

or absent reflexes in the lower extremities, and neurogenic bowel or bladder dysfunction).

With the herniation of a lower cervical disk, paresthesias and pain are present in the upper arm, forearm, and hand in the affected nerve root distribution. Neck motion and straining, including coughing and sneezing, may increase neck and nerve root pain. Neck range of motion is diminished. Slight weakness and atrophy of biceps or triceps may occur; the biceps or triceps reflex may decrease. Occasionally signs of corticospinal and sensory tract impairments appear. These include motor weakness of the lower extremities, sensory disturbances in the lower extremities, and presence of a Babinski reflex.

◆**EVALUATION AND TREATMENT.** Diagnosis of a herniated intervertebral disk is made through the history and physical examination, spinal x-ray films, electromyelography, CT scan, MRI, myelography, diskography, and nerve conduction studies. Evidence-based practice guidelines have been published to guide treatment options.[68] Most herniated disks heal spontaneously over time and do not require surgery. A surgical approach is indicated if there is evidence of severe compression (weakness or decreased deep tendon, bladder, or bowel reflexes) or if a conservative approach is unsuccessful.[69] Cauda equina syndrome requires emergency surgical evaluation[70] (see Table 18.4).

Cerebrovascular Disorders

Cerebrovascular disease is the most frequently occurring neurologic disorder, accounting for more than 50% of persons admitted to general hospitals with neurologic problems. Any abnormality of the brain caused by a pathologic process in the blood vessels is referred to as a *cerebrovascular disease*. Included in this category are lesions of the vessel wall (e.g., aneurysm or malformations); occlusion of the vessel lumen by thrombus or embolus; rupture of the vessel; and alteration in blood quality, such as increased blood viscosity or clotting.

The brain abnormalities induced by cerebrovascular disease are either (1) ischemia with or without infarction (death of brain tissues) or (2) hemorrhage. The common clinical manifestation of cerebrovascular disease is a cerebrovascular accident or stroke. The symptoms occur suddenly and are usually focal (i.e., slurred speech, difficulty swallowing, limb weakness, or paralysis). In its mildest form, a cerebrovascular accident is so minimal that it is almost unnoticed. In its most severe form, hemiplegia, coma, and death result.

Cerebrovascular Accidents (Stroke Syndromes)

Cerebrovascular accidents (CVAs) are the leading cause of disability, the third cause of death in women, and the fifth leading cause of death in men in the United States. About 75% of CVAs occur among those older than 65 years. There has been a decline in ischemic strokes among whites but not blacks. The yearly incidence of new and recurrent stroke is 795,000; approximately 185,000 of these are recurrent and there are about 128,932 deaths each year, a decline of 18.2% from 2003 to 2013. The incidence of stroke is about 150% greater in blacks than whites. Stroke tends to run in families. Of all strokes, 87% are ischemic (thrombotic or embolic), 10% are intracerebral hemorrhagic, and 3% are subarachnoid hemorrhagic.[71] Strokes in children are presented in Chapter 20.

Cerebrovascular accidents (stroke syndromes) are classified pathophysiologically as ischemic, hemorrhagic, or cryptogenic. If no identifiable cause can be established by conventional diagnostic tests in ischemic strokes, they are classified as "undetermined" or "cryptogenic." Risk factors for stroke include the following:[72]

- Poorly or uncontrolled arterial hypertension
- Smoking, which increases the risk of stroke by 50%
- Insulin resistance and diabetes mellitus
- Polycythemia and thrombocythemia

- High total cholesterol or low high-density lipoprotein (HDL) cholesterol, elevated lipoprotein-a
- Congestive heart disease and peripheral vascular disease
- Hyperhomocysteinemia
- Atrial fibrillation
- Physical inactivity
- Family history and genetics
- Sleep apnea
- *Chlamydia pneumoniae* infection[73]
- Sickle cell disease
- Postmenopausal hormone therapy
- High sodium intake, >2300 mg; low potassium intake, <4700 mg
- Obesity
- Depression

Ischemic Stroke. Ischemic stroke occurs when there is obstruction to arterial blood flow to the brain from thrombus formation, an embolus associated with atherosclerosis, or hypoperfusion related to decreased blood volume or heart failure. The inadequate blood supply results in ischemia (inadequate cellular oxygen) and can progress to infarction (death of tissue).

Transient ischemic attacks (TIAs) are episodes of neurologic dysfunction lasting no more than 1 hour and resulting from focal cerebral ischemia. The clinical manifestations of a TIA may include weakness, numbness, sudden confusion, loss of balance, loss of vision, or sudden severe headache resulting from focal cerebral ischemia. The use of brain imaging modalities often reveals a brain infarction. About 3% to 17% of individuals experiencing a TIA will have a stroke within 90 days.[74] Risk stratification for early stroke is enhanced when imaging is combined with a risk stratification score (e.g., the ABCD[3] and ABCD[3]-I) which considers age, blood pressure, neurologic symptoms, symptom duration, and diabetes.[75] Guidelines are available for the prevention of future strokes.[76]

Thrombotic strokes (cerebral thrombosis) arise from arterial occlusions caused by thrombus formation in large or small arteries supplying the brain or intracranial vessels. Conditions causing increased coagulation or inadequate cerebral perfusion (e.g., dehydration, hypotension, prolonged vasoconstriction from malignant hypertension) increase the risk of thrombosis. Cerebral thrombosis develops most often from atherosclerosis and inflammatory disease processes that damage arterial walls. It may take as long as 20 to 30 years for obstruction (stenosis) to develop at the branches and curvatures found in the cerebral circulation (see Chapter 33 for a discussion of atherogenesis). The smooth stenotic area can degenerate, forming an ulcerated area of vessel wall. Platelets and fibrin adhere to the damaged wall, and clots form, gradually occluding the artery. The thrombus may enlarge both distally and proximally in the vessel. Thrombotic strokes occur when portions of the clot detach, travel upstream, and obstruct blood flow, causing acute ischemia.

Embolic stroke involves fragments that break from a thrombus formed outside the brain usually in the heart, aorta, or common carotid artery. Other sources of embolism include fat, air, tumor, bacterial clumps, and foreign bodies. The embolus usually involves small brain vessels and obstructs at a bifurcation or other point of narrowing, thus causing ischemia. An embolus may obstruct the lumen entirely and remain in place or shatter into fragments and become part of the vessel's blood flow. Risk factors for an embolic stroke are atrial fibrillation (15% to 25% of strokes), left ventricular aneurysm or thrombus, left atrial thrombus, recent myocardial infarction, rheumatic valvular disease, mechanical prosthetic valve, nonbacterial thrombotic endocarditis, bacterial endocarditis, patent foramen ovale, and primary intracardiac tumors.[77] In persons who experience an embolic stroke, a second stroke usually follows at some point because the source of emboli continues to exist. Embolization is usually in the distribution of the middle cerebral

artery (the largest cerebral artery). Ischemic strokes in children are associated with congenital heart disease, cerebral arteriovenous malformations, and sickle cell disease.

Lacunar strokes (lacunar infarcts or small vessel disease) are usually caused by perivascular edema, thickening and inflammation of the arteriolar wall in a deep perforating artery that supplies small penetrating subcortical vessels (small vessel disease). The ischemic lesions (0.5 to 15 mm) or lacunes are predominantly in the basal ganglia, internal capsules, and pons. They are associated with hyperlipidemia, smoking,[78] hypertension, and diabetes mellitus. These strokes represent about 25% of ischemic strokes and, because of the location and small area of infarction, may have pure motor or sensory deficits.[79]

Hemodynamic stroke (brain hypoperfusion) is associated with *systemic hypoperfusion* caused by cardiac failure, pulmonary embolism, or bleeding that results in inadequate blood supply to the brain. Stroke may occur more readily if there is carotid artery occlusion. Symptoms usually are bilateral and diffuse.[80]

◆ **PATHOPHYSIOLOGY.** Cerebral infarction results when an area of the brain loses its blood supply because of vascular occlusion. Causes include (1) abrupt vascular occlusion (e.g., embolus or thrombi), (2) gradual vessel occlusion (e.g., atheroma), and (3) vessels that are stenosed but not completely occluded. Cerebral thrombi and cerebral emboli most commonly produce occlusion, but atherosclerosis and hypotension are the dominant underlying processes.

There is a central core of irreversible ischemia and necrosis or cerebral infarction. The central core is surrounded by a zone of borderline ischemic tissue, the ischemic penumbra. Ischemia in the penumbra is not severe enough to result in structural damage. Prompt restoration of perfusion in the penumbra by injection of thrombolytic agents promotes perfusion and may prevent necrosis and loss of neurologic function. The window of opportunity for protecting the penumbra is about 3 hours.

Cerebral infarctions are ischemic or hemorrhagic. In *ischemic infarcts,* the affected area becomes pale and softens 6 to 12 hours after the occlusion (white infarct). Necrosis, swelling around the insult, and mushy disintegration appear by 48 to 72 hours after infarction. There is infiltration of macrophages and phagocytosis of necrotic tissue. The necrosis resolves by about the second week, ultimately leaving a cavity surrounded by glial scarring.

After occlusion of a cerebral artery, anastomoses connecting the distal segments of the middle cerebral artery with distal branches of the anterior and posterior cerebral arteries (known as *leptomeningeal* or *pial collaterals*) can partially maintain blood flow in the ischemic penumbra and delay or prevent cell death in some individuals. Vascular remodeling (angiogenesis) can occur with new arterioles sprouting from penumbra vessels that penetrate the ischemic core to reestablish collateral circulation. Efforts are in progress to enhance and promote collateral circulation following acute ischemic stroke (i.e., inhaled nitric oxide, transient suprarenal aortic occlusion, and electrical stimulation of the parasympathetic sphenopalatine ganglion).[81]

In *hemorrhagic infarcts,* bleeding occurs into the infarcted area through leaking vessels when the embolic fragments resolve and reperfusion begins to occur. Hemorrhagic transformation of ischemic infarct (red infarct) may be exacerbated by thrombolytic therapy.[82] Unfortunately, reperfusion can compromise recovery by accelerating the sequence of metabolically damaging events, including oxidative stress (reperfusion injury) (see Chapter 2).

◆ **CLINICAL MANIFESTATIONS.** Clinical manifestations of thrombotic or embolic ischemic stroke vary, depending on the distribution of the artery obstructed. Different sites of vessel obstruction create different occlusion syndromes. Table 18.5 summarizes the various stroke syndromes. Contralateral sensory and motor manifestations occur on the

TABLE 18.5	STROKE SYNDROMES SECONDARY TO OCCLUSION OR STENOSIS	
LOCATION/VESSEL	**AREA OF BRAIN INFARCTED**	**SIGNS AND SYMPTOMS NOTED**
Anterior and Central Circulation		
Note: The internal carotid artery enters the circle of Willis and supplies the lateral anterior and central portions of the cerebral hemispheres through the middle cerebral artery and the paramedial frontal lobe superior to the corpus callosum through the anterior cerebral artery; penetrating branches serve the deeper layers of the hemispheres.		
Internal carotid	If collateral circulation is intact, there is commonly no infarction; if infarcted, it is in the same area of the middle cerebral artery	• Arterial pressure may be low in the retina • Bruits over the internal carotid artery • Possible retinal emboli • History of transient ischemic attacks (TIAs) • Positive noninvasive studies
Middle cerebral artery (MCA) (most common area); either stem or branches of MCA	Cortical motor area (face, arm, leg) and/or posterior limb, internal capsule, corona radiata	• **Motor:** contralateral hemiparesis or hemiplegia, greater in face and arm than leg
	Cortical sensory area (face, arm, leg) and/or posterior limb of internal capsule	• **Sensation:** contralateral loss in same distribution as motor loss
	Broca area and deep fibers in the dominant hemisphere	• **Speech:** expressive (motor) disorder with anomia (left hemisphere most commonly affected) with nonfluent aphasia and some comprehension defects
	Broca area and deep fibers in the nondominant hemisphere	• **Speech:** dysarthria
	Optic radiations deep in the temporal lobe	• **Vision:** contralateral homonymous hemianopsia or quadranopsia
	Location not known	• **Motor:** mirror movements • **Respirations:** Cheyne-Stokes respirations, contralateral hyperhidrosis, occasional mydriasis
	Posterior limb or internal capsule and adjacent corona radiate	• **Motor:** pure motor hemiplegia
	Penetrating branches of MCA (lenticulostriate branches) into the basal nuclei	• **Motor:** varying degrees of contralateral weakness of face, arm, or leg • **Sensory:** little or no loss; if present, contralateral following the motor distribution • **Speech:** transcortical sensory aphasia (communicating pathways are interrupted) • **Perception:** transient visual and sensory neglect on the left if a right lesion
Anterior cerebral artery (ACA) (least common)	Proximal segment: corona radiata (rarely)	• **Motor:** when present, a mild contralateral hemiparesis, greater in leg; with bilateral occlusion of ACA, cerebral paraplegia in both legs can occur
	Main stem (complete occlusion is uncommon, thus areas affected differ and collateral circulation may alleviate signs or symptoms); medial aspect of frontal lobes, caudate nucleus, and corpus callosum are supplied by the ACA	• **Motor:** contralateral paralysis or paresis (greater in foot and thigh); mild upper extremity weakness • **Sensory:** mild contralateral lower extremity deficiency with loss of vibratory and/or position sense, loss of two-point discrimination • **Speech:** may have transcortical motor and sensory aphasia if left hemisphere • Frontal lobe releasing signs (grasp, snout, root, and suck reflexes) • Apraxia
Posterior Circulation		
Note: The posterior circulation includes the posterior cerebral artery, the vertebral arteries, and the basilar artery; the anatomic territory covered includes the posterior aspects of the hemispheres, the central areas of the thalamus and midbrain, and the brainstem; occlusion of the vessels is most commonly by emboli; effects of infarct in these vessels and their penetrating vessels can be specific or devastatingly global; many complex syndromes have been identified.		
Vertebral arteries	Medulla and spinal cord tracts, anterior spinal artery and penetrating branches (medial medullary syndrome)	• **Motor:** contralateral hemiparesis (face spared) and/or impaired contralateral proprioception; flaccid weakness or paralysis of the tongue and/or dysarthria

Continued

TABLE 18.5   STROKE SYNDROMES SECONDARY TO OCCLUSION OR STENOSIS—cont'd

LOCATION/VESSEL	AREA OF BRAIN INFARCTED	SIGNS AND SYMPTOMS NOTED
Basilar artery (three sets of branches)	Midline structures of pons (paramedian branches); three general areas of infarction are common: (1) medial inferior pontine syndrome, (2) medial midpontine syndrome, and (3) medial superior pontine syndrome	• **Motor:** contralateral hemiparesis or hemiplegia, ipsilateral lower motor neuron facial palsy, "locked-in syndrome" • **Sensory:** contralateral loss of vibratory sense, sense of position with dysmetria, loss of two-point discrimination, impaired rapid alternating movements • **Visual:** inferior pontine: diplopia; impaired abduction of ipsilateral eye: internuclear ophthalmoplegia; medial superior; diplopia, internuclear ophthalmoplegia, skewed deviation
	Corticospinal and corticobulbar tracts in pons, sensory tracts of medial and lateral lemnisci, vestibular nuclei, inferior and middle cerebellar peduncles, cranial nerve nuclei and/or fibers, cerebellar connections in tectum, descending sympathetic pathways, central brainstem, pontine tegmentum (vertebrobasilar syndrome)	• **Motor:** upper motor neuron type of weakness: paralysis in combinations involving face, tongue, throat, and extremities; dysphagia, facial weakness, dysmetria, ataxia (either trunk or extremities), weak mastication muscles • **Sensation:** combinations of impaired sensation (vibratory, two-point, position sense, pain, temperature), facial hypesthesia, anesthesia of cranial nerve V
Posterior cerebral artery (PCA)	Central territory (thalamic area, dentothalamic tract, cerebral peduncle, red nucleus, subthalamic nucleus, and cranial nerve III)	• **Motor:** contralateral hemiplegia with possible dysmetria, dyskinesia, hemiballism or choreoathetosis, dystaxia, cerebellar ataxia, and tremor; contralateral upper motor neuron palsy; several syndromes are associated: (1) Weber: cranial nerve III palsy and contralateral hemiplegia; (2) thalamoperforate syndrome: superior crossed cerebellar ataxia or inferior crossed cerebellar ataxia with cranial nerve III palsy (Claude syndrome); (3) decerebrate attacks • **Sensory:** contralateral sensory loss of all modalities without agraphia • **Function:** prosopagnosia (inability to recognize familiar faces), topographic disorientation, memory deficits, alexia, inability to read, color anomia • **Level of consciousness:** in bilateral PCA syndromes, coma with absent doll's eyes reflex or loss of alertness may occur; if tegmentum of midbrain near hypothalamus and third ventricle is damaged, akinetic mutism may occur

Small Vessel Disease

Note: Small penetrating vessels in brain parenchyma that supply areas near the basal ganglia are most vulnerable to infarction, although any small vessels can occlude deep in the brain and cause injury, producing neurologic signs or symptoms; such infarcts are commonly called *lacunes* (small pit or hollow), a term that is changing in meaning; they can be caused by emboli but are most commonly associated with microatheromas; although they can be found in otherwise healthy people, those with concurrent atherosclerosis, arterial hypertension, and/or diabetes have a higher incidence of this type of infarct.

	Internal capsule, most commonly	• **Motor:** contralateral hemiparesis on a single side, with equal deficit in face, arm, and leg; often unaccompanied by detectable signs of sensory, visual, and speech loss, depending on location; old term is *pure motor stroke*, although evidence suggests that other neurologic signs are present but overlooked because of low intensity
	Thalamus, most commonly	• **Sensory:** complete or partial loss in face, arm, trunk, and leg that appears exactly midline; may be accompanied by pain, hyperesthesias, and uncomfortable sensations (hemisensory stroke)
	Pons	• Dysarthria, clumsy hand
	Pons, midbrain, capsule or parietal white matter	• Hemiparesis, ataxia on same side

Modified from Barker E: *Neuroscience nursing*, St Louis, 1994, Mosby.

opposite side of the body from the location of the brain lesion because motor tracts originate in the cortex and most cross over in the medulla. Sensory tracts originate in the periphery and cross over in the spinal cord. Ipsilateral manifestations occur on the same side as the brain lesion for tracts that do not cross over.

◆ **EVALUATION AND TREATMENT.** Imaging is used to diagnose the different subtypes of ischemic stroke (i.e., MRI and CT imaging). Treatment of ischemic stroke is focused on (1) restoring brain perfusion in a timeframe that does not contribute to reperfusion injury, (2) counteracting the ischemic cascade pathways, (3) lowering cerebral metabolic demand so that the susceptible brain tissue is protected against impaired perfusion, (4) preventing recurrent ischemic events, and (5) promoting tissue restoration. Intravenous thrombolysis (i.e., recombinant tissue plasminogen activator [rtPA]) given within 3 and up to 4.5 hours of onset of symptoms increases independent ambulation at 6 months when the diagnosis of ischemic stroke has been confirmed and contraindications are eliminated. Endovascular intraarterial thrombectomy can be used in combination with rtPA or alone as an approach to endovascular reperfusion.[83] Intracranial hemorrhage can be a complication of rTPA administration.[84] The American Heart Association and American Stroke Association provide guidelines for the early management of acute ischemic stroke.[85]

Acute ischemic stroke frequently presents with hypertension, but the systemic blood pressure should not be treated unless the systolic pressure is 150 to 220 mmHg or mean arterial pressure exceeds 150 mmHg. Overly aggressive treatment of hypertension can compromise collateral perfusion of the ischemic penumbra. When the pathophysiology of stroke is stabilized, all individuals should receive blood pressure (BP)-lowering therapy to maintain BP lower than 140/90 mmHg or 130/90 mmHg if there are comorbidities, such as diabetes or chronic kidney disease.[86] Hypothermia has been used for neuroprotection in ischemic stroke with some promising results, but additional studies are needed to determine best methods and clinical practice guidelines.[87]

Neuroprotective agents have not been shown to significantly reduce the risk of poor outcome including death with ischemic stroke. New neuroprotective agents are continuing to be evaluated for neuroprotection and to improve neuroplasticity and remodeling, including cell transplantation and neurostimulation.[88] Arresting the disease process by control of risk factors is critical to prevention of stroke and to reduce associated morbidity and costs.

Hemorrhagic Stroke. **Hemorrhagic stroke (spontaneous intracranial hemorrhage [ICH])** is the third most common cause of CVA. Hemorrhagic stroke can occur within the brain tissue (intraparenchymal) or in the subarachnoid or subdural spaces. The primary cause of intraparenchymal hemorrhagic stroke is hypertension with other causes including tumors; coagulation disorders; trauma; or illicit drug use, particularly cocaine. Hypertensive causes of hemorrhagic stroke evolve over several years. They involve primarily smaller arteries and arterioles, resulting in thickening of the vessel walls and increased cellularity of the vessels. Necrosis may be present with vessel rupture. Microaneurysms in these smaller vessels or arteriolar necrosis may precipitate bleeding. Prevention or control of hypertension reduces the incidence of hemorrhagic stroke. Subarachnoid hemorrhage is associated with ruptured aneurysms, arteriovenous malformations or cavernous angioma or brain trauma. Subdural hemorrhage (hematoma) is usually associated with brain trauma.

◆ PATHOPHYSIOLOGY. A mass of blood is formed as bleeding occurs into the brain tissue (Fig. 18.18). Adjacent brain tissue is deformed, compressed, and displaced producing ischemia, edema, IICP, and necrosis. Rupture or seepage of blood into the ventricular system often occurs and is associated with higher mortality. Hemorrhages are described as massive, small, slit, or petechial. Massive hemorrhages are several centimeters in diameter, small hemorrhages are 1 to 2 cm in diameter, a slit hemorrhage occurs in small penetrating vessels in the subcortical area leaving a slitlike cavity, and a petechial hemorrhage is the size of a pinhead. The most common sites for hypertensive hemorrhages are in the putamen of the basal ganglia, the thalamus, the cortex and subcortex, the pons, the caudate nucleus, and the cerebellar hemispheres.

Because neurons surrounding the ischemic or infarcted areas undergo changes that disrupt plasma membranes, cellular edema results, causing further compression of capillaries. In massive intracerebral hemorrhage (volume greater than 150 mL), cerebral perfusion falls to zero and cerebral blood flow stops, resulting in death. In strokes with less than massive hemorrhage, adjacent brain tissue is displaced and compressed. Maximal cerebral edema develops in approximately 72 hours and takes about 2 weeks to subside. An inflammatory reaction in surrounding brain tissue appears rapidly and peaks in several days. Fig. 18.19 illustrates additional detail. Most persons survive an initial hemispheric ischemic stroke unless there is massive cerebral edema, which is nearly always fatal. The cerebral hemorrhage resolves through reabsorption; macrophages and astrocytes clear blood from the area; and a cavity forms surrounded by a dense gliosis (glial scar) after removal of the blood.

◆ CLINICAL MANIFESTATIONS. The clinical manifestations of hemorrhagic stroke are similar to those for embolic and thrombotic stroke and depend on the location and size of the bleed. Once a deep unresponsive state occurs, the immediate prognosis is grave, and the individual rarely survives. If the person survives, however, recovery of function frequently is possible.

Individuals experiencing intracranial hemorrhage from a ruptured or leaking aneurysm have one of three sets of symptoms: (1) onset of an excruciating generalized headache with an almost immediate lapse into an unresponsive state; (2) headache, but with consciousness maintained; and (3) sudden lapse into unconsciousness. If the hemorrhage is confined to the subarachnoid space, there may be no local signs. If bleeding spreads into the brain tissue, hemiparesis/paralysis, dysphasia, or homonymous hemianopsia may be present. Warning signs of an impending aneurysm rupture include headache, transient unilateral weakness, transient numbness and tingling, and transient speech disturbance. Such warning signs are often absent.

◆ EVALUATION AND TREATMENT. Clinical guidelines for the management of spontaneous intracerebral hemorrhage have been published by the American Heart Association/American Stroke Association.[89]

Diagnosis of hemorrhagic stroke considers the health history, clinical presentation, laboratory tests, and neuroimaging procedures (CT and MRI). Treatment needs to be initiated within 3 to 4 hours of symptom onset for reversibility of brain ischemia. Care in multidisciplinary stroke rehabilitation units appears to be most effective at reducing disability, dependency, and length of hospital stay for all stroke syndromes.[90]

Treatment of a hemorrhagic stroke, regardless of cause, is focused on (1) stopping or reducing the bleeding, (2) controlling cerebral edema and IICP, (3) preventing a rebleed, (4) preventing vasospasm, and (5) promoting tissue restoration and preventing or controlling seizures. Known coagulopathies should be corrected and oral anticoagulation reversed.[91]

Hypertension management is individualized. Elevated blood pressure can expand the hematoma, and low blood pressure can contribute to ischemia. Lowering systolic blood pressure to no lower than 130 mmHg is probably beneficial but requires more evaluative studies.[86,92] Intracranial

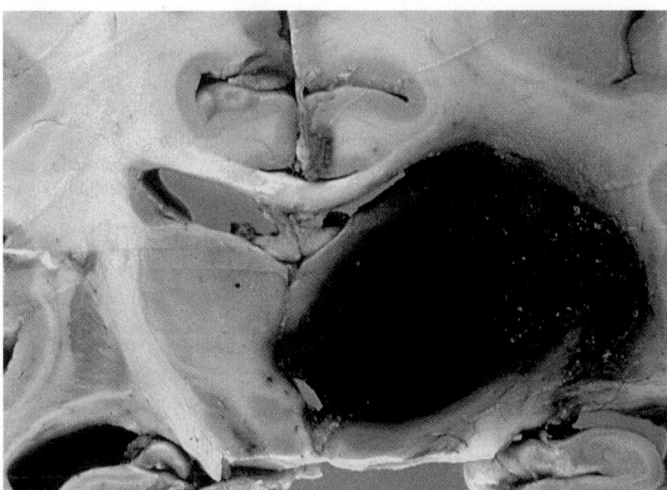

FIGURE 18.18 Hypertensive Intracerebral Hemorrhage. Cross section of the pons showing a hypertensive intracerebral hemorrhage. (From Damjanov I: *Pathology for the health professions*, Philadelphia, 2012, Saunders.)

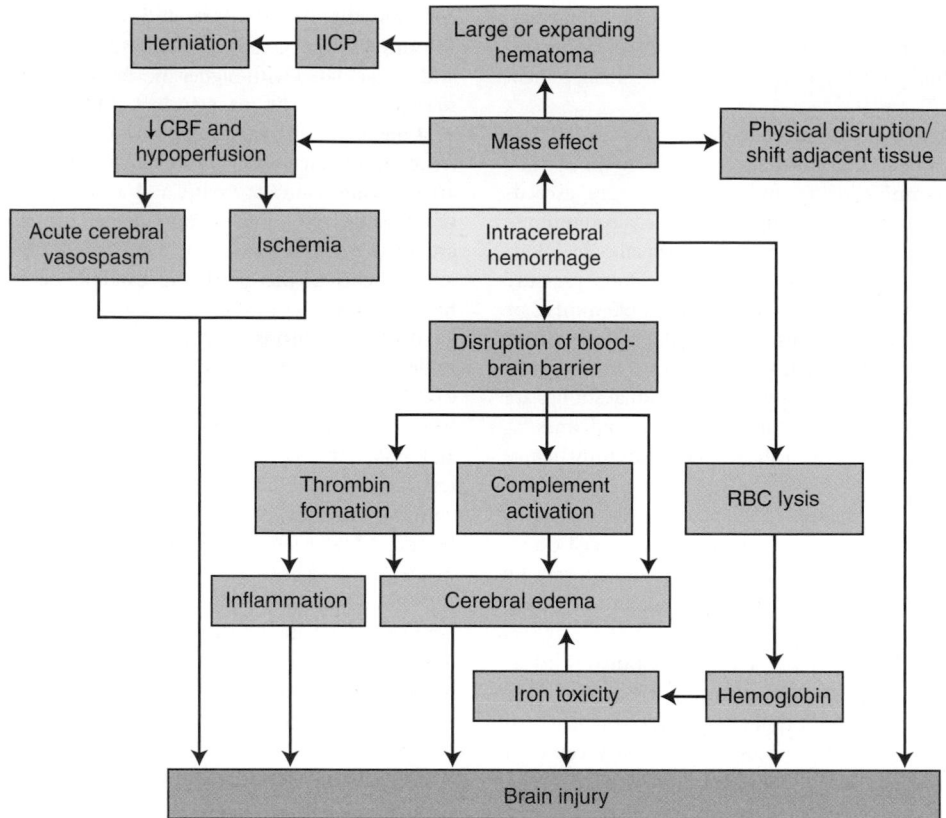

FIGURE 18.19 Injury Mechanisms Promoted by Intracerebral Hemorrhage. Hemorrhages can induce neuronal injury through mass effect, particularly in large hematomas that can cause increased intracranial pressure and herniation. Hemorrhages may also cause tissue damage through cerebral edema and secondary "neurotoxic" mechanisms caused by activation of the coagulation cascade and inflammation. Not all potential interactions are shown (e.g., thrombin may potentiate iron-induced injury; the complement and inflammatory systems overlap; and several factors contribute to cerebral edema). *CBF,* Cerebral blood flow; *IICP,* increased intracranial pressure; *RBC,* red blood cell. (Data from Mocco J, et al: *Neurosurg Focus* 15:22[5]:E7, 2007; Schubert GA, Thome C: *Front Biosci* 13:1594–1603, 2008; Xi G, Keep RF, Hoff JT: *Lancet Neurol* 5[1]:53–63, 2006.)

hemorrhage and hemorrhagic transformation of ischemic stroke are risk factors for early seizures, and cortical involvement is associated with late seizures. Routine prophylactic treatment of seizures that may be associated with stroke is controversial and requires more investigation.[93]

Disruption of the blood-brain barrier results in cerebral edema and IICP. Osmotic therapies (e.g., mannitol) are used for the treatment of IICP and cerebral edema in hemorrhagic stroke.[94] Medical therapies to control clot expansion have not shown significant effects on improving mortality. There are some attempts to drain blood in a cerebral bleed, but the benefit is not documented in studies. Microsurgical interventions are under investigation. Surgical treatments are options for ruptured aneurysms, vascular malformations, and subarachnoid hemorrhage.[95,96] Supportive care is provided for airway management; respiratory function; blood pressure control; avoidance of fever; and maintenance of fluids, glucose, electrolytes, and nutrition.

Intracranial Aneurysm. Intracranial aneurysms (weak bulging areas of an arterial vessel wall) may result from arteriosclerosis, congenital abnormality, cocaine use, trauma, inflammation, and vascular shear wall stress. The size of the aneurysm may vary from 2 mm to 3 cm. Aneurysms may be single; however, more than one is present in 20% to 25% of cases. The aneurysms may be unilateral or bilateral in these instances. Peak incidence of rupture occurs in persons 50 to 59 years of age, with the incidence in postmenopausal women slightly higher than that in men.

◆ PATHOPHYSIOLOGY. No single pathologic mechanism exists. A combination of genetic, congenital, and acquired factors (hypertension) is usually present. Abnormalities in multiple layers of the blood vessel are found. The endothelial layer is thin, the internal elastic lamina is not present or fragmented, and the muscularis layer of the media ends at the aneurysm. Inflammatory cells are recruited, inducing apoptosis and remodeling of the vascular wall. Atherosclerotic changes are found. Aneurysm development is attributed to hemodynamic and wall shear stress and flow turbulence, particularly at bifurcations, such as in or near the circle of Willis, in the vertebrobasilar arteries, or within the carotid artery system (see Figs. 15.20 and 15.21). They are symptoms of underlying vascular disease. Hypertension and certain connective tissue disorders in which there are abnormalities in the extracellular matrix exacerbate aneurysm formation.[98] Aneurysms may be classified on the basis of shape and form (Fig. 18.20).

Saccular aneurysms (berry aneurysms) occur frequently (in approximately 2% of the population) and are the result of a combination of a congenital abnormality in the media of the arterial wall with loss of smooth muscle cells, inflammation, thrombus formation, and degenerative changes. The sac expands over time.[99] A saccular aneurysm may be (1) round with a narrow stalk connecting it to the parent artery (Fig. 18.21), (2) broad based without a stalk, or (3) cylindrical. Saccular aneurysms are rare in childhood; their highest incidence of rupturing or bleeding is among people 20 to 50 years of age.

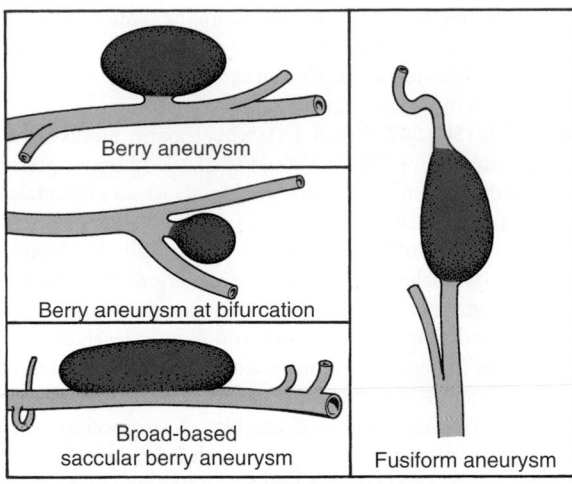

FIGURE 18.20 Types of Aneurysms.

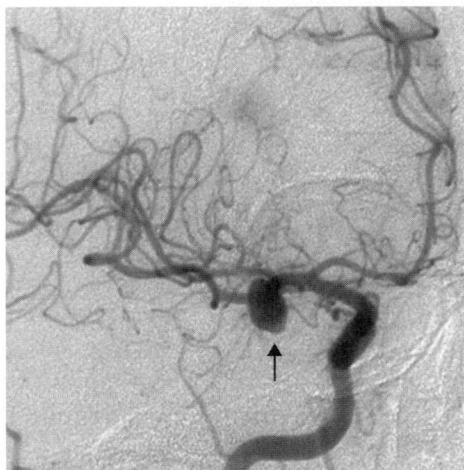

FIGURE 18.21 Berry Aneurysm, Angiogram. This lateral view, with contrast filling a portion of the cerebral arterial circulation, shows a berry aneurysm *(arrow)* involving the middle cerebral artery of the circle of Willis at the base of the brain. (From Klatt EC: *Robbins and Cotran atlas of pathology,* ed 3, Philadelphia, 2015, Saunders.)

Fusiform aneurysms (giant aneurysms), by definition greater than 25 mm in diameter, make up 5% of all intracranial aneurysms. They occur as a result of diffuse arteriosclerotic changes and are found most commonly in the basilar arteries or terminal portions of the internal carotid arteries. They act as space-occupying lesions and often present as an ischemic stroke. **Mycotic aneurysms** are rare and result from arteritis caused by bacterial emboli (e.g., associated with bacterial endocarditis); these aneurysms are uncommon. **Traumatic (dissecting) aneurysms** are a weakening of the arterial wall caused by a fracture line, a penetrating missile, or after neurosurgical or imaging (e.g., angiographic) procedures.

What causes an aneurysm to rupture is not known.[100] Aneurysms rupture through thin areas, often at bifurcation sites, and cause hemorrhage into the subarachnoid space (subarachnoid hemorrhage) (see the Subarachnoid Hemorrhage section) with rapid spread, producing localized changes in the cerebral cortex and focal irritation of nerves and arteries. Because of compression, bleeding ceases with the formation of a fibrin-platelet plug at the point of rupture. Blood undergoes reabsorption through arachnoid villi within 3 weeks.

◆ **CLINICAL MANIFESTATIONS.** Aneurysms are often asymptomatic. Of all persons undergoing routine autopsy, 5% are found to have one or more intracranial aneurysms. Clinical manifestations may arise from cranial nerve compression, but the signs vary, depending on the location and size of the aneurysm. Most often, cranial nerves III, IV, V, and VI are affected (see Table 15.6). Unfortunately the most common first indication is a ruptured aneurysm causing acute subarachnoid hemorrhage, intracerebral hemorrhage, or combined subarachnoid-intracerebral hemorrhage.

◆ **EVALUATION AND TREATMENT.** Diagnosis before a bleeding episode is made using arteriography. Intracranial aneurysms may be found incidentally during CT or MRI imaging for other conditions. After a subarachnoid or an intracerebral hemorrhage, a tentative diagnosis of an aneurysm that has bled is based on clinical manifestations, history, and imaging. Modifiable risk factors include smoking, alcohol use, and hypertension. Treatments for intracranial aneurysm are both medical (i.e., control of hypertension) and surgical (i.e., microvascular clipping or placement of endovascular coils). The mortality rate following rupture is 50%, and 50% of survivors are disabled, often severely.[101]

Vascular Malformations

Vascular malformations are rare, congenital vascular lesions that usually occur sporadically. An **arteriovenous malformation (AVM)** is a mass of dilated vessels between the arterial and venous systems (arteriovenous fistula) that lack a muscularis layer and have the absence of an intervening capillary bed. They can cause hemorrhagic stroke, epilepsy, chronic headache, or focal neurologic deficits.[102]

Four types of vascular malformation exist: arteriovenous malformation, cavernous angioma, capillary telangiectasis, and venous angioma.[103] They usually rupture in the second and third decades of life. **Cavernous angiomas (malformations)** are rare sinusoidal collections of blood vessels without interspersed normal brain tissue. They rarely hemorrhage and comprise 2% to 4% of hemorrhagic strokes. A **capillary telangiectasis** is dilated capillaries with interspersed normal brain tissue found deep in the brain, particularly in the brainstem; hemorrhage is rare. These vascular malformations are associated with Rendu-Osler-Weber disease (AVM in various areas of the body). **Venous angioma,** the most common vascular malformation found at autopsy (3% of cases), is considered a subset of developmental venous anomalies that occur secondary to arrested development. The result is primitive embryologic veins in a radial pattern feeding a central vein. These rarely hemorrhage.[104]

◆ **PATHOPHYSIOLOGY.** AVMs are developmental abnormalities that represent persistence of embryonic patterns of blood vessels. The vessels are abnormally thin and have complex growth and remodeling patterns[105] (Fig. 18.22). Their size is variable. The direct shunting of arterial blood into the venous vasculature without the dissipation of the arterial blood pressure increases risk for rupture. One or several arteries may feed the AVM, and over time, they become tortuous and dilated. With moderate to large AVMs, sufficient blood is shunted into the malformation to deprive surrounding tissue of adequate blood perfusion.

◆ **CLINICAL MANIFESTATIONS.** Twenty percent of persons with an AVM have a characteristic chronic, nondescript headache, although some experience migraine. Fifty percent of persons experience seizures. The other 50% experience an intracerebral, subarachnoid, or subdural hemorrhage with progressive neurologic deficits.[106] Bleeding from an AVM into the subarachnoid space causes clinical manifestations identical to those associated with a ruptured aneurysm. If bleeding is into the brain tissue, focal signs progress over a short period of time. Ten percent of persons experience hemiparesis or other focal signs. Hemiparesis usually is caused by compression or rupture. At times, noncommunicating hydrocephalus (see Chapters 17 and 20) develops with a large AVM that extends into the ventricle lining. AVMs account for up to 1% of all sudden deaths.

◆**EVALUATION AND TREATMENT.** A systolic bruit over the carotid in the neck, the mastoid process, or (in a young person) the eyeball is almost diagnostic of an AVM. Confirming diagnosis is made by CT and MRI followed by magnetic resonance angiography (MRA). Treatment options include direct surgical excision, endovascular embolization, or radiotherapy.[107]

Subarachnoid Hemorrhage

Subarachnoid hemorrhage (SAH) is the escape of blood from a defective or injured vasculature into the subarachnoid space (Fig. 18.23). Individuals at risk for SAH are those with intracranial aneurysm, intracranial arteriovenous malformation, hypertension, a family history of SAH, and those who have sustained head injuries. Subarachnoid hemorrhages often recur, especially from a ruptured intracranial aneurysm. Other

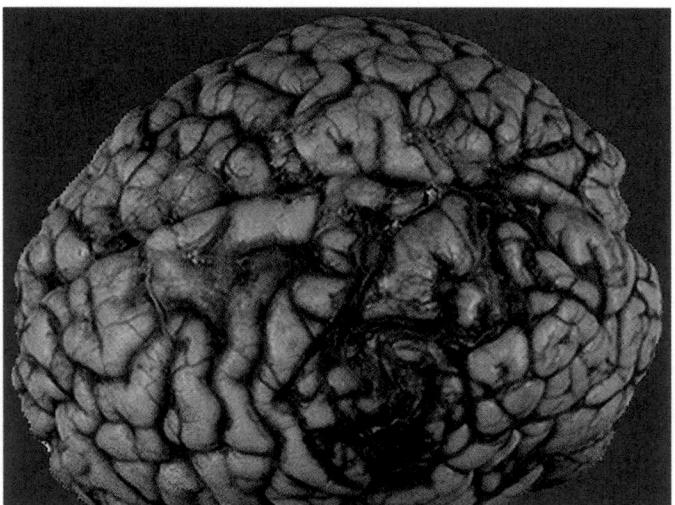

FIGURE 18.22 Vascular Malformation, Gross. A vascular malformation represented by a mass of irregular tortuous vessels over the left posterior parietal region of the brain. (From Klatt EC: *Robbins and Cotran atlas of pathology*, ed 3, Philadelphia, 2015, Saunders.)

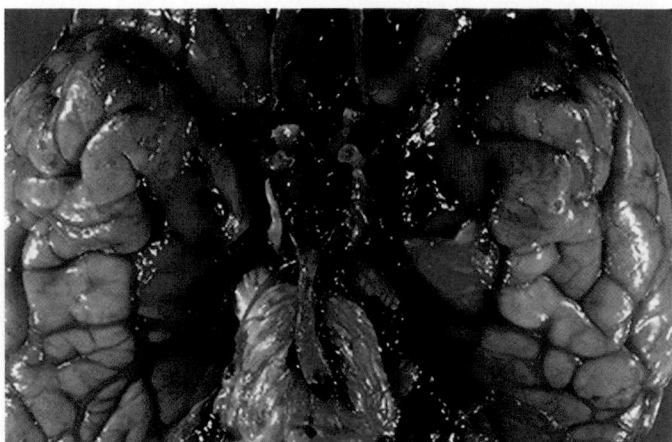

FIGURE 18.23 Subarachnoid Hemorrhage, Gross. Subarachnoid hemorrhage resulting from rupture of a berry aneurysm. (From Klatt EC: *Robbins and Cotran atlas of pathology*, ed 3, Philadelphia, 2015, Saunders.)

risk factors include heavy alcohol use, smoking, anticoagulation use, and oral contraceptive use. Mortality is approximately 50%, and about one-third of survivors require dependent care. SAHs often recur, especially from a ruptured intracranial aneurysm.[108]

◆**PATHOPHYSIOLOGY.** When a vessel is leaking, blood oozes into the subarachnoid space. When a vessel tears, blood under pressure is pumped into the subarachnoid space. The blood increases the intracranial volume, is extremely irritating to the meningeal and other neural tissues, and produces an inflammatory reaction. Additionally, the blood coats nerve roots, clogs arachnoid granulations (impairing CSF reabsorption), and clogs foramina within the ventricular system (impairing CSF circulation). ICP immediately increases to almost diastolic levels. ICP returns to near baseline in about 10 minutes. Autoregulation of blood flow is impaired and there is a compensatory increase in systolic blood pressure.[109] The expanding hematoma acts like a space-occupying lesion, compressing and displacing brain tissue with IICP, decreased cerebral perfusion pressure, decreased cerebral blood flow, blood-brain barrier breakdown, brain edema, inflammation, and cell death. Secondary brain injury can occur as described for TBI.

Delayed cerebral ischemia (DCI), a syndrome of progressive neurologic deterioration, is associated with *cerebral artery vasospasm.* From 40% to 60% of persons with a subarachnoid hemorrhage experience vasospasms in adjacent and, occasionally, in nonadjacent vessels. Vasospasm may occur because of leukocyte–endothelial cell interactions or the effects of inflammatory vasoactive substances (e.g., calcium, prostaglandins, serotonin, catecholamines, endothelin-1) on the arteries of the subarachnoid space. Edema, medial necrosis, and proliferation of the tunica intima have been found. Vasospasm causes decreased cerebral blood flow, ischemia, and possibly infarct and can lead to delayed ischemic injury and death 3 to 14 days after the initial hemorrhage.[110]

◆**CLINICAL MANIFESTATIONS.** Early manifestations associated with leaking vessels are episodic and include headache; changes in mental status or level of consciousness; nausea or vomiting; and focal neurologic defects, such as visual or speech disturbances, cranial nerve palsies, or stiff neck. A ruptured vessel causes a sudden throbbing, "explosive" headache accompanied by nausea and vomiting, visual disturbances, motor deficits, and loss of consciousness related to a dramatic rise in ICP. Meningeal irritation and inflammation often occur, causing neck stiffness (nuchal rigidity), photophobia, blurred vision, irritability, restlessness, and low-grade fever. A positive Kernig sign (straightening the knee with the hip and knee in a flexed position produces pain in the back and neck regions) and a positive Brudzinski sign (passive flexion of the neck produces neck pain and increased rigidity) may appear. No localizing signs are present if the bleed is confined completely to the subarachnoid space. Hyponatremia is common and related to cerebral salt wasting or syndrome of inappropriate antidiuretic hormone. Several scales have been developed for grading SAH.[111] One of the commonly used is the Hunt and Hess grading system combined with the Glasgow Coma Score (see Table 18.1). The Hunt and Hess SAH grading system is based on description of the clinical manifestations (Table 18.6). Rebleeding is a significant risk with a high mortality (up to 70%). The period of greatest risk is the first 6 hours after an SAH in association with high systolic blood pressure and higher Hunt and Hess grade (III-IV), larger-sized aneurysm (>10 mm), and large posterior hematomas.[112] Rebleeding is manifested by a sudden increase in blood pressure and ICP, along with a deteriorating neurologic status.

Seizures occur in 25% of persons with an SAH. Granulation tissue is formed and scarring of the meninges, with resulting impairment of CSF reabsorption leads to secondary hydrocephalus in about 20% of cases. Hypothalamic dysfunction, manifested by salt wasting, hyponatremia, and ECG changes, is common.

◆ **EVALUATION AND TREATMENT.** The diagnosis of an SAH is based on the clinical presentation, imaging, and CSF evaluation. Treatment is directed at controlling ICP, improving cerebral perfusion pressure, preventing ischemia and hypoxia of neural tissues, and avoiding rebleeding episodes. Surgical intervention is common, including surgical clipping of the aneurysm and endovascular placement of coils to occlude the aneurysm. Nimodipine (a calcium channel blocker) is used to prevent vasospasm, and magnesium, phosphodiesterase 3 inhibitors, and therapeutic hypothermia are being evaluated.[113] Treatment guidelines are available to direct therapy.[114]

Primary Headache Syndromes

Headache is a common neurologic disorder and is usually a benign symptom. However, it can be associated with serious disease, such as brain tumor, meningitis, giant cell arteritis, and cerebrovascular disease (secondary headaches). The primary headache syndromes discussed here are the chronic, recurring type not associated with structural abnormalities or systemic disease and include migraine, cluster, paroxysmal hemicrania, and tension headaches. Characteristics of the major types of headache syndromes are summarized in Table 18.7.

TABLE 18.6	SUBARACHNOID HEMORRHAGE CLASSIFICATION SCALE
CATEGORY	**DESCRIPTION**
Grade I	Neurologic status intact; mild headache, slight nuchal rigidity
Grade II	Neurologic deficit evidenced by cranial nerve involvement; moderate to severe headache with more pronounced meningeal signs (e.g., photophobia, nuchal rigidity)
Grade III	Drowsiness and confusion with or without focal neurologic deficits; pronounced meningeal signs
Grade IV	Stuporous with pronounced neurologic deficits (e.g., hemiparesis, dysphasia); nuchal rigidity
Grade V	Deep coma state with decerebrate posturing and other brainstem dysfunction

From Hunt WE, Hess RM: *J Neurosurg* 28(1):14-20, 1968.

Migraine

Migraine is an episodic neurologic disorder whose marker is headache lasting 4 to 72 hours. It is diagnosed when any two of the following features occur: unilateral head pain, throbbing pain, pain worsens with activity, moderate or severe pain intensity; *and* at least one of the following: nausea and/or vomiting, or photophobia and phonophobia.[115] Migraine is broadly classified as (1) *migraine with aura* with visual, sensory, or motor symptoms; and, more commonly, (2) *migraine without aura* (most common) and (3) *chronic migraine.*[116]

Migraine occurs in about 18% of women, 6% of men, and about 10% of children in the United States. It is more common in those 25 to 55 years of age. There often is a family history of migraine. In susceptible women, migraine occurs most frequently before and during menstruation and is decreased during pregnancy and menopause. The cyclic withdrawal of estrogen and progesterone may trigger attacks of migraine.[117]

Migraine is caused by a combination of multiple genetic and environmental factors. Persons with migraine have an increased risk for epilepsy, depression, anxiety disorders, cardiovascular disease, and ischemic stroke.[119] Migraine may be precipitated by triggers. Individuals with migraine are likely to have a genetically determined reduced threshold for triggers. Triggers can include endogenous factors (e.g., altered sleep patterns [becoming tired or too much sleep], missed meals, overexertion, weather change, stress or relaxation from stress, hormonal changes [such as menstrual periods], excess afferent stimulation [bright lights, strong smells], and chemicals [alcohol or nitrates]).[120]

The pathophysiologic basis for migraine is complex and not clearly established. There is no identifiable pathology, but there are associated changes in brain metabolism and blood flow. Current theories include neurologic, vascular, hormonal, and neurotransmitter components. Migraine aura is associated with cortical spreading depression (CSD). CSD is a spontaneous, self-propagating wave of glial and neuronal depolarization resulting in hyperactivity that starts in the occipital region and spreads across the cortex.[121] CSD initiates the headache phase with release of neurotransmitters that activate the trigeminal vascular system (afferent projections from cranial nerve V), stimulating vasodilation of dural blood vessels, activation of inflammation, peripheral and central sensitization of pain receptors (hypersensitivity to pain), and activation

TABLE 18.7	CHARACTERISTICS OF COMMON HEADACHES			
	MIGRAINE		**CLUSTER HEADACHE/ PROXIMAL HEMICRANIA**	**TENSION TYPE OF HEADACHE**
	WITHOUT AURA	**WITH AURA (25%-30%)**		
Age of onset	Childhood, adolescence, or young adulthood	Childhood, adolescence, or young adulthood	Young adulthood, middle age	Young adulthood, middle age
Sex	Higher in females	Higher in females	Male	Not sex specific
Family history of headaches	Yes	Yes	No	Yes
Onset and evolution	Slow to rapid	Slow to rapid	Rapid	Slow to rapid
Time course	Episodic	Episodic	Clusters in time	Episodic, may become constant
Quality	Usually throbbing	Usually throbbing	Steady	Steady
Location	Variable, unilateral to bilateral	Variable, unilateral to bilateral	Orbit, temple, cheek	Variable
Associated features	Prodrome, vomiting	Aura: visual, sensory, language, and motor disturbance Prodrome, vomiting	Lacrimation, rhinorrhea, Horner syndrome	None

of areas of the brainstem and forebrain that modulate pain. Release of inflammatory mediators with sterile meningeal inflammation and edema of blood vessels may be an important component of migraine pain. Vasodilation of blood vessels is not sufficient to account for the pain of migraine. Calcitonin gene–related peptide (CGRP) release by the trigeminal vascular system is related to migraine pain. The mechanism is not clear, but CGRP antagonists prevent the headache. Glutamate (an excitatory neurotransmitter) concentration is increased and 5-hydroxytryptamine (5-HT, serotonin) concentration is decreased. 5-HT causes vasoconstriction and antagonizes CGRP. Consequently, 5-HT(1B/1D) receptor agonists (i.e., triptans) and CGRP receptor and glutamate receptor antagonists have been used for the acute treatment of severe migraine.[122]

The clinical phases of a migraine attack are as follows:

1. *Premonitory phase:* Up to one-third of persons have premonitory symptoms hours to days before onset of aura or headache. These symptoms may include tiredness, irritability, loss of concentration, stiff neck, and food cravings.
2. *Migraine aura:* Up to one-third of persons have aura symptoms at least some of the time that may last up to 1 hour. Symptoms can be visual, sensory, or motor. There are no associated focal neurologic symptoms in migraine without aura.
3. *Headache phase:* Throbbing pain usually begins on one side and spreads to include the entire head. Headache may be accompanied by fatigue, nausea, and vomiting or dizziness. There may be hypersensitivity to anything touching the head. Symptoms may last from 4 to 72 hours (usually about a day).
4. *Recovery phase:* Irritability, fatigue, or depression may take hours or days to resolve.

The diagnosis of migraine is made from medical history and physical examination. Differential diagnosis is confirmed by imaging and EEG. Functional neuroimaging and genetic studies are advancing the understanding of the mechanisms involved in migraine attacks and individual variants involved with disease susceptibility.[123] The management of migraine includes avoidance of triggers (e.g., darkening the room, applying ice). Sleeping can provide some relief with the onset of acute migraine. Pharmacologic management for the treatment and prevention of migraine is available and individualized.[124] A transcutaneous electrical stimulation device providing trigeminal neurostimulation has been approved by the Food and Drug Administration for the prevention of migraine.[125]

Chronic migraines usually begin as episodic migraines that increase in frequency over time. Chronic migraine occurs at least 15 days in a month (can occur daily or on a near-daily basis) for more than 3 months. Chronic migraines are associated with overuse of analgesic migraine medications (sometimes called rebound headaches), obesity, and caffeine overuse. Treatment is similar to that for episodic migraine. Injections with botulinum toxin A are approved for preventing chronic migraine.[126] Individuals with chronic migraine unresponsive to medical treatment should be evaluated for intracranial hypertension without papilledema and the possibility of sinus venous stenosis.[127]

Cluster Headache

Cluster headaches are one of a group of rare disorders referred to as trigeminal autonomic cephalagia.[128] They occur in one side of the head primarily in men between 20 and 50 years of age. The pain may alternate sides with each headache episode and is severe, stabbing, and throbbing. These uncommon headaches occur in clusters (up to eight attacks per day) and last for minutes to hours for a period of days, followed by a long period of spontaneous remission. Cluster headache has an episodic and a chronic form with extreme pain intensity and short duration. If the cluster of attacks occurs more frequently without sustained spontaneous remission, they are classified as *chronic cluster headaches* (10% to 20% of cases) (see Table 18.7). Triggers are similar to those that cause migraine headache.

Trigeminal activation occurs, but the mechanism is unclear. Functional imaging indicates a role for concomitant posterior hypothalamic and pain neuromatrix activation with opioid system involvement.[129] The pathogenic mechanism for pain is related to the release of vasoactive peptides and the formation of neurogenic inflammation. Autonomic dysfunction is characterized by sympathetic underactivity and parasympathetic activation. The headache attack usually begins without warning. There is unilateral trigeminal distribution of severe pain with ipsilateral autonomic manifestations, including tearing on the affected side, ptosis of the ipsilateral eye, and congestion of the nasal mucosa. Pain often is referred to the midface and teeth. Prophylactic drugs and avoidance of triggers are used to treat cluster headache. Acute attacks are managed with oxygen inhalation, sumatriptan or inhaled ergotamine administration, and nerve stimulation. New drugs are under investigation.[131]

Chronic paroxysmal hemicrania (CPH) is a cluster-type headache with unilateral head pain associated with autonomic features (lacrimation or rhinorrhea) that occurs with more daily frequency (4 to 12 times per day) but with shorter duration (20 to 120 minutes). The remission phases are often shorter. The attacks occur in both men and women beginning at 30 to 40 years of age. The symptoms are similar to cluster headache. As with cluster headache, there is an episodic and a chronic form. The pathophysiology involves a disorder of sympathetic hyperactivity, but the mechanism is different from that of cluster headache because there is effective relief of symptoms with indomethacin.[132]

Tension-Type Headache

Tension-type headache (TTH) is the most prevalent type of recurrent headache. It is not a vascular or migrainous headache. The average age of onset is during the second decade of life. It is usually a mild to moderate bilateral headache with a sensation of a tight band or pressure around the head. The onset of pain is usually gradual. *Episodic tension-type headache* occurs less than 15 days per month and may last for several hours or several days. It is not aggravated by physical activity and may be triggered by sleep disorders (insomnia). *Chronic tension-type headache* evolves from episodic TTH and occurs at least 15 days per month for at least 3 months. Many individuals have both tension-type and migraine headaches.

Both central and peripheral mechanisms operate in causing tension headache. The central mechanism probably involves hypersensitivity of pain fibers from the trigeminal nerve that leads to central sensitization with deficits in the descending inhibitory pain pathways within the brainstem. The peripheral sensitization of myofascial sensory afferents may contribute to muscular hypersensitivity and the development of chronic TTH. Headache sufferers have more localized pain and tenderness of pericranial muscles.[133]

Mild headaches are treated with ice, and more severe forms are treated with aspirin or other nonsteroidal antiinflammatory drugs. Chronic TTHs are best managed with a tricyclic antidepressant and behavioral and relaxation therapy. Some individuals benefit from injection of botulinum toxin A. Long-term use of analgesics or other drugs, such as muscle relaxants, antihistamines, tranquilizers, caffeine, and ergot alkaloids, should be avoided.[134]

Infection and Inflammation of the Central Nervous System

The CNS may be infected by bacteria, viruses, fungi, parasites, and mycobacteria. The infecting microorganisms gain entry to the nervous system by (1) spreading through arterial blood vessels or (2) direct extension from another site of infection. Neurologic infections produce disease by several mechanisms: direct neuronal or glial infection, mass lesion formation, inflammation with subsequent edema, interruption of CSF pathways, neuronal or vascular damage, and secretion of neurotoxins. An immune process initiates an inflammatory reaction.

Syndromes are acute and subacute bacterial meningitis, epidural and brain abscess, encephalitis, peripheral neuropathy, or neurosyphilis, depending on the infecting microorganism. Signs and symptoms are produced because of (1) interference with the function of the nervous system tissue being invaded or compressed or (2) the inflammatory response produced by the body in response to infection. The cardinal signs of CNS infection are fever, head or spine pain, and generalized or focal neurologic dysfunction.[135]

Meningitis

Meningitis is inflammation of the brain or spinal cord. Infectious meningitis may be caused by bacteria, viruses, fungi, parasites, or toxins. (The pathophysiology of infection is discussed in Chapter 10.) The infection may be acute, subacute, or chronic with the pathophysiology, clinical manifestations, and treatment differing for each type of microorganism.

Bacterial Meningitis.
Bacterial meningitis is primarily an infection of the pia mater and arachnoid villi, the subarachnoid space, the ventricular system, and the CSF. About 5 to 10 per 100,000 persons are affected annually.[136] Meningococcus (Neisseria meningitidis) and pneumococcus (Streptococcus pneumoniae) are the most common pathogens. An increase of drug-resistant strains of S. pneumoniae is an emerging problem worldwide. Meningococcus has been identified worldwide, and there are six serogroups: A, B, C, W-135, X, and Y. Most cases are sporadic and occur predominantly in children younger than 1 year of age and adolescents. Local outbreaks may occur in dormitories, military bases, or sub-Saharan Africa. Young persons and those more than 40 years of age are mostly affected with pneumococcal meningitis. Predisposing conditions are otitis or sinusitis (25%), immunocompromised status (16%), and pneumonia (12%).[136] The disease is spread by respiratory droplets and contact with contaminated saliva or respiratory tract secretions (kissing, coughing, and sneezing or sharing utensils, food, and drink).[138] Carriers of the meningococcal bacteria do not develop meningitis but may pass it on to others.

Bacterial meningococci and pneumococci are inhaled and attach to epithelial cells in the nasopharynx where they evade immune defenses, cross the mucosal barrier, enter the bloodstream, travel to cerebral blood vessels, cross the blood-brain barrier, and infect the meninges (Fig. 18.24). Bacteria multiply in the subarachnoid space and attract large numbers of neutrophils. Release of cytotoxic inflammatory agents and bacterial endotoxin alter the blood-brain barrier, cause cerebral edema, and damage brain tissue. The inflammatory exudate thickens the CSF and interferes with normal CSF flow around the brain and spinal cord, possibly obstructing arachnoid villi and producing hydrocephalus. Meningeal cells become edematous, and the combined exudate and edematous cells increase ICP. Engorged blood vessels and thrombi can disrupt blood flow, causing further injury[139] (Fig. 18.25). The cortical neurons also show some changes, including an increase in the number of microglia and astrocytes. Acute infectious purpura fulminans is a rare, rapidly progressive syndrome of hemorrhagic infarction of the skin and disseminated intravascular coagulation that can lead to multiple organ failure, ischemic necrosis of digits and limbs with amputation required, and death. It is caused by bacterial endotoxin and inflammatory cytokines associated with meningitis.

The clinical manifestations of bacterial meningitis can be grouped into infectious signs, meningeal inflammatory signs, and neurologic signs. The clinical manifestations of systemic infection include fever,

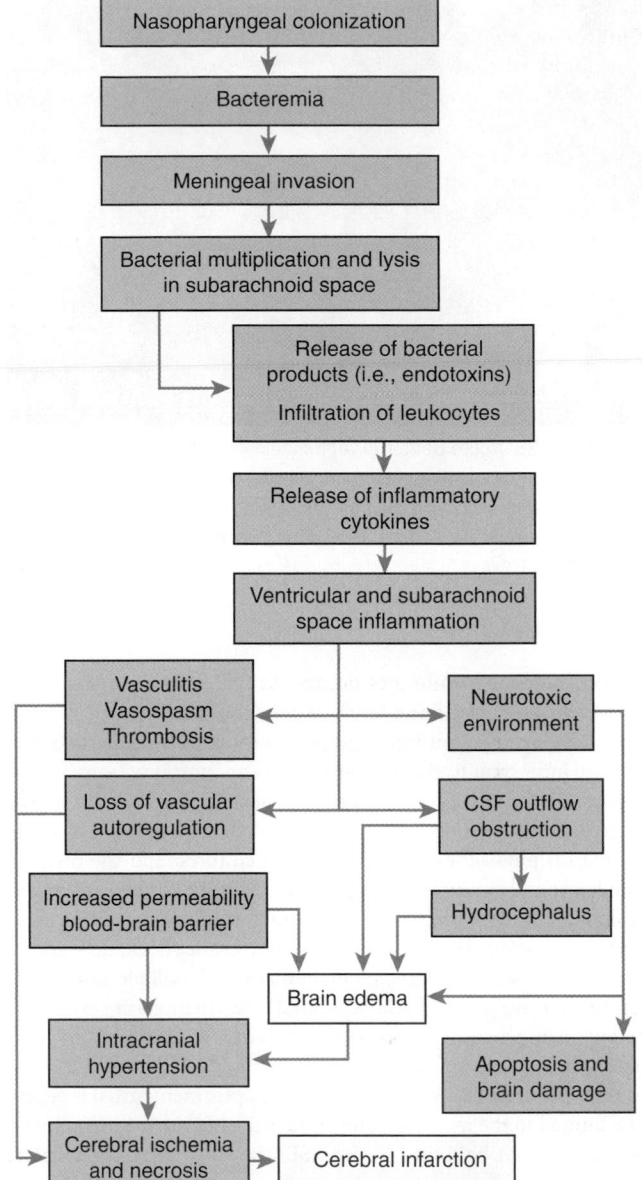

FIGURE 18.24 Pathogenesis of Meningitis. (Adapted from Cohen J, Powderly WG: *Infectious diseases*, ed 2, Mosby, 2004, Edinburgh.)

tachycardia, and chills. The clinical manifestations of meningeal irritation are a severe throbbing headache, severe photophobia, nuchal rigidity, and positive Kernig and Brudzinski signs. The neurologic signs include a decrease in consciousness, focal neurologic deficits (such as hemiparesis/hemiplegia and ataxia), and seizures. The irritation and damage to the cranial nerves produced by the inflamed sheaths manifest as follows:

Cranial nerve II: papilledema, blindness
Cranial nerves III, IV, and VI: ptosis, visual field deficits, diplopia
Cranial nerve V: photophobia
Cranial nerve VII: facial paresis
Cranial nerve VIII: deafness, tinnitus, vertigo

Neck stiffness and pain, and possibly head retraction, reflect the irritability of spinal accessory and cervical spinal nerves. Often the vomiting center is irritated, causing projectile vomiting. Confusion and decreasing responsiveness are evidence of cortical involvement. In meningococcal meningitis, petechial or purpuric rash involving the

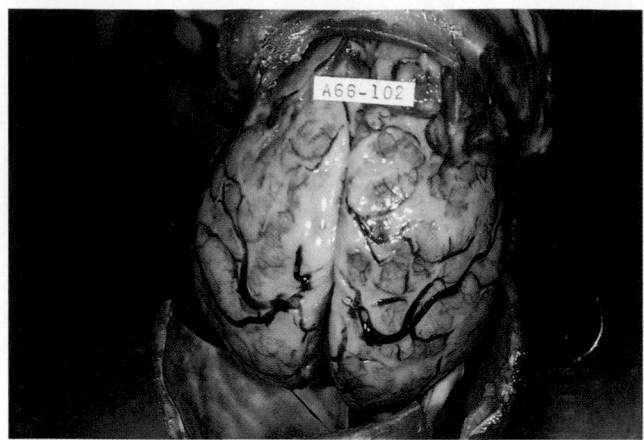

FIGURE 18.25 Acute Bacterial Leptomeningitis. The leptomeninges contain abundant creamy, purulent exudate, most prominently over the superior surface of the cerebrum. The underlying brain is swollen, and the vessels are congested. (From Kumar V, Cotran RS, Robbins SL: *Robbins basic pathology*, ed 7, Philadelphia, 2003, Saunders.)

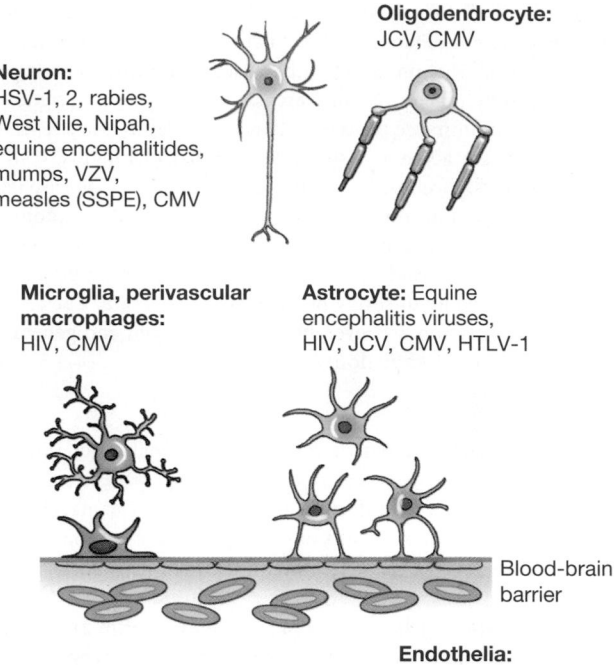

FIGURE 18.26 Viral Infection of Specific Cells in the Central Nervous System (CNS). Viruses infect specific cell types within the CNS depending on the specific properties of the virus together with individual cell-membrane proteins expressed on permissive cell types. Normally the brain is protected from circulating pathogens and toxins by the blood-brain barrier. *CMV,* Cytomegalovirus; *HIV,* human immunodeficiency virus; *HSV,* herpes simplex virus; *HTLV-1,* human T-cell lymphotropic virus type 1 (causes T-cell leukemia); *JCV,* John Cunningham virus (a polyomavirus causing progressive multifocal leukoencephalopathy); *SSPE,* subacute sclerosing panencephalitis; *VZV,* varicella-zoster virus. (Adapted from Power C, Noorbakhsh G: Central nervous system viral infections: clinical aspects and pathogenic mechanisms. In Gilman S, editor: *Neurobiology of disease*, Burlington, MA, 2007, Elsevier, p 488.)

skin and mucous membranes occurs. As ICP increases, papilledema may develop with declining levels of consciousness.

Rapid diagnosis, antibiotic administration, and supportive treatment are important to prevent morbidity and mortality from bacterial meningitis. Dexamethasone therapy has been implemented as adjunctive treatment of adults with pneumococcal meningitis.[139] Diagnosis is based on physical examination, blood cultures, and the results of nasopharyngeal smear and antigen tests. CSF analysis and cultures are required to diagnose fungal meningitis. Other supportive measures may be needed. Serious complications, including septic shock, disseminated intravascular coagulation, purpura fulminans, and multiple organ failure, require intensive multidisciplinary care.[140] Vaccinations are available to prevent meningococcal, pneumococcal, and *Haemophilus influenzae* meningitis.

Viral Meningitis. Viral meningitis (aseptic meningitis) is believed to be limited to the meninges and an identifiable bacterium or specific pathogen cannot be found in the CSF. The most at-risk populations and the time of year when occurrences are seen depend on the virus and on the immune status of the individual. Viral meningitis produces a variety of symptoms and is caused by a variety of viruses. Viruses infecting specific cell types are presented in Fig. 18.26. Viruses causing acute and chronic CNS infections are listed in Table 18.8.

In viral meningitis, the virus reaches the CNS by hematogenous spread (Fig. 18.27). The virus enters the brain either directly or indirectly, through infected migrating leukocytes, and then infects vascular endothelial cells. The virus then enters the subarachnoid space, leading to meningitis. The immune response leads to release of inflammatory cytokines with increased permeability of the blood-brain barrier and entry of circulating immunoglobulins that combat the virus.

The clinical manifestations of viral meningitis are mild compared with those associated with bacterial meningitis. Mild generalized throbbing headache, mild photophobia, mild neck pain, stiffness, fever, and malaise are manifestations of viral meningitis. Treatment is primarily supportive and the disease usually resolves within 7 to 10 days.

Fungal Meningitis. Fungal meningitis is a chronic condition that is much less common than bacterial or viral meningitis. The most common fungal infections of the nervous system are histoplasmosis, cryptococcosis, coccidioidomycosis, mucormycosis, candidiasis, and aspergillosis. It develops insidiously, usually over days or weeks.

Fungi in the nervous system usually produce a granulomatous reaction with formations of granulomas or gelatinous masses. These usually develop in the meninges at the base of the brain. Fungi also may extend along the perivascular sites in the subarachnoid space and into the brain tissue, producing arteritis with thrombosis, infarction, and communicating hydrocephalus. Meningeal fibrosis develops later in the inflammatory process. Cranial nerve dysfunction, caused by compression, often results from the granulomas and fibrosis.

The first manifestations are often those of dementia or communicating hydrocephalus (see Chapter 17). The individual is characteristically afebrile. Cryptococcal meningitis occurs in immunosuppressed hosts, including organ transplant recipients and individuals with HIV/AIDS.[142] *Candida* and *Aspergillus* are less common infections. Antifungal treatments are organism-specific and effective.[143]

Tubercular Meningitis. Tubercular meningitis is a common and serious form of CNS tuberculosis, especially in immunosuppressed persons or those with acquired immunodeficiency syndrome (AIDS). Mycobacteria are acquired through inhalation of aerosolized droplet nuclei. The miliary tubercles form in the brain and meninges. At some point the tuberculomas erode the pia mater, and the mycobacteria enter the CSF, producing a hypersensitivity reaction that results in a purulent exudate involving the basal meninges, cerebrum, and spinal nerves. Cerebral ischemia and infarction occur from vasculitis. Symptoms are

TABLE 18.8   VIRUSES CAUSING ACUTE AND CHRONIC CNS DISEASES

VIRUS	FAMILY	NUCLEIC ACID	CNS DISEASE	CELL TROPISM	NONHUMAN HOST	ROUTE OF ENTRY TO CNS	TREATMENT
Viruses Causing Acute CNS Diseases							
Herpes simplex viruses 1 and 2	Herpesviridae	DNA	Meningoencephalitis	Neuron	ND	Intraneuronal	Acyclovir
Rabies virus	Rhabdoviridae	RNA	Encephalomyelitis	Neuron	Carnivores	Intraneuronal	Postexposure prophylaxis; RIG and vaccine
West Nile virus	Flaviviridae	RNA	Meningoencephalomyelitis	Neuron	Birds, horses	Hematogenous	IVIg, interferon-alpha
Mumps virus	Paramyxoviridae	RNA	Meningitis, encephalitis, myelitis	Neuron, ependymal cell	ND	Hematogenous	IVIg
Nipah virus	Paramyxoviridae	RNA	Encephalitis	Neuron, endothelia	Pigs, fruit bats	Hematogenous	Ribavirin
Rubella virus	Togaviridae	RNA	Meningitis, encephalitis	Not specified	ND	Hematogenous	Plasmapheresis
Equine encephalitis viruses	Togaviridae	RNA	Meningitis, encephalitis	Neuron, astrocytes	Horses	Hematogenous	Supportive care
Coxsackievirus, echovirus	Picornaviridae	RNA	Meningitis, meningoencephalitis, myelitis	Neuron	ND	Hematogenous	Pleconaril
Poliovirus	Picornaviridae	RNA	Meningitis, myelitis	Neuron	ND	Hematogenous	Pleconaril
California encephalitis virus	Bunyaviridae	RNA	Meningitis, encephalitis	Neuron	Small mammals	Hematogenous	Ribavirin
Viruses Causing Chronic CNS Disease							
Human immunodeficiency virus	Retroviridae	RNA	Encephalitis, meningitis, myelitis	Microglia, macrophage, astrocytes	ND	Hematogenous	HAART and neuroprotective agents
Human T-cell leukemia viruses 1 and 2	Retroviridae	RNA	Myelitis	Astrocyte, leukocyte	ND	Hematogenous	Zidovudine, lamivudine, glucocorticoids
JC virus	Polyomaviridae	DNA	Progressive multifocal leukoencephalopathy	Oligodendrocyte, astrocyte	ND	Hematogenous	Interferon-alpha, cidofovir
Measles virus	Paramyxoviridae	RNA	Encephalitis; SSPE	Neuron	ND	Hematogenous	Ribavirin, interferon-alpha, isoprinosine
Varicella-zoster virus	Herpesviridae	DNA	Leukoencephalitis, cerebellitis, meningitis, myelitis	Neurons, satellite cell	ND	Hematogenous	Acyclovir, valacyclovir
Cytomegalovirus	Herpesviridae	DNA	Encephalitis	Neuron, ependymal cell, oligodendrocyte, monocytoid cell, endothelia	ND	Hematogenous	Foscarnet, ganciclovir, cidofovir, fomivirsen, valganciclovir
Epstein-Barr virus	Herpesviridae	DNA	Encephalitis, meningitis, myelitis	Infiltrating mononuclear cells	ND	Hematogenous	Acyclovir, ganciclovir (?)

CNS, Central nervous system; *DNA*, deoxyribonucleic acid; *HAART*, highly active antiretroviral therapy; *IVIg*, intravenous immunoglobulin; *JC*, John Cunningham; *ND*, not determined; *RIG*, rabies immune globulin; *RNA*, ribonucleic acid; *SSPE*, subacute sclerosing panencephalitis.

From Lindquist L, Vapalahti O: *Lancet* 371(9627):1861-1871, 2008; Power C, Noorbakhsh F: Central nervous system viral infections: clinical aspects and pathogenic mechanism. In Gilman S, editor: *Neurobiology of disease*, Burlington, MA, 2007, Elsevier, pp 487-488.

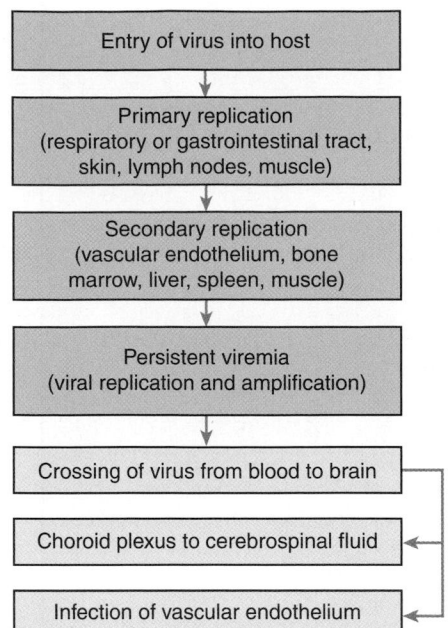

FIGURE 18.27 Hematogenous Spread of Viral Pathogens to the Central Nervous System. (Adapted from Cohen J, Powderly WG: *Infectious diseases*, Mosby, 2007, Edinburgh.)

nonspecific, making early diagnosis difficult. Symptoms include headache, low-grade fever, nausea and vomiting, irritability, difficulty sleeping, and fatigue.[144] These signs and symptoms increase to confusion, stiff neck, significant behavioral changes, and seizures. Hydrocephalus and cranial nerve palsies or cerebral infarcts may occur. Recovery rate is 90% with early diagnosis and treatment with appropriate antituberculosis therapy. Treatment is difficult in resource-poor countries.[145]

Brain or Spinal Cord Abscess

Abscesses are localized collections of pus within the parenchyma of the brain or spinal cord and are rare. Immunosuppressed persons are particularly at risk.

Brain abscesses are classified as extradural, subdural, or intracerebral. Extradural brain abscesses (empyemas) are associated with osteomyelitis in a cranial bone. Subdural brain abscesses (empyemas) arise from a sinus infection or a vascular source. Intracerebral brain abscesses arise from a vascular source. Brain abscesses progress from localized inflammation to a necrotic core with the formation of a connective tissue capsule, usually within 14 days or longer.[146] Existing abscesses also tend to spread and form daughter abscesses. Spinal cord abscesses are rare and classified as epidural or intramedullary. Epidural spinal abscesses usually originate as osteomyelitis in a vertebra or as a bacterial meningitis; the infection then spreads into the epidural space.[147]

PATHOPHYSIOLOGY. Microorganisms gain entrance to the CNS from adjacent sites by direct extension from trauma, mastoiditis, sinusitis, or dental infection. Blood vessels carry infective emboli from distant sites, such as the heart, lungs, pelvic organs, skin, tonsils, abscessed teeth, osteomyelitis (with the exception of cranial bones), and dirty needles (especially in immune-compromised hosts). *Streptococci, Staphylococci,* and *Bacteroides,* often in combination with anaerobes, are the most common bacteria that cause abscesses; however, yeast and fungi also have been found in CNS abscesses. *Toxoplasma gondii* is producing an ever-increasing number of CNS abscesses in persons with AIDS. Most CNS abscesses are located in the frontal and temporal lobes (Fig. 18.28).

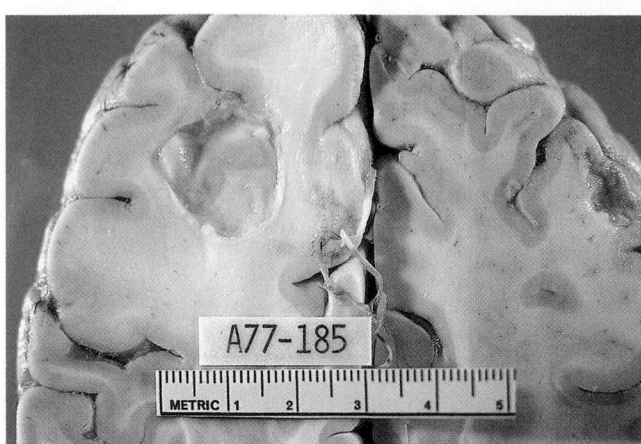

FIGURE 18.28 Brain Abscess. The abscess is sharply demarcated, indicating that it has been present for some time. Purulent exudate is visible in the center of the abscess. Because antibiotics penetrate very poorly into abscesses, surgical drainage is often necessary to treat such lesions. (From Kumar V, Cotran RS, Robbins SL: *Robbins basic pathology*, ed 7, Philadelphia, 2003, Saunders.)

Brain abscesses evolve through four stages regardless of infecting microorganism, except in the immunosuppressed host where the process may be incomplete. The stages are as follows:

1. *Early cerebritis* (days 1 to 3): A localized inflammatory process develops in which perivascular infiltration and inflammatory cells, composed of neutrophils, plasma cells, and mononuclear cells, surround a central core of coagulative necrosis; marked cerebral edema surrounds the area.
2. *Late cerebritis* (days 4 to 9): The necrotic center is surrounded by an inflammatory infiltrate of macrophages and fibroblasts; rapid new blood vessels form around the abscess; a thin capsule of fibroblasts and reticular fibers gradually develops; the area is still surrounded by cerebral edema.
3. *Early capsule formation* (days 10 to 13): The necrotic center decreases in size; the inflammatory infiltrate changes in character and contains an increasing number of fibroblasts and macrophages; mature collagen evolves, forming a capsule.
4. *Late capsule formation* (days 14 and longer): A well-formed necrotic center surrounded by a dense collagenous capsule develops.[148]

CLINICAL MANIFESTATIONS. Early manifestations include low-grade fever, headache (most common symptom), nausea and vomiting, neck pain and stiffness, confusion, drowsiness, sensory deficits, and communication deficits. Later manifestations are associated with an expanding mass and include decreased attention span, memory deficits, decreased visual acuity and narrowed visual fields, papilledema, ocular palsy, ataxia, cognitive deficits, and seizures. The development of symptoms may be very insidious, often making an abscess difficult to diagnose.

Extradural brain abscesses are associated with localized pain, purulent drainage from the nasal passages or auditory canal, fever, localized tenderness, and neck stiffness; occasionally the individual experiences a focal seizure. Clinical manifestations of spinal cord abscesses have four stages: (1) spinal aching; (2) root pain, which is usually severe, accompanied by spasms of the back muscles and limited vertebral movement because of pain and spasm; (3) weakness caused by progressive cord compression; and (4) paralysis.[150]

EVALUATION AND TREATMENT. The diagnosis is suggested on the basis of clinical features and confirmed with MRI or contrast-enhanced CT. Stereotactic surgical aspiration is usually indicated for identification of the pathogen and for decompression of the abscess. Antibiotics are initiated when there is clinical suspicion of an abscess. Multiple or surgically inaccessible abscesses are treated with antibiotics, often in conjunction with corticosteroid therapy to treat the cerebral edema. In addition, ICP or hydrocephalus, or both, require management.[148] Because decompression is necessary, spinal cord abscesses are treated with surgical excision or aspiration. Antibiotic administration and supportive therapy are instituted.

Encephalitis

Encephalitis is an acute febrile illness, usually of viral origin, with nervous system involvement. The most common forms are caused by bites of mosquitos, ticks, or flies. Herpes simplex type 1 is the most common sporadic cause of encephalitis. Etiologic agents for viral encephalitis are presented in Table 18.8. Referred to as *infectious viral encephalitides,* encephalitis also may occur as a complication of systemic viral diseases such as poliomyelitis, rabies, mononucleosis, rubella, or rubeola. Encephalitis also may follow vaccination with a live attenuated virus vaccine if the vaccine has an encephalitis component. Such vaccines include measles, mumps, rubella; varicella; rotavirus; and yellow fever. Typhus, trichinosis, malaria, and schistosomiasis also are associated with encephalitis. Toxoplasmosis may acutely reactivate in immunosuppressed hosts when the once-dormant parasite in cyst form disseminates in brain tissues.[151]

With the exception of the California viral encephalitis, which is endemic, the arthropod-borne encephalitides occur in epidemics, varying in geographic and seasonal incidence (Table 18.9). Eastern equine encephalitis is the most serious but least common of the encephalitides.[152] West Nile virus is presented in Box 18.1.

◆ **PATHOPHYSIOLOGY.** Viruses gain access to the CNS through the bloodstream, olfactory bulb, or choroid plexus or through an intraneuronal route from peripheral nerves. Meningeal involvement is present in all encephalitides. The arthropod-borne viral encephalitides cause widespread nerve cell degeneration. Edema and areas of necrosis with or without hemorrhage develop. IICP develops and may progress to herniation. Large degenerative injuries are found in eastern equine encephalitis, whereas the other arthropod-borne viral encephalitides have microscopic areas of injury and degeneration. Infectious encephalitis may result from a postinfectious autoimmune response to the virus or from direct invasion of the CNS by the virus. Herpes simplex type 1 has a tendency to infect the inferomedial surfaces of the temporal and frontal lobes and causes hemorrhagic necrosis.

◆ **CLINICAL MANIFESTATIONS.** Encephalitis may range from a mild infectious disease to a life-threatening disorder. The dramatic clinical manifestations of encephalitis are fever (minor criterion), altered mental status, delirium, or confusion progressing to unconsciousness, seizure activity, cranial nerve palsies, paresis and paralysis, involuntary movement, and abnormal reflexes. Signs of marked ICP may be present.

◆ **EVALUATION AND TREATMENT.** Diagnosis is based on health history and clinical presentation aided by CSF examination and culture, serologic examination, white blood cell (WBC) count, CT scan, or MRI. (Treatment available for the viral encephalitides is listed in Table 18.8.) Antiviral or immune therapy is initiated as well as supportive therapy for cerebral edema, status epilepticus, and thrombocytopenia.[153]

Neurologic Complications of Acquired Immunodeficiency Syndrome

Approximately 40% to 60% of all persons with AIDS have neurologic complications (see Chapter 10 for the pathophysiology of AIDS). On postmortem examination, 75% have nervous system pathologic findings. The CNS pathologic findings result from (1) the primary human immunodeficiency virus (HIV) infection, which seeds the CNS soon after primary infection when CD4+ T cells are depressed; (2) the immune dysregulation of early HIV infection and progressive immunosuppression in late HIV infections resulting in opportunistic infections, neoplasms, and systemic illness; and (3) the complications of therapy.[154]

Human Immunodeficiency Virus–Associated Neurocognitive Disorders (HANDs). A variety of names have been used for human immunodeficiency virus–associated neurocognitive disorders (HANDs), including HIV-associated dementia (HAD), HIV-associated

TABLE 18.9	CLASSIFICATION AND CHARACTERISTICS OF ARTHROPOD-BORNE VIRUSES (ARBOVIRUS) CAUSING ENCEPHALITIS					
VIRUSES	INCUBATION PERIOD (DAYS)	VIRUS	LOCATION	VECTOR	SEASON	AFFECTED POPULATION
Eastern equine encephalitis	5–10	Togaviridae *Alphavirus* (formerly group A arbovirus)	Swampy areas of eastern United States and Michigan	Mosquito	June to October	Infants, children, and adults >50 years
Western equine encephalitis	5–10	Same as above	All parts of United States: eastern, central, and western	Mosquito	July to October	All ages
Venezuelan equine encephalitis	2–5	Same as above	Texas, Florida, Mexico; Central and South America	Mosquito	All year	Infants and young children
St. Louis encephalitis	4–21	Flaviviridae *Flavivirus*	All parts of United States: eastern, central, and western	Mosquito	June to October	Adults >40 years; older adults more often affected than younger ages
La Cross encephalitis including California	5–15	Bunyaviridae *Bunyavirus* (California virus serogroup)	Midwestern United States, eastern seaboard, and Canada	Woodland mosquito	July to September	Children <15 years
West Nile encephalitis	3–14	Flaviviridae *Flavivirus*	Lower 48 states of United States	Mosquito	Summer and fall	Older adults most seriously

BOX 18.1　WEST NILE VIRUS

West Nile virus (WNV), a *Flavivirus* transmitted predominantly by the *Culex* mosquito, emerged in New York state in 1999. By the end of 2004, human cases had been found in the 48 contiguous states. Humans and horses, as well as other mammals, are incidental hosts. Birds and mosquitoes are life cycle hosts. Summer and fall are peak times of infection incidence. The highest amount of virus carried by mosquitoes is in early fall. Besides mosquito transmission, WNV can be transmitted through blood transfusions and organ transplants. Health experts believe transmission from mother to unborn child and through breast milk is possible.

The human incubation period is 2 to 14 days; however, most individuals develop no symptoms. About 20% of those infected have mild symptoms that last 4 to 6 days and generally include fever, headache, skin rash, and lymphadenopathy. Less than 1% of affected persons develop severe illness, including *WNV encephalitis* marked by headache, disorientation, stupor, coma, seizures, and movement disorders, including tremor, ataxia, extrapyramidal signs, and paralysis. *WNV meningitis* is characterized by meningeal signs of severe headache, high fever, and nuchal rigidity. Myelitis and polyradiculitis also may be present. Abnormalities in the thalamus, basal ganglia, and cerebellum are often seen on MRI in people with severe infection. Identifiable risk factors are very young children or those with advanced age, immunocompromised individuals, and pregnant women.

A preliminary diagnosis is made if WNV-specific IgM for the virus is found in serum or CSF. A rapid test became available in 2007. Plaque reduction neutralization assay (PRNA) is the confirmatory test. MRI may show abnormalities in the basal ganglia, thalamus, and brainstem in those with encephalitis. Treatment is supportive care. No WNV vaccine has been developed for humans. Environmental control and prevention of mosquito bites are the best protection. Since 2003, all blood banks use blood-screening tests for West Nile virus.

CSF, Cerebrospinal fluid; *IgM,* immunoglobulin M; *MRI,* magnetic resonance imaging.
Data from Brandler S, Tangy F: *Viruses* 5(10):2384-2409, 2013; Centers for Disease Control and Prevention: *West Nile virus,* updated February 12, 2015, Available at: www.cdc.gov/westnile/index.html; Petersen LR et al: *J Am Med Assoc* 310(3):308-315, 2013; Pierce KK et al: *J Infect Dis* 215(1):52-55, 2017.

BOX 18.2　CLINICAL MANIFESTATIONS OF HIV-RELATED DEMENTIA

Early Stages

- *Cognitive impairments*
  Short-term memory deficit
  Decreased concentration/attention
  Confusion and disorientation
  Visuospatial perception deficits
- *Changes in personality or behavior*
  Apathy, depression
  Impaired judgment, erratic behavior
  Social withdrawal
  Rigidity of thought
  Speech impairment

- *Psychotic symptoms*
  Hallucinations and delusions
  Suspiciousness and delusions
  Agitation and inappropriate behavior
- *Motor symptoms*
  Ataxia, loss of coordination, weakness
  Tremors
- *Generalized systemic symptoms*
  Fatigue, sleep changes (hypersomnia)
  Anorexia, weight loss
  Enuresis
  Hypersensitivity to drugs and alcohol

Advanced Stages

- *Cognitive symptoms*
  Global cognitive impairment
  Impaired social relationship
  Disorientation
  Psychomotor retardation, decreased spontaneity
  Agitation (e.g., nighttime delusions)
  Coma, vegetative state

- *Motor symptoms*
  Ataxia
  Spastic weakness
  Paraplegia, quadriparesis
  Hyperreflexia, myoclonus, seizures
  Bladder and bowel incontinence

Data from Clark C: Psychiatric aspects of AIDS. In Jacobson JL, Jacobson AM, editors: *Psychiatric secrets,* ed 2, Philadelphia, 2001, Hanley & Belfus; Stern TA et al: *Massachusetts General Hospital comprehensive clinical psychiatry,* St Louis, 2008, Mosby.

---

cognitive dysfunction, HIV encephalopathy, subacute encephalitis, HIV-associated dementia complex, HIV cognitive motor complex, AIDS encephalopathy, AIDS dementia complex, or AIDS-related dementia. Both adults and children may be affected with progressive cognitive dysfunction in conjunction with motor and behavioral alterations. The syndrome typically develops later in the disease but may be an early or a singular manifestation. The syndrome is more prevalent in drug users with HIV and among those with reduced highly active antiretroviral therapy adherence (HAART).[156] HAART with more efficient CNS drug penetration has reduced the prevalence and improved survival for severe HAND, but milder forms of the disease persist because of longer life.[157]

The neurologic syndromes develop from properties of the virus, genetic characteristics of the host, and interactions with the environment (including treatment). At the time of primary HIV infection, HIV infects the perivascular macrophages, microglial cells, and astrocytes, particularly in the basal ganglia and deep white matter. Affected macrophages, macrophage-derived multinucleated cells, and microglia cause an immune-mediated demyelination process in white matter. Focal and diffuse demyelination of white matter and spongy changes of the spinal cord are present.

HAND is insidious in onset and unpredictable in its course. Most individuals experience a steady progression of mental decline characterized by abrupt accelerations of signs over several months to more than 1 year, although some experience an abrupt onset or an accelerated course. The triad of clinical manifestations are neurocognitive impairment, behavioral disturbance, and motor abnormalities. Clinical manifestations are summarized in Box 18.2.

Diagnosis is difficult, especially in early stages. The individual's health history, along with physical examination findings and supporting CSF analysis, CT, and MRI data, helps establish the diagnosis, although the brain may appear normal until there is advanced disease. Research is continuing to evaluate the best treatment protocols and the possible neurotoxicity of HAART.[159]

HIV Myelopathy. HIV myelopathy involving diffuse degeneration of the spinal cord may occur with HIV. Vacuolar myelopathy is believed to be a direct consequence of HIV. The lateral and posterior columns of the lumbar spinal cord are affected. A progressive spastic paraparesis with ataxia is the predominant clinical manifestation. Leg weakness, upper motor neuron signs, incontinence, and posterior column sensory loss may be present. Diagnosis is made on the basis of history, physical findings, and supporting data from diagnostic procedures. Vacuolar myelopathy is treated supportively and does not respond to antiretrovirals.[160]

HIV-Associated Peripheral Neuropathy. Some HIV-associated peripheral neuropathies occur early, may coincide with seroconversion, are immune-mediated, and respond to standard immunotherapies. Other peripheral neuropathies primarily develop with advanced HIV infection and immunocompromised states and are facilitated by HIV replication, neurotoxicity from antiretroviral therapies, and coinfection with opportunistic pathogens.

HIV neuropathy may have one or a combination of several presentations: a predominantly sensory neuropathy, an autonomic neuropathy, a mononeuritis multiplex, an inflammatory demyelinating polyneuropathy (e.g., a Guillain-Barré–like syndrome), and a myopathy. The peripheral nervous system may sustain injury in HIV, manifesting as a peripheral neuropathy or radiculopathy. A progressive radiculopathy of predominantly the dorsal roots of the lumbar and sacral nerves may occur, involving severe myelin and axonal loss.

HIV-associated distal symmetric polyneuropathy, a sensory neuropathy occurring late in the disease, is the most commonly occurring neuropathy, with slowly progressive numbness and paresthesias and burning sensations in the extremities and feet. Weakness may be present, and distal reflexes may be decreased or absent.[161] The most common myopathy is polymyositis; it may be present initially or develop later. Inflammation leads to muscle cell degeneration and necrosis resulting in weakness of extremities with myalgia and fatigue.

HIV Meningitis. Some people develop an acute viral meningitis at approximately the time of seroconversion. This may well represent the initial infection of the nervous system by HIV. Symptoms include headache, fever, and meningismus.

Opportunistic Infections and HIV. Opportunistic infections may be bacterial, fungal, protozoal, or viral in origin and produce nervous system disease.[162] Cytomegalovirus encephalitis and tuberculosis meningitis have high incidence rates in African countries.[163] Typically bacterial infections are caused by unusual microorganisms. Cryptococcal infection is the most common fungal disorder and the most common cause of meningitis in HIV. In *Cryptococcus neoformans,* small granulomas and cysts are found in the cerebral cortex and later may be present in deep cerebral tissues. The symptoms are vague, such as fever, headache, malaise, and meningismus. Herpes encephalitis and herpes varicella-zoster radiculitis may develop. Polyomavirus (especially John Cunningham virus [JCV]) in the immunocompromised person with HIV may produce a demyelinating disorder called *progressive multifocal leukoencephalopathy (PML).* This virus is found in 90% of healthy persons but is dormant. The virus reactivates to cause PML in 15% of persons with HIV. Sensory and motor deficits, aphasia, and apraxia are common clinical manifestations. The condition is progressive, and there is no effective treatment.

Toxoplasmosis (a protozoan infection) is the most common opportunistic infection and occurs in one-third of persons with HIV. CNS toxoplasmosis typically manifests as focal encephalitis. *Toxoplasma gondii,* a protozoan, is thought to reactivate from latent lesions to produce a well-demarcated necrotizing process. Lesions may be multiple and exist throughout the cerebral hemispheres. Clinical manifestations of CNS toxoplasmosis are focal but highly variable and include clumsiness to hemiplegia, aphasia, seizures, ataxia, cognitive changes, and constitutional symptoms. Fever, headache, and confusion are common initial symptoms. Toxoplasmosis is difficult to diagnose but is treated effectively with pyrimethamine, sulfadiazine plus leucovorin (folinic acid) for 6 to 8 weeks.[164]

HIV-Associated Central Nervous System Neoplasms. HIV-associated CNS neoplasms have declined significantly with HAART, particularly primary CNS lymphoma. Other neoplasms associated with HIV include systemic non-Hodgkin lymphoma and metastatic Kaposi sarcoma. Metastasis of a Kaposi sarcoma to the CNS is uncommon.[165]

Demyelinating Disorders

Demyelinating disorders are the result of damage to the myelin nerve sheath and affect neural transmission. They can occur in either the central (e.g., multiple sclerosis) or the peripheral (e.g., Guillain-Barré syndrome) nervous system. Contributing factors include genetics, infections, autoimmune reactions, environmental toxins, and unknown factors.

Multiple Sclerosis

Multiple sclerosis (MS) is a chronic inflammatory disease involving degeneration of CNS myelin, scarring (sclerosis or plaque formation), and loss of axons. MS is caused by an autoimmune response to self or microbial antigens in genetically susceptible individuals. The onset of MS is usually between 20 and 40 years of age and is more common in women. Men may have a more severe progressive course. The prevalence rate is higher in northern latitudes. Risk factors that may be involved include smoking, vitamin D deficiency, and Epstein-Barr virus infection.[166] An estimated 2.3 million people worldwide live with MS. Life expectancy is not greatly altered by MS, and the disease course often extends over 30 years. The etiology of MS is unknown.[167]

The first demyelinating event, or "clinically isolated syndrome" (CIS), is a single episode of neurologic dysfunction lasting greater than 24 hours that can be a prelude to MS. Characteristic episodes include optic neuritis, solitary brainstem lesions, and transverse myelitis.[168]

◆ PATHOPHYSIOLOGY. MS is a diffuse and progressive CNS inflammatory autoimmune disease that affects white and gray matter. Autoreactive T and B cells and macrophages breach the blood-brain barrier of the brain and spinal cord in association with upregulation of adhesion molecules and inflammatory cytokines. These cells recognize myelin autoantigens and produce myelin-specific antibodies triggering inflammatory demyelination. There is subsequent loss of oligodendrocytes, and the hallmark plaque of MS is characterized by loss of myelin sheaths, relative preservation of axons, and glial (astrocytic) scar formation (Fig. 18.29). Activated macrophages and microglial cells (brain macrophages) are found in active MS lesions. Loss of myelin disrupts nerve conduction leading to symptom presentation. There is at least partial myelin repair during relapse of symptoms. There is, ultimately, death of neurons and brain atrophy in the most progressive forms of the disease.[170]

MS is characterized not only by focal inflammatory changes but also by diffuse injury throughout the CNS (MS lesions) (Fig. 18.30). MS lesions may occur anywhere in white or gray matter.[172] A paucity of immune cells and iron deposits are found, particularly in gray matter, and the pathologic significance may be associated with mitochondrial and oxidative injury.[173] Research is in progress to determine if cerebral hypoperfusion is a pathogenic factor in MS.[174]

◆ CLINICAL MANIFESTATIONS. *Clinically isolated syndrome*, an acute neurologic episode, is the first manifestation of the disease. There is no evidence of previous episodes of demyelination. Symptoms last more than 24 hours; occur in the absence of fever, infection, or encephalopathy; and are caused by inflammation and demyelination in the CNS. Symptoms can be multifocal, including paresthesias of the face, trunk, or limbs; weakness; impaired gait; visual disturbances; or urinary incontinence, indicating diffuse CNS involvement. Monofocal symptoms are caused by a single lesion and include optic neuritis, spinal cord syndrome, and brainstem and cerebellar syndromes. *Optic neuritis* is a common presentation in one eye with progressive blurring of vision and pain with eye movement. *Spinal cord syndrome* can involve both sensory and motor tracks starting on one side and progressing to the other. *Brainstem syndromes* can involve facial sensory loss or weakness, vertigo, or double vision. *Cerebellar syndromes* demonstrate lack of coordination, tremor, gait instability, and ataxia. Lesions in the cerebrum present as hemifacial weakness, pain, and motor impairments. Cognitive deficits, including memory and attention problems, are common later in the disease as well as psychiatric disorders, depression, and dementia. Individuals with CIS may or may not progress to MS. MS is diagnosed by MRI-detected brain or spinal cord lesions. The initial syndrome depends on the portion of the CNS that is most involved. After years

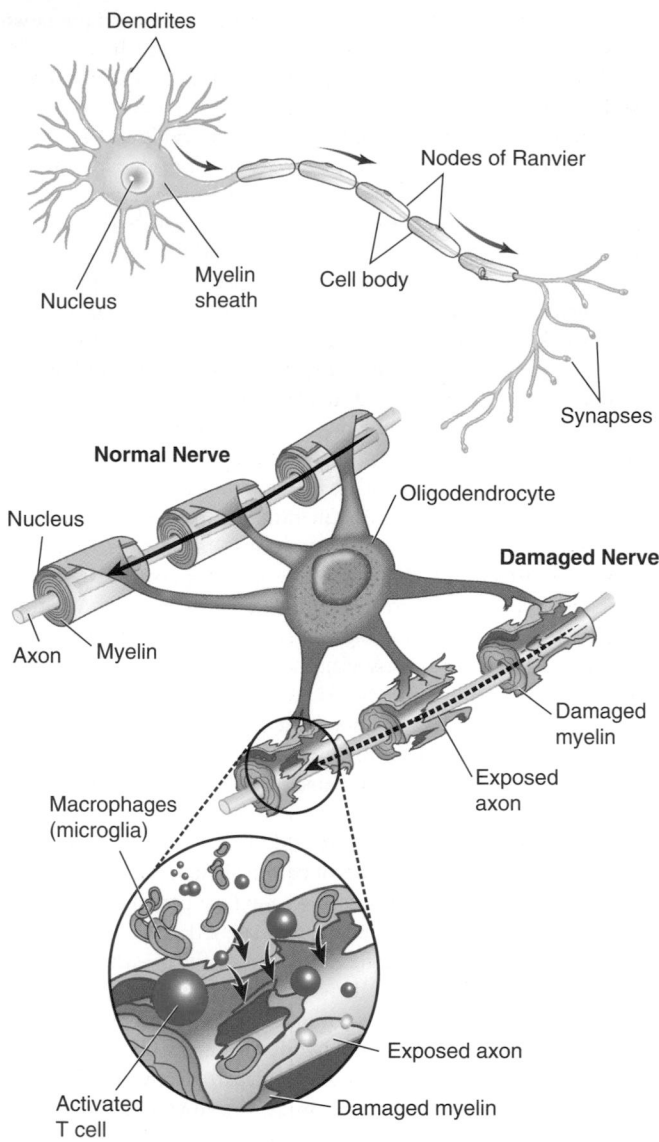

FIGURE 18.29 Pathogenesis of Multiple Sclerosis.

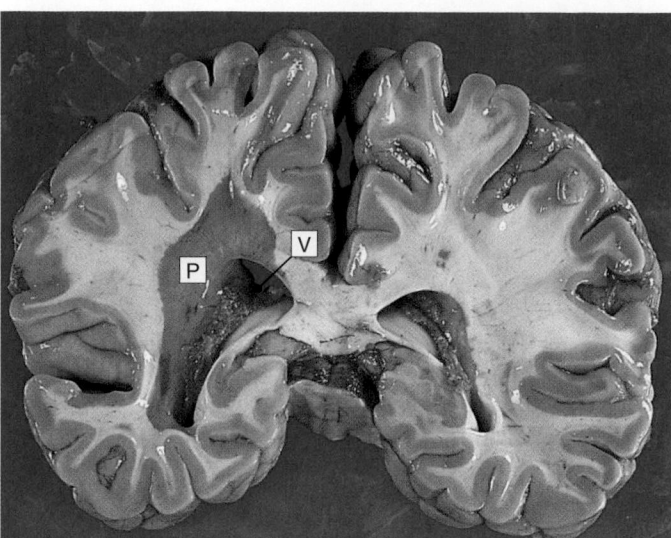

FIGURE 18.30 Multiple Sclerosis, Gross. Seen here in periventricular white matter is a large "plaque" *(P)* of demyelination that has a sharp border with adjacent normal white matter. Such plaques have a gray-tan appearance and are typically associated with the clinical appearance of transient or progressive loss of neurologic function in multiple sclerosis (MS). Because MS is often multifocal, and the lesions appear in various white matter locations in the central nervous system over time, the clinical course and findings can be quite varied. *V,* ventricle. (From Stevens A, et al: *Core pathology,* ed 3, London, 2009, Mosby.)

of disease, 50% of individuals appear to have established syndromes of multifocal involvement.[175]

The four symptom subtypes of MS are:[176]

Relapsing/remitting: This subtype is the most common type of MS and is characterized by relapses or exacerbations (flares) of previous symptoms or worsening of neurologic symptoms. After a relapse, a period of full or partial recovery lasts for days, weeks, or months. It is more common in women.

Primary progressive MS: This subtype is the least common and characterized by a gradual progression of the disease without periods of remission. Men and women seem to be equally affected, with the most common age of onset between late 30s and early 40s. Disease activity is more prevalent in the spinal cord and is less likely than other forms to affect cognitive function. There is gradual loss of power in the lower limbs that can be asymmetric, and bowel and bladder symptoms. Symptom acuity has the potential to level off.

Secondary progressive MS: This subtype follows an initial period of relapsing/remitting MS followed by a gradual worsening of the symptoms between relapses. Although there may be short intervals

of symptom remission, these periods decrease over time and are often accompanied by more severe symptoms.

Progressive relapsing multiple sclerosis (PRMS): This subtype is also characterized by steadily worsening symptoms from the onset with clear acute relapses but often with more severe symptoms.

◆ **EVALUATION AND TREATMENT.** There is no single test available to diagnose or rule out MS, and many conditions can mimic MS clinically and radiologically, particularly early in the disease process. The diagnostic criteria for MS were revised in 2010 and are known as the *McDonald criteria.* The criteria include the clinical examination in combination with MRI to demonstrate MS lesions in time and space. MRI is the most sensitive and available method of detecting demyelinated plaques and monitoring disease (Table 18.10) and quantifying macrophage infiltration and abnormal iron deposition.[177] Evoked potential (EP) testing aids diagnosis by detecting decreased conduction velocity in visual, auditory, and somatosensory pathways. Further studies are needed to confirm the diagnostic value of CSF findings.[178]

The treatment goal in MS is to prevent exacerbations, decrease MRI lesion burden, and control symptoms. Disease-modifying drugs are initiated with diagnosis and include corticosteroids, immunosuppressants, and immune system modulators. They suppress circulating immune cells, inhibit passing the blood brain barrier (BBB), and decrease the inflammatory responses.[179] Continuous monitoring is important because of the increased risk for infection when taking these drugs. Acute relapses are treated with corticosteroids to speed recovery. Both oral and injectable immunosuppressant and immune system modulators (i.e., monoclonal antibodies) are used to decrease the number of relapses, promote remyelination and repair, prevent demyelination, suppress selective B-cell and T-cell function, and prevent disability. New agents are under investigation.[180] Vitamin D supplementation may reduce the risk of MS and promote a more favorable progression.[181] Stem cell therapy is under investigation.[182]

TABLE 18.10	DIAGNOSTIC EVALUATION FOR MULTIPLE SCLEROSIS
FINDINGS IN MULTIPLE SCLEROSIS	
Clinical Signs and Symptoms	Signs and symptoms indicating disease of the brain or spinal cord not attributable to another diagnosis with two or more episodes lasting at least 24 hours and occurring at least 1 month apart
Tests	
Dissemination in space	
Magnetic resonance imaging (MRI), T2 weighted	Demyelinated plaques, both active and inactive; two of the following:
	Periventricular: three or more lesions
	Cortical-juxtacortical: one or more lesions
	Infratentorial: one or more lesions
	Spinal cord: one or more lesions
	Optic nerve: one or more lesions
Dissemination in time	
Gadolinium-enhanced MRI	A new lesion when compared to a previous scan (irrespective of timing)
MRI, T2 weighted	Presence of enhancing lesion and a nonenhancing T2 bright lesion on any one scan
Cerebrospinal fluid analysis	Oligoclonal bands of immunoglobulin G
	Elevated immunoglobulin G index
Evoked potentials	Slowed nerve impulse conduction

Data from Filippi M, Rocca MA, Ciccarelli O: *Lancet Neurol* 15(3):292–303, 2016; Polman CH et al: *Ann Neurol* 69(2):292-302, 2011.

Symptom management for fatigue, weakness, vertigo, ataxia, tremor, heat intolerance, spasticity, bladder dysfunction, bowel dysfunction, sexual dysfunction, sensory sensations, pain, cognitive difficulties, depression, and psychosocial issues is essential to improve quality of life. Many treatments are only partially effective, particularly for fatigue and spasticity. Supportive and rehabilitative management is directed toward preventing the complications of immobility, especially pressure sores and infections of the pulmonary and genitourinary systems. Interdisciplinary inpatient rehabilitation may improve function in the short term.[183] Supportive care includes participation in a regular exercise program, cessation of smoking, and avoidance of overwork, extreme fatigue, and heat exposure.

Guillain-Barré Syndrome

Guillain-Barré syndrome (GBS) (Landry-Guillain-Barré syndrome, idiopathic polyneuritis, acute inflammatory demyelinating polyradiculopathy, acute autoimmune neuropathy) is a rare demyelinating disorder caused by a humoral (antibody) and cell-mediated immunologic reaction directed at the peripheral nerves. The subtypes and their features are presented in Table 18.11. GBS usually occurs after a respiratory tract or gastrointestinal infection, and has been associated with surgery, immunization, and viral infections including the Zika virus.[184] In axonal forms of GBS, it is proposed that molecular mimicry of pathogen-borne antigens (i.e., *Campylobacter jejuni*) leads to generation of cross-reactive antibodies that target axonal gangliosides at nodes of Ranvier, activate complement, and disrupt nerve conduction in peripheral motor nerves.

The clinical manifestations can vary from ascending flaccid paresis starting in the legs to complete quadriplegia, respiratory insufficiency, and autonomic nervous system instability. Diagnostic criteria include progressive weakness of more than two limbs, areflexia, and progression

for no more than 4 weeks. Intravenous immunoglobulin or plasmapheresis is used during the acute phase and followed by aggressive rehabilitation. A monoclonal antibody to human complement is under investigation.[185] Recovery occurs within weeks to months or up to 2 years. About 30% of individuals have residual weakness.[186]

PERIPHERAL NERVOUS SYSTEM AND NEUROMUSCULAR JUNCTION DISORDERS

Peripheral Nervous System Disorders
Neuropathies

Neuropathies are disease processes that may injure axons traveling to and from the brainstem and spinal cord neuronal cell bodies.[187] The injury may affect distinct anatomic areas of the axon, or the spinal nerves may be injured at the roots, at the plexus before peripheral nerve formation, or at the peripheral nerves themselves. The cranial nerves do not have roots or plexuses so are affected only within themselves. Autonomic nerve fibers may be injured as they travel in certain cranial nerves or emerge through the ventral root and plexuses to pass through the peripheral nerves of the body.

Neuropathies can be classified as (1) generalized symmetric polyneuropathies, (2) generalized neuropathies, and (3) focal or multifocal neuropathies. Generalized symmetric polyneuropathies are characterized by symmetric involvement of sensory, motor, or autonomic fibers, although, with clinical signs, one type of fiber may predominate. Generalized symmetric polyneuropathies further subdivide into distal axonal polyneuropathy and demyelinating polyneuropathy. Distal axonal polyneuropathy affects peripheral axons and is the generalized peripheral neuropathy commonly seen. The clinical feature of distal axonal polyneuropathy is initial involvement of the longest nerves of the body, those going to the feet. Sensory impairment is greater than motor impairment. Symptoms are burning pain, tingling, and numbness of the feet. Small nerve fiber damage produces decreased pain and temperature sensation, as well as burning, numbness, and tingling. Large nerve fiber injury causes decreased light touch, vibration, and position sense. The two most common causes are diabetes mellitus and alcohol abuse; occasionally, neurotoxic therapeutic agents also are the cause. Within the classification of distal axonal neuropathies is another group of neuropathies called *autonomic neuropathy*. This neuropathy can involve virtually any sympathetic or parasympathetic nerve fiber with impairment of cardiovascular, gastrointestinal, urogenital, thermoregulatory, sudomotor, and pupillomotor autonomic function. Autonomic neuropathies have a progressive course and are usually reversible. The myelin or Schwann cells are affected in demyelinating polyneuropathy, which occurs far less frequently. Weakness is the predominant sign with far less sensory impairment. Acute and chronic inflammatory demyelinating neuropathies make up this group, of which Guillain-Barré syndrome is the most widely recognized disorder (see previous discussion).

Generalized neuropathies affect the cell body of only one type of peripheral neuron. The dorsal root ganglion cell is affected in sensory neuropathies, producing numbness that may begin in a focal or asymmetric distribution or in a distal symmetric pattern. Sensory neuropathies are seen in leprosy, some industrial solvent poisonings, some hereditary disorders, and chloramphenicol toxicity. Motor neuropathies are caused by anterior horn cell disease, such as amyotrophic lateral sclerosis or paralytic poliomyelitis. There is weakness or paralysis that may be symmetric or asymmetric.

Focal neuropathy (mononeuropathies) or multifocal neuropathies affect sensory and motor fibers (i.e., asymmetric limb weakness) in one or more nerves, as is seen in common compression neuropathies such as carpal tunnel syndrome (median nerve compression), ulnar

TABLE 18.11 EXPANDED CLASSIFICATION OF GUILLAIN-BARRÉ SYNDROME (GBS)

SUBTYPES	CLINICAL FEATURES	PATHOLOGY	PATHOGENESIS
Acute inflammatory demyelinating polyneuropathy (AIDP; accounts for most cases of GBS)	Ascending paralysis with typically distant start Early sensory symptoms Loss of deep tendon reflexes	Macrophages invade myelin sheaths and denude axons Lymphocytic inflammation Demyelination Endoneurial edema Some degree of axon loss (all findings most prominent in the spinal roots and nerve terminals) CD4 and CD8 lymphocytes and macrophages are present Complement is deposited on the outermost Schwann cell plasmalemma	T-cell–mediated lymphocytic infiltration into nerves is common Antibody-mediated pathogenesis not yet demonstrated
Acute motor axonal neuropathy (AMAN)	Acute progressive weakness with no sensory impairment	Autoantibodies invade nodes of Ranvier; activate complement and disrupt sodium-channel clusters and axoglial junctions; leads to nerve conduction failure and muscle weakness; leaves the myelin sheath intact (absence of demyelination) Axonal degeneration in ventral root in severe cases Lymphocyte infiltration sparse	Immunoglobulin G (IgG)-mediated attack on nodes of Ranvier Associated with *Campylobacter jejuni* enteritis GM1 autoantibodies play a direct pathogenic role through molecular mimicry
Acute motor and sensory axonal neuropathy (AMSAN)	Ascending paralysis Early sensory symptoms	Similar to AMAN Absence of demyelination Evidence of axonal loss in dorsal and ventral roots Lymphocytic infiltration sparse Extensive sensory nerve fiber degeneration	Undetermined
Miller Fisher syndrome (MFS) (5% of cases of GBS)	In purist form have ophthalmoparesis, areflexia, and ataxia In atypical MFS also have features of AIDP Infections are common triggers for MFS (*Campylobacter jejuni* enteritis)	Pathologic features similar to those in AIDP, but are atypical MFS Deposition of antiganglioside antibodies initially causes reversible conduction block followed by axonal degeneration	Antibodies to ganglioside GQ1b measured in serum in 90% of cases Anti-GQ1b antibodies cross-react with other gangliosides (typically GT1a, but in many cases with GD3, GD1b, and GT1b)

Data from Hosokawa T et al: *J Neurol* 261(10):1986-1993, 2014; Arcila-Londono X, Lewis RA: *Semin Neurol* 32(3):179-186, 2012.

nerve compression (at the elbow), peroneal nerve compression, or sciatic nerve compression. Focal neuropathies can involve one or more cranial nerves. Plexus injuries and radiculopathies also fall into this category.

◆ **PATHOPHYSIOLOGY.** Although distinct pathophysiologic processes are recognized in a neuropathy, these are not disease specific and may exist simultaneously in any one neuropathy. Pathologic processes that may be present include *wallerian degeneration*, in which the axon and myelin distal to the site of axonal interruption degenerate (see Chapter 15). This type of degeneration is characteristic of a traumatic nerve injury in which the nerve is severed. *Axonal degeneration* is caused by metabolic failure within an axon or vascular ischemia. In axonal degeneration, distal degeneration of the axon occurs first and is followed by degeneration of the myelin and the axis cylinder. This results in "stocking and glove" sensory or motor symptoms. In *demyelinating neuropathies*, the axon may be spared and only the myelin degenerates. Electromyography and ultrasound can assist in differentiating axonal from demyelination neuropathies.[188] Many pathologic processes may give rise to neuropathy, and one or more nerves may be involved.

◆ **CLINICAL MANIFESTATIONS.** When the axons are affected, muscle strength, muscle tone, and muscle mass also are affected. Whole muscles or groups of muscles are paretic or paralyzed, and the muscles of the feet and legs often are affected first and more severely. These long, large axons are thought to (1) be more vulnerable to injury because of their size and length, (2) have more Schwann cells available to be injured, and (3) exhibit a "dying back" phenomenon caused by difficulty of the nerve cell body in maintaining the terminal portion of the axon. If unchecked, the pathologic process tends to involve the hands and arms because these have the next longest and largest axons.

Tone and the deep tendon reflexes in the affected muscles generally are decreased in a neuropathy. Atrophy is distributed according to the peripheral nerves involved. The degree and distribution of the atrophy probably depend on the extent of the injury. Fasciculation may be present, especially with associated ventral root or motor neuron changes, or both, as in Guillain-Barré syndrome, diabetic neuropathy, and porphyric neuropathy. Mild fatigue may be experienced. A few disorders, notably Guillain-Barré syndrome, produce a pattern of paresis and paralysis that involves all limbs, the trunk, and the neck. Peripheral bifacial and other cranial nerve palsies may be seen with a variety of disorders. Tenderness of the nerve trunks and associated sensory alterations help to distinguish neuropathy from amyotrophy. These include paresthesias and dysesthesias as well as decreased or absent primary sensations (e.g., of temperature, touch, light pain, position, or vibration). Ataxia of gait or limb may arise from the loss of position and vibratory sensations (i.e., proprioceptive sensory loss) and may be enhanced by motor weakness.

Reflexes may be altered. Reflex-mediated autonomic nervous system functions, such as sweating, pupillary size, bladder, gastric, intestinal, and cardiovascular function, may be affected. Neuropathies associated with autonomic disturbances include diabetes mellitus, alcoholism and related nutritional neuropathies, amyloidosis, porphyria, Guillain-Barré syndrome, Riley-Day syndrome, and familial sensory neuropathy. In many chronic polyneuropathies, the feet, hands, and spine become deformed. Metabolic changes may arise secondary to nerve dysfunction.

◆ **EVALUATION AND TREATMENT.** The diagnostic workup to determine the cause of a neuropathy is often extensive. Early diagnosis and treatment before irreversible neuronal cell damage ensues are of paramount importance. Although axonal regrowth and recovery of function may take months, many neuropathies can be reversed. The therapeutic management is directed first at elimination of the cause, if possible. At least the primary disorder, such as diabetes mellitus, should be controlled. Further damage to the axon must be prevented by avoiding (1) trauma from premature demand for reuse of the nerve, (2) accidents that cause tissue damage, and (3) hypoxia and ischemia or other deprivation of essential substrates.

Radiculopathies

Radiculopathies are disorders of spinal nerve roots. As the spinal roots emerge from or enter the vertebral canal, they may be injured or damaged by compression, infection, inflammation, ischemia, or direct trauma whereby the roots are stretched or torn. Cervical and lumbar nerve roots are more commonly affected. Radiculitis (radiculoneuritis) refers to an inflammatory disorder of the spinal nerve roots. One or more roots may be affected.

◆ **PATHOPHYSIOLOGY.** Many different pathologic conditions may cause tearing, compression, or inflammation of nerve roots.[189] Roots may be traumatized by a forceful tearing of a nerve, termed *avulsion*, often associated with injuries to the head and shoulders. An acute intervertebral disk prolapse (herniated disk), degenerative spondyloarthropathies, or a benign tumor may compress nerve roots. Metastatic tumors of the lung, breast, and gastrointestinal tract may produce a carcinomatous meningitis, causing compression and inflammatory changes in nerve roots. Other causes of inflammatory changes in nerve roots are chronic meningitis, neurosyphilis, sarcoidosis, and inflammatory arachnoiditis produced by myelography and lumbar punctures.[190]

◆ **CLINICAL MANIFESTATIONS.** The strength, tone, and bulk of the muscles innervated by the involved roots are affected. The pattern and distribution of weakness and atrophy are similar to those of the amyotrophies. Tone and deep tendon reflexes are decreased, but rarely absent, because the involved muscles are usually innervated by two or more spinal roots. Fasciculations often are present, and mild fatigue may be experienced. Because pathologic processes usually affect the ventral as well as the dorsal roots, sensory alterations are common.

Diseases that involve spinal roots typically produce local pain; pain on local percussion; pain and paresthesias in the sensory root distribution (called radicular pain and radicular paresthesia); increased pain with movement, stretching of the root, and maneuvers that transiently increase CSF pressure; sensory loss in a radicular pattern; and spasms of the muscles surrounding the vertebral column (i.e., paravertebral muscle spasms).

◆ **EVALUATION AND TREATMENT.** Diagnostic measures may include physical examination, spinal films, nerve conduction studies, electromyelogram (EMG), lumbar puncture with CSF examination, myelography, and biopsy of tumor masses.[191]

Treatment is directed at the cause of the injury and may take the form of surgical intervention, antibiotic administration, removal of the injurious agent, corticosteroid use, and radiation therapy and chemotherapy. Supportive management may include control of the discomfort, protection from further injury, prevention of complications, and rehabilitation when appropriate.

Nerve Plexus Injuries

Plexus injuries involve the nerve plexus distal to the spinal roots but proximal to the formation of the peripheral nerves. Such injuries may be caused by trauma, compression (entrapment), or infiltration, or they may be iatrogenic, caused by positioning during surgery or by an intramuscular injection. Clinical manifestations include motor weakness, muscle atrophy, and sensory loss in affected areas. Paralysis can occur with complete plexus lesions.[192]

The diagnosis is made on the basis of history and clinical manifestations. Therapeutic treatment is directed at removal of the cause, surgical repair and approximation of nervous tissue, nerve transfers, growth factors, prevention of further injury, control of discomfort, prevention of complications, and rehabilitation when appropriate.

Neuromuscular Junction Disorders

Transmission of the nerve impulse at the neuromuscular junction requires the release of adequate amounts of neurotransmitter from the presynaptic terminals of the axon and effective binding of the released transmitter to the receptors on the membranes of muscle cells (see Fig. 15.16).

Botulism is a food poisoning resulting from the botulinum neurotoxins being released from *Clostridium botulinum*. The toxins are the most potent known and act at the myoneural junction, inhibiting release of acetylcholine (ACh) and causing severe flaccid paralysis including respiratory paralysis and death. Other forms include *C. botulinum*–contaminated wounds, infant and adult intestinal botulism released from spores that grow in the intestine after eating contaminated food, and iatrogenic botulism from accidental overdose of botulinum toxin. The endospores are resilient and resistant to heat. All forms are life-threatening and require emergency treatment. Treatments include supportive care with mechanical ventilation and antitoxin.[193]

Neuromuscular junction disorders (NMJDs), whose pathogenesis is caused by autoantibodies, include myasthenia gravis and Lambert-Eaton myasthenic syndrome. In addition, there are rare inherited (congenital) myasthenic syndromes that result from mutations in different key proteins for the postsynaptic nicotinic acetylcholine receptor, ion channels, and motor end plates at the neuromuscular junction.

Myasthenia Gravis

Myasthenia gravis is a chronic autoimmune disease mediated by acetylcholine receptor (AChR) antibodies that act at the neuromuscular junction (Fig. 18.31 and Table 18.12). About 20,000 to 70,000 people in the United States have the disease. Myasthenia gravis is associated with an increased incidence of other autoimmune diseases, including systemic lupus erythematosus, rheumatoid arthritis, polymyositis, and thyrotoxicosis. (Autoimmune mechanisms are discussed in Chapter 9.) The etiology of myasthenia gravis is unknown. Some persons have genetic susceptibility related to variants in AChR genes, as well as the major histocompatibility genes, and they can present with varying clinical phenotypes.[194] Presynaptic autoimmune diseases are rare and include

A
B

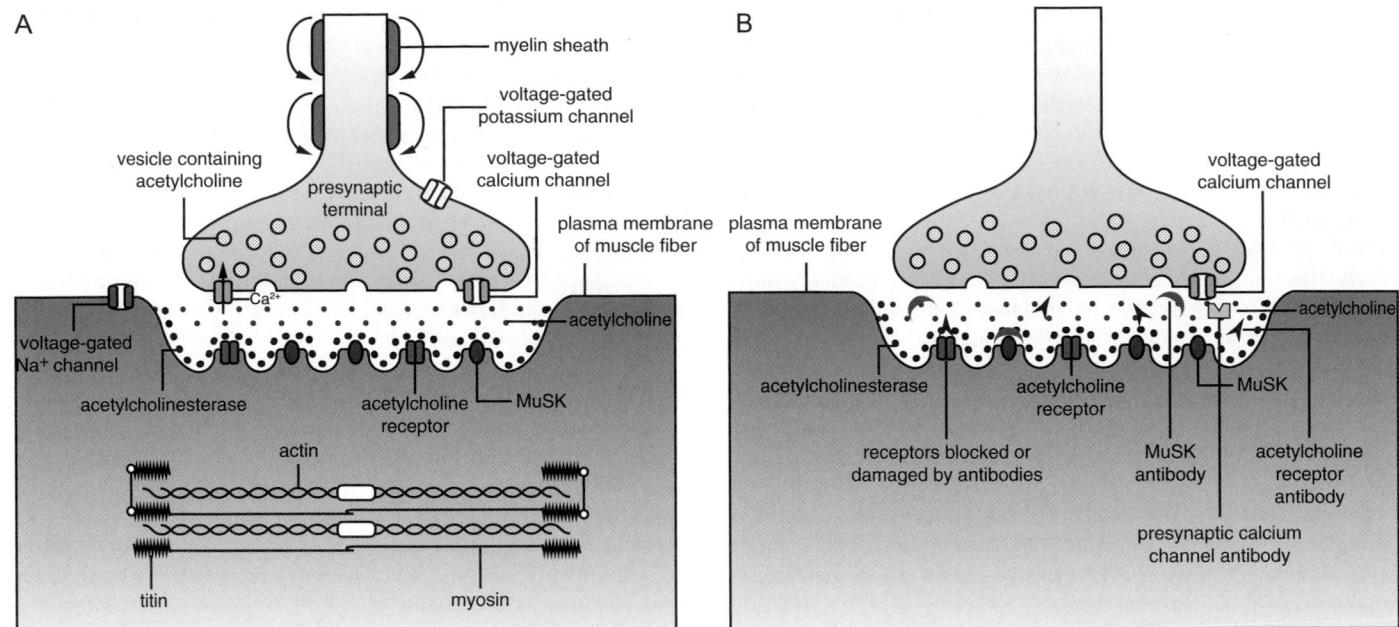

FIGURE 18.31 Antibodies and Myasthenia Gravis. Schematic diagrams of **(A)** a normal neuromuscular junction illustrating locations of the presynaptic vesicles, acetylcholine within the synapse, and the postsynaptic acetylcholine receptors, as well as **(B)** a neuromuscular junction affected by myasthenia gravis, with antibodies that interfere with the binding or structure, or both, of the acetylcholine receptors and muscle-specific kinase (MuSK). (Note that antibodies to both proteins are not typically present in the same individual, though this phenomenon has been reported on occasion.) Presynaptic calcium channel antibodies occur with Lambert-Eaton myasthenic syndrome. (From Darras BT et al: *Neuromuscular disorders of infancy, childhood, and adolescence,* ed 2, London, 2015, Academic Press.)

TABLE 18.12   ANTIBODIES AND MECHANISMS OF ACTION AT NEUROMUSCULAR JUNCTION

FEATURES	MYASTHENIA GRAVIS (MG)	MUSCLE-SPECIFIC KINASE MG	LAMBERT-EATON MYASTHENIC SYNDROME	NEUROMYOTONIA
Target	AChR	MuSK	α1A VGCC	VGKC
Principal subclass of antibody	IgG1, IgG3 (autoantibodies against AChR) Autoantibodies against LRP4, an agrin receptor critical for NMJ formation found in AChR and MuSK-negative MG	IgG4 (autoantibody against MuSK)	Autoantibodies to voltage-gated calcium channel	IgG4 (autoantibody against voltage-gated K+ channels)
Principal mechanisms of action at NMJ	Postsynaptic antibody destruction of nicotinic AChR	Not clear yet; complement not activated; may involve mutations in end-plate protein Dok-7	Presynaptic antibody destruction of voltage-gated calcium channels inhibit fusion of ACh at presynaptic membrane	Increased turnover
Compensatory mechanisms identified	Increased presynaptic ACh release, increased postsynaptic AChR synthesis	Not clear yet	Involvement of other VGCCs in release process	Probable up-regulation of other VGKCs

ACh, acetylcholine; *AChR,* Acetylcholine receptor; *Ig,* immunoglobulin; *LRP4,* low-density lipoprotein receptor–related protein 4; *MuSK,* muscle-specific kinase; *NMJ,* neuromuscular junction; *VGCC,* voltage-gated calcium channel; *VGKC,* voltage-gated potassium channel.
Data from Oger J, Frykman H: *Clin Chim Acta* 449:43-48, 2015.

Lambert-Eaton myasthenic syndrome with autoantibodies to calcium channels on presynaptic nerve terminals, which presents with muscle weakness and is commonly associated with small-cell lung carcinoma (see Fig. 18.31).[195]

The subtypes of autoimmune myasthenia gravis are generalized AChR, ocular, and neonatal. Generalized AChR myasthenia gravis is further subdivided based on age and thymic pathology into the following categories:
1. Early onset: young persons, mostly female, with thymomas; generally begins with ocular weakness followed by generalized weakness
2. Late onset: males over 60 years without thymomas
3. Persons of both sexes with thymomas

Generalized AChR myasthenia involves the proximal musculature throughout the body and has several courses: (1) a course with periodic remissions, (2) a slowly progressive course, (3) a rapidly progressive course, or (4) a fulminating course. Classification by disease severity is as follows:[196]

Class I: Any eye muscle weakness, possible ptosis, no other evidence of muscle weakness elsewhere

Class II: Eye muscle weakness of any severity, mild weakness of other muscles

Class II a: Predominantly limb or axial muscles

Class II b: Predominantly bulbar or respiratory muscles, or both

Class III: Eye muscle weakness of any severity, moderate weakness of other muscles

Class III a: Predominantly limb or axial muscles

Class III b: Predominantly bulbar and/or respiratory muscles

Class IV: Eye muscle weakness of any severity, severe weakness of other muscles

Class IV a: Predominantly limb or axial muscles

Class IV b: Predominantly bulbar or respiratory muscles, or both (can also include feeding tube without intubation)

Class V: Intubation needed to maintain airway

In **neonatal myasthenia**, transitory signs of myasthenia gravis are present in 10% to 15% of infants born to mothers with myasthenia gravis. The signs appear 1 to 3 days after birth and persist for a few days to a few weeks. Myasthenia immunoglobulin is transferred from the mother to the neonate through the placenta. **Ocular myasthenia**, which is more common in males, involves weakness of the eye muscles and eyelids and may include swallowing difficulties and slurred speech as well.

◆ **PATHOPHYSIOLOGY.** Myasthenia gravis results from a defect in nerve impulse transmission at the neuromuscular junction. The main defect is T-cell–dependent formation of autoantibodies (an IgG antibody) against nicotinic AChR (90% of cases), muscle-specific kinase (MuSK), lipoprotein-related protein 4 (LRP4), or agrin in the postsynaptic membrane at the neuromuscular junction. Agrin is a component of MuSK receptor function. The autoantibodies destroy the AChR through antibody-mediated complement activation (see Fig. 18.31).[197] The cause of this autosensitization is unknown. Destruction of receptor sites occurs, decreasing the number of receptors on the plasma membrane and causing diminished transmission of nerve impulses across the neuromuscular junction. Muscle depolarization is incomplete or unsuccessful. About 10% to 15% of individuals with myasthenia gravis do not have AChR antibodies on testing but have MuSK antibodies (an IgG4). This is now subtyped as MuSK antibody–associated myasthenia gravis.

◆ **CLINICAL MANIFESTATIONS.** Myasthenia gravis has an insidious onset. The variable distribution of ACh receptor sites or the number of and different isoforms of antibodies may determine when and which muscle groups are affected first—usually the muscles of the eyes, face, mouth, throat, and neck. The extraocular (eye) muscles and the levator muscles are most affected. Manifestations include diplopia, ptosis, and ocular palsies. The muscles of facial expression, mastication, swallowing, and speech are the next most involved. The results are facial droop and an expressionless face; difficulty chewing and swallowing associated with dietary changes and weight loss; drooling; episodes of choking and aspiration; and a nasal, low-volume but high-pitched monotonous speech pattern.

The muscles of the neck, shoulder girdle, and hip flexors are less frequently affected, but muscle fatigue is common after exercise and there can be progressive weakness. The respiratory muscles of the diaphragm and chest wall become weak, with impaired ventilation.

Impairment in deep breathing and coughing predisposes the individual to atelectasis and congestion. MuSK antibody type MG often involves severe swallowing and breathing (bulbar) problems

Clinical manifestations may first appear during pregnancy, during the postpartum period, or in conjunction with the administration of certain anesthetic agents. The progression of myasthenia gravis varies, appearing first as a mild case that spontaneously remits with a series of relapses and symptom-free intervals ranging from weeks to months. Over time, the disease can progress, and all muscles are weak.

Myasthenic crisis occurs when severe muscle weakness causes extreme quadriparesis or quadriplegia, respiratory insufficiency with shortness of breath and a markedly decreased tidal volume and vital capacity, and extreme difficulty in swallowing. The individual in myasthenic crisis is in danger of respiratory arrest.

Cholinergic crisis may arise from anticholinesterase drug toxicity with increased intestinal motility, episodes of diarrhea and complaints of intestinal cramping, bradycardia, pupillary constriction, increased salivation, and diaphoresis. The clinical picture resembles that of myasthenic crisis but the weakness occurs 30 to 60 minutes after taking anticholinergic medication. The clinical manifestations are caused by the smooth muscle hyperactivity secondary to excessive accumulation of acetylcholine at the neuromuscular junctions and excessive parasympathetic-like activity. As in myasthenic crisis, the individual is in danger of respiratory arrest.

◆ **EVALUATION AND TREATMENT.** The diagnosis of myasthenia gravis is made on the basis of a response to edrophonium chloride (Tensilon), results of results of EMG studies, and detection of AChR and MuSK antibodies. With the intravenous administration of the drug, immediate demonstrable improvement in muscle strength usually persists for several minutes. Mediastinal tomography and MRI help determine whether a thymoma is present.

Treatment of myasthenia gravis is individualized. Anticholinesterase drugs, corticosteroids, immunosuppressant drugs (e.g., rituximab, chimeric monoclonal antibody against the protein CD20 primarily found on the surface of B cells, azathioprine, cyclosporine, and mycophenolate mofetil) are used to treat myasthenia gravis and myasthenic crisis. Plasmapheresis may be lifesaving during myasthenic crisis, before and after thymectomy, and at the start of immunosuppressant therapy. For individuals with cholinergic crisis, treatment is to withhold anticholinergic drugs until blood levels fall out of the toxic range while providing ventilatory support and preventing respiratory complications. Thymectomy is the treatment of choice for a thymoma.[198] Complement inhibitors are being evaluated. Current treatments for myasthenia gravis have improved prognosis, including in those individuals who have ocular myasthenia.

TUMORS OF THE CENTRAL NERVOUS SYSTEM

Central nervous system (CNS) tumors include brain and spinal cord tumors. The incidence of CNS tumors increases to age 70 years and then decreases. CNS tumors are the second most common group of tumors occurring in children. Approximately 70% to 75% of all intracranial tumors in children are located infratentorially (see Chapter 20), and 70% are located supratentorially in adults. Peripheral nerve tumors are rare in children and common in adults. Carcinogenesis is discussed in Chapter 12, pituitary tumors are discussed in Chapter 22, and cerebral tumors in children are discussed in Chapter 20.

Brain Tumors

Primary brain tumors (both malignant [32%] and nonmalignant) had an estimated incidence rate of 80,000, with about 17,000 deaths in the United States in 2017.[199] Tumors within the cranium can be either primary or metastatic. *Primary (intracerebral) brain tumors* originate from brain substance (neuroepithelium), including neuroglia, neurons, cells of blood vessels, and connective tissue. *Extracerebral tumors* originate outside substances of the brain and include meningiomas, acoustic nerve tumors, and tumors of pituitary and pineal glands. *Metastatic (secondary) brain tumors* arise in organ systems outside the brain and spread to the brain. Sites of intracranial tumors are illustrated in Fig. 18.32.

Intracranial brain tumors do not metastasize as readily as tumors in other organs because there are no lymphatic channels within the brain substance. If metastasis does occur, it is usually through seeding of cerebral blood, through CSF, during cranial surgery, or through artificial shunts.

Cranial tumors cause local and generalized clinical manifestations. The local effects are caused by the destructive action of the tumor itself on a particular site in the brain and compression causing decreased cerebral blood flow. The effects are varied and include seizures, visual disturbances, unstable gait, and cranial nerve dysfunction. The generalized effects result from IICP (Fig. 18.33). IICP may occur because of obstruction of the ventricular system, hemorrhages occurring in and around the tumor, cerebral edema caused by tumors, or expansion of the tumor mass.

Primary Brain (Intracerebral) Tumors

Primary brain tumors constitute about 2% of all cancers in the United States. Gliomas comprise about 25% of all adult primary brain tumors and 74.6% of malignant brain tumors. Gliomas include astrocytomas, oligodendrogliomas, mixed oligoastrocytomas, and glioblastoma multiforme. The World Health Organization (WHO) divides gliomas into four grades based on histopathologic features, cellular density, atypia, mitotic activity, microvascular proliferation, and necrosis (Table 18.13). Grades I and II are generally benign or slow growing, and well to moderately differentiated. Grades III and IV are malignant tumors and poorly differentiated. Other CNS tumors include meningiomas, ependymomas, nerve sheath tumors (schwannomas), and neurofibromas. Etiology for primary brain tumors is not clearly known. Ionizing radiation is the only known environmental risk factor. The association between mobile phone use and gliomas and acoustic neuromas is controversial.[201]

Molecular characteristics of gliomas include mutation of the isocitrate dehydrogenase 1 *(IDH1)* gene, or, less commonly, mutation of the related *IDH2* gene identified in the vast majority of World Health Organization (WHO) grades II and III astrocytic, oligodendroglial, and oligoastrocytic gliomas. Silencing of the *MGMT* gene (methylated-DNA-protein-cysteine

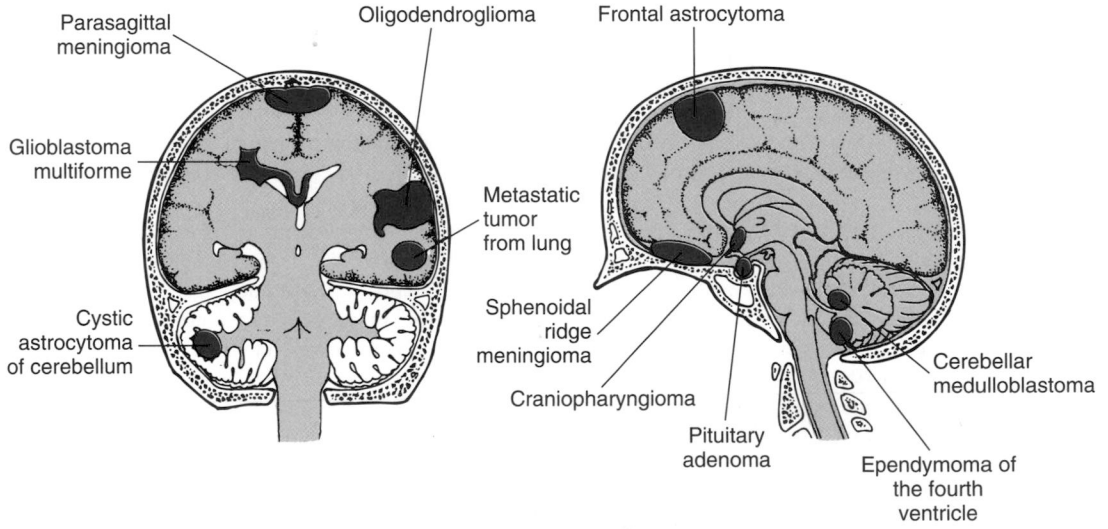

FIGURE 18.32 Common Sites of Intracranial Tumors.

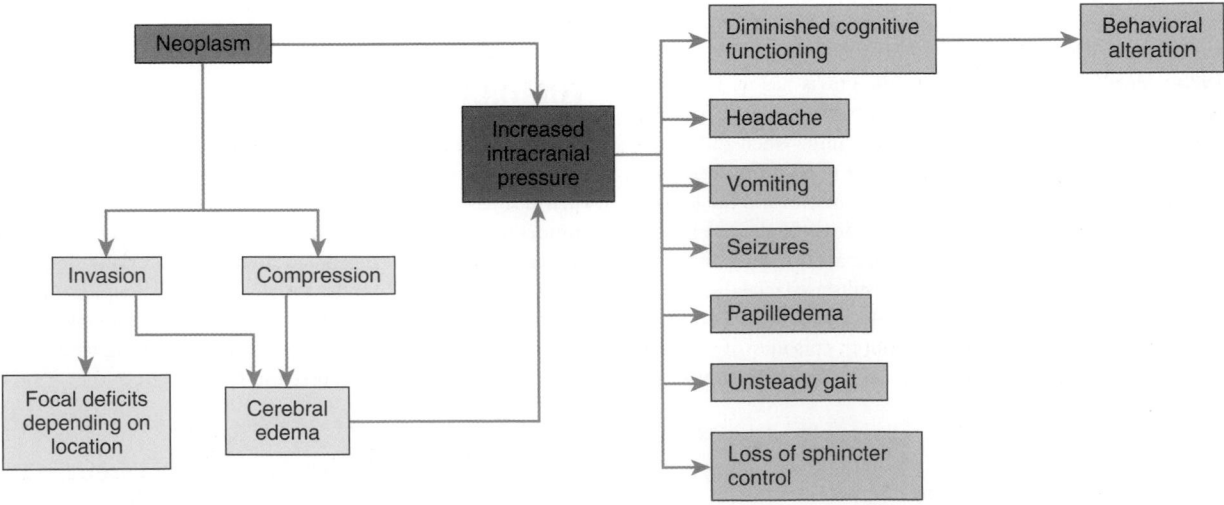

FIGURE 18.33 Origin of Clinical Manifestations Associated with an Intracranial Neoplasm.

TABLE 18.13 BRAIN AND SPINAL CORD TUMORS

NEOPLASM	LOCATION	CHARACTERISTICS	CELL OF ORIGIN
Gliomas			
Astrocytomas			
Pilocytic astrocytoma (grade I)	Anywhere in brain or spinal cord	Slow growing, well circumscribed Common in children and young adults and people with neurofibromatosis type 1; common in cerebellum	Astrocytes
Diffuse astrocytoma (grade II)	Anywhere in brain	Slow growing; marked cellular differentiation; infiltrative; undergoing malignant progression over time	Astrocytes
Anaplastic astrocytoma (grade III)	Anywhere in brain or spinal cord, but predominantly in cerebral hemispheres	Malignant; many cells undergoing mitosis; infiltrates adjacent tissue; frequently recurs at higher grade	Astrocytes
Glioblastoma multiforme (grade IV astrocytoma)	Predominantly in cerebral hemispheres	Poorly differentiated neoplastic cells; extensive cellular heterogeneity; well-developed microvascular proliferation; necrosis	Astrocytes
Oligodendroglioma; anaplastic oligodendroglioma (grades II and III)	Most commonly in frontal lobes deep in white matter; may arise in brainstem, cerebellum, and spinal cord	Well differentiated; diffusely infiltrative; well-demarcated borders; increased mitotic activity, often associated with microvascular proliferation and necrosis	Oligodendrocytes
Oligoastrocytoma (grades II and III)	Same as with diffuse astrocytoma and oligodendroglioma	Most common mixed glioma	At least two distinct populations of neoplastic cell types—astrocytes and oligodendrocytes
Anaplastic oligoastrocytoma (grade III)	Same as with anaplastic astrocytoma	Same as anaplastic astrocytoma or anaplastic oligodendroglioma	Astrocytes and oligodendrocytes
Ependymoma (grade II)	Intramedullary: wall of ventricles, may arise in caudal tail of spinal cord	More common in children, variable growth rates; more malignant, invasive form is called *ependymoblastoma*; may extend into ventricle or invade brain tissue	Ependymal cells
Neuronal Cell			
Medulloblastoma	Posterior cerebellar vermis, roof of fourth ventricle	Well demarcated, rapid growing, fills fourth ventricle	Embryonic cells
Mesodermal Tissue			
Meningioma	Intradural, extramedullary: sylvian fissure region, superior parasagittal surface of frontal and parietal lobes, olfactory groove, wing of sphenoid bone, superior surface of cerebellum, cerebellopontine angle, spinal cord	Slow growing, circumscribed, encapsulated, sharply demarcated from normal tissues, compressive in nature	Arachnoid cells, may be from fibroblast
Choroid Plexus			
Papillomas	Choroid plexus of ventricular system, lateral ventricle in children, fourth ventricle in adults	Usually benign, slow expansion inducing hemorrhage and hydrocephalus; malignant tumor is rare	Epithelial cells
Cranial Nerves and Spinal Nerve Roots			
Schwannoma (neuroma, neurolemma)	Cranial nerves (most commonly vestibular division of cranial nerve VIII)	Slow growing	Sheath of Schwann cells
Neurofibroma (NF1 and NF2)	NF1 primarily PNS, occasionally CNS NF2 primarily CNS	Both types slow growing	Nerve sheath
Pituitary Tumors	Pituitary gland; may extend to or invade floor of third ventricle	Age linked, several types, slow growing, macroadenomas and microadenomas	Pituitary cells, pituitary chromophobes, basophils, eosinophils

Continued

TABLE 18.13   BRAIN AND SPINAL CORD TUMORS—cont'd

NEOPLASM	LOCATION	CHARACTERISTICS	CELL OF ORIGIN
Germ Cell Tumors	Neurohypophysis, hypothalamus, pineal region	Rare, 0.5% of all primary brain tumors; primarily in adolescents; male more common than female; variable prognosis	Several types: germinoma, embryonal carcinoma, yolk sac tumor, choriocarcinoma, teratoma, mixed germ cell tumor, with different cell origins
Blood Vessel Tumors			
Angioma	Predominantly in posterior cerebral hemispheres	Slow growing	Arising from congenitally malformed arteriovenous connections
Hemangioblastomas	Predominantly in cerebellum	Slow growing	Embryonic vascular tissue

CNS, Central nervous system; *PNS,* peripheral nervous system.

methyltransferase, a DNA repair enzyme) is found in astrocytomas. Mutant epidermal growth factor vIII (EGFRvIII) amplification is found in most subtype gliomas. Chromosome 1p and 19q deletions are associated with oligodendrogliomas,[202] and gliomas may arise from cancer-initiating resident stem cells.[204]

The principal treatment for cerebral tumors is surgical or radiosurgical excision or surgical decompression if total excision is not possible. Chemotherapy, radiation therapy, or their combination may be used. The blood-brain barrier is an obstacle to the delivery of chemotherapeutic agents. New methods are in progress for penetration of this barrier, including nanoparticle drug carriers and focused ultrasound combined with microbubbles.[205,206]

Specificity of treatment is advancing with the development of vaccines (i.e., tumor-specific peptides), cell therapy (T cells and antibodies), reshaping of the tumor microenvironment (i.e., transforming growth factor β [TGFβ] inhibition), immune checkpoint inhibitors,[207] and modified polio virus.[209] (Cancer treatment is discussed in Chapter 12.)

Astrocytoma. Astrocytomas are the most common glioma (about 75% of all tumors of the brain and spinal cord)[210] (see Table 18.13). These tumor cells develop from astrocytes and are believed to have lost normal growth restraint and thus proliferate uncontrollably. Astrocytomas are graded I through IV. They may occur anywhere in the brain or spinal cord and are generally located in the cerebrum, hypothalamus, or pons. Low-grade astrocytomas tend to be located laterally or supratentorially in adults and in the posterior fossa in children.

Headache and subtle neurobehavioral changes may be early signs, with other neurologic symptoms evolving slowly and IICP occurring late in the tumor's course. Onset of a focal seizure disorder between the second and sixth decade of life suggests an astrocytoma. Low-grade astrocytomas are treated with surgery or by external radiation, and at least 50% of persons survive 5 years when surgery is followed by radiation therapy (RT).[210,211]

Grades III and IV astrocytomas are found predominantly in the frontal lobes and cerebral hemispheres, although they may occur in the brainstem, cerebellum, and spinal cord (Figs. 18.34 and 18.35). Men are twice as likely to have astrocytomas as women; in the 15- to 34-year-old age group they are the third most common brain cancer, whereas in the 35- to 54-year-old age group they are the fourth most common.

Grade IV astrocytoma, **glioblastoma multiforme (GBM),** is the most lethal and common type of primary brain tumor. GBM is highly vascular and extensively irregular and infiltrative, making them difficult to remove surgically. Fifty percent of glioblastomas are bilateral or at least occupy more than one lobe at the time of death. The typical clinical presentation for a glioblastoma multiforme is that of diffuse, nonspecific clinical

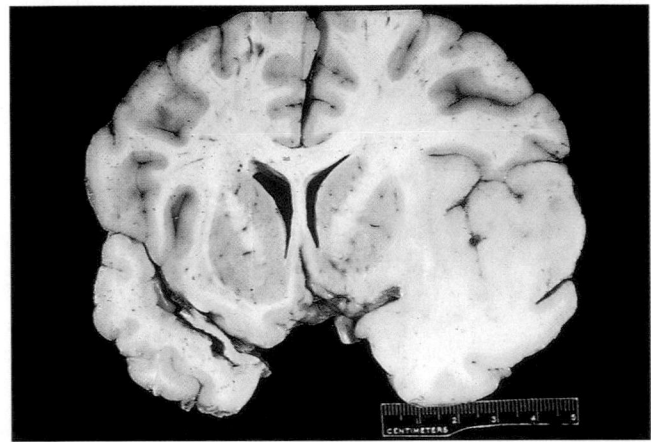

FIGURE 18.34 Well-Differentiated Infiltrating Astrocytoma. The right temporal lobe contains an infiltrative, homogeneous lesion that has expanded the lobe and obscured the normal boundaries between gray and white matter (compare to left temporal lobe). Because of the ill-defined borders, surgical resection rarely removes all of the tumor in such cases. (From Kumar V, Cotran RS, Robbins SL: *Robbins basic pathology,* ed 7, Philadelphia, 2003, Saunders.)

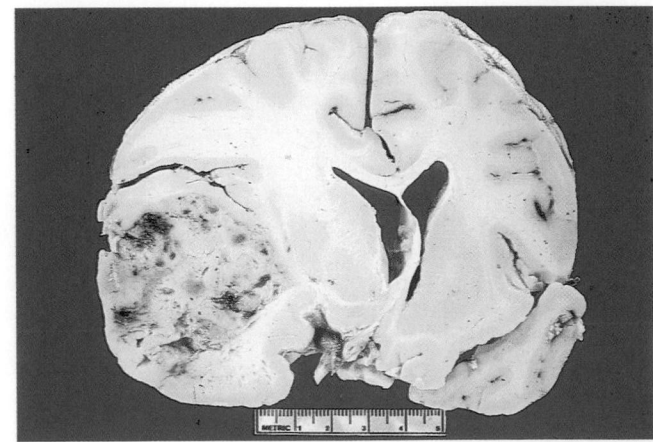

FIGURE 18.35 Glioblastoma Multiforme. In contrast to the well-differentiated infiltrating astrocytoma in Fig. 18.34, this glioblastoma contains irregular areas of discoloration and cystic change, reflecting the presence of necrosis and hemorrhage. These lesions are widely infiltrative and associated with considerable mass effect. Note the shift of midline structures to the right. (From Kumar V, Cotran RS, Robbins SL: *Robbins basic pathology,* ed 7, Philadelphia, 2003, Saunders.)

signs, such as headache, irritability, and "personality changes" that progress to more clear-cut manifestations of IICP, including headache on position change, papilledema, vomiting, or seizure activity. Symptoms may progress to include definite focal signs, such as hemiparesis, dysphasia, dyspraxia, cranial nerve palsies, and visual field deficits. Treatment for newly diagnosed GBM is radiotherapy with temozolomide (alkylating agent) following maximal surgical resection. Adjuvant immunotherapy may be beneficial.[212] Survival at 5 years for grades III and IV astrocytomas is about 5% to 10%.

Oligodendroglioma. Oligodendrogliomas constitute about 2% of all primary brain tumors and 10% to 15% of all gliomas. They are typically slow-growing tumors; most oligodendrogliomas are macroscopically indistinguishable from other gliomas and may be a mixed type of oligodendroglioma and astrocytoma (oligoastrocytoma). The majority are found in the frontal and temporal lobes, often in the deep white matter, but they are also found in other parts of the brain and spinal cord. Many are found in young adults with a history of temporal lobe epilepsy. Malignant degeneration occurs in approximately one-third of persons with oligodendrogliomas (a grade II tumor), and the tumors are then referred to as anaplastic oligodendroglioma (a grade III tumor).

More than 50% of individuals experience a focal or generalized seizure as the first clinical manifestation. Only half of those with an oligodendroglioma have IICP at the time of diagnosis or surgery, and only one-third develop focal manifestations. Those with 1p19q codeletion experience a benefit from adding chemotherapy to radiation.[213]

Ependymoma. Ependymomas are nonencapsulated gliomas that arise from ependymal cells that form the walls of the ventricles or the spinal canal (Fig. 18.36, and see Table 18.13). They are rare in adults, usually occurring in the spinal cord. They comprise about 6% of all primary brain tumors in adults and 10% in children and adolescents, usually occurring in intracranial locations. Approximately 70% of these tumors occur in the fourth ventricle, with others found in the third and lateral ventricles and caudal portion of the spinal cord. Approximately 40% of infratentorial ependymomas occur in children younger than 10 years of age. Cerebral (supratentorial) ependymomas occur at all ages.

Fourth ventricle ependymomas present with difficulty in balance, unsteady gait, uncoordinated muscle movement, and difficulty with fine motor movement. The clinical manifestations of a lateral and third

ventricle ependymoma that involves the cerebral hemispheres are seizures, visual changes, and hemiparesis. Blockage of the CSF pathway produces hydrocephalus and presents with headache, nausea, and vomiting.

Ependymomas are treated with surgical resection and adjuvant radiotherapy and chemotherapy.[214] About 20% to 50% of persons survive 5 years. Some persons benefit from a shunting procedure when the ependymoma has caused a noncommunicating hydrocephalus.

Primary Extracerebral Tumors

Meningioma. Meningioma constitutes about 36% of all primary brain tumors and is more common in women. Predisposing factors include neurofibromatosis (NF) type 2 (NF2; see Nerve Sheath Tumors) and undergoing ionizing radiation after a several-decade latency period. Formation of benign meningiomas has been linked to *NF2* gene mutation and chromosome 22q12–2 loss along with *DAL-1* loss on chromosome 18. Atypical and anaplastic meningiomas have been linked to additional gene alterations involving other multiple chromosomes. They are resistant to treatment.[215]

A meningioma is sharply circumscribed and adapts to the shape it occupies. It may extend to the dural surface and erode the cranial bones or produce an osteoblastic reaction. A few meningiomas exhibit malignant, invasive qualities (Fig. 18.37).

Meningiomas are slow growing, and clinical manifestations occur when they reach a certain size and begin to indent the brain parenchyma. Focal seizures are often the first manifestation, and IICP is less common than with gliomas. Other symptoms are related to the site of tumor location:

1. *Sphenoidal wing:* ophthalmoplegia, mild proptosis, and involvement of the ophthalmic division of the trigeminal nerve
2. *Olfactory groove:* anosmia, personality change, and visual failure
3. *Parasagittal:* focal seizures of a focal motor or sensory deficit
4. *Parasellar:* evidence of chiasmatic compression; urinary incontinence; dementia; gradual paraparesis, hormonal failure; optic atrophy; bitemporal hemianopia
5. *Lateral convexity:* variable depending on structures compressed, including slow hemiparesis, speech abnormalities

Because of the extremely slow-growing nature of most meningiomas, IICP is less common than with gliomas. Diagnosis is made using contrast-enhanced CT, MRI, or both. The primary treatment is surgical resection. Stereotactic radiotherapy is used with incomplete resection or recurrence (20% rate).[216]

Nerve Sheath Tumors. Nerve sheath tumors are either neurofibromas or schwannomas (neuroma, neurolemma). Neurofibromas

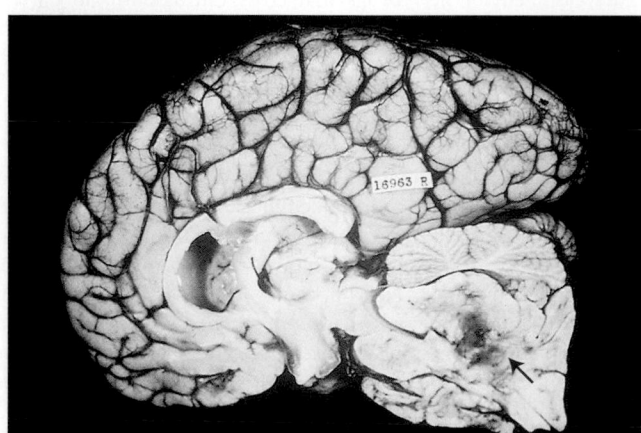

FIGURE 18.36 Ependymoma. These tumors may arise in both the intracranial compartment and the spine. Intracranial tumors typically originate from a ventricular surface, as in the case of this large lesion arising in the fourth ventricle *(arrow).* (From Kumar V, Cotran RS, Robbins SL: *Robbins basic pathology,* ed 7, Philadelphia, 2003, Saunders.)

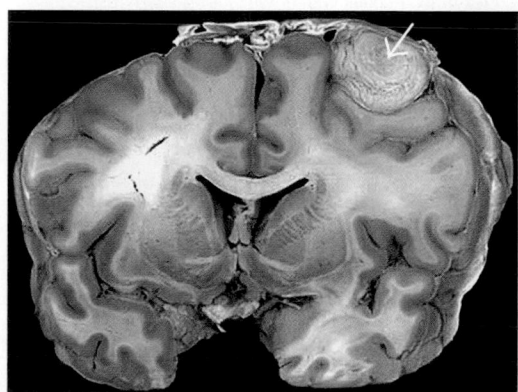

FIGURE 18.37 Meningioma, Gross. Meningioma beneath the dura with compression of underlying cerebral hemisphere. (From Klatt EC: *Robbins and Cotran atlas of pathology,* ed 3, Philadelphia, 2015, Saunders.)

(benign nerve sheath tumors) are a group of autosomal dominant disorders of the nervous system. They include neurofibromatosis type 1 (NF1, previously known as *von Recklinghausen disease*) and neurofibromatosis type 2 (NF2); NF1 and NF2 are also known as *peripheral* and *central neurofibromatosis,* respectively.

Neurofibromatosis type 1 is the most prevalent with an incidence of about 1 in 3500 people and causes multiple cutaneous neurofibromas; cutaneous macular lesions (café-au-lait spots and freckles); and, less commonly, bone and soft tissue tumors. Inactivation of the *NF1* gene (chromosome 17q11.2) results in loss of function of neurofibromin in Schwann cells and promotes tumorigenesis (neurofibromas). Learning disabilities are present in about 50% of affected individuals.[217]

Neurofibromatosis type 2 is rare and occurs in about 1 in 60,000 people. The *NF2* gene (chromosome 22 q12–2) product is neurofibromin 2 (merlin), a tumor-suppressor protein. Mutations promote development of central nervous system tumors, particularly schwannomas, although other tumor types can occur (meningiomas, ependymomas, astrocytomas, and neurofibromas). Benign bilateral schwannomas of the vestibular nerves present with hearing loss progressing to deafness, dizziness and balance problems, tinnitus, and facial nerve paralysis. Other symptoms may include loss of balance and dizziness. Schwannomas also may develop in other cranial, spinal, and peripheral nerves, and cutaneous signs are less prominent. Intracranial meningiomas can involve the optic nerve with loss of visual acuity and cataracts or can be intraspinal with formation of ependymomas.[218]

Genetic testing is available for the management of families susceptible to NF, and prenatal diagnosis is possible. Diagnosis is based on clinical manifestations and neuroimaging studies. Criteria for the diagnosis of neurofibromatosis types 1 and 2 are presented in Box 18.3.[219,220]

BOX 18.3　NIH DIAGNOSTIC CRITERIA FOR NEUROFIBROMATOSIS

Criteria for the Diagnosis of NF1

Two of the following seven criteria:

- Six or more café-au-lait macules greater than 5 mm in greatest diameter in prepubertal individuals and greater than 15 mm in greatest diameter in postpubertal individuals (adults)
- Multiple axillary or inguinal freckles
- One plexiform neurofibroma or two or more neurofibromas of any type
- Optic glioma
- Two or more Lisch nodules (iris hamartomas)
- A distinctive osseous lesion such as sphenoid dysplasia or thinning of the cortex of long bones with or without pseudarthrosis
- A first-degree relative with NF1 by the above criteria

Criteria for the Diagnosis of NF2

Either one of the following criteria:

- Bilateral masses of the eighth cranial nerve seen with appropriate imaging techniques (e.g., CT or MRI)
- A first-degree relative with NF2 and either:
  a. Unilateral mass of the eighth cranial nerve or
  b. Two of the following:
     1. Neurofibroma
     2. Meningioma
     3. Glioma
     4. Schwannoma
     5. Juvenile posterior subcapsular lenticular opacity

CT, Computed tomography; *MRI,* magnetic resonance imaging; *NF,* neurofibromatosis; *NIH,* National Institutes of Health.

Surgery is the major treatment. Individuals with NF2 have extensive morbidity and reduced life expectancy, particularly with early age of onset. Molecular targeted therapies (i.e., angiogenesis and epidermal growth factor inhibitors) are likely to provide personalized treatment for both of these devastating conditions.[221]

Metastatic Brain Tumors. Metastatic brain tumors from systemic cancers are approximately 10 times more common than primary brain tumors. Ten percent to 20% of persons with cancer have metastasis to the brain. Lung (40% to 50%) and breast cancer (15% to 20%) are the most common tumors to have brain metastases within 1 to 3 years, followed by malignant melanoma, renal cell carcinoma, and, less commonly, gastrointestinal and reproductive tract cancers. Metastasis to the brain is believed to be through vascular channels.

The brain metastatic process requires a series of sequential events called the metastatic cascade[222] (see Chapter 12 and Fig. 12.19). Peripheral cancer cells degrade the extracellular matrix, invade blood vessels and lymph nodes, migrate, extravasate, and colonize at their new locations forming a metastatic niche. Tumor cells reach the brain vasculature by attaching themselves to endothelial cells of brain microvessels in the blood-brain barrier. Using enzymes, they disrupt the epithelial basement membrane and extravasate into the brain parenchyma. They can attach platelets that protect them from immune defenses. Local brain invasion requires cell motility, adhesion, survival, and proliferation. They induce blood vessel development (angiogenesis) and proliferate in response to growth factors, cytokines, and chemokines.[223] The cerebrum is the most common site of seeding.[224]

Metastatic brain tumors produce signs resembling those of glioblastomas, although several unusual syndromes do exist. Carcinomatous (metastatic cancer) encephalopathy causes headache, nervousness, depression, trembling, confusion, forgetfulness, and gait disorder. In carcinomatosis of the cerebellum, headache, dizziness, and ataxia are found. Carcinomatosis of the craniospinal meninges (also called carcinomatous meningitis) manifests with headache, confusion, and symptoms of cranial or spinal nerve root dysfunction.

Contrast-enhanced CT and MRI imaging techniques are the most sensitive imaging procedures for metastatic brain tumors. Treatment is guided by the pathology of the original tumor; number, size, and location of the brain metastasis; and prior cancer treatments. Corticosteroids and antiepileptic drugs can help relieve symptoms. One to four lesions are treated with stereotactic radiosurgery. Chemotherapy is considered when surgery or radiation therapy is not possible. With the development of new drugs that cross the blood-brain barrier, chemotherapy is increasingly recommended.[226] Survival with treatment is about a year.

Spinal Cord Tumors

Primary spinal cord tumors are rare and represent about 2% of CNS tumors. They are histologically classified as extradural, intradural extramedullary, or intradural intramedullary. Extramedullary tumors originate from tissues outside the spinal cord. Extramedullary tumors are either peripheral nerve sheath tumors (neurofibromas or schwannomas) or meningiomas. Neurofibromas are generally found in the thoracic and lumbar region, whereas meningiomas are more evenly distributed through the spine. Complete resection of these tumors can be curative. Other extramedullary tumors are sarcomas, vascular tumors, chordomas, and epidermoid tumors.

Intramedullary tumors are least common (5% to 10% of all spinal tumors) and originate within the neural tissues of the spinal cord. Intramedullary tumors are primarily gliomas (astrocytomas, ependymomas, hemangioblastomas). Gliomas are difficult to resect completely, and radiotherapy is required. Spinal ependymomas may be completely resected and are more common in adults.[227]

Metastatic spinal cord tumors are usually carcinomas (i.e., from breast, lung, or prostate cancer), lymphomas, or myelomas. Their location is often extradural, having proliferated to the spine through direct extension from tumors of the vertebral structures or from extraspinal sources extending through the interventricular foramen or bloodstream. They are three to four times more common than primary spinal cord tumors.

◆ **PATHOPHYSIOLOGY.** Extramedullary spinal cord tumors produce dysfunction by compression of adjacent tissue, not by direct invasion. The spinal cord is compressed by the tumor from without, and destruction of the white matter tracts occurs. The spinal canal around the cord becomes filled by tumor.

Intramedullary spinal cord tumors produce dysfunction by invasion and compression. The cord enlarges as a result of the tumor that is enlarging inside the cord. In addition, distortion of adjacent white matter tracts occurs. Metastases from spinal cord tumors occur from seeding through the CSF; medulloblastomas and ependymomas establish distant implants in this manner.

◆ **CLINICAL MANIFESTATIONS.** Clinical manifestations depend on growth rate, location, and longitudinal extent of the tumor. An acute onset suggests a vascular occlusion of vessels supplying the spinal cord, whereas gradual and progressive symptoms suggest compression with dural distention and irritation. Pain is usually a presenting symptom. The compressive syndrome (sensorimotor syndrome) involves both the anterior and the posterior spinal tracts and nerve roots, and motor function and sensory function are affected as the tumor grows, with weakness, spasticity, and clumsiness and a decrease in pain and temperature sensation.

The irritative syndrome (radicular syndrome) combines the clinical manifestations of cord compression with radicular pain that occurs in the sensory root distribution and indicates root irritation. The segmental manifestations include segmental sensory changes, such as paresthesias and impaired pain and touch perception; motor disturbances, including cramps, atrophy, fasciculations, and decreased or absent deep tendon reflexes; and continuous spinal pain.

◆ **EVALUATION AND TREATMENT.** The diagnosis of a spinal cord tumor is made using MRI techniques, bone scan, PET, CT-guided needle biopsy, or open biopsy. Involvement of specific cord segments is established. Any metastases also are identified. Spinal tumors are not staged but can be classified as slow growing (low-grade) or rapidly growing (high-grade). Treatment varies depending on the nature of the tumor and the person's clinical status, but surgery is essential for all spinal cord tumors.[228] Radiotherapy, chemotherapy, hormonal therapy, and pain management protocols may be appropriate.[229]

SUMMARY REVIEW

Central Nervous System Disorders

1. Traumatic brain injury (TBI) is an alteration in brain function or other evidence of brain pathology caused by an external force.
2. Primary brain injury is caused by an impact and can be focal or diffuse with open- or closed-head injury.
3. Severity of TBI is graded using the Glasgow Coma Score.
4. Focal brain injury includes coup and contrecoup, contusion (bruising of the brain), laceration (tearing of brain tissue), extradural hematoma (accumulation of blood above the dura mater), subdural hematoma (blood between the dura mater and arachnoid membrane), intracerebral hematoma (bleeding into the brain), and open-head trauma.
5. Open-head injury involves a skull fracture with exposure of the cranial vault to the environment. The types of skull fracture include compound fracture or perforated fracture and linear, comminuted, and basilar skull fracture.
6. Closed-head injuries occur in a precise location, and most are mild. More severe damage includes contusions and epidural, subdural, subarachnoid, and intracerebral hemorrhage.
7. Diffuse axonal injury (DAI) results from mechanical forces of acceleration, deceleration, and rotation that cause stretching and shearing of axons and can only be seen microscopically. The injury can be mild, moderate, or severe.
8. Secondary neuronal injury occurs as an indirect result of primary brain injury. Systemic processes include hypotension, hypoxia, anemia, hypoglycemia, hyperglycemia, and hypercapnia or hypocapnia. Cerebral contributions include inflammation, oxidative stress, alterations in the blood-brain barrier, excitotoxicity, cerebral edema, increased intracranial pressure (IICP), decreased cerebral perfusion pressure, cerebral ischemia, and brain herniation.
9. Complications of TBI include postconcussion syndrome, posttraumatic seizures, and chronic and traumatic encephalopathy.
10. Spinal cord and vertebral injuries occur most often in young men who sustain various kinds of injuries (recreational or travel-related) and older adults because of preexisting degenerative vertebral disorders.
11. Vertebral injuries include fractures, dislocations, compressions, and penetrating bone fragments from shearing and compression force. Fractures can be simple, compressed, or comminuted.
12. Primary spinal cord injury involves damage to vertebral or neural tissues from shearing, compression, or traction forces.
13. Secondary spinal cord injury is related to edema, ischemia, excitotoxicity, inflammation, oxidative damage, and activation of necrotic and apoptotic cell death and begins within minutes after injury and continues for weeks.
14. Spinal cord injury often causes spinal shock with cessation of all motor, sensory, reflex, and autonomic functions below any transected area. Loss of motor and sensory function depends on the level of injury.
15. Neurogenic shock (vasogenic shock) occurs with cervical or upper thoracic cord injury above T5 and may be seen in addition to spinal shock. There is loss of sympathetic activity and unopposed vagal parasympathetic activity with symptoms of hypotension, bradycardia, and hypothermia.
16. Paralysis of the lower half of the body with both legs involved is called *paraplegia*. Paralysis involving all four extremities is called *quadriplegia*.
17. Return of spinal neuron excitability occurs slowly. Reflex activity can return in 1 to 2 weeks in most people with acute spinal cord injury. A pattern of flexion reflexes emerges, involving first the toes and then the feet and legs. Eventually reflex voiding and bowel elimination appear, and mass reflex (flexor spasms accompanied by profuse sweating, piloerection, and automatic bladder emptying) may develop.
18. Autonomic hyperreflexia (dysreflexia) is a syndrome of sudden massive reflex sympathetic discharge associated with spinal cord injury at level T5-T6 or above and can cause life-threatening hypertension.

19. The pathologic findings in degenerative disk disease (DDD) include disk protrusion, spondylosis and/or subluxation, degeneration of the vertebrae (spondylolisthesis), and spinal stenosis.

20. Low back pain is pain between the lower rib cage and gluteal muscles and often radiates into the thigh.

21. Most causes of low back pain are unknown; however, some secondary causes are disk prolapse, tumor, bursitis, synovitis, degenerative disk disease, osteoporosis, hyperparathyroidism, fracture, inflammation, and sprain.

22. Degenerative disk disease is part of normal aging as a response to continuous vertical compression of the spine, usually in the lumbar region. Both genetic and environmental factors contribute to loss of disk connective tissue. Disks can tear and herniate, pinching nerves and straining the spine. In addition there may be changes in the vertebral body with spondylolysis or spondylolisthesis, or both, degeneration of vertebrae, and spinal stenosis.

23. Spondylolysis is a structural defect in the pars interarticularis of the vertebral arch with anterior displacement (sliding) of the deficient vertebra (spondylolisthesis) and is a cause of low back pain.

24. Cervical spondylolysis is facet hypertrophy and disk degeneration with narrowing in the cervical spine predominantly at C5-C6 and C6-C7 and can cause radiculopathy and myelopathy with numbness and tingling in the arms, occipital headache, difficulty walking, altered sensation in the feet, and sphincter disturbances.

25. Spinal stenosis is narrowing of the spinal canal that causes pressure on the spinal cord and is associated with trauma or arthritis. Symptoms include pain, numbness, and weakness in the areas of affected spinal nerves.

26. Herniation of an intervertebral disk is a protrusion of part of the nucleus pulposus, most commonly at L5-S1 and L4-L5. The extruded pulposus compresses the nerve root, causing pain that radiates along the sciatic nerve.

27. Cerebrovascular disease is the most frequently occurring neurologic disorder. Any abnormality of the blood vessels of the brain is referred to as *cerebrovascular disease* and includes vessel wall abnormalities and vascular malformations, thrombotic or embolic occlusion, and increased blood viscosity or clotting.

28. Cerebrovascular disease causes (a) ischemia with or without infarction and (b) hemorrhage. The common clinical manifestation is a cerebrovascular accident (CVA) or stroke syndrome. Hypertension is the greatest risk factor followed by other preventable risks.

29. CVAs are classified according to pathophysiology and include ischemic (thrombotic, embolic, and hypoperfusion), lacunar (small vessel disease), and hemorrhagic strokes.

30. A transient ischemic attack is a transient episode of neurologic dysfunction resulting from focal cerebral ischemia with risk for progressing to stroke.

31. Ischemic strokes result from interruption in brain blood flow with a core of irreversible ischemia and necrosis or infarction that appears pale (white infarct). The zone around the infarction has reversible ischemia, is called the *ischemic penumbra*, and can regain neurologic function, particularly with thrombolytic treatment. Leaking blood vessels can develop in the infarcted area, resulting in a hemorrhagic transformation (a red infarct) that can be exacerbated by thrombolytic therapy.

32. Reperfusion injury can occur with ischemic stroke.

33. Intracerebral hemorrhagic stroke is primarily associated with vessel disease related to hypertension. Subarachnoid hemorrhage is associated with ruptured aneurysms, arteriovenous malformations (AVMs), or cavernous angioma.

34. Intracranial aneurysms result from defects and weakness in the vascular wall and are classified on the basis of form and shape. They are commonly asymptomatic, but the signs vary according to the location and size of the aneurysm.

35. An AVM is a tangled mass of dilated blood vessels. Although sometimes present at birth, AVM exhibits a delayed age of onset with symptoms ranging from headache and dementia to seizures and ICH or SAH. Vasospasm and delayed cerebral ischemia are serious complications.

36. Subarachnoid hemorrhage is bleeding into the subarachnoid space commonly associated with intracranial aneurysms, AVM, and hypertension. The expanding hematoma increases ICP, compresses brain tissue, reduces cerebral perfusion, disrupts the blood-brain barrier, and causes inflammation and neuronal death. Secondary brain injury follows. Seizures and hydrocephalus can accompany neurologic deficits.

37. Migraine is an episodic disorder whose marker is headache lasting 4 to 72 hours. Migraine is classified as a headache with and without aura and chronic migraine (migraines 15 days in a month for more than 3 months). Migraine may be precipitated by a triggering event. The aura is associated with cortical spreading depression, which initiates the release of neurotransmitters, particularly CGRP, that stimulate vasodilation in the trigeminal vascular system, inflammation, and sensitization of pain receptors. Glutamate is increased and serotonin is decreased.

38. Cluster headaches (trigeminal autonomic cephalalgia) occur in episodes several times during a day for a period of days at different times of the year, primarily in men. The pain is unilateral, intense, tearing, and burning and associated with ptosis, lacrimation, reddening of the eye, and nausea. The cause of trigeminal activation is unknown. There is sympathetic nervous system underactivity and parasympathetic overactivity with trigger events similar to migraine. The two forms are acute and chronic.

39. Chronic paroxysmal hemicranias are a cluster-type headache that occurs 4 to 12 times per day for 20 to 120 minutes in both men and women. There is sympathetic activity different from that in cluster headache, as it is relieved with indomethacin.

40. Tension-type headache (TTH) is the most common type of headache. Both central and peripheral pain mechanisms are associated with the etiology. The headache is bilateral, with the sensation of a tight band around the head. The pain may last for hours or days. There are acute and chronic forms.

41. Infection and inflammation of the CNS can occur by bacteria, viruses, fungi, parasites, and mycobacteria (i.e., tuberculosis). The resulting infection by bacteria is pus-producing, or pyogenic.

42. Meningitis is inflammation of the brain or spinal cord. Bacterial meningitis is primarily an infection of the pia mater and arachnoid villi and of the fluid of the subarachnoid space. Viral meningitis is believed to be limited to the meninges. Fungal and tubercular meningitis are less common, and immunosuppressed individuals are at greatest risk.

43. The meningeal vessels become hyperemic, and neutrophils migrate into the subarachnoid space with bacterial meningitis. An inflammatory reaction occurs, and exudation ensues and increases, rapidly producing edema and brain injury.

44. Brain abscesses can be extradural, subdural, or intracerebral and often originate from infections outside the CNS. Microorganisms gain access to the CNS from adjacent sites or spread along the wall

SUMMARY REVIEW—cont'd

of a vein. A localized inflammatory process develops with exudate formation, vessel thrombosis, and leukocyte degeneration. After a few days the infection becomes delimited, with a center of pus and a wall of granular tissue that forms a capsule.

45. Encephalitis is an acute febrile illness of viral origin with nervous system involvement. The most common encephalitides are caused by arthropod-borne viruses and herpes simplex virus. The infection causes widespread brain edema and necrosis. Meningeal involvement appears in all encephalitides.

46. The common neurologic complications of AIDS are HIV-associated neurocognitive disorder (HAND), HIV neuropathy, HIV myelopathy, opportunistic infections, cytomegalovirus infection, parasitic infection, and neoplasms. Pathologically, there may be diffuse CNS involvement, focal pathologic findings, and obstructive hydrocephalus. Neurologic involvement associated with HIV has declined with HARRT.

47. MS is a chronic inflammatory disease involving degeneration of CNS myelin in genetically susceptible individuals. The cause is unknown and autoreactive T and B cells recognize myelin auto-antigens and produce myelin-specific antibodies triggering inflammatory demyelination with loss of oligodendrocytes and plaque formation leading to disruption of nerve conduction.

48. The clinical manifestations of MS involve different types: relapsing-remitting, primary progressive, secondary progressive, and progressive-relapsing.

49. Guillain-Barré syndrome is a rare demyelinating disorder caused by an antibody and cell-mediated immunologic reaction directed against peripheral nerves that causes weakness or paralysis and can have irreversible effects. Different subtypes have been identified, and clinical manifestations depend on the subtype.

Peripheral Nervous System and Neuromuscular Junction Disorders

1. Neuropathies result when there is injury to peripheral nerves and can involve sensory, motor, and autonomic pathways. Axon and myelin degeneration may be present. Neuropathies are classified as generalized symmetric polyneuropathies, generalized neuropathy, and focal or multifocal neuropathies.

2. Radiculopathies are disorders of spinal cord nerve roots. The roots may be compressed, inflamed, or torn. Cervical and lumbar nerve roots are more commonly affected.

3. Plexus injuries involve the nerve plexus distal to the spinal roots but proximal to the formation of the peripheral nerves and are caused by trauma, compression, or infiltration with motor and/or sensory loss, weakness, and muscle atrophy.

4. Botulism is poisoning by botulinum toxin released by *Clostridium botulinum* that acts by inhibiting release of ACh at the myoneural junction causing life-threatening flaccid paralysis.

5. Myasthenia gravis results from a defect in nerve impulse transmission at the neuromuscular junction with generalized, ocular, or neonatal subtypes. Autoantibodies, complement deposits, and membrane attack complex destroy the acetylcholine receptor (AChR) sites, causing decreased transmission of nerve impulses, leading to muscle weakness, including ocular and systemic muscles. There can be childhood and adult onset.

Tumors of the Central Nervous System

1. Tumors that occur within the cranium are either primary or metastatic (secondary). Primary tumors arise from brain tissue and are classified as intracerebral or extracerebral. Metastatic tumors to the brain arise in organs outside the brain and are much more common than primary brain tumors.

2. Primary brain tumors include astrocytomas, oligodendrogliomas, mixed oligoastrocytomas, glioblastoma multiforme (grade IV astrocytoma), and ependymomas. Other CNS tumors include meningiomas, nerve sheath tumors (schwannomas), and neurofibromas.

3. Metastatic brain tumors invade brain tissue by attaching to endothelial cells of microvessels and use enzymes to cross the blood-brain barrier and extravasate into the brain parenchyma.

4. Spinal cord tumors are classified as intramedullary (within the neural tissues) or extramedullary (outside the spinal cord). Metastatic spinal cord tumors are usually carcinomas, lymphomas, or myelomas.

5. Extramedullary spinal cord tumors produce dysfunction by compression of adjacent tissue, not by direct invasion. Intramedullary spinal cord tumors produce dysfunction by invasion and compression.

KEY TERMS

Arteriovenous malformation (AVM), 571
Astrocytoma, 590
Autonomic hyperreflexia (dysreflexia), 559
Bacterial meningitis, 575
Botulism, 585
Brain abscess, 578
Capillary telangiectasis, 571
Cavernous angioma (malformation), 571
Cerebrovascular accident (CVA), 565
Cholinergic crisis, 587
Chronic migraine, 574
Chronic paroxysmal hemicrania (CPH), 574
Chronic traumatic encephalopathy (CTE), 557
Closed (blunt) trauma, 552
Closed head injury, 552
Cluster headache, 574
Compressive syndrome (sensorimotor syndrome), 593
Contrecoup injury, 552
Contusion, 552

Coup injury, 552
Degenerative disk disease (DDD), 563
Delayed cerebral ischemia (DCI), 572
Demyelinating polyneuropathy, 583
Diffuse axonal injury (DAI), 555
Distal axonal polyneuropathy, 583
Embolic stroke, 566
Encephalitis, 579
Ependymoma, 591
Epidural (extradural) hematoma, 552
Extradural brain abscess (empyema), 578
Extramedullary tumor, 592
Focal brain injury, 552
Focal neuropathy (mononeuropathy), 583
Fungal meningitis, 576
Fusiform aneurysm (giant aneurysm), 571
Generalized AChR myasthenia, 587
Generalized neuropathy, 583
Generalized symmetric polyneuropathy, 583
Glioblastoma multiforme (GBM), 590

Glioma, 588
Guillain-Barré syndrome (GBS) (Landry-Guillain-Barré syndrome, idiopathic polyneuritis, acute inflammatory demyelinating polyradiculopathy, acute autoimmune neuropathy), 583
Hemodynamic stroke (brain hypoperfusion), 566
Hemorrhagic stroke (spontaneous intracranial hemorrhage [ICH]), 569
HIV-associated peripheral neuropathy, 580
HIV myelopathy, 580
HIV neuropathy, 581
Human immunodeficiency virus–associated neuro-cognitive disorder (HAND), 579
Inherited (congenital) myasthenic syndrome, 585
Intracerebral brain abscess, 578
Intracerebral hematoma, 553
Intracranial aneurysm, 570
Intramedullary tumor, 592
Irritative syndrome (radicular syndrome), 593
Ischemic penumbra, 566

KEY TERMS—cont'd

Lacunar stroke (lacunar infarct), 566
Lambert-Eaton myasthenic syndrome, 586
Low back pain (LBP), 561
Mass reflex, 561
Meningioma, 591
Meningitis (nonpurulent meningitis, lymphocytic meningitis), 575
Metastatic brain tumor, 592
Migraine, 573
Mild traumatic brain injury (mild concussion), 556
Moderate traumatic brain injury (moderate cerebral concussion), 556
Motor neuropathy, 583
Multifocal neuropathy, 583
Multiple sclerosis (MS), 581
Myasthenia gravis, 585
Myasthenic crisis, 587
Mycotic aneurysm, 571
Neonatal myasthenia, 587
Neurofibroma (benign nerve sheath tumor), 591
Neurofibromatosis type 1, 592

Neurofibromatosis type 2, 592
Neurogenic shock, 559
Neuropathy, 583
Ocular myasthenia, 587
Oligodendroglioma, 591
Open brain trauma, 554
Open head injury, 552
Open (penetrating) trauma, 552
Plexus injury, 585
Postconcussion syndrome, 557
Posttraumatic seizure (epilepsy), 557
Primary spinal cord injury, 557
Primary spinal cord tumor, 592
Purpura fulminans, 575
Radicular pain, 585
Radicular paresthesia, 585
Radiculitis (radiculoneuritis), 585
Radiculopathy, 564
Saccular aneurysm (berry aneurysm), 570
Secondary brain injury, 556
Secondary spinal cord injury, 557

Sensory neuropathy, 583
Severe traumatic brain injury (severe concussion), 556
Spinal cord abscess, 579
Spinal shock, 559
Spinal stenosis, 563
Spondylolisthesis, 563
Spondylolysis, 563
Subarachnoid hemorrhage (SAH), 572
Subdural brain abscess (empyema), 578
Subdural hematoma, 552
Thrombotic stroke (cerebral thrombosis), 566
Toxoplasmosis, 581
Transient ischemic attack (TIA), 566
Traumatic (dissecting) aneurysm, 571
Traumatic brain injury (TBI), 550
Tubercular meningitis, 576
Vacuolar myelopathy, 580
Venous angioma, 571
Viral meningitis (aseptic meningitis), 576

REFERENCES

1. Centers for Disease Control and Prevention: *TBI: get the facts.* Available at: http://www.cdc.gov/traumaticbraininjury/get_the_facts.html.
2. McGinn MJ, Povlishock JT: Pathophysiology of traumatic brain injury. *Neurosurg Clin N Am* 27(4):397–407, 2016.
3. Tagliaferri F, et al: A systematic review of brain injury epidemiology in Europe. *Acta Neurochir (Wien)* 148(3):255–268, 2006.
4. Zakaria Z, et al: Extradural haematoma—to evacuate or not? Revisiting treatment guidelines. *Clin Neurol Neurosurg* 115(8):1201–1205, 2013.
5. Johnson VE, et al: Axonal pathology in traumatic brain injury. *Exp Neurol* 246:35–43, 2013.
6. Su E, Bell M: Diffuse axonal injury. In Laskowitz D, Grant G, editors: *Translational research in traumatic brain injury,* Boca Raton, FL, 2016, CRC Press/Taylor and Francis Group.
7. Sharp DJ, Scott G, Leech R: Network dysfunction after traumatic brain injury. *Nat Rev Neurol* 10(3):156–166, 2014.
8. Echemendia RJ, Giza CC, Kutcher JS: Developing guidelines for return to play: consensus and evidence-based approaches. *Brain Inj* 29(2):185–194, 2015.
9. Giza CC, et al: Summary of evidence-based guideline update: evaluation and management of concussion in sports: report of the Guideline Development Subcommittee of the American Academy of Neurology. *Neurology* 80(24):2250–2257, 2013.
10. Harmon KG, et al: American Medical Society for Sports Medicine position statement: concussion in sport. *Br J Sports Med* 47(1):15–26, 2013.
11. Malec JF, et al: The Mayo classification system for traumatic brain injury severity. *J Neurotrauma* 24(9):1417–1424, 2007.
12. McCrory P, et al: Consensus statement on concussion in sport: the 4th International Conference on Concussion in Sport held in Zurich, November 2012. *Br J Sports Med* 47(5):250–258, 2013.
13. Sharp DJ, Jenkins PO: Concussion is confusing us all. *Pract Neurol* 15(3):172–186, 2015.

14. Currie S, et al: Imaging assessment of traumatic brain injury. *Postgrad Med J* 92(1083):41–50, 2016.
15. Koerte IK, et al: Advanced neuroimaging of mild traumatic brain injury. In Laskowitz D, Grant G, editors: *Translational research in traumatic brain injury,* Boca Raton, FL, 2016, CRC Press/Taylor and Francis Group.
16. Shan R, et al: A new panel of blood biomarkers for the diagnosis of mild traumatic brain injury/concussion in adults. *J Neurotrauma* 33(1):49–57, 2016.
17. Wintermark M, et al: Imaging evidence and recommendations for traumatic brain injury: conventional neuroimaging techniques. *J Am Coll Radiol* 12(2):e1–e14, 2015.
18. Levin HS, Diaz-Arrastia RR: Diagnosis, prognosis, and clinical management of mild traumatic brain injury. *Lancet Neurol* 14(5):506–517, 2015.
19. Jagoda AS: Mild traumatic brain injury: key decisions in acute management. *Psychiatr Clin North Am* 33(4):797–806, 2010.
20. Meares S, et al: Validation of the abbreviated Westmead post-traumatic amnesia scale: a brief measure to identify acute cognitive impairment in mild traumatic brain injury. *Brain Inj* 25(12):1198–1205, 2011.
21. Reis C, et al: What's new in traumatic brain injury: update on tracking, monitoring and treatment. *Int J Mol Sci* 16(6):11903–11965, 2015.
22. National Institute for Health and Care Excellence: *Triage, assessment, investigation and early management of head injury in children, young people and adults,* June 2017. Available at: www.nice.org.uk/guidance/CG176.
23. Quillinan N, Herson PS, Traystman RJ: Neuropathophysiology of brain injury. *Anesthesiol Clin* 34(3):453–464, 2016.
24. Hiebert JB, et al: Traumatic brain injury and mitochondrial dysfunction. *Am J Med Sci* 350(2):132–138, 2015.
25. Corps KN, Roth TL, McGavern DB: Inflammation and neuroprotection in traumatic brain injury. *JAMA Neurol* 72(3):355–362, 2015.

26. Karve IP, Taylor JM, Crack PJ: The contribution of astrocytes and microglia to traumatic brain injury. *Br J Pharmacol* 173(4):692–702, 2016.
27. Wan H, AlHarbi BM, Macdonald RL: Mechanisms, treatment and prevention of cellular injury and death from delayed events after aneurysmal subarachnoid hemorrhage. *Expert Opin Pharmacother* 15(2):231–243, 2014.
28. Kabadi SV, Faden AI: Neuroprotective strategies for traumatic brain injury: improving clinical translation. *Int J Mol Sci* 15(1):1216–1236, 2014.
29. Loane DJ, Stoica BA, Faden AI: Neuroprotection for traumatic brain injury. *Handb Clin Neurol* 127:343–366, 2015.
30. Scrimgeour AG, Condlin ML: Nutritional treatment for traumatic brain injury. *J Neurotrauma* 31(11):989–999, 2014.
31. Ling H, Hardy J, Zetterberg H: Neurological consequences of traumatic brain injuries in sports. *Mol Cell Neurosci* 66(Pt B):114–122, 2015.
32. American College of Emergency Physicians: *Updated mild traumatic brain injury guideline for adults.* Available at: https://www.cdc.gov/traumaticbraininjury/mtbi_guideline.html.
33. Brain Trauma Foundation: Guidelines for the acute medical management of severe traumatic brain injury in infants, children, and adolescents—second edition. *Pediatr Crit Care Med* 13(1):S1–S82, 2012. Available at: https://braintrauma.org/uploads/03/15/guidelines_pediatric2_2.pdf.
34. Ontario Neurotrauma Foundation: *Guidelines for diagnosing and managing pediatric concussion,* ed 1, Toronto, 2014, Author. Available at: http://onf.org/system/attachments/266/original/GUIDELINES_for_Diagnosing_and_Managing_Pediatric_Concussion_Recommendations_for_HCPs__v1.1.pdf.
35. Harmon KG, et al: American Medical Society for Sports Medicine position statement: concussion in sport. *Br J Sports Med* 47(1):15–26, 2013. Review erratum in *Br J Sports Med* 47(3):184, 2013.
36. Rathbone AT, et al: A review of the neuro- and systemic inflammatory responses in

postconcussion symptoms: introduction of the "post-inflammatory brain syndrome" PIBS. *Brain Behav Immun* 46:1–16, 2015.

37. Christensen J: The epidemiology of posttraumatic epilepsy. *Semin Neurol* 35(3):218–222, 2015.

38. Rao VR, Parko KL: Clinical approach to posttraumatic epilepsy. *Semin Neurol* 35(1):57–63, 2015.

39. McKee AC, Alosco ML, Huber BR: Repetitive head impacts and chronic traumatic encephalopathy. *Neurosurg Clin N Am* 27(4):529–535, 2016.

40. 24 National Spinal Cord Injury Statistical Center: *Spinal cord injury facts and figures at a glance*, Birmingham AL, 2016, University of Alabama at Birmingham. Available at: https://www.nscisc.uab.edu/Public/Facts%202016.pdf.

41. Oyinbo CA: Secondary injury mechanisms in traumatic spinal cord injury: a nugget of this multiply cascade. *Acta Neurobiol Exp (Wars)* 71(2):281–299, 2011.

42. Perry EC, 3rd, Ahmed HM, Origitano TC: Neurotraumatology. *Handb Clin Neurol* 121:1751–1772, 2014.

43. Yokobori S, et al: Acute diagnostic biomarkers for spinal cord injury: review of the literature and preliminary research report. *World Neurosurg* 83(5):867–878, 2015.

44. Zhang B, Gensel JC: Is neuroinflammation in the injured spinal cord different than in the brain? Examining intrinsic differences between the brain and spinal cord. *Exp Neurol* 258:112–120, 2014.

45. Ju KL, Harris MG: Initial evaluation of the spine in trauma patients. In Browner BD, et al, editors: *Skeletal trauma: basic science, management and reconstruction*, Philadelphia, 2015, Saunders, pp 303–312.

46. Hagen EM: Acute complications of spinal cord injuries. *World J Orthop* 6(1):17–23, 2015.

47. Wan D, Krassioukov AV: Life-threatening outcomes associated with autonomic dysreflexia: a clinical review. *J Spinal Cord Med* 37(1):2–10, 2014.

48. Sezer N, Akkuş S, Uğurlu FG: Chronic complications of spinal cord injury. *World J Orthop* 6(1):24–33, 2015.

49. Rogers WK, Todd M: Acute spinal cord injury. *Best Pract Res Clin Anaesthesiol* 30(1):27–39, 2016.

50. Martirosyan NL, et al: The role of therapeutic hypothermia in the management of acute spinal cord injury. *Clin Neurol Neurosurg* 154:79–88, 2017.

51. Kabu S, et al: Drug delivery, cell-based therapies, and tissue engineering approaches for spinal cord injury. *J Control Release* 219:141–154, 2015.

52. Raspa A, et al: Recent therapeutic approaches for spinal cord injury. *Biotechnol Bioeng* 113(2):253–259, 2016.

53. Department of Health and Human Services (DHHS), Centers for Disease Control and Prevention (CDC), National Center for Health Statistics (NCHS): Summary health statistics for U.S. adults: National Health Interview Survey 2010. *Vital Health Stat 10* (252):7, 2012. Available at: www.cdc.gov/nchs/data/series/sr_10/sr10_252.pdf.

54. Hoy D, et al: The global burden of low back pain: estimates from the Global Burden of Disease 2010 study. *Ann Rheum Dis* 73(6):968–974, 2014.

55. Balagué F, et al: Non-specific low back pain. *Lancet* 379(9814):482–491, 2012.

56. Hoy D, et al: The epidemiology of low back pain. *Best Pract Res Clin Rheumatol* 24(6):769–781, 2010.

57. Golob AL, Wipf JE: Low back pain. *Med Clin North Am* 98(3):405–428, 2014.

58. Ito K, Creemers L: Mechanisms of intervertebral disk degeneration/injury and pain: a review. *Global Spine J* 3(3):145–152, 2013.

59. Chou R, et al: Diagnosis and treatment of low back pain: a joint clinical practice guideline from the American College of Physicians and the American Pain Society. *Ann Intern Med* 147(7):478–491, 2007.

60. Koes BW, et al: An updated overview of clinical guidelines for the management of non-specific low back pain in primary care. *Eur Spine J* 19(12):2075–2094, 2010.

61. Casazza BA: Diagnosis and treatment of acute low back pain. *Am Fam Physician* 85(4):343–350, 2012.

62. Deyo RA, et al: Opioids for low back pain. *Br Med J* 350:g6380, 2015.

63. Hooten WM, Cohen SP: Evaluation and treatment of low back pain: a clinically focused review for primary care specialists. *Mayo Clin Proc* 90(12):1699–1718, 2015.

64. Jiang SD, Jiang LS, Dai LY: Degenerative cervical spondylolisthesis: a systematic review. *Int Orthop* 35(6):869–875, 2011.

65. Leone A, et al: Lumbar spondylolysis: a review. *Skeletal Radiol* 40(6):683–700, 2011.

66. Chan WC, et al: Structure and biology of the intervertebral disk in health and disease. *Orthop Clin North Am* 42(4):447–464, vii, 2011.

67. Deyo RA, Mirza SK: Clinical practice. Herniated lumbar intervertebral disk. *N Engl J Med* 374(18):1763–1772, 2016.

68. Agency for Healthcare Research and Quality (AHRQ), National Guideline Clearing House: *Clinical guidelines for diagnosis and treatment of lumbar disc herniation with radiculopathy.* Available at: http://www.guideline.gov/content.aspx?f=rss&id=46414.

69. Jacobs WC, et al: Evidence for surgery in degenerative lumbar spine disorders. *Best Pract Res Clin Rheumatol* 27(5):673–684, 2013.

70. Todd NV, Dickson RA: Standards of care in cauda equina syndrome. *Br J Neurosurg* 30(5):518–522, 2016.

71. Writing Group Members, et al: Heart disease and stroke statistics—2016 update: a report from the American Heart Association. *Circulation* 133(4):e38–e360, 2016.

72. Sherzai AZ, Elkind MS: Advances in stroke prevention. *Ann N Y Acad Sci* 1338:1–15, 2015.

73. Bandaru VC, et al: Outcome of *Chlamydia pneumoniae* associated acute ischemic stroke in elderly patients: a case-control study. *Clin Neurol Neurosurg* 114(2):120–123, 2012.

74. Gupta HV, et al: Transient ischemic attacks: predictability of future ischemic stroke or transient ischemic attack events. *Ther Clin Risk Manag* 10:27–35, 2014.

75. Kiyohara T, et al: ABCD3 and ABCD3-I scores are superior to ABCD2 score in the prediction of short- and long-term risks of stroke after transient ischemic attack. *Stroke* 45(2):418–425, 2014.

76. Kernan WN, et al: Guidelines for the prevention of stroke in patients with stroke and transient ischemic attack: a guideline for healthcare professionals from the American Heart Association/American Stroke Association. *Stroke* 45(7):2160–2236, 2014.

77. Freeman WD, Aguilar MI: Prevention of cardioembolic stroke. *Neurother* 8(3):488–502, 2011.

78. Ihle-Hansen H, et al: Risk factors for and incidence of subtypes of ischemic stroke. *Funct Neurol* 27(1):35–40, 2012.

79. Bailey EL, et al: Pathology of lacunar ischemic stroke in humans—a systematic review. *Brain Pathol* 22(5):583–591, 2012.

80. Klijn CJ, Kappelle LJ: Haemodynamic stroke: clinical features, prognosis, and management. *Lancet Neurol* 9(10):1008–1017, 2010.

81. Winship IR: Cerebral collaterals and collateral therapeutics for acute ischemic stroke. *Microcirculation* 22(3):228–236, 2015.

82. Jickling GC, et al: Hemorrhagic transformation after ischemic stroke in animals and humans. *J Cereb Blood Flow Metab* 34(2):185–199, 2014.

83. Prabhakaran S, Ruff I, Bernstein RA: Acute stroke intervention: a systematic review. *JAMA* 313(14):1451–1462, 2015.

84. Karaszewski B, et al: What causes intracerebral bleeding after thrombolysis for acute ischaemic stroke? Recent insights into mechanisms and potential biomarkers. *J Neurol Neurosurg Psychiatry* 86(10):1127–1136, 2015.

85. Jauch EC, et al: Guidelines for the early management of patients with acute ischemic stroke: a guideline for healthcare professionals from the American Heart Association/American Stroke Association. *Stroke* 44(3):870–947, 2013.

86. Feldstein CA: Early treatment of hypertension in acute ischemic and intracerebral hemorrhagic stroke: progress achieved, challenges, and perspectives. *J Am Soc Hypertens* 8(3):192–202, 2014.

87. Lee JH, Zhang J, Yu SP: Neuroprotective mechanisms and translational potential of therapeutic hypothermia in the treatment of ischemic stroke. *Neural Regen Res* 12(3):341–350, 2017.

88. Azad TD, Veeravagu A, Steinberg GK: Neurorestoration after stroke. *Neurosurg Focus* 40(5):E2, 2016.

89. Hemphill JC, 3rd, et al: Guidelines for the management of spontaneous intracerebral hemorrhage: a guideline for healthcare professionals from the American Heart Association/American Stroke Association. *Stroke* 46(7):2032–2060, 2015.

90. Langhorne P, Bernhardt J, Kwakkel G: Stroke rehabilitation. *Lancet* 377(9778):1693–1702, 2011.

91. Naidech AM: Diagnosis and management of spontaneous intracerebral hemorrhage. *Continuum (Minneap Minn)* 21(5 Neurocritical Care):1288–1298, 2015.

92. Ma J, et al: Effects of intensive blood pressure lowering on intracerebral hemorrhage outcomes: a meta-analysis of randomized controlled trials. *Turk Neurosurg* 25(4):544–551, 2015.

93. Sykes L, Wood E, Kwan J: Antiepileptic drugs for the primary and secondary prevention of seizures after stroke. *Cochrane Database Syst Rev* (1):CD005398, 2014.

94. Helbok R, et al: Effect of mannitol on brain metabolism and tissue oxygenation in severe haemorrhagic stroke. *J Neurol Neurosurg Psychiatry* 82(4):378–383, 2011.

95. Beynon C, et al: Minimally invasive endoscopic surgery for treatment of spontaneous intracerebral haematomas. *Neurosurg Rev* 38(3):421–428, 2015.

96. Fiorella D, et al: Intracerebral hemorrhage: a common and devastating disease in need of better treatment. *World Neurosurg* 84(4):1136–1141, 2015.

97. Deleted in page proofs.

98. Hosaka K, Hoh BL: Inflammation and cerebral aneurysms. *Transl Stroke Res* 5(2):190–198, 2014.

99. Hokari M, et al: Pathological findings of saccular cerebral aneurysms-impact of subintimal fibrin

deposition on aneurysm rupture. *Neurosurg Rev* 38(3):531–540, 2015.

100. Ajiboye N, et al: Unruptured cerebral aneurysms: evaluation and management. *ScientificWorldJournal* 2015:954954, 2015.

101. Manhas A, et al: Comprehensive overview of contemporary management strategies for cerebral aneurysms. *World Neurosurg* 84(4):1147–1160, 2015.

102. Ajiboye N, et al: Cerebral arteriovenous malformations: evaluation and management. *ScientificWorldJournal* 2014:649036, 2014.

103. Brouillard P, Vikkula M: Genetic causes of vascular malformations. *Hum Mol Genet* 16(Spec 2):R140–R149, 2007.

104. San Millán Ruíz D, Gailloud P: Cerebral developmental venous anomalies. *Childs Nerv Syst* 26(10):1395–1406, 2010.

105. Mouchtouris N, et al: Biology of cerebral arteriovenous malformations with a focus on inflammation. *J Cereb Blood Flow Metab* 35(2):167–175, 2015.

106. Novakovic RL, et al: The diagnosis and management of brain arteriovenous malformations. *Neurol Clin* 31(3):749–763, 2013.

107. Gross BA, Du R: Diagnosis and treatment of vascular malformations of the brain. *Curr Treat Options Neurol* 16(1):279, 2014.

108. Zacharia BE, et al: Epidemiology of aneurysmal subarachnoid hemorrhage. *Neurosurg Clin N Am* 21(2):221–233, 2010.

109. Dority JS, Oldham JS: Subarachnoid hemorrhage: an update. *Anesthesiol Clin* 34(3):577–600, 2016.

110. Miller BA, et al: Inflammation, vasospasm, and brain injury after subarachnoid hemorrhage. *Biomed Res Int* 2014:384342, 2014.

111. Rosen DS, Macdonald RL: Subarachnoid hemorrhage grading scales: a systematic review. *Neurocrit Care* 2(2):110–118, 2005.

112. Tang C, Zhang TS, Zhou LF: Risk factors for rebleeding of aneurysmal subarachnoid hemorrhage: a meta-analysis. *PLoS ONE* 9(6):e99536, 2014.

113. Gruenbaum SE, Bilotta F: Postoperative ICU management of patients after subarachnoid hemorrhage. *Curr Opin Anaesthesiol* 27(5):489–493, 2014.

114. Connolly ES, Jr, et al: Guidelines for the management of aneurysmal subarachnoid hemorrhage: a guideline for healthcare professionals from the American Heart Association/American Stroke Association. *Stroke* 43:1711–1737, 2012.

115. International Headache Society (IHS): *IHS classification ICHD-II 1. Migraine*. Available at: https://www.ichd-3.org/1-migraine/.

116. Headache Classification Committee of the International Headache Society (IHS): The international classification of headache disorders, ed 3 (beta version). *Cephalalgia* 33(9):629–808, 2013. Available at: http://www.ihs-classification .org/_downloads/mixed/International-Headach e-Classification-III-ICHD-III-2013-Beta.pdf.

117. Allais G, et al: Migraine in perimenopausal women. *Neurol Sci* 36(Suppl 1):79–83, 2015.

118. Deleted in page proofs.

119. Sacco S, Kurth T: Migraine and the risk for stroke and cardiovascular disease. *Curr Cardiol Rep* 16(9):524, 2014.

120. Bigal ME, Lipton RB: The epidemiology, burden, and comorbidities of migraine. *Neurol Clin* 27(2):321–334, 2009.

121. Burstein R, Noseda R, Borsook D: Migraine: multiple processes, complex pathophysiology. *J Neurosci* 35(17):6619–6629, 2015.

122. Akerman S, Goadsby PJ: Pathophysiology of migraine. In Aminoff JF, Daroff RB, editors: *Encyclopedia of the neurological sciences*, ed 2, London, 2014, Academic Press, pp 67–71.

123. Cutrer FM, Smith JH: Human studies in the pathophysiology of migraine: genetics and functional neuroimaging. *Headache* 53(2):401–412, 2013.

124. Becker WJ: Acute migraine treatment in adults. *Headache* 55(6):778–793, 2015.

125. US Food and Drug Administration (US FDA): *FDA news release: FDA allows marketing of first medical device to prevent migraine headaches*, March 11, 2014. Available at: https://www .meddeviceonline.com/doc/fda-marketing-medical -device-prevent-migraine-headaches-0001.

126. Whitcup SM, et al: Development of onabotulinumtoxinA for chronic migraine. *Ann N Y Acad Sci* 1329:67–80, 2014.

127. De Simone R, et al: Intracranial pressure in unresponsive chronic migraine. *J Neurol* 261(7):1365–1373, 2014.

128. May A: Diagnosis and clinical features of trigemino-autonomic headaches. *Headache* 53(9):1470–1478, 2013.

129. Iacovelli E, et al: Neuroimaging in cluster headache and other trigeminal autonomic cephalalgias. *J Headache Pain* 13(1):11–20, 2012.

130. Deleted in page proofs.

131. Robbins MS, Starling AJ, Pringsheim TM, et al: Treatment of cluster headache: the American headache society evidence-based guidelines. *Headache* 2016;56(7):1093–1106.

132. Prakash S, Patell R: Paroxysmal hemicrania: an update. *Curr Pain Headache Rep* 18(4):407, 2014.

133. Bernstein JA, et al: Headache and facial pain: differential diagnosis and treatment. *J Allergy Clin Immunol Pract* 1(3):242–251, 2013.

134. Freitag F: Managing and treating tension-type headache. *Med Clin North Am* 97(2):281–292, 2013.

135. Roos KL: Nonviral infections. In Goetz CG, editor: *Textbook of clinical neurology*, ed 2, Philadelphia, 2003, Saunders.

136. Thigpen MC, et al: Emerging Infections Programs Network. Bacterial meningitis in the United States, 1998-2007. *N Engl J Med* 364(21):2016–2025, 2011.

137. Deleted in page proofs.

138. Coureuil M, et al: Pathogenesis of meningococcemia. *Cold Spring Harb Perspect Med* 3(6):2013.

139. Heckenberg SG, Brouwer MC, van de Beek D: Bacterial meningitis. *Handb Clin Neurol* 121:1361–1375, 2014.

140. Liechti FD, Grandgirard D, Leib SL: Bacterial meningitis: insights into pathogenesis and evaluation of new treatment options: a perspective from experimental studies. *Future Microbiol* 10(7):1195–1213, 2015.

141. Deleted in page proofs.

142. Franco-Paredes C, et al: Management of Cryptococcus gattii meningoencephalitis. *Lancet Infect Dis* 15(3):348–355, 2015.

143. Murthy JM, Sundaram C: Fungal infections of the central nervous system. *Handb Clin Neurol* 121:1383–1401, 2014.

144. Garcia-Monco JC: Tuberculosis. *Handb Clin Neurol* 121:1485–1499, 2014.

145. van Toorn R, Solomons R: Update on the diagnosis and management of tuberculous meningitis in children. *Semin Pediatr Neurol* 21(1):12–18, 2014.

146. Alvis Miranda H, et al: Brain abscess: current management. *J Neurosci Rural Pract* 4(Suppl 1):S67–S81, 2013.

147. Tihan T: Pathologic approach to spinal cord infections. *Neuroimaging Clin N Am* 25(2):163–172, 2015.

148. Brouwer MC, et al: Brain abscess. *N Engl J Med* 371(5):447–456, 2014.

149. Deleted in page proofs.

150. Honda H, Warren DK: Central nervous system infections: meningitis and brain abscess. *Infect Dis Clin North Am* 23(3):609–623, 2009.

151. Rust RS: Human arboviral encephalitis. *Semin Pediatr Neurol* 19(3):130–151, 2012.

152. Centers for Disease Control and Prevention: *Eastern equine encephalitis*. Updated April 5, 2016. Available at: www.cdc.gov/EasternEquine Encephalitis/tech/epi.html.

153. Halperin JJ: Diagnosis and management of acute encephalitis. *Handb Clin Neurol* 140:337–347, 2017.

154. Price RW, et al: Evolving character of chronic central nervous system HIV infection. *Semin Neurol* 34(1):7–13, 2014.

155. Deleted in page proofs.

156. Kamal S, et al: The presence of human immunodeficiency virus-associated neurocognitive disorders is associated with a lower adherence to combined antiretroviral treatment. *Open Forum Infect Dis* 4(2):ofx070, 2017.

157. Brew BJ, Chan P: Update on HIV dementia and HIV-associated neurocognitive disorders. *Curr Neurol Neurosci Rep* 14(8):468, 2014.

158. Deleted in page proofs.

159. Underwood J, Robertson KR, Winston A: Could antiretroviral neurotoxicity play a role in the pathogenesis of cognitive impairment in treated HIV disease? *AIDS* 29(3):253–261, 2015.

160. Singer EJ, et al: Neurologic presentations of AIDS. *Neurol Clin* 28(1):253–275, 2010.

161. Stavros K, Simpson DM: Understanding the etiology and management of HIV-associated peripheral neuropathy. *Curr HIV/AIDS Rep* 11(3):195–201, 2014.

162. Albarillo F, O'Keefe P: Opportunistic neurologic infections in patients with acquired immunodeficiency syndrome (AIDS). *Curr Neurol Neurosci Rep* 16(1):10, 2016.

163. Chang CC, et al: HIV and co-infections. *Immunol Rev* 254(1):114–142, 2013.

164. Bilgrami M, O'Keefe P: Neurologic diseases in HIV-infected patients. *Handb Clin Neurol* 121:1321–1344, 2014.

165. Malfitano A, et al: Human immunodeficiency virus-associated malignancies: a therapeutic update. *Curr HIV Res* 10(2):123–132, 2012.

166. Belbasis L, et al: Environmental risk factors and multiple sclerosis: an umbrella review of systematic reviews and meta-analyses. *Lancet Neurol* 14(3):263–273, 2015.

167. National Multiple Sclerosis Society: *Multiple sclerosis: just the facts*, 2016. Available at: http:// www.nationalmssociety.org/NationalMSSociety/ media/MSNationalFiles/Brochures/Brochure -Just-the-Facts.pdf.

168. Miller E: Multiple sclerosis. *Adv Exp Med Biol* 724:222–238, 2012.

169. Deleted in page proofs.

170. Mallucci G, et al: The role of immune cells, glia and neurons in white and gray matter pathology in multiple sclerosis. *Prog Neurobiol* 127-128:1–22, 2015.

171. Deleted in page proofs.

172. Zeis T, Schaeren-Wiemers N: Lame ducks or fierce creatures? The role of oligodendrocytes in multiple sclerosis. *J Mol Neurosci* 35(1):91–100, 2008.

173. Prins M, et al: Pathological differences between white and grey matter multiple sclerosis lesions. *Ann N Y Acad Sci* 1351:99–113, 2015.

174. D'haeseleer M, et al: Cerebral hypoperfusion: a new pathophysiologic concept in multiple sclerosis? *J Cereb Blood Flow Metab* 35(9): 1406–1410, 2015.

175. Brownlee WJ, Miller DH: Clinically isolated syndromes and the relationship to multiple sclerosis. *J Clin Neurosci* 21(12):2065–2071, 2014.

176. Joanna P, et al: Evolution of diagnostic criteria for multiple sclerosis. *Neurol Neurochir Pol* 49(5): 313–321, 2015.

177. Filippi M, Preziosa P, Rocca MA: Multiple sclerosis. *Handb Clin Neurol* 135:399–423, 2016.

178. Files DK, et al: Multiple sclerosis. *Prim Care* 42(2):159–175, 2015.

179. Dolati S, et al: Multiple sclerosis: therapeutic applications of advancing drug delivery systems. *Biomed Pharmacother* 86:343–353, 2017.

180. Pawate S, Bagnato F: Newer agents in the treatment of multiple sclerosis. *Neurologist* 19(4):104–117, 2015.

181. Burton JM, Costello FE: Vitamin D in multiple sclerosis and central nervous system demyelinating disease—a review. *J Neuroophthalmol* 35(2):194–200, 2015.

182. Xiao J, et al: Mesenchymal stem cells and induced pluripotent stem cells as therapies for multiple sclerosis. *Int J Mol Sci* 16(5):9283–9302, 2015.

183. Toosy A, Ciccarelli O, Thompson A: Symptomatic treatment and management of multiple sclerosis. *Handb Clin Neurol* 122:513–562, 2014.

184. Li H, et al: The neurobiology of zika virus. *Neuron* 92(5):949–958, 2016.

185. Wakerley BR, Yuki N: Guillain-Barré syndrome. *Expert Rev Neurother* 15(8):847–849, 2015.

186. Wijdicks EF, Klein CJ: Guillain-Barré syndrome. *Mayo Clin Proc* 92(3):467–479, 2017.

187. Hanewinckel R, Ikram MA, Van Doorn PA: Peripheral neuropathies. *Handb Clin Neurol* 138:263–282, 2016.

188. Grimm A, et al: Ultrasound differentiation of axonal and demyelinating neuropathies. *Muscle Nerve* 50(6):976–983, 2014.

189. Tsao B: The electrodiagnosis of cervical and lumbosacral radiculopathy. *Neurol Clin* 25(2): 473–494, 2007.

190. Corey DL, Comeau D: Cervical radiculopathy. *Med Clin North Am* 98(4):791–799, 2014.

191. De Luigi AJ, Fitzpatrick KF: Physical examination in radiculopathy. *Phys Med Rehabil Clin N Am* 22(1):7–40, 2011.

192. Fox IK, Mackinnon SE: Adult peripheral nerve disorders: nerve entrapment, repair, transfer, and brachial plexus disorders. *Plast Reconstr Surg* 127(5):105e–118e, 2011.

193. Chalk CH, Benstead TJ, Keezer M: Medical treatment for botulism. *Cochrane Database Syst Rev* (2):CD008123, 2014.

194. Berrih-Aknin S: Myasthenia gravis: paradox versus paradigm in autoimmunity. *J Autoimmun* 52:1–28, 2014.

195. Ha JC, Richman DP: Myasthenia gravis and related disorders: pathology and molecular pathogenesis. *Biochim Biophys Acta* 1852(4): 651–657, 2015.

196. Myasthenia Gravis Foundation of America: *Clinical classification of myasthenia gravis.* Available at: http://mystheniagravis.wix.com/ mgravis#!classification/c211a.

197. Guptill JT, Soni M, Meriggioli MN: Current treatment, emerging translational therapies, and new therapeutic targets for autoimmune myasthenia gravis. *Neurother* 13(1):118–131, 2016.

198. Gilhus NE: Myasthenia gravis. *N Engl J Med* 375(26):2570–2581, 2016.

199. American Brain Tumor Association: *Brain tumor statistics.* Last updated January 2017. Available at: www.abta.org/about-us/news/brain-tumor -statistics/.

200. Deleted in page proofs.

201. Morgan LL, et al: Mobile phone radiation causes brain tumors and should be classified as a probable human carcinogen (2A) (review). *Int J Oncol* 46(5):1865–1871, 2015.

202. Siegal T: Clinical relevance of prognostic and predictive molecular markers in gliomas. *Adv Tech Stand Neurosurg* 43:91–108, 2016.

203. Deleted in page proofs.

204. Lathia JD, et al: Cancer stem cells in glioblastoma. *Genes Dev* 29(12):1203–1217, 2015.

205. Burgess A, Hynynen K: Microbubble-assisted ultrasound for drug delivery in the brain and central nervous system. *Adv Exp Med Biol* 880: 293–308, 2016.

206. Ferroni L, et al: Novel nanotechnologies for brain cancer therapeutics and imaging. *J Biomed Nanotechnol* 11(11):1899–1912, 2015.

207. Dutoit V, et al: Immunotherapy of brain tumors. *Prog Tumor Res* 42:11–21, 2015.

208. Deleted in page proofs.

209. Brown MC, Gromeier M: Oncolytic immunotherapy through tumor-specific translation and cytotoxicity of poliovirus. *Discov Med* 19(106):359–365, 2015.

210. Grier JT, Batchelor T: Low grade gliomas in adults. *Oncologist* 11:681–693, 2006.

211. Venur VA, et al: Current medical treatment of glioblastoma. *Cancer Treat Res* 163:103–115, 2015.

212. Okonogi N, et al: Topics in chemotherapy, molecular-targeted therapy, and immunotherapy for newly-diagnosed glioblastoma multiforme. *Anticancer Res* 35(3):1229–1235, 2015.

213. Jaeckle KA: Oligodendroglial tumors. *Semin Oncol* 41(4):468–477, 2014.

214. Asaid M, et al: Ependymoma in adults: local experience with an uncommon tumour. *J Clin Neurosci* 22(9):1392–1396, 2015.

215. Cimino PJ: Malignant progression to anaplastic meningioma: neuropathology, molecular pathology, and experimental models. *Exp Mol Pathol* 99(2):354–359, 2015.

216. Mehdorn HM: Intracranial meningiomas: a 30-year experience and literature review. *Adv Tech Stand Neurosurg* 43:139 184, 2016.

217. Gutmann DH, et al: Neurofibromatosis type 1. *Nat Rev Dis Primers* 3:17004, 2017.

218. Kresak JL, Walsh M: Neurofibromatosis: a review of NF1, NF2, and schwannomatosis. *J Pediatr Genet* 5(2):98–104, 2016.

219. DeBella K, et al: Use of the National Institutes of Health criteria for diagnosis of neurofibromatosis 1 in children. *Pediatrics* 105(3 Pt 1):608–614, 2000.

220. Slattery WH: Neurofibromatosis type 2. *Otolaryngol Clin North Am* 48(3):443–460, 2015.

221. Karajannis MA, Ferner RE: Neurofibromatosis-related tumors: emerging biology and therapies. *Curr Opin Pediatr* 27(1): 26–33, 2015.

222. Liu W, et al: Microenvironmental influences on metastasis suppressor expression and function during a metastatic cell's journey. *Cancer Microenviron* 7(3):117–131, 2014.

223. Weidle UH, et al: Dissection of the process of brain metastasis reveals targets and mechanisms for molecular-based intervention. *Cancer Genomics Proteomics* 13(4):245–258, 2016.

224. Svokos KA, Salhia B, Toms SA: Molecular biology of brain metastasis. *Int J Mol Sci* 15(6):9519–9530, 2014.

225. Deleted in page proofs.

226. Lin X, DeAngelis LM: Treatment of brain metastases. *J Clin Oncol* 33(30):3475–3484, 2015.

227. Samartzis D, et al: Intramedullary spinal cord tumors: part I—epidemiology, pathophysiology, and diagnosis. *Global Spine J* 5(5):425–435, 2015.

228. Tredway TL: Minimally invasive approaches for the treatment of intramedullary spinal tumors. *Neurosurg Clin N Am* 25(2):327–336, 2014.

229. Samartzis D, et al: Intramedullary spinal cord tumors: part II—management options and outcomes. *Global Spine J* 6(2):176–185, 2016.

Neurobiology of Schizophrenia, Mood Disorders, Anxiety Disorders, and Obsessive-Compulsive Disorder

Lorey K. Takahashi

⊖volve WEBSITE

CHAPTER OUTLINE

Mental illnesses are common and found in different cultures and across the socioeconomic spectrum. When left untreated, the consequences can be devastating. This chapter provides an introduction to the neurobiology of schizophrenia, mood disorders, and some anxiety disorders. The etiology and pathophysiology of mental illnesses are diverse and complex. Diagnostic criteria are constantly being updated to more precisely diagnose and effectively treat the disorders. Every mental disorder manifests a range of symptoms that vary in intensity. Symptom variations likely reflect individual differences in pathologic brain structures and functions which affect treatment. Risk factors, such as exposure to uncontrollable psychosocial stress, may precipitate the onset of mental disorders and point to the challenge in understanding how diseased genes and environmental factors interact.

The development of visual and quantitative structural and functional neuroimaging techniques provides insight into the pathophysiologic basis of mental disorders. In schizophrenia, neuroanatomic, functional, and neurochemical alterations associated with this debilitating illness have uncovered abnormal brain regions along with a host of candidate genes that confer risk. Similarly, in mood and anxiety disorders, brain scans are revealing structural and functional abnormalities. Notably, many brain regions implicated in normal cognitive and emotional processing are found in schizophrenia, mood, and anxiety disorders. The future lies in unraveling how the highly interconnected brain

structures modulated by neurotransmitters, neuropeptides, and hormones operate in normal to abnormal mental states.

Knowledge of the pathophysiology associated with a specific mental illness has guided the development of new psychopharmacologic medications with fewer side effects. However, some individuals with mental disorders do not respond to current medications or may relapse after a period of treatment. The use of psychotherapies alone or as an adjunct to pharmacotherapy also may be effective in treating some disorders by making the person aware of potential environmental factors that trigger stress and the onset of the illness. Learning to cope with these triggers offers hope for alleviating psychiatric symptoms or attenuates pathophysiologic functions.

SCHIZOPHRENIA

Schizophrenia is a serious psychiatric illness that strikes 1% of the world's population. The illness is equally prevalent in males and females and emerges in young adults during the late teens and early twenties, with a slightly earlier onset in males than in females. Schizophrenia is the term coined originally by Eugen Bleuler in 1911 to describe a collection of illnesses characterized by thought disorders, which reflect a break in reality or splitting of the cognitive from the emotional side of one's personality. A schizophrenic individual may exhibit a feeling of happiness when recollecting a terrible event or emotional indifference when describing a joyful occasion. Today, disorganized thought in schizophrenia is characterized by positive and negative symptoms including auditory hallucinations, paranoid delusions, and cognitive deficits that have devastating effects on the individual and the individual's family.

◆Etiology and Pathophysiology
Genetic Predisposition

Schizophrenia is a heritable disorder. In monozygotic twins, the concordance rate varies from 30% to 50%. This variability may stem from different diagnostic criteria and methodologic or sampling differences across studies. In dizygotic twins and siblings the concordance rate decreases to 12%, which is still considerably higher than the 1% figure found in the general population.

Nonetheless, schizophrenia is not a simple genetic disorder in which inherited disease alleles will always lead to illness. Schizophrenia likely involves several genes located on different chromosomes and differs from mendelian disorders, in which genes are fully penetrant and recognized as the primary cause of disease (e.g., genes for Huntington disease). As indicated by the 50% concordance rate in monozygotic twins, the genes for schizophrenia show reduced penetrance, resulting in individuals who carry the disease genes without manifesting the illness. Further complicating the search for the specific genes that confer risk of schizophrenia is the variability in biologic and phenotypic traits among individuals who manifest the illness. Ongoing studies based on protein interactions may be valuable in identifying novel gene associations.[1]

Prenatal and Perinatal Vulnerability Factors. Because the concordance rate of schizophrenia in monozygotic twins is never 100% as in mendelian disorders, environmental factors likely play an important role in increasing the risk of developing the disorder. A leading hypothesis suggests that early environmental factors interfere with genetically programmed neural developmental alterations that eventually compromise normal brain structures and functions.[2] An early brain defect may remain silent and not dramatically affect the individual until subsequent development requires adaptive use of brain structures.[3] Several hypothesized early environmental factors that may alter brain development and increase the risk of developing schizophrenia include exposure to prenatal infection, prenatal nutritional deficiencies, perinatal complications (such as birth defects and neonatal hypoxia), and upbringing in an urban environment.[4]

Neuroanatomic and Functional Abnormalities

Neuroanatomic Alterations. Advanced neuroimaging techniques have revealed structural brain abnormalities in schizophrenia.[5,6] A consistent finding is the enlargement of the lateral and third ventricles and the widening of frontocortical fissures and sulci (Fig. 19.1). Schizophrenics with cerebral ventricular enlargement often exhibit cognitive impairments and negative symptoms and respond poorly to treatment. Other studies reported a reduction in the thalamus and temporal lobe areas (e.g., amygdala, hippocampus, and parahippocampal gyrus).[7] A reduction in thalamus size may disrupt neurotransmission between the frontal cortex and primary sensory and motor areas. Hippocampal volume loss in the first years of the illness is another consistent finding, and hippocampal volume reduction accelerates in schizophrenics more than 50 years of age.[8] This hippocampal atrophy is strongly associated with global cognitive and socio-occupational functional impairments, which also may reflect a fronto-hippocampal disconnection in socio-cognitive processing.

The amygdala plays a central role in the social brain emotional processing network.[9] Abnormal amygdala connectivity is widely reported

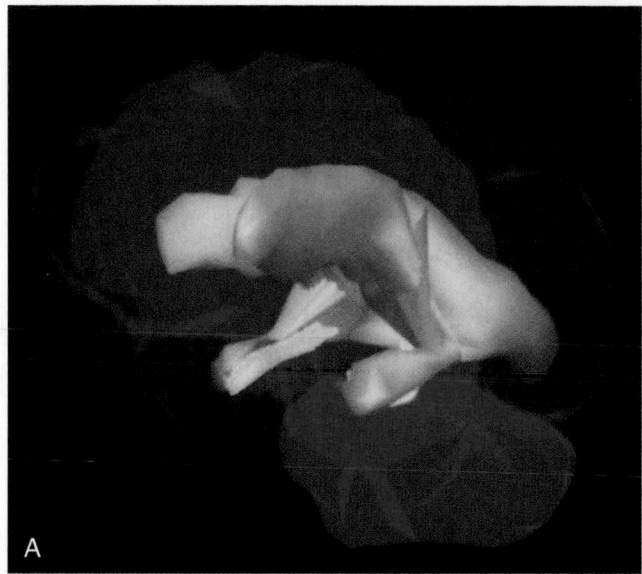

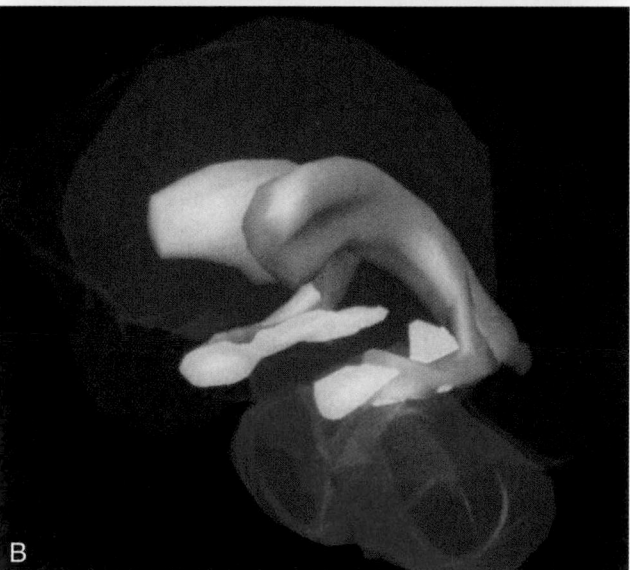

FIGURE 19.1 Magnetic Resonance Imaging (MRI) Comparison of Normal Brain and Brain with Schizophrenia. Three-dimensional MRI reconstructions showing **A,** the cerebral ventricles *(gray regions)* and hippocampus *(yellow regions)* of a schizophrenic patient, and **B,** those of a healthy individual. Note the enlarged cerebral ventricles and reduced hippocampal volume of the brain of the schizophrenic individual. (From Gershon ES, Rieder RO: *Sci Am* 267:128, 1992. Original illustrations by Nancy C. Andreason, University of Iowa.)

in schizophrenia and hypothesized to represent the basis underlying pronounced difficulties for schizophrenics to make appropriate social judgments as found in tests of facial identity, affect recognition, and in emotional processing.[10] Reported amygdala abnormalities in schizophrenia include reduced volume[7] and abnormal functional activation patterns for social and emotion processing.[11] The induction of abnormal amygdala projections to brain regions such as the hippocampus during late adolescence and young adulthood may be linked to the onset of schizophrenia.

Brain imaging studies in adolescents with early-onset schizophrenia reveal progressive loss of cortical gray matter in temporal lobes, somatosensory and motor cortices, and the dorsolateral cortex (Fig. 19.2). Of clinical concern is the loss of cortical tissue, which is evident

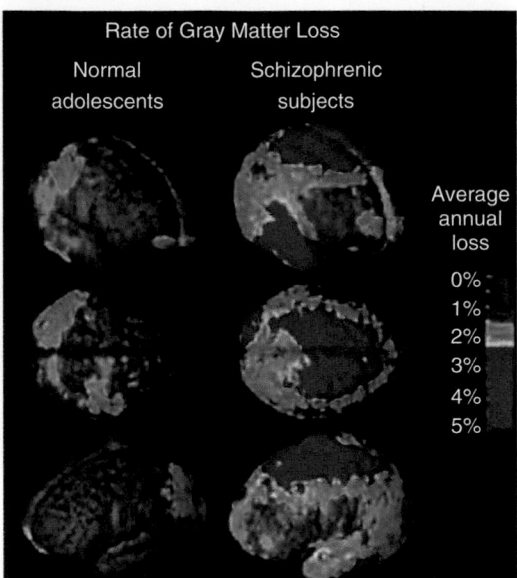

FIGURE 19.2 Accelerated Gray Matter Loss in Brains of Early-Onset Schizophrenic Adolescents. Annual gray matter loss ranging from 2% to 5% was found in 13- to 18-year-old schizophrenics—compared with age-matched healthy adolescents. (From Thompson PM et al: *Proc Natl Acad Sci U S A* 98:11650, 2001.)

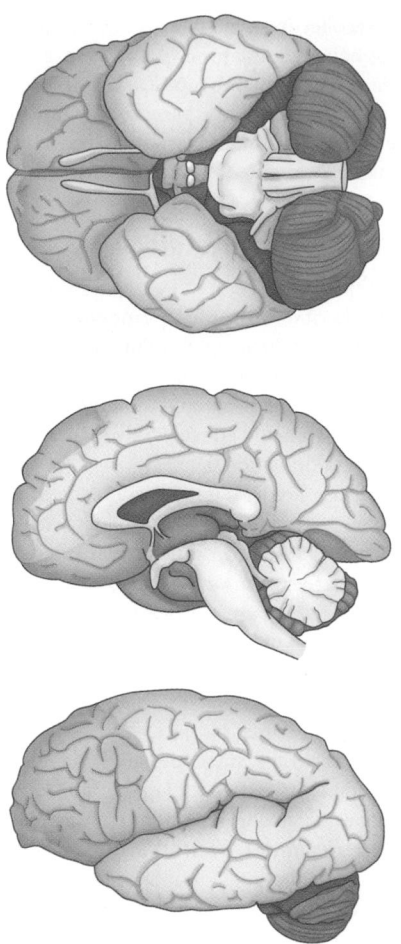

FIGURE 19.3 The Prefrontal Cortex. The prefrontal cortex consists of a dorsolateral *(blue)* and an orbitofrontal *(green)* region.

by the time the individual seeks treatment and continues throughout the course of the illness despite the use of antipsychotic medication.[12] The progressive loss in frontal lobe volume is accompanied by increased severity of negative symptoms and further reductions in cognitive functioning. These results highlight the ineffectiveness of current medications for schizophrenia to attenuate or reverse the loss of frontal brain tissue.

Brain abnormalities in schizophrenia are believed to originate in the prenatal period of cell proliferation and migration. Reelin, an extracellular matrix protein involved in neuronal migration during development and in synaptic function during adulthood, is reduced in the prefrontal cortex and hippocampus of schizophrenic individuals.[13,14] Reelin is concentrated in interneurons that contain gamma-aminobutyric acid (GABA), the most widespread inhibitory neurotransmitter. Furthermore, in the dorsal prefrontal cortex of schizophrenic brains, the level of glutamic acid decarboxylase, the major enzyme in GABA biosynthesis, is reduced, which likely impairs normal cognitive/emotional functions.

Pathophysiologic changes in the dorsal prefrontal cortex are believed to contribute to the production of negative symptoms in schizophrenia (Fig. 19.3). In particular, the dorsolateral prefrontal cortex (DLPFC) (Brodmann areas 9, 10, 46, 47) is intricately involved in the initiation and maintenance of goal-directed activities and in solving cognitive problems related to working memory. Working memory involves the brief storage and use of information to complete cognitive tasks such as language comprehension, learning, and reasoning. Blood flow and metabolism normally increase in the DLPFC during working memory processing but not in schizophrenics, who also perform poorly in tests of working memory. Thus the dorsolateral prefrontal cortex appears to be hypoactive in schizophrenia.

Neurotransmitter Alterations. The onset of schizophrenia was initially hypothesized to stem from abnormally high concentrations of the brain neurotransmitter dopamine. This dopamine hypothesis of schizophrenia was proposed on the basis of pharmacologic studies showing that antipsychotic drugs were potent blockers of brain dopamine receptors. A strong positive correlation was found between the clinical potencies of first-generation antipsychotic drugs (e.g., chlorpromazine, fluphenazine, and haloperidol) and their affinity for the dopamine D_2 receptor. In addition, drugs at high doses that dramatically increased dopaminergic transmission—such as levodopa (L-dopa), cocaine, and amphetamine—produced schizophrenic-like psychosis, which was reversed by dopamine blockers.

A current view of the dopamine hypothesis of schizophrenia is that brain dopamine pathways are altered in different ways (Fig. 19.4). For example, the negative symptoms and cognitive alterations in schizophrenia are proposed to result from reduced dopaminergic neurotransmission in the mesocortical dopamine pathway.[15] This hypodopaminergic transmission in the prefrontal cortex contrasts with the hypothesized hyperdopaminergic secretion in mesolimbic brain regions that may contribute to the production of positive schizophrenic symptoms. The mesolimbic dopamine pathway innervates temporal lobe structures including the hippocampal formation and amygdala, as well as the nucleus accumbens and anterior cingulate cortex.

Another neurotransmitter system that may underlie the pathogenesis of schizophrenia is the excitatory neurotransmitter glutamate and its actions on the N-methyl-D-aspartate (NMDA) receptor subtype. The glutamate hypothesis of schizophrenia proposes that underactivation of glutamate receptors contributes to schizophrenia.[16] In schizophrenia, glutamate concentrations in the cerebrospinal fluid (CSF) are reduced along with a decrease in cortical glutamate synthesis. Furthermore, in unaffected individuals, blocking the glutamate NMDA receptor with antagonists, such as phencyclidine (PCP) and ketamine, facilitates the positive and negative symptoms of schizophrenia. PCP users report auditory hallucinations and disorientation and may become violent from their delusions. In monkeys, chronic PCP treatment impairs cognitive performance in a test associated with prefrontal cortical damage.[17]

◆Clinical Manifestations

The symptoms of schizophrenia are currently divided into three broad categories of positive, negative, and cognitive symptoms (Box 19.1).

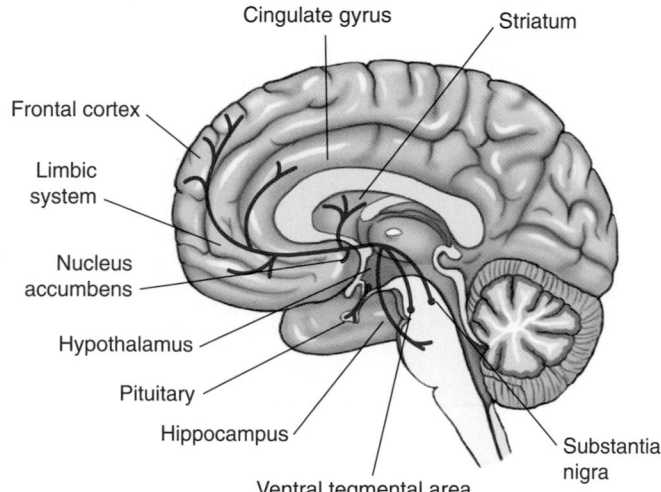

FIGURE 19.4 The Dopamine System. Dopamine cell bodies are located in the substantia nigra, where they project to the stratum (nigrostriatal pathway); and in the ventral tegmental area, where they project to the frontal and cingulate cortex (mesocortical pathway), the striatum, the hippocampus, and other limbic structures (mesolimbic pathway). Dopamine nuclei are also located in the hypothalamus and project to the pituitary.

Positive symptoms frequently occur during a psychotic episode, when an individual loses touch with reality and experiences something that should be absent (e.g., hallucinations). *Negative symptoms* are characterized by disruptions in normal emotional states and expressions. Cognitive symptoms are fairly common and involve problems with thought processes that severely impair the ability to perform routine daily tasks that involve attention, planning, and social skills. According to the 5th edition of the *Diagnostic and Statistical Manual of Mental Disorders (DSM-5)*,[18] the diagnosis of schizophrenia begins by eliminating other mental disorders and symptoms not caused by substance abuse, medication, or medical condition. The individual will then be diagnosed with schizophrenia when at least two of the following symptoms (1) delusions, (2) hallucinations, (3) disorganized speech, (4) disorganized or catatonic behavior, and (5) negative symptoms are experienced most of the time during a 1-month period with some disturbance present over 6 months. In addition, one of the symptoms must be delusions, hallucinations, or disorganized speech.

Psychotic Dimension

Psychotic dimension refers to hallucinations and delusions and reflects a person's confusion or loss of touch with the external world. Hallucinations and delusions are classified as positive symptoms and are the most common in schizophrenia.

Hallucinations. A hallucination is a perception experienced without external stimulation of the sense organs. Sensory hallucinations can be auditory, tactile, visual, gustatory, and olfactory. For example, the schizophrenic individual may hear voices, experience touch or electrical sensations, report images of animate and inanimate objects, or complain of unpleasant tastes and odors. These hallucinations may occur alone or together.

Delusions. A delusion is a persistent belief contrary to the educational and cultural background of the individual. Delusions may involve grandiose, nihilistic, persecutory, somatic, sexual, and religious themes. Paranoid beliefs are common and may involve spying, conspiracy, persecution, and ridicule. Delusions also may be referential in that particular stimuli or events become highly personalized, such as believing a television talk show host is directing information specifically at them.

BOX 19.1 MAJOR SYMPTOMS OF SCHIZOPHRENIA

Positive Symptoms
Hallucinations
Auditory
Olfactory
Somatic-tactile
Visual
Voices commenting
Voices conversing

Delusions
Delusions of being controlled
Delusions of mind reading
Delusions of reference
Grandiosity
Guilt
Persecutory
Religious
Somatic
Thought broadcasting
Thought insertion
Thought withdrawal

Positive Formal Thought Disorder
Circumstantiality
Derailment
Distractible speech
Illogicality
Incoherence
Pressure of speech
Tangentiality

Bizarre Behavior
Aggressive, agitated
Clothing, appearance
Repetitive, stereotyped
Social, sexual behavior

Negative Symptoms
Affective Flattening
Affective nonresponsivity
Decreased spontaneous movements
Inappropriate affect

Lack of vocal inflections
Paucity of expressive gestures
Poor eye contact
Unchanging facial expression

Alogia
Blocking
Increase in response latency
Poverty of speech
Poverty of speech content

Anhedonia-Asociality
Few recreational interests
Few social relationships
Impaired intimacy
Little sexual interest

Attention
Social inattentiveness
Inattentiveness during testing

Avolition-Apathy
Impaired personal hygiene
Lack of persistence
Physical anergia

Cognitive Symptoms
Inability to understand information and make proper decision to complete a task
Difficulty paying attention
Problems with working memory or the inability to use recently learned information
Lack of insight

Disorganized Behavior

Disorganized behavior includes disorganized speech and disorganized or bizarre behavior. Incongruity of affect is another dimension of disorganized behavior.

Disorganized Speech. A common form of disorganized speech is formal thought disorder, which involves fluent speech that is difficult to comprehend. The speech often moves from one topic to another unexpectedly (loose associations) and illogically, and the person becomes easily distracted when talking.

Another form of disorganized speech is called poverty of content. Here, the use of vocabularies to convey information is severely retarded despite a fair amount of spoken words. For instance, the same phrases are used repeatedly throughout a conversation.

Disorganized Behavior. Disorganized (or bizarre) behavior is the conceptual equivalent of disorganized speech. The individual has difficulty engaging in goal-directed activities. Repetitive (e.g., stereotyped rocking) or aimless behavior and poor personal hygiene are exhibited. Another feature is the incongruity of affect or the manifestation of inappropriate situational affect as exemplified by hostility without provocation or child-like silliness in sober situations.

Negative Dimensions

Negative dimensions reflect a deficit in normal functioning and are characterized by affective flattening, anhedonia, alogia (poverty of speech), and avolition. Affective flattening is the near absence of emotional or facial expressions throughout a conversation or in different situations. In anhedonia, individuals are unable to experience emotions such as pleasure or pain and report a sense of detachment from the environment. Alogia is the absence of spontaneous speech production for the purpose of answering questions or expressing oneself. Avolition is a deficit in spontaneous or goal-directed behavior, such as completing simple daily tasks.

◆Treatment

The use of chlorpromazine in the mid-1950s dramatically altered the treatment of schizophrenia, which previously required extensive institutional hospitalization. The drug was especially effective in reducing positive symptoms such as hallucinations and delusions as well as thought disorders and hyperactivity. The beneficial effects of chlorpromazine and similar first-generation antipsychotic drugs such as haloperidol on positive symptoms were believed to stem from their ability to block the dopamine D_2-receptor subtype, especially in the overly active mesolimbic dopamine pathways.

However, D_2-receptor blockade, such as in the striatum, produces a notable neurologic side effect resembling Parkinson disease—a disorder associated with degeneration of dopamine cell bodies in the substantia nigra that project to the striatum. A related side effect of conventional antipsychotics that develops in 15% to 20% of schizophrenics after several years of treatment is a condition called tardive dyskinesia. This condition is characterized by tic-like jerky movements, such as smacking the lips or flicking the tongue, unsteady gait, or rocking back and forth when seated. Other side effects may include sedation, hypotension, akathisia (motor restlessness), constipation, weight gain, amenorrhea, and, less frequently, hepatotoxicity and electrocardiographic changes.

Although the majority of schizophrenic individuals obtained some positive symptom relief from the first-generation or conventional antipsychotics, approximately 20% failed to respond to D_2-blocking drugs (Table 19.1), especially those with pronounced symptoms of apathy, disorientation, and social withdrawal. However, some of these treatment-resistant individuals responded to a second generation of drugs that became known as *atypical antipsychotic drugs*.[19] Atypical

TABLE 19.1	MEDICATIONS USED IN THE TREATMENT OF SCHIZOPHRENIA
GENERIC NAME	**BRAND NAME**
Conventional Antipsychotics	
Chlorpromazine	Thorazine
Fluphenazine	Prolixin
Haloperidol	Haldol
Perphenazine	Trilafon
Pimozide	Orap
Prochlorperazine	Compazine
Thioridazine	Mellaril
Thiothixene	Navane
Trifluoperazine	Stelazine
Second-Generation Atypical Antipsychotics	
Aripiprazole	Abilify
Clozapine	Clozaril
Loxapine	Loxitane
Lurasidone	Latuda
Molindone	Moban
Olanzapine	Zyprexa
Paliperidone	Invega
Quetiapine	Seroquel
Risperidone	Risperdal
Ziprasidone	Geodon

antipsychotics also were shown to have superior efficacy in reducing not only the positive but also the negative symptoms in comparison with conventional antipsychotics. For example, clozapine improves some cognitive functions (such as verbal fluency, verbal learning, and memory) and some physical functions (such as psychomotor speed). In addition, the notable neurologic side effects that accompany the use of the conventional antipsychotics were diminished.

Unlike conventional antipsychotics, atypical drugs appear to work by blocking a range of neurotransmitter receptors. For example, clozapine blocks not only D_2 receptors but also D_1, D_3, D_4, and D_5 receptors and serotonin (5-hydroxytryptamine, i.e., HT_2, $5-HT_6$, $5-HT_7$); norepinephrine; and cholinergic and histamine receptors. Risperidone and ziprasidone have higher affinity for blocking $5-HT_2$ than D_2 receptors. The higher $5-HT_2/D_2$-receptor–binding ratio of atypical antipsychotics in comparison with conventional drugs may reflect a normalization of serotonin-dopamine interactions leading to clinical efficacy not observed with D_2-receptor blockade alone.

Atypical antipsychotics are not without adverse effects, most notably metabolic abnormalities including regulation of glucose and lipid levels and weight gain. For example, long-term clozapine or olanzapine treatment increases body weight gain, which becomes a risk factor for diabetes and cardiovascular disease. Schizophrenics treated with clozapine also are at risk of developing agranulocytosis, a potentially lethal blood disorder involving the loss of white blood cells and a compromised immune system.

In conjunction with antipsychotic medication, psychosocial therapy can facilitate the management of schizophrenia. Psychosocial relationships assist the individual in developing coping strategies and in identifying stressors and relapse symptoms. Cognitive-behavioral therapy (CBT), a talking therapy that initiates cognitive and behavioral change based on an individualized reappraisal of the person's faulty beliefs, is effective in treating schizophrenics with stabilized antipsychotic medications.[20]

An important benefit of psychosocial and family support is the encouragement of compliance with antipsychotic medication that requires a period before the emergence of clinical efficacy.

MOOD DISORDERS: DEPRESSION AND BIPOLAR DISORDER

Mood refers to a sustained emotional state as opposed to brief emotional feelings, which are termed *affective states*. Healthy individuals are normally capable of experiencing a variety of affective states including euphoria, joy, surprise, fear, sadness, anxiety, and depression. When emotional states, such as sadness, become chronic and uncontrollable, individuals may be diagnosed with a mood disorder called *depression*. The two major classifications of mood disorder are (1) unipolar or major depressive disorder, also known as *major depression* or *clinical depression*; and (2) bipolar disorder, which is further classified into bipolar I and bipolar II disorders. Major (unipolar) depressive disorder consists of depressed mood, loss of interest/pleasure, changes in activity, guilt/worthlessness, death/suicide, fatigue/loss of energy, decreased concentration, and changes in sleep, appetite, or weight. In addition, two new specifiers were added in *DSM-5*. One specifier with mixed symptoms allows for the occurrence of manic symptoms as part of the diagnosis in depressed people who do not meet the criteria for a manic episode. Another specifier with anxious distress was added because anxiety may affect treatment choices for major depressive disorder. A manic episode consists of elevated, expansive, and irritable mood, as well as changes in energy and activity levels. In bipolar I disorder, the person experienced at least one manic episode that may be preceded or followed by hypomanic or major depressive episodes. Mania symptoms may significantly impair the individual, trigger psychosis, and require hospitalization. In bipolar II disorder, the individual experiences one major depressive episode for at least 2 weeks and at least one hypomanic episode for at least 4 days. Box 19.2 presents the major criteria of major depression and bipolar disorder according to the American Psychiatric Association's *DSM-5*.[18]

Major (unipolar) depressive disorder is the most common mood disorder and the leading cause of disability in the United States and throughout the world.[21] Unipolar depression appears in all age groups including young children. In the United States, the lifetime prevalence rate is 16.2% of the population with a twofold greater risk in women than men after adolescence. In children and adolescents, 2% to 6% suffer from depression. The prevalence of bipolar disorder ranges from 3% to 5% in the general population. Bipolar I disorder occurs equally in men and women in comparison with bipolar II disorder, which afflicts more women than men. When left untreated, a number of depressed and bipolar individuals are at risk of developing a host of medical illnesses, including cardiovascular disease, obesity, diabetes, and thyroid disease.

◆Etiology and Pathophysiology
Genetic Predisposition and Environmental Influences

Family and twin studies indicate a strong basis for mood disorders. Concordance rates for bipolar disorder ranged up to 62% and 42% for monozygotic and dizygotic twins, respectively.[22] Concordance rates of 62% and 28% for unipolar disorder were reported in monozygotic and dizygotic twins, respectively. Even among adoptees with a biologic family history of mood disorders, the incidence of developing major depression or manic-depressive illness is higher than among control adoptees. The strong tendency for mood disorders to run in families has encouraged a search for the abnormal gene or genes. Interestingly, loci on chromosomes 18 and 22 have been linked to both bipolar disorder and

---

BOX 19.2 MAJOR SYMPTOMS OF DEPRESSION AND MANIA

Symptoms of Depression*
Depressed or irritable mood
Loss of interests and pleasure
Significant (>5%) weight gain or loss in a month
Insomnia or hypersomnia
Psychomotor agitation or retardation
Fatigue or loss of energy
Feelings of worthlessness or excessive guilt
Poor concentration or indecisiveness
Recent thoughts of death or suicide

Symptoms of Manic Episode†
Elevated mood
Irritable mood
Inflated self-esteem
Decreased need for sleep
Excessive talking
Racing/crowded thoughts
Distractibility
Increase in goal-directed activity
Excessive risky activities

*Five or more of the symptoms are present in a 2-week period and at least one of the symptoms is either depressed mood or loss of interests or pleasure.
†Three or more symptoms (four if the mood is only irritable) during a distinct period of abnormally and persistently elevated, expansive, or irritable mood occurring for at least 1 week.

---

schizophrenia. Bipolar individuals, who may exhibit psychotic behavior, have deficits in reelin expression linked to genetic loci, located on chromosome 22, which confers susceptibility to schizophrenia (see preceding section on Schizophrenia). However, the large variation in clinical symptoms suggests that developmental and environmental factors are as important as genetic factors in contributing to the etiology of mood disorders.

Neurochemical Dysregulation

Modern theories of mood disorders began with the important observations that drugs such as imipramine that elevated norepinephrine levels within the synapse reduced depression whereas drugs that depleted monoamine levels (e.g., reserpine) increased depression. These studies led to the dominant monoamine hypothesis of depression, in which a deficit in the concentration of brain norepinephrine, dopamine, and/or serotonin is the underlying cause of depression, in contrast to mania, which results from elevated concentrations of monoamines. Three major classes of antidepressant drugs were initially developed and included monoamine oxidase inhibitors (MAOIs), tricyclic antidepressants (TCAs), and selective serotonin reuptake inhibitors (SSRIs). These antidepressants shared the common property, albeit through different mechanisms, that increasing monoamine neurotransmitter levels within the synapse is the basis for their antidepressant effects (Fig. 19.5).

Additional support for the monoamine hypothesis of depression came from studies showing a reduction of monoamine metabolites in the cerebral spinal fluid (CSF) of depressed people. Other work demonstrated that dietary depletion of tryptophan, the precursor of serotonin synthesis, or alpha-methylparatyrosine (AMPT), a drug that inhibits dopamine and norepinephrine synthesis, produced a rapid return to depression in individuals successfully treated with antidepressants.[23]

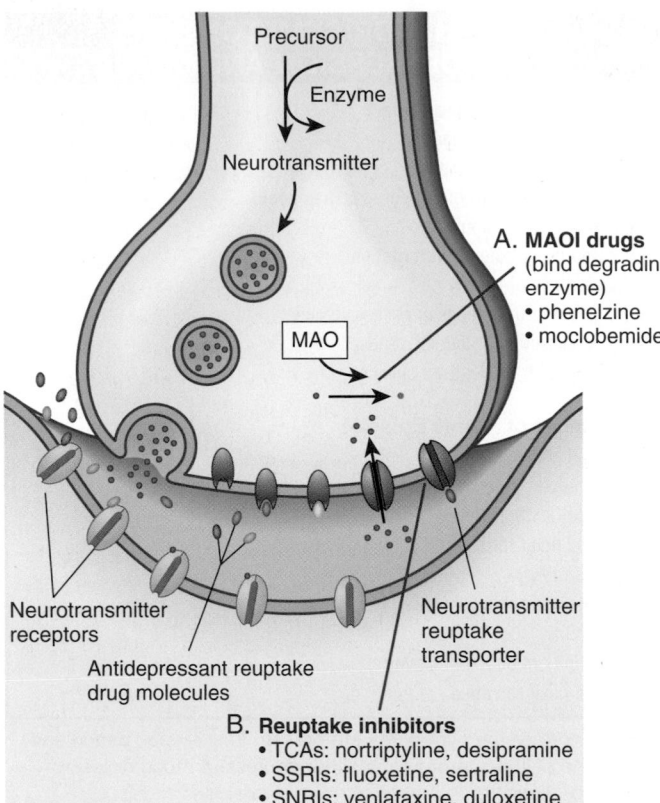

A. **MAOI drugs**
(bind degrading enzyme)
• phenelzine
• moclobemide

MAO

Neurotransmitter receptors

Antidepressant reuptake drug molecules

Neurotransmitter reuptake transporter

B. **Reuptake inhibitors**
• TCAs: nortriptyline, desipramine
• SSRIs: fluoxetine, sertraline
• SNRIs: venlafaxine, duloxetine

FIGURE 19.5 Schematic Diagrams Showing the Sites of Actions of Antidepressants and Their Effects on Neurotransmitter Levels. **A,** MAO inhibitors (MAOIs) act by blocking the enzyme that normally degrades neurotransmitters, such as norepinephrine and serotonin increasing their presynaptic concentration. **B,** The tricyclic antidepressants (TCAs), selective serotonin reuptake inhibitors (SSRIs), and serotonin-norepinephrine reuptake inhibitors (SNRIs) act by reducing the uptake of neurotransmitters from the synapse, which leads to increased neurotransmitter levels.

Neuroendocrine Dysregulation

Stress and Hypothalamic-Pituitary-Adrenal System Dysregulation. The hypothalamic-pituitary-adrenal (HPA) system plays an essential role in an individual's ability to cope with stress (see Chapter 11). However, chronic stress-induced activation of the HPA system and elevated glucocorticoid secretion are found in a large percentage (30% to 70%) of people with major depression, suggesting that mechanisms responsible for increased HPA hormone secretion contribute to the pathophysiology of depression.[24] Notably, antidepressant drugs effective in normalizing the HPA system are associated with a good clinical response, whereas persistent dysregulation of the HPA system is related to continued depression or relapse. Psychosocial stress-induced activation of the immune system increases secretion of proinflammatory cytokines, such as interleukin-1α (IL-1α) and IL-β, tumor necrosis factor-alpha (TNF-α), and IL-6, which modulates signaling pathways throughout the periphery and brain and augments further secretion of HPA hormones and monoamine metabolism. Evidence suggests that inflammation is another risk factor that triggers the onset of depression. For example, a study involving 73,131 Danish individuals from the general population reported elevated levels of C-reactive protein, a commonly used marker of inflammatory disease, was associated with increased risk of psychologic distress and depression.[25] Another study reported that depressed people treated with antidepressants, a combination of antidepressants and psychotherapy, or psychotherapy alone initially exhibited elevated

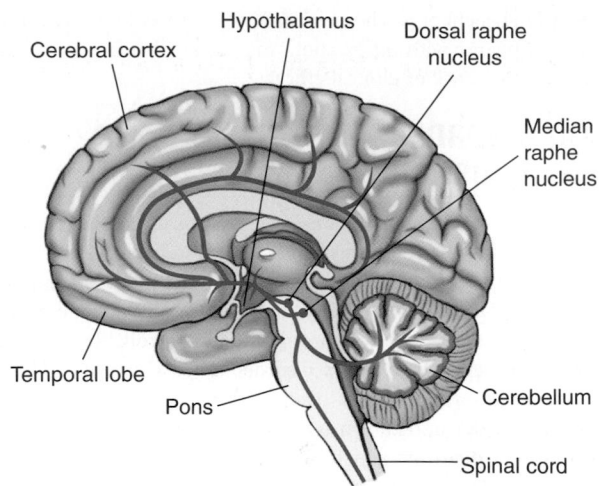

FIGURE 19.6 The Serotonin System. Serotonin neurons are located in the brainstem raphe nuclei. They project diffusely to all regions of the cortex, temporolimbic regions, hypothalamus, basal ganglia, cerebellum, the brainstem, and spinal cord.

cytokine levels that returned to normal levels after recovery from depression.[26] These studies suggest that cytokines are involved in the pathophysiology of depression (see *What's New?* Inflammatory Cytokines Are Linked to Diverse Mental Illnesses).

Increasing evidence from animal models of stress-induced depression shows that depression-like behavior is accompanied by atrophy of neurons in the hippocampus, a reduction in the development of new hippocampal neurons (i.e., neurogenesis), and a deficit in hippocampal brain-derived neurotrophic factor (BDNF) levels.[27,28] Consistent with animal studies, human postmortem work indicates low hippocampal BDNF levels in depression. Because the growth factor BDNF supports the survival of neurons and facilitates neurogenesis from hippocampal stem cells, a neurotrophic hypothesis of depression has been proposed as an extension of the monoamine hypothesis of depression to broadly account for the pathophysiologic basis of depression. That is, stress-induced depression and the accompanying reduction in levels of monoamines are caused by deficits in neurogenesis and BDNF levels. Of clinical relevance, administration of antidepressants to animals reverses the depression-like state and increases the development of neurogenesis and BDNF levels.

Hypothalamic-Pituitary-Thyroid System Dysregulation. Alterations in thyroid function and mental illnesses, particularly major depression and anxiety disorders, have long been recognized. People with hyperthyroidism often manifest symptoms of dysphoria, anxiety, irritability, emotional lability, and cognitive impairments. On the other hand, individuals with severe hypothyroid exhibit features of major depression, apathy, psychomotor slowing, and dementia.[29] Notably, although thyroid dysfunction may be linked to symptoms of depression and anxiety, people diagnosed with primary depression generally have normal thyroid function.[30] The causal mechanisms or basis underlying altered thyroid secretion and depression remain to be determined.

Neuroanatomic and Functional Abnormalities

The dorsal and median raphe nuclei, located in the central gray matter of the caudal mesencephalon and rostral pons, contain a large group of serotonin-synthesizing neurons that project extensively to all regions of the cortex, basal ganglia, limbic system, hypothalamus, cerebellum, and brainstem (Fig. 19.6). Postmortem and/or brain imaging studies of depressed individuals revealed a widespread decrease in serotonin

WHAT'S NEW?

Inflammatory Cytokines Are Linked to Diverse Mental Illnesses

Inflammation plays a major role in the pathophysiology of many chronic diseases, such as cardiovascular disease, diabetes, rheumatoid arthritis, asthma, multiple sclerosis, and chronic pain. A growing body of evidence now suggests that psychologic and social stressors increase inflammatory cytokine production that contribute to the pathophysiology of mental illnesses including schizophrenia, depression, bipolar disorder, and anxiety disorders, such as posttraumatic stress disorder. Although normal brain function requires low levels of inflammatory cytokines, derived from the brain's resident innate immune cells called microglia, elevated cytokine levels in the brain appear to facilitate neuronal damage, atrophy, and loss of spine synapses. In addition, peripheral cytokines may contribute to microglia functional alterations by entering the brain through the circumventricular organs and also compromise the protective role of the blood-brain barrier resulting in direct trafficking of cells and inflammatory molecules between the periphery and brain to enhance brain inflammation. The peripheral cytokines, such as interleukin 6 (IL-6) may also bind to vagus nerve receptors to activate a pathway that reaches hypothalamic brain nuclei to further stimulate microglia secretion of proinflammatory cytokines, chemokines, and proteases.

In schizophrenia, studies found increased blood concentrations of inflammatory cytokines in subjects with first-episode, drug-naive psychosis suggesting an association independent of the effects of antipsychotic medications. People diagnosed with schizophrenia also have higher cytokine levels, especially during periods of symptomatic exacerbation, than controls, but not during periods of clinical stability. Studies further suggest that inflammatory cytokines may predict subsequent relapse.

Similarly, high levels of inflammation appear to increase the risk of developing depression. For example, elevations in IL-6 and C-reactive protein predict the eventual onset of depressive symptoms. Of particular interest is that selective serotonin reuptake inhibitor treatment is shown to decrease the production of the proinflammatory cytokines, tumor necrosis factor-alpha (TNF-α), and interleukin-1 (IL-1). However, depressed people with heightened plasma inflammatory markers respond poorly when treated with antidepressant medications. Studies further found significant elevations of proinflammatory cytokines in symptom severity and manic episodes in medication-free bipolar disorder.

The role of inflammation in depression also extends to posttraumatic stress disorder (PTSD). A strong comorbidity exists between depression and PTSD and people with this comorbidity show higher inflammatory responses than those with PTSD or depression alone. As in depression, the inflammatory marker C-reactive protein was found to be a predictor of PTSD onset in a study of war zone-deployed soldiers. Recent evidence further showed inflammation in PTSD is associated with reduced volume of the hippocampus, a structure that processes memory. The severity of stress and trauma and the association between PTSD and smoking, obesity/metabolic syndrome, and sleep disorders may further exacerbate the activation of immuno-inflammatory pathways in PTSD or comorbid PTSD and depression.

Future research will likely yield insights into the basis of inflammation that promotes the pathophysiology of diverse mental illnesses. New treatments that reduce inflammation and attenuate the adverse effects of proinflammatory cytokines could have a major impact on alleviating serious psychiatric disorders.

Data from Khandaker GM et al: *Lancet Psychiatry* 2:258-270, 2015; Kiecolt-Glaser JK et al: *Am J Psychiat* 172:1075-1091, 2015; Kirkpatrick B, Miller BJ: *Schizophrenia Bull* 39:1174-1179, 2013; Miller AH, Raison CL: *Nat Rev Immunol* 16:22-34, 2016; Modabbernia A et al: *Biol Psychiatry* 74:15-25, 2013; O'Donovan A et al: *Psychoneuroendocrinology* 51:557-566, 2015.

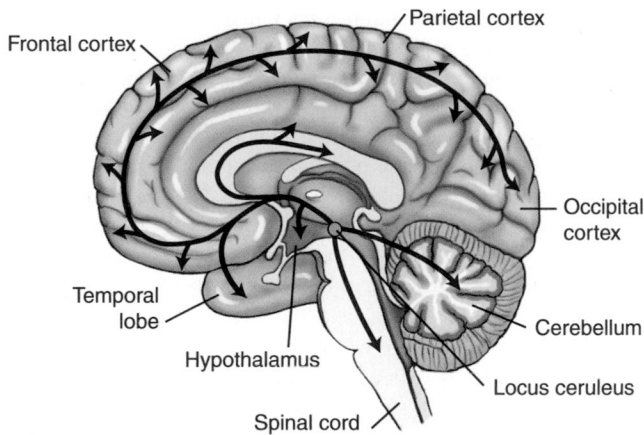

FIGURE 19.7 The Norepinephrine System. The norepinephrine cell bodies originate in the locus ceruleus and project throughout the brain, including the hypothalamus, the temporal lobe, the entire cortex, the cerebellum, and spinal cord.

5-HT$_{1A}$ receptor subtype binding in the frontal, temporal, and limbic cortex as well as serotonin transporter binding in the cerebral cortex and hippocampus. Mood disorders in some people may reflect a dysfunctional raphe-serotonin system, which normally modulates homeostasis, emotionality, and tolerance to aversive experiences.

A group of norepinephrine-containing cells located in the locus ceruleus of the rostral pons project to vast areas of the forebrain, brainstem, and spinal cord (Fig. 19.7). The locus ceruleus–norepinephrine

system is implicated in global psychologic processes including attention, vigilance, and orientation to novel, aversive, or threatening stimuli. Activation of the locus ceruleus–norepinephrine system is also capable of inhibiting the raphe-serotonin system, suggesting an indirect role in modulating serotonin functions. Norepinephrine receptor alterations (e.g., α- and β-adrenergic receptor subtypes) are found in the frontal cortex of some suicide victims with major depression. Alterations in norepinephrine systems may be linked to attention or concentration difficulties as well as sleep and arousal disturbances in depression.

Functional abnormalities associated with mood disorders are found in frontal and limbic regions such as the amygdala.[31,32] Postmortem studies report a reduction in glial cell numbers in people with unipolar and bipolar disorders. There are also reports of reduced frontal lobe volume in depressed individuals and decreased or asymmetric temporal lobe volume in individuals with bipolar illness and depression.

Functional neuroimaging studies indicate decreased cerebral blood flow and glucose metabolism in the dorsolateral and dorsomedial prefrontal cortex of individuals affected by major depression or bipolar disorder. Dorsolateral prefrontal abnormalities in depression may be responsible for the retardation in cognitive processing and speech deficits similar to those found in schizophrenia. Dorsomedial frontal dysfunction may be associated with mnemonic and attentional impairments that accompany mood disorders. Other frontocortical regions, including the ventrolateral, ventromedial, and orbital areas, exhibit increased blood flow and metabolism in unipolar depression (Fig. 19.8). These frontal brain areas have extensive interconnections with the amygdala, and increased blood flow and metabolism, especially in the right amygdala, are positively related to negative affect in depressed individuals. These functional changes in brain activity begin to normalize with successful

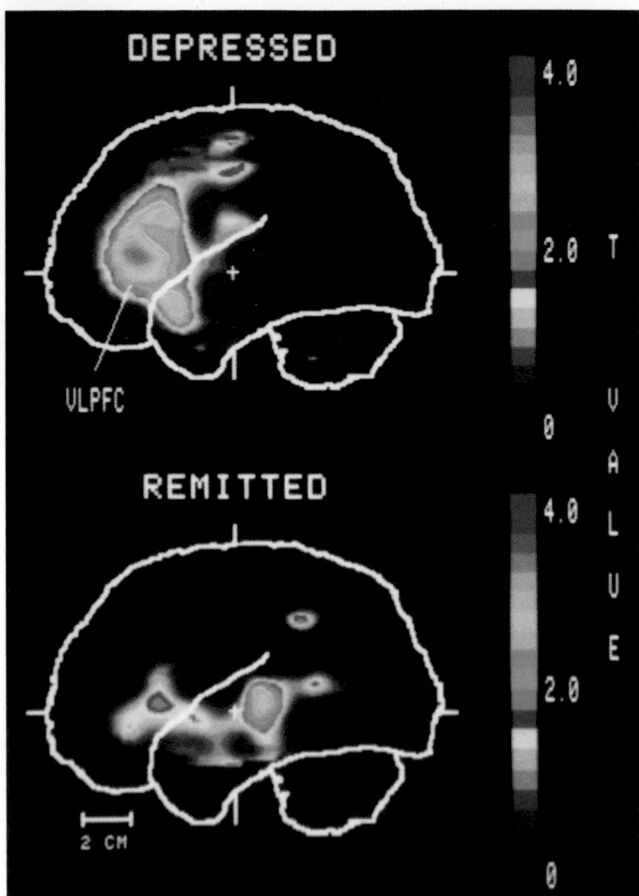

FIGURE 19.8 Positron-Emission Tomography (PET) Comparison of Brain Activity in Depression and in Remittance. PET scan showing increased activity in the left prefrontal cortex in a depressed person but not in the remitted person. *VLPFC,* Ventrolateral prefrontal cortex. (From Drevets WC et al: *J Neurosci* 12:3628, 1992. Copyright ©1992 by the Society for Neuroscience.)

antidepressant treatments, suggesting they are state rather than trait related.

Hippocampal volume reduction in major depression is a widely reported finding, especially in people with a history of recurrent major depression.[33] Similar to the hippocampus, the amygdala is reduced in volume after experiencing a number of major depression episodes and a family history of depression, albeit enlarged in first episode depression.[34] The cumulative effects of stress may be responsible of a reduction in hippocampal and amygdala volume. MRI studies showed increased volume of the amygdala in bipolar illness and larger lateral ventricles in people suffering multiple bipolar episodes compared to those with only a single episode or healthy controls.[35] Ventricular enlargement suggests progressive brain tissue loss resulting from multiple bipolar episodes.

The Glutamate System. Because of the delayed onset of action of current antidepressants and poor remission rates, investigators are constantly searching for new drugs with novel mechanisms of actions. An emerging body of evidence suggests that elevated cortical levels of glutamate, the major excitatory neurotransmitter in the central nervous system, may be involved in the pathophysiology of major depression. A potential promising target is the glutamate N-methyl-D-aspartate (NMDA) receptor. At nontoxic doses, the glutamate receptor antagonist ketamine was found in animal models to rapidly increase synaptic density and signaling in cortical neurons. Of clinical relevance, a few studies reported ketamine was effective in inducing rapid but transient anti-

depressant effects in treatment-resistant depressed people.[36,37] Further research on unraveling the mechanism of action of ketamine and on the long-term safety and efficacy of ketamine will be required before this drug can be recommended as an alternative innovative treatment for depression.

Clinical Manifestations
Depression

Major depression is characterized by unremitting feelings of sadness and despair (see Box 19.2). The dysphoric mood or intensely painful mood is accompanied frequently by insomnia, loss of appetite and body weight, and reduced interest in pleasurable activities and interpersonal relationships. Sleep disturbances may include difficulty in initially falling asleep and awakening in the middle of the night, lying awake for several hours with an inability to subsequently fall asleep. Individuals may have reduced motor activity and suffer marked fatigue. Others complain of restlessness and agitation. Feelings of worthlessness and guilt are common, and pessimistic or negative outcomes are often perceived even in routine situations. The ability to function (e.g., work) and concentrate is greatly diminished. Depressive episodes may occur or recur suddenly or gradually and continue from a few weeks to months, and 20% may exhibit a chronic form of depression.

Suicidal risk increases in depression. Factors such as living alone or being divorced, having a prior history of drug abuse or suicide attempt, or having depression at midlife or older ages contribute to suicide in 10% to 15% of depressed individuals.

Bipolar Disorder: Mania

Manic individuals experience elevated levels of euphoria and self-esteem and feelings of grandiosity. Energy levels are greatly enhanced even after only a few hours of sleep each night. The increased energy, however, does not lead to organized plans and thoughts. The individual may show poor judgment in spending money, may become hypersexual, or may make poor business commitments. Other hallmarks of mania are excessive, rapid, loud, and pressured speech. The manic person frequently skips from one topic of conversation to another and is easily distracted both when speaking and when performing tasks. Approximately 50% of manic individuals develop psychotic symptoms, such as delusions or hallucinations, which require hospitalization. The onset and termination of manic symptoms (see Box 19.2) are usually abrupt and may last for a few days or months followed by depression. The risk of recurrence of bipolar disorder is high, especially without immediate treatment.

Treatment
Depression

Approximately 80% of depressed persons will respond to antidepressant drugs such as MAOIs, TCAs, and SSRIs (Table 19.2); psychotherapy; or a combination of both treatment modalities. Although SSRIs have become the standard first-line treatment for major depression, initial selection of an antidepressant often includes an assessment of the person's symptoms and age as well as the side effects, safety, cost, and convenience of the prescribed medication. For example, medications that produce sedation may be helpful for the treatment of sleep disturbances. Approximately 50% of depressed individuals may not show a favorable response during initial treatment to an antidepressant drug, and 10% to 20% may continue to exhibit symptoms after 2 years. Individuals who are nonresponsive to a specific antidepressant during a 2-month period may be given another antidepressant medication. Atypical antidepressants, such as nefazodone, trazodone, and mirtazapine, presumably produce their clinical effects by blocking specific receptors (e.g.,

TABLE 19.2 FDA-APPROVED MEDICATIONS USED IN THE TREATMENT OF DEPRESSION AND ANXIETY DISORDERS

GENERIC NAME	BRAND NAME
Monoamine Oxidase Inhibitors	
Isocarboxazid	Marplan
Phenelzine	Nardil
Tranylcypromine	Parnate
Selegiline	Emsam
Tricyclics	
Amitriptyline	Elavil, Endep, Levate
Amoxapine	Asendin
Clomipramine	Anafranil
Desipramine	Norpramin, Pertofrane
Doxepin	Adapin, Sinequan
Imipramine	Tofranil
Maprotiline	Ludiomil
Nortriptyline	Aventyl, Pamelor
Protriptyline	Vivactil
Trimipramine	Surmontil
Selective Serotonin Reuptake Inhibitors	
Citalopram	Celexa
Escitalopram	Lexapro
Fluoxetine	Prozac
Fluvoxamine	Luvox
Paroxetine	Paxil
Sertraline	Zoloft
Serotonin and Norepinephrine Reuptake Inhibitors	
Desvenlafaxine	Pristiq
Duloxetine	Cymbalta
Levomilnacipran	Fetzima
Venlafaxine	Effexor, Effexor XR
Serotonin Reuptake Inhibitor and 5-HT$_{1A}$ Receptor Partial Agonist	
Vilazodone	Viibryd
Norepinephrine and Specific Serotonergic Modulator	
Mirtazapine	Remeron
Norepinephrine–Dopamine Reuptake Inhibitor	
Bupropion	Wellbutrin, Zyban
Serotonin Modulator	
Nefazodone	Serzone
Trazodone	Desyrel, Oleptro
Vortioxetine	Trintellix

5-HT$_{2A}$). A new generation of antidepressants that selectively block serotonin and norepinephrine reuptake is available in the United States (e.g., venlafaxine) and Europe (i.e., milnacipran, reboxetine). At present, there are no criteria to determine whether selection of the next antidepressant will be efficacious. Among children and adolescents, only fluoxetine is currently approved for use in children by the U.S. Food and Drug Administration (FDA)[38] (Box 19.2).

In bipolar depression, antidepressant medications may lead to cycle acceleration or induction of mania. However, SSRIs and bupropion may be less likely to induce these effects than MAOIs or TCAs.

A number of side effects are reported with MAOIs, TCAs, and SSRIs. Commonly reported side effects of MAOIs include sedation or agitation, insomnia, dry mouth, impotence, and weight gain. MAOIs also may induce acute and heightened elevations in blood pressure (e.g., hypertensive crisis) after intake of tyramine-rich foods, such as aged cheeses, sour cream, pods of broad beans, pickled herring, liver, canned figs, raisins, and avocados. In addition, MAOI interactions with TCAs, SSRIs, stimulants, and over-the-counter flu medications are dangerous and should be avoided. Because of these adverse side effect issues, MAOIs are used less often than other antidepressants.

TCAs may produce sedation, insomnia, orthostatic hypotension, seizures, and weight gain. Some TCAs have moderate anticholinergic side effects, including constipation, urinary hesitancy or retention, dry mouth, blurred vision, and memory impairment. These side effects may be an issue when considering TCA treatment of older adults, in which case the TCAs desipramine and nortriptyline may be preferred because of their reduced anticholinergic, cardiovascular, and sedating effects.

Common side effects of SSRIs include sleep disturbances (e.g., insomnia) and nausea. However, agitation, allergic skin reactions, dry mouth, anxiety, altered appetite, and sexual dysfunction have been reported. Unlike MAOIs and TCAs, SSRIs do not have pronounced effects on the cardiovascular or cholinergic systems. SSRIs are potent inhibitors of cytochrome P-450 isoenzymes, which are involved in drug metabolism. Therefore SSRIs may lead to dangerous elevations in blood concentrations of other psychiatric medications when taken together. SSRIs should not be taken with MAOIs or immediately after discontinuing MAOI treatment. A serotonin syndrome characterized by excitement or autonomic hyperactivity, abdominal pain, rigidity, and hyperthermia may develop, leading to coma or death.

Side effects of atypical antidepressants may include sedation, dry mouth, weight gain, and constipation. Nefazodone and trazodone have been associated with hepatic toxicity. Venlafaxine and reboxetine lack many of the serious side effects associated with TCAs; however, sweating, dry mouth, and some sedation may occur. Electroconvulsive therapy (ECT) may be used when individuals fail to respond to antidepressants or when they are severely depressed, pregnant, suicidal, or psychotic. ECT effectively alleviates depressive symptoms in about 50% to 80% of people, who may then begin to respond to antidepressant medications. Recent work suggests that ECT increases the volume of the hippocampus and amygdala, brain structures linked to emotion, mood, and cognitive functions.[39] Depressed people with relatively small hippocampal volumes were most likely to show hippocampal volume increases and improved clinical response after ECT. Neurotrophic processes activated by ECT, including neurogenesis, may underlie these structural changes and clinical benefits.

Deep brain stimulation (DBS) is another treatment showing promise to alleviate major depression in people resistant to current antidepressant medications, ECT, and psychotherapy.[40,41] The treatment involves implanting electrodes during neurosurgery into brain regions such as the subcallosal cingulate gyrus (SCG [Brodmann area 25 and parts of 24 and 32]) and the nucleus accumbens.[42] This SCG region was targeted because abnormal SCG brain activity, a suggested pathophysiologic

BOX 19.3   COMPREHENSIVE TREATMENT OF RISK FACTORS MAY PROMOTE RESILIENCE AND RAPID RECOVERY FROM DEPRESSION

Environmental stressors and genetic predisposition

	Depression risk factors	Therapeutic intervention	Resilience protective factors
Cognitive/behavioral	Weak executive function: weak coping self-efficiency; negative attention bias; cognitive inflexibility	Cognitive behavioral therapy with cognitive reappraisal; positive emotion exercises, coping skill development, and training; well-being therapy	Strong executive function; high coping self-efficacy; positive emotions; realistic optimism; cognitive flexibility
Emotion regulation	Weak regulation (e.g., anhedonia; slow stress recovery)	Mindfulness; training; antidepressant medications	Strong regulation (e.g., delay gratification; rapid stress recovery)
Social	Weak social skills; minimal social network; no resilient role models	Social emotional training; network support treatment	Strong social skills; diverse social network; resilient role models
Physical health	Sleep deprivation; poor cardiovascular fitness; poor nutrition; obesity	Teach sleep hygiene; exercise regimen; improve diet	Strong sleep habits; physically fit; good nutrition
Neurobiology	Dysregulated HPA axis and SNS in response to stress; attenuated prefontal cortical executive function and stress-induced limbic system hyperactivity	Neural circuit training; novel medications (corticotropin-releasing factor, NPY, GABA, glutamate)	Effective regulation of HPA axis and SNS in response to stress; robust prefrontal cortical executive function and capacity to regulate limbic reactivity to stress

From Southwick SM, Charney DS: *Science* 338(6103):79-82, 2012.

Genetic and environmental factors, such as uncontrollable stress, interact to increase the risk of developing major depression. These factors interact in complex ways that are not fully understood to dysregulate neurobiologic systems that compromise adaptive cognitive, emotional, social, and physiologic/health functions. For example, exaggerated stress-induced arousal of sympathetic and neuroendocrine systems may be due, in part, to genetic polymorphisms in serotonin, endocrine, and neuropeptide systems. However, the extent to which a genetic predisposition contributes to severe depression also may arise from the individual's inability to cope with stressors, inexperience in exhibiting flexible psychosocial and emotional skills, and lack of physical health, among others. Identifying and addressing these varied genetic and cognitive/behavioral/socioemotional/health risk factors of depression may open new doors to effective treatment. In particular, combined treatments or behavioral programs that promote resilience, the ability to recover from adversity—such as cognitive-behavioral therapy; social support; and improved diet, sleep, and exercise used in conjunction with current or novel drug medications that lessen or reverse the neuropathophysiology associated with heightened activation of stress systems—may quickly lead to remission. Although in its early stages, the development of comprehensive resilience programs holds promise not only for treating depressed individuals but also for proactively serving to diminish or prevent the risk of acquiring stress-related disorders.

GABA, Gamma-aminobutyric acid; *HPA,* hypothalamic pituitary adrenal axis; *NPY,* neuropeptide Y; *SNS,* sympathetic nervous system.
Data from Karatsoreos IN, McEwen BS: *Trends Cogn Neurosci* 15(12):576-584, 2011; Southwick SM, Charney DS: *Science* 338(6103):79-82, 2012.

cause of major depression, is reversed by effective antidepressant treatment. A 3- to 6-year follow-up study of 20 treatment-resistant depressed individuals who received DBS in the SCG found that more than half eventually returned to work and improved their quality of life.[43] Preliminary work with DBS in the nucleus accumbens, a region involved in rewarding experiences, was shown to reverse treatment-resistant depression in people unresponsive to pharmacotherapy, psychotherapy, and ECT.[42] Pathophysiology in the nucleus accumbens may be linked to impairments in reward processing and underlie the anhedonic symptom of depression. Preclinical studies suggest that the mechanism responsible for reversing the anhedonic state of depression is caused by the rapid increase in monoamine release in the prefrontal cortical areas following DBS stimulation in the nucleus accumbens.[44]

Another therapy for treatment-resistant depression is transcranial magnetic stimulation (TMS). This FDA-approved treatment involves noninvasive focal brain stimulation—unlike DBS, which requires neurosurgery, or ECT seizure induction. The procedure uses an electromagnetic coil to create a magnetic field that passes from the scalp to the brain, where the electrical current flow stimulates neurons. Daily repeated left prefrontal TMS was shown to induce acute antidepressant effects with few side effects and remission in 30% to 40% of depressed people.[45]

A weakness of many antidepressant treatments is that, even among individuals who receive the gold standard of antidepressant pharmacotherapy with psychotherapy, at least 50% of people who recover from a first episode of depression will, nonetheless, experience another one or more depression episodes in their lifetime (see *What's New?* Are Nutraceuticals Effective in the Treatment of Depression?). The recurrence rate of depression increases to approximately 80% in those with a history of two episodes.[46] One contributing factor for relapse is the failure of people to continue with their treatment plan by stopping their therapy sessions or drug medications. Another related factor is low social support and perceived loneliness. Studies reported low social support predicts poor response to depression treatment, early drop-out, and heightened

WHAT'S NEW?

Are Nutraceuticals Effective in the Treatment of Depression?

Although many pharmacologic medications were developed to treat depression, effective therapeutic drugs remain a challenge. Recent interest has begun to focus on alternative treatments, such as nutraceuticals or pharmaceutical-grade nutrients, which have the potential to modulate neurochemical systems involved in depression without adverse side effects. For instance, some studies reported beneficial effects of zinc supplementation as an adjunct to antidepressant treatment. Zinc is an essential trace element and serves diverse functions, such as growth, development, immune response, neurotransmission, and hormone storage and release. In the brain, zinc is found in glutamatergic neurons that modulate the circuitry involving the cortex, amygdala, and hippocampus to affect mood and cognitive functions. Serum zinc is reduced in major depression, which may contribute to the symptomatology and pathophysiology (e.g., monoamine deficiency, inflammation, stress hormone hypersecretion) of the disorder. Zinc deficiency also may serve as a state marker and risk factor of treatment-resistant depression. Another nutraceutical of considerable interest in the treatment of major depression is the omega-3 polyunsaturated fatty acid (n-3 PUFA) eicosapentaenoic acid (EPA). Omega-3 fatty acids are well known to be derived through consumption of fatty cold-water fish. Studies reported that omega-3 fatty acid deficiency is associated with depression and omega-3 fatty acid supplementation alone or as an adjunct to antidepressant medications may be more effective in the treatment of depression than placebo or antidepressant medication. Of interest, a subset of depressed people with high inflammation biomarkers (e.g., IL-6, high-sensitivity C-reactive protein) are more likely to benefit from EPA than placebo. Omega-3 fatty acids are known to suppress cytokine production, and their antiinflammatory effects may contribute to the efficacy of EPA treatment in depressed people with high inflammatory biomarkers. Zinc and omega-3 fatty acids are two from a growing list of potential nutraceuticals, including S-adenosylmethionine, tryptophan, and vitamin D_3, which are generally well tolerated with low dropout rates. Data from large-scale studies that reliably replicate the antidepressant effects of nutraceuticals for depression are needed.

Data from Hegartya B, Parker G: *Curr Opin Psychiatry* 26:33-40, 2013; Rapaport MH et al: *Mol Psychiatry* 21:71-79, 2016; Sarris J et al: *Am J Psychiatry* 173:575-587, 2016; Swardfager W et al: *Neurosci Biobehav Rev*, 37:911-929, 2013.

risk of relapse.[47,48] Interventions aimed at increasing social interactions may prove to be valuable in reducing depression symptoms and relapse.[49]

Bipolar Disorder

FDA-approved treatments are available for bipolar disorders.[50] Individuals with bipolar I disorder are usually treated with lithium, the first choice of treatment to control mania and rapid cycling and to reduce the risk of suicide. In some cases, lithium in combination with SSRIs is used to treat bipolar disorder. In addition to lithium, several medications are used, including anticonvulsants (e.g., carbamazepine, valproate, gabapentin, lamotrigine, or topiramate) or atypical antipsychotics (e.g., clozapine, risperidone, ziprasidone, quetiapine, or a combination of olanzapine with the SSRI fluoxetine). Some bipolar individuals benefit from thyroid augmentation (levothyroxine). As in depression, ECT is administered when manic individuals fail to respond to medication, are pregnant, or have cardiovascular disease.

Frequently reported side effects of lithium treatment include increased thirst, tremors, diarrhea, and weight gain, which diminish over time. A potentially serious side effect is lithium toxicity. Lithium is normally removed from the kidneys; however, when the body is sodium depleted, the kidneys will reabsorb sodium along with lithium. Individuals receiving lithium treatment are advised to avoid physically demanding activities that may dehydrate the body and to seek medical attention during fever or other conditions that may increase sweating. Anticonvulsant treatment may produce unsteadiness, dizziness, tremors, nausea, and blurry vision.

In addition to pharmacotherapy, psychotherapy can be beneficial for those who have difficulty with psychosocial stressors, such as low self-esteem, legal problems, fear of recurrence, and interpersonal conflicts. Treatment is effective when the individual becomes aware of the bipolar disorder, copes with psychosocial stressors, engages in drug compliance, and monitors symptom recurrences.

Unlike treatment of mania in bipolar I disorder, a major focus in the treatment of bipolar II disorder, the less severe form of mania, is on the recurrent depressive symptoms. Here, antidepressants alone (e.g., escitalopram, fluoxetine, venlafaxine) are reported to be effective in treating bipolar II disorder.

The treatment of bipolar II in children has raised concerns because of complications with its diagnosis. For example, bipolar II and attention-deficit/hyperactivity disorder (ADHD) share the common features of elevated behavioral activity levels, excessive talking, restlessness, and distractibility. Misdiagnosing bipolar II as ADHD has negative consequences for treatment because the stimulant drugs Ritalin and Adderall, which are frequently used to treat ADHD, will potentially exacerbate the symptoms of a child with bipolar II disorder. On the other hand, when ADHD is misdiagnosed as bipolar disorder, the child may begin an ineffective treatment regimen. To reduce misdiagnosis of children with bipolar and other similar symptomatic characteristics, such as ADHD as well as conduct disorder and oppositional defiant disorder, the *DSM-5*[18] now includes a category called *disruptive mood dysregulation disorder*. This diagnosis will be used to describe a young child (6 to 10 years of age) who exhibits only some of the symptoms of bipolar II, such as frequent temper outbursts, irritability, and bad moods. This category is hoped to exclude children from being diagnosed with bipolar disorder and reduce possible unwarranted treatment with strong medications.[51]

ANXIETY DISORDERS

Fear and anxiety are normal feelings expressed in threatening or harmful situations. The symptoms may include arousal, tenseness, and increased autonomic activity such as heart rate, blood pressure, and respiration. In addition, individuals often engage in protective behavioral responses such as flight or avoidance. These physiologic and behavioral responses allowed humans to adapt and cope under a variety of situational challenges. However, when fear and anxiety become too intense and undermine the ability to function on a daily basis, the individual may develop an anxiety disorder. Anxiety disorders are the most prevalent psychiatric illness, occurring in approximately 10% to 30% of the general population. Notably, many individuals with anxiety disorders develop major depression, and the high comorbidity of anxiety disorders and depression suggests a common neural pathophysiologic basis linking these two mental illnesses. This section presents an overview of several anxiety disorders, including panic disorder, social anxiety disorder, generalized anxiety disorder, and posttraumatic stress disorder, which in *DSM-5* is listed in the chapter on Trauma- and Stressor-Related Disorders.[18]

Panic Disorder

Panic disorder consists of multiple disabling panic attacks and is characterized by intense autonomic arousal involving a wide variety of symptoms, including lightheadedness, a rapid heart rate (tachycardia), difficulty breathing, chest discomfort, generalized sweating, general weakness, trembling, abdominal distress, and chills or hot flashes. Between panic attacks the individual often worries about future panic attacks and fear of losing control and dying. Symptoms originally occur spontaneously and vary in length from several minutes to an hour.

A notable complication of panic disorder is the development of agoraphobia or phobic avoidance of places or situations where escape or help is not readily available. The agoraphobic individual will avoid being away from home, standing in line or in a crowd, or traveling in a train, plane, or automobile. Severely agoraphobic individuals become housebound.

◆Etiology and Pathophysiology

Genetic factors play a major role in panic disorder. The risk is nearly 20% among first-degree relatives, and the prevalence of panic disorder is about 1.5% in men and up to 3.0% in women with no family history of the illness. Some studies suggest that the cholecystokinin (CCK) receptor gene on chromosome 11p may be linked to panic disorder.[52]

The etiology of panic disorder is not known, but the ability to elicit physical symptoms of panic attacks by chemicals, called *panicogens*, provides insight into its pathophysiology. Panic-prone individuals respond to panicogens that include carbon dioxide, caffeine, cholecystokinin, sodium lactate, and adrenergic receptor agonists, such as yohimbine. Carbon dioxide and sodium lactate, two well-studied panicogens, alter brain pH balance that panic-prone people are sensitive in detecting. Brain pH chemosensors are located in the brainstem medulla and pons, the midbrain serotonergic raphe neurons, the hypothalamus, and the amygdala. Heightened pH sensitivity in the amygdala may play a key role in generating fearful perceptions and activating the cerebral cortex and neural circuits in the temporal lobe and brainstem, which further facilitates the production of panic symptoms (see Figs. 19.7 and 19.9).[53] Exaggerated activation of physiologic and behavioral arousal stemming from the noradrenergic locus ceruleus neurons also may enhance the symptoms of panic. Thus panic-prone people appear especially sensitive in detecting pH alterations in brain sites that modulate fear and arousal.

Panic disorder also may involve the GABA-benzodiazepine (BZ) receptor system. BZ increases the $GABA_A$ ion channel response to GABA, thereby elevating chloride ion influx and producing a neuronal inhibitory effect. Brain imaging work reveals a reduction in BZ receptor binding in brain regions including the hippocampus, insular, and prefrontal cortex.[54] Drugs that block the benzodiazepine receptor are reported to increase panic attacks and feelings of anxiety, suggesting that an alteration in inhibitory neuromodulation contributes to panic disorder.

◆Treatment

Up to 80% of individuals affected by panic disorder respond to CBT and antidepressant drugs, either separately or in combination. In CBT, the individual learns that the physical symptoms are not fatal and attempts to exert control over the anxiety and panic. For example, breathing exercises to control hyperventilation serve to lessen the intense physiologic symptoms of panic, such as elevated heart and respiration rates. Another benefit of CBT is awareness of compliance with drug medications. However, for individuals with mild agoraphobia, CBT alone may be effective.

Antidepressants such as SSRIs are considered first-line medications for panic disorder. Among the SSRIs, paroxetine and sertraline have received FDA approval specifically for panic disorder. Venlafaxine, a serotonin-norepinephrine reuptake blocker, also is effective.

BZs, such as alprazolam and clonazepam, are other medications for treating panic disorder. These drugs also serve as an adjunct or augmentation therapy for individuals who do not fully respond to SSRIs. Short-term effects of BZs include sedation, ataxia, and cognitive impairments. Long-term BZ treatment may lead to potential physiologic and psychologic dependence. Abrupt BZ withdrawal induces a withdrawal syndrome of heightened reemergence of anxiety, insomnia, photophobia, and diarrhea. A gradual reduction in BZ medication or adjunct CBT may reduce the reliance and withdrawal symptoms of BZs.

Social Anxiety Disorder

Social anxiety disorder (SAD), also known as *social phobia*, is characterized by fear and avoidance of social situations. For example, the anxious person may feel very uncomfortable having a conversation or interacting with others and very conscious of being scrutinized and humiliated or rejected by others. A person diagnosed with SAD suffers significant distress or impairment that interferes with ordinary routines in everyday social settings, at work or at school.[18] Epidemiologic surveys indicate that SAD is one of the most common psychiatric disorders with 12-month and lifetime prevalence rates of 6.8% and 12.1%, respectively.[55] The onset of SAD often occurs during adolescence.[56] As with adults, children with SAD exhibit fear of speaking, reading, and eating in public; going to parties; speaking to authority figures; and engaging in informal social interactions.

◆Etiology and Pathophysiology

A prominent finding from brain imaging work with SAD people is the increased activity found in limbic and frontal cortical areas. Exposure to facial expressions of threat, which hypersensitive SAD people are likely to perceive as extreme dislike, rejection, or criticism, often implicates the amygdala and its connections to other brain regions. Heightened anxiety in SAD may arise from deficits in an inhibitory tone from prefrontal cortical areas to the amygdala resulting in increased amygdala activation and a fear bias in threat-related processing.[57] Support of abnormal signaling comes from work showing decreased white matter connectivity between amygdala and orbitofrontal cortex.[58]

Neuroimaging studies have also implicated neurotransmitter systems. One study in SAD people noted altered serotonergic neurotransmission,[59] which may be caused by a reduction in the serotonin 5-HT1A-binding protein in the amygdala, anterior cingulate, and insula. Another study found a reduction in GABA in the thalamus of SAD people.[60] Impaired GABAergic function may contribute to amygdala hyperactivity observed in SAD.

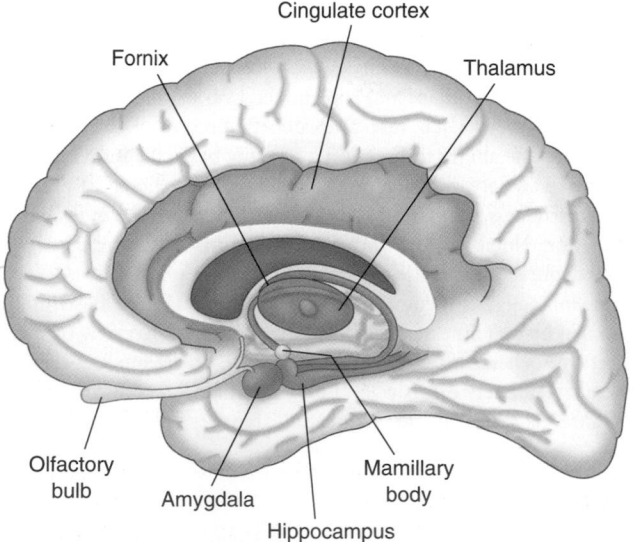

Cingulate cortex

Fornix

Thalamus

Olfactory bulb

Amygdala

Mamillary body

Hippocampus

FIGURE 19.9 The Limbic System. Structures of the limbic system play important roles in emotion, learning, and memory. Pathophysiology in limbic structures is frequently found in mental disorders.

The neuropeptide oxytocin (OXT) has attracted considerable research attention. OXT is produced in the hypothalamic paraventricular and supraoptic nuclei and secreted by the posterior pituitary gland. OXT is well known to be secreted during childbirth and lactation. In addition, an increasing body of work indicates that OXT secretion has antianxiety effects by reducing HPA activation; promoting social, attachment, and maternal behavior; and increasing empathy and trust.

Of relevance to SAD, OXT plasma levels are reduced in SAD people before and after playing a trust game, which normally increases OXT levels and promotes cooperation and reciprocation in control groups.[61] The reduction on OXT may account for the amygdala hyperactivity accompanied by excessive social avoidance and fear in SAD.[62] Indeed, intranasal OXT administration is reported to attenuate amygdala reactivity to threatening facial expressions,[63] perhaps by promoting GABAergic inhibition in the amygdala.[64] Intranasal OXT also improves self-reported speech performance compared with placebo.[65] The oxytocin system is further implicated in SAD on a genetic level. An OXT receptor single nucleotide polymorphism was found to be associated with negative emotionality[66] and moral judgments.[67] On the basis of these studies, the oxytocin system is a promising target to potentially develop treatments for SAD and disorders related to social dysfunctioning, such as autism.[68]

◆Treatment

The antidepressant SSRIs that include fluoxetine, paroxetine, sertraline, and fluvoxamine along with the serotonin norepinephrine reuptake inhibitor (SNRI) venlafaxine are considered first-line pharmacotherapies for SAD. These drugs shared similar efficacy profiles and are approved by the FDA for treatment of SAD. However, drug-related side effects, such as agitation and sexual dysfunction, can be distressing for some SAD people. Also, discontinuation of medication increases the risk for relapse. One study reported that 60% of people with SAD relapsed after discontinuation of sertraline treatment.[69]

Alternatives to SSRI and SNRI treatments may include psychologic or cognitive and group behavioral therapies.[70,71] People with SAD are reported to respond well to CBT compared to placebo. The choice between pharmacotherapy and CBT may depend on the person's preference and access to treatment. Of note, psychologic interventions at the end of acute drug treatment appear beneficial in continuing to alleviate the symptoms of SAD and may lower the side effects of long-term drug treatment.

Generalized Anxiety Disorder

Excessive and persistent worries are the hallmarks of generalized anxiety disorder (GAD). The individual worries about life events such as marital relationships, job performance, health, money, or social status. The lifetime prevalence rates of GAD range from 4.1% to 6.6%, with somewhat higher rates in women than in men. GAD usually emerges in the early twenties, but can occur in childhood. Six major symptoms of GAD have been identified and include restlessness, muscle tension, irritability, being easily fatigued, difficulty concentrating, and difficulty sleeping. The individual startles easily and frequently suffers from depression and panic attacks. The severity of symptoms fluctuates over time and may be linked to the changing nature of stress. Although GAD tends to be chronic, the symptoms may lessen with age. A frequent complication of GAD is substance abuse, which may result from self-medication with alcohol or drugs to relieve anxiety symptoms.

◆Etiology and Pathophysiology

Female twin studies suggest a concordance rate of 30%, but disease genes linked to specific chromosomes have yet to be identified. Abnormalities in the norepinephrine and serotonin systems were reported in GAD.[72] For example, there is a reduction in α_2-adrenergic receptor binding, a decrease in serotonin levels in CSF, and reduced platelet binding of paroxetine, an SSRI. Another reported alteration in GAD is a reduction of BZ binding in the left temporal hemisphere.[73]

Two functional magnetic resonance imaging (fMRI) studies have revealed alterations in specific brain regions in adults and adolescents with GAD. One study in GAD adults showed that increased anticipatory anxiety was associated with elevated cingulate cortex activity, and both the heightened anxiety and cingulate cortex activation were reduced after 8 weeks of treatment with venlafaxine, a serotonin and norepinephrine reuptake inhibitor.[74] This study suggests that a decrease in pathophysiologic cingulate cortex activity is a predictor of GAD treatment efficacy. In children and adolescents with GAD, brief exposure to masked angry faces induced heightened right amygdala activation, which correlated positively with severity of anxiety.[75] This study underscores the role of abnormal amygdala activity in attentional bias or vigilance to threats in GAD.

◆Treatment

GAD is diagnosed when a person spends at least 6 months worrying excessively and engages in at least three of the six major symptoms.[17] 5-HT/norepinephrine (NE) reuptake inhibitors, such as venlafaxine or the SSRIs paroxetine and escitalopram, have become first-line therapeutics for managing GAD. These medications may produce relief of GAD symptoms within 1 week and are effective in treating comorbid symptoms of depression. Buspirone, which has an affinity for serotonin receptors (5-HT$_{1A}$), is another treatment option, although the onset of clinical efficacy may take 2 weeks. The primary side effects of buspirone, which lessen over time, include dizziness, headaches, nausea, and mild nervousness. GAD nonresponders to 5-HT/NE reuptake inhibitors or buspirone may be treated with BZs. However, because GAD tends to be chronic, and comorbid with depression or other anxiety disorders,[76] BZs are usually limited to uncomplicated cases of GAD. In addition to drug therapy, behavioral therapy is used to acquire relaxation techniques that control anxiety.

Posttraumatic Stress Disorder

Exposure to a terrifying or life-threatening event may produce posttraumatic stress disorder (PTSD).[77,78] Although the disorder was initially described in combat situations and called "shell shock," "war neurosis," or "traumatic neurosis," PTSD does not develop only from exposure to traumatic experiences in the battlefield. PTSD may develop after exposure to threat of death, serious injury, or sexual violation. The disorder may develop within hours of the traumatic experience or after several months or years. The DMS-5 criteria for PTSD list four diagnostic clusters described as re-experiencing, avoidance, negative cognitions and mood, and arousal. Re-experiencing refers to spontaneous recollection of the traumatic event, recurrent nightmares, flashbacks, or other intense or chronic psychologic distress. Avoidance refers to distressing memories, feelings, or external reminders of the traumatic event. Negative cognitions and mood may occur from a persistent and distorted sense of blame of self or others, from estrangement from others or diminished interest in activities, or from an inability to remember key aspects of the event. Arousal is marked by aggressive, reckless, or self-destructive behavior, sleep disturbances, hypervigilance, or related problems. The "flight" or "fight" behavioral aspects also are associated with the arousing nature of PTSD.

The lifetime prevalence rate of PTSD is 7% to 8%. In men, PTSD is usually found among combat veterans, whereas PTSD in women is often related to rape or assault. Abused children also may develop PTSD. Individuals with a history of psychiatric illness (major depression, panic disorder) or those lacking strong social support appear more sensitive to the effects of traumatic stress.

◆Etiology and Pathophysiology

The primary etiology of PTSD is exposure to a terrifying life-threatening event and likely involves stress-induced alterations in several neural structures and neurotransmitter systems. The amygdala and prefrontal cortex are highly involved in the pathophysiology of PTSD because these brain structures normally play important roles in how fearful memories are stored, retrieved, and extinguished. Individuals with PTSD who are exposed to trauma-related stimuli generally exhibit increased activity in the amygdala and diminished activity in prefrontal cortical areas. Persistent dysregulation of this fear-based memory system may underlie chronic PTSD—that is, the failure of prefrontal cortical inhibition to control amygdala-induced activation of fear compromises the extinction of fear memory.[79] Structural brain imaging studies show that combat-exposed PTSD victims also have a smaller hippocampus, a brain structure involved in endocrine functions and memory formation. Pediatric PTSD studies reveal a more generalized effect of trauma on reducing total brain volume. Other brain sites exhibiting increased activity in PTSD are the dorsal anterior cingulate cortex and insula, albeit similar findings were reported in other anxiety disorders (e.g., GAD, obsessive-compulsive disorder)[80] (see *What's New? A Stress-Related Protein Kinase in the Prefrontal Cortex Is Downregulated in Post-traumatic Stress Disorder*).

WHAT'S NEW?

A Stress-Related Protein Kinase in the Prefrontal Cortex Is Downregulated in Posttraumatic Stress Disorder

Posttraumatic stress disorder (PTSD) develops after exposure to traumatic experiences, such as combat-related trauma, domestic violence, rape, or natural disasters. Although the pathophysiology of PTSD is not fully understood, preclinical and clinical research have identified at least two brain structures, the amygdala and prefrontal cortex (PFC), that are reciprocally connected and suggested to play major roles underlying the debilitating effects of the disorder. The amygdala is necessary in detecting threat and in modulating associative emotional or conditioned fear. Animal and human laboratory studies demonstrate that under normal circumstances one important function of the PFC is to exert an inhibitory influence on amygdala activation of conditioned fear and allow fear extinction to occur. Lessening amygdala activation of the fear experience enables the individual to acquire coping skills. Clinical studies, however, revealed that many PTSD subjects exhibit impairments in prefrontal cortical inhibitory control of amygdala. Thus increased activity in the amygdala is accompanied by uncontrolled recollection of the traumatic experience with heightened fear expression and deficits in fear extinction. The potential mechanism contributing to this pathophysiologic PFC-amygdala connection was not clear until a recent study using whole genome microarray analysis examined the expression of genes in the postmortem PFC of people diagnosed with PTSD. The investigators in this study reported that serum and glucocorticoid regulated kinase 1 (SGK1), a protein kinase involved in cellular responses to stress, was dramatically down-regulated in the PFC. To support an important function of SGK1 in PTSD, the investigators further demonstrated in an animal model that inhibition of SGK1 in the PFC induced a behavioral phenotype that mimics that effects of traumatic stress. The authors concluded that down-regulation of PFC SGK1 in people may be a major factor responsible for the eventual development of PTSD. Further characterization of SGK1 could lead to a clearer understanding of the molecular pathophysiology of PTSD and development of novel medications for the disorder.

Data from Licznerski P et al: *PLoS Biol* 13(10):e1002282, 2015; Mahan AL, Ressler KJ: *Trends Neurosci* 35:24-35, 2012; Pitman RK et al: *Nat Rev Neurosci* 13:769-787, 2012.

As in panic disorder, BZ binding is altered in PTSD as indicated by a reduced distribution of BZ receptor binding in the prefrontal cortex compared with healthy controls.[81] This reduction in prefrontal BZ receptor distribution was not found in other brain regions.

◆Treatment

Chronic PTSD lasting for years may occur in 30% of diagnosed individuals. Paroxetine and sertraline are considered first-line SSRI medications for chronic PTSD because of their tendency to lessen the recurrent nightmares and flashbacks and to treat the high accompanying prevalence of depression and substance abuse. Other antidepressants, such as the TCAs (amitriptyline and imipramine), have moderate effects and are second-line drugs; drugs such as nefazodone and bupropion may provide benefits. BZs may be used in the aftermath of a traumatic event to control hyperarousal symptoms such as irritability, insomnia, and muscle tension. However, there is no clear evidence that BZs have clinical efficacy or provide prophylaxis against the development of chronic PTSD, and BZs should be carefully monitored among individuals with a history of drug abuse.

OBSESSIVE-COMPULSIVE DISORDER

Obsessive-compulsive disorder (OCD) is a chronic, disabling illness characterized by the two core symptoms of obsessions and compulsions. Obsessions are recurrent, intrusive thoughts or impulses that provoke an intense anxiety that leads the individual to perform compulsive repetitive behavioral acts to alleviate the anxiety activated by the obsessions. Although *DSM-5* no longer classifies OCD as an anxiety disorder,[18] obsessions are associated with significant distress and compulsions that are consciously performed to reduce the obsession-related anxiety. OCD is a time-consuming illness that significantly impairs a range of everyday functions, such as social relationships, job performance, and academic success.

Examples of obsessions may include preoccupation with contamination, doubting, religious or sexual themes, or the belief that a negative outcome will occur if a specific act is not performed. Compulsions are ritualized acts such as washing, cleaning, checking, counting, organizing, and repeating specific thoughts or prayers. Performing the compulsions may provide temporary relief of the anxiety but also reinforces the dysfunctional thoughts and neural circuits that underlie the negative obsessions that generate the compulsive anxiety.

The lifetime prevalence rates of OCD range from 2% to 3% with a slightly higher onset in males during childhood or adolescence. In many cases, the OCD individual also is diagnosed with major depression, panic disorder, or GAD.[82] Among children with OCD, common comorbid disorders include Tourette syndrome, oppositional defiant disorder, attention-deficit/hyperactivity disorder, and depression[83]; 30% to 50% of adults report experiencing OCD in childhood.[84]

◆Etiology and Pathophysiology

Family and twin studies demonstrate that OCD involves polygenetic and environmental risk factors.[85] First-degree relatives of affected adults also are at increased risk (4.6%) of Tourette syndrome and tics in comparison with control relatives (1%). Thus OCD and Tourette syndrome may share common genes and pathophysiology.

Functional brain imaging studies have identified a pathologic brain circuit consisting of increased metabolism in the anterior thalamus, orbitofrontal cortex, dorsal anterior cingulate cortex, and especially in the basal ganglia (Fig. 19.10) subregions of the caudate and putamen.[86,87] Abnormalities in caudate volume in OCD also are found using structural neuroimaging techniques. This neural circuit is activated in OCD people by symptom provocation and reduced by effective pharmacotherapy

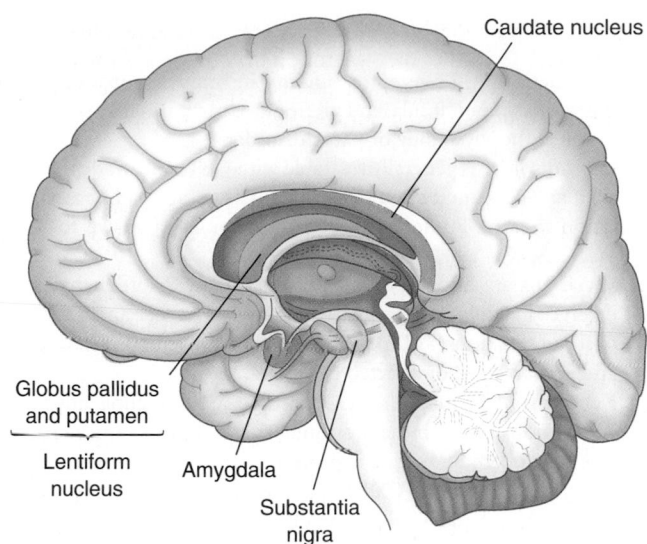

FIGURE 19.10 Basal Ganglion. Structures of the basal ganglion, which include the caudate nucleus, putamen, globus pallidus, and substantia nigra, are important in movement.

or psychotherapy. Genetic studies further indicate that genes affecting the serotonergic, dopaminergic, and glutamate systems play a major role in the pathophysiologic basis of this OCD neural circuit.[85]

One particular abnormality in the neural circuit of OCD is the dorsal anterior cingulate cortex (dACC). Several functional neuroimaging studies reported hyperactivity of the dACC in OCD people compared to controls. Furthermore, electrophysiologic studies showed altered biomarkers of cognitive control in the dACC. The dACC is hypothesized to be a key center that receives negative emotional and reinforcing information and integrates that information to direct motivated behavior.[88,89]

◆Treatment

SSRIs, including citalopram, fluvoxamine, paroxetine, and sertraline, are the first drugs of choice for OCD.[90] Approximately 70% to 80% of OCD individuals show a partial positive response that may be further improved by other medications. For example, clonazepam, a BZ, is found to improve the effects of fluoxetine and clomipramine therapy. The tricyclic antidepressant clomipramine is also used if SSRIs are not effective or are not tolerated by the OCD person. The therapeutic effects of SSRIs and clomipramine may be the result of blocking serotonin reuptake and increasing serotonin availability to postsynaptic receptors to stimulate serotonergic neurotransmission in dysfunctional serotonin neurons in the brain of OCD people.

Antipsychotic drugs (e.g., haloperidol, risperidone, olanzapine, or quetiapine) in combination with SSRIs also are effective, especially in comorbid OCD and tic disorders. Here, the normalization of dysfunctional serotonin and dopamine brain systems in OCD may underlie the therapeutic effects of SSRIs and dopamine receptor–related drugs.

Psychotherapy involves verbal interactions between a therapist and the individual to overcome the mental disorder. Several types of psychotherapy are available, but CBT and response preventive therapy are effective in treating OCD. CBT is a problem-focused, goal-directed, and time-limited treatment of the abnormal learned obsessions and compulsive actions. Response prevention therapy involves exposure to cues that elicit distress followed by preventing the individual from engaging in compulsive rituals for at least an hour or until the anxiety subsides. CBT employing response prevention therapy is found to produce long-term symptom remission.[91]

Because of the chronic nature of OCD, treatment in adults may involve pharmacotherapy, psychotherapy, a combination of pharmacotherapy and psychotherapy, brain modulation, or invasive brain methods.[92] In children, the American Academy of Child and Adolescent Psychiatry (AACAP)[93] recommends a combination of SSRI and CBT for those with moderate or severe OCD. However, recent meta-analysis studies find no strong evidence for the superiority of SSRI and CBT combination treatment in comparison to CBT alone for children with OCD.[94,95]

In people with severe OCD who are resistant to pharmaco- or psychotherapy, electroconvulsive therapy[96] and transcranial magnetic stimulation[97] may be used to provide some relief of OCD symptoms. An alternative, promising treatment for OCD is deep brain stimulation, which also is used for intractable depression.[97] Deep brain stimulation in the anterior limb of internal capsule, striatum/ventral capsule, nucleus accumbens, subthalamic nucleus, and inferior thalamic peduncle is effective in alleviating some OCD symptoms.[98,99] Stimulating these brain regions may be reducing abnormal neuronal firing in the neuroanatomic circuitry linked to OCD. The long-term treatment effects of deep brain stimulation are still under investigation.

Another invasive treatment for people with severe treatment-resistant OCD is neurosurgery. One focus of neurosurgery is to disconnect the basal ganglia from the frontal cortex.[100] Dorsal anterior cingulotomy also is used in the treatment of refractory OCD.[101] Neurosurgery offers significant relief of obsessions and compulsions in nearly 50% of treatment-resistant OCD individuals.

▌ SUMMARY REVIEW

Schizophrenia

1. Schizophrenia is characterized by thought disorders that reflect a break between the cognitive and the emotional sides of one's personality.
2. Schizophrenic symptoms are classified into positive, negative, and cognitive categories. Positive symptoms include hallucinations, delusions, formal thought disorder, and bizarre behavior. Negative symptoms include flattened affect, alogia, anhedonia, attention deficits, and apathy. Cognitive symptoms are the inability to perform daily tasks requiring attention and planning.
3. Schizophrenia has a strong genetic predisposition, and environmental factors (e.g., viral infection, nutritional deficiencies, prenatal birth complications, urban upbringing) may interfere with genetically programmed neural development to alter brain structure and function.
4. Brain imaging studies reveal structural brain abnormalities including an enlargement of the cerebral ventricles and widening of the fissures and sulci in the frontal cortex. In addition, there is a reduction in the volumes of both the thalamus, which may disrupt communication among cortical brain regions, and the temporal lobe, which may be responsible for the manifestations of positive symptoms.
5. In schizophrenia the frontal lobe shows a progressive loss in volume and a worsening of negative symptoms despite the use of antipsychotic medications. Blood flow and metabolism are reduced in the

dorsolateral prefrontal cortex, which compromises the ability to engage in goal-directed and cognitive problem-solving behavior.

6. Neurochemical abnormalities in dopamine and glutamate systems are found in schizophrenia.

7. The first generation of antipsychotic drugs blocks the dopamine D_2 receptor. The second generation, called atypical antipsychotics, blocks not only D_2 receptors but also dopamine, serotonin, and other neurotransmitter receptors. Antipsychotic medications, however, are not always effective in treating schizophrenic individuals with severe negative symptoms. Talk therapies are used to increase drug compliance and to encourage coping strategies.

Mood Disorders: Depression and Bipolar Disorder

1. Major depression and bipolar disorder are two common mood disorders. Major depression is characterized by an intense and sustained unpleasant state of sadness and hopelessness. In bipolar disorder, individuals show recurrent patterns of depression and mania, the latter characterized by extreme levels of energy and euphoria.

2. Environmental triggers such as psychosocial stress appear to facilitate the onset of depression in individuals with a genetic vulnerability.

3. A reduction in brain monoamine neurotransmission is linked to depression, whereas an elevated monoamine level is associated with mania.

4. Exposure to uncontrollable stress elevates secretion of the stress hormone cortisol, which increases both the secretion of proinflammatory cytokines and the risk of developing depression. Abnormalities involving thyroid hormones also are found in depression.

5. Stress-induced depression is accompanied by deficits in brain-derived neurotrophic factor (BDNF) and neurogenesis in the hippocampus. In animal models, stress-induced depression-like behavior and the accompanying deficits in hippocampal BDNF and neurogenesis are reversed by antidepressant treatment.

6. The frontal lobe and limbic system volumes are reduced in major depression and bipolar illness. In addition, blood flow is altered in prefrontal and limbic brain regions that include the amygdala, a structure implicated in emotional behavior.

7. Pharmacotherapy involves the use of MAOIs, TCAs, SSRIs, and atypical antidepressants. Manic and bipolar individuals are treated with lithium or mood stabilizers. Severely depressed and manic people may be administered ECT. Deep brain stimulation is another promising treatment for intractable depression.

Anxiety Disorders

1. When normal fear and anxiety mental states persist and become uncontrollable, an individual may develop an anxiety disorder. PD, SAD, GAD, and PTSD are examples of uncontrollable fear and anxiety states that require medical attention.

2. Panic disorder consists of panic attacks characterized by intense autonomic arousal that occurs spontaneously and is accompanied by symptoms including lightheadedness, tachycardia, and difficulty breathing. In addition, the intense occurrence of autonomic responses is accompanied by heightened fear and anxiety that often continue between panic attacks.

3. Panic-prone people are sensitive in detecting pH alterations in the amygdala, a brain structure that modulates fear. An activated amygdala recruits the cerebral cortex and neural circuits in the temporal lobe and brainstem, which may further exacerbate symptoms of panic.

4. A reduction in BZ receptor binding in brain regions, including the hippocampus, insula, and prefrontal cortex, also may contribute to the pathophysiology of panic disorder.

5. Panic disorder is generally treatable with CBT and antidepressants such as TCAs and SSRIs. BZs are used as an adjunct or augmentation therapy for individuals who are nonresponsive to SSRIs or TCAs.

6. Social anxiety disorder is a common anxiety disorder that often emerges in adolescence and is characterized by fear and avoidance of social situations. SAD people are very sensitive in being evaluated and embarrassed or rejected by others.

7. Neuroimaging studies in SAD people are revealing abnormal connections between the prefrontal cortex and the amygdala.

8. The neuropeptide oxytocin promotes social behavior, empathy, and trust. Secretion of OXT is reduced in SAD people, and a single nucleotide polymorphism of an OXT receptor gene is found to be altered in SAD, both of which suggest that OXT plays a major role in the pathophysiology of SAD.

9. SAD treatment may involve SSRI or SNRI drug or cognitive therapies.

10. GAD is characterized by excessive and persistent worries about life events. Individuals exhibit varying levels of motor disturbances, irritability, and fatigue that may be linked to fluctuations in psychosocial stress. Many GAD individuals manifest symptoms of depression.

11. Pathophysiologic changes in the cingulate cortex and amygdala may have prominent roles in stimulating anticipatory anxiety and attentional bias to threats in people with GAD.

12. Treatment of GAD usually involves a combination of behavioral therapy and drug medications, especially 5-HT/NE reuptake inhibitors.

13. PTSD develops after exposure to a life-threatening or traumatic experience. Individuals experience recurring thoughts and flashbacks and nightmares of the terrifying event.

14. In PTSD structural and/or functional alterations exist in the amygdala, prefrontal cortex, and hippocampus, which likely contribute to dysfunction in an emotional fear memory system.

15. Treatment of chronic PTSD is difficult and involves psychotherapy and SSRI pharmacotherapy.

Obsessive-Compulsive Disorder

1. OCD is a chronic illness characterized by irrational obsessions and ritualized acts that impair normal functioning and cause severe distress. It is a chronic disabling illness.

2. OCD is a time-consuming illness, which significantly impairs everyday functions, such as social relationships, job performance, and academic success. Examples of obsessions include preoccupation with doubting, religious or sexual themes, or the belief that a negative outcome will occur if a specific act is not performed.

3. A pathophysiologic brain circuit consisting of the anterior thalamus, orbitofrontal cortex, dorsal anterior cingulate cortex, and especially in the basal ganglia subregions of the caudate and putamen is involved in OCD.

4. OCD requires long-term treatment that may include psychotherapy and pharmacotherapy. However, people with severe OCD who are resistant to these treatments may require neurosurgery to disconnect regions of pathophysiologic brain circuit to provide relief of OCD symptoms. Deep brain stimulation may be another option for uncontrollable OCD.

KEY TERMS

Affective flattening, 604
Agoraphobia, 612
Agranulocytosis, 604
Alogia, 604
Anhedonia, 604
Anxiety disorder, 611
Avolition, 604
Bipolar disorder, 605
Brain-derived neurotrophic factor (BDNF), 606
Delusion, 603
Depression, 608
Dopamine hypothesis, 602
Dorsolateral prefrontal cortex (DLPFC), 602

Dysphoric mood, 608
Formal thought disorder, 604
Gamma-aminobutyric acid (GABA), 602
Generalized anxiety disorder (GAD), 613
Glutamate hypothesis, 602
Hallucination, 603
Inflammation, 606
Major (unipolar) depressive disorder, 605
Manic, 608
Monoamine hypothesis of depression, 605
Mood, 605
Neurogenesis, 606
Obsessive-compulsive disorder (OCD), 614

Panic disorder, 611
Posttraumatic stress disorder (PTSD), 613
Poverty of content, 604
Psychotic episode, 603
Schizophrenia, 600
Social anxiety disorder (SAD), 612
Social brain emotional processing network, 601
Tardive dyskinesia, 604
Thought disorder, 600
Unipolar or major depressive disorder, 605
Working memory, 602

REFERENCES

1. Ganapathiraju MK, et al: Schizophrenia interactome with 504 novel protein-protein interactions. *NPJ Schizophr* 2:16012, 2016.
2. Lewis DA, Levitt P: Schizophrenia as a disorder of neurodevelopment. *Annu Rev Neurosci* 25: 409–432, 2002.
3. Marenco S, Weinberger DR: The neurodevelopmental hypothesis of schizophrenia: following a trail of evidence from cradle to grave. *Dev Psychopathol* 12(3):501–527, 2000.
4. Réthelyi JM, Benkovits J, Bitter I: Genes and environments in schizophrenia: the different pieces of a manifold puzzle. *Neurosci Biobehav Rev* 37:2424–2437, 2013.
5. Berman KF, Meyer-Lindenberg A: Functional brain imaging studies in schizophrenia. In Charney DS, Nestler EJ, editors: *Neurobiology of mental illness*, ed 2, New York, 2004, Oxford.
6. Shenton LD, et al: A review of MRI findings in schizophrenia. *Schizophr Res* 49(1-2):1–52, 2001.
7. Ross CA, et al: Neurobiology of schizophrenia. *Neuron* 52(1):139–153, 2006.
8. Pujol N, et al: Hippocampal abnormalities and age in chronic schizophrenia: morphometric study across the adult lifespan. *Br J Psychiatry* 250: 369–375, 2014.
9. Bickart KC, Dickerson BC, Barrett LF: The amygdala as a hub in brain networks that support social life. *Neuropsychologia* 63:235–248, 2014.
10. Mukherjee P, et al: Altered amygdala connectivity within the social brain in schizophrenia. *Schizophr Bull* 40:152–160, 2014.
11. Aleman A, Kahn RS: Strange feelings: do amygdala abnormalities dysregulate the emotional brain in schizophrenia? *Prog Neurobiol* 77:283–298, 2005.
12. Ho BC, et al: Progressive structural brain abnormalities and their relationship to clinical outcome. *Arch Gen Psychiatry* 60:585–594, 2003.
13. Costa E, et al: Dendritic spine hypoplasticity and downregulation of reelin and GABAergic tone in schizophrenia vulnerability. *Neurobiol Dis* 8(5): 723–742, 2001.
14. Fatemi SH, Earle JA, McMenomy T: Reduction in reelin immunoreactivity in hippocampus of subjects with schizophrenia, bipolar disorder and major depression. *Mol Psychiatry* 5(6):654–663, 2000.
15. Duncan GE, Sheitman BB, Lieberman JA: An integrated view of pathophysiological models of schizophrenia. *Brain Res Brain Res Rev* 29(2-3): 250–264, 1999.
16. Coyle JT, Tsai G, Goff D: Converging evidence of NMDA receptor hypofunction in the pathophysiology of schizophrenia. *Ann N Y Acad Sci* 1003:318–327, 2003.
17. Jentsch JD, et al: Enduring cognitive deficits and cortical dopamine dysfunction in monkeys after long-term administration of phencyclidine. *Science* 277:953–955, 1997.
18. American Psychiatric Association (APA): *Diagnostic and statistical manual of mental disorders (DSM-5)*, ed 5, Washington DC, 2013, Author.
19. Tamminga CA: Principles of the pharmacotherapy of schizophrenia. In Charney DS, Nestler EJ, editors: *Neurobiology of mental illness*, ed 2, New York, 2004, Oxford.
20. Tai S, Turkington D: The evolution of cognitive behavior therapy for schizophrenia: current practice and recent developments. *Schizophr Bull* 35(5):865–873, 2009.
21. World Health Organization (WHO): *Depression*, Geneva, 2017, Author.
22. Shih RA, Belmonte PL, Zandi PP: A review of the evidence from family, twin and adoption studies for a genetic contribution to adult psychiatric disorders. *Int Rev Psychiatry* 16:260–283, 2004.
23. Heninger GR, et al: The revised monoamine theory of depression: a modulatory role for monoamines, based on new findings from monoamine depletion experiments in humans. *Pharmacopsychiatry* 29(1):2–11, 1996.
24. Holsboer F: The corticosteroid receptor hypothesis of depression. *Neuropsychopharmacology* 23:477, 2000.
25. Wium-Andersen MK, et al: Elevated C-reactive protein levels, psychological distress, and depression in 73131 individuals. *JAMA Psychiatry* 70:176–184, 2013.
26. Dahl J, et al: The plasma levels of various cytokines are increased during ongoing depression and are reduced to normal levels after recovery. *Psychoneuroendocrinology* 45:77–86, 2014.
27. Masi G, Brovedani P: The hippocampus, neurotrophic factors and depression. Possible implications for the pharmacotherapy of depression. *CNS Drugs* 25(11):913–931, 2012.
28. Pittenger C, Duman RS: Stress, depression, and neuroplasticity: a convergence of mechanisms. *Neuropsychopharmacology* 33:88–109, 2008.
29. Bauer M, et al: The thyroid-brain interaction in thyroid disorders and mood disorders. *J Neuroendocrinol* 20:1101–1114, 2008.
30. Hage MP, Azar ST: The link between thyroid function and depression. *J Thyroid Res* 2012: 590648, 2012.
31. Drevets WC: Prefrontal cortical-amygdalar metabolism in major depression. *Ann N Y Acad Sci* 877:614–637, 1999.
32. Rajkowska G: Depression: what we can learn from postmortem studies. *Neuroscientist* 9(4):273–284, 2003.
33. Frodl T, O'Keane V: How does the brain deal with cumulative stress? A review with focus on developmental stress, HPA axis function and hippocampal structure in humans. *Neurobiol Dis* 52:24–37, 2013.
34. Saleh K, et al: Impact of family history and depression on amygdala volume. *Psychiatry Res* 203:24–30, 2012.
35. Maletic C, Raison C: Integrative neurobiology of bipolar disorder. *Front Psychiatry* 5:99, 2014.
36. Duman RS, Aghajanian GK: Synaptic dysfunction in depression: potential therapeutic targets. *Science* 338:68–72, 2012.
37. Newport DJ, et al: Ketamine and other NMDA antagonists: early clinical trials and possible mechanisms in depression. *Am J Psychiatry* 172:950–966, 2015.
38. Whittington CJ, et al: Selective serotonin reuptake inhibitors in childhood depression: systematic review of published versus unpublished data. *Lancet* 363(9418):1341–1345, 2004.
39. Joshi SH, et al: Structural plasticity of the hippocampus and amygdala induced by electroconvulsive therapy in major depression. *Biol Psychiatry* 79:282–292, 2016.
40. Goodman WK, Alterman RL: Deep brain stimulation for intractable psychiatric disorders. *Annu Rev Med* 63:511–524, 2012.
41. Hamani C, et al: The subcallosal cingulate gyrus in the context of major depression. *Biol Psychiatry* 69:301–308, 2011.
42. Schlaepfer TE, et al: Deep brain stimulation to reward circuitry alleviates anhedonia in refractory major depression. *Neuropsychopharmacology* 33:368–377, 2008.
43. Kennedy SH, et al: Deep brain stimulation for treatment-resistant depression: follow-up after 3 to 6 years. *Am J Psychiatry* 168:502–510, 2011. .
44. van Dijk A, et al: Deep brain stimulation of the accumbens increases dopamine, serotonin, and noradrenaline in the prefrontal cortex. *J Neurochem* 123:897–903, 2012.
45. George MS, Taylor JJ, Short EB: The expanding evidence base for rTMS treatment of depression. *Curr Opin Psychiatry* 26:13–18, 2013.
46. Boland RJ, Keller MB: The course of depression. In Davis KL, Charney D, Coyle JT, et al, editors:

Neuropsychopharmacology: the fifth generation of progress, Philadelphia, 2002, Lippincott Williams & Wilkins.

47. Backs-Dermott BJ, Dobson KS, Jones SL: An evaluation of an integrated model of relapse in depression. *J Affect Disord* 124(1-2):60–67, 2010.
48. Trivedi MH, et al: What moderator characteristics are associated with better prognosis for depression? *Neuropsychiatr Dis Treat* 1(1):51–57, 2005.
49. Cruwys T, et al: Social group memberships protect against future depression, alleviate depression symptoms and prevent depression relapse. *Soc Sci Med* 98:179–186, 2013.
50. Goldberg JF: What psychotherapists should know about pharmacotherapies for bipolar disorder. *J Clin Psychol* 63(5):475–490, 2007.
51. Parens E, Johnston J: Controversies concerning the diagnosis and treatment of bipolar disorder in children. *Child Adolesc Psychiatry Ment Health* 4:9, 2010.
52. Kennedy JL, et al: Investigation of cholecystokinin system genes in panic disorder. *Mol Psychiatry* 4(3):284, 1999.
53. Wemmie JA: Neurobiology of panic and pH chemosensation in the brain. *Dialogues Clin Neurosci* 13:475–483, 2011.
54. Malizia AL, et al: Decreased brain GABA$_A$-benzodiazepine receptor binding in panic disorder. *Arch Gen Psychiatry* 55(8):715–720, 1998.
55. Kessler RC, et al: Lifetime prevalence and age-of-onset distributions of DSM-IV disorders in the National Comorbidity Survey Replication. *Arch Gen Psychiatry* 62:593–602, 2005.
56. Wittchen HU, Fehm L: Epidemiology, patterns of comorbidity, and associated disabilities of social phobia. *Psychiatr Clin North Am* 24:617–641, 2001.
57. Akirav I, Maroun M: The role of the medial prefrontal cortex-amygdala circuit in stress effects on the extinction of fear. *Neural Plast* 2007:30873, 2007.
58. Fouche J-P, et al: Recent advances in the brain imaging of social anxiety disorder. *Hum Psychopharmacol* 28:102–105, 2013.
59. Lanzenberger RR, et al: Reduced serotonin-1A receptor binding in social anxiety disorder. *Biol Psychiatry* 61:1081–1089, 2007.
60. Pollack MH, et al: High-field MRS study of GABA, glutamate and glutamine in social anxiety disorder: response to treatment with levetiracetam. *Prog Neuropsychopharmacol Biol Psychiatry* 32:739–743, 2008.
61. Hoge EA, et al: Plasma oxytocin immunoreactive products and response to trust in patients with social anxiety disorder. *Depress Anxiety* 29:924–930, 2012.
62. Gorka SM, et al: Oxytocin modulation of amygdala functional connectivity to fearful faces in generalized social anxiety disorder. *Neuropsychopharmacology* 40:278–286, 2015.
63. Domes G, et al: Oxytocin attenuates amygdala responses to emotional faces regardless of valence. *Biol Psychiatry* 62:1187–1190, 2007.
64. Huber D, Veinante P, Stoop R: Vasopressin and oxytocin excite distinct neuronal populations in the central amygdala. *Science* 308:245–248, 2005.
65. Guastella A-J, et al: A randomized controlled trial of intranasal oxytocin as an adjunct to exposure therapy for social anxiety disorder. *Psychoneuroendocrinology* 34:917–923, 2009.

66. Montag C, et al: Interaction of 5-HTTLPR and a variation on the oxytocin receptor gene influences negative emotionality. *Biol Psychiatry* 69:601–603, 2011.
67. Walter NT, et al: Ignorance is no excuse: moral judgments are influenced by a genetic variation on the oxytocin receptor gene. *Brain Cogn* 78:268–273, 2012.
68. Meyer-Lindenberg A, et al: Oxytocin and vasopressin in the human brain: social neuropeptides for translational medicine. *Nat Rev Neurosci* 12:524–538, 2011.
69. Koen N, Stein DJ: Pharmacotherapy of anxiety disorders: a critical review. *Dialogues Clin Neurosci* 13:423–437, 2011.
70. Barkowski S, et al: Efficacy of group psychotherapy for social anxiety disorder: A meta-analysis of randomized-controlled trials. *J Anxiety Disord* 39:44–64, 2016.
71. Mayo-Wilson E, et al: Psychological and pharmacological interventions for social anxiety disorder in adults: a systematic review and network meta-analysis. *Lancet Psychiatry* 1:368–376, 2014.
72. Jetty PV, et al: Neurobiology of generalized anxiety disorder. *Psychiatr Clin North Am* 24(1):75, 2001.
73. Tiihonen J, et al: Cerebral benzodiazepine receptor binding and distribution in generalized anxiety disorder. *Mol Psychiatry* 2(6):463–471, 1997.
74. Nitschke JB, et al: Anticipatory activation in the amygdala and anterior cingulate in generalized anxiety disorder and prediction of treatment response. *Am J Psychiatry* 166:302–310, 2009.
75. Monk CS, et al: Ventrolateral prefrontal cortex activation and attentional bias in response to angry faces in adolescents with generalized anxiety disorder. *Am J Psychiatry* 163:1091–1097, 2006.
76. Bruce SE: Infrequency of "pure" GAD: impact of psychiatric comorbidity on clinical course. *Depress Anxiety* 14(4):219–225, 2001.
77. Charney DS, et al: Psychobiologic mechanisms of posttraumatic stress disorder. *Arch Gen Psychiatry* 50(4):294–305, 1993.
78. Southwick SM, et al: Neurotransmitter alterations in PTSD: catecholamines and serotonin. *Semin Clin Neuropsychiatry* 4(4):242–248, 1999.
79. Bremner JD, et al: Structural and functional plasticity of the human brain in posttraumatic stress disorder. *Prog Brain Res* 167:171–186, 2008.
80. Shin LM, Liberzon I: The neurocircuitry of fear, stress, and anxiety disorders. *Neuropsychopharmacology* 35(1):169–191, 2010.
81. Bremner JD, et al: Structural and functional plasticity of the human brain in posttraumatic stress disorder. *Prog Brain Res* 167:171–186, 2008.
82. Fireman B, et al: The prevalence of clinically recognized obsessive-compulsive disorder in a large health maintenance organization. *Am J Psychiatry* 158(11):1904–1910, 2001.
83. Geller DA, et al: Fluoxetine treatment for obsessive-compulsive disorder in children and adolescents: a placebo-controlled clinical trial. *J Am Acad Child Adolesc Psychiatry* 40:773–779, 2001.

84. Rasmussen SA: Epidemiology of obsessive compulsive disorder. *J Clin Psychiatry* 51(Suppl S):10–13, 1990.
85. Pauls DL, et al: Obsessive-compulsive disorder: an integrative genetic and neurobiological perspective. *Nat Rev Neurosci* 15:410–424, 2014.
86. Rauch SL, et al: Probing striato-thalamic function in obsessive-compulsive disorder and Tourette syndrome using neuroimaging methods. *Adv Neurol* 85:207–224, 2001.
87. Rosenberg DR, et al: Brain anatomy and chemistry may predict treatment response in paediatric obsessive-compulsive disorder. *Int J Neuropsychopharmacol* 4:179–190, 2001.
88. McGovern RA, Sheth SA: Role of the dorsal anterior cingulate cortex in obsessive-compulsive disorder: converging evidence from cognitive neuroscience and psychiatric neurosurgery. *J Neurosurg* 126(1):132–147, 2017.
89. Shackman AJ, et al: The integration of negative affect, pain and cognitive control in the cingulate cortex. *Nat Rev Neurosci* 12:154–167, 2011.
90. Swedo SE, Snider LA: The neurobiology and treatment of obsessive-compulsive disorder. In Charney DS, Nestler EJ, editors: *Neurobiology of mental illness,* ed 2, New York, 2004, Oxford.
91. McKay D, et al: Efficacy of cognitive-behavioral therapy for obsessive-compulsive disorder. *Psychiatry Res* 227:104–113, 2015.
92. Koran LM, et al: Practice guideline for the treatment of patients with obsessive-compulsive disorder. *Am J Psychiatry* 164(7 Suppl):5–53, 2007.
93. American Academy of Child and Adolescent Psychiatry (ACAP): Practice parameter for the assessment and treatment of children and adolescents with obsessive-compulsive disorder. *J Am Acad Child Adolesc Psychiatry* 51:98–113, 2012.
94. Ivarsson T, et al: The place of and evidence for serotonin reuptake inhibitors (SRIs) for obsessive compulsive disorder (OCD) in children and adolescents: views based on a systematic review and meta-analysis. *Psychiatry Res* 227:93–103, 2015.
95. Öst L-G, et al: Cognitive behavioral and pharmacological treatments of OCD in children: a systematic review and meta-analysis. *J Anxiety Disord* 43:58–69, 2016.
96. Whittington CJ, et al: Selective serotonin reuptake inhibitors in childhood depression: systematic review of published versus unpublished data. *Lancet* 363(9418):1341–1345, 2004.
97. Goodman WK, Alterman RL: Deep brain stimulation for intractable psychiatric disorders. *Annu Rev Med* 63:511–524, 2012.
98. de Koning PP, et al: Current status of deep brain stimulation for obsessive-compulsive disorder: a clinical review of different targets. *Curr Psychiatry Rep* 13:274–282, 2011.
99. Holtzheimer PE, Mayberg HS: Deep brain stimulation for psychiatric disorders. *Annu Rev Neurosci* 34:289–307, 2011.
100. Greenberg BD, Murphy DL, Rasmussen SA: Neuroanatomically based approaches to obsessive-compulsive disorder. *Psychiatr Clin North Am* 23(3):671–686, 2000.
101. Schlösser RGM, et al: Fronto-cingulate effective connectivity in obsessive compulsive disorder: a study with fMRI and dynamic causal modeling. *Hum Brain Mapp* 31:1834–1850, 2010.

Alterations of Neurologic Function in Children

Russell J. Butterfield, Sue E. Huether

CHAPTER OUTLINE

Neurologic disorders in children can arise any time before birth through adolescence and include congenital malformations, genetic defects in metabolism, brain injuries, infection, tumors, and other disorders that affect neurologic structure and function. The symptoms, diagnosis, and management of neurologic disorders in children are often different from those of adults, even with similar disorders.

DEVELOPMENT OF THE NERVOUS SYSTEM IN CHILDREN

Both genetics and environment shape development of the nervous system. Because brain development starts in the first days of embryonic development, maternal factors, including lifestyle, nutrition, exposure to toxins or infection, and state of health, have crucial effects on the developing nervous system.

The nervous system develops from embryonic ectoderm through a complex and sequential process, including (1) formation of the neural tube (3 to 4 weeks' gestation), (2) development of the forebrain from the neural tube (2 to 3 months' gestation), (3) neuronal proliferation and migration (3 to 5 months' gestation), (4) formation of network connections and synapses (5 months' gestation to many years postnatally), and (5) myelination (birth to many years postnatally). Formation of the neural tube begins between 3 and 4 weeks' gestation as the neural plate folds to form a neural groove and neural folds. The neural groove deepens and closes dorsally to form the neural tube, which gives rise to the entire central nervous system (CNS). The neural tube closes first in the cervical region and then "zippers" in two directions—cranially and caudally (Fig. 20.1).

The caudal end of the neural tube forms the brain, and the remainder develops into the spinal cord. The lumen of the neural tube becomes the ventricles of the brain and the central canal of the spinal cord (Fig. 20.2). Some neuroectodermal cells separate from the neural tube but remain between the tube and the surface ectoderm, creating the neural crest. This cellular band develops into the *peripheral nervous system*. On either side of the neural tube's inner surface is a longitudinal groove (sulcus limitans). Anterior to this region (basal plate) the gray matter

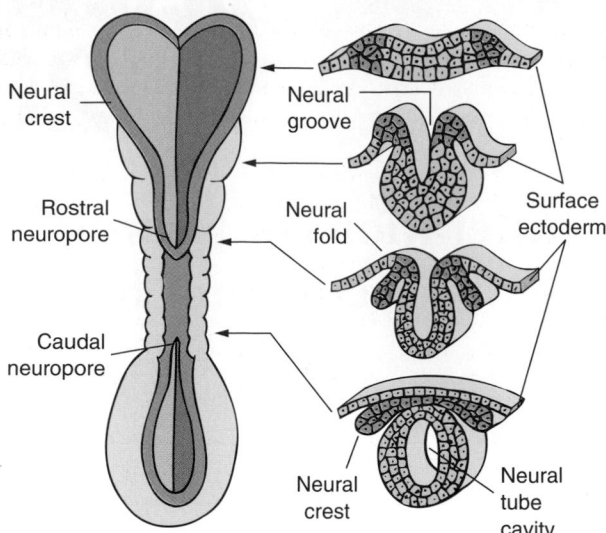

FIGURE 20.1 Neural Tube at 3 Weeks' Gestation. Neural folds have begun to fuse at the cervical level of the future spinal cord. *Right,* Cross sections of the neural tube at four different levels; at any given level the embryonic central nervous system (CNS) goes through a series of stages resembling these four cross sections. Total length of neural tube at this time is about 2.5 mm.

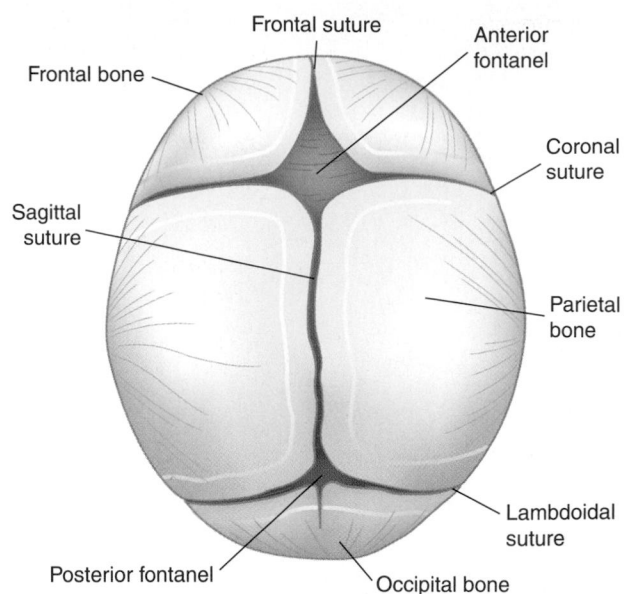

FIGURE 20.3 Cranial Sutures and Fontanels in Infancy. Fibrous union of suture lines and interlocking of serrated edges (occurs by 6 months; solid union requires approximately 12 years).

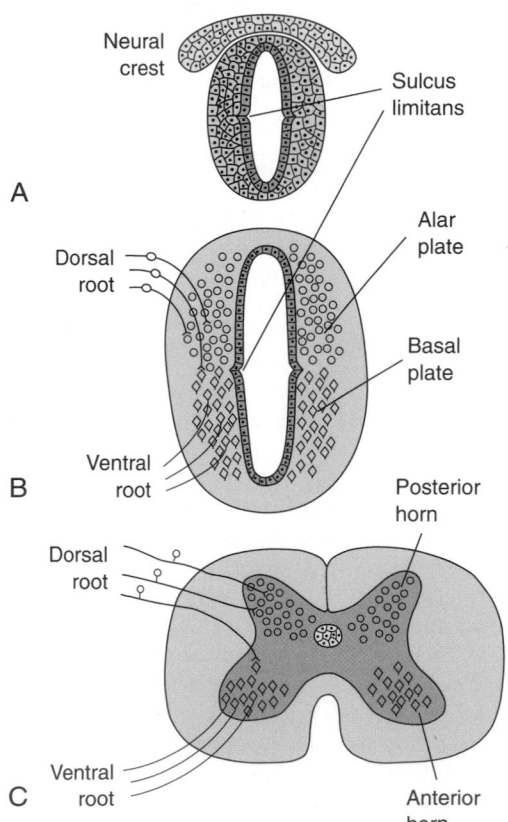

FIGURE 20.2 Sulcus Limitans and Alar and Basal Plates. A, Neural tube during the fourth week of gestation. **B,** Embryonic spinal cord during the sixth week of gestation; dorsal root ganglion cells, derived from the neural crest, send their central processes into the spinal cord to terminate mainly in alar plate cells; basal plate cells become motor neurons, whose axons exit in the ventral roots. **C,** Adult spinal cord.

differentiates into the nuclei of the lower motor neurons. The region posterior to the sulcus (**alar plate**) differentiates into the sensory nuclei of the spinal cord.

The growth and development of the brain occurs rapidly during the third and fourth months of gestation and again from the fifth month of gestation through the first year of life, reflecting the proliferation of neurons and glial cells. Although most of the neurons that an individual will have are present at birth, development of skills, such as walking, talking, and thinking, depends on these neurons making correct connections with other neurons and on myelination of the axons making those connections. The head is the fastest-growing body part during infancy. One half of postnatal brain growth is achieved by the first year and is 90% complete by age 6 years. The cortex thickens with maturation and the sulci deepen as a result of rapid expansion of the surface area of the brain. Cerebral blood flow and oxygen consumption during these years are about twice those of the adult brain. Structures arising from mesoderm (**somite**) include blood vessels, microglial cells, dural and arachnoid layers of the meninges, the capsule of some peripheral sensory nerve endings, and peripheral nerve coverings.

The bones of the infant's skull are separated at the suture lines, forming two **fontanels** or "soft spots": one diamond-shaped anterior fontanel and one triangular-shaped posterior fontanel. The unclosed sutures allow for expansion of the rapidly growing brain. The posterior fontanel may be open until 2 to 3 months of age; the anterior fontanel normally does not fully close until 18 months of age (Fig. 20.3). Head growth almost always reflects brain growth. Monitoring the fontanels and careful measurement of the head circumference on standardized growth charts are essential elements of the pediatric examination.

Because of the immaturity of much of the human forebrain at birth, neurologic examination of the infant detects mostly reflex responses that require an intact spinal cord and brainstem. Some of these reflex patterns are inhibited as cerebral cortical function matures; these patterns disappear at predictable times during infancy (Table 20.1).

Absence of expected reflex responses at the appropriate age indicates general depression of central or peripheral motor function. Asymmetric

TABLE 20.1 REFLEXES OF INFANCY

REFLEX	AGE AT APPEARANCE OF REFLEX	AGE AT WHICH REFLEX SHOULD NO LONGER BE OBTAINABLE
Stepping	Birth	6 weeks
Moro	Birth	3 months
Sucking	Birth	4 months awake 7 months asleep
Rooting	Birth	4 months awake 7 months asleep
Palmar grasp	Birth	6 months
Plantar grasp	Birth	10 months
Tonic neck	2 months	5 months
Neck righting	4-6 months	24 months
Landau	3 months	24 months
Parachute reaction	9 months	Persists for life

responses may indicate lesions in the motor cortex on the contralateral side of the brain or may occur with fractures of bones after traumatic delivery or postnatal injury. As the infant matures, the primitive reflexes disappear in a predictable order as voluntary motor functions supersede them. Abnormal persistence of these reflexes is seen in infants with developmental delays or with central nervous system lesions.

STRUCTURAL MALFORMATIONS

CNS malformations are a common cause of significant morbidity and mortality in the first year of life. Malformations include defects of neural tube closure (anencephaly, spina bifida, myelomeningocele), formation of the skull and surrounding structures (craniosynostosis), neuronal migration (lissencephaly, microcephaly), and flow of CSF (hydrocephalus).

Defects of Neural Tube Closure

Neural tube defects (NTDs) are the most common anomaly of the CNS. They occur in about 3000 pregnancies in the United States each year, although there are significant regional differences in prevalence.[1] Maternal folate deficiency had been associated with significant risk for NTD. These defects originate during the first month of embryonic development when the neural tube fails to close completely. Fetal death often occurs in the more severe cases, thereby reducing the actual prevalence of neural defects at birth.[2,3] In 1996 the United States mandated folate fortification in many foods, and since that time neural tube defects have decreased by 20% to 30%[4] Guidelines are available for folic acid supplementation for women at high risk for neural tube defects.[5]

Defects of neural tube closure are divided into two categories: anterior midline defects (ventral induction) and posterior defects (dorsal induction). Anterior midline defects may cause brain and face abnormalities in the holoprosencephaly spectrum, with the most extreme form being cyclopia, in which the child has a single midline orbit and eye with a protruding noselike proboscis above the orbit. Posterior defects result from failure of closure of the neural tube and result in a variety of myelodysplasias depending on the level of the failure. Although myelodysplasia is defined as a defect in formation of the spinal cord, the term is used to refer to anomalies of both the vertebral column and the spinal cord. Spina bifida (split spine) is the most common neural tube defect and includes anencephaly, encephalocele, meningocele, and myelomeningocele. Disorders of embryonic neural development are summarized in Fig. 20.4.

Anencephaly (an, "without"; enkephalos, "brain") is an anomaly in which the soft, bony component of the skull and part of the brain are missing. This is a relatively common disorder, with an incidence of approximately 1 per 4859 live births in the United States each year.[2] These infants are stillborn or die within a few days after birth. The pathologic mechanism is unknown. Diagnosis is often made prenatally using ultrasound or evaluating maternal serum α_1-fetoprotein (AFP).[6]

Encephalocele refers to a herniation or protrusion of various amounts of brain and meninges through a defect in the skull, resulting in a saclike structure (Fig. 20.5). The incidence is approximately 1 in 10,000 live births in the United States each year.[7] Encephalocele occurs during the first weeks of pregnancy. When the defect contains only meninges, it is referred to as a cranial meningocele. Most encephaloceles, which contain neural tissue as well as meninges, occur in the occipital area, with the remainder found in the frontal, parietal, or nasopharyngeal regions. If the defect is located in the nasopharynx, no external anomaly is visible but the child may experience nasal airway obstruction. On examination with a nasal speculum, a smooth, round mass will be visible in the nasal passages. A frontal encephalocele may extend into the orbit of the eye and produce proptosis on the affected side. An occipital encephalocele may be associated with other findings, such as blindness and cognitive impairment. The size, location, and involvement of the encephalocele help determine a child's development and intellectual outcome.

Meningocele is a saclike cyst of meninges filled with spinal fluid and is a mild form of spina bifida. It develops during the first 4 weeks of pregnancy when the neural tube fails to close completely. The cystic dilation of meninges protrudes through a defect in the posterior arch of the vertebra. The vertebral defect does not involve the spinal cord or nerve roots and may produce no neurologic deficit or symptoms. Meningoceles occur with equal frequency in the cervical, thoracic, and lumbar spine. With cranial meningocele, surgical repair of the cranial defect affords a good prognosis for most affected infants whose intellectual and motor functioning is usually normal.

Myelomeningocele (meningomyelocele; spina bifida cystica) is a hernial protrusion of a saclike cyst (containing meninges, spinal fluid, and a portion of the spinal cord with its nerves) through a defect in the posterior arch of a vertebra (Fig. 20.6). Myelomeningocele is one of the most common developmental anomalies of the nervous system, with an incidence ranging from 0.5 to 1.0 per 1000 pregnancies.[8] Eighty percent of myelomeningoceles are located in the lumbar and lumbosacral regions, the last regions of the neural tube to close.

Meningocele and myelomeningoceles are evident at birth as a pronounced skin defect on the infant's back. The bony prominences of the unfused neural arches can be palpated at the lateral border of the defect. The defect is usually covered by a transparent membrane that may have neural tissue attached to its inner surface. This membrane may be intact at birth or may leak cerebrospinal fluid (CSF), thereby increasing the risks of infection and neuronal damage.

The spinal cord and nerve roots are malformed below the level of the lesion, resulting in loss of motor, sensory, reflex, and autonomic functions. A brief neurologic examination concentrating on motor function in the legs, reflexes, and sphincter tone is usually sufficient to determine the level above which spinal cord and nerve root function is preserved (Table 20.2). This is useful to predict if the child will ambulate, require bladder catheterization, or be at high risk for developing scoliosis (see Chapter 46).

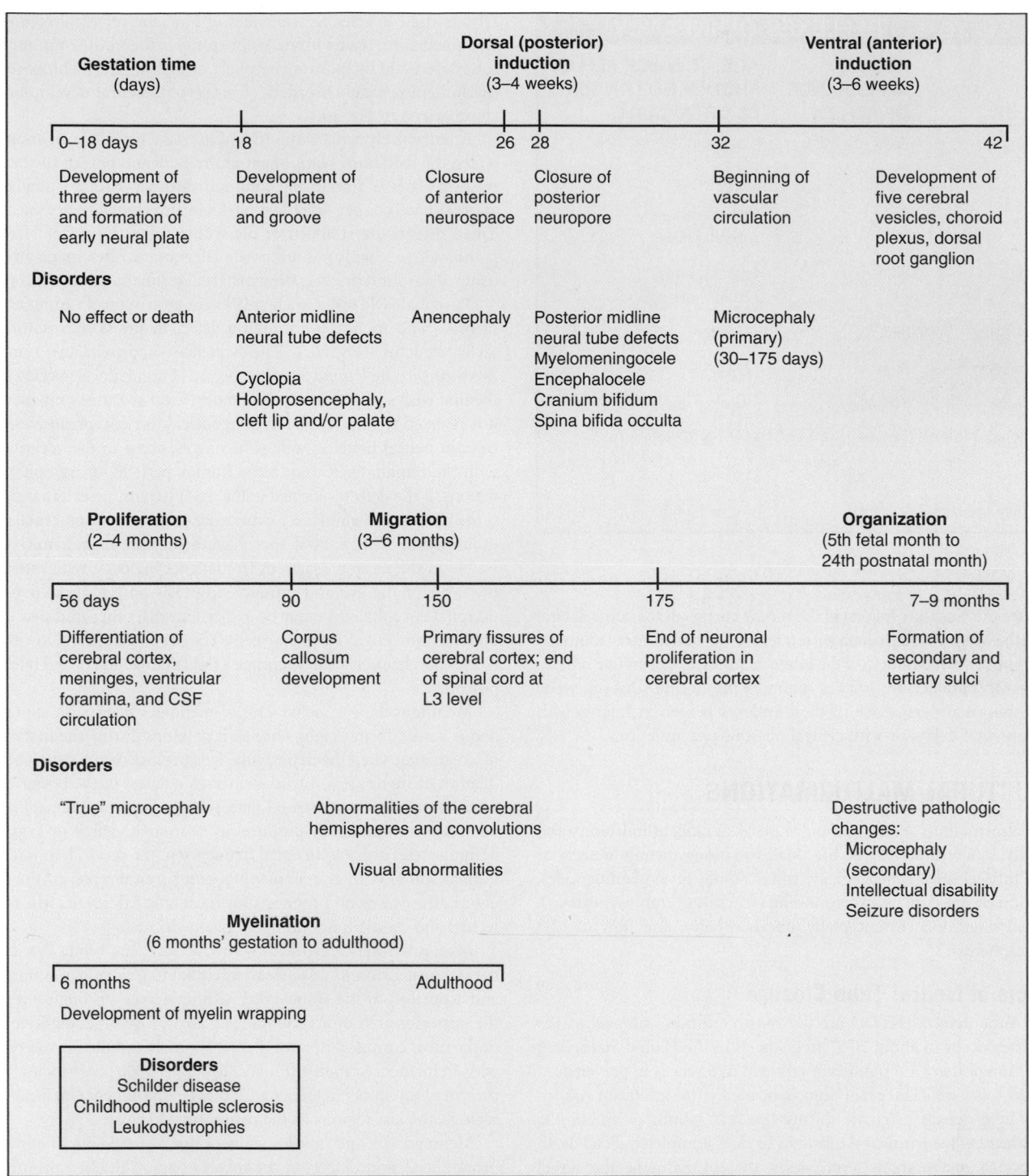

FIGURE 20.4 Disorders Associated with Specific Stages of Embryonic Development. *CSF,* Cerebrospinal fluid.

Hydrocephalus occurs in 85% of infants with myelomeningocele.[9] Seizures also occur in 30% of those with myelodysplasia. Visual and perceptual problems, including ocular palsies, astigmatism, and visuoperceptual deficits, are common. Motor and sensory functions below the level of the lesions are altered. Often these problems worsen as the child grows and the cord ascends within the vertebral canal, pulling primary scar tissue and tethering the cord.

Myelomeningoceles are almost always associated with a brain malformation known as type II **Arnold-Chiari malformation.**[9] This is a complex malformation of the brainstem and cerebellum in which the cerebellar tonsils are displaced downward into the cervical spinal canal, the upper medulla and lower pons are elongated and thin, and the medulla also is displaced downward and sometimes has a "kink" (Fig. 20.7). The Chiari II malformation is associated with hydrocephalus from pressure that blocks the flow of cerebrospinal fluid and syringomyelia, an abnormality causing cysts at multiple levels within the spinal canal. Cognitive and motor deficits are common.[10] Symptomatic Chiari II malformations require surgical decompression or placement of

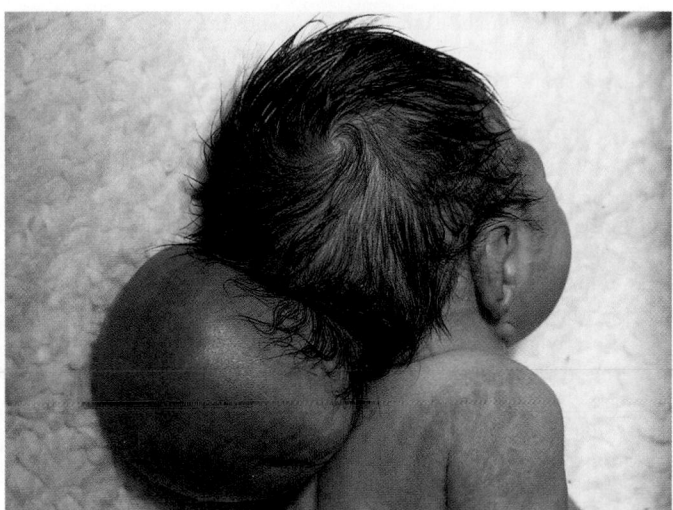

FIGURE 20.5 Meningoencephalocele of the Occipital Region. (From Gilbert-Barness: *Potter's pathology of the fetus, infant and child,* ed 2, Philadelphia, 2007, Mosby.)

TABLE 20.2	FUNCTIONAL ALTERATIONS IN MYELODYSPLASIA (NEURAL TUBE DEFECTS) RELATED TO LEVEL OF LESION
LEVEL OF LESION	**FUNCTIONAL IMPLICATIONS**
Thoracic	Flaccid paralysis of lower extremities; variable weakness in abdominal trunk musculature; high thoracic level may mean respiratory compromise; absence of bowel and bladder control
High lumbar	Voluntary hip flexion and adduction; flaccid paralysis of knees, ankles, and feet; may walk with extensive braces and crutches; absence of bowel and bladder control
Midlumbar	Strong hip flexion and adduction; fair knee extension; flaccid paralysis of ankles and feet; absence of bowel and bladder control
Low lumbar	Strong hip flexion, extension, and adduction and knee extension; weak ankle and toe mobility; may have limited bowel and bladder function
Sacral	Normal function of lower extremities; normal bowel and bladder function

Data from Martin RJ, Fanaroff AA, Walsh MC: *Fanaroff and Martin's neonatal-perinatal medicine*, Philadelphia, 2015, Saunders.

cerebrospinal fluid shunts, or both. The type I Chiari malformation does not involve the brainstem and may be asymptomatic. In type III, the brainstem or cerebellum extends into a high cervical myelomeningocele. Type IV is characterized by lack of cerebellar development.

Most cases of meningocele and myelomeningocele are diagnosed prenatally by a combination of maternal serologic testing (α-fetoprotein) and prenatal ultrasound. In these cases, the fetus is usually delivered by elective cesarean section to minimize trauma during labor. Surgical repair is critical and can be performed by in utero fetal surgery or during the first 72 hours of life.[11]

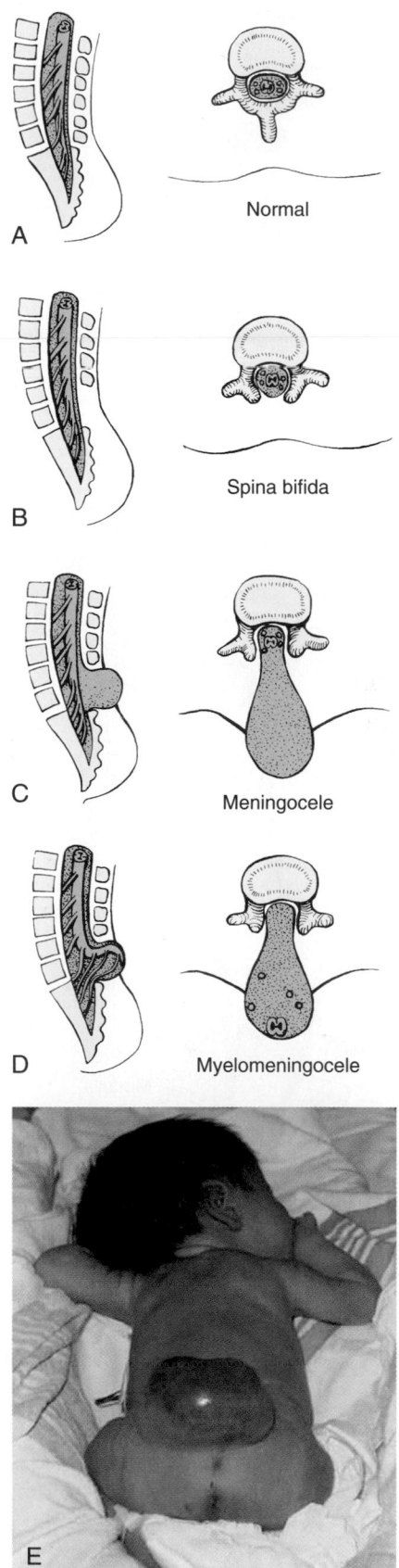

FIGURE 20.6 Normal Spine, Spina Bifida, Meningocele, and Myelomeningocele. (From Nockenberry MJ, Wilson D: *Wong's nursing care of infants and children,* ed 10, St Louis, 2015, Mosby.)

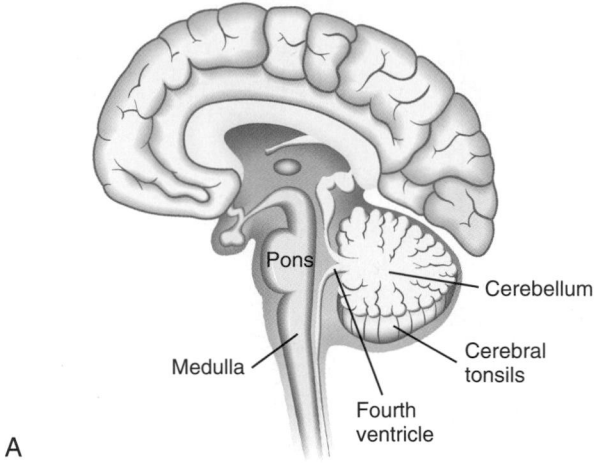

A

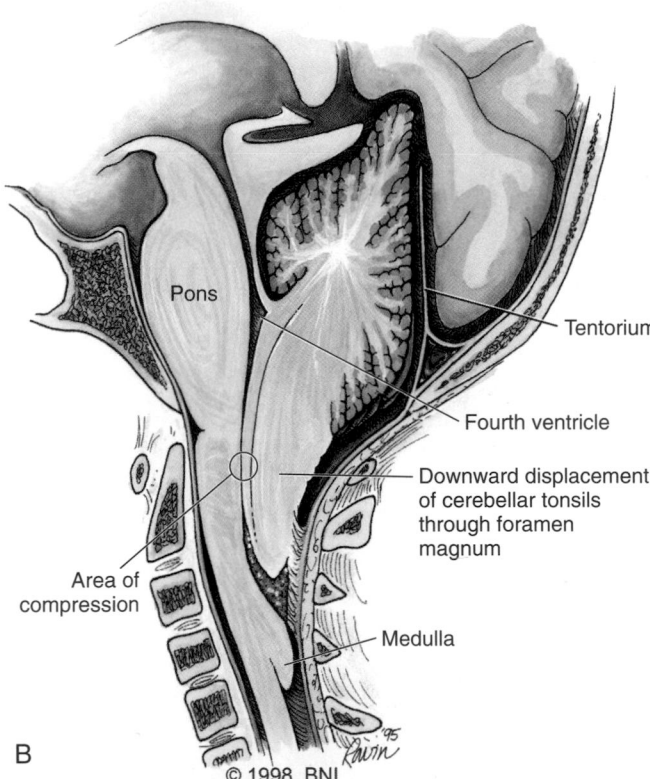

B

© 1998, BNI

FIGURE 20.7 Normal Brain and Chiari Type II Malformation. **A,** Normal brain. **B,** Chiari II malformation with downward displacement of cerebellar tonsils and medulla through foramen magnum causing compression and obstruction to flow of CSF. (**B** modified from Barrow Neurological Institute of St. Joseph's Hospital and Medical Center, Phoenix, Arizona. Reprinted with permission.)

It is possible for a defect to occur without any visible exposure of meninges or neural tissue. This defect, termed spina bifida occulta, is common and occurs to some degree in 10% to 25% of infants. Spina bifida occulta usually causes no neurologic dysfunction because the spinal cord and spinal nerves are normal. Surgical treatment is usually directed at associated intraspinal abnormalities that occur with growth of the child (tethered cord, sacral lipoma, or dermoid cyst). Tethered cord syndrome may develop after surgical correction for myelomeningocele.[12] In these cases, the cord becomes abnormally attached or tethered

as a result of scar tissue as the cord transcends the vertebral canal with growth. Traction decreases blood flow and impairs oxidative metabolism. The cord can be untethered surgically.[12]

Craniosynostosis

Skull malformations range from minor, insignificant defects to major defects that are incompatible with life. Craniosynostosis (craniostenosis) is the premature closure of one or more of the cranial sutures (sagittal, coronal, lambdoid, metopic) during the first 18 to 20 months of an infant's life. The incidence of craniosynostosis is 1 in 2000 to 2500 live births.[13] Males are affected twice as often as females. Fusion of a cranial suture prevents growth of the skull perpendicular to the suture line, resulting in an asymmetric shape of the skull. The general term *plagiocephaly*, meaning "misshapen skull," is used to describe deformities that result from craniosynostosis or from asymmetric head posture (positional). When a single coronal suture fuses prematurely, the head is flattened on that side in front. When the sagittal suture fuses prematurely, the head is elongated in the anteroposterior direction and is termed *scaphocephaly*[14] (Fig. 20.8). Diagnosis of craniosynostosis is made on the basis of physical examination, head circumference, and radiologic examination. Single-suture craniosynostosis is usually only a cosmetic issue. Rarely, when multiple sutures fuse prematurely, brain growth may be restricted and surgical repair may prevent neurologic dysfunction (Fig. 20.9). Syndromic craniosynostosis involves deformities in other systems (i.e., the heart, limbs, and central nervous system).

Malformations of Brain Development

Structural malformations of the brain are a diverse group of disorders caused by abnormal neuronal migration, abnormal neuronal, or glial proliferation. Reduced proliferation or accelerated apoptosis causes congenital microcephaly (small brain) and increased proliferation causes megalencephaly (abnormally large brain). Malformations can occur any time during fetal development or after birth. There are specific genetic defects for some of these disorders; others are multifactorial or acquired (i.e., intrauterine trauma or infection). Most brain malformations increase the risk for seizures, developmental delay, and motor dysfunction. Diagnosis is made by clinical history, family history, and magnetic resonance imaging (MRI) of the brain. Genetic testing is done for diagnosis to assess risk in other family members and to guide prospective therapy.[15]

Microcephaly is a defect in brain growth as a whole (see Fig. 20.8). Cranial size is significantly below average for the infant's age, sex, race, and gestation. The small size of the skull reflects a small brain (microencephaly, head circumference two standard deviations below the mean for age and sex). *Primary microcephaly* is caused by an autosomal recessive genetic defect in 1 of as many as 16 or more different genes. *Secondary (acquired) microcephaly* is associated with various causes, including infection, trauma, metabolic disorders, toxin or radiation exposure, maternal anorexia experienced during the third trimester of pregnancy, and the presence of other genetic syndromes (Box 20.1). Maternal infection with Zika virus causes microcephaly and other congenital malformations known as *congenital Zika syndrome*. The current theory is that the virus crosses the placental barrier and blood-brain barrier inducing neural cell death and inhibiting brain tissue development.[16]

Cortical dysplasias are a heterogeneous group of disorders caused by defects in brain development These disorders may range from a small area of abnormal tissue (e.g., heterotopia, which are areas of gray matter that did not migrate to their normal position in the cortex) to an entire brain that is smooth without the normal gyri and sulci of a developed brain (lissencephaly) (Fig. 20.10). Specific genetic defects are known for some of these disorders; others are multifactorial or acquired (e.g., intrauterine trauma or infection). Cortical dysplasias

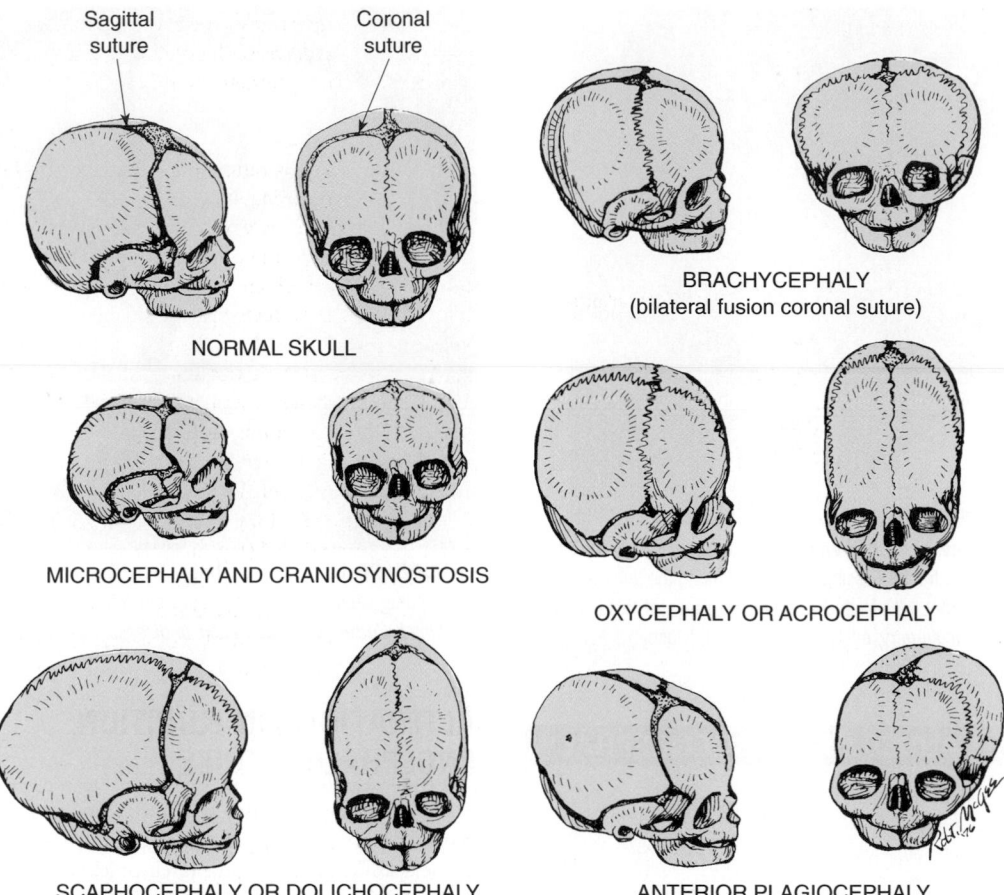

Sagittal suture   Coronal suture

NORMAL SKULL

BRACHYCEPHALY
(bilateral fusion coronal suture)

MICROCEPHALY AND CRANIOSYNOSTOSIS

OXYCEPHALY OR ACROCEPHALY

SCAPHOCEPHALY OR DOLICHOCEPHALY

ANTERIOR PLAGIOCEPHALY

FIGURE 20.8 Types and Frequency of Craniosynostosis. Abnormal head configuration resulting from premature closing of cranial sutures. *Normal skull:* Bones separated by membranous seams until sutures gradually close. *Microcephaly and craniosynostosis:* Microcephaly is head circumference more than two standard deviations below the mean for age, sex, race, and gestation and reflects a small brain; craniosynostosis is premature closure or fusion of sutures. *Scaphocephaly or dolichocephaly* (frequency 56%): Premature closure of sagittal suture, resulting in restricted lateral growth. *Brachycephaly:* Premature closure of coronal suture, resulting in excessive lateral growth. *Oxycephaly or acrocephaly* (frequency 5.8% to 12%): Premature closure of all coronal and sagittal sutures, resulting in accelerated upward growth and small head circumference. *Anterior plagiocephaly* (frequency 13%): Unilateral premature closure of coronal suture, resulting in asymmetric growth. (From Hockenberry JH, Wilson D: *Wong's nursing care of infants and children,* ed 10, St Louis, 2015, Mosby.)

increase the risk for seizures that are difficult to control and cause developmental delay and motor dysfunction.[17] Genetic testing assists diagnosis, assesses risk in other family members, and guides therapy.

Congenital hydrocephalus is present at birth and characterized by increased CSF pressure. It may be caused by obstruction within the ventricular system, an imbalance in the production, or reabsorption of CSF. *Obstructive hydrocephalus* is most commonly caused by congenital aqueductal stenosis. The cerebral aqueduct, which connects the third ventricle to the fourth ventricle, is narrowed or replaced by multiple channels that end blindly. In a small number of children the stenosis is transmitted as an X-linked recessive trait that affects brain growth and development or as nonsyndromic autosomal recessive hydrocephalus.[18] The increased pressure within the ventricular system dilates the ventricles and compresses the brain tissue against the skull (Fig. 20.11). When hydrocephalus develops before fusion of the cranial sutures, the skull has the capacity to increase its size to accommodate this additional space-occupying volume (progressive macrocephaly) (Fig. 20.12) and

to preserve neuronal function. The overall incidence of hydrocephalus is approximately 1 to 3 per 1000 live births.[19] The incidence of hydrocephalus that is not associated with myelomeningocele is approximately 0.5 to 1 per 1000 live births, with aqueductal stenosis as the cause for approximately one-third of these cases.[20] (Types of hydrocephalus are discussed in Chapter 17.)

Congenital hydrocephalus may cause fetal death in utero, or the increased head circumference may require cesarean delivery of the infant. Symptoms depend directly on the cause and rate of progression. When there is separation of the cranial sutures, a resonant note sounds when the skull is tapped, a manifestation termed Macewen sign or "cracked pot" sign. Typically, the fontanels enlarge and become full and bulging. The eyes may assume a staring expression, with sclera visible above the cornea, called *sunsetting*. Cognitive impairment in children with hydrocephalus is often related to associated brain malformations, episodes of shunt failure, or infection. Approximately 30% to 40% of children with uncomplicated congenital hydrocephalus complete schooling and

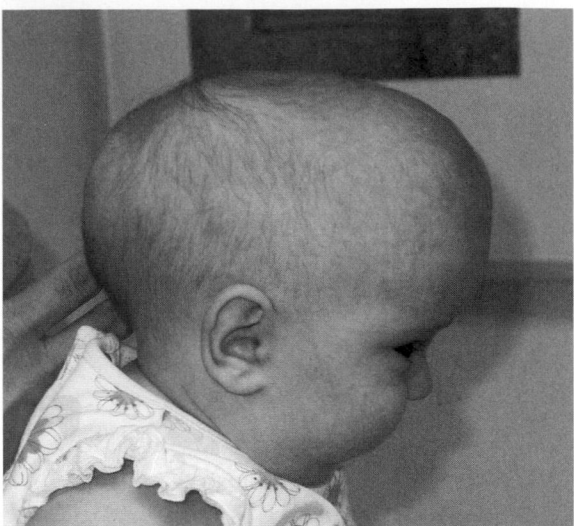

FIGURE 20.9 Lateral View of a Child with Scaphocephaly Resulting from Sagittal Synostosis. Note the frontal bossing, elongation along the anteroposterior (AP) axis, and prominent occiput, all of which are characteristic of this condition. (From Coran A et al: *Pediatric surgery,* ed 7, St Louis, 2012, Mosby.)

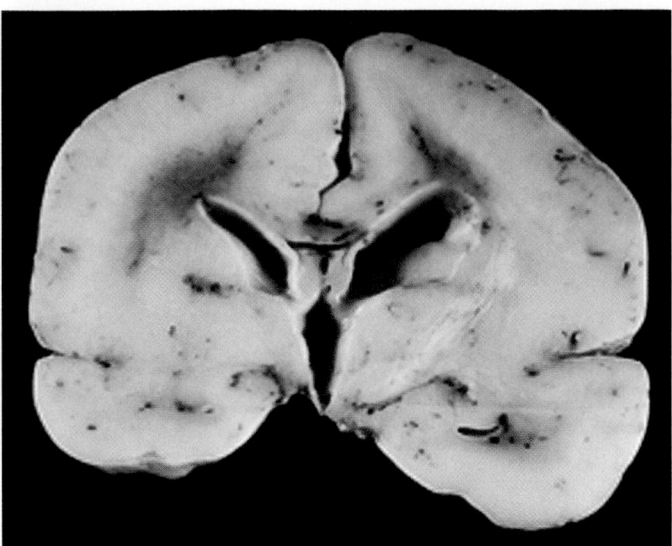

FIGURE 20.10 Lissencephaly. The absence of cortical gyri defines this abnormality, seen here in the brain from a full-term infant. (From Kumar V et al: *Robbins & Cotran pathologic basis of disease,* ed 8, Saunders, 2010, Philadelphia.)

BOX 20.1	CAUSES OF MICROENCEPHALY

Defects in Brain Development
Hereditary (recessive) microcephaly
Down syndrome and other trisomy syndromes
Fetal ionizing radiation exposure
Maternal phenylketonuria
Seckel syndrome
Cornelia de Lange syndrome
Rubinstein-Taybi syndrome
Smith-Lemli-Opitz syndrome
Fetal alcohol syndrome

Intrauterine Infections
Congenital rubella
Cytomegalovirus infection
Congenital toxoplasmosis
Congenital syphilis
Congenital Zika virus

Perinatal and Postnatal Disorders
Intrauterine or neonatal anoxia
Severe malnutrition in early infancy
Neonatal herpesvirus infection

ALTERATIONS IN FUNCTION: ENCEPHALOPATHIES

Encephalopathy, meaning dysfunction of overall brain function, is a general category that includes a large number of syndromes and diseases. These disorders may be acute or chronic, as well as static or progressive. Some common neurologic disorders with a genetic basis are summarized in Table 20.3.

Static Encephalopathies

Static or nonprogressive encephalopathy describes a neurologic condition caused by a fixed lesion without active and ongoing disease. Causes include brain malformations or brain injury that may occur during gestation or birth, or at any time during childhood. The degree of neurologic impairment is directly related to the extent of the injury or malformation. Anoxia, trauma, and infections are the most common factors that cause injury to the nervous system in the perinatal period. Infections, metabolic disturbances (acquired or genetic), trauma, toxins, and vascular disease may injure the nervous system in the postnatal period. The clinical manifestations of a static encephalopathy depend on the site and extent of the injury, as well as the age of the child and stage of development at the time of injury.

Cerebral palsy (CP) is a disorder of movement, muscle tone, or posture that is caused by injury or abnormal development in the immature brain, before, during, or after birth up to 1 year of age. CP is one of the most common disorders of childhood, affecting nearly 500,000 children in the United States alone. Although the exact incidence is unknown, studies suggest that the prevalence is approximately 1 in 323 children in the United States.[22] Risk factors include prenatal or perinatal cerebral hypoxia, hemorrhage, infection, genetic abnormalities, or low birth weight (Table 20.4). Severity of CP depends on the gestational age at the time of the injury and the type and degree of injury sustained. CP can be classified on the basis of neurologic signs and motor symptoms, with the major types involving spasticity (increased tone), dystonia, ataxia, or a combination of these symptoms (mixed). Diplegia, hemiplegia, or tetraplegia may be present.

Pyramidal/spastic cerebral palsy results from damage to corticospinal pathways (upper motor neurons) and is associated with increased muscle

are employed when treated successfully with shunting or endoscopic third ventriculostomy and choroid plexus cauterization.[18]

Hydrocephalus caused by CSF obstructions within the ventricular system can result from Dandy-Walker malformation (DWM) brain tumors, cysts, trauma, arteriovenous malformations, blood clots, infections, and the Chiari malformations (see the Defects of Neural Tube Closure section). DWM is a congenital defect of the cerebellum characterized by a large posterior fossa cyst that communicates with the fourth ventricle and an atrophic, upwardly rotated, cerebellar vermis.[21] DWM is commonly associated with hydrocephalus caused by compression of the aqueduct of Sylvius.

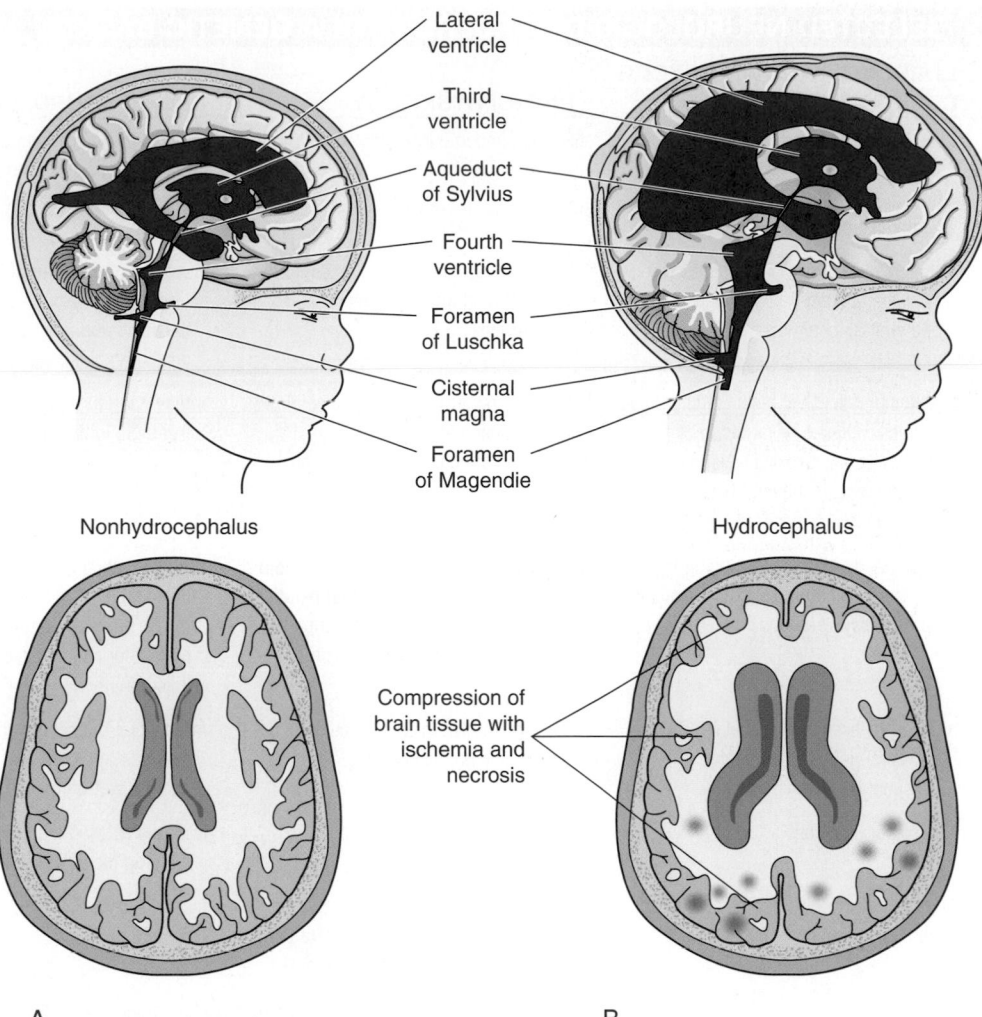

FIGURE 20.11 Hydrocephalus. Fluid accumulation in the brain because of blockage in the flow of cerebrospinal fluid (CSF). **A,** Patent cerebrospinal fluid circulation. **B,** Enlarged lateral and third ventricles caused by obstruction of circulation of CSF—stenosis of aqueduct of Sylvius.

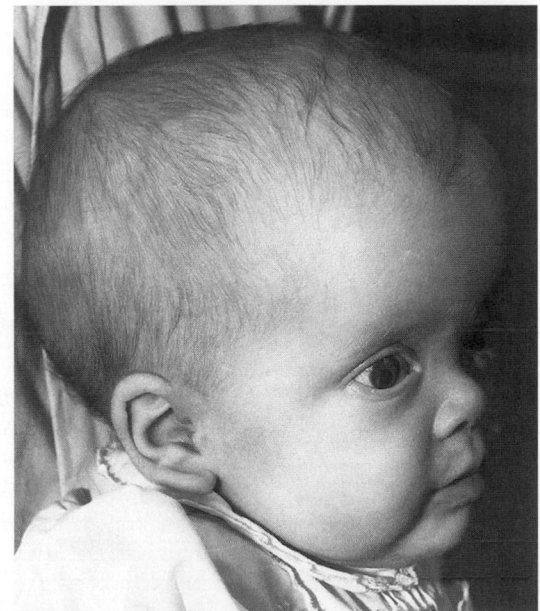

FIGURE 20.12 Child with Enlarged Head Caused by Hydrocephalus. (From McLaurin DC: *Pediatric neurosurgery,* ed 2, Philadelphia, 1989, Saunders.)

tone, persistent primitive reflexes, hyperactive deep tendon reflexes, clonus, rigidity of the extremities, scoliosis, and contractures. This accounts for 70% to 80% of cerebral palsy cases.[23] **Extrapyramidal/nonspastic cerebral palsy** is caused by damage to cells in the basal ganglia, thalamus, or cerebellum and includes two subtypes: dyskinetic and ataxic. **Dyskinetic (dystonic and athetoid) cerebral palsy** results in movements that are stiff, uncontrolled, abrupt, and can be repetitive resulting in extreme difficulty in fine motor coordination and purposeful movements. Dyskinetic CP accounts for 10% to 20% of cases. **Ataxic cerebral palsy** manifests with gait disturbances and reflects cerebellar involvement. The infant with this form of CP may have hypotonia at birth, but stiffness of the trunk muscles develops by late infancy. Persistence of increased tone in truncal muscles affects the child's gait and ability to maintain balance. Ataxic CP accounts for 5% to 10% of cases. A child may have symptoms of each of these cerebral palsy types, which leads to a mixed disorder accounting for approximately 13% of cases.[24]

Children with CP often have associated neurologic disorders, such as seizures (about 50%) and intellectual impairment ranging from mild to severe (about 67%). Other complications include visual impairment, communication disorders, difficulty swallowing, respiratory problems, bowel and bladder problems, malnutrition, and orthopedic disabilities.[25] The management of children with CP varies with age, type, severity of involvement, and associated disorders. Thus the scope of care required

TABLE 20.3	SELECTED NEUROLOGIC DISORDERS WITH A GENETIC BASIS		
SYNDROME/ DISORDERS	**CURRENTLY KNOWN GENETIC COMPONENTS**	**PATHOPHYSIOLOGY**	**MAJOR NEUROLOGIC FEATURES**
Angelman syndrome	Microdeletion on chromosome 15 leading to loss of function of the *UBE3A* gene (ubiquitin protein ligase); can be acquired from mother	Protein, important in degradation of proteins in the brain	Little to no verbal language, intellectual disability, seizure disorder, sleep disorder, movement/balance disorder
Batten disease	Autosomal recessive; mutation of the *CLN3* gene (ceroid-lipofuscinosis, neuronal 3) (chromosome 16)	Lysosomal storage defect resulting in abnormal storage of cerebral lipofuscins	Develops normally until 6 months to 2 years of age when progressive brain disease becomes apparent; seizures, intellectual disability, blindness, and death
Branched-chain ketoaciduria (maple syrup urine disease)	Autosomal recessive; most common type is classic caused by mutation of the *BCKDHA* gene (2-oxoisovalerate dehydrogenase subunit alpha, a mitochondrial enzyme) (chromosome 19)	All types result in inability to metabolize three amino acids; these acids accumulate and are toxic at high levels	Intellectual disability, seizures, and death; treatable with early diagnosis
Cri du chat syndrome	Autosomal dominant; deletion on the short arm of chromosome 5 (also called *5p minus syndrome*)	Deletion of multiple genes responsible for phenotype; evidence that deletion of telomerase reverse transcriptase gene contributes to phenotype	High-pitched cry; intellectual disability, microcephaly, low birth weight, failure to thrive; widely spaced eyes (ocular hypertelorism), unusually small jaw (micrognathia)
Lesch-Nyhan syndrome	X-linked recessive; mutation of the *HPRT* gene (hypoxanthine phosphoribosyltransferase 1)	Metabolism disturbance of purines; excessive production of uric acid	Intellectual disability, progressive neurologic disorder, compulsively bitten lips and fingers; self-mutilating
Neurofibromatosis (NF)	Autosomal dominant	Variable expressivity	Multiple café-au-lait spots, neurofibromas, learning disability, seizure disorder
NF1 (von Recklinghausen disease)	Mutation of the *NF1* gene (neurofibromin) (chromosome 17)	A large, complex protein; this protein may act as a switch to regulate cell growth; mutation may lessen or inhibit the normal output of this protein and allow irregular cell growth that may lead to tumor development	Increased risk for nerve sheath tumors and brain tumors
NF2 (bilateral acoustic NF)	Autosomal dominant: mutation of either the *NF2* gene (merlin; moesin-ezrin-radixin-like protein or schwannomin) (chromosome 22)	A tumor-suppressor protein (merlin or schwannomin)	Multiple tumors (schwannomas) on cranial and spinal nerves, acoustic neuromas, hearing loss
Progressive myoclonic epilepsy (Unverricht-Lundborg disease)	Autosomal recessive; mutation *CSTB* gene (cystatin B, a cysteine protease inhibitor) (chromosome 21)	This protein regulates enzymes that break down other proteins	Onset at age 6–15 years, severe incapacitating stimulus-sensitive progressive myoclonus, tonic-clonic epileptic seizures, and characteristic abnormalities on electroencephalogram; also may develop other neurologic symptoms such as ataxia, incoordination, and dysarthria
Lafora disease	Autosomal recessive; mutation of the *EMP2A* gene (epilepsy, progressive myoclonus type 2A or laforin) and *EMP2B* gene (malin) (chromosome 6)	Concentric amyloid (Lafora) bodies found in neurons, liver, skin, bone, and muscle; defects in protein degradation and clearance	Grand mal seizures and/or myoclonus at about age 15; rapid and severe motor and coordination impairments, rapid mental deterioration, often with psychotic features; survival is short, less than 10 years after onset
Rett syndrome	X-linked dominant; appears to occur only in girls; defective *MECP2* gene (methyl CpG binding protein 2) (X-chromosome)	Protein involved in regulation of gene expression; defects in this gene allow other genes to be expressed at inappropriate times in development	Progressive neurologic disorder; develops normally in first year of life, then loss of mental capacity and motor skills begins; loss of purposeful hand movements; stereotypical hand wringing and flapping

TABLE 20.3 SELECTED NEUROLOGIC DISORDERS WITH A GENETIC BASIS—cont'd

SYNDROME/ DISORDERS	CURRENTLY KNOWN GENETIC COMPONENTS	PATHOPHYSIOLOGY	MAJOR NEUROLOGIC FEATURES
Tay-Sachs disease	Autosomal recessive; mutation of the HEXA gene (chromosome 15)	Caused by a deficiency of hexosaminidase, an enzyme, which results in accumulation of a material that damages the brain	Failure to thrive, blindness, seizures, progressive paralysis; usually death by age 4
Tuberous sclerosis	Autosomal dominant; mutation of either the TSC1 gene (hamartin) (chromosome 9) or the TSC2 gene (tuberin) (chromosome 16)	These proteins act as tumor growth suppressors	Develops in early childhood; seizures, intellectual disability, skin and eye lesions; multiple benign tumors in brain and other vital organs

TABLE 20.4 CEREBRAL PALSY: PREDISPOSING FACTORS AND KNOWN CAUSES

RISK FACTORS	ASSOCIATED CAUSES
Prenatal	
Maternal	Metabolic diseases
	Nutritional deficiencies (e.g., anemia)
	Twin or multiple births
	Bleeding
	Toxemia
	Blood incompatibilities
	Exposure to radiation
	Infection (e.g., rubella, toxoplasmosis, cytomegalic inclusion disease)
	Premature labor
Prematurity	Asphyxia leading to cerebral hemorrhage
Genetic factors	Absence of corpus callosum, aqueductal stenosis, cerebellar hypoplasia
Congenital anomalies of the brain	Unknown causes not evident on clinical examination
Perinatal	Anesthesia or analgesia during labor and delivery
	Mechanical trauma or hypoxia during delivery
	Immaturity at birth
	Metabolic disorders (e.g., hyperbilirubinemia, hypoglycemia, amino acid disorders, hyperosmolality)
	Electrolyte disturbances (e.g., hypernatremia, hypoglycemia)
Postnatal	Head trauma
	Infections (e.g., meningitis, encephalitis)
	Cerebrovascular accidents
	Toxicosis
	Environmental toxins (e.g., lead ingestion, methyl mercury ingestion from contaminated fish)

by the child and family includes ongoing medical, social, and educational intervention and a family-focused multidisciplinary team approach.[26,27]

Inherited Metabolic Disorders of the Central Nervous System

A large number of inherited metabolic disorders have been identified leading to diffuse brain dysfunction. Inborn errors of metabolism are present at birth, including defects in amino acid and lipid and, more rarely, carbohydrate metabolism. Most cause disturbances of the nervous system, although they may not manifest until childhood or even adulthood. Early diagnosis and treatment is vital if these infants are to survive without severe neurologic problems. Newborn screening is recommended for 35 different genetic and metabolic conditions and has led to many of these children being identified before symptoms develop. The following website contains a list of the newborn metabolic screening tests: www.marchofdimes.com/professionals/bringinghome_screening.html.

Table E 20.1 (on Evolve) lists some of these inherited metabolic disorders

Defects in Amino Acid Metabolism. Biochemical defects in amino acid metabolism include (1) those in which the transport of an amino acid is impaired; (2) those involving an enzyme or cofactor deficiency; and (3) those encompassing certain chemical components, such as branched chain or sulfur-containing amino acids.[28] Most of the disorders are caused by genetic defects resulting in a lack of a normal protein and absence of enzymatic activity.

Phenylketonuria (PKU), an inborn error in the metabolism of amino acids, is characterized by phenylalanine hydroxylase deficiency and results in the inability of the body to convert the essential amino acid phenylalanine to tyrosine. PKU is an autosomal recessive disorder characterized by mutations of the phenylalanine hydroxylase *(PAH)* gene. PKU has an incidence of about 1 per 10,000 to 15,000 live births in the United States.[29] Statistical prevalence varies widely on the basis of geographic and ethnic differences.[30]

Most natural food proteins contain about 15% phenylalanine, an essential amino acid. Phenylalanine hydroxylase controls the conversion of this essential amino acid to tyrosine in the liver. Tyrosine is essential for the biosynthesis of proteins, melanin, thyroxine, and the catecholamine neurotransmitters in the brain and adrenal medulla. Phenylalanine hydroxylase deficiency causes an accumulation of phenylalanine in the serum. Elevated serum phenylalanine levels result in developmental abnormalities of the cerebral cortical layers, defective myelination, and cystic degeneration of the gray and white matter (Fig. 20.13). Unfortunately, brain damage occurs before the metabolites can be detected in the urine and damage continues as long as phenylalanine levels remain high. Nonselective newborn screening is used to detect PKU in the United States and in more than 30 other countries. Treatment, consisting of reduction of dietary phenylalanine (PKU diet), is effective and allows for normal development. Treatment must be continued for life, and strict adherence to the diet is especially important for pregnant women with PKU so that damage does not occur prenatally to the fetus.

Mutations in the *PAH* gene are the most common cause of PKU.[31] In one such variation, there is impaired synthesis of cofactors (e.g., tetrahydrobiopterin [BH$_4$]) which contributes to elevated levels of phenylalanine. Individuals with impaired synthesis of BH$_4$ have a positive

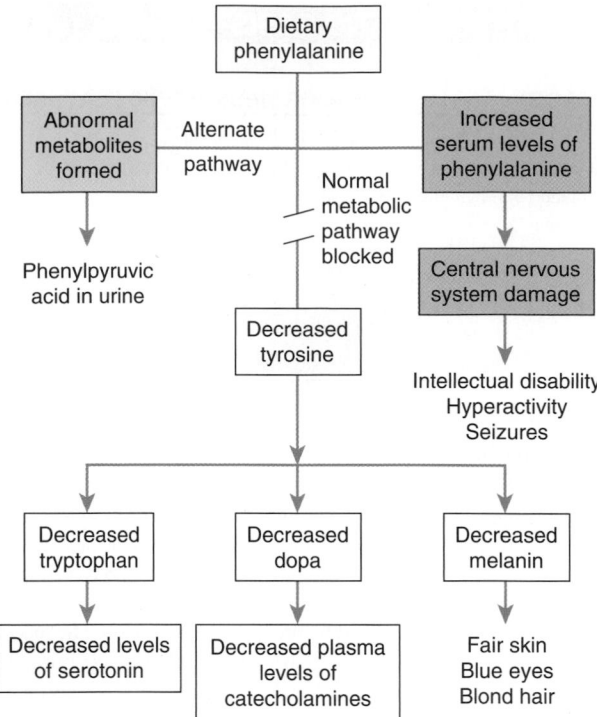

FIGURE 20.13 Metabolic Errors and Consequences in Phenylketonuria. (Redrawn from Hockenberry MJ et al: *Wong's nursing care of infants and children,* ed 9, St Louis, 2011, Mosby.)

BOX 20.2	**COMMON POISONS**	
PHARMACOLOGIC AGENTS	**HEAVY METALS**	**MISCELLANEOUS AGENTS**
Acetaminophen	Lead	Botulinum toxin
Amphetamines	Acute	Alcohols
Anticonvulsants	Chronic	Ethyl, isopropyl, methyl
Antidepressants	Mercury	Pesticides
Antihistamines	Thallium	Organophosphates
Atropine	Arsenic	Chlorinated hydrocarbons
Barbiturates	Cadmium	Mushrooms
Methadone		Venoms
Phencyclidine		Snake bite
Salicylates		Tick paralysis
Tranquilizers		Ethylene glycol
		Aliphatic hydrocarbons (e.g., gasoline, kerosene, lamp oil)

Data from Swaiman KF et al: *Swaiman's pediatric neurology: principles and practice,* vol 2, ed 5, St Louis, 2012, Mosby.

response when sapropterin, a synthetic form of tetrahydrobiopterin, is included in their treatment.[32] Because of the lack of tyrosine and its relationship to the biosynthesis of melanin, untreated children with PKU have a characteristic phenotype that includes blond hair, blue eyes, and fair skin. Children with genetically darker complexions may be red haired or brunette in contrast to their parents.

Storage Diseases. Disorders of lipid metabolism are termed lysosomal storage diseases because each disorder in this group can be traced to a missing lysosomal enzyme. Lysosomal storage disorders include more than 50 known genetic disorders, including sphingolipidoses (i.e., Gaucher disease, Fabry disease, Tay-Sachs disease), mucopolysaccharidoses (lack of enzymes to break down glycosaminoglycans), and oligosaccharidoses (lack of enzymes to break down glycoproteins). They occur in 7.7 to 23.5 per 100,000 live births.[33]

Lipids include oils, fatty acids, waxes, steroids (such as cholesterol and estrogen), and other related compounds. Although these compounds accumulate to some extent in cells, excess amounts are broken down in lysosomes (vesicles within the cell whose primary function is to degrade the breakdown products of cellular metabolism as discussed in Chapter 1). A genetic defect resulting in a missing or defective enzyme, such as lysosomal hydrolase, causes an excessive accumulation of the enzyme's substrate, which alters cell function. These disorders cause an excessive accumulation of a particular cell product, occurring in the brain, liver, spleen, bone, and lung, thus involving several organ systems. Generally, these disorders have not been included in newborn screening, but support for screening is growing. Some of these disorders may be treated with enzyme replacement therapy, which is effective in peripheral organs but cannot cross the blood-brain barrier to prevent neurodegeneration.[34]

Perhaps the best known of the lysosomal storage disorders is Tay-Sachs disease (GM₂ gangliosidosis), an autosomal recessive disorder (*HexA* gene on chromosome 15) caused by a deficiency of the lysosomal enzyme hexosaminidase A (HexA), an enzyme that degrades GM_2 gangliosides (fatty acids) within nerve cell lysosomes. Accumulation of gangliosides (gangliosidosis) causes toxicity to nerve cells, particularly in the CNS. Because of a founder effect, approximately 80% of individuals diagnosed are of Jewish ancestry, although sporadic cases appear in the non-Jewish population. Onset of this disease usually occurs when the infant is 4 to 6 months old. Symptoms of Tay-Sachs include an exaggerated startle response, seizures, developmental regression, dementia, and blindness. Death from this disease is almost universal and occurs by 5 years of age. Screening for carriers of the gene defect concomitant with genetic counseling has been a successful approach to prevent disease transmission.[35]

Acute Encephalopathies
Intoxications of the Central Nervous System

Drug-induced encephalopathies must always be considered a possibility in the child with unexplained neurologic changes. Such encephalopathies may result from accidental ingestion, therapeutic overdose, intentional overdose, or ingestion of environmental toxins (the most commonly ingested poisons are listed in Box 20.2). Approximately 42.6 children younger than 6 years/1000 persons were exposed to poisons, and approximately 1.1% of these children died in the United States in 2014.[36]

Lead poisoning results in high blood lead levels. No level of lead in the blood is safe. If lead poisoning is untreated, lead encephalopathy results and is responsible for serious and irreversible neurologic damage[37,38] Those at greatest risk are children less than 72 months of age, those with pica, or those living in lead-contaminated environments. It is a global health concern in children. Pica is the habitual, purposeful, and compulsive ingestion of nonfood substances such as clay, dirt, or paint chips. Lead intoxication also may occur from long-term exposure to smelters, sniffing of lead-containing solvents, exposure to lead-based paint, and ingestion of airborne lead or contaminated food and water.[39]

An estimated 535,000 U.S. children (2.6%) had excessive amounts of lead in their blood (>5 µg/dL) based on 2010 census data.[40] Excessive amounts cause varying degrees of intellectual disability depending on level and length of exposure. Young children are more likely to be exposed to lead-containing materials than older children because of mouthing behavior, and they absorb lead more easily than older children and adults. Levels continue to be highest among non-Hispanic black children, Mexican American, and non-Hispanic white children, with the greatest

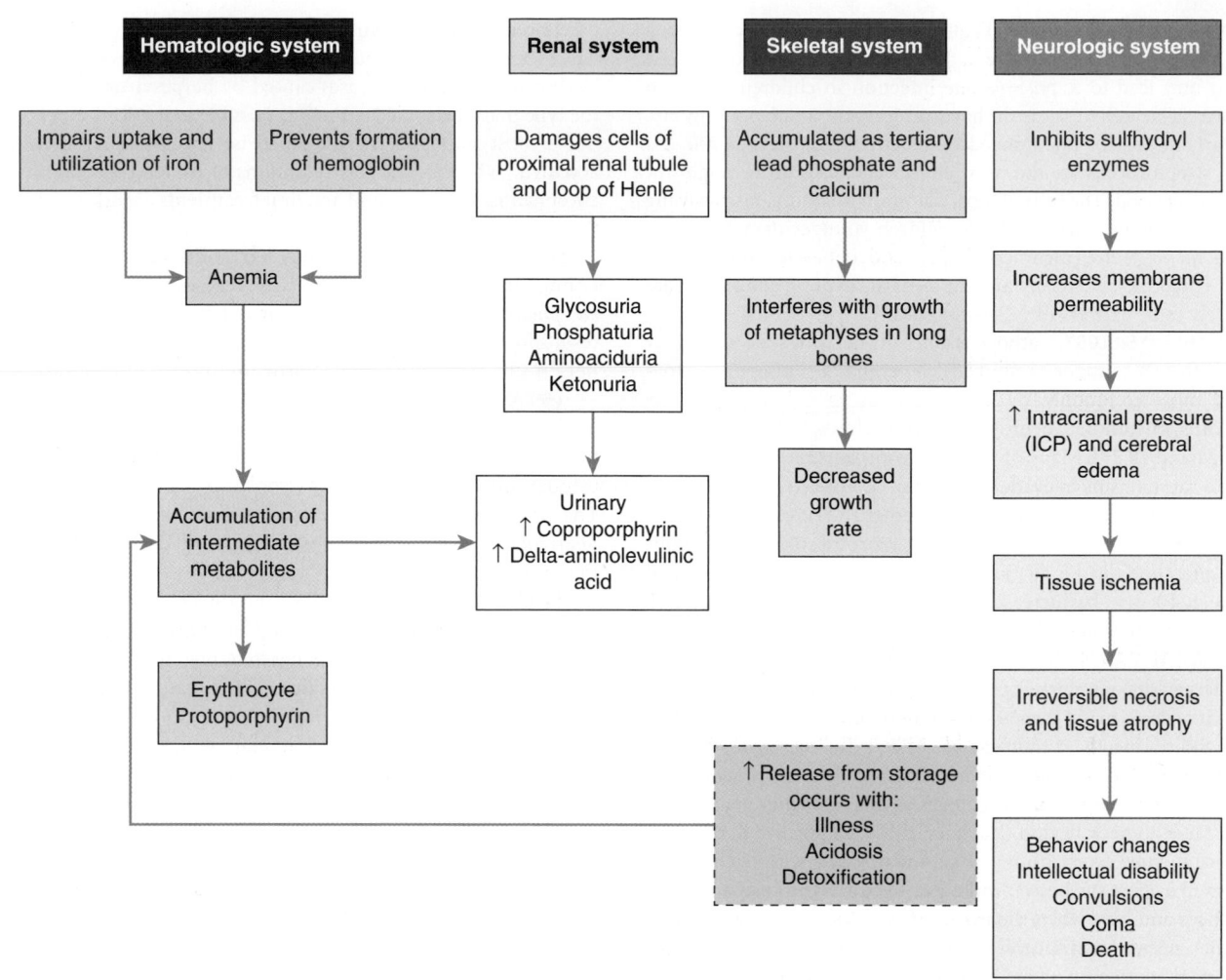

FIGURE 20.14 Systemic Effects of Increased Lead Absorption in Children.

risk being in the non-Hispanic black population.[41] The toxic effects of lead are summarized in Fig. 20.14 (also see Table 2.6, Table 2.7, and Fig. 2.20). The neurologic effects include developmental delays and encephalopathy with ataxia, stupor, coma, seizures, and death.[42] Guidelines are available for the treatment of lead exposure in children and include decontamination and chelation therapy.[43]

Infections of the Central Nervous System

Meningitis is infection of the meninges and subarachnoid space of the brain and spinal cord, whereas the word encephalitis reflects inflammation within the brain. In many infections of the meninges, encephalitis also is present and the term *meningoencephalitis* is used. Such inflammation and acute encephalopathy can be caused by bacteria, viruses, or other microorganisms. Aseptic meningitis has no evidence of bacterial infection but may be associated with viral infection, systemic disease, or drugs.

Bacterial Meningitis. Acute bacterial meningitis is one of the most serious infections to which infants and children are susceptible. In the United States approximately 4100 cases of bacterial meningitis occurred each year between 2003 and 2007, including 500 deaths.[44] About half of these cases occurred in children younger than 18 years of age. The most common microorganisms accountable for bacterial meningitis in children are summarized in Table 20.5.

The introduction of conjugate vaccines against *Haemophilus influenzae* type B, *Streptococcus pneumoniae,* and *Neisseria meningitidis* (menin-

TABLE 20.5	CAUSES OF BACTERIAL MENINGITIS
AGE GROUP	**COMMON BACTERIAL PATHOGENS**
Newborns	Group B *Streptococcus, Escherichia coli, Listeria monocytogenes*
Infants and children	*Streptococcus pneumoniae, Neisseria meningitidis, Haemophilus influenzae* type b
Adolescents and young adults	*Neisseria meningitidis, Streptococcus pneumoniae*

gococcus) has greatly decreased the incidence of bacterial meningitis. Vaccines for *H. influenzae* and *S. pneumoniae* are available for young children, and a vaccine for serogroup B *N. meningitidis* is available for individuals 10 to 25 years of age.[45] Meningitis is still prevalent in countries without access to these vaccines.[44] (Note that although many families are worried about potential side effects from giving their infants vaccines, the introduction of these vaccines has resulted in a drastic reduction of these serious illnesses; bacterial meningitis is just one example.)

Group B *Streptococcus* causes lethal meningitis and sepsis in neonates and is transmitted to the child from the mother's birth canal. *S. pneumoniae* is the most common cause for meningitis in children 1 to 23 months of age. Staphylococcal or streptococcal meningitis can occur in children of any age but shows a predilection for children who have had neurosurgical procedures, skull fracture, or systemic bacterial infection. Infections that originate in the middle ear, sinuses, or mastoid cells also may lead to *S. pneumoniae* infection in children. Children who have sickle cell disease or have undergone a splenectomy are particularly at risk for pneumococcal infection.[46] *Escherichia coli* and group B streptococcus are the most common causes of meningitis in the newborn period. The second most common microorganism causing bacterial meningitis, particularly in children younger than 4 years, is *Neisseria meningitidis* (meningococcus), and it has the potential to occur in epidemics, especially among teens and young adults who are more likely to be carriers of *N. meningitidis*.[47]

◆**PATHOPHYSIOLOGY.** Pathogens enter the nervous system by direct extension from a contiguous source (i.e., paranasal sinuses or mastoid cells) or, more commonly, by hematogenous spread (e.g., infective endocarditis, pneumonia, neurosurgical procedures, severe burns) (see Figs. 18.24 and 18.27). Many of these microorganisms have developed successful mechanisms to evade the normal defenses (see Chapter 10). Pathogens cross the blood-brain barrier, enter the cerebrospinal fluid, and multiply.[48] Bacterial toxins increase cerebrovascular permeability, causing alterations in blood flow and edema. Increased intracranial pressure (ICP) may be increased further by obstruction to the CSF circulation. Herniation of the brainstem causes death.

◆**CLINICAL MANIFESTATIONS.** Acute bacterial meningitis often is preceded by an upper respiratory tract or a gastrointestinal tract infection. Inflammation leads to the general symptoms of fever, headache, vomiting, and irritability. Specific symptoms of concern for meningitis include photophobia, nuchal and spinal rigidity, decreased level of consciousness, and seizures. Irritation of the meninges and spinal roots causes pain and resistance to neck flexion (nuchal rigidity), a positive Kernig sign (resistance to knee extension in the supine position with the hips and knees flexed against the body), and a positive Brudzinski sign (flexion of the knees and hips when the neck is flexed forward rapidly). With severe meningeal irritation the child may demonstrate opisthotonic posturing (rigid arching of the back with the head extended). Infants may have bulging fontanels. Meningococcal meningitis can produce a characteristic purpuric rash, particularly when there is sepsis.

◆**EVALUATION AND TREATMENT.** A definitive diagnosis is made by examination of CSF obtained from a lumbar puncture and by CSF and blood cultures. The principles of treatment are similar to those followed for adults (see Chapter 18) and are based on the culture results in which the causative microorganism is identified. Empirical antibiotic therapy should be initiated and continued until CSF cultures are negative or changed if the empirical therapy is not correct for the bacteria cultured from the CSF.[49] Bacterial lysis induced by antibiotics can cause sub-arachnoid inflammation; the severity may be reduced with corticosteroid treatment.[50] The factors that influence outcomes are the age of the child (mortality is highest in infants younger than 1 year), the infective microorganisms (the lowest mortality is in meningococcal meningitis and the highest in meningitis caused by gram-negative enteric micro-organisms), and the duration and extent of inflammation before treatment. Approximately 8% of children with *H. influenzae* meningitis die; 35% of the survivors have serious and permanent sensory or motor dysfunction caused by pressure on the peripheral nerves during the early phases of the illness. Approximately 5% of the children who survive meningitis have hearing deficits; 15% to 30% have cerebral damage, hydrocephalus, motor deficits, or sensory impairments.[51,52]

Viral Meningitis. Viral meningitis may result from direct infection by a virus, or it may be secondary to disease, such as measles, mumps, herpes, or leukemia. The hallmark of viral meningitis is a mononuclear pleocytosis in the CSF and the presence of normal blood glucose level.

The clinical manifestations are similar to those in bacterial meningitis, although usually milder. Isolation of the specific virus is difficult. An exception is when the virus responsible is the herpes simplex virus, which can occur in infants after exposure to herpesvirus type 2 in the birth canal, or sporadic cases caused by herpesvirus type 1, which is the type that causes cold sores. It is possible to test for herpesvirus and, unlike most of the other viruses, there is a specific antiviral medication, acyclovir. When a child has symptoms of bacterial or viral meningo-encephalitis, antibiotic and antiviral treatments are administered until the cause is determined.[53]

Human Immunodeficiency Virus Encephalopathy. Human immunodeficiency virus type 1 (HIV-1) causes a syndrome called *HIV-1 encephalopathy* (see Chapter 10 for details of HIV infection, which results in developmental delays and impaired brain growth in children not directly related to opportunistic infections in the brain).

◆**PATHOPHYSIOLOGY.** The CNS is a distinct reservoir for HIV-1, but the pathogenesis of HIV encephalopathy in children is not clearly understood. HIV-1 invades the CNS early in infection, primarily through infected monocytes/macrophages and CD4+ T lymphocytes. The presence of viral products and inflammatory mediators induce neurotoxicity that leads to neuronal injury and death, particularly in the immature brain.[54]

◆**CLINICAL MANIFESTATIONS.** The 1994 revised classification from the Centers for Disease Control and Prevention (CDC) requires one of the following progressing findings to be present for at least 2 months,[55] in the absence of a concurrent illness other than HIV that could explain the findings:

1. Failure to attain or loss of developmental milestones, or loss of intellectual ability, verified by standard developmental scale or neuropsychologic tests
2. Impaired brain growth or acquired microcephaly demonstrated by head circumference measurements or brain atrophy established by CT or MRI, with serial imaging required in children younger than 2 years
3. Acquired symmetric motor deficits manifested by two or more of the following: paresis, pathologic reflexes, ataxia, or gait disturbances

The onset of progressive encephalopathy may be a prognostic indicator of a poor outcome, and it may be difficult to completely differentiate the effects of HIV infection on the CNS from the effects of prenatal and perinatal exposures. In addition, other insults, such as drug exposure, prematurity, and chronic illness, may accompany HIV in a young child and affect growth and development.

◆**EVALUATION AND TREATMENT.** A definite diagnosis of HIV is made by patient history, viral culture, and clinical manifestations. Monitoring CD8+ T lymphocytes and monocytes, in addition to CD4+ T lympho-cytes, has been suggested for predicting risk for progressive encepha-lopathy. Decreases in CD8+ T lymphocytes diminish defenses against viral infection and facilitate infected monocytes to cross the blood-brain barrier. In general, treatment is focused on preservation and maintenance of the immune system, aggressive response to opportunistic infections, and support and relief of symptomatic occurrences by administration of highly active antiretroviral therapy (HAART). (HIV treatment is discussed in Chapter 10.) Progressive HIV encephalopathy is an infrequent and reversible complication of HIV infection because the disease responds to HAART.[56]

CEREBROVASCULAR DISEASE IN CHILDREN

Perinatal Stroke

Perinatal stroke is estimated to occur in about 1 to 2 in 5000 live births. Strokes can be either ischemic or hemorrhagic. Neonatal ischemic strokes occur between 20 weeks of fetal life and the 28th postnatal day and are confirmed by neuroimaging or neuropathologic studies. The cause is usually secondary to arterial or cerebral venous thrombosis or embolization.[57] Intraventricular hemorrhage (IVH) is a common complication of prematurity and is related to the fragility of an immature vasculature and the hemodynamic and respiratory instability associated with prematurity. Prenatal glucocorticoids are the most effective means of preventing IVH. Fifty percent to 75% of premature infants with IVH develop hydrocephalus, cerebral palsy, and/or intellectual disability.[58]

Children with perinatal stroke may not be diagnosed until later in infancy or childhood when it becomes apparent that the child is not moving one side of the body as much as the other. Early signs may consist of the family noticing that one hand is preferred over the other at an early age—typical "handedness" does not usually occur until 16 to 18 months of age—or one foot is dragging. An MRI is often performed at this point and is most likely to show evidence of a previous middle cerebral artery stroke. The clinical pattern that usually results from this type of stroke is contralateral hemiplegia, with the arm more affected than the leg. Children with hemiplegia caused by perinatal stroke (hemiplegic CP) are prone to seizures, although they generally do well cognitively. Testing for abnormalities in blood-clotting mechanisms, such as antithrombin enzyme activity, protein C and protein S deficiencies, or abnormal factor V Leiden, is often performed in children with prenatal stroke. Although often normal, abnormalities in these clotting mechanisms should be assessed because they may make the child prone to further vascular events.

Childhood Stroke

Childhood stroke occurs in about 1 to 13 per 100,000 live births (Box 20.3).[59]

Ischemic Stroke

Ischemic stroke is rare in children and may result from embolism, arteriopathy, or, rarely, sinovenous thrombosis leading to a decreased flow of blood and oxygen to areas of the brain. Children with arterial ischemic stroke do not have the typical adult risk factors, such as atherosclerosis and hypertension. Approximately 40% of children with ischemic stroke have no identifiable underlying risk factors. Sickle cell disease, cerebral arteriopathies, cardiac anomalies, and brain infections are the most common disorders that lead to arterial ischemic stroke.[60]

Hemorrhagic Stroke

Congenital cerebral arteriovenous malformations are the most common cause of intracranial bleeding and hemorrhagic stroke in children.[61] Hemorrhagic stroke may result from vascular anomalies that lead to rupture, such as aneurysm, or from congenital arteriovenous malformations (pial arteriovenous malformations, vein of Galen malformations, and arteriovenous fistulae). The rupture of a cerebral aneurysm is rare in children younger than 19 years. Intraventricular hemorrhage associated with premature birth is related to immature blood vessels and unstable blood pressure. There is a high risk of developing posthemorrhagic hydrocephalus.[62]

Moyamoya Disease

Moyamoya disease is a rare, chronic, progressive stenosis of the anterior circulation, such as the internal carotid arteries and middle cerebral arteries. *Moyamoya* is a Japanese term that means "puff of smoke," which describes the vascular appearance on cerebral angiogram. The disease is more common among the east Asian population. *Moyamoya* results from fibrocellular thickening of the intima of the arterial wall of large cerebral vessels. Obstruction of arterial flow to the brain occurs slowly, and neovascularization and increased collateral blood flow to ischemic areas develop. Moyamoya vasculopathy may be idiopathic, associated with certain genetic or metabolic syndromes, or develop as a result of cranial radiation therapy. Complications are developmental delay/intellectual disability, recurrent ischemic strokes, and cerebral hemorrhage. Treatment is surgical bypass of the ischemic region.[63] Symptoms of ischemic or hemorrhagic stroke may include degrees of hemiplegia (flaccid, spastic), weakness, seizures, headache, high fever, nuchal rigidity, hemianopia, sensory changes, facial palsy, and temporary aphasia.

Diagnosis of cerebrovascular disease is made through a series of tests, including imaging studies, particularly MRI. The most important factor in diagnosis is the recognition that children can have strokes, but this possibility is often not recognized. History of evolving neurologic symptoms (seizures, altered mental status, weakness, numbness on one side of body or face, expressive or sensory aphasia) for less than 12 hours and medical history are of vital importance in attaining an accurate diagnosis of stroke etiology, although causative factors often cannot be determined.[64] There is no evidence-based treatment for pediatric stroke. Prophylactic medications may be prescribed in those children who have suffered an ischemic stroke (e.g., aspirin, but Reye syndrome must be considered).[60] Arteriovenous malformations that may leak and cause hemorrhagic stroke vary in size, location, and symptoms, and these factors determine treatment. If a malformation is present, treatment options include endovascular, surgical, and radiosurgical techniques for embolic occlusion or resection of the malformation.[65] Excellent collateral circulation in the child's brain allows for more rapid recovery of motor function than in adults. The developing brain, however, may suffer more global, long-term effects leading to intellectual disability, behavior disorders, and seizures.

EPILEPSY AND SEIZURE DISORDERS IN CHILDREN

Epilepsy is defined as the occurrence of at least two unprovoked seizures more than 24 hours apart.[66] The incidence of epilepsy varies greatly with age, geographic location, and study design. The highest incidence is in children younger than 2 years of age and adults older than 65 years. Approximately 150,000 persons in the United States are newly

---

BOX 20.3 STROKE IN CHILDREN

- Risk factors different from those for adult (i.e., hypertension, atherosclerosis, diabetes, smoking, obesity)
- Important risk factors (causes) include:
  Ischemic stroke—heart disease or congenital cardiac disorders (most common), blood disorders, clotting or coagulation disorders, sickle cell anemia, infections (chickenpox, meningitis, encephalitis, Moyamoya disease), and arterial dissection
  Hemorrhagic stroke—vascular malformations, including arteriovenous malformations (AVMs) and aneurysms; blood disorders, including thrombocytopenia and leukemia; and malignancy, including intracranial tumors; head and neck trauma
- Vascular occlusion occurs more often in intracranial vessels (cerebral arteriopathy), including internal carotid, middle cerebral, and basilar arteries; infarcts more often limited to deep regions of the cerebral hemispheres, mostly basal ganglion and internal capsule areas.
- Intracerebral hemorrhage and subarachnoid hemorrhage account for a much higher percentage of strokes in children.
- Risk for recurrence and mortality appear to be low for neonatal and childhood stroke.

From Kirton A, deVeber G: *Lancet Neurol* 14(1):92-102, 2015; Lo WD, Kumar R: *Continuum (Minneap Minn)* 23(1, Cerebrovascular Disease):158-180, 2017; Numis AL, Fox CK: *Curr Neurol Neurosci Rep* 14(1):422, 2014; Moraitis E, Ganesan V: *Curr Cardiol Rep* 16(9):527, 2014.

diagnosed each year.[67] The focus of content in this section is related to children. Chapter 17 contains a general discussion of seizures and epilepsy and content related to adults.

Seizures are the abnormal autonomous discharge of electrical activity within the brain (an epileptogenic focus). When a sufficient number of neurons become overexcited, they discharge abnormally, which sometimes results in clinical manifestations (seizures) with alterations in motor function, sensation, autonomic function, behavior, and consciousness. Dysregulation of inhibitory $GABA_A$ neurotransmission with imbalance of glutamatergic excitatory mechanisms is speculated to be a cause of early childhood seizures. Dysregulation of other types of voltage- and ligand-gated ion channels (i.e., sodium, calcium, potassium, and chloride) is associated with genetically determined epileptic syndromes.[68] If seizures develop, the specific physical activity that occurs depends on the origin of the electrical activity and its extent within the brain. If a child has more than one unprovoked seizure, that child is said to have epilepsy, although there are a few exceptions—one example being febrile seizures. Seizures can be the result of an underlying disorder (e.g., meningitis or a brain tumor), or seizures themselves may be the primary disorder; the latter may have a genetic or a familial predisposition (for instance, childhood absence epilepsy and juvenile myoclonic epilepsy) (see later and Table 17.16 and Table 17.17). Nearly half of childhood epilepsy is of unknown etiology.[69]

Seizures and seizure patterns may change as a child grows and develops. The differences between the immature and mature nervous systems may help explain the changing patterns of clinical seizures with age. For example, febrile seizures manifest in children 6 months to 3 years of age, and juvenile myoclonic epilepsy is first noted in adolescence. The immature nervous system has a reduced capacity for sustaining well-organized seizures and, therefore, infants are prone to have seizures that occur only in small parts of the body compared to generalized tonic-clonic seizures in older children. This is because intracortical connections are poorly developed in children and the sending of impulses throughout the cortex is limited. At the cellular level, neurons are less capable of firing in repetitive high-frequency bursts. The excitatory output of a seizure focus is further diminished because the affected neurons do not act synchronously. In addition, changing neurotransmitters, immaturity of cells, and ongoing postnatal factors affect seizure expression in children.

During the newborn period, asphyxia, intracranial hemorrhage, CNS infection, injury, electrolyte imbalances, and inborn errors of metabolism may cause seizures. Despite an extensive search for a cause, the etiology often remains unknown. Infants and children may have seizures based on earlier brain damage (e.g., cerebral palsy) or may manifest specific epilepsy syndromes (childhood absence epilepsy, Lennox-Gastaut syndrome). Adolescents may have seizures caused by juvenile myoclonic epilepsy or because of other underlying conditions. There is an association between autism spectrum disorder and seizures; however, the mechanisms are unclear.[70]

The clinical manifestations at the time of the seizures vary depending on the primary cause and the extent and involvement of abnormal electrical discharges within the neuronal tissue. Because of the diversity and complexity that seizure activity invariably displays, an international classification system was adopted. This classification system groups seizures with similar clinical manifestations (see Table 17.17). Its general purpose is to assist the clinician with the type of evaluation needed, the identification of the most appropriate treatment, and the evaluation of the individual's response to treatment.[71]

Focal seizures are characterized by seizure activity that begins in and usually is limited to one part of either the left or the right hemisphere, and may occur with or without loss of consciousness. The clinical activity displayed is contingent on the particular part of the cortex from which the seizure is generated. For example, focal seizures may result in abnormal motor activity, such as twitching or loss of tone, or sensory changes, such as tingling or numbness (see Table 17.17).

Focal seizures may evolve into a generalized tonic, clonic, or atonic seizures. Focal seizures are more likely to be caused by an abnormality in a specific part of the brain, and thus brain imaging is usually performed in children whose seizures have started in a localized manner, even if they generalize later. Possibilities include brain tumors, small areas of localized brain damage, and other causes.

Generalized seizures are those in which the first clinical manifestations indicate that the seizure activity starts in or involves both cerebral hemispheres. Because both hemispheres are involved, the clinical manifestations are almost always bilateral. Consciousness may be impaired in this grouping of seizures. The clinical manifestations may include convulsive activity (tonic-clonic, tonic, clonic, myoclonic, myoclonic-atonic, or epileptic spasms) or absence seizures (nonconvulsive activity). Generalized seizures are more likely than focal seizures to have a genetic component; although the genetics of some of the epilepsy syndromes have been identified, many appear to have a multifactorial genetic etiology.[72]

Childhood absence epilepsy (also called *petit mal seizures* or *nonconvulsive epilepsy*) is a type of generalized epilepsy. The age of onset is 4 to 10 years. The genetic causes are unknown and probably multifactorial; it also can be sporadic. Mutations in inhibitory gamma-aminobutyric acid A ($GABA_A$) receptor subunit genes and ion channel genes are associated with absence seizures. The seizures are initiated at a cortical site and spread to other cortical areas and to the thalamus. The electroencephalogram (EEG) shows a characteristic bilateral 3-Hz spike-wave discharge. The characteristic absence seizure is of sudden onset and sudden termination, with impairment of consciousness and unresponsiveness usually lasting less than 10 seconds with no residual deficits. There is interruption of ongoing voluntary activity accompanied by staring, mild eyelid fluttering, or myoclonic jerks. There is no aura. Pallor is common. Seizures may be provoked by about 3 minutes of hyperventilation. Hundreds of seizures can occur per day, disrupting schoolwork and socialization. Behavioral, cognitive, and linguistic impairment is common. Antiepileptic drugs provide beneficial treatment.[73]

Epilepsy Syndromes

Epilepsy syndromes are seizure disorders that display a common group of signs and symptoms that occur in a recognizable pattern. Several syndromes associated with epilepsy occur in infants and children: neonatal seizure, febrile seizures, infantile spasms, Lennox-Gastaut syndrome, and juvenile myoclonic epilepsy.

Neonatal seizures have activity that includes rhythmic eye movements, chewing, and swimming movements. These seizures are more often associated with hypoxic-ischemic encephalopathy, transient metabolic disturbance, infection, stroke, or intracranial hemorrhage rather than neonatal-onset epilepsies, which may stem from malformation, prior injury, or genetic causes. The immature brain is hyperexcitable and vulnerable to seizure activity. Meticulous efforts are required for diagnosis, and there are no standardized treatment guidelines. Some seizures are self-limiting.[74,75]

Febrile seizures are defined as seizures associated with fever in the absence of central nervous system infection. They are divided into two types: simple febrile seizures and complex febrile seizures. Simple febrile seizures occur in 2% to 5% of children. They are benign and the most common childhood seizure.

The pathogenesis of simple febrile seizures is unknown. A familial incidence of simple febrile seizures indicates a genetic predisposition. Factors that contribute to susceptibility include age, degree and rate of temperature elevation, and nature of the particular fever-inducing illness.

Any disorder producing a high fever may provoke benign febrile seizures in susceptible children.

The following characteristic features distinguish simple febrile seizures from complex seizures precipitated by fever:

1. Simple febrile seizures usually occur between 3 months and 5 years of age.
2. The convulsion occurs with a rise in temperature to greater than 39°C (102.2°F).
3. An acute respiratory tract or ear infection usually is present, with no evidence of CNS infection or inflammation.
4. Most seizures occur during the first 24 hours of the illness.
5. The convulsion is short (15 minutes or less), generalized, and predominantly tonic.
6. Interictal (period between seizures) EEG is normal.
7. The seizure usually does not recur during the same infection.
8. No acute systemic metabolic disorder is present.

Complex febrile seizures have characteristic features similar to those of simple febrile seizures except that (1) they have a longer duration than do benign febrile seizures, usually longer than 15 minutes; (2) they have focal characteristics, confined to one side of the child's body; and (3) they usually occur more than once in a 24-hour period. The link between complex febrile seizures and the development of epilepsy continues to be evaluated.[76]

For febrile seizures, the cause of the child's fever should be determined, and meningitis should be considered in the differential diagnosis. Medications for preventing recurrence of simple febrile seizures are rarely used because side effects outweigh benefits.[77]

Infantile spasms (also known as West syndrome) are a severe form of epilepsy characterized by a variety of clinical manifestations. Children with infantile spasms have episodes consisting of sudden flexion or extension involving the neck, trunk, and extremities. Infantile spasms in some children are caused by underlying brain abnormalities such as intrauterine stroke or tuberous sclerosis, whereas others may be caused by mutations in one of several genes. Clinical manifestations of the resulting spasms may range from subtle head nods to violent body contractions, commonly referred to as *jackknife seizures*. Onset of infantile spasms usually is between 4 and 8 months of age and may be idiopathic or may occur in response to a CNS insult. An EEG will display the classic hypsarrhythmic pattern on a slow, disorganized background. After infantile spasms begin, there is usually a typical clinical course. The "spasms" usually occur in clusters and happen 5 to 150 times per day. They are usually worse when the infant is waking up or falling asleep. Once begun, the seizure activity increases in intensity and severity over time. Invariably, a loss of developmental milestones and disability is associated with this syndrome. A short-term course of adrenocorticotropic hormone or prednisolone is effective in many cases of infantile spasms.[78]

Infantile spasms are present in about 30% of children with tuberous sclerosis complex (TSC). TSC develops from autosomal dominant mutations in hamartin (*TSC1*) found on chromosome 9q34 or tuberin (*TSC2*) genes found on chromosome 16p13. *Tubers* are cortical developmental malformations in the brain; they also form in other organs (i.e., skin, heart, lung, kidneys). Epilepsy associated with TSC is often difficult to treat. Steroids or vigabatrin, which may cause vision defects, are the medications of choice for children with infantile spasms attributable to tuberous sclerosis because they seem to be particularly effective in these children.[79] Epilepsy surgery (resection of the epileptogenic zone of brain tissue or severing of the corpus callosum for intractable generalized epilepsy) also may be effective.[80]

Lennox-Gastaut syndrome is an epileptic syndrome characterized by an onset of seizures early in childhood; it occurs in males more often than females and begins between 1 and 8 years of age. This syndrome includes a variety of generalized seizures—predominantly tonic-clonic, atonic (drop attacks), akinetic, absence, and myoclonic activity and a specific pattern on EEG (slow spike and wave). Seizures associated with this syndrome are usually very difficult to treat. Children may be prescribed multiple medications and alternative therapies, such as a ketogenic diet (see *Nutrition & Disease*: Ketogenic Diet in Children with Epilepsy), vagal nerve stimulation, or epilepsy surgery. Although children may be developmentally on track when the seizures begin, development is usually affected and the future manifestation of intellectual disability is common.[81]

NUTRITION & DISEASE
Ketogenic Diet in Children with Epilepsy

The goal of the ketogenic diet is to maintain a state of ketosis, which appears to facilitate reduced seizure frequency and severity for difficult-to-control (medically refractory, nonsurgical) seizures in children. The diet may be helpful to children who do not respond to conventional therapy or have intolerable side effects from antiepileptic medications. Seizure reduction can occur within 5 to 14 days of initiating the diet and usually within 6 months with beneficial effects after discontinuation. Two basic approaches to the ketogenic diet are: (1) a traditional approach with four parts fat to one part carbohydrate/protein in the diet, and (2) the medium-chain triglyceride (MCT) approach, in which MCTs make up about 50% to 70% of the diet. Either diet may be unpalatable and difficult to follow, particularly if the child has free access to food. Carbohydrates can be added by 5-g increments after 3 to 6 months if there has been no seizure activity, provided ketosis is maintained. Both dietary approaches include adequate protein for growth. A medium-chain triglyceride diet, modified Atkins diet, or low glycemic index treatment can also induce ketosis and does not restrict protein, fluid, or calories. The mechanisms are not clearly understood, but enhanced mitochondrial respiration, adenosine triphosphate (ATP) production, and reduced reactive oxygen species formation may influence the dynamics of excitatory and inhibitory neurotransmitter systems in the brain and may be neuroprotective. Side effects can include acidosis, kidney stones, hypoglycemia, gastrointestinal distress, dehydration, lethargy, and poor growth. Most side effects are treatable.

Data from Agarwal et al: *SAGE Open Med* 5:2050312117712887, 2017; Lin A et al: *Pediatr Neurol* 68:35-39, 2017; Sampaio LPB, Takakura G, Manreza MLG: *Arq Neuropsiquiatr* 75(4):234-237, 2017.

Juvenile myoclonic epilepsy (JME) is a primary, generalized epilepsy that usually affects adolescents and young adults. Genetic factors are complex and are still being clarified. JME is a relatively benign form of epilepsy involving myoclonic jerks of the neck, shoulders, and arms as well as generalized tonic-clonic seizures. Myoclonic jerks typically occur after awakening. The seizures may occur singularly or repetitively. This form of epilepsy is commonly associated with a normal neurologic examination, normal intelligence, and a family history of seizures. Cognitive impairment and psychiatric disorders have been reported. Because clinical features can be subtle, JME is likely to be underdiagnosed. Children with this syndrome will usually need to take medications for life, but with appropriate treatment, seizures are well controlled.[82]

CHILDHOOD TUMORS
Brain Tumors

Brain tumors are the most common solid tumor and cause of cancer death in children[83] (see *What's New?* Childhood Brain Cancer Deaths). Approximately 45% of primary brain tumors in children are nonmalignant.[84] Overall, primary brain tumors account for nearly 26% of all childhood cancers, with an annual incidence of 5.37 per 100,000 for

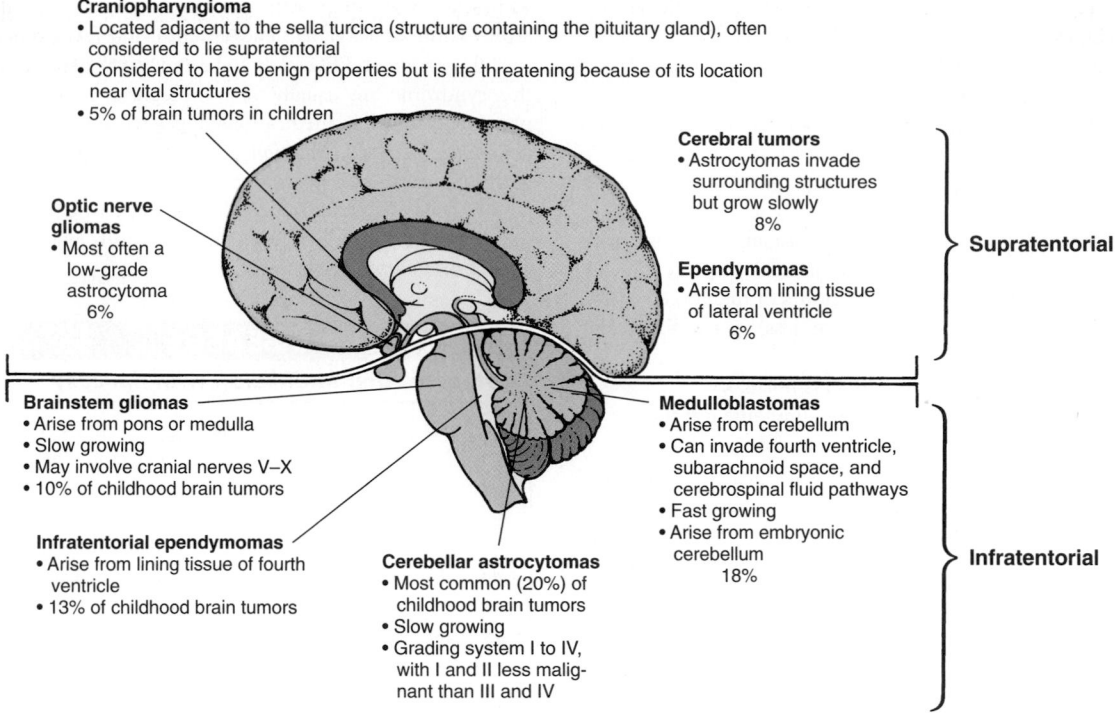

Craniopharyngioma
- Located adjacent to the sella turcica (structure containing the pituitary gland), often considered to lie supratentorial
- Considered to have benign properties but is life threatening because of its location near vital structures
- 5% of brain tumors in children

Optic nerve gliomas
- Most often a low-grade astrocytoma 6%

Cerebral tumors
- Astrocytomas invade surrounding structures but grow slowly 8%

Ependymomas
- Arise from lining tissue of lateral ventricle 6%

Supratentorial

Brainstem gliomas
- Arise from pons or medulla
- Slow growing
- May involve cranial nerves V–X
- 10% of childhood brain tumors

Infratentorial ependymomas
- Arise from lining tissue of fourth ventricle
- 13% of childhood brain tumors

Cerebellar astrocytomas
- Most common (20%) of childhood brain tumors
- Slow growing
- Grading system I to IV, with I and II less malignant than III and IV

Medulloblastomas
- Arise from cerebellum
- Can invade fourth ventricle, subarachnoid space, and cerebrospinal fluid pathways
- Fast growing
- Arise from embryonic cerebellum 18%

Infratentorial

FIGURE 20.15 Location and Approximate Percentage of Brain Tumors in Children.

primary malignant and nonmalignant tumors in the United States; approximately 4,630 new cases will be diagnosed in 2016. Many nonmalignant brain and CNS tumors are not histologically confirmed, and reporting varies across cancer registries. Survival at 5 years for primary malignant brain tumor for ages 0 to 19 years of age is 73.9%, varying significantly by tumor type, and there is often significant morbidity.[85]

Primary brain tumors arise from brain tissue and do not metastasize outside the brain. The cause of brain tumors is largely unknown, although genetic, environmental, and immune factors have been investigated. Exposure to ionizing radiation has been the only environmental factor consistently related to the development of brain tumors.[86]

◆PATHOPHYSIOLOGY. Brain tumors can arise from any CNS cell and are classified by cell type. Medulloblastoma, ependymoma, astrocytoma, brainstem glioma, craniopharyngioma, and optic nerve glioma constitute

approximately 75% to 80% of all pediatric brain tumors.[85] Germ cell tumors are rare. Two-thirds of all pediatric brain tumors in children are located in the posterior fossa (Fig. 20.15). Brain tumors spread by direct invasion or dissemination of cells through CSF. Specific characteristics, treatment strategies, and prognoses are listed in Table 20.6.

Brain tumors, by virtue of their location, have unique characteristics that distinguish them from tumors found elsewhere in the body. A number of brain tumors in children may be considered histologically benign yet clinically malignant and life threatening because of their location. For example, a tumor located in the brainstem may appear benign under the microscope, but the clinical presentation threatens and all too often overrides the vital functions of the brainstem.

◆CLINICAL MANIFESTATIONS. The location of the brain tumor, cell type, and rate of growth dictate the presenting signs and symptoms (discussed in greater detail with each particular brain tumor type). The ability of the brain and intracranial cavity to compensate for tumor growth is directly related to the rate of its growth. This compensatory mechanism allows the components of the intracranial space (blood, brain, and CSF) to adapt temporarily to slow changes in increased intracranial pressure. Therefore slow-growing tumors can grow to enormous size before signs and symptoms are apparent. Conversely, fast-growing tumors allow little time for compensation of the space-occupying lesion, and clinical symptoms occur quickly. Clinical symptoms may range from changes in personality to paralysis, depending on the location of the tumor.

Signs and symptoms of brain tumors in children vary from generalized and vague to those that are localized and related specifically to the area of the brain involved. If the tumor is located in the posterior fossa, the fourth ventricle may become blocked, which leads to obstructive hydrocephalus and signs of increased ICP. The symptoms of increased ICP include headache, vomiting, lethargy, and irritability. If a young child complains of repeated and worsening headache, a thorough investigation should take place because headache is an uncommon complaint in young children. Headache caused by increased ICP usually

TABLE 20.6   BRAIN TUMORS IN CHILDREN

TYPE	CHARACTERISTICS	TREATMENT	PROGNOSIS
Astrocytoma	Arises from astrocytes, often in cerebellum or lateral cerebral hemisphere Slow growing, solid or cystic Often very large before diagnosed Varies in degree of malignancy	*Cerebellar astrocytoma* Surgery; possibly curative Radiation and chemotherapy not proved successful but may delay recurrence *Cerebral astrocytoma* Surgery used if resection is possible Radiation useful for all grades of astrocytoma Chemotherapy beneficial in higher grade tumors but further study required	*Cerebellar astrocytoma* 90%–100% 5-year survival rate if pilocytic type (most common); if tumor recurs, it does so very slowly *Cerebral astrocytoma* 75% 5-year survival rate with lower grade tumors 20% 5-year survival rate if high-grade tumor
Optic pathway glioma	Arises from optic chiasm or optic nerve (association with neurofibromatosis type 1) Slow-growing, low-grade astrocytoma	In setting of visual impairment or progression (increase in size), chemotherapy is usual initial treatment Radiation therapy for tumors that progress or recur in spite of chemotherapy Surgery for large tumors, or hydrocephalus, or other complications; rarely for diagnosis	100% 5-year survival when confined to optic nerve 70% 5-year survival for tumor progression beyond optic chiasm
Medulloblastoma (infiltrating glioma)	Often located in cerebellum, extending into fourth ventricle and spinal fluid pathway Can extend outside central nervous system Rapidly growing malignant tumor	Type of treatment is age and tumor type dependent Surgery, primarily as partial resection to relieve increased intracranial pressure and "debulk" tumor Radiation as primary treatment; may include spinal radiation Chemotherapy showing some promise in conjunction with craniospinal radiation	65%–85% 5-year survival rate depending on stage/type
Brainstem glioma	Arises from pons Numerous cell types Compresses cranial nerves V through X	Surgery, resection occasionally possible Radiation, primarily palliative treatment Chemotherapy not yet proven beneficial, but new protocols being studied	20%–40% 5-year survival rate
Ependymoma	Arises from ependymal cells lining ventricles Circumscribed, solid, nodular tumors	Tumor possibly indolent for many years Surgery rarely curative; risk of resecting an infratentorial tumor too great Radiation for palliation (current controversy over whether local or craniospinal radiation is best) Chemotherapy used for recurrent disease but with disappointing results	20%–80% 5-year survival rate dependent on total resection
Craniopharyngioma	Arises near pituitary gland, optic chiasm, and hypothalamus Cystic and solid tumors that affect vision, pituitary, and hypothalamic functions	Surgery possibly successful when complete resection is performed (partial resection usually requires further treatment) Radiation after partial surgical resection Chemotherapy not commonly used	80%–95% 5-year survival rate

is worse in the morning and gradually improves during the day when the child is upright and venous drainage is enhanced. The frequency of headache and other symptoms increases as the tumor grows. Irritability or possible apathy and increased somnolence also may result from increased ICP. Like headache, vomiting occurs more commonly in the morning. It is often *not* preceded by nausea and may become projectile, differing from a gastrointestinal disturbance in that the child may be ready to eat immediately after vomiting. Other signs and symptoms that can accompany increased ICP include increased head circumference with bulging fontanels in children younger than 2 years, cranial nerve palsies, and papilledema.

Localized findings relate to the degree of disturbance in physiologic functioning in the area where the tumor is located. Children with infratentorial tumors exhibit localized signs of impaired coordination and balance, including ataxia, gait difficulties, truncal ataxia, and loss of balance. Medulloblastoma and ependymoma are embryonal tumors.

Medulloblastoma is the most common, develops in the vermis of the cerebellum, and may extend into the fourth ventricle. Angiogenesis is the hallmark of progressive medulloblastomas. Subclassifications based on histopathology and genomics are contributing to targeted therapy.[87] **Ependymoma** develops in the fourth ventricle and arises from the ependymal cells that line the ventricular system. Because both tumors are located in the posterior fossa region along the midline, presenting signs and symptoms are similar, and they are more likely to spread throughout the neuraxis. In contrast, cerebellar astrocytomas are located on the surface of the right or left cerebellar hemisphere and cause unilateral symptoms (occurring on the same side as the tumor), such as head tilt, limb ataxia, and nystagmus when the eyes are turned toward the side with the tumor.

Brainstem gliomas often cause a combination of cranial nerve involvement (facial weakness, limitation of horizontal eye movement), ataxia, and corticospinal tract dysfunction. A common clinical pattern includes unilateral paralysis of cranial nerves with contralateral paralysis of the arm and leg, hyperreflexia, and extensor plantar responses. Increased ICP can occur if there is expansion of the pons.[88]

The area of the sella turcica, the structure containing the pituitary gland, is the site of several childhood brain tumors. Most common in this group is **craniopharyngioma**. This tumor originates from the pituitary gland or hypothalamus. Usually slow growing, it may be quite large at the time of diagnosis with compression of the pituitary gland and hypothalamus and increased intracranial pressure. Symptoms include headache, seizures, diabetes insipidus, early onset of puberty, and growth delay. Other tumors located in this region of the brain include **optic gliomas**. Optic nerve gliomas are associated with neurofibromatosis type 1, a neurocutaneous condition characterized by café-au-lait macules on the skin and benign tumors of the skin. Tumors that involve the optic tract may cause complete unilateral blindness and hemianopia of the other eye. Optic atrophy is another common finding.

Supratentorial tumors of the cerebral hemispheres are more common in neonates and adolescents.[89] **Pilocytic astrocytomas** are the most common supratentorial tumors. These are localized (grade I) slow-growing, cyst-filled gliomas that are often completely removed surgically with very high survival rates. Tumors located in the cortex may cause focal cerebral dysfunction, weakness, hemiparesis, seizures, and visual changes. Involvement of particular lobes may result in more specific localized symptoms. For example, a tumor located in the frontal lobe may cause changes in affect and behavior, and a tumor in the occipital lobe may cause cortical blindness or blindness in half of the visual field.

◆**EVALUATION AND TREATMENT.** A child with signs and symptoms of a brain tumor requires a complete workup, including a neurologic, developmental, and ophthalmic examination. CT with contrast enhancement allows direct visualization of the tumor mass. MRI provides advanced, high-resolution examination of the brain and neoplasms. Small low-grade tumors not seen on CT may be detected by MRI. Magnetic resonance angiography (MRA) is very helpful in assessing the vascularity of the tumor and its relationship to major blood vessels. Spine MRI examination may be used to evaluate tumor dissemination along the spinal column. Lumbar puncture to examine CSF for tumor cells also may be performed. Histochemical and molecular genetic analysis of tumor tissue assists with tumor classification.

The most useful treatment for brain tumors is surgical resection. Surgery is important to establish the diagnosis, reduce tumor size, and relieve tumor compression and obstructive hydrocephalus when present. Some brain tumors, such as low-grade cerebellar astrocytomas, may be cured with complete resection alone. Contraindications to such interventions are tumors in which surgical resection and biopsy carry a high risk of mortality or serious morbidity (brainstem gliomas). In these instances, diagnosis is made on the basis of radiologic evidence and clinical manifestations.

Most brain tumors require additional radiation and chemotherapy. Although these treatments are essential for potential eradication of the brain tumor, radiation to a young child's brain is associated with significant morbidity, including acute- and long-term sequelae. Prognosis varies according to the type, classification, location of the brain tumor, and age of the child (see Table 20.6). Historically, survival rates have been low; however, advances have been made with the combination of surgery, radiation therapy, and chemotherapy. High-dose chemotherapy with autologous stem cell rescue has been used for treatment of resistant tumors.[90] Advances are being made in areas of immunotherapy and targeted molecular therapy.[91] Comprehensive care and management of these children and their families are vital. Multidisciplinary teams enhance the continuity and consistency needed to care for these children and their families.[92]

Neuroblastoma

Neuroblastoma is an embryonal tumor derived from neural crest cells that form the adrenal medulla and the sympathetic nervous system. Neuroblastoma involves a defect of embryonic tissue and is the most common extra-cranial solid tumor in infants less than 1 year of age. Seventy-five percent of neuroblastomas are found before the child is 5 years old, and onset after 10 years of age is rare. Occasionally, these tumors have been diagnosed at birth, with metastasis apparent in the placenta. The incidence is about 10.54 per million per year in children younger than 15 years. Black children are more likely to have high-risk disease and fatal outcomes. Approximately 70% of children with neuroblastoma have metastatic disease at diagnosis.[93] Neuroblastomas are heterogeneous and can spontaneously regress or become highly metastatic with low, intermediate, or high risk for recurrence. Prognosis is worse for children older than 2 years of age with disseminated disease. Neuroblastoma is sporadic in most children. Familial cases of neuroblastoma (1% to 2% of cases) are considered to have an autosomal dominant pattern of inheritance (mechanisms of inheritance are discussed in Chapter 4).

Ganglioneuroblastomas are localized tumors of an intermediate level of cellular differentiation composed of mature ganglion and myelin sheath. The most differentiated tumor is a **ganglioneuroma**, which is considered benign and does not metastasize. They are usually surgically removed.

◆**PATHOPHYSIOLOGY.** Neuroblastomas arise from neural crest tissue, and the mechanisms are not clearly understood. Both genetic and epigenetic events are involved. The most common location of neuroblastoma is in the retroperitoneal region (65% of cases), most often the adrenal medulla. The tumor is evident as an abdominal mass and may cause anorexia, bowel and bladder alteration, and sometimes spinal cord compression. The second most common location of neuroblastoma is the mediastinum (15% of cases), where the tumor may cause dyspnea or infection related to airway obstruction. Less commonly, neuroblastoma may arise from the cervical sympathetic ganglion (3% to 4% of cases). Cervical neuroblastoma often causes Horner syndrome, which consists of miosis (pupil contraction), ptosis (drooping eyelid), enophthalmos (backward displacement of the eyeball), and anhidrosis (sweat deficiency). Neuroblastoma presents with a neurologic syndrome called *opsoclonus-myoclonus syndrome* (jerky movements of the limbs, ataxia, and chaotic eye movements in all directions).[94]

◆**CLINICAL MANIFESTATIONS.** A number of systemic signs and symptoms are characteristic of neuroblastoma, including weight loss, irritability, fatigue, and fever. Intractable diarrhea occurs in 7% to 9% of children and is caused by tumor secretion of a hormone called *vasoactive intestinal polypeptide (VIP)*. More than 90% of children with neuroblastoma have increased amounts of catecholamines and associated metabolites in their urine. High levels of urinary catecholamines and serum ferritin are associated with a poor prognosis.

◆**EVALUATION AND TREATMENT.** Initial diagnostic studies are dictated by the location of the primary tumor. Diagnosis begins with a complete physical and neurologic examination. Laboratory analyses include measurement of levels of urinary catecholamines; plasma ferritin; serum neuron-specific enolase (NSE), an enzyme produced by neuronal tissues; and gangliosides, lipid molecules that may be shed from the surface of tumor cells; and bone marrow biopsy. Imaging studies assist with localization. The diagnosis of neuroblastoma is confirmed by surgical biopsy and histopathologic results. Antenatal ultrasound may detect the tumor in the antenatal period.[95]

Treatment is based on the extent of the disease and prognostic markers, such as age, *MYCN* copy numbers (a proto-oncogene), chromosome 11q status, DNA ploidy, and high serum ferritin or NSE levels.

Low-risk disease is treated surgically. Chemotherapy is used if there is recurrence. Intermediate-risk tumors are treated with surgery and chemotherapy. High-risk neuroblastomas are treated with high-dose chemotherapy and radiotherapy followed by transplantation of purged autologous bone marrow. Monoclonal antibody–based immunotherapy has been shown to be effective for high-risk tumors.[96] Approximately 50% of children with high-risk disease will die despite intensive therapy, although this percentage is improving.[97]

Retinoblastoma

Retinoblastoma is a rare congenital eye tumor of young children that originates in the retina of one or both eyes. Retinoblastoma can be either inherited and acquired. The inherited form of the disease generally is diagnosed during the first year of life. The acquired disease is most commonly diagnosed in children 2 to 3 years of age and involves unilateral disease.[98] Approximately 40% of retinoblastomas are inherited as an autosomal dominant trait with incomplete penetrance. The remaining 60% are acquired. About 200 to 300 children are diagnosed in the United States each year and 1 in 4 cases involves both eyes.[99]

◆**PATHOPHYSIOLOGY.** In the early 1970s, Knudson proposed the "two-hit" hypothesis to explain the occurrence of both hereditary and acquired forms of the disease.[100] This hypothesis predicts that two separate transforming events, or "hits," must occur in a normal retinoblast cell to cause the cancer. Further, it proposes that in the inherited form, the first hit or mutation occurs in the germ cell (inherited from either parent), and the mutation is contained in every cell of the child's body. Only a second, random mutation in a retinoblast cell is needed to transform that cell into cancer. Multiple tumors are observed in the inherited form because these second mutations are likely to occur in several of the approximately 1 to 2 million retinoblast cells. In contrast, the acquired form of retinoblastoma requires two independent hits or mutations to occur in the same somatic cell (after the egg is fertilized) for the transformation to cancer. This is much less likely to happen. Fig. 20.16 illustrates the two-mutation model for these two patterns of mutation.

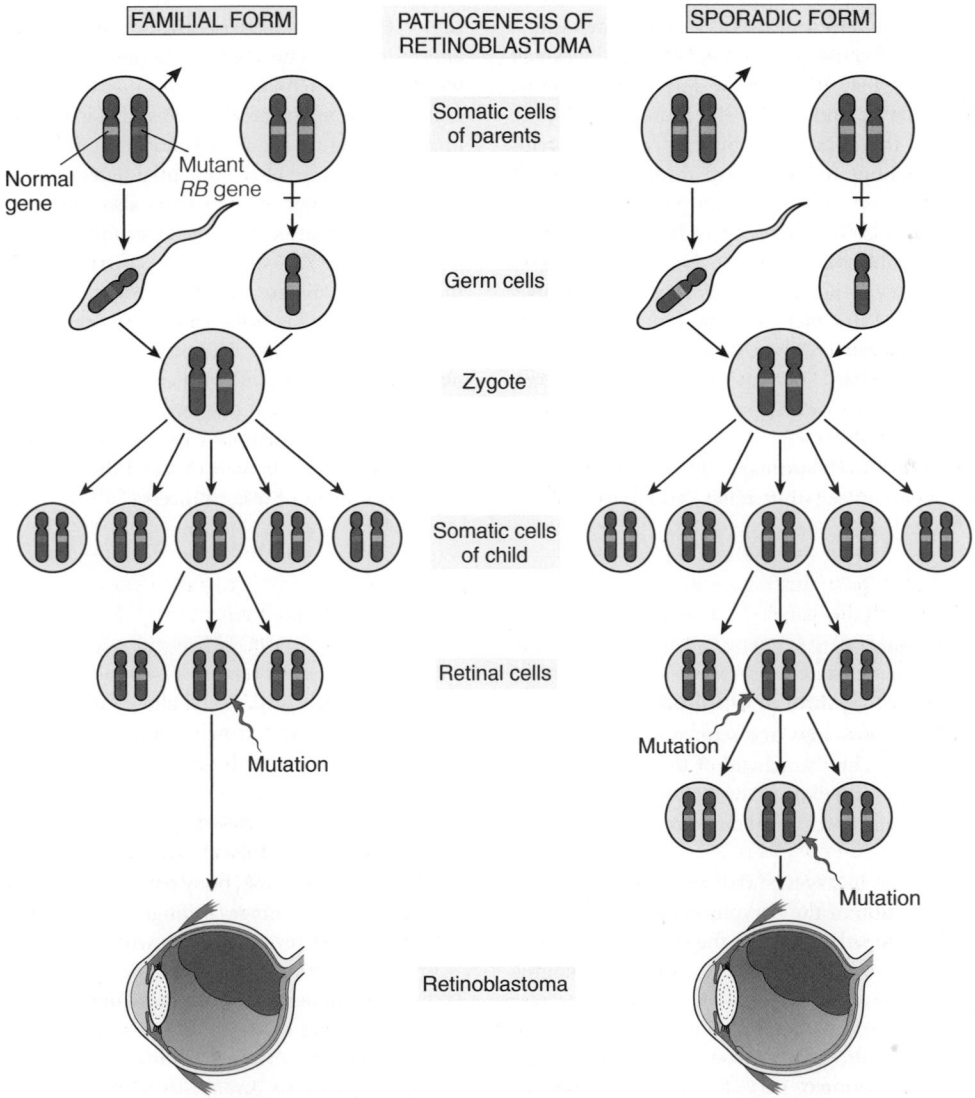

FIGURE 20.16 The Two-Mutation Model of Retinoblastoma Development. In inherited (familial) retinoblastoma, mutations of the *RB1* gene on chromosome 13q14 lead to neoplastic proliferation of retinal cells. The first mutation is transmitted through the germline of an affected parent. The second mutation occurs somatically in a retinal cell, leading to development of the tumor. In sporadic retinoblastoma, development of a tumor requires two somatic mutations. (From Kumar V, Cotran RS, Robbins SL: *Robbins basic pathology*, ed 8, Philadelphia, 2010, Saunders.)

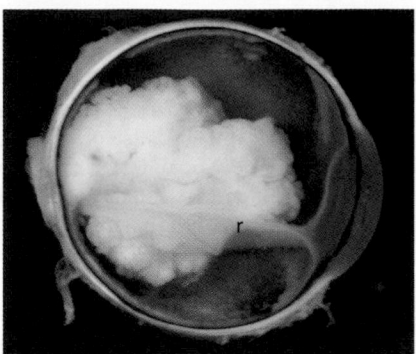

FIGURE 20.17 Retinoblastoma. Presence of white mass surrounding the detached retina *(r)*. (From Roberts F: *Semin Diagn Pathol* 33(3):114-121, 2016.)

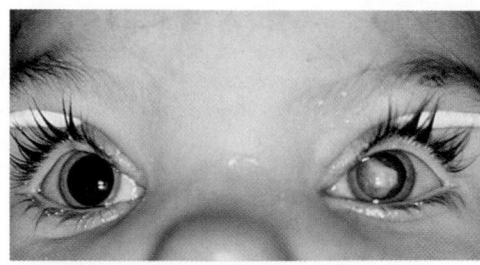

FIGURE 20.18 Retinoblastoma. The tumor occupies a large portion of the inside of the globe. (From Damjanov I: *Pathology for the health professions*, ed 3, St Louis, 2006, Saunders. Courtesy Dr. Walter Richardson and Dr. Jamsheed Khan, Kansas City, Kansas.)

Tumor formation usually begins with mutation in both alleles of the retinoblastoma tumor suppressor gene *RB1*, which codes for retinoblastoma protein. Retinoblastoma grows as one or more tumors in the retina and extends into the vitreous humor. Free-floating, small tumors in the vitreous humor may attach to the surface of the retina in multiple areas and proliferate and detach the retina (Fig. 20.17). The tumor also can invade the optic nerve by infiltrating the cribriform plate of the ethmoid bone or can spread through the sheath around the nerve. In either case the tumor can gain access to the subarachnoid space and the CNS. The tumor spreads into the choroid in 25% of children with retinoblastoma. Because the choroid is highly vascular, metastasis by means of hematogenous spread is possible. When hematogenous spread occurs, metastatic sites include the bone marrow, long bones, lymph nodes, and liver. If the tumor invades the orbit, lymphatic spread is possible. Spontaneous regression occurs, although infrequently, and may be caused by the tumor outgrowing its blood supply.[101]

◆ **CLINICAL MANIFESTATIONS.** The primary sign of retinoblastoma is leukocoria, a white pupillary reflex (white reflex) also called *cat's eye reflex*, which is caused by the mass behind the lens (see Fig. 20.18). This easy-to-identify sign can be missed. Other signs and symptoms include strabismus; a red, painful eye; and limited vision.

◆ **EVALUATION AND TREATMENT.** Because retinoblastoma is a treatable tumor, the priorities are saving the child's life, preservation of the eye, and restoring useful vision. Diagnostic evaluation for retinoblastoma includes documentation of family history; complete ophthalmologic examination; and metastatic studies that include bone marrow aspiration, lumbar puncture for spinal fluid examination, bone scan, and MRI scanning. Because of the potential hereditary risk to a child's siblings, all siblings younger than 4 years also should receive ophthalmologic evaluations. Treatment is related to tumor stage, number of tumor foci and unilateral (75% of cases, 10% carry *RB1* gene) or bilateral (carries the *RB1* gene) disease, vitreous seeding, and age of the child. The need for enucleation has been significantly reduced with the use of intra-arterial chemotherapy. The prognosis for most children with retinoblastoma is excellent, with greater than 90% long-term survival, although children with bilateral or metastatic disease at diagnosis have a poor prognosis. Approximately 75% of children have useful vision in the treated eye. Children with bilateral disease need to be monitored for the development of other cancers.[102,103]

▮ SUMMARY REVIEW

Development of the Nervous System in Children

1. The central nervous system develops in a sequential process from the ectodermal neural tube. The cranial end of the tube forms the brain, and the spinal cord is formed from the remainder of the tube.
2. The cranial and spinal ganglia (peripheral nervous system) develop from the neural crest.
3. The nervous system develops in stages, and disruption of any of the stages can lead to malfunction of the nervous system.
4. The bones of the skull are joined by sutures; the wide, membranous junctions of the sutures, known as *fontanels*, close by 20 months of age.
5. Myelin is a sheath that develops around axons to facilitate speed of nerve impulse conduction. Progressive development of reflexes corresponds to normal maturation of nerve tissue and development of voluntary movement.
6. Neurologic functioning at birth is at the subcortical level with reflex patterns mediated by the brainstem and spinal cord. With maturation, neonatal reflexes disappear and voluntary motor functions develop.

7. The fontanels of the skull allow for cranial expansion because the head is the fastest-growing body part during infancy. Sutures close by 5 to 8 years after birth.

Structural Malformations

1. Defects of neural tube closure include anencephaly (absence of part of the brain and soft, bony part of skull), encephalocele (protrusion of brain and meninges through a skull defect), and myelodysplasias: meningocele (cystlike defect with protrusion of spinal fluid–filled meninges through a vertebral defect), myelomeningocele (a defect like meningocele only also containing the spinal cord), and spina bifida (failure of the vertebrae to close with protrusion of neural tube contents with intact skin).
2. Craniosynostosis (craniostenosis) is premature closure of one or more of the cranial sutures and prevents normal skull expansion, causing compression of growing brain tissue.
3. Microcephaly is lack of brain growth and retarded mental and motor development.

SUMMARY REVIEW—cont'd

4. Cortical dysplasias are a heterogeneous group of disorders caused by defects in neuronal cell migration and subsequent abnormalities in connections between cells.

5. Congenital hydrocephalus results from an imbalance between the production and reabsorption of cerebrospinal fluid.

Alterations in Function: Encephalopathies

1. Static encephalopathies (i.e., cerebral palsy and epilepsy) are non-progressive disorders of the brain that can occur during gestation, birth, or childhood and can be caused by trauma or genetic factors.

2. Cerebral palsy (CP) is a group of nonprogressive syndromes that can be caused by prenatal cerebral hypoxia or perinatal or postnatal trauma with symptoms of intellectual disability, seizure disorders, or developmental disabilities. CP can be extrapyramidal/nonspastic or pyramidal/spastic.

3. Inherited disorders that damage the nervous system include metabolic defects in amino acid metabolism (phenylketonuria) and storage diseases.

4. Storage diseases, including lysosomal storage disease, are linked to a missing lysosomal enzyme, such as Tay-Sachs disease (GM_2 gangliosidosis). Both inherited disorders and storage diseases result in abnormal behavior, seizures, and deficient psychomotor development.

5. Poisonings from a variety of toxins can cause serious neurologic damage, including drugs and lead poisoning.

6. Infections of the nervous system include bacterial and viral infections, or aseptic meningitis.

7. Bacterial meningitis is commonly caused by *Haemophilus influenzae* type B, *S. pneumoniae*, or *N. meningitidis* and may result from respiratory tract or gastrointestinal tract infections with symptoms of fever, headache, photophobia, seizure, rigidity, and stupor.

8. Viral meningitis presents similar to bacterial meningitis, and the specific virus is often unknown.

9. HIV-1 encephalopathy is a CNS infection that can occur in infants and children.

Cerebrovascular Disease in Children

1. Perinatal strokes can be either ischemic or hemorrhagic and occur between the 20th week of fetal life and 28th postnatal day, usually secondary to arterial or cerebral venous thrombosis, embolization, or intraventricular hemorrhage.

2. Ischemic stroke is rare in children and may result from embolism, arteriopathy, or, rarely, sinovenous thrombosis.

3. Hemorrhagic stroke results from congenital arteriovenous malformations that rupture and cause intracranial bleeding.

Epilepsy and Seizure Disorders in Children

1. Epilepsy is the occurrence of seizures. Seizures are the abnormal discharge of electrical activity within the brain. Seizure disorders are associated with numerous nervous system disorders and more often are a generalized rather than a focal type of seizure.

2. Generalized forms of seizures involve both brain hemispheres and include tonic-clonic, myoclonic, atonic, akinetic, and infantile spasms.

3. Focal seizures suggest more localized brain dysfunction.

4. Childhood absence epilepsy (petit mal seizures or nonconvulsive epilepsy) is a type of generalized epilepsy.

5. Epilepsy syndromes include febrile seizures, infantile spasms, Lennox-Gastaut syndrome, and juvenile myoclonic epilepsy.

6. Unclassified epileptic seizure that do not fit neatly into a classified grouping include neonatal seizures and febrile seizures.

Childhood Tumors

1. Brain tumors are the most common primary neoplasm and cause of cancer death in children. They are classified by cell type as medulloblastoma, ependymoma, gliomas (astrocytoma, brainstem glioma, and optic nerve glioma), and craniopharyngioma.

2. Tumors in children are most often located below the tentorial membrane in the posterior fossa.

3. Fast-growing tumors produce symptoms early in the disease, whereas slow-growing tumors may become very large before symptoms appear.

4. Symptoms of brain tumors may be generalized or localized. The most common general symptom is increased ICP (headache, irritability, vomiting, somnolence, and bulging of fontanels).

5. Localized signs of infratentorial tumors in the cerebellum include impaired coordination and balance. Cranial nerve signs occur with tumors near the brainstem.

6. Supratentorial tumors may be located near the cortex or deep in the brain. Symptoms depend on the specific location of the tumor.

7. Neuroblastoma is an embryonal tumor of the sympathetic nervous system and can be located anywhere there is sympathetic nervous tissue. It is the most common type of solid tumor occurring in the first year.

8. Symptoms are related to tumor location and size and site of metastasis.

9. Retinoblastoma is a rare, congenital eye tumor of young children that originates in the retina of one or both eyes and may be inherited or acquired.

KEY TERMS

Acute bacterial meningitis, 631
Alar plate, 620
Anencephaly, 621
Arnold-Chiari malformation, 622
Arterial ischemic stroke, 633
Aseptic meningitis, 631
Ataxic cerebral palsy, 627
Basal plate, 619
Brainstem glioma, 637
Cerebellar astrocytoma, 637
Cerebral palsy (CP), 626
Childhood absence epilepsy, 634
Complex febrile seizure, 635
Congenital hydrocephalus, 625

Cortical dysplasia, 624
Cranial meningocele, 621
Craniopharyngioma, 638
Craniosynostosis (craniostenosis), 624
Cyclopia, 621
Dandy-Walker malformation (DWM), 626
Dyskinetic (dystonic and athetoid) cerebral palsy, 627
Encephalitis, 631
Encephalocele, 621
Encephalopathy, 626
Ependymoma, 637
Epilepsy, 633
Epileptogenic focus, 634

Extrapyramidal/nonspastic cerebral palsy, 627
Febrile seizure, 634
Focal seizure, 634
Fontanels, 620
Ganglioneuroblastoma, 638
Ganglioneuroma, 638
Gangliosidosis, 630
Generalized seizure, 634
Hemorrhagic stroke, 633
Infantile spasms (West syndrome), 635
Juvenile myoclonic epilepsy (JME), 635
Lennox-Gastaut syndrome, 635
Lysosomal storage disease, 630
Medulloblastoma, 637

KEY TERMS—cont'd

Meningitis, 631
Meningocele, 621
Microcephaly, 624
Moyamoya disease, 633
Myelodysplasia, 621
Myelomeningocele, 621
Neonatal seizure, 634
Neural crest, 619
Neural tube, 619

Neural tube defect (NTD), 621
Neuroblastoma, 638
Optic glioma, 638
Phenylketonuria (PKU), 629
Pica, 630
Pilocytic astrocytoma, 638
Pyramidal/spastic cerebral palsy, 626
Retinoblastoma, 639
Seizure, 634

Somite, 620
Spina bifida (split spine), 621
Spina bifida occulta, 624
Sulcus limitans, 619
Syndromic craniosynostosis, 624
Tay-Sachs disease (GM_2 gangliosidosis), 630
Tethered cord syndrome, 624
Tuberous sclerosis complex (TSC), 635
Viral meningitis, 632

REFERENCES

1. National Center on Birth Defects and Developmental Disabilities: *Folic acid: reducing folic acid-preventable neural tube defects.* Updated April 2, 2012. Available at: www.cdc.gov/ncbddd/aboutus/birthdefects-folicacid.html.
2. Centers for Disease Control and Prevention (CDC): *Facts about anencephaly,* Updated March 26, 2013. Available at: www.cdc.gov/ncbddd/birthdefects/anencephaly.html.
3. De Marco P, et al: Human neural tube defects: genetic causes and prevention. *Biofactors* 37(4): 261–268, 2011.
4. Williams J, et al: Updated estimates of neural tube defects prevented by mandatory folic acid fortification—United States, 1995-2011. *MMWR Morb Mortal Wkly Rep* 64(1):1–5, 2015.
5. US Preventive Service Task Force: *Folic acid to prevent neural tube defects: preventive medication,* released May 2009, current as of July 2015. Available at: http://www.uspreventiveservicestaskforce.org/Page/Document/UpdateSummaryFinal/folic-acid-to-prevent-neural-tube-defects-preventive-medication.
6. Krantz DA, Hallahan TW, Sherwin JE: Screening for open neural tube defects. *Clin Lab Med* 30(3): 721–725, 2010.
7. Centers for Disease Control and Prevention (CDC): *Facts about encephalocele,* Updated February 25, 2011. Available at: www.cdc.gov/ncbddd/birthdefects/encephalocele.html.
8. Shaer CM, Chescheir N, Schulkin J: Myelomeningocele: a review of the epidemiology, genetics, risk factors for conception, prenatal diagnosis, and prognosis for affected individuals. *Obstet Gynecol Surv* 62(7):471–479, 2007.
9. Tamburrini G, et al: Myelomeningocele: the management of the associated hydrocephalus. *Childs Nerv Syst* 29(9):1569–1579, 2013.
10. Salman MS: Posterior fossa decompression and the cerebellum in Chiari type II malformation: a preliminary MRI study. *Childs Nerv Syst* 27(3): 457–462, 2011.
11. Keller BA, Farmer DL: Fetal surgery for myelomeningocele: history, research, clinical trials, and future directions. *Minerva Pediatr* 67(4): 341–356, 2015.
12. Mehta VA, et al: Spinal cord tethering following myelomeningocele repair. *J Neurosurg Pediatr* 6(5):498–505, 2010.
13. Di Rocco F, Arnaud E, Renier D: Evolution in the frequency of nonsyndromic craniosynostosis. *J Neurosurg Pediatr* 4(1):21–25, 2009.
14. Governale LS: Craniosynostosis. *Pediatr Neurol* 53(5):394–401, 2015.
15. Desikan RS, Barkovich AJ: Malformations of cortical development. *Ann Neurol* 80(6):797–810, 2016.

16. Alvarado MG, Schwartz DA: Zika virus infection in pregnancy, microcephaly, and maternal and fetal health: what we think, what we know, and what we think we know. *Arch Pathol Lab Med* 141(1):26–32, 2017.
17. Crino PB: Focal cortical dysplasia. *Semin Neurol* 35(3):201–208, 2015.
18. Kahle KT, et al: Hydrocephalus in children. *Lancet* 387(10020):788–799, 2016.
19. Garton HJ, Platt JH, Jr: Hydrocephalus. *Pediatr Clin North Am* 51(2):305–325, 2004.
20. Jackson PL: Hydrocephalus. In Jackson PL, Vessey JA, editors: *Primary care of the child with a chronic condition,* ed 4, St Louis, 2003, Mosby.
21. Gandolfi Colleoni G, et al: Prenatal diagnosis and outcome of fetal posterior fossa fluid collections. *Ultrasound Obstet Gynecol* 39(6): 625–631, 2012.
22. Centers for Disease Control and Prevention (CDCP): *Cerebral palsy (CP).* Updated July 31, 2015. Available at: http://www.cdc.gov/ncbddd/cp/data.html.
23. Jones MW, et al: Cerebral palsy: introduction and diagnosis (part I). *J Pediatr Health Care* 21(3): 146–152, 2007.
24. Krigger KW: Cerebral palsy: an overview. *Am Fam Physician* 73(1):91–100, 2006.
25. Chan G, Miller F: Assessment and treatment of children with cerebral palsy. *Orthop Clin North Am* 45(3):313–325, 2014.
26. Jones KB, et al: Care of adults with intellectual and developmental disabilities: cerebral palsy. *FP Essent* 439:26–30, 2015.
27. Novak I, et al: Clinical prognostic messages from a systematic review on cerebral palsy. *Pediatrics* 130(5):e1285–e1312, 2012.
28. Gleason CA, Devaskar S: *Avery's diseases of the newborn,* ed 9, Philadelphia, 2012, Saunders.
29. March of Dimes: *PKU (phenylketonuria) in your baby.* Available at: http://www.marchofdimes.org/baby/phenylketonuria-in-your-baby.aspx.
30. Blau N, van Spronsen FJ, Levy HL: Phenylketonuria. *Lancet* 376(9750):1417–1427, 2010.
31. Blau N: Genetics of phenylketonuria: then and now. *Hum Mutat* 37(6):508–515, 2016.
32. Somaraju UR, Merrin M: Sapropterin dihydrochloride for phenylketonuria. *Cochrane Database Syst Rev* (3):CD008005, 2015.
33. Kingma SD, Bodamer OA, Wijburg FA: Epidemiology and diagnosis of lysosomal storage disorders; challenges of screening. *Best Pract Res Clin Endocrinol Metab* 29(2):145–157, 2015.
34. Scarpa M, et al: Neuronopathic lysosomal storage disorders: approaches to treat the central nervous system. *Best Pract Res Clin Endocrinol Metab* 29(2):159–171, 2015.

35. Lew RM, et al: Tay-Sachs disease: current perspectives from Australia. *Appl Clin Genet* 8:19–25, 2015.
36. Poison Control National Capital Poison Center: *Poison statistics national data,* 2014. Available at: http://www.poison.org/poison-statistics-national.
37. Abelsohn AR, Sanborn M: Lead and children: clinical management for family physicians. *Can Fam Physician* 56(6):531–535, 2010.
38. Bellinger DC: Very low lead exposures and children's neurodevelopment. *Curr Opin Pediatr* 20(2):172–177, 2008.
39. Keller B, et al: Epidemiologic characteristics of children with blood lead levels ≥45 µg/dL. *J Pediatr* 180:229–234, 2017.
40. Centers for Disease Control and Prevention (CDC): Blood levels in children aged 1–5 years—United States. *MMWR Morb Mortal Wkly Rep* 62(13):245–248, 2012.
41. Jones RL, et al: Trends in blood lead levels and blood lead testing among U.S. children aged 1 to 5 years, 1988-2004. *Pediatrics* 123(3):e376–e385, 2009.
42. Dapul H, Laraque D: Lead poisoning in children. *Adv Pediatr* 61(1):313–333, 2014.
43. Newman N, et al: *Fact sheet: recommendations on medical management of childhood lead exposure and poisoning.* Pediatric Environmental Health Specialty Unit (PEHSU) Network, June 2013 update. Available at: http://www.pehsu.net/_Childhood_Lead_Exposure.html.
44. Thigpen MC, et al: Bacterial meningitis in the United States, 1998-2007. *N Engl J Med* 364(21): 2016–2025, 2011.
45. Centers for Disease Control and Prevention (CDC): *Meningococcal vaccination.* Available at: http://www.cdc.gov/meningococcal/vaccine-info.html.
46. Ramakrishnan M, et al: Increased risk of invasive bacterial infections in African people with sickle-cell disease: a systematic review and meta-analysis. *Lancet Infect Dis* 10(5):329–337, 2010.
47. Gabutti G, Stefanati A, Kuhdari P: Epidemiology of Neisseria meningitidis infections: case distribution by age and relevance of carriage. *J Prev Med Hyg* 56(3):E116–E120, 2015.
48. Wang S, et al: Pathogenic triad in bacterial meningitis: pathogen invasion, NF-κB activation, and leukocyte transmigration that occur at the blood brain barrier. *Front Microbiol* 7:148, 2016.
49. Bosis S, Mayer A, Esposito S: Meningococcal disease in childhood: epidemiology, clinical features and prevention. *J Prev Med Hyg* 56(3): E121–E124, 2015.
50. Ogunlesi TA, Odigwe CC, Oladapo OT: Adjuvant corticosteroids for reducing death in neonatal

bacterial meningitis. *Cochrane Database Syst Rev* (11):CD010435, 2015.

51. Lepage P, Dan B: Infantile and childhood bacterial meningitis. *Handb Clin Neurol* 112:1115–1125, 2013.

52. Sabatini C, et al: Clinical presentation of meningococcal disease in childhood. *J Prev Med Hyg* 53(2):116–119, 2012.

53. Nigrovic LE: Aseptic meningitis. *Handb Clin Neurol* 112:1153–1156, 2013.

54. Donald KA, et al: Neurologic complications of pediatric human immunodeficiency virus: implications for clinical practice and management challenges in the African setting. *Semin Pediatr Neurol* 21(1):3–11, 2014.

55. Centers for Disease Control and Prevention (CDC): 1994 revised classification system for human immunodeficiency virus infection in children less than 13 years of age. *MMWR Morb Mortal Wkly Rep* 43(12):1, 1994. Available at: www.cdc.gov/mmwr/preview/mmwrhtml/00032890.htm.

56. Luzuriaga K: Early combination antiretroviral therapy limits HIV-1 persistence in children. *Annu Rev Med* 67:201–213, 2016.

57. Saxonhouse MA: Thrombosis in the neonatal intensive care unit. *Clin Perinatol* 42(3):651–673, 2015.

58. Ballabh P: Pathogenesis and prevention of intraventricular hemorrhage. *Clin Perinatol* 41(1):47–67, 2014.

59. Mallick AA, O'Callaghan FJ: The epidemiology of childhood stroke. *Eur J Paediatr Neurol* 14(3): 197–205, 2010.

60. Rosa M, et al: Paediatric arterial ischemic stroke: acute management, recent advances and remaining issues. *Ital J Pediatr* 41:95, 2015.

61. Beslow LA, Jordan LC: Pediatric stroke: the importance of cerebral arteriopathy and vascular malformations. *Childs Nerv Syst* 26(10): 1263–1273, 2010.

62. Toma AK, et al: Cerebral arteriovenous shunts in children. *Neuroimaging Clin N Am* 23(4):757–770, 2013.

63. Bang OY, Fujimura M, Kim SK: The pathophysiology of Moyamoya disease: an update. *J Stroke* 18(1):12–20, 2016.

64. Bernard TJ, et al: Preparing for a "pediatric stroke alert". *Pediatr Neurol* 56:18–24, 2016.

65. Gross BA, et al: Microsurgical treatment of arteriovenous malformations in pediatric patients: the Boston Children's Hospital experience. *J Neurosurg Pediatr* 15(1):71–77, 2015.

66. Fisher RS: ILAE official report: a practical clinical definition of epilepsy. *Epilepsia* 55(4):475–482, 2014.

67. Epilepsy Foundation: *About epilepsy: incidence and prevalence.* Reviewed March 2014. Available at: http://www.epilepsy.com/learn/epilepsy-statistics.

68. Orsini A, Zara F, Striano P: Recent advances in epilepsy genetics. *Neurosci Lett* 2017 May 10. [Epub ahead of print].

69. Berg AT, et al: Revised terminology and concepts for organization of seizures and epilepsies: report of the ILAE Commission on Classification and Terminology, 2005-2009. *Epilepsia* 51(4):676–685, 2010.

70. Frye RE, et al: Neuropathological mechanisms of seizures in autism spectrum disorder. *Front Neurosci* 10:192, 2016.

71. Fisher RS: The new classification of seizures by the International League Against Epilepsy. *Curr Neurol Neurosci Rep* 17(6):48–2017, 2017.

72. Staley K: Molecular mechanisms of epilepsy. *Nat Neurosci* 18(3):367–372, 2015.

73. Matricardi S, et al: Current advances in childhood absence epilepsy. *Pediatr Neurol* 50(3):205–212, 2014.

74. Glass HC: Neonatal seizures: advances in mechanisms and management. *Clin Perinatol* 41(1):177–190, 2014.

75. Shetty J: Neonatal seizures in hypoxic-ischaemic encephalopathy—risks and benefits of anticonvulsant therapy. *Dev Med Child Neurol* 57(Suppl 3):40–43, 2015.

76. Patel AD, Vidaurre J: Complex febrile seizures: a practical guide to evaluation and treatment. *J Child Neurol* 28(6):762–767, 2013.

77. Mastrangelo M, Midulla F, Moretti C: Actual insights into the clinical management of febrile seizures. *Eur J Pediatr* 173(8):977–982, 2014.

78. Go CY, et al: Evidence-based guideline update: medical treatment of infantile spasms. Report of the Guideline Development Subcommittee of the American Academy of Neurology and the Practice Committee of the Child Neurology Society. *Neurology* 78(24):1974–1980, 2012.

79. Song JM, et al: Efficacy of treatments for infantile spasms: a systematic review. *Clin Neuropharmacol* 40(2):63–84, 2017.

80. Overwater IE, et al: Epilepsy in children with tuberous sclerosis complex: chance of remission and response to antiepileptic drugs. *Epilepsia* 56(8):1239–1245, 2015.

81. Al-Banji MH, Zahr DK, Jan MM: Lennox-Gastaut syndrome. Management update. *Neurosciences (Riyadh)* 20(3):207–212, 2015.

82. Wolf P, et al: Juvenile myoclonic epilepsy: a system disorder of the brain. *Epilepsy Res* 114:2–12, 2015.

83. Centers for Disease Control and Prevention, National Center for Health Statistics: *Declines in cancer death rates among children and adolescents in the United States, 1999–2014,* NCHS Data Brief N 257, September, 2016. Available at: http://www.cdc.gov/nchs/products/databriefs/db257.htm.

84. Kohler BA, et al: Annual report to the nation on the status of cancer, 1975-2007, featuring tumors of the brain and other nervous system. *J Natl Cancer Inst* 103(9):714–736, 2011.

85. Central Brain Tumor Registry of the United States: *2015 CBTRUS fact sheet.* Available at: http://www.cbtrus.org/factsheet/factsheet.html.

86. McNeill KA: Epidemiology of brain tumors. *Neurol Clin* 34(4):981–998, 2016.

87. Samkari A, White JC, Packer RJ: Medulloblastoma: toward biologically based management. *Semin Pediatr Neurol* 22(1):6–13, 2015.

88. PDQ Pediatric Treatment Editorial Board: Childhood brain stem glioma treatment (PDQ®): health professional version, 2017 Jun 2. *PDQ cancer information summaries [Internet]*, Bethesda, MD, 2017, National Cancer Institute. Available from: http://www.ncbi.nlm.nih.gov/books/NBK65812/.

89. Zamora C, Huisman TA, Izbudak I: Supratentorial tumors in pediatric patients. *Neuroimaging Clin N Am* 27(1):39–67, 2017.

90. Ajeawung NF, Wang HY, Kamnasaran D: Progress from clinical trials and emerging non-conventional therapies for the treatment of Medulloblastomas. *Cancer Lett* 330(2):130–140, 2013.

91. Esparza R, et al: Glioblastoma stem cells and stem cell-targeting immunotherapies. *J Neurooncol* 123(3):449–457, 2015.

92. Abdel-Baki MS, Hanzlik E, Kieran MW: Multidisciplinary pediatric brain tumor clinics: the key to successful treatment? *CNS Oncol* 4(3):147–155, 2015.

93. National Cancer Institute: *General information about neuroblastoma.* Updated January 14, 2016. Available at: http://www.cancer.gov/types/neuroblastoma/hp/neuroblastoma-treatment-pdq#link/_866.

94. Singhi P, et al: Clinical profile and outcome of children with opsoclonus-myoclonus syndrome. *J Child Neurol* 29(1):58–61, 2014.

95. Newman EA, Nuchtern JG: Recent biologic and genetic advances in neuroblastoma: implications for diagnostic, risk stratification, and treatment strategies. *Semin Pediatr Surg* 25(5):257–264, 2016.

96. Croce M, et al: New immunotherapeutic strategies for the treatment of neuroblastoma. *Immunotherapy* 7(3):285–300, 2015.

97. Matthay KK, et al: Neuroblastoma. *Nat Rev Dis Primers* 2:16078, 2016.

98. Rodriguez-Galindo C, et al: Retinoblastoma. *Pediatr Clin North Am* 62(1):201–223, 2015.

99. American Cancer Society (ACS): *What are the key statistics about retinoblastoma?* Last revised August 16, 2012. Available at: www.cancer.org/Cancer/Retinoblastoma/DetailedGuide/retinoblastoma-key-statistics.

100. Knudson AG, Jr: Mutation and cancer: a statistical study of retinoblastoma. *Proc Natl Acad Sci USA* 68(4):820–823, 1971.

101. Mendoza PR, Grossniklaus HE: The biology of retinoblastoma. *Prog Mol Biol Transl Sci* 134: 503–516, 2015.

102. Chantada G, Schaiquevich P: Management of retinoblastoma in children: current status. *Paediatr Drugs* 17(3):185–198, 2015.

103. Rodriguez-Galindo C, Orbach DB, VanderVeen D: Retinoblastoma. *Pediatr Clin North Am* 62(1): 201–223, 2015.

CHAPTER
21

Mechanisms of Hormonal Regulation

Valentina L. Brashers, Sue E. Huether

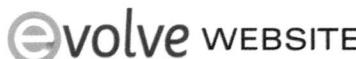
WEBSITE

http://evolve.elsevier.com/McCance/
- Content Updates
- Chapter Summary Review
- Review Questions
- Case Studies
- Animations

CHAPTER OUTLINE

The endocrine system is composed of various glands located throughout the body (Fig. 21.1). These glands synthesize and release special chemical messengers called **hormones**. In addition, numerous hormones are synthesized and released from endocrine cells within the upper and lower gastrointestinal tract (i.e., incretins). The endocrine system has five general functions:

1. Differentiation of the reproductive and central nervous systems in the developing fetus
2. Stimulation of sequential growth and development during childhood and adolescence
3. Coordination of the male and female reproductive systems, which makes sexual reproduction possible
4. Maintenance of an optimal internal environment throughout the life span

5. Initiation of corrective and adaptive responses when emergency demands occur

The endocrine, nervous, and immune systems work together to regulate responses to the internal and external environments. Hormones convey specific regulatory information among cells and organs and are integrated with the nervous system to maintain communication and control. The mechanisms of communication and control occur within a cell *(autocrine)*, between local cells *(paracrine)*, and between cells located remotely from each other *(endocrine)*.

MECHANISMS OF HORMONAL REGULATION

Endocrine glands respond to specific signals by synthesizing and releasing hormones into the circulation, which then trigger intracellular responses.

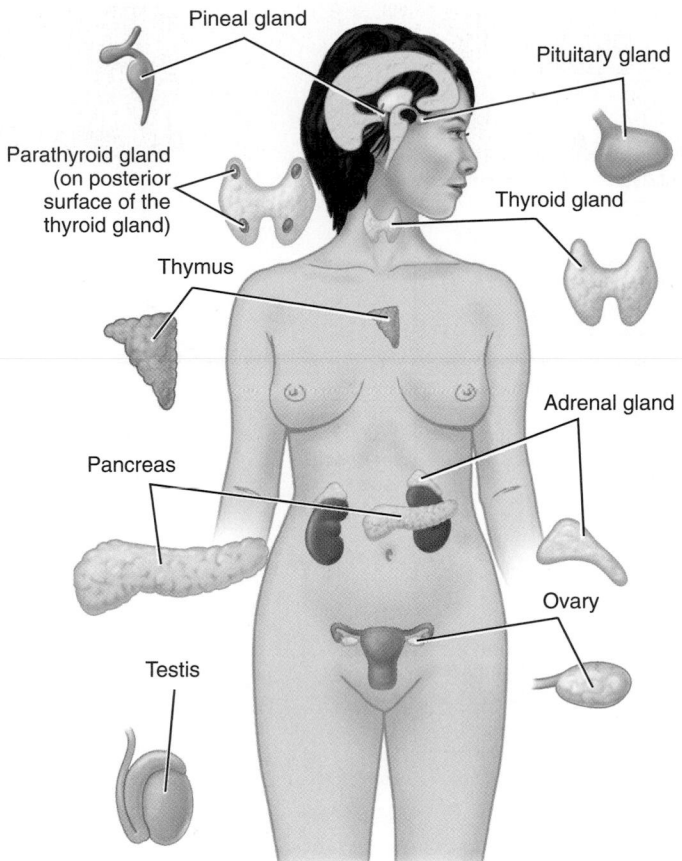

FIGURE 21.1 Major Endocrine Glands. (From Applegate E: *The anatomy and physiology learning system*, ed 4, St Louis, 2011, Saunders.)

TABLE 21.1	STRUCTURAL CATEGORIES OF HORMONES
STRUCTURAL CATEGORY	**EXAMPLES**
Water Soluble	
Peptides	Growth hormone
	Insulin
	Leptin
	Parathyroid hormone
	Prolactin
Glycoproteins	Follicle-stimulating hormone
	Luteinizing hormone
	Thyroid stimulating hormone
Polypeptides	Adrenocorticotropic hormone
	Antidiuretic hormone
	Calcitonin
	Endorphins
	Glucagon
	Hypothalamic hormones
	Lipotropins
	Melanocyte-stimulating hormone
	Oxytocin
	Somatostatin
	Thymosin
	Thyrotropin-releasing hormone
Amines	Epinephrine
	Norepinephrine
Lipid Soluble	
Thyroxine (an amine but lipid soluble)	Thyroxine (both thyroxine [T_4] and triiodothyronine [T_3])
Steroids (cholesterol is a precursor for all steroids)	Estrogens
	Glucocorticoids (cortisol)
	Mineralocorticoids (aldosterone)
	Progestins (progesterone)
	Testosterone
Derivatives of arachidonic acid (autocrine or paracrine action)	Leukotrienes
	Prostacyclins
	Prostaglandins
	Thromboxanes

Although a wide variety of hormones function within the body, they share certain general characteristics:

1. Hormones have specific rates and rhythms of secretion. Three basic secretion patterns are: (1) circadian or diurnal patterns, (2) pulsatile and cyclic patterns, and (3) patterns that depend on levels of circulating substrates (e.g., calcium, sodium, potassium, or the hormones themselves).
2. Hormones operate within feedback systems, either positive or negative, to maintain an optimal internal environment.
3. Hormones affect only cells with appropriate receptors and then act on those cells to initiate specific cell functions or activities.
4. Steroid hormones are either excreted directly by the kidneys or metabolized (conjugated) by the liver, which inactivates them and renders the hormone more water soluble for renal excretion. Peptide hormones are catabolized by circulating enzymes and eliminated in the feces or urine.

Hormones may be classified according to their structure, gland of origin, effects, or chemical composition. (Table 21.1 categorizes hormones based on structure.) The secretion and mechanisms of action of hormones represent an extremely complex system of integrated responses.

Regulation of Hormone Release

Hormone release occurs either in response to an alteration in the cellular environment or in the process of maintaining a regulated level of certain hormones or certain substances. Hormone release is regulated by one or more of the following mechanisms: (1) chemical factors (i.e., blood glucose or calcium levels); (2) endocrine factors (a hormone from one endocrine gland controlling another endocrine gland); and (3) neural

control. An example of chemical regulation is seen when insulin is secreted following chemical stimulation by increased plasma glucose levels. Cortisol from the adrenal cortex is an endocrine factor that regulates and stimulates insulin secretion from beta cells within the pancreas. Neural control occurs when the autonomic nervous system directly stimulates the insulin-secreting cells of the pancreas.

Feedback systems provide precise monitoring and control of the cellular environment. Both negative and positive feedback systems are important for maintaining hormone levels within physiologic ranges. Negative feedback is the most common and occurs when a changing chemical, neural, or endocrine response decreases the subsequent synthesis and secretion of a hormone. Positive feedback occurs when a neural, chemical, or endocrine response increases the synthesis and secretion of a hormone. Fig. 21.2 illustrates both positive and negative feedback within the hypothalamus-pituitary-target organ axis. Positive feedback also occurs when an increased hormone level further increases the synthesis and secretion of that same hormone. An example of this

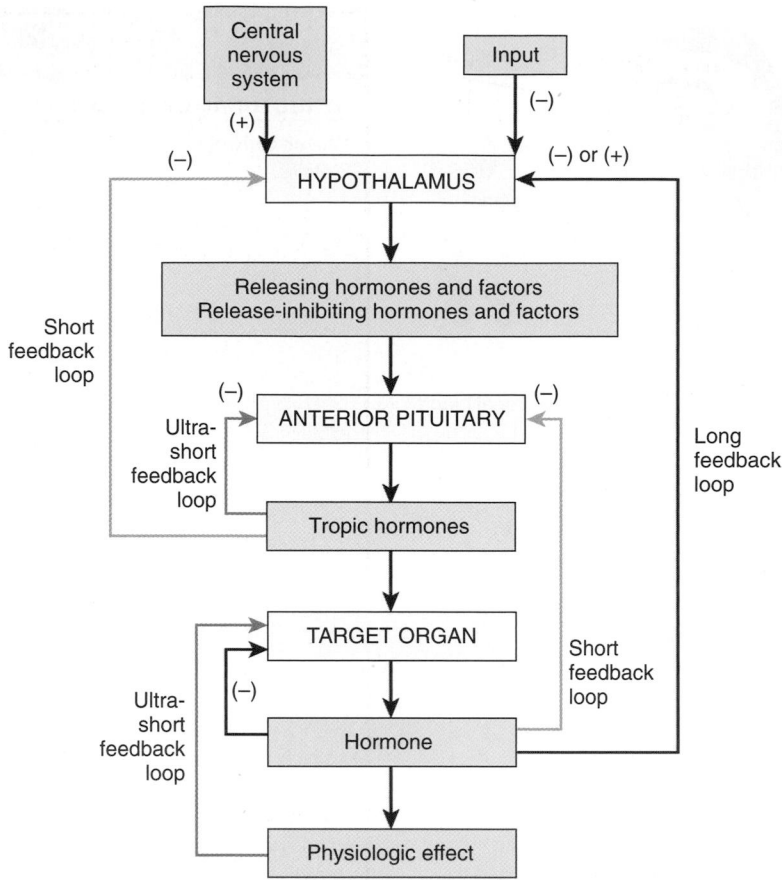

FIGURE 21.2 Feedback Loops. General model for control and negative feedback to hypothalamic-pituitary target organ systems. Negative-feedback regulation is possible at three levels: target organ (ultra-short feedback), anterior pituitary (short feedback), and hypothalamus (long feedback).

kind of positive feedback is found in the female reproductive system. The cyclic rise of estradiol levels provides positive feedback on the anterior pituitary and hypothalamus, causing a subsequent increase in gonadotropin-releasing hormone and follicle-stimulating hormone (see Fig. 24.3).

Hormone Transport

Once hormones are released into the circulatory system, they are distributed throughout the body. The protein (peptide) hormones (Table 21.2) are water soluble and generally circulate in free (unbound) forms. Water-soluble hormones generally have a short half-life of seconds to minutes because they are catabolized by circulating enzymes. For example, insulin has a half-life of 3 to 5 minutes and is catabolized by insulinases. Lipid-soluble hormones (see Table 21.2), such as cortisol and adrenal androgens, are transported bound to a carrier protein and can remain in the blood for hours to days. Only free hormones (those not bound to the carrier protein) can initiate changes within a target cell. At the cell membrane, lipid-soluble hormones dissociate from their carrier protein and diffuse into the cell. Because there is equilibrium between the concentrations of free hormones and hormones bound to plasma proteins, a significant change in the concentration of binding proteins can affect the concentration of free hormones in the plasma (see Table 21.2). (Mechanisms of hormone binding are discussed in Chapter 1.)

Hormone Receptors

Although a hormone is distributed throughout the body, only target cells with specific receptors for that hormone are affected. Target cell

TABLE 21.2	BINDING PROTEINS, THEIR HORMONES, AND VARIABLES THAT AFFECT THEIR CIRCULATING LEVELS		
BINDING PROTEIN	**HORMONE**	**FACTORS THAT INCREASE BINDING PROTEIN LEVELS**	**FACTORS THAT DECREASE BINDING PROTEIN LEVELS**
Corticosteroid-binding globulin	Cortisol Progesterone	Estrogen	Liver disease
Sex hormone–binding globulin	Dihydrotestosterone Testosterone Estradiol	—	Androgens Hypothyroidism Liver disease
Thyroid-binding globulin	Thyroxine (T_4) Triiodothyronine (T_3)	Estrogen Hyperthyroidism	Testosterone Glucocorticoids Liver disease
Albumin	All lipid-soluble hormones	Estrogen	Liver disease Malnutrition Renal disease

Upregulation

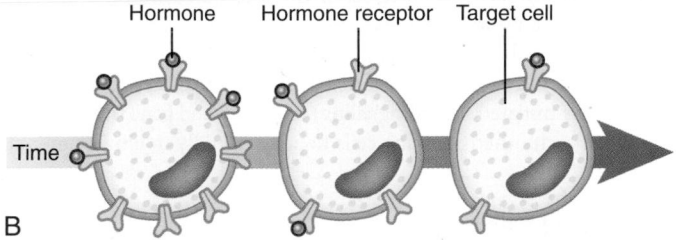

Downregulation

FIGURE 21.3 Regulation of Target Cell Sensitivity. **A,** Low hormone level and upregulation, or an increase in the number of receptors. **B,** High hormone level and downregulation, or a decrease in the number of receptors.

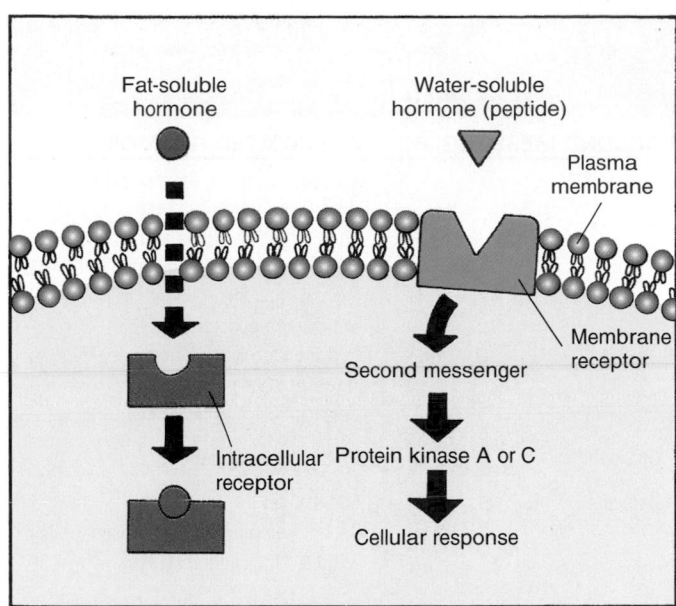

FIGURE 21.4 Hormone Binding at Target Cell.

response depends on blood levels of the hormone, the concentration of target cell receptors, and affinity of the receptor for the hormone. *Hormone receptors* of the target cell have two main functions: (1) to recognize and bind with high affinity to their particular hormones and (2) to initiate a signal to appropriate intracellular effectors. See Chapter 1 for cell signaling pathways, particularly Figs. 1.20 and 1.21.

The sensitivity or affinity of the target cell to a particular hormone is related to the concentration of receptors per cell: the more receptors, the higher the affinity or the more sensitive the cell is to the stimulating effects of the hormone. Low concentrations of hormone increase the number of receptors per cell, called upregulation (Fig. 21.3, *A*). High concentrations of hormone decrease the number or affinity of receptors, called downregulation (see Fig. 21.3, *B*). Thus the cell can adjust its sensitivity to the concentration of the signaling hormone. The receptors on the plasma membrane are continuously synthesized and degraded, so that changes in receptor concentration may occur within hours. Various physiochemical conditions also can affect both the receptor number and the affinity of the hormone for its receptor. Some of these physiochemical conditions are the fluidity and structure of the plasma membrane, pH, temperature, ion concentration, diet, and the presence of other chemicals (e.g., drugs). Finally, mutations in receptor structure can affect target cell activation such that normal cellular responses are increased or decreased. For example, mutations in thyroid-stimulating hormone receptors can lead to resistance to thyroid hormone and can contribute to defective thyroid hormone production.[1]

Hormone receptors may be located in or on the plasma membrane or in the intracellular compartment of the target cell (Fig. 21.4). Water-soluble hormones (see Table 21.1) are proteins that are polarized with a high molecular weight and cannot diffuse across the lipid layer of the cell (plasma) membrane. They interact or bind with receptors in or on the cell membrane and activate a second messenger to mediate short-acting responses. Most lipid-soluble steroids diffuse freely across the plasma and nuclear membranes and bind the cytosolic or nuclear receptors (see Fig. 21.4), although receptors for some lipid-soluble hormones are also located in or on the plasma membrane.

Water Soluble Hormone Receptors

Water-soluble hormone binding with the plasma membrane receptor initiates a complex cascade of intracellular effects. In this cascade, the hormone is termed the first messenger. The hormone-receptor interaction initiates a signal that generates a small molecule inside the cell, called the second messenger. The second messenger conveys the signal from the receptor to the cytoplasm and nucleus of the cell and mediates the effect of the hormone on the target cell (e.g., membrane permeability alterations, protein synthesis, inhibition of specific metabolic pathways, enzyme activation, or cellular growth) (Table 21.3 and Fig. 21.5). Second messengers include (1) cyclic adenosine monophosphate (cAMP), (2) cyclic guanosine monophosphate (cGMP), calcium, (3) inositol triphosphate (IP_3) and membrane-associated diacylglycerol (DAG), and (4) the tyrosine kinase system (see Table 21.3).

When first messengers (i.e., adrenocorticotropic hormone and thyroid-stimulating hormone) from the anterior pituitary gland bind to a cell membrane receptor, intracellular levels of cAMP increase. Second-messenger cAMP activates protein kinases, leading to phosphorylation of cellular proteins. This either activates or deactivates intracellular enzymes, thus directing the actions or products of specific cells. For example, binding of epinephrine to a β-adrenergic receptor subtype activates (through a stimulatory G protein [G_s]) the enzyme adenylyl cyclase. Adenylyl cyclase catalyzes the conversion of adenosine triphosphate (ATP) to the second messenger 3',5'-cAMP. Elevation of cAMP activates the enzyme cAMP-dependent protein kinase A (PKA). PKA phosphorylates and activates nuclear transcription factors (cAMP response element–binding [CREB] proteins) that influence numerous cellular functions.[2] Alterations in CREB activity have been implicated in many disease states including diabetes and cancer.[3,4] The actions of cAMP are terminated by the enzyme phosphodiesterase (PDE) III, which hydrolyzes cAMP into inactive adenosine monophosphate (AMP).

cGMP also functions as a second messenger following receptor binding of first messengers (e.g., atrial natriuretic peptide and nitric oxide). These hormones and signaling molecules play crucial roles in cardiovascular and pulmonary health and disease; thus drugs, such as phosphodiesterase inhibitors that sustain the action of cGMP, are being explored for the treatment of vascular and pulmonary hypertension and cognitive dysfunction (i.e., phosphodiesterase inhibitors).[5,6]

TABLE 21.3 SECOND MESSENGERS IDENTIFIED FOR SPECIFIC HORMONES

SECOND MESSENGER	ASSOCIATED HORMONES
Cyclic AMP	Adrenocorticotropic hormone (ACTH)
	Luteinizing hormone (LH)
	Human chorionic gonadotropin (hCG)
	Follicle-stimulating hormone (FSH)
	Thyroid-stimulating hormone (TSH)
	Antidiuretic hormone (ADH)
	Thyrotropin-releasing hormone (TRH)
	Parathyroid hormone (PTH)
	Glucagon
Cyclic GMP	Atrial natriuretic peptide
Calcium	Angiotensin II
	Gonadotropin-releasing hormone (GnRH)
	Antidiuretic hormone (ADH)
IP_3 and DAG	Angiotensin II
	Antidiuretic hormone (ADH)
	Luteinizing hormone–releasing hormone (LHRH)
Tyrosine phosphorylation	
Tyrosine kinase	Insulin
JAK-STAT	Growth hormone
	Leptin
	Prolactin

AMP, Adenosine monophosphate; *DAG,* diacylglycerol; *GMP,* guanosine monophosphate; IP_3, inositol triphosphate; *JAK,* Janus family of tyrosine kinases; *STAT,* signal transducers and activators of transcription.

Hormone receptor binding of first-messenger angiotensin II and antidiuretic hormone (ADH) results in generation of second messengers DAG or IP_3 and triggers a release of intracellular calcium, as another second messenger. Increased intracellular calcium levels can lead to the formation of the calcium-calmodulin complex, which mediates the effects of calcium on intracellular activities that are crucial for cell metabolism and growth. For example, calmodulin-dependent protein kinases control intracellular contractile components (myosin and actin, which cause muscle contraction), alter plasma membrane permeability to calcium, and regulate the intracellular enzyme activity that promotes hormone secretion.

Some hormone first messengers, such as insulin, growth hormone, and prolactin, bind to surface receptors in the cell membrane that have a transmembrane domain and directly activate second messengers of the tyrosine kinase family (a subgroup of protein kinases). These tyrosine kinases transfer a phosphate group from ATP to a protein in a cell, including the Janus family of tyrosine kinases (JAK) and signal transducers and activators of transcription (STAT)—the JAK/STAT pathway. They regulate a wide range of intracellular processes that contribute to cellular metabolism, immunity, growth, apoptosis, and oncogenesis and are targeted for inhibition in treatments for tuning down immune-mediated responses, as in rheumatoid arthritis and cancer.

Steroid (Lipid-Soluble) Hormone Receptors

With the exception of thyroid hormones, the lipid-soluble hormones are synthesized from cholesterol (giving rise to the term "steroid"). These include glucocorticoids, androgens, estrogens, progestins, miner-alocorticoids, vitamin D, and retinoid. Because they are relatively small, nonpolar, lipophilic, hydrophobic molecules, steroid hormones can cross the plasma and nuclear membranes by simple diffusion (see Chapter 1). They bind with cytosolic or nuclear receptors (Fig. 21.6), which keeps them from diffusing back out of the cell. Examples of cytosolic steroid hormone receptors include those for glucocorticoids and androgens, whereas progesterone has nuclear receptors.[7] The hormone-receptor complex then binds to a specific region in the deoxyribonucleic acid (DNA) which initiates transcription of specific genes to form messenger ribonucleic acid (mRNA) with translation at the ribosome for protein synthesis.[8] Modulation of gene expression can take hours to days.

In addition, lipid hormone receptors for estrogen, thyroid hormone, and aldosterone are also located in the plasma membrane and are associated with rapid responses (seconds or minutes). These receptors, when activated, have primarily intracellular nongenomic (membrane initiated steroid signaling) effects. Through crosstalk, nongenomic (membrane-initiated steroid signaling) responses and gene transcription modulate each other, allowing cells to adapt rapidly to environmental changes.[9,10]

Hormone Effects

The binding of hormones with their receptors stimulates three general types of effects by:
1. Acting on preexisting channel-forming proteins to alter membrane channel permeability
2. Activating preexisting proteins through a second-messenger system
3. Activating genes to cause protein synthesis

Hormones affect target cells directly or permissively. **Direct effects** are the obvious changes in cell function that specifically result from stimulation by a particular hormone. **Permissive effects** are less obvious hormone-induced changes that facilitate the maximal response or functioning of a cell. For example, insulin has a direct effect on skeletal muscle cells, causing increased glucose transport into these cells and a permissive effect on mammary cells, facilitating their response to the direct effects of prolactin.

Some hormones have biphasic effects that are dependent on the concentration or secretion pattern of the hormone. For example, low or physiologic levels of antidiuretic hormone (ADH; or arginine-vasopressin) stimulate renal tubular reabsorption of sodium and water. However, at supraphysiologic levels (i.e., those that can be achieved by exogenous administration), ADH acts as a vasoconstrictor.

STRUCTURE AND FUNCTION OF THE ENDOCRINE GLANDS

Hypothalamic-Pituitary Axis

The hypothalamic-pituitary axis (HPA) forms the structural and functional basis for central integration of the neurologic and endocrine systems, creating what is called the **neuroendocrine system**. The HPA produces a number of releasing/inhibitory hormones and tropic hormones that affect a number of diverse body functions (Fig. 21.7), including thyroid, adrenal, and reproductive functions.

Hypothalamus

The hypothalamus is located at the base of the brain. It is connected to the pituitary gland by the infundibulum (pituitary stalk) (Fig. 21.8), to the anterior pituitary through hypophysial portal blood vessels (Fig. 21.9), and to the posterior pituitary through a nerve tract referred to as the *hypothalamohypophysial tract* (Fig. 21.10). These connections are vital to the functioning of the hypothalamic-pituitary system.[11] The hypothalamus contains special neurosecretory cells that are like other

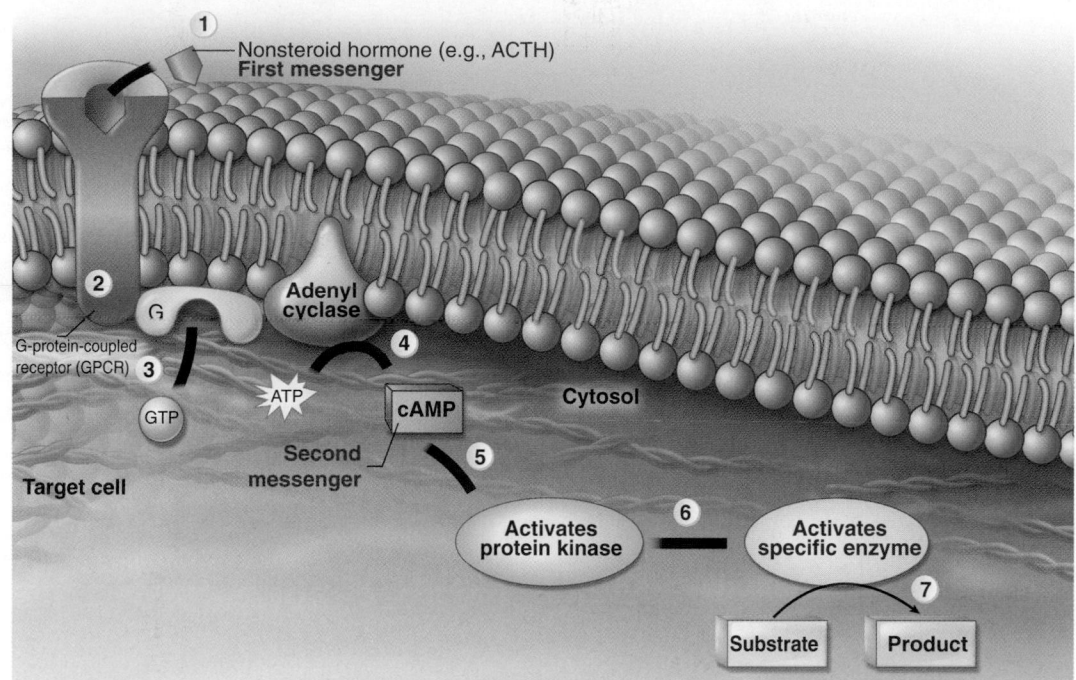

FIGURE 21.5 Examples of First- and Second-Messenger Signaling. A nonsteroid hormone (first messenger) binds to a fixed receptor of the target cell **(1)**. The hormone-receptor complex activates the G protein **(2)**. The activated G protein *(G)* reacts with guanosine triphosphate *(GTP)*, which in turn activates the membrane-bound enzyme adenylyl cyclase **(3)**. Adenylyl cyclase catalyzes the conversion of adenosine triphosphate *(ATP)* to cyclic adenosine monophosphate (*cAMP*; second messenger) **(4)**. cAMP activates protein kinase **(5)**. Protein kinases activate specific intracellular enzymes **(6)**. These activated enzymes then influence specific cellular reactions and metabolic pathways, thus producing the target cell's response to the hormone **(7)**. *ACTH,* Adrenocorticotropic hormone. (From Patton KT, Thibodeau GA: *Anatomy & physiology,* ed 9, St Louis, 2016, Mosby.)

neurons in that they have similar electrical properties, organelles, membranes, and synapses. Hypothalamic neurosecretory cells, however, can synthesize and secrete the hypothalamic-releasing hormones that regulate the release of hormones from the anterior pituitary. In addition, these cells synthesize the hormones ADH and oxytocin that are then stored and released from the posterior pituitary gland.

ADH and oxytocin travel to the posterior pituitary by way of the hypothalamohypophysial nerve tract. Releasing and inhibitory hormones also are synthesized in the hypothalamus and are secreted into the portal blood vessels, through which they travel to their target tissues within the anterior pituitary and control the release of tropic hormones. These releasing/inhibitory hormones from the hypothalamus include prolactin-inhibiting hormone (PIH), prolactin-releasing hormone (PRH), thyrotropin-releasing hormone (TRH), gonadotropin-releasing hormone (GnRH), hypothalamic somatostatin, growth hormone–releasing hormone (GHRH), corticotropin-releasing hormone (CRH), and substance P. These hormones are summarized in Table 21.4.

The Anterior Pituitary

The anterior pituitary (adenohypophysis) accounts for 75% of the total weight of the pituitary gland. It is composed of three regions: (1) the pars distalis, (2) the pars tuberalis, and (3) the pars intermedia. The pars distalis is the major component of the anterior pituitary and the source of the anterior pituitary hormones. The pars tuberalis is a thin layer of cells on the anterior and lateral portions of the pituitary stalk. The pars intermedia lies between the two. In the adult the distinct intermediate lobe disappears, and the individual cells are distributed

diffusely throughout the pars distalis and pars nervosa (neural lobe), which are part of the posterior pituitary. The anterior pituitary is composed of two main cell types: (1) the chromophobes, which appear to be nonsecretory; and (2) the chromophils, which are considered the secretory cells of the adenohypophysis. The chromophils are subdivided into seven secretory cell types, each type secreting one or more specific tropic hormones (Table 21.5).

The tropic hormones secreted by the chromophils affect the physiologic function of specific target organs (see Fig. 21.7). These hormones can be grouped into three categories: corticotropin-related hormones (adrenocorticotropic hormone [ACTH] and melanocyte-stimulating hormone [MSH]), glycoproteins (luteinizing hormone [LH], follicle-stimulating hormone [FSH], and thyroid-stimulating hormone [TSH]), and somatotropins (growth hormone [GH] and prolactin). The corticotropin-related hormones are all derived from the precursor pro-opiomelanocortin (POMC). Melanocyte-stimulating hormone (MSH) promotes the pituitary secretion of melanin, which darkens skin color. β-Lipotropin and β-endorphins are corticotropic hormones also released from the anterior pituitary. β-Lipotropin plays a role in fat catabolism, and β-endorphins impact pain perception, body temperature, and food and water intake. The glycoprotein hormones follicle-stimulating hormone (FSH) and luteinizing hormone (LH) influence reproductive function and are discussed in Chapter 24. Adrenocorticotropic hormone (ACTH) regulates the release of cortisol from the adrenal cortex. Thyroid-stimulating hormone (TSH) regulates the activity of the thyroid gland. The roles of ACTH and TSH are discussed later in this chapter.

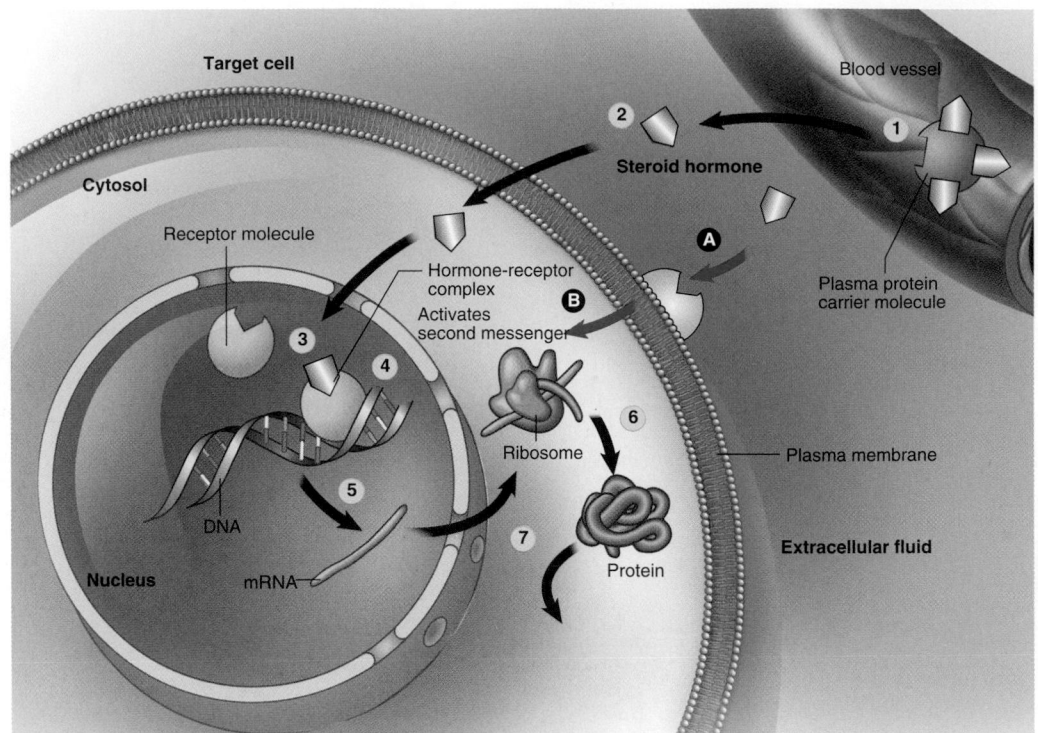

FIGURE 21.6 Steroid Hormone Signaling Mechanism. Lipid-soluble steroid hormone molecules detach from the carrier protein **(1)** and pass through the plasma membrane **(2)**. Hormone molecules then diffuse into the nucleus, where they bind to a receptor to form a hormone-receptor complex **(3)**. This complex then binds to a specific site on a DNA molecule **(4)**, triggering transcription of the genetic information encoded there **(5)**. The resulting messenger ribonucleic acid *(mRNA)* molecule moves to the cytosol, where it associates with a ribosome, initiating synthesis of a new protein **(6)**. This new protein—usually an enzyme or channel protein—produces specific effects on the target cell **(7)**. The classic genomic action is typically slow *(red arrows)*. Steroids also may exact rapid effects by binding to receptors on the plasma membrane **(A)** and activating an intercellular second messenger **(B)**. (Modified from Patton KT, Thibodeau GA: *Anatomy & physiology*, ed 9, St Louis, 2016, Mosby.)

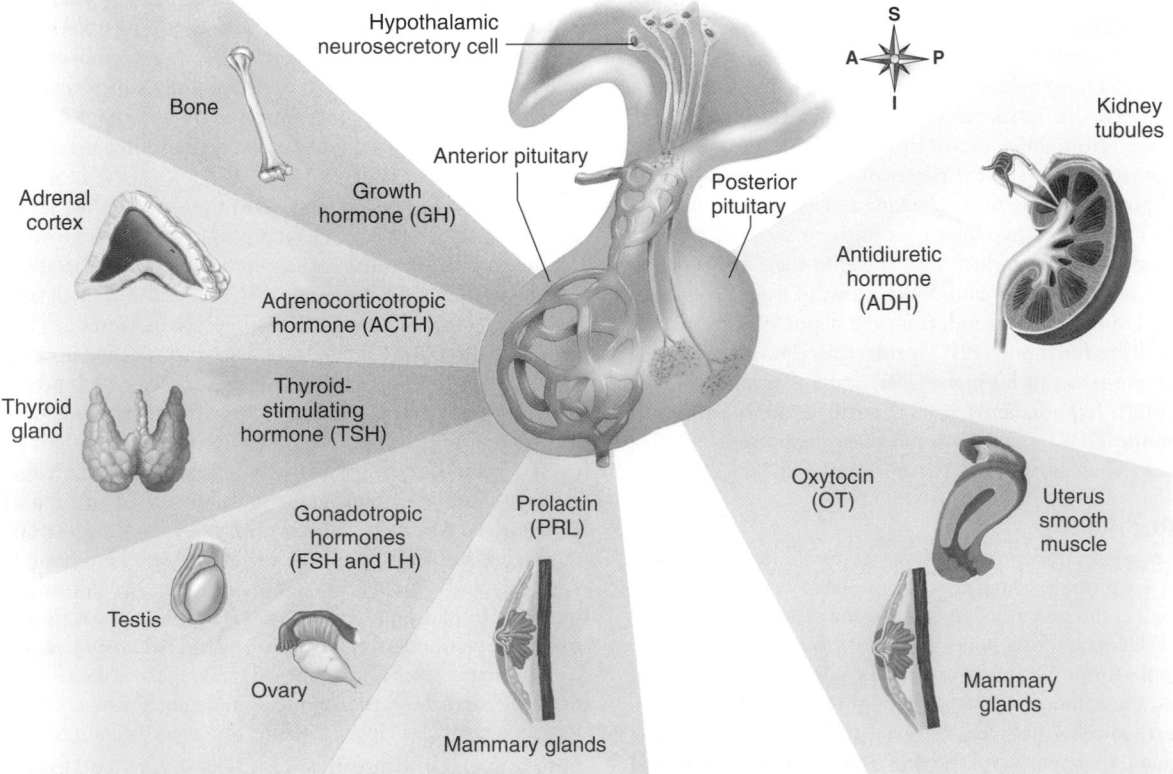

FIGURE 21.7 Pituitary Hormones and Their Target Organs. *FSH,* Follicle-stimulating hormone; *LH,* luteinizing hormone. (From Patton KT, Thibodeau GA: *The human body in health & disease*, ed 7, St Louis, 2018, Elsevier.)

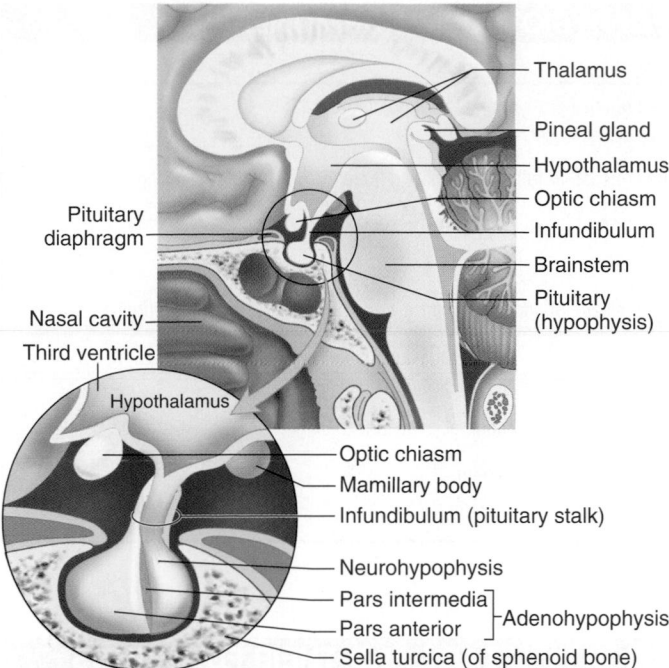

FIGURE 21.8 Location and Structure of the Pituitary Gland (Hypophysis). The pituitary gland is located within the sella turcica of the skull's sphenoid bone and is connected to the hypothalamus by a stalklike infundibulum. The infundibulum passes through a gap in the portion of the dura mater that covers the pituitary (the pituitary diaphragm). The inset shows that the pituitary is divided into an anterior portion, the adenohypophysis, and a posterior portion, the neurohypophysis. The adenohypophysis is further subdivided into the pars anterior and pars intermedia. The pars intermedia is almost absent in the adult pituitary. (Modified from Patton KT, Thibodeau GA: *Anatomy & physiology*, ed 9, St Louis, 2016, Mosby.)

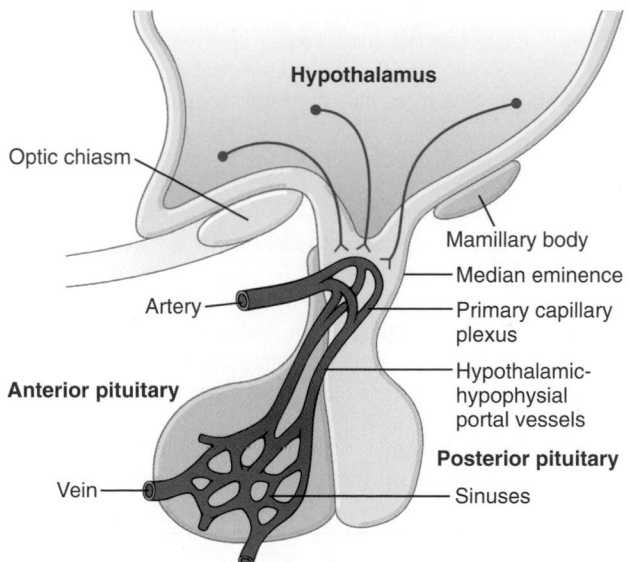

FIGURE 21.9 Hypophysial Portal System. (From Hall JE: *Guyton and Hall textbook of medical physiology*, ed 13, Philadelphia, 2016, Saunders.)

Growth hormone (GH) and prolactin are called the *somatotropic hormones* and have diverse effects on body tissues. GH secretion is controlled by two hormones from the hypothalamus: growth hormone–releasing hormone (GHRH), which increases GH secretion; and somatostatin, which inhibits GH secretion. GH is essential to normal

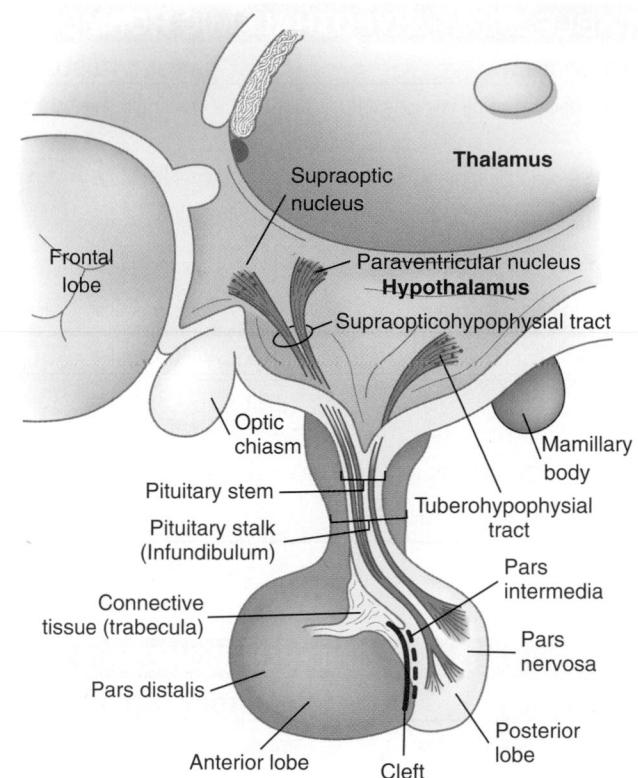

FIGURE 21.10 Nerve Tracts from Hypothalamus to Posterior Lobe of Pituitary Gland.

tissue growth and maturation and peaks during adolescence. GH also impacts aging, sleep, nutritional status, stress, and reproductive hormones. In the bone, GH stimulates epiphyseal growth and increases osteoclast and osteoblast activity, resulting in increased bone mass. GH also increases amino acid transport in muscles. Other functions of GH include lipolysis and enhancement of hepatic protein synthesis. Many of the anabolic functions of GH are mediated, at least in part, by the insulin-like growth factors (IGFs), which are also known as the *somatomedins* (promote cell growth and division).

There are two primary forms of IGF: IGF-1 and IGF-2, of which IGF-1 is the most biologically active. They both circulate bound to a group of IGF-binding proteins (IGFBPs) modulating their availability. IGF-1 binds to IGF-1 receptors, mediating the anabolic effects of GH. IGF-1 also binds to insulin receptors, providing an insulin-like effect on skeletal muscle. IGF-2 has important effects on fetal growth, but suppresses GH in the adult. Because of the anabolic effects of GH and IGF-1, they can be used to treat growth disorders, increase muscle mass, and potentially slow the aging process; however, their use also has been linked to increased rates of cancer.[12,13]

Prolactin primarily functions to induce milk production during pregnancy and lactation. It has immune stimulatory effects and modulates immune and inflammatory responses with both physiologic and pathologic reactions.[14] Its synthesis and release are increased by stimulation of the nipples and mammary gland during nursing. Vasoactive intestinal polypeptide, serotonin, and growth factors also stimulate the synthesis of prolactin, while its release is inhibited by dopamine.

The Posterior Pituitary

The embryonic **posterior pituitary (neurohypophysis)** is derived from the hypothalamus and is composed of three parts: (1) the median

TABLE 21.4   HYPOTHALAMIC HORMONES (HYPOPHYSIOTROPIC HORMONES)

HORMONE	TARGET TISSUE	ACTION
Thyrotropin-releasing hormone (TRH)	Anterior pituitary	Stimulates release of thyroid-stimulating hormone (TSH) Modulates prolactin secretion
Gonadotropin-releasing hormone (GnRH)	Anterior pituitary	Stimulates release of follicle-stimulating hormone (FSH) and luteinizing hormone (LH)
Somatostatin	Anterior pituitary	Inhibits release of growth hormone (GH) and TSH
Growth hormone–releasing hormone (GHRH)	Anterior pituitary	Stimulates release of GH
Corticotropin-releasing hormone (CRH)	Anterior pituitary	Stimulates release of adrenocorticotropic hormone (ACTH) and β-endorphin
Substance P	Anterior pituitary	Inhibits synthesis and release of ACTH Stimulates secretion of GH, FSH, LH, and prolactin
Dopamine	Anterior pituitary	Inhibits synthesis and secretion of prolactin
Prolactin-releasing hormone (PRH)	Anterior pituitary	Stimulates secretion of prolactin
Prolactin-inhibiting hormone (PIH)	Anterior pituitary	Inhibits secretion of prolactin

TABLE 21.5   TROPIC HORMONES OF THE ANTERIOR PITUITARY AND THEIR FUNCTIONS

HORMONE	SECRETORY CELL TYPE	TARGET ORGANS	FUNCTIONS
Adrenocorticotropic hormone (ACTH)	Corticotropic	Adrenal gland (cortex)	Increased steroidogenesis (cortisol and androgenic hormones) Synthesis of adrenal proteins contributing to maintenance of the adrenal gland
Melanocyte-stimulating hormone (MSH)	Melanotropic	Anterior pituitary	Promotes secretion of melanin and lipotropin by anterior pituitary; makes skin darker
Somatotropic Hormones			
Growth hormone (GH)	Somatotropic	Muscle, bone, liver	Regulates metabolic processes related to growth and adaptation to physical and emotional stressors, muscle growth, increased protein synthesis, increased liver glycogenolysis, increased fat mobilization
		Liver	Induces formation of somatomedins, or insulin-like growth factors (IGFs) that have actions similar to insulin
Prolactin	Lactotropic	Breast	Milk production
Glycoprotein Hormones			
Thyroid-stimulating hormone (TSH)	Thyrotropic	Thyroid gland	Increased production and secretion of thyroid hormone Increased iodide uptake Promotes hypertrophy and hyperplasia of thymocytes
Luteinizing hormone (LH)	Gonadotropic	In women: granulosa cells In men: Leydig cells	Ovulation, progesterone production Testicular growth, testosterone production
Follicle-stimulating hormone (FSH)	Gonadotropic	In women: granulosa cells In men: Sertoli cells	Follicle maturation, estrogen production Spermatogenesis
β-Lipotropin	Corticotropic	Adipose cells	Fat breakdown and release of fatty acids
β-Endorphins	Corticotropic	Adipose cells Brain opioid receptors	Analgesia; may regulate body temperature, food and water intake

eminence located at the base of the hypothalamus; (2) the pituitary stalk; and (3) the infundibular process, also known as the *pars nervosa* or *neural lobe*. The median eminence is composed largely of the nerve endings of axons that arise primarily in the ventral hypothalamus. It often is designated as part of the posterior pituitary but contains at least 10 biologically active hypothalamic-releasing hormones, as well as the neurotransmitters dopamine, norepinephrine, serotonin, acetylcholine, and histamine. The pituitary stalk contains the axons of neurons that originate in the supraoptic and paraventricular nuclei of the hypothalamus. Axons originating in the hypothalamus terminate in the pars nervosa, which secretes the hormones of the posterior pituitary (see Fig. 21.10).

The posterior pituitary secretes two polypeptide hormones: (1) ADH, also called *arginine-vasopressin*; and (2) oxytocin. These hormones differ by only two amino acids. They are synthesized along with their binding proteins, the neurophysins, in the supraoptic and paraventricular nuclei of the hypothalamus (see Fig. 21.10). They are packaged in secretory vesicles and are moved down the axons of the pituitary stalk to the pars nervosa for storage. The posterior pituitary thus can be seen as a site for both storing and releasing hormones synthesized in the hypothalamus. The release of ADH and oxytocin is mediated by cholinergic and adrenergic neurotransmitters. The major stimulus to both ADH and oxytocin release is glutamate, whereas the major inhibitory input is through gamma-aminobutyric acid (GABA). Before release into the circulatory system, ADH and oxytocin are split from the neurophysins and are secreted in unbound form.

Antidiuretic Hormone. The major homeostatic function of the posterior pituitary is the control of plasma osmolality, as regulated by ADH (see Chapter 3). At physiologic levels, ADH acts on the vasopressin 2 (V2) receptors of the renal tubular cells to increase their permeability (see Chapter 38). This increased permeability leads to increased water reabsorption into the blood, thus concentrating the urine and reducing serum osmolality. These effects may be inhibited by hypercalcemia, prostaglandin E, and hypokalemia.

The secretion of ADH is regulated primarily by the osmoreceptors of the hypothalamus, located near or in the supraoptic nuclei. As plasma osmolality increases, these osmoreceptors are stimulated, the rate of ADH secretion increases, more water is reabsorbed from the kidney, and the plasma is diluted to its set-point osmolality (approximately 280 mOsm/kg). ADH has no direct effect on electrolyte levels, but with increasing water reabsorption, serum electrolyte concentrations may decrease because of a dilutional effect.

ADH secretion also is increased by changes in intravascular volume, which are monitored by baroreceptors in the left atrium and in the carotid arteries and aortic arch. A volume loss of 7% to 25% acts through these receptors to stimulate ADH secretion. Stress, trauma, pain, exercise, nausea, nicotine, exposure to heat, and drugs such as morphine also increase ADH secretion. ADH secretion decreases with a decrease in plasma osmolality; an increase in intravascular volume; hypertension; an increase in estrogen, progesterone, and angiotensin II levels; and alcohol ingestion.

Physiologic levels of ADH do not significantly affect vessel tone. However, at pathophysiologically high serum levels, ADH acts on vasopressin 1 (V1) receptors causing vasoconstriction resulting in an increase in arterial blood pressure. For example, high doses of ADH (given as the drug vasopressin) may be administered to achieve hemostasis during hemorrhage and to raise blood pressure in shock states.[15]

Oxytocin. Oxytocin is responsible for contraction of the uterus and milk ejection in lactating women and may affect sperm motility in men. In both sexes, oxytocin has an antidiuretic effect similar to that of ADH. In women, oxytocin is secreted in response to suckling and mechanical distention of the female reproductive tract. Oxytocin binds to its receptors on myoepithelial cells in the mammary tissues and causes contraction of those cells which increases intramammary pressure and milk expression ("let down" reflex). Oxytocin also acts on the uterus to stimulate contractions. Uterine contractions act in a positive feedback loop to further increase oxytocin secretion. Oxytocin functions near the end of labor to enhance the effectiveness of contractions, promote delivery of the placenta, and stimulate postpartum uterine contractions, thereby preventing excessive bleeding. The function of this hormone is discussed in more detail in Chapter 24.

Pineal Gland

The pineal gland is located near the center of the brain (see Fig. 21.1) and is composed of melatonin-secreting photoreceptive cells. It is innervated by noradrenergic sympathetic nerve terminals controlled by pathways within the hypothalamus. Melatonin release is stimulated by exposure to dark and inhibited by light exposure. It is synthesized from tryptophan, which is first converted to serotonin and then to melatonin. Melatonin regulates circadian rhythms and reproductive systems, including the secretion of gonadotropin-releasing hormones and the onset of puberty. It also plays an important role in immune regulation and is postulated to affect the aging process. Further effects of melatonin include increasing nitric oxide release from blood vessels, removing toxic oxygen free radicals, and decreasing insulin secretion. Melatonin has been used therapeutically in humans to help with sleep disturbances, jet lag, and inflammatory and psychologic disorders. Its utility for numerous other disorders including anti-cancer therapy is being explored.[16]

Thyroid and Parathyroid Glands

The thyroid gland, located in the neck just below the larynx, produces hormones that control the rates of metabolic processes throughout the body. The four parathyroid glands are located near the posterior side of the thyroid and function to control serum calcium levels (Fig. 21.11).

Thyroid Gland

The two lobes of the **thyroid gland** lie on either side of the trachea, inferior to the thyroid cartilage, and are joined by a small band of tissue termed the **isthmus** which crosses the anterior surface of the trachea and larynx at the cricoid cartilage (see Fig. 21.11). The **pyramidal lobe** is superior to the isthmus. The normal thyroid gland is not visible on inspection, but it may be palpated on swallowing, which causes it to be displaced upward. The thyroid gland consists of **follicles** that contain follicular cells surrounding a viscous substance called *colloid* (Fig. 21.12). The follicular cells synthesize and secrete thyroid hormones. Neurons of the autonomic nervous system terminate on blood vessels within the thyroid gland and on the follicular cells themselves. Acetylcholine, catecholamines, and other peptides directly affect secretory activity of the follicular cells and thyroid blood flow. Approximately a 2-month supply of thyroid hormone is stored in the gland.

Also found in the tissue of the thyroid are parafollicular cells, or C cells (see Fig. 21.12). C cells secrete various regulatory peptides, including **calcitonin**, and, in much smaller quantities, the neuropeptides ghrelin,

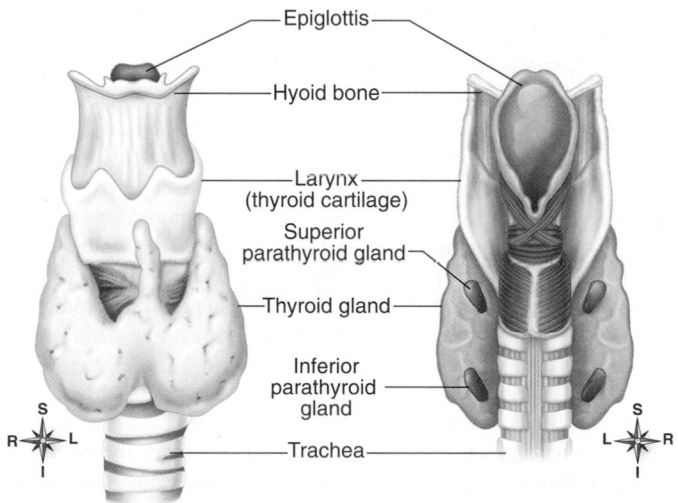

FIGURE 21.11 Thyroid and Parathyroid Glands. Note the relationship of the thyroid and parathyroid glands to each other, to the larynx (voice box), and to the trachea. (From Patton KT, Thibodeau GA: *The human body in health & disease,* ed 7, St Louis, 2018, Elsevier.)

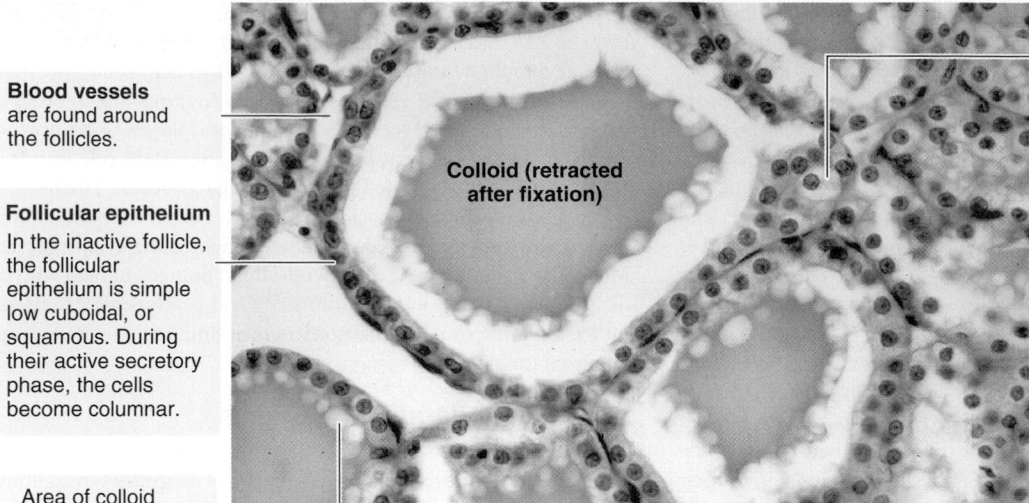

Blood vessels are found around the follicles.

Follicular epithelium In the inactive follicle, the follicular epithelium is simple low cuboidal, or squamous. During their active secretory phase, the cells become columnar.

Area of colloid resorption

Colloid (retracted after fixation)

A **C cell** can be distinguished from surrounding follicular cells by its pale cytoplasm.
Two more effective identification approaches are:
1. Immunocytochemistry, using an antibody to calcitonin.
2. Electron microscopy, to visualize calcitonin-containing cytoplasmic granules.

FIGURE 21.12 Thyroid Follicle Cells.

serotonin, and somatostatin. At high levels, calcitonin, also called *thyrocalcitonin,* lowers serum calcium levels by inhibiting bone-resorbing osteoclasts. However, in humans the metabolic consequences of calcitonin deficiency or excess do not appear to be significant (bone resorption is described in Chapter 44). Calcitonin is used therapeutically to treat a number of bone disorders, including osteoporosis, osteoarthritis, Paget bone disease, hypercalcemia, osteogenesis imperfecta, and metastatic cancer of the bone. The precursor molecule to calcitonin, called *procalcitonin,* is a stress hormone that is elevated in infectious and inflammatory disorders, and its measurement can aid in the diagnosis of these serious diseases.[17,18]

Regulation of Thyroid Hormone Secretion. Thyroid hormone (TH) is regulated through a negative-feedback loop involving the hypothalamus, the anterior pituitary, and the thyroid gland (Fig. 21.13). This loop is initiated by TRH, which is synthesized and stored within the hypothalamus. TRH is released into the hypothalamic-pituitary portal system and circulates to the anterior pituitary, where it stimulates the release of TSH. TRH levels increase with exposure to cold or stress and from decreased levels of T_4.

Thyroid-stimulating hormone (TSH) is a glycoprotein hormone synthesized and stored within the anterior pituitary. It circulates to bind with TSH receptor sites located on the plasma membrane of the thyroid follicular cells. The primary effects of TSH on the thyroid gland include: (1) an immediate increase in the release of stored thyroid hormones, (2) an increase in iodide uptake and oxidation, (3) an increase in thyroid hormone synthesis, and (4) an increase in the synthesis and secretion of prostaglandins by the thyroid. TSH also increases growth of the thyroid gland by stimulating thymocyte hyperplasia and hypertrophy and decreasing apoptosis.[19] As TH levels rise, there is a negative-feedback effect on the HPA to inhibit TRH and TSH release, which then results in decreased TH synthesis and secretion. TH synthesis also is controlled by serum iodide levels and by circulating selenium-dependent enzymes, called *deiodinases,* which inactivate the precursor molecule thyroxine.[20] Thyroid gland hormones and their regulation and function are summarized in Table 21.6.

Synthesis of Thyroid Hormone. Thyroid hormone synthesis is summarized in the following steps:
1. Uniodinated thyroglobulin (a large glycoprotein) is produced by the endoplasmic reticulum of the follicular cells.

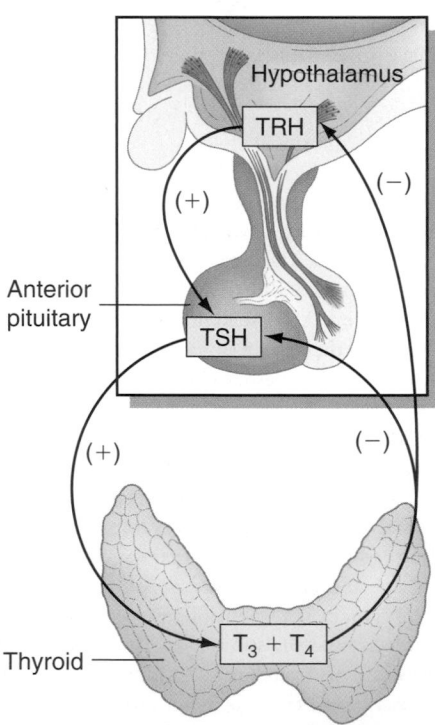

FIGURE 21.13 Feedback Loops for the Thyroid Gland. *TRH,* Thyrotropin-releasing hormone; *TSH,* thyroid-stimulating hormone; T_3, triiodothyronine; T_4, tetraiodothyronine (thyroxine).

2. Tyrosine is incorporated into the thyroglobulin as it is synthesized.
3. Iodide (the inorganic form of iodine) is actively transferred (pumped) from the blood into the colloid by carrier proteins located in the outer membrane of the follicular cells. This active transport system is called the *iodide trap* and is very efficient at accumulating the trace amounts of iodide from the blood.
4. Iodide is oxidized and quickly attaches to tyrosine within the thyroglobulin molecule.
5. Coupling of iodinated tyrosine forms thyroid hormones. Triiodothyronine (T_3) is formed from coupling of monoiodotyrosine (one

TABLE 21.6	THYROID GLAND HORMONES AND THEIR REGULATION AND FUNCTIONS	
HORMONE	**REGULATION**	**FUNCTIONS**

Thyroxine (T_4) and triiodothyronine (T_3)	T_4 and T_3 levels are controlled by TSH
	Released in response to metabolic demand
	Influences on amount secreted:
	  Sex
	  Pregnancy
	  Gonadal and adrenocortical-increased steroids = ↑ levels
	  Exposure to extreme cold = ↑ levels
	  Nutritional state
	  Chemicals
	  GHIH = ↓ levels
	  Dopamine = ↓ levels
	  Catecholamines = ↑ levels
		Regulates protein, fat, and carbohydrate catabolism in all cells
		Regulates metabolic rate of all cells
		Regulates body heat production
		Insulin antagonist
		Maintains growth hormone secretion, skeletal maturation
		Affects CNS development
		Necessary for muscle tone and vigor
		Maintains cardiac rate, force, and output
		Maintains secretion of GI tract
		Affects respiratory rate and oxygen utilization
		Maintains calcium mobilization
		Affects RBC production
		Stimulates lipid turnover, free fatty acid release, and cholesterol synthesis

Calcitonin	Elevated serum calcium—major stimulant for calcitonin
	Other stimulants
	  Gastrin
	  Calcium-rich foods (regardless of serum Ca^{++} levels)
	  Pregnancy
	Lowered serum calcium—suppresses calcitonin release
		Lowers serum calcium by opposing bone-resorbing effects of PTH, prostaglandins, and calciferols by inhibiting osteoclastic activity
		Lowers serum phosphate levels
		May also decrease calcium and phosphorus absorption in GI tract

From Monahan FD et al: *Phipps' medical-surgical nursing: health and illness perspectives*, ed 8, St Louis, 2007, Mosby.
CNS, Central nervous system; *GHIH,* growth hormone–inhibiting hormone; *GI,* gastrointestinal; *PTH,* parathyroid hormone; *RBC,* red blood cell; *TSH,* thyroid-stimulating hormone.

iodine atom and tyrosine) and diiodotyrosine (two iodine atoms and tyrosine). Tetraiodothyronine (T_4), commonly known as *thyroxine,* is formed from coupling of two diiodotyrosines.

6. Thyroid hormones are stored attached to thyroglobulin within the colloid until they are released into the circulation.

The thyroid gland normally produces 90% T_4 and 10% T_3. Once released into the circulation, T_3 and T_4 are primarily transported bound to one of three carrier proteins: thyroxine-binding globulin (though some TH is transported by thyroxine-binding prealbumin [transthyretin]), albumin, or lipoproteins. The bound form serves as a reservoir, whereas the unbound form is active. In the body tissues, most of the T_4 is converted to T_3, which acts on the target cell. T_3 binds with three different receptors (TRα1, TRβ1, and TRβ2).

Actions of Thyroid Hormone. TH has a significant effect on the growth, maturation, and function of cells and tissues throughout the body. TH is essential for normal growth and neurologic development in the fetus and infant and affects metabolic, neurologic, cardiovascular, and respiratory functioning across the life span. In addition, TH is required for the metabolism and function of blood cells, as well as normal muscle functioning and the integrity of skin, nails, and hair. Similar to some steroid hormones, thyroid hormones bind to intracellular receptor complexes and then influence the genetic expression of specific proteins. They also may bind to receptors in the plasma membrane, mitochondria, or cytoplasm and mediate nongenomic (membrane-initiated signaling) effects.[21] Thyroid hormones affect cell metabolism by altering protein, fat, and glucose metabolism and, as a result, heat production and oxygen consumption are increased.

TH has permissive effects throughout the body, optimizing the actions of other hormones and neurotransmitters. These effects can become very pronounced when there are either high or low levels of circulating thyroid hormones. For example, in the heart, T_3 stimulates the synthesis of specific contractile proteins (e.g., α-myosin heavy chain), sarcolemmal

ion pumps (Na^+-K^+ ATPase pump, Ca^{++} ATPase pump), and membrane receptors (β-adrenergic receptors). Therefore in hyperthyroidism, which is associated with elevated levels of thyroid hormones, cardiac effects include increased heart rate and cardiac output, as well as the development of cardiomyopathy. Thyroid hormones also affect the respiratory center, contributing to the normal hypoxic and hypercapnic drives. In severe hypothyroidism, ventilation can become very depressed. Thyroid hormone also stimulates bone resorption, and hyperthyroidism is associated with osteopenia, hypercalcemia, and hypercalciuria.

Parathyroid Glands

Normally, two pairs of parathyroid glands are present behind the upper and lower poles of the thyroid gland (see Fig. 21.11), but the number may range from two to six. The parathyroid glands produce **parathyroid hormone (PTH)**, which is the single most important factor in the regulation of serum calcium concentration.[22] The overall effect of PTH secretion is to increase serum calcium concentration and decrease the concentration of serum phosphate. A decrease in serum-ionized calcium level stimulates PTH secretion. On release, PTH enters the circulation in unbound form. The hormone attaches to plasma membrane receptors in target tissues, where the biologic effects of PTH are mediated primarily by activation of the adenylyl cyclase system (see Chapter 1). To achieve regulation of serum calcium concentration, PTH acts directly on bone with at least two effects. In acute hypocalcemia, PTH secretion stimulates osteoblasts to release receptor activator for nuclear factor κB (NF-κB), receptor activator of nuclear factor κB ligand (RANKL), and macrophage-colony stimulating factor (M-CSF), which results in osteoclast proliferation, maturation, and release of acidic enzymes, such as cathepsin. These enzymes mobilize calcium release from bone (bone resorption), which increases the serum calcium level (Fig. 21.14). There is bone remodeling with chronic stimulation by PTH, a process in which bone is broken down and re-formed. Paradoxically, when PTH

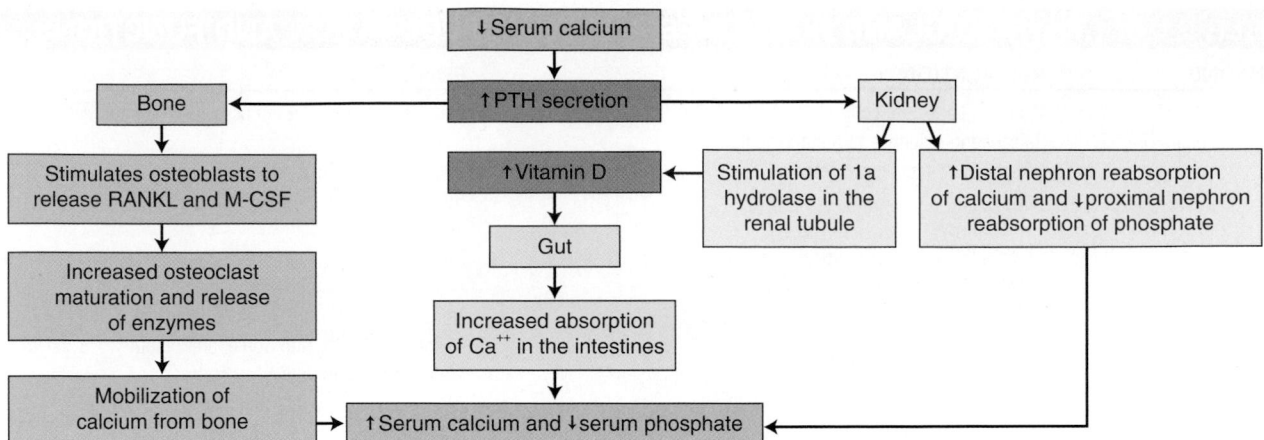

FIGURE 21.14 Normal Calcium Metabolism Regulated by PTH and Vitamin D. *M-CSF,* Macrophage-colony stimulating factor; *PTH,* parathyroid hormone; *RANKL,* receptor activator of NF-κB ligand.

is administered intermittently and at a low dose, it stimulates bone formation. This observation led to the use of PTH for treatment of osteoporosis.[23]

PTH also acts on the kidney to increase calcium reabsorption while phosphate reabsorption is decreased. PTH acts on its plasma membrane receptor in the distal tubules of the nephron to increase reabsorption of calcium. It acts on the proximal tubules to decrease reabsorption of phosphorus and bicarbonate. The resultant increase in serum calcium concentration inhibits PTH secretion. In renal cells, PTH also stimulates the activity of 1α-hydroxylase, which mediates a step in the formation of the biologically active form of vitamin D, or **1,25-dihydroxy-vitamin D₃**. Vitamin D works as a cofactor with PTH to promote calcium and phosphate absorption in the gut and enhance bone mineralization. Vitamin D also plays an important role in metabolic processes and controlling inflammation. It has been found to be deficient in the majority of individuals in the United States and many other countries.[24]

Magnesium and phosphate concentrations also affect PTH secretion. Hypomagnesemia in persons with normal calcium levels acts as a mild stimulant to PTH secretion, whereas in hypocalcemic individuals, hypomagnesemia decreases PTH secretion. Hyperphosphatemia leads to hypocalcemia because of calcium phosphate precipitation in soft tissue and bone. Alterations in serum phosphate levels therefore may indirectly influence PTH secretion by affecting serum calcium levels.

Another hormone that plays an important role in calcium and bone physiology is parathyroid hormone–related protein (PTHrP). This hormone is synthesized in many adult and fetal tissues and affects tissues around it in a paracrine fashion. It has similar biologic properties to PTH and uses the same receptors but has other actions mediated by different regions within the molecule. It is important for endochondral bone formation and bone remodeling. It was discovered as the primary hormone involved in malignancy-related hypercalcemia.[25]

Endocrine Pancreas

The **pancreas** is both an endocrine gland that produces hormones and an exocrine gland that produces digestive enzymes. (The exocrine pancreas is discussed in Chapter 41.) The pancreas is located behind the stomach, between the spleen and the duodenum and houses the **islets of Langerhans**. The islets of Langerhans have four types of hormone-secreting cells: **alpha cells**, which secrete glucagon; **beta cells**, which secrete insulin and amylin; **delta cells**, which secrete gastrin and somatostatin; and **F (or PP) cells**, which secrete pancreatic polypeptide that stimulates gastric secretion and antagonizes cholecystokinin. These hormones regulate carbohydrate, fat, and protein metabolism. (The

pancreas is illustrated in Fig. 21.15.) Nerves from both the sympathetic and the parasympathetic divisions of the autonomic nervous system innervate the pancreatic islets.

The perfusion of the anterior lobe of the pancreas, where alpha, beta, and delta cells are most numerous, comes from branches of the superior mesenteric artery. The posterior lobe is perfused by branches of the celiac artery. The pancreatic islets receive 10% of the pancreatic blood flow but represent only 1% of pancreatic mass. This is necessary for oxygenation and delivery of islet hormones to target cells.

Insulin

The beta cells of the pancreas synthesize **insulin** from the precursor proinsulin, which is formed from a larger and earlier precursor molecule, preproinsulin. Proinsulin is composed of an A peptide and a B peptide connected by a C peptide and two disulfide bonds. C peptide is cleaved by proteolytic enzymes, leaving the bonded A and B peptide chains that become insulin. Insulin circulates freely in the plasma and is not bound to a carrier. C peptide can be measured in the blood as an indirect measure of serum insulin synthesis.

Secretion of insulin is regulated by chemical, hormonal, and neural control. Insulin secretion is pulsatile, increasing when the beta cells are stimulated by the parasympathetic nervous system, usually before eating a meal. Other factors stimulating insulin secretion include increased blood levels of glucose, amino acids (leucine, arginine, and lysine), and gastrointestinal hormones (glucagon, gastrin, cholecystokinin, secretin). Insulin secretion diminishes in response to low blood levels of glucose (hypoglycemia), high levels of insulin (through negative feedback to the beta cells), and sympathetic stimulation of the beta cells in the islets. Prostaglandins also inhibit insulin secretion.

At the target cell, insulin binds with an enzyme-linked plasma membrane receptor that contains tyrosine kinase on the cytosolic surface found on cells throughout the body. Insulin receptor binding sends a cascade of signals to activate glucose transporters (GLUT) for entry of glucose into the cell. The primary GLUT is called GLUT4. It is stored in cellular vesicles until activated by the insulin receptor and is then translocated to the cell surface where it facilitates the diffusion of glucose into the cell. Translocation of GLUT4 to the cell surface is associated with a 10- to 21-fold increase in glucose diffusion into the cell, particularly in skeletal and cardiac muscle, liver, and adipose cells (Fig. 21.16). Insulin sensitivity, denoting the biological responsiveness to insulin, is affected by age, weight, abdominal fat, and physical activity. Insulin resistance, a subnormal biological response to normal insulin concentrations, has been implicated in numerous diseases, including hypertension, heart

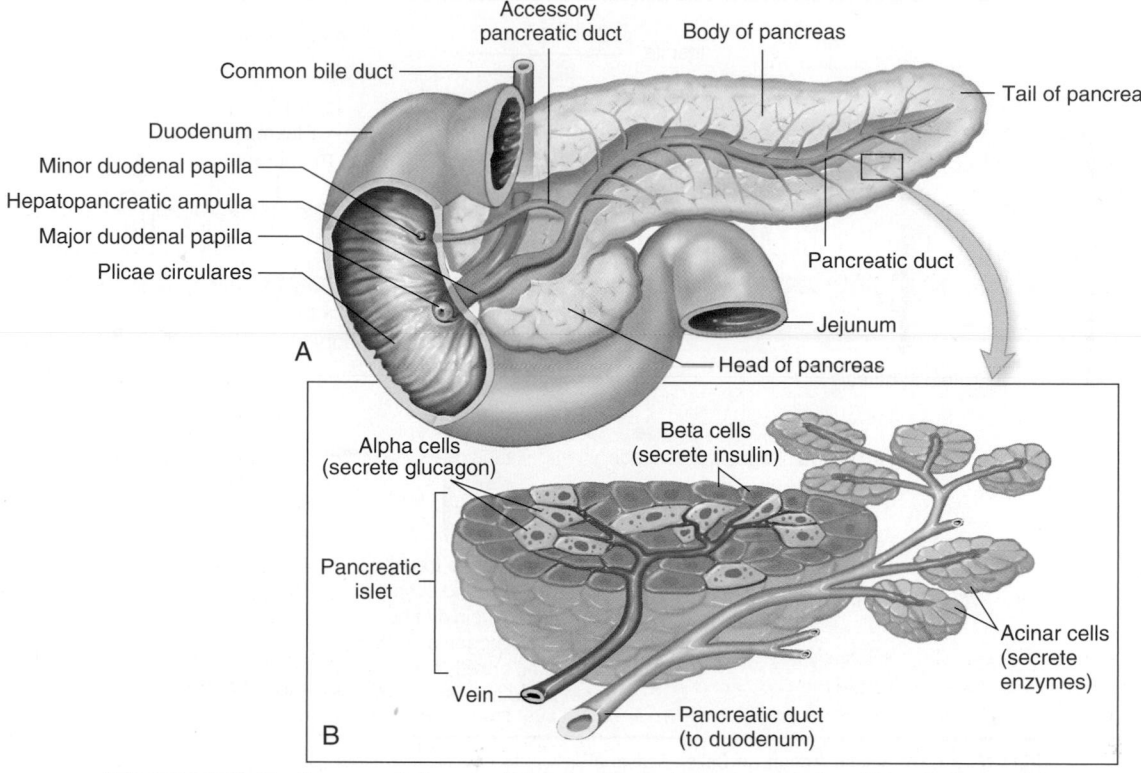

FIGURE 21.15 The Pancreas. **A,** Pancreas dissected to show main and accessory ducts. The main duct may join the common bile duct, as shown here, to enter the duodenum by a single opening at the major duodenal papilla, or the two ducts may have separate openings. The accessory pancreatic duct is usually present and has a separate opening into the duodenum. **B,** Exocrine glandular cells (around small pancreatic ducts) and endocrine glandular cells of the pancreatic islets (adjacent to blood capillaries). Exocrine pancreatic cells secrete pancreatic juice, alpha endocrine cells secrete glucagon, and beta cells secrete insulin. (Adapted from Patton KT, Thibodeau GA: *The human body in health & disease*, ed 7, St Louis, 2018, Elsevier.)

disease, and type 2 diabetes mellitus. Adipocytes release a number of hormones that are altered in obesity and have an important adverse effect on insulin sensitivity. The most effective measures shown to improve insulin sensitivity in humans are weight loss and exercise.[26]

Insulin is an anabolic hormone that promotes glucose uptake primarily in liver, muscle, and adipose tissue. It also increases the synthesis of proteins, carbohydrates, lipids, and nucleic acids. Table 21.7 summarizes the actions of insulin. The net effect of insulin in these tissues is to stimulate protein and fat synthesis and decrease blood glucose level. The brain, red blood cells, kidney, and lens of the eye do not require insulin for glucose transport. Insulin also facilitates the intracellular transport of potassium (K^+), phosphate, and magnesium. Insulin is metabolized in the liver and kidney by enzymes that split disulfide bonds. Very little insulin is excreted unchanged in the urine.

Amylin

Amylin (islet amyloid polypeptide) is a peptide hormone cosecreted with insulin by beta cells in response to nutrient stimuli. It regulates blood glucose concentration by delaying gastric emptying and suppressing glucagon secretion after meals. Amylin also has a satiety effect which reduces food intake. Through these mechanisms, amylin has an antihyperglycemic effect.[27]

Glucagon

Glucagon is produced by the alpha cells of the pancreas and by cells lining the gastrointestinal tract. Glucagon is an antagonist to insulin and

TABLE 21.7 INSULIN ACTIONS

ACTIONS	SITES OF INSULIN-PROMOTED SYNTHESIS		
	LIVER CELLS	**MUSCLE CELLS**	**ADIPOSE CELLS**
Glucose uptake	Increased	Increased	Increased
Glucose use	—	—	Increased glycerol phosphate
Glycogenesis	Increased	Increased	—
Glycogenolysis	Decreased	Decreased	—
Glycolysis	Increased	Increased	Increased
Gluconeogenesis	Increased	—	—
Other	Increased fatty acid synthesis	Increased amino acid uptake	Increased fat esterification
	Decreased ketogenesis	Increased protein synthesis	Decreased lipolysis
	Decreased urea cycle activity	Decreased proteolysis	Increased fat storage

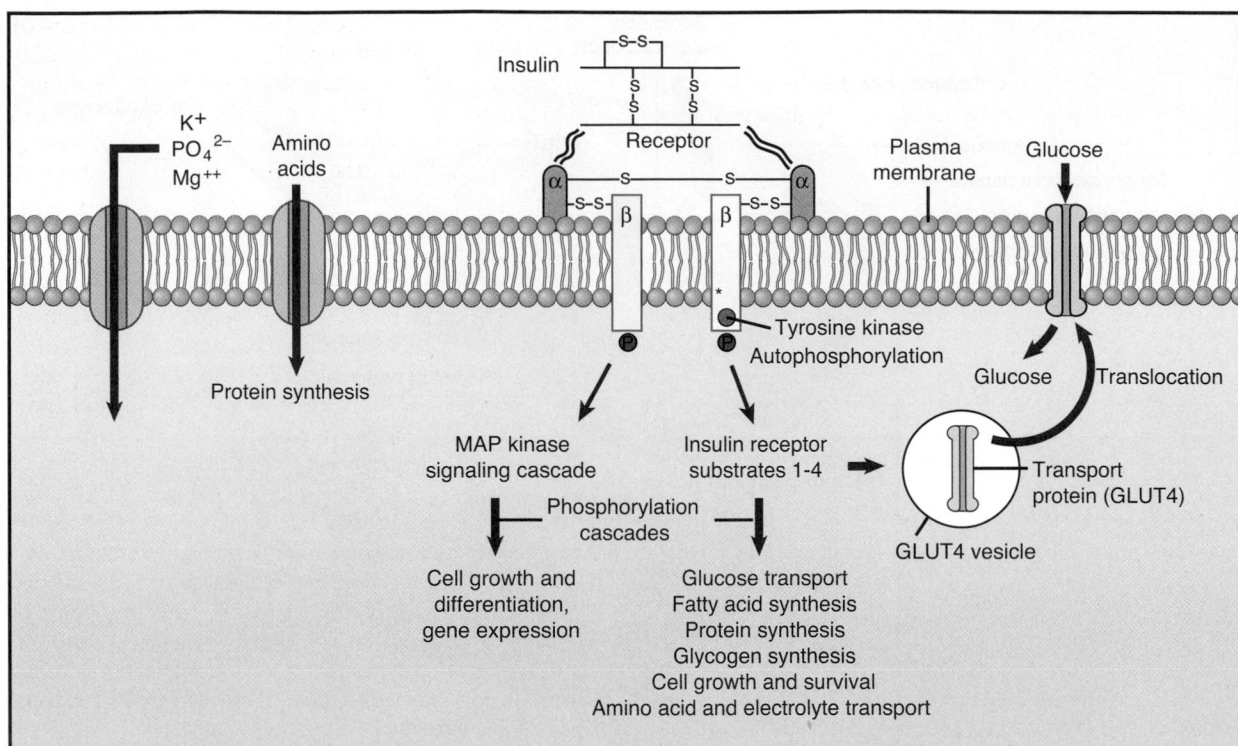

FIGURE 21.16 Insulin Action on Cells. Binding of insulin to its receptor causes autophosphorylation of the receptor, which then itself acts as a tyrosine kinase that phosphorylates insulin receptor substrate 1. Numerous target enzymes, such as protein kinase B and MAP kinase, are activated, and these enzymes have a multitude of effects on cell function. The glucose transporter, GLUT4, is recruited to the plasma membrane, where it facilitates glucose entry into the cell. The transport of amino acids, potassium, magnesium, and phosphate into the cell is also facilitated. The synthesis of various enzymes is induced or suppressed, and cell growth is regulated by signal molecules that modulate gene expression. *MAP*, Mitogen-activated protein. (Redrawn from Levy MN, Koeppen BM, Stanton BA: *Principles of physiology*, ed 4, St Louis, 2006, Mosby.)

acts to increase blood glucose during fasting, exercise, and hypoglycemia. It acts primarily in the liver to increase blood glucose concentration by stimulating glycogenolysis. Glucagon also stimulates gluconeogenesis in the kidneys and lipolysis in adipose tissue. Muscle glucagon is used only by muscle and not systemically. High glucose levels cause glucagon release to be inhibited; low glucose levels and sympathetic stimulation promote glucagon release. Amino acids, such as alanine, glycine, and asparagine, also stimulate glucagon secretion. A protein-rich meal has the same effect. Glucagon also stimulates lipolysis, which has a ketogenic effect caused by the metabolism of free fatty acids in the liver. These effects have led to the hypothesis that impaired glucagon secretion is as important as insulin insufficiency in the pathogenesis of diabetes.[28]

Pancreatic Somatostatin

Pancreatic somatostatin is produced by delta cells of the pancreas in response to food intake and is a hormone essential in carbohydrate, fat, and protein metabolism. It differs from hypothalamic somatostatin, which inhibits release of growth hormone and TSH. Pancreatic somatostatin is involved in regulating alpha-cell and beta-cell function within the islets by inhibiting secretion of insulin, glucagon, and pancreatic polypeptide.

Incretins

The incretin hormones are secreted from endocrine cells in the gastrointestinal tract in the presence of carbohydrates, proteins, and fats. The major incretin hormones are glucagon-like peptide-1 (GLP-1) and glucose-dependent insulinotropic polypeptide (GIP). They control postprandial glucose levels by promoting glucose-dependent insulin secretion, inhibiting glucagon synthesis, promoting hepatic glucose secretion, and delaying gastric emptying. Incretins also enhance beta-cell mass and replenish intracellular stores of insulin. Incretins are broken down by an enzyme called *dipeptidyl peptidase 4 (DPP-4)*, and drugs that inhibit this enzyme (called *gliptins*) increase incretin levels. The gliptins are incretin agonists used for the treatment of type 2 diabetes.[29]

Gastrin, Ghrelin, and Pancreatic Polypeptide

Gastrin is released by G cells in the stomach and stimulates the secretion of gastric acid. Ghrelin is an intestinal hormone and stimulates GH secretion, controls appetite, and plays a role in obesity and the regulation of insulin sensitivity and glucose tolerance.[30] Pancreatic polypeptide is released by PP cells (gamma cells) in response to hypoglycemia and protein-rich meals. It promotes gastric secretion, antagonizes cholecystokinin, and is frequently increased in pancreatic tumors and in diabetes.[31]

Adrenal Glands

The adrenal glands are paired pyramid-shaped organs located behind the peritoneum and close to the upper pole of each kidney. Each gland is surrounded by a capsule embedded in fat and well supplied with blood from the phrenic and renal arteries and the aorta. Venous return from the left adrenal gland is to the renal vein and from the right is to the inferior vena cava.

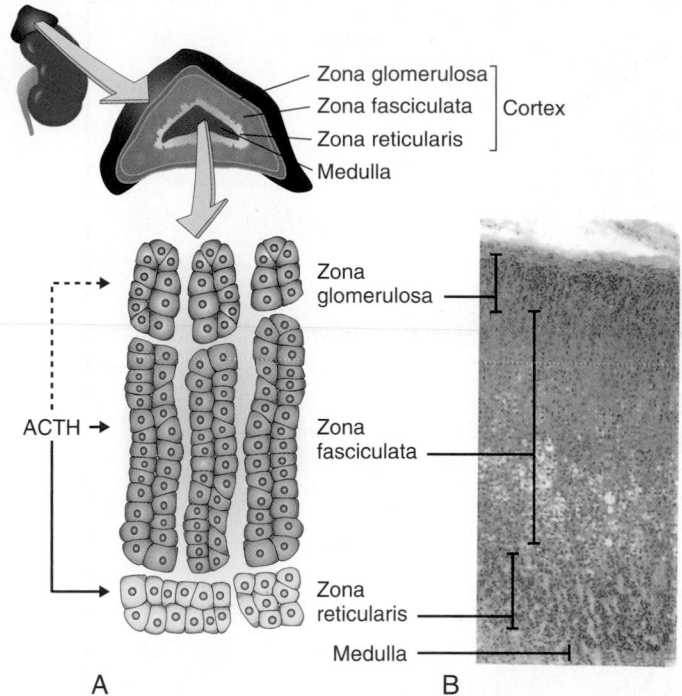

FIGURE 21.17 Structure of the Adrenal Gland Showing Cell Layers (Zones) of the Cortex. **A,** Adrenal glands. Each gland consists of cortex and medulla. The cortex has three layers: zona glomerulosa, zona fasciculata, and zona reticularis. **B,** A portion of the medulla is visible at the lower right in the photomicrograph (×35) and at the bottom of the drawing. *ACTH,* Adrenocorticotropic hormone. (**A** from Damjanov I: *Pathophysiology,* Philadelphia, 2008, Saunders; **B** from Kierszenbaum A: *Histology and cell biology,* St Louis, 2002, Mosby.)

Each adrenal gland consists of two separate portions: an outer cortex and an inner medulla. These two portions have different embryonic origins, different structures, and different hormonal functions. The adrenal cortex and medulla function like two separate but interrelated glands (Fig. 21.17).

Adrenal Cortex

The adrenal cortex accounts for 80% of the weight of the adult gland. The cortex is histologically subdivided into the following three zones:
1. The zona glomerulosa, the outer layer, constitutes about 15% of the cortex and primarily produces the mineralocorticoid aldosterone.
2. The zona fasciculata, the middle layer, constitutes 78% of the cortex and secretes the glucocorticoids cortisol, cortisone, and corticosterone.
3. The zona reticularis, the inner layer, constitutes 7% of the cortex and secretes mineralocorticoids (aldosterone), adrenal androgens and estrogens, and glucocorticoids.

The cells of the adrenal cortex are stimulated by the anterior pituitary hormone ACTH. All hormones of the adrenal cortex are synthesized from low-density lipoprotein cholesterol. The best-known pathway of steroidogenesis involves the conversion of cholesterol to pregnenolone, which is then converted to the major corticosteroids.[32]

Glucocorticoids. The glucocorticoids are steroid hormones and have metabolic, neurologic, antiinflammatory, immunosuppressive, and growth-suppressing effects (Fig. 21.18). They are released under stress conditions.[33] They act through nuclear (genomic) and nongenomic (membrane-initiated steroid signaling) pathways in the cell. The term *glucocorticoid* refers to those steroid hormones that have direct effects on carbohydrate metabolism. These hormones increase blood glucose concentration by promoting gluconeogenesis in the liver and conserving glucose by decreasing uptake of glucose into muscle cells, adipose cells, and lymphatic cells by antagonizing insulin. This results in increased glucose for the brain during stress.[34] In extrahepatic tissues, the glucocorticoids stimulate protein catabolism and inhibit amino acid uptake and protein synthesis. The ultimate effect on the body is protein catabolism and muscle wasting.

The glucocorticoids act at several sites to suppress immune and inflammatory reactions (described in Chapters 7 and 9).[35] They affect innate immunity through several pathways, including inhibition of antigen presentation by dendritic cells and decreased activity of pattern recognition receptors on the surface of macrophages (see Chapter 7). They decrease the proliferation of T lymphocytes, primarily T-helper lymphocytes. There is a greater adverse effect on T-helper 1 cell cytokine production (including antiviral interferons) than there is on T-helper 2 cell cytokine production and therefore greater depression of cellular immunity than humoral immunity (see Chapter 8). Glucocorticoids also decrease immune and inflammatory responses by decreasing natural killer cell activity; by blocking phospholipase A and the synthesis of prostaglandins, thromboxanes, and leukotrienes; and by inhibiting inflammatory gene expression. In addition, glucocorticoids suppress the synthesis, secretion, and actions of chemical mediators involved in inflammatory and immune responses, including histamine, adhesion molecules, inducible cyclooxygenase, and inducible nitric oxide synthase.[36]

Glucocorticoids increase resistance to the severe inflammatory response to lipopolysaccharide (LPS, a bacterial endotoxin) through the inhibition of cytokines, chemokines, certain hormones, and neurotransmitters. In addition, glucocorticoids stimulate antiinflammatory cytokines (e.g., interleukin-10 [IL-10] and transforming growth factor-beta). Lysosomal membranes are also stabilized, decreasing the release of proteolytic enzymes. This suppression of innate and adaptive immunity by glucocorticoids means that infection and poor wound healing are some of the most problematic complications of the use of glucocorticoids in the treatment of disease. Similarly, psychologic and physiologic stress increases glucocorticoid production, which provides a pathway for the well-described decrease in immunity seen in both acute and chronic stress conditions (see Chapter 11).[37,38]

Other effects of glucocorticoids include inhibition of bone formation, inhibition of ADH secretion, and stimulation of gastric acid secretion. Glucocorticoids appear to potentiate the effects of catecholamines, including sensitizing the arterioles to the vasoconstrictive effects of norepinephrine. Thyroid hormone and growth hormone effects on adipose tissue also are potentiated by glucocorticoids. A metabolite of cortisol may act like a barbiturate and depress nerve cell function in the brain, accounting for the noted effects on mood associated with steroid level fluctuation in disease or stress.

Pathologically high levels of glucocorticoids increase the number of circulating erythrocytes (leading to polycythemia), increase the appetite, promote fat deposition in the face and cervical areas, increase uric acid excretion, decrease serum calcium levels (possibly by inhibiting gastrointestinal absorption of calcium), suppress the secretion and synthesis of ACTH, and interfere with the action of growth hormone so that somatic growth is inhibited.[39]

The most potent of the naturally occurring glucocorticoids is cortisol. It is the main secretory product of the adrenal cortex and is needed to maintain life and regulate the body during both positive and negative stress (see Chapter 11, particularly Fig. 11.2). Cortisol has a biologic half-life of approximately 90 minutes, with the liver primarily responsible for its deactivation.

Cortisol secretion is regulated primarily by the hypothalamus and the anterior pituitary gland (Fig. 21.19). Corticotropin-releasing hormone

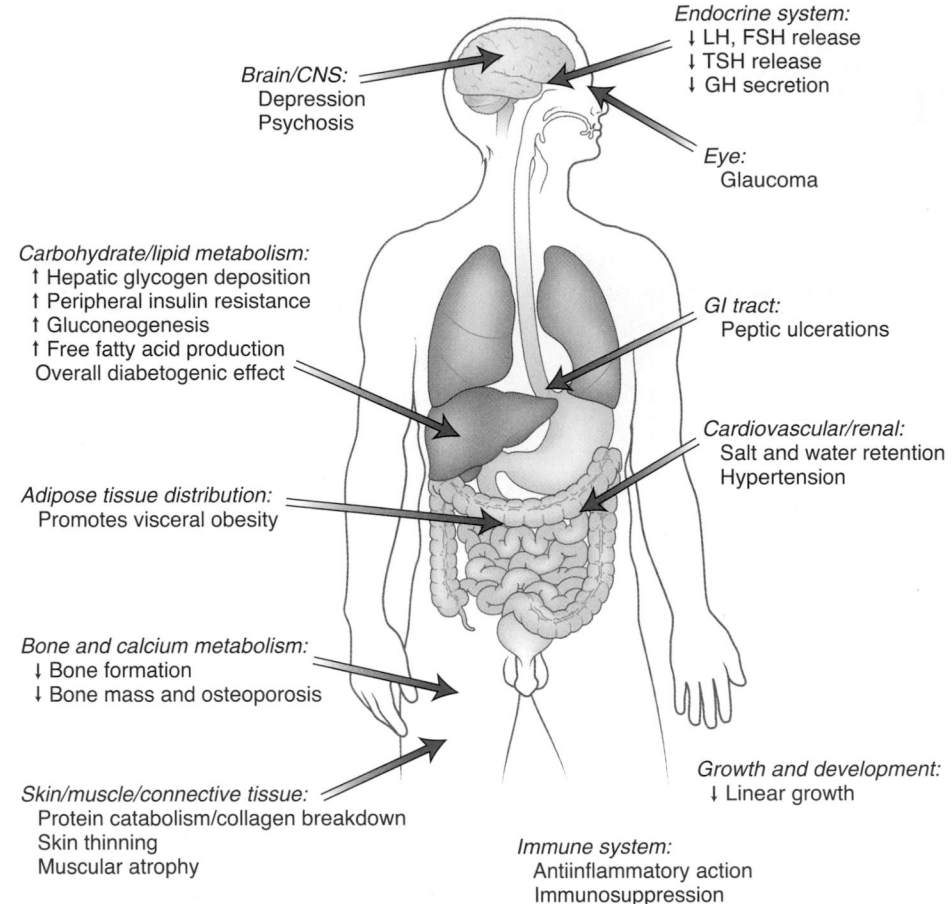

Brain/CNS:
Depression
Psychosis

Endocrine system:
↓ LH, FSH release
↓ TSH release
↓ GH secretion

Eye:
Glaucoma

Carbohydrate/lipid metabolism:
↑ Hepatic glycogen deposition
↑ Peripheral insulin resistance
↑ Gluconeogenesis
↑ Free fatty acid production
Overall diabetogenic effect

GI tract:
Peptic ulcerations

Cardiovascular/renal:
Salt and water retention
Hypertension

Adipose tissue distribution:
Promotes visceral obesity

Bone and calcium metabolism:
↓ Bone formation
↓ Bone mass and osteoporosis

Skin/muscle/connective tissue:
Protein catabolism/collagen breakdown
Skin thinning
Muscular atrophy

Growth and development:
↓ Linear growth

Immune system:
Antiinflammatory action
Immunosuppression

FIGURE 21.18 Effects of Glucocorticoids on the Body. *CNS,* Central nervous system; *FSH,* follicle-stimulating hormone; *GH,* growth hormone; *GI,* gastrointestinal; *LH,* luteinizing hormone; *TSH,* thyroid-stimulating hormone. (From Steward PM, Newell-Price JDC: The adrenal cortex. In Melmed S et al, editors: *Williams textbook of endocrinology,* ed 13, Philadelphia, 2016, Saunders.)

is produced in several nuclei in the hypothalamus and stored in the median eminence. Once released, CRH travels through the portal vessels to stimulate the production of ACTH, β-lipotropin, γ-lipotropin, endorphins, and enkephalins by the anterior pituitary. ACTH is the main regulator of cortisol secretion and adrenocortical growth.

The precursor from which ACTH is synthesized is proopiomelanocortin (POMC). Three factors appear to be primarily involved in regulating the secretion of ACTH: (1) negative feedback effects of high circulating levels of cortisol and synthetic glucocorticoids suppress both CRH and ACTH, whereas low cortisol levels stimulate their secretion; (2) diurnal rhythms affect ACTH and cortisol levels (in persons with regular sleep-wake patterns, ACTH peaks 3 to 5 hours after sleep begins and declines throughout the day; and cortisol levels follow a similar pattern, peaking just before awakening); and (3) psychologic and physiologic (e.g., hypoxia, hypoglycemia, hyperthermia, exercise) stress increases ACTH secretion, leading to increased cortisol levels.[40] (Neurologic mechanisms regulating sleep are discussed in Chapter 16.)

There also is evidence that there is synthesis and secretion of glucocorticoids from extra-adrenal tissue including the thymus, lung, intestine, skin, brain, and possibly heart in response to immune stimulation. This is thought to provide autocrine and paracrine immune regulation and control of inflammation.[41,42]

When ACTH is secreted, it binds to specific plasma membrane receptors on the cells of the adrenal cortex and on other extra-adrenal tissues. Because both adrenal and extra-adrenal tissues have ACTH

BOX 21.1   EFFECTS OF ADRENOCORTICOTROPIC HORMONE

Adrenal
Maintenance of gland size
Depletion of ascorbic acid
Activation of adenylyl cyclase
Conversion of cholesterol to pregnenolone
Maintenance of enzymes active in converting pregnenolone to other steroids
Accumulation of cholesterol for steroid hormone synthesis
Secretion of cortisol and adrenal androgens

Extra-Adrenal
Stimulation of melanocytes
Activation of tissue lipase

receptors, a number of effects result from stimulation by ACTH (these effects are summarized in Box 21.1).[43]

Once ACTH stimulates the cells of the adrenal cortex, cortisol synthesis and secretion immediately occur. In the healthy person, the secretory patterns of ACTH and cortisol are nearly identical. After secretion, most cortisol circulates in bound form: 15% to 30% is bound

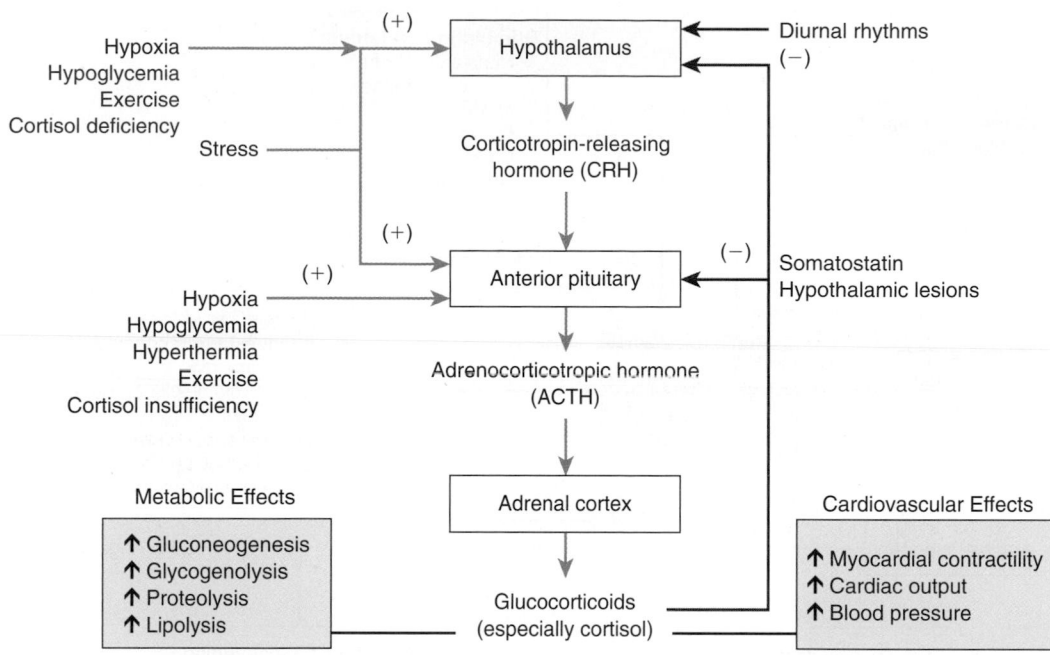

FIGURE 21.19 Feedback Control of Glucocorticoid Synthesis and Secretion.

to albumin, 55% to 75% is tightly but reversibly bound to a plasma glycoprotein called *transcortin,* and 10% to 15% is unbound. The levels of transcortin play a role in the HPA feedback system controlling cortisol secretion. Transcortin levels are significantly elevated by increased estrogen levels that occur with pregnancy and hormone therapy. The unbound portion is free to diffuse into cells, but only those cells with specific intracellular glucocorticoid receptors respond to cortisol stimulation. ACTH is rapidly inactivated in the circulation, and the liver and kidneys remove the deactivated hormone.

Mineralocorticoids: Aldosterone. Mineralocorticoid steroids directly affect ion transport by epithelial cells, causing sodium retention and potassium and hydrogen loss. Aldosterone is the most potent of the naturally occurring mineralocorticoids and acts to conserve sodium by increasing the activity of the sodium pump of the epithelial cells in the nephron. (The sodium pump is described in Chapter 1.)

The initial stages of aldosterone synthesis occur in the adrenal zona fasciculata and zona reticularis. The final conversion of corticosterone to aldosterone occurs in the zona glomerulosa. Aldosterone synthesis and secretion are regulated primarily by the renin-angiotensin-aldosterone system (described in Chapter 3 and Chapter 38; see Figs. 3.4 and 38.10), although other factors also may be involved. The renin-angiotensin system is activated by sodium and water depletion, increased potassium levels, and a diminished effective blood volume (Fig. 21.20). Angiotensin II is the primary stimulant of aldosterone synthesis and secretion; however, increases in serum potassium concentration also directly stimulate aldosterone secretion. ACTH acutely stimulates aldosterone secretion but is secondary to angiotensin II and potassium.[44]

When sodium and potassium levels are within normal limits, approximately 50 to 250 mg of aldosterone is secreted daily. Of the secreted aldosterone, 50% to 75% binds to plasma proteins. The proportion of unbound aldosterone contributes to its rapid metabolic turnover in the liver, its low plasma concentration, and its short half-life (about 15 minutes). Aldosterone is degraded in the liver and is excreted by the kidney.

Aldosterone maintains extracellular volume and blood pressure by acting on distal nephron epithelial cells to increase sodium reabsorption and potassium and hydrogen excretion.[45] The renal effect takes from

90 minutes to 6 hours. Other effects of aldosterone include enhancement of cardiac muscle contraction, stimulation of ectopic ventricular activity through secondary cardiac pacemakers in the ventricles, stiffening of blood vessels with increased vascular resistance, and decreased fibrinolysis. Pathologically elevated levels of aldosterone have been implicated in the myocardial changes associated with heart failure.[46]

Adrenal Estrogens and Androgens. The healthy adrenal cortex secretes small amounts of estrogen and androgens. ACTH appears to be the major regulator. Some of the weak androgenic substances secreted by the cortex (dehydroepiandrosterone [DHEA], androstenedione) are converted by peripheral tissues to stronger androgens, such as testosterone, thus accounting for some androgenic effects initiated by the adrenal cortex. Peripheral conversion of adrenal androgens to estrogens is enhanced in aging or obese persons, as well as in those with liver disease or hyperthyroidism. The biologic effects and metabolism of the adrenal sex steroids do not vary from those produced by the gonads (see Chapter 24).

Adrenal Medulla

The adrenal medulla, together with the sympathetic division of the autonomic nervous system, is embryonically derived from neural crest cells. Chromaffin cells (pheochromocytes) are the cells of the adrenal gland that store and secrete the catecholamines epinephrine (adrenaline) and norepinephrine. Both are synthesized from the amino acid phenylalanine (Fig. 21.21). Only 30% of circulating epinephrine comes from the adrenal medulla; the other 70% is released from nerve terminals. The medulla is only a minor source of norepinephrine.[47] The adrenal medulla functions as a sympathetic ganglion without postganglionic processes. Sympathetic cholinergic preganglion fibers terminate on the chromaffin cells and secrete catecholamines directly into the bloodstream. The catecholamines are, therefore, hormones and not neurotransmitters.

Physiologic stress to the body (e.g., traumatic injury, hypoxia, hypoglycemia, and many others) triggers release of adrenal catecholamines through acetylcholine (from the preganglionic sympathetic fibers), which depolarizes the chromaffin cells. Depolarization causes exocytosis of storage granules from the chromaffin cells with release of epinephrine and

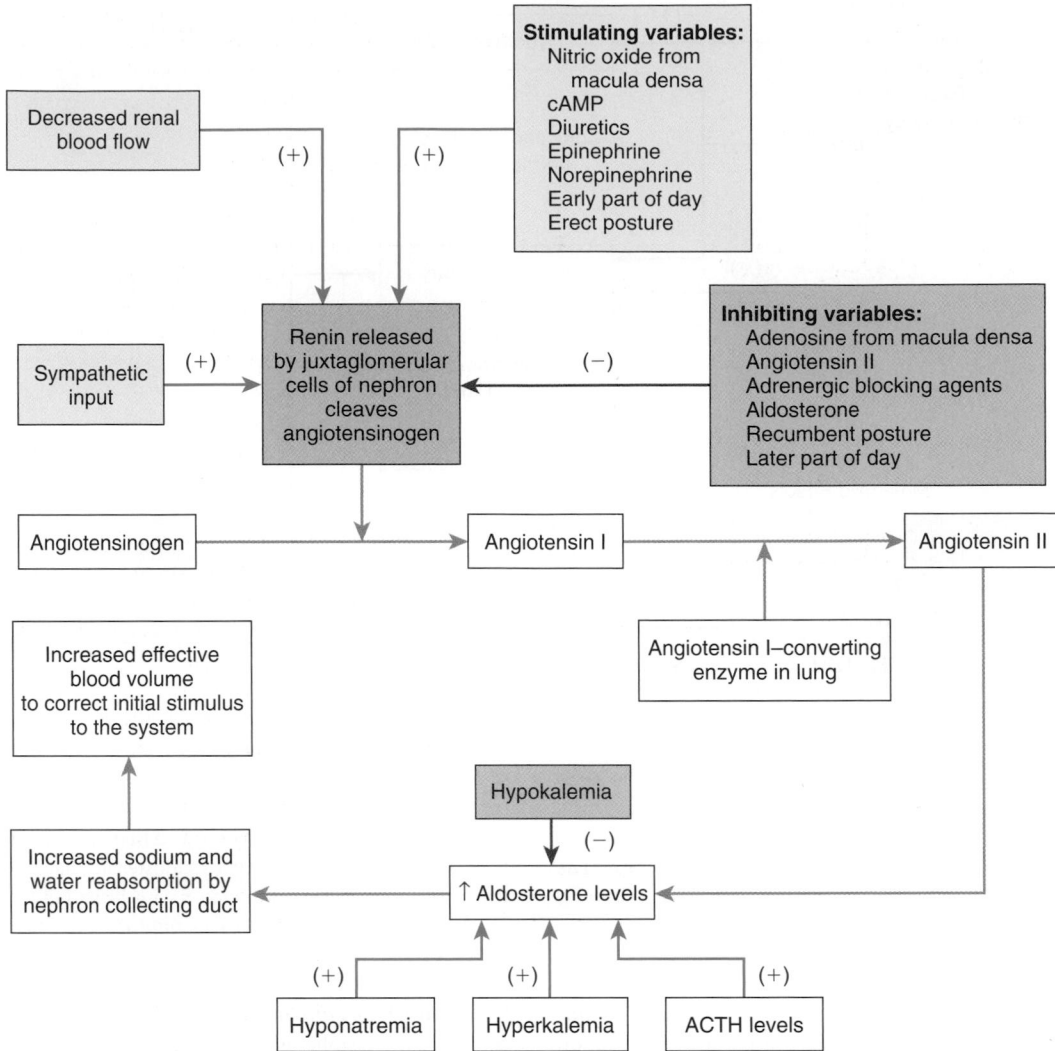

FIGURE 21.20 Feedback Mechanisms Regulating Aldosterone Secretion. *ACTH,* Adrenocorticotropic hormone; *cAMP,* cyclic adenosine monophosphate.

norepinephrine into the bloodstream. Secretion of adrenal catecholamines is also increased by ACTH and the glucocorticoids.

Once released, the catecholamines remain in the plasma for only seconds to minutes. The catecholamines exert rapid biologic effects after binding to a plasma membrane receptor (α_1, α_2, β_1, β_2, β_3) in target cells and activating the adenylyl cyclase system (see Table 15.7). Catecholamines are rapidly removed from the plasma by neurons for storage in new cytoplasmic granules, or they may be metabolically inactivated and excreted in the urine.

Catecholamines have diverse effects on the entire body. Their release and the body's response have been characterized as the "fight or flight" response (see Chapter 11 and Table 11.1). In general, the effects of catecholamines activate adrenergic receptors on cell membranes of all visceral organs and smooth muscles and promote hyperglycemia.[48]

Tests of Endocrine Function

Evaluation of the endocrine system is challenging because of (1) the complexity of the clinical presentation as a result of multiple organ system involvement, (2) the nonspecific nature of complaints frequently associated with endocrine dysfunction, and (3) the inappropriate use of laboratory test interpretations.

Tests of the endocrine system involve several general types of clinical evaluation. Measurement of hormone level is accomplished by radioimmunoassay, by enzyme-linked immunosorbent assay, and less commonly by bioassay. **Radioimmunoassay (RIA)**, a technique for measuring the minute quantities of hormones in the blood, uses antibodies and radiolabeled hormones to determine the quantity of hormone in the plasma. **Enzyme-linked immunosorbent assay (ELISA)** also is used to determine circulating hormone levels. This method is similar to that of RIA but is less expensive and easier to conduct. Instead of radiolabeled hormones, an enzyme-labeled hormone is used. A **bioassay** involves the use of graded doses of hormone in a reference preparation and then comparison of the results with an unknown sample. Bioassays are used more commonly in investigative endocrinology than in clinical laboratories. If the serum level is greater or less than the reference values, more definitive tests are required to determine the source of the problem.

Measurement of individual hormones does not always permit differentiation between normal and abnormal values when hormone levels are changing over time. For an accurate interpretation, the broad normal range of some hormones requires knowledge of previous hormonal levels and timed sampling. Stimulation and suppression tests that

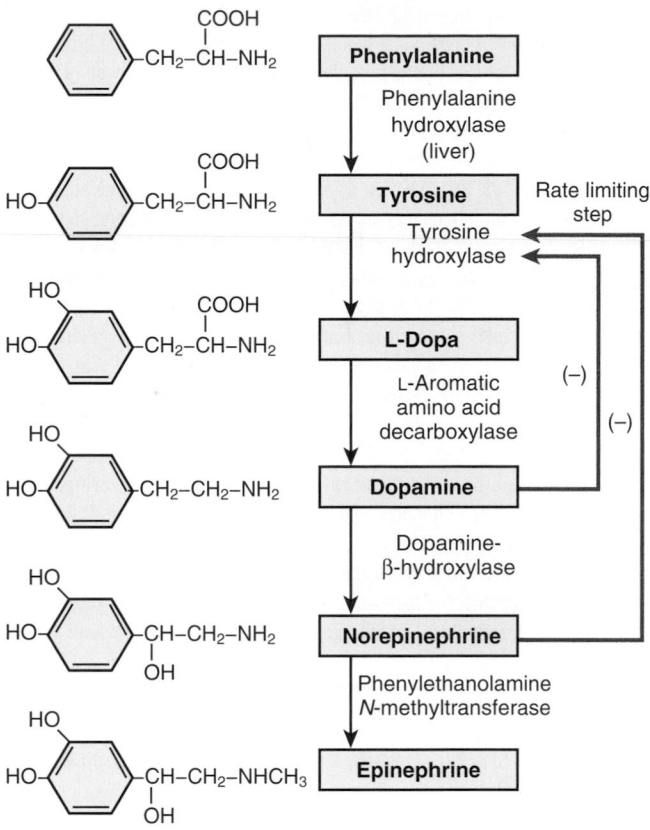

FIGURE 21.21 Synthesis of Catecholamines.

determine the response to exogenous stimulants or inhibitors can help to decipher some of these complexities.

Indirect assessment of hormonal function often includes measurement of concentrations of serum glucose and electrolytes that are affected by the endocrine process. Evaluation of hormonal function also may include radiographic imaging of specific glands.

AGING AND THE ENDOCRINE SYSTEM

The precise relationship between aging and the endocrine system is not clear. Perhaps most important, the question of whether changes in endocrine function are a consequence or a cause of aging has yet to be resolved. These relationships have been difficult to identify, in part because of a number of age-related variables that may coexist, such as acute and chronic nonendocrine disease; use of medications; alterations in diet, body composition, and weight; and changes in sleep-wake cycles. However, the endocrine system is so integral to health that changes in endocrine function have been used as "biomarkers" for unhealthy aging.

Investigation into the role of the endocrine glands and their interactions in the aging process has generated much data, although the evidence is contradictory. There are complex changes within the HPA; altered biologic activity of hormones, altered circulating levels of hormones, altered secretory response of the endocrine glands, altered metabolism of hormones, loss of circadian control of hormone secretion, and effects of oxidative stress and inflammation are among the findings. Changes in secretion of hypothalamic regulatory factors and hormones or changes in hypothalamic feedback sensitivity may contribute to alterations in control of an optimal internal environment.[49]

The dynamic equilibrium of the endocrine system also may be affected by altered secretion of neurotransmitters within certain areas of the brain, affecting hypothalamic and pituitary function. Such alterations may include an excess or deficit in secretion of pituitary hormones and loss of appropriate secretory pattern of those hormones. Loss of endocrine steady states may be associated with or contribute to aging.[50]

The most studied changes in hormone function with aging affect the levels of reproductive hormones and gonadotropins (menopause and andropause) (discussed in Chapter 24). Two of the most important endocrine changes associated with aging affect the thyroid gland and the pancreas. Other important hormone changes associated with aging include a decline in serum levels of growth hormone and IGF-1, parathyroid hormone, dehydroepiandrosterone, and ADH.

Thyroid Gland

Changes in thyroid structure and function occur with aging.[51] Structurally, some glandular atrophy and fibrosis occur with nodularity and increasing inflammatory infiltrates. These infiltrative changes may reflect age-related autoimmune damage. Clinical signs of thyroid disease are more difficult to detect in older adults. Overall, it is estimated that there is some evidence of thyroid dysfunction in 5% to 10% of older adult women. The presence of thyroid nodules increases after the age of 70 years. Changes relative to thyroid hormone and its function are more difficult to assess and much of the available data are contradictory. Overall, TSH secretion is thought to increase slightly, but there is controversy regarding whether this is normal aging or the presence of hypothyroidism with risk for adverse consequences.[52]

Treatment for thyroid deficiency is also affected by aging. The appropriate dose for TH replacement is often lower in older adults because the peripheral metabolism of TH decreases with age. In addition, TH must be replaced slowly in older adults with coronary artery disease to prevent angina and myocardial infarction.[51]

The Endocrine Pancreas

It is estimated that 40% to 50% of individuals older than age 65 have impaired glucose tolerance or diabetes and there is an age-dependent decline in beta-cell function.[53] With aging, pancreatic cell regeneration declines and there is increased distribution of fat tissue.[54]

Dysfunction of the pancreas with decreased insulin secretion of beta cells and insulin receptors and increased insulin resistance have all been documented and may be related to changes in adipokine physiology.[55] These changes have significant implications for many target organs, particularly the cardiovascular system, which is increasingly at risk for both vascular (hypertension, atherosclerosis, glomerulosclerosis) and cardiac (infarction, failure) disorders.

Growth Hormone and Insulin-Like Growth Factors

The amounts of GH and IGF decline with aging, a process that has been called the *somatopause*.[56] This decline in anabolic stimuli is linked to decreases in muscle size and function, decreased amounts of fat and bone mass, and changes in reproductive and cognitive function.[57] Some studies have shown that growth hormone resistance and declines in GH are associated with longevity in animals, but this has not been confirmed in humans.[58]

Parathyroid Glands

An age-related alteration in PTH secretion has been proposed to explain alterations in calcium homeostasis that have been noted in older adults.[59] Calcium intake, especially in women, tends to decrease with aging and may contribute to osteoporosis (see Chapter 45). The average daily intake of 450 to 500 mg/day causes a negative calcium balance greater than 40 mg/day and may be related to the absolute bone loss of approximately 1.5% per year. Older adults show decreased intestinal adaptation to variations in calcium intake. Hyperparathyroidism may occur secondary to calcium malabsorption and hypocalcemia with increased bone remodeling that results in cortical bone thinning and porosity. Elevated levels of parathyroid hormone have been linked with an increase in mortality in older adults, many of whom also have a mild, persistent hypercalciuria, which indicates a defective renal mechanism for responding to decreased calcium intake. Decreased circulating levels of vitamin D are common in older adults, especially those in long-term care institutions. Vitamin D deficiency has been linked to not only osteoporosis but also cancer, autoimmune diseases, diabetes, cardiovascular disease, and mental health disorders. The parathyroid gland, kidney, and choroid plexus secrete the Klotho protein, which, when overexpressed, has antiaging effects (see *What's New?* Klotho Protein and Aging).

Adrenal Glands

The adrenal cortex loses some weight and has more fibrous tissue after the age of 50 years. Age does not appear to affect the feedback mechanisms involved in maintaining glucocorticoid levels, but there is an age-related decrease in the metabolic clearance rate of the glucocorticoids.

The metabolic clearance of cortisol decreases with an age-related decline in liver and kidney function. Further, less cortisol appears to be used by the body when aging is accompanied by a loss of lean body mass. Decreased clearance and reduced use of cortisol contribute to higher circulating cortisol levels, but diurnal variation is maintained. Because feedback mechanisms are intact, the higher cortisol levels cause a decrease in cortisol secretion. Circadian patterns of ACTH and cortisol secretion may change with aging.

Plasma levels of the adrenal androgens, as well as urinary excretion of the metabolic end products, decrease gradually but dramatically with age, to as much as 50% to 70% of the young adult level. This change in adrenal function has been called the *adrenopause* and is correlated with decreased synthesis activity of DHEA.[60]

This change appears to reflect a decline in the function of the zona reticularis. In postmenopausal women, this decline in adrenal androgen secretion is especially important because nearly all sex steroids after menopause come from adrenal and ovarian production of androgen precursors converted to estrogens in the periphery. In older adult men, adrenal androgen production accounts for more than half of circulating testosterone levels.

WHAT'S NEW?

Klotho Protein and Aging

Klotho is a protein known to have antiaging effects and is expressed in parathyroid glands, kidney distal tubules, and choroid plexus of the brain. The transmembrane form of Klotho protein functions as an obligatory co-receptor for FGF23, which is important for the regulation of vitamin D metabolism and subsequently blood phosphate levels. In addition, the extracellular domain of the protein is secreted into the blood, cerebrospinal fluid, and urine. This suggests that Klotho may function as an endocrine or paracrine hormone, but the mechanisms are not clearly known. Decreased plasma, urinary, and renal Klotho levels are associated with normal aging, chronic kidney disease, salt-sensitive hypertension, cancers, osteoporosis, atherosclerosis, coronary artery disease, and increased mortality. Klotho also is known to have a tumor suppressor function. In contrast, overexpression of the Klotho gene results in longevity and reversal of the aging process in animals. It is postulated that Klotho extends life by attenuating generation of reactive oxygen species, cytokines, and growth factors, including insulin, insulin-like growth factor-1 (IGF-1), transforming growth factor-β (TGF-β), and interferon-γ (IFN-γ). Finally, the Klotho protein is a powerful regulator of a wide variety of cellular transport systems, including ion channels, transport proteins, and the Na^+-K^+-ATPase pump. These functions can be stimulatory or inhibitory, and more research is needed to determine how these processes have antiaging effects and how their disruption contributes to disease. Recombinant human Klotho protein has been developed, and efforts are in progress to target its function in both health and disease.

Data from Kim JH et al: *J Lifestyle Med* 5(1):1-6, 2016; Sopjani M, Dërmaku-Sopjani M: *Vitam Horm* 101:59-84, 2016; Sopjani M et al: *Curr Mol Med* 15(1):27-37, 2015; Tang X et al: Klotho: *Lab Invest* 96(2):197-205, 2016.

Antidiuretic Hormone

Although hyponatremia is a common finding in older adults, it appears related to changes in renal function or sensitivity rather than to ADH-related mechanisms. Morphologic studies have not shown significant age-related degenerative changes in the neuroendocrine pathways that regulate the synthesis and secretion of ADH. However, it appears that ADH secretion is augmented when stimulated by changes in osmotic concentration, whereas baroreceptor-mediated ADH secretion is reduced producing the syndrome of inappropriate ADH secretion (SIADH), common in older adults.[61]

SUMMARY REVIEW

Mechanisms of Hormonal Regulation

1. The endocrine system has diverse functions, including reproductive and CNS differentiation, sequential growth and development, coordination of reproductive systems, continuous maintenance of the body's internal environment, and adaptive responses to stress.
2. Hormones are chemical messengers synthesized by endocrine glands and released into the circulation; they work with the nervous and immune systems to maintain communication and control.
3. Hormones have specific negative- and positive-feedback mechanisms. Most hormone levels are regulated by negative feedback, in which tropic hormone secretion raises the level of a specific hormone. The elevated level of the specific hormone then causes negative feedback, decreasing secretion of the tropic hormone. Positive feedback systems, in which elevated hormone levels increase a response which then further increases hormone secretion, is seen most often in reproductive hormones.
4. In addition to negative and positive feedback systems, endocrine feedback is described in terms of the levels of feedback (long and short feedback loops).
5. Endocrine communications occur within cells (autocrine), between cells (paracrine), and between remote cells (endocrine).
6. Water-soluble hormones circulate throughout the body in unbound form, whereas lipid-soluble hormones (i.e., steroid and thyroid hormones) circulate throughout the body bound to carrier proteins.
7. Hormones affect only cells with appropriate receptors (target cells) and then act on those cells to initiate specific cell functions or activities.

8. Hormones have two general types of effects on cells: direct effects, or obvious changes in cell function; and permissive effects, or less obvious changes that facilitate cell function.

9. Receptors for hormones are large proteins and may be located either on or in the plasma membrane, in the cytosol, or in the nucleus of the target cell. Receptors include those that are G-protein linked, enzyme linked, or ion gated channels.

10. Water-soluble hormones act as first messengers, binding to specific receptors on the cell's plasma membrane. The signals initiated by hormone-receptor binding are then transmitted into the cell by the action of second messengers.

11. Second messengers that have been identified include cAMP, cGMP, and calcium. Calcium associates with IP_3 and DAG to produce physiologic effects.

12. For cells that have cAMP as their second messenger, a series of interactions within the plasma membrane take place, activating adenylyl cyclase.

13. Cells that have cGMP as their second messenger are activated by the enzyme guanylyl cyclase.

14. For cells that have calcium as their second messenger, an increase in intracellular calcium concentration causes calcium to bind with calmodulin, a regulatory protein. This step then initiates other intracellular processes.

15. Lipid-soluble hormones (including steroid and thyroid hormones) may have rapid (nongenomic) effects by binding to a plasma membrane or receptor or crossing the plasma membrane through diffusion. These hormones then either bind to cytoplasmic proteins or diffuse directly into the cell nucleus and bind to nuclear receptors.

Structure and Function of the Endocrine Glands

1. The hypothalamic-pituitary axis (HPA) forms the structural and functional basis for central integration of the neurologic and endocrine systems

2. The pituitary gland, consisting of anterior and posterior portions, is connected to the central nervous system through the hypothalamus.

3. The hypothalamus regulates anterior pituitary function by secreting releasing hormones into the portal circulation.

4. Hypothalamic hormones include dopamine, which inhibits prolactin secretion; TRH, which affects release of thyroid hormones; CRH, which facilitates release of ACTH and endorphins; and substance P, which inhibits ACTH release and stimulates release of a variety of other hormones. ADH and oxytocin are synthesized in the hypothalamus and stored and secreted by the posterior pituitary.

5. The posterior pituitary stores and secretes oxytocin and ADH, also called arginine-vasopressin.

6. ADH controls serum osmolality, increases the permeability of the renal tubules to water, and causes vasoconstriction when administered pharmacologically in high doses. ADH also may regulate some central nervous system functions.

7. Oxytocin causes uterine contraction and lactation in women and may have a role in sperm motility in men. In men and women, oxytocin has an antidiuretic effect similar to that of ADH.

8. The majority of the hormones of the anterior pituitary are regulated by (1) secretion of hypothalamic-releasing hormones or factors, (2) negative feedback from hormones secreted by target organs, and (3) mediating effects of neurotransmitters. Prolactin is regulated by a positive feedback system.

9. Hormones of the anterior pituitary include ACTH, MSH, somatotropic hormones (GH and prolactin), and glycoprotein hormones (FSH, LH, and TSH).

10. Growth hormone stimulates bone growth, increased protein metabolism in muscles, and lipolysis. Its anabolic effects are mediated in part by IGFs, of which IGF-1 is the most biologically active.

11. Prolactin functions to produce milk during pregnancy and lactation.

12. The pineal gland produces melatonin, which affects sleep, circadian rhythms, secretion of GHRH onset of puberty, immune function, and aging.

13. The two-lobed thyroid gland contains follicles, which secrete the thyroid hormones, and parafollicular cells (C cells), which secrete calcitonin and, in smaller quantities, the neuropeptides ghrelin, serotonin, and somatostatin.

14. Regulation of TH levels is complex and involves the hypothalamus (TRH), anterior pituitary (TSH), thyroid gland, and numerous biochemical variables.

15. TH secretion is regulated by TRH through a negative-feedback loop that involves the anterior pituitary and hypothalamus.

16. TSH, which is synthesized and stored in the anterior pituitary, stimulates secretion of TH by activating intracellular processes, including uptake of iodine necessary for the synthesis of TH.

17. Synthesis of TH depends on the glycoprotein thyroglobulin, which contains a precursor of TH, tyrosine. Tyrosine then combines with iodide to form precursor molecules of the thyroid hormones T_4 and T_3.

18. When released into the circulation, T_3 and T_4 are bound by carrier proteins in the plasma that store these hormones and provide a buffer for rapid changes in hormone levels.

19. Thyroid hormones alter protein synthesis and have a wide range of metabolic effects on proteins, carbohydrates, lipids, and vitamins. TH is responsible for growth, maturation, and function of cells and body systems throughout the body and across the life span.

20. The paired parathyroid glands normally are located behind the upper and lower poles of the thyroid gland. These glands secrete PTH, the single most important regulator of serum calcium and phosphate levels.

21. PTH secretion is regulated by levels of ionized calcium in the plasma and by cAMP within the cell. Some other substances—hormones, neurotransmitters, and ions—affect PTH secretion by inhibiting cAMP or by changing calcium levels.

22. In bone, PTH causes bone breakdown and resorption. In the kidney, PTH increases reabsorption of calcium, decreases reabsorption of phosphorus and bicarbonate, and stimulates synthesis of the active form of vitamin D. Paradoxically, low-dose PTH, administered intermittently, stimulates bone formation.

23. Parathyroid hormone–related peptide (PTHrP) has properties similar to those of PTH and plays a role in placental calcium transport, lactation, and fetal tooth development.

24. The endocrine pancreas contains the islets of Langerhans, which secrete hormones responsible for much of the carbohydrate metabolism in the body.

25. The islets of Langerhans consist of alpha cells, beta cells, delta cells, and F cells.

26. Alpha cells produce glucagon, which is secreted inversely to blood glucose concentrations and stimulates glycogenolysis, gluconeogenesis, and lipolysis.

27. Beta cells synthesize insulin, a hormone that regulates blood glucose concentrations and overall body metabolism of fat, protein, and

▌ SUMMARY REVIEW—cont'd

carbohydrates. Secretion of insulin is regulated by chemical, hormonal, and neural control. Biological responsiveness to insulin is affected by age, weight, abdominal fat, and physical activity.

28. Beta cells also secrete amylin, which promotes glucose-dependent insulin secretion, inhibits glucagon synthesis, and delays gastric emptying, producing an antihyperglycemic effect.

29. Delta cells secrete pancreatic somatostatin, which inhibits secretion of glucagon, insulin, and polypeptide.

30. F cells secrete pancreatic polypeptide, which stimulates Y receptors, promotes gastric secretion, and antagonizes cholecystokinin.

31. Incretin hormones are produced by endocrine cells of the gastrointestinal tract and promote glucose-dependent insulin secretion, inhibit glucagon synthesis, and delay gastric emptying.

32. The paired adrenal glands are situated on the kidneys. Each gland consists of an adrenal medulla, which secretes catecholamines, and an adrenal cortex, which secretes steroid hormones.

33. The steroid hormones secreted by the adrenal cortex are all synthesized from cholesterol. These hormones include glucocorticoids, mineralocorticoids, and adrenal androgens and estrogens.

34. Glucocorticoids directly affect carbohydrate metabolism by increasing blood glucose concentration through gluconeogenesis in the liver and by decreasing use of glucose. Glucocorticoids also inhibit immune and inflammatory responses, inhibit bone formation and ADH secretion, and stimulate gastric secretion.

35. Cortisol secretion is related to secretion of ACTH, which is stimulated by CRH. ACTH binds with receptors of the adrenal cortex, which activates intracellular mechanisms (specifically cAMP) and leads to cortisol release.

36. Mineralocorticoids, especially aldosterone, are steroid hormones that directly affect ion transport by epithelial cells, causing sodium retention and potassium and hydrogen loss.

37. Aldosterone secretion is controlled by the renin-angiotensin-aldosterone system and acts by binding to a site on the cell nucleus and altering protein production within the cell. Its principal site of action is the kidney, where it causes sodium reabsorption and potassium and hydrogen excretion.

38. Androgens and estrogens secreted by the adrenal cortex act in the same way as those secreted by the gonads.

39. The adrenal medulla secretes the catecholamines epinephrine and norepinephrine. Catecholamines are synthesized from the amino acid phenylalanine. Their release is stimulated by sympathetic nervous system stimulation, ACTH, and glucocorticoids.

40. Catecholamines bind with various target cells and are taken up by neurons or excreted in the urine. They cause a range of metabolic effects that generally are characterized as the "fight or flight" response.

41. The endocrine system acts together with the nervous and immune systems to respond to stressors, providing an integrated and protective response.

42. Several assay methods are used to measure levels of hormones in the plasma. RIA compares the proportion of radiolabeled and nonradiolabeled hormone against standard reference curves.

43. ELISA is a method similar to RIA, but uses a radiolabeled enzyme rather than a radiolabeled hormone.

44. Bioassays use graded doses of hormone in a reference preparation and then compare the results with an unknown sample to determine the hormone level.

Aging and the Endocrine System

1. Endocrine changes that may be associated with aging include altered biologic activity of hormones, altered circulating levels of hormones, altered secretory responses of endocrine glands, altered metabolism of hormones, loss of circadian control of hormone release, and changes in secretion of hypothalamic regulatory hormones.

2. Cellular damage associated with aging, genetically programmed cell change, and chronic wear and tear may contribute to endocrine gland dysfunction or alterations in the responsiveness of target organs.

3. Aging apparently causes atrophy of the thyroid gland and is associated with infiltrative glandular changes. Secretion of thyroid hormones may diminish with age.

4. Aging causes pancreatic fat deposition and is associated with a decrease both in insulin secretion and in insulin sensitivity. In addition, there is an age-dependent decline in beta-cell function.

5. Growth hormone levels decrease with aging, leading to decreased bone and muscle mass.

6. Aging is associated with alterations in calcium steady states, which may be related to alterations in PTH secretion from the parathyroid glands.

7. Age-related changes in adrenal function include decreased clearance of glucocorticoids and a decrease in levels of adrenal androgens. The effects of these changes, however, are offset by feedback mechanisms that maintain glucocorticoid levels and by gonadal secretion of androgens.

8. The kidney, choroid plexus, and parathyroid gland secrete the Klotho protein, which has antiaging effects.

▌ KEY TERMS

1,25-Dihydroxy-vitamin D$_3$, 656
Adrenal cortex, 659
Adrenal gland, 658
Adrenal medulla, 661
Adrenocorticotropic hormone (ACTH), 649
Aldosterone, 661
Alpha cell, 656
Amylin, 657
Anterior pituitary, 649
Beta cell, 656
Bioassay, 662
C cell, 653
Calcitonin, 653
Chromaffin cell (pheochromocyte), 661
Chromophil, 649

Chromophobe, 649
Corticotropin-releasing hormone (CRH), 649
Cortisol, 659
Delta cell, 656
Direct effect, 648
Downregulation, 647
Enzyme-linked immunosorbent assay (ELISA), 662
F (or PP) cell, 656
First messenger, 647
Follicle, 653
Follicle-stimulating hormone (FSH), 649
Ghrelin, 658
Glucagon, 657
Glucocorticoid, 659

Gonadotropin-releasing hormone (GnRH), 649
Growth hormone (GH), 651
Growth hormone–releasing hormone (GHRH), 649
Hormone, 644
Hypothalamic somatostatin, 649
Insulin, 656
Islets of Langerhans, 656
Isthmus, 653
Klotho protein, 664
Lipid-soluble steroid, 647
Luteinizing hormone (LH), 649
Median eminence, 652
Melanocyte-stimulating hormone (MSH), 649
Melatonin, 653

KEY TERMS—cont'd

REFERENCES

1. Narumi S, Hasegawa T: TSH resistance revisited. *Endocr J* 62(5):393–398, 2015.
2. Lefrancois-Martinez AM, et al: Transcriptional control of adrenal steroidogenesis: novel connection between Janus kinase (JAK) 2 protein and protein kinase A (PKA) through stabilization of cAMP response element-binding protein (CREB) transcription factor. *J Biol Chem* 286(38):3276–3285, 2011.
3. Cho EC, Mitton B, Sakamoto KM: CREB and leukemogenesis. *Crit Rev Oncog* 16(1-2):37–46, 2011.
4. Wang YW, et al: Understanding the CREB1-miRNA feedback loop in human malignancies. *Tumour Biol* 37(7):8487–8502, 2016.
5. Mergia E, Stegbauer J: Role of phosphodiesterase 5 and cyclic GMP in hypertension. *Curr Hypertens Rep* 18(5):39, 2016.
6. Knott EP, et al: Phosphodiesterase inhibitors as a therapeutic approach to neuroprotection and repair. *Int J Mol Sci* 18(4):2017.
7. Zheng Y, Murphy L: Regulation of steroid hormone receptors and coregulators during the cell cycle highlights potential novel function in addition to roles as transcription factors. *Nucl Recept Signal* 14:e001, 2016.
8. Yen PM: Classical nuclear hormone receptor activity as a mediator of complex biological responses: a look at health and disease. *Best Pract Res Clin Endocrinol Metab* 29(4):517–528, 2015.
9. Hammes SR, Davis PJ: Overlapping nongenomic and genomic actions of thyroid hormone and steroids. *Best Pract Res Clin Endocrinol Metab* 29(4):581–593, 2015.
10. Kow LM, Pfaff DW: Rapid estrogen actions on ion channels: a survey in search for mechanisms. *Steroids* 111:46–53, 2016.
11. Clarke IJ: Hypothalamus as an endocrine organ. *Compr Physiol* 5(1):217–253, 2015.
12. Christopoulos PF, Msaouel P, Koutsilieris M: The role of the insulin-like growth factor-1 system in breast cancer. *Mol Cancer* 14:43, 2015.
13. Heidegger I, et al: The insulin-like growth factor (IGF) axis as an anticancer target in prostate cancer. *Cancer Lett* 367(2):113–121, 2015.
14. Suarez AL, et al: Prolactin in inflammatory response. *Adv Exp Med Biol* 846:243–264, 2015.
15. Jentzer JC, et al: Pharmacotherapy update on the use of vasopressors and inotropes in the intensive care unit. *J Cardiovasc Pharmacol Ther* 20(3):249–260, 2015.
16. Reiter RJ, et al: Melatonin, a full service anti-cancer agent: inhibition of initiation, progression and metastasis. *Int J Mol Sci* 18(4):pii:E843, 2017.
17. Huang MY, et al: Serum procalcitonin and procalcitonin clearance as a prognostic biomarker in patients with severe sepsis and septic shock. *Biomed Res Int* 2016:1758501, 2016.

18. Kim J, et al: Procalcitonin as a diagnostic and prognostic factor for tuberculosis meningitis. *J Clin Neurol* 12(3):332–339, 2016.
19. Gordon DF, et al: Thyroid-stimulating hormone: physiology and secretion. In Jameson JL, Degroot LJ, editors: *Endocrinology*, ed 6, Philadelphia, 2010, Saunders.
20. Verloop H, et al: Genetics in endocrinology: genetic variation in deiodinases: a systematic review of potential clinical effects in humans. *Eur J Endocrinol* 171(3):R123–R135, 2014.
21. Davis PJ, Goglia F, Leonard JL: Nongenomic actions of thyroid hormone. *Nat Rev Endocrinol* 12(2):111–121, 2016.
22. Kumar R, Thompson JR: The regulation of parathyroid hormone secretion and synthesis. *J Am Soc Nephrol* 22(2):216–224, 2011.
23. Bellido T, Saini V, Pajevic PD: Effects of PTH on osteocyte function. *Bone* 54(2):250–257, 2013.
24. Souberbielle JC: Epidemiology of vitamin-D deficiency. *Geriatr Psychol Neuropsychiatr Vieil* 14(1):7–15, 2015.
25. Martin TJ: Parathyroid hormone-related protein, its regulation of cartilage and bone development, and role in treating bone diseases. *Physiol Rev* 96(3):831–871, 2016.
26. Conn VS, et al: Insulin sensitivity following exercise interventions: systematic review and meta-analysis of outcomes among healthy adults. *J Prim Care Community Health* 5(3):211–222, 2014.
27. Hayes MR, et al: Incretins and amylin: neuroendocrine communication between the gut, pancreas, and brain in control of food intake and blood glucose. *Annu Rev Nutr* 34:237–260, 2014.
28. Campbell JE, Drucker DJ: Islet α cells and glucagon—critical regulators of energy homeostasis. *Nat Rev Endocrinol* 11(6):329–338, 2015.
29. Dey J: SGLT2 inhibitor/DPP-4 inhibitor combination therapy—complementary mechanisms of action for management of type 2 diabetes mellitus. *Postgrad Med* 129(4):409–420, 2017.
30. Tong J, et al: Ghrelin impairs prandial glucose tolerance and insulin secretion in healthy humans despite increasing GLP-1. *J Clin Endocrinol Metab* 101(16):2405–2414, 2016.
31. Walther C, Morl K, Beck-Sickinger AG: Neuropeptide Y receptors: ligand binding and trafficking suggest novel approaches in drug development. *J Pept Sci* 17(4):233–246, 2011.
32. Turcu AF, Auchus RJ: Adrenal steroidogenesis and congenital adrenal hyperplasia. *Endocrinol Metab Clin North Am* 44(2):275–296, 2015.
33. Oakley RH, Cidlowski JA: The biology of the glucocorticoid receptor: new signaling mechanisms in health and disease. *J Allergy Clin Immunol* 132(5):1033–1044, 2013.
34. Kuo T, et al: Regulation of glucose homeostasis by glucocorticoids. *Adv Exp Med Biol* 872:99–126, 2015.

35. Xavier AM, et al: Gene expression control by glucocorticoid receptors during innate immune responses. *Front Endocrinol (Lausanne)* 7:31, 2016.
36. Ingawale DK, Mandlik SK, Patel SS: An emphasis on molecular mechanisms of anti-inflammatory effects and glucocorticoid resistance. *J Complement Integr Med* 12(1):1–13, 2015.
37. Barnes PJ: How corticosteroids control inflammation: Quintiles prize lecture 2005. *Br J Pharmacol* 148(3):245–254, 2006.
38. Mitre-Aguilar IB, Cabrera-Quintero AJ, Zentella-Dehesa A: Genomic and non-genomic effects of glucocorticoids: implications for breast cancer. *Int J Clin Exp Pathol* 8(1):1–10, 2015.
39. Mazziotti G, Giustina A: Glucocorticoids and the regulation of growth hormone secretion. *Nat Rev Endocrinol* 9(5):265–276, 2013.
40. Keller-Wood M: Hypothalamic-pituitary-adrenal axis—feedback control. *Compr Physiol* 5(3):1161–1182, 2015.
41. Kostadinova F, et al: Why does the gut synthesize glucocorticoids? *Ann Med* 46(7):490–497, 2014.
42. Talabér G, Jondal M, Okret S: Extra-adrenal glucocorticoid synthesis: immune regulation and aspects on local organ homeostasis. *Mol Cell Endocrinol* 380(1-2):89–98, 2013.
43. Gallo-Payet N: Gallo-Payet N: 60 years of POMC: adrenal and extra-adrenal functions of ACTH. *J Mol Endocrinol* 56(4):T135–T156, 2016.
44. Bollag WB: Regulation of aldosterone synthesis and secretion. *Compr Physiol* 4(3):1017–1055, 2014.
45. Toney GM, Vallon V, Stockand JD: Intrinsic control of sodium excretion in the distal nephron by inhibitory purinergic regulation of the epithelial Na$^+$ channel. *Curr Opin Nephrol Hypertens* 21(1):52–60, 2012.
46. Le HH, et al: Impact of aldosterone antagonists on sudden cardiac death prevention in heart failure and post-myocardial infarction patients: a systematic review and meta-analysis of randomized controlled trials. *PLoS ONE* 11(2):e0145958, 2016.
47. Pacak K, Timmers HJLM, Eisenhofer G: Pheochromocytoma. In Jameson JL, Degroot LJ, editors: *Endocrinology*, ed 6, Philadelphia, 2010, Saunders.
48. Tank AW, Lee Wong D: Peripheral and central effects of circulating catecholamines. *Compr Physiol* 5(1):1–15, 2015.
49. Diamanti-Kandarakis E, et al: Mechanisms in Endocrinology: aging and anti-aging: a combo-endocrinology overview. *Eur J Endocrinol* 176(6):R283–R308, 2017.
50. Vitale G, Salvioli S, Franceschi C: Oxidative stress and the ageing endocrine system. *Nat Rev Endocrinol* 9(4):228–240, 2013.
51. Mitrou P, Raptis SA, Dimitriadis G: Thyroid disease in older people. *Maturitas* 70(1):5–9, 2011.

52. Tabatabaie V, Surks MI: The aging thyroid. *Curr Opin Endocrinol Diabetes Obes* 20(5):455–459, 2013.

53. Barker CJ, et al: β-Cell Ca²⁺ dynamics and function are compromised in aging. *Adv Biol Regul* 57:112–119, 2015.

54. Kalyani RR, Egan JM: Diabetes and altered glucose metabolism with aging. *Endocrinol Metab Clin North Am* 42(2):333–347, 2013.

55. Gulcelik NE, et al: Adipocytokines and aging: adiponectin and leptin. *Minerva Endocrinol* 38(2):203–210, 2013.

56. Di Somma C, et al: Somatopause: state of the art. *Minerva Endocrinol* 36(3):243–255, 2011.

57. Bartke A: Pleiotropic effects of growth hormone signaling in aging. *Trends Endocrinol Metab* 22(11):437–442, 2011.

58. Bartke A, Sun LY, Longo V: Somatotropic signaling: trade-offs between growth, reproductive development, and longevity. *Physiol Rev* 93(2):571–598, 2013.

59. Chapurlat RD, Delmas PD, Genant HK: Bone density and imaging of osteoporosis. In Jamerson JL, Degroot LJ, editors: *Endocrinology*, ed 6, Philadelphia, 2010, Saunders.

60. Samaras N, et al: A review of age-related dehydroepiandrosterone decline and its association with well-known geriatric syndromes: is treatment beneficial? *Rejuvenation Res* 16(4):285–294, 2013.

61. Cowen LE, Hodak SP, Verbalis JG: Age-associated abnormalities of water homeostasis. *Endocrinol Metab Clin North Am* 42(2):349–370, 2013.

Alterations of Hormonal Regulation

Valentina L. Brashers, Robert E. Jones, Sue E. Huether

evolve WEBSITE

CHAPTER OUTLINE

The function of the endocrine system involves complex interrelationships and interactions that maintain dynamic steady-states, provide growth and reproductive capabilities, and allow for adaptive changes in times of stress. Alterations in function are caused by either hypersecretion or hyposecretion of the various hormones, leading to abnormal hormone concentrations in the blood and abnormal receptor function or from altered intracellular response to the hormone-receptor complex.

MECHANISMS OF HORMONAL ALTERATIONS

Significantly elevated or depressed hormone levels may result from a variety of causes (Box 22.1). Dysfunction of an endocrine gland may involve the gland's failure to produce adequate amounts of biologically free or active hormone forms (hyposecretion). This failure may occur when the secretory cells are unable to produce or obtain an adequate quantity of required hormone precursors or when they are unable to convert the precursors to the active hormone. Once hormones are released into the circulation, they may be degraded at an altered rate or inactivated by antibodies before reaching the target cell. Other causes

of decreased hormone delivery to the target cell include an inadequate blood supply to the gland or target tissues or an abnormal amount of the appropriate carrier proteins in the serum. A gland also may synthesize or release excessive amounts of hormone (hypersecretion). For example, feedback systems that recognize the need for a particular hormone may fail to function properly or may respond to inappropriate signals. Ectopic sources of hormones (hormones produced by nonendocrine tissues) may result also in abnormally elevated hormone levels without benefit of the normal feedback system for hormone control. In these cases the ectopic hormone production is said to be *autonomous*. There also may be alterations in the expression/function of hormone receptors, thus affecting hormone action.

Target cells may fail to appropriately respond to hormonal stimulation *(hormone insensitivity)* (see Box 22.1). Two general types of target cell insensitivity to hormones are cell surface receptor–associated disorders and intracellular disorders:

1. *Cell surface receptor–associated disorders.* These disorders have been identified primarily in water-soluble hormones, such as insulin. They may involve (1) a decrease in the number of receptors, leading to

BOX 22.1 MECHANISMS OF HORMONE ALTERATIONS

INAPPROPRIATE AMOUNTS OF HORMONE DELIVERED TO TARGET CELL	INAPPROPRIATE RESPONSE BY TARGET CELL
Inadequate Hormone Synthesis Inadequate quantity of hormone precursors Secretory cell unable to convert precursors to active hormone	**Cell Surface Receptor–Associated Disorders** Decrease in the number of receptors Impaired receptor function (altered affinity for hormones) Presence of antibodies against specific receptors Unusual expression of receptor function
Failure of Feedback Systems Do not recognize positive feedback leading to inadequate hormone synthesis Do not recognize negative feedback leading to excessive hormone synthesis	
Inactive Hormones Inadequate biologically free hormone Hormone degraded at an altered rate Circulating inhibitors	**Intracellular Disorders** Acquired defects in postreceptor signaling cascades Inadequate synthesis of a second messenger Intracellular enzymes or proteins are altered Alterations in nuclear co-regulators Altered protein synthesis
Dysfunctional Delivery System Inadequate blood supply Inadequate carrier proteins Ectopic production of hormones	

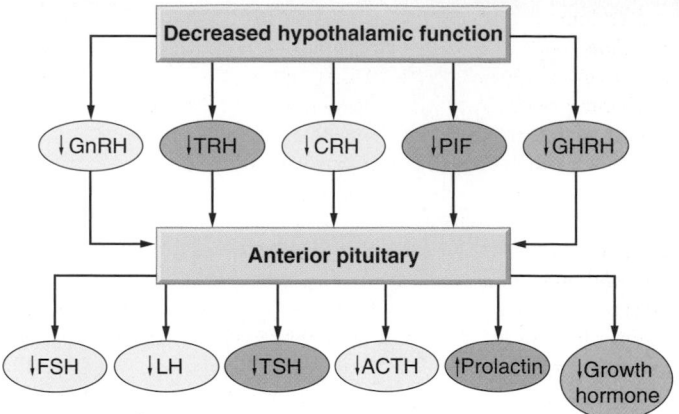

FIGURE 22.1 Loss of Hypothalamic Hormones. *ACTH,* Adrenocorticotropic hormone; *CRH,* corticotropin-releasing hormone; *FSH,* follicle-stimulating hormone; *GHRH,* growth hormone–releasing hormone; *GnRH,* gonadotropin-releasing hormone; *LH,* luteinizing hormone; *PIF,* prolactin inhibitor factor; *TRH,* thyrotropin-releasing hormone; *TSH,* thyroid-stimulating hormone.

decreased or defective hormone-receptor binding; (2) impairment of receptor function, resulting in insensitivity to the hormone; (3) presence of antibodies against specific receptors that either reduce available binding sites or mimic hormone action suppressing or exaggerating, respectively, the target cell response; or (4) unusual expression of receptor function, as occurs in some tumor cells.

2. *Intracellular disorders.* These disorders involve acquired defects in postreceptor signaling cascades or inadequate synthesis of a second messenger, such as cyclic adenosine monophosphate (cAMP), needed to transduce the hormonal signal into intracellular events. The target cell for water-soluble hormones may have a faulty response to hormone-receptor binding and thus fail to generate the required second messenger, or the cell also may have an abnormal response to the second messenger if levels of intracellular enzymes or proteins are altered. (Second messengers for various hormones are listed in Table 21.3.) As a result, the target cell fails to express the usual hormonal effect (e.g., see pseudohypoparathyroidism under Hypoparathyroidism).

Pathogenic mechanisms affecting target cell response for lipid-soluble hormones, such as thyroid hormone or glucocorticoids, are recognized less often than those affecting the water-soluble hormones. When they do occur, the mechanisms are similar to those for water-soluble hormones, including changes in the number and binding affinity of intracellular receptors or altered generation of new messenger ribonucleic acid (mRNA) and substrates for new protein synthesis. In other cases, hormone responsiveness may be linked to alterations in nuclear co-regulators, or transcription factors, which are proteins (such as cAMP response element–binding protein [CREB]; see Chapter 21) that facilitate or inhibit the transcription of the target gene.[1,2]

ALTERATIONS OF THE HYPOTHALAMIC-PITUITARY SYSTEM

Perhaps the most common cause of apparent hypothalamic dysfunction is interruption of the pituitary stalk, which can be caused by destructive lesions, rupture after head injury, surgical transection, or tumor. In these cases, the absence of hypothalamic releasing or inhibiting hormones (Fig. 22.1) causes a variety of manifestations that present clinically as pituitary disease. For example, if there is an absence of gonadotropin-releasing hormone (GnRH) from the hypothalamus, then there is a lack of stimulation of gonadotropin follicle–stimulating hormone (FSH) and luteinizing hormone (LH) from the pituitary; thus menses cease in women and spermatogenesis is impaired in men. Adrenocorticotropic hormone (ACTH) response to low serum cortisol levels is decreased because of the absence of corticotropin-releasing hormone (CRH). Hypothalamic hypothyroidism is caused by the absence of thyrotropin-releasing hormone (TRH). Low levels of growth hormone–releasing hormone (GHRH) result in growth hormone (GH) deficiency and growth failure in children. Hyperprolactinemia is caused by an absence of the usual inhibitory control of prolactin secretion by dopamine.

Diseases of the Posterior Pituitary

Diseases of the posterior pituitary usually cause abnormal secretion of antidiuretic hormone (ADH, arginine vasopressin). An excess amount of this hormone results in water retention and a hypoosmolar state, whereas deficiency in the amount or response to ADH results in serum hyperosmolarity (see Chapters 1 and 3). Changes in both ADH and oxytocin release and function are increasingly linked to changes in social behavior, particularly during stress.[3] Thus these complex pathophysiologic states not only have significant clinical effects on the modulation of body fluids and electrolytes, but also affect cognitive, emotional, and behavioral responses to stress.

Syndrome of Inappropriate Antidiuretic Hormone Secretion

Syndrome of inappropriate antidiuretic hormone (SIADH) secretion is characterized by high levels of ADH in the absence of normal physiologic stimuli for its release. A common cause of SIADH is the ectopic production of ADH by tumors, such as small cell carcinoma of the duodenum, stomach, and pancreas; cancers of the bladder, prostate, and endometrium; lymphomas; and sarcomas. Pulmonary disorders associated with SIADH include pneumonia (e.g., tuberculosis), small cell carcinoma, asthma, cystic fibrosis, and respiratory failure requiring mechanical ventilation. Central nervous system disorders that may cause SIADH include encephalitis, meningitis, intracranial hemorrhage, tumors, and trauma including neurosurgery. A nephrogenic form of SIADH involves an X-linked mutation in arginine vasopressin (AVP) genes leading to chronic activation of tubular V2 receptor and resulting in excessive free water reabsorption and concentrated urine.[4] Any surgery can result in an increased ADH secretion for as long as 5 to 7 days. The precise mechanism is uncertain but is likely related to fluid and volume changes following surgery, the amount and type of intravenous fluids given, and the use of narcotic analgesics. Transient SIADH is especially common after pituitary surgery because stored ADH is released in an unregulated fashion.[5]

Medications are an important cause of SIADH, especially in the elderly. These include hypoglycemic medications (e.g., chlorpropamide), antidepressants, antipsychotics, narcotics, general anesthetics, chemotherapeutic agents, nonsteroidal antiinflammatory drugs, and synthetic ADH. These drugs either stimulate ADH release, enhance the physiologic effects of ADH, or have a biologic action similar to that of ADH.[6]

◆PATHOPHYSIOLOGY. The pathophysiologic features of SIADH are the result of enhanced renal water retention. ADH increases renal collecting duct permeability to water by inducing the insertion of aquaporin-2, a water channel protein, into the tubular luminal membrane, which increases water reabsorption by the kidneys.[7] This results in an expansion of extracellular fluid volume that leads to dilutional hyponatremia (low serum sodium concentration), hypoosmolarity, and urine that is inappropriately concentrated with respect to serum osmolarity, because water is reabsorbed that normally would be excreted.

◆CLINICAL MANIFESTATIONS. The symptoms of SIADH result from hypotonic (dilutional) hyponatremia and are associated with hypervolemia and weight gain. The severity and rapidity of onset determine the extent of the symptoms. Thirst, impaired taste, anorexia, dyspnea on exertion, fatigue, and dulled sensorium occur when the serum sodium level decreases rapidly from 140 to 130 mEq/L. Peripheral edema is usually absent. Gastrointestinal symptoms, including vomiting and abdominal cramps, occur with a drop in sodium concentration from 130 to 120 mEq/L. There is weight gain from water retention, even with nausea and vomiting. Even if hyponatremia develops slowly, serum sodium levels less than 110 to 115 mEq/L cause confusion, lethargy, muscle twitching, and seizures; severe and sometimes irreversible neurologic damage may occur. Symptoms resolve with correction of hyponatremia (see Chapter 3).

◆EVALUATION AND TREATMENT. A diagnosis of SIADH includes the following manifestations: (1) serum hypoosmolality (<280 mOsm/kg) and hyponatremia (serum sodium level <135 mEq/L); (2) urine hyperosmolarity (i.e., the osmolality of the urine is always higher than the concurrent serum osmolality); (3) urine sodium excretion that matches sodium intake; (4) normal renal, adrenal, and thyroid function; and (5) absence of conditions that can alter volume status (e.g., recent diuretic use, heart or liver failure, hypervolemia from any cause, or renal insufficiency). ADH is difficult to measure in the serum. Copeptin, an ADH precursor molecule, may be used as a surrogate marker.[8] Individuals with neurologic injury also may develop hyponatremia caused by cerebral salt wasting syndrome. This can be differentiated from SIADH because cerebral salt wasting is characterized by hyponatremia, hypovolemia, and weight loss. In addition, urine sodium levels are elevated.[9]

The treatment of SIADH involves the correction of any underlying causal problems and fluid restriction (when feasible) with careful monitoring of sodium level status and neurologic symptoms. In severe SIADH, emergency correction of severe hyponatremia involves careful administration of hypertonic saline and, most importantly, fluid restriction to 800 to 1000 mL/day. Resolution usually occurs within 3 days, with a 2- to 3-kg weight loss resulting from enhanced free water clearance and correction of hyponatremia and salt wasting. If hyponatremia is corrected too rapidly, a severe neurologic syndrome called *central pontine myelinolysis* can ensue. Demeclocycline, which causes the renal tubules to develop resistance to ADH, may be used to treat resistant or chronic SIADH. Vasopressin receptor antagonists, known as *vaptans,* are effective in treating SIADH.[10]

Diabetes Insipidus

Diabetes insipidus (DI) is an insufficiency of ADH, leading to polyuria (frequent urination) and polydipsia (frequent drinking). There are two forms: neurogenic or central (hypothalamic) and nephrogenic (renal).[11]

Neurogenic or central DI is caused by insufficient secretion of ADH. It occurs when any organic lesion of the hypothalamus, pituitary stalk, or posterior pituitary interferes with ADH synthesis, transport, or release. Causative lesions include primary or metastatic brain tumors, hypophysectomy, aneurysms, thrombosis, infections, and immunologic disorders. Neurogenic DI is a well-recognized complication of traumatic brain injury or pituitary surgery in which DI can be transient or permanent. Neurogenic DI can be a complication of pregnancy. In rare cases, it also can be caused by hereditary disorders that affect ADH genes or result in structural changes in the pituitary gland.

Nephrogenic DI is caused by inadequate response of the renal tubules to ADH and is usually acquired or may be genetic, including genes that code for vasopressin V2 receptor (AVPR2) and aquaporin 2 (AQP2) proteins. Acquired nephrogenic DI is generally related to disorders and drugs that damage the renal tubules or inhibit the generation of cAMP in the tubules. These disorders include pyelonephritis, amyloidosis, destructive uropathies, polycystic disease, and intrinsic renal disease, all of which lead to irreversible DI. Drugs that may induce a reversible form of nephrogenic DI include lithium carbonate, colchicines, amphotericin B, loop diuretics, general anesthetics (such as methoxyflurane), and demeclocycline.[12]

Gestational DI is a rare form associated with pregnancy in which the level of the vasopressin-degrading enzyme vasopressinase is increased. Clinical manifestations are usually mild and do not require treatment.[13]

Dipsogenic or primary polydipsia may be confused with DI. It occurs when excessive fluid intake lowers the plasma osmolarity to the point that it falls below the threshold for ADH secretion. This condition may be associated with psychiatric disorders but also has been found in individuals who have a low osmotic threshold for inducing thirst. It is caused by chronic ingestion of extremely large quantities of fluid that wash out the renal medullary concentration gradient, which results in a partial resistance to ADH. This condition resolves with decreased fluid ingestion. Psychogenic causes of polydipsia must be differentiated from true DI because administering an ADH analog to an individual with psychogenic DI will result in severe hypoosmolality.

◆PATHOPHYSIOLOGY. Individuals with diabetes insipidus have a partial to total inability to concentrate urine. Insufficient ADH activity causes excretion of large volumes of dilute urine, leading to increased plasma osmolality. In conscious individuals, the thirst mechanism is stimulated and induces polydipsia—usually a craving for cold drinks. Dehydration develops rapidly without ongoing fluid replacement. If the individual with DI cannot conserve as much water as is lost in the urine, serum hypernatremia and hyperosmolality occur. Concentrations of other serum electrolytes generally are not affected.

◆CLINICAL MANIFESTATIONS. The clinical manifestations of DI include polyuria, nocturia, continuous thirst, and polydipsia. Urine

TABLE 22.1	Signs and Symptoms of Diabetes Insipidus (DI) and Syndrome of Inappropriate Antidiuretic Hormone (SIADH) Secretion	
SIGNS AND SYMPTOMS	**DI**	**SIADH**
Urine output	High	Low (no hypovolemia)
Urine osmolality	Low (<100–200 mOsm/L)	High (>800 mOsm/L)
Urine specific gravity	Low (<1.010)	High (>1.020)
Serum sodium	Hypernatremia (>145 mEq/L)	Hyponatremia (<135 mEq/L)
Serum osmolality	Hyperosmolar (>300 mOsm/L)	Hypoosmolar (<285 mOsm/L)
Symptoms	Polyuria, thirst, high urine output, signs of dehydration	Water retention, low urine output, nausea, vomiting, mental changes

output is varied but can increase from the normal output of 1 to 2 L/day to as much as 8 to 12 L/day, and can be higher than daily fluid intake. Individuals with long-standing DI may develop a large bladder capacity and hydronephrosis (see Chapter 39). Neurogenic DI usually has an abrupt onset, and many individuals can specifically recall the date of onset of their symptoms. Nephrogenic DI usually has a more gradual onset. Table 22.1 compares the signs and symptoms of DI and SIADH.

◆**EVALUATION AND TREATMENT.** DI must be distinguished from other polyuric states, including diabetes mellitus, osmotically induced diuresis, and psychogenic polydipsia. The criteria for the diagnosis of DI include polyuria, polydipsia, low urine specific gravity (<1.010), low urine osmolality (<200 mOsm/kg), hypernatremia, high serum osmolality (300 mOsm or more depending on adequate water intake), and continued diuresis despite a serum sodium level of 145 mEq/L or greater.

The first step in the diagnosis of DI uses water deprivation with measurement of serum osmolarity and plasma ADH levels. Water deprivation is a useful test because individuals without DI respond with a rapid decrease in urine volume and an increase in urine osmolality, whereas those with DI have no decrease in urine volume or increase in urine osmolality. In individuals with severe DI, water deprivation testing can be hazardous. If the individual loses more than 3% of the pretest body weight, circulatory collapse and shock can ensue. Neurogenic DI can be differentiated from nephrogenic DI by measuring the response to administered desmopressin. Neurogenic DI will respond with an increased ability to concentrate the urine, whereas nephrogenic DI will not respond. The diagnosis of dipsogenic polyuria can be extremely difficult, and differentiation from nephrogenic DI is based on plasma ADH levels. Copeptin, an ADH precursor molecule, is a reliable surrogate measurement for ADH secretion and can be used for the diagnosis of dipsogenic polyuria.[14]

Treatment for nephrogenic DI is based on the extent of the ADH deficiency and on the individual's age, endocrine and cardiovascular status, and lifestyle. Some individuals require ADH replacement, but fluid replacement using oral or intravenous routes is usually adequate. ADH replacement therapy for symptomatic central or neurogenic diabetes insipidus includes intravascular or, more commonly, oral or intranasal administration of the synthetic vasopressin analog DDAVP (desmopressin).[15] Management of nephrogenic DI requires treatment of any reversible underlying disorders, discontinuation of etiologic medications,

and correction of associated electrolyte disorders. Surprisingly, thiazide diuretics may improve renal tubular salt and water retention in individuals with moderate nephrogenic DI. Drugs that potentiate the action of otherwise insufficient amounts of endogenous ADH, such as chlorpropamide, carbamazepine, and clofibrate, may be used in individuals with incomplete ADH deficiency. New treatments aimed at reversing aquaporin-2 dysfunction are being developed.[16]

Diseases of the Anterior Pituitary

Disorders of the anterior pituitary may involve either hypofunction or hyperfunction of the gland.

Hypopituitarism

Hypopituitarism is the absence or deficiency of one or more anterior pituitary hormones or the complete failure of all anterior pituitary hormone functions. Hypopituitarism results from an inadequate supply of hypothalamic-releasing hormones, damage to the pituitary stalk, or an inability of the gland to produce hormones. The most common causes of hypopituitarism are pituitary adenoma, pituitary surgery or radiotherapy, pituitary infarction resulting from severe shock; pituitary apoplexy; aneurysms; or sickle cell disease. Pituitary infarction may occur in women during the postpartum period (Sheehan syndrome) because of blood loss (hemorrhage, not common in developed countries) and hypovolemic shock.[17] Traumatic brain injury is increasingly recognized as an important cause of hypopituitarism and can have a significant impact on acute and long-term recovery in children and adults.[18] Other causes of hypopituitarism include infections (e.g., meningitis, syphilis, tuberculosis), sarcoidosis, autoimmune hypophysitis, or certain drugs (e.g., bexarotene, carbamazepine).[19] Immune checkpoint inhibitors, such as ipilimumab, have been associated with hypophysitis in up to 11% of individuals treated for melanoma.[20] A rare form of hypopituitarism is characterized by combined hormonal deficiencies and is related to mutations of the thyroid-stimulating hormone (TSH) biosynthetic pathway or early or late transcription factors involved in early embryonic pituitary development.[21]

◆**PATHOPHYSIOLOGY.** The pituitary gland is highly vascular and relies heavily upon portal blood flow from the hypothalamus. Therefore it is extremely vulnerable to ischemia and infarction. Infarction results in tissue necrosis and edema with swelling of the gland. Expansion of the pituitary within the fixed compartment of the sella turcica further impedes blood supply to the pituitary. Over time, fibrosis of pituitary tissue occurs and the symptoms of hypopituitarism develop. Adenomas and aneurysms may compress otherwise normal secreting pituitary cells and lead to compromised hormonal output.

◆**CLINICAL MANIFESTATIONS.** The signs and symptoms of hypofunction of the anterior pituitary are variable and depend on which hormones are affected. In panhypopituitarism, all hormones are deficient and the individual suffers from multiple complications including cortisol deficiency from lack of ACTH, thyroid deficiency from lack of TSH, and loss of secondary sex characteristics from lack of FSH and LH. Low levels of GH and insulin-like growth factor-1 (IGF-1) affect growth in children and can cause physiologic and psychologic symptoms in adults. Postpartum women cannot lactate because of decreased or absent prolactin.

ACTH deficiency, with associated loss of cortisol, is a potentially life-threatening disorder. ACTH deficiency is usually encountered with generalized pituitary hypofunction. It rarely occurs as an isolated event.[22] Within 2 weeks of the complete absence of ACTH, symptoms of cortisol insufficiency develop, including nausea, vomiting, anorexia, fatigue, and weakness. Hypoglycemia results from increased insulin sensitivity, decreased glycogen reserves, and decreased gluconeogenesis associated with hypocortisolism. ACTH deficiency also limits maximum aldosterone secretion, although the renin-angiotensin system can stimulate some aldosterone secretion. The glomerular filtration rate decreases, causing decreased urine output.

TSH deficiency is rarely seen in isolation but occurs in conjunction with other pituitary hormone deficiencies. Symptoms develop 4 to 8 weeks after hypothyrotropinemia occurs and includes cold intolerance, skin dryness, mild myxedema, lethargy, and decreased metabolic rate. The symptoms are usually less severe than those associated with primary hypothyroidism.

The onset of FSH and LH deficiencies in women of reproductive age is associated with amenorrhea and with atrophy in the vagina, uterus, and breasts. In postpubertal males, the testicles atrophy and facial hair growth is diminished. Both men and women experience a decrease in body hair and diminished libido.

GH deficiency occurs in children and adults. As described previously, GH deficiency may result from any of the causes of hypopituitarism. Several genetic defects have been identified in the GH axis in children, including a recessive mutation in the *GH* gene, resulting in a failure of growth hormone secretion. These include a recessive mutation in the *GHRH* gene, resulting in a failure of GH secretion, and mutations that cause GH insensitivity by affecting the GH receptor, IGF-1 biosynthesis, IGF-1 receptors, or defects in GH signal transduction.[21]

GH deficiency in children is manifested by growth failure and a condition known as *hypopituitary dwarfism* (Fig. 22.2); however, not all children with short stature have growth hormone deficiency because there is wide variation in normal growth patterns. Another feature of GH deficiency in children is fasting hypoglycemia, likely attributable to impaired substrate mobilization for gluconeogenesis and enhanced insulin sensitivity.[23] Symptoms of chronic adult GH deficiency syndrome include increased body fat; decreased muscle bulk and lean body mass; osteoporosis; reduced sweating; dry skin; and psychologic problems, including depression, social withdrawal, fatigue, loss of motivation, and

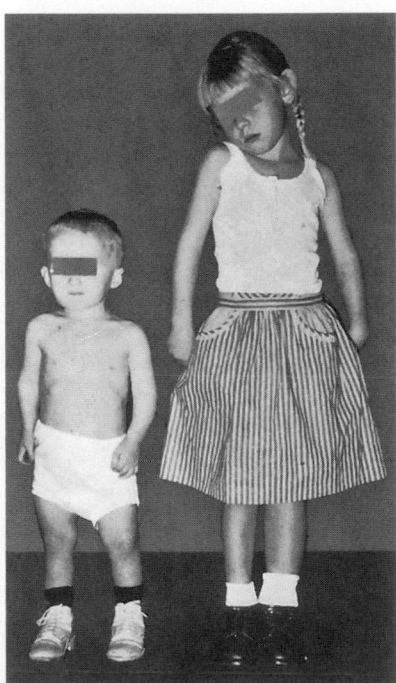

FIGURE 22.2 Hypopituitary Dwarfism. A 4-year-old boy whose height is 25 inches. The girl is also 4 years old and has a normal height of 39 inches. Dwarf has a normal face, as well as head, trunk, and limbs of approximately normal proportions. (From Brashear HR, Raney RB: *Shands' handbook of orthopaedic surgery,* ed 10, St Louis, 1986, Mosby.)

a diminished feeling of well-being. Without adequate GH replacement, increased mortality can occur as a result of myocardial infarction and stroke associated with dyslipidemias and atherosclerosis.[24]

◆EVALUATION AND TREATMENT. The diagnostic evaluation of suspected pituitary disease is often challenging and must be carefully interpreted together with the individual's signs and symptoms. Simultaneous measurements of the tropic hormones from the pituitary and target endocrine glands are crucial and, in some cases, dynamic testing of the various axes is indicated, particularly GH and ACTH.[25]

Radiographic assessment of the pituitary (magnetic resonance imaging [MRI] or computed tomography [CT] scans) may demonstrate enlargement of the pituitary, abnormal areas of enhancement suggestive of an adenoma, deviation of the pituitary stalk, or evidence of a locally aggressive tumor.

Management of hypopituitarism is individualized and requires correction of the underlying disorder as quickly as possible. Replacement of target gland hormones that are deficient because of lack of tropic anterior pituitary hormones is essential (such as cortisol, thyroid hormone, growth hormone, and sex-specific steroid hormones). In cases of circulatory collapse, immediate therapy with glucocorticoids and intravenous fluids is critical. Treatment adaptations are made during pregnancy and in transition from childhood to adulthood. Treatment of adult GH deficiency improves quality of life, metabolism, body composition, and physical performance in some individuals.[19]

Hyperpituitarism: Primary Adenoma

Pituitary adenomas are usually benign slow-growing tumors that arise from cells of the anterior pituitary. The cause of pituitary adenomas is not known and most occur sporadically. Altered gene expression is commonly detected and familial pituitary adenomas occur as part of syndromes affecting other organs, such as multiple endocrine neoplasia type 1.[26] Microadenomas (≤10 mm) are found only on postmortem examinations or incidentally discovered on MRI examinations. The majority of pituitary microadenomas are hormonally silent and do not pose significant hazards to the individual. Macroadenomas (≥10 mm) and giant adenomas (≥40 mm) are associated with morbidity and mortality attributable to alterations in hormone secretion or to invasion or impingement of structures surrounding the pituitary.[27] The pathogenesis of pituitary adenomas includes hypothalamic and intrapituitary factors, including altered expression of pituitary cell cycle genes, activation of pituitary selective oncoproteins, or loss of pituitary suppressor factors.[26] Several associated gene mutations have been identified, including isolated growth hormone deficiency and those associated with multiple endocrine neoplasia (MEN) syndromes.[28] Primary pituitary carcinomas are rare, representing about 0.2% of all pituitary tumors.

◆PATHOPHYSIOLOGY. Local expansion of pituitary adenomas may impinge on the optic chiasm and cause various visual disturbances, depending on the area of the optic nerve that is compressed. If the tumor is locally aggressive, invasion of the cavernous sinuses may occur, resulting in compromise of the oculomotor, trochlear, abducens, and trigeminal nerves with attending symptoms. Extension to the hypothalamus disturbs control of wakefulness, thirst, appetite, and temperature. Benign, slow-growing adenomas can transform to aggressive adenomas or carcinomas.[26]

Hormonal effects of adenomas include hypersecretion from the adenoma itself, and hyposecretion from surrounding pituitary cells. The adenomatous tissue secretes the hormone of the cell type from which it arose, without regard to physiologic needs and without benefit of regulatory feedback mechanisms. Because of the pressure exerted by the tumor in the unexpandable bony sella turcica, hyposecretion from those cells is most sensitive to common pressure (GH-, FSH-, and LH-secreting cells).[29]

◆**CLINICAL MANIFESTATIONS.** The clinical manifestations of pituitary adenomas are related to tumor growth and hormone hypersecretion or hyposecretion. Increased tumor size causes headache and fatigue, neck pain or stiffness, and seizures. Visual changes include visual field impairments (often beginning in one eye and progressing to the other) and temporary blindness. If the tumor infiltrates other cranial nerves, neurologic function is affected.

Pituitary adenomas are most often associated with increased secretion of GH and prolactin (see Hypersecretion of Growth Hormone: Acromegaly and Hypersecretion of Prolactin: Prolactinoma in this chapter). Gonadotropic hyposecretion results in menstrual irregularity in women, decreased libido, and receding secondary sex characteristics in both men and women. If the tumor exerts sufficient pressure, thyroid and adrenal hypofunction may occur because of lack of TSH and ACTH resulting in the symptoms of hypothyroidism and hypocortisolism, respectively.

◆**EVALUATION AND TREATMENT.** Diagnosis of pituitary adenoma involves physical and laboratory evaluations, including pertinent hormone assays and radiographic examination of the skull (MRI [preferred] or contrast-enhanced CT). The goal of treatment is to protect the individual from the effects of tumor growth and manage hormone hypersecretion or hyposecretion while minimizing damage to appropriately secreting portions of the pituitary. Depending on the tumor size and type, individuals may be treated by administration of specific medications to suppress tumor growth, transsphenoidal tumor resection, or radiation therapy including stereotactic treatments. Observation and close follow-up are commonly employed for individuals who have no evidence of hormonal alterations and no suggestion of anatomic aggressiveness. Chemotherapy with temozolomide is considered for those individuals who are still uncontrolled.

Hypersecretion of Growth Hormone: Acromegaly

Acromegaly results from continuous exposure to high levels of GH and IGF-1. It almost always is caused by a GH-secreting pituitary adenoma and rarely results from the ectopic production of GHRH.[30] Acromegaly usually occurs in adults in the 40–59-year-old age group, although it is often present for years before diagnosis because of the insidious nature of the disease. Consequently, there are systemic complications at diagnosis leading to increased mortality and premature death. Deaths from acromegaly are caused by heart disease secondary to hypertension and coronary artery disease, stroke, diabetes mellitus, or malignancy (colon or lung cancers).

◆**PATHOPHYSIOLOGY.** With a GH-secreting adenoma, the usual GH baseline secretion pattern and sleep-related GH peaks are lost, and an unpredictable secretory pattern ensues. However, GH levels in acromegalics are never completely suppressed. Only slight elevations of GH and IGF-1 levels can stimulate growth. In children and adolescents whose epiphyseal plates have not yet closed, the effect of increased GH levels causes excessive skeletal growth, with some individuals becoming 8- or 9-feet tall, termed **giantism** (Fig. 22.3). In the adult, epiphyseal closure has occurred and increased amounts of GH and IGF-1 cause connective tissue proliferation and increased cytoplasmic matrix, as well as bony proliferation that results in the characteristic appearance of acromegaly (Figs. 22.4 and 22.5).

GH also has significant effects on glucose, lipid, and protein metabolism. Hyperglycemia results from inhibition of peripheral glucose uptake, and increased hepatic glucose production followed by compensatory hyperinsulinism. Adipose tissue inflammation and impaired adipogenesis contribute to insulin resistance.[31] Diabetes mellitus occurs when the pancreas cannot secrete enough insulin to offset the effects of GH. Excessive levels of GH and IGF-1 also affect the cardiovascular system. Although the associated pathophysiology is not clearly understood,

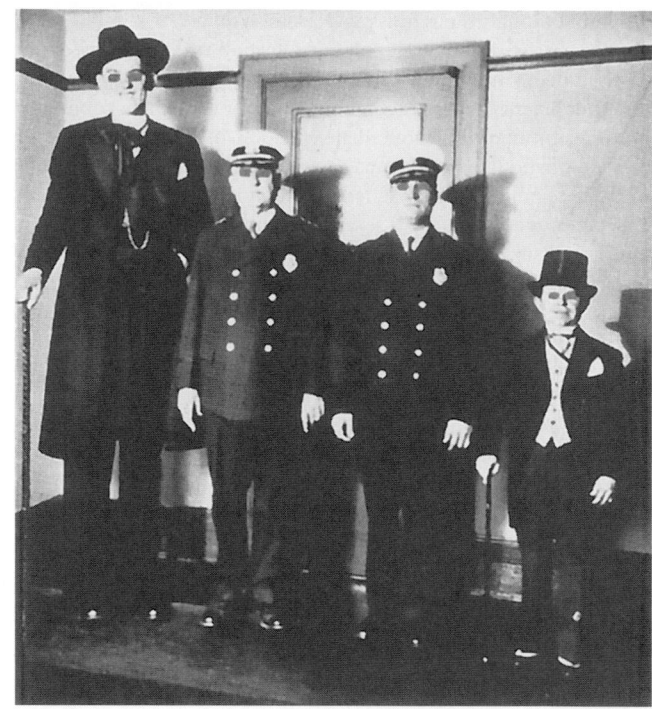

FIGURE 22.3 Giantism. A pituitary giant and dwarf contrasted with normal-size men. Excessive secretion of growth hormone by the anterior lobe of the pituitary gland during the early years of life produces giants of this type, whereas deficient secretion of this hormone produces well-formed dwarfs. (From Patton K, Thibodeau GA: *Anatomy & physiology*, ed 8, St Louis, 2013, Mosby.)

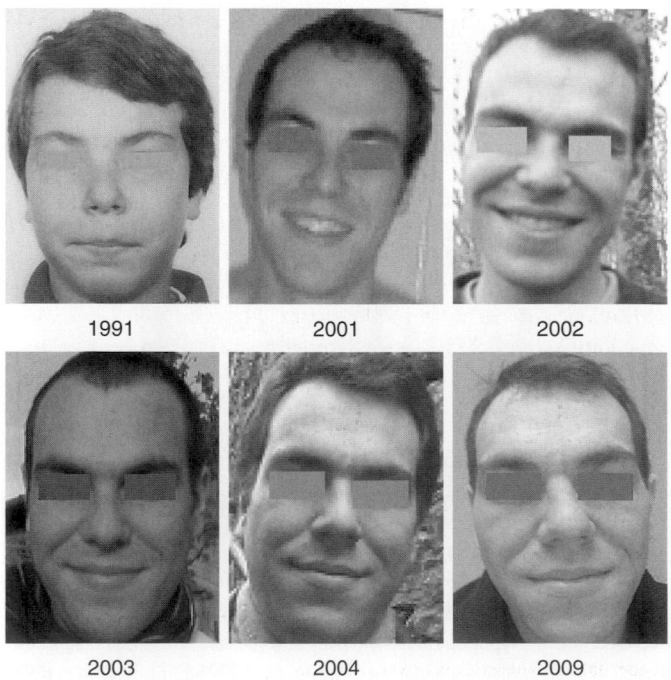

1991   2001   2002

2003   2004   2009

FIGURE 22.4 Acromegaly in a Male. Chronologic sequence of photographs showing slow development of acromegaly. (From Chanson P et al: *Best Pract Res Clin Endocrinol Metab* 23[5]:555–574, 2009.)

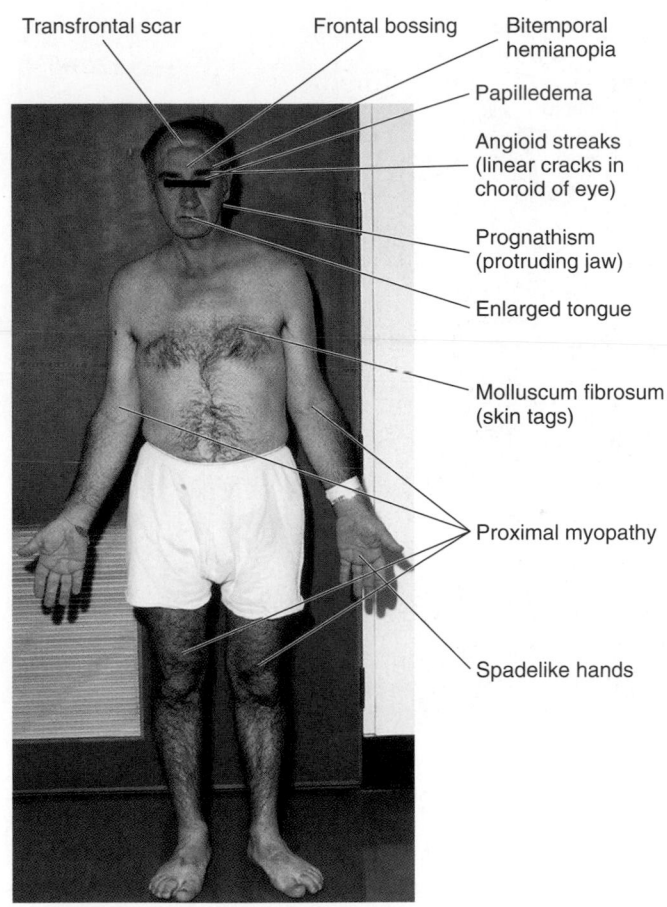

Transfrontal scar
Frontal bossing
Bitemporal
hemianopia
Papilledema
Angioid streaks
(linear cracks in
choroid of eye)
Prognathism
(protruding jaw)
Enlarged tongue
Molluscum fibrosum
(skin tags)
Proximal myopathy
Spadelike hands

FIGURE 22.5 Acromegaly. (From Talley NJ, O'Connor S: *Clinical examination*, ed 7, Australia, 2014, Churchill Livingstone.)

hypertension and left heart failure are seen in one-third to one-half of individuals with acromegaly. Cardiomyopathy associated with progressive and unrestrained myocardial growth is a significant factor. Valvular heart disease and arrhythmias can occur.[32] GH also acts on the renal tubules to increase phosphate reabsorption, leading to mild hyperphosphatemia. Because the adenoma increasingly becomes a space-occupying lesion, hypopituitarism may occur because of compression of surrounding hormone-secreting cells.

◆**CLINICAL MANIFESTATIONS.** With connective tissue proliferation, individuals with acromegaly have enlarged tongues, interstitial edema, enlarged and overactive sebaceous and sweat glands (leading to increased body odor), and coarse skin and body hair. Bony proliferation involves large joint arthropathy, periosteal vertebral growth, and enlargement of the bones of the face, hands, and feet. As a result, decreased joint range of motion, kyphosis, and lower jaw and forehead protrusion are common (see Figs. 22.4 and 22.5). Increased IGF-1 levels stimulate cartilaginous growth and cause ribs to elongate at the bone-cartilage junction, leading to a barrel-chest appearance, and increased proliferation of cartilage in the spine and joints, which causes backache and arthralgias. With continued bony and soft tissue overgrowth, entrapment of nerves may occur, leading to peripheral nerve damage as manifested by weakness, muscular atrophy, footdrop, and sensory changes in the hands (carpal tunnel syndrome). Sleep-disordered breathing is common and may exacerbate cardiovascular dysfunction.

Symptoms of diabetes mellitus, such as polyuria and polydipsia, may occur because of decreased insulin sensitivity in an individual who cannot mount adequate compensatory hyperinsulinemia. Acromegaly-associated hypertension is usually asymptomatic until heart failure symptoms develop. Increased tumor size results in central nervous system symptoms of headache, seizure activity, visual field disturbances, and papilledema. If compression hypopituitarism occurs, gonadotropin secretion may be affected, causing amenorrhea in women and sexual dysfunction in men. Hyperprolactinemia can occur in 30% to 40% of individuals with acromegaly.[33] Recent reports have documented mutations in the aryl hydrocarbon–interacting protein gene *(AIP)* in sporadic cases of familial acromegaly, polymorphisms in the somatostatin receptor type 5 gene, and GTP-binding (G) protein receptor mutations.[34]

◆**EVALUATION AND TREATMENT.** Diagnosis is confirmed by the appearance of clinical features of the disease, visual field testing, MRI scans, and elevated levels of IGF-1.[35] GH level is typically elevated and not suppressed with oral glucose tolerance testing. The goals of treatment are to normalize GH and IGF-1 serum levels to age range, restoring normal pituitary function and relieving or preventing complications related to tumor expansion. The treatment of choice for acromegaly is transsphenoidal surgery for removal of the GH-secreting adenoma. Treatment by stereotactic radiation therapy may be effective when rapid control of GH levels is not essential, when the individual is not a good surgical candidate, or when hyperfunction persists after subtotal resection. Somatostatin analogs, such as octreotide, octreotide acetate, and lanreotide, normalize IGF-1 levels and lower growth hormone levels. Pegvisomant can be used to supplement somatostatin analogs and is an effective drug that induces tissue insensitivity to GH by blocking the GH receptor.[33] Dopaminergic agonists, such as cabergoline, also may be helpful, especially if the tumor also secretes prolactin. Diagnostic and therapeutic clinical practice guidelines are available to support management during pregnancy and long-term management.[36] Cardiovascular, metabolic, and symptoms of tumor compression often improve with treatment. Skeletal abnormalities are irreversible.

Hypersecretion of Prolactin: Prolactinoma

Pituitary tumors that secrete prolactin, prolactinomas, are the most common of the hormonally active pituitary adenomas.

Other conditions or medications can elevate prolactin level in the absence of a pituitary pathologic condition. For example, renal failure, polycystic ovarian disease, breast stimulation, or even the stress of venipuncture can increase prolactin levels. Prolactin is under tonic inhibitory hypothalamic control through the secretion of dopamine (prolactin inhibitor factor [PIF]). Thus medications that block the effects of dopamine can increase prolactin production and stimulate proliferation of prolactin-secreting cells (lactotropes). These include antipsychotics (risperidone, chlorpromazine), metoclopramide, tricyclic antidepressants, and methyldopa. Any process that interferes with the delivery of dopamine from the hypothalamus to the lactotropes (pituitary stalk tumor, pituitary stalk transection, or compressive pituitary tumor) also results in hyperprolactinemia. Because TRH stimulates prolactin secretion, in addition to enhancing TSH release, prolactin concentration may be elevated in individuals with primary hypothyroidism.

◆**PATHOPHYSIOLOGY.** The hallmark of a prolactinoma is sustained increases in serum prolactin concentration. These tumors can be classified as microprolactinomas (<1 cm in size) or macroprolactinomas (>1 cm in size). Microprolactinomas are usually encapsulated and noninvasive, whereas macroprolactinomas commonly expand into the optic chasm, invade local structures, and are more difficult to treat.[37] Because the adenoma can become an increasingly space-occupying lesion, hypopituitarism may occur because of compression of surrounding hormone-secreting cells. Central nervous system symptoms may develop because of growth and pressure of the adenoma within the sella turcica.

◆**CLINICAL MANIFESTATIONS.** The physiologic actions of prolactin include breast development during pregnancy, postpartum milk production, and suppression of ovarian function in nursing women. Pathologic elevation of prolactin levels inhibits the pulsatile secretion of gonadotropin-releasing hormone, alters the pattern of release of luteinizing hormone and follicle-stimulating hormone, and suppresses gonadal steroidogenesis, thereby resulting in hypogonadotropic hypogonadism in both sexes. This causes amenorrhea, infertility, nonpuerperal milk production (galactorrhea), and hirsutism in women. If not detected until after many years, estrogen deficiency may result in osteopenia or osteoporosis. Hyperprolactinemia in men causes erectile dysfunction, infertility, and osteopenia. Symptoms related to the increasing size of the adenoma include headache or visual impairment.[38]

◆**EVALUATION AND TREATMENT.** The diagnostic evaluation of hyperprolactinemia includes a careful history to exclude medications or other diseases that may cause elevations in prolactin level. Symptoms of hypothyroidism should be elicited, and screening with a serum TSH measurement is mandatory. MRI scanning of the pituitary is indicated to determine the size and location of an adenoma. If prolactin concentration is less than 50 ng/mL, a careful search for a nonpituitary cause should be pursued.

The goals of treatment are to restore normal gonadal function and fertility and reduce tumor size. Dopaminergic agonists (cabergoline) are the treatment of choice for prolactinomas, and their use is often associated with both a rapid reduction in the size of the tumor and a reversal of the gonadal effects of hyperprolactinemia. Restoration of fertility in previously anovulatory women is common. In individuals resistant or intolerant to these medications, transsphenoidal surgery and radiotherapy are options. New chemotherapeutic and targeted molecular therapies are being explored.[38]

ALTERATIONS OF THYROID FUNCTION

Disorders of thyroid function develop as a result of primary dysfunction or disease of the thyroid gland or, secondarily, as a result of pituitary or hypothalamic alterations. **Primary thyroid disorders** result in alterations of thyroid hormone (TH) levels with secondary feedback effects on pituitary TSH levels. For example, when there are primary elevations in TH level, TSH level will secondarily decrease because of negative feedback. When TH level is decreased because of a condition affecting the thyroid gland, TSH level will be elevated. Thyroid disease also can present with no or minimal symptoms but with abnormal laboratory values. This is known as *subclinical thyroid disease*. Central (secondary) thyroid disorders are related to disorders of pituitary gland TSH production. When there is excessive TSH production, TH level is elevated secondary to the primary elevation of TSH level. The reverse is true with inadequate TSH production. Exposure to iodinated contrast media has been shown to be associated with development of both hyperthyroidism and hypothyroidism

Thyrotoxicosis/Hyperthyroidism

◆**PATHOPHYSIOLOGY.** **Thyrotoxicosis** is a condition that results from any cause of increased amounts of TH levels. **Hyperthyroidism** is a form of thyrotoxicosis in which excess amounts of TH are secreted from the thyroid gland. The terms *thyrotoxicosis* and *hyperthyroidism* are often used interchangeably. The prevalence of hyperthyroidism is estimated to be 0.7% to 2.1% in the United States, of which 0.7% is subclinical and is more prevalent in women and in iodine-deficient geographical areas.[39] Thyroid hormones are regulated by a negative feedback loop involving the hypothalamus, pituitary gland, and thyroid gland (see Fig. 21.13). Common diseases that cause **primary hyperthyroidism** include Graves disease, toxic multinodular goiter, a solitary toxic adenoma (Fig. 22.6), and, very rarely, follicular thyroid carcinoma. **Central (secondary) hyperthyroidism** is less common and is caused

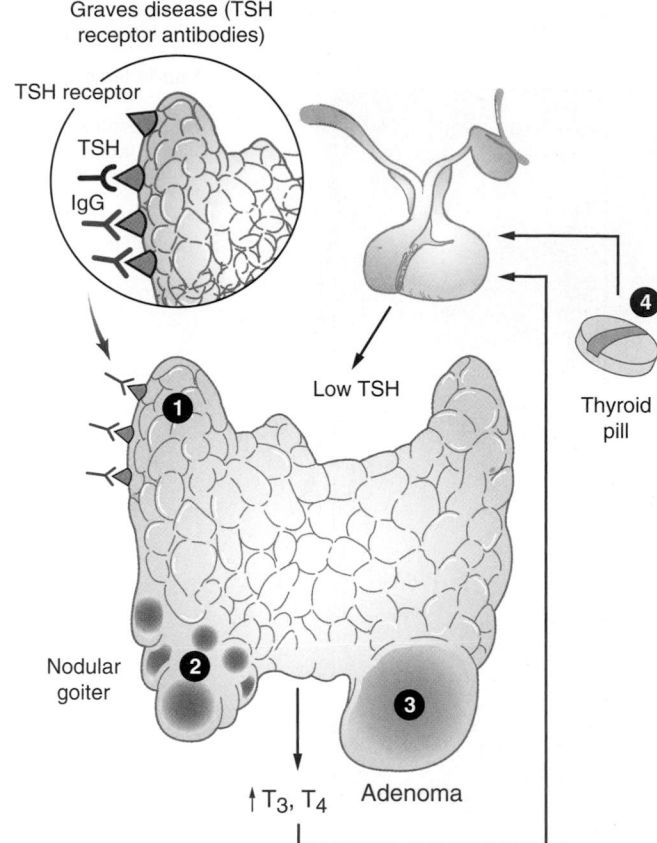

FIGURE 22.6 Causes of Hyperthyroidism. Hyperthyroidism may have several causes, among them: **1,** Graves disease; **2,** toxic multinodular goiter; **3,** follicular adenoma; **4,** thyroid medication. *IgG,* Immunoglobulin G; *T_3,* triiodothyronine; *T_4,* tetraiodothyronine; *TSH,* thyroid-stimulating hormone; *TSI,* thyroid-stimulating immunoglobulin. (Adapted from Damjanov I: *Pathology for the health professions,* ed 4, St Louis, 2012, Saunders.)

by TSH-secreting pituitary adenomas. Thyrotoxicosis not associated with hyperthyroidism includes ectopic thyroid tissue or ingestion of excessive TH, and low thyroid radioactive iodine uptake. Each condition is associated with specific pathophysiology, manifestations, and treatments. However, all forms of thyrotoxicosis share some common characteristics.[40]

◆**CLINICAL MANIFESTATIONS.** The clinical features of thyrotoxicosis are attributable to the metabolic effects of increased circulating levels of TH (Fig. 22.7). This usually results in an increased metabolic rate with heat intolerance and increased tissue sensitivity to stimulation by the sympathetic division of the autonomic nervous system. The major manifestations are summarized in Table 22.2. Enlargement of the thyroid gland (goiter) is common in hyperthyroid conditions caused by stimulation of TSH receptors.

◆**EVALUATION AND TREATMENT.** Elevated serum tetraiodothyronine (thyroxine) (T_4) and triiodothyronine (T_3) levels and decreased serum TSH levels are diagnostic for primary hyperthyroidism. By contrast, central (secondary) hyperthyroidism caused by TSH-secreting pituitary tumors is characterized by normal to increased TSH levels despite elevated thyroid hormone concentrations. Radioactive iodine is used to test for increased uptake in primary hyperthyroidism (Fig. 22.8).

Treatment is directed at controlling excessive TH production, secretion, or action and includes antithyroid drug therapy (methimazole or propylthiouracil), radioactive iodine therapy (absorbed only by thyroid tissue, causing death of cells), and surgery. Guidelines for the treatment

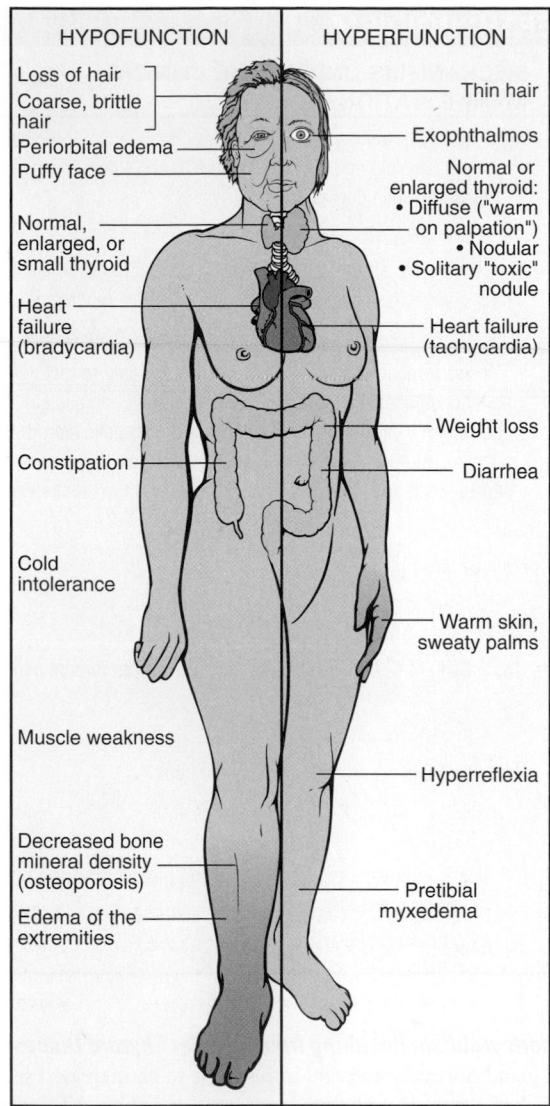

FIGURE 22.7 Clinical Manifestations of Hyperthyroidism and Hypothyroidism. (From Damjanov I: *Pathology for the health professions*, ed 4, St Louis, 2012, Saunders.)

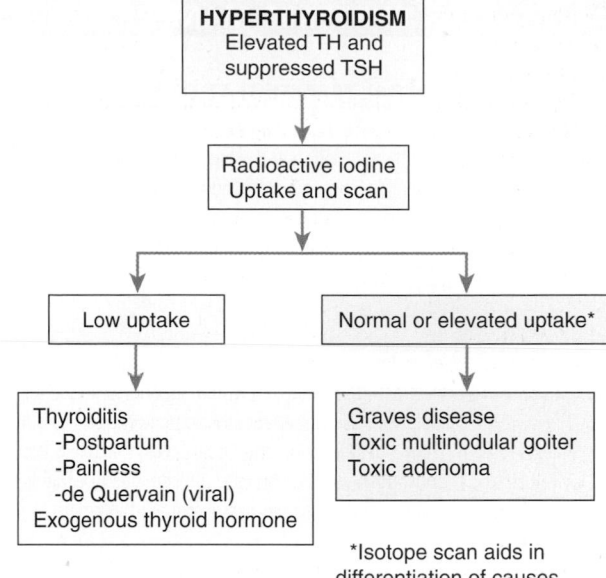

FIGURE 22.8 Evaluation of Hyperthyroidism. Radioactive iodine is used in the differential diagnosis of hyperthyroidism. *TH*, Thyroid hormone; *TSH*, thyroid-stimulating hormone.

in hyperplasia of the gland (goiter) and increased synthesis of TH, especially of T_3. Increased levels of TH affect every physiologic system and result in the classic signs and symptoms of hyperthyroidism illustrated in Fig. 22.8. TSH production by the pituitary is inhibited through the usual negative feedback loop.

TSIs also contribute to two major distinguishing clinical manifestations of Graves disease: ophthalmopathy and dermopathy (pretibial myxedema and acropachy). Two categories of ophthalmopathy associated with Graves disease are (1) functional abnormalities resulting from hyperactivity of the sympathetic division of the autonomic nervous system (lag of the globe on upward gaze or a lag of the upper lid on downward gaze) and (2) infiltrative changes involving the orbital contents with enlargement of the ocular muscles. The infiltrative changes possibly result from TSH receptor autoantibodies reacting with receptors on orbital fibroblasts (Fig. 22.9, *A*). These changes affect more than half of individuals with Graves disease. Increased secretion of hyaluronic acid, adipogenesis, inflammation, and edema of the orbital contents result in exophthalmos (protrusion of the eyeball), periorbital edema, and extraocular muscle weakness leading to strabismus and diplopia (double vision). The individual may experience irritation, pain, lacrimation, photophobia, blurred vision, decreased visual acuity, papilledema, visual field impairment, exposure keratosis, and corneal ulceration.[44] Smoking exacerbates the disease.

A small number of individuals with Graves disease and very high levels of TSI experience pretibial myxedema (Graves dermopathy), characterized by subcutaneous swelling on the anterior portions of the legs and by indurated and erythematous skin (see Fig. 22.9, *B*). Graves dermopathy is associated with thyrotropin receptor antigens on fibroblasts and recruited T lymphocytes that stimulate excess amounts of hyaluronic acid production in the dermis and subcutaneous tissue. The manifestations occasionally appear on the hands, giving the appearance of clubbing of the fingers (thyroid acropachy).[45]

Therapy for Graves disease includes antithyroid drugs, radioactive iodine ablation (used with caution in Graves ophthalmopathy because it may worsen the condition), or surgery. Smoking cessation is necessary. Unfortunately, current treatment for Graves disease does not reverse

of hyperthyroidism and thyrotoxicosis have been published.[41] Treatment of subclinical hyperthyroidism is based on lower levels of TSH with free T_4 and T_3 concentrations within the reference range and clinical symptoms.[42] A major complication of all forms of treatment for hyperthyroidism is hypothyroidism.

Hyperthyroid Conditions

Graves Disease. Graves disease is the underlying cause of 50% to 80% of cases of hyperthyroidism and has a prevalence of approximately 3.0% of women and 0.5% of men in the United States.[43] Although the cause of Graves disease is not known, genetic factors interacting with environmental triggers play an important role in the pathogenesis. Graves disease is classified as an autoimmune disease and results from a form of type II hypersensitivity (see Chapter 9) in which there is infiltration of lymphocytes and stimulation of the thyroid by autoantibodies directed against the TSH receptor. These autoantibodies, called *thyroid-stimulating immunoglobulins* (TSIs; also called *thyroid-stimulating antibodies [TSAbs]* or *thyroid receptor antibodies [TRAbs]*), override normal negative feedback mechanisms. The TSI stimulation of TSH receptors in the gland results

TABLE 22.2   SYSTEMIC MANIFESTATIONS OF HYPERTHYROIDISM

SYSTEM	CLINICAL MANIFESTATIONS	MECHANISMS UNDERLYING CLINICAL MANIFESTATIONS
Endocrine	Enlarged thyroid gland (goiter) (97%–99% of cases); systolic or continuous bruit over thyroid; increased cortisol degradation; hypercalcemia and decreased parathyroid hormone (PTH) secretion; diminished sensitivity to exogenous insulin	Hyperactivity of the thyroid gland; excess bone resorption leading to hypercalcemia and a disruption of PTH-regulating mechanisms; increased insulin degradation
Reproductive	Oligomenorrhea or amenorrhea; erectile dysfunction and decreased libido; increased serum estradiol and estrone levels but lower than normal levels of free estradiol and estrone	Menstrual cycle alterations that may be related to hypothalamic or pituitary disturbances; increase in sex hormone–binding globulin
Gastrointestinal	Weight loss; increased peristalsis leading to less formed and more frequent stools; nausea, vomiting, anorexia, abdominal pain; increased use of hepatic glycogen stores and of adipose and protein stores; decrease in serum lipid levels (including triglycerides, phospholipids, and cholesterol); changes in vitamin metabolism leading to decrease in tissue stores of vitamins	Increased catabolism leading to the body's inability to meet its metabolic needs; increased glucose absorption; increase in cholesterol excretion in feces and cholesterol conversion to bile salts; impaired conversion of B vitamins to their coenzymes, causing increased need for water-soluble and fat-soluble vitamins
Integumentary	Excessive sweating, flushing, and warm skin; heat intolerance; hair fine, soft, and straight; temporary hair loss; nails that grow away from nail beds, palmar erythema	Hyperdynamic circulatory state
Sensory (eyes)	Ocular manifestations including elevated upper eyelid leading to decreased blinking and a staring quality; fine tremor of lid; infiltrative ocular changes associated with Graves disease	Overactivity of Müller muscle; inflammation of retroorbital contents
Cardiovascular	Increased cardiac output and decreased peripheral resistance; tachycardia at rest; loud heart sounds; supraventricular dysrhythmias, left ventricular dilation and hypertrophy	Hypermetabolism and need to dissipate heat
Nervous	Restlessness; short attention span; compulsive movement; fatigue; tremor; insomnia; increased appetite; emotional lability	Not clearly defined; alterations in cerebral metabolism resulting from excess thyroid hormone
Pulmonary	Dyspnea; reduced vital capacity	Weakness of respiratory muscles

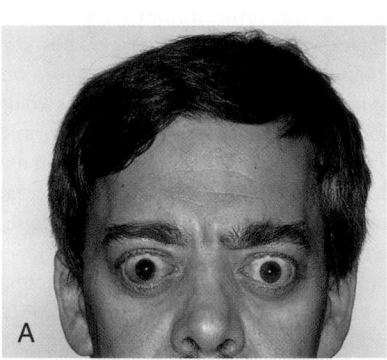
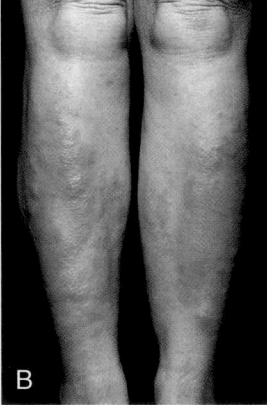

FIGURE 22.9 Thyrotoxicosis (Graves Disease). **A,** Exophthalmos (large and protruding eyeballs often in association with a large goiter). **B,** Pretibial myxedema associated with Graves disease; note lumpy and swollen appearance from accumulation of connective tissue and pinkish-purple discoloration. (**A** from Belchetz P, Hammond P: *Mosby's color atlas and text of diabetes and endocrinology,* Edinburgh, 2003, Mosby; **B** from Habif T: *Clinical dermatology,* ed 5, St Louis, 2009, Mosby.)

the infiltrative ophthalmopathy or the pretibial myxedema. Surgical orbital decompression and glucocorticoids can help many individuals with progressive ophthalmopathy. Immunosuppressive drugs, such as rituximab, are being evaluated.[43] Skin lesions rarely require treatment, but if they are symptomatic they may respond to topical glucocorticoids.[45]

Hyperthyroidism Resulting from Nodular Thyroid Disease. The thyroid gland normally enlarges in response to an increased secretion of TSH that occurs in puberty, pregnancy, or iodine deficiency, and from immunologic, viral, or genetic disorders. The increased number of follicles is a compensatory mechanism in response to increased TSH levels. When the condition requiring increased TH resolves, TSH secretion normally subsides and the thyroid gland returns to its original size.

Irreversible changes may occur in some follicular cells; thus these cells function autonomously and produce excessive amounts of TH. On the other hand, some follicular cells may cease to function. The balance between the amount of TH produced by hyperfunctioning nodules and that produced by the remainder of the gland determines whether an individual becomes euthyroid (nontoxic nodular goiter) or hyperthyroid. Nontoxic nodular goiter is more common in iodine-deficient regions and may require decompression when associated with airway, esophageal, or venous obstruction.[46] Toxic multinodular goiter occurs when there are several hyperfunctioning nodules leading to hyperthyroidism. If only one nodule becomes hyperfunctioning it is termed solitary toxic adenoma. Unlike Graves disease, there is absence of an autoimmune stimulus. The classic clinical manifestations of hyperthyroidism (see Fig. 22.7) usually develop slowly, and exophthalmos and pretibial myxedema do not occur. Nodules may be palpable on physical examination and there is increased uptake of radioactive iodine. The incidence of malignancy in toxic multinodular goiter is more likely in single nodules so most individuals should undergo a fine-needle aspiration biopsy of suspicious nodules before treatment.[47] Treatment consists of a combination of radioactive iodine, surgery, or antithyroid drugs.

Thyrotoxic Crisis (Thyroid Storm). Thyrotoxic crisis (thyroid storm) is a rare but dangerous worsening of the thyrotoxic state, in which death can occur within 48 hours without treatment. The condition may develop spontaneously, but it usually occurs in individuals who have undiagnosed or partially treated severe hyperthyroidism and who are subjected to excessive stress from other causes. These causes may include infection, pulmonary or cardiovascular disorders, trauma, burns, seizures, surgery (especially thyroid surgery), obstetric complications, emotional distress, or dialysis. The symptoms of thyroid crisis are caused by the sudden release and increased action of thyroxine (T_4) and tri-iodothyronine (T_3) exceeding metabolic demands.[48]

The systemic symptoms of thyrotoxic crisis include hyperthermia; tachycardia, especially atrial tachydysrhythmias; high-output heart failure; agitation or delirium; and nausea, vomiting, or diarrhea, contributing to fluid volume depletion. Treatment includes (1) the use of drugs that block TH synthesis (i.e., propylthiouracil or methimazole), (2) the use of beta-blockers for control of cardiovascular symptoms, (3) administration of corticosteroids or (4) iodine (e.g., saturated solution of potassium iodide [SSKI]), and (5) supportive care. Plasma exchange or thyroidectomy may be used when medical treatment fails.[49]

Hypothyroidism

Hypothyroidism results from deficient production of TH by the thyroid gland. Hypothyroidism is the most common disorder of thyroid function; it affects between 0.1% and 2% of the U.S. population and is more common in women and the elderly. It may be primary or secondary. Primary hypothyroidism accounts for 99% of all cases. Central (secondary) hypothyroidism, which is much less common, is related to either pituitary or hypothalamic failure.

◆**PATHOPHYSIOLOGY.** Loss of thyroid function in *primary hypothyroidism* leads to a decreased production of TH and increased secretion of TSH and TRH. The most common causes in adults include autoimmune thyroiditis (Hashimoto disease), iatrogenic loss of thyroid tissue after surgical or radioactive treatment for hyperthyroidism, head and neck radiation therapy, medications, and endemic iodine deficiency. Infants and children may present with hypothyroidism because of congenital defects in the pituitary or thyroid glands. *Central (secondary) hypothyroidism* is caused by the pituitary's failure to synthesize adequate amounts of TSH or a lack of TRH. Pituitary tumors that compress surrounding pituitary cells or the consequences of their treatment are the most common causes of **secondary hypothyroidism**. Other causes include traumatic brain injury, subarachnoid hemorrhage, or pituitary infarction. Hypothalamic dysfunction results in low levels of TRH, TSH, and TH (Fig. 22.10). **Subclinical hypothyroidism** is mild thyroid failure and is estimated to occur in 4% to 8% of U.S. adults. It is defined as an elevation in TSH level with normal levels of circulating TH.[50]

◆**CLINICAL MANIFESTATIONS.** Hypothyroidism generally affects all body systems and occurs insidiously over months or years. The extent of the symptoms is closely related to the degree of TH deficiency (see Fig. 22.7). The decrease in TH level lowers energy metabolism and heat production. The individual develops a low basal metabolic rate, cold intolerance, lethargy, tiredness, and slightly lowered basal body temperature and also may have diastolic hypertension. Many organ systems are affected (Table 22.3). The decrease in the level of TH can lead to excessive TSH production, which stimulates thyroid tissue and causes goiter.

The characteristic sign of severe or long-standing hypothyroidism is **myxedema**, which results from altered composition of the dermis and other tissues. The connective fibers are separated by an increased amount of protein and mucopolysaccharides. This protein-mucopolysaccharide complex binds water, producing nonpitting, boggy edema, especially around the eyes, hands, and feet and in the supraclavicular fossae. The

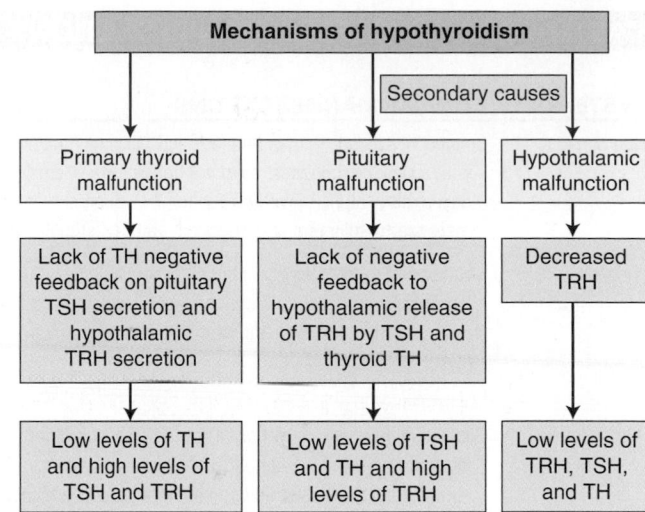

FIGURE 22.10 Mechanisms of Primary and Central (Secondary) Hypothyroidism. *TH,* Thyroid hormone; *TRH,* thyroid-releasing hormone; *TSH,* thyroid-stimulating hormone.

tongue and laryngeal and pharyngeal mucous membranes thicken, producing thick, slurred speech and hoarseness.

Myxedema coma, a medical emergency, is a diminished level of consciousness associated with severe hypothyroidism. Most individuals are not unconscious. Precipitating events include infections, discontinuation of thyroid supplements, overuse of narcotics or sedatives, or a consequence of an acute illness in individuals who have hypothyroidism. Older individuals with comorbid conditions, such as pulmonary or urinary tract infections, congestive heart failure, or cerebrovascular accident, and with moderate or untreated hypothyroidism are particularly at risk. Signs and symptoms include hypothermia without shivering, hypoventilation, hypotension, hypoglycemia, lactic acidosis, and coma. Symptoms of hypothyroidism in older adults should not be attributed to normal aging changes.[51]

◆**EVALUATION AND TREATMENT.** The diagnosis of primary hypothyroidism is made by documentation of the clinical symptoms of hypothyroidism and by measurement of increased levels of TSH and decreased levels of TH (total T_3 and both total and free T_4). When hypothyroidism is caused by pituitary deficiencies, serum TSH levels are decreased or are inappropriately normal in the face of low levels of TH. Hormone replacement therapy with the hormone levothyroxine is the treatment of choice for hypothyroidism. Treatment of subclinical hypothyroidism is related to elevated levels of TSH and clinical symptoms. The restoration of normal TH levels should be timed appropriately; a regimen of hormonal therapy depends on the individual's age, the duration and severity of the hypothyroidism, and the presence of other disorders, particularly cardiovascular disorders. Pregnant women need to be evaluated for thyroid function.[52] Treatment of myxedema coma with TH, combined with circulatory and ventilatory support and management of hyponatremia and hypothermia, is usually effective. Mortality can be as high as 25%.[48]

Hypothyroid Conditions

Primary Hypothyroidism. **Primary hypothyroidism** has several causes. **Iodine deficiency (endemic goiter)** is the most common cause worldwide, but is relatively rare in the United States because of the use of iodized table salt and fortified foods.[53]

The most common cause of hypothyroidism in the United States is **autoimmune thyroiditis (Hashimoto disease, chronic lymphocytic thyroiditis),** which results in gradual inflammatory destruction of thyroid

TABLE 22.3   SYSTEMIC MANIFESTATIONS OF HYPOTHYROIDISM

SYSTEM	CLINICAL MANIFESTATIONS	MECHANISMS UNDERLYING CLINICAL MANIFESTATIONS
Neurologic	Confusion, syncope, slowed speech and thinking, memory loss; lethargy, headaches, hearing loss, night blindness; slow, clumsy movements; cerebellar ataxia; slow alpha-wave activity and loss of amplitude in EEG; reduced cAMP response to epinephrine, glucagons, and PTH stimulation; decreased appetite	Decreased cerebral blood flow leading to cerebral hypoxia; reduced intracellular processes caused by decreased β-adrenergic activity that may be related to a decrease in the number of β-adrenergic receptor sites
Endocrine	Increased TSH production in primary hypothyroidism; enlarged pituitary thyrotropes, increase in serum prolactin levels with galactorrhea; decreased rate of cortisol turnover but with normal serum cortisol levels	Impaired TH synthesis or defects in iodide trapping leading to compensatory TSH production; chronic overstimulation of thyrotropes of TRH and by TSH synthesis; stimulation of lactotropes by TRH related to increased prolactin levels; decreased deactivation of cortisol
Reproductive	Decreased androgen secretion in men, increased estriol formation in women; low total hormone values but with increased amounts of unbound hormone; anovulation, decreased libido, menorrhagia, and a high incidence of spontaneous abortion in women; erectile dysfunction, decreased libido, and oligospermia in men	Altered metabolism of estrogens and androgens; decreased levels of sex hormone–binding globulin
Hematologic	Decrease in red cell mass leading to normocytic, normochromic anemia; macrocytic anemia associated with vitamin B_{12} deficiency and inadequate folate or iron absorption in the gastrointestinal tract	Decreased basal metabolic rate and reduced oxygen requirements; decreased production of erythropoietin; possible relationship between TH and optimal hematologic response to vitamin B_{12}
Cardiovascular	Reduction in stroke volume and heart rate causing lowered cardiac output; increased peripheral vascular resistance to maintain systolic blood pressure can cause hypertension; normal response to exercise but with alterations in circulatory system at rest (prolonged circulation time and decreased blood flow to tissues); cool skin and cold tolerance; enlarged heart; decreased intensity of heart sounds and variety of ECG changes (sinus bradycardia, prolonged PR interval, depressed P waves, flattened or inverted T waves, and low-amplitude QRS complexes); cardiac tamponade (although rare) (see Chapter 33)	Decreased metabolic demands and loss of regulatory and rate-setting effects of TH; protein-mucopolysaccharide–rich fluid in the pericardial sac associated with enlarged heart; pericardial effusions associated with heart sounds and ECG changes Increases in peripheral vascular resistance and increased blood volume can cause hypertension
Pulmonary	Dyspnea; myxedematous changes in respiratory muscles leading to hypoventilation and carbon dioxide retention, which contribute to myxedema coma	Pleural effusions associated with dyspnea, although effusions may be asymptomatic
Renal	Reduced renal blood flow and glomerular filtration rate leading to decreased renal excretion of water; increase in total body water and dilutional hyponatremia; reduced production of erythropoietin	Hemodynamic alterations associated with reduced blood flow and filtration; increased total body water related to decreased excretion and mucinous deposits in tissue
Gastrointestinal	Constipation, weight gain, and fluid retention; decreased absorption of most nutrients; decreased protein metabolism leading to retarded skeletal and soft tissue growth and slightly positive nitrogen balance; edema; decreased glucose absorption and delayed glucose uptake; elevated serum lipid values	Reduced intake and reduced peristaltic activity that may progress to fecal impaction; water absorption related to prolonged transit time; fluid retention associated with myxedematous changes; edema associated with high concentrations of exchangeable albumin in the extravascular space caused by increased capillary permeability to proteins; depressed insulin degradation; depressed lipid synthesis and degradation
Musculoskeletal	Muscle aching and stiffness; slow movement and slow tendon jerk reflexes; decreased bone formation and resorption, increased bone density; aching and stiffness in joints	Decreased rate of muscle contraction and relaxation contributing to slow movement and reflexes
Integumentary	Dry, flaky skin; dry, brittle head and body hair; reduced growth of nails and hair; slow wound healing	Reduced sweat and sebaceous gland secretion
	Myxedema	Accumulation of hyaluronic acid, which binds water and causes a puffy appearance
	Cool skin	Decreased circulation to skin

cAMP, Cyclic adenosine monophosphate; *ECG,* electrocardiogram; *EEG,* electroencephalogram; *PTH,* parathyroid hormone; *TH,* thyroid hormone; *TRH,* thyrotropin-releasing hormone; *TSH,* thyroid-stimulating hormone.

tissue. Hashimoto disease occurs in genetically predisposed individuals and epigenetic mechanisms are probably involved.[54] Variants in major histocompatibility complex (MHC) antigens have been associated with autoimmune thyroiditis that are different from those found in Graves disease. Infiltration of thyroid autoantibodies (antithyroid peroxidase and antithyroglobulin antibodies), autoreactive T lymphocytes, natural killer cells, and inflammatory cytokines, and induction of apoptosis are involved in the tissue destruction seen in Hashimoto thyroiditis. Goiter formation is commonly observed. Hashimoto disease is commonly associated with other autoimmune conditions. Autoimmune thyroiditis is diagnosed by the presence of thyroperoxidase and thyroglobulin antibodies. Treatment is symptomatic and requires thyroid hormone replacement.[55]

Subacute thyroiditis (subacute granulomatous thyroiditis, or de Quervain thyroiditis) is an uncommon nonbacterial inflammation of the thyroid often preceded by a viral infection. It is accompanied by fever, tenderness, and enlargement of the thyroid. The inflammatory process initially results in elevated levels of TH caused by release of stored thyroglobulin, which is then followed by transient hypothyroidism before the gland recovers normal activity. Thyroid antibodies are not present in the blood. Symptoms may last 2 to 4 months and nonsteroidal antiinflammatory drugs or corticosteroids usually resolve symptoms. Painless (silent) thyroiditis (silent or subacute lymphocytic thyroiditis) has a course similar to that of subacute thyroiditis but is pathologically identical to Hashimoto disease. Iatrogenic hypothyroidism results from radioiodine thyroid ablation, thyroidectomy, and medications (lithium and amiodarone). Postpartum thyroiditis is pathologically related to Hashimoto disease and generally occurs within 6 to 12 months of delivery with a course similar to that of painless thyroiditis. A hyperthyroid phase (with a low thyroid radioiodine uptake) precedes the hypothyroid phase in typical cases of subacute, painless, or postpartum thyroiditis. Spontaneous recovery occurs in 95% of these conditions.[56]

Congenital Hypothyroidism.
Congenital hypothyroidism in infants occurs when thyroid tissue is absent (thyroid dysgenesis) or with hereditary defects in TH synthesis.[57] Thyroid dysgenesis occurs more often in female infants, with permanent abnormalities in 1 of every 4000 live births. Congenital central hypothyroidism in children is caused by defects in thyroid-stimulating hormone (TSH) synthesis.[58] Because TH is essential for embryonic growth, particularly of brain tissue, the infant will be cognitively disabled if there is no thyroxine during fetal life. The fetus is dependent on maternal thyroxine for the first 20 weeks of gestation. Hypothyroidism may not be evident at birth since there is transplacental passage of some maternal thyroid hormone. Symptoms may include high birth weight, hypothermia, delay in passing meconium, and neonatal jaundice. Cord blood can be examined in the first days of life for measurement of T_4 and TSH levels. The probability of normal growth and intellectual function is high if treatment with levothyroxine is started before the child is 3 or 4 months old. The earlier thyroid hormone replacement therapy is initiated, the better the child's outcome.[59]

Without early screening, hypothyroidism may not be evident until after 4 months of age. Symptoms include difficulty eating, hoarse cry, and protruding tongue caused by myxedema of oral tissues and vocal cords; hypotonic muscles of the abdomen with constipation, abdominal protrusion, and umbilical herniation; subnormal temperature; lethargy; excessive sleeping; slow pulse rate; and cold, mottled skin. Skeletal growth is stunted because of impaired protein synthesis, poor absorption of nutrients, and lack of bone mineralization. The individual will become dwarfed, with short limbs, if not treated (cretinism) (Fig. 22.11). Dentition is often delayed. Cognitive disability varies with the severity of hypothyroidism and the length of delay before initiation of treatment. Treatment is required for life.

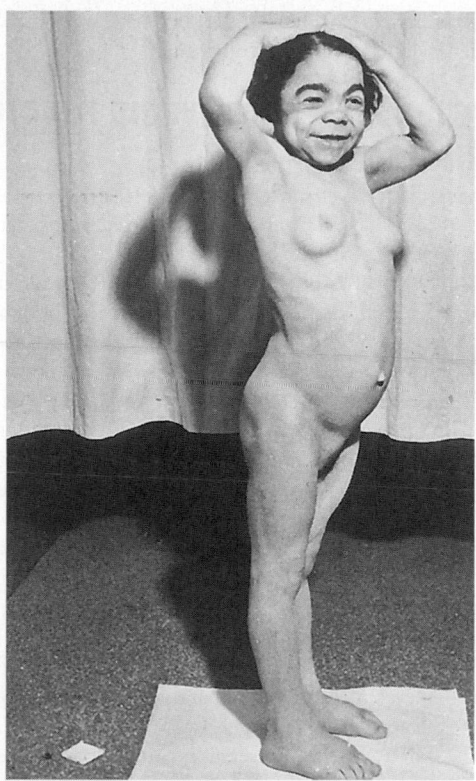

FIGURE 22.11 Adult Cretin. Note characteristic facial features, dwarfism (44 inches), absent axillary and scant pubic hair, poorly developed breasts, potbelly, and small umbilical hernia. (From Schneeberg NG: *Essentials of clinical endocrinology,* St Louis, 1970, Mosby.)

Thyroid Carcinoma.
Thyroid carcinoma accounts for 56,870 estimated new cases and 2010 estimated cancer deaths in 2017 in the United States.[60] Although it is the most common endocrine malignancy, it constitutes less than 4% of all neoplasms. Exposure to ionizing radiation, especially during childhood, is the most consistent causal factor.[61] Papillary and follicular thyroid carcinomas are the most frequent (80% to 85%) and are usually well differentiated. Medullary (occurs in C cells and secretes calcitonin and carcinoembryonic antigen) and anaplastic thyroid carcinomas are less common.

Most individuals with thyroid carcinoma have normal T_3 and T_4 levels and are therefore euthyroid. Thyroid cancer typically is discovered as a small thyroid nodule or as a metastatic tumor most commonly occurring in the regional lymph nodes, lungs, brain, or bone. Changes in voice and swallowing and difficulty in breathing are related to tumor growth impinging on the trachea or esophagus. Ultrasonographic characteristics may be suggestive of malignancy, but are neither sensitive nor specific. The diagnosis of thyroid carcinoma is generally made by fine-needle aspiration of a thyroid nodule.[62]

Treatment for well-differentiated thyroid carcinoma remains somewhat controversial mainly because of its protracted nature and the relatively low mortality regardless of the method of treatment. Treatment of well-differentiated tumors includes surgical dissection (e.g., a near-total or total thyroidectomy), postoperative radioactive iodine therapy to treat any microscopic residual tumor, and suppression of TSH with levothyroxine to replace TH and suppress TSH on any tumor cells.[63] Anaplastic thyroid carcinoma carries a grave prognosis, and palliation with surgical debulking, external beam radiotherapy, and chemotherapy may be offered. New insights into the molecular pathogenesis of thyroid carcinoma are leading to new therapies, including immunotherapy and oncolytic virotherapy.[64]

ALTERATIONS OF PARATHYROID FUNCTION

Hyperparathyroidism

Hyperparathyroidism is characterized by greater than normal secretion of parathyroid hormone (PTH) and hypercalcemia. Hyperparathyroidism is classified as primary, secondary, or tertiary.

◆**PATHOPHYSIOLOGY.** *Primary hyperparathyroidism* is characterized by inappropriate excess secretion of PTH by one or more of the parathyroid glands. It is one of the most common endocrine disorders: 80% to 85% of cases are caused by parathyroid adenomas, another 10% to 15% result from parathyroid hyperplasia, and approximately 1% of cases are caused by parathyroid carcinoma.[65] In addition, primary hyperparathyroidism may be caused by a variety of genetic causes (about 5% of cases), especially the genes that cause multiple endocrine neoplasia (*MEN-1* and *MEN-2a*).[65]

In primary hyperparathyroidism, PTH secretion is increased and is not under the usual feedback control mechanisms. The calcium level in the blood increases because of increased bone resorption and gastrointestinal absorption of calcium, but fails to inhibit PTH secretion at normal levels of calcium because the feedback threshold for calcium is set at a higher level in the abnormal parathyroid tissue. Hypercalcemia and hypophosphatemia are the hallmarks of primary hyperparathyroidism. The effects of excessive PTH secretion and primary hyperparathyroidism on various organ systems are summarized in Table 22.4.

Normocalcemic hyperparathyroidism is a phenotype of primary hyperparathyroidism characterized by increased levels of PTH, normal total and ionized serum calcium concentrations, normal activated vitamin D levels, and no underlying etiology. Increased PTH screening for osteoporosis has led to the development of this diagnosis. There may be tissue resistance to PTH or the elevated level of PTH may represent an early phase of primary hyperparathyroidism as, ultimately, there is development of hypercalcemia.[66]

Secondary hyperparathyroidism is a compensatory response of the parathyroid glands to chronic hypocalcemia, which is a common complication of chronic kidney disease (see Chapter 39) or vitamin D deficiency. Secretion of PTH is elevated, but PTH cannot achieve normal calcium levels because of insufficient levels of activated vitamin D.[67] Other causes of secondary hyperparathyroidism include chronic vitamin D or calcium deficiency; decreased intestinal absorption of vitamin D or calcium; and ingestion of drugs, such as phenytoin, phenobarbital, and laxatives, which either accelerate the metabolism of vitamin D or decrease the intestinal absorption of calcium.

Tertiary hyperparathyroidism can develop after any long-standing period of hypocalcemia, such as those seen with chronic dialysis or gastrointestinal malabsorption. In these individuals, prolonged hypocalcemia causes parathyroid chief cell hyperplasia and excess PTH production. It is most commonly seen after renal transplantation. After correction of the renal failure by renal transplant, the hypertrophied parathyroid tissue continues to over-secrete PTH. Consequently, serum calcium levels are normal or even elevated in these individuals because the hyperplastic glands function autonomously despite withdrawal of calcium and calcitriol. New drugs are being used to inhibit the synthesis of PTH. Surgical removal of one or more of the parathyroid glands is completed when there is no response to medical treatment.[68]

Familial hypocalciuric hypercalcemia (FHH) is a benign autosomal dominant condition that can mimic hyperparathyroidism and is characterized by a high serum calcium level, low serum phosphate level, and low urine calcium excretion. It is caused by a mutation in the calcium-sensing receptor in the parathyroid gland. It can be differentiated from primary hyperparathyroidism by measurement of 24-hour urine calcium excretion, which is very low in FHH.[69]

TABLE 22.4   MANIFESTATIONS OF PRIMARY HYPERPARATHYROIDISM

SYMPTOMS	RESPONSIBLE DERANGEMENTS	MECHANISMS
Renal colic, nephrolithiasis, recurrent urinary tract infections, renal failure	Hypercalciuria, hyperphosphaturia, proximal renal tubular bicarbonate leak, urine pH >6	Calcium phosphate salts precipitate in alkaline urine, renal pelvis, and collecting ducts; calcium oxalate stones also formed
Abdominal pain, peptic ulcer disease	Hypercalcemia-stimulated hypergastrinemia	Elevated hydrochloric acid secretion
Pancreatitis	Hypercalcemia	Etiology of relationship unknown
Bone disease, osteitis fibrosa and osteitis cystica, osteoporosis	Parathyroid hormone (PTH)-stimulated bone resorption, metabolic acidosis	Osteoporosis now more commonly encountered, but other disorders are more specific for hyperparathyroidism
Muscle weakness, myalgia	PTH excess, possible direct effect on striated muscle and on nerves	Characteristic myopathic changes in muscle histology (neuropathy of type I and type II muscle fibers)
Neurologic and psychiatric problems (impaired memory, confusion, depression, anxiety, psychosis)	Hypercalcemia	Neuropathy; electroencephalographic changes present
Polyuria, polydipsia	Hypercalcemia	Direct effect on renal tubule to decrease responsiveness to antidiuretic hormone
Constipation	Hypercalcemia	Decreased peristalsis of gastrointestinal tract
Anorexia, nausea, and vomiting	Hypercalcemia	Central stimulation of vomiting center
Hypertension	Renal disease, direct effect of calcium on arterial smooth muscle, pheochromocytoma	Plasma renin activity elevated or normal
Arthralgia and arthritis	Gout, pseudogout, periarticular classification	Hyperuricemia, chronic renal failure with high calcium phosphate product

Data from Flint PW et al: *Cummings otolaryngology: head & neck surgery,* ed 5, St Louis, 2010, Mosby.

◆CLINICAL MANIFESTATIONS. Hypercalcemia and hypophosphatemia are the hallmarks of primary hyperparathyroidism and may be discovered incidentally. Hypercalcemia and hypophosphatemia may be asymptomatic or affected individuals may present with symptoms related to the muscular, nervous, and gastrointestinal systems, including fatigue, headache, depression, anorexia, and nausea and vomiting. Excessive osteoclastic and osteocytic activity resulting in bone resorption may cause pathologic fractures, kyphosis of the dorsal spine, and compression fractures of the vertebral bodies. (Bone resorption is discussed in Chapter 44.)

The increased renal filtration load of calcium leads to hypercalciuria. Hypercalcemia also affects proximal renal tubular function, causing metabolic acidosis and production of an abnormally alkaline urine. PTH hypersecretion enhances renal phosphate excretion and results in hypophosphatemia and hyperphosphaturia. The combination of these three variables—hypercalciuria, alkaline urine, and hyperphosphaturia—predisposes the individual to the formation of calcium stones, particularly in the renal pelvis or in the renal collecting ducts. These may be associated with infections.[70] Hypercalcemia also impairs the concentrating ability of the renal tubule by decreasing its response to ADH. Chronic hypercalcemia of hyperparathyroidism is associated with mild insulin resistance, necessitating increased insulin secretion to maintain normal glucose levels.[71]

Secondary hyperparathyroidism caused by renal disease presents clinically not only with bone resorption but also with the symptoms of hypocalcemia and hyperphosphatemia. Hypocalcemia can cause many significant clinical problems (see Chapter 3). Hyperphosphatemia can cause deleterious effects on the cardiovascular system (i.e., increased calcification).

◆EVALUATION AND TREATMENT. The concurrent findings of increased ionized calcium concentration in the face of elevated PTH concentration are suggestive of primary hyperparathyroidism. PTH levels also may be inappropriately within the normal range because hypercalcemia should completely suppress PTH production. Observation of asymptomatic individuals with mild hypercalcemia is recommended; these individuals are advised to avoid dehydration and limit dietary calcium intake. Definitive treatment of severe primary hyperparathyroidism involves surgical removal of a solitary adenoma or, in the case of hyperplasia, complete removal of three and partial removal of the fourth hyperplastic parathyroid glands. Imaging procedures are used to localize adenomas before surgery. In those individuals who fail surgery, other treatments, such as bisphosphonates and calcimimetics (e.g., cinacalcet), may be considered. Calcimimetics increase the parathyroid calcium receptor sensitivity, thus lowering PTH levels.

If hypercalcemia is documented but PTH levels are low, the differential diagnosis shifts to hypercalcemia of malignancy, granulomatous diseases (sarcoidosis), excessive calcium ingestion, or hypervitaminosis A or D. Treatment of these conditions depends on the underlying cause.

If serum calcium level is low but PTH level is elevated, secondary hyperparathyroidism is likely. Evaluation for renal function frequently documents chronic renal disease. Treatment for secondary hyperparathyroidism in chronic kidney disease requires calcium replacement, dietary phosphate restriction and phosphate binders, and vitamin D replacement. Treatment also may include calcimimetics but adverse effects must be considered.[72]

Hypoparathyroidism

Hypoparathyroidism (abnormally low PTH levels) most commonly is caused by damage to or removal of the parathyroid glands during thyroid surgery and occurs because of the anatomic proximity of the parathyroid glands to the thyroid (see Fig. 21.11).[70] Hypoparathyroidism also is associated with genetic syndromes, including familial hypopara-

thyroidism and DiGeorge syndrome (velocardiofacial syndrome), and an idiopathic or autoimmune form of the disease.[73] Hypomagnesemia also can cause a decrease in PTH secretion and function. There is an inherited condition associated with hypocalcemia with normal to elevated levels of PTH called pseudohypoparathyroidism. Individuals with this condition are resistant to PTH in the proximal renal tubule and cannot produce cAMP in response to PTH (a postreceptor defect in PTH action).[74]

◆PATHOPHYSIOLOGY. A lack of circulating PTH causes depressed serum calcium levels and increased serum phosphate levels. In the absence of PTH, resorption of calcium from bone and regulation of calcium reabsorption from the renal tubules are impaired. Therefore phosphate reabsorption by the renal tubules is increased, causing decreased renal phosphate excretion and hyperphosphatemia.

Hypomagnesemia inhibits PTH secretion. When serum magnesium levels return to normal, however, PTH secretion returns to normal, as does the responsiveness of peripheral tissues to PTH. Hypomagnesemia may be related to chronic alcoholism, malnutrition, malabsorption, increased renal clearance of magnesium caused by the use of aminoglycoside antibiotics or certain chemotherapeutic agents, or prolonged magnesium-deficient parenteral nutritional therapy.

◆CLINICAL MANIFESTATIONS. Symptoms associated with hypoparathyroidism are primarily those of hypocalcemia. Hypocalcemia causes a lowered threshold for nerve and muscle excitation so that a nerve impulse may be initiated by a slight stimulus anywhere along the length of a nerve or muscle fiber. This creates perioral numbness, paresthesias, tingling, and tetany caused by muscle spasms, hyperreflexia, tonic-clonic convulsions, laryngeal spasms, and, in severe cases, death from asphyxiation. Chvostek and Trousseau signs may be used to evaluate for neuromuscular irritability. Chvostek sign is elicited by tapping the cheek, resulting in twitching of the upper lip. Trousseau sign is elicited by sustained inflation of a sphygmomanometer placed on the upper arm to a level above the systolic blood pressure with resultant painful carpal spasm. Other symptoms of hypocalcemia include dry skin, loss of body and scalp hair, hypoplasia of developing teeth, horizontal ridges on the nails, cataracts, basal ganglia calcifications (which may be associated with a parkinsonian syndrome), and bone deformities, including brachydactyly and bowing of the long bones.

Phosphate retention caused by increased renal reabsorption of phosphate is associated also with hypoparathyroidism. Hyperphosphatemia results from PTH deficiency and, in turn, hyperphosphatemia further lowers calcium concentration by inhibiting the activation of vitamin D, thereby lowering the gastrointestinal absorption of calcium.

◆EVALUATION AND TREATMENT. A low serum calcium level and a high phosphorous level in the absence of renal failure, intestinal disorders, nutritional deficiencies, or in individuals who have had thyroidectomy suggest hypoparathyroidism. PTH levels are low in hypoparathyroidism, and measurement of serum magnesium and urinary calcium excretion can help in diagnosis. Treatment is directed toward the alleviation of hypocalcemia. In acute states this involves parenteral administration of calcium, which corrects serum calcium concentration within minutes. Maintenance of serum calcium level is achieved with pharmacologic doses of an active form of vitamin D and oral calcium. Hypoplastic dentition, cataracts, bone deformities, and basal ganglia calcifications do not respond to the correction of hypocalcemia, but the other symptoms of hypocalcemia are reversible. PTH hormone replacement therapy with recombinant human parathyroid hormone (rhPTH[1–84]) is safe and effective with reduced requirements for supplemental calcium and vitamin D.[75]

As serum calcium levels return to normal, phosphaturia usually is stimulated with a return to normal serum phosphate levels. In some individuals, however, the absence of the phosphaturic effect of PTH causes a persistent hyperphosphatemia, which should be treated with drugs that inhibit gastrointestinal absorption of phosphate (i.e., non–calcium-containing phosphate binders).

DYSFUNCTION OF THE ENDOCRINE PANCREAS: DIABETES MELLITUS

Diabetes mellitus (DM) is a group of metabolic diseases characterized by hyperglycemia resulting from defects in insulin secretion, insulin action, or both. In 2015 in the United States, an estimated 30.3 million people (9.4%) had diabetes and 7.2 million were estimated to be undiagnosed. DM was the seventh leading cause of death in 2015.[76]

The American Diabetes Association (ADA)[77] classifies four categories of diabetes mellitus (see details in Table 22.5) as follows:
1. Type 1 beta-cell destruction, usually leading to absolute insulin deficiency
2. Type 2: ranging from predominantly insulin resistance with relative insulin deficiency to predominantly an insulin secretory defect with insulin resistance
3. Other specific types
4. Gestational diabetes

The diagnosis of diabetes mellitus is based on glycosylated hemoglobin (HbA_{1c}) levels, fasting plasma glucose (FPG) levels, 2-hour plasma glucose level during oral glucose tolerance testing (OGTT) using a

TABLE 22.5 CLASSIFICATION AND CHARACTERISTICS OF DIABETES MELLITUS

NAME	CHARACTERISTICS
Type 1 Beta-cell destruction leading to absolute insulin deficiency; immune-mediated diabetes is most common form (≈90%)	Cellular-mediated autoimmune destruction of pancreatic beta cells Individual prone to ketoacidosis Little or no insulin secretion Insulin dependent 75% of individuals develop before 30 years of age; can occur up to the tenth decade Usually not obese
Idiopathic (≈10%)	No defined etiologies; absolute requirement for insulin replacement therapy in affected individuals may be sporadic
Type 2 Progressive loss of b-cell insulin secretion frequency on the background of insulin resistance	Usually not insulin dependent but may be insulin requiring Individual not ketosis prone (but may form ketones under stress) Obesity common in the abdominal region Generally occurs in those older than 40 years, but the frequency is rapidly increasing in children Strong genetic predisposition Often associated with hypertension and dyslipidemia
Other Specific Types Genetic defects of beta-cell function	Genetic abnormalities that decrease the ability of the beta cell to secrete insulin: 1. Maturity-onset diabetes of youth (MODY) includes six specific autosomal dominant mutations including genes for hepatocyte nuclear factor-1α (HNF-1α; *MODY 3*), glucokinase (*MODY 2*), HNF-4α (*MODY 1*), insulin-promoter factor-1(IPF-1; *MODY 4*), HNF-1β (*MODY 5*), and NeuroD1 (*MODY 6*) 2. Defects in mitochondrial deoxyribonucleic acid (DNA) 3. Other (including an inability to convert proinsulin to insulin)
Genetic defects in insulin action	Mutations in the insulin receptor with hyperinsulinism or hyperglycemia or severe diabetes
Diseases of the exocrine pancreas	Any process that diffusely injures the pancreas, including pancreatitis, neoplasia, and cystic fibrosis
Endocrinopathies	Endocrine disorders including acromegaly, Cushing syndrome, glucagonoma, pheochromocytoma, hyperthyroidism, somatostatinoma, and aldosteronoma
Drug- or chemical-induced beta-cell dysfunction	Commonly associated drugs include glucocorticoids, treatment of HIV/AIDS, and after organ transplantation although many others may be implicated
Infections	Beta-cell destruction by viruses including cytomegalovirus, congenital rubella
Uncommon forms of immune-mediated diabetes mellitus	Anti–insulin receptor antibodies Reported with "stiff man syndrome" and individuals receiving interferon-α
Other genetic syndromes sometimes associated with diabetes mellitus	Down, Klinefelter, Turner, and Wolfram syndromes
Gestational Diabetes Mellitus (GDM) Any degree of glucose intolerance with onset or first recognition during pregnancy	Insulin resistance combined with inadequate insulin secretion in relation to hyperglycemia Women who are obese, older than 25 years of age, have a family history of diabetes, have a history of previous GDM, or are of certain ethnic groups (Hispanic, Native American, Asian, or black) are at increased risk of developing GDM The metabolic stress of pregnancy may uncover a genetic tendency for type 2 diabetes mellitus

Data from American Diabetes Association: *Diabetes Care 40*(Suppl 1): S11–S24, 2017.

BOX 22.2 DIAGNOSTIC CRITERIA FOR DIABETES MELLITUS

1. HbA$_{1c}$ (as measured in a DCCT-referenced assay) ≥6.5%
   OR
2. FPG ≥126 mg/dL (7.0 mmol/L); fasting is defined as no caloric intake for at least 8 hr
   OR
3. 2-hr plasma glucose ≥200 mg/dL (11.1 mmol/L) during an OGTT
   OR
4. In a patient with classic symptoms of hyperglycemia or hyperglycemic crisis, a random plasma glucose ≥200 mg/dL (11.1 mmol/L)

Categories of Increased Risk for Diabetes (Prediabetes)
1. FPG 100 to 125 mg/dL
2. 2-hr PG in the range of 140 to 199 mg/dL during an OGTT
3. HbA$_{1c}$ 5.7% to 6.4%

DCCT, Diabetes Control and Complications Trial; *FPG,* fasting plasma glucose; *HbA$_{1c}$,* hemoglobin A$_{1c}$; *hr,* hour(s); *OGTT,* oral glucose tolerance test; *PG,* plasma glucose.
From American Diabetes Association (ADA): *2016 guidelines.* Available at http://www.ndei.org/ADA-diabetes-management-guidelines-diagnosis-A1C-testing.aspx.

75-g oral glucose load, or random glucose levels in an individual with symptoms (Box 22.2). Glycosylated hemoglobin refers to the permanent attachment of glucose to hemoglobin molecules and reflects the average plasma glucose exposure over the life of a red blood cell (approximately 120 days). It provides a more accurate measure for monitoring long-term control of blood glucose levels. This test is critically dependent upon the method of measurement and must be related to established standards.

The ADA classification categories of increased risk for diabetes (or prediabetes)[77] describe nondiabetic elevations of HbA$_{1c}$, FPG, or the 2-hour plasma glucose value during OGTT (see Box 22.2). The Centers for Disease Control and Prevention (CDC) estimates that 37% of U.S. adults aged 20 years or older have prediabetes (86 million people) including 51% of those aged 65 years or older.[76] This classification includes impaired glucose tolerance (IGT), which results from diminished insulin secretion, and impaired fasting glucose (IFG), which is caused by enhanced hepatic glucose output secondary to hepatic insulin resistance. Individuals with IGT and IFG are at increased risk of cardiovascular disease and premature death and carry a 15% to 50% 5-year risk of developing diabetes, particularly type 2 diabetes.[78] Thus prevention of diabetes with lifestyle interventions is essential.[77]

Types of Diabetes Mellitus
Type 1 Diabetes Mellitus

Type 1 diabetes mellitus (DM) is the most common pediatric chronic disease and affects 0.17% of U.S. children, and the incidence is increasing.[76] Between 10% and 13% of individuals with newly diagnosed type 1 DM have a first-degree relative (parent or sibling) with type 1 DM. There is a 50% concordance rate in twins.[79] Diagnosis is rare during the first 9 months of life and peaks at 12 years of age. Two distinct types of type 1 DM have been identified: autoimmune (type 1A) and idiopathic or nonimmune (type 1B). Type 3c DM is associated with chronic pancreatitis and is discussed in Chapter 42. Table 22.6 summarizes the epidemiology of type 1 and type 2 DM.

PATHOPHYSIOLOGY. In autoimmune-mediated DM, environmental-genetic factors are thought to trigger cell-mediated destruction of pancreatic beta cells. A specific cause is still unknown. Idiopathic or nonimmune type 1 DM is far less common than autoimmune and does not have an autoimmune basis for beta-cell destruction. It occurs secondary to other diseases, such as pancreatitis, and mostly in people of Asian or African descent. Affected individuals have varying degrees of insulin deficiency, lack islet autoantibodies and HLA association, and have intermittent proneness to ketosis. It also is described as ketosis prone type 2 DM.[80]

Gene/Environmental Factors. Interactions between environmental factors and susceptibility genes are thought to have a significant contribution to the development of type 1 DM but the mechanisms are still poorly defined. The strongest genetic association is with major histocompatibility complex, or MHC (histocompatibility leukocyte antigen [HLA] class II alleles HLA-DR3-DQ2 or HLA-DR4-DQ8 haplotypes, or both). Numerous other mutations involving single genes both within and outside of the MHC complex have been associated with an increased risk of type 1 DM.[81] Various epigenetic modifications of gene expression also have been postulated. Environmental factors, including viral infections, particularly enteroviruses, coxsackievirus, other infectious microorganisms (such as *Helicobacter pylori*); exposure to cow's milk proteins; a relative lack of vitamin D; air pollution; vaccinations; stress; gut microbial flora; and family density also have been implicated but more research is needed.[82]

Immunologically Mediated Destruction of Beta Cells. Autoimmune type 1 DM is a slowly progressive autoimmune T-cell–mediated disease that destroys beta cells of the pancreas and occurs in genetically susceptible individuals (Fig. 22.12 and see Chapter 9). There is a deficient immune tolerance linked to abnormalities in immune cells and changes in beta-cell antigens.[83] Gene-environment interactions result in the loss of tolerance to self-antigens with formation of autoantigens that are expressed on the surface of pancreatic beta cells and circulate in the bloodstream and lymphatics. Cellular immunity (T-cytotoxic cells and macrophages) and humoral immunity (autoantibodies) are stimulated, resulting in beta-cell destruction and apoptosis.

The destruction of beta cells progresses through the following stages:
1. *Lymphocyte and macrophage infiltration of the islets resulting in inflammation (insulinitis) and islet beta-cell death.* Autoantigens are expressed on the surface of pancreatic islet cells and circulate in the bloodstream and lymphatics (see Fig. 22.12). Circulating autoantigens are ingested by antigen-presenting cells that activate CD4+ T helper 1 (Th1) lymphocytes. The activated T helper lymphocytes secrete interleukin-2 (IL-2) that activates beta-cell autoantigen-specific T cytotoxic lymphocytes, causing them to proliferate and attack islet cells through secretion of toxic perforins and granzymes.[84] T helper lymphocytes also secrete interferon that activates macrophages and stimulates the release of inflammatory cytokines (including IL-1, and tumor necrosis factor [TNF]), which cause further beta-cell destruction and apoptosis.[85]
2. *Production of autoantibodies against islet cells, insulin, glutamic acid decarboxylase (GAD), and other cytoplasmic proteins.* Activated T helper 2 (Th2) lymphocytes produce IL-4, which stimulates B lymphocytes to proliferate and produce antibodies (see Fig. 22.12). Islet cell autoantibodies (ICAs) precede evidence of beta-cell deficiency and can be found in the serum years before symptoms occur.[86] Beta-cell destruction also is mediated by the production of autoantibodies against insulin, glutamic acid decarboxylase (GAD), and tyrosine phosphatase.[85] Finally, another islet antigen against which antibodies are produced in type 1 and type 2 DM is the zinc transporter 8 (Znt8) protein. It can be measured in the serum and is associated with variation in disease progression.[87]

TABLE 22.6	EPIDEMIOLOGY AND ETIOLOGY OF DIABETES MELLITUS IN THE UNITED STATES	
	TYPE 1 DIABETES: PRIMARY BETA-CELL DEFECT OR FAILURE	**TYPE 2 DIABETES: INSULIN RESISTANCE WITH INADEQUATE INSULIN SECRETION**
Incidence		
Frequency	One of the most common childhood diseases (≈5% of all cases of diabetes mellitus) Prevalence rate is ≈0.17%	Accounts for most cases (≈90–95%) *Incident rates for all diabetes (e.g., type 1 and type 2):* women, 11.7%; men, 12.7%. For women and men ages 18–44 yr, 4%; ages 45–64, 17%; ages >65 yr, 25.2%.
Change in incidences	No documented increase in incidence in the United States	Incidence in all age groups increased 382% from 1988 to 2014
Characteristics		
Age at onset	Peak onset at age 11–13 yr (slightly earlier for girls than for boys) Rare in children younger than 1 yr and adults older than 30 yr	Risk of developing diabetes increases after age 40 yr; in general, incidence increases with age into the 70s; among Pima Indians, incidence peaks between ages 40 and 50 yr, then falls
Sex	Similar in males and females	Similar in males and females overall, although black females have the highest incidence and prevalence of all groups
Racial distribution	Rates for whites 1.5–2 times higher than those for nonwhites Higher rates for those of Scandinavian descent than for those of central or southern European descent	*For all diabetes (e.g., type 1 and type 2):* American Indians/Alaska Natives 15.1%; black, non-Hispanic 12.7%; Hispanic 12.1%; Asian, non-Hispanic 8.0%; white, non-Hispanic 7.4%
Obesity	Generally normal or underweight	Frequent contributing factor to precipitate type 2 diabetes among those susceptible; a major factor in populations recently exposed to westernized environment Increased risk related to duration, degree, and distribution of obesity
Etiology		
Common theory	*Autoimmune:* Genetic and environmental factors, resulting in gradual process of autoimmune destruction in genetically susceptible individuals *Nonautoimmune:* Unknown Strong association with *HLA-DQA* and *HLA-DQB* genes	Disease results from genetic susceptibility (polygenic) combined with environmental determinants and other risk factors; inherited defects in beta-cell mass and function combined with peripheral tissue insulin resistance Associated with long-duration obesity
Heredity	Risk to sibling: 5%–10% Risk to offspring: 2%–5%	Risk to first-degree relative (child or sibling): 10%–15%
Presence of antibody	Islet cell autoantibodies (ICAs) and/or autoantibodies to insulin, and autoantibodies to glutamic acid decarboxylase (GAD_{65}) and tyrosine phosphatases IA-2 and IA-2β are present in 85%–90% of individuals when fasting; hyperglycemia is initially detected	Islet cell antibodies not prevalent
Insulin resistance	Insulin resistance at diagnosis is unusual, but insulin resistance may occur as the individual ages and gains weight	Insulin resistance is generally caused by altered cellular metabolism and an intracellular postreceptor defect
Insulin secretion	Severe insulin deficiency or no insulin secretion at all	Typically increased at time of diagnosis, but progressively declines over the course of the illness

Data from Centers for Disease Control and Prevention (CDC): *Diabetes public health resource, diagnosed diabetes,* last updated Dec 1, 2015. Available at: http://www.cdc.gov/diabetes/statistics/prevalence_national.htm; Centers for Disease Control and Prevention (CDC). *National diabetes statistics report, 2017.* Atlanta, GA, 2017, US Department of Health and Human Services. Available at: https://www.cdc.gov/diabetes/pdfs/data/statistics/national-diabetes-statistics-report.pdf. Satterfield D et al: *MMWR Suppl* 65(1):4–10, 2016.

3. *Relative inactivity of T regulatory cells that contribute to a decrease in beta-cell mass and insulin production.* Normally these T lymphocytes serve to inhibit the immune response and maintain self-tolerance.[88]

For insulin synthesis to decline enough such that hyperglycemia occurs, 80% to 90% of the insulin-secreting beta cells of the islet of Langerhans must be destroyed. Insulin normally suppresses secretion of glucagon and, thus, hypoinsulinemia leads to a marked increase in glucagon secretion. Glucagon, a hormone produced by the alpha cells of the islets, acts in the liver to increase blood glucose level by stimulating glycogenolysis and gluconeogenesis. In addition to the decline in insulin secretion, there is decreased secretion of amylin, another beta-cell hormone. One of the critical actions of amylin is to suppress glucagon release from the alpha cells. Thus both alpha-cell and beta-cell functions are abnormal and both a lack of insulin and a relative excess of glucagon contribute to hyperglycemia in type 1 DM.[89]

◆CLINICAL MANIFESTATIONS. The onset of type 1 DM involves a long preclinical period with gradual destruction of beta cells, eventually leading to insulin deficiency and hyperglycemia. Generally, this latent

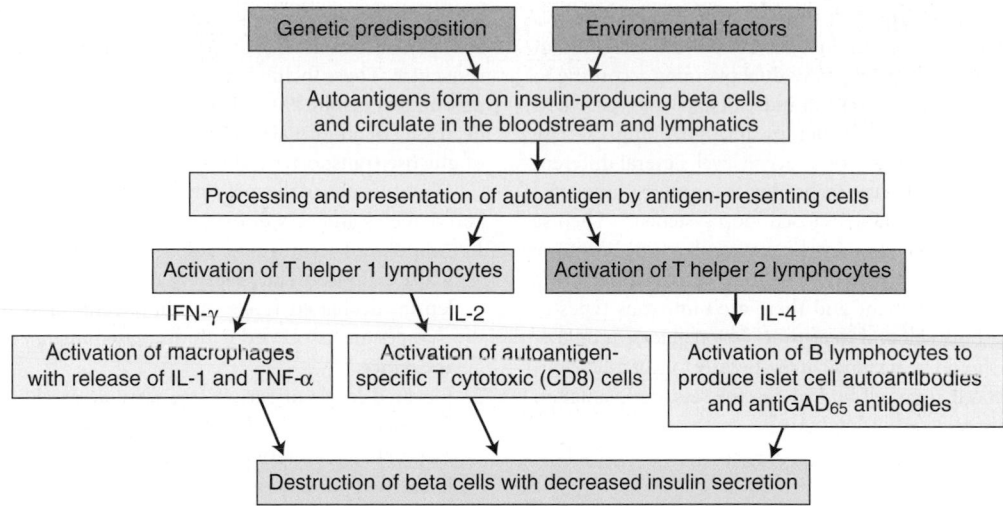

FIGURE 22.12 Pathophysiology of Type 1 Diabetes Mellitus. *GAD₆₅,* Glutamic acid decarboxylase; *IFN-γ,* interferon-gamma; *IL,* interleukin; *TNF-α,* tumor necrosis factor-alpha.

period is longer in older individuals with type 1 DM and often results in misclassification of those affected as having type 2 DM. This is sometimes called *latent autoimmune diabetes of adults (LADA).*

Type 1 DM affects the metabolism of fat, protein, and carbohydrates. Glucose accumulates in the blood and appears in the urine as the renal threshold for glucose is exceeded, producing an osmotic diuresis manifested as polyuria and thirst. Wide fluctuations in blood glucose levels occur. In addition, protein and fat breakdown occurs because of the lack of insulin, resulting in weight loss. Increased hepatic metabolism of fat leads to high levels of circulating ketones, causing diabetic ketoacidosis (DKA) (Table 22.7, and see Diabetic Ketoacidosis).

Currently half of individuals with type 1 DM are obese and there is an increasing number of individuals who have both type 1 DM and the clinical manifestations of metabolic syndrome, including dyslipidemia and hypertension. This is because, in part, of successful intensive insulin therapy that promotes weight gain and also, in part, because of lifestyle factors, including lack of exercise and poor nutrition. This creates a high risk of synergistic effects for chronic complications of DM, including heart disease and stroke,[90,91] and adjunctive noninsulin antihyperglycemic therapies are under investigation.[92]

◆**EVALUATION AND TREATMENT.** The criteria for diagnosis of type 1 DM are the same as those for type 2 DM (see Box 22.2). The diagnosis of DM is not difficult when the symptoms of polydipsia, polyuria, polyphagia, weight loss, and hyperglycemia are present in fasting and postprandial states. Many children are first diagnosed when they present with the signs and symptoms of DKA. It reflects lack of awareness by parents and primary care providers of the evolving symptoms of type 1 DM. In DKA, acetone (a volatile form of ketones) is exhaled by hyperventilation and gives the breath a sweet or "fruity" odor. Occasionally, diabetic coma is the initial symptom of the disease.[93] C-peptide, a component of proinsulin released during insulin production, can be measured in the serum as a surrogate for insulin levels and is indicative of residual beta-cell mass and function. The zinc transporter 8 autoantibody (ZnT8Ab) test has been approved to help differentiate type 1 from type 2 DM.[94] Currently, measurement of autoantibodies remains the best way to identify diabetes and to distinguish type 1 DM from other forms of diabetes. Having two or more islet autoantibodies confers a 100% risk of diabetes development.[95] Other important aspects of evaluation include assessing for evidence of the chronic complications of diabetes (see Chronic Complications of Diabetes Mellitus).

TABLE 22.7	CLINICAL MANIFESTATIONS AND RATIONALE FOR TYPE 1 DIABETES MELLITUS
MANIFESTATIONS	**RATIONALE**
Polydipsia	Because of elevated blood glucose levels, water is osmotically attracted from body cells, resulting in intracellular dehydration and hypothalamic stimulation of thirst
Polyuria	Hyperglycemia acts as an osmotic diuretic; the amount of glucose filtered by the glomeruli of the kidneys exceeds the amount that can be reabsorbed by the renal tubules; glycosuria results, accompanied by large amounts of water lost in the urine
Polyphagia	Depletion of cellular stores of carbohydrates, fats, and protein results in cellular starvation and a corresponding increase in hunger
Weight loss	Weight loss occurs because of fluid loss in osmotic diuresis and the loss of body tissue as fat and proteins are used for energy as a result of the effects of insulin deficiency
Fatigue	Metabolic changes result in poor use of food products, contributing to lethargy and fatigue; sleep loss from severe nocturia also contributes to fatigue

There are no approved therapies for preserving beta-cell mass. Many different kinds of approaches are being tested to prevent the autoimmune destruction of beta cells that is characteristic of type 1 DM. Avoidance of cow's milk, utilization of a gluten-free diet, and increased intake of omega-3 fatty acids and vitamin D are all being explored.[95] Pharmacologic prevention trials include immunosuppression and immunomodulation therapies (antigen-specific therapies, monoclonal antibodies, fusion proteins, alternate Treg effectors, and oral or intranasal insulin)[96] (see *What's New?* Immunomodulation in the Prevention and Treatment of Type 1 Diabetes on Evolve).

Treatment regimens are designed to achieve optimal glucose control (as measured by the HbA$_{1c}$ value) without causing episodes of significant hypoglycemia. Management requires individual planning according to type of disease, age, and activity level. All individuals with type 1 DM require some combination of insulin therapy, meal planning, exercise program, and self-monitoring of blood glucose level. Several different types of insulin preparations and new technologies for more physiologic insulin delivery systems are available (closed loop systems).[97] The use of pramlintide, a synthetic analog of amylin, can replace this hormone in individuals with type 1 and type 2 DM.[98] Blood glucose monitoring is an essential part of management and there are numerous types of monitoring devices for both self and "real-time" blood glucose monitoring.[99] Individuals also should be screened at least yearly for complications of diabetes. Finally, islet cell, stem cell, and whole pancreas transplantation have been successful in selected individuals.

Type 2 Diabetes Mellitus

Type 2 diabetes mellitus (DM) affects 9.3% of adults in the United States.[76] Prevalence is highest among American Indians and Alaska Natives (16%) and lowest among non-Hispanic whites (7.6%). There also is an increased prevalence of type 2 DM in children, especially in obese children[76] (see Table 22.6).

A genetic-environmental interaction appears to be responsible for type 2 DM.[100,101] The most well-recognized risk factors are age, obesity, hypertension, physical inactivity, and family history. There is increasing evidence that diet, including diet during pregnancy, influences the long-term risk of type 2 DM in children and adults.[102] More than 65 genes have been identified that are associated with type 2 DM, including those that code for beta-cell mass, beta-cell function (ability to sense blood glucose levels, insulin synthesis, and insulin secretion), proinsulin and insulin molecular structures, insulin receptors, hepatic synthesis of glucose, glucagon synthesis, and cellular responsiveness to insulin stimulation.[103] Metabolic syndrome is a constellation of disorders (central obesity, dyslipidemia, prehypertension, and an elevated fasting blood glucose level) that together confer a high risk of developing type 2 DM and associated cardiovascular complications (Box 22.3). The metabolic syndrome develops during childhood, is highly prevalent among overweight children and adolescents, and affects millions of adults. Metabolic syndrome is characterized by many of the same genetic and environmental risks as type 2 DM and individuals should be screened on a regular basis. Early recognition and treatment, including vigorous lifestyle changes, are critical to reducing cardiovascular events and improving clinical outcomes.[104]

◆PATHOPHYSIOLOGY. Many organs contribute to insulin resistance, chronic hyperglycemia, and the consequences of type 2 DM (Fig. 22.13). The combination of genetic, and environmental influences results in the basic pathophysiologic mechanisms of type 2 DM (Fig. 22.14).

Insulin resistance is defined as a suboptimal response of insulin-sensitive tissues (especially liver, muscle, and adipose tissue) to insulin

and is associated with obesity. Several mechanisms are involved in abnormalities of the insulin signaling pathway and contribute to insulin resistance. These include an abnormality of the insulin molecule, high amounts of insulin antagonists, downregulation of the insulin receptor, decreased or abnormal activation of postreceptor kinases, and alteration of glucose transporter (GLUT) proteins.

Obesity is one of the most important contributors to insulin resistance and diabetes and acts through several important mechanisms:

1. Adipokines (leptin and adiponectin) are hormones produced in white adipose tissue. Obesity results in increased serum levels of leptin, decreased levels of adiponectin, and inflammation These changes are associated with decreased insulin synthesis and insulin resistance.[105]
2. Elevated levels of serum free fatty acids (FFAs) and intracellular deposits of triglycerides and cholesterol are found in obese individuals. These changes interfere with intracellular insulin signaling, decrease tissue responses to insulin, alter incretin action, promote inflammation, and cause apoptotic beta-cell death. This is known as *lipotoxicity*.[106]
3. Obesity causes release of inflammatory cytokines (TNF-α, IL-6) from intraabdominal adipocytes or adipocyte-associated mononuclear cells and from activated macrophages that release inflammatory cytokines. These cytokines induce insulin resistance through a postreceptor mechanism and play an important role in the genesis of fatty liver, atherosclerosis, and dyslipidemia.[107]
4. Alterations in oxidative phosphorylation in cellular mitochondria have been documented, resulting in reduced insulin-stimulated mitochondrial activity and insulin resistance, especially in skeletal muscle and hepatocytes. However, the mechanisms are not clearly defined.[108]
5. Obesity is correlated with hyperinsulinemia and impaired insulin receptor signaling.[109]

Compensatory hyperinsulinemia prevents the clinical appearance of diabetes for many years. Eventually, however, beta-cell dysfunction develops and leads to a relative deficiency of insulin activity. The islet dysfunction is caused by a combination of a decrease in beta-cell mass and a reduction in beta-cell function. A progressive decrease in the weight and number of beta cells occurs and many of the remaining cells develop "exhaustion" from increased demand for insulin biosynthesis.

Glucagon concentration is increased in type 2 DM because pancreatic alpha cells become less responsive to glucose inhibition, resulting in an increase in glucagon secretion. These abnormally high levels of glucagon increase blood glucose level by stimulating glycogenolysis and gluconeogenesis. As was discussed under type 1 DM, type 2 DM also is associated with a deficiency in amylin, further increasing glucagon levels.

Amylin (islet amyloid polypeptide) is another beta-cell hormone that is decreased in both type 1 and type 2 DM. Amylin increases satiety and suppresses glucagon release from the alpha cells. Amylin contributes to islet cell destruction through the deposition of abnormal (misfolded) amyloid polypeptide within the pancreas.[110] As in type 1 DM, pramlintide, a synthetic analog of amylin, is used for treatment in type 2 DM.

Hormones released from the gastrointestinal (GI) tract play a role in insulin resistance, beta-cell function, and diabetes.[98] Ghrelin is a peptide produced in the stomach and pancreatic islets that regulates food intake, energy balance, and hormonal secretion. Decreased levels of circulating ghrelin have been associated with insulin resistance and increased fasting insulin levels. Its use as a potential treatment for type 2 DM is being investigated.[111] The incretins are a class of peptides that are released from the GI tract in response to food intake and function to increase synthesis and secretion of insulin and beta-cell proliferation and regeneration, and protection against beta-cell damage. The most studied incretin is glucagon-like peptide 1 (GLP-1), and studies have

---

BOX 22.3   CRITERIA FOR THE DIAGNOSIS OF METABOLIC SYNDROME

Three of the following five traits:
- Increased waist circumference (>40 inches in men; >35 inches in women)
- Plasma triglycerides ≥150 mg/dL
- Plasma high-density lipoprotein (HDL) cholesterol <40 mg/dL (men) or <50 mg/dL (women)
- Blood pressure ≥130/85 mmHg
- Fasting plasma glucose ≥100 mg/dL

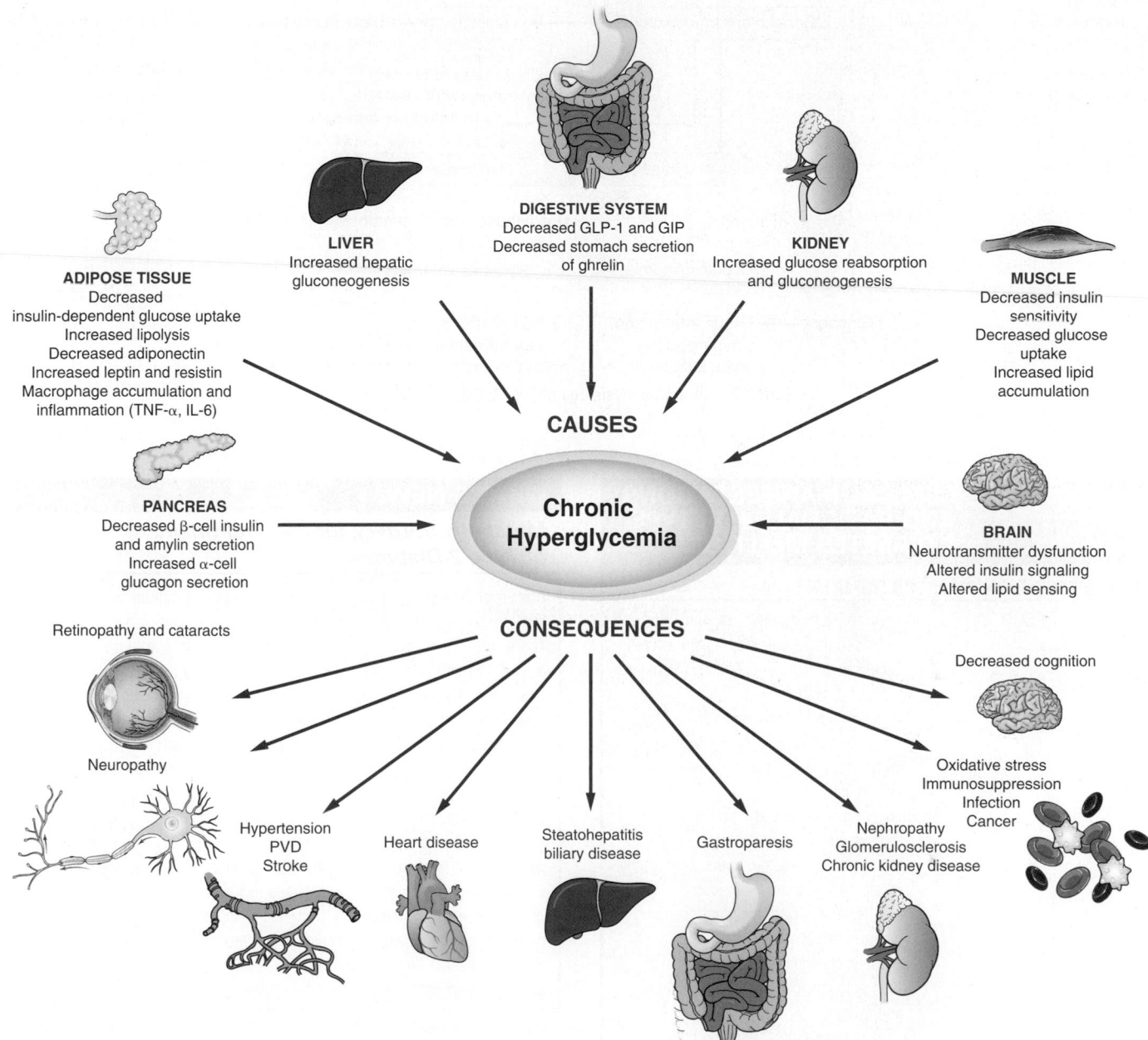

FIGURE 22.13 Multiorgan Causes and Common Consequences of Chronic Hyperglycemia in Type 2 Diabetes Mellitus. *GIP,* Gastrifc inhibitory peptide; *GLP-1,* glucagon-like peptide-1; *IL,* interleukin; *PVD,* peripheral vascular disease; *TNF,* tumor necrosis factor.

demonstrated that beta-cell responsiveness to GLP 1 is reduced both in prediabetes and in type 2 diabetes.[112]

◆**CLINICAL MANIFESTATIONS.** Clinical manifestations of type 2 DM are nonspecific. The affected individual often is overweight, dyslipidemic, hyperinsulinemic, and hypertensive. Classic symptoms of polyuria and polydipsia may present, but more often individuals will have nonspecific symptoms such as fatigue, pruritus, recurrent infections, visual changes, or symptoms of neuropathy (paresthesias or weakness) (Table 22.8). In those whose diabetes has progressed without treatment, symptoms related to coronary artery, peripheral artery, and cerebrovascular disease may develop.

◆**EVALUATION AND TREATMENT.** The diagnostic criteria for type 2 DM are the same as those for type 1. The diagnostic criteria for prediabetes also have been defined (see Box 22.2). Prevention of type 2 DM,

especially in those individuals with prediabetes, hinges on diet and exercise although there is increasing support for the use of some diabetes medications in high-risk individuals.[113]

As with type 1 DM, the goal of treatment for individuals with type 2 DM is the restoration of near-euglycemia (a normal blood glucose level) and correction of related metabolic disorders. Weight loss results in improved insulin sensitivity and glucose tolerance, preserves beta-cell function, and has an inhibitory effect on progression to type 2 DM. Diet should match activity levels and include more complex carbohydrates (rather than simple sugars), foods low in fats, adequate protein, and fiber. Bariatric surgery may be indicated for individuals with morbid obesity who are unresponsive to diet and exercise interventions, although long-term studies are needed to evaluate sustained effectiveness[114] (see *What's New?* Metabolic Surgery for the Treatment of Type 2 Diabetes).

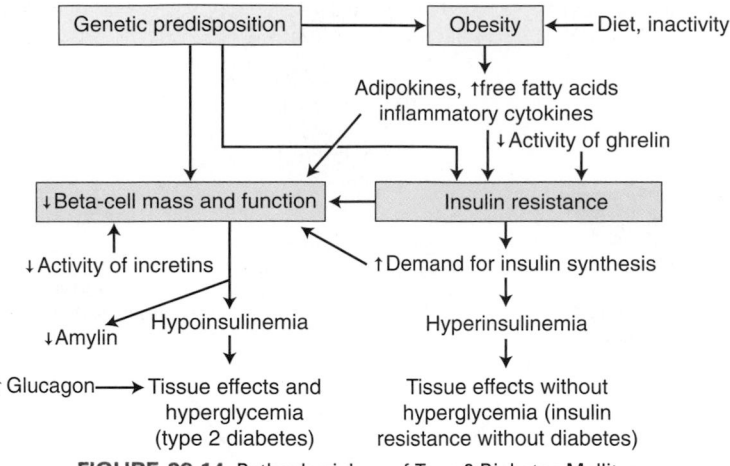

FIGURE 22.14 Pathophysiology of Type 2 Diabetes Mellitus.

TABLE 22.8	CLINICAL MANIFESTATIONS AND RATIONALE FOR TYPE 2 DIABETES MELLITUS*
MANIFESTATION	**RATIONALE**
Recurrent infections (e.g., boils and carbuncles; skin infections) and prolonged wound healing	Growth of microorganisms is stimulated by increased glucose levels; impaired blood supply hinders healing; decline in immune protection
Genital pruritus	Hyperglycemia and glycosuria favor fungal growth; candidal infections, resulting in pruritus, are a common presenting symptom in women
Visual changes	Blurred vision occurs as water balance in the eye fluctuates because of elevated blood glucose levels; diabetic retinopathy is another cause of visual loss
Paresthesias	Paresthesias are common manifestations of diabetic neuropathies
Fatigue	Metabolic changes result in poor use of food products, contributing to lethargy and fatigue
Acanthosis nigricans	Brown to black pigmentation in body folds associated with insulin resistance

*Type 2 diabetes mellitus also can have symptoms of polyuria, polydipsia, polyphagia, and weight loss as in type 1 diabetes mellitus.

Exercise reduces postprandial blood glucose levels, diminishes insulin requirements, lowers triglyceride and cholesterol levels, and increases the level of high-density lipoprotein (HDL) cholesterol.[115] Hypoglycemia may result, however, when the exercising individual receives sulfonylurea or insulin therapy. Exercise also can be associated with a decreasing response of counter-regulatory hormones to hypoglycemia.[116]

For individuals who require further intervention, oral hypoglycemic agents are indicated. Currently, there are nine classes of oral agents available (Table 22.9). Metformin is considered the primary pharmacologic choice for the treatment of type 2 DM and a second oral agent, a GLP-1 receptor agonist, or basal insulin is added if the HbA$_{1c}$ target is not maintained over 3 months.[117] A combination of drugs may be required. Insulin therapy may be needed in the later stage of type 2

WHAT'S NEW?

Metabolic Surgery for the Treatment of Type 2 Diabetes

After over 20 years of study, international recommendations were issued in 2016 for the use of metabolic surgery for the treatment of type 2 diabetes. These recommendations state that surgery is indicated in those with either class III obesity (BMI ≥40 kg/m²) or class II obesity (BMI 35.0–39.9 kg/m²) when hyperglycemia is inadequately controlled by lifestyle and optimal medical therapy. Surgery can be considered for persons with diabetes who have a BMI of 30.0–34.9 kg/m² if hyperglycemia is inadequately controlled despite optimal treatment with either oral or injectable medications. Postoperatively, caloric restriction along with anatomic rearrangement of the intestinal tract and rapid gastric emptying initiate a series of complex changes in gut hormone physiology, neural inputs, and alterations in the gut microbiome. Changes have been documented in bile acid metabolism and GI tract nutrient sensing and absorption. Peptides associated with these changes include peptide YY, GIP, GLP-1 and -2, FGF-19, and oxyntomodulin. Systemic changes following surgery include decreased hepatic glucose production, enhanced insulin sensitivity, and improved beta-cell function. Long disease duration, insulin use, and low C-peptide levels are associated with higher rates of diabetes nonremission following surgery.

Data from Argyropoulos G: *Curr Diab Rep* 15(4):15, 2015; Batterham R, Cummings D: *Diabetes Care* 39(6):893–901, 2016; Corcelles R, Daigle CR, Schauer PR: *Eur J Endocrinol* 174(1):R19–R28, 2016; de Heide LJ, de Vries F, Lalmohamed A: *JAMA Surgery* 150(12):1126–1133, 2015; Esposito K et al: *Endocrine* 48(2):417–421, 2015; Holst J et al: *Diabetes Care* 39(6):884–892, 2016; Malkani S: *Curr Opinion Endocrinol Diabetes Obes* 22(2):98–105, 2015; Rubino F et al: *Diabetes Care* 39(6):861–877, 2016; Yska JP et al: *JAMA Surgery* 150(10):940, 2015.

DM because of the loss of beta-cell function, which is progressive over time. Renal reabsorption of glucose through the sodium-glucose cotransporter 2 (SGLT2) is an important controller of serum glucose levels, and new medications aimed at blocking it have resulted in decreased measurements of blood glucose level, weight, blood pressure, and uric acid level. However, there is increased risk for ketoacidosis and the safety profile continues to be evaluated[118] (see *What's New?* Selective Sodium-Glucose Cotransporter 2 [SGLT2] Inhibitors for Type 2 Diabetes Mellitus Therapy). There are standards of care to guide the management of type 2 DM.[119]

TABLE 22.9 TYPES OF ORAL HYPOGLYCEMIC DRUGS

DRUG TYPE	MECHANISMS OF METABOLIC CONTROL
α-Glycosidase inhibitor (miglitol and voglibose)	Delays carbohydrate absorption in gut by inhibiting disaccharidases
Biguanide (metformin)	Decreases hepatic glucose production and increases insulin sensitivity and peripheral glucose uptake
Meglitinides (glinides; repaglinide and nateglinide)	Stimulate insulin release from pancreatic beta cells
Sulfonylureas (glyburide, glipizide, gliclazide, glimepiride)	Stimulate insulin release from pancreatic beta cells
Peroxisome proliferator–activated receptor-gamma agonists (thiazolidinediones, pioglitazone, and rosiglitazone)	Increase insulin sensitivity, particularly in adipose tissue
Bile acid sequestrant (colesevelam)	Unknown; theories include decreased hepatic glucose production, increased insulin secretion, and increased incretin release
GLP-1 receptor agonists (exenatide and liraglutide)	Increase insulin secretion, decrease glucagon secretion, decrease rate of gastric emptying, decrease appetite, weight loss
DPP-IV inhibitors (sitagliptin, saxagliptin, vildagliptin, and linagliptin)	Increase insulin secretion, decrease glucagon secretion, decrease rate of gastric emptying, decrease appetite
Amylin mimetics (pramlintide)	Decrease glucagon secretion, decrease rate of gastric emptying, and decrease appetite
SGLT2 inhibitor (sodium-glucose cotransporter 2); In clinical trials: canagliflozin, dapagliflozin, empagliflozin	Inhibits proximal tubular renal transport of glucose, decreasing glucose reabsorption and increasing renal excretion of glucose independent of insulin
Bromocriptine mesylate	Increases CNS dopamine, reducing sympathetic nervous activity, hepatic glucose production, and lipolysis

CNS, Central nervous system; *DPP-IV,* dipeptidyl peptidase-IV; *GLP-1,* glucagon-like peptide-1; *SGLT2,* sodium-glucose cotransporter 2.
Data from Brietzke SA: *Med Clin North Am* 99(1):87–106, 2015; Tran L et al: *Ann Pharmacother* 49(5):540–556, 2015.

WHAT'S NEW?

Selective Sodium-Glucose Cotransporter 2 (SGLT2) Inhibitors for Type 2 Diabetes Mellitus Therapy

Under normal conditions, the kidneys act to filter, reabsorb, and return to the circulation almost all of the glucose in the blood. Filtered glucose is actively reabsorbed by specific transporters located on the apical membrane of proximal tubular cells. These transporters are termed sodium-glucose cotransporters 1 and 2 (SGLT1 and -2). Approximately 90% of glucose is reabsorbed in the proximal renal tubule by SGLT2. The remaining 10% is reabsorbed lower in the tubule by SGLT1. Glucose reabsorption by SGLT2 continues even when plasma glucose levels are abnormally elevated, and glucose begins to be excreted in the urine only once the renal threshold is exceeded (at about 180 to 200 mg/dL). Inhibition of SGLT2 prevents renal reabsorption of glucose and facilitates its excretion in the urine. With an increase in glucose excretion, individuals with type 2 diabetes experience weight loss and serum glucose levels fall independently of insulin levels or beta-cell function. SGLT2 inhibitors currently approved for use in the United States for type 2 diabetes include canagliflozin, empagliflozin, and dapagliflozin, either as monotherapy or as adjunctive therapy. Reduced drug effectiveness occurs in older individuals as well as individuals with impaired renal function, since the mode of action depends upon normal renal glomerular-tubular function. FDA warnings have been issued regarding adverse effects including ketoacidosis, serious urinary tract infections, increased rates of toe amputation, and increased risk of lowered bone density and fractures.

Data from Cefalu WT, Riddle MC: *Diabetes Care* 38(3):352–354, 2015; FDA: Available at: http://www.fda.gov/Drugs/DrugSafety/PostmarketDrugSafetyInformationforPatientsandProviders/ucm446852.htm, 2016; Fioretto P, Giaccari A, Sesti G: *Cardiovasc Diabetol* 14:142, 2015; Hattersley AT, Thorens B: *N Eng J Med* 373(10):974–976, 2015; Kasichayanula S et al: *Clin Pharmacokinet* 53(1):17–27, 2014; Kasichayanula S et al: *Clin Pharmacokinet* 53(1):17–27, 2014; Kuecker C, Vivian E: *Diabetes Metab Syndr Obes* 9:25–35, 2016; Mikhail N: *South Med J* 108(2):91–96, 2015; Mudaliar S et al: *Diabetes Care* 38(12):2344–2353, 2015; Solini A: *Acta Diabetol* 53(6):863-870, 2016; Vallon V: *Annu Rev Med* 66:255–270, 2015; Whalen K, Miller S, Onge ES: *Clin Ther* 37(6):1150–1166, 2015; Wu JH et al: *Lancet Diabetes Endocrinol* 4(5):411–419, 2016.

Other Specific Types of Diabetes Mellitus and Gestational Diabetes Mellitus

As listed in Table 22.5, the American Diabetes Association (ADA) classification of DM mellitus encompasses not only the most common forms of diabetes (type 1 and type 2) but also "other specific types of DM" and "gestational DM." Other specific types of diabetes include genetic defects in beta-cell function, genetic defects in insulin action, diseases of the exocrine pancreas (i.e., cystic fibrosis), endocrinopathies, drug- or chemical-induced beta-cell dysfunction, infections, and other uncommon autoimmune and inherited disorders that are associated with diabetes. The best-described of these other specific types of diabetes is termed maturity-onset diabetes of youth (MODY).[120] MODY classically presents as non–insulin-requiring diabetes in lean individuals typically younger than 25 with evidence of autosomal dominant inheritance.

MODY is a monogenic form of diabetes and accounts for 1% to 2% of diabetes and should be considered in children who lack beta-cell antibodies. It also may account for up to 5% of individuals diagnosed with gestational diabetes.[121] MODY includes six specific autosomal dominant mutations, including genes for hepatocyte nuclear factor-1α/4a (HNF-1α/4a; *MODY 3* and *MODY 1*), glucokinase (*MODY 2*), and less commonly insulin promoter factor-1 (IPF-1; *MODY 4*), HNF-1β (*MODY 5*), and NeuroD1 (*MODY 6*) important for the development or function of beta cells.[122] The clinical diagnosis of MODY is based on the following criteria: family history of diabetes with an autosomal dominant mode of inheritance, insulin independence (nonketotic diabetes mellitus), and age at onset younger than 25 years. Genetic testing confirms the diagnosis. Management is similar to those techniques used for type 2 DM.

Gestational diabetes mellitus (GDM) has been defined as any degree of glucose intolerance with onset or first recognition during pregnancy. However, this definition meant that many women with previously undiagnosed type 1 or type 2 DM were diagnosed with GDM, and many of them had progressive disease after diagnosis. Therefore the American Diabetes Association (ADA) recommends that high-risk women found to have diabetes at their initial prenatal visit receive a diagnosis of type 1 or type 2 DM (FPG level >126 mg/dL [7.0 mmol/L] or a casual plasma glucose >200 mg/dL [11.1 mmol/L]) and not GDM.[123]

GDM complicates approximately 7% of all pregnancies. The exact mechanism of GDM is unknown, but insulin resistance and inadequate insulin secretion are contributing factors both before and during pregnancy. Insulin sensitivity declines with advancing gestation in normal pregnancy, but euglycemia is maintained by increased insulin secretion.[124] The ADA recommends that pregnant women with risk factors be screened for type 2 DM at their first prenatal visit. Those without a history of DM also should be screened with an oral glucose tolerance test at 24 to 28 weeks' gestation. Often there are no symptoms and careful glucose level control prenatally, during pregnancy, and after delivery is essential. Women who had a pregnancy affected by GDM and normal results on postpartum screening should be screened at 6 to 12 weeks after delivery with repeat testing every 1 to 3 years depending on risk factors.[123] GDM results in increased risk for type 2 DM and long-term metabolic and cardiovascular complications later in life for both mother and baby.[124]

Acute Complications of Diabetes Mellitus

The major acute complications of DM are hypoglycemia, diabetic ketoacidosis, and hyperosmolar hyperglycemic nonketotic syndrome. Table 22.10 contains a comparison of complications of DM. Morning hyperglycemia in diabetic subjects may be caused by the Somogyi effect, the dawn phenomenon, or poor glycemic control. The Somogyi effect

TABLE 22.10 COMMON ACUTE COMPLICATIONS OF DIABETES MELLITUS (DM)

HYPOGLYCEMIA IN PERSONS WITH DM	DIABETIC KETOACIDOSIS	HYPERGLYCEMIC NONKETOTIC SYNDROMES
Synonyms		
Insulin shock, insulin reaction	Diabetic coma syndrome	Hyperosmolar hyperglycemia nonketotic coma
Persons at Risk		
Individuals taking insulin	Individuals with type 1 diabetes	Older adults or very young individuals with
Individuals with rapidly fluctuating blood glucose levels	Individuals with nondiagnosed diabetes	type 2 diabetes, nondiabetic individuals with predisposing factors, such as pancreatitis;
Individuals with type 2 diabetes taking sulfonylurea agents		individuals with undiagnosed diabetes
Predisposing Factors		
Excessive insulin or sulfonylurea agent intake, lack of sufficient food intake, excessive physical exercise, abrupt decline in insulin needs (e.g., renal failure, immediately postpartum), simultaneous use of insulin-potentiating agents or beta-blocking agents that mask symptoms	Stressful situation such as infection, accident, trauma, emotional stress; omission of insulin; medications that antagonize insulin	Infection, medications that antagonize insulin, comorbid condition
Typical Onset		
Rapid	Slow	Slowest
Presenting Symptoms		
Adrenergic reaction: pallor, sweating, tachycardia, palpitations, hunger, restlessness, anxiety, tremors. Neurogenic reaction: fatigue, irritability, headache, loss of concentration, visual disturbances, dizziness, hunger, confusion, transient sensory or motor defects, convulsions, coma, death	Malaise, dry mouth, headache, polyuria, polydipsia, weight loss, nausea, vomiting, pruritus, abdominal pain, lethargy, shortness of breath, Kussmaul respirations, fruity or acetone odor to breath	Polyuria, polydipsia, hypovolemia, dehydration (parched lips, poor skin turgor), hypotension, tachycardia, hypoperfusion, weight loss, weakness, nausea, vomiting, abdominal pain, hypothermia, stupor, coma, seizures
Laboratory Analysis		
Serum glucose <30 mg/dL in newborn (first 2–3 days) and <55–60 mg/dL in adults	Glucose levels >250 mg/dL, reduction in bicarbonate concentration; increased anion gap; increased plasma levels of β-hydroxybutyrate, acetoacetate, and acetone	Glucose levels >600 mg/dL, lack of ketosis, serum osmolarity >320 mOsm/L, elevated blood urea nitrogen and creatinine

is the occurrence of hypoglycemia at about 3:00 AM caused by too much intermediate-acting insulin (i.e., NPH insulin) given at dinner time followed by rebound hyperglycemia caused by normal early morning secretion of counter-regulatory hormones (epinephrine, GH, corticosteroids), which are stimulated by hypoglycemia and cause gluconeogenesis. Excessive carbohydrate intake may contribute to the rebound hyperglycemia. The treatment is to decrease evening insulin level. The Somogyi effect is becoming much less common because of the increasing use of long-acting bioengineered insulins. The **dawn phenomenon** is an early morning rise in blood glucose concentration caused by nocturnal elevations of GH, which decreases metabolism of glucose by muscle and fat. Increasing the dose of evening insulin manages the problem.

Hypoglycemia

Hypoglycemia occurs when blood glucose levels are less than 47 mg/dL in newborns for the first 48 hours of life (clinical signs should also be considered)[125] and less than 70 mg/dL in children and adults. Its causes may be exogenous (medications, alcohol, or exercise), endogenous (tumors of the pancreas or inherited disorders), or functional (hyperalimentation, spontaneous, or liver disease). Hypoglycemia in diabetes is sometimes called *insulin shock* or *insulin reaction.* Individuals with type 2 diabetes are at less risk for hypoglycemia than those with type 1 diabetes because they retain relatively intact glucose counter-regulatory mechanisms. However, hypoglycemia does occur in type 2 DM when treatment involves SGLT2 inhibitors, GLP-1 receptor agonists, sulfonylureas, thiazolidinediones, and exogenous insulin, particularly when used in combination (see Table 22.9).

Symptoms of hypoglycemia result either from activation of the sympathetic nervous system (neurogenic adrenergic symptoms) or from an abrupt cessation of glucose delivery to the brain (neuroglycopenic symptoms), or both.[126,127] Neurogenic reactions occur when the decrease in blood glucose level is rapid and presents with tachycardia, palpitations, diaphoresis, tremors, pallor, and arousal anxiety. Other symptoms include headache, dizziness, blurred vision, irritability, fatigue, poor judgment, confusion, hunger, seizures, and coma. Hypoglycemia unawareness is

a phenomenon that occurs in individuals without appropriate autonomic warning symptoms, and recovery from hypoglycemia may be delayed because of impaired glycogenolysis and hampered delivery of gluconeogenic substrates to the liver.

Treatment requires immediate replacement of glucose either orally or intravenously. Glucagon for home use can be prescribed for individuals who are at high risk.[128] Prevention is achieved with individualized management of medications and diet, monitoring of blood glucose levels, and education.

Diabetic Ketoacidosis

Diabetic ketoacidosis (DKA) is a serious complication related to a deficiency of insulin and an increase in the levels of insulin counter-regulatory hormones (catecholamines, cortisol, glucagon, growth hormone). DKA occurs in approximately 30% of children with type 1 DM and 5% of children with type 2 DM.[129] DKA is most common in individuals with type 1 DM because insulin is more deficient. It rarely occurs in those with type 2 DM (called *ketosis-prone type 2 diabetes [KPD]*) and occurs most frequently in obese non-Hispanic blacks.[130] The most common precipitating factor for DKA is intercurrent illness, such as infection, trauma, surgery, or myocardial infarction. Poor adherence to insulin treatment or interruption of insulin administration also may result in DKA. Factors associated with increased risk are type 1 DM, poor glycemic control, younger or older age, diagnostic error, ethnic minority, lack of health insurance in the United States, lower body mass index, preceding infection, and delayed treatment.[131]

PATHOPHYSIOLOGY. The most important pathophysiologic mechanisms for DKA are insulin deficiency and an increase in counter-regulatory hormones, including catecholamines, cortisol, glucagon, and GH. The counter-regulatory hormones normally antagonize insulin by increasing glucose production and decreasing tissue use of glucose. Profound insulin deficiency results in decreased glucose uptake, increased fat mobilization with release of fatty acids, and accelerated gluconeogenesis, glycogenesis, and ketogenesis[132] (Fig. 22.15). In the absence of insulin, the release of free fatty acids from adipocytes increases production of ketone bodies (acetoacetate, hydroxybutyrate, and acetone) by the

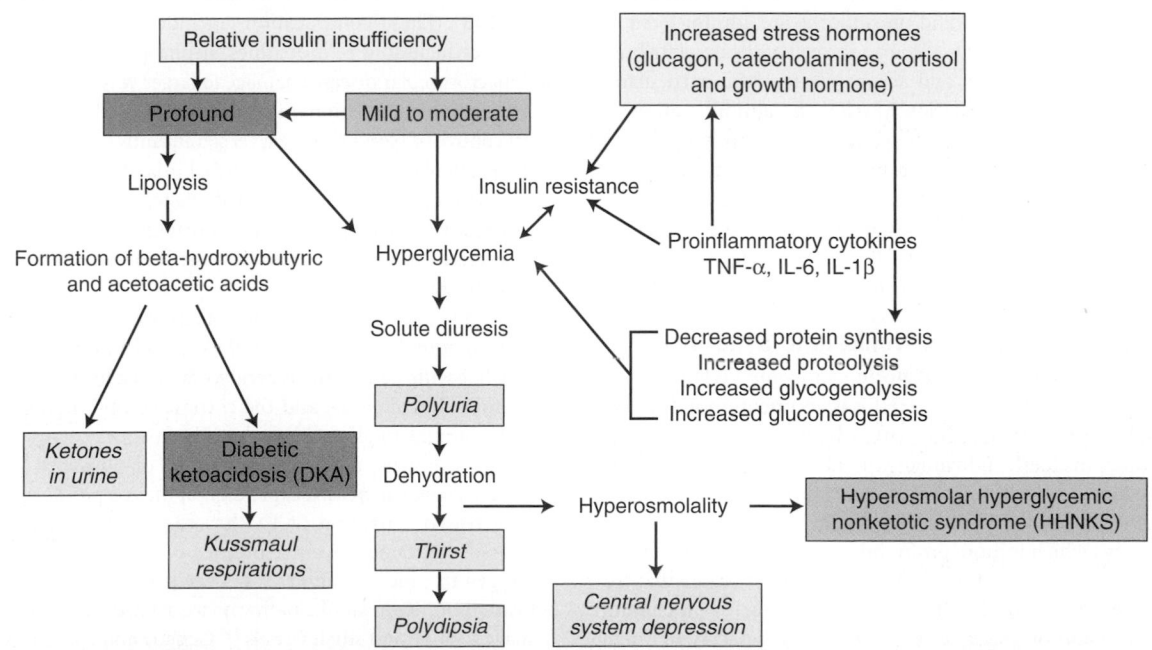

FIGURE 22.15 Pathophysiology of DKA and HHNKS in Diabetes Mellitus. See text for details. *DKA,* Diabetic keto-acidosis; *HHNKS,* hyperosmolar hyperglycemic non-ketotic syndrome; *IL-6,* interleukin-6; *IL-1β,* interleukin-1β; *TNF-α,* tumor necrosis factor-a.

mitochondria of the liver at a rate that exceeds peripheral use. Accumulation of ketone bodies causes a drop in pH and triggers the buffering system associated with metabolic acidosis. DKA caused by increased levels of circulating ketones in the absence of the antilipolytic effect of insulin occurs. Relatively increased glucagon levels also contribute to activation of the gluconeogenic (glucose-forming) and ketogenic (ketone-forming) pathways in the liver. Ordinarily ketones are used by tissues as an energy source to regenerate bicarbonate. This balances the loss of bicarbonate, which occurs when the ketone is formed. Hyperketonemia (increased blood ketone levels) may result from impaired use of ketones by peripheral tissue, which permits strong organic acids to circulate freely. Bicarbonate buffering then does not occur, and the individual develops a metabolic acidosis.

◆**CLINICAL MANIFESTATIONS.** The signs and symptoms of DKA include Kussmaul respirations (hyperventilation in an attempt to compensate for the acidosis), postural dizziness, central nervous system depression, ketonuria, anorexia, nausea, vomiting, abdominal pain, an acetone odor on the breath, dehydration, thirst, and polyuria (see Table 22.10). Polyuria and dehydration result from the osmotic diuresis associated with hyperglycemia. In this case, the plasma glucose level is higher than the individual's renal threshold, allowing significant amounts of glucose to be lost in the urine. Deficits of sodium, phosphorus, and magnesium are common. The most important electrolyte disturbance is a marked deficiency in the level of total body potassium. Although the serum potassium concentration may appear normal or elevated because of volume contraction and a shift of potassium out of the cell and into the blood caused by metabolic acidosis, the total body deficiency of potassium may reach 3 to 5 mEq/kg.

◆**EVALUATION AND TREATMENT.** The diagnosis of DKA is suggested when individuals have symptoms described earlier. The American Diabetes Association criteria for the diagnosis of DKA are (1) a serum glucose level >250 mg/dL, (2) a serum bicarbonate level <18, (3) a serum pH <7.30, (4) the presence of an anion gap, and (5) the presence of urine and serum ketones.[133]

Treatment of DKA involves administration of insulin to decrease glucose levels. Fluids are administered to replace lost fluid volume. Electrolyte deficits become apparent as fluid volume is replaced, and intravenous sodium, potassium, and phosphorus are administered as needed. Potassium moves with insulin into the cell and can contribute to hypokalemia. Volume status and serum electrolytes, particularly potassium, should be monitored closely. After the administration of insulin, the concentration of β-hydroxybutyrate promptly begins to decrease and, after a slight increase, acetoacetate concentration also begins to decrease. A persistent ketonuria may be observed for several days after treatment. Continuous monitoring of the individual is essential to ensure an uncomplicated recovery from DKA. Health teaching emphasizes predisposing factors and strategies for avoiding DKA.

Hyperosmolar Hyperglycemic Nonketotic Syndrome

Hyperosmolar hyperglycemic nonketotic syndrome (HHNKS), or hyperglycemic hyperosmolar state (HHS), is an uncommon but significant complication of type 2 DM with a high overall mortality. It occurs more often in elderly individuals who have other comorbidities, including infections or cardiovascular or renal disease.

◆**PATHOPHYSIOLOGY.** HHNKS differs from DKA in the degree of insulin deficiency (which is more profound in DKA) and the elevation of glucose levels and degree of fluid deficiency (which are more marked in HHNKS) (see Fig. 22.15). HHNKS has synergistic factors, including insulin deficiency and increased levels of counter-regulatory or stress hormones (glucagon, catecholamines, cortisol, and growth hormone), with increased gluconeogenesis and glycogenolysis and inadequate use of glucose by peripheral tissues, primarily muscle, characterized by a

lack of ketosis. Proinflammatory mediators (TNF-α, IL-6, IL-1β) also promote insulin resistance and release of counter-regulatory hormones contributing to insulin resistance and hyperglycemia. Because the amount of insulin required to inhibit fat breakdown is less than that needed for effective glucose transport, insulin levels are sufficient to prevent excessive lipolysis but not to use glucose properly.[134]

◆**CLINICAL MANIFESTATIONS.** Glycosuria and polyuria in HHNKS result from the extreme serum glucose level elevation. As much as 19 g of glucose per hour may be lost in diuresis, which causes severe volume depletion, increased serum osmolarity, intracellular dehydration, and loss of electrolytes including potassium. Neurologic changes, such as stupor, correlate with the degree of hyperosmolarity and are common in HHNKS; thus this syndrome is sometimes called *hyperosmolar hyperglycemic coma.*

◆**EVALUATION AND TREATMENT.** The diagnostic features of HHNKS include a very high serum glucose concentration (often more than 600 mg/dL), a near-normal serum bicarbonate level and pH, a serum osmolarity that is usually greater than 320 mOsm/L, and either absent or low levels of ketones in the urine and in the serum (lack of ketoacidosis). DKA and HHNKS show considerable overlap in symptoms and treatment. Insulin infusion should be combined with fluid repletion over 24 hours. An important distinction, however, is that the dehydration in HHNKS is far more severe than that in DKA. Thus fluid replacement, with both crystalloids and colloids, is more rapid. Potassium deficits may be extreme and require several days of treatment. Phosphorus and sodium also may be needed. HHNKS is a significant risk factor for infection, sepsis, and venous thrombosis. Mortality is between 10% and 20% and is related to the age of the individual and comorbid conditions, including the severity of the precipitating illness[134] (see Table 22.10 for a comparison of the three acute complications described thus far).

Chronic Complications of Diabetes Mellitus

A number of serious complications are associated with any type of poorly controlled DM. Insulin resistance or deficit, chronic hyperglycemia (also known as *glucose toxicity*), accumulation of advanced glycation end products and activation of metabolic pathways that cause tissue damage result in the chronic complications of diabetes mellitus (see Fig. 22.13). These complications include microvascular (damage to capillaries including retinopathies, nephropathies, and neuropathies) and macrovascular disease (damage to larger vessels, including coronary artery disease, and peripheral vascular and cerebral vascular disease). Strict control of blood glucose level significantly reduces some complications, particularly nonfatal myocardial infarction. Strict control is not recommended for high-risk individuals with type 2 DM because it is associated with increased all-cause mortality, cardiovascular mortality, and severe hypoglycemia. However, the individual risk/benefit profile should be considered.[135]

Oxidative stress (overproduction of reactive oxygen species), activation of several complex metabolic pathways and inflammation have been associated with persistent hyperglycemia, insulin resistance, hyperinsulinemia, dyslipidemia, and the chronic complications of DM. They include shunting of glucose into the polyol pathway, activation of protein kinase C isoforms, increased formation of advanced glycation end products (AGEs), increased expression of the receptor for AGEs (RAGE), and increased activation of the hexosamine pathway.[136] It has been proposed that hyperglycemia induces mitochondrial overproduction of oxygen free radicals and this is a key pathologic mechanism for the activation of the metabolic pathways associated with atherogenesis and damage to large and small vessels.[136] Genetic and epigenetic factors also contribute to complications of DM.[137]

Tissues that do not require insulin for glucose transport, such as the kidney, red blood cells (RBCs), blood vessels, eye lens, and nerves, cannot down-regulate the cellular uptake of glucose. Consequently, with hyperglycemia, intracellular glucose is shunted into an alternate metabolic pathway for glucose metabolism known as the polyol pathway. Overactivation of the polyol pathway results in two processes that may contribute to the complications of diabetes. One is the excessive accumulation of sorbitol (a polyol-sugar alcohol) through the action of the enzyme aldose reductase. The accumulated sorbitol increases intracellular osmotic pressure and attracts water in tissue. Swelling occurs along with visual changes and predisposition to cataracts in the lens of the eye. Sorbitol interferes with ion pumps in the nerves, damages Schwann cells, and disrupts nerve conduction. RBCs become swollen and stiff and interfere with perfusion. Second, activation of the polyol pathway reduces glutathione, an important antioxidant, contributing to oxidative injury in cells and tissues, particularly blood vessels. Aldose reductase inhibitors are being evaluated for treatment of these complications.[138]

Protein kinase C (PKC) is a family of intracellular signaling proteins that can become inappropriately activated in different tissues by hyperglycemia. Intracellular hyperglycemia increases the second-messenger diacylglycerol (DAG)–PKC pathway, which in turn activates protein kinase C. Various consequences have been observed, including insulin resistance, extracellular matrix and cytokine production, vascular cell proliferation, enhanced contractility, angiogenesis, and increased permeability. These effects may contribute to the microvascular complications of diabetes.[139]

Glycation is a normal nonenzymatic process that involves the reversible attachment of glucose to proteins, lipids, and nucleic acids. With recurrent or persistent hyperglycemia, glucose becomes irreversibly bound to collagen and other proteins in red blood cells (e.g., glycated hemoglobin [HbA$_{1c}$] is used as a biomarker for diabetes), blood vessel walls, interstitial tissue, and within cells. The products of this binding are known as advanced glycation end products (AGEs), and their receptor (RAGE). A number of properties may cause tissue injury or pathologic conditions associated with diabetes, such as:

1. Cross-linking and trapping of proteins, including albumin, low-density lipoprotein (LDL), immunoglobulin, and complement, with thickening of the basement membrane or increased permeability in small blood vessels and nerves
2. Binding to cell receptors, such as macrophages and glomerular mesangial cells, inducing release of inflammatory cytokines and growth factors that stimulate cellular proliferation in the glomeruli, smooth muscle of blood vessels, and collagen synthesis with fibrosis
3. Induction of lipid oxidation, oxidative stress, and inflammation
4. Inactivation of nitric oxide with loss of vasodilation and diminished endothelial function
5. Procoagulant changes on endothelial cells with promotion of platelet adhesion and reduced fibrinolysis, and/or
6. Promotion of beta-cell apoptosis and insulin resistance
Pharmacologic agents that inhibit AGE formation or block their receptor (RAGE) are used to treat type 2 DM.[140,141]

Chronic intracellular hyperglycemia causes shunting of excess intracellular glucose into the hexosamine pathway and leads to O-linked glycosylation (an enzymatic process) of several proteins with alteration in signal transduction pathways and oxidative stress. The O-linked attachment of N-acetylglucosamine (O-GlcNAc) on serine and threonine residues of nuclear and cytoplasmic proteins is associated with insulin resistance, oxidative stress, and vascular complications of DM.[142]

Microvascular Disease

Diabetic microvascular complications (disease in capillaries) are a leading cause of blindness, end-stage kidney failure, and various neuropathies. Characteristics of diabetic microangiopathy include occlusion of capillaries with thickening of the capillary basement membrane, endothelial cell hyperplasia, thrombosis, and pericyte degeneration. Hypoxia and ischemia accompany microvascular disease, especially in the eye, kidney, and nerves. The frequency and severity of lesions appear to be proportional to the duration of the disease (more than 10 years) and the status of glycemic control. Many individuals with type 2 DM present with microvascular complications because of the long duration of asymptomatic hyperglycemia that generally precedes diagnosis. This underscores the need to screen for diabetes.

Diabetic Retinopathy. Diabetic retinopathy is a leading cause of blindness worldwide. The retina is the most metabolically active structure per weight of tissue in the body. Thus the retina is a vulnerable target for neurovascular disease in DM.[143] In comparison to type 1 DM, retinopathy seems to develop more rapidly in individuals with type 2 DM because of the likelihood of long-standing hyperglycemia before diagnosis. Most individuals with diabetes will eventually develop retinopathy and they also are more likely to develop cataracts and glaucoma (see Chapter 16).

Diabetic retinopathy results from damage to retinal blood vessels and red blood cells (RBCs), platelet aggregation, relative hypoxemia and hypertension. Three stages of retinopathy lead to loss of vision: nonproliferative (stage I), characterized by thickening of the retinal capillary basement membrane and an increase in retinal capillary permeability, vein dilation, microaneurysm formation, and superficial (flame-shaped) and deep (blot) hemorrhages; preproliferative (stage II), a progression of retinal ischemia with areas of poor perfusion that culminate in infarcts; and proliferative (stage III), the result of neovascularization (angiogenesis) and fibrous tissue formation within the retina or optic disc (see Figs. 22.16 and 22.17, and Table 22.11 for details). Traction of the new vessels on the vitreous humor may cause retinal detachment or hemorrhage into the vitreous humor with severe blurring or loss of vision. Macular edema (fluid accumulation and retinal thickening near the center of the macula) is the leading cause of visual impairment (blurring) among persons with diabetes. Blurring of vision also can be a consequence of hyperglycemia and sorbitol accumulation in the lens. Dehydration of the lens, aqueous humor, and vitreous humor also reduces visual acuity.[144] In addition to the ocular vasculopathy associated with hyperglycemia, activation of inflammatory cells (i.e., retinal glial and immune cells) and release of inflammatory mediators contribute to chronic neuroinflammation with injury to retinal sensory cells and loss of vision (optic neuropathy).[145] Cataracts and defects in eye muscle function also are associated with the chronic complications of hyperglycemia and diabetes mellitus.

Diabetic Kidney Disease. Diabetic kidney disease is the most common cause of chronic kidney disease and end-stage kidney disease. Approximately 50% of individuals with DM develop diabetic kidney disease.[146] Hyperglycemia leads to activation of the polyol pathway, the hexosamine pathway, protein kinase C, and inflammation, and the production of advanced glycation end products (AGEs). All contribute to kidney tissue injury; yet the exact process responsible for destruction of kidneys in diabetes is not clear.

The glomeruli are injured by protein denaturation, hyperglycemia with high renal blood flow (hyperfiltration), activation of the renin-angiotensin system, and production of angiotensin II resulting in intraglomerular hypertension exacerbated by systemic hypertension. Renal glomerular changes can occur early in diabetes mellitus and occasionally may precede the overt manifestations of the disease (Fig. 22.18). Progressive changes include glomerular enlargement, glomerular basement membrane thickening with proliferation of mesangial cells, and proliferation of the mesangial matrix. Later in the disease, this results in diffuse and nodular glomerulosclerosis (Kimmelstiel-Wilson nodule), loss of podocytes, resistance to glomerular capillary blood

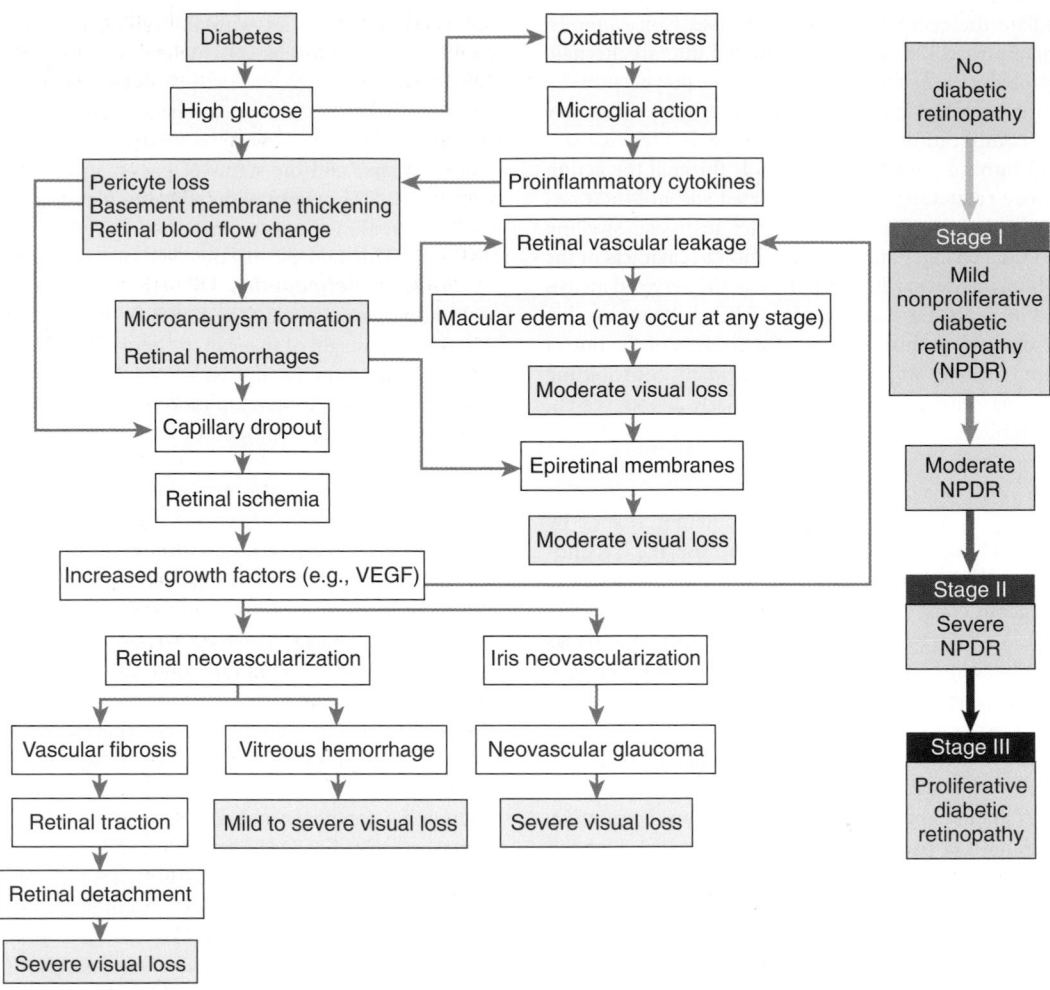

FIGURE 22.16 Pathophysiology of Diabetic Retinopathy. *VEGF,* Vascular endothelial growth factor. (Adapted from Mehlmed S et al: *Williams textbook of endocrinology,* ed 12, Philadelphia, 2012, Saunders.)

TABLE 22.11	FINDINGS IN DIABETIC RETINOPATHY
STAGES OF RETINOPATHY	**PATHOLOGIC FINDINGS**
Nonproliferative Retinopathy (Stage I)	
Venous abnormalities	Increased tortuosity, dilation with irregular constriction; frequency increases with increased severity of retinopathy
Microaneurysms	Mostly thin walled; 15–50 mcg in diameter; pathogenesis controversial
Interretinal hemorrhage	Circular and small; may take several months to resorb
Macular edema	Caused by serum leakage through incompetent vessel walls; may resorb in several weeks
Hard exudates	Characteristically "hard" exudates with pattern of exudation irregular in shape and sharply defined may appear and disappear over months to years; common with hypertension; "soft" exudates may appear and disappear more often; related to increased retinal capillary permeability
Preproliferative Diabetic Retinopathy (Stage II)	
Cotton-wool patches	Infarcts of the nerve fiber layer caused by retinal ischemia
Intraretinal microvascular shunts	Tortuous shunts between patent and occluded retinal vessels
Proliferative Diabetic Retinopathy (Stage III)	
Neovascularization	New vessels surrounded by connective tissue; five distinct groups representing different hazards to the eye
Glial proliferation	Often produced to reinforce neovascularization; may occur on optic disc and along vascular arcades
Vitreoretinal traction hemorrhage; retinal detachment	Traction occurring from the vitreous jelly; eventually causes small blood vessels to hemorrhage and retinal detachment to occur

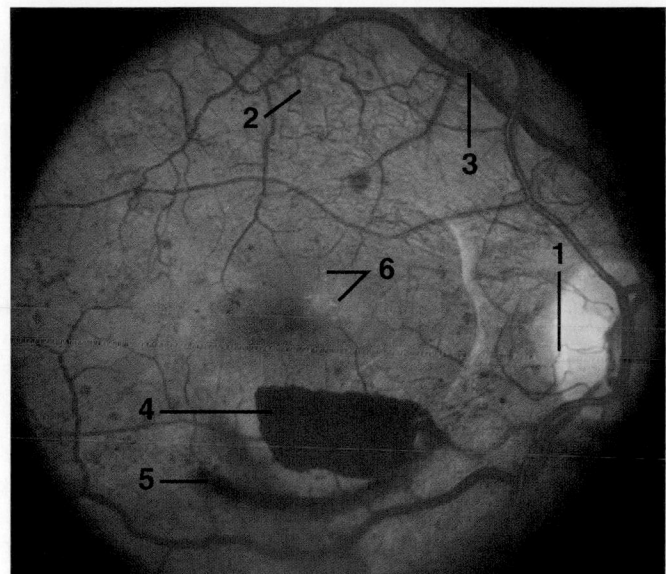

FIGURE 22.17 Proliferative Diabetic Retinopathy. Neovascularization is present at the optic nerve **(1)** and along the vascular arcades **(2)**. Retinal veins are engorged **(3)**, and a preretinal hemorrhage **(4)** is present inferior to the fovea. This boat-shaped hemorrhage blocks the view of the retinal vessels. A more diffuse hemorrhage **(5)** is present in an arcuate pattern just inferior to the preretinal hemorrhage that represents a mild vitreous hemorrhage. A few small, hard exudates are visible in the fovea **(6)**. (From Palay D, Krachmer J: *Ophthalmology*, ed 2, St Louis 2005, Mosby.)

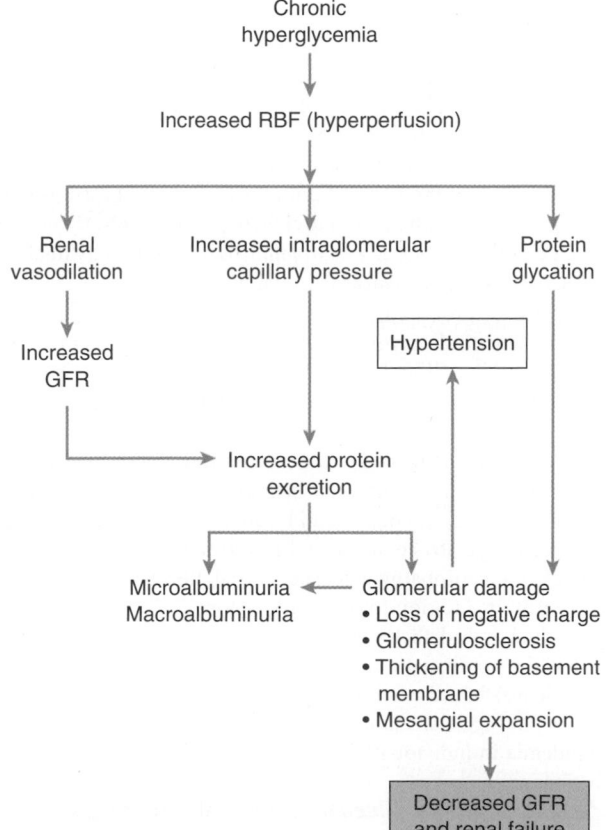

FIGURE 22.18 Diabetic Kidney Disease. *GFR*, Glomerular filtration rate; *RBF*, renal blood flow.

flow, and decreased glomerular filtration rates (GFRs). Alterations in glomerular membrane permeability occur with loss of negative charge and albuminuria. Tubular and interstitial fibrosis contributes to loss of function.[147] The proximal tubule is particularly vulnerable because of its aerobic metabolism and high energy requirements.[148]

Microalbuminuria (30 to 300 mg/day) is the first manifestation of diabetic kidney dysfunction and develops within 5 to 10 years of disease. Before proteinuria, no clinical signs or symptoms of progressive glomerulosclerosis are likely to be evident. Later, hypoproteinemia, reduction in plasma oncotic pressure, fluid overload, anasarca (generalized body edema), and hypertension may occur. As renal function continues to deteriorate, individuals with type 1 DM may experience hypoglycemia (because of loss of renal insulin metabolism), which necessitates a decrease in insulin therapy. As the glomerular filtration rate drops below 10 mL/minute, uremic signs, such as nausea, lethargy, acidosis, anemia, and uncontrolled hypertension, occur (see Chapter 39 for a discussion of renal failure). Glomerular filtration rate can decline independently of albuminuria, particularly in type 1 DM.[149] Macroalbuminuria (greater than 300 mg per day) is strongly correlated with morbidity and mortality from cardiovascular disease, particularly in type 2 DM. Early diagnosis and control of hypertension and hyperglycemia decrease the severity of nephropathy and delay the onset of end-stage kidney disease.[150]

The development of more sensitive tests has permitted the detection of microalbuminuria. Earlier intervention with tight glucose control and angiotensin-converting enzyme (ACE) inhibitors or angiotensin II receptor blockers can reduce proteinuria and slow the progression of nephropathy. Newer agents are being evaluated, including renin inhibitors or aldosterone blockers and antiinflammatory agents.[151] Aggressive treatment of hypertension is another therapeutic intervention definitively shown to decrease albuminuria of established renal disease, but it has not reduced progression to end-stage renal disease and the need for renal replacement therapy.[152]

Diabetic Neuropathies. Diabetic neuropathy is the most common cause of neuropathy in the Western world and is probably the most common complication of diabetes. Nerves do not require insulin for glucose transport and are particularly vulnerable to the pathologic effects of chronic hyperglycemia. Peripheral neuropathy affects up to 50% of individuals with diabetes and is more common in type 2 DM.[153] The American Diabetes Association has published a guideline to assist clinicians with the prevention, diagnosis, and management of diabetic neuropathy.[154]

The underlying pathologic mechanism includes both metabolic and vascular factors related to chronic hyperglycemia with inflammation, ischemia, oxidative stress, advanced glycation end products, and increased formation of polyols contributing to demyelination, nerve degeneration, and delayed conduction[155] (Fig. 22.19). The earliest morphologic change is axonal degeneration that preferentially involves sensory nerve fibers, particularly the smaller polymodal unmyelinated peripheral C fibers and the larger myelinated Aδ fibers. The metabolic activity of Schwann cells is disturbed, causing segmental loss of myelin and a characteristic pattern of demyelination and remyelination observed in long-term diabetic neuropathy. Nerve degeneration begins in the periphery, but the pathologic condition also can include the spinal cord and the posterior root ganglia. These changes may occur alone or in combination. Both somatic and peripheral nerve cells show diffuse or focal damage resulting in polyneuropathy. Sensory deficits generally precede motor involvement. The extremities are involved first in a "stocking and glove" pattern.

Distal symmetric polyneuropathy (sensory, autonomic, and motor nerve involvement) is the most common neuropathy with involvement of both large and small nerve fibers (Table 22.12). Loss of small nerve fiber function includes neuropathic pain and loss of sensation, and carries high risk for development of foot ulceration with subsequent

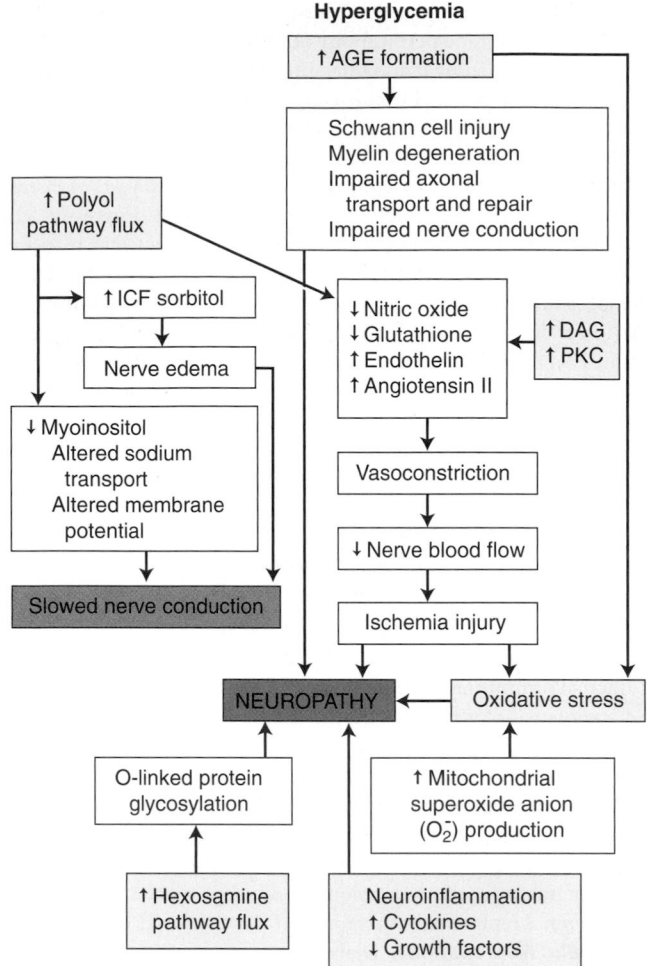

Hyperglycemia

FIGURE 22.19 Multifactorial Pathogenesis of Diabetic Neuropathy. The yellow boxes represent the consequences of chronic hyperglycemia in the development of neuropathy. *AGE,* Advanced glycation end product; *DAG,* diacylglycerol; *ICF,* intracellular fluid; *PKC,* protein kinase C.

gangrene and amputation. Large nerve fiber involvement results in sensory loss of proprioception and vibration with ataxia, loss of coordination, and risk for falls and fractures. Motor involvement is less common and occurs later in the disease with weakness and muscle atrophy, particularly in the lower legs and feet.[156]

Autonomic neuropathies can occur early, affecting gastrointestinal enteric nerves (nausea, bloating, gastroparesis, diarrhea, or constipation), bladder and sexual function (loss of bladder sensation, urine retention, recurrent infection, erectile dysfunction), sweating, and body temperature regulation. Cardiovascular autonomic neuropathy is a serious complication with heart rate variability, changes in baroreceptor reflexes, postural hypotension, dysrhythmias, exercise intolerance, painless myocardial infarction, and sudden death.[157]

Alterations in cognitive function and increased risk for dementia may accompany long-term complications in the brain, particularly in persons with type 2 diabetes. The specific neurodegenerative mechanisms are not clear.[158]

Charcot neuroarthropathy (Charcot joint) is the progressive degeneration and structural disorganization of a joint, particularly in the foot and ankle of individuals affected by long-term diabetes. The pathogenesis may be related to inflammation, loss of sensation, and neurally mediated vascular alterations with osteoclastic bone resorption.[159]

Macrovascular Disease

Diabetic macrovascular disease (lesions in large and medium-sized arteries) increases morbidity and mortality and increases risk for hypertension, accelerated atherosclerosis, cardiovascular disease, stroke, and peripheral vascular disease, particularly among individuals with type 2 DM. Children with poorly controlled diabetes, particularly type 2 DM, have high risk for macrovascular disease within one or two decades.[160] Unlike microangiopathy, atherosclerotic disease is unrelated to the severity of diabetes and is often present in those with insulin resistance and impaired glucose tolerance.[161] The premature atherosclerosis of diabetes has many contributing factors, including hyperinsulinemia (insulin resistance), hyperglycemia, hypertriglyceridemia, low levels of high-density lipoprotein (HDL), high levels of low-density lipoprotein (LDL), lipoprotein oxidation, and platelet abnormalities. Advanced glycosylated end products attach to their receptor (RAGE) in the walls of blood vessels, promoting oxidative stress, inflammation, endothelial and vascular smooth muscle dysfunction, and thrombosis (Fig. 22.20). The process tends to be more severe and accelerated with the presence of other risk factors, including hyperlipidemia, hypertension, and smoking.[162]

Cardiovascular Disease. Cardiovascular disease is the ultimate cause of death in up to 68% of people with diabetes, with higher risk for women.[163] Hypertension often coexists with DM, is more prevalent than in the nondiabetic population, and can have many causes. In type 1 DM, hypertension is associated with the development of microalbuminuria. In type 2 DM, hypertension is associated with metabolic syndrome (see Box 22.3). Hypertension increases the risk for coronary artery disease and stroke. Coronary artery disease (CAD) is the most common cause of morbidity and mortality in individuals with DM (heart disease is described in Chapter 33). In general, the prevalence of CAD increases with the duration but not the severity of diabetes and the onset can be silent. Myocardial infarction (death of heart muscle as a result of coronary artery occlusion) is the cause of death in up to 75% of those with diabetes. Individuals with diabetes mellitus have a higher mortality during the acute phase of myocardial infarctions than do nondiabetic individuals because they are often asymptomatic as a result of sensory and autonomic neuropathy.[164] Guidelines have been developed to reduce the risk and improve treatment of cardiovascular and coronary artery disease in individuals with diabetes.[165]

The incidence of *congestive heart failure* is higher in individuals with diabetes, even without myocardial infarction. This may be related to oxidative stress, proinflammatory factors that result in myocardial remodeling and cardiomyopathy with increased amounts of collagen in the ventricular wall, and ventricular hypertrophy. There is reduced mechanical compliance of the heart during filling with diastolic and, eventually, systolic failure.[166]

Stroke. Stroke is twice as common in those with diabetes (particularly type 2 DM) as in the nondiabetic population and more common in diabetic women.[167] Ischemic and lacunar stroke are more common than hemorrhagic stroke and may be related to autonomic nervous system (ANS) neuropathy-associated atrial fibrillation and platelet coagulopathy, in addition to other risk factors.[168] The survival rate for an individual with diabetes after a massive stroke is typically shorter than that for nondiabetic individuals. Hypertension, hyperglycemia, hyperlipidemia, thrombosis, and sleep apnea are risk factors (see Chapters 16 and 33), and aggressive management of blood pressure, hyperglycemia, and lipidemia in individuals with diabetes has been shown to reduce the incidence of stroke.[169]

Peripheral Artery Disease. Peripheral vascular disease is an atherosclerotic occlusive disease of the lower extremity. DM increases the incidence of peripheral artery disease (PAD) with claudication (pain from reduced blood flow during exercise), ulcers, gangrene, and

TABLE 22.12   CLASSIFICATION OF DIABETIC NEUROPATHIES

TYPE OF NEUROPATHY	CHARACTERISTICS
Hyperglycemic neuropathy	Hyperesthesia, tingling and pain associated with hyperglycemia that resolves with glycemic control
Distal symmetric polyneuropathy (sensorimotor neuropathy)	Symmetric loss of large and small myelinated and unmyelinated nerve fibers Longest nerves affected first with numbness, tingling, and pain (sharp, burning, aching) in toes and feet and then ascending to hands (stocking and glove pattern); loss of vibration and proprioception (large nerve fiber); loss of sensory light touch and temperature and pain (small nerve fiber) Motor nerves affected later with weakness, depressed reflexes, and gait disturbances
Autonomic neuropathy	Cardiovascular: postural hypotension; exercise intolerance; silent myocardial infarction Gastrointestinal: decreased esophageal motility, gastroparesis and delayed gastric emptying, diabetic constipation or diarrhea Genitourinary tract: neurogenic bladder, urine retention, erectile dysfunction and retrograde ejaculation in men Sudomotor: anhidrosis, gustatory sweating Cranial nerve III: pain and ptosis and may spare the pupil
Mononeuropathies (focal neuropathies)	Compression and entrapment syndromes: carpel tunnel syndrome, radial nerve (wristdrop), peroneal nerve (footdrop), femoral nerve Cranial neuropathies: cranial nerve III, pain and ptosis and may spare the pupil Truncal mononeuropathy: abdominal or lower chest pain or hyperesthesia, abdominal muscle weakness Asymmetric lower limb neuropathy (diabetic amyotrophy; diabetic polyradiculopathy): involvement of lower thoracic and lumbar nerve roots (upper leg weakness, upper leg muscle atrophy, diminished knee and ankle tendon reflexes); may have paresthesia, hyperesthesia, pain
Prediabetic neuropathy	Same presentation as distal symmetric polyneuropathy primarily involving the feet and ankles and occurring in individuals with prediabetes; may predate the onset of clinical diabetes by several years

amputation[170] (see Chapter 33). Age, duration of diabetes, glycemic control, genetics, and additional risk factors (smoking, hyperlipidemia, hypertension) influence the development and management of PAD.[171] Occlusions of the small arteries and arterioles, particularly below the knee, cause most of the gangrenous changes of the lower extremities and occur in patchy areas of the feet and toes. The lesions begin as ulcers and progress to osteomyelitis or gangrene requiring amputation. Peripheral neuropathies and increased risk for infection advance the disease. Fig. 22.21 illustrates how foot lesions of diabetes can lead to amputation. Significant morbidity and mortality are associated with major amputation.[172]

Infection

Increased morbidity and mortality from infectious agents have been documented in those with diabetes.[173] The individual with diabetes is at increased risk for infection for several reasons:

1. *The senses.* Impaired vision caused by retinal changes and impaired touch caused by sensory neuropathy lead to loss of protection with injury.
2. *Hypoxia.* Once skin integrity is compromised, tissues' susceptibility to infection increases as a result of vascular disease and hypoxia. In addition, the glycosylated hemoglobin in the RBCs impedes the release of oxygen to tissues.
3. *Pathogens.* Some pathogens proliferate rapidly because of increased levels of glucose in body fluids, which provides an excellent source of energy.
4. *Blood supply.* Decreased blood supply results from vascular changes and autonomic dysfunction, which decreases the supply of white blood cells to the affected area.
5. *Suppressed immune response.* Chronic hyperglycemia impairs both the innate and the adaptive immune responses, including abnormal chemotaxis, vasoactive responses, and defective phagocytosis. Clinical signs of infection may be absent.
6. *Delayed wound healing.* Slower collagen synthesis and decreased angiogenesis increase the opportunity for infection.

The risk of infection is especially high for individuals who take immunosuppressant medications, who have comorbidities, or who are undergoing surgery.[174-176]

ALTERATIONS OF ADRENAL FUNCTION

Disorders of the Adrenal Cortex

Disorders of the adrenal cortex are related to either hyperfunction or hypofunction. Hyperfunction that causes increased secretion of cortisol (hypercortisolism) leads to Cushing disease or Cushing syndrome. Hyperfunction that causes increased secretion of adrenal androgens and estrogens leads to virilization or feminization. Hyperfunction that causes increased levels of aldosterone leads to hyperaldosteronism, which may be primary or secondary. These syndromes often have overlapping features. Hypofunction of the adrenal cortex leads to Addison disease.

Hypercortical Function: Cushing Disease, Cushing Syndrome

Cushing syndrome refers to the clinical manifestations resulting from chronic exposure to excess endogenous cortisol and is more common in women. Cushing disease refers to excess endogenous secretion of ACTH (corticotropin).[177] *ACTH-dependent hypercortisolism* (about 80%) results from overproduction of pituitary ACTH by a pituitary adenoma (most common and can occur at any age) or by an ectopic secreting nonpituitary tumor, such as a small cell carcinoma of the lung (more common in older adults). *ACTH-independent hypercortisolism* (about 20%) is caused by cortisol secretion from a rare benign or malignant tumor of one or both adrenal glands (more common in children). A Cushing-like syndrome may develop as a side effect of long-term pharmacologic administration of glucocorticoids.

◆**PATHOPHYSIOLOGY.** With ACTH-dependent hypercortisolism, the excess ACTH stimulates excess production of cortisol and there is loss of feedback control of ACTH secretion. Whatever the cause, two observations consistently apply to individuals with Cushing syndrome: (1) they do not have diurnal or circadian secretion patterns of ACTH

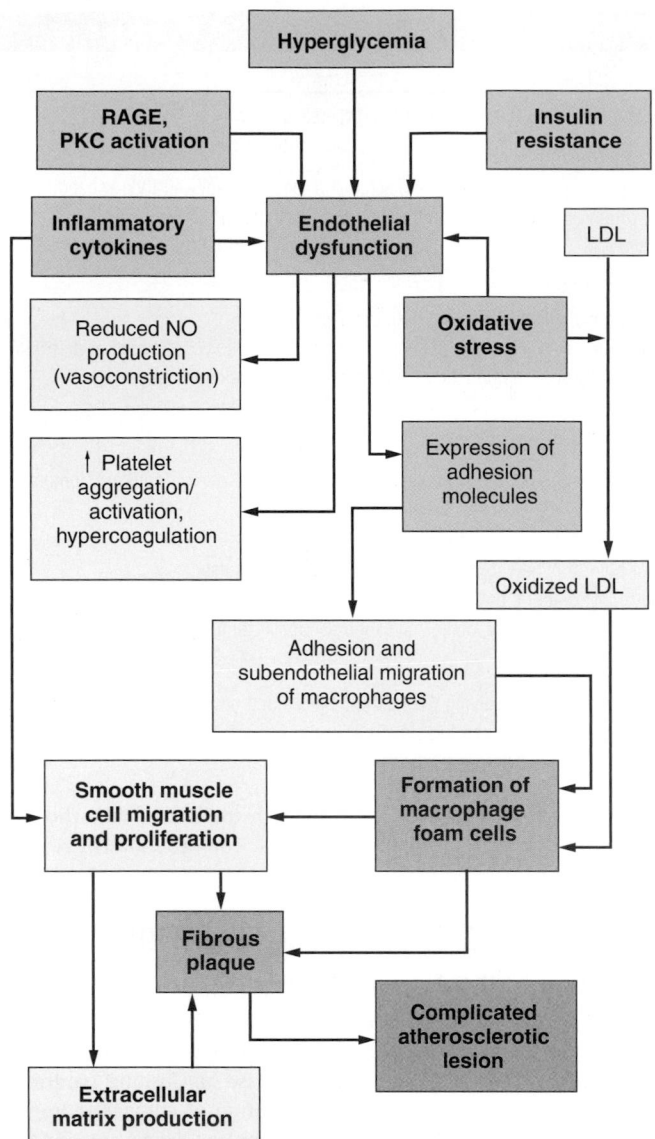

FIGURE 22.20 Diabetes Mellitus and Atherosclerosis. Diabetes with its associated hyperglycemia, relative hypoinsulinemia, oxidative stress, and proinflammatory state contributes to atherogenesis by causing arterial endothelial dysfunction (impaired vasodilation and adhesion of inflammatory cells), dyslipidemia, and smooth muscle proliferation. *LDL,* Low-density lipoprotein; *NO,* nitric oxide; *PKC,* protein kinase; *RAGE,* receptor for advanced glycation end product. (Data from D'Souza A et al: *Mol Cell Biochem* 331[1–2]:89–116, 2009; Stratmann B, Tschoepe D: *Best Pract Res Clin Endocrinol Metab* 23[3]:291–303, 2009.)

and cortisol, and (2) they do not increase ACTH and cortisol secretion in response to a stressor.[178] In individuals with ACTH-dependent hypercortisolism, secretion of both cortisol and adrenal androgens is increased, and corticotropin-releasing hormone (CRH) secretion is inhibited.

ACTH-independent secreting tumors of the adrenal cortex, however, generally secrete only cortisol. Elevated cortisol levels suppress CRH and ACTH secretion from the hypothalamus and anterior pituitary, respectively, which leads to low levels of ACTH. Low levels of ACTH cause atrophy of the remaining normal portions of the adrenal cortex, which over time will alter the cortisol-secreting activity of normal cells. When the secretion of cortisol by the tumor exceeds normal cortisol levels, symptoms of hypercortisolism develop.[179]

◆**CLINICAL MANIFESTATIONS.** Weight gain is the most common feature and results from the accumulation of adipose tissue in the trunk, facial, and cervical areas. These characteristic patterns of fat deposition have been described as "truncal [central] obesity," "moon face," and "buffalo hump" (Figs. 22.22 and 22.23). Transient weight gain from sodium and water retention may be present because of the mineralo-corticoid effects of cortisol, exhibited when cortisol is present in high levels.

Glucose intolerance occurs because of cortisol-induced insulin resistance and increased gluconeogenesis and glycogen storage by the liver. Overt diabetes mellitus develops in approximately 20% of individuals with hypercortisolism. Polyuria is a manifestation of hyperglycemia and resultant glycosuria.

Protein wasting is caused by the catabolic effects of cortisol on peripheral tissues. Muscle wasting leads to muscle weakness and is especially obvious in the muscles of the extremities, with thinning of the limbs. In bone, loss of the protein matrix and increases in bone resorption lead to osteoporosis and can result in pathologic fractures, vertebral compression fractures, bone and back pain, kyphosis, and reduced height. Hypercalciuria may result in renal stones, which are experienced by approximately 20% of individuals with this disease. Loss of collagen also leads to thin, weakened integumentary tissues through which capillaries are more visible; the tissues are easily stretched by adipose deposits. Together these changes account for the characteristic purple striae most often observed in the truncal area. Loss of collagenous support around small vessels makes them susceptible to rupture, leading to easy bruising, even with minor trauma. Thin, atrophied skin is also easily damaged, leading to skin breaks and ulcerations. Bronze or brownish hyperpigmentation of the skin, mucous membranes, and hair occurs when there are very high levels of ACTH. This is caused by increased levels of melanocyte-stimulating hormones resulting from excess conversion of pro-opiomelanocortin when ACTH concentration is elevated.[180]

With elevated cortisol levels, vascular sensitivity to catecholamines is increased significantly, leading to vasoconstriction and hypertension. Metabolic syndrome with abdominal obesity, hypertension, glucose intolerance, and dyslipidemias is a common complication (see Box 22.3). Individuals with hypercortisolism are at increased risk for cardiovascular complications (CAD, heart failure, and stroke).[181,182] Chronically elevated cortisol levels also cause suppression of the immune system, increased susceptibility to infections, and poor wound healing.

Approximately 50% of individuals with hypercortisolism experience alterations in their mental status, caused by the effects of cortisol on hippocampal neurons and the subsequent implications on learning, memory, and other neurologic functions when cortisol levels are elevated. These may range from irritability and depression to severe psychiatric disturbances, such as schizophrenia, which improve with treatment.[183,184]

Females may experience symptoms of increased adrenal androgen levels, increased hair growth (especially facial hair), acne, and oligo-menorrhea. Rarely do androgen levels become high enough to cause changes of the voice, recession of the hairline, and hypertrophy of the clitoris unless an adrenal carcinoma is involved. Infertility is more common among women.[185]

◆**EVALUATION AND TREATMENT.** A variety of laboratory tests must be used to diagnose hypercortisolism to determine the underlying disorder and differentiate ACTH-dependent (ACTH measurable) from ACTH-independent (ACTH not measurable) Cushing disease. These tests include urinary and serum cortisol and serum ACTH concentration. Other tests include the dexamethasone suppression test and bilateral inferior petrosal sinus sampling. Late night salivary cortisol levels are used as a screening test and to document alterations in the diurnal variation of cortisol level. Routine laboratory examinations may reveal

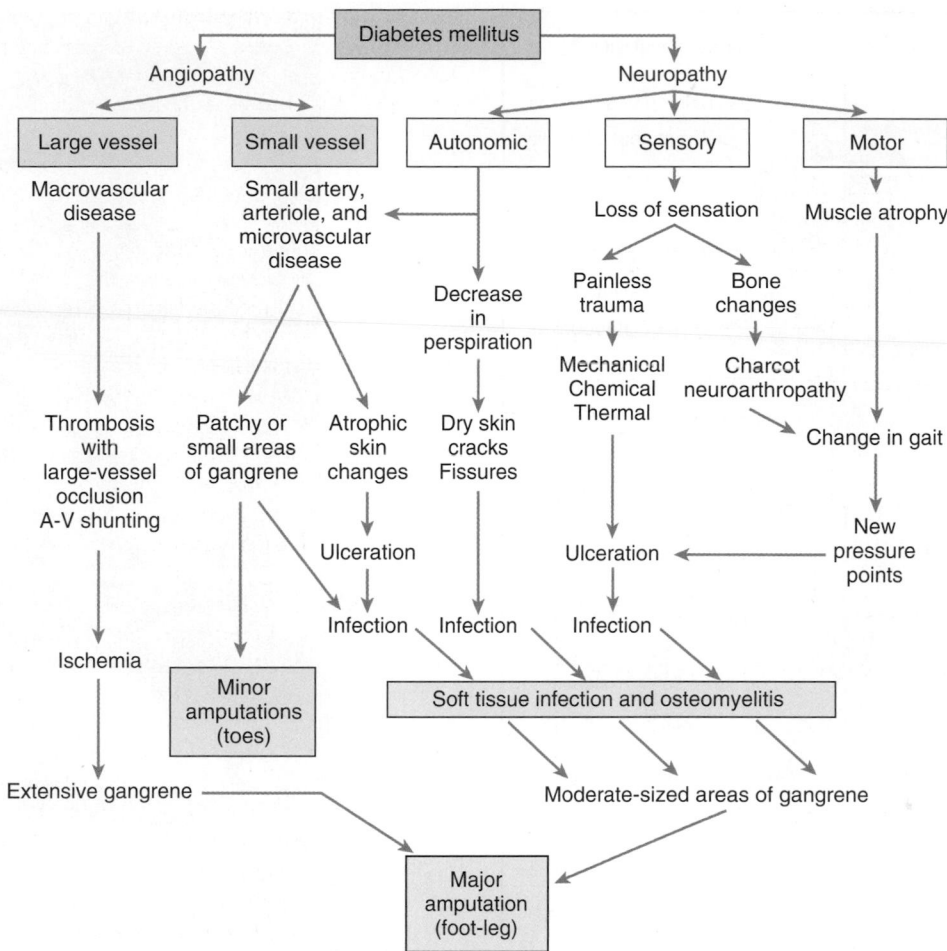

FIGURE 22.21 How Foot Lesions of Diabetes Can Lead to Amputation. *A-V,* Arteriovenous. (From Levin ME, O'Neal LW, Bowker JH: *The diabetic foot,* ed 5, St Louis, 1993, Mosby.)

hyperglycemia, glycosuria, hypokalemia, and metabolic alkalosis. Tumors are diagnosed using imaging procedures.[186]

Treatment is specific for the cause of hypercorticoadrenalism and includes medication, radiation, and surgery. Differentiation among pituitary, ectopic, and adrenal causes is essential for effective treatment. Without treatment, approximately 50% of individuals with Cushing syndrome die within 5 years of onset as a result of overwhelming infection, suicide, complications from generalized arteriosclerosis, and hypertensive disease. Guidelines are available for the treatment of Cushing syndrome.[187]

Congenital Adrenal Hyperplasia

Congenital adrenal hyperplasia is an autosomal recessive disorder that causes the deficiency of an enzyme that is critical in cortisol biosynthesis. Because cortisol production is low, ACTH concentration increases and causes trophic adrenal hyperplasia. The most common form is a 21-hydroxylase deficiency (90%) that results in both mineralocorticoid and glucocorticoid deficiency and adrenal androgen synthesis. Affected female infants are virilized and infants of both sexes exhibit salt wasting. Neonatal screening includes measurement of 17-hydroxyprogesterone. Treatment includes avoidance of glucocorticoid overtreatment and management of sex steroid excess.[188]

Hyperaldosteronism

Hyperaldosteronism is characterized by excessive aldosterone secretion by the adrenal cortex. There are both primary and secondary forms of hyperaldosteronism. Primary hyperaldosteronism (Conn syndrome, primary aldosteronism) is caused by excessive secretion of aldosterone from an abnormality of the adrenal cortex. Secondary hyperaldosteronism (secondary aldosteronism) involves excessive aldosterone secretion from an extra-adrenal stimulus.

◆**PATHOPHYSIOLOGY.** Primary hyperaldosteronism (Conn syndrome, primary aldosteronism) is usually the result of a unilateral benign aldosterone-producing adrenal adenoma (Fig. 22.24). Bilateral adrenal nodular hyperplasia and adrenal carcinomas account for the remainder of cases. The incidence is estimated to be about 10% of all hypertensive individuals; however, approximately 33% of people with resistant hypertension will have evidence of primary hyperaldosteronism.[189] Excessive autonomous secretion of aldosterone without its principal regulator, angiotensin II, causes hypokalemia and induces insulin resistance; promotes inflammation, endothelial dysfunction, and cardiovascular remodeling (increased left ventricular wall and carotid intima thickness); and affects adipose tissue differentiation and function.[190] Thus primary hyperaldosteronism can influence the features of the metabolic syndrome, including hypertension (most common cause of secondary hypertension), obesity, dyslipidemia, insulin resistance, and hyperglycemia.

Secondary hyperaldosteronism (secondary aldosteronism) involves excessive aldosterone secretion from the action of angiotensin II through a renin-dependent mechanism. (Factors that affect normal renin and aldosterone secretion are summarized in Table 22.13.) Examples include decreased circulating blood volume (e.g., in dehydration, shock, or

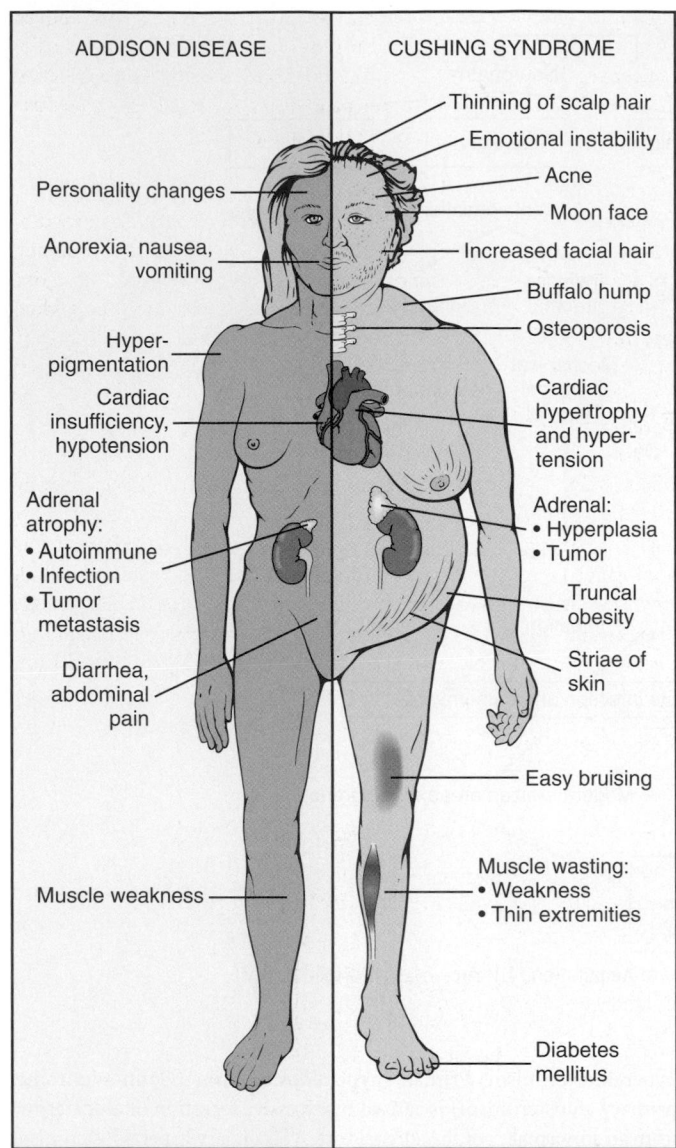

ADDISON DISEASE | CUSHING SYNDROME

- Personality changes
- Anorexia, nausea, vomiting
- Hyper-pigmentation
- Cardiac insufficiency, hypotension
- Adrenal atrophy:
  • Autoimmune
  • Infection
  • Tumor metastasis
- Diarrhea, abdominal pain
- Muscle weakness

- Thinning of scalp hair
- Emotional instability
- Acne
- Moon face
- Increased facial hair
- Buffalo hump
- Osteoporosis
- Cardiac hypertrophy and hyper-tension
- Adrenal:
  • Hyperplasia
  • Tumor
- Truncal obesity
- Striae of skin
- Easy bruising
- Muscle wasting:
  • Weakness
  • Thin extremities
- Diabetes mellitus

FIGURE 22.22 Symptoms of Addison and Cushing Diseases. (From Goodman CC, Kelly Snyder TE: *Differential diagnosis for physical therapists,* ed 5, Philadelphia, 2013, Saunders.)

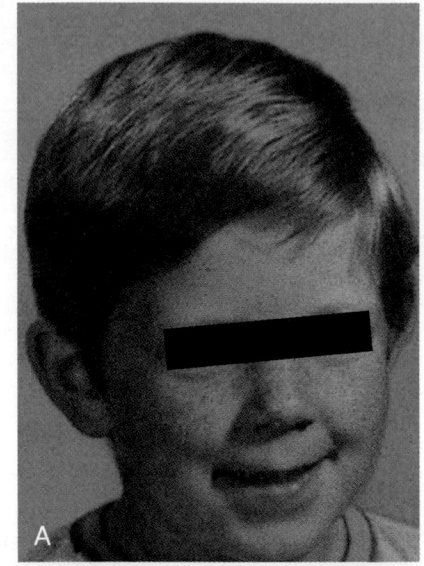
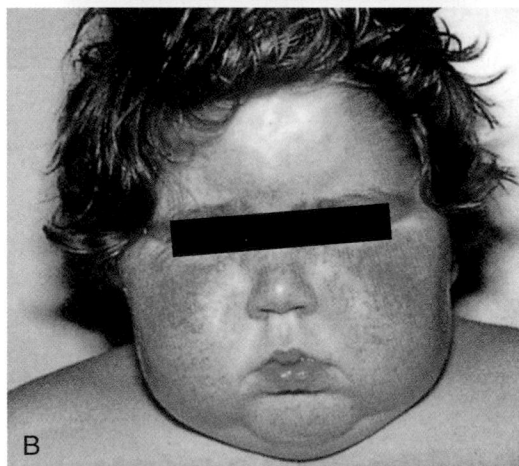

FIGURE 22.23 Cushing Syndrome. **A,** Patient before onset of Cushing syndrome. **B,** Patient 4 months later. Moon facies is clearly demonstrated. (From Zitelli BJ, McIntire SC, Nowalk AJ: *Zitelli and Davis' atlas of pediatric physical diagnosis,* ed 6, London, 2012, Saunders.)

TABLE 22.13	PHYSIOLOGIC FACTORS AFFECTING RENIN AND ALDOSTERONE SECRETION
FACTORS	**RENIN SECRETION**
Age	Highest in infants; lowest in older adults
Menstrual cycle	Highest in luteal phase (see Chapter 24)
Sodium intake	Increased by salt restriction
	Decreased by salt loading
Potassium status	Increased by K+ excess
Posture	Increased with erect posture
Sympathetic nervous system	Renin increased by catecholamine stimulation
Time of sampling	Highest before noon; lowest in evening

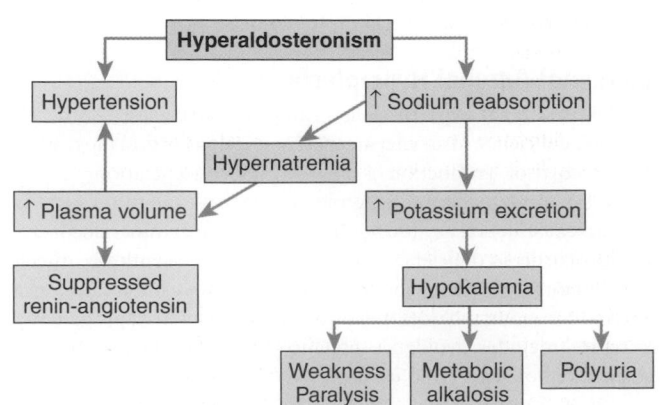

FIGURE 22.24 Pathophysiology of Primary Hyperaldosteronism. (From Bonow RO et al: *Braunwald's heart disease: a textbook of cardiovascular medicine,* ed 9, Philadelphia, 2012, Saunders.)

hypoalbuminemia) and decreased delivery of blood to the kidneys (e.g., renal artery stenosis, heart failure, or hepatic cirrhosis). Here, the activation of the renin-angiotensin system and subsequent aldosterone secretion may be seen as compensatory, although in some instances (e.g., congestive heart failure) the increased circulating volume further worsens the condition. Other causes of secondary hyperaldosteronism are Bartter syndrome, a renal tubular defect causing hypokalemia, and renin-secreting tumors of the kidney.

◆**CLINICAL MANIFESTATIONS.** Hypertension, hypokalemia, and hypervolemia, because of increased sodium reabsorption (without peripheral edema) and metabolic alkalosis, are the hallmarks of hyperaldosteronism.[189] Hypertension is resistant to treatment and may result from increased intravascular volume from a state of aldosterone-mediated vasoconstriction, although the latter mechanism requires very high levels of aldosterone. If hypertension is sustained, the long-term effects of elevated arterial pressure become evident, which include the development of left ventricular dilation and hypertrophy, vascular disease, and renal disease. In primary hyperaldosteronism, renin secretion is typically suppressed because of the autonomous production of aldosterone, although it is elevated in secondary hyperaldosteronism, which provides a means to clearly differentiate between these conditions.

Edema usually does not occur with primary aldosteronism. Sodium loss and water loss are maintained by hypervolemia-induced atrial natriuretic factor release, pressure natriuresis, and aldosterone escape (spontaneous diuresis). The escape phenomenon changes or resets the rate of sodium excretion in the proximal tubules and prevents more severe sodium retention. Although this mechanism provides protection from excessive sodium reabsorption and edema, it can increase urinary losses of potassium and cause hypokalemia.

Aldosterone-stimulated potassium loss can be variable. Serum potassium levels less than 3.0 mEq/L result in the typical manifestations of hypokalemia (see Chapter 3). Hypokalemic metabolic alkalosis is caused by the movement of potassium from the intercellular to extracellular space in exchange for hydrogen ions as well as renal loss of hydrogen ions to facilitate sodium reabsorption.

◆**EVALUATION AND TREATMENT.** Various clinical and laboratory measurements are useful in the assessment of hyperaldosteronism and include the following:

1. Measurement of blood pressure: hypertension is usually present.
2. Serum and urinary electrolyte levels: serum sodium level is normal or slightly elevated, serum potassium level is normal or depressed, and urinary potassium level is elevated; metabolic alkalosis may be present.
3. Plasma aldosterone-to-renin ratio increases.
4. Aldosterone suppression testing is performed using either salt loading or fludrocortisone acetate (Florinef) if the aldosterone-to-renin ratio is increased.
5. Imaging techniques may be used to localize an aldosterone-secreting adenoma.

Serum aldosterone and plasma renin activity both must be measured under controlled situations and after careful dietary regulation of sodium and potassium intake and withdrawal of hypertensive agents, if feasible. Table 22.13 summarizes normal physiologic factors that affect renin and aldosterone secretion.

Imaging techniques, such as CT and nuclear magnetic resonance (NMR), may be used to localize an autonomous aldosterone-secreting adenoma. Sampling from both adrenal veins also is useful. Renography can be used to diagnose secondary hyperaldosteronism.

Treatment includes management of hypertension and hypokalemia, as well as correction of any underlying causal abnormalities. If an aldosterone-secreting adenoma is present, it is generally approached surgically. Medical management with aldosterone receptor antagonists,

such as spironolactone or eplerenone (a drug without the side effects of spironolactone), is a viable option in selected cases. Angiotensin-converting enzyme (ACE) inhibitors, angiotensin receptor blockers (ARBs),[191] and revascularization procedures for renal artery stenosis are used to treat secondary hyperaldosteronism.

Hypersecretion of Adrenal Androgens and Estrogens

Hypersecretion of adrenal androgens and estrogens may be caused by adrenal tumors, either adenomas or carcinomas; endogenous hypercortisolism; or defects in steroid synthesis. The clinical syndrome that is manifested depends on the hormone secreted, the sex of the individual, and the ages at which the hypersecretion is initiated. Hypersecretion of estrogens causes *feminization*, the development of female sex characteristics. Hypersecretion of androgens causes *virilization*, the development of male sex characteristics (Fig. 22.25).

The effects of an estrogen-secreting tumor are most evident in males and result in gynecomastia (98% of cases), testicular atrophy, and decreased libido. In female children, such tumors may lead to early development of secondary sex characteristics. The effects of an androgen-secreting tumor are more easily observed in females and include excessive face and body hair growth (hirsutism), clitoral enlargement, deepening of the voice, amenorrhea, acne, and breast atrophy. In children, virilizing tumors promote precocious sexual development and bone aging. Treatment of androgen-secreting tumors usually involves surgical excision.

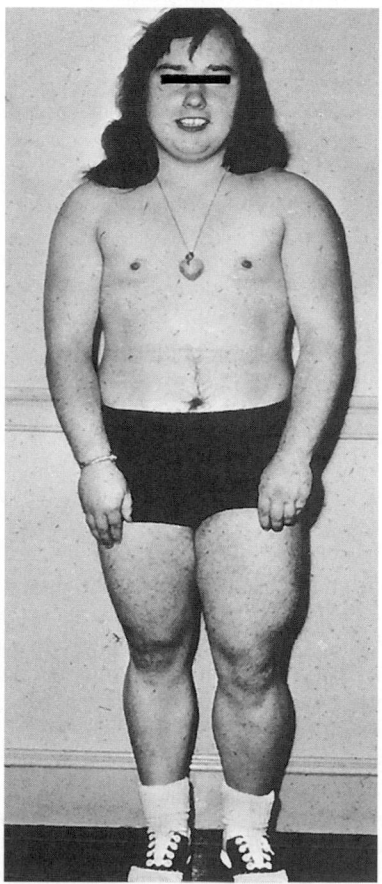

FIGURE 22.25 Virilization. Virilization of a young girl by an androgen-secreting tumor of the adrenal cortex. Masculine features include lack of breast development, increased muscle bulk, and hirsutism. (From Thibodeau GA, Patton KT: *The human body in health & disease*, ed 4, St Louis, 2010, Mosby.)

Adrenocortical Hypofunction

Hypocortisolism (low levels of cortisol secretion) can be primary, secondary, or tertiary. Primary hypocortisolism (Addison disease) develops because of a primary inability of the adrenals to produce and secrete the adrenocortical hormones. Secondary hypocortisolism develops because of inadequate stimulation of the adrenal glands by ACTH. Sometimes there is partial dysfunction of the adrenal cortex, so only synthesis of cortisol or aldosterone or the adrenal androgens is affected because the adrenal cortex has three distinct zones, which secrete the various hormones. Tertiary hypocortisolism is commonly caused by abrupt withdrawal of exogenous glucocorticoids or as a complication of treatment for Cushing syndrome. High levels of glucocorticoids (endogenous or exogenous) decrease hypothalamic corticotropin-releasing hormone (CRH) synthesis and secretion and also block the trophic and ACTH-secretagogue actions of CRH on anterior pituitary cells, resulting in loss of ACTH and its actions on the adrenal gland. Symptoms and management are similar to those for secondary hypocortisolism.[192]

Primary Adrenal Insufficiency.

Primary adrenal insufficiency (hypocortisolism and hypoaldosteronism) is often termed Addison disease. Addison disease is relatively rare, occurring most often in adults 30 to 60 years of age, although it may appear at any time. The most common cause of Addison disease in the United States is autoimmune destruction of the adrenal cortex and it is more common in women. Other causes include infections (tuberculosis, fungal infections, human immunodeficiency virus [HIV]), infiltrative diseases (amyloidosis, metastatic carcinoma), or bilateral adrenal hemorrhage. Adrenoleukodystrophy and adrenomyeloneuropathy are two rare types of X-linked adrenal deficiency that lead to symptoms of hypocortisolism and progressive neurologic symptoms.

◆PATHOPHYSIOLOGY. Addison disease is characterized by inadequate corticosteroid and mineralocorticoid synthesis and elevated serum ACTH levels (loss of negative feedback). Before clinical manifestations of hypocortisolism are evident, more than 90% of total adrenocortical tissue must be destroyed.

Idiopathic Addison disease (organ-specific autoimmune adrenalitis) causes adrenal atrophy and hypofunction and is an organ-specific autoimmune disease. (Autoimmunity is discussed in Chapter 9.) It may occur in childhood (type 1) or adulthood (type 2). 21-Hydroxylase autoantibodies and autoreactive T cells specific to adrenal cortical cells are present in 50% to 70% of individuals with idiopathic Addison disease; this percentage increases in younger persons and in those with other autoimmune diseases. This deficiency allows the proliferation of immunocytes directed against specific antigens within the adrenocortical cells.

The adrenal glands in idiopathic Addison disease are smaller than normal and may be misshapen. Several genes have been identified. Idiopathic Addison disease often is associated with other autoimmune diseases and in such cases is known as autoimmune polyendocrine syndrome (APS). APSI (APS type I) is inherited as autosomal recessive with childhood onset and includes Addison disease, hypoparathyroidism, mucocutaneous candidiasis, and other less common symptoms. APSII (APS type II) is more common and involves Addison disease, immune thyroid disease, diabetes mellitus, celiac disease, and hypogonadism.[193] (Mechanisms of inheritance are described in Chapter 4.)

◆CLINICAL MANIFESTATIONS. The symptoms of Addison disease are primarily a result of hypocortisolism and hypoaldosteronism and are often vague and not well-defined (see Fig. 22.22). With mild to moderate hypocortisolism, symptoms usually begin with weakness and easy fatigability. Skin changes, including hyperpigmentation and vitiligo, may occur. As the condition progresses, anorexia, nausea, vomiting, and diarrhea may develop. Symptoms of mineralocorticoid deficiency include hypovolemia, postural hypotension and dizziness, dehydration, hyperkalemia, and salt craving. Of greatest concern is the development of hypotension that can progress to complete vascular collapse and shock. This is known as adrenal crisis or addisonian crisis, and develops with undiagnosed disease, acute withdrawal of glucocorticoid therapy, or the occurrence of infection or other comorbid stressful events.[194]

Decreased adrenal androgen secretion is usually not clinically obvious in men because the adrenals are not a major source of male androgens; however, hypogonadism can occur. Women may experience a loss of some secondary sexual characteristics, such as pubic and axillary hair, normally maintained by the adrenal androgens.[195] Some studies also have reported an associated low functional ovarian reserve.[196] Disturbances in mood and motivation are common. The symptoms of Addison disease are summarized in Table 22.14.

◆EVALUATION AND TREATMENT. Serum and urine levels of cortisol are depressed with primary hypocortisolism, and ACTH levels are increased. Because of dehydration, blood urea nitrogen levels may increase. Serum glucose concentration is low. Eosinophil and lymphocyte counts are often elevated. Hyperkalemia is seen in Addison disease and may cause mild metabolic alkalosis (see Chapter 3). The ACTH

TABLE 22.14	CLINICAL MANIFESTATIONS AND PATHOPHYSIOLOGIC MECHANISMS OF ADDISON DISEASE	
CLINICAL MANIFESTATIONS	**PATHOPHYSIOLOGIC MECHANISM**
Weakness and easy fatigability that worsen as the day progresses, seen especially after exposure to stressors	Not known; may be related to hypoglycemia, hypotension, decreased metabolism of proteins
Gastrointestinal disturbances: anorexia, nausea, vomiting, diarrhea, abdominal pain, weight loss	May be associated with celiac disease or electrolyte abnormalities
Hypoglycemia, manifested by fatigue, mental confusion, apathy, psychosis	Absence of cortisol leads to decreased gluconeogenesis, decreased glycogen storage by liver, decreased metabolism of proteins, increased insulin sensitivity
Hyperpigmentation	Elevations of ACTH that lead to stimulation of melanocytes
Vitiligo (white patchy areas of depigmented skin)	Autoimmune destruction of melanocytes
Addisonian crisis: severe hypotension and vascular collapse	Combined effects of hypocortisolism, hypoaldosteronism, extracellular volume depletion, and some precipitating stressor (e.g., infection, vomiting, diarrhea); decreased vasomotor tone caused by cortisol deficiency

ACTH, Adrenocorticotropic hormone.

stimulation short test (250 µg) may be used to evaluate serum cortisol levels or, if not possible, the measurement of morning plasma ACTH and cortisol levels. Measurement of serum 21-hydroxylase (anti-adrenal) autoantibodies and a baseline serum 17-hydroxyprogesterone level also may be diagnostic.[197]

The treatment of Addison disease involves lifetime glucocorticoid and mineralocorticoid replacement therapy, together with dietary modifications and correction of any underlying disorders. Efforts are in progress to replace cortisol in a physiologic manner using modified-release formulations of hydrocortisone.[198] With acute stressors (e.g., infection, surgery, or trauma), additional cortisol must be administered to approximate the amount of cortisol that might be expected to be secreted if normal adrenal function were present (approximately 100 to 300 mg/day);[199] and this is called *stress dosing*. The individual's diet should include at least 150 mEq of sodium per day, with sodium intake increased in the event of excessive sweating or diarrhea.

Secondary Hypocortisolism.

Secondary hypocortisolism commonly results from prolonged administration of exogenous glucocorticoids and effective treatment of endogenous hypercortisolism. The consequence is suppression of ACTH secretion that causes adrenal atrophy and results in inadequate corticosteroidogenesis once the exogenous glucocorticoids are withdrawn. Decreased ACTH secretion also can result from pituitary infarction, pituitary tumors that compress ACTH-secreting cells, or hypophysectomy. In all instances of low ACTH levels, adrenal atrophy occurs and endogenous adrenal steroidogenesis is depressed. Clinical manifestations of secondary hypocortisolism are similar to those of Addison disease, although hyperpigmentation usually does not occur because melanocyte-stimulating hormone is also deficient. The renin-angiotensin system usually is normal, so aldosterone and potassium levels also tend to be normal and hypotension is less prominent. Recovery of adrenal function is possible with correction of the primary problem.

Tumors of the Adrenal Medulla

Hyperfunction of the adrenal medulla is caused by pheochromocytomas (chromaffin cell tumors) or sympathetic paragangliomas of the adrenal medulla that continuously secrete catecholamines (norepinephrine and epinephrine) (Fig. 22.26). These are rare neuroendocrine tumors and are usually sporadic, although up to 40% of them can be inherited. Familial forms are associated with mutations in the neurofibromatosis type 1 gene *(NF1)*, von Hippel-Lindau *(VHL)* gene, and multiple endocrine neoplasia type 2 *(RET)*. Any of the succinate dehydrogenase complex *(SDHA)* subunit genes can lead to pheochromocytoma and paragangliomas.[200] About 10% to 20% of pheochromocytomas are malignant. Those that are malignant metastasize to the lungs, liver, bones, or paraaortic lymph nodes.

PATHOPHYSIOLOGY. Pheochromocytomas and sympathetic paragangliomas cause uncontrolled production of norepinephrine, although large tumors also secrete epinephrine. Approximately 5% of people with pheochromocytomas have no symptoms because the tumor appears to be nonfunctioning. Such tumors can, however, release catecholamines in response to stressors, such as surgery.

CLINICAL MANIFESTATIONS. The clinical manifestations of a pheochromocytoma and sympathetic paragangliomas are related to the chronic effects of catecholamine secretion and include persistent hypertension, headache, sweating palpitations, tachycardia, palpitations, and pallor. Hypertension results from increased peripheral vascular resistance and may be sustained or paroxysmal. An acute episode of hypertension related to hypersecretion of catecholamines may follow specific events, such as exercise, excessive ingestion of tyrosine-containing foods (aged cheese, red wine, beer, yogurt), ingestion of caffeine-

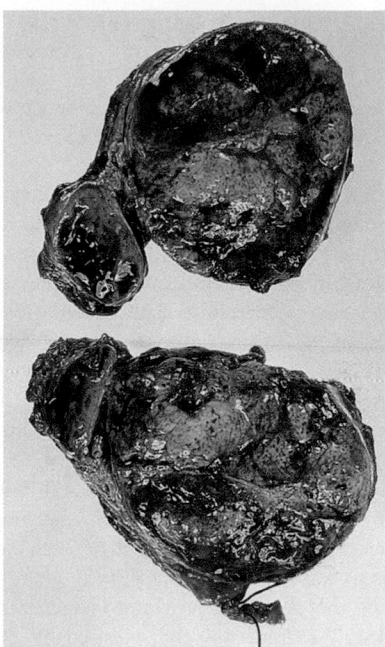

FIGURE 22.26 Pheochromocytoma. Gross appearance of adrenal pheochromocytoma. (From Rosai J: *Rosai and Ackerman's surgical pathology*, ed 10, Philadelphia, 2011, Mosby.)

containing foods, external pressure on the tumor, and induction of anesthesia. Hypertension unresponsive to drug therapy is often the first indication of a pheochromocytoma. Headaches appear because of sudden changes in catecholamine levels in the blood, affecting cerebral blood flow. Hypermetabolism and sweating are related to chronic activation of sympathetic receptors in adipocytes, hepatocytes, and other tissues. Glucose intolerance may occur because of catecholamine-induced inhibition of insulin release by the pancreas. Complaints of warmth, heat intolerance, weight loss, and constipation are common despite a normal or an increased appetite. These tumors tend to be extremely vascular and can rupture, causing massive and potentially fatal hemorrhage.

EVALUATION AND TREATMENT. Symptoms of pheochromocytoma can be insidious or intermittent and difficult to diagnose. A diagnosis of pheochromocytoma is made when increased catecholamines are found in the blood or urine. Plasma-free metanephrines and urinary fractionated metanephrine levels are highly sensitive diagnostic indicators when these laboratory techniques are available. The site of the tumor is determined using abdominal imaging techniques. Because of the possibility of metastasis, whole-body scanning may be done. Genetic testing is commonly completed and can guide therapy.[201]

Management of catecholamine excess is essential to prevent hypertensive emergencies and requires the use of α- and β-adrenergic blockers and calcium channel blockers that are typically initiated several weeks before surgery. The usual treatment of pheochromocytoma is laparoscopic surgical excision of the tumor, although open resection is still completed for large tumors or when metastasis is suspected. Medical therapy is continued to stabilize blood pressure before, during, and after surgery. Malignant pheochromocytoma is rarely curable and is usually managed by a combination of surgical debulking of the tumor combined with chemotherapy.[202]

SUMMARY REVIEW

Mechanisms of Hormonal Alterations

1. Abnormalities in endocrine function may be caused by hypersecretion or hyposecretion of hormones or alterations in transport molecules.

2. Endocrine abnormalities also may be caused by alterations in receptor function through a variety of mechanisms: (a) a decrease in the number of receptors, (b) receptor insensitivity to the hormone, (c) the presence of antibodies against specific receptors, and (d) defects in second-messenger generation or postreceptor defects.

3. Abnormally high levels of circulating hormones sometimes are caused by hormone release from tissues outside the endocrine system (ectopic foci) that may not respond to normal feedback mechanisms, in which case they are said to function autonomously.

Alterations of the Hypothalamic-Pituitary System

1. Dysfunction in the release of hypothalamic hormones probably is related to interruption of the connection between the hypothalamus and pituitary—namely, the pituitary stalk.

2. Disorders of the posterior pituitary include SIADH secretion and DI. SIADH secretion is characterized by abnormally high ADH secretion; DI is characterized by abnormally low ADH secretion.

3. In SIADH, high ADH levels interfere with renal free water clearance, leading to hyponatremia and hypoosmolality. SIADH secretion is associated with certain forms of cancer, apparently because of ectopic secretion of ADH by tumor cells.

4. DI may be neurogenic, caused by insufficient amounts of ADH, or nephrogenic, caused by an inadequate response to ADH. Its principal clinical features are failure to concentrate urine with polyuria and polydipsia. Dipsogenic polyuria occurs when excessive fluid intake lowers the plasma osmolarity to the point that it falls below the threshold for ADH secretion.

5. Hypopituitarism is dysfunction of the anterior pituitary that causes failure of hormonal functions. Symptoms may be mild to severe.

6. Causes of hypopituitarism include pituitary infarction, space-occupying lesions such as tumor or aneurysm, surgical removal, or infections. Symptoms are variable depending on which hormones are deficient (e.g., TSH, ACTH, or GH).

7. Hyperpituitarism is caused by pituitary adenomas. These are usually benign slow-growing tumors that arise from cells of the anterior pituitary.

8. Expansion of a pituitary adenoma causes neurologic and secretory effects. Pressure from the expanding tumor causes hyposecretion of cells, dysfunction of the optic chiasm (leading to visual disturbances), and dysfunction of the hypothalamus and some cranial nerves.

9. Hypersecretion of GH causes acromegaly in adults and giantism in children. Pituitary adenoma is the most common cause of acromegaly.

10. Prolonged, abnormally high levels of GH lead to proliferation of body and connective tissues. Renal, thyroid, cardiovascular, and reproductive dysfunctions develop slowly, together with a change in bony proportions and insulin resistance.

11. GH deficiency in children results in growth failure and fasting hypoglycemia. Adult GH deficiency results in fatigue, osteoporosis, and increased mortality.

12. Pituitary prolactinomas, renal failure, and medications can result in increased levels of prolactin and affect reproductive organs and function in both men and women.

Alterations of Thyroid Function

1. Thyrotoxicosis is a general condition in which TH levels are elevated and produce an exaggerated physiologic response in tissues. The condition can be primary, secondary, or subclinical.

2. Hyperthyroidism has a range of endocrine, reproductive, gastrointestinal, integumentary, and ocular manifestations. These are caused by increased circulating levels of TH and by stimulation of the sympathetic division of the autonomic nervous system.

3. Graves disease, the most common form of hyperthyroidism, is caused by thyroid-stimulating immunoglobulins that stimulate thyroid TSH receptors, resulting in thyroid hyperplasia and increased synthesis of TH.

4. Manifestations of Graves disease can include symptoms of hyperthyroidism, diffuse thyroid enlargement, and disorders of the skin and eyes.

5. The cutaneous manifestation of Graves disease is pretibial myxedema, a condition characterized by subcutaneous swelling of the legs and, occasionally, the hands.

6. Ocular manifestations of Graves disease are caused by hyperactivity of the sympathetic division of the autonomic nervous system and by immune-induced infiltration of extraocular muscles, orbital fat accumulation, and edema (exophthalmos).

7. Toxic multinodular goiter and solitary toxic adenoma occur when some hyperplastic, hyperfunctioning thyroid nodules autonomously secrete TH, causing hyperthyroidism and producing symptoms similar to those of Graves disease.

8. Toxic multinodular goiters result from multiple functioning adenomas.

9. Thyrotoxic crisis (thyroid storm) is a severe form of hyperthyroidism that often is associated with physiologic stress. Without treatment, death occurs quickly.

10. Hypothyroidism is caused by deficient production of TH by the thyroid gland. The condition may be primary, secondary, or subclinical.

11. Causes of primary hypothyroidism include iodine deficiency, autoimmune thyroiditis, subacute or painless thyroiditis, silent or subacute lymphocytic thyroiditis, iatrogenic hypothyroidism, and postpartum thyroiditis.

12. Autoimmune thyroiditis (Hashimoto disease) is associated with lymphocyte infiltration, antibody activation of natural killer cells, induction of apoptosis with gradual loss of thyroid function, and hypothyroidism.

13. Subacute thyroiditis, a form of hypothyroidism, is a self-limited nonbacterial inflammation of the thyroid gland. The inflammatory process damages follicular cells, causing leakage of triiodothyronine (T_3) and tetraiodothyronine (thyroxine) (T_4). Hyperthyroidism then is followed by transient hypothyroidism, which is corrected by cellular repair and a return to normal levels in the thyroid.

14. Secondary hypothyroidism is caused by hypothalamic-pituitary dysfunction in which TRH and TSH are not produced in sufficient amounts.

15. Thyroid carcinoma is a relatively rare cancer. The most consistent causal risk factor associated with thyroid carcinoma is exposure to ionizing radiation, especially in childhood.

16. Hypothyroidism affects all body systems. Symptoms depend on the degree of TH deficiency. Common manifestations include decreased energy metabolism and loss of heat production.

17. Myxedema is the characteristic sign of hypothyroidism. Myxedema is caused by alterations in connective tissue with water-binding proteins. The excess water leads to thickened mucous membranes

SUMMARY REVIEW—cont'd

and edema, particularly around the eyes and in the hands and feet.

18. Myxedema coma is a severe form of hypothyroidism, which may be life-threatening without emergency medical treatment.

19. Congenital hypothyroidism is TH deficiency at birth; it occurs with thyroid agenesis and results in hypothyroidism, growth failure, and intellectual disability from absence of thyroxine.

20. Papillary and follicular thyroid carcinomas are the most common thyroid malignancies probably caused by exposure to ionizing radiation, particularly during childhood. Thyroid nodules are present with normal thyroxine levels.

Alterations of Parathyroid Function

1. Hyperparathyroidism may be primary, secondary, or tertiary and is characterized by greater than normal secretion of PTH.

2. Primary hyperparathyroidism is usually caused by a parathyroid adenoma with interruption of the normal mechanisms that regulate calcium and PTH levels. Manifestations include chronic hypercalcemia, increased bone resorption, and hypercalciuria.

3. Secondary hyperparathyroidism is a compensatory response to hypocalcemia and often occurs with chronic renal failure or chronic vitamin D deficiency.

4. Tertiary hyperparathyroidism is excessive secretion of PTH and hypercalcemia that occurs after long-standing hypocalcemia.

5. Pseudohypoparathyroidism and familial hypocalciuric hypercalcemia are inherited conditions. In pseudohypoparathyroidism there is resistance to PTH.

6. Hypoparathyroidism, defined by abnormally low PTH levels, is caused by thyroid surgery, autoimmunity, or genetic mechanisms.

7. The lack of circulating PTH in hypoparathyroidism causes depressed serum calcium levels, increased serum phosphate levels, decreased bone resorption, and eventual hypocalciuria.

Dysfunction of the Endocrine Pancreas: Diabetes Mellitus

1. Diabetes mellitus is a group of diseases characterized by hyperglycemia resulting from defects in insulin secretion or insulin action, or both. The two most common types of diabetes mellitus are type 1 and type 2.

2. A diagnosis of diabetes mellitus is based on glycosylated hemoglobin (HbA_{1c}) levels, fasting plasma glucose (FPG) levels, and 2-hour plasma glucose levels during oral glucose tolerance testing (OGTT).

3. Type 1 diabetes mellitus includes an autoimmune (most common) and a nonimmune type. The immune type (type 1A) is associated with genetic susceptibility, environmental factors, and autoantibody, T-cell, and macrophage destruction of pancreatic beta cells with loss of insulin production and a relative excess of glucagon. Antibodies also can be formed against glutamic acid decarboxylase and insulin.

4. Nonimmune type diabetes (type 1B) occurs secondary to other disease.

5. Type 2 diabetes mellitus is caused by genetic susceptibility that is triggered by environmental factors. The most compelling environmental risk factor is obesity. Insulin production continues but the weight and number of beta cells decrease.

6. Several mechanisms of insulin resistance (hyperinsulinemia) cause reduced glucose uptake and metabolism in type 2 diabetes. These mechanisms include alteration in the production of adipokines by adipose tissue (i.e., leptin resistance), elevated levels of serum free fatty acids and intracellular lipid deposits, release of inflammatory cytokines from adipose tissue, reduced insulin-stimulated mitochondrial activity, and obesity-associated insulin resistance.

7. In type 2 diabetes, amylin deficiency results in increased glucagon secretion and hyperglycemia.

8. Decreased ghrelin and amylin levels and decreased beta-cell response to glucagon-like peptide have been associated with insulin resistance and type 2 diabetes.

9. Other specific types of diabetes mellitus include MODY associated with autosomal dominant gene mutations and gestational diabetes associated with onset of glucose intolerance during pregnancy.

10. Acute complications of diabetes mellitus include hypoglycemia, DKA, HHNKS, the Somogyi effect, and the dawn phenomenon.

11. Hypoglycemia is a lowered blood glucose level that may be related to exogenous (i.e., insulin shock or insulin reaction), endogenous, or functional causes.

12. Symptoms of hypoglycemia are divided into adrenergic, caused by activation of the sympathetic nervous system; and neuroglycopenic, reflecting defective central nervous system metabolism resulting from impaired energy generation.

13. DKA develops when there is an absolute or relative deficiency of insulin and an increase in the amounts of insulin counter-regulatory hormones of catecholamines, cortisol, glucagon, and GH; increased lipolysis; and accelerated gluconeogenesis and ketogenesis. It is most common in type 1 diabetes, but also occurs in type 2.

14. HHNKS is pathophysiologically similar to DKA, although levels of FFAs are lower in HHNKS and lack of ketosis indicates that some level of insulin is present. The hyperosmolar state can cause osmotic diuresis and profound dehydration, causing coma.

15. The Somogyi effect is a combination of hypoglycemia with rebound hyperglycemia caused by effects of counter-regulatory hormones. It is most common in persons with type 1 diabetes mellitus and in children.

16. The dawn phenomenon is an early morning rise in glucose levels caused by nocturnal elevations of GH concentration.

17. Chronic complications of diabetes mellitus are related to chronic hyperglycemia and include microvascular disease (e.g., retinopathy, nephropathy, and neuropathy), macrovascular disease (e.g., CAD, stroke, and peripheral vascular disease), and infection. Metabolic changes contributing to complications include oxidative stress, shunting of glucose to the polyol pathway, activation of protein kinase C, formation of AGEs, and accumulation of hexosamines.

18. Microvascular complications are associated with vascular alterations in the endothelium and the basement membrane as well as thrombosis.

19. Diabetic retinopathy is caused by several mechanisms including microvascular changes and thrombosis that lead to microvascular occlusion, retinal ischemia, increased vascular permeability, microaneurysm formation, hemorrhages, and neovascularization with loss of vision.

20. Diabetic nephropathy is related to hyperglycemia, hyperperfusion, oxidative stress, and inflammation with glomerular enlargement and glomerular basement membrane thickening, diffuse intercapillary glomerulosclerosis, expansion of the mesangial matrix, and progressive renal failure.

21. Diabetic neuropathies may be caused by vascular and metabolic mechanisms, or by a combination of both, with axonal and Schwann cell degeneration and abnormalities in sensory and motor nerve conduction velocity, and involvement of the autonomic nervous system.

SUMMARY REVIEW—cont'd

22. Macrovascular disease associated with diabetes mellitus is associated with hyperglycemia, hyperlipidemia, inflammation, and altered endothelial function.

23. The incidence of coronary heart disease, peripheral vascular disease, and stroke is greater in persons with diabetes than in nondiabetic individuals.

24. CAD and stroke in diabetes are a consequence of accelerated atherosclerosis, hypertension, and increased risk for thrombus formation.

25. Peripheral artery disease is a consequence of neuropathy and occlusion of large and small arteries with an increased risk of ischemia, necrosis, and amputation.

26. Individuals with diabetes are at risk for a variety of infections related to sensory impairment, vascular complications, impaired white blood cells and suppressed immunity, rapid proliferation of pathogens, and delayed wound healing.

Alterations of Adrenal Function

1. Disorders of the adrenal cortex are related to hyperfunction or hypofunction. No known disorders are associated with hypofunction of the adrenal medulla, but medullary hyperfunction causes clinically defined syndromes.

2. Hypercortisolism is divided into ACTH-dependent (Cushing disease or ectopic ACTH syndrome) and ACTH-independent (adrenal adenoma or adenocarcinoma) mechanisms.

3. Cushing disease is excessive anterior pituitary ACTH production most commonly by an ACTH-secreting pituitary microadenoma.

4. Cushing syndrome occurs whenever there is an excessive level of cortisol regardless of cause. Exogenous forms result from exogenous administration of glucocorticoids. Endogenous forms are either corticotropin dependent (most common and caused by an ACTH-secreting pituitary tumor) or corticotropin independent (usually caused by an adrenal cortical tumor).

5. Individuals with Cushing disease lose diurnal and circadian patterns of ACTH and cortisol secretion, and they lack the ability to increase secretion of these hormones in response to a stressor. Individuals experience weight gain, glucose intolerance, protein wasting, bone disease, hyperpigmentation, and immunosuppression.

6. Congenital adrenal hyperplasia is an autosomal recessive disorder with inadequate synthesis of cortisol and increased levels of ACTH that cause adrenal hyperplasia and overproduction of mineralo-corticoids or androgens.

7. Primary hyperaldosteronism is a disorder of excessive aldosterone secretion usually caused by an adrenal cortical adenoma or bilateral nodular hyperplasia. The condition is characterized by hypertension, hypokalemia, renal potassium wasting, and neuromuscular manifestations.

8. Secondary hyperaldosterone secretion is related to a variety of conditions associated with elevated renin release and activation of angiotensin II. These include decreased circulating blood volume, decreased renal blood supply, elevated estrogen levels, Bartter syndrome, and renin-secreting tumors.

9. Adrenal tumors, either adenomas or carcinomas, can autonomously secrete androgens or estrogens.

10. Hypofunction of the adrenal cortex can affect glucocorticoid or mineralocorticoid secretion or both. Hypofunction can be caused by a deficiency of ACTH or by a primary deficiency in the gland itself.

11. Hypocortisolism (low levels of cortisol) is caused by inadequate adrenal stimulation by ACTH or by primary cortisol hyposecretion. Primary adrenal insufficiency is termed Addison disease.

12. Addison disease is characterized by elevated ACTH levels with inadequate corticosteroid synthesis and output. Causes include idiopathic autoimmune disease, tuberculosis of the adrenal gland, familial adrenal insufficiency, amyloidosis, metastatic destruction of the adrenal glands, and adrenal hemorrhage.

13. Manifestations of Addison disease are related to hypocortisolism and hypoaldosteronism. Symptoms include weakness, fatigability, hypoglycemia and related metabolic problems, lowered response to stressors, vitiligo, hyperpigmentation, and manifestations of hypovolemia and hyperkalemia.

14. Secondary hypercortisolism is characterized by low to absent ACTH levels, leading to inadequate adrenal stimulation, adrenal atrophy, and decreased corticosteroidogenesis. The most common cause is withdrawal of exogenous administration of glucocorticoids. Manifestations are similar to those of Addison disease only without hyperpigmentation.

15. Hyperfunction of the adrenal medulla is caused by a pheochromocytoma, which is a catecholamine-producing tumor. Symptoms of catecholamine excess are related to their sympathetic nervous system effects and include hypertension, palpitations, tachycardia, glucose intolerance, excessive sweating, and constipation.

KEY TERMS

Acromegaly, 674
ACTH deficiency, 672
Advanced glycation end product (AGE), 695
Aldose reductase, 695
Amylin, 686
Autoimmune thyroiditis (Hashimoto disease, chronic lymphocytic thyroiditis), 679
Autonomic neuropathy, 698
Central (secondary) hyperthyroidism, 676
Charcot neuroarthropathy (Charcot joint), 698
Congenital adrenal hyperplasia, 701
Congenital hypothyroidism, 681
Cushing disease, 699
Cushing-like syndrome, 699
Cushing syndrome, 699
Dawn phenomenon, 693
Diabetes insipidus (DI), 671
Diabetes mellitus (DM), 684

Diabetic ketoacidosis (DKA), 693
Diabetic kidney disease, 695
Diabetic macrovascular disease, 698
Diabetic microvascular complication, 695
Diabetic neuropathy, 697
Diabetic retinopathy, 695
Distal symmetric polyneuropathy, 697
Exophthalmos, 677
Familial hypocalciuric hypercalcemia (FHH), 682
Feminization, 703
FSH deficiency, 673
Gestational diabetes mellitus (GDM), 692
GH deficiency, 673
Ghrelin, 688
Giantism, 674
Glucagon, 686
Glycation, 695
Graves disease, 677

Hexosamine pathway, 695
Hyperaldosteronism, 701
Hypercortisolism, 699
Hyperglycemic hyperosmolar state (HHS), 694
Hyperosmolar hyperglycemic nonketotic syndrome (HHNKS), 694
Hyperparathyroidism, 682
Hyperthyroidism, 676
Hypocortisolism, 704
Hypoglycemia, 693
Hypoparathyroidism, 683
Hypopituitarism, 672
Hypothyroidism, 679
Iatrogenic hypothyroidism, 681
Idiopathic Addison disease (organ-specific autoimmune adrenalitis), 704
Incretin, 688
Insulin resistance, 688

KEY TERMS—cont'd

REFERENCES

1. Lonard DM, O'Malley BW: Nuclear receptor coregulators: modulators of pathology and therapeutic targets. Nat Rev Endocrinol 8(10):598–604, 2012.
2. Ortega-Martínez S: A new perspective on the role of the CREB family of transcription factors in memory consolidation via adult hippocampal neurogenesis. Front Mol Neurosci 8:46, 2015.
3. Albers HE: Oxytocin, vasopressin, and the motivational forces that drive social behaviors. Curr Top Behav Neurosci 27:51–103, 2016.
4. Vandergheynst F, et al: Lack of responsiveness to 1-desamino-D arginine vasopressin (desmopressin) in male patients with nephrogenic syndrome of inappropriate antidiuresis: from bench to bedside. Eur J Clin Invest 42(3):254–259, 2012.
5. Janneck M, et al: Hyponatremia after trans-sphenoidal surgery. Minerva Endocrinol 39(1):27–31, 2014.
6. Ramos-Levi AM, et al: Drug-induced hyponatremia: an updated review. Minerva Endocrinol 39(1):1–12, 2014.
7. Kortenoeven ML, Fenton RA: Renal aquaporins and water balance disorders. Biochim Biophys Acta 1840(5):1533–1549, 2014.
8. Bolignano D, et al: Copeptin (CTproAVP), a new tool for understanding the role of vasopressin in pathophysiology. Clin Chem Lab Med 52(10):1447–1456, 2014.
9. Morley JE: Dehydration, hypernatremia, and hyponatremia. Clin Geriatr Med 31(3):389–399, 2015.
10. Cuesta M, Thompson CJ: The syndrome of inappropriate antidiuresis (SIAD). Best Pract Res Clin Endocrinol Metab 30(2):175–187, 2016.
11. Kalra S, et al: Diabetes insipidus: the other diabetes. Indian J Endocrinol Metab 20(1):9–21, 2016.
12. Bockenhauer D, Bichet DG: Pathophysiology, diagnosis and management of nephrogenic diabetes insipidus. Nat Rev Nephrol 11(10):576–588, 2015.
13. Marques P, Gunawardana K, Grossman A: Transient diabetes insipidus in pregnancy. Endocrinol Diabetes Metab Case Rep 2015:150078, 2015.
14. de Fost M, et al: The water deprivation test and a potential role for the arginine vasopressin precursor copeptin to differentiate diabetes insipidus from primary polydipsia. Endocr Connect 4(2):86–91, 2015.
15. Oiso Y, et al: Clinical review: treatment of neurohypophyseal diabetes insipidus. J Clin Endocrinol Metab 98(10):3958–3967, 2013.
16. Moeller HB, et al: Nephrogenic diabetes insipidus: essential insights into the molecular background and potential therapies for treatment. Endocrinol Rev 34(2):278–301, 2013.
17. Matsuwaki T, et al: Evaluation of obstetrical factors related to Sheehan syndrome. J Obstet Gynaecol Res 40(1):46–52, 2014.
18. Tanriverdi F, et al: Pituitary dysfunction after traumatic brain injury: a clinical and pathophysiological approach. Endocr Rev 36(3):305–342, 2015.
19. Higham CE, Johannsson G, Shalet SM: Hypopituitarism. Lancet 388(10058):2403–2415, 2016.
20. Fage AT, et al: Ipilimumab-induced hypophysitis: a detailed longitudinal analysis in a large cohort of patients metastatic melanoma. J Clin Endocrinol Metab 99:4078–4085, 2014.
21. Schoenmakers N, et al: Recent advances in central congenital hypothyroidism. J Endocrinol 227(3):R51–R71, 2015.
22. Hannon MJ, O'Halloran DJ: Isolated acquired ACTH deficiency and primary hypothyroidism: a short series and review. Pituitary 14(4):358–361, 2011.
23. Elijah IE, et al: The GH/IGF-1 system in critical illness. Best Pract Res Clin Endocrinol Metab 25(5):759–767, 2011.
24. van Bunderen CC, et al: Efficacy and safety of growth hormone treatment in adults with growth hormone deficiency: a systematic review of studies on morbidity. Clin Endocrinol (Oxf) 81(1):1–14, 2014.
25. Kim SY: Diagnosis and treatment of hypopituitarism. Endocrinol Metab (Seoul) 30(4):443–455, 2015.
26. Syro LV, et al: Progress in the diagnosis and classification of pituitary adenomas. Front Endocrinol (Lausanne) 6:97, 2015.
27. Molitch ME: Diagnosis and treatment of pituitary adenomas: a review. JAMA 317(5):516–524, 2017.
28. Birla S, et al: Identification of novel GHRHR and GH1 mutations in patients with isolated growth hormone deficiency. Growth Horm IGF Res 29:50–56, 2016.
29. Samarasinghe S, et al: Neurology of the pituitary. Handb Clin Neurol 120:685–701, 2014.
30. Dineen R, Stewart PM, Sherlock M: Acromegaly. QJM 2016. Feb 12, [Epub ahead of print].
31. Olarescu NC, Bollerslev J: The impact of adipose tissue on insulin resistance in acromegaly. Trends Endocrinol Metab 27(4):226–237, 2016.
32. Powlson AS, Gurnell M: Cardiovascular disease and sleep-disordered breathing in acromegaly. Neuroendocrinology 103(1):75–85, 2016.
33. Andersen M: Management of endocrine disease: GH excess: diagnosis and medical therapy. Eur J Endocrinol 170(1):R31–R41, 2014.
34. Ramos-Levi AM, et al: Genetic predictors of response to different medical therapies in acromegaly. Prog Mol Biol Transl Sci 138:85–114, 2016.
35. Capatina C, Wass JA: 60 years of neuroendocrinology, acromegaly. J Endocrinol 226(2):T141–T160, 2015.
36. Katznelson L, et al: Acromegaly: an endocrine society clinical practice guideline. J Clin Endocrinol Metab 99(11):3933–3951, 2014.
37. Oh MC, et al: Medical versus surgical management of prolactinomas. Neurosurg Clin N Am 23(4):669–678, 2012.
38. Glezer A, Bronstein MD: Prolactinomas. Endocrinol Metab Clin North Am 44(1):71–78, 2015.
39. Seigel SC, Hodak SP: Thyrotoxicosis. Med Clin North Am 96(2):175–201, 2012.
40. De Leo S, Lee SY, Braverman LE: Hyperthyroidism. Lancet 388(10047):906–918, 2016.
41. National Guideline Clearing House: Hyperthyroidism and other causes of thyrotoxicosis: management guidelines of the American Thyroid Association and American Association of Clinical Endocrinologists, Last updated Sept 18, 2015. Available at: http://www.guideline.gov/content.aspx?id=36623.
42. Palmeiro C, et al: Subclinical hyperthyroidism and risk: recommendations for treatment. Cardiol Rev 21(6):300–308, 2013.
43. Burch HB, Cooper DS: Management of Graves disease: a review. JAMA 314(23):2544–2554, 2015.
44. Khong JJ, et al: Pathogenesis of thyroid eye disease: review and update on molecular mechanisms. Br J Ophthalmol 100(1):142–150, 2016.

45. Bartalena L, Fatourechi V: Extrathyroidal manifestations of Graves' disease: a 2014 update. *J Endocrinol Invest* 37(8):691–700, 2014.

46. Rayes N, Seehofer D, Neuhaus P: The surgical treatment of bilateral benign nodular goiter: balancing invasiveness with complications. *Dtsch Arztebl Int* 111(10):171–178, 2014.

47. Brito JP, et al: Prevalence of thyroid cancer in multinodular goiter versus single nodule: a systematic review and meta-analysis. *Thyroid* 23(4):449–455, 2013.

48. Klubo-Gwiezdzinska J, Wartofsky L: Thyroid emergencies. *Med Clin North Am* 96(2):385–403, 2012.

49. Chiha M, Samarasinghe S, Kabaker AS: Thyroid storm: an updated review. *J Intensive Care Med* 30(3):131–140, 2015.

50. Baumgartner C, Blum MR, Rodondi N: Subclinical hypothyroidism: summary of evidence in 2014. *Swiss Med Wkly* 144:w14058, 2014.

51. Dubbs SB, Spangler R: Hypothyroidism: causes, killers, and life-saving treatments. *Emerg Med Clin North Am* 32(2):303–317, 2014.

52. Springer D, et al: Thyroid in pregnancy: from physiology to screening. *Crit Rev Clin Lab Sci* 54(2):102–116, 2017.

53. Doggui R, El Atia J: Iodine deficiency: physiological, clinical and epidemiological features, and pre-analytical considerations. *Ann Endocrinol (Paris)* 76(1):59–66, 2015.

54. Pyzik A, et al: Immune disorders in Hashimoto's thyroiditis: what do we know so far? *J Immunol Res* 2015:979167, 2015.

55. Caturegli P, De Remigis A, Rose NR: Hashimoto thyroiditis: clinical and diagnostic criteria. *Autoimmun Rev* 13(4-5):391–397, 2014.

56. Samuels MH: Subacute, silent, and postpartum thyroiditis. *Med Clin North Am* 96(2):223–233, 2012.

57. Szinnai G: Clinical genetics of congenital hypothyroidism. *Endocr Dev* 26:60–78, 2014.

58. García M, Fernández A, Moreno JC: Central hypothyroidism in children. *Endocr Dev* 26:79–107, 2014.

59. Van Vliet G, Deladoëy J: Diagnosis, treatment and outcome of congenital hypothyroidism. *Endocr Dev* 26:50–59, 2014.

60. American Cancer Society: *Cancer facts & figures 2017*, Atlanta, 2017, Author.

61. Marcello MA, et al: The influence of the environment on the development of thyroid tumors: a new appraisal. *Endocr Relat Cancer* 21(5):T235–T254, 2014.

62. Paschou SA, Vryonidou A, Goulis DG: Thyroid nodules: a guide to assessment, treatment and follow-up. *Maturitas* 96:1–9, 2017.

63. Yoo JY, Stang MT: Current guidelines for postoperative treatment and follow-up of well-differentiated thyroid cancer. *Surg Oncol Clin N Am* 25(1):41–59, 2016.

64. Cabanillas ME, McFadden DG, Durante C: Thyroid cancer. *Lancet* 388(10061):2783–2795, 2016.

65. Duan K, Gomez Hernandez K, Mete O: Clinicopathological correlates of hyperparathyroidism. *J Clin Pathol* 68(10):771–787, 2015.

66. Yener Ozturk F, et al: Patients with normocalcemic primary hyperparathyroidism may have similar metabolic profile as hypercalcemic patients. *Endocr J* 63(2):111–118, 2016.

67. Portillo MR, Rodríguez-Ortiz ME: Secondary hyperparathyroidism: pathogenesis, diagnosis, preventive and therapeutic strategies. *Rev Endocr Metab Disord* 18(1):79–95, 2017.

68. Cocchiara G, et al: The medical and surgical treatment in secondary and tertiary hyperparathyroidism. Review. *Clin Ter* 168(2):e158–e167, 2017.

69. Mrgan M, Nielsen S, Brixen K: Familial hypocalciuric hypercalcemia and calcium sensing receptor. *Acta Clin Croat* 53(2):220–225, 2014.

70. Monis EL, Mannstadt M: Hypoparathyroidism—disease update and emerging treatments. *Ann Endocrinol (Paris)* 76(2):84–88, 2015.

71. Anderson JL, et al: Parathyroid hormone, vitamin D, renal dysfunction, and cardiovascular disease: dependent or independent risk factors? *Am Heart J* 162(2):331–339, e2, 2011.

72. Sekercioglu N, et al: Cinacalcet versus standard treatment for chronic kidney disease: a systematic review and meta-analysis. *Ren Fail* 38(6):857–874, 2016.

73. Betterle C, Garelli S, Presotto F: Diagnosis and classification of autoimmune parathyroid disease. *Autoimmun Rev* 13(4-5):417–422, 2014.

74. Thiele S, et al: From pseudohypoparathyroidism to inactivating PTH/PTHrP signalling disorder (iPPSD), a novel classification proposed by the EuroPHP network. *Eur J Endocrinol* 175(6):P1–P17, 2016.

75. Rubin MR, et al: Therapy of hypoparathyroidism with PTH(1-84): a prospective six year investigation of efficacy and safety. *J Clin Endocrinol Metab* 101(7):2742–2750, 2016.

76. Centers for Disease Control and Prevention (CDC): National diabetes statistics report, 2017: estimates of diabetes and its burden in the United States. Available at: https://www.cdc.gov/diabetes/pdfs/data/statistics/national-diabetes-statistics-report.pdf.

77. American Diabetes Association (ADA): Standards of medical care in diabetes—2015 abridged for primary care providers. *Clin Diabetes* 33(2):97–111, 2015.

78. Pyram R, et al: Primary hyperparathyroidism: skeletal and non-skeletal effects, diagnosis and management. *Maturitas* 70(3):246–255, 2011.

79. Ferrannini E, et al: Progression to diabetes in relatives of type 1 diabetic patients: mechanisms and mode of onset. *Diabetes* 59(3):679–685, 2010.

80. Umpierrez GE, Kitabchi AE: Ketosis-prone type 2 diabetes mellitus. *Ann Intern Med* 144:350–357, 2006.

81. Pociot F, Lernmark Å: Genetic risk factors for type 1 diabetes. *Lancet* 387(10035):2331–2339, 2016.

82. Butalia S, et al: Environmental risk factors and type 1 diabetes: past, present, and future. *Can J Diabetes* 40(6):586–593, 2016.

83. Atkinson MA, et al: Type 1 diabetes. *Lancet* 383(9911):69–82, 2014.

84. Graham KL, et al: Pathogenic mechanisms in type 1 diabetes: the islet is both target and driver of disease. *Rev Diabet Stud* 9(4):148–168, 2012.

85. Szablewski L: Role of immune system in type 1 diabetes mellitus pathogenesis. *Int Immunopharmacol* 22(1):182–191, 2014.

86. Nakayama M, Simmons KM, Michels AW: Molecular interactions governing autoantigen presentation in type 1 diabetes. *Curr Diab Rep* 15(12):113, 2015.

87. Yi B, Huang G, Zhou Z: Different role of zinc transporter 8 between type 1 diabetes mellitus and type 2 diabetes mellitus. *J Diabetes Investig* 7(4):459–465, 2016.

88. ElEssawy B, Li XC: Type 1 diabetes and T regulatory cells. *Pharmacol Res* 98:22–30, 2015.

89. Campbell JE, Drucker DJ: Islet α cells and glucagon—critical regulators of energy homeostasis. *Nat Rev Endocrinol* 11(6):329–338, 2015.

90. Islam ST, Srinivasan S, Craig ME: Environmental determinants of type 1 diabetes: a role for overweight and insulin resistance. *J Paediatr Child Health* 50(11):874–879, 2014.

91. Leroux C, et al: Lifestyle and cardiometabolic risk in adults with type 1 diabetes: a review. *Can J Diabetes* 38(1):62–69, 2014.

92. Bode BW, Garg SK: The emerging role of adjunctive noninsulin antihyperglycemic therapy in the management of type 1 diabetes. *Endocr Pract* 22(2):220–230, 2016.

93. Jefferies CA, et al: Preventing diabetic ketoacidosis. *Pediatr Clin North Am* 62(4):857–871, 2015.

94. U.S. Food and Drug Administration (FDA): *FDA allows marketing of first ZnT8Ab autoantibody test to help diagnose type 1 diabetes*, Aug 20, 2014. Available at: http://www.fda.gov/NewsEvents/Newsroom/PressAnnouncements/ucm410830.htm.

95. Simmons K, Michels AW: Lessons from type 1 diabetes for understanding natural history and prevention of autoimmune disease. *Rheum Dis Clin North Am* 40(4):797–811, 2014.

96. Davis IC, Randell J, Davis SN: Immunotherapies currently in development for the treatment of type 1 diabetes. *Expert Opin Investig Drugs* 24(10):1331–1341, 2015.

97. Rege NK, Phillips NFB, Weiss MA: Development of glucose-responsive 'smart' insulin systems. *Curr Opin Endocrinol Diabetes Obes*. 2017. May 15, [Epub ahead of print].

98. Hay DL, et al: Amylin: pharmacology, physiology, and clinical potential. *Pharmacol Rev* 67(3):564–600, 2015.

99. Garvey K, Wolfsdorf JI: The impact of technology on current diabetes management. *Pediatr Clin North Am* 62(4):873–888, 2015.

100. Bouret S, Levin BE, Ozanne SE: Gene-environment interactions controlling energy and glucose homeostasis and the developmental origins of obesity. *Physiol Rev* 95(1):47–82, 2015.

101. Kahn SE, Cooper ME, Del Prato S: Pathophysiology and treatment of type 2 diabetes: perspectives on the past, present, and future. *Lancet* 383(9922):1068–1083, 2014.

102. Bruce KD: Maternal and in utero determinants of type 2 diabetes risk in the young. *Curr Diab Rep* 14(1):446, 2014.

103. Hivert MF, Vassy JL, Meigs JB: Susceptibility to type 2 diabetes mellitus—from genes to prevention. *Nat Rev Endocrinol* 10(4):198–205, 2014.

104. Sperling LS, et al: The CardioMetabolic Health Alliance: working toward a new care model for the metabolic syndrome. *J Am Coll Cardiol* 66(9):1050–1067, 2015.

105. Andrade-Oliveira V, Câmara NO, Moraes-Vieira PM: Adipokines as drug targets in diabetes and underlying disturbances. *J Diabetes Res* 2015:681612, 2015.

106. Sears B, Perry M: The role of fatty acids in insulin resistance. *Lipids Health Dis* 14:121, 2015.

107. Lee BC, Lee J: Cellular and molecular players in adipose tissue inflammation in the development of obesity-induced insulin resistance. *Biochim Biophys Acta* 1842(3):446–462, 2014.

108. Zamora M, Pardo R, Villena JA: Pharmacological induction of mitochondrial biogenesis as a therapeutic strategy for the treatment of type 2 diabetes. *Biochem Pharmacol* 98(1):16–28, 2015.

109. Keane KN, et al: Molecular events linking oxidative stress and inflammation to insulin resistance and β-cell dysfunction. *Oxid Med Cell Longev* 2015:181643, 2015.

110. Akter R, et al: Islet amyloid polypeptide: structure, function, and pathophysiology. *J Diabetes Res* 2016:2798269, 2016.

111. Allas S, Abribat T: Clinical perspectives for ghrelin-derived therapeutic products. *Endocr Dev* 25:157–166, 2013.

112. Chon S, Gautier JF: An update on the effect of incretin-based therapies on β-cell function and mass. *Diabetes Metab J* 40(2):99–114, 2016.

113. Bansal N: Prediabetes diagnosis and treatment: a review. *World J Diabetes* 6(2):296–303, 2015.

114. Corcelles R, Daigle CR, Schauer PR: Management of endocrine disease: metabolic effects of bariatric surgery. *Eur J Endocrinol* 174(1): R19–R28, 2016.

115. Cox DJ, et al: Glycemic load, exercise, and monitoring blood glucose (GEM): a paradigm shift in the treatment of type 2 diabetes mellitus. *Diabetes Res Clin Pract* 111:28–35, 2016.

116. Davis SN, Tate D, Hedrington MS: Mechanisms of hypoglycemia and exercise-associated autonomic dysfunction. *Trans Am Clin Climatol Assoc* 125:281–291, 2014.

117. Tomlinson B, et al: An overview of new GLP-1 receptor agonists for type 2 diabetes. *Expert Opin Investig Drugs* 25(2):145–158, 2016.

118. Scheen AJ: SGLT2 inhibitors: benefit/risk balance. *Curr Diab Rep* 16(10):92, 2016.

119. National Guideline Clearinghouse: Standards of medical care in diabetes-2016: summary of revisions. *Diabetes Care* 39(Suppl 1):S4–S5, 2016.

120. American Diabetes Association (ADA): Classification and diagnosis of diabetes. *Diabetes Care* 39:S13–S22, 2016.

121. Konig M, Shuldiner AR: The genetic interface between gestational diabetes and type 2 diabetes. *J Matern Fetal Neonatal Med* 25(1):36–40, 2012.

122. Anik A, et al: Maturity-onset diabetes of the young (MODY): an update. *J Pediatr Endocrinol Metab* 28(3-4):251–263, 2015.

123. American Diabetes Association: Management of diabetes in pregnancy. *Diabetes Care* 39:S94–S98, 2016.

124. Baz B, Riveline JP, Gautier JF: Endocrinology of pregnancy: gestational diabetes mellitus: definition, aetiological and clinical aspects. *Eur J Endocrinol* 174(2):R43–R51, 2016.

125. Tin W: Defining neonatal hypoglycaemia: a continuing debate. *Semin Fetal Neonatal Med* 19(1):27–32, 2014.

126. Beall C, Ashford ML, McCrimmon RJ: The physiology and pathophysiology of the neural control of the counterregulatory response. *Am J Physiol Regul Integr Comp Physiol* 302(2): R215–R223, 2012.

127. McCrimmon RJ: Update in the CNS response to hypoglycemia. *J Clin Endocrinol Metab* 97(1):1–8, 2012.

128. American Diabetes Association: Standards of medical care in diabetes—2015. *Diabetes Care* 38:S1–S93, 2015.

129. Dabelea D, et al: Trends in the prevalence of ketoacidosis at diabetes diagnosis: the SEARCH for diabetes in youth study. *Pediatrics* 133(4): e938–e945, 2014.

130. Umpierrez GE, Smiley D, Kitabchi AE: Narrative review: ketosis-prone type 2 diabetes mellitus. *Ann Intern Med* 144(5):350–357, 2006.

131. Jefferies CA, et al: Preventing diabetic ketoacidosis. *Pediatr Clin North Am* 62(4): 857–871, 2015.

132. Nyenwe EA, Kitabchi AE: The evolution of diabetic ketoacidosis: an update of its etiology, pathogenesis and management. *Metabolism* 65(4): 507–521, 2016.

133. Westerberg DP: Diabetic ketoacidosis: evaluation and treatment. *Am Fam Physician* 87(5):337–346, 2013.

134. Pasquel FJ, Umpierrez GE: Hyperosmolar hyperglycemic state: a historic review of the clinical presentation, diagnosis, and treatment. *Diabetes Care* 37(11):3124–3131, 2014.

135. Sardar P, et al: Effect of intensive versus standard blood glucose control in patients with type 2 diabetes mellitus in different regions of the world: systematic review and meta-analysis of randomized controlled trials. *J Am Heart Assoc* 4(5):e001577, 2015.

136. Yan LJ: Pathogenesis of chronic hyperglycemia: from reductive stress to oxidative stress. *J Diabetes Res* 2014:137919, 2014.

137. Ahlqvist E, et al: The genetics of diabetic complications. *Nat Rev Nephrol* 11(5):277–287, 2015.

138. Grewal AS, et al: Updates on aldose reductase inhibitors for management of diabetic complications and non-diabetic diseases. *Mini Rev Med Chem* 16(2):120–162, 2016.

139. Kizub IV, Klymenko KI, Soloviev AI: Protein kinase C in enhanced vascular tone in diabetes mellitus. *Int J Cardiol* 174(2):230–242, 2014.

140. Litwinoff E, et al: Emerging targets for therapeutic development in diabetes and its complications: the RAGE signaling pathway. *Clin Pharmacol Ther* 98(2):135–144, 2015.

141. Nowotny K, et al: Advanced glycation end products and oxidative stress in type 2 diabetes mellitus. *Biomolecules* 5(1):194–222, 2015.

142. Adeshara KA, Diwan AG, Tupe RS: Diabetes and complications: cellular signaling pathways, current understanding and targeted therapies. *Curr Drug Targets* 17(11):1309–1328, 2016.

143. Safi SZ, et al: Molecular mechanisms of diabetic retinopathy, general preventive strategies, and novel therapeutic targets. *Biomed Res Int* 2014: 801269, 2014.

144. Romero-Aroca P: Managing diabetic macular edema: the leading cause of diabetes blindness. *World J Diabetes* 2(6):98–104, 2011.

145. Yu Y, Chen H, Su SB: Neuroinflammatory responses in diabetic retinopathy. *J Neuroinflammation* 12:141, 2015.

146. Tuttle KR, et al: Diabetic kidney disease: a report from an ADA consensus conference. *Am J Kidney Dis* 64(4):510–533, 2014.

147. Blantz RC, Singh P: Glomerular and tubular function in the diabetic kidney. *Adv Chronic Kidney Dis* 21(3):297–303, 2014.

148. Gilbert RE: Proximal tubulopathy: prime mover and key therapeutic target in diabetic kidney disease. *Diabetes* 66(4):791–800, 2017.

149. Krolewski AS: Progressive renal decline: the new paradigm of diabetic nephropathy in type 1 diabetes. *Diabetes Care* 38(6):954–962, 2015.

150. Mora-Fernández C, et al: Diabetic kidney disease: from physiology to therapeutics. *J Physiol* 592(18):3997–4012, 2014.

151. Quiroga B, Arroyo D, de Arriba G: Present and future in the treatment of diabetic kidney disease. *J Diabetes Res* 2015:801348, 2015.

152. Joven MH, Anderson RJ: Update on blood pressure control and renal outcomes in diabetes mellitus. *Curr Diab Rep* 15(7):44, 2015.

153. Tesfaye S, Selvarajah D: Advances in the epidemiology, pathogenesis and management of diabetic peripheral neuropathy. *Diabetes Metab Res Rev* 28(Suppl 1):8–14, 2012.

154. Pop-Busui R, et al: Diabetic neuropathy: a position statement by the American Diabetes Association. *Diabetes Care* 40(1):136–154, 2017.

155. Singh R, Kishore L, Kaur N: Diabetic peripheral neuropathy: current perspective and future directions. *Pharmacol Res* 80:21–35, 2014.

156. Juster-Switlyk K, Smith AG: Updates in diabetic peripheral neuropathy. *F1000Res* 5:2016.

157. Balcıoğlu AS, Müderrisoğlu H: Diabetes and cardiac autonomic neuropathy: clinical manifestations, cardiovascular consequences, diagnosis and treatment. *World J Diabetes* 6(1): 80–91, 2015.

158. Moheet A, Mangia S, Seaquist ER: Impact of diabetes on cognitive function and brain structure. *Ann N Y Acad Sci* 1353:60–71, 2015.

159. Jeffcoate WJ: Charcot foot syndrome. *Diabet Med* 32(6):760–770, 2015.

160. White NH: Long term outcomes in youths with diabetes mellitus. *Pediatr Clin North Am* 62(4): 889–909, 2015.

161. Patel TP, et al: Insulin resistance: an additional risk factor in the pathogenesis of cardiovascular disease in type 2 diabetes. *Heart Fail Rev* 21(1): 11–23, 2016.

162. Rafieian-Kopaei M, et al: Atherosclerosis: process, indicators, risk factors and new hopes. *Int J Prev Med* 5(8):927–946, 2014.

163. Lyon A, et al: Sex-specific differential in risk of diabetes-related macrovascular outcomes. *Curr Diab Rep* 15(11):85, 2015.

164. Soma P, Pretorius E: Interplay between ultrastructural findings and atherothrombotic complications in type 2 diabetes mellitus. *Cardiovasc Diabetol* 14:96, 2015.

165. Task Force on Diabetes, Pre-diabetes, and Cardiovascular Diseases of the European Society of Cardiology (ESC), et al: ESC guidelines on diabetes, pre-diabetes, and cardiovascular diseases developed in collaboration with the EASD— summary. *Diab Vasc Dis Res* 11(3):133–173, 2014.

166. Varga ZV, et al: Interplay of oxidative, nitrosative/ nitrative stress, inflammation, cell death and autophagy in diabetic cardiomyopathy. *Biochim Biophys Acta* 1852(2):232–242, 2015.

167. Samai AA, Martin-Schild S: Sex differences in predictors of ischemic stroke: current perspectives. *Vasc Health Risk Manag* 11:427–436, 2015.

168. Yang S, et al: Biomarkers associated with ischemic stroke in diabetes mellitus patients. *Cardiovasc Toxicol* 16(3):213–222, 2016.

169. Hill MD: Stroke and diabetes mellitus. *Handb Clin Neurol* 126:167–174, 2014.

170. Gibbons GW, Shaw PM: Diabetic vascular disease: characteristics of vascular disease unique to the diabetic patient. *Semin Vasc Surg* 25(2):89–92, 2012.

171. Faglia E: Characteristics of peripheral arterial disease and its relevance to the diabetic population. *Int J Low Extrem Wounds* 10(3): 152–166, 2011.

172. Chin JA, Sumpio BE: Diabetes mellitus and peripheral vascular disease: diagnosis and management. *Clin Podiatr Med Surg* 31(1):11–26, 2014.

173. Dryden M, et al: Pathophysiology and burden of infection in patients with diabetes mellitus and peripheral vascular disease: focus on skin and soft-tissue infections. *Clin Microbiol Infect* 21(Suppl 2):S27–S232, 2015.

174. Jafar N, Edriss H, Nugent K: The effect of short term hyperglycemia on the innate immune system. *Am J Med Sci* 351(2):201–211, 2016.

175. Knapp S: Diabetes and infection: is there a link? A mini-review. *Gerontology* 59(2):99–104, 2013.

176. Shilling AM, Raphael J: Diabetes, hyperglycemia, and infections. *Best Pract Res Clin Anaesthesiol* 22(3):519–535, 2008.

177. Witek P, et al: Ectopic Cushing's syndrome in light of modern diagnostic techniques and treatment options. *Neuro Endocrinol Lett* 36(3):201–208, 2015.

178. Castinetti F, et al: Cushing's disease. *Orphanet J Rare Dis* 7:41, 2012.

179. Nieman LK: Cushing's syndrome: update on signs, symptoms and biochemical screening. *Eur J Endocrinol* 173(4):M33–M38, 2015.

180. Newell-Price J: Proopiomelanocortin gene expression and DNA methylation: implications for Cushing's syndrome and beyond. *Endocrinology* 177(3):365–372, 2003.

181. Isidori AM, et al: The hypertension of Cushing's syndrome: controversies in the pathophysiology and focus on cardiovascular complications. *J Hypertens* 33(1):44–60, 2015.

182. Ferraù F, Korbonits M: Metabolic comorbidities in Cushing's syndrome. *Eur J Endocrinol* 173(4): M133–M157, 2015.

183. Bratek A, et al: Psychiatric disorders associated with Cushing's syndrome. *Psychiatr Danub* 27(Suppl 1):S339–S343, 2015.

184. Starkman MN: Neuropsychiatric findings in Cushing syndrome and exogenous glucocorticoid administration. *Endocrinol Metab Clin North Am* 42(3):477–488, 2013.

185. Unuane D, et al: Endocrine disorders & female infertility. *Best Pract Res Clin Endocrinol Metab* 25(6):861–873, 2011.

186. Loriaux DL: Diagnosis and differential diagnosis of Cushing's syndrome. *N Engl J Med* 376(15): 1451–1459, 2017.

187. Nieman LK, et al: Treatment of Cushing's syndrome: an Endocrine Society practice guideline. *Clin Endocrinol Metab* 100(8):2807–2831, 2015.

188. El-Maouche D, Arlt W, Merke DP: Congenital adrenal hyperplasia. *Lancet* 2017. May 30, [Epub ahead of print].

189. Galati SJ: Primary aldosteronism: challenges in diagnosis and management. *Endocrinol Metab Clin North Am* 44(2):355–369, 2015.

190. Vaidya A, Dluhy R: Hyperaldosteronism. In De Groot LJ, et al, editors: *Endotext [Internet]*, South Dartmouth, MA, 2000-2017, MDText.com, Inc. Available at: http://www.ncbi.nlm.nih.gov/books/NBK279065/.

191. Gyamlani G, et al: Primary aldosteronism: diagnosis and management. *Am J Med Sci* 352(4): 391–398, 2016.

192. Charmandari E, Nicolaides NC, Chrousos GP: Adrenal insufficiency. *Lancet* 383(9935): 2152–2167, 2014.

193. Husebye ES, et al: Consensus statement on the diagnosis, treatment and follow-up of patients with primary adrenal insufficiency. *J Intern Med* 275(2):104–115, 2014.

194. Smans LC, et al: Incidence of adrenal crisis in patients with adrenal insufficiency. *Clin Endocrinol (Oxf)* 84(1):17–22, 2016.

195. Nieman LK, Chanco Turner ML: Addison's disease. *Clin Dermatol* 24(4):276–280, 2006.

196. Gleicher N, et al: The importance of adrenal hypoandrogenism in infertile women with low functional ovarian reserve: a case study of associated adrenal insufficiency. *Reprod Biol Endocrinol* 14:23, 2016.

197. Bornstein SR, et al: Diagnosis and treatment of primary adrenal insufficiency: an Endocrine Society clinical practice guideline. *J Clin Endocrinol Metab* 101(2):364–389, 2016.

198. Mallappa A, Debono M: Recent advances in hydrocortisone replacement treatment. *Endocr Dev* 30:42–53, 2016.

199. Betterle C, Morlin L: Autoimmune Addison's disease. *Endocr Dev* 20:161–172, 2011.

200. Baysal BE, Maher ER: 15 years of paraganglioma: genetics and mechanism of pheochromocytoma-paraganglioma syndromes characterized by germline SDHB and SDHD mutations. *Endocr Relat Cancer* 22(4):T71–T82, 2015.

201. Fishbein L: Pheochromocytoma and paraganglioma: genetics, diagnosis, and treatment. *Hematol Oncol Clin North Am* 30(1):135–150, 2016.

202. Kiernan CM, Solórzano CC: Pheochromocytoma and paraganglioma: diagnosis, genetics, and treatment. *Surg Oncol Clin North Am* 25(1): 119–138, 2016.

Obesity and Disorders of Nutrition

Sue E. Huether

CHAPTER OUTLINE

ADIPOSE TISSUE

Adipose tissue provides insulation and mechanical support and is the body's major energy reserve to fuel other tissues. As an endocrine organ, white adipose tissue (WAT) contributes to the regulation of energy homeostasis by secretion of adipokines that function like hormones with autocrine, paracrine, and endocrine actions necessary for metabolic function and immune responses.[1] Adipocytes are fat-storing cells and store excess energy in the form of triglycerides (triglycerol), synthesize triglycerides from glucose, and mobilize energy in the form of free fatty acids (FFAs) and glycerol. Adipokines include all of the biologically active substances synthesized by WAT, which function in the control of food intake and energy expenditure, lipid storage, insulin sensitivity, immune and inflammatory responses, coagulation, fibrinolysis, angiogenesis, fertility vascular homeostasis, blood pressure regulation, and bone metabolism. Excess WAT causes dysregulation of the adipokines, contributing to the comorbidities of obesity. The most common adipokines are summarized in Box 23.1.

Adipose tissue is classified according to color as WAT, brown adipose tissue (BAT), and beige adipose tissue (bAT). These tissue types are found in different locations, have different gene expression patterns, different rates of lipogenesis and lipolysis, and different origins.[2,3] The origins of different adipose tissue depots are complex and unclear and likely associated with the heterogeneous function of their different locations.[4]

Most adipose tissue in the body is WAT. WAT is located in visceral (central) and subcutaneous (peripheral) stores. WAT also is found in muscle groups providing mechanical protection and sliding of muscle bundles, and bone marrow. WAT has a stromal structure that contains macrophages, mast cells, neutrophils, fibroblasts, endothelial cells, blood vessels, nerves, and precursor adipocytes. White adipocytes contain a single triglyceride fat droplet or vacuole (unilocular). Visceral adipocytes store fat as triglycerides primarily in the form of very-low-density lipoprotein (VLDL), derived from hepatic and dietary sources. A low nutritional state, stimulation of the β-adrenergic sympathetic nervous system, and release of catecholamines (epinephrine and norepinephrine) activate hormone-sensitive lipase, triggering lipolysis in WAT to release FFAs and glycerol into the circulation.[2] Pancreatic insulin can inhibit lipolysis by activation of insulin receptors in adipocytes. With obesity adipocytes are resistant to insulin lipolysis.

When energy balance is positive, excess fat is stored in mature white adipocytes, which undergo hypertrophy and adipogenesis (hyperplasia, formation of new fat cells from preadipocytes). Chronic positive energy balance can overwhelm adipogenesis, and fat storage then depends only on hypertrophy. Visceral WAT is more likely to store fat by adipose tissue hypertrophy; produce more adiponectin, less leptin, and more inflammatory cytokines; and result in central (visceral) obesity. Visceral WAT hypertrophy is associated with release of numerous adipokines, greater macrophage infiltration, increased vascularity, insulin resistance,

BOX 23.1   MAJOR ADIPOKINES SECRETED BY ADIPOSE TISSUE

Adipokines
Increased in Obesity
Acylation-Stimulating Protein (Also Known as Complement 3a desArg)
- Stimulates triacylglycerol synthesis in adipocytes
- Inhibits action of hormone-sensitive lipase (triglycerol lipase)
- Promotes glucose transport
- Inhibited by insulin

Angiopoietin-Related Protein 2 (A Vascular Endothelial Growth Factor)
- Promotes insulin resistance
- Promotes inflammation

Angiotensinogen, Angiotensin Type 1 and Type 1 Receptors, Renin, and Angiotensin Converting Enzyme
- Promotes vasoconstriction
- Promotes inflammation
- Promotes lipogenesis
- Increases insulin resistance

Leptin (Primarily from Subcutaneous White Adipose Tissue [WAT] [Leptin Resistance])
- Inhibits appetite and stimulates energy expenditure
- Promotes satiety (hunger/appetite suppression) and regulation of eating behavior by hypothalamus
- Promotes sympathoactivation
- Is insulin sensitizing in liver and skeletal muscle
- Plays a modulating role in reproduction, angiogenesis, immune response, blood pressure control, and osteogenesis
- Promotes inflammation (a harmful effect)

Resistin (Increased in Obesity; Action Still Being Clarified)
- Expressed by macrophages in adipose tissue
- Promotes insulin resistance and increased blood glucose levels
- Inhibits adipocyte differentiation and may function as a feedback regulator of adipogenesis
- Promotes inflammation

Retinol-Binding Protein 4 (RBP4) (From Visceral WAT, Role Not Clear)
- Promotes insulin resistance in muscle
- Promotes angiogenesis

Serum Amyloid A (An Acute Phase Protein)
- Promotes systemic inflammation
- Promotes atherosclerosis

Vaspin (From Visceral WAT, Role Not Clear)
- Suppresses appetite
- Is insulin sensitizing
- Is antiinflammatory

Visfatin (From Visceral WAT)
- Mimics insulin and binds to insulin receptors and promotes insulin sensitivity
- Promotes adhesion of monocytes to endothelial cells and promotes plaque instability (harmful in cardiac disease)

Decreased in Obesity
Adiponectin (Primarily from Subcutaneous WAT)
- Is insulin sensitizing
- Is antiinflammatory
- Is antiatherogenic

Apelin (Role Not Clear)
- Improves insulin sensitivity in muscle
- Promotes vasodilation by blocking angiotensin
- Promotes cardiac contractility

Regulators of Lipoprotein Metabolism
- Adipocyte apolipoprotein E (increases adipocyte triglyceride content)
- Hormone-sensitive lipase (promotes lipolysis)
- Lipoprotein lipase (promotes hypertriglyceridemia)
- Lipotransin (transfers hormone-sensitive lipase to lipid droplet)

Proinflammatory Cytokines: **Increased in Obesity**
Interleukin-6
- Promotes insulin resistance
- Inhibits adipogenesis
- Decreases adiponectin secretion
- Promotes inflammation

Monocyte Chemoattractant Protein 1
- Attracts macrophages
- Promotes insulin resistance
- Promotes atherogenesis

Macrophage Products
Plasminogen activator inhibitor 1 (from visceral WAT)
- Promotes clot formation (inhibits fibrinolysis) by inhibiting tissue plasminogen activator and urokinase (also released by endothelial cells)
- Promotes insulin resistance
Prostaglandin E2 and leukotriene B4
- Promote inflammation
Tumor necrosis factor-alpha
- Promotes insulin resistance
- Promotes inflammation

Data from Fasshauer M, Blüher M: *Trends Pharmacol Sci* 36(7):461–470, 2015; Jung UJ, Choi MS: *Int J Mol Sci* 15(4):6184–6223, 2014; Leal Vde O, Mafra D: *Clin Chim Acta* 419:87–94, 2013.

a chronic proinflammatory state, and altered lipid metabolism, all characteristics of the metabolic syndrome associated with obesity.[5,6] Insulin resistance results in type 2 diabetes mellitus, and excess lipolysis leads to increased release of FFAs into the circulation. With chronic increased energy intake, the increase in adipocyte size in visceral WAT exceeds the supporting vascular supply, resulting in hypoxia and inflamed and fibrotic adipose tissues. Excess FFAs are distributed to nonadipose cells, and when their utilization capacity is exceeded cellular dysfunction or death occurs (lipotoxicity). The increase in FFAs and inflammation contributes to cardiovascular disease, nonalcoholic steatohepatitis (NASH), and other disorders associated with obesity, including carcinogenesis.

Subcutaneous fat is more likely to store fat by adipogenesis (hyperplasia), with smaller adipocytes and greater fat storage capacity. Subcutaneous fat has higher leptin production, lower adiponectin production, lower production of inflammatory cytokines, lower association with insulin resistance, and is a healthier expansion of fat tissue. Thus the complications of obesity are related to where fat is stored, not just the accumulation of fat stores.

Estrogen and estrogen receptors have a role in fat metabolism and enhance the deposition of fat in the subcutaneous tissue and inhibit it in visceral tissue. Estradiol increases α_2-adrenergic receptors in subcutaneous adipose tissue but not in visceral adipose tissue. The ratio of α_2-adrenergic receptors to β-adrenergic receptors in the subcutaneous adipose tissue in premenopausal women is increased and accounts for the lower lipolytic response to epinephrine and norepinephrine as compared to adipocytes from men. This ratio is reversed in visceral adipose tissue in women. This may explain the higher incidence of peripheral obesity among premenopausal women and the increase in central obesity with menopause and in men.[7]

Brown adipocytes have multiple lipid droplets or vacuoles (multilocular) and are rich in mitochondria that contain iron, giving them a brown color. Exposure to cold, activation of the sympathetic nervous system and catecholamines, and activation of triiodothyronine (T_3) stimulate BAT to rapidly generate heat through the activation of uncoupling protein 1 (UCP1) (nonshivering thermogenesis). UCP1 promotes mitochondrial respiration and dissipates chemical energy as heat from increased glucose and free fatty acid (FFA) oxidation. This occurs at a rate 50-fold greater than that in WAT and protects against obesity and metabolic syndrome.[8] Estrogen-related receptors also participate in the induction of UCP1 in response to cold adrenergic stimulation in BAT.[9]

Neonates generate body heat from BAT primarily located in the interscapular and perirenal regions. It was traditionally thought that brown adipose tissue did not persist into adult life. However, using positron emission tomography (PET) scanning methods it is now known that adults also have UCP1-positive BAT. It is most common in lean individuals, usually located in the neck, supraclavicular, axillary, paravertebral, and perirenal regions.[10] Muscle myokines, irisin and fibroblast growth factor-21, also promote thermogenesis and protect against obesity.

Leptin and adiponectin are minimally produced by BAT so there is little effect on appetite and satiety. There also is an inverse relationship between the amount of BAT, body mass index, and age. Interindividual differences in BAT-mediated thermogenesis may explain some of the variability in obesity susceptibility and the increased prevalence of obesity with aging. Variation in BAT and "brite" adipocytes (bATs) also may participate in natural regulation of weight reduction.

Located within WAT, particularly in subcutaneous fat depots, are beige or bAT (from "brown in white"), a subpopulation of white adipocytes that also contains multiple mitochondria and UCP1 but not in amounts associated with BAT. **Beige adipocytes** are thermogenic and emerge within WAT with chronic exposure to cold, with exercise, and with exposure to the synthetic ligand of peroxisome proliferator–activated receptor-γ (PPARγ), such as thiazolidinedione (TZD).[11] This is known as the "beiging" of WAT. They disappear with elevated ambient temperatures.[12] Chronic exposure to cold also stimulates WAT transdifferentiation to bAT, which is thermogenic. With warm adaptation, bAT reverts to WAT. Exercise also promotes browning of white adipose tissue, and several myokines are involved in the crosstalk between adipose and muscle tissue.[13] Leptin and insulin together promote bAT, increasing energy expenditure and weight loss. bAT is diminished in obesity. Since

"beiging" or "browning" of adipose tissue protects against obesity and metabolic syndrome, efforts are in progress to discover if there is a way to stimulate synthesis and activity of BAT and bAT as an approach to preventing or treating obesity and diabetes mellitus.[8,14]

Bone marrow adipose tissue (MAT) is found in all bones, but in greater numbers in long bones. MAT releases adipokines with autocrine, paracrine, and endocrine effects. MAT has paracrine effects associated with both osteoblast function and endocrine actions that affect distant organs, including the cardiovascular system. In general, excessive MAT is associated with osteoporosis.[15] Obesity and alterations in adipokines, activation of macrophages, and release of inflammatory mediators are associated with rheumatoid arthritis.[16] Loss of visceral and subcutaneous adipose tissue as occurs in anorexia nervosa results in the accumulation of MAT and osteoporosis. The mechanism is associated with a decrease in myokine, delta homolog 1 protein (DLK1) (inhibits adipogenesis), and hypoleptinemia, resulting in increased adipocyte and osteoblast differentiation.[17]

OBESITY

Obesity is an increase in body adipose tissue and an endocrine and metabolic disorder that has become epidemic worldwide. Obesity develops when caloric intake exceeds caloric expenditure in genetically susceptible individuals.[18] The incidence among U.S. adults was 36.5% between 2011 and 2014 (women 38.3% and men 34.3%) and 17% among children and adolescents between ages 2 and 19 years. Children tend to become obese adults. There are ethnic differences in rates of obesity: non-Hispanic blacks have the highest age-adjusted rate at 48.1% followed by Hispanics (42.5%), non-Hispanic whites (34.5%), and non-Hispanic Asians (11.7%).[19] It is projected that 42% of people in the United States will be obese by 2030.[20] Obesity is defined as a body mass index (BMI) that exceeds 30 kg/m^2 in adults and a BMI greater than or equal to the age- and sex-specific 95th percentile of the 2000 Centers for Disease Control and Prevention growth charts in children.[19]

Obesity is the fifth leading cause of death in the United States and accounts for high healthcare costs worldwide.[21] Three leading causes of death in the United States are associated with obesity: cardiovascular disease, type 2 diabetes mellitus, and cancer (liver, advanced prostate, ovarian, gallbladder, kidney, colorectal, esophageal [adenocarcinoma], postmenopausal breast, pancreatic, endometrial, and stomach [cardia])[22] Obesity also is a risk factor for hypertension, stroke, hyperlipidemia, gallstones, nonalcoholic steatohepatitis, gastroesophageal reflux, hiatal hernia, osteoarthritis, infectious disease, asthma, obstructive sleep apnea, and chronic kidney disease. However, some studies have shown that mild obesity in older individuals is associated with lower mortality (the obesity paradox) but the mechanisms are not clear.[23] The causes and consequences of obesity are multiple and complex and there is rapidly advancing research regarding causal mechanisms, complications, and treatment. Genotype and gene-environment interactions are important predisposing factors[24] (see *What's New? Obesogens*). Single-gene defects (monogenic) are rare, and obesity is usually polygenic and associated with other phenotypes such as endocrine disorders (i.e., diabetes and hypothyroidism) and intellectual disability (i.e., Down and Prader-Willi syndromes). Single-gene defects include the melanocortin-4 receptor gene, leptin gene (also known as the *obesity gene*), and leptin-receptor gene. All single-gene defects are directly or indirectly related to leptin and melanocortin pathways (decrease appetite and regulate energy homeostasis).[25,26] Metabolic abnormalities contributing to obesity include Cushing syndrome, Cushing disease, polycystic ovary syndrome, growth hormone deficiency, hypothyroidism, and hypothalamic injury. Contributing environmental factors include socioeconomic status (both high and low incomes), food intake (low-nutrient, energy-dense foods),

WHAT'S NEW?
Obesogens

Obesogens are exogenous chemicals that contribute to the development of obesity. These are molecules that stimulate adipogenesis and fat storage and interfere with neuroendocrine control of appetite and satiety. Developmental exposure to environmental obesogens is proposed to contribute to the epidemic of obesity in addition to high caloric intake, a sedentary lifestyle, and genetic predisposition. In early life, these substances are included in the maternal diet (i.e., phytoestrogens) or are associated with exposure to pesticides (i.e., organophosphates), plastics (phthalates, bisphenol-A), personal care products, and household and other consumer products that can cross the placental barrier or be transmitted, or both, through breast milk. Epigenetic changes in gene regulation and expression affect adipocyte differentiation, adipogenesis, and lipid metabolism, resulting in obesity in later life. Animal studies indicate these genetic changes can be transmitted through generations of families.

Data from Janesick AS, Blumberg B: *Am J Obstet Gynecol* 214(5):559–565; 2016; Nappi F et al: *Int J Environ Res Public Health* 13(8):765, 2016; Stel J, Legler J: *Endocrinology* 156(10):3466–3472, 2015.

and physical inactivity. Obesity also is associated with adverse social and psychologic consequences, including depression and mood disorders.[27]

◆**PATHOPHYSIOLOGY.** The pathophysiology of obesity is complex and involves the interaction of peripheral and central pathways, numerous adipokines, hormones, and neurotransmitters (Fig. 23.1). The adipocyte is the cellular basis of obesity and most of the adipocytes are white.[28] In the periphery, white adipocytes increase in size and number, store triglyceride, and secrete adipokines. Adipokines and other hormones participate in regulation of food intake, energy metabolism, and other functions as previously described. Adipokines circulate in the blood at concentrations that increase or decrease in relation to body fat mass (see Box 23.1) and provide signals to the hypothalamus, brainstem, autonomic nervous system, and other centers to regulate hunger, satiety, and energy balance.[29] Visceral WAT accumulation causes dysfunction in the regulation and interaction of this signaling system and contributes to the complications and consequences of obesity.[30] The following section summarizes the mechanisms controlling food intake and energy balance.

Food Intake and Energy Balance

Centrally, the arcuate nucleus (ARC) in the hypothalamus regulates food intake and energy metabolism by balancing the opposing effects of two sets of neurons. One set of neurons produces agouti-related protein (AgRP) and neuropeptide Y (NPY), collectively known as *AgRP/NPY neurons*. These neurons promote appetite, stimulate eating, and decrease metabolism (anabolic). They are known as *orexigenic neurons* and are stimulated by molecules called *orexins*. Another set of neurons synthesize pro-opiomelanocortin–producing (POMC-producing) peptide and cocaine-and-amphetamine–regulated transcript (CART), collectively known as *POMC/CART neurons*. These neurons suppress appetite, inhibit eating, and increase metabolism. They are known as *anorexigenic neurons* and are stimulated by molecules called *anorexins* (Box 23.2). The orexin and anorexin signaling pathways are transmitted through the autonomic nervous and endocrine systems to regulate appetite, food intake, energy metabolism, and body temperature.[31] The hypothalamus also communicates with higher brain centers related to reward, pleasure, memory, and addictive behavior. These centers can override hypothalamic control of food intake and satiety, increasing consumption of highly palatable foods, resulting in increased fat stores.[32-34]

BOX 23.2   EXAMPLES OF HORMONES AND NEUROPEPTIDES THAT INFLUENCE EATING BEHAVIOR

Orexins (Appetite Stimulants)
Neuropeptide Y (NPY)
Melanin-concentrating hormone (MCH)
Agouti-related protein (AgRP)
Ghrelin
Galanin
Orexins A and B
Endocannabinoids
Cortisol

Anorexins (Appetite Suppressants)
Leptin
Insulin
Cholecystokinin (CCK)
Glucagon-like peptide 1 (GLP-1)
Peptide YY (PYY)
Corticotropin-releasing factor (CRF)
Urocortin (a CRF satiety signaling hormone)
Cocaine- and amphetamine-regulated transcript (CART)
Alpha-melanocyte–stimulating hormone (α-MSH)
Bombesin
Serotonin
Calcitonin

Adipokines and hormones released from the gastrointestinal tract and pancreas interact with brain centers (adipose tissue-gut-brain axis), and play a significant role in the pathophysiology of obesity. The major adipokines and hormones are reviewed next.

Leptin is a product of the obesity gene (*Ob* gene) and expressed primarily by adipocytes.[35] High leptin levels in the normally fed state act on the hypothalamus to inhibit orexigenic AgRP/NPY neurons and stimulate anorexigenic POMC/CART neurons to suppress appetite and increase energy expenditure. At low leptin levels (i.e., during fasting), leptin stimulates food intake and reduces energy expenditure. This balance regulates body weight and energy expenditure within a fairly narrow range. Leptin levels increase as the number of adipocytes increases. However, high leptin levels are ineffective at decreasing appetite and energy expenditure, a condition known as central *leptin resistance*.

Leptin resistance fails to inhibit orexigenic hypothalamic satiety signaling and promotes overeating and excessive weight gain. Leptin also regulates hepatic gluconeogenesis, insulin sensitivity, and glucose and lipid metabolism in liver, muscle, and adipose tissue. Peripheral leptin resistance results in hyperglycemia, hyperinsulinemia, and hyperlipidemia, and stimulates macrophages and endothelial cells to produce proinflammatory mediators. The cause of leptin resistance is unknown. It may be related to a defect in leptin transport, an inability of leptin to cross the blood-brain barrier, an alteration in the permissive effect of leptin, or a defect in or suppression of the leptin receptor. The low-grade inflammation accompanying obesity also is thought to contribute to leptin resistance.[36] Chronic hyperleptinemia also stimulates the sympathetic nervous system, oxidative stress, chronic low-grade inflammation, and ventricular hypertrophy and contributes to the pathogenesis of hypertension, atherosclerosis, cardiovascular disease, and cancer associated with obesity.[37-39]

Decreased beta-cell function and insulin resistance are associated with obesity. The mechanisms are not clear, but there is an association

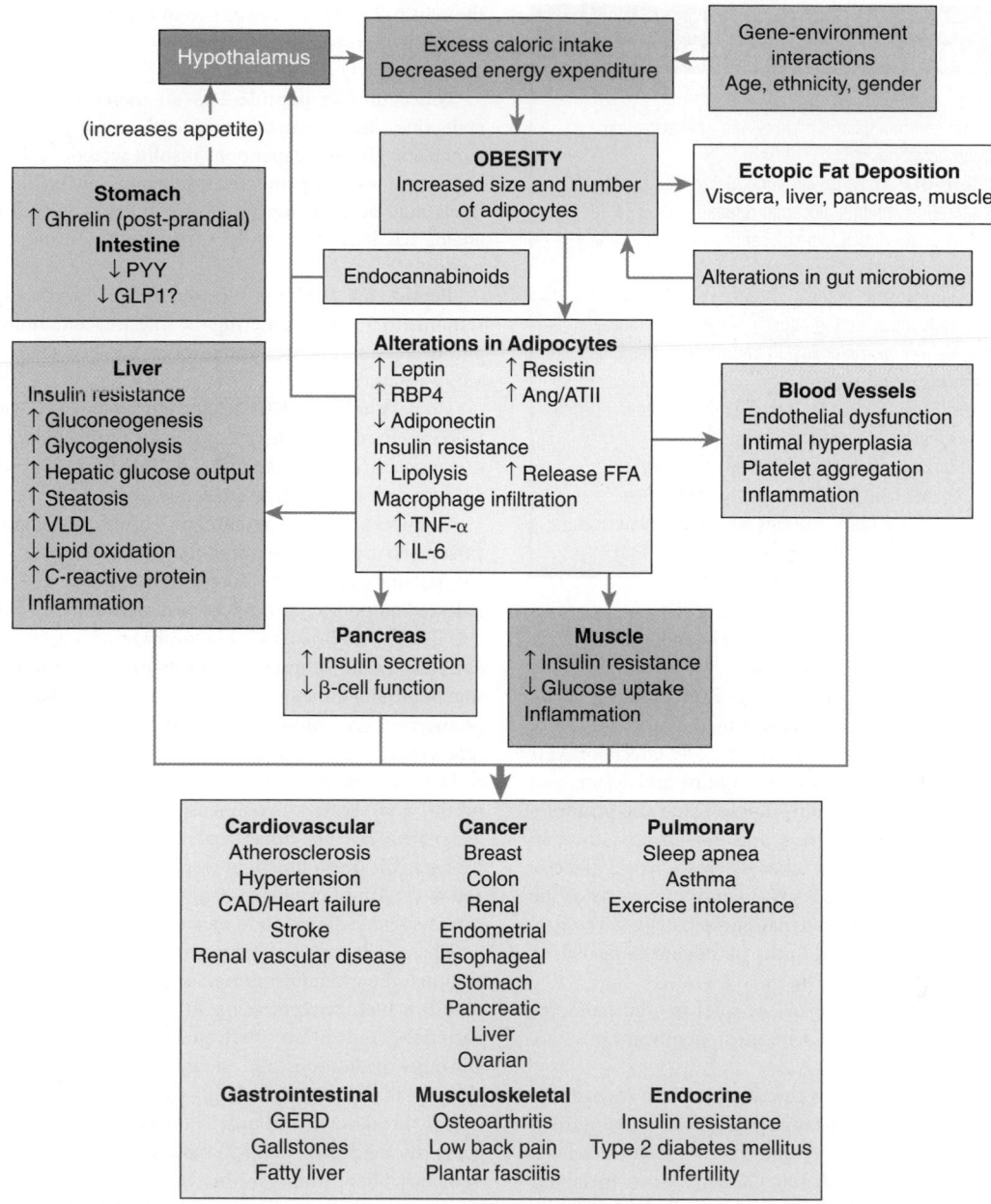

FIGURE 23.1 Pathophysiology and Common Complications of Obesity. See text for details. *Ang/ATII*, Angiotensinogen/angiotensin II; *CAD*, coronary artery disease; *FFA*, free fatty acids; *GERD*, gastroesophageal reflux disease; *GLP1*, glucagon-like peptide 1; *IL-6*, interleukin-6; *PYY*, intestinal peptide YY; *RBP4*, retinol-binding protein 4; *TNF-α*, tumor necrosis factor-alpha; *VLDL*, very-low-density lipoprotein.

between hyperlipidemia and fat storage, macrophages and inflammation, and alterations in adipokines. Leptin resistance and decreased adiponectin contribute to insulin resistance.[40] Insulin resistance results in hyperinsulinemia, hyperglycemia, and a predisposition to type 2 diabetes mellitus. Retinol-binding protein 4 (binds vitamin A) is an adipocytokine produced both in the liver and by adipocytes. It is increased in visceral adiposity and contributes to inflammation and insulin resistance in liver and muscle and is associated with hepatic steatosis and cardiovascular disease.[41,42]

Adiponectin is produced primarily by visceral adipose tissue but is also produced by cardiomyocytes and skeletal muscle. It has insulin-sensitizing and antiinflammatory properties, and plasma levels decrease with visceral obesity, contributing to insulin resistance and type 2 diabetes mellitus.[43] Decreased adiponectin levels are associated with increased

hepatic gluconeogenesis, decreased skeletal muscle glucose uptake, and increased levels of inflammatory mediators, such as interleukin-6 (IL-6) and tumor necrosis factor-alpha (TNF-α). Adiponectin may serve as an antiinflammatory and antiatherogenic plasma protein; it has an important role in vascular remodeling and is cardioprotective.[44] Decreased levels of adiponectin are associated with increased risk for coronary artery disease resulting from hyperlipidemia, hypertension, and factors that promote thrombosis and inflammation.[45,46]

Endocannabinoids (i.e., anandamide) are arachidonic acid derivatives expressed in both the brain and the peripheral nerve tissues, and have effects on endocannabinoid (CB) receptors in orexigenic pathways. They increase appetite, enhance nutrient absorption, stimulate lipogenesis, and increase white adipose tissue accumulation by acting at both central (CB1 receptor) and peripheral sites (CB2 receptor). They also inhibit energy expenditure and thermogenesis. An increase in endocannabinoids is proposed to be associated with obesity.[47,48]

Angiotensinogen (AGT) is produced in the liver and adipocytes and is increased in obesity. AGT is the precursor to angiotensin I (ATI), which is then converted to angiotensin II (ATII). The effects of ATII include vasoconstriction, renal retention of sodium and water, and release of aldosterone. Increased ATII from adipose tissue also promotes inflammation, lipogenesis, oxidative stress, and insulin resistance, all of which contribute to the hypertension, atherosclerosis, type 2 diabetes mellitus, and cancer associated with obesity.[49] Paracrine effects of the renin-angiotensin system in the brain also may participate in the control of energy balance and may be involved in the pathogenesis of obesity and obesity-related hypertension.[50]

Gastrointestinal hormones also play a role in the complex pathophysiology of obesity (Box 23.3). The most significant ones are reviewed next.

Ghrelin is produced by the stomach gastric mucosa in response to hunger and stimulates food intake through activation of the ghrelin receptor (GHS-R) located on neuropeptide Y (NPY)/agouti-related peptide (AgRP) neurons in the hypothalamus. Ghrelin induces metabolic changes leading to an increase in body weight and body fat mass. Ghrelin also stimulates release of growth hormone (GH) from anterior pituitary cells, release of gastric acid, gastrointestinal motility, and pancreatic secretion of insulin. An elevation in the levels of free fatty acids and growth hormone after eating decreases release of ghrelin. It also has satiety, vasodilatory, cardioprotective, and antiproliferative effects.[51,52] In lean individuals, ghrelin levels increase with hunger and fall during the postprandial interval. In people with diet-induced obesity, circulating ghrelin levels tend to be lower with blunted meal-related fluctuations. An obesity-induced central ghrelin resistance has been observed in neural circuits. However, the causative mechanisms relating ghrelin with obesity have yet to be clearly defined.[53]

Signals from leptin and ghrelin are complementary yet antagonistic signals reflecting acute and chronic changes in energy balance, the effects of which are mediated by hypothalamic neuropeptides, such as NPY and AgRP. In obesity, plasma ghrelin level does not decrease after eating. Endocrine and vagal afferent pathways also are involved in the actions of ghrelin and leptin, adding to the complexity of mechanisms that can affect obesity.[54] Ghrelin is thought to have antilipolytic effects and stimulates lipogenesis in visceral WAT.[55] However, with obesity there is

thought to be ghrelin resistance in the hypothalamus. Thus although ghrelin is increased with obesity, its role in contributing to obesity is yet to be clearly defined.[53]

Glucagon-like peptide 1 is an incretin secreted from intestinal endocrine cells when nutrients enter the small intestine. GLP-1 stimulates pancreatic glucose–dependent insulin secretion, delays gastric emptying, suppresses appetite, and increases energy expenditure. GLP-1 levels may be decreased in obese individuals, and a GLP-1 receptor analog has been approved to treat both obesity and type 2 diabetes mellitus.[56,57]

Peptide YY (PYY) is released from intestinal endocrine cells in response to nutrients entering the intestine and inhibits gastric motility and decreases appetite. The level of PYY decreases with increases in adiposity, and decreased PYY level is associated with obesity.[29,58]

Cholecystokinin (CCK) is secreted by proximal small intestinal cells following food intake. Its actions include gallbladder contraction, release of pancreatic enzymes and insulin, satiation, and reduced food intake. CCK secretion is reduced in obesity.[59]

Obesity produces a state of chronic, low-grade inflammation (metabolic triggered inflammation) in WAT. Macrophages, lymphocytes (proinflammatory CD8+ T cells), neutrophils, and mast cells infiltrate enlarged adipocytes and release inflammatory cytokines (e.g., TNF-α, and IL-6)[60] (see Box 23.1). Macrophages change their phenotype from antiinflammatory expression of cytokines (M2 macrophages) to expression of proinflammatory cytokines (M1 macrophages). The mechanisms of macrophage infiltration are thought to be related to adipocyte senescence, necrosis, and death. The inflammatory state is supported by increased levels of leptin and resistin and decreased levels of adiponectin, and escalation of eicosanoid-generating prostaglandins and leukotriene B4. The inflammatory state and accelerated lipolysis contribute to the development of insulin resistance and metabolic syndrome, and to the complications of obesity, particularly type 2 diabetes mellitus, cardiovascular disease, and cancer.[61-64]

Changes in the intestinal microbiome also are associated with obesity, although the mechanisms are not clear. Microbes (mostly bacteria) are found in high concentration in the lower gastrointestinal tract, and bacterial composition is affected by genetics, diet, use of antibiotics and other medications, and energy balance. These bacteria have considerable variability among individuals and participate in complex carbohydrate breakdown and nutrient absorption, inflammatory responses, gut permeability, and bile acid metabolism.[65] Gut microbial fermentation of dietary fiber produces short-chain fatty acids (acetate, butyrate, and propionate) that function as energy sources and signaling molecules that affect host energy metabolism and inflammation. Gut microbiota transplanted from obese mice into germ-free mice or from an obese human twin have shown that the gut microbiota may have a causal role in the development of obesity and insulin resistance.[66] More studies are needed to determine how changes in the microbiota contribute to body weight regulation, metabolism, low-grade inflammation and increased adiposity, and how manipulation of the gut microbiota can assist in preventing or treating obesity.[67,68]

CLINICAL MANIFESTATIONS. Obesity usually presents with two different forms or phenotypes of adipose tissue distribution: visceral and peripheral.[69,70] Visceral obesity (also known as *intraabdominal, central,* or *masculine obesity*) occurs when the distribution of body fat is localized around the abdomen and upper body, resulting in an apple shape. Visceral obesity is associated with accelerated lipolysis and has an increased risk for chronic systemic inflammation, metabolic syndrome, obstructive sleep apnea syndrome, type 2 diabetes mellitus, cardiovascular complications, osteoarthritis, and cancer. Visceral venous blood drains into the portal vein, contributing to higher liver synthesis of plasma lipids. Lipids also are located in intracellular liposomes. In the liver,

---

BOX 23.4 METABOLICALLY HEALTHY OBESITY

Metabolically healthy obesity (MHO, also known as the *obesity paradox*) describes a phenotype of about 10% to 30% of individuals who are obese but have no metabolic-obesity–associated complications (i.e., high insulin sensitivity, absence of metabolic syndrome, high level of cardiorespiratory fitness, adequate inflammatory profile [high adiponectin level, low C-reactive protein, tumor necrosis factor-alpha, and IL-6 levels]) and decreased risk for morbidity and mortality. However, there is no standard definition for this phenotype, and complications related to pulmonary function and to orthopedic and other disorders are often not described. MHO is more prevalent among those with absence of visceral fat accumulation, among women, and among those who are more physically active. Research is in progress to better understand the genetics, body fat distribution patterns, metabolic pathways, adipocyte differentiation, lifestyle practices, age-related adverse outcomes and patterns of morbidity and mortality, and therapeutic options for these individuals.

Data from Gonçalves CG, Glade MJ, Meguid MM: *Nutrition* 32(1):14–20, 2016; Muñoz-Garach A, Cornejo-Pareja I, Tinahones FJ: *Nutrients* 8(6), 2016; Phillips CM: *Ann N Y Acad Sci* 1391(1):85-100, 2016.

---

liposomes can increase in size (steatosis). Increased fat in the liver increases the risk for nonalcoholic fatty liver disease, steatohepatitis, and cirrhosis.[28,71]

Peripheral obesity (also known as *subcutaneous, gluteal-femoral,* or *feminine obesity*) occurs when the distribution of body fat is extraperitoneal and distributed around the thighs and buttocks and through the muscle, resulting in a pear shape; it is more common in premenopausal women. Peripheral and subcutaneous fat is less metabolically active and lipolytic and releases fewer adipocytokines (particularly adiponectin) than visceral fat. Risk factors are still present for the complications of obesity, but they are less severe than those for visceral obesity.[2]

Normal weight obesity (NWO) describes a phenotype of individuals with normal body weight and BMI with percent of body fat greater than 30%. These individuals are at risk for metabolic dysregulation, increases in inflammatory cytokines, insulin resistance, increased risk for cardiovascular disease, and other complications of obesity, and higher mortality.[72] NWO is estimated to occur in 2% to 28% of women and 3% of men.[73] Another phenotype associated with obesity is metabolically healthy obesity (Box 23.4).

◀**EVALUATION AND TREATMENT.** All children and adults should be screened for obesity.[74] There are several methods for estimating or measuring the amount of adipose tissue: anthropometric measurements including weight, height, and circumferences of various body diameters (i.e., waist-to-hip ratios and waist circumference); skinfold thickness (measured via skinfold calipers); ultrasound to measure peripheral body fat; and bioelectric impedance and underwater hydrostatic weighing to calculate total body fat. The only method for directly measuring total body fat is via the DEXA scans (dual energy x-ray absorptiometry).[75]

In clinical practice, anthropometric and body diameter measures are most commonly used to calculate the body mass index because they are the easiest to measure and most cost-effective. Body mass indices have been established based on height, weight, age, gender, and ethnicity. Overweight is defined as a BMI greater than 25 kg/m² and obesity is a BMI greater than 30 kg/m². BMI charts are available for children ages 2 to 20 years; these can be used for comparison during adulthood because obese children generally become obese adults.

However, BMI does not measure the amount and distribution of body fat. Waist circumference (more than 40 inches [102 cm] for men and more than 35 inches [88 cm] for women) adds information to assist with disease risk assessment in general practice. Obesity risk

assessment is available from the American Association of Clinical Endocrinologists and the American College of Endocrinology.[76] No specific diagnostic criteria for obesity have been established.

Obesity is a chronic disease for which various treatment approaches have been used, including correction of metabolic abnormalities and implementation of individually tailored lifestyle interventions, such as weight-reduction diets and exercise programs. Additional treatments include psychotherapy, behavioral modification, self-motivation, and support systems.[77]

Several drugs have been approved for the pharmacologic management of obesity.[78] Currently, bariatric surgical procedures (i.e., the Roux-en-Y gastric bypass, adjustable gastric banding, and sleeve gastrectomy) offer the most significant reduction in weight, reduction in comorbidities, and decrease in insulin resistance for treatment of obesity[78,79] (see *What's New?* Outcomes of Bariatric Surgery). Efforts are continuing to identify the molecular and neuroendocrine causes of obesity. This will lead to more specific and personalized prevention and treatment strategies.[80,81]

WHAT'S NEW?
Outcomes of Bariatric Surgery

Bariatric surgery (BS) includes malabsorptive procedures, such as Roux-en-Y gastric bypass, biliary pancreatic diversion (BPD), intra-gastric balloon (to restrict the gastric volume), and duodenal-jejunal bypass liner; and restrictive procedures, such as vertical sleeve gastrectomy or adjustable gastric banding. BS results in caloric restriction, sustained weight loss (reduction in BMI), glycemic control, reduced inflammation and complex changes in neuroendocrine and immune signals emanating from the gut. BS is performed for individuals with severe obesity, including extremely obese children and adolescents, and improves quality of life compared to other treatments. Improvements in cognitive function, including attention, executive function, and memory, have been documented and may be related to improved cardiovascular function, correction of sleep apnea, reduced insulin resistance, and improved glycemic control. Depression and anxiety also have improved. Physical functioning improves but may be related to efficiency and not absolute improvement in cardiorespiratory or muscle function. Bariatric surgery–induced weight loss improves secretion of glucagon-like peptide 1 (GLP-1) and insulin sensitivity, and it can result in remission of type 2 diabetes, hypertension, hyperlipidemia, obstructive sleep apnea, gastroesophageal reflux, and degenerative joint disease. More data are needed to understand long-term complications, long-term survival, microvascular and macrovascular events, remission of type 2 diabetes, and psychologic responses. There also are changes in hypothalamic signaling with increases in anorexigenic signals and decreases in orexigenic signals; however, more research is needed to understand these mechanisms of change in energy homeostasis. Changes in the intestinal microbiota also have been observed after BS, but the specific changes that may promote or inhibit weight loss are to be determined.

Data from Anhê FF et al: *Can J Diabetes* 2017 May 25 [Epub ahead of print]; Inge et al: *Lancet Diabetes Endocrinol* 5(3):165-173, 2017; Jumbe S, Hamlet C, Meyrick J: *Curr Obes Rep* 6(12):71-78, 2017; Labrecque J et al: *Can J Diabetes* 2017 Mar 29 [Epub ahead of print]; Nguyen NT, Varela JE: *Nat Rev Gastroenterol Hepatol* 14(3):160-169, 2017; Thiara G et al: *Psychosomatics* 58(3):217-227, 2017.

ANOREXIA NERVOSA, BULIMIA NERVOSA, AND BINGE EATING DISORDER

Anorexia nervosa, bulimia nervosa, and binge eating disorder are psychiatric disorders related to a distorted body image with a desire

BOX 23.5   DIAGNOSTIC CRITERIA FOR EATING DISORDERS

Anorexia Nervosa

Persistent restriction of energy intake leading to significantly low body weight (in context of what is minimally expected for age, sex, developmental trajectory, and physical health).

Either an intense fear of gaining weight or of becoming fat, or persistent behavior that interferes with weight gain (even though significantly low weight).

Disturbance in the way one's body weight or shape is experienced, undue influence of body shape and weight on self-evaluation, or persistent lack of recognition of the seriousness of the current low body weight.

Subtypes:

    Restricting type

    Binge-eating/purging type

Bulimia Nervosa

Recurrent episodes of binge eating. An episode of binge eating is characterized by both of the following:

    Eating, in a discrete period of time (e.g., within any 2-hour period), an amount of food that is definitely larger than most people would eat during a similar period of time and under similar circumstances.

    A sense of lack of control over eating during the episode (e.g., a feeling that one cannot stop eating or control what or how much one is eating).

Recurrent inappropriate compensatory behavior in order to prevent weight gain, such as self-induced vomiting; misuse of laxatives, diuretics, or other medications; fasting; or excessive exercise.

The binge eating and inappropriate compensatory behaviors both occur, on average, at least once a week for 3 months.

Self-evaluation is unduly influenced by body shape and weight.

The disturbance does not occur exclusively during episodes of anorexia nervosa.

Binge Eating Disorder*

Recurrent episodes of binge eating. An episode of binge eating is characterized by both of the following:

    Eating, in a discrete period of time (e.g., within any 2-hour period), an amount of food that is definitely larger than most people would eat during a similar period of time and under similar circumstances.

    A sense of lack of control over eating during the episode (e.g., a feeling that one cannot stop eating or control what or how much one is eating).

The binge eating episodes are associated with three or more of the following:

    Eating much more rapidly than normal.

    Eating until feeling uncomfortably full.

    Eating large amounts of food when not feeling physically hungry.

    Eating alone because of feeling embarrassed by how much one is eating.

    Feeling disgusted with oneself, depressed, or very guilty afterward.

    Marked distress regarding binge eating is present.

    Binge eating occurs, on average, at least once a week for 3 months.

    Binge eating is not associated with the recurrent use of inappropriate compensatory behaviors as in bulimia nervosa and does not occur exclusively during the course of bulimia nervosa or anorexia nervosa methods to compensate for overeating, such as self-induced vomiting.

***NOTE:** Binge eating disorder is less common but much more severe than overeating. Binge eating disorder is associated with more subjective distress regarding the eating behavior, and commonly other co-occurring psychologic problems.
Data from American Psychiatric Association (APA): *DSM-5: diagnostic and statistical manual of mental disorders,* ed 5, Arlington, VA, 2013, Author, pp. 338-345.

---

for thinness and a fear of fatness that result in extreme restrictions in eating habits. These psychiatric disorders are included in the Diagnostic and Statistical Manual of Mental Disorders-5 (*DSM-5*) classification of eating disorders by the American Psychiatric Association (Box 23.5). They occur in as many as 1% of young women and adolescent girls in the United States and rarely occur in black women. Only 5% to 10% of cases are men.[82,83] However, eating disorders also may occur in children and women ages 45 to 50 years.[84] Risk factors include genetic, epigenetic, familial, biologic, psychologic, and social factors.[85-90]

Complications of chronic and severe eating disorders are related to malnutrition, and weight changes involve all organ systems and can be life-threatening. Most complications are reversible with treatment (Box 23.6). However, refeeding syndrome can increase morbidity (Box 23.7). The death rate is highest among women with anorexia nervosa, particularly those with a psychiatric comorbidity.[83,91]

STARVATION

Malnutrition is lack of nourishment from inadequate amounts of calories, protein, vitamins, or minerals and is caused by improper diet, alterations in digestion or absorption, chronic disease, or a combination of these factors. **Starvation** is a reduction in energy intake leading to weight loss. Short-term starvation and long-term starvation have different effects. Therapeutic short-term starvation is part of many weight-reduction programs because it causes an initial rapid weight

loss that reinforces the individual's motivation to diet. Therapeutic long-term starvation is used in medically controlled environments to facilitate rapid weight loss in morbidly obese individuals. Pathologic long-term starvation can be caused by poverty; chronic diseases of the cardiovascular, pulmonary, hepatic, and digestive systems; malabsorption syndromes; human immunodeficiency virus (HIV) infection; and cancer.[92]

Short-term starvation, or extended fasting, consists of several days of total dietary abstinence or deprivation. The body responds with mechanisms to protect protein mass. For 4 to 6 hours after the last meal, the body is in a well-fed state and its energy requirements are supplied by glucose from recently ingested carbohydrates. Once all available energy has been absorbed from the intestine, glycogen in the liver is converted to glucose through glycogenolysis, the splitting of glycogen into glucose. This process peaks within 4 to 8 hours, and gluconeogenesis begins. Gluconeogenesis is the formation of glucose from noncarbohydrate molecules: lactate, pyruvate, amino acids, and the glycerol portion of fats from lipolysis. Like glycogenolysis, gluconeogenesis takes place within the liver. Both of these processes deplete stored nutrients and thus cannot meet the body's energy needs indefinitely. Proteins continue to be catabolized to a minimal degree, providing carbon for the synthesis of glucose.[93]

Long-term starvation begins after several days of dietary abstinence and eventually causes death. Absolute deprivation of food causes marasmus or protein-energy malnutrition (loss of muscle mass and

BOX 23.6 COMPLICATIONS OF SEVERE ANOREXIA NERVOSA/BULIMIA

Anorexia Nervosa

Gastrointestinal

Dysphagia related to weakened pharyngeal muscles

Slowed gastric emptying, early satiety, nausea and bloating; gastric dilation is a serious complication

Constipation related to slowed peristalsis

Apoptosis of liver cells related to malnutrition; elevated transaminases

Cardiac

Dysrhythmias: prolonged QT interval, ventricular arrhythmias, and cardiac syncope

Left ventricular atrophy and mitral valve prolapse

Sudden cardiac death

Pulmonary

Complications are rare, but can include aspiration pneumonitis

Hematologic

Anemia, leukopenia, and thrombocytopenia

Delayed response to infection

Musculoskeletal

Osteoporosis: decreased bone formation and increased bone resorption

Increased risk for stress fractures

Endocrine

Hypogonadal: related to reduced pulsed hypothalamic gonadotropin-releasing hormone secretion

Females: low estrogen, loss of menses

Males: low testosterone, low libido, loss of potency and muscle strength

Hypothyroidism: euthyroid sick syndrome, low blood pressure, cold intolerance

Hypercortisolism

Hypoglycemia: depleted liver glycogen stores

Impaired temperature regulation

Neurologic

Brain atrophy and impaired cognitive function

Dermatologic

Xerosis, hair thinning, acrocyanosis

Bulimia

Self-Induced Vomiting

Persistent gastric acid reflux, dysphagia, and dyspepsia: chronic induced vomiting

Electrolyte and acid-base disorders: metabolic alkalosis, hypokalemia

Tooth erosion

Inflammation of vocal cords and hoarse voice

Parotid gland enlargement

Laxative Abuse

Hypokalemic metabolic alkalosis

Diarrhea, hemorrhoids, rectal prolapse

Hyperphosphatemia: use of laxatives containing sodium phosphate

Data from Donaldson AA, Gordon CM: *Metabolism* 64(9):943–951, 2015; Sangvai D: *Prim Care* 43(2):301-312, 2016; Sato Y, Fukudo S: *Clin J Gastroenterol* 8(5):255–263, 2015; Westmoreland P, Krantz MJ, Mehler PS: *Am J Med* 129(1):30–37, 2016.

body fat depletion). Protein deprivation in the presence of carbohydrate intake is called *kwashiorkor* (loss of muscle mass with sustained body fat). Marasmic kwashiorkor (edematous, severe childhood malnutrition) is a combination of chronic energy deficiency and chronic or acute protein deficiency and inadequate micronutrients.[94] These conditions are described in Chapter 43. Anorexia nervosa is a psychologic cause of long-term starvation (see Box 23.5). Cachexia (also known as *cytokine-induced malnutrition*) is physical wasting with loss of weight and muscle atrophy, fatigue, and weakness. Inflammatory mediators (i.e., TNF-α, interferon-γ, IL-1, IL-6) and an increased catabolic response are associated with the cachexia of advanced cancer.[95-97] Cancer, AIDS, tuberculosis, and other major chronic progressive diseases contribute to cachexia. Anorexia and cachexia often occur together. Cachexia is not the same as food deprivation starvation. A healthy person's body can adjust to starvation by slowing the metabolic rate; however, in cachexia, the body does not make this adjustment.

The major characteristic of long-term starvation is a decreased dependence on gluconeogenesis and an increased use of ketone bodies (products of lipid and pyruvate metabolism) as a cellular energy source. During long-term starvation, depressed insulin levels and increased levels of glucagon, cortisone, epinephrine, and growth hormones promote lipolysis in adipose tissue. Lipolysis liberates fatty acids, which supply energy to cardiac and skeletal muscle cells, and ketone bodies, which sustain brain tissue. Fatty acid, or ketone body, oxidation meets most of the energy needs of the cells. (Some glucose is still needed as fuel for brain tissue.) Once the supply of adipose tissue is depleted, proteolysis begins. The breakdown of muscle and visceral protein is the last process the body engages to supply energy for life. Death results from severe alterations in electrolyte balance and loss of renal, pulmonary, and cardiac function.[98]

Adequate ingestion of appropriate nutrients is the obvious treatment for starvation. In medically induced starvation the body is maintained in a ketotic state until the desired amount of adipose tissue has been lysed. Starvation imposed by chronic disease, long-term illness, malabsorption syndromes, and chronic eating disorders is treated with enteral or parenteral nutrition. Perioperative or critical care management of nutrition is necessary to prevent unnecessary starvation.[99] Care must be taken to prevent refeeding syndrome (see Box 23.7) during the treatment of long-term starvation.

ANOREXIA OF AGING

Anorexia of aging is defined as a decrease in appetite or food intake in older adults, and can occur in illness-free individuals and in the presence of an adequate food supply. The resulting undernutrition leads to adverse outcomes and may affect up to 20% to 30% of elders.[100] The anorexia of aging results from multiple age-related changes, including reduced energy needs, waning hunger, diminished senses of smell and taste, decreased production of saliva, altered gastrointestinal satiety control mechanisms, and the presence of comorbidities. Centrally, aging is associated with decreased orexigenic signals (e.g., levels of ghrelin or ghrelin resistance and reduced NPY or NPY receptors, or both) and increased anorexigenic signals (e.g., decreased levels of leptin, insulin, PPY, and CCK), which lead to loss of appetite and diminished food intake. Chronic low-grade inflammation with elevated cytokines also can contribute to delayed gastric emptying and decreased motility of

---

BOX 23.7 **REFEEDING SYNDROME**

Refeeding syndrome occurs in severely malnourished individuals when parenteral or enteral nutritional therapy is initiated. During starvation, loss of body minerals causes the movement of phosphate, magnesium, and potassium ions out of the cells and into the plasma. When refeeding starts, an increase in insulin levels stimulates the movement of glucose and these ions back into the cells, and the plasma concentrations can decrease to dangerously low levels, causing hypophosphatemia, hypomagnesemia, hypokalemia, hyponatremia, hypocalcemia, and vitamin deficiency. Rapid expansion of the extracellular fluid volume also can occur with carbohydrate refeeding and may cause fluid overload. Hypophosphatemia contributes to alterations in red blood cell shape and function, contributing to tissue hypoxia and increased respiratory drive. The consequences of these alterations include life-threatening dysrhythmias, congestive heart failure, muscle weakness (including respiratory muscles), and death. Individuals at greatest risk are those with starvation from any cause including anorexia nervosa, chronic alcoholism, morbid obesity with massive weight loss, and prolonged fasting. Refeeding syndrome is prevented by slowly reinstituting feeding (about 20 kcal/kg/day for the first few days) and monitoring plasma levels of phosphate, potassium, magnesium, and calcium during the change from catabolic to anabolic metabolism. Some studies have recommended higher caloric feedings (≥1400 kcal/d).

Data from Crook MA: *Nutrition* 30(11–12):1448–1455, 2014; Garber et al: *Int J Eat Disord* 49(3):293-310, 2016; Sachs K et al: *Eat Disord* 2015;23(5):411–421, 2015.

---

the small intestine. Risk factors for anorexia of aging include functional impairments and deficiencies (e.g., loss of vision, poor dentition, inability to prepare foods); medical and psychiatric conditions (such as malabsorption syndromes and depression); loneliness and grief; medications, including polypharmacy; social isolation; and abuse or neglect.[101] The consequences of anorexia of aging include malnutrition, physical frailty, mitochondrial dysfunction, reduced regenerative capacity, increased oxidative stress, and imbalanced hormonal levels. There are no currently used specific treatments for the anorexia of aging, though numerous supportive strategies are used (e.g., improved food access and appearance, dental and eye care, social stimulation). Death rates have been shown to be higher in those with anorexia of aging and unintentional weight loss.[102]

SUMMARY REVIEW

Adipose Tissue

1. Adipose tissue provides insulation and tissue support and is the body's major energy reserve, storing triglycerides and glycerol.
2. Adipose tissue is an endocrine organ that secretes hormones called adipokines with autocrine, paracrine, and endocrine actions necessary for metabolic function and immune responses.
3. WAT has a stromal structure that contains macrophages, mast cells, neutrophils, fibroblasts, endothelial cells, blood vessels, nerves, and precursor adipocytes.
4. WAT is the largest fat depot and is located in visceral (central) and subcutaneous (peripheral) sites. It also is located in muscle and bone marrow.
5. White adipocytes store fat as a single lipid droplet or vacuole.
6. With positive energy balance, WAT storage increases by adipocyte hypertrophy (more common in visceral fat) and adipogenesis (more common in subcutaneous fat).
7. Estrogen enhances the deposition of subcutaneous fat compared to visceral fat.
8. BAT has multiple lipid droplets and is rich in mitochondria containing iron, giving BAT a brown color. Exposure to cold, sympathetic activation and release of catecholamines, and activation of T_3 generate heat through activation of UCP1 and free fatty acid oxidation (nonshivering thermogenesis).
9. Both neonates and adults have BAT, but not in the amounts of WAT.
10. bAT emerges within WAT with exposure to cold, exercise, and synthetic ligands of PPARγ. This is known as the *"beiging" of WAT*.
11. BAT and bAT both protect against obesity and metabolic syndrome.
12. In muscle, the myokines irisin and fibroblast growth factor-21, respectively, activate BAT and bAT for thermogenesis and protect against obesity.
13. Bone marrow adipose tissue also releases adipokine, and there is crosstalk with osteoclasts to maintain bone structure.

Obesity

1. Obesity is an epidemic that has occurred worldwide in both adults and children and is the fifth leading cause of death in the United States. Three leading causes of death in the United States are associated with obesity: cardiovascular disease, type 2 diabetes mellitus, and certain cancers. Obesity also increases the risk for numerous other systemic disorders.
2. Obesity is defined as a BMI greater than 30 kg/m² in adults and a BMI greater than or equal to the age- and sex-specific 95th percentile of the 2000 Centers for Disease Control and Prevention growth charts in children and usually results from energy intake exceeding expenditure.
3. Single-gene (rare) and polygenetic disorders and metabolic disorders are associated with obesity, as well gene-environment interactions.
4. Regulation of food intake and energy expenditure is coordinated centrally by the hypothalamus and higher brain centers. Two opposing sets of neurons in the arcuate nucleus of the hypothalamus regulate appetite and energy metabolism: orexigenic neurons, which promote appetite, stimulate eating, and decrease metabolism; and anorexigenic neurons, which suppress appetite, inhibit eating, and increase metabolism.
5. Brain centers related to reward, pleasure, and memory can override hypothalamic control of food intake and satiety, causing increased fat stores by increasing consumption of highly palatable foods.
6. Adipokines and gastrointestinal hormones are altered with obesity and contribute to associated complications.
7. Leptin levels increase with obesity (leptin resistance), promoting overeating, insulin resistance and hyperinsulinemia, and hyperlipidemia, and stimulating adipocyte endothelial cells and macrophages to release inflammatory mediators contributing to the complications of obesity.
8. RBP4 levels are increased in visceral adiposity and promote insulin resistance and hepatic steatosis.

■ SUMMARY REVIEW—cont'd

9. Adiponectin levels decrease with obesity, contributing to insulin resistance, inflammation, and hyperlipidemia.

10. Endocannabinoids are increased in obesity and promote food intake and lipogenesis and inhibit energy expenditure.

11. Angiotensin I and angiotensin II increase in obesity, promoting vasoconstriction, inflammation, lipogenesis, oxidative stress, and insulin resistance.

12. Ghrelin increases with obesity and stimulates food intake, promotes release of growth hormone, and stimulates lipogenesis. It also has satiety, vasodilatory, cardioprotective, and antiproliferative effects; its role in obesity is not clear.

13. Glucagon-like peptide 1 promotes insulin secretion, delays gastric emptying, suppresses appetite, and increases energy expenditure, and is decreased with obesity.

14. Peptide YY inhibits gastric motility, decreases appetite, and is decreased with obesity.

15. Obesity is a state of chronic low-grade inflammation caused by expansion of adipocyte macrophages, neutrophils, and lymphocytes that release inflammatory mediators.

16. The chronic inflammation, alterations in adipokine action, and accelerated lipolysis related to excessive fat contribute to the complications of obesity, particularly insulin resistance, type 2 diabetes mellitus, cardiovascular disease, and cancer.

17. Changes in the intestinal microbiome also contribute to obesity, but the mechanisms need to be defined.

18. Obesity has two major phenotypes: visceral, or central obesity; and peripheral, or subcutaneous obesity. Visceral obesity has the greatest risk for accelerated lipolysis, chronic inflammation, insulin resistance, and associated complications.

19. Treatment of obesity may include correction of metabolic abnormalities, and individually tailored lifestyle interventions (diets, exercise, behavioral modifications, self-motivation) and psychotherapy. The current most effective treatment for extreme obesity is bariatric surgery.

20. New drugs are being developed that target specific molecules and will provide a personalized approach to treatment.

Anorexia Nervosa, Bulimia Nervosa, and Binge Eating Disorder

1. Eating disorders include anorexia nervosa, bulimia nervosa, and binge eating disorder. They are psychogenic disorders that can lead to malnutrition.

2. Complications of chronic and severe eating disorders lead to malnutrition and weight changes, involve all organ systems, and can be life-threatening. Most complications are reversible with treatment.

Starvation

1. The body responds to short-term starvation with mechanisms to protect protein mass, using the processes of glycogenolysis and gluconeogenesis. Neither of these processes can meet the body's energy needs indefinitely since they deplete stored nutrients.

2. Long-term starvation results in an initial decreased dependence on gluconeogenesis and an increased use of ketone bodies as a cellular energy source, followed by lipolysis in adipose tissue. In the absence of adequate nutrition, long-term starvation results in proteolysis with death resulting from severe alterations in electrolyte balance and loss of renal, pulmonary, and cardiac function.

Anorexia of Aging

1. Anorexia of aging is a decrease in appetite or food intake in older adults leading to undernutrition and resulting in a decline in function and increased risk for morbidity and mortality.

2. Contributing factors related to aging include diminished sensory functions, poor dentition, decreased gastric emptying, decreased hunger and satiety, effects of medications, social isolation, and neglect.

■ KEY TERMS

Arcuate nucleus (ARC), 716
Adiponectin, 717
Adipose tissue, 713
Anorexia of aging, 721
Angiotensinogen (AGT), 718
Beige adipocyte, 715

Brown adipocyte, 715
Cholecystokinin (CCK), 718
Endocannabinoid, 717
Ghrelin, 718
Glucagon-like peptide 1, 718
Leptin, 716

Malnutrition, 720
Obesity, 715
Peptide YY (PYY), 718
Retinol-binding protein 4, 717
Starvation, 720
White adipose tissue (WAT), 713

REFERENCES

1. Booth A, et al: Adipose tissue: an endocrine organ playing a role in metabolic regulation. *Horm Mol Biol Clin Investig* 26(1):25–42, 2016.

2. Kwok KH, Lam KS, Xu A: Heterogeneity of white adipose tissue: molecular basis and clinical implications. *Exp Mol Med* 48:e215, 2016.

3. Park A, Kim WK, Bae KH: Distinction of white, beige and brown adipocytes derived from mesenchymal stem cells. *World J Stem Cells* 6(1):33–42, 2014.

4. Sanchez-Gurmaches J, Guertin DA: Adipocyte lineages: tracing back the origins of fat. *Biochim Biophys Acta* 1842(3):340–351, 2014.

5. DiSpirito JR, Mathis D: Immunological contributions to adipose tissue homeostasis. *Semin Immunol* 27(5):315–321, 2015.

6. Zhang M, et al: Associations of different adipose tissue depots with insulin resistance: a systematic review and meta-analysis of observational studies. *Sci Rep* 5:18495, 2015.

7. Palmer BF, Clegg DJ: The sexual dimorphism of obesity. *Mol Cell Endocrinol* 402:113–119, 2015.

8. Kiefer FW: Browning and thermogenic programing of adipose tissue. *Best Pract Res Clin Endocrinol Metab* 30(4):479–485, 2016.

9. Gantner ML, et al: Complementary roles of estrogen-related receptors in brown adipocyte thermogenic function. *Endocrinology* 157(12):4770–4781, 2016.

10. Virtanen KA: The rediscovery of BAT in adult humans using imaging. *Best Pract Res Clin Endocrinol Metab* 30(4):471–477, 2016.

11. Sakai J, Kajimura S: Transcriptional and epigenetic control of brown and beige adipose cell fate and function. *Nat Rev Mol Cell Biol* 17(8):480–495, 2016.

12. Cereijo R, Giralt M, Villarroya F: Thermogenic brown and beige/brite adipogenesis in humans. *Ann Med* 47(2):169–177, 2015.

13. Rodríguez A, et al: Crosstalk between adipokines and myokines in fat browning. *Acta Physiol (Oxf)* 219(2):362–381, 2017.

14. McMillan AC, White MD: Induction of thermogenesis in brown and beige adipose tissues: molecular markers, mild cold exposure and novel therapies. *Curr Opin Endocrinol Diabetes Obes* 22(5):347–352, 2015.

15. Lecka-Czernik B, Rosen CJ: Skeletal integration of energy homeostasis: translational implications. *Bone* 82:35–41, 2016.

16. Del Prete A, Salvi V, Sozzani S: Adipokines as potential biomarkers in rheumatoid arthritis. *Mediators Inflamm* 2014:425068, 2014.

17. Devlin MJ, Rosen CJ: The bone-fat interface: basic and clinical implications of marrow adiposity. *Lancet Diabetes Endocrinol* 3(2):141–147, 2015.

18. González-Muniesa P, et al: Obesity. *Nat Rev Dis Primers* 3:17034, 2017.

19. Ogden CL, et al: *Prevalence of obesity among adults and youth: United States, 2011–2014, National Center for Health Statistics (NCHS) data brief, no. 219*, Hyattsville, MD, 2015, National Center for Health Statistics. Available at: https://www.cdc.gov/nchs/data/databriefs/db219.pdf.

20. Finkelstein EA, et al: Obesity and severe obesity forecasts through 2030. *Am J Prev Med* 42(6):563–570, 2012.

21. Smith KB, Smith MS: Obesity statistics. *Prim Care* 43(1):121–135, 2016.

22. Lauby-Secretan B, et al: Body fatness and cancer—viewpoint of the IARC Working Group. *N Engl J Med* 375:794–798, 2016.

23. Roth J, et al: Obesity paradox, obesity orthodox, and the metabolic syndrome: an approach to unity. *Mol Med* 22:873–885, 2016.

24. Huang T, Hu FB: Gene-environment interactions and obesity: recent developments and future directions. *BMC Med Genomics* 8(Suppl 1):S2, 2015.

25. Albuquerque D, et al: Current review of genetics of human obesity: from molecular mechanisms to an evolutionary perspective. *Mol Genet Genomics* 290(4):1191–1221, 2015.

26. Cheung WW, Mao P: Recent advances in obesity: genetics and beyond. *ISRN Endocrinol* 2012:536905, 2012.

27. Jantaratnotai N, et al: The interface of depression and obesity. *Obes Res Clin Pract* 11(1):1–10, 2017.

28. Heymsfield SB, Wadden TA: Mechanisms, pathophysiology, and management of obesity. *N Engl J Med* 376(3):254–266, 2017.

29. Mishra AK, Dubey V, Ghosh AR: Obesity: an overview of possible role(s) of gut hormones, lipid sensing and gut microbiota. *Metabolism* 65(1):48–65, 2016.

30. Choe SS, et al: Adipose tissue remodeling: its role in energy metabolism and metabolic disorders. *Front Endocrinol (Lausanne)* 7:30, 2016.

31. Yu JH, Kim MS: Molecular mechanisms of appetite regulation. *Diabetes Metab J* 36(6):391–398, 2012.

32. Jauch-Chara K, Oltmanns KM: Obesity—a neuropsychological disease? Systematic review and neuropsychological model. *Prog Neurobiol* 114:84–101, 2014.

33. Münzberg H, et al: Neural control of energy expenditure. *Handb Exp Pharmacol* 233:173–194, 2016.

34. Murray S, et al: Hormonal and neural mechanisms of food reward, eating behaviour and obesity. *Nat Rev Endocrinol* 10(9):540–552, 2014.

35. Park H-K, Ahima RS: Physiology of leptin: energy homeostasis, neuroendocrine function and metabolism. *Metabolism* 64(1):24–34, 2015.

36. Santoro A, Mattace Raso G, Meli R: Drug targeting of leptin resistance. *Life Sci* 140:64–74, 2015.

37. Feijóo-Bandín S, et al: 20 years of leptin: role of leptin in cardiomyocyte physiology and physiopathology. *Life Sci* 140:10–18, 2015.

38. Mullen M, Gonzalez-Perez RR: Leptin-induced JAK/STAT signaling and cancer growth. *Vaccines (Basel)* 4(3):2016.

39. Sáinz N, et al: Leptin resistance and diet-induced obesity: central and peripheral actions of leptin. *Metabolism* 64(1):35–46, 2015.

40. Yadav A, Katarina MA, Saini V: Role of leptin and adiponectin in insulin resistance. *Clin Chim Acta* 417:80–84, 2013.

41. Liu Y, et al: Retinol-binding protein 4 induces hepatic mitochondrial dysfunction and promotes hepatic steatosis. *J Clin Endocrinol Metab* 101(11):4338–4348, 2016.

42. Noy N, et al: Is retinol binding protein 4 a link between adiposity and cancer? *Horm Mol Biol Clin Investig* 23(2):39–46, 2015.

43. Shehzad A, et al: Adiponectin: regulation of its production and its role in human diseases. *Hormones (Athens)* 11(1):8–20, 2012.

44. Ghantous CM, et al: Differential role of leptin and adiponectin in cardiovascular system. *Int J Endocrinol* 2015:534320, 2015.

45. Ebrahimi-Mamaeghani M, et al: Adiponectin as a potential biomarker of vascular disease. *Vasc Health Risk Manag* 11:55–70, 2015.

46. Ohashi K, et al: Adiponectin as a target in obesity-related inflammatory state. *Endocr Metab Immune Disord Drug Targets* 15(2):145–150, 2015.

47. Mazier W, et al: The endocannabinoid system: pivotal orchestrator of obesity and metabolic disease. *Trends Endocrinol Metab* 26(10):524–537, 2015.

48. Quarta C, et al: Energy balance regulation by endocannabinoids at central and peripheral levels. *Trends Mol Med* 17(9):518–526, 2011.

49. Ramalingam L, et al: The renin angiotensin system, oxidative stress and mitochondrial function in obesity and insulin resistance. *Biochim Biophys Acta* 1863(5):1106–1114, 2016.

50. Littlejohn NK, Grobe JL: Opposing tissue-specific roles of angiotensin in the pathogenesis of obesity, and implications for obesity-related hypertension. *Am J Physiol Regul Integr Comp Physiol* 309(12):R1463–R1473, 2015.

51. Perello M, et al: Functional implications of limited leptin receptor and ghrelin receptor coexpression in the brain. *J Comp Neurol* 520(2):281–294, 2012.

52. Sato T, et al: Physiological roles of ghrelin on obesity. *Obes Res Clin Pract* 8(5):e405–e413, 2014.

53. Zigman JM, Bouret SG, Andrews ZB: Obesity impairs the action of the neuroendocrine ghrelin system. *Trends Endocrinol Metab* 27(1):54–63, 2016.

54. McKenney RL, Short DK: Tipping the balance: the pathophysiology of obesity and type 2 diabetes mellitus. *Surg Clin North Am* 91(6):1139–1148, vii, 2011.

55. Rodríguez A, et al: Acylated and desacyl ghrelin stimulate lipid accumulation in human visceral adipocytes. *Int J Obes* 33(5):541–552, 2009.

56. Burcelin R, Gourdy P: Harnessing glucagon-like peptide-1 receptor agonists for the pharmacological treatment of overweight and obesity. *Obes Rev* 18(1):86–98, 2016.

57. Deacon CF, Ahrén B: Physiology of incretins in health and disease. *Rev Diabet Stud* 8(3):293–306, 2011.

58. Karra E, Chandarana K, Batterham RL: The role of peptide YY in appetite regulation and obesity. *J Physiol* 587(Pt 1):19–25, 2009.

59. Miller LJ, Desai AJ: Metabolic actions of the type 1 cholecystokinin receptor: its potential as a therapeutic target. *Trends Endocrinol Metab* 27(9):609–619, 2016.

60. Chatzigeorgiou A, Chavakis T: Immune cells and metabolism. *Handb Exp Pharmacol* 233:221–249, 2016.

61. Bai Y, Sun Q: Macrophage recruitment in obese adipose tissue. *Obes Rev* 16(2):127–136, 2015.

62. Harwood HJ, Jr: The adipocyte as an endocrine organ in the regulation of metabolic homeostasis. *Neuropharmacol* 63(1):57–75, 2012.

63. Titos E, Clària J: Omega-3-derived mediators counteract obesity-induced adipose tissue inflammation. *Prostaglandins Other Lipid Mediat* 107:77–84, 2013.

64. Vieira-Potter VJ: Inflammation and macrophage modulation in adipose tissues. *Cell Microbiol* 16:1484–1492, 2014.

65. Rosenbaum M, Knight R, Leibel RL: The gut microbiota in human energy homeostasis and obesity. *Trends Endocrinol Metab* 26(9):493–501, 2015.

66. Komaroff AL: The microbiome and risk for obesity and diabetes. *JAMA* 317(4):355–356, 2016.

67. Gérard P: Gut microbiota and obesity. *Cell Mol Life Sci* 73(1):147–162, 2016.

68. Sze MA, Schloss PD: Looking for a signal in the noise: revisiting obesity and the microbiome. *MBio* 7(4):pii:e01018, 2016.

69. Ibrahim MM: Subcutaneous and visceral adipose tissue: structural and functional differences. *Obes Rev* 11(1):p11–18, 2010.

70. Karpe F, Pinnick KE: Biology of upper-body and lower-body adipose tissue—link to whole-body phenotypes. *Nat Rev Endocrinol* 11(2):90–100, 2015.

71. Lopes HF, et al: Visceral adiposity syndrome. *Diabetol Metab Syndr* 8:40, 2016.

72. Franco LP, Morais CC, Cominetti C: Normal-weight obesity syndrome: diagnosis, prevalence, and clinical implications. *Nutr Rev* 74(9):558–570, 2016.

73. Marques-Vidal P, et al: Prevalence of normal weight obesity in Switzerland: effect of various definitions. *Eur J Nutr* 47(5):251–257, 2008.

74. Kushner RF, Ryan D: Answers to clinical questions in the primary care management of people with obesity: screening and diagnosis. *J Fam Pract* 65(7 Suppl):S2–S4, 2016.

75. Andreoli A, et al: Body composition in clinical practice. *Eur J Radiol* 85(8):1461–1468, 2016.

76. Garvey WT, et al: American Association of Clinical Endocrinologists and American College of Endocrinology position statement on the 2014 advanced framework for a new diagnosis of obesity as a chronic disease. *Endocr Pract* 20:977–989, 2014.

77. Kelley CP, Sbrocco G, Sbrocco T: Behavioral modification for the management of obesity. *Prim Care* 43(1):159–175, 2016.

78. Bray GA, et al: Management of obesity. *Lancet* 387(10031):1947–1956, 2016.

79. Dixon JB: Obesity in 2015: advances in managing obesity. *Nat Rev Endocrinol* 12(2):65–66, 2016.

80. Jackson VM, et al: Latest approaches for the treatment of obesity. *Expert Opin Drug Discov* 10(8):825–839, 2015.

81. Maksimov ML, et al: Approaches for the development of drugs for treatment of obesity and metabolic syndrome. *Curr Pharm Des* 22(7):895–903, 2016.

82. Raevuori A, Keski-Rahkonen A, Hoek HW: A review of eating disorders in males. *Curr Opin Psychiatry* 27(6):426–430, 2014.

83. Smink FR, van Hoeken D, Hoek HW: Epidemiology of eating disorders: incidence, prevalence and mortality rates. *Curr Psychiatry Rep* 14(4):406–414, 2012.

84. Baker JH, Runfola CD: Eating disorders in midlife women: a perimenopausal eating disorder? *Maturitas* 85:112–116, 2016.

85. Bakalar JL, et al: Recent advances in developmental and risk factor research on eating disorders. *Curr Psychiatry Rep* 17(6):42, 2015.

86. Dubosc A, et al: Early adult sexual assault and disordered eating: the mediating role of posttraumatic stress symptoms. *J Trauma Stress* 25(1):50–56, 2012.

87. Fischer S, Stojek M, Hartzell E: Effects of multiple forms of childhood abuse and adult sexual assault on current eating disorder symptoms. *Eat Behav* 11(3):190–192, 2010.

88. Helder SG, Collier DA: The genetics of eating disorders. *Curr Top Behav Neurosci* 6:157–175, 2011.

89. Pjetri E, et al: Epigenetics and eating disorders. *Curr Opin Clin Nutr Metab Care* 15(4):330–335, 2012.

90. Reyes-Rodríguez ML, et al: Posttraumatic stress disorder in anorexia nervosa. *Psychosom Med* 73(6):491–497, 2011.

91. Kask J, et al: Mortality in women with anorexia nervosa: the role of comorbid psychiatric disorders. *Psychosom Med* 78(8):910–919, 2016.

92. Jensen GL, Wheeler D: A new approach to defining and diagnosing malnutrition in adult critical illness. *Curr Opin Crit Care* 18(2):206–211, 2012.

93. Finn PF, Dice JF: Proteolytic and lipolytic responses to starvation. *Nutrition* 22(7-8):830–844, 2006.

94. Tierney EP, Sage RJ, Shwayder T: Kwashiorkor from a severe dietary restriction in an 8-month infant in suburban Detroit, Michigan: case report and review of the literature. *Int J Dermatol* 49(5):500–506, 2010.

95. Esposito A, et al: Mechanisms of anorexia-cachexia syndrome and rational for treatment with selective ghrelin receptor agonist. *Cancer Treat Rev* 41(9):793–797, 2015.

96. Kim HJ, et al: Pathophysiological role of hormones and cytokines in cancer cachexia. *J Korean Med Sci* 27(2):128–134, 2012.

97. Petruzzelli M, Wagner EF: Mechanisms of metabolic dysfunction in cancer-associated cachexia. *Genes Dev* 30(5):489–501, 2016.

98. Berkley JA, et al: Prognostic indicators of early and late death in children admitted to district hospital in Kenya: cohort study. *BMJ* 326(7385): 361, 2003.

99. Hiesmayr M: Nutrition risk assessment in the ICU. *Curr Opin Clin Nutr Metab Care* 15(2): 174–180, 2012.

100. Sanford AM: Anorexia of aging and its role in frailty. *Curr Opin Clin Nutr Metab Care* 20(1): 54–60, 2017.

101. Landi F, et al: Anorexia of aging: risk factors, consequences and potential treatments. *Nutrients* 8(2):69, 2016.

102. Wysokiński A, et al: Mechanisms of the anorexia of aging—a review. *Age (Dordr)* 37(4):9821, 2015.

CHAPTER

24

Structure and Function of the Reproductive Systems

George W. Rodway, Sue E. Huether

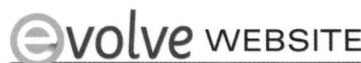

http://evolve.elsevier.com/McCance/
- Content Updates
- Chapter Summary Review
- Review Questions
- Case Studies
- Animations

CHAPTER OUTLINE

The male and female reproductive systems have several anatomic and physiologic features in common. Most obvious is their major function, reproduction, through which a 23-chromosome female gamete, the ovum, and a 23-chromosome male gamete, the spermatozoon (sperm cell), unite to form a 46-chromosome zygote that is capable of developing into a new individual. The male reproductive system produces sperm and delivers them to the female reproductive tract. The female reproductive system produces the ovum and, if it is fertilized, can nurture and protect it (at that point called the embryo and developing fetus) and expel it at birth. These functions are determined not only by anatomic structures but also by complex hormonal, neurologic, and psychogenic factors.

DEVELOPMENT OF THE REPRODUCTIVE SYSTEMS

The structure and function of the male and female reproductive systems depend on steroid hormones called sex hormones and their precursors. Cholesterol is the precursor for steroid hormones, including the sex hormones. Other hormones support reproduction. The actions of both sex and reproductive hormones are summarized in Table 24.1. Sex hormones, like all hormones, act on target tissues by binding with cellular receptors (see Chapter 21). Hormonal effects on the reproductive systems begin well before birth and continue for life.

TABLE 24.1   SUMMARY OF FEMALE AND MALE SEX AND REPRODUCTIVE HORMONES

HORMONE (SOURCE)	ACTION IN FEMALES	ACTION IN MALES
Dehydroepiandrosterone (DHEA) (adrenal gland, ovary, other tissues)	Converted to androstenedione and then to estrogens, testosterone, or both	Converted to androstenedione and then to estrogens, testosterone, or both
Estrogens (estrone, estradiol, estriol) function through estrogen receptors alpha and beta (ovary and placenta, small amounts in other tissues)	Stimulates development of female sexual characteristics: maturation of breast, uterus, and vagina; promotes proliferative development of endometrium during menstrual cycle; during pregnancy promotes mammary gland development, fetal adrenal gland function, and uteroplacental blood flow	Growth at puberty, growth plate fusion in bone, prevention of apoptosis of germ cells
Testosterone (adrenal glands from DHEA, ovaries)	Libido, learning, sleep, protein anabolism, growth of muscle and bone; growth of pubic and axillary hair; activation of sebaceous glands, accounting for some cases of acne during puberty	Stimulates spermatogenesis, stimulates development of primary and secondary sexual characteristics, promotes growth of muscle and bone (anabolic effect); growth of pubic and axillary hair; activates sebaceous glands, accounting for some cases of acne during puberty; maintains libido
Gonadotropin-releasing hormone (GnRH) (hypothalamus-neuroendocrine cells)	Stimulates secretion of gonadotropins (FSH and LH) from anterior pituitary	Stimulates secretion of gonadotropins (FSH and LH) from anterior pituitary
Follicle-stimulating hormone (FSH) (anterior pituitary, gonadotroph cells)	Gonadotropin; promotes development of ovarian follicle; stimulates estrogen secretion	Gonadotropin; promotes development of testes and stimulates spermatogenesis by Sertoli cells
Luteinizing hormone (LH) (anterior pituitary, gonadotroph cells)	Gonadotropin; triggers ovulation; promotes development of corpus luteum	Gonadotropin; stimulates testosterone production by Leydig cells of testis
Inhibin (ovary and testes)	Inhibits FSH production in anterior pituitary (perhaps by limiting GnRH)	Inhibits FSH production in anterior pituitary
Human chorionic gonadotropin (hCG) (placenta)	Supports corpus luteum, which secretes estrogen and progesterone during first 7 weeks of pregnancy	
Activin (ovary)	Stimulates secretion of FSH and pituitary response to GnRH and FSH binding in dominant granulosa cells	
Progesterone (ovary and placenta)	Promotes secretory changes in endometrium during luteal phase of menstrual cycle; quiets uterine myometrium (muscle) activity and prevents lactogenesis during pregnancy	
Relaxin (corpus luteum, myometrium, and placenta)	Inhibits uterine contractions during pregnancy and softens pelvic joints and cervix to facilitate childbirth	

Sexual Differentiation and Hormone Production In Utero

Initially in embryonic development, the reproductive structures of male and female embryos are homologous (the same) or undifferentiated. They consist of one pair of primary sex organs, or **gonads**, and two pairs of ducts: the mesonephric ducts (wolffian ducts) and the paramesonephric ducts (müllerian ducts). The müllerian ducts are the precursor of the internal female sex organs (oviducts, uterus, cervix, and upper vagina). Müllerian ducts are initially formed regardless of genotypic sex and require no sex-determining region on the Y chromosome *(SRY)* signaling for development. *SRY* signaling is required in males to cause regression of the müllerian ducts, which in turn prevents the development of the female reproductive tract. The wolffian ducts are the precursors of male internal sex organs (secrete testosterone and promote development of the male sex organs) (Fig. 24.1). Both pairs of ducts empty into an opening called the *urogenital sinus*.

The first sign of development of reproductive organs (male or female) occurs during the fifth week of gestation. Between 6 and 7 weeks' gestation, the male embryo will differentiate under the influence of testes-determining factor (TDF), a protein expressed by a gene in the SRY. When the *SRY* gene is expressed, male gonadal development prevails. TDF stimulates the male gonads to develop into the two testes and by 8 weeks of gestation testosterone secretion begins. Müllerian inhibitory hormone (MIH), secreted by Sertoli cells in the testes, promotes degeneration of the müllerian ducts. Without MIH, the müllerian ducts would develop and the wolffian ducts would degenerate with loss of male sex organ development. By 9 months' gestation, the male gonads (testes) have descended into the scrotum. The testes produce sperm after puberty.

Female gonadal development occurs in the absence of *SRY* expression and with the expression of other genes.[1] The presence of *estrogen* and the absence of *testosterone* and MIH cause a loss of the wolffian system

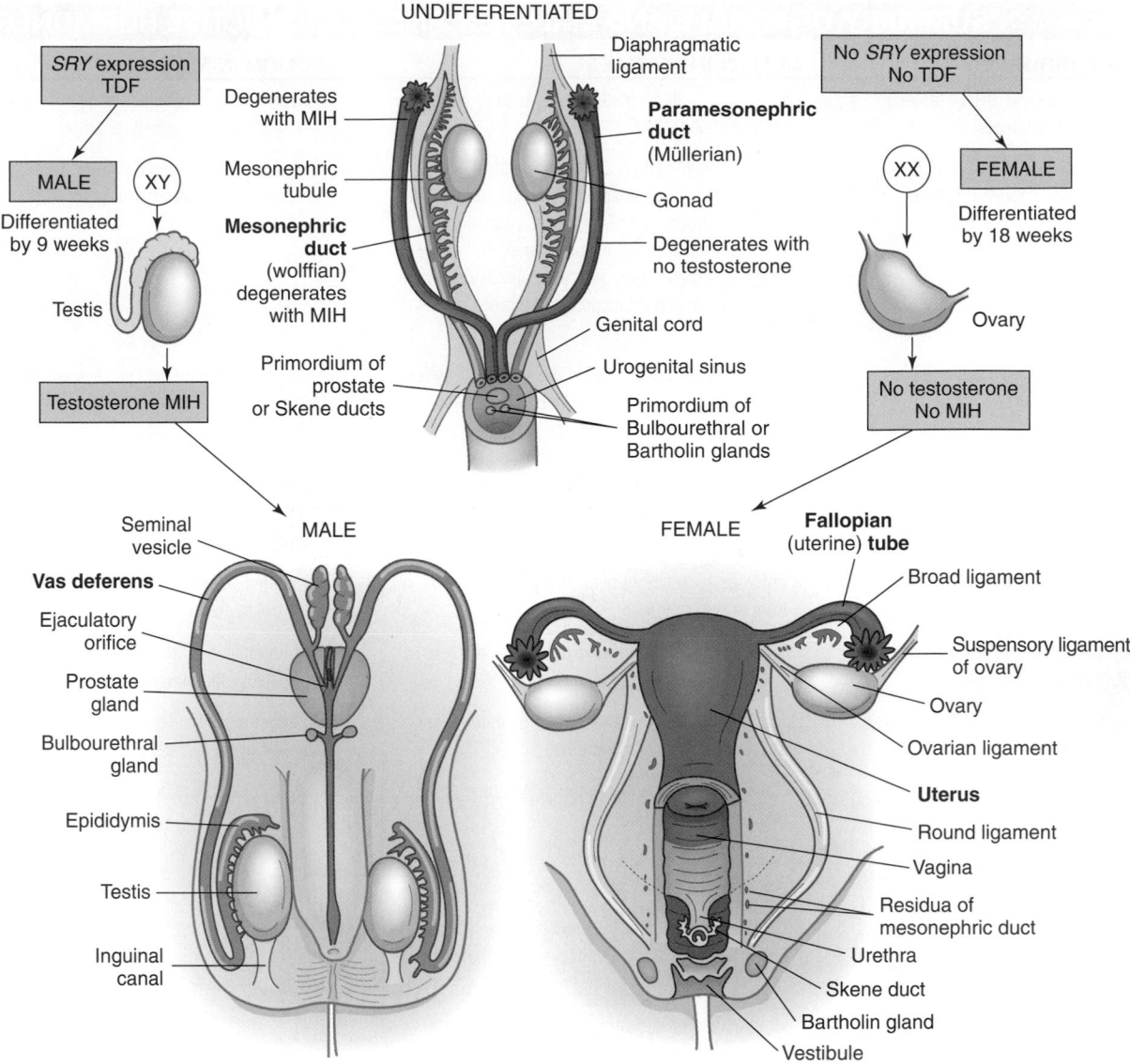

FIGURE 24.1 Internal Genitalia Development. Embryonic and fetal development of the internal genitalia. *MIH,* Müllerian inhibitory hormone; *TDF,* testes-determining factor.

and, at 6 to 8 weeks' gestation, the two female gonads develop into ovaries, which will produce ova. By the tenth week, the mesonephric ducts deteriorate and the upper ends of the paramesonephric ducts become the fallopian tubules whereas the lower ends join to become the uterus, cervix, and upper two-thirds of the vagina (see Fig. 24.1). The fallopian tubes carry ova from the ovaries to the uterus during a woman's reproductive years. Lack of testosterone and the presence of estrogen promote the development of external genitalia (lower end of vagina, labia, and clitoris).

Like the internal reproductive structures, the external structures develop from homologous embryonic tissues. During the first 7 to 8 weeks of gestation, both male and female embryos develop an elevated structure called the *genital tubercle* (Fig. 24.2). Testosterone is necessary for the genital tubercle to differentiate into male genitalia; otherwise, female genitalia develop, which may occur even in the absence of ovaries, possibly because of the presence of placental estrogens.

Anterior pituitary gland development begins between the fourth and fifth weeks of fetal life, and the vascular connection between the hypothalamus and the pituitary is established by the 12th week. Gonadotropin-releasing hormone (GnRH) is produced in the hypothalamus by 10 weeks' gestation and controls the production of two gonadotropins by the anterior pituitary gland: luteinizing hormone (LH), and follicle-stimulating hormone (FSH). In the female fetus, high levels of FSH and LH are excreted. FSH and LH stimulate the production of estrogen and progesterone by the ovary. The production of FSH and LH rises until about 28 weeks' gestation, when the production of estrogen and progesterone by the ovaries and placenta is high enough to result in the decline of gonadotropin production. Production of primitive female gametes (ova) occurs solely during fetal life. From puberty to menopause, one female gamete matures per menstrual cycle. Production of the male gametes (sperm) begins at puberty; after that millions are produced daily, usually for life.

By the end of pregnancy a sensitive negative-feedback system, which includes the gonadostat (also known as the gonadotropin-releasing hormone pulse generator), is operative in the human fetus. The gonadostat responds to high placental estrogen levels by releasing low levels of GnRH. Soon after birth steroid hormones levels drop because of withdrawal of maternal placental hormones. Hypothalamic pulsatile GnRH is secreted and gonadotropins LH and FSH are released. Their levels peak at 3 to 6 months for boys and at 12 to 18 months for girls,

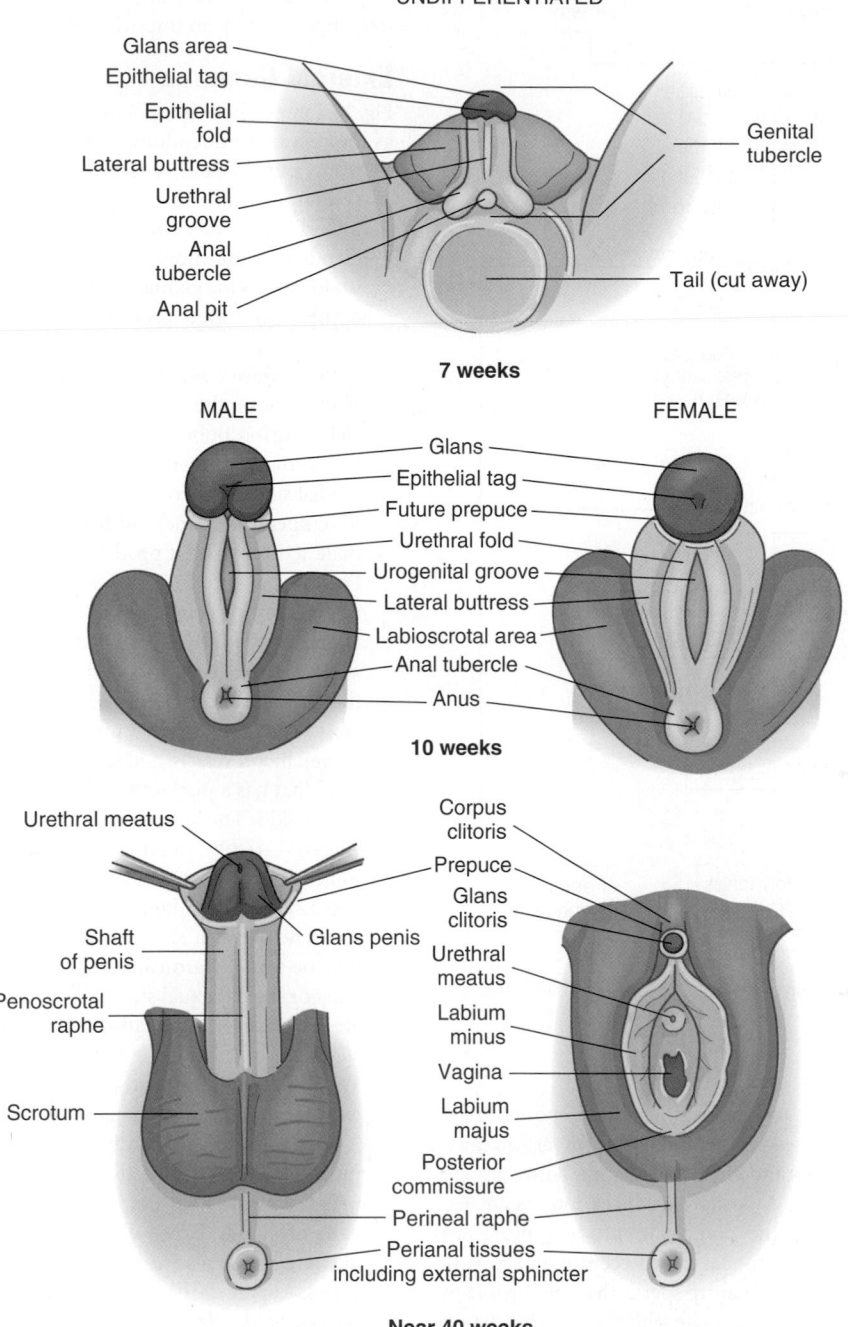

UNDIFFERENTIATED

Glans area
Epithelial tag
Epithelial fold
Lateral buttress
Urethral groove
Anal tubercle
Anal pit
Genital tubercle
Tail (cut away)

7 weeks

MALE   FEMALE

Glans
Epithelial tag
Future prepuce
Urethral fold
Urogenital groove
Lateral buttress
Labioscrotal area
Anal tubercle
Anus

10 weeks

Urethral meatus
Shaft of penis
Glans penis
Penoscrotal raphe
Scrotum

Corpus clitoris
Prepuce
Glans clitoris
Urethral meatus
Labium minus
Vagina
Labium majus
Posterior commissure
Perineal raphe
Perianal tissues including external sphincter

Near 40 weeks

FIGURE 24.2 External Genitalia Development. Embryonic and fetal development of the external genitalia.

and then fall steadily. The gonadotropins will be suppressed until the onset of puberty.

Puberty and Reproductive Maturation

Puberty is the onset of sexual maturation and differs from adolescence. Adolescence is the stage of human development between childhood and adulthood and includes social, psychologic, and biologic changes. In girls, puberty begins at about ages 8 to 9 years with thelarche (breast development). In boys, it begins later—at about age 11 years—but occurs earlier with increased weight and body mass index.[2] Genetics, environment, ethnicity, general health, and nutrition can influence the timing of puberty. There is an association between obesity and earlier puberty in girls, perhaps from higher estrogen levels related to

gonadotropin and estrogen secretion.[3] Girls who have low body fat and reduced body weight and perform intense exercise may experience delayed maturation.[5] Although leptin is not the trigger for puberty onset, it plays an important permissive role.

Reproductive maturation involves the hypothalamic-pituitary-gonadal (HPG) axis, the central nervous system, and the endocrine system (Fig. 24.3). There is a sequential series of hormonal events that promote sexual maturation as puberty approaches. About 1 year before puberty in girls, nocturnal pulses of gonadotropin secretion (i.e., LH and FSH) and an increased response in the pituitary to GnRH occur. This, in turn, stimulates gonadal maturation (**gonadarche**) with estradiol secretion in girls and testosterone secretion in boys. Estradiol causes development of the breasts (thelarche), maturation of the reproductive

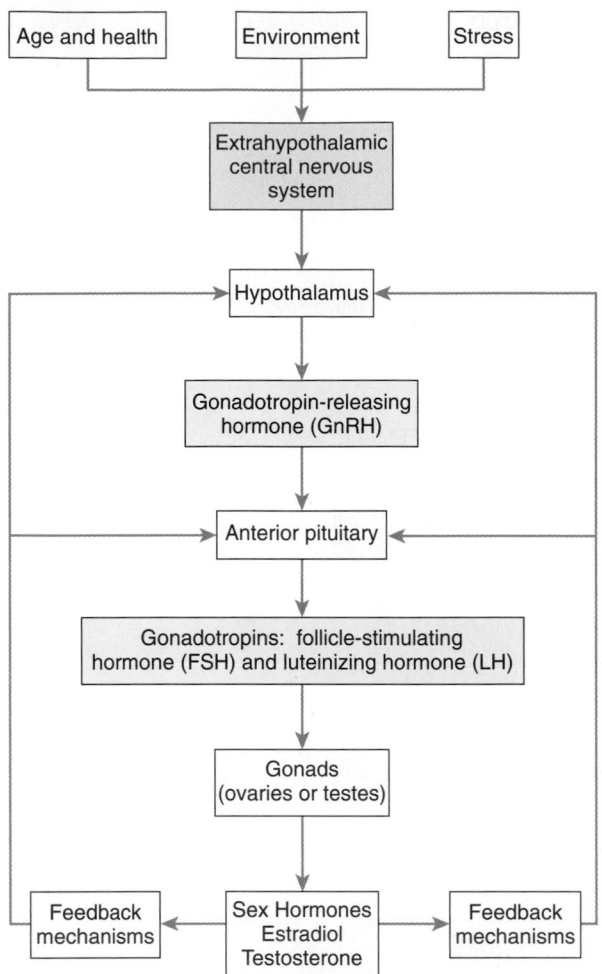

FIGURE 24.3 Hormonal Stimulation of the Gonads. The hypothalamic-pituitary-gonadal axis.

organs (vagina, uterus, ovaries), and deposition of fat deposits in the hips of girls. Estrogen and increased production of growth factors cause rapid skeletal growth in both boys and girls. Testosterone causes growth of the testes, scrotum, and penis. A positive-feedback loop is created with gonadotropins stimulating the gonads to produce more sex hormones. The most important hormonal effects occur in the gonads. In males the testes begin to produce mature sperm that are capable of fertilizing an ovum. Male puberty is complete with the first ejaculation that contains mature sperm. In females, the ovaries begin to release mature ova. Female puberty is complete with the first ovulatory menstrual period; however, this can take up to 1 to 2 years after menarche. Adrenarche is the increased production of adrenal androgens (dehydroepiandrosterone and androstenedione, which is converted to testosterone and estrogen) before puberty, which occurs in both sexes, and is manifested by growth of axillary and pubic hair and activation of sweat and sebaceous glands. Puberty is complete when an individual is capable of reproduction.

THE FEMALE REPRODUCTIVE SYSTEM

The function of the reproductive system is to produce mature ova; if fertilization occurs, the female reproductive system provides protection and nourishment of the fetus until it is expelled at birth. The most important internal reproductive organs in females are the ovaries,

fallopian tubes, uterus, and vagina. The external genitalia protect body openings and play an important role in sexual functioning.

External Genitalia

Fig. 24.4 shows the external female genitalia, which are known collectively as the vulva, or pudendum. The major structures are as follows:

- Mons pubis *(mons veneris)*—a fatty layer of tissue over the pubic symphysis (joint formed by union of the pubic bones). During puberty it becomes covered with pubic hair and sebaceous and sweat glands become more active. Estrogen causes fat to be deposited under the skin, giving the mons pubis a moundlike shape. This cushion of tissue protects the pubic symphysis during sexual intercourse.
- Labia majora *(singular,* labium majus*)*—two folds of skin arising at the mons pubis and extending back to the fourchette, forming a cleft. During puberty the amount of fatty tissue increases, pubic hair grows on lateral surfaces, and sebaceous glands on hairless medial surfaces secrete lubricants. This structure is highly sensitive to temperature, touch, pressure, and pain; it is homologous to the male scrotum and it protects the inner structures of the vulva (see Figs. 24.1 and 24.2).
- Labia minora *(singular,* labium minus*)*—two smaller, thinner, asymmetric folds of skin within the labia majora that form the clitoral hood (prepuce) and frenulum, and then split to enclose the vestibule and converge near the anus to form the fourchette. The labia minora are hairless, pink, and moist and are well supplied with nerves, blood vessels, and sebaceous glands that secrete a bactericidal fluid that has a distinctive odor and lubricates and waterproofs the vulvar skin. The labia swell with blood during sexual arousal.
- Clitoris—richly innervated, erectile organ between the labia minora. It is a small, cylindrical structure having a visible glans and a shaft that lie beneath the skin. The clitoris is homologous to the male penis. It secretes smegma, which has a unique odor that may be sexually arousing to the male. Like the penis the clitoris is a major site of sexual stimulation and orgasm. With sexual arousal, erectile tissues in the clitoris fill with blood, causing it to enlarge slightly.
- Vestibule—an area protected by the labia minora and contains the external opening of the vagina, called the introitus, or vaginal orifice. A thin, perforated membrane called the hymen may cover the introitus. The vestibule also contains the opening of the urethra, or urinary meatus (orifice). These structures are lubricated by two pairs of glands: Skene glands and Bartholin glands. The ducts of Skene glands (also called the lesser vestibular or paraurethral glands) open on both sides of the urinary meatus. The ducts of Bartholin glands (greater vestibular or vulvovaginal glands) open on either side of the introitus. In response to sexual stimulation, Bartholin glands secrete mucus that lubricates the inner labial surfaces, as well as enhances the viability and motility of sperm. Skene glands help lubricate the urinary meatus and the vestibule. Secretions from both sets of glands facilitate coitus. In response to sexual excitement, the highly vascular tissue just beneath the vestibule fills with blood and becomes engorged.
- Perineum—an area with less hair, skin, and subcutaneous tissue lying between the vaginal orifice and anus. Unlike the rest of the vulva, this area has little subcutaneous fat so that the skin is close to the underlying muscles. The perineum covers the muscular perineal body, a fibrous structure that consists of elastic fibers and connective tissue, and serves as the common attachment for the bulbocavernosus, the external anal sphincter, and the levator ani muscles (see Fig. 24.4). The perineum varies in length from 2 to 5 cm or more and stretches remarkably. The length of the perineum and the elasticity

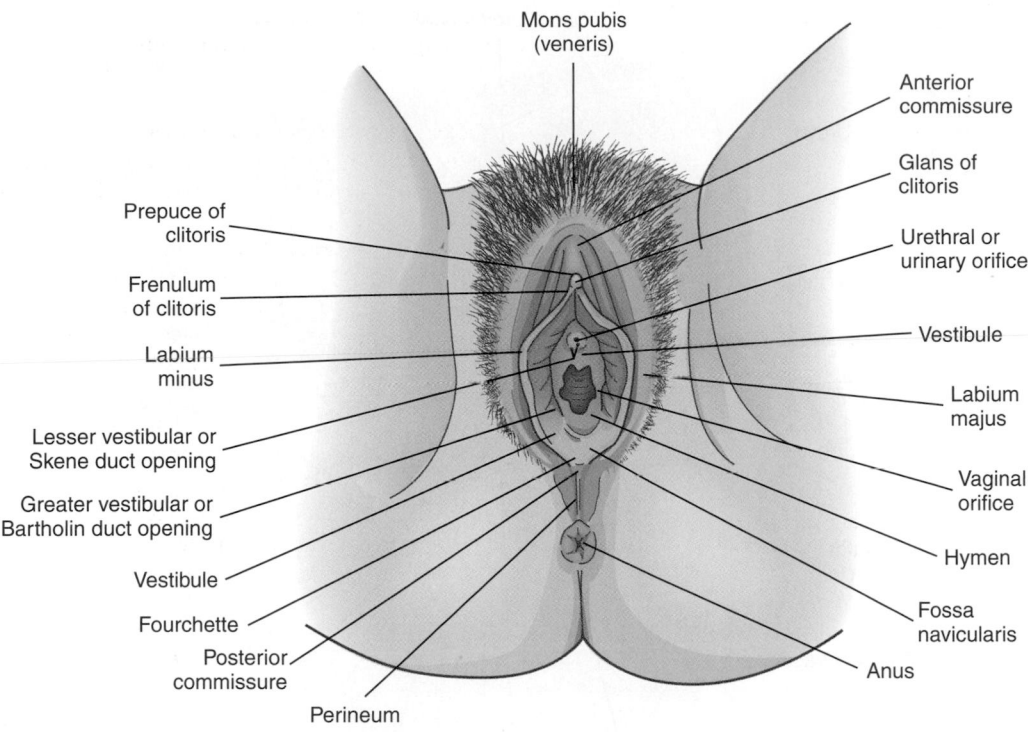

FIGURE 24.4 External Female Genitalia.

of the perineal body influence tissue resistance and injury during childbirth.

Internal Genitalia
Vagina

The vagina is an elastic fibromuscular canal, 9 to 10 cm long in a reproductive-aged female. It extends up and back from the introitus to the lower portion of the uterus. As Fig. 24.5 shows, the vagina lies between the urethra (and part of the bladder) and the rectum. Mucosal secretions from the upper genital organs, menstrual fluids, and products of conception leave the body through the vagina, which also receives the penis during coitus. During sexual excitement the vagina lengthens and widens and the lower third becomes congested with blood.

The vaginal wall is composed of four layers:

1. Mucous membrane lining of squamous epithelial cells that thickens and thins in response to hormones, particularly estrogen. The squamous epithelial membrane is continuous with the membrane that covers the lower part of the uterus. In women of reproductive age, the mucosal layer is arranged in transverse wrinkles, or folds, called rugae (*singular, ruga*) that permit stretching during coitus and childbirth.
2. Fibrous connective tissue containing numerous blood and lymphatic vessels
3. Smooth muscle
4. Connective tissue and a rich network of blood vessels

The upper part of the vagina surrounds the cervix, the lower end of the uterus (see Fig. 24.5). The recessed space around the cervix is called the fornix of the vagina. The posterior fornix is "deeper" than the anterior fornix because of the angle at which the cervix meets the vaginal canal. In most women this angle is about 90 degrees. A pouch called the cul-de-sac separates the posterior fornix and the rectum.

Its elasticity and relatively sparse nerve supply enhance the vagina's function as the birth canal. During sexual arousal the vaginal wall becomes engorged with blood, like the labia minora and clitoris. Engorgement pushes some fluid to the surface of the mucosa, enhancing lubrication. The vaginal wall does not contain mucous-secreting glands; rather, secretions drain into the vagina from the endocervical glands or enter from the vestibule, from the Bartholin and Skene glands.

Two factors help maintain the self-cleansing action of the vagina and defend it from infection, particularly during the reproductive years. They are (1) an acid-base balance that discourages the proliferation of most pathogenic bacteria and (2) the thickness of the vaginal epithelium. Before puberty, the vaginal pH is about 7 (neutral) and the vaginal epithelium is thin. At puberty the pH becomes more acidic (4 to 5) and the squamous epithelial lining thickens. These changes are maintained until menopause (cessation of menstruation), at which time the pH rises again to more alkaline levels and the epithelium thins. Therefore protection from infection is greatest during the years when a woman is most likely to be sexually active. Between puberty and menopause, vulnerability to infection varies somewhat with cyclic changes in pH and epithelial thickness. Both defenses are greatest when estrogen levels are high and the vagina contains a normal population of *Lactobacillus acidophilus,* a harmless resident bacterium that helps maintain the pH at acidic levels. Any condition that causes the vaginal pH to rise; such as douching or use of vaginal sprays or deodorants, the presence of low estrogen levels, or destruction of *L. acidophilus* by antibiotics; lowers vaginal defenses against infection.

Uterus

The uterus is a hollow pear-shaped organ whose lower end opens into the vagina. It anchors and protects a fertilized ovum, provides an optimal environment while the ovum develops, and expels the fetus at birth. In addition, the uterus plays an important role in sexual response and conception. During sexual excitement the opening of the uterus (the cervix) dilates slightly. At the same time, the uterus increases in size and moves upward and backward, creating a tenting effect in the

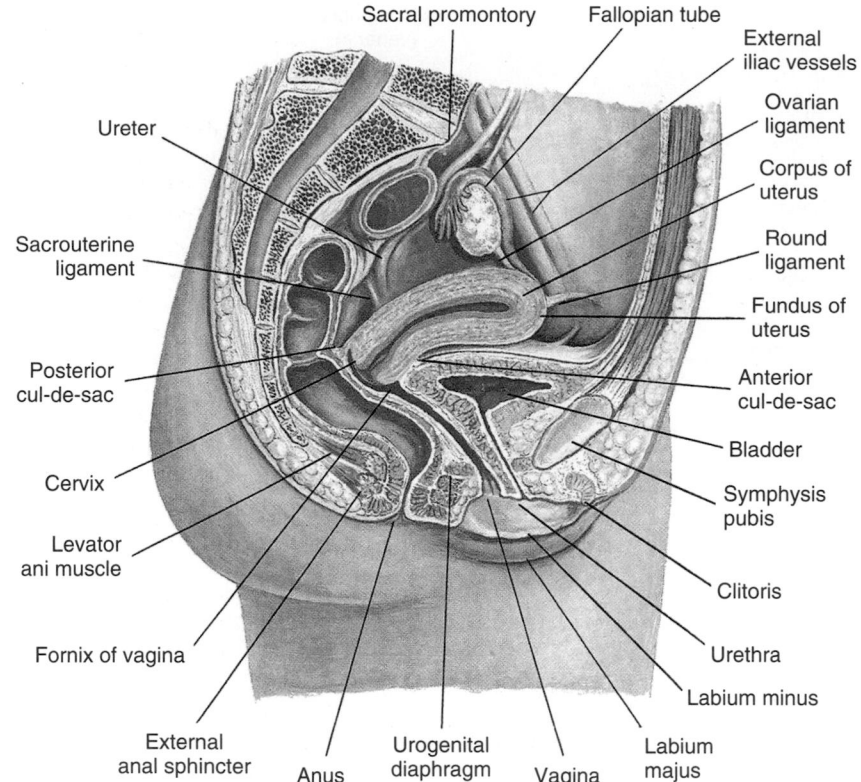

Sacral promontory   Fallopian tube

External
iliac vessels

Ovarian
ligament

Corpus of
uterus

Round
ligament

Fundus of
uterus

Anterior
cul-de-sac

Bladder

Symphysis
pubis

Clitoris

Urethra

Labium minus

Labium
majus

Vagina

Urogenital
diaphragm

Anus

External
anal sphincter

Fornix of vagina

Levator
ani muscle

Cervix

Posterior
cul-de-sac

Sacrouterine
ligament

Ureter

FIGURE 24.5 Internal Female Genitalia and Other Pelvic Organs. Midsagittal view. (Modified from Ball JW et al: *Seidel's guide to physical examination,* ed 8, St Louis, 2015, Mosby.)

midvagina that results in the cervix "sitting" in a pool of semen. During orgasm, rhythmic contractions facilitate movement of sperm through the cervical os while also enhancing physical pleasure.

At puberty the uterus attains its adult size and proportions and descends from the abdomen to the lower pelvis, between the bladder and the rectum (see Fig. 24.5). The uterus of a mature, nonpregnant female is approximately 7 to 9 cm long and 6.5 cm wide, with muscular walls 3.5 cm thick. It is held loosely in position by ligaments, peritoneal tissue folds, and the pressure of adjacent organs, especially the urinary bladder, sigmoid colon, and rectum. In most women the uterus is anteverted; that is, it is tipped forward so that it rests on the urinary bladder. However, it may be retroverted, or tipped backward. Various degrees of flexion are normal (Fig. 24.6).

The uterus has two major parts (Fig. 24.7): the body, or corpus, and the cervix. The top of the corpus, above the insertion of the fallopian tubes, is called the fundus. The diameter of the uterine cavity is widest at the fundus and narrowest at the isthmus, just above the cervix. The cervix, or "neck of the uterus," extends from the isthmus to the vagina. The passageway between the cervix's upper opening (the internal os) and its lower opening (the external os) is called the endocervical canal. The entire uterus, like the upper vagina, is innervated exclusively by motor and sensory fibers of the autonomic nervous system.

The uterine wall is composed of three layers (see Fig. 24.7). The perimetrium (parietal peritoneum) is the outer serous membrane that covers the uterus. The myometrium is the thick muscular middle layer. It is thickest at the fundus, apparently to facilitate birth. The endometrium, or uterine lining, is composed of a functional layer (superficial compact layer and spongy middle layer) and a basal layer. The functional layer of the endometrium is responsive to the sex hormones

estrogen and progesterone. This layer proliferates and sloughs off monthly between puberty and menopause. The basal layer, which is attached to the myometrium, regenerates the functional layer after shedding (menstruation).

The endocervical canal does not have an endometrial layer but is lined with columnar epithelial cells. It is continuous with the lining of the outer cervix and vagina, which are lined with squamous epithelial cells. The point at which the two types of cells meet is called the *transformation zone,* or the squamous-columnar junction. The transformation zone is vulnerable to human papillomavirus (HPV), especially HPV types 16 and 18, which can lead to cervical dysplasia or carcinoma in situ. Cells of the transformation zone are removed for examination during a Papanicolaou (Pap test) smear, which may be combined with an HPV DNA test.[6]

The cervix acts as a mechanical barrier to infectious microorganisms from the vagina. The external cervical os is a very small opening that contains thick, sticky mucus (the *mucous plug*) during the luteal phase of the menstrual cycle and all of pregnancy. During ovulation the mucus changes under the influence of estrogen and forms watery strands, or spinnbarkeit mucus, to facilitate the transport of sperm into the uterus. In addition, the downward flow of cervical secretions moves microorganisms away from the cervix and uterus. In women of reproductive age, the pH of these secretions is inhospitable to most bacteria. Furthermore, mucosal secretions contain enzymes and antibodies (mostly immunoglobulin A [IgA]) of the secretory (humoral) immune system (see Chapter 8). Uterine pathophysiologic disorders include infection, displacement of the uterus within the pelvis, benign growths (fibroids) of the uterine wall, hyperplasia of the endometrium, endometriosis, and cancer (see Chapter 25).

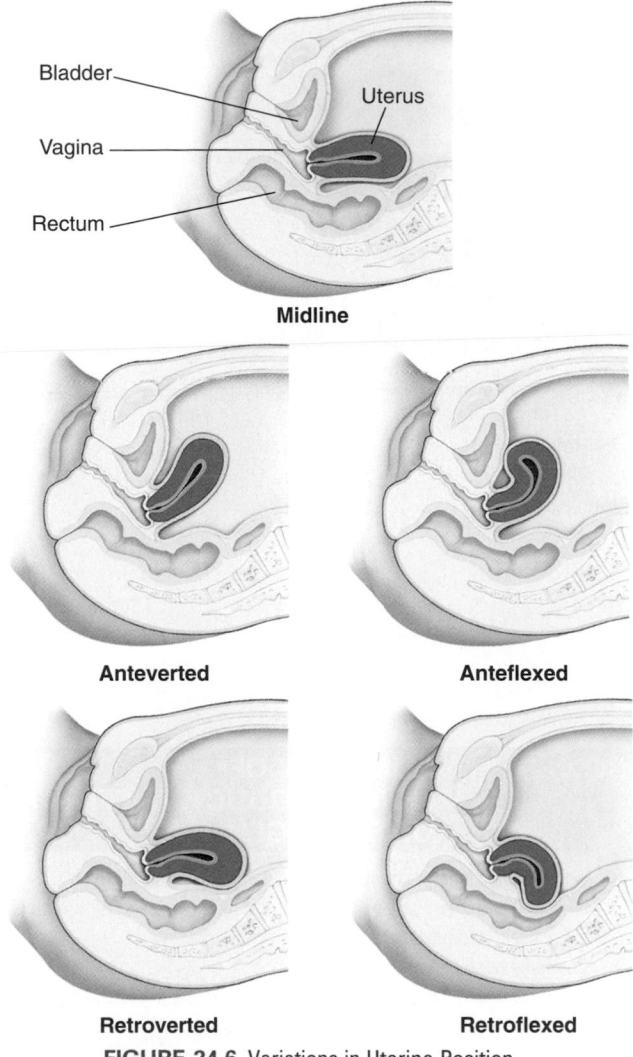

Bladder

Uterus

Vagina

Rectum

Midline

Anteverted

Anteflexed

Retroverted

Retroflexed

FIGURE 24.6 Variations in Uterine Position.

Fallopian Tubes

The two fallopian tubes (oviducts, uterine tubes) enter the uterus bilaterally just beneath the fundus (see Fig. 24.7). Their function is to conduct the ova from the spaces around the ovaries to the uterus. From the uterus the fallopian tubes curve up and over the two ovaries. Each tube is 8 to 12 cm long and about 1 cm in diameter, except at its ovarian end, which flares out like the bell of a trumpet. This widened end, called the infundibulum, is fringed or fimbriated. The fimbriae (*singular, fimbria*) (fringes) move, creating a current that draws the ovum into the infundibulum. Once the ovum has entered the fallopian tube, cilia and peristalsis (muscle contractions) keep it moving toward the uterus.

The ampulla, or distal third, of the fallopian tube is the usual site of fertilization (see Fig. 24.7). Sperm released into the vagina travel upward through the endocervical canal and uterine cavity and enter the fallopian tubes. If an ovum is present in either tube, fertilization can occur. Whether or not the ovum encounters sperm, it continues to travel through the fallopian tube to the uterus. If fertilized, the ovum (then called a *blastocyst*) implants itself in the endometrial layer of the uterine wall. If not fertilized, the ovum breaks down within 12 to 24 hours. Disorders that affect the fallopian tubes (e.g., congenital malformations, infection, and inflammation) can block the path of sperm and ovum and cause infertility or ectopic (tubal) pregnancy.

Ovaries

The ovaries, the female gonads, are the primary female reproductive organs. Their two main functions are secretion of female sex hormones and development and release of female gametes, or ova.

The almond-shaped ovaries are located on both sides of the uterus and are suspended and supported by the mesovarian portions of the broad ligament, ovarian ligaments, and suspensory ligaments (see Fig. 24.7). The ovaries are smaller than their male homologs, the testes. In women of reproductive age, each ovary is 3 to 5 cm long, 2.5 cm wide, and 2 cm thick and weighs 4 to 8 g. Size and weight vary somewhat from phase to phase of the menstrual cycle (see the section titled The Menstrual [Ovarian] Cycle).

Fig. 24.8, *A*, shows a cross section of an ovary. The central part, or medulla, is composed of connective tissue and contains many small arteries, veins, and lymphatics that enter at the hilum. Surrounding the medulla is the cortex. At birth the cortex of each ovary contains approximately 2 million ova within primordial (immature) ovarian follicles. Follicles grow and undergo atresia continuously and irrevocably throughout a woman's life. By puberty the number ranges between 300,000 and 500,000 ova. Between puberty and menopause the ovarian cortex always contains follicles and ova in various stages of development, including the primary and secondary follicles (see Fig. 24.8, *A*). Once every menstrual cycle (about every 28 days), usually only one of the follicles reaches maturation (see Fig. 24.8, *B* and *C*) and discharges its ovum through the ovary's outer covering, the germinal epithelium. During the reproductive years, 400 to 500 ovarian follicles mature completely and release an ovum (ovulation). The remaining follicles either fail to develop at all or degenerate without maturing completely and are known as *atretic follicles* (Fig. 24.8).

After release of the mature ovum (ovulation), the follicle develops into another structure, the corpus luteum (see Fig. 24.8). The immediate fate of the corpus luteum depends on whether the ejected ovum is fertilized. If fertilization occurs, the corpus luteum enlarges and begins to secrete hormones that maintain and support pregnancy. If fertilization does not occur, the corpus luteum secretes these hormones for approximately 14 days and then degenerates, which triggers the maturation of another follicle. The ovarian cycle—the process of follicular maturation, ovulation, corpus luteum development, and corpus luteum degeneration—is continuous from puberty to menopause, except during pregnancy or hormonal contraceptive use. At menopause this process ceases and the ovaries atrophy to the point that they cannot be felt during pelvic examination.

Sex hormones are secreted by cells present within the ovarian cortex including two types of cells in the ovarian follicle (theca cells [produce androgens that migrate to granulosa cells] and granulosa cells [convert androgens to estradiol]) and cells of the corpus luteum that primarily secrete progesterone, estrogen, and inhibin (see Fig. 24.8). These cells all contain receptors for the gonadotropins (LH, FSH) or for the sex hormones, which are discussed in the next section.

Female Sex Hormones

The sex hormones are all steroid hormones and are synthesized from cholesterol (see Chapter 21). Male and female sex hormones are present in all adults. However, the female body contains low levels of testosterone and other androgens, and the male body contains low levels of estrogen. Individual effects of sex hormones depend on their amount and concentration in the blood.

The dominant female sex hormones, estrogen and progesterone, are produced primarily by the ovaries (see Table 24.1). During fetal development, infancy, and childhood, sex hormone production is low. At puberty, hormone production surges, triggering sexual maturation and development of secondary sex characteristics. From puberty to menopause,

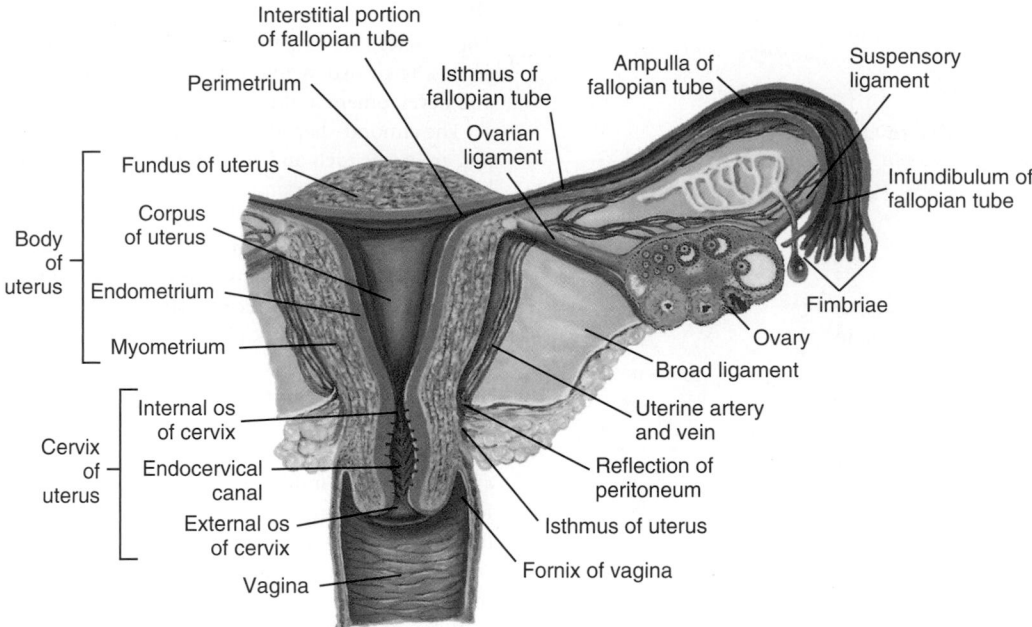

FIGURE 24.7 Cross Section of Uterus, Fallopian Tube, and Ovary. (From Seidel HM et al: *Mosby's guide to physical examination*, ed 7, St Louis, 2011, Mosby.)

the sex hormones control the menstrual cycle and are produced cyclically; that is, production surges and diminishes monthly, creating the ovarian and uterine changes associated with the menstrual cycle. These hormones also are produced in higher levels during pregnancy by the placenta, inhibiting ovulation. Androgens are produced in small amounts by the ovaries and the adrenals and have important functions in women.

Estrogens and Androgens

Estrogen is a generic term for three similar hormones: estradiol, estrone, and estriol. Estradiol (E_2) is the most potent and plentiful of the three and is principally produced (95%) by the ovaries (ovarian follicle and corpus luteum). Limited amounts are secreted by the cortices of the adrenal glands and the placenta during pregnancy. Androgens are converted to estrone in ovarian and peripheral adipose tissue. Estriol is the peripheral metabolite of estrone and estradiol.

Estrogen has numerous biologic effects, many of which involve interactions with other hormones, and is needed for maturation of reproductive organs, development of secondary sex characteristics (differentiating male and female physical characteristics that are not directly related to reproduction), growth, and maintenance of pregnancy. Nonreproductive effects of estrogen include closure of long bones after the pubertal growth spurt (in both males and females), maintenance of bone and skin, and systemic organ function (Box 24.1). After menopause, the ovaries dramatically reduce production of estradiol and secretion of estrone (see Menopause, under Aging and the Female Reproductive System). At this time the majority of estradiol is derived from intracellular synthesis in peripheral tissues. Estradiol acts locally to meet physiologic needs according to cell type and is then inactivated without systemic effects.[7]

Like other steroid hormones, estrogens are derived from cholesterol in a complex, enzyme-mediated series of reactions. (Mechanisms of hormone synthesis and action are described in Chapter 21.) The hypothalamus secretes GnRH in a pulsatile manner that stimulates gonadotropin (LH and FSH) release from the anterior pituitary. Gonadotropins trigger ovarian production of estrogen. The primary function of LH is to stimulate theca cells of the ovarian follicle to

---

BOX 24.1   SUMMARY OF NONREPRODUCTIVE EFFECTS OF ESTROGEN

- Estrogens (including estrone, estradiol, estriol) function through estrogen receptors alpha and beta, have different roles in different cells and tissues, and have paracrine or intracrine function.
- Maintains bone density.
- Acts in liver to decrease cholesterol level, increase high-density lipoprotein (HDL) level, and decrease low-density lipoprotein (LDL) level (antiatherosclerotic); promotes fat deposition.
- Maintains nervous system (neurotrophic and neuroprotective); facilitates memory and cognition.
- Increases collagen content, dermal thickness, elasticity, water content, and healing ability of skin.
- Protects against chronic kidney disease in individuals without diabetes.
- Prevents vascular injury and early atheroma formation through endothelial mechanisms.
- Inhibits platelet adhesiveness.
- Can promote inflammation and have variable effects on immunity.
- Estrogen associated with pregnancy or use in contraceptive pills promotes clotting and increased risk of thromboembolism.

---

produce androgens, mainly androstenedione. (Androgens are discussed further under the section titled Male Sex and Reproductive Hormones.) Some of these androgens are converted to estrogen by the theca cells themselves, and others diffuse into the granulosa cells. Within the granulosa layer, FSH induces conversion (aromatization) of androgens to estrogens. Estrogens are then released into the bloodstream. Estrogen and FSH together increase FSH receptors in the follicle, stimulating additional granulosa cells until a dominant follicle is determined.

Although androgens are primarily male sex hormones produced by the testes, small amounts are produced in the adrenal cortex in both men and women and in the ovaries in women. Some androgens

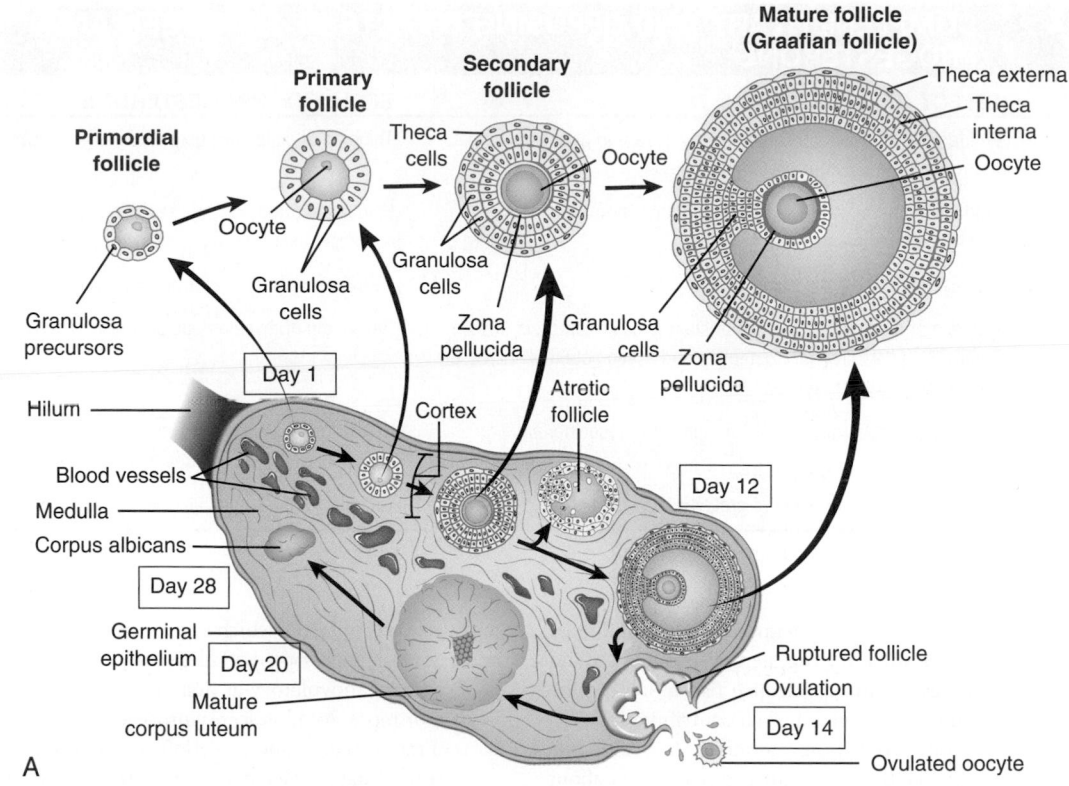

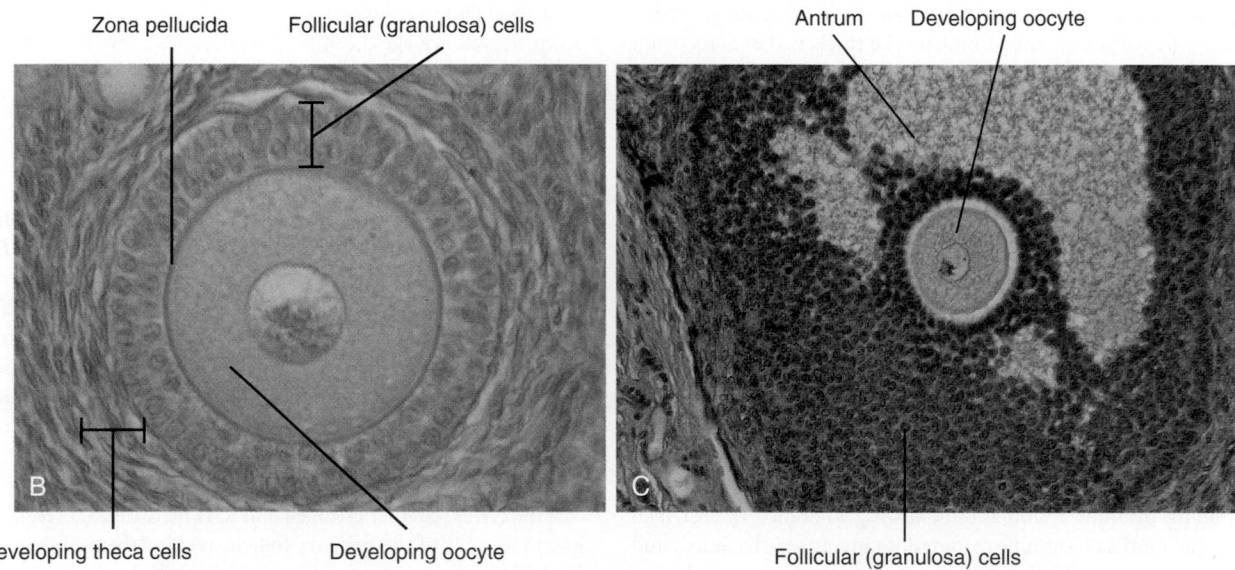

FIGURE 24.8 Cross Section of Ovary and Development of an Ovarian Follicle. A, Schematic representation (not to scale) of the structure of the ovary, showing the various stages in the development of the follicle and its successor structure, the corpus luteum. **B,** A developing oocyte surrounded by hormone-secreting follicular (granulosa) cells. **C,** A more mature ovarian follicle has a fluid-filled cavity called the *antrum*. (**A** Adapted from Berne RM, Levy MN, editors: *Physiology,* ed 5, St Louis, 2003, Mosby. **B** and **C** From Patton KT, Thibodeau GA: *Anatomy & physiology,* ed 9, St Louis, 2016, Mosby.)

(dehydroepiandrosterone and its metabolite androstenedione) are precursors of estrogens (estrone, estradiol). At puberty, androgens contribute to the skeletal growth spurt and cause growth of pubic and axillary hair. The androgens also activate sebaceous glands, accounting for some cases of acne during puberty, and play a role in libido.

Progesterone

Luteinizing hormone (LH) from the anterior pituitary stimulates the corpus luteum to secrete progesterone, the second major female sex hormone. With estrogen, progesterone controls the ovarian menstrual cycle. LH surge occurs when there is a peak level of estrogen, about 24

TABLE 24.2	COMPLEMENTARY AND OPPOSING EFFECTS OF ESTROGEN AND PROGESTERONE	
STRUCTURE	EFFECT OF ESTROGEN	EFFECT OF PROGESTERONE
Vaginal mucosa	Proliferation of squamous epithelium; increase in glycogen content of cells; layering (cornification) of cells	Thinning of squamous epithelium; decornification
Cervical mucosa	Production of abundant fluid secretions that favor survival and enhance motility of sperm	Production of thick, sticky secretions that tend to "plug" the cervical os
Fallopian tube	Increase of motility and ciliary action	Decrease of motility and ciliary action
Uterine muscle	Increase of blood flow; increase of contractile proteins and uterine muscle and myometrial excitability and action potential; increase of sensitization to oxytocin	Relaxation of myometrium; decrease of sensitization to oxytocin
Endometrium	Stimulation of growth; increase in number of progesterone receptors	Activation of glands and blood vessels; accumulation of glycogen and enzymes; decrease in number of estrogen receptors
Breasts	Growth of ducts; promotion of prolactin effects	Growth of lobules and alveoli; inhibition of prolactin effects

to 36 hours before ovulation. LH promotes luteinization of the granulosa in the dominant follicle and results in progesterone production and the development of blood vessels and connective tissue. During the follicular phase, the ovary and adrenal glands each contribute approximately 50% of the progesterone production. Conversely, large amounts are secreted from the ovary while the corpus luteum is active for about 9 to 13 days after ovulation. The opposing and complementary effects of progesterone and estrogen are listed in Table 24.2. Progesterone secreted by the corpus luteum stimulates the thickened endometrium to become more complex in preparation for implantation of a blastocyst. If conception and implantation do occur, the corpus luteum persists and secretes progesterone (and estrogen) until the placenta is well established at approximately 8 to 10 weeks' gestation and undertakes progesterone production.

Progesterone is sometimes called the *hormone of pregnancy.* Progesterone's effects in pregnancy include (1) maintaining the thickened endometrium; (2) relaxing smooth muscle in the myometrium, which prevents premature contractions and helps the uterus expand; (3) thickening (hypertrophy) the myometrium, which prepares it for the muscular work of labor; (4) promoting growth of lobules and alveoli in the breast in preparation for lactation but preventing lactation until the fetus is born and then promoting lactation in collaboration with prolactin after birth; (5) preventing additional maturation of ova by way of suppressing FSH and LH, thereby stopping the menstrual cycle; (6) providing immune modulation, allowing tolerance against fetal antigens (the mother's immune system does not attack the fetus); and (7) preventing preterm birth.[8]

The Menstrual (Ovarian) Cycle

In addition to pregnancy the obvious manifestation of female reproductive functioning is menstrual bleeding (the menses), which starts with menarche (first menstruation) and ends with menopause (cessation of menstrual flow for 1 year). In the United States, the median age of first menstruation is about 12.14 years in black females, 12.25 years in Latina or Hispanic females, and 12.6 years in white females, with a range from 9 to 13.5 years.[9] Menarche appears to be related to body weight, especially percentage of body fat (ratio of fat to lean tissue), which may trigger a change in the metabolic rate and lead to hormonal changes associated with early menarche. There is increased circulating leptin (a regulatory hormone of appetite and energy metabolism), which promotes the secretion of kisspeptin from the hypothalamus and leads

to the release of GnRH, which in turn enhances release of FSH and LH and estradiol, triggering ovulation and the onset of puberty.

Cycles are anovulatory at first and may vary in length from 10 to 60 days or more. As adolescence proceeds into adulthood, regular patterns of menstruation and ovulation are established at intervals ranging from 21 to 45 days.[11] Menstruation continues to recur in a recognizable and characteristic pattern during adulthood, with the length of the menstrual cycle varying considerably among women. The commonly accepted cycle average is 28 (27 to 30) days, with rhythmic intervals of 21 to 35 days considered normal. Approximately 2 to 8 years before menopause, cycles begin to lengthen again with variation related to changing hormone levels.[12]

Phases of the Menstrual Cycle

The menstrual (ovarian) cycle (Fig. 24.9) consists of two phases: the follicular/proliferative phase (postmenstrual) followed by the luteal/secretory phase (premenstrual). During menstruation (menses), the functional layer of the endometrium disintegrates and is discharged through the vagina. Menstruation is followed by the follicular/proliferative phase. During the follicular/proliferative phase, GnRH and a balance between activin and inhibin from the granulosa cells contribute to the rise of FSH levels, which stimulates a number of follicles. The pulsatile secretion of FSH from the anterior pituitary gland rescues a dominant ovarian follicle from apoptosis by days 5 to 7 of the cycle. Together estrogen and FSH increase FSH receptors in the granulosa cells of the primary follicle, making them more sensitive to FSH. FSH and estrogen combine to induce production of LH receptors on the granulosa cells, thus promoting LH stimulation to combine with FSH stimulation, causing a more rapid secretion of follicular estrogen. As estrogen levels increase, FSH levels drop because of an increase in inhibin-B secreted by the granulosa cells in the dominant follicle. This drop in FSH level decreases the growth of less-developed follicles (see Fig. 24.9). Estrogen causes cells of the endometrium to proliferate and stimulates production of LH. A surge in both FSH and LH levels is required for final follicular growth and ovulation. An increase in stromal tissue in the late follicular phase is associated with a rise in androgen levels. Androgen production enhances the process of follicle atresia although there may be a dose-dependent support of follicle maturation.[13]

Ovulation is the release of an ovum from a mature follicle and marks the beginning of the luteal/secretory phase of the menstrual

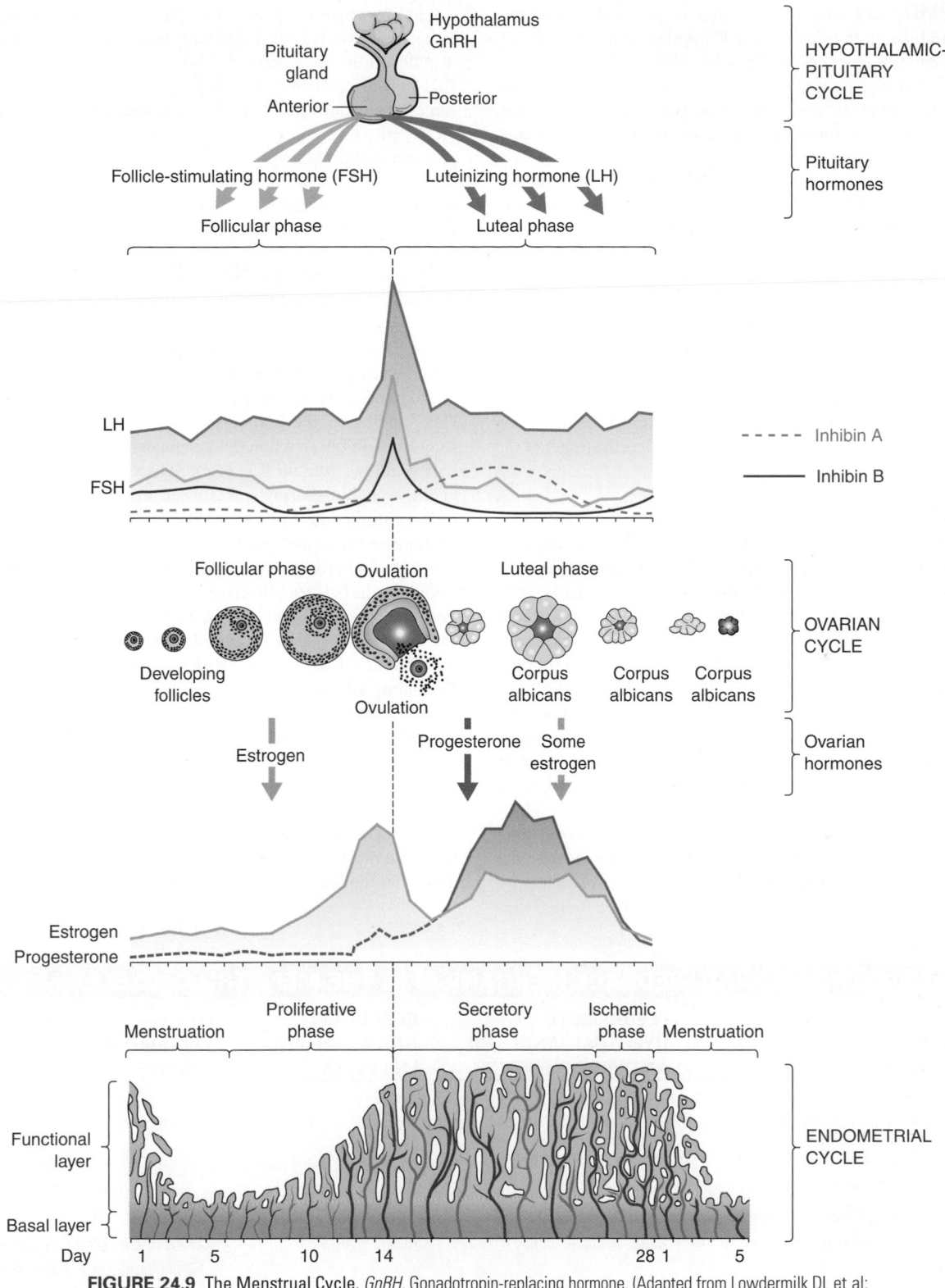

FIGURE 24.9 The Menstrual Cycle. *GnRH,* Gonadotropin-replacing hormone. (Adapted from Lowdermilk DL et al: *Maternity and women's health care,* ed 10, St Louis, 2012, Mosby.)

cycle. The ovarian follicle begins its transformation into a corpus luteum (see Fig. 24.8, *A*), hence the name *luteal phase.* Pulsatile secretion of LH from the anterior pituitary stimulates the corpus luteum to secrete progesterone, which in turn initiates the secretory phase of endometrial development. Glands and blood vessels in the endometrium branch and curl throughout the functional layer, and the glands begin to secrete a thin glycogen-containing fluid, the *secretory phase.* If conception occurs, the nutrient-laden endometrium is ready for implantation. Human chorionic gonadotropin (HCG) is secreted 3 days after fertilization by the blastocytes and maintains the corpus luteum once implantation occurs at about day 6 or 7. HCG can be detected in maternal blood and urine 8 to 10 days after ovulation. The production of estrogen and progesterone continues until the placenta can adequately maintain hormonal production. If conception and implantation do not occur, the corpus luteum degenerates and ceases production of progesterone and estrogen. Without progesterone or estrogen to maintain it, the endometrium becomes ischemic ("blood-starved") and disintegrates, hence the name ischemic/menstrual phase. Menstruation then occurs, marking the beginning of another cycle.

Ovulatory cycles appear to have a minimum length of 24 to 26.5 days: the primary ovarian follicle requires 10 to 12.5 days to develop, and the luteal phase appears relatively fixed at 14 days (±3 days). Menstrual blood flow usually lasts 3 to 7 days, but it may last as long as 8 days or stop after 1 to 2 days and still be considered within normal limits. Bleeding is consistently scant to heavy and varies from 30 to 80 mL, with most blood loss occurring during the first 3 days of menses. Menstrual discharge consists of blood, mucus, and desquamated endometrial tissue and does not clot under normal circumstances. It is usually dark and produces a characteristic musty odor on oxidation. Environmental factors such as severe emotional stress, illness, malnutrition, obesity, and seasonal variation may affect the length of the menstrual cycle.[14,15]

Hormonal Control

Hormonal control of the menstrual cycle depends on complex interactions among the hypothalamus, the anterior pituitary, and the ovaries (or hypothalamic-pituitary-ovarian [HPO] axis) (Table 24.3). Hormonal control is dependent on negative and positive ovarian feedback mechanisms. In the hypothalamus, kisspeptin (also known as *metastin*) activates the release of GnRH to stimulate the gonadotropin production of FSH and LH. The constant and pulsatile release of GnRH is critical to the timing of the menstrual cycle. GnRH is secreted into the hypophyseal portal system and travels to the anterior pituitary, where it stimulates the secretion of LH and FSH. FSH and LH are released from the anterior pituitary in pulses that correspond to the pulsatile secretion of GnRH.

During the early follicular phase, estrogen levels rise steadily and, through negative feedback, suppress FSH and positively increase the production of LH. During the late follicular phase, the preovulatory rise in progesterone concentration facilitates the positive feedback of estrogen; estrogen levels begin to increase, stimulating a surge of LH secretion from the anterior pituitary. The midcycle surge of LH and FSH induces ovulation. A nonsteroidal ovarian factor, gonadotropin surge–attenuating factor (GnSAF), may antagonize the effect of estrogen on the pituitary and regulate the surge of LH at midcycle.[17] Rising estrogen and progesterone levels during the luteal phase may inhibit the anterior pituitary, and thus reduce LH and FSH secretion. Just before the onset of menstruation, FSH and LH levels begin to increase slightly, probably because of declining estrogen and progesterone levels (see Fig. 24.9).

A variety of growth factors and autocrine/paracrine peptides influence hormonal control and follicular response. During the early follicular stage, FSH stimulates FSH receptors and LH receptors and the release of insulin-like growth factor 1, as well as the production of inhibin and activin in the ovary. Activin from granulosa cells stimulates the secretion of FSH and increases the pituitary response to GnRH, and increases FSH binding in the granulosa cells in the dominant follicle. FSH stimulates inhibin secretion from granulosa cells and it in turn suppresses FSH synthesis. Inhibin B is primarily secreted in the follicular phase of the cycle but sharply spikes when ovulation occurs. Inhibin A is secreted in the luteal phase and further suppresses FSH. Inhibin also restrains prolactin and growth hormone release, interferes with GnRH receptors, and promotes breakdown of intracellular gonadotropins. In summary, the balance between activin and inhibin regulates FSH secretion. Follistatin inhibits activin and boosts inhibin activity. Inhibin and activin also regulate LH stimulation of androgen synthesis (required for ovarian estrogen biosynthesis) in theca cells.[19] Fig. 24.9 depicts fluctuating estrogen, progesterone, gonadotropin, and inhibin levels. Research continues to advance understanding of the function and structural complexity of these polypeptides and their interaction with GnRH, gonadotropins, and sex hormones.[20]

Ovarian Cycle

By stimulating follicles, gonadotropins initiate their growth and maturation. The most important hormonal event is a rise in FSH levels. The decline in the late luteal phase of estrogen, progesterone, and inhibin

PHASE OF CYCLE AND OVARIAN HORMONE LEVELS	FEEDBACK TO HYPOTHALAMUS AND ANTERIOR PITUITARY	RESULTANT GNRH, FSH, AND LH LEVELS	OVARIAN AND MENSTRUAL EVENTS
Early follicular phase: estrogen levels low; minute amount of progesterone secreted	Negative and inhibitory	All low	Ovarian follicle develops; endometrium proliferates
Late follicular (preovulatory) phase: estrogen levels high; progesterone increases with small surge before ovulation	Positive and stimulatory	All surge; LH dominates	Process of ovulation begins; endometrial proliferation complete
Ovulatory phase: estrogen levels dip; progesterone levels begin to rise	Negative and inhibitory	All fall sharply	Corpus luteum begins to develop; endometrium enters secretory phase
Early luteal phase: estrogen and progesterone levels high; progesterone dominates	Negative and inhibitory	All continue to decline, but gradually	Corpus luteum fully developed; endometrium ready for implantation
Late luteal phase: estrogen and progesterone levels fall sharply	Negative and inhibitory; feedback lessens slightly	All rise slightly	Corpus luteum regresses; endometrium breaks down; menstruation begins
Menstrual phase: estrogens levels low; minute amount of progesterone secreted	Negative and inhibitory	All low	More ovarian follicles begin to develop; functional layer of endometrium is shed

TABLE 24.3   HORMONAL FEEDBACK MECHANISM IN THE MENSTRUAL CYCLE

FSH, Follicle-stimulating hormone; *GnRH*, gonadotropin-releasing hormone; *LH*, luteinizing hormone.

secretion allows FSH levels to rise; concurrently there is a slight increase in LH levels (see Fig. 24.9). FSH stimulates granulosa cell growth and initiates estrogen production in these cells in the next cycle. At this time a group of ovarian follicles is recruited and begins to mature; the exact number depends on the remaining pool of inactive follicles. As the follicles mature, granulosa cells multiply, increasing estradiol secretion. Within a few days of the cycle, one follicle becomes dominant and the others atrophy. The mechanism for follicular recruitment or dominance is unknown.[21] The dominant follicle begins to secrete progressively larger amounts of estrogen (estradiol), which exerts an increase in GnRH receptor concentration and an increase in pituitary sensitivity to GnRH, creating a positive-feedback effect causing an FSH and LH surge. Ovulation generally occurs 1 to 2 hours before the final progesterone surge, or about 12 to 36 hours after the onset of the FSH and LH surge. Progesterone, proteolytic enzymes, and prostaglandins (E and F series) trigger mechanisms controlling follicular rupture and release of the ovum into the fallopian tube.[22] The FSH and LH surge also transforms the granulosa cells of the ovulatory follicle into the corpus luteum. The corpus luteum secretes estrogen and progesterone in amounts that depend in part on adequate development of the follicle before ovulation. Progesterone acts centrally and locally within the ovary to suppress new follicular growth during the early and midluteal phases. If pregnancy does not occur, the corpus luteum persists for 11 to 14 days, and then regresses and eventually disappears. An increase in pulse frequency of GnRH from a low level of estrogen and progesterone reactivates hormonal control of the menstrual cycle and FSH secretion increases.

Uterine Phases

Uterine phases of the menstrual cycle—the follicular/proliferative phase, the luteal/secretory phase, and menstruation—involve cyclic changes that occur in the endometrium controlled by estrogen and progesterone. Hormonal effects are influenced by the presence of receptors and numerous growth factors, peptides, and enzymes that act as intermediaries between the sex steroids and the endometrium. During the midfollicular phase, increasing levels of estrogen contribute to endometrial repair and proliferation, thus increasing endometrial thickness (luteal phase). Once ovulation occurs and serum progesterone levels increase, the endometrial tissue develops secretory characteristics (secretory phase). If implantation of a fertilized ovum does not take place, endometrial tissue begins to break down approximately 11 days after ovulation (ischemic phase of menstruation) (see Fig. 24.9). Sloughing of tissue (menstrual bleeding) begins about 14 days after ovulation.

Cervical mucus also undergoes cyclic changes. During the proliferative phase the cervical mucus is thin and watery. Peak estrogen levels occur just before ovulation and maximally stimulate the cervical glands to produce mucus. Cervical mucus becomes abundant and more elastic (spinnbarkeit). In the presence of estrogen, tiny channels develop in the mucus, which allows sperm access to the interior of the uterus. Changes in the consistency of cervical mucus can be used to identify fertile intervals. After ovulation, the ovary begins to secrete progesterone under the influence of the corpus luteum. The amount of cervical mucus is reduced, becomes thicker and stickier, and blocks sperm migration.

Vaginal Response

The vaginal endothelium also responds to cyclic hormonal changes of the menstrual cycle. Under the influence of estrogen, cells of the vagina epithelium grow maximally during the follicular/proliferative phase. After ovulation, layers of keratinized cells overgrow the basal epithelium, a process known as cornification. Near the end of the luteal phase, leukocytes invade vaginal epithelium, removing the outer layers in a process termed decornification.

Body Temperature

Basal body temperature (BBT) undergoes characteristic biphasic changes during menstrual cycles in which ovulation occurs. During the follicular phase the BBT fluctuates around 37°C (98°F). After the LH surge, the average temperature increases by 0.2°C to 0.5°C (0.4°F to 1°F). At the end of the luteal phase, 1 to 3 days before the onset of menstruation, BBT declines to follicular-phase levels. The shift in temperature is related to ovulation, corpus luteum formation, and increased serum progesterone levels. Progesterone probably acts on the thermoregulatory center of the hypothalamus to increase body temperature. Changes in BBT are used to document ovulatory cycles, but when used alone are not the best method to predict the exact timing of ovulation.[24]

STRUCTURE AND FUNCTION OF THE BREAST

The adult breast lies on the ventral surface of the thorax, within the superficial fascia of the chest wall, extending vertically from the second rib to the sixth or seventh intercostal space and laterally from the side of the sternum to the midaxillary line. Breast tissue also may extend into the axilla; this tissue is known as the *tail of Spence.*

The Female Breast

The female breast is composed of 15 to 20 pyramid-shaped lobes that are separated and supported by suspensory (Cooper) ligaments (Fig. 24.10). Each lobe contains 20 to 40 lobules. The lobules subdivide further into many functional units called acini (*singular,* acinus). Each acinus is lined with a layer of epithelial cells capable of secreting milk and an underlying layer of myoepithelial cells capable of contracting to squeeze milk from the acinus. Biochemical signaling and density within the extracellular matrix are essential for differentiation and function of the acini glandular epithelium. The acini empty into a network of lobular collecting ducts, which empty into interlobular collecting and ejecting ducts. Collagen fiber alignment is required for ductal elongation and organized branching.[25] The ducts reach the skin through openings (pores) in the nipple. The lobes and lobules are surrounded and separated by muscle strands and fatty connective tissue. The amount of fatty connective tissue varies among individuals, depending on weight and genetic and endocrine factors, and contributes to the diversity of breast size and shape and to the function of the mammary epithelium. Fat increases in the breast after menopause.[26]

Fetal and early postnatal breast tissue development does not depend on hormones, although fetal breast tissue becomes progressively responsive to hormonal stimulation. The neonatal breasts are rudimentary, containing 10 to 12 branching ducts. During childhood, breast growth is latent and growth of the nipple and areola keep pace with other body tissues. (Male breast development normally does not progress any further.) At the onset of puberty in the female, growth hormone, insulin-like growth factor-1 (IGF-1), and estrogen stimulate mammary growth. Breast development, or thelarche, is usually the first sign of puberty in the female. Full differentiation and maturation of breast tissue occur over approximately 4 years and are mediated by the levels of a variety of hormones, including estrogen, progesterone, prolactin, growth hormone, thyroid and parathyroid hormones, insulin, and cortisol. Estrogen promotes the increase in size of the breast by the formation of a mass of tissue under the areola, increases the size and pigmentation of the areola, and promotes development of the lobular ducts. The breast cells of parous women are different than those of women who never become pregnant as expansion of acini only occurs with pregnancy when the mammary gland prepares for lactation. During menopause the lobules of the parous breast involute to prepregnancy composition and become identical to the nulliparous breast.[27] Variations in breast development are listed in Box E 24-1 found on Evolve.

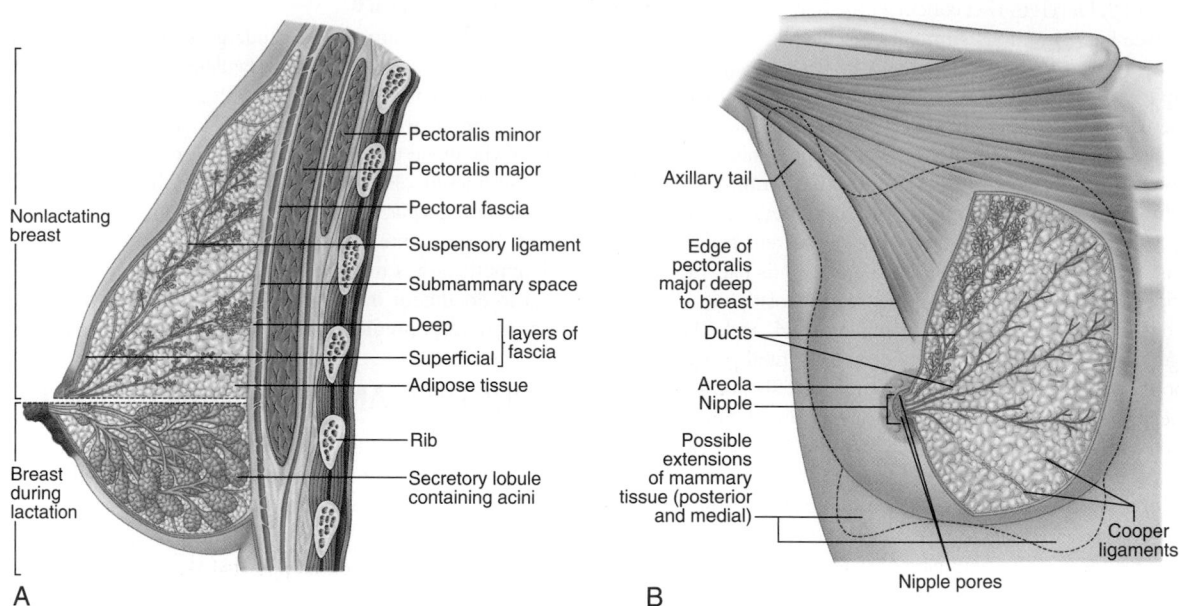

FIGURE 24.10 Schematic Diagram of Breast. **A,** Lactating breast. **B,** Structures of the breast. (From Shah P: Breast. In Standring S, editor: *Gray's anatomy*, ed 40, London, 2009, Elsevier Churchill Livingstone.)

During the reproductive years the breast undergoes cyclic changes in response to changes in the levels of estrogen and progesterone associated with the menstrual cycle. Estrogen promotes development of the lobular ducts; progesterone stimulates development of cells lining the acini. Lactation (milk production) occurs after childbirth in response to increased levels of prolactin. Prolactin secretion, in turn, increases by continued breast-feeding. Oxytocin, another hormone released from the hypothalamus after delivery, controls milk ejection (let-down) from acini cells. During the follicular/proliferative phase of the menstrual cycle, high estradiol levels increase the vascularity of breast tissue and stimulate proliferation of ductal and acinar tissue. This effect is sustained into the luteal/secretory phase of the cycle. During this phase, progesterone levels increase and contribute to the breast changes induced by estradiol. Specific effects of progesterone include dilation of the ducts and conversion of the acinar cells into secretory cells. Most women experience some degree of premenstrual breast fullness, tenderness, and increased nodularity. Breast volume may increase as much as 10 to 30 mL. Because the length of the menstrual cycle does not allow for complete regression of new cell growth, breast growth continues at a slow rate until approximately 35 years of age. Because of the cyclic changes that occur in breast tissue, clinical breast examination is recommended at the conclusion of or a few days after the menstrual cycle when hormonal effects are minimal and breasts are at their smallest and least tender.

During pregnancy the breast remodels into a milk-secreting organ and reaches its ultimate mature developmental stage. With increased levels of estrogen, the lobules further differentiate. Progesterone stimulates development of cells lining the alveoli to produce milk. Lactation (milk production) occurs after childbirth in response to increased levels of prolactin. Prolactin secretion, in turn, increases by continued breast-feeding. Milk is continuously secreted into the alveolar lumen and is stored there until the myoepithelial cells are stimulated by suckling stimulation of oxytocin, which triggers the let-down reflex. The alveoli empty into a network of lactiferous ducts. These ducts reach the skin through 9 or 10 openings (pores) in the nipple. After pregnancy, the milk is continuously secreted into the alveolar lumen and is stored there until the myoepithelial cells are stimulated by oxytocin to contract,

which triggers the let-down reflex. The alveoli empty into a network of lactiferous ducts. These ducts reach the skin through 9 or 10 openings (pores) in the nipple.

The breast has the capacity to regress to a resting state after cessation of lactation and then undergo the same cycle of expansion and regression in subsequent pregnancies, a process possibly maintained by stem cells.[30] This remarkable plasticity of the breast suggests tight hormonal control and dramatic tissue-stromal and lobular restructuring.[31]

An extensive capillary network surrounds the acini and is supplied by perforating branches of the internal mammary, the thoracoacromial, the internal and lateral thoracic, and the intercostal arteries. Venous return follows arterial supply, with relatively rapid emptying into the superior vena cava. The breasts receive sensory innervation from branches of the second through sixth intercostal nerves and the cervical plexus. This accounts for the fact that breast pain may be referred to the chest, back, scapula, medial arm, and neck. Lymphatic drainage from the subareolar plexus occurs largely through axillary nodes but there may be a predominance of superficial mammary routes with resultant asymmetry between a person's breasts (Fig. 24.11).[26]

The nipple is a pigmented, cylindrical structure usually located at the fourth or fifth intercostal space. On its surface lie multiple openings, one from each lobe. It measures 0.5 to 1.3 cm in diameter and is approximately 10 to 12 mm in height when erect. The areola is the pigmented circular area in the center of the breast surrounding the nipple. It may be 15 to 60 mm in diameter. A number of sebaceous glands, the glands of Montgomery, are located within the areola and aid in lubrication of the nipple during lactation. The nipple and areola contain smooth muscles that receive motor innervation from the sympathetic nervous system. Breast-feeding, sexual stimulation, and exposure to cold cause the nipple to become erect.

The function of the female breast is primarily to provide a source of nourishment for the newborn. Physiologically, breast milk is the most appropriate nourishment for newborns. Colostrum, produced in low quantities in the first few days postpartum, is rich in immunologic components, including secretory IgA, lactoferrin, leukocytes, and developmental factors, such as epidermal growth factor. The nutrient composition changes over time to meet the changing digestive capabilities

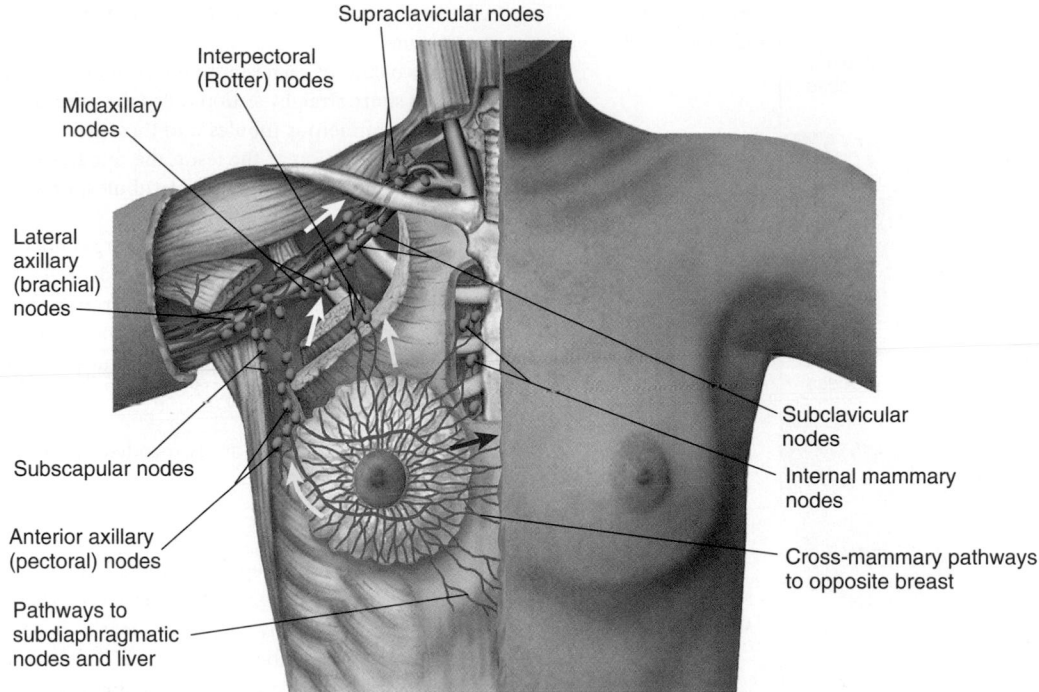

FIGURE 24.11 Lymphatic Drainage of the Female Breast. Arrows indicate the direction of lymphatic drainage. (From Ball JW et al: *Seidel's guide to physical examination,* ed 8, St Louis, 2015, Mosby.)

and nutritional requirements of the infant. Secretory IgA and nonspecific antimicrobial factors, such as lysosomes and lactoferrin, protect the infant against infection.[32] During lactation, high prolactin levels interfere with hypothalamic-pituitary hormones that stimulate ovulation. This mechanism suppresses the menstrual cycle and can prevent ovulation.[33] In some parts of the world, breast-feeding is the major means of contraception (lactational amenorrhea method).[35] However, it is not absolute that ovulation will not occur and this method will not ensure that pregnancy will not occur. Breasts also are a source of pleasurable sexual sensation and in Western cultures have become a sexual symbol.

The Male Breast

Until puberty, development of the male breast is similar to that of the female breast. In the absence of sufficiently high levels of estrogen and progesterone, the male breast does not develop any further. The normal male breast consists of a small underdeveloped nipple, some fatty and fibrous tissue, and a few ductlike structures in the subareolar area. The male breast may appear enlarged in obese men because of accumulation of fatty tissue. During puberty, some males experience benign gynecomastia (benign proliferation of male breast glandular tissue), a condition in which the breasts enlarge temporarily as a result of hormonal fluctuations, and should be differentiated from any underlying systemic disorders.[36]

THE MALE REPRODUCTIVE SYSTEM

The external genitalia in men perform the major functions of reproduction. Sperm are produced in the male gonads, the testes, and delivered by the penis to the female vagina. The internal male genitalia consist of conducting tubes and fluid-producing glands, all of which aid in the transport of sperm from the testes to the urethral opening of the penis. The male reproductive and urinary structures are shown in Fig. 24.12.

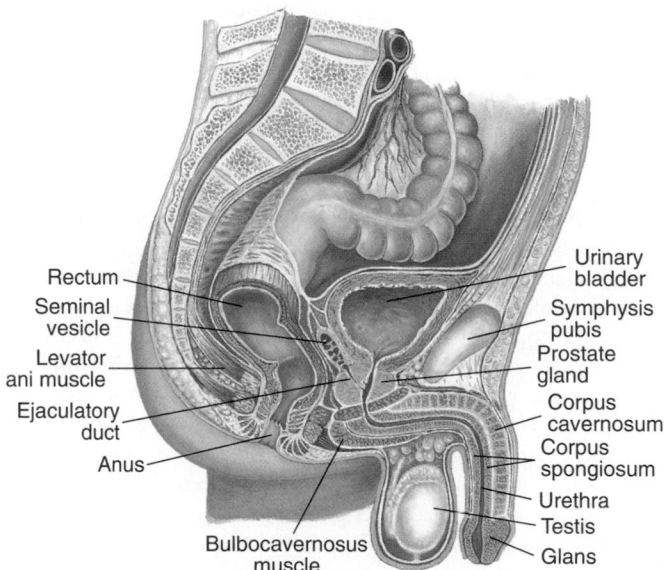

FIGURE 24.12 Structure of the Male Reproductive Organs. (From Ball JW et al: *Seidel's guide to physical examination,* ed 8, St Louis, 2015, Mosby.)

External Genitalia

Testes

In men the **testes** (*singular,* **testis**) are the essential organs of reproduction. Like the ovaries, the testes have two functions: (1) production of gametes (i.e., sperm) and (2) production of sex hormones (i.e., androgens and testosterone).

During embryonic and fetal life, the testes develop within the abdomen (see Fig. 24.1). About 3 months before birth, the testes start

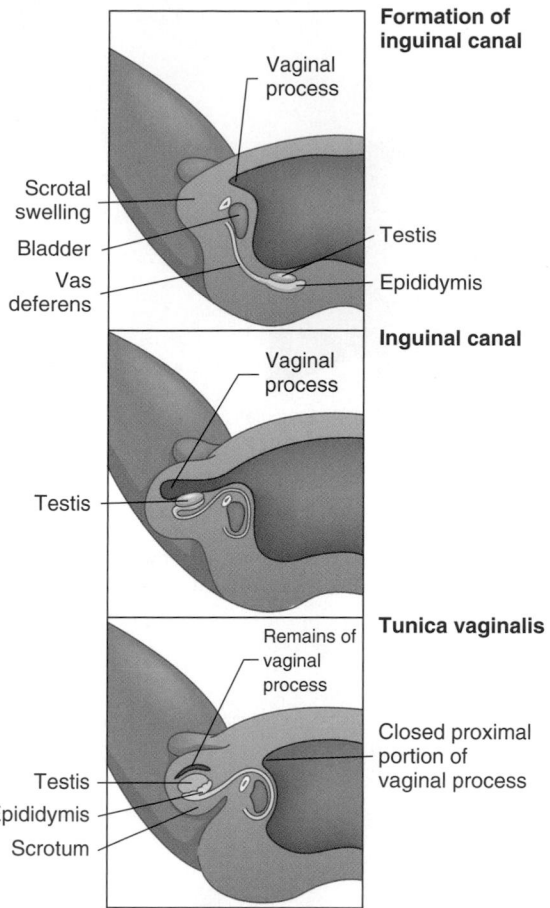

Formation of inguinal canal

Vaginal process

Scrotal swelling
Bladder
Vas deferens

Testis

Epididymis

Inguinal canal

Vaginal process

Testis

Tunica vaginalis

Remains of vaginal process

Closed proximal portion of vaginal process

Testis
Epididymis
Scrotum

FIGURE 24.13 Descent of a Testis. The testes descend from the abdominal cavity to the scrotum during the last 3 months of fetal development.

to descend toward the developing scrotum. About 1 month before birth they enter twin passageways called inguinal canals. The inguinal canals are vaginal processes created by outpouchings of the peritoneum (lining of the abdominal cavity). The descent of a testis is shown in Fig. 24.13. Each testis moves down outside the peritoneum until it is suspended in the scrotal sac by its supply lines: the ducts, blood vessels, lymphatic vessels, and nerves of the spermatic cord. When descent is complete, the abdominal end of each vaginal process closes and the inguinal canal disappears. If peritoneal closure at the site of the inguinal canal is incomplete or weak, an inguinal hernia may occur later in life. The scrotal end of each vaginal process becomes the outer covering of the testis, the tunica vaginalis. Failure of the testes to descend through the inguinal canal is known as *cryptorchidism.*

Fig. 24.14 shows a sagittal section of a mature testis. The adult testis is ovoid and varies considerably in length (3 to 6 cm), width (2 to 3.5 cm), depth (3 to 4 cm), and weight (10 to 40 g). The testis is almost entirely surrounded by an outer covering, the tunica vaginalis, which separates the testis from the scrotal wall, and an inner covering, the tunica albuginea. Inward extensions of the tunica albuginea form septa that separate the testis into about 250 compartments, or lobules, each of which contains several tortuously coiled ducts called seminiferous tubules. The seminiferous tubules constitute the bulk (80%) of testicular volume and are the site of sperm production. Spermatogenesis is described under the section titled Spermatogenesis. Tissue surrounding these ducts contains blood and lymphatic vessels, fibroblastic support cells, macrophages, mast cells, and Leydig

cells. Leydig cells occur in clusters and produce androgens, chiefly testosterone.

The two ends of each seminiferous tubule join and leave the lobule through a short, straight section called the tubulus rectus. Sperm travel from the seminiferous tubules into these straight sections, which lead to the central portion of the testis, the rete testis. From the rete testis, sperm move through the efferent tubules, or vasa efferentia, to the epididymis, where they mature.

The testes are innervated by adrenergic fibers, whose sole function is to regulate blood flow to the Leydig cells. Arterial blood from the internal spermatic and differential arteries flows over the surface of the testes before entering the parenchyma (functional tissues). Surface flow cools the blood to temperatures that promote spermatogenesis, approximately 2°C to 7°C (3.6°F to 12.6°F) below body core temperature.[37]

Additionally, the testes are suspended outside the pelvic cavity to facilitate cooling.

Epididymis

The epididymis (*plural,* epididymides) is a comma-shaped structure that curves over the posterior portion of each testis (see Fig. 24.14). It consists of a single highly packed and markedly coiled duct measuring 5 to 7 cm in length (about 6 meters in length when uncoiled). The epididymis has structural and physiologic functions. Its structural function is to conduct sperm from the efferent tubules to the vas deferens, whereas physiologic functions include sperm maturation, mobility, and fertility. When sperm enter the head of the epididymis, they are not fully mature or motile, nor are they capable of fertilizing an ovum. During the 12 days (or more) sperm take to travel the length of the epididymis, they receive nutrients and testosterone from the epididymal epithelium, and their capacity for fertilization is enhanced.[38] After traveling the length of the epididymis, sperm are stored in the epididymal tail, which is continuous with the vas deferens. The vas deferens (ductus deferens) is a duct with muscular layers capable of powerful peristalsis that transports sperm toward the urethra. The vas deferens enters the pelvic cavity through the spermatic cord (see Fig. 24.14).

Scrotum

The testes, epididymides, and spermatic cord are enclosed and protected by the scrotum—a skin-covered fibromuscular sac that is homologous to the female labia majora (see Fig. 24.2). The skin of the scrotum is thin and has rugae (wrinkles or folds) that enable it to enlarge or relax away from the body. At puberty the scrotal skin darkens, develops active sebaceous glands, and becomes sparsely covered with hair. Just under the skin lies a layer of connective tissue (fascia) and smooth muscle, the tunica dartos (see Fig. 24.14). The tunica dartos also forms a septum that separates the two testes. Exposure to cold temperatures causes the tunica dartos to contract, pulling the testes close to the warm body. In warm temperatures the tunica dartos relaxes, suspending the testes away from body heat. These mechanisms promote optimal temperatures for spermatogenesis. In addition, scrotal sensitivity to touch, pressure, temperature, and pain protects the testes against potential harm. During sexual excitement the scrotal skin and tunica thicken, the scrotum tightens and lifts, and the spermatic cords shorten, partially elevating the testes toward the body. As excitement plateaus, the engorged testes increase 50% in size, rotate anteriorly, and flatten against the body, signaling impending ejaculation.

Penis

The penis has two main functions: delivery of sperm to the female vagina and elimination of urine. (Urine formation and excretion are

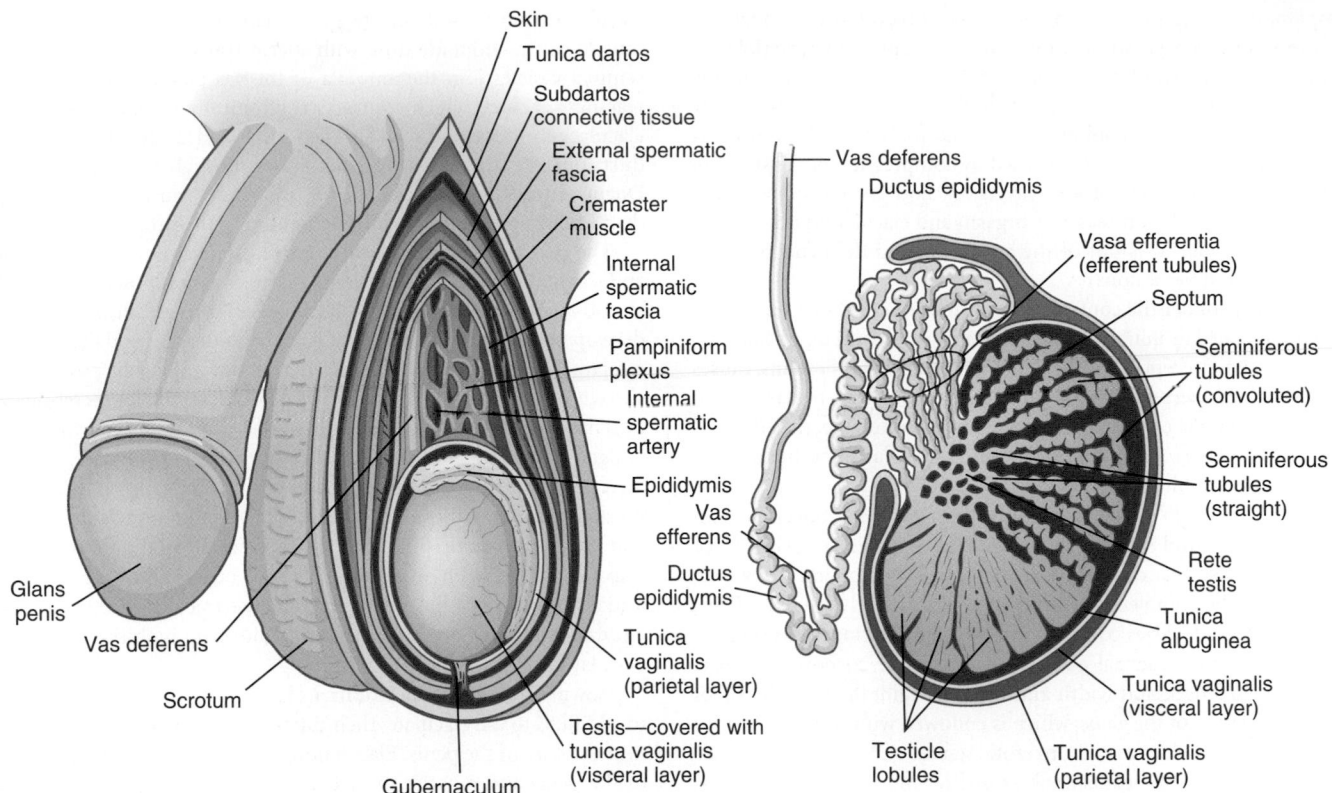

FIGURE 24.14 The Testes. External and sagittal views showing interior anatomy. (From Seidel HM et al: *Mosby's guide to physical examination,* ed 6, St Louis, 2006, Mosby.)

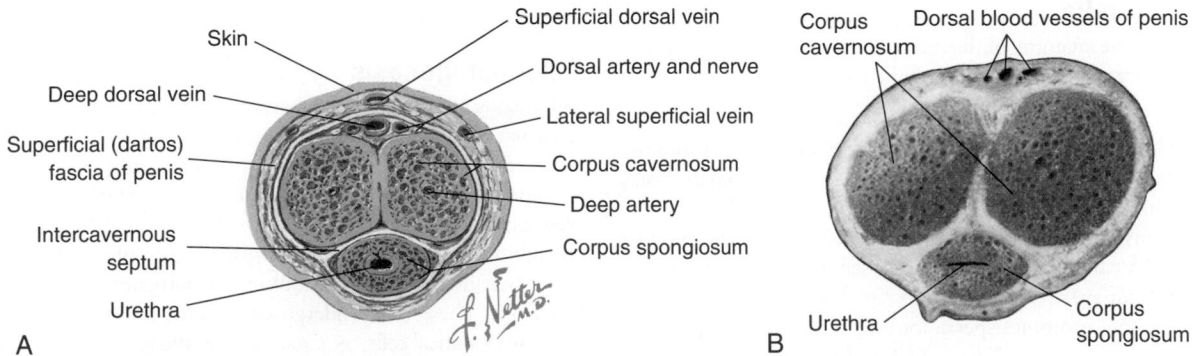

FIGURE 24.15 The Penis. A, Cross section of the penis. **B,** Cross section of the shaft of the penis showing three columns of erectile, or cavernous, tissue. (**A** From Netter illustration from www.netterimages.com. Copyright Elsevier Inc. All rights reserved. **B** From Vidic B, Suarez RF: *Photographic atlas of the human body,* St Louis, 1984, Mosby.)

the subjects of Chapter 38.) Embryonically, the penis is homologous to the female clitoris (see Fig. 24.2).

Fig. 24.12 shows a sagittal section of the adult penis and its anatomic relation to other urogenital structures. Externally the penis consists of a shaft with a tip, the **glans,** that contains the opening of the urethra (see Figs. 24.14 and 24.15). The skin of the glans folds over the tip of the penis, forming the prepuce, or **foreskin (prepuce).** At birth, the foreskin is adhered to the glans. Penile erections, which commonly occur, cause the adhesions to break so that by age 3 years the foreskin becomes completely retractable. The skin of the penis is continuous with that of the groin, scrotum, and inner thighs. It is hairless, movable, and darker than the surrounding skin.

Internally the penis consists of the urethra and three compartments: two **corpora cavernosa** (*singular,* **corpus cavernosum**) and the **corpus spongiosum** (see Fig. 24.15) separated by Buck fascia. Like the testes, these compartments are enclosed by the fibrous tunica albuginea. The **urethra** passes through the corpus spongiosum and ends at a sagittal slit in the glans.

Penetration of the female vagina is made possible by the **erectile reflex,** a process in which erectile tissues within the corpora cavernosa and corpus spongiosum become engorged with blood, generally 20 to 50 mL. The erectile tissues consist of vascular spaces, or chambers, that are supplied with blood by arterioles (small arteries). Typically, the arterioles are constricted through tonic noradrenaline release from sympathetic nerves so that small amounts of blood flow through the erectile tissues. Sexual stimulation, however, causes the arterioles to dilate through release of nitric oxide and fill with blood, expanding the erectile tissues and causing an erection. Other central transmitters, such as dopamine and acetylcholine, are facilitators of erectile control, as well. Erection apparently is maintained by compression or constriction of veins that drain the corpora cavernosa and corpus spongiosum. When sexual stimulation ceases or orgasm and ejaculation occur, these veins open, blood flows out of the arterioles, and the penis becomes flaccid (soft and pendulous).

Erection is under the control of the autonomic nervous system but can be stimulated or inhibited by central nervous system input. Stimulation of mechanoreceptors of the penis, particularly of the glans, causes parasympathetic nerves of the autonomic nervous system to relax smooth muscle in the walls of penile arterioles. At the same time, the effects of sympathetic nerves, which normally cause arteriolar smooth muscle to constrict, are inhibited.

Erections begin in utero and continue throughout life, but ejaculation does not occur until sperm production begins at puberty. Growth of the penis and scrotal contents continues well past puberty, however, and may not be complete until the late teens or early twenties. Penis size, when flaccid, varies considerably; with an erection, differences in penis size diminish. Sexual excitement causes the corpora cavernosa to increase in length and width and become rigid; the penis becomes erect. Stimulation of the glans, which is endowed with copious sensitive nerve endings, provides maximum erotic sensation. With sexual arousal, skin color deepens, the glans doubles in size, and the urethral meatus dilates. Ejaculation occurs with frequent, strong contractions of the vas deferens, epididymis, seminal vesicles, prostate, urethra, and penis. Erection and ejaculation can occur independently of each other, but it is not common.[39]

Internal Genitalia

Fig. 24.13 shows the anatomy of the internal genitalia and their relation to other pelvic organs. The internal genitalia consist of ducts and glands as follows:

Ducts—consist of two vasa deferentia, the ejaculatory duct, and the urethra—conduct sperm and glandular secretions from the testes to the urethral opening of the penis

Glands—consist of the prostate gland, two seminal vesicles, and two Cowper (or bulbourethral) glands—secrete fluids that serve as a vehicle for sperm transport and create an alkaline, nutritious medium that promotes sperm motility and survival

Together the sperm and the glandular fluids comprise semen.

Sperm leave the epididymides and travel rapidly through the internal ducts in a process called emission. Emission occurs just seconds before ejaculation, at the moment when sexual arousal peaks. It always leads to ejaculation.

Emission occurs as smooth muscle in the walls of the epididymides and vasa deferentia begins to contract rhythmically, pushing sperm and epididymal secretions through the vasa deferentia. Each vas deferens is a firm, elastic fibromuscular tube that begins at the tail of the epididymis, enters the pelvic cavity within the spermatic cord, loops up and over the bladder, and ends in the prostate gland (Fig. 24.16; see also Fig. 24.12). Sperm are moved along by peristaltic contractions of smooth muscle in the walls of the vas deferens.

As sperm leave the ampulla (wide portion) of the vas deferens, the seminal vesicles secrete a nutritive glucose-rich fluid into the ejaculate (semen). The seminal vesicles are a pair of glands, each about 4 to 6 cm long, that lie behind the urinary bladder and in front of the rectum. The seminal vesicles provide fructose as a source of energy for

ejaculated sperm, and secrete prostaglandins that promote smooth muscle contraction, assisting with sperm transport. The ducts of the seminal vesicles join the ampulla of the vas deferens to become the ejaculatory duct, which contracts rhythmically during emission and ejaculation. As can be seen in Figs. 24.12 and 24.16, the ejaculatory duct joins the urethra, where both pass through the prostate gland. During emission and ejaculation a sphincter (muscle surrounding a duct) closes, preventing urine from entering the prostatic urethra.

The prostate gland is about the size of a walnut, has three zones, and surrounds the urethra (see Fig. 24.16). It is composed of glandular alveoli and ducts embedded in fibromuscular tissue. Prostate growth, development, and function are regulated by androgens and the androgen receptor. Nerves required for penile erection travel along the posterolateral surface of the prostate. Included in prostate epithelial secretions are prostate-specific antigen (PSA), cytokeratins, prostate-specific membrane antigen (PSMA), and prostate-specific acid phosphatase. Prostate secretions contribute to the ejaculate. While semen moves through the prostatic portion of the urethra, the prostate gland contracts rhythmically and secretes prostatic fluid into the mixture. Prostatic fluid is a thin, milky substance with an alkaline pH that helps sperm survive in the acid environment of the female reproductive tract. In addition, clotting enzymes and fibrinolysin in prostatic fluids help mobilize sperm after ejaculation.

Cowper glands (bulbourethral glands) are the last pair of glands to add fluid to the ejaculate; their ducts secrete mucus into the urethra near the base of the penis. Ejaculation occurs as semen reaches the base of the penis and muscles there begin the rhythmic contractions that expel semen. A man normally ejaculates between 2 and 6 mL of semen, containing 75 million to 400 million sperm. About 98% of the ejaculate consists of glandular fluids; 60% to 70% of volume originates from the seminal vesicles and 20% from the prostate. Therefore the ejaculate of a man who has undergone a vasectomy (a surgical procedure that prevents sperm from entering the vas deferens) is reduced by about 2%.

Spermatogenesis

Spermatogenesis begins at puberty and continues for life. In this respect, spermatogenesis differs markedly from oogenesis (production of primordial ova), which occurs during fetal life only.

Spermatogenesis (the production of sperm) takes place within the seminiferous tubules of the testes (see Fig. 24.14). The basement membrane of each seminiferous tubule is lined with diploid (46-chromosome) germ cells called spermatogonia (*singular*, spermatogonium). These cells undergo continuous mitotic division (division into two identical cells, see Chapter 1). Some spermatogonia move away from the basement membrane and mature, becoming primary spermatocytes (Fig. 24.17). These undergo meiosis, cell division that results in two haploid (23-chromosome) cells called secondary spermatocytes. (Meiosis is described and illustrated in Chapter 4.) The secondary spermatocytes also undergo meiosis, resulting in four spermatids. The spermatids differentiate into spermatozoa, or sperm, each of which contains 23 chromosomes (Fig. 24.18).

The development of spermatids into sperm depends on the presence of Sertoli cells (nondividing support cells) within the seminiferous tubules. Spermatids attach themselves to the Sertoli cells, from which they receive nutrients and hormonal signals (i.e., testosterone) needed to develop into sperm.[41] The process of spermatogenesis, from mitotic division of a spermatogonium to maturation of the spermatids, takes about 70 to 80 days. Mature sperm migrate from the seminiferous tubules to the epididymis, where their capacity for fertilization continues to develop. Although they are completely mature by the time they are ejaculated, the sperm do not become motile (capable of movement) until they are activated by biochemicals in semen and in the female reproductive tract.

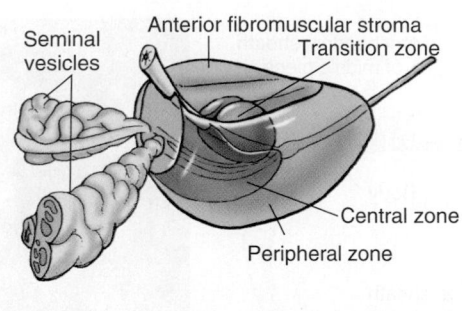

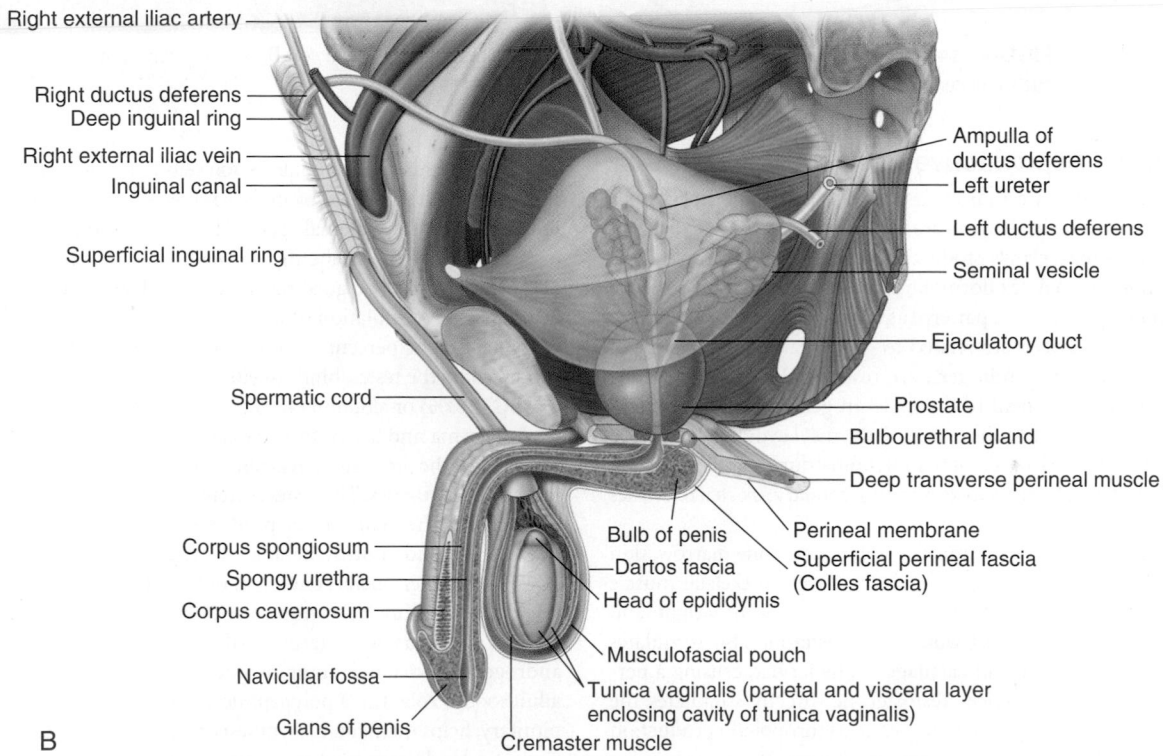

FIGURE 24.16 Zones of the Prostate Gland and Seminal Vesicles. **A,** Zones of the prostate. The peripheral zone, accounting for 70% of the prostate gland, is the site of origin of ≤70% of prostate cancers; the central zone, approximately 25% of the prostate gland, gives rise to only 1% to 5% of prostate cancers; and the transition zone, approximately 5% to 10% of the prostate gland, gives rise to 20% of prostate cancers and is the site of origin of benign prostatic hyperplasia (BPH). **B,** Prostate gland within the male reproductive system. (**A** Copyright Baylor College of Medicine, Houston, TX. **B** From Drake et al: *Gray's atlas of anatomy*, Philadelphia, 2008, Churchill Livingstone.)

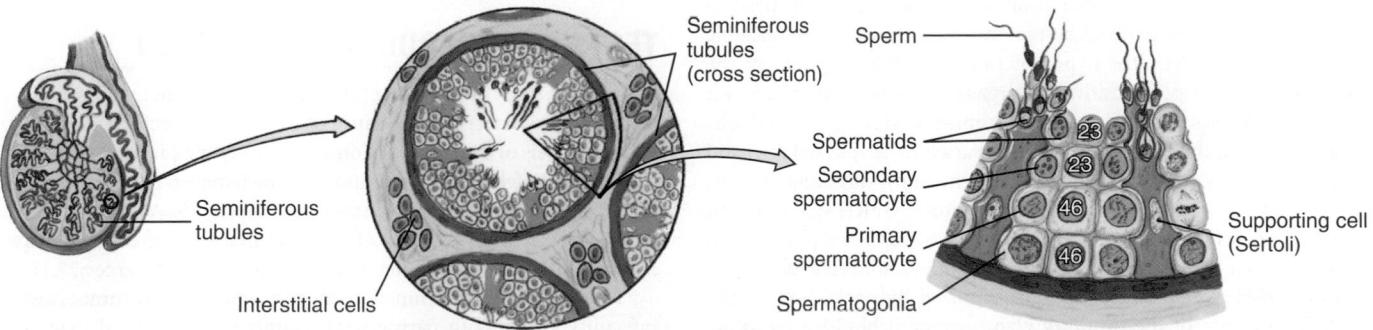

FIGURE 24.17 Seminiferous Tubule and Spermatogenesis. Cross section of a seminiferous tubule showing the different cell types. Interstitial cells that produce testosterone are between the seminiferous tubules. Spermatids in the lumen become sperm by a process called spermatogenesis. The numbers in white represent the number of chromosomes. (From Applegate E: *The anatomy and physiology learning system*, ed 4, St Louis, 2011, Saunders.)

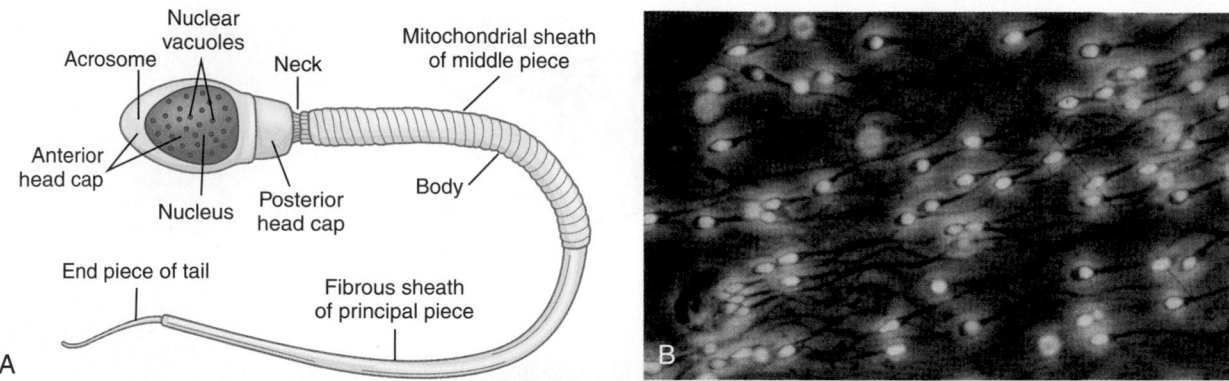

FIGURE 24.18 Mature Sperm Cell (Spermatozoon). **A,** Anatomy of mature sperm cell. **B,** Human sperm with nuclear material glowing with a fluorescent dye. (**B** From Lennart Nilsson.)

Male Sex and Reproductive Hormones

The male sex hormones are androgens. Testosterone, the primary male sex hormone, and other androgens are produced mainly by Leydig cells of the testes. The adrenal glands produce testosterone and other androgens in lesser amounts. In men, sex hormone production is relatively constant and does not occur in a cyclic pattern, as it does in women. The physiologic actions of androgen are related to growth and development of male tissues and organs. Androgens are responsible for the fetal differentiation and development of the male urogenital system and have some effects on the fetal brain. After birth, the Leydig cells become quiescent until activated by the gonadotropins during puberty. Then androgens cause the sex organs to grow and secondary sex characteristics to develop.

Testosterone affects nervous and skeletal tissues, bone marrow, skin and hair, and sex organs. It has an anabolic effect on skeletal muscle tissue, thereby contributing to the difference in body weight and composition between men and women. Testosterone also stimulates growth of the musculature and cartilage of the larynx, causing a permanent deepening of the voice. Testosterone directly stimulates the bone marrow and indirectly stimulates renal erythropoietin production to achieve increased hemoglobin and hematocrit levels. Because sebaceous gland activity is stimulated by testosterone, acne may develop. In the presence of testosterone, hair becomes coarser in texture, and facial hair, axillary hair, and pubic hair grow in male patterns. Testosterone is required for spermatogenesis and for secretion of fluid by the prostate gland, seminal vesicles, and Cowper glands. Testosterone is also associated with an increase in libido (sex drive). Other, less-understood, effects of testosterone include regulatory proteins involved in glycolysis, glycogen synthesis, insulin action, and lipid and cholesterol metabolism.[43]

The regulation of androgen production and spermatogenesis is achieved by a complex feedback system involving the extrahypothalamic central nervous system, the hypothalamus, the anterior pituitary, the testes, and the androgen-sensitive end organs. These relationships, which are essentially the same in women, are summarized in Fig. 24.3. Extrahypothalamic influences include such variables as physiologic and psychologic stress, which may inhibit or augment hypothalamic activity. In the hypothalamus, neurotransmitters regulate GnRH synthesis and pulsatile release (about every 3 hours) into the hypophyseal portal veins. Norepinephrine stimulates GnRH secretion, and serotonin and dopamine inhibit GnRH secretion. GnRH is transported by portal flow to the median eminence of the pituitary gland, where it binds to receptors and stimulates the synthesis and secretion of the gonadotropins LH and FSH. These gonadotropins are named for their effects in the female reproductive system, but have important effects on the male system as well. LH acts on the Leydig cells to regulate testosterone secretion. FSH acts on the seminiferous tubule Sertoli cells to promote spermatogenesis. FSH secretion is inhibited by inhibin secreted by the Sertoli cells. Similar to their action in the female gonad, inhibin functions as an autocrine/paracrine regulator in the male gonad. Inhibin inhibits proliferation of spermatogonia by regulating pituitary FSH levels. In addition, inhibin facilitates LH stimulation of androgen biosynthesis in Leydig cells.[44]

Ninety-eight percent of testosterone, the major steroid hormone produced by the testes, binds to either sex hormone–binding globulin (SHBG) (40%) or albumin (48%). The remaining 2% remains unbound in the plasma and is free to enter cells and wield its metabolic effects. Changes in the amount of available SHBG affect the amount of testosterone within tissues. The testes secrete only 25% of circulating estrogen (estradiol). The majority is produced by peripheral conversion of testosterone and androstenedione. Estrogens help regulate GnRH and LH secretion. Peripheral conversion of testosterone by 5-alpha-reductase also produces dihydrotestosterone (DHT), another potent androgen. DHT is necessary for external virilization during embryogenesis and androgen activity beginning at puberty and continuing throughout adulthood. Prolactin, a polypeptide synthesized and secreted from the pituitary, helps maintain biosynthesis of testosterone. However, elevated prolactin levels may suppress biosynthesis.[45]

In summary, hormones secreted at each level of the hypothalamic-pituitary-testicular (HPT) axis control and coordinate testicular function (Fig. 24.19). This control is exerted through positive and negative feedback signals by (1) sex steroids that inhibit hypothalamic GnRH secretion and pituitary LH responsiveness to GnRH; and (2) testicular inhibin that inhibits pituitary FSH and, possibly, circulating estrogens (E_2). Any disruption along the HPT axis may lead to hypogonadism or infertility.

TESTS OF REPRODUCTIVE FUNCTION

Diagnostic tests of the male and female reproductive systems are performed to determine the cause of infertility, detect the presence of endometriosis or cancerous lesions, or identify the presence of sexually transmitted infections.[46] (Alterations of the female reproductive system including carcinoma are discussed in Chapter 25. Alterations of the male reproductive system including carcinoma are discussed in Chapter 26. Sexually transmitted infections are discussed in Chapter 27.)

Tests of reproductive function are performed most commonly when infertility exists. Both partners are examined, and several diagnostic evaluations may be completed. The types of tests and their normal values are summarized in Tables 24.4 and 24.5. The man is evaluated for number, amount, structure, and motility of sperm and obstruction along the reproductive tract. Tests for women determine whether (1)

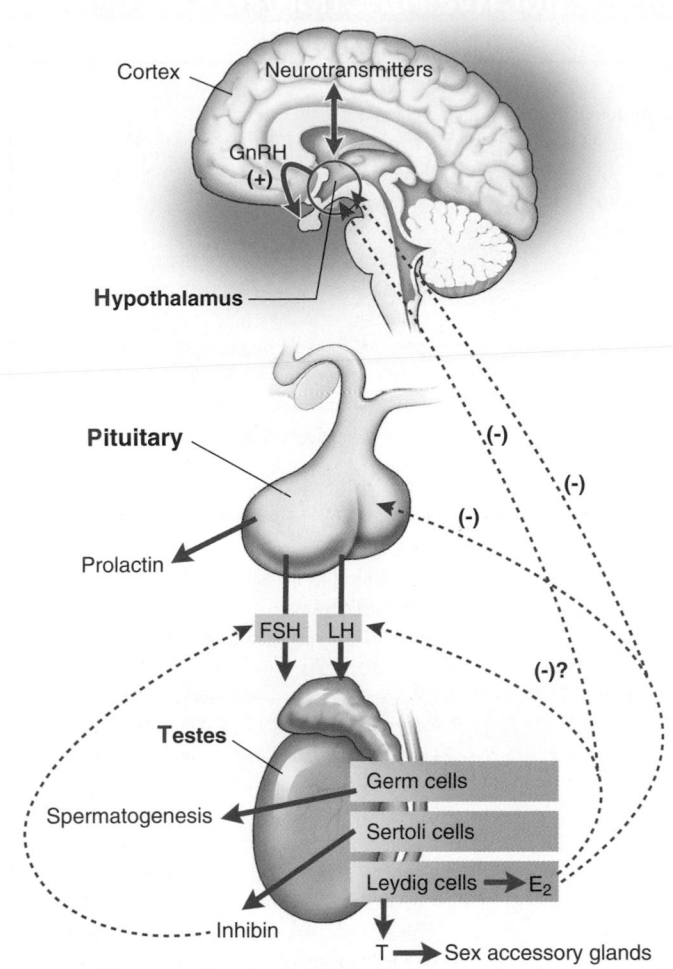

FIGURE 24.19 Schematic Representation of Activity Along the Hypothalamus-Pituitary-Testicular (HPT) Axis. *E₂,* Estrogen; *FSH,* follicle-stimulating hormone; *GnRH,* gonadotropin-releasing hormone; *LH,* luteinizing hormone; *T,* testosterone.

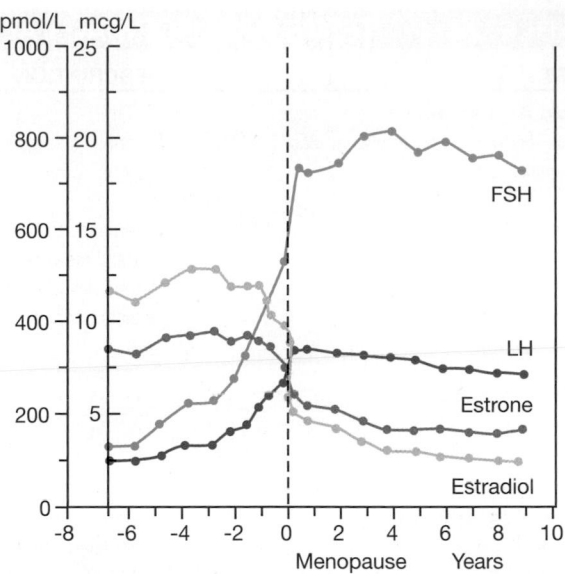

FIGURE 24.20 The Perimenopausal Hormone Transition. Mean circulating hormone levels. *FSH,* Follicle-stimulating hormone; *LH,* luteinizing hormone.

the reproductive tract (cervix, uterus, fallopian tubes) is adequately patent to allow for passage of ovum and sperm, (2) ovulation occurs normally, (3) the endometrium is responding normally to hormones, and (4) reproductive tissues are free of tumors or infections. Hormonal assays evaluate the adequacy of pituitary function and target organ response. The position and size of organs or the presence of tumors can be detected by direct observation procedures using a laparoscope or by ultrasound, radiographic studies, such as plain films, computerized scans, or tomography.[47]

AGING AND REPRODUCTIVE FUNCTION

Aging and the Female Reproductive System

Natural menopause is the cessation of ovulation and menses caused by ovarian failure. It is a normal developmental event marking the end of reproduction. Menopause is universally experienced by midlife women at the average age of 50.5 to 51.4 years in North America with variability between 40 and 60 years.[48,49] Premature menopause is cessation of ovulation before 40 years of age. A number of factors are thought to influence the age of menopause, including genetics, socioeconomic status, race, parity, oral contraceptive use, and lifestyle, such as smoking

or weight.[50] It can occur 2 years sooner on average for smokers; thinner women also tend to experience menopause at a slightly younger age. Genetics accounts for about 50% of the variation in age at menopause.[51] The term "climacteric" refers to gradual changes of ovarian function that start before menopause and result in the symptoms associated with loss of ovarian function.[52] For clarity, the term *menopause* will be used here. The primary changes of menopause are as follows:

- *Perimenopause:* This is the transitional period between reproductive and nonreproductive years, a transition lasting 2 to 8 years. About 5 to 10 years before menopause, approximately 90% of women note mild to extreme variability in frequency and quality of menstrual flow. Changes in hormones occur during this time including erratically higher estradiol levels, decreased progesterone levels (in normal ovulatory, short luteal phase, or anovulatory cycles), and a disturbed ovarian-pituitary-hypothalamic feedback relationship with higher LH levels. A decrease in the sensitivity of the target tissue receptors and the development of perimenopausal symptoms commonly are experienced. Symptoms usually begin with a lengthening of the menstrual cycle, which correlates with anovulatory cycles. Unpredictable or irregular ovulation uniformly precedes menopause. The perimenopause experience varies among women and from cycle to cycle in the same woman. Estradiol levels remain in the normal to slightly elevated range until about 1 year before menopause.
- *Menopause:* Menopause is defined by the point that marks 12 consecutive months of amenorrhea and is determined retrospectively after a woman has not had a menstrual period for 1 year. It is characterized by loss of ovarian function, low estrogen and progesterone levels, and high FSH and LH levels (Fig. 24.20). Early menopause is the 5 years after menopause onset. Late menopause follows and continues until death.[54]
- *Ovarian changes:* Beginning in utero, the number of follicles steadily decreases through activation, maturation, and atresia. Around 37 to 38 years of age, women experience accelerated follicular loss, which ends when the supply of follicles is depleted at menopause. This accelerated loss is correlated with increased FSH stimulation, slightly elevated estradiol levels, declining inhibin B production (normally maintain folliculogenesis and estradiol secretion), and decreasing amounts of anti-müllerian hormone (normally decreases FSH effects). Attenuated LH surges are associated with impaired

TABLE 24.4	TESTS AND NORMAL VALUES OF REPRODUCTIVE FUNCTION/FERTILITY	
TEST	**DESCRIPTION**	**NORMAL VALUE**
Basic Assessment		
Semen analysis (two samples at least 2 weeks apart)	Determines number, motility, and structure of sperm cells	Volume = 2–6 mL Number = >20 million/mL Motility = >50% with forward progression
Sperm DNA fragmentation	Determines the percentage of sperm DNA strand breaks and likelihood of infertility	Less than 15%–25%
White blood cells	Determines presence of bacteria/leukocytes	Morphology = >50% normal shape
Immunologic tests	Detects antibody to sperm	Immunobead test = <20% with adherent particles Sperm MAR test (mixed antiglobulin reaction) = <10% with adherent particles $<10^6$ WBC/mL No sperm agglutinins present
Other Assessments		
Basal body temperature	Determines whether ovulation has occurred	Decrease in basal body temperature before ovulation followed by a rise in temperature at the time of ovulation
FSH level	Day 2–3 of cycle to measure ovarian reserve	Lab specific results
Estradiol	Day 2–3 of cycle to measure ovarian reserve	Low FSH in conjunction with low estradiol—lab specific results
Progesterone	Midluteal phase—1 week before menses	Lab specific results—low level associated with decreased or absent ovulation.
Prolactin	Day 3 of cycle	Lab specific results—high levels can interfere with ovulation
TSH level	Day 3 of cycle	Lab specific results—elevated value associated with hypothyroidism
Urinary LH	Day 11 of cycle	Identifies LH surge and indirect evidence of ovulation: if positive should ovulate in 24–36 hours; high false negative and positive rates
Cervical mucus	Evaluates presence of ovulation from estrogenic effects at ovulation; mucus also may be examined for pH, glucose, or proteins or cultured for presence of infection	Fern pattern appears when cervical mucus dries on a clean slide; mucus is clear, watery, and elastic (spinnbarkeit ≥8–10 cm) with no inflammatory cells
Postcoital cervical mucus (Sims-Huhner test)	Tests ability of sperm to penetrate and maintain motility in cervical mucus 2–4 hours after coitus approximately 1 day before ovulation	≥10 motile sperm in each high-power field; motility in one direction; previous sperm analysis normal
Zona binding test or hamster penetration test	Nonliving oocytes are surgically removed and bisected; sperm added to the hemi-oocyte to test fertilizing capability	Bonding <30% predicted failed fertilization 70% of the time Bonding >30% predicted successful fertilization 85% of the time Results may vary with lab
Ultrasound vaginal scanning	Provides superior quality resolution of the uterine, fallopian, and ovarian structures; also can be used to study folliculogenesis, ovulation, and luteogenesis to detect abnormalities	Normal structures visualized
More Specialized Tests		
Endometrial biopsy	Determines whether ovulation has occurred by obtaining endometrial tissue on day 26 of 28-day menstrual cycle (or postovulatory day 12)	Finding is "secretory-type" endometrium if ovulation has occurred; read in conjunction with day of cycle and serum progesterone levels

TABLE 24.4	TESTS AND NORMAL VALUES OF REPRODUCTIVE FUNCTION/ FERTILITY—cont'd	
TEST	**DESCRIPTION**	**NORMAL VALUE**
Hysterosalpingogram	Assessment of uterus and fallopian tubes for obstructions using transuterine injection of contrast material and radiography; performed 1–2 days after cessation of menses	No obstruction evident
Laparoscopy (pelvic endoscopy)	Visualization of reproductive organs using a laparoscope inserted within the pelvic cavity through the abdomen to assess structure or determine presence of adhesions, endometriosis, tumors, or infection	Normal structure and position of organs
Hysteroscopy	Visualization of uterine cavity using modified cystoscope inserted through cervical os; best done during first 14 days of cycle	Absence of intrauterine lesions
Transvaginal ultrasound	Identifies endometrial development	Shows size and numbers of developing follicles and evidence of ovulation – low counts associated with infertility

FSH, Follicle-stimulating hormone; *TSH,* thyroid-stimulating hormone; *WBC,* white blood cell.

TABLE 24.5	SERUM HORMONE VALUES
HORMONE	**VALUE**
Serum progesterone	Normal = >10 ng/dL, presumptive evidence of ovulation; draw level between days 20 and 25 of 28-day cycle or 6–10 days postovulation <10 ng/mL = inadequate luteal function <3 ng/mL suggests anovulation
Serum testosterone	Normal = 300–1200 ng/dL; must be interpreted with serum LH and FSH levels
Resulting from diurnal and pulsatile pattern, need serial blood draws	Low values in male hypogonadism
Serum FSH and LH	FSH = <22 international units/L
Resulting from diurnal and pulsatile pattern, need serial blood draws	LH = 4–24 international units/L High levels in males indicate primary testicular disease; low levels in males indicate hypogonadism caused by hypothalamic-pituitary dysfunction

FSH, Follicle-stimulating hormone; *LH,* luteinizing hormone.

BOX 24.2   CHANGES IN OVARIAN FOLLICULOGENESIS DURING THE PERIMENOPAUSE LEADING TO ENDOGENOUS OVERSTIMULATION

- ↑ FSH → ovarian hyperstimulation → ↑ number of follicles recruited (net effect of follicular depletion) → ↑ estradiol
- ↓ Follicular reserve → ↓ inhibin and ↑ activin in FP and LP → ↑ FSH → ↑ number of follicles recruited, partial development, infrequent ovulation → ↑ estrogen (E_2) and ↓ progesterone

FP, Follicular phase; *FSH,* follicle-stimulating hormone; *LP,* luteal phase.

---

hypothalamic responses to estradiol positive feedback (see Fig. 24.20 and Box 24.2). The ovarian response to high FSH recruits increasing numbers of follicles; these follicles only partially develop, with a net effect of irregular ovulation, lower progesterone levels, depleted follicle reserve, and infertility. The ovaries begin to decrease in size around age 30; this decrease accelerates after age 60. Of the 500,000 follicles present at the onset of puberty, the number dwindles to between 100 and 1000 with menopause.[55] Table 24.6 summarizes endocrine events occurring during the perimenopause. Table 24.7 provides a template to visualize the complex physiology of the perimenopause and the dynamic changes that occur during this time.

- *Uterine changes:* Uterine changes occur primarily in the endometrium. The increase in anovulatory cycles allows for proliferative growth of the endometrium. The longer exposure to estrogen alone results in greater thickness of the endometrium, and 50% of perimenopausal women will experience dysfunctional uterine bleeding that is heavy and unpredictable. Increased endometrial bleeding is correlated with a change from ovulatory to anovulatory cycles and is associated with unopposed high estrogen levels the week before menses. Estrogen causes endometrial tissue to thicken. However, without corresponding stromal support from progesterone, estrogen production leads to heavier periods, menometrorrhagia (excessive bleeding often caused by submucosal myomas and endometrial polyps), or metrorrhagia (midcycle bleeding) (Table 24.8). In the past this has put women at high risk for hysterectomy or endometrial ablation. Medical and hormonal management is the first line of therapy if the uterus is normal.[56]
- *Breast tissue changes:* Glandular breast tissue becomes involuted, fat deposits and connective tissue increase, and breasts are reduced in size and firmness. There can be an increase in white adipose tissue inflammation with elevated aromatase levels (decreases circulating estrogen).[57]
- *Genitourinary tract changes:* The ovaries shrink; the uterus atrophies; the vagina shortens, narrows, and loses some elasticity. Lubrication

TABLE 24.6 ENDOCRINE EVENTS ASSOCIATED WITH PERIMENOPAUSE

HORMONE CHANGES	EFFECTS
Estradiol (E₂) levels	Erratic and intermittent increase
Mean FP level 1 greater than mean FP level in younger women	First in FP (inverse relationship between length of FP and estradiol level)
FP level may be greater than midcycle peak level in fertile women	Later during premenstrual phase
Ovulatory cycles	Short or insufficient LP (decreased fertility)
Progesterone levels	Decreased in ovulatory cycle; minimal during anovulatory cycles
Anovulatory cycles	Increased to about 50%; perhaps more in later perimenopause
FSH levels	Variable, then increased
LH levels	Normal initially, then increased
Inhibin levels	Correlate with progesterone levels

FP, Follicular phase; *FSH,* follicle-stimulating hormone; *LH,* luteinizing hormone; *LP,* luteal phase.

of the vagina diminishes and vaginal pH increases, creating higher incidence of vaginitis. The cervix atrophies and the cervical os shrinks; vaginal epithelium atrophies; labia majora and minora become less prominent; some pubic hair is lost; urethral tone declines along with muscle tone throughout the pelvic area; urinary frequency or urgency, urinary tract infections, and incontinence may occur. Regular sexual activity and orgasm may diminish some of these changes. Sexually active women have less vaginal atrophy.

- *Skeletal changes:* Bone mass is reduced, leading to increased brittleness and porosity, which increases the risk of osteoporosis and fracture, particularly in the lumbar spine and femoral neck.[58]
- *Cardiovascular changes:* The risk of cardiovascular disease (CVD) increases significantly and is the leading cause of death in post-menopausal women. Blood pressure and total and LDL-cholesterol increase and HDL-cholesterol decreases. There is increased risk for metabolic syndrome.[60]
- *Systemic changes:* **Vasomotor flushes** are characterized by a rise in skin temperature, dilation of peripheral blood vessels, increased blood flow in the hands, increased skin conductance, and a transient increase in heart rate followed by a temperature drop and profuse perspiration over the area of flush distribution. This usually occurs in the face and neck and may radiate into the chest and other parts of the body. Night sweats, dizziness, nausea, headaches, or palpitations may accompany the flush. These flushes can vary in frequency, intensity, and duration and are experienced by up to 85% of peri-menopausal to postmenopausal women from 1 to 15 years (mean 1 to 5 years). The physiology of vasomotor flushes is poorly understood. One theory proposes that rapid changes in estrogen levels may result in loss of negative feedback over hypothalamic noradrenaline synthesis, the primary neurotransmitter involved in

TABLE 24.7 POSTULATED PERIMENOPAUSAL TRANSITION TIME LINE

PHASE	MENSTRUAL PHYSIOLOGY	HORMONAL CHANGES	SYMPTOMATOLOGY
A	Regular, ovulatory cycles; Short cycles, short FP	Intermittent ↑ E₂; FSH usually normal; Intermittent ↑ FP FSH; Low inhibin	Increased breast tenderness, mood swings, fluid retention, premenstrual symptoms; Early morning night sweats (vasomotor symptoms); Weight gain, migraine headaches, heavy flow
B	Regular cycles with disturbances in ovulation; Short LP; Insufficient LP; Anovulatory cycles	Intermittent ↑ FP FSH; E₂ often ↑; Inhibin inappropriately low	Heavy flow; ↑ Premenstrual symptoms; ↑ Dysmenorrhea; Predictable or ↑ vasomotor symptoms before flow
C	Onset of perimenopause; Alternating short, long, or skipped cycles	E₂ often quite ↑; E₂ normal or low; ↑ FSH (slight); ↑ LH; Low inhibin	Vasomotor symptoms during waking hours; Vasomotor symptoms more persistent, remain cyclic before flow
D	Onset of oligomenorrhea; 50% of cycles anovulatory; Heavy flow may predict onset of oligomenorrhea	↑ Progesterone with ovulation; Persistent ↓ FSH; ↑ LH; ↑ E₂; Low inhibin	↑ Vasomotor symptoms; ↑ Signs/symptoms of high estrogen after long periods without flow; Flow light but unpredictable
E	Final menstrual period plus 1 year	↑ FSH and LH; ↓ or normal E₂; Consistent low inhibin; ↓ Progesterone	↑ Intensity and frequency of vasomotor symptoms (although vasomotor symptoms may disappear); ↓ Cramps and premenstrual-type symptoms without subsequent flow; ↓ Breast, mood, and fluid symptoms

E₂, Estradiol; *FP,* follicular phase; *FSH,* follicle-stimulating hormone; *LP,* luteal phase.

TABLE 24.8	IMPACT OF HIGH ESTROGEN LEVELS ON MENSTRUAL CYCLE AND SYMPTOMATOLOGY
ASSOCIATED PHYSIOLOGIC CHANGE	**SIGNS/SYMPTOMS**
Short follicular phase (FP)	Short cycles
Long FP	Long cycles
Thickened endometrium	Heavy, long, or unpredictable flow (including clotting and flooding)*
Increase in glandular cells without stromal support produced by progesterone → unstable endometrium	Midcycle spotting Menorrhagia
Possible increased production of prostaglandins within endometrial tissue	Metrorrhagia Dysmenorrhea Breast tenderness, modularity, enlargement Water retention Emotional stress; new or unpredictable mood swings Weight gain Vasomotor symptoms New onset of migraine headaches; exacerbation of headaches Increased premenstrual symptoms

*Symptoms aggravated by anovulatory cycles; leads to dysfunctional uterine bleeding (see Chapter 25).

thermoregulation.[61] Estrogen modulates adrenergic receptors. The decrease in estrogen level in menopause is thought to decrease the number of receptors leading to increased noradrenaline levels and hot flushes. Interestingly, emerging evidence shows that the intensity of vasomotor flushes may be associated with increased risk for cardiovascular disease.[62]

- *Other changes:* Emotional stress with unpredictable mood swings, weight gain, migraine headaches, insomnia, and depression often accompany the change in estrogen levels.[63]
- Lower estrogen levels decrease skin thickness and diminish skin elasticity, thereby causing increased skin dryness and wrinkling. Alopecia and unwanted facial hair are common.[64]

Aging and the Male Reproductive System

Men maintain reproductive capacity longer than women. There is no known discrete event, comparable to menopause, that characterizes aging of the male reproductive system, although the term andropause is sometimes used to describe the changes associated with male aging and lower levels of testosterone. Gradual changes do occur, and aging

in the male reproductive system is characterized by hypogonadism, testosterone deficiency, erectile dysfunction, and proliferative disorders of the prostate gland (see Chapter 26). Aging changes are also influenced by chronic diseases and use of medications.[65]

Components of male sexual behavior include both sexual drive and erectile and ejaculatory capacity. Libido, or sexual drive, is a complex phenomenon that requires a baseline hormonal milieu but is influenced significantly by health status and environmental, social, and psychologic factors. In men older than 40 years, organic factors and chronic disease (e.g., vascular, endocrine, and neurologic disorders) are involved in more than half of the cases of male sexual dysfunction. Aging causes specific physical changes that may influence erectile and ejaculatory capabilities. Alterations in sexual response include the need for longer stimulation to achieve full erection; slower and less forceful ejaculation, with less pelvic muscle involvement; decreased vasocongestive response; and longer refractory period (time during which erection and ejaculation are not possible), up to 24 hours in some men.

The testes undergo several age-related structural changes, including decreased weight, atrophy, and softening. Degenerative changes in the seminiferous tubules may include thickening of the basement membrane; increase in lumen size; germ cell (spermatogonium) arrest and a decrease in spermatogenic activity; and collapse of tubules, followed by complete obstruction caused by sclerosis and fibrosis. Areas of mild to severe degenerative change may be interspersed with areas having intact tubules. These morphologic changes may result from atherosclerosis (arterial clogging) in the testicular vascular bed. Alterations of the seminiferous tubules do not appear to diminish sperm counts (20 million sperm per milliliter of semen is estimated as the minimum concentration for fertility) but they do reduce fertility because a greater percentage of the sperm lack motility or have structural abnormalities.

About 20% of healthy men more than 60 years of age and 30% to 50% older than 80 years of age have testosterone levels below the reference range and about 2% have hypogonadism. Aging can cause changes in the production of male sex hormones, levels of SHBG, and responsiveness of target tissue receptors. Hormone synthesis by the testes and testicular responsiveness to the gonadotropins (FSH and LH) are diminished, and pituitary secretion of these gonadotropins is elevated. The reduced levels of testosterone may be related to alterations in the Leydig cells, the testosterone producers of the testes. The number of Leydig cells and their function decrease as age increases, perhaps because of decreased arterial perfusion of the testes, and varicoceles and decreased LH or responsiveness to LH.

Even if testosterone levels are not decreased, older men may have less unbound testosterone in their blood, decreasing the amount of unbound hormone available to stimulate target tissues. Decreased testosterone levels have several effects, including functional deterioration of the accessory sex organs (the prostate gland, seminal vesicles, epididymis, and ductus deferens); loss of muscle mass, strength, and endurance; increased visceral fat, osteopenia, and cognitive decline; and, in many men, decrease in libido. This last effect also may be caused by alterations in other variables that affect libido. Modifiable risk factors for low testosterone level and symptoms of androgen deficiency include health status and waist circumference.

■ SUMMARY REVIEW

Development of the Reproductive Systems

1. Differentiation of female and male genitalia begins around weeks 7 to 8 of embryonic development, when the gonads of genetically male embryos begin secretion of male sex hormones, primarily testosterone; expression of testes-determining factor (TDF); and

expression of the *SRY* gene. Until that time the primitive reproductive organs of males and females are homologous (the same).

2. The structure and function of male and female reproductive systems are controlled by the hypothalamic-pituitary-gonadal (HPG) axis, a set of complex neurologic and hormonal interactions that accelerate

at puberty and lead to sexual maturation and reproductive capability.

3. Extrahypothalamic factors cause the hypothalamus to secrete GnRH, which stimulates the anterior pituitary to secrete gonadotropins—FSH and LH—that stimulate the gonads (ovaries or testes) to secrete female or male sex hormones. Paracrine hormones (inhibin, activin, and follistatin) influence the positive and negative feedback loops that occur along the HPG axis.

4. Production of primitive female gametes (ova) occurs solely during fetal life. From puberty to menopause, one female gamete matures per menstrual cycle. Production of the male gametes (sperm) begins at puberty; after that, millions are produced daily, usually for life. Females release a mature ova at the time of puberty.

The Female Reproductive System

1. The function of the female reproductive system is to produce mature ova and, when fertilized, to protect and nourish them through embryonic and fetal life, and expel them at birth.

2. The external female genitalia are the mons pubis, labia majora, labia minora, clitoris, vestibule (urinary and vaginal openings), Bartholin glands, and Skene glands.

3. The internal female genitalia are the vagina, uterus, fallopian tubes, and ovaries.

4. The vagina is a fibromuscular canal that receives the penis during sexual intercourse and is the exit route for menstrual fluids and products of conception. The vagina leads from the introitus (its external opening) to the cervical portion of the uterus.

5. The uterus is the hollow, muscular organ in which a fertilized ovum develops. The uterine walls have three layers: the endometrium (lining), myometrium (muscular layer), and perimetrium (outer covering, which is continuous with the pelvic peritoneum). The endometrium proliferates (thickens) and sloughs off in response to cyclic hormonal changes. The cervix is the narrow, lower portion of the uterus that opens into the vagina.

6. The two fallopian tubes extend from the uterus to the ovaries. Their function is to conduct ova from the spaces around the ovaries to the uterus. Fertilization normally occurs in the distal third of the fallopian tubes.

7. From puberty to menopause, the ovaries are the site of (a) ovum maturation and release and (b) production of female sex (estrogen and progesterone) and male (androgens) hormones. Female sex hormones predominate and are involved in sexual differentiation and development, the menstrual cycle, pregnancy, and lactation. Androgens in women contribute to prepubertal growth spurt, pubic and axillary hair growth, and activation of sebaceous glands.

8. Developing ovarian follicles (structures that enclose the ovum) produce estrogen (primarily estradiol). The corpus luteum, the structure that develops from the ruptured ovarian follicle after ovulation or ovum release, produces progesterone. Androgens in women are produced within the ovarian follicle, adrenal glands, and adipose tissue.

9. The average menstrual cycle lasts 27 to 30 days and consists of three phases, which are named for ovarian and endometrial changes: the follicular/proliferative phase, the luteal/secretory phase, and the ischemic/menstrual phase.

10. Ovarian events of the menstrual cycle are controlled by gonadotropins. High FSH levels stimulate follicle and ovum maturation (follicular phase), and then a surge of LH causes ovulation, which is followed by development of the corpus luteum (luteal phase).

11. Ovarian hormones control the uterine (endometrial) events of the menstrual cycle. During the follicular/proliferative phase of the ovarian cycle, estrogen produced by the follicle causes the endometrium to proliferate (proliferative phase) and induces the LH surge and progesterone production in the granulosa layer. During the luteal/secretory phase, estrogen maintains the thickened endometrium, and progesterone causes it to develop blood vessels and secretory glands (secretory phase). As the corpus luteum degenerates, production of both hormones drops sharply, and the "starved" endometrium degenerates and sloughs off, causing menstruation, the ischemic/menstrual phase.

12. Cyclic changes in hormone levels also cause thinning and thickening of the vaginal epithelium, thinning and thickening of cervical secretions, and changes in basal body temperature.

Structure and Function of the Breast

1. Until puberty the female and male breasts are similar, consisting of a small underdeveloped nipple, some fatty and fibrous tissue, and a few ductlike structures under the areola. At puberty, however, a variety of hormones (estrogen, progesterone, prolactin, growth hormone, insulin, cortisol) cause the female breast to develop into a system of glands and ducts that is capable of producing and ejecting milk.

2. The basic functional unit of the female breast is the lobe, a system of ducts that branches from the nipple to milk-producing units called lobules. The lobules contain alveolar cells, which are convoluted spaces lined with epithelial cells that secrete milk and subepithelial cells that contract, moving the milk into the system of ducts that leads to the nipple.

3. Each breast contains 15 to 20 lobes, which are separated and supported by Cooper ligaments.

4. Milk production occurs in response to prolactin, a hormone that is secreted by alveolar epithelial cells in larger amounts after childbirth. Milk ejection is under the control of oxytocin, which causes contraction of myoepithelial cells.

5. During the reproductive years breast tissue undergoes cyclic changes in response to hormonal changes of the menstrual cycle.

6. Prior to puberty the male breast development is similar to female development. Lack of high levels of estrogen and progesterone prevents further development of the male breast.

The Male Reproductive System

1. The function of the male reproductive system is to produce male gametes (sperm) and deliver them to the female reproductive tract.

2. The external male genitalia are the testes, epididymides, scrotum, and penis. The internal genitalia are the vas deferens, ejaculatory duct, prostatic and membranous sections of the urethra, seminal vesicles, prostate gland, and Cowper glands.

3. The testes (male gonads) are paired glands suspended within the scrotum. The testes have two functions: spermatogenesis (sperm production) and production of male sex hormones (androgens, chiefly testosterone).

4. The epididymis is a long coiled tube arranged in a comma-shaped compartment that curves over the top and rear of the testis. The epididymis receives sperm from the testis and stores them while they develop further. Sperm travel the length of the epididymis and then are ejaculated into the vas deferens.

5. The scrotum is a skin-covered fibromuscular sac that encloses the testes and epididymides, which are suspended within the scrotum by the spermatic cord. The scrotum keeps these organs at optimal

SUMMARY REVIEW—cont'd

temperatures for sperm survival (about 1°C to 2°C [33.8°F to 35.6°F] lower than body temperature) by contracting in cold environments and relaxing in warm environments.

6. The penis is a cylindrical organ consisting of three longitudinal compartments (two corpora cavernosa and one corpus spongiosum) and the urethra. The urethra runs through the corpus spongiosum. The corpora cavernosa and corpus spongiosum consist of erectile tissue. Externally the penis consists of a shaft and a tip, which is called the *glans*. The glans contains sebaceous glands and the opening of the urethra and is covered by a flap of skin (the foreskin).

7. The penis has two functions: delivery of sperm to the female vagina and elimination of urine. These two fluids are never in the urethra at the same time.

8. Sexual intercourse is made possible by the erectile reflex, in which tactile or psychogenic stimulation of the parasympathetic nerves causes arterioles in the corpora cavernosa and corpus spongiosum to dilate and fill with blood, causing the penis to enlarge and become firm.

9. Emission, which occurs at the peak of sexual arousal, is the movement of semen from the epididymides to the penis. Ejaculation, which is a continuation of emission, is the pulsatile ejection of semen from the penis. Both emission and ejaculation involve rhythmic contractions of smooth muscle within the internal glands and ducts.

10. The prostate gland is about the size of a walnut and surrounds the urethra. Prostatic secretions are alkaline and contribute to the ejaculate.

11. Cowper glands (bulbourethral glands) secrete mucus in the urethra and add fluid to the ejaculate.

12. Spermatogenesis is a continuous process because spermatogonia, the primitive male gametes, undergo continuous mitosis within the seminiferous tubules of the testes. Some of the spermatogonia develop into primary spermatocytes, which divide meiotically into secondary spermatocytes and then spermatids. The spermatids develop into sperm with the help of nutrients and hormonal signals from Sertoli cells.

13. Production of the male sex hormones is controlled (like production of the female sex hormones) by the HPG axis and by complex feedback mechanisms. The male hormones are produced steadily, with diurnal variations.

Tests of Reproductive Function

1. Diagnostic tests are performed to evaluate fertility.

2. Evaluation of fertility includes reproductive hormone assays and assessment of structural alteration or infections and the determination of normal ovulation or adequate sperm motility and count.

Aging and Reproductive Function

1. In women the transition from fertility to menopause (perimenopause) starts about 2 to 8 years before the last menstrual period and ends the following year. During this transition period the ovaries produce erratic and high levels of estrogen that contribute to such symptoms as hot flashes, breast tenderness and nodularity, and migraine headaches. Menstrual cycles shorten and then become irregular as anovulation occurs. Menstruation ceases, and women move into menopause.

2. Men maintain reproductive capacity into their later years. In some men there are gradual changes with testosterone deficiency, hypogonadism, proliferative disorders of the prostate, and erectile dysfunction.

KEY TERMS

Activin, 738
Adrenarche, 730
Androgen, 734
Areola, 740
Bartholin gland (greater vestibular or vulvovaginal gland), 730
Breast, 739
Bulbocavernosus, 730
Cervix (neck of the uterus), 732
Clitoris, 730
Cornification, 739
Corpora cavernosa (*singular*, corpus cavernosum), 743
Corpus luteum, 733
Corpus of the uterus (body of uterus), 732
Corpus spongiosum, 743
Cowper gland (bulbourethral gland), 744
Cul-de-sac, 731
Decornification, 739
Developing fetus, 726
Dihydrotestosterone (DHT), 746
Efferent tubule, 742
Ejaculatory duct, 744
Embryo, 726
Emission, 744
Endocervical canal, 732
Endometrium, 732
Epididymis (*plural*, epididymides), 742
Erectile reflex, 743
Estradiol (E₂), 734
Estrogen, 734

Fallopian tube (oviduct, uterine tube), 733
Fimbriae (*singular*, fimbria), 733
Follicle-stimulating hormone (FSH), 728
Follicular/proliferative phase, 736
Follistatin, 738
Foreskin (prepuce), 743
Fornix, 731
Fundus of the uterus, 732
Glands of Montgomery, 740
Glans, 743
Gonad, 727
Gonadarche, 729
Gonadostat, 728
Gonadotropin-releasing hormone (GnRH), 728
Gonadotropin-releasing hormone pulse generator, 728
Granulosa cell, 733
Hymen, 730
Infundibulum, 733
Inguinal canal, 742
Inhibin, 738
Introitus, 730
Ischemic/menstrual phase, 738
Isthmus of the uterus, 732
Labia majora (*singular*, labium majus), 730
Labia minora (*singular*, labium minus), 730
Leptin, 736
Leydig cell, 742
Libido, 746
Luteal/secretory phase, 736
Luteinizing hormone (LH), 735

Menarche, 736
Menopause, 736
Menstruation (menses), 736
Mons pubis, 730
Myometrium, 732
Natural menopause, 747
Nipple, 740
Ovarian cycle, 733
Ovarian follicle, 733
Ovary, 733
Ovulation, 736
Ovum, 726
Oxytocin, 740
Penis, 742
Perimetrium (parietal peritoneum), 732
Perineal body, 730
Perineum, 730
Primary spermatocyte, 744
Progesterone, 735
Prolactin, 746
Prostate gland, 744
Puberty, 729
Rete testis, 742
Rugae (*singular*, ruga; pertains to vagina and testes), 731
Scrotum, 742
Secondary spermatocyte, 744
Semen, 744
Seminal vesicle, 744
Seminiferous tubule, 742
Sertoli cell (nondividing support cell), 744

KEY TERMS—cont'd

Sex hormone, 726
Sex hormone–binding globulin (SHBG), 746
Skene gland (lesser vestibular or paraurethral gland), 730
Spermatic cord, 742
Spermatid, 744
Spermatogenesis, 744
Spermatogonia (*singular,* spermatogonium), 744
Spermatozoon (sperm cell), 726

Squamous-columnar junction, 732
Testes (*singular,* testis), 741
Testosterone, 746
Theca cell, 733
Thelarche, 739
Tubulus rectus, 742
Tunica albuginea, 742
Tunica dartos, 742
Tunica vaginalis, 742

Urethra, 743
Urinary meatus, 730
Uterus, 731
Vagina, 731
Vas deferens (ductus deferens), 742
Vasomotor flush, 750
Vestibule, 730
Vulva, 730

REFERENCES

1. Larney C, et al: Switching on sex: transcriptional regulation of the testis-determining gene *Sry. Development* 141(11):2195–2205, 2014.
2. Tomova A, et al: Influence of the body weight on the onset and progression of puberty in boys. *J Pediatr Endocrinol Metab* 28(7-8):859–865, 2015.
3. Elizondo-Montemayor L, et al: Gynecologic and obstetric consequences of obesity in adolescent girls. *J Pediatr Adolesc Gynecol* 30(2):156–168, 2017.
4. Removed in pages.
5. Muñoz-Calvo MT, Argente J: Nutritional and pubertal disorders. *Endocr Dev* 29:153–173, 2016.
6. Practice Bulletin No. 157 Summary: Cervical Cancer Screening and Prevention. *Obstet Gynecol* 127(1): 185–187, 2016.
7. Labrie F: All sex steroids are made intracellularly in peripheral tissues by the mechanisms of intracrinology after menopause. *J Steroid Biochem Mol Biol* 145C:133–138, 2015.
8. Di Renzo GC, et al: Progesterone in normal and pathological pregnancy. *Horm Mol Biol Clin Investig* 27(1):35–48, 2016.
9. Euling SY, et al: Examination of US puberty-timing data from 1940 to 1994 for secular trends: panel findings. *Pediatrics* 121(Suppl 3):S172–S191, 2008.
10. Removed in pages.
11. Rosenfeld RL: Clinical review: adolescent anovulation: maturational mechanisms and implications. *J Clin Endocrinol Metab* 98(9): 3572–3583, 2013.
12. Hall JE: Endocrinology of the menopause. *Endocrinol Metab Clin North Am* 44(3):485–496, 2015.
13. Gleicher N, Weghofer A, Barad DH: The role of androgens in follicle maturation and ovulation induction: friend or foe of infertility treatment? *Reprod Biol Endocrinol* 9:116s, 2011.
14. Pandey S, Bhattacharya S: Impact of obesity on gynecology. *Womens Health (Lond)* 6(1):107–117, 2010.
15. Scheid JL, De Souza MJ: Menstrual irregularities and energy deficiency in physically active women: the role of ghrelin, PYY and adipocytokines. *Med Sport Sci* 55:82–102, 2010.
16. Removed in pages.
17. Messinis IE, Messini CI, Dafopoulos K: Novel aspects of the endocrinology of the menstrual cycle. *Reprod Biomed Online* 28(6):714–722, 2014.
18. Removed in pages.
19. Palaniappan M, Menon KM: Luteinizing hormone/ human chorionic gonadotropin-mediated activation of mTORC1 signaling is required for androgen synthesis by theca-interstitial cells. *Mol Endocrinol* 26(10):1732–1742, 2012.
20. Knight PG, Satchell L, Glister C: Intra-ovarian roles of activins and inhibins. *Mol Cell Endocrinol* 359(1-2):53–65, 2012.
21. Son WY, et al: Mechanisms of follicle selection and development. *Minerva Ginecol* 63(2):89–102, 2011.

22. Nunes C, et al: Signalling pathways involved in oocyte growth, acquisition of competence and activation. *Hum Fertil (Camb)* 18(2):149–155, 2015.
23. Removed in pages.
24. Manders M, et al: Timed intercourse for couples trying to conceive. *Cochrane Database Syst Rev* (3):CD011345, 2015.
25. Barnes C, et al: From single cells to tissues: interactions between the matrix and human breast cells in real time. *PLoS ONE* 9(4):e93325, 2014.
26. Jesinger RA: Breast anatomy for the interventionalist. *Tech Vasc Interv Radiol* 17(1):3–9, 2014.
27. Macias H, Hinck L: Mammary gland development. *Wiley Interdiscip Rev Dev Biol* 1(4):533–557, 2012.
28. Removed in pages.
29. Removed in pages.
30. Inman JL, et al: Mammary gland development: cell fate specification, stem cells and the microenvironment. *Development* 142(6):1028–1042, 2015.
31. Jindal S, et al: Postpartum breast involution reveals regression of secretory lobules mediated by tissue-remodeling. *Breast Cancer Res* 16(2):R31, 2014.
32. Palmeira P, Carneiro-Sampaio M: Immunology of breast milk. *Rev Assoc Med Bras (1992)* 62(6): 584–593, 2016.
33. Bachelot A, Binart N: Reproductive role of prolactin. *Reproduction* 133(2):361–369, 2007.
34. Removed in pages.
35. Romero-Gutiérrez G, et al: Actual use of the lactational amenorrhoea method. *Eur J Contracept Reprod Health Care* 12(4):340–344, 2007.
36. Limony Y, et al: Pubertal gynecomastia coincides with peak height velocity. *J Clin Res Pediatr Endocrinol* 3:142–144, 2013.
37. Garolla A, et al: Twenty-four-hour monitoring of scrotal temperature in obese men and men with a varicocele as a mirror of spermatogenic function. *Hum Reprod* 30(5):1006–1013, 2015.
38. Dacheux JL, Dacheux F: New insights into epididymal function in relation to sperm maturation. *Reproduction* 147(2):R27–R42, 2013.
39. Clement P, Giuliano F: Anatomy and physiology of genital organs—men. *Handb Clin Neurol* 130:19–37, 2015.
40. Removed in pages.
41. Walker WH: Molecular mechanisms of testosterone action in spermatogenesis. *Steroids* 74(7):602–607, 2009.
42. Removed in pages.
43. Kelly DM, Jones TH: Testosterone: a metabolic hormone in health and disease. *J Endocrinol* 217(3): R25–R45, 2013.
44. Schlatt S, Ehmcke J: Regulation of spermatogenesis: an evolutionary biologist's perspective. *Semin Cell Dev Biol* 29:2–16, 2014.
45. Maggi M, et al: Hormonal causes of male sexual dysfunctions and their management

(hyperprolactinemia, thyroid disorders, GH disorders, and DHEA). *J Sex Med* 10(3):661–677, 2013.
46. Practice Committee of the American Society for Reproductive Medicine: Diagnostic evaluation of the infertile female: a committee opinion. *Fertil Steril* 103(6):e44–e50, 2015.
47. Lenz GM, et al: *Comprehensive gynecology,* ed 8, St Louis, 2013, Mosby.
48. Gold EB: The timing of the age at which natural menopause occurs. *Obstet Gynecol Clin North Am* 38(3):425–440, 2011.
49. Palacios S, et al: Age of menopause and impact of climacteric symptoms by geographical region. *Climacteric* 13(5):419–428, 2010.
50. Takahashi TA, Johnson KM: Menopause. *Med Clin North Am* 99(3):521–534, 2015.
51. Laven JS: Genetics of early and normal menopause. *Semin Reprod Med* 33(6):377–383, 2015.
52. Blümel JE, et al: Menopause or climacteric, just a semantic discussion or has it clinical implications? *Climacteric* 17(3):235–241, 2014.
53. Removed in pages.
54. Gold EB: The timing of the age at which natural menopause occurs. *Obstet Gynecol Clin North Am* 38(3):425–440, 2011.
55. Hall JE: Endocrinology of the menopause. *Endocrinol Metab Clin North Am* 44(3):485–496, 2015.
56. Bradley LD, Gueye NA: The medical management of abnormal uterine bleeding in reproductive-aged women. *Am J Obstet Gynecol* 214(1):31–44, 2016.
57. Iyengar NM, et al: Menopause is a determinant of breast adipose inflammation. *Cancer Prev Res (Phila)* 8(5):349–358, 2015.
58. Lupsa BC, Insogna K: Bone health and osteoporosis. *Endocrinol Metab Clin North Am* 44(3):517–530, 2015.
59. Removed in pages.
60. Stefanska A, Bergmann K, Sypniewska G: Metabolic syndrome and menopause: pathophysiology, clinical and diagnostic significance. *Adv Clin Chem* 72:1–75, 2015.
61. Vilar-González S, Pérez-Rozos A, Cabanillas-Farpón R: Mechanism of hot flashes. *Clin Transl Oncol* 13(3):143–147, 2011.
62. Sassarini J, Lumsden MA: Vascular function and cardiovascular risk factors in women with severe flushing. *Maturitas* 80(4):379–383, 2015.
63. Roberts H, Hickey M: Managing the menopause: an update. *Maturitas* 86:53–58, 2016.
64. Blume-Peytavi U, et al: Skin academy: hair, skin, hormones and menopause—current status/ knowledge on the management of hair disorders in menopausal women. *Eur J Dermatol* 22(3):310–318, 2012.
65. McBride JA, Carson CC, 3rd, Coward RM: Testosterone deficiency in the aging male. *Ther Adv Urol* 8(1):47–60, 2016.

Alterations of the Female Reproductive System

Kathleen E. Danhausen, Julia C. Phillippi, Kathryn L. McCance

http://evolve.elsevier.com/McCance/
- Content Updates
- Chapter Summary Review
- Review Questions
- Case Studies
- Animations

CHAPTER OUTLINE

Alterations of the reproductive system have a wide range of clinical presentations, from delayed sexual development and suboptimal sexual performance to structural and functional abnormalities. Many common reproductive disorders carry potentially serious physiologic or psychologic consequences. Sexual or reproductive dysfunction, such as impotence or infertility, can dramatically affect self-concept, relationships, and overall quality of life. Conversely, organic and psychosocial problems, such as alcoholism, depression, situational stressors, chronic illness, and medications, can affect ovulation and menstruation, sexual performance, and fertility, and may be risk factors for the development of some types of reproductive tract cancers.[1,2] Diagnosis and treatment of reproductive system disorders are complicated by the stigma and symbolism associated with the reproductive organs and the emotion-laden beliefs and behaviors related to reproductive health and fertility. Treatment and diagnosis for related problems may be delayed because of embarrassment, guilt, fear, or denial.[3]

ABNORMALITIES OF REPRODUCTIVE TRACT DEVELOPMENT

As discussed in Chapter 24, normal development of the female reproductive tract requires absence of testosterone during embryonic/fetal life.

The resulting fusion of the two paramesonephric (müllerian) ducts produces the normal cervix and the uterus with an internal cavity. The distal portions of the paramesonephric ducts remain independent and form the two fallopian/uterine tubes. Alterations in the normal process include errors in cellular sensitivity to testosterone (androgen insensitivity) or failures of cell line migration, resulting in changes in the structure of the reproductive organs.

Androgen insensitivity occurs in its most extreme form in about 1 in 20,000 people[4] and is discussed briefly in this chapter because of the often resulting female phenotype, despite a male genotype. This syndrome is caused by an X-linked genetic mutation in cellular androgen receptors that results in an end-organ insensitivity to testosterone, which normally acts as the catalyst for the development of the male reproductive system in embryonic development.[5] Complete androgen insensitivity syndrome (CAIS) is characterized by external female genitalia with a 46,XY genotype, whereas partial androgen insensitivity syndrome (PAIS) presents with ambiguous genitalia and varying genotype.[6] Children with CAIS often have testes within the labia majora, inguinal ring, or abdominal cavity that produce testosterone (and estrogen) in normal-range levels. Breast development may be normal, but pubic and axillary hair is often sparse and the cervix, uterus, and ovaries are absent. A short vagina that ends without a cervix also may be present. These individuals are often undiagnosed until puberty when menarche does not occur.[5] Both CAIS and PAIS carry an increased risk of gonadal tumors and malignancies. Gonadectomy and hormone replacement therapy are recommended for all individuals with CAIS and those with PAIS who are living as females. There remains controversy about the optimal timing of gonadectomy.[6]

Other abnormalities of the uterus, cervix, and fallopian/uterine tubes are caused by müllerian duct abnormalities. These have multifactorial origins, often the result of an interaction between genetic predisposition and environmental factors.[7] Some medications, chemicals, and toxins have been implicated as a direct cause of uterine abnormalities. For instance, diethylstilbestrol (DES) was prescribed from 1938 until 1971 as a drug to prevent miscarriages.[8] Although it was not effective at preventing miscarriage, DES affected cell development, causing abnormal internal reproductive anatomy that resulted in uterine malformations and a predisposition to cancer.

Disorders of müllerian tube development include agenesis, a complete absence of uterus and fallopian tubes, or fusion abnormalities resulting in a duplicate, bicornuate, or septate uterus[7] (Fig. 25.1). About 7% of the general female population has some sort of uterine abnormality, but the rate is much higher in populations of women who have experienced infertility or miscarriage.[9] Uterine abnormalities are often diagnosed when the woman has menstrual abnormalities or presents with sexual dysfunction. In other cases, these abnormalities are diagnosed during the diagnostic work-up for infertility, because the uterus is capable of menstruation but may have difficulty supporting a fetus.[9]

During pregnancy, uterine malformations are usually diagnosed by ultrasound or with magnetic resonance imaging (MRI). The prognosis of these pregnancies depends on the severity of the malformation and the location and size of the placenta and fetus. Some abnormalities can be surgically corrected to improve the outcome of subsequent pregnancies.[9] Abnormalities of the lower genital tract can also result in women having two vaginas or a vaginal septum (a thin membrane dividing the vaginal vault). For most women this does not create functional problems but can be surgically corrected if needed.[7]

ALTERATIONS OF SEXUAL MATURATION

The process of sexual maturation, or puberty, is marked by the development of secondary sexual characteristics, rapid growth of the body, and, ultimately, the ability to reproduce. A variety of congenital and endocrine disorders can disrupt the timing of sexual maturation, causing

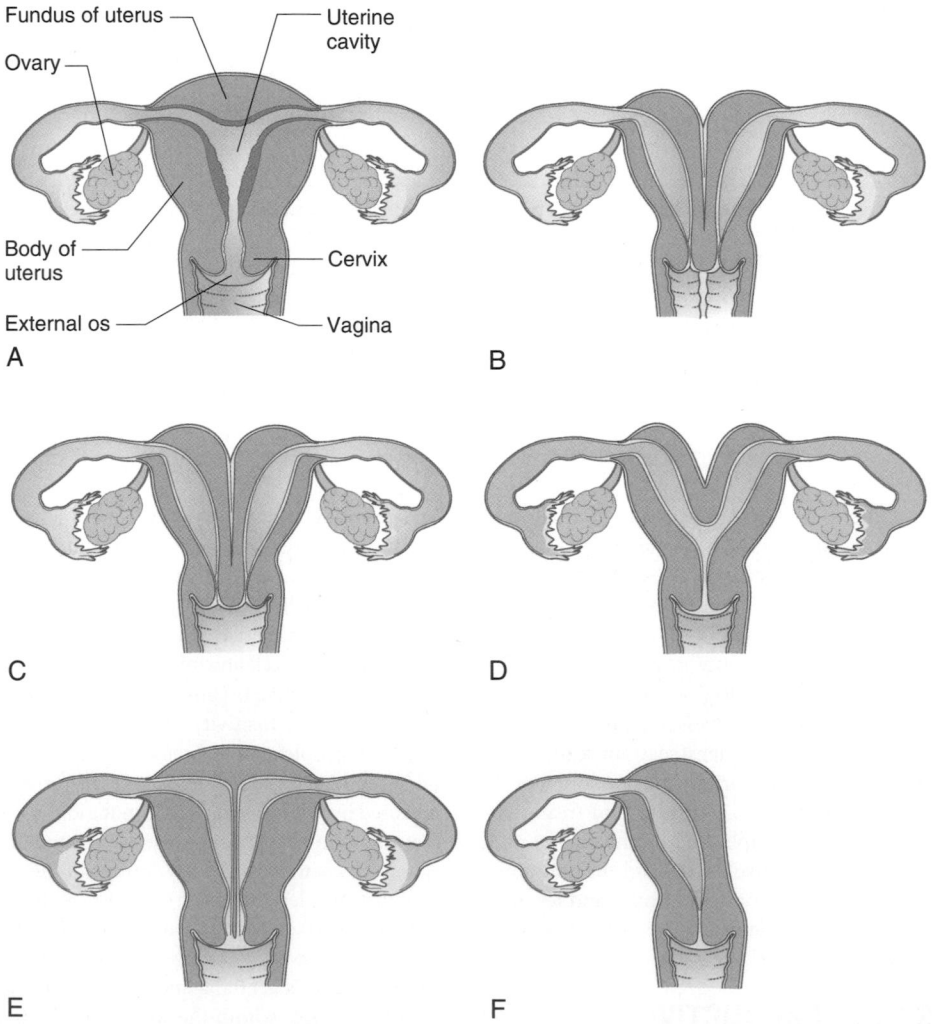

FIGURE 25.1 Uterine Malformations. Congenital uterine abnormalities. **A,** The normal configuration of the uterus and the ovaries. **B,** Double uterus with a double vagina and **C,** a single vagina. **D,** Bicornuate uterus. **E,** A uterus with a midline septum. **F,** Unicornuate uterus. (From de Bruyn R: *Pediatric ultrasound,* ed 2, London, 2010, Churchill Livingstone.)

puberty to occur too late (delayed puberty) or too early (precocious puberty). Both scenarios involve a disrupted onset of sex hormone production by the gonads.

The age of puberty is multifactorial, involving genetic and environmental components. The normal range for the onset of puberty is now 8 to 13 years of age and appears to be decreasing for girls. Girls of African descent and Hispanic/Latina girls may begin puberty up to 1 year sooner than the average young female.[10,11] This earlier onset appears primarily in breast development, not age of menarche, and 5% of white and 15% of all girls will begin puberty before age 8.[10] Both precocious puberty and delayed puberty have implications for the child's social interactions and self-esteem.[12] In addition, obesity has been shown to accelerate the onset of puberty, making it difficult to determine the impact of race on pubertal timing.

Delayed Puberty

About 2% of children in North America experience delayed development of secondary sex characteristics.[13] In girls, the onset of puberty is usually marked by *thelarche*, or breast development, which normally begins by age 13. Delayed puberty is diagnosed if there is no breast development by age 13, which is 2 to 2.5 standard deviations greater than the mean age of pubertal onset. Pubic hair may be present, because that is largely dependent on adrenal rather than gonadal function. Clinical diagnosis can be made in the absence of menarche by age 15 or 16.[14] Although delayed, puberty may have significant psychosocial implications and carries a risk of inadequate skeletal development and mineralization. Puberty is a time of rapid skeletal growth, with the majority of bone development and mineralization achieved during adolescence. Estrogen plays a major role in this process, and a lack of circulating estrogen puts individuals at risk for inadequate bone density in adulthood.[15]

In most cases, delayed puberty is a physiologic (constitutional) delay in which hormonal levels are normal and the hypothalamic-pituitary-gonadal (HPG) axis is intact, but maturation is happening slowly. This physiologic delay tends to be familial, less common in girls than boys, and is frequently diagnosed retrospectively once pubertal progression is complete. Although the exact incidence of this constitutional delay in growth and puberty (CDGP) is unknown, the sentinel and leading study on the issue reported that approximately 30% of girls with delayed puberty ultimately progressed through normal and spontaneous puberty. An additional 19% of girls had functional hypogonadotropic hypogonadism (FHH), essentially an underlying condition or illness (unrelated to gonadal function) responsible for the delayed development (e.g., anorexia nervosa)[16] (Table 25.1). Treatment of FHH includes a correction of the underlying condition, with a possible initiation of hormone therapy if a prolonged recovery is projected. Treatment for CDGP includes expectant management or initiation of hormone therapy in small doses to promote pubertal development and diminish the risk of poor skeletal growth and mineralization.

In other cases, a disruption in the HPG axis is the primary cause of delayed puberty. Human gonadal function is partially controlled by luteinizing hormone (LH) and follicle-stimulating hormone (FSH), the release of which is regulated by the pulsatile secretion of hypothalamic gonadotropin-releasing hormone (GnRH).[17] The G-protein–coupled receptor 54 (GPR54) has been identified as the gatekeeper gene for activation of the GnRH axis. GPR54 is required for the normal function of this axis, and data suggest that the ligand kisspeptin-1 may act as a neurohormonal regulator of the GnRH axis.[17]

The mechanisms of childhood inhibition of GnRH release and activation are poorly understood but appear to involve feedback inhibition by sex steroids and presumably other central nervous system (CNS) pathways.[14] Given the numerous etiologies contributing to the occurrence of delayed puberty, a thorough evaluation should be conducted that includes physical examination and medical and family history that specifically targets known contributors to delayed puberty. Laboratory workup may consist of x-ray studies for bone age, measurement of thyroid function, determination of serum levels of prolactin and adrenal and gonadal steroids, radioimmunoassay of plasma gonadotropins, and screening for systemic disorders. Adolescents with high gonadotropin levels require a karyotype to rule out genetic causes, and those with low levels need skull imaging (lateral skull film, computed tomography [CT], or MRI) to rule out pituitary or other CNS infiltrate or tumor. Treatment of delayed puberty depends on the cause; the goal of treatment is the development of secondary sex characteristics and fertility, and the promotion of bone growth and mineralization.[13] Insufficient sex hormone secretion can be corrected by hormone replacement therapy, such as estrogen. Idiopathic hypogonadotropic hypogonadism is treated with synthetic GnRH or sex hormone administration, or both, and may be lifelong.[14]

Precocious Puberty

Precocious puberty is a rare event, affecting about 29 in 100,000 girls.[18] Precocious puberty is defined as the onset of clinical signs of puberty (breast or pubic hair development) before age 8. However, some endocrinologists have recommended that the criteria be changed to reflect the trend toward an earlier onset of puberty, suggesting that pubertal changes before age 6 in black girls or age 7 in white girls are

TABLE 25.1	FREQUENCY AND COMMON CAUSES OF DELAYED PUBERTY OTHER THAN CONSTITUTIONAL DELAY OF GROWTH AND PUBERTY		
DELAYED PUBERTY	HYPERGONADOTROPIC HYPOGONADISM	PERMANENT HYPOGONADOTROPIC HYPOGONADISM	FUNCTIONAL HYPOGONADOTROPIC HYPOGONADISM
Frequency (%)			
Boys	5–10	10	20
Girls	25	20	20
Common causes	Turner syndrome, gonadal dysgenesis, chemotherapy, radiation therapy	Tumors or infiltrative diseases of the central nervous system, GnRH deficiency (isolated hypogonadotropic hypogonadism, Kallmann syndrome), combined pituitary-hormone deficiency, chemotherapy, or radiation therapy	Systemic illness (inflammatory bowel disease, celiac disease, anorexia nervosa, or bulimia), hypothyroidism, excessive exercise

GnRH, Gonadotropin-releasing hormone.
From Palmert MR, Dunkel L: *N Engl J Med* 366(5):443–453, 2012.

BOX 25.1   CAUSES OF PRECOCIOUS PUBERTY

Central (Gonadotropin-Releasing Hormone [GnRH] Dependent)
Idiopathic
Central nervous system (CNS) disorders
    Congenital anomalies (hydrocephalus)
    Hypothalamic hamartoma
    Postinflammatory/infectious condition
    Trauma
    Tumors (hypothalamic, pineal, other)
    Imprinted gene *(MKRN3)*

Peripheral Puberty (GnRH Independent)
Adrenal hyperplasia or tumor
Environmental endocrine disruptors
Exogenous sex steroid exposure
Exogenous anabolic steroids
Familial Leydig cell hyperplasia
Gonadal tumors or cysts
Human chorionic gonadotropin (hCG)–secreting tumors (hepatoblastomas, intracranial lesions)
Hypothyroidism (severe)
McCune-Albright syndrome
Testotoxicosis

Data from Fuqua JS: *J Clin Endocrinol Metab* 98(6):2198–2207, 2013; Rosenfield RL et al: Puberty and its disorders in the female. In Sperling MA, editor: *Pediatric endocrinology,* Philadelphia, PA, 2014, Elsevier Health Sciences; Schoelwer M, Eugster EA: *Endocr Dev* 29:230–239, 2016.

BOX 25.2   PRIMARY FORMS OF PRECOCIOUS PUBERTY

Complete Precocious Puberty
Premature development of appropriate characteristics for the child's sex
Hypothalamic-pituitary-ovarian axis working normally but prematurely
In about 10% of cases, lethal central nervous system tumor may be the cause

Partial Precocious Puberty
Partial development of appropriate secondary sex characteristics
Premature thelarche (breast budding) seen in girls between 6 months and 2 years of age
Does not progress to complete puberty (ovulation and menstruation)
Premature adrenarche (growth of axillary and pubic hair) tends to occur between 5 and 8 years of age
Can progress to complete precocious puberty; may be caused by estrogen-secreting neoplasms or may be a variant of normal pubertal development

Mixed Precocious Puberty
Causes the child to develop some secondary sex characteristics of the opposite sex
Common causes: adrenal hyperplasia or androgen-secreting tumors

Data from Burchett MLR et al: Endocrine and metabolic diseases. In Burns CE et al, editors: *Pediatric primary care,* St Louis, 2009, Saunders; Rosenfield RL et al: Puberty and its disorders in the female. In Sperling MA, editor: *Pediatric endocrinology,* Philadelphia, PA, 2014, Elsevier Health Sciences.

WHAT'S NEW?

Precocious Puberty

Studies implicate obesity, leptin, ghrelin, and environmental endocrine disruptor chemicals (EDCs) as possible contributors to precocious puberty in girls. Obesity may affect the production and secretion of leptin and ghrelin, powerful communicators of satiety, hunger, metabolic rate, and in timing of puberty. EDCs may mimic, block, or alter the normal signaling systems involved in sex hormone secretion, uptake, and use. EDCs include agrochemicals, widespread industrial compounds, and persistent pollutants.

Data from Buluş AD et al: *Toxicol Mech Methods* 26(7):493–500, 2016; Rosenfield RL, Cooke DW, Radovick S: Puberty and its disorders in the female. In Sperling Mark A, editor: *Pediatric endocrinology,* pp 569–663, Philadelphia, PA, 2014, Elsevier Health Sciences; Sørensen K et al: *Horm Res Paediatr* 77(3):137–145, 2012; Trotman GEL: *Curr Opin Obstet Gynecol* 28(5):366–372, 2016; Willemsen RH, Dunger DB: *Endocr Dev* 29:17–35, 2016.

more reflective of abnormal development.[19] Others are concerned that lowering the age of precocious puberty will miss those individuals who present after the age cut-off with a pathologic underlying condition causing early puberty. There have been many postulated causes of precocious puberty (Box 25.1), including alterations in genetic factors, an increase in obesity, an increase in protein consumption,[20,21] and the growing prevalence of molecular compounds known as *endocrine disruptors* in common household products[22] (see *What's New?* Precocious Puberty). Besides the premature development of secondary sex characteristics, precocity causes premature closure of the epiphysis of long bones, which results in lifelong short stature,[23] and often carries profound psychosocial consequences.[24] Because precocious puberty can be a sign of pathologic conditions, all cases of precocious puberty require thorough evaluation.

Precocious puberty may be partial, complete, or mixed types (Box 25.2) and can be further categorized into central (GnRH dependent) and peripheral (GnRH independent) (see Box 25.1). **Central precocious puberty** is GnRH dependent and occurs when the HPG axis is working normally but prematurely.[23] Central precocious puberty results from failure of central inhibition of the GnRH pulse generator (the gonadostat), often because of CNS abnormality. Although most cases are idiopathic, mutations in the imprinted gene *MKRN3* were recently reported as a cause of central precocious puberty.[25]

The diagnosis of central precocious puberty is one of exclusion.[19] Because a CNS lesion may be missed, children with presumed central precocious puberty require long-term surveillance. Peripheral puberty is GnRH independent and develops when sex hormones are produced by some mechanism other than stimulation by the gonadotropins and is either genetic or exogenous.[26] Sex steroid–producing tumors (i.e.,

gonadal tumors), testotoxicosis, and exposure to exogenous sex steroids (i.e., hormonal contraceptives and environmental endocrine disruptors) are some of the causes (see Box 25.1).

Partial precocious puberty is the partial early development of appropriate secondary sex characteristics alone or in combination. A girl with incomplete precocious puberty might undergo thelarche or pubarche and, rarely, premature menarche. Premature thelarche can be seen as early as 2 to 24 months of age, and in very small children breast development often reverses. Thelarche is considered premature if it occurs before age 8 years, but is usually a variation of normal and represents the higher end of prepubertal hormone release. Skeletal growth and menarche in these girls occur during the normal timeframe.[27] Premature pubarche tends to occur between ages 5 and 8 years. Premature

BOX 25.3	CAUSES OF MIXED PRECOCIOUS PUBERTY	
Female (Virilization)	**Male (Feminization)**	
Congenital adrenal hyperplasia	Estrogen-producing tumors	
Androgen-secreting tumors	Adrenal	
Adrenal	Teratoma	
Ovarian	Hepatoma	
Teratoma	Testicular	
Exogenous androgens	Exogenous estrogens	
	Increased peripheral conversion of androgens to estrogens	

Data from Rosenfield RL et al: Puberty and its disorders in the female. In Sperling MA, editor: *Pediatric endocrinology*, Philadelphia, PA, 2014, Elsevier Health Sciences.

pubarche is usually the consequence of an early increase in the adrenal androgens that leads to early growth of pubic hair and possibly a transient acceleration in growth and bone maturation that has no significant effect on timing of puberty or final height. Sparse hair growth on the genitalia, in the absence of thelarche or menarche, does not represent precocious puberty.[27] Girls with premature pubarche and thelarche should be followed through puberty to ensure normal progression; occasionally pathologic conditions may contribute to premature development.

Complete precocious puberty refers to the onset and progression of all pubertal features (i.e., thelarche, pubarche, and menarche). Mixed precocious puberty (virilization of a girl or feminization of a boy) causes the child to develop some secondary sex characteristics of the opposite sex. This condition is usually evident at birth and is rare in older children (Box 25.3).

The diagnosis and cause of premature development are often straightforward.[18] A thorough history and physical examination are done to determine the velocity of the process and to rule out life-threatening CNS, ovarian, or adrenal neoplasms. A history of family occurrence helps exclude tumors. Children with precocious puberty also have a tendency toward obesity.[21]

Treatment for all forms of precocious puberty includes identifying and removing the underlying cause or administering appropriate hormones (see Boxes 25.1 and 25.2). If needed, precocious puberty can be reversed. Management goals include diagnosing and treating intracranial disease, arresting maturation until developmentally appropriate, maximizing eventual adult height, and reducing emotional problems. The most common form, central precocious puberty, is usually treated with potent GnRH agonist analogs, which induce reversible, selective suppression of the HPG axis.[18] Because many of these children are obese and childhood obesity is predictive of morbidity in adolescence and adulthood, it is important for clinicians to include assessment and management of obesity as a component of the treatment for central precocious puberty.

DISORDERS OF THE FEMALE REPRODUCTIVE SYSTEM

Hormonal and Menstrual Alterations

Primary Dysmenorrhea

Primary dysmenorrhea is painful menstruation associated with the release of prostaglandins in ovulatory cycles, but not with pelvic disease. Approximately 90% of all women experience dysmenorrhea, 15% of whom are incapacitated for 1 to 3 days because of pain severity. Primary dysmenorrhea usually begins with the onset of ovulatory cycles with

prevalence highest during adolescence.[28] In contrast, secondary dysmenorrhea is related to pelvic pathologic disorders (i.e., ovarian cysts, adenomyosis, endometriosis) that manifest in later reproductive years and may occur any time in the menstrual cycle.[29]

◆**PATHOPHYSIOLOGY.** Primary dysmenorrhea is attributed to excessive endometrial prostaglandin production, primarily released during the first 48 hours of menstruation, when symptoms are the most intense.[28] Women with painful periods produce 10 times as much prostaglandin F ($PGF_2\alpha$), a potent myometrial stimulant and vasoconstrictor, as asymptomatic women. Elevated levels of prostaglandins (especially $PGF_2\alpha$ and $PGE_2\alpha$) cause uterine hypercontractility, decreased blood flow to the uterus, and increased nerve hypersensitivity, resulting in pain.[29] Women with dysmenorrhea may have up-regulated cyclooxygenase (COX) enzyme activity, which contributes to increased synthesis of prostaglandins. Furthermore, leukotriene production is elevated, further contributing to increased levels of pain.[29] Women are more likely to report primary dysmenorrhea if they are younger than 30; have not given birth; have a history of pelvic inflammatory disease, sexual assault, premenstrual syndrome, or sterilization; are heavy tobacco or alcohol users; have a family history of dysmenorrhea; or have a body mass index (BMI) less than 20.[29] Women who experience severe primary dysmenorrhea appear to have a heightened pain sensitivity; emerging research suggests an alteration in their pain modulating system, putting them at higher risk for functional pain disorders (e.g., fibromyalgia) in later life.[30] Women who are anovulatory because they use oral contraceptives rarely have primary dysmenorrhea.[29]

Secondary dysmenorrhea results from disorders such as endometriosis (the most common cause), endometritis (infection), adenomyosis, pelvic inflammatory disease, obstructive uterine or vaginal anomalies, uterine fibroids, polyps, tumors, ovarian cysts, pelvic congestion syndrome, or nonhormonal intrauterine devices (IUDs).[28]

◆**CLINICAL MANIFESTATIONS.** The chief symptom of dysmenorrhea is pelvic pain associated with the onset of menses. The pain often radiates into the groin and may be accompanied by backache, anorexia, vomiting, diarrhea, syncope, insomnia, and headache. The latter symptoms are caused by entry of prostaglandins and prostaglandin metabolites into the systemic circulation. Usually the discomfort associated with primary dysmenorrhea begins shortly before the onset of menstruation and persists for the first 1 to 3 days of menstrual flow.[28]

◆**EVALUATION AND TREATMENT.** Primary dysmenorrhea can be differentiated from secondary dysmenorrhea by a thorough history and pelvic examination. Administration of nonsteroidal antiinflammatory drugs (NSAIDs, e.g., ibuprofen) is the treatment of choice because these medications reduce COX enzyme activity, and thus prostaglandin production. NSAIDs work in the majority of women with primary dysmenorrhea and are most effective if started at the first sign of bleeding or cramping.[31] In women who desire contraception or do not respond to NSAIDs, dysmenorrhea may be relieved with hormonal contraceptives, such as combined estrogen-progestin pills or the progestin-only intrauterine device (IUD).[32] Hormonal contraception stops ovulation and creates an atrophic endometrium, thereby decreasing prostaglandin synthesis and myometrial contractility. Other treatment approaches with some evidence of effectiveness in pain relief include transdermal nitroglycerin patches to diminish uterine contractility, local application of heat, acupuncture, transcutaneous electrical nerve stimulation (TENS), increased physical activity, stress reduction through meditation, additional sleep, and supplements such as thiamine, vitamin E, and herbal treatments.[29]

Amenorrhea

Amenorrhea means lack of menstruation, and the most common causes (aside from pregnancy) are chromosomal abnormalities, hypothalamic dysfunction, polycystic ovarian syndrome, hyperprolactinemia, hypothyroidism, malnutrition, and ovarian failure.[33] **Primary amenorrhea** is the failure of menarche and the absence of menstruation by age 13 years, without the development of secondary sex characteristics, or by age 15 regardless of the presence of secondary sex characteristics (see the Alterations of Sexual Maturation section for a discussion of delayed puberty).[34] Primary amenorrhea differs from delayed puberty in that most cases of delayed puberty require only reassurance, but when the diagnosis of primary amenorrhea is reached, a thorough evaluation is needed. **Secondary amenorrhea** is the absence of regular menses for 3 months or irregular menses for 6 months in women who have previously menstruated. Pregnancy is the most common condition to exclude before further evaluation.

◆**PATHOPHYSIOLOGY.** There are numerous classifications of the etiologies of primary amenorrhea. One approach to understanding the pathophysiology is through compartmentalization. *Compartment IV disorders* include CNS disorders, in particular hypothalamic disorders. In some of the congenital syndromes that cause primary amenorrhea, the hypothalamic-pituitary-ovarian (HPO) axis is dysfunctional. The hypothalamus is unable to synthesize GnRH, so the pituitary fails to secrete LH and FSH. Therefore the ovary does not receive the hormonal signals required to stimulate estrogen production, and ovulation and menstruation do not occur. Because the ovarian hormones are absent, estrogen-dependent sex characteristics do not develop. CNS tumors can cause these disruptions in the hypothalamic-pituitary-ovarian axis. Other etiologies of amenorrhea caused by a dysfunction in the hypothalamus can include malnutrition (e.g., anorexia nervosa), stress, infection (e.g., meningitis, syphilis), or traumatic brain injury.[33]

Compartment III disorders are disorders of the anterior pituitary gland including tumors. Some anatomic defects of the CNS, whether congenital or acquired, impinge on the hypothalamic-pituitary unit so as to interfere with, or interrupt, the secretion of GnRH or FSH and LH. Examples of such defects include hydrocephalus, craniopharyngiomas, and other space-occupying lesions of the CNS. Again the target organ, the ovary, does not receive the necessary signals and ovulation and menstruation do not occur. In some cases, these lesions develop between the onset and conclusion of puberty. Therefore skeletal growth may occur and secondary sex characteristics may develop, but sexual maturation is interrupted before menarche. Autoimmune disease, hyperprolactinemia, and some medications also can affect the pituitary and disrupt normal menstruation.

Compartment II disorders involve the ovary and are often linked with genetic abnormalities. These include gonadal dysgenesis (Turner syndrome) or androgen insensitivity syndrome (AIS). Turner syndrome involves the lack of two functional and complete X chromosomes in at least some body tissues (45,X/46,XX; structural X or Y abnormalities; mosaicism),[33] which results in the ovaries lacking gametes and ovarian failure. Without primitive gametes and follicles, follicular development and estrogen secretion cannot occur. Lack of estrogen accounts for failure of secondary sex characteristic development and amenorrhea, although there are high levels of circulating FSH and LH.[33]

As mentioned previously, an individual with AIS is male genetically and their body produces testosterone. However, their cells do not have a receptor for testosterone, which is needed to activate the development of male genitalia.[34] Because target tissues have estrogen receptors, most individuals with AIS have female external genitalia and female secondary sex characteristics. With the exception of a small vagina, internal female genitalia are absent, accounting for amenorrhea and infertility.[34]

Compartment I disorders are anatomic defects of the outflow tract associated with primary amenorrhea. They include congenital absence of the vagina and uterus and congenital uterine hypoplasia. Genetically

normal females without a uterus or vagina usually have normal ovarian function. Therefore skeletal growth occurs and secondary sex characteristics develop in the proper sequence, but menstruation does not occur because the uterus is too small or malformed to produce substantial endometrium.

◆**CLINICAL MANIFESTATIONS.** The major clinical manifestation of primary amenorrhea is the absence of the first menstrual period. The cause of the amenorrhea determines whether secondary sex characteristics and height are affected.

◆**EVALUATION AND TREATMENT.** Diagnosis of primary amenorrhea is based on history and physical examination and determination of whether secondary sexual characteristics are present or absent. Absence of these sexual characteristics indicates that a female has never been exposed to estrogen. If ovarian steroid hormone levels are low, the individual has the appearance of an immature female. Physical examination may show structural or physiologic alterations of the reproductive tract as outlined at the beginning of the chapter. Laboratory studies may be required to document karyotype, abnormal levels of gonadotropins, thyroid and prolactin levels, and ovarian hormones. Diagnostic imaging is used to document structural abnormalities[35] (see Fig. 25.1).

Treatment involves correction of any underlying disorders and use of hormone replacement therapy to induce the development of secondary sex characteristics as necessary (see the section on Alterations of Sexual Maturation for a discussion of delayed puberty). Although surgical alteration of the genitalia may be undertaken to correct structural abnormalities, surgery should be delayed until the individual can make a truly informed decision. Hormonal manipulation or embryo transplantation may make pregnancy possible for women with primary amenorrhea who have a normal uterus.

Secondary Amenorrhea

A wide variety of disorders and physiologic conditions are associated with secondary amenorrhea. Besides disease, secondary amenorrhea can be triggered by dramatic weight loss, whether the loss results from malnutrition or excessive exercise. Secondary amenorrhea is common during early adolescence and the perimenopausal period, pregnancy, and lactation. The most common causes (after pregnancy) are thyroid disorders (e.g., hypothyroidism), hyperprolactinemia, HPO interruption secondary to excessive exercise, stress, weight loss, and polycystic ovary syndrome (PCOS). The factors leading to secondary amenorrhea also may cause primary amenorrhea in a young woman who has not begun to menstruate.

◆**PATHOPHYSIOLOGY.** The causes of secondary amenorrhea are summarized in Fig. 25.2. In women with normal ovarian steroid hormone levels, secondary amenorrhea may be caused by structural abnormalities (müllerian anomalies), Asherman syndrome (removal of the endometrial decidua basalis), or removal of the uterus. In women with elevated ovarian steroid hormone levels, inhibited ovulation leads to amenorrhea. An excess of ovarian hormones disrupts feedback relationships within the HPO axis, preventing ovulation. Depressed ovarian hormone levels, which are associated with a variety of clinical disorders, also cause amenorrhea by preventing ovulation. Lack of ovulation, termed **anovulation**, may result from increased levels of prolactin, decreased levels of gonadotropins, irregular secretion of gonadotropins, or abnormally low levels of CNS neurotransmitters (i.e., dopamine and GnRH). Any of these variables alters the feedback effects that the ovarian hormones have on the hypothalamus and pituitary.

High levels of prolactin are physiologic during lactation because it increases milk production and suppresses ovulation, preventing closely spaced pregnancies. However, high levels of prolactin not related to lactation are abnormal and will disrupt the menstrual cycle. **Hyperprolactinemia** (overproduction of prolactin by the pituitary)

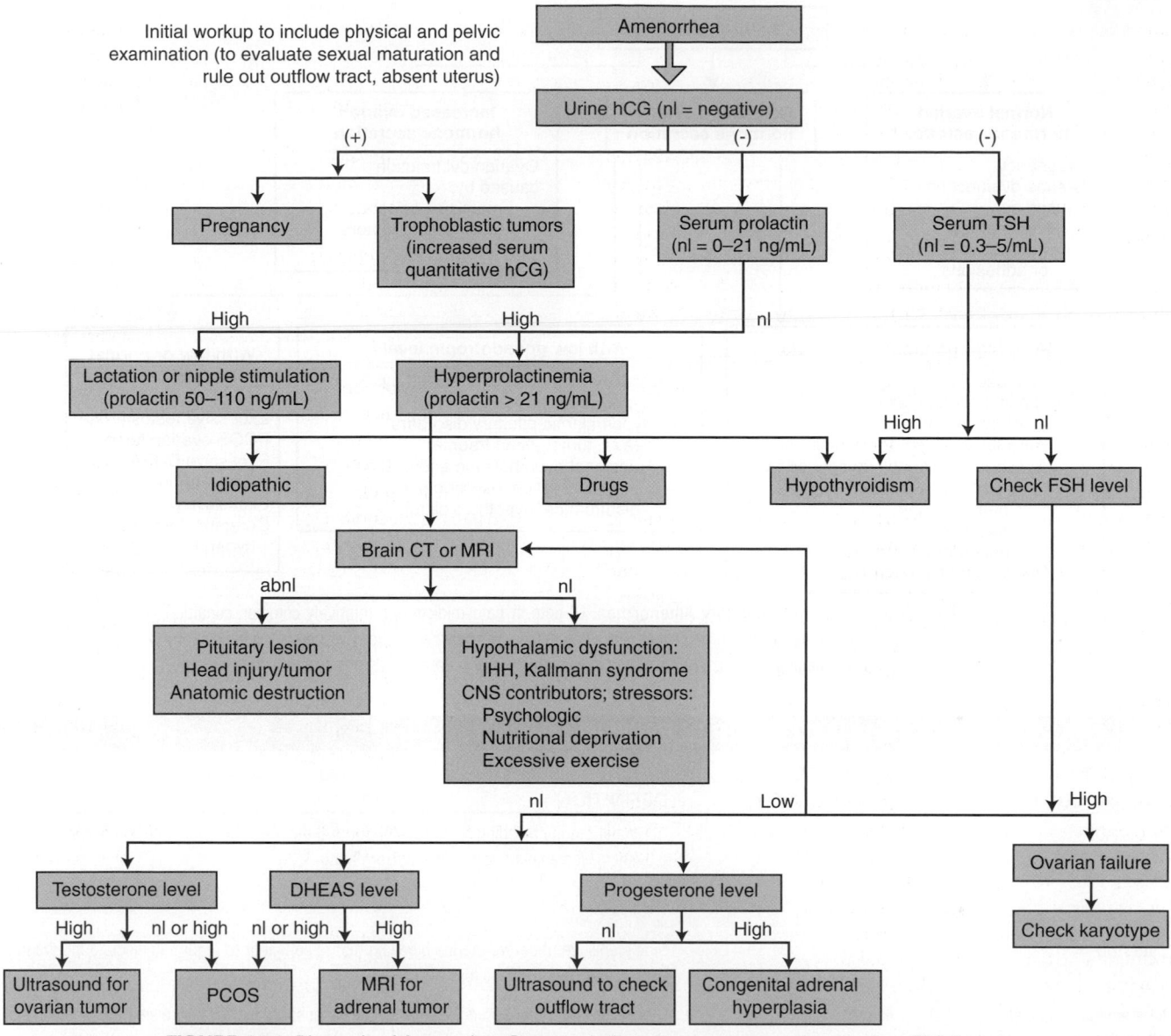

Initial workup to include physical and pelvic examination (to evaluate sexual maturation and rule out outflow tract, absent uterus)

FIGURE 25.2 Diagnosis of Amenorrhea. Pregnancy is the most common cause of amenorrhea. *CNS,* Central nervous system; *CT,* computed tomography; *DHEAS,* dehydroepiandrosterone sulfate; *FSH,* follicle-stimulating hormone; *hCG,* human chorionic gonadotropin; *IHH,* idiopathic hypogonadotropic hypogonadism; *MRI,* magnetic resonance imaging; *nl,* normal; *PCOS,* polycystic ovary syndrome; *TSH,* thyroid-stimulating hormone. (Adapted from Hoffman BL et al, editors: *Williams gynecology,* ed 3, New York, 2016, McGraw-Hill.)

may have indirect effects that lead to decreased secretion of GnRH by the hypothalamus. The result is a reduction in FSH and LH secretion followed by anovulation and secondary amenorrhea. Hyperprolactinemia should be diagnosed through blood testing for both normal-size and large molecular prolactin (macroprolactin). Hyperprolactinemia can have many causes including medication side effects, hypothyroidism, excessive nipple stimulation, and pituitary tumors.[36]

◆**CLINICAL MANIFESTATIONS.** The major manifestation of secondary amenorrhea is the absence of menses after previous menstrual periods. Infertility, vasomotor flushes, vaginal atrophy, acne, osteopenia, and hirsutism (abnormal hairiness) also may be present, depending on the underlying cause of the amenorrhea.

◆**EVALUATION AND TREATMENT.** Pregnancy is the most common cause of amenorrhea and must be ruled out before other evaluations. The menstrual cycle also may stop or become irregular in response to

stress, extreme exercise, large dietary changes, eating disorders, or sleep abnormalities. A thorough history of the woman's life and stressors is important in assessing amenorrhea. Diagnosis of the organic cause of secondary amenorrhea involves the identification of underlying hormonal or anatomic alterations. A woman with secondary amenorrhea and normal secondary sex characteristics should have a complete history and physical examination. After ruling out pregnancy and performing an in-depth history, initial laboratory evaluation includes measurement of thyroid-stimulating hormone (TSH) and prolactin levels (Fig. 25.3). Elevated prolactin levels warrant further investigation, including a complete medication history, TSH level measurement, and brain CT or MRI if warranted.[33] If these initial tests are normal, further testing would include measurement of gonadotropins (FSH), estrogen and testosterone, ultrasonography of the outflow tract and ovaries or adrenal MRI, or both.

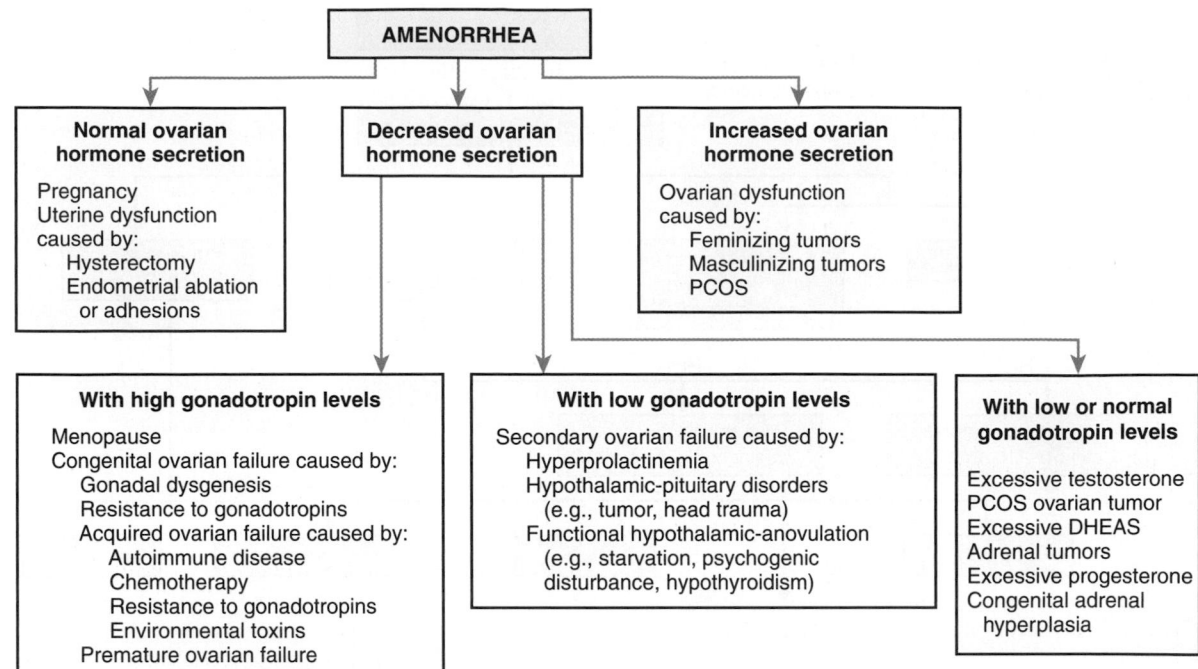

FIGURE 25.3 Causes of Secondary Amenorrhea. Of note, hypothyroidism is a relatively common condition and should be ruled out as the cause of hyperprolactinemia before more extensive evaluation (i.e., computed tomography or magnetic resonance imaging) occurs. *DHEAS,* Dehydroepiandrosterone sulfate; *PCOS,* polycystic ovary syndrome.

TABLE 25.2	ABNORMAL UTERINE BLEEDING	
CURRENT TERMINOLOGY	**OUTDATED TERMINOLOGY**	**DEFINITION**
Chronic AUB	Menometrorrhagia Menorrhagia Menorrhea Polymenorrhea	Abnormal uterine bleeding for at least 4 out of 6 months; abnormal bleeding is characterized by increased amount, regularity, and/or timing
Acute AUB		Single episode of severe uterine bleeding that is sufficient to require immediate intervention to prevent further blood loss
Intermenstrual bleeding (AUB/IMB)	Metrorrhagia	Uterine bleeding that occurs between regular menstrual cycles; intermenstrual bleeding can be random or predictable.
Heavy menstrual bleeding (HMB/AUB)	Hypermenorrhea	Increased menstrual volume that interferes with a woman's physical, emotional, and social quality of life

AUB, Abnormal uterine bleeding.
Data from Fraser IS et al: *Semin Reprod Med* 29(5):383–390, 2011; Munro MG et al: *Int J Gynecol Obstet* 113(1):3–13, 2011.

Treatment of amenorrhea depends on the cause and the woman's psychologic need for cycle stability. Treatments may include replacing deficient hormones (e.g., estrogens, thyroid hormone, glucocorticoids, gonadotropins) or correcting underlying pathologic conditions (e.g., tumor removal).[34] A diagnosis of PCOS might be treated with an insulin-sensitizing agent, such as metformin, as well as ovulation-inducing drugs if fertility is desired (a discussion of PCOS is in the section on Disorders of the Female Reproductive System).

Some treatments for amenorrhea prevent pregnancy, whereas others may restore fertility. The choice of treatment may be influenced by the woman's childbearing plans. After pathologic conditions have been corrected and the menstrual cycle stabilized, fertility may return. Occasionally, women with secondary amenorrhea may need additional ovulation-inducing drugs to assist conception, whereas others are able to conceive naturally.[34]

Abnormal Uterine Bleeding

Menstrual irregularity or abnormal bleeding patterns (Table 25.2) account for approximately 33% of all gynecologic visits. For many years, these abnormal patterns were poorly and inconsistently defined, and in 2010 the International Federation of Gynecology and Obstetrics (FIGO) developed a new system of definition and classification that has been adopted in the United States. The outdated definitions remain commonly used and are included in Table 25.2. Abnormal uterine bleeding (AUB) is bleeding that is abnormal in duration, volume, frequency, or regularity; and has been present for the majority of the previous 6 months.[37] AUB may be acute or chronic and is classified by the cause of bleeding using an internationally recognized PALM-COEIN system. PALM-COEIN stands for **p**olyp, **a**denomyosis, **l**eiomyoma, and **m**alignancy and hyperplasia; and **c**oagulopathy, **o**vulatory dysfunction, **e**ndometrial, **i**atrogenic, and **n**ot-yet classified (Fig. 25.4). The first group, PALM, consists of

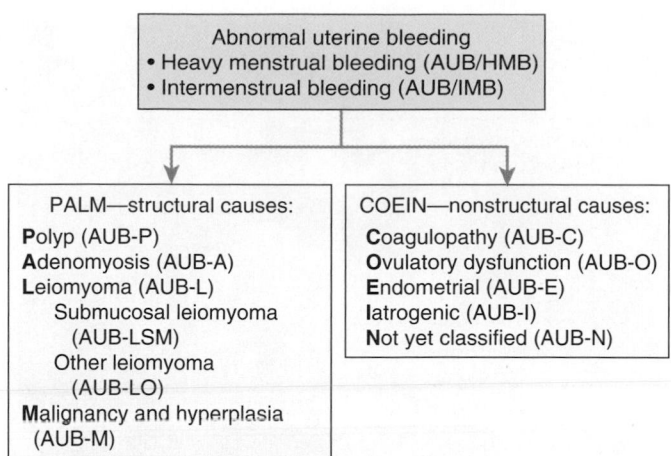

FIGURE 25.4 PALM-COEIN System for Classification of Abnormal Uterine Bleeding. *AUB,* Abnormal uterine bleeding. (From Committee Opinion No. 557, American College of Obstetricians and Gynecologists: *Obstet Gynecol* 121:891–896, 2013.)

disorders of tissue or structure that are diagnosed through imaging or biopsy. The second group, COEIN, consists of nonstructural causes of AUB. More than one etiology may contribute to a woman's AUB.[38]

In premenstrual or menopausal women, any bleeding is considered abnormal. For reproductive-aged women, normal uterine bleeding is every 28 days with variation up to 7 days. Therefore bleeding more frequently than every 21 days, or less frequently than every 35 days, is considered abnormal. Menstrual bleeding for longer than 7 days also is considered abnormal.[39] Studies show that 10% to 30% of women will experience AUB in their lifetime.[40] Approximately one-third of all gynecologic visits for premenopausal women and three-quarters of all visits for perimenopausal and menopausal women are because of AUB.[41] AUB (all etiologies) is the leading reason for hysterectomy in the United States.[42] Perimenopausal women are most commonly affected by AUB.

◆**PATHOPHYSIOLOGY.** The majority of abnormal uterine bleeding is due to lack of ovulation.[41] Normal, regular periods are the result of a complex interplay between the hypothalamus, pituitary, ovary, and the uterine endometrium (see Chapter 24). Disruptions in this system can affect the amount and structure of the uterine endometrium, causing it to shed irregularly or heavily. Although anovulatory AUB may occur at any time during the reproductive years, it tends to occur in adolescents and perimenopausal women more frequently, because women at the edges of the reproductive years are more likely to ovulate irregularly. The formation of a follicle and its rupture to release an ovum are important components of the menstrual cycle. As the follicle forms, it produces estrogen, which causes proliferation of the endometrium. Following ovulation, the remaining portions of the follicle, known as the *corpus luteum,* release progesterone. The progesterone acts on the proliferating endometrium to limit growth and cause changes in the vasculature of the endometrium, which limits bleeding during endometrial shedding.

If a follicle forms but never releases the ovum, the follicle may continue to produce estrogen (estradiol [E_2]), encouraging endometrial proliferation beyond the normal 14-day time window. In addition, the lack of progesterone causes the thickened endometrium to be unable to shed in a predictable fashion without excessive blood loss. Women who fail to ovulate experience irregularities in their menstrual bleeding related to the lack of progesterone and, in some cases, an excess of estrogen.

Many conditions are associated with irregular ovulation, including physiologic changes of aging (e.g., adolescent and perimenopausal

women); PCOS, in which follicles begin to form but never reach maturation and rupture; obesity because adipose tissue excretes estrogen, which can suppress the HPG axis; hyperthyroidism and hypothyroidism; and estrogen-secreting ovarian neoplasms.

Without ovulation, menstrual flow may become irregular, excessive, or both, resulting from the large quantity of tissue available for bleeding and the random breakdown of tissue that results in exposure of vascular channels. In the absence of adequate progesterone levels, usual endometrial control mechanisms are missing, such as vasoconstrictive rhythmicity, tight coiling of spiral vessels, and orderly collapse, and stasis does not occur. Unopposed estrogen induces a progression of endometrial responses beginning with proliferation, hyperplasia, and adenomatous hyperplasia. Over a course of many years, unopposed estrogen may end with atypia and carcinoma.

Abnormal menstrual bleeding also can result from defects of the corpus luteum, resulting in progesterone deficiencies, or from abnormalities of the uterus or cervix, such as endometrial polyps, uterine fibroids, or even uterine or cervical cancers. (These conditions are covered in more detail later in the chapter.) Coagulation defects also can cause heavy and abnormal uterine bleeding and should be suspected in younger women with a history of extensive bruising or bleeding during dental procedures. Iatrogenic AUB can be caused by intrauterine devices or long-acting contraceptive implants or medications, such as anticoagulants, steroids, digitalis, phenytoin, or hypothalamic depressants.

◆**CLINICAL MANIFESTATIONS.** Abnormal uterine bleeding is characterized by unpredictable and variable bleeding. Especially during perimenopause, abnormal bleeding also may involve increased menstrual flow and the passage of large clots, leading to excessive blood loss. Excessive bleeding can lead to iron deficiency anemia and associated symptoms (fatigue, shortness of breath). AUB also may cause pain, decreased productivity, and sexual dysfunction.

◆**EVALUATION AND TREATMENT.** The first step in assessing abnormal bleeding is to determine the cause of bleeding. If an organic cause can be found, the focus is on eliminating the pathologic disorder or mitigating its effects. To determine the cause of the bleeding, a complete and thorough history and physical examination, including transvaginal ultrasound, is needed. The woman's age and risk factors for other abnormal conditions are important in assessing the likely cause of the bleeding. Initial laboratory evaluation includes a complete blood count, measurement of thyroid-stimulating hormone levels, and coagulation studies if indicated. If no cause can be found, it is usually assumed that the bleeding is caused by lack of regular ovulation. Treatment goals include preventing or controlling abnormal bleeding, identifying underlying disease, and inducing regular menstrual cycles. Treatment varies greatly by the age of the woman and her desire for current and future fertility.

NSAIDs, such as ibuprofen and naproxen, are often first-line treatments for excessive menstrual bleeding because they reduce prostaglandin synthesis within the endometrial tissues, which causes vasoconstriction and decreased menstrual blood loss. NSAIDs can reduce menstrual bleeding significantly with minimal side effects.[43] For best effect, they should be taken in the few days preceding the beginning of the menstrual period and be continued through the days of heaviest bleeding. NSAIDs are not as effective in controlling menstrual blood loss as hormonal therapies, but they are readily available without a prescription.

Young women and those of childbearing age with abnormal bleeding are often treated with hormonal therapies to override the HPG axis and mimic normal menstrual bleeding or suppress it entirely. Common treatments include oral contraceptive pills that contain both estrogen and progesterone, long-term treatment with medroxyprogesterone (Depo-Provera) (although the U.S. Food and Drug Administration [FDA] black box warning about potential bone loss has drastically curtailed the use of this therapy), and the levonorgestrel intrauterine device (LNG-IUD). The LNG-IUD has a dual indication from the FDA for both birth control and suppression of abnormal menstrual bleeding. The device releases a steady amount of progesterone into the uterus to stabilize and suppress the uterine lining. In addition, the progesterone suppresses the HPG axis, preventing ovulation. There is no strong evidence to differentiate whether estrogen and progesterone or progesterone alone is superior in the treatment of abnormal uterine bleeding; the woman should be allowed to select a treatment regimen that is compatible with lifestyle and needs.[43]

Women who are greater than 35 years old and smoke cigarettes may not be candidates for oral contraceptive pills because the estrogen increases their risk of cardiovascular incidents, such as myocardial infarction. However, the LNG-IUD can still be used because it contains only progesterone. The LNG-IUD is widely used as a first step in controlling perimenopausal bleeding because it can be inserted in a clinic office and is easily removed. The LNG-IUD decreases blood loss by 86% to 97% by decreasing endometrial proliferation and has similar success rates as more invasive procedures, such as ablation or hysterectomy.[44] Women who do not wish to have future pregnancies also can opt for treatments that permanently suppress their uterine lining. These treatments include ablation, where the lining is burned to prevent future proliferation of the endometrial cells, and complete removal of the uterus in hysterectomy.[39]

If a woman is menopausal, and has not had a menstrual period for more than 1 year, all vaginal bleeding should be investigated to rule out uterine and other cancers. Appropriate initial evaluation includes ultrasound and endometrial biopsy to exclude uterine cancer.[39]

Women with coagulation disorders may have excessive menstrual bleeding because they have a predisposition to bleeding or because they are taking anticoagulant medications to overcome a genetic predisposition to excessive clotting.[38] To control their menstrual bleeding, these women can opt for cycle suppression. Provision of birth control for these women is important because pregnancy may be a risk to their health.[44]

Polycystic Ovary Syndrome

Polycystic ovary syndrome (PCOS) is the most common cause of anovulation and ovulatory dysfunction in women. Although PCOS presents in a variety of ways, it is defined as having at least two of the following three features: irregular ovulation, elevated levels of androgens (e.g., testosterone), and the appearance of polycystic ovaries on ultrasound.[45] Polycystic ovaries do not have to be present to diagnose PCOS, and conversely their presence alone does not establish the diagnosis. The diagnosis is one of exclusion, and all other disorders potentially responsible for the clinical findings also must be ruled out, including thyroid dysfunction, hyperprolactinemia, and congenital adrenal hyperplasia.[46] PCOS is associated with metabolic dysfunction, including dyslipidemia, insulin resistance, and obesity. PCOS remains one of the most common endocrine disturbances affecting women, especially young women, and is a leading cause of infertility in the United States, where prevalence rates are estimated at between 5% and 15% of women.[47]

There is a strong genetic component to PCOS, and various features of the syndrome may be differentially inherited.[48] Confusing the issue is the frequency, expression, and timing of PCOS symptoms and diagnosis. From 22% to 30% of women have polycystic ovaries on ultrasound, with 80% having one or more symptoms of the syndrome; 80% of women with normal ovaries also experience one or more PCOS symptoms. Signs and symptoms of women with PCOS may change over time, with metabolic syndrome becoming more prominent with age. In addition, polycystic ovaries may be associated with Cushing syndrome, acromegaly, premature ovarian failure, simple obesity, congenital adrenal hyperplasia, thyroid disease,

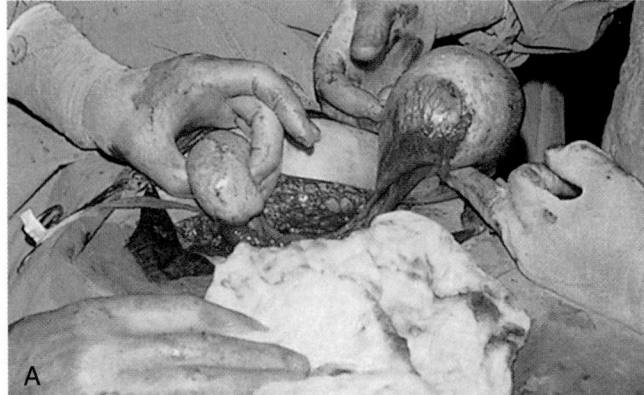
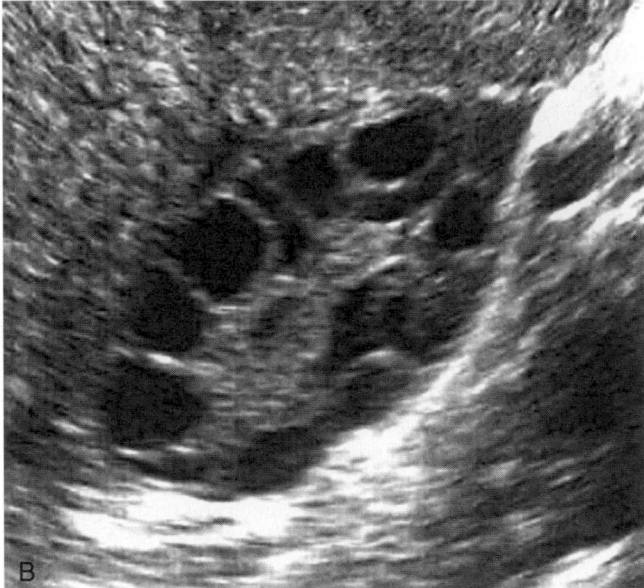

FIGURE 25.5 Polycystic Ovary. **A,** Surgical view of polycystic ovaries. **B,** Ultrasound of polycystic ovary. (**A** From Symonds EM, Macpherson MBA: *Diagnosis in color: obstetrics and gynecology,* London, 1997, Mosby-Wolfe. **B** From King J: *J Midwifery Womens Health* 51[6]:415–422, 2006. Reprinted with permission.)

androgen-producing adrenal tumors or ovarian tumors (Fig. 25.5), and syndromes with hyperprolactinemia.[46]

PATHOPHYSIOLOGY. Although the underlying cause of PCOS is unknown, a genetic basis is suspected. Initial identification of genes involved in steroid biosynthesis, androgen biosynthesis, and insulin receptors within the ovary indicates genetic involvement. No single factor fully accounts for the abnormalities of PCOS.[48] A hyperandrogenic state is a cardinal feature in the pathogenesis of PCOS. However, glucose intolerance/insulin resistance (IR) and hyperinsulinemia often run parallel to and markedly aggravate the hyperandrogenic state, thus contributing to the severity of signs and symptoms of PCOS.[47] Women with PCOS are three times as likely to have insulin resistance. This number is even higher among obese women, who account for approximately 60% of women with PCOS.[49]

Insulin stimulates androgen secretion by the ovarian stroma and reduces serum sex hormone–binding globulin (SHBG) directly and independently. The net effect is an increase in free testosterone levels. Excessive androgens affect follicular growth, and insulin affects follicular decline by suppressing apoptosis and enabling follicles to persist[49] (Fig. 25.6). Further, there appears to be a genetic ovarian defect in PCOS, which makes the ovary either more susceptible to or sensitive to insulin's

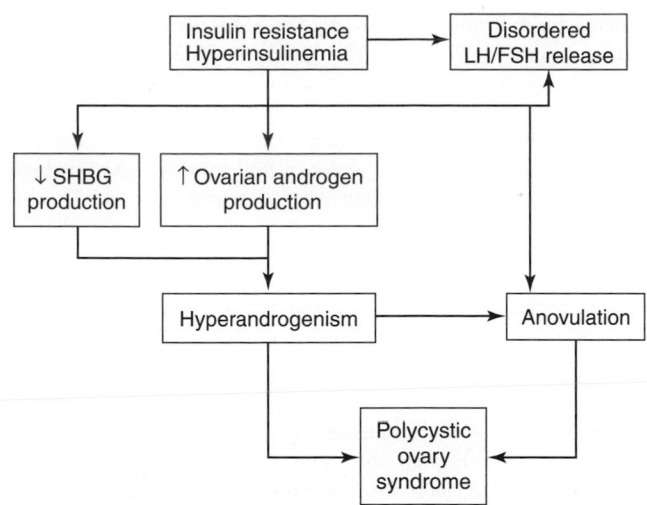

FIGURE 25.6 Insulin Resistance and Hyperinsulinemia in Polycystic Ovary Syndrome (PCOS). See text. *FSH*, Follicle-stimulating hormone; *LH*, luteinizing hormone; *SHBG*, sex hormone–binding globulin. (From Franks S, Berga SL: *Fertil Steril* 97[1]:2–6, 2012.)

stimulation of androgen production. Recent research suggests that decreased intraovarian receptors for estrogen receptor-α or insulin-like growth factor 1 (IGF-1), increased leptin levels, or direct infrared radiation within selective ovarian cells (fibroblasts) may contribute to this phenomenon.[49] Intrauterine and early childhood environments may also contribute to the development of PCOS (see *What's New? Early Programming for PCOS?*).

WHAT'S NEW?

Early Programming for PCOS?

A fetal environment containing abnormal levels of pollutants, hormones, and other factors yet undefined can induce epigenetic modifications of the DNA and increased risk for adult disease. Female fetuses exposed to testosterone at levels normally found with male fetuses appear programmed to develop altered TGF-β signaling and increased risk of hyperinsulinemia and hyperandrogenism related to PCOS.

Data from Diamanti-Kandarakis E, Dunaif A: *Endocr Rev* 33(6):981–1030, 2012.

Weight gain tends to aggravate symptoms, whereas weight loss may ameliorate some of the endocrine and metabolic events and thus decrease symptoms. Women with PCOS tend to have increased leptin levels (leptin levels are increased in thin as well as overweight women with PCOS).[48] Leptin influences the hypothalamic pulsatility of GnRH and consequent interaction along the entire HPO axis. Feedback from the polycystic ovary is disturbed because of changes in ovarian steroid and nonsteroidal (inhibins and related proteins) hormones.

In PCOS there is dysfunction in ovarian follicle development.[50] Inappropriate gonadotropin secretion triggers the beginning of a vicious cycle that perpetuates anovulation. Typically, levels of FSH are low or below normal and LH levels and LH bioactivity are elevated. An increased frequency of GnRH pulses appears to cause increased frequency of LH pulses.[48,50] Persistent LH elevation causes an increase in the levels of androgens (dehydroepiandrosterone sulfate [DHEAS] from the adrenal glands and testosterone, androstenedione, and DHEAS from the ovary). Androgens are converted to estrogen in peripheral tissues, and increased testosterone levels cause a significant reduction (approximately 50%)

in SHBG, which in turn causes increased levels of free estradiol. Elevated estrogen levels trigger a positive-feedback response in LH and a negative-feedback response in FSH. Because FSH levels are not totally depressed, new follicular growth is continuously stimulated, but not to full maturation and ovulation. The accumulation of follicular tissue in various stages of development allows an increased and relatively constant production of steroids in response to gonadotropin stimulation. Thus PCOS is characterized by excessive production of both androgen and estrogen.

Increased androgen secretion by the ovaries contributes to premature follicular failure (atresia) and persistent anovulation. In turn, persistent anovulation causes enlarged polycystic ovaries characterized by a smooth, pearly white capsule. This characteristic appearance is caused by an increase of surface area and increased volume of up to 2.8 times, doubling of growing and atretic follicles, thickening of the tunica (outermost area) by 50%, increasing cortical stromal thickening by one-third and a fivefold increase in subcortical stroma, and escalating hyperplasia. With advancing age, menstrual irregularities may improve while the incidence of metabolic syndrome and type 2 diabetes mellitus increases. Women with PCOS have a three times greater incidence of uterine cancer in later life than normally cycling women related to the anovulatory lack of progesterone in PCOS. Without treatment for anovulation, women with PCOS have a 9% lifetime risk for endometrial cancers related to the effects of unopposed estrogen.[47]

CLINICAL MANIFESTATIONS. Clinical manifestations of PCOS usually appear within 2 years of puberty but may present after a variable period of normal menstrual function and, possibly, pregnancy. The symptoms are related to anovulation, hyperandrogenism, and insulin resistance and include dysfunctional bleeding or amenorrhea, hirsutism, acne, acanthosis nigricans, and infertility. Approximately 60% of women with PCOS are obese.[51] Box 25.4 contains a list of signs and symptoms, summary of hormonal disturbances, and complications of PCOS. In addition, women with PCOS are more likely to experience sleep apnea than unaffected women, which results in impaired sleep and may reduce their overall quality of life.[52]

EVALUATION AND TREATMENT. Diagnosis of PCOS is based on evidence of androgen excess, chronic anovulation, and sonographic evidence of polycystic ovaries with at least two of the three criteria present. Tests for impaired glucose tolerance are recommended. As stated, polycystic ovaries do not have to be present and, conversely, their presence alone does not establish the diagnosis. Because of the normalcy of anovulatory cycles in adolescence, evidence of hyperandrogenism (in the setting of irregular menses) must be present before PCOS is diagnosed in an adolescent female.[46] Goals of treatment include reversing signs and symptoms of androgen excess, instituting cyclic menstruation, restoring fertility, and ameliorating any associated metabolic or endocrine, or both, disturbances.[47] First-line treatment of PCOS includes combined oral contraceptives (COCs) for management of symptoms (e.g., hirsutism, acne) and to establish regular menses. For those women with PCOS who are overweight or obese, lifestyle modifications, including regular exercise and weight loss, also are considered first-line treatments. Women with insulin resistance, or those women who do not respond to contraceptive therapy, may benefit from the insulin sensitizer metformin.[46,47] If COCs are not used and pregnancy is not desired, progesterone therapy is recommended to oppose estrogen's effects on the endometrium and as a means to initiate monthly withdrawal bleeding (at the expense of continued hirsutism).

For overweight or obese infertile women desiring pregnancy, lifestyle modifications are first-line therapy. Even a small reduction of weight restores ovulation and increases insulin sensitivity by 71% in obese women with PCOS. Reduction of insulin by loss of abdominal fat appears crucial in restoring ovulation.[53]

BOX 25.4   CLINICAL MANIFESTATIONS OF POLYCYSTIC OVARY SYNDROME

Presenting Signs and Symptoms (% of Women Affected)
Obesity (41%)
Menstrual disturbance (70% [i.e., dysfunctional uterine bleeding])
Oligomenorrhea (47%)
Amenorrhea (19%)
Regular menstruation (48%)
Hyperandrogenism (69% to 74%)
Infertility (73% of anovulatory infertility)
Asymptomatic (20% of those with PCOS)

Hormonal Disturbances
Increased insulin (independent of obesity)
Decreased SHBG
Increased androgens (testosterone, androstenedione)
Increased DHEA (occurs in 50% of women)
Increased LH (genetic variant LH-β subunit)
Increased prolactin
Increased leptin, especially in obesity (independent of insulin)
Suggested decreased insulin-like growth factor (IGF-1) receptors on theca cells
Possible decreased estrogen receptors (intraovarian and along hypothalamic-pituitary axis)

Possible Late Sequelae
Dyslipidemia: increased low-density lipoproteins, decreased high-density lipoproteins, increased triglycerides
Diabetes mellitus (30% of women with or without obesity develop type 2 diabetes mellitus by age 30)
Cardiovascular disease; hypertension
Endometrial hyperplasia and carcinoma (anovulatory women are hyperestrogenic)

Other
Women with PCOS are at increased risk of gestational diabetes mellitus, pregnancy-induced hypertension, preterm birth, and perinatal mortality

DHEA, Dehydroepiandrosterone; *LH*, luteinizing hormone; *PCOS*, polycystic ovary syndrome; *SHBG*, sex hormone–binding globulin.
Data from Azziz R et al: *Fertil Steril* 91(2):456–488, 2009; Boomsma CM et al: *Semin Reprod Med* 26(1):2008; Diamanti-Kandarakis E: *Expert Rev Mol Med* 10(2):e3, 2008; Simoni M et al: *Hum Reprod Update* 14(5):459–484, 2008.

Clomiphene citrate, an antiestrogen, can be used to facilitate ovulation[46] and can be combined with metformin for improved outcomes.[46] Management of PCOS is a nearly lifelong process because the effects of the syndrome persist past childbearing years. Appropriate primary care is needed to control the systemic features of PCOS so that it has minimal impact on a woman's life and health outcomes.

Premenstrual Disorders

Premenstrual syndrome (PMS) and **premenstrual dysphoric disorder (PMDD)** are the cyclic recurrence (in the luteal phase of the menstrual cycle) of distressing physical, psychologic, or behavioral changes that impair interpersonal relationships or interfere with usual activities and resolve after menstruation. The prevalence of PMS and PMDD is difficult to determine, in part because of the wide-ranging nature of accepted symptoms, but it is estimated that 12% of menstruating women are significantly affected by these disorders, with 3% to 8% meeting criteria for PMDD.[54,55] Symptoms of PMS and PMDD begin after ovulation during the luteal phase and persist up to 4 days into the menstrual cycle.[55]

◆PATHOPHYSIOLOGY. The psychologic and physiologic changes of PMS/PMDD occur in the luteal phase of ovulatory cycles and are linked with the complex hormonal changes of the menstrual cycle. There are many theories on the cause(s) of the disorder, including that the drop in estrogen level following ovulation and the immediate rise in progesterone level interact with hormones and neurotransmitters to cause symptoms.[56] However, the mechanisms involved are not known and may include an individual sensitivity to hormone levels. Furthermore, the neurotransmitters serotonin, gamma-aminobutyric acid (GABA), and noradrenaline may have mediating or moderating roles on symptom manifestation. These neurotransmitters have demonstrated interactions with estrogen and progesterone and *all* of these are neuroactive with known mood and behavior effects, including negative mood, irritability, aggression, and impulse control.[56] Sex steroids also interact with the renin-angiotensin-aldosterone system (RAAS), which explains some PMS/PMDD signs and symptoms (e.g., water retention, bloating, weight gain). There is a predisposition of PMS to occur in families, perhaps because of genetics or shared environment; however, no genes have been identified.

◆CLINICAL MANIFESTATIONS. The pattern of symptom frequency and severity is more important than specific complaints. Nearly 300 physical, emotional, and behavioral symptoms have been attributed to PMS/PMDD. Emotional symptoms, particularly depression, anger, irritability, and fatigue, have been reported as the most prominent and the most distressing, whereas physical symptoms seem to be the least prevalent and problematic. Physical symptoms include breast tenderness, abdominal bloating, headache, and swelling of extremities. In addition, underlying physical or psychologic disease may be aggravated premenstrually and must be diagnosed and treated independently from PMS/PMDD.

◆EVALUATION AND TREATMENT. Diagnosis of PMS/PMDD is based on prospective health history and symptoms, with completion of a 2-month prospective symptom questionnaire, which is considered the gold standard. Diagnostic criteria for PMDD are presented in Box 25.5. Because the cause of PMS is not known and cannot be reduced to a single biologic explanation, and because the occurrence and severity of PMS are mediated by lifestyle and social and psychologic factors, treatment for PMS is symptomatic. Initial treatment focuses on validating the premenstrual experience, relieving the physical and psychologic symptoms, and eliminating contributing factors, as well as treatment of coexisting or underlying disorders.

Nonpharmacologic methods are first-line treatments for women who have mild symptoms or do not desire medication. These include acupuncture, herbal or mineral supplements, and lifestyle modifications. Lifestyle changes include regular exercise, appropriate sleep, and stress reduction during the premenstrual period. Calcium supplementation has been shown to decrease symptoms, although it is not as effective as pharmacologic treatment.[57] Vitamin B6, vitamin D, and vitamin E also have been studied, but sample sizes are small and no clear evidence exists regarding their efficacy. Several studies of the herbal preparations vitex agnus-castus and ginkgo biloba have shown a reduction in symptoms as compared with a placebo.[58] Finally, cognitive-behavioral therapy, which assists individuals in identifying and restructuring thought or behavior patterns, has been effective in improving coping in the context of other chronic pain conditions; several small trials have shown positive effects in individuals with PMS/PMDD.[59]

If nonpharmacologic methods fail or symptoms are severe, medical therapy is indicated. Two major forms of pharmacologic treatment include the use of hormonal cycle regulation and use of selective serotonin

BOX 25.5 DIAGNOSTIC CRITERIA FOR PREMENSTRUAL DYSPHORIC DISORDER

A. ≥5 symptoms below: occur in most cycles during the week before menses onset, improve within a few days after menses onset, and diminish in the week postmenses
B. One (or more) of the following symptoms must be present:
   a. Marked affective lability
   b. Marked irritability or anger or increased interpersonal conflicts
   c. Marked anxiety, tension
C. One (or more) of the following symptoms must also be present:
   a. Decreased interest
   b. Difficulty concentrating
   c. Easy fatigability, low energy
   d. Increase or decrease in sleep
   e. Feelings of being overwhelmed
   f. Physical symptoms such as breast tenderness, muscle or joint aches, "bloating" or weight gain

   NOTE: Criteria A–C must be present for most menstrual cycles in the preceding year
D. Symptoms are associated with significant distress or interferences with work, school, relationships
E. The disturbance is not merely an exacerbation of another disorder such as major depression, panic disorder, persistent depressive disorder, or a personality disorder
F. Criterion A should be confirmed by prospective daily ratings in at least two symptomatic cycles
G. The symptoms are not due to physiological effects of a substance or another medical condition

Data from American Psychiatric Association: *Diagnostic and statistical manual of mental disorders*, ed 5, Washington, 2013, Author.

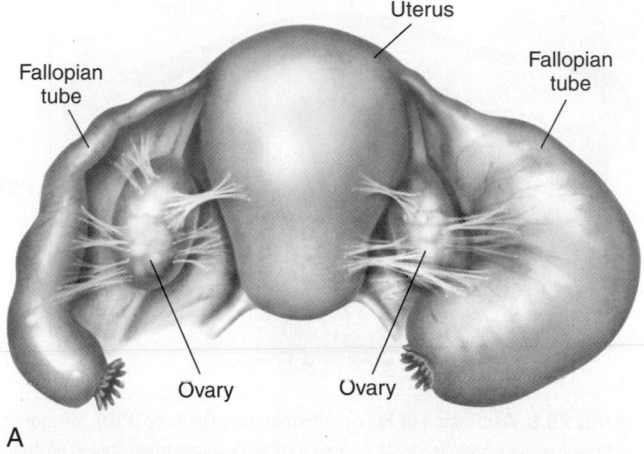

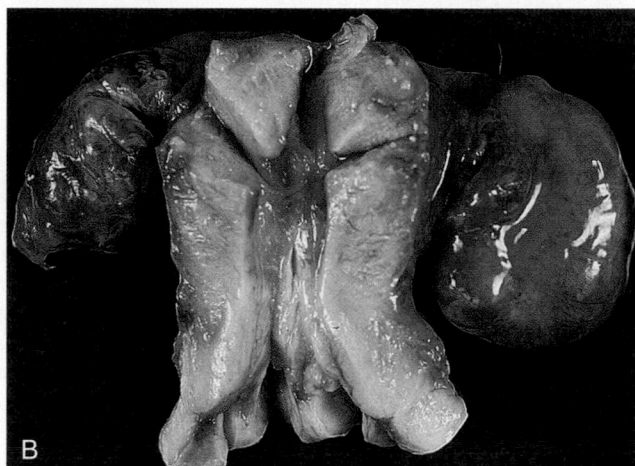

FIGURE 25.7 Salpingitis. **A,** Advanced pyosalpinx. Note the swollen fallopian tubes. **B,** Bilateral, retort-shaped, swollen, sealed tubes and adhesions of ovaries are typical of salpingitis. (**A** From Seidel HM et al: *Mosby's guide to physical examination*, ed 7, St Louis, 2011, Mosby. **B** From Damjanov I, Linder J, editors: *Anderson's pathology*, ed 10, St Louis, 1996, Mosby.)

reuptake inhibitor (SSRI) antidepressants. If a woman does not desire immediate fertility, COCs may regulate her menstrual cycle and decrease levels of circulating steroidal hormones. The oral contraceptive pill containing estrogen and progesterone has shown benefits in decreasing PMS/PMDD, in particular bloating, breast tenderness, and headache.[58,60] Oral contraceptive pills also can be used continuously for up to 3 months to decrease the frequency of menstrual periods and PMS/PMDD.[55]

SSRIs have been well studied for use in prevention and treatment of PMS/PMDD and are first-line therapy for severe symptomatology.[58] They are used to treat psychologic symptoms and also have a beneficial effect on physical symptoms.[31] These medications are effective when taken either continuously or limited to the luteal phase of the menstrual cycle. They may have undesired side effects, such as nausea, fatigue, or decreased libido, but these are largely dose-dependent.[31] Serotonin-norepinephrine reuptake inhibitors (SNRIs) and the antipsychotic medication Seroquel (quetiapine fumarate) also have been shown to improve symptomatology; however, more research is needed.[55]

Infection and Inflammation

Infections of the genital tract may result from exogenous or endogenous microorganisms. Exogenous pathogens are most often sexually transmitted (see Chapter 27). Endogenous causes of infection include microorganisms that are normally present in the vagina, bowel, or vulva. Infection occurs if these microorganisms overproliferate or migrate to a new location or if the immune system and other defense mechanisms are impaired.

A number of skin disorders also can affect the vulva. They include reactive dermatitis, contact dermatitis, psoriasis, and impetigo. (See Chapter 47 for a discussion of skin disorders.) Many infectious disorders that affect the vulva and vagina are sexually transmitted; these disorders are described in Chapter 27.

Pelvic Inflammatory Disease

Pelvic inflammatory disease (PID) is an acute inflammatory process caused by infection and affects an estimated 800,000 to 1,000,000 women per year.[61,62] PID may involve any or all organs in the upper genital tract—the uterus, fallopian tubes, or ovaries—and, in its most severe form, the entire peritoneal cavity. Inflammation of the fallopian tubes is termed salpingitis (Fig. 25.7); inflammation of the ovaries is called oophoritis. Most cases of PID are caused by sexually transmitted microorganisms, such as chlamydia and gonorrhea, that migrate from the vagina to the uterus, fallopian tubes, and ovaries. The ascension of these microorganisms into the upper genital tract may be facilitated by disruptions in the normal vaginal flora.[63,64]

Pelvic inflammatory disease is very common in the United States and around the world and has both immediate and long-term health implications for women. Infections of the upper reproductive tract cause changes to the delicate cells of the fallopian/uterine tubes, which can affect fertility and increase the risk of ectopic pregnancy.[65]

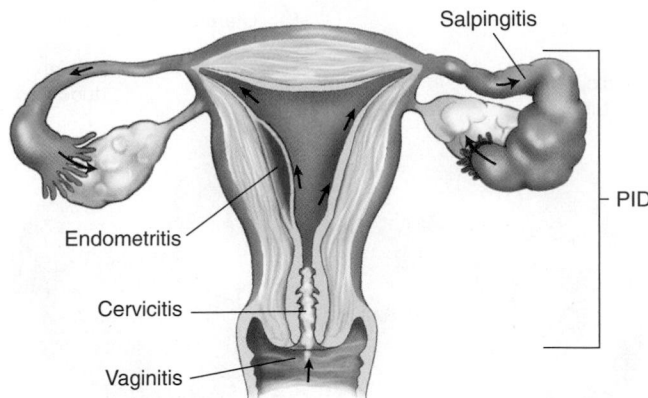

Salpingitis

PID

Endometritis

Cervicitis

Vaginitis

FIGURE 25.8 Ascension of Pelvic Inflammatory Disease (PID). Microorganisms from the lower genital tract ascend into the endometrium, fallopian tubes, and peritoneum to cause endometritis-salpingitis-peritonitis (pelvic inflammatory disease). The *arrows* indicate the "flow" of microorganisms from the lower genital tract to the upper genital tract. This is noted as an ascending infection in the text. (Adapted from Brooks ML: *Exploring medical language,* ed 8, St Louis, 2012, Mosby.)

◆PATHOPHYSIOLOGY. The development of upper genital tract infections is mediated by the failure of a number of defense mechanisms that usually are effective in preventing PID. Virulence of the organism, size of the inoculum, and defense status of the individual determine whether an infectious process results. Gonorrhea and chlamydia are the main infectious causes of PID.[66] These microorganisms can infect the vagina and cervix but do not usually ascend into the upper genital tract and cause PID (Fig. 25.8). However, when the normal vaginal microbial flora is disrupted, the pathogens can more easily ascend through the cervix.

Many anaerobic bacteria have been implicated in increasing the risk of PID because they alter the pH of the vaginal environment and may decrease the integrity of the mucus blocking the cervical canal.[63] Bacterial vaginosis (BV) is present in up to 66% of women with PID; and other anaerobes, such as *Bacteroides, Gardnerella vaginalis,* and *Haemophilus influenzae,* and genital tract mycoplasmas (*Mycoplasma hominis, Mycoplasma genitalis,* and *Ureaplasma urealyticum*) are frequently isolated from women with PID (see Chapter 27 for further discussion of BV). *Escherichia coli* may contribute to pelvic infections in older women. Therefore although gonorrhea and chlamydia are the main pathogens in PID, the disease is really polymicrobial and is treated with a broad spectrum of antibiotics to ensure that all the causative agents are eliminated.[63,66]

Once the infection is established within the uterus and fallopian/uterine tubes, the infection may induce changes in the columnar epithelium lining the upper reproductive tract, causing permanent damage. The resultant inflammatory response causes localized edema and, occasionally, obstruction or necrosis of the area. Gonorrhea gonococci attach to the fallopian tubes and excrete a substance toxic to the tubal mucosa, causing further inflammation and damage. Chlamydia enters the tubal cells and replicates, bursting the cell membrane as it reproduces, causing permanent scarring. Gonorrhea and chlamydia can spread to the abdominal cavity through the openings of the fallopian/uterine tubes. Other mechanisms that may contribute to PID include lymphatic drainage with parametrial spread of the infection, sexual intercourse, and retrograde menstruation.[67]

The rate of mortality from PID in the United States is fairly low. However, PID infection results in permanent changes to the ciliated epithelium of the fallopian or uterine tubes. Studies suggest that approximately 20% to 50% of women with PID subsequently struggle

---

BOX 25.6 **DIAGNOSTIC CRITERIA FOR PELVIC INFLAMMATORY DISEASE (PID)**

Minimum Criteria (One or More Needed for Diagnosis)
Cervical motion tenderness, *or*
Uterine tenderness, *or*
Adnexal tenderness

Additional Criteria That Increase Specificity of Diagnosis
Fever >38.3°C (>101°F)
Mucopurulent cervical or vaginal discharge, or cervical friability
Numerous white blood cells on saline wet prep
Elevated C-reactive protein
Elevated erythrocyte sedimentation rate
Documented infection with *Chlamydia trachomatis* or *Neisseria gonorrhoeae*

Definitive Criteria (*Not* Needed for Treatment)
Transvaginal ultrasound, magnetic resonance imaging, *or* Doppler studies showing thickened and fluid-filled tubes
Laparoscopic visualization of PID-related abnormalities
Endometrial biopsy with evidence of endometritis

From Centers for Disease Control and Prevention (CDC): *Pelvic inflammatory disease (PID) treatment and care,* Atlanta, GA, 2015, U.S. Department of Health and Human Services.

---

with infertility.[65] A recent study found that one episode of mild, sub-clinical PID resulted in a 40% decrease in later pregnancy rates, and multiple episodes of PID further increase the risk of infertility.[68] Scarring caused by PID greatly increases the risk of later ectopic pregnancy by up to 10-fold because the mobility of an egg through the fallopian tubes is slowed by damaged cilia.[67] Scarring and adhesions also can result in chronic pelvic pain and, potentially, an increased risk of later uterine cancer.[67]

◆CLINICAL MANIFESTATIONS. The clinical manifestations of PID vary from sudden, severe abdominal pain with fever to no symptoms at all. An asymptomatic cervicitis with or without discharge may be present for some time before PID develops. The first sign of the ascending infection may be the onset of low bilateral abdominal pain, most often characterized as dull and steady with a gradual onset.[66] Symptoms are more likely to develop during or immediately after menstruation. The pain of PID may worsen with walking, intercourse, or other activities involving movement. Other manifestations of PID include dysuria (difficult or painful urination), dyspareunia (pain with sexual intercourse), and irregular bleeding.[67]

◆EVALUATION AND TREATMENT. PID often has limited or vague clinical symptoms, leading to undertreatment and subsequent long-term health effects.[62] Because PID is a substantial health risk to a woman, the Centers for Disease Control and Prevention (CDC) encourage clinicians to consider PID as a likely diagnosis when a sexually-active woman has abdominal or pelvic tenderness and *one* of the following: cervical motion tenderness, uterine tenderness, or adnexal tenderness.[66] Box 25.6 lists the diagnostic criteria for PID. No laboratory tests or studies are needed to begin treatment; however, additional information can improve the specificity of diagnosis.[66] Abdominal pain in women can have many causes, and it is important to rule out other diagnoses (Fig. 25.9); however, further studies to rule out other diagnoses can be done while treating for PID.[66]

Because of the significance of the complications of PID, rapid treatment is recommended even before the causative pathogen can be

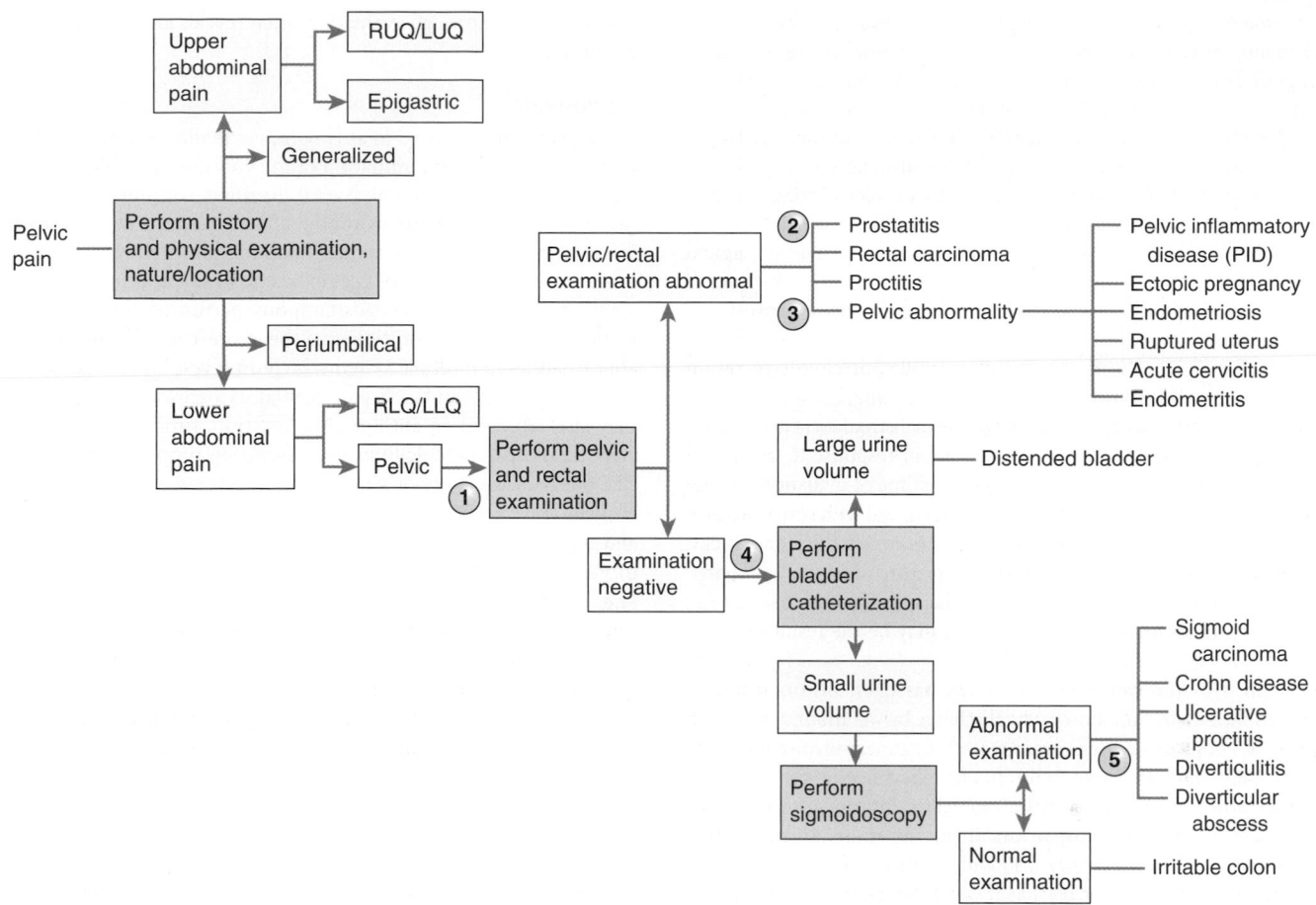

FIGURE 25.9 Diagnostic Algorithm for Pelvic Pain. *LLQ,* Left lower quadrant; *LUQ,* left upper quadrant; *RLQ,* right lower quadrant; *RUQ,* right upper quadrant.

BOX 25.7	CDC RECOMMENDED ORAL TREATMENT FOR PELVIC INFLAMMATORY DISEASE

Ceftriaxone: 250 mg IM in a single dose
Doxycycline: 100 mg orally twice a day for 14 days
WITH or WITHOUT
Metronidazole: 500 mg orally twice a day for 14 days

Data from Centers for Disease Control and Prevention (CDC): *Pelvic inflammatory disease (PID) treatment and care,* Atlanta, GA, 2015, U.S. Department of Health and Human Services.

---

identified. Because treatment is empiric, it needs to be effective against a broad range of pathogens, especially chlamydia, gonorrhea, and anaerobic bacteria.[66] Treatment is usually conducted in an outpatient setting unless the woman has symptoms of advanced infection, cannot take oral medications, or is pregnant; or if other pathologic conditions cannot be excluded. The CDC-recommended outpatient regimen is shown in Box 25.7.[66] Although alternative treatment regimens are available, the growing antibiotic resistance of gonorrhea limits antibiotic choices. The CDC is closely monitoring gonorrhea's antibiotic sensitivity and updates treatment guidelines periodically to reflect new information.[66] The most up-to-date treatment guidelines can be found on the CDC website.

Sexual partners of women with PID also should also receive treatment, even if they are asymptomatic. Women receiving treatment should be reevaluated by their care provider in 3 days to ensure antibiotic treatment is effective.[66] Because women with a history of PID are at increased risk for ectopic pregnancy, they should seek care as soon as they know they are pregnant because ectopic pregnancy is a major cause of maternal mortality.[62] Additionally, all sexually-active women younger than age 25 should receive minimal annual screening for chlamydia and gonorrhea, as well as women older than age 25 with a new sexual partner, more than one sexual partner, a partner who has been diagnosed with a sexually transmitted infection (STI), or a partner with more than one sexual partner.

Vaginitis

Vaginitis is irritation of the vagina that can be caused by a variety of microorganisms, irritants, or pathologies, or by a disruption of the normal flora of the vagina. Vaginitis is characterized by complaints of vaginal irritation, itching, burning, odor, or abnormal discharge. Clinically, an increase in the number of white blood cells or abnormal or foreign cells, or both, is observed on saline wet prep examination. The major causes of vaginitis are overgrowth of normal flora, sexually transmitted diseases, and vaginal irritation related to low estrogen levels during menopause (a condition known as *atrophic vaginitis*). The primary forms of vaginitis are vulvovaginal candidiasis or yeast vaginitis, bacterial vaginosis, or trichomoniasis.[69,70]

The irritation of vaginitis is related to an alteration in the vaginal environment, including changes in skin integrity, immune reaction, and particularly vaginal pH. The pH of the vagina depends on cervical secretions and the presence of normal flora that help maintain an acidic environment. A neutral or alkaline pH normally occurs before puberty, after menopause, and during pregnancy. The acidic nature of vaginal secretions during the reproductive years provides protection against a variety of sexually transmitted pathogens and establishes a healthy microflora in the vagina (see Chapter 27). Changes in the vaginal pH may predispose a woman to infection. Many substances and conditions can alter vaginal pH including exposure to soaps, spermicides, douches, feminine hygiene sprays, semen, or deodorant menstrual pads or tampons; and conditions associated with increased glycogen content of vaginal secretions, such as pregnancy or diabetes. Antibiotics can destroy normal vaginal flora, facilitating overgrowth of *Candida albicans,* causing a yeast vaginitis.

Normally vaginal discharge is a clear, milky, or cloudy secretion with a slippery or clumpy texture. It is nonirritating, has a mild smell, and may yellow after drying. Throughout the menstrual cycle the amount and texture of a woman's discharge change in response to hormonal fluctuation. Vaginal secretions increase at the time of ovulation, during pregnancy (because of increased estrogen levels), and with sexual arousal; just before menstruation, vaginal discharge becomes thick and sticky. Unusual changes in the amount, color, or texture of vaginal discharge may signal an infection, especially if the discharge is copious, malodorous, or irritating. Irritation of the vaginal area may be the result of many factors.

Diagnosis of the cause of vaginitis is based on history, physical examination, and examination of the discharge by wet mount; treatment by physical symptoms alone is inadequate.[70] Treatment involves developing and maintaining an acidic environment, relieving symptoms (usually pruritus), and administering antimicrobial or antifungal medications to eradicate the infectious organism. If the infection can be sexually transmitted, a woman's partner also will be treated. Research suggests that probiotics, especially *Lactobacillus rhamnosus,* can encourage normal vaginal flora and decrease the incidence of vaginitis in women at risk for vaginitis.[71,72]

Cervicitis

Cervicitis is a nonspecific term used to describe inflammation of the cervix. The CDC defines cervicitis as having two diagnostic signs: a purulent or mucopurulent discharge from the cervical os or endocervical bleeding, or both, induced by gently introducing a cotton swab into the cervix.[73] Cervicitis can have infectious or noninfectious causes, with approximately half of all cases caused by sexually transmitted pathogens.[74,75] Chemicals and substances introduced into the vagina can cause cervicitis in addition to disrupting the normal vaginal flora. Age and risk factors are important in assessing a woman with cervicitis. Younger women are at risk for sexually transmitted infections (STIs) and should be tested for chlamydia, gonorrhea, and *Trichomonas.* Older women with cervicitis may have STIs but are more likely to have irritation from abnormal vaginal flora related to low vaginal estrogen levels. In cases where no infectious agent is found, pharmacologic therapy may still be effective. Surgery may be an option or necessary for unresponsive and chronic cases.[74]

Mucopurulent cervicitis (MPC) usually is caused by one or more sexually transmitted pathogens, such as *Trichomonas, Gonorrhea, Chlamydia, Mycoplasma,* or *Ureaplasma.* Infection causes the cervix to become red and edematous. A mucopurulent (mucus- and pus-containing) exudate drains from the external cervical os, and the individual may report pelvic pain, bleeding, or dysuria. The cervix often becomes friable, bleeding easily during sexual intercourse or with pelvic examinations and Papanicolaou (Pap) smears. Because mucopurulent cervicitis is a symptom of PID, women at risk for STIs, especially those less than 25 years old, should receive treatment for PID while awaiting results of microbial testing.[73] If the woman is not at

risk for STIs, a thorough evaluation often reveals another cause for the inflammation.

Vulvodynia

Vulvodynia (also referred to as *vulvitis, vestibulitis,* or *vulvovestibulitis*) is chronic pain and inflammation of the vulva or vestibule, or both. In many cases it may represent several disorders without an identifiable cause. Vulvodynia is fairly common, affecting up to 16% of women at some point in life.[76] Whereas the inflammation of vulvodynia may be caused by contact dermatitis (i.e., exposure to soaps, detergents, lotions, sprays, shaving, menstrual pads/tampons, perfumed toilet paper, tight-fitting clothes), the condition may be more complex and represent abnormalities in multiple systems, including vestibular mucosa, pelvic floor musculature, and CNS pain regulatory pathways.[76] The condition may also represent an autoimmune reaction, similar to fibromyalgia. Genetic and psychologic links have also been proposed and studied.[77] The mechanisms are poorly understood; thus vulvodynia is difficult to evaluate and treat. Vulvodynia can be classified as generalized or localized and as provoked and unprovoked.[77] Vulvodynia may increase susceptibility to vaginal infection; likewise, it may be caused by vaginal infections (e.g., candidiasis, trichomoniasis) that spread to the labia, where they cause inflammation and edema. Other skin diseases, such as tinea cruris, psoriasis, lichen sclerosus, and inflammation of the apocrine (sweat) glands, can involve the vulva (see Chapter 47). Assessment includes excluding and treating conditions that may contribute to or cause vulvar inflammation (e.g., *Candida,* STI, seborrhea, psoriasis, lichen sclerosus, and contact dermatitis), and gently probing the vagina (e.g., labia majora and minora, vestibule, interlabial sulcus, clitoris) with a cotton-tipped swab to assess whether the pain is generalized or local to one region and how the pain is perceived in terms of quality (e.g., sharp, burning) and severity.

Treatment is focused on identifying and treating any infectious cause or comorbid contributor and using a multidisciplinary approach to address both the physical and the emotional aspects of the disorder. Women are advised to avoid potential irritants and to wear loose cotton clothing, use mild soaps, and apply a vaginal emollient (e.g., coconut or vegetable oil) after bathing. Studies on treatments are limited but suggest that women may benefit from topical lidocaine (Xylocaine) or estrogen cream; topical or systemic antidepressants or anxiolytics; Botox injections into the affected nerve; dietary modifications; physical therapy; behavioral or sexual counseling, or both; acupuncture; nerve blocks; or vestibulectomy.[76]

Bartholinitis

Bartholinitis, or Bartholin cyst, is an inflammation of one or both of the ducts that lead from the introitus (vaginal opening) to the Bartholin/greater vestibular glands (Fig. 25.10). The usual causes of bartholinitis are microorganisms that infect the lower female reproductive tract, such as streptococci, staphylococci, and sexually transmitted pathogens.

Infection or trauma causes inflammatory changes that narrow the distal portion of the duct, leading to obstruction and stasis of glandular secretions. The obstruction, or cyst, varies from 1 to 8 cm in diameter and is located in the posterolateral portion of the vulva. The cyst may be reddened and painful, and pus may be visible at the opening of the duct. Any exudate should be tested for gonorrhea and chlamydia. The individual may have symptoms of the initiating infection, fever, and malaise. Diagnosis of a Bartholin cyst is based on the clinical manifestations and the identification of infectious microorganisms.

Most Bartholin cysts are asymptomatic and require no treatment in women younger than age 40.[78] However, if they are uncomfortable or show signs of infection, treatment is advised to prevent abscess formation.

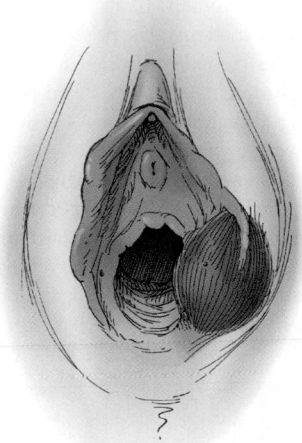

FIGURE 25.10 Inflammation of Bartholin Gland. (Modified from Gershenson DM et al: *Operative gynecology*, ed 2, Philadelphia, 2001, W.B. Saunders. In Fuller JK: *Surgical technology*, ed 6, Philadelphia, 2013, Saunders.)

Treatment is controversial but involves broad-spectrum antibiotics for suspected infection.[78] Some clinicians also attempt to drain the cyst using hot soaks, needle aspiration, insertion of a catheter, or marsupialization of the infected gland. No one treatment has proved to be superior in symptom relief and prevention of recurrence. In women older than 40, drainage and biopsy are advised to rule out carcinoma.[78]

Pelvic Organ Prolapse

The bladder, urethra, and rectum are supported by the endopelvic fascia and the perineal muscles, particularly the levator ani group. This muscular and fascial tissue loses tone and strength with aging and may not maintain the pelvic organs in the proper position. The pelvic area contains many organs and has the force of gravity and the abdominal contents pushing down on it. If the pelvic fascia and musculature are not firm, the pelvic organs may move to fill any space voids. With weak support, the bladder and rectum tend to push into the vagina and vaginal wall. The vagina is an opening in the pelvic musculature for intercourse and childbirth. (Chapter 24 contains a discussion of pelvic support structures.) However, as gravity acts on the pelvis, this opening becomes a weakness in the musculature support of the entire pelvic cavity. Without proper support from the vaginal muscles and fascia, the uterus and bulging vaginal walls can begin to herniate through the vaginal opening.

Pelvic organ prolapse (POP) is the descent of one or more of the following into the vaginal space: the vaginal wall, the uterus, or the apex of the vagina (after a hysterectomy).[79] Up to 50% of women have some version of POP on physical examination. However, most women have no symptoms, and there is no need for intervention. As the degree of prolapse increases, women feel more vaginal pressure. Bulging of the organs beyond the hymenal ring or vaginal entrance is commonly used as the clinical indicator for significant prolapse.[79] When prolapse becomes severe, the function of the surrounding organs can be altered. For instance, as the bladder is pulled posteriorly, incontinence and incomplete voiding become more common. As the bowel bulges into the vaginal space, defecation becomes more difficult. The severity of POP and its symptoms increase with age, and half of women older than age 50 have symptoms of POP.[79]

POP is multifactorial, but several factors contribute to the weakening the pelvic fascia that support the female reproductive tract. Trauma is the most common risk factor, including vaginal birth (especially with

BOX 25.8	RISK FACTORS ASSOCIATED WITH PELVIC ORGAN PROLAPSE

Menopause	Obesity
Aging	Prolonged standing or lifting
Hypoestrogenism	Pelvic floor trauma
Chronically increased	Vaginal childbirth
Intraabdominal pressure	Hysterectomy
Pregnancy	Genetic factors
Coughing (lung disease)	Connective tissue disorders
Constipation	Spina bifida

From Barber MD: *Br Med J* 354:i3853, 2016; Schaefer JI: Pelvic organ prolapse. In Hoffman BL et al, editors: *Williams gynecology*, ed 3, pp 538–561, New York, 2016, McGraw-Hill.

BOX 25.9	PHYSICAL EXAMINATION TERMS FOR DESCRIPTION OF SUPPORT ABNORMALITIES

Anterior vaginal wall prolapse	Cervical prolapse
Apical vaginal wall prolapse	Perineal prolapse
Posterior vaginal wall prolapse	Rectal prolapse

Data from Schaefer JI: Pelvic organ prolapse. In Hoffman BL et al, editors: *Williams gynecology*, ed 3, New York, 2016, McGraw-Hill, pp 538–561.

a large baby or forceps) and hysterectomy.[79] Both of these events can cause disruption or tearing of the pelvic fascia. Chronic stress on the pelvic fascia also contributes to risk. Pregnancy, obesity, prolonged standing, and chronic constipation are associated with stretching of the fascia and prolapse over time. Women with connective tissue disorders are also at risk, so there is a strong genetic/familial component. In addition, risk of prolapse increases with age because of cumulative effects of stress on the pelvic floor. Because estrogen improves vascularity of the pelvic area, postmenopausal women are at risk since their fascia and pelvis musculature lose resilience with diminished estrogen levels.[79] A list of risk factors is contained in Box 25.8.

The trend is to use terminology that describes physical examination findings, thus avoiding assumptions about structural involvement (Box 25.9). The terms *cystocele* and *rectocele* may be used when the structures involved (bladder and rectum, respectively) have been definitively identified (i.e., an anterior vaginal wall prolapse may or may not be a cystocele involving the urinary bladder) (see Fig. 25.12). Examining the woman in multiple positions and while straining maximally provides the best information about the degree of pelvic organ relaxation.[79] Physical examination may be augmented with imaging by ultrasound, or magnetic resonance. Several systems are used to describe prolapse. One in widespread clinical use is based on physical examination findings (see Box 25.9) and uses a grading system to describe the extent of the prolapse (Box 25.10). Subjective reports regarding the symptoms and effects of POP can be assessed through direct questioning or by using questionnaires such as the Pelvic Floor Impact Questionnaire or the Pelvic Floor Distress Inventory.

Uterine prolapse is descent of the cervix or entire uterus into the vaginal canal (Fig. 25.11). In severe cases the uterus falls completely through the vagina and protrudes from the introitus. Symptoms of other pelvic floor disorders also may be present.

Fig. 25.12 shows vaginal prolapse caused by cystocele and rectocele. **Cystocele** is descent of a portion of the posterior bladder wall and trigone into the vaginal canal. In severe cases, the bladder and anterior vaginal wall bulge outside the introitus. Occasionally a cystocele causes significant residual urine and an increased rate of bladder infections.

A rectocele is the bulging of the rectum and posterior vaginal wall into the vaginal canal. Although most rectoceles are asymptomatic, larger ones cause vaginal pressure, rectal fullness, and incomplete bowel evacuation. If rectoceles are severe, defecation is difficult and can be facilitated by applying manual pressure to the posterior vaginal wall.

An enterocele is herniation of the rectouterine pouch into the rectovaginal septum (between the rectum and posterior vaginal wall). It can be congenital or acquired. Congenital enteroceles rarely cause symptoms or progress in size. Enteroceles also can result from a muscular weakness caused by previous surgery, especially surgeries through the vagina, or by pelvic relaxation disorders, such as uterine prolapse, cystocele, and rectocele. Most large enteroceles are found in grossly obese and older adults and can be complicated by rupture or complete eversion of the vagina with trophic ulceration, edema, and fibrosis. Treatment is surgical. Box 25.11 summarizes the symptoms and treatments of POP.

Treatment of POP depends on the severity of symptoms and the physical condition of the woman. Treatment is often progressive with less aggressive treatments tried first. The pelvic fascia may be strengthened through Kegel exercises (repetitive isometric tightening and relaxing of the pubococcygeal muscles) or by estrogen therapy in menopausal women. Maintaining a healthy body mass index (BMI), preventing constipation, and treating chronic cough or constipation may help as well. A common treatment is a pessary, which is a removable device that, when placed in the vagina, holds the uterus in position.[80] Surgical repair with or without hysterectomy is the treatment of last resort. Women should be active participants in the decision-making surrounding treatment because they need to balance expectations for improvement with potential side effects[79] (see *What's New?* Vaginal Mesh).

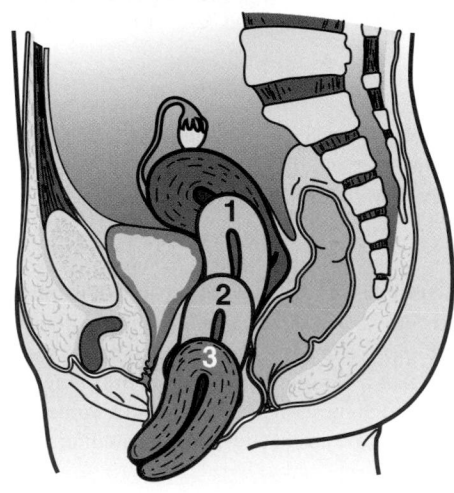

FIGURE 25.11 Degrees of Uterine Prolapse. **Grade 1** is minimal and rarely requires correction; **Grade 2** prolapse has moderate symptoms, and **Grade 3** prolapse is severe. The uterus is so low that the cervix protrudes from the vagina. (From Phillips N: *Berry & Kohn's operating room technique,* ed 12, Philadelphia, 2013, Mosby.)

BOX 25.10	**EVALUATION OF PELVIC ORGAN PROLAPSE (BADEN-WALKER HALFWAY SCORING SYSTEM)**

Grade 0: Normal position, no prolapse
Grade 1: Descent halfway to the hymen
Grade 2: Descent reaches the hymen
Grade 3: Descent halfway past hymen
Grade 4: Maximum possible descent for each site

NOTE: Any type of prolapse (posterior, apical, anterior vaginal, uterine, etc.) can be graded using this system.
From Baden WF, Walker TA: *Clin Obstet Gynecol* 15:1070–1072, 1972.

BOX 25.11	**PELVIC ORGAN PROLAPSE: SYMPTOMS AND TREATMENTS**

SYMPTOMS	**TREATMENT**

Urinary
Sensation of incomplete emptying of bladder
Urinary incontinence
Urinary frequency/urgency
Bladder "splinting" to accomplish voiding
	Depending on age of woman and cause and severity of the condition:
	  Isometric exercise to strengthen the pubococcygeal muscle (Kegels)
	  Estrogen to improve tone and vascularity of fascial support (postmenopausal)
	  Pessary (a removable device) to hold pelvic organs in place
	  Weight loss
	  Avoidance of constipation
	  Treatment of cough/lung conditions

Bowel Constipation or feeling of rectal fullness or blockage Difficult defecation Stool or flatus incontinence	**Surgical** Reconstructive: autologous grafts; synthetic mesh/sling Obliterative (most extreme)
Urgency Manual "splinting" of posterior vaginal wall to accomplish defecation	
Pain and Bulging Vaginal, bladder, rectum Pelvic pressure, bulging, pain Lower back pain	
Sexual Dyspareunia Decreased sensation, lubrication, arousal	

WHAT'S NEW?

Vaginal Mesh

Because pelvic organ prolapse is often a result of weakened pelvic fascia and musculature, a surgical mesh was developed to improve pelvic support. This mesh was designed to be placed surgically along the area needing support. The goal was to have the woman's tissues grow through the mesh and provide consistent, long-term support. However, women who received the surgical mesh had a high rate of complications, including infection and persistent postoperative pain. In many cases the mesh eroded through the tissue, protruding into the vagina and perforating other organs. In addition, the mesh may shrink over time, causing vaginal shortening, tightening, and pain. The U.S. Food and Drug Administration (FDA) has issued several warnings about the mesh to caution women and practitioners and encourage fully informed consent about the risks and benefits of mesh placement, and the FDA has reclassified the surgical mesh based on the lack of data about the safety of implanted mesh.

Data from U.S. Food and Drug Administration: Reclassification of surgical mesh for transvaginal pelvic organ prolapse repair and surgical instrumentation for urogynecologic surgical mesh procedures: designation of special controls for urogynecologic surgical mesh instrumentation 2014, 2015. Available at: https://www.federalregister.gov/documents/2014/05/01/2014-09907/reclassification-of-surgical-mesh for-transvaginal -pelvic-organ-prolapse-repair-and-surgical. Accessed Sept 19, 2016.

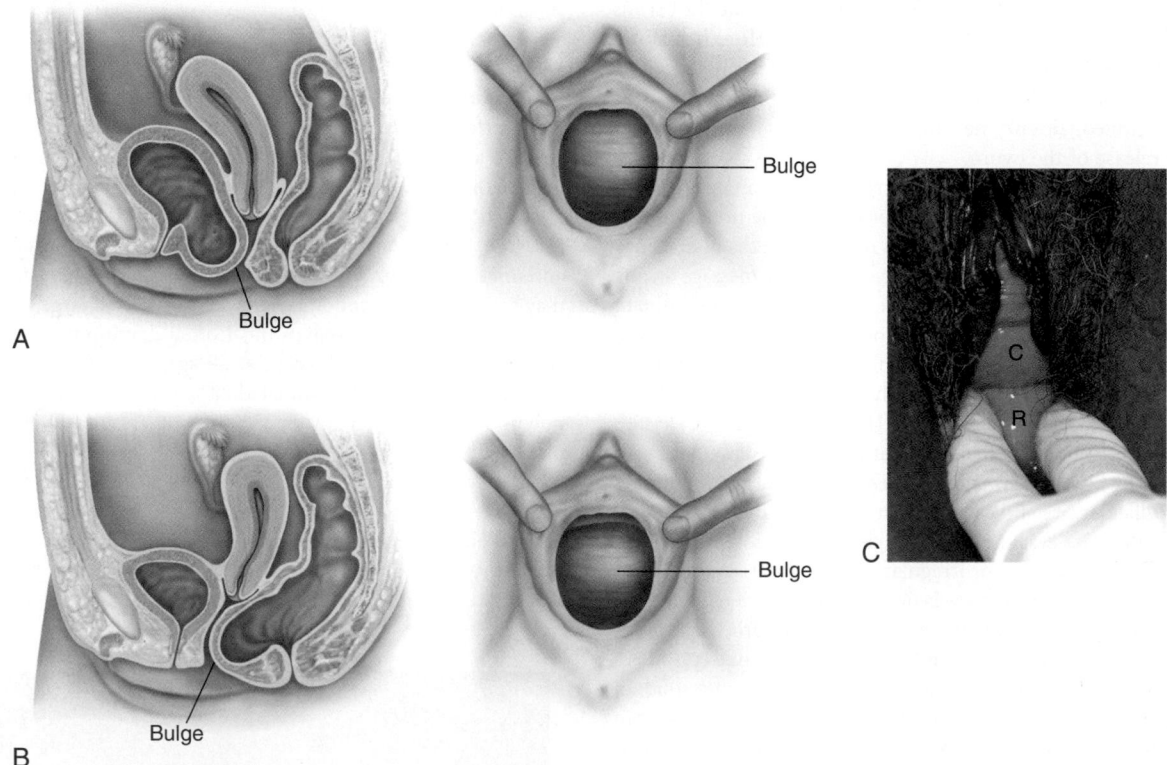

FIGURE 25.12 Cystocele and Rectocele. A, Grade 2: anterior vaginal wall prolapse. **B,** Grade 2: posterior wall prolapse. **C,** Photo showing cystocele *(C)* and rectocele *(R)*. (**A** and **B** From Seidel H et al: *Mosby's guide to physical examination,* ed 4, St Louis, 1999, Mosby. **C** From Seidel HM et al: *Mosby's guide to physical examination,* ed 7, St Louis, 2011, Mosby.)

Benign Growths and Proliferative Conditions
Benign Ovarian Cysts

Benign cysts of the ovary may occur at any time during the life span, but are most common during the reproductive years and, in particular, at the extremes of those years (Fig. 25.13). An increase in benign ovarian cysts occurs when hormonal imbalances are more likely (e.g., during puberty and menopause).[81] However, ovarian masses can occur during fetal development and throughout childhood as well.[82]

Benign ovarian cysts are quite common and are the fourth leading diagnosis for gynecologic hospital admissions.[83] Two common causes of benign ovarian enlargement in ovulating women are follicular cysts and corpus luteum cysts. These cysts are called functional cysts because they are caused by variations of normal physiologic events. Follicular

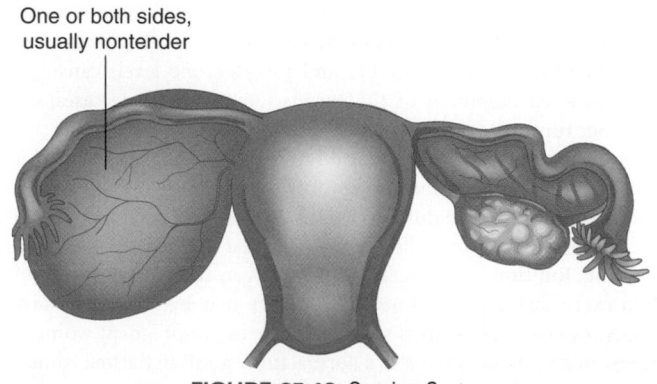

FIGURE 25.13 Ovarian Cyst.

and corpus luteum cysts are usually unilateral. They are typically 5 to 6 cm in diameter but can grow as large as 8 to 10 cm. Most women are asymptomatic. Any ovarian mass greater than 6 cm or noted for a period longer than 12 weeks should be referred to a gynecologist.[84]

Benign cysts of the ovary are produced when a follicle or a number of follicles are stimulated but no dominant follicle develops and completes the maturity process. Every month about 120 follicles are stimulated, but in most cycles only 1 follicle succeeds in ovulating a mature ovum. Normally, during the early follicular phase of the menstrual cycle, follicles of the ovary respond to hormonal signals from the pituitary gland. The pituitary produces FSH to mature follicles in the ovary. As the follicles enlarge, granulosa cells in the follicle multiply and secrete estradiol (a form of estrogen). As a dominant follicle develops, it secretes higher levels of estradiol, which stimulates the LH surge that comes from the pituitary. A small cyst on the ovary during the follicular phase is normal. The LH surge stimulates the follicle to rupture, releasing the ovum and transforming the granulosa cells of the dominant follicle into the corpus luteum. If the dominant follicle develops properly before ovulation, the corpus luteum becomes vascularized and secretes progesterone. Progesterone arrests development of other follicles in both ovaries in that cycle. LH, proteolytic enzymes, and prostaglandins trigger follicular rupture and release of the ovum.

Follicular cysts can be caused by a transient condition in which the dominant follicle fails to rupture or one or more of the nondominant follicles fail to regress. This disturbance is not well understood. It may be that the hypothalamus does not receive or send a message strong enough to increase FSH levels needed to develop or mature a dominant follicle. The hypothalamus monitors blood levels of estradiol and progesterone; when FSH level is low, estradiol does not increase enough to stimulate LH. Evidence indicates that when progesterone is not being produced, the hypothalamus releases GnRH to increase the FSH level.[85] FSH continues to stimulate follicles to mature, and the granulosa cells grow and, presumably, estradiol increases. This abnormal cycle continues to stimulate follicular size and causes follicular cysts to develop. Clinical symptoms of follicular cysts or even a single cyst are bloating, swollen and tender breasts, and heavy or irregular menses. After several subsequent cycles in which hormone levels once again follow a regular cycle and progesterone levels are restored, cysts usually are absorbed or regress.

Follicular cysts can vary in size and symptoms from one episode to the next and often can recur. Most are fluid filled; the more solid an ovarian cyst, the greater the chance of malignancy. Follicular cysts can be treated with combined estrogen-progestin oral contraceptives because they block the HPG axis, effectively quieting the ovary. Progestin-only contraceptives, however, increase the likelihood of developing follicular cysts because ovarian function is diminished, but not suppressed, leading to an increased number of immature follicles.[81]

A **corpus luteum cyst** is normally formed by the granulosa cells left behind after ovulation. This cyst is highly vascularized but limited in size and spontaneously regresses as part of the normal menstrual cycle. However, an abnormal or hemorrhagic cyst may develop because of a hormonal imbalance in low LH and progesterone levels causing an inadequate development of the corpus luteum. In some cases, large cysts can rupture, causing hemorrhage.[82]

Corpus luteum cysts are less common than follicular cysts, but luteal cysts typically cause more symptoms, particularly if they rupture. Manifestations include dull, unilateral pelvic pain and amenorrhea or delayed menstruation, followed by irregular or heavier than usual bleeding. Rupture occasionally occurs and can cause massive bleeding with excruciating pain; immediate surgery may be required. Corpus luteum cysts usually regress spontaneously in nonpregnant women. A persistent corpus luteum cyst is a normal finding within the first trimester of pregnancy since the corpus luteum produces progesterone to support

the pregnancy until the placenta is established.[81] Following the development of a large, painful, or hemorrhagic cyst, oral contraceptives can be used to suppress ovarian function and prevent future cysts.

Dermoid cysts are ovarian teratomas that contain elements of all three germ layers; they are common ovarian neoplasms. These growths may contain mature tissue including skin, hair, sebaceous and sweat glands, muscle fibers, cartilage, teeth, and bone. Dermoid cysts are usually asymptomatic and are found incidentally on pelvic examination. However, these cysts should be carefully evaluated for removal because they have malignant potential.[81]

Torsion of the ovary is a rare complication of ovarian cysts or tumors or enlargement of the ovary and can occur in girls or women. If a cyst is large enough it can cause the ovary to twist on its ligaments, pinching off blood supply to the ovary and causing extreme pain. Ovarian torsion is rare but is a gynecologic emergency. Individuals present with acute, severe unilateral abdominal or pelvic pain. Ovarian torsion is treated surgically.[86]

Endometrial Polyps

An **endometrial polyp** is a benign mass of endometrial tissue, covered by a surface epithelium, and contains a variable amount of glands, stroma, and blood vessels. Endometrial polyps can occur anywhere within the uterus. Polyps are morphologically diverse and usually classified as hyperplastic, atrophic (or inactive), or functional. In the last case, the surface epithelium may be "out of phase" with other endometrial tissue. Hyperplastic polyps are often pedunculated and may be mistaken for endometrial hyperplasia or, if large, adenosarcoma (Fig. 25.14). Although polyps most often develop in women between ages 40 and 50, they can occur at all ages. These are often related to estrogen stimulation. An estimated 20% to 25% of women have uterine polyps, including as many as 35% of women with abnormal uterine bleeding.[82]

Endometrial polyps are a common cause of intermenstrual or excessive menstrual bleeding. Diagnosis is made by transvaginal sonography or hysteroscopy. Risk factors include advanced age; obesity; nulliparity; early menarche or late menopause, or both; diabetes;

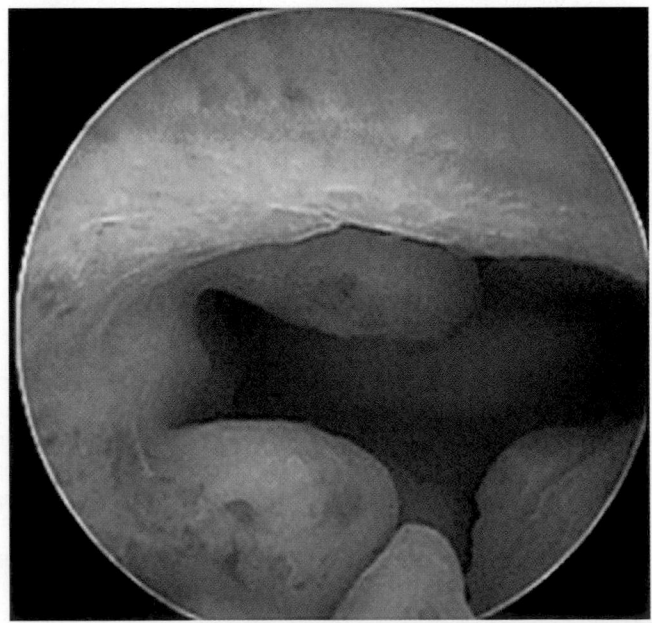

FIGURE 25.14 Uterine Polyps Visible Through Hysteroscopy. (From Cheng C et al: *J Minim Invasive Gynecol* 16[6]:739–742, 2009.)

tamoxifen use; hypertension; and estrogenic states (i.e., anovulatory cycles and unopposed estrogen). Malignancy is rare (up to 4.8% of polyps have evidence of malignancy); however, polyps that cause abnormal bleeding have twice the rate of malignancy of asymptomatic polyps.[87] Coexistence of a separate endometrial atypical hyperplasia or adenocarcinoma is common. Uterine polyps have a high rate of spontaneous resolution but have been associated with suboptimal fertility.[82,88] Polypectomy can be performed through hysteroscopy for symptomatic women, for those at risk for malignancy, or for women who are struggling to conceive.[89]

Leiomyomas

Leiomyomas, commonly called myomas or uterine fibroids, are benign smooth muscle tumors in the myometrium (Fig. 25.15). Leiomyomas are the most common benign tumors of the uterus, affecting as many as 70% to 80% of all women, and most remain small, asymptomatic, and clinically insignificant.[90] Prevalence increases in women ages 30 to 50 but decreases with menopause. The incidence of leiomyomas in black and Asian women is two to five times higher than that in white women, and the age of onset for black women is, on average, 10 years earlier than that for white women.[91] Complications related to leiomyomas are the primary reason for gynecologic hospitalizations and account for 30% of all hysterectomies in women less than 40 years of age.[83,91]

The cause of uterine leiomyomas is unknown, although their size appears to be related to estrogen, progesterone, growth factors, angiogenesis, and apoptosis. There is a genetic component to fibroids, and the leiomyomas exhibit chromosomal changes within their tissues.[92] Leiomyomas are estrogen- and progesterone-sensitive and are found to have increased numbers of estrogen receptors.[82] Uterine leiomyomas are not seen before menarche, and those that develop during the reproductive years generally decrease in size after menopause. Occurrence is multifactorial but often linked with estrogen exposure. Tumors in pregnant women may enlarge rapidly but often decrease in size after the end of the pregnancy. Risk factors for fibroids include nulliparity, obesity, PCOS, black race, postmenopausal hormone use, and hypertension.[92]

◆**PATHOPHYSIOLOGY.** Most leiomyomas occur in multiples in the fundus of the uterus, although they may occur singly and throughout the uterus. Leiomyomas are classified as subserous, submucous, or intramural according to their location within the various layers of the uterine wall (Fig. 25.16). Uterine leiomyomas are usually firm and surrounded by a connective tissue layer. Unlike cancer, leiomyomas are unable to cause blood vessel proliferation to support their growth. Degeneration and necrosis may occur when a large leiomyoma outgrows its blood supply; the ensuing tissue necrosis causes pain.

◆**CLINICAL MANIFESTATIONS.** The major clinical manifestations of leiomyomas are abnormal uterine bleeding, pain, and symptoms related to pressure on nearby structures. The leiomyoma may distort the uterine cavity and increase the endometrial surface area. This increase may account for the increased menstrual bleeding that is associated with leiomyomas. Pain is not an early symptom but tends to occur with the devascularization of larger leiomyomas. It is also associated with blood vessel compression that limits blood supply to adjacent structures. Symptoms of abdominal pressure are slow to develop, apparently because the tumor is relatively slow growing, enabling adjacent structures to adapt to pressure. Pressure on the bladder may contribute to urinary frequency, urgency, and dysuria. Pressure on the ureter may cause it to become distended "upstream" from the pressure point; rectosigmoid pressure may lead to constipation. A sensation of abdominal or genital heaviness may be felt with larger tumors. Fibroids also may contribute to infertility and subfertility.

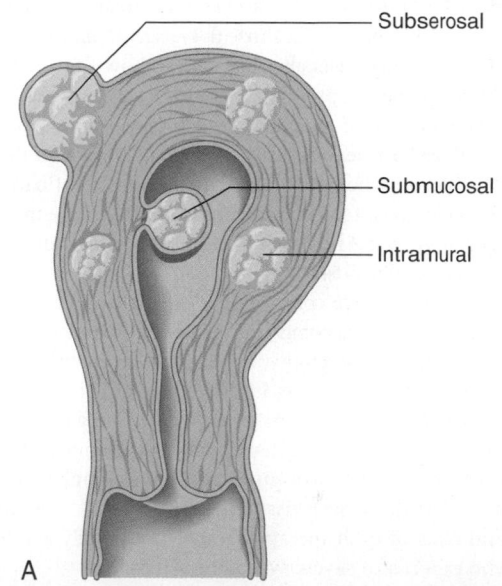

A

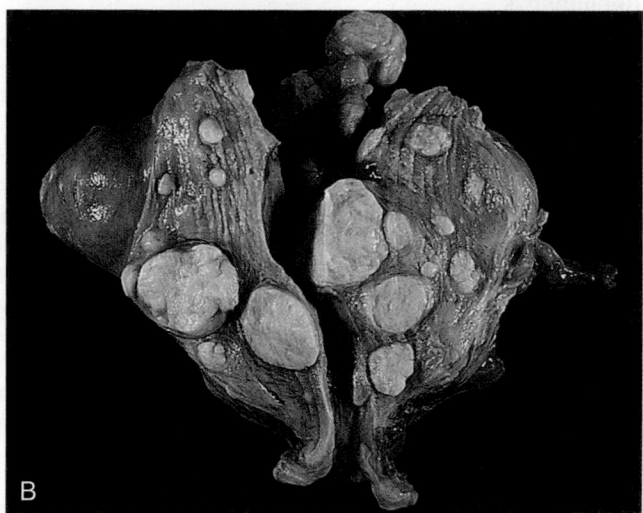

B

FIGURE 25.16 Leiomyomas. **A,** Uterine section showing whorl-like appearance and locations of leiomyomas, which are also called *uterine fibroids.* **B,** Multiple leiomyomas in sagittal section. Typical, well-circumscribed, solid, light gray nodules distort uterus. (**B** From Damjanov I, Linder J: *Pathology: a color atlas,* St Louis, 2000, Mosby.)

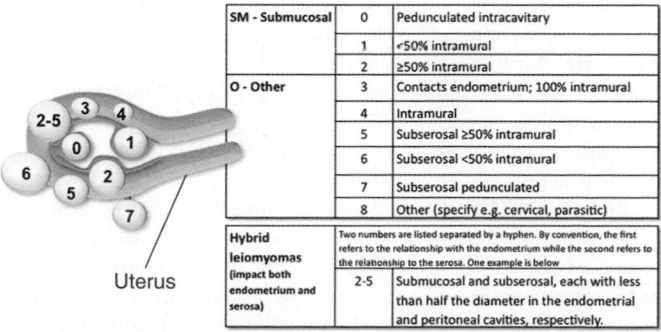

SM - Submucosal	0	Pedunculated intracavitary
	1	<50% intramural
	2	≥50% intramural
O - Other	3	Contacts endometrium; 100% intramural
	4	Intramural
	5	Subserosal ≥50% intramural
	6	Subserosal <50% intramural
	7	Subserosal pedunculated
	8	Other (specify e.g. cervical, parasitic)
Hybrid leiomyomas (impact both endometrium and serosa)		Two numbers are listed separated by a hyphen. By convention, the first refers to the relationship with the endometrium while the second refers to the relationship to the serosa. One example is below
	2-5	Submucosal and subserosal, each with less than half the diameter in the endometrial and peritoneal cavities, respectively.

FIGURE 25.15 Leiomyoma (Fibroid) Classification System. (From Munro M et al: *Int Gynaecol Obstet* 113[1]:3–13, 2011.)

◆**EVALUATION AND TREATMENT**. Uterine leiomyomas are suspected when the bimanual examination discloses uterine enlargement and irregular, nontender nodularity of the uterus. Pelvic sonography or MRI confirms diagnosis.[82] Treatment depends on the symptoms, tumor size, age, reproductive status, overall health of the individual, and the woman's preference.[93] Most myomas are asymptomatic and can be managed by observation only. Medical treatment for symptomatic women not desiring pregnancy is aimed at shrinking the myoma, or reducing symptoms, or both. Some leiomyomas shrink in response to oral contraceptives; however, oral contraceptive pills (OCPs) may enhance growth, so they should be monitored carefully. An LNG-IUD (progestin-only) may be helpful for women who wish to reduce their bleeding and decrease the size of the tumors, if their uterine cavity is not completely blocked by large fibroids. GnRH agonists are usually a temporary management for those close to menopause or as a presurgical treatment. GnRH side effects related to decreased levels of estrogen, including hot flashes and osteoporosis, limit its usefulness. Various selective estrogen receptor modulators have been studied alone and in conjunction with GnRH agonists and appear effective, although more research is needed, especially because these agents may decrease bone density.[93] GnRH antagonists also have been shown to reduce fibroid volume. Progesterone receptor agonists, such as mifepristone (RU486) and ulipristal acetate, also have shown some effectiveness in shrinking leiomyomas; these have been approved for use in Europe for the purpose of shrinking fibroids before surgery. Promising nonpharmacologic therapies include green tea extract, curcumin (the active ingredient in turmeric), vitamin D, and herbal preparations used in Chinese medicine specifically to treat fibroids.[93]

Surgical treatments are commonly used but may be decreasing in frequency. Hysterectomy is commonly performed for bleeding and pain related to fibroids. Myomectomy, or removal of the fibroid from the muscle of the uterus, may be less invasive than a full hysterectomy and remains the standard of treatment for women wishing to preserve their fertility. Newer less-invasive treatments that show promise include uterine artery embolization, and MRI-guided ultrasonography to coagulate areas of the fibroid, causing tissue destruction and involution. The benefits and risks of each therapy should be carefully explored with women who experience severe symptoms.[93]

Adenomyosis

Adenomyosis is the presence of endometrial tissue within the uterine myometrium. Endometrial cells migrate into the myometrial layer through an unknown mechanism. Estrogen and progesterone likely play a role and, perhaps, metaplasia of müllerian tissue. Unlike endometriosis, this tissue does not respond to cyclic hormone changes. It is more commonly found during the late reproductive years; however, because adenomyosis is generally diagnosed after hysterectomy, time of diagnosis may not correspond with incidence. Adenomyosis has been found in up to 30% to 60% of hysterectomy specimens from otherwise normal women; rates are higher for women taking tamoxifen.[82] Parity also increases the risk for adenomyosis, as does any history of uterine surgery. While women diagnosed with adenomyosis are often out of their childbearing years, those with adenomyosis who become pregnant are at risk for poor outcomes, including preterm labor, preterm premature rupture of membranes, and low birth weight.[82]

Adenomyosis may be asymptomatic or may be associated with abnormal menstrual bleeding, dysmenorrhea, dyspareunia, uterine enlargement, uterine tenderness during menstruation, chronic pelvic pain, and infertility.[94] Secondary dysmenorrhea becomes increasingly severe as disease progresses. On bimanual examination the uterus is diffusely enlarged (two to three times the expected size), globular, and most tender just before or after menstruation. Diagnosis is confirmed

with ultrasound or MRI.[94] Treatment is symptomatic and first-line therapies include NSAIDs, combined oral contraceptives, and the LNG-IUD. Other promising medical treatments include selective estrogen receptor modulators, high-dose progestins, selective progesterone receptor modulators, aromatase inhibitors, and GnRH agonists.[95] Surgical treatment includes resection of localized areas of adenomyosis (though this is difficult) or, if severe, hysterectomy. Uterine artery embolization and uterine ablation have shown good initial results but need further testing. In addition, there is an emerging body of research looking at the use of high-intensity ultrasound and other interventional radiology treatments.[95] Decisions are based on managing symptoms and whether future fertility is desired.

Endometriosis

Endometriosis is the presence of functioning endometrial tissue or implants outside the uterus. Like normal endometrial tissue, the ectopic (out of place) endometrium responds to the hormonal fluctuations of the menstrual cycle. Common sites of implantation include the pelvic peritoneum, ovaries, and uterosacral ligaments. Endometriosis primarily affects younger (premenopausal) women, with peak incidence in the third decade. However, the overall incidence of endometriosis is difficult to determine, particularly in asymptomatic adolescent and fertile women. It is estimated that 11% of asymptomatic women have endometriosis; however, as many as 50% of women evaluated for pelvic pain, infertility, or a pelvic mass are diagnosed as having endometriosis.[96] It is the third most common reason for hysterectomy.[97] In addition, women with endometriosis are at greater risk for cancers, especially ovarian cancer.[98]

The cause of endometriosis is not known, but multiple theories have been proposed. One commonly accepted theory was proposed in 1927,[99] and suggested that endometriosis is caused by the implantation of endometrial cells during retrograde menstruation, in which menstrual fluids move through the fallopian tubes and into the pelvic cavity. Indeed, there is a higher incidence of endometriosis in women who have an obstructed menstrual flow.[97] However, it is now known that although retrograde menstruation occurs in almost all women, not all women develop endometriosis.

Another theory is that women with endometriosis have impaired cellular and humoral immunity. Alterations in cytokine and growth factor signaling have been identified. Cytotoxic T-cell and natural killer (NK) cell activity has been found to be depressed. At the same time, increased numbers of macrophages appear to be stimulating endometrial cell proliferation outside the uterus. An autoimmune response is also suspected.[100] Such alterations may cause the body to tolerate ectopic implantation of endometrial cells. Researchers also have proposed that endometrial cells spread through the lymphatic or vascular systems or that multipotential cells in the epithelial coverings of reproductive organs are somehow stimulated to develop into endometrial and metaplastic cells. Another theory, supported by recent findings of endometriosis found in female fetuses,[101] is that endometrial cells may spread outside the uterus during fetal organogenesis. A genetic predisposition to endometriosis has been documented, and genetic polymorphisms have been identified; emerging research also suggests that there may be a disruption in gene expression during embryogenesis that is responsible for the generation of endometriosis.[102]

◆**PATHOPHYSIOLOGY**. Endometrial implants can occur throughout the body but generally occur in the pelvic and abdominal cavities. The most common sites of implantation are the ovaries, uterine ligaments, rectovaginal septum, and pelvic peritoneum (Fig. 25.17). Other sites of implantation are the sigmoid colon, small intestine, rectum, appendix, bladder, uterus, vulva, vagina, cervix, lymph nodes, extremities, pleural cavity, lungs, laparotomy scars, and hernial sacs. Indeed, pathologic

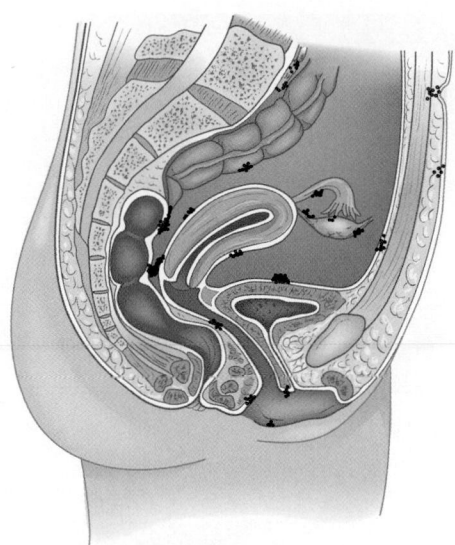

FIGURE 25.17 Pelvic Sites of Endometrial Implantation. Endometrial cells may enter the pelvic cavity during retrograde menstruation.

studies have found endometriosis on all organs of the body except the spleen.[103]

The growth of endometrial lesions depends on estrogen exposure. Endometriosis lesions are affected by ovarian hormones in the same manner as endometrial tissue within the uterus, with the exception of marked progesterone resistance of the endometriosis cells. Cyclic changes depend on the vascularity and blood supply of the lesion and the presence of glandular and stromal cells. Given that blood supply is sufficient, the ectopic endometrium proliferates, breaks down, and bleeds with the normal menstrual cycle. The bleeding causes inflammation, triggering a cascade of cellular inflammatory mediators, including cytokines, chemokines, growth factors, and protective factors such as secretory leukocyte protease inhibitor and superoxide dismutase.[100] The inflammation may lead to fibrosis, scarring, adhesions, and pain.

◆**CLINICAL MANIFESTATIONS.** The clinical manifestations of endometriosis can mimic other disease processes (i.e., PID, irritable bowel syndrome, ovarian cysts). Symptoms are variable in frequency and severity and most commonly include pain and infertility. Women with endometriosis report progressive dysmenorrhea, dysuria, dyschezia (pain on defecation), and dyspareunia (pain on intercourse); they may also report constipation and abnormal vaginal bleeding. If implants are located within the pelvis they can cause an asymptomatic pelvic mass having irregular, movable nodules and a fixed, retroverted uterus. Most symptoms of endometriosis can be explained by the proliferation, breakdown, and bleeding of the ectopic endometrial tissue with subsequent formation of adhesions. In most instances, however, the degree of endometriosis is not related to the frequency or severity of symptoms.[97] Dysmenorrhea, for example, does not appear to be related to the degree of endometriosis. With involvement of the rectovaginal septum or the uterosacral ligaments, dyspareunia develops. Dyschezia occurs with bleeding of ectopic endometrium in the rectosigmoid musculature and subsequent fibrosis.

Approximately 25% to 40% of women with infertility have endometriosis. The link between endometriosis and infertility is strong, yet the degree of disease and infertility is not as closely associated. That is, women with untreated minimal to mild disease may have high pregnancy rates or may experience infertility.[100] The exact mechanism for infertility in women with endometriosis is unknown. Infertility may result from mechanical interference with ovulation or ovum transport through the fallopian tube because of adhesions and the effects of inflammation and cytokine activity. However, the infertility also could be a result of the underlying autoimmune disorder that caused the endometriosis.[96] There are conflicting reports regarding the effect of endometriosis on sperm activity. An increased phagocytosis of spermatozoa by macrophages has been observed. The uterine endometrium in women with endometriosis appears to have an overactive response to estrogen and an underactive response to progesterone, impairing the endometrial receptivity to blastocyst implantation, decreasing the chance of successful pregnancy.[104] Women with endometriosis who achieve pregnancy naturally or through in vitro fertilization (IVF) also seem to be at higher risk for poor obstetric outcomes, including preterm birth, small-for-gestational-age babies, and placental complications.[105]

◆**EVALUATION AND TREATMENT.** A presumptive diagnosis can be made based on clinical manifestations, but laparoscopy is required for definitive diagnosis of endometriosis. A uniform classification system that includes both extent and severity has been developed but still does not correlate well with a woman's symptoms. Treatment is aimed at preventing or decreasing progression and spread, alleviating pain, and restoring fertility. Current therapies include suppression of ovulation with continuous estrogen-progestin COCs, danazol (which diminishes the midcycle LH surge), GnRH agonists/analogs in oral or depot formulations (to suppress ovarian hormones), and the antiprogestins gestrinone, mifepristone (RU486), and dienogest (inhibit ovulation and disrupt endometrial integrity); and atrophy of the endometrium with progestins, including medroxyprogesterone acetate (DMPA), oral progestins, the etonogestrel rod, or an LNG-IUD.[106,107] Conservative surgical treatment includes laparoscopic removal of ectopic endometrium with conventional or laser techniques. Effectiveness may be increased when medical regimens are combined with surgical techniques. All treatments have risks or side effects, and recurrent symptoms develop in the majority of women within a few years, even with surgical treatments. Women should be fully informed about all options and carefully weigh the risk-to-benefit ratio of nonreversible treatments.[108]

Cancer

Malignant tumors of the female reproductive system are common. Cancers of the female reproductive tract can often grow large before causing pain because the pelvis and abdomen are poorly innervated and designed to accommodate a growing fetus. Reproductive tract cancers are more likely to be diagnosed early if there are symptoms. Uterine cancer is the third leading cancer diagnosis in women (behind breast and lung cancers) but is only the seventh leading cause of death, in part because symptoms of vaginal bleeding prompt women to seek treatment. Ovarian cancer, on the other hand, occurs less frequently, at 2.6% of new cancer diagnoses in women, but is the sixth leading cause of death from cancer related to its lack of symptoms and lack of clear screening or diagnostic testing.[1] Cervical cancer is also generally asymptomatic until the cancer has progressed, but early detection is possible with routine screening. Two percent of cancers in women begin in the cervix, but the death rate from cervical cancer has declined by half since the advent of screening techniques.[1]

Cervical Cancer

Cancer of the cervix is the leading cancer-related death in most of Africa, Central America, and South-Central Asia; however, it has a lower prevalence in the United States.[1,109] In the United States, rates of cervical cancer incidence and mortality have declined by half since 1975, largely because of the increased prevalence and frequency of cervical cancer screening with the Papanicolaou (Pap) test. In 2016, the American Cancer Society estimated 12,990 new cases of invasive cervical cancer and 4120 cervical cancer deaths.[1]

◆**PATHOPHYSIOLOGY.** It is established that cervical cancer is almost exclusively caused by cervical human papillomavirus (HPV) infection. Infection with "high-risk" (oncogenic) types of HPV is a necessary precursor to development of cervical dysplasia, otherwise known as the *precancerous cell changes that lead to invasive cancer* (also see Chapter 12). Precancerous dysplasia, also called *cervical intraepithelial carcinoma (CIN)* and *cervical carcinoma in situ (CIS),* is a more advanced form of these cell changes. Importantly, cervical dysplasia can be detected noninvasively through examination of the cervical cells. If dysplasia is detected early, treatment is available to prevent invasive cancer.

Most sexually active women will contract HPV at some point in their lifetime; most of these infections are asymptomatic and resolve spontaneously. However, high-risk HPV may persist and cause abnormal cellular changes that can become cancerous[110] (also see Chapter 27). HPV strains 16 and 18 are most often implicated as causing 70% of all cervical cancers and also contribute to many vaginal, vulvar, penile, anal, and oropharyngeal cancers.[111] Most HPV infections are cleared by the immune system; the vast majority of infections do not cause cervical cancer. For this reason, screening for cervical cancer before age 21 is not recommended. Previous efforts at early screening resulted in many young women receiving treatments on their cervix that may have been unnecessary. These treatments destroyed or removed cervical cells and in many cases altered the structural integrity of the cervix, resulting in an increase in preterm births in women treated without substantially decreasing the later rates of cervical cancer.[112]

It is unknown why some women are able to clear HPV infection and others cannot. Women with multiple sexual partners are more likely to be exposed to high-risk HPV, but women with only one lifetime sexual partner also can become infected. Smoking has been shown to increase the risks of persistent infection and later development of cervical cancer; in addition, women who have had many children, have a long history of oral contraceptive use, and are immunocompromised also are at higher risk of cervical cancer.[1] Women who use vaginal douches also seem to be at increased risk of HPV infection, likely caused by the alteration in the cervico-vaginal microbiome;[113] on the contrary, women with healthy vaginal microbiomes, marked by adequate quantities of lactobacilli, seem to have a decreased prevalence and increased clearance of HPV.[114] Anything that affects the integrity of the immune system may affect the later risk of cervical cancer, including tobacco use, poor nutrition, chronic stress, and immunosuppressant medications.[115,116] HIV infection greatly increases the risk that women infected with HPV will develop cervical cancer, and women with HIV should be screened for cervical cancer more frequently than women without HIV.[117] In addition, high-risk HPV is found more frequently in women who are coinfected with chlamydia or gonorrhea, suggesting that those infectious processes may support the persistence of HPV in those women.[118,119] It is hoped that the widespread use of the HPV vaccine in boys and girls will decrease rates of invasive cervical, genital, and anal cancers over the next several decades.[1]

There are two main cell types of the cervix: squamous epithelium cells and columnar epithelial cells. The line where the two cells types meet, known as the transformation zone, is very vulnerable to the oncogenic effects of HPV, and this is where carcinoma in situ is most likely to develop (Fig. 25.18). In this zone, columnar epithelium is constantly being replaced by squamous epithelium in a process known as *metaplasia.* Metaplasia is thought to be affected by hormonal levels; change in cervical epithelium is not understood as well as endometrial tissue change in response to fluctuating hormones. Because metaplastic cells are at increased risk of incorporating foreign or abnormal genetic material, neoplastic changes are most common in the transformation zone.

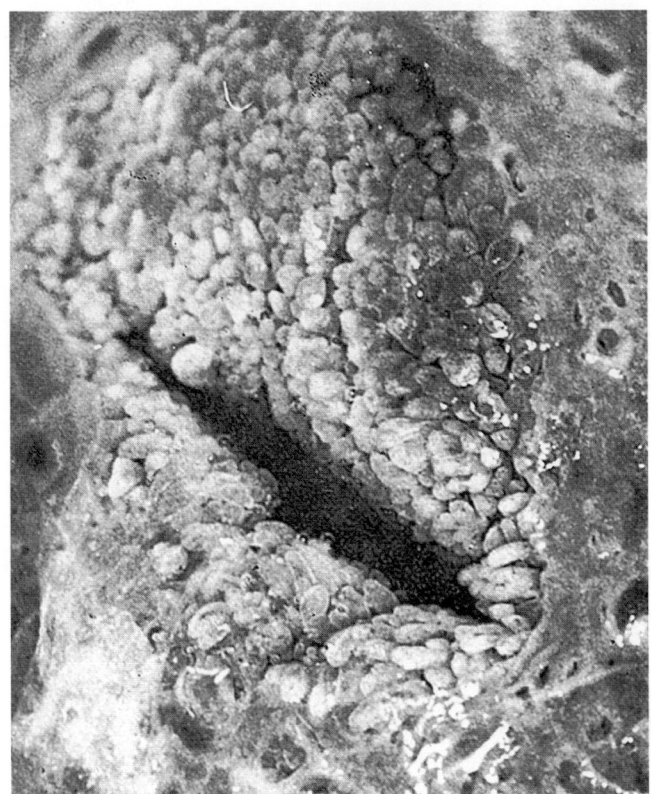

FIGURE 25.18 Cervical Carcinoma in Situ. Typical transformation zone, where the columnar (grapelike) epithelium is replaced by metaplastic epithelium. At its outer edge the metaplastic epithelium adjoins the squamous epithelium, which extends into the vagina. (From Coppleson M, Pixley E, Reid B: *Colposcopy: a scientific approach to the cervix in health and disease,* Springfield, IL, 1971, Charles C Thomas.)

Young women are especially vulnerable to HPV because of their cervical anatomy. Squamous epithelial cells in older women cover the portions of the cervix that protrude into the vagina, and columnar epithelial cells line the inner portions of the cervical canal. The location of the transformation zone changes as girls and women age and in response to estrogen and vaginal pH changes. In girls and young women, a large portion of their cervix is covered with columnar epithelium, a condition known as *squamous metaplasia.*[111] As women age, the transformation zone moves as the squamous epithelium covers the surface of the cervix. Therefore the younger a woman is when she contacts HPV, the more sensitive cervical cells are exposed. This is one reason vaccinations against HPV are aimed at women before the initiation of sexual activity.[111] Many chromosomes may contain genes that relate to HPV-linked cervical cancer.[120] Like other cancers, cervical cancer requires the accumulation of genetic alterations for carcinogenesis to occur. Several genetic mutations have been identified, including some that have not been seen in other cancers.[120] Several chromosome regions with recurrent loss of heterozygosity (LOH) have been identified (also see Chapter 12). In addition, other genes may influence a woman's receptivity to HPV.[121] For instance, HPV may up-regulate the E6 oncoprotein in certain gene sequences, causing a greater production of vascular epidermal growth factor, which allows the tumor to promote blood vessel growth toward the proliferating cells, fueling growth.[120,121] Moreover, mutations in genes regulating the immune response have also been identified as playing a role in the development of cervical cancer.[120]

◆**CLINICAL MANIFESTATIONS.** Cervical neoplasms are predominantly asymptomatic; therefore regular Pap test or HPV screening is necessary

WHAT'S NEW?

Cervical Cancer Screening in the Developing World

The problem with the use of the conventional Papanicolaou (Pap) test in screening for cervical cancer is the low sensitivity of the test, which ranges between 44% and 77%. This means that a large number of cervical abnormalities (23% to 56%) can be missed with a single test! Thus the success of Pap test screening in reducing cervical cancer in the United States lies in the frequency of screenings and that cervical cancer is a slowly progressive condition. However, a high frequency of Pap test screenings is often not feasible, either economically, socially, culturally, or logistically, in many countries and in some regions leads to much higher rates of invasive cervical cancer for women in such populations or locales. Multiple, large, well-conducted studies have demonstrated that human papillomavirus (HPV) testing is considerably more sensitive (between 97% and 98%) than either conventional or liquid-based Pap testing. HPV infection is known to be the required precursor to cervical cancer. With sensitive HPV tests now widely available, requiring less frequent screening (every 3 to 5 years), the future of cervical cancer screening may rely on HPV screening, not on conventional cervical cytology testing.

In settings where there is not even adequate infrastructure for HPV testing, several studies have shown that simple visualization with acetic acid (VIA) can be used to diagnosis women with HPV infection and then immediately provide onsite cryotherapy to reduce rates of later cervical cancer. Although not ideal, this approach shows promise in low-resources settings, especially when the baseline rate of HIV infection is high, because it allows women to be screened and treated on the same visit.

Data from Campos NG et al: *Int J Cancer* 2015 137(9):2208–2219, 2015.

TABLE 25.3   CERVICAL EPITHELIAL CELL ABNORMALITIES (PRECANCEROUS CERVICAL NEOPLASIAS)

CYTOLOGY REPORT	TYPE OF INTRAEPITHELIAL LESION
Atypical squamous cells of undetermined significance (ASC-US)	Suggestive of but do not meet criteria for LSIL (mild dysplasia)
Atypical squamous cells— cannot exclude HSIL (ASC-H)	Do not meet criteria for HSIL but do not preclude HSIL (potentially CIN I/II; moderate to severe dysplasia)
LSIL	CIN 1 (mild dysplasia)
HSIL	CIN 2 and 3 (moderate to severe dysplasia and CIS)

CIN, Cervical intraepithelial neoplasia; *CIS,* carcinoma in situ; *HSIL,* high-grade squamous intraepithelial lesion; *LSIL,* low-grade squamous intraepithelial lesion.

then sent to a laboratory for analysis. When dysplasia is detected, further testing is indicated for diagnosis. Colposcopy involves examining the cervix visually and taking needed biopsies. An acetic acid (vinegar) solution is applied to the cervix, making areas of HPV infection stand out in a white color, known as *aceto-white*. The cervix is then viewed under magnification for aceto-white areas, changes in the epithelium, and the presence of abnormal vascular patterns.[123] Abnormal areas of the cervix are biopsied. Because the vulnerable transformation zones move into the cervical canal as a woman ages, the endocervix is sampled using curettage for diagnosis (Table 25.3).

The progressive neoplastic changes of cervical cells are classified on a continuum from cervical intraepithelial neoplasia (dysplasia), to cervical carcinoma in situ (full epithelial thickness of the cervix is involved), to invasive carcinoma (see Tables 25.3 and 25.4). Various terms are used to describe the cellular changes in the cervix based on how the cells were obtained. Screening for cervical cancer is done with a Pap test, and the cytology report describes test findings; these terms are outlined on the left side of Table 25.3. If a Pap test has abnormal findings, a biopsy of the affected tissue is taken during a colposcopy. The biopsy reveals the actual extent of the lesion within the cervix. Terminology used in pathology reports is listed on the right side of Table 25.3. Pathology reports that involve cancerous changes begin with the abbreviation *CIN* or *CIS*; cervical intraepithelial neoplasia and carcinoma in situ, respectively.

Cervical dysplasia is replacement of some epithelial cells by atypical neoplastic cells, and is "staged" depending on the depth of epithelial involvement (Fig. 25.19). Risk of progression to invasive carcinoma rises steadily with the severity of dysplasia; however, women with intact immune systems are likely to resolve dysplasia on their own. At least a third or more of all cervical intraepithelial lesions persist without progression or regression. Women with CIN 1 (low-grade squamous intraepithelial lesion [LSIL] or mild dysplasia) have an 11% chance of progression to CIS and a 1% chance of progression to cervical invasion. Women with CIN 2 have a 22% chance of progression to CIS and a 5% chance of invasive lesions. In cervical CIN 3 or HSIL (high-grade squamous intraepithelial lesion), all or most of the cervical epithelium shows cellular features of carcinoma; however, underlying tissue is not affected. At least 12% of women with CIN 3 (CIS) progress to cervical invasion.

for early detection (see Chapter 27 for screening frequency guidelines). About 90% of cervical cancer cases can be detected through early use of regular screening tests (see *What's New? Cervical Cancer Screening in the Developing World*). If symptoms exist, they may include vaginal bleeding or abnormal discharge. Bleeding is variable and may occur after intercourse or between menstrual periods. Vaginal discharge is a less common presenting symptom and may be serosanguineous or yellowish with a foul odor. Bleeding and discharge are subtle and are likely to be disregarded by premenopausal women. Postmenopausal women are more likely to seek medical attention if these signs appear. Advanced disease may cause urinary or rectal symptoms and pelvic or back pain along with anemia.

EVALUATION AND TREATMENT. Women should be screened for cervical cancer and risk for future cervical cancer through Pap and HPV testing.[122] For women aged 30 to 65 years, HPV testing is now recommended at the same time as the Pap test because it is noninvasive and identifies women at later risk for cellular abnormalities leading to cancer; indeed, HPV is often detectable for more than a decade before any noticed cellular changes. For women aged 21 to 29, HPV testing is only indicated if the Pap test is abnormal, which is known as *reflex HPV testing*.[122] Recent studies suggest that HPV testing alone may be as effective but less expensive than co-testing or reflex testing. The WHO recommends HPV testing in settings where HPV tests are available but Pap tests are not.

A Pap test involves the noninvasive collection of cellular samples from the surface of the cervix during a pelvic examination, using a speculum to allow for visualization of the cervix. Cervical cytologic examination is most accurate if cells are obtained from both the endocervix and the ectocervix, which involves placing the collection device (a small brush or broom) into the cervical os. These cells are

TABLE 25.4	CLINICAL STAGING FOR CANCER OF THE CERVIX
STAGE	**CHARACTERISTICS**
0	Cancer in situ, intraepithelial carcinoma; earliest stage of cancer; cancer confined to its original site
I	Carcinoma confined to cervix (extension to corpus disregarded)
IA	Earliest form of stage I; there is very small amount of cancer, which is visible only under a microscope
IA1	Area of invasion is <3 mm (about $\frac{1}{8}$ inch) deep and <7 mm (about $\frac{1}{3}$ inch) wide
IA2	Area of invasion is between 3 and 5 mm (about $\frac{1}{5}$ inch) deep, and <7 mm (about $\frac{1}{3}$ inch) wide
IB	Includes cancers that can be seen without a microscope; also includes cancers seen only with a microscope that have spread deeper than 5 mm (about $\frac{1}{5}$ inch) into connective tissue of the cervix or are wider than 7 mm
IB1	IB cancer that is no larger than 4 cm (about $1\frac{1}{3}$ inches)
IB2	IB cancer that is >4 cm
II	Cancer has spread beyond the cervix to the upper part of the vagina; cancer does not involve the lower third of the vagina
IIA	Cancer has spread beyond the cervix to the upper part of the vagina; cancer does not involve the lower third of the vagina
IIB	Cancer has spread to the tissue next to the cervix, called the *parametrial tissue*
III	Cancer has spread to the lower part of the vagina or the pelvic wall; cancer may be blocking the ureters (tubes that carry urine from the kidneys to the bladder)
IIIA	Cancer has spread to the lower third of the vagina but not to the pelvic wall
IIIB	Cancer extends to the pelvic wall, blocks urine flow to the bladder, or both
IV	Most advanced stage of cervical cancer; cancer has spread to other parts of the body
IVA	Cancer has spread to the bladder or rectum, which are organs close to the cervix
IVB	Cancer has spread to distant organs beyond the pelvic area, such as the lungs

Reprinted from the American Cancer Society's Cancer Information Database with permission.

CIS is generally a precursor of invasive carcinoma of the cervix. A number of factors, including tumor type, contribute to the rate at which CIS becomes invasive. Because of the ease of Pap test screening, invasive cervical cancer is rare within the United States but much more common in the developing world, where screening is not available. **Invasive carcinoma of the cervix** consists of cancer invasion into adjacent tissues and metastasis. Adjacent tissues most often involved are the ureters and structures of the lateral pelvic wall, the vaginal stroma and epithelium, and the lower uterine segment and myometrium. The internal, external, and common iliac lymph nodes and the obturator nodes are common sites of lymphatic involvement. Invasive cervical cancer is most often discovered through Pap tests, tentatively diagnosed with a biopsy during a colposcopy, and then further diagnosed using surgery and lymphangiography, CT scan, MRI, ultrasonography, or radioimmunodetection methods. The staging system for carcinoma of the cervix is shown in Table 25.4.

Treatment depends on the degree of neoplastic change, the size and location of the lesion, and the extent of metastatic spread. For premalignant cellular changes and CIS, the goal is to kill or remove abnormal cells; these procedures can be done in a clinic with the administration of a local anesthetic. Invasive carcinoma requires surgery, including removal of the cervix and other affected tissues.

Common treatments can be classified as ablative, when the cells are killed without being removed, or excisional, in which the abnormal cells are physically removed from the cervix. Ablative therapies are appropriate for lower levels of cervical dysplasia because they leave the cervix intact, which may be beneficial for later childbearing. However, they do not provide a tissue sample for testing. Ablative surgeries include cryotherapy and cold coagulation in which extreme cold is applied to the surface of the cervix. Carbon dioxide laser and electrocoagulation also are used to kill abnormal cells and coagulate vessels supporting their growth. Excisional therapies are appropriate if a more advanced lesion is suspected because they produce tissue for analysis. Excisional therapies include conization, in which a cone-shaped portion of the cervix is removed, and the loop electrosurgical excision procedure (LEEP), in which a small looped wire with electric current generates heat and destroys cancer cells. Heat, cold, or lasers are used in excisional procedures to simultaneously excise the tissue and obliterate abnormal blood vessels.

For invasive cervical carcinoma, treatment depends on the stage of the tumor. Surgical intervention may include a hysterectomy, pelvic lymphadenectomy, or pelvic exenteration (radical removal of the contents of the body cavity). Multidrug chemotherapy regimens also have been used alone or in combination with radiation, and emerging treatments targeting specific cancer genes show promise.[124] Smokers tend to have a higher stage of disease at diagnosis, and their cancer is more resistant to radiation treatment.

With early detection and treatment, prognosis is excellent. Overall, the 5-year survival rate is 92% for stage IA or lower (e.g., early detection). For women diagnosed with cervical carcinoma, the 5-year survival rate is 68%.[1] The prevention of HPV infection may be the key to substantially reducing the risk of cervical cancer. There are currently three licensed HPV vaccines available in the United States: one that protects against two strains of HPV (16 and 18), four strains of HPV (6, 11, 16, and 18), and nine strains of HPV (6, 11, 16, 18, 31, 33, 45, 52, and 58).[110] It is recommended that all young men and women be vaccinated[125] (Table 25.5). More recent studies indicate that 63% of girls have received at least one dose of the vaccine[110] and 42% are fully vaccinated; and that rates of HPV infection in young women have been cut in half.[126] As vaccine uptake increases and longitudinal studies persist, further reductions are likely to be seen in cervical cancer–related mortality and morbidity over the next 20 years.

Vaginal Cancer

Cancer of the vagina is the rarest of the female genital cancers and accounts for less than 2% of gynecologic cancers.[127] In 2016, there were an estimated 4620 diagnoses of vaginal cancer, and 950 deaths.[127] Vaginal and cervical cancers are thought to have similar epidemiology. Both start as intraepithelial lesions, occur in women who have been sexually active, and are associated with HPV infection. Prior carcinoma of the cervix or uterus places a woman at higher risk for developing vaginal cancer.[128] In utero exposure to nonsteroidal estrogens is a risk factor: It has been estimated that 100,000 to 160,000 women were exposed in utero to such nonsteroidal estrogens as DES, dienestrol, or hexestrol from 1960 to 1971.[129] Exposure to such hormones during the first 3 months of gestation inhibits the normal replacement of columnar epithelium by squamous epithelium in the vagina of the fetus. The columnar epithelium, which is not normally found in the

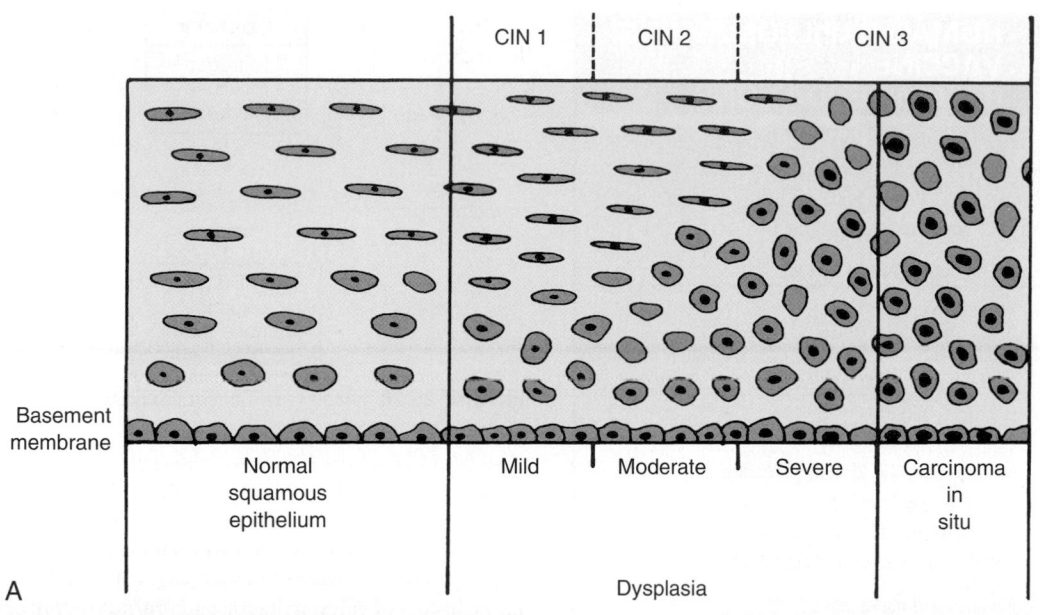

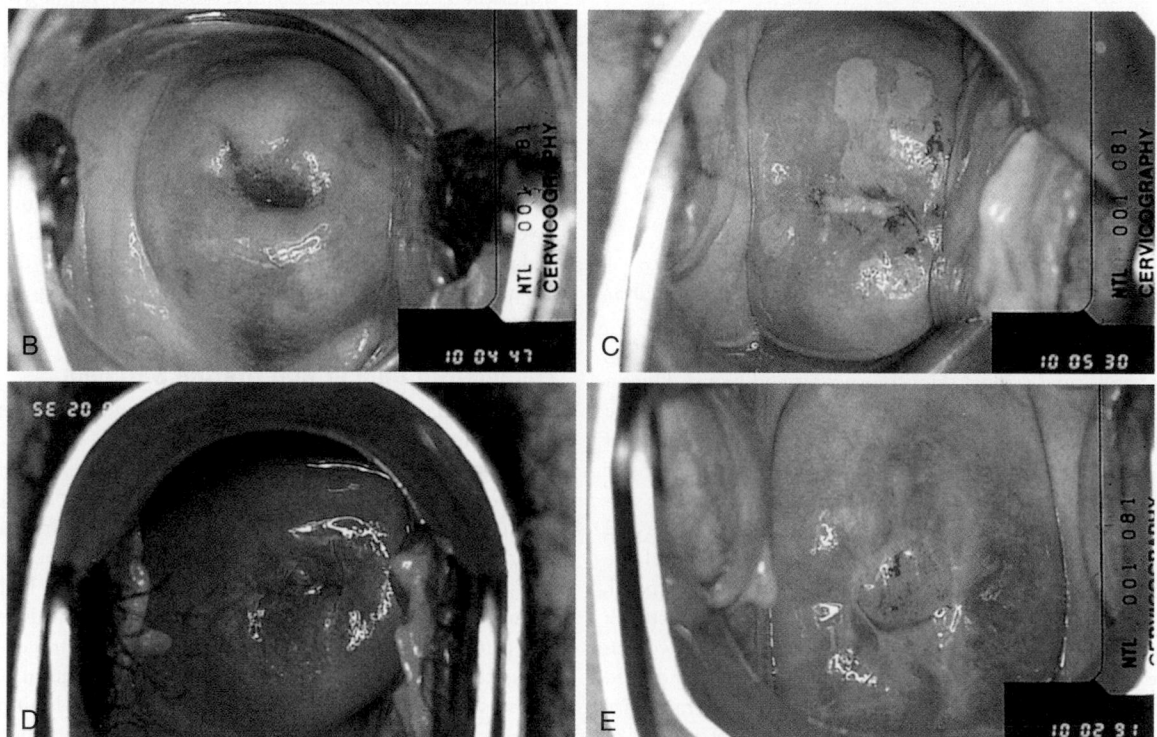

FIGURE 25.19 Cervical Intraepithelial Neoplasia (CIN). **A,** Diagram of cervical endothelium showing progressive degrees of CIN. **B,** Normal multiparous cervix. **C,** CIN stage 1. Note the white appearance of part of the anterior lip of the cervix associated with neoplastic changes. **D,** CIN stage 2. Lesions reflected in distant capillaries. **E,** CIN stage 3. Lesion predominantly around the external os. (**A** From Herbst AL et al: *Comprehensive gynecology,* ed 2, St Louis, 1992, Mosby. **B–E** From Symonds EM, Macpherson MBA: *Color atlas of obstetrics and gynecology,* London, 1994, Mosby-Wolfe.)

vagina, may then undergo malignant transformation. Not all women exposed to DES in utero develop neoplastic changes in the vagina, however.[129]

Vaginal cancer is usually diagnosed in women in their 60s and 70s, but the cellular changes begin many years before the appearance of clinically apparent disease.[127] The most common type of vaginal cancer is squamous cell carcinoma. About 90% of tumors are squamous cell–type

cancers; the remaining 10% are adenocarcinomas, sarcomas (rare), and melanomas (rare). Nonsquamous types of cancer are more common in younger women. Vaginal sarcomas can develop in children younger than 5 years, and adenocarcinomas are the most common in women less than 30 years old.[127]

Vaginal cancer is generally asymptomatic until fairly late in the disease process. The major symptom of invasive cancer is vaginal bleeding or

TABLE 25.5	HUMAN PAPILLOMAVIRUS VACCINE RECOMMENDATIONS

Eligible individuals: 11- or 12-year old girls and boys; females aged 13–26 who have not already been vaccinated; males aged 13–21 who have not been vaccinated; males aged 21–26 who have not been vaccinated and are immunocompromised or who have sex with men.

VACCINE TYPE	RECOMMENDED FOR
Cervarix	Females ages 11–12
(HPV #16, 18)	Females ages 13–26 who have not been previously vaccinated
Gardasil	Females and males ages 11–12
(HPV #6, 11, 16, 18)	Females ages 13–26 and males ages 13–21 who have not been previously vaccinated Unvaccinated males ages 22–26 who have sex with men or who are immunocompromised
Gardasil 9	Females and males ages 11–12
(HPV #6, 11, 16, 18, 31, 33, 45, 52, 58)	Females ages 13–26 and males ages 13–21 who have not been previously vaccinated Unvaccinated males ages 22–26 who have sex with men or who are immunocompromised

Data adapted from Centers for Disease Control and Prevention: *HPV vaccine information for clinicians.* Available at https://www.cdc.gov/hpv/hcp/need-to-know.pdf.

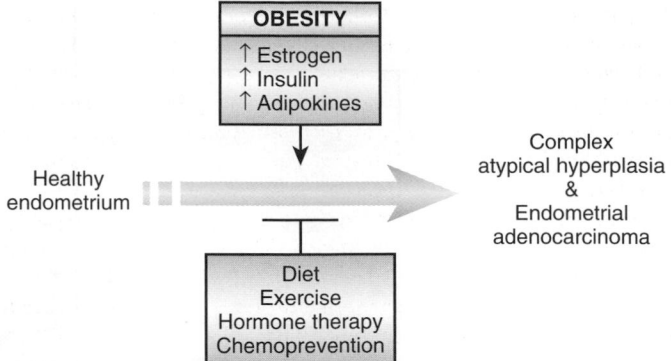

FIGURE 25.20 Endometrial Cancer. Overview of the contribution of obesity to endometrial cancer progression and preventive strategies. (From Schmandt RE et al: *Am J Obstet Gynecol* 205[6]:518–525, 2011.)

bloody discharge. Other symptoms can include vaginal discharge, vulvar pruritus, rectal or bladder symptoms, pain, or leg edema.

Several mechanisms can be used to diagnose vaginal cancer including Pap testing of abnormal vaginal skin, colposcopy, and biopsy. Once a diagnosis of cancer is established, the size and extent of the lesion are determined using MRI, before surgery.[130] Like cervical neoplasms, vaginal cancers are classified as intraepithelial neoplasia (dysplasia), CIS, or invasive carcinoma and are staged based on extension into local tissues and metastasis to distant organs. Treatment depends on the type and extent of the cancer and the overall health and expectations of the woman.[130] Potential treatment modalities include laser therapy or removal, or both, of the affected tissues (vagina, uterus, bladder, and rectum); excision of lymph nodes; radiation; and chemotherapy. Many women with invasive vaginal cancer develop recurrent pelvic cancer and need intensive monitoring for recurrence. Recurrence and survival rates vary greatly by the type and extent of cancer and the aggressiveness of the treatment regimen.[130] HPV vaccination is the primary form of prevention.[128]

Vulvar Cancer

Cancer of the vulva is responsible for about 3% to 5% of all gynecologic cancers; however, there has been a steady increase in the incidence of vulvar cancers over the last 30 years. There were an estimated 5950 new diagnoses and 1110 deaths in 2016. The majority (90%) are squamous cell carcinomas, although melanoma (5%), Bartholin gland carcinoma (2%), sarcoma (2%), and adenosquamous carcinoma (1%) may occur. A history of HPV infection related to 20% to 80% of vulvar cancers, depending on type; interestingly, HPV-related lesions have a better prognosis than those that are not positive for HPV.[131] Previous squamous dysplasia of the vagina or cervix also is a major risk factor, as are smoking and HIV infections.[132] Although it usually affects postmenopausal women

(median age of presentation is women in their 60s), vulvar cancer has been diagnosed in women between ages 30 and 90.[132] Usually women have a history of vulvar irritation and pruritus (70%); urinary symptoms and discharge are less common. In addition, there may be a hard ulcerated area of the vulva, large cauliflower lesions, or lesions similar to those of chronic dermatitis. Biopsy confirms the diagnosis. Treatment options include primarily ablative or excisional surgery, and sometimes radiation with or without chemotherapy. Less extensive removal of vulvar tissue is being studied to decrease postsurgical morbidity and maintain function.[133] Prognosis depends on lesion size and location, histology, and lymph involvement; risk of metastasis increases with tumor size. The 5-year survival rate depends on the extent of the lesion, the treatment, and the overall health of the woman. Cancer caught in the early stages has a greater than 90% 5-year survival rate with progressively poorer prognosis with advancing stages.[133,134]

Endometrial Cancer and Uterine Sarcoma

Endometrial carcinomas arise within the glandular epithelium of the uterine lining. Estimates include 60,050 new cases in 2016, with approximately 10,470 deaths.[1] Most cases occur in postmenopausal women (Fig. 25.20), with peak incidence occurring in the late 50s to early 60s.[135] Women have a 3% lifetime risk of developing uterine cancer. Although incidence rates are higher in white than in black women, mortality rates in black women are nearly twice as high, primarily because cancers are more likely to be diagnosed in advanced stages.[1] The primary risk factor is prolonged exposure to estrogen without the presence of progesterone. Estrogen causes endometrial proliferation, whereas progesterone changes the uterine lining to limit proliferation and encourage normal shedding. Estrogen without the presence of progesterone is known as *unopposed estrogen* because its proliferating effects are not restrained. Exposure to unopposed estrogen includes estrogen-only hormone replacement therapy, tamoxifen use, early menarche, late menopause, never having children, and a failure to ovulate (i.e., PCOS and anovulatory cycles typical of the late reproductive years). Obesity also is a known source of endogenous estrogen and is a risk factor for endometrial cancer (see Fig. 25.20).[136] Other risk factors not directly related to estrogen include diabetes, gallbladder disease, and hypertension, though obesity may be a mediating factor for these risks. A family history of colon, endometrial, or ovarian cancer could signal hereditary nonpolyposis colorectal cancer (HNPCC); women with this family history may wish to explore genetic testing and more aggressive screening.[137]

Although estrogen and obesity increase the risk of endometrial cancer, several interventions have been shown to decrease the risk of cancer.

A review of modifiable risk factors and prevention for endometrial hyperplasia and cancer indicates that controlling obesity, hypertension, and diabetes may reduce an individual's risk of endometrial cancer.[138,139] Exposure to progesterone also decreases the risk of endometrial cancer both immediately and long term. Large amounts of progesterone are released during pregnancy. Smaller, but still effective, amounts of progesterone are in OCPs and the progestin-containing IUD. The use of birth control pills can decrease the risk of endometrial cancer by 80%, even more than a decade after use.[135] The progestin-containing IUD is used to prevent endometrial abnormalities in women who need to take tamoxifen as part of breast cancer prevention[140] and has shown promise in protecting the endometria of obese women[141] with an estimated 50% reduction in endometrial cancer incidence among obese women using a LNG-IUD.

About 75% of endometrial cancers are adenocarcinomas. Abnormal vaginal bleeding caused by disruption of the endometrial surface by neoplastic processes is the most common clinical manifestation of endometrial cancer. Pain and weight loss are symptoms of late disease.

Screening methods for early detection of endometrial cancer are as effective as those for cervical cancer. Pap tests, highly effective in detecting cervical dysplasia, are ineffective in detecting early endometrial cancer. Transvaginal ultrasound (TVUS) may be used to measure endometrial thickness and screen postmenopausal and high-risk premenopausal women. If the endometrium is abnormally thick (defined as >5 mm), then further testing, such as endometrial biopsy, is warranted to rule out cancer, especially in high-risk women.[142] Endometrial biopsies can be performed in a normal clinic with minimal additional equipment. The biopsy involves placement of a small thin tube through the cervix to collect a specimen of the endometrium for analysis.[142] Once cancer is confirmed by biopsy, a laparoscopy and MRI may be performed to determine stage of disease.

Uterine cancers can be divided into two types by histology. Type I tumors are by far the most common and result from estrogen exposure leading to endometrial hyperplasia. Type II cancers make up 10% of endometrial cancers but are more likely to be invasive into the uterine muscle and metastasize beyond their original location, resulting in a much greater risk for death.[142] Treatment is based on the cancer type and the extent of the disease. For women with simple hyperplasia, progestin therapy (orally or through LNG-IUD) may often suffice. However, treatment for atypical hyperplasia or invasive disease usually includes surgical intervention, such as curettage for carcinoma in situ, total abdominal hysterectomy with bilateral salpingo-oophorectomy, and lymphadenectomy.[143] Chemotherapy and radiation also may be used. The 5-year relative survival rate is 82%. There are health disparities in survival rates; the 5-year survival rate for white women is 84% compared to 62% in black women, partly because white women are likely to be diagnosed at earlier stages of the disease.[1]

Uterine sarcomas are rare neoplasms that arise from mesenchymal tissues of and near the uterus, including myometrial smooth muscle, endometrial stroma, or adjacent connective tissues. Uterine sarcomas are rare, constituting up to 3% of all genital tract cancers and 3% to 5% of all uterine malignancies. The average age at diagnosis is the early 50s, though some sarcomas can form in childhood. Uterine sarcomas can be divided into endometrial stromal sarcoma, leiomyosarcoma, and adenosarcoma based on the involved tissue types. The very low occurrence and diversity of cellular composition of these tumors explain the lack of epidemiologic and treatment data.[144] Thus relatively few risk factors have been identified. However, prior pelvic radiation therapy, chronic excess estrogen exposure, use of tamoxifen, and black race have been cited as risks. Symptoms include abnormal uterine bleeding, awareness of a mass, and pelvic pressure or pain. Vaginal discharge may be profuse and foul. Gastrointestinal and genitourinary complaints are common. Treatment consists of total hysterectomy, which may include bilateral salpingo-oophorectomy and selective lymphadenectomy followed by radiation therapy or chemotherapy, or both. Molecularly targeted therapies are also under investigation.[145,146] Five-year survival rates range from 50% in early disease to 5% in advanced disease. Like most cancers, stage and histopathologic analyses are the most important determinants of prognosis. The survival rate at 5 years for stage I disease is 50%. Few women survive advanced-stage disease.[145]

Ovarian Cancer

The incidence of ovarian cancer is estimated at 22,280 women in the United States in 2016. In 2013 ovarian cancer accounted for 3% of all cancers among women and 21% of gynecologic cancers; it caused more deaths (14,240) than any other female reproductive cancer. From 2003 to 2012, the incidence declined at a rate of 0.9% per year.[1] Ovarian cancer in women older than 40 years is associated with conditions associated with increased ovulation over the lifetime, such as early menarche, late menopause, and nulliparity.[147-149] A history of endometriosis also increases risk.[150] There is a genetic component to ovarian cancer and women with a *BRCA1* or *BRCA2* mutation have a 40% to 60% lifetime risk of ovarian cancer. Women who have this gene tend to be diagnosed approximately 10 years before women without the genetic predisposition.[147] Factors that suppress ovulation decrease the risk of ovarian cancer and include pregnancies, prolonged lactation, and the use of hormonal contraceptives that limit ovulation, including the birth control pill.[149] Tubal ligation and hysterectomy, and specifically the prevention of retrograde menses around the ovary, also have been shown to decrease risk.[151]

◆**PATHOPHYSIOLOGY.** There is controversy about the pathogenesis of ovarian cancer. The great majority of ovarian cancers are sporadic and not associated with a known pattern of inheritance.[152] Of the approximately 20% of cancers that are familial, the majority are associated with the breast cancer susceptibility gene 1 *(BRCA1)* and a smaller number with mutations of *BRCA2* or mismatched repair genes (HNPCC syndrome). Various pathways have been proposed. Women and families who are more susceptible to cancer may have errors in the ability to repair cellular DNA, related to abnormalities in several genes responsible for repair of damaged DNA.[153] In sporadic ovarian cancer, *BRCA1* and *BRCA2* are rarely mutated. A newer theory proposes that many spontaneous, nonhereditary ovarian tumors arise from the migration of cells from tissues of mesoderm origin to the surface of the ovary.[147,154] Cells from a variety of intraabdominal locations, including endometrial tissue and epithelium of the fallopian/uterine tubes, can attach to the ovary (Fig. 25.21). The local ovarian environment, including the ovarian stroma, may then interact with the transplanted cells to enhance cellular growth and encourage metastasis[147,154] (Fig. 25.22).

The two major types of ovarian cancer are epithelial ovarian neoplasms and germ-cell neoplasms. Most ovarian malignancies are epithelial ovarian neoplasms that usually develop from the surface epithelium of the ovary or the epithelium that lines cysts immediately beneath the ovarian surface, or may be cells that have migrated from precursor lesions in the fallopian/uterine tubes.[147,154] Most epithelial cancers seem to arise from a single cell (i.e., clonal) because of a loss of tumor-suppressor genes and activation of oncogenes (see Chapter 12). Epithelial ovarian tumors may have cellular similarities to other tissues within the abdomen, including the lining of the fallopian/uterine tubes, or the endometrium, or be undifferentiated. Tumors are often classified as type I (low grade) and type II (high grade) based on their cellular type. Type I tumors grow more slowly and are genetically stable. Type II tumors often grow rapidly and aggressively and often have genetic mutations; type II tumors have a poorer prognosis[155] (Fig. 25.23). The 5-year survival rate is 92% if treated in stage I; however, only 15% of

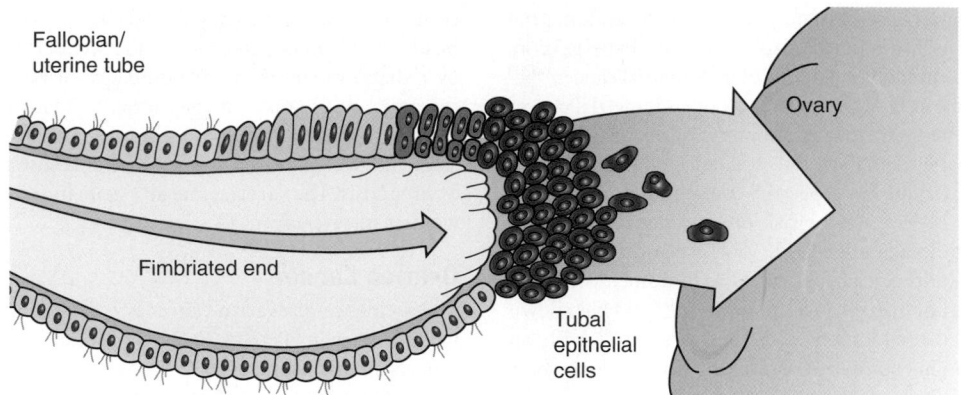

FIGURE 25.21 Migration of Epithelial Cells from the Fallopian/Uterine Tubes to the Ovary. (Adapted from Kurman RJ, Shih IM: *Am J Surg Pathol* 34[3]:433, 2010.)

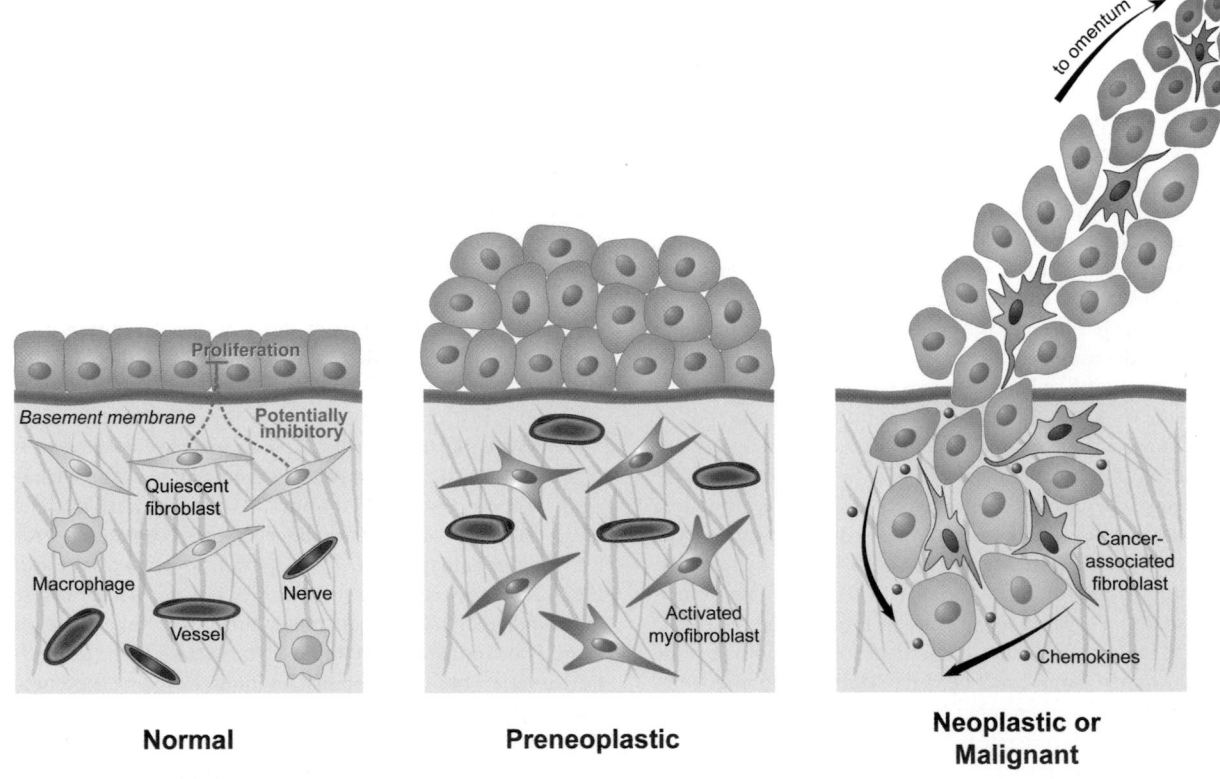

FIGURE 25.22 Ovarian Stroma. The ovarian stroma interacts with precancerous and cancerous cells within the ovary. (From Schauer IG et al: *Neoplasia* 13[5]:393, 2011.)

ovarian cancers are diagnosed this early. The 5-year survival rate varies by age at diagnosis, with women younger than 65 having a 58% rate compared to 28% survival in women older than 65.[1]

Germ-cell tumors are derived from the primitive germ cells (gametes) of the embryonic gonad and may be malignant or benign. The benign cystic teratoma accounts for approximately 10% of all ovarian tumors. These tumors represent an error in meiosis that results in the formation of ectoderm, endoderm, and mesoderm cell lines. Hair, teeth, and skin can be visualized within cystic teratomas. If the germ-cell tumor is malignant, it tends to be highly aggressive and rapidly growing with a poor prognosis. Cystic hygromas and other germ-cell tumors can occur on the ovaries of girls and women. Germ-cell tumors in children can be particularly aggressive.

CLINICAL MANIFESTATIONS. Ovarian cancer is commonly asymptomatic until the tumors have grown very large. Given the location of the ovaries, assessing abnormalities on routine gynecologic examination poses difficulty, especially in obese women. There is no sensitive and specific test for ovarian cancer for screening low-risk women, and routine screening of women without risk factors has not been shown to be beneficial and may cause harm because more women have unnecessary surgical procedures.[148]

Common first symptoms of ovarian cancer are vague and include persistent abdominal distention, loss of appetite due to early satiety, and pelvic pain. Screening is warranted if women have a new onset of these symptoms that persist for more than 12 days each month. However, many women fail to notice the very first signs of ovarian cancer because

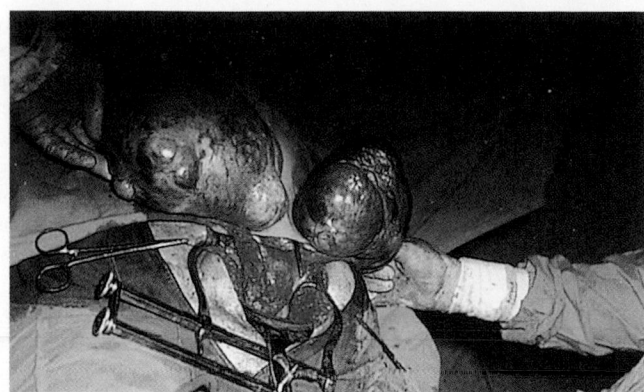

FIGURE 25.23 Ovarian Tumors. Bilateral multicystic ovarian tumors. (From Symonds EM, Macpherson MBA: *Color atlas of obstetrics and gynecology,* London, 1994, Mosby-Wolfe.)

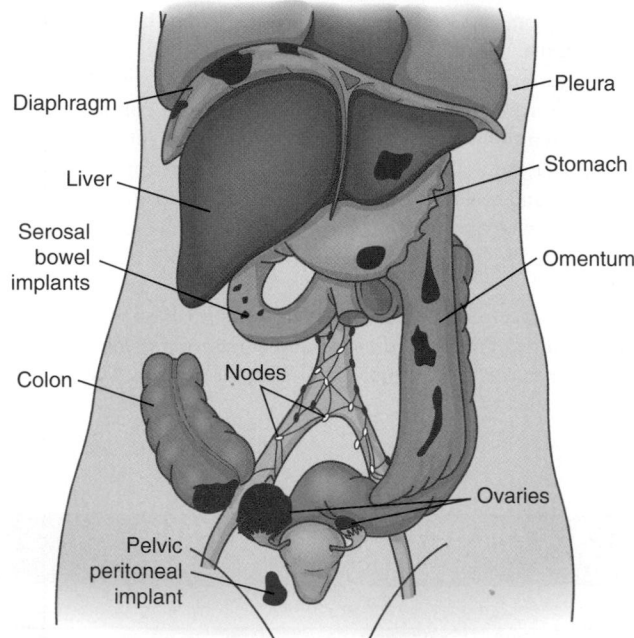

Labels: Diaphragm, Liver, Serosal bowel implants, Colon, Pelvic peritoneal implant, Nodes, Pleura, Stomach, Omentum, Ovaries

FIGURE 25.24 Large Malignant Ovarian Tumor and Metastasis of Ovarian Cancer. Pattern of spread for epithelial cancer of the ovary.

STAGE	CHARACTERISTICS
I	Growth limited to the ovaries
IA	Growth limited to one ovary
IB	Growth limited to both ovaries; no ascites
IC	Tumor either stage IA or stage IB, with ruptured capsule, ascites present, or with positive peritoneal washings
II	Growth involving one or both ovaries with pelvic extension
IIA	Extension and/or metastases to the uterus and/or tubes
IIB	Extension to other pelvic tissues
IIC	Tumor either stage IIA or stage IIB but with ruptured capsule, with ascites present, or with positive peritoneal washings
III	Growth involving one or both ovaries, with metastasis into the abdomen, and/or to the lymph nodes
IIIA	Microscopic involvement of abdominal peritoneal surfaces
IIIB	Disease up to 2-cm diameter
IIIC	Disease greater than 2-cm diameter, with or without regional lymph nodes
IV	Distant metastasis excluding peritoneal metastases
IVA	Pleural effusion with positive cytology; parenchymal metastases and metastases to extraabdominal organs

TABLE 25.6 **FIGO STAGING OF CARCINOMA OF THE OVARY**

FIGO, International Federation of Gynecologists and Obstetricians. Data from Prat J: *Int J Gynaecol Obstet* 124(1):1–5, 2014.

they are vague and fairly common in older women. The disease is most commonly diagnosed after metastasis has occurred. Consequently, ovarian cancer is often termed the *silent killer.* Symptoms of advanced disease include pain and abdominal swelling from the primary ovarian mass or ascites and abdominal distention (Fig. 25.24). Gastrointestinal manifestations may include dyspepsia, vomiting, and alterations in bowel habits caused by mechanical obstruction. Abnormal vaginal bleeding may occur if the postmenopausal endometrium is stimulated by a hormone-secreting tumor. The tumor also may cause ulcerations through the vaginal wall that result in bleeding. There also can be a feeling of pressure in the pelvis and leg pain.

Tumor obstruction of vascular channels can cause venous and, occasionally, arterial thrombosis. Alterations in coagulability also occur, contributing to clot formation. Metastasis often causes pleural effusion.

EVALUATION AND TREATMENT. Because ovarian cancer has no early symptoms and there is no cost-effective screening technique for

early detection, disease usually is advanced by the time treatment is sought. Screening procedures including gynecologic assessment, vaginal ultrasound, and CA-125 assay have low predictive value in women without special risk factors.[156] Women with symptoms of disease, as outlined earlier, should be assessed with minimally-invasive tests first. Screening commonly begins with a CA-125 blood test looking for specific cancer markers and a transvaginal ultrasound.[147] Increased CA-125 levels are found in about 78% to 80% of nonmucinous ovarian cancers; however, elevated levels are produced in 29% of nongynecologic tumors and in a variety of noncancerous conditions, for example, endometriosis, PID, benign ovarian cysts, myomas, and pregnancy.

Women less than 40 years of age are more likely to have nonepithelial cell tumors and should be assessed with blood tests to look for the CA-125 marker α-fetoprotein (AFP), and for β-human chorionic growth hormone to screen for tumors of nonepithelial cell origin.[157] Some types of germ cells and, rarely, adenocarcinoma may be associated with increased levels of AFP, hCG, or CA-125.

If initial tests are suspicious for a cancerous mass, diagnosis is confirmed by biopsy and extent of the disease is determined by ultrasound, CT, MRI, or other imaging techniques. Women undergoing surgery for ovarian cancer staging receive a thorough assessment for metastasis. The International Federation of Gynecologists and Obstetricians (FIGO) staging system is described in Table 25.6. Other studies may be used to determine the extent of metastasis. These include an upper gastrointestinal series, barium enema, intravenous pyelogram (IVP), mammography, and lymphography.

The initial approach to treatment is surgery, which is performed to determine the stage of disease and to remove as much of the tumor as possible. Future treatment is then customized based on the clinical stage of the cancer, the woman's desires, and the cell type and sensitivity of the cancer cells. Ideally, treatment plans are developed and implemented by a multidisciplinary team from a variety of disciplines including surgeons, pathologists, and oncologists.[157]

Radiation therapy and chemotherapy with an agent containing platinum are common treatments.[147] Even after initially effective treatment, 55% to 75% of women relapse, and less than 20% survive long-term with stage III or IV disease. New therapies under investigation include small-molecular-weight inhibitors, monoclonal antibodies, epidermal growth factor receptors, and gene therapy.[147] Survivors of ovarian cancer should be monitored with serial CA-125 testing. Prophylactic removal of the ovaries and fallopian tubes is associated with increased survival rates among those carrying a *BRCA* mutation, and is considered for those women who do not desire fertility.[158]

Sexual Dysfunction

Sexual dysfunction is the lack of satisfaction with sexual function resulting from pain or a deficiency in sexual desire, arousal, or orgasm/climax.[159,160] Moreover, in order to meet diagnostic criteria, these symptoms should cause distress and persist for at least 3 months. Sexual function and dysfunction result from a complex interplay of the individual, culture, and physiology.[160] Sexual problems are multifaceted and often difficult to diagnose; adequate research is still needed. Sexual dysfunction can have organic or psychogenic causes or, more commonly, be a combination of both.[160] Studies show that at any given time up to 40% to 50% of adult women have some form of sexual dysfunction.[161]

The sexual response cycle is complex, involving the brain/mind, sympathetic and parasympathetic nervous systems, the systemic and local vasculature, and local innervation. Any disruption in these systems can affect sexual response. Chronic medical conditions can greatly affect both sexual desire and sexual function (Table 25.7). Acute illness and infections also can affect the woman's desire and ability to engage in fulfilling sexual activity. Vaginal infections are especially problematic because they can lead to vaginal irritation and pain with friction. Medications also can disrupt the sexual response cycle. Antihypertensives and antidepressants are commonly associated with sexual problems.[162]

Surgeries on the genital area can disrupt nerve pathways and hysterectomy may affect sexual function because the uterus, cervix, and vagina are involved in sexual response and orgasm. The mind is a large component of sexual response, and any stressor that affects the woman can affect her sexual response, including her feelings about her sexuality and relationship, as well as past sexual abuse.[163] A thorough history is needed to assess for sexual dysfunction, and testing is appropriate to assess for organic dysfunction (Fig. 25.25). The American College of Obstetricians and Gynecologists divides sexual dysfunction into four categories: disorders of desire, arousal, orgasm, and sexual pain.[159]

Disorders of desire (hypoactive sexual desire, decreased libido) are the most common sexual dysfunction in women.[163] The prevalence of hypoactive sexual desire increases with age and may be a biologic manifestation of depression, alcohol or other substance abuse, prolactin-secreting pituitary tumors, or testosterone deficiency. β-Adrenergic blockers used for heart disease also may inhibit sexual desire. A promising medication, flibanserin, has emerged that activates dopamine and norepinephrine in the brain and has been shown to increase sexual desire. In addition, treatment with exogenous testosterone, the antidepressant bupropion, and sexual and psychologic therapy have all shown to increase sexual desire in women.[163]

Anorgasmia, or **orgasmic dysfunction**, is the inability of the woman to reach or achieve orgasm. Dysfunction follows a continuum from difficulty in arousal to lack of orgasm. Any chronic illness may affect arousal. Diabetes, alcoholism, neurologic disturbances, hormonal deficiencies, and pelvic disorders (such as infections, trauma, and surgical scarring) may block orgasm. Narcotics, tranquilizers, antidepressants (especially SSRIs), and antihypertensive medications also can inhibit orgasm.[160]

Dyspareunia (painful intercourse) is common. Women may experience pain during arousal, at the initiation of intercourse, midway during intercourse, at the time of orgasm, or after intercourse. The pain may

TABLE 25.7	POSSIBLE EFFECTS OF CHRONIC DISEASE ON SEXUAL FUNCTIONING IN WOMEN	
DISEASE	**SEXUAL FUNCTION**
Cerebral palsy	Intact genital sensations, decreased lubrication; difficulty with sexual activity/positioning because of muscle spasticity, rigidity, and/or weakness; pain with positioning caused by contracture of knees and hips or because of increased spasms with arousal
Cerebrovascular accident (CVA)	Difficulties in sexual positioning and sensitivity because of impaired motor strength, coordination, or paralysis; decreased sex drive with stroke on the dominant side of the brain
Diabetes	Diminished intensity of orgasm and gradual decline in ability to achieve orgasm; decreased lubrication and/or recurrent vaginal infections with resultant dyspareunia
Chronic renal failure	Decreased arousal; increasingly rare and less intense orgasms; decreased lubrication
Rheumatoid arthritis (RA)	Painful sexual activity/positions because of swollen, painful joints, muscular atrophy and joint contracture; decreased sex drive because of pain, fatigue, and/or medication; genital sensations remain intact
Systemic lupus erythematosus (SLE)	Similar to RA; decreased lubrication and vaginal lesions result in painful penetration
Myocardial infarction (MI)	Most literature male oriented; problems related to medications
Multiple sclerosis (MS)	Diminished genital sensitivity; decreased lubrication; declining orgasmic ability; difficulty with sexual activity because of muscle weakness, pain, or incontinence
Spinal cord injury	Reflex sexual response with injury above sacral area; disrupted response with lesion at or below sacrum; loss of sensation, decreased lubrication; spasticity, incontinence, or pain with arousal; continued orgasmic sensations or sensations diffused in general or to specific body parts, such as breast or lips

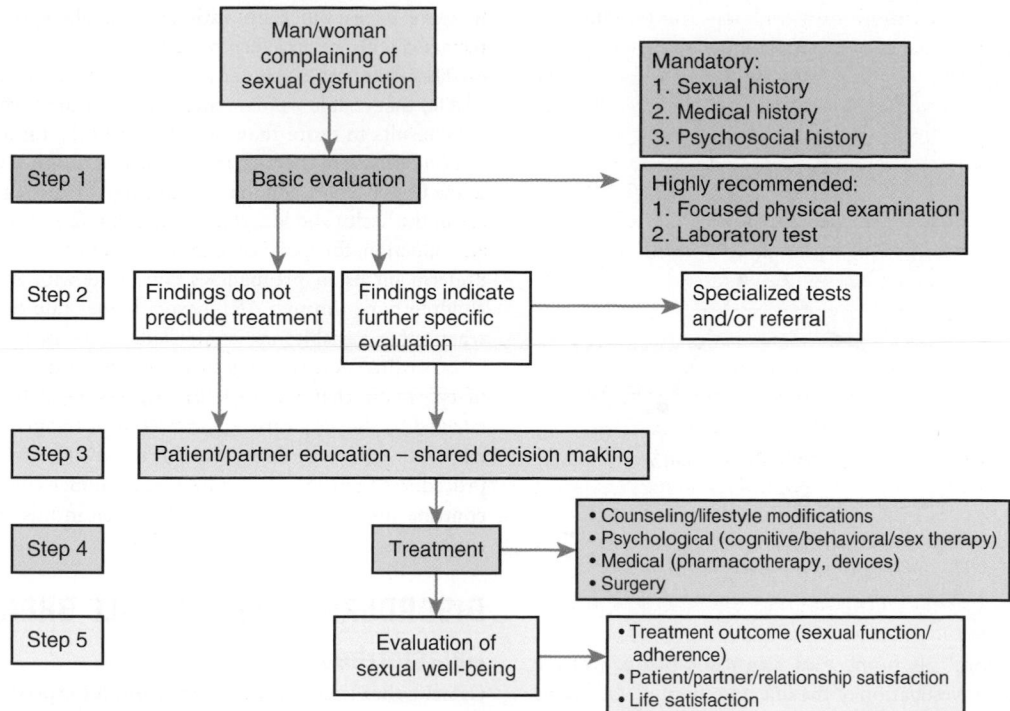

FIGURE 25.25 Diagnostic and Treatment Algorithm for Sexual Dysfunction. The International Consultation in Sexual Medicine stepwise diagnostic and treatment algorithm for sexual dysfunction in men and women. (From Hatzichristou D et al: *J Sex Med* 7[1pt2]:337–348, 2010.)

have a burning, sharp, searing, or cramping quality and may be described as external, vaginal, deep abdominal, or pelvic. A variety of psychosocial and organic causes have been identified.

Inadequate lubrication may make penetration or intercourse difficult or painful. Low estrogen levels, as are common with menopause and lactation, can decrease vaginal lubrication. Drugs with a drying effect, such as antihistamines, certain tranquilizers, and marijuana, can decrease lubrication. Infections and skin problems of the vulva and vagina are a frequent cause of acute onset dyspareunia. The use of products such as spermicides and fragrances on the sensitive vaginal mucosa may increase the risk of irritation. Disorders of the vaginal opening, such as scarring from female genital mutilation, episiotomy, or an intact hymen, also can be problematic. Deep pelvic disorders such as infection, tumors, and cervical or uterine abnormalities can cause pain with intercourse.

Vaginismus is an involuntary muscle spasm in response to attempted penetration. Vaginismus is often a response to previous painful penetration. Common causes include prior sexual trauma or fear of sex; organic causes are less common and are similar to those that cause dyspareunia, including vulvovestibulitis. Even after the underlying organic problem is detected and successfully treated, vaginismus may persist.

Sexual dysfunction may develop as a coping mechanism. Women with a history of sexual trauma—rape, incest, or molestation—often have problems of desire, arousal, or orgasm or experience pain with sexual activity. In extreme cases total sexual aversion may develop.[164] At other times, sexual dysfunction may be a symptom of marital or relationship problems. Because sexual dysfunction has many causes, assessment and treatment should be holistic and culturally sensitive.

Impaired Fertility

Infertility affects approximately 15% of all couples and is defined as the inability to conceive after 1 year of unprotected intercourse with the same partner. However, many sources believe that medical intervention is indicated for women who are older than 35 years if they fail to conceive after 6 months of unprotected intercourse.[165] The rate of infertility may be increasing because of an increase in sexually transmitted disease and environmental exposures, and a delay in the start of childbearing; but the increase in incidence rates may also reflect the greater utilization of medical services for infertility.[166,167] Fertility can be impaired by factors in the man or the woman or both partners. Causes include ovulatory disorder, abnormal semen, blockage of the fallopian tubes, endometriosis, and unexplained infertility.[168] The majority of cases of infertility involve the female, caused in part by the complexity of the female reproductive cycle and tract. Ovulatory factors account for 40% of female infertility.[167] Regular ovulation occurs as a result of a functioning hypothalamic/pituitary axis. Ovulation can be disrupted by a wide variety of factors, including imbalances in a diversity of hormones (e.g., TSH, estrogen, progesterone), chronic conditions, and stress. Age is a major factor in female fertility because the regularity of ovulation and the quality of ova decrease with age (Fig. 25.26). Abnormalities of the reproductive tract, including tubal pathologies, cause another 20% of cases of infertility.[167] Endometriosis and adhesions and scarring from PID are major contributors to blockages within the female reproductive tract. The remaining 20% of female infertility is caused by rare conditions or unknown etiology.[167]

Male infertility has a variety of causes, many of which can be corrected, and contributes to approximately 40% of cases of infertility.[167] Hormonal disorders, such as thyroid disturbances or low testosterone levels, can be diagnosed and corrected.[169] Throughout the 82 days of their creation and maturation, the sperm must be kept cooler than body temperature.[169] Elevations in temperature caused by illness, abnormal placement of the testes, varicoceles near the testes, or exposure to high temperatures in hot tubs or saunas may kill or disable sperm. Male infertility is also linked to abnormalities of the seminal tract and sexual dysfunction

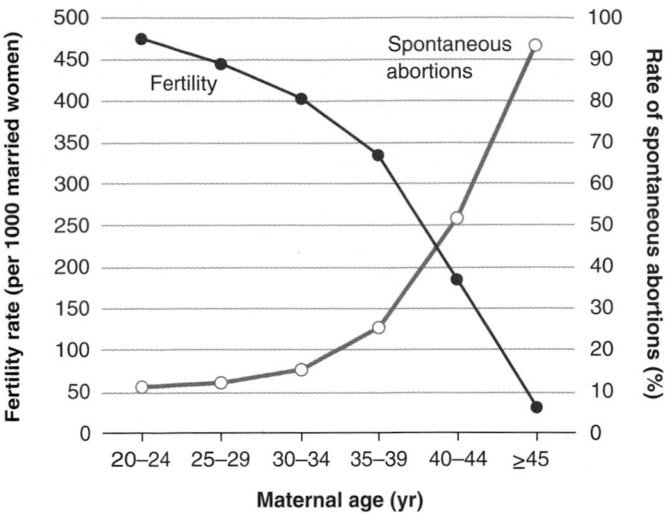

FIGURE 25.26 Relationship of Fertility and Miscarriage with Maternal Age. (From Heffner LJ: *N Engl J Med* 351[19]:1927–1929, 2004.)

that disrupts ejaculation.[169] A number of diagnostic procedures are required in the routine investigation of the infertile couple[165] (see Table 24.4). In many instances no cause may be identified.

Fertility Tests

Before the performance of even basic fertility tests, a complete history should be obtained that includes (1) coital (sex) timing and frequency in relation to the menstrual cycle, (2) an in-depth assessment and charting of the menstrual cycle, (3) a reproductive history including all previous pregnancies from both partners and their outcome, (4) a medical history of systemic disease, (5) current medications, (6) past surgeries, (7) a sexual history including any previous STIs, and (8) any exposure to toxins.[165] The history allows the clinician to focus on the most useful tests. Testing starts with the least invasive test or procedure and increases in invasiveness and complexity as the duration of infertility increases. The types of tests and their normal values are summarized in Table 24.4.

The most common test for male infertility is the basic semen analysis. A sample of fresh semen is evaluated for volume and the concentration, morphology, and forward motility of sperm.[165] More advanced semen analysis also examines the function of the sperm including their ability to bind to and penetrate eggs. In-depth analysis also may analyze the sperm's DNA for number, fragmentation, and ability to merge with the egg's DNA.[169]

Tests for women determine whether (1) ovulation occurs normally, (2) the endometrium is responding normally to hormones, (3) reproductive tissues are free of tumors or infections, (4) the woman does not have any chronic conditions interfering with fertilization or implantation, and (5) the reproductive tract (cervix, uterus, fallopian tubes) is adequately patent to allow for passage of ovum and sperm. Hormonal assays can be useful to detecting underlying abnormalities. The position and size of organs or the presence of tumors can be assessed by pelvic examination, ultrasound, or hysterosalpingogram that injects contrast dye into the reproductive tract to look for normal anatomy and fallopian/uterine tube patency. Chromosomal analysis of the couple may reveal mutations or translocations that result in very early embryo loss.[167]

Treatment of infertility aims at correcting underlying pathologies or overriding the deficient system. Male infertility can be overcome through injection of the male DNA directly into the uterus or even the ovum. Anovulation in the female can be overcome with ovulation-

inducing drugs. Blockages within the female reproductive tract can be bypassed with in vitro fertilization.

There has been a proliferation in assisted reproductive technologies (ARTs) that enable women and couples to conceive and bear children. ART results in more than 50,000 live births (and more than 60,000 infants because of the higher incidence of multiple gestations) per year in the United States, and the rate is rising.[170] However, there are questions about the health and long-term safety of infants conceived with assisted reproduction, for instance, concerns about the high rate of twins and preterm births in pregnancies conceived with ARTs.[171] In addition, children born through ART have a higher rate of birth defects, even when other variables are controlled.[172] The many theories about the cause of this increase suggest that the birth defects may be the result of epigenetic changes when the expression of the embryo's DNA is affected by the very early environment of the blastocysts, though it is not clear if damage done through the fertilization and implantation procedures themselves is caused by an underlying medical condition contributing to the infertility.[172] Research in this area and the field of epigenetics is ongoing.[172]

DISORDERS OF THE FEMALE BREAST

Galactorrhea

Galactorrhea (inappropriate lactation) is the persistent and sometimes excessive secretion of a milky fluid from the breasts of a woman who is not pregnant or nursing an infant. It can occur in men, may involve one or both breasts, and is not associated with breast cancer.

Incidence is difficult to estimate because of differences among definitions of the condition, examination techniques, and populations of women who have been studied. Prevalence has been documented as 0.1% to 32% of all women.

◆**PATHOPHYSIOLOGY.** Galactorrhea is a manifestation of pathophysiologic processes in the body, rather than a breast disorder. These processes are chiefly hormone imbalances caused by hypothalamic/pituitary disturbances, pituitary tumors, or neurologic damage. Exogenous causes include drugs, estrogen, and manipulation of the nipples. When caused by hyperprolactinemia, it is manifested by the spontaneous appearance of a milky secretion from multiple duct openings, usually from both breasts. Galactorrhea caused by oral contraceptives (OCs) is more likely to occur with high-dose use; is characterized by clear, serous, or milky discharge from multiple ducts; and is noticeable during the drug-free interval between OC packets. In premenopausal women, unilateral or bilateral spontaneous multiple duct discharge that increases before menstruation often is caused by fibrocystic change. Unilateral, spontaneous, serous, or serosanguineous discharge from a single duct usually is caused by an intraductal papilloma. Bloody discharge suggests cancer; bilateral, sticky, multicolored discharge from multiple ducts is often caused by ductal ectasia; and purulent discharge indicates a subareolar abscess.[173]

The most common cause of galactorrhea is nonpuerperal hyperprolactinemia, or excessive amounts of prolactin (the pituitary hormone that stimulates milk production) in the blood not related to pregnancy or childbirth. Nonpuerperal hyperprolactinemia can be caused by any factor that (1) stimulates or overstimulates the prolactin-secreting units of the pituitary gland; (2) interferes with production of prolactin-inhibiting factor (PIF), a neurotransmitter (probably dopamine) that inhibits prolactin secretion; or (3) interferes with pituitary receptors for PIF. A variety of exogenous agents (such as drugs) and disorders can trigger one of these three mechanisms, thereby causing hyperprolactinemia (Box 25.12).

Hypothyroidism causes increased secretion of hypothalamic TSH that stimulates prolactin release from the pituitary. Hypothyroidism

BOX 25.12 COMMON CAUSES OF HYPERPROLACTINEMIA

Physiologic Causes
Exercise
Idiopathic
Pregnancy and postpartum period
Sleep (rapid eye movement [REM] phase)
Stress (trauma, surgery)
Suckling

Drug Causes
Amoxapine
Amphetamines
Anesthetic agents
Butyrophenones
Cimetidine
Estrogens
Hydroxyzine
Methyldopa
Metoclopramide
Narcotics

Phenothiazines
Progestins
Reserpine
Tricyclic antidepressants
Verapamil

Pathophysiologic Causes
Acromegaly
Chronic chest wall stimulation (e.g., post-thoracotomy, postmastectomy, herpes zoster)
Cirrhosis
Hypothalamic disease
Hypothyroidism
Pressure on pituitary stalk
Prolactin-secreting tumors
Pseudocyesis (false pregnancy)
Renal failure (especially with zinc deficiency)
Spinal cord lesions

also is associated with reduced metabolic clearance of prolactin, which prolongs its effects.

Many types of pituitary tumors cause hyperprolactinemia. Prolactinomas cause hyperprolactinemia by secreting prolactin, decreasing production of PIF, or putting pressure on the pituitary stalk such that delivery of PIF to the anterior pituitary is prevented. Growth hormone–secreting pituitary tumors may cause galactorrhea through the intrinsic lactogenic effect that growth hormone appears to have on mammary tissue. Prolactin-secreting lung and kidney tumors also cause hyperprolactinemia.

Chronic stress may cause hyperprolactinemia by inhibiting PIF release. Cervical spinal injuries, head trauma, encephalitis, meningitis, herpes zoster, or thoracotomy scars may stimulate the afferent portion of the suckling reflex arc, which is carried in the second to sixth thoracic nerves. The suckling reflex increases prolactin secretion.

CLINICAL MANIFESTATIONS. A small amount of breast milk expressed from the nipples of parous women usually is not a concern, and normal breast milk color can be other than white. Inappropriate lactation is manifested by the appearance of a milky breast secretion in nonpregnant, nonlactating women from one or both breasts. Most women with galactorrhea also experience menstrual abnormalities. If a pituitary process is involved, the woman usually experiences hirsutism and infertility; if a hypothalamic lesion is present, she may report such CNS symptoms as intractable headache, visual field disturbances, sleep disturbances, and abnormal temperature, thirst, or appetite.

EVALUATION AND TREATMENT. Galactorrhea requires evaluation when it (1) occurs in nulliparous women or in parous women who have not been pregnant or have not breast-fed for 12 months, or (2) is associated with amenorrhea, headache, visual field abnormalities, or other symptoms implying systemic illness. Evaluation includes a variety of diagnostic tests. When amenorrhea accompanies galactorrhea, the assessment is the same as that for amenorrhea. Breast secretions are examined for fat globules and neoplastic cells to verify their source. Serum prolactin levels are measured. Because such variables as eating,

sleeping, stress, and breast examinations increase prolactin levels, at least two positive results are needed for a diagnosis of hyperprolactinemia. Prolactin levels greater than 25 to 30 ng/mL (by radioimmunoassay) are elevated. Those in the range of 75 to 100 ng/mL are considered to be caused by a pituitary tumor until proved otherwise. Serum thyroxine and TSH levels are measured to rule out hypothyroidism, and LH and FSH levels are obtained if the individual is amenorrheic. MRI may assist in locating adenomas.

Treatment is specific to the underlying cause and occurs after identification of the cause. Medical therapy is usual and surgery or radiation therapy is rarely required.

Benign Breast Disease

Benign breast disease (BBD) is a range of noncancerous changes in the breast of different components of the breast (epithelial, stromal, adipocytes, or vascular). Numerous benign alterations in ducts and lobules occur in the breast, including irregular lumps, cysts, sensitive nipples, and itching. The most common symptoms reported by women are pain, palpable mass, or nipple discharge; the majority of these prove to have a benign cause. After a diagnosis of BBD, however, major determinants of breast cancer risk include degree of family history, histologic or biologic features (or both), and results of previous biopsy.[174] The College of American Pathologists has classified biopsy tissue according to breast cancer risk. Benign epithelial lesions can be broadly classified according to their risk of developing breast cancer as (1) nonproliferative breast lesions, (2) proliferative breast disease, and (3) atypical (atypia) hyperplasia. The majority of nonproliferative benign lesions are not precursors of cancer and generally not associated with an increased risk of breast cancer.[175] Examples of other benign conditions are summarized in Table 25.8.

Nonproliferative Breast Lesions

Nonproliferative epithelial breast lesions are usually not associated with an increased risk of breast cancer. The nonproliferative lesions include: (1) simple breast cysts, (2) papillary apocrine change, and (3) mild hyperplasia of the usual type. Terms such as fibrocystic changes (FCCs) (or physiologic nodularity and cysts), fibrocystic disease, chronic cystic mastitis, and mammary dysplasia refer to nonproliferative lesions that are not clinically definitive because they encompass a heterogeneous group of diagnoses.[174] Simple cysts (fluid-filled sacs) are the most common nonproliferative breast lesion and are a specific type of lump that commonly occurs in women in their 30s, 40s, and early 50s. Cysts feel "squishy" when they occur close to the surface of the breast but when deeply embedded they can feel hard (Fig. 25.27). An estimated 50% to 80% of women normally experience some of these changes. The prevalence of fibrocystic lesions is probably related to systemic factors, particularly hormones, through their receptors to produce signal pathways that result in cell regulation and stimulation. These events are affected by genetic background, age, parity, history of lactation, caffeine consumption, and use of exogenous hormones.[176] Calcifications, found in cysts and adenosis or an increase in the number of acini per lobule, can form mammographically suspicious alterations.[175] Cysts also can be associated with unilateral nipple discharge. A variety of substances are secreted into cyst fluid, including polypeptide hormones and male and female sex steroid hormones. Cysts often rupture with release of secretory material into the adjacent tissue. The resulting chronic inflammation and scarring fibrosis contribute to the palpable firmness of the breast.[175] Fibrous tissue increases progressively until menopause and regresses thereafter.

Papillary apocrine (glandular) change is an increase in ductal epithelial cells that has apocrine changes or an eosinophilic cytoplasm. Mild hyperplasia of the usual type is an increase in the number of

TABLE 25.8   OTHER BENIGN BREAST CONDITIONS

TYPE	COMMENT
Developmental	
Milk-line remnants	Increase in number of nipples or breasts results from persistent epidermal thickening along the milk line
Accessory axillary breast tissue	Ductal system may extend into subcutaneous tissue of the chest wall and axillary region; this tissue can undergo lactational changes and give rise to tumors
Congenital nipple inversion	Is common and may be unilateral; can spontaneously correct during pregnancy; can be confused with retraction of nipple, which is sometimes part of invasive cancer or inflammation
Macromastia	Juvenile hypertrophy may be caused by unusual tissue response to hormonal stimulus
Iatrogenic	
Reconstruction or augmentation	Breast tissue can be replaced or augmented by skin and muscle flaps for synthetic prostheses; silicone implants, the most common, are rubbery silicone filled with either silicone gel or saline; a common complication of implants is formation of a thick fibrous capsule (i.e., chronic inflammatory responses) that can cause cosmetic deformity; the capsule can limit the spread of a ruptured implant but if the capsule ruptures, silicone gel can escape; long-term consequences of rupture are unknown
Inflammation	
Acute mastitis	Inflammatory diseases of the breast are rare; acute mastitis is confined to the lactating period of nursing; the nipples can become dry, cracked, and fissured, increasing risk of bacterial infection; infection may lead to abscess formation
Periductal mastitis	Women or men present with a painful subareolar mass thought to be infectious; not associated with lactation; 90% of individuals are smokers; vitamin A deficiency associated with smoking may alter the differentiation of the ductal epithelium; keratin is trapped within the ductal system causing dilation and rupture; antibiotic therapy and surgery are usually indicated
Mammary duct ectasia	Affects 50- and 60-year-olds, usually multiparous women, not associated with smoking; dilation of ducts with chronic granulomatous inflammatory reaction; fibrosis may eventually lead to skin and nipple retraction, thus mistaken for cancer; may have white nipple secretions
Fat necrosis	Painless, palpable mass, skin thickening or retraction; mammographic density or calcification; may have hemorrhage; most women will give a history of prior surgery or trauma; can be confused with breast carcinoma
Lymphocytic mastopathy	Single or multiple hard, palpable masses; can be so hard that interferes with biopsy; lesion includes collagenized stroma surrounding atrophic ducts and lobules; the breast membrane is frequently thickened; a prominent lymphocytic infiltrate surrounds epithelium and blood vessels; most common in women with type 1 diabetes or autoimmune thyroid disease

Data from Lester SC: The breast. In Kumar V, Abbas AK, Fausto N, editors: *Robbins & Cotran pathologic basis of disease,* ed 7, Philadelphia, 2005, Saunders.

epithelial cells within a duct that is more than two, but not more than four, cells in depth.[174]

Proliferative Breast Lesions without Atypia

These disorders are characterized by proliferation of ductal epithelium or stroma, or both, without cellular signs of abnormality (atypia or deviation from normal). The following structurally diverse lesions are included: (1) usual ductal hyperplasia, (2) intraductal papillomas, (3) sclerosing adenosis, (4) radial scar, and (5) simple fibroadenoma.[174]

Criteria for the diagnosis of intraductal proliferative lesions have been the subject of much research and controversy and include the following structurally diverse lesions:

1. Usual ductal hyperplasia (UDH) is additional or proliferating epithelial cells that fill and distend the ducts and lobules. They retain features of benign cells, but the cells can vary in size and shape.[174] They are usually found as an incidental result from mammography. No additional treatment is needed and chemoprevention is not recommended.[174]
2. Intraductal papillomas can occur as solitary or multiple lesions. *Solitary papillomas* are a monotonous (sameness) array of papillary

cells that grow from the wall of a cyst into the lumen of the duct. Growth occurs within a dilated duct often near or beside the nipple, causing benign nipple discharge (Fig. 25.28). Epithelial hyperplasia and apocrine metaplasia are frequently present.[175] Diffuse papillomatosis (multiple papillomas) may present as breast masses (densities or calcifications on mammogram), nodules on ultrasound, or the cause of nipple discharge. Diffuse papillomatosis is defined as a minimum of five papillomas within a localized segment of breast tissue.[175] It is controversial whether papillary lesions require surgical excision after core needle biopsy.[177]

3. Sclerosing adenosis is a lobular lesion with increased fibrous tissue and scattered glandular cells.[174] Calcification is commonly present within the lumens; however, the normal lobular arrangement is maintained. It can present as a mass or suspicious finding from mammogram but requires no treatment. Occasionally, stromal fibrosis may mimic the appearance of invasive carcinoma.[175]
4. Radial scar (RS) refers to an irregular, radial proliferation of ductlike small tubules entrapped in a densely fibrotic stroma (Fig. 25.29). The term *scar* refers to the structural appearance only because these lesions are not associated with scarring and fibrosis from a prior

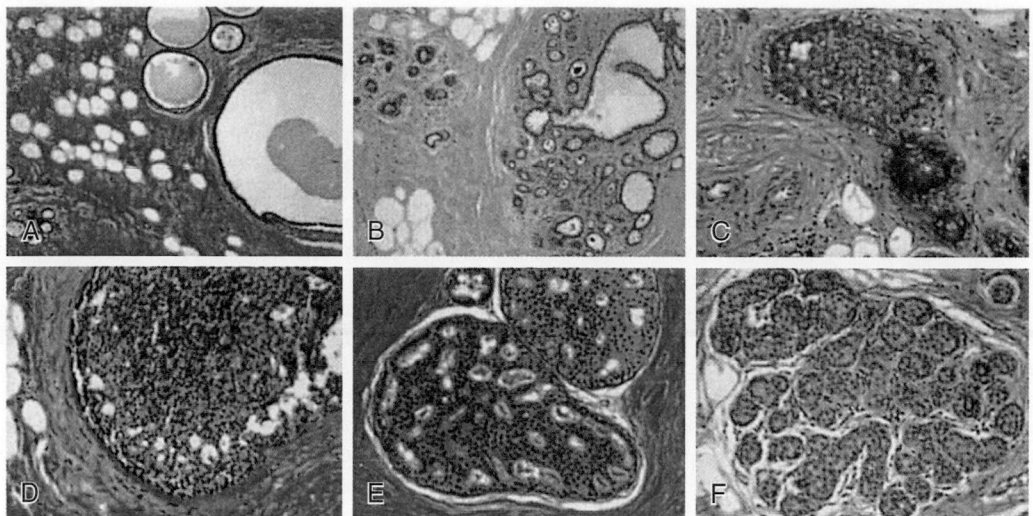

FIGURE 25.27 Benign Breast Disease. **A,** *Nonproliferative fibrocystic changes:* The architecture of the terminal-duct lobular unit is distorted by the formation of microcysts, associated with interlobular fibrosis. **B,** *Proliferative hyperplasia without atypia:* This is adenosis, a distinctive form of hyperplasia characterized by the proliferation of lobular acini, forming crowded glandlike structures. For comparison, a normal lobule is on the left side. **C,** *Proliferative hyperplasia without atypia:* There is moderate ductal hyperplasia, which is characterized by a duct that is partially distended by hyperplastic epithelium within the lumen. **D,** *Proliferative hyperplasia without atypia, which is florid ductal hyperplasia:* The involved duct is greatly expanded by a crowded, jumbled-appearing epithelial proliferation. **E,** *Atypical ductal hyperplasia:* These proliferations are complex and partially formed secondary lumens and mild nuclear hyperchromasia in the epithelial cell population. The peripheral spaces are irregular and slitlike. **F,** *Atypical lobular hyperplasia:* Monomorphic, small, rounded loosely cohesive cells fill the lumens of partially distended acini in this terminal-duct lobular unit (hematoxylin and eosin). (From Elmore JG, Gigerenzer G: *N Engl J Med* 353[3]:231, 2005.)

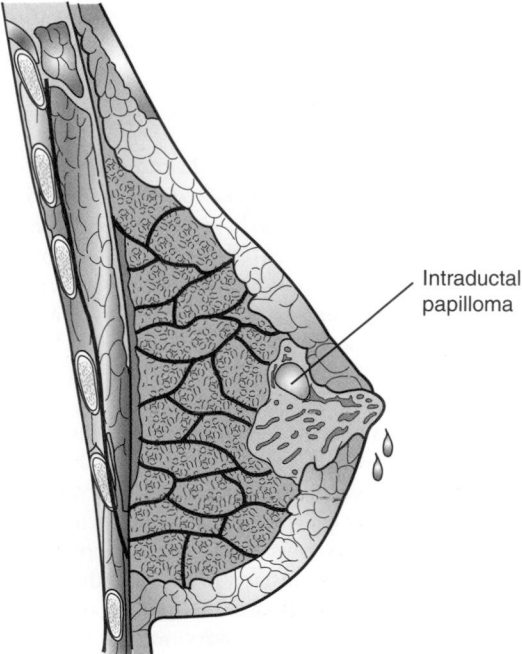

Intraductal papilloma

FIGURE 25.28 Intraductal Papilloma.

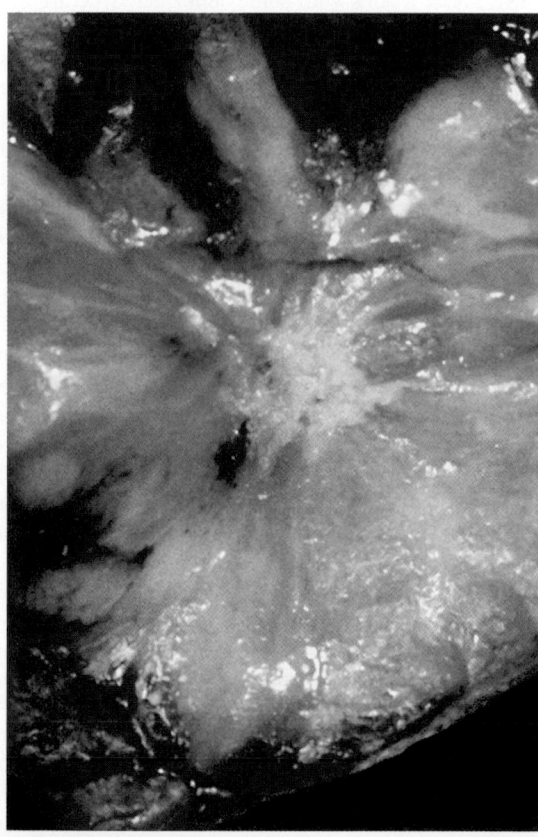

FIGURE 25.29 Radial Scar. Gross pathologic specimen of radial scar. (From the Armed Forces Institute of Pathology.)

injury, biopsy, or surgery. RS also has been called *radial sclerosing lesions* and *sclerosing papillary proliferation*. RSs are usually discovered when a breast lesion or radiologic abnormality is biopsied or removed. Controversy exists about the need for surgical excision when RSs are found.

5. **Simple fibroadenomas** are benign solid lumps or masses composed of both stromal and glandular tissue.[178] Fibroadenomas *usually* present as a well-defined mobile mass, smooth and hard like a marble on physical examination, or as a well-defined solid mass on ultrasound. Fibroadenomas are common, and regression or resolution is frequent. There is no increased risk of breast cancer in the majority of women with a simple fibroadenoma. If the fibroadenoma is *complex* with adjacent proliferative disease or if there is a family history of breast cancer, the risk of breast cancer is slightly elevated. Multiple fibro-adenomas occur in the same breast or bilaterally in about 20% of cases.[178] Fibroadenomas are found most commonly in women between the ages of 15 and 35 years but they can occur at any age, especially in older women receiving hormone therapy.[179] The etiology is unknown, but a hormonal role is likely because they persist during the reproductive years, increase in size during pregnancy or with estrogen therapy, and usually regress after menopause. Not all biopsy-proven lesions require surgical excision. Disadvantages of excisional surgery include scarring at the incision site, dimpling of the breast from the removal of the tumor, damage to the breast's duct system, and mammographic changes (e.g., architectural distortion, skin thickening, increased focal density).[175] If a biopsy-proven fibroadenoma is asymptomatic, then it can be left in place, although some women wish to have the mass excised so that they will not worry further.[175]

Proliferative Breast Lesions with Atypia

Proliferative breast lesions with some abnormal structure or *atypia* include **atypical ductal hyperplasia (ADH)**, or abnormal proliferating cells in breast ducts (Fig. 25.30, *A*), and **atypical lobular hyperplasia (ALH)**, or abnormal proliferating cells in the lumen of lobular units (see Fig. 25.30, *B*).[175] ALH may lie between the ductal basement membrane and overlying normal luminal cells.[175] **Atypical hyperplasia (AH)** is an increase in the number of cells with some variation in cellular structure. Unlike ductal carcinoma in situ (DCIS), ADH only partially fills involved ducts.[175] Studies continue to indicate that women with atypical hyperplasia (AH) have an increased risk (about three- or fourfold) of breast cancer compared with women who have nonproliferative lesions.[180-183] About 60% of the subsequent breast cancers in women with AH occur in the ipsilateral breast (same side) as the biopsy.[180,184,185] As mentioned earlier from long-term follow-up studies, atypical hyperplasia has been shown to confer a relative risk of 4 for future breast cancer and recently the *absolute risk* has been better defined with a cumulative incidence of breast cancer about 30% at 25 years of follow-up.[182,186] It appears that menopausal status at the time of benign breast biopsy influences the magnitude of subsequent breast cancer risk. For women who were premenopausal at the time of their breast biopsy, the risk of breast cancer was greater in those with ALH than among women with ADH.[185] Overall, the younger a woman is when she receives a diagnosis of atypical hyperplasia the higher the risk that breast cancer will develop.[180,182] Among women who were postmenopausal at the time of benign breast biopsy, the risk was similar with ALH and women with ADH.[185] Two independent cohorts of women found the *extent* of atypia stratified the long-term risk of breast cancer for ADH and ALH[187]; however, from the Nurses' Health Study the extent of ADH or ALH did not significantly contribute to breast cancer risk.[188] The discrepant findings are important to clarify for breast cancer risk and because of concerns about overdiagnosis and overtreatment of high-risk breast lesions.[189,190] Overall, ADH

and ALH are viewed best as "markers" of a generalized bilateral increase in breast cancer risk.[185]

◆**EVALUATION AND TREATMENT.** Breast problems are diagnosed from a multimodal approach that combines physical examination, mammography, ultrasonography, thermography, possibly MRI, and biopsy. The dense breast tissue often seen in young women can make mammographic interpretation extremely difficult (*What's New? Breast Cancer Screening Mammography*). Ultrasonography (ultrasound) is used to differentiate a solid mass from a cystic (fluid-filled) mass, which is generally benign.

Treatment consists largely of relieving symptoms. Reduction in the consumption of caffeinated beverages (e.g., cola) and chocolate, which can cause overstimulation for some women, may reduce pain and nodularity. Research for primary prevention of AH is weak. The roles of regular exercise, dietary factors, and sleep and the avoidance of psychologic stress are unknown. Given time, the cysts may disappear without treatment.

Certain selective estrogen modulators, such as tamoxifen and raloxifene, or an aromatase inhibitor may be considered for chemoprevention after a thorough discussion of risks and benefits. Although still controversial, isoflavone exposure was associated with a decreased risk of proliferative benign fibrocystic changes, nonproliferative changes, and breast cancer.[191,192] Genistein, a soy isoflavone, has been reported to down-regulate an enzyme important in cancer progression (i.e., telomerase) and contributes to inhibition in both breast benign and cancer cells.[193] Toxicologists conclude soy supplement intake will not induce proliferation of normal breast tissue and may even inhibit proliferation.[194] The North American Menopause Society (NAMS) found that soy foods generally appear to be breast protective and recommended moderate lifelong soy consumption.[195] Another preventive factor may be iodine.[196] Investigators report that povidone-iodine (PVP-1), Lugol solution, and a combination of iodide and molecular iodine (I_2) may be potent agents for use in development of antitumor strategies.[197] Drugs used to treat severe breast pain are listed in Table 25.9.

Cancer

Except for skin cancer, breast cancer is the most common cancer in American women.[198] It is estimated that 246,660 women and 2600 men will be diagnosed with breast cancer, and 40,450 women and 440 men will die from breast cancer in 2016.[1] Age and the chance of being diagnosed with breast cancer are presented in Table 25.10. The age-adjusted death rate based on years 2009 to 2013 cases and deaths in the United States is 21.5 per 100,000 women per year.[199] Using Centers for Disease Control and Prevention (CDC) data from 2013 in the United States, white women had the highest rate of getting breast cancer followed by black, Hispanic, Asian/Pacific Islander, and American Indian/Alaska Native women. Dying from breast cancer varies by race and ethnicity. In 2013, black women were more likely to die of breast cancer than other groups, followed by white, Hispanic, Asian/Pacific Islander, and American Indian/Alaska Native women.[200] Globally, breast cancer is the second most common cancer in the world.[201] It is the most frequent cancer of women with an estimated 1.67 million new cancer cases diagnosed in 2012.[201] Incidence rates vary nearly fourfold across the world regions with rates ranging from 27 per 100,000 in Middle Africa and Eastern Asia to 92 in North America.[201]

More than two-thirds of breast cancer cases occur in women older than 55 years. From 2005 to 2009, the median age for breast cancer diagnosis was 61 years of age. The median age at death for breast cancer was 68 years of age.[202] Because ductal carcinoma in situ (DCIS) is almost exclusively detected by mammography, the large increase in incidence of DCIS over the past 20 years can be attributed to screening (see

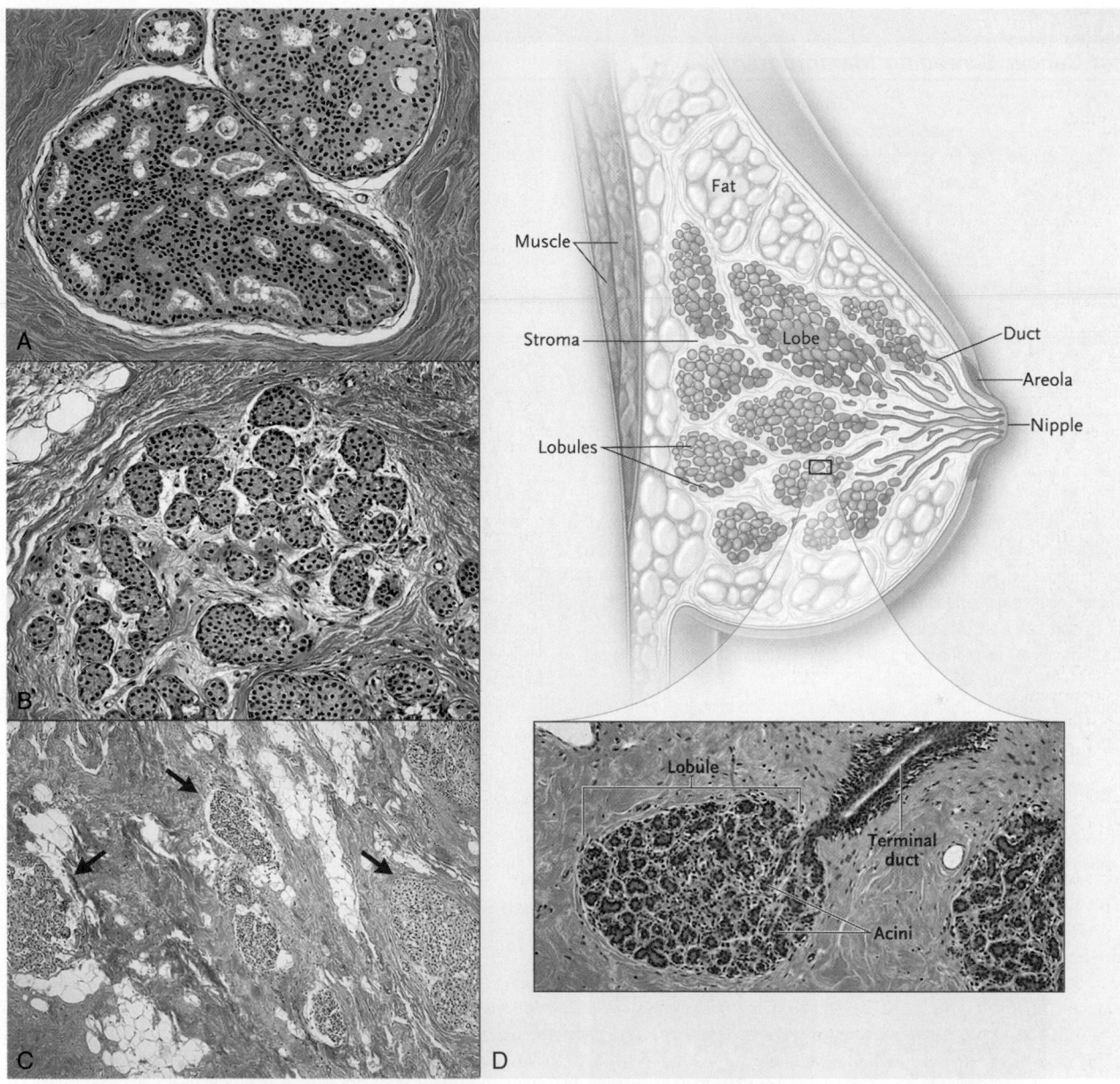

FIGURE 25.30 Anatomic and Histologic Features of Atypical Hyperplasias. **A,** shows atypical ductal hyperplasia with proliferation of monotonous cells in architecturally complex patterns, including secondary lumens and micropapillary formations. **B,** shows atypical lobular hyperplasia, with expanded acini filled with monotonous polygonal cells and a loss of acinar lumen. **C,** shows multifocal atypical hyperplasia (in this case atypical lobular hyperplasia). Atypical lobular hyperplasia is present in more than one terminal duct lobular unit, and units are clearly separated from one another by interlobular mammary stroma *(arrows)*. **D,** is an illustration of the microanatomy of the breast, including a photomicrograph of a terminal duct lobular unit. (From Hartmann LC, Degnim AC, Santen RJ, et al: *N Engl J Med* 372[1]:1271–1272, 2015.)

pp. 794 and 820). Some women younger than age 45 may have a higher risk for getting breast cancer compared with other women their age if they have the following risks factors: (1) close relatives (parents, siblings, or children) who were diagnosed with breast or ovarian cancer when they were younger than 45, especially if more than one relative was diagnosed or a male relative had breast cancer; (2) alterations in certain breast genes (*BRCA1* and *BRCA2*), or having close relatives with these alterations; (3) Ashkenazi Jewish heritage; (4) treatment with radiation therapy to the breast or chest during childhood or early adulthood; (5) have been diagnosed with breast cancer or other breast health problems, such as lobular carcinoma in situ (LCIS), DCIS, atypical ductal hyperplasia, or typical lobular hyperplasia; and (6) high breast density.[203] A high-risk breast cancer condition is postpartum breast cancer with immune suppression and delayed involution (see Reproductive Factors: Pregnancy).[204]

Although breast cancer is a multifactorial disease involving a complex web of interacting factors, risk is related to timing, duration, and pattern of exposures. Risk factors and possible causes of breast cancer can be classified as reproductive, hormonal, environmental and lifestyle, and familial (Table 25.11). Two factors emerging as important are postpartum involution of the mammary gland, a reproductive factor, and breast density, which is not as easily classified.

Breast Cancer Screening Mammography

Joann G. Elmore, MD, MPH

Programs intended to screen the entire population of a country for disease usually require extensive resources. Possible harms of screening are important to consider, because screening at a population level involves testing healthy individuals. It must be made certain that the disease is not too rare, the test has a high level of accuracy, the potential costs and disadvantages are reasonable, and the treatment is effective for individuals who are diagnosed through screening.

Women have been encouraged to undergo breast cancer screening for many decades. The idea behind screening healthy women for breast cancer is to diagnose the disease early, when more treatment options are available and when they can positively impact their lives. Early screening programs encouraged women to perform breast self-examinations and also to have their clinician perform a breast examination in the office. Research has since shown that these screening techniques lead to false-positive examinations and are not associated with a reduction in mortality.

Most guidelines continue to recommend mammography screening for breast cancer, although the benefits of mammography are less than hoped, and more is being learned about potential harms. A mammogram is an x-ray examination that takes images of each breast (see Figure). The recommended age for a first mammogram and the suggested frequency of mammography screening vary among guidelines and between countries. The U.S. Preventive Services Task Force periodically reviews the evidence and publishes mammography guidelines to aid discussions with women about screening.

Mammography, like any medical test, is imperfect. The benefits, harms, and accuracy of screening depend on numerous factors, including a woman's age, breast density, and time interval between mammograms. About 10% of screening mammograms in the United States are interpreted as "abnormal," requiring additional testing. The great majority of women with an "abnormal" mammogram do not have breast cancer; this is called a *false-positive* mammogram. False-positive examinations lead to additional diagnostic testing, which may increase anxiety and morbidity. It is estimated that at least 50% of women who are screened annually for a decade will experience at least one false-positive mammogram. Most abnormal mammograms are evaluated with additional imaging and less frequently require biopsies. Some women think that a breast biopsy will provide an immediate and definitive diagnosis, but this is not always the case. For example, studies have shown that pathologists disagree on the diagnoses of breast atypia and ductal carcinoma in situ (DCIS).

As more women undergo mammography screening, there has been a sharp increase in the number of women *diagnosed* with DCIS and early-stage breast cancer. By definition, DCIS is confined to the breast milk duct and is *not* an immediately threatening, invasive carcinoma, although it is most often treated like an early-stage invasive breast cancer. Women with DCIS are at increased risk for a subsequent invasive breast cancer diagnosis, even though the majority of women with DCIS are never diagnosed with invasive cancer. Furthermore, treatment of DCIS does not alter mortality; women with DCIS have the same mortality rates as women without DCIS.

Another potential harm of screening mammography is *overdiagnosis*—a *diagnosis* of cancer that would never have harmed the woman during her lifetime. Overdiagnosis can lead to overtreatment. This can occur either with a preinvasive lesion, such as DCIS, or with invasive breast cancer. Unfortunately, it is not possible to identify which individual women with a new diagnosis of DCIS or invasive breast cancer have a lesion that is so low-risk it will never harm them. Most women diagnosed with breast cancer undergo treatment with either mastectomy or with lumpectomy plus radiation therapy. This is considered *overtreatment* if the DCIS or invasive cancer was *overdiagnosed*. Published estimates of the prevalence of overdiagnosis range from <10% to 50%, and further research on this topic is needed.

Balancing the potential benefits and harms of breast cancer screening is not easy for women or their clinicians. Every woman should be encouraged to make informed decisions about participation in screening for breast cancer.

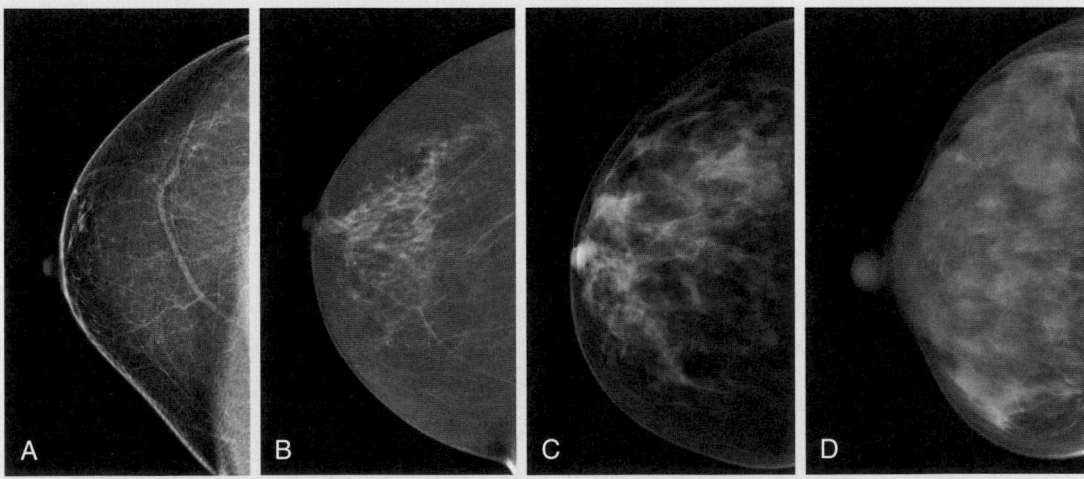

FIGURE Mammograms. Mammograms depicting varying breast densities from a craniocaudal view: **A,** almost entirely fat; **B,** scattered fibroglandular densities; **C,** heterogeneously dense; and **D,** extremely dense. (Images provided by Christoph I. Lee, MD, MSHS. From Fuller MS et al: *Med Clin North Am* 99[3]:451–468, 2015.)

Data from Elmore JG et al: *JAMA* 313(11):1122–1132, 2015; Fuller MS et al: *Med Clin North Am* 99(3):451–468, 2015; Katz DL et al: *Jekel's epidemiology, biostatistics, preventive medicine, and public health*, ed 4, Philadelphia, 2013, Elsevier Saunders; Welch HG et al: *N Engl J Med* 375(15), 2016; Elmore JG: *N Engl J Med* 375(15), 2016; U.S. Preventive Services Task Force: *Final update summary: breast cancer screening*, Jan 2016. Available at: https://www.uspreventiveservicestaskforce.org/Page/Document/UpdateSummaryFinal/breast-cancer-screening, accessed January 30, 2017; U.S. Preventive Services Task Force: *Ann Intern Med* 151(10):716–726, 2009.

TABLE 25.9   DRUGS USED TO TREAT SEVERE BREAST PAIN (MASTALGIA)

AGENTS	COMMENTS
Definitely Effective	
Danazol	Causes a decrease in cyclic pain and nodularity believed to reduce estrogen; also used for endometriosis; some side effects include changes in menstrual cycle regularity, weight gain, acne, and flushing
Bromocriptine	Decreases cyclic pain, nodularity, and tenderness; decreases prolactin levels and may alter dopamine receptors; is also used to suppress lactation after childbirth; can cause nausea, vomiting, hypotension, and dizziness
Tamoxifen	As an antiestrogen it can decrease cyclic pain, increase clot formation (phlebitis, emboli, strokes), and cause hot flashes, amenorrhea, weight gain, and increased risk of uterine cancers
Evening primrose oil (linoleic acid)	Can decrease cyclic pain, nodularity, and tenderness; women with mastalgia believed to have low levels of breast linoleic acid; reduces PGE_2 prostaglandins and inflammation; too much oil, however, has been associated with increasing inflammation (>1000 mg/day)
Possibly Effective	
Iodine	Can decrease cyclic pain and nodularity (see *Nutrition & Disease:* Premenstrual Syndrome, p. 813)
Vaginal progesterone	Decrease in cyclic pain and tenderness; not as effective for decreasing tenderness; antagonist to estrogen; can cause weight gain
Insufficiently Studied	
Progestins	May decrease estrogenic effects; however, related to endothelial vasospasms, weight gain, and increased risk of breast cancer

TABLE 25.10   CHANCE OF BEING DIAGNOSED WITH BREAST CANCER*

BY AGE (YEARS)	BY RATIO
30–39	1 in 238
40–49	1 in 69
50–59	1 in 38
60–69	1 in 27
Ever†	1 in 8
Never	7 in 8

*NOTE: These calculations are averages. An individual's risk may be higher or lower depending on several factors (e.g., family history, reproductive history, race/ethnicity, and others).

†Absolute lifetime risk.

Data from Reis LAG et al: *Cancer statistics review,* 1975–2005, Bethesda, MD, 2008, National Cancer Institute. Available at: http://seer.cancer.gov/csr/1975_2005. Based on November 2007 SEER data, posted SEER website, 2008.

Reproductive Factors: Pregnancy

A clearer understanding of mammary gland structure (morphology) and function from fetal development, to puberty, pregnancy, and aging will help elucidate fundamental changes to breast development and disease. A key element is "branching morphogenesis," in which the mammary gland produces and delivers copious amounts of milk by forming a rootlike network of branched ducts from a rudimentary epithelial bud.[205] Branching morphogenesis begins in fetal development, pauses after birth, starts again in response to estrogens at puberty, and is modified by cyclic ovarian hormonal action. This systemic hormonal action elicits local paracrine interactions between the developing epithelial ducts and their adjacent mesenchyme (embryonic) or postnatal stroma. The local cellular crosstalk then directs the tissue remodeling, ultimately producing a mature ductal tree.[205] The gland is unique because it undergoes most of its branching during adolescence and not fetal development. This allows experimental manipulation of the gland not possible with any other organ.[206]

A woman's age when her first child is born affects her risk for developing breast cancer—the younger she is, the lower the risk. Overall, lifetime risk of breast cancer is reduced in parous women compared to nulliparous women, but pregnancy must occur at a young age[207] (see *What's New?* Potential Mechanisms Underlying Protective Effect of Pregnancy and Implications for Prevention of Breast Cancer). The protective factor is especially observed in the years of peak incidence, the postmenopausal years.[208] The risk reduction is limited to hormone receptor–positive breast cancer.[209] The influence of pregnancy on the risk of breast cancer also depends on family history, lactation postpartum, and overall parity.[210] Paradoxically, women of all ages have a transient *increase* in breast cancer risk with a recent pregnancy and after each subsequent pregnancy.[210,211] Pregnancy-associated breast cancer (PABC) is defined as breast cancer diagnosed up to 5 years after a completed pregnancy; however, risk may persist for a decade.[210,212] Delayed childbearing observed in the United States and all developing countries is expected to show a rise in diagnosed breast cancers.[210] (see *What's New?* Potential Mechanisms Underlying Protective Effect of Pregnancy and Implications for Prevention of Breast Cancer). The transient increase in breast cancer risk for all parous women includes events associated with pregnancy, including pregnancy-related hormones, such as estrogen, progesterone, and growth hormone, that promote or initiate cancer cells; immune suppressive effects of pregnancy; and breast tissue involution.[210] Breast gland *involution* after pregnancy and lactation uses some of the same tissue remodeling pathways activated during wound healing (i.e., proinflammatory pathways). The proinflammatory environment, although physiologically normal, promotes tumor progression. One mechanism identified links fibrillar collagen deposition, noted during normal involution, to high levels of COX-2 expression in tumor cells and subsequent tumor cell metastasis.[210] This alteration provides support to the tissue change in stroma for driving carcinogenesis.[213] The presence of macrophages in the involuting mammary gland contributes to carcinogenesis.[212,214] Immature macrophages are capable of suppressing cytotoxic T-cell function, causing an immunosuppressive stroma conducive to tumor cell promotion (see pp. 798 and 799).

TABLE 25.11   FACTORS ASSOCIATED WITH INCREASED RISK OF BREAST CANCER*

CATEGORY	RISK FACTOR	RELATIVE RISK[†]
Race	Blacks have higher incidence up to age 40 yr; whites have higher incidence after age 40 yr	1.1–1.9
Family history	Breast cancer in first-degree relative before age 60 yr	2–3
	Premenopausal or bilateral breast cancer	>4
	Postmenopausal in first-degree relative	≤2
	Breast cancer in two first-degree relatives,	4–6
	BRCA1 or BRCA2	≤4
	TP53 (Li-Fraumeni syndrome)	≤4
Previous medical history	Moderate or florid mammary hyperplasia	1.5–2
	Mammary papilloma	1.5–2
	Atypical mammary hyperplasia	4–5
	DCIS, LCIS[‡]	8–10
Estrogen exposure	Early menarche (before age 12 yr)	1.1–1.9
	Late menopause (after age 55 yr)	1.1–1.9
	Postmenopausal hormone therapy	1.4
	Oral contraceptive use	1.5
Pregnancy	Nulliparous or late first pregnancy (after age 35 yr)	1.1–1.9
Radiation	Atomic bomb	3
	Repeated fluoroscopy	1.5–2[§]
Obesity and stature	Postmenopausal	1.2
	Tallness	≤2
Dietary/alcohol	High alcohol consumption	1.4–2
	High energy intake	≤2
	Advanced age	2–4
	Xenobiotics	≤2
Social	Smoking	2–4
	Higher socioeconomic status	≤2
	Low physical activity	≤2
Environmental	Excess radiation to breasts	??[‡]
	Chemical carcinogens	≤2–??
	Infectious agents	≤2–??

*Normal lifetime risk in white non-Hispanic women: 1 in 8.
[†]Relative risk is defined and discussed in Chapter 5.
[‡]Data from Lester SC: The breast. In Kumar V, Abbas AK, Fausto N, editors: Robbins & Cotran pathologic basis of disease, ed 7, Philadelphia, 2005, Saunders.
[§]Currently debated.
DCIS, Ductal carcinoma in situ; LCIS, lobular carcinoma in situ.

The main mechanisms for the *protective* effect of pregnancy are controversial including (1) induction of breast differentiation with lasting protective phenotypic (morphologic) changes; (2) altered cell fate with removal or modification of vulnerable cells, possibly stem cells; (3) enhancement of the ability for DNA repair or apoptosis, or

WHAT'S NEW?

Potential Mechanisms Underlying Protective Effect of Pregnancy and Implications for Prevention of Breast Cancer

The most effective modifiable breast cancer prevention method is an early age (before 20 years) first-full-term birth (FFTB). An historic landmark case-control study of 17,022 women in 7 regions worldwide found that compared to nulliparous women, women who had their FFTB before the age of 20 had a risk reduction of 50%. Others have replicated this study with reproducible findings. From the same early study, women who gave birth for the first time older than age 33 were no longer protected against breast cancer compared to nulliparous women. These women were now at an increased risk compared to nulliparous women. The average age at FFTB in the United States has been increasing over time with those who gave birth for the first time between the ages of 30 and 34 rising 28% and those older than 35 years of age rising 23% between 2000 and 2014. The protective effect has been replicated in animal models including mice and rats. Ongoing research is needed to understand the stage of the pregnancy cycle (i.e., pregnancy, lactation, or involution) most important in reducing breast cancer risk. Investigators are concentrating on potential mechanisms of parity-induced protection against breast cancer (see text for discussion) and now include the insulin-like growth factor (IGF) system and effects of long-lasting reprogramming of the epigenome. Newer data on the genomic profile of parous women have shown pregnancy induces a long-lasting "genomic signature" that reveals chromatin remodeling derived from the early first pregnancy. The chromatin modifications are accompanied by higher expression of genes related to cell adhesion and differentiation, and genes only activated during the first 5 years after pregnancy may contribute to increased risk but the long-lasting genetic signature may explain pregnancy's preventive effect.

Data from Barton M et al: *Front Endocrinol (Lausanne)* 5:213, 2014; Horne HN et al: *Breast Cancer Res* 18(1):24, 2016; Katz TA: *Front Oncol* 6:228, 2016; MacMahon B et al: *Bull World Health Organ* 43:209–221, 1970; Mathews TJ, Hamilton BE: *NCHS Data Brief* 232:1–8, 2016.

both; (4) altered systemic hormonal regulation and possible persistent changes in intracellular pathways regulating proliferation; (5) decreased proliferation in the parous involuted gland; and (6) early-life hormonal and dietary exposures[208,215] (see *What's New?* Potential Mechanisms Underlying Protective Effect of Pregnancy and Implications for Prevention of Breast Cancer).

Lobular Involution and Age and Postlactational Involution

Part of the uniqueness of the mammary gland is its profound physiologic changes throughout the phases of a woman's life: puberty, pregnancy, lactation, postlactational involution, and aging. The human breast is organized into 15 to 20 major lobes, each with terminal lobules containing milk-forming acini (see Fig. 24.10). **Terminal duct lobular units (TDLUs)**, also called *lobules*, are epithelial structures within the breast that produce milk during lactation and are the major source of most breast cancers (Fig. 25.31). With aging, breast lobules regress or involute with a decrease in the number and size of acini per lobule and replacement of the intralobular stroma with the denser collagen of connective tissue.[216] With time, the glandular elements and collagen are replaced with fatty tissue. This process is called **lobular involution**, and over many years the parenchymal elements progressively decrease in size and function and disappear. The first study of its kind found lobular involution was associated with reduced risk of breast cancer. Breast cancer risk decreased with increasing extent of involution

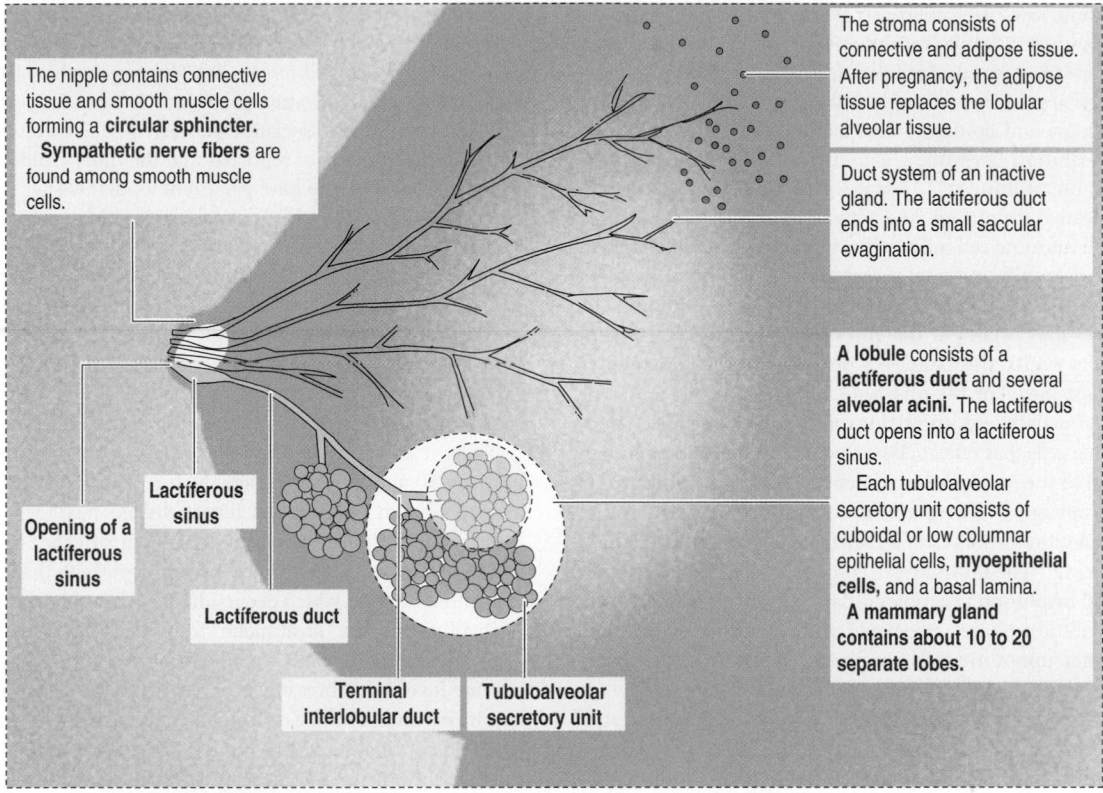

The nipple contains connective tissue and smooth muscle cells forming a **circular sphincter**. **Sympathetic nerve fibers** are found among smooth muscle cells.

The stroma consists of connective and adipose tissue. After pregnancy, the adipose tissue replaces the lobular alveolar tissue.

Duct system of an inactive gland. The lactiferous duct ends into a small saccular evagination.

A lobule consists of a **lactiferous duct** and several **alveolar acini.** The lactiferous duct opens into a lactiferous sinus.

Each tubuloalveolar secretory unit consists of cuboidal or low columnar epithelial cells, **myoepithelial cells,** and a basal lamina. **A mammary gland contains about 10 to 20 separate lobes.**

Opening of a lactiferous sinus

Lactíferous sinus

Lactiferous duct

Terminal interlobular duct

Tubuloalveolar secretory unit

A

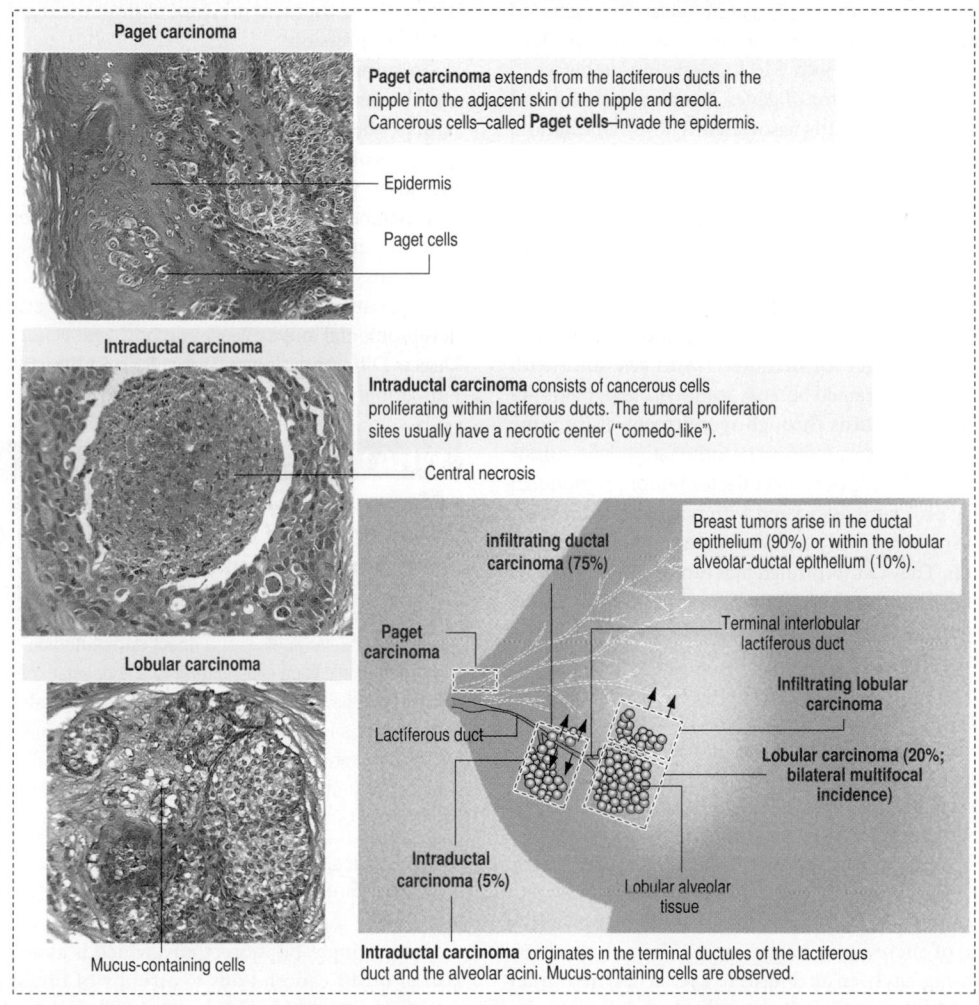

Paget carcinoma

Paget carcinoma extends from the lactiferous ducts in the nipple into the adjacent skin of the nipple and areola. Cancerous cells–called **Paget cells**–invade the epidermis.

Epidermis

Paget cells

Intraductal carcinoma

Intraductal carcinoma consists of cancerous cells proliferating within lactiferous ducts. The tumoral proliferation sites usually have a necrotic center ("comedo-like").

Central necrosis

Lobular carcinoma

Mucus-containing cells

Breast tumors arise in the ductal epithelium (90%) or within the lobular alveolar-ductal epithelium (10%).

infiltrating ductal carcinoma (75%)

Terminal interlobular lactíferous duct

Paget carcinoma

Infiltrating lobular carcinoma

Lactiferous duct

Lobular carcinoma (20%; bilateral multifocal incidence)

Intraductal carcinoma (5%)

Lobular alveolar tissue

Intraductal carcinoma originates in the terminal ductules of the lactiferous duct and the alveolar acini. Mucus-containing cells are observed.

B

FIGURE 25.31 Normal Breast and Breast Cancer. **A,** Normal breast. **B,** Breast cancer. (From Kierszenbaum AL: *Histology and cell biology: an introduction to pathology,* ed 2, Philadelphia, 2007, Mosby.)

in both high- and low-risk subgroups defined by family history of breast cancer, epithelial atypia, reproductive history, and age. Recent data suggest breast cancer susceptibility from single nucleotide polymorphisms (SNPs) may not strongly influence TDLU involution.[217] Based on histologic and epidemiologic factors, investigators propose that *delayed* involution (persistent glandular epithelium) is a major risk factor for breast cancer.[216] Tissue involution involves massive epithelial cell death; recruitment and activation of fibroblasts; stromal remodeling; and immune cell infiltration, including macrophages with similarities to microenvironments present during wound healing and tumor progression.[218] Post-lactational involution is involution of the mammary gland that occurs at the end of every period of lactation and is essential to return the gland to a prepregnant state in readiness for the next pregnancy. For the first time, investigators, using murine postpartum mammary gland, showed involution is characterized by an influx of immune cells that reflect classic wound healing and mammary tumors exposed to the involution microenvironment are infiltrated by immature macrophages.[204] These macrophages inhibit T-cell activation ex vivo and involution tumors have a growth edge that is interleukin-10 (IL-10) dependent.[204] The immune cell composition across postpartum mammary gland involution resembles inflammation, proliferation, and remodeling/resolution phases associated with classic wound healing. Importantly, when apoptotic cells are phagocytosed by macrophages, macrophages are stimulated to an immune-suppressive phenotype, with transforming growth factor-beta (TGF-β) and IL-10 expression.[204] Phagocytosis is crucial for the remodeling process, removal of cell debris, and residual milk in the second phase of involution.[219] Additionally, other investigators in a first study in rodent models demonstrated *Nucling,* a novel apoptosis-associated protein that plays an important role in involution by regulating NF-κβ STAT3 signaling pathways.[220] An important transcriptional regulator of genes, signal transducer and activator of transcription 3 (Stat3) is associated with inflammation, wound healing, mammary macrophages, and mast cells. Stat3 appears to have an important role in modulating cell death and involution.[221] Regulatory T cells (Tregs) provide a checkpoint against inflammation during wounding by suppressing multiple cell types including CD4+ and CD8+ T cells, B cells, natural killer cells, and antigen-presenting cells.[204] All of these data are suggestive of classic wound resolution. The association between wound healing and tumor promotion has been recognized as a therapeutic target for decades.[222] This relevance with breast cancer has been recently obtained because mammary gland biopsies in rodents promote lung metastasis through recruitment of immune cells, and a skin wound adjacent to a mammary tumor stimulates tumor progression.[223] Therefore studies support potential for tumor promotional effects of wound healing programs associated with normal gland involution. Investigators developed an immune-competent murine model of postpartum breast cancer. They demonstrated that tumor size is increased sixfold in the involution microenvironment compared to nulliparous hosts.[204] In the postpartum group, mammary tumors have high levels of immature macrophages and reduced cytotoxic T-cell levels, a pattern predictive of poor prognosis in individuals with human breast cancer.[224] Importantly, because involution macrophages have been proposed to be associated with the poor prognosis of postpartum breast cancer, macrophages may be a therapeutic target for blocking the tumor-promotional characteristics of the involuting gland (Fig. 25.32). Additionally, in rodents, circulating estrogens are responsible for recruiting estrogen receptor alpha (ERα) bone marrow cells that promote mammary tumor growth.[225,226]

Widely appreciated is that as women age, their risk of breast cancer increases. But the *rate* of increase of breast cancer *slows* at about 50 years of age.[227] This slowing has been attributed to a reduction in ovarian hormone production. Milanese and colleagues[216] observed a definite increase in the process of involution at about 50 years of age with complete involution present in 5.8% of women ages 40 to 49 years and in 21.6% of women ages 50 to 59 years. Investigators propose that involution may contribute to this slowing in the rate of increase of breast cancer among women older than 50 years. Importantly, investigators found an inverse association between lobular involution and parity.[216] Other investigators have reported that the more children a woman has, the more likely she is to have persistent lobular tissue,[228] which Milanese and colleagues[216] found was associated with increased risk of breast cancer. However, multiparity also has been found to reduce risk of breast cancer.[229,230] This apparent contradiction may be explained by studies documenting that full-term pregnancies after 35 years of age are correlated with an increased risk of breast cancer.[231] In the Milanese study, the age of the mother at each child's birth was unknown.

Henson and colleagues[232] propose that late pregnancy with its concomitant increase in the proliferation of the ductal-alveolar epithelium is likely to interrupt the process of involution, which typically begins between 30 and 40 years of age. Failure to undergo TDLU involution among women with benign breast disease has been associated with progression to breast cancer, independent of other breast cancer risk factors.[233] The activated stromal environment (with the influx of immune cells similar to that which occurs during wound healing) in the process of involution is the "ideal niche" for carcinogenesis.

Major signaling pathways involved in mammary gland involution also are involved in breast cancer.[234] Certain proteases activated during involution modify the extracellular matrix and are implicated in loss of cell anchoring, providing a microenvironment for tumor growth.[234] Further, the normal involuting gland may be in an immunosuppressed state with the transient presence of immune regulating cells that promote T-cell suppression.[204]

In summary, an increase in breast cancer risk following pregnancy may be caused by the *process* of mammary gland involution, which returns the tissue back to its prepregnant state and is co-opted by processes of wound healing resulting in a proinflammatory environment that although physiologically normal can promote carcinogenesis.[214] The extracellular matrix (ECM) is very different between nulliparous, lactating, and involuting glands as shown in Fig. 25.33. Understanding the factors from the microenvironment that control cell function, differentiation, and stem cell renewal is the crux—*the bottom line*—of developmental and cancer biology[235] (see *What's New?* Mammary ECM Directs Differentiation of Testicular and Embryonic Stem Cells to Form Functional Mammary Glands In Vivo).

WHAT'S NEW?

Mammary ECM Directs Differentiation of Testicular and Embryonic System Cells to Form Functional Mammary Glands In Vivo

Investigators tested whether acellular mammary extracellular matrix (mECM) preparations are sufficient to direct differentiation of testicular-derived cells and embryonic stem cells to form functional mammary epithelial trees in vivo. Incredibly, they found that mECMs from mice and rats were sufficient to redirect testicular-derived cells to produce normal mammary epithelial trees within mammary fat-pads. This study, to the best of current knowledge, is the first to demonstrate tissue-specific ECM drives differentiation of cells to form functional tissue in vivo.

ECM, Extracellular matrix.
Data from Bruno RD et al: *Sci Rep* 7:40196, 2017.

Interestingly, oophorectomy, which is associated with a decrease in risk of breast cancer, leads to atrophy of breast parenchyma in young women as is noted in older women. Thus the risk reduction of oophorectomy may be caused by an accelerated involution.[232]

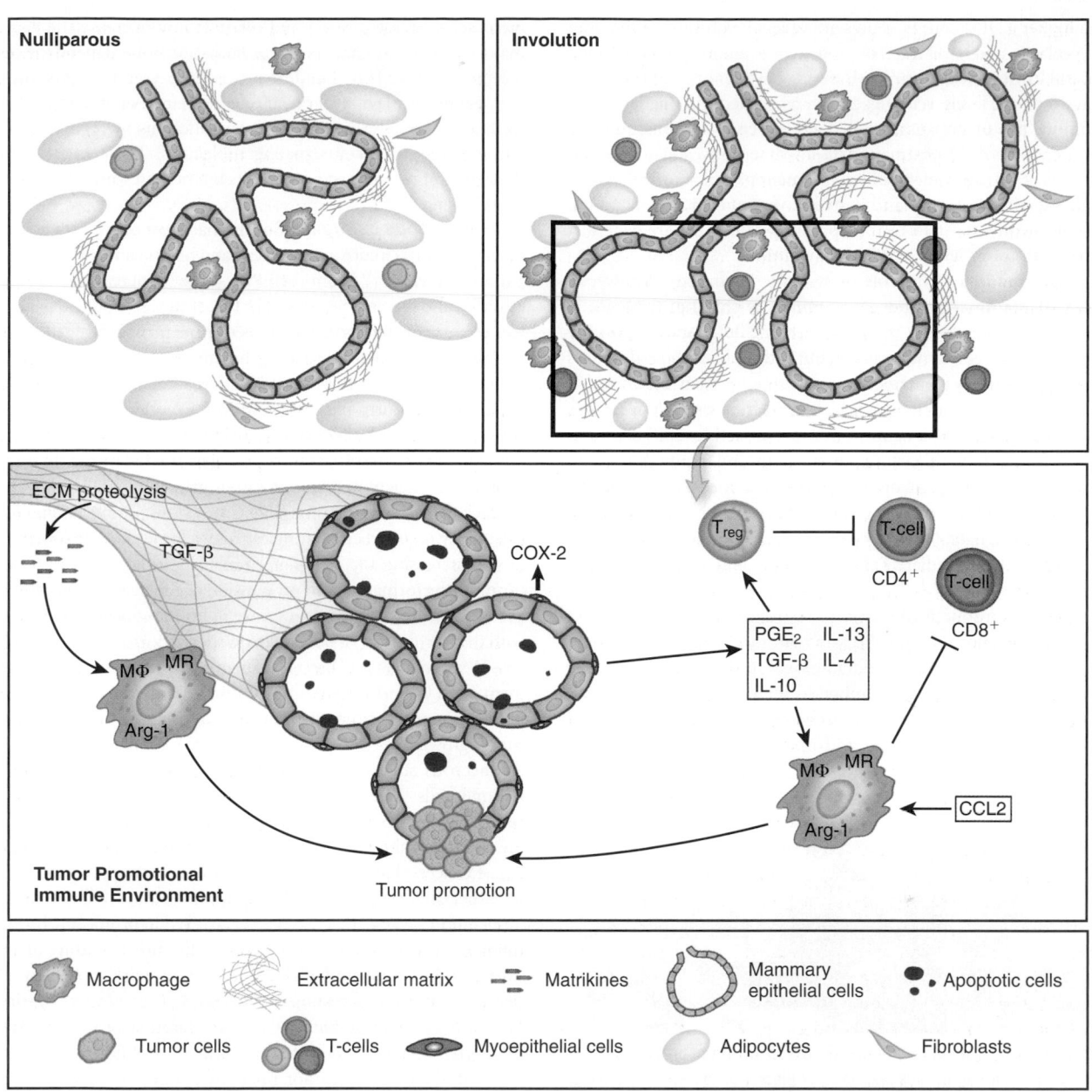

Nulliparous

Involution

ECM proteolysis

TGF-β

COX-2

Tᵣₑ𝓰 — T-cell

CD4⁺ T-cell

CD8⁺

PGE₂ IL-13
TGF-β IL-4
IL-10

CCL2

MΦ MR
Arg-1

MΦ MR
Arg-1

Tumor Promotional Immune Environment

Tumor promotion

Macrophage Extracellular matrix Matrikines Mammary epithelial cells Apoptotic cells

Tumor cells T-cells Myoepithelial cells Adipocytes Fibroblasts

FIGURE 25.32 Macrophages as Instigators of a Tumor Promotional Environment? Macrophages are proposed as the orchestrators of a tumor promotional immune environment during postpartum mammary involution. Also proposed is activated macrophages increase in the mammary gland during involution. Involution macrophages may contribute to tumor promotion through the production of growth factors, such as epidermal growth factor (EGF), and indirectly suppress antitumor immunity. Involution macrophage recruitment and activation are hypothesized as promoted by extracellular matrix (ECM) components, cytokines, growth factors, and prostaglandins, all of which may be immunotherapeutic targets. *Arg-1*, Arginase-1; *CD*, cluster of differentiation; *COX-2*, cyclooxygenase-2; *IL*, interleukin; *MR*, macrophage mannose receptor; *MΦ*, mouse; *PGE₂*, prostaglandin E2; *TGF-β*, transforming growth factor-beta. (Adapted from Fornetti J et al: *J Mammary Gland Biol Neoplasia* 19[2]:213–228, 2014.)

Hormonal Factors

The link between breast cancer and hormones is based on six factors that affect risk: (1) the protective effect of an early (i.e., in the 20s) first pregnancy; (2) the protective effect of removal of the ovaries and pituitary gland; (3) the increased risk associated with early menarche, late menopause, and nulliparity; (4) the relationship between types of fat, free estrogen levels, and oxidative changes in estrogen metabolism; (5) the hormone-dependent development and differentiation of mammary gland structures; and (6) the efficacy of anti–hormone therapies for treatment and prevention of breast cancer. Throughout its existence, the mammary gland epithelium proceeds through critical "exposure periods" of rapid growth or cycles of proliferation, including neonatal growth, pubertal development, pregnancy, lactation, and involution (after pregnancy and postmenopause; see the sections on Lobular Involution and Age and Postlactational Involution).[214,236] Importantly, lack of TDLU involution has been associated with increased breast cancer risk, but the role of sex hormone levels and TDLU assessments is only beginning. Investigators suggest that hormone levels may act, in part, to delay age-appropriate TDLU involution, resulting in a higher quantity of at-risk epithelium.[233] These investigators found significant associations between higher TDLU counts, representing less involution with higher levels of prolactin and lower levels of progesterone among premenopausal women, and higher levels of estradiol, among postmenopausal women.[233] Higher testosterone levels were suggestively associated with higher TDLU counts among postmenopausal women. From a cross-sectional study (*n* = 94 premenopausal; 92 postmenopausal women) investigators found higher levels of estrogen metabolites (premenopausal = unconjugated estradiol, 2-hydroxyestrone, and 4-hydroxyestrone; postmenopausal conjugated estrone and two to four pathway catechols) are generally associated with lower levels of TDLU involution.[237]

The understanding of the role of systemic hormones as powerful regulators of mammary gland development is shifting. Evidence is pointing to the wide-ranging effects of systemic hormones as possibly not due to their *direct* hormone action but rather their *induced* actions from multiple secondary paracrine effectors—thus the term *hierarchical*.[205] Unraveling is a complex model of hormone, paracrine, possibly autocrine, and adhesion molecule–signaling pathways affecting epithelial and stromal cell fate in breast development and cancer. Despite differences between the organized process of development and the less, even chaotic, environment of invasive cancer, both processes share many identical mechanisms and signaling pathways. Key is *tissue remodeling* that applies to pubertal growth, immediately after pregnancy and during involution (see previous section).[214,238,239]

The female reproductive hormones (estrogens, progesterone, and prolactin) have a major role and effect on mammary gland development and breast cancer (Fig. 25.34). Epidemiologic studies show that breast cancer risk increases with the number of menstrual cycles a woman has during her lifetime.[240] Early menarche, late menopause, and short menstrual cycles all increase risk, and menopause (slows the *rate* of

increase of breast cancer) and ovariectomy decrease the risk. A vast majority of breast cancers are *initially* hormone dependent (estrogen receptor positive [ER+] and/or progesterone receptor positive [PR+]), with estrogens playing a crucial role in their development.[241] Estrogens control processes critical for cellular functions by regulating activities and expression of key signaling molecules. These processes include regulation of receptor activity and its interaction with other intracellular proteins and DNA.[241]

Endogenous Estrogen. Substantial prospective data have accrued on endogenous circulating estrogens and breast cancer risk in postmenopausal women.[242-244] From the EPIC study,[245] increasing blood levels of estradiol also increased the risks for breast cancer. Updated analyses from two cohorts of the pooled analysis of nine prospective studies provide strong evidence that circulating hormones are an important marker of increased risk in postmenopausal women and not a result of the production of hormones by a tumor.[246] Emerging data reveal estrogen acting on cells of hematopoietic origin.[225] Coinjection of tumor cells and bone marrow isolated from estrogen-treated mice into nulliparous hosts was sufficient to promote tumor growth.[225] In this model, despite the lack of estrogen receptor (ER) expression, tumors arising following pregnancy required circulating estrogens for their formation.[225] Importantly, increasing the levels of circulating estrogens was sufficient to promote the formation and progression of ER-negative cancers. This was accompanied by a systemic increase in host angiogenesis and coincided with the recruitment of bone marrow–derived stromal cells[225] (see *What's New?* Mammary ECM Directs Differentiation of Testicular and Embryonic Stem Cells to Form Functional Mammary Glands In Vivo). Moreover, bone marrow cells from estrogen-treated mice were sufficient to promote tumor growth. The progression of normal mammary epithelium toward a cancerous state depends on diverse functions of the surrounding stromal cells. The many different mesenchymal cells appear to be recruited into developing tumor masses. Circulating levels of estrogen are at their highest in women during pregnancy, and the majority of breast cancers that develop during this time lack appreciable expression of either ERs or progesterone receptors (PRs).[247,248] This significant observation suggests that estrogen is involved in promoting breast cancer following pregnancy and not through the direct binding of receptors expressed by breast epithelial cells.[225] Recent work shows that estrogen may promote the progression of ER-negative breast cancer by stimulating cancer-associated fibroblasts (CAFs) to secrete stromal-derived factor-1 (SDF-1α), which can recruit bone marrow myeloid-derived suppressor cells (MDSCs) to the tumor microenvironment, which exerts tumor promoting effects.[249]

Evidence for estrogens in modulating the immune environment of the mammary gland comes from studies showing changes in macrophage number and phenotype in the mammary gland across the estrous cycle and with treatment with estradiol and progesterone.[250] In a wound–healing model, estradiol and progesterone promoted an alternative

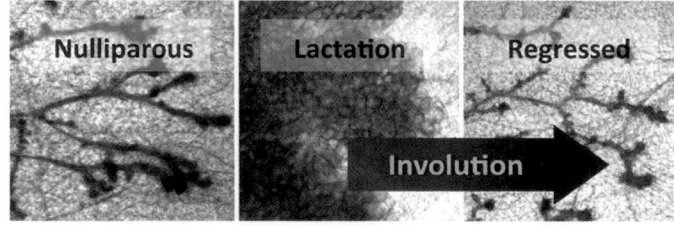

FIGURE 25.33 Extracellular Matrix (ECM) Is Different in Nulliparous, Lactating, and Involuting Glands. Several ECM differences between nulliparous, lactational, and involuting mammary glands are related to collagen-fiber organization, cell motility and attachment, and cytokine regulation in a rodent model. Many protumorigenic ECM proteins are mediators of breast cancer progression specific to the involutional window, and systemic ibuprofen experimental treatment during involution decreases its tumor promotional changes. (From O'Brien JH et al: *J Proteome Res* 11:4894–4905, 2012.)

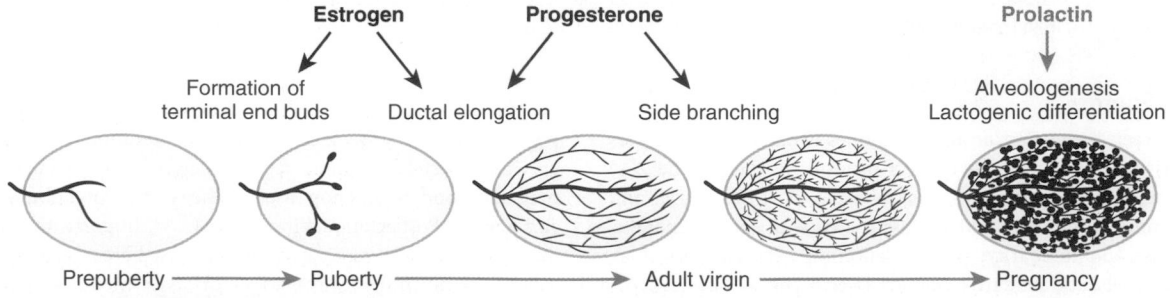

FIGURE 25.34 Mammary Gland Development in the Mouse. Schematic representation of distinct stages of postnatal mammary gland development. (From Brisken C, Hess K, Jeitziner R: *Endocrinology* 156[10]:3442–3450, 2015.)

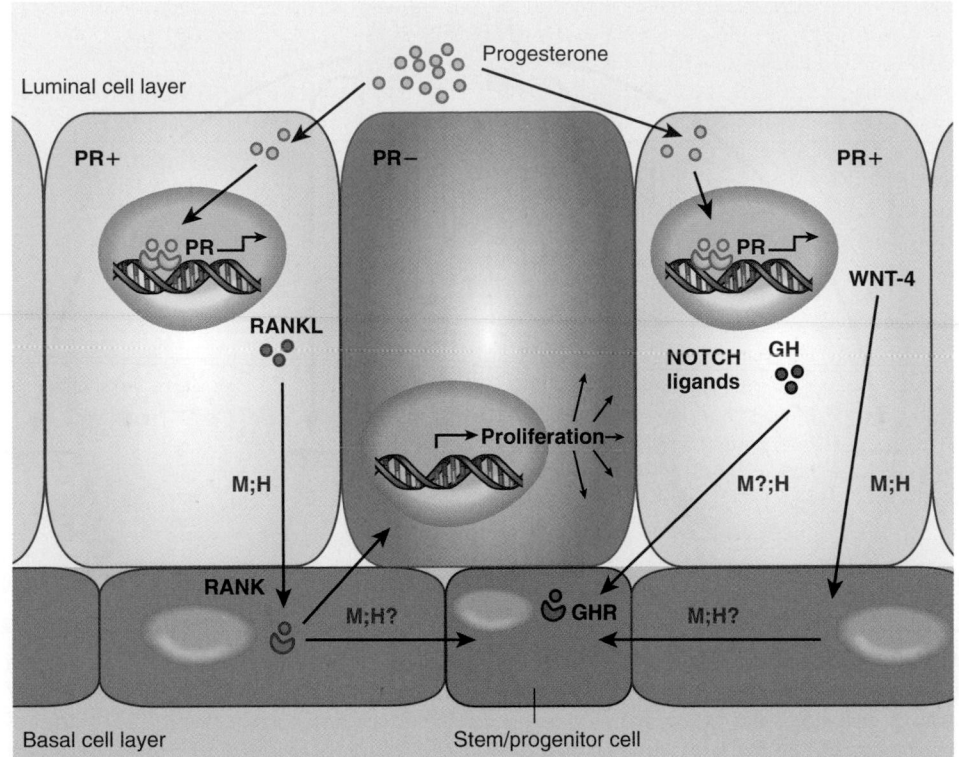

FIGURE 25.35 Working Model How Progesterone Promotes Proliferation in Human Breast Epithelium. After progesterone (P) exposure, P enters a PR+ luminal cell *(blue)* and binds to progesterone receptor (PR). PR moves laterally on the cell membrane (dimerizes) and transcribes target genes (e.g., RANKL, WNT-4, NOTCH ligands, GH). These signaling pathways then stimulate proliferation of neighboring PR− luminal cells *(red)*, possibly also involving cells in the basal cell layer *(purple)*. Not all of these pathways have been shown to be active in both mouse mammary gland and human breast. *GHR*, Growth hormone releaser; *H*, human gland; *M*, mouse gland; *PR+*, progesterone receptor positive; *PR−*, progesterone receptor negative; *RANKL*, receptor activator of nuclear factor kappa-β ligand; *WNT*, wingless-related integration site. (Adapted from Hilton HN, Graham JD, Clarke CL: *Mol Endocrinol* 29[9]:1230–1242, 2015.)

phenotype in macrophages.[251] Estradiol can promote a proinflammatory phenotype in macrophages.[252] In response to estrogen and progesterone, mast cells up-regulate chemokine receptors, maturation markers, and degranulate.[253,254] T and B cells can be directly regulated by estrogen.[255] Estrogen signaling drives the mobilization of MDSCs and enhances their immunosuppressive effects in vivo.[256] More simply, estrogen promotes immunosuppression by promoting the mobilization and accumulation of the immunosuppressive action of MDSCs.[256] Investigators found that removing the ovaries, and thus estrogen production, from mice boosted the antitumor immune response and blocked malignant progression.[256] Estrogen signaling is a critical mechanism underlying pathologic myelopoiesis in cancer.[256]

Endogenous Progesterone. The role of progesterone receptor (PR) signaling in breast cancer is complex and controversial. See the section on Menopausal Hormone Therapy (MRT) and Breast Cancer Risk: Estrogen Plus Progesterone and Estrogen Only (ET) on treatment effects with progesterone. Several types of evidence show that repeated exposure to the luteal phase, and therefore endogenous increased serum progesterone (P) levels, increases breast cancer risk.[257] Confusion exists about the term "proliferative" phase in the first part of the menstrual cycle, the follicular phase. The breast is quiet (quiescent) during the follicular phase. The term proliferative phase is based on changes that occur in the uterus; the endometrium proliferates before ovulation.[257] Postovulatory secretion of P has antiproliferative effects on the endometrium and induces differentiation in the uterine lining.[257] In the breast, cell proliferation occurs during the luteal phase and is accompanied

by changes in the stroma, or microenvironment.[258,259] Moreover, proliferation happens in the TDLUs where breast cancers originate.[257] Data from cancer models show P is now recognized as a major proliferative hormone in both the mouse mammary gland and the normal human breast epithelium.[260] The understanding of how P promotes proliferation in the human breast has grown over the years, mainly from animal studies (Fig. 25.35).

P is required to promote the wave of proliferation, which occurs in early pregnancy.[260] Ovariectomy causes endogenous levels of estrogen and progesterone to decrease significantly. As a result, cell proliferation in mammary epithelium ceases and the epithelium becomes atropic.[257] Emerging from mouse studies is the mechanism by which progesterone triggers cell proliferation, activates progenitor cells, induces branching morphogenesis, affects immune cells, and controls the blood vessels to enable increased blood flow during the luteal phase and pregnancy (Fig. 25.36).[257]

Endogenous Prolactin. Prolactin, produced by the pituitary gland, travels through the blood and exerts multiple metabolic and reproductive effects, especially on the breast as the key regulator of lactation. Prolactin is also produced in other tissues, including the breast (known as *extrapituitary prolactin*).[261,262] Recently, investigators reported that autocrine prolactin is required for terminal mammary epithelial differentiation during pregnancy and production is regulated by the signaling pathway Pten-PI3K-Akt.[261] Although this finding is critical for normal breast development, differentiation, and lactation, it may also be important in breast carcinogenesis because the PI3K-Akt signaling

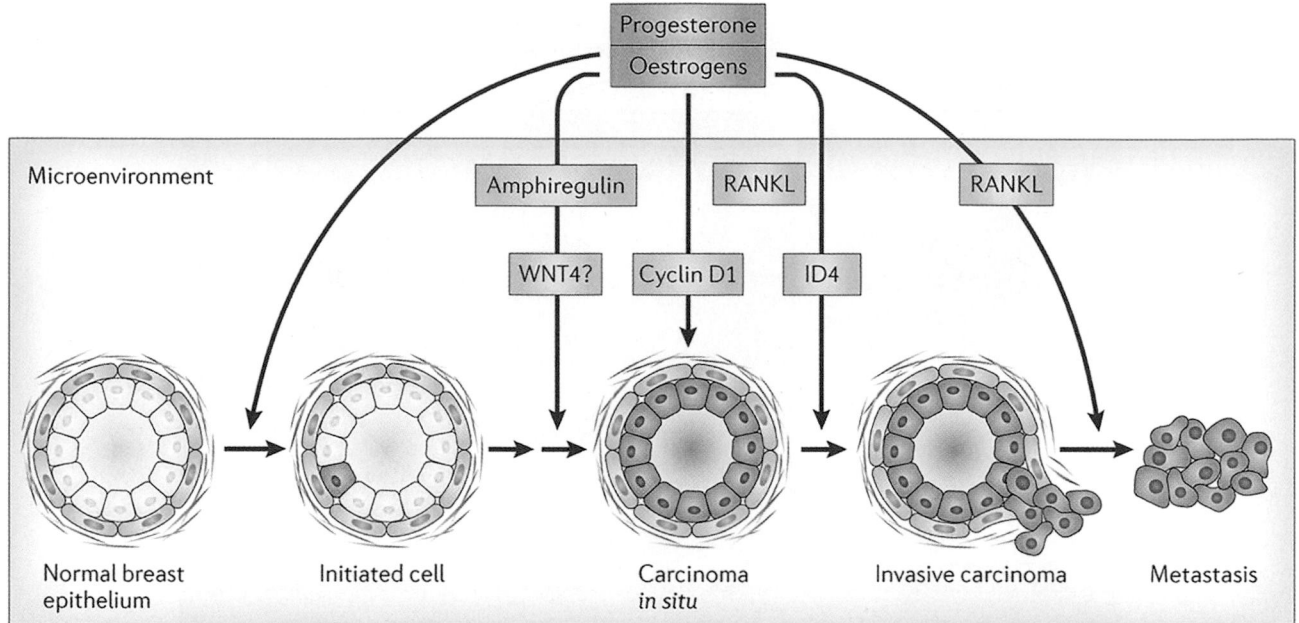

FIGURE 25.36 Working Model of Breast Carcinogenesis and Hormonal Involvement. Cross sections of a milk duct with luminal *(beige)* and outer myoepithelial cells *(green)* are surrounded by a basement membrane *(pink)*. Although early stages of breast carcinogenesis are incompletely characterized, hormones impinge on all stages of breast cancer development. Progesterone signaling is important in determining whether preexisting lesions progress to invasive and metastatic breast cancer. Progesterone changes the microenvironment and activates a number of signaling pathways implicated in the development of different subtypes of breast cancer in the mouse model. Recently developed ex vivo models of the human breast have shown that progesterone promotes cell proliferation. Progesterone promotes stem cell activation in the adult mammary gland. Investigators hypothesize that repeated activation of these pathways during the luteal phase of the menstrual cycles promotes breast carcinogenesis. Some of the factors involved include amphiregulin, receptor activator of nuclear factor-κβ (NF-κβ) ligand (RANKL), and inhibitor of DNA binding 4 (ID4) have been implicated in distinct breast cancer subtypes. (From Brisken C: *Nat Rev Cancer* 13[6]:385–396, 2013; with data from Brisken C, Hess K, Jeitziner R: *Endocrinology* 156[10]:3442–3450, 2015; Tanos T et al: *Sci Transl Med* 5[182]:182ra55, 2013; Wang J et al: *Sci Trans Med* 5[215]:215le4, 2013.)

pathway is commonly activated in human cancers. This suggests the important possibility that autocrine prolactin may play a role in breast cancer. A recent meta-analysis of seven studies supports a positive association between plasma prolactin levels and the risk of breast cancer.[263] Prolactin may inhibit a major tumor-suppressive function of *BRCA1* by interfering with p21.[264] From the Nurses' Health Study, the association with prolactin was more modest than with estradiol;[265] the association was stronger among postmenopausal women and for ER-positive tumors.

Endogenous Testosterone: Androgen Receptor. From the combination of prospective studies, case-control studies, and laboratory data the association between circulating testosterone in postmenopausal women and subsequent risk of breast cancer is now well established.[266-269] Unclear is whether the association with testosterone is direct or indirect (i.e., enzyme conversion by aromatase of testosterone to estradiol) (Fig. 25.37).

The androgen receptor (AR) has been implicated in prostate cancer, and now in the development and progression of breast cancer.[270] The question of whether ARs are harmful or beneficial for individuals with breast cancer is complex and may differ by breast cancer subtype and menopausal status. Investigators used breast cancer cell lines and found that treatment of breast cancer cells with 5α-dihydrotestosterone (DHT) promotes cell proliferation and decreases apoptosis.[270] The reduction of testosterone levels in women with oophorectomy or hysterectomy may also be a protective factor.[271]

Serum Estrogen, Progesterone, Androgens, and Prolactin. Substantial evidence supports a positive association of circulating estrogens, androgens, and prolactin with postmenopausal breast cancer risk.[268] From the Nurses' Health Study the inclusion of endogenous hormones (testosterone, estrone sulfate, and prolactin) to both the Gail score and the original Rosner-Colditz model significantly improved risk prediction for breast cancer among postmenopausal women.[265] Measurements of endogenous hormones improve risk prediction for invasive breast cancer.[268] A recent reanalysis of 13 prospective studies showed that circulating concentrations of sex hormones are associated with several of the established or suspected risk factors for breast cancer.[272] Data identify mammary stem cells (MaSCs) as critical targets for ovarian hormones, especially progesterone surges during the normal reproductive cycle and pregnancy increasing the proliferation of mammary stem cells.[273-276] A key aspect of MaSCs is cytoskeletal function that facilitates cell shape and mobility.[277]

Local in Situ Estrogens (Paracrine). The formation of estrogens in breast tumors may be significant for the growth and survival of estrogen-dependent breast cancer in postmenopausal women. The rationale is based on the following evidence: (1) estradiol (E$_2$) levels in breast tumors are equivalent to those in premenopausal women, despite plasma E$_2$ levels being lower after menopause; (2) E$_2$ concentrations in breast tumors of postmenopausal women are at least 10 times higher than serum levels; and (3) biosynthesis of estrogens in breast tumors

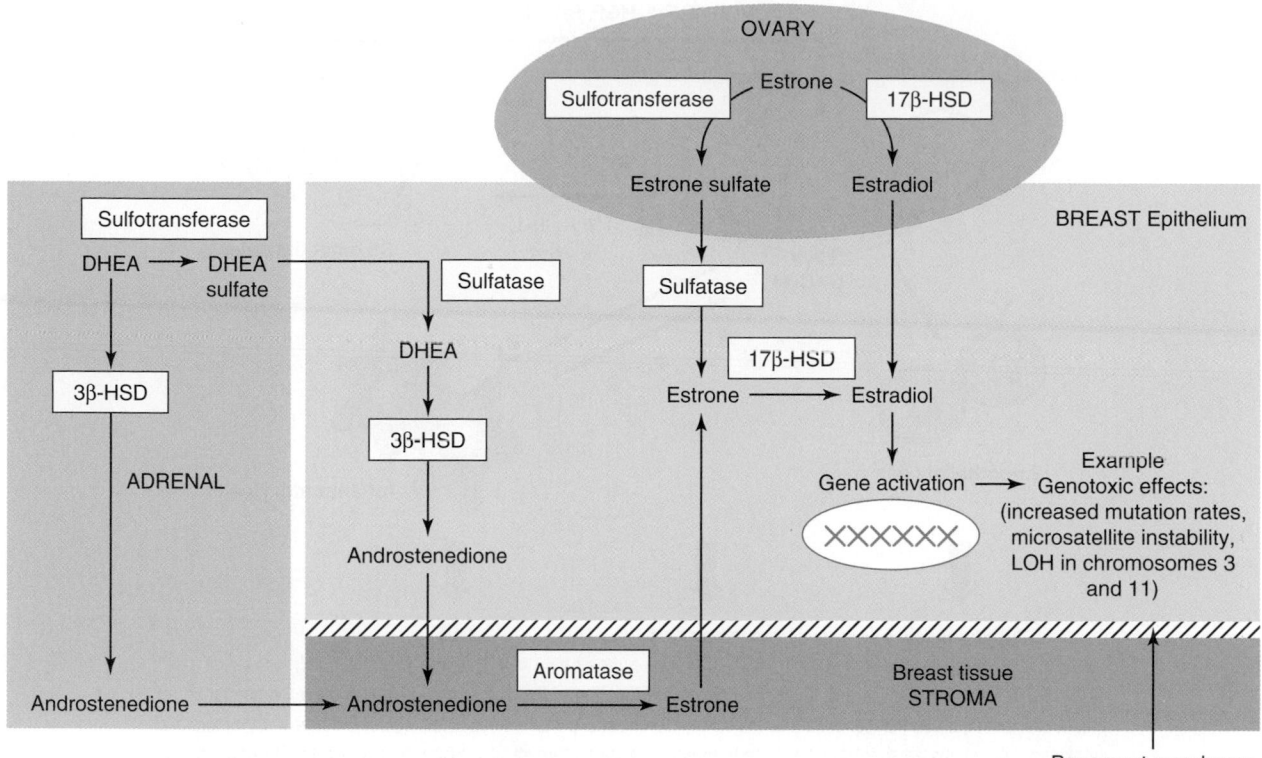

FIGURE 25.37 Local Biosynthesis of Estrogens. Three main enzyme complexes *(yellow)* involved in estrogen formation in breast tissue, including aromatase, sulfatase, and 17β-estradiol hydroxysteroid dehydrogenase *(17β-HSD).* Thus despite low levels of circulating estrogens in postmenopausal women with breast cancer, the tissue levels are severalfold higher than those in plasma, suggesting tumor accumulation of these estrogens. Data suggest that most abundant is sulfatase in both premenopausal and postmenopausal women with breast cancer. Numerous agents can block the aromatase action. Exploration of progesterone and various progestins to inhibit sulfatase and 17β-HSD or stimulate sulfotransferase (i.e., breast cancer cells cannot inactivate estrogens because they lack sulfotransferase) may provide new possibilities for treatment. *LOH,* Loss of heterozygosity (see Chapter 12); *DHEA,* dehydroepiandrosterone. (Adapted from Russo J, Russo I: *Molecular basis of breast cancer: prevention and treatment,* Berlin, Heidelberg, New York, 2004, Springer-Verlag.)

occurs through two different routes: the aromatase pathway and the steroid sulfate (STS) pathway[241] (see Fig. 25.36).

Investigators measured levels of breast sex steroids in both benign and cancerous tissue.[278] Estrogen and androgen concentrations varied greatly in both tissue and blood levels in benign and cancerous tissue.[278] The estradiol/estrone ratio was lowest in premenopausal benign tissue and much higher in premenopausal cancerous tissue and postmenopausal benign and cancerous tissue. Estradiol and estrone levels were substantially higher in tissue than in plasma in both premenopausal and postmenopausal women.[278] Hormone levels in breast adipose tissue revealed high levels of androstenedione and testosterone and significant estrone and estradiol levels in breast adipocytes from postmenopausal breast cancer patients, consistent with an obesity-inflammation-aromatase axis (obesity with inflammation, COX elevation, and increased aromatase, which converts androgens to estrogen) occurring locally in breast tissue.[278] Crown-like structures (CLSs; microscopic foci of dying adipocytes surrounded by macrophages) are proposed as sites of increased aromatization of androgens to estrogen. CLSs were more frequently identified in the breast fat of obese women and were associated with increased ratios of select estrogens/androgens in the blood and tissues but not with individual hormones.[279]

Evidence suggests that the site of conversion of androgens to estrogens in breast cancer is the stroma and not the malignant epithelial cells.[280] Stromal fibroblasts adjacent to the tumor express aromatase and actively induce local estrogen production and signal crosstalk between estrogen and growth factors affecting the progression of breast carcinomas (Fig. 25.38). In the presence of estrogen in mice studies, fibroblasts provided cancer cells (MCF7S1 cell) additional growth capacity.[281] Breast tissue also contains high sulfatase activity and produces estrone through the hydrolysis of estrone sulfate (see Fig. 25.36). Thus quantitatively estrone sulfate may be the most important circulating estrogen in women; it increases the reservoir for the production of estrone and, ultimately, estradiol. It was found that E_2, itself, has antisulfatase action. This paradoxical effect of estradiol could be related to some studies that have found estrogen replacement therapy (ERT) either to have no effect or to decrease breast cancer mortality in postmenopausal women.[282,283]

Estrogen metabolism from oxidation of the parent estrogens, estrone, and estradiol occurs at the 2, 4, or 16 position of the carbon skeleton to yield 2-hydroxylated, 4-hydroxylated, or 16-hydroxylated estrogens, respectively. The 4- and 16α-hydroxylated pathways are potentially tumor promoting; conversely, the 2-hydroxylated pathway has been demonstrated to be less tumor promoting and, possibly, inhibiting.[284] A recent prospective case-control study found nearly all estrogens, estrogen metabolites, and metabolic pathway groups were associated with an increased risk of breast cancer, especially unconjugated estradiol. These investigators found more extensive 2-hydroxylation of estrogens is associated with lower risk and less methylation of the potentially genotoxic 4-hydroxylation pathway with a higher risk of breast cancer

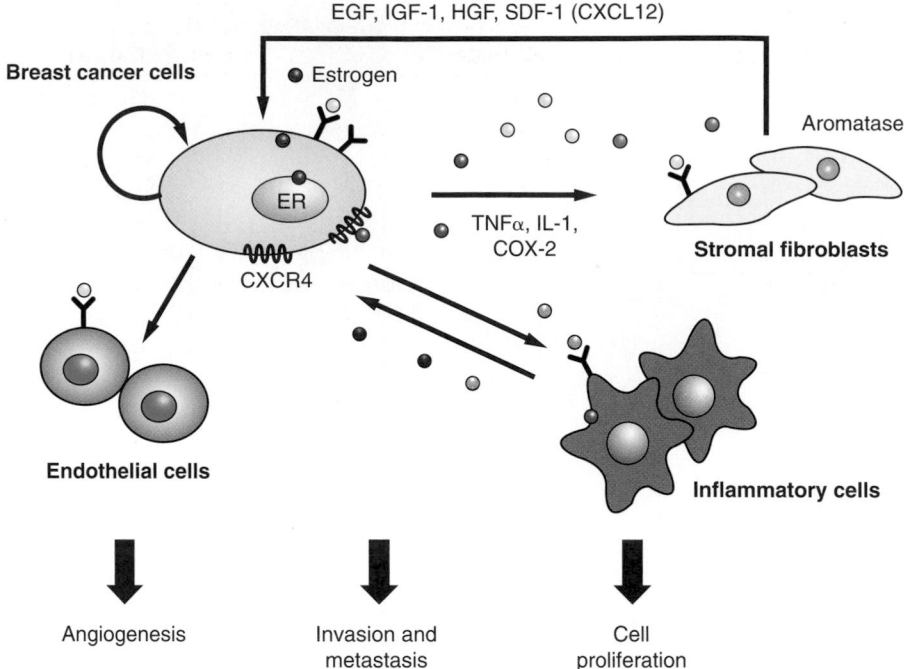

FIGURE 25.38 Breast Cancer Cells and Stromal Fibroblasts Produce Estrogen. In the microenvironment of breast carcinoma, breast cancer cells interact with different stromal cells through the secretion of growth factors and cytokines. Fibroblasts adjacent to cancer cells produce estrogen through the expression of the enzyme aromatase, which is induced by several factors including tumor necrosis factor-alpha *(TNFα)*, interleukin-1 *(IL-1)*, and cyclooxygenase-2 *(COX-2)*. *EGF*, Epidermal growth factor; *ER*, estrogen receptor; *HGF*, hepatocyte growth factor; *IGF-1*, insulin-like growth factor 1; *SDF-1*, stromal-derived factor 1 also known as *CXCL12* or chemokine 12. These interactions lead to cancer cell proliferation, angiogenesis, and metastasis. (Adapted from Yamaguchi Y, Hayashi S: *Endocr J* 56[1], 2009.)

in postmenopausal women.[285] From the Nurses' Health Study a comprehensive nested case-control study found that women who excrete more parent estrogens are at reduced breast cancer risk.[286]

Overall, two main mechanisms of carcinogenicity of estrogens involve (1) a receptor-mediated hormonal activity shown to stimulate cellular proliferation, resulting in increased opportunities for accumulation of genetic damage; and (2) oxidative catabolism of estrogens mediated by various cytochrome complexes (P450 [CYP] system) that eventually activate and generate reactive oxygen species (ROS) that can cause oxidative stress and genomic damage directly. Oxidative metabolites of estrogens can develop ultimate carcinogens that react with DNA to cause mutations leading to carcinogenesis. Thus imbalances in estrogen metabolites in breast tissue correlate with the development of tumors and suggest possible biomarkers related to the risk of developing breast cancer (see *Nutrition & Disease:* Sustained Proliferation in Cancer and Dietary Substances to Block Cancer Proliferation).

Menopausal Hormone Therapy (MHT) and Breast Cancer Risk: Estrogen Plus Progesterone and Estrogen Only (ET).
The Nurses' Health Study (NHS) is one of the largest cohort studies with comprehensive knowledge on hormone therapy (HT) use for more than four decades.[287] Table 25.12 summarizes postmenopausal hormone use and risk of cancer and cardiovascular disease from the NHS and NHSII from 1976 to 2016. Most epidemiologic studies have found an increase in breast cancer risk related to MHT with combined estrogen and progestogens[287-289] (Table 25.13). Evidence comes from observational studies and clinical trials showing an increase in breast cancer risk with MHT current use, stronger among those with longer duration of use, and breast cancer risk disappearing a few years after treatment discontinuation.[290-295]

Similar to the findings of the intervention phase of the Women's Health Initiative (WHI), current use of unopposed estrogen therapy for 5.0 to 9.9 years was not associated with a higher risk of breast cancer in the NHS among postmenopausal women who had undergone a hysterectomy.[290,296] However, longer duration of use, which could not be examined in the WHI, was associated with a trend toward higher risk: use for 20 years or more was associated with a 42% higher risk of breast cancer, especially for those positive for estrogen receptor and progesterone receptor.[287,297] Longer use in animal studies has been linked with increasing cell proliferation, angiogenesis, and inhibition of apoptosis.[298] Longer use of ET that may increase breast cancer risk was found in combined data of 16 studies and another analysis of 52,705 women with breast cancer.[299,300] In these studies and the Million Women Study, leaner women had an even higher risk of breast cancer.[301]

From the NHS, as with the WHI, current use of MHT was associated with a higher risk of invasive breast cancer.[287] The NHS was one of the first studies to quantify the relationship between other types of HT formulations and breast cancer risk.[287] During 14 years of follow-up studies, the use of estrogens (other than conjugated estrogens) or progestins alone was associated with adjusted relative risks for breast cancer.[291] These data from women in the United States confirm the data from European studies.[291] Moreover, with 10 additional years of follow-up, the risk of breast cancer was found to be nearly 2.5 times higher among current users of estrogen plus testosterone than among those who had never used these hormones.[302] Additional support for MHT to increase breast cancer risk was the *reduction* in risk reported by several countries with discontinuation of MHT use.[289,303] The risks associated with transdermal, intranasal, or "natural" estrogens have insufficient data and hypotheses remain unsubstantiated.

NUTRITION & DISEASE

Sustained Proliferation in Cancer and Dietary Substances to Block Cancer Proliferation

Some of the leading natural compounds used in cancer therapy and in chemoprevention are presented below. Early steps in tumor development are associated with a fibrogenic response and hypoxic environment that favors the survival and proliferation of cancer stem cells. Once tumors appear, hormones support growth and metastases (in hormonally-dependent cancers) by promoting angiogenesis, by undergoing **epithelial to mesenchymal transition**, by triggering autophagy, and by taking cues from surrounding stroma. A number of natural compounds

(e.g., curcumin, resveratrol, indole-3-carbinaol, brassinin, sulforaphane, epigallocatechin-3-gallate, genistein, ellagitannins, lycopene, and quercetin) have been found to inhibit one or more pathways that contribute to proliferation (e.g., hypoxia-inducible factor 1, nuclear factor-$\kappa\beta$, phosphoinositide-3 kinase/Akt, insulin-like growth factor receptor 1, WNT, and cell cycle–associated proteins, as well as androgen and estrogen receptor signaling).

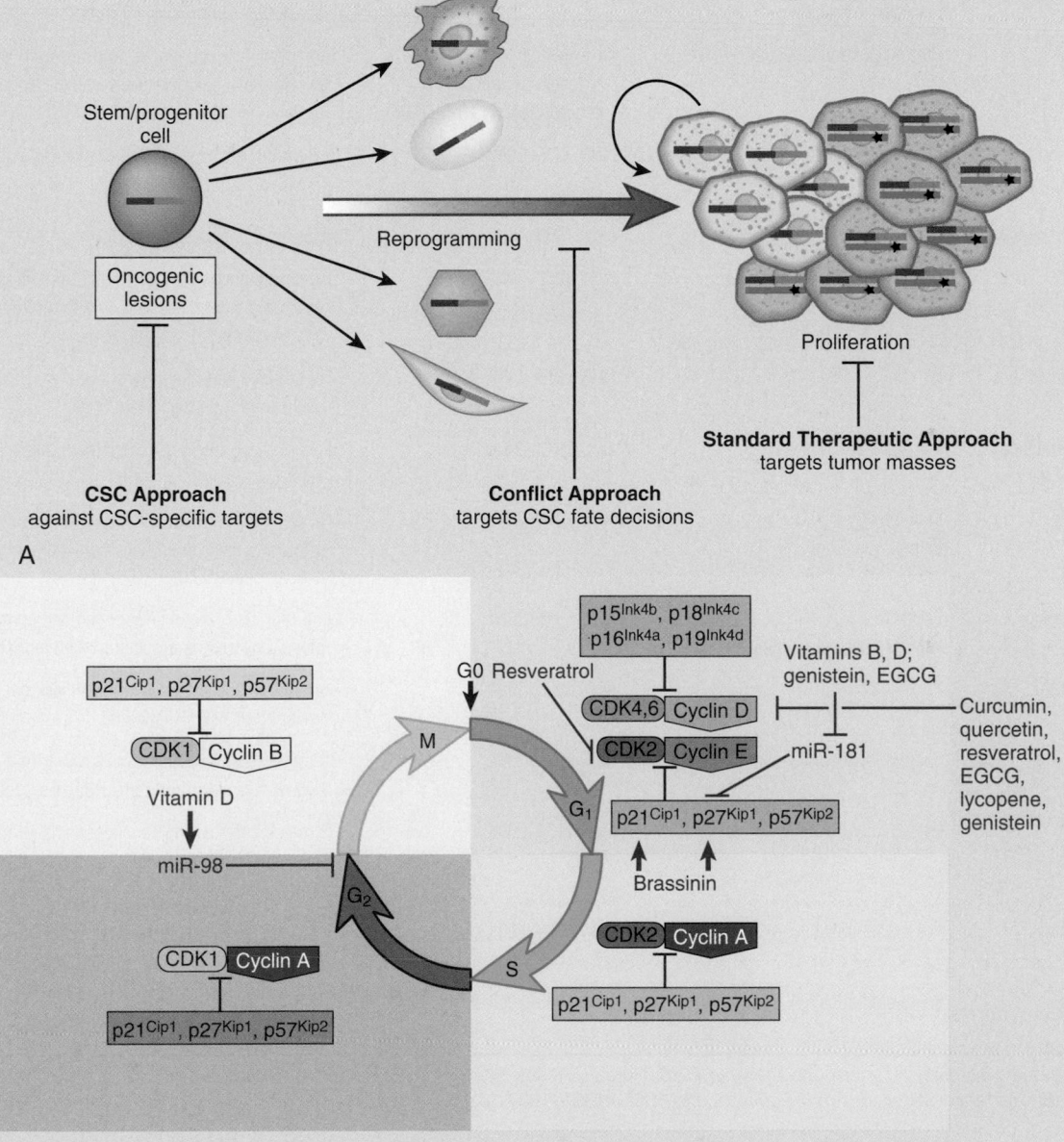

FIGURE Cancer Stem Cells, Proliferation, and Natural Products That Block Cell Cycle Progression.
A, Cancer stem cells (CSCs) arise from tissue stem or progenitor cells that have undergone reprogramming or changes in gene expression as a result of epigenetic mechanisms or oncogenic mutations. These CSCs proliferate and differentiate into tumor cells. CSCs are resistant to most therapies that are effective against the bulk of the tumor. Thus blocking the reprogramming and proliferation of stem cells will be essential to contribute to cancer chemoprevention. **B,** Selected natural products that block cell cycle progression. *CDK,* Cyclin-dependent kinase; *EGCG,* epigallocatechin gallate; *miR,* micron RNA; *p15, p16, p18, p19, p21, p27, p57,* cell cycle regulatory genes. (Adapted from Feitelson MA et al: *Semin Cancer Biol* 35[suppl]:S25–S54, 2015.)

TABLE 25.12   POSTMENOPAUSAL HORMONE USE AND RISK OF CARDIOVASCULAR DISEASE AND CANCER: NHS AND NHS II, UNITED STATES 1976–2016

OUTCOME	EXPOSURE OR HORMONE FORMULATION	POPULATION	SUMMARY OF FINDINGS
Cardiovascular Disease			
CHD	Estrogen / Estrogen + progestin	NHS 1976–2000	Initiation of HT near menopause (<4 yr since onset) associated with lower CHD risk; initiation of HT ≥10 yr after menopause onset not associated CHD risk; current use of estrogen + progestin not associated with risk
Stroke	Estrogen / Estrogen + progestin	NHS 1976–2004	Use associated with higher risk that does not appear to be related to timing of HT initiation
Recurrent CHD	Current postmenopausal HT use	NHS women with previous myocardial infarction or atherosclerosis 1976–1996	Short-term use appears to be associated with higher risk of recurrent major coronary events; longer-term use associated with lower risk
Pulmonary embolism	Postmenopausal HT use	NHS 1976–1992	Current but not past HT use associated with higher risk
Cancer			
Invasive breast cancer	Current HT use	NHS 1980–1996	Higher risk of breast cancer
Invasive breast cancer	Conjugated equine estrogens	NHS 1980–2002	Use associated with higher risk of breast cancer but only after longer-term use and only for estrogen receptor and progesterone receptor cancers
Invasive breast cancer	HT use	NHS 1976–1992	Use of conjugated estrogens alone or with progestins associated with higher risk
Invasive breast cancer	Estrogen + testosterone	NHS 1978–2002	Higher risk with use of testosterone alone or with estrogen
Ovarian cancer	Estrogen / Estrogen + progestin	NHS 1976–2002	Use of unopposed estrogen, but not estrogen plus progestin, associated with significantly higher epithelial ovarian cancer risk
Endometrial cancer	Estrogen / Estrogen + progesterone	NHS 1976–2004	Long-term use (≥5 yr) of estrogen and combined estrogen plus progesterone associated with higher risk
Colorectal cancer	Postmenopausal HT use	NHS 1980–1994	Current use associated with lower risk but apparent lowering of risk disappeared on cessation
Colorectal cancer	Postmenopausal HT use	NHS 1980–2006	Current HT use associated with lower risk for CDKN1A-nonexpressed but not for CDKN1A-expressed tumors
Lung cancer	Postmenopausal HT use	NHS 1984–2006	HT may influence lung carcinogenesis although association is likely modest and altered by smoking status
Renal cell cancer	Postmenopausal HT use	NHS 1976–2004	Current use of estrogen alone or with progesterone not associated with risk
Bladder cancer	Postmenopausal HT use	NHS 1976–2002	Current use of estrogen or with progestin not associated with bladder cancer risk

CHD, Coronary heart disease; HT, hormone therapy; NHS, Nurse's Health Study.
Adapted from Bhupathiraju SN et al: Am J Public Health 106(9):1631–1637, 2016.

The International Agency for Research on Cancer lists estrogen-progestogen menopausal therapy and estrogen-progestogen contraceptives as carcinogenic agents with sufficient evidence in humans for breast cancer (see Table 25.13). Evidence from the Agency for Healthcare Research and Quality (AHRQ, Rockville, MD) published a systematic review from 283 trials comparing effectiveness of treatments for menopausal symptoms.[304] From this report, they state, "Over the long term, estrogen combined with progestogen has both beneficial effects (fewer osteoporotic fractures) and harmful effects (increased risk of breast cancer, gallbladder disease, venous thromboembolic events, and stroke). Estrogens given alone do not appear to increase breast cancer risk, although endometrial cancer risk is increased."

Insulin and Insulin-Like Growth Factors. IGFs regulate cellular functions involving cell proliferation, migration, differentiation, and apoptosis. IGF-1 is a protein hormone with a structure similar to that of insulin. IGF-1 is a potent mitogen after binding to the IGF-1R

TABLE 25.13 HORMONAL TREATMENTS ASSESSED BY THE IARC MONOGRAPH WORKING GROUP

GROUP 1 AGENT	CANCER ON WHICH SUFFICIENT EVIDENCE IN HUMANS IS BASED	SITES WHERE CANCER RISK IS REDUCED	ESTABLISHED MECHANISTIC EVENTS	OTHER LIKELY MECHANISTIC EVENTS
Diethylstilbestrol	Breast (exposure during pregnancy), vagina and cervix (exposure in utero); limited evidence: testis (exposure in utero), endometrium	–	Estrogen receptor–mediated events (vagina, cervix), genotoxicity	Epigenetic programming
Estrogen-only menopausal therapy	Endometrium, ovary; limited evidence: breast	–	Estrogen receptor–mediated events	Genotoxicity
Combined estrogen-progestogen menopausal therapy	Endometrium (risk decreases with number days/month of progestogen use), breast	–	Receptor-mediated events	Estrogen genotoxicity
Combined estrogen-progestogen oral contraceptives	Breast, cervix, liver	Endometrium, ovary	Receptor-mediated events	Estrogen genotoxicity, hormone-stimulated expression of human papillomavirus genes
Tamoxifen	Endometrium	Breast	Estrogen receptor–mediated events, genotoxicity	

From IARC Special Report: *Lancet* 10:13–14, 2009.
Adapted from Cogliano et al: Last updated March 23, 2015; available at: http://jnci.oxfordjournals.org/content/ early/2011/12/11/jnci.djr483. short?rss=1. World Health Organization (WHO): A review of human carcinogens. B. Biological agents IARC monographs on the evaluation of carcinogenic risks to humans, *IARC Monographs,* vol 100(B), Geneva, Switzerland, 2015, Author.

(receptor) triggers a signaling cascade leading to proliferation and antiapoptosis.[305] The growth hormone–IGF-1 axis can stimulate proliferation of both breast cancer and normal breast epithelial cells.[306] A pooled analysis of 17 studies showed a significant association of IGF-1 with breast cancer risk.[307] Interestingly, no significant difference was found according to menopausal status. Joint associations of IGF-1 and estradiol together showed they were related to risk and those women in the top thirds of estradiol and IGF-1 levels had the highest risk. Estradiol increases IGF-1 activity in the breast.[308] Agents to target IGF-1R in triple-negative breast cancer (TNBC) may induce cell protective autophagy.[309] Investigators suggest that elevated IGF levels may define a subgroup of women with high mammographic density and limited TDLU involution, two markers related to increased breast cancer risk.[310] Insulin and IGF-1 receptor family are now known to have a role in macronutrient intake and cancer, diabetes and cancer, and obesity and cancer.[311]

Diabetes is associated with a complex physiology of insulin resistance; increased insulin, estrogen, and growth hormone levels; increased inflammatory levels; and signaling pathways leading to an increased risk of breast cancer.[312] Insulin therapy and sulfonylurea were found to be mildly associated with increased breast cancer risk.[312] A United Kingdom study showed women treated with insulin glargine were not associated with breast cancer risk in the first 5 years; however, longer use may increase the risk.[313] Metformin appears to have a protective role. Much more investigation is needed to understand the role of insulin, insulin-like growth factors, and diabetes mellitus and their associated risk of breast cancer and recurrence of breast cancers. A recent study found women with multiple gestational diabetes mellitus (GDM) pregnancies had a higher incidence of breast cancer.[314]

Melatonin as a regulator of circadian rhythm is the main focus of shift-work and light at night and breast cancer risk. However, tumor growth (in vivo) can be accelerated by light at night (LAN), in part from continuous activation of IGF-1 receptor (IGF-1R) signaling.[308] A recent case-control study of 1679 women exposed to LAN during sleep was significantly associated with breast cancer risk.[315] This study was the first to identify bedroom light intensity and breast cancer risk. Although inconclusive, shift-work and its disruptive effects on circadian rhythms and sleep deprivation at night have been suggested as a risk factor for breast cancer.[316]

Human Chorionic Gonadotropin. Human chorionic gonadotropin (hCG) level increases during the first trimester and then rapidly declines to a steady state throughout pregnancy. Data from rat studies indicate that measurement of hCG levels may be useful in developing new therapies because it has antiproliferative and antiinvasive effects.[317] However, insufficient data exist on the safety of hCG; its role in carcinogenesis is complex and much research needs to be done.[318]

Oral Contraceptives. The International Agency for Research on Cancer (IARC) group confirmed that combined estrogen-progestogen oral contraceptives (OCs) increase the risk for breast, cervix, and liver cancers.[289,319] A recent meta-analysis of 66 studies showed current use of oral contraceptives, nulliparity, and maternal age of 30 years or older at first birth were associated with a 1–1.5-fold increased risk of breast cancer.[320] Current OC use appears to be associated with a higher risk of invasive breast cancer, but risk differs by hormone fluctuations and age.[287] From the NHS, older women's (40 years and older) use of OCs for 10 or more years and past OC use before a first full-term pregnancy were not associated significantly with breast cancer.[321] OC formulations were prescribed in the 1990s in the younger NHSII cohort but current OC use is associated with a 33% higher risk of breast cancer. A higher risk was not observed in past users.[322] Hormones are discussed further in the Pathophysiology section.

Mammographic Breast Density

Mammographic breast density (MBD) is the radiologic appearance of the breast (largely stromal and epithelial tissues) reflecting variations in breast tissue composition (Fig. 25.39). Mammographic breast density appears white or dense on a mammogram, is expressed as a percentage

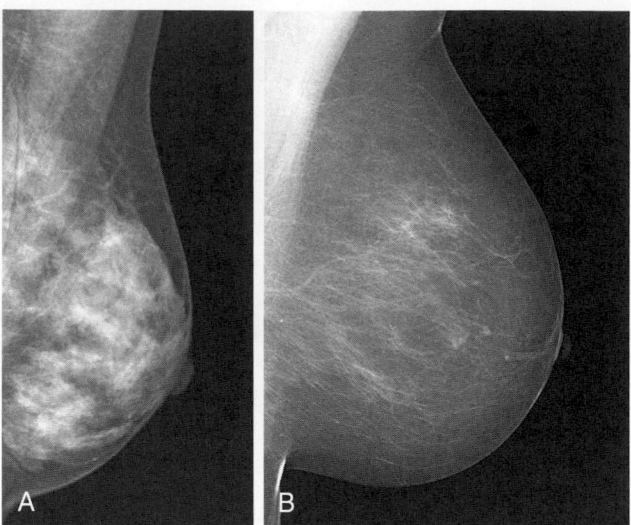

FIGURE 25.39 Breast Density Varies Among Women. The sensitivity of mammography for detecting malignancy is significantly reduced if the breast consists of a high proportion of fibroglandular (dense) breast tissue **(A)** compared to a breast that is fatty **(B)**. (From O'Malley FP, Pinder SE, Mulligan AM: *Breast pathology*, ed 2, Philadelphia, 2011, Saunders.)

of the mammogram (percent mammographic density), and is a strong and consistent risk factor for breast cancer.[265,323,324] A recent prospective study (sample size of 18,437 women) revealed breast density was the most prevalent risk factor for both premenopausal and postmenopausal women and had the largest effect on the population-attributable risk proportion (PARP).[325] Percent mammographic density (PMD) estimates the proportion of stromal and epithelial tissues in relation to fat tissue in the breast. Internationally, studies done in the United States, Canada, and Europe all found that a significant increase in risk is associated with more extensive PMD; risk persisted for 8 to 10 years from the date of the mammogram, and increased with increasing PMD. Extensive PMD is associated with a markedly increased risk of invasive breast cancer.[323] PMD is inversely associated with age, weight, age of menopause, and use of tamoxifen and directly associated with height, parity, family history of breast cancer, and combined hormone therapy.[326] High breast density correlates with collagen level.[327] Investigators suggest that COX-2 has a direct role in modulating tumor progression in tumors arising within collagen-dense microenvironments.[327] CC-chemokine ligand 2 (CCL2) is an inflammatory cytokine that recruits macrophages to sites of injury.[328] CCL2 by mouse mammary epithelium induces a state of low-level chronic inflammation that increases stromal density.[328] Investigators hypothesize that CCL2-driven inflammation contributes to the increased breast cancer in women with high MBD.[328]

Environmental Factors and Lifestyle

The environmental causes of breast cancer possibly affect the breast the most during critical phases or "windows" of development including early differential stages—that is, undifferentiated cells to alveolar buds and then lobules, puberty, pregnancy and lactation, involution, and menopause. During early phases, mitotic activity and cell division are greater than later in life.

Radiation. Ionizing radiation is a known mutagen and established carcinogen for breast cancer. To date, only accidentally or medically induced radiation has been demonstrated to exert a carcinogenic effect on the breast. The Institute of Medicine (IOM) reports that the two most strongly associated environmental factors are exposure to ionizing radiation and combined postmenopausal HT.[329] There are many sources

of ionizing radiation, including x-rays, CT scans, fluoroscopy, and other medical radiologic procedures. Although only about 10% of diagnostic radiologic procedures in large U.S. hospitals are CTs, they contribute an estimated 65% of the effective radiation dose to the public from all medical x-ray examinations.[330] The IOM conclusion of a causal relationship between radiation exposure in the same range as CT and cancer is consistent from a large varied literature.[331] The IOM makes it clear that *avoidance* of medical imaging is an important and concrete step that women (girls) can take to reduce their risk of breast cancer.[332] Scientists and clinicians also have expressed concern about the increasing number of CT scans performed, including on children.[332,333] Radiologic exposure of the upper spine, heart, ribs, lungs, shoulders, and esophagus also exposes breast tissue to radiation. Breast tissue may be exposed from abdominal CT scans. X-rays and fluoroscopy of infants may constitute whole-body irradiation. Epidemiologic studies have shown that adolescent and young women are at increased risk of developing breast cancer following exposure to ionizing radiation compared with older women, and the risk is dose-dependent.[334] The duration of increased risk from radiation is unknown, but increased risk appears to have lasted at least 35 years in women treated for mastitis, those treated with fluoroscopy, and those who survived the atom bomb. Breast cancer rates in atomic bomb survivors in Japan were highest among women younger than 20 years of age at time of exposure; importantly, those who had early full-term pregnancies were at significantly lower risk than those who had not.[335] Thus interacting factors can modulate the risks from radiation. Similarly, young women exposed to high levels of diagnostic radiation have an elevated risk of breast cancer.[334] In women treated with radiotherapy for Hodgkin lymphoma, there is a linear relationship between radiation exposure and breast cancer risk, and women younger than age 20 years at the time of exposure had the highest risk of developing subsequent breast cancer.[336]

Cancer induction and exposure to low doses and low-energy x-rays are controversial and the topic of much debate and research. Biologic understanding related to low doses of radiation is presented in Chapters 2 and 13. Delivered dose and specific low-dose effects are main concerns in radiologic breast imaging.[337] Conventional x-ray mammography is one of the most valuable diagnostic tools for imaging of the breast. Today much use is with full-field digital mammography (FFDM). Continuous technical development has led to several new imaging techniques, including digital breast tomosynthesis (DBT), phase-contrast x-ray imaging, computed tomography of the breast, as well as ultrasound and magnetic resonance imaging (MRI). Despite technical innovations, except for ultrasound and MRI, these modalities require exposure of breast tissue to ionizing radiation and the breast is considered the most radiosensitive organ in the body.[337,338] Therefore it is critical to compare delivered radiation doses to the breast and measure x-ray–induced DNA damage, as well as other biologic effects. A technique for the detection and quantification of in vivo DNA damage has been developed. DNA double-strand breaks (DSBs) are the most relevant lesion induced by ionizing irradiation.[338] After induction of DSBs, the phosphorylation of the histone variant H2AX, named γ-H2AX, is the second most source of DNA damage. γ-H2AX is a visible focus and a reliable and sensitive tool for the determination of DNA damage. Investigators found mammography induces a slight but significant increase of γ-H2AX foci in systemic blood lymphocytes. A clear induction of DNA lesions was found both by FFDM and by DBT.[338] Investigators assessed in vitro mammographic radiation-induced DNA damage in mammary epithelial cells from 30 women with low (LR) or high (HR) family risk of breast cancer.[339] They found the existence of double-strand breaks (DSBs) induced by mammography and revealed by γ-H2AX assay with two radiobiologic effects: a low-dose effect and a low and repeated dose (LORD) effect.[339] These effects were greater in high-risk patients.[339,340]

TABLE 25.14 BENEFITS AND HARMS OF SCREENING MAMMOGRAPHY: SUMMARY OF THE EVIDENCE FROM THE NATIONAL CANCER INSTITUTE

Benefit

- Screening mammography in women ages 40 to 70 years decreases breast cancer mortality (see Magnitude of Effects below). The benefit is higher for older women, in part because their breast cancer risk is higher.

Evidence

- Study design: Meta-analysis of individual data from four randomized controlled trials (RCTs) and three additional RCTs.
- Internal validity: Validity of RCTs varies from poor to good; internal validity of meta-analysis is good.
- Overall consistency: Fair.
- Magnitude of effects on health outcomes: Relative breast cancer–specific mortality is decreased by 15% for follow-up analysis and 20% for evaluation analysis. Absolute mortality benefit for women screened annually starting at age 40 is 4 per 10,000 women screened over 10.7 years. The comparable number for women screened annually starting at age 50 years is approximately 50 per 10,000. Overall, the absolute benefit is approximately 1%, but depends on inherent breast cancer risk, which increases with age.

HARM	STUDY DESIGN	INTERNAL VALIDITY	CONSISTENCY	MAGNITUDE OF EFFECTS	EXTERNAL VALIDITY
Treatment of insignificant cancers (overdiagnosis, true positives) can result in breast deformity, lymphedema, thromboembolic events, or chemotherapy-induced toxicities	Descriptive population based, autopsy series, and series of mammary reduction specimens	Good	Good	Approximately 33% of breast cancers detected by screening mammograms represent overdiagnosis	Good
Additional testing (false-positives)	Descriptive population based	Good	Good	Estimated to occur in 50% of women screened annually for 10 years, 25% of whom will have biopsies	Good
False sense of security, delay in cancer diagnosis (false-negatives)	Descriptive population based	Good	Good	6% to 46% of women with invasive cancer will have negative mammograms, especially if young, with dense breasts, or with mucinous, lobular, or fast-growing cancers	Good
Radiation-induced mutations can cause breast cancer, especially if exposed before age 30 years; latency is more than 10 years, and the increased risk persists lifelong	Descriptive population based	Good	Good	Between 9.9 and 32 breast cancers per 10,000 women exposed to a cumulative dose of 1 Sv; risk is higher for younger women	Good

Data from National Cancer Institute: *Summary of evidence.* Available at: www.cancer.gov/cancertopics/pdq/screening/breast/healthprofessional/page1update 03/30/2012; Nystrom L et al: *Lancet* 359(9310):909–919, 2002.

In agreement with these findings was a low and repeated dose effect and a lack of DNA repair of DNA damage.[341] Investigators from international studies have concluded that diagnostic chest irradiation or radiation therapy for benign or malignant diseases increases the risk of breast cancer for cumulative doses as low as 130 mGy. The breast cancer risk did not decrease when increasing the number of radiologic treatment fractions for delivering the same total dose, but the risk decreased greatly with increasing age of exposure to ionizing radiation.[339] International agencies are assessing the utility of screening MRI and mammography in these high-risk populations. The risk of secondary lung malignancy (SLM) is an important concern for women treated with whole-breast radiation therapy after breast-conserving surgery for early-stage breast cancer.[342] According to a Cochrane review, radiation therapy as a treatment for breast cancer increases deaths from heart disease by more than 25% and much higher for deaths from lung cancer.[343] Investigators studied SLM risk associated with several common methods of delivering whole-breast radiation therapy (RT). Compared with supine whole-breast irradiation (WBI), prone breast irradiation is associated with a significantly lower predicted risk of secondary lung malignancy.[342] These data will be important to compare different breast imaging techniques. The United States Preventive Services Task Force (USPSTF) has updated the recommendations for mammography because of overdiagnosis and overtreatment issues related to screening mammography (also see *What's New?* Breast Cancer Screening Mammography). Table 25.14 presents benefits and harms of screening mammography from randomized controlled trials.

Investigators are looking for markers that are activated by DNA damage. One new marker may be caveolin-1 (CAV1) protein (see Chapter 1 for a discussion on caveolin protein). Caveolin proteins acts as a sensor and early mediator in response to DNA damage and may be important as a biomarker for radiosensitivity.[344]

The pathogenesis of radiogenic breast cancer is unclear. Evidence shows that cancers that develop after radiation exposure have genotypic and phenotypic features that distinguish them from other breast cancers.

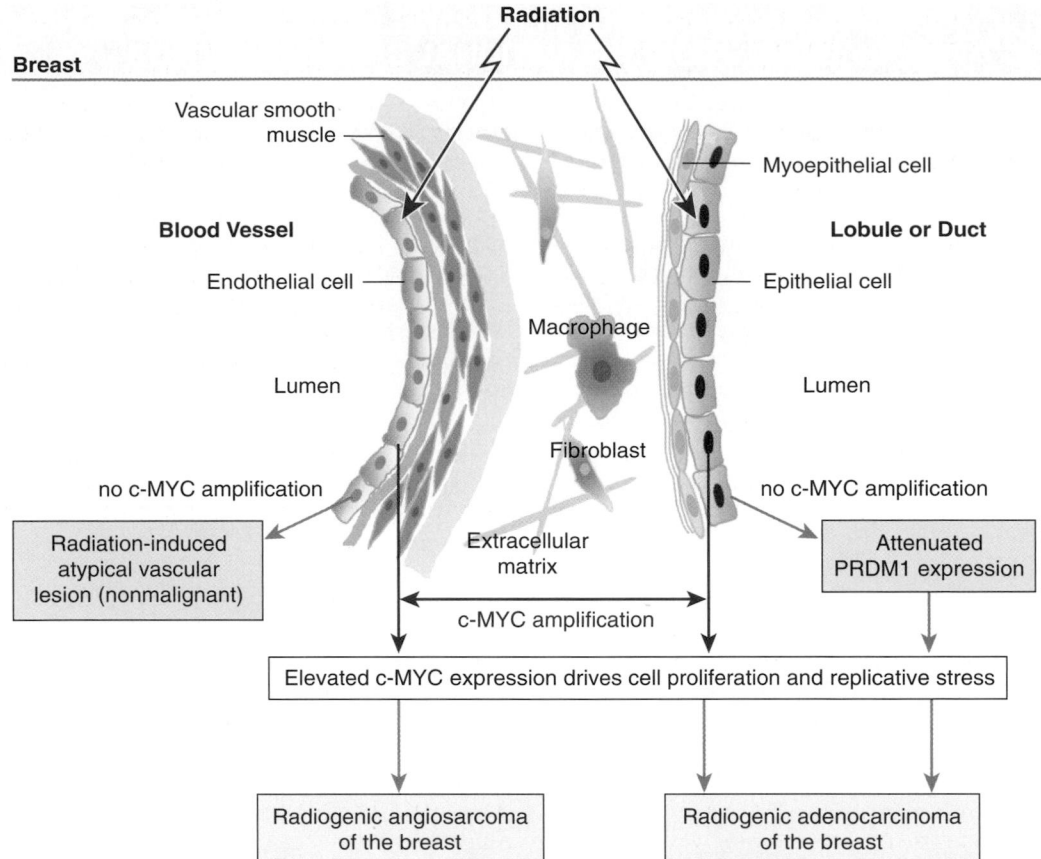

FIGURE 25.40 Working Model of Possible Mechanisms of Radiogenic Carcinogenesis in the Breast. Radiation-induced c-MYC amplifications *(red arrows)* in epithelial cells of the ductal/lobular tissue and in endothelial cells of the vascular tissue (blood/lymphatics) drive the evolving development of radiogenic adenocarcinoma and radiogenic angiosarcoma of the breast. c-MYC amplification of the breast suggests that dysregulation of this proto-oncogene is an early and necessary event in the development of radiogenic angiosarcoma. c-MYC amplification is an early event in the pathogenesis of radiogenic breast adenocarcinoma. (Adapted from Wade MA et al: *Mol Cell Oncol* 3[1]:e1010950, 2015.)

Specific alterations have been implicated in radiogenic breast transformation.[334] These cancers are more likely to be of the human epidermal growth factor receptor 2 (HER2) or basal-like subtypes.[344] Radiogenic breast cancers have a higher degree of genetic instability, such as a higher frequency of allelic loss of chromosome bands 6q13 and 9p21.[345,346] Investigators identified numerous alterations of c-MYC with high levels of c-MYC amplifications.[334] c-MYC protein expression is significantly higher in breast cancers after radiotherapy exposure. Radiogenic breast cancers reveal extensive intratumor heterogeneity with respect to c-MYC copy number, which suggests continuous evolution at this locus during pathogenesis and progression.[334] These data implicate c-MYC as an oncogenic transcription factor in the etiology of radiogenic breast cancer. Elevated c-MYC expression drives cell proliferation and replicative stress (Fig. 25.40).

The interplay between two factors that together may increase breast cancer risk is ionizing radiation and elevated estrogen levels.[347] For the first time, a study was done in rat mammary gland tissue with ionizing radiation combined with elevated levels of estrogen. Combined exposures caused a significant induction of p24/44 MAPK (mitogen-activated protein kinase) and p38 signaling pathways that was paralleled by elevated levels of H3S10 phosphorylation, a well-established biomarker of genome and chromosome instability.[347]

Diet. Prospective epidemiologic studies on diet and breast cancer risk fail to show an association that is consistent, strong, and statistically significant except for alcohol intake, being overweight, and weight gain after menopause (see following discussion).[348,349] Diet has been postulated as important for breast cancer risk because of the international correlations of consumption of specific dietary factors (e.g., fats) and breast cancer incidence and mortality, and because migrant studies show greater incidence of breast cancer among descendants who relocated to another country compared with those in the country of origin. International variations also can occur because of differences in reproductive history, physical activity, obesity, and other factors. Animal models have identified the influence of diet on mammary carcinogenesis.[348]

Dietary Fat. Dietary fat and breast cancer risk is the subject of much study, controversy, and debate. Potential biologic mechanisms between fat intake and breast cancer risk include: (1) that fat may stimulate endogenous steroid hormone production (also affect weight gain, age of menarche), (2) that fat interferes with immune or inflammatory function, and (3) that fat influences gene expression. Animal studies reveal obesity induced by high-fat diets increases the risk of several cancers, including breast cancer.[350] Evidence from large, prospective cohort studies has been mostly unsupportive, and clinical trials have not supported a strong association with total fat intake.[351] Cohort studies, however, suggest a modest positive association between fat intake and the risk of breast cancer;[352] but so far more than 70 studies of the consumption of dietary fat during midlife on risk of breast cancer show the relationship is likely to be small. After 8.1 years of follow-up, the largest randomized controlled dietary trial conducted in the United States showed no significant difference in the number of newly diagnosed breast cancer cases in the women in the treatment group (intervention of a low-fat diet) compared with the control group (usual fat intake).[353] The World Cancer Research Fund/American Institute for Cancer Research (WCRF/AICR) report indicated that although the evidence is limited, there was an increase in breast cancer risk among postmenopausal women consuming higher fat diets.[354] The hypothesis that exposures that occur between menarche and first pregnancy are especially important in determining subsequent risk of breast cancer is supported by several lines of evidence. A first prospective study of 39,268 premenopausal women observed a modest direct association between adolescent intake of fat and breast cancer.[355] This association persisted after adjusting for adult fat intake. Subtypes of fat were not significantly related to invasive breast cancer. Additionally, from this same study, milk, dairy, and total carbohydrate intake in adolescence, as well as the quality of carbohydrate as assessed by glycemic load, glycemic index, and dietary fiber, was not associated with breast cancer. A large prospective study (90,655 subjects) with an 8-year follow-up found that dietary fat does increase the risk of breast cancer recurrence or death in premenopausal women.[356] Concern also has been that any association with fat intake may be because of total energy intake.

A meta-analysis of 57 international and national studies indicates that saturated fat intake was associated with an increased risk for postmenopausal disease, polyunsaturated fats were associated with increased risk regardless of menopausal status, and monounsaturated fats had no significant correlation with risk.[357] Breast cancer risk may be determined earlier in life before the period of investigations.

Red Meat. Another area of study is how consumption of red meat could increase breast cancer risk. The hypotheses range from available iron content, growth-promoting hormones used in the cattle industry, and carcinogenic heterocyclic amines released from cooking the fatty acid content. Case-control and cohort studies have shown a modest association of red meat intake with breast cancer incidence but no association in a pooled analysis of prospective studies.[358] Researchers reported an increased risk with red meat consumption.[359-361] However, a 2010 meta-analysis supported the WCRF/AICR report that suggested there was no conclusive evidence that red meat or processed meat acts as an independent risk factor for breast cancer.[354,362]

Fiber. Fiber intake could affect breast cancer risk by several mechanisms, including stimulation of the intestinal microflora and reduction of the enterohepatic estrogen circulation that could reduce overall body estrogen concentrations.[363,364] Dietary fiber has been shown to modify estrogen concentrations.[365] A recent meta-analysis of prospective cohort studies showed that every 10-g/day increment in dietary fiber was associated with a significant reduction in breast cancer risk.[366] A meta-analysis of prospective case-control studies also found an inverse association between dietary fiber intake and breast cancer risk.[367] Data from the NHS support the hypothesis that higher fiber intake reduces breast cancer risk and suggests intake during adolescence and early adulthood may be especially important.[368]

Similar in structure to estrogens, lignans are biphenolic compounds in plant foods.[369] Primarily found in fiber-rich foods (seeds, grains, vegetables, and fruits), lignans are the major source of phytoestrogens in Western populations.[363,364] Plant lignans are converted in the human gut by intestinal bacteria to the enterolignans, enterolactone, and enterodiol, which are bioactive and are subsequently absorbed.[363] Enterolignans may protect against cancer and several mechanisms have

been proposed and include: (1) they have weak estrogenic activity, and therefore may bind to estrogen receptors (thus preventing other more powerful estrogens from binding to ERs); (2) they inhibit tumor growth; (3) they stimulate apoptosis; and (4) they stimulate production of the carrier SHBG (which presumably lowers circulating free estrogen levels).[369] Two meta-analyses found lignans to be associated with a small risk reduction in postmenopausal breast cancer but not premenopausal,[370,371] and from a follow-up study those postmenopausal women with higher enterolignan levels may have better survival.[369]

Soy. Soy products are a hot topic because of their consumption in Asian countries that have low rates of cancer. Soybeans are the main source of isoflavones. The isoflavone compounds, including daidzein and genistein, can bind estrogen receptors but are far less potent than estradiol. Soy may act like other antiestrogens, such as tamoxifen, by blocking the action of endogenous estrogens to reduce breast cancer risk. Thus depending on the estradiol concentration and the timing of administration, soy exhibits weak estrogenic or antiestrogenic activity. Isoflavones act through various mechanisms by which they may be cancer protective including antiproliferative effects, tyrosine kinase inhibition, induction of apoptosis, and inhibition of angiogenesis. They modulate enzyme activities, as well as signal transduction, and have antioxidant properties. Researchers found that rats fed genistein before puberty had activated T-cell immune response before they started treatment with tamoxifen. Genistein improved response of mammary tumors in rats by reduced activity of unfolded protein response (UPR), prosurvival autophagy signaling, and increased antitumor immunity.[372]

Soy is one of the few plant foods with all the amino acids to make necessary protein.[373] In 2011 the North American Menopause Society held a symposium to review the latest evidence-based science on the role of soy and found that soy foods generally appear to be breast protective and recommended moderate lifelong soy consumption.[195] Specific recommendations for breast cancer survivors and soy or iso-flavone consumption could not be reached, because animals studies indicate potential for risk and studies in humans imply a null or protective effect.[195,374] A recent large study of both American and Chinese women, however, suggested that moderate intake of soy ($\geq$10 mg of isoflavones/day) had a significant reduction in breast cancer recurrence as well as a nonsignificant trend toward reduced all-cause mortality.[375] In addition, soy may optimize extrarenal $1,25(OH)_2$-cholecalciferol or vitamin D_3 (a prodifferentiating vitamin D metabolite), which could result in growth control and, conceivably, inhibition of tumor progression.[376]

Iodine deficiency is hypothesized as contributing to the development of breast pathology and cancer.[377,378] Iodine plays a significant role in breast health.[378-381] Evidence reveals that iodine is an antioxidant and antiproliferative agent contributing to the integrity of normal mammary tissue.[382] Seaweed, which is iodine-rich, is an important dietary item in Asian communities and has been associated with the *low* evidence of benign and breast cancer disease in Japanese women.[382] Molecular iodine (I_2) supplementation exerts an inhibitory effect on the development and size of benign and cancerous tissue.[383] A study in mice showed molecular iodine (I_2) with zoledronate (Zol) as a potent adjuvant therapeutic target for triple negative breast cancer. Combined therapy reduced metalloproteinases 2 and 9, inhibited invasion/migration of cells, and prevented growth of tumor in mice.[384] Nutrition remains a critical area of study.

Data on *dietary patterns* are emerging. The Mediterranean diet includes high intake of vegetables, legumes, fruits, nuts, and minimally processed cereals; moderately high intake of fish; and high intake of monounsaturated lipids coupled with low intake of saturated fat, low to moderate intake of dairy products, low intake of meat products, and moderate intake of alcohol. The Mediterranean pattern was recently reported (EPIC study) to lower overall cancer risk.[385] A case-control study among Greek-Cypriot women found the Mediterranean diet may favorably influence the risk of breast cancer.[385] The Western pattern includes higher intake of red and processed meats, refined grains, sweets and desserts, and high-fat dairy products.

Evidence exists that alcohol consumption increases breast cancer risk. In a report on carcinogens, the National Toxicology Program of the U.S. Department of Health and Human Services lists consumption of alcoholic beverages as a known human carcinogen. The IARC also lists alcohol with sufficient evidence in humans as a carcinogenic agent for cancer of the breast as well as other cancers. More than 100 epidemiologic studies have looked at the association between alcohol consumption and the risk of breast cancer in women.[386] These studies have consistently found an increase in breast cancer risk with increasing alcohol intake. A meta-analysis of 53 studies with a large sample size found that woman who drank more than 45 grams of alcohol per day (approximately 3 drinks) had 1.5 times the risk of developing breast cancer as nondrinkers (a modest increased risk).[387] The Million Women Study in the United Kingdom produced a slightly higher estimate of breast cancer risk at low to moderate levels of alcohol consumption: every 10 grams of alcohol consumed per day was associated with a 12% increase in the risk of breast cancer.[388]

The mechanisms by which alcohol intake increases the risk of breast cancer are unknown; however, proposed mechanisms include: (1) acetaldehyde is a toxic chemical and can damage DNA and proteins; (2) generation of ROS; (3) impaired nutrition decreasing absorption of certain vitamins (vitamin A; nutrients in vitamin B complex, such as folate; vitamins C, D, and E; and carotenoids); (4) alcoholic beverages may contain carcinogenic contaminants (nitrosamines, asbestos fibers, phenols, and hydrocarbons); and (5) physiologic studies have reported an estrogen level increase in women taking menopausal hormone therapy (MHT) and IGF-1 level increases with alcohol intake. Alcohol may increase breast cancer risk through increasing mammographic breast density especially in women at high risk.[389] It is not known whether reducing or discontinuing alcohol consumption in midlife decreases the risk of breast cancer.

Obesity. Excess body fatness is known to increase cancer risk from cellular pathways that involve hormonal regulation, cellular proliferation, and immunity.[390] Obesity, measured as body mass index (BMI), has been associated with a *reduced* risk of *premenopausal* breast cancer. Recently reported (from the Nurses' Health Studies I and II), however, was that weight gain or weight loss since age 18 did not significantly decrease the risk of premenopausal breast cancer.[391] Other data measuring adiposity using waist/hip ratio (WHR) have not found a reduced risk, but rather no association (null) nor an increased risk. Excess adiposity is positively associated with breast cancer recurrence and breast cancer specific mortality among both premenopausal and postmenopausal women.[392]

In 2002 the International Agency for Research on Cancer (IARC) concluded that excess body weight (EBW) increased the risk of developing postmenopausal breast, colorectum, endometrium, kidney, and esophageal adenocarcinoma.[393] Numerous studies have observed increasing adult BMI and postmenopausal breast cancer, particularly for estrogen-receptor positive tumors.[394] The World Cancer Research Fund (WCRF) concluded that evidence is convincing and that a probable association exists between body fat and postmenopausal breast cancer.[354]

Weight gain may be more strongly related to postmenopausal breast cancer risk than attained weight.[393-399] A meta-analysis of 11 studies suggests that adult weight gain is predictive of a twofold increase in the risk for ER+, as well as ER+/PR+, breast tumors with a greater risk in postmenopausal women.[400] Premenopausal and postmenopausal weight gain also is associated with higher estradiol and estrone levels

and lower SHBG levels as a transporter protein; low levels cause higher bioavailable estrogen.[395] This increase in estrogens, particularly estradiol, is from aromatization in the adipose tissue. Second, use of exogenous hormones postmenopausally obscures the variation in endogenous estrogens caused by adiposity and elevates breast cancer risk regardless of body weight.[396] Excess body fat and weight gain are stronger risk factors for women who do not use hormone therapy. However, a prospective study found weight gained at multiple time points throughout adulthood of 44 to 63 lb was associated with a 56% higher risk of breast cancer, and weight gain of 88 to 108 lb doubled the risk of breast cancer among hormone users.[401] A recent animal study showed obese animals deposited excess calories into the tumors themselves.[402] These tumors from obese animals had an increased expression of progesterone receptors.[402]

Obesity is associated with poor survival among women with breast cancer, and the association of obesity with mortality from breast cancer appears to be stronger than its association with incidence.[396,398] The increase in breast cancer risk with increasing BMI among postmenopausal women is most likely the result of increases in levels of estrogens by aromatase activity in adipose tissue.[354] However, studies of hormones secreted by adipose tissue, *leptin* and *adiponectin,* may underlie the association between obesity and breast cancer risk. Increasing BMI and central fat deposition are associated with increased risk for breast cancer in prospective studies, and in vitro studies have shown leptin-stimulated breast carcinogenesis.[403,404] From molecular mechanism studies, leptin enhances breast cancer cell proliferation by inhibiting cell death (proapoptosis) signaling pathways and by increasing in vitro sensitivity to estrogens.[405] Leptin secreted by adipocytes and fibroblasts in the microenvironment act on breast cancer cells in a paracrine manner.[406] Adiponectin has been shown to exert antiproliferative effects in vitro on human breast cancer cells.[405] Additionally, factors that may be related to recurrence of breast cancer in women with excess adiposity at the time of diagnosis include cytokines, IGF or immune function, or both.[390]

Synthetic Chemicals. Evidence for linking synthetic chemicals to the cause of breast cancer is difficult to obtain. It is challenging because it is a life history of exposure that is important, not just a single chemical but also complex mixtures of chemicals and their interaction with endogenous hormones. The highest rates of breast cancer are found in superindustrialized countries—North America and Europe—and the lowest rates in central Africa and Asia. With industrial development, breast cancer rates increase. An estimated 100,000 synthetic chemicals are registered for use today in the United States, another 1000 or more are added each year, and toxicologic screening for these chemicals is minimal—only about 7%.[407] In 2006, more than 34 million metric tons of chemicals were produced or imported into the United States every day and chemical production is projected to double over the next 25 years.[408] Current approaches to chemical screening are being reenvisioned. Several major federal research initiatives were instigated, including the EPA, ToxCast, the National Toxicology Program (NTP) High Throughput Screening Initiative, and the Interagency Tox21 Initiative.[409] New important end points will include altered mammary gland development, Her2 activation, progesterone receptor activity, prolactin effects, and aspects of estrogen receptor β activity.[409]

Chemicals persist in the environment, accumulate in adipose tissue, interact with local adipose tissue physiology in an endocrine-paracrine manner, and remain in breast tissue for decades. Some of these chemicals are known human carcinogens and many have been linked to mammary tumors in animals. Women who emigrate to the United States from Asian countries experience an enormous percent increase in risk within one generation. A generation later their daughters' risk approaches that of women born in the United States. This change in risk suggests that in utero exposures affect subsequent disease risk. However, it is difficult to know whether these changes in risk are derived from nutritional content, pollutants, cosmetics, food additives, or other factors.

Xenoestrogens are synthetic chemicals that mimic the actions of estrogens and are found in many pesticides, fuels, plastics, detergents, and drugs. Because many factors correlated with breast cancer (e.g., early menarche, delayed pregnancy and breast-feeding, and late menopause) are associated with lifetime exposure to estrogens, investigators reasoned that environmental chemicals affect estrogen metabolism and contribute to breast cancer. The most significant chemicals may be polychlorinated biphenyls (PCBs), pesticides, BPA (pervasive in polycarbonate plastics), tobacco smoke (active and passive), dioxins (vehicle exhaust, incineration, contaminated food supply), alkylphenols (detergents and cleaning products), metals, phthalates (makes plastics flexible, some cosmetics), parabens (antimicrobials), food additives (recombinant bovine somatotropin [rBST] and zeranol to enhance growth in cattle and sheep), MHT (i.e., HRT), and others. Bisphenol A treatment of breast epithelial cells cultured from premalignant biopsied tissue elicited a genetic expression profile associated with large, high–histologic-grade breast tumors.[410] Some chemicals are fat soluble and the estrogenic effect would require either that they bind to the nuclear estrogen receptor and then cause cell division or gene transcription or that they activate reactive oxygen species through oxidative catabolism of estrogens (see the section on Hormonal Factors) (Table 25.15).

Physical Activity. Physically active individuals have lower rates of many cancers and improved cancer outcomes.[411,412] Activity also may reduce the invasiveness of breast cancer.[413] A sedentary lifestyle may increase cancer risk through several mechanisms including increased insulin resistance, increased inflammation, and decreased immune function.[414] Epidemiologic studies demonstrated that physical activity lowered the risk of breast cancer mortality in breast cancer survivors and improved their physiologic and immune functions.[414] In a 2013 meta-analysis of 31 prospective studies, the average breast cancer risk reduction with physical activity was 12%.[415] Although the evidence is stronger for postmenopausal women, physical activity has been associated with reduced risk in both premenopausal and postmenopausal women.[416] Mechanisms for this protective effect are not known but include

alterations in endogenous free radical formation and oxidative damage, effects on DNA repair capacity, changes in circulating insulin and insulin-related pathways, inflammation, alteration in carcinogen-metabolizing enzymes, increased intestinal transit times (i.e., reduced exposures to carcinogens), weight loss, and changes in endogenous sex hormone levels and possibly immune cell levels.

Inherited Cancer Syndromes, Genes, Epigenetic Considerations

The causes of breast cancer have been difficult to define because each woman has a different genetic profile called genetic heterogeneity.[417] Genetic heterogeneity is common among individuals but also at the level of the tumor itself, involving both genetic and epigenetic processes. Phenotypic heterogeneity is the result of tumor cell plasticity and together with the genetic background of the tumor determines whether cells resist environmental stress, such as microenvironmental stressors (for example, becoming hypoxic, entering dormancy [see Chapter 12]) and metastasizing.[418] The genetic factors interact with environmental factors. These facts are sobering and make the understanding of the genetic driving force behind tumor initiation, progression, and metastasis very complicated. Driver mutations are causally implicated in tumor development. Investigators examined the genomes of 100 tumors for somatic mutations and found they varied markedly between individual tumors.[417] Several new driver mutations were identified, including AKT2, ARIDIB, CASP8, CDKN1B, MAP3K1, MAP3K13, NCOR1, SMARCD1, and TBX3 (Fig. 25.41). A novel 95-gene signature of residual breast cancer risk, which integrates lymph nodal status, has better clinical utility for early recurrence than the currently available multiparametric tests.[419]

A history of breast cancer in first-degree relatives (mother or sister) increases a woman's risk about 2 to 3 times. Risk increases even more if two first-degree relatives are involved, especially if the disease occurred before menopause and was bilateral. A small total proportion of breast cancers (5% to 10%, although the prevalence is significant) is the result of highly penetrant dominant genes (i.e., hereditary breast cancers). The most important of the dominant genes are the breast cancer susceptibility genes (BRCA1, BRCA2). BRCA1 (breast cancer 1 gene), located on chromosome 17, is a tumor-suppressor gene; therefore any

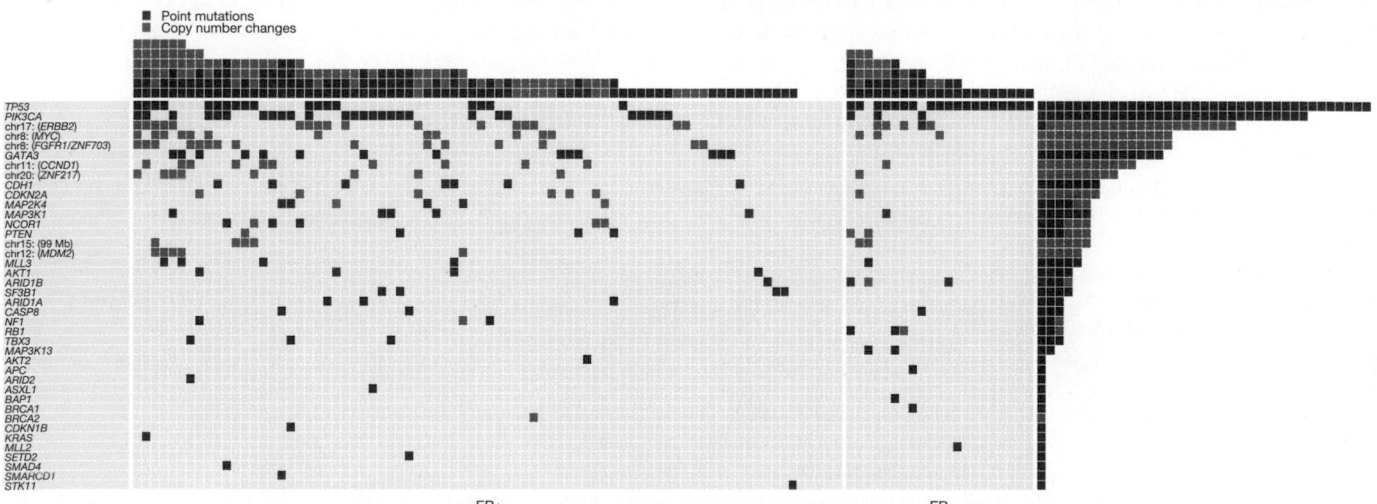

FIGURE 25.41 Driver Mutations and Copy Number Changes in Breast Cancer. The left side identifies each of the 40 cancer genes in which a driver mutation or copy number change has been identified. From investigation of 100 tumors, the number of mutations in each gene is shown (rows) as is the number of driver mutations in each breast cancer (columns). Point mutations are red and copy number changes are blue. (From Stephens PJ et al: *Nature* 486:400–404, 2012.)

TABLE 25.15　SELECTED CHEMICALS AND RISK OF BREAST CANCER

CHEMICAL	COMMENTS
Bisphenol-A (BPA)	Studies have shown altered reproductive systems and breast tissue when exposed to BPA in utero[1] BPA is commonly found in plastics[2]
Polyvinyl chloride (PVC)	Used in food packaging, medical products, appliances, cars, toys, credit cards, rainwear[3] Has been found in the air near waste sites, landfills, and tobacco smoke Has been linked to increased mortality from breast and liver cancer among manufacturing workers[4,5]
Pesticides: aldrin and dieldrin (organochlorines)	Used in crops like corn and cotton from 1950s to 1970s Banned by the EPA in 1975 except for termite control; completely banned in 1987 In vitro assays showed estrogenic activity and dieldrin found in 78% of women diagnosed with breast cancer[6] High incidence of breast cancer in Massachusetts study found associations with higher income and regular use of lawn services, termite treatments, and home pesticides[7]
Household products: methylene chloride	Spray paints and paint removers may contain methylene chloride, documented breast cancer in laboratory animals[8]
Diethylstilbestrol (DES)	Prescribed for women to avert miscarriages between 1941 and 1971 Exposed daughters known to have higher rates of vaginal cancer; and in the mothers, slight increased risk of breast cancer[9,10] Daughters now known to have slight increased risk of breast cancer[11]
Solvents (e.g., benzene, toluene, trichloroethylene, chlorinated organic solvents)	Used in manufacture of computers, also some in cosmetics In 2003 a Taiwanese study documented increased risk of breast cancer among electronic workers exposed to chlorinated organic solvents[12] A Danish study of women 22 to 55 years of age employed in industries (fabricated metal, lumber, furniture, printing, textiles) using solvents doubled the risk of breast cancer[13]
Styrene, carbon tetrachloride, formaldehyde	A 1995 study suggested increased risk with occupational exposure—validation in Finland, Sweden, and Italy[14–17]
Ethylene glycol methyl ether (EGME)	A Duke University study found it acts as a hormone sensitizer in vivo and in vitro.[18,19] Compounds are found in semiconductor industry, varnishes, paints, dyes, and fuel additives
Valproic acid (anticonvulsant medication)	Found to be hormone-sensitizing and prescribed for migraines and bipolar disorder[18,19]
1,3-butadiene	Air pollutant and synthetic rubber product and some fungicides and tobacco smoke Causes mammary and ovarian tumors in female mice and rats[20,21]
Aromatic amines (heterocyclic, polycyclic, monocyclic)	Found in plastics, tobacco smoke, grilled meats and fish, combustion of wood chips and rubber Exposure in adolescence before full-term pregnancy may increase risk[22]
Dichlorodiphenyltrichloroethane (DDT) and polychlorinated biphenyls (PCBs)	PCB used in manufacture of electrical equipment[23] PCB and DDT are banned in the United States since 1970s but are still found in body fat, as well as breast milk[24] DDT was used as pesticide for insects on farms and swamps PCB deteriorates slowly in soil PCB is difficult to study because it is a diverse class of compounds A 1999 in vitro study showed PCBs proliferate in breast cancer cells[25] Conflicting results; several large studies failed to show relationship with PCBs
Polycystic aromatic hydrocarbons (PAHs, including tobacco)	Found in soot and fumes from fuels Increased DNA damage (DNA adducts) implicated from the Long Island Breast Cancer Study Project[26] Tobacco smoke also contains PAHs Smokers who began smoking as adolescents have an increased risk of breast cancer[27–29] In 2004 the California EPA concluded that environmental tobacco smoke (ETS) increases the risk of breast cancer, and the association appears stronger for premenopausal women[30] Tobacco smoke also contains the carcinogens polonium-210, vinyl chloride, benzene, and 1,3-butadiene[31]
Dioxin	Products containing PVC, PCBs, or other chlorinated compounds release dioxin from incineration Declared a known carcinogen by the EPA in 2000 It may be the most prevalent of all toxic chemicals Occurs in meat, poultry, dairy products, and human breast milk A United Kingdom study linked dioxin to the development of mammary tumors in mice[32] A study in Seveso, Italy, connected dioxin with breast cancer[33]
Ethylene oxide	Used to sterilize surgical instruments and in some cosmetics Linked to breast cancer in women exposed to ethylene oxide in commercial sterilization facilities[34]

TABLE 25.15   SELECTED CHEMICALS AND RISK OF BREAST CANCER—cont'd

References

1 Markey CM et al: *Biol Reprod* 65(4):1215–1223, 2001.

2 Infante PF, Pesak J: *J Occup Med* 36(8):826–831, 1994.

3 Chiazze L Jr, Ference LD: *Env Health Perspect* 41:137–143, 1981.

4 Hoyer AP et al: *Lancet* 352(9143):1816–1820, 1998.

5 Maxwell NI et al: *Newton breast cancer study*, Newton, MA, 1999, Silent Spring Institute.

6 National Toxicology Program (NTP): *Chemicals associated with site-specific tumor induction in mammary glands*, 2003. Available at: http://ntp-server.niehs.nih.gov/htdocs/sites/MAMM.html.

7 Colton T et al: *JAMA* 269(16):2096–2100, 1993.

8 Herbst AL, Scully RE: *Cancer* 25(4):745–757, 1970.

9 Palmer JR et al: *Cancer Causes Control* 13(8):753–758, 2002.

10 Chang YM et al: *Indust Health* 41(2):77–87, 2003.

11 Hansen J: *Am J Ind Med* 36(1):43–47, 1999.

12 Belli S et al: *Scand J Work Environ Health* 18(1):64–67, 1992.

13 Walrath J et al: *Am J Public Health* 75(8):883–885, 1985.

14 Weiderpass E et al: *Am J Ind Med* 36(1):48–53, 1999.

15 Wennborg H et al: *Am J Ind Med* 35(4):382–389, 1999.

16 Almekinder JL et al: *Fund Appl Toxicol* 38(2):191–194, 1997.

17 Jansen MS et al: *Proc Natl Acad Sci U S A* 101(18):7199–7204, 2004.

18 Melnick RL et al: *Carcinogenesis* 20(5):867–878, 1999.

19 National Toxicology Program (NTP), *U.S. Department of Health and Human Services: Toxicology and carcinogenesis studies of 1,3-butadiene (CAS No 106-99-0) in B6C3F1 mice (inhalation studies)*, NTP TR 434, NIH Pub No 93-3165, Research Triangle Park, NC, 1993, National Institutes of Health.

20 DeBruin LS, Josephy PD: *Environ Health Perspect* 110(S1):119–128, 2002.

21 Evans N: *State of the evidence: what is the connection between the environment and breast cancer?* ed 3, San Francisco, 2004, Breast Cancer Fund.

22 Zheng T et al: *Am J Epidemiol* 150(5):453–458, 1999.

23 Hatakeyama M, Matsumura F: *J Biochem Molec Toxicol* 13(6):296–302, 1999.

24 Gammon MD et al: *Cancer Epidemiol Biomark Prev* 11(8):677–685, 2002.

25 Band PR et al: *Lancet* 360(9339):1044–1049, 2002.

26 Calle EE et al: *Am J Epidemiol* 139(10):1001–1007, 1994.

27 Johnson KC, Hu J, Mao Y: *Cancer Causes Control* 11(3):211–221, 2000.

28 California Environmental Protection Agency: *Draft Report Part B, chap* 7:147, 2004.

29 Kilthau GF: *Radiol Tech* 67(3):217–222, 1996.

30 Brown NM et al: *Carcinogenesis* 19(9):1623–1629, 1998.

31 Warner MB et al: *Environ Health Perspect* 110(7):625–628, 2002.

32 Steenland K et al: *Cancer Causes Control* 14(6):531–539, 2003.

33 Dorn J et al: *Med Sci Sports Exercise* 35(2):278–285, 2003.

34 Friedenreich CM, Orenstein MR: *J Nutr* 132(11 Suppl):3464S–3465S, 2002.

mutation in the gene may inhibit or retard its suppressor function, leading to uncontrolled cell proliferation. *BRCA2* (breast cancer 2 gene) is located on chromosome 13. A family history of both breast cancer and ovarian cancer increases the risk that an individual with breast cancer carries a *BRCA1* mutation.[420] Carriers of the *BRCA1* gene also are at higher risk for ovarian cancer. The risks for breast or ovarian cancer, or both, however, are not equal in all mutation carriers and have been found to vary by several factors, including type of cancer, age at onset, and position of mutation.[420] This observed variation in penetrance has led to the hypothesis that other genetic and/or environmental factors modify cancer risk in mutation carriers. Men who develop breast cancer are more likely to have a *BRCA2* mutation than a *BRCA1* mutation (see Chapter 26). Options for those who have a positive test for *BRCA1* or *BRCA2* mutation include surveillance to find cancers early, prophylactic surgery (i.e., bilateral salpingo-oophorectomy), risk factor avoidance, promotion of breast-feeding, and chemoprevention. Several other genetic alterations can increase the risk of breast cancer.

◆PATHOPHYSIOLOGY. Most breast cancers are adenocarcinomas and first arise from the ductal/lobular epithelium as carcinoma in situ. Carcinoma in situ is an early-stage, noninvasive, proliferation of epithelial cells that is confined to the ducts and lobules, by the basement membrane. (Ductal carcinoma in situ [DCIS] and lobular carcinoma in situ [LCIS] are discussed next.) Breast cancer is a heterogeneous—not a single—disease with diverse molecular, genetic, phenotypic, and pathologic changes[421] (Table 25.16). Tumor heterogeneity results from the genetic, epigenetic, and microenvironmental influences (selective pressure) that tumor cells undergo during cancer progression. Cellular subpopulations from different sections of the same tumor vary in many ways including growth rate, immunogenicity, ability to metastasize, and drug response, demonstrating significant heterogeneity.[422] The biologic attributes of a tumor as a whole are strongly influenced by its subpopulation of cells with cellular populations communicating through paracrine or contact-dependent signaling (juxtacrine) from ligands and mediated from components of the microenvironment such as blood vessels, immune cells, and fibroblasts.[422] The rich microenvironment of breast tumors

TABLE 25.16 TYPES OF BREAST CARCINOMAS AND MAJOR DISTINGUISHING FEATURES

HISTOLOGIC TYPE	DISTINGUISHING FEATURES
Carcinoma of Mammary Ducts	
Papillary	Well-delineated cystic masses in multiple areas; hemorrhage often present; majority appear in 40- to 60-year age group; often involves skin
Intraductal (comedo)	Often accompanied by evidence of inflammation; well-circumscribed tumors within duct; well-differentiated tumor cells; rarely ulcerates skin
Infiltrating Carcinoma	
Ductal (no specific type [NST])	Fibrous, firm, glistening, gray-tan mass with chalky streaks, mixture of patterns; may cause discharge from nipple; represents about 70%–80% of all breast cancers
Mucinous	Usually large (>3 cm in diameter), circumscribed, and encapsulated; glistening appearance; varies in color; two types: pure and mixed; pure tumor is surrounded by mucin; infrequent; found in lateral half of breast; tends to occur in women after age 70 years
Medullary	Encapsulated and grows very large (7–8 cm in diameter); commonly surrounded by lymphocytic inflammatory infiltrate; occurs after age 50 years
Tubular	Well-differentiated with orderly tubules in center (stroma) of mass; can be associated with noninfiltrating ductal carcinoma; occurs in women about 50 years of age; nodal metastasis infrequent; occurrence rare
Adenoid cystic	Very rare; well-circumscribed, painless mass arising from nipple and areola
Metaplastic	Involves cartilage or bone, mixed tumors or osteogenic sarcomas
Squamous cell	Frequent in blacks; originates in ductal epithelium
Carcinoma of Mammary Lobules	
Lobular carcinoma in situ	Found in individuals with fibrocystic disease; localized to upper breast quadrants; 15%–35% risk of becoming invasive; occurs frequently in mid-40s; infiltrating variety occurs in early 50s
Infiltrating lobular	Infiltrates from duct; firm mass with chalky streaks
Paget disease	Eczema of nipple that extends to areola; cancer usually found underneath nipple; poorly circumscribed; large Paget cells arise from duct and directly invade nipple; history of scaly, red rash spreading from nipple; lesion palpable beneath nipple, often bilateral; occurs in middle age
Inflammatory carcinoma	Not a histologic type; fairly diffuse within breast tissue, diffuse edema of overlying skin; extremely undifferentiated, very rare; most metastasize to axilla
Sarcoma of the Breast	
Cystosarcoma phyllodes	Usually large (>17 cm in diameter); mostly localized but can rupture through skin; rarely metastasizes to lymph nodes; history of painless nodule present for years before it forms a large mass; ulceration and bleeding of skin often present; occurs in wide age range (13–77 years)
Fibrosarcoma	Well-circumscribed, firm, and usually does not involve skin or nipple; well-differentiated to extremely undifferentiated; arises from connective tissue; extremely rare (e.g., liposarcoma, angiosarcoma)

is highly dynamic and heterogeneous.[422-424] Cancer cells behave as communities, and the cooperative behaviors of these subclones can influence cancer progression.[422] Recent research suggests that breast cancer is heterogeneous from its initial preinvasive stages[425] and within the same tumor.

Despite heroic efforts, this heterogeneity has greatly challenged the understanding of breast cancer evolution and the development of therapeutic strategies. Gene expression profiling studies have identified major subtypes classified as luminal A, luminal B, HER2+, basal-like, Claudin-low, and normal breast.[426] These subtypes have different prognoses and responses to therapy.[427] Tumors can be stratified with gene expression profiles such as Oncotype Dx, Prosigna, and MammaPrint on the basis of genomic profiles.[427] This information helps personalize breast cancer treatment and determine which women need aggressive systemic treatment for high-risk cancers versus close surveillance for indolent tumors.[427]

Many models of breast carcinogenesis have been suggested and the expanding themes include (1) gene addiction, (2) phenotype plasticity, (3) cancer stem cells, and (4) hormonal outcomes affecting cell turnover of mammary epithelium, stem cells, extracellular matrix, and immune function (see previous sections Reproductive Factors: Pregnancy, Lobular Involution, and Age and Postlactational Involution and Hormonal Factors).

Cancer gene addiction includes oncogene addiction, whereby these driver genes play key roles in breast cancer development and progression, and non–oncogene addiction, whereby these genes may not initiate cancer but play roles in cancer development and progression.[428] Examples of key driver genes include *HER2* and MYC, and examples of

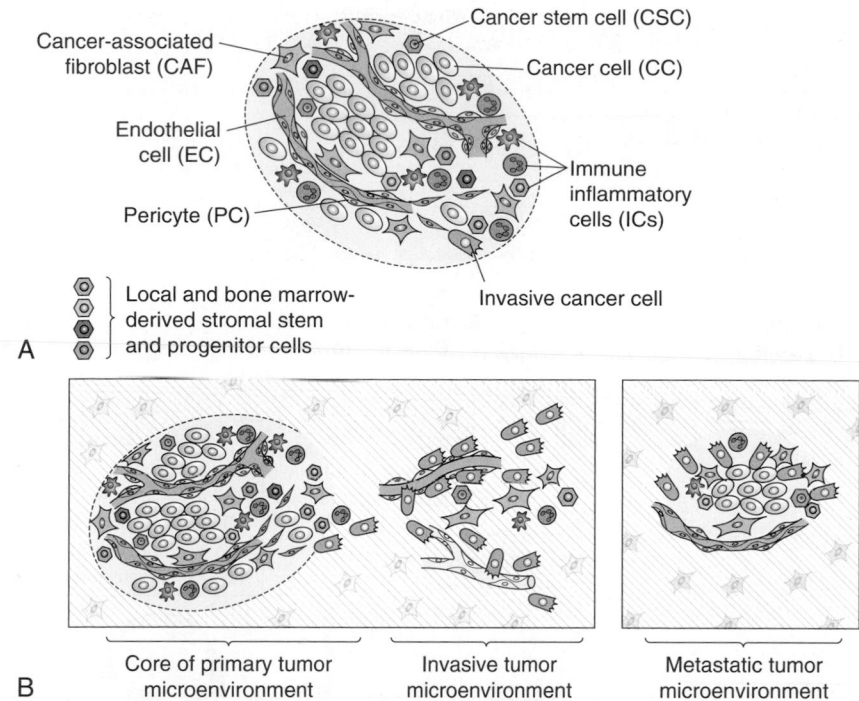

FIGURE 25.42 Cells of the Tumor Microenvironment. A, Distinct cell types constitute most solid tumors including breast tumors. Both the main cellular tissue, called *parenchyma*, and the surrounding tissue, or stroma of tumors, contain cell types that enable tumor growth and progression. For example, the immune-inflammatory cells present in tumors can include both tumor-promoting and tumor-killing subclasses of cells. **B,** The microenvironment of tumors. Multiple stromal cell types create a succession of tumor microenvironments that change as tumors invade normal tissue, eventually seeding and colonizing distant tissues. The organization, numbers, and phenotypic characteristics of the stromal cell types and the extracellular matrix *(hatched background)* evolve during progression and enable primary, invasive, and metastatic growth. (Not shown are the premalignant stages.) (Data from Hanahan D, Weinberg R: *Cell* 144:646–674, 2011.)

tumor-suppressor genes include *TP53*, *BRCA1*, and *BRCA2*. Once a founding tumor clone is established, genomic instability may assist through the establishment of other subclones and contribute to both tumor progression and therapy resistance.[175]

Phenotypic plasticity is exemplified by a distinctive phenotype called *epithelial-to-mesenchymal transition (EMT)* (see Chapter 12). EMT is involved in the generation of tissues and organs during embryogenesis, is essential for driving tissue plasticity during development, and is hijacked during cancer progression.[429] The EMT-associated reprogramming is involved in many cancer cell characteristics, including suppression of cell death or apoptosis and senescence, is reactivated during wound healing, and is resistant to chemotherapy and radiation therapy.[430] Remodeling or reprogramming of the breast during postpregnancy involution is important because it involves inflammatory and "wound healing-like" tissue reactions known as **reactive stroma** or **inflammatory stroma**. The reactive stroma releases various signals and interleukins that affect nearby carcinoma cells, inducing these cells to activate their previously silent EMT programs. The activation is typically reversible (i.e., plasticity) and those EMT programs may revert through mesenchymal-epithelial (MET) to the previous phenotypic state before induction of the EMT program[429] (see Chapter 12). Reactive stroma increases the risk for tumor invasion and may facilitate the transition of carcinoma in situ to invasive carcinoma. Activation of an EMT program during cancer development often requires signaling between cancer cells and neighboring stromal cells.[431] In advanced primary carcinomas,

cancer cells recruit a variety of cell types into the surrounding stroma, including fibroblasts, myofibroblasts, granulocytes, macrophages, mesenchymal stem cells, and lymphocytes (Fig. 25.42). Overall, increasing evidence suggests that interactions of cancer cells with adjacent tumor-associated stromal cells induce malignant cell phenotypes (Fig. 25.43). Several types of carcinoma cells are reported to acquire tumor-initiating capability after induction of the EMT program.[429] The tumor-initiating traits are depicted as cancer stem cells (CSCs). Tissues with residing carcinoma cells in the CSC state seem critical for progression through the invasion-metastasis cascade as founders of new metastatic colonies.[429] With increasing acquisition of mesenchymal traits, as driven by an EMT program, it is reported to increase the resistance of carcinoma cells to both radiation and chemotherapy.[429]

Invasion by primary tumor cells typically involves the collective migration of large, cohesive groups of cells into adjacent tissue rather than the scattering of individual carcinoma cells (Fig. 25.44).[432] Still unknown are the precise events occurring at the invasive edge. Critical to understand is the process of invasion as it relates to treatment. The possibility of displacing tumor cells into the biopsy needle track is a concern.[433] Although reported as a low incidence, mechanical disruption from surgery can lead to displacement and seeding of tumor cells. Dormant carcinoma cells appear to perpetuate carcinogenesis and form the precursors of eventual metastatic relapse and, sometimes, rapid cancer recurrence.[434,435] These dormant cells are called **minimal residual disease (MRD)** and may remain after initial chemotherapy, radiotherapy,

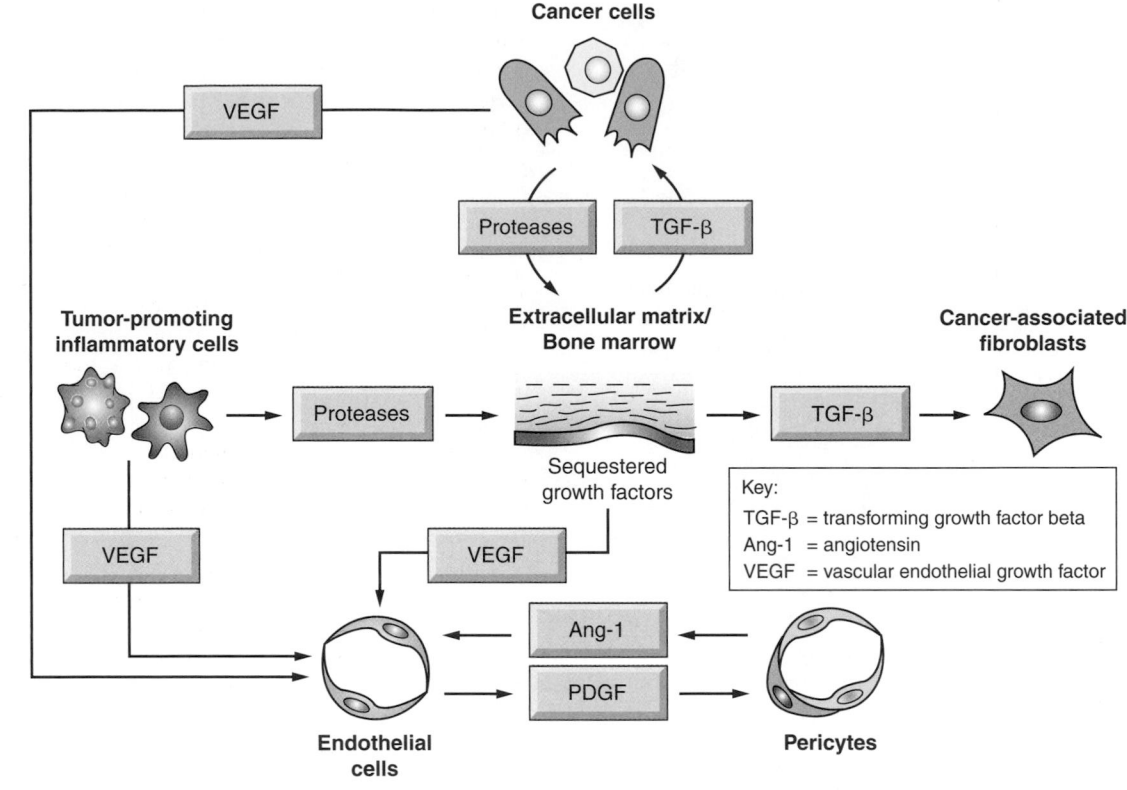

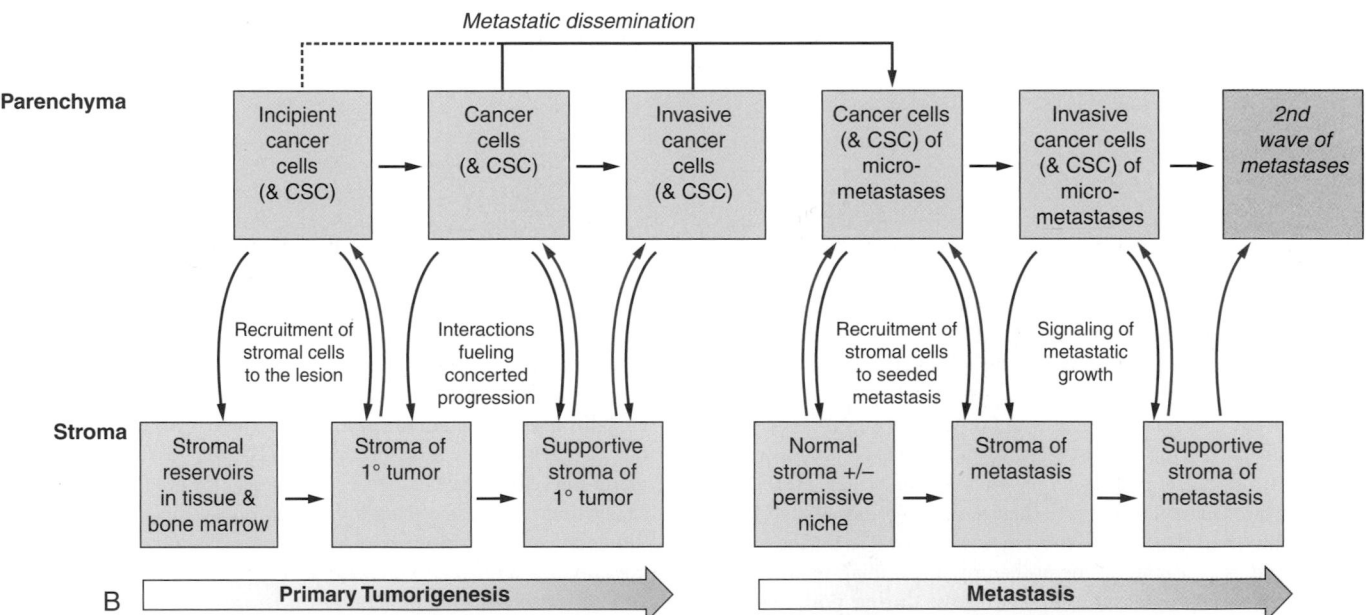

FIGURE 25.43 Signaling Interactions in the Tumor Microenvironment During Malignant Progression. **A,** Numerous cell types constitute the tumor microenvironment and are orchestrated and maintained by reciprocal interactions. **B,** The reciprocal interactions between the breast main tissue or parenchyma and the surrounding stroma are important for cancer progression and growth. Certain organ sites of "fertile soil" or "metastasis niches" facilitate metastatic seeding and colonization. Cancer stem cells are involved in some or all stages of tumor development and progression. *CSC,* Cancer stem cells. (Adapted from Hanahan D, Weinberg R: *Cell* 144:646–674, 2011.)

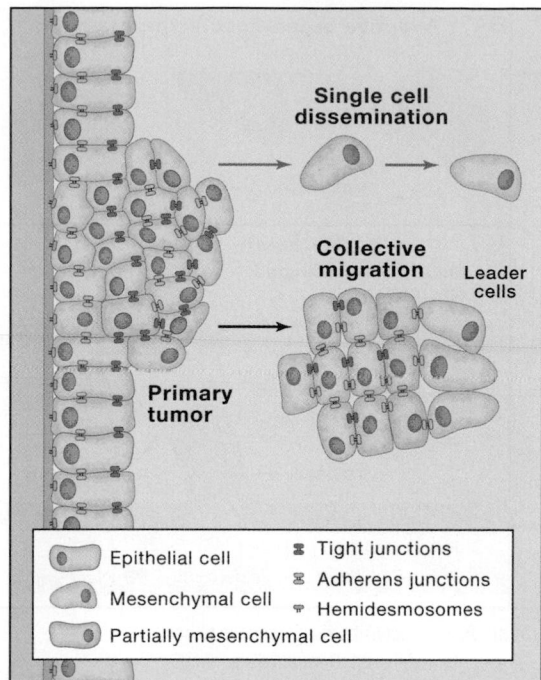

FIGURE 25.44 Invasion. Invasion of carcinoma cells occurs through two mechanisms: single cell dissemination through an epithelial-mesenchymal transition (EMT) *(gray arrow)*, or the collective dissemination of a tumor cluster of cells. Emerging evidence suggests that the leader cells of tumor groups or clusters undergo EMT-associated phenotypic changes. Clusters of migrating cells are commonly noted at the borders of invasive carcinomas and are best documented in breast and lungs. (Adapted from Lambert AW, Pattabiraman DR, Weinberg RA: *Cell* 168[4]:670–691, 2017.)

and surgery. Dormant cells have exited the cell cycle; thus they are not proliferating, and current treatments preferentially kill proliferating cells rendering dormant cells intrinsically more resistant to almost all current treatments.[429] The benefit of surgery is reducing the numbers of cancer cells and diversity of neoplastic cells and perhaps increasing the chance of getting rid of therapy-resistant cells.[429]

A large number of reports identify the existence of the partial EMT state and its ability to enhance tumor progression and metastasis.[429] The phenotypic plasticity associated with the epithelial-mesenchymal spectrum appears critical to the founding of metastatic colonies.[429] Invasive clusters or individual invasive carcinoma cells eventually invade into the vasculature of either adjacent normal tissue or the neovasculature that has been assembled within the tumors themselves.[429] The resulting intravasation is an avenue for circulating tumor cells (CTCs) to distant sites.

Using a mouse model of tumor heterogeneity, investigators demonstrate that different clones of mammary tumor cell lines possess different abilities to the formation of metastasis.[436] More simply, different clones within the heterogeneous population had distinct properties, such as an ability to dominate the primary tumor, or to contribute to metastatic populations, or to enter the lymphatic or vascular systems.[437] The expression of two proteins, Serpine2 and Slpi, correlates with lung metastases and similar associations were observed in human datasets. Serpine2 and Slpi act as anticoagulants and allow tumor cells to undergo *vascular mimicry*, whereby the tumor cells themselves form part of blood vessels and contribute to increased intravasation by building more leaky blood vessels.[436] Vascular mimicry was first detailed in 1999 in aggressive melanomas, and involves the formation of vascular-like networks by aggressive tumor cells that have similar characteristics to the endothelial cells that line normal blood vessels. These networks are rich in extracellular matrix and allow perfusion of blood and fluid through tumor tissues (Fig. 25.45).

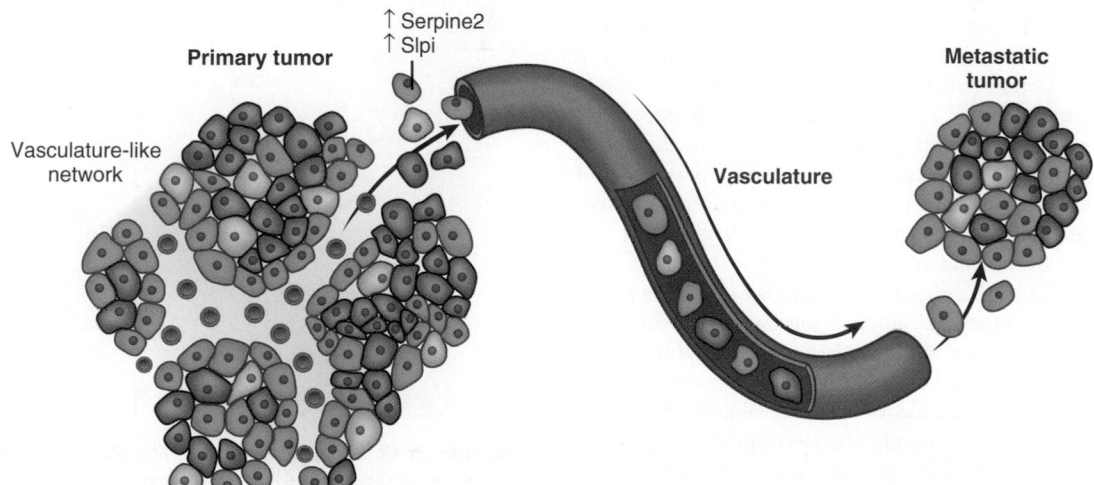

FIGURE 25.45 Vascular Mimicry Drives Metastasis. The steps to accomplish metastasis include *intravasation,* in which tumor cells escape from the primary tumor into the vasculature and move through the bloodstream; or *extravasation,* in which tumor cells escape from the vasculature to colonize in distant tissue. Metastasis is promoted by vascular mimicry, whereby tumor cells adopt characteristics similar to those of the endothelial cells that line blood vessels, and mimic vascular-like networks within tumors and between tumors and blood vessels. Wagenblast and colleagues found that two proteins, Serpine2 and Slpi, promoted metastasis by stimulating vascular mimicry. Tumor cells expressing these proteins *(green)* form the vascular-like network that allows other tumor cells *(purple, blue)* to move to secondary sites. (Adapted from Hendrix MJC: *Nature* 520:300–302, 2015; Wagenblast E et al: *Nature* 520:358–362, 2015.)

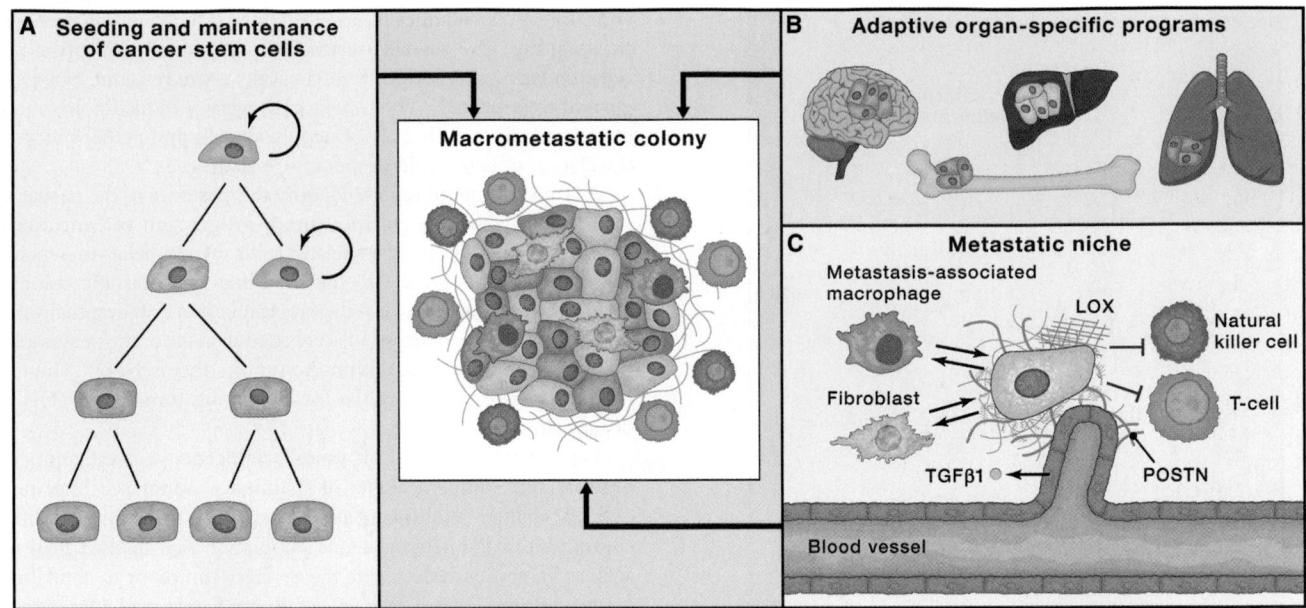

FIGURE 25.46 The Three Requirements for Metastatic Colonization. **A,** The necessity of cancer cells to seed (spread) and maintain a population of cancer stem cells. These cells can reinitiate tumor growth. Dormant disseminating tumor cells (DTCs) also exhibit key cancer stem cell competencies that possibly contribute to persistence in a quiescent (resting) state and can eventually develop a metastatic colony. **B,** Cancer stem cells must be capable to thrive in a foreign tissue microenvironment. **C,** During many stages of metastases, cancer cells have the ability to crosstalk with the microenvironment and stromal cells, including endothelial cell, fibroblasts, and cells of the immune system. The microenvironment is a component of the niche and can be modified to support the metastatic cascade. *LOX,* Lysyl oxidase; *POSTN,* periostin; *TGF,* transforming growth factor. (Data from Lambert AW, Pattabiraman DR, Weinberg RA: *Cell* 168[4]:670–691, 2017.)

Carcinoma cells may promote the growth of lymphatic vessels through the process of lymphangiogenesis;[438] this process is correlated with disease progression.[439] It is not yet defined what specific factors determine the efficiency of clinical metastatic disease and why some patients present with metastasis and other patients experience years before a relapse and present with metastasis.[429] The emergent evidence supports three main prerequisites that must be met in order for metastatic colonization to succeed:[429] (1) the capacity to seed and maintain a population of tumor-initiating cancer stem cells; (2) the ability to create adaptive, organ-specific colonization programs; and (3) the development of a supportive microenvironmental niche (Fig. 25.46).

Traditionally, metastases have been considered a late event in multistep tumor progression. Recent reports, however, suggest that dissemination can occur early during the process of neoplastic transformation.[429] One explanation has been attributed to the presence of preneoplastic cells residing within inflammatory microenvironments that through signaling can activate EMT programs causing the development of invasive phenotypes.[440] Additionally, from murine models of HER2+ breast cancer and in early stages of primary tumor formation, a migratory and stemlike program predominates before the proliferative pathways occur during the later stages of tumor growth.[441,442] In other cases, however, metastases appear to be a late event.[429]

Ductal Carcinoma in Situ

Ductal carcinoma in situ (DCIS) is a heterogeneous group of proliferative lesions clinically, radiologically, morphologically, and genetically. DCIS is limited to breast ducts and lobules without invasion of the basement membrane (Fig. 25.47). When DCIS breaches the basement membrane

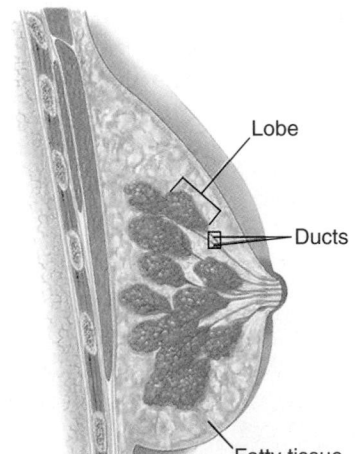
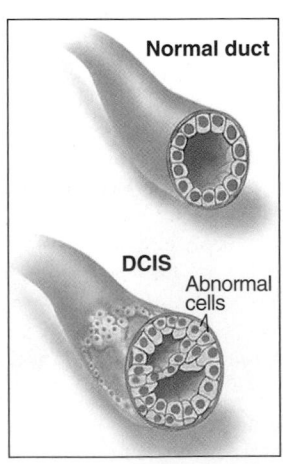

FIGURE 25.47 Ductal Carcinoma in Situ (DCIS). Illustration showing the location of DCIS. Given the low breast cancer mortality, new approaches to managing DCIS are needed. (From National Cancer Institute: *Risk of breast cancer death is low after a diagnosis of ductal carcinoma in situ,* Bethesda, MD, 2015, Author. With permission from Terese Winslow.)

and invades adjacent stroma to a depth of 1 mm or less, microinvasion (MI) is said to be present. About 84% of all in situ disease is DCIS; the remainder is mostly LCIS disease.[443] DCIS occurs predominantly in women but can occur in men. DCIS has a wide spectrum of risk for invasive cancers.[442] Since 1980, the widespread adoption of screening mammography has led to an epidemic of diagnoses of DCIS.[444] With the introduction of screening mammography, there has been a 500% increase in the diagnosis of DCIS, which represents about 25% of mammographically detected breast lesions.[442] Since 1983 there has been a 290% increase in DCIS among women younger than 50 years, and the incidence is still increasing.[444] Because of the large numbers of cases diagnosed yearly in the United States, the debate is whether mammography is causing the overdiagnosis of potential pseudodisease; for example, the Canadian National Breast Screening Study-2 of women aged 50 to 59 years found a fourfold increase in DCIS cases in those screened by clinical breast examination (CBE) plus mammography compared with those screened by CBE alone, with no difference in breast cancer mortality.[444,445]

The perspectives on DCIS are changing. The cells of DCIS look like invasive cancer both pathologically and molecularly, and therefore the presumption was that these lesions were the precursors of cancer and that early removal and treatment would reduce cancer incidence and mortality.[446] Long-term epidemiologic studies have demonstrated that the removal of 50,000 to 60,000 DCIS lesions annually has not been accompanied by a reduction in the incidence of invasive cancer.[447] Contrarily, the removal of colonic polyps and of intraepithelial neoplasia lesions of the cervix and precursor lesions has led to a decrease in the incidence of colon and cervical cancer, respectively.[448] It is now known that breast cancer has a range of behaviors, aggressive to indolent, and screening mammography increases the likelihood of indolent lesions surfacing.[446]

New data from Narod and colleagues[449] add to the growing concern to rethink the strategy for the detection and treatment of DCIS. In a large observational study of 100,000 women with a diagnosis of DCIS, the risk of dying from breast cancer is low.[449,450] Less than 1% of women in this 20-year study died of breast cancer (compared to 5% of women who died of other causes). Surprisingly, the overall death rate for women with DCIS is lower than that for women in the population as a whole.[175,451] Aggressive treatment of almost all DCIS does not lead to a reduction in breast cancer mortality, confirming the conclusions from the NSABP trials.[452] Because of these findings, some argue that the term DCIS is misleading and should be replaced by *ductal intraepithelial neoplasia*, similar to the term used in prostate cancer, and that breast cancer statistics should exclude those DCIS cases with invasive breast cancer statistics.[451] This very critical news suggests a treatment change as an alternative to surgery and radiation.[446] A study of 6 months of letrozole therapy is one example of a new approach along with observation and may increase clinical trials of observation and endocrine risk–reducing therapy.[446] Prevention or risk-reducing strategies are discussed next and need initiation and study. Stratification of risk is mandated to avoid overtreatment, unnecessary morbidity, and the same treatment as invasive cancer. Factors to help risk stratification of DCIS include grade and comedonecrosis; however, these factors are not predictive.[427] Molecular tests, such as the Oncotype DCIS Score, have been shown to predict the 10-year risk of invasive cancer following surgical excision alone.[427] Therefore some direction in solving the overtreatment dilemma is emerging. For example, if the emerging data suggest that it is safe to eliminate radiation for luminal A invasive tumors in postmenopausal women, then radiation should not be routine in low-grade or low-risk DCIS.[427] The majority of DCIS is detected in women from screening and who are recalled for biopsy of calcifications. Importantly, to minimize risk of overdiagnosis or overtreatment, or both, reassessment of whether clustered amorphous calcifications should be a target for screening, recall, and biopsy, especially in older women.[453]

Increased mortality risk from DCIS is associated with risk factors: age at diagnosis; ethnicity; and DCIS characteristics, such as estrogen receptor status, grade, size (>5 cm), and comedonecrosis.[446] DCIS lesions diagnosed before 35 or 40 years of age do pose an increased risk of breast cancer mortality.[446] These lesions are likely different from those found from mammography, since screening before age 40 is rare, and may be associated with a symptomatic event, such as a mass, or bloody nipple discharge. Black women (who have a higher risk for hormone receptor–negative, or HER2+, DCIS) should continue with today's aggressive standards.[446] In total, these higher risk groups account for about 20% of the total population of women with DCIS.

Although DCIS may remain stable and never progress (or may regress), for invasive DCIS the cells within the DCIS *breach* the myoepithelial layer and the basement membrane, defining the moment when an invasive carcinoma is formed[454] (Fig. 25.48). Importantly, the layer of myoepithelial cells is thought to be natural "tumor suppressors" and critical to maintaining tissue polarity (cell directional orientation) (see Fig. 1.10), a role that is lost in invasive breast carcinomas. Investigators and clinicians are intensely studying this key step, or breach, in terms of cellular alterations because of tumor biology or iatrogenic stimuli, or both.

DCIS represents an opportunity to alter the breast environment. Alteration may be done with increased exercise, decreased alcohol intake, and avoidance of postmenopausal hormone therapy with progesterone-containing regimens.[446] Stratification of DCIS lesions may be accomplished through available tools such as Oncotype DCIS; unfortunately, according to one population-based study, only half of such women are tested with genetic testing.[455]

In summary, based on large numbers and long-term follow-up, given the low breast cancer mortality risk, DCIS is not an emergency. The detection and treatment of nonpalpable DCIS often represent overdiagnosis and overtreatment.[451] Data now suggest the following:

1. Much of DCIS should be considered a "risk factor" for invasive cancer and targeting for preventive strategies.
2. Radiation therapy should not be routinely offered after lumpectomy for DCIS lesions that are not high-risk because it does not affect mortality.
3. Low- and intermediate-grade DCIS does not need to be a target for screening or early detection.
4. Continuing study is needed both of the biologic nature of the highest-risk DCIS (large, high grade, hormone receptor negative, and HER2 positive, especially in very young and black women) and of target approaches to reduce death from breast cancer.[446]

Lobular Carcinoma in Situ

Lobular carcinoma in situ (LCIS) originates from the terminal duct–lobular unit (see Fig. 25.31, *B*). Unlike DCIS, LCIS has a uniform appearance (i.e., the cells expand but do not distort involved spaces); thus the lobular structure is preserved. The cells grow in noncohesive (discohesive) clusters, typically because of a loss of the tumor-suppressive adhesion protein E-cadherin.[175] Also unlike DCIS, LCIS is found as an incidental lesion from a biopsy and not from mammography because it is not associated with calcifications or stromal reactions that produce mammographic densities. LCIS has an incidence of about 1% to 6% of all carcinomas and did not increase with mammographic screening.[175] With biopsies in both breasts, LCIS is bilateral in 20% to 40% of cases, compared with 10% to 20% of cases of DCIS.[175] The cells of atypical hyperplasia, LCIS, and invasive lobular carcinoma are structurally identical.[175] Dysfunction of E-cadherin results in loss of cellular adhesion, and lesions have a rounded shape without attachment to adjacent cells, increasing the risk of invasion.

Invasive carcinoma from LCIS develops in 25% to 35% of women over a period of 20 to 30 years. Unlike DCIS, the risk is almost as high

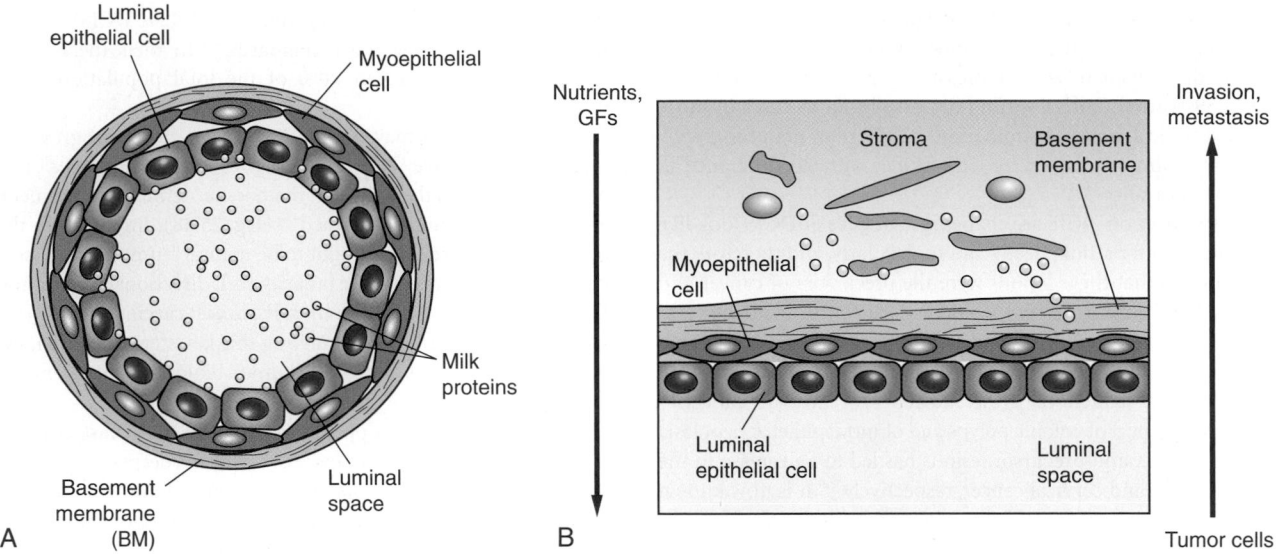

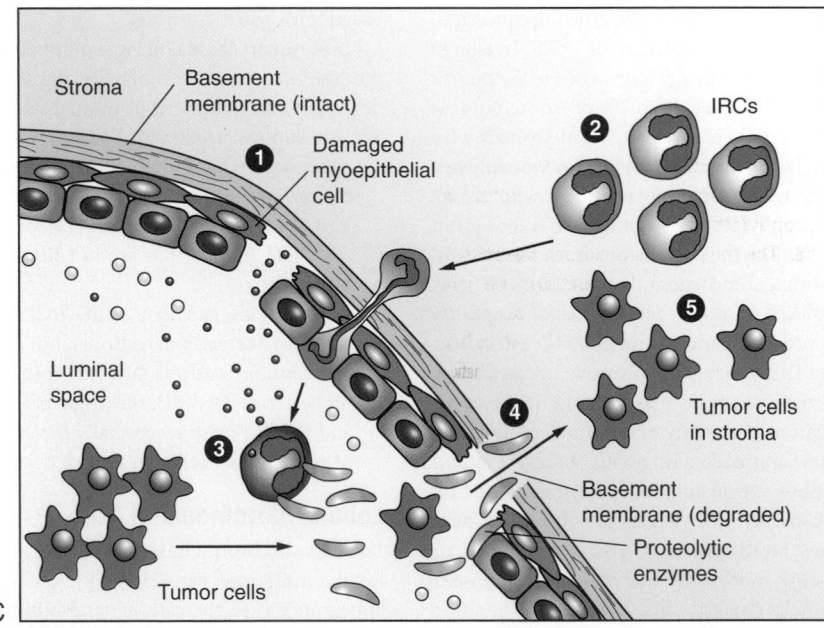

FIGURE 25.48 The Role of Myoepithelial Cells in Invasive Breast Cancer. **A,** Cross section of a normal mammary gland. **B,** Schematic of the anatomic relationship between mammary gland duct cells, basement membrane (BM), and stroma. **C,** With degradation of the normal "tumor-suppressing" basement membrane, tumor cells invade the stroma; **(1)** myoepithelial cells are damaged by various factors and release their inner contents (for example, diffusible molecules and chemoattractants); **(2)** immunoreactive cells (IRCs) are drawn to the luminal space by these chemoattractants; **(3)** IRCs become activated after contact with chemoattractants and secrete various proteolytic enzymes; **(4)** these enzymes then degrade the basement membrane resulting in gaps; and **(5)** tumor cells enter the stromal region through these gaps. *GF,* Growth factor. (Data and adapted figures from Pandey PR, Saidou J, Watabe K: *Front Biosci* 15:226–236, 2011.)

TABLE 25.17 CLINICAL MANIFESTATIONS OF BREAST CANCER

CLINICAL MANIFESTATION	PATHOPHYSIOLOGY
Chest pain	Metastasis to the lung
Dilated blood vessels	Obstruction of venous return by a fast-growing tumor; obstruction dilates superficial veins
Dimpling of the skin	Can occur with invasion of the dermal lymphatics because of retraction of Cooper ligament or involvement of the pectoralis fascia
Edema	Local inflammation or lymphatic obstruction
Edema of the arm	Obstruction of lymphatic drainage in the axilla
Hemorrhage	Erosion of blood vessels
Local pain	Local obstruction caused by the tumor
Nipple/areolar eczema	Paget disease
Nipple discharge in a nonlactating woman	Spontaneous and intermittent discharge caused by tumor obstruction
Nipple retraction	Shortening of the mammary ducts
Pitting of the skin (similar to the surface of an orange [peau d'orange])	Obstruction of the subcutaneous lymphatics, resulting in the accumulation of fluid
Reddened skin, local tenderness, and warmth	Inflammation
Skin retraction	Involvement of the suspensory ligaments
Ulceration	Tumor necrosis

Data from Griffiths MJ, Murray KH, Russo PC: *Oncology nursing: pathophysiology, assessment, and intervention*, New York, 1984, Macmillan.

in the contralateral breast as in the ipsilateral breast. Treatments include close clinical follow-up and mammographic screening, tamoxifen administration, and bilateral prophylactic mastectomy.

CLINICAL MANIFESTATIONS. The upper outer quadrant, where most of the glandular tissue of the breast is located, is where the majority of carcinomas of the breast occur. The lymphatic spread of cancer to the opposite breast, to lymph nodes in the base of the neck, and to the abdominal cavity is caused by obstruction of the normal lymphatic pathways or destruction of lymphatic vessels by surgery or radiotherapy (see Fig. 24.11). The less common inner quadrant tumors may spread to mediastinal nodes or Rotter nodes, which are located between the pectoral muscles (see Fig. 24.11). Other common sites of metastasis include the internal mammary chain nodes. Metastases from the vertebral veins can involve the vertebrae, pelvic bones, ribs, and skull. The lungs, kidneys, liver, adrenal glands, ovaries, and pituitary gland also are sites of metastasis.

The first sign of breast cancer is usually a painless lump. Lumps caused by breast tumors do not have any classic characteristics. Other presenting signs include palpable nodes in the axilla, retraction of tissue (dimpling) (Fig. 25.49), or bone pain caused by metastasis to the vertebrae. Table 25.17 summarizes the clinical manifestations of breast cancers. Manifestations vary according to the type of tumor and stage of disease.

EVALUATION AND TREATMENT. Clinical breast examination, mammography, ultrasound, thermography, MRI, biopsy, hormone receptor assays, and gene expression profiling are used in evaluating breast alterations and cancer.

Treatment is based on the extent or stage of the cancer. The extent of the tumor at the primary site, the presence and extent of lymph node metastasis, and the presence of distant metastases are all evaluated to determine the stage of disease. Treatment includes surgery,

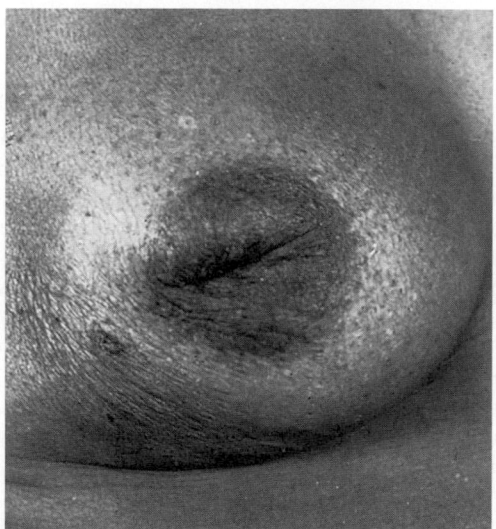

FIGURE 25.49 Retraction of Nipple Caused by Carcinoma. (From del Regato JA, Spjut HJ, Cox JD: *Ackerman and del Regato's cancer: diagnosis, treatment, and prognosis*, ed 6, St Louis, 1985, Mosby.)

radiation, chemotherapy, hormone therapy, and biologic therapy. Strategies for risk reduction of breast cancer are evolving and include implementation of a modified diet including decreased alcohol consumption, utilization of an exercise program, and avoidance of postmenopausal hormone therapy with progesterone-containing regimens, and possibly others.

SUMMARY REVIEW

Abnormalities of Reproductive Tract Development

1. Abnormalities of the female reproductive tract have multifactorial causes, including genetics and environmental factors. Common abnormalities include uterine agenesis or structural malformations of the vagina, uterus, and fallopian tubes.

Alterations of Sexual Maturation

1. Sexual maturation, or puberty, should begin in girls between ages 8 and 13 years. Delayed puberty is the onset of sexual maturation after these ages; precocious puberty is onset before these ages. The average age of puberty has been occurring earlier than in previous generations.

2. Alterations of sexual maturation can be idiopathic or caused by a disease or congenital anomaly. In most cases of delayed puberty, the hypothalamic-pituitary-gonadal (HPG) axis is intact but the surge of activity that stimulates puberty is delayed. Precocious puberty, more common in girls, also can be caused by mistiming of the stimulatory surge in a child whose HPG system is otherwise normal. Obesity is associated with younger pubertal age.

3. Precocious puberty can be complete (sex appropriate), mixed (not sex appropriate), or partial (development of one secondary sex characteristic only). Causes of delayed or incomplete puberty can be divided into categories based on gonadotropic secretion: hypergonadotropism (increased levels of FSH and LH) and hypogonadotropism (decreased LH and FSH levels).

Disorders of the Female Reproductive System

1. The female reproductive system can be altered by hormonal imbalances, infectious microorganisms, inflammation, structural abnormalities, and benign or malignant proliferative conditions.

2. Menstrual disorders usually involve some disruption of the HPG axis and subsequent alteration of hormone production, reception by target organs, or feedback mechanisms.

3. Primary dysmenorrhea is painful menstruation not associated with pelvic disease. It often results from excessive synthesis of prostaglandins (or sensitivity to prostaglandins), which cause the myometrium to contract and constrict blood vessels, resulting in ischemic pain.

4. Primary amenorrhea is the continued absence of menarche and menstrual function by 13 years of age without the development of secondary sex characteristics, or by age 15 years if these changes have occurred.

5. Secondary amenorrhea is the absence of regular menses for 3 months, or 6 months of irregular menses in women who have previously menstruated. Secondary amenorrhea is usually associated with anovulation.

6. Amenorrhea is divided into compartments that reflect the underlying disorder: compartment I, disorders of the outflow tract or uterine target organ; compartment II, disorders of the ovary; compartment III, disorders of the anterior pituitary; and compartment IV, disorders of the CNS or hypothalamic factors.

7. Abnormal uterine bleeding (AUB) is bleeding that is abnormal in duration, volume, frequency, regularity, or some combination of these factors.

8. Polycystic ovary syndrome (PCOS) is a difficult syndrome to diagnose because several factors are involved. It is a syndrome in which at least two of the following are present: irregular ovulation or anovulation; elevated levels of androgens, or clinical signs of hyperandrogenism; and polycystic ovaries. Prolonged anovulation often leads to infertility, menstrual bleeding disorders, hirsutism,

acne, endometrial hyperplasia, cardiovascular disease, and diabetes mellitus in women with hyperinsulinemia.

9. PMS is the cyclic recurrence of physical, psychologic, or behavioral changes distressing enough to disrupt normal activities or interpersonal relationships. Approximately 300 emotional, physical, and behavioral symptoms have been attributed to PMS. Emotional symptoms, particularly depression, anger, irritability, and fatigue, are reported as the most distressing; physical symptoms tend to be less problematic. Treatment is symptomatic and includes self-help techniques, lifestyle changes, counseling, and selective serotonin reuptake inhibitors (SSRIs).

10. Infection and inflammation of the female genitalia may result from exogenous pathogens, most often sexually transmitted, or from overproliferation of microorganisms that normally populate the genital tract.

11. Pelvic inflammatory disease (PID) is an acute ascending polymicrobial infection of the upper genital tract and is often caused by sexually transmitted pathogens that are allowed to ascend because of disruptions in the normal vaginal flora.

12. Vaginitis, or vaginal infection, can be caused by a variety of microorganisms or irritants, or disruptions in the vaginal pH, and involves vaginal irritation, itching, burning, odor, or abnormal discharge. The primary forms are vulvovaginal candidiasis, bacterial vaginosis, or trichomoniasis.

13. Cervicitis, which is inflammation of the cervix, can be acute (mucopurulent cervicitis) or chronic.

14. Vulvovestibulitis is an inflammation of the skin of the vulva. It can be caused by chemical and mechanical irritants, allergens, skin disorders, nerve problems, or vaginal infections, such as candidiasis.

15. Bartholinitis, also called Bartholin cyst, is an inflammation of the ducts that lead from the Bartholin glands to the surface of the vulva. Inflammation blocks the glands, preventing the outflow of glandular secretions, and is caused by trauma or infection.

16. Pelvic organ prolapse—uterine prolapse, cystocele, rectocele, and urethrocele—is caused by loss of support provided by the pelvic muscles and fascia. Age and pelvic trauma are associated. Women with a familial or genetic predisposition have a higher risk.

17. Benign growths and proliferative conditions of the female reproductive tract tend to affect the ovaries (benign ovarian cysts) or uterine tissues (endometrial polyps, leiomyomas, and endometriosis).

18. Benign ovarian cysts develop from mature ovarian follicles that do not release their ova (follicular cysts) or from a corpus luteum that persists abnormally instead of degenerating (corpus luteum cyst). Cysts usually regress spontaneously.

19. Endometrial polyps are overgrowths of endometrial tissue and often cause abnormal bleeding.

20. Leiomyomas, also called *uterine fibroids,* are tumors arising from the muscle layer of the uterus, the myometrium. Prevalence increases in women between ages 30 and 50; most myomas remain small and asymptomatic.

21. Adenomyosis is the presence of endometrial glands and stroma within the uterine myometrium.

22. Endometriosis is the presence of functional endometrial tissue (i.e., tissue that responds to hormonal stimulation) at sites outside the uterus. Endometriosis causes an inflammatory reaction at the site of implantation and is a cause of pain and infertility.

23. Most cancers of the female genitalia involve the uterus (particularly the cervix) and the ovaries. Cancer of the vagina is rare.

24. Infection with high-risk HPV, a sexually transmitted infection, is a necessary precursor to developing CIN and cervical cancer.

SUMMARY REVIEW—cont'd

Smoking, immunosuppression, and poor nutrition are cofactors. HPV vaccination can substantially reduce the risk of cervical cancer.

25. Cervical cancer arises from the cervical epithelium. The progressively serious neoplastic alterations are: (1) cervical intraepithelial neoplasia (cervical dysplasia), (2) cervical carcinoma in situ, and (3) invasive cervical carcinoma.

26. Risk factors for vaginal cancer are in utero diethylstilbestrol (DES) exposure and prior or concurrent cervical cancer. Like cervical cancers, vaginal cancers arise from the epithelium and are identified as intraepithelial neoplasia (dysplasia), carcinoma in situ, or invasive carcinoma. Most are secondary in nature.

27. The major risk for vulvar cancer is a history of HPV infection or squamous dysplasia of the vagina or cervix. Symptoms include chronic vulvar irritation, pruritus, bloody discharge, and a hard, ulcerated area of the vulva or large cauliflower-like lesions. Peak incidence is in postmenopausal women, but younger women can be affected.

28. Endometrial cancer is the most common cancer of the pelvic region. Risk factors for endometrial cancer include unopposed estrogen exposure, obesity, infertility, failure to ovulate, early menarche or late menopause, and tamoxifen. Oral contraceptive use protects against endometrial and ovarian cancers. Peak incidence occurs at 58 to 60 years of age.

29. Risk factors for ovarian cancer include an increased number of total lifetime ovulations including early menarche, late menopause, nulliparity, use of fertility drugs. *BRCA1, BRCA2,* and HNPCC gene abnormalities also are linked with ovarian cancer. Ovarian cancer causes more deaths than any other genital cancer in women.

30. Awareness of sexual dysfunction is relatively new. Chronic illness, medications, infection, sexual trauma, and a variety of psychosocial concerns have been implicated as causes.

31. Infertility, or the inability to conceive after 1 year of unprotected intercourse, affects approximately 15% of all couples. Women's fertility decreases with age, and older women may opt for intervention sooner than younger women. Fertility can be impaired by factors in the male, female, or both partners. Treatment depends on the cause of the infertility; ovulation disorders and tubal blockages are the most common pathologies.

Disorders of the Female Breast

1. Most disorders of the breast are disorders of the mammary gland, that is, the female breast.

2. Galactorrhea, or inappropriate lactation, is the persistent secretion of a milky substance by one or both breasts in nonpregnant, nonlactating women. It can occur in men. Its most common cause is nonpuerperal hyperprolactinemia, a rise in serum prolactin levels that is not associated with pregnancy and childbirth. Hyperprolactinemia can be caused by medications, pituitary tumors, hypothyroidism, chronic stress, or persistent and repeated suckling.

3. Numerous benign conditions occur in ducts and lobules in the breast. Benign breast disease is a spectrum of noncancerous changes in the breast. Benign lesions are broadly classified as (1) nonproliferating breast lesions, (2) proliferative breast disease, and (3) atypical (atypia) hyperplasia.

4. The term *nonproliferative lesions* is used to discriminate such lesions from the "proliferative" changes associated with increased risk of breast cancer. The nonproliferative lesions include simple breast cysts, papillary apocrine change, and mild hyperplasia of the usual type.

5. Fibrocystic changes or physiologic nodularity and cysts are not clinically definitive because they include a heterogeneous group of disorders and refer to nonproliferative lesions. Symptoms affect women ages 30 to 50 and include cyclic bilateral breast tenderness and transient breast lumps.

6. Proliferative breast lesions without atypia are characterized by proliferation of ductal epithelium and/or stroma. Criteria for the diagnosis of intraductal proliferative lesions have been the subject of much research and controversy and include the following structurally diverse lesions: (1) usual ductal hyperplasia, (2) intraductal papillomas, (3) sclerosing adenosis, (4) radial scar, and (5) simple fibroadenoma.

7. Proliferative breast lesions with atypia include ADH and ALH. ADH is abnormal proliferating cells in breast ducts. ALH is abnormal proliferating cells in the lumen of lobular units.

8. Except for skin cancer, breast cancer is the most common form of cancer in American women. Most breast cancer occurs in women older than 50 years. The major risk factors for breast cancer are classified as reproductive, such as nulliparity and pregnancy-associated breast cancer; familial, such as inherited gene syndromes; and environmental and lifestyle, such as hormonal factors and radiation exposure. Other important factors are delayed involution of the mammary gland and increased breast density.

9. Overall, lifetime risk of breast cancer is reduced in parous women compared to nulliparous women, but pregnancy must occur at a young age. The influence of pregnancy on the risk of breast cancer also depends on family history, lactation postpartum, and overall parity.

10. Breast gland involution after pregnancy and lactation uses some of the same tissue remodeling pathways activated during wound healing. The presence of macrophages in the involuting mammary gland contributes to carcinogenesis.

11. Most breast cancers are adenocarcinomas and first arise from the ductal/lobular epithelium as carcinoma in situ. Carcinoma in situ is an early stage, noninvasive proliferation of epithelial cells confined to the ducts and lobules by the basement membrane.

12. Breast cancer is a heterogeneous disease with diverse molecular, biologic, phenotypic, and pathologic changes. Breast cancer is heterogeneous *within* the same tumor. Cellular subpopulations from different sections of the same tumor vary in growth rate, immunogenicity, ability to metastasize, and drug response. Biologic attributes of a tumor are influenced by the surrounding neighborhood or microenvironment.

13. Cancer cells behave as communities, and the cooperative behaviors of subclones can influence cancer progression.

14. Epithelial-to-mesenchymal transition (EMT) is involved in the generation of tissues and organs during embryogenesis, is essential for driving tissue plasticity during development, and is hijacked during cancer progression.

15. EMT-associated reprogramming is involved in many cancer cell characteristics, including suppression of cell death and senescence, and is reactivated during wound healing.

16. Invasion by primary tumor cells typically involves the collective migration of large, cohesive groups into adjacent tissue rather than the scattering of individual carcinoma cells. However, still unknown are the precise events occurring at the invasive edge.

17. Emerging evidence supports three main prerequisites that must be met for metastatic colonization to succeed: the capacity to seed and maintain a population of tumor-initiating stem cells; the ability

SUMMARY REVIEW—cont'd

to create adaptive, organ-specific colonization programs; and the development of a supportive microenvironmental niche.

18. Metastases also may occur early in the process of neoplastic transformation.

19. DCIS refers to a heterogeneous group of proliferative lesions limited to ducts and lobules without invasion to the basement membrane. Preinvasive lesions do not invariably progress to invasive malignancy. LCIS originates from the terminal duct-lobular unit.

20. The first clinical manifestation of breast cancer is usually a small, painless lump in the breast. Other manifestations include palpable lymph nodes in the axilla, dimpling of the skin, nipple and skin retraction, nipple discharge, ulcerations, reddened skin, and bone pain associated with bony metastases.

21. Treatment is based on the extent or stage of the cancer and includes surgery, radiation, chemotherapy, hormone therapy, and biologic therapy.

KEY TERMS

Abnormal uterine bleeding (AUB), 762
Adenomyosis, 776
Amenorrhea, 759
Anorgasmia (orgasmic dysfunction), 786
Anovulation, 760
Atypia, 790
Atypical ductal hyperplasia (ADH), 792
Atypical hyperplasia (AH), 792
Atypical lobular hyperplasia (ALH), 792
Bartholinitis (Bartholin cyst), 770
Benign breast disease (BBD), 789
Central precocious puberty, 758
Cervical dysplasia, 779
Cervicitis, 770
Complete precocious puberty, 759
Corpus luteum cyst, 774
Cyst, 789
Cystocele, 771
Dermoid cyst, 774
Diffuse papillomatosis (multiple papilloma), 790
Disorders of desire (hypoactive sexual desire, decreased libido), 786
Ductal carcinoma in situ (DCIS), 820
Dyspareunia (painful intercourse), 786
E-cadherin, 821
Endometrial polyp, 774
Endometriosis, 776
Enterocele, 772
Epithelial to mesenchymal transition, 805
Fibrocystic change (FCC), 789

Follicular cyst, 774
Functional cyst, 773
Galactorrhea (inappropriate lactation), 788
Genetic heterogeneity, 813
Hirsutism, 761
Hyperprolactinemia, 760
Infertility, 787
Intraductal papilloma, 790
Invasive breast carcinoma, 821
Invasive carcinoma of the cervix, 780
Leiomyoma (myoma, uterine fibroid), 775
Lobular carcinoma in situ (LCIS), 821
Lobular hyperplasia, 793
Lobular involution, 796
Mammographic breast density (MBD), 807
Mild hyperplasia of the usual type, 789
Minimal residual disease (MRD), 817
Mixed precocious puberty, 759
Mucopurulent cervicitis (MPC), 770
Nonpuerperal hyperprolactinemia, 788
Oophoritis, 767
Papillary apocrine (glandular) change, 789
Partial precocious puberty, 758
Pelvic inflammatory disease (PID), 767
Pelvic organ prolapse (POP), 771
Percent mammographic density (PMD), 808
Pessary, 772
Phenotypic heterogeneity, 813
Polycystic ovary syndrome (PCOS), 764
Post-lactational involution, 798

Precocious puberty, 757
Pregnancy-associated breast cancer (PABC), 795
Premenstrual dysphoric disorder (PMDD), 766
Premenstrual syndrome (PMS), 766
Primary amenorrhea, 760
Primary dysmenorrhea, 759
Prolactin-inhibiting factor (PIF), 788
Radial scar (RS), 790
Radiogenic breast cancer, 809
Reactive stroma (inflammatory stroma), 817
Rectocele, 772
Retrograde menstruation, 776
Salpingitis, 767
Sclerosing adenosis, 790
Secondary amenorrhea, 760
Secondary dysmenorrhea, 759
Simple fibroadenoma, 792
Signal transducer and activator of transcription 3 (Stat3), 798
Terminal duct lobular unit (TDLU), 796
Transformation zone, 778
Usual ductal hyperplasia (UDH), 790
Uterine prolapse, 771
Uterine sarcoma, 783
Vaginismus, 787
Vaginitis, 769
Vulvodynia, 770
Xenoestrogen, 813

REFERENCES

1. American Cancer Society (ACS): *Cancer facts & figures—2017*, Atlanta, 2017, Author.
2. Eisenberg ML, et al: Increased risk of incident chronic medical conditions in infertile men: analysis of United States claims data. *Fertil Steril* 105(3):629–636, 2016.
3. Winkelman WD, et al: The sexual impact of infertility among women seeking fertility care. *Sex Med* 4(3):e190–e197, 2016.
4. Mongan NP, et al: Androgen insensitivity syndrome. *Best Pract Res Clin Endocrinol Metab* 29(4):569–580, 2015.
5. Hughes IA, et al: Consensus statement on management of intersex disorders. *J Pediatr Urol* 2(3):148–162, 2006.
6. Patel V, Casey RK, Gomez-Lobo V: Timing of gonadectomy in patients with complete androgen insensitivity syndrome—current recommendations and future directions. *J Pediatr Adolesc Gynecol* 29(4):320–325, 2016.
7. Acién P, Acién M: The presentation and management of complex female genital malformations. *Hum Reprod Update* 22(1):48–69, 2016.

8. Scsukova S, et al: Impact of endocrine disrupting chemicals on onset and development of female reproductive disorders and hormone-related cancer. *Reprod Biol* 16(4):243–254, 2016.
9. Venetis CA, et al: Clinical implications of congenital uterine anomalies: a meta-analysis of comparative studies. *Reprod Biomed Online* 29(6):665–683, 2014.
10. Kaplowitz P, et al: Evaluation and referral of children with signs of early puberty. *Pediatrics* 137(1):1–6, 2016.
11. Marcovecchio ML, Chiarelli F: Obesity and growth during childhood and puberty. *World Rev Nutr Diet* 106:135–141, 2013.
12. Palmert MR, Dunkel L: Clinical practice. Delayed puberty. *N Engl J Med* 366(5):443–453, 2012.
13. Abitbol L, Zborovski S, Palmert MR: Evaluation of delayed puberty: what diagnostic tests should be performed in the seemingly otherwise well adolescent? *Arch Dis Child* 101(8):767–771, 2015.
14. Trotman GE: Delayed puberty in the female patient. *Curr Opin Obstet Gynecol* 28(5):366–372, 2015.

15. Cattran AM, et al: Bone density and timing of puberty in a longitudinal study of girls. *J Pediatr Adolesc Gynecol* 28(3):170–172, 2015.
16. Sedlmeyer IL, Palmert MR: Delayed puberty: analysis of a large case series from an academic center. *J Clin Endocrinol Metab* 87(4):1613–1620, 2002.
17. Colvin CW, Abdullatif H: Anatomy of female puberty: the clinical relevance of developmental changes in the reproductive system. *Clin Anat* 26(1):115–129, 2013.
18. Fuqua JS: Treatment and outcomes of precocious puberty: an update. *J Clin Endocrinol Metab* 98(6):2198–2207, 2013.
19. Sørensen K, et al: Recent secular trends in pubertal timing: implications for evaluation and diagnosis of precocious puberty. *Horm Res Paediatr* 77(3):137–145, 2012.
20. Cheng G, et al: Beyond overweight: nutrition as an important lifestyle factor influencing timing of puberty. *Nutr Rev* 70(3):133–152, 2012.
21. Willemsen RH, Dunger DB: Normal variation in pubertal timing: genetic determinants in relation

to growth and adiposity. *Endocr Dev* 29:17–35, 2016.

22. Buluş AD, et al: The evaluation of possible role of endocrine disruptors in central and peripheral precocious puberty. *Toxicol Mech Methods* 25:1–8, 2016.
23. Bertelloni S, et al: Central precocious puberty: adult height in girls treated with quarterly or monthly gonadotropin-releasing hormone analog triptorelin. *Horm Res Paediatr* 84(6):396–400, 2015.
24. Roberts C: Psychosocial dimensions of early-onset puberty and its treatment. *Lancet Diabetes Endocrinol* 4(3):195–197, 2016.
25. Macedo DB, et al: Central precocious puberty that appears to be sporadic caused by paternally inherited mutations in the imprinted gene *makorin ring finger 3. J Clin Endocrinol Metab* 99(6):E1097–E1103, 2014.
26. Schoelwer M, Eugster EA: Treatment of peripheral precocious puberty. *Endocr Dev* 29:230–239, 2016.
27. Rosenfield RL, Cooke DW, Radovick S: Puberty and its disorders in the female. In Sperling M, Mark A, editors: *Pediatric endocrinology*, Philadelphia, PA, 2014, Elsevier Health Sciences, pp 569–663.
28. Menditta V: Primary and secondary dysmenorrhea, premenstrual syndrome, and premenstrual dysphoric disorder. In Lobo RA, et al, editors: *Comprehensive gynecology*, Philadelphia, PA, 2017, Elsevier, pp 815–828.
29. Iacovides S, Avidon I, Baker FC: What we know about primary dysmenorrhea today: a critical review. *Hum Reprod Update* 21(6):762–778, 2015.
30. Wei SY, et al: Changes in functional connectivity of pain modulatory systems in women with primary dysmenorrhea. *Pain* 157(1):92–102, 2016.
31. Marjoribanks J, et al: Nonsteroidal anti-inflammatory drugs for dysmenorrhea. *Cochrane Database Syst Rev* (7):CD001751, 2015.
32. Lethaby A, et al: Progesterone or progestogen-releasing intrauterine systems for heavy menstrual bleeding. *Cochrane Database Syst Rev* (4):CD002126, 2015.
33. Klein DA, Poth MA: Amenorrhea: an approach to diagnosis and management. *Am Fam Physician* 87(11):781–788, 2013.
34. Lobo R: Primary and secondary amenorrhea and precocious puberty. In Lobo RA, et al, editors: *Comprehensive gynecology*, Philadelphia, PA, 2017, Elsevier, pp 829–852.
35. Marsh CA, Grimstad FW: Primary amenorrhea: diagnosis and management. *Obstet Gynecol Surv* 69(10):603–612, 2014.
36. DiVall SA, Rosenfield RL: Menstrual disorders and hyperandrogenism in adolescence. In Radovick S, MacGillivray MH, editors: *Pediatric endocrinology: a practical clinical guide*, New York, 2013, Springer Science + Business Media, pp 441–464.
37. Munro MG, et al: FIGO classification system (PALM-COEIN) for causes of abnormal uterine bleeding in nongravid women of reproductive age. *Int J Gynaecol Obstet* 113(1):3–13, 2011.
38. Munro MG: Practical aspects of the two FIGO systems for management of abnormal uterine bleeding in the reproductive years. *Best Pract Res Clin Obstet Gynaecol* 40:3–22, 2017.
39. Ryntz T, Lobo RA: Abnormal uterine bleeding: etiology and management of acute and chronic excessive bleeding. In Lobo R, et al, editors: *Comprehensive gynecology*, Philadelphia, PA, 2017, Elsevier, pp 621–634.
40. Matteson KA, et al: Abnormal uterine bleeding, health status, and usual source of medical care: analyses using the Medical Expenditures Panel

Survey. *J Womens Health (Larchmt)* 22(11):959–965, 2013.
41. Matthews ML: Abnormal uterine bleeding in reproductive-aged women. *Obstet Gynecol Clin North Am* 42(1):103–115, 2015.
42. Whiteman MK, et al: Inpatient hospitalization for gynecologic disorders in the United States. *Am J Obstet Gynecol* 202(6):541, 2010.
43. Deneris A: PALM-COEIN nomenclature for abnormal uterine bleeding. *J Midwifery Womens Health* 61(3):376–379, 2016.
44. Bradley LD, Gueye NA: The medical management of abnormal uterine bleeding in reproductive-aged women. *Am J Obstet Gynecol* 214(1):31–44, 2016.
45. Chang RJ: Polycystic ovary syndrome and hyperandrogenic states. In Strauss JF, Barbieri RL, editors: *Yen and Jaffe's reproductive endocrinology*, ed 7, Philadelphia, PA, 2014, Elsevier, pp 485–511.
46. Legro RS, et al: Diagnosis and treatment of polycystic ovary syndrome: an Endocrine Society clinical practice guideline. *J Clin Endocrinol Metab* 98(12):4565–4592, 2013.
47. Ecklund LC, Usadi RS: Endocrine and reproductive effects of polycystic ovarian syndrome. *Obstet Gynecol Clin North Am* 42(1):55–65, 2015.
48. Wilson EE: Polycystic ovarian syndrome and hyperandrogenism. In Hoffman BL, et al, editors: *Williams gynecology*, ed 3, New York, 2016, McGraw-Hill, pp 386–404.
49. Diamanti-Kandarakis E, Dunaif A: Insulin resistance and the polycystic ovary syndrome revisited: an update on mechanisms and implications. *Endocr Rev* 33(6):981–1030, 2012.
50. Rosenfield RL, Ehrmann DA: The pathogenesis of polycystic ovary syndrome (PCOS): the hypothesis of PCOS as functional ovarian hyperandrogenism revisited. *Endocr Rev* 37(5):467–520, 2016.
51. Lim SS, et al: Overweight, obesity and central obesity in women with polycystic ovary syndrome: a systematic review and meta-analysis. *Hum Reprod Update* 18(6):618–637, 2012.
52. Franik G, et al: Sleep disturbances in women with polycystic ovary syndrome. *Gynecol Endocrinol* 32(12):1014–1017, 2016.
53. Chang RJ: Polycystic ovary syndrome and hyperandrogenic states. In Strauss JF, Barbieri RL, editors: *Yen and Jaffe's reproductive endocrinology*, ed 7, Philadelphia, PA, 2014, Elsevier, pp 485–511.
54. Bradshaw KD, Brandon AR: Psychosocial issues and female sexuality. In Hoffman BL, et al, editors: *Williams gynecology*, ed 3, New York, 2016, McGraw-Hill, pp 297–317.
55. Hofmeister S, Bodden S: Premenstrual syndrome and premenstrual dysphoric disorder. *Am Fam Physician* 94(3):236–240, 2016.
56. Hantsoo L, Epperson CN: Premenstrual dysphoric disorder: epidemiology and treatment. *Curr Psychiatry Rep* 17(11):87, 2015.
57. Shehata NA: Calcium versus oral contraceptive pills containing drospirenone for the treatment of mild to moderate premenstrual syndrome: a double blind randomized placebo controlled trial. *Eur J Obstet Gynecol Reprod Biol* 198:100–104, 2016.
58. Kelderhouse K, Taylor JS: A review of treatment and management modalities for premenstrual dysphoric disorder. *Nurs Womens Health* 17(4):294–305, 2013.
59. Lustyk MK, et al: Cognitive-behavioral therapy for premenstrual syndrome and premenstrual dysphoric disorder: a systematic review. *Arch Womens Ment Health* 12(2):85–96, 2009.

60. Lopez LM, Kaptein AA, Helmerhorst FM: Oral contraceptives containing drospirenone for premenstrual syndrome. *Cochrane Database Syst Rev* (2):CD006586, 2012.
61. Centers for Disease Control and Prevention (CDC): *Sexually transmitted diseases treatment guidelines*, Atlanta, GA, 2015, Author.
62. Das BB, Ronda J, Trent M: Pelvic inflammatory disease: improving awareness, prevention, and treatment. *Infect Drug Resist* 9:191–197, 2016.
63. Haggerty CL, et al: Identification of novel microbes associated with pelvic inflammatory disease and infertility. *Sex Transm Infect* 92(6):441–446, 2016.
64. Jatlaoui TC, Riley HE, Curtis KM: The safety of intrauterine devices among young women: a systematic review. *Contraception* 95(1):17–39, 2016.
65. Chayachinda C, Rekhawasin T: Reproductive outcomes of patients being hospitalised with pelvic inflammatory disease. *J Obstet Gynaecol* 37(2):228–232, 2017.
66. Centers for Disease Control and Prevention (CDC): *Pelvic inflammatory disease (PID) treatment and care*, Atlanta, GA, 2015, Author.
67. Brunham RC, Gottlieb SL, Paavonen J: Pelvic inflammatory disease. *N Engl J Med* 372(21):2039–2048, 2015.
68. Wiesenfeld HC, et al: Subclinical pelvic inflammatory disease and infertility. *Obstet Gynecol* 120(1):37–43, 2012.
69. Gardella C, Eckert LO, Lentz GM: Genital tract infections. In Lobo RA, et al, editors: *Comprehensive gynecology*, Philadelphia, PA, 2017, Elsevier, pp 524–565.
70. McCord E, Rahn D: Gynecologic infection. In Hoffman BL, et al, editors: *Williams gynecology*, ed 3, New York, 2016, McGraw-Hill, pp 50–85.
71. Palmeira-de-Oliveira R, Palmeira-de-Oliveira A, Martinez-de-Oliveira J: New strategies for local treatment of vaginal infections. *Adv Drug Deliv Rev* 92:105–122, 2015.
72. Recine N, et al: Restoring vaginal microbiota: biological control of bacterial vaginosis. A prospective case–control study using *Lactobacillus rhamnosus* BMX 54 as adjuvant treatment against bacterial vaginosis. *Arch Gynecol Obstet* 293(1):101–107, 2016.
73. Workowski KA, Bolan GA: Sexually transmitted diseases treatment guidelines 2015. *MMWR Recomm Rep* 64(RR-3):1–137, 2015.
74. Mattson SK, Polk JP, Nyirjesy P: Chronic cervicitis: presenting features and response to therapy. *J Low Genit Tract Dis* 20(3):e30–e33, 2016.
75. Taylor SN, et al: Prevalence and treatment outcome of cervicitis of unknown etiology. *Sex Transm Dis* 40(5):379–385, 2013.
76. Stockdale CK, Lawson HW: 2013 vulvodynia guideline update. *J Low Genit Tract Dis* 18(2):93–100, 2014.
77. De Andres J, et al: Vulvodynia—an evidence-based literature review and proposed treatment algorithm. *Pain Pract* 16(2):204–236, 2016.
78. Lee MY, et al: Clinical pathology of Bartholin's glands: a review of the literature. *Curr Urol* 8(1):22–25, 2015.
79. Barber MD: Pelvic organ prolapse. *BMJ* 354:i3853, 2016.
80. Bugge C, et al: Pessaries (mechanical devices) for pelvic organ prolapse in women. *Cochrane Database Syst Rev* (2):CD004010, 2013.
81. Hoffman BL: Pelvic mass. In Hoffman BL, et al, editors: *Williams gynecology*, ed 3, New York, 2016, McGraw-Hill, pp 202–229.

82. Dolan MS, Hill C, Valea FA: Benign gynecologic lesions. In Lobo RA, et al, editors: *Comprehensive gynecology*, Philadelphia, PA, 2017, Elsevier, pp 370–422.

83. Whiteman MK, et al: Inpatient hospitalization for gynecologic disorders in the United States. *Am J Obstet Gynecol* 202(6):541, 2010.

84. Biggs WS, Marks ST: Diagnosis and management of adnexal masses. *Am Fam Physician* 93(8): 676–681, 2016.

85. Bulun SE: Physiology and pathology of the female reproductive axis. In Melmed S, et al, editors: *Williams textbook of endocrinology*, Philadelphia, 2016, Elsevier.

86. Eskander R, Berman M, Keder L: Practice bulletin No. 174: evaluation and management of adnexal masses. *Obstet Gynecol* 128(5):e210–e226, 2016.

87. Bueloni-Dias FN, et al: Metabolic syndrome as a predictor of endometrial polyps in postmenopausal women. *Menopause* 23(7): 759–764, 2016.

88. Cholkeri-Singh A, Sasaki KJ: Hysteroscopy for infertile women: a review. *J Minim Invasive Gynecol* 22(3):353–362, 2015.

89. Hamani Y, et al: The clinical significance of small endometrial polyps. *Eur J Obstet Gynecol Reprod Biol* 170(2):497–500, 2013.

90. Fuldeore M, et al: Healthcare utilization and costs among women diagnosed with uterine fibroids: a longitudinal evaluation for 5 years pre- and post-diagnosis. *Curr Med Res Opin* 31(9): 1719–1731, 2015.

91. Wise LA, Laughlin-Tommaso SK: Epidemiology of uterine fibroids: from menarche to menopause. *Clin Obstet Gynecol* 59(1):2–24, 2016.

92. Styer AK, Rueda BR: The epidemiology and genetics of uterine leiomyoma. *Best Pract Res Clin Obstet Gynaecol* 34:3–12, 2016.

93. Bartels CB, et al: An evidence-based approach to the medical management of fibroids: a systematic review. *Clin Obstet Gynecol* 59(1):30–52, 2016.

94. Pontis A, et al: Adenomyosis: a systematic review of medical treatment. *Gynecol Endocrinol* 23(9): 696–700, 2016.

95. Abbott JA: Adenomyosis and abnormal uterine bleeding (AUB-A)—pathogenesis, diagnosis, and management. *Best Pract Res Clin Obstet Gynaecol* 40:68–81, 2017.

96. Hoffman BL: Endometriosis. In Hoffman BL, et al, editors: *Williams gynecology*, ed 3, New York, 2016, McGraw-Hill, pp 230–248.

97. Taylor R, Lebovic DI: Endometriosis. In Strauss JF, Barbieri RL, editors: *Yen and Jaffe's reproductive endocrinology*, ed 7, Philadelphia, PA, 2014, Elsevier, pp 565–585.

98. Mogensen JB, et al: Endometriosis and risks for ovarian, endometrial and breast cancers: a nationwide cohort study. *Gynecol Oncol* 143(1): 87–92, 2016.

99. Sampson JA: Peritoneal endometriosis due to the menstrual dissemination of endometrial tissue into the peritoneal cavity. *Am J Obstet Gynecol* 14:422, 1927.

100. Burney RO, Giudice LC: Pathogenesis and pathophysiology of endometriosis. *Fertil Steril* 98(3):511–519, 2012.

101. Signorile PG, et al: Embryologic origin of endometriosis: analysis of 101 human female fetuses. *J Cell Physiol* 227(4):1653–1656, 2012.

102. Signorile PG, Baldi A: New evidence in endometriosis. *Int J Biochem Cell Biol* 60:19–22, 2015.

103. Markham SM, et al: Extrapelvic endometriosis. *Obstet Gynecol Clin North Am* 16(1):193–219, 1989.

104. Lessey BA, Young SL: Pathophysiology of infertility in endometriosis. In Giudice LC, Evers JLH, Healy DL, editors: *Endometriosis: science and practice*, Oxford, UK, 2012, Wiley-Blackwell.

105. Vannuccini S, et al: Infertility and reproductive disorders: impact of hormonal and inflammatory mechanisms on pregnancy outcome. *Hum Reprod Update* 22(1):104–115, 2016.

106. Kodaman PH: Current strategies for endometriosis management. *Obstet Gynecol Clin North Am* 42(1):87–101, 2015.

107. Vercellini P, et al: Estrogen-progestins and progestins for the management of endometriosis. *Fertil Steril* 106(7):1552–1571, 2016.

108. Johnson NP, Hummelshoj L: World Endometriosis Society Montpellier Consortium. Consensus on current management of endometriosis. *Hum Reprod* 28(6):1552–1568, 2013.

109. Singh GK, Azuine RE, Siahpush M: Global inequalities in cervical cancer incidence and mortality are linked to deprivation, low socioeconomic status, and human development. *Int J MCH AIDS* 1(1):17–30, 2012.

110. Centers for Disease Control and Prevention (CDC): *Sexually transmitted disease surveillance 2015*, Atlanta, 2016, U.S. Department of Health and Human Services.

111. Frieden TR, et al: Sexually transmitted diseases treatment guidelines 2015. *MMWR Recomm Rep* 64(3):84–90, 2015.

112. Vesco KK, et al: *Screening for cervical cancer: a systematic evidence review for the U.S. Preventive Services Task Force [Internet]*, Rockville, MD, 2011, Agency for Healthcare Research and Quality.

113. Bui TC, et al: Association between vaginal douching and genital human papillomavirus infection among women in the United States. *J Infect Dis* 214(9):1370–1375, 2016.

114. Mitra A, et al: The vaginal microbiota, human papillomavirus infection and cervical intraepithelial neoplasia: what do we know and where are we going next? *Microbiome* 4(1):58, 2016.

115. Bittoni MA, Fisher JL, Weier R: The influence of lifestyle risk factors on the occurrence of gynecological cancers: a review of the evidence and opportunities for prevention and management. *Int J Cancer Stud Res* S2(001):1–8, 2015.

116. Dugué PA, et al: Immunosuppression and risk of cervical cancer. *Expert Rev Anticancer Ther* 13(1):29–42, 2013.

117. Panel on Opportunistic Infections in HIV-Infected Adults and Adolescents: *Guidelines for the prevention and treatment of opportunistic infections in HIV-infected adults and adolescents: recommendations from the Centers for Disease Control and Prevention, the National Institutes of Health, and the HIV Medicine Association of the Infectious Diseases Society of America*. Available at: https://aidsinfo.nih.gov/contentfiles/lvguidelines/Adult_OI.pdf.

118. Bianchi S, et al: *Chlamydia trachomatis* infection and HPV/*Chlamydia trachomatis* co-infection among HPV-vaccinated young women at the beginning of their sexual activity. *Arch Gynecol Obstet* 294(6):1227–1233, 2016.

119. de Abreu AL, et al: Association of human papillomavirus, *Neisseria gonorrhoeae* and *Chlamydia trachomatis* co-infections on the risk of high-grade squamous intraepithelial cervical lesion. *Am J Cancer Res* 6(6):1371–1383, 2016.

120. Ojesina AI, et al: Landscape of genomic alterations in cervical carcinomas. *Nature* 506(7488):371–375, 2014.

121. Hu Z, et al: Human papillomavirus 16 oncoprotein regulates the translocation of β-catenin via the activation of epidermal growth factor receptor. *Cancer* 121(2):214–225, 2015.

122. Massad LS, et al: 2012 updated consensus guidelines for the management of abnormal cervical cancer screening tests and cancer precursors. *Obstet Gynecol* 121(4):829–846, 2013.

123. Salcedo MP, Baker ES, Schmeler K: Interepithelial neoplasia of the lower genital tract. In Lobo RA, et al, editors: *Comprehensive gynecology*, Philadelphia, PA, 2017, Elsevier, pp 655–665.

124. Pfaendler KS, Tewari KS: Changing paradigms in the systemic treatment of advanced cervical cancer. *Am J Obstet Gynecol* 214(1):22–30, 2016.

125. Committee opinion No. 641: human papillomavirus vaccination. *Obstet Gynecol* 126(3):e38–e43, 2015.

126. Berenson AB, Laz TH, Rahman M: Reduction in vaccine-type human papillomavirus prevalence among adult females in the United States, 2009–2012. *J Infect Dis* 214(12):1961–1964, 2016.

127. PDQ Adult Treatment Editorial Board: Vaginal cancer treatment (PDQ): health professional version, 2016 Feb 9. *PDQ cancer information summaries [Internet]*, Bethesda, MD, National Cancer Institute. Available at: http://www-ncbi-nlm-nih-gov.proxy.library.vanderbilt.edu/books/NBK65801/.

128. Shrivastava SB, et al: Management of vaginal cancer. *Rev Recent Clin Trials* 10(4):289–297, 2015.

129. Goodman A, Schorge J, Greene MF: The long-term effects of in utero exposures—the DES story. *N Engl J Med* 364(22):2083–2084, 2011.

130. Bodurka DC, Frumovitz M: Malignant diseases of the vagina. In Lobo RA, et al, editors: *Comprehensive gynecology*, Philadelphia, PA, 2017, Elsevier, pp 704–713.

131. Wakeham K, et al: HPV status and favorable outcome in vulvar squamous cancer. *Int J Cancer* 140(5):1134–1146, 2017.

132. PDQ Adult Treatment Editorial Board: Vulvar cancer treatment (PDQ): health professional version, 2016 Feb 11. *PDQ cancer information summaries [Internet]*, Bethesda, MD, National Cancer Institute. Available at: http://www-ncbi-nlm-nih-gov.proxy.library.vanderbilt.edu/books/NBK65760/.

133. Committee opinion No. 675: management of vulvar intraepithelial neoplasia. *Obstet Gynecol* 128(4):e178–e182, 2016.

134. Soderini A, Aragona A, Reed N: Advanced vulvar cancers: what are the best options for treatment? *Curr Oncol Rep* 18(10):64, 2016.

135. PDQ Screening and Prevention Editorial Board: Endometrial cancer prevention (PDQ®): health professional version, 2016 Jun 30. *PDQ cancer information summaries [Internet]*, Bethesda, MD, National Cancer Institute. Available at: http://www-ncbi-nlm-nih-gov.proxy.library.vanderbilt.edu/books/NBK66042/.

136. Onstad MA, Schmandt RE, Lu KH: Addressing the role of obesity in endometrial cancer risk, prevention, and treatment. *J Clin Oncol* 34(35): 4225–4230, 2016.

137. Brosens LA, Offerhaus GJ, Giardiello FM: Hereditary colorectal cancer: genetics and screening. *Surg Clin North Am* 95(5):1067–1080, 2015.

138. Beavis AL, Smith AJ, Fader A: Lifestyle changes and the risk of developing endometrial and ovarian cancers: opportunities for prevention and management. *Int J Womens Health* 8:151–167, 2016.

139. Staff S, et al: Endometrial cancer risk factors among Lynch syndrome women: a retrospective cohort study. *Br J Cancer* 115(3):375–381, 2016.

140. Dominick S, et al: Levonorgestrel intrauterine system for endometrial protection in women with breast cancer on adjuvant tamoxifen. *Cochrane Database Syst Rev* (12):CD007245, 2015.

141. Dottino JA, et al: Levonorgestrel intrauterine device as an endometrial cancer prevention strategy in obese women: a cost-effectiveness analysis. *Obstet Gynecol* 128(4):747–753, 2016.

142. Soliman PT, Lu KH: Neoplastic diseases of the uterus. In Lobo RA, et al, editors: *Comprehensive gynecology*, Philadelphia, PA, 2017, Elsevier, pp 714–732.

143. Mørch LS, et al: The influence of hormone therapies on type I and II endometrial cancer: a nationwide cohort study. *Int J Cancer* 138(6):1506–1515, 2016.

144. Nathenson MJ, et al: Uterine adenosarcoma: a review. *Curr Oncol Rep* 18(11):68, 2016.

145. PDQ Adult Treatment Editorial Board: Uterine sarcoma treatment (PDQ): health professional version, 2015 Jul 15. *PDQ cancer information summaries [Internet]*, Bethesda, MD, National Cancer Institute. Available at: http://www-ncbi -nlm-nih-gov.proxy.library.vanderbilt.edu/books/ NBK65888/.

146. Wais M, et al: A multi-center retrospective review of clinical characteristics of uterine sarcoma. *J Minim Invasive Gynecol* 22(6S):S93, 2015.

147. Jayson GC, et al: Ovarian cancer. *Lancet* 384(9951):1376–1388, 2014.

148. PDQ Screening and Prevention Editorial Board: Ovarian, fallopian tube, and primary peritoneal cancer prevention (PDQ): health professional version, 2016 Nov 18. *PDQ cancer information summaries [Internet]*, Bethesda, MD, National Cancer Institute. Available at: http:// www-ncbi-nlm-nih-gov.proxy.library.vanderbilt.edu/ books/NBK65898/.

149. Wentzensen N, et al: Ovarian cancer risk factors by histologic subtype: an analysis from the Ovarian Cancer Cohort Consortium. *J Clin Oncol* 34(24):2888–2898, 2016.

150. Nezhat FR, et al: New insights in the pathophysiology of ovarian cancer and implications for screening and prevention. *Am J Obstet Gynecol* 213(3):262–267, 2015.

151. Rice MS, Hankinson SE, Tworoger SS: Tubal ligation, hysterectomy, unilateral oophorectomy, and risk of ovarian cancer in the Nurses' Health Study. *Fertil Steril* 102(1):192–198, 2014.

152. Rebbeck TR, et al: Association of type and location of *BRCA1* and *BRCA2* mutations with risk of breast and ovarian cancer. *JAMA* 313(13):1347–1361, 2015.

153. Ramus SJ, et al: Germline mutations in the *BRIP1*, *BARD1*, *PALB2*, and *NBN* genes in women with ovarian cancer. *J Natl Cancer Inst* 107(11):2015. pii: djv214. doi:10.1093/jnci/djv214.

154. Karnezis AN, et al: The disparate origins of ovarian cancers: pathogenesis and prevention strategies. *Nat Rev Cancer* 17(1):65–74, 2016.

155. Prahm KP, et al: The prognostic value of dividing epithelial ovarian cancer into type I and type II tumors based on pathologic characteristics. *Gynecol Oncol* 136(2):205–211, 2015.

156. National Cancer Institute (NCI): *PDQ ovarian epithelial, fallopian tube, and primary peritoneal cancer treatment*, Bethesda, MD, 2017, Health Professional National Cancer Institute, National Institutes of Health, U.S. Dept of Health and Human Services.

157. Coleman RL, Ramirez PT, Gershenson DM: Neoplastic diseases of the ovary. In Lobo RA, et al, editors: *Comprehensive gynecology*, Philadelphia, PA, 2017, Elsevier, pp 733–780.

158. Ludwig KK, et al: Risk reduction and survival benefit of prophylactic surgery in *BRCA* mutation carriers, a systematic review. *Am J Surg* 212(4):660–669, 2016.

159. American College of Obstetricians and Gynecologists (ACOG): *Female sexual dysfunction*, Washington, DC, 2011, Author.

160. Levin RJ, et al: The physiology of female sexual function and the pathophysiology of female sexual dysfunction (Committee 13A). *J Sex Med* 13(5):733–759, 2016.

161. Nappi PR, et al: Female sexual dysfunction (FSD): prevalence and impact on quality of life (QoL). *Maturitas* 94:87–91, 2016.

162. Dean J: Medication and sexual dysfunction. In Wylie K, editor: *ABC of sexual health*, West Sussex, UK, 2015, John Wiley & Sons, pp 51–54.

163. Parish SJ, Hahn SR: Hypoactive sexual desire disorder: a review of epidemiology, biopsychology, diagnosis, and treatment. *Sex Med Rev* 4(2):103–120, 2016.

164. Carreiro AV, et al: Sexual dysfunction risk and quality of life among women with a history of sexual abuse. *Int J Gynaecol Obstet* 134(3):260–263, 2016.

165. Lindsay TJ, Vitrikas KR: Evaluation and treatment of infertility. *Am Fam Physician* 91(5):308–314, 2015.

166. Barbieri RL: Female infertility. In Strauss JF, Barbieri RL, editors: *Yen and Jaffe's reproductive endocrinology*, ed 7, Philadelphia, PA, 2014, Elsevier, pp 512–517.

167. Marshburn PB: Counseling and diagnostic evaluation for the infertile couple. *Obstet Gynecol Clin North Am* 42(1):1–14, 2015.

168. Dickey RP: Evaluation of women with unexplained infertility. In Schattman G, Perelman RO, Esteves SC, editors: *Unexplained infertility*, New York, 2015, Springer, pp 213–221.

169. Turek PJ: Male infertility. In Strauss JF, Barbieri RL, editors: *Yen and Jaffe's reproductive endocrinology*, ed 7, Philadelphia, PA, 2014, Elsevier, pp 538–550.

170. Sunderum S, et al: Assisted reproductive technology surveillance—United States, 2013. *MMWR Surveill Summ* 64(11):1–25, 2015.

171. Stern JE, et al: Adverse pregnancy and birth outcomes associated with underlying diagnosis with and without assisted reproductive technology treatment. *Fertil Steril* 103(6):1438–1445, 2015.

172. Boulet SL, et al: Assisted reproductive technology and birth defects among liveborn infants in Florida, Massachusetts, and Michigan, 2000–2010. *JAMA Pediatr* 170(6):e154934, 2016.

173. Harney KA, Smith LF: The breast. In DeCherney AH, Pernoll ML, editors: *Current obstetric and gynecologic diagnosis and treatment*, ed 8, Norwalk, CT, 1994, Appleton & Lange.

174. Sabel MS: *Overview of benign breast disease*, 2015. Available at: www.uptodate.com.

175. Lester S: The breast. In Kumar V, Abbas AK, Fausto N, editors: *Robbins and Cotran pathologic basis of disease*, ed 9, Philadelphia, 2015, Elsevier Saunders.

176. Friedenreich C, et al: Risk factors for benign proliferative breast disease. *Int J Epidemiol* 29(4):634, 2000.

177. Murray M: Pathologic high-risk lesions, diagnosis and management. *Clin Obstet Gynecol* 59(4):727–732, 2016.

178. Costarelli L, et al: Intraductal proliferative lesions of the breast—terminology and biology matter: premalignant lesions or preinvasive cancer? *Int J Surg Oncol* 2012:501905, 2012.

179. Love SM, Lindsey K: *Dr. Susan Love's breast book*, ed 5, Philadelphia, 2010, Merloyd Lawrence, Da Capo Press.

180. Dupont WD, Page DL: Risk factors for breast cancer in women with proliferative breast disease. *N Engl J Med* 312:146–151, 1985.

181. Hartmann LC, et al: Benign breast disease and the risk of breast cancer. *N Engl J Med* 353:229–237, 2005.

182. Hartmann LC, et al: Understanding the premalignant potential of atypical hyperplasia through its natural history: a longitudinal cohort study. *Cancer Prev Res (Phila)* 7:211–217, 2014.

183. Zhou WB, et al: The influence of family history and histological stratification on breast cancer risk in women with benign breast disease: a meta-analysis. *J Cancer Res Clin Oncol* 137(7):1053–1060, 2011.

184. Page DL, et al: Atypical hyperplastic lesions of the female breast. A long-term follow-up study. *Cancer* 55:2698–2708, 1985.

185. Sanders M, et al: Continued observation of the natural history of low-grade ductal carcinoma in situ reaffirms proclivity for local recurrence even after more than 30 years of follow-up. *Mod Pathol* 28(5):662–669, 2015.

186. Page DL, et al: Atypical lobular hyperplasia as a unilateral predictor of breast cancer risk: a retrospective cohort study. *Lancet* 361(9352):125–129, 2003.

187. Degnim AC, et al: Extent of atypical hyperplasia stratifies breast cancer risk in 2 independent cohorts of women. *Cancer* 122(19):2971–2978, 2016.

188. Collins LC, et al: Breast cancer risk by extent and type of atypical hyperplasia: an update from the Nurses' Health Studies. *Cancer* 122(4):515–520, 2016.

189. Calhoun BC, Livasy CA: Mitigating overdiagnosis and overtreatment in breast cancer. *Arch Pathol Lab Med* 138:1428–1431, 2014.

190. Esserman LJ, et al: Addressing overdiagnosis and overtreatment in cancer: a prescription for change. *Lancet Oncol* 15(6):e234–e242, 2014.

191. Lampe JW, et al: Plasma isoflavones and fibrocystic breast conditions and breast cancer among women in Shanghai, China. *Cancer Epidemiol Biomarkers Prev* 16(12):2579–2586, 2007.

192. Guha N, et al: Soy isoflavones and risk of cancer recurrence in a cohort of breast cancer survivors: the Life after Cancer Epidemiology Study. *Breast Cancer Res Treat* 118:395–405, 2009.

193. Li Y, et al: Genistein depletes telomerase activity through cross-talk between genetic and epigenetic mechanism. *Int J Cancer* 125(2):286–296, 2009.

194. Islam MA, et al: Deconjugation of soy isoflavone glucuronides needed for estrogenic activity. *Toxicol In Vitro* 29(4):706–715, 2015.

195. North American Menopause Society (NAMS): The role of soy isoflavones in menopausal health: report of The North American Menopause Society/Wulf H. Utian Translational Science Symposium in Chicago, IL. *Menopause* 18(7):732–753, 2011.

196. National Cancer Institute (NCI): *Radiation risks and pediatric computed tomography (CT): a guide for health care providers*, 2002. Available at: www.cancer.gov.

197. Rösner H, et al: Antiproliferative/cytotoxic effects of molecular iodine, povidone-iodine and Lugol's

solution in different carcinoma cell lines. *Oncol Lett* 12(3):2159–2162, 2016.

198. Centers for Disease Control and Prevention (CDC): *Breast cancer: what you need to know,* Atlanta, GA, 2016, National Center for Chronic Disease Prevention and Health Promotion, Division of Cancer Prevention and Control.

199. National Cancer Institute (NCI): *Cancer stat facts: female breast cancer,* Bethesda, MD, 2016, National Cancer Institute Surveillance, Epidemiology, and End Results Program.

200. Centers for Disease Control and Prevention (CDC): *Breast cancer rates by race and ethnicity,* Atlanta, 2016, Author.

201. International Agency for Research on Cancer (IARC): *GLOBOCAN 2012: estimated cancer incidence, mortality and prevalence worldwide in 2012,* Geneva, 2016 International Agency for Research on Cancer, World Health Organization.

202. Howlader N, et al: *SEER cancer statistics review, 1975–2009 (vintage 2009 populations),* Bethesda, MD, 2012, National Cancer Institute. Available at: http://seer.cancer.gov/csr/1975_2009_pops09.

203. Centers for Disease Control and Prevention (CDC): *Risk factors for breast cancer in young women,* Atlanta, GA, 2014, Author.

204. Martinson HA, et al: Wound healing-like immune program facilitates postpartum mammary gland involution and tumor progression. *Int J Cancer* 136(8):1803–1813, 2015.

205. Sternlicht MD, et al: Hormonal and local control of mammary branching morphogenesis. *Differentiation* 74:365–381, 2006.

206. Medina D: Mammary developmental fate and breast cancer risk. *Endocr Relat Cancer* 12:483–495, 2005.

207. Lyons TR, et al: Postpartum mammary gland involution drives progression of ductal carcinoma in situ through collagen and COX-2. *Nat Med* 17:1109–1115, 2011.

208. Medina D: Breast cancer: the protective effect of pregnancy. *Clin Cancer Res* 10(1 Pt 2):380S–384S, 2004.

209. Lord SJ, et al: Breast cancer risk and hormone receptor status in older women by parity, age of first birth, and breastfeeding: a case-control study. *Cancer Epidemiol Biomarkers Prev* 17(7):1723–1730, 2008.

210. Lyons TR, Schedin PJ, Borges VF: Pregnancy and breast cancer: when they collide. *J Mammary Gland Biol Neoplasia* 14:87–98, 2009.

211. O'Brien J, et al: Alternatively activated macrophages and collagen remodeling characterize the postpartum involuting mammary gland across species. *Am J Pathol* 176(3):1241–1255, 2010.

212. Schedin P: Pregnancy-associated breast cancer and metastasis. *Nat Rev Cancer* 6:281–291, 2006.

213. Fornetti J, et al: Emerging targets for the prevention of pregnancy-associated breast cancer. *Cell Cycle* 11(4):639–640, 2012.

214. Schedin P, et al: Microenvironment of the involuting mammary gland mediates mammary cancer progression. *J Mammary Gland Biol Neoplasia* 12:71–82, 2007.

215. Barton M, Santucci-Pereira J, Russo J: Molecular pathways involved in pregnancy-induced prevention against breast cancer. *Front Endocrinol (Lausanne)* 5:213, 2014.

216. Milanese TR, et al: Age-related lobular involution and risk of breast cancer. *J Natl Cancer Inst* 98(2):1600–1607, 2006.

217. Bodelon C, et al: Association between breast cancer genetic susceptibility variants and terminal duct lobular unit involution of the breast. *Int J Cancer* 140(4):825–832, 2016.

218. Jindal S, et al: Postpartum breast involution reveals regression of secretory lobules mediated by tissue-remodeling. *Breast Cancer Res* 16(2):R31, 2014.

219. Watson CJ: Involution: apoptosis and tissue remodeling that convert the mammary gland from milk factory to a quiescent organ. *Breast Cancer Res* 8(2):203, 2006.

220. Van Dang H, et al: Nucling, a novel apoptosis-associated protein, controls mammary gland involution by regulating NF-κB and STAT3. *J Biol Chem* 290(40):24626–24635, 2015.

221. Hughes K, et al: Conditional deletion of Stat3 in mammary epithelium impairs the acute phase response and modulates immune cell numbers during post-lactational regression. *J Pathol* 227(1):106–117, 2012.

222. Dvorak HP: Tumors: wounds that do not heal. Similarities between tumor stroma generation and wound healing. *N Engl J Med* 315:1650–1659, 1989.

223. Hobson J, et al: Acute inflammation induced by the biopsy of mouse mammary tumors promotes the development of metastasis. *Breast Cancer Res Treat* 139:391–401, 2013.

224. DeNardo DG, et al: Leukocyte complexity predicts breast cancer survival and functionally regulates response to chemotherapy. *Cancer Discov* 1(1):54–67, 2011.

225. Gupta PB, et al: Systemic stromal effects of estrogen promote the growth of estrogen receptor-negative cancers. *Cancer Res* 67:2062–2071, 2007.

226. Iyer V, et al: Estrogen promotes ER-negative tumor growth and angiogenesis through mobilization of bone marrow-derived monocytes. *Cancer Res* 72:2705–2713, 2012.

227. Cutler SY, Young JL: Third National Cancer Survey: incidence data. *Natl Cancer Inst Monogr* 41, 1975.

228. Vorrherr H, editor: *The breast: morphology, physiology, and lactation,* New York, 1974, Academic Press.

229. Kelsey JL, Gammon MD, John EM: Reproductive factors and breast cancer. *Epidemiol Rev* 15:36–47, 1993.

230. Ursin G, et al: Reproductive factors and subtypes of breast cancer defined by hormone receptor and histology. *Br J Cancer* 93:364–371, 2005.

231. Trichopoulos D, et al: Age at any birth and breast cancer risk. *Int J Cancer* 31:701–704, 1983.

232. Henson DE, Tarone RE, Nsouli H: Lobular involution: the physiologic prevention of breast cancer. *J Natl Cancer Inst* 98(22):1589–1590, 2006.

233. Khodr ZG, et al: Circulating sex hormones and terminal duct lobular unit involution of the normal breast cancer. *Cancer Epidemiol Biomarkers Prev* 23(12):2765–2773, 2014.

234. Zaragoza R, et al: Involvement of different networks in mammary gland involution after the pregnancy/lactation cycle: implications in breast cancer. *IUBMB Life* 67(4):227–238, 2015.

235. Bruno RD, et al: Mammary extracellular matrix directs differentiation of testicular and embryonic stem cells to form functional mammary glands in vivo. *Sci Rep* 7:40196, 2017.

236. Reis LAG, et al: *Cancer statistics review, 1975–2005,* Bethesda, MD, 2008, National Cancer Institute. Available at: http://seer.cancer.gov/csr/1975_2005.

237. Oh H, et al: Relation of serum estrogen metabolites with terminal duct lobular unit involution among women undergoing diagnostic image-guided breast biopsy. *Horm Cancer* 7(5):305–315, 2016.

238. Fenton SE: Endocrine-disrupting compounds and mammary gland development: early exposure and later life consequences. *Endocrinology* 147(Suppl 6):S18–S24, 2006.

239. Lanigan F, et al: Molecular links between mammary gland development and breast cancer. *Cell Mol Life Sci* 64:3161–3184, 2007.

240. Pike MC, et al: 'Hormonal' risk factors, 'breast tissue age' and the age-incidence of breast cancer. *Nature* 303(5920):767–770, 1983.

241. Cheskis BJ, et al: Signaling by estrogens: mini review. *J Cell Physiol* 213(3):610–617, 2007.

242. Key TJ: Endogenous oestrogens and breast cancer risk in premenopausal and postmenopausal women. *Steroids* 76(8):812–815, 2011.

243. Toniolo PG: Endogenous estrogens and breast cancer risk: the case for prospective cohort studies. *Environ Health Perspect* 105(Suppl 3):587–592, 1997.

244. Zeleniuch-Jacquotte A, et al: Premenopausal levels of oestrogen, androgen, and SHBG and breast cancer: long term results of a prospective study. *Br J Cancer* 90:153–159, 2004.

245. Key T, et al: Endogenous sex hormones and breast cancer in postmenopausal women; reanalysis of nine prospective studies. *J Natl Cancer Inst* 94:606–616, 2002.

246. Key TJ, et al: A prospective study of urinary oestrogen excretion and breast cancer risk. *Br J Cancer* 73:1615–1619, 1996.

247. Hildreth NG, et al: Differences in breast cancer risk factors according to the estrogen receptor level of the tumor. *J Natl Cancer Inst* 70(6):1027–1031, 1983.

248. Ruder AM, et al: Estrogen and progesterone receptors in breast cancer patients. Epidemiologic characteristics and survival differences. *Cancer* 64(1):196–202, 1989.

249. Ouyang L, et al: Estrogen-induced SDF-1α production promotes the progression of ER-negative breast cancer via the accumulation of MDSCs in the tumor microenvironment. *Sci Rep* 6:39541, 2016.

250. Chua AC, et al: Dual roles for macrophages in ovarian cycle-associated development and remodeling of the mammary gland epithelium. *Development* 137(24):4229–4238, 2010.

251. Hodson IJ, et al: Macrophage phenotype in the mammary gland fluctuates over the course of the estrous cycle and is regulated by ovarian steroid hormones. *Biol Reprod* 89(3):65, 2013.

252. Calippe B, et al: 17beta-estradiol promotes TLR4-triggered proinflammatory mediator production through direct estrogen receptor alpha signaling in macrophages in vivo. *J Immunol* 185(2):1169–1176, 2010.

253. Jensen F, et al: Estradiol and progesterone regulate the migration of mast cells from the periphery to the uterus and induce their maturation and degranulation. *PLoS ONE* 5(12):e14409, 2010.

254. Zaitsu M, et al: Estradiol activates mast cells via a non-genomic estrogen receptor-alpha and calcium influx. *Mol Immunol* 44(8):1977–1985, 2007.

255. Lelu K, et al: Estrogen receptor alpha signaling in T lymphocytes is required for estrogen-mediated inhibition of Th1 and Th17 cell differentiation and protection against experimental autoimmune encephalomyelitis. *J Immunol* 187(5):2386–2393, 2011.

256. Svoronos N, et al: Tumor cell-independent estrogen signaling drives disease progression through mobilization of myeloid-derived suppressor cells. *Cancer Discov* 7(1):72–85, 2017.

257. Brisken C: Progesterone signalling in breast cancer: a neglected hormone coming into the limelight. *Nat Rev Cancer* 13(6):385–396, 2013.

258. Longacre TA, Bartow SA: A correlative morphologic study of human breast and

endometrium in the menstrual cycle. *Am J Surg Pathol* 10:382–393, 1986.

259. Masters JR, Drife JO, Scarisbrick JJ: Cyclic variation of DNA synthesis in human breast epithelium. *J Natl Cancer Inst* 58:1263–1265, 1977.

260. Hilton HN, Graham JD, Clarke CL: Minireview: progesterone regulation in the normal human breast and in breast cancer: a tale of two scenarios. *Mol Endocrinol* 29(9):1230–1242, 2015.

261. Chen CC, et al: Autocrine prolactin induced by the Pten-Akt pathway is required for lactation initiation and provides a direct link between the Akt and Stat5 pathways. *Genes Dev* 26(19): 2154–2168, 2012.

262. McHale K, et al: Altered expression of prolactin receptor-associated signaling proteins in human breast carcinoma. *Mod Pathol* 21(5):565–571, 2008.

263. Wang M, et al: Plasma prolactin and breast cancer risk: a meta-analysis. *Sci Rep* 6:25998, 2016.

264. Chen KH, Walker AM: Prolactin inhibits a major tumor-suppressive function of wild type *BRCA1*. *Cancer Lett* 375(2):293–302, 2016.

265. Rice MS, et al: Breast cancer research in the Nurses' Health Studies: exposures across the life course. *Am J Public Health* 106(9):1592–1598, 2016.

266. Hankinson SE, Eliassen H: Endogenous estrogen, testosterone, and progesterone levels in relation to breast cancer risk. *J Steroid Biochem Mol Biol* 106(1-5):24–30, 2007.

267. Stanczyk FZ, et al: Relationships of sex steroid hormone levels in benign and cancerous breast tissue and blood: a critical appraisal of current science. *Steroids* 99(Pt A):91–102, 2015.

268. Tworoger SS, et al: Inclusion of endogenous hormone levels in risk prediction models of postmenopausal breast cancer. *J Clin Oncol* 32(28):3111–3117, 2014.

269. World Health Organization: *A review of human carcinogens. B. Biological agents: IARC monographs on the evaluation of carcinogenic risks to humans, IARC Monographs, vol 100(B)*, Geneva, Switzerland, 2015, Author.

270. Mehta J, et al: A molecular analysis provides novel insights into androgen receptor signaling in breast cancer. *PLoS ONE* 10(3):e0120622, 2015.

271. Kotsssopoulos J, et al: The relationship between bilateral oophorectomy and plasma hormone levels in postmenopausal women. *Horm Cancer* 6(1):54–63, 2015.

272. Endogenous Hormones and Breast Cancer Collaborative Group et al: Circulating sex hormones and breast cancer risk factors in postmenopausal women: reanalysis of 13 studies. *Br J Cancer* 105(5):709–722, 2011.

273. Asselin-Labat ML, et al: Control of mammary stem cell function by steroid hormone signaling. *Nature* 465(7299):798–802, 2010.

274. Danovi SA: Tumorigenesis: hormonally driven. *Nat Rev Cancer* 10(7):451, 2010.

275. Joshi PA, et al: Progesterone induces adult mammary stem cell expansion. *Nature* 465(7299):803–807, 2010.

276. Manjer J, et al: Postmenopausal breast cancer risk in relation to sex steroid hormones, prolactin and SHBG (Sweden). *Cancer Causes Control* 14(2003):599–607, 2003.

277. Soady KJ, et al: Mouse mammary stem cells express prognostic markers for triple-negative breast cancer. *Breast Cancer Res* 17:31, 2015.

278. Stanczyk FZ, Mathews BW, Sherman ME: Relationships of sex steroid hormone levels in benign and cancerous breast tissue and blood: a

critical appraisal of current science. *Steroids* 99(Pt A):92–102, 2015.

279. Mullooly M, et al: Relationship between crown-like structures and sex-hormones in breast adipose tissue and serum among postmenopausal breast cancer patients. *Breast Cancer Res* 19:8, 2017.

280. Pasqualini JR, Chetrite GS: Recent insight on the control of enzymes involved in estrogen formation and transformation in human breast cancer. *J Steroid Biochem Mol Biol* 93(2-5): 221–236, 2005.

281. Olsen CJ, et al: Human mammary fibroblasts stimulate invasion of breast cancer cells in a three-dimensional culture and increase stroma development in mouse xenografts. *BMC Cancer* 10:444, 2010.

282. Cavalieri E, Rogan E: Catechol quinines of estrogen in the initiation of breast, prostate, and other cancers: keynote lecture. *Ann N Y Acad Sci* 1089:286–301, 2006.

283. Sasano H, et al: *In situ* estrogen production and its regulation in human breast carcinoma: from endocrinology to intracrinology. *Pathol Int* 59:777–789, 2009.

284. Cogliano V, et al: Carcinogenicity of combined estrogen-progestogen contraceptives and menopausal treatment. *Lancet Oncol* 6:552–553, 2005.

285. Fuhrman BJ, et al: Estrogen metabolism and risk of breast cancer in postmenopausal women. *J Natl Cancer Inst* 104(4):326–339, 2012.

286. Eliassen AH, et al: Urinary estrogens and estrogen metabolites and subsequent risk of breast cancer among premenopausal women. *Cancer Res* 72(3): 696–706, 2012.

287. Bhupathiraju SN, et al: Exogenous hormone use: oral contraceptives, postmenopausal hormone therapy, and health outcomes in the Nurses' Health Study. *Am J Public Health* 106(9): 1631–1637, 2016.

288. International Agency for Research on Cancer (IARC) Special Report: Policy: a review of human carcinogens—part A: pharmaceuticals. *Lancet* 10:13–14, 2009.

289. Chlebowski RT, et al: Breast cancer after use of estrogen plus progestin in postmenopausal women. *N Engl J Med* 360:573–587, 2009.

290. Chen WY, et al: Use of postmenopausal hormones, alcohol, and risk for invasive breast cancer. *Ann Intern Med* 137(1):798–804, 2002.

291. Colditz GA, et al: The use of estrogens and progestins and the risk of breast cancer in postmenopausal women. *N Engl J Med* 332(24): 1589–1593, 1995.

292. Collaborative Group on Hormonal Factors in Breast Cancer: Breast cancer and hormone replacement therapy: collaborative reanalysis of data from 51 epidemiological studies of 52,705 women with breast cancer and 108,411 women without breast cancer. *Lancet* 350(9084):1047–1059, 1997.

293. Rossouw JE, et al: Risks and benefits of estrogen plus progestin in healthy postmenopausal women: principal results from the Women's Health initiative randomized controlled trial. *N Engl J Med* 288(3):321–333, 2002.

294. Shah NR, Borenstein J, Dubois RW: Postmenopausal hormone therapy and breast cancer: a systematic review and meta-analysis. *Menopause* 12:668–678, 2005.

295. Sisti JS, et al: Reproductive risk factors in relation to molecular subtypes of breast cancer: results from the Nurses' Health Studies. *Int J Cancer* 138(10):2346–2356, 2016.

296. Anderson GL, et al: Effects of conjugated equine estrogen in postmenopausal women with hysterectomy: the Women's Health Initiative randomized controlled trial. *JAMA* 291(14):1701–1712, 2004.

297. Chen WY, et al: Unopposed estrogen therapy and the risk of invasive breast cancer. *Arch Intern Med* 166(9):1027–1032, 2006.

298. Beral V, et al: Breast cancer risk in relation to the interval between menopause and starting hormone therapy. *J Natl Cancer Inst* 103(4): 296–305, 2011.

299. Jordan VC, Ford LG: Paradoxical clinical effect of estrogen on breast cancer risk: a "new" biology of estrogen-induced apoptosis. *Cancer Prev Res (Phila)* 4(5):633 637, 2011.

300. Ariazi EA, et al: Estrogen induces apoptosis in estrogen deprivation-resistant breast cancer through stress responses as identified by global gene expression across time. *Proc Natl Acad Sci USA* 108(47):18879–18886, 2011.

301. Jungheim ES, Colditz GA: Short-term use of unopposed estrogen. *J Am Med Assoc* 305(13): 1354–1355, 2011.

302. Tamimi RM, et al: Combined estrogen and testosterone use and risk of breast cancer in postmenopausal women. *Arch Intern Med* 166(14):1483–1489, 2006.

303. Fournier A: Should transdermal rather than oral estrogens be used in menopausal hormone therapy? A review. *Menopause Int* 16(1):23–32, 2010.

304. Grant MD, et al: *Menopausal symptoms: comparative effectiveness of therapies Blue Cross and Blue Shield Association technology evaluation center, evidence-based practice center*, Rockville, MD, 2015, Agency for Healthcare Research and Quality.

305. Christopoulos PF, Msaouel P, Koutsillieris M: The role of insulin-like growth factor-1 system in breast cancer. *Mol Cancer* 14(1):43, 2015.

306. Endogenous Hormones and Breast Cancer Collaborative Group et al: Insulin-like growth factor-1 (IGF1), IGF binding protein 3 (IGFBP3), and breast cancer risk: pooled individual data analysis of 17 prospective studies. *Lancet Oncol* 11:530–542, 2010.

307. Kleinberg DL, Feldman M, Ruan W: IGF-1: an essential factor in terminal end bud formation and ductal morphogenesis. *J Mammary Gland Biol Neoplasia* 5(1):7–17, 2000 (review).

308. Wu J, et al: Light at night activates IGF-1R/PDK1 signaling and accelerates tumor growth in human breast cancer xenografts. *Cancer Res* 71(7): 2622–2631, 2011.

309. Wu W, et al: Co-targeting IGF-1R and autophagy enhances the effects of cell growth suppression and apoptosis induced by the IGF-1R inhibitor NVP-AEW541 in triple-negative breast cancer cells. *PLoS ONE* 12(1):e0169229, 2017.

310. Horne HN, et al: Circulating insulin-like growth factor-1, insulin-like growth factor binding protein-3 and terminal unit involution of the breast: a cross-sectional study of women with benign breast disease. *Breast Cancer Res* 18(1):24, 2016.

311. Pollak M: The insulin and insulin-like growth factor receptor family in neoplasia: an update. *Nat Rev Cancer* 12(3):159–169, 2012.

312. Ahmadieh H, Azar ST: Type 2 diabetes oral diabetic medications, insulin therapy, and overall breast cancer risk. *ISRN Endocrinol* 2013:181240, 2013.

313. Suissa S, et al: Long-term effects of insulin glargine on the risk of breast cancer. *Diabetologia* 54(9):2254–2262, 2011.

314. Park YM, et al: Gestational diabetes mellitus may be associated with increased risk of breast cancer. *Br J Cancer* 116(7):960–963, 2017.

315. Wang XS, et al: Shift work and chronic disease: the epidemiological evidence. *Occup Med (Lond)* 61(2):78–89, 2011.

316. Wennbo H, Tornell J: The role of prolactin and growth hormone in breast cancer. *Oncogene* 19(8):1072–1076, 2000.

317. Iles RK, Delves PJ, Butler SA: Does hCG or hCGβ play a role in cancer cell biology review? *Mol Cell Endocrinol* 329(1-2):62–70, 2010.

318. Gehring C, et al: The controversial role of human chorionic gonadotropin in the development of breast cancer and other types of tumors. *Breast* 26:135–140, 2016.

319. Grosse Y, et al: A review of human carcinogens—Part A: pharmaceuticals. *Lancet Oncol* 10(1):13–14, 2009.

320. Nelson HP, et al: Risk factors for breast cancer for women aged 40 to 49 years: a systematic review and meta-analysis. *Ann Intern Med* 156(9):635–648, 2012.

321. Hankinson SE, et al: A prospective study of oral contraceptive use and risk of breast cancer (Nurses' Health Study, United States). *Cancer Causes Control* 8(1):65–72, 1997.

322. Hunter DJ, et al: Oral contraceptive use and breast cancer: a prospective study of young women. *Cancer Epidemiol Biomarkers Prev* 19(10):2496–2502, 2010.

323. Boyd NF, et al: Mammographic density and breast cancer risk: current understanding and future prospects. *Breast Cancer Res* 13(6):223, 2011.

324. Krishnan K, et al: Longitudinal study of mammographic density measures that predict breast cancer risk. *Cancer Epidemiol Biomarkers Prev* 26(4):651–660, 2017.

325. Engmann NJ, et al: Population-attributable risk proportion of clinical risk factors for breast cancer. *JAMA Oncol* 2017 Feb 2. [Epub ahead of print].

326. Boyd NF: Mammographic density and risk of breast cancer. *Am Soc Clin Oncol Educ Book* 2013, doi:10.1200/EdBook_AM.2013.33.e57.

327. Esbona K, et al: COX-2 modulates mammary tumor progression in response to collagen density. *Breast Cancer Res* 18(1):35, 2016.

328. Sun X, et al: CCL2-driven inflammation increases mammary gland stromal density and cancer susceptibility in a transgenic mouse model. *Breast Cancer Res* 19(1):4, 2017.

329. Institute of Medicine of the National Academies: *Breast cancer and the environment: a life course approach*, Washington, DC, 2011, The National Academies Press.

330. National Cancer Institute (NCI): *Radiation risks and pediatric computed tomography (CT): a guide for health care providers*, 2002. Available at: www.cancer.gov.

331. Ginsburg ON, et al: Mammographic density, lobular involution, and risk of breast cancer. *Br J Cancer* 4(99):1369–1374, 2008.

332. Smith-Bindman R: Environmental causes of breast cancer and radiation from medical imaging. *Arch Intern Med* 172(13):1023–1027, 2012.

333. Brenner DJ, Hall EJ: Computed tomography—an increasing source of radiation exposure. *N Engl J Med* 357(22):2277–2284, 2007.

334. Wade MA, et al: c-MYC is a radiosensitive locus in human breast cells. *Oncogene* 1734(38):4985–4994, 2015.

335. Land CD: Radiation and breast cancer risk. *Prog Clin Biol Res* 396:115–124, 1997.

336. Travis LB, et al: Breast cancer following radiotherapy and chemotherapy among women with Hodgkin disease. *JAMA* 290:465–475, 2003.

337. Colin C, et al: Updated relevance of mammographic screening modalities in women previously treated with chest irradiation for Hodgkin disease. *Radiology* 265(3):669–676, 2012.

338. Schwab SA, et al: X-ray induced formation of γ-H2AX foci after full-field digital mammography and digital breast tomosynthesis. *PLoS ONE* 8(7):e70660, 2013.

339. Colin C, et al: DNA double-strand breaks induced by mammographic screening procedures in human mammary epithelial cells. *Int J Radiat Biol* 87(11):1103–1112, 2011.

340. Colin C, Foray N: DNA damage induced by mammography in high family risk patients: only one single view in screening. *Breast* 21:409–410, 2012.

341. Grudzenski S, et al: Inducible response required for repair of low-dose radiation damage in human fibroblasts. *Proc Natl Acad Sci USA* 107(32):14205–14210, 2010.

342. Ng J, et al: Predicting the risk of secondary lung malignancies associated with whole-breast radiation therapy. *Int J Radiat Oncol Biol Phys* 83(4):1101–1106, 2012.

343. Gotzsche PC, Nielsen M: Screening for breast cancer with mammography. *Cochrane Database Syst Rev* (1):CD001877, 2011.

344. Pucci M, et al: Caveolin-1, breast cancer and ionizing radiation. *Cancer Genomics Proteomics* 12(3):143–152, 2015.

345. Behrens C, et al: Molecular changes in second primary lung and breast cancers therapy for Hodgkin's disease. *Cancer Epidemiol Biomarkers Prev* 9:1027–1035, 2000.

346. Oikawa M, et al: Significance of genomic instability in breast cancer in atomic bomb survivors: analysis of microarray-comparative genomic hybridization. *Radiat Oncol* 6:168, 2011.

347. Kutanzi K, Kovalchuk O: Exposure to estrogen and ionizing radiation causes epigenetic dysregulation, activation of mitogen-activated protein kinase pathways, and genome instability in the mammary gland of ACI rats. *Cancer Biol Ther* 14(7):564–573, 2013.

348. Ferrini K, et al: Lifestyle, nutrition and breast cancer: facts and presumptions for consideration. *Ecancermedicalscience* 9:557, 2015.

349. Michels KB, et al: Diet and breast cancer: a review of the prospective observational studies. *Cancer* 109(Suppl 12):2712–2749, 2007.

350. Khandekar MJ, Cohen P, Spiegelman BM: Molecular mechanisms of cancer development in obesity. *Nat Rev Cancer* 11:886–895, 2011.

351. Mahoney MC, et al: Opportunities and strategies for breast cancer prevention through risk reduction. *CA Cancer J Clin* 58(6):347–371, 2008.

352. Smith-Warner SA, Stampfer MJ: Fat intake and breast cancer revisited. *J Natl Cancer Inst* 99(6):418–419, 2007.

353. Prentice RL, et al: Low-fat dietary pattern and risk of invasive breast cancer: the Women's Health Initiative Randomized Controlled Dietary Modification Trial. *JAMA* 295(6):629–642, 2006.

354. World Cancer Research Fund/American Institute for Cancer Research (WCRF/AICR): *Food, nutrition, physical activity, and prevention of cancer: a global perspective*, ed 2, Washington, DC, 2007, Author.

355. Linos E, et al: Adolescent diet in relation to breast cancer risk among premenopausal women. *Cancer Epidemiol Biomarkers Prev* 19(3):689–696, 2010.

356. Cho E, et al: Premenopausal fat intake and risk of breast cancer. *J Natl Cancer Inst* 95(14):1079–1085, 2001.

357. Turner LB: Meta-analysis of fat intake, reproduction, and breast cancer risk: an evolutionary perspective. *Am J Hum Biol* 23:601–608, 2011.

358. Missner SA, et al: Meat and dairy food consumption and breast cancer: a pooled analysis of cohort studies. *Int J Epidemiol* 31:78–85, 2002.

359. Cho E, et al: Red meat intake and risk of breast cancer among premenopausal women. *Arch Intern Med* 166:2258–2259, 2006.

360. Taylor EF, et al: Meat consumption and risk of breast cancer in the UK Women's Cohort Study. *Br J Cancer* 96:1139–1146, 2007.

361. Egeberg R, et al: Meat consumption, N-acetyl transferase 1 and 2 polymorphism and risk of breast cancer in Danish postmenopausal women. *Eur J Cancer Prev* 17:39–47, 2008.

362. Alexander DD, et al: A review and meta-analysis of red and processed meat consumption and breast cancer. *Nutr Res Rev* 23(2):349–365, 2010.

363. Aldercreutz H: Ligans and human health. *Rev Clin Lab Sci* 44(5-6):483–525, 2007.

364. Sonestedt E, Wirfält E: Enterolactone and breast cancer: methodological issues may contribute to conflicting results in observational studies. *Nutr Res* 30:667–677, 2010.

365. Rock CL, et al: Effects of a high-fiber, low-fat diet intervention on serum concentrations of reproductive steroid hormones in women with a history of breast cancer. *J Clin Oncol* 22(12):2379–2387, 2004.

366. Dong JY, et al: Dietary fiber intake and risk of breast cancer: a meta-analysis of prospective cohort studies. *Am J Clin Nutr* 94(3):900–905, 2011.

367. Aune D, et al: Dietary fiber and breast cancer risk: a systematic review and meta-analysis of prospective studies. *Ann Oncol* 23(6):1394–1402, 2012.

368. Farvid MS, et al: Dietary fiber intake in young adults and breast cancer risk. *Pediatrics* 137(3): e20151226, 2016.

369. Buck K, et al: Estimated enterolignans, lignan-rich foods, and fibre in relation to survival after postmenopausal breast cancer. *Br J Cancer* 105(8):1151–1157, 2011.

370. Buck K: Meta-analyses of lignans and enterolignans in relation to breast cancer risk. *Am J Clin Nutr* 92:141–153, 2010.

371. Velentzis LS, et al: Lignans and breast cancer risk in pre-post-menopausal women: meta-analyses of observational studies. *Br J Cancer* 100:1492–1498, 2009.

372. Zhang X, et al: Lifetime genistein intake increases the response of mammary tumors to tamoxifen in rats. *Clin Cancer Res* 23(3):814–824, 2017.

373. World Cancer Research Fund/American Institute for Cancer Research (WCRF/AICR): *Foods that fight cancer: soy*, Washington, DC, 2017, Author.

374. Bedell S, Nachtigall M, Naftolin F: The pros and cons of plant estrogens for menopause. *J Steroid Biochem Mol Biol* 139:225–236, 2014.

375. Nechuta SJ, et al: Soy food intake after diagnosis of breast cancer and survival: an in-depth analysis of combined evidence from cohort studies of U.S. and Chinese women. *Am J Nutr* 96(1):123–132, 2012.

376. Cross HS, et al: Phytoestrogens and vitamin D metabolism: a new concept for the prevention and therapy of colorectal, prostate, and mammary carcinomas. *J Nutr* 134(5):1207S–1212S, 2004.

377. Iodine Monograph. *Altern Med Rev* 15(3): 273–278, 2010.

378. Aceves C, et al: Is iodine a gatekeeper of the integrity of the mammary gland? *J Mammary Gland Biol Neoplasia* 10(2):189–196, 2005.

379. Cann SA, et al: Hypothesis: iodine, selenium and the development of breast cancer. *Cancer Causes Control* 11:121–127, 2000.

380. Eskin BA, et al: Different tissue responses for iodine and iodide in rat thyroid and mammary glands. *Biol Trace Elem Res* 49:9–19, 1995.

381. Ghent WR, et al: Iodine replacement in fibrocystic disease of the breast. *Can J Surg* 36:453–460, 1993.

382. Funahashi H, et al: Seaweed prevents breast cancer. *Jpn J Cancer Res* 92(5):483–487, 2001.

383. Smyth PP: Role of iodine in antioxidant defense in thyroid and breast disease. *Biofactors* 19(3-4): 121–130, 2003.

384. Tripathi R, et al: Zoledronate and molecular iodine synergistic cell death in triple negative breast cancer through endoplastic reticulum stress. *Nutr Cancer* 68(4):679–688, 2016.

385. Demetriou CA, et al: The Mediterreanean dietary pattern and breast cancer risk in Greek-Cypriot women: a case-control study. *BMC Cancer* 12:113, 2012.

386. National Cancer Institute (NCI): *Alcohol and cancer risk*, Bethesda, MD, 2013, National Cancer Institute, National Institutes of Health, U.S. Department of Health and Human Services.

387. Hamajima N, et al: Alcohol, tobacco and breast cancer—collaborative reanalysis of individual data from 53 epidemiological studies, including 58,515 women with breast cancer and 95,067 women without the disease. *Br J Cancer* 87(11): 1234–1245, 2002.

388. Allen NE, et al: Moderate alcohol intake and cancer incidence in women. *J Natl Cancer Inst* 101(5):296–305, 2009.

389. Trinh T, et al: Background risk of breast cancer influences the association between alcohol consumption and mammographic density. *Br J Cancer* 113(1):159–165, 2015.

390. Byers T, Sedjo RL: Body fatness as a cause of cancer: epidemiologic clues to biologic mechanisms. *Endocr Relat Cancer* 22(3): R125–R134, 2015.

391. Michels KB, et al: Adult weight change and incidence of premenopausal breast cancer. *Int J Cancer* 130(4):902–909, 2012.

392. Protani M, et al: Effect of obesity on survival of women with breast cancer: systematic review and meta-analysis. *Breast Cancer Res Treat* 123(3): 627–635, 2010.

393. Vaino H, Kaaks R, Bianchini F: Weight control and physical activity in cancer prevention: international evaluation of the evidence. *Eur J Cancer Prev* 11(Suppl 2):S94–S100, 2002.

394. Renehan AG, et al: Body-mass index and incidence of cancer: a systematic review and meta-analysis of prospective observational studies. *Lancet* 371:569–578, 2008.

395. Endogenous Hormones Breast Cancer Collaborative Group: Body mass index, serum sex hormones, and breast cancer risk in postmenopausal women. *J Natl Cancer Inst* 95(6):1218–1226, 2003.

396. Holmes MD, Willett WC: Does diet affect breast cancer risk? *Breast Cancer Res* 6(4):170–178, 2004.

397. Le Marchand L, et al: Body size at different periods of life and breast cancer risk. *Am J Epidemiol* 128(1):137–152, 1998.

398. Morimoto LM, et al: Obesity, body size, and risk of postmenopausal breast cancer: the Women's Health Initiative (United States). *Cancer Causes Control* 13(8):741–751, 2002.

399. Trentham-Diaz A, et al: Weight change and risk of postmenopausal breast cancer (United States). *Cancer Causes Control* 11(6):533–542, 2000.

400. Vrieling A, et al: Adult weight gain in relation to breast cancer risk by estrogen and progesterone receptor status: a meta-analysis. *Breast Cancer Res Treat* 123:641–649, 2010.

401. Ahn J, et al: Adiposity, adult weight gain, and postmenopausal breast cancer risk. *Arch Intern Med* 167:2091–2102, 2007.

402. Giles ED, et al: Obesity and overfeeding affecting both tumor and systemic metabolism activates the progesterone receptor to contribute to postmenopausal breast cancer. *Cancer Res* 72(24):6490–6501, 2012.

403. Korner A, et al: Total and high molecular weight adiponectin in breast cancer: in vitro and in vivo studies. *J Clin Endocrinol Metab* 92(3):1041–1048, 2007.

404. Surmacz E: Obesity hormone leptin: a new target in breast cancer? *Breast Cancer Res* 9(1):301, 2007.

405. Jarde T, et al: Molecular mechanism of leptin and adiponectin in breast cancer. *Eur J Cancer* 47:33–43, 2011.

406. Andó S, et al: The multifaceted mechanism of leptin signaling within tumor microenvironment in driving breast cancer growth and progression. *Front Oncol* 4:340, 2014.

407. *EPAsScience matters: the future of toxicity testing is here*, 2011. Available at: www.EPA.Gov/Research.

408. Wilson MP, Schwarzman MR: Toward a new U.S. chemicals policy: rebuilding the foundation to advance new science, green chemistry, and environmental health. *Environ Health Perspect* 117(8):1202–1209, 2009.

409. Schwarzman MR, et al: Screening for chemical contributions to breast cancer: a case study for chemical safety evaluation. *Environ Health Perspect* 123(12):1255–1264, 2015.

410. Dairkee SH, et al: Bisphenol A induces a profile of tumor aggressiveness in high-risk cells from breast cancer patients. *Cancer Res* 68:2076–2080, 2008.

411. Loprinzi PD, et al: Physical activity and the risk of breast cancer recurrence: a literature review. *Oncol Nurs Forum* 39(3):269–274, 2012.

412. Winzer BM, et al: Physical activity and cancer prevention: a systematic review of clinical trials. *Cancer Causes Control* 22(6):811–826, 2011.

413. Sprague BL, et al: Lifetime recreational and occupational physical activity and risk of in situ and invasive breast cancer. *Cancer Epidemiol Biomarkers Prev* 16(2):236–243, 2007.

414. Kim J, et al: The effects of physical activity on breast cancer survivors after diagnosis. *J Cancer Prev* 18(3):193–200, 2013.

415. Wu Y, Zhang D, Kang S: Physical activity and risk of breast cancer: a meta-analysis of prospective studies. *Breast Cancer Res Treat* 137(3):869–882, 2013.

416. National Cancer Institute (NCI): *Physical activity and cancer*, Bethesda, MD, 2017, National Cancer Institute, National Institutes of Health.

417. Stephens PJ, et al: The landscape of cancer genes and mutational processes in breast cancer. *Nature* 486:400–404, 2012.

418. Senft D, Ronai ZE: Adaptive stress responses during tumor metastasis and dormancy. *Trends Cancer* 2(8):429–442, 2016.

419. Bayani J, Yao CQ, Quintayo MA: Molecular stratification of early breast cancer identifies drug targets to drive stratified medicine. *Breast Cancer* 15(3):3, 2017, doi:10.1038/s41523-016-0003-5.

420. National Cancer Institute (NCI): *PDQ genetics of breast and gynecologic cancers*, Bethesda, MD, 2017, Author. Updated March 3, 2017. Available at: www.cancer.gov/types/breast/hp/breast-ovarian-genetics-pdq.

421. Marusyk A, et al: Non-cell-autonomous driving of tumour growth supports sub-clonal heterogeneity. *Nature* 514(7520):54–58, 2014.

422. Tabassum DP, Polyak K: Tumorigensis: it takes a village. *Nat Rev Cancer* 15(8):473–483, 2015.

423. Beca F, Polyak K: Intratumor heterogeneity in breast cancer. *Adv Exp Med Biol* 882:169–189, 2016.

424. Kim J, et al: Heterogeneous perivascular cell coverage affects breast cancer metastasis and response to chemotherapy. *JCI Insight* 1(21): e90733, 2016.

425. Damonte P, et al: Mammary carcinoma behavior is programmed in the precancer stem cell. *Breast Cancer Res* 10(3):R50, 2008.

426. Eroles P, et al: Molecular biology in breast cancer: intrinsic subtypes and signaling pathways. *Cancer Treat Rev* 38:698–707, 2012.

427. Hosseini A, Khoury AL, Esserman LJ: Precision surgery and avoiding over-treatment. *Eur J Surg Oncol* 43(5):938–943, 2017.

428. Cardiff RD, et al: Three interrelated themes in current breast cancer research: gene addiction, phenotypic plasticity, and cancer stem cells. *Breast Cancer Res* 13:216, 2011.

429. Lambert AW, Pattabiraman DR, Weinberg RA: Emerging biological principles of metastasis. *Cell* 168(4):670–691, 2017.

430. Craene DB, Berx G: Regulatory networks defining EMT during cancer initiation and progression. *Nat Rev Cancer* 13(2):97–110, 2013.

431. Chaffer CL, Weinberg RA: A perspective on cancer cell metastasis. *Science* 331(6024):1559–1564, 2011.

432. Friedl P, et al: Classifying collective cancer cell invasion. *Nat Cell Biol* 14:777–783, 2012.

433. Loughran CF, Keeling CR: Seeding of tumor cells following breast biopsy: a literature review. *Br J Radiol* 84:869–874, 2011.

434. Enderling H, et al, editors: *System biology of tumor dormancy advances in experimental medicine and biology*, New York, 2013, Springer Science.

435. Kim Y, Boushaba K: Regulation of tumor dormancy and role of microenvironment: a mathematical model. In Enderling H, et al, editors: *System biology of tumor dormancy advances in experimental medicine and biology*, New York, 2013, Springer Science.

436. Wagenblast E, et al: A model of breast cancer heterogeneity reveals vascular mimicry as a driver of metastasis. *Nature* 520:358–362, 2015.

437. Hendrix MJC: Cancer: an extravascular route for tumor cells. *Nature* 520:300–302, 2015.

438. Karaman S, Detmar M: Mechanisms of lymphatic metastasis. *J Clin Invest* 124:922–928, 2014.

439. Skobe M, et al: Induction of tumor lymphangiogenesis by VEGF-C promotes breast cancer metastasis. *Nat Med* 7:192–198, 2001.

440. Rhim AD, et al: EMT and dissemination precede pancreatic tumor formation. *Cell* 148:349–361, 2012.

441. Harper KL, et al: Mechanism of early dissemination and metastases in Her2+ mammary cancer. *Nature* 2016 Dec 14. [Epub ahead of print].

442. Hosseini H, et al: Early dissemination seeds metastasis in breast cancer. *Nature* 2016 Dec 16. [Epub ahead of print].

443. Lee RJ, et al: Ductal carcinoma in situ of the breast. *Int J Surg Oncol* 2012:123549, 2012.

444. Kerlikowske K: Epidemiology of ductal carcinoma in situ. *J Natl Cancer Inst Monogr* 41:139–141, 2010.

445. Miller AB, et al: Canadian National Breast Screening Study: 2. Breast cancer detection and death rates among women aged 50 to 59 years. *CMAJ* 147(10):1477–1488, 1992.

446. Esserman L, Yau C: Rethinking the standard for ductal carcinoma in situ treatment. *JAMA Oncol* 1(7):881–883, 2015.

447. Lin C, et al: The majority of locally advanced breast cancers are interval cancers. *J Clin Oncol* 27:1503, 2009.

448. Ozanne EM, et al: Characterizing the impact of 25 years of DCIS treatment. *Breast Cancer Res Treat* 129(1):165–173, 2011.

449. Narod SA, et al: Breast cancer mortality after a diagnosis of ductal carcinoma in situ. *JAMA Oncol* 1(7):888–896, 2015.

450. National Cancer Institute (NCI): *Risk of breast cancer death is low after a diagnosis of ductal carcinoma in situ*, Bethesda, MD, 2015, Author.

451. National Cancer Institute (NCI): *PDQ breast cancer screening*, Bethesda, MD, 2015, Author. Date last modified May 14, 2015. Available at: www.cancer.gov/types/breast/hp/breast -screening-pdq.

452. Wapnir IL, et al: Long-term outcomes of invasive ipsilateral breast tumor recurrences after lumpectomy in NSABP B-17 and B-24 randomized clinical trials for DCIS. *J Natl Cancer Inst* 103(6):478–488, 2011.

453. Ayvaci MU, et al: Predicting invasive breast cancer versus DCIS in different age groups. *BMC Cancer* 14(584):584, 2014.

454. Boudreau A, van't Veer LJ, Bissell M: An "elite hacker:" breast tumors exploit the normal microenvironment program to instruct their progression and biological diversity. *Cell Adh Migr* 6(3):236–248, 2012.

455. Kurian AW, Griffith KA, Hamilton AS: Genetic testing and counseling among patients with newly diagnosed breast cancer. *JAMA* 317(5):531–534, 2017.

Alterations of the Male Reproductive System

George W. Rodway, Kathryn L. McCance

evolve WEBSITE

http://evolve.elsevier.com/McCance/
- Content Updates
- Chapter Summary Review
- Review Questions
- Case Studies
- Animations

CHAPTER OUTLINE

Alterations of the reproductive system span a wide range of concerns, from delayed sexual development and suboptimal sexual performance to structural and functional abnormalities. Many common male reproductive disorders carry potentially serious physiologic or psychologic consequences. Sexual or reproductive dysfunction, such as impotence or infertility, can dramatically affect self-concept, relationships, and overall quality of life. Conversely, organic and psychosocial problems, such as alcoholism, depression, situational stressors, chronic illness, and medications, can affect sexual performance and fertility and may be risk factors for the development of some types of reproductive tract cancers. Prostate cancer is the second leading cause of cancer death in men and is the most frequently diagnosed cancer in men aside from skin cancer. About 6 in 10 cases of prostate cancer are diagnosed in men aged 65 or older; it is rare before age 40. Incidence rates for prostate cancer changed substantially between the mid-1980s and mid-1990s and have since fluctuated widely from year to year, in large part reflecting changes in prostate cancer screening with the prostate-specific antigen (PSA) blood test. The decline in rates since 2000 has accelerated in recent years, likely because of recommendations against routine PSA screening beginning in 2008. From 2009 to 2013, the rate decreased by about 8% per year.[1] Diagnosis and treatment of male reproductive system disorders are, like female reproductive system disorders, complicated because of the stigma and symbolism associated with the reproductive organs and the emotion-laden beliefs and behaviors related to reproductive health. Treatment and diagnosis for related problems may be delayed because of embarrassment, guilt, fear, or denial.

ALTERATIONS OF SEXUAL MATURATION

The process of sexual maturation, or puberty, is marked by the development of secondary sexual characteristics, rapid growth, and, ultimately, the ability to reproduce. A variety of congenital and endocrine disorders can disrupt the timing of puberty, or sexual maturation. These disorders may cause puberty to occur too late (delayed puberty) or too early (precocious puberty). Both types involve a disrupted onset of sex hormone production by the gonads. While the average age of pubertal onset appears to be decreasing for girls, the age of pubertal onset has remained essentially unchanged for boys.

Delayed Puberty

About 3% of children in North America experience delayed development of secondary sex characteristics.[2] Normally, boys tend to mature later than girls, around 14 to 14.5 years of age. In boys the first sign is enlargement of the testes and thinning of the scrotal skin. Puberty is considered delayed if there are no clinical signs of puberty by age 14 in boys (2 standard deviations [SDs] above the mean age of pubertal onset). Boys especially tend to be embarrassed by sexual immaturity[3]; therefore early diagnosis and treatment are recommended, as well as reassurance for boys as well as girls.

In 95% of cases delayed puberty is a physiologic delay; that is, hormonal levels are normal and the hypothalamic-pituitary-gonadal (HPG) axis is intact, but maturation is occurring slowly.[4] This constitutional delay tends to be familial and is much more common in boys than in girls. Physiologic delay is difficult to distinguish from isolated gonadotropin deficiency and is usually diagnosed retrospectively once pubertal progression is complete.

Delayed puberty also may be related to consequences of any chronic condition that delays bone aging (e.g., lung disease, renal failure, cystic fibrosis) (Box 26.1).[5] Many clinicians recommend intervention (e.g., exogenous sex steroid administration) in physiologic cases of delayed puberty to reduce the psychologic effects (e.g., self-esteem issues, embarrassment) often associated with delayed puberty.[4]

The other 5% of cases of delayed puberty are caused by a disruption of the HPG axis of various etiologies (see Box 26.1).[6] Human gonadal function is partially controlled by luteinizing hormone (LH) and follicle-stimulating hormone (FSH), the release of which is regulated by the pulsatile secretion of hypothalamic gonadotropin-releasing hormone (GnRH).[4,6] Most recently, the G-protein–coupled receptor 54 (GPR54) has been identified as the gatekeeper gene for activation of the GnRH axis based on loss of function studies in mice and humans. GPR54 is required for the normal function of this axis, and data suggest that the ligand kisspeptin-1 acts by stimulating neurons expressing gonadotropin-releasing hormone (GnRH).[7,8] The mechanisms of childhood inhibition of GnRH release and activation are poorly understood but appear to involve feedback inhibition by sex steroids and presumably other central nervous system (CNS) pathways.[9] Given the myriad etiologies contributing to the occurrence of delayed puberty, a thorough evaluation should be conducted that includes physical examination and medical and family history. Such evaluation should specifically target known contributors to delayed puberty.[4] Laboratory workup generally consists of x-ray studies for determination of bone age; measurement of thyroid function and serum levels of prolactin and adrenal and gonadal steroids; radioimmunoassay of plasma gonadotropins; and screening for systemic disorders. Adolescents with high gonadotropin levels require a karyotype to rule out genetic causes, and those with low levels need skull imaging (lateral skull film, computed tomography [CT], or magnetic resonance imaging [MRI]) to rule out pituitary or other CNS infiltrate or tumor.[5] Although several genes involved in the HPG maturation cascade have been characterized from familial or sporadic cases of primitive isolated hypogonadotropic hypogonadism, many genes regulating puberty onset remain undetermined. Treatment of delayed puberty depends on the cause; the goal of treatment is the development of secondary sex characteristics and fertility, when possible. Insufficient sex hormone secretion can be corrected by hormone replacement therapy, such as testosterone for boys.[10] Idiopathic hypogonadotropic hypogonadism is treated with synthetic GnRH or sex hormone administration, or both, and may be lifelong.[4,5,10]

Precocious Puberty

Precocious puberty is a rare event in boys, affecting less than 1 in 50,000. Precocious puberty in boys has been redefined as sexual maturation before age 9.[11] One study has noted observed mean ages of beginning male genital and pubic hair growth and early testicular volumes tending toward younger ages than earlier studies have suggested, although this seems to be dependent on race and ethnicity.[12] For instance, black boys are showing significantly earlier mean ages for stages 2 to 4 genital development and stages 2 to 4 pubic hair than white and Hispanic boys. All cases of precocious puberty require thorough evaluation.

Precocious puberty may be partial, complete, or mixed (heterosexual) types (Box 26.2) and can be further categorized into central (GnRH-dependent) and peripheral (GnRH-independent) (Box 26.3). Central precocious puberty is GnRH-dependent and occurs when the HPG axis is working normally but prematurely. It mimics physiologic pubertal development, although at an inappropriate chronological age (before 8 years in girls and 9 years in boys).[13] Besides the premature development of secondary sex characteristics, precocity causes premature closure of the epiphysis of long bones, which results in shorter stature. Central precocious puberty results from failure of central inhibition of the GnRH pulse generator (the gonadostat). The diagnosis of central precocious puberty is one of exclusion. Because of the possibility of a central nervous system (CNS) lesion, children with presumed central precocious puberty require long-term surveillance. Peripheral puberty is GnRH-independent and develops when sex hormones are produced by some mechanism other than stimulation by the gonadotropins. Sex steroid–producing tumors such as gonadal tumors, testotoxicosis, and exposure

---

BOX 26.1 CAUSES OF DELAYED OR ABSENT PUBERTY

Chronic or Systemic Conditions
- Chronic renal disease
- Cystic fibrosis
- Diabetes mellitus
- Excessive exercise
- Hematologic diseases
- Hypothyroidism
- Irritable bowel diseases
- Poor nutrition (eating disorders, GI diseases, poverty)
- Gonadal dysgenesis
  - Turner syndrome (genetic karyotype 45,XO)
- Bilateral gonadal failure
  - Autoimmune
  - Congenital anorchia
  - Postsurgical, postirradiation, postchemotherapy
  - Traumatic or infectious

Hypogonadotropic Hypogonadism (Deficient FSH/LH)
- Central nervous system defects (GnRH deficiency)
  - Craniopharyngioma
  - GPR54 mutations
  - Hemochromatosis
  - Hypopituitarism
  - Kallmann syndrome, Bardet-Biedl syndrome, Prader-Willi syndrome
  - Marijuana use
  - Pituitary adenoma/tumor
  - Prolactinomas

Disordered Puberty

FSH, Follicle-stimulating hormone; *GI*, gastrointestinal; *GnRH*, gonadotropin-releasing hormone; *LH*, luteinizing hormone.
Data from Burchett MLR, Hanna CE, Steiner RD: Endocrine and metabolic diseases. In Burns CE, Brady MA, Dunn AM, editors: *Pediatric primary care*, ed 4, St Louis, 2009, Saunders; Jospe N: Disorders of pubertal development. In Osborne LM et al, editors: *Pediatrics*, Philadelphia, 2005, Mosby; Karagiannis A, Harsoulis F: *Eur J Endocrinol* 152(4):501–513, 2005.

BOX 26.2   PRIMARY FORMS OF PRECOCIOUS PUBERTY

Complete Precocious Puberty

Premature development of appropriate characteristics for the child's sex

Hypothalamic-pituitary-ovarian axis working normally but prematurely

In about 10% of cases, lethal central nervous system tumor may be the cause

Partial Precocious Puberty

Partial development of appropriate secondary sex characteristics

Premature thelarche (breast budding) seen in girls between 6 months and 2 years of age

Does not progress to complete puberty (ovulation and menstruation)

Premature adrenarche (growth of axillary and pubic hair) tends to occur between 5 and 8 years of age

Can progress to complete precocious puberty; may be caused by estrogen-secreting neoplasms or may be a variant of normal pubertal development

Mixed Precocious Puberty

Causes the child to develop some secondary sex characteristics of the opposite sex

Common causes: adrenal hyperplasia or androgen-secreting tumors

Data from Burchette MLR, Hanna CE, Steiner RD: Endocrine and metabolic diseases. In Burns CE et al, editors: *Pediatric primary care,* St Louis, 2009, Saunders; Jospe N: Disorders of pubertal development. In Osborne LM et al, editors: *Pediatrics,* Philadelphia, 2005, Mosby.

BOX 26.3   CAUSES OF PRECOCIOUS PUBERTY

Central (Gonadotropin-Releasing Hormone [GnRH] Dependent)

Idiopathic

Central nervous system (CNS) disorders

    Congenital anomalies (hydrocephalus)

    Hypothalamic hamartoma

    Postinflammatory/infectious condition

    Trauma

    Tumors (hypothalamic, pineal, other)

Hypothyroidism (severe)

Peripheral Puberty (GnRH Independent)

Adrenal hyperplasia or tumor

Environmental endocrine disruptors

Exogenous sex steroid exposure

Exogenous anabolic steroids

Familial Leydig cell hyperplasia

Gonadal tumors or cysts

Human chorionic gonadotropin (hCG)–secreting tumors (hepatoblastomas, intracranial lesions)

McCune-Albright syndrome

Testotoxicosis

From Bhagavath B, Layman LC: *Semin Reprod Med* 25(4):272–286, 2007; Burchett MLR, Hanna CE, Steiner RD: Endocrine and metabolic diseases. In Burns CE et al, editors: *Pediatric primary care,* St Louis, 2009, Saunders; Caserta DL et al: *Hum Reprod Update* 14(1):59–72, 2008; Cesario SK, Hughes LA: *J Obstetr Gynecol Neonatal Nurs* 36(3):263–274, 2007; Jospe N: Disorders of pubertal development. In Osborne LM et al, editors: *Pediatrics,* Philadelphia, 2005, Mosby.

to exogenous sex steroids (e.g., hormonal contraceptives and environmental endocrine disruptors) are some of the causes (see Box 26.3).

Complete precocious puberty refers to the onset and progression of all pubertal features. **Partial precocious puberty** is the partial development of appropriate secondary sexual characteristics alone or in combination. Premature pubarche tends to occur between ages 5 and 8 years. Premature pubarche is usually the consequence of an early increase in the adrenal androgens that leads to early growth of pubic hair and possibly a transient acceleration in growth and bone maturation that has no significant effect on timing of puberty or final height.

The diagnosis and cause of premature development are often obvious. A thorough history and physical examination is done to determine the velocity of the process and to rule out life-threatening CNS or adrenal neoplasms. Family occurrence helps exclude tumors. Children with precocious puberty also have a tendency toward obesity.[9] In addition, excess body weight early in life can actually influence growth patterns. There is evidence suggesting that excess adiposity during childhood influences growth patterns and pubertal development.[14]

Treatment for all forms of precocious puberty includes identifying and removing the underlying cause (see Boxes 26.2 and 26.3) or administering appropriate hormones. In many cases precocious puberty can be reversed. Management goals include diagnosing and treating intracranial disease; arresting maturation until early teen years; maximizing eventual adult height; reducing emotional problems; and providing contraception, if necessary. The most common form, central precocious puberty, is usually treated with potent GnRH agonist analogs, which induce reversible, selective suppression of the HPG axis. Treatment does not seem to affect body composition or increase obesity in children with central precocious puberty. Because many of these children are obese and childhood obesity is predictive of morbidity in adolescence and adulthood, it is important for clinicians to include assessment and management of obesity as part of the treatment for central precocious puberty.

Mixed precocious puberty, such as feminization of a boy, causes the child to develop some secondary sexual characteristics of the opposite sex. This condition is usually evident at birth and is rare in older children (Box 26.4).

BOX 26.4   CAUSES OF MIXED PRECOCIOUS PUBERTY

Female (Virilization)

Congenital adrenal hyperplasia

Androgen-secreting tumors

    Adrenal

    Ovarian

    Teratoma

    Exogenous androgens

Male (Feminization)

Estrogen-producing tumors

    Adrenal

    Teratoma

    Hepatoma

    Testicular

Exogenous estrogens

Increased peripheral conversion of androgens to estrogens

Data from Jospe N: Disorders of pubertal development. In Osborn LM et al, editors: *Pediatrics,* Philadelphia, 2005, Mosby.

DISORDERS OF THE MALE REPRODUCTIVE SYSTEM

Disorders of the Urethra

Urethritis and urethral strictures are common disorders of the male urethra. Urethral carcinoma occurs in men older than 60 years, but it is an extremely rare form of cancer.

Urethritis

Urethritis is an inflammatory process of the urethra without concurrent bladder infection that is usually, but not always, caused by a sexually transmitted microorganism. Biologic agents associated with infectious urethritis in males include *Neisseria gonorrhoeae* and *Chlamydia trachomatis, Ureaplasma urealyticum,* and other, less common, mycobacteria; parasites (e.g., *Trichomonas vaginalis*); and viruses (herpes simplex virus [HSV]).[15,16] Infectious urethritis caused by *N. gonorrhoeae* often is called *gonococcal urethritis (GU);* infection caused by other microorganisms is called *nongonococcal urethritis (NGU).*[17] (Sexually transmitted urethritis is described in Chapter 27.) Nonsexual origins of urethritis include inflammation or infection as a result of urologic procedures, insertion of foreign bodies into the urethra, anatomic abnormalities, or trauma.

Noninfectious urethritis is rare and is associated with the ingestion of wood alcohol, ethyl alcohol, or turpentine. It is seen also with Reiter syndrome, which involves a number of mucocutaneous lesions.

Symptoms of urethritis include urethral tingling, itching, or burning sensation on urination (dysuria) and urinary frequency and urgency. The individual may note a purulent or clear mucous-like discharge from the urethra. Nucleic acid detection amplification tests allow easy detection of *N. gonorrhoeae* and *C. trachomatis* in first-void urine.[17,18] Treatment consists of appropriate antibiotic therapy for infectious urethritis and avoidance of future chemical or mechanical irritation.

Urethral Stricture

A urethral stricture is a fibrotic narrowing of the urethra caused by scarring. The scars may be congenital but can be present at any age and have a wide range of etiologic factors, including untreated urethral infection (e.g., from long-term use of indwelling urinary catheters), trauma, and urologic instrumentation. It can present at any age and has a wide range of etiologic factors, including infection, trauma, and instrumentation. Large catheters and instruments cause internal trauma and ischemia, whereas external trauma, such as pelvic fracture, can partially or completely sever the urethra and cause severe and complex strictures.[19] In addition, a report has concluded that stricture may occur decades after initial hypospadias surgery.[20] Urethral carcinoma is a less common cause of urethral stricture. Prostatitis and infection secondary to urinary stasis are common complications. Severe and prolonged obstruction can result in hydronephrosis and renal failure. In addition, chronic, severe strictures may lead to urethral fistulae and periurethral abscesses.[19,21]

The clinical manifestations of urethral stricture are caused by bladder outlet obstruction. Urethral stricture often manifests itself as lower urinary tract symptoms or urinary tract infections with significant impairment in the quality of life. The primary symptom is diminished force and caliber of the urinary stream; other symptoms include urinary frequency and hesitancy, mild dysuria, double urine stream or spraying, and postvoid dribbling. Symptoms of acute urinary retention may occur in the presence of infection or urinary obstruction. Induration at the stricture site may be palpable. Tender, enlarged masses along the urethra usually indicate periurethral abscesses. Urethral stricture often manifests itself as lower urinary tract symptoms or urinary tract infections with significant impairment in the quality of life.

Urethral stricture is diagnosed on the basis of history, physical examination, urinary flow rates, voiding cystourethrogram, and urethroscopy; biopsy confirms carcinoma. Treatment is usually surgical and may involve urethral dilation, urethrotomy, or a variety of open surgical techniques. The choice of surgical intervention depends on the age of the individual and the severity of the problem. Strictures may recur up to 1 year after treatment. Follow-up is necessary during this time; urinary flow measurements and a urethrogram help determine the extent of residual obstruction.

Disorders of the Penis
Phimosis and Paraphimosis

Phimosis and paraphimosis are disorders in which the foreskin (prepuce) is "too tight" to be moved easily over the glans penis. Phimosis is a condition in which the foreskin cannot be retracted back over the glans, whereas paraphimosis is the opposite: the foreskin is retracted and cannot be moved forward (reduced) to cover the glans (Fig. 26.1). Both conditions can cause penile pathologic conditions.

The inability to retract the foreskin is normal in infancy and is caused by congenital adhesions. During the first 3 years of life these adhesions separate naturally with penile erections and are not an indication for circumcision. Although most cases occur in uncircumcised males, stenosis and resultant phimosis can occur in males with excessive skin remaining after circumcision.[21] Phimosis can occur at any age and is caused most commonly by poor hygiene and chronic infection. Chronic balanoposthitis (inflammation of the glans and prepuce) predisposes older diabetic men to phimosis. It rarely occurs with normal foreskin.

Edema, erythema, and tenderness of the prepuce and purulent discharge are usually the reasons for seeking treatment; inability to retract the foreskin is a less common complaint. Circumcision, if needed, is performed after infection has been eradicated. Complications of phimosis include inflammation of the glans (balanitis) or prepuce (posthitis) and paraphimosis. There is a higher incidence of penile carcinoma in uncircumcised males, which is associated with morbidity and mortality, but chronic infection, most likely with human papillomavirus (HPV), is usually the underlying factor in such cases. HPV infection can result in a spectrum of genitourinary manifestations ranging from genital warts to cancer. Approximately 40% of invasive penile carcinomas are attributable to HPV.[21,22]

Paraphimosis, in which the foreskin is retracted, can constrict the penis, causing edema of the glans. If edema is such that the foreskin cannot be reduced manually, surgery must be performed to prevent necrosis of the glans caused by constricted blood vessels. Severe paraphimosis is a surgical emergency, and phimosis may require immediate release if there is urinary obstruction.

Peyronie Disease

Peyronie disease (bent nail syndrome) is a fibrotic condition of the tunica albuginea of the penis resulting in varying degrees of curvature and sexual dysfunction. It is an underdiagnosed condition with prevalence in the male population as high as 9%[23] (Fig. 26.2). Peyronie disease develops slowly and is characterized by tough, fibrous thickening of the fascia in the erectile tissue of the corpora cavernosa. A dense fibrous plaque is usually palpable on the dorsum of the penile shaft. The problem usually affects middle-age men and is associated with painful erection, painful intercourse (for both partners), and poor erection distal to the involved area. In some cases, impotence or unsatisfactory penetration occurs. There is no pain when the penis is flaccid.

Although the exact cause is unknown, a local vasculitis-like inflammatory reaction occurs and decreased tissue oxygenation results in fibrosis and calcification. Peyronie disease is associated with Dupuytren

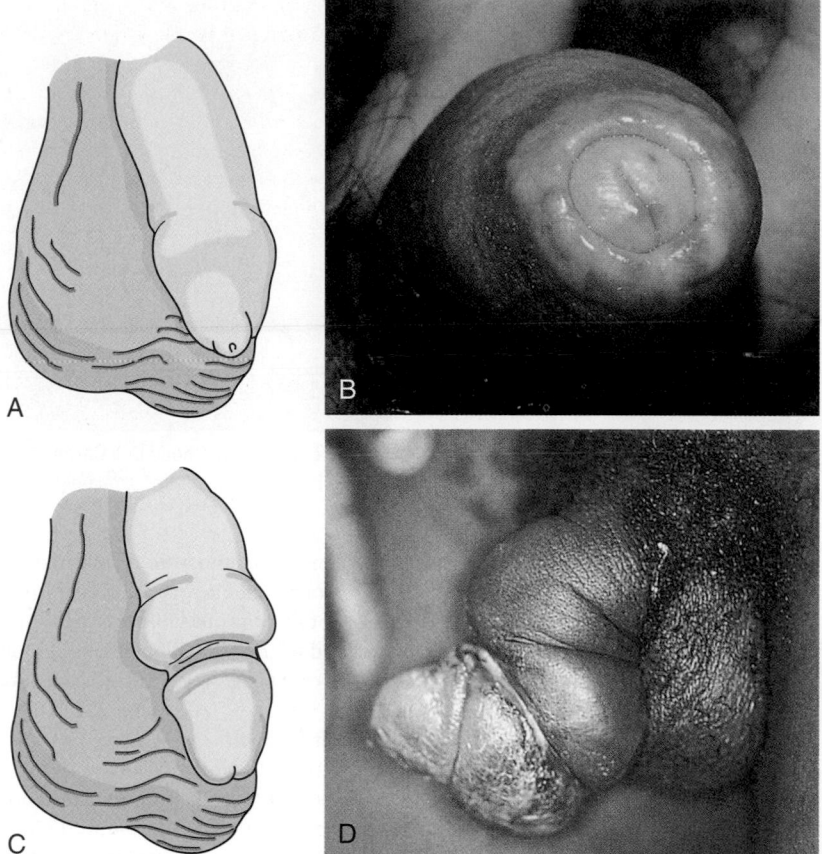

FIGURE 26.1 Phimosis and Paraphimosis. **A,** Phimosis: the foreskin has a narrow opening that is not large enough to permit retraction over the glans. **B,** Lesions on the prepuce secondary to infection cause swelling, and retraction of foreskin may be impossible. **C,** Paraphimosis: the foreskin is retracted over the glans but cannot be reduced to its normal position. Here it has formed a constricting band around the penis. **D,** Ulcer on the retracted prepuce with edema. (**A** and **C** From Monahan FD et al: *Phipps' medical-surgical nursing*, ed 8, St Louis, 2007, Mosby; **B** from Taylor PK: *Diagnostic picture tests in sexually transmitted diseases*, London, 1995, Mosby-Wolfe; **D** from Morse SA, Holmes KK, Ballard RC: *Atlas of sexually transmitted diseases and AIDS*, ed 4, London, 2011, Saunders.)

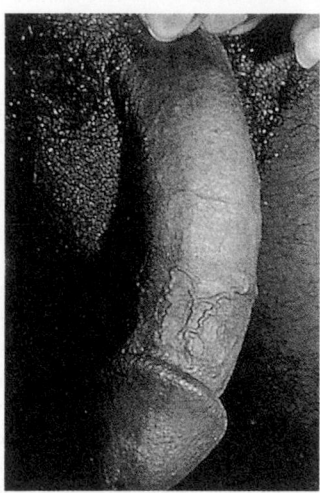

FIGURE 26.2 Peyronie Disease. (From Taylor PK: *Diagnostic picture tests in sexually transmitted diseases*, London, 1995, Mosby-Wolfe.)

contracture (a flexion deformity of the fingers or toes caused by shortening or fibrosis of the palmar or plantar fascia), diabetes, tendency to develop keloids, and, in rare cases, use of beta-blocker medications.

There is no definitive treatment for Peyronie disease. Spontaneous remissions occur in as many as 50% of cases. Treatment with pharmacologic therapies includes colchicine, aminobenzoate potassium (Potaba), L-carnitine, and liposomal superoxide dismutase. Men suffering with Peyronie disease who have significant penile deformity precluding successful coitus can be appraised for surgical correction. In men with adequate erectile function tunical plication or incision/partial excision, or both, and grafting can be offered depending on the degree of curvature or the presence of destabilizing deformity, or both. Surgery is considered the gold standard and includes the measures mentioned in the previous sentence, in addition to penile prosthesis–related procedures.[17,23]

Priapism

Priapism is an uncommon condition of prolonged penile erection, and is defined as a persistent and painful erection lasting longer than 4 hours without sexual stimulation (Fig. 26.3). Priapism is idiopathic in 60% of cases; the remaining 40% of cases are associated with spinal cord trauma, sickle cell disease, leukemia, pelvic tumors or infections, or penile trauma. Priapism also has been associated with cocaine use.[24,25] Intracavernous injection therapy for impotence seems to be the most

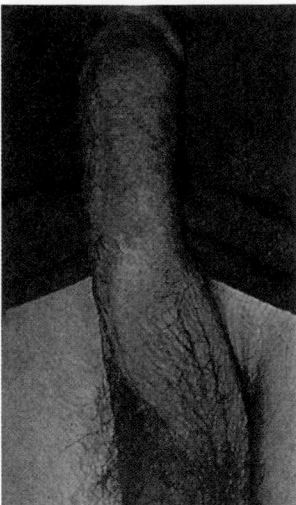

FIGURE 26.3 Priapism. (From Lloyd-Davies RW, Gow JG, Davies DR: *Color atlas of urology*, ed 2, London, 1994, Mosby-Wolfe.)

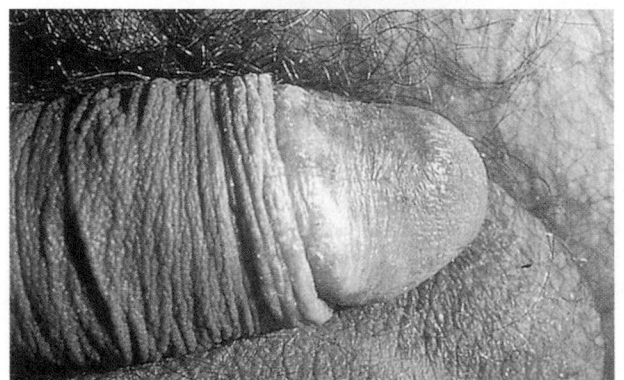

FIGURE 26.4 Balanitis. (From Taylor PK: *Diagnostic picture tests in sexually transmitted diseases*, London, 1995, Mosby-Wolfe.)

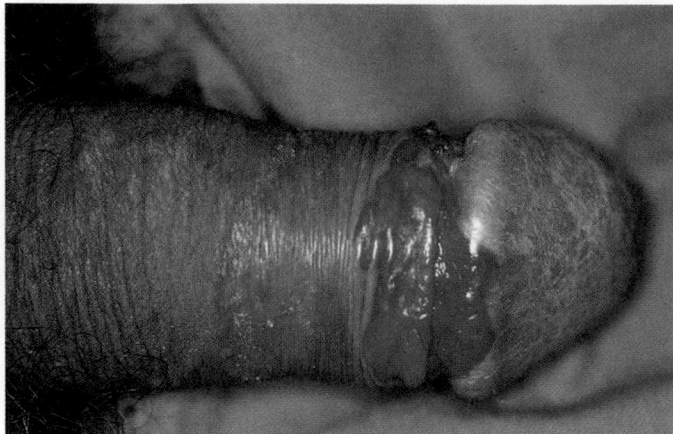

FIGURE 26.5 Squamous Cell Carcinoma Involving the Glans Penis. (From Callen JP et al: *Color atlas of dermatology*, Philadelphia, 1993, Saunders.)

common cause. Prolonged sexual stimulation often is associated with initial development of the idiopathic type.[21] The two corpora cavernosa within the erect penis are filled with blood and are tender to palpation; neither the corpus spongiosum nor the glans is engorged. The vascular congestion is thought to be associated with venous obstruction. If the erection remains over a period of days, edema and fibrosis develop, leading to erectile dysfunction (impotence).

Priapism is a urologic emergency. Treatment within hours is effective and prevents impotence. Conservative approaches include iced saline enemas, ketamine administration, and spinal anesthesia. Needle aspiration of blood from the corpus through the dorsal glans is often effective and is followed by catheterization and pressure dressings to maintain decompression. More aggressive surgical treatments include the creation of vascular shunts to maintain blood flow. Erectile dysfunction results in up to 50% of prolonged cases.

Balanitis

Balanitis is an inflammation of the glans penis (Fig. 26.4) and usually occurs in conjunction with posthitis, an inflammation of the prepuce. It is associated with poor hygiene and phimosis. The accumulation under the foreskin of glandular secretions (smegma), sloughed epithelial cells, and *Mycobacterium smegmatis* can irritate the glans directly or lead to infection. Skin disorders (e.g., psoriasis, lichen planus, eczema)

and candidiasis must be differentiated from inflammation resulting from poor hygienic practices. Balanitis is seen most commonly in men with poorly controlled diabetes mellitus and candidiasis. Antimicrobials are used to treat infection. Circumcision can prevent recurrences and can be considered after the inflammation has subsided.

Penile Cancer

In the United States, carcinoma of the penis is rare and affects about 1 in 100,000 men. The American Cancer Society estimates for penile cancer in the United States for 2017 are approximately 2120 cases and 360 deaths.[26] Although rare in North America and Europe, where it accounts for about 0.2% of cancers and 0.1% of cancer deaths in men, penile cancer may account for up to 10% of cancers in African and South American men.

In the United States, about four out of five cases of the disease are diagnosed in men older than age 55 years. Major risk factors include infection with HPV (mainly serotypes 16 and 18), smoking, and psoriasis treated with a combination involving the drug psoralen and ultraviolet (UV) light. Men circumcised at birth have less than half the chance of getting penile cancer than those who were not. Penile cancer is more common in men with phimosis and those with acquired immunodeficiency syndrome (AIDS). About two-thirds of men with penile cancer are diagnosed at more than 65 years of age.[26]

Before the development of penile cancer, signs of premalignant cancer or epidermal cancer in situ are present.[27] These include thick white plaque (leukoplakia) that typically involves the meatus; red, inflamed areas of Paget disease; red, velvety, ulcerative lesions of erythroplasia of Queyrat that usually involve the glans; large, invasive, scaly growths of Buschke-Löwenstein tumor; red plaque with encrustations of Bowen disease; and in situ carcinoma that generally affects the penile shaft. Men with leukoplakia or erythroplasia of Queyrat may have concurrent invasive penile carcinoma.[28,29] Pain and bleeding are late signs of penile cancer. Condylomata (genital warts) caused by HPV may be involved in the development of precancerous lesions[22] (see Chapter 27 for a discussion of HPV). At times the penis might be the site of metastatic spread of solid tumors from the bladder, prostate, rectum, or kidney. Early squamous cell carcinoma and premalignant epidermal lesions are easily treated but are often ignored. Delays in seeking treatment are attributed to denial, embarrassment, failure to detect lesions under a phimotic foreskin, fear, guilt, and ignorance.

Penile cancer is mostly squamous cell carcinoma, which usually begins as a small, fat, ulcerative or papillary lesion on the glans or foreskin that grows to involve the entire penile shaft (Fig. 26.5). Extensive lesions are associated with metastases and a poor prognosis. These lesions are not as painful as the amount of tissue involvement would seem to indicate. The regional femoral and iliac nodes are common metastatic sites. Rarely the urethra and bladder are involved. Weight loss, fatigue, and malaise accompany chronic suppurative lesions. Untreated, progressive disease causes death within 2 years.[29]

The specific diagnosis is made by biopsy after examination to document the location, size, and fixation of the lesion. After a positive biopsy the extent of cancer spread is determined by imaging tests such as ultrasound, CT, or MRI. Fine-needle aspiration of lymph tissue confirms the absence or presence of regional adenopathy. About 30% of penile cancers spread to lymph nodes before diagnosis. Distant metastases occur in less than 10% of cases and may involve lung, liver, bone, or brain.[24] The following stages are used for penile cancer: stage 0 (carcinoma in situ), stage I, stage II, stage III, and stage IV.[30]

Penile carcinoma is primarily managed with surgery. Newer, innovative surgical techniques can preserve as much penile tissue as possible without compromising cancer control. For invasive penile carcinoma, complete excision leaving adequate tumor-free margins is the goal. A simple circumcision may be sufficient for localized lesions of the prepuce. If the primary site is the glans and distal shaft, removal of the penis may be necessary. Although conventional radical surgery continues to be an effective approach, the emasculating nature of the treatment has serious psychologic and sexual consequences. Recent studies have challenged the conventional belief that a 2-cm margin was required for adequate cancer control.[27] Newer innovative surgical techniques can preserve as much penile tissue and functional integrity as possible without compromising cancer control. Inguinal lymph nodes also are removed if metastasis to these structures is known or suspected. Palliative treatment with radiation or chemotherapy may be used when the disease is inoperable and bulky inguinal metastases have occurred. Options for individuals with carcinoma in situ include local excision, radiation, laser surgery, cryosurgery, chemosurgery, or chemotherapy with topical (5%) 5-fluorouracil (5-FU). Differentiation, tumor stage, and age influence prognosis.[29,31] For cancers that are still confined to the penis (e.g., stage I and II cancers), the 5-year relative survival rate is around 85%. If the cancer has spread to nearby tissues or lymph nodes (e.g., stage III and some stage IV cancers), the 5-year relative survival rate is approximately 59%.[26]

Disorders of the Scrotum, Testis, and Epididymis
Disorders of the Scrotum

Men may seek treatment for painful or painless scrotal masses. Masses may be serious (cancer or torsion) or benign (hydrocele or cyst) and may require immediate surgical intervention or allow for careful observation.[32] Varicocele, hydrocele, and spermatocele are common intrascrotal disorders.[33-35] A varicocele is an abnormal dilation of a vein within the spermatic cord and is classically described as a "bag of worms" (Fig. 26.6). Most (95%) occur on the left side and may be painful or tender. Varicocele occurs in 10% of males and is seen most often after puberty. Sudden development of a varicocele in an older man is a late sign of renal tumor.[36,37] Unilateral right-sided varicoceles are rare and result from compression or obstruction of the inferior vena cava by a tumor or thrombus. Color Doppler ultrasonography is used to confirm the diagnosis.[27,35]

The cause of a varicocele is incompetent or congenitally absent valves in the spermatic veins. The valves that normally prevent backflow are absent or do not close adequately, permitting blood to pool in the veins rather than flow into the venous system. A varicocele decreases blood flow through the testis. This interferes with spermatogenesis and is a cause of infertility.[35,38] If infertility is a problem, treatment consists of ligation of the spermatic vein or occlusion of the vein by percutaneous methods, such as balloon catheter and sclerosing fluids.[38] If the varicocele is mild and fertility is not an issue, a scrotal support usually is sufficient to relieve symptoms of scrotal heaviness or "dragging."

A hydrocele is a collection of fluid within the tunica vaginalis[39,40] (Fig. 26.7). It is the most common cause of scrotal swelling. Hydroceles occur in 6% of male newborns and are congenital malformations (patent processus vaginalis) that often resolve spontaneously in the first year of life. Surgical ligation is recommended if the hydrocele persists after age 1 year.[34] Hydroceles in adults may be caused by an imbalance between

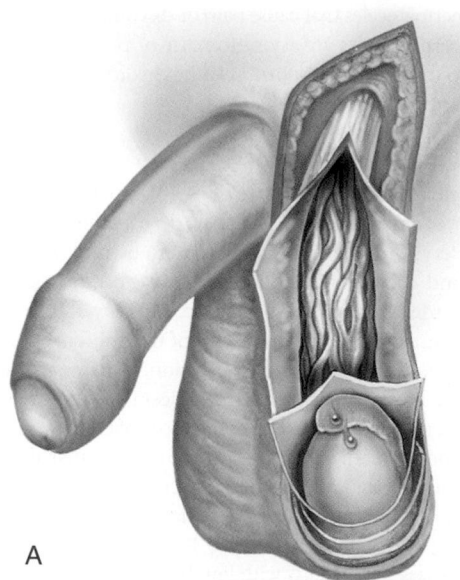
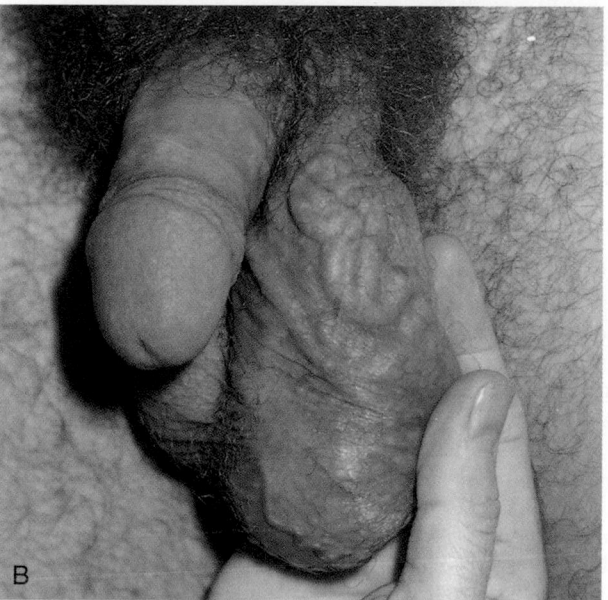

FIGURE 26.6 Varicocele. A, Dilation of veins within the spermatic cord. **B,** Varicocele on physical examination. (**A** From Ball JW et al: *Seidel's guide to physical examination,* ed 8, St Louis, 2015, Mosby. **B** From Swartz MH: *Textbook of physical diagnosis,* ed 6, Philadelphia, 2010, Saunders.)

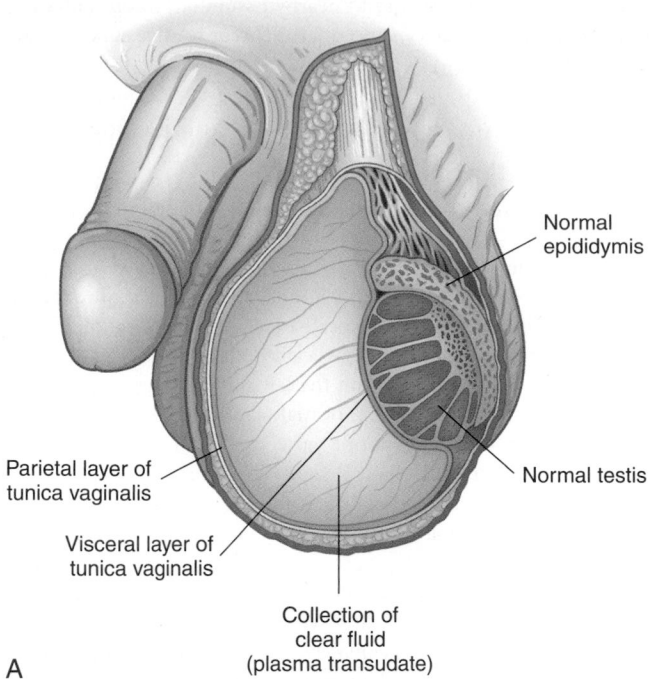

Normal epididymis

Parietal layer of tunica vaginalis

Normal testis

Visceral layer of tunica vaginalis

Collection of clear fluid (plasma transudate)

A

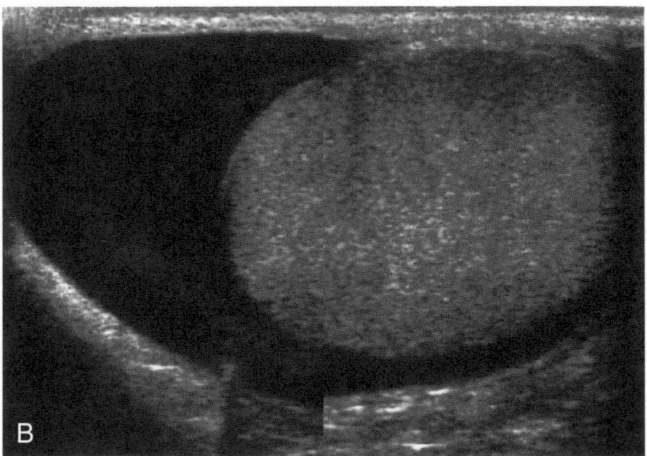

B

FIGURE 26.7 Depiction of a Hydrocele. **A,** Accumulation of clear fluid between the visceral (inner) and parietal (outer) layers of the tunica vaginalis. **B,** The appearance of a hydrocele on ultrasound examination. (**B** From Adam A et al: *Grainger & Allison's diagnostic radiology,* ed 6, London, 2008, Churchill Livingstone.)

the secreting and absorptive capacities of scrotal tissues. Hydroceles range in size from slightly larger than the testes to the size of a grapefruit or larger and may be flaccid or tense. Compression of testicular blood supply may lead to atrophy.

The exact mechanism of idiopathic hydrocele development is unknown. A secondary hydrocele may result from trauma or infection of the testis or epididymis or from a testicular tumor. Rapid accumulation of fluid occurs after local injury, radiotherapy, or infection (epididymitis or orchitis), or it may accompany testicular neoplasm. Chronic hydroceles are more common and occur in men older than 40 because of an imbalance between fluid secretion and reabsorption in the tunica vaginalis. A painless, extratesticular mass that easily transilluminates is found on physical examination. Ultrasonography of a large hydrocele, which may conceal a testicular tumor, is recommended. Treatment is usually not required unless a large, bulky hydrocele causes considerable

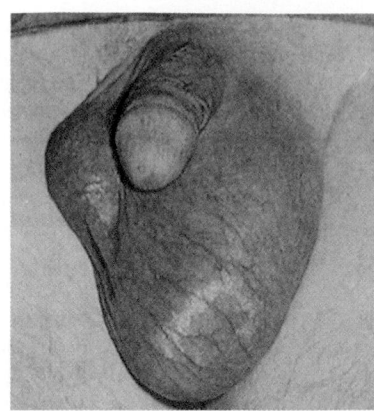

FIGURE 26.8 Spermatocele. Retention cyst of the head of the epididymis or of an aberrant tubule or tubules of the rete testis. The spermatocele lies outside the tunica vaginalis; therefore, on palpation it can be readily distinguished and separated from the testis. (From Lloyd-Davies RW, Gow JG, Davies DR: *Color atlas of urology,* ed 2, London, 1994, Mosby-Wolfe.)

physical discomfort or undesirable cosmetic appearance.[39] Treatment for uncomplicated hydrocele is aspiration of the fluid and injection of a sclerosing agent into the scrotal sac.[40-42] The goal of treatment is to remove the hydrocele and prevent recurrence by sclerosing or excising the tunica vaginalis.

Spermatoceles (epididymal cysts) are benign cystic collections of fluid of the epididymis located between the head of the epididymis and the testis. Efferent ducts of the epididymis have potential for cystic dilation to form a spermatocele[40-42] (Fig. 26.8). Spermatoceles are filled with milky fluid that contains sperm. A spermatocele is differentiated from a hydrocele in that aspiration of the hydrocele recovers a clear, yellow fluid, and unlike a hydrocele, a spermatocele does not cover the entire anterior surface of the testis.

Spermatoceles manifest as discrete, firm, freely mobile masses distinct from the testis that may be transilluminated. Epididymal cysts do not require treatment.[40,41] A spermatic cord tumor may feel like a tense spermatocele but does not contain fluid and will not transilluminate.[32] Spermatoceles that cause pain or discomfort are excised. Usually, however, spermatoceles are asymptomatic or produce mild discomfort that is relieved by scrotal support.[42] Neither hydroceles nor spermatoceles are associated with infertility.

Cryptorchidism and Ectopy

Cryptorchidism is a condition of testicular maldescent, whereas an ectopic testis has strayed from the normal pathway of descent. The etiology of cryptorchidism is considered to be multifactorial (genetic, maternal, and environmental factors) and it occurs most often as an isolated disorder with no obvious cause.[43] Ectopy may be caused by an abnormal connection at the distal end of the gubernaculum testis that leads the gonad to an abnormal position, usually at the superficial inguinal site. In cryptorchidism the descent of one or both testes is arrested, with unilateral arrest occurring more often than bilateral arrest.[42] The testes may remain in the abdomen, or testicular descent may be arrested in the inguinal canal or the penoscrotal junction. Cryptorchidism is a common pathologic condition that occurs in 3% of full-term newborns and it decreases to 0.8% to 1.2% at 1 year of age.[44] However, this rate increases significantly with low-birth-weight infants; for instance, the rate of cryptorchidism at 3 months has been found to be 7.7% for infants with birth weights less than 2000 g, 2.5% for birth weights of 2000 to 2500 g, and 1.41% for birth weights of 2500 g or more.[42,45,46]

The incidence of cryptorchidism in adults is 0.7% to 0.8%.[38] Cryptorchidism is commonly associated with vasal or epididymal abnormalities. These congenital anomalies affect about one-third to two-thirds of newborns with cryptorchidism. Other structural anomalies include posterior urethral valves (less than 5%), upper tract abnormalities (less than 5%), and hypospadias. The presence of hypospadias as well as cryptorchidism raises the suspicion of mixed gonadal dysgenesis (intersex infant). It has been hypothesized that cryptorchidism may result from an absence or abnormality of the gubernaculum, a cordlike structure that extends from the lower pole of the testis to the scrotum; a congenital gonadal or dysgenetic defect that makes the testes insensitive to gonadotropins (a likely explanation for unilateral cryptorchidism); or a lack of maternal gonadotropins (a likely explanation for bilateral cryptorchidism of prematurity).[38] Mechanical possibilities include a short spermatic cord, fibrous bands or adhesions in the normal path of the testes, or a narrowed inguinal canal. Chromosomal studies do not support a genetic component. Physiologic cryptorchidism, also called *retractile* or *migratory testis,* is an involuntary retraction of the testes out of the scrotum that occurs with excitement, physical activity, or exposure to cold and is caused by the small mass of prepubertal testis and the strength of the cremaster muscle. This is a common phenomenon that is self-limiting (descent occurs at puberty).

Physical examination discloses the absence of one or both testes in the scrotum and an atrophic scrotum on the affected side. If the undescended testis is in a vulnerable position, for example, over the pubic bone, an individual may complain of severe pain secondary to trauma. The adult male with bilateral cryptorchidism may be infertile. Ultrasonography, CT, or MRI can be used to locate an intraabdominal or nonpalpable testis.

Testicular cancer is also a well-established complication of cryptorchidism. In men with a history of unilateral cryptorchidism, neoplasms also develop more commonly in the contralateral testis. This finding suggests cryptorchidism affects the testes and is a process more significant than simply the position of the testis in childhood.[38,47] The risk of testicular cancer is 35 to 50 times greater for men with cryptorchidism or a history of cryptorchidism than for the general male population. Because definite histologic change (decreased Leydig cells, loss of germ cells, and peritubular fibrosis) occurs in the cryptorchid testis by 1 year of age, surgical correction is recommended earlier.[43,48] Treatment often

begins with administration of GnRH or human chorionic gonadotropin (hCG), hormones that may initiate descent, making surgery unnecessary. GnRH is given as a nasal spray in Europe and may enhance germ cell counts even when the testis does not descend.[48] If hormonal therapy is not successful, the testis is located and moved surgically (orchiopexy) in young children or removed (orchiectomy) in adults and children older than 10 years.[43,48] The testis that is properly placed in the scrotum provides adequate hormonal function and gives the scrotum a normal appearance. A successful operation does not ensure fertility if the testis is congenitally defective. Approximately 20% of males with unilateral undescended testis remain infertile even though orchiopexy is performed by age 1 year; most individuals with treated or untreated bilateral testicular maldescent have poor fertility. In addition, placement of the cryptorchid testis into the scrotal sac does not decrease the potential for malignancy; it does facilitate examination and tumor detection.

Torsion of the Testis

Torsion of the testis is rotation of a testis, which twists blood vessels in the spermatic cord. It causes an acute scrotum, which is testicular pain and swelling (Fig. 26.9). Differentiation between testicular torsion and two other common causes of an acute scrotum is based on physical examination and history[49] (Table 26.1). This event is most common among neonates and pubertal adolescents, but it can occur in males at any age.[34,50] Onset may be spontaneous or follow physical exertion or trauma. Torsion twists the arteries and veins in the spermatic cord, reducing or stopping circulation to the testis. Vascular engorgement and ischemia develop, causing scrotal swelling and pain. These manifestations are not relieved by scrotal elevation (Prehn sign), rest, or scrotal support. On physical examination, men have a tender high-riding testis, a thickened spermatic cord, and an absent cremasteric reflex. Unlike epididymitis, the epididymis cannot be differentiated from the testis.[49] Diagnostic testing includes urinalysis (to rule out infection) and color Doppler ultrasonography.[38] Torsion of the testis is a surgical emergency. If the torsion cannot be reduced manually, surgery must be performed within 6 hours after the onset of symptoms to preserve normal testicular function. Surgery includes untwisting the spermatic cord and anchoring both testes in correct position within the scrotum to prevent recurrences. With successful manual detorsion, surgical fixation should be done within a few days.

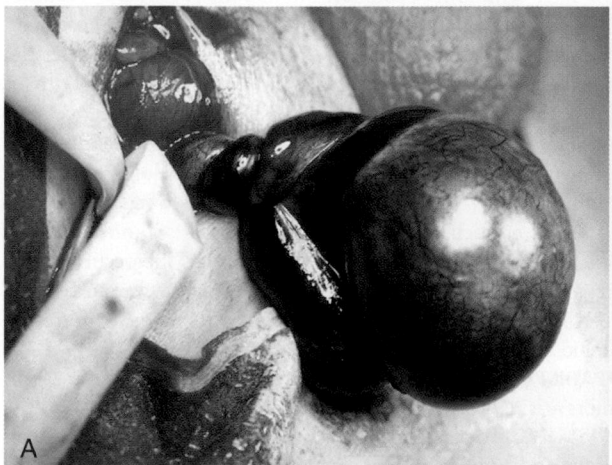
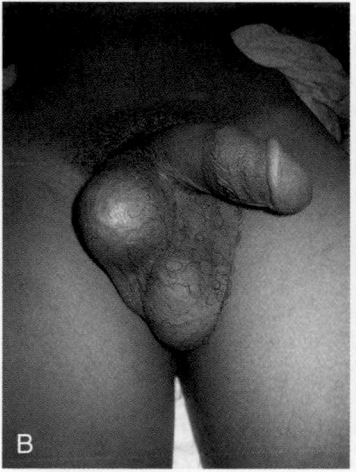
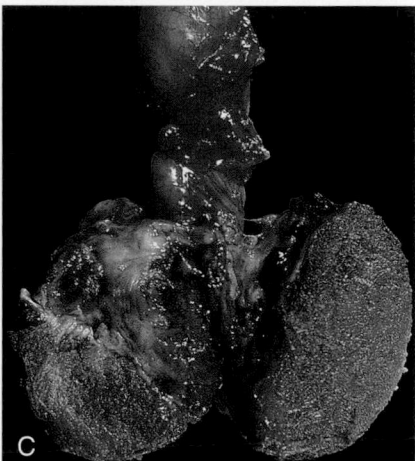

FIGURE 26.9 Torsion of the Testes. **A,** Left testicular torsion in an adolescent with acute scrotum; the testis is necrotic. **B,** Late phase torsion in an adolescent with severe testicular pain 1 month previously. Note the absence of inflammation and the high position of the testis in the scrotum. **C,** The testes appear dark red and partially necrotic owing to hemorrhagic infarction. (**A** and **B** From Kliegman RM et al: *Nelson's textbook of pediatrics,* ed 19, Philadelphia, 2011, Saunders. **C** From Damjanov I, Linder J, editors: *Anderson's pathology,* ed 10, St Louis, 1996, Mosby.)

TABLE 26.1		DIAGNOSIS OF SELECTED CONDITIONS RESPONSIBLE FOR THE ACUTE SCROTUM				
CONDITION	**ONSET OF SYMPTOMS**	**AGE**	**TENDERNESS**	**URINALYSIS**	**CREMASTERIC REFLEX**	**TREATMENT**
Testicular torsion	Acute	Early puberty	Diffuse	Negative	Negative	Surgical exploration
Appendiceal torsion	Subacute	Prepubertal	Localized to upper pole	Negative	Positive	Bed rest and scrotal elevation
Epididymitis	Insidious	Adolescence	Epididymal	Positive or negative	Positive	Antibiotics

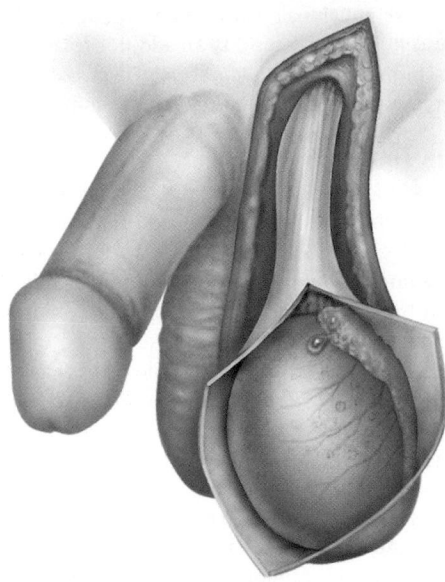

FIGURE 26.10 Orchitis. Inflammation of the testicle with enlargement or swelling. (From Ball JW et al: *Seidel's guide to physical examination,* ed 8, St Louis, 2015, Mosby.)

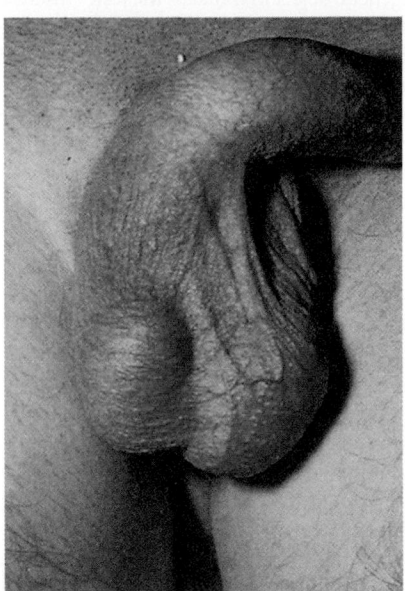

FIGURE 26.11 Testicular Tumor. (From Wolfe J: *400 Self-assessment picture tests in clinical medicine,* London, 1984, Mosby.)

Orchitis

Orchitis is an acute infection of the testes (Fig. 26.10) and is uncommon except as a complication of systemic infection or as an extension of an associated epididymitis.[51] Infectious microorganisms may reach the testes through the blood or the lymphatics or, most commonly, by ascent through the urethra, vas deferens, and epididymis. Most cases of orchitis are actually cases of epididymo-orchitis. Occasionally, in middle-age men, a nonspecific, apparently noninfectious, inflammatory process (called *granulomatous orchitis*) occurs. It seems to be an autoimmune disease that triggers a granulomatous response to spermatozoa.

Mumps is the most common infectious cause of orchitis and usually affects postpubertal males. The onset is sudden, occurring 3 to 4 days after the onset of parotitis. Signs and symptoms include high fever, reaching 40°C (104°F), marked prostration, bilateral or unilateral erythema, edema and tenderness of the scrotum, and leukocytosis. An acute hydrocele may develop. Urinary signs and symptoms, which accompany epididymitis, are absent. Atrophy with irreversible damage to spermatogenesis may result in 30% of affected testes. Bilateral orchitis does not affect androgenic function but may cause permanent sterility.

Treatment is supportive and includes bed rest, scrotal support, scrotal elevation, hot or cold compresses, and analgesic agents for relief of pain. If an acute hydrocele develops, it is aspirated. Testicular abscess usually requires orchiectomy (removal of the testis). Appropriate antimicrobial drugs should be used for bacterial orchitis, and corticosteroids are indicated in proved cases of nonspecific granulomatous orchitis.

Cancer of the Testis

Testicular cancer is a highly treatable, usually curable, cancer that most often develops in young and middle-aged men. For men with seminoma (all stages combined), the cure rate exceeds 90%. For those with low-stage seminoma or nonseminoma, the cure rate approaches 100%.[52] Overall, testicular cancers are rare, yet they are the most common form of cancer in young men between ages 15 and 35. The American Cancer Society's estimates for testicular cancer in the United States for 2017 suggest approximately 8850 new cases of testicular cancer will be diagnosed, and about 410 deaths will result from testicular cancer.[1] In the United States, the lifetime probability of developing testicular cancer is 0.2% for white men, an incidence that is 4 times higher than that for blacks. Testicular tumors are slightly more common on the right side than on the left, a pattern that parallels the occurrence of cryptorchidism; about 1% to 2% of primary testicular cancers are bilateral (Fig. 26.11), and 50% of these tumors arise from treated or untreated cryptorchid testes.[53]

◆**PATHOPHYSIOLOGY.** Ninety percent of testicular cancers are germ cell tumors arising from the male gametes. Germ cell tumors constitute 90% of testicular cancers and can be broadly classified into two types: seminomas and nonseminomas. Seminomas are the most common, are the least aggressive, and make up about 30% to 35% of testicular cancers. Nonseminomas include embryonal carcinomas, teratomas, and choriocarcinomas, which are the most aggressive but rare (less than 1%) form of testicular cancer. Testicular cancers can include a mix of types.[54] In addition, testicular tumors can arise from specialized cells of the gonadal stroma. These tumors, which are named for their cellular origins, are Leydig cell, Sertoli cell, granulosa cell, and theca cell tumors and constitute less than 10% of all testicular cancers.[55]

The cause of testicular neoplasms is unknown. A genetic predisposition is suggested by the fact that the incidence is higher among brothers, identical twins, and other close male relatives. Genetic predisposition is supported further by statistics showing that the disease is relatively rare among black Africans, black Americans, Asians, and native New Zealanders. Familial testicular germ cell tumors may be associated with transgenerational inheritance of epigenetic events.[56] Risk factors include history of cryptorchidism, abnormal testicular development, human immunodeficiency virus (HIV) and AIDS, Klinefelter syndrome, and history of testicular cancer.[53]

CLINICAL MANIFESTATIONS. Painless testicular enlargement is usually the first sign of testicular cancer. Enlargement is usually gradual and may be accompanied by a sensation of testicular heaviness or dull ache in the lower abdomen.[54] Occasionally, acute pain occurs because of rapid growth, resulting in hemorrhage and necrosis. Approximately 10% of affected men have epididymitis, 10% have hydroceles,[42] and 5% have gynecomastia or hydroceles. The incidence of gynecomastia increases considerably (30% to 45%) in men with Sertoli or Leydig tumors. Approximately 10% of individuals already have symptoms related to metastases at the time of initial diagnosis, which correlates with the typical delay of 3 to 6 months from initial recognition to definitive treatment. Lumbar pain may be present and usually is caused by retroperitoneal node metastasis. Signs of metastasis to the lungs include cough, dyspnea, and bloody sputum (hemoptysis). Supraclavicular node involvement may cause difficulty swallowing (dysphagia) and neck swelling. Alterations in vision or mental status, papilledema, and seizures may be experienced with metastasis to the CNS. Approximately 10% of affected individuals are asymptomatic; the tumor may be detected by the man's sexual partner or incidentally following trauma.

EVALUATION AND TREATMENT. An incorrect diagnosis at the initial examination occurs in as many as 25% of men with testicular cancer. Epididymitis and epididymo-orchitis are the most common misdiagnoses; others include hydrocele and spermatocele. Evaluation begins with careful physical examination, including palpation of the scrotal contents with the individual in the erect and supine positions. The abdomen and lymph nodes are palpated to rule out metastases. Signs of testicular cancer include abnormal consistency, induration, nodularity, or irregularity of the testis. A firm, nontender testicular mass or diffuse enlargement is found in the majority of cases. Primary testicular cancer can be assessed rapidly and accurately by scrotal ultrasonography. Tumor markers are higher than normal in the presence of a tumor and may help detect a tumor that is too small to be palpated during physical examination or seen on imaging.[49] Tumor type is identified after inguinal biopsy or orchiectomy. Scrotal incisions may cause dissemination of the tumor and increase the risk of local recurrence and therefore are avoided. Chest x-ray, lymphangiogram, intravenous pyelogram (IVP), abdominal ultrasound, and CT are used in clinical staging of the disease. Treatment is based on type of tumor, stage of disease, general health, and age. Besides surgery, treatment involves radiation and chemotherapy singly or in combination. A number of factors influence the prognosis (Table 26.2). They include the histology of the tumor, the stage of the

TABLE 26.2	**TESTICULAR TUMORS OF GERM CELL ORIGIN**		
CELL TYPES	**OCCURRENCE**	**METASTATIC PATTERN**	**PROGNOSIS/REMISSION RATE**
A. Seminoma (germinoma)	30%–35% of all testicular tumors	Rarely to retroperitoneal lymph nodes	Excellent; tumor usually remains localized and is responsive to radiation; cure rate stages I and II >95%; stages III and IV >80%
B. Nonseminomatous tumors	60% of all testicular tumors		
1. Single cell			
a. Embryonal carcinoma	20%–25% of all testicular tumors; most common testicular tumor in infants and children	Earlier to regional lymphatics; also lung, liver, bone	Good; complete remission rate stages I and II >95%; stages III and IV >70%–80%
b. Teratoma	5%–10% of all testicular tumors (occurs in children and adults)	Through lymphatics and bloodstream; affects same organ systems as embryonal type	Fair
c. Choriocarcinoma	<1% of all testicular tumors	Earliest and widest, initially through bloodstream	Poor; early metastasis
2. Mixed tumors	30%–40% of all testicular tumors		
a. Teratocarcinoma	20%–25% of all testicular tumors	Mixed pattern; depends on cell types	Variable; prognosis becomes that of the most malignant element
b. Other i. Teratocarcinoma with seminoma ii. Embryonal cancer with seminoma iii. Teratoma with seminoma iv. Any combination with choriocarcinoma	10%–15% of all testicular tumors	Mixed pattern; depends on cell types	Variable; prognosis becomes that of the most malignant element
3. Non–germ cell tumors (Leydig cell, Sertoli cell, granulosa cell, and thecal cell tumors)	<10%		

Data from American Cancer Society: *Cancer response system document #10029,* New York, 1995, The Society; Cancer Net: *Cancer facts: questions and answers about testicular cancer,* National Cancer Institute, 2000. Available at: http://www.cancernet.nci.nih.gov.

disease, and the selection of appropriate treatment. Serum markers, such as alpha fetoprotein (AFP), β-hCG, and lactate dehydrogenase, are useful for detecting metastases and assessing responses to therapy. With appropriate treatment survival rates from testicular cancer are excellent, although some affected men have persistent paresthesias, Raynaud phenomenon, or infertility. According to the National Cancer Institute, the overall 5-year survival rate from testicular cancer was 95.4% between 2006 and 2012. If the cancer was confined to the testis at the time of diagnosis, the survival rate was 99.3% and dropped only slightly to 96.1% with regional extension. For those with distant metastases, the survival rate was 73.9%.[49,55] Orchiectomy does not affect sexual function, but infertility can result from chemotherapy or surgical removal of affected abdominal lymph nodes if the nerves necessary for ejaculation are severed. After orchiectomy, testicular silicone implants may be used to restore "normal" scrotal appearance.

Epididymitis

Epididymitis, or inflammation of the epididymis, generally occurs in sexually active young males (younger than 35 years) and is rare before puberty (Fig. 26.12). In young men the usual cause is a sexually transmitted microorganism, such as *N. gonorrhoeae* or *C. trachomatis*. Men who practice unprotected anal intercourse may acquire sexually transmitted epididymitis because of *Escherichia coli*, *Haemophilus influenzae*, tuberculosis (especially in regions where the incidence of pulmonary tuberculosis is high), *Cryptococcus*, or *Brucella*.[41,42] In men older than 35 years, Enterobacteriaceae (intestinal bacteria) and *Pseudomonas aeruginosa* associated with urinary tract infections and prostatitis also may cause epididymitis. Besides an infectious etiology, epididymitis may result from a chemical inflammation caused by the reflux of sterile urine into the ejaculatory ducts.[41] It is associated with urethral strictures, congenital posterior valves, and excessive physical straining in which increased abdominal pressure is transmitted to the bladder. Chemical epididymitis is usually self-limiting and does not require evaluation or intervention unless it persists.

◆**PATHOPHYSIOLOGY.** The pathogenic microorganism usually reaches the epididymis by ascending the vasa deferentia from an already infected urethra or bladder. The presence of bacteria initiates the inflammatory response, causing symptoms of bacterial epididymitis. Epididymitis caused by heavy lifting or straining results from reflux of urine from the bladder into the vas deferens and epididymis. Urine is extremely irritating to the epididymis and initiates an inflammatory response called *chemical epididymitis*.

◆**CLINICAL MANIFESTATIONS.** Pain is the main symptom of epididymitis. Scrotal or inguinal pain is caused by inflammation of the epididymis and surrounding tissues. The pain is usually acute and severe. Flank pain may occur if, as the urethra passes over the spermatic cord, edematous swelling of the cord obstructs the urethra. The individual may have pyuria and bacteriuria and a history of urinary symptoms, including urethral discharge. The scrotum on the involved side is red and edematous as a result of inflammatory changes. The tail of the epididymis near the lower pole of the testes usually swells first; then swelling ascends to the head of the epididymis. The spermatic cord also may be swollen and tender.

Complications of epididymitis include abscess formation, infarction of the testis, recurrent infection, and infertility. Infarction probably is caused by thrombosis (obstruction by blood clots) of the prostatic vessels secondary to severe inflammation. Recurrent epididymitis may result from inadequate initial treatment or failure to identify or treat predisposing factors. Chronic epididymitis can cause scarring of the epididymal endothelium. Once scarring has occurred, treatment with antibiotics is ineffective because adequate antibiotic levels cannot be achieved within the epididymis.[41]

◆**EVALUATION AND TREATMENT.** A history of recent urinary tract infection or urethral discharge suggests the diagnosis of epididymitis. The relief of pain when the inflamed testis and epididymis are elevated (Prehn sign) is also diagnostic. Definitive diagnosis is based on culture or Gram stain of a urethral swab. Epididymal aspiration may be necessary to obtain a specimen, especially if the individual has been taking antibiotics and has sterile urine.

Treatment includes antibiotic therapy for the infection itself (see Chapter 27). Analgesics, ice, and scrotal elevation can provide symptomatic relief. If the individual does not steadily improve, he should be reevaluated for possible complications, such as abscess formation, sepsis, or continued infection.[41] Bed rest and scrotal elevation are recommended until the scrotum is no longer tender. Scrotal elevation facilitates maximal lymphatic and venous drainage. Abscess formation is rare with antibiotic therapy. If an abscess occurs and persists, it is drained surgically and an orchiectomy may be indicated. Complete resolution of swelling and pain may take several weeks to months. The individual's sexual partner should be treated with antibiotics if the causative microorganism is a sexually transmitted pathogen.

Disorders of the Prostate Gland
Benign Prostatic Hyperplasia

Benign prostatic hyperplasia (BPH), also called benign prostatic hypertrophy, is the enlargement of the prostate gland (Fig. 26.13). Because the major prostatic changes are caused by hyperplasia, not hypertrophy, benign prostatic hyperplasia is the preferred term. This condition becomes problematic as prostatic tissue compresses the urethra, where it passes through the prostate, resulting in frequency of lower urinary tract symptoms. The prevalence among U.S. men 60 years and older is about 50% and among men 70 years or older 90%.[57] BPH is common and involves a complex pathophysiology with several endocrine and local factors and a remodeled microenvironment. Its relationship to aging is well documented. At birth the prostate is pea sized, and growth of the gland is gradual until puberty. A period of rapid development continues until the third decade of life, when the prostate reaches adult size. Around 40 to 45 years of age, benign hyperplasia begins and continues slowly until death. Although dihydrotestosterone (DHT) is necessary for normal prostatic development, its role in BPH remains unclear. Among all androgen-metabolizing enzymes within the human

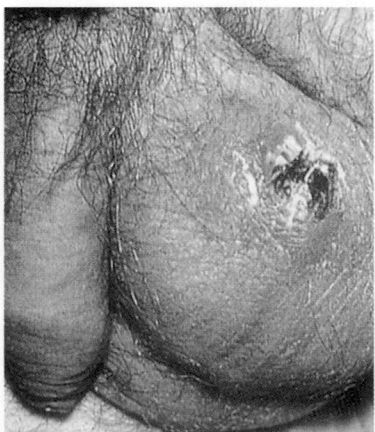

FIGURE 26.12 Epididymitis Secondary to Gonorrhea or Nongonococcal Urethritis. This infection spread to the testes, and rupture through the scrotal wall is threatened. (From Taylor PK: *Diagnostic picture tests in sexually transmitted diseases*, London, 1995, Mosby-Wolfe.)

Prostate zones

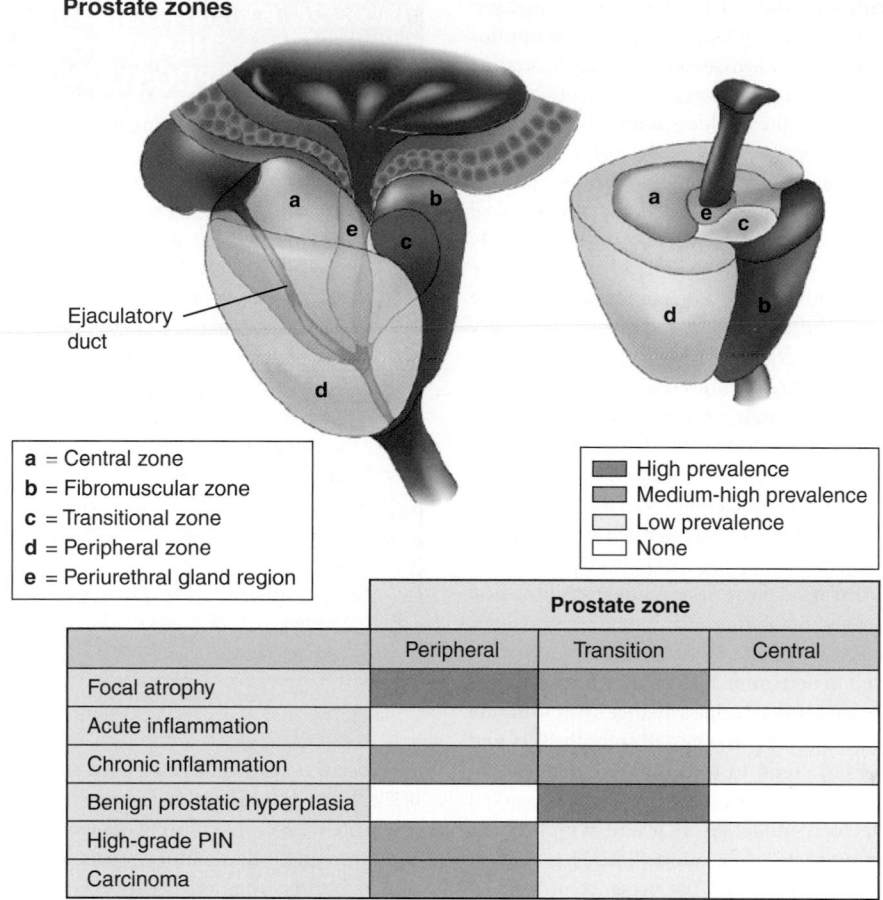

a = Central zone
b = Fibromuscular zone
c = Transitional zone
d = Peripheral zone
e = Periurethral gland region

Ejaculatory duct

■ High prevalence
■ Medium-high prevalence
☐ Low prevalence
☐ None

	Prostate zone		
	Peripheral	Transition	Central
Focal atrophy			
Acute inflammation			
Chronic inflammation			
Benign prostatic hyperplasia			
High-grade PIN			
Carcinoma			

FIGURE 26.13 Prostate Zones, Benign Prostatic Hyperplasia (BPH), and Prostate Cancer Locations. BPH occurs in the peripheral zone of the prostate gland that can enlarge (not shown). BPH nodules and atrophy are associated with inflammation in the transition zone. Most cancer lesions occur in the peripheral zone. Carcinoma can involve the central zone but rarely occurs in isolation, suggesting that prostatic intraepithelial neoplasia (PIN) lesions do not easily progress to carcinoma in this region. (Adapted from De Marzo AM et al: *Nat Rev Cancer* 7:256–269, 2007.)

prostate, 5α-reductase is the most powerful. The level of this reductase positively corresponds to the age-dependent DHT level. Therefore although 5α-reductase and DHT levels decrease with age in the epithelium, they remain relatively constant in the stroma of the prostate gland.

◆PATHOPHYSIOLOGY. Current causative theories of BPH focus on levels and ratios of endocrine factors such as androgens, estrogens, gonadotropins, and prolactin and changes in the balance between autocrine/paracrine growth-stimulatory and growth-inhibitory factors. These factors include insulin-like growth factors (IGFs), epidermal growth factor, nerve growth factor, fibroblast factors, IGF binding proteins, and transforming growth factor-beta (TGF-β).[58]

Aging and circulating androgens are associated with BPH and enlargement. These factors are predisposed as disrupting the *balance* of growth factor signaling pathways and stromal/epithelial interactions, creating a growth-promoting and tissue-remodeling microenvironment. However, BPH is a multifactorial disease, and not all men respond well to available treatments, suggesting factors other than androgens are involved. Testosterone, the primary circulating androgen in men, also can be metabolized through CYP19/aromatase into the potent estrogen, estradiol-17β. The prostate is an estrogen target tissue, and estrogens directly and indirectly affect growth and differentiation of the prostate. The precise role of endogenous and exogenous estrogens in directly affecting prostate growth and differentiation in the context of BPH is an understudied area. Estrogens and selective estrogen receptor modulators have been shown to promote or inhibit prostate proliferation, illustrating their potential roles in the development of BPH as therapy.[59] Taken together, these interactions lead to an increase in prostate volume. The remodeled stroma promotes local inflammation with altered cytokine, reactive oxygen/nitrogen species, and chemoattractants.[60] The resultant increased oxygen demands of proliferating cells causes a local hypoxia that induces angiogenesis and changes to fibroblasts. Functional and phenotypic changes (transdifferentiation) of fibroblasts to the myofibroblasts is a hallmark of the remodeled microenviroment.[58]

BPH begins in the periurethral glands, which are the inner glands or layers of the prostate. The prostate enlarges as nodules form and grow (nodular hyperplasia) and glandular cells enlarge (hypertrophy). The development of BPH occurs over a prolonged period, and changes within the urinary tract are slow and insidious.

◆CLINICAL MANIFESTATIONS. Preclinical studies demonstrate that the activation of a chronic inflammatory prostatic response plays an important role in the pathogenesis and progression of BPH and prostate cancer. Approximately 40% to 70% of men with BPH-related lower urinary tract symptoms harbor chronic inflammation at the time of pathologic evaluation.[58] As nodular hyperplasia and cellular hypertrophy progress, tissues that surround the prostatic urethra usually compress it, but do not always cause bladder outflow obstruction. These symptoms are sometimes called the spectrum of lower urinary tract symptoms (LUTSs). Symptoms include the urge to urinate often, a delay in starting urination, and decreased force of the urinary stream. As the obstruction progresses, often over several years, the bladder cannot empty all the urine and the increasing volume leads to long-term urine retention. The volume of urine retained may be great enough to produce uncontrolled "overflow incontinence" with any increase in intraabdominal pressure. At this stage the force of the urinary stream is significantly reduced, and much more time is required to initiate and complete voiding. Hematuria, bladder or kidney infection, bladder calculi, acute urinary retention (hydroureter), hydronephrosis, and renal insufficiency are common complications.[61]

Some men initially have signs of uremia and renal failure. On digital rectal examination the hyperplastic prostate is a soft or firm enlargement with a smooth mucosal surface and no discernible distinction between lobes; asymmetry is common. The palpated prostate does not always reflect the degree of BPH because a substantial portion of the enlargement is intravesicular.[62] Thirty percent of men with mild to moderate symptoms improve with watchful waiting.

◆**EVALUATION AND TREATMENT.** Diagnosis is made from a medical history, physical examination, and laboratory tests including urinalysis. Careful review of symptoms is necessary. Digital rectal examination (DRE) and PSA are conducted to determine hyperplasia. Measurement of PSA level alone, however, cannot determine whether symptoms are caused by BPH because the level of PSA is elevated in both BPH and prostate cancer. Annual DREs are used to screen men older than 40 years of age for BPH, sooner in high-risk men.[63] If there is marked enlargement of the prostate or if moderate to severe symptoms or complications are present, transrectal ultrasound (TRUS) is used to determine bladder and prostate volume and the presence of residual urine. Urinalysis, measurements of serum creatinine and blood urea nitrogen levels, uroflowmetry, determination of postvoid residual (PVR) urine, pressure-flow study, cystometry, and cystourethroscopy are used to determine kidney and bladder function.[61] BPH has been treated successfully with drugs. α_1-Adrenergic blockers (prazosin and tamsulosin) are used to relax the smooth muscle of the bladder and prostate. Antiandrogen agents, such as finasteride (Proscar), selectively block androgens at the prostate cellular level and cause the prostate gland to shrink.[63] By shrinking the prostate, these drugs have been shown to improve BPH-related symptoms and reduce the risk of future urinary retention and BPH-related surgery. α_1-Adrenergic blockers do not affect PSA level and have no effect on prostate cancer risk.[63]

Newer minimally invasive procedures include interstitial laser therapy, transurethral radiofrequency procedure (TUNA), cooled Thermo Therapy, and prostate artery embolization. When necessary, the hyperplastic tissue may be removed surgically to prevent the serious consequences of urethral obstruction. A permanent indwelling catheter is inserted if the individual cannot tolerate surgery. It also should be noted that new techniques in genomics, proteomics, and epigenetics have led to the discovery of aberrant signaling pathways, novel biomarkers, DNA methylation signatures, and potential gene-specific targets. As such, the ability to risk stratify men with symptomatic benign prostatic hyperplasia, identify those at higher risk for progression, and seek alternative therapies for those in whom conventional options are likely to fail will become the standard of targeted therapy in the future.[64]

Prostatitis

Prostatitis is an inflammation of the prostate. Some degree of prostatic inflammation is present in 4% to 36% of the male population, increasing to 50% in older men. Inflammation is usually limited to a few of the gland's excretory ducts.

BOX 26.5 NATIONAL INSTITUTES OF HEALTH CLASSIFICATION OF PROSTATITIS SYNDROMES

This system, developed for clinical research purposes, can be simplified for use in primary care practice.

Category I, or acute bacterial prostatitis (ABP), is an acute infection of the prostate and is manifested by systemic signs of infection and a positive urine culture.

Category II, or chronic bacterial prostatitis (CBP), is a chronic bacterial infection in which bacteria are recovered in significant numbers from a purulent prostatic fluid. These bacteria are thought to be the most common cause of recurrent urinary tract infection in men.

Category III, or chronic pelvic pain syndrome (CPPS), is diagnosed when no pathogenic bacteria can be localized to the prostate (culture of expressed prostatic fluid or postprostatic massage urine specimen) and is further divided into IIIa and IIIb. Category IIIa refers to inflammatory CPPS in which a significant number of white blood cells (WBCs) are localized to the prostate, whereas category IIIb is noninflammatory.

Category IV refers to asymptomatic inflammatory prostatitis in which bacteria or WBCs are localized to the prostate, but individuals are asymptomatic.

Prostatitis syndromes have been classified by the National Institutes of Health as (1) acute bacterial prostatitis (ABP), (2) chronic bacterial prostatitis (CBP), (3) chronic pelvic pain syndrome (CPPS), and (4) asymptomatic inflammatory prostatitis (Box 26.5). ABP and CBP are caused mostly by gram-negative Enterobacteriaceae and *Enterococci* species, which originate in the gastrointestinal flora. The most common microorganism is *E. coli,* which is identified in the majority of infections.[65] *Klebsiella* species, *P. aeruginosa*, and *Serratia* species are common gram-negative cultured microorganisms. Nonbacterial prostatitis (CP/CPPS) syndromes are caused by a cascade of inflammatory, immunologic, neuroendocrine, and neuropathic mechanisms in which the initiating cause is unknown.

Bacterial Prostatitis. Acute bacterial prostatitis (ABP, category I) is an ascending infection of the urinary tract that tends to occur in men between the ages of 30 and 50 years but also is associated with BPH in older men. Infection stimulates an inflammatory response in which the prostate becomes enlarged, tender, firm, or boggy. The onset of prostatitis may be acute and unrelated to previous illnesses or it may follow catheterization or cystoscopy.

Clinical manifestations of acute bacterial prostatitis are those of urinary tract infection or pyelonephritis. Sudden onset of malaise, low back and perineal pain, high fever (up to 40°C [104°F]), and chills is common, as are dysuria, inability to empty the bladder, nocturia, and urinary retention. The individual also may have symptoms of lower urinary tract obstruction, such as a slow, small, "narrowed" urinary stream, which may be a medical emergency. Acute inflammatory prostatic edema can compress the urethra, causing urinary obstruction. Systemic signs of infection include sudden onset of a high fever, fatigue, arthralgia, and myalgia. Prostatic pain may occur, especially when the individual is in an upright position, because the pelvic floor muscles tighten with standing and the prostate gland is compressed. Some individuals experience low back pain, painful ejaculation, and rectal or perineal pain. Palpation discloses an enlarged, extremely tender and swollen prostate that is firm, indurated, and warm to the touch.

Because ABP is usually associated with a bladder infection caused by the same microorganism, urine cultures disclose its identity. Prostatic massage may express enough secretions from the urethra for direct bacterial examination, but massage may be painful and increases the risk that the infection will ascend to adjacent structures or enter the bloodstream and cause septicemia.

To resolve the infection and control its spread, individuals may require antibiotics. In severe cases, the individual is hospitalized and treated with intravenous antibiotics, followed by oral antibiotics. Analgesics, antipyretics, bed rest, and adequate hydration also are therapeutic. Complications include urinary retention that resolves with antibiotic therapy; prostatic abscess that may rupture into the urethra, rectum, or perineum; epididymitis; bacteremia; and septic shock. Urinary retention requiring drainage is best managed with a suprapubic catheter. Foley catheterization is contraindicated during acute infection.

Chronic bacterial prostatitis (CBP, category II) is characterized by recurrent urinary tract symptoms and persistence of pathogenic bacteria (usually gram negative) in urine or prostatic fluid. This form of prostatitis is the most common recurrent urinary tract infection in men. Symptoms may be similar to those of an acute bladder infection, such as frequency, urgency, dysuria, perineal discomfort, low back pain, myalgia, arthralgia, and sexual dysfunction. The prostate may only be slightly enlarged or boggy but it may be fibrotic because repeated infections can cause it to be firm and irregular in shape.

When the initial urine sample is bacteria-free, prostatic massage is used to express secretions. Subsequently, the first 10 mL of voided urine is collected and examined microscopically. Prostatic secretions showing more than 10 white blood cells (WBCs) per high-power field and macrophages containing fat are indicative of bacterial infection; diagnosis is confirmed by culture. A pelvic x-ray or TRUS may show prostatic calculi.

Treatment of chronic bacterial prostatitis is difficult because it is often caused by prostatic calculi. Calculi are silent and are found in up to 50% of men with prostatitis, and infected calculi can serve as a source of bacterial persistence and relapsing urinary tract infection.[66] Calculi harbor pathogens within the stone, and consequently pathogens cannot be eradicated from the urinary tract. Permanent cure is achieved by surgical intervention.

Chronic Prostatitis/Chronic Pelvic Pain Syndrome.
Chronic prostatitis/chronic pelvic pain syndrome (CPPS, category III) is diagnosed when no pathogenic bacteria can be localized to the prostate and is further divided into subcategories IIIa and IIIb (see Box 26.5). Category IIIa refers to inflammatory chronic pelvic pain syndrome where WBCs are elevated and localized to the prostate. Symptoms tend to be milder but are persistent and annoying. Presumably, noninfectious prostatitis or pain is caused by reflux of sterile urine into the ejaculatory ducts because of high-pressure voiding.[65] Reflux may be triggered by spasms of the external or internal sphincters. Category IIIb is noninflammatory; in category IV, individuals are asymptomatic but have an increase in the number of bacteria and WBCs localized to the prostate. Microorganisms suspected of causing CP/CPPS include *E. coli*, *Enterobacter*, *P. aeruginosa*, and *Helicobacter pylori*, a new suspect.[65]

Men with nonbacterial prostatitis may complain of pain or a dull ache that is continuous or spasmodic in the suprapubic, infrapubic, scrotal, penile, or inguinal area. Other symptoms are pain on ejaculation and urinary symptoms, such as frequency of urination. The prostate gland generally feels normal on palpation.

Nonbacterial prostatitis is a diagnosis of exclusion. Digital examination of the prostate, bacterial cultures of the urogenital tract, microscopic examination of expressed prostatic fluid, urethroscopy, and urodynamic studies are used to verify the diagnosis of nonbacterial prostatitis.

There is no generally accepted treatment for nonbacterial prostatitis. Hot sitz baths, bed rest, alpha-blockers, anticholinergics, and antiinflammatory drugs can relieve symptoms.

Cancer of the Prostate

Prostate cancer is the most commonly diagnosed non–skin cancer in men in the United States, with a lifetime risk for diagnosis currently estimated at 15.9%, according to the 2012 United States Preventive Services Task Force screening recommendation document.[67] The incidence varies greatly worldwide[68] (Fig. 26.14), but it is still considered to be the second most frequently diagnosed cancer and the sixth leading cause of death worldwide. Importantly, incidence rates vary by more than 25-fold worldwide, and the highest rates recorded mostly in developed countries include Oceania, Europe, and North America, largely because of the wide use or overuse of PSA testing.[69] Screening with PSA can amplify the incidence of prostate cancer by allowing detection of prostate lesions that although meeting the pathologic criteria for malignancy, may have low potential (e.g., latent, indolent, preclinical) for growth and metastasis. In countries with higher use of PSA testing, such as the United States, Canada, Australia, and the Nordic countries, trends in incidence rates follow similar patterns.[68]

Different from Western countries, incidence and mortality rates are rising in several Asian (including Japan) and Central and Eastern European countries.[69] Death rates have been decreasing in several countries including Australia, Canada, the United Kingdom, the United States, Italy, and Norway, in part from improved treatment. Males of African descent in the Caribbean have the highest mortality rates from prostate cancer in the world. Most cases of prostate cancer have a good prognosis even without treatment but some cases are aggressive; the lifetime risk for dying of prostate cancer is 2.8%. Prostate cancer is rare before age 50 years and very few men die from it before 60 years of age. Indeed, more than 75% of all prostate cancer is diagnosed in men older than 65.[67] With aging, most of the androgen-metabolizing enzymes undergo significant alteration and older age, race (black), and family history remain the well-established risk factors.[69]

Dietary Factors.
Although evidence exists for a dietary role in prostate cancer, the epidemiologic evidence is inconsistent. The problem has been confounded by a lack of biomarkers for certain nutrients, difficulties in measuring and quantifying diet, and a limitation of clinical trials to study diet over time. Important are the effects of diet on signaling pathways, hormones, oxidative stress, and reactive oxygen species (ROS). The nutrients in the epidemiology of prostate cancer that have received the most attention include carotenoids, fat, vitamin E, vitamin D/calcium, and selenium. Less studied are isoflavones, curcumin, lycopene, zinc, green tea, omega-3 polyunsaturated fats, and sulforaphane (see *Nutrition & Disease: Diet for Prostate Cancer*). Associations between obesity and prostate cancer are not clear, with some research inconsistencies, but obesity seems to be negatively associated with more indolent prostate cancer and positively associated with more aggressive disease and a worse outcome.[70,71] In process is a randomized clinical trial of diet and early-stage prostate cancer, Men's Eating and Living Study (MEAL). The hypothesis for MEAL is that a change in diet from a high intake of animal products to the consumption of more fruits and vegetables will slow the progression of the indolent form to the aggressive form of prostate cancer.[71] Likewise, a recent systematic review found that physical activity does not significantly reduce the risk of prostate cancer; however, the authors noted that vigorous exercise may reduce the risk of an aggressive tumor.[70] Because adipose tissue is increasingly being regarded as hormonally active tissue, high body fat and obesity need in-depth exploration to understand the associated risk of prostate problems. Adipose tissue is now known to affect circulating levels of several bioactive messengers and therefore could affect the risk of developing prostate problems in addition to several other well-recognized health problems.[72] High energy intake (consumption of excess calories) indicates that this may indeed increase insulin levels and insulin-like

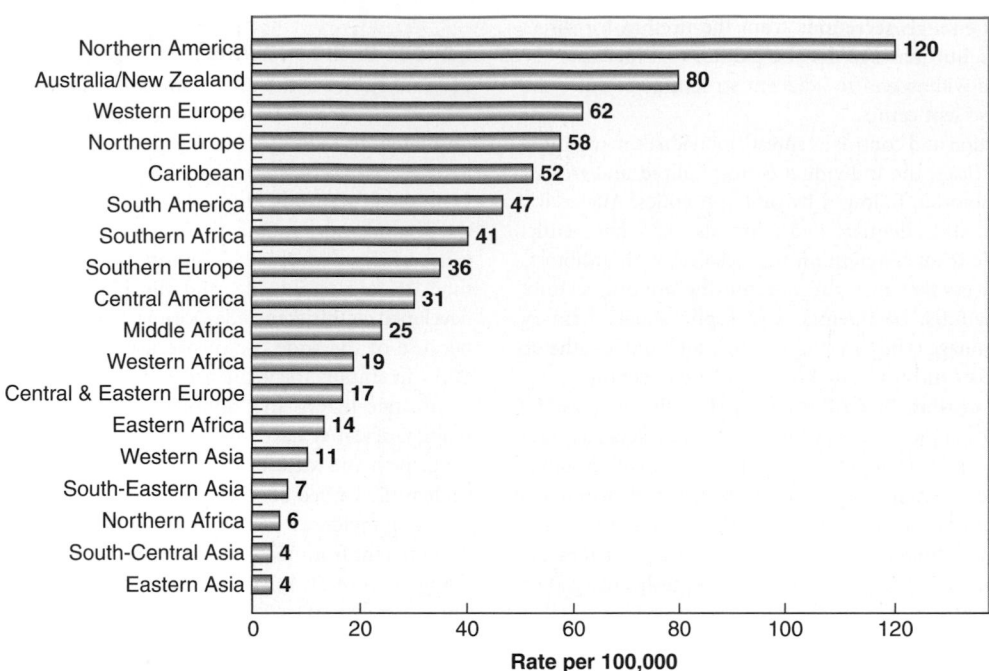

FIGURE 26.14 Selected World Population Age-Standardized (to the World Population) Incidence Rates of Prostate Cancer. (Modified from Jemal A et al: *Biomark Prev* 19:1893, 2010.)

NUTRITION & DISEASE

Diet for Prostate Cancer

- Epidemiologic studies have found total fat intake, animal and saturated fat, red meat, and dairy products are associated with an increase in prostate cancer risk.
- Obesity is linked to advanced and aggressive prostate cancer.
- High body mass index (BMI) is associated with more aggressive disease and a worse outcome.
- Calorie-dense or excessive carbohydrate intake and obesity, independent of dietary fat intake, may increase the risk of developing prostate cancer.
- Dietary fat may increase androgens, increase oxidative stress, and increase reactive oxygen species (ROS).
- Monounsaturated fats may decrease the risk of prostate cancer.
- High levels of linoleic acid (e.g., found in corn oil; safflower) tend to act as a proinflammatory eicosanoid, which is implicated in promotion of cell proliferation and angiogenesis as well as inhibition of apoptosis.
- The Western diet has increased omega-6/omega-3 ratios and therefore is proinflammatory.
- Cooking meat at high temperatures produces heterocyclic amines and aromatic hydrocarbons that are carcinogenic.
- A pooled analysis of 15 prospective cohort studies did not support a strong role of fruits, vegetables (including cruciferous vegetables and tomato products [few studies assessed tomato sources of more bioavailable lycopene]) or mature beans in prostate cancer. The MEAL (The Men's Eating and Living) Study, a randomized trial of diet to alter disease, is assessing a diet-based intervention to increase vegetable and fruit consumption to see if it can slow prostate cancer progression for men with low-grade prostate cancer.
- A systematic review and meta-analysis concluded that IGF-1 is a potential mechanism underlying observed associations between milk intake and prostate cancer risk.
- Carcinogenic nitrosamines are formed after consumption of processed meat that contains nitrites and from heme iron present in large quantities of red meat.

- Vitamin E has long been considered a candidate for prostate cancer prevention from in vitro and in vivo animal studies. Vitamin E belongs to the family of tocopherols and tocotrienols that exist as α, β, γ, and δ isoforms. Among these, δ-tocopherol is the major dietary isoform, whereas supplements contain α-tocopherol. Vitamin E is a fat-soluble vitamin obtained from vegetable oils, nuts, and egg yolk. It is a potent intracellular antioxidant known to inhibit peroxidation and DNA damage. The Alpha-Tocopherol, Beta-Carotene Cancer Prevention (ATBC) Study showed supplementation with vitamin E could reduce the incidence of prostate cancer among men who smoked. In vitro studies demonstrate that γ-tocopherol and δ-tocopherol induce cell cycle arrest in human prostate cancer cells (i.e., induce apoptosis) and inhibit the androgen receptor. Mouse studies show vitamin E can inhibit the growth-promoting effects of a high-fat diet; however, vitamin E in combination with selenium does not reduce the incidence of prostate cancer in lady mice models. In the prospective large clinical trial SELECT, the study found no apparent benefit of administering vitamin E.
- Selenium is a trace mineral and exists in food as selenomethionine and selenocysteine. It is essential for the functioning of many antioxidant enzymes and proteins in the body. Humans receive selenium in their diet through plant (dependent on soil concentrations) and animal products. Several large prospective studies reported 50% to 65% reductions in prostate cancer risk with high levels versus low levels of selenium as measured in toenails and plasma. The Nutritional Prevention of Cancer (NPC) trial reported a 50% reduction in risk of developing prostate cancer. No potential benefit was found in the SELECT trial, whereas a small insignificant increase was noted for type 2 diabetes. From these two trials, two different forms of selenium were used—the NPC trial used selenized yeast and the SELECT trial used selenomethionine. A meta-analysis of 12 studies with 13,254 subjects and 5007 cases of prostate cancer showed that the risk of prostate cancer decreased with increasing plasma/serum selenium up to 170 ng/mL. Selenium has several modes of

NUTRITION & DISEASE—cont'd

Diet for Prostate Cancer

action depending on its form. Selenomethionine inhibits cell proliferation and induces cell cycle arrest of human prostate cells (i.e., apoptosis) and inhibits angiogenesis mediated in part by the androgen receptor. This also is true of methylseleninic acid. Sodium selenite's anticancer effects are mediated through cellular antioxidants, leading to increased apoptosis and sensitizing cells to radiation-induced killing. Selenium and its derivatives can activate both intrinsic and extrinsic pathways of apoptosis. Selenium intervention may depend on individual genotype.

- Vitamin D may play an important role in prostate cancer prevention.
- Soy contains isoflavones purported to have anticancer properties including inhibition of cell proliferation and angiogenesis and reduction in prostate-specific antigen (PSA) and androgen receptor levels.
- Tomatoes or tomato products ingested daily seem to reduce prostate cancer risk. In vitro studies show lycopene inhibits DNA strand breaks. Unresolved is whether lycopene itself or a metabolic product is responsible for its biologic effect. In clinical studies, tomato paste, which is high in lycopene, reduced plasma PSA levels in those men with benign prostatic hyperplasia. Lycopene administration is associated with cell cycle arrest (apoptosis) and growth factor signaling. In 2007 the U.S. Food and Drug Administration (FDA) evaluated 13 available studies and found the relationship between lycopene and reduced risk of prostate cancer inadequate. A Cochrane review found that given only three randomized controlled trials were included in the analysis and a high risk of bias was found in two, there is insufficient evidence to support or refute lycopene for the prevention of prostate cancer.
- Vegetables including broccoli, cabbage, cauliflower, brussels sprouts, Chinese cabbage, and turnips (all crucifers) may be protective (several epidemiologic studies) against prostate cancer. In particular, a diet high in broccoli reduced cancer risk. By contrast, four studies revealed no

cancer preventive effects. Crucifers have anticancer properties mediated by the phytochemicals phenethyl isothiocyanate, sulforaphane, and indole-3-carbinol. Sulforaphane is a naturally occurring isothiocyanate that was first isolated in broccoli. It protects against carcinogen-induced cancer in many rodents. Mice given 240 mg of broccoli sprouts per day showed a significant reduction in growth of prostate cancer cells. Sulforaphane treatment lowered androgen receptor protein and gene expression.

- Green tea contains polyphenols, including epigallocatechin gallate (EGCG). Green tea consumption has been associated with a reduced incidence of several cancers including prostate cancer. Green tea consumed within a balanced controlled diet in humans improved overall antioxidant potential. The anticancer effect potential of green tea from in vitro and experimental studies shows polyphenols bind directly to carcinogens and induce phase II enzymes that inhibit heterocyclic amines. EGCG administration decreased NF-$\kappa\beta$ activity. Green tea was shown to inhibit IGF-1 and increase IGFBP3, leading to inhibition of prostate cancer development and progression. Yet, in two small randomized studies in individuals with high-grade prostatic neoplasia, it showed no effects. In a population prospective large study ($n = 27,293$), green tea did not protect against prostate cancer and black tea showed a positive association with prostate cancer.
- Curcumin has anticarcinogenic potential with well-characterized antiinflammatory, antiangiogenic, and antioxidant properties. Recent studies report curcumin modulates the wingless signaling pathway (Wnt) that supports its antiproliferative potential.
- Overall, multiple signaling pathways are involved in prostate cancer development and progression, many of which are affected by dietary and lifestyle factors.

Data from Astog P: *Cancer Causes Control* 15:367–386, 2004; Beier R et al: *EMBO J* 19(21):5813–5823, 2000; Dagnelie PC et al: *BJ Int* 98(8):1139–1150, 2004; Demark-Wahnefried W, Moyad MA: *Curr Opin Urol* 17:168–174, 2007; Freedland SJ, Aronson WJ: *Urology* 65:433–439, 2005; Giovannucci E et al: *Int J Cancer* 121:1571–1578, 2007; Greenwald P: *J Nutr* 234(12 suppl):3507S–3512S, 2004; Hill P et al: *Cancer Res* 39:5101–5104, 1979; Hurst R et al: *Am J Clin Nutr* 96(1):111–122, 2012; Khan N, Mukhtar H: *Biochem Pharmacol* 85(5):667–672, 2014; Kim DJ et al: *Cancer Causes Control* 11:65–77, 2000; Kobayashi N et al: *Clin Cancer Res* 12(15):4660–4670, 2006; Kolonel LN: *Epidemiol Rev* 23:72–81, 2001; Llic D, Forbes KM, Hassed C: *Cochran Database Syst Rev* (11):CD008007, 2011; Lloyd JC et al: *J Urol* 183:1619–1624, 2010; Matsumura K et al: *Anticancer Res* 28:709–714, 2008; Montague JA et al: *Cancer Causes Control* 23(10):1635–1641, 2012; Ngo TH et al: *Cancer Causes Control* 13:929–935, 2002; Ngo TH et al: *Clin Cancer Res* 9:2734–2743, 2003; Ni J, Yeh S: *Vitam Horm* 76:493–518, 2007; Parsons JK et al: *BJU Int* 2017 Apr 24, [Epub ahead of print]; Petimar J et al: *Cancer Epidemiol Biomarkers Prev* 2017 Apr 26, [Epub ahead of print]; Rodriguez C et al: *Cancer Epidemiol Biomarker Prev* 16:63–69, 2007; Sinha R et al: *Am J Epidemiol* 170:1165–1177, 2009; Teiten M et al: *Int J Oncol* 38:603–611, 2011; Yang CD, Suh N, Kong AN: *Cancer Prev Res (Phil)* 5(5):701–705, 2012.

growth factor 1 (IGF-1), a powerful carcinogenic agent[73] (see Pathophysiology). A meta-analysis found IGF-1 as a *potential* mechanism for the associations between milk intake and prostate cancer risk.[74] Investigators suggest a positive association between high-fat milk intake and prostate cancer progression among individuals diagnosed with localized prostate cancer.[75] Although epidemiologic studies have revealed some dietary factors modulate the risk of advanced prostate cancer,[76] there is a lack of definitive evidence supporting the preventive role of diet against prostate cancer. More robust, high-quality research trials are needed to guide understanding of the complex relationship between diet and prostate cancer.

Hormones. Prostate cancer develops in an androgen-dependent epithelium and is usually androgen sensitive. Androgens are synthesized not only in the testis, accounting for 50% to 60% of the total testosterone in the prostate, but also in the prostate gland itself. In a process called intraprostatic conversion, the hormone dehydroepiandrosterone (DHEA) produced by the adrenal glands[77,78] is converted to testosterone

and then into DHT in the prostate (Fig. 26.15). Additionally, prostate cancer cells have been reported to make androgens from cholesterol (i.e., de novo).[79] However, these overall relative contributions from intratumoral sources remain to be determined. Population studies have not, however, provided clear and convincing patterns involving associations between circulating hormone concentrations (e.g., not tissue concentrations) and prostate cancer risk.[80-82] A recent case-control study found the risk of aggressive prostate cancer was strongly inversely associated with estradiol/testosterone ratios and positively associated with 2-hydroxyestrone/16α-hydroxyestrone ratios.[83] These findings suggest that sex steroid hormones, specifically the estrogen-androgen balance, may be important in the development of aggressive prostate cancer.[83] Thus there is universal agreement that androgens are important for prostatic growth, development, and maintenance of tissue balance but their role in cancer is still controversial. As such, it also has been hypothesized that reducing the concentration of active hormones in the systemic circulation may be insufficient to block cancer progression,

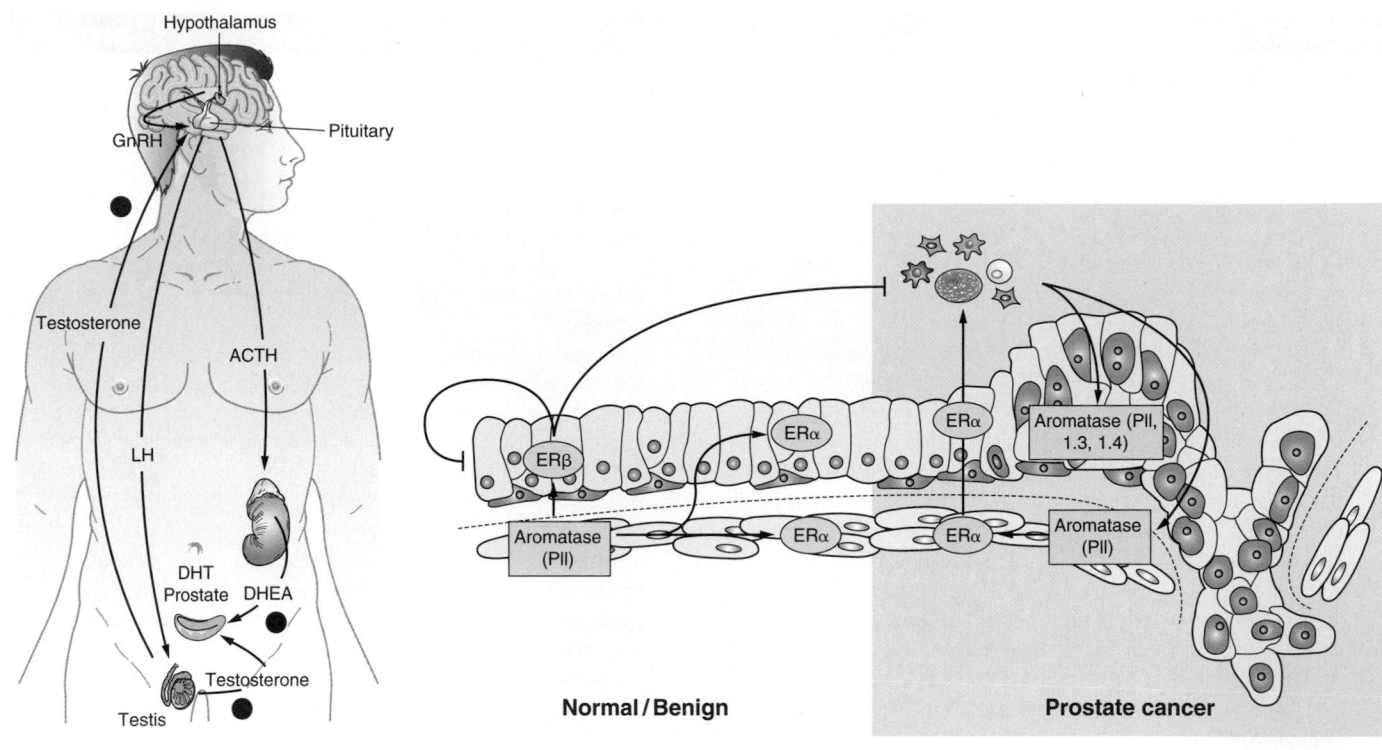

FIGURE 26.15 Sources of Androgens and Aromatase and Estrogen Signaling in the Prostate. **A,** Body sources of androgens in the prostate gland. Hypothalamic GnRH causes the release of LH from the anterior pituitary gland. LH stimulates the testes to produce testosterone, which then accumulates in the blood. Pituitary ACTH release stimulates the adrenal glands, which secrete the androgen precursor DHEA into the blood. DHEA is converted into testosterone and then into DHT in the prostate. **B,** Aromatase and estrogen signaling in the prostate. In normal and benign tissue, aromatase is expressed within the stroma and regulated by promoter PII. Estrogen then exerts its effects in an autocrine fashion through the stromal ER-α receptor and also in a paracrine fashion through both ER-α and ER-β receptors. With prostate cancer, aromatase is now expressed within the tumor cells and in stromal cells, and regulated by aromatase promoters 1.3, 1.4, and PII. Thus estrogen exerts its effects in an autocrine way through stromal and epithelial ER-α and ER-β. Consequently, the increased levels of estrogen and abnormal ER-α signaling promote inflammation, which increases aromatase expression and the development of a positive feedback cycle. Inflammation drives aromatase expression, thus increasing estrogen, which in turn promotes further inflammation. *ACTH,* Adrenocorticotropic hormone; *DHEA,* dehydroepiandrosterone; *DHT,* dihydrotestosterone; *GnRH,* gonadotropin-releasing hormone; *LH,* luteinizing hormone. (**A** Adapted from Labrie F: *Nat Rev Urol* 8:73–80, 2011; **B** from Ellem SJ, Risbridger GP: *J Steroid Biochem Mol Biol* 118[4–5]:246–251, 2010.)

because this action selects for tumor cells that can generate active steroids from circulating precursors.[77,84] Evidence for involvement of 5α-reductase activity, which is critical in androgen activity in the prostate, is contradictory and inconsistent[80,82] (see Fig. 26.15). A prevention study has provided some of the strongest hormonal data with the drug finasteride, which inhibits 5α-reductase. The 7-year intervention study reduced prostate cancer risk in healthy men by about 25%.[85] Important, however, was that more high-grade tumors were found in those men who developed prostate cancer while taking the drug. In men younger than 50 years, circulating levels of androgens and estrogens appear to be higher in men of African descent than in European-American men.

Despite the well-documented importance of androgens, their pathophysiologic process in prostate diseases is incomplete.[82,84] Identifying cellular signaling pathways that become corrupted and facilitate metastases in the presence of androgens is the focus of recent work. Investigators suggest that inhibition of CXCR7 (chemokine receptor 7) function might decrease metastatic potential by altering cell motility.[86] Androgens also are metabolized to estrogens (see Figs. 26.17 and 25.37)

through the action of the enzyme aromatase, and a growing body of evidence implicates estrogens (estrogen receptor–mediated effects, estrogen metabolites, and estrogen genotoxicity) in the etiology of prostate disease (see Pathophysiology under Prostate Cancer). Importantly, the aberrant expression of aromatase has been implicated in other tissues, such as the breast and endometrium.[84]

Only a few associations with prostate cancer risk have been observed consistently (in at least three studies), and their associations are weak: (1) slightly higher circulating testosterone and estrogen levels and lower DHEA (sulfate) levels in high-risk black men as compared with lower-risk European-American men; and (2) a cytosine-adenine-guanine (CAG) repeat-length polymorphism in the androgen receptor gene associated with increased risk and increased receptor activity (androgen receptor). Moreover, in a more recent collaborative analysis of existing worldwide epidemiologic data (18 prospective studies), the Endogenous Hormones and Prostate Cancer Collaborative Group found no associations between the risk of prostate cancer and serum concentrations of testosterone, calculated free testosterone, dihydrotestosterone, dehydroepiandrosterone sulfate, androstenedione, androstanediol glucuronide, estradiol, or calculated free estradiol.[87]

As the results of the above-mentioned Endogenous Hormones and Prostate Cancer Collaborative Group suggest, investigations directed at understanding the hormonal basis of prostate carcinogenesis have numerous problems. Understanding the complexities of interacting hormones and differentiating the effects of a single hormone are profound. In addition, only single *blood* samples are generally available; *tissue* hormone samples important for paracrine signaling are not consistently measured, and within-subject variations over time and differences in circadian rhythms cannot be adequately measured. The results of several animal studies do support elevation of the levels of bioavailable and bioactive androgens in the circulation and in target tissue as an important risk factor. Animal studies also indicate that increased biologic activity of the androgen receptor may be associated with prostate cancer. See the Pathophysiology section for prostate cancer for a more thorough discussion of the role of hormones in the pathogenesis of prostate cancer.

Vasectomy.   Vasectomy has been identified as a possible risk factor for prostate cancer in case-controlled and cohort studies.[88-90] Three mechanisms by which vasectomy could increase risk are (1) elevation of the levels of circulating androgens; (2) immunologic mechanisms involving anti–sperm antibodies; and (3) reduction of seminal fluid levels of 5α-dihydrotestosterone, the active metabolite of testosterone in the prostate, in vasectomized men. These results suggest an elevation of circulating free testosterone level following vasectomy. However, with these combined mechanisms it is unlikely that vasectomy plays a causal role.[91] In fact, a recent systematic review and meta-analysis of cohort studies indicated that vasectomy may not contribute to the risk of prostate cancer.[92]

Chronic Inflammation.   Data from the Medical Therapy of Prostatic Symptoms (MTOPS) study suggest the risk of BPH progression and acute urinary retention is greater in men with prostatic inflammation.[93,94] Preclinical studies have claimed that inflammatory mediators are involved in prostate cancer development and, therefore, suggested these as attractive targets for intervention. However, among the many proinflammatory mediators, there is no consensus regarding the identity of the primary one(s).[95,96] In a 5-year longitudinal study of the influence of chronic inflammation on prostate cancer, 33 of 144 men presented with chronic inflammation in their initial biopsy.[97] The investigators also found prostatic hyperplasia and proliferative inflammatory atrophy in those with chronic inflammation. Upon repeat biopsy, 29 new cancers were diagnosed, representing a new cancer incidence of 20%.[97] In contrast, of the 33 men initially showing no inflammation, 2 (6%) were found to have adenocarcinoma. Certain metabolic comorbidities, including obesity, diabetes, sleep apnea, and erectile dysfunction, may be linked to both BPH and inflammation.[98] The causes of chronic inflammation are unknown (possible causes are shown in Fig. 26.16). Thus chronic inflammation may be an important risk factor for prostatic adenocarcinoma.

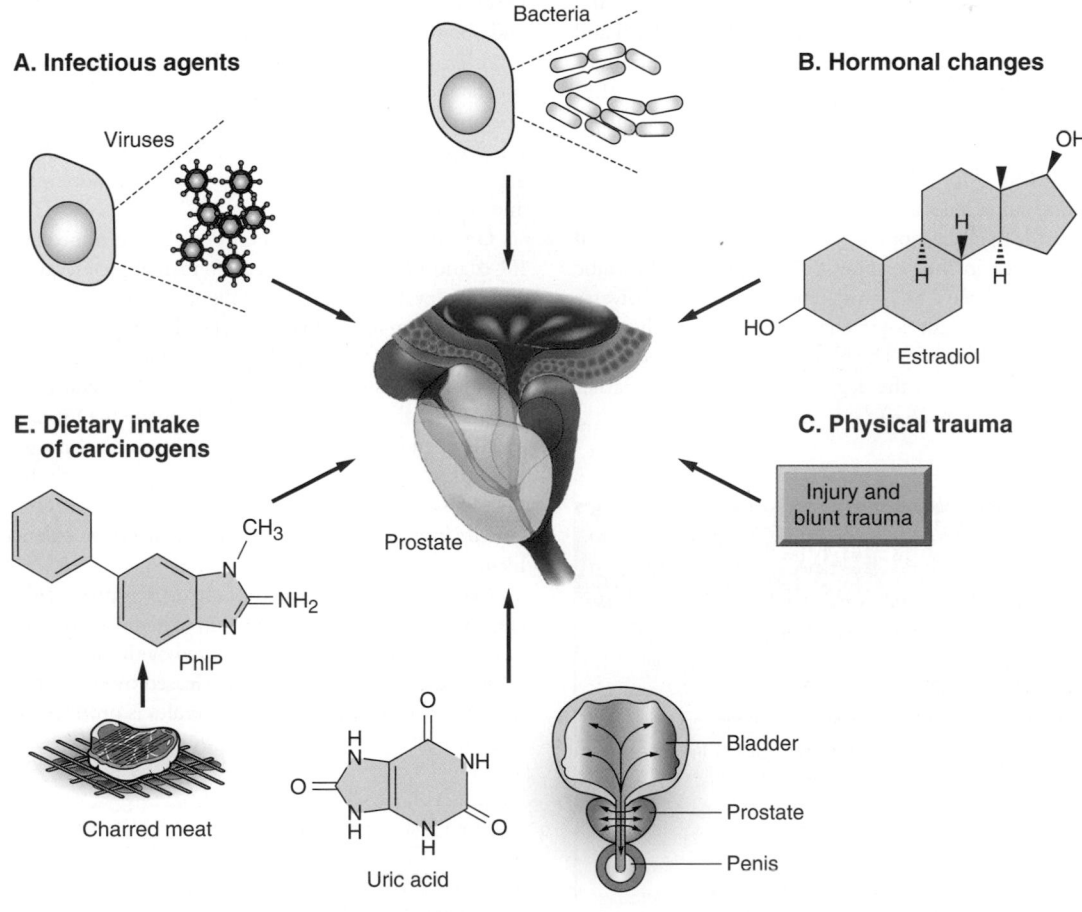

FIGURE 26.16 Possible Causes of Prostate Inflammation. **A,** Infection, including viruses, bacteria, fungi, and parasites. **B,** Hormones, for example, estrogen at key times during development. **C,** Physical trauma, any type of blunt physical injury. **D,** Urine reflux. **E,** Certain dietary factors (see text).

Genetic and Epigenetic Factors. Other possible causes are genetic predisposition (familial and hereditary forms). Genetic studies suggest that strong familial predisposition may be responsible for 5% to 10% of prostate cancers.[1] Compared with men with no family history, those with one first-degree relative with prostate cancer have twice the risk and those with two first-degree relatives have 5 times the risk.[99] Germline mutations in the breast cancer predisposition gene 2 *(BRCA2)* are the genetic events known to date that confer the highest risk of prostate cancer (8.6-fold in men ≤65 years). Although the role of *BRCA2* and *BRCA1* in prostate tumorigenesis remains unrevealed, deleterious mutations in both genes have been associated with more aggressive disease and poor clinical outcomes.[100] The strongest predictors are the *BRCA2* mutations and the highly penetrant G84E mutation in HOXB13.[101] Men with *BRCA2* germline mutations have a 20-fold increase in risk for prostate cancer.[102] Using previously estimated population carrier frequencies, investigators have recently found that deleterious *BRCA1* mutations confer a relative risk of prostate cancer of approximately 3.75-fold, translating to an 8.6% cumulative risk by age 65.[103] A common type of somatic mutation that gives rise to chromosomal rearrangements is the *ETS* gene. The most common epigenetic alteration in prostate cancer is hypermethylation of the glutathione *S*-transferase *(GST-P1)* gene. This gene is located on chromosome 11 and is part of the pathway that helps protect against carcinogen damage. More than 30 independent peer-reviewed studies have reported a consistently high sensitivity and specificity of *GST-P1* hypermethylation in prostatectomy or biopsy tissue.[104] A number of other epigenetic modifications found on tumor-suppressor genes include *PTEN, RB, p16/INK4α, MLH1, MSH21,* and *APC.*[105,106] There is no clear evidence of a causal link between BPH and prostate cancer even though they may often occur together. Variations in several other genes related to inflammatory pathways might affect the probability of developing prostate cancer. The presence of multiple risk alleles is more highly predictive than a single allele.[102,107]

◆**PATHOPHYSIOLOGY.** More than 95% of prostatic neoplasms are histologically similar to adenocarcinomas and rely on androgen-dependent signaling for their development and progression.[108-110] Most of these neoplasms occur in the periphery of the prostate. Prostatic adenocarcinoma is a heterogeneous group of tumors with a diverse spectrum of molecular and pathologic characteristics, and therefore clinical behaviors and challenges.[111] The biologic aggressiveness of the neoplasm appears to be related to the degree of differentiation rather than the size of the tumor (Box 26.6).

Hormonal Levels. Just as the testicles are the male equivalent of the female ovaries, the prostate is the male equivalent of the female uterus; in both situations, they originate from the same embryonic cells. This may be important in understanding the role of the associated hormones testosterone (T), DHT, and estrogens in prostate carcinogenesis. Testicular testosterone synthesis and serum testosterone levels usually fall as men age, however, the levels of estradiol do not decline.[112] The relationship between hormones and the pathophysiology of prostate carcinogenesis is incomplete and controversial. The main issues and controversies include (1) the sources of androgen production outside of the testes, or extratesticular sources (e.g., from adrenal DHEA and from prostate cholesterol [de novo], itself); (2) the role of prostatic androgen receptor (AR); (3) the role of estrogens (e.g., genotoxicity), aromatase enzyme, and the estrogen receptors (ERs) ER-α and ER-β; and (4) the role of the surrounding microenvironment or stroma.

The hormone concentrations in prostate tissue are important, and there is little evidence that circulating hormone levels are associated with future risk of prostate cancer.[81,113,114] Testicular testosterone provides the main source of androgens in the prostate (see Fig. 26.15) and is the major circulating androgen, whereas DHT predominates in prostate tissue and binds to the AR with greater affinity than does T.[115,116] The adrenal cortex contributes the far less potent DHEA that promotes synthesis of androgens in the prostate. In the target tissues and, to a lesser extent, in the testes themselves, testosterone is converted to DHT by the enzyme 5α-reductase (Fig. 26.17). Thus DHT is the most potent intraprostatic androgen. About half of circulating testosterone is bound to sex hormone–binding globulin (SHBG), about half binds to albumin, and about 1% to 2% exists in a free state. Free testosterone, including testosterone disassociated from albumin and possibly SHBG, enters the prostate cell, where it is converted to DHT.[115,116] DHT is a paracrine hormone because it affects the local environment or stroma. Several intraprostatic enzymes encoded by genes, *HSD3A* and *HDS3B,* are activated by DHT and are important components of intraprostatic androgen regulation.

One mechanistic effect of estrogen is determined by the two receptors ER-α and ER-β. ER-α leads to abnormal proliferation, inflammation, and the development of premalignant lesions. Increased expression of ER-α has been found to be associated with prostate cancer progression, metastasis, and the so-called castration-resistant (medical treatment that suppresses androgens) phenotype.[117] A specific oncogene is regulated by ERs, and those hormones that stimulate the ER-α receptor–like (i.e., agonists) endogenous estrogens can stimulate oncogene expression.[118] In contrast, ER-β leads to antiproliferative and antiinflammatory effects, differentiation and maturation of prostatic epithelial cells, and potentially anticarcinogenic effects that act in concert or balance the actions of ER-α and androgens.[115,119]

Normally a small amount of estrogen is produced per day—estrone and estradiol—by the aromatization of androstenedione and testosterone, respectively. This reaction is catalyzed by the aromatase enzyme system. A small quantity of estradiol is released by the testes (see Fig. 26.17); the remainder of the estrogens in males is produced by adipose tissue,

---

BOX 26.6	**DETERMINING THE GRADE OF PROSTATE CANCER WITH THE GLEASON SCORE**

Grade 1: The cancer cells closely resemble normal cells. They are small, uniformly shaped, evenly spaced, and well differentiated (i.e., they remain separate from one another).

Grade 2: The cancer cells are still well differentiated, but they are arranged more loosely and are irregular in shape and size. Some of the cancer cells have invaded the neighboring prostate tissue.

Grade 3: This is the most common grade. The cells are less well differentiated (some have fused into clumps) and are more variable in shape.

Grade 4: The cells are poorly differentiated and highly irregular in shape. Invasion of the neighboring prostate tissue has progressed further.

Grade 5: The cells are undifferentiated. They have merged into large masses that no longer resemble normal prostate cells. Invasion of the surrounding tissue is extensive.

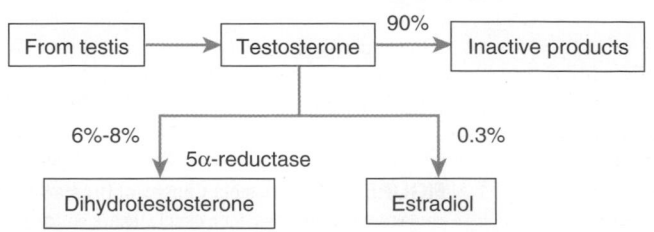

FIGURE 26.17 Testosterone and Conversion to Dihydrotestosterone (DHT).

liver, skin, brain, and other nonendocrine tissue. Thus testosterone is a precursor of the two hormones DHT and estradiol.

Studies show aromatase is expressed in stromal tissue in the benign human prostate gland. Thus it appears that both normal prostate and benign prostate have the capacity to locally metabolize androgens to estrogens through aromatase. Investigators have demonstrated altered aromatase expression in prostate cancer[120,121] (see Fig. 26.15, B). Data, mostly from animal studies, suggest that for androgens to cause prostate cancer they must be aromatized to estrogen and act in concert with these estrogen metabolites. The androgen receptor–mediated activity of androgens and the estrogen receptor–mediated effects of estrogen metabolites are likely to be necessary, but estrogen genotoxicity appears to be a probable critical factor as well. Prostate carcinogenesis can occur only when all these mechanisms are active.[81]

The effects of progesterone are underinvestigated. Stromal progesterone/PR signaling may play a role in prostate cancer development and progression.[122]

Chronic exposure to arsenic, as well as estrogen, is a known risk factor for prostate cancer. Though the evidence suggests that exposure to arsenic or estrogens can disrupt normal DNA methylation patterns and histone modifications, the mechanisms by which these chemicals induce epigenetic changes are not fully understood. Moreover, the epigenetic effects of coexposure to these two chemicals are not well-known. Investigators have revealed that exposure to arsenic, estrogen, and their combination alters the expression of epigenetic regulatory genes and changes global DNA methylation and histone modification patterns.[123]

Most of the androgen-metabolizing enzymes undergo a significant age-dependent alteration. In epithelium, both the 5α-reductase activity and the DHT level decrease with age, whereas in stroma (prostate) not only the 5α-reductase activity but also the stromal DHT level is rather constant over the lifetime. In contrast to the relatively unaltered DHT level over time, the estrogen concentration follows an age-dependent increase. Thus the age-dependent decrease of the DHT accumulation in epithelium and the concomitant increase of the estrogen accumulation in stroma lead to a tremendous increase with age of the estrogen/androgen ratio in the human prostate. In animal studies, chronic exposure to testosterone plus estradiol is strongly carcinogenic, whereas testosterone alone is weakly carcinogenic.[80,81] In mice studies elevated testosterone level in the absence of estrogen leads to the development of hypertrophy and hyperplasia but not malignancy. High estrogen and low testosterone levels have been shown to lead to inflammation with aging and the emergence of precancerous lesions.[120] The mechanism is not clearly understood and may involve estrogen-generated oxidative stress and DNA toxicity, and it requires androgen-mediated and estrogen receptor–mediated processes, such as changes in sex steroid metabolism and receptor status.[80] In addition, there are changes in the balance between autocrine/paracrine growth-stimulatory and growth-inhibitory factors, such as the insulin-like growth factors (IGFs).[124] When exogenous estradiol is added to testosterone treatment of rats, prostate cancer incidence is markedly increased, and even a short course of estrogen treatment results in a high incidence of prostate cancer.[80]

Androgen Receptor Signaling. The androgenic hormone responses in the normal prostate and in prostate cancer are mediated by AR signaling. Exactly how AR drives the growth of prostate cancer cells is not fully known. Several mechanisms have been suggested,[125,126] and specific pathways of signaling are important because they can provide novel therapeutic targets. A study using animal models found that loss of androgen receptor function prevented prostatic carcinogenesis, malignant transformation, and metastasis. Tissue-specific evaluation of androgen hormone action demonstrated that epithelial androgen receptor was not necessary for prostate cancer progression, whereas stromal androgen receptor was essential for prostate cancer progression, malignant transformation, and metastasis.[127-130]

Changes in AR signaling in the surrounding stroma can significantly affect tumor cell behavior.[131] Emerging is the mechanism of AR function in prostate stroma. In the benign prostate, the chief stromal cells are smooth muscle cells and a majority express AR. In tumor stroma, the chief stromal cells are myofibroblasts.[131] Recent work involves the identification of AR signaling in fibroblasts/myofibroblasts in prostate stroma.[131] Key is the role of mesenchymal hormone signaling in the development of both male and female reproductive organs, with expression of the appropriate hormone receptors in adjacent stroma necessary for organ-specific responses to estrogen, progesterone, and testosterone.[132-134] Stromal AR activity has been investigated in animal models in early-stage cancer and AR signaling in tumor formation. Evidence supports stromal AR signaling to induce prostate cancer cell proliferation and the possibility of this signaling in early prostate carcinogenesis.[131] Importantly, studies are ongoing to define the events (genetic, epigenetic, paracrine factors) and the potential role of loss or decreased stromal AR (lost stromal AR signaling is related to cancer progression) in cancer progression and metastases (Fig. 26.18).

AR signaling in fibroblasts regulates growth factors, chemoattractants (inflammatory mediators), cytokines, and extracellular matrix (ECM) production.[131] AR regulates growth factors creating a favorable environment for cancer, and with loss of AR the local environment may drive cancer cells to metastasize elsewhere. One hypothesis is that by regulating cytokine production, AR signaling in fibroblasts influences immune responses that affect tumor cells. The declining mesenchymal AR signaling and decreased local availability of paracrine mediators could result in dedifferentiation or epithelial-mesenchymal transition (EMT), or both, and a less hospitable environment for epithelial cells driving pathways

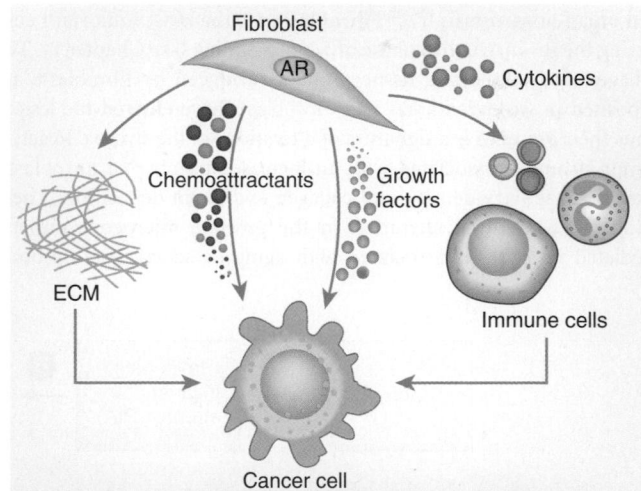

FIGURE 26.18 Working Model Mechanism for Fibroblast Androgen Receptor (AR) on Prostate Cancer Outcomes. AR signaling in stromal fibroblasts regulates growth factors, chemoattractants, cytokines, and extracellular matrix (ECM) production. The regulation of growth factors by AR creates a favorable environment for cancer, and the loss of AR is hypothesized to drive cancer cells to metastasize elsewhere. Disruption of chemoattractant production regulated by AR may induce the migratory capacity of cancer cells. AR signaling in fibroblasts and regulation of cytokine production may influence immune responses that have important effects on tumor cells. AR signaling in fibroblasts regulates production of ECM, and with loss of AR it is hypothesized that ECM becomes dysregulated, enhancing the migratory potential of cancer cells. (Data and illustration adapted from Leach DA, Buchanan G: *Cancers [Basel]* 9[1], 2017.)

for cell mobility and metastases.[131] The emerging significance of tumor stroma is shaping the understanding of prostate development, cancer, and metastases.

Prostate Epithelial Neoplasia. A precursor lesion, prostatic epithelial neoplasia (PIN), has been described. PIN may be more concentrated in prostates containing cancer and is noted in proximity to cancer.[105] However, the final fate of PIN is unknown, including the possibilities of latency, invasion, and even regression. The current working model of prostate carcinogenesis suggests that repeated cycles of injury and cell death occur to the prostate epithelium as a result of damage (e.g., from oxidative stress) from inflammatory responses.[135] There is growing evidence that chronic inflammation is involved in the regulation of cellular events in prostate carcinogenesis, including disruption of the immune response and regulation of the tumor microenvironment.[136] The direct injury is hypothesized as a response to infections; autoimmune disease; circulating carcinogens or toxins, or both, from the diet; or urine that has refluxed into the prostate (see Fig. 26.16). The resultant manifestation of this injury is focal atrophy or prostatic intraepithelial atrophy (PIA). Biologic responses cause an increase in proliferation and a massive increase in the number of epithelial cells that possess a phenotype intermediate between basal cells and mature luminal cells (Fig. 26.19).[135,136] In a small subset of cells, some may contain "stem cell" or tumor-initiating properties and telomere shortening (see Chapter 12). A subset of PIN cells may activate telomerase enzyme, causing the cells to become immortal.[137] Molecular, genetic, and epigenetic changes can increase genetic instability that might progress to high-grade PIN and early prostate cancer formation. This model of prostate carcinogenesis needs much more research.

Stromal Environment. The prostate gland is composed of secretory luminal epithelium, basal epithelium, neuroendocrine cells, and various cell types comprising supportive tissue or stroma. Stroma, or tissue microenvironment, produces autocrine/paracrine factors, as well as structural supporting molecules that help regulate normal cell behavior and organ homeostasis.[138,139] Fibroblasts are the most important cells during the reconstructive phase of wound healing (see Chapter 7). The collagen and connective tissue proteins produced by fibroblasts are deposited in wounded areas after fibroblasts have entered the lesion. Thus their presence is a signature of alterations in the stroma. Reactive tumor stroma is associated with an increased number of fibroblasts, increased capillary density, and collagen and fibrin deposition. These findings suggest that alteration in the prostate microenvironment, mediated by changes associated with aging or senescence, or both,

promote epithelial responses that contribute to diseases. In animal studies, investigators have noted that the microenvironment has an increased number of cells that promote inflammation and a collapsed appearance of the smooth muscle cells within adjacent glandular stroma.[138,139] Fibroblast spreading has been proposed as indicative of decreased mechanical tension because of a lack of direct association of the fibroblasts with aged fragmented collagen fibrils.[140,141] These alterations in mechanical tension and cell shape are suggested as determinants in altering gene expression and cellular function. These alterations in aged prostate stroma for mice and men include significant enhancement for inflammation pathways (e.g., NF-κβ, collagens).[140,141] Inflammation can induce cell stress, and stressed mesenchymal cells can secrete inflammatory mediators (chemoattractants); however, it remains to be determined whether inflammatory infiltrates are a cause of or response to the alterations of aged stroma.[142] Evidence supports that inflammation has a role in the pathogenesis of prostate cancer.[135,136,143] Investigators have found that disruption of fibroblast growth factor signaling pathways leads to strongly activated and atypical stroma that preceded the development of mice PIN (mPIN).

Epithelial-mesenchymal transition (EMT) was first described in embryonic development, and is observed in a number of solid tumors[144,145] (also see Chapter 12). Cells that undergo EMT become more migratory and invasive and gain access to vascular vessels.[146] Numerous studies have shown that these transition states (EMT and mesenchymal-epithelial transition [MET]) are a consequence of tumor-stroma interactions.[146-148]

Investigators studying prostate cancer cells in vitro correlated EMT with increased growth, migration, and invasion. These investigators demonstrated that the microenvironment is a critical site for the transition of human prostate cancer cells from epithelial to mesenchymal structure, resulting in increased metastatic potential for bone and the adrenal gland.[149]

Prostate cancer is known to be diverse and composed of multiple genetically distinct cancer cell clones. Studies, however, indicate that most metastatic cancers arise from a single precursor cancer cell.[150] Various research models have been proposed to understand EMT (MET) and invasion and metastasis.[151]

In summary, the following multifactorial general hypothesis of prostate carcinogenesis emerges from all of these observations: (1) androgens act as strong tumor promoters through androgen receptor–mediated mechanisms to enhance the carcinogenic activity of strong endogenous DNA toxic carcinogens, including reactive estrogen metabolites and estrogen, and prostate-generated reactive oxygen species; (2) alterations

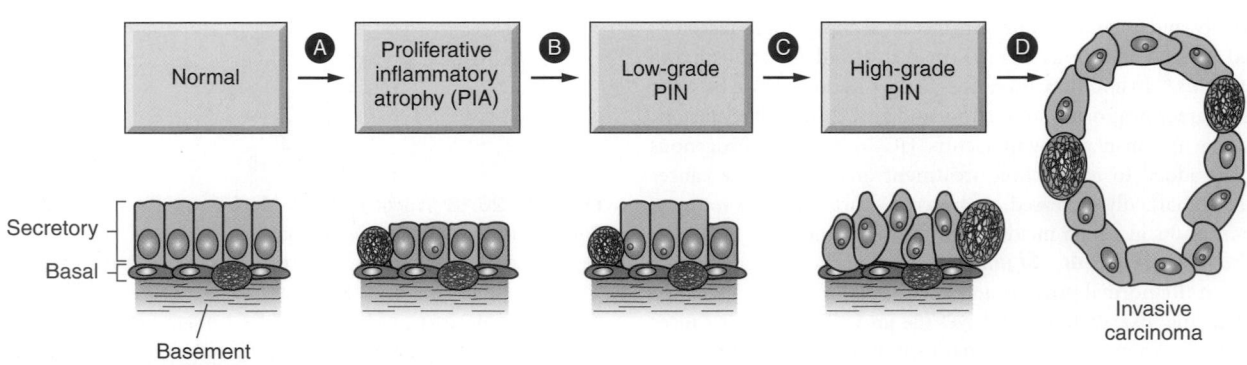

FIGURE 26.19 Cellular and Molecular Model of Early Prostate Neoplasia Progression. **A,** This stage includes infiltration of lymphocytes, macrophages, and neutrophils caused by repeated infections, dietary factors, urine reflux, injury, onset of autoimmunity (which triggers inflammation), and wound healing. **B,** Epigenetic alterations mediate telomere shortening. **C,** Genetic instability and accumulation of genetic alterations. **D,** Continued proliferation of genetically unstable cells leading to cancer progression. *PIN,* Prostatic intraepithelial neoplasia.

in autocrine/paracrine growth-stimulating and growth-inhibiting factors between the prostate tumor cells and microenvironment influence cancer pathogenesis; and (3) possibly unknown environmental-lifestyle carcinogens may contribute to prostate cancer. All of these factors are modulated by diet and genetic determinants, such as hereditary susceptibility genes and polymorphic genes, which encode receptors and enzymes involved in the metabolism and action of steroid hormones.[80]

The most common sites of distant metastasis are the lymph nodes, bones, lungs, liver, and adrenals. The pelvis, lumbar spine, femur, thoracic spine, and ribs are the most common sites of bone metastasis. Local extension is usually posterior, although late in the disease the tumor may invade the rectum or encroach on the prostatic urethra and cause bladder outlet obstruction (Fig. 26.20). The spread of cancer through blood vessels is illustrated in Fig. 26.21.

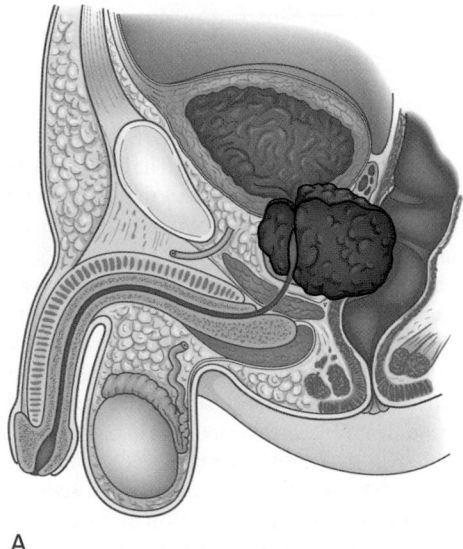

A

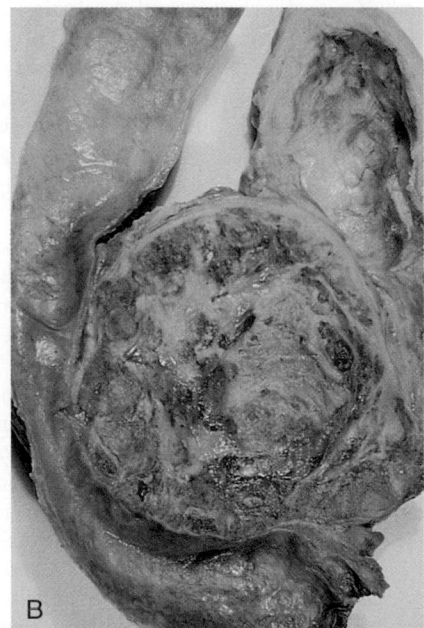

B

FIGURE 26.20 Carcinoma of the Prostate. **A,** Schematic of carcinoma of the prostate. **B,** Carcinoma of the prostate extending into the rectum and urinary bladder. (**B** From Damjanov I, Linder J, editors: *Pathology: a color atlas,* St Louis, 2000, Mosby.)

◆**CLINICAL MANIFESTATIONS.** Prostatic cancer often causes no symptoms until it is far advanced. The first manifestations of disease are those of bladder outlet obstruction: slow urinary stream, hesitancy, incomplete emptying, frequency, nocturia, and dysuria. Unlike the symptoms of obstruction caused by BPH, the symptoms of obstruction caused by prostatic cancer are progressive and do not remit. Local extension of prostatic cancer can obstruct the upper urinary tract ureters as well. If rectal obstruction occurs, a man may experience a large-bowel obstruction or difficulty in defecation. Symptoms of late disease include bone pain at sites of bone metastasis, edema of the lower extremities, enlargement of lymph nodes, enlargement of the liver, development of pathologic bone fractures, and mental confusion associated with brain metastases.

◆**EVALUATION AND TREATMENT.** Screening for prostatic cancer includes DRE, PSA blood tests, and TRUS. The most significant test used in the diagnosis and management of prostate cancer is measurement of the level of **prostate-specific antigen (PSA)**. DRE may detect early prostatic carcinomas but it has low sensitivity and specificity.[105] Cancer diagnosis is confirmed through tissue biopsy and microscopic examination of tissue. Lymphography, bone scans, MRI, and CT scans also may be used to determine metastasis to lymph, bone, or other adjacent tissue. Important for treatment is to accurately measure the size of the index (longest) tumor and its percentage Gleason grade of differentiation.[152,153]

PSA screening for prostate cancer has led to considerable controversy. A review of the evidence from the 2012 U.S. Preventive Services Task Force (USPSTF) regarding screening for prostate cancer concluded that PSA-based screening results in small or no reduction in prostate cancer–specific mortality and is associated with harmful consequences related to subsequent evaluation and treatments, some of which may be unnecessary. However, additional evidence published since the 2012 recommendation statement suggests increased confidence in the benefits of screening: slightly more than 1 man per 1000 who is offered screening may avoid death from prostate cancer.[154] There also is new evidence that 3 men per 1000 offered screening may avoid metastatic disease.[155] The USPSTF assigned a grade of D (recommending against screening) for men aged ≥75 years in 2008 and for men of all ages in 2012; however, USPSTF *draft* recommendations in 2017 recommend against PSA-based screening for prostate cancer only in men age 70 years and older. Furthermore, the 2017 USPSTF draft recommendations now suggest that clinicians inform men ages 55 to 69 years about the potential benefits and detriments of PSA–based screening for prostate cancer;

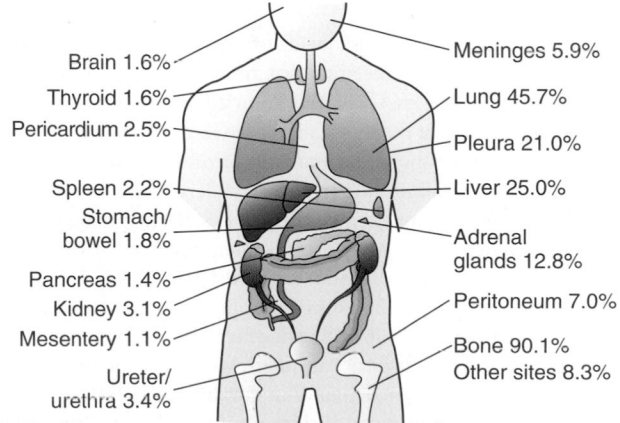

Brain 1.6%
Thyroid 1.6%
Pericardium 2.5%
Spleen 2.2%
Stomach/bowel 1.8%
Pancreas 1.4%
Kidney 3.1%
Mesentery 1.1%
Ureter/urethra 3.4%

Meninges 5.9%
Lung 45.7%
Pleura 21.0%
Liver 25.0%
Adrenal glands 12.8%
Peritoneum 7.0%
Bone 90.1%
Other sites 8.3%

FIGURE 26.21 Distribution of Hematogenous Metastases in Prostate Cancer. Study of 556 individuals with metastatic prostate cancer. (Adapted from Budendorf L et al: *Hum Pathol* 31:578, 2000.)

thus making the decision about whether to be screened for prostate cancer is an individual choice for each man. Choosing to screen (or not to screen) should be based on each man's values and preferences after an informed discussion with his clinician.[156] This approach may be particularly important for men who have had immediate family members diagnosed with prostate cancer. Nonetheless, convincing evidence used to formulate the 2012 U.S. Preventive Services Task Force guidelines demonstrated that the PSA test unfortunately often produces false-positive results. Men who have a false-positive test are more likely to have additional testing, including one or more biopsies. Over a 10-year span, approximately 15% to 20% of men will have a PSA test result that triggers a biopsy, depending on the PSA threshold and testing interval used.[67] In addition, because PSA level is organ specific and not cancer specific, its measurement can increase and overlap with BPH, prostatitis, infarct, manipulation from instrumentation, and ejaculation.[105] Since the 2012 recommendation, rates of PSA screening decreased by 3% to 10% in all age groups and across most geographical regions of the United States. Rates of prostate biopsy and prostate cancer incidence have declined in unison, with a shift towards tumors being of higher grade and stage upon detection (i.e., reduced incidence of detecting early-stage prostate cancer). The implications of this are being considered as more data are obtained.[157,158]

The annual rate by which PSA level rises is known as **PSA velocity** or doubling time (generally described as *PSA kinetics*). Its calculation has been judged to be far from straightforward. More than 20 different methods for calculation have been proposed, and many of these give divergent results. Evidence clearly shows that PSA kinetics are critical for understanding prognosis in advanced or relapsed prostate cancer. However, PSA kinetics have questionable value for men with an untreated prostate; neither PSA velocity nor doubling time has an established role in diagnosing prostate cancer or providing a prognosis for men before treatment.[159,160] In fact, investigators recently evaluated guidelines on the use of PSA velocity in prostate cancer detection and found that change in PSA levels over time is such a poor predictor of prostate cancer (in a previously untreated prostate) that it is highly likely many unnecessary biopsies have been performed.[161] It is thus somewhat doubtful at this juncture that PSA velocity adds any additional predictive accuracy to PSA level measurement alone or positive digital rectal examination, or both, for purposes of prostate cancer screening. For instance, a systematic review found that even when definitions are rigorously applied, PSA velocity calculation does not significantly enhance the clinical performance of PSA alone.[159] As such, it should be noted a recent study found that PSA levels in midlife strongly predict future lethal prostate cancer in a U.S. cohort subjected to opportunistic screening.[162]

Older age is the strongest risk factor for the development of prostate cancer. However, neither screening nor treatment trials show benefit in men older than 70 years. Given this knowledge, recent recommendations from a task force of the International Society of Geriatric Oncology suggest that older men should be managed according to their individual health status and not according to age. Fit elderly men should receive the same treatment as younger men on the basis of international recommendations.[163] Across age ranges, black men and men with a family history of prostate cancer have an increased risk of developing and dying of prostate cancer.[164] Black men are approximately twice as likely to die of prostate cancer compared with other men in the United States, and the reason for this disparity in unknown. Black men represent a very small minority of participants in randomized clinical trials of screening and, thus, no firm conclusions can be made about the balance of benefits and detriments of PSA-based screening in this population. As such, it is a questionable practice to selectively recommend PSA-based screening for black men in the absence of data that support a more

---

BOX 26.7   RETHINKING SCREENING FOR PROSTATE CANCER AND BREAST CANCER

In essence, it has become necessary to rethink screening for both prostate cancer and breast cancer because since screening was introduced the incidence of both prostate cancer and breast cancer increased and never returned to prescreening levels; in addition, the absolute number of advanced prostate and breast cancers diagnosed during this period has not decreased as predicted. Furthermore, whereas colon and cervical cancer screening detects precancerous treatable conditions, prostate and breast cancer screening detects so-called early cancers that may not be destined to grow or become lethal. Thus it is possible that prostate and breast cancer screening may be increasing the burden of low-risk cancers without any significant reduction of burden associated with aggressive lesions, thereby not resulting in the anticipated reduction in breast and prostate cancer mortality.

Data from Esserman L, Shieh Y, Thompson I: *J Am Med Assoc* 302(15):1685–1920, 2000.

---

favorable balance of risks and benefits.[67,156] The ability to predict cancer rises significantly when TRUS is added to the annual DRE and PSA testing. Researchers are studying microRNAs as potential new biomarkers for prostate cancer.

Prostate cancer is now detected in greater numbers of men at lower stages of disease and is amenable to multiple forms of efficacious treatment. However, there is a lack of conclusive data demonstrating a definitive mortality benefit from this earlier diagnosis and treatment of prostate cancer. This is likely because of the treatment of a large proportion of indolent cancers that would have had little adverse effect on health or life span if left untreated (Box 26.7).

Because of this "over-treatment" phenomenon, active surveillance with delayed intervention is gaining traction as a viable management approach in contemporary practice. The ability to distinguish clinically insignificant cancers from those with a high risk of progression or lethality, or both, is critical to the appropriate selection of surveillance protocols versus immediate intervention[165] (Box 26.8). Mounting evidence also suggests that intermittent PSA testing may decrease the costs and detriments of screening while preserving the benefits of annual testing.[166] The most important observation for pathologists to make to facilitate cure of any man with prostate cancer is that of accurately measuring the size of the index (longest) tumor and determining the Gleason score (degree of differentiation) (see Box 26.6).[167]

Treatment of prostatic cancer depends on the stage of the neoplasm (see Box 26.6); the anticipated effects of treatment; and the age, general health, and life expectancy of the individual. Options include (1) no treatment; (2) surgical treatments, such as total prostatectomy, transurethral resection of the prostate (TURP), and cryotherapy; (3) nonsurgical treatments, such as radiation therapy, hormone therapy, or chemotherapy; (4) watchful waiting; and (5) any combination of these.[67] In addition, new approaches are using immunotherapy. Palliative treatment is aimed at relieving urinary, bladder outlet, or colon obstruction; spinal cord compression; and pain. Prognosis and survival rates have improved steadily since the early 1960s. According to the most recent data, 10- and 15-year relative survival rates are 98% and 95%, respectively.[1] A study examining 10-year outcomes after monitoring, surgery, or radiotherapy for localized prostate cancer found that at a median of 10 years, prostate cancer–specific mortality was low regardless of the treatment assigned, with no significant difference among treatments. Surgery and radiotherapy were associated with lower incidences of disease progression and metastases than was active monitoring.[168]

BOX 26.8   PROSTATE SPECIFIC ANTIGEN-BASED SCREENING FOR PROSTATE CANCER*

Why not screen for prostate cancer?

Screening may benefit a small number of men but will result in harm to many others. A person choosing to be screened should believe that the possibility of benefit is more important than the risk for harm. The U.S. Preventive Services Task Force assessment of the balance of benefits and harms in a screened population is that the benefits do not outweigh the harms.

What are the benefits and harms of screening 1000 men ages 55 to 69 years[†] with a prostate-specific antigen (PSA) test every 1 to 4 years for 10 years?

Possible Benefits of Screening:	Men, >*n*
Reduced 10-year risk for dying of prostate cancer:	
Die of prostate cancer with no screening	5 in 1000
Die of prostate cancer with screening	4–5 in 1000
Do not die of prostate cancer because of screening	0–1 in 1000

Harms of Screening:	
At least one false-positive screening PSA test result:	
Most positive test results lead to biopsy. Of men having biopsy, up to 33% will have moderate or major bothersome symptoms, including pain, fever, bleeding, infection, and temporary urinary difficulties; 1% will be hospitalized.	100–120 in 1000
Prostate cancer diagnosis:	
Although a diagnosis of prostate cancer may not be considered a harm, currently 90% of diagnosed men are treated and thus are at risk for the harms of treatment. A large majority of the men who are being treated would do well without treatment. A substantial percentage of these men would have remained asymptomatic for life.	110 in 1000
Complications of treatment (among persons who are screened)[‡]:	
Develop serious cardiovascular events because of treatment	2 in 1000
Develop deep venous thrombosis or pulmonary embolus because of treatment	1 in 1000
Develop erectile dysfunction because of treatment	29 in 1000
Develop urinary incontinence because of treatment	18 in 1000
Die because of treatment	<1 in 1000

*Calculations of the estimated benefits and harms rely on assumption and are, by nature, somewhat imprecise. Estimates should be considered in the full context of clinical decision making and used to stimulate shared decision making.
[†]The best evidence of possible benefit of PSA screening is in men ages 55 to 69 years.
[‡]The rate of complications depends on the proportion of men having treatment and the method of treatment. The preceding data reflect a distribution of 60% surgical treatment, 30% radiation treatment, and 10% observation. Other harms of radiation, such as bowel damage, are not shown.
Data from Moyer VA, U.S. Preventive Services Task Force: *Ann Intern Med* 157(2):120–124, 2012; also see Esserman L, Shieh Y, Thompson I: *J Am Med Assoc* 302(15):1685–1910, 2009, for further reading on this matter. A brief summary of the thinking of Esserman and colleagues is provided in the Prostate Cancer Evaluation and Treatment section.

Treatment for prostate cancer may lead to loss of urinary control, which may or may not return to normal after several weeks or months. Stress incontinence can occur after surgery, and mild urge incontinence can occur after radiation therapy. Prostate cancer and its treatment can affect sexual functioning. Sensation of orgasm is not usually affected, but smaller amounts of ejaculate will be produced or men may experience a "dry" ejaculate because of retrograde ejaculation.

Sexual Dysfunction

In men the normal sexual response involves three processes: erection, emission, and ejaculation. Sexual dysfunction is the impairment of any or all of these processes. Impairment can be caused by a number of physiologic and psychologic factors.

Until the late 1970s, most cases of male sexual dysfunction were thought to be psychogenic. Studies of this problem indicate that in men older than 40 years, organic factors are involved in more than 50% of cases. The causes of organic sexual dysfunction include (1) vascular, endocrine, and neurologic disorders; (2) chronic disease, including renal failure and diabetes mellitus; (3) penile diseases and penile trauma; and (4) iatrogenic factors, such as surgery and pharmacologic therapies. Most of these disorders cause erectile dysfunction.

◆**PATHOPHYSIOLOGY AND CLINICAL MANIFESTATIONS.** Vascular disorders can prevent erection. Some arterial diseases diminish or interrupt circulation to the penis. This prevents engorgement of erectile tissues in the corpora cavernosa and corpus spongiosum. Rarely, excessive venous drainage of the corpora cavernosa prevents erection.

Endocrine disorders that reduce testosterone production affect sexual function and libido. The reduction may be caused by inadequate secretion of the gonadotropins caused by pituitary dysfunction or hyperprolactinemia. Feminizing tumors and estrogen therapy reduce relative levels of testosterone. Testicular atrophy from any cause also decreases testosterone levels and contributes to sexual dysfunction.

Neurologic disorders can interfere with the important sympathetic, parasympathetic, and CNS mechanisms required for erection, emission, and ejaculation. They include spinal cord injury or tumor, multiple sclerosis, and disorders that cause peripheral neuropathies, such as diabetes mellitus and chronic renal failure. Spinal cord injuries or tumors can alter one or more components of the sexual response, depending on the location of the lesion. For example, in most men with upper motor neuron lesions, reflexogenic erection is possible, but emission and ejaculation (i.e., orgasm) are not possible. Lesions affecting the lower motor neurons usually prevent erection. In approximately 40% of such cases, emission and ejaculation are prevented.

Many chronic diseases are associated with sexual dysfunction. In some conditions the sexual dysfunction has a specific physiologic cause. Diabetes mellitus, for example, causes peripheral vascular and neurologic pathology that can lead to erectile dysfunction. Impotence occurs in about 50% of men undergoing dialysis because of decreased testosterone levels, autonomic neuropathy, accelerated vascular disease, multiple medications, worsening of primary disease, and psychologic stress. Potency may be restored by successful renal transplantation, except in bilateral transplantation if arterial flow is diminished or interrupted. Cirrhosis of the liver, scleroderma, chronic debilitation, and cachexia also are known to cause impotence. Emotional and psychologic response to chronic illness, such as anxiety, depression, and loss of self-esteem, can affect sexual functioning. In other chronic conditions, sexual dysfunction is associated with low energy levels and loss of libido. The pathophysiologic mechanisms responsible for such changes are not known.

Priapism causes fibrosis of trabeculae (erectile tissues) within the corpora cavernosa, making erection difficult. The penile curvature caused by Peyronie disease does not make erection impossible but may make it extremely painful and intercourse impossible. Penile trauma can damage the erectile tissue, disrupt the posterior urethra, and disrupt the pudendal arteries or nerves.

Iatrogenic factors, including drugs and surgery, have a significant effect on erectile function. The following surgical procedures carry the risk of erectile dysfunction: radical pelvic surgery; radical prostatectomy; transurethral, suprapubic, or simple retropubic prostatectomy; and aortoiliac surgery. Erectile dysfunction is caused by the severing of small nerve branches that are essential for erection. Aortoiliac surgery, retroperitoneal lymphadenectomy, and sympathectomy cause the loss of ejaculation capacity in some individuals.

A few pharmacologic agents enhance the sexual response, but most have the opposite effect. Men who are taking antihypertensives, antidepressants, antihistamines, antispasmodics, sedatives or tranquilizers, barbiturates, diuretics, sex hormone preparations, narcotics, or psychoactive drugs may experience some degree of sexual dysfunction. Drug-induced sexual dysfunction consists of decreased desire, decreased erectile ability, or decreased ejaculatory ability. Ethyl alcohol may induce alcoholic neuropathy or increased levels of estrogens because of hepatic dysfunction; marijuana depresses testosterone levels; and cigarette smoking contributes to vasoconstriction and venous leakage. A number of pharmacologic agents also diminish the quality or quantity of sperm. A few may cause priapism. Drugs can assist in maintaining an erection.

◆**EVALUATION AND TREATMENT.** Evaluation of sexual dysfunction includes a physical examination, with particular attention to the genitalia, prostate, and nervous system, and basic laboratory tests to identify the presence of endocrinopathies or other underlying disorders that can cause the dysfunction. If no physiologic cause is found and the condition does not improve with psychotherapy, the man is referred for further investigation of organic causes. Psychologic evaluation is indicated for younger men with a sudden onset of sexual dysfunction or men of any age who are able to achieve but not maintain an erection.

Sophisticated diagnostic techniques can be used to assess penile blood flow, erectile tissue anatomy, nervous system function, and occurrence of erection or emission during sleep (nocturnal emission). Penile blood flow is measured by Doppler techniques and penile arteriography. Corpus cavernosography, in which contrast material is injected into the corpora cavernosa, provides anatomic information about the erectile tissue of the penis. Neuropathic causes of sexual dysfunction are evaluated by measuring the speed of the bulbocavernosus reflex. Nocturnal penile tumescence monitoring measures the frequency of nocturnal erections. Depending on the equipment used, this information may be correlated to rapid eye movement (REM) or non-REM sleep.

Treatments for organic sexual dysfunction include medical and surgical interventions. Nonsurgical interventions include correction of underlying disorders, particularly drug-induced dysfunction and endocrinopathy-related (e.g., reduced testosterone level associated with

chronic renal failure) dysfunction. Use of vasodilators and cessation of smoking can benefit individuals with vasculogenic erectile dysfunction. Surgical interventions include penile implants, penile revascularization, and correction of other anatomic defects contributing to sexual dysfunction.

Impairment of Sperm Production and Quality

Spermatogenesis requires adequate secretion of FSH and LH by the pituitary; sufficient secretion of testosterone by the Leydig cells; sufficient function of the Sertoli cells, including secretion of androgen-binding protein, growth factors, inhibin B, and a number of other important (but poorly understood) peptides; and adequate spermatogonia.[38,169] The Leydig cells are located in the testicular interstitium *between* the tubules, and the Sertoli cells and spermatogonia are located *within* the seminiferous tubules. The Sertoli cells extend from the basement membrane to the lumen, display tight junctions between adjacent cells, and form the blood-testis barrier. Inadequate secretion of gonadotropins may be caused by hypothyroidism, hyperadrenocortisolism, hyperprolactinemia, or hypogonadotropic hypogonadism. In these situations, gonadotropin levels are low because of feedback inhibition or idiopathic hyposecretion. In the absence of adequate gonadotropin levels, the Leydig cells are not stimulated to secrete testosterone and sperm maturation is not promoted in the Sertoli cells. Spermatogenesis depends not only on appropriate stimulation by the gonadotropins but also on an appropriate response by the testes. Defects in testicular response to the gonadotropins result in decreased secretion of testosterone and inhibin B and, as a result of normal feedback mechanisms, high levels of circulating gonadotropins. In the absence of adequate testosterone levels, spermatogenesis is impaired. Newer research demonstrates the significance of inhibin B as an important marker of the competence of Sertoli cells and spermatogenesis. Inhibin B is strongly correlated with the severity of spermatogenic effects. A positive correlation exists between serum inhibin B levels and sperm concentration and testicular volume, and lower levels have been associated with azoospermia, testicular disorders, and infertility.[169]

Impaired spermatogenesis also can be caused by genetic disorders (such as Klinefelter syndrome), myotonic dystrophy, or testicular trauma. Other conditions associated with impaired spermatogenesis include systemic illness, such as renal failure, hepatic disease, or sickle cell disease; exposure to gonadotoxins, such as chemotherapy or radiation; varicocele; and cryptorchidism.

Fertility is adversely affected if spermatogenesis is normal but the sperm are chromosomally or morphologically abnormal or are produced in insufficient quantities. Chromosomal abnormalities are caused by genetic factors and by external variables, such as exposure to radiation or toxic substances. Ongoing research using small ribonucleic acids (RNAs) is elucidating the molecular mechanisms regulating spermatogenesis.[170] A sperm count of 20 million sperm per milliliter of semen has been suggested as the minimum concentration required for fertility. Average fertile men have 50 to 100 million sperm per milliliter.[38]

Sperm motility is another important variable affecting fertility. Motility appears to be affected by the sperm's chemical environment, that is, the characteristics of semen. Prostatic dysfunction, excessive semen viscosity, presence of drugs or toxins in the semen, and presence of anti–sperm antibodies are associated with impaired sperm motility. Approximately 3% to 7% of infertile males have anti–sperm antibodies in their semen. Anti–sperm antibodies may develop as a result of epididymitis or other inflammation of the genitourinary tract, testicular injury or torsion, a previous vasectomy or biopsy, and cryptorchidism. Anti–sperm antibodies may be (1) cytotoxic antibodies, which attack sperm and reduce their number in the semen; or (2) sperm-immobilizing antibodies, which impair sperm motility and reduce their ability to

---

BOX 26.9 EVALUATION OF MALE PARTNER OF INFERTILE COUPLES

Thorough history and physical examination, including imaging for varicocele

Two semen analyses and quantification of serum FSH, LH, testosterone levels, and prolactin if indicated

Semen and urethral cultures

Serum assays or monoclonal antibody testing for white blood cells

Immunobead monoclonal antibody test

Postcoital testing of semen activity and function

Sperm penetration assay

Inhibin B assays or testicular biopsy

Vasogram, TRUS, or other imaging studies

FSH, Follicle-stimulating hormone; *LH*, luteinizing hormone; *TRUS*, transrectal ultrasonography.

traverse the endocervical canal. Intrinsic, biologic factors leading to the production of anti–sperm antibodies seem to play a greater role than extrinsic factors. The exact mechanism remains unclear.[38]

A male factor contributes to the cause of up to 50% of cases of infertility. As understanding of the male factor in infertility increases, evaluation becomes more complex and essential to appropriate treatment (Box 26.9). Treatment for impaired spermatogenesis involves correction of any underlying disorders and avoidance of radiation or toxins. Androgens, human gonadotropins, and antiestrogens (e.g., clomiphene citrate, tamoxifen citrate) may enhance spermatogenesis. Semen can be modified to improve sperm motility. If conception is desired, the semen is obtained by masturbation (or mechanical device),[38] after which it can be diluted, concentrated, or washed to remove anti–sperm antibodies. These alterations are followed by artificial insemination.

DISORDERS OF THE MALE BREAST

Gynecomastia

Gynecomastia is the overdevelopment of breast tissue in a male. Gynecomastia accounts for approximately 85% of all masses that develop in the male breast and affects 32% to 40% of the male population. If only one breast is involved, it is typically the left. Incidence is greatest among adolescents and men older than 50 years.

Gynecomastia results from hormonal alterations, which may be idiopathic or caused by systemic disorders, drugs, or neoplasms. It usually involves an imbalance of the estrogen/testosterone ratio, which can be altered in one of two ways. First, estrogen levels may be excessively high although testosterone levels are normal, as in drug-induced and tumor-induced cases of hyperestrogenism. Second, testosterone levels may be extremely low although estrogen levels are normal, as is the case in hypergonadism. Gynecomastia also can be caused by alterations in breast tissue responsiveness to hormonal stimulation. Breast tissue may have increased responsiveness to estrogen or decreased responsiveness to androgens. Alterations of responsiveness may cause many cases of idiopathic gynecomastia.

Besides puberty and aging, estrogen-testosterone imbalances are associated with hypogonadism, Klinefelter syndrome, and testicular neoplasms. Hormone-induced gynecomastia is usually bilateral. Pubertal gynecomastia is a self-limiting phenomenon that usually disappears within 4 to 6 months. Senescent gynecomastia usually regresses spontaneously within 6 to 12 months.

Systemic disorders associated with gynecomastia include obesity, cirrhosis of the liver, infectious hepatitis, chronic renal failure, chronic obstructive lung disease, hyperthyroidism, tuberculosis, and chronic malnutrition. It may be that these disorders ultimately alter the estrogen/testosterone ratio, initiating gynecomastia.

Gynecomastia is often seen in men receiving estrogen therapy, in preparation either for a sex-change operation or for prostatic carcinoma. Other drugs that can cause gynecomastia include digitalis, cimetidine, spironolactone, reserpine, thiazide, isoniazid, ergotamine, tricyclic antidepressants, amphetamines, vincristine, and busulfan. Recent data reveal that the use of 5α-reductase inhibitors for BPH increased the risk of gynecomastia.[171]

Malignancies of the testes, adrenals, or liver can cause gynecomastia if they alter the estrogen/testosterone ratio. Pituitary adenomas and lung cancer also are associated with gynecomastia.

◆ **PATHOPHYSIOLOGY.** The breast enlargement consists of hyperplastic stroma and ductal tissue. Hyperplasia results in a firm, palpable mass, at least 2 cm in diameter located beneath the areola.

◆ **EVALUATION AND TREATMENT.** The diagnosis of gynecomastia is based on physical examination. Identification and treatment of the cause are likely to be followed by resolution of the gynecomastia. The man should be taught to perform breast self-examination and is examined at 6- and 12-month intervals if the gynecomastia persists. All unilateral breast enlargement in men warrants an evaluation for malignancy; workup includes fine-needle aspiration, cytology, mammography, ultrasound, and biopsy.

Cancer

Male breast cancer (MBC) is rare. MBC accounts for 1% of all male cancers and less than 1% of all breast cancers. Global incidence rates were generally less than 1 per 100,000 man-years in contrast to much higher rates in females (see Chapter 25). The highest incidence rate for MBC is in Israel with 1.24 per 100,000, and the lowest incidence rates for males (0.16) and females (18.0) were observed in Thailand.[172] The mean age of diagnosis is between 60 and 70 years, although men of all ages can be affected.[173] Risk factors for MBC include radiation exposure, estrogen administration, and diseases associated with hyperestrogenism, such as cirrhosis or Klinefelter syndrome.[173] An increased incidence is reported in men with a number of female relatives with breast cancer; there is an increased incidence in families with *BRCA2* mutations.[173]

Similar to female breast cancer, infiltrating ductal cancer is the most common tumor type.[173] Intraductal cancer, inflammatory carcinoma, and Paget disease of the nipple have been diagnosed in men. Patterns of metastasis are similar to those in females.

The diagnosis of cancer is confirmed by biopsy, but because of delays in seeking treatment male breast cancer may be advanced at the time of diagnosis. Main treatments include chemotherapy and surgery.

▮ SUMMARY REVIEW

Alterations of Sexual Maturation

1. Sexual maturation, or puberty, should begin in boys between 9 and 14 years of age. Delayed puberty is the onset of sexual maturation after these ages; precocious puberty is onset before these ages. While the average age of pubertal onset appears to be decreasing for girls,

the age of pubertal onset has remained essentially unchanged for boys.

2. Alterations of sexual maturation can be idiopathic or caused by a disease or congenital anomaly. In most cases of delayed puberty, the hypothalamic-pituitary-gonadal (HPG) axis is intact but the surge

▊ SUMMARY REVIEW—cont'd

of activity that stimulates puberty is delayed. This situation is common in boys. Precocious puberty also can be caused by mistiming of the stimulatory surge in a child whose HPG system is otherwise normal.

3. Precocious puberty can be complete (sex appropriate), mixed (not sex appropriate), or partial (development of one secondary sex characteristic only). Causes of delayed or incomplete puberty can be divided into categories based on gonadotropic secretion: hypergonadotropism (increased levels of FSH and LH) and hypogonadotropism (decreased LH and FSH levels).

Disorders of the Male Reproductive System

1. Disorders of the urethra include urethritis (inflammation of the urethra) and urethral strictures (narrowing or obstruction of the urethral lumen caused by scarring). Urethral stricture often manifests itself as lower urinary tract symptoms or urinary tract infections with significant impairment in the quality of life.

2. Although noninfectious urethritis can occur, most cases of urethritis result from sexually transmitted pathogens. Symptoms of urethritis include dysuria, frequency, urgency, urethral tingling or itching, and clear or purulent discharge. Treatment consists of appropriate antibiotic therapy and avoidance of future chemical or mechanical irritation.

3. Acquired or congenital scarring that causes urethral stricture can be caused by trauma or by severe or untreated urethral infection. The primary symptom is diminished force and caliber of the urinary stream; other symptoms include urinary frequency and hesitancy, mild dysuria, double urine stream or spraying, and postvoid dribbling. Treatment is usually surgical.

4. Phimosis and paraphimosis are penile disorders involving the foreskin (prepuce). In phimosis the foreskin cannot be retracted over the glans. In paraphimosis the foreskin is retracted and cannot be returned to its normal anatomic position over the glans. Phimosis is caused by poor hygiene and chronic infection and can lead to paraphimosis. Paraphimosis can constrict the penile blood vessels, preventing circulation to the glans.

5. Peyronie disease consists of fibrosis that affects the corpora cavernosa, which causes penile curvature during erection. Fibrosis prevents engorgement on the affected side, causing a lateral curvature that can prevent intercourse. Peyronie disease is an underdiagnosed condition with a prevalence as high as 9% in the male population.

6. Priapism, a prolonged painful erection not stimulated by sexual arousal, is a urologic emergency. The corpora cavernosa (but not the corpus spongiosum) fills with blood that does not drain, probably because of venous obstruction. Priapism is associated with spinal cord trauma, sickle cell disease, leukemia, and pelvic tumors. It can also be idiopathic and can occur with cocaine use.

7. Balanitis is an inflammation of the glans penis and usually occurs in conjunction with posthitis. It is associated with phimosis, inadequate cleansing under the foreskin, skin disorders, and infections.

8. Cancer of the penis is rare; major risk factors include HPV, smoking, and consequences of treatment for psoriasis. Penile carcinoma in situ tends to involve the glans; invasive carcinoma of the penis involves the shaft as well.

9. A varicocele is an abnormal dilation of the veins within the spermatic cord caused by either congenital absence of valves in the internal spermatic vein or acquired valvular incompetence.

10. A hydrocele is a collection of fluid between the testicular and scrotal layers of the tunica vaginalis. Hydroceles can be idiopathic or caused by trauma or infection of the testes.

11. A spermatocele is a cyst located between the testis and epididymis that is filled with fluid and sperm.

12. Cryptorchidism is a condition in which one or both testes fail to descend into the scrotum. The etiology of cryptorchidism is considered to be multifactorial (genetic, maternal, and environmental factors) and occurs most often as an isolated disorder with no obvious cause. Uncorrected cryptorchidism is associated with infertility and a significantly increased risk of testicular cancer.

13. Testicular torsion is the rotation of a testis, which twists blood vessels in the spermatic cord. This interrupts blood supply to the testis, resulting in edema and, if not corrected within 4 to 6 hours, necrosis and atrophy of testicular tissues.

14. Orchitis is an acute infection of the testes. Pathogenic organisms may reach the testes through the blood or the lymphatics; most commonly, they reach the testes by ascending through the vas deferens and epididymis. Complications of orchitis include hydrocele and atrophy. Granulomatous orchitis, an autoimmune disease, is a nonspecific, noninfectious, inflammatory process that occurs in middle-aged men.

15. Testicular cancer is the most common malignancy in males 15 to 35 years of age. Although its cause is unknown, high androgen levels, genetic predisposition, and a history of cryptorchidism, trauma, or infection may contribute to tumorigenesis. Most testicular neoplasms are germ cell tumors.

16. Epididymitis, inflammation of the epididymis, is usually caused by a sexually transmitted pathogen that ascends through the vasa deferentia from an already infected urethra or bladder.

17. Benign prostatic hyperplasia (BPH) is enlargement of the prostate gland. This condition becomes symptomatic as the enlarging prostate compresses the urethra, causing symptoms of bladder outlet syndrome and urine retention. Studies demonstrate that the activation of a chronic, inflammatory prostatic response plays an important role in the pathogenesis and progression of BPH and prostate cancer.

18. Prostatitis is inflammation of the prostate. Prostate syndromes have been classified by the National Institutes of Health as (a) acute bacterial prostatitis (ABP), (b) chronic bacterial prostatitis (CBP), (c) chronic pelvic pain syndrome (CPPS), and (d) asymptomatic inflammatory prostatitis.

19. Prostate cancer is the most common cancer in American men, and the incidence varies greatly worldwide. Possible causes include genetic predisposition, environmental and dietary factors, inflammation, and alterations in levels of hormones (testosterone, dihydrotestosterone, and estradiol) and growth factors. Incidence is greatest among northwestern European and North American men (particularly blacks) older than 65 years of age.

20. Most cancers of the prostate are adenocarcinomas that develop at the periphery of the gland.

21. Sexual dysfunction in males can be caused by any physical or psychologic factor that impairs erection, emission, or ejaculation.

22. Spermatogenesis (sperm production by the testes) can be impaired by disruptions of the HPG axis that reduce testosterone secretion and by testicular trauma or atrophy from any cause. Sperm production is also impaired by neoplastic disease, cryptorchidism, or any factor that causes testicular temperature to rise.

23. Sperm quality is impaired by chromosomal abnormalities resulting from genetic factors, irradiation, or toxins. Sperm motility can be impaired by unfavorable constituents or characteristics of semen.

▌ SUMMARY REVIEW—cont'd

Disorders of the Male Breast

1. Gynecomastia is the overdevelopment (hyperplasia) of breast tissue in a male resulting from hormonal alterations, which may be idiopathic or caused by systemic disorders, drugs, or neoplasms. It usually involves an imbalance of the estrogen/testosterone ratio.

2. Gynecomastia affects 32% to 40% of the male population. The incidence is greatest among adolescents and men older than 50 years.

3. Gynecomastia is caused by hormonal or breast tissue alterations that cause estrogen to dominate. These alterations can result from systemic disorders, drugs, neoplasms, or idiopathic causes.

4. Breast cancer is relatively uncommon in males, but it has a poor prognosis because men tend to delay seeking treatment until the disease is advanced. The mean age at diagnosis is between 60 and 70 years of age.

5. Most breast cancers in men are estrogen positive.

▌ KEY TERMS

Acute bacterial prostatitis (ABP, category I), 848
Balanitis, 840
Benign prostatic hyperplasia (BPH) (benign prostatic hypertrophy), 846
Bladder outflow obstruction, 848
Central precocious puberty, 836
Chronic bacterial prostatitis (CBP, category II), 849
Chronic prostatitis/chronic pelvic pain syndrome (CPPS, category III), 849
Complete precocious puberty, 837
Cryptorchidism, 842
Ectopic testis, 842

Epididymitis, 846
Fibroblast, 856
Gynecomastia, 861
Hydrocele, 841
Intraprostatic conversion, 851
Mixed precocious puberty, 837
Nonbacterial prostatitis, 849
Orchitis, 844
Paraphimosis, 838
Partial precocious puberty, 837
Peyronie disease (bent nail syndrome), 838
Phimosis, 838
Precocious puberty, 836

Priapism, 839
Prostate-specific antigen (PSA), 857
Prostatitis, 848
PSA velocity, 858
Sexual dysfunction, 859
Spermatocele, 842
Stroma, 856
Torsion of the testis, 843
Urethral stricture, 838
Urethritis, 838
Varicocele, 841

REFERENCES

1. American Cancer Society (ACS): *Cancer facts & figures—2017*, Atlanta, 2017, Author.

2. Jospe N: Disorders of pubertal development. In Osborn LM, et al, editors: *Pediatrics*, Philadelphia, 2005, Mosby.

3. Healtheon/WebMD: *Hypothalamic disorders. Scientific American Medicine*, 1999. Available at: www.samed.com/sam/forms/index.htm.

4. Smaldone A, et al: Endocrine and metabolic diseases. In Burns CE, et al, editors: *Pediatric primary care*, St Louis, 2016, Saunders.

5. Abitbol L, Zborovski S, Palmert MR: Evaluation of delayed puberty: What diagnostic tests should be performed in the seemingly otherwise well adolescent? *Arch Dis Child* 101(8):767–771, 2016.

6. Veldhuis JD, Keenan DM, Pincus SM: Regulation of complex pulsatile and rhythmic neuroendocrine systems: the male gonadal axis as a prototype. *Prog Brain Res* 181:79–110, 2010.

7. Pineda R, et al: Physiological roles of the kisspeptin/GPR54 system in the neuroendocrine control of reproduction. *Prog Brain Res* 181:55–77, 2010.

8. Higo S, Iijima N, Ozawa H: Characterization of Kiss1r (Gpr54)-expressing neurons in the arcuate nucleus of the female rat hypothalamus. *J Neuroendocrinol* 29(2):2017.

9. Sørensen K, et al: Recent secular trends in pubertal timing: implications for evaluation and diagnosis of precocious puberty. *Horm Res Paediatr* 77:137–145, 2012.

10. Fenichel P: Delayed puberty. *Endocr Dev* 22:138–159, 2012.

11. Euling SY, et al: Examination of US puberty-timing data from 1940 to 1994 for secular trends: panel findings. *Pediatrics* 121(Suppl 3):S172–S191, 2008.

12. Herman-Giddens ME, et al: Secondary sexual characteristics in boys: data from the pediatric research in office settings network. *Pediatrics* 130(5):e1058–e1068, 2012.

13. Latronico AC, Brito VN, Carel JC: Causes, diagnosis, and treatment of central precocious puberty. *Lancet Diabetes Endocrinol* 4(3):265–274, 2016.

14. Marcovecchio ML, Chiarelli F: Obesity and growth during childhood and puberty. *World Rev Nutr Diet* 106:135–141, 2013.

15. Rey-Ladino J, Ross AG, Cripps AW: Immunity, immunopathology, and human vaccine development against sexually transmitted *Chlamydia trachomatis. Hum Vaccin Immunother* 10(9):2664–2673, 2014.

16. Schollum JB, Walker RJ: Adult urinary tract infection. *Br J Hosp Med (Lond)* 73(4):218–223, 2012.

17. Moi H, Blee K, Horner PJ: Management of non-gonococcal urethritis. *BMC Infect Dis* 15:294, 2015.

18. Brill JR: Diagnosis and treatment of urethritis in men. *Am Fam Physician* 81(7):873–878, 2010.

19. Smith TG, 3rd: Current management of urethral stricture disease. *Indian J Urol* 32(1):27–33, 2016.

20. Tang SH, et al: Adult urethral stricture disease after childhood hypospadias repair. *Adv Urol* 2008:150315, 2008.

21. McAninch JW: Disorders of the penis and male urethra. In McAninch JW, Lue TF, editors: *Smith and Tanagho's general urology*, ed 18, Norwalk, CT, 2012, McGraw-Hill Lange.

22. Stratton KL, Culkin DJ: A contemporary review of HPV and penile cancer. *Oncology (Williston Park)* 30(3):245–249, 2016.

23. Yafi FA, et al: Therapeutic advances in the treatment of Peyronie's disease. *Andrology* 3(4):650–660, 2015.

24. Altman AL, et al: Cocaine associated priapism. *J Urol* 161(6):1817–1818, 1999.

25. Shigehara K, Namiki M: Clinical management of priapism: a review. *World J Mens Health* 34(1):1–8, 2016.

26. American Cancer Society (ACS): *Penile cancer resource center*, 2017. Available at: http://www.cancer.org/cancer/penilecancer/index.

27. Letendre J, Saad F, Lattouf JB: Penile cancer: What's new? *Curr Opin Support Palliat Care* 5(3):185–191, 2011.

28. Presti JC: Genital tumors. In McAninch JW, Lue TF, editors: *Smith and Tanagho's general urology*, ed 18, Norwalk, CT, 2012, McGraw-Hill Lange.

29. Spiess PE, et al: Current concepts in penile cancer. *J Natl Compr Canc Netw* 11(5):617–624, 2013.

30. Mossanen M, et al: 15 Years of penile cancer management in the United States: an analysis of the use of partial penectomy for localized disease and chemotherapy in the metastatic setting. *Urol Oncol* 34(12):530.e1–530.e7, 2016.

31. Gupta S, Sonpavde G: Emerging systemic therapies for the management of penile cancer. *Urol Clin North Am* 43(4):481–491, 2016.

32. Montgomery JS, Bloom DA: The diagnosis and management of scrotal masses. *Med Clin North Am* 95(1):235–244, 2011.

33. Davis JE, Silverman M: Scrotal emergencies. *Emerg Med Clin North Am* 29(3):469–484, 2011.

34. Günther P, Rübben I: The acute scrotum in childhood and adolescence. *Dtsch Arztebl Int* 109(25):449–457, 2012.

35. Marmar JL: The evolution and refinements of varicocele surgery. *Asian J Androl* 18(2):171–178, 2016.

36. Chen SS: Differences in the clinical characteristics between young and elderly men with varicocele. *Int J Androl* 35(5):695–699, 2012.

37. Hart RJ, et al: Testicular function in a birth cohort of young men. *Hum Reprod* 30(12):2713–2724, 2015.

38. Walsh TJ, Smith JF: Male infertility. In McAninch JW, Lue TF, editors: *Smith and Tanagho's general urology*, ed 18, Norwalk, CT, 2012, McGraw-Hill Lange.

39. Doudt AD, et al: Abdominoscrotal hydrocele: a systematic review. *J Pediatr Surg* 51(9):1561–1564, 2016.

40. Rioja J, et al: Adult hydrocele and spermatocele. *BJU Int* 107(11):1852–1864, 2011.

41. Crawford P, Crop JA: Evaluation of scrotal masses. *Am Fam Physician* 89(9):723–727, 2014.

42. Wampler SM, Llanes M: Common scrotal and testicular problems. *Prim Care* 37(3):613–626, 2010.

43. Kollin C, Ritzén EM: Cryptorchidism: a clinical perspective. *Pediatr Endocrinol Rev* 11(Suppl 2):240–250, 2014.

44. Sepúlveda X, Egaña PL: Current management of non-palpable testes: a literature review and clinical results. *Transl Pediatr* 5(4):233–239, 2016.

45. Fantasia J, et al: Undescended testes: a clinical and surgical review. *Urol Nurs* 35(3):117–126, 2015.

46. John Radcliffe Hospital Cryptorchidism Study Group: Cryptorchidism: a prospective study of 7500 consecutive male births, 1984–8. *Arch Dis Child* 67:892–899, 1992.

47. Kathrins M, Kolon TF: Malignancy in disorders of sex development. *Transl Androl Urol* 5(5):794–798, 2016.

48. Walsh TJ, et al: Prepubertal orchiopexy for cryptorchidism may be associated with lower risk of testicular cancer. *J Urol* 178(4 Pt 1):1440–1446, 2007.

49. Ludvigson AE, Beaule LT: Urologic emergencies. *Surg Clin North Am* 96(3):407–424, 2016.

50. Bowlin PR, Gatti JM, Murphy JP: Pediatric testicular torsion. *Surg Clin North Am* 97(1):161–172, 2017.

51. Nguyen HT: Bacterial infections of the genitourinary tract. In McAninch JW, Lue TF, editors: *Smith and Tanagho's general urology*, ed 18, Norwalk, CT, 2012, McGraw-Hill Lange.

52. Filippou P, Ferguson JE, 3rd, Nielsen ME: Epidemiology of prostate and testicular cancer. *Semin Intervent Radiol* 33(3):182–185, 2016.

53. Saab MM, Landers M, Hegarty J: Testicular cancer awareness and screening practices: a systematic review. *Oncol Nurs Forum* 43(1):E8–E23, 2016.

54. National Cancer Institute (NCI): *Testicular cancer information*, 2017. Available at: https://seer.cancer.gov/statfacts/html/testis.html.

55. Shala C, Tripathi R, Mishra DP: Male germ cell apoptosis: regulation and biology. *Philos Trans R Soc Lond B Biol Sci* 365(1546):1501–1515, 2010.

56. Mirabello L, et al: Promotor methylation of candidate genes associated with familial testicular cancer. *Int J Mol Epidemiol Genet* 3(3):213–227, 2012.

57. Egan KB: The epidemiology of benign prostatic hyperplasia associated with lower urinary tract symptoms: prevalence and incident rates. *Urol Clin North Am* 43(3):289–297, 2016.

58. Gandaglia G, et al: The role of prostatic inflammation in the development and progression of benign and malignant diseases. *Curr Opin Urol* 27(2):99–106, 2017.

59. Wynder JL, et al: Estrogens and male lower urinary tract dysfunction. *Curr Urol Rep* 16(9):61, 2015.

60. Chughtai B, et al: Inflammation and benign prostatic hyperplasia: clinical implications. *Curr Urol Rep* 12(4):274–277, 2011.

61. Bachmann A, de la Rosette J, editors: *Benign prostatic hyperplasia and lower urinary tract symptoms in men*, New York, 2012, Oxford University Press.

62. Cooperberg MR, et al: Neoplasms of the prostate gland. In McAninch JW, Lue TF, editors: *Smith and Tanagho's general urology*, ed 18, Norwalk, CT, 2012, McGraw-Hill Lange.

63. Unnikrishnan R, Almassi N, Fareed K: Benign prostatic hyperplasia: evaluation and medical management in primary care. *Cleve Clin J Med* 84(1):53–64, 2017.

64. Bechis SK, et al: Personalized medicine for the management of benign prostatic hyperplasia. *J Urol* 192(1):16–23, 2014.

65. Krieger JN, Thumbikat P: Bacterial prostatitis: bacterial virulence, clinical outcomes, and new directions. *Microbiol Spectr* 4(1):2016.

66. Wagenlehner FM, et al: Bacterial prostatitis. *World J Urol* 31(4):711–716, 2013.

67. Moyer VA, U.S. Preventive Services Task Force: Screening for prostate cancer: U.S. Preventive Services Task Force recommendation statement. *Ann Intern Med* 157(2):120–134, 2012.

68. Khazaei S, et al: Global prostate cancer incidence and mortality rates according to the Human Development Index. *Asian Pac J Cancer Prev* 17(8):3793–3796, 2016.

69. Torre LA, et al: Global cancer incidence and mortality rates and trends—an update. *Cancer Epidemiol Biomarkers Prev* 25(1):16–27, 2016.

70. Kruk J, Aboul-Enein H: What are the links of prostate cancer with physical activity and nutrition? A systematic review article. *Iran J Public Health* 45(12):1558–1567, 2016.

71. Marshall JR: Diet and prostate cancer prevention. *World J Urol* 30(2):157–165, 2012.

72. Tewari R, et al: Diet, obesity, and prostate health: Are we missing the link? *J Androl* 33(5):763–776, 2012.

73. Fair AM, Montgomery K: Energy balance, physical activity, and cancer risk. *Methods Mol Biol* 472:57–88, 2009.

74. Harrison S, et al: Does milk intake promote prostate cancer initiation or progression via effects on insulin-like growth factors (IGFs)? A systematic review and meta-analysis. *Cancer Causes Control* 28(6):497–528, 2017.

75. Downer MK, et al: Dairy intake in relation to prostate cancer survival. *Int J Cancer* 140(9):2060–2069, 2017.

76. Gathirua-Mwangi WG, Zhang J: Dietary factors and risk of advanced prostate cancer. *Eur J Cancer Prev* 23(2):96–109, 2014.

77. Capper CP, Rae JM, Auchus RJ: The metabolism, analysis, and targeting of steroid hormones in breast and prostate cancer. *Horm Cancer* 7(3):149–164, 2016.

78. Labrie F: Blockage of testicular and adrenal androgens in prostate cancer treatment. *Nat Rev Urol* 8:73–80, 2011.

79. Hagberg Thulin M, et al: Osteoblasts promote castration-resistant prostate cancer by altering intratumoral steroidogenesis. *Mol Cell Endocrinol* 422:182–191, 2016.

80. Bosland MC: Sex steroids and prostate carcinogenesis: integrated, multifactorial working hypothesis. *Ann N Y Acad Sci* 1089:168–176, 2006.

81. Bosland MC: A perspective on the role of estrogen in hormone-induced prostate carcinogenesis. *Cancer Lett* 334(1):28–33, 2013.

82. Ricke WA, Wang Y, Cunha GR: Steroid hormones and carcinogenesis of the prostate: the role of estrogens. *Differentiation* 75(9):871–882, 2007.

83. Black A, et al: Sex steroid hormone metabolism in relation to risk of aggressive prostate cancer. *Cancer Epidemiol Biomarkers Prev* 23(11):2374–2382, 2014.

84. Ellem SJ, Risbridger GP: The dual, opposing roles of estrogen in the prostate. *Ann N Y Acad Sci* 1155:174–186, 2009.

85. Thompson IM, et al: The influence of finasteride on the development of prostate cancer. *N Engl J Med* 349:215–224, 2003.

86. Hsiao JJ, et al: Androgen receptor and chemokine receptors 4 and 7 form a signaling axis to regulate CXCL12-dependent cellular motility. *BMC Cancer* 15:204, 2015.

87. Endogenous Hormones and Prostate Cancer Collaborative Group et al: Endogenous sex hormones and prostate cancer: a collaborative analysis of 18 prospective studies. *J Natl Cancer Inst* 100(3):170–183, 2008.

88. Ganesh B, et al: Risk factors for prostate cancer: a hospital-based case-control study from Mumbai, India. *Indian J Urol* 27(3):345–350, 2011.

89. Perdana NR, et al: The risk factors of prostate cancer and its prevention: a literature review. *Acta Med Indones* 48(3):228–238, 2016.

90. van Leeuwen PJ, et al: Critical assessment of prebiopsy parameters for predicting prostate cancer metastasis and mortality. *Can J Urol* 6:6018–6024, 2011.

91. Köhler TS, Fazili AA, Brannigan RE: Putative health risks associated with vasectomy. *Urol Clin North Am* 36(3):337–345, 2009.

92. Liu LH, et al: Vasectomy and risk of prostate cancer: a systematic review and meta-analysis of cohort studies. *Andrology* 3(4):643–649, 2015.

93. McConnell JD, et al: The long-term effect of doxazosin, finasteride, and combination therapy on the clinical progression of benign prostatic hyperplasia. *N Engl J Med* 349(25):2387–2398, 2003.

94. McVary KT: A review of combination therapy in patients with benign prostatic hyperplasia. *Clin Ther* 29(3):387–398, 2007.

95. Jiang M, et al: Disruption of PPAR gamma signaling results in mouse prostatic intraepithelial neoplasia involving active autophagy. *Cell Death Differ* 17:469–481, 2010.

96. Thapa D, Ghosh R: Chronic inflammatory mediators enhance prostate cancer development and progression. *Biochem Pharmacol* 94(2):53–62, 2015.

97. MacLennan GT, et al: The influence of chronic inflammation in prostatic carcinogenesis: a 5-year follow-up study. *J Urol* 176(3):1012–1016, 2006.

98. Wang JY, Fu YY, Kang DY: The association between metabolic syndrome and characteristics of benign prostatic hyperplasia: a systematic review and meta-analysis. *Medicine (Baltimore)* 95(19):e3243, 2016.

99. Albright F, et al: Significant evidence for a heritable contribution to cancer predisposition: a review of cancer familiality by site. *BMC Cancer* 12:138, 2012.

100. Castro E, Eeles R: The role of BRCA1 and BRCA2 in prostate cancer. *Asian J Androl* 14(3):409–414, 2012.

101. Stott-Miller M, et al: HOXB13 mutations in a population-based, case-control study of prostate cancer. *Prostate* 73(6):634–641, 2013.

102. Lynch HT, et al: Screening for familial and hereditary prostate cancer. *Int J Cancer* 138(11):2579–2591, 2016.

103. Leongamornlert D, et al: Germline BRCA1 mutations increase prostate cancer risk. *Br J Cancer* 106(10):1697–1701, 2012.

104. Van Neste L, et al: The epigenetic promise for prostate cancer diagnosis. *Prostate* 72(11): 1248–1261, 2012.

105. Epstein JI: The lower urinary tract and male genital system. In Kumar V, Abbas AK, Fausto N, editors: *Robbins & Cotran pathologic basis of disease*, ed 8, Philadelphia, 2009, Saunders.

106. Rubin MA: ETS rearrangements in prostate cancer. *Asian J Androl* 14(3):393–399, 2012.

107. De Nunzio C, et al: The controversial relationship between benign prostatic hyperplasia and prostate cancer: the role of inflammation. *Eur Urol* 60(1): 106–117, 2011.

108. Fisher KW, et al: Molecular foundations for personalized therapy in prostate cancer. *Curr Drug Targets* 16(2):103–114, 2015.

109. Lumen N, et al: Screening and early diagnosis of prostate cancer: an update. *Acta Clin Belg* 67(4): 270–275, 2012.

110. Morgan T, Palapattu G, Wei J: Screening for prostate cancer-beyond total PSA, utilization of novel biomarkers. *Curr Urol Rep* 16(9):63, 2015.

111. Mackinnon AC, et al: Molecular biology underlying the clinical heterogeneity of prostate cancer: an update. *Arch Pathol Lab Med* 133(7): 1033–1040, 2009.

112. Kowalska K, Piastowska-Ciesielska AW: Oestrogens and oestrogen receptors in prostate cancer. *Springerplus* 5:522, 2016.

113. Eaton NE, et al: Endogenous sex hormones and prostate cancer: a quantitative review of prospective studies. *Br J Cancer* 80:930–934, 1999.

114. Roddam AW, et al: Endogenous sex hormones and prostate cancer: a collaborative analysis of 18 prospective studies. *J Natl Cancer Inst* 100: 170–183, 2008.

115. Parnes HL, Thompson IM, Ford LG: Review article: prevention of hormone-related cancers: prostate cancer. *J Clin Oncol* 23(2):368–377, 2005.

116. Pastuszak AW, et al: Testosterone therapy and prostate cancer. *Transl Androl Urol* 5(6):909–920, 2016.

117. Bonkhoff H, et al: Progesterone receptor expression in human prostate cancer: correlation with cancer progression. *Prostate* 48(4):285–291, 2001.

118. Setlur SR, et al: Estrogen-dependent signaling in a molecular distinct subclass of aggressive prostate cancer. *J Natl Cancer Inst* 100:815–825, 2008.

119. Kawashima H, Nakatani T: Involvement of estrogen receptors in prostatic diseases. *Int J Urol* 19(6):512–522, 2012.

120. Ellem SJ, Risbridger GP: Aromatase and regulating the estrogen: androgen ratio in the prostate gland. *J Steroid Biochem Mol Biol* 118(4-5):246–251, 2010.

121. Quintar AA, Maldonado CA: Androgen regulation of host defenses and response to inflammatory stimuli in the prostate gland. *Cell Biol Int* 2017 Feb 28. [Epub ahead of print].

122. Chen R, Yu Y, Dong X: Progesterone receptor in the prostate: a potential suppressor for benign prostatic hyperplasia and prostate cancer. *J Steroid Biochem Mol Biol* 166:91–96, 2017.

123. Treas JN, Tvagi T, Singh KP: Effects of chronic exposure to arsenic and estrogen on epigenetic regulatory genes expression and epigenetic code in human prostate epithelial cells. *PLoS ONE* 7(8): e43880, 2012.

124. Bosland MC, Mahmoud AM: Hormones and prostate carcinogenesis: androgens and estrogens. *J Carcinog* 10:33, 2011.

125. Deng Q, Tang DG: Androgen receptor and prostate cancer stem cells: biological mechanisms and clinical implications. *Endocr Relat Cancer* 22(6):T209–T220, 2015.

126. Vander Griend DJ, et al: Cell autonomous intracellular androgen signaling drives the growth of human prostate cancer-initiating cells. *Prostate* 70(1):90–99, 2010.

127. Nieto CM, Rider LC, Cramer SD: Influence of stromal-epithelial interactions on androgen action. *Endocr Relat Cancer* 21(4):T147–T160, 2014.

128. Ricke EA, et al: Androgen hormone action in prostatic carcinogenesis: stromal androgen receptors mediate prostate cancer progression, malignant transformation and metastasis. *Carcinogenesis* 33(7):1391–1398, 2012.

129. Singh M, et al: Stromal androgen receptor in prostate development and cancer. *Am J Pathol* 184:2598–2607, 2014.

130. Wen S, et al: Stromal androgen receptor roles in the development of normal prostate, benign prostate hyperplasia, and prostate cancer. *Am J Pathol* 185:293–301, 2015.

131. Leach DA, Buchanan G: Stromal androgen receptor in prostate cancer development and progression. *Cancers (Basel)* 9(1):2017.

132. Cooke PS, Young P, Cunha GR: Androgen receptor expression in developing male reproductive organs. *Endocrinology* 128(6):2867–2873, 1991.

133. Cooke PS, et al: Estrogen receptor expression in developing epididymis, efferent ductules, and other male reproductive organs. *Endocrinology* 128(6):2874–2879, 1991.

134. Kurita T, et al: Stromal progesterone receptors mediate the inhibitory effects of progesterone on estrogen-induced uterine epithelial cell deoxyribonucleic acid synthesis. *Endocrinology* 139(11):4708–4713, 1998.

135. DeMarzo AM, et al: Inflammation in prostate carcinogenesis. *Nat Rev Cancer* 7:256–269, 2007.

136. Taverna G, et al: Inflammation and prostate cancer: friends or foe? *Inflamm Res* 64(5):275–286, 2015.

137. Marian CO, Shay JW: Prostate tumor initiating cells: a new target for telomerase inhibition therapy? *Biochim Biophys Acta* 1792:289–296, 2009.

138. Bianchi-Frias D, et al: The effects of aging on the molecular and cellular composition of the prostate microenvironment. *PLoS ONE* 5(9): e12501, 2010.

139. Montico F, et al: Reactive stroma in the prostate during late life: the role of microvasculature and antiangiogenic therapy influences. *Prostate* 75(14):1643–1661, 2015.

140. DeMagalhaes JP, Curado J, Church GM: Meta-analysis of age-related gene expression profiles identifies common signatures of aging. *Bioinformatics* 25:875–881, 2009.

141. Kim SK: Common aging pathways in worms, flies, mice and humans. *J Exp Biol* 210:1607–1612, 2007.

142. Kuilman T, et al: Oncogene-induced senescence relayed by an interleukin-dependent inflammatory network. *Cell* 133:1019–1031, 2008.

143. Paapatto GS, et al: Prostate carcinogenesis and inflammation: emerging insights. *Carcinogenesis* 26:1170–1181, 2005.

144. Thiery JP: Epithelial-mesenchymal transitions in tumor progression. *Nat Rev Cancer* 2(6):441–454, 2002.

145. Yadavalli S, et al: Data-driven discovery of extravasation pathway in circulating tumor cells. *Sci Rep* 7:43710, 2017.

146. Josson S, et al: Tumor-stromal interaction influence radiation sensitivity in epithelial versus mesenchymal-like prostate cancer cell. *J Oncol* 2010:232831, 2010.

147. Bhowmick NA, Moses HL: Tumor-stromal interactions. *Curr Opin Genet Dev* 15(1):97–101, 2005.

148. Friedlander TW, Premasekharan G, Paris PL: Looking back, to the future of circulating tumor cells. *Pharmacol Ther* 142(3):271–280, 2014.

149. Xu J, et al: Prostate cancer metastasis: role of the host microenvironment in promoting epithelial to mesenchymal transition and increase bone adrenal gland metastasis. *Prostate* 66: 1664–1673, 2006.

150. Liu W, et al: Copy number analysis indicates monoclonal origin of lethal metastatic prostate cancer. *Nat Med* 15(5):559–565, 2009.

151. Celia-Terrassa T, et al: Epithelial-mesenchymal transition can suppress major attributes of human epithelial tumor-initiating cells. *J Clin Invest* 122(5):1849–1868, 2012.

152. Fitzpatrick JM, Banu E, Oudard S: Prostate-specific antigen kinetics in localized and advanced prostate cancer. *BJU Int* 103(5):578–587, 2009.

153. Stamey TA: The era of serum prostate antigens as a marker for biopsy of the prostate and detecting prostate cancer is now over in the USA. *BJU Int* 94(7):963–964, 2004.

154. Schröder FH, et al: Screening and prostate cancer mortality: results of the European Randomised Study of Screening for Prostate Cancer (ERSPC) at 13 years of follow-up. *Lancet* 384(9959): 2027–2035, 2014.

155. Schröder FH, et al: Screening for prostate cancer decreases the risk of developing metastatic disease: findings from the European Randomized Study of Screening for Prostate Cancer (ERSPC). *Eur Urol* 62(5):745–752, 2012.

156. U.S. Preventive Services Task Force (USPSTF): *Screening for prostate cancer*, 2017. Available at: http://www.screeningforprostatecancer.org.

157. Fleshner K, Carlsson SV, Roobol MJ: The effect of the USPSTF PSA screening recommendation on prostate cancer incidence patterns in the USA. *Nat Rev Urol* 14(1):26–37, 2017.

158. Jemal A, et al: Prostate cancer incidence and PSA testing patterns in relation to USPSTF screening recommendations. *JAMA* 314(19):2054–2061, 2015.

159. Loughlin KR: PSA velocity: a systematic review of clinical applications. *Urol Oncol* 32(8):1116–1125, 2014.

160. Vickers AJ, Brewster SF: PSA velocity and doubling time in diagnosis and prognosis of prostate cancer. *Br J Med Surg Urol* 5(4):162–168, 2012.

161. Vickers AJ, et al: An empirical evaluation of guidelines on prostate-specific antigen velocity in prostate cancer detection. *J Natl Cancer Inst* 103(6):462–469, 2011.

162. Preston MA, et al: Baseline prostate-specific antigen levels in midlife predict lethal prostate cancer. *J Clin Oncol* 34(23):2705–2711, 2016.

163. Droz JP, et al: Management of prostate cancer in elderly patients: recommendations of a Task Force of the International Society of Geriatric Oncology. *Eur Urol* 2017 Jan 11. [Epub ahead of print].

164. Benjamins MR, et al: Racial disparities in prostate cancer mortality in the 50 largest US cities. *Cancer Epidemiol* 44:125–131, 2016.

165. Nguyen CT, Kattan MW: Formalized prediction of clinically significant prostate cancer: Is it possible? *Asian J Androl* 14(3):349–354, 2012.

166. Shoag JE, Mittal S, Hu JC: Reevaluating PSA testing rates in the PLCO trial. *N Engl J Med* 374(18):1795–1796, 2016.

167. Boorjian SA, et al: The impact of discordance between biopsy and pathological Gleason scores on survival after radical prostatectomy. *J Urol* 181(1):95–104, 2009.

168. Hamdy FC, et al: 10-year outcomes after monitoring, surgery, or radiotherapy for localized prostate cancer. *N Engl J Med* 375(15):1415–1424, 2016.

169. Toulis KA, et al: Inhibin B and anti-Müllerian hormone as markers of persistent spermatogenesis in men with non-obstructive azoospermia: a meta-analysis of diagnostic accuracy studies. *Hum Reprod Update* 16(6):713–724, 2010.

170. Yadav RP, Kotaja N: Small RNAs in spermatogenesis. *Mol Cell Endocrinol* 382(1): 498–508, 2014.

171. Hapberg KW, et al: Risk of gynecomastic and breast cancer associated with the use of 5-alpha reductase inhibitors for benign prostatic hyperplasia. *Clin Epidemiol* 19:83–91, 2017.

172. Ly D, et al: An international comparison of male and female breast cancer incidence rates. *Int J Cancer* 132(8):1918–1926, 2013.

173. National Cancer Institute (NCI): *Male breast cancer treatment (PDQ) health professional version*, Bethesda, MD, 2017.

Sexually Transmitted Infections

Julia C. Phillippi, Kathleen E. Danhausen

evolve WEBSITE

CHAPTER OUTLINE

Newly acquired sexually contracted infections affect more than 20 million Americans per year, and half of those individuals are younger than 25 years of age[1] (see *What's New?* Sexually Transmitted Infection [STI] Statistical Summary from 2015 CDC). **Sexually transmitted infections (STIs)** account for nearly $16 billion dollars in healthcare costs in the United States. They have been called the *hidden epidemic* by the CDC[1] because they are so prevalent, yet rarely discussed. Complications of STIs include short- and long-term morbidity and even mortality that can affect physical, emotional, and financial well-being.

In the past, an infection transmitted through sexual intercourse was called a *venereal disease*. However, the term venereal disease has been replaced with STI. STIs are contracted by genital contact or through contact with infected blood or body fluids. Infections can be transmitted directly through touch or the infectious agent can be transmitted by an object, known as a **fomite**. STIs also can be transmitted from mother to child during pregnancy and birth, a process known as **vertical transmission**.

Many infected individuals are not screened for STIs because symptoms are absent, minor, or transient, or because health services are inaccessible, unaffordable, or culturally insensitive. When individuals do not know they have an STI, they often fail to prevent transmission to others. With adequate screening and early treatment and education, the prevalence and sequelae of STIs can be greatly reduced.

Behaviors are the greatest risk factor for STI acquisition. Individuals who have unprotected intercourse or genital/oral contact, especially with nonmonogamous or multiple partners, are at the greatest risk. Certain populations as defined by age, behaviors, geographic location, traits, or race/ethnicity have a higher incidence of STIs. This increase is usually a result of increased risky behaviors by individuals in this group, but it can also be due to physical or cultural characteristics that contribute to transmission. For example, rates of gonorrhea, chlamydia, vaginitis, cervical condyloma, genital warts, and pelvic inflammatory disease (PID) are highest in adolescents and decline exponentially with increasing age (Fig. 27.1). Adolescents more often engage in risky behaviors and have a greater number of sexual partners than older adults. People entering correctional facilities, such as jails, also have higher rates of STI prevalence related to their risky behaviors before incarceration.[1]

Some populations are at greater risk because of the pathophysiology of STI transmission. Transmission of many STIs is enhanced when the infectious agent contacts mucous membranes, such as the mouth, oropharynx, vagina, rectum, and the inner foreskin, which provide a more favorable environment for transmission than skin. Therefore women, uncircumcised men, and men who are the receptive partner in oral or anal sex are at increased risk.[1] In addition, prolonged contact with infectious body fluids also increases transmission, which occurs when semen is deposited in the vagina or rectum. Young women also are at greater risk for STI acquisition when compared with older women,

Sexually Transmitted Infection (STI) Statistical Summary From 2015 CDC Report

Each year in the United States:

- 20 million individuals contract a sexually transmitted infection; half of those infected are younger than 25 years.
- 16 billion dollars are spent on STIs, not including long-term healthcare costs.
- Only half of people who need STI screening receive needed services.

Chlamydia cases:

- 1.4 million cases were reported and treated, but an estimated 1 million of additional cases remain untreated.

Gonorrhea cases:

- 350,062 cases were reported in 2014, a 5% increase in 1 year.
- Increasing antibiotic resistance means that gonorrhea may soon become resistant to all known treatments.

Syphilis cases:

- There was a 15% overall increase in cases reported since 2013.
- The syphilis rate is highest among men who have sex with men.

Viral STIs affect more than 70 million people in the United States:

- The use of the HPV vaccine is already demonstrating positive effects on the rates of HPV acquisition in the United States.
- 50 million people are estimated to have genital herpes.
- 1.2 million adults in the United States live with an HIV infection.

Data from Centers for Disease Control and Prevention (CDC): *Sexually transmitted disease surveillance 2014,* Washington, DC, 2015, U.S. Department of Health and Human Services.

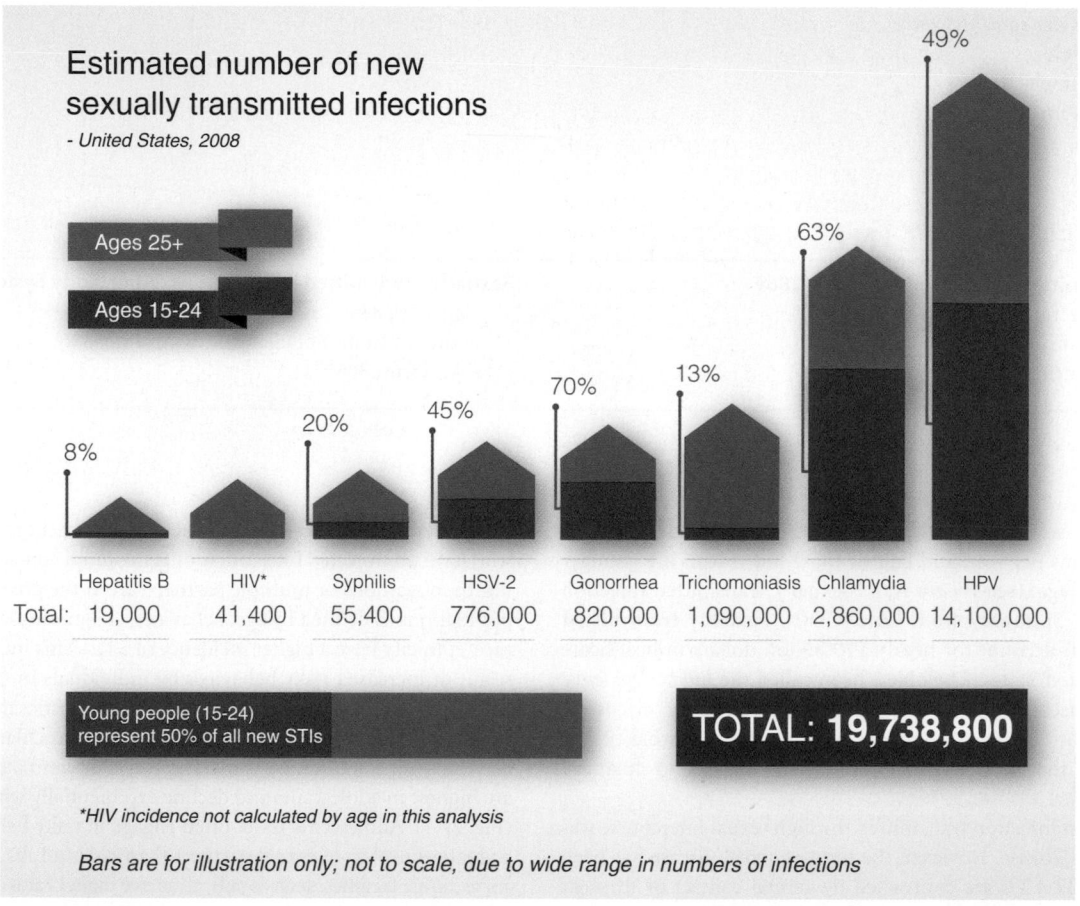

FIGURE 27.1 Incidence of Sexually Transmitted Infections by Age. (From Centers for Disease Control and Prevention [CDC]: *CDC fact sheet: sexually transmitted infections among young Americans,* 2013. Available at: http://www.cdc.gov/std/products/infographics.htm.)

which is related to the position of susceptible cells on the surface of their cervix.

STI transmission is enhanced when the infectious agent has contact with broken skin or blood vessels; therefore sexual contact that is damaging to the genitals increases STI acquisition. This is the case with rectal-penile sex, as well as forced genital contact. Broken or friable skin caused by genital infections or trauma also can increase the risk of STI acquisition. As a result, if an individual has one STI, he or she is more susceptible to acquisition when exposed to other STIs.

Race and ethnicity are not direct factors in STI acquisition. STIs are prevalent in all socioeconomic and racial/ethnic groups. Publicly available data suggest a greater prevalence in minority groups or among people with low socioeconomic status, which may be a reflection of greater STI reporting from public clinics that serve marginalized groups when compared with private providers who are not required to report all infections to authorities. Race and ethnicity alone do not alter STI risk, but rather act as risk markers that correlate with other more fundamental determinants of health status, such as (1) poverty, (2) access to quality care, and (3) health-seeking behavior. In some geographic areas racial, ethnic, or socioeconomic groups may be more or less likely to engage in at-risk behaviors such as intravenous drug use and unprotected sex. Healthcare providers should provide risk-appropriate screening based on behaviors and physiologic risk factors without racial profiling. To assist clinicians the CDC regularly publishes a comprehensive guideline detailing STI screening, evaluation, and treatment that specifies current at-risk groups. This guide and its corresponding smartphone app are the best sources of current information on STI screening and treatment since this area of clinical care changes rapidly.

An STI can be caused by bacteria, viruses, protozoa, parasites, or fungi (Table 27.1). Transmission rates and prevalence depend on the characteristics of the pathogen and complex factors associated with behavioral and societal factors. Bacterial, protozoan, parasitic, and fungal STIs can be successfully treated once diagnosed, but viral STIs cannot be cured by pharmacologic means alone and, depending on the virus, affected individuals have the potential to carry or transmit the virus throughout their life.

Treatment or symptom management of STIs depends on the causative pathogen. Treatments change frequently based on drug resistance and availability of medications, and are personalized on the basis of the individual's medical needs and personal preferences. Treatment of the person and his or her sexual partner(s) is often complicated by inadequate access to medical care, drug cost, and privacy concerns.[1] Many states have enacted legislation to allow sexual partners to be treated without having to go to a clinic for an examination and prescription.[2]

Prevention of STI acquisition involves a multifaceted approach including encouraging behavioral changes to decrease transmission, such as decreasing the number of sexual partners or using condoms. Preexposure vaccines, including vaccines for hepatitis and human papillomavirus (HPV), have been used to protect populations against viral STIs before exposure.[3] Medications also may be used to prevent acquisition of STIs as preexposure and postexposure prophylaxis, especially in the prevention of human immunodeficiency virus (HIV) acquisition.[3] Early treatment of STIs prevents transmission to new hosts and decreases the risk of additional STI acquisition for the index person. Testing and treatment are especially helpful in preventing vertical transmission.

SEXUALLY TRANSMITTED UROGENITAL INFECTIONS

Bacterial Infections

Gonorrhea

Gonorrhea is caused by gonococci (singular, gonococcus), microorganisms of the species *Neisseria gonorrhoeae*. First identified in 1879, gonorrhea became the most widely reported STI in the United States before entering a decline because of widespread availability of testing and treatment. After reaching a record low in 2009, the rates for gonorrhea have increased 10.5% since 2010, in part because of widespread testing using more accurate nucleic acid amplification tests (NAATs).[4]

The risk of developing gonorrhea from intercourse with an infected male partner is 50% to 80% for women, and with an infected female partner, it is 20% to 30% for men. The risk increases threefold to fourfold for men after four exposures to an infected partner. Men who have sex

TABLE 27.1	CURRENTLY RECOGNIZED SEXUALLY TRANSMITTED INFECTIONS
CAUSAL MICROORGANISM	**INFECTION**
Bacteria	
Campylobacter	Campylobacter enteritis
Calymmatobacterium granulomatis	Granuloma inguinale
Chlamydia trachomatis	Urogenital infections; lymphogranuloma venereum
Polymicrobial	
Gardnerella vaginalis interaction with anaerobes (*Bacteroides* and *Mobiluncus* spp.) and genital mycoplasmas	Bacterial vaginosis
Haemophilus ducreyi	Chancroid
Mycoplasma	Mycoplasmosis
Neisseria gonorrhoeae	Gonorrhea
Shigella	Shigellosis
Treponema pallidum	Syphilis
Viruses	
Cytomegalovirus	Cytomegalic inclusion disease
Hepatitis B virus (HBV)	Hepatitis
Hepatitis C virus (HCV)	Hepatitis
Herpes simplex virus (HSV)	Genital herpes
Human immunodeficiency virus (HIV)	Acquired immunodeficiency syndrome (AIDS)
Human papillomavirus (HPV)	Condylomata acuminata, cervical dysplasia, and cervical cancer
Molluscum contagiosum virus	Molluscum contagiosum
Zika virus	Zika virus disease
Protozoa	
Entamoeba histolytica	Amebiasis; amebic dysentery
Giardia lamblia	Giardiasis
Trichomonas vaginalis	Trichomoniasis
Ectoparasites	
Pthirus pubis	Pediculosis pubis
Sarcoptes scabiei	Scabies
Fungus	
Candida albicans	Candidiasis

with infected men have a greater risk of contracting gonorrhea if they are the receptive partner.[5]

Transmission of gonococcal infection generally requires contact of epithelial (mucosal) surfaces, such as occurs during vaginal, oral, or anal intercourse, and infection in adults can be maintained in the vagina, rectum, oropharynx, or urethra.[4] A pregnant woman also can transmit gonorrhea to her fetus through infected cervical and vaginal secretions contacting the baby's mucosal surfaces during birth. Following vertical transmission, the newborn eyes can be infected and can result in blindness if untreated.

Treatment for gonorrhea is becoming more difficult because of rapidly developing resistance to available antibiotics. Both the CDC and the World Health Organization (WHO) advise dual drug treatment for gonorrhea to effectively treat infection and staunch increasing resistance.[3] This antibiotic resistance is increased in populations that frequently have oral or anal receptive intercourse, such men who have sex with men (MSM). The CDC states that it is reasonable to expect that gonorrhea may become resistant to all known antibiotics in the near future.[3]

Pathophysiology

Humans are the only natural hosts for *N. gonorrhoeae,* an aerobic, non–spore-forming, oxidase-positive gram-negative coccal (round) microorganism that usually appears in pairs (diplococci), with adjacent, slightly-flattened sides. Hairlike filaments, called *pili,* appear to help the microorganisms attach themselves to host cells: the epithelial cells of mucous membranes (Fig. 27.2). Columnar, transitional, and stratified squamous epithelial cells are most often infected. First, the microorganisms become attached to the plasma membranes (cell walls) of these cells, and then they invade the cells and begin to damage the mucosa. Generally, a quick leukocytic (inflammatory) response and exudation at the site of infection occur.

In women, the endocervical canal (inner portion of the cervix) is a common site of initial gonococcal infection, although urethral colonization and infection of glands (paraurethral [Skene] glands and greater vestibular [Bartholin] glands) near the urethra and vagina also are common. Several factors facilitate ascent of gonococci into the uterus and the fallopian tubes, where they can cause PID. Among these factors are (1) disintegration of the cervical mucous plug and an increase in vaginal pH to >4.5 during menstruation, (2) uterine contractions that may cause retrograde menstruation into the fallopian/uterine tubes, and (3) various microbes that possess virulent potentiating factors for chlamydia or gonococcal PID. Bacteria *(N. gonorrhoeae, Chlamydia*

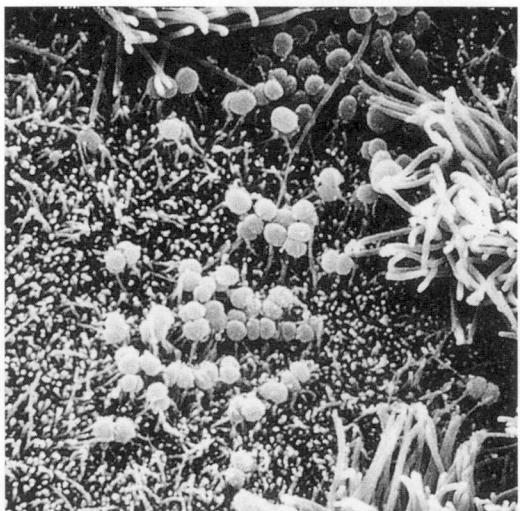

FIGURE 27.2 Gonococci. Scanning electron microscopy showing gonococci attaching to the nonciliated cells of human uterine/fallopian tube mucosa. (From Morse SA et al, editors: *Atlas of sexually transmitted diseases and AIDS,* ed 3, London, 2003, Mosby.)

trachomatis) also may adhere to sperm and be transported to the fallopian/uterine tubes. Once gonococci are in the fallopian/uterine tubes, progressive mucosal and submucosal invasion of the tissues causes sloughing of normal, ciliated tubal epithelium and a marked inflammatory response causing the tubes to fill with exudate (see Chapter 26 for more on PID).

In men, the gonococci typically infect the urethra or rectum. Untreated urethral infection can cause epididymitis in men, and potentially lead to urethral stricture, fistula formation, and sterility. However, a few men maintain asymptomatic infections for long periods of time.[3]

Concurrent or isolated oropharyngeal and anorectal infection can be found in infected men and women and may be difficult to detect with common testing mechanisms.[5] These sites are associated with greater antibiotic resistance than urethral or vaginal infection and may need additional treatment and monitoring.[5] One hypothesis for the increase in resistant strains in populations with a high prevalence of oral and anal intercourse is that the oral and rectal mucosae normally contain many nonpathogenic forms of *Neisseria* bacteria. These bacteria are often exposed to antibiotics used for other non–STI conditions; however, instead of being eliminated, they develop antibiotic resistance. Gonococci frequently share plasmids and DNA across species, facilitating the transfer of antibiotic resistance.[4] When the oropharynx and the rectum are infected by *N. gonorrhoeae,* the pathogens come in contact with antibiotic-resistant bacteria that share plasmids and DNA. As the *N. gonorrhea* proliferate, they can acquire antibiotic resistance before being spread to new individuals through orosexual contact.[4]

Clinical Manifestations

The clinical manifestations of gonorrhea can be categorized as local or systemic and uncomplicated or complicated. Uncomplicated local infections include urethral infections in men and urogenital infections in women. While infection can initially be asymptomatic, the majority of infected men will develop painful urination or purulent penile discharge, or both, within a week of infection.[3] These severe symptoms encourage most men in developed countries to seek treatment.[3] However, some men only have a little discharge or urethral itching (pruritus), and 5% to 10% never have signs or symptoms. Most cases of untreated gonococcal urethritis resolve spontaneously after several weeks, and more than 95% of individuals are asymptomatic by 6 months after infection (although they may still be infectious).

In women, the incubation period varies but those who develop symptoms usually manifest within 10 days of exposure or 1 to 2 days after the next menstrual period. More than half of gonorrhea infections in women are initially asymptomatic. Symptoms often do not appear until the infection has spread to the upper reproductive tract (uterus, fallopian/uterine tubes, and ovaries). Symptoms can include dysuria, increased vaginal discharge, abnormal menses (increased flow or dysmenorrhea), dyspareunia, lower abdominal/pelvic pain, and fever. Physical examination may disclose cervical friability and erythema (redness) and mucopurulent discharge from the cervical os (Fig. 27.3). There may be discharge from the paraurethral (Skene) or greater vestibular (Bartholin) glands if these sites are involved.

Anorectal gonorrhea occurs more commonly in MSM, but also is found in women both as an isolated finding and with coexisting urogenital gonorrhea.[1] Symptoms of anorectal gonorrhea range from mild anal pruritus (itching), mucopurulent rectal discharge, and slight rectal bleeding to severe rectal pain, tenesmus (painful and ineffectual straining at stool), and constipation. Physical examination findings include anal erythema and discharge and evidence of mucosal damage to the anus and rectum, such as friability, edema, and purulent exudate.

Gonococcal pharyngitis occurs after oral sexual contact with an infected partner. Symptomatic pharyngitis is indistinguishable from

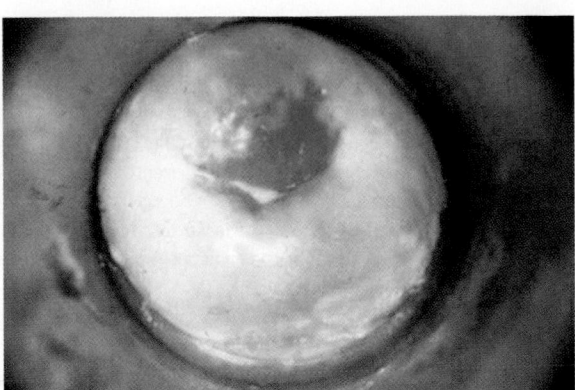

FIGURE 27.3 Gonococcal Cervicitis. The cervix is involved in 85% to 90% of cases in women, but discharge is profuse enough to be recognized in only 10%. (From Centers for Disease Control and Prevention [CDC]: *STD clinical slides [website]*. Available at: www.cdc.gov/std/training/clinicalslides/slides-dl.htm. Accessed April 27, 2017.)

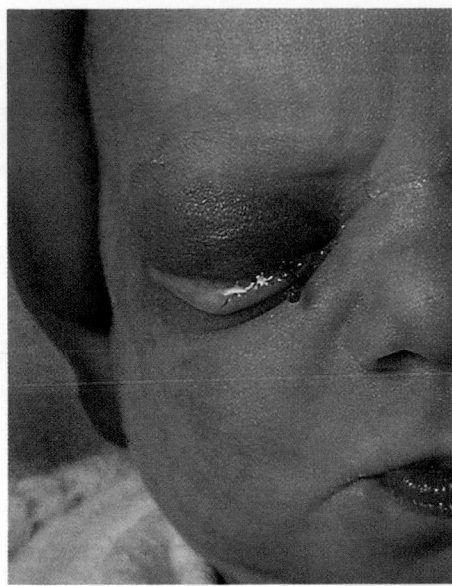

FIGURE 27.4 Gonococcal Ophthalmia Neonatorum. Examiner should be gloved. (From McMillan A, Scott GR: *Sexually transmitted infections,* ed 2, London, 2000, Churchill Livingstone.)

any other bacterial pharyngitis and can include fever, lymphadenopathy, and tonsillitis. However, 60% of people with oropharyngeal infections are asymptomatic.[3] In addition, many clinicians neglect to test for oropharyngeal gonorrhea because they do not screen for unprotected oral sex. Cure rates for this type of gonorrhea are much lower because of inadequate antibiotic concentrations in oral tissue.[4] Other sites of uncomplicated local infections include the eyes, leading to conjunctivitis; this condition occurs almost exclusively in newborns born vaginally to infected mothers. Primary cutaneous infection also has been reported and is usually manifested as a localized ulcer of the genitalia, perineum, proximal lower extremities, or fingers.

Complicated gonococcal infections include prostatitis, epididymitis, lymphangitis, and urethral stricture in men, and salpingitis, PID, and bartholinitis in women. Infections spread from the site of infection further into the genital tract, causing severe inflammation and scarring. In women, infection of the uterus, uterine tubes, and eventually the peritoneum is known as *PID*. The onset of PID symptoms may be rapid and usually occurs during menses.[6] Women may experience chills, fever, nausea, vomiting, and lower abdominal/pelvic pain that worsens with movement, such as walking, coughing, sneezing, or intercourse. Abdominal palpation often discloses bilateral lower quadrant tenderness and rebound tenderness from peritoneal irritation.[3] Marked tenderness of the internal genitalia is often noted during pelvic examination.

PID resulting from any pathogen contributes to infertility through a variety of mechanisms. During infection, the delicate ciliated epithelium of the uterine tubes is permanently damaged and the lack of regular cilia movement can impair the transit of sperm and fertilized ova.[6] Scarring and adhesions of the tubes may further impair fertility. Up to 18% of women who have been diagnosed with PID experience later infertility, and ectopic pregnancy rates in this population are as high as 9% because of slowed motility of the cilia in the fallopian tubes.[6]

Disseminated gonococcal infection (DGI) is a rare systemic complication caused by the spread of infection through the bloodstream. Symptoms of this life-threatening condition include a generalized rash, severe joint pain, and even meningitis and endocarditis.[3] Gonococcal strains that can cause DGI may cause genital inflammation before systemic dissemination.[3]

If a mother has gonorrhea at the time of birth, she can transmit the infection to her child. Most states require that all infants receive prophylactic ophthalmic antibiotics to prevent gonococcal eye infection (ophthalmia neonatorum) (Fig. 27.4). Topical antibiotics may not be effective in eliminating neonatal infection, and systemic treatment is indicated for all newborns with known exposure.[3] Untreated infection causes bilateral corneal ulceration, with a profuse yellow or gray purulent exudate, and is followed by necrosis, scarring, and blindness. Newborns born to infected mothers also may develop gonorrheal rhinitis, anorectal infection, or an abscess at the site of electrode placement for fetal monitoring. Onset of symptoms generally occurs 1 to 12 days after birth.[3]

Evaluation and Treatment

Because of the large percentage of infected women without symptoms, routine genital tract screening for at-risk women (i.e., those younger than age 25, pregnant, or with a new sexual partner) is recommended. Men should be screened according to risk factors and symptoms.[3] Clinical signs and symptoms are not sufficient for the differential diagnosis. The test that is used should be selected on the basis of the suspected site of infection. Nucleic acid hybridization tests can be used on samples collected from the vagina and urethra (of adult males and females; female children but not male children), as well as urine (except in boys).[3] Culture should be used to diagnose infections of the rectum, oropharynx, and conjunctiva of both sexes and all ages, as well as any site on boys.[3] Microscopic evaluation of Gram-stained slides of specimens from symptomatic men also can be used for diagnosis, and it is deemed positive for *N. gonorrhoeae* if gram-negative diplococci with typical "kidney bean" morphology are seen inside polymorphonuclear leukocytes.

N. gonorrhoeae has developed resistance to many antibiotics and has the real potential to become resistant to all current treatments.[3] There is currently only one CDC recommended drug (ceftriaxone) to treat gonorrhea, although less-effective alternatives are available.[3] To prevent further drug resistance, the CDC and the WHO recommend a multidrug treatment for gonorrhea that also is effective against chlamydia.[3] The CDC is closely observing the drug resistance of gonorrhea through monitoring of samples obtained at clinics around the country. CDC treatment guidelines are updated regularly and the most recent edition, found on the CDC website or app, should be used. Current CDC treatment guidelines for uncomplicated gonorrheal

BOX 27.1   **OUTPATIENT TREATMENT FOR UNCOMPLICATED GONORRHEA* INFECTION OF THE CERVIX, URETHRA, RECTUM, AND PHARYNX**

- One of the following:
  Ceftriaxone, 250 mg IM in a single dose
- *AND* to prevent drug resistance and treat potential infection with chlamydia:
  Azithromycin, 1 g PO in a single dose

*Antibiotic resistance is rapidly increasing for this pathogen; please check current guidelines at the Centers for Disease Control and Prevention website at https://www.cdc.gov and search "gonorrhea." *IM,* Intramuscularly; *PO,* orally.
Data from Workowski KA, Bolan GA: *MMWR Recommend Rep* 64(RR-03):1–137, 2015.

BOX 27.2   **PROGRESSION OF UNTREATED SYPHILIS**

Stage I, primary syphilis—local invasion: *Treponema pallidum* multiplies in epithelium, producing granulomatous tissue reaction (chancre); lymph-containing microorganisms drain into adjacent lymph nodes and stimulate immune responses
Stage II, secondary syphilis—systemic disease: blood-borne bacteria spread to all major organ systems; immune system suppresses infection and symptoms regress spontaneously
Stage III, latent syphilis—silent infection: transmission of infection possible even though there are no clinical signs of infection
Stage IV, tertiary syphilis—noninfectious disease: significant morbidity and mortality occur; destructive skin, bone, and soft tissue lesions, or gummas, result from severe hypersensitivity; cardiovascular complications (aneurysms, heart valve insufficiency, heart failure) and neurosyphilis develop

infections are listed in Box 27.1. Complicated infections require intravenous antibiotic therapy and possibly hospitalization.

Sexual partners also are assessed and treated according to these protocols, and sexual contact is avoided until treatment is completed. Condoms for all genital contact, including oral sex, are strongly recommended to prevent future infection.

Syphilis

Syphilis, a disease with local and systemic manifestations that stretch over years, has been well-known throughout history. Many famous figures from the ancient world and royal families were thought or known to have had syphilis. With the advent of antibiotics and intensive public health efforts during and after World War II, the prevalence of syphilis declined sharply. Rates of syphilis reached a record low in 2000.[7] However, since this all-time low, the rate of syphilis in the United States has doubled to 5.3 cases per 100,000. Men account for nearly 91% of all new cases of syphilis, whereas rates between sexes were equivalent two decades ago.[7] Data suggest this increase is driven by transmission of syphilis among MSM and accounts for over 89% of new cases.[1]

Congenital syphilis, caused by vertical transmission of the spirochete, also has experienced resurgence in the United States. After years of decline, the rate of congenital syphilis increased by 38% between 2012 and 2014 to 11.6 per 100,000 births.[8] During pregnancy, untreated early syphilis results in perinatal death in as many as 40% of cases and may lead to perinatal complications in more than 70% of cases because the spirochete can cross the placental membrane to infect the fetus.[9] However, simple treatment with penicillin is 98% effective at preventing vertical transmission.[8] Therefore all pregnant women should be screened at their first prenatal visit, and women at risk should be screened again in the third trimester and at the time of delivery.[8]

◆Pathophysiology

Treponema pallidum, the cause of syphilis, is an anaerobic spirochete bacterium that can grow in any human organ or tissue but cannot be cultured in vitro. When viewed through dark-field microscopy, the *Treponema* (individual microorganism) resembles a corkscrew, with regular, tight spirals and a rotary motion.

Because the bacterium is present in exudate from moist mucosal or cutaneous lesions, the spirochete is usually transmitted to others during the first few years of infection.[3] Transmission generally occurs through minor abrasions during sexual intercourse but can occur extragenitally

as well. Although condoms can decrease the likelihood of infection, if lesions are present on areas not covered during intercourse, transmission can occur even with safer sex practices.

The course of untreated syphilis consists of four stages based on clinical findings: primary, secondary, latent, and tertiary (Box 27.2); the division between stages is not always apparent and the drug of choice is the same for all stages.[3]

Primary syphilis begins at the site of bacterial invasion (Fig. 27.5), where *T. pallidum* multiplies in the epithelium and produces a granulomatous tissue reaction called a chancre. Some microorganisms drain with lymph into adjacent lymph nodes. Within the nodes and at the site of the chancre, the cell-mediated and humoral immune responses are stimulated.

Secondary syphilis is systemic. During this stage, blood-borne bacteria spread to all major organ systems. The secondary stage is followed by a period during which the immune system is able to suppress the infection. Even without treatment, spontaneous resolution of the skin lesions occurs and the individual enters the latent stage of infection.

Latent syphilis may be subdivided into early and late stages; however, no specific criteria delineate one from the other.[3] Medical history and serologic studies can show that syphilis is present, but the individual has no clinical manifestations. Transmission remains possible during this phase.

Tertiary syphilis is the most severe stage, involving significant morbidity and mortality. The pathogenesis of syphilitic manifestations at this stage remains unclear. The destructive skin, bone, and soft tissue lesions (called gummas) of tertiary syphilis probably are caused by a severe hypersensitivity reaction to the microorganism. Within the cardiovascular system, infection with *T. pallidum* may cause aneurysms, heart valve insufficiencies, and heart failure.

Congenital syphilis (CS) is caused by vertical transmission and is estimated to cause 500,000 fetal and neonatal deaths every year worldwide.[9] Syphilis becomes a systemic disease shortly after maternal infection and can be transmitted to the fetus as early as the ninth week of gestation because the spirochete can pass through the placenta. Intrauterine infection causes fetal or perinatal death in 40% of affected infants, and many live-born infants have permanent, lifelong morbidity, including congenital abnormalities.[9] The risk of CS is estimated at up to 80% in primary syphilis and declines with advancing stages of the disease.[9] Penicillin is very effective in decreasing morbidity and mortality if the disease can be diagnosed early in fetal development.[10]

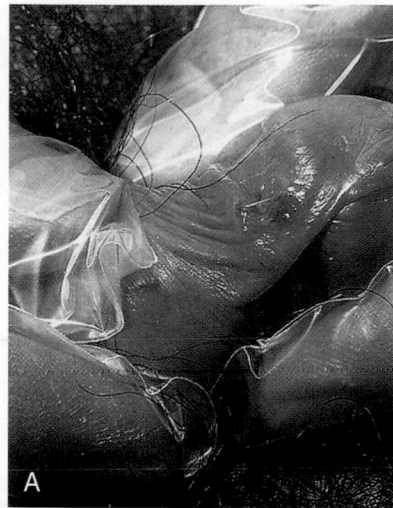

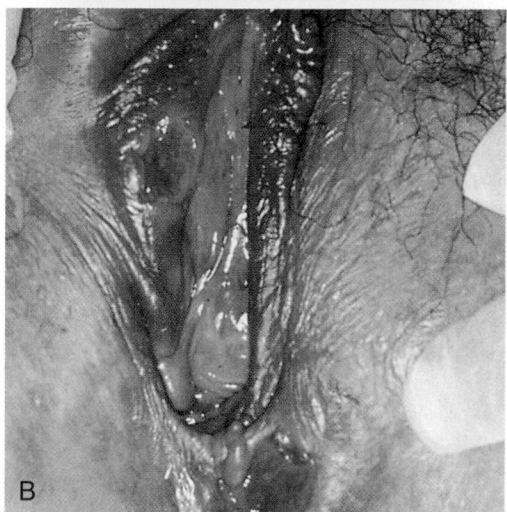

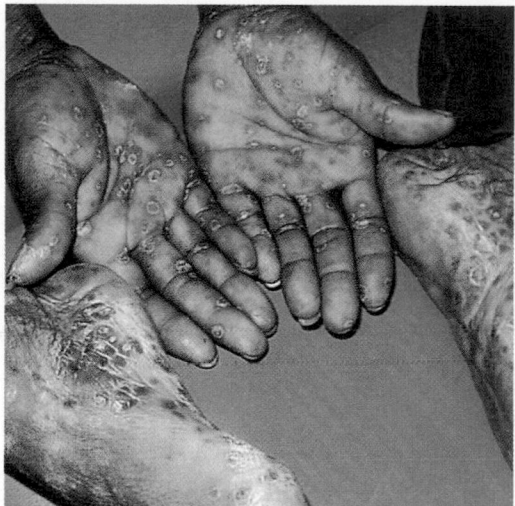

FIGURE 27.6 Secondary Syphilis. Secondary syphilis to the palms and plantar surfaces. (From Morse S et al, editors: *Atlas of sexually transmitted diseases and AIDS,* ed 4, London, 2013, Saunders.)

FIGURE 27.5 Primary Syphilis. **A,** Penile chancre. **B,** Vulval chancres; the labia and perineum show induration and edema of chancres. (**A** From McMillan A, Scott GR: *Sexually transmitted infections,* ed 2, London, 2000, Churchill Livingstone; **B** courtesy Barbara Romanowski, MD, from Morse SA et al, editors: *Atlas of sexually transmitted diseases and AIDS,* ed 4, London, 2013, Saunders.)

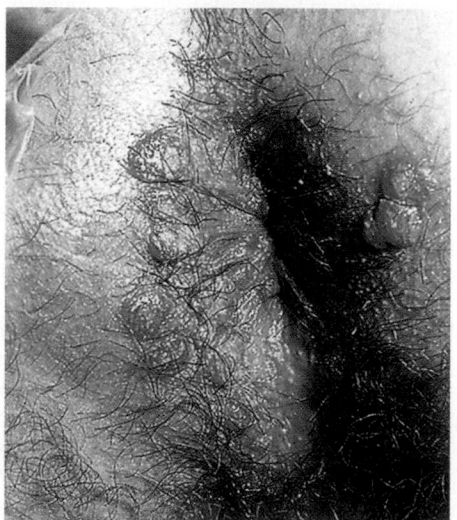

FIGURE 27.7 Condylomata Lata. Broad-based, moist, dark-field–positive condylomata lata of the perineum. (From McMillan A, Scott GR: *Sexually transmitted infections,* ed 2, London, 2000, Churchill Livingstone.)

◆Clinical Manifestations
Primary Stage

In adults, the incubation period of syphilis ranges from 12 days to 12 weeks after exposure and averages 3 weeks. A sore, or *hard chancre,* develops at the site of treponemal entry. Typically the chancre is an eroded, painless, firm, and indurated (hard) ulcer up to 2 cm in diameter. Firm, enlarged, and nontender regional lymph nodes accompany chancres. Typical chancres of the penis and vulva are shown in Fig. 27.5. Syphilitic chancres are not always typical and syphilis should be considered in the presence of any open lesion. Secondary infection can cause chancres to become necrotic and painful, and lesions on the fingers may be dry, scaly, and papular or moist and vegetative. If left untreated, the chancre of primary syphilis heals in 2 to 8 weeks and then spontaneously disappears, usually without leaving a scar.

Secondary Stage

Clinical manifestations of secondary syphilis usually develop 6 weeks after the first appearance of the chancre but may overlap with those of

the primary stage. Systemic symptoms are variable and can include low-grade fever, malaise, sore throat, hoarseness, anorexia, generalized adenopathy, headache, joint pain, and skin or mucous membrane lesions or rashes. Cutaneous (skin) rashes are generally papulosquamous (raised and scaly), but any variation or combination of macular (flat), papular (raised), and pustular (pus-filled) lesions may be seen. Lesions are often widespread and bilateral, appearing on the palms and soles (Fig. 27.6). Some lesions become hypertrophied, flat, moist, and wartlike or vegetative (e.g., cauliflower-like). These lesions, called condylomata lata, are highly contagious and develop on the perineum, vulva, and groin of women (Fig. 27.7), and around the inner thigh and anal area in men and women. Besides skin sores, oral mucous membrane lesions (known as *mucous patches*), lymphadenopathy, pruritus, and alopecia are common. Some individuals develop anemia, leukocytosis, increased sedimentation rate, hepatitis, transitory proteinuria, arthritis, electrocardiographic abnormalities, and central nervous system (CNS) symptoms. Regardless of treatment, cutaneous lesions generally heal in 2 to 10 weeks. Within the CNS, the presence of *T. pallidum* in cerebrospinal fluid may cause the manifestations of neurosyphilis, including altered mental status and meningitis, which can occur within any stage of syphilis infection but are more common in early stages of infection.[3]

Latent and Tertiary Stages

The asymptomatic, latent stage of syphilis may be as short as 1 year or as long as a lifetime. After the latent stage, tertiary syphilis may present with gummas, cardiovascular lesions, and neurosyphilis manifestations, including tabes dorsalis and general paresis.[3] Tertiary syphilis is rare because of the widespread availability of antibiotics.

Congenital Syphilis

Congenital syphilis (CS) is caused by the passage of the spirochete across the placental membrane to affect any or all fetal tissues. The infection can cause fetal death or growth abnormalities, including changes in the fetal bones, teeth, and neurologic system. Affected newborns can have a variety of manifestations of the disease, including growth abnormalities, rashes, hepatosplenomegaly, jaundice, and CNS involvement, including blindness and deafness.[8] A classically reported late manifestation of congenital syphilis is notched incisors. While now rare, this stigma is used in historical studies of syphilis.

◆Evaluation and Treatment

Numerous dermatologic disorders can mimic the skin lesions of secondary syphilis, making differential diagnosis difficult. Laboratory confirmation is important. Two categories of serologic testing exist: nontreponemal antigen tests and treponemal antibody tests.[3] Nontreponemal antigen tests, which demonstrate the presence of *reagin* (a group of antibodies present in syphilis) in serum, provide indirect evidence of infection. Examples of nontreponemal analysis are the Venereal Disease Research Laboratory (VDRL) antigen and the rapid plasma reagin (RPR) tests (Box 27.3). These tests yield a positive result (presence of reagin) in more than 50% of individuals with primary syphilis and in 100% of individuals in the secondary phase of disease and can be useful in screening and assessing response to treatment.[3]

Because the VDRL and RPR tests have high rates of false positives, a treponemal test is performed if the screening test is positive. Treponemal tests are serologic-specific tests that are used to assess antibody response to *T. pallidum* and include enzyme immunoassays (EIAs), chemoluminescence immunoassays, the fluorescent treponemal antibody absorption (FTA-ABS) test, and the passive particle agglutination (TP-PA) assay.[3]

Preferred treatment for all stages of syphilis is parenteral injection of benzathine penicillin G, because other types of penicillin are not as effective. If the individual has manifested signs of the disease for less than 1 year, a single intramuscular dose is appropriate. If signs have been present for more than 1 year or they are asymptomatic and assumed to be in late latent syphilis, the treatment is three weekly injections. The CDC is the best source for current information on treatment regimens.[3] Penicillin therapy also is appropriate for pregnant women to prevent vertical transmission.[3] There is no evidence to date that *T. pallidum* has developed resistance to penicillin. In fact, it is highly sensitive; but because of the slow replication time, serum levels must be maintained for 7 to 14 days. Men and nonpregnant women who are allergic to penicillin may receive oral doxycycline, 100 mg twice daily for 14 days, or tetracycline, 500 mg every day for 14 days. Pregnant women with a penicillin allergy should be desensitized and then treated with benzathine penicillin G as recommended by the CDC because the other available antibiotics cause lifelong discoloration of the forming teeth of the fetus.[3]

BOX 27.3   FALSE-POSITIVE SEROLOGIC TESTS FOR SYPHILIS

Reasons for False-Positive, Nontreponemal Reactions (VDRL, RPR)
Transient Reactions (<6 Months)
  Technical error (low titer)
  Mycoplasma pneumonia
  Enterovirus infections
  Infectious mononucleosis
  Pregnancy
  Narcotic abuse
  Advanced tuberculosis
  Scarlet fever
  Viral and atypical pneumonia
  Brucellosis
  Rat-bite fever
  Leptospirosis
  Measles
  Mumps
  Lymphogranuloma venereum
  Malaria
  Trypanosomiasis
  Varicella

Chronic Reactions (>6 Months)
  Malaria
  Leprosy
  Systemic lupus erythematosus
  Narcotic abuse
  Other connective tissue diseases
  Elderly population
  Hashimoto thyroiditis
  Rheumatoid arthritis
  Reticuloendothelial malignancy
  Familial false-positive reaction
  Idiopathic

Reasons for False-Positive, Treponemal-Specific Reactions (FTA-ABS)
  Technical error
  Inefficient sorbents
  Healthy individuals without syphilis
  Genital herpes simplex
  Pregnancy
  Lupus erythematosus (skin only or systemic)
  Alcoholic cirrhosis
  Scleroderma
  Mixed connective tissue disease

FTA-ABS, Fluorescent treponemal antibody absorption; *RPR,* rapid plasma reagin; *VDRL,* Venereal Disease Research Laboratory.

Repeated assessment of VDRL or RPR titers is used to determine effectiveness of treatment. Titers should decrease fourfold if treatment was successful. Sexual partners also are tested and treated, and the use of condoms is recommended until effective treatment is verified.

Newborns of mothers with documented syphilis need careful evaluation after birth. Definitive diagnosis of congenital syphilis is complicated by the presence of maternal antibodies in the newborn's blood. Treatment decisions are made based on maternal status, clinical symptoms of congenital syphilis, and also comparison of maternal and neonatal titers.[3]

If the infant requires treatment, penicillin is the drug of choice with carefully titrated dosing depending on fetal weight and the day of treatment, and the CDC is the best source of current information.[3]

Chancroid

Chancroid, or soft chancre, is an acute infectious disease that was first differentiated from syphilis in 1852. It is caused by *Haemophilus ducreyi*, a gram-negative bacillus. The incidence of chancroid is decreasing worldwide, and it is infrequently seen in the United States.[1] Sporadic outbreaks occur throughout the world and tend to be associated with prostitution and illicit drug use, when individuals continue to engage in intercourse in spite of a painful genital lesion.[11] Chancroid is a risk factor for HIV acquisition, and existing HIV infection is a risk factor for chancroid infection with exposure.[5]

◆ Pathophysiology

H. ducreyi is a gram-negative bacillus with rounded ends. It is commonly observed in small chains or clusters along mucous strands under a microscope. Transmission can occur through sexual contact and autoinoculation, but there is no evidence for vertical transmission.[3] Chancroid lesions are found throughout the genital area. Initially, the papule enlarges; it then erodes into a soft, circumscribed ulcer containing a superficial exudate of varying size and presentation.[11] Beneath the ulcer is a lesion characterized by edema, endothelial proliferation, and a base of granulation tissue. Adjacent lymph nodes are acutely inflamed and full of polymorphonuclear leukocytes and necrotic cells.

◆ Clinical Manifestations

Chancroid has an incubation period of 3 to 10 days.[11] Women are generally asymptomatic but, depending on the site of infection, can present with less obvious symptoms (dysuria, dyspareunia, vaginal discharge, pain on defecation, or rectal bleeding). Constitutional symptoms are unusual. An initial vesicopustule lesion forms at the site of inoculation and erodes into a soft ulcer with a necrotic base; surrounding erythema; and a ragged, serpiginous (spreading) border (Fig. 27.8). Unilateral, painful, local lymphadenopathy presents in about half of infected individuals. Inguinal buboes (unilocular abscess of the inguinal lymph nodes) develop 7 to 10 days after the initial chancre and fill with exudate. In 25% to 60% of cases, the buboes spontaneously rupture out onto the skin, spreading the infection through autoinoculation.

Ulcers on the prepuce may lead to phimosis or paraphimosis. Other complications of chancroid include balanitis, secondary infections, necrosis, and fistula formation. Lesions may take months or years to heal and cause scarring.[3]

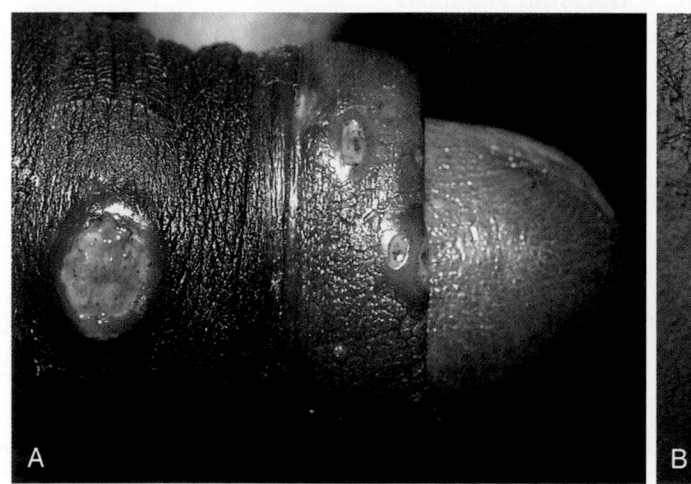

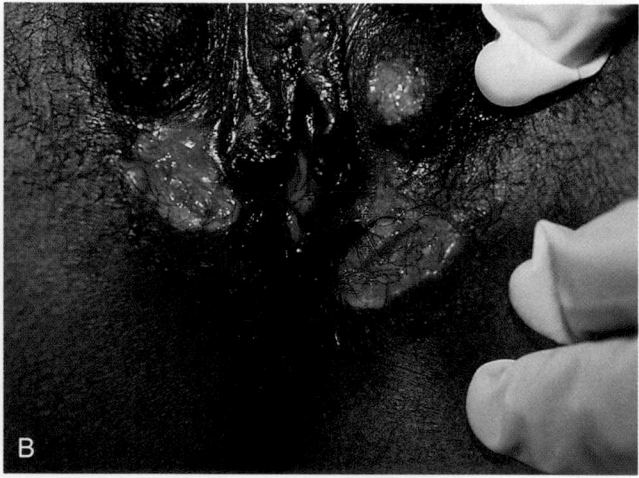

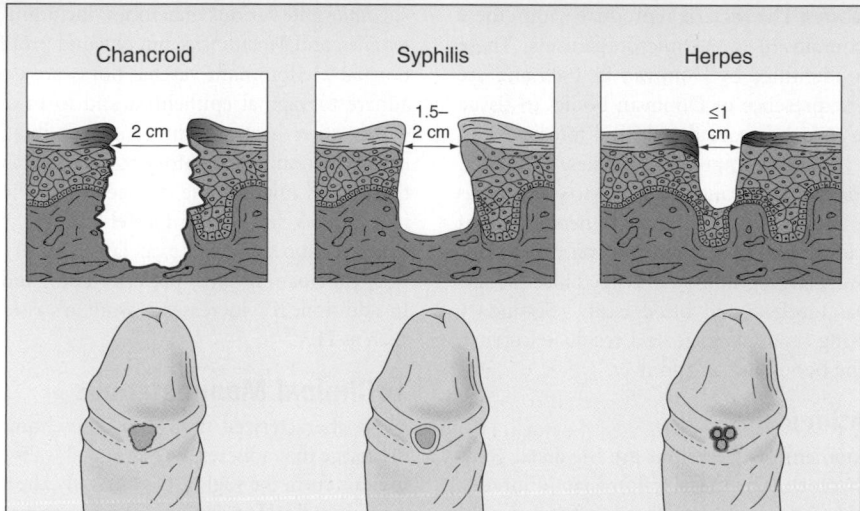

FIGURE 27.8 Chancroid. A, Ulcers on the penile shaft. **B,** Multiple vulvar lesions. **C,** Differences in clinical appearance among chancroid, syphilis, and genital herpes. (From Morse SA et al, editors: *Atlas of sexually transmitted diseases and AIDS,* ed 4, London, 2013, Saunders.)

❖Evaluation and Treatment

Chancroid is easily confused with other types of genital ulcers, particularly those of syphilis, genital herpes, and granuloma inguinale (see Fig. 27.8). Unlike the syphilitic ulcer, chancroidal ulcer is painful, tender, and nonindurated and inguinal lymphadenopathy is pronounced. Microscopic analysis of a Gram-stained smear from the chancroid helps to identify the microorganism. Definitive diagnosis depends on recovery of *H. ducreyi* from cultured specimens; however, the culture medium is not commercially available.[3] Diagnosis depends on the clinical presentation of a painful genital ulcer with inguinal lymphadenopathy and with negative testing for syphilis and herpes simplex virus.[3] In addition, HIV testing is recommended because chancroid is a cofactor for transmission of HIV.

Resistance to recommended antibiotics has emerged in isolated instances worldwide. Recent treatment recommendations include a single intramuscular injection of ceftriaxone (250 mg) or a single dose of oral azithromycin (1 g). Effective oral multiple-dose regimens include ciprofloxacin, 500 mg orally twice daily for 3 days; or erythromycin, 500 mg 3 times daily for 7 days. Persons infected with HIV and uncircumcised men have higher rates of treatment failure and may require a longer treatment regimen. Treatment failure requires more intensive assessment for coinfection with other diseases.[3] Simultaneous treatment of sexual partners and use of condoms are recommended to prevent reinfection.

Granuloma Inguinale

Granuloma inguinale (donovanosis) is a chronic, progressively destructive bacterial infection caused by *Klebsiella granulomatis*. Although sexually transmitted, granuloma inguinale has a low transmission rate between sexual partners.[11] Infection through fecal contamination and autoinoculation also is possible.[11] As with all genital ulcerative diseases, granuloma inguinale plays a role in HIV transmission.[11] Granuloma inguinale very rarely occurs in the United States[11]; it is more prevalent in some tropical and subtropical parts of the world (India, New Guinea, Africa, central Australia, and to a lesser extent the Caribbean and Brazil).

❖Pathophysiology

C. granulomatis is a gram-negative, nonsporing, nonmotile, encapsulated rod not easily cultured in the laboratory. After an individual is infected, bacteria survive and multiply within vacuoles of large histiocytic cells or polymorphonuclear leukocytes. The bacteria reproduce within these cells, and a vacuole may contain 20 to 30 microorganisms. These bacteria-filled vacuoles were identified by Donovan in 1905 and are termed Donovan bodies. The presence of Donovan bodies in tissue smears of material from the lesions is considered ideal for diagnosis, but this test is difficult even in well-equipped laboratories.[3]

The incubation period of granuloma inguinale is 8 to 80 days. As lesions begin to form, single lesions often coalesce with nearby lesions or form new lesions by autoinoculation of nearby skin surfaces. Progression from the initial nodule to a large, granuloma-heaped ulcer occurs slowly. These lesions are vascularized and bleed easily.[3] Secondary infection may occur, increasing tissue damage and residual scarring. The disease may spread to the bones, joints, and liver.

❖Clinical Manifestations

The primary sites for development of the lesions are the distal penis in men and the introitus in women. The initial lesion is an indurated, sharply defined, painless, subcutaneous nodule that is often preceded and accompanied by itching. Nodules bleed easily and contain abundant red, beefy-looking granulation tissue. These lesions spread as the disease progresses. Secondary infection may occur, increasing tissue damage

and residual scarring. Although systemic symptoms are rare, the disease may spread to the bones, joints, and liver. In some cases, infection spreads to the inguinal area and produces pseudobuboes. In these instances, the affected lymph nodes are not directly affected, but the surrounding area may be infected and abscessed.

❖Evaluation and Treatment

Although the clinical manifestations of this disease are important for diagnosis, confirmation involves microscopic examination for Donovan bodies in a smear or biopsy specimen. Currently, there is not an FDA-approved laboratory test for detection of *K. granulomatis*.[3]

Many antibiotics successfully treat *K. granulomatis*. With effective antibiotic treatment, lesions begin to heal in 7 days, but treatment is continued for at least 3 weeks and until all lesions are healed. Oral therapy includes doxycycline, 100 mg twice a day; azithromycin, 1 g once a week for 3 weeks, and until lesions are healed; ciprofloxacin, 750 mg twice a day for at least 3 weeks; erythromycin base, 500 mg 4 times a day for at least 3 weeks; or trimethoprim-sulfamethoxazole, 160 mg/800 mg, double-strength tablet twice a day for at least 3 weeks.[3] Relapses can occur 6 to 18 months later despite effective initial therapy; thus prolonged follow-up is necessary as is treatment of sexual partners. Because other STIs frequently coexist, individuals should be tested for chlamydia, gonorrhea, syphilis, hepatitis B, and HIV.

Bacterial Vaginosis

Bacterial vaginosis (BV) (previously called nonspecific vaginitis, nonspecific vaginosis, or *Haemophilus*, *Corynebacterium*, or *Gardnerella* vaginitis) is a sexually associated condition, but is not necessarily considered an STI. The condition is associated with sexual contact, including genital touching and digital penetration, oral sex, and penile penetration. Although BV occurs mostly in sexually active women of reproductive age, it can affect women, especially menopausal women, who are not sexually active. BV is diagnosed by the presence of characteristic symptoms and clinical findings. Prevalence rates vary from 17% among women in family planning clinics to 37% among some groups of pregnant women. Fifty percent of women clinically diagnosed with BV state they are asymptomatic.[3]

❖Pathophysiology

The exact etiology of BV is unknown but is thought to be a dysbiosis of normal vaginal flora that is associated with sexual contact. *Gardnerella vaginalis* and various anaerobes, including *Mycoplasma hominis*, *Bacteroides*, and *Mobiluncus*, interact and proliferate when lactobacilli (the normal predominant vaginal flora) are decreased or absent. Bacteria adhere to vaginal epithelium and form a scaffolding-like biofilm to which other bacteria can adhere, facilitating their proliferation and causing a noninflammatory response in the surrounding tissues.[12] As the vaginal microbiome changes, catabolic enzymes degrade proteins into amines. In turn, amines elevate the vaginal pH and produce the characteristic fishy odor associated with BV. BV has been implicated in PID, chorioamnionitis, preterm labor, and postpartum endometritis. In addition, BV increases a woman's risk of contracting other STIs, such as HIV.[3]

❖Clinical Manifestations

BV is characterized by a thin, gray, homogeneous, and malodorous discharge that adheres to the vaginal walls but is often copious enough to drain from the vagina. Occasionally, the discharge is bubbly or frothy. The vaginal pH is usually 5 to 5.5, and women often complain of a strong, foul, fishy vaginal odor, particularly after intercourse and during menses. Odor is intensified by contact with alkaline secretions, including semen and menstrual discharge. Male and female partners of infected women may harbor the microorganisms responsible for BV but have no signs or symptoms.

Evaluation and Treatment

Diagnosis of BV can be made on the basis of the presence of three of four of the following criteria, known as *Amsel criteria:* (1) the presence of homogeneous, adherent gray or white vaginal discharge; (2) a vaginal pH greater than 4.5; (3) a positive amine odor in the presence of an alkali, such as potassium hydroxide, known as the *whiff test;* and (4) the presence of clue cells on wet mount.[3] *Clue cells* are considered pathognomonic for BV. They are vaginal epithelial cells that are covered with bacteria, causing them to look as if they were sprinkled with pepper. The saline wet mount also may show the absence of lactobacilli and few or no leukocytes. There also is a commercially available test, Affirm VPIII, that uses DNA hybridization to detect *G. vaginalis.* Cultures for BV are not recommended; however, high-risk individuals should be screened for gonorrhea and chlamydia.[3]

The most commonly used treatment for BV is a course of oral metronidazole (Flagyl), 500 mg twice daily for 7 days; 0.75% vaginal gel, once daily for 5 days; or clindamycin cream 2% applied vaginally for 7 days.[3] Alternative regimens include tinidazole, 2 g orally once daily for 2 days or 1 g orally for 5 days; oral clindamycin, 300 mg twice daily for 7 days; or clindamycin ovules, 100 mg intravaginally for 7 days.[3] Treatment for BV should be personalized based on the woman's needs and behaviors. For example, metronidazole and tinidazole strongly react with alcohol and should not be used by women who cannot or will not eliminate alcohol ingestion for the full duration of treatment plus an additional 24 hours. In addition, the ovules can weaken latex condoms and diaphragms.[3]

BV treatment in women infected with HIV is the same as that in individuals who are HIV-negative. The CDC currently recommends treatment of BV in pregnancy to reduce the risk of poor perinatal outcomes, including preterm birth.[3]

Chlamydia

Chlamydia is the common name for infections caused by *Chlamydia trachomatis* (CT). *C. trachomatis* is responsible for a variety of syndromes, including acute urethral syndrome, nongonococcal urethritis (NGU), mucopurulent cervicitis, and PID. Chlamydia is the most common reportable STI in the United States and is a leading cause of preventable infertility and ectopic pregnancy. In 2014, more than 1.4 million cases of chlamydial infections were reported,[1] the greatest number of cases ever reported in a single year. Rates of chlamydia infections are increasing in all age groups, areas of the country, and racial/ethnic groups. This increase probably reflects the continued expansion of screening efforts and the increased use of more sensitive diagnostic tests, as well as an actual increase in incidence.[3] The majority of reported cases of chlamydia are in people younger than 26 years old, but the incidence in older adults is increasing.[1] Up to 90% of women with CT infection are asymptomatic, which can delay diagnosis and increase the risk of long-term health sequelae.[3] Without timely treatment, 10% to 20% of women will have the infection spread to the uterus and uterine tubes.[3]

Risk groups for chlamydia include age younger than 26, recent new sexual partner, and drug use or other risky behaviors.[1] Like gonorrhea, *Chlamydia* infection can be transmitted from mother to infant during birth and can cause eye infections and pneumonia in affected newborns.[3]

Pathophysiology

C. trachomatis is an obligate, gram-negative intracellular bacterium that lacks the ability to reproduce without a host cell. It is differentiated from other bacteria by its unique two-part growth cycle. The first part

consists of an elementary body that is small and resilient and is able to survive extracellularly.[13] Once this elementary body attaches itself to a receptor host cell, it is able to enter by endocytosis. Once inside the cell, the second part of the cycle begins and the microorganism becomes a metabolically active parasite, reproducing within the cell until the cell is destroyed and ruptures, disseminating up to 1000 new elementary bodies. Infection with *C. trachomatis* produces an inflammatory reaction that results in permanent scarring of tissues.[13]

Chlamydia microorganisms are always pathogens; they are not part of the normal flora of the urogenital tract, despite the fact that infection is often asymptomatic. Numerous serotypes, or strains, of *C. trachomatis* have been identified. Some cause urogenital infection; some, blindness; and others, lymphogranuloma venereum, which is discussed in the next section.[13] The strains of *C. trachomatis* that cause urogenital infection require squamous-columnar and columnar-epithelial cells as hosts. *C. trachomatis* infects and disrupts superficial tissues, causing damage and scarring, but does not seem to invade or destroy deeper tissues.[14]

In newborns, several sites may be inoculated with *Chlamydia* during passage through the infected maternal cervix. These include the eye, nasopharynx, rectum, and vagina. The infant also may aspirate infected secretions with its first breaths, resulting in chlamydial pneumonitis and substantial newborn morbidity.[3]

Clinical Manifestations

Chlamydial infections are asymptomatic in up to 90% of adults.[3] Urogenital infections caused by *Chlamydia* closely parallel those caused by gonorrhea. Both microorganisms infect superficial genital tract tissues, such as mucosa of the urethra and cervix, and both can invade the epididymides, the fallopian/uterine tubes, and (rarely) the hepatic capsule. Table 27.2 lists the pathophysiologic similarities of chlamydial and gonococcal infections. Men and women have different responses to the infection.

TABLE 27.2	SIMILARITY OF CLINICAL SYNDROMES CAUSED BY *Neisseria gonorrhoeae* AND *Chlamydia trachomatis*	
SITE OF INFECTION	**CLINICAL SYNDROME**	
	N. gonorrhoeae	*C. trachomatis*
Men		
Urethra	Urethritis	Urethritis
Epididymis	Epididymitis	Epididymitis
Rectum	Proctitis	Proctitis
Conjunctiva	Conjunctivitis	Conjunctivitis
Systemic	Disseminated gonococcal infection	Reiter syndrome
Women		
Urethra	Acute urethral syndrome	Acute urethral syndrome
Bartholin gland	Bartholinitis	Bartholinitis
Cervix	Cervicitis	Cervicitis; cervical atypia
Fallopian tube	Salpingitis	Salpingitis
Conjunctiva	Conjunctivitis	Conjunctivitis
Liver capsule	Perihepatitis	Perihepatitis
Systemic	Disseminated gonococcal infection	Arthritis-dermatitis syndrome

Data from Stamm WE, Holmes KK: *Chlamydia trachomatis* infections in the adult. In Holmes KK et al, editors: *Sexually transmitted diseases,* ed 2, New York, 1990, McGraw-Hill.

The rate of chlamydial infection in men appears to be rising, with a 22% increase in diagnoses from 2010 to 2014. This increase may be an expression of increased testing as a result of easier screening methods. Rates of diagnosis are highest in adolescent men who have sex with women.[1]

Although most men do not have symptoms even while contagious, chlamydial infection can cause nongonococcal urethritis. Clinically, urethritis caused by gonorrhea and chlamydia cannot be differentiated: both have a 7- to 21-day incubation period and cause dysuria. Although urethral discharge in men may be similar in the two infections, chlamydial discharge tends to be more clear and gonococcal discharge more purulent. Men might note a clear, mucous discharge or mild burning with urination.

Chlamydial epididymitis can accompany urethritis in men and is characterized by fever and a unilaterally painful, swollen scrotum. Chlamydial infection also causes proctitis (rectal inflammation) in people who have receptive anal intercourse. Chlamydial proctitis is generally mild, although it may, like gonorrheal proctitis, cause rectal bleeding, mucous discharge, and diarrhea. Reiter syndrome (urethritis, conjunctivitis, arthritis, and characteristic mucocutaneous lesions) is also associated with untreated urogenital tract infections.

C. trachomatis can cause asymptomatic urethral infection or acute urethral syndrome (dysuria, urinary frequency, and presence of sterile pus in the urine) in infected women. Chlamydial infection of Bartholin/greater vestibular glands can cause purulent discharge leading to a Bartholin cyst. Women with chlamydial cervicitis may be asymptomatic or may have a yellow mucopurulent discharge from the cervical os and a hypertrophic, edematous, and friable area of cervical ectopy. The woman also may report intermenstrual or postcoital spotting. Although ectopy alone does not indicate a pathologic condition, an erythematous, raw, and friable cervix is suggestive of chlamydial cervicitis (Fig. 27.9).

Chlamydia infection is the leading cause of tubal infertility in women because of infectious damage to the fallopian tubes similar to that which may occur with gonorrhea. Risk factors for infertility include the duration and severity of infection and the lifetime number of chlamydial infections. Even women with asymptomatic salpingitis have a risk of subsequent infertility.[3]

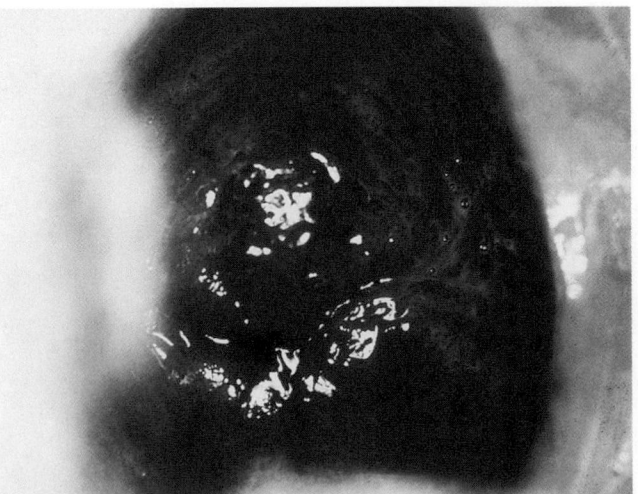

FIGURE 27.9 Chlamydial Cervicitis. Beefy red mucosa of columnar epithelium of cervix. (Courtesy Paul Weisner. From Morse SA et al, editors: *Atlas of sexually transmitted diseases and AIDS*, ed 4, London, 2013, Saunders.)

The most common manifestations of chlamydial infections in the newborn are conjunctivitis and pneumonia. Prophylactic treatment with antibiotic eye ointment at birth does not provide complete protection against neonatal conjunctivitis and does not protect against neonatal pneumonia. Intravenous (IV) antibiotics are needed for any child at risk of acquisition. Chlamydial conjunctivitis begins between 5 and 14 days after delivery when the infant's eyes begin to water. This discharge may become purulent, and both eyes may become red and swollen.

Scarring of the conjunctivae may result, but this infection does not cause blindness. Infants with chlamydial pneumonia develop staccato coughing spells, nasal congestion, and fever at 3 to 11 weeks of age.

◆Evaluation and Treatment

Since most infections are asymptomatic, the CDC recommends widespread screening of at-risk groups. A complete detailing of groups needing annual screening can be found in their treatment guideline, on their website, or through their smartphone app. All sexually active women who are less than 26 years old should be screened annually. In addition, the CDC recommends that all women, regardless of age, be screened if they have a new sexual partner or their partner is not monogamous. Pregnant women should be routinely screened for *Chlamydia* at least once during pregnancy.[3]

Methods for diagnosing chlamydial infections include tissue culture, direct chlamydial enzyme immunoassay, fluorescein-labeled monoclonal antibody tests, and nucleic acid amplification testing (NAAT). Currently, tests using chlamydia-specific nucleic acid sequences are the most sensitive and cost-effective tests available. In addition, they are easy to use with a variety of specimen types.[3] Concurrent testing for gonorrhea can be done using the same swab. NAAT can be performed on samples taken from the vagina, endocervix, or urethra; or urine specimens can be used. The person should be tested in all the locations of genital contact. The ease of NAAT testing means that screening can be performed without a clinician, if needed, because the individual can collect the specimen following basic instructions.[3]

C. trachomatis is susceptible to inexpensive, readily accessible antibiotics, and treatment should begin as soon as possible to prevent complications. Treatment includes antibiotic therapy for infected individuals and all sexual contacts; abstinence or use of condoms during treatment and for 7 days after treatment is recommended. The CDC recommends observed, on-site treatment for both partners when feasible.[3]

Azithromycin is given 1 g orally, as a single dose, or a 7-day course of oral doxycycline is administered, 100 mg twice daily. Single-dose azithromycin is preferred if adherence to a multiple-dose, multiple-day regimen is not feasible for the individual. Alternative regimens include a 7-day course of oral erythromycin, 500 mg 4 times a day; or erythromycin E, 800 mg 4 times daily for 7 days. Ofloxacin, 300 mg twice daily; and levofloxacin, 500 mg once daily for 7 days, also are effective alternatives.[3] Azithromycin is the drug of choice in pregnancy. A test of cure is only needed if there is concern that treatment of both partners was not successful. However, treatment failures are common, especially with multidose regimens and when the partner is not immediately provided with a prescription.[3]

Lymphogranuloma Venereum

C. trachomatis (invasive serovars of strains L1, L2, or L3) can cause a chronic STI known as lymphogranuloma venereum (LGV), which may be confused with syphilis, herpes, or chancroid. LGV was previously rare in the developed world but now is increasingly found in men who have sex with men and may spread to other populations.[1] The infection is acquired during sexual intercourse or through contact with contaminated exudate from active lesions. HIV infection increases the likelihood of acquisition and the severity of symptoms.[15]

◆Pathophysiology

The strain of *C. trachomatis* that causes LGV probably penetrates skin and mucous membranes through tiny abrasions. LGV spreads to genital and rectal lymphatic tissue, where it causes marked inflammation, necrosis, buboes, abscesses of inguinal lymph nodes, and infection of surrounding tissues. Healing occurs by fibrosis after several weeks or months and results in scarring and damaging the lymph nodes and disrupting their function. LGV can cause permanent lymphatic disruption and genital disfigurement. Affected nodes become chronically swollen, hardened, and enlarged. *C. trachomatis* also spreads systemically through the bloodstream and can enter the CNS.[3]

◆Clinical Manifestations

The primary lesion of LGV appears after an incubation period of 5 to 21 days. The lesion is most commonly a herpetiform (multivesicular) ulcer, but it can assume various forms. The ulcer generally is asymptomatic and inconspicuous and heals rapidly, leaving no scar. However, when contracted through receptive anal intercourse (a common current mode of transmission), the ulcer is never visible. When rectal infection occurs, LGV can cause an inflammatory response that mimics inflammatory bowel disease or proctocolitis.[3] Other signs of primary LGV include a large, tender lymphatic nodule (especially unilateral) or bubo; urethritis; and cervicitis. While historically this infection resulted in three clinical stages, anorectal infection has become the most common location of infection and results in symptoms that mimic other primary care conditions.[11]

Clinical symptoms of anorectal infection mimic other inflammatory bowel conditions and include irregular bowel movements, multiple ulcerations of the rectal mucosa, mucopurulent rectal discharge, and rectovaginal fistulae in women. Individuals may have fever, rectal pain, and tenesmus. Rectal strictures, perirectal abscesses, and anal fissures may develop with untreated infection.[3]

◆Evaluation and Treatment

Clinical manifestations, history of sexual intercourse, and laboratory tests are used for LGV diagnosis. LGV is diagnosed with NAAT testing at the suspected site of infection. If clinical symptoms match LGV presentation, pharmacologic treatment should begin while waiting definitive diagnosis with test results.[3] LGV is treated with oral doxycycline, 100 mg twice daily for 21 days. A 21-day course of erythromycin (500 mg) also is effective. Sexual partners within the past 60 days should be treated.[3]

Viral Infections
Genital Herpes

Genital herpes, which causes painful blisters (cold sores), is the most common infectious cause of genital ulcerations in the United States. In fact, genital infection with herpes simplex virus (HSV) is an epidemic in the United States. HSV is not a reportable disease so national statistics are not available. However, HSV infections are estimated to affect 1 million new individuals each year. Recurrent infections are mostly asymptomatic (50% to 70%) and affect an estimated 50 million Americans annually.[1] Eighty percent of infected individuals do not know they have herpes. Genital herpes can be caused by either of the two serotypes of HSV: HSV-1 or HSV-2. Historically, HSV-1 lesions were more common around the mouth while HSV-2 lesions were more frequently found in the genital area. However, HSV-1 is increasingly found in the anogenital area.[1] HSV-2 outbreaks are more frequent and more severe, so serologic testing to determine the HSV subtype is warranted at diagnosis to guide suppression efforts.[3]

HSV infection is transmitted through contact with HSV-infected fluids or skin as occurs with genital skin or mucosal contact with a person shedding the virus. There is even the possibility that saliva alone can transmit the virus when placed on mucous membranes or genitals for lubrication.[16] Persons without symptoms probably transmit most infections. Asymptomatic viral shedding is common. Transmission rates are not well identified. However, women and men who are the receptive partner for men are more susceptible to contracting herpes related to prolonged semen contact with the vaginal or rectal mucosa. Any type of rough intercourse that causes breaks in the skin surface increases transmission as well. It is estimated that a woman has an 80% to 90% risk of developing genital herpes after being exposed to an infected man.

Condoms reduce the risk of transmission, especially from males to females.[17] However, if lesions or shedding occur outside the area covered by the condom, transmission can still occur.[17] Female condoms offer a bit more protection from HSV because they cover and protect the vulva, but they do not eliminate risk. HSV infection greatly increases the risk of HIV acquisition. People with HSV are 4 times more likely to contract HIV if exposed, potentially because of skin splits that occur as a result of HSV infection.[3]

Neonatal infections can begin in utero or, more commonly, during the intrapartum or postpartum period. The risk of transmission of HSV to the neonate varies from <1% among women with recurrence of known herpes at term to up to 30% to 50% in women who acquire HSV near term.[1] Perinatal transmission can cause extensive morbidity and mortality. Intrauterine transmission is rare (only 5% of neonatal infections) but can occur through transplacental or ascending infection and can cause fetal malformations.[18]

Eighty-five percent of infections are transmitted during the intrapartum period.[18] Infants are at greatest risk if the mother has a primary infection acquired near the time of delivery rather than a recurrent infection or an infection acquired during the first half of pregnancy.[1] Ruptured membranes have a role in the development of HSV. Rupture of membranes for more than 4 hours increases the risk of the fetus for contracting HSV. Internal fetal monitoring devices also increase the risk of vertical transmission because they break the fetal skin. Infants also may be exposed after birth through mouth-to-mouth kissing by family members; there have been several cases of infants exposed during ritual circumcision involving direct orogenital suction.[19]

◆Pathophysiology

After initial exposure and entry of the virus at mucocutaneous sites or abraded skin, the virus undergoes replication locally in the dermis and epidermis. This leads to cell destruction, transudation, and vesicle formation. The virus spreads to contiguous cells and eventually into sensory nerves. This process often causes a systemic, inflammatory, immune response, especially with HSV-2 infection, that includes fever and malaise. In rare cases, the herpes can cause CNS manifestations. Painful lesions can last from days to weeks. Eventually, the virus is transported intraaxonally to the dorsal root, where it remains in a latent stage until it becomes reactivated. After oral infection, the latent virus resides in the trigeminal ganglion; after genital infection, it resides in the dorsal sacral nerve roots. During the latent period, the viral genome is maintained in the host cell nucleus without causing cell death.

Latent infections can become reactivated, often during times of physical or emotional stress, and cause a recurrent infection. Compared to HSV-1 infections, reactivation of the HSV-2 infection is twice as common, and the likelihood of HSV-2 recurrent infections is 8 to 10 times that of HSV-1. Reactivation of HSV is not well understood but may be attributable to physical, hormonal, and immunologic stimuli.

During reactivation, the viral genomes are transported through the peripheral sensory nerves back to the dermal surface.

Shedding of the virus occurs during outbreaks, and also may occur when the person is asymptomatic, increasing the likelihood of transmission. Antiviral medications decrease asymptomatic viral shedding and should be considered as an adjunct to safe sex practices.

◆Clinical Manifestations

Three distinct syndromes associated with HSV infection are first-episode primary genital infection, first-episode non–primary HSV, and recurrent infections. The manifestations of each one depend on the individual's immune state. First-episode primary genital infection occurs when an individual has no antibodies to HSV-1 or HSV-2. Many primary infections with HSV are asymptomatic, or the symptoms are not severe enough to warrant medical attention. If symptoms occur, the individual may have small (1 to 2 mm), multiple, vesicular lesions at the site of infection, usually on the labia minora, fourchette, penis, or mouth (Fig. 27.10). They also may appear on the cervix, buttocks, and thighs and are often painful and pruritic. These lesions usually last about 10 to 20 days. The lesions of HSV-1 and HSV-2 can be very small and almost indistinguishable to the naked eye or fairly large and clustered into raw areas. These wet lesions actively shed virus for about 10 to 14 days, after which they heal by reepithelialization. Small lesions may coalesce into larger ulcers and become secondarily infected.

Systemic manifestations often accompany primary HSV infection, and an individual may experience fever, malaise, myalgia, lymphadenopathy, and urinary retention. Pharyngitis, aseptic meningitis, and hepatitis also may accompany primary HSV infection. Fig. 27.11 illustrates the clinical course of primary genital HSV.

First-episode non–primary HSV occurs in individuals who have preexisting antibodies. In some individuals, the primary infection may not have had any clinical manifestations, but the HSV virus has become latent in the nerve root and can reactivate later in life. Compared with primary infection, the first episode of non–primary HSV is often milder with fewer lesions that are less painful and heal faster. Fewer systemic manifestations occur and viral shedding is of shorter duration. However, the symptoms may be severe if the second infection occurs during a period of immunocompromised health status.

Recurrent infections usually produce mild local symptoms. The number of lesions is greatly reduced and the lesions are less painful. Lesions are often unilateral, with crusting within 4 to 5 days. Recovery and healing are usually complete within 10 days. Asymptomatic viral shedding can occur with both HSV-1 and HSV-2, but is more common with HSV-2.[3]

Individuals infected with HSV-2 are more likely to experience recurrent infections. Recurrent infections occur on an average of 5 to 8 times per year but may be more frequent in the first few years of infection. Individuals may experience prodromal symptoms (e.g., pruritus, tingling, dysesthesias) a few hours to 2 days before the eruption of lesions. Women may experience a vaginal discharge and dysuria, and 44% of men have dysuria.

Symptomatic HSV infection of the newborn may occur any time in the first month of life. Manifestations range from a local infection of the eyes, skin, or mucous membranes to a severe disseminated infection with CNS involvement. About 70% of affected infants present with skin lesions. CNS involvement includes seizures and is associated with a mortality of more than 50% and extensive neurologic sequelae in survivors.[18]

◆Evaluation and Treatment

Genital HSV infection is suggested if typical genital lesions are present; painful genital lesions alone are enough to begin treatment. The CDC

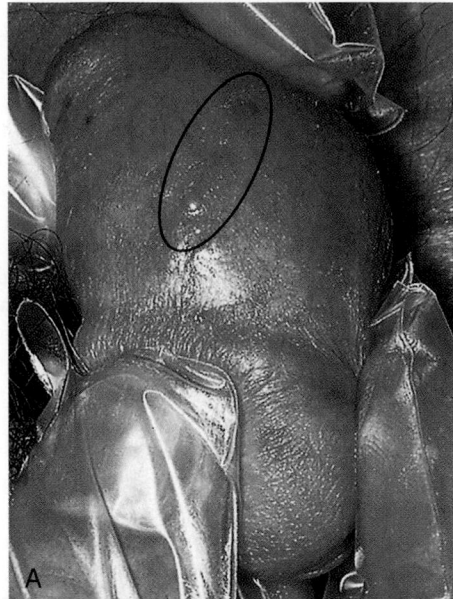

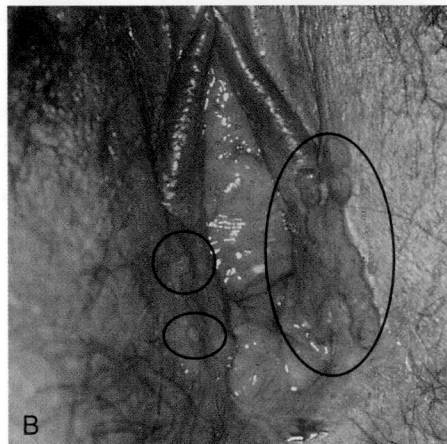

FIGURE 27.10 Herpes Lesions. **A,** Herpetic vesicles on the penis. **B,** Herpetic ulceration of the vulva. (**A** From McMillan A, Scott GR: *Sexually transmitted infections,* ed 2, London, 2000, Churchill Livingstone. **B** From Morse SA et al, editors: *Atlas of sexually transmitted diseases and AIDS,* ed 4, London, 2013, Saunders.)

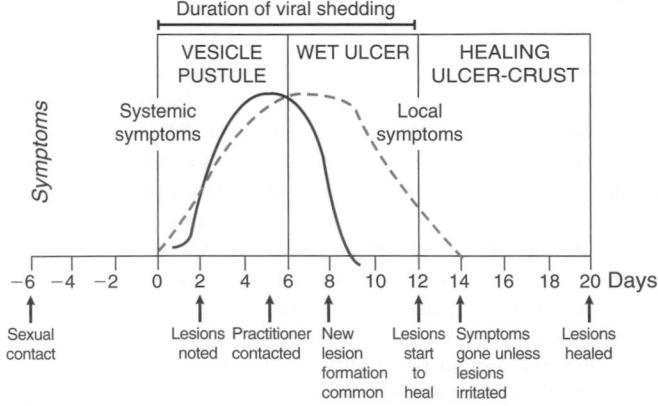

FIGURE 27.11 Clinical Course of Primary Genital Herpes. (From Corey L: Genital herpes. In Holmes KK et al, editors: *Sexually transmitted diseases,* ed 2, New York, 1990, McGraw-Hill.)

recommends serologic testing for diagnosis and to determine the virus subtype because the prognosis and the risk of transmission differ.[3] Viral cultures have been used in the past but their sensitivity is low, especially if lesions have crusted over and begun healing.

There is no cure for HSV, only symptom management and viral suppression treatments. All primary outbreaks should be treated with antiviral medications to prevent complications and speed healing.[3] Oral acyclovir, valacyclovir, penciclovir, and famciclovir are used for primary and periodic outbreaks and to prevent recurrences. Acyclovir has a better safety profile for pregnant and nursing women, but there is ongoing research supporting the safety of valacyclovir as well. Intravenous acyclovir is reserved for very ill or severely immunocompromised individuals.[3]

Suppressive treatment is recommended for individuals with frequent or severe outbreaks[3] and pregnant women at term with a history of herpes.[20] Suppressive treatment also may reduce asymptomatic viral shedding, decreasing transmission to sexual partners and vaginally-born infants. Although there are few side effects with suppression drugs, the decision to take daily medication is complex for many individuals. Although male and female condoms offer some protection, individuals with HSV should refrain from all genital or oral contact when prodromal or symptomatic and understand that an undetermined risk of transmission exists even during asymptomatic periods.

Human Papillomavirus Infection

Human papillomavirus (HPV) infection is the most common symptomatic viral STI in the United States. Although more than 5.5 million cases are diagnosed yearly, the prevalence is considered underestimated because HPV infection is often subclinical. More sensitive measures of HPV indicate that 50% of all sexually active people are infected with the virus at some point in their lives, although these numbers are expected to decrease sharply in response to widespread vaccination. The virus is easily transmissible through direct contact with lesions or infected secretions. Vertical transmission in utero and during vaginal birth also is possible.[21]

More than 120 different types of HPV have been identified. More than 40 serotypes are unique to the stratified squamous epithelia of the anogenital area, although research is finding these same subtypes also may infect the oropharynx.[22] These are divided into high-risk serotypes (which have a high risk of causing cancer) and low-risk serotypes (which are associated with benign genital lesions or warts: *condylomata acuminata* of the vulva, vagina, penis, and perianal areas).

Serotypes 6 and 11 are associated with 90% of genital warts. These low-risk, or nononcogenic, subtypes, can coexist with the high-risk types but do not cause cancer independently. Genital warts are very contagious, with transmission rates among individuals estimated to be between 38% and 95%. Such a wide range is attributable to the subclinical nature of some infections and various influencing factors that include number of exposures, HPV type, location of lesions, and cellular immunity response.

High-risk, or oncogenic, types 16 and 18 are the most common, causing up to 70% of anogenital cancers, and are highly associated with oropharyngeal cancers[1] (see Chapters 12, 13, and 25). HPV-related cancers of the anogenital and oropharynx areas are more common than ovarian cancer in women and more common than brain cancer in men. In future generations, most of these cancers can be prevented through vaccination before HPV exposure.[22]

HPV infection is closely associated with multiple sexual partners and early onset of sexual activity, and is most common in teens and young adults 16 to 25 years of age. Fortunately, most cases of HPV are transient and 70% of healthy individuals will spontaneously eliminate the virus.[23] The persistence of the virus and the immune response play

a role in the development of cancer following HPV exposure. Behaviors and conditions that affect overall health status affect the body's ability to clear HPV infection. Alcohol use, smoking, and HIV infection are strongly correlated with persistent HPV infection.[24]

Several vaccines are available to protect against HPV. All approved vaccines use noninfectious virus-like particles to induce an immune response, and newer vaccines protect against a greater number of subtypes. Approved vaccines induce protection against 2 (bivalent vaccine), 4 (quadrivalent vaccine), or 9 (9-valent vaccine) subtypes and increase in cost with greater protection. The CDC advises using the 9-valent vaccine because of greater prevention capability and cost-effectiveness.[25]

HPV vaccination is recommended for females 11 to 26 years of age and for nonimmunocompromised males ages 11 to 21, but vaccination is recommended until 26 years of age for immunocompromised males and men who have sex with men. Originally released as a three-dose series, the CDC now advises two doses are sufficient for protection from the most dangerous HPV strains.[25,26] Prevention of HPV acquisition in young adults is important because they are more likely than older adults to contract STIs and the cervices of younger women are more vulnerable to HPV. Public health officials are hopeful that vaccination of boys and girls before they become sexually active will decrease the burden of HPV infection in the future. Preliminary data suggest the effects of widespread vaccination that began in 2006 are already becoming apparent[27] (see *What's New?* Human Papillomavirus Vaccine). There are even some reports that vaccination of pregnant women can decrease vertical transmission during vaginal birth because maternal antibodies to HPV cross the placenta.[28]

The immune system is prepared to eliminate the virus through the immune response when previously vaccinated. When an individual has not been vaccinated, he or she may or may not be able to clear this viral infection. Although most HPV subtypes are not associated with abnormal cellular growth, high-risk HPV subtypes cause cellular changes that can lead to cell proliferation, causing warts or cancer.

Pathophysiology

HPV is a nonenveloped, circular, double-stranded DNA virus, one of the papovaviruses, that belongs to the Papovaviridae family.[24] Transmission of the virus occurs through close physical contact with infected skin, mucosa, or fluids; however, the exact transmissibility of the virus into the cell is unknown. The initial infection follows trauma to the epithelium that allows the virus to reach and infect the basal cells of the epithelium, which appear to be supportive of viral propagation. Such minor trauma may occur during sexual intercourse. HPV may enter the nuclear DNA and change the expression of cell proteins, leading either to increased but noncancerous cell growth (e.g., warts) or to unchecked cell growth (e.g., cancer). It is not known exactly why some HPV serotypes are cleared from cells whereas other serotypes cause cellular transformations, but immune response and other cofactors play a role.[24] HPV infection may occur months to years before symptoms appear, such as warts or precancerous lesions.

Clinical Manifestations

Genital warts, condylomata acuminata, are soft, skin-colored, whitish pink to reddish brown discrete growths. They may occur singly or in clusters, may be broad at the base or pedunculated, and may be feathery or smooth. Sometimes the warts enlarge to form cauliflower-like masses on the male frenulum, glans, foreskin, urinary meatus, shaft, scrotum, or anus and on the female labia, clitoris, perineum, vagina, or anus (Fig. 27.12). Although the lesions are usually not painful, they may cause dyspareunia (painful intercourse) and may be friable and bleed easily. Some individuals complain of pruritus. Common locations for condylomata are the on the vaginal introitus, on the shaft of the penis,

WHAT'S NEW?

Human Papillomavirus Vaccine

Every year in the United States:

- Nearly 1 in 4 adults have at least one strain of HPV.
- About 12,000 women are diagnosed with HPV-related cervical cancer.
- Almost 4000 women die from HPV-related cervical cancer.
- About 1900 men are diagnosed with HPV-related penile or anal cancer.

Vaccines are available in the United States to vaccinate 2, 4, or 9 strains of high-risk human papillomavirus (HPV):

- Vaccines are recommended for females and males beginning at age 11 years and up to age 26 depending on gender and risk factors.
- The CDC now recommends children ages 11 to 12 years receive two doses of HPV vaccine rather than the previously recommended three doses; the second dose should be given 6 to 12 months after the first dose.
- Vaccines are highly effective in preventing high-risk HPV types associated with cervical cancer; they have been proven safe and effective by the Centers for Disease Control and Prevention (CDC), with ongoing safety monitoring.
- Vaccines are not recommended for pregnant women because their safety is not yet established, but preliminary reports suggest that HPV vaccination in pregnancy may decrease vertical transmission during vaginal birth.
- Vaccinated women still need cervical cancer screening at regular intervals.
- The three-injection vaccine series is covered by most insurance plans, Medicaid, and the Vaccines for Children (VFC) program if individuals meet eligibility requirements, including age and financial need.

For more information, visit the Centers for Disease Control and Prevention (CDC) STD website at http://www.cdc.gov/std/default.htm. Data from Centers for Disease Control and Prevention (CDC): *Human papillomavirus (HPV)*, Atlanta, GA, 2017, U.S. Department of Health and Human Services. Available at: https://www.cdc.gov/mmwr/volumes/65/wr/mm6549a5.html, updated January 25, 2017; Centers for Disease Control and Prevention (CDC): *Multi-, routine-, & non-routine-vaccine VISs*, Atlanta, GA, 2016, U.S. Department of Health and Human Services. Available at: http://www.cdc.gov/vaccines/hcp/vis/index.html.

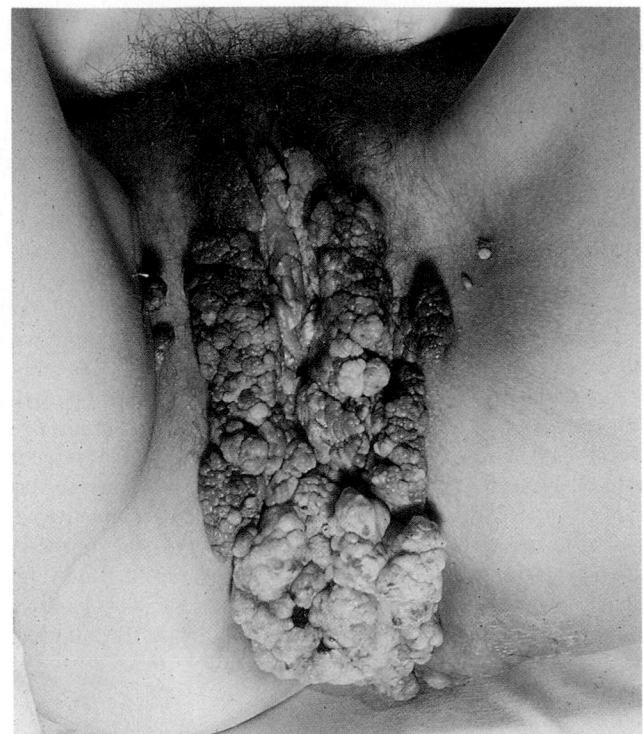

FIGURE 27.12   Condylomata Acuminata—Vulva and Perineum. The clinical diagnosis was giant condylomata. Such large and confluent lesions should be carefully examined and multiple biopsies obtained to rule out underlying malignancy. (From Morse SA et al, editors: *Atlas of sexually transmitted diseases and AIDS*, ed 4, London, 2013, Saunders.)

and under the foreskin. However, warts can be in any location infected by HPV along the reproductive tract, anus, and oropharynx.[3,12] Laryngeal papillomas can occur in infants and children whose mothers had genital warts at the time of delivery. Clinical manifestations of laryngeal warts include stridor, hoarseness, abnormal cry, cough, and respiratory distress.[28]

Precancerous changes related to HPV often do not have any visible manifestations and are not painful, hampering early detection. In addition, cervical and anal cancers may not cause symptoms until late into the disease process. Routine screening for cervical cancer (see below) was begun to increase early detection since clinical symptoms are minimal.

◆ Evaluation and Treatment

Generally, diagnosis of condylomata acuminata is made on the basis of clinical manifestations. Verrucose, fleshy pink lesions caused by HPV must be differentiated from condylomata lata (the whitish gray, flat lesions) of secondary syphilis. Because HPV infection often accompanies other STIs, gonorrhea culture, chlamydia culture, serologic test for syphilis, and wet mount for other vaginal microorganisms also should be performed.

Treatments for external genital warts are considered cosmetic—not curative—and include patient-applied therapies (podofilox, imiquimod, and sinecatechins) and provider-administered therapies (cryotherapy, podophyllin resin, trichloroacetic acid [TCA], bichloroacetic acid [BCA], and surgery). Vaginal, urethral, or anal warts are treated in the clinic using topical medications, cryotherapy, or surgical excision; the CDC provides specific guidance on therapies based on wart location and pregnancy status. Cervical and anal warts require additional screening to exclude more extensive lesions.[3] Success of treatment depends on response of the immune system. Surgical excision is the treatment for laryngeal warts in infants.

Evaluation of infection with oncogenic strains is more difficult since infection is often asymptomatic until cancer is advanced. This is especially true for cervical cancer because of poor innervation of the upper pelvis, allowing cancerous masses to grow large before causing symptoms. The development of the Papanicolaou, or "Pap," smear helped reduce deaths related to cervical cancer by 80% since the 1950s.[29] Ideally, persistent HPV infections can be identified to encourage greater screening for abnormal cellular changes. The appropriate screening for HPV infection is controversial because there are no guidelines delineating who should be screened for anal and oropharyngeal infection. There are guidelines on screening for cervical cancer in women, and these guidelines change frequently in response to new evidence and testing techniques.

Following the development of the Pap smear, women were advised to have yearly Pap tests to detect cancer. Over time, however, it became apparent that while younger women often had abnormal Pap tests, they were often able to clear HPV infection and resolve cellular changes without treatment. Treatment of women less than 20 years of age provides little to no benefit in reducing later rates of cervical cancer but results in pain, anxiety, and increased healthcare costs. Therefore the United States Preventive Services Health Task Force, the American College of Obstetricians and Gynecologists, and many other national cancer agencies recommended that Pap smear testing begin only after 21 years of age.[30,31]

Women ages 21 to 29 should receive just Pap testing every 3 years, whereas women 30 to 65 years of age may receive Pap testing with HPV screening every 5 years (preferred) or Pap testing alone every 3 years. After 65 years of age, Pap testing and HPV screening are no longer recommended for women with previous normal testing results since the risk of new malignancy is low. Women who have had a hysterectomy with removal of the uterine cervix for a noncancerous condition do not need Pap smears or HPV testing for the rest of their lives. Although the HPV vaccine does reduce the risk for cervical cancer, it does not change the frequency or need for Pap and HPV testing at this time.

If the results of a Pap test are abnormal, the woman's cervix will be further evaluated using colposcopy, which involves applying acetic acid (vinegar) and using magnification to examine the cervix for changes indicative of cancer or precancerous lesions. HPV-infected cells will appear white when exposed to acetic acid. In some developing countries with limited laboratory facilities, this test alone is used to screen for cervical cancer (see *What's New? Cervical Cancer Screening in the Developing World* in Chapter 25). Following visual investigation of the cervix during colposcopy, the clinician biopsies suspicious areas for further investigation. Treatment of precancerous and cancerous lesions varies and involves removal or destruction of the affected cells through excision or ablation so they cannot continue to divide.

Although infection with high-risk HPV strains is a risk factor for development of anogenital cancers, as well as cervical cancer, there is not a consensus on screening for rectal and anal cancers.[22] Anyone who engages in receptive anal intercourse is at risk for rectal acquisition of HPV and subsequent development of anal cancer. Women are about twice as likely as men to develop anal cancer, but men who have sex with men remain at risk.[22] Hopefully, the need for treatment of HPV-related genital conditions will decrease as more children and young adults receive the HPV vaccine before becoming sexually active.[25]

Molluscum Contagiosum

Molluscum contagiosum is a benign viral infection of the skin in children and adults. For detailed information, see Chapter 47. In adults, the disease is more commonly sexually transmitted and affects the lower abdomen, genitalia, and perianal area.[11] Molluscum contagiosum in adults is most common in men 20 to 29 years of age and in those with multiple sexual partners. Treatment for sexually transmitted molluscum contagiosum is the same as that for the nonsexually transmitted form of the disease; the CDC also includes information in their regularly updated guidelines.[3]

Parasitic Infections
Trichomoniasis

Trichomonas vaginalis, commonly known as *trich*, affects more than 3.5 million people in the United States and 11% of women older than 40, and is the most common non–viral STI in this region.[1] The high rate of asymptomatic infection aids the spread of this pathogen. Male-female vaginal intercourse is the most common route of transmission.[1] Although sexual transmission is clearly the most common means of disease spread, transmission through fomites is theoretically possible.

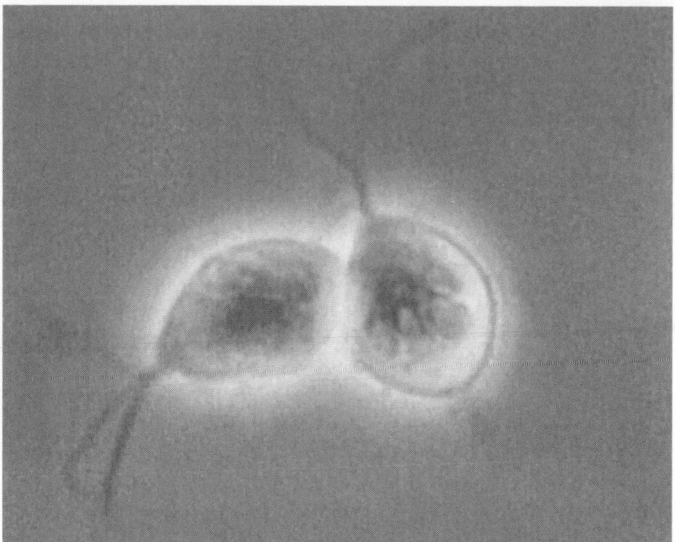

FIGURE 27.13 *Trichomonas vaginalis.* (From CDC Public Health Information Library [PHIL].)

Pathophysiology

T. vaginalis is an anaerobic, unicellular, flagellated, parasitic protozoan that adheres to and damages squamous epithelial cells (Fig. 27.13). It is primarily spread through penal-vaginal sex, although anal sex and oral sex could be potential routes of infection.[3] Because this protozoan selectively affects squamous epithelia, the vaginal and urethral tissues in women are often infected, as are periurethral (Skene) and greater vestibular (Bartholin) glands. The endocervical canal is not affected because it is lined with columnar epithelium. In men, the urethra is the most common site of infection, although the protozoa, called trichomonads, also can infect the epididymis and (rarely) the prostate. Uncircumcised men are more likely to become infected after exposure than circumcised men.[3] There are no conclusive data that the rectum or the oropharynx is a reservoir for infection.[3]

Clinical Manifestations

Manifestations of vaginal trichomoniasis range from none to severe. Up to 85% of those infected have minimal or no symptoms.[3] Vaginal discharge and internal pruritus are the most common manifestations of infection. Dyspareunia and dysuria also are fairly common. Some women report an increase in symptoms immediately after menses. Vaginal secretions can be copious, frothy, malodorous, and yellow-green to gray-green. On examination, the vaginal walls may appear erythematous and sore. Small, punctate red marks, sometimes called *strawberry spots*, are sometimes visible on the vaginal walls and cervix. Most men with trichomoniasis are asymptomatic but may have scant intermittent discharge, slight pruritus, and mild dysuria.[3]

Evaluation and Treatment

All women reporting abnormal vaginal discharge should be tested for trichomoniasis.[3] Nucleic acid amplification testing (NAAT) is the most sensitive and specific method for detection of *T. vaginalis* infection. Samples for testing can be obtained from the woman's endocervix, vagina, or urine. Samples for men ideally come from the penile meatus, but urine is acceptable as well. Self-collection of samples is acceptable; some tests have even been shown to be accurately used in self-testing,[3] which can aid diagnosis, especially in cases of recurrence. A microscopic examination of vaginal fluid mixed with saline was previously widely used to detect the presence of this protozoan but, with a sensitivity of just greater than 50%, it is much less accurate than NAAT-based tests.[3] However, this method can be used when other tests are unavailable or cost-prohibitive. On microscopic examination, the ovoid microorganism is slightly larger than a polymorphonuclear leukocyte and has one rounded, flagellated end and one slightly pointed, flagellated end. The flagella give the trichomonads their characteristic twisting motility. When women are infected, their vaginal secretions have a pH higher than 4.5 and when mixed with 10% potassium hydroxide (KOH) emit a "fishy" odor related to amine release, known as a positive *whiff test*.

The treatment of choice for trichomoniasis is a single 2-gram dose of tinidazole or metronidazole (Flagyl) with tinidazole, achieving better cure rates.[3] These drugs have intense side effects when taken with alcohol; thus individuals must be able to abstain from all alcohol products for 3 days after treatment. Sexual partners, even if asymptomatic, also should be treated. There are high rates of reinfection and the CDC advises a 3-month follow-up after treatment for a test of cure.[3]

T. vaginalis infection in pregnant women is associated with an increased risk of preterm birth through unknown mechanisms that may be linked with inflammation.[32] The 2-gram single dose of metronidazole can be used to treat pregnant women. However, it is not clear if treatment improves outcomes and metronidazole therapy may actually increase the rate of preterm delivery.[33] An alternative dosing regimen is available for lactating women, or the woman can abstain from breastfeeding for 12 to 24 hours after taking the drug.

Scabies

Scabies is a common parasitic infection that can be spread by skin-to-skin and sexual contact.[34] Transmission of scabies requires close skin-to-skin contact, which occurs between sexual partners.[34] Scabies is more common in children and the elderly than in adults.[34] (Detailed information on scabies is contained in Chapter 48.) However, sexual transmission is the most frequent cause of infection in adults.[3]

◆Pathophysiology

The discussion of scabies is presented in Chapter 48.

◆Clinical Manifestations

The classic symptom of scabies is intense pruritus, which increases at night. Pruritus is a result of a reaction to the presence of the *Sarcoptes scabiei* mite. This reaction may take weeks with initial infection, but only 24 hours if the person has been previously infected. The groin and buttocks are common locations for sexually transmitted scabies. Fig. 27.14 shows the typical sites of scabies burrows. The typical burrow of *S. scabiei* is a short, linear, curved, or S-shaped line (Fig. 27.15). There may be small, erythematous, excoriated larval papules near the burrows. Secondary infections are common and are caused by scratching. Even after successful treatment, some individuals will continue to experience pruritus for several weeks.[3]

◆Evaluation and Treatment

The diagnosis of scabies is often made clinically when risk factors are present. Microscopic identification of the mite, eggs, larvae, or feces is ideal because the symptoms of scabies can imitate many dermatologic conditions. Superficial scrapings from an intact papule or burrow can be observed under the microscope and KOH application facilitates mite visualization.

Preferred treatment is topical application of 5% permethrin massaged into the skin and left for 8 to 14 hours or ivermectin 1% dosed at 200 mcg/kg orally and repeated again in 2 weeks.[3] Lindane (1%) lotion or cream also is effective if applied thinly to all areas of the body below the neck and washed thoroughly 8 hours after application.[3] Close

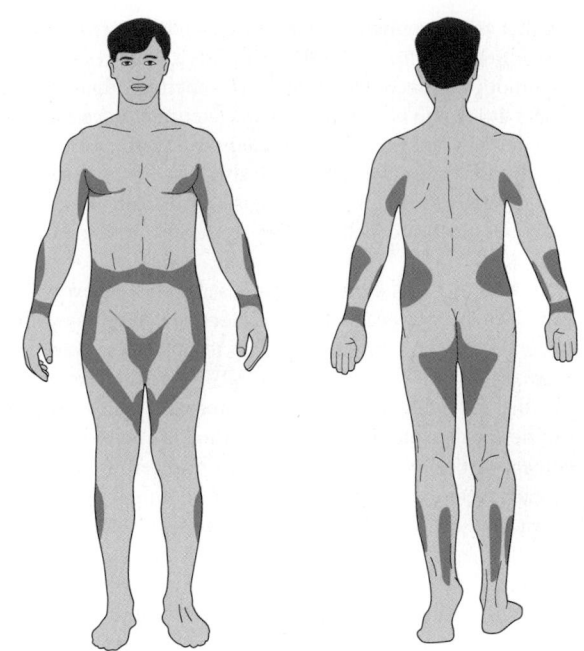

FIGURE 27.14 Distribution of Skin Lesions of *Sarcoptes scabiei* Infestation. Unshaded areas are rarely affected in healthy adults. (From Morse SA et al, editors: *Atlas of sexually transmitted diseases and AIDS*, ed 3, London, 2003, Mosby.)

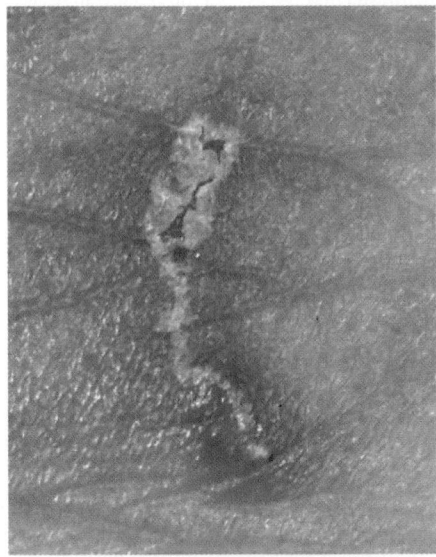

FIGURE 27.15 Scabies Burrow. An S-shaped burrow with a tiny vesicle at one end. (From Marks JG, Miller JJ: *Lookingbill and Marks' principles of dermatology*, ed 4, St Louis, 2006, Saunders.)

household and sexual contacts should be examined and treated if infected.[3] Pregnant women should be treated with permethrin.[3] To prevent reinfestation, clothing and bed linens should be washed and dried in a machine at high temperatures or kept away from body contact for 72 hours.[3]

Pediculosis Pubis

Pthirus pubis, the crab louse, is one of three species of lice that infest humans. *P. pubis* is commonly transmitted sexually and causes pediculosis pubis, or "crabs." *P. pubis* is transmitted primarily by intimate sexual contact or by contact with infected linens. It is highly contagious; there is a 95% chance of contracting lice during a single sexual encounter.

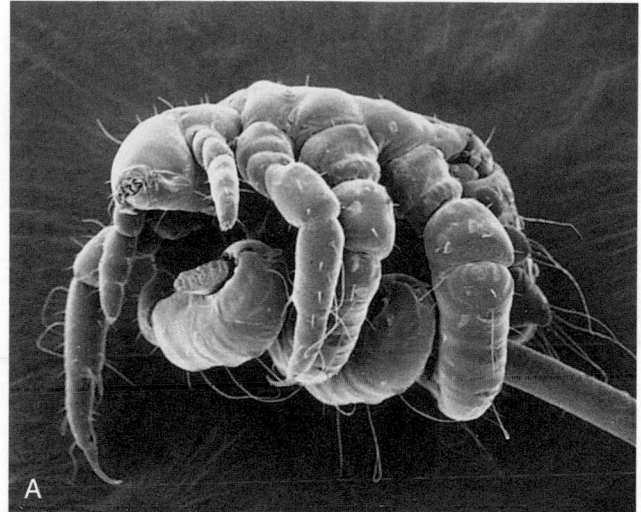
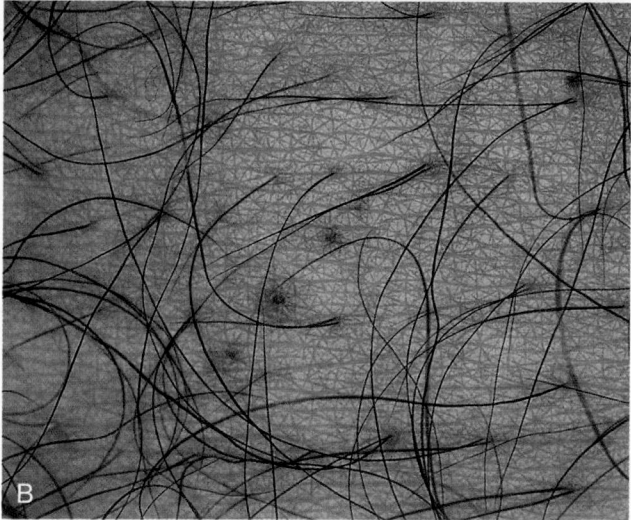

FIGURE 27.16 Pubic Louse and Crab Louse. A, Pubic louse *(Pthirus pubis)* encircling a pubic hair; the clawlike legs produce a firm grip. **B,** Crab louse bites *(P. pubis).* (From Morse SA et al, editors: *Atlas of sexually transmitted diseases and AIDS,* ed 4, London, 2013, Saunders.)

Fomites are a common method of infection because crabs can live away from the body for several days. The transfer of lice from pubic hair is probably mechanical, assisted by scratching, fingernails, and towels rather than by self-propulsion. Pubic lice usually infect the perineal and axillary hair and occasionally the hair of the trunk, beard, scalp, and eyelashes.

◆Pathophysiology

The crab louse has a 25- to 30-day life cycle that consists of five stages: an egg (or nit) stage; three nymphal stages; and an adult stage, all of which occur on the host. The nits of crab lice are found "glued" to hairs; they are oval, 0.8 by 0.3 mm in length, and whitish, and they hatch in 5 to 10 days (Fig. 27.16). In the adult stage, pubic lice are grayish, are approximately 1 mm in length, and have a segmented body and claws to cling to hairs. They bite into the host's skin to feed on blood, causing itching and pain.

◆Clinical Manifestations

The mites are visible, facilitating self-identification of infestation.[3] Symptoms range from mild pruritus to severe, intolerable itching,

depending on the individual's sensitivity to louse bites. Allergic sensitization occurs in about 5 days, when itching, erythema, and inflammation may worsen. Excessive scratching may lead to secondary infection.

◆Evaluation and Treatment

The individual usually presents with a history of itching in the infected area. Because the lice and nits are visible to the naked eye, a thorough clinical examination permits definitive diagnosis. Pediculosis pubis is treated either with 1% permethrin cream rinse and 1% lindane lotion, cream, or shampoo or with over-the-counter pyrethrin or piperonyl butoxide. For nonocular infections, the pediculicide is applied to infested and adjacent hairy areas and washed off after a specified time. Remaining nits can be removed with a fine-toothed comb. Permethrin is the first-line treatment. However, drug resistance is widespread and increasing. Malathion and ivermectin are alternative regimens, although ivermectin does not adequately kill the eggs and requires a second dose, and malathion has multiple contraindications.[3] Lindane is a higher-level treatment and cannot be used by pregnant women because of risk of toxicity.[3] Sexual contacts from the past month should be treated regardless of symptoms, and household contacts should be examined and treated if needed. Clothing and bed linens should be machine washed and dried at high temperatures or kept away from body contact for 72 hours.[3]

SEXUALLY TRANSMITTED INFECTIONS OF OTHER BODY SYSTEMS

The effects of some STIs extend beyond the urogenital tract. Many disorders have varied methods of transmission that may include nonsexual means. Although the major mode of transmission may be by oral ingestion or by direct contact with blood or body fluids (e.g., sharing of needles among drug users, blood transfusions, vertical transmission from mother to baby, health worker exposures), infection can be transmitted through intimate sexual contact as well. Anal contact and physically damaging sex can increase the transmission of many of these infections.

Among the most serious of these infections are acquired immunodeficiency syndrome (AIDS) caused by the human immunodeficiency virus (HIV) and hepatitis (all types). Worldwide, the main mode of transmission of HIV and hepatitis B is through sexual intercourse (primarily male-female), but nonsexual exposure to infected blood and body fluids, especially through needle sharing, contributes to infection rates. The epidemiology, modes of transmission, pathophysiology, clinical manifestations, and evaluation and treatment of AIDS and hepatitis are discussed in detail in Chapters 10 and 42, respectively.

Sexual transmission of less serious but often debilitating infections, such as shigellosis and giardiasis, and systemic diseases, such as Epstein-Barr virus and cytomegalovirus infections, also can occur, although nonsexual transmission is more common. Table 27.3 provides a list of several gastrointestinal and systemic infections that are known to be transmitted by intimate sexual contact, but in which the mode of transmission is primarily through other routes.

Hepatitis

Hepatitis is a liver infection that can be caused by six types of viruses: hepatitis A, hepatitis B, hepatitis C, hepatitis D, hepatitis E, and hepatitis G. Each virus causes a syndrome of acute, icteric (jaundice-producing) liver inflammation. Additional information about hepatitis is found in Chapter 42. Of the three most common types, A, B, and C, the **hepatitis B virus (HBV)** is most commonly sexually transmitted. Hepatitis A, like most other predominantly enteric infections, may be considered an STI because of anal-oral transmission, and vaccination is advised for men who have sex with men.[3] Although hepatitis C virus (HCV)

TABLE 27.3	INFECTIONS WITH KNOWN SEXUAL TRANSMISSIBILITY: MAIN MODE OF TRANSMISSION BY OTHER MEANS
INFECTION/DISEASE	**MAIN ROUTE OF TRANSMISSION**
Gastrointestinal Infections	
Shigellosis caused by *Shigella* bacteria	Contact with infected feces Hand-to-mouth
Campylobacter enteritis caused by *Campylobacter jejuni* bacteria	Primarily an animal pathogen Hand-to-mouth
Giardiasis caused by *Giardia lamblia* protozoa	Contaminated drinking water Hand-to-mouth
Amebiasis caused by *Entamoeba histolytica* protozoa	Contaminated drinking water Hand-to-mouth
Hepatitides A and C (liver infection and inflammation)	Hepatitis A: contact with infected feces; hand-to-mouth Hepatitis C: blood-borne pathogen; direct exposure to contaminated blood; sexual transmission very uncommon
Systemic Diseases	
Epstein-Barr virus	Mucous membrane (oral) exposure
Cytomegalovirus	Body fluids; exposure via close interpersonal contact or direct transfer
Zika virus	Primary spread through bites from infected mosquitos but may be transmitted sexually and across the placental membrane

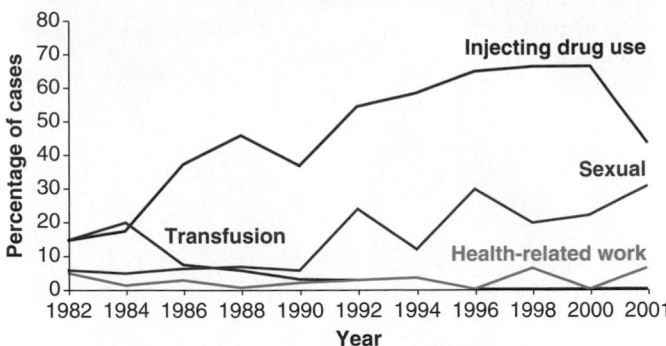

Reported Cases of Acute Hepatitis C by Selected Risk Factors, United States, 1982–2001*

*1982–1990 based on non-A, non-B hepatitis

FIGURE 27.17 Risk for Hepatitis C Exposure. Comparison of injecting drug use *(blue)*, transfusions *(purple)*, health-related work *(green)*, and sexual exposure *(red)*. Note the rise in sexually transmitted incidences. (From Centers for Disease Control and Prevention [CDC]: *Hepatitis C: what clinicians and other health professionals need to know, 2000.* Available at: www.cdc.giv/ncid/diseases/hepatitis/c _training/edu/intro.)

is not recognized as an STI, the CDC has listed sexual exposure, particularly for individuals with multiple partners, as a potential risk factor (Fig. 27.17).

Hepatitis B prevalence varies dramatically worldwide with some geographic areas having more than 10% of the population infected with the virus.[35] There are an estimated 19,000 new cases of HBV infection in the United States each year, and more than 2.2 million people are chronically infected.[36] Those at risk for HBV infection in the United States are infants born to hepatitis-infected mothers, healthcare workers, individuals who have sex with HBV-infected persons, people with diabetes, and immigrants from areas of high HBV prevalence.[36] Widespread screening of pregnant women and vaccination of all infants since 1991 have decreased the rate of infection in the United States by more than 80% and are expected to have lasting effects into future decades.[37] Vaccination of healthcare workers also has decreased infection rates.[38]

Transmission of HBV can occur through needle puncture, blood transfusion, cuts or abrasions in the skin, and absorption by mucosal surfaces. Direct contact with infected body fluids, such as semen and vaginal fluid, may transmit the infection. HBV can survive dry and outside the body for up to 1 week, making it easily infectious on fomites.

In the United States, seropositivity generally increases with age.[36] This is a function of more time for exposure as well as the lack of routine vaccination before the 1990s. However, the younger a person is when he or she contracts the virus, the greater likelihood of chronic

infection.[35] Perinatal transmission of HBV is relatively common, especially in developed countries without routine screening of pregnant women. Neonates whose mothers are infectious have a 90% chance of becoming chronically infected with HBV during labor or delivery if they do not receive treatment, but a 1% risk if they receive adequate treatment.[38] Infants of infected mothers should receive HBV vaccine and immunoglobulin against hepatitis within 12 hours of birth to reduce risk. The vaccine and immunoglobulin combination successfully prevents chronic carrier status in 99% of infants.[38] Although HBV is in many maternal body fluids, it is not found in breast milk and breast-feeding is still encouraged for mothers with HBV.[39] More information about the pathology, diagnosis, and treatment of hepatitis is covered in Chapter 42.

Acquired Immunodeficiency Syndrome

Epidemiology, modes of transmission, pathophysiology, clinical manifestations, and evaluation and treatment of AIDS are discussed in detail in Chapter 10.

Zika Virus

Zika virus is a single-stranded RNA virus from the Flaviviridae family, genus *Flavivirus*. The virus is predominantly transmitted through bites from infected mosquitos (see Chapter 10 for additional information). However, vertical transmission easily occurs in infected women, and sexual transmission also has been confirmed. At this time, the exact mechanism of sexual transmission is not known, although shedding of the virus in semen is suspected.[40] The Centers for Disease Control and Prevention is investigating the issue and advises safer sex precautions for all sexual contact (including vagina, anal, and oral sex) between an infected person and his or her partners, especially if a female partner is pregnant or plans on becoming pregnant.[40]

Infection with zika virus during pregnancy has been associated with severe fetal infection and associated CNS abnormalities. The zika virus is able to infect human placental tissue and multiply within these tissues, spreading virus to the fetus, especially early in gestation.[41] Although the exact pathophysiology is still unclear, postmortem studies of affected fetuses demonstrate a high level of zika virus within fetal brain tissue, even higher than levels found in other tissues or in adult serum.[42] It is thought that the presence of zika virus within fetal central nervous system tissues disrupts normal cell developmental pathways, resulting in stunted brain and cranium formation and causing the characteristic microcephaly (abnormally small head) associated with this infection.[42] Microcephaly is a permanent birth defect that results in lifelong disability because of an inadequately developed brain. The WHO and the CDC are actively studying the disease, and scientists are working to understand the exact mechanisms of zika transmission and cellular disruption.

SUMMARY REVIEW

Sexually Transmitted Urogenital Infections

1. Sexually transmitted diseases many be more common in certain populations related to increased physiologic risk for acquisition (such as with younger women or with men who have sex with men) or insufficient access to quality health care (such as with lower socioeconomic groups, racial/ethnic minorities, and marginalized groups).

2. Gonorrhea is a sexually transmitted communicable disease that can be local or systemic. Complications include PID, sterility, and disseminated infection.

3. Gonorrhea can be passed to the fetus from the mother and typically manifests as an eye infection 1 to 12 days after birth. Ophthalmic antibiotic prophylaxis alone is not sufficient to prevent vertical transmission.

4. Gonorrhea is rapidly becoming resistant to available antibiotics. Multidrug therapy is now recommended to decrease drug resistance.

5. Syphilis is an STI that becomes systemic shortly after infection. The four stages of the disease are (a) primary syphilis with a chancre at the site of infection; (b) secondary syphilis with systemic spread to all body systems; (c) latent syphilis with minimal symptoms or the development of skin lesions; and (d) tertiary syphilis, the most severe stage, with destruction of bone, skin, and soft and neurologic tissues.

6. Congenital syphilis contributes to prematurity of the newborn with bone marrow depression, CNS involvement, renal failure, and intrauterine growth retardation.

7. Syphilis is diagnosed with serologic testing and is treated with injectable penicillin.

8. With chancroid infection, women are generally asymptomatic and men may develop inflamed, painful genital ulcers and inguinal buboes. The incubation period is 1 to 14 days. Single-dose therapy with injectable ceftriaxone or oral azithromycin for both partners is recommended. Persons with HIV may require a longer treatment regimen.

9. Granuloma inguinale (donovanosis) is rare in the United States. The bacteria are gram negative and survive within macrophages. Localized nodules coalesce to form granulomas and ulcers on the penis in men and on the labia in women. Antibiotics provide effective treatment.

10. Bacterial vaginosis (BV) is a sexually associated condition caused by an overgrowth of anaerobic bacteria that produce aromatic amines and raise the pH of the vagina, promoting further bacterial growth (without an inflammatory response) and a fishy odor. "Clue cells" are found on the wet mount. Metronidazole (Flagyl) provides effective treatment. BV has been associated with PID, chorioamnionitis, preterm labor, and postpartum endometritis. Treatment of male sexual partners is not recommended.

11. Chlamydia is the most common bacterial STI in the United States and a leading preventable cause of infertility and ectopic pregnancy. The causative organism, *C. trachomatis,* localizes to epithelial tissue and can spread throughout the urogenital tract or pass from the infected mother to the eyes and respiratory tract of newborn infants during birth. *C. trachomatis* is susceptible to inexpensive, readily accessible antibiotics. Single-dose azithromycin is the drug of choice for infected individuals and all sexual contacts. Because of the asymptomatic nature of chlamydia and the potential sequelae of infection, widespread screening is recommended by the CDC.

12. Lymphogranuloma venereum is a chronic STI uncommon in the United States. The lesion begins as a skin infection and spreads to the lymph tissue, causing inflammation, necrosis, buboes, and abscesses of the inguinal lymph nodes. Primary lesions appear on the penis and scrotum in men and on the cervix, vaginal wall, and labia in women. Secondary lesions involve inflammation and swelling of the lymph nodes with formation of large buboes that rupture and drain. A 21-day or longer course of oral doxycycline or erythromycin is needed for treatment. Treatment of sexual partners is recommended.

13. Genital herpes is the most common genital ulceration in the United States and is caused by either HSV-1 or HSV-2. Lesions initially appear as groups of vesicles that progress to ulceration with pain, lymphadenopathy, and fever. Herpes simplex virus can pass from mother to fetus; thus women with active lesions should give birth by cesarean section to avoid vertical transmission.

14. Herpes simplex virus (HSV) infection is lifelong and can result in an initial outbreak and subsequent outbreaks. Individuals are contagious during outbreaks and episodes of asymptomatic viral shedding. Acyclovir reduces symptoms but does not cure the disease. Recurrent infections are most often attributable to HSV-2 and are generally milder and of shorter duration.

15. Human papillomavirus (HPV) is associated with the development of cervical dysplasia and cancer as well as condylomata acuminata. The high-risk strains of HPV (HR-HPV) that are precursors to the development of cervical cancer do not cause genital warts. Testing is available to detect HR-HPV and a vaccine is now available for the HPV types with highest risk for cervical cancer.

16. Condylomata acuminata (genital warts) are sexually transmitted and highly contagious. The velvety cauliflower-like lesions occur in the genital and anal areas, vagina, and cervix and are painless. They can be transmitted to the infant at birth.

17. Molluscum contagiosum is a benign viral infection of the skin. It is transmitted by skin-to-skin contact in children and adults. In adults, it tends to occur on the genitalia and be transmitted by sexual contact.

18. Trichomoniasis *(T. vaginalis)* causes vaginitis in women and urethritis in men. Both partners usually are infected. Women usually have a copious, malodorous, gray-green discharge with pruritus. Men usually are asymptomatic. Metronidazole is the treatment for both sexes.

19. Scabies is a parasitic infection that spreads by skin-to-skin and sexual contact. The scabies mite burrows through the skin, depositing eggs, causing intense pruritus, especially at night. Treatment consists of topical application of a pediculicide.

20. Pediculosis pubis (crabs) is commonly transmitted sexually and is caused by the crab louse, *P. pubis.* The lice bite into the skin for

SUMMARY REVIEW—cont'd

nutrition. Symptoms include mild and severe pruritus. Topical application of prescription or over-the-counter pediculicides is effective treatment.

Sexually Transmitted Infections of Other Body Systems

1. Systemic diseases known to be sexually transmitted include AIDS (see Chapter 10), cytomegalovirus infection, and Epstein-Barr virus.
2. Transmission of HBV can occur through needle puncture, blood transfusion, cuts in the skin, and contact with infected body fluids.
3. Hepatitis B infection poses significant health risks including chronic liver disease and hepatocellular cancer. Immunization against hepatitis B is the most effective means of preventing transmission. Universal vaccination of infants and children is recommended, as well as vaccination of high-risk adults.
4. The risk of perinatal transmission of HBV is high for infants of HBV-infected mothers unless they receive immunoglobulin and are vaccinated.
5. Hepatitis C is generally transmitted percutaneously but sexual transmission appears possible.
6. Although normally transmitted through mosquito bites, zika virus can be transmitted through sexual contact with infected body fluids or through vertical transmission. Zika virus sequesters in fetal brain tissue, disrupting brain growth and causing persistent, lifelong microcephaly.

KEY TERMS

Acute urethral syndrome, 878
Bacterial vaginosis (BV), 876
Buboes, 875
Chancre, 872
Chancroid, 875
Chlamydia, 877
Condylomata acuminata, 881
Condylomata lata, 873
Congenital syphilis (CS), 872
Disseminated gonococcal infection (DGI), 871
Donovan body, 876
Fomite, 867

Genital herpes, 879
Gonococci (*singular,* gonococcus), 869
Gonorrhea, 869
Granuloma inguinale (donovanosis), 876
Gummas, 872
Hepatitis B virus (HBV), 885
Human papillomavirus (HPV), 881
Latent syphilis, 872
Lymphogranuloma venereum (LGV), 878
Molluscum contagiosum, 883
Nononcogenic, 881
Ophthalmia neonatorum, 871

Oncogenic, 881
Pediculosis pubis, 884
Primary syphilis, 872
Pseudobuboes, 876
Scabies, 884
Secondary syphilis, 872
Sexually transmitted infection (STI), 867
Syphilis, 872
Tertiary syphilis, 872
Trichomonad, 883
Vertical transmission, 867
Zika virus, 886

REFERENCES

1. Centers for Disease Control and Prevention (CDC): *Sexually transmitted disease surveillance, 2014,* Washington, DC, 2015, U.S. Department of Health and Human Services, pp 4–39.
2. Cramer R, et al: The legal aspects of expedited partner therapy practice: do state laws and policies really matter? *Sex Transm Dis* 40(8):657–662, 2013.
3. Workowski KA, Bolan GA, Centers for Disease Control and Prevention (CDC): Sexually transmitted diseases treatment guidelines, 2015. *MMWR Recomm Rep* 64(RR-03):1–137, 2015.
4. Lewis D: Will targeting oropharyngeal gonorrhoea delay the further emergence of drug-resistant Neisseria gonorrhoeae strains? *Sex Transm Infect* 91(4):234–237, 2015.
5. Patton ME, et al: Extragenital gonorrhea and chlamydia testing and infection among men who have sex with men—STD Surveillance Network, United States, 2010–2012. *Clin Infect Dis* 58(11): 1564–1570, 2014.
6. Brunham RC, Gottlieb SL, Paavonen J: Pelvic inflammatory disease. *N Engl J Med* 372(21): 2039–2048, 2015.
7. Patton ME, et al: Primary and secondary syphilis—United States, 2005–2013. *MMWR Morb Mortal Wkly Rep* 63(18):402–406, 2014.
8. Bowen V, et al: Increase in incidence of congenital syphilis–United States, 2012–2014. *MMWR Morb Mortal Wkly Rep* 64:1241–1245, 2015.
9. Gomez GB, et al: Untreated maternal syphilis and adverse outcomes of pregnancy: a systematic review and meta-analysis. *Bull World Health Organ* 91(3): 217–226, 2013.
10. Benatar S, et al: Midwifery care at a freestanding birth center: a safe and effective alternative to conventional maternity care. *Health Serv Res* 48(5): 1750–1768, 2013.

11. Basta-Juzbašić A, Čeović R: Chancroid, lymphogranuloma venereum, granuloma inguinale, genital herpes simplex infection, and molluscum contagiosum. *Clin Dermatol* 32(2):290–298, 2014.
12. Verstraelen H, Swidsinski A: The biofilm in bacterial vaginosis: implications for epidemiology, diagnosis and treatment. *Curr Opin Infect Dis* 26(1):86–89, 2013.
13. Elwell C, Mirrashidi K, Engel J: Chlamydia cell biology and pathogenesis. *Nat Rev Microbiol* 14(6): 385–400, 2016.
14. Quayle A: The innate and early immune response to pathogen challenge in the female genital tract and the pivotal role of epithelial cells. *J Reprod Immunol* 57(1):61–79, 2002.
15. Van der Bij AK, et al: Diagnostic and clinical implications of anorectal lymphogranuloma venereum in men who have sex with men: a retrospective case-control study. *Clin Infect Dis* 42(2):186–194, 2006.
16. Kaufman HE, et al: HSV-1 DNA in tears and saliva of normal adults. *Invest Ophthalmol Vis Sci* 46(1): 241–247, 2005.
17. Magaret AS, et al: Effect of condom use on per-act HSV-2 transmission risk in HIV-1, HSV-2-discordant couples. *Clin Infect Dis* 62(4):456–461, 2016.
18. James SH, Kimberlin DW: Neonatal herpes simplex virus infection: epidemiology and treatment. *Clin Perinatol* 42(1):47–59, 2015.
19. Madan RP, et al: Neonatal herpes infection associated with direct orogenital suction during ritual Jewish circumcision. *J Pediatric Infect Dis Soc* 4(3):283–284, 2015.
20. American College of Obstetricians and Gynecologists (ACOG): *Management of herpes in pregnancy, 2016.* Available from Agency for

Healthcare Research and Quality, Rockville, MD, U.S. Department of Health and Human Services, at: https://www.guideline.gov?summaries/summary/11430/management-of-herpes-in -pregnancy.
21. Trottier H, et al: Human papillomavirus (HPV) perinatal transmission and risk of HPV persistence among children: design, methods and preliminary results of the HERITAGE study. *Papillomavirus Res* 2:145–152, 2016.
22. Centers for Disease Control and Prevention (CDC): Human papillomavirus-associated cancers – United States, 2004–2008. *MMWR Morb Mortal Wkly Rep* 61:258, 2012.
23. Moreira ED, et al: Incidence, clearance, and disease progression of genital human papillomavirus infection in heterosexual men. *J Infect Dis* 210(2): 192–199, 2014.
24. Pytynia KB, Dahlstrom KR, Sturgis EM: Epidemiology of HPV-associated oropharyngeal cancer. *Oral Oncol* 50(5):380–386, 2014.
25. Petrosky E, et al: Use of 9-valent human papillomavirus (HPV) vaccine: updated HPV vaccination recommendations of the advisory committee on immunization practices. *MMWR Morb Mortal Wkly Rep* 64(11):300–304, 2015.
26. Meites E, Kemp A, Markowitz LE: Use of a 2-dose schedule for human papillomavirus vaccination—updated recommendations of the Advisory Committee on Immunization Practices. *MMWR Morb Mortal Wkly Rep* 65(49):1405–1408, 2016.
27. Hariri S, et al: Monitoring effect of human papillomavirus vaccines in US population, Emerging Infections Program, 2008–2012. *Emerg Infect Dis* 21(9):1557–1561, 2015.
28. Shah KV: A case for immunization of human papillomavirus (HPV) 6/11–infected pregnant

women with the quadrivalent HPV vaccine to prevent juvenile-onset laryngeal papilloma. *J Infect Dis* 209(9):1307–1309, 2013.

29. Siegel RL, Miller KD, Jemal A: Cancer statistics, 2015. *CA Cancer J Clin* 65(1):5–29, 2015.

30. American College of Obstetricians and Gynecologists (ACOG): ACOG practice bulletin: clinical management guidelines for obstetrician-gynecologists, number 45, August 2003, cervical cytology screening (replaces committee opinion 152, March 1995). *Obstet Gynecol* 102(2):417–427, 2003.

31. Moyer VA: Screening for cervical cancer: US Preventive Services Task Force recommendation statement. *Ann Intern Med* 156(12):880–891, 2012.

32. Silver BJ, et al: *Trichomonas vaginalis* as a cause of perinatal morbidity: a systematic review and meta-analysis. *Sex Transm Dis* 41(6):369–376, 2014.

33. Gülmezoglu AM, Azhar M: Interventions for trichomoniasis in pregnancy. *Cochrane Database Syst Rev* (5):CD000220, 2011.

34. Romani L, et al: Prevalence of scabies and impetigo worldwide: a systematic review. *Lancet Infect Dis* 15(8):960–967, 2015.

35. Ott J, et al: Global epidemiology of hepatitis B virus infection: new estimates of age-specific HBsAg seroprevalence and endemicity. *Vaccine* 30(12):2212–2219, 2012.

36. Centers for Disease Control Prevention (CDC): *Surveillance for viral hepatitis – United States, 2011*, Atlanta, GA, 2014, Author. Available at: http://www.cdc.gov/hepatitis/statistics/2011surveillance/pdfs/2011surveillance/index.htm.

37. Schillie S, et al: Update: shortened interval for postvaccination serologic testing of infants born to Hepatitis B-infected mothers. *MMWR Morb Mortal Wkly Rep* 64(39):1118–1120, 2015.

38. Schillie S, et al: CDC guidance for evaluating health-care personnel for hepatitis B virus protection and for administering postexposure management. *MMWR Recomm Rep* 62(10):1–19, 2013.

39. Chen X, et al: Breastfeeding is not a risk factor for mother-to-child transmission of hepatitis B virus. *PLoS ONE* 8(1):e55303, 2013.

40. Oster AM: Update: interim guidance for prevention of sexual transmission of Zika virus—United States, 2016. *MMWR Morb Mortal Wkly Rep* 65(12):323–325, 2016.

41. Tabata T, et al: Zika virus targets different primary human placental cells, suggesting two routes for vertical transmission. *Cell Host Microbe* 20(2):155–166, 2016.

42. Mlakar J, et al: Zika virus associated with microcephaly. *N Engl J Med* 374(10):951–958, 2016.

CHAPTER

28

Structure and Function of the Hematologic System

Sue E. Huether, Neal S. Rote, Kathryn L. McCance

evolve WEBSITE

CHAPTER OUTLINE

All the body's tissues and organs require oxygen and nutrients to survive. These essential needs are provided by the blood that flows through miles of vessels throughout the human body. The red blood cells provide the oxygen and remove carbon dioxide, and the fluid portion of the blood carries the nutrients and ions for proper acid-base balance. The blood also cleans discarded waste from the tissues; transports hormones; conveys white blood cells, platelets, and other ingredients that are necessary for protecting the entire body from injury and infection and initiating healing; and provides thermal regulation to maintain organs and tissues within an acceptable range of temperatures.

COMPONENTS OF THE HEMATOLOGIC SYSTEM

Composition of the Blood

Blood consists of various cells that circulate in the cardiovascular system suspended in a solution of protein and inorganic materials (plasma), which is approximately 92% water and 8% dissolved substances (solutes) (Fig. 28.1). The blood volume amounts to about 6 quarts (5.5 L) in adults. The continuous movement of blood guarantees that critical components are available to all parts of the body to carry out their

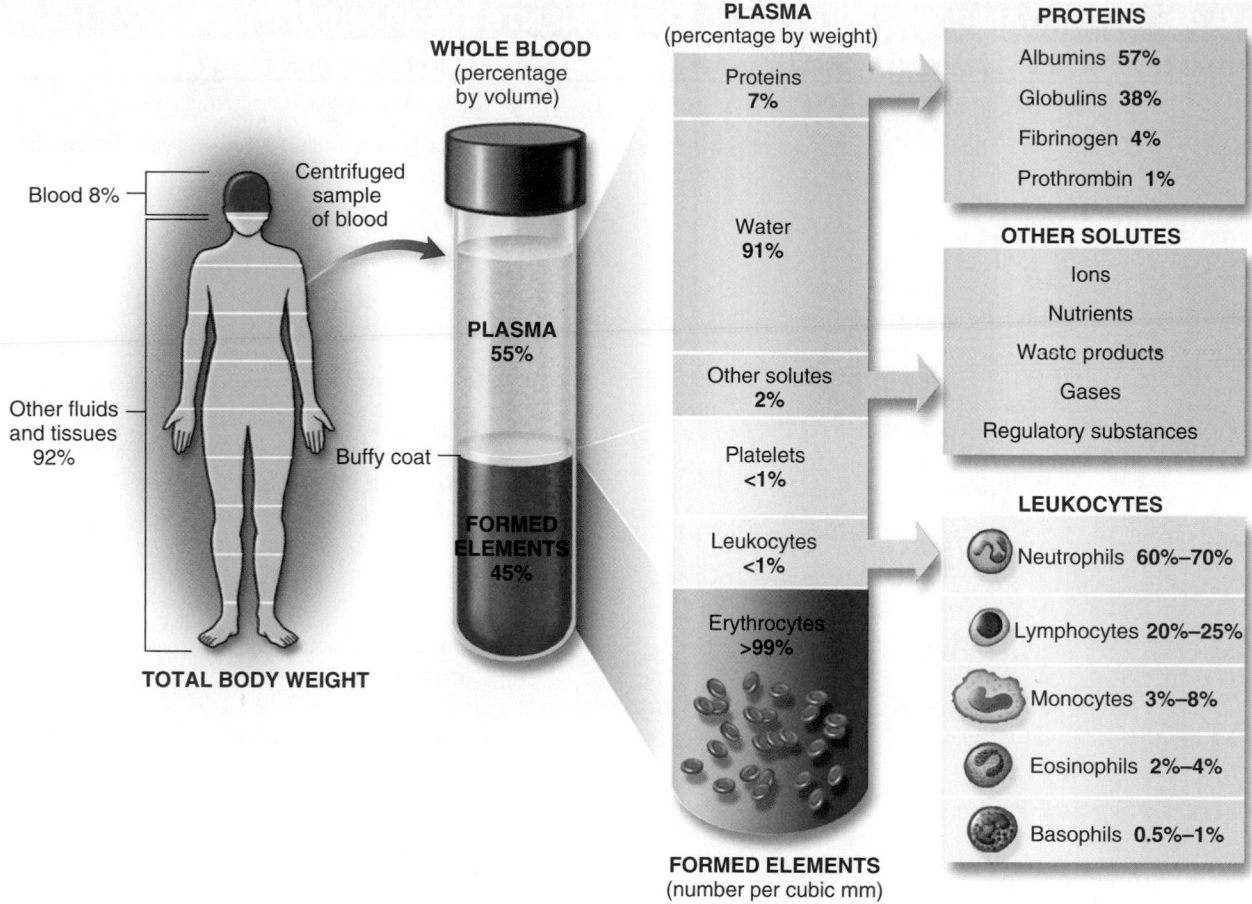

FIGURE 28.1 Composition of Whole Blood. Approximate values for the components of blood in a normal adult. (Adapted from Patton KT, Thibodeau GA: *The human body in health & disease,* ed 7, St Louis, 2018, Mosby.)

chief functions: (1) delivery of substances needed for cellular metabolism in the tissues, (2) removal of the wastes of cellular metabolism, (3) defense against invading microorganisms and injury, and (4) maintenance of acid-base balance. Fetal and neonatal hematopoiesis and blood composition are presented in Chapter 30.

Plasma and Plasma Proteins

In adults, plasma accounts for 50% to 55% of blood volume. Plasma is a complex aqueous liquid containing a variety of organic and inorganic elements (Table 28.1). The concentration of these elements varies depending on diet, metabolic demand, hormones, and vitamins. Plasma differs from serum in that serum is plasma that has been allowed to clot in the laboratory in order to remove fibrinogen and other clotting factors that may interfere with some diagnostic tests.

The plasma contains a large number of proteins (plasma proteins) that constitute about 7% of the total plasma weight. These vary in structure and function and can be classified into two major groups, albumin and globulins. Most plasma proteins are produced by the liver. The major exception is antibodies (immunoglobulins), which are produced by plasma cells in the lymph nodes and other lymphoid tissues (see Chapter 8).

Albumin (about 57% of total plasma protein at a concentration of about 4 g/dL) serves as a carrier molecule for normal components of blood as well as drugs that have low solubility in water (e.g., free fatty acids, lipid-soluble hormones, thyroid hormones, bile salts). Its most essential role is regulation of the passage of water and solutes through the capillaries. Albumin molecules are large and do not diffuse freely

through the vascular endothelium, and thus they maintain the critical colloidal osmotic pressure (or oncotic pressure) that regulates the passage of water and solutes into the surrounding tissues (see Chapters 1 and 3). Water and solute particles tend to diffuse out of the arterial portions of the capillaries because the blood pressure is greater in arterial than in venous blood vessels (see Chapter 3). Water and solutes move from tissue cells into the venous portions of the capillaries where the pressures are reversed, oncotic pressure being greater than intravascular pressure or hydrostatic pressure. In the case of decreased production of albumin (e.g., cirrhosis, other diffuse liver diseases, protein malnutrition) or excessive loss of albumin (e.g., certain kidney diseases, extensive burns), the reduced oncotic pressure leads to excessive movement of fluid and solutes into the tissue and decreased blood volume.

The remaining plasma proteins, or globulins, are often classified by their properties in an electric field (serum electrophoresis). Under the normal conditions used to perform serum electrophoresis, albumin is the most rapidly moving protein. The globulins are classified by their movement relative to albumin: alpha (α) globulins (those moving most closely to albumin), beta (β) globulins, and gamma (γ) globulins (those with the least movement). Depending on the electrophoretic procedure, the α- and β-globulins may be subdivided into subregions (α_1-, α_2-, β_1-, or β_2-globulins). Fibrinogen is a major plasma protein (about 4% of total plasma protein) that would move between the beta and gamma regions but is removed during the formation of serum. The γ-globulin region consists primarily of immunoglobulin G (IgG) (see Chapter 8).

Plasma proteins can also be classified into groups by function: clotting, defense, transport, or regulation. The clotting factors promote

TABLE 28.1	ORGANIC AND INORGANIC COMPONENTS OF ARTERIAL PLASMA	
CONSTITUENT	**AMOUNT/CONCENTRATION**	**MAJOR FUNCTIONS**
Water	91% of plasma weight	Medium for carrying all other constituents
Electrolytes	Total <1% of plasma weight	Maintain H_2O in extracellular compartment; act as buffers; function in membrane excitability
Na$^+$	142 mEq/L (142 mM)	
K$^+$	4 mEq/L (4 mM)	
Ca^{++}	5 mEq/L (2.5 mM)	
Mg^{++}	3 mEq/L (1.5 mM)	
Cl$^-$	103 mEq/L (103 mM)	
HCO$_3^-$	27 mEq/L (27 mM)	
Phosphate (mostly)	2 mEq/L (1 mM)	
Sulfate	1 mEq/L (0.5 mM)	
Proteins	7.3 g/dL (2.5 mM)	Provide colloid osmotic pressure of plasma; act as buffers; bind other plasma constituents (lipids, hormones, vitamins, minerals, etc.); clotting factors; enzymes; enzyme precursors; antibodies (immunoglobulins); hormones; transporters
Albumin	4.5 g/dL	
Globulins	2.5 g/dL	
Fibrinogen	0.3 g/dL	
Transferrin	250 mg/dL	
Ferritin	15–300 mcg/L	
Gases		
CO$_2$ content	22–32 mmol/L plasma	Byproduct of oxygenation; most CO_2 content is from HCO$_3^-$ and acts as a buffer
O$_2$	PaO$_2$ 80 torr or greater (arterial); PvO$_2$ 30–40 torr (venous)	Oxygenation
N$_2$	0.9 mL/dL	Byproduct of protein catabolism
Nutrients		Provide nutrition and substances for tissue repair
Glucose and other carbohydrates	100 mg/dL (5.6 mM)	
Total amino acids	40 mg/dL (2 mM)	
Total lipids	500 mg/dL (7.5 mM)	
Cholesterol	150–250 mg/dL (4–7 mM)	
Individual vitamins	0.0001–2.5 mg/dL	
Individual trace elements	0.001–0.3 mg/dL	
Iron	50–150 mcg/dL	
Waste products		
Urea (blood urea nitrogen [BUN])	7–18 mg/dL (5.7 mM)	End product of protein catabolism
Creatinine (from creatine)	1 mg/dL (0.09 mM)	End product from energy metabolism
Uric acid (from nucleic acids)	5 mg/dL (0.3 mM)	End product from protein metabolism
Bilirubin (from heme)	0.2–1.2 mg/dL (0.003–0.018 mM)	End product of red blood cell destruction
Individual hormones	0.000001–0.05 mg/dL	Functions specific to target tissue

PaO$_2$, Partial pressure of oxygen in arterial blood.
Data from Vander AJ, Sherman JH, Luciano DS: *Human physiology: the mechanisms of body function*, ed 8, New York, 2001, McGraw-Hill.

coagulation and stop bleeding from damaged blood vessels (see Function of Clotting Factors under Mechanisms of Hemostasis). Fibrinogen is the most plentiful of the clotting factors and is the precursor of the fibrin clot (see Fig. 7.9). Proteins involved in defense, or protection, against infection include antibodies and complement proteins (see Chapters 7 and 8). Transport proteins specifically bind and carry a variety of inorganic and organic molecules, including iron (transferrin), copper (ceruloplasmin), steroid hormones, and vitamins (e.g., retinol-binding protein). The plasma lipids, triglycerides, phospholipids, cholesterol, and fatty acids are carried through the blood as complexes with plasma proteins; they are known as *lipoproteins* (see Chapters 1 and 33). Regulatory proteins include a variety of enzymatic inhibitors (e.g., α_1-antitrypsin) that protect the tissues from damage, precursor molecules (e.g., kininogen) that are converted into active biologic molecules when needed, and protein hormones (e.g., cytokines) that communicate between cells.

Plasma also contains several charged inorganic ions (electrolytes) that regulate cell function, osmotic pressure, and blood pH. (Electrolytes are described in Chapters 1 and 3.)

Cellular Components of the Blood

The cellular elements of the blood are broadly classified as red blood cells (RBCs) (i.e., erythrocytes), white blood cells (WBCs) (i.e., leukocytes), and platelets (thrombocytes). The components of the blood are listed in Table 28.2.

Erythrocytes. Erythrocytes (red blood cells [RBCs]) are the most abundant cells of the blood, occupying approximately 48% of the blood volume in men and about 42% in women. Erythrocytes are primarily responsible for tissue oxygenation. The erythrocyte contains hemoglobin, which carries the gases, and electrolytes, which regulate diffusion through a cell's plasma membrane. The mature erythrocyte lacks a nucleus and cytoplasmic organelles (e.g., mitochondria), so it cannot synthesize

TABLE 28.2	CELLULAR COMPONENTS OF THE BLOOD			
CELL	**STRUCTURAL CHARACTERISTICS***	**NORMAL AMOUNTS OF CIRCULATING BLOOD**	**FUNCTION**	**LIFE SPAN**
Erythrocyte (red blood cell)	Nonnucleated cytoplasmic disk containing hemoglobin	4.2–6.2 million/mm^3	Gas transport to and from tissue cells and lungs	80–120 days
Leukocyte (white blood cell)	Nucleated cell	5000–10,000/mm^3	Body defense mechanisms	See below
Lymphocyte	Mononuclear immunocyte	25%–33% of leukocyte count (leukocyte differential)	Humoral and cell-mediated immunity (see Chapter 7)	Days or years depending on type
Monocyte and macrophage	Large kidney-shaped mononuclear phagocyte	3%–7% of leukocyte differential	Phagocytosis; mononuclear phagocyte system	Months or years
Neutrophil	Segmented polymorphonuclear granulocyte with granules stainable by neutral staining	57%–67% of leukocyte differential	Phagocytosis, particularly during early phase of inflammation, bacterial killing	4 days
Basophil	Lobate nuclear granulocyte with granules stainable by basic dyes	0%–0.75% of leukocyte differential	Similar to mast cell; secretes inflammatory mediators (e.g., histamine, chemotactic factors for eosinophils and neutrophils); involved with allergic reactions	Few hours to days
Eosinophil	Segmented polymorphonuclear granulocyte with granules stainable by eosin dyes	1%–4% of leukocyte differential	Phagocytosis; response to parasites, control of allergic reactions	8–12 days
Platelet	Irregularly shaped cytoplasmic fragment (not a cell)	140,000–340,000/mm^3	Hemostasis following vascular injury; normal coagulation and clot formation/retraction	8–11 days

*See bottom row of Fig. 28.12 for illustrations of cells.

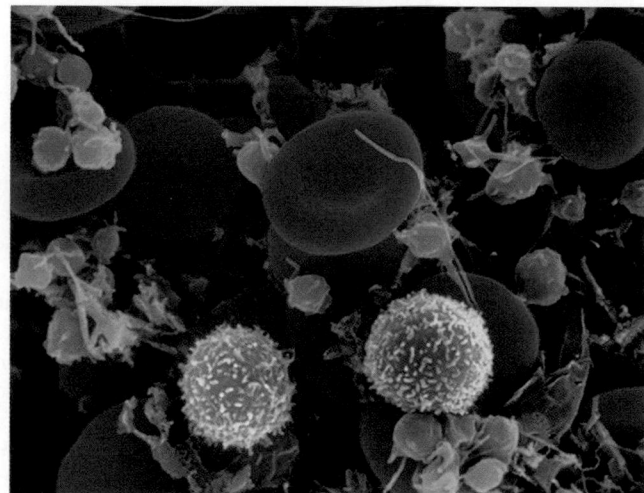

FIGURE 28.2 Blood Cells. Leukocytes are spherical and have irregular surfaces with numerous extending pili (appear as yellow). Erythrocytes are flattened spheres with a depressed center. Activated platelets are green. (Copyright Dennis Kunkel Microscopy, Inc.)

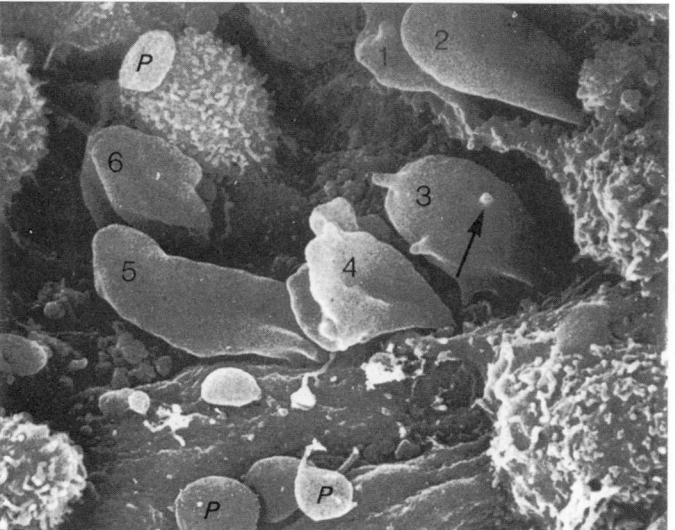

FIGURE 28.3 Red Cells in the Spleen. Scanning electron micrograph of spleen demonstrating erythrocytes (numbered **1** through **6**) squeezing through the fenestrated wall in transit from the splenic cord to the sinus. The view shows the endothelial lining of the sinus wall, to which platelets *(P)* adhere, along with "hairy" white cells, probably macrophages. The *arrow* shows a protrusion on a red blood cell (×5000). (From Weiss L: *Blood* 43:665, 1974; reprinted with permission.)

protein or carry out oxidative reactions. Because it cannot undergo mitotic division, the erythrocyte has a limited life span (approximately 100 to 120 days), ages, and is removed from the circulation, primarily in the spleen, to be replaced by new erythrocytes.

The erythrocyte's size and shape are ideally suited to its function as a gas carrier. An RBC is a small disk with two unique properties: (1) a *biconcave* shape and (2) the capacity to be *reversibly deformed* (Fig. 28.2 and Fig. 28.3). The flattened, biconcave shape provides a

surface area/volume ratio that is optimal for gas diffusion into and out of the cell and for deformity. During its life span, the erythrocyte, which is 6 to 8 μm in diameter, repeatedly circulates through splenic sinusoids and capillaries that are only 2 μm in diameter (see Fig. 28.3). Reversible deformity enables the erythrocyte to assume a more compact

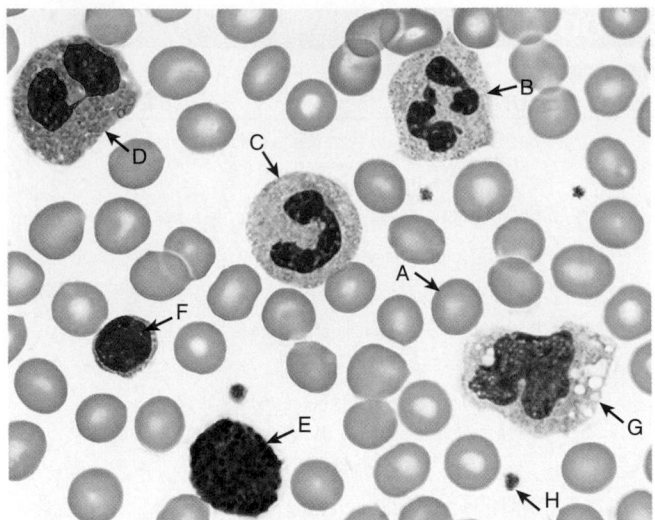

FIGURE 28.4 Leukocytes. Normal cells in peripheral blood: **A,** erythrocyte (red blood cell); **B,** neutrophil (segmented); **C,** neutrophil (banded); **D,** eosinophil; **E,** basophil; **F,** lymphocyte; **G,** monocyte; **H,** platelet. (From Keohane E, Smith L, Walenga J: *Rodak's hematology,* ed 5, St Louis, 2016, Saunders.)

torpedo-like shape, squeeze through the microcirculation, and return to normal shape.

Leukocytes. Leukocytes (white blood cells [WBCs]) defend the body against microorganisms that cause infection and remove debris, including dead or injured cells of all kinds (see Fig. 28.2). The leukocytes act primarily in the tissues but are transported in the circulation. The average adult has approximately 5000 to 10,000 leukocytes/mm³ of blood.

Leukocytes are classified according to structure as either granulocytes or agranulocytes and according to function as either phagocytes or immunocytes. Granulocytes include neutrophils, basophils, and eosinophils and all are phagocytes. (Phagocytic action is described in Chapter 7.) Mast cells also are classified as granulocytes. Of the agranulocytes, the monocytes and macrophages are phagocytes, whereas the lymphocytes are immunocytes (cells that create immunity; see Chapter 8) (Fig. 28.4).

Granulocytes. Granulocytes have many membrane-bound granules in their cytoplasm. These granules contain enzymes capable of killing microorganisms and catabolizing debris ingested during phagocytosis. The granules also contain powerful biochemical mediators with inflammatory and immune functions. These mediators, along with the digestive enzymes, are released from granulocytes in response to specific stimuli. The biochemical mediators have vascular and intercellular effects, and the enzymes participate in the breakdown of debris from sites of infection or injury. Granulocytes are capable of amoeboid movement, by which they migrate through vessel walls (diapedesis) and then to sites where their action is needed (see Chapter 7).

The neutrophil (polymorphonuclear neutrophil [PMN]) is the most numerous and best understood of the granulocytes (see Fig. 28.4, *B* and *C*, and Table 28.2). Neutrophils constitute about 57% to 67% of the total leukocyte count in adults. The cytoplasm of neutrophils contains small lysosomal granules and a central nucleus with two to five distinct lobes.[1] Immature neutrophils are called *bands* or *stabs.* Mature neutrophils are called *segmented neutrophils* because of the characteristic appearance of their nucleus. Neutrophils reach a fully mature state in the bone marrow, and these mature neutrophils are called the *marrow neutrophil reserve.* Normally it takes about 14 days for neutrophils to develop from early precursors, but this process is accelerated by infection and treatment with colony-stimulating factors.

Neutrophils are the chief phagocytes of early inflammation. Soon after bacterial invasion or tissue injury, neutrophils migrate out of the capillaries and into the inflamed site, where they ingest and destroy microorganisms and debris and then die in 1 or 2 days. The dissolution of dead neutrophils releases digestive enzymes from their cytoplasmic granules. These enzymes dissolve cellular debris and prepare the site for healing. (This final function, called *débridement,* is described in Chapter 7.)

Eosinophils have large, coarse granules and constitute only 1% to 4% of the normal leukocyte count in adults (see Fig. 28.4, *D,* and Table 28.2). Like neutrophils, eosinophils are capable of amoeboid movement and phagocytosis. Using a spectrum of pattern-recognition receptors, eosinophils ingest antigen-antibody complexes and viruses and are induced by mast cell chemotactic factors to attack parasites and other pathogens.[2] Eosinophil secondary granules contain toxic chemicals (e.g., major basic protein, eosinophil cationic protein, eosinophil peroxidase, eosinophil-derived neurotoxin) that are highly destructive to parasites and viruses. The eosinophil granules contain a variety of enzymes (e.g., histaminase) that help to control inflammatory processes. (Their function in inflammation and defense against parasites and other pathogens is described in Chapters 7 and 8.) Eosinophils process antigen and also release leukotrienes, prostaglandins, platelet-activating factor (PAF), and a variety of cytokines (e.g., interleukin-1 [IL-1], IL-6, tumor necrosis factor-alpha [TNF-α], granulocyte-macrophage colony–stimulating factor [GM-CSF]) and chemokines (e.g., IL-8) that augment the inflammatory response. Type I hypersensitivity allergic reactions and asthma are characterized by high numbers of circulating eosinophils that may be involved in a dual role: regulation of inflammation and contribution to the destructive inflammatory processes observed in the lungs of persons with asthma (see Chapters 9 and 36).

Basophils, which comprise less than 1% (0.01% to 0.3%) of the leukocytes, contain cytoplasmic granules that have an abundant mixture of biochemical mediators, including histamine, chemotactic factors, proteolytic enzymes (e.g., elastase, lysophospholipase), and an anticoagulant (heparin) (see Fig. 28.4, *E*). Stimulation of basophils also induces synthesis of vasoactive lipid molecules (e.g., leukotrienes) and cytokines. Basophils produce IL-6, which induces IL-10 by T helper 1 (Th1) cells and also induces Th2 cells that favor B-cell differentiation.[3] Basophils also are a particularly rich source of the cytokine IL-4,[4] which preferentially guides B-cell differentiation toward plasma cells that secrete IgE (see Chapter 8).

The numbers of basophils are often increased at sites of allergic inflammatory reactions and parasitic infection, particularly ectoparasites (e.g., ticks). IgE receptors on the basophil would induce degranulation at sites of IgE-mediated hypersensitivity reactions and contribute to the local inflammatory response.

Mast cells are highly similar to basophils, but are generated from a different set of precursor cells in the bone marrow, from which they migrate in an immature form into tissues.[5] They reside in vascularized connective tissues just beneath body epithelial surfaces, including the submucosal tissues of the gastrointestinal and respiratory tracts and the dermal layer that lies just below the surface of the skin. Mast cells play a central role in inflammation, and their activation and degranulation affect a great number of cells, including those involved in inflammation (e.g., vascular endothelial cells, smooth muscle cells, circulating platelets and leukocytes, nerves) and healing (e.g., fibroblasts), as well as glandular cells and cells of the immune system. Their activation contributes greatly to increased permeability of blood vessels and synthesis of mediators producing smooth muscle contraction (see Fig. 7.11).

Agranulocytes. The agranulocytes—monocytes, macrophages, and lymphocytes—differ from the granulocytes in that they contain

TABLE 28.3	MONONUCLEAR PHAGOCYTE SYSTEM*	
NAME OF CELL	**LOCATION**	
Committed Stem Cells[†]	Bone marrow	
Monoblasts	Bone marrow	
Promonoblasts	Bone marrow	
Monocytes	Bone marrow and peripheral blood	
Macrophages	Tissue	
Kupffer cells	Liver macrophages	
Alveolar macrophages	Lung	
Histiocytes	Connective tissue	
Macrophages	Bone marrow	
Fixed and free macrophages	Spleen and lymph nodes	
Pleural and peritoneal macrophages	Serous cavities	
Adipose macrophages	Adipose (fat) tissue	
Microglial cells	Nervous system	
Mesangial cells	Kidney	
Osteoclasts	Bone	
Langerhans cells	Skin	
Dendritic cells	Lymphoid tissue, lining of respiratory and gastrointestinal tracts	

*Formerly called the *reticuloendothelial system.*
[†]Development of blood cells from stem cells in the marrow is described on this page and illustrated in Fig. 28.12.
Modified from Kumar V et al: *Robbins & Cotran pathologic basis of disease,* ed 9, Philadelphia, 2015 Saunders.

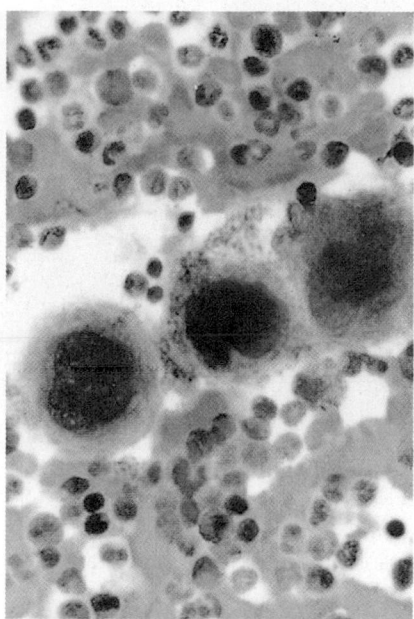

FIGURE 28.5 Megakaryocyte and Platelets. Note the large number of platelets *(purple)* that have budded from the surrounding large megakaryocytes in the center. (From Miale JB: *Laboratory medicine: hematology,* ed 6, St Louis, 1982, Mosby.)

relatively fewer granules in their cytoplasm. Monocytes and macrophages make up the mononuclear phagocyte system.

The mononuclear phagocyte system (MPS), also known as the *reticuloendothelial system* or *macrophage system,* consists of specialized endothelial cells in the bone marrow, spleen, and lymph nodes: promonocytes and their precursors in the bone marrow; monocytes in the peripheral blood; and a portion of macrophages that reside in the tissues, remaining there for months or perhaps years.[6] Cells of the MPS ingest and destroy (by phagocytosis) unwanted materials, such as foreign protein particles, circulating immune complexes, microorganisms, debris from dead or injured cells, defective or injured erythrocytes, and dead neutrophils. Recently, the osteoclast was classified as a true member of the MPS. Macrophages stimulate formation of osteoclasts, multinucleated macrophage-like cells specialized for the function of lacunar bone resorptions and remodeling, in addition to phagocytosis.[7] Table 28.3 lists the various names given to macrophages localized in specific tissues.

Monocytes are the largest normal blood cell and have a horseshoe-shaped nucleus (see Fig. 28.4, G). They are formed and released by the bone marrow into the bloodstream. Monocytes migrate into a variety of tissues and fully mature into tissue macrophages and myeloid dendritic cells (see Table 28.3). Other monocytes may mature into macrophages in the circulation and migrate out of the vessels in response to infection or inflammation. Macrophages are generally larger and are more active as phagocytes than monocytes. Dendritic cells frequently extend projections *(dendrites)* into the tissue and assume a "neuron-like" appearance. The origin and turnover of many of the tissue macrophages are not precisely known. It seems clear that once monocytes leave the circulation, they do not return. They can survive many months or even years.

The normal role of macrophages is to remove old and damaged cells and large molecular substances from the blood. Cellular targets of macrophage phagocytosis include circulating senescent or damaged erythrocytes and platelets (removed primarily in spleen), dead neutrophils (in the circulation and at sites of inflammation), and cells undergoing

apoptosis. Noncellular targets include antigen-antibody complexes, cellular debris, products of coagulation, and macromolecules (such as lipids and carbohydrates synthesized by the body as the result of faulty metabolism, as in storage diseases). Macrophages remove and kill contaminating microorganisms in the blood (mostly in the liver and spleen) and at sites of infection. Macrophages and, particularly, dendritic cells are the major "antigen-processing" and "antigen-presenting" cells that initiate immune responses (see Chapter 8). Macrophages initiate wound healing and tissue remodeling and if activated by cytokines from T cells secrete a large array of biologically active chemicals that if uncontrolled result in chronic inflammation and tissue injury (see Chapter 7).

Lymphocytes constitute approximately 25% to 33% of the total leukocyte count and are the primary cells of the immune response (see Fig. 28.4, F, and Table 28.2; also see Chapter 8). Most lymphocytes transiently circulate in the blood and eventually reside in secondary lymphoid tissues as mature T cells, B cells, or plasma cells. The lymphocytes do not contain any enzyme-filled digestive vacuoles. The life span of the lymphocyte can be days, months, or years, depending on its type and subtype. (Lymphocyte function and dysfunction are described in detail in Unit III.)

Natural killer (NK) cells, which resemble large granular lymphocytes, kill some types of tumor cells (in vitro) and some virus-infected cells without being induced by previous exposure to these antigens (see Chapters 7 and 8). Hence they are named *natural killer cells* to differentiate them from T-cytotoxic cells, which are induced by antigen. NK cells also have the capacity to activate T cells and phagocytes and produce a variety of cytokines that can regulate immune responses. The predominant form of NK cells develops in the bone marrow and circulates in the blood, where it accounts for 5% to 10% of the circulating lymphoid pool, and is found mainly in the peripheral blood and spleen. NK cells develop independent of a thymus, although some NK precursors are found in the thymus and may develop into NK T cells that have markers of both NK and T cells.

Platelets. Platelets (thrombocytes) are not true cells but irregularly shaped cytoplasmic fragments that are essential for blood coagulation

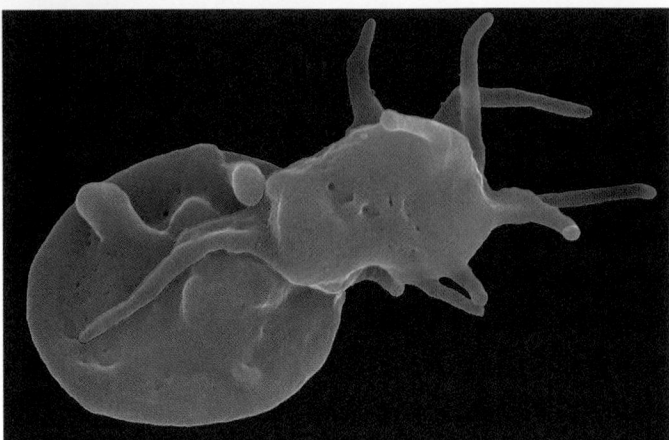

FIGURE 28.6 Colored Micrograph of Platelets. The platelet on the left is moderately activated, with a generally round shape and the beginning of formation of pseudopodia (footlike extensions from the membrane). The platelet on the right is fully activated, with extensive pseudopodia that increase its surface area. (Copyright Dennis Kunkel, Microscopy, Inc.)

and control of bleeding. They are formed in the bone marrow by fragmentation of very large (40 to 100 μm in diameter) cells known as megakaryocytes (Fig. 28.5), a process that takes 7 to 10 days. They lack a nucleus and deoxyribonucleic acid (DNA), and are incapable of mitotic division. They do, however, contain cytoplasmic granules (i.e., dense granules, alpha granules, and lysosomes) capable of releasing biochemical mediators when stimulated by injury to a blood vessel. These mediators are generally proinflammatory (e.g., adenosine diphosphate [ADP], adenosine triphosphate [ATP], calcium, serotonin, and histamine). The alpha granules contain a mixture of coagulation factors, growth and angiogenic factors (e.g., platelet-derived growth factor [PDGF], vascular endothelial growth factor [VEGF], and basic fibroblast growth factor), and angiogenesis inhibitors (e.g., platelet factor 4, thrombospondin, and inhibitors of metalloproteinases). Depending upon the particular stimulus, platelets may selectively release promoters or inhibitors of angiogenesis.[8] Activation also stimulates synthesis of arachidonic acid pathway products (e.g., thromboxane A_2) (see Chapter 7). Platelets can assume different shapes with pseudopodia and adhere to collagen fibers in damaged vascular walls, plugging vascular openings (the platelet plug) to control bleeding (Fig. 28.6).

There are approximately 140,000 to 340,000 platelets/mm³ of circulating blood. An additional one-third of the body's available platelets are in a reserve pool in the spleen. A platelet circulates for approximately 8 to 11 days, ages, and is removed by macrophages of the MPS, mostly in the spleen.

Lymphoid Organs

The lymphoid system is closely integrated with the circulatory system. The lymphoid organs, some of which are merely aggregations of lymphoid tissue, are classified as primary or secondary. The primary lymphoid organs are the thymus and the bone marrow. The secondary lymphoid organs consist of the spleen, lymph nodes, tonsils, and Peyer patches in the ileum of the small intestine. All of the lymphoid organs link the hematologic and immune systems in that they are sites of residence, proliferation, differentiation, or function of lymphocytes and mononuclear phagocytes (monocytes and macrophages). (The liver, which also has hematologic functions, is primarily a digestive organ and is described in Chapter 41.)

Spleen

The spleen is the largest of the secondary lymphoid organs. It is a site of fetal hematopoiesis, filters blood-borne antigens and cleanses the blood through the action of mononuclear phagocytes, initiates immune responses to blood-borne microorganisms (particularly bacteria), destroys aged erythrocytes, and serves as a reservoir for blood.[9] The spleen is a concave, encapsulated organ that weighs approximately 150 g and is about the size of a fist. It is located in the left upper abdominal cavity, curved around a portion of the stomach (see Fig. 8.3). Strands of connective tissue (trabeculae) extend from the capsule, dividing the spleen into compartments (Fig. 28.7). The compartments contain masses of lymphoid tissue called *splenic pulp* (white and red) with the white pulp embedded within the red pulp. The spleen is interlaced with many blood vessels, some of which are capable of distending to store blood. Blood that circulates through the spleen comes from the splenic artery, which branches from the descending aorta and reenters the circulatory system through the splenic vein and into the portal vein.

Arterial blood that enters the spleen first encounters the white splenic pulp, which consists of masses of lymphoid tissue containing macrophages and lymphocytes, primarily T lymphocytes in proximity to the arterioles (the periarterial lymphoid sheath) (see Fig. 28.7). Cellular clumps (lymphoid follicles) are formed in the white pulp around the splenic arterioles. The lymphoid follicles consist primarily of B lymphocytes. These are the chief sites of immune function within the spleen. Here blood-borne antigens encounter lymphocytes, initiating the immune response and the conversion of lymphoid follicles into germinal centers where B cells proliferate and differentiate during the humoral immune response (see Chapter 8).

Some of the blood that enters the terminal capillaries continues through the microcirculation and enters highly distensible storage areas called *venous sinuses* in the red pulp of the spleen. The venous sinuses are capable of storing more than 300 mL of blood. Passive dilation of the venous sinuses enables the spleen to increase its storage capacity as needed by the body. Sudden reductions in blood pressure cause the sympathetic nervous system to stimulate constriction of the sinuses, resulting in expulsion of as much as 200 mL of blood into the venous circulation, which helps restore blood volume and increases the hematocrit by as much as 4%.

The endothelial lining of the venous sinuses is discontinuous (having gaps between endothelial cells) and therefore extremely permeable so that blood cells are allowed to exit the circulation. The red pulp contains a system of loosely interconnected resident macrophages that provide the principal site of splenic filtration. Because of the slow circulation in the sinuses (Fig. 28.8), the macrophages easily phagocytose old, damaged, or dead blood cells of all kinds (but chiefly erythrocytes), microorganisms, macromolecules, and particles of debris. Hemoglobin from phagocytosed erythrocytes is catabolized, and heme (iron) is stored in the cytoplasm of the macrophages or released back into the blood to support hemoglobin synthesis[10] (see Fig. 28.18). The macrophages also can remove particulate inclusions containing denatured hemoglobin (Heinz bodies) from erythrocytes without harming the cells themselves. Blood that filters through the red pulp also finds its way into the venous sinuses and hence into the portal circulation.

The spleen is not absolutely necessary for life or for adequate hematologic function. However, splenic absence from any cause (atrophy, traumatic injury, or removal because of disease) has several secondary effects on the body. For example, leukocytosis (high levels of circulating leukocytes) often occurs after splenectomy, suggesting that the spleen exerts some control over the rate of proliferation of leukocyte stem cells in the bone marrow or their release into the bloodstream. Circulating levels of iron may also decrease, reflecting the spleen's role in the iron

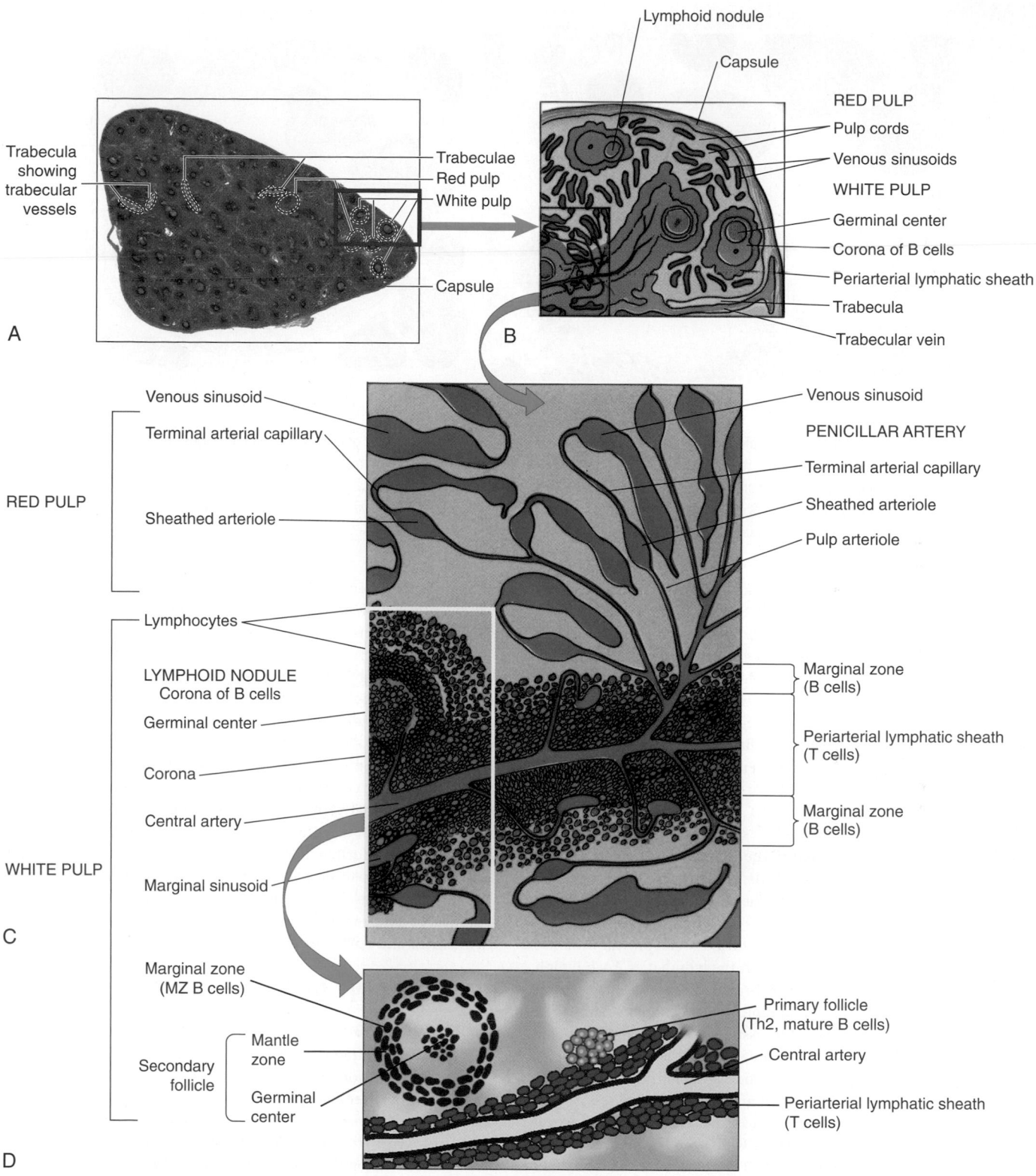

FIGURE 28.7 Splenic Architecture. A, Cross section of the spleen. The spleen is enclosed in a capsule with the interior pulp divided into compartments by strands of connective tissue. The splenic pulp contains regions that are rich in lymphocytes (white pulp) and those containing erythrocytes (red pulp). **B,** Subcapsular splenic structures. **C,** Magnified view of red and white pulp structures. **D,** The splenic artery branches into trabecular arteries and then to central arteries frequently surrounded by a periarterial lymphoid sheath, primarily containing T cells. The secondary lymphoid follicles contain B cells that are proliferating in response to antigen. *Th2,* T-helper 2 cells. (**A** From Telser AG, Young JK, Baldwin KM: *Elsevier's integrated histology,* St Louis, 2007, Mosby; **B** and **C** from Gartner LP, Hiatt JL: *Color textbook of histology,* ed 3, Philadelphia, 2007, Elsevier; **D** from Hoffman R et al: *Hematology: basic principles and practice,* ed 6, Philadelphia, 2013, Churchill Livingstone.)

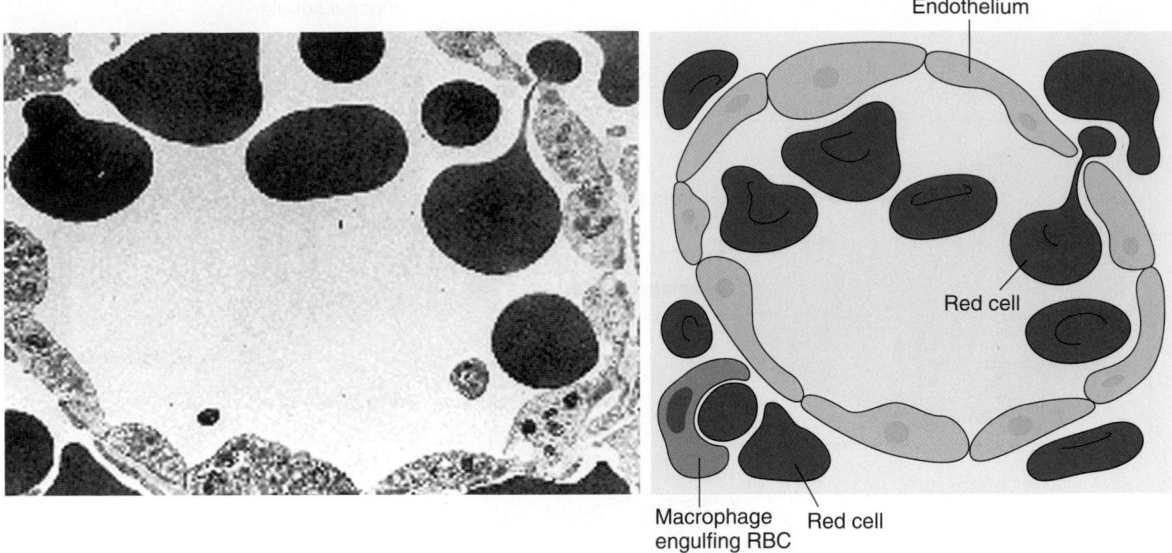

FIGURE 28.8 Splenic Sinus. Transmission electron micrograph and schematic of erythrocytes in the process of squeezing from the red pulp cords into the sinus lumen. Note the degree of deformability required for red cells to pass through the wall of the sinus. *RBC,* Red blood cell. (From Damjanov I, Linder J, editors: *Anderson's pathology,* ed 10, St Louis, 1996, Mosby. Schematic from Kumar V, Fausto N, Abbas A: *Robbins & Cotran pathologic basis of disease,* ed 7, St Louis, 2005, Saunders.)

cycle. The immune response to encapsulated bacteria (e.g., *Streptococcus pneumoniae* [pneumococcus], *Neisseria meningitidis* [meningococcus], *Haemophilus influenzae*), which is primarily an IgM response, may be severely diminished, resulting in increased susceptibility to disseminated infections and sepsis.[11] Loss of the spleen results in an increase in morphologically defective blood cells in the circulation, as well as senescent platelets, confirming the spleen's role in removing old or damaged red blood cells and platelets. Thrombocytosis and thrombosis are complications of splenectomy and can require anticoagulation therapy for 3 to 6 months.[12]

Lymph Nodes

Structurally, lymph nodes are part of the lymphatic system. Lymphatic vessels collect interstitial fluid from the tissues and transport it, as lymph, through vessels of increasing size to the thoracic duct, which drains into the superior vena cava and returns the lymph to the circulation. Lymph nodes are distributed throughout the body and provide filtration of the lymph during its journey through the lymphatics. Each lymph node is enclosed in a fibrous capsule, branches of which (trabeculae) extend inward to partition the node into several compartments (Fig. 28.9). Reticular fibers of connective tissue divide the compartments into a meshwork throughout the lymph node. The node consists of outer (cortex) and inner (paracortex) cortical areas and an inner medulla. Lymph enters through multiple small afferent lymphatic vessels into the subcapsular sinus, just beneath the capsule; drains into the cortical sinuses to the medullary sinuses, from which the lymph is collected; and leaves the node by way of the efferent lymphatic vessel. Blood flows into the lymph nodes through the lymphatic artery, which ends in groups of postcapillary venules distributed throughout the outer cortex. The blood is drained through the lymphatic vein.

Functionally, lymph nodes are part of the hematologic and immune systems and are the primary site for the first encounter between antigen and lymphocytes. Lymphocytes enter the lymph node from the blood through the postcapillary venules by means of diapedesis across the endothelial lining. B lymphocytes tend to migrate preferentially to nodes in the cortex and medulla, whereas T lymphocytes predominantly migrate

to the paracortex (see Fig. 28.9). Macrophages reside in the lymph node; help filter the lymph of debris, foreign substances, and microorganisms; and provide antigen-processing functions. The dendritic cells encounter and process antigens and microorganisms in other tissues, enter the lymph node through the afferent lymph vessels, and migrate throughout the nodes. The reticular network provides adhesive surfaces for trapping large numbers of phagocytes and lymphocytes and facilitating their organization into follicles or primary nodules. The presence of antigen, either removed from the lymph by macrophages or presented on the surface of dendritic cells, results in the production of secondary nodules containing germinal centers. In the germinal centers, lymphocytes, particularly B cells, respond to antigenic stimulation by undergoing proliferation and further differentiation, including class-switch, into memory cells and plasma cells (see Chapter 8). Plasma cells migrate to the medullary cords. The B-lymphocyte proliferation in response to a great deal of antigen (e.g., during infection) may result in lymph node enlargement and tenderness (reactive lymph node).

DEVELOPMENT OF BLOOD CELLS

Hematopoiesis

The typical human requires about 100 billion new blood cells per day. Blood cell production, termed hematopoiesis, is constantly ongoing, occurring in the liver and spleen of the fetus and only in bone marrow (*medullary hematopoiesis*) after birth. These cells carry out functions including oxygen transport, immunity, and tissue remodeling. The process of hematopoiesis involves the biochemical stimulation of populations of relatively undifferentiated cells to undergo mitotic division (i.e., proliferation) and maturation (i.e., differentiation) into mature hematologic cells (Table 28.4). Although proliferation and differentiation are usually sequential, certain blood cells proliferate and differentiate simultaneously. Erythrocytes and granulocytes generally differentiate fully before entering the blood, but monocytes and lymphocytes continue to mature in the blood and in secondary lymphatic organs.

Hematopoiesis continues throughout life, increasing in response to a need to replenish aged RBCs or destroyed circulating cells (e.g., during

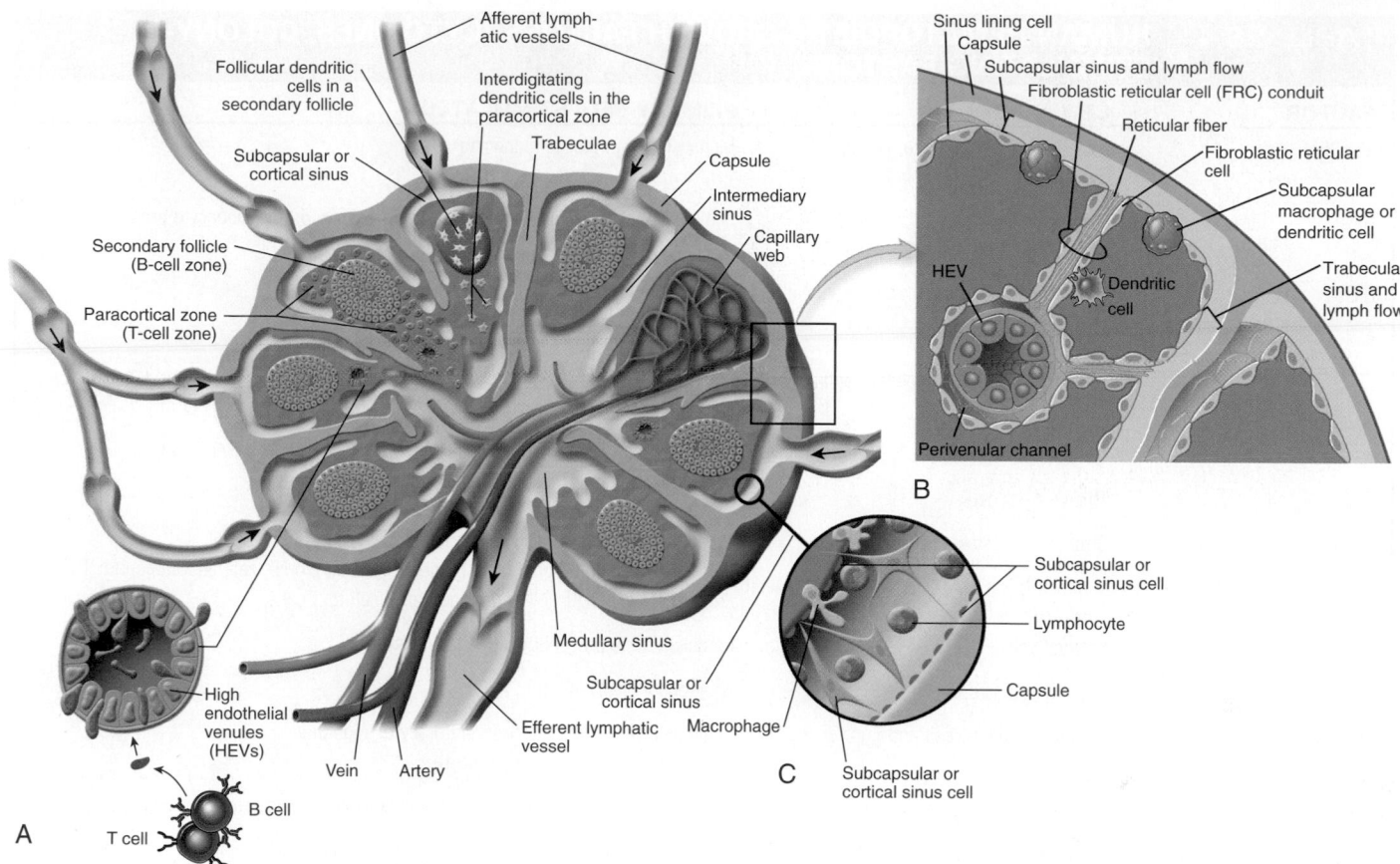

FIGURE 28.9 Lymph Node Architecture. **A,** Cross section showing ingoing and outgoing lymph vessels (afferent and efferent), blood supply, compartmentalization of the B-cell region (secondary follicle), T-cell region (paracortical zone) with precapillary or high endothelium venules, follicular interdigitating dendritic cells, medullary sinus, intermediate sinus, and subcapsular or cortical sinus. Naive B and T lymphocytes enter through the high endothelial venule (HEV), shown in cross section, and are drawn to different areas of the node by chemokines that are produced in these areas and bind selectively to either cell type. **B,** Cellular composition of the lymph node cortex depicting the route of lymph drainage from the subcapsular sinus, through fibroreticular cell conduits, to the perivenular channel around the high endothelial venule (HEV). Dendritic cells pick up antigen from peripheral sites of antigen entry and enter the lymph node through the afferent lymph vessels and migrate to the T-cell region of the node. **C,** Cellular composition of subcapsular sinus. (**A** and **C** From Paulsen F: *Sobottta atlas of human anatomy,* vol 1, ed 15, Philadelphia, 2013, Elsevier; **B** from Abbas AK, Pillai S: *Cellular and molecular immunology,* ed 9, Philadelphia, 2015, Saunders.)

hemorrhage, hemolytic anemia [peripheral destruction of erythrocytes], consumptive thrombocytopenia) or in response to infection. In general, long-term stimuli, such as chronic diseases, cause a greater increase in hematopoiesis than acute conditions, such as hemorrhage.

Various abnormalities in medullary hematopoiesis have been identified and are discussed in Chapter 29. Extramedullary hematopoiesis—blood cell production in tissues other than bone marrow—of apparently normal blood cells has been reported in the spleen, liver, and, less frequently, lymph nodes, adrenal glands, cartilage, adipose tissue, intrathoracic areas, and kidneys. In adults, however, extramedullary hematopoiesis is usually a sign of disease, occurring in pernicious anemia, sickle cell anemia, thalassemia, hemolytic disease of the newborn (erythroblastosis fetalis), hereditary spherocytosis, and certain leukemias.

Bone Marrow

Bone marrow is confined to the cavities of bone and is the primary site of residence of hematopoietic stem cells (Fig. 28.10). Adults have two kinds of bone marrow: red marrow (active or hematopoietic marrow; also called myeloid tissue) and yellow marrow (inactive marrow). The large quantity of fat in marrow is responsible for its yellow appearance. Not all bones contain active marrow. In adults, active marrow is found primarily in the flat bones of the pelvis (34%), vertebrae (28%), cranium and mandible (13%), and sternum and ribs (10%), and in the extreme proximal portions of the humerus and femur (4% to 8%). Inactive marrow predominates in cavities of other bones. (Bones are discussed further in Chapter 44.)

At least two populations of stem cells are found in bone marrow niches. Hematopoietic stem cells (HSCs) are progenitors of all hematologic cells. Both populations of stem cells undergo continuous proliferation and self-renewal in the microenvironment of the bone marrow so that additional HSCs are produced to replace those undergoing differentiation. Mesenchymal stem cells (MSCs) are stromal cells and have a role in maintaining HSCs. They can differentiate into a variety of cells, including osteoblasts (produce bone), adipocytes (store fat), and chondrocytes (produce cartilage).

The hematologic compartment of the bone marrow consists of a variety of cellular and molecular microenvironments, called niches. Niches simultaneously contain stem cells, precursor cells, and terminally

TABLE 28.4   HUMAN HEMATOPOIETIC GROWTH FACTORS (CYTOKINES, COLONY-STIMULATING FACTORS)

FACTOR	CELL ORIGIN	PRIMARY CELL STIMULATED
M-CSF	Macrophage, lymphocyte, fibroblast, endothelial cell, osteoblast	Monocyte progenitor to monocyte
GM-CSF	Macrophage, T cell, endothelial cell, fibroblast, mast cell	Common myeloid progenitor to granulocyte progenitor and monocyte progenitor
G-CSF	Macrophage, fibroblast, endothelial cell	Granulocyte progenitor to neutrophil
IL-2	Th cell	T-cell progenitor to T cell
IL-3	T cell, monocyte/macrophage, stromal cell	Common myeloid progenitor to progenitors for megakaryocyte, erythroid, granulocyte, and monocyte series
IL-4	Th cell	B-cell progenitor to B cell
IL-5	Th cell, mast cell	Common myeloid progenitor to eosinophil
IL-7	Stromal cell, intestinal epithelium	Hematopoietic stem cell to common lymphoid progenitor Common lymphoid progenitor to progenitor B cell, pro NK cell, and progenitor T cell Progenitor T cell to T cell and progenitor B cell to B cell
IL-11	Stromal cell	Megakaryocyte progenitor to megakaryocyte
IL-15	Monocyte/macrophage	NK progenitor to NK cell
Erythropoietin	Peritubular kidney cell and Kupffer cell	Common myeloid progenitor to erythrocyte progenitor Erythrocyte progenitor to erythrocyte
Thrombopoietin	Liver, kidney, skeletal muscle	All cells in megakaryocyte lineage from common myeloid progenitor to platelet
Stem cell factor (steel factor)	Stromal cell in bone marrow and many other cells	Hematopoietic progenitor to common myeloid progenitor Common myeloid progenitor to progenitors for megakaryocyte, erythroid, granulocyte, and monocyte series

G-CSF, Granulocyte colony-stimulating factor; *GM-CSF,* granulocyte-macrophage colony–stimulating factor; *IL,* interleukin; *M-CSF,* macrophage colony-stimulating factor; *NK,* natural killer; *pro,* progenitor; *Th,* T helper.

differentiated cells and provide a coordinated signaling network necessary to regulate the self-renewal, differentiation, and maintenance of HSCs[13] (Fig. 28.11). They protect HSCs by maintaining quiescence, limiting their entry into the cell cycle, and preventing exhaustion or errors in DNA replication. The niches of the bone marrow are commonly described as endosteal (at the interface of bone and bone marrow) and vascular (endothelial and perivascular cells), but this is an oversimplification of the complexity that is emerging with more investigation. There is more likely an array of niches that harbor the cells and cytokines that support hematopoiesis.[14] Niches also have a role in metastasis related to the microenvironment of dormant disseminated cancer cells.[15]

The cellular composition of niches includes osteoclasts, osteoblasts, sinusoidal endothelial cells, fibroblasts, adipocytes, and other stromal cells. Osteoblasts are derived from fibroblasts and are responsible for construction of bone. Osteoclasts are multinucleate cells of monocytic origin that remodel bone by resorption. Both cells are located near the endosteum and can produce cytokines that affect proliferation and maintenance of hematopoietic cells. Megakaryocytes and macrophages promote HSC migration and proliferation in the niches. Adipocytes suppress HSC numbers. The area is innervated through the sympathetic nervous system.

Hematopoietic marrow is vascularized by the primary arteries of the bones. Arterial vessels enter the bone, branch near the endosteum into smaller arterioles and capillaries, and drain into venous sinusoids (see Fig. 28.11). These sinuses coalesce into a large central sinus in the central cavity. Hematopoietic marrow and fat (yellow marrow) fill the spaces surrounding the network of venous sinuses. Newly produced blood cells traverse narrow openings between endothelial cells in the venous sinus walls and thus enter the circulation. Dormant or quiescent HSCs localize near small arterioles of the endosteal region that are ensheathed by pericytes, which express high levels of nestin and act together with sympathetic nerves to promote HSC maintenance and retention. The low blood flow of the arteriole/sinusoid network limits gas exchange, creates a relatively hypoxic microenvironment, and maintains quiescence.[16] Active HSCs are located near the sinusoids, which are likely more diverse in their influence for self-renewal, proliferation, and differentiation.[17]

Hematopoietic niches are affected by direct cell-to-cell signaling and by soluble mediators produced by cells within the niches. Niches contain two specialized MSCs: CXCL12-abundant sinusoidal reticular (CAR) cells and periarteriolar and sinusoidal nestin-expressing cells.[18] These cells closely interact with HSCs and provide intercellular signaling through several HSC regulatory molecules important for retention, expansion, maintenance, and quiescence of HSCs. These molecules include chemokine ligand 12 (CXCL12, promotes retention and expansion of HSCs), stem cell factor (SCF, stimulates hematopoiesis), vascular cell adhesion molecule 1 (VCAM-1, promotes HSC retention), and secreted protein angiopoietin 1 (ANG1, promotes quiescence or HSC stemness or ability to self-replicate). The CAR cell is the predominant cell in the sinusoids.[13] The sympathetic nervous system regulates HSC mobilization through circadian release of β_3-norepinephrine (adrenergic signaling), which down-regulates CXCL12 expression in the bone marrow. Nestin-expressing MSCs express large amounts of the protein nestin and, particularly, SCF and VCAM-1. Transforming growth factor-beta (TGF-β) also plays an important role in regulating HSC behavior, particularly quiescence and self-renewal.[19]

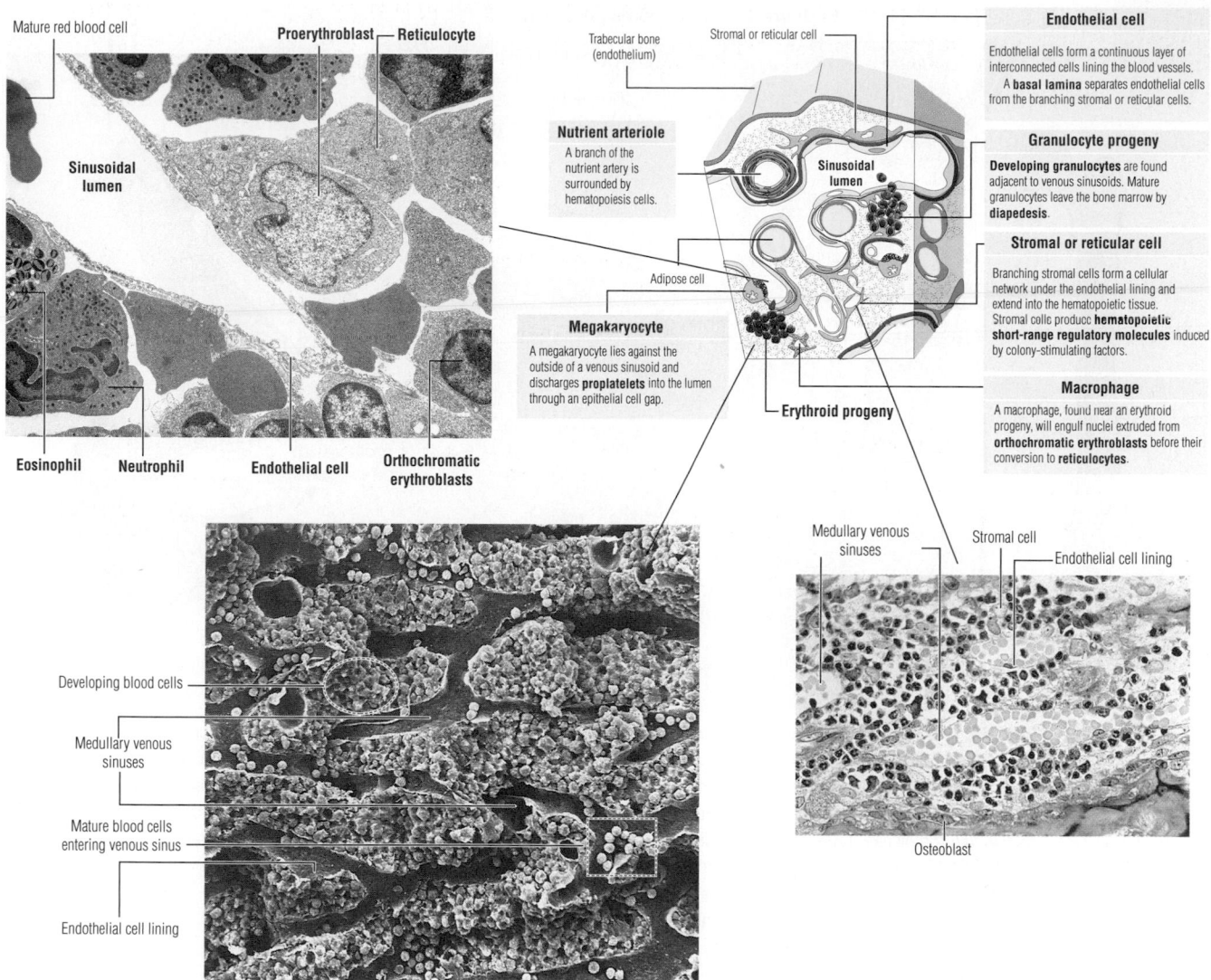

FIGURE 28.10 Bone Marrow: Structure and Vascularization. (From Kierszenbaum A, Tres L: *Histology and cell biology: an introduction to pathology,* ed 4, Philadelphia, 2016, Mosby. Scanning electron micrograph from Kessel RG, Kardon RH: *Tissues and organs,* New York, 1979, WH Freeman.)

Cellular Differentiation

All humans originate from a single cell (the fertilized egg) that has the capacity to proliferate and eventually differentiate into the huge diversity of cells of the human body. After fertilization, the egg divides over a 5-day period to form a hollow ball (blastocyst) that implants on the uterus. Until about 3 days after fertilization, each cell (blastomere) is undifferentiated and retains the capacity to differentiate into any cell type. In the 5-day blastocyst, the outer layer cells have undergone differentiation and commitment to become the placenta. Cells of the inner cell mass *(embryonic stem cells),* however, continue to have unlimited differentiation potential (currently referred to as being *pluripotent*) and can grow into different kinds of tissue—blood, nerves, heart, bone, and so forth. After implantation, cells of the inner cell mass begin differentiation into other cell types. Differentiation is a multistep process and results in intermediate groups of stem cells *(multipotent stem cells)* with more limited, but still impressive, abilities to differentiate into many different types of cells[20] (Fig. 28.12).

Within the bone marrow niches, each type of blood cell originates from hematopoietic stem cells that proliferate and differentiate under the control of a variety of cytokines and growth factors (see Fig. 28.12 and Table 28.4). During this process some hematopoietic stem cells undergo alternative paths of differentiation into more differentiated stem cells that are committed to a particular line of blood cells.

As with all stem cells, the hematopoietic stem cells are self-renewing (they have the ability to proliferate without further differentiation) so that a relatively constant population of stem cells is available. Some hematopoietic stem cells will continue differentiation into hematopoietic progenitor cells. Progenitor cells retain proliferative capacity but are committed to possible further differentiation into particular types of hematologic cells: lymphoid (lymphocytes, NK cells), granulocyte-monocyte (granulocytes, monocytes, macrophages), and megakaryocyte-erythroid (platelets, erythrocytes) progenitor cells (see Fig. 28.12).

In addition to intercellular signaling events between HSCs and cells in the osteoblastic and vascular niches, several cytokines participate in hematopoiesis, particularly **colony-stimulating factors (CSFs or hematopoietic growth factors)**, which stimulate the proliferation of progenitor cells and their progeny and initiate the maturation events necessary to produce fully mature cells (see Fig. 28.12). Multiple cell types in the hematopoietic organs, including endothelial cells, fibroblasts, and lymphocytes, produce the necessary CSFs (Box 28.1).

Endosteal area   Vascular area

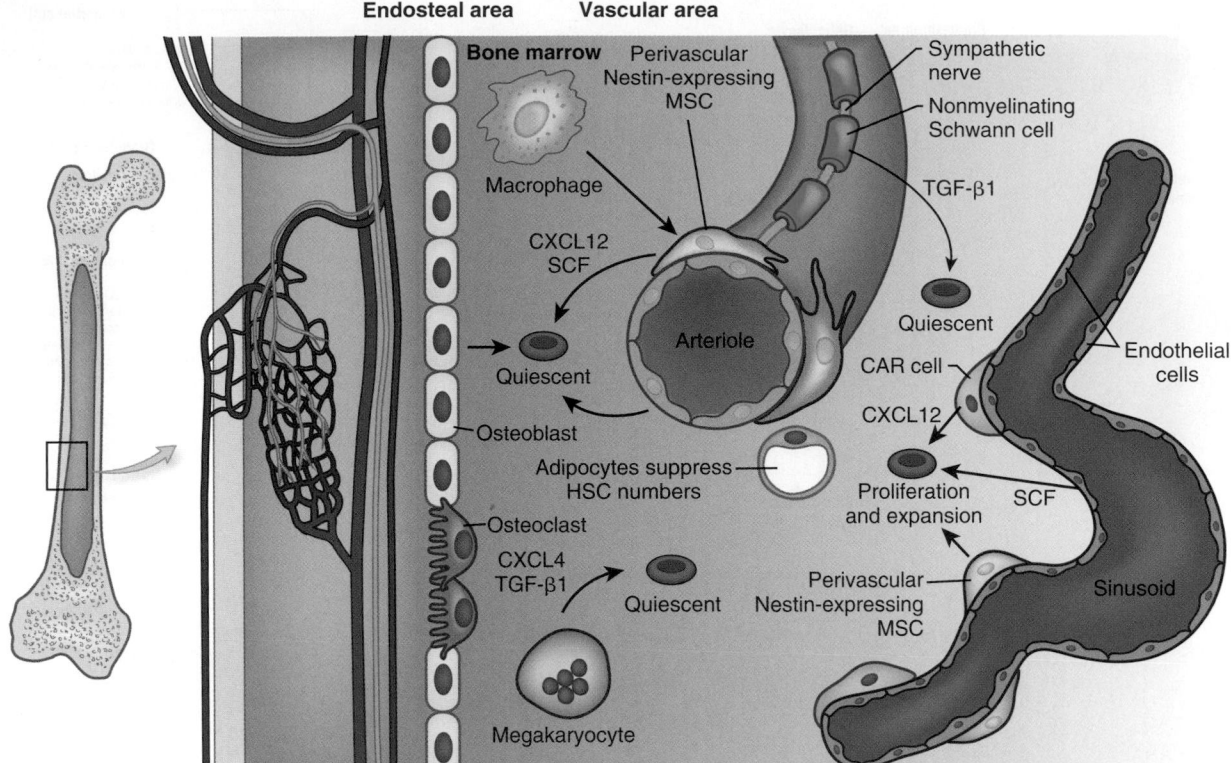

FIGURE 28.11 Bone Marrow Stem Cell Niches. Stem cell niches are microenvironments where stem cells undergo hematopoiesis into all forms of blood cells. Stem cell niches retain and maintain adult quiescent hematopoietic stem cells (HSCs) and are activated to promote cell self-renewal, proliferation, and differentiation to form new cells. The fate of individual HSCs is determined by interactions (intercellular adherence, cytokines, chemokines) with specialized cells within the niches. *CAR*, CXCL12-abundant reticular cells; *CXCL4*, chemokine ligand 4 (also known as *platelet factor 4*); *CXLC12*, chemokine ligand 12; *MSC*, mesenchymal stem cells; *SCF*, stem cell factor; *TGF-β1*, transforming growth factor-beta 1. (Adapted from Boulais PE, Frenette PS: *Blood* 125[17]:2621–2629; Schepers K, Campbell TB, Passegué E: *Cell Stem Cell* 16[3]:254–267, 2015.)

Hematopoiesis in the bone marrow occurs in two separate pools: the stem cell pool and the bone marrow pool (Fig. 28.13). The stem cell pool is the product of self-renewal that maintains the number of pluripotent stem cells and partially committed progenitor cells. The bone marrow pool contains cells that are proliferating and maturing in preparation for release into the circulation and mature cells that are stored for later release into the peripheral blood. The peripheral blood also contains two pools of cells: those in the circulation and those stored around the walls of the blood vessels (often called the **marginating storage pool**). The marginating storage pool primarily consists of neutrophils that adhere to the endothelium in vessels where the blood flow is relatively slow. These cells can rapidly move into tissues and mucous membranes when needed (i.e., during an inflammatory response).

Under certain conditions of rapid depletion of the circulating pool, the circulating hematologic cells need to be rapidly replenished. Medullary hematopoiesis can be accelerated by any or all of three mechanisms: (1) conversion of yellow bone marrow, which does not produce blood cells, to hematopoietic red marrow by the actions of **erythropoietin** (a hormone that stimulates erythrocyte production); (2) faster differentiation of progenitor cells; and (3) faster proliferation of stem cells into progenitor cells (see Table 28.4).

Development of Erythrocytes

For almost 100 years it was believed that erythrocytes developed from lymphocytes that were transformed in the spleen. It was not

until the 1850s that the bone marrow was identified as the site of erythropoiesis.

Erythropoiesis

Erythropoiesis is the development of red blood cells. In the confines of the bone marrow, erythroid progenitor cells proliferate and differentiate into large, nucleated **proerythroblasts**, which are committed into producing cells of the erythroid series (Fig. 28.14). All stages of erythroid development are referred to as the *erythron*. The proerythroblast, which has ribosomes and can produce protein, differentiates through several intermediate forms of **erythroblast** while synthesizing hemoglobin and progressively eliminating most intracellular structures, including the nucleus. Thus the maturing erythroblast becomes more compact and progressively assumes the shape and characteristics of an erythrocyte. Hemoglobin is readily apparent and increases in quantity as nuclear size shrinks throughout the basophilic and polychromatophilic stages. The orthochromatic erythroblast (**normoblast**) is the smallest of the nucleated erythrocyte precursors.

The last immature form of the erythroblast is the **reticulocyte**, which is anuclear and contains a meshlike (reticular) network of ribosomal ribonucleic acid (rRNA) that is visible microscopically after being stained with certain dyes. The reticulocyte contains polyribosomes (for globin synthesis) and mitochondria (for oxidative metabolism and heme synthesis). The reticulocyte matures into an erythrocyte within 24 to 48 hours. During this period, mitochondria and ribosomes disappear

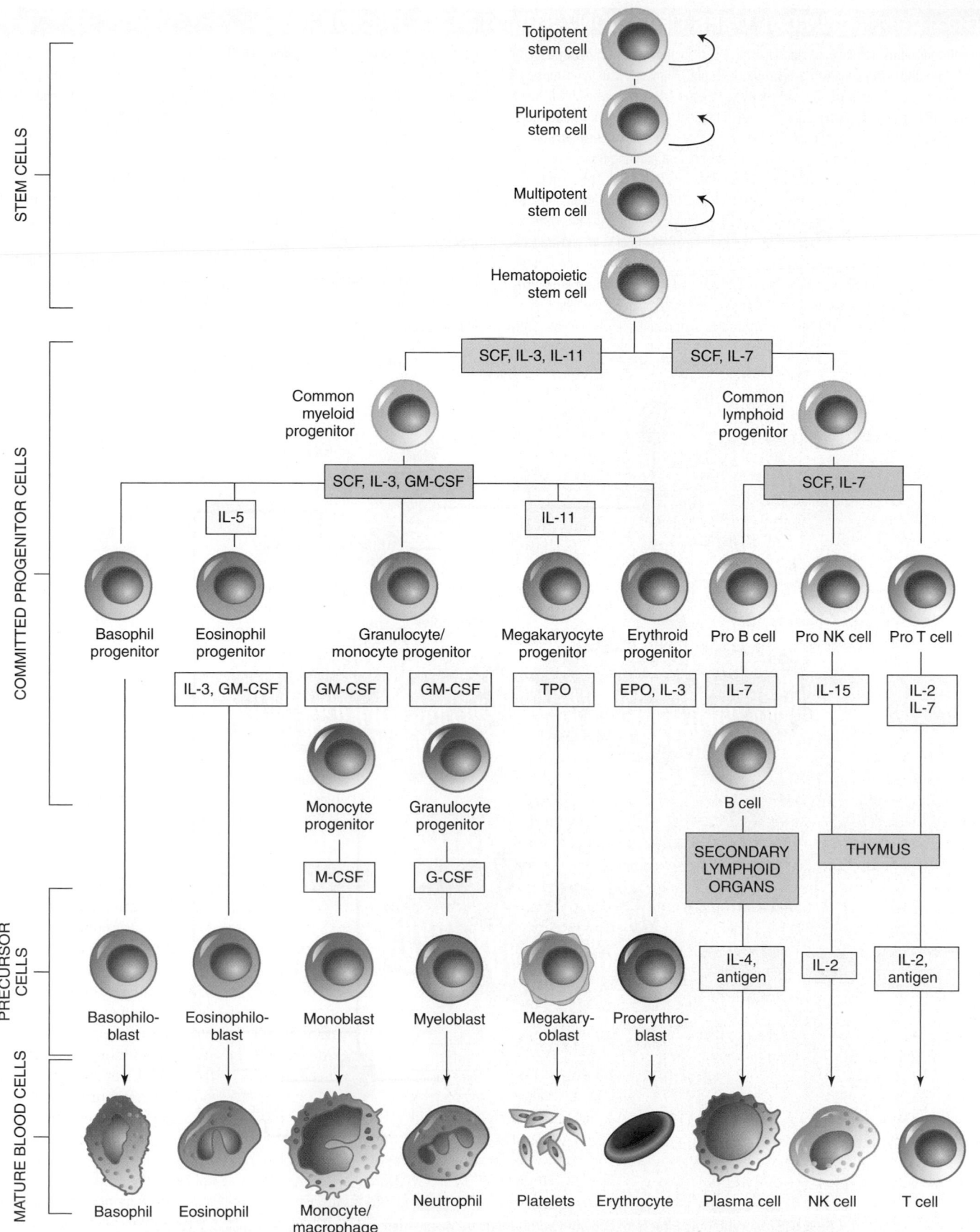

FIGURE 28.12 Differentiation of Hematopoietic Cells. Curved arrows indicate proliferation and expansion of prehematopoietic stem cell populations. *EPO,* Erythropoietin; *G-CSF,* granulocyte colony-stimulating factor; *GM-CSF,* granulocyte-macrophage colony–stimulating factor; *IL,* interleukin; *M-CSF,* macrophage colony-stimulating factor; *NK,* natural killer; *SCF,* stem cell factor; *TPO,* thrombopoietin.

BOX 28.1 CLINICAL USES OF COLONY-STIMULATING FACTOR (CSF)

Neutrophils are normally present in the blood in the range of 4000 to 6000 cells/μL, and in response to a bacterial infection, numbers usually increase to 10,000 to 20,000 cells/μL. Susceptibility to infection develops when levels drop below 1000 cells/μL, such as during congenital neutropenia or as a consequence of cytotoxic therapy for cancer. Similarly, normal levels of other hematologic cells may be suppressed (e.g., congenital or acquired immune deficiencies and anemia or myelodysplastic syndromes) (see Chapters 9 and 29). The numbers of circulating hematologic cells are under the control of CSFs (see Table 28.4). CSF therapy can stimulate increases in circulating granulocyte-monocyte populations, but the degree of response depends on the available numbers of stem and progenitor cells that have survived chemotherapy or the effects of disease (see Figure).

Administration of CSFs has been approved for use when neutropenia is <1500/μL, and current guidelines recommend their use when the risk for febrile neutropenia is >20%.[1] The results of CSF use to prevent neutropenia in individuals with cancer have been variable. In a review of 633 individuals receiving myelosuppressive chemotherapy and treated with granulocyte CSF (G-CSF) to prevent neutropenia for nonmyeloid malignancies, adverse events occurred in about 27% of individuals, including bone pain, myalgia, and asthenia.[2] A recent study reported improved prognosis using CSF therapy for prevention of febrile neutropenia associated with chemotherapy in adult acute lymphoblastic leukemia.[3] Results of other studies using prophylactic granulocyte colony-stimulating factors to prevent febrile neutropenia in adult acute leukemia and stem cell transplants have been disappointing.[4] An analysis of 19 trials in which CSFs were administered postchemotherapy to those with acute myelogenous leukemia detected no effect on overall survival or infections.[5] Using CSF prophylactically to avoid neutropenia in individuals undergoing chemotherapy for breast cancer has shown low to modest benefit.[6] An analysis of randomized trials of prophylactic use of GM-CSF and G-CSF in individuals undergoing chemotherapy for metastatic breast cancer indicated a

FIGURE Morphologic Effects of Growth Factor. Marrow aspirate from a patient receiving granulocyte colony-stimulating factor (G-CSF) showing an early neutrophil response. There is a marked shift toward immaturity in the neutrophils with the majority at the promyelocyte and early myelocyte stages of maturation (Wright-Giemsa stain). (From Damjanov I, Linder J, editors: *Anderson's pathology*, ed 10, St Louis, 1996, Mosby.)

BOX 28.1   CLINICAL USES OF COLONY-STIMULATING FACTOR (CSF)—cont'd

significant effect on prevention of febrile neutropenia and a decrease of general mortality and need for hospital care.[7] However, no effect was observed on the incidence of severe neutropenia, infections, or infection-related mortality. There is substantial lack of data to encourage the use of G-CSF and GM-CSF for the prevention of infection in cases of neutropenia associated with myelodysplastic syndromes.[8] In severe congenital neutropenia, treatment with G-CSF increases the absolute neutrophil count but use of GM-CSF is not effective.[9] CSF treatment can result in shorter periods of intensive nursing and hospitalization but the cost of use must be considered in relation to outcome benefit and healthcare policy. Recombinant or biosimilar CSFs (e.g., G-CSF, GM-CSF, erythropoietin) are being mass-produced for therapeutic use.[10]

References

1. Mehta HM, Malandra M, Corey SJ: G-CSF and GM-CSF in neutropenia. *J Immunol* 195(4):1341–1349, 2015.
2. Pettengell R, et al: Clinical safety of tbo-filgrastim, a short-acting human granulocyte colony-stimulating factor. *Support Care Cancer* 24(6):2677–2684, 2016.
3. Ye SG, et al: Colony-stimulating factors for chemotherapy-related febrile neutropenia are associated with improved prognosis in adult acute lymphoblastic leukemia. *Mol Clin Oncol* 3(3):730–736, 2015.
4. K Hockings J, et al: Impact of recommended weight-based dosing of granulocyte-colony stimulating factors in acute leukemia and stem cell transplant patients. *Support Care Cancer* 25(6), 2017.
5. Gurion R, et al: Colony-stimulating factors for prevention and treatment of infectious complications in patients with myelogenous leukemia. *Cochrane Database Syst Rev* (6):CD008238, 2012.
6. Agiro A, et al: Risk of neutropenia-related hospitalization in patients who received colony-stimulating factors with chemotherapy for breast cancer. *J Clin Oncol* 34(32):3872–3879, 2016.
7. Renner P, et al: Primary prophylactic colony-stimulating factors for the prevention of chemotherapy-induced febrile neutropenia in breast cancer patients. *Cochrane Database Syst Rev* (10):CD007913, 2012.
8. Hutzschenreuter F, et al: Granulocyte and granulocyte-macrophage colony stimulating factors for newly diagnosed patients with myelodysplastic syndromes. *Cochrane Database Syst Rev* (2):CD009310, 2016.
9. Koch C, et al: GM-CSF treatment is not effective in congenital neutropenia patients due to its inability to activate NAMPT signaling. *Ann Hematol* 96(3):345–353, 2017.
10. Schulz M, Bonig H: Update on biosimilars of granulocyte colony-stimulating factor—when no news is good news. *Curr Opin Hematol* 23(1):61–66, 2016.

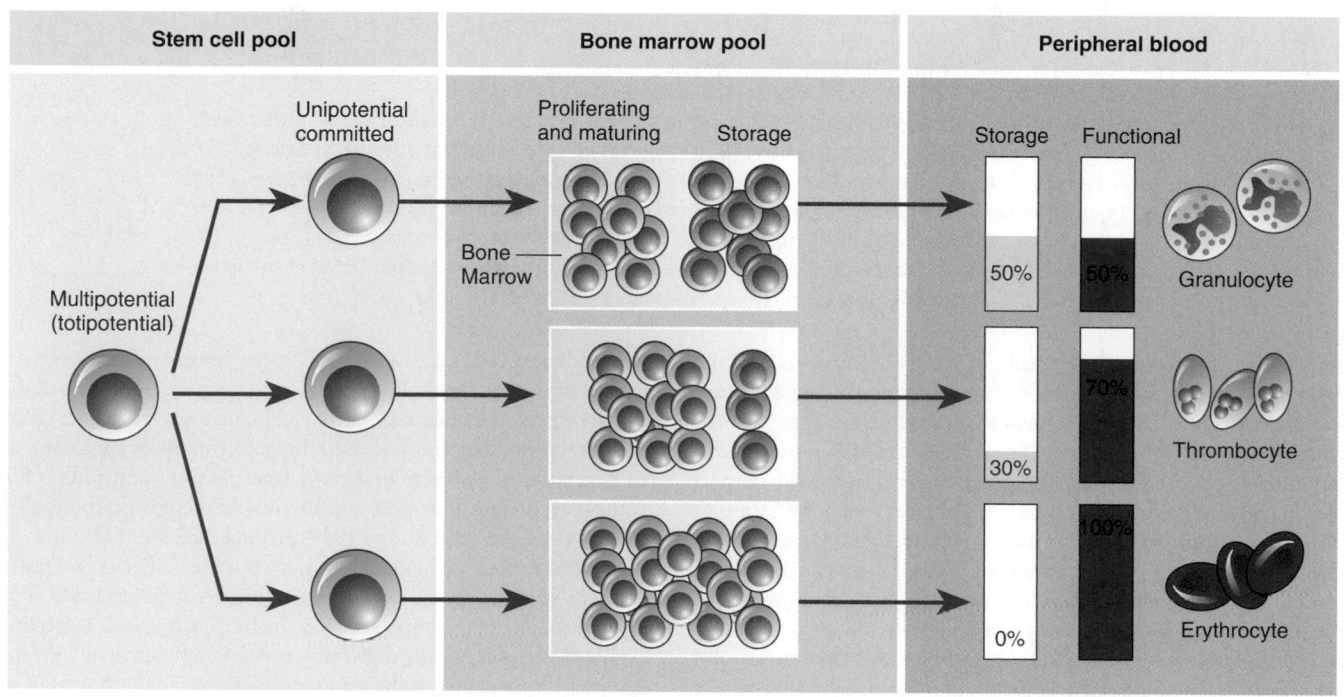

FIGURE 28.13 Hematopoiesis. Hematopoiesis from the stem cell pool; activity occurs mainly in the bone marrow and in the peripheral blood. (Modified from Harmening DM, editor: *Clinical hematology and fundamentals of hemostasis,* ed 3, Philadelphia, 1997, FA Davis.)

and the cell becomes smaller and more disklike. With these final changes, the erythrocyte loses its capacity for hemoglobin synthesis and oxidative metabolism. Reticulocytes remain in the marrow approximately 1 day and are released into the venous sinuses. They continue to mature in the bloodstream and may travel to the spleen for several days of additional maturation. The normal reticulocyte count is 1% of the total red blood cell count. Approximately 1% of the body's circulating erythrocyte mass normally is generated every 24 hours. Therefore the reticulocyte count is a useful clinical index of erythropoietic activity and indicates whether new red cells are being produced.

Regulation of Erythropoiesis

In healthy individuals, the total volume of circulating erythrocytes remains surprisingly constant. Most steps of erythropoiesis are primarily under the control of a feedback loop involving the glycoprotein erythropoietin (see Table 28.4). In conditions of tissue hypoxia, erythropoietin

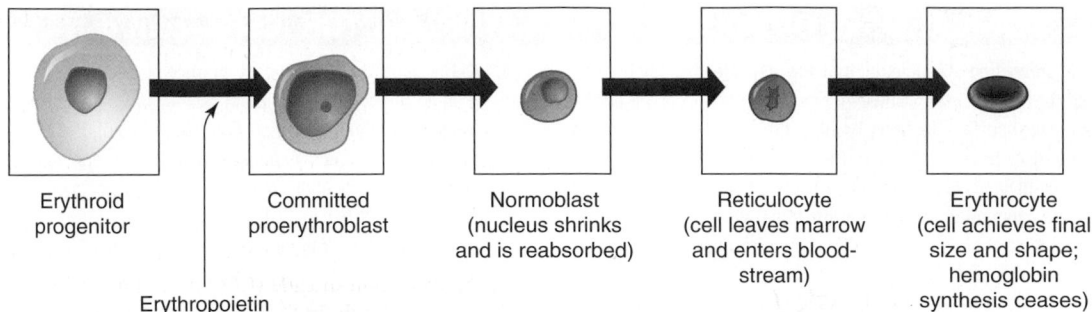

FIGURE 28.14 Erythrocyte Differentiation. Erythrocyte differentiation from large nucleated progenitor cells to small nonnucleated erythrocytes.

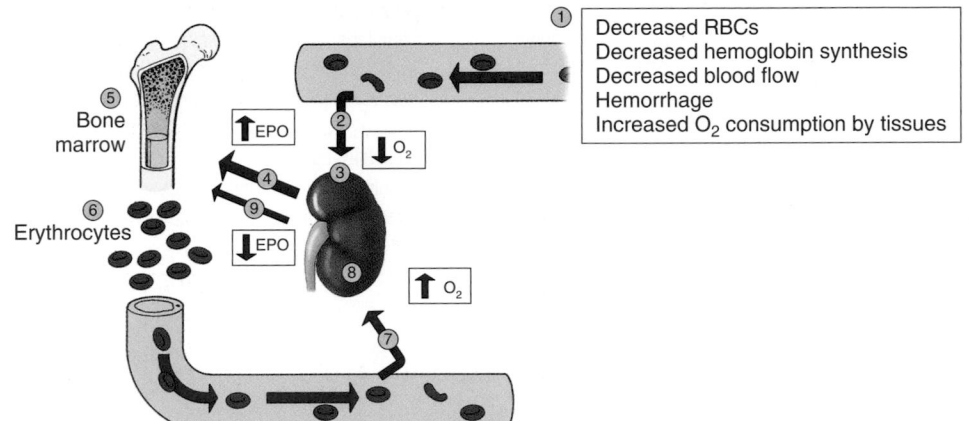

FIGURE 28.15 Role of Erythropoietin in Regulation of Erythropoiesis. (1) Decreased arterial oxygen levels result in **(2)** decreased tissue oxygen (hypoxia) that **(3)** stimulates the kidney to increase **(4)** production of erythropoietin. Erythropoietin is carried to the bone marrow **(5)** and binds to erythropoietin receptors on proerythroblasts, resulting in increased red cell production and maturation and expansion of the erythron **(6)**. The increased release of red cells into the circulation frequently corrects the hypoxia in the tissues **(7)**. **(8)** Perception of normal oxygen levels by the kidney causes **(9)** diminished production of erythropoietin (negative feedback) and return to normal levels of erythrocyte production. *EPO*, Erythropoietin; O_2, oxygen in the blood and tissue; *RBCs*, red blood cells.

is secreted by the liver and, primarily, by the peritubular cells of the kidney[21] (Fig. 28.15). Rising levels of circulating erythropoietin cause a compensatory increase in proliferation and differentiation of pro-erythroblasts in the bone marrow. The density of cellular erythropoietin receptor decreases progressively during erythroid maturation to almost undetectable levels on reticulocytes. The normal steady-state rate of production of approximately 2.5 million erythrocytes per second can increase to 17 million per second during anemia or under conditions of low oxygen concentration, such as high-altitude environments or pulmonary disease. Thus the body responds to reduced oxygenation of blood in two ways: (1) stimulation of chemoreceptors of the carotid body and aortic arch that signals the brain to increase oxygen intake through increased ventilation; and (2) stimulation of receptors on the kidney peritubular cells to increase erythropoietin synthesis and release, thus increasing the oxygen-carrying capacity of the blood.

Recombinant human erythropoietin (r-HuEPO) is used in individuals with anemia secondary to decreased erythropoietin production from chronic renal failure. An immediate effect of increased endogenous or exogenous erythropoietin is an increase in the blood reticulocyte count, followed by increasing levels of erythrocytes. The most significant side effect associated with r-HuEPO is increased blood pressure.

Hemoglobin Synthesis

Hemoglobin (Hb), the oxygen-carrying protein of the erythrocyte, constitutes approximately 90% of the cell's dry weight. Hemoglobin-

packed blood cells take up oxygen in the lungs and exchange it for carbon dioxide in the tissues. A single erythrocyte can contain as many as 300 hemoglobin molecules. Hemoglobin increases the oxygen-carrying capacity of blood by 100-fold. Each hemoglobin molecule is composed of two pairs of polypeptide chains (the globins) and four colorful complexes of iron plus protoporphyrin (the hemes), responsible for blood's ruby-red color and oxygen-carrying capacity (Fig. 28.16).

Several variants of hemoglobin exist, but they differ only slightly in primary structure based on the use of different polypeptide chains: alpha, beta, gamma, delta, epsilon, or zeta (α, β, γ, δ, ε, or ζ, respectively) (Table 28.5). Each polypeptide chain contains approximately 150 amino acids and is arranged in the knotted-sausage configuration shown in Fig. 28.16. The chains assemble to form a tetrahedron containing two pairs of identical chains. Hemoglobin A, the most common type in adults, is composed of two α- and two β-polypeptide chains ($\alpha_2\beta_2$). A normal variant, fetal hemoglobin (hemoglobin F), is a complex of two α- and two γ-polypeptide chains ($\alpha_2\gamma_2$) that binds oxygen with a much greater affinity than adult hemoglobin.

Heme is a large, flat, iron-protoporphyrin disk that is synthesized in the mitochondria and can carry one molecule of oxygen (O_2). Thus an individual hemoglobin molecule with its four hemes can carry four oxygen molecules. If all four oxygen-binding sites are occupied by oxygen, the molecule is said to be saturated. Through a series of complex biochemical reactions, protoporphyrin, a complex four-ringed molecule, is produced and bound with ferrous iron (Fe^{++}). It is crucial that the

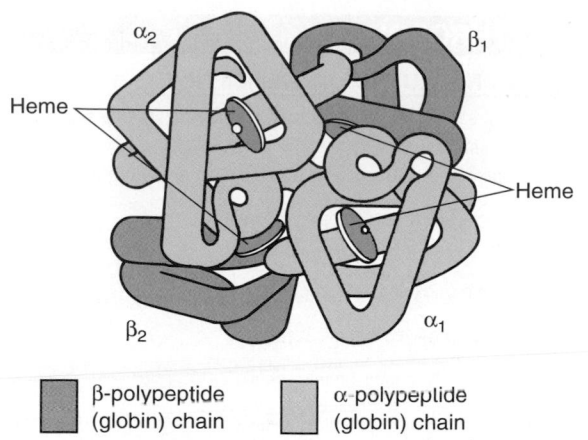

β-polypeptide
(globin) chain

α-polypeptide
(globin) chain

FIGURE 28.16 Molecular Structure of Hemoglobin. Hemoglobin is a spherical tetramer weighing approximately 64,500 daltons. It contains two α subunits, two β subunits, and an iron-containing heme group for each protein subunit. Each heme group can bind four oxygen molecules.

TABLE 28.5 STRUCTURE OF NORMAL HEMOGLOBIN MOLECULES

TYPE OF HEMOGLOBIN (Hb)	IDENTITY OF POLYPEPTIDE CHAIN	SIGNIFICANCE
HbA	$\alpha_2\beta_2$	92% of adult Hb
HbA$_{1c}$	α_2 (β-*NH*-glucose)	5% of adult Hb; increased in diabetes (see Chapter 22)
HbA$_2$	$\alpha_2\delta_2$	2% of adult Hb; increased in β-thalassemia (see Chapter 31)
HbF	$\alpha_2\gamma_2$	Major fetal Hb from the third through ninth month of gestation; promotes oxygen transfer across platelets; increased in β-thalassemia
Hb Gower I	ϵ_4 or $\zeta_2\beta_2$	Present in early embryo; function unknown
Hb Gower II	$\alpha_2\epsilon_2$	Present in early embryo; function unknown
Hb Portland	$\zeta_2\gamma_2$	Present in early embryo; function unknown

NH, Amine.

iron be correctly charged; reduced ferrous iron (Fe^{++}) can bind oxygen in the lungs and release it in the tissues, where oxygen concentration is less, whereas ferric iron (Fe^{+++}) cannot. Binding of oxygen to ferrous iron (**oxyhemoglobin**) temporally oxidizes Fe^{++} to Fe^{+++}, but after the release of oxygen the body reduces the iron to Fe^{++} (**deoxyhemoglobin** [reduced hemoglobin]) and reactivates the hemoglobin's capacity to bind oxygen. Without reactivation by methemoglobin reductase, the Fe^{+++}-containing hemoglobin (**methemoglobin**) cannot bind oxygen. An excess of ferric iron occurs with certain drugs and chemicals, such as nitrates and sulfonamides, and reduces oxygen-carrying capacity. Hemoglobin also undergoes a conformational change when binding oxygen. When one of the iron molecules binds oxygen, the porphyrin ring changes shape, increasing the exposure of the three remaining iron atoms to oxygen. This greatly increases the affinity for the oxygen-carrying capacity of hemoglobin, as occurs in the lungs. When oxygen is unloaded from hemoglobin, the oxygen-carrying capacity of hemoglobin is low, facilitating the transport of carbon dioxide back to the lungs.

Several other molecules can competitively bind to deoxyhemoglobin. Carbon monoxide (CO) directly competes with oxygen for binding to ferrous ion with an affinity that is about 200-fold greater than that of oxygen. Thus even a small amount of CO can dramatically decrease the ability of hemoglobin to bind and transport oxygen. Hemoglobin also binds carbon dioxide (CO_2), but at a binding site separate from where oxygen binds. In the lungs, CO_2 is released, allowing hemoglobin to bind oxygen.

Erythrocytes may play a role in the maintenance of vascular relaxation. Nitric oxide (NO) produced by blood vessels is a major mediator of relaxation and dilation of the vessel walls. In the lungs, hemoglobin can concurrently bind oxygen to the ferrous ion and NO to cysteine residues in the globins. As hemoglobin transfers its oxygen to tissue, it may also shed small amounts of nitric oxide, contributing to dilation of the blood vessels and helping the oxygen gain access to tissues.

Nutritional Requirements for Erythropoiesis

Normal development of erythrocytes and synthesis of hemoglobin depend on an optimal biochemical milieu and adequate supplies of the necessary building blocks, including protein, vitamins, and minerals (Table 28.6). If these components are lacking for a prolonged time, erythrocyte production slows and anemia (insufficient numbers of functional erythrocytes) may result (see Chapter 29).

Erythropoiesis cannot proceed in the absence of vitamins, especially B_{12} (cobalamin), folate (folic acid), B_6, riboflavin, pantothenic acid, niacin, ascorbic acid, and vitamin E. Dietary vitamin B_{12} is a large molecule that requires a protein secreted by parietal cells into the stomach (intrinsic factor [IF]) for transport across the ileum. Once absorbed, vitamin B_{12} is stored in the liver and used as needed in erythropoiesis. Defects in IF production lead to decreased B_{12} absorption and pernicious anemia.

Folate is the second most important vitamin for erythrocyte production and maturation. Folate is necessary for DNA synthesis, being a component of three of the four DNA bases (thymine, adenine, and guanine), and RNA synthesis. Folate absorption occurs principally in the upper small intestine and it is stored in the liver. Folate deficiency is more common than vitamin B_{12} deficiency and occurs more rapidly. Folate stores can be depleted within a few months, whereas vitamin B_{12} depletion can take years. Folate supplements are prescribed for pregnant women because pregnancy increases the demand for folate and may cause anemia. Supplements can protect against neural tube defects and may prevent anemia.

Normal Destruction of Senescent Erythrocytes

After about 100 to 120 days in the circulation, old erythrocytes are removed by tissue macrophages, primarily in the spleen. Although mature erythrocytes lack nuclei, mitochondria, and the endoplasmic reticulum, they do have cytoplasmic enzymes capable of glycolysis (anaerobic glucose metabolism) and production of small quantities of ATP, which provides the energy needed to maintain cell function and membrane pliability. Metabolic processes diminish as the erythrocyte ages, so less ATP is available to maintain plasma membrane function. Disruption of the anchorage between the cytoskeleton and the plasma membrane results in the senescent red cell becoming increasingly fragile and losing its reversible deformability, and thus becoming susceptible to rupture while passing through narrowed regions of the microcirculation.

Additionally, the plasma membrane of senescent red cells undergoes phospholipid rearrangement (movement of the phospholipid

TABLE 28.6	NUTRITIONAL REQUIREMENTS FOR ERYTHROPOIESIS	
NUTRIENT	**ROLE IN ERYTHROPOIESIS**	**CONSEQUENCE OF DEFICIENCY**
Protein (amino acids)	Structural component of plasma membrane	Decreased strength, elasticity, and flexibility of membrane; hemolytic anemia
	Synthesis of hemoglobin	Decreased erythropoiesis and life span of erythrocytes
Cobalamin (vitamin B_{12})	Synthesis of DNA, maturation of erythrocytes, facilitator of folate metabolism	Macrocytic (megaloblastic) anemia
Folate (folic acid)	Synthesis of DNA and RNA, maturation of erythrocytes	Macrocytic (megaloblastic) anemia
Vitamin B_6 (pyridoxine)	Heme synthesis	Microcytic-hypochromic anemia
Vitamin B_2 (riboflavin)	Oxidative reactions	Normocytic-normochromic anemia
Vitamin C (ascorbic acid)	Iron metabolism; acts as a reducing agent to maintain iron in its ferrous (Fe^{++}) form	Normocytic-normochromic anemia
Pantothenic acid	Heme synthesis	Unknown in humans*
Niacin	None, but needed for respiration in mature erythrocytes	Unknown in humans
Vitamin E	Heme synthesis (?); protection against oxidative damage in mature erythrocytes	Hemolytic anemia with increased cell membrane fragility; shortens life span of erythrocytes in individuals with cystic fibrosis
Iron	Hemoglobin synthesis	Iron deficiency anemia
Copper	Required for optimal mobilization of iron from tissues to plasma	Microcytic-hypochromic anemia

*NOTE: Although pantothenic acid is important for optimal synthesis of heme, experimentally induced deficiency *failed* to produce anemia or other hematopoietic disturbances.
DNA, Deoxyribonucleic acid; *RNA*, ribonucleic acid.
Data from Ames BN, Atamna H, Killilea DW: *Mol Aspects Med* 26(4–5):367–378, 2005; Strine-Martin EA, Lotspeich-Steininger CA, Koepke JA: *Clinical hematology: principles, procedures, correlations,* ed 2, Philadelphia, 1998, Lippincott.

phosphatidylserine from the cytoplasmic surface of the membrane to the external surface) that is recognized by receptors for phosphatidylserine on macrophages (primarily in the spleen) that selectively remove and sequester the red cells.[22] If the spleen is dysfunctional or absent, macrophages in the liver (Kupffer cells) become responsible for this process. The erythrocytes are digested by proteolytic and lipolytic enzymes in the phagolysosomes (digestive vacuoles) of the macrophage. The heme and globin of methemoglobin dissociate easily, and the globin is broken down into its component amino acids. The iron in hemoglobin is oxidized, forming Fe^{+++} (methemoglobin), and recycled (see following section).

Porphyrin is reduced to bilirubin, which is transported to the liver, conjugated, and finally excreted in the bile as glucuronide (Fig. 28.17). Approximately 6 g of hemoglobin is catabolized daily, producing 200 mg of bilirubin. Bacteria in the intestinal lumen transform conjugated bilirubin into urobilinogen. Although a small portion is reabsorbed for further metabolism by the liver or excreted by the kidney into the urine, most urobilinogen is excreted in feces. Conditions causing accelerated erythrocyte destruction increase the load of bilirubin for hepatic clearance, leading to increased serum levels of unconjugated bilirubin and increased urinary excretion of urobilinogen. Gallstones (cholelithiasis) can result from a chronically elevated rate of bilirubin excretion.

Iron Cycle

Approximately 67% of total body iron is bound to heme in erythrocytes (hemoglobin) and muscle cells (**myoglobin**), and approximately 30% is stored in mononuclear phagocytes (i.e., macrophages) and hepatic parenchymal cells as either ferritin or hemosiderin. The remaining 3% (less than 1 mg) is lost daily by expelling urine, sweat, or bile; sloughing epithelial cells from the skin and intestinal mucosa; and minor bleeding. Approximately 25 mg of iron is required daily for erythropoiesis; only

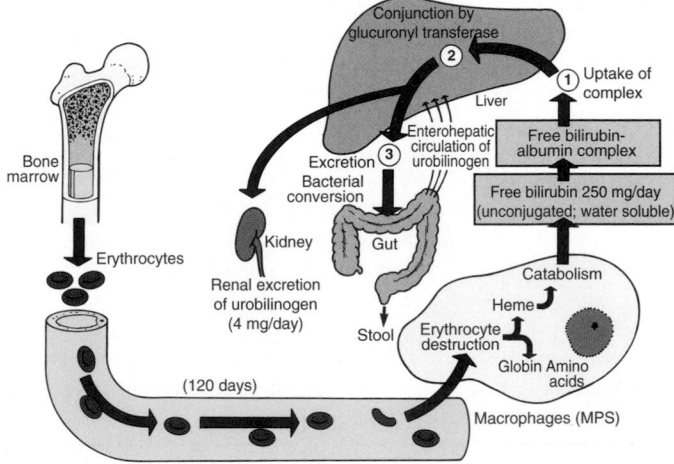

FIGURE 28.17 Metabolism of Bilirubin Released by Heme Breakdown. *MPS,* Mononuclear phagocyte system.

1 to 2 mg of iron is dietary and the remainder is obtained from iron recycling of erythrocytes.

The methemoglobin released from the breakdown of senescent or damaged erythrocytes (see preceding section) is dissociated by the enzyme heme oxygenase, and the iron is released into the bloodstream, where it is free to bind again to transferrin or be stored in the macrophage's cytoplasm as ferritin or hemosiderin (Fig. 28.18). A minute amount of iron is stored in muscle cells by the heme-containing protein myoglobin. Unavailable stores of iron are present in cytochromes, catalases, and peroxidase enzymes.

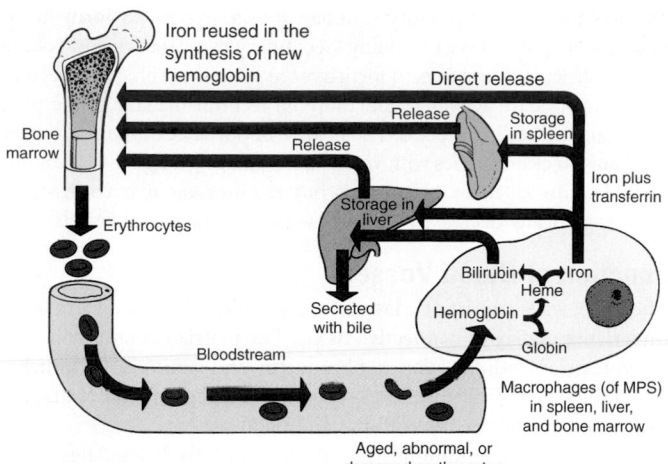

FIGURE 28.18 Iron Cycle. Iron released from gastrointestinal epithelial cells circulates in the bloodstream associated with its plasma carrier, transferrin. It is delivered to erythroblasts in bone marrow, where most of it is incorporated into hemoglobin. Mature erythrocytes circulate for approximately 120 days, after which they become senescent and are removed by the mononuclear phagocyte system *(MPS)*. Macrophages of MPS (mostly in spleen) break down ingested erythrocytes and return iron to the bloodstream directly or after storing it as ferritin or hemosiderin.

The protein ferritin is the major intracellular iron storage protein. Apoferritin, which is ferritin without attached iron, can store thousands of atoms of iron. Several apoferritin complexes combine to form the micelle ferritin. Large aggregates of micelles (if a large amount of iron is present) produce numerous ferritin micelles, known as hemosiderin. Hemosiderin is visible as an iron-based pigment under a light microscope as cell inclusions. The iron within deposits of hemosiderin is poorly available to supply iron when needed. The most common cause of hemosiderin deposition is simple bruising. Hemosiderin in small amounts within iron-rich tissues (i.e., spleen, liver, bone marrow) is considered normal. Large aggregates or its presence in tissue such as the lungs or subcutaneous tissue suggests a pathologic condition.

Iron acquired by utilization of dietary sources, release of iron stores, or catabolism of erythrocytes is transported in the blood bound to apotransferrin, thus becoming transferrin. Under normal conditions, only one-third of the iron-binding sites on transferrin molecules are occupied. Apotransferrin is a glycoprotein synthesized primarily by hepatocytes in the liver but also produced in small quantities by tissue macrophages, submaxillary and mammary glands, and ovaries or testes. Iron for hemoglobin production is carried by transferrin to the bone marrow, where it binds to transferrin receptors on erythroblasts. Transferrin receptors are on the plasma membrane of all nucleated cells, although they are at particularly high levels on erythroid precursors and rapidly proliferating cells (e.g., lymphocytes), and are thought to be the only route of cellular entry for transferrin-attached iron. Transferrin is recycled (transferrin cycle) by intracellular dissociation of the iron with secretion of the resultant apotransferrin into the bloodstream.

The iron is transported to the erythroblast's mitochondria (the site of hemoglobin production), where the enzyme heme synthetase inserts ferrous iron into protoporphyrin to form heme. Heme then is bound to globin to form hemoglobin. Iron not used in erythropoiesis is stored temporarily as ferritin or hemosiderin and later excreted.

Splenic red pulp macrophages are specialized for iron recycling with increased expression of proteins for the uptake of hemoglobin, the

breakdown of heme, and the export of iron.[23] The body's iron homeostasis is primarily controlled by the hormone hepcidin. Hepcidin is synthesized in the liver and released as a 25–amino acid peptide, most of which is bound in the plasma with high affinity to α_2-macroglobulin and relatively lower affinity to albumin. Hepatocellular hepcidin production is regulated physiologically by the body's dietary absorption of iron, rate of erythropoiesis, and level of oxygen saturation.[24] Hepatocytes sense levels of circulating iron by means of receptors for transferrin, the major transporter of iron in the plasma. Excess iron is stored in hepatocytes and macrophages. Hepatocytes sense these levels by means of bone morphogenetic protein (BMP), most likely BMP-6, which is a growth factor produced to a large extent by bone marrow sinusoid endothelial cells and the mother against the decapentaplegic (SMAD) protein pathway (BMP-SMAD pathway). Hepcidin production also can be induced by inflammation through IL-6.

Hepcidin regulates iron levels through its binding capacity to ferroportin, which is a transmembrane iron exporter found in the plasma membrane of cells that transport or store iron, including macrophages, hepatocytes, and enterocytes. The body's total iron balance is maintained through controlled absorption rather than excretion. Dietary iron (primarily as Fe^{++}) is transported directly across the membranes of epithelial cells (enterocytes) in the duodenum and proximal jejunum. (Transport mechanisms are described in Chapter 1.) Hepcidin induces internalization and degradation of ferroportin, thus leading to increased intracellular iron stores, decreased dietary iron absorption, and decreased levels of circulating iron.[25] Decreased production of hepcidin leads to release of stored iron and increased dietary absorption. Thus if the body's iron stores are low or the demand for erythropoiesis increases, dietary iron is transported rapidly through the epithelial cell and into the plasma. If body stores are high and erythropoiesis is not increased, iron transport is stopped, although iron can cross the plasma membranes of epithelial cells and be stored as ferritin.

Development of Leukocytes

Leukocytes consist of lymphocytes, granulocytes, and monocytes. Most of the leukocytes arise from stem cells in the bone marrow (their pathways of differentiation are shown in Fig. 28.12). Hematopoietic stem cells differentiate into two populations of progenitor cells: common lymphoid progenitors and common myeloid progenitors. Lymphoid progenitors that remain in the bone marrow undergo differentiation into the B-cell lineage, after which they are released into the circulation and undergo further maturation in the peripheral lymphoid organs (described in Chapter 8; see Fig. 8.3). The common myeloid progenitors further differentiate into progenitors for basophils, mast cells, eosinophils, and megakaryocytes, and into granulocyte/monocyte progenitors. The granulocyte/monocyte progenitors further differentiate into monocyte progenitors and granulocyte progenitors, which develop into monocytes/ macrophages and neutrophils, respectively. Development from hematopoietic stem cells to common granulocyte-monocyte progenitors primarily is under the control of stem cell factor, IL-3, and GM-CSF, whereas further differentiation into granulocytic and monocytic progenitors is controlled by G-CSF and M-CSF, respectively (see Table 28.4).

Monocytic progenitors undergo development into monocytes within 24 hours and are released into the circulation. Monocytes mature into various forms of macrophages, a process that is usually completed within 1 or 2 days after their release (see Tables 28.3 and 28.4).

Progenitor cells for granulocytes normally fully mature in the bone marrow into neutrophils, eosinophils, and basophils. The ultimate phenotype is determined by relative local bone marrow concentrations of early- and late-acting cytokines, including GM-CSF, G-CSF, IL-3, IL-5, stem cell factor, and others (see Table 28.4). Granulocytes are released into the blood within 14 days of development. The bone marrow selectively retains immature granulocytes as a reserve pool that can be rapidly mobilized in response to the body's needs.

Most leukocytes exist in the body from days to years, depending on type. Maintenance of optimal levels of granulocytes and monocytes in the blood depends on the availability of pluripotent stem cells in the marrow, induction of these into committed stem cells, timely release of new cells from the marrow, and mobilization of the granulocyte reserve pool. Leukocyte production increases in response to infection, to the presence of steroids, and to reduction or depletion of reserves in the marrow. It is also associated with strenuous exercise, convulsive seizures, heat, intense radiation, paroxysmal tachycardias, pain, nausea and vomiting, and anxiety.

Development of Platelets

Platelets (thrombocytes) are derived from stem cells and progenitor cells that differentiate into megakaryocytes. During thrombopoiesis, the megakaryocyte progenitor is programmed to undergo an endomitotic cell cycle (endomitosis) during which DNA replication occurs, but anaphase and cytokinesis are blocked. Thus the megakaryocyte nucleus enlarges and becomes extremely polyploidy (up to 100-fold or more of the normal amount of DNA) without cellular division. Concurrently, the numbers of cytoplasmic organelles (e.g., internal membranes, granules) increase, and the cell develops cell surface proplatelet elongations into the sinusoidal blood vessels. These branches progressively fragment into platelets. A single large (30 to 100 μm) megakaryocyte may produce thousands of smaller platelets (2 to 3 μm). Like erythrocytes, platelets released from the bone marrow lack nuclei.

About two-thirds of platelets enter the circulation and the remainder reside in the splenic pool. Platelets circulate in the bloodstream for about 8 to 10 days before losing their ability to perform thrombogenic activity and biochemical reactions. Senescent platelets are sequestered and destroyed in the spleen by mononuclear cell phagocytosis.

An adequate level of committed platelet precursors (megakaryoblasts) in the bone marrow and differentiation into circulating platelets are controlled by specific interactions between megakaryocyte progenitors and stromal cells in the bone marrow as well as thrombopoietin (TPO, a hormonal growth factor primarily produced by the liver) and various cytokines and colony-stimulating factors and interleukins (see Table 28.4). Platelets express high-affinity receptors for TPO, and when circulating platelet levels are normal, TPO is adsorbed onto the platelet surface and prevented from accessing the bone marrow and initiating further platelet production. TPO stimulates committed cells at further stages of differentiation to differentiate faster so that rates of megakaryocyte development, endomitosis, and platelet release are increased.[26] During inflammation, IL-6 induces increased synthesis of TPO, which increases production of newly formed platelets, which are more thrombogenic.

MECHANISMS OF HEMOSTASIS

Hemostasis is the arrest of bleeding by the formation of blood clots at sites of vascular injury (Fig. 28.19). As a result of hemostasis, damaged blood vessels maintain a relatively steady-state of blood volume, pressure, and flow. Three equally important interactive components of hemostasis are the vasculature (endothelial cells and subendothelial matrix), platelets, and blood proteins (clotting factors). The general sequence of events in hemostasis is the following: (1) vascular injury leads to a transient arteriolar vasoconstriction to limit blood flow to the affected site; (2) damage to the endothelial cell lining of the vessel exposes prothrombogenic subendothelial connective tissue matrix, leading to platelet adherence and activation and formation of a *hemostatic plug* to prevent further bleeding (primary hemostasis); (3) tissue factor, produced by the endothelium, collaborates with secreted platelet factors and activated

platelets to activate the clotting (coagulation) system to form fibrin clots and further prevent bleeding (secondary hemostasis); and (4) the fibrin/platelet clot contracts to form a more permanent plug, and regulatory pathways are activated (fibrinolysis) to limit the size of the plug and begin the healing process. The relative importance of the hemostatic mechanisms clearly varies with vessel size. Damage to large vessels cannot easily be controlled by hemostasis but requires vascular contraction and dramatically decreased blood flow into the damaged vessels.

Function of Blood Vessels

The vessel walls consist of a layer of endothelial cells that adhere to an underlying matrix of connective tissue. The matrix contains a variety of proteins, including collagen, fibronectin, and laminins. Endothelial cells adhere to the matrix and to each other through receptors that are expressed only on the intercellular and basal surfaces.

Under normal conditions the endothelium actively regulates blood flow and prevents spontaneous activation of platelets and the clotting system (see Fig. 28.19). Endothelial cells produce nitric oxide (NO) from L-arginine and synthesize prostacyclin (prostaglandin I$_2$ [PGI$_2$]) from arachidonic acid. Both NO, through cGMP, and PGI$_2$ are vasodilators that work in concert with endothelin (a vasoconstrictor) to modulate blood flow and pressure.[27] NO and PGI$_2$ also inhibit platelet adhesion and aggregation. Synergism between PGI$_2$ and NO is significant. PGI$_2$ production varies a great deal in response to stimuli, whereas NO is released continually to regulate vascular tone. NO has other biologic functions including cell signaling, free radical production, and possibly others. Endothelium also produces adenosine diphosphatase, which degrades adenosine diphosphate (ADP, a potent activator of platelets).

The endothelial cell surface contains antithrombotic molecules, such as glycosaminoglycans (e.g., heparan sulfate), thrombomodulin, and plasminogen activators. These limit platelet activation and fibrin deposition. Although thrombomodulin and plasminogen activators help control hemostasis in normal vessels, their effects are magnified during vascular damage and clot formation; therefore further information is provided on these molecules in the section Control of Hemostatic Mechanisms.

As a result of damage to the vessels, the endothelial cell barrier is frequently compromised, the remaining endothelial cells are activated by products of tissue damage, and the underlying subendothelial matrix is exposed. Endothelial cells contain intracellular structures (Weibel-Palade bodies) that contain von Willebrand factor (vWF) that is released during vascular injury and activates platelets.[28]

Function of Platelets

Platelets normally circulate freely, suspended in plasma, in an unactivated state. The roles of platelets are to (1) contribute to regulation of blood flow into a damaged site by induction of vasoconstriction (vasospasm); (2) initiate platelet-platelet interactions, resulting in formation of a platelet plug to stop further bleeding; (3) activate the coagulation (or clotting) cascade to stabilize the platelet plug; and (4) initiate repair processes including clot retraction and clot dissolution (fibrinolysis). The normal platelet count ranges from 140,000 to 340,000/mm³. Thrombocytopenia (abnormally low numbers of platelets) develops if the platelet count drops below 100,000/mm³. The individual may experience prolongation of normal clotting but is usually not at risk for spontaneous major bleeding episodes unless the platelet count falls below 20,000/mm³. If platelet numbers are elevated (thrombocytosis), the risk for spontaneous blood clots (thrombosis), stroke, or heart attack is increased.

The state of platelet activation is primarily under the control of endothelial cells lining the vessels. Damage to the vessel initiates a process of platelet activation: (1) increased platelet *adhesion* to the damaged

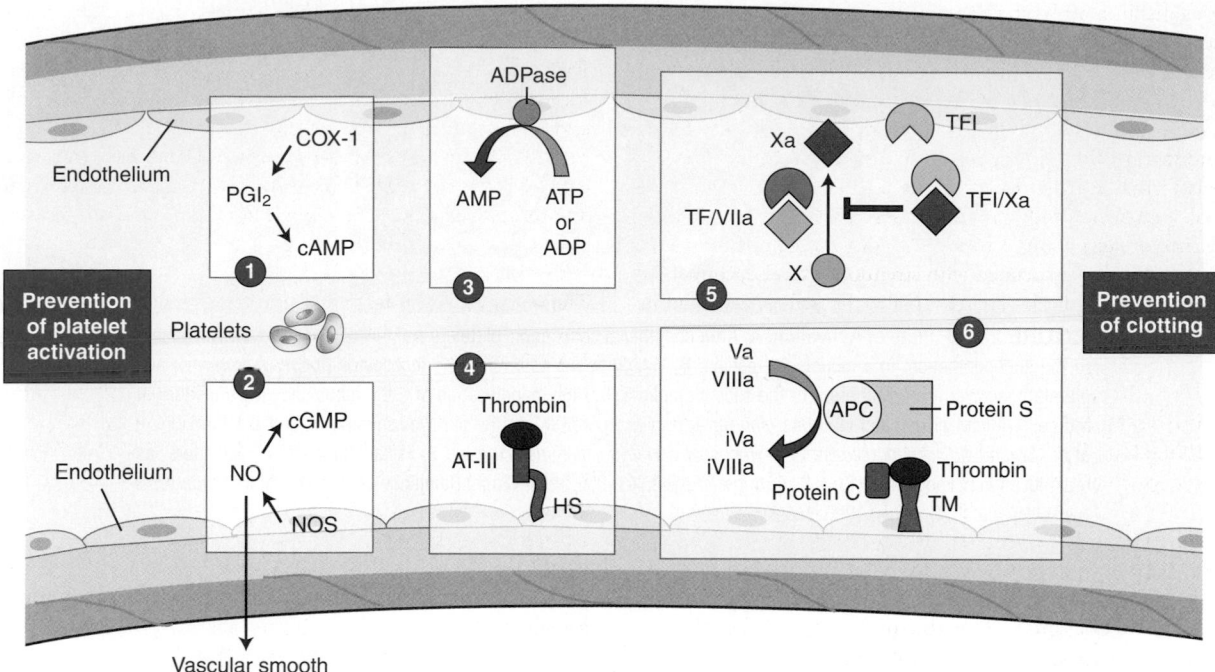

FIGURE 28.19 Hemostasis. Endothelium controls hemostasis by preventing platelet activation **(1–3)** and preventing activation of the clotting system **(4–6)**. **(1)** *Prostacyclin production:* Injury activates inflammation (*COX-1*, [cyclooxygenase-1] arachidonic acid). Enzymes convert arachidonic acid into prostacyclin (prostaglandin I_2 *[PGI$_2$]*) in endothelial cells. PGI$_2$ eventually increases intracellular cyclic adenosine monophosphate *(cAMP)*; cAMP inhibits platelet aggregation and induces vasodilation. Nitric oxide *(NO)* formation is induced by NO synthases *(NOS)* and NO causes increased cyclic guanosine monophosphate *(cGMP)*. **(2)** *Nitric oxide system:* Endothelial cell NOS produces NO, which controls platelet activation through cGMP-mediated signaling. **(3)** *Adenosine diphosphatase (ADPase):* Endothelial cells express a surface-bound ADPase (CD39) that converts circulating ADP (adenosine diphosphate) and ATP (adenosine triphosphate) to AMP (adenosine monophosphate). **(4)** *Antithrombin III–heparan sulfate system:* Antithrombin III (*AT-III*) inhibits thrombin slowly when heparan sulfate *(HS)* is absent. When HS is present, it quickly activates thrombin because it binds to a specific site on AT-III that causes an instant conformational change in AT-III, allowing it to quickly activate thrombin. **(5)** *Tissue factor inhibitor (TFI) system:* Expression of TFI on the endothelial cells and secreted into the circulation complexes with factor IXa to form a competitive inhibitor of the tissue factor/factor VIIa complex *(TF/VIIa)* and prevent further activation of factor X to Xa. **(6)** *Protein C/protein S pathway (thrombomodulin):* Thrombin in the circulation binds to thrombomodulin (TM) on the endothelial cell, creating a complex that can bind and activate protein C to activated protein C *(APC)* that complexes in the blood or on the surface of active platelets with protein S. This complex degrades circulating clotting factors Va and VIIIa to inactive forms *(iVa, iVIIIa)* to prevent further activation of clotting.

vascular wall; (2) *activation* leading to platelet degranulation, which stimulates changes in platelet shape and biochemistry; (3) *aggregation* as platelet–vascular wall and platelet-platelet adherence increases;[29] and (4) activation of the clotting system and development of an immobilizing meshwork of platelets and fibrin (Fig. 28.20).

Adhesion

Normally, platelets are generally observed "rolling" along the margins of vessels. At sites of vessel injury, however, platelets become adherent to the site of endothelial damage, where the subendothelial matrix is exposed and endothelial cells have released von Willebrand factor and decreased their antithrombotic activities (Fig. 28.21). **Platelet adhesion** is mostly mediated by the binding of platelet surface receptor glycoprotein Ib (GPIb) (in a complex with clotting factors IX and V) to **von Willebrand factor (vWF)**.[30] The vWF protein is found in the subendothelial matrix and is released by endothelial cells and platelets. Platelet adhesion narrows the diameter of the blood vessel, resulting in increasing shear forces that could strip platelets off the vessel surface. However, those same forces induce conformational changes in the vWF

molecule that result in increased affinity with GPIb, thus stabilizing the adherent platelet.

Platelet adhesion is also facilitated by other interactions between platelet receptors and exposed molecules of the subendothelial matrix. For instance, adhesion is increased through binding of the platelet collagen receptors GPVI and integrin $\alpha_2\beta_1$ to exposed collagen in the matrix.

Activation

As a result of interactions with the endothelium or the subendothelial matrix, as well as exposure to inflammatory mediators produced by the endothelium and other cells, the platelets are activated. Activation results in reorganization of the platelet cytoskeleton, leading to dynamic changes in platelet shape from smooth spheres to those with spiny projections (increases surface area) and degranulation (also called the **platelet-release reaction**) and resulting in the release of various potent biochemicals[8] (see Fig. 28.6).

Platelets contain three types of granules: dense bodies, alpha granules, and lysosomes.[31] The contents of the dense bodies and alpha granules

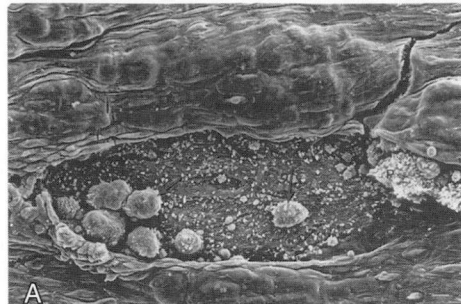 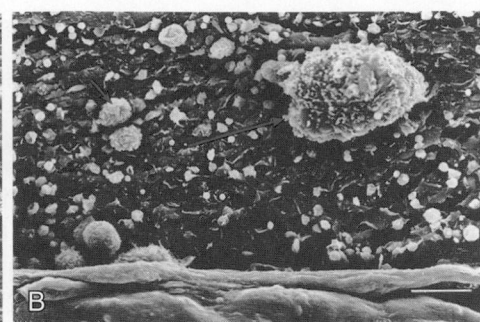 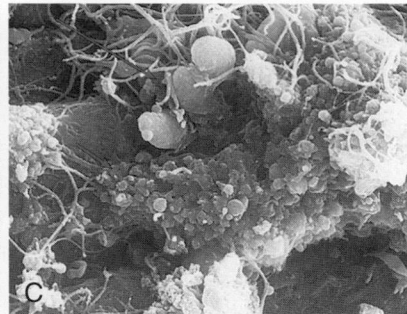

FIGURE 28.20 Platelet Activation. **A,** After endothelial denudation, platelets and leukocytes *(blue arrows)* adhere to the subendothelium in a monolayer fashion. **B,** Higher-power view showing leukocytes *(longer blue arrow)* and platelets *(shorter arrow)* adherent to the subendothelium. **C,** High magnification of a thrombus showing a mixture of red cells *(longer arrow)* and platelets *(shorter arrow)* incorporated into the fibrin meshwork. (**A** and **B** From Libby P et al: *Braunwald's heart disease: a textbook of cardiovascular medicine,* ed 8, Philadelphia, 2007, Saunders, as reproduced from Faggiotto A, Ross R: *Arteriosclerosis* 4:341–356, 1984; **C** from Damjanov I, Linder J, editors: *Anderson's pathology,* ed 10, St Louis, 1996, Mosby.)

are particularly important in hemostasis. The dense bodies contain ADP, serotonin, and calcium. ADP recruits and activates other platelets through specific receptors. During activation the platelet plasma membrane experiences several important changes, including becoming ruffled and sticky; undergoing cellular spreading to make tight contacts between neighboring platelets, causing the platelet plug to seal the injured endothelium; and externalizing the phospholipid phosphatidylserine, which provides a matrix for activation of clotting factors (see Fig. 28.21). Serotonin is a vasoactive amine that functions like histamine and increases vasodilation and vascular permeability. Calcium is necessary for many of the adhesive interactions as well as for intracellular signaling mechanisms that control platelet activation.

Alpha granules contain a mixture of clotting factors (e.g., fibrinogen, factor V), growth and angiogenic factors (e.g., platelet-derived growth factor [PDGF], vascular endothelial growth factor [VEGF], basic fibroblast growth factor), and angiogenesis inhibitors (e.g., platelet factor 4, thrombospondin, inhibitors of metalloproteinases). Platelet factor 4 also is a heparin-binding protein and enhances clot formation at the site of injury. Depending upon the particular stimulus, platelets may selectively release promoters or inhibitors of angiogenesis. Many of these mediators either promote or inhibit platelet activity and the eventual process of clot formation. PDGF stimulates smooth muscle cells and promotes tissue repair.

Platelet lysosomes have a role in the digestion of phagocytic and cytosolic components, similar to that in nucleated cells. Lysosomal contents also may have important extracellular functions, such as supporting receptor cleavage, fibrinolysis and degradation of extracellular matrix components, and remodeling of the vasculature.[8]

Platelets also initiate production of the prostaglandin derivative thromboxane A_2 (TXA_2), which counters the effects of PGI_2 produced by endothelial cells (see Fig. 28.21). TXA_2 causes vasoconstriction and promotes the degranulation of platelets, increases expression of platelet fibrinogen receptors, and stimulates platelet aggregation; whereas PGI_2 promotes vasodilation and inhibits platelet degranulation. An isoform of cyclooxygenase (COX-1) converts arachidonic acid to TXA_2 in platelets. Aspirin at low doses specifically and irreversibly inactivates COX-1, decreasing production of TXA_2 and decreasing platelet activation and aggregation.[32] Daily intake of low doses of aspirin leads to more than 95% inhibition of TXA_2 in just a few days.

Other stimuli of platelet activation include epinephrine, thrombin, and collagen. Thrombin and collagen are particularly strong stimuli. Thrombin cleaves the extracellular domain of G-protein–coupled protease-activated receptors (PARs), thereby initiating transmembrane signaling.

Aggregation

Platelet aggregation is stimulated primarily by TXA_2 and ADP, which induce functional fibrinogen receptors on the platelet. The glycoprotein IIb/IIIa (GPIIb/IIIa) complex (also called *integrin $\alpha IIb\beta_3$*) undergoes a conformational change during activation to become a calcium-dependent receptor for fibrinogen (see Fig. 28.21). It is a member of the integrin receptor family and binds other matrix proteins (e.g., fibronectin, fibrinogen, thrombospondin). Defects in expression of the GPIIb/IIIa complex (Glanzmann thrombasthenia) result in a failure to aggregate and diminished clotting times.[33] Although the GPIIb/IIIa complex is the most abundant fibrinogen receptor on the platelet, receptors for vWF (GPIb) and collagen (GPVI) also contribute to the process. Interplatelet aggregation and clot retraction, which forms the *primary hemostatic plug*, are facilitated by fibrinogen bridges between receptors on the platelets. The GPIIb/IIIa–fibrinogen pathway is essential for the formation of a thrombus and as such is an important therapeutic target for blockage by antiplatelet drugs. In addition, fibrin strands within the clot shorten and become denser and stronger, helping the clot to approximate the edges of the injured vessel wall and sealing the site of injury. Contraction of myosin and actin filaments in the platelet cytoskeleton mediates *platelet contraction* and fusion of the platelet mass into a *secondary hemostatic plug*. Contraction expels serum from the fibrin meshwork, resulting in greater packing and increased strength. This process usually begins within a few minutes after a clot has formed, and most of the serum is expelled within 20 to 60 minutes.[34]

If blood vessel injury is minor, primary hemostasis is achieved by formation of the platelet plug within 3 to 5 minutes of injury. Platelet plugs seal the many minute ruptures that occur daily in the microcirculation, particularly in capillaries. With too few platelets, numerous small hemorrhagic areas called *purpuras* develop under the skin and throughout the tissues (see Chapter 30). If primary hemostasis is inadequate to prevent further bleeding, the process proceeds through secondary hemostasis to create a larger complex of more tightly interactive platelets within a matrix created by activation of the clotting system.

Function of Clotting Factors

A blood clot is a meshwork of protein strands that stabilizes the platelet plug and traps other cells, such as erythrocytes, phagocytes, and microorganisms. The strands are made of fibrin, which is produced by

I. Subendothelial exposure

- Occurs after endothelial sloughing
- Platelets begin to fill endothelial gaps
- Promoted by thromboxane A_2 (TXA_2)
- Inhibited by prostacyclin I_2 (PGI_2)
- Platelet function depends on many factors, especially calcium

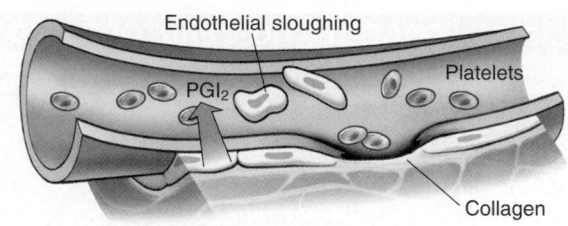

II. Adhesion

- Adhesion is initiated by loss of endothelial cells (or rupture or erosion of atherosclerotic plaque), which exposes adhesive glycoproteins such as collagen and von Willebrand factor (vWF) in the subendothelium. vWF and, perhaps, other adhesive glycoproteins in the plasma deposit on the damaged area. Platelets adhere to the subendothelium through receptors that bind to the adhesive glycoproteins (GPIb, GPIa/IIa, GPIIb/IIIa).

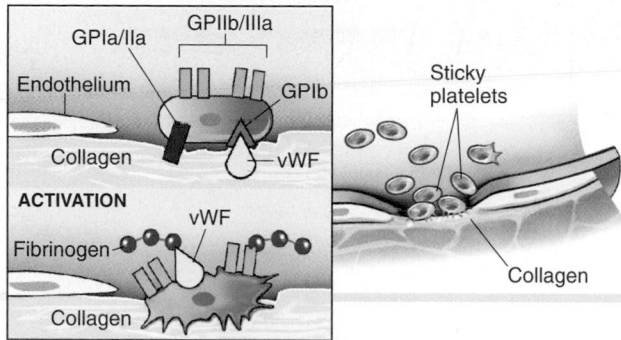

III. Activation

- After platelets adhere they undergo an activation process that leads to a conformational change in GPIIb/IIIa receptors, resulting in their ability to bind adhesive proteins, including fibrinogen and vWF
- Changes in platelet shape
- Formation of pseudopods
- Activation of arachidonic pathway

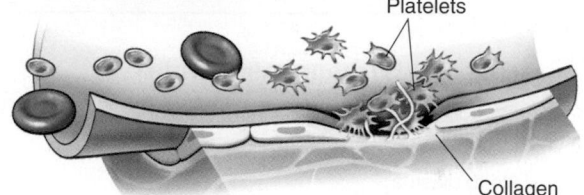

IV. Aggregation

- Induced by release of TXA_2
- Adhesive glycoproteins bind simultaneously to GPIIb/IIIa on two different platelets
- Stabilization of the platelet plug (blood clot) occurs by activation of coagulation factors, thrombin, and fibrin
- Heparin neutralizing factor enhances clot formation

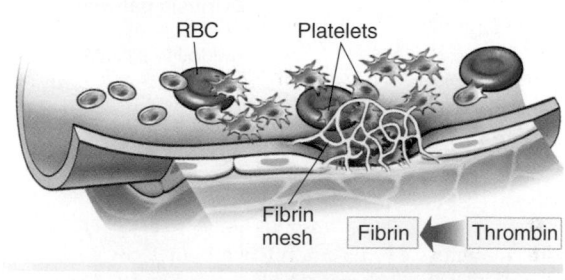

V. Platelet plug formation

- RBCs and platelets enmeshed in fibrin

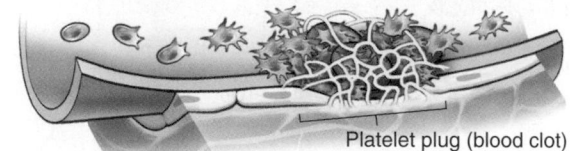

VI. Clot retraction and clot dissolution

- Clot retraction, using large number of platelets, joins the edges of the injured vessel
- Clot dissolution is regulated by thrombin and plasminogen activators

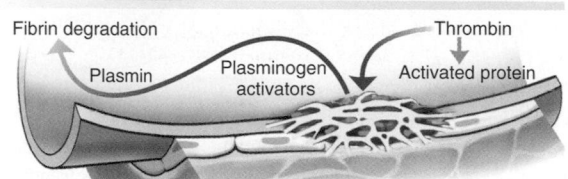

FIGURE 28.21 Blood Vessel Damage, Platelet Activation, Blood Clot, and Clot Dissolution.

the clotting (coagulation) system. The clotting system was described in Chapter 7 and consists of a family of proteins that circulate in the plasma of the blood in inactive forms (proenzymes). Initiation of the system results in sequential enzymatic activation (pathway) of multiple members of the system until a fibrin clot is created (Table 28.7).

Based on laboratory evaluation, the clotting system is commonly presented as two pathways of initiation: the extrinsic pathway (also known as the *tissue factor pathway*) and the intrinsic pathway (also known as the *contact activation pathway* or the *plasma kallikrein-kinin system*). These pathways join in a common pathway with activation of factor X, which proceeds to thrombin, fibrin, and clot formation (Fig. 28.22). These pathways are controlled by anticoagulant proteins. The in vivo understanding of the clotting pathways has developed from the clinical disorders that result from deficiency of clotting factors. The extrinsic pathway is activated when there is vascular injury and blood escapes into tissue with activation of tissue factor. It is the normal mechanism of hemostasis and plug breaks in capillaries that occur with activities of daily living.[35] Tissue factor (TF) (also called tissue thromboplastin) is abundant in vascular subendothelium and adventitial cells surrounding larger blood vessels and body organs, particularly

TABLE 28.7 COAGULATION FACTORS AND SYNONYMS

FACTOR	SYNONYM	PRIMARY FUNCTION
I	Fibrinogen	Source of fibrin to form clot
II	Prothrombin	Source of thrombin that activates fibrinogen, V, VII, VIII, XI, XIII, protein C, platelets
Tissue factor (thromboplastin)	Previously called *factor III*	Cofactor for factor VIIa
Calcium	Previously called *factor IV*	Cofactor for clotting factor binding to phosphatidylserine
V	Labile factor	Va is cofactor in prothrombinase complex
VII	Stable factor, proconvertin	VIIa forms complex with tissue factor and activates factors IX and X
VIII	Antihemophilic factor	VIIIa is component of tenase complex
IX	Christmas factor	IXa is component of tenase complex, activates factor X
X	Stuart-Prower factor	Xa is component of prothrombinase complex, activates prothrombin
XI	Plasma thromboplastin antecedent	XIa activates factor IX
XII	Hageman (contact) factor	XIIa activates factor XI
XIII	Fibrin-stabilizing factor	XIIIa cross-links fibrin

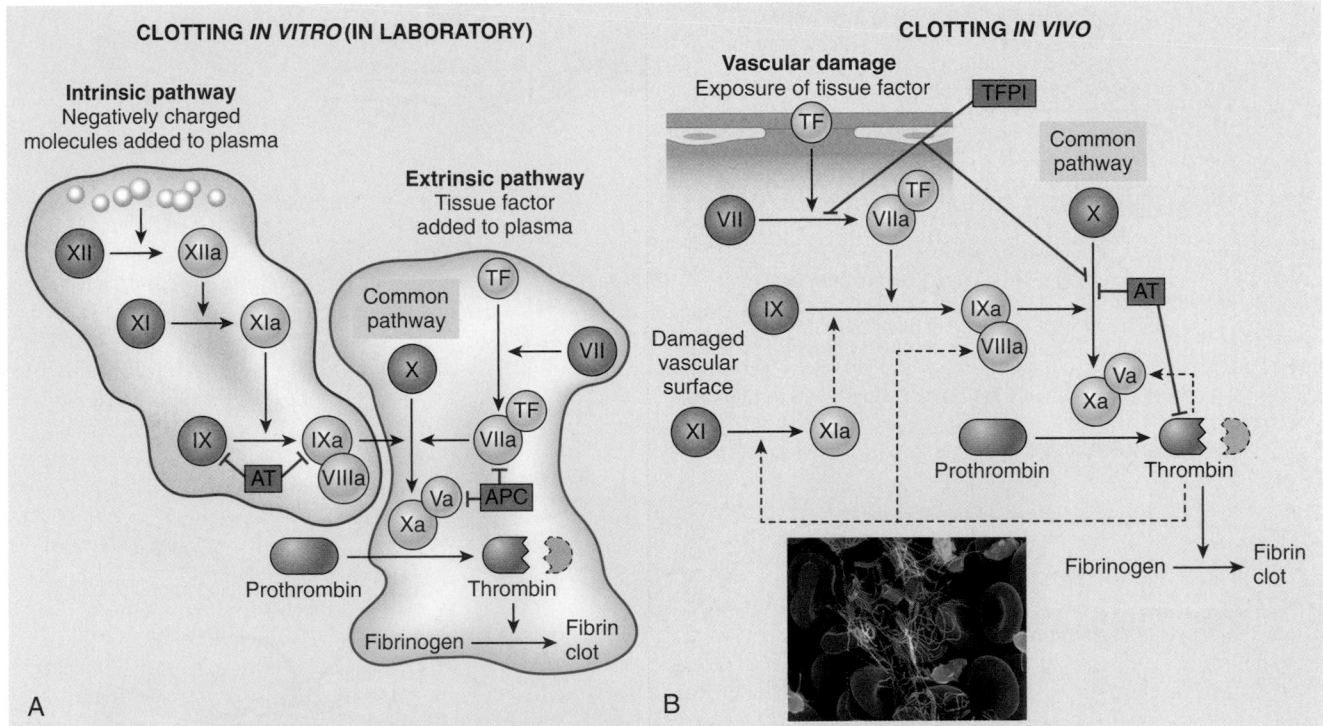

FIGURE 28.22 The Clotting Pathways and Control Proteins. The coagulation pathways in vitro (in the laboratory) and in vivo. **A,** Clotting evaluation of the intrinsic (contact) pathway (within the pink cloud) is initiated in the laboratory by adding phospholipids, calcium, and a negatively charged substance (such as silica or glass beads) and is measured as the activated partial thromboplastin time (aPTT, time for a fibrin clot to form). The extrinsic pathway (within the light blue cloud) is measured as prothrombin time (PT, time for a fibrin clot to form). **B,** In vivo, tissue factor is the major initiator of coagulation, which is amplified by feedback loops involving thrombin *(dotted lines)*. The red polypeptides are inactive factors, the dark green polypeptides are active factors, and the light green polypeptides correspond to cofactors. The orange boxes represent control proteins. Electron micrograph *inset* shows entrapped red blood cells (RBCs) and platelets *(blue)* in a fibrin clot *(yellow strands)*. **NOTE:** Factor XII is not a clotting factor for maintaining normal hemostasis. In experiments, factor XI is thought to be involved in thrombus formation occurring with intrinsic vascular damage. Thrombin also can activate factor XI (as well as factors V and VIII), a feedback mechanism *(dotted lines)* that amplifies the coagulation cascade. *APC,* Activated protein C (protein C is activated by binding to the thrombomodulin-thrombin complex with protein S as a cofactor); *AT,* antithrombin; *TF,* tissue factor; *TFPI,* tissue factor pathway inhibitor. (Adapted from Kumar V, Abbas AK, Aster JC: *Robbins & Cotran pathologic basis of disease*, ed 9, Philadelphia, 2015, Saunders. Inset Copyright Dennis Kunkel Microscopy, Inc.)

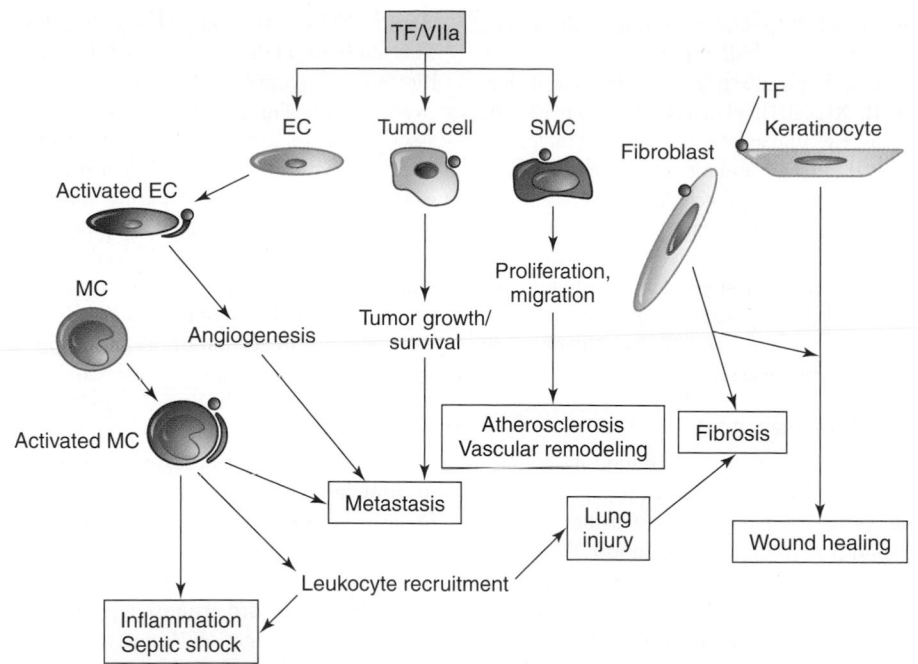

FIGURE 28.23 Factor VIIa Signaling Through Tissue Factor (TF) Expressed on the Surface of Cells Mediates Changes in Disease-Related Cellular Activities. *EC,* Endothelial cell; *MC,* monocyte/macrophage; *SMC,* smooth muscle cell. (Modified from Rao LV, Pendurthi UR: *Arterioscler Thromb Vasc Biol* 25[1]:47–56, 2005.)

the skin, brain, lungs, kidney, and placenta. There also are receptors for TF on activated monocytes. With vessel trauma and bleeding, TF binds with high affinity to circulating activated factor VII (TF/VIIa), initiating the clotting pathway. TF is a transmembrane protein that exists in an inactive form but is activated into an active enzyme with factors IX and X as substrates.[36] TF mediates a number of changes in disease-related activities, including inflammation, tumor angiogenesis metastasis, cell migration, and clotting associated with atherosclerosis (Fig. 28.23). The extrinsic pathway is evaluated in vitro by adding TF to a sample of plasma and measuring the prothrombin time (time to form a fibrin clot).

Factor XIIa (Hageman factor), prekallikrein (PK), and high-molecular-weight kininogen (HK; activates factor XII) initiate the intrinsic coagulation pathway through activation of the downstream substrate factor XI. The terms *intrinsic* or *contact* mean that the pathway is activated within the blood vessel by contact with anionic surfaces (i.e., exposure of subendothelial collagen from vessel damage) or other substances without the action of TF. The intrinsic pathway is not a significant pathway for normal hemostasis but is a pathophysiologic surface defense mechanism against foreign proteins, microbial pathogens, and artificial materials. Individuals with deficiencies in intrinsic pathway components (i.e., factor XI, factor XII) do not have disruption of hemostasis or prolonged bleeding with the exception of hemophilia C (deficiency of factor XI that usually causes mild bleeding). Consequently, factor XII and factor XI are being investigated for targeted anticoagulant strategies with lower risk for bleeding tendencies than anticoagulants that target thrombin and/or factor Xa.[37]

The activation of the intrinsic pathway has been investigated using in vitro techniques. For example, in the laboratory negatively charged substances are introduced to activate factor XII (contact activation) for the diagnostic plasma clotting test known as the *activated partial thromboplastin time* (aPTT). Factor XIIa recruits HK that is complexed with prekallikrein (PK). Factor XIIa activates PK to kallikrein, which in turn generates more factor XIIa and amplifies the pathway. Factor

XIIa also activates HK to release bradykinin (a proinflammatory mediator). This reaction is prevented from occurring in the plasma by the presence of C1 inhibitor (C1-INH) (see Chapter 7 and Figs. 7.8 and 7.9). Other exogenous artificial surfaces also can activate factor XII (i.e., use of tubing for blood flow during hemodialysis, cardiopulmonary bypass, or extracorporeal membrane oxygenation) and require anticoagulation therapy. More recently it has been discovered that naturally occurring polyphosphates (i.e., RNA and DNA from injury in arterioles, such as ruptured plaque[38] or dying cells), activated platelets, neutrophil extracellular traps, and cell membranes from bacteria can activate the intrinsic pathway and promote thrombin formation and thrombosis. Factor XIa also is able to activate coagulation factors X, V, and VIII and inhibit the anticoagulant tissue factor pathway inhibitor (TFPI).[39] Thus factor XI may have a role in thrombus formation and is thought to be a risk factor for deep vein thrombosis and ischemic stroke. The role of factors XII and XI in myocardial infarction is not clear.[40,41] In mice factor XII or factor XI, deficiency results in fragmented unstable thrombi prone to embolization. Consequently, the intrinsic pathway also may be essential for stabilization of thrombi and prevention of embolism.[42] It is important to recognize that factor XIa and factor IXa can be generated by routes independent of factor XIIa (i.e., thrombin also can activate factor XI, as well as factors V and VIII). Thrombin activation of XI and IX is a feedback mechanism that amplifies the coagulation pathway (see dotted lines in Fig. 28.22) and maintains the clot over time. Thus the older intrinsic pathway nomenclature has fallen out of use, to some extent, because of preference for contact activation pathway nomenclature.[41]

Activated platelets are important participants in clotting. The phosphatidylserine-rich surface produced during activation provides a matrix on which several important complexes of clotting factors are formed. These include the intrinsic pathway's *tenase complex* (factor X and activated factors VIII and IX) that activates factor X and the *prothrombinase complex* (prothrombin and activated factors X and V) that activates prothrombin into thrombin (see Fig. 28.22). Thrombin then converts fibrinogen into fibrin, which polymerizes into a fibrin clot. Thrombin has broad reactivity in the inflammatory response.[43] In addition to producing fibrin, thrombin is an activator of other coagulation proteins (e.g., factors V, VIII, XI, XIII), platelets (e.g., aggregation, degranulation), endothelial cells (e.g., upregulation of adhesion molecules for leukocytes, increased NO, PGI_2, PDGF), and monocytes (e.g., cytokine secretion, increased receptors for endothelial cells).

Vitamin K–dependent clotting factors include prothrombin (factor II) factors VII, IX, and X, and the anticoagulation proteins (C and cofactors S and Z). These proteins undergo vitamin K–dependent γ-carboxylation of glutamic acid residues that enables them to bind calcium and other divalent cations and participate in the clotting pathways. Vitamin K is antagonized by the anticoagulant drug warfarin.[44]

Control of Hemostatic Mechanisms

The intact endothelium prevents thrombosis by inhibiting platelet aggregation, preventing coagulation activation and propagation, and enhancing fibrinolysis. Blood normally remains fluid despite the continual presence of clotting factors and platelets in the circulation. The major regulatory factors that control hemostasis reside where the greatest probability of clotting would occur: on the endothelial cell surface (see Fig. 28.19). The primary anticoagulant mechanisms include thrombin inhibitors (e.g., antithrombin III), tissue factor inhibitors (e.g., tissue factor pathway inhibitor), and mechanisms for degrading activated clotting factors (e.g., protein C). Antithrombotic mechanisms are listed in Table 28.8. When the endothelium is damaged, it transitions to the hemostatic action (vasoconstriction, platelet and clotting factor activation) described previously.

Antithrombin III (AT-III) is a circulating plasma serine protease inhibitor produced by the liver. Specifically, it inhibits thrombin and several activated clotting factors (e.g., VIIa, IXa, Xa, XIa, XIIa). AT-III is produced by the liver and binds with heparan sulfate found naturally on the surface of endothelial cells, or with heparin administered clinically to prevent thrombosis. Heparin induces a change in AT-III that greatly enhances its capacity to inhibit thrombin and other activated clotting factors. Under normal conditions the presence of endothelial cell heparan sulfate and the available AT-III in the circulation cooperate to protect the vessels from the effects of spontaneously activated thrombin (see Fig. 28.19). Acquired AT-III deficiencies can result from infection with bacteria that produce AT-III inhibitors, sepsis, liver disease, and nephrotic syndrome and lead to venous thrombosis and pulmonary embolism.

Tissue factor pathway inhibitor (TFPI) is produced by endothelial cells and platelets and is the primary inhibitor of the initiation of blood clotting. TFPI forms complexes with and reversibly inhibits factor Xa. The resultant TFPI/Xa complex inhibits TF/VIIa complex and prothrombinase (converts prothrombin to thrombin) and thus inhibits clotting[45] (see Fig. 28.19). Although the majority of TFPI remains associated with endothelial or platelet surfaces, about 20% circulates in plasma with lipoproteins. Heparin increases plasma levels of TFPI, which may contribute to heparin's antithrombotic effects.

Thrombomodulin is a transmembrane thrombin-binding protein on the surface of endothelial cells and a receptor for thrombin. When thrombin binds to thrombomodulin, it no longer serves as a procoagulant and cannot activate platelets, convert fibrinogen to fibrin, or amplify fibrin generation. **Protein C** in the circulation binds to the thrombomodulin-thrombin complex and is rapidly converted to activated protein C[46] (see Fig. 28.19). Activated protein C in association with a cofactor (**protein S**) inactivates factors Va and VIIIa, inhibits fibrin formation, and inhibits coagulation. Deficiencies of AT-III, protein C, or protein S are important inherited causes of hypercoagulation (increased clotting).[47] Expression of thrombomodulin and the endothelial cell protein C receptor is down-regulated by cytokines and other products of inflammation (e.g., IL-1α, tumor necrosis factor-alpha [TNF-α], endotoxin). Decreased expression prevents protein C activation, thereby enhancing clot formation. Activated protein C inhibits the adhesion of neutrophils to the endothelium, but during inflammation neutrophil elastase enzymatically removes thrombomodulin from the endothelial cell surface.[48] Protein Z is a cofactor for the inhibition of factor Xa through protein Z–dependent protease inhibitor.[49]

Lysis of Blood Clots

Concurrent with activation of coagulation is the activation of pathways that limit the size of the clot and remove the clot after bleeding has ceased and repair has begun. The primary mechanism for lysis (breakdown) of blood clots is the **fibrinolytic system (plasminogen-plasmin system)**, a cascade of serine proteases that produce plasmin. The **plasmin** (also called *fibrinase* or *fibrinolysin*) degrades fibrin polymers in clots.[50] The inactive precursor of plasmin is **plasminogen**, which is produced in the liver (Fig. 28.24). Plasminogen activation may occur by several

TABLE 28.8	ANTITHROMBOTIC MECHANISMS OF ENDOTHELIAL CELLS
FUNCTION REGULATED	**SUBSTANCES INVOLVED**
Clotting cascade	Tissue factor pathway inhibitor
	Antithrombin III
	Heparan sulfate
	Thrombomodulin/protein C/protein S/protein Z
Vessel and platelet activity	Covering of prothrombotic intercellular matrix molecules
	Prostacyclin (PGI_2)
	Nitric oxide (NO)
	Adenosine diphosphate
Eliminate fibrin clot	Plasminogen activators

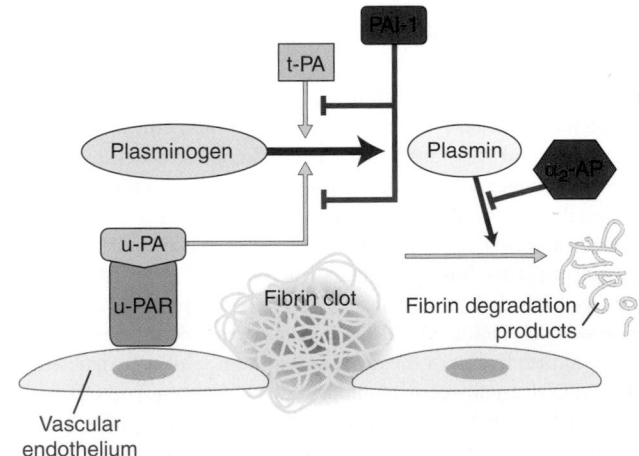

FIGURE 28.24 The Fibrinolytic System. Fibrinolysis is initiated by the binding of plasminogen to fibrin. Although tissue plasminogen activator *(t-PA)* initiates intravascular fibrinolysis, urokinase plasminogen activator *(u-PA)* is the major activator of fibrinolysis in tissue (extravascular). Inhibitors (indicated by red lines) of fibrinolysis include α₂-antiplasmin *(α₂-AP)*, which inhibits plasmin, and plasminogen activator inhibitor 1 *(PAI-1)*, which inhibits t-PA. Plasmin digests the fibrin into smaller soluble pieces *(Fibrin degradation products)*. *u-PAR*, Urokinase-like plasminogen activator receptor.

means, although the most physiologically important is by the action of **tissue plasminogen activator (t-PA)**. Endothelial cells at a site of vascular injury express t-PA, which is also a serine protease that reaches maximal enzymatic activity after binding to fibrin and proteolytically activates plasminogen to plasmin. Another activator of plasminogen is **urokinase-like plasminogen activator (u-PA)**. The u-PA is a serine protease that can bind to a specific cellular u-PA receptor (u-PAR), causing activation of plasminogen and resulting in plasmin generation. This urokinase is the major activator of fibrinolysis in the *extravascular* or tissue compartment, whereas t-PA is largely involved in *intravascular* fibrinolysis. Both t-PA and u-PA have been used clinically to treat diseases associated with a blood clot (e.g., pulmonary embolism, myocardial infarction, or stroke).

As with most components of inflammation, plasmin interacts greatly with other factors. In addition to activation by t-PA and u-PA, plasminogen is activated to plasmin by thrombin, fibrin, factor XIIa, factor XIa, and kallikrein. Plasmin is proteolytic to several substrates, including activation of collagenases, complement components C1 and C3, and factor XII, and cleaves fibronectin, fibrin, thrombospondin, laminin, and vWF. Plasmin activity is usually controlled directly by the serine protease inhibitor α_2-antiplasmin or by inhibiting plasminogen activation by specific plasminogen activator inhibitors (PAIs).

Cross-linked fibrin is deposited in tissues around wounds, inflammatory sites, and tumors. Fibrin removal is an important biologic process, for intravascular and extravascular spaces, with various controlling mechanisms that can lead to abnormalities of fibrin accumulation and thrombotic events and can be a structural barrier to tumor invasion.

Products of fibrinolysis include **fibrin degradation products (FDPs)** (see Fig. 28.24). A major FDP is D-dimer. D-dimer is two D domains from adjacent fibrin monomers that are cross-linked by factor XIIIa and released as a result of enzymatic cleavage by plasmin. Measurement of levels of circulating D-dimer has been used for diagnosis of deep venous thrombosis (DVT) or pulmonary embolism (PE). Despite extensive literature, the diagnostic role of D-dimer is unclear because of the use of multiple D-dimer assays with different sensitivities and variabilities.[51]

CLINICAL EVALUATION OF THE HEMATOLOGIC SYSTEM

Tests of Bone Marrow Function

The bone marrow is the soft spongy tissue found within bones, especially the sternum, pelvis, and femur. Several abnormal conditions in the numbers or morphology of circulating blood cells or suspected infection of the marrow may justify further investigation of the bone marrow.

Usually bone marrow is aspirated from the sternum or pelvis using a needle. In children a bone marrow aspirate can be obtained from the vertebrae or the femur. The aspirate is examined microscopically and may be cultured if infection (e.g., fungi, mycobacteria, brucellosis, typhoid fever) is suspected. Microscopic evaluation may also include flow cytometry, chromosome analysis, or polymerase chain reaction (PCR) related to the presence of atypical cells, the presence of atypical numbers of normal cells, and the absence of particular cell types. A normal bone marrow aspirate contains stromal cells (fibroblasts, macrophages, osteoblasts, adipocytes), stem cells (hematopoietic, mesenchymal, and endothelial), and immature and mature forms of blood cells (erythrocytes, leukocytes, platelets) (Fig. 28.25). The differential cell count of a bone marrow aspirate involves examining approximately 400 nucleated cells under oil-immersion magnification and counting populations of cells differentiated on the basis of morphology. The relative number of each type of stem cell is expressed as a fraction of 400 (Table 28.9).

Bone marrow iron stores, primarily in macrophages, can be examined using special stains (e.g., Prussian blue) for iron-containing granules. A direct measure of iron stores also can be obtained only from liver biopsy specimens, although bone marrow is preferred because it is a safer procedure and because bone marrow is the immediate source of iron destined for erythrocyte production.

Bone marrow aspiration is an important diagnostic test for severe central defects in hematopoiesis (e.g., aplastic anemia, metabolic anemias arising from insufficient iron or inadequate erythropoietin, thrombocytopenia, neutropenia; see Chapters 29 and 31.) Examination of the bone marrow is also useful to diagnose B-lymphocyte immune deficiencies (see Chapter 9), nonmalignant myeloproliferative disorders (e.g., polycythemia vera), and lymphoid/monocytic malignancies (e.g., leukemias, myelomas, lymphomas; see Chapters 30 and 31). This test can also be used to monitor the effects of chemotherapy on malignancies that have invaded the bone marrow (see Fig. 28.25). A marrow aspirate that is richly cellular implies normal or increased hematopoiesis but does not indicate whether marrow activity is effective.

Results from bone marrow aspiration are sometimes limited because this technique disturbs the architecture of the marrow and only provides an analysis of the general cellularity (numbers of constituent cells) of the marrow. On occasion, analysis of an aspirate may only suggest the presence of a malignancy or a central defect in hematopoiesis without being clearly confirmatory, or the sample may be inadequate for diagnosis of bone marrow fibrosis. In these cases the need for a bone marrow biopsy may be indicated.

During a biopsy, a special needle is used to obtain a "core" or cylindrical sample of bone and marrow in which the three-dimensional structure of the marrow is preserved. The biopsy specimens provide the most reliable and complete information about marrow cellularity (see Fig. 28.25). Obtaining a bone marrow biopsy is, however, usually more painful and expensive than aspiration. Therefore biopsy is not performed unless insufficient information is obtained from aspiration.

Blood Tests

Blood tests provide information about the absolute and relative numbers of blood cells in a specimen of blood, as well as various structural and functional characteristics of the cells, and usually provide the initial justification for performing a bone marrow aspiration. Deviations from the normal differential distribution and the presence of abnormal or immature cells can reflect disease, physiologic states (e.g., pregnancy, infancy, old age), injury, or dysfunction in almost any part of the body. Blood tests that reflect chiefly hematologic disorders are listed in Table 28.10.

PEDIATRICS AND THE HEMATOLOGIC SYSTEM

Blood cell counts tend to rise above adult levels at birth and then decline gradually throughout childhood. Table 28.11 lists normal ranges during infancy and childhood. The immediate rise in values is the result of accelerated hematopoiesis during fetal life, increased numbers of cells that result from the trauma of birth, and cutting of the umbilical cord.

Average blood volume in the full-term neonate is 85 mL/kg of body weight. The premature infant has a slightly larger blood volume of 90 mL/kg of body weight, with the mean increasing to 150 mL/kg during the first few days after birth. In both full-term and premature infants, blood volume decreases during the first few months. Thereafter the average blood volume is 75 to 77 mL/kg, which is similar to that of older children and adults.

The hypoxic intrauterine environment stimulates erythropoietin production in the fetus and accelerates fetal erythropoiesis, producing

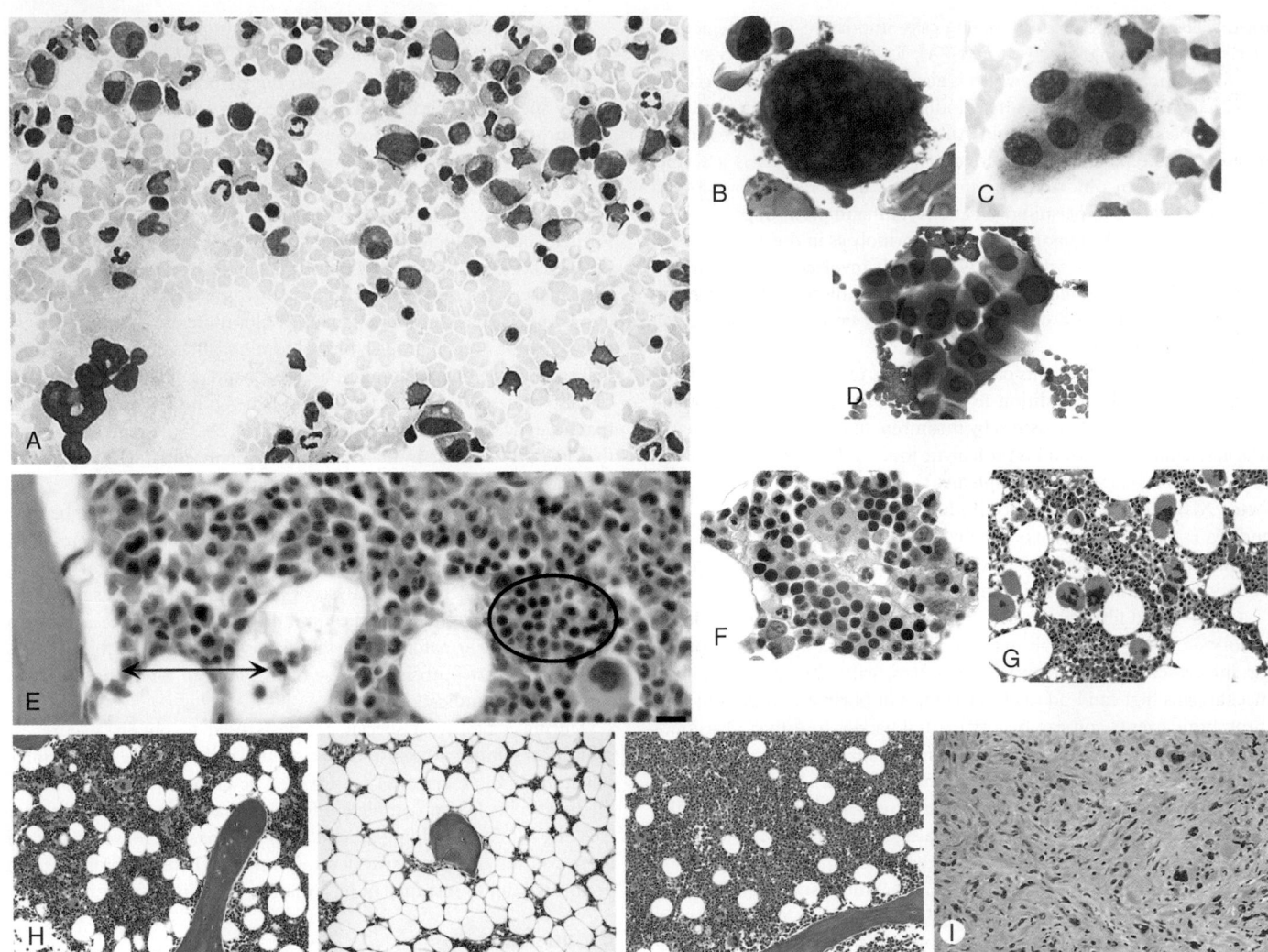

FIGURE 28.25 Bone Marrow Samples. Images **A** through **D** contain bone marrow aspirates; images **E** through **I** contain bone marrow biopsy specimens. **A,** Normal bone marrow aspirate stained by the May-Grünwald/Giemsa technique. **B,** Normal megakaryocyte with budding platelets at the plasma membrane (Wright stain). **C,** Osteoclasts containing multiple nuclei that are separated by cytoplasm. These cells may be confused with megakaryocytes. **D,** Metastatic adenocarcinoma of the breast. **E,** Normal bone marrow biopsy with paratrabecular space with immature myeloid cells *(two-headed arrow)* and circled erythron (site of erythrocyte production). **F,** Normal erythroid island in which several erythroid precursors cluster. **G,** Essential thrombocytopenia with normal cellularity, but increased numbers of large megakaryocytes. **H,** Bone marrow biopsies representing conditions of normal cellularity *(left),* hypocellularity *(middle)* as would be seen in conditions of bone marrow depletion such as aplastic anemia, and hypercellularity *(right)* as seen in malignant conditions. **I,** Advanced chronic idiopathic myelofibrosis marked by extensive replacement of the normal marrow stroma by fibrous tissue (stained pink; hematoxylin-eosin stain). (Sources for photographs: **A, C** from Hoffbrand V et al: *Color atlas of clinical hematology,* ed 4, Philadelphia, 2013, Mosby; **B** from Rodak BF et al: *Hematology,* ed 4, Philadelphia, 2012, Saunders; **D–H** from Jaffe E: *Hematology,* Philadelphia, 2010, Saunders; **E** from Young NS, Gerson SL, High KA: *Clinical hematology,* ed 1, St Louis, 2005, Mosby; **I** from Cleveland Clinic: *Current clinical medicine,* ed 2, Philadelphia, 2010, Saunders.)

TABLE 28.9 DIFFERENTIAL CELL COUNTS IN BONE MARROW WITH AGE*

DEVELOPING CELLS IN MARROW	BIRTH	1 Month–1 Year	1–4 Years	4–12 Years	ADULT
Erythrocytic series	14	8	19	21	20
Lymphocytic series	14	47	22	18	17
Eosinophilic series	3	3	6	3	3
Neutrophilic series	60	33	50	52	57
Myeloid/erythroid ratio	4:3	4:0	1:3	2:5	1:3

*NOTE: Values are percentages of cell types counted during examination of a marrow specimen containing approximately 400 nucleated cells.

TABLE 28.10 **BLOOD TESTS FOR HEMATOLOGIC DISORDERS**

CELL TYPE AND TEST	PROPERTY EVALUATED BY TEST	POSSIBLE HEMATOLOGIC CAUSE OF ABNORMAL FINDINGS
Erythrocytes		
Red cell count	Number (in millions) of erythrocytes/μL of blood	Altered erythropoiesis, anemias, hemorrhage, Hodgkin disease, leukemia
Mean corpuscular volume	Size of erythrocytes	Anemias, thalassemias
Mean corpuscular hemoglobin (MCH)	Amount of hemoglobin in each erythrocyte (by weight)	Anemias, hemoglobinopathy
Mean corpuscular hemoglobin concentration (MCHC)	Concentration of hemoglobin in each erythrocyte (percentage of erythrocyte occupied by hemoglobin)	Anemias, hereditary spherocytosis
Hemoglobin determination	Amount of hemoglobin (by weight)/dL of blood	Anemias
Hematocrit determination	Percentage of a given volume of blood that is occupied by erythrocytes	Hemorrhage, polycythemia, erythrocytosis, anemias, leukemia
Reticulocyte count	Number of reticulocytes/μL of blood (also expressed as percentage of reticulocytes in total red cell count)	Hyperactive or hypoactive bone marrow function
Erythrocyte osmotic fragility test	Cellular shape (biconcavity), structure of plasma membrane	Anemias, hemolytic disease caused by ABO or Rh blood group incompatibility, Hodgkin disease, polycythemia vera, thalassemia major
Hemoglobin electrophoresis	Relative percentage of different types of hemoglobin in erythrocytes	Sickle cell disease, sickle cell trait, hemoglobin C disease, hemoglobin C trait, thalassemias
Sickle cell test	Presence of hemoglobin S in erythrocytes	Sickle cell trait, sickle cell anemia
Glucose-6-phosphate dehydrogenase (G6PD) deficiency test	Deficiency of G6PD in erythrocytes	Hemolytic anemia
Hemoglobin Metabolism		
Serum ferritin determination	Depletion of body iron (potential deficiency of heme synthesis)	Iron deficiency anemias
Total iron-binding capacity (TIBC)	Amount of iron in serum plus amount of transferrin available in serum (mcg/dL)	Hemorrhage, iron deficiency anemia, hemochromatosis, hemosiderosis, iron overload, anemias, thalassemias
Transferrin saturation	Percentage of transferrin that is saturated with iron	Acute hemorrhage, hemochromatosis, hemosiderosis, sideroblastic anemia, iron deficiency anemia, iron overload, thalassemias
Porphyrin analysis (protoporphyrin analysis)	Concentration of protoporphyrin in erythrocytes (mcg/dL); an indicator of iron-deficient erythropoiesis	Megaloblastic anemia, congenital erythropoietic porphyria
Direct antiglobulin test (DAT)	Antibody binding to erythrocytes	Hemolytic disease of the newborn, autoimmune hemolytic anemia, drug-induced hemolytic anemia, transfusion reaction
Antibody screen (indirect Coombs test)	Detection of antibodies to erythrocyte antigens (other than the ABO antigens)	Same as for DAT
Leukocytes		
Differential white cell count (absolute number of a type of leukocyte/μL of blood)	See below	See below
Neutrophil count	Neutrophils/μL	Myeloproliferative disorders, hematopoietic disorders, hemolysis, infection, immune deficiency
Lymphocyte count	Lymphocytes/μL	Infectious lymphocytosis, infectious mononucleosis, hematopoietic disorders, anemias, leukemia, lymphosarcoma, Hodgkin disease, primary immune deficiency
Plasma cell count	Plasma cells/μL	Infectious mononucleosis, lymphocytosis, plasma cell leukemia, primary immune deficiency
Monocyte count	Monocytes/μL	Hodgkin disease, infectious mononucleosis, monocytic leukemia, non-Hodgkin lymphoma, polycythemia vera, primary immune deficiency

Continued

TABLE 28.10   BLOOD TESTS FOR HEMATOLOGIC DISORDERS—cont'd

CELL TYPE AND TEST	PROPERTY EVALUATED BY TEST	POSSIBLE HEMATOLOGIC CAUSE OF ABNORMAL FINDINGS
Eosinophil count	Eosinophils/μL	Hematopoietic disorders
Basophil count	Basophils/μL	Chronic myelogenous leukemia, hemolytic anemias, Hodgkin disease, polycythemia vera

Platelets and Clotting Factors*

CELL TYPE AND TEST	PROPERTY EVALUATED BY TEST	POSSIBLE HEMATOLOGIC CAUSE OF ABNORMAL FINDINGS
Platelet count	Number of circulating platelets (in thousands)/μL of blood	Anemias, multiple myeloma, myelofibrosis, polycythemia vera, leukemia, disseminated intravascular coagulation (DIC), hemolytic disease of the newborn, idiopathic thrombocytopenic purpura, transfusion reaction, lymphoproliferative disorders
Bleeding time	Duration of bleeding following a standardized superficial puncture wound of the skin, integrity of the platelet plug; measured in minutes following puncture	Leukemia, anemias, DIC, fibrinolytic activity, purpuras, hemorrhagic disease of the newborn, infectious mononucleosis, multiple myeloma, clotting factor deficiencies, thrombasthenia, thrombocytopenia, von Willebrand disease
Clot retraction test	Platelet number and function, fibrinogen quantity and use; measured in hours, which is required for expression of serum from a clot incubated in a test tube	Acute leukemia, aplastic anemia, factor XIII deficiency, increased fibrinolytic activity, Hodgkin disease, hyperfibrinogenemia or hypofibrinogenemia, idiopathic thrombocytopenic purpura, multiple myeloma, polycythemia vera, secondary thrombocytopenia, thrombasthenia
Platelet adhesion studies	Ability of platelets to adhere to foreign surfaces	Anemia, macroglobulinemia, Bernard-Soulier syndrome, multiple myeloma, myeloid metaplasia, plasma cell dyscrasias, thrombasthenia, thrombocytopathy, von Willebrand disease
Platelet aggregation tests	Ability of platelets to adhere to one another	Afibrinogenemia, Bernard-Soulier syndrome, thrombasthenia, hemorrhagic thrombocythemia, myeloid metaplasia, plasma cell dyscrasias, platelet-release defects, polycythemia vera, preleukemia, sideroblastic anemia, von Willebrand disease, Waldenström macroglobulinemia, hypercoagulability
Whole blood clotting time (Lee-White coagulation time)	Overall ability of blood to clot; measured in minutes in a test tube	Afibrinogenemia, clotting factor deficiencies, excessive fibrinolysis, hemorrhagic disease of the newborn, hypofibrinogenemia, hypoprothrombinemia, leukemia
Circulating anticoagulants (immunoglobulin G [IgG] or M [IgM] antibodies that inhibit coagulation)	Presence of antibodies that neutralize clotting factors and inhibit coagulation, as indicated by prolonged clotting time, prothrombin time, or partial thromboplastin time	Afibrinogenemia, presence of fibrin-fibrinogen degradation products, macroglobulinemia, multiple myeloma, DIC, plasma cell dyscrasias
Partial thromboplastin time (PTT)	Effectiveness of clotting factors (except factors VII and VIII), effectiveness of intrinsic pathway of coagulation cascade; measured in seconds in a test tube	Presence of circulating anticoagulants, DIC, clotting factor deficiencies, excessive fibrinolysis, hemorrhagic disease of the newborn, hypofibrinogenemia and afibrinogenemia, prothrombin deficiency, von Willebrand disease, acute hemorrhage
Prothrombin time (PT)	Effectiveness of activity of prothrombin, fibrinogen, and factors V, VII, and X; effectiveness of vitamin K–dependent coagulation factors of the extrinsic and common pathways of the coagulation cascade; measured in seconds in a test tube	Hypofibrinogenemia, dysfibrinogenemia, and afibrinogenemia; presence of circulating anticoagulants; DIC; deficiency of factors V, VII, or X; presence of fibrin degradation products, increased fibrinolytic activity, hemolytic jaundice, hemorrhagic disease of the newborn; acute leukemia, polycythemia vera, prothrombin deficiency, multiple myeloma
Thrombin time	Quantity and activity of fibrinogen; measured in seconds in a test tube	Hypofibrinogenemia, dysfibrinogenemia, and afibrinogenemia; presence of circulating anticoagulants; hemorrhagic disease of the newborn; polycythemia vera; increase in fibrin-fibrinogen degradation products; increased fibrinolytic activity
Fibrinogen assay	Amount of fibrinogen available for fibrin formation	Acute leukemia, congenital hypofibrinogenemia or afibrinogenemia, DIC, increased fibrinolytic activity, severe hemorrhage
Fibrin-fibrinogen degradation products (fibrin-fibrinogen split products)	Fibrinogenic activity as measured by levels of fibrin-fibrinogen degradation products (in mcg/mL of blood)	Transfusion reactions, DIC, internal hemorrhage in the newborn, deep vein thrombosis, pulmonary embolism

*NOTE: See Fig. 28.23 and Table 28.7 for information about clotting factors and their sequence of activation in the coagulation cascade.
Data from Garrels M, Oatis CS: *Laboratory and diagnostic testing in ambulatory care: a guide for health care professionals*, ed 3, St Louis, 2015, Saunders; Hudnall D: *Hematology: a pathophysiologic approach*, St Louis, 2012, Mosby.

TABLE 28.11 **HEMATOLOGIC VALUES DURING INFANCY AND CHILDHOOD**

| AGE | HEMOGLOBIN (g/dL) | HEMATOCRIT (%) | RETICULOCYTES (%) | LEUKOCYTES (WBCs/mm³) | DIFFERENTIAL COUNTS* | | | | | PLATELETS (×10³/mm³) |
					NEUTROPHILS (%)	LYMPHOCYTES (%)	EOSINOPHILS (%)	MONOCYTES (%)	
Cord blood	16.8	55	5.0	18,000	61	31	2	6	290
2 wk	16.5	50	1.0	12,000	40	48	3	9	252
3 mo	12.0	36	1.0	12,000	30	63	2	5	140–340
6 mo–6 yr	12.0	37	1.0	10,000	45	48	2	5	140–340
7–12 yr	13.0	38	1.0	8000	55	38	2	5	140–340
Adult	13.0	40	1.0	8000	55	35	2	5	140–340
Female	14	41	0.8–4.1	7400	54–62	25–33	1–4	3–7	140–340
Male	16	47	0.8–2.5	7400	54–62	25–33	1–4	3–7	140–340

*All values are means except for platelets.
WBCs, White blood cells.

polycythemia (excessive proliferation of erythrocyte precursors) of the newborn. After birth the oxygen from the lungs saturates arterial blood, and more oxygen is delivered to the tissues. In response to the change from a placental to a pulmonary oxygen supply during the first few days of life, levels of erythropoietin and the rate of blood cell formation decrease.

The very active rate of fetal erythropoiesis results in a large number of immature erythrocytes (reticulocytes) in the peripheral blood of full-term neonates. After birth the number of reticulocytes decreases about 50% every 12 hours so that it is rare to find an elevated reticulocyte count after the first week of life. During this period of rapid growth, the rate of erythrocyte destruction is greater than that in later childhood and adulthood. In full-term infants, normal erythrocyte life span is 60 to 80 days; in premature infants, it may be as short as 20 to 30 days; and in children and adolescents, it is the same as that in adults—100 to 120 days.

The postnatal decrease in hemoglobin and hematocrit values is more marked in premature infants than in the full-term infant. In the preschool and school-age child, hemoglobin, hematocrit, and red blood cell counts gradually rise. Metabolic processes within the erythrocytes of neonates differ significantly from those of erythrocytes in the normal adult. Among other differences, the relatively young population of erythrocytes in the newborn consumes greater quantities of glucose than do erythrocytes in adults.

Most coagulation factors (both procoagulants and anticoagulants) in children reach adult levels by 6 months of age, and some not until adolescence. Children have quantitative and qualitative differences in clotting factors that result in decreased risk for thrombosis without increased risk for bleeding (developmental hemostasis) because the reduction of procoagulant and anticoagulant proteins is balanced.[52] Laboratory values for hemostasis (i.e., prothrombin time and activated partial thromboplastin time) are referenced by the testing laboratory.[53]

At birth, the lymphocyte count is high and continues to rise during the first year of life, and then steadily declines until lower adult values are reached. The lymphocytes of children also tend to have more cytoplasm and less compact nuclear chromatin than do the lymphocytes of adults. A possible explanation is that children tend to have more frequent viral infections, some of which are subclinical, and are receiving vaccinations, both of which are associated with atypical lymphocytes.

The neutrophil count, like the lymphocyte count, is high at birth and rises during the first days of life. After 2 weeks the neutrophil count falls to within or below the normal adult range. By approximately 4 years of age, the neutrophil count is the same as that of an adult. The eosinophil count is high in the first year of life and higher in children than in teenagers or adults. Monocyte counts also are high in the first year of life but then decrease to adult levels. Platelet counts in full-term neonates are comparable with platelet counts in adults and remain so throughout infancy and childhood.

AGING AND THE HEMATOLOGIC SYSTEM

Blood composition changes little with age. Erythrocyte life span in older adults is normal, although erythrocytes are replenished more slowly after bleeding, probably because of iron depletion. Values of total serum iron, total iron-binding capacity, and intestinal iron absorption are all decreased in older adults. Iron deficiency is often responsible for the low hemoglobin levels noted in older adults. The plasma membranes of erythrocytes become increasingly fragile, presumably because of physical trauma inflicted during circulation. Chronic inflammation and the presence of chronic disease, including diabetes mellitus, chronic heart disease, chronic renal insufficiency, and Parkinson disease, are associated with suppressed erythropoiesis and anemia occurring in older adults.[54]

Lymphocyte function decreases with age (see Chapters 8 and 9), causing changes in cellular immunity with some decline in T-cell function. The humoral immune system is less able to respond to antigenic challenge and to vaccination.[55] No changes in platelet numbers or structure have been observed in elderly persons, yet platelet adhesiveness probably increases and may be related to oxidative stress.[56] Levels of fibrinogen and factors V, VII, and IX and also levels of vWF tend to be increased in older adults. In addition, thrombin generation and platelet activation are enhanced in older adults. Consequently, there is an increased incidence of venous thromboembolism.[57]

SUMMARY REVIEW

Components of the Hematologic System

1. Blood consists of cells suspended in a solution of about 91% water and 8% solutes. In adults the total blood volume is approximately 5.5 L.
2. Plasma, the liquid portion of the blood (50% to 55% of blood volume), contains two major groups of proteins: albumins and globulins.
3. The cellular elements of blood are the erythrocytes (red blood cells), leukocytes (white blood cells), and platelets (thrombocytes).
4. Erythrocytes are the most abundant cells of the blood, occupying approximately 48% of the blood volume in men and approximately 42% in women. Erythrocytes are responsible for tissue oxygenation.
5. Leukocytes are fewer in number than erythrocytes and constitute approximately 5000 to 10,000 mm³ of blood. Leukocytes defend the body against infection and remove dead or injured host cells.
6. Leukocytes are classified as either granulocytes (neutrophils, basophils, eosinophils) or agranulocytes (monocytes, macrophages, lymphocytes).
7. Macrophages remove old and damaged cells and large molecular substances from the blood by phagocytosis.
8. The neutrophil is the most abundant leukocyte (approximately 55% of the leukocytes) and is the primary granulocyte that defends against infections.
9. Lymphocytes are the primary cells of the immune response.
10. Platelets are not cells—they are disk-shaped cytoplasmic fragments. Platelets are essential for blood coagulation and control of bleeding.
11. The lymphoid organs are classified as primary (thymus and bone marrow) or secondary (spleen, lymph nodes, tonsils, and Peyer patches of the small intestine).
12. The lymphoid organs are sites of residence, proliferation, differentiation, and function of lymphocytes and mononuclear phagocytes.
13. The spleen is the largest of the secondary lymphoid organs and functions as the site of hematopoiesis in the fetus, filters and cleanses the blood, and is a reservoir for lymphocytes and other blood cells.
14. The lymph nodes are the site of development or activity of large numbers of lymphocytes, monocytes, and macrophages.
15. The MPS is composed of macrophages in tissue and lymphoid organs.
16. The MPS is the main line of defense against bacteria in the bloodstream and cleanses the blood by removing old, injured, or dead blood cells; antigen-antibody complexes; and macromolecules.

▮ SUMMARY REVIEW—cont'd

Development of Blood Cells

1. Hematopoiesis, or blood cell production, occurs in the liver and spleen of the fetus and in the bone marrow after birth.

2. Hematopoiesis involves two stages: (a) proliferation and (b) maturation.

3. Hematopoiesis continues throughout life to replace blood cells that grow old and die, are killed by disease, or are lost through bleeding.

4. Bone marrow consists of red (hematopoietic) marrow (blood vessels, mononuclear phagocytes, stem cells, blood cells in various stages of differentiation, stromal cells) and yellow marrow (fatty tissue).

5. The bone marrow contains multiple populations of *stem cells;* mesenchymal stem cells develop into fibroblasts, osteoclasts, and adipocytes; and hematopoietic stem cells develop into blood cells.

6. Regulation of hematopoiesis occurs in specialized microenvironments (niches) in the bone marrow (an osteoblastic niche and a vascular niche) in which hematopoietic stem cells are signaled to undergo differentiation through the effects of multiple cytokines and chemokines and through direct contact with osteoblasts (osteoblastic niche) or vascular endothelial cells (vascular niche), as well as several other specialized cells, including CAR cells and nestin-expressing cells.

7. Specific hematopoietic growth factors (e.g., colony-stimulating factors) are necessary for the adequate production of myeloid, erythroid, lymphoid, and megakaryocytic lineages.

8. Erythropoiesis (production of erythrocytes) is regulated by erythropoietin. Erythropoietin is secreted by the kidneys in response to tissue hypoxia and causes a compensatory increase in erythrocyte production if the oxygen content of the blood decreases because of anemia, high altitude, or pulmonary disease.

9. Hemoglobin, the oxygen-carrying protein of the erythrocyte, enables the blood to transport 100 times more oxygen than could be transported dissolved in plasma alone.

10. The iron cycle reutilizes iron released from old or damaged erythrocytes. Iron binds to transferrin in the blood, is transported to macrophages of the MPS, and is stored in the cytoplasm as ferritin.

11. Iron homeostasis is controlled by hepcidin, a small hormone produced by hepatocytes, which regulates ferroportin, the principal transporter of iron from stores in hepatocytes and macrophages and from intestinal cells that take up dietary iron.

12. Granulocytes and monocytes in the blood develop from common myeloid progenitor cells in the bone marrow under the direction of several growth factors, including stem cell factor, IL-3, and GM-CSF.

13. Platelets develop from megakaryocytes by a process called *endomitosis,* which is controlled by thrombopoietin. During endomitosis the megakaryocytes undergo mitosis but not cell division and the cytoplasm and plasma membrane fragment into platelets.

Mechanisms of Hemostasis

1. Hemostasis, or arrest of bleeding in damaged vessels, involves (a) vasoconstriction, (b) damage to the endothelium and exposure of connective tissue resulting in formation of a platelet plug, (c) activation of the clotting cascade, (d) formation of a blood clot, and (e) activation of fibrinolysis for clot retraction and clot dissolution.

2. Platelet activation involves three linked processes: (a) adhesion, (b) activation, and (c) aggregation.

3. A blood clot is a meshwork of protein strands that stabilizes the platelet plug. The strands are made of fibrin. Fibrin is the end product of the coagulation cascade.

4. The pathways of hemostasis include the intrinsic pathway (also known as the *contact pathway*) and extrinsic pathway. The extrinsic pathway is the major pathway of normal hemostasis initiated by TF that forms a complex with the TF/VIIa complex. The intrinsic (contact) pathway is activated by artificial negative surfaces and also functions in thrombotic states.

5. The endothelium prevents the formation of spontaneous clots in normal vessels by several anticoagulant mechanisms, including production of NO and PGI_2, thrombin inhibitors (antithrombin III), and tissue factor inhibitors (tissue factor pathway inhibitors); and degradation of activated clotting factors (thrombomodulin–protein C).

6. Fibrinolysis (breakdown of blood clots) is the function of the plasminogen-plasmin system. Plasmin is a degrading enzyme of fibrin clots. It is produced from plasminogen by activation of plasminogen activators (t-PA, u-PA), thrombin, fibrin, factor XIIa, factor XIa, and kallikrein.

7. Products of fibrinolysis include fibrin degradation products, such as D-dimer.

Clinical Evaluation of the Hematologic System

1. Tests of bone marrow function include bone marrow aspiration and bone marrow biopsy.

2. Cells contained in the marrow specimen are assessed with respect to (a) relative numbers of stem cells and their developing daughter cells, and (b) morphologic structure.

Pediatrics and the Hematologic System

1. Blood cell counts rise above adult levels at birth and then gradually decline throughout childhood.

2. The average blood volume of an infant is 75 to 77 mL/kg, which is similar to that of older children and adults.

3. In response to the change from a placental to a pulmonary oxygen supply during the first few days of life, levels of erythropoietin and the rate of blood cell formation decrease.

4. The normal erythrocyte life span is 60 to 80 days in full-term infants, 20 to 30 days in premature infants, and 120 days in children, adolescents, and adults.

5. The lymphocyte count is high at birth, rises further during the first year of life, and steadily declines until lower adult volumes are reached.

6. The neutrophil count is very high at birth, falls to adult ranges after 2 weeks, and is the same as that for adults by 4 years of age.

7. The eosinophil count is high in the first year of life and is higher in children than in adolescents and adults. Monocyte counts are high in the first year of life and decrease to adult levels.

8. Platelet counts in full-term infants are comparable with those in adults and remain so throughout childhood.

Aging and the Hematologic System

1. Blood composition changes little with age. A delay in erythrocyte replenishment may occur after bleeding, presumably because of iron deficiency.

2. Lymphocyte function appears to decrease with age. Particularly affected is a decrease in cellular immunity.

3. Platelet adhesiveness probably increases with age, as do clotting factors increasing risk for thromboembolism.

KEY TERMS

Agranulocyte, 894
Albumin, 891
Antithrombin III (AT-III), 916
Apoferritin, 909
Apotransferrin, 909
Basophil, 894
Blood clot, 912
Bone marrow, 899
Clotting (coagulation) system, 913
Clotting factor, 891
Colony-stimulating factor (CSF, hematopoietic growth factor), 901
Cyclooxygenase 1 (COX-1), 912
D-dimer, 917
Dendritic cell, 895
Deoxyhemoglobin, 907
Endomitosis, 910
Eosinophil, 894
Erythroblast, 902
Erythrocyte (red blood cell [RBC]), 892
Erythropoiesis, 902
Erythropoietin, 902
Extramedullary hematopoiesis, 899
Fibrin degradation product (FDP), 917
Fibrinolysis, 910
Fibrinolytic system (plasminogen-plasmin system), 916
Globin, 906
Globulin, 891

Glycoprotein IIb/IIIa (GPIIb/IIIa) complex, 912
Granulocyte, 894
Hematopoiesis, 898
Hematopoietic stem cell (HSC), 899
Heme, 906
Hemoglobin (Hb), 906
Hemosiderin, 909
Hemostasis, 910
Hepcidin, 909
Immunocyte, 894
Leukocyte (white blood cell [WBC]), 894
Lymph node, 898
Lymphocyte, 895
Macrophage, 895
Marginating storage pool, 902
Mast cell, 894
Megakaryocyte, 896
Mesenchymal stem cell (MSC), 899
Methemoglobin, 907
Monocyte, 895
Mononuclear phagocyte system (MPS), 895
Myeloid tissue, 899
Myoglobin, 908
Natural killer (NK) cell, 895
Neutrophil (polymorphonuclear neutrophil [PMN]), 894
Niche, 899
Normoblast, 902

Oxyhemoglobin, 907
Phagocyte, 894
Plasma, 891
Plasma protein, 891
Plasmin, 916
Plasminogen, 916
Platelet (thrombocyte), 895
Platelet adhesion, 911
Platelet aggregation, 912
Platelet-release reaction, 911
Primary lymphoid organ, 896
Proerythroblast, 902
Prostacyclin (prostaglandin I_2 [PGI_2]), 910
Protein C, 916
Protein S, 916
Protoporphyrin, 906
Reticulocyte, 902
Secondary lymphoid organ, 896
Serum, 891
Thrombomodulin, 916
Thrombopoietin, 910
Thromboxane A_2 (TXA_2), 912
Tissue factor (TF, tissue thromboplastin), 913
Tissue factor pathway inhibitor (TFPI), 916
Tissue plasminogen activator (t-PA), 917
Transferrin, 909
Urokinase-like plasminogen activator (u-PA), 917
von Willebrand factor (vWF), 911

REFERENCES

1. Selders GS, et al: An overview of the role of neutrophils in innate immunity, inflammation and host-biomaterial integration. *Regen Biomater* 4(1):55–68, 2017.
2. Ravin KA, Loy M: The eosinophil in infection. *Clin Rev Allergy Immunol* 50(2):214–227, 2016.
3. Merluzzi S, et al: Mast cells, basophils and B cell connection network. *Mol Immunol* 63(1):94–103, 2015.
4. Yamanishi Y, Karasuyama H: Basophil-derived IL-4 plays versatile roles in immunity. *Semin Immunopathol* 38(5):615–622, 2016.
5. Reber LL, Frossard N: Targeting mast cells in inflammatory diseases. *Pharmacol Ther* 142(3):416–435, 2014.
6. Jenkins SJ, Hume DA: Homeostasis in the mononuclear phagocyte system. *Trends Immunol* 35(8):358–367, 2014.
7. Lampiasi N, Russo R, Zito F: The alternative faces of macrophage generate osteoclasts. *Biomed Res Int* 2016:9089610, 2016.
8. Heijnen H, van der Sluijs P: Platelet secretory behaviour: as diverse as the granules … or not? *J Thromb Haemost* 13(12):2141–2151, 2015.
9. Steiniger BS: Human spleen microanatomy: why mice do not suffice. *Immunology* 145(3):334–346, 2015.
10. Soares MP, Hamza I: Macrophages and iron metabolism. *Immunity* 44(3):492–504, 2016.
11. Luoto TT, Pakarinen MP, Koivusalo A: Long-term outcomes after pediatric splenectomy. *Surgery* 159(6):1583–1590, 2016.
12. Buzelé R, et al: Medical complications following splenectomy. *J Vasc Surg* 153(4):277–286, 2016.
13. Boulais PE, Frenette PS: Making sense of hematopoietic stem cell niches. *Blood* 125(17):2621–2629, 2015.
14. Beerman I, et al: The evolving view of the hematopoietic stem cell niche. *Exp Hematol* 50:22–26, 2017.

15. Price TT, et al: Dormant breast cancer micrometastases reside in specific bone marrow niches that regulate their transit to and from bone. *Sci Transl Med* 8(340):340ra73, 2016.
16. Spencer JA, et al: Direct measurement of local oxygen concentration in the bone marrow of live animals. *Nature* 508(7495):269–273, 2014.
17. Calvi LM, Link DC: The hematopoietic stem cell niche in homeostasis and disease. *Blood* 126(22):2443–2451, 2015.
18. Tamma R, Ribatti D: Bone niches, hematopoietic stem cells, and vessel formation. *Int J Mol Sci* 18(1):2017.
19. Blank U, Karlsson S: TGF-β signaling in the control of hematopoietic stem cells. *Blood* 125(23):3542–3550, 2015.
20. *Stem cell information*, Bethesda, MD, 2010, National Institutes of Health, U.S. Department of Health and Human Services. Available at: http://stemcells.nih.gov/info.
21. Ingley E: Integrating novel signaling pathways involved in erythropoiesis. *IUBMB Life* 64(5):402–410, 2012.
22. Klei TR, et al: From the cradle to the grave: the role of macrophages in erythropoiesis and erythrophagocytosis. *Front Immunol* 8:73, 2017.
23. Ganz T: Macrophages and iron metabolism. *Microbiol Spectr* 4(5):2016.
24. Rishi G, Wallace DF, Subramaniam VN: Hepcidin: regulation of the master iron regulator. *Biosci Rep* 35(3):2015.
25. Vyoral D, Petrak J: Therapeutic potential of hepcidin—the master regulator of iron metabolism. *Pharmacol Res* 115:242–254, 2017.
26. Kaushansky K: Thrombopoiesis. *Semin Hematol* 52(1):4–11, 2015.
27. Campia U, et al: The vascular endothelin system in obesity and type 2 diabetes: pathophysiology and

therapeutic implications. *Life Sci* 118(2):149–155, 2014.
28. Lö A, et al: Biophysical approaches promote advances in the understanding of von Willebrand factor processing and function. *Adv Biol Regul* 63:81–91, 2017.
29. Bye AP, Unsworth AJ, Gibbins JM: Platelet signaling: a complex interplay between inhibitory and activatory networks. *J Thromb Haemost* 14(5):918–930, 2016.
30. Ruggeri ZM, Mendolicchio GL: Interaction of von Willebrand factor with platelets and the vessel wall. *Hamostaseologie* 35(3):211–224, 2015.
31. Gremmel T, Frelinger AL, 3rd, Michelson AD: Platelet physiology. *Semin Thromb Hemost* 42(3):191–204, 2016.
32. Patrono C: The multifaceted clinical readouts of platelet inhibition by low-dose aspirin. *J Am Coll Cardiol* 66(1):74–85, 2015.
33. Poon MC, et al: New insights into the treatment of Glanzmann thrombasthenia. *Transfus Med Rev* 30(2):92–99, 2016.
34. de Witt SM, et al: Insights into platelet-based control of coagulation. *Thromb Res* 133(Suppl 2):S139–S148, 2014.
35. Smith SA, Travers RJ, Morrissey JH: How it all starts: initiation of the clotting cascade. *Crit Rev Biochem Mol Biol* 50(4):326–336, 2015.
36. Foley JH, Conway EM: Cross talk pathways between coagulation and inflammation. *Circ Res* 118(9):1392–1408, 2016.
37. Weitz JI: Factor XI and factor XII as targets for new anticoagulants. *Thromb Res* 141(Suppl 2):S40–S45, 2016.
38. Kuijpers MJE, et al: Factor XII regulates the pathological process of thrombus formation on ruptured plaques. *Arterioscler Thromb Vasc Biol* 34:1674–1680, 2014.
39. Puy C, et al: Activated factor XI increases the procoagulant activity of the extrinsic pathway by

inactivating tissue factor pathway inhibitor. *Blood* 125(9):1488–1496, 2015.

40. Puy C, Rigg RA, McCarty OJ: The hemostatic role of factor XI. *Thromb Res* 141(Suppl 2):S8–S11, 2016.

41. Wheeler AP, Gailani D: The intrinsic pathway of coagulation as a target for antithrombotic therapy. *Hematol Oncol Clin North Am* 30(5):1099–1114, 2016.

42. Weitz JI, Fredenburgh JC: Factors XI and XII as targets for new anticoagulants. *Front Med (Lausanne)* 4:19, 2017.

43. Levi M, van der Poll T: Coagulation in patients with severe sepsis. *Semin Thromb Hemost* 41(1): 9–15, 2015.

44. Smith SA, Travers RJ, Morrissey JH: How it all starts: initiation of the clotting cascade. *Crit Rev Biochem Mol Biol* 50(4):326–336, 2015.

45. Mast AE: Tissue factor pathway inhibitor: multiple anticoagulant activities for a single

protein. *Arterioscler Thromb Vasc Biol* 36(1):9–14, 2016.

46. Spronk HM, Borissoff JI, ten Cate H: New insights into modulation of thrombin formation. *Curr Atheroscler Rep* 15(11):363, 2013.

47. Franchini M, Martinelli I, Mannucci PM: Uncertain thrombophilia markers. *Thromb Haemost* 115(1): 25–30, 2016.

48. Jackson CJ, Xue M: Activated protein C—an anticoagulant that does more than stop clots. *Int J Biochem Cell Biol* 40(12):2692–2697, 2008.

49. Almawi WY, et al: Protein Z, an anticoagulant protein with expanding role in reproductive biology. *Reproduction* 146(2):R73–R80, 2013.

50. Draxler DF, Medcalf RL: The fibrinolytic system-more than fibrinolysis? *Transfus Med Rev* 29(2):102–109, 2015.

51. Linkins LA, Takach Lapner S: Review of D-dimer testing: good, bad, and ugly. *Int J Lab Hematol* 39(Suppl 1):98–103, 2017.

52. Jaffray J, Young G: Developmental hemostasis: clinical implications from the fetus to the adolescent. *Pediatr Clin North Am* 60(6):1407–1417, 2013.

53. Toulon P: Developmental hemostasis: laboratory and clinical implications. *Int J Lab Hematol* 38(Suppl 1):66–77, 2016.

54. Röhrig G: Anemia in the frail, elderly patient. *Clin Interv Aging* 11:319–326, 2016.

55. Stervbo U, et al: Effects of aging on human leukocytes (part I): immunophenotyping of innate immune cells. *Age (Dordr)* 37(5):92, 2015.

56. Fuentes E, Palomo I: Role of oxidative stress on platelet hyperreactivity during aging. *Life Sci* 148:17–23, 2016.

57. Sepúlveda C, Palomo I, Fuentes E: Primary and secondary haemostasis changes related to aging. *Mech Ageing Dev* 150:46–54, 2015.

Alterations of Erythrocyte, Platelet, and Hemostatic Function

Kathryn L. McCance, Neal S. Rote

evolve WEBSITE

CHAPTER OUTLINE

Alterations of erythrocyte function involve either insufficient or excessive numbers of red blood cells (RBCs) in the circulation or normal numbers of cells with abnormal components. Anemias occur when there is an inadequate number of RBCs or an insufficient volume or mass of RBCs in the blood, while polycythemias develop when the number or volume of RBCs is excessive. Each of these conditions has many causes and is a pathophysiologic manifestation of a variety of disease states.

The primary role of clotting (hemostasis) is to stop bleeding through an interaction among vascular endothelium, platelets, and the clotting system. Many disease states are associated with clinically significant aberrations in any of these three necessary components of clotting. This chapter discusses alterations of platelets and various components of clotting and their control systems.

ANEMIA

Anemia is a reduction in the total circulating red cell mass or a decrease in the quality or quantity of hemoglobin. Anemias commonly result from (1) blood loss (acute or chronic), (2) impaired erythrocyte production, (3) increased erythrocyte destruction, or (4) a combination of these factors. Total circulating red blood cell mass is reflected by changes in plasma volume caused by dehydration and fluid retention. For example, decreased plasma volume from dehydration (less water intake, prolonged vomiting,

diarrhea, excessive use of diuretics) with a normal red blood cell mass may indicate a *relative polycythemia* or abnormally elevated red cell count because of hemoconcentration. Severe dehydration can correlate with increased hematocrit and hemoglobin levels. Fluid retention is associated with hemodilution rather than a true decrease in red blood cell mass.

Classification and General Characteristics

There are several ways to classify anemias. A useful way is by the underlying main mechanism (Table 29.1). Another way to classify anemias is based on changes that affect the erythrocyte's size or hemoglobin content. The terminology reflects these characteristics: terms that end in "-cytic" refer to cell size, whereas "-chromic" refers to hemoglobin content. Microcytic-hypochromic anemias are caused by disorders of hemoglobin synthesis, particularly iron deficiency. Macrocytic anemias arise commonly from abnormalities that hinder the maturation of erythroid precursors in the bone marrow. Various etiologies occur in normocytic-normochromic anemias, and the specific shapes of the red blood cell can help determine the cause. Additional descriptors of erythrocytes associated with some anemias include **anisocytosis** (assuming various sizes) or **poikilocytosis** (assuming various shapes) (Fig. 29.1).

The main physiologic manifestation of anemia is a reduced oxygen-carrying capacity of the blood resulting in tissue hypoxia. Symptoms of anemia vary, depending on the body's ability to compensate for

TABLE 29.1	CLASSIFICATION OF ANEMIA ACCORDING TO UNDERLYING MECHANISM
MECHANISM	**SPECIFIC EXAMPLES**
Blood Loss	
Acute blood loss	Trauma
Chronic blood loss	Gastrointestinal tract lesions, gynecologic disturbances*
Increased Red Cell Destruction (Hemolysis)	
Inherited Genetic Defects	
Red cell membrane disorders	Hereditary spherocytosis, hereditary elliptocytosis
Enzyme deficiencies	
Hexose monophosphate shunt enzyme deficiencies	G6PD deficiency, glutathione synthetase deficiency
Glycolytic enzyme deficiencies	Pyruvate kinase deficiency, hexokinase deficiency
Hemoglobin abnormalities	
Deficient globin synthesis	Thalassemia syndromes
Structurally abnormal globins (hemoglobinopathies)	Sickle cell disease, unstable hemoglobins
Acquired Genetic Defects	
Deficiency of phosphatidylinositol-linked glycoproteins	Paroxysmal nocturnal hemoglobinuria
Antibody-mediated destruction	Hemolytic disease of the newborn (Rh disease), transfusion reactions, drug-induced, autoimmune disorders
Mechanical trauma	
Microangiopathic hemolytic anemias	Hemolytic uremic syndrome, disseminated intravascular coagulation, thrombotic thrombocytopenia purpura
Cardiac traumatic hemolysis	Defective cardiac valves
Repetitive physical trauma	Bongo drumming, marathon running, karate chopping
Infections of red cells	Malaria, babesiosis
Toxic or chemical injury	Clostridial sepsis, snake venom, lead poisoning
Membrane lipid abnormalities	Abetalipoproteinemia, severe hepatocellular liver disease
Sequestration	Hypersplenism
Decreased Red Cell Production	
Inherited Genetic Defects	
Defects leading to stem cell depletion	Fanconi anemia, telomerase defects
Defects affecting erythroblast maturation	Thalassemia syndromes
Nutritional Deficiencies	
Deficiencies affecting DNA synthesis	B$_{12}$ and folate deficiencies
Deficiencies affecting hemoglobin synthesis	Iron deficiency anemia
Erythropoietin deficiency	Renal failure, anemia of chronic disease
Immune-mediated injury of progenitors	Aplastic anemia, pure red cell aplasia
Inflammation-mediated iron sequestration	Anemia of chronic disease
Primary hematopoietic neoplasms	Acute leukemia, myelodysplasia, myeloproliferative disorders
Space-occupying marrow lesions	Metastatic neoplasms, granulomatous disease
Infections of red cell progenitors	Parvovirus B19 infection
Unknown mechanisms	Endocrine disorders, hepatocellular liver disease

*The usual cause of anemia is iron deficiency, not actual bleeding.
G6PD, Glucose-6-phosphate dehydrogenase.
From Kumar V, Abbas A, Aster JC: *Robbins & Cotran pathologic basis of disease,* ed 9, Philadelphia, 2015, Saunders.

reduced oxygen-carrying capacity (Fig. 29.2). Anemia that is mild and develops gradually is usually easier to compensate and may cause problems for the individual only during physical exertion. As the reduction in the number of red blood cells (RBCs) continues, symptoms become more pronounced and alterations of specific organs and compensatory effects become more apparent. Compensation generally involves the cardiovascular, respiratory, and hematologic systems. (Hematologic findings associated with various anemias are listed in Table 29.2 and progression and manifestations of anemias are shown in Fig. 29.2.)

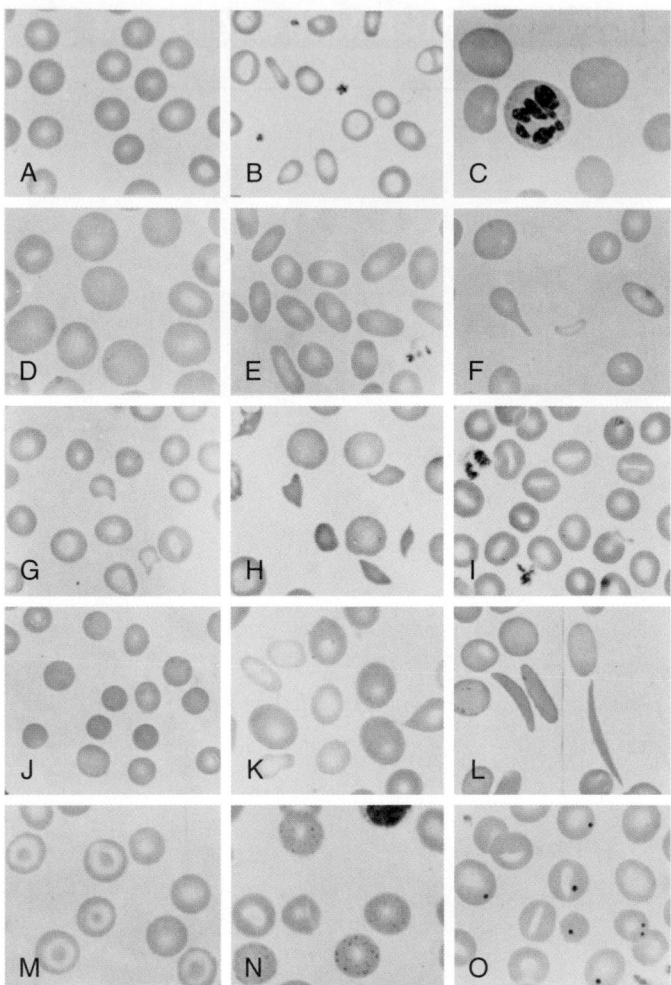

FIGURE 29.1 Appearance of Red Blood Cells in Various Disorders.
A, Normal blood smear. **B,** Microcytic-hypochromic anemia (iron deficiency).
C, Macrocytic anemia (pernicious anemia). **D,** Macrocytic anemia in pregnancy.
E, Hereditary elliptocytosis. **F,** Myelofibrosis (teardrop). **G,** Hemolytic anemia
associated with prosthetic heart valve. **H,** Microangiopathic anemia. **I,** Stomatocytes.
J, Spherocytes (hereditary spherocytosis). **K,** Sideroblastic anemia; note the double
population of red blood cells. **L,** Sickle cell anemia. **M,** Target cells (after splenectomy).
N, Basophil stippling in case of unexplained anemia. **O,** Howell-Jolly bodies (after
splenectomy). (From Wintrobe MM et al: *Clinical hematology*, ed 8, Philadelphia,
1981, Lea & Febiger.)

A reduction in the number of blood cells in the blood causes a reduction in the consistency and volume of blood. Compensation for a reduced blood volume causes interstitial fluid to move into the intravascular space, expanding plasma volume. This movement maintains adequate blood volume, but the viscosity (thickness) of the blood decreases. The diluted blood flows faster and more turbulently than normal blood, causing a hyperdynamic circulatory state. This hyperdynamic state creates cardiovascular changes—increased stroke volume and heart rate. These changes may lead to cardiac dilation and heart valve insufficiency if the underlying anemic condition is not corrected.

Hypoxemia, reduced oxygen levels in the blood, further contributes to cardiovascular dysfunction by causing dilation of arterioles, capillaries, and venules, thus leading to decreased vascular resistance and increased flow. Increased peripheral blood flow and accelerated venous return further contribute to an increase in heart rate and stroke volume in a continuing effort to meet normal oxygen demand and prevent

cardiopulmonary congestion. These compensatory mechanisms may lead to heart failure.

Tissue hypoxia creates additional demands and compensatory actions on the pulmonary and hematologic systems. The rate and depth of breathing increase in an attempt to increase the availability of oxygen. These demands are accompanied by an increase in the release of oxygen from hemoglobin. (Mechanisms of oxygen transport and release by hemoglobin are described in Chapter 28.) All of these compensatory mechanisms may cause individuals to experience shortness of breath (dyspnea); a rapid, pounding heartbeat (palpitations); dizziness; and fatigue. In mild, chronic conditions, these symptoms might be present only when the demand for oxygen is increased (e.g., during physical exertion), but in severe conditions they may be experienced at rest.

Manifestations of anemia may be observed in other parts of the body. The skin, mucous membranes, lips, nail beds, and conjunctivae become pale as a result of reduced hemoglobin concentration. If anemia is caused by RBC destruction (hemolysis), the skin may become yellowish because of accumulation of the products of hemolysis. Tissue hypoxia of the skin results in impaired healing and loss of elasticity, as well as thinning and early graying of the hair. Nervous system manifestations can occur if the anemia is caused by a vitamin B_{12} deficiency. Myelin degeneration may occur, causing a loss of nerve fibers in the spinal cord and producing paresthesias (numbness), gait disturbances, extreme weakness, spasticity, and reflex abnormalities. Decreased oxygen supply to the gastrointestinal (GI) tract often produces abdominal pain, nausea, vomiting, and anorexia. A low-grade fever of less than 38.5°C (less than about 101°F) occurs in some anemic individuals and may result from the release of leukocyte pyrogens from ischemic tissues.

When the anemia is severe or acute in onset (e.g., hemorrhage), the initial compensatory mechanism is peripheral blood vessel constriction, diverting blood flow to vital organs. Decreased blood flow detected by the kidneys activates the renal renin-angiotensin response, causing salt and water retention in an attempt to increase blood volume. These situations are emergencies and require immediate intervention to correct the underlying problem that caused the acute loss of blood; therefore long-term compensatory mechanisms do not develop.

Therapeutic interventions for slowly developing anemic conditions require treatment of the underlying disorder and palliation of associated symptoms. Therapies include provision of transfusions, correction of dietary imbalances, and administration of supplemental vitamins or iron. Effective management of an individual's blood is described in *What's New?* Patient-Centered Blood Management.

Anemias of Blood Loss
Acute Blood Loss

Posthemorrhagic anemia is a normocytic-normochromic anemia (NNA) caused by acute blood loss. Acute blood loss is mainly a loss of intravascular volume and the effects depend on the rate of hemorrhage that can lead to cardiovascular collapse, shock, and death. A major

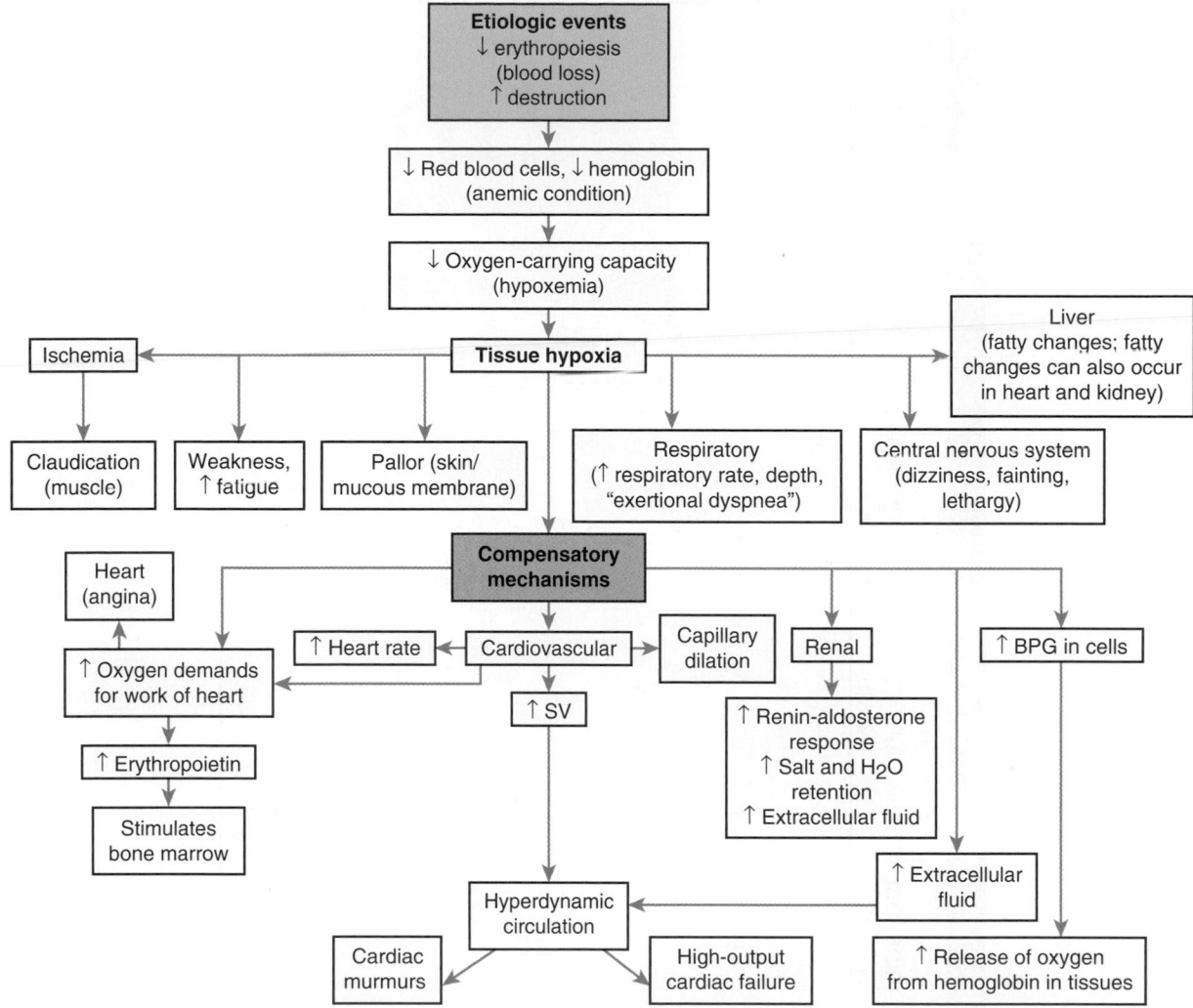

FIGURE 29.2 Progression and Manifestations of Anemia. *BPG,* Bisphosphoglycerate; *SV,* stroke volume.

cause of acute blood loss is **trauma**. Severe trauma is a rising global problem.[1] Traumatic injury results in an annual worldwide death of more than 5.8 million people, or 1 in 10 mortalities.[1,2] Uncontrolled posttraumatic bleeding is the leading cause of potentially preventable death among injured individuals.[1] The pathophysiologic mechanisms associated with traumatic injury is an evolving field of study (see *What's New?* Traumatic Injury, Bleeding, and Coagulopathy). Table 29.3 presents classification of estimated blood loss for a 70-kg man based on initial presentation, as developed by the American College of Surgeons Advanced Trauma Life Support (ATLS).[1] The overall reliability and validity of the ATLS classification are still undergoing study.

Volume loss reduces mean systemic filling pressure, resulting in decreased venous return. The initial manifestations (increased sympathetic nerve activation and a reduction in blood pressure, cardiac output, and central venous pressure) are caused by cardiovascular adaptations to blood volume depletion. Indexes to predict the risk of hemorrhagic shock are proposed as useful to provide prompt and appropriate treatment.[1]

If the acute blood loss is not severe (does not cause the preceding manifestations), complete recovery is possible. Within 24 hours of blood loss, lost plasma is replaced by mobilizing water and electrolytes from tissues and interstitial spaces into the vascular system. The hemodilution that results lowers the hematocrit value; concurrently, there is often a rapid elevation of circulating neutrophils and platelets. Neutrophils can rise to levels between 10,000 and 30,000/μL within a few hours as

a result of a shift of marginated leukocytes into the circulation and a release of leukocytes from the bone marrow. The platelet count can rise to levels of about 1 million/μL. In severe blood loss, more immature cells—metamyelocytes, myelocytes, and nucleated red blood cells—may enter the circulation. Reduction in tissue oxygenation stimulates production of erythropoietin and increasing production of erythrocytes (reticulocytes) in the bone marrow. Iron recovery from destroyed erythrocytes may occur if the acute blood loss is internal; however, if blood is lost externally, iron stores may be depleted and erythropoiesis may be impeded. Hemorrhage that is chronic (occult [i.e., bleeding ulcer or neoplasm]) produces adaptations that are less prominent, but the individual may experience an iron deficiency anemia (IDA) when iron reserves become depleted. Initial treatment for acute blood loss is restoration of blood volume by intravenous administration of saline, dextran, albumin, or plasma. Large volume losses may require transfusion of fresh whole blood.

Successful therapy is first indicated by a return of erythrocytes to their normal size and shape. As the bone marrow begins to produce more erythrocytes, an increase in the number of reticulocytes (10% to 15% after 7 days) is seen. Changes in the appearance of erythrocytes (polychromatophilia and macrocytosis) associated with reticulocytosis may give the impression that an underlying hemolytic process is occurring. A normal erythrocyte count is usually noted in 4 to 6 weeks, but hemoglobin restoration may take 6 to 8 weeks.

TABLE 29.2 LABORATORY FINDINGS FOR VARIOUS ANEMIAS

TEST	PERNICIOUS ANEMIA	FOLATE DEFICIENCY ANEMIA	IRON DEFICIENCY ANEMIA	SIDEROBLASTIC ANEMIA	APLASTIC ANEMIA	POSTHEMORRHAGIC ANEMIA	HEMOLYTIC ANEMIA	ANEMIA OF CHRONIC DISEASE
Hemoglobin	Low	Low	Low	Low	Low or normal	Normal or low	Low	Low
Hematocrit	Low	Low	Low	Low	Low or normal	Normal or low	Low	Low
Reticulocyte count	Low	Low	Normal or slightly high or low	Normal or slightly high	Low	Increased	High	Normal
Mean corpuscular volume	High	High	Low	Low	Normal or slightly high	Slightly low	Normal or high	Normal or low
Plasma iron	High	High	Low	High	High	Normal	Normal or high	Low
Total iron-binding capacity	Normal	Normal	High	Normal	Normal	Normal	Normal	Low
Ferritin	High	High	Low	High	Normal	Normal	Normal	Normal
Serum B$_{12}$	Low	Normal	Normal	Normal	Normal	Normal	Normal	Normal
Folate	Normal	Low	Normal	Normal	Normal	Normal	Normal	Normal
Bilirubin	Slightly high	Slightly high	Normal	High	Normal	Normal	Slightly high	Normal
Free erythrocyte protoporphyrin	Normal	Normal	High	Increased or normal	High	Normal	Normal	Normal or slightly high
Transferrin	Slightly high	Slightly high	Low	High	Normal	Normal	Normal	Slightly low

TABLE 29.3 CLASSIFICATION OF ESTIMATED BLOOD LOSS*

	CLASS I	CLASS II	CLASS III	CLASS IV
Blood loss (mL)	Up to 750	750–1500	1500–2000	>2000
Blood loss (% blood volume)	Up to 15	15–30	30–40	>40
Pulse rate (beats/min)	<100	100–120	120–140	>140
Systolic blood pressure	Normal	Normal	Decreased	Decreased
Pulse pressure	Normal or increased	Decreased	Decreased	Decreased
Respiratory rate (breaths/min)	14–20	20–30	30–40	>35
Urine output (mL/hr)	>30	20–30	5–15	Negligible
Central nervous system/mental state	Slightly anxious	Mildly anxious	Anxious, confused	Confused, lethargic
Initial fluid replacement	Crystalloid	Crystalloid	Crystalloid and blood	Crystalloid and blood

*For a 70 kg man.
Data from Rossaint R et al: *Crit Care* 20:100, 2016.

WHAT'S NEW?

Traumatic Injury, Bleeding, and Coagulopathy

Emerging is the understanding that about one-third of all persons with bleeding trauma are already showing signs of coagulopathy upon hospital admission. The presence of coagulopathy is related to an increased risk of multiple organ failure and death (see Chapter 49). Acute coagulopathy associated with traumatic injury is now recognized as a multifactorial condition caused by bleeding-induced shock, tissue-related thrombin-thrombomodulin complex generation, and activation of anticoagulant and fibrinolytic pathways (see Figure). The severity of the coagulopathy disorder is impacted by preexisting and treatment factors that contribute to acidosis, hypothermia, hemodilution, hypoperfusion, and coagulation factor consumption. Coagulopathy is modified by brain injury, age, genetic background, comorbidities, inflammation, medications (especially oral anticoagulants), and prehospital fluid administration. New terms for trauma-associated coagulopathic physiology include acute traumatic coagulopathy, early coagulation of trauma, acute coagulopathy of trauma-shock, trauma-induced coagulopathy, and trauma-associated coagulopathy. New guidelines recommend that individuals be transferred directly to trauma centers to improve outcomes.

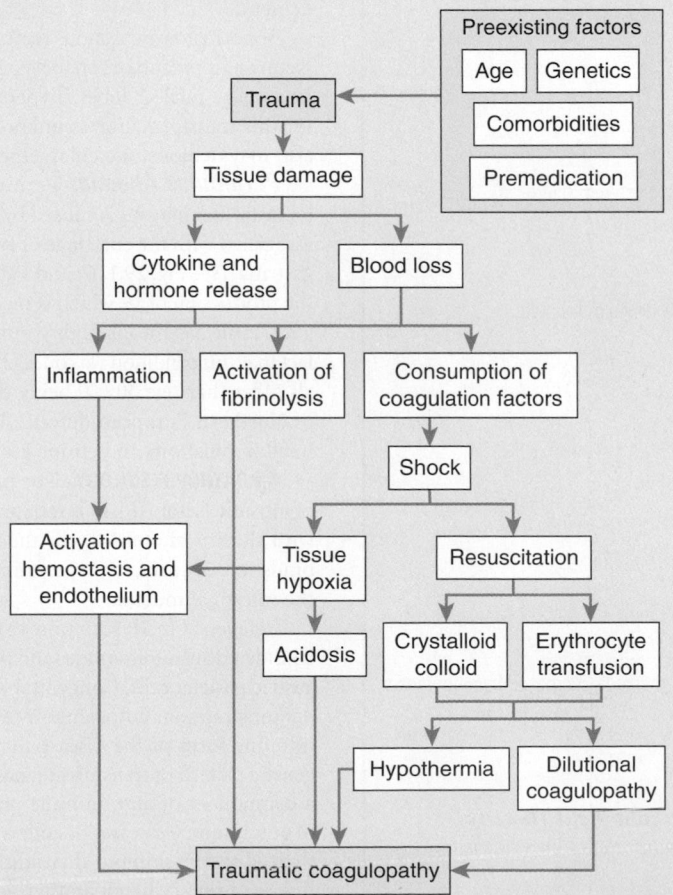

FIGURE Traumatic Coagulopathy. Preexisting and trauma-related factors contribute to coagulopathy. (Box data from Firth D et al: *J Thromb Haemost* 8(9):1919–1925, 2010; MacLeod JB et al: *J Trauma* 55(1):39–44, 2003; Maegele M et al: *Injury* 38(3):298–304, 2007; Rossaint R et al: *Crit Care* 20:100, 2016. Figure adapted from Rossaint R et al: *Crit Care* 20:100, 2016.)

Chronic Blood Loss

Anemia from chronic blood loss only occurs if the loss is greater than the replacement capacity of the bone marrow. If iron stores are depleted, iron deficiency anemia can occur.

Anemias of Diminished Erythropoiesis

The anemias of diminished red cell production are heterogeneous and can be classified according to the underlying mechanism (see Table 29.1). The most common anemias of diminished red cell production are the result of ineffective erythrocyte DNA synthesis, commonly caused by nutritional deficiencies of vitamin B_{12} (cobalamin) or folate (folic acid), coenzymes that are required for nuclear maturation and DNA synthesis.[3] These anemias, also called macrocytic (megaloblastic) anemias, are characterized by abnormally large erythroid precursors (megaloblasts) in the marrow that mature into large erythrocytes (macrocytes). Box 29.1 lists the various causes of megaloblastic anemia. Other anemias from underproduction of red cells are secondary to renal failure and chronic inflammation.

BOX 29.1	CAUSES OF MEGALOBLASTIC ANEMIA

Vitamin B_{12} Deficiency
Decreased Intake
   Inadequate diet, vegetarianism

Impaired Absorption
Intrinsic factor deficiency
   Pernicious anemia
   Gastrectomy
Malabsorption states
Diffuse intestinal disease (e.g., lymphoma, systemic sclerosis)
Ileal resection, ileitis
   Competitive parasitic uptake
   Fish tapeworm infestations
Bacterial overgrowth in blind loops and diverticula of bowel

Folic Acid Deficiency
Decreased Intake
Inadequate diet, alcoholism, infancy
Impaired absorption
Malabsorption states
Intrinsic intestinal disease
Anticonvulsants, oral contraceptives
Increased loss
Hemodialysis

Increased Requirement
Pregnancy, infancy, disseminated cancer, markedly increased hematopoiesis

Impaired Utilization
Folic acid antagonists

Unresponsive to Vitamin B_{12} or Folic Acid Therapy
Metabolic inhibitors of DNA synthesis and/or folate metabolism (e.g., methotrexate)

From Kumar V, Abbas A, Aster JC: *Robbins & Cotran pathologic basis of disease,* ed 9, Philadelphia, 2015, Saunders.

Megaloblastic Anemias

With megaloblastic anemias the cells are challenged to make DNA; however, RNA production proceeds normally. The cells have slow-maturing nuclei but have normal maturing cytoplasm. Therefore megaloblastic erythroid precursors grow large before the larger nuclei become mature enough to signal division (causing the cell to be larger than normal). Examination shows the nucleus to be more immature than the cytoplasm, hence the term *"nuclear-cytoplasmic asynchrony."* The overall nuclear-cytoplasmic asynchrony from the ineffective DNA synthesis produces megaloblastic changes in the bone marrow with resulting anemia. These defective erythrocytes die prematurely, called eryptosis, which decreases their numbers in the circulation and causes anemia. Damaged erythrocytes undergo cell shrinkage, membrane changes (blebbing), and rearrangement of plasma membrane phospholipid distribution with efflux of phosphatidylserine (PS). Macrophages have receptors that recognize surface PS and remove the damaged erythrocytes from the circulation.

Dietary cause of vitamin B_{12} deficiency is decreased intake. Vitamin B_{12}, known as *cobalamin,* is dependent on dietary vitamin B_{12} intake. Plants and vegetables contain little cobalamin and strictly vegetarian and macrobiotic diets do not provide adequate amounts.[4] Another important cause that results in megaloblastic anemia is pernicious anemia, caused by autoimmune destruction of parietal cells that make intrinsic factor.[3] Intrinsic factor (IF) is a protein transporter necessary for absorption of vitamin B_{12} in the intestine. The prevalence of folate deficiency has decreased because of food fortification with folate; however, it does occur among the poor, elderly, and alcoholics, especially in countries without folate fortification. Vitamin B_{12} deficiency also can result from malabsorption or increased cell turnover and increased demand.[3]

Abnormal asynchronous maturation may affect the neutrophil series. Neutrophil precursors create giant metamyelocytes with a tendency to have more nuclear lobes (hypersegmented) than normal. The reason for this transformation is unknown. Other cells throughout the body also may demonstrate enlargement and nuclear abnormalities.

Pernicious Anemia. Pernicious anemia (PA) is a type of megaloblastic anemia and is caused by vitamin B_{12} deficiency, which is often associated with the end stage of type A chronic atrophic (autoimmune) gastritis[5] (see Fig. 29.1, *C*; and Fig. 29.3). Autoimmune gastritis impairs the production of IF, which is required for vitamin B_{12} uptake from the gut. *Pernicious* means highly injurious or destructive and reflects the fact that this condition was once fatal. It most commonly affects individuals older than age 30 (60 being the median age of diagnosis) who are of Northern European descent; however, it has now been recognized in all populations and ethnic groups.

◆PATHOPHYSIOLOGY. The principal disorder in PA is an absence of intrinsic factor (IF). IF is secreted by gastric parietal cells and complexes with dietary vitamin B_{12} in the small intestine. The B_{12}-IF complex binds to cell surface receptors in the ileum and is transported across the intestinal mucosa.

Deficiency in IF secretion may be congenital; however, it is often considered an autoimmune (and possibly innate) process directed against gastric parietal cells. Congenital IF deficiency is a genetic disorder that demonstrates an autosomal recessive inheritance pattern.[6] The autoimmune form of the disease may have a genetic component, but no genetic pattern of transmission has been identified.[4] PA is also frequently a component of autoimmune polyendocrinopathy, which is a cluster of autoimmune diseases of endocrine organs (e.g., chronic autoimmune thyroiditis [Hashimoto thyroiditis], type 1 diabetes mellitus, Addison disease, primary hypoparathyroidism, Graves disease, and myasthenia gravis) that frequently present as comorbidities. Autoimmune thyroiditis and type 1 diabetes mellitus, in particular, are associated with PA. Other

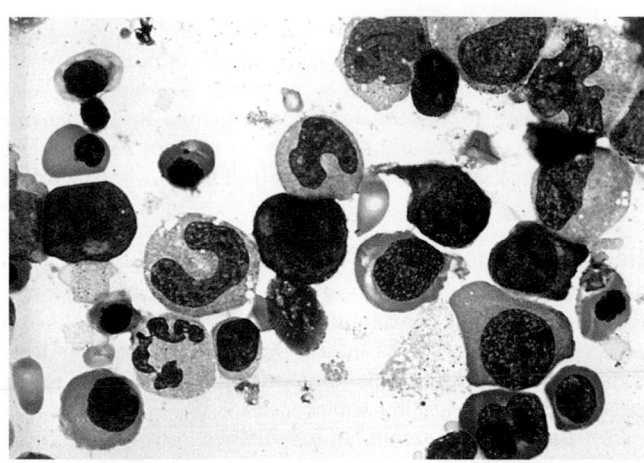

FIGURE 29.3 Bone Marrow Aspirate from Individual with Pernicious Anemia. Bone marrow aspirate smear from an individual with megaloblastic red blood cell precursors and giant metamyelocytes. The chromatin in the red blood cell nuclei is more dispersed than that in normal red blood cell precursors at comparable stages of maturation; the giant metamyelocytes have dispersed nuclear chromatin in contrast to a normal metamyelocyte, which has condensed chromatin (Wright-Giemsa stain). (From Damjanov I, Linder J, editors: *Anderson's pathology,* ed 10, St Louis, 1996, Mosby.)

causes include surgical removal of the stomach, resection of the ileum, and infestation with tapeworms; in addition, various conditions related to increased demand for vitamin B_{12}, such as pregnancy, hyperthyroidism, chronic infection, and disseminated cancer, are associated with PA (see Box 29.1). Environmental conditions also may contribute to chronic gastritis. These include excessive alcohol or hot tea ingestion and smoking. Drugs known as *proton pump inhibitors (PPIs)* are used to decrease gastric acidity, but also may decrease cobalamin absorption, although it is not believed that they actually cause PA. Although PA is a benign disorder, individuals with type A chronic gastritis also are at risk for developing gastric adenocarcinoma and gastric carcinoid type I. The incidence of carcinoma in these individuals is 2% to 3%.

The presence of PA with autoimmune gastritis (type A chronic gastritis) leads to gastric atrophy from destruction of parietal and zymogenic cells. Individuals with PA commonly have autoantibodies against the gastric H^+-K^+ ATPase, which is the major protein constituent of parietal cell membranes. Early in the disease process the gastric submucosa becomes infiltrated with inflammatory cells, including autoreactive T cells. It appears that the T-cell response initiates gastric mucosal injury and triggers the formation of autoantibodies.[4] The susceptibility to develop PA (as well as other autoimmune disorders) is linked to genetic variants involving the inflammasome, which suggests a relationship to innate immunity.[4] Eventually, the parietal and zymogenic cells are destroyed and replaced by mucous-containing cells (intestinal metaplasia). Gastric mucosal atrophy, in which gastric parietal cells are destroyed, results in a deficiency of all secretions of the stomach—hydrochloric acid, pepsin, and IF.

Initiation of the autoimmune process may be secondary to a past infection with *Helicobacter pylori*.[7-9] Although active infection with *H. pylori* is rare in individuals with PA, more than half of these individuals possess circulating antibodies against this microorganism, suggesting a history of infection. The current opinion is that in genetically prone individuals, antigens expressed by *H. pylori* mimic the parietal cell H^+-K^+ ATPase, resulting in production of an antibody that binds and damages

the parietal cell (see Chapter 9 for a discussion of antigenic mimicry and autoimmune disease).

◆**CLINICAL MANIFESTATIONS.** PA develops slowly (possibly over 20 to 30 years); 60 years of age is the median age at time of diagnosis. Because of the slow onset of symptoms, PA is usually severe by the time the individual seeks treatment. Early symptoms are often ignored because they are nonspecific and vague and include infections, mood swings, and gastrointestinal, cardiac, or kidney ailments. When the hemoglobin level has decreased significantly (7 to 8 g/dL), the individual experiences the classic symptoms of anemia—weakness, fatigue, paresthesias of the feet and fingers, difficulty walking, loss of appetite, abdominal pains, weight loss, and a sore tongue that is smooth and beefy red secondary to atrophic glossitis. The skin may become "lemon yellow" (sallow) as a result of a combination of pallor and icterus. Hepatomegaly, indicating right-sided heart failure, may be present in the elderly along with splenomegaly, which is nonpalpable.

Neurologic manifestations result from nerve demyelination that may produce neuronal death. The posterior and lateral columns of the spinal cord also may be affected, causing a loss of position and vibration sense, ataxia, and spasticity. The cerebrum also may be involved with manifestations of affective disorders, most commonly of the depressive types. Low levels of vitamin B_{12} have been associated with neurocognitive disorders. Overall, the consequences of vitamin B_{12} deficiency can include encephalopathy, myelopathy, and peripheral and optic neuropathy. An increased prevalence of serum vitamin B_{12} deficiency has been reported among individuals with Alzheimer disease. Individuals with atrophy and metaplasia of the gastric mucosa associated with PA have an increased risk of gastric carcinoma.[4]

◆**EVALUATION AND TREATMENT.** Diagnosis of PA is based on clinical manifestations and a variety of test results (see Table 29.2), including blood tests, bone marrow aspiration, serologic studies, and gastric biopsy. The following tests are used to diagnose PA: (1) moderate to severe megaloblastic anemia, (2) leukopenia with hypersegmented granulocytes, (3) low levels of serum vitamin B_{12}, (4) elevated serum levels of homocysteine and methylmalonic acid, and (5) an outpouring of reticulocytes and an increase in hematocrit level after about 5 days of parenteral administration of vitamin B_{12}.[4] The presence of circulating antibodies against parietal cells and intrinsic factor is also useful in diagnosis.[10] Gastric biopsy reveals total achlorhydria (absence of hydrochloric acid), which is diagnostic for PA because it occurs only in the presence of this gastric lesion.

Replacement of vitamin B_{12} (cobalamin) is the treatment of choice. Initial injections of vitamin B_{12} are administered weekly until the deficiency is corrected, followed by monthly injections for the remainder of the individual's life. The effectiveness of cobalamin replacement therapy is determined by a rising reticulocyte count. Conventional wisdom and practice assumed that oral preparations were ineffective because there was no IF to facilitate absorption of vitamin B_{12}. However, recent experience has shown that higher doses of orally administered vitamin B_{12} are absorbed across the small bowel and are beneficial.

Untreated PA is fatal, usually because of heart failure. Death occurs after a course of remissions and exacerbations lasting from 1 to 3 years. Since 1926, when replacement therapy began, mortality has been reduced significantly. Today, death from PA is rare, and any relapses that occur are usually the result of noncompliance with therapy.

Folate Deficiency Anemia. A deficiency of folic acid results in a megaloblastic anemia having the same pathologic consequences as those caused by vitamin B_{12} deficiency.[4] Folate (folic acid) is an essential vitamin for RNA and DNA synthesis within the maturing erythrocyte. Folates are coenzymes required for the synthesis of thymine and purines (adenine and guanine) and the conversion of homocysteine to methionine. Deficient production of thymine, in particular, affects cells undergoing rapid division (e.g., bone marrow cells undergoing erythropoiesis). Humans are totally dependent on folate dietary intake to meet the daily requirement of 50 to 200 mcg/day. Increased amounts are required for pregnant and lactating females. Absorption of folate occurs primarily in the upper small intestine and does not depend on the presence of any other facilitating factor, such as IF. After absorption, folate circulates through the liver, where it is stored. Folate deficiency is more common than B_{12} deficiency, particularly in alcoholics and individuals with chronic malnourishment. Alcohol interferes with folate metabolism in the liver, causing a profound depletion of folate stores. Fad diets and diets low in vegetables also may cause folate deficiency because of the absence of plant sources of folate. It is estimated that at least 10% of North Americans have a folate deficiency, although the incidence has been on the decrease in the United States since the fortification of foods with folate and the increased use of folate supplements. Box 29.1 lists the various causes of folic acid deficiency including (1) decreased intake, (2) increased requirement, and (3) impaired utilization.

◆**PATHOPHYSIOLOGY.** Impaired DNA synthesis secondary to folate deficiency results in megaloblastic cells with clumped nuclear chromatin. Anemia may result from apoptosis of erythroblasts in the late stages of erythropoiesis. In addition to anemia, folate deficiency in pregnant women is associated with neural tube defects of the fetus. Folate is necessary for the reduction of circulating levels of homocysteine, a risk factor for the development of atherosclerosis (see Chapter 33); thus a folate deficiency increases the risk for developing coronary artery disease. A deficiency of folate also is implicated in the development of cancers, specifically colorectal cancers.

◆**CLINICAL MANIFESTATIONS.** Clinical manifestations are similar to the cachectic, malnourished appearance of individuals with PA. Specific symptoms include severe cheilosis (scales and fissures of the lips and corners of the mouth), stomatitis (inflammation of the mouth), and painful ulcerations of the buccal mucosa and tongue, characteristic of burning mouth syndrome. Burning mouth syndrome may be secondary to a large number of disorders (e.g., extremely dry mouth, infection, autoimmune disease, nutritional deficiencies, and other conditions). The mechanisms underlying folate deficiency as a cause remain unknown. Gastrointestinal (GI) symptoms may be present and include dysphagia (difficulty swallowing), flatulence, and watery diarrhea, as well as histologic and roentgenographic changes of the GI tract suggestive of sprue (a chronic malabsorption syndrome). Undiagnosed inflammatory bowel disease (e.g., Crohn disease, ulcerative colitis) may be the underlying cause of folate malabsorption in some individuals, and folate deficiency may suppress proliferation of the intestinal mucosa, leading to exacerbation of gastrointestinal damage. Neurologic manifestations, such as those that occur in PA, are generally not seen in folate deficiency anemia. Any neurologic symptoms are usually caused by a thiamine deficiency, which often accompanies folate deficiency.

◆**EVALUATION AND TREATMENT.** Evaluation of folate deficiency is based on measurement of serum folate levels and documentation of symptoms. Treatment requires daily oral administration of folate preparations until adequate blood levels are obtained and clinical symptoms are reduced or eliminated; 1 mg daily is sufficient for most individuals, although persons with alcoholism may require 5 mg/day. Prophylactic dosages of 0.1 to 0.4 mg/day are sometimes given during pregnancy. Parenteral administration of folic acid (citrovorum factor or leucovorin) generally is not used except in situations in which an individual has been using drugs that inhibit dihydrofolate reductase. After administration of folate, the manifestations of anemia disappear within 1 to 2 weeks.

After the folate deficiency has been corrected, long-term treatment with folate is not necessary if the appropriate dietary adjustments are made to maintain adequate intake. An intake of folate (400 mcg/day) is recommended as a measure to reduce the risk of heart disease and stroke. The symptoms of vitamin B_{12} deficiency also respond to folate therapy; however, it is essential to exclude vitamin B_{12} deficiency as the cause of anemia because folate does not prevent the neurologic deficits (and may even exacerbate symptoms) found with vitamin B_{12} deficiency.[4]

Microcytic-Hypochromic Anemias

The microcytic-hypochromic anemias are characterized by abnormally small erythrocytes that contain unusually reduced amounts of hemoglobin (see Fig. 29.1, *B*). The most common nutritional disorder of microcytic-hypochromic anemia—iron deficiency anemia—is discussed here; others are discussed in Chapter 31.

Iron Deficiency Anemia. Iron deficiency anemia (IDA) is the most common type of nutritional disorder worldwide, occurring in both developing and developed countries and affecting as many as one-fifth of the world population. The prevalence of IDA is higher in developing countries, but IDA is common in the United States, particularly in toddlers, adolescent girls, and women of childbearing age.[4] Populations also at increased risk for IDA include individuals living in poverty; infants consuming cow's milk, which has poor bioavailability of iron; older individuals ingesting restricted diets; and teenagers eating poor (junk-food) diets. The daily requirement of iron is 7 to 10 mg for adult men and 7 to 20 mg for adult women. The bioavailability of iron is especially important because only about 10% to 15% of ingested iron is absorbed.[4] Men typically ingest more iron than women, and premenopausal women, particularly during pregnancy, have an increased requirement. Increased requirement is an important cause of iron deficiency in growing infants, children, and adolescents. The causes of IDA include (1) dietary deficiency, (2) impaired absorption, (3) increased requirement, and (4) chronic blood loss. Impaired absorption can occur in sprue, disorders involving alterations of fat absorption, and chronic diarrhea.[4] Other causes for both genders include use of medications that cause GI bleeding (such as aspirin or nonsteroidal antiinflammatory drugs [NSAIDs]); surgical procedures that decrease stomach acidity, intestinal transit time, and absorption (e.g., gastric bypass); and eating disorders, such as pica, which is the craving and eating of nonnutritional substances, such as dirt, chalk, and paper. The clinical manifestations are mostly related to the reduction in adequate levels of hemoglobin.

Females have a higher incidence of hypoferremia (13.9%) than do males (8.3%), as well as IDA (4% to 6% in females and 4% in males). The incidence peaks in females during their reproductive years and decreases after menopause. Those at highest risk are black females living in urban poverty.[11] Males have a higher incidence during childhood and adolescence, with a decrease occurring during young adulthood and an increase during late adulthood. An increased prevalence of iron deficiency has been observed in overweight children, adolescents, women, and those undergoing bariatric surgery.[12]

In developed countries, pregnancy and a continuous loss of blood are the most common causes of IDA. A blood loss of 2 to 4 mL/day (1 to 2 mg of iron) is enough to cause IDA. Menorrhagia (excessive menstrual bleeding) causes primary IDA in females. Males may experience bleeding as a result of ulcers, hiatal hernia, esophageal varices, cirrhosis, hemorrhoids, ulcerative colitis, or cancer. An occult bleeding source, such as gastrointestinal cancer or other lesion, can lead to IDA; the astute clinician who understands the cause of IDA may be a cancerous lesion can save a life.

Children in developing countries often are affected by chronic parasite infestations that result in intestinal blood and iron loss that outpaces dietary intake.[13] Treatment of helminth infections results in an improvement in the anemia as well as in appetite and growth. *H. pylori* infections also have been found to cause IDA of unknown origin, although *H. pylori* impairs iron uptake. Iron deficiency anemia is associated with an increased absorption of other elements such as lead (Pb) and cadmium (Cd).[14] Heavy exposure to Pb and Cd causes hypochromic-microcytic anemia.[15] Treatment of the iron deficiency is associated with a decrease in lead levels. Deficiencies in vitamins C, B_1, and B_6 may enhance sensitivity toward Cd and Pb toxicity.[16]

◆**PATHOPHYSIOLOGY.** IDA is a hypochromic-microcytic anemia. Anemia occurs when iron stores are depleted. With inadequate dietary intake or excessive blood loss, there is no intrinsic dysfunction in iron metabolism; however, both conditions deplete iron stores and reduce hemoglobin synthesis. With metabolic or functional iron deficiency, various metabolic disorders lead to either insufficient iron delivery to bone marrow or impaired iron use within the marrow. Paradoxically, iron stores may be sufficient but delivery is inadequate to maintain heme synthesis, thus producing a functional or relative iron deficiency.

Iron in the form of hemoglobin is in constant demand by the body. Iron is recyclable; therefore the body maintains a balance between iron that is contained in hemoglobin and iron that is in storage and available for future hemoglobin synthesis (see Chapter 28). Blood loss disrupts this balance by creating a need for more iron, thus depleting the iron stores more rapidly to replace the iron lost from bleeding.

Iron also contributes to immune function by regulating immune effector mechanisms (i.e., cytokine activities [interferon-gamma (IFN-γ)], nitric oxide formation, and T-cell proliferation). Acquired hypoferremia may be part of the body's response to infection. Anemia can be part of the nonspecific acute phase response to any type of inflammation of sufficient degree. Many pathogens require iron for survival; thus hypoferremia would hamper their growth. However, the precise benefits or detriments of iron deficiency and immunity are still controversial.

IDA occurs when the demand for iron exceeds the supply and develops slowly through three overlapping stages. In stage I, the body's iron stores are depleted. Erythropoiesis proceeds normally, with the hemoglobin content of erythrocytes remaining normal. In stage II, iron transportation to bone marrow is diminished, resulting in iron-deficient erythropoiesis. Stage III begins when the small hemoglobin-deficient cells enter the circulation to replace the normal aged erythrocytes that have been removed from the circulation. The manifestations of IDA appear in stage III when there is depletion of iron stores and diminished hemoglobin production.

◆**CLINICAL MANIFESTATIONS.** Symptoms of IDA begin gradually, and individuals usually do not seek medical attention until hemoglobin levels have decreased to about 7 to 8 g/dL. Early symptoms are nonspecific and include fatigue, weakness, shortness of breath, and pale earlobes, palms, and conjunctivae (Fig. 29.4, *A*).

As the condition progresses and becomes more severe, structural and functional changes occur in epithelial tissue (see Fig. 29.4). The fingernails become brittle, thin, coarsely ridged, and "spoon-shaped" or concave (koilonychia) as a result of impaired capillary circulation (Fig. 29.4, *B*). IDA also is associated with unexplained burning mouth syndrome, as was discussed for folate deficiency. Tongue papillae atrophy and cause soreness along with redness and burning (glossitis) (Fig. 29.4, *C*). The degree of pain experienced is directly associated with the amount of iron deficiency, and these changes can be reversed within 1 to 2 weeks of iron replacement therapy. Individuals also experience dryness and soreness in the epithelium at the corners of the mouth, known as *angular stomatitis*. Difficulty in swallowing is associated with an esophageal "web," a thin, concentric, smooth extension of normal esophageal tissue consisting of mucosa and submucosa at the juncture between the hypopharynx and esophagus. The duration of iron deficiency required for web formation is uncertain. Dysphagia also is exacerbated by hyposalivation. The pathophysiology associated with these epithelial

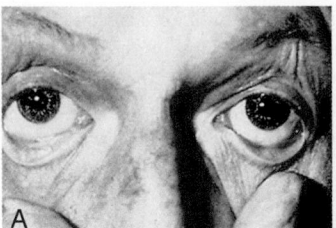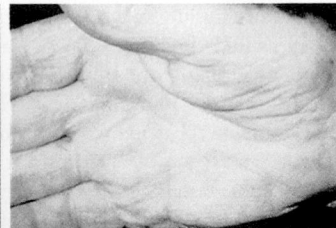
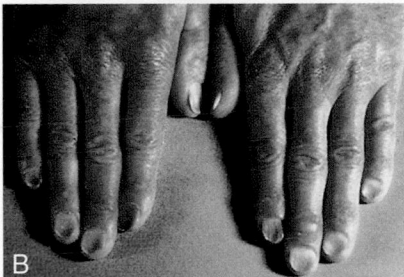
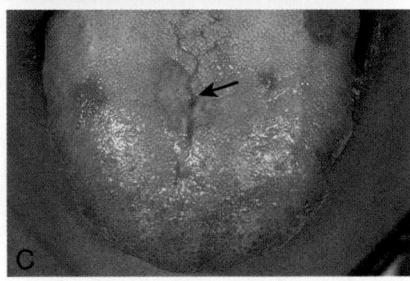

FIGURE 29.4 Manifestations of Iron Deficiency Anemia. **A,** Pallor and iron deficiency. Pallor of the skin, mucous membranes, and palmar creases in an individual with a hemoglobin level of 9 g/dL. Palmar creases become as pale as the surrounding skin when the hemoglobin level approaches 7 g/dL. **B,** Koilonychia. The nails are concave, ridged, and brittle. **C,** Glossitis. Tongue of individual with iron deficiency anemia has bald, fissured appearance caused by loss of papillae and flattening. (From Hoffbrand AV, Pettit JE, Vyas P: *Color atlas of clinical hematology,* ed 4, London, 2009, Mosby; **B** courtesy Dr. S.M. Knowles.)

lesions is not well understood, but the lesions have the potential to become cancerous.

Nonheme iron is a component of many enzymes in the body (e.g., cytochromes, myoglobin, catalases, peroxidases), particularly those involved in the metabolism of amine neurotransmitters, the reduction of nucleotides, and the biosynthesis of methionine. Abnormalities and deficiencies of iron-dependent enzymes may account for many of the clinical manifestations of IDA. Individuals with IDA also exhibit gastritis, neuromuscular changes, irritability, headache, numbness, tingling, and vasomotor disturbances. Gait disturbances are rare. The pathogenesis of neurologic symptoms is unknown but may be caused by hypoxia in already compromised cerebral vessels. In the elderly, mental confusion, memory loss, and disorientation are often associated with anemia and may be wrongly perceived as "normal" events related to aging.

Iron deficiency in children is associated with numerous adverse health-related manifestations, especially cognitive impairment, which may be long-lasting and even irreversible (see Chapter 31). Teens with a history of iron deficiency as infants are likely to score lower on cognitive and motor tests, even if the iron deficiency was identified and treated in infancy.

◆**EVALUATION AND TREATMENT.** Initial evaluation is based on clinical symptoms and decreased levels of hemoglobin and hematocrit. Anemia appears only when iron stores are depleted and is accompanied by lower than normal serum iron, ferritin, and transferrin saturation levels.[4]

Laboratory findings for IDA are included in Table 29.2. Iron stores may be measured directly by bone marrow biopsy and iron staining or indirectly by laboratory tests for serum ferritin level, transferrin saturation, or total iron-binding capacity. Serum ferritin is a widely accepted and available measurement of iron status that has been used for the past 25 years; 1 mcg/L serum ferritin corresponds to 8 to 10 mg or 120 mcg of storage iron per kilogram body weight. A limitation on interpretation of serum ferritin levels is that values may be elevated independently of iron status during acute or chronic inflammation, malignancy, liver disease, or alcoholism. A sensitive indicator of heme synthesis is the amount of free erythrocyte protoporphyrin (FEP) within erythrocytes. A test that determines the concentration of soluble fragment transferrin receptor differentiates primary IDA from IDA that is associated with chronic disease.

An indicator of iron levels is the level of serum transferrin receptor (sTfR). Transferrin receptors are membrane glycoproteins that bind circulating transferrin for transport into cells. Soluble forms of the receptor are found in serum. The ratio of serum levels of transferrin receptor to ferritin (R/F) estimates body iron stores and differentiates primary IDA from anemia secondary to chronic disease. A major drawback, however, is the lack of proper standardization for the sTfR assay.

The first step in treatment of IDA is to identify and eliminate sources of blood loss.[17] With ongoing bleeding, any replacement therapy is likely to be ineffective. Iron replacement therapy is required and very effective. Initial doses are 150 to 200 mg/day. Hematocrit levels should improve within 1 to 2 months of therapy; however, the serum ferritin level is a more precise measurement of improvement and total body stores of iron. Once the serum ferritin level reaches 50 mcg/L, adequate replacement of iron has occurred. A rapid decrease in fatigue, lethargy, and other associated symptoms is generally seen within the first month of therapy. Replacement therapy usually continues for 6 to 12 months after the bleeding has stopped but may continue for as long as 24 months. Menstruating females may need daily oral iron replacement therapy (325 mg/day) until menopause.

Parenteral iron replacement is used in instances of uncontrolled blood loss, intolerance to oral iron, intestinal malabsorption, or poor adherence to oral therapy. Iron dextran has been the only parenteral agent available in the United States. Intramuscular injection is the recommended method; however, intravenous (IV) administration is generally preferred because of the ability to administer larger doses. A significant concern in the use of IV dextran is the potential for severe anaphylactic reaction. Delayed allergic reactions are also major concerns.

Medications that have recently been approved for parenteral therapy in treating IDA are sodium ferric gluconate complex in sucrose (Ferrlecit) and iron sucrose injection (Venofer). Iron dextran is recommended as the first choice in spite of its higher rate of adverse reactions. For individuals who are intolerant of iron dextran, the two newer agents are safe and effective alternatives. Drawbacks to their use include higher cost and the need for multiple infusions.

Anemia of Chronic Disease

Anemia of chronic disease (ACD, also called anemia of inflammation [AI]) is a mild to moderate anemia resulting from decreased erythropoiesis and impaired iron utilization in individuals with conditions of chronic systemic disease or inflammation (e.g., infections, cancer, and chronic inflammatory or autoimmune diseases). ACD is a common type of anemia in hospitalized individuals. Table 29.4 lists the possible causes of ACD. This form of anemia also is commonly noted in the presence of congestive heart failure (CHF). The anemia develops after 1 to 2 months of disease activity. The initial severity is related to that of the underlying disorder but, although persistent, it usually does

TABLE 29.4	UNDERLYING CAUSES OF ACD	
ASSOCIATED DISEASES	**ESTIMATED PREVALENCE (%)**
Infections	18–95
Acute and chronic; viral infections including HIV infection, bacterial, parasitic, fungal	
Cancer	30–77
Hematologic, solid tumor	
Autoimmune	8–71
Rheumatoid arthritis, systemic lupus erythematosus and connective tissue diseases, vasculitis, sarcoidosis, inflammatory bowel disease	
Chronic rejection after solid-organ transplantation	8–70
CKD and inflammation	25–30

ACD, Anemia of chronic disease; *CKD,* chronic kidney disease. Data from Weiss G, Goodnough LT: *N Engl J Med* 352(10):1011–1023, 2005.

not progress. Individuals may be asymptomatic or the anemia may be a coincidental clinical finding. ACD shares features observed in individuals with chronic obstructive pulmonary disease; in persons with critical illnesses after acute events such as major surgery, severe trauma, myocardial infarction, and sepsis; and in the elderly. It shares some features with anemia noted in multiple myeloma and malignant lymphoma.[18]

ACD is one of the most common conditions encountered in medicine and is probably only secondary to IDA in overall incidence. In individuals older than age 65, anemia is present in 10% of those who live in the community and in more than 50% of those who reside in nursing homes, with two-thirds of these cases being ACD or unexplained anemia. The elderly may be predisposed to ACD related to age-associated hematopoietic restriction and generally have increased concentrations of inflammatory cytokines, which play a significant role in the development of ACD. The elderly who present with characteristics of ACD without an underlying malignancy or inflammatory condition are described as having primary defective iron utilization syndrome.

◆**PATHOPHYSIOLOGY.** ACD results from a combination of (1) decreased erythrocyte life span, (2) suppressed production of erythropoietin, (3) ineffective bone marrow erythroid progenitor response to erythropoietin, and (4) altered iron metabolism and iron sequestration in macrophages.[19] During chronic inflammation a large variety of cytokines are released by lymphocytes, macrophages, and the affected tissue.[20] These include tumor necrosis factor-alpha (TNF-α), IFN-γ, interleukin-1β (IL-1β), IL-3, and IL-6[21] (also see Chapters 7 and 8).

Impaired iron metabolism is partially the result of iron sequestration.[22] IL-6 in particular affects hepatocytes and increases the release of the peptide hepcidin, which regulates the activity of ferroportin. Ferroportin is the primary transporter for the export of iron from macrophages to the plasma, and increased levels of hepcidin result in decreased ferroportin activity and suppression of iron release (Fig. 29.5).

Erythrocyte destruction is the result of eryptosis (described earlier in this chapter). Most of the diseases responsible for ACD damage erythrocytes, resulting in increased efflux of plasma membrane phosphatidylserine and susceptibility to removal by macrophages. Normal iron transport by transferrin also may be decreased as a result of competitive iron binding by inflammation-related increases in the levels of circulating lactoferrin and apoferritin. Lactoferrin is a member of

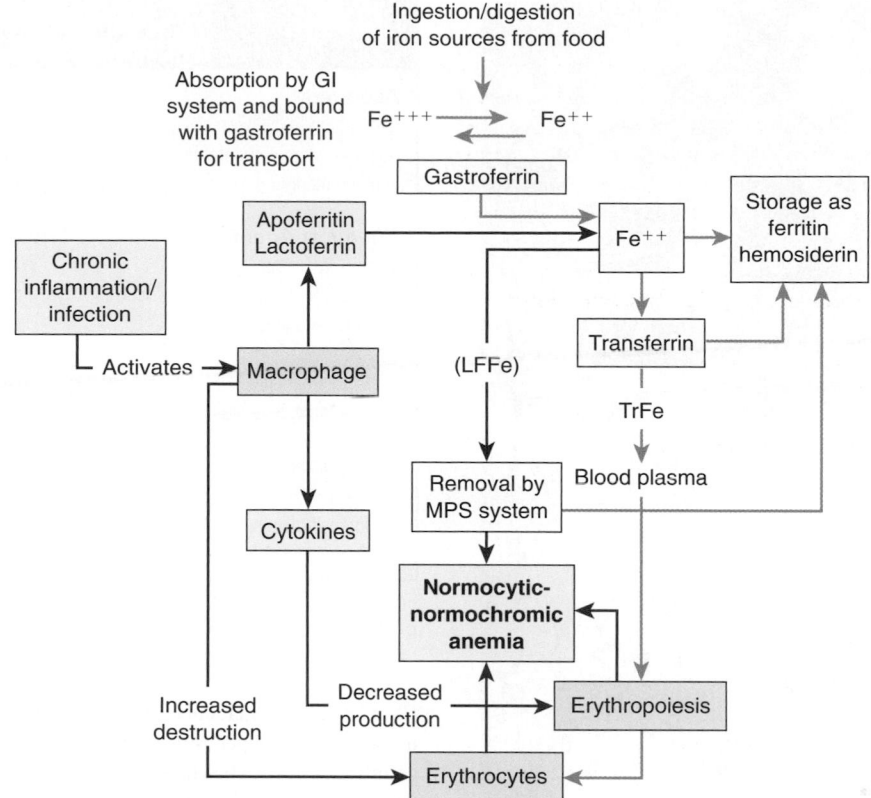

FIGURE 29.5 Pathophysiology of Anemia of Chronic Disease. Normal iron metabolism is indicated by the blue arrows. Abnormal mechanisms that are instrumental in the development of anemia of chronic inflammation are indicated by red arrows. See discussion in text. *GI,* Gastrointestinal; *LFFe,* lactoferrin bound to iron; *MPS,* mononuclear phagocyte system; *TrFe,* transferrin bound to iron.

the transferrin family of nonheme iron-binding glycoproteins, and under normal conditions is present in the blood in only small amounts. During inflammation neutrophils release lactoferrin to bind iron and reduce its availability for bacteria. However, the affinity of iron for lactoferrin is 260 times greater than that for transferrin. Lactoferrin-bound iron is removed by the mononuclear-phagocyte system and converted into ferritin, the storage form of iron. **Apoferritin** also has a higher affinity for iron and affects available iron in a similar manner.

The erythropoietic defect in ACD is failure to increase erythropoiesis in response to decreased numbers of erythrocytes. In part, decreased erythropoiesis results from diminished production of erythropoietin by the kidneys. The kidney is frequently affected by chronic inflammatory processes caused by circulating immune complexes and other factors that deposit in the kidney and activate secondary inflammatory mechanisms. In addition, the failure in erythropoiesis may reflect decreased responsiveness of erythroid progenitors to erythropoietin. Decreased availability of iron would diminish the rate of erythropoiesis. Proliferation of erythroid cells is also inhibited by proinflammatory cytokines, especially TNF-α, IFN-γ, and IL-1β. TNF-α also directly induces apoptosis of erythroid progenitors, thus diminishing the number of responsive cells. In individuals who had anemia secondary to rheumatoid arthritis, the bone marrow contained elevated levels of IL-3, which correlated with diminished expression of integrins on the surface of cells of the erythroid series.[23] Loss of integrins may prevent adequate interaction with stromal cells and matrix proteins and inhibit erythropoiesis.

Anemia associated with chronic renal failure may result from a variety of simultaneous mechanisms. Damage to the kidney affects the secretion of erythropoietin, a necessary hormone for production of erythrocytes

in the bone marrow, thus resulting in diminished bone marrow erythropoiesis.[24] Uremic toxins (e.g., uric acid, sulfates, phosphates) that increase in the blood secondarily to renal failure may suppress bone marrow function and damage erythrocytes, which undergo eryptosis. Platelet function also may be defective in these individuals, which results in chronic bleeding and loss of erythrocytes.

Anemia may arise from the direct action of bacterial toxins. For example, *Clostridium perfringens* (gas gangrene and a cause of food poisoning) produces an alpha toxin. This toxin has enzymatic activity (phospholipase C, sphingomyelinase) that disrupts the membrane of cells. If the cells are erythrocytes, hemolysis will result.

◆**CLINICAL MANIFESTATIONS.** The anemia of ACD is usually in the mild to moderate range, with few additional complications. If hemoglobin levels drop significantly, clinical manifestations of IDA appear.

◆**EVALUATION AND TREATMENT.** Morphologically, ACD is initially normocytic-normochromic, but as the condition persists it becomes hypochromic and microcytic. ACD is characterized by abnormal iron metabolism with low levels of circulating iron (less than 60 mcg/dL) and reduced levels of transferrin. The most significant finding of ACD is very high total body iron storage, although inadequate iron is released from the bone marrow for erythropoiesis. Very often the first indication of ACD is a failure to respond to conventional iron replacement therapy. Levels of erythropoietin are generally lower than expected for the degree of anemia. The affected individuals also frequently present with low or normal total iron-binding capacity (TIBC), normal or high serum ferritin levels, and low concentrations of soluble transferrin receptor (blood test findings are listed in Table 29.2). Occasionally it may be difficult to differentiate ACD from IDA; however, measurement of sTfR (key receptor

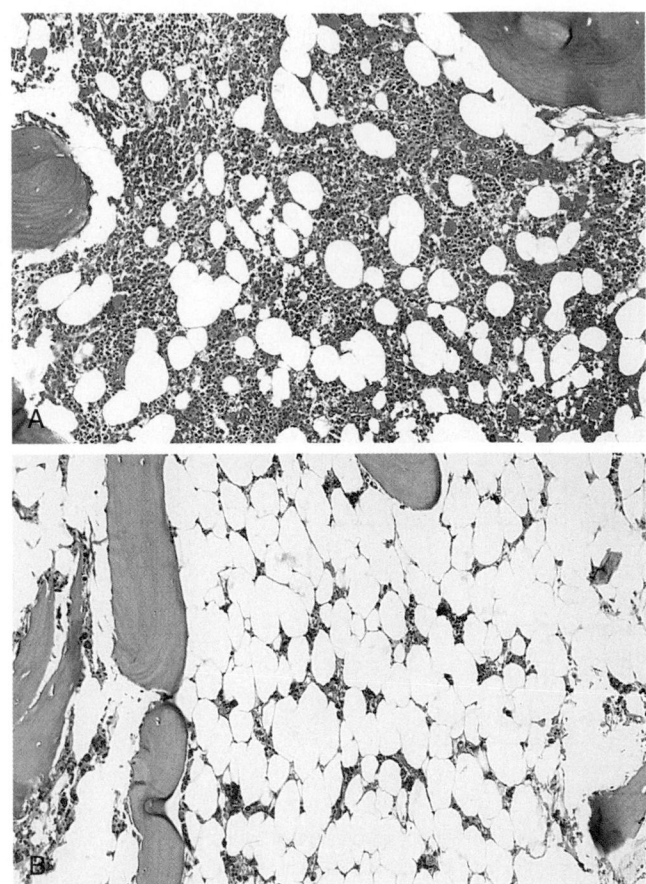

From Kumar V, Abbas A, Aster JC: *Robbins & Cotran pathologic basis of disease*, ed 9, Philadelphia, 2015, Saunders.

BOX 29.2 — MAJOR CAUSES OF APLASTIC ANEMIA

Acquired
Idiopathic
Acquired stem cell defects
Immune mediated

Chemical Agents
Dose Related
Alkylating agents
Antimetabolites
Benzene
Chloramphenicol
Inorganic arsenicals

Idiosyncratic
Chloramphenicol
Phenylbutazone
Organic arsenicals

Methylphenylethylhydantoin
Carbamazepine
Penicillamine
Gold salts

Physical Agents
Whole-body irradiation
Viral infections
Hepatitis (unknown virus)
Cytomegalovirus infections
Epstein-Barr virus infections
Herpes zoster (varicella zoster)

Inherited
Fanconi anemia
Telomerase defects

FIGURE 29.6 Aplastic Anemia. **A,** Normal bone marrow of an adult. Hematopoietic cells account for approximately 40% of marrow's cellularity. **B,** There is a marked reduction in hematopoietic cells with expansion of fat cells. (From Damjanov I, Linder J: *Pathology: a color atlas,* St Louis, 2000, Mosby.)

for iron acquisition by erythroid cells) may be useful. Levels of sTfR do not respond to iron supplementation in ACD but do so in IDA.

Use of erythropoietin in treatment of ACD associated with arthritis, malignancies, and acquired immunodeficiency syndrome (AIDS) has met with limited success. Individuals with severe anemia secondary to chronic kidney disease (CKD) can be treated successfully with erythropoietin and treatments to increase iron stores.[25] However, the optimal degree of restoration of hemoglobin levels (a measure of anemia) has not been determined; achievement of normal levels increases the risk of hypertension, stroke, and death.[26] Transfusion of critically ill individuals may worsen the outcome and increase morbidity and mortality.[27] The principal treatment is alleviation of the underlying disorder. Individuals who have ACD but demonstrate no evidence of inflammatory or infectious conditions are screened for the presence of malignancies.

Aplastic Anemia

Aplastic anemia (AA) is a hematopoietic failure or bone marrow aplasia characterized by reduction in the effective production of mature cells by the bone marrow, causing peripheral pancytopenia (anemia, neutropenia, and thrombocytopenia), which is a reduction or absence of all three blood cell types (Fig. 29.6). Although the pathogenesis is not clearly defined, mechanisms include immune-mediated destruction of hematopoietic stem cells or their progenitors at various stages of differentiation.[28]

The known causes of AA are from chemicals and drugs, physical agents, or unpredictable exposures; AA can be inherited or idiosyncratic

(Box 29.2). The incidence of AA is relatively rare (annual rate of two to five new cases per million per year). The incidence in developing countries is somewhat higher and may be related to greater exposure to certain chemicals known to cause AA. The incidence is bimodal, with one peak occurring between 15 and 25 years of age and a second peak occurring in individuals older than age 60. AA is equally distributed between genders.

AAs are the most common type of bone marrow aplasia, with *idiopathic AA* (primary acquired) accounting for approximately 75% of all confirmed cases and being an autoimmune disease. *Secondary AA,* which accounts for approximately 15% of cases, is caused by a variety of known chemical agents and ionizing radiation. Chemical agents and drug effects are included in Table 29.5. The development of AA with use of these agents is generally dose related, and the effect can be controlled with diminished dosages. In other instances, AA might develop after the use of small amounts of these drugs (idiosyncratic), with the anemia following a severe, rapid, irreversible progression. Liver disease (seronegative hepatitis) is also recognized as a cause of AA.

AA is constitutional or familial in origin or is associated with one or more somatic abnormalities in approximately 5% to 10% of affected individuals. A subset of these is found to have defective telomerase RNA, resulting in shortened telomeres. This abnormality also is found in some individuals with idiopathic AA.

Total body irradiation also causes AA and in certain instances may be used therapeutically for this effect. Infections are also known to cause AA, with viruses being the most common agent. These include infections with the human immunodeficiency virus (HIV), Epstein-Barr virus (EBV), and hepatitis (non-A, non-B, non-C, and non-G forms of the virus). Persistent parvovirus B19 infection also has been identified as producing bone marrow failure resulting in AA. Parvovirus B19 has been identified as the cause of aplastic crisis in children who have sickle cell hemoglobinopathies and hereditary spherocytosis.

Another condition associated with AA is pure red cell aplasia (PRCA), in which only the erythrocytes are affected. PRCA is a rare disorder and has been associated with autoimmune, viral, and neoplastic (leukemias) disorders; infiltrative disorders of the bone marrow (myelofibrosis); renal failure; hepatitis; mononucleosis; and systemic lupus erythematosus. It also is a well-recognized but infrequent complication of allogeneic bone

TABLE 29.5   ANEMIAS SECONDARY TO DRUG EFFECTS

DRUG	HEMOLYTIC	MEGALOBLASTIC	SIDEROBLASTIC	APLASTIC
Antibiotics				
Amphotericin B				X
Trimethoprim-sulfamethoxazole (Bactrim)		X		
Chloramphenicol (Chloromycetin)			XX	XXXX
Erythromycin	X			X
Sulfisoxazole (Gantrisin)				X
Penicillin	XXX			X
Sulfanilamide/Sulfonamides	XX			X, X*
Streptomycin	X			X
Anticonvulsants				
Phenytoin (Dilantin)		XXX		XXX, X*
Mephenytoin		XXX		XXX
Primidone (Mysoline)		XX		
Phenobarbital		XX		
Trimethadione (Tridione)				XXX
Antiinflammatories				
ASA (aspirin)				X*
Colchicine		X?		
Gold compounds				XX
Ibuprofen (Motrin)	X			X
Indomethacin (Indocin)				X
Phenacetin	XXX			X
Phenylbutazone				XX, X*
Antihypertensives/Diuretics				
Methyldopa (Aldomet)	XXX			
Acetazolamide (Diamox)				X
Thiazides	X			
Tranquilizers				
Chlordiazepoxide (Librium)				X
Chlorpromazine (Thorazine)	XX			X
Meprobamate				X
Oral Hypoglycemics				
Chlorpropamide (Diabinese)	X			
Tolbutamide (Orinase)				X, X*
Immunosuppressants				
Azathioprine (Imuran)			X	X*
Cyclosporine	X			

Continued

TABLE 29.5	ANEMIAS SECONDARY TO DRUG EFFECTS—cont'd			
DRUG	**HEMOLYTIC**	**MEGALOBLASTIC**	**SIDEROBLASTIC**	**APLASTIC**
Miscellaneous Agents				
Benzene	XX			XX
Cimetidine (Tagamet)				X
Heparin				X*
Potassium perchlorate				XX
Quinine/quinidine	XX			
Acetaminophen (Tylenol)	X			X
Antituberculosis Agents				
INH (isoniazid)	XX			
PASA (*para*-aminosalicylic acid)	XX	X		
Pyridium (phenazopyridine HCl)				XX

ASA, Acetylsalicylic acid; *X*, rare number of reported cases; *XXXX*, substantial number of reported cases; *XX* and *XXX*, intermediate number of reported cases; *X**, "pure red cell" aplasia; *X?*, uncertain.

marrow transplantation, particularly when there is donor-recipient ABO mismatch. A thymoma often is found in association with PRCA and is also present in Diamond-Blackfan syndrome, a congenital disorder.

A very small percentage of AA cases are linked to genetic alterations. Fanconi anemia is a rare genetic anemia characterized by pancytopenia resulting from defects in DNA repair.[29] This anemia develops early in life and is accompanied by multiple congenital anomalies.

◆**PATHOPHYSIOLOGY.** The characteristic lesion of AA is a hypocellular bone marrow that has been replaced with fat. The pathogenesis of AA is not certain. Two etiologies and mechanisms are observed: an extrinsic immune-mediated suppression of bone marrow progenitor cells and an intrinsic abnormality of stem cells.[4] The primary mechanism of acquired AA involves immune-mediated destruction directed against hematopoietic stem cells (HSCs).[28,30] Several immune abnormalities are found in individuals including dysregulated CD4+, CD8+, and Th-17 T-cell responses and reduced numbers of regulatory T cells.[28] Additionally, many people have elevations of circulating levels of inflammatory or myelosuppressive cytokines, such as interferon-gamma (IFN-γ), tumor necrosis factor-alpha (TNF-α), and transforming growth factor-beta (TGF-β).[28,31] Although efforts have identified circulating antibodies in acquired AA individuals, the identification of autoantigens capable of eliciting cytotoxic T-cell responses and causing stem cell destruction has been challenging.[28] Laboratory studies have focused on a working model where activated T cells suppress HSCs. Stem cells may be altered from exposure to drugs, infectious agents, or other unknown environmental factors. In many cases no initiating factor can be identified and therefore this type of AA belongs in the idiopathic category. A genetic predisposition may involve polymorphisms in human leukocyte antigens (HLAs) and inhibitory cytokines (e.g., TNF-α, TGF-β, and IFN-γ).[31] An emerging understanding suggests that the initial immune response may be triggered by pathogens, drugs, or chemicals, or by neoantigens through epigenetic mechanisms.[28,32-34] It is interesting that transient and persistent bone marrow hypoplasia has been linked to many microorganisms, and the interaction and alterations between the gut microbiota and immune system is hypothesized as an initial insult in the development of bone marrow failure syndromes such as AA[28] (Fig. 29.7).

The evidence supporting an autoimmune process includes the response of AA to immunosuppressive therapy including depletion of T cells by antithymocyte antibodies. Cytotoxic T cells (Tc cells) appear to be the main culprits, although the causative antigen has yet to be identified. Th1 cytokines (involved in the differentiation of Tc cells), such as IFN-γ and TNF-α, as well as cellular contact with Tc cells through FasL, induce apoptosis of CD34+ target cells, which includes most of the hematopoietic progenitors. The presence of stem cell abnormalities is supported by the existence of abnormal karyotypes, short telomeres, and the low incidence of transformation of AA into myeloid neoplasms.[4]

◆**CLINICAL MANIFESTATIONS.** The onset of symptoms is insidious and related to the rapidity with which the bone marrow is destroyed and replaced. AA affects both males and females at any age. Approximately 50% of AA cases progress rapidly, with a high risk of death from overwhelming infection or bleeding. In some cases the rate of decline is slow and the individual may adapt progressively to a new level of hematologic function. This condition is referred to as *hypoplastic anemia* rather than aplastic anemia.

Initial symptoms depend on which cell line is affected. Rapidly progressing disease is usually associated with hypoxemia, pallor (occasionally with a brownish pigmentation of the skin), and weakness along with fever and dyspnea with rapidly developing signs of hemorrhaging if platelets are affected (e.g., unexplained bruising, nosebleeds, bleeding gums, bleeding in the GI tract, prolonged bleeding at sites of minor injury). A slower onset over weeks or months is characterized by progressive weakness and fatigue with developing signs of hemorrhaging. Major hemorrhage may occur from any organ; however, it is generally observed in the late stages and is often secondary to other events. Menorrhagia and purpura also may be evident; however, purpura is not necessarily a classic indication of AA and may not be representative of the degree of thrombocytopenia. In both rapid onset and slow onset AA, diminished leukocyte production may result in a progressive frequency and prolongation of infections.

Late manifestations of the condition include ulcerations of the mouth and pharynx or a low-grade cellulitis in the neck. Splenomegaly is extremely rare; if it is present, however, other conditions that may imitate AA should be excluded. Neurologic changes are only evident when hemorrhages have occurred within the system; however, some individuals have complained of paresthesias.

◆**EVALUATION AND TREATMENT.** Diagnosis is made by blood tests and bone marrow biopsy. AA is suspected if levels of circulating

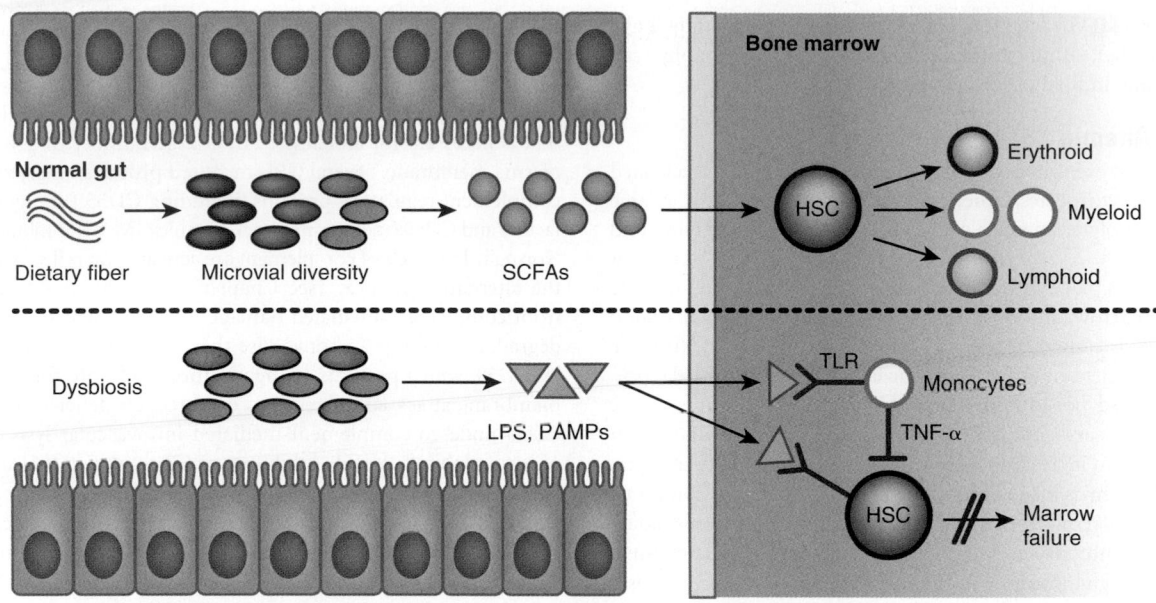

FIGURE 29.7 Working Model: Microbes, Microbiota, Hematopoiesis, and Immune Response. Microbes can participate in a symbiotic relationship (commensal) with hosts to maintain hematopoietic stem cells (HSCs) and precursor myeloid cells. Defects in innate immune cell populations, including neutrophils, monocytes, and macrophages, can occur with deficient commensal microbes. Experiments feeding mice diets rich in fiber changed the ratio of firmicutes to bacteroidetes and bifidobacteriaceae. Gut microbiota metabolize fiber, increasing short-chain fatty acids (SCFAs) and promoting the growth of bone marrow myeloid precursors (not affecting lymphoid progenitors). With dysbiosis (disrupted microbiosis; microbial imbalance or maladaptation) pathologic microbes may increase and provide a source of chronic low-grade inflammation mediated by lipopolysaccharides (LPSs) and other pathogen-associated molecular patterns (PAMPs). These factors continuously stimulate hematopoietic stem progenitor cells (HSPCs) through pathogen recognition receptors like TLRs, resulting in hematopoiesis inhibition. The LPS stimulation of toll-like receptors (TLRs) on monocytes causes tumor necrosis factor-alpha (TNF-α) secretion and with continuous stimulation of HSPCs may eventually inhibit hematopoiesis through exhaustion. (Adapted from Espinoza JL, Kotecha R, Nakao S: *Front Immunol* 8:186, 2017.)

erythrocytes, leukocytes, and platelets are diminished: a granulocyte count less than 500/μL, a platelet count less than 20,000/μL, and an absolute reticulocyte count less than or equal to 40×10^9/L. The diagnosis is confirmed by bone marrow biopsy. The bone marrow usually has reduced cellularity (i.e., less than 25% normal cellularity). The morphology of the few remaining hematopoietic cells is usually normal. Occasionally the erythrocytes are macrocytic, with anisocytosis and poikilocytosis, and may appear immature.

Marrow biopsied from individuals with typical AA contains yellowish white material consisting mainly of fat, fibrous tissue, and lymphocytes. Pancytopenia is usually characterized by decreased stem cell and progenitor cell populations to approximately 1% or less of normal.

Up until 20 years ago, treatment involved determination of the cause, removal of the potential causative agent, implementation of transfusions, and prevention and treatment of infection and hemorrhage. Stimulation of blood cell production also was used, and in some instances splenectomy was recommended. The prognosis with these forms of treatment was extremely poor. In acute cases, 25% of individuals succumbed within 4 months, and approximately 70% died within 5 years; only about 10% experienced complete recovery. Newer forms of treatment, such as bone marrow transplant (BMT), immunosuppression, and identification of high-risk individuals, have decreased mortality significantly.[35]

Bone marrow and, most recently, peripheral blood stem cell transplantation from a histocompatible sibling often cures the underlying bone marrow failure.[36] Survival rates of 75% to 80% have been reported, and death rates within the first 100 days have decreased. Before transplantation the recipient usually receives radiation or chemotherapy to

deplete the bone marrow of disease-causing lymphocytes. Thus an unsuccessful transplantation may leave the recipient with a depleted immune system and an increased vulnerability to infection. Graft-versus-host (GVH) disease remains a risk and is a major contributor to premature death.[37] Children demonstrate higher survival rates than adults.

For those individuals unable to undergo bone marrow transplantation or who lack a suitable sibling donor, immunosuppression remains the treatment of choice. Antithymocyte globulin (ATG) specifically suppresses lymphocytes, including those autoreactive lymphocytes destroying the bone marrow cells. Drugs like cyclosporine, which is often used in combination with ATG, broadly suppress the activity of immune cells. Response rates (i.e., increased blood cell counts) of 40% to 50% may occur in individuals who receive ATG. The addition of cyclosporine has increased the response and survival rates to as much as 70% to 80%, with a 5-year survival rate between 80% and 90%. Cyclosporine as a single therapeutic agent is not as effective. Corticosteroids are often used concurrently with ATG and cyclosporine. Cyclophosphamide also has been used as an immunosuppressive agent and has produced the same effects as ATG; however, its use has been discontinued because of its toxicity. The addition of recombinant hematopoietic growth factors, such as granulocyte-macrophage colony–stimulating factor (GM-CSF), IL-6, and epoetin, to immunosuppressive therapy has produced significant additional benefit in both children and adults.

Immunosuppressive therapy is not without risk. Individuals receiving immunosuppressive therapy are at risk of experiencing treatment failure or late clonal/malignant conditions, or both. Late clonal/malignant conditions include paroxysmal nocturnal hemoglobinuria (PNH), myelodysplasia (MDS), acute leukemia, or solid tumor. Although quite rare (less than 3%), administration of ATG may cause an anaphylactic reaction in some individuals.

Hemolytic Anemia

The predominant event in hemolytic anemias is premature accelerated destruction of erythrocytes, either episodically or continuously. A large majority of hemolytic anemias occur within phagocytes in lymphoid tissue, called *extravascular hemolysis*. The destruction of senescent erythrocytes takes place within macrophages typically abundant in the spleen, bone marrow, and liver. Less common is *intravascular* (blood vessels) *hemolysis* caused by mechanical injury, complement fixation, intracellular parasites, or exogenous toxic factors (e.g., clostridial sepsis, snake venom, lead poisoning). The consequences of the anemia are elevated levels of erythropoietin to induce accelerated production of erythrocytes and an increase in the products of hemoglobin catabolism.

Hemolytic anemias may be either congenital or acquired. Congenital hemolytic anemias result from intrinsic defects in erythrocytes, including the red cell membrane (e.g., hereditary spherocytosis, paroxysmal nocturnal hemoglobinuria), enzymatic pathways (e.g., glucose-6-phosphate dehydrogenase deficiency), and hemoglobin synthesis (e.g., the thalassemia syndromes, sickle cell anemia). (Glucose-6-phosphate dehydrogenase deficiency, thalassemia, and sickle cell disease are discussed in Chapter 31.) Acquired hemolytic anemias are usually immunologic (immune hemolytic anemias), such as erythrocyte destruction caused by autoantibodies against erythrocyte antigens (e.g., autoimmune hemolytic anemia), isohemagglutinins (e.g., mismatched erythrocyte transfusions), or allergic reactions against drug antigens adsorbed onto the erythrocyte surface (drug-induced hemolytic anemia). (Isohemagglutinins, erythrocyte antigens, autoantibodies, and allergic reactions are discussed in Chapter 9.) Acquired hemolytic anemia may also be secondary to erythrocyte damage caused by cardiac valve prostheses or by increased shear stresses in narrowed small vessels (e.g., during disseminated intravascular coagulation). Causes of acquired and hereditary hemolytic anemias are listed in Table 29.6.

◆**PATHOPHYSIOLOGY.** Extravascular hemolysis appears to be initiated by age-related changes in erythrocyte surface proteins leading to their recognition and phagocytosis. Erythrocytes continuously circulate through the spleen, passing through the thin-walled splenic cords into the splenic sinusoids, a spongelike labyrinth of macrophages. Normally, erythrocytes are able to alter their shape to allow passage through openings in the splenic cords. Macrophages will phagocytose erythrocytes with structural alterations of the membrane surface, or erythrocytes may become more rigid and therefore incapable of maneuvering through this network. In some cases, IgG antibodies or complement component C3b can coat erythrocytes without causing hemolysis, but can function as opsonins that are recognized by macrophages.

Intravascular hemolysis is caused by physical destruction of erythrocytes in the circulation, frequently by antibody and complement. As mentioned earlier, other forms of destruction include mechanical injury, such as shear stresses in narrowed microcirculation; repetitive physical trauma (karate chopping, bongo drumming, marathon running); or trauma caused by cardiac valves. Intracellular parasites such as *Plasmodium falciparum* malaria can cause intravascular hemolysis because infection may generate early elimination of normal or nonparasitized RBCs, lysis of parasitized RBCs, and impairment of erythropoiesis.[38] Toxic injury, such as from snake venom, contains hemolytic toxins and clostridial sepsis results in the release of enzymes that digest the erythrocyte membrane.

Paroxysmal nocturnal hemoglobinuria, although rare, is the only hemolytic anemia caused by an acquired genetic defect that is manifested by complement-mediated hemolysis. It may be congenital or acquired

secondarily to acquired aplastic anemia. The disease results from a mutation in the X-linked gene for phosphatidylinositol glycan—class A *(PIG-A)*, which results in a defect in expression of glycosylphosphatidylinositol (GPI) in hematologic stem cells.[39] GPI is a lipid anchor that is necessary for attachment of a large number of proteins to the plasma membrane. Several GPI-anchored proteins on erythrocytes are complement regulatory proteins, including CD55 (decay-accelerating factor) and CD59 (membrane attack complex [MAC] inhibitory protein). Normally low levels of complement are activated on cell surfaces through the alternative pathway (see Chapter 7). Erythrocytes are protected from complement-mediated damage by CD55, which accelerates the degradation of any C3 convertase that forms on the cell surface, and by CD59, which prevents C9 aggregation and pore formation by the membrane attack complex. Thus erythrocytes deficient in CD55 and CD59 undergo complement-mediated intravascular lysis and release of hemoglobin.[40] Peptide inhibitors of C3 activation that may prevent hemolysis are under investigation.[41] In addition to anemia and hemoglobinuria, affected individuals also present with severe fatigue, abdominal pain, and thrombosis.[42] The cause of death is usually thrombosis of the abdominal or cerebral veins.[43] Thrombosis most likely results from a depletion of vascular nitric oxide (NO) by free hemoglobin, which has a high affinity for NO. The result is dysregulation of normal hemostasis and increased platelet vascular adherence and clot formation (see Chapter 28).

Immunohemolytic anemias, also called autoimmune hemolytic anemias (AIHAs), are acquired disorders caused by autoantibodies or complement, or both, on red cells against antigens normally on the surface of erythrocytes.[4,44] Immunohemolytic anemia is the preferred term because in some instances the immune reaction is initiated by an ingested drug.[4] Three types of AIHAs have been described: (1) warm reactive antibody type, (2) cold agglutinin type, and (3) cold hemolysin type (paroxysmal cold hemoglobinuria). This classification is based on the optimal temperature at which the antibody binds to erythrocytes and the mechanism of erythrocyte destruction.

Warm autoimmune hemolytic anemia is uncommon (incidence of about 1 per 80,000 population annually), although it is the most common form of AIHA (80% to 90% of cases), and generally occurs in individuals older than the age of 40.[45] Approximately half of the cases are secondary to other diseases, especially lymphomas but also chronic lymphocytic leukemia, other neoplastic disorders, or systemic lupus erythematosus (SLE). The anemia is caused by IgG that binds optimally to erythrocytes at normal body temperature (37°C [98.6°F]). Most cases are related to antibody against Rh-related antigens other than the D epitope (Rh antigens are discussed in Chapter 9). The spectrum of antibody specificities includes antibodies against the e, E, or c antigens of the Rh complex. Other cases are caused by IgG antibodies against erythrocyte antigens outside the Rh complex and include antibodies against Wr[b], En[a], the Kell blood group, and many others. The warm reactive IgG antibodies usually do not activate complement because of the rather sparse distribution of antigens on the erythrocyte surface. (Activation of complement by antibody is discussed in Chapters 7, 8, and 9.) Erythrocyte destruction is caused by extravascular processes. The IgG-coated erythrocytes bind to the Fc receptors on monocytes and splenic macrophages and are removed by phagocytosis.

Cold agglutinin autoimmune hemolytic anemia is mediated by immunoglobulin M (IgM) antibodies and occurs less often than warm antibody hemolysis, affecting mostly middle-aged and older adults. Cold antibodies optimally bind to erythrocytes at colder temperatures (lower than 31°C [87.8°F]) with maximal binding capacity at 4°C (39.2°F). Cold agglutinin autoantibodies may appear acutely during recovery of certain infectious disorders, particularly infectious mononucleosis, *Mycoplasma pneumoniae*, and disseminated tuberculosis.[46] Individuals

TABLE 29.6	CAUSES OF HEMOLYTIC ANEMIAS	
TYPE OF HEMOLYTIC DISORDER	**PRIMARY CAUSE OR ASSOCIATED DISORDER**	**MECHANISMS OF ERYTHROCYTE DESTRUCTION**
Acquired Forms		
Immune system–mediated hemolysis	Transfusion reaction Hemolytic disease of the newborn (see Chapter 31) Autoimmune hemolytic anemia (see text)	Antibody-mediated: intravascular hemolysis by activation of complement system; extravascular hemolysis by phagocytosis of antibody-coated erythrocytes in spleen (see Chapter 9)
Traumatic hemolysis	Presence of prosthetic heart valves Structural abnormalities of the heart Hemolytic uremic syndrome Disseminated intravascular coagulation Hemodialysis	Physical destruction of erythrocytes by "mechanical" means (trauma)
Infectious hemolysis	Bacterial infection Viral infection Protozoal infection Helminthic infection	Bacterial hemolysins (e.g., *Escherichia coli* 0157:H7 shiga toxin; *Clostridium perfringens* toxin) Initiates autoimmune hemolysis (e.g., *Mycoplasma pneumoniae*: cold agglutinin) Affects erythrocytes (e.g., parvovirus B19: infects erythroid progenitors) Infects erythrocytes (e.g., malaria) Causes intestinal bleeding (e.g., hookworm)
Drug or toxic (chemical) hemolysis	Exposure to toxic chemical agents Hemodialysis or uremia Venoms	Chemical injury of erythrocytes (see Chapter 2)
Physical hemolysis	Burns Radiation	Heat or radiation injury (see Chapter 2)
Hypophosphatemic hemolysis	Hypophosphatemia (phosphate deficiency in plasma; see Chapter 3)	Diminished cellular production of substances required for erythrocyte life and function
Hereditary Forms		
Structural defects	Plasma membrane defects	Fragility of the erythrocyte
Plasma membrane protein mutation	Deficient complement regulatory proteins (i.e., paroxysmal nocturnal hemoglobinuria)	Complement activation on erythrocyte surface, intravascular lysis
Enzyme deficiencies	Deficiency of glycolytic enzymes Deficiency of metabolic enzymes (i.e., glucose-6-phosphate dehydrogenase deficiency)	Diminished cellular function
Defects of globin synthesis or structure	Sickle cell anemia	Increased membrane fragility and deformation during sickle crises
	Thalassemia	Defective hemoglobin structure and function
	Miscellaneous hemoglobin defects	Defective hemoglobin structure and function

From Lee GR et al: *Wintrobe's clinical hematology*, ed 9, Philadelphia, 1993, Lea & Febiger.

with these conditions are usually younger than those with primary disease; the anemia may be severe but may be self-limiting. Chronic cold agglutinin AIHAs also can occur in association with lymphoid neoplasm and other unknown or idiopathic conditions.[47]

The IgM autoantibody is usually monoclonal and directed against erythrocyte carbohydrate antigens of the I system (i.e., i, I) or the P system (i.e., Pr).[48] In the colder areas of the body (e.g., fingers, toes, nose, ears, exposed skin), particularly during cold weather, the IgM autoantibodies bind to circulating erythrocytes. The IgM is rapidly released when the blood recirculates and warms. IgM is an extremely efficient activator of complement, resulting in the stable deposition of C3b on the cell surface. If an adequate amount of complement is deposited, the erythrocytes become vulnerable to recognition and rapid phagocytosis by mononuclear phagocytes in the liver and spleen (also

see Chapter 9). The severity of hemolysis is variable and may result in a progressive chronic anemia. If the level of antibody is high or has particularly strong binding, hemagglutination may occur in the capillaries of exposed sites, such as fingers, toes, and ears, when temperatures are below 30°C (86°F). Obstruction of blood flow caused by erythrocyte agglutination may lead to a bluish discoloration of the skin (acrocyanosis) that resolves as the skin is warmed. Prolonged exposure to the cold may lead to gangrene.

Cold hemolysin autoimmune hemolytic anemia (paroxysmal cold hemoglobinuria) is a disorder in which exposure to cold initiates acute and severe intravascular hemolysis that, unlike cold agglutinin anemia, results in hemoglobinuria. The chronic form of this anemia is extremely rare, but an acute form of paroxysmal cold hemoglobinuria is frequently observed (30% to 40% of cases) in AIHA of childhood. The acute form occurs primarily in children younger than the age of 10 years and is usually preceded by an upper respiratory tract infection or flulike symptoms. Infections with measles, mumps, *Mycoplasma* (pneumonia), and *Varicella* have also been linked to an onset of paroxysmal cold hemoglobinuria. The anemia may be rapidly progressing and severe and associated with fever, reddish brown urine, hemoglobinuria, jaundice, abdominal pains, and pallor, with about 25% of individuals presenting with hepatomegaly and splenomegaly.

Paroxysmal cold hemoglobinuria is generally caused by IgG autoantibodies against the P blood group antigen. Antibody binding occurs in the colder portions of the body. As the erythrocyte recirculates, enzymes of the complement cascade are activated, and cells are destroyed in the vasculature by complement-mediated lysis. The involved antibody, also called *Donath-Landsteiner antibody,* was first recognized in individuals with anemia secondary to chronic syphilis infection. A transfusion reaction is an example of alloimmune hemolytic anemia (also see Chapter 9). Transfused blood that is mismatched for ABO antigens is destroyed by preexisting isohemagglutinins in the recipient. Isohemagglutinins, which are generally IgM antibodies, activate complement, resulting in a rapid intravascular hemolysis. The individual may immediately experience fever, chills, dyspnea, and hypotension and may progress to shock. In some cases the hemolytic reaction may be delayed and develop 3 to 10 days after transfusion. The delayed reaction is caused by a low titer of preexisting antibodies to minor erythrocyte antigens.

Drug-induced hemolytic anemia is a form of immune hemolytic anemia usually resulting from an allergic reaction against foreign antigens (e.g., antibiotics)[49] (also see Chapter 9). Usually the drug is low molecular weight, functions as a hapten, and binds to proteins on the surface of erythrocytes. This is sometimes called the *hapten model* and is based on anemia caused by penicillin, cephalosporins (more than 90% of cases), and hydrocortisone[50] (Fig. 29.8, *A*). IgG antibody against the drug or against the unique antigen formed by the interface of the drug and erythrocyte protein is formed and binds to the erythrocyte at normal body temperature. Hemolysis is usually extravascular because the opsonized erythrocytes are removed by phagocytes in the spleen and liver, although complement-dependent intravascular hemolysis may occur in some individuals. This form of drug-induced anemia usually follows a large intravenous infusion of an antibiotic and occurs 1 to 2 weeks after the initiation of therapy. Cessation of administration of the drug results in rapid resolution of the anemia.

The erythrocyte plasma membrane contains receptors of components of the complement system, such as C3b, and can bind circulating immune complexes that have activated the complement cascade (see Chapter 9 for a discussion of immune complexes). This forms the basis for the *immune complex model* of drug-induced hemolytic anemia and was first described for anemia resulting from administration of the drug quinidine (Fig. 29.8, *B*). The drug or a metabolite of the drug, both of which are haptens, initially binds to plasma proteins and becomes immunogenic (see Chapter 8). The circulating drug-protein complex reacts with the resultant antibody (usually IgM, although IgG complexes have also been described) and activates the complement system, resulting in the deposition of C3b into the complex. Binding of the immune complexes to the erythrocyte surface results in further complement activation and intravascular hemolysis. This mechanism also may explain some of the anemia observed in other immune complex conditions, such as SLE.

In at least one instance, administration of the drug α-methyldopa induces an immune response against normal erythrocyte antigens and thus initiates a true AIHA *(autoimmune model)* (Fig. 29.8, *C*). The autoantibody is usually against Rh blood group antigens. It is estimated that 20% of individuals taking α-methyldopa develop detectable antibodies, but only 1% actually develop clinically significant anemia. The mechanism by which α-methyldopa induces autoantibodies against the erythrocytes is unknown.

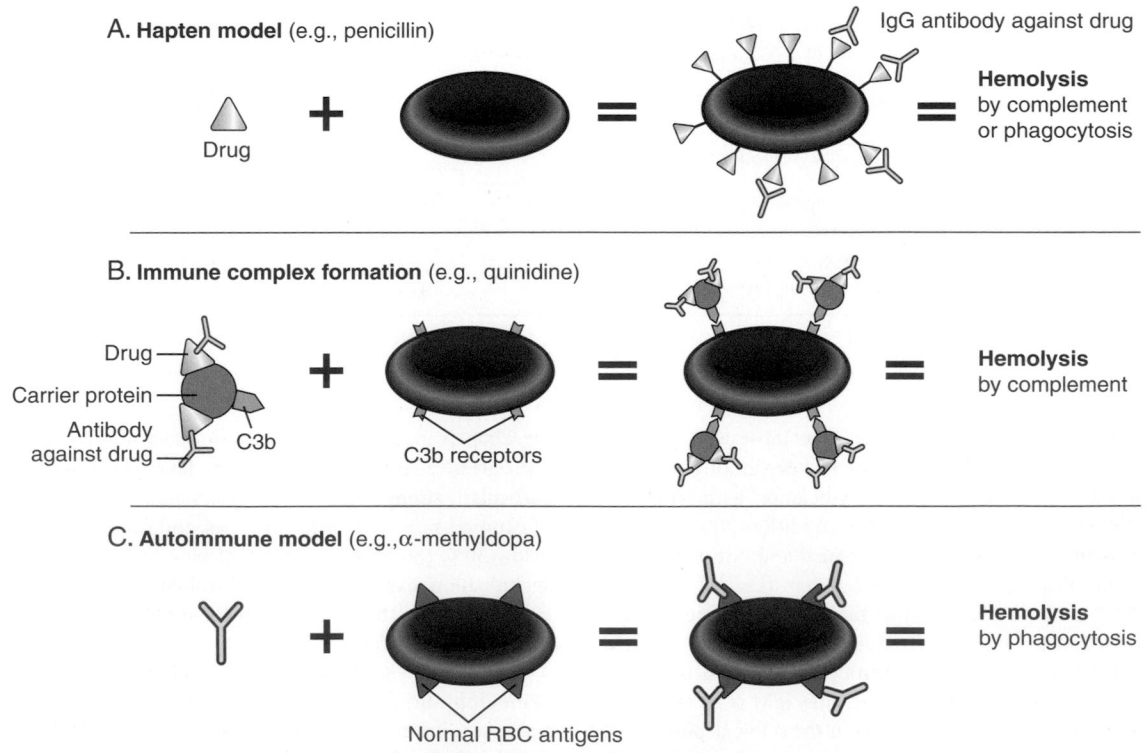

A. Hapten model (e.g., penicillin)

Drug + = IgG antibody against drug = Hemolysis by complement or phagocytosis

B. Immune complex formation (e.g., quinidine)

Drug / Carrier protein / Antibody against drug / C3b + C3b receptors = = Hemolysis by complement

C. Autoimmune model (e.g., α-methyldopa)

+ Normal RBC antigens = = Hemolysis by phagocytosis

FIGURE 29.8 Models of Drug-Induced Hemolytic Anemia. See discussion in text. *IgG,* Immunoglobulin G; *RBC,* red blood cell.

CLINICAL MANIFESTATIONS. The presence and severity of signs and symptoms of hemolytic anemia depend on the degree of anemia and hemolysis and the success of compensatory erythropoiesis. Adaptation to red cell destruction is facilitated by increased red cell production. Bone marrow is capable of increasing red cell production up to eight times its normal rate. Accelerated erythrocyte production that is incapable of keeping up with destruction develops into a true hemolytic anemia.

The severity of anemia varies widely among individuals, even in those who have the same illness. Severe disease is commonly diagnosed shortly after birth or within the first year of life. Mild to moderate anemia is more common because the shortened erythrocyte survival time is offset by increased erythropoiesis. Some individuals have no symptoms of anemia, and the underlying hemolytic process remains undetected unless some other complications develop during the course of the disease.

Jaundice (icterus) is present when heme destruction exceeds the liver's ability to conjugate and excrete bilirubin. Jaundice is first noticed in the neonatal period. Children and adults with congenital hemolytic anemia may not have icterus, or it may be mild enough that it remains unnoticed. In some individuals, faint scleral icterus may be the only indication of hemolytic disease.

Acute conditions that disrupt the delicate equilibrium of accelerated erythropoiesis and erythrocyte destruction may precipitate a crisis. The most common type of crisis is aplastic and results from failure of bone marrow erythrocyte production. The most common cause of aplastic crisis is human parvovirus B19 infection.

Commonly, individuals with congenital hemolytic disorders demonstrate splenomegaly, which is often only mild in nature. In some cases the spleen may become quite enlarged and may cause discovery of the underlying hemolytic disorder. Another underlying condition that may be the cause of inadvertently determining the presence of the anemic disorder is the development of gallstones.

Children who have hemolytic anemia often demonstrate skeletal abnormalities caused by expansion of erythroid bone marrow during the active phase of growth and development. These alterations are more pronounced in the bony structures of the face and skull and may result in pathologic fractures (see Chapter 31). Cardiovascular and respiratory manifestations vary with the degree of anemia. In spite of the disorder being characterized as hemolytic in nature, thromboembolism may occur. Pulmonary embolism is a common finding during autopsies of individuals with immune hemolytic anemia.

EVALUATION AND TREATMENT. Diagnosis is based on clinical manifestations, bone marrow studies, and blood tests (see Table 29.2). Abnormally increased numbers of erythrocyte stem cells are found in the marrow, a finding termed *erythroid hyperplasia*. Accelerated erythropoiesis causes large numbers of fragile and immature erythrocytes (stem cells and reticulocytes) to be released prematurely into the circulation. These cells are observed in blood smears. If the bone marrow is able to consistently maintain adequate compensation, the hemoglobin may remain stable. The mean corpuscular volume, however, may be decreased in the presence of reticulocytes. A blood smear is helpful in determining the presence of spherocytes or schistocytes, as well as examining white blood cells and platelets for coexisting hematologic or malignant conditions.

Acquired hemolytic anemias are treated by removing the cause or treating the underlying disorder. Corticosteroids are used for initial treatment. Approximately 75% of individuals initially respond to treatment with corticosteroids, but many of these patients relapse within a year. The most commonly used second-line treatments are splenectomy and administration of rituximab. Splenectomy is performed if the spleen is the major site of hemolysis and splenomegaly is significant. Analysis of multiple studies confirms that some response (complete or partial) is achieved in between 59% and 100% of individuals.[51] Although some individuals relapse after splenectomy, most achieve long-term remission.

The therapeutic use of monoclonal antibody has proven beneficial in individuals who relapse or are resistant to the effects of corticosteroids. Rituximab is a monoclonal antibody directed against the CD20 antigen and specifically depletes or suppresses B cells throughout the body. CD20 is expressed on most cells in the B-cell lineage, except hematopoietic stem cells and plasma cells. Rituximab is used to treat a variety of leukemias and lymphomas and autoimmune diseases (e.g., rheumatoid arthritis, idiopathic thrombocytopenia, multiple sclerosis, type 1 diabetes mellitus, systemic lupus erythematosus). It is used successfully in several types of immune hemolytic anemias. Eculizumab is a monoclonal antibody against complement protein C5, which blocks the enzymatic activation of C5 to C5a and C5b, and thus may be useful to treat paroxysmal nocturnal hemoglobinuria. Treatment with eculizumab prevents the formation of the membrane attack complex and complement-mediated cell lysis.

Acute fulminating hemolytic anemia (hemolytic crisis) is treated with fluid and electrolyte replacement to prevent shock and renal damage, which may be caused by erythrocyte debris clogging the kidney tubules. Transfusions of blood products sometimes are given. Folate also is used in treating chronic hemolytic disease to prevent megaloblastic crisis because long-term erythrocyte turnover increases folate requirements.

MYELOPROLIFERATIVE RED BLOOD CELL DISORDERS

Hematologic dysfunction results from an overproduction of cells as well as a deficiency. One or more hematopoietic lines may be overproduced in the marrow in response to exogenous (e.g., exposure to radiation, drugs) or endogenous (e.g., physiologic compensatory responses, immune disorders) signals. Excessive red blood cell production is classified as polycythemia. Polycythemia exists in two forms: relative and absolute. Relative polycythemia results from hemoconcentration of the blood associated with dehydration that may be caused by decreased water intake, diarrhea, excessive vomiting, or increased use of diuretics. Its development is usually of minor consequence and resolves with fluid administration or treatment of the underlying condition.

Absolute polycythemia consists of two forms: primary or secondary. *Secondary polycythemia*, the more common type, is a physiologic response resulting from increased erythropoietin secretion in response to chronic hypoxia. This hypoxia is noted in individuals who live at higher altitudes (i.e., higher than 10,000 feet), smokers with increased levels of carbon monoxide (CO), and individuals with chronic obstructive pulmonary disease or congestive heart failure, or both. Abnormal types of hemoglobin (e.g., hemoglobin San Diego or hemoglobin Chesapeake), which have a greater affinity for oxygen, also can cause secondary polycythemia, as does secretion of erythropoietin by certain tumors (e.g., renal cell carcinoma, hepatoma, and cerebral hemangioblastoma).

Polycythemia Vera

Polycythemia vera (PV) (also known as *primary polycythemia*) is one of several disorders collectively known as *chronic myeloproliferative disorders* (CMPDs).[52] Others in this group include essential thrombocytosis, chronic idiopathic myelofibrosis, chronic myeloid leukemia, chronic neutrophilic leukemia, and chronic eosinophilic leukemia. All result from abnormal regulation of the multipotent hematopoietic stem cells. The major characteristics shared by these disorders are (1) involvement of a multipotent hematopoietic progenitor cell, (2) overproduction of one or more of the formed elements of the blood in the absence of a defined stimulus, (3) dominance of a transformed progenitor cell over the nontransformed progenitor cells, (4) marrow hypercellularity or fibrosis, (5) cytogenetic abnormalities, (6) predisposition to thrombus formation and hemorrhage, and (7) spontaneous transformation to acute leukemia.

PV is quite rare with an estimated incidence of 2.3 per 100,000 individuals; peak incidence is between the ages of 60 and 80 years, with a median incidence in individuals ages 55 to 60. However, PV has been observed in individuals younger than the age of 40. Males are twice as likely as females to develop PV. PV is more common in whites than in blacks, particularly in whites of Eastern European Jewish ancestry. PV is rarely found in children or in multiple members of a single family; however, an autosomal dominant form exists that is characterized by increased production of erythropoietin.

PATHOPHYSIOLOGY. PV is a chronic neoplastic, nonmalignant condition characterized by overproduction of red blood cells (frequently with increased levels of white blood cells [leukocytosis] and platelets [thrombocytosis]) and splenomegaly. Erythrocytosis is the essential component of PV. Clonal proliferation of erythroid progenitors occurs in the bone marrow independent of erythropoietin, although the cells express a normal erythropoietin receptor. However, more than 95% of individuals with PV possess an acquired point mutation (e.g., V617F) in the *Janus kinase 2* gene *(JAK2)*, a cytoplasmic tyrosine kinase, on chromosome 9.[53] *JAK2* increases the activity of the erythropoietin receptor and is self-regulatory so that *JAK2* activity diminishes over time. The mutation associated with PV negates the self-regulatory activity of *JAK2* so that the erythropoietin receptor is constitutively active regardless of the level of erythropoietin.[54] These red blood cell precursors also demonstrate sensitivity to other growth factors, such as interleukin-3 (IL-3), granulocyte-macrophage colony–stimulating factor (GM-CSF), or insulin-like growth factor. Very recent data suggest that erythropoietin could stimulate the proliferation of cells expressing *JAK2* and that phosphorylation of three tyrosine residues in the erythropoietin receptor underlie *JAK2* point mutation (V617F) induced tumorigenesis.[55]

CLINICAL MANIFESTATIONS. Almost every individual initially presents with an enlarged spleen, frequently with abdominal pain and discomfort. As the disease progresses many of the symptoms are related to the increased blood cellularity and viscosity. Increased viscosity, as well as thrombocythemia and increased platelet dysfunction, leads to a hypercoagulable state with formation of venous and arterial thrombosis and vessel occlusion.[56] Endothelial cells carrying the $JAK2^{V617F}$ mutation suggest that endothelial cells are involved in the pathogenesis of the myeloproliferative neoplasms.[57] Thrombi with occlusion of major and minor blood vessels lead to tissue and/or organ injury (ischemia) and death (infarction). Extreme thrombocythemia (greater than 1,500,000/mm^3 of blood) increases the risk for excessive bleeding, rather than thrombosis.

Increased blood viscosity results in a variety of circulatory alterations in PV, such as plethora (ruddy, red color of the face, hands, feet, ears, and mucous membranes) and engorgement of the retinal and cerebral veins. Individuals also may experience headache, drowsiness, delirium, mania, psychotic depression, chorea, and visual disturbances. Death from cerebral thrombosis is increased approximately fivefold in individuals with PV.

Cardiac workload and output remain essentially unchanged; however, increased blood volume may lead to elevated blood pressure. Coronary blood flow may be affected, precipitating angina, although cardiovascular infarctions are relatively rare. Other evidence of cardiovascular involvement is the development of Raynaud phenomenon and thromboangiitis obliterans.

Additionally, gastrointestinal gastric and duodenal thrombosis may occur with resultant hemorrhaging. The development of mesenteric thrombosis requires immediate medical intervention. Splenomegaly and hepatomegaly result from pooling of blood in these organs; consequently, individuals may develop portal hypertension. The respiratory system is generally not affected by PV, unless thrombosis and embolization occur.

A unique feature of PV, one helpful in diagnosis, is the development of intense, painful itching that is intensified by heat or exposure to water (aquagenic pruritus), particularly warm water when bathing or showering. The intensity of the itching is related to the concentration of mast cells in the skin and is generally not responsive to antihistamines or topical lotions.

EVALUATION AND TREATMENT. PV is frequently suspected on the basis of clinical features, such as a thrombotic event, splenomegaly, or aquagenic pruritus. Diagnosis of PV is made from blood and laboratory findings. An absolute increase in the number of red blood cells and in total blood volume confirms the diagnosis. The hemoglobin concentration ranges from 14 to 28 g/dL, and the hematocrit is usually 60% or higher.[4] Erythrocytes appear normal but anisocytosis may be present. A bone marrow examination may be done but is not very valuable unless performed in association with cytogenetic and molecular studies for relevant mutations in *JAK2*.[58] The presence of a *JAK2* mutation confirms the diagnosis.[59] Typically the marrow is hypercellular but not in such a manner as to differentiate it from other myeloproliferative disorders. Additional observations of abnormal megakaryocyte morphologies, formation of clusters of abnormal cells, and increased fibrosis add more specificity and usefulness to bone marrow analysis. Elevated serum levels of erythropoietin are not helpful because most individuals with PV have normal or low levels.

Treatment of PV is challenging and directed toward minimizing the risk of thrombosis and preventing progression to myelofibrosis and acute leukemia. In low-risk individuals (e.g., those younger than age 60 or with no history of thrombosis and without risk factors for cardiovascular disease), the recommended therapy is phlebotomy (300 to 500 mL at a time to reduce erythrocytosis and blood volume) and low-dose aspirin. Initial phlebotomies are done 2 or 3 times a week until the hematocrit drops sufficiently and repeated every 3 to 4 months to maintain a safe hematocrit level (less than 45%). Aspirin is used for its antithrombotic (decrease in thromboxane) properties.

Hydroxyurea, an antimetabolite that blocks DNA synthesis and reduces vascular cellularity, is the drug of choice for myelosuppression. Unlike other similar drugs, hydroxyurea reduces the risk of thrombotic complications, but does not increase the risk for developing leukemia.[60] Radioactive phosphorus (^{32}P) has been used to suppress erythropoiesis. Its effects may last up to 18 months. Side effects of ^{32}P treatment include suppression of hematopoiesis resulting in anemia, leukopenia, or thrombocytopenia. Acute leukemia also is a side effect, although most often it occurs after 7 or more years of treatment, making this therapy more useful in the elderly.

Interferon-alpha (IFN-α) has been used when other forms of treatment have failed. Interferon inhibits the growth of the abnormal progenitors and inhibits the actions of cytokines that may lead to the development of myelofibrosis. Therapy with IFN-α is complicated by its proinflammatory activities; thus fever, flulike symptoms, and more severe complications are common. IFN-α is not consistently effective in high-risk adult cases, but is considered in individuals who are intolerant to hydroxyurea, younger individuals, and individuals who are pregnant.

Treatment with inhibitors of the *JAK2* pathway has resulted in the reduction of many associated disease symptoms (e.g., thrombosis) and a significant improvement in the quality of life.[61] However, the optimal target defining successful treatment (hematocrit level) and the effects on life span have not yet been determined. Recent studies comparing the effects of phlebotomy or hydroxyurea, or both, concluded that a goal of maintaining a hematocrit of less than 45% was preferable to the goal of 45% to 50%.[62] The lower target goal resulted in a significantly lower rate of death from cardiovascular causes or major thrombotic events.

Survival for 10 to 15 years is common. However, without proper treatment, 50% of individuals with PV die within 18 months of the onset of initial symptoms. The primary cause of death is thrombosis, which is more prevalent in elderly individuals and those with prior vascular complications. Death because of hemorrhage is rare but more common in individuals with high platelet counts and those taking antiplatelet drugs. Conversion to acute myeloid leukemia (AML) occurs spontaneously in 10% of individuals within 15 years, increasing to 50% within 20 years. This leukemia is generally refractory to conventional treatment. Conversion to AML is most likely related to treatment with cytotoxic myelosuppressive agents, such as chlorambucil.[59] Those individuals treated only with IFN-α or hydroxyurea had the same incidence of conversion as those who received no treatment. Although PV is a chronic disorder, appropriate therapy results in remissions and prevention of significant morbidity.

Iron Overload

Iron overload can be primary, as in hereditary hemochromatosis, or secondary. The secondary causes of iron overload include parenteral iron overload in conditions such as anemias with inefficient erythropoiesis (e.g., aplastic anemia), dietary iron overload, or other conditions that require repeated blood transfusions or iron dextran injections.

Hereditary hemochromatosis (HH) is a common inherited, autosomal recessive disorder of iron metabolism and is characterized by increased gastrointestinal iron absorption with subsequent tissue iron deposition. Excess iron is deposited in the liver, pancreas, heart, joints, and endocrine glands, causing tissue damage that can lead to diseases such as cirrhosis, diabetes, heart failure, arthropathies, and impotence.[63]

HH is caused by two genetic base pair alterations, C282Y and H63D. These are mutations in the *HFE* gene on chromosome 6. Homozygosity of C282Y is the most common genotype and accounts for 82% to 90% of HH cases. The remaining cases appear to be caused by environmental factors or other genotypes. *HFE* mutations are common in the United States with 1 in 10 white individuals heterozygous for the *HFE* C282Y mutation and 4.4 in 1000 homozygous for the C282Y mutation. C282Y homozygosity is much lower among Hispanics (0.27 in 1000), Asian Americans (<0.001 per 1000), Pacific Islanders (0.12 per 1000), and blacks (0.14 per 1000).

◆**PATHOPHYSIOLOGY.** Studies in mice have confirmed that the *HFE* gene (high Fe gene) is responsible for the majority of adult form HH. HFE protein, found in the crypt cells of the duodenum, facilitates transferrin receptor–dependent iron uptake into crypt cells. The HFE protein regulates the production of the protein hepcidin, considered the "master" regulator of iron.[64] The C282Y mutation prevents the altered HFE protein from reaching the cell surface, preventing interaction with hepcidin and transferrin receptors. The deficiency results in an increase in the expression of an iron transport protein, divalent metal ion transporter 1 (DMT-1), which is responsible for dietary iron absorption in the villus cells of the small intestine. This inappropriate intestinal iron absorption leads to iron overload and, eventually, end-organ damage that can result in cirrhosis, diabetes mellitus, hypothyroidism, cardiomyopathies, and arthritis.

Although the natural history of HH is emerging, there appears to be a long latent period with individual variation in biochemical expression modified by environmental factors, such as blood loss from menstruation or donation, alcohol intake, and diet. Cirrhosis is a late-stage development of HH that can shorten life expectancy. Cirrhosis also is a risk factor for hepatocellular carcinoma that occurs in individuals between the ages of 40 and 60 years. Cirrhosis prevention is a major goal of HH screening and treatment.

◆**CLINICAL MANIFESTATIONS.** Clinical manifestations of HH include symptoms such as fatigue, malaise, abdominal pain, arthralgias, and sometimes amenorrhea in women and loss of libido or impotence in men. Clinical findings of HH include hepatomegaly, abnormal levels of liver enzymes, bronzed skin, altered glucose homeostasis or diabetes, and cardiac dysfunction (dysrhythmias, cardiomegaly). Many individuals are diagnosed as a result of serum iron studies as part of a health-screening panel. Most individuals (>75%) are asymptomatic and have a low frequency (<25%) of cirrhosis, diabetes, or skin pigmentation.

◆**EVALUATION AND TREATMENT.** Laboratory findings in individuals with HH show elevations in serum iron levels, transferrin saturation, and ferritin levels. Documentation of iron overload relies on quantitative phlebotomy with calculation of the amount of iron removed, or liver biopsy with determination of quantitative hepatic iron. With the advent of genetic testing, no further workup is necessary in individuals who are C282Y homozygous or compound heterozygous, are less than 40 years old, and have normal liver function.

Treatment of HH is simple and consists of phlebotomy of 550 mL of whole blood, which is equivalent to 200 to 250 mg of iron. Frequency of phlebotomy depends on ferritin levels and should continue until the ferritin level is between 20 and 50 ng/mL. Initially, phlebotomy may be needed weekly but once therapeutic ferritin levels are reached, phlebotomy may only be needed every 2 to 3 months. Blood banks now accept blood donations from persons with documented HH. Iron chelating agents are sometimes used in addition to phlebotomy, but this is not the mainstay of treatment. Individuals with HH should be instructed to refrain from taking iron and vitamin C supplements and consuming raw shellfish; in addition, alcohol should be used in moderation. Family screening is recommended and necessary for all first-degree relatives of a person with HH.

ALTERATIONS OF PLATELETS AND COAGULATION

Hemostasis is dependent on adequate numbers of platelets and levels of coagulation factors. Diminished or excessive levels may lead to defective hemostasis or spontaneous and unnecessary activation of clotting. (Hemostasis is described in Chapter 28.) Diminished hemostasis results in either internal or external hemorrhage. Diffuse hemorrhage into skin tissues that is visible through the skin causes a red-purple discoloration identified as a purpura. Purpuric disorders occur when there are not enough normal platelets to plug damaged vessels or prevent leakage from the many minute tears that occur daily in normal capillaries. Disorders of the clotting system tend to result in more serious internal bleeding than platelet defects and are usually caused by a deficiency of one or several clotting factors. Disorders that result in spontaneous clotting can result from genetic disorders of clotting system components or from acquired diseases that activate clotting. These disorders are known collectively as thromboembolic disease.

Disorders of Platelets

Quantitative or qualitative abnormalities of platelets can interrupt normal blood coagulation and prevent hemostasis.[65] The quantitative abnormalities are thrombocytopenia (a decrease in the number of circulating platelets) and thrombocythemia (an increase in the number of platelets). Qualitative disorders affect the structure or function of individual platelets and can coexist with the quantitative disorders. Qualitative disorders usually prevent platelet adherence and aggregation, preventing formation of a platelet plug.

Thrombocytopenia

Thrombocytopenia is defined as a platelet count less than 150,000 platelets/mm^3 of blood, although most healthcare providers do not consider the decrease of significance unless the count falls to less than 100,000 platelets/mm^3.[4] Hemorrhage resulting from minor trauma does not usually occur until the count falls below 50,000/mm^3. Spontaneous bleeding without apparent trauma can occur with counts between 10,000 and 15,000/mm^3, resulting in petechiae, ecchymoses, larger purpuric spots, or frank bleeding from mucous membranes. Severe spontaneous bleeding may result if the count is less than 10,000/mm^3 and can be fatal if it occurs in the gastrointestinal tract, respiratory system, or central nervous system (CNS).

Before the diagnosis of thrombocytopenia is made, **pseudothrombocytopenia** must be ruled out. This phenomenon occurs in approximately 1 in 1000 to 1 in 10,000 laboratory samples and is an in vitro artifact that may occur when a blood sample is analyzed by an automated cell counter. Platelets in the sample may become nonspecifically agglutinated by immunoglobulins in the presence of ethylenediaminetetraacetic acid (EDTA), a preservative in banked blood. The agglutinated platelets are not counted, thus giving an apparent, but false, thrombocytopenia. Thrombocytopenia also may be falsely diagnosed because of a dilutional effect observed after massive transfusion of platelet-poor packed cells to treat a hemorrhage. This occurs when more than 10 units of blood have been transfused within a 24-hour period. The hemorrhage that necessitated the transfusion also accelerates the loss of platelets, which further contributes to the pseudothrombocytopenic state. Splenic sequestering of platelets secondary to hypersplenism (congestive) induces an apparent thrombocytopenia, as does hypothermia (less than 25°C [77°F]), which is reversed when temperatures return to normal, suggesting an increased platelet sequestration in response to chilling.

PATHOPHYSIOLOGY. Thrombocytopenia results from decreased platelet production, increased consumption, or both. The condition also may be congenital or acquired and primary or secondary to other acquired or congenital conditions. Thrombocytopenia secondary to congenital conditions occurs in a large number of different diseases, although each is relatively rare. These include thrombocytopenia with absence of radius (TAR) syndrome, Wiskott-Aldrich syndrome (see Chapter 9), various forms of *MYH9* gene mutation (e.g., May-Hegglin syndrome), X-linked thrombocytopenia, and many other examples.

Acquired thrombocytopenia is more common and may occur as a result of decreased platelet production secondary to viral infections (e.g., EBV, rubella, cytomegalovirus [CMV], HIV), drugs (e.g., thiazides, estrogens, quinine-containing medications, chemotherapeutic agents, ethanol), nutritional deficiencies (vitamin B$_{12}$ or folic acid in particular), chronic renal failure, bone marrow hypoplasia (e.g., aplastic anemia), radiation therapy, or bone marrow infiltration by cancer. Most common forms of thrombocytopenia are the result of increased platelet consumption. Examples include heparin-induced thrombocytopenia, idiopathic (immune) thrombocytopenic purpura, and thrombotic thrombocytopenic purpura.

Heparin-Induced Thrombocytopenia. Heparin is a common cause of drug-induced thrombocytopenia. Approximately 4% of individuals treated with unfractionated heparin develop **heparin-induced thrombocytopenia (HIT)**. The incidence is lower (about 0.1%) with the use of low-molecular-weight heparin. HIT is an immune-mediated, adverse drug reaction caused by IgG antibodies against the heparin–platelet factor 4 complex leading to platelet activation through platelet FcγIIa receptors (Fig. 29.9).[66] The release of additional platelet factor

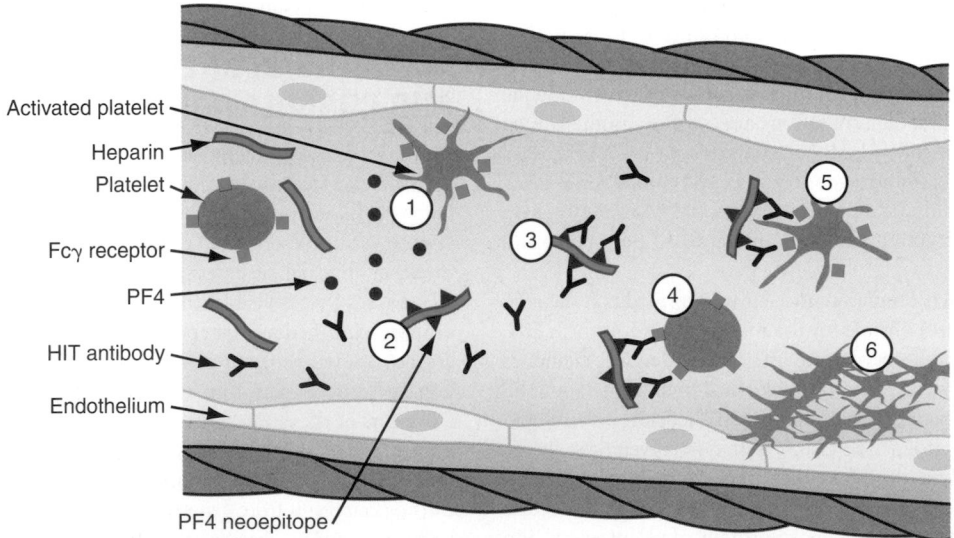

FIGURE 29.9 Pathogenesis of Heparin-Induced Thrombocytopenia (HIT). **(1)** Activated platelets release procoagulant proteins from α-granules, including platelet factor 4 *(PF4)*. Administered heparin binds PF4 **(2),** which undergoes a conformational change and expresses a new antigen (neoepitope). Individuals with HIT produce an immunoglobulin G (IgG) antibody that specifically reacts **(3)** with multiple identical neoepitopes on the heparin-PF4 complex. The reaction forms heparin-PF4-IgG immune complexes. Platelets express FcγRIIa receptors (Fcγ receptor) that react **(4)** with the Fc portion of IgG in immune complexes. Cross-linking of Fc receptors **(5)** results in FcγRIIa-dependent platelet activation. The activated platelets mediate a series of events that lead to further activation of the coagulation cascade, resulting in thrombin generation. Further release of PF4 from newly activated platelets leads to a cycle of continuing platelet activation and **(6)** formation of a primary clot. The reaction can be enhanced by the release of platelet-derived microparticles that are rich in surface phosphatidylserine and increase activation of coagulation and by the binding of heparin-PF4 complexes and HIT-IgG to the vascular endothelium (not shown).

4 from activated platelets and activation of thrombin lead to increased platelet consumption and a decrease in platelet counts beginning 5 to 10 days after administration of heparin.

◆**CLINICAL MANIFESTATIONS.** The hallmark of HIT is thrombocytopenia. A decrease of approximately 50% in the platelet count is seen in more than 95% of individuals. However, 30% or more of those with thrombocytopenia also are at risk for venous or arterial thrombosis.[66] Venous thrombosis is most common and results in deep venous thrombosis and pulmonary emboli. Arterial thromboses affect the large arteries of the lower extremities, causing acute limb ischemia. Arterial thrombosis also may lead to cerebrovascular accidents and myocardial infarctions. Other major arteries (renal, mesenteric, upper limb) also may be affected. Bleeding is uncommon in HIT, even with low platelet counts.

◆**EVALUATION AND TREATMENT.** Diagnosis is primarily based on clinical observations.[67] The individual presents with dropping platelet counts after 5 days or longer of heparin treatment. On average, platelet counts may reach 60,000/mm^3. Because most individuals are postsurgery and the onset of symptoms, including thrombosis, may be delayed until after release from the hospital, other possible causes of thrombocytopenia (e.g., infection, other drug reactions) must be considered.

Tests are available to measure antibodies against heparin–platelet factor 4.[68] The test sensitivity is extremely high (more than 90%), but the specificity is less because of false-positive reactions (e.g., those on dialysis). HIT antibody titers may be measured, but the titers must be evaluated in the context of the clinical presentation. If HIT is not recognized and treated, intravascular aggregation of platelets causes rapid development of arterial and venous thrombosis. Although rare, heparin antibodies have caused anaphylactic shock.

Treatment is the withdrawal of heparin and use of alternative anticoagulants. A switch to low-molecular-weight heparin is not indicated, and warfarin should not be used until the symptoms of HIT have resolved because of an increased risk of initiating skin necrosis. The thrombocytopenia should progressively resolve. The chance of spontaneous blood clots can be diminished using thrombin inhibitors (e.g., lepirudin, argatroban).[67]

Immune Thrombocytopenic Purpura. The most common cause of thrombocytopenia secondary to increased platelet destruction is immune thrombocytopenic purpura (ITP). The incidence of ITP is estimated to be 5.8 to 6.6 per 100,000 in the general population. ITP was formerly known as *idiopathic thrombocytopenic purpura;* however, it is widely recognized now as an immune process, hence the change from idiopathic to immune.[69] ITP may be acute or chronic. The acute form is frequently observed in children and typically lasts 1 to 2 months with a complete remission. In some instances it may last for up to 6 months, and some children (7% to 28%) may progress to the chronic condition. Acute ITP is usually secondary to infections (particularly viral) or other conditions that lead to large amounts of antigen in the blood, such as drug allergies or systemic lupus erythematosus (SLE) (see Chapter 9). Under these conditions the antigen usually forms immune complexes with circulating antibody, and it is thought that the immune complexes bind to Fc receptors on platelets, leading to their destruction in the spleen. The acute form of ITP usually resolves as the source of antigen is removed (e.g., the viral infection resolves).

Chronic ITP is associated with autoantibodies against platelet-specific antigens. This form is more commonly observed in adults, with the highest prevalence in women between 20 and 40 years old, although it can develop at most any age. The chronic form tends to get progressively worse.

The autoantibodies are generally of the IgG class, although IgA and IgM antibodies also have been identified. They react against one or more of several platelet glycoproteins (e.g., GPIIb/IIIa, GPIb/IX, GPIa/

IIa)[70] (see Chapter 28). The antibody-coated platelets are removed from the circulation by mononuclear phagocytes in the spleen through the Fc receptor.

◆**CLINICAL MANIFESTATIONS.** Initial manifestations are usually minor bleeding problems (development of petechiae and purpura) that occur over the course of several days and progress to major hemorrhage from mucosal sites (epistaxis, hematuria, menorrhagia, bleeding gums). Rarely will an individual present with intracranial bleeding or internal bleeding at other sites.

During pregnancy, an individual with ITP may have a newborn that is also thrombocytopenic. In most individuals the antiplatelet antibody is an IgG that readily crosses the placenta (see Chapters 8 and 9). If the fetal platelets express the same antigen as the mother, the maternal antibody will coat the platelets, potentially resulting in thrombocytopenia in utero. A variant of neonatal thrombocytopenia (neonatal alloimmune thrombocytopenia) occurs when the mother does not have ITP, but makes IgG antibodies against an antigen inherited from the father and found on fetal platelets but not on maternal platelets.[70] Alloimmune neonatal thrombocytopenia occurs in 1 of 2000 pregnancies. The most common antibody in this condition is against the human platelet antigen-a (HPA-a) antigen on the GPIIIa protein. Neonatal thrombocytopenia, either secondary to maternal autoimmune thrombocytopenia or as alloimmune thrombocytopenia, may occur to various degrees. The most severe form results in fetal platelet counts below 20,000/mm^3 with a high associated risk of intracranial hemorrhage.

◆**EVALUATION AND TREATMENT.** Diagnosis of ITP is based on a history of bleeding and associated symptoms, such as weight loss, fever, and headache. Physical examination includes notations on the types of bleeding, location, and severity. Assessment includes determination of a history of infections (bacteria, HIV, and other viruses) as well as medication history and family history; evidence of thrombosis also is assessed. Diagnostic tests include complete blood count (CBC) and peripheral blood smear. Unlike some other forms of thrombocytopenia, splenectomy is rarely observed. Testing for antiplatelet antibodies is usually not helpful. Although most cases of ITP are associated with elevated levels of IgG on platelets, other forms of thrombocytopenia also have a high incidence of platelet-associated antibodies; thus the specificity is low (50% to 65%).[71] In addition, some cases of ITP will not present with elevated platelet-associated antibodies; the sensitivity is 75% to 94%, so that a negative test does not completely rule out ITP.

The acute form of ITP usually resolves without major clinical consequences. As with most autoimmune diseases, the course of the chronic form is variable, with multiple remissions and exacerbations. For many individuals the platelet count may remain adequate enough to avoid clinically serious bleeding. However, the presence of spontaneous bleeding suggests more severe disease and requires immediate attention. Treatment is initiated when platelet counts are less than 30,000/mm^3 or less than 50,000/mm^3 with evidence of bleeding from mucous membranes or when the individual is at high risk to develop bleeding.

Treatment is palliative, not curative, focusing on prevention of platelet destruction. Initial therapy for ITP is infusion of glucocorticoids (e.g., prednisone), which suppresses the production of antiplatelet antibodies and prevents sequestering and further destruction of platelets. If platelet counts do not increase appropriately, other medications may be tried. Treatment with intravenous immunoglobulin (IVIG) is used to prevent major bleeding. The response rate is 80%, but the effects are transient, lasting only days or a few weeks. Anti-Rh$_o$(D) immune globulin (anti-D), which is a preparation of antibody against the D antigen of the Rh blood group, has been used with limited success to treat individuals who are Rh-positive.

Newer treatments include romiplostim (trade name Nplate) and eltrombopag (trade name Promacta in the United States, Revolade in the European Union). Both drugs are thrombopoiesis-stimulating Fc-peptide fusion proteins (peptibody). Romiplostim is administered subcutaneously and eltrombopag is taken orally. These drugs increase platelet counts and decrease bleeding. Romiplostim is often used as a second-line treatment after IVIG or in individuals who experience relapse postsplenectomy.

If all other therapies are ineffective, splenectomy is considered to remove the primary site of platelet destruction.[72] The response rate (resolution of the thrombocytopenia) is 60% to 70%; however, the procedure is not without risk. Approximately 10% to 20% of individuals who undergo splenectomy suffer a relapse and require further treatment. It is thought that other reticuloendothelial organs, particularly the liver, can become major sites for platelet destruction. If splenectomy is unsuccessful and life-threatening thrombocytopenia persists, more aggressive immunosuppressive medications (e.g., azathioprine, cyclophosphamide) may be used. Because of potential major complications, these medications are reserved for individuals who are severely thrombocytopenic and refractory to other therapies.

Thrombotic Thrombocytopenic Purpura. Thrombotic thrombocytopenic purpura (TTP; also known as Moschcowitz disease) is characterized by the concomitant occurrence of often severe thrombocytopenia and thrombotic microangiopathy in which platelets aggregate and cause occlusion of arterioles and capillaries within the microcirculation[73,74] (Fig. 29.10). Aggregation may lead to increased platelet consumption and organ ischemia, particularly in the brain, heart, and kidneys.[73]

TTP is relatively uncommon, occurring in about 5 per 1 million individuals per year. The incidence is increasing, which appears to be an actual increase in the number of affected individuals rather than a result of improved recognition. There are two forms of TTP: familial or acquired idiopathic. The familial form is more rare and is usually chronic, relapsing, and is seen in children. The child experiences predictable recurring episodes at approximately 3-week intervals that are responsive to treatment. Acquired TTP is more common, as well as more acute and severe. It occurs mostly in females in their thirties and is rarely observed in infants or older adults.

Platelet aggregation and microthrombi formation are found throughout the entire vascular system, causing damage to multiple organs.

Although the organs most susceptible to damage are the kidney, brain, and heart, other organs often affected are the pancreas, spleen, and adrenal glands. The thrombi are primarily composed of platelets with minimal fibrin and red cells, differentiating them from thrombi secondary to intravascular coagulation. Most cases of TTP are related to a decrease or dysfunction of the plasma disintegrin and metalloprotease ADAMTS13[73] (see Fig. 29.10). This enzyme is responsible for digesting large precursor molecules of von Willebrand factor (vWF), which is produced by endothelial cells, into smaller molecules. A lack of ADAMTS13 enzyme activity alters the balance between bleeding and clotting.[75] Decreases or defects in ADAMTS13 result in expression of large-molecular-weight vWF on the endothelial cell surface and formation of large aggregates of platelets. The aggregates may detach and form occlusions in smaller vessels. Most individuals with TTP (about 80%) have less than 5% of normal plasma ADAMTS13 levels. TTP also is commonly associated with an IgG autoantibody against ADAMTS13 that is able to neutralize the enzyme's activity and accelerate its clearance from the plasma.

◆**CLINICAL MANIFESTATIONS.** The rare familial chronic relapsing TTP observed in children is usually recognized and successfully treated. The acquired acute idiopathic TTP is much more common and more severe.[74] Early diagnosis and treatment are important because the disease may be fatal within 90 days of onset. TTP is clinically related to and must be distinguished from other thrombotic microangiopathic conditions, including hemolytic uremic syndrome, malignant hypertension, preeclampsia, or the pregnancy-induced HELLP (hemolysis, elevated liver enzymes, low platelet count) syndrome. Hemolytic uremic syndrome (HUS) shares many of the clinical characteristics of TTP; however, HUS often follows a hemorrhagic, diarrheal illness.

◆**EVALUATION AND TREATMENT.** Acute idiopathic TTP is characterized by a "pathognomonic pentad" of symptoms. However, only 20% to 30% of people present with the classic pentad. These include extreme thrombocytopenia (less than 20,000 platelets/mm³), intravascular hemolytic anemia, ischemic signs and symptoms most often involving the CNS (about 65% present with memory disturbances, behavioral irregularities, headaches, or coma), kidney failure (affecting about 65% of individuals), and fever (present in about 33% of individuals with

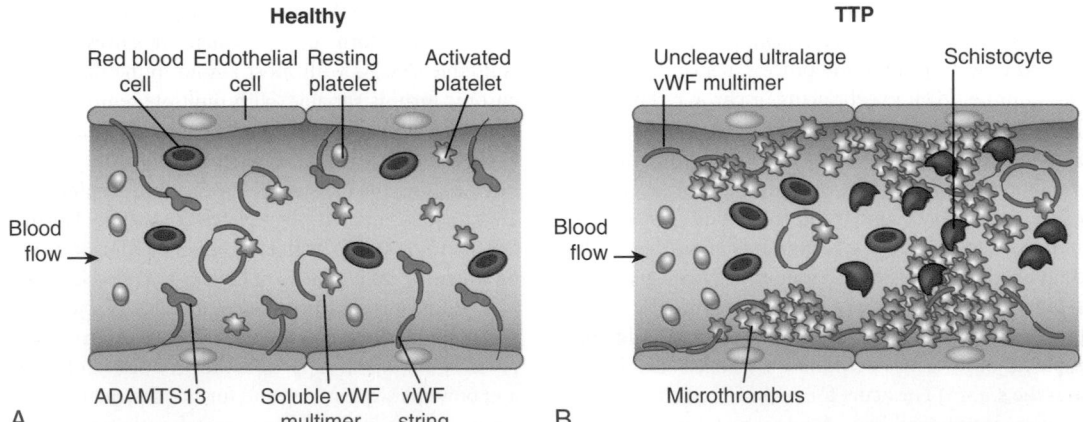

FIGURE 29.10 Thrombotic Thrombocytopenic Purpura. **A,** A microvessel (arteriole or capillary) in a healthy individual. Normal proteolysis by ADAMTS13 of ultralarge von Willebrand factor *(vWF)* strings anchored to or secreted from stimulated microvascular endothelial cells. **B,** A microvessel in thrombotic thrombocytopenic purpura *(TTP).* Cleavage of secreted or anchored ultralarge vWF is severely reduced when ADAMTS13 activity is less than 10% of normal level. The results include excessive microthrombi formation, shear stress injury to red blood cells (schistocytes) flowing through microvessels that are partially occluded by platelet clumps (producing hemolysis), and perhaps damage from activation of the alternative complement pathway on the uncleaved ultralarge vWF strings. (From Kremer Hovinga JA et al: *Nat Rev Dis Primers* 3:17020, 2017.)

TTP).[74] It is not mandatory that all five be present to begin treatment. A routine blood smear usually reveals fragmented red cells (*schizocytes; schistocytes*) produced by shear forces when red cells are in contact with the fibrin mesh in clots that form in the vessels. As a result of tissue injury, serum levels of lactate dehydrogenase (LDH) may be very high, and low-density lipoprotein (LDL) levels may be elevated. Tests for antibody on red cells are negative, excluding immune hemolytic anemia.

Untreated acute TTP has a death rate of 90%, which can be reduced to 10% to 20% with prompt treatment. Plasma exchange with fresh frozen plasma replenishes functional ADAMTS13 and is the treatment of choice, achieving a response rate of 70% to 85%. Additionally, steroids (glucocorticoids) are administered. In the absence of major organ damage, this approach may lead to complete recovery with no long-term complications. The anti-CD20 monocolonal antibody rituximab has shown some activity in people who are refractory to plasma exchange.[76] Caplacizumab, an anti-vWF, has demonstrated platelet-protective effects and an increased tendency toward bleeding as compared to placebo.[77] Relapses do occur at a rate of 13% to 36%, and recurrences have been reported, some as far out as 9 years. Individuals who do not respond to conventional treatment may be candidates for splenectomy; however, postoperative hemorrhage remains a dangerous complication. Immunosuppressive (azathioprine) therapy has been successful in some individuals.

Thrombocythemia

Thrombocythemia (also called thrombocytosis) is defined as a platelet count greater than 450,000/mm^3 of blood.[78] Thrombocythemia may be primary or secondary (reactive) and is usually asymptomatic until the count exceeds 1 million/mm^3 of blood. Then intravascular clot formation (thrombosis), hemorrhage, or other abnormalities can occur.

◆**PATHOPHYSIOLOGY.** Secondary thrombocythemia may occur after splenectomy because platelets that normally would be stored in the spleen remain in circulating blood. The increase in platelets may be gradual, with thrombocythemia not occurring for up to 3 weeks after splenectomy. Reactive thrombocythemia may occur from infections and during some inflammatory conditions, such as rheumatoid arthritis and cancers. In these conditions, excessive production of some cytokines (e.g., IL-6, IL-11) may induce increased production of thrombopoietin in the liver, resulting in increased megakaryocyte proliferation. Reactive thrombocythemia also may occur during a variety of physiologic conditions, such as after exercise. Because of the relatively self-resolving nature of secondary thrombocythemia, the remaining discussion will focus on the more severe primary form.

Essential (primary) thrombocythemia (ET) is a chronic myeloproliferative disorder characterized by excessive platelet production resulting from a defect in bone marrow megakaryocyte progenitor cells.[79] The overall incidence of ET is 0.8 per 100,000 in the United Kingdom, 2.53 in the United States, and 0.59 in Denmark. It is more common in middle-age individuals, with the majority of cases occurring between ages 50 and 60 years. There is no known gender preference. There also is a rare hereditary type of ET called *familial essential thrombocythemia (FET)* that is inherited in an autosomal dominant pattern.

The thrombocythemia is secondary to increased plasma thrombopoietin levels resulting from defects in the thrombopoietin receptor. The defective receptor cannot adequately bind and remove thrombopoietin from the blood; thus circulating levels remain high. Along with increased platelet levels, there may be a concomitant increase in the level of red cells, indicating a myeloproliferative disorder; however, the increase in red cell level is not to the extent seen in polycythemia vera. The bone marrow of affected individuals with ET is characterized by hyperplasia of megakaryocytes. The platelets of affected individuals appear to have a normal survival time, compatible with a defect in production rather than an increase in platelet life span.

RBCs in ET tend to aggregate and contribute to the blockage of flow in the microvasculature and altered interactions between platelets and the vascular endothelium.[80] Increased adherence of erythrocytes to the endothelium appears to result from a mutation in an erythrocyte Janus kinase 2 gene *(JAK2)* that is responsible for phosphorylation of the erythrocyte receptor for endothelial laminin.[81,82] The frequency of *JAK2* mutations in ET is about 30%. Increased platelet aggregation arises from several mutations that result in altered platelet membrane glycoproteins, particularly resulting in increased expression of GPIV, and increased secretion of thromboxane.

◆**CLINICAL MANIFESTATIONS.** Clinical manifestations vary significantly among individuals. Those with ET are at risk for large-vessel arterial or venous thrombosis, although the most common complication is microvasculature thrombosis leading to ischemia in the fingers, toes, or cerebrovascular regions.[80] The primary presenting symptoms of microvasculature thrombosis are erythromelalgia, headache, and paresthesias. Erythromelalgia is characterized by unilateral or bilateral warm, congested, red hands and feet with painful burning sensations, particularly in the forefoot sole and one or more toes. The lower extremities are affected more often, and only one side may be involved. The pain is initiated by standing, exercise, or warmth and relieved by elevation and cooling. In extreme situations, acrocyanosis and gangrene may result.

Arterial thrombosis is more common than venous thrombosis and may involve the coronary and renal arteries. The carotid, mesenteric, and subclavian arteries also may be affected. Myocardial ischemia and infarction have occurred without clear evidence of coronary artery disease. Deep venous thrombosis of the lower extremities and pulmonary embolism are the major sites for venous involvement. Common sites of intraabdominal venous thrombosis are in the portal and hepatic circulation. People older than 60 years of age or those with prior history of thrombotic events have as much as a 25% chance of developing a cerebral, cardiac, or peripheral arterial thrombus. Conversion to acute leukemia is found in less than 10% of affected individuals.[83]

Microvascular thrombosis in the CNS is usually associated with headache and dizziness, with paresthesias, transient ischemic attacks, strokes, visual disturbances, and seizures also being reported. Major thrombotic events, not directly related to the platelet count, occur in about 20% to 30% of individuals with ET. Prior history of thrombotic events, advanced age, and duration of thrombocytosis are predictors of future thrombotic complications. Individuals older than age 60 are at greatest risk.

Although thrombosis is the most common symptom, hemorrhage can also occur. Sites for bleeding include the GI tract, skin, mucous membranes, urinary tract, gums, tooth sockets (after extraction), joints, eyes, and brain. GI bleeding may be mistaken for a duodenal ulcer. Hemorrhage is not severe and generally occurs in the presence of very high platelet counts, occasionally requiring transfusion. It is important to recognize that bleeding and clotting may exist simultaneously and individuals will not necessarily be "bleeders" or "clotters."

◆**EVALUATION AND TREATMENT.** Initial diagnosis is not difficult; as many as two-thirds of affected individuals are diagnosed from a routine CBC. Secondary thrombocytosis may present as a moderate rise in the platelet count that resolves with treatment or resolution of the underlying condition. The World Health Organization (WHO) criteria for the diagnosis of ET require the following four conditions be met: (1) sustained platelet count of at least 450 × 10^9/L; (2) bone marrow biopsy showing proliferation of enlarged mature megakaryocytes and no increase of granulocyte or erythrocyte precursors; (3) person does not meet the criteria of polycythemia vera, myelofibrosis, chronic myeloid leukemia (CML), or other myelodysplastic syndrome; and (4) presence of *JAK2*^{V617F} or another clonal marker or evidence of reactive thrombocytosis.[84]

After diagnosis, these individuals may recall events related to thrombosis or hemorrhage. Manifestations of ET may be mistaken for CML; therefore differentiation of the two is important because treatment varies significantly. Identification of the Philadelphia chromosome is recommended in all cases of ET.

Treatment of ET is directed toward preventing thrombosis or hemorrhage.[85] The reduction of platelet count remains a significant treatment issue. Historically, treatment of ET relied on the use of alkylating agents (busulfan) or radiophosphorus (^{32}P) to suppress platelet production. Hydroxyurea, a nonalkylating myelosuppressive agent, has been the drug of choice to suppress platelet production; however, long-term use may cause progression to other myelodysplastic disorders, particularly AML or myelofibrosis.[85] Conversion to myelofibrosis occurs approximately 8% of the time and conversion to AML occurs approximately 3.5% of the time when treated with hydroxyurea as a single cytotoxic agent, but increases to 14% when more than one cytotoxic agent is used.

Interferon (IFN) also may be used and has a response rate of 80%. IFN may not work for everyone because it has many side effects and 20% of individuals may be intolerant. Anagrelide is now considered to be the drug of choice. Anagrelide specifically interferes with platelet maturation rather than production, thus not affecting erythropoiesis or leukopoiesis.

Aspirin also is used in the treatment of ET; however, its action is not to reduce the platelet count but to prevent adherence of platelets to each other and prevent thrombus formation. Early studies with aspirin found hemorrhage to be a major contraindication for its use; however, in lower doses (80 to 160 mg/daily) it effectively alleviates erythromelalgia and transient neurologic manifestations. Vitamin K antagonists (VKAs) are used for secondary prevention of thrombosis in those with ET.[86]

Prognosis and survival of individuals with ET have been somewhat difficult to establish. ET is not necessarily considered life-threatening; however, in persons who are older than age 60 and have a history of previous incidences of thrombosis, complications are more common and have a higher risk of mortality.

Alterations of Platelet Function

Qualitative alterations in platelet function occur with an increased bleeding time in the presence of a normal platelet count. Associated clinical manifestations include spontaneous petechiae and purpura and bleeding from the GI tract, genitourinary tract, pulmonary mucosa, and gums. Congenital alterations in platelet function (thrombocytopathies) are quite rare and may be categorized into several types of disorders: (1) platelet–vessel wall adhesion, (2) platelet-platelet interactions, (3) platelet granules and secretion, (4) arachidonic acid pathways, and (5) membrane phospholipid regulation (coagulation protein–platelet interactions).[87]

Disorders of platelet–vascular wall adhesion result from aberrations of the platelet membrane glycoprotein GPIb/IX/V (Bernard-Soulier syndrome), anomalies of the collagen receptor GPVI, or deficiencies of vWF. The GPIb protein is the most commonly mutated protein in individuals with Bernard-Soulier syndrome. Lack of these proteins prevents platelets from adhering to collagen, resulting in impaired hemostasis and clinical hemorrhage.

Disorders of platelet-platelet interactions result in failure of platelets to aggregate in response to adenosine diphosphate (ADP), collagen, epinephrine, or thrombin because of a deficiency in the glycoprotein (αIIbβ_3) that acts as a receptor for fibrinogen, vWF, and fibronectin (Glanzmann thrombasthenia). Lack of this glycol protein results in a failure to build "fibrinogen bridges" between platelets (see Fig. 28.21). Defects also can occur in platelet receptors for platelet activators. These include mutations in the receptors for thromboxane or ADP.

Disorders of platelet granules and secretion and disorders of arachidonic pathways are characterized by initial normal platelet aggregation with collagen or ADP; however, subsequent processes fail, specifically secretion of prostaglandins and release of granules. Defective α-granule numbers or release (gray platelet syndrome) results from mutations in several aspects of granule function, including biosynthesis or loading of proteins normally found in these granules. Defects in dense granules include Hermansky-Pudlak syndrome, Chédiak-Higashi syndrome, and delta-storage pool disease. These usually result from mutations in proteins involved in formation of dense granules or their movement to the plasma membrane. Defects in the thromboxane pathway prevent the release of this mediator.

Externalization of plasma membrane phosphatidylserine (PS) is necessary for effective platelet function. In Scott syndrome, the enzyme responsible for PS efflux is defective; thus platelets are unable to support the activation of factor X and prothrombin. The reverse of Scott syndrome is Stormorken syndrome, in which platelets constitutively externalize PS.

Acquired disorders of platelet function are more common than the congenital disorders and may be categorized into three principal causes: (1) drug effects, (2) systemic inflammatory conditions, and (3) hematologic conditions.

Multiple drugs are known to affect platelet function in several ways: inhibition of platelet membrane receptors, inhibition of prostaglandin pathways, and inhibition of phosphodiesterase activity. Aspirin is the most commonly used drug that affects platelets and the only drug specifically used for its platelet effects. It irreversibly inhibits cyclooxygenase function for several days after administration. Nonsteroidal antiinflammatory drugs also affect cyclooxygenase, although in a reversible fashion.

Systemic disorders that affect platelet function are chronic renal disease, liver disease, cardiopulmonary bypass surgery, severe deficiencies of iron or folate, and the presence of antiplatelet antibodies associated with autoimmune disorders. Hematologic disorders that cause platelet dysfunction are chronic myeloproliferative disorders, multiple myeloma, leukemias, myelodysplastic syndromes, and dysproteinemias.

Disorders of Coagulation

Disorders of coagulation usually are caused by defects or deficiencies of one or more of the clotting factors. (Normal function of the clotting factors is described in Chapter 28.) Qualitative or quantitative abnormalities of clotting factors interfere with or prevent the enzymatic reactions that transform circulating clotting proteins into a stable fibrin clot (see Fig. 28.22).

Some clotting factor defects are inherited and usually involve a single factor, such as hemophilias and von Willebrand disease, caused by deficiencies of specific clotting factors (see Chapter 31). Other coagulation defects are acquired and tend to result from deficient synthesis of clotting factors by the liver. Causes include liver disease and dietary deficiency of vitamin K.

Other coagulation disorders are attributed to pathologic conditions that trigger coagulation inappropriately. For example, any cardiovascular abnormality that alters normal blood flow by accelerating, decelerating, or obstructing it can result in spontaneous coagulation within the vessels. Coagulation is also stimulated by the presence of tissue factor, which is released by damaged or dead tissues. Vasculitis, or inflammation of the blood vessels, as well as vessel damage, activates platelets, which in turn activates the coagulation cascade. In extensive or prolonged vasculitis, blood clot formation can suppress mechanisms that normally control clot formation and breakdown, leading to clogging of the vessels. In each of these acquired conditions, normal hemostatic function proves detrimental to the body by consuming coagulation factors excessively or by overwhelming the normal control of clot formation and breakdown (fibrinolysis).

Impaired Hemostasis

Impaired hemostasis, or the inability to promote coagulation and the development of a stable fibrin clot, is commonly associated with liver disorders, resulting either from the lack of vitamin K or from specific diseases of the liver.

Vitamin K Deficiency. Vitamin K, a fat-soluble vitamin, is necessary for synthesis and regulation of prothrombin, procoagulant factors (VII, IX, X), and anticoagulant regulators (proteins C and S) within the liver.[88] Vitamin K is found in green leafy vegetables, which is its primary dietary source. Vitamin K also is synthesized by intestinal flora, but its contribution to the overall supply of vitamin K is uncertain. The most common cause of vitamin K deficiency is parenteral nutrition in combination with broad-spectrum antibiotics that destroy normal gut flora. Rarely is a deficiency caused by lack of dietary intake; however, bulimia can suppress vitamin K–dependent activity. Clinical manifestations of vitamin K deficiency are caused by a reduction of vitamin K–dependent proteins. The severity of manifestations is related to the degree of deficiency and ranges from laboratory abnormalities to significant hemorrhage.

Parenteral administration of vitamin K is the treatment of choice and usually results in correction of the deficiency. Improvement of clotting tests is usually noted within 8 to 12 hours. Fresh frozen plasma may be administered but usually is reserved for individuals with life-threatening hemorrhages or who require emergency surgery.

Liver Disease. Individuals who have liver disease (e.g., acute or chronic hepatocellular diseases, cirrhosis, vitamin K deficiency) or major liver surgery present with a broad range of hemostasis derangements that may be characterized by defects in the clotting or fibrinolytic systems or in platelet function.[88] The hepatic parenchymal cells produce most of the factors involved in hemostasis. Thus damage to the liver frequently results in diminished production of factors involved in clotting, usually in proportion to the degree of hepatic parenchymal cell damage. For instance, factor VII is most sensitive to liver damage because of its rapid turnover. Factor IX levels are less affected and do not decline until liver destruction is well advanced. The liver is also a major site for production of plasminogen and α_2-antiplasmin of the fibrinolytic system, as well as thrombopoietin and the metalloprotease ADAMTS13. Diminished levels of thrombopoietin may lead to thrombocytopenia from decreased platelet production. Decreased production of ADAMTS13 results in increased levels of large precursor molecules of vWF, which leads to the formation of large aggregates of platelets.

In conditions of severe liver disease (e.g., cirrhosis), circulating levels of most clotting factors are significantly depressed. Concurrently, production of clotting system regulators (e.g., antithrombin, protein C, protein S) and of fibrinogen is diminished. The fibrinolytic system is commonly active because of decreased levels of plasmin inhibitor and unaffected levels of fibrinolytic activators (e.g., tissue plasminogen activator [tPA], urokinase-like plasminogen activator [uPA]). The affected individuals also are thrombocytopenic because of diminished production of thrombopoietin and ADAMTS13, as well as increased platelet sequestration in the spleen, which is frequently enlarged in cirrhosis and is associated with portal hypertension. Thus individuals with cirrhosis may appear to have a condition similar to DIC (see Consumptive Thrombohemorrhagic Disorders).

Treatment of hemostatic alterations in liver disease must be comprehensive to cover all aspects related to platelet, clotting, and fibrinolytic dysfunctions. Fresh frozen plasma administration is the treatment of choice, but not all individuals tolerate the volume needed to adequately replace all deficient factors. Alternative modalities include the addition of exchange transfusions and platelet concentration to plasma administration.

Consumptive Thrombohemorrhagic Disorders

Consumptive thrombohemorrhagic disorders are a heterogeneous group of conditions that demonstrate the entire range of hemorrhagic and thrombotic pathologic conditions. Symptoms range from subtle to devastating and generally are considered to be intermediary disease processes that complicate many primary disease states. These disorders also are characterized by confusion and controversy regarding diagnosis, treatment, and management. No one definition can cover all possible varieties of these disorders; however, disseminated intravascular coagulation is the most common term used in the clinical setting to describe a pathologic condition associated with hemorrhage and thrombosis.

Disseminated Intravascular Coagulation. Disseminated intravascular coagulation (DIC) is an acquired clinical syndrome characterized by widespread activation of coagulation resulting in formation of fibrin clots in medium and small vessels (microvasculature) throughout the body. Disseminated clotting may lead to blockage of blood flow to organs, resulting in multiple organ failure. The magnitude of clotting may result in consumption of platelets and clotting factors leading to severe bleeding. The Subcommittee on DIC of the International Society on Thrombosis and Haemostasis (ISTH) defined DIC as "An acquired syndrome characterized by the intravascular activation of coagulation with loss of localization arising from different causes. It can originate from and cause damage to the microvasculature, which if sufficiently severe, can produce organ dysfunction."[89] The ISTH has contributed to defining better criteria and clinical management strategies.[90]

The clinical course of DIC largely is determined by the intensity of the stimulus, host response, and comorbidities, and it ranges from an acute, severe, life-threatening process that is characterized by massive hemorrhage and thrombosis to a chronic low-grade condition. The chronic condition is characterized by subacute hemorrhage and diffuse microcirculatory thrombosis. DIC may be localized to one specific organ or generalized, involving multiple organs.

Because of the complexity and wide variations in manifestations of DIC, diagnosis has been challenging. Diagnostic criteria have been established and include a systemic thrombohemorrhagic disorder with laboratory evidence of (1) clotting activation, (2) fibrinolytic activation, (3) coagulation inhibitor consumption, and (4) biochemical evidence of end-organ damage or failure.

DIC is secondary to a wide variety of well-defined clinical conditions, specifically those capable of activating the clotting cascade (Box 29.3). These include (1) arterial hypotension, frequently accompanying shock; (2) hypoxemia; (3) acidemia; and (4) stasis of capillary blood flow.

Sepsis is the most common condition associated with DIC. Gram-negative microorganisms (as well as some gram-positive microorganisms), fungi, protozoa (malaria), and viruses (influenza, herpes) are capable of precipitating DIC by causing damage to vascular endothelium. Gram-negative endotoxins are the primary cause of endothelial damage; DIC may occur in up to 50% of individuals with gram-negative sepsis. DIC occurs in approximately 10% to 20% of individuals with metastatic cancer or acute leukemia. Direct tissue damage (ischemia and necrosis, surgical manipulation, crushing injury) also results in release of tissue factor (TF) by the endothelium. Severe trauma, especially to the brain, can induce DIC. DIC occurs in about two-thirds of individuals with a systemic inflammatory response to trauma. Some complications of pregnancy also are associated with DIC; incidence ranges from 50% for women with placental abruptions to less than 10% for severe preeclampsia. Other causes of DIC have been identified, most notably blood transfusion. Transfused blood dilutes the clotting factors, as well as circulating naturally occurring antithrombins. In hemolytic transfusion reactions, the endothelium is damaged by complement-mediated reactions.

BOX 29.3   CLINICAL CONDITIONS ASSOCIATED WITH DISSEMINATED INTRAVASCULAR COAGULATION

SEPSIS OR SEVERE INFECTION
Potentially from any microorganism, including malaria

TRAUMA
Serious head injury
Head injury
Fat metabolism
Burns

LIVER DISEASES
Fulminant hepatitis
Severe liver cirrhosis

HEAT STROKE

ORGAN DESTRUCTION
Severe pancreatitis

MALIGNANCY
Solid tumors
Hematologic cancers

OBSTETRIC CALAMITIES
Preeclampsia or eclampsia
Placental abruption

Amniotic fluid embolism
HELLP (hemolysis, elevated liver enzymes, and low platelet count) syndrome
Acute fatty liver
Sepsis during pregnancy

VASCULAR ABNORMALITIES
Hemangioma
Leaking or ruptured aneurysm (such as in the aorta)
Aortic aneurysm
Kasabach-Merritt syndrome
Other vascular malformations

SEVERE TOXIC OR IMMUNOLOGIC REACTIONS
Snake bite
Recreational drug use
Severe transfusion reaction
Transplant rejection

Data from Gando S, Levi M, Toh CH: *Nat Rev Dis Primers* 2:16037, 2016.

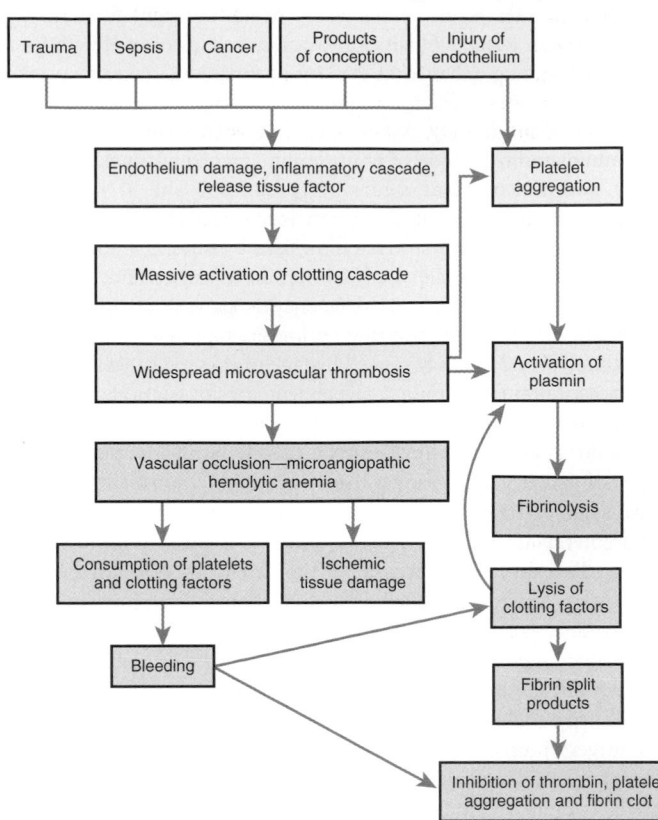

Disseminated Intravascular Coagulation (DIC)

FIGURE 29.11 Pathophysiology of Disseminated Intravascular Coagulation. See text.

◆ PATHOPHYSIOLOGY. The coagulation system is designed to function at local areas of vascular damage, resulting in cessation of bleeding and activation of repair to the vessels. DIC results from abnormally widespread and ongoing activation of clotting (Fig. 29.11). A variety of conditions are associated with DIC (see Box 29.3). The common pathway for DIC appears to be excessive and widespread exposure of TF.[91] This may occur by several mechanisms. Widespread damage to the vascular endothelium results in exposure of subendothelial TF. Several types of cells, either produced after stimulation by cytokines or occurring constitutively, express TF on their surfaces. Normally, endothelial cells and monocytes do not express surface TF unless stimulated by inflammatory cytokines (particularly IL-6 and TNF-α).[92] Many tumors express surface TF or produce cytokines that stimulate TF expression by the endothelium or monocytes, or both.[93] These cytokines are abundantly produced during many of the conditions listed in Box 29.3. Endotoxin, in particular, triggers the release of multiple cytokines that play a significant role in the development and maintenance of DIC. Proinflammatory cytokines (TNF-α, interleukins [IL-1, IL-6, IL-8], and platelet-activating factor [PAF]) are responsible for the clinical signs and symptoms associated with sepsis. They also contribute to the development of DIC by activating endothelial cells, causing release of TF and vWF, increasing plasminogen activator inhibitor-1 (PAI-1) synthesis and tissue factor activity, and decreasing thrombomodulin expression, thereby promoting development of thrombi. TF also may be released directly into the bloodstream from circulating white blood cells (monocyte/endotoxin interaction).[91]

TF binds clotting factor VII, which leads to conversion of prothrombin to thrombin and formation of fibrin clots (see Fig. 28.22). This pathway appears to be the primary route by which DIC is initiated; inhibition of TF or factor VIIa completely prevents the generation of thrombi by gram-negative bacterial endotoxin in animal models of DIC.

Not only is the clotting system extensively activated in DIC, but levels of the predominant natural anticoagulants (tissue factor inhibitor, antithrombin III [AT-III], protein C) are also greatly diminished (see Fig. 28.19). During DIC the activation of clotting is prolonged both by the increased rate of consumption of clotting factors and platelets, because of persistent thrombin production as well as decreased synthesis of the natural anticoagulants and protein S, and by the cytokine-mediated decreased expression of thrombomodulin on the endothelial cell surface. Hepatic dysfunction in sepsis results in decreased antithrombin synthesis and extravascular leakage of this protease inhibitor because of capillary leakage. Additionally, antithrombin is degraded by elastase released by activated neutrophils, and clotting is initiated concurrently with loss of regulation of the extent of thrombosis; thus the amount of thrombin produced during DIC exceeds the ability of the body's naturally occurring anticoagulants to regulate it.

The rate of fibrinolysis is also diminished in DIC. The primary component of fibrinolysis is plasmin, which exists in the circulation as an inactive precursor, plasminogen (see Fig. 28.24). Plasminogen is activated to plasmin that digests fibrin clots, thus controlling the extent of fibrin deposition in the vessels. During DIC the activity of plasmin is diminished by increased production of its natural inhibitor, PAI-1. Although some fibrinolytic activity remains, the level is inadequate to control the systemic deposition of fibrin. The slow breakdown of fibrin by plasmin produces fibrin degradation products (FDPs) that are released into the blood. These are potent anticoagulants that are normally removed from blood by fibronectin and macrophages. FDPs, along with thrombin, induce further cytokine release from monocytes, contributing to endothelial damage and TF release. During DIC the presence of fibrin degradation products is prolonged, probably because of diminished production of fibronectin. Fibronectin is a glycoprotein with adhesive properties that mediate removal of particulate matter (e.g., fibrin clumps). Low levels of fibronectin suggest a poor prognosis.

Although thrombosis is generalized and widespread, individuals with DIC are paradoxically at risk for hemorrhage. Hemorrhage is secondary to the abnormally high consumption of clotting factors and platelets, as well as the anticoagulant properties of FDPs, which interfere with polymerization of fibrin monomers. Both thrombin and FDPs have a high affinity for platelets and cause platelet activation and aggregation—an event that occurs early in the development of DIC and that facilitates microcirculatory coagulation and obstruction in the initial phase. However, platelet consumption exceeds production, resulting in a thrombocytopenia that increases bleeding.

Activation of clotting also leads to activation of other inflammatory pathways, including the kallikrein-kinin and complement systems (see Chapter 7). Factor XIIa, generated in DIC, converts prekallikrein to kallikrein, ultimately resulting in conversion to circulating kinins. Activation of these systems contributes to increased vascular permeability, hypotension, and shock. Activated complement components also induce platelet destruction, further contributing initially to the thrombosis and later to the thrombocytopenia.

The deposition of fibrin clots in the circulation interferes with blood flow, causing widespread organ hypoperfusion. This condition may lead to ischemia, infarction, and necrosis, further potentiating and complicating the existing DIC process by causing additional release of TF and eventually organ failure.

In addition to initiation of clotting by TF, DIC may be precipitated by direct proteolytic activation of factor X. This has been described as "thrombin mimicry" and is the result of activated factor X directly converting fibrinogen to fibrin. The proteases that activate factor X may come from snake venom, some tumor cells, or the pancreas and liver, where they are released during episodes of pancreatitis and various stages of liver disease. Direct proteolytic activity appears to be independent of any type of damage to the endothelium or tissue.

Vascular obstruction results from circulatory deposition of thrombin and clot formation that impedes blood flow, causing widespread organ hypoperfusion that can lead to tissue ischemia, infarction, and necrosis. The resulting tissue damage further potentiates and complicates the existing DIC process. Because organ perfusion is drastically impaired, manifestations of multisystem organ dysfunction and failure ultimately result. Multisystem organ dysfunction and failure are discussed in Chapter 49. Whatever initiates the process of DIC, the cycle of thrombosis and hemorrhage persists until the underlying cause of the DIC is removed or appropriate therapeutic interventions are used.

CLINICAL MANIFESTATIONS. Clinical signs and symptoms of DIC present a wide spectrum of possibilities, depending on the underlying disease process that initiates DIC and whether the DIC is acute or chronic (Box 29.4). Most symptoms are the result of either hemorrhage or thrombosis. Acute DIC presents with rapid development of hemorrhaging, such as oozing from venipuncture sites, arterial lines, and surgical wounds, or development of ecchymotic lesions (purpura, petechiae) and hematomas. Other sites of bleeding include the eyes (sclera and conjunctiva), the nose (epistaxis), and the gums. Most individuals with DIC demonstrate bleeding at three or more unrelated sites, and any combination may be observed. Shock of variable intensity, out of proportion to the amount of apparent blood loss, also may be

---

BOX 29.4   CLINICAL MANIFESTATIONS ASSOCIATED WITH DISSEMINATED INTRAVASCULAR COAGULATION (DIC)

Integumentary System
Widespread hemorrhage and vascular lesions
Oozing from puncture sites, incisions, mucous membranes
Acrocyanosis (irregularly shaped cyanotic patches)
Gangrene

Central Nervous System
Subarachnoid hemorrhage
Altered state of consciousness (from slight confusion to convulsions and coma)

Gastrointestinal System
Occult bleeding to massive gastrointestinal bleeding
Abdominal distention
Malaise
Weakness

Pulmonary System
Pulmonary infarctions
Acute respiratory distress syndrome (ARDS)
Cyanosis
Tachypnea
Hypoxemia

Renal System
Hematuria
Oliguria
Renal failure

Modified from Bailes BK: *AORN J* 55(2):517–529, 1992.

---

observed. Hemorrhaging into closed compartments of the body also can occur and may precede the development of shock.

DIC has been conceptualized as a systemic hemorrhagic disorder because bleeding, sometimes very extensive, is usually the initial observation. Symptoms of thrombosis are not always as evident, even though it is often the first pathologic alteration to occur and ultimately determines the degree of morbidity and risk for death. A large amount of microvascular and macrovascular occlusion may occur that is not clinically obvious. Several organ systems are susceptible to microvascular thrombosis that affects their function; these include the cardiovascular, pulmonary, central nervous, renal, and hepatic systems. Quick and accurate clinical diagnosis is critical to preventing further progression of DIC that may lead to multisystem organ dysfunction or failure. Indicators of multisystem failure include changes in level of consciousness, behavior, and mentation; confusion; seizure activity; oliguria; hematuria; hypoxia; hypotension; hemoptysis; chest pain; and tachycardia. Symmetrical cyanosis of the fingers and toes ("blue finger/toe syndrome") and, in some instances, of the nose and breasts may be present. Symmetrical parts are often affected and are indicative of microvascular thrombosis. This may progress to infarction and gangrene, requiring amputation. Jaundice also may be present and is believed to result from red blood cell destruction rather than hepatic dysfunction.

Individuals with chronic or low-grade DIC do not present with overt manifestations of hemorrhaging and thrombosis but instead have subacute bleeding and diffuse thrombosis and are described as having

BOX 29.5   LABORATORY DIAGNOSTIC CRITERIA FOR DISSEMINATED INTRAVASCULAR COAGULATION (DIC)*

Group I Tests (Indicators of Procoagulant Activation)
1. Elevated prothrombin fragment 1+2
2. Elevated fibrinopeptide A
3. Elevated fibrinopeptide B
4. Elevated thrombin-antithrombin (TAT) complex
5. Elevated D-dimer

Group II Tests (Indicators of Fibrinolytic Activity)
1. Elevated D-dimer
2. Elevated fibrin degradation products (FDPs)
3. Elevated plasmin
4. Elevated plasmin-antiplasmin (PAP) complex

Group III Tests (Indicators of Inhibitor Consumption)
1. Decreased antithrombin III
2. Decreased α_2-antiplasmin
3. Decreased heparin cofactor II
4. Decreased protein C or S
5. Elevated TAT complex
6. Elevated PAP complex

Group IV Tests (Indicators of End-Organ Damage/Failure)
1. Elevated lactic dehydrogenase (LDH)
2. Elevated creatinine
3. Decreased pH
4. Decreased PaO_2

*Satisfactory criteria for laboratory diagnosis of DIC require one abnormality in each of groups I through III and at least two abnormalities in group IV.
Data from Bick RL: *Semin Thromb Hemost* 24(1):3, 1998.

a **compensated DIC**, or non–overt DIC. The major characteristic of this state is an increased turnover and decreased survival time of the components of hemostasis: platelets and clotting factors. Occasionally, diffuse or localized thrombosis develops, but this is infrequent.

◆**EVALUATION AND TREATMENT.** No single laboratory test can be used to effectively diagnosis DIC. Diagnosis is based primarily on clinical symptoms and confirmed by a combination of laboratory tests. The individual must present with a clinical condition that is known to be associated with DIC. The most commonly used combination of laboratory tests usually confirms thrombocytopenia or a rapidly decreasing platelet count on repeated testing, prolongation of clotting times, the presence of fibrin degradation products, and decreased levels of coagulation inhibitors. The relationships among these criteria are summarized in Box 29.5. Platelet counts less than 100,000/mm³ or a progressive decrease in platelet counts is very sensitive for DIC, although not greatly specific. These changes usually indicate consumption of platelets.

The standard coagulation tests (e.g., prothrombin time [PT], activated partial thromboplastin time [aPTT]) also have a high degree of sensitivity, but they are not highly specific for DIC. As a result of consumption of circulating clotting factors, these tests are usually abnormal, ranging from shortened to prolonged times. However, conditions other than DIC may prolong clotting times. Assays of specific clotting factors do not contribute meaningful diagnostic information.

Detection of various fibrin degradation products is more specific for DIC; of these tests the detection of D-dimers is the most widely used, reliable, and specific test.[94] A D-dimer is a molecule produced by plasmin degradation of cross-linked fibrin in clots. D-dimers in the blood can be quantified using enzyme-linked immunosorbent assay (ELISA) tests that include commercially available and highly specific monoclonal antibody against the D-dimer. Agglutination tests for other fibrin degradation products are available. Levels of fibrin degradation products, in general, are elevated in the plasma in 95% to 100% of cases; however, concentrations of FDPs are less specific and only document the presence of plasmin and its action of fibrin, whereas detection of D-dimers measures a specific DIC-related product.

ELISAs for markers of thrombin activity are sometimes used. Normal conversion of prothrombin to thrombin produces an inactive prothrombin fragment 1.2 (PF1+2).[94] This fragment is released from the prothrombin molecule, generating an intermediate factor, prethrombin 2. Once generated, prethrombin 2 can either split to produce thrombin, which can then proteolyze fibrinogen and thus liberate fibrinopeptide A (FPA), or can combine with its major antagonist (antithrombin) and form a stable inactive enzyme–inhibitor complex, the thrombin-antithrombin (TAT) complex. Assays of these factors (PF1+2, FPA, TAT) are now generally available to quantify their blood levels, providing evidence of excessive factor Xa (PF1+2) and thrombin (FPA) generation.

Levels of coagulation inhibitors (e.g., AT-III, protein C) can be measured by assays that rely on function or by ELISAs that quantify the amount of the specific inhibitor. AT-III levels can provide key information for diagnosing and monitoring therapy for DIC. Initial levels of functional AT-III are low in DIC because thrombin is irreversibly complexed with activated clotting factors and AT-III.

Treatment of DIC is directed toward (1) eliminating the underlying pathology, (2) controlling ongoing thrombosis, and (3) maintaining organ function. Elimination of the underlying pathology is the initial intervention in the treatment phase in order to eliminate the trigger for activation of clotting. Once the stimulus is gone, production of coagulation factors in the liver leads to restoration of normal plasma levels within 24 to 48 hours.

Control of thrombosis is more difficult to attain. Heparin has been used for this; however, its use is controversial because its mechanism of action is binding to and activating AT-III, which is deficient in many types of DIC. Currently heparin is indicated only in certain situations related to DIC. For instance, heparin seems to be effective in DIC caused by a retained dead fetus or associated with acute promyelocytic leukemia. Organ function is compromised by microthrombi, and there is a risk of losing an extremity because of vascular occlusion; thus heparin is also indicated in these conditions. Heparin's usefulness, however, for DIC that is precipitated by septic shock has not been established and so is contraindicated in that instance; heparin is also contraindicated when there is evidence of postoperative bleeding, peptic ulcer, or CNS bleeding.

Replacement therapy (interventions based on restoring the balance of coagulation factors, deficient coagulation factors, platelets, and other coagulation elements) is gaining recognition as an effective treatment modality. Components used in replacement therapy include platelets, fresh frozen plasma, and cryoprecipitate. Platelets are given for thrombocytopenia, plasma provides volume and replaces clotting factors, and cryoprecipitate replaces fibrinogen. Their use is not without controversy, however, because of the possible risk of adding components that will increase the rate of thrombosis. Clinical judgment is the key factor in determining whether replacement is to be used as a treatment modality.

Several clinical trials are evaluating replacement of anticoagulants (i.e., AT-III, protein C). Studies assessing the use of anticoagulants are presented in the review by Gando and colleagues.[91] Antifibrinolytic drugs also are used in treatment but are limited to instances of life-threatening bleeding that have not been controlled by blood component replacement therapy. Maintenance of organ function is achieved by

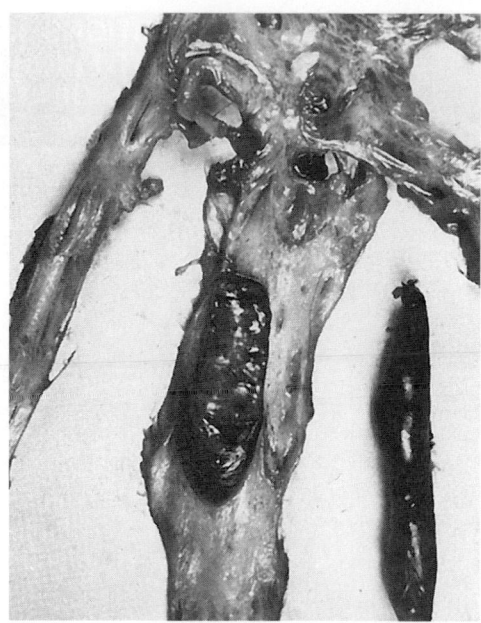

FIGURE 29.12 Thrombus. Thrombus arising in valve pocket at upper end of superficial femoral vein. Postmortem clot on the right is shown for comparison. (From McLachlin J, Paterson JC: *Surg Gynecol Obstet* 93:1, 1951.)

fluid replacement to sustain adequate circulating blood volume and to maintain optimal tissue and organ perfusion. Fluids may be required to restore blood pressure, cardiac output, and urine output to normal parameters.

Thromboembolic Disease

Certain conditions within the blood vessels predispose an individual to develop clots spontaneously.[95] A stationary clot attached to the vessel wall is called a **thrombus** (Fig. 29.12). A thrombus is composed of fibrin and blood cells and can develop in either the arterial or the venous system. **Arterial thrombi** form under conditions of high blood flow and are composed mostly of platelet aggregates held together by fibrin strands. **Venous thrombi** form in conditions of low flow and are composed mostly of red cells with larger amounts of fibrin and few platelets.

A thrombus may eventually grow large enough to reduce or obstruct blood flow to tissues or organs, such as the heart, brain, or lungs, depriving them of essential nutrients critical to survival. A thrombus also has the potential of detaching from the vessel wall and circulating within the bloodstream (referred to as an **embolus**). The embolus may become lodged in smaller blood vessels, blocking blood flow into the local tissue or organ and leading to ischemia. The potential for episodes of thromboembolism to become life-threatening depends on the site of vessel occlusion.

Therapy consists of removal or breakdown of the clot and provision of supportive measures. Anticoagulant therapy is effective in treating or preventing venous thrombosis; it is not as useful in treating or preventing arterial thrombosis. Parenteral heparin is the major anticoagulant used to treat thromboembolism. Oral coumarin drugs also are widely used, particularly for individuals not hospitalized. More aggressive therapy may be indicated for such conditions as pulmonary embolism, coronary thrombosis, or thrombophlebitis. Streptokinase and urokinase activate the fibrinolytic system and are administered to accelerate the lysis of known thrombi. Thrombolytic therapy has limited uses and is prescribed with a high degree of caution because it can cause hemorrhagic complications.

The risk for developing spontaneous thrombi is related to several factors, referred to as the **Virchow triad**: (1) injury to the blood vessel endothelium, (2) abnormalities of blood flow, and (3) hypercoagulability of the blood.

Vascular endothelial injury can result from atherosclerosis (plaque deposits on arterial walls). Atherosclerosis initiates platelet adhesion and aggregation, promoting the development of atherosclerotic plaques that enlarge, causing further damage and occlusion. Other causes of vessel endothelial injury may be related to hemodynamic alterations associated with hypertension and turbulent blood flow. Injury also is caused by radiation injury, exogenous chemical agents (toxins from cigarette smoke), endogenous agents (cholesterol), bacterial toxins or endotoxins, or immunologic mechanisms. Whatever the precipitating cause of endothelial injury, it is a potent thrombogenic agent.

Turbulent blood flow in the arteries and stasis of blood flow in the veins are at-risk conditions for thrombus formation. In areas of turbulence, platelets and endothelial cells may be activated, leading to thrombosis. In sites of stasis, platelets may remain in contact with the endothelium for prolonged times, and clotting factors that would normally be diluted with fresh-flowing blood are not diluted and may become activated. The most common clinical conditions that predispose to venous stasis and subsequent thromboembolic phenomena are major surgery (e.g., orthopedic surgery), acute myocardial infarction, congestive heart failure, limb paralysis, spinal injury, malignancy, advanced age, the postpartum period, and bed rest longer than 1 week. Turbulence and stasis occur with ulcerated atherosclerotic plaques (myocardial infarction), hyperviscosity (polycythemia), and conditions with deformed red cells (sickle cell anemia).

Hypercoagulability, or **thrombophilia**, is the condition in which an individual is at risk for thrombosis. Hypercoagulability is differentiated according to whether it results from primary (hereditary) or secondary (acquired) causes. Primary causes include defects in proteins involved in hemostasis. Secondary causes include a variety of clinical disorders or conditions (Box 29.6). It is not well understood why there is not a greater incidence of thrombosis formation in hypercoagulable states associated with various disease states and conditions.

Hereditary Thrombophilias. A large number of inherited conditions have been identified that increase the risk of developing thrombosis. Most are autosomal dominant; thus individuals who are homozygous for the mutation are at greatest risk for thrombosis. These include mutations in coagulation proteins, fibrinolytic proteins, platelet receptors, and other factors. The mutations most strongly linked as risk factors for venous thrombosis or for arterial thrombosis leading to coronary artery disease or stroke include those that affect prothrombin (G20210A variant) and factor V (factor V Leiden) of the coagulation system. Other inherited thrombophilias are reviewed in Box 29.6.

Factor V Leiden results from a single nucleotide mutation of guanine to adenine at nucleotide 1691 (G1691A). Activated factor V (Va) is usually inactivated by protein C, but this single mutation results in a change in amino acid 506 from arginine to glutamine. The change alters the site where protein C would cleave factor Va and confers partial resistance, resulting in prolonged high levels of Va and prolongation of clot formation.[96] Although this mutation increases the risk for thrombosis, most individuals with factor V Leiden do not have clinically relevant thrombotic events. It is the most common hereditary thrombophilia and is found in about 30% of individuals presenting with deep venous thrombosis (DVT) or pulmonary embolism. It is primarily observed in individuals of European ancestry and in about 5% of whites in the United States and Europe.

The second most common inherited form of thrombophilia (after factor V Leiden) is a mutation in the *F2* gene. The mutation that causes prothrombin thrombophilia results in an overactive *F2* gene that causes

BOX 29.6 HYPERCOAGULABLE STATES

Primary (Genetic)

Common

Factor V mutation (Arg to Glu substitution in amino acid residue 506 leading to resistance to activated protein C; factor V Leiden)

Prothrombin mutation (G20210A noncoding sequence variant leading to increased prothrombin levels)

Increased levels of factors VIII, IX, XI, or fibrinogen (genetics unknown)

Rare

Antithrombin III deficiency

Protein C deficiency

Protein S deficiency

Very Rare

Fibrinolysis defects

Homozygous homocystinuria (deficiency of cystathionine β-synthetase)

Secondary (Acquired)

High Risk for Thrombosis

Prolonged bed rest or immobilization

Myocardial infarction

Atrial fibrillation

Tissue injury (surgery, fracture, burn)

Cancer

Prosthetic cardiac valves

Disseminated intravascular coagulation

Heparin-induced thrombocytopenia

Antiphospholipid antibody syndrome

Lower Risk for Thrombosis

Cardiomyopathy

Nephrotic syndrome

Hyperestrogenic states (pregnancy and postpartum)

Oral contraceptive use

Sickle cell anemia

Smoking

From Kumar V, Abbas A, Aster JC: *Robbins & Cotran pathologic basis of disease*, ed 9, Philadelphia, 2015, Saunders.

BOX 29.7 CLINICAL CONDITIONS ASSOCIATED WITH HIGH RISK FOR THROMBOSIS OR THROMBOEMBOLISM

ARTERIAL	VENOUS
Atherosclerosis	General surgery
Cigarette smoking	Orthopedic surgery
Hypertension	Arthroscopy
Diabetes mellitus	Trauma
LDL cholesterol	Malignancy
Hypertriglyceridemia	Immobility
Positive family history	Sepsis
Left ventricular failure	Congestive heart failure
Oral contraceptives	Nephrotic syndrome
Estrogens	Obesity
Lipoprotein A	Varicose veins
Polycythemia	Postphlebitic syndrome
Hyperviscosity syndrome	Oral contraceptives
Leukostasis syndrome	Estrogens
Thrombocythemia	Thrombocythemia

LDL, Low-density lipoprotein.

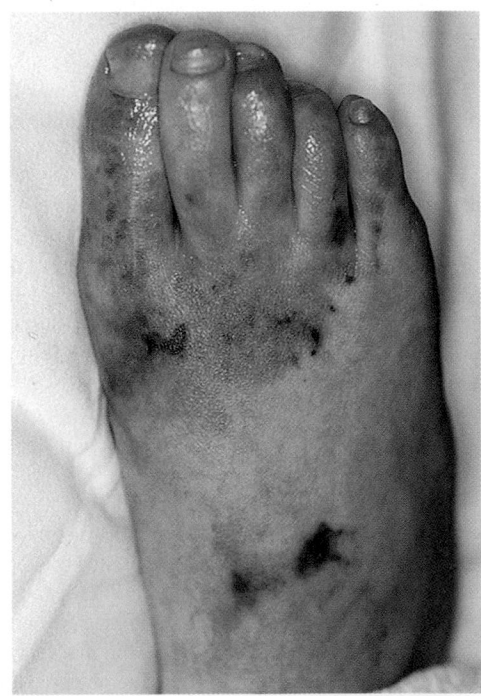

FIGURE 29.13 Arterial Thrombosis Associated with Antiphospholipid Antibodies. A 12-year-old girl with systemic lupus erythematosus and antiphospholipid antibodies with painful cutaneous vasculitis of the right foot. Arterial thrombosis documented by angiography resulted in cyanosis of the large toe. Symptoms resolved with treatment with heparin and corticosteroids. (From Kliegman R et al: *Nelson textbook of pediatrics*, ed 18, Philadelphia, 2007, Saunders.)

too much prothrombin to be produced.[97] An increase in prothrombin levels leads to more thrombin which promotes the formation of blood clots.[97] Other factors that increase the risk of blood clots include increasing age, obesity, trauma, surgery, smoking, use of oral contraceptives or hormone replacement therapy, and pregnancy. Other mutations in genes involved in blood clotting also can influence risk.[97]

Acquired Hypercoagulability. The acquired thrombophilias are often multifactorial (Box 29.7). An example of an acquired hypercoagulable state is antiphospholipid syndrome (APS), an autoimmune syndrome characterized by autoantibodies against plasma membrane phospholipids and phospholipid-binding proteins. As with most autoimmune diseases, the predominantly affected individual is female and of reproductive age. Those with APS are at risk for arterial and venous thrombosis and a variety of obstetric complications, including pregnancy loss and preeclampsia or eclampsia (Fig. 29.13).[98] In severe cases the person may die from recurrent major thrombus formation.[99] The pathophysiology is related to autoantibodies directly reacting with platelets or endothelial cells (increasing the risk for thrombosis) or the placental surface (resulting in damage to the placenta). The predominant diagnostic tests measure prolongation of laboratory blood coagulation tests related to an antibody inhibitor (lupus anticoagulant) and specific ELISAs for antibodies against phospholipids (e.g., anticardiolipin antibody) or proteins that bind to phospholipids (e.g., β$_2$-glycoprotein I).[100,101] Highly effective therapy (i.e., unfractionated or low-molecular-weight heparin with low-dose aspirin) is available to prevent the obstetric complications.[102]

SUMMARY REVIEW

Anemia

1. Anemia is defined as a reduction in the total circulating red cell mass or a decrease in the quality or quantity of hemoglobin. Polycythemias are excessive levels or volumes of RBCs.
2. Anemias can result from blood loss, impaired erythrocyte production, increased erythrocyte destruction, and a combination of these factors.
3. Total circulating red blood cell mass is reflected by changes in plasma volume caused by dehydration and fluid retention.
4. Anemias can be classified in several ways and a useful way is by the main underlying mechanism.
5. Clinical manifestations of anemia may be demonstrated in all organs and tissues (tissue hypoxia) throughout the body. Decreased oxygen delivery to tissues causes fatigue, dyspnea, syncope, angina, compensatory tachycardia, and organ dysfunction.
6. Posthemorrhagic anemia is a normocytic-normochromic anemia caused by acute blood loss. A major cause of acute blood loss is trauma, a rising global problem.
7. Anemia from chronic blood loss occurs if the loss is greater than the replacement capacity of the bone marrow. If iron stores are depleted, iron deficiency anemia can occur.
8. Macrocytic (megaloblastic) anemias are characterized by larger than normal erythroid precursors (megaloblasts) in the bone marrow that mature into large erythrocytes. They most commonly are caused by deficiency of vitamin B_{12} or folate.
9. PA results from inadequate vitamin B_{12} absorption because autoimmune gastritis impairs the production of IF, which is required for vitamin B_{12} uptake from the gut. Folate deficiency anemia is caused by inadequate dietary intake of folate. Both anemias respond to replacement therapy.
10. Microcytic-hypochromic anemias are characterized by abnormally small erythrocytes with insufficient hemoglobin content. The anemias result from disorders of (a) iron metabolism (IDA), (b) porphyrin and heme synthesis (SAs), or (c) globin synthesis (thalassemia).
11. IDA is the most common type of nutritional disorder worldwide. It is usually a result of dietary deficiency. Other major causes are impaired absorption, increased requirement, and chronic blood loss. IDA usually develops slowly, with a gradual insidious onset of symptoms, which include fatigue, weakness, dyspnea, alteration of various epithelial tissues, and vague neuromuscular complaints result.
12. Individuals at highest risk for developing IDA include older adults, women, infants, teenagers eating poor diets, and those living in poverty. Once the source of blood loss is identified and corrected, oral iron replacement therapy can be initiated.
13. ACD, also called *anemia of inflammation,* results from decreased erythropoiesis and impaired iron utilization in people with chronic systemic disease or inflammation. ACD is common among hospitalized individuals.
14. Examples of mechanisms associated with ACD include (1) decreased erythrocyte life span, (2) reduced production of erythropoietin, (3) ineffective bone marrow response to erythropoietin, and (4) iron sequestration in macrophages. In particular, the proinflammatory cytokine IL-6 increases hepatocyte release of hepcidin which suppresses ferroportin transport of iron out of macrophages.
15. AA is a critical condition characterized by a reduction or absence of all three blood cell types (pancytopenia). Unless the cause is determined, bone marrow aplasia results in death.
16. Hemolytic anemia is a result of excessive destruction of erythrocytes and may be acquired or hereditary. Common, acquired forms are autoimmune reaction (immunohemolytic) and drug-induced hemolysis.
17. AIHAs include (a) warm reactive antibody type, (b) cold agglutinin type, and (c) cold hemolysin type (paroxysmal cold hemoglobinuria).
18. Examples of mechanisms associated with ACD include (a) decreased erythrocyte life span, (b) reduced production of erythropoietin, (c) ineffective bone marrow response to erythropoietin, and (d) iron sequestration in macrophages. In particular, the proinflammatory cytokine IL-6 increases hepatocyte release of hepcidin, which suppresses ferroportin transport of iron out of macrophages.

Myeloproliferative Red Blood Cell Disorders

1. Polycythemia vera is a myeloproliferative disorder characterized by excessive proliferation of erythrocyte precursors, frequently with increased levels of white blood cells and platelets, in the bone marrow and splenomegaly. Signs and symptoms result directly from increased blood volume and viscosity and a predisposition to thrombosis.
2. Therapeutic phlebotomy to remove excessive blood volume and the use of hydroxyurea have been helpful in decreasing the excessive erythrocyte population.

Alterations of Platelets and Coagulation

1. Thrombocytopenia is characterized by a platelet count less than $150,000/mm^3$ of blood; a count less than $50,000/mm^3$ increases the potential for hemorrhage associated with minor trauma.
2. Thrombocytopenia may be congenital or acquired and primary or secondary to other acquired or congenital conditions. Acquired thrombocytopenia is associated with autoimmune diseases, viral infections, nutritional deficiencies, chronic renal failure, bone marrow hypoplasia, radiation therapy, and bone marrow infiltration by cancer. Most common forms of thrombocytopenia are the result of increased platelet consumption
3. Heparin-induced thrombocytopenia develops in approximately 4% of individuals receiving unfractionated heparin.
4. Immune thrombocytopenic purpura (ITP) is a major cause of platelet destruction, often affecting females, and results in hemorrhaging that ranges from petechiae to bleeding from mucosal sites.
5. Thrombotic thrombocytopenic purpura (TTP) causes platelet aggregation leading to microcirculatory occlusion.
6. Thrombocythemia is characterized by a platelet count more than $450,000/mm^3$ of blood and is symptomatic when the count exceeds 1 million/mm^3, which increases the risk for intravascular clotting (thrombosis).
7. Essential or primary thrombocythemia is caused by excessive platelet production in the bone marrow secondary to increased plasma thrombopoietin levels resulting from defects in the thrombopoietin receptor.
8. Qualitative alterations in normal platelet adherence or aggregation prevent platelet plug formation and may result in prolonged bleeding times.
9. Prolonged bleeding can result from alterations in platelet function, including adhesion between platelets and the vessel wall, platelet-platelet adhesion, platelet granule secretion, arachidonic acid pathway activity, and membrane phospholipid regulation.
10. Disorders of coagulation are usually caused by defects or deficiencies of clotting factors.
11. Coagulation is impaired when there is a deficiency of vitamin K because of insufficient production of prothrombin and synthesis

SUMMARY REVIEW—cont'd

of clotting factors II, VII, IX, and X, often associated with liver diseases.

12. DIC is a complex syndrome that results from a variety of clinical conditions that release tissue factor, causing an increase in fibrin and thrombin activity in the blood and producing augmented clot formation and accelerated fibrinolysis. Sepsis is often associated with DIC.

13. DIC is characterized by a cycle of intravascular clotting followed by active bleeding caused by the initial consumption of coagulation factors and platelets and diffuse fibrinolysis.

14. Diagnosis of DIC is based on dysfunctional coagulation activity. Treatment is complex, nonstandardized, and focused on removing the primary cause, restoring hemostasis, and preventing further organ damage.

15. Thromboembolic disease results from a fixed (thrombus) or moving (embolus) clot that blocks flow within a vessel, denying nutrients to tissues distal to the occlusion; death can result when clots obstruct blood flow to the heart, brain, or lungs.

16. Hypercoagulability is the result of deficient anticoagulation proteins. Secondary causes are conditions that promote venous stasis.

17. The term *Virchow triad* refers to three factors that can cause thrombus formation: (1) vessel wall injury, (2) blood flow abnormalities, and (3) altered blood constituents leading to hypercoagulability.

18. Autoantibodies against phospholipids result in a state of acquired hypercoagulability, an increased risk for venous or arterial thrombosis, and a higher incidence of pregnancy complications.

KEY TERMS

Absolute polycythemia, 945
Acute idiopathic TTP, 950
Anemia, 926
Anemia of chronic disease (ACD; anemia of inflammation [AI]), 936
Anisocytosis, 926
Aplastic anemia (AA), 938
Apoferritin, 937
Arterial thrombi (*singular,* thrombus), 957
Autoimmune hemolytic anemia (AIHA), 942
Chronic relapsing TTP, 950
Cold agglutinin autoimmune hemolytic anemia, 942
Cold hemolysin autoimmune hemolytic anemia (paroxysmal cold hemoglobinuria), 943
Compensated DIC, 956
Consumptive thrombohemorrhagic disorder, 953
D-dimer, 956
Disseminated intravascular coagulation (DIC), 953
Drug-induced hemolytic anemia, 944
Embolus (*plural,* emboli), 957
Eryptosis, 932

Erythromelalgia, 951
Essential (primary) thrombocythemia (ET), 951
Fanconi anemia, 940
Folate (folic acid), 933
Hemolytic anemia, 942
Heparin-induced thrombocytopenia (HIT), 948
Hereditary hemochromatosis (HH), 947
Hypercoagulability (thrombophilia), 957
Hypoxemia, 928
Immune thrombocytopenic purpura (ITP), 949
Immunohemolytic anemia, 942
Impaired hemostasis, 953
Intrinsic factor (IF), 932
Iron deficiency anemia (IDA), 934
Janus kinase 2 gene (JAK2), 946
Lactoferrin, 936
Macrocytic (megaloblastic) anemia, 932
Microangiopathy, 950
Microcytic-hypochromic anemia, 934
Microvasculature thrombosis, 951
Normocytic-normochromic anemia (NNA), 928
Pancytopenia, 938

Paroxysmal nocturnal hemoglobinuria, 942
Pernicious anemia (PA), 932
Poikilocytosis, 926
Polycythemia, 945
Polycythemia vera (PV), 945
Posthemorrhagic anemia, 928
Pseudothrombocytopenia, 948
Pure red cell aplasia (PRCA), 938
Purpura, 947
Relative polycythemia, 945
Thrombocythemia (thrombocytosis), 951
Thrombocytopenia, 948
Thromboembolic disease, 947
Thrombotic thrombocytopenic purpura (TTP; Moschcowitz disease), 950
Thrombus (*plural,* thrombi), 957
Trauma, 929
Vasculitis, 952
Venous thrombi (*singular,* thrombus), 957
Virchow triad, 957
Warm autoimmune hemolytic anemia, 942

REFERENCES

1. Rossaint R, et al: The European guideline on management of major bleeding and coagulopathy following trauma: fourth edition. *Crit Care* 20:100, 2016.

2. World Health Organization (WHO): *Injuries and violence: the facts*, 2010. Available at: http://whqlibdoc.who.int/publications/2010/9789241599375_eng.pdf.

3. Green R, Mitra AD: Megaloblastic anemias. *Med Clin North Am* 101(2):297–317, 2017.

4. Kumar V, Abbas A, Aster JC: *Robbins & Cotran pathologic basis of disease,* ed 9, Philadelphia, 2015, Saunders.

5. Stabler SP: Vitamin B12 deficiency. *N Engl J Med* 368(2):149–160, 2013.

6. Banka S, et al: Pernicious anemia—genetic insights. *Autoimmun Rev* 10(8):455–459, 2011.

7. Gowdappa HB, et al: *Helicobacter pylori* associated vitamin B12 deficiency, pernicious anemia and subacute combined degeneration of the spinal cord. *BMJ Case Rep* 2013, doi:10.1136/bcr-2013-200380.

8. Perez-Perez GI: Role of *Helicobacter pylori* infection in the development of pernicious anemia. *Clin Infect Dis* 25:1020–1022, 1997.

9. Toh BH, et al: Cutting edge issues in autoimmune gastritis. *Clin Rev Allergy Immunol* 42(3):269–278, 2012.

10. Vojdani A: Antibodies as predictors of complex autoimmune diseases. *Int J Immunopathol Pharmacol* 21(2):267–278, 2008.

11. Killip S, Bennett JM, Chambers MD: Iron deficiency anemia. *Am Fam Physician* 75(5):671–678, 2007.

12. Aigner E, Feldman A, Datz C: Obesity as an emerging risk factor for iron deficiency. *Nutrients* 6(9):3587–3600, 2014.

13. West AR, Oates PS: Mechanisms of heme iron absorption: current questions and controversies. *World J Gastroenterol* 14(26):4101–4110, 2008.

14. Hegazy AA, et al: Relation between anemia and blood levels of lead, copper, zinc and iron among children. *BMC Res Notes* 3:133, 2010.

15. Sebahat T, et al: Interaction between anemia and blood levels of iron, copper, cadmium and lead in children. *Indian J Pediatr* 74:827–830, 2007.

16. Zhai Q, Narbad A, Chen W: Dietary strategies for the treatment of cadmium and lead toxicity. *Nutrients* 7(1):552–571, 2015.

17. Alleyne M, Horne MK, Miller JL: Individualized treatment for iron-deficiency anemia in adults. *Am J Med* 121(11):943–948, 2008.

18. Nairz M, et al: Iron deficiency or anemia of inflammation? *Wien Med Wochenschr* 166(13):411–423, 2016.

19. Ganz T, Nemeth E: Iron homeostasis in host defense and inflammation. *Nat Rev Immunol* 15:500–510, 2015.

20. Kwaan HC: Infection and anemia. *Infect Disord Drug Targets* 11(1):40–44, 2011.

21. Zarychanski R, Houston DS: Anemia of chronic disease: a harmful disorder or an adaptive, beneficial response? *Can Med Assoc J* 179(4):333–337, 2008.

22. Tussing-Humphreys L, et al: Rethinking iron regulation and assessment in iron deficiency, anemia of chronic disease, and obesity: introducing hepcidin. *J Acad Nutr Diet* 112(3):391–400, 2012.

23. Jaworski J, et al: Decreased expression of integrins by hematopoietic cells in patients with rheumatoid arthritis and anemia: relationship with bone marrow cytokine levels. *J Investig Allergy Clin Immunol* 18(1):17–21, 2008.

24. Portolés J, et al: The development of anemia is associated to poor prognosis in NKF/KDOQI stage 3 chronic kidney disease. *BMC Nephrol* 14(1):2, 2013.

25. Drüeke TB: Anemia treatment in patients with chronic kidney disease. *N Engl J Med* 368(4):387–389, 2013.

26. Jing Z, et al: Hemoglobin targets for chronic kidney disease patients with anemia: a systematic review and meta-analysis. *PLoS ONE* 7(8):1–9, 2012.

27. Asare K: Anemia of critical illness. *Pharmacotherapy* 28(10):1267–1282, 2008.

28. Espinoza JL, Kotecha R, Nakao S: Microbe-induced inflammatory signals triggering acquired bone marrow failure syndromes. *Front Immunol* 8:186, 2017.

29. Kee Y, D'Andrea AD: Molecular pathogenesis and clinical management of Fanconi anemia. *J Clin Invest* 122(11):3799–3806, 2012.

30. Bacigalupo A: Aplastic anemia: pathogenesis and treatment. *Hematology* 2007:23–28, 2007.

31. Mavroudi I, Papadaki HA: Genetic associations in acquired immune-mediated bone marrow failure syndromes: insights in aplastic anemia and chronic idiopathic neutropenia. *Clin Dev Immunol* 2012:1–7, 2012. Article ID 123789.

32. Ogawa S: Clonal hematopoiesis in acquired aplastic anemia. *Blood* 28(3):337–347, 2016.

33. Young NS: Current concepts in pathophysiology and treatment of aplastic anemia. *Hematology Am Soc Hematol Educ Program* 2013:76–81, 2013.

34. Zeng Y, Katsanis E: The complex pathophysiology of acquired aplastic anaemia. *Clin Exp Immunol* 180:361–370, 2015.

35. Scheinberg P, Young NS: How I treat acquired aplastic anemia. *Blood* 120(6):1185–1196, 2012.

36. Armand P, Antin JH: Allogeneic stem cell transplantation for aplastic anemia. *Biol Blood Marrow Transplant* 13(5):505–516, 2007.

37. Davies JK, Guinan EC: An update on the management of severe idiopathic aplastic anaemia in children. *Br J Haematol* 136(4):549–564, 2007.

38. Totino PRR, Daniel-Ribeiro CT, Ferreira-da-Cruz M: Evidencing the role of erythrocytic apoptosis in malarial anemia. *Front Cell Infect Microbiol* 6:176, 2016.

39. Brodsky RA: Narrative review: paroxysmal nocturnal hemoglobinuria: the physiology of complement-related hemolytic anemia. *Ann Intern Med* 148(8):587–595, 2008.

40. Risitano AM: Paroxysmal nocturnal hemoglobinuria and the complement system: recent insights and novel anticomplement strategies. *Adv Exp Med Biol* 735:155–172, 2013.

41. Risitano AM, et al: Peptide inhibitors of C3 activation as a novel strategy of complement inhibition for the treatment of paroxysmal nocturnal hemoglobinuria. *Blood* 123(13):2094–2101, 2014.

42. Ziakas PD, Poulou LS, Pomont A: Thrombosis in paroxysmal nocturnal hemoglobinuria at a glance: a clinical review. *Curr Vasc Pharmacol* 6(4):347–353, 2008.

43. Brodsky R: Advances in the diagnosis and therapy of paroxysmal nocturnal hemoglobinuria. *Blood Rev* 22(2):65–74, 2008.

44. Valent P, Lechner K: Diagnosis and treatment of autoimmune haemolytic anaemias in adults: a clinical review. *Wien Klin Wochenschr* 120(5-6):136–151, 2008.

45. Packman CH: Hemolytic anemia due to warm autoantibodies. *Blood Rev* 22(1):17–31, 2008.

46. Wu B, Rong R: Cold agglutinin syndrome with severe haemolytic anaemia in a patient diagnosed of disseminated tuberculosis and concomitant *Mycoplasma pneumoniae* infection. *Transfus Med* 22(2):151–152, 2012.

47. Berentsen S, Belske K, Tjønnfjord GE: Primary chronic cold agglutinin disease: an update on pathogenesis, clinical features and therapy. *Hematology* 12(5):361–370, 2007.

48. Petz LD: Cold antibody autoimmune hemolytic anemias. *Blood Rev* 22(1):1–15, 2008.

49. Garratty G: Immune hemolytic anemia caused by drugs. *Expert Opin Drug Saf* 11(4):635–642, 2012.

50. Martinengo M, et al: The first case of drug-induced immune hemolytic anemia due to hydrocortisone. *Transfusion* 48(9):1925–1929, 2008.

51. Crowther M, et al: Evidence-based focused review of the treatment of idiopathic warm immune hemolytic anemia in adults. *Blood* 118(15):4036–4040, 2013.

52. Levine RL, Gilliland DG: Myeloproliferative disorders. *Blood* 112(6):2190–2198, 2008.

53. Kravolics R, et al: A gain of function mutation of JAK2 in myeloproliferative disorders. *N Engl J Med* 352(17):1779–1790, 2005.

54. Chen G, Prchal JT: Polycythemia vera and its molecular basis: an update. *Best Pract Res Clin Haemotol* 19(3):387–397, 2006.

55. Ueda F, et al: Three tyrosine residues in the erythropoietin receptor are essential for Janus kinase 2 V617F mutant-induced tumorigenesis. *J Biol Chem* 292(5):1826–1846, 2016.

56. Landolfi R, Cipriani MC, Novarese L: Thrombosis and bleeding in polycythemia vera and essential thrombocythemia: pathogenetic mechanisms and prevention. *Best Pract Res Clin Haematol* 19(3):617–633, 2006.

57. Lin CH, Kaushansky K, Zhan H: JAK2V617F-mutant vascular niche contributes to JAK2V617F clonal expansion in myeloproliferative neoplasms. *Blood Cells Mol Dis* 62:42–48, 2016.

58. Tefferi A: The diagnosis of polycythemia vera: new tests and old dictums. *Best Pract Res Clin Haematol* 19(3):455–469, 2006.

59. Tefferi A: Polycythemia vera and essential thrombocythemia: 2012 update on diagnosis, risk stratification, and management. *Am J Hematol* 87(3):285–293, 2012.

60. Finazzi G, Barbui T: Evidence and expertise in the management of polycythemia vera and essential thrombocythemia. *Leukemia* 22(8):1494–1502, 2008.

61. Tibes R, Bogenberger JM, Mesa RA: JAK inhibition: the key to treating myeloproliferative neoplasm? *Expert Rev Hematol* 5(6):583–585, 2012.

62. Marchioli R, et al: Cardiovascular events and intensity of treatment in polycythemia vera. *N Engl J Med* 368(1):22–33, 2013.

63. Crownover BK, Covey CJ: Hereditary hemochromatosis. *Am Fam Physician* 87(3):183–190, 2013.

64. National Institutes of Health (NIH) Genetics Home Reference: *HFE gene hemochromatosis*, Bethesda, MD, 2017, U.S. National Library of Medicine, National Institutes of Health. Available at: https://ghr.nlm.nih.gov.

65. Ioannou A, Kannan L, Tsokos GC: Platelets, complement and tissue inflammation. *Autoimmunity* 46(1):1–5, 2013.

66. Selleng K, Selleng S, Greinacher A: Heparin-induced thrombocytopenia in intensive care patients. *Semin Thromb Hemost* 34(5):425–438, 2008.

67. Shaikh N: Heparin-induced thrombocytopenia. *J Emerg Trauma Shock* 4(1):97–102, 2011.

68. Warkentin TE, Sheppard J-AI: Testing for heparin-induced thrombocytopenia antibodies. *Transfus Med Rev* 20(4):259–272, 2006.

69. Lakshmanan S, Cuker A: Contemporary management of primary immune thrombocytopenia (ITP) in adults. *J Thromb Haemost* 10(10):1988–1998, 2012.

70. Kuhne T, Imback P: Management of children and adolescents with primary immune thrombocytopenia: controversies and solutions. *Vox Sang* 104(1):55–66, 2013.

71. Bennett CM, de Jong JLO, Neufeld EJ: Targeted ITP strategies: do they elucidate the biology of ITP and related disorders? *Pediatr Blood Cancer* 47(Suppl 5):706–709, 2006.

72. Gomez-Almaguer D: Monoclonal antibodies in the treatment of immune thrombocytopenic purpura (ITP). *Hematology* 17(Suppl 1):S25–S27, 2012.

73. Kremer Hovinga JA, et al: Thrombotic thrombocytopenic purpura. *Nat Rev Dis Primers* 3:17020, 2017.

74. Zoller B, et al: Autoimmune disease and venous thromboembolism: a review of the literature. *Am J Cardiovasc Dis* 2(3):171–183, 2012.

75. National Institutes of Health (NIH) Genetics Home Reference: *Thrombotic thrombocytopenia purpura*, Bethesda, MD, 2017, U.S. National Library of Medicine, National Institutes of Health. Available at: https://ghr.nlm.nih.gov.

76. Scully M, et al: A phase 2 study of the safety and efficacy of rituximab with plasma exchange in acute acquired thrombotic thrombocytopenic purpura. *Blood* 118(7):1746–1753, 2011.

77. Peyvandi F, et al: Capalacizumab for acquired thrombotic thrombocytopenic purpura. *N Engl J Med* 374(6):511–522, 2016.

78. National Institutes of Health (NIH): *Thrombocytopenia & thrombocytosis*, Bethesda, MD, 2008, National Institutes of Health, U.S. Department of Health and Human Services. Available at: www.nhlbi.nih.gov/health/dci/Diseases/thrm/thrm_all.html.

79. Cervantes F: Management of essential thrombocythemia. *Hematology Am Soc Hematol Educ Program* 2011:214–221, 2011.

80. Landolfi R, Fi Gennaro L: Thrombosis in myeloproliferative and myelodysplastic syndromes. *Hematology* 17(Suppl 1):S174–S176, 2012.

81. Santos FP, Verstovsek S: Breakthroughs in myeloproliferative neoplasms. *Hematology* 17(Suppl 1):S55–S58, 2012.

82. Tefferi A, Elliott M: Thrombosis in myeloproliferative disorders: prevalence, prognostic factors, and the role of leukocytes and JAK2V617F. *Semin Thromb Hemost* 33(4):313–320, 2007.

83. Wolanskyj AP, et al: Essential thrombocythemia beyond the first decade: life expectancy, long-term complication rates, and prognostic factors. *Mayo Clin Proc* 81(2):159–166, 2006.

84. Tefferi A, Thiele J, Vardiman JW: The 2008 World Health Organization classification system for myeloproliferative neoplasms: order out of chaos. *Cancer* 115(17):3842–3847, 2009.

85. Barbui T, Finazzi MC, Finazzi G: Front-line therapy in polycythemia vera and essential thrombocythemia. *Blood Rev* 26(5):205–211, 2012.

86. Hernandez-Boluda JC, et al: Oral anticoagulation to prevent thrombosis recurrence in polycythemia vera and essential thrombocythemia. *Ann Hematol* 94(6):911–918, 2015.

87. Salles II, et al: Inherited traits affecting platelet function. *Blood Rev* 22(3):155–172, 2008.

88. Lisman T, et al: Hemostasis and thrombosis in patients with liver disease: the ups and downs. *J Hepatol* 53(2):362–371, 2010.

89. Taylor FB, Jr, et al: Towards definition, clinical and laboratory criteria, and a scoring system for disseminated intravascular coagulation. *Thromb Haemost* 86:1327–1330, 2001.

90. Wad H, et al: Guidance for diagnosis and treatment of DIC from harmonization of the recommendations from three guidelines. *J Thromb Haemost* 11:761–767, 2013.

91. Gando S, Levi M, Toh C: Disseminated intravascular coagulation. *Nat Rev Dis Primers* 2:16037, 2016.

92. Kwaan HC, Vicuna B: Incidence and pathogenesis of thrombosis in hematologic malignancies. *Semin Thromb Hemost* 33(4):303–312, 2007.

93. Palumbo JS: Mechanisms linking tumor cell-associated procoagulant function to tumor dissemination. *Semin Thromb Hemost* 34(2):154–160, 2008.

94. Tripodi A: D-dimer testing in laboratory practice. *Clin Chem* 57(9):1256–1262, 2011.

95. Sorensen B, et al: Clinical review: prothrombin complex concentrates—evaluation of safety and thrombogenicity. *Crit Care* 15(1):201, 2011.

96. Baglin T: Inherited and acquired risk factors for venous thromoembolimsm. *Semin Respir Crit Care Med* 33(2):127–137, 2012.

97. National Institutes of Health (NIH): *Genetics home reference: prothrombin thrombophilia*, Bethesda, MA, 2017, National Institutes of Health, National Library of Medicine.

98. McNamee K, Dawood F, Farquharson R: Recurrent miscarriage and thrombophilia: an update. *Curr Opin Obstet Gynecol* 24(4):229–234, 2012.

99. Aksu K, Donmez A, Keser G: Inflammation-induced thrombosis: mechanisms, disease associations and management. *Curr Pharm Des* 18(11):1478–1493, 2012.

100. Wahl D, et al: Definition and significance of high positivity aCL ELISA. *Lupus* 21(7):725–726, 2012.

101. Willis R, Harris EN, Pierangeli SS: Current international initiatives in antiphospholipid antibody testing. *Semin Thromb Hemost* 38(4):360–374, 2012.

102. Heilmann L, et al: Pregnancy outcome in women with antiphospholipid antibodies: report on a retrospective study. *Semin Thromb Hemost* 34(8):794–802, 2008.

Alterations of Leukocyte and Lymphoid Function

Kathryn L. McCance, Neal S. Rote

evolve WEBSITE

CHAPTER OUTLINE

Disorders involving leukocytes range from deficiencies in the quality and quantity of leukocytes (leukopenia) to increased numbers of leukocytes (leukocytosis) in response to infections or proliferative disorders, such as leukemia. Many hematologic disorders are malignancies, and many nonhematologic malignancies act like malignancies and can metastasize to bone marrow, affecting leukocyte production. Because of the complexity of hematologic disorders a large portion of this chapter is devoted to malignant disease.

ALTERATIONS OF LEUKOCYTE FUNCTION

Leukocyte function is affected if too many or too few white cells are present in the blood or if the cells that are present are structurally or functionally defective. Quantitative leukocyte disorders, such as infections and leukemias, result from decreased production in the bone marrow or accelerated destruction of cells in the circulation. Other quantitative alterations, however, occur in response to infections.

Qualitative leukocyte disorders consist of disruptions of leukocyte function. Phagocytic cells (granulocytes, monocytes, macrophages) may lose their phagocytic capacity to function. Lymphocytes may lose their capacity to respond to antigens. (Qualitative disruptions of inflammatory and immune processes caused by leukocyte disorders are described in

Chapter 9.) Other leukocyte alterations include infectious mononucleosis and cancers of the blood—leukemia and multiple myeloma.

Quantitative Alterations of Leukocytes

Leukocytosis is a leukocyte count that is higher than normal; conversely, leukopenia is a count that is lower than normal. Leukocytosis or leukopenia may affect all cell types or only a specific type of leukocyte and may result from a variety of physiologic conditions and alterations.

Leukocytosis occurs as a normal protective response to physiologic stressors, such as infection, strenuous exercise, emotional changes, temperature changes, anesthesia, surgery, pregnancy, and some drugs, hormones, and toxins. It is also caused by pathologic conditions, such as malignancies and hematologic disorders. Leukopenia is never normal and is defined as an absolute blood cell count less than 4000 cells/μL. Leukopenia is associated with a decrease in the number of neutrophils, which increases the risk for infection. The absolute neutrophil count (ANC) is calculated by multiplying the white blood cell count by the percent of band and segmented neutrophils. The ANC is classified as mild (1000 to 1500 cells/μL), moderate (500 to 1000 cells/μL), or severe (<500 cells/μL). When the ANC is less than 500/μL, the possibility for life-threatening infections is high. Leukopenia can be caused by radiation, anaphylactic shock, autoimmune disease (e.g., systemic lupus erythematosus), immune deficiencies (see Chapter 9), and exposure to certain drugs such as glucocorticoids and chemotherapeutic agents.

Granulocytes and Monocytes

Increased numbers of circulating granulocytes (neutrophils, eosinophils, basophils) and monocytes are primarily a response to infection. Increased numbers also occur as a result of myeloproliferative disorders (i.e., polycythemia vera, chronic myelogenous leukemia, chronic neutrophilic leukemia, chronic eosinophilic leukemia) that increase stem cell proliferation in bone marrow.

Decreased numbers occur when infectious processes exhaust the supply of circulating granulocytes and monocytes by drawing them out of the circulation and into infected tissues faster than they can be replaced. Decreases also can be caused by disorders that suppress marrow function.

Granulocytosis—an increase in the number of granulocytes (neutrophils, eosinophils, basophils)—begins with the release of stored leukocytes from the venous sinuses of the marrow. Neutrophilia is another term that may be used to describe *granulocytosis* because neutrophils are the most numerous of the granulocytes (Table 30.1). Neutrophilia occurs in the early stages of infection or inflammation and is established when the absolute neutrophil count exceeds 7500/μL. Stored neutrophils are approximately 20 to 40 times greater in number than circulating neutrophils. On rare occasions when the neutrophil count increases significantly—more than 100,000/μL (usually seen only in those with myelocytic leukemia)—the blood viscosity may increase considerably so that thrombosis or occlusion of blood vessels occurs. Release and depletion of stored neutrophils from the venous sinuses stimulate granulopoiesis to replenish neutrophil reserves. Specific conditions associated with neutrophilia are identified in Table 30.1.

When the demand for circulating mature neutrophils exceeds the supply, the marrow begins to release immature neutrophils (and other leukocytes) into the blood. Premature release of the immature white cells is responsible for the phenomenon known as a shift-to-the-left or leukemoid reaction. This refers to the microscopic detection of disproportionate numbers of immature leukocytes in peripheral blood smears. Many diagrams present cellular differentiation and maturation progressing from left to right within the drawing, instead of vertically as shown in Fig. 28.12. When immature leukocytes are released prematurely they cause a shift in the distribution of cells in the blood toward the left side, or immaturity side, of the diagram. This phenomenon is also seen in the blood smear of individuals with leukemia as well, hence the term *leukemoid reaction*. As infection or inflammation diminishes and as granulopoiesis replenishes circulating granulocytes, a shift back to normal occurs.

Neutropenia is a condition associated with a reduction in the number of circulating neutrophils. Clinically, neutropenia exists when the neutrophil count is less than 2000/μL.[1] The absolute neutrophil count reflects not only the degree of neutropenia but also the risk for infection (see preceding discussion of leukocytosis). A reduction in the number of neutrophils can occur in severe, prolonged infections when production of granulocytes cannot keep up with demand. Severe neutropenia, granulocytopenia (less than 500/μL) or agranulocytosis (complete absence of granulocytes in blood), is usually secondary to arrested hematopoiesis in the bone marrow or massive cell destruction in the circulation. Chemotherapeutic agents used to treat hematologic and other malignancies cause generalized bone marrow suppression. Several other drugs and large doses of ionizing radiation cause agranulocytosis, which occurs rarely but carries a high death rate (10% to 50%). Clinical manifestations of agranulocytosis include recurrent and persistent life-threatening infection (particularly of the respiratory system) leading to septicemia, general malaise, fever, tachycardia, and ulcers in the mouth and colon. If untreated, sepsis caused by agranulocytosis results in death within 3 to 6 days.

Other causes of neutropenia, in the absence of infection, may be (1) decreased neutrophil production or ineffective granulopoiesis, (2) reduced neutrophil survival, and (3) abnormal neutrophil distribution and sequestration. Neutropenia also is categorized as primary or secondary; primary disorders are further identified as congenital or acquired (Box 30.1).

Congenital defects in neutrophil production include cyclic neutropenia and neutropenia with congenital immunodeficiency diseases, as well as multiple syndromes (e.g., Kostmann, Shwachman-Diamond, Diamond-Blackfan, Griscelli, Chédiak-Higashi, and Barth syndromes). Primary acquired neutropenia is associated with multiple conditions, for example, hypoplastic anemia or aplastic anemia, leukemia (acute myelogenous leukemia [AML]/chronic lymphocytic leukemia [CLL]), lymphomas (Hodgkin, non-Hodgkin), and myelodysplastic syndrome (MDS). The megaloblastic anemias (vitamin B_{12} and folate deficiency) as well as starvation and anorexia nervosa cause neutropenia because of an inadequate supply of vitamins and nutrients for protein production.

Reduced neutrophil survival and abnormal distribution and sequestration are usually secondary to other disorders. Neutropenia occurs in a variety of immunologic disorders, particularly systemic lupus erythematosus, rheumatoid arthritis, Felty and Sjögren syndromes, splenomegaly, and drug-related causes.

Eosinophilia is an absolute increase (more than 450/μL) in the total numbers of circulating eosinophils. Allergic disorders (type I hypersensitivity) associated with asthma, hay fever, and drug reactions, as well as parasitic infections (particularly with metazoal parasites), are often cited as causes. Hypersensitivity reactions and the normal defense against parasites trigger the release of eosinophil chemotactic factor of anaphylaxis (ECF-A) from mast cells, attracting eosinophils to the area. (These processes are described and illustrated in Chapters 8 and 9.) Tissues with abundant mast cells, such as the respiratory and gastrointestinal tracts, are particularly common sites for eosinophil invasion. Mast cells also release interleukin-5 (IL-5), which stimulates the bone marrow to produce and release more eosinophils into the blood. Eosinophilia may also be associated with dermatologic disorders, such as atopic dermatitis, eczema, and pemphigus. Various types of eosinophilic scleroderma-like diseases also have been reported to occur in association with hemato-oncogenic disorders (i.e., eosinophilic cellulitis [Wells syndrome] and eosinophilic fasciitis [Shulman syndrome]). Increased numbers of eosinophils have been observed in individuals with eosinophilia-myalgia syndrome (EMS), which is associated with ingestion of the supplement L-tryptophan. EMS may develop in individuals with fibromyalgia syndrome as an allergic reaction to L-tryptophan.[2]

Eosinopenia, a decrease in circulating numbers of eosinophils, generally is caused by migration of eosinophils into inflammatory sites. It also may be seen in Cushing syndrome and as a result of stress caused by surgery, shock, trauma, burns, or mental distress. Other conditions causing eosinopenia are detailed in Table 30.1.

Basophilia, an increase in circulating numbers of basophils, is rare and generally is a response to inflammation and immediate hypersensitivity reactions. Basophils contain histamine that is released during an allergic reaction. An increase in the levels of basophils is seen also in myeloproliferative disorders, such as chronic myeloid leukemia and myeloid metaplasia. Other conditions associated with basophilia are listed in Table 30.1.

Basopenia (also known as *basophilic leukopenia*), a decrease in circulating numbers of basophils, is seen in hyperthyroidism, acute infection, and long-term therapy with steroids. A decrease in the number of basophils may be seen during ovulation and pregnancy. Other conditions associated with basopenia are listed in Table 30.1.

TABLE 30.1 OTHER CONDITIONS ASSOCIATED WITH NEUTROPHILS, EOSINOPHILS, BASOPHILS, MONOCYTES, AND LYMPHOCYTES

CONDITION	CAUSE	EXAMPLE
Neutrophil		
Neutrophilia (granulocytosis)	Inflammation or tissue necrosis	Surgery, burns, MI, pneumonitis, rheumatic fever, rheumatoid arthritis
	Infection	Bacterial: gram positive (staphylococci, streptococci, pneumococci), gram negative (*Escherichia coli, Pseudomonas* species)
	Physiologic	Exercise, extreme heat or cold, third-trimester pregnancy, emotional distress
	Hematologic	Acute hemorrhage, hemolysis, myeloproliferative disorder, chronic granulocytic leukemia
	Drugs or chemicals	Epinephrine, steroids, heparin, histamine, endotoxin
	Metabolic	Diabetes (acidosis), eclampsia, gout, thyroid storm
	Neoplasm	Liver, GI tract, bone marrow
Neutropenia	Decreased marrow production	Radiation, chemotherapy, leukemia, aplastic anemia, abnormal granulopoiesis
	Increased destruction	Splenomegaly, hemodialysis, autoimmune disease
	Infection	Gram negative (typhoid), viral (influenza, hepatitis B, measles, mumps, rubella), severe infections, protozoal infections (malaria)
Eosinophil		
Eosinophilia	Allergy	Asthma, hay fever, drug sensitivity
	Infection	Parasites (trichinosis, hookworm), chronic (fungal, leprosy, TB)
	Malignancy	CML, lung, stomach, ovary, Hodgkin disease
	Dermatosis	Pemphigus, exfoliative dermatitis (drug-induced)
	Drugs	Digitalis, heparin, streptomycin, tryptophan (eosinophilia-myalgia syndrome), penicillins, propranolol
Eosinopenia	Stress response	Trauma, shock, burns, surgery, mental distress
	Drugs	Steroids (Cushing syndrome)
Basophil		
Basophilia	Inflammation	Infection (measles, chickenpox), hypersensitivity reaction (immediate)
	Hematologic	Myeloproliferative disorders (CML, polycythemia vera, Hodgkin lymphoma, hemolytic anemia)
	Endocrine	Myxedema, antithyroid therapy
Basopenia	Physiologic	Pregnancy, ovulation, stress
	Endocrine	Graves disease
Monocyte		
Monocytosis	Infection	Bacterial (subacute bacterial endocarditis, TB), recovery phase of infection
	Hematologic	Myeloproliferative disorders, Hodgkin disease, agranulocytosis
	Physiologic	Normal newborn
Monocytopenia	Rare	
Lymphocyte		
Lymphocytosis	Physiologic	4 months to 4 years
	Acute infection	Infectious mononucleosis, CMV infection, pertussis, hepatitis, mycoplasma pneumonia, typhoid
	Chronic infection	Congenital syphilis, tertiary syphilis
	Endocrine	Thyrotoxicosis, adrenal insufficiency
	Malignancy	ALL, CLL, lymphosarcoma cell leukemia
Lymphocytopenia	Immunodeficiency syndrome	AIDS, agammaglobulinemia
	Lymphocyte destruction	Steroids (Cushing syndrome), radiation, chemotherapy, Hodgkin lymphoma, CHF, renal failure, TB, SLE, aplastic anemia

AIDS, Acquired immunodeficiency syndrome; *ALL,* acute lymphocytic leukemia; *CHF,* congestive (left) heart failure; *CLL,* chronic lymphocytic leukemia; *CML,* chronic myelogenous leukemia; *CMV,* cytomegalovirus; *GI,* gastrointestinal; *MI,* myocardial infarction; *SLE,* systemic lupus erythematosus; *TB,* tuberculosis.

BOX 30.1 CLASSIFICATION OF NEUTROPENIA

Congenital
Severe infantile agranulocytosis (Kostmann syndrome)
Shwachman-Diamond-Oski syndrome
Myelokathexis/neutropenia with tetraploid nuclei
Cyclic neutropenia
Chédiak-Higashi syndrome
Reticular dysgenesis
Dyskeratosis congenita

Acquired
Postinfectious neutropenia
Drug-induced neutropenia
Complement activation (hemodialysis, leukapheresis, ARDS)
Immune neutropenia
    Isoimmune neonatal neutropenia
    Alloimmune neutropenia (transfusion reaction)
    Autoimmune neutropenia—primary
        Beginning of childhood
        Adult chronic form
    Autoimmune neutropenia—secondary
        Autoimmune diseases
        Large granular lymphocyte
    Pure white cell aplasia
Chronic idiopathic neutropenia
Hypersplenism
Nutritional deficiency (vitamin B_{12} or folate deficiency)
Diseases affecting the bone marrow
    Postchemotherapy
    Aplastic anemia
    Fanconi anemia
    Myelodysplastic syndrome
    Acute and chronic leukemias

ARDS, Acute respiratory distress syndrome.
Data from Capsoni F, Sarzi-Puttini P, Zanella A: *Arthritis Res Ther* 7(5):208–214, 2005.

Monocytosis is an increase (generally greater than 800/µL) in numbers of circulating monocytes. The condition is often transient and not related to a dysfunction of monocyte production. When present, it most commonly occurs with neutropenia associated with bacterial infections, particularly in the late stages or recovery stage, when monocytes are needed to phagocytize surviving microorganisms and debris. Monocytosis often is seen in chronic infections, usually with intracellular bacteria, such as tuberculosis (TB), brucellosis, listeriosis, and subacute bacterial endocarditis (SBE). Peripheral monocytosis has been found to correlate with the extent of myocardial damage following myocardial infarction. Increased numbers of monocytes also may indicate marrow recovery from agranulocytosis. Other conditions associated with monocytosis are identified in Table 30.1.

Monocytopenia, a decrease in numbers of circulating monocytes, is rare, and not much is known about this condition because of the small numbers of monocytes generally present in the blood. Monocytopenia, however, has been identified with hairy cell leukemia and prednisone therapy.

Lymphocytes

Quantitative alteration of lymphocytes occurs when lymphocytes are activated by antigenic stimuli, usually microorganisms (see Chapter 8).

Lymphocytosis (absolute lymphocytosis) is an increase in the number or proportion of lymphocytes in the blood. It is rare in acute bacterial infections and occurs most commonly in acute viral infections, particularly those caused by the Epstein-Barr virus (EBV), a causative agent in infectious mononucleosis. Other specific disorders associated with lymphocytosis are listed in Table 30.1.

Lymphocytopenia is a decrease in the number of circulating lymphocytes in the blood. It may be attributable to (1) abnormalities of lymphocyte production associated with neoplasias and immune deficiencies and (2) destruction by drugs, viruses, or radiation. It also can occur in individuals for no apparent reason. Other conditions associated with lymphocytopenia are identified in Table 30.1. The lymphocytopenia associated with heart failure and other acute illnesses may be caused by elevated levels of cortisol. Lymphocytopenia is a major problem in acquired immunodeficiency syndrome (AIDS) in which the human immunodeficiency virus (HIV) is cytopathic for T helper lymphocytes. (For a more detailed discussion of AIDS, see Chapter 10.)

Infectious Mononucleosis

Infectious mononucleosis (IM) is a benign, acute, self-limiting, lymphoproliferative clinical syndrome characterized by acute viral infection of B lymphocytes (B cells). It is associated with several human tumors, most commonly specific lymphomas and nasopharyngeal carcinoma.[3] The most common etiologic agent is EBV, a ubiquitous, lymphotrophic, gamma-group herpesvirus, which was first recognized as the causative agent of IM in the late 1960s. EBV accounts for approximately 85% of all IM cases. Other etiologic agents that may cause symptoms resembling IM are viruses (cytomegalovirus [CMV], adenovirus, HIV, hepatitis A, influenzas A and B, and rubella), as well as the bacteria *Toxoplasma gondii, Corynebacterium diphtheriae,* and *Coxiella burnetii.* IM caused by CMV is generally noted in older individuals, with fever and malaise the major complaints; the major manifestations of EBV-induced IM are the classic triad of symptoms of pharyngitis, lymphadenopathy, and fever.

Approximately 50% to 85% of children are infected with EBV by age 4, and more than 90% of adults have indications of subclinical EBV infections. These early infections are usually asymptomatic and provide immunity to EBV; thus early EBV infections rarely develop into IM. IM may arise when the initial infection occurs during adolescence or later, but still only results in IM in 35% to 50% of these individuals. Symptomatic IM usually affects young adults between ages 15 and 35 years, with the peak incidences occurring between 15 and 24 years; males have a later peak (18 to 24 years) than females. The overall incidence rate for the 15- and 24-year age group is 6 to 8 cases per 1000 persons per year. Children from low socioeconomic environments are particularly susceptible to infections with EBV. IM is uncommon in individuals older than age 40; but if it does occur, it is more commonly caused by CMV.

Transmission of EBV is usually by saliva through personal contact (e.g., kissing, hence the term "kissing disease"). The virus also may be present in other mucosal secretions of the genitalia, rectum, and respiratory tract, as well as blood. No evidence of aerosol transmission through sneezing or coughing has been documented. The disease begins with widespread infection of B lymphocytes, all of which possess receptors for EBV. The virus initially infects the oropharynx, nasopharynx, and salivary epithelial cells with later spread to the lymphoid tissue and B cells. Infection of B cells permits the virus to enter the bloodstream, which spreads the infection systemically.

◆PATHOPHYSIOLOGY. In the immunocompetent individual, unaffected B cells produce antibodies (IgG, IgM, IgA) against the virus. Concomitantly, there is a massive activation and proliferation of cytotoxic

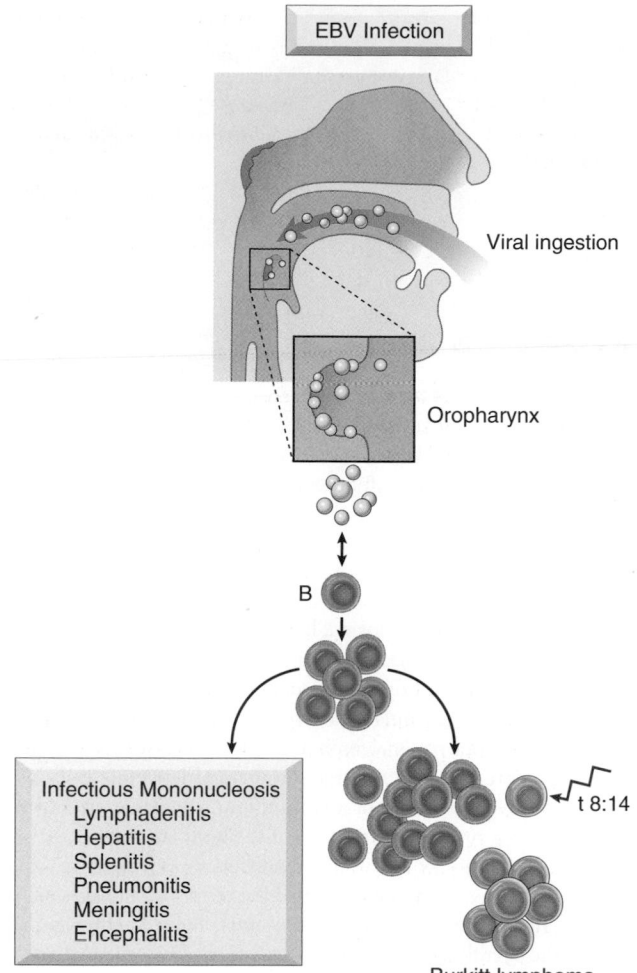

FIGURE 30.1 Outcomes of Epstein-Barr Virus (EBV). In individuals with normal immune function, infection is typically asymptomatic or leads to mononucleosis. With immunodeficiency, proliferation of B cells may be uncontrolled and progress to the development of B-cell neoplasms. Individuals without evidence of immunodeficiency can also develop EBV-positive neoplasms. In Burkitt lymphoma, the individual's susceptibility to EBV causes B cells to undergo genetic alterations (usually an 8;14 chromosomal translocation). EBV also is implicated in Hodgkin lymphoma, nasopharyngeal carcinoma, and other rare non-Hodgkin lymphomas. (From Kumar V, Abbas A, Aster JC: *Robbins & Cotran pathologic basis of disease,* ed 9, Philadelphia, 2015, Saunders.)

T cells (CD8) directed against EBV-infected cells; CD8 lymphocytes can account for greater than 50% of the total circulating lymphocytes. The immune response against EBV-infected cells (cellular infiltration, cytokine production) is largely responsible for the cellular proliferation in the lymphoid tissues (lymph nodes, spleen, tonsils, occasionally liver). Sore throat and fever, two of the earliest manifestations, are caused by inflammation at the site of viral entry and initial infection (the mouth and throat). Outcomes of EBV infection are presented in Fig. 30.1.

◆**CLINICAL MANIFESTATIONS.** The incubation period of IM is approximately 30 to 50 days (4 to 8 weeks) followed by a 3- to 5-day prodrome of fever, malaise, and arthralgias that are often attributed to viral infection, although some individuals remain asymptomatic. These symptoms may vary in severity for the next 7 to 20 days. At the time of diagnosis the individual usually has the classic triad of symptoms: fever, pharyngitis, and lymphadenopathy of the cervical lymph nodes.

The pharyngitis is usually diffuse and often accompanied by a whitish or grayish green, thick exudate. It also is quite painful and is the symptom that most often causes the individual to seek treatment. IM is usually self-limiting, and recovery occurs in a few weeks. Fatigue may last for 1 to 2 months after resolution of the infection.

Although severe clinical complications are rare, as the condition progresses generalized lymph node enlargement may develop and enlargement of the spleen and liver also may occur. Splenomegaly is clinically evident 50% of the time and is demonstrated radiologically 100% of the time. Difficulty in detecting splenomegaly with physical examination contributes to the underestimation of actual enlargement. Splenic rupture is rare (only 0.1% to 0.5% of all cases) and can occur spontaneously as a result of mild trauma, occurring primarily in men younger than 25 years of age and between days 4 and 21 after the onset of symptoms. It is the most common cause of death related to IM. Other causes of fatalities are hepatic failure, extensive bacterial infection, or viral myocarditis.

Other organ systems are rarely involved, but such involvement may result in additional symptoms, such as meningitis, encephalitis, Guillain-Barré syndrome, Bell palsy, optic neuritis, mental impairment, transverse myelitis, cerebellar ataxia, and demyelinating diseases. Ocular manifestations may include eyelid and periorbital edema, dry eyes, keratitis, uveitis, conjunctivitis, retinitis, oculoglandular syndrome, choroiditis, papillitis, and ophthalmoplegia. In children, Reye syndrome also has been associated with EBV infection.

Pulmonary involvement is rare, but when present may include hilar and mediastinal lymphadenopathy, interstitial pneumonitis, and pleural effusion. Pneumonia and respiratory failure have been documented; however, they are more likely to develop in immunocompromised individuals. Approximately 3% to 10% of adults older than 40 years of age have never been infected with EBV and are susceptible to IM later in life. In these individuals the classic symptoms are not generally present, making diagnosis more difficult. If an older individual has an elevated temperature that cannot be explained and persists for more than 2 weeks, EBV infection should be suspected, particularly in the presence of abnormal liver function tests with hepatomegaly and jaundice. Other neurologic manifestations that may be present include peripheral neuropathy and Guillain-Barré syndrome.

◆**EVALUATION AND TREATMENT.** Children commonly present with fever, sore throat, lymphadenitis, and the manifestations discussed earlier. The presentation in young adults includes malaise, fatigue, and lymphadenopathy and often a fever of unknown origin. The blood of affected individuals contains an increased number of atypical lymphocytes (Fig. 30.2). Diagnosis of IM is commonly based on Hoagland's criteria of at least 50% lymphocytes and at least 10% atypical lymphocytes in the blood in the presence of fever, pharyngitis, and adenopathy confirmed by a positive serologic test. Serologic tests are used to determine a heterophile antibody response.[4] Heterophile antibodies are a heterogeneous group of immunoglobulin M (IgM) antibodies that are agglutinins against nonhuman red blood cells (e.g., sheep, horse) and are detected by qualitative (Monospot) or quantitative methods (heterophile antibody test).

The Monospot test is limited because other infections (e.g., CMV, adenovirus) and toxoplasmosis also produce heterophilic antibodies. Thus 5% to 15% of Monospot tests yield false-positive results. Levels of heterophilic antibodies in the blood increase as the condition progresses, although some individuals and children younger than age 4 years do not produce them. These individuals give a false-negative result. Specificity for diagnosis of EBV infection may be increased with viral-specific serologic tests that identify EBV-specific antibodies (e.g., IgG or IgM against the viral capsid antigen [VCA], or IgG against the EBV nuclear antigen [EBNA]). These tests are more expensive and labor

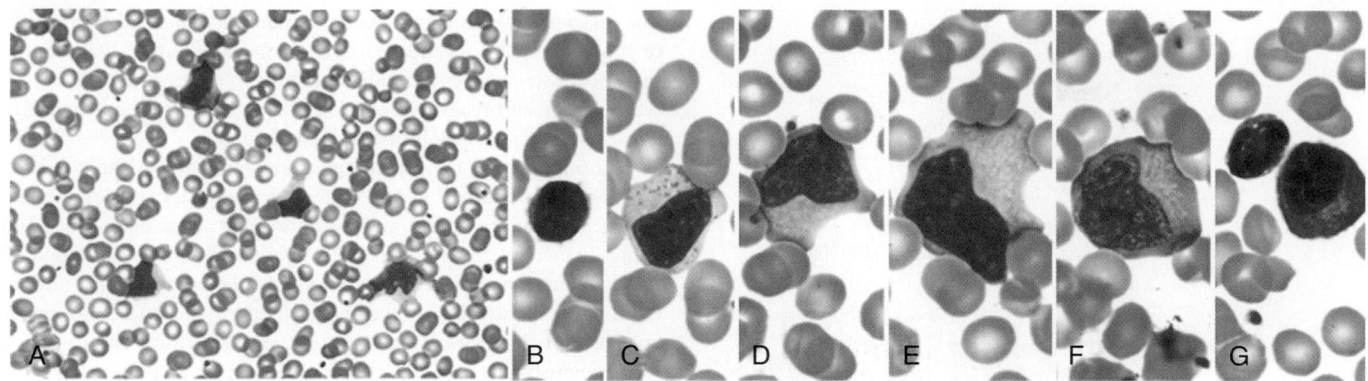

FIGURE 30.2 Peripheral Blood Smear in Infectious Mononucleosis. Low power **(A)** shows moderately high white blood cell count and a high number of reactive, or "atypical," lymphocytes. Higher power **(B–G)** illustrates the spectrum of lymphoid morphology, including small resting lymphocytes **(B)** for comparison, large granular lymphocytes **(C)**, atypical forms **(D–F)** (also referred to as *reactive lymphs*), and circulating plasma cells **(G)**. (From Hoffman R et al: *Hematology: basic principles and practice,* ed 6, Philadelphia, 2013, Churchill Livingstone.)

intensive; therefore they are reserved for instances in which the Monospot test is not appropriate.

Because IM is usually self-limiting, medical intervention is rarely required. Treatment of IM is supportive and includes rest and alleviation of symptoms with analgesics and antipyretics. Ibuprofen, *not aspirin,* is used with children and adolescents because of the reported incidence of Reye syndrome associated with EBV infection. Pharyngitis of streptococcal origin, which occurs in 20% to 30% of cases, is treated with penicillin or erythromycin. Ampicillin is contraindicated because it causes a rash in most individuals with IM.

Bed rest and avoidance of strenuous activity should be included in the therapy. Steroids may be used, but only in the presence of severe complications (e.g., impending airway obstruction) or other organ system involvement (e.g., nervous system manifestations, thrombocytopenic purpura, myocarditis, pericarditis). Acyclovir has been used with immunosuppressed individuals; however, clinical improvement has been minimal and therefore it is not recommended for standard treatment.

In the rare event of splenic rupture, the treatment has been removal of the spleen and continues to be the choice in hemodynamically unstable individuals. However, new research is suggesting that it may be better to repair the spleen to avoid overwhelming postsplenectomy infection (OPSI). Children are at greater risk of OPSI than adults. Postsplenectomy vaccinations for *Streptococcus pneumoniae, Haemophilus influenzae,* and *Meningococcus* are essential because these microorganisms are responsible for 92% of fatal infections. Treatment may also be necessary for airway obstruction from massive edema of the Waldeyer ring or for autoimmune hemolytic anemia, which occurs in approximately 3% to 5% of cases.

Fatal IM also is expressed with the inherited X-linked lymphoproliferative (XLP) syndrome (Duncan disease). Duncan disease is a rare disorder characterized by severe dysregulation of the immune system, often in response to EBV. The underlying cause leading to death is the absence of a functional SAP protein that allows for the unregulated proliferation of cytotoxic T cells and the concomitant production and release of cytokines.

Lymphoid Neoplasm: Leukemias

Leukemia is a clonal malignant disorder of leukocytes in the bone marrow and usually, but not always, of the blood. The common feature of all forms of leukemia is an uncontrolled proliferation of malignant leukocytes, causing an overcrowding of bone marrow and decreased production and function of normal hematopoietic cells. Thus leukemia has been termed an *accumulation* disorder, as well as a *proliferation* disorder. In the majority of cases, leukemic cells are ejected into the blood where they accumulate. These cells also may infiltrate and accumulate in the liver, spleen, lymph nodes, and other organs throughout the body. The presentation of large numbers of leukemic cells in the blood may be one of the most dramatic indicators of leukemia; however, leukemia is still a primary disruption of the bone marrow.

The first description of a "leukemic" individual was written by Velpeau in 1827.[5] Virchow, a pathologist, coined the term *white blood (Weissus blut)* and later originated the term *leukemia.* Since Virchow's initial discovery, the overall classification of leukemia has become increasingly complex and undergone several permutations. With increased understanding, the *distinct* divisions between *leukemia* and *lymphoma* has become indistinct or blurred. Many entities known as "lymphoma" that arise as a discrete tissue mass sometimes have "leukemic" presentations, and evolution to leukemia is not unusual during the progression of incurable lymphomas.[3] The current World Health Organization (WHO) classification scheme uses morphologic, immunophenotypic, genotypic, and clinical features to group the lymphoid neoplasms into five broad categories, which are sorted according to the cell of origin[3]:

1. Precursor B-cell neoplasms (immature B cells)
2. Peripheral B-cell neoplasms (mature B cells)
3. Precursor T-cell neoplasms (immature T cells)
4. Peripheral T-cell and NK-cell neoplasms (mature T cells and NK cells
5. Hodgkin lymphoma (Reed-Sternberg cells and variants)

Most lymphoid neoplasms relate to stages of differentiation of B-cell or T-cell differentiation (Fig. 30.3, *A*). Fig. 30.3, *B* provides a simple schematic overview of the main types of leukemia.

Acute leukemia is characterized by undifferentiated or immature cells, usually a blast cell, and the onset of disease is abrupt and rapid with a short survival time. In chronic leukemia the predominant cell is more differentiated but does not function normally, with a relatively slow progression. There are four general types of leukemia: acute lymphocytic (ALL), acute myelogenous (AML), chronic lymphocytic (CLL), and chronic myelogenous (CML).

Leukemia occurs with varying frequencies at different ages and is more common in adults than children (Fig. 30.4). Worldwide, the number of new leukemia cases is estimated at 351,965 and deaths of 265,471 for 2012.[6] In the United States it is estimated that more than

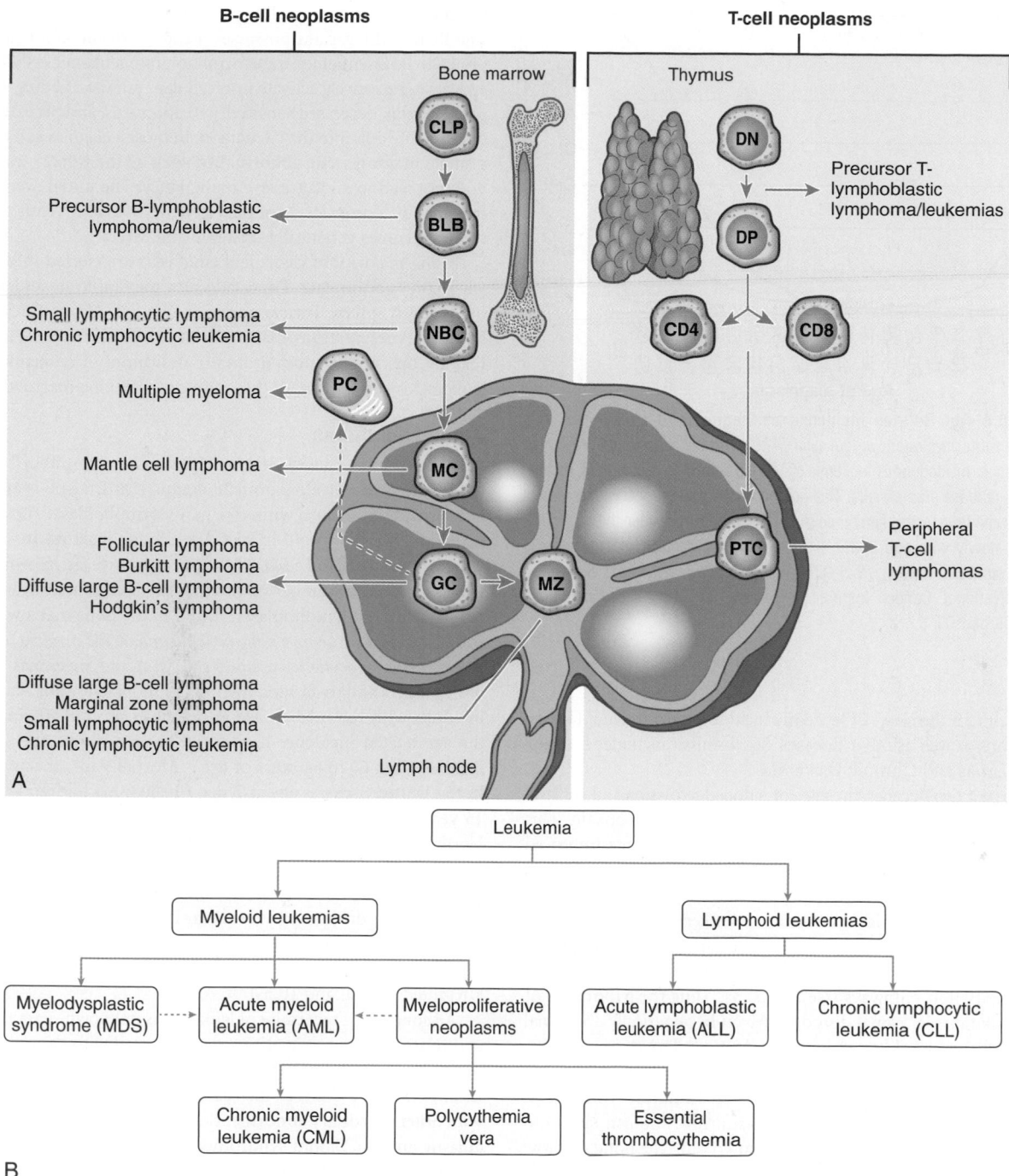

FIGURE 30.3 Origin of Lymphoid Neoplasms. A, Specific lymphoid tumors emerge from stages of B- and T-cell differentiation. **B,** Overview of main types of leukemia. Acute myeloid lymphoma (AML) may arise *de novo* or be preceded by myelodysplastic phase. Not all cases of myelodysplastic syndrome (MDS) evolve to AML (dashed line). Some myelodysplastic neoplasms can transform into AML, although very rarely (dotted line). *BLB,* Pre-B lymphoblast; *CLP,* common lymphoid precursor; *DN,* CD4/CD8 double-negative pro-T cell; *DP,* CD4/CD8 double-positive pre-T cell; *GC,* germinal-center B cell; *MC,* mantle B cell; *MZ,* marginal zone B cell; *NBC,* naïve B cell; *PTC,* peripheral T cell. (**A,** From Kumar V, Abbas A, Aster JC: *Robbins & Cotran pathologic basis of disease,* ed 9, Philadelphia, 2015, Saunders; **B,** from Khwaja A et al: Acute myeloid leukemia, *Nat Rev Dis Pimers* 2:16010, 2016.)

62,100 new cases of leukemia were diagnosed and 24,500 deaths occurred in 2017,[7] with males having a slightly higher incidence than females. In all types of leukemia males have a higher incidence rate as do Americans of European descent. White children have higher rates of leukemia than children of other groups. ALL is the least common type overall, but is the most common in children (approximately 66% of ALL cases are diagnosed before the age of 20). Leukemia accounts for about 29% of all childhood cancers, and ALL accounts for a majority of all new cases of leukemia in children. CLL and AML are the most common types in adults. CML is found mostly in adults.

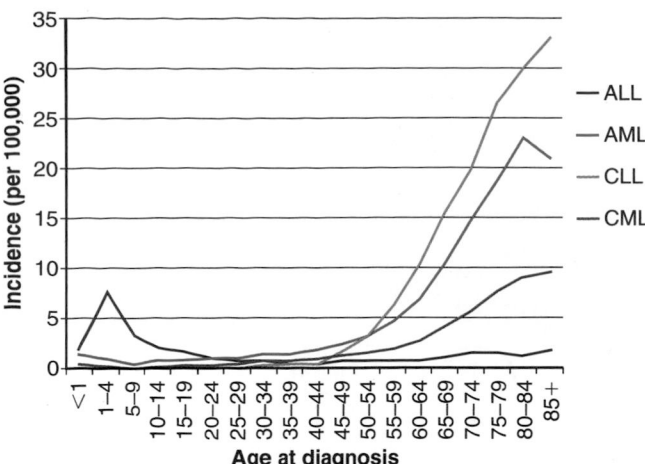

FIGURE 30.4 Age-Related Incidence at Diagnosis of Leukemias. The incidences of acute myelogenous leukemia *(AML)*, chronic lymphocytic leukemia *(CLL)*, and chronic myelogenous leukemia *(CML)* are relatively stable until middle age and then increase dramatically. The incidence of acute lymphocytic leukemia *(ALL)* peaks in childhood, and then diminishes until middle age when the incidence begins rising slowly with age. (Data obtained from Howlander N et al, editors: *SEER cancer statistics review, 1975-2009 [vintage 2009 populations]*, Bethesda, MD, 2012, National Cancer Institute. Available at http://seer.cancer.gov/csr/1975_2005/pops09/.)

Risk factors for the onset of leukemia include environmental factors, genetic factors, as well as other diseases. See discussions under sections Acute Leukemias and Chronic Leukemias.

Over the past two decades, the rates of induced remission and survival in most forms of leukemia have increased, sometimes dramatically. This progress is the result of more effective chemotherapeutic agents, improved blood product and antimicrobial support, and specialized nursing care. Chemotherapy and bone marrow transplants have significantly increased the survival time for individuals with acute leukemia.

◆PATHOPHYSIOLOGY. All leukemias have certain pathophysiologic features in common. Most lymphoid neoplasms arise from B-cell and T-cell differentiation pathways (see Fig. 30.3). Thus the hypothesis of origin for leukemias is "clonal disorders driven by genetically abnormal progenitor cells or stemlike cancer cells (SLCC)."[8] The majority (85% to 90%) of lymphoid neoplasm are of B-cell origin, followed by T-cell tumors, and NK-cell tumors rarely.[3] Abnormal immature white blood cells, called leukemic blasts, fill the bone marrow and can spill into the blood. The leukemic blasts literally "crowd out" the bone marrow and cause cellular proliferation of the other cell lines to cease. Normal granulocytic-monocytic, lymphocytic, erythrocytic, and megakaryocytic progenitor cells can cease to function, leading to pancytopenia (a reduction in all cellular components of the blood). Almost 90% of ALLs have chromosomal changes that correlate with immunophenotyping and sometime confer prognostic significance. Genetic translocations (mitotic errors) are observed in leukemic cells. The most common genetic abnormality is the reciprocal translocation between chromosomes 9 and 22—t(9;22)(q34;q11), the Philadelphia chromosome.[9]

The Philadelphia chromosome was first observed in persons with CML, and is present in 95% of those with CML, 3% of individuals with AML, and 25% to 30% of adults with ALL and 2% to 10% of children with ALL.[10] This translocation results in the novel fusion of the *BCR1* gene region from chromosome 22 and the proto-oncogene *ABL1* from chromosome 9 (Fig. 30.5). The *BCR-ABL1* joining results in the expression of a unique fused oncoprotein, BCR-ABL1.[9] The ABL1 protein is a

tyrosine kinase in the signaling pathway that promotes cell proliferation. The BCR-ABL1 variant possesses greater tyrosine kinase activity and proves to be essential for transformation into leukemic cells. BCR-ABL1 appears to excessively activate intracellular pathways, leading to increased proliferation, decreased sensitivity to apoptosis, and premature release of immature cells into the circulation. In most leukemias and lymphomas a single major genetic abnormality, such as the t(9;22) translocation, does not lead to an aggressive malignancy. The initial event is usually followed by a series of secondary genetic changes.[11] Thus the original tumor becomes genetically unstable and diverse.

In the majority of cases, leukemic cells are ejected into the blood, where they accumulate. These cells also may infiltrate and accumulate in the liver, spleen, lymph nodes, and other organs throughout the body. The presentation of large numbers of leukemic cells in the blood may be one of the most dramatic indicators of leukemia; however, leukemia is still a primary disruption of the bone marrow.

Acute Leukemias

Acute leukemias consist of two types: acute lymphocytic leukemia (ALL) and acute myelogenous leukemia (AML). ALL is an aggressive fast-growing leukemia with too many lymphoblasts (i.e., immature white blood cells) found in blood and bone marrow. It is also called *acute lymphoblastic leukemia.* AML is an aggressive fast-growing leukemia with an excessive number of myeloblasts (i.e., immature white blood cells that are not lymphoblasts) found in the bone marrow and blood. It is also called *acute myeloblastic leukemia, acute myeloid leukemia,* or *acute nonlymphocytic leukemia (ANLL).* Acute leukemias are seen in both genders and in all ages. AML is the more common acute leukemia in adults with the median age at diagnosis around 70 years, a rise in the age-related incidence around 40 to 50 years of age, and a steep increase from 60 to 64 years of age.[12] Mortality for all acute leukemias in the United States is about 7 per 100,000. In children younger than 15 years, leukemia accounts for one-third of all deaths from cancer. North American and Scandinavian countries have the highest mortality; Eastern European countries, Asia (except Japan), and Central America have the lowest mortality. Japan's higher mortality is the result of the atomic bombs dropped in World War II. Blacks have consistently shown a lower mortality than whites. More than 5970 new cases of ALL and 21,380 cases of AML are estimated in 2017, with more than 1440 deaths attributed to ALL and 10,590 to AML.[7]

Although the exact cause of leukemia is unknown, several risk factors and related genetic aberrations are associated with the onset of malignancy. There is a statistically significant tendency for leukemia to reappear in families. There also is an increased incidence of leukemia in association with other hereditary abnormalities, such as Down syndrome, Fanconi aplastic anemia, Bloom syndrome, trisomy 13 (Patau syndrome), and some immune deficiencies (i.e., ataxia-telangiectasia, Wiskott-Aldrich syndrome, and congenital X–linked agammaglobulinemia) (see Chapter 9). Increased risk in adults has been linked to exposure to cigarette smoke, benzene, and ionizing radiation. Large doses of ionizing radiation particularly result in an increased incidence of myelogenous leukemia. There is growing concern about the effect of low-dose radiation on subsequent risk of leukemia.[13] Infections with HIV or hepatitis C virus increase the risk for lymphoid neoplasms, and it is now widely accepted that some types of leukemia are caused by infection with the human T-cell leukemia/lymphoma virus-1 (HTLV-1). Drugs that cause bone marrow depression (e.g., chloramphenicol, phenylbutazone, and certain alkylating agents, such as cytoxan) also can predispose an individual to leukemia. AML is the most frequently reported secondary cancer after high doses of chemotherapy for Hodgkin lymphoma, non-Hodgkin lymphoma, multiple myeloma, ovarian cancer, and breast cancer. Acute leukemia also may develop secondary to certain acquired disorders,

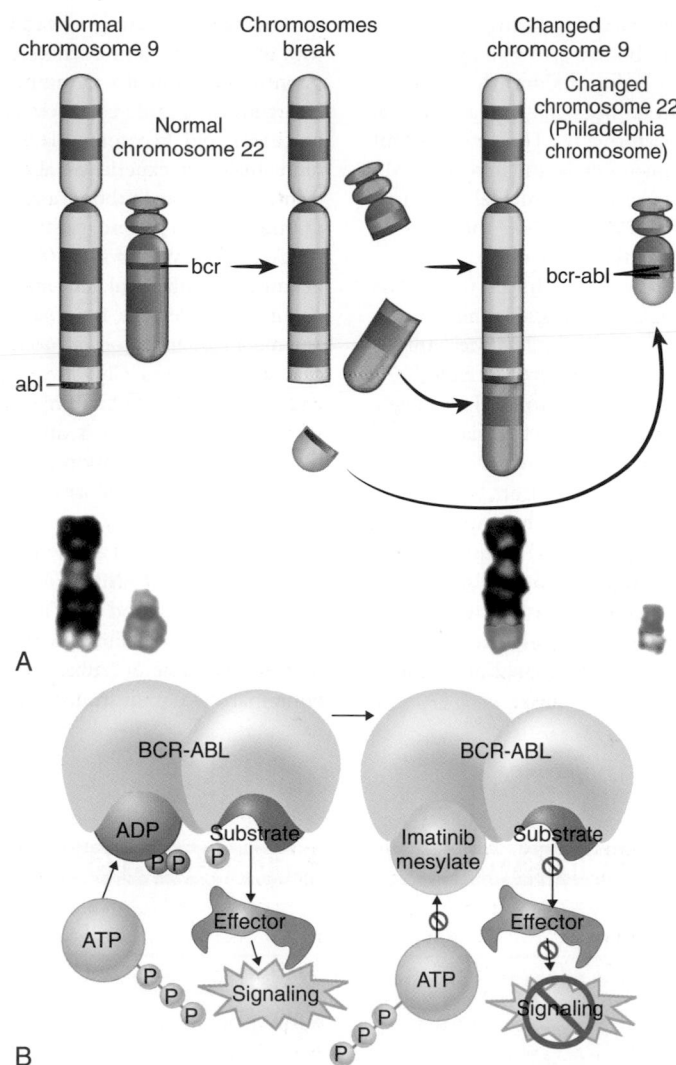

FIGURE 30.5 **Philadelphia Chromosome.** The Philadelphia chromosome is an example of a reciprocal chromosomal translocation that results in an abnormal gene product responsible for a clinical disorder. **A,** An exchange occurs between the long arm of chromosome 9 (black chromosome) and the long arm of chromosome 22 (blue chromosome); t(9;22)(q34;q11). **B,** Mechanism of action of imatinib. By occupying the ATP-binding pocket of the ABL kinase domain, imatinib prevents substrate phosphorylation and downstream activation of signals, thus inhibiting the leukemogenic effects of BCR-ABL1 on cells in chronic myelogenous leukemia. *ADP,* Adenosine diphosphate; *ATP,* adenosine triphosphate; *BCR-ABL,* Breakpoint cluster region-Abelson; *P,* phosphate group. (**A,** Top portion from Rakel R, Bope E: *Conn's current therapy 2008,* Philadelphia, 2008, Saunders; lower portion from Yanoff M, Duker J: *Ophthalmology,* ed 3, Edinburgh, 2009, Mosby. **B** From Goldman L, Schafer AI: *Goldman's Cecil medicine,* ed 24, Philadelphia, 2012, Saunders.)

including CML, CLL, polycythemia vera, myelofibrosis, Hodgkin lymphoma, multiple myeloma, ovarian cancer, and sideroblastic anemia. A unique characteristic of ALL, unlike other forms, is that ALL develops at different rates in different geographic locations, although the reason for this is unclear. Individuals in developed countries and in higher socioeconomic categories have an increased incidence of ALL.

◆**PATHOPHYSIOLOGY.** Chromosomal alterations in ALL cause alterations of expression and function of transcription factors necessary for normal B- and T-cell development.[3] All of the varied mutations present in B- and T-cell development interrupt the normal differentiation of lymphoid precursors and stop (arrest) maturation, causing an increased proliferation or self-renewal of a stem cell–like phenotype.[3] A similar process occurs in AML. ALL of B-cell origin occurs mainly in children and has diverse chromosomal translocations, such as translocation [t(12;21)] involving gene mutations required for B-cell development, including *ETV6* and *RUNX1*. ALL of T-cell origin involves diverse chromosomal translocations with, for example, mutations in *NOTCH1*, a gene required for T-cell development found in approximately 50% to 70% of cases, mostly in adolescent males. Adult ALL is a mixture of cancers of precursor B- and T-cell origin. The identity of mutations found in ALL is ongoing and includes mutations that drive cell growth (e.g., *RAS* signaling) and mutations that increase tyrosine kinase activity. ALL is a progressive neoplasm defined by the presence of greater than 30% lymphoblasts in the bone marrow or blood.

Genetic aberrations in AML alter genes encoding transcription factors needed for normal myeloid differentiation; consequently, differentiation becomes arrested. These mutations affect the epigenome, suggesting that epigenetic alterations are key in AML.[3] Mutations may lead to proliferation by activating growth factor signaling, as well as a decreased rate of apoptosis. Therefore, the bone marrow and peripheral blood are characterized by leukocytosis and a predominance of blast cells. As the immature blasts increase in number, they replace normal myelocytic cells, megakaryocytes, and erythrocytes. This displacement eventually leads to complications of bleeding, anemia, and infection. AML subtypes are classified on the basis of the developmental stage that myeloblasts have reached at the time of diagnosis. The incidence of AML increases with age, peaking in the sixth decade of life.

◆CLINICAL MANIFESTATIONS. More prevalent with ALL, within days to a few weeks, is an abrupt stormy onset. The clinical manifestations of all the varieties of acute leukemia are generally similar. (Mechanisms associated with common manifestations are summarized in Table 30.2.) Signs and symptoms related to bone marrow depression include fatigue caused by anemia, bleeding resulting from thrombocytopenia (reduced numbers of circulating platelets), and fever caused by infection. Sites of infection include the oral cavity, throat, respiratory tract, lower colon, urinary tract, and skin. Common organisms include the gram-negative bacilli *Escherichia coli, Pseudomonas aeruginosa,* and *Klebsiella pneumoniae.* Fever is an early sign, often accompanied by chills. Bleeding can occur in skin, gums, mucous membranes, and gastrointestinal and genitourinary tracts. Visible signs of bleeding include petechiae and ecchymosis, as well as discoloration of the skin, gingival bleeding, hematuria, and midcycle or heavy menstrual bleeding.

Anorexia can occur in all varieties of acute leukemia and is associated with weight loss, diminished sensitivity to sour and sweet tastes, muscle atrophy, and difficulty in swallowing. Liver, spleen, and lymph node enlargement is more common in ALL than in AML (Fig. 30.6). Splenomegaly and hepatomegaly usually occur together. The leukemic individual often experiences abdominal pain and tenderness and breast tenderness. Pain in the bones and joints is thought to result from leukemia infiltration with secondary stretching of the periosteum.

Central nervous system (CNS) involvement is common and may be caused by either leukemic infiltration or cerebral bleeding. Headache, vomiting, papilledema, facial palsy, blurred vision, auditory disturbances, and meningeal irritation can occur if leukemic cells infiltrate the cerebral or spinal meninges. CNS involvement at the time of diagnosis is rare, and less than 5% of children and less than 10% of adults are affected. Without CNS prophylaxis, approximately one-third of individuals will develop CNS complications. Interventions associated with CNS prophylaxis include cranial irradiation, chemotherapy, and high doses of systemic chemotherapy. Specific treatment modalities or combinations of treatment vary and are determined by age and risk status.

◆EVALUATION AND TREATMENT. The diagnosis is made through examination of blood cells and bone marrow. A stained peripheral blood smear will exhibit low red blood cell and platelet counts along with the presence of leukemic blast cells (Fig. 30.7). Examination of bone marrow demonstrates hypercellularity with 60% to 100% blast

TABLE 30.2   CLINICAL MANIFESTATIONS AND RELATED PHYSIOLOGY IN LEUKEMIA

CLINICAL MANIFESTATIONS	LABORATORY ABNORMALITIES	CAUSE	COMMENTS
Anemia	Key is the relative *proportion* of erythroblasts to total count (decreased in anemia)	Decreased stem cell input or ineffective erythropoiesis, or both	In acute leukemia, anemia is usually present from the beginning, often the first symptom noticed, and severe; mild form without symptoms is common in CML and CLL; hemorrhage common in acute forms, occasional in CML, and rare in CLL
Bleeding (purpura, petechiae, ecchymosis, hemorrhage)	Decreased and possibly abnormal platelets	Reduction in megakaryocytes leading to thrombocytopenia	Bleeding more common in acute than in chronic leukemia
Infection	Increased multisegmented neutrophils	Opportunistic organisms; decreased protection resulting from granulocytopenia or immune deficiency secondary to chemotherapy, corticosteroids, and the disease process	Major sites of infection: oral cavity, throat, lower colon, urinary tract, lungs, and skin; prevention of infection focuses on restoring host defenses, decreasing invasive procedures, and reducing colonization of organisms
Weight loss	Decreased 24-hr urinary creatinine excretion; hypoalbuminemia	Condition can be attributed to pain, depression, chemotherapy, radiation therapy, loss of appetite, and alterations in taste	Severe weight loss may be related to excess production of TNF-α
Bone pain	Often no radiographic evidence of bone problems	Result of bone infiltration by leukemic cells or intramedullary infection	If combination drug regimens are ineffective, radiation therapy is used
Liver, spleen, and lymph node enlargement	Biopsy abnormal for liver and spleen	Leukemic cell infiltration; lymph nodes also undergo leukemia proliferation in CLL	
Elevated uric acid	Normal excretion of uric acid is 300–500 mg/day; leukemic individual can excrete 50 times more	Increased catabolism of protein and nucleic acid; urate precipitation increased from dehydration caused by anorexia or fever and drug therapy	Hyperuricemia is present in both acute leukemia and CML; increasing urine pH or decreasing acid production with the drug allopurinol

CLL, Chronic lymphocytic leukemia; *CML,* chronic myelogenous leukemia; *TNF-α,* tumor necrosis factor-alpha.

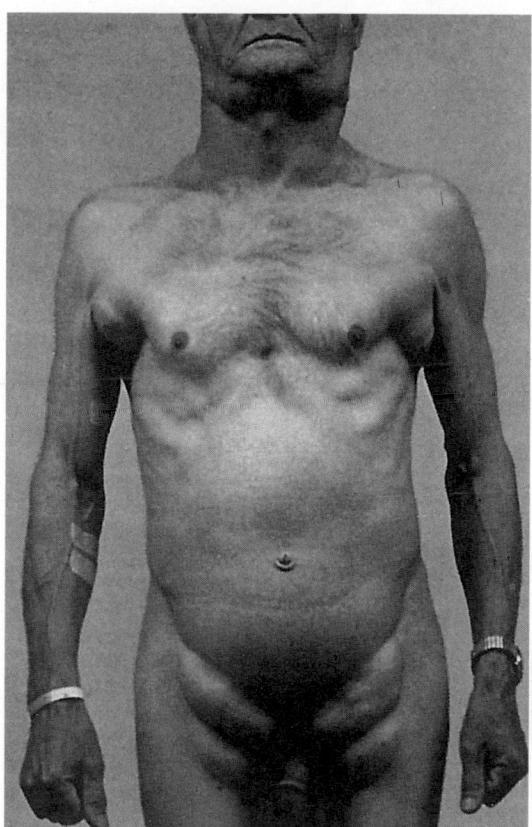

FIGURE 30.6 Lymphadenopathy. Individual with lymphocyte leukemia with extreme but symmetric lymphadenopathy. (Courtesy Dr. A.R. Kagan, Los Angeles. From del Regato JA, Spjut HJ, Cox JD: *Ackerman and del Regato's cancer*, ed 2, St Louis, 1985, Mosby.)

cells, an occasional normal myeloid, precursor and erythroid precursors, and few to no megakaryocytes. For ALL, diagnostic confusion with AML, hairy cell leukemia, and malignant lymphoma is not uncommon.[14] It is critical to obtain an accurate diagnosis because of the differences in both the treatment and prognosis of ALL and AML.[14] The examination of bone marrow aspirates should be done by an experienced oncologist, hematologist, hematopathologist, or general pathologist experienced in interpreting conventional and specially stained specimens.[14]

Successful treatment of AML depends on control of bone marrow and systemic disease.[14] Treatment is divided into two phases: remission induction (to attain remission) and postremission (to maintain remission). Historically, maintenance therapy for AML was administered for several years but is not included in most current treatment clinical trials in the United States, except for promyelocytic leukemia.[14] Standard treatment during the remission induction phase depends on the subtype of AML. Postremission therapy appears to be more effective when given immediately after remission is achieved.[14] Since only 5% of individuals with AML develop CNS disease, prophylactic treatment is not indicated.[14]

Chemotherapy, used in varying combinations, is the treatment of choice for leukemia.[15-17] Supportive measures include blood transfusions, antibiotics, antifungals, and antivirals. Stem cell transplantation is now considered standard therapy for selected individuals with leukemia. It is critical that stem cell transplants be done at hospitals with very experienced staff for both the procedure and the recovery phase.

All-trans-Retinoic acid (ATRA;atRA) is made in the body from vitamin A and helps cells grow and differentiate (e.g., differentiation therapy). In the leukemia arena, experiments with retinoic acid propels cells to develop into functional cells and thereby alleviate the disease. It is a chemotherapeutic agent used to treat some forms of leukemia. Although there were five deaths in a study performed by Hu and colleagues, the 5-year event-free survival rate was 89%, a remarkable improvement over historically bleak survival rates.[18] A recent study showed the rate of relapse in those administered ATRA+As$_2$O$_3$ was significantly lower than in those administered ATRA+chemotherapy maintenance.[19] The relative effectiveness of ATRA may depend on the microenvironment's ability to inactivate ATRA.[20]

The 5-year survival rate for those with leukemia is 38%, largely because of poor survival rates of individuals with certain types of leukemia (e.g., acute myelogenous). Since the 1970s, 5-year survival rates for those with ALL have increased from 38% to 65% for adults and from 53% to 85% for children. Factors influencing increased survival rate include the use of combined and multimodality treatment methods, improvement in supportive services such as blood banking and nutritional support, and implementation of antimicrobial treatment. The presence of the Philadelphia chromosome (observed in about 5% of children with ALL, in 30% of adults with ALL, and occasionally in AML) is a poor prognostic indicator.

Myelosuppression is both a consequence of leukemia and its treatment. Hematologic support with blood products and granulocyte colony-stimulating factor (G-CSF) or granulocyte-macrophage colony–stimulating factor (GM-CSF) has effectively shortened the time of neutropenia and improved survival by reducing the reducing risk for infection.

Chronic Leukemias

The two main types of chronic leukemia are (1) chronic myelogenous leukemia (CML) and (2) chronic lymphocytic leukemia (CLL). In adults, CLL is the most common leukemia in the western world.[3] CLL is a slow-growing cancer in which too many immature lymphocytes are found mostly in the blood and bone marrow. CLL and small lymphocytic lymphoma (SLL; also CLL/SLL) differ only in the degree of proliferation of peripheral blood lymphocytes.[3] Several forms of CML can occur, depending on the lineage of the malignant cells (e.g., chronic neutrophilic leukemia [CNL], chronic eosinophilic leukemia [CEL]). Unlike cells in acute leukemia, chronic leukemic cells are well differentiated and can be readily identified. CML is mostly a disease of adults but can occur in children or adolescents. The peak incidence is in the fifth to sixth decades. Individuals with chronic leukemia have a longer life expectancy, usually extending several years from the time of diagnosis.

It is estimated that in 2017 more than 20,110 cases of CLL and 8950 cases of CML will be newly diagnosed in the United States.[7] CML is a member of the family of myeloproliferative disorders that also includes polycythemia vera (see Chapter 29), essential thrombocythemia, chronic idiopathic myelofibrosis (invasion of bone marrow by fibrous tissue), chronic neutrophilic leukemia, and chronic eosinophilic leukemia.

The etiology of CLL is unknown. A familial tendency suggests a genetic linkage; first-degree relatives have a three times greater risk of developing the disease. It is rare in individuals younger than 45 years of age and, when diagnosed, 95% of individuals are older than age 50. Genetic anomalies occur in approximately 90% of cases, frequently as deletions, although none have been linked to the etiology of CLL. The only known cause of CML is exposure to ionizing radiation.

◆**PATHOPHYSIOLOGY.** CML is clonal and thought to arise from a hematopoietic stem cell. The cells observed in CML are heterogeneous in differentiation, depending on the stage of the disease. During the chronic phase, the predominant cell is a long-lasting hematopoietic stem cell. A leukemic granulocyte-monocyte progenitor cell is seen. The Philadelphia chromosome is present in more than 95% of persons diagnosed with CML, and the presence of the BCR-ABL1 protein is

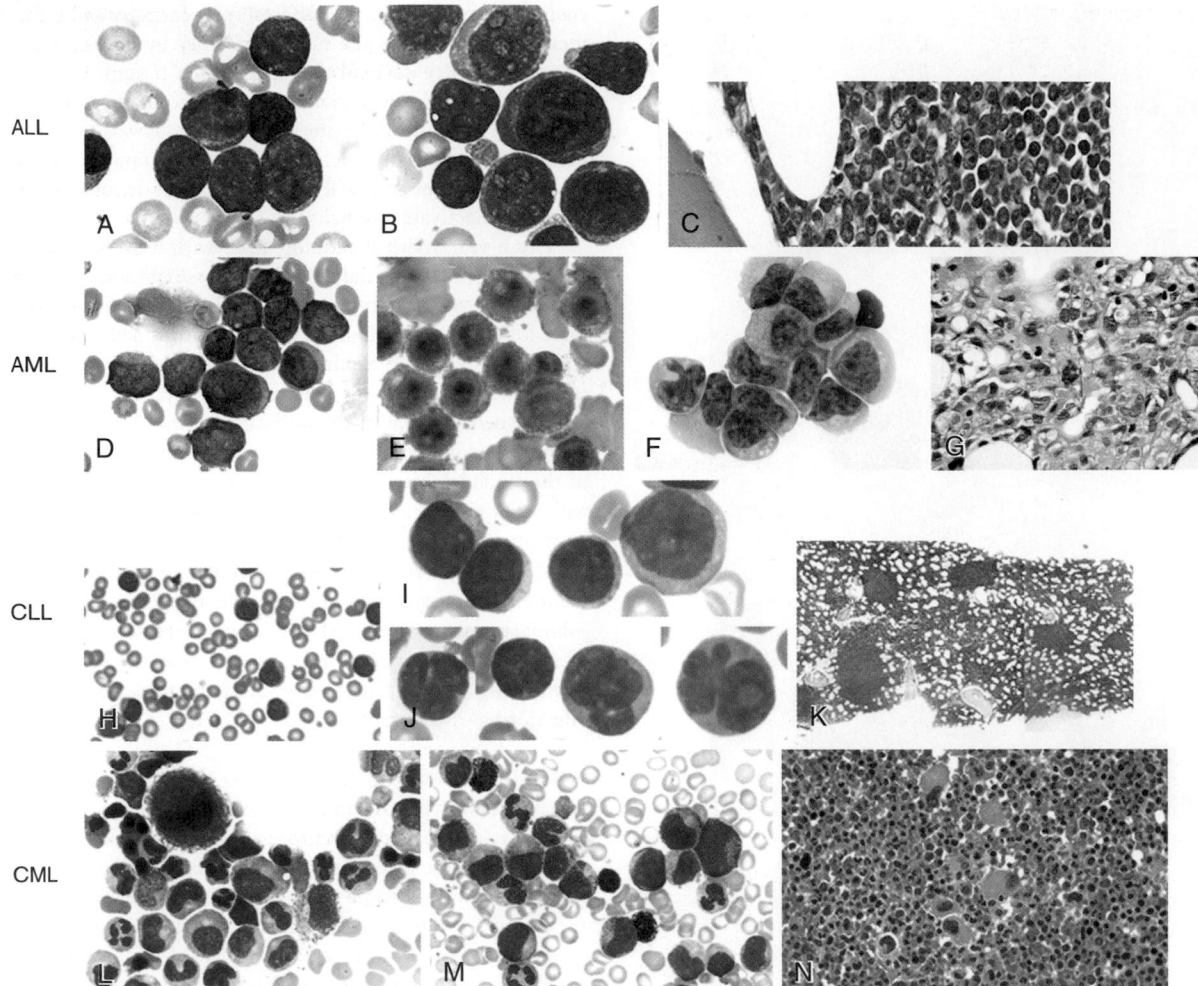

FIGURE 30.7 Morphologic Aspects of Leukemia Cells. *Acute lymphoblastic leukemia (ALL)* **(A–C). A,** Typical uniform lymphoblasts with intermediate-sized nuclei, fine but "smudgy" chromatin, absence of nucleoli, and scant cytoplasm. **B,** Lymphoblasts with more cytologic variation, including variability in size, number of nucleoli, and amount of cytoplasm. **C,** Histologic features of ALL in bone core biopsy. *Acute myeloid leukemia (AML)* **(D–G). D,** Acute myeloblastic leukemia with minimal or no maturation. The cells are myeloblasts with dispersed chromatin and variable amounts of agranular cytoplasm. Some display medium-sized, poorly defined nucleoli. **E,** Acute monoblastic leukemia; characteristic monoblasts with round nuclei and delicate chromatin and prominent nucleoli. Cytoplasm is abundant. **F,** Acute monocytic leukemia with most of the cells in this field being promonocytes. Monoblasts and an abnormal monocyte also are present. **G,** Marrow biopsy of acute megakaryoblastic leukemia containing large and small blasts and atypical megakaryocytes. *Chronic lymphocytic leukemia (CLL)* **(H–K). H,** Peripheral blood smear typically shows lymphocytosis. Cytologic features of CLL cells differ. **I,** Classic cells have a small nucleus with a "soccer ball" chromatin pattern. **J,** Some cases have increased large cells, or prolymphocytes, with more open chromatin and prominent "punched-out" nucleoli (prolymphocyte, right side). **K,** The bone marrow can show nodular infiltrates of CLL cells. *Chronic myelogenous leukemia (CML)* **(L–N). L,** Peripheral smear shows marked leukocytosis attributable to a granulocytic proliferation of all stages with particularly increased myelocytes and absolute basophilia. **M,** Bone core biopsy illustrates markedly hypercellular marrow attributable to granulocytic proliferation and increased small hypolobated megakaryocytes. **N,** Bone marrow aspirate shows granulocytic proliferation and small, "dwarf" megakaryocyte. **(A–C, H–N** from Hoffman R et al: *Hematology: basic principles and practice,* ed 6, Philadelphia, 2013, Churchill Livingstone. **D–G** from Abeloff M et al: *Abeloff's clinical oncology,* ed 4, Philadelphia, 2008, Churchill Livingstone.)

responsible for initiation of CML (Fig. 30.8). The presence of the chimeric *BCR-ABL* fusion gene distinguishes CML from other myeloproliferative disorders. In advanced disease, the accumulation of additional mutations leads to the more aggressive leukemic phenotype.

CLL involves malignant transformation and progressive accumulation of monoclonal B lymphocytes; rarely (less than 5%) are CLL malignancies of T-cell origin. The characteristic immunophenotype is expression of CD5, CD19, and CD23 molecules and low amounts of surface membrane Ig, CD20, and CD22 molecules.[21] CD5 is a signal transduction molecule linked to the B-cell receptor (BCR); CD19 is a low-affinity antigen receptor expressed on maturing B cells, but is lost in plasma cells; and CD23 is a low-affinity receptor for the Fc portion

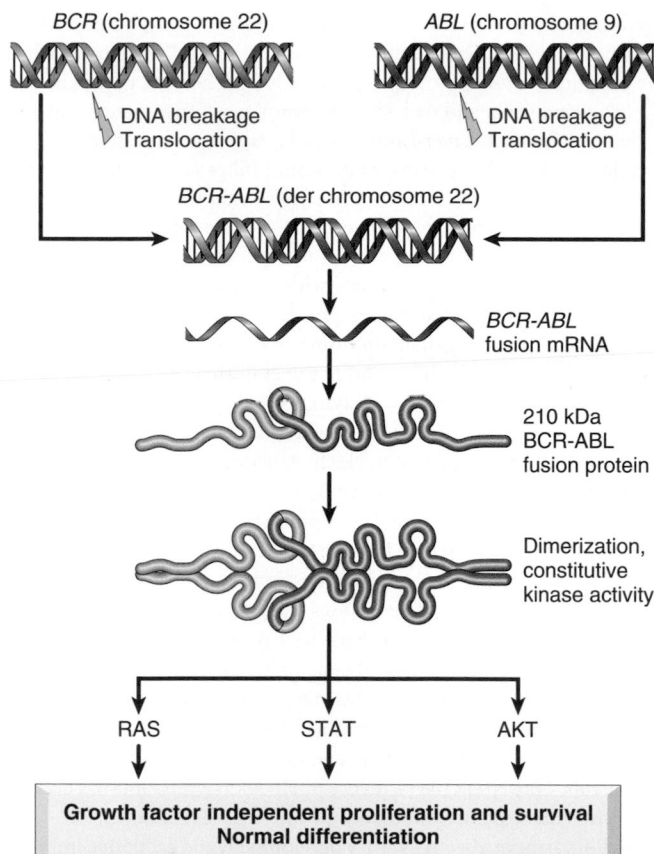

FIGURE 30.8 Pathogenesis of Chronic Myeloid Leukemia. The breakage and joining of *BCR* and *ABL* creates the chimeric fusion gene *BCR-ABL*. *BCR-ABL* genetically encodes an active BCR-ABL intracellular tyrosine kinase (an enzyme that controls intracellular "on-off" switches). The ABL kinase in turn induces signaling through the same pro-growth and pro-survival pathways that are activated by normal hematologic growth factors. Altogether the activation of many downstream pathways drives growth factor–independent proliferation and survival of bone marrow progenitors. *der chromosome* is a structurally rearranged chromosome. *AKT,* Serine/threonine kinases; *BCR-ABL,* breakpoint cluster region-Abelson; *RAS,* rat sarcoma; *STAT,* signal transducer and activator of transcription. (From Kumar V, Abbas A, Aster JC: *Robbins & Cotran pathologic basis of disease,* ed 9, Philadelphia, 2015, Saunders.)

of IgE. CLL is derived from a transformation of a partially mature B cell that has not yet encountered antigen. The gene for the variable region of the antibody heavy chain *(IGHV)* is frequently mutated (30% to 40% of persons). (See Chapter 8 for discussion of immunoglobulin heavy-chain structure.) Individuals with a mutated *IGHV* gene tend to have a more benign condition with a more slowly developing and less malignant disease. Significant numbers of this mutation are associated with a median survival in excess of 20 to 25 years, whereas the absence of mutations is associated with a poorer survival rate (median survival 8 to 10 years).[22]

CLL cells that accumulate in the marrow do not interfere with normal blood cell production to the extent found in acute leukemias. This is a significant feature explaining the reduced severity in the beginning stage of disease. Accumulation of malignant B cells is the result of cell cycle arrest in the G_0/G_1 phase. CLL cells tend to express increased levels of proapoptotic proteins (e.g., BCL2) and suppress antiapoptotic proteins (e.g., BCL2L1), which reduces their sensitivity to apoptosis. Because the major pathophysiologic deficit in CLL is the failure of B cells to

mature into plasma cells that synthesize immunoglobulin, this often results in hypogammaglobulinemia (60% of individuals).

◆**CLINICAL MANIFESTATIONS.** Chronic leukemia advances slowly and insidiously. Approximately 70% of individuals with CLL are asymptomatic at the time of diagnosis. When symptoms do appear, the most common finding is lymphadenopathy. The most significant effect of CLL is suppression of humoral immunity and increased infection with encapsulated bacteria. Frequently the level of neutrophils is depressed, which adds to the risk of infection. Invasion of most organ cells is uncommon but infiltration does occur in lymph nodes, liver, spleen, and salivary glands. CNS involvement is rare. Approximately 10% of individuals develop a more aggressive malignancy, usually a diffuse, large B-cell lymphoma. In these individuals, extreme fatigue, weight loss, night sweats, low-grade fever, elevated levels of the enzyme lactic dehydrogenase, hypercalcemia, anemia, and thrombocytopenia are common.

Individuals with CML may progress through three phases of the disease: a chronic phase lasting 2 to 5 years during which symptoms may not be apparent; an accelerated phase of 6 to 18 months during which the primary symptoms develop; and a terminal blast phase ("blast crisis") with a survival of only 3 to 6 months. The accelerated phase is characterized by excessive proliferation and accumulation of malignant cells. Splenomegaly is the most common finding, which may be prominent and painful, but lymphadenopathy generally is not present. Liver enlargement also occurs, but liver function is rarely altered. Hyperuricemia is common and produces gouty arthritis. Infections, fever, and weight loss also are frequent. The terminal blast phase is characterized by rapid and progressive leukocytosis with an increase in the number of basophils. In the later stages of the terminal phase, which then resembles AML, blast cells or promyelocytes predominate, and the individual experiences a blast crisis.

The acute effects of CML resemble those of acute leukemia but with more prominent and painful splenomegaly. Liver function rarely is altered despite enlargement, and lymphadenopathy generally is found only in the acute phase of the disease. Hyperuricemia invariably is present and produces gouty arthritis. Infections, fever, and weight loss are common findings in individuals with CML.

◆**EVALUATION AND TREATMENT.** Diagnosis of chronic leukemia depends on laboratory analyses of peripheral blood and bone marrow samples. Diagnosis of CLL is based on detection of a monoclonal B-cell lymphocytosis in the blood. The cells must have the immunophenotype characteristic of CLL (CD5+, CD19+, CD20 [weak], CD23+), at levels in excess of 5000 cells/µL, over a sustained period of time (usually 4 weeks). Bone marrow may contain more than 30% lymphocytes and be normocellular or hypercellular.

Treatment is frequently based on prognostic indicators and ranges from observation with treatment of infection, hemorrhage, or immune complications; to a variety of drug options, including steroids, alkylating agents, purine analogs, and monoclonal antibodies; to combination chemotherapy and transplant options.[23] Because this disease typically occurs in the elderly and the rate of progression is slow, it is often simply observed until the disease progresses. Meta-analysis of randomized trials shows no survival advantage for immediate versus delayed treatment of those individuals with early stage disease.[24] For individuals with progressing CLL, treatment with conventional doses of chemotherapy is not curative; selected individuals treated with allogeneic stem cell transplantation have achieved prolonged disease-free survival.[23] Antileukemic therapy is frequently unnecessary in uncomplicated early disease.[23] From older clinical trials (1970s to 1990s), the median survival for all individuals ranges from 8 to 12 years.[23] A large variation in survival, however, exists among individuals, ranging from several months to a normal life expectancy. Treatment must be individualized based on the clinical behavior of the disease.[23] Complications of pancytopenia, including hemorrhage and infection, are a major cause of death.

Typically, individuals with CLL survive 10 years or more. However, those with certain risk markers have a more aggressive disease that shortens survival to less than 3 years. Markers of high risk include anemia, thrombocytopenia, and absence of mutations in the *IGHV* gene. Mutations in *IGHV* correlate very closely with levels of intracellular ZAP-70, detection of which may be substituted for tests of *IGHV* mutation. ZAP-70 is a tyrosine kinase that is linked to the T-cell receptor (see Chapter 8). ZAP-70 negativity is associated with improved mean survival.[25] It is not normally detected in CLL cells with mutated *IGHV*, but is easily detectable by immunohistologic studies in cells with an unmutated *IGHV*.

Current treatment modalities for CML do not cure the disease or prevent blastic transformation. Standard treatment consists of combined chemotherapy, biologic response modifiers, and allogeneic stem cell transplantation. Although transplantation is potentially curative, its use is limited by donor availability and high toxicity in older adults, thus limiting use to those older than 65 years. Traditional chemotherapy agents used are hydroxyurea and busulfan. The development and introduction of the first tyrosine kinase inhibitor imatinib mesylate (Gleevec) as a treatment modality lead to changes in the management of CML. Other tyrosine kinase inhibitors have been developed; however, concerns regarding disease persistence and resistance still exist.[26] Imatinib mesylate is highly specific for CML and suppression of BCR-ABL kinase activity and produces a complete cytogenetic response in more than 80% of newly diagnosed persons; however, it does not cure CML because it does not kill leukemia stem cells (LSCs) both in vitro and in vivo.[27-30] New targets or drugs have been reported to inhibit LSCs in cultured CD34+ CML cells or in mouse models. These drugs include the Alox5 pathway inhibitor, Hsp90 inhibitors, omacetaxine, hedgehog inhibitor, and BMS-214662. Some suggest targeting LSCs but not normal stem cells is a correct strategy for anticancer therapies in the future.[28]

ALTERATIONS OF LYMPHOID FUNCTION

Lymphadenopathy

Lymphadenopathy is characterized by enlarged lymph nodes. Lymph node enlargement is caused by an increase in size and number of its germinal centers caused by proliferation of lymphocytes and monocytes or invasion by malignant cells. Normally, lymph nodes are not palpable or are barely palpable. Enlarged lymph nodes are characterized by being palpable and often also may be tender or painful to touch, although not in all situations (see Fig. 30.6).

Localized lymphadenopathy usually indicates drainage of an area associated with an inflammatory process or infection (reactive lymph nodes). Generalized lymphadenopathy is usually a result of malignant or nonmalignant disease, particularly in adults. Palpable nodes, however, do not always indicate serious disease and may indicate only a reaction to minor trauma or infection of a specific structure. The location and size of the enlarged nodes are important factors in diagnosing the cause of the lymphadenopathy, as are the individual's age, gender, and geographic location. Generalized lymphadenopathy occurs with non-Hodgkin lymphomas, chronic lymphocytic leukemia, histiocytosis, and disorders that produce lymphocytosis. In general, lymphadenopathy results from one of four types of conditions: (1) neoplastic disease, (2) immunologic or inflammatory conditions, (3) endocrine disorders, or (4) lipid storage diseases. Diseases of unknown cause, including reactions to drugs, also may lead to generalized lymphadenopathy.

Malignant Lymphomas

Lymphomas consist of a diverse group of neoplasms that develop from the proliferation of malignant lymphocytes in the lymphoid system. The classification of lymphomas was published by the WHO and is derived from the Revised European-American Lymphoma (REAL) classification. This classification is based on the cell type from which the lymphoma probably originated (Box 30.2). The basic groups include *Hodgkin lymphoma* and *non-Hodgkin lymphoma*. Two groups that were previously classified as *non-Hodgkin lymphoma* are now classified as B-cell neoplasms, T-cell neoplasms, and natural killer (NK) cell neoplasms. With the new classification, multiple myeloma, which was previously classified independently, is included as a B-cell lymphoma. Non-Hodgkin lymphoma can be further divided into cancers that have an *indolent* or slow-growing course and those with an *aggressive* or fast-growing course. These different subtypes progress and respond to treatment differently. Both Hodgkin lymphoma and non-Hodgkin lymphoma occur in children and adults, and the overall treatment and prognosis depend on the stage and type of lymphoma.

Globally, the incidence of lymphoma exhibits a significant geographic variation; it is more prevalent in North America, Australia/New Zealand, and Europe whereas it is less common in Asia and Africa, except where Burkitt lymphoma is endemic.[31] Lymphoma is the most common blood cancer in the United States. Incidence rates of lymphoma differ with respect to age, gender, geographic location, and socioeconomic class. The estimated number of new cases of lymphoma for 2017 is more than 80,500 individuals with estimated deaths at 21,210.[7] Since the early 1970s, the incidence of non-Hodgkin lymphoma has nearly doubled. The exact reason for this increase remains a mystery; however, a modest portion of the increase is attributed to lymphomas developing in association with immune deficiencies, including AIDS and organ transplants. Conversely, the incidence of Hodgkin lymphoma has declined over the same time period, especially among older adults.

Factors associated with country development and economic improvement include changes in diet (e.g., overnutrition), increases in anthropometric measurements (e.g., metabolic syndrome), improvements in hygiene, changes in family size (i.e., smaller families), adoption of sedentary lifestyles, advancements in medical access and care, increases in life span, and exposure to environmental carcinogens associated with industrialization.[31] In general, lymphomas are the result of genetic mutations or viral infection. These factors are related to an aging world population and increasing adoption of cancer-causing behaviors.[31] Malignant transformation produces a cell with uncontrolled and excessive growth that accumulates in the lymph nodes and other sites, producing tumor masses. Lymphomas usually start in the lymph nodes or lymphoid tissues of the stomach or intestines.

Hodgkin Lymphoma

Hodgkin lymphoma (HL) is a malignant lymphoma first characterized by Thomas Hodgkin in 1832. HL progresses from one group of lymph nodes to another and includes the development of systemic symptoms and the presence of B cells called **Reed-Sternberg (RS) cells** (Fig. 30.9). It is estimated that more than 8260 individuals will be newly diagnosed with HL in 2017 with estimated deaths of 1070.[7] The incidence of HL is higher in males, and the median age of diagnosis is 64 years. Incidence rates for HL have declined, especially among older adults. The decrease in incidence in older adults is attributed to improved diagnostic accuracy. The incidence is greater in whites than blacks. Denmark, the Netherlands, and the United States have the highest incidence of HL, and Japan and Australia have the lowest incidence. HL peaks at two different ages: early in life in the second and third decades and later in life during the sixth and seventh decades.

◆**PATHOPHYSIOLOGY.** It is widely accepted that the RS cell represents the malignant transformed lymphocyte. RS cells are often large and binucleate, with occasional mononuclear variants; these cells are the hallmark of HL and are necessary for the diagnosis of HL. However, they are not specific to HL. In rare instances, cells resembling RS cells

BOX 30.2   WORLD HEALTH ORGANIZATION CLASSIFICATION OF LYMPHOID NEOPLASMS

B-Cell Neoplasms
Precursor B-Cell Neoplasms
   Precursor B-lymphoblastic leukemia/lymphoma
   Precursor B-cell acute lymphoblastic leukemia

Mature (Peripheral) B-Cell Neoplasms
   B-cell chronic lymphocytic leukemia/small lymphocytic lymphoma
   B-cell prolymphocytic leukemia
   Lymphoplasmacytoid lymphoma
   Splenic marginal zone B-cell lymphoma (with/without villous lymphocytes)
   Hairy cell leukemia
   Plasma cell myeloma/plasmacytoma
   Extranodal marginal zone B-cell lymphoma of mucosa-associated lymphoid (MAL type) tissue
   Nodal marginal zone B-cell lymphoma (with/without monocytoid B cells)
   Follicular lymphoma
   Mantle-cell lymphoma
   Diffuse large B-cell lymphoma
       Mediastinal large B-cell lymphoma
       Primary effusion lymphoma
   Burkitt lymphoma/Burkitt cell leukemia

T-Cell and NK-Cell Neoplasms
Precursor T-Cell Neoplasms
   Precursor T-lymphoblastic lymphoma/leukemia
   Precursor T-cell acute lymphoblastic leukemia

Mature (Peripheral) T-Cell Neoplasms
   T-cell prolymphocytic leukemia
   T-cell granular lymphocytic leukemia
   Aggressive NK-cell leukemia
   Adult T-cell lymphoma/leukemia (HTLV-1 positive)
   Extranodal NK/T-cell lymphoma, nasal type
   Enteropathy-type T-cell lymphoma
   Hepatosplenic gamma-delta T-cell lymphoma
   Subcutaneous panniculitis-like T-cell lymphoma
   Mycosis fungoides/Sézary syndrome
   Anaplastic large-cell lymphoma, T/null cell, primary cutaneous type
   Peripheral T-cell lymphoma, not otherwise characterized
   Angioimmunoblastic T-cell lymphoma
   Anaplastic large-cell lymphoma, T/null cell, primary systemic type

Hodgkin Lymphoma (Hodgkin Disease)
   Nodular lymphocyte predominant Hodgkin lymphoma
   Classic Hodgkin lymphoma
       Nodular sclerosis Hodgkin lymphoma (grades 1 and 2)
       Lymphocyte-rich classic Hodgkin lymphoma
       Mixed cellularity Hodgkin lymphoma
       Lymphocyte depletion Hodgkin lymphoma

HTLV, Human T-cell leukemia virus; *NK,* natural killer.
From National Institutes of Health, National Cancer Institute: *Surveillance Epidemiology and End Results (SEER) Program.* Available at: http://training.seer.cancer.gov/module_coding_primary/table_who_class_hemo_2.html.

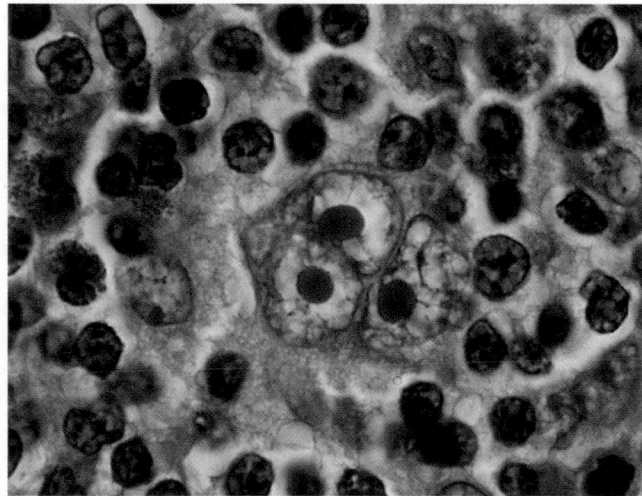

FIGURE 30.9 Reed-Sternberg Cell. A large, multinucleated or multilobed cell (center of photograph) with inclusion body–like nucleoli surrounded by a halo of clear nucleoplasm. (From Damjanov I, Linder J, editors: *Anderson's pathology,* ed 10, St Louis, 1996, Mosby.)

can be found in benign illnesses, as well as in other forms of cancer, including non-Hodgkin lymphomas and solid tissue cancers and in infectious mononucleosis.

The triggering mechanism for the malignant transformation of cells remains unknown. Classic HL appears to be derived from a B cell in the germinal center that has not undergone successful immunoglobulin gene rearrangement (see Chapter 8) and would normally be induced to undergo apoptosis. Survival of this cell may be linked to infection with EBV. Laboratory and epidemiologic studies have linked HL with EBV infections and EBV DNA. RNA and proteins are frequently observed in HL cells. The RS cells secrete and release cytokines (e.g., IL-10, transforming growth factor-beta [TGF-β]) that result in the accumulation of inflammatory cells that produces the local and systemic effects. HL is subcategorized into two main types: classic Hodgkin and nodular lymphocyte–predominant Hodgkin. Classic HL is subclassified into four types (Table 30.3) based on the morphology of RS cells, and the characteristics of the inflammatory cell infiltrate in the tumor. Nodular lymphocyte–predominant HL presents with earlier stage disease, longer survival, and fewer treatment failures than classic HL.[32] However, despite a more favorable prognosis, in approximately 10% of people nodular lymphocyte–predominant HL has a tendency to histologically transform into diffuse large B-cell lymphoma.[33]

The molecular events causing malignant transformation remain controversial; although RS cells are apparently from B-cell lineage, they express very few B-cell markers and express markers normally not found on B cells. For instance, RS cells do not express immunoglobulin, but do express CD15 (a carbohydrate adhesion molecule found on neutrophils), TARC (a Th2-cell–specific chemokine), and T-cell–associated antigens (e.g., β-chain of the T-cell receptor).[34] The precise genetic defects leading to development of HL are unknown, although several have been suggested. These generally include defects in immunoglobulin variable region gene rearrangement or defects in other B-cell–specific differentiation genes.

TABLE 30.3   SUBTYPES OF HODGKIN LYMPHOMA

SUBTYPE	INCIDENCE	PRESENTATION
Nodular sclerosis Hodgkin lymphoma (HL)	Most common subtype in developing countries Found in all ages but most common in adolescents and young adults (median age of onset is about 28 years) Incidence in females exceeds that in males	Large tumor nodules with RS cells surrounded by collagen and fibrous bands
Mixed cellularity HL	Second most common subtype Incidence in males exceeds that in females	RS cells with mixed inflammatory cell (lymphocytes, monocytes/macrophages, eosinophils, plasma cells) infiltrates
Lymphocyte-rich classic HL	Uncommon subtype Found in all ages but most common in adults Incidence in males exceeds that in females	Few RS cells and predominantly lymphocytic infiltration Usually localized at diagnosis Survival is long with or without treatment
Lymphocyte depletion HL	Uncommon subtype Most common type in older adults, HIV-positive individuals, and persons in nonindustrialized countries Incidence in males exceeds that in females	Large number of RS cells with less additional cellular infiltrate Usually widespread disease: abdominal lymphadenopathy; spleen, liver, and bone marrow involvement, without peripheral lymphadenopathy Stage is usually more advanced at diagnosis

HIV, Human immunodeficiency virus; *RS,* Reed-Sternberg.

BOX 30.3   CLINICAL MANIFESTATIONS OF HODGKIN LYMPHOMA

Physical Findings
Adenopathy
Mediastinal mass
Splenomegaly
Abdominal mass

Symptoms
Fever, weight loss, night sweats
Pruritus

Laboratory Findings
Thrombocytosis
Leukocytosis
Eosinophilia
Elevated erythrocyte sedimentation rate (ESR)
Elevated alkaline phosphatase
Paraneoplastic syndromes

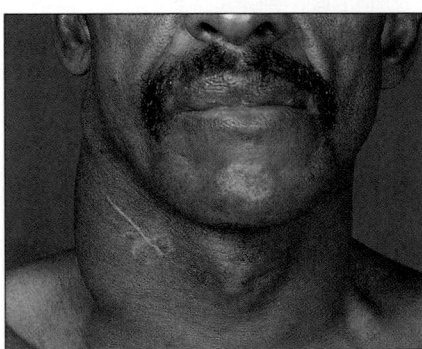

FIGURE 30.10 Hodgkin Lymphoma and Enlarged Cervical Lymph Node. Typical enlarged cervical lymph node in the neck of a man with Hodgkin lymphoma. The scar of a previous biopsy incision is well healed. (From Hoffbrand AV, Petit JE, Vyas P: *Color atlas of clinical hematology,* ed 4, Philadelphia, 2009, Mosby Elsevier.)

CLINICAL MANIFESTATIONS. Many of the characteristic clinical features (Box 30.3) of HL can be explained by the complex action of cytokines and other growth factors that are secreted by the malignant cells. These substances induce infiltration and proliferation of inflammatory cells, resulting in an enlarged, painless lymph node in the neck (often the first sign of HL) (Fig. 30.10). The discovery of an asymptomatic mediastinal mass on routine chest x-ray is not uncommon and is often an initial sign of HL. The cervical, axillary, inguinal, and retroperitoneal lymph nodes are commonly affected in HL (Fig. 30.11). Local symptoms caused by pressure and obstruction of the lymph nodes are the result of the lymphadenopathy.

About one-third of individuals will have some degree of systemic symptoms.[35] Intermittent fever, without other symptoms of infection, drenching night sweats, itchy skin (pruritus), and fatigue are relatively common. These constitutional symptoms accompanied by weight loss are associated with a poor prognosis. The Cotswold staging classification

system used for HL is able to establish a correlation between the anatomic extent of the disease and the prognosis (Table 30.4). This classification system is based on the individual's medical history and physical examination (presence of symptoms and palpable lymph nodes) as well as other radiologic and hematologic results. Prognostic indicators include clinical stage, histologic type, tumor cell concentration and tumor burden, constitutional symptoms, and age.

Although HL rarely arises in the lung, mediastinal and hilar node adenopathy can cause secondary involvement of the trachea, bronchi, pleura, or lungs. Retroperitoneal nodes can involve vertebral bodies and nerves, causing displacement of ureters. Spinal cord involvement is more common in the dorsal and lumbar regions than in the cervical region. Although uncommon, skin manifestations include psoriasis and eczematoid lesions, causing itching and scratching.

As a result of direct invasion from mediastinal lymph nodes, pericardial involvement can cause pericardial friction rub, pericardial effusion, and engorgement of the neck veins. The gastrointestinal (GI) tract and urinary tract rarely are involved. Anemia often is found in individuals with HL, accompanied by a low serum iron level and decreased iron-binding capacity. Other laboratory findings include

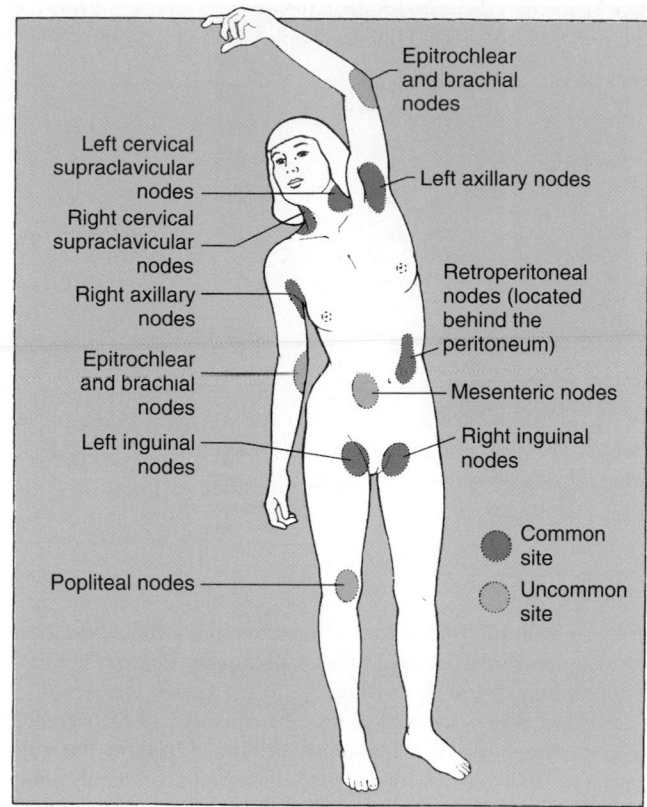

FIGURE 30.11 Common and Uncommon Involved Lymph Node Sites for Hodgkin Lymphoma.

TABLE 30.4	**COTSWOLD STAGING CLASSIFICATION SYSTEM**
STAGE	**CRITERIA**
I	Involvement of a single lymph node region or single extranodal organ or site
II	Involvement of two or more lymph node regions on the same side of the diaphragm or a single extranodal organ or site and its regional lymph nodes
III	Involvement of lymph node regions or structures on both sides of the diaphragm
IV	Disseminated involvement of one or more extralymphatic organs or an isolated extralymphatic organ with distant nodal involvement
	Modifying characteristics for all four stages:
	A: No B symptoms
	B: Unexplained fever of >38°C (100.4°F), drenching night sweats, unexplained loss of >10% of body weight in the 6 months preceding diagnosis
	E: Large mediastinal mass with direct extension into extranodal sites

Data from Lister TA, Crowther D: *Semin Oncol* 17:696, 1990.

elevated sedimentation rate, leukocytosis, and eosinophilia. Leukopenia occurs in advanced states of HL.

Splenic involvement of HL depends on histopathologic type (see Table 30.3). The spleen is involved in 60% of cases of mixed cellularity and lymphocytic depletion types. With lymphocyte predominance and nodular sclerosis types, only 34% of cases reveal splenic involvement.

◆**EVALUATION AND TREATMENT.** Because of the variability in symptoms, early definitive detection may be difficult. Asymptomatic lymphadenopathy can progress undetected for several years. Careful evaluation, including chest x-rays, lymphangiography, and biopsy, should be carried out for individuals with fever of unknown origin and peripheral lymphadenopathy.[35] A lymph node biopsy with scattered RS cells and a cellular infiltrate is highly indicative of HL. The effectiveness of treatment is related to the age of the individual and the extent of the disease. Approximately 75% of individuals diagnosed with HL are cured, largely because of successful combined treatment with radiation therapy and chemotherapy (Fig. 30.12). Over the past 50 years, the death rate has fallen more rapidly for HL than for any other malignancy. More recent treatments include high-dose chemotherapy in conjunction with bone marrow or stem cell transplantation. Monoclonal antibodies also are being developed and nonmyeloablative allogeneic stem cell transplantation has been found to help certain individuals, even though this treatment is still under development.

The 5-year survival rate varies depending on the stage that is identified at diagnosis. The 5-year survival rate for stages I and II is 90% to 95%, 80% to 85% for stage III, and 75% for stage IV. Those with stage I or II disease are candidates for chemotherapy, radiation therapy, or a combination of these treatment modalities. Individuals with stage III or IV disease, bulky disease (more than 10-cm mass or mediastinal disease with a transverse diameter exceeding 33% of the transthoracic

diameter), or the presence of B symptoms require combined chemotherapy with or without additional radiation treatment. Other factors, if present, have an influence on survival. Poorer survival is related to a high white blood cell count (greater than 15,000/μL) or a low hemoglobin (Hb) level (less than 10.5 g/dL); low lymphocyte count (less than 600/μL); and male gender. Cure for HL can be achieved in 75% of cases with current therapies.

Non-Hodgkin Lymphoma

The non-Hodgkin lymphomas (NHLs) are a heterogeneous group of neoplasms arising from lymphoid tissue, with varied biologic and clinical features. Worldwide, NHLs account for about 3% of the cancer burden with global variations in patterns of occurrence.[36] NHL incidence in developed countries was 8.6/100,000 compared to 3.6/100,000 in less developed countries, whereas HL incidence in developed countries was 2.1/100,000 compared to 0.6/100,000 in less developed countries.[6] In the United States, NHLs account for 4.3% of all new cancer cases and HLs account for about 0.5% of all new cancer cases.[37] NHL incidence rates increased worldwide from 1950 to 2000, tripling in adults older than 65 years.[38] The previously used generic classification of non-Hodgkin lymphoma (NHL) has been reclassified in the WHO/REAL scheme into (1) B-cell neoplasms, which include a variety of lymphomas including myelomas that originate from B cells at various stages of differentiation, and (2) T-cell and NK-cell neoplasms, which include lymphomas that originate from either T cells or NK cells. These cancers are differentiated from HL by lack of RS cells and other cellular changes not characteristic of HL.

More than 72,240 cases of NHL with 20,140 deaths are predicted in the United States for 2017.[7] The median age of diagnosis is 67 years. The highest incidence of NHL is in North America, Europe, Oceania, and several African countries.[39] NHL affects more men than women. For unknown reasons, the incidence increased in many high-income countries between the 1950s and 1990s and no further increase has been observed during the last decade.[39] Part of the increased incidence has been attributed to diagnostic improvements as well as increases in the number of AIDS-related cancers following the HIV epidemic.[39]

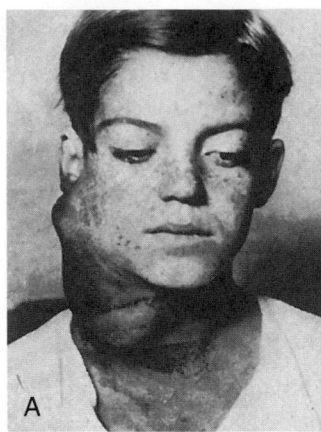 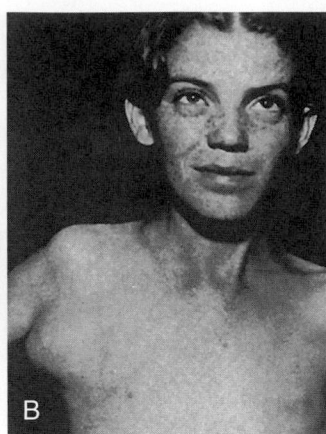 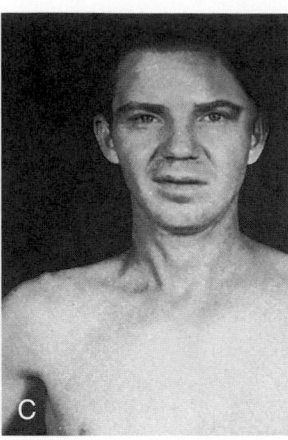

FIGURE 30.12 Cervical Hodgkin Lymphoma (Extreme Case). A, Young boy with extensive cervical Hodgkin lymphoma. **B,** Appearance several years later and after treatment, when axillary manifestations developed. **C,** Appearance 23 years after initial treatment with radiation. (From del Regato JA, Spjut HJ, Cox JD: *Ackerman and del Regato's cancer,* ed 2, St Louis, 1985, Mosby.)

Mortality from NHL has declined since 1997.[40] It is thought that newer treatment modalities are improving survival rates.

Risk factors include a family history of the disease, exposure to a variety of mutagenic chemicals (e.g., certain occupations) or to irradiation, infection with certain cancer-related viruses (e.g., EBV, human herpesvirus-8, HIV, HTLV-1, hepatitis C), and immune suppression related to organ transplantation. Gastric infection with *Helicobacter pylori* increases the risk for gastric lymphomas. NHL is a disease of middle age, usually found in individuals more than 50 years old.

◆**PATHOPHYSIOLOGY.** NHL is best described as a progressive clonal expansion of B cells, T cells, or NK cells. B cells account for 85% to 90% of NHLs, with most of the remaining cases of NHL attributable to T cells and, rarely, NK cells. A very small percentage originates from macrophages. Chromosomal translocations may activate oncogenes, or the tumor-suppressor loci may be inactivated by deletion or mutation of chromosomes. Certain subtypes may have altered genomes by oncogenic viruses. The genetic lesions affecting proto-oncogenes or tumor-suppressor genes result in cell immortalization and the resultant increase in the number of malignant cells. The various subtypes of NHL may be identified by specific diagnostic markers related to various cytogenic lesions.

Lymphomas most likely originate from mutations in cellular genes (many of which are environmentally induced) in a single cell that lead to loss of control of proliferation and other aspects of cell growth. The most common type of chromosomal alteration in NHL is translocation, which disrupts the genes encoded at the breakpoints.

NHL tumors are categorized by the level of differentiation, cell of origin, and rate of cellular proliferation. Tumor aggressiveness of many B-cell NHLs may be predicted by the pattern of cell growth and size. Tumors with a characteristic nodular pattern, vaguely resembling lymphoid follicular structures, are generally less aggressive than lymphomas, with a diffuse pattern of proliferation. Small lymphocyte lymphomas are less aggressive than large-cell lymphomas, which are generally intermediate to high grade in aggressiveness. However, small cells are characteristic of some subtypes of high-grade lymphomas.

◆**CLINICAL MANIFESTATIONS.** Clinical manifestations of NHL usually begin as localized or generalized lymphadenopathy, similar to HL. The cervical, axillary, inguinal, and femoral chains are the most commonly affected sites. Generally, the swelling is painless and the nodes have enlarged and transformed over a period of months or years. Other sites of involvement are the nasopharynx, GI tract, bone, thyroid, testes, and soft tissue. Some individuals have retroperitoneal and abdominal masses with symptoms of abdominal fullness, back pain, ascites (fluid in the peritoneal cavity), and leg swelling.

Lymphomas are classified as low, intermediate, or high grade. A low-grade lymphoma, which also may be termed *indolent,* has a slow progression. Individuals with low-grade lymphoma commonly present with a painless, peripheral adenopathy. Spontaneous regression of these nodes may occur, mimicking the presence of an infection. Night sweats with an elevated temperature (more than 38°C [100.4°F]) and weight loss, as well as extranodular involvement, are not typically present in the early stages but are common in advanced or end stages of the disease. Cytopenia, reflective of bone marrow involvement, is often observed. Hepatomegaly is common; however, splenomegaly is present in approximately 40% of individuals. Fatigue and weakness are more prevalent with advanced stages.

Intermediate- and high-grade lymphomas, which are more aggressive, have a more varied clinical presentation. A high-grade lymphoma also may be termed *aggressive.* Adenopathy is common with more than one-third of individuals having extranodal involvement. Common sites are the GI tract, skin, bone marrow, sinuses, genitourinary (GU) tract, thyroid, and CNS. Night sweats, with an increased temperature (more than 38°C [100.4°F]), as well as weight loss (more than 10% from baseline within 6 months) are present in approximately 30% to 40% of individuals. Some individuals have retroperitoneal and abdominal masses with symptoms of abdominal fullness, back pain, ascites (fluid in the peritoneal cavity), and leg swelling. Hepatomegaly and splenomegaly are often present. Differences in clinical features are noted in Table 30.5.

◆**EVALUATION AND TREATMENT.** Biopsy is considered the primary means for diagnosis of NHL. Staging of NHL is necessary to identify treatment and make a prognosis. In addition to biopsy, computed tomography (CT) scans of the neck, chest, abdomen, and pelvis, as well as bilateral bone marrow aspirate examination, are performed. Data from all three procedures are necessary for appropriate staging. A common finding in NHL is noncontiguous lymph node involvement, which is not common in HL. The Ann Arbor staging system is most commonly used to stage NHL (Table 30.6).

Treatment for NHL is quite diverse and depends on cell type (B or T), tumor stage, histologic status (low, intermediate, or high grade), symptoms, age, and presence of comorbidities. Depending on the cell type (B or T) of the tumor, the stage of the disease, and the aggressiveness

TABLE 30.5	CLINICAL DIFFERENCES BETWEEN NON-HODGKIN LYMPHOMA AND HODGKIN LYMPHOMA	
CHARACTERISTIC	**NON-HODGKIN LYMPHOMA**	**HODGKIN LYMPHOMA**
Nodal involvement	Multiple peripheral nodes	Localized to single axial group of nodes (i.e., cervical, mediastinal, paraaortic)
	Mesenteric nodes and Waldeyer ring commonly involved	Mesenteric nodes and Waldeyer ring rarely involved
Spread	Noncontiguous	Orderly spread by contiguity
B symptoms*	Uncommon	Common
Extranodal involvement	Common	Rare
Extent of disease	Rarely localized	Often localized

*Fever, weight loss, night sweats.

TABLE 30.6	ANN ARBOR STAGING FOR HODGKIN LYMPHOMA
STAGE	**CRITERIA**
I	Involvement of single lymph node
II	Involvement of two or more lymph node regions
III	Involvement of lymph nodes on both sides of diaphragm
IV	Diffuse involvement of one or more extralymphatic organs with or without associated lymph node involvement
	SUBCLASSIFICATIONS
E	Involvement of adjacent extralymphatic site
S	Involvement of spleen
A	Asymptomatic
B	Fever, night sweats, weight loss

of the tumor, treatment is usually initiated at the time of diagnosis. However, because treatment is not curative for some low-grade indolent lymphomas that are widely disseminated, observation without treatment may be the most appropriate choice. These indolent tumors are often asymptomatic for the individual and this approach improves quality of life. In some cases the disease may be so slow growing that treatment is not needed for an extended period of time.

Success of treatment is dependent on several parameters, including the type of lymphoma, stage of disease, type of cell, involvement of organs outside the lymph nodes, age of the person, and severity of the body's reaction to the disease (e.g., fever, night sweats, weight loss). Treatment with chemotherapy alone may be adequate in many cases, although radiation therapy is frequently included. Low-dose chemotherapy has been followed by autologous stem cell transplantation in some NHLs or for recurrent disease. Treatment of B-cell lymphomas with rituximab has proven effective. Rituximab is a commercial monoclonal antibody against antigen CD20, which is expressed on the surface of all B cells, including those that are malignant. Administration of rituximab depletes most B cells and allows the replenishment of normal B cells from the lymphoid stem cell pool. It has also proven useful in a variety of autoimmune diseases, including immune thrombocytopenic purpura, autoimmune anemias, systemic lupus erythematosus, and rheumatoid arthritis.

Radioimmunotherapy, a newer treatment approach, combines radiation therapy with monoclonal antibody therapy and is used to improve rates of complete remission both in indolent forms of lymphoma (follicular and marginal zone) and in aggressive forms, including large B-cell and mantle cell lymphomas. Studies suggest improved complete remission rates and longer disease-free survival in persons with these types of lymphomas.

Individuals with NHL can survive for extended periods.[41] A partial remission may be achieved in some cases in which evidence of the disease remains but the disease does not progress. Survival with nodular lymphoma ranges up to 15 years, but those with diffuse disease generally do not survive as long. Overall, the survival rates of NHL are less than those for Hodgkin lymphoma. For NHL, the survival rates are 1 year, 77%; 5 years, 59%; and 10 years, 42%. Many investigators believe that

more aggressive treatment increases the cure rate. High-grade NHL is seen with increasing frequency in persons with AIDS and has an extremely poor prognosis.

Burkitt Lymphoma

Burkitt lymphoma is a B-cell non-Hodgkin lymphoma with unique clinical and epidemiologic features and it accounts for 30% of childhood lymphomas worldwide. It is highly aggressive and is the fastest growing human tumor. There are three main types of Burkitt lymphoma (*endemic, sporadic,* and *immunodeficiency-related*). *Endemic* Burkitt lymphoma commonly occurs in Africa and is linked to the EBV, and *sporadic* Burkitt lymphoma occurs worldwide.[41] *Immunodeficiency-related* Burkitt lymphoma is most often seen in individuals with AIDS. Burkitt lymphoma occurs most often in children and young adults. *Endemic* cases, usually from Africa, involve a rapidly growing tumor of the jaw and facial bones (Fig. 30.13). In the United States, Burkitt lymphoma is rare, usually involves the abdomen, and is characterized by extensive bone marrow invasion and replacement.

◆**PATHOPHYSIOLOGY.** EBV is associated with almost all cases (more than 90%) of Burkitt lymphoma. It is suspected that suppression of the immune system by other illnesses (e.g., HIV infection, chronic malaria) increases the individual's susceptibility to EBV. B cells are particularly sensitive because of specific surface receptors for EBV. As a result, the B cell undergoes chromosomal translocations that result in overexpression of the *C-MYC* proto-oncogene and loss of control of cell growth (Fig. 30.14). The most common translocation (75% of individuals) is between chromosomes 8 (containing the *C-MYC* gene) and 14 (containing the immunoglobulin heavy-chain genes). Other translocations have been reported between chromosome 8 and chromosomes 2 or 22, which contain genes for immunoglobulin light chains.

◆**CLINICAL MANIFESTATIONS.** In non-African Burkitt lymphoma the most common presentation is abdominal swelling. Manifestations of most tumors occur at extranodal sites. More advanced disease may involve the eye, ovaries, kidneys, or glandular tissue (breast, thyroid, tonsils), and presents with type B symptoms (night sweats, fever, weight loss). Common manifestations may include nausea and vomiting; loss of appetite or change in bowel habits, or both; gastrointestinal bleeding, symptoms of an acute abdominal condition; intestinal perforation; and renal failure.

◆**EVALUATION AND TREATMENT.** The presence of tumors in the jaw and facial bones, enlarged lymph nodes, and bone marrow containing malignant B cells is usually indicative of Burkitt lymphoma. The mainstay of treatment is aggressive multidrug regimens, such as combination chemotherapy. Adjuvant monoclonal antibody therapy with rituximab (anti-CD20) may be a promising agent for improving outcomes.[42]

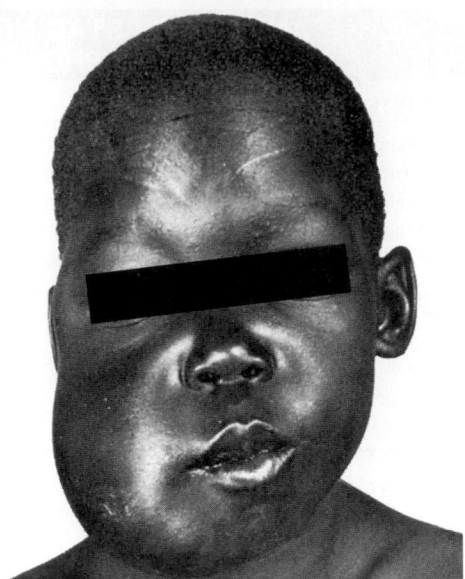

FIGURE 30.13 Burkitt Lymphoma. Burkitt lymphoma involving the jaw in a young African boy. (Courtesy I. Mcgrath, MD, Bethesda, MD. From Zitelli BJ, McIntire SC, Norwalk AJ: *Zitelli and Davis' atlas of pediatric physical diagnosis,* ed 6, Philadelphia, 2012, Saunders.)

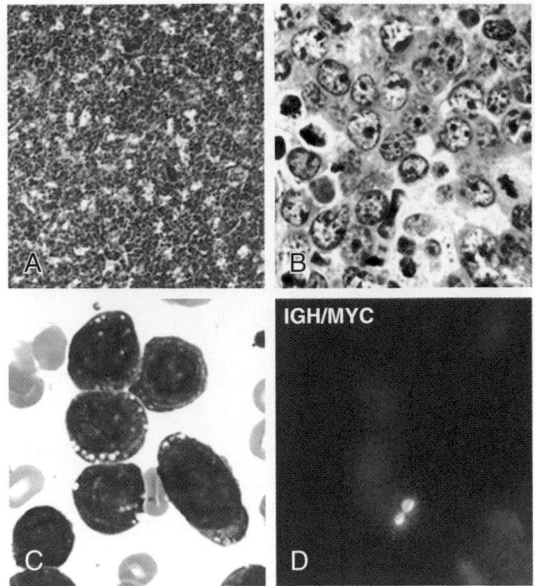

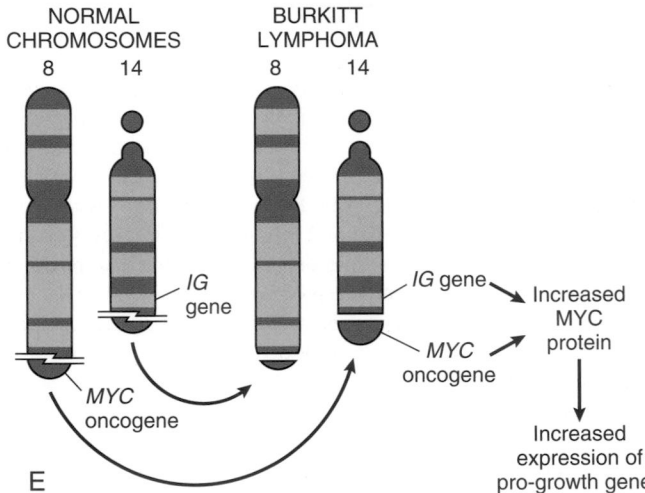

FIGURE 30.14 Burkitt Lymphoma Cells. A, A case of Burkitt lymphoma illustrated at low power showing the "starry sky" appearance. This is due to the dense proliferating cells producing the dark sky, and the scattered lighter-staining tingible body macrophages *(stars)* phagocytizing dying cells. B, Higher magnification illustrating the syncytia of intermediate-sized cells with coarse chromatin and multiple nucleoli. Note the tingible body macrophage with abundant light cytoplasm and ingested debris *(center bottom).* C, Burkitt cells as seen on a Wright-stained bone marrow aspirate in a person with Burkitt leukemia. Note the deep blue cytoplasm with numerous vacuoles. D, Fluorescence in situ hybridization (FISH) with probes to MYC and IGH illustrates the IGH/MYC fusion. E, The 8;14 chromosomal transloca-tion and associated oncogenes in Burkitt lymphoma. *IGH,* Immunoglobulin heavy chain loci; *MYC,* protooncogene. (A–D Courtesy Dr. Y. Zhang, University of Chicago. From Hoffman R et al: *Hematology: basic principles and practice,* ed 6, Philadelphia, 2013, Churchill Livingstone. E From Kumar V, Abbas A, Aster JC: *Robbins & Cotran pathologic basis of disease,* ed 9, Philadelphia, 2015, Saunders.)

Lymphoblastic Lymphoma

Lymphoblastic lymphoma (LL) is a relatively rare variant of NHL (2% to 4%) but accounts for about 20% of cases of NHL in children and adolescents, with a male predominance. It is a fast-growing type of NHL in which increased numbers of lymphoblasts are found in the lymph nodes and the thymus gland. Lymphoblasts also can spread to other areas of the body. The vast majority of cases of LL (more than 85%) are of T-cell origin, and the remainder of LL cases arise from B cells. LL is similar to acute lymphoblastic leukemia and may be considered a variant of that disease.

◆PATHOPHYSIOLOGY. The disease arises from a clone of relatively immature T cells that becomes malignant in the thymus. As with most lymphoid tumors, LL is frequently associated with translocations, primar-ily of the chromosomes that encode for the T-cell receptor (chromosomes 7 and 14). These aberrations result in increased expression of a variety of transcription factors and loss of growth control.

◆CLINICAL MANIFESTATIONS. The first sign of LL is usually a painless lymphadenopathy in the neck. Peripheral lymph nodes in the chest become involved in about 70% of individuals, mostly above the dia-phragm. LL is a very aggressive tumor that presents as stage IV in most people. T-cell LL is associated with a unique mediastinal mass (up to 75%) because of the apparent origin of the tumor in the thymus.

The mass results in chest pain and may cause compression of bronchi or the superior vena cava. The tumor may infiltrate the bone marrow in about half of those affected, and suppression of bone marrow hematopoiesis leads to increased susceptibility to infections. Other organs, including the liver, kidney, spleen, and brain, may also be affected. Many individuals express type B symptoms (fever, night sweats, and significant weight loss).

◆EVALUATION AND TREATMENT. The most common therapeutic approach is combined chemotherapy with multiple drugs. In early stages of the disease, the response rate is high with increased survival; the 5-year survival in children is 80% to 90%, and 45% to 55% in adults. Although LL is easily treated, there is a high relapse rate: 40% to 60% of adults.

Conditions That Mimic Lymphomas

Certain other clinical conditions mimic the malignant lymphomas. These conditions include tuberculosis (TB), syphilis, systemic lupus erythematosus, lung cancer, and bone cancer. An important distinction between lymphomas and other conditions is that lymphomas usually

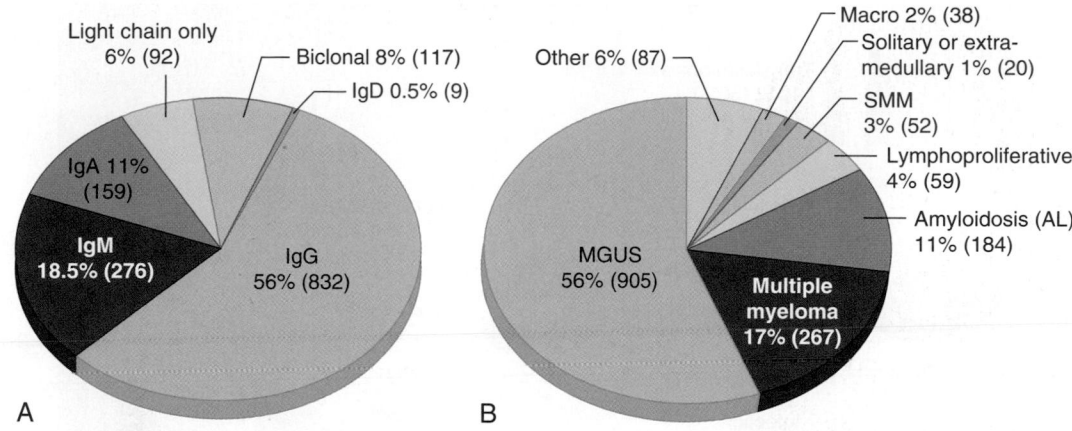

FIGURE 30.15 Distribution of Monoclonal Gammamopathy Types. **A,** Distribution of serum monoclonal proteins in 1485 patients seen at the Mayo Clinic during 2008. **B,** Diagnoses in 1612 cases of monoclonal gammopathy seen at the Mayo Clinic during 2008. *Ig,* Immunoglobulin; *MGUS,* monoclonal gammopathy of undetermined significance; *SMM,* smoldering multiple myeloma. (From Goldman L, Schafer AI: *Goldman's Cecil medicine,* ed 24, Philadelphia, 2012, Saunders.)

involve localized lymphadenopathy. Infectious precursors of malignant lymphomas are characterized by more generalized lymphadenopathy with systemic signs and symptoms.

Plasma Cell Malignancies

The plasma cell is the end-stage cell of the humoral immune response (see Chapter 8). Immunocompetent B cells presented with antigen and stimulated with cytokines from T helper cells will undergo proliferation and differentiation into antibody-producing plasma cells. Antigen-reactive B cells have undergone rearrangement of immunoglobulin heavy-chain variable region genes *(V, D, J)* and express surface IgM or IgD, or both. After stimulation with antigen, the B cells may not undergo any further genetic rearrangement; instead, they may develop into plasma cells that secrete IgM or selectively rearrange the immunoglobulin heavy-chain genes to irreversibly switch to secretion of IgG, IgA, or IgE. During this process some cells may undergo malignant transformation, leading to one of several types of plasma cell malignancies (Fig. 30.15). The most common and most aggressive plasma cell tumor is multiple myeloma. Examples of other diseases in this classification include precursors to malignant myeloma (smoldering myeloma, monoclonal gammopathy of undetermined significance [MGUS]), solitary plasmacytoma of the bone, and Waldenström macroglobulinemia. A common characteristic of these tumors is secretion of complete or partial immunoglobulin molecules.

Multiple Myeloma

Multiple myeloma (MM; *plasma cell myeloma)* is a clonal plasma cell cancer characterized by the slow proliferation of tumor cell masses in the bone marrow associated with lytic bone lesions. Uncommon variants include *solitary myeloma (plasmacytoma)* with a single mass in bone or soft tissue and *smoldering myeloma,* which is defined by a lack of symptoms and a high plasma abnormal antibody called the **M protein.** Most MMs secrete large amounts of monoclonal proteins that resemble intact immunoglobulins. MM is the third most common blood cancer (after lymphoma and leukemia) in the United States. For unknown reasons, the reported incidence of myeloma has doubled in the past two decades. The number of new cases in the United States is estimated at greater than 30,280 with more than 12,590 deaths for 2017.[7] Multiple myeloma occurs in all races, but the incidence in blacks is about twice

that of whites. It rarely occurs before the age of 40 years—the peak age of incidence is between 65 and 70 years. It is slightly more common in men than women. Other risk factors include exposure to radiation or certain chemicals including pesticides, and a history of monoclonal gammopathy of undetermined significance (MGUS, see Clinical Manifestations) or plasmacytoma.[43,44] Neoplastic cells of multiple myeloma reside in the bone marrow and are usually not found in the peripheral blood. Occasionally it may spread to other tissues, especially in very advanced stages of the disease.

◆PATHOPHYSIOLOGY. Multiple myeloma is a biologically complex disease with significant heterogeneity reflected by a wide range of genetic alterations and individual differences in clinical response and survival of individuals receiving the same treatment.[45] The genetic mutations in different pathways alter the intrinsic biology of the plasma cell, generating the features of myeloma.[46] The genetic mutations may affect genes that impact cell growth and division, causing excessive proliferation of plasma cells. Many myelomas are aneuploidy, with chromosomal numbers ranging from 44 chromosomes to near tetraploid. Chromosomal translocations (breakpoints) are responsible for development of myeloma in most individuals. The primary translocation involves the immunoglobulin heavy chain on chromosome 14 that relocates to sites containing genes that cell-cycle (cyclins) on chromosomes 11(q13), 12(p13), and 6(p21); oncogenes on chromosomes 16(q23), 8(q24), and 20; and fibroblast growth factor receptor on chromosome 4(p16).[10] A progression of further secondary genetic alterations causes development to an aggressive MM (Fig. 30.16). The molecular pathogenesis of multiple myeloma also involves proto-oncogene mutations and, more rarely, inactivation of tumor-suppressor genes. The precise timing and reason for the genetic alteration and accumulation are unknown, but probably occur initially late in B-cell development after exposure to antigen. Investigators are studying various epigenetic alterations in multiple myeloma, for example, microRNAs and global changes in chromatin.[47] Epigenetic aberrations play an important role in the pathogenic events leading to MM, and further studies are warranted to identify the precise mechanisms.[45]

Malignant plasma cells arise from one clone of B cells that produce abnormally large amounts of one class of immunoglobulin (usually IgG, occasionally IgA, and rarely IgD or IgE). The malignant transformation may begin early in B-cell development, possibly before encountering

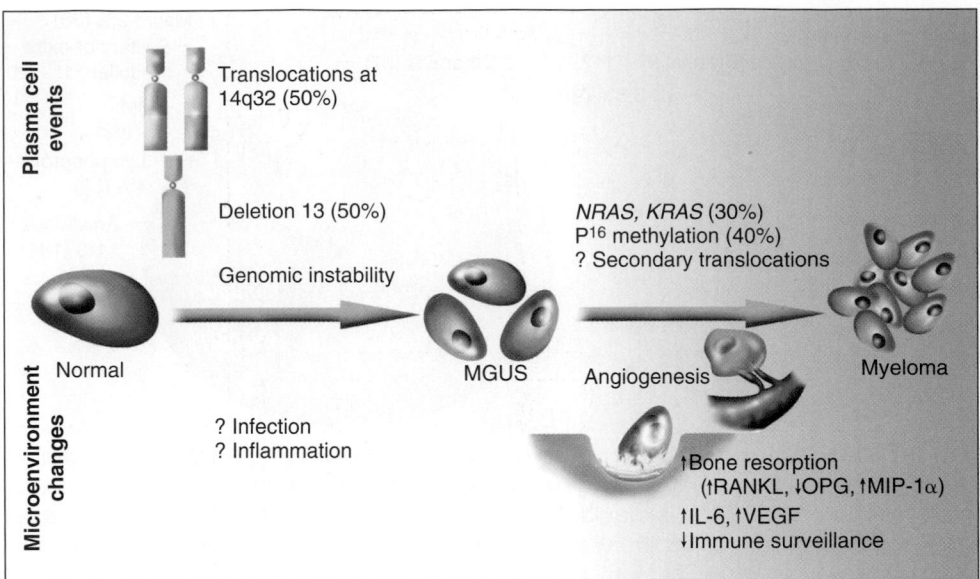

FIGURE 30.16 Myeloma Cell Proliferation and Disease Progression. Development of malignant myeloma results from multiple genetic changes, initially a translocation involving the immunoglobulin heavy-chain genes on chromosome 14 or a deletion in chromosome 13. The intermediate phenotype is frequently genetically unstable, leading to further mutations that result in a myeloma. Interactions between myeloma cells and extracellular matrix proteins further increase adhesion molecule expression, antiapoptotic pathways, angiogenesis, bone resorption, and cytokine secretion. *IL-6,* Interleukin-6; *KRAS,* V-Ki-ras Z Kirsten rat sarcoma viral oncogene homolog; *MGUS,* monoclonal gammopathy of undetermined significance; *MIP-1α,* macrophage inflammatory protein-1α; *NRAS,* neuroblastoma RAS viral (v-ras) oncogene homolog; *OPG,* osteoprotegerin; *RANKL,* receptor activator of nuclear factor-κB ligand; *VEGF,* vascular endothelial growth factor. (From Abeloff M et al: *Abeloff's clinical oncology,* ed 4, Philadelphia, 2008, Churchill Livingstone.)

antigen in the secondary lymphoid organs. The myeloma cells return either to the bone marrow or to other soft tissue sites. Cell adhesion molecules help them target favorable sites that promote continued expansion and maturation.

Myeloma cells in the bone marrow directly secrete hepatocyte growth factor and parathyroid hormone–related peptide and adhere to stromal cells, inducing their production of several cytokines (e.g., IL-6, IL-1, TNF-α, TNF-β, IL-11, macrophage inflammatory protein). (Lymphocytes and cytokines are described in Chapter 8.) These factors, particularly IL-6, act as an osteoclast-activating factor and stimulate osteoclasts to reabsorb bone. This process results in bone lesions and hypercalcemia attributable to release of calcium from the breakdown of bone.

The antibody produced by the transformed plasma cell is usually defective, containing truncations, deletions, and other abnormalities, and is frequently referred to as a *paraprotein* (abnormal protein in the blood). Because of the large number of malignant plasma cells, M protein becomes the most prominent protein in the blood in 80% of individuals with myeloma (Fig. 30.17). Suppression of normal plasma cells by the myeloma results in diminished or absent normal antibodies. The excessive amount of M protein also may contribute to many of the clinical manifestations of the disease. The myeloma may produce free immunoglobulin light chain (Bence Jones protein) that is present in the blood and urine in approximately 80% of individuals and contributes to damage of renal tubular cells.

◆**CLINICAL MANIFESTATIONS.** The common presentation of MM is characterized by elevated levels of calcium in the blood (hypercalcemia) (13% of persons), renal failure (19%), anemia (72% of persons), and bone lesions (80% of persons).[48] The hypercalcemia and bone lesions result from infiltration of the bone by malignant plasma cells and

stimulation of osteoclasts to reabsorb bone. This process results in the release of calcium (hypercalcemia) and the development of "lytic lesions" (round, "punched-out" regions of bone) (Fig. 30.18). Destruction of bone tissue causes pain, the most common presenting symptom, and pathologic fractures. The pain may be felt in a single bone of the entire skeleton, and the bones most commonly involved, in decreasing order of frequency, are the vertebrae, ribs, skull, pelvis, femur, clavicle, and scapula. Spinal cord compression, because of the weakened vertebrae, occurs in about 10% of individuals. The pain is initially aching and intermittent, and is aggravated by weightbearing activities. As the disease progresses, pain becomes severe and prolonged. It is common for those with myeloma to be treated for a slipped vertebral disc or arthritis before the correct diagnosis of myeloma is established. The individual may complain of weakness, fatigue, weight loss, anorexia, easy bruising or bleeding, and trouble breathing in addition to pain.

Antibody proteins can increase in number and stick together, called *amyloidosis,* in peripheral nerves and organs, such as the heart and kidneys. Amyloidosis causes the nerves and organs to become stiff, and the manifestations include extreme exhaustion, purple spots on the skin, enlarged tongue, diarrhea, edema, and tingling and numbness in the legs and feet.

Proteinuria is observed in 90% of individuals. Renal failure may be either acute or chronic and is usually secondary to the hypercalcemia. Bence Jones protein may lead to damage of the proximal tubules. Anemia is usually normocytic and normochromic and results from inhibited erythropoiesis caused by tumor cell infiltration of the bone marrow.

The high concentration of paraprotein in the blood may lead to hyperviscosity syndrome. The increased viscosity interferes with blood circulation to various sites (brain, kidneys, extremities). Hyperviscosity

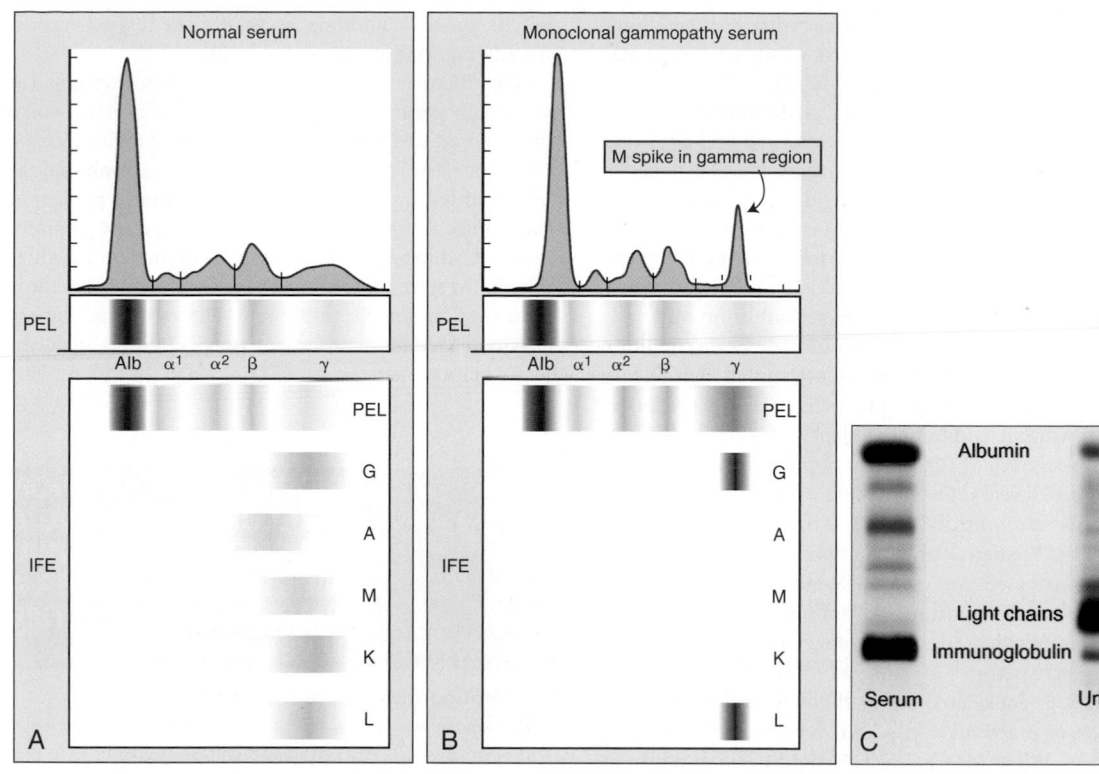

FIGURE 30.17 M Protein. Serum protein electrophoresis *(PEL)* is used to screen for M proteins in multiple myeloma. **A,** In normal serum the proteins separate into several regions between albumin *(Alb)* and a broad band in the gamma (γ) region, where most antibodies (gamma globulins) are found. Immunofixation *(IFE)* can identify the location of IgG *(G)*, IgA *(A)*, IgM *(M)*, and kappa *(K)* and lambda *(L)* light chains. **B,** Serum from an individual with multiple myeloma contains a sharp M protein *(M spike)*. The M protein is monoclonal and contains only one heavy chain and one light chain. In this instance the IFE identifies the M protein as an IgG containing a lambda light chain. **C,** Serum and urine protein electrophoretic patterns in a client with multiple myeloma. Serum demonstrates an M protein *(Immunoglobulin)* in the gamma region, and the urine has a large amount of the smaller-sized light chains with only a small amount of the intact immunoglobulin. (**A** and **B** From Abeloff M et al: *Abeloff's clinical oncology,* ed 4, Philadelphia, 2008, Churchill Livingstone. **C** From McPherson R, Pincus M: *Henry's clinical diagnosis and management by laboratory methods,* ed 22, Edinburgh, 2012, Saunders.)

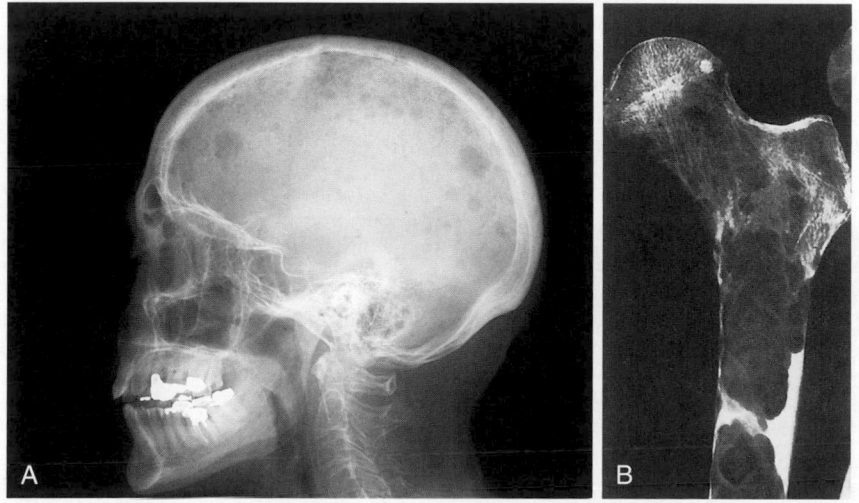

FIGURE 30.18 Osteolytic Lesions in Individuals with Multiple Myeloma. A, Radiograph showing skull lesions in a client with myeloma. **B,** Roentgenogram of femur showing extensive bone destruction caused by tumor. Note absence of reactive bone formation. (**A** From Abeloff M et al: *Abeloff's clinical oncology,* ed 4, Philadelphia, 2008, Churchill Livingstone. **B** From Kissane JM, editor: *Anderson's pathology,* ed 9, St Louis, 1990, Mosby.)

syndrome is observed in up to 20% of individuals with MM. Additional neurologic symptoms (e.g., confusion, headaches, blurred vision) may occur secondary to hypercalcemia or hyperviscosity.

Suppression of the humoral (antibody-mediated) immune response results in repeated infections, primarily pneumonias and pyelonephritis. The most commonly involved organisms are encapsulated bacteria that are particularly sensitive to the effects of antibody, such as pneumonia caused by *Streptococcus pneumoniae*, *Staphylococcus aureus*, or *Klebsiella pneumoniae* or pyelonephritis caused by *Escherichia coli* or other gram-negative organisms. Cell-mediated (T-cell) function is relatively normal. Overwhelming infection is the leading cause of death from MM.

MM is a progressive disorder and is often preceded by a condition known as monoclonal gammopathy of undetermined significance (MGUS). MGUS is diagnosed by the presence of an M protein in the blood or urine without additional evidence of MM.[48] MGUS is present in approximately 1% of the general population and in 3% of individuals older than 70 years. The herbicide Agent Orange contains 2,3,7,8-tetrachlorodibenzo-*p*-dioxin (TCDD), a human carcinogen, and was sprayed during the Vietnam War. Operation Ranch Hand veterans have a significantly increased risk of MGUS, supporting an association between Agent Orange exposure and multiple myeloma.[49] From occupational studies, pesticides (i.e., insecticides, herbicides, fungicides) are associated with increased risk of MM and MGUS.[49]

Although MGUS is considered nonpathologic and requires no treatment, about 2% of individuals with MGUS progress to malignant plasma cell disorders. When MM is preceded by MGUS, it advances first to asymptomatic MM and then to symptomatic MM. Asymptomatic MM also may be referred to as smoldering myeloma and indolent myeloma.[48] Smoldering myeloma is usually characterized by the presence of an M protein and clonal bone marrow plasma cells, but with no indication of end-organ damage.

Most cases of symptomatic plasma cell tumors are multiple myeloma (about 94%). The remaining 6% of cases are divided equally between solitary plasmacytomas and extramedullary plasmacytomas.[50] Solitary plasmacytoma is characterized by a solitary tumor of malignant plasma cells that may result in a single lytic bone lesion or may develop in the tissues (extramedullary plasmacytoma).[48] Extramedullary plasmacytoma can be found in a variety of soft tissues, but commonly in those of the upper respiratory tract (e.g., tonsils, nasopharynx, sinuses). Additionally, MM is staged to help determine prognosis and appropriate treatment (Table 30.7).

◆EVALUATION AND TREATMENT. Diagnosis of MM is made by symptom assessment, radiographic and laboratory studies, and bone marrow biopsy. The International Myeloma Working Group consensus updated the disease definition of MM to include validated biomarkers and the existing requirements of CRAB features (hypercalcemia, renal failure, anemia, and bone lesions).[51] The revised criteria for MM and smoldering MM are presented in Box 30.4.

Quantitative measurements of immunoglobulins (IgG, IgM, IgA) are usually performed. Typically, one class of immunoglobulin (the M protein produced by the myeloma cell) is significantly expressed whereas the other classes are suppressed. Serum electrophoretic analysis reveals increased levels of M protein. Because the M protein is monoclonal, each molecule has the same electric charge and migrates to about the same site during electrophoresis, resulting in a highly concentrated protein (M spike). Bence Jones protein is observed in the urine or serum by using immunoelectrophoretic analysis or in the serum by using enzyme-linked immunosorbent assay (ELISA). Usually individuals with Bence Jones protein also have M protein in their blood. However, variants

BOX 30.4   REVISED INTERNATIONAL MYELOMA WORKING GROUP DIAGNOSTIC CRITERIA FOR MULTIPLE MYELOMA AND SMOLDERING MULTIPLE MYELOMA

Definition of Multiple Myeloma

Clonal bone marrow plasma cells ≥10% or biopsy-proven bony or extramedullary plasmacytoma* and any one or more of the following myeloma-defining events:

Evidence of end-organ damage that can be attributed to the underlying plasma cell proliferative disorder, specifically:

Hypercalcemia: serum calcium >0.25 mmol/L (>1 mg/dL) higher than the upper limit of normal or >2.75 mmol/L (>11 mg/dL)

Renal insufficiency: creatinine clearance >40 mL/min† or serum creatinine >177 μmol/L (>2 mg/dL)

Anemia: hemoglobin value of >20 g/L below the lower limit of normal, or hemoglobin value <100 g/L

Bone lesions: one or more osteolytic lesions on skeletal radiography, CT, or PET-CT‡

Any one or more of the following biomarkers of malignancy:

Clonal bone marrow plasma cell percentage* ≥60%

Involved/uninvolved serum-free light-chain ratio§ ≥100

>1 focal lesion on MRI studies¶

Definition of Smoldering Multiple Myeloma

Both criteria must be met:

Serum monoclonal protein (IgG or IgA) ≥30 g/L or urine monoclonal protein ≥500 mg/24 hr and/or clonal bone marrow plasma cells 10% to 60%

Absence of myeloma-defining events or amyloidosis

*Clonality should be established by showing κ/λ-light-chain restriction on flow cytometry, immunohistochemistry, or immunofluorescence. Bone marrow plasma cell percentage should preferably be estimated from a core biopsy specimen; in case of disparity between the aspirate and core biopsy, the highest value should be used.
†Measured or estimated by validated equations.
‡If bone marrow has less than 10% clonal plasma cells, more than one bone lesion is required to distinguish from solitary plasmacytoma with minimal marrow involvement.
§These values are based on the serum Freelite assay (The Binding Site Group, Birmingham, U.K.). The involved free light chain must be ≥100 mg/L.
¶Each focal lesion must be 5 mm or more in size.
PET-CT, 18F-Labeled fluorodeoxyglucose PET with CT.
From Rajkumar SV et al: *Lancet Oncol* 15(12):e538–e548, 2014.

TABLE 30.7   INTERNATIONAL STAGING SYSTEM FOR MULTIPLE MYELOMA

STAGE	CRITERIA
I	Serum β₂-microglobulin <3.5 mg/L
	Serum albumin ≥3.5 g/dL
II	Not stage I or III*
III	Serum β₂-microglobulin ≥5.5 mg/L

*There are two categories for stage II: serum β₂-microglobulin <3.5 mg/L but serum albumin <3.5 g/dL; or serum β₂-microglobulin 3.5 to <5.5 mg/L irrespective of the serum albumin level.
From Greipp PR et al: *J Clin Oncol* 23(15):3412–3420, 2005.

of MM include individuals in which only free light chain is produced and a rare variant that produces only free heavy chain, and approximately 1% of variants are nonsecretory so that neither M protein nor Bence Jones protein is produced. The amount of M protein in the blood may be used as a measure of the extent of the disease or as a measure of response to therapy. The serum level of another protein, free β_2-microglobulin, is a useful indicator of prognosis or effectiveness of therapy.

A bone marrow biopsy is performed to confirm the presence of myeloma cells in the marrow (Fig. 30.19). Radiographic studies include x-ray, CT scans, and magnetic resonance imaging (MRI) to document the presence of bone lesions and areas of destruction. Diagnosis is based on findings and the degree of involvement (see Box 30.4).

Treatment options include combinations of chemotherapy, other drug therapy, targeted therapy, high-dose chemotherapy with stem cell transplant, biologic therapy, radiation therapy (bone lesions of the spine), and sometimes surgery. Supported therapy includes plasmapheresis (exchange) if the blood becomes thick with increased antibody proteins and interferes with circulation. Conventional combinations of chemotherapeutic agents have included melphalan and prednisone (MP); MP with vincristine, carmustine, and cyclophosphamide; vincristine, doxorubicin, and dexamethasone; and thalidomide and dexamethasone. The drug thalidomide disrupts the stromal marrow–MM cell interaction by modulating cell surface adhesion molecules and inhibiting angiogenesis. In addition, it increases apoptosis and G_1 growth arrest (i.e., the cell cycle gap 1; see Chapter 1) of MM cells. New therapies called *proteasome inhibitors* are emerging. Myeloma cells are sensitive to inhibitors of the proteasome because the proteasome degrades unwanted and misfolded proteins and myeloma cells are prone to the accumulation of misfolded, unpaired Ig chains. Proteasome inhibitors induce cell death and retard bone resorption through effects on stromal cells.[3]

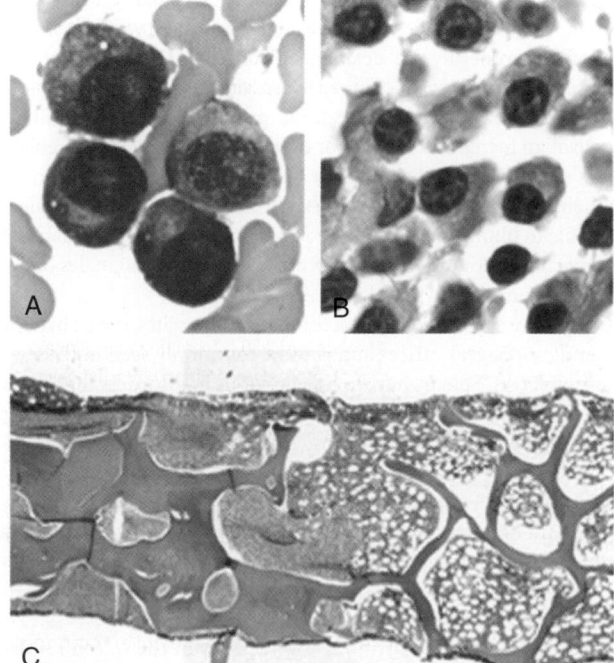

FIGURE 30.19 Myeloma Cells. The typical myeloma type has fairly mature appearing plasma cells with eccentric nuclei on bone marrow aspirate **(A)** and biopsy **(B). C,** Osteosclerotic myeloma in which the left side of the photograph shows bone sclerosis and the marrow cavity replaced by myeloma. (From Hoffman R et al: *Hematology: basic principles and practice,* ed 6, Philadelphia, 2013, Churchill Livingstone.)

Dose intensification improves the outcomes in younger persons; however, long-term remissions are obtained in a minority of individuals. Thus intensive research measuring the effect of novel new therapies is the objective of ongoing trials.

Gene expression profiling (GEP) helps improve the treatment of MM because it identifies prognostic subgroups and defines the molecular pathways associated with these subgroups. Newer agents (e.g., bortezomib, lenalidomide) have broadened the therapeutic regimens for end-stage myeloma. Lenalidomide is related to thalidomide; however, it increases treatment efficacy while avoiding the adverse effects associated with thalidomide. In combination with dexamethasone, lenalidomide is now an approved second-line treatment for MM. The FDA has approved daratumumab for people who have received at least three prior treatments. Ixazomib has been approved for the treatment of relapsed multiple myeloma in individuals who have received at least one prior treatment, and elotuzumab has been approved for those who have received one to three prior therapies.

High-dose chemotherapy followed by blood-forming stem cell transplantation (SCT) has become standard treatment for younger individuals (up to 70 years old in some trials).[50,52] Survival is increased with SCT compared with chemotherapy alone. SCT uses the client's own blood-forming stem cells (autologous) or a donor's cells (allogeneic). Survival may be prolonged by performing a second autologous transplant, called a *tandem transplant,* within 6 to 12 months after the first transplant.

Radiation with high-energy x-rays is used more for a localized, rather than system, effect. It is most often used to treat areas of the bone that have been damaged and are not responding to chemotherapy. In addition, it may be used to treat sites where tumor has led to collapse of vertebrae and spinal cord compression.

Additional interventions are used to prevent and treat complications arising from progression of the disease. Drugs that inhibit bone resorption—bisphosphonates—reduce the incidence of skeletal damage, which also reduces hypercalcemia and decreases bone pain. Hydration and diuretics may be used to maintain a high urine output, and antibiotics to treat recurring infections.

The median survival for all stages of MM is 3 years. Individuals with multiple bone lesions, if untreated, rarely survive more than 6 to 12 months. Individuals with inactive (indolent) myeloma, however, can survive for many years. With chemotherapy and aggressive management of complications, median survival may increase to 24 to 30 months, with a 10-year survival rate of 3%. With the approval of new drugs, the management of MM has changed and research for survival improvement is ongoing.

Waldenström Macroglobulinemia

Waldenström macroglobulinemia (WM), also called lymphoplasmacytic lymphoma, is a rare type of slow-growing plasma cell tumor that secretes a monoclonal IgM molecule. Approximately 1500 new cases are diagnosed yearly in the United States; the median age of diagnosis is 63 years of age.[53] WM shares a great deal of similarity with multiple myeloma regarding its plasma cell origin, diagnosis, and treatment. However, the overproduction of the macromolecule IgM leads to certain unique clinical characteristics.

PATHOPHYSIOLOGY. WM arises from plasma cells that have undergone genetic rearrangement of the variable region genes *(V, D, J),* but have not undergone class-switch. Therefore, the principal secretory product of the tumor is IgM. Although no definitive genetic defect has been identified, WM may originate from aberrant B-cell maturation and class-switch.

Most of the pathology is associated with the production of large amounts of IgM, a high-molecular-weight protein (about 900,000 daltons). Excessive production leads to thickening of the blood and abnormally high blood viscosity (hyperviscosity syndrome). The increased viscosity interferes with circulation to various sites (e.g., eyes, brain, kidneys, extremities). IgM paraprotein may also result in the formation of cryoglobulins (i.e., proteins that precipitate from the blood at lower than body temperature). Hyperviscosity syndrome is observed in up to 20% of individuals with WM.

◆**CLINICAL MANIFESTATIONS.** Many individuals with WM are asymptomatic. The most common symptoms include weakness and fatigue, bleeding (from gums and nose), weight loss, and bruising. Bleeding may result secondary to formation of complexes among the macroglobulin, clotting factors, and platelets that diminish hemostatic capacity. If hyperviscosity syndrome occurs, the individual may develop neurologic problems (e.g., blurred vision, loss of vision, headaches, dizziness, vertigo). The macromolecules may also precipitate in colder regions of the body (cryoglobulins), leading to Raynaud phenomenon.

Although the malignant plasma cells invade the bone marrow, erosion of the bone is not commonly observed; less than 5% of individuals have lytic bone lesions. The tumor often disseminates to other organs, including the spleen, lymph nodes, and liver. Anemia occurs in about 10% of individuals, secondary to tumor infiltration of the bone marrow. Peripheral hemolysis can also result from production of cold agglutinins.

◆**EVALUATION AND TREATMENT.** Diagnosis is made on the basis of high levels of monoclonal IgM in the blood and the identification of malignant cells in bone marrow aspirates. Other hematologic abnormalities may be observed, especially anemia (80% of people with symptomatic WM) but also thrombocytopenia and leukopenia. Bence Jones protein may be observed in almost half of individuals with WM.

Therapy includes combined chemotherapy with nucleoside analogs, alkylating agents, and monoclonal antibody (e.g., rituximab). Bone marrow stem cell transplantation has also proven effective in some individuals.

ALTERATIONS OF SPLENIC FUNCTION

The spleen has been an organ of mystery and perplexity in the study of medicine. Its relationship to other organs and disease processes, particularly the immune and hematologic systems, was not identified until the eighteenth century. The complexities of splenic function are not totally understood, and its mysteries are still being explored. The spleen is a useful organ, but its functions overlap those of other organs so that one is capable of living a normal, healthy life without the spleen. The relationship between asplenia and a higher risk for infection was not recognized until the early 1950s.

In the past, splenomegaly (enlargement of the spleen) was associated with various disease states. It is now recognized that splenomegaly is not necessarily pathologic; an enlarged spleen may be present in certain individuals without any evidence of disease. However, splenomegaly may be one of the first physical signs of underlying conditions, and its presence should not be ignored. In conditions in which splenomegaly is present, the normal functions of the spleen may become overactive, producing a condition known as hypersplenism.

Current criteria indicating the presence of hypersplenism include (1) cytopenias (anemia, leukopenia, thrombocytopenia, or combinations of these); (2) cellular bone marrow; (3) splenomegaly; and (4) improvement after splenectomy. Some individuals may seek treatment for problems even though they have not met all these clinical criteria; therefore, the relevance and significance of hypersplenism are still uncertain. Primary hypersplenism is recognized when no etiologic factor has been identified; secondary hypersplenism occurs in the presence of another condition.

BOX 30.5   DISEASES RELATED TO CLASSIFICATION OF SPLENOMEGALY

Inflammation or Infection
Acute: viral (hepatitis, infectious mononucleosis, cytomegalovirus), bacterial (*Salmonella*, gram negative), parasitic (typhoid)
Subacute or chronic: bacterial (subacute bacterial endocarditis, tuberculosis), parasitic (malaria), fungal (histoplasmosis), Felty syndrome, systemic lupus erythematosus, rheumatoid arthritis, thrombocytopenia

Congestive
Cirrhosis, heart failure, portal vein obstruction (portal hypertension), splenic vein obstruction

Infiltrative
Gaucher disease, amyloidosis, diabetic lipemia

Tumors or Cysts
Malignant: polycythemia vera, chronic or acute leukemias, Hodgkin lymphoma, metastatic solid tumors
Nonmalignant: hamartoma
Cysts: true cysts (lymphangiomas, hemangiomas, epithelial, endothelial); false cysts (hemorrhagic, serous, inflammatory)

◆**PATHOPHYSIOLOGY.** Splenomegaly without a specific etiology is seen in 7% to 15% of individuals who are being evaluated for primary splenomegaly and is generally a diagnosis of exclusion. Specific conditions causing secondary splenomegaly and resulting hypersplenism are numerous and are related to all other categories of disease that affect individuals. Secondary splenomegaly may be classified according to the underlying cause. Specific conditions related to these various classifications of splenomegaly are detailed in Box 30.5. Different pathologic processes that produce splenomegaly are described briefly.

Acute inflammatory or infectious processes cause splenomegaly because of an increased demand for defensive activities. Acutely enlarged spleens secondary to infection may become so filled with erythrocytes that their natural rubbery resilience is lost and they become fragile and vulnerable to blunt trauma. Splenic rupture is a complication associated with infectious mononucleosis; rupture occurs mostly in males between the fourth and twenty-first day of acute illness.

Congestive splenomegaly is accompanied by ascites, portal hypertension, and esophageal varices and is most commonly seen in those with hepatic cirrhosis. Splenic hyperplasia develops in disorders that increase splenic workload and is associated most commonly with various types of anemia (hemolytic) and chronic myeloproliferative disorders (i.e., polycythemia vera).

Infiltrative splenomegaly is caused by engorgement by the macrophages with indigestible materials associated with various "storage diseases." Tumors and cysts cause actual growth of the spleen. Metastatic tumors in the spleen are rare and may result from primary tumors of the skin, lung, breast, and cervix.

◆**CLINICAL MANIFESTATIONS.** Overactivity of the spleen results in hematologic alterations that affect all blood components. Sequestering of red blood cells, granulocytes, and platelets causes a reduction in the number of all circulating blood cells. The spleen may sequester up to 50% of the red blood cell population, thereby upsetting the normal physiologic concentration of red blood cells in the circulation. The rate of splenic pooling is directly related to the size of the spleen and the degree of increased blood flow through it. Sequestering exposes the red blood cells to splenic conditions that accelerate destruction, further contributing to the decreased red blood cell concentration. Anemia is the result of these combined activities. Anemia may be further potentiated by an increase in blood volume, which produces a dilutional effect on the already reduced concentration of red blood cells. The dilutional effect, as well as the removal and destruction of red blood cells, depends primarily on the degree of splenomegaly.

White blood cells and platelets also are affected by sequestering, although not to the same degree as the red blood cell. Again, the size of the spleen is the determining factor in the number of cells sequestered.

◆**EVALUATION AND TREATMENT.** Treatment for hypersplenism is splenectomy; however, it is not always the treatment of choice. A splenectomy should be performed when its removal is considered necessary to alleviate the destructive effects on red blood cells. Clinical indicators should determine the need for splenectomy, not necessarily the specific condition. Splenectomy for splenic rupture no longer is considered mandatory in light of the possibility of overwhelming sepsis after removal. Repair and preservation of the ruptured spleen are now considered before the decision to remove the spleen. Splenectomy also may be performed as treatment for hairy cell leukemia, Felty syndrome,

agnogenic myeloid metaplasia, thalassemia major, Gaucher disease, hemodialysis, splenomegaly, splenic venous thrombosis, and thrombotic thrombocytopenic purpura (TTP).

Individuals are able to lead normal lives after splenectomy, but hematologic abnormalities often exist after removal of the spleen. The red blood cells become thinner, broader, and wrinkled as a result of increases in surface area and membrane lipids. The white blood cell count increases dramatically 1 week after removal and then stabilizes to approximately 40% greater than normal. Platelet numbers also rise immediately after surgery and then equilibrate to above-normal levels for the duration of the individual's life. Increased platelet levels have been implicated in ischemic heart disease in males because of increased thrombocytosis and hypercoagulability.

A major postoperative complication following splenectomy is overwhelming postsplenectomy infection (OPSI). Unless treated in time, OPSI may rapidly progress to septic shock and possibly disseminated intravascular coagulation (DIC). Initial statistics indicate a death rate of 50% to 70%, with most deaths occurring within the first 48 hours after hospitalization. Prompt medical attention can reduce the death rate to 10%.

▮ SUMMARY REVIEW

Alterations of Leukocyte Function

1. Quantitative alterations of leukocytes (too many or too few) can be caused by bone marrow dysfunction or premature destruction of cells in the circulation. Many quantitative changes in leukocytes occur in response to invasion by microorganisms.

2. Leukocytosis is a leukocyte count higher than normal and is usually a response to physiologic stressors, malignancies and hematologic disorders, and invasion of microorganisms.

3. Leukopenia is a leukocyte count lower than normal, is associated with neutropenia and infection, and is caused by physiologic stressors and by pathologic conditions such as malignancies and hematologic disorders.

4. Granulocytosis (particularly as a result of an increase in the number of neutrophils) occurs in response to infection. The marrow releases immature cells, causing a shift-to-the-left when responding to an infection that has created a demand for neutrophils that exceeds the supply in the circulation.

5. Eosinophilia results most commonly from parasitic invasion and ingestion or from inhalation of toxic foreign particles.

6. Basophilia is seen in hypersensitivity reactions because of the high content of histamine and subsequent release.

7. Monocytosis occurs during the late or recuperative phase of infection when macrophages (mature monocytes) phagocytose surviving microorganisms and debris. Monocytosis is often seen in chronic infections, usually with intracellular bacteria, such as tuberculosis (TB), brucellosis, listeriosis, and subacute bacterial endocarditis (SBE). Peripheral monocytosis has been found to correlate with the extent of myocardial damage following myocardial infarction. Increased numbers of monocytes also may indicate marrow recovery from agranulocytosis.

8. Granulocytopenia, a significant decrease in the number of neutrophils, can be a life-threatening condition if sepsis occurs; it is often caused by chemotherapeutic agents, severe infection, and radiation.

9. The number of lymphocytes is decreased (lymphocytopenia) in most acute infections and in some immunodeficiency syndromes.

10. Lymphocytosis occurs in viral infections (IM and infectious hepatitis, in particular), leukemia, lymphomas, and some chronic infections.

11. Infectious mononucleosis is an acute infection of B lymphocytes most commonly associated with EBV, a type of herpesvirus. Transmission of EBV is by personal contact, commonly through saliva (e.g., kissing, hence its nickname "kissing disease").

12. Two of the earliest manifestations of mononucleosis are sore throat and fever caused by inflammation at the primary site of viral entry. It is self-limiting and treatment consists of rest and relief of symptoms.

13. EBV is associated with several tumors including lymphomas and nasopharyngeal carcinoma.

14. Leukemia is a clonal disorder of leukocytes in the bone marrow, and usually of the blood. The common pathologic feature of all forms of leukemia is an uncontrolled proliferation of leukocytes and overcrowding of the bone marrow, causing a decreased production and function of the other blood cell lines.

15. All leukemias are classified by the cell type involved: B cells, T cells, and NK cells. They are differentiated by onset: acute or chronic. Overall, there are four major types of leukemia: ALL, CLL, AML, and CML. With increased understanding, the distinct divisions between leukemia and lymphoma have become indistinct and blurred. Conditions known as "lymphoma" that arise as a discrete tissue mass sometimes have "leukemic" presentations and progression to leukemia is not unusual during the progression of incurable lymphomas.

16. Although the exact cause of leukemia is unknown, it is considered a clonal disorder. A higher incidence of acute leukemias and CLL is reported in certain families, suggesting a possible genetic predisposition. Risk factors have been linked to exposure to cigarette smoke, benzene, and ionizing radiation.

17. The most common genetic abnormality in adult ALL is the Philadelphia chromosome.

18. Genetic aberrations in AML alter genes encoding transcription factors needed for normal myeloid differentiation and arrest differentiation. These mutations affect the epigenome, suggesting that epigenetic alterations are key in AML.

19. The major clinical manifestations of leukemia include fatigue caused by anemia, bleeding caused by thrombocytopenia, fever secondary to infection, anorexia, and weight loss. Chronic leukemias

■ SUMMARY REVIEW—cont'd

progress differently than acute leukemias, advancing slowly and without warning. The presence of the Philadelphia chromosome is a diagnostic marker for CML.

20. Chemotherapy is the treatment of choice for leukemia. New targets or drugs have been reported to inhibit leukemia stem cells both in vitro and in vivo.

Alterations of Lymphoid Function

1. The number of lymphocytes is decreased (lymphocytopenia) in most acute infections and in some immunodeficiency syndromes.

2. Lymphocytosis occurs in viral infections (IM and infectious hepatitis, in particular), leukemia, lymphomas, and some chronic infections.

3. Lymphomas are tumors of primary lymphoid tissue (thymus, bone marrow) or secondary lymphoid tissue (lymph nodes, spleen, tonsils, intestinal lymphoid tissue). The two major types of malignant lymphomas are Hodgkin lymphoma (HL) and non-Hodgkin lymphoma (NHL).

4. Reed-Sternberg (RS) cells in lymph nodes are classically associated with HL. The RS cell is derived from a malignant B cell that usually becomes binucleate.

5. A virus might be involved in the pathogenesis of HL. Some familial clustering suggests an unknown genetic mechanism.

6. An enlarged painless mass or swelling, most commonly in the neck, is an initial sign of HL. Local symptoms are produced by lymphadenopathy, usually caused by pressure or obstruction.

7. Treatment of HL includes radiation therapy and chemotherapy.

8. The cause of lymph node enlargement and cancerous transformation in NHL is unknown. Factors associated with industrialization and economic improvement may be linked to the incidence of lymphoma, geographically. In general, lymphomas are the result of genetic mutations or viral infection. Immunosuppressed persons have a higher incidence of NHL, suggesting an immune mechanism.

9. Generally, with NHL the swelling of lymph nodes is painless, and the nodes enlarge and transform over months or years.

10. Individuals with NHL can survive for long periods. Treatment is chemotherapy.

11. Burkitt lymphoma involves the jaw and facial bones and occurs in children from east-central Africa and New Guinea. In the United States, Burkitt lymphoma is rare, usually involves the abdomen, and is characterized by extensive bone marrow invasion and replacement.

12. Multiple myeloma (MM) is a neoplasm of B cells (immature plasma cells) and mature plasma cells. It is characterized by multiple malignant tumors of plasma cells scattered throughout the skeletal system and occasionally in soft tissue.

13. Myeloma cells usually secrete monoclonal protein (M protein) that is an abnormal antibody molecule. The myeloma cell may also secrete free antibody light chain that is excreted in the urine (Bence Jones protein).

14. The exact cause of MM is unknown. Risk factors include exposure to radiation or certain chemicals and a history of monoclonal gammopathy of undetermined significance (MGUS).

15. The major clinical manifestations for MM include recurrent infections caused by suppression of the humoral immune response and renal disease as a result of Bence Jones proteinuria.

16. Chemotherapy is the treatment of choice for MM. Other therapies include stem cell transplantation, biologic therapy, radiation therapy, and sometimes surgery.

17. Waldenström macroglobulinemia is a rare type of slow-growing plasma cell tumor that secretes a monoclonal IgM molecule.

Alterations of Splenic Function

1. Splenomegaly (enlargement of the spleen) may be considered normal in certain individuals, but its presence should not be ignored.

2. Splenomegaly results from (1) acute inflammatory or infectious processes, (2) congestive disorders, (3) infiltrative processes, and (4) tumors or cysts.

3. Splenomegaly causes hypersplenism (overactivity of the spleen). Hypersplenism results in blood cell sequestration, causing destruction of red blood cells and development of anemia.

■ KEY TERMS

Acute leukemia, 968
Acute lymphocytic leukemia (ALL), 970
Acute myelogenous leukemia (AML), 970
Agranulocytosis, 964
Basopenia, 964
Basophilia, 964
B-cell neoplasm, 979
Bence Jones protein, 984
β_2-Microglobulin, 987
Burkitt lymphoma, 981
Chronic leukemia, 968
Chronic lymphocytic leukemia (CLL), 973
Chronic myelogenous leukemia (CML), 973
Congestive splenomegaly, 988
Eosinopenia, 964
Eosinophilia, 964
Granulocytopenia, 964
Granulocytosis, 964
Heterophile antibody, 967

Hodgkin lymphoma (HL), 976
Hypersplenism, 988
Infectious mononucleosis (IM), 966
Infiltrative splenomegaly, 988
Leukemia, 968
Leukemic blast, 970
Leukemoid reaction, 964
Leukocytosis, 963
Leukopenia, 963
Lymphadenopathy, 976
Lymphoblastic lymphoma (LL), 982
Lymphocytopenia, 966
Lymphocytosis (absolute lymphocytosis), 966
Lymphoplasmacytic lymphoma, 987
Monoclonal gammopathy of undetermined significance (MGUS), 986
Monocytopenia, 966
Monocytosis, 966
M protein, 983

Multiple myeloma (MM), 983
Neutropenia, 964
Neutrophilia, 964
NK-cell neoplasm, 979
Non-Hodgkin lymphoma (NHL), 979
Pancytopenia, 970
Philadelphia chromosome, 970
Qualitative leukocyte disorder, 963
Quantitative leukocyte disorder, 963
Reed-Sternberg (RS) cell, 976
Shift-to-the-left, 964
Small lymphocyte lymphoma (SLL; CLL/SLL), 973
Smoldering myeloma, 986
Solitary plasmacytoma, 986
Splenomegaly, 988
T-cell neoplasm, 979
Waldenström macroglobulinemia (WM), 987

REFERENCES

1. Dubos F, Delebarre M, Martinot A: Predicting the risk of severe infection in children with chemotherapy-induced febrile neutropenia. *Curr Opin Hematol* 19(1):39–43, 2012.

2. Schwartz MJ, et al: Evidence for an altered tryptophan metabolism in fibromyalgia. *Neurobiol Dis* 11(3):434–442, 2002.

3. Kumar V, Abbas A, Aster JC: *Robbins & Cotran pathologic basis of disease*, ed 9, Philadelphia, 2015, Saunders.

4. Hanna B: Re: the diagnosis of infectious mononucleosis. *Clin Otolaryngol* 37(1):80–81, 2012.

5. Gunz FW: The dreaded leukemias and the lymphomas: their nature and their prospects. In Wintrobe MM, editor: *Blood, pure and eloquent: a story of discovery, of people, and of ideas*, New York, 1980, McGraw-Hill.

6. Ferlay J, et al: *GLOBOCAN 2012 v1.0: Cancer incidence and mortality worldwide: IARC CancerBase No. 11 [Internet]*, Lyon, France, 2013, International Agency for Research on Cancer. Available at: http://globocan.iarc.fr.

7. American Cancer Society (ACS): *Cancer facts & figures 2017*, Atlanta, 2017, Author.

8. Radivoyevitch T, Li H, Sachs RK: Etiology and treatment of hematological neoplasms: stochastic mathematical models. *Adv Exp Med Biol* 844:317–346, 2014.

9. Druker BJ: Translation of the Philadelphia chromosome into therapy for CML. *Blood* 112(13):4808–4817, 2008.

10. Talpaz M, et al: Dasatinib in imatinib-resistant Philadelphia chromosome-positive leukemias. *N Engl J Med* 354(24):2531–2541, 2006.

11. Dick JE: Stem cell concepts renew cancer research. *Blood* 112(13):4793–4807, 2008.

12. Khwaja A, et al: Acute myeloid leukaemia. *Nat Rev Dis Primers* 2:16010, 2016.

13. Wakeford R, Little MP, Kendall GM: Risk of childhood leukemia after low-level exposure to ionizing radiation. *Expert Rev Hematol* 3(3):251–254, 2010.

14. PDQ® Adult Treatment Editorial Board: *PDQ adult acute lymphoblastic leukemia treatment*, Bethesda, MD, National Cancer Institute. Updated 03/16/2017. Available at: https://www.cancer.gov/types/leukemia/hp/adult-all-treatment-pdq.

15. *Childhood acute lymphoblastic leukemia treatment: health professional version*, Bethesda, MD, 2008, National Institutes of Health, U.S. Department of Health and Human Services. Available at: www.cancer.gov/cancertopics/pdq/treatment/childALL/healthprofessional.

16. *Adult acute lymphoblastic leukemia treatment: health professional version*, Bethesda, MD, 2008, National Institutes of Health, U.S. Department of Health and Human Services. Available at: www.cancer.gov/cancertopics/pdq/treatment/adultALL/healthprofessional.

17. PDQ® Adult Treatment Editorial Board: *PDQ adult acute myeloid leukemia treatment*, Bethesda, MD, National Cancer Institute. Updated 01/20/2017. Available at: https://www.cancer.gov/types/leukemia/hp/adult-aml-treatment-pdq. (Accessed 08 March 2017). [PMID: 26389432].

18. Hu J, et al: Long-term efficacy and safety of all-trans retinoic acid/arsenic trioxide-based therapy in newly diagnosed acute promyelocytic leukemia. *Proc Natl Acad Sci USA* 106(9):3342–3347, 2009.

19. Liang B, et al: Maintenance therapy with all-trans retinoic acid and arsenic trioxide improves relapse-free survival in adults with low-to intermediate-risk acute promyelocytic leukemia who have achieved complete remission after consolidation therapy. *Onco Targets Ther* 10:2305–2313, 2017.

20. Su M, et al: All-trans retinoic acid activity in acute myeloid leukemia: role of cytochrome P450 enzyme expression by the microenvironment. *PLoS ONE* 10(6):e0127790, 2015.

21. Ivancevic TD, et al: The role of immunophenotyping in differential diagnosis of chronic lymphocytic leukemia. *Srp Arh Celok Lek* 142(3-4):197–203, 2014.

22. Ouillette P, et al: Acquired genomic copy number aberrations and survival in chronic lymphocytic leukemia. *Blood* 118(1):3051–3061, 2011.

23. National Cancer Institute: *PDQ® chronic lymphocytic leukemia treatment*, Bethesda, MD, Author. Date last modified 01/20/2017. Available at: http://www.cancer.gov/cancertopics/pdq/treatment/CLL/HealthProfessional.

24. Friese CR, et al: Timeliness and quality of diagnostic care for Medicare recipients with chronic lymphocytic leukemia. *Cancer* 117(7):1470–1477, 2011.

25. Orchard JA, et al: ZAP-70 expression and prognosis in chronic lymphocytic leukaemia. *Lancet* 363(9403):105–111, 2004.

26. Helgason GV, Young GAR, Holyoake TL: Targeting chronic myeloid leukemic stem cells. *Curr Hematol Malig Rep* 5(2):81–87, 2010.

27. Arock M, Mahon F, Valent P: Characterization and targeting of neoplastic stem cells in Ph+ chronic myeloid leukemia. *Int J Hematol Oncol* 4(4):151–165, 2015, doi:10.2217/ijh.15.16.

28. Chen Y, et al: Novel therapeutic agents against cancer stem cells of chronic myeloid leukemia. *Anticancer Agents Med Chem* 10(2):111–115, 2010.

29. Kinstrie R, Copland M: Targeting chronic myeloid leukemia stem cells. *Curr Hematol Malig Rep* 8(1):14–21, 2013.

30. Ma W, et al: Modulating the growth and imatinib sensitivity of chronic myeloid leukemia stem/progenitor cells with pullulan/microRNA nanoparticles in vitro. *J Biomed Nanotechnol* 11(11):1961–1974, 2015.

31. Huh J: Epidemiologic overview of malignant lymphoma. *Korean J Hematol* 47(2):92–104, 2012.

32. Nogová L, et al: Lymphocyte-predominant and classic Hodgkin's lymphoma: a comprehensive analysis from the German Hodgkin Study Group. *J Clin Oncol* 26(3):434–439, 2008.

33. Al-Mansour M, et al: Transformation to aggressive lymphoma in nodular lymphocyte-predominant Hodgkin's lymphoma. *J Clin Oncol* 28(5):793–799, 2010.

34. Bakshi N, Maghfoor I: The current lymphoma classification: new concepts and practical applications triumphs and woes. *Ann Saudi Med* 32(3):296–305, 2012.

35. *What you need to know about Hodgkin lymphoma*, Bethesda, MD, 2008, National Institutes of Health, U.S. Department of Health and Human Services. Available at: http://cancer.gov/cancertopics/wyntk/hodgkin.

36. Kleinstern G: Ethnic variation in medical and lifestyle risk factors for B cell non-Hodgkin lymphoma: a case-control study among Israelis and Palestinians. *PLoS ONE* 12(2):e0171709, 2017.

37. *SEER Cancer Stat Facts: Hodgkin lymphoma and non-Hodgkin lymphoma*, Bethesda, MD, 2017, National Cancer Institute Surveillance, Epidemiology, and End Results Program, National Institutes of Health, US Department of Health and Human Services. Available at: https://seer.cancer.gov/statfacts/.

38. Howlader N, et al: *SEER cancer statistics review, 1975-2011*, Bethesda, MD, 2013, National Cancer Institute Surveillance, Epidemiology, and End Results Program, National Institutes of Health, U.S. Department of Health and Human Services. Available at: https://seer.cancer.gov/statfacts/. Based on November 2013 SEER data submission.

39. Boffetta P: Epidemiology of adult non-Hodgkin lymphoma. *Ann Oncol* 22(4):1v27–1v31, 2011.

40. National Cancer Institute: *A snapshot of lymphoma*, Bethesda, MD, 2014, National Cancer Institute, U.S. Department of Health and Human Services.

41. PDQ® Adult Treatment Editorial Board: *PDQ adult non-Hodgkin lymphoma treatment*, Bethesda, MD, 2017, National Cancer Institute. Updated 05/12/2017. Available at: https://www.cancer.gov/types/lymphoma/hp/adult-nhl-treatment-pdq. [PMID: 26389492].

42. Hoelzer D, et al: Improved outcome of adult Burkitt lymphoma/leukemia with rituximab and chemotherapy: report of a large prospective multicenter trial. *Blood* 124(26):3870–3879, 2014.

43. PDQ® Adult Treatment Editorial Board: *PDQ plasma cell neoplasms (including multiple myeloma) treatment*, Bethesda, MD, National Cancer Institute. Updated 03/23/2017. Available at: https://www.cancer.gov/types/myeloma/patient/myeloma-treatment-pdq. [PMID: 26389437].

44. Presutti R, et al: Pesticide exposures and the risk of multiple myeloma in men: an analysis of the North American Pooled Project. *Int J Cancer* 139(7):1703–1714, 2016.

45. Dimopoulos K, Gimsing P, Grønbaek K: The role of epigenetics in the biology of multiple myeloma. *Blood Cancer J* 4:e207, 2014.

46. Morgan GJ, et al: The genetic architecture of multiple myeloma. *Nat Rev Cancer* 12:335–348, 2012.

47. Min DJ, et al: MMSET stimulates myeloma cell growth through micro-RNA mediated modulation of c-MYC. *Leukemia* 27(3):686–694, 2013.

48. Rajkumar SV, Melini G, San Miguel JF: Haematological cancer: redefining myeloma. *Nat Rev Clin Oncol* 9(9):494–496, 2012.

49. Landgren O, et al: Agent Orange exposure and monoclonal gammopathy of undetermined significance: an Operation Ranch Hand veteran cohort study. *JAMA Oncol* 1(8):1061–1068, 2015.

50. *Multiple myeloma and other plasma cell neoplasms treatment: health professional version*, Bethesda, MD, 2008, National Institutes of Health, U.S. Department of Health and Human Services. Available at: www.cancer.gov/cancertopics/pdq/treatment/adult-non-hodgkins/healthprofessional.

51. Rajkumar SV, et al: International Myeloma Working Group updated criteria for the diagnosis of multiple myeloma. *Lancet Oncol* 15(12):e538–e548, 2014.

52. Eshaghian S, Berenson JR: Multiple myeloma: improved outcomes with new therapeutic approaches. *Curr Opin Support Palliat Care* 6(3):330–336, 2012.

53. *Waldenström macroglobulinemia: questions and answers: fact sheet*, Bethesda, MD, 2008, National Institutes of Health, U.S. Department of Health and Human Services. Available at: http://cancer.gov/cancertopics/factsheet/Sites-Types/WM.

Alterations of Hematologic Function in Children

Lauri A. Linder, Kathryn L. McCance

evolve WEBSITE

http://evolve.elsevier.com/McCance/
- Content Updates
- Chapter Summary Review
- Review Questions
- Case Studies
- Animations

CHAPTER OUTLINE

This chapter briefly explains fetal and neonatal hematopoiesis and postnatal changes in blood as a foundation for understanding the pathophysiology of specific blood disorders in childhood. Among the diseases that affect erythrocytes are acquired disorders, such as iron deficiency anemia, hemolytic disease of the newborn, and anemia of infectious disease; and inherited disorders, such as glucose-6-phosphate dehydrogenase (G6PD) deficiency, hereditary spherocytosis, sickle cell disease, and the thalassemias. Disorders of coagulation and platelets include inherited hemorrhagic diseases, such as the hemophilias, and antibody-mediated hemorrhagic diseases, which include immune thrombocytopenia, autoimmune neonatal thrombocytopenias, and autoimmune vascular purpuras. Finally, leukocyte disorders, such as leukemia and the lymphomas (non-Hodgkin lymphoma as well as Hodgkin lymphoma), are discussed.

FETAL AND NEONATAL HEMATOPOIESIS

As the developing embryo becomes too large for oxygenation of tissues by simple diffusion, the production of erythrocytes begins within the vessels of the yolk sac. Shortly after 2 weeks of gestation, circulating erythrocytes play a major role in delivering oxygen to the tissues. At approximately the eighth week of gestation, the site of erythrocyte production shifts from the vessels to the liver sinusoids, and the production of leukocytes and platelets begins in the liver and spleen. Erythropoiesis in the liver and, to a lesser extent, in the spleen and lymph nodes, reaches a peak at approximately 4 months. Hepatic blood formation declines steadily thereafter but does not disappear entirely during the remainder of gestation. By the fifth month of gestation, hematopoiesis begins to occur in the bone marrow and increases rapidly until hematopoietic (red) marrow fills the entire bone marrow space. By the time of delivery, the marrow is the only significant site of hematopoiesis.

In neonates and young infants, hematopoietic marrow progressively fills the bony cavities of the entire axial skeleton (skull, vertebrae, ribs, sternum), the long bones of the limbs, and many intramembranous bones. (These structures are described in Chapter 46.) Fatty (yellow) marrow gradually replaces hematopoietic marrow in some bones. During childhood, hematopoietic tissue retreats centrally to the vertebrae, ribs, sternum, pelvis, scapulae, skull, and proximal ends of the femur and humerus.

In diseases characterized by hemolysis, erythrocyte production can increase as much as eight times the normal level because erythropoietin causes hematopoietic marrow to increase in volume. Initially, hematopoietic marrow expands from the ends of the long bones toward the middle of the shafts, replacing fatty marrow. Next, blood cell production begins

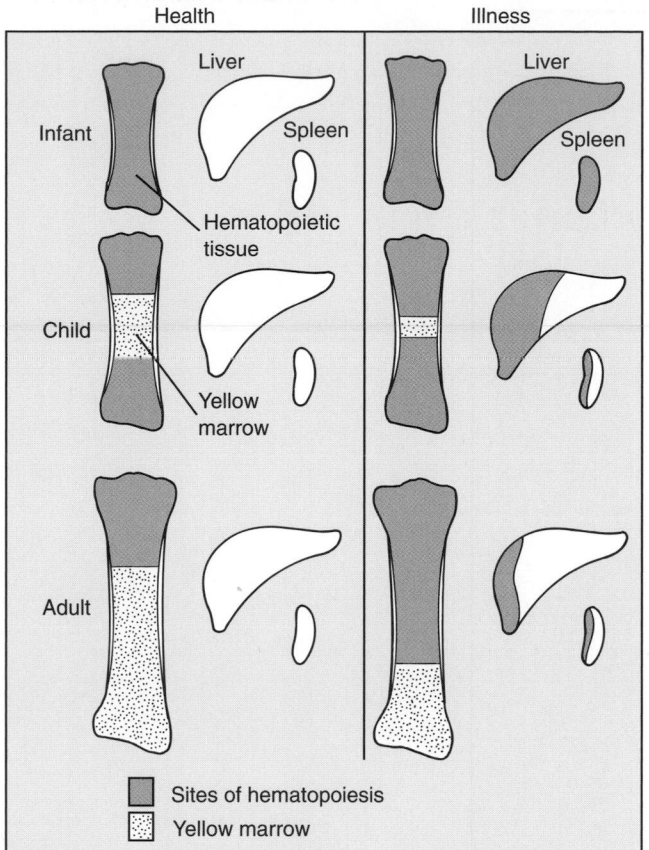

FIGURE 31.1 Sites of Hematopoiesis in Health and Illness. With normal maturation, red marrow is partly replaced by yellow marrow in the shafts of the long bones. In adults, red marrow is largely restricted to the proximal ends of the femur and humerus. In response to hemolysis, red marrow replaces yellow marrow in the long bones. In infants, whose long bones already are filled with red marrow, additional hematopoiesis takes place in the liver and spleen. In children and adults, red marrow can replace yellow marrow in response to hemolysis, necessitating less hematopoiesis in the liver and spleen.

to occur outside the marrow cavities, especially in the liver and spleen. Extramedullary hematopoiesis is more likely to occur in children than in adults because the bony cavities of children already are filled with red marrow (Fig. 31.1). This is why hemolytic disease causes especially pronounced enlargement of the spleen and liver in children.

The erythrocytes undergo striking changes during gestation, particularly during the first two trimesters, at which time they nearly double in numbers and in hemoglobin content. A proportionate increase in hematocrit level also occurs. By the end of gestation the erythrocyte count has more than tripled but the size of each erythrocyte has decreased.

A biochemically distinct type of hemoglobin is synthesized during fetal life. The three **embryonic hemoglobins (Gower 1, Gower 2, and Portland)** and the **fetal hemoglobin (HbF)** are composed of two α and two γ chains of polypeptides, whereas the adult hemoglobins (HbA and HbA$_2$) are composed of two α chains and two β chains. (The structure of an adult hemoglobin molecule is illustrated in Fig. 28.16, and types of hemoglobin are defined in Table 28.5.) Some unknown regulatory mechanism promotes γ-chain synthesis and inhibits β- and δ-chain synthesis in utero. This results in production of embryonic or fetal hemoglobin. After birth, γ-chain synthesis is inhibited, whereas β- and δ-chain synthesis is facilitated, resulting in production of adult hemoglobins.

Fetal hemoglobin has greater affinity for oxygen than does adult hemoglobin because it interacts less readily with an enzyme (2,3-diphosphoglycerate [2,3-DPG]) that inhibits hemoglobin-oxygen binding. The decreased inhibitory effects of 2,3-DPG enable fetal blood to transport oxygen despite the relative lack of oxygen in the uterine environment. The increased affinity for oxygen enables HbF to bind with maternal oxygen in the placental circulation.

During the first trimester nearly all of the hemoglobin in the fetus is embryonic, but some HbA can be detected. Therefore it is possible to identify as early as 16 to 20 weeks of gestation some disorders of adult hemoglobin, such as sickle cell anemia and thalassemia major. In the 6-month fetus, HbF constitutes 90% of the total. This percentage then begins to decline. At birth, neonatal hemoglobin consists of 70% HbF, 29% HbA, and 1% HbA$_2$. Between 6 and 12 months of age, normal adult hemoglobin percentages are established (see Chapter 28).

POSTNATAL CHANGES IN THE BLOOD

Blood cell counts tend to rise higher than adult levels at birth and then decline gradually throughout childhood. Table 31.1 lists normal ranges during infancy and childhood. The immediate rise in values is the result of the accelerated hematopoiesis during fetal life, the increased numbers of cells that result from the trauma of birth, and the cutting of the umbilical cord. These events surrounding the birth also are accompanied by the presence of large numbers of immature erythrocytes and leukocytes (particularly granulocytes) in peripheral blood (see Chapter 28). As the infant develops over the first 2 to 3 months of life, the numbers of these immature blood cells decrease.

Average blood volume in the full-term neonate is 85 mL/kg of body weight. The premature infant has a proportionately larger blood volume of 90 to 100 mL/kg of body weight. In both full-term and premature infants, blood volume relative to body weight decreases during the first few months. By 3 years of age, a child's average blood volume is 75 to 77 mL/kg, which is similar to that of older children and adults.

Erythrocytes

The hypoxic intrauterine environment stimulates erythropoietin production in the fetus. This accelerates fetal erythropoiesis, producing polycythemia (excessive proliferation of erythrocyte precursors) of the newborn. After birth the oxygen from the lungs saturates arterial blood, and the amount of oxygen delivered to the tissues increases. In response to the change from a placental to a pulmonary oxygen supply during the first few days of life, levels of erythropoietin and the rate of blood cell formation decrease. The very active rate of fetal erythropoiesis is reflected by the large numbers of immature erythrocytes (reticulocytes) in the peripheral blood of full-term neonates. The number of reticulocytes decreases abruptly during the first few days after birth, which is associated with decreased erythropoietin production.[1] Finding an elevated reticulocyte count after the first week of life is rare. A decrease in extramedullary hematopoiesis also occurs at this time. In the peripheral blood the erythrocyte count drops for 6 to 8 weeks after birth. During this period of rapid growth the rate of erythrocyte destruction is greater than that in later childhood and adulthood. In full-term infants, the normal erythrocyte life span is 60 to 80 days; in premature infants it may be as short as 20 to 30 days; and in children and adolescents, it is the same as that in adults—120 days. (Mechanisms of hemolysis are described in Chapter 28.)

In the premature infant, the postnatal decrease in hemoglobin and hematocrit values is more marked than in the full-term infant. In the preschool and school-age child, hemoglobin, hematocrit, and red blood cell (RBC) count values rise gradually. In males and females, these values first begin to diverge in adolescence. In the female, the gradual

TABLE 31.1 HEMATOLOGIC VALUES DURING INFANCY AND CHILDHOOD

AGE	HEMOGLOBIN (g/dL)		HEMATOCRIT (%)		RETICULOCYTES (%) MEAN	MCV (fl) LOWEST	LEUKOCYTES (WBC/mm³)		NEUTROPHILS (%)		LYMPHOCYTES (%) MEAN*	EOSINOPHILS (%) MEAN	MONOCYTES (%) MEAN
	MEAN	RANGE	MEAN	RANGE			MEAN	RANGE	MEAN	RANGE			
Cord blood	16.8	13.7–20.1	55	45–65	5	110	18,000	(9000–30,000)	61	(40–80)	31	2	6
2 wk	16.5	13–20	50	42–66	1		12,000	(5000–21,000)	40		63	3	9
3 months	12	9.5–14.5	36	31–41	1		12,000	(6000–18,000)	30		48	2	5
6 months to 6 yr	12	10.5–14	37	33–42	1	70–74	10,000	(6000–15,000)	45		48	2	5
7–12 yr	13	11–16	38	34–40	1	76–80	8,000	(4500–13,500)	55		38	2	5
Adult													
Female	14	12–16	42	37–47	1.6	80	7,500	(5000–10,000)	55	(35–70)	35	3	7
Male	16	14–18	47	42–52		80							

*Relatively wide range.

fl, Femtoliters; MCV, mean corpuscular volume; WBC, white blood cells.

From Behrman R et al, editors: Nelson textbook of pediatrics, ed 17, Philadelphia, 2004, Saunders.

hemoglobin level increase continues into early puberty, at which time it stabilizes. In the male, the hemoglobin level increase keeps pace with growth and maturation and eventually surpasses that of the female. This higher value of hemoglobin level in the mature male is related to androgen secretion.

Metabolic processes within the erythrocytes of neonates differ significantly from those of erythrocytes in the normal adult. The relatively young population of erythrocytes in the newborn consumes greater quantities of glucose than do erythrocytes in adults. Several enzymes that regulate glucose consumption are increased in the erythrocytes of neonates, with a subsequent increase in the rate of glycolysis.

Leukocytes and Platelets

The lymphocytes of children tend to have more cytoplasm and less compact nuclear chromatin than do the lymphocytes of adults. The significance of these differences is unknown. One possible explanation is that children tend to have more frequent viral infections, which are associated with atypical lymphocytes. Even minor infections, in which the child fails to exhibit clinical manifestations of illness, or administration of immunizations may result in lymphocyte changes.[2]

The lymphocyte count is high at birth and continues to rise in some healthy infants during the first year of life. A steady decline occurs throughout childhood and adolescence until lower adult values are reached. Whether these developmental variations are physiologic or are a pathologic response to frequent viral infections and immunizations in children is not known.

In healthy neonates, the neutrophil count peaks at 6 to 12 hours after birth and then declines over the next few days of life.[3] Neutrophil counts also are slightly higher in female neonates compared with males. After 2 weeks of life, neutrophil counts fall to within or below normal adult ranges. By approximately 4 years of age, the neutrophil count is similar to that of an adult. White children have slightly higher counts than black children.[4]

The eosinophil count is elevated in the first year of life relative to children, teenagers, or adults.[5,6] Monocyte counts are elevated through the preschool years and then decrease to adult levels. No relationship between age and basophil count has been found. Platelet counts in full-term neonates are comparable to platelet counts in adults and remain so throughout infancy and childhood.[5]

DISORDERS OF ERYTHROCYTES

Anemia is the most common blood disorder in children. Although not a disease state in and of itself, the presence of anemia may be associated with an underlying pathophysiologic process. Like anemia in adults, the anemias of childhood are caused by ineffective erythropoiesis or premature destruction of erythrocytes. The most common cause of insufficient erythropoiesis is iron deficiency, which may result from insufficient dietary intake or chronic loss of iron caused by bleeding. The hemolytic anemias of childhood may be divided into two large categories. The first category consists of disorders that result from premature destruction caused by intrinsic abnormalities of the erythrocytes, and the second category consists of disorders that result from damaging extra-erythrocytic factors. The hemolytic anemias can be inherited, congenital, or both.

The most dramatic form of acquired congenital hemolytic anemia is *hemolytic disease of the fetus and newborn (HDFN)* an alloimmune disorder in which maternal blood and fetal blood are antigenically incompatible, causing the mother's immune system to produce antibodies against fetal erythrocytes. Fetal erythrocytes that have been bound to maternal antibodies are recognized as foreign or defective by the fetal mononuclear phagocyte system and are removed from the circulation

by phagocytosis, usually in the fetal spleen. (For a complete discussion of HDFN, see Hemolytic Disease of the Fetus and Newborn.) Other acquired hemolytic anemias—some of which begin in utero—include those caused by infections or the presence of toxins.

The inherited forms of hemolytic anemia result from intrinsic defects of the child's erythrocytes, any of which can lead to erythrocyte destruction by the mononuclear phagocyte system. Structural defects include abnormal red blood cell size and abnormalities of plasma membrane structure (spherocytosis). Intracellular defects include enzyme deficiencies, the most common of which is G6PD deficiency; and defects of hemoglobin synthesis, which manifest as sickle cell disease or thalassemia, depending on which component of hemoglobin is defective. These and other causes of childhood anemia, some more common than others, are listed in Table 31.2.

Acquired Disorders
Iron Deficiency Anemia

Iron is *critical* to the developing child, especially for normal brain development, and without it the damage from the periods of iron deficiency anemia (IDA) in children is irreversible. IDA is the most common nutritional disorder worldwide with the highest incidence occurring between 6 months and 2 years of age. IDA is common in the United States where prevalence is higher in toddlers, adolescent girls, and women of childbearing age, and causes clinical manifestations mostly related to inadequate hemoglobin synthesis.[7] Its incidence is not related to gender or race; however, socioeconomic factors are important because they affect nutrition.

IDA can result from (1) dietary insufficiencies, (2) absorption problems, (3) blood loss, and (4) increased requirement of iron. Inadequate intake is the most common cause of IDA during the first few years of life and blood loss is the most common cause during childhood and adolescence, and for adults in the Western world. Chronic IDA from occult (hidden) blood loss may be caused by a gastrointestinal lesion, parasitic infestation, or hemorrhagic disease. A reasonable hypothesis for infants and young children who develop IDA is they have chronic intestinal blood loss induced by exposure to a heat-labile protein in cow's milk. Such exposure causes an inflammatory gastrointestinal reaction that damages the mucosa and results in diffuse microhemorrhage. Growing evidence indicates that cellular components of both innate and adaptive immunity play significant roles during the pathogenesis of cow's milk allergy.[8] Dietary lack is not common in developed countries where iron is in the readily absorbed form from heme that comes from meat. IDA has declined in the United States; however, a recent study in the United States found toddlers are vulnerable to IDA, especially those consuming excessive quantities of whole cow's milk.[9] Increased consumption of iron-fortified infant foods, including formula, is hypothesized to have contributed to the overall decline in IDA.[10] However, bioavailability of iron from breast milk is higher than that from cow's milk. At this point, only low-quality evidence for use of micronutrient powders in pregnant women is available.[11] Impaired absorption is found in chronic diarrhea, fat malabsorption, and celiac disease. Evidence also is emerging regarding genetic polymorphisms that may contribute to altered iron absorption in cases of refractory IDA with a familial component.[12]

Children in developing countries are often affected by chronic parasite infestations that result in blood and iron loss greater than dietary intake.[13] Treatment of helminth infections results in improvement in appetite, growth, and in the anemia. Controversial is the association of IDA with lead (Pb) poisoning. Newer areas of investigation include iron deficiency in overweight children and the association of *H. pylori* infection with IDA.[14]

TABLE 31.2 ANEMIAS OF CHILDHOOD

CAUSE	ANEMIC CONDITION
Deficient Erythropoiesis or Hemoglobin Synthesis	
Decreased stem cell population in marrow (congenital or acquired pure red cell aplasia)	Normocytic-normochromic anemia
Decreased erythropoiesis despite normal stem cell population in marrow (infection, inflammation, cancer, chronic renal disease, congenital dyserythropoiesis)	Normocytic-normochromic anemia
Deficiency of a factor or nutrient needed for erythropoiesis	
Cobalamin (vitamin B$_{12}$), folate	Megaloblastic anemia
Iron	Microcytic-hypochromic anemia
Increased or Premature Hemolysis	
Alloimmune disease (maternal-fetal Rh, ABO, or minor blood group incompatibility)	Hemolytic disease of the newborn (HDN)
Autoimmune disease (idiopathic autoimmune hemolytic anemia, symptomatic systemic lupus erythematosus, lymphoma, drug-induced autoimmune processes)	Autoimmune hemolytic anemia
Inherited defects of plasma membrane structure (spherocytosis, elliptocytosis, stomatocytosis) or cellular size or both (pyknocytosis)	Hemolytic anemia
Infection (bacterial sepsis, congenital syphilis, malaria, cytomegalovirus infection, rubella, toxoplasmosis, disseminated herpes)	Hemolytic anemia
Intrinsic and inherited enzymatic defects (deficiencies of glucose-6-phosphate dehydrogenase [G6PD], pyruvate kinase, 5'-nucleotidase, glucose phosphate isomerase)	Hemolytic anemia
Inherited defects of hemoglobin synthesis	Sickle cell anemia Thalassemia
Disseminated intravascular coagulation (see Chapter 29)	Hemolytic anemia
Galactosemia	Hemolytic anemia
Prolonged or recurrent respiratory or metabolic acidosis	Hemolytic anemia
Blood vessel disorders (cavernous hemangioma, large vessel thrombus, renal artery stenosis, severe coarctation of the aorta) (see Chapter 33)	Hemolytic anemia

◆PATHOPHYSIOLOGY. Regardless of the cause, a deficiency of iron produces a hypochromic-microcytic anemia.[7] Progressive depletion of blood and low serum levels of ferritin and transferrin saturation eventually lead to a lowering of hemoglobin and hematocrit values. In early stages an adaptive increase in red blood cell activity in the bone marrow may prevent the development of anemia. Anemia develops when the iron stores are depleted with accompanying important laboratory indicators. (Mechanisms of iron depletion are described in Chapter 28.)

◆CLINICAL MANIFESTATIONS. The symptoms of mild anemia—lethargy and listlessness—usually are not clearly evident in infants and young children, who are unable to describe these symptoms. Therefore parents usually do not notice any change in the child's behavior or appearance until moderate anemia has developed. General irritability, decreased activity tolerance, weakness, and lack of interest in play are nonspecific indications of anemia. In mild to moderate IDA (hemoglobin level of 6 to 10 g/dL), compensatory mechanisms of tissue oxygenation, such as increased amounts of 2,3-DPG within erythrocytes and a shift of the oxyhemoglobin dissociation curve, may be so effective that few clinical manifestations are apparent. When the hemoglobin level falls below 5 g/dL, however, pallor, tachycardia, and systolic murmurs often occur.

Clinical manifestations of chronic IDA include splenomegaly; widened skull sutures; decreased physical growth and developmental delays; and *pica*, a behavior in which non–food substances such as clay, paper, or ice are eaten. Weight is not necessarily an indicator of IDA because children may be obese, underweight, or of normal weight.

Consequences of IDA are significant and may include altered neurologic and intellectual function, especially involving attention span, alertness, and learning ability.

◆EVALUATION AND TREATMENT. Laboratory tests confirm the diagnosis of IDA. Laboratory tests include measurements of hemoglobin, hematocrit, serum iron, ferritin, and the total iron-binding capacity. A thorough history of present illness, a dietary history, and a physical examination are essential. Evaluation and treatment of IDA in children are similar to evaluation and treatment in adults (see Chapter 29). Oral administration of simple ferrous salts usually is satisfactory, and additional vitamin C helps promote absorption.[15] Iron in a liquid form should be administered through a straw because it can stain teeth. Iron therapy is continued for at least 2 months after erythrocyte indexes have returned to normal in order to replenish iron stores.[16]

Dietary modification is required to prevent recurrences of IDA. Intake of iron-rich foods is increased and the intake of cow's milk may be restricted, with the exact amount restricted to 16 to 32 ounces per day depending on the child's age. Limiting milk intake makes the child hungrier for other iron-rich foods and prevents gastrointestinal blood loss in children whose anemia is aggravated or caused by inflammatory reactions to proteins in cow's milk.

Hemolytic Disease of the Fetus and Newborn

Hemolytic disease of the fetus and newborn (HDFN) can occur only if antigens on fetal erythrocytes differ from antigens on maternal erythrocytes. The antigenic properties of erythrocytes are determined genetically: they may be type A, B, or O and may or may not include Rh antigen D. Erythrocytes that express Rh antigen D are Rh-positive; those that do not are Rh-negative. The frequency of Rh negativity is higher in whites (15%) than in blacks (5%), and is rare in Asians. Maternal-fetal incompatibility exists if mother and fetus differ in ABO blood type or if the fetus is Rh-positive and the mother is Rh-negative. (The antigenic properties of erythrocytes are described in Chapter 9.)

ABO incompatibility occurs in about 20% to 25% of all pregnancies, but only 1 in 10 cases of ABO incompatibility results in HDFN. Rh incompatibility occurs in less than 10% of pregnancies and rarely causes HDFN in the first incompatible fetus. Even after five or more pregnancies, only 5% of women have babies with hemolytic disease. Typically, erythrocytes from the first incompatible fetus cause the mother's immune system to produce antibodies that affect the fetuses of subsequent incompatible pregnancies. Most cases of HDFN are caused by ABO incompatibility, and only one in three cases is caused by Rh incompatibility.

◆PATHOPHYSIOLOGY. HDFN will result from the following: (1) if the mother's blood contains preformed antibodies against erythrocytes or produces antibodies on exposure to fetal erythrocytes, (2) if sufficient amounts of antibody (usually immunoglobulin G [IgG]) cross the placenta and enter fetal blood, and (3) if IgG binds with sufficient numbers of fetal erythrocytes to cause widespread antibody-mediated hemolysis or splenic removal. (Antibody-mediated red blood cell destruction is discussed in Chapter 9.)

Maternal antibodies may be formed against type B fetal erythrocytes if the mother is type A or against type A fetal erythrocytes if the mother is type B. Usually, however, the mother is type O and the fetus is A or B. ABO incompatibility can cause HDFN even if fetal erythrocytes do not escape into the maternal circulation during pregnancy. This occurs because the blood of most adults already contains anti-A or anti-B antibodies, which are produced on exposure to certain foods or infection by gram-negative bacteria. (Anti-O antibodies do not exist because type O erythrocytes are not antigenic.) Therefore IgG against type A or B erythrocytes is usually preformed in maternal blood and can enter the fetal circulation throughout the first incompatible pregnancy.

Anti-Rh antibodies, on the other hand, are formed *only* in response to the presence of incompatible (Rh-positive) erythrocytes in the blood of an Rh-negative mother. Sources of exposure include fetal blood that is mixed with the mother's blood at the time of delivery, transfused blood, and, rarely, previous sensitization of the mother by her own mother's incompatible blood (Fig. 31.2).

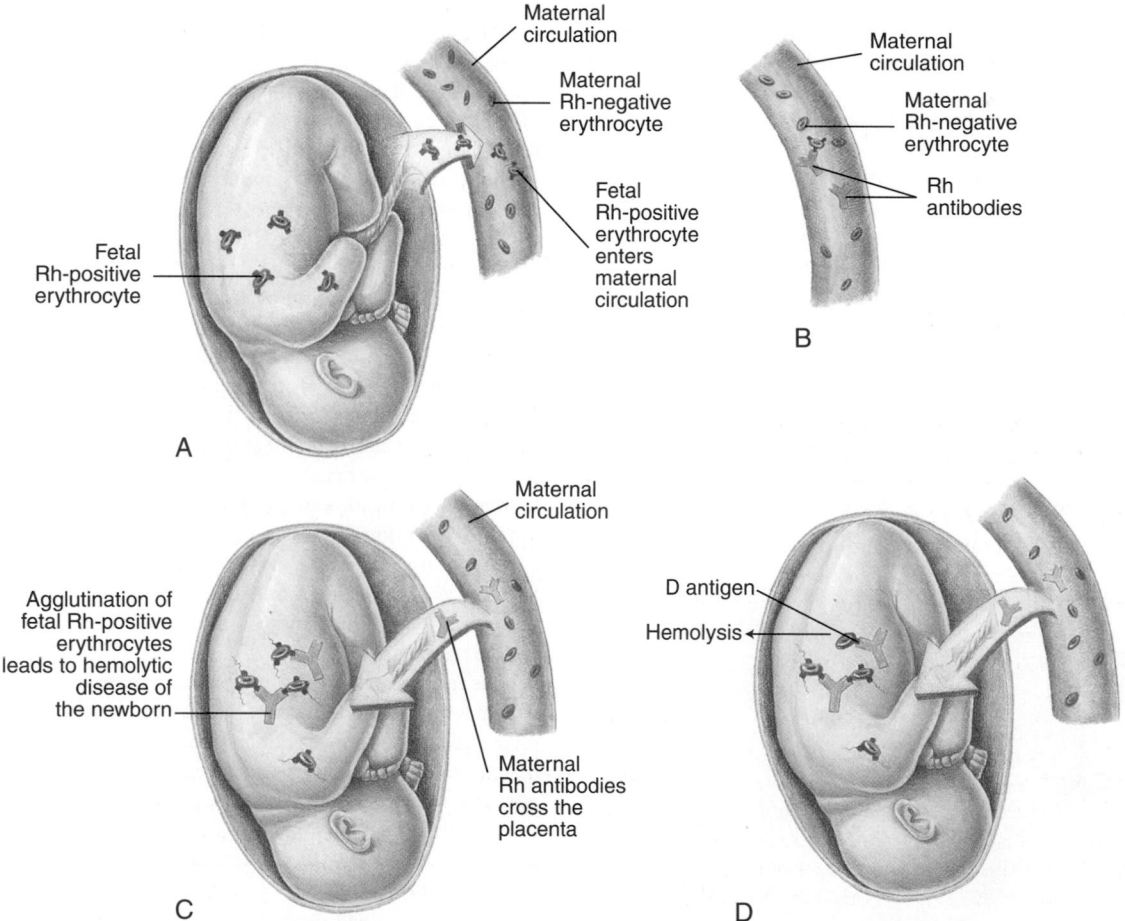

FIGURE 31.2 Hemolytic Disease of the Fetus and Newborn (HDFN). A, Before or during delivery, Rh-positive erythrocytes from the fetus enter the blood of an Rh-negative woman through a tear in the placenta. **B,** The mother is sensitized to the Rh antigen and produces Rh antibodies. Because this usually happens after delivery, there is no effect on the fetus in the first pregnancy. **C,** During a subsequent pregnancy with an Rh-positive fetus, Rh-positive erythrocytes cross the placenta, enter the maternal circulation, and **(D)** stimulate the mother to produce antibodies against the Rh antigen. The Rh antibodies from the mother cross the placenta, using agglutination and hemolysis of fetal erythrocytes, and HDFN develops. (Modified from Seeley RR, Stephens TD, Tate P: *Anatomy and physiology,* ed 3, St Louis, 1995, Mosby.)

The first Rh-incompatible pregnancy usually presents no difficulties because very few fetal erythrocytes cross the placental barrier during gestation. However, when the placenta detaches at birth, large numbers of fetal erythrocytes usually enter the mother's bloodstream. If the mother is Rh-negative and the fetus is Rh-positive, the mother produces anti-Rh antibodies. The capacity of the mother's immune system to produce anti-Rh antibodies depends on many factors, including her genetic capacity to make antibodies against the Rh antigen D, the amount of fetal-to-maternal bleeding, and the occurrence of any bleeding earlier in the pregnancy. Anti-Rh antibodies persist in the bloodstream for a very long time, and if the next offspring is Rh-positive, the mother's anti-Rh antibodies can enter the fetus's bloodstream and destroy the erythrocytes. Antibodies against Rh antigen D are of the IgG class and easily cross the placenta.

IgG-coated fetal erythrocytes are destroyed through extravascular hemolysis, primarily by mononuclear phagocytes in the spleen. As hemolysis progresses, the fetus becomes anemic. Erythropoiesis accelerates, particularly in the liver and spleen, and immature nucleated cells (erythroblasts) are released into the bloodstream, hence the name erythroblastosis fetalis (Fig. 31.3). The degree of anemia depends on the length of time the antibody has been in the fetal circulation, the concentration of antibody, and the ability of the fetus to compensate for increased hemolysis. Unconjugated (indirect) bilirubin, which is formed during breakdown of hemoglobin, is transported across the placental barrier into the maternal circulation and is excreted by the mother. Hyperbilirubinemia, an increase in bilirubin concentration in the blood, occurs in the neonate after birth because excretion of lipid-soluble unconjugated bilirubin through the placenta no longer is possible.

The pathophysiologic effects of HDFN are more severe in Rh incompatibility than in ABO incompatibility. ABO incompatibility may resolve after birth without life-threatening complications. Maternal-fetal incompatibility in which a mother with type O blood has a child with type A or B blood usually is so mild that it does not require treatment.

Rh incompatibility is more likely than ABO incompatibility to cause severe or even life-threatening anemia, death in utero, or damage to the central nervous system (CNS). Severe anemia alone can cause death as a result of cardiovascular complications (see Chapter 29). Extensive hemolysis also results in increased levels of unconjugated bilirubin in the circulation. If bilirubin levels exceed the liver's ability to conjugate and excrete bilirubin, some of it is deposited in the brain, causing

cellular damage and eventually death, if exchange transfusions are not administered.

Fetuses that do not survive anemia in utero usually are stillborn, exhibiting gross edema throughout the entire body, a condition called hydrops fetalis. Death can occur as early as 17 weeks of gestation and results in spontaneous abortion.

◆ **CLINICAL MANIFESTATIONS.** Neonates with mild HDFN may appear healthy or slightly pale, with slight enlargement of the liver and spleen. Pronounced pallor, splenomegaly, and hepatomegaly indicate severe anemia, which predisposes the neonate to cardiovascular failure and shock. Life-threatening Rh incompatibility is rare today, largely because of maternal testing and the routine use of Rh immune globulin.

Because maternal antibodies remain in the neonatal circulation after birth, erythrocyte destruction can continue. This causes hyperbilirubinemia and icterus neonatorum (neonatal jaundice) that occurs shortly after birth. Without replacement transfusions, in which the child receives Rh-negative erythrocytes, the bilirubin is deposited in the brain, causing a condition termed kernicterus. Kernicterus produces cerebral damage and usually causes death (icterus gravis neonatorum). Infants who do not die may have significant developmental delay, cerebral palsy, or high-frequency deafness.[17]

◆ **EVALUATION AND TREATMENT.** Routine evaluation for HDFN includes the Coombs test. The indirect Coombs test measures antibody in the mother's circulation and indicates whether the fetus is at risk for HDFN. The direct Coombs test measures antibody already bound to the surfaces of fetal erythrocytes and is used primarily to confirm the diagnosis of antibody-mediated HDFN. Determining prior history of fetal hemolytic disease, as well as diagnostic tests, may help predict the severity of the disorder. Diagnostic measures include maternal antibody titers, fetal blood sampling, amniotic fluid spectrophotometry, and ultrasound fetal assessment.[18]

The key to treatment of HDFN resulting from Rh incompatibility lies in prevention (immunoprophylaxis). Rh immune globulin (RhoGAM), a preparation of antibody against Rh antigen D (anti-D Ig) administered within 72 hours of exposure to Rh-positive erythrocytes, ensures that the mother will not produce antibody against the D antigen, and that the next Rh-positive baby will be protected (see Fig. 31.2). Updated recommendations also state that if anti-D Ig is not given within 72 hours every effort should still be made to administer the anti-D Ig within 10 days. The newer updates on the use of anti-D Ig as prophylaxis to prevent sensitization to the D antigen *during* pregnancy or at *delivery* for the prevention of HDFN can be found at the National Guideline Clearinghouse at http://www.guideline.gov/content.aspx?id=34964# Section420 for the use of anti-D immunoglobulin for rhesus D prophylaxis and from the British Committee for Standards in Haematology (BCSH) guidelines.[19]

The injected (anti-D Ig) antibodies remain in the mother's bloodstream long enough to prevent her immune system from producing its own anti-Rh antibodies but not long enough to affect subsequent offspring. The mother must be given Rh immune globulin injections after the birth of each Rh-positive baby and after a miscarriage. The mother also must be especially careful not to receive a transfusion containing Rh-positive blood, because this would stimulate production of anti-Rh antibodies.

If antigenic incompatibility of the mother's erythrocytes is not discovered in time to administer Rh immune globulin and a child is born with HDFN, treatment consists of exchange transfusions in which the neonate's blood is replaced with new Rh-positive blood that is not contaminated with anti-Rh antibodies. This treatment is instituted during the first 24 hours of extrauterine life to prevent kernicterus. Phototherapy also is used to reduce the toxic effects of unconjugated bilirubin.

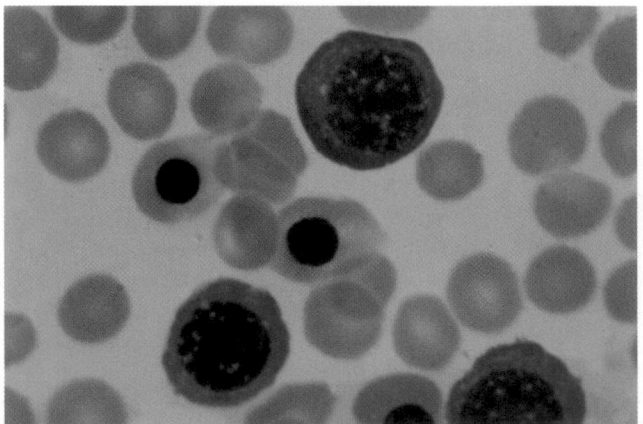

FIGURE 31.3 Rh Incompatibility in Hemolytic Disease of the Newborn. This micrograph shows immature red blood cells not normally found in blood. Large purple cells are erythroblasts; nucleated red blood cells are normoblasts. Normal red blood cells also are shown (×500). (Copyright Ed Reschke.)

Jaundice and indirect hyperbilirubinemia are reduced when the infant is exposed to high-intensity light in the visible spectrum from 460 to 490 nm.[20] Bilirubin in the skin absorbs light energy, which, by photoisomerization, converts the toxic unconjugated bilirubin into conjugated isomers that are excreted in the bile. Phototherapy also causes autosensitization that results in oxidation reactions. Breakdown products from the oxidation reactions are excreted by the liver and kidney without need for conjugation. The therapeutic effect of phototherapy depends on the light energy emitted in the effective wavelengths, the distance between the infant and the light source, and the amount of skin exposed; the rate of hemolysis and the infant's ability to excrete bilirubin also are factors in determining the effectiveness of phototherapy in lowering serum bilirubin levels.

Anemia of Infectious Disease

Infections of the newborn, often initially acquired by the mother and transmitted to the fetus, may result in a hemolytic anemia with clinical manifestations similar to those of HDFN. Congenital syphilis, toxoplasmosis, cytomegalic inclusion disease, rubella, coxsackievirus B infection, herpesvirus infection, and bacterial sepsis can cause hemolytic anemia in the neonate.

The exact mechanism of anemia caused by congenital infections is unclear. In some instances, it is related to direct injury of erythrocyte membranes or erythrocyte precursors by the infectious microorganism. In other instances, it results from traumatic destruction of erythrocytes during their passage through inflamed capillaries.

Anemia in Critically Ill Children

Anemia is a common occurrence in critically ill children (see Chapter 50). The causes are numerous and include decreased erythropoietin activity, poor iron use by the body, and blood loss from diverse conditions and consequences of treatment. A topic of ongoing discussion is whether transfusion of blood products, particularly packed RBCs, improves outcomes in critically ill children because of problems related to blood storage. New research is ongoing and needed to understand these problems, the development of new blood transfusion strategies, and blood substitutes.[21]

Inherited Disorders

A number of inherited and intrinsic erythrocyte defects are known to cause hemolytic disease or increased hemolysis (see Table 31.2). These defects may result from enzymatic abnormalities that disrupt metabolic processes and prevent normal biochemical balance within the cell, alterations of hemoglobin structure or synthesis, or plasma membrane defects accompanied by changes in erythrocyte size or shape.

Glucose-6-Phosphate Dehydrogenase Deficiency

Glucose-6-phosphate dehydrogenase (G6PD) deficiency is an inherited disorder caused by a genetic defect in the RBC enzyme G6PD, which is involved in the normal processing of carbohydrates. The enzyme G6PD is responsible for the first step in a pathway that converts glucose to ribose-5-phosphate. The chemical reactions usually produce nicotinamide adenine dinucleotide phosphate (NADPH), which helps in protecting cells from oxidative stress from reactive oxygen species (ROS). G6PD deficiency is the most common disorder of RBCs, estimated to affect 200 to 400 million people worldwide. The enzyme deficiency leads to damaged RBCs that can rupture and break down prematurely, causing hemolysis. The deficiency occurs most often in tropical and subtropical regions of the Eastern Hemisphere including Europe, Africa, and Asia. G6PD deficiency is an X-linked recessive disorder, most fully expressed in homozygous males, although partial expression is possible in heterozygous females because of mosaicism resulting from X-

inactivation. (X-linked inheritance is discussed in Chapter 4.) Several genetic variants of G6PD are identified but most are harmless.[7] Two variants, G6PD and G6PD Mediterranean, cause most of the significant hemolytic anemias.[7] The deficiency is present in 10% of American blacks, and the G6PD Mediterranean variant is prevalent in Middle East populations.

PATHOPHYSIOLOGY. Deficient or abnormal enzyme function can cause abnormalities in the hexose monophosphate shunt or glutathione metabolism that impairs the ability of RBCs to protect themselves against oxidative stress injuries that lead to hemolysis. One of the most important enzymes is G6PD. Oxidants cause both an intravascular and an extravascular hemolysis in G6PD-deficient individuals. G6PD enables erythrocytes to maintain normal metabolic processes despite injury from oxidative stressors, such as exposure to certain classes of drugs (sulfonamides, nitrofurantoins, antimalarial agents, salicylates, or naphthaquinolones), ingestion of fava beans (a dietary staple in some Mediterranean areas), hypoxemia, infection, fever, or acidosis. Therefore G6PD deficiency is usually asymptomatic unless one of these events occurs. Commonly, infections can initiate hemolysis, especially viral hepatitis, pneumonia, and typhoid fever. The fava bean is often ingested in Mediterranean cultures, causing "favism," and in some parts of Africa. Erythrocyte damage in affected children begins after intense or prolonged exposure to one of these stressors (substances or conditions) and ceases when the stressors are removed. In black males, the G6PD defect becomes more pronounced as the erythrocyte ages, and in other populations the defect is profound even in young erythrocytes. A pregnant woman may cause an episode of hemolysis in a fetus with G6PD deficiency by ingesting a substance with oxidant properties, such as a salicylate (aspirin).

In the absence of G6PD, oxidative stressors damage hemoglobin and the plasma membranes of erythrocytes and possibly interfere with the activities of other enzymes within the cell. Hemoglobin is oxidized progressively to methemoglobin, sulfmethemoglobin, and denatured globin-glutathione complexes. Exposure to oxidizing substances results in the precipitation of insoluble hemoglobin inclusions, called *Heinz bodies*, within the cell. Plasma damage and the presence of Heinz bodies cause hemolysis, primarily in the spleen.

CLINICAL MANIFESTATIONS. In infants, G6PD deficiency may present as icterus neonatorum. The most common clinical manifestation of G6PD deficiency is acute hemolytic anemia, usually after infections or the ingestion of certain oxidative drugs. The fava bean produces a severe hemolytic reaction in children with G6PD deficiency.

Hemolytic episodes are characterized by pallor, icterus, dark urine, back pain, and, in severe cases, shock, cardiovascular collapse, and death. Between hemolytic episodes, the child does not have anemia and erythrocyte survival is normal.

EVALUATION AND TREATMENT. Reduced G6PD activity in erythrocytes is required for diagnosis. Immediately after a hemolytic episode, reticulocytes and young erythrocytes are evident. Because young erythrocytes have significantly higher enzyme activity than do older cells, laboratory evaluation should be performed shortly after a crisis so that a low level of enzyme activity can be demonstrated. G6PD activity that is within the low normal range in the presence of a high reticulocyte count suggests G6PD deficiency. G6PD deficiency also can be detected by electrophoretic analysis.

Prevention of hemolysis is the most important therapeutic measure. Prevention includes avoiding medications and dietary substances associated with hemolysis. Because of the high frequency of G6PD deficiency in areas of the world that are endemic for malaria, the World Health Organization currently recommends testing for G6PD deficiency before administration of antimalarial medications in these regions.[22] When hemolysis occurs, supportive treatment may include blood transfusions and oral iron therapy. Spontaneous recovery generally follows treatment.

Hereditary Spherocytosis

Hereditary spherocytosis (HS) is an inherited disorder caused by defects in the membrane skeleton of RBCs. The changes cause RBCs to become spherical, less deformable, and vulnerable to destruction. HS is caused by genetic mutations in at least five genes (*ANK1*, *EPB42*, *SLC4A1*, *SPTA1*, and *SPTB*). These genes provide proteins for producing RBC membranes. These proteins act as transporters for molecules in and out of the cells, attach to other proteins, and maintain cell shape. Thus these proteins help the cells to be flexible for RBC mobility from large blood vessels to capillaries. Mutations in RBC membranes result in changes in shape, becoming more spherical instead of a flattened disc shape, and rigid. The misshapen cells, or spherocytes, are removed from circulation and end in the spleen for destruction. In the spleen, the spherocytes break down and undergo hemolysis.

◆**PATHOPHYSIOLOGY.** HS is transmitted as an autosomal dominant trait in about 75% of cases. The defect results from properties of its specialized membrane skeleton, which lies close to the internal surface of the plasma membrane.[7] The affected proteins include spectrins and ankyrin, and their intrinsic defects in the membrane cause less deformability and increased vulnerability to splenic sequestration and destruction.

The spleen is intimately involved in the hemolytic process. The spherocyte is relatively rigid and passes with difficulty through the small openings between the splenic cords and sinuses initiating macrophage response. Circulation of blood to the spleen creates repeated circulation through a metabolic environment that results in sequestration and destruction of spherocytes.

◆**CLINICAL MANIFESTATIONS.** The presenting signs of HS are anemia, jaundice, and splenomegaly. Anemia may be mild or absent in some cases depending on the individual's physiologic compensation. In these cases, the reticulocyte count will be elevated. Splenomegaly is usually mild. HS can present at any age, from the neonatal period until older adulthood. If HS presents during the newborn period, it is typically more severe with the infant developing signs of hemolytic anemia and hyperbilirubinemia.[23] These children, therefore, may have life-threatening anemia with clinical symptoms ranging from difficulty feeding, cir-cumoral pallor, tachycardia, nasal flaring, and diaphoresis to lethargy. They also are at increased risk for gallstones because of the presence of extra bile pigment. Infection (specifically parvovirus),[24] fever, and stress stimulate the spleen to destroy more RBCs than usual, leading to a worsening anemia in a child with baseline anemia.

◆**EVALUATION AND TREATMENT.** Ascertaining a family history of spherocytosis is important. Laboratory findings include spherocytes in the peripheral blood smear (*spherocytosis*), elevated reticulocyte count (with or without anemia), indirect hyperbilirubinemia, and a positive osmotic fragility test. An osmotic fragility test is performed by placing RBCs in a saline solution for 24 hours. Spherocytes do not tolerate saline solutions; as a result, they burst more readily than normal RBCs. Treatment of HS is based on disease severity. Although some children with HS will have severe anemia, blood transfusions are rarely required. Treatment before the age of 5 years consists of daily folic acid supplementation to increase production of healthy RBCs. In the past, splenectomy was the first line of treatment. Currently, however, splenectomy is only recommended for those children more than 5 years of age with severe disease or those who develop symptomatic gallstones. Partial splenectomy, in which only a portion of the spleen is removed, is being performed on children with HS in an attempt to decrease the risk of postsplenectomy complications.[25]

Sickle Cell Disease

Sickle cell disease (SCD) is a group of disorders that affects hemoglobin characterized by the presence of an atypical form of hemoglobin—*hemoglobin S (HbS; sickle hemoglobin)*—within the erythrocytes. It is a common hereditary hemoglobinopathy where HbS is formed by a genetic point mutation (missense) in β-globin that leads to the replacement of one glutamate amino acid with a valine amino acid (Fig. 31.4). Abnormal versions of β-globin can distort erythrocytes into a sickle shape. Hemoglobin consists of four protein subunits called α-globin and two subunits called β-globin. The hemoglobin B (*HbB*) gene provides instructions for making protein β-globin. Other mutations in the *HbB* gene lead to other versions of β-globin, such as hemoglobin C (HbC) and hemoglobin E (HbE). *HbB* gene mutations also can affect the quantity of β-globin, such as low levels of β-globin found in β-thalassemia. Sickle cell disease affects millions of people worldwide and is most common among individuals with ancestors from Africa and less so

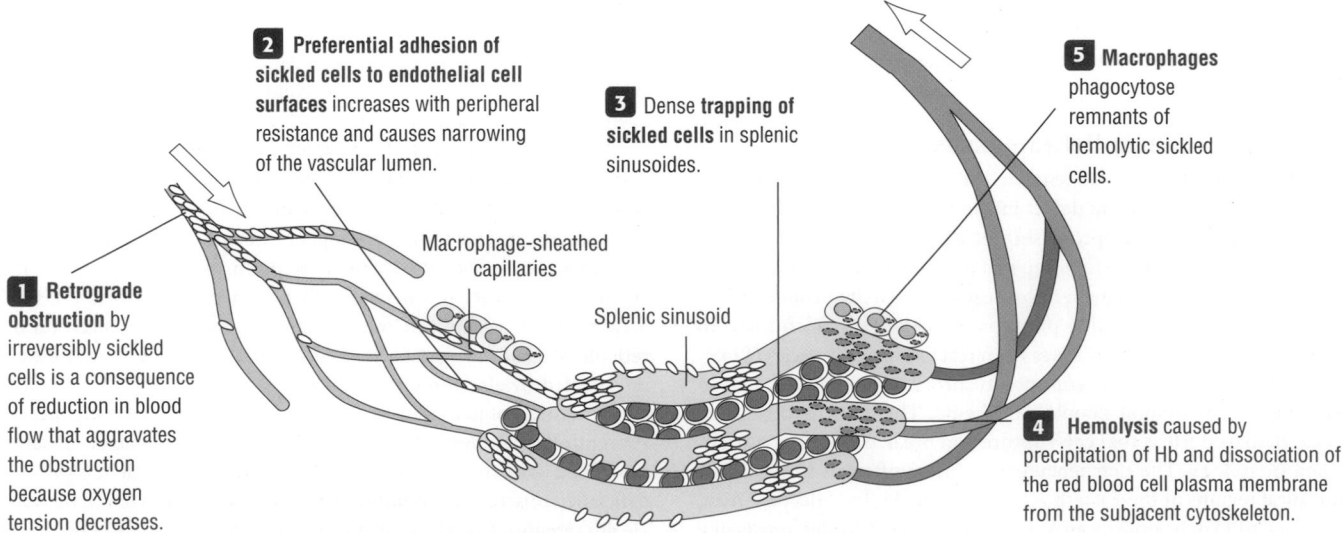

2 Preferential adhesion of sickled cells to endothelial cell surfaces increases with peripheral resistance and causes narrowing of the vascular lumen.

3 Dense trapping of sickled cells in splenic sinusoides.

5 Macrophages phagocytose remnants of hemolytic sickled cells.

Macrophage-sheathed capillaries

Splenic sinusoid

1 Retrograde obstruction by irreversibly sickled cells is a consequence of reduction in blood flow that aggravates the obstruction because oxygen tension decreases.

4 Hemolysis caused by precipitation of Hb and dissociation of the red blood cell plasma membrane from the subjacent cytoskeleton.

FIGURE 31.4 Sickle Cell Hemoglobin. Brief summary of sickle cell. (From Kierzenbaum AL, Tres LL: *Histology and cell biology: an introduction to pathology*, ed 4, Philadelphia, 2015, Saunders.)

from the Mediterranean countries, such as Greece, Turkey, and Italy; the Arabian peninsula; India; and Spanish-speaking regions in South America, Central America, and parts of the Caribbean.[26] Most infants with SCD born in the United States are now identified by routine neonatal screening. Between 1 and 3 million Americans and more than 100 million individuals worldwide are estimated to be heterozygous carriers for the sickle cell trait (HbAS).[27] It is estimated that between 70,000 and 100,000 Americans have SCD.[28]

Cycles of deoxygenation and oxygenation cause the HbS molecule to polymerize and stiffen. These polymers can damage the RBC structure, leading to sickle-shaped RBCs. This change causes a variety of pathologic consequences; the sickle-shaped RBCs die prematurely leading to hemolytic anemia, microvascular obstruction, and ischemic tissue damage. SCD is inherited in an autosomal recessive pattern where each parent carries one copy of the mutated gene. Sickle cell anemia (SCA; HbSS), a homozygous form, is the most severe. Sickle cell trait (HbAS), in which the child inherits HbS from one parent and normal hemoglobin (HbA) from the other, is a heterozygous carrier state and not a form of SCD. The most prevalent SCD genotypes include homozygous hemoglobin SS (HbSS, or sickle cell anemia) and the compound heterozygous conditions hemoglobin Sβ^0-thalassemia (Hbβ^0-thalassemia), hemoglobin Sβ-thalassemia (HbSβ^+-thalassemia), and hemoglobin SC disease (HbSC).[28] HbSS and HbSβ^0-thalassemia are clinically similar and are, therefore, commonly referred to as *sickle cell anemia (SCA);* these genotypes are associated with the most severe clinical manifestations.[28] All forms of SCD are lifelong conditions. Two effective disease therapies for SCD are hydroxyurea and chronic transfusion.[28] Hope for a cure is use of hematopoietic stem cell transplantation (HSCT); however, it is infrequently performed and needs significant investigation.[28]

◆PATHOPHYSIOLOGY. Pathogenesis of sickling includes erythrocyte derangement, chronic hemolysis (hemolytic anemia), microvascular occlusions, and tissue damage. Deoxygenation is probably the most important variable in determining the occurrence of sickling. Other significant variables that affect sickling include interaction of HbS with other types of hemoglobin in the cell, mean cell hemoglobin concentration (MCHC), intracellular pH, and transit times of erythrocytes through the microcirculation.[7] In heterozygotes with sickle cell trait, the presence of other types of Hb prevents sickling except under conditions of severe hypoxia. Intracellular dehydration increases the MCHC, which increases sickling. A decrease in pH reduces the oxygen affinity of hemoglobin, resulting in an increase in the quantity of deoxygenated HbS at any oxygen tension and increasing sickling. Inflammation in the microcirculation will slow erythrocyte transit times because blood flow is sluggish with adhesion of leukocytes to activated endothelial cells. Increased osmolality of the plasma draws water out of the erythrocytes. This promotes sickling by raising the relative HbS content in erythrocytes. Investigators are studying the optimal intravenous fluid to increase erythrocyte deformability and biomechanical properties.[29] To simplify, sickling as an occasional, intermittent phenomenon can be triggered or sustained by one or more of the following stressors: decreased oxygen tension (Po$_2$) of the blood (i.e., hypoxemia), acidosis (decreased pH), increased plasma osmolality, decreased plasma volume, and low temperature (Fig. 31.5). Low temperatures precipitate sickle crisis, presumably because of vasoconstriction.[30]

Sickling causes damage to erythrocytes through several mechanisms, including (1) *membrane derangements* occur because as HbS units (polymers) grow they protrude through the membrane skeleton by only the lipid layer, causing changes in membrane structure: (2) membrane derangement leads to *changes in ionic flow* with an influx in Ca^{++} ions, which induces cross-linking of membrane proteins and activation of an ion channel that induces the efflux of K$^+$ and H$_2$O; and (3) with time the damaged *cells are converted to end-stage,* nondeformable

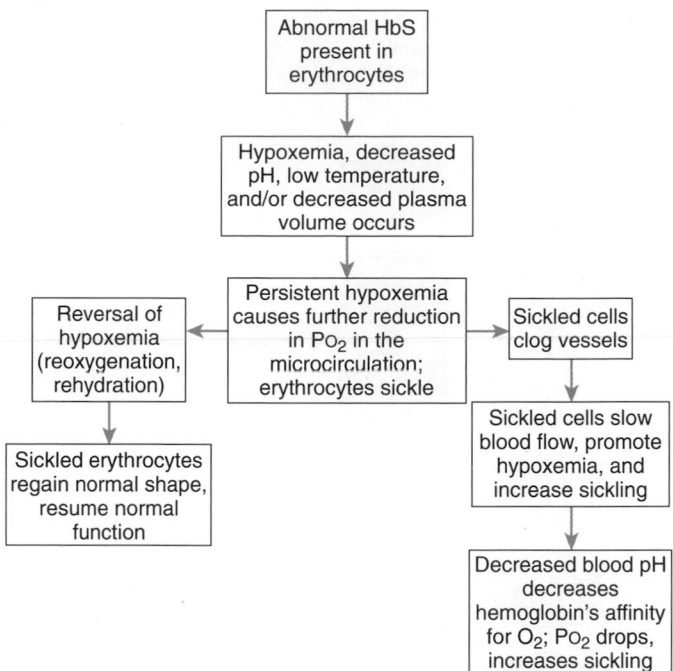

FIGURE 31.5 Sickling of Erythrocytes.

or stiff and irreversibly sickled cells (Fig. 31.6). Recent studies have shown that elevated red cell levels of the enzyme *sphingosine kinase 1 (SPH1)* underlie sickling and disease progression by increasing *sphingosine 1-phosphate (S1P)* production in the blood.[31] S1P level, a bioactive lipid enriched in red cells, is elevated in red cells and plasma of mice and humans with SCD.[31] S1P also is a signaling molecule that regulates diverse biologic functions including inflammation.[32] Additionally, investigators demonstrated that the compound 5C can inhibit *SPHK1* and, thus, has antisickling properties.[33] These data are important for identifying the structure of the sickling process to assess potential new therapeutics.

The cells remain sickled even with full oxygenation and some cells are vulnerable to hemolysis. Polymerization of sickled hemoglobin is central to the disorder. Polymerization stiffens the sickled erythrocyte, changing it from a flexible, beneficial cell to an inflexible one where HbS molecules stack into polymers that starve and damage tissues. The pathogenesis of SCD totally derives from the tendency of HbS molecules to stack into polymers when deoxygenated and assemble into needle-like fibers within cells, producing the distorted crescent-like sickle or holly-leaf shape (Fig. 31.7). Sickled cells undergo hemolysis in the spleen or become sequestered there, causing blood pooling and infarction of splenic vessels. The anemia that follows triggers erythropoiesis in the marrow and, in extreme cases, in the liver.[34,35]

However, the pathogenesis of microvascular occlusions, a main feature of SCD not fully understood, is responsible for the most serious and urgent manifestations. Microvascular occlusions are not related to the quantity of irreversibly sickled cells in the blood but are dependent on understated RBC membrane damages and other local factors, such as inflammation or vasoconstriction, that tends to decrease blood flow or arrest red cells through the microcirculation.[7] Investigators are studying the microvasculature from a developed model and mathematics of the microvasculature to allow the understanding of the rheology of sickle cell blood.[36,37] Sickle RBCs express higher than normal amounts of adhesion molecules and are sticky. During inflammatory reactions, leukocyte release of mediators increases the

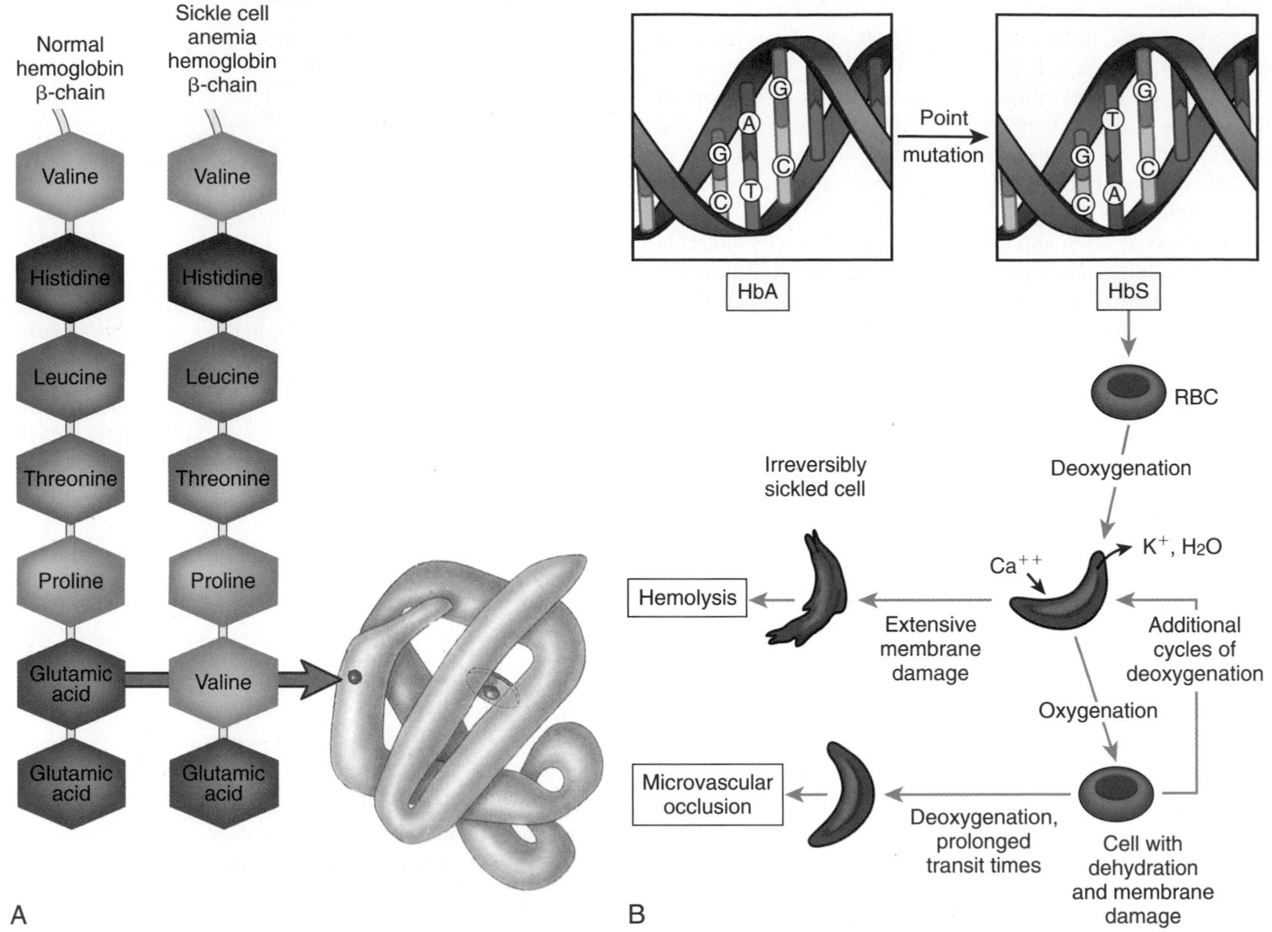

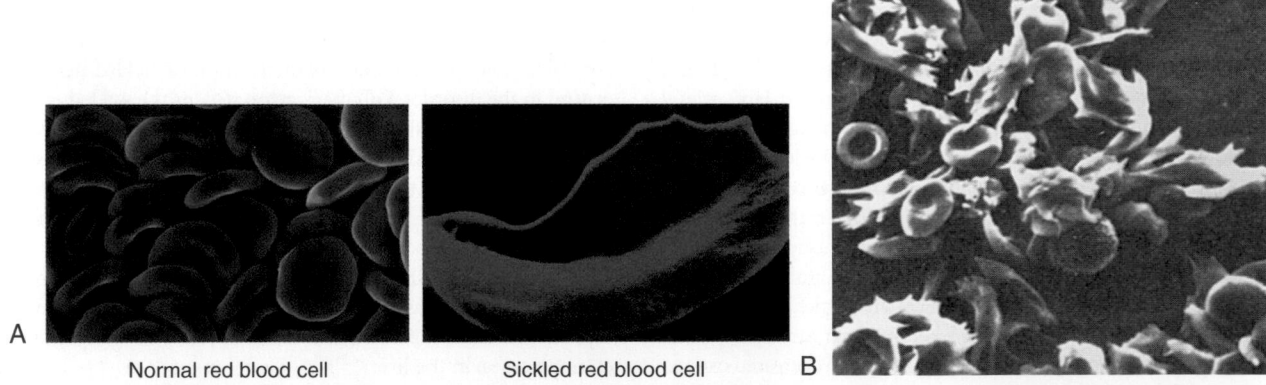

FIGURE 31.6 Sickle Cell Disease Pathogenesis. See text for discussion. (**B** adapted from Kumar V, Abbas AK, Aster JC: *Robbins and Cotran pathologic basis of disease,* ed 9, Philadelphia, 2015, Elsevier Saunders.)

FIGURE 31.7 Normal and Sickle-Shaped Blood Cells. **A,** Color-enhanced electron micrograph shows normal erythrocytes and sickled blood cell. **B,** Scanning electron micrograph of normal and sickle-shaped red blood cells together. The irregularly shaped cells are the sickle cells; the circular cells are the normal blood cells. (From Raven PH, Johnson GB: *Biology,* ed 3, St Louis, 1992, Mosby.)

expression of adhesion molecules on endothelial cells. These reactions further promote sickled erythrocytes to become arrested during movement through the microvasculature.[7] The sluggish and stagnant red cells within the inflamed vascular vessels result in extended exposure to low oxygen tension, sickling, and vascular obstruction.[7] Lysed sickle erythrocytes release hemoglobin and free hemoglobin can bind and inactivate nitric oxide (NO), which is a powerful vasodilator and inhibitor of platelet aggregation. Decreased blood pH reduces hemoglobin's affinity for oxygen leading to an increasing fraction of deoxygenated HbS at any oxygen tension and predisposition to sickling. As less oxygen is taken up by hemoglobin in the lungs, the Po_2 drops promoting additional sickling.

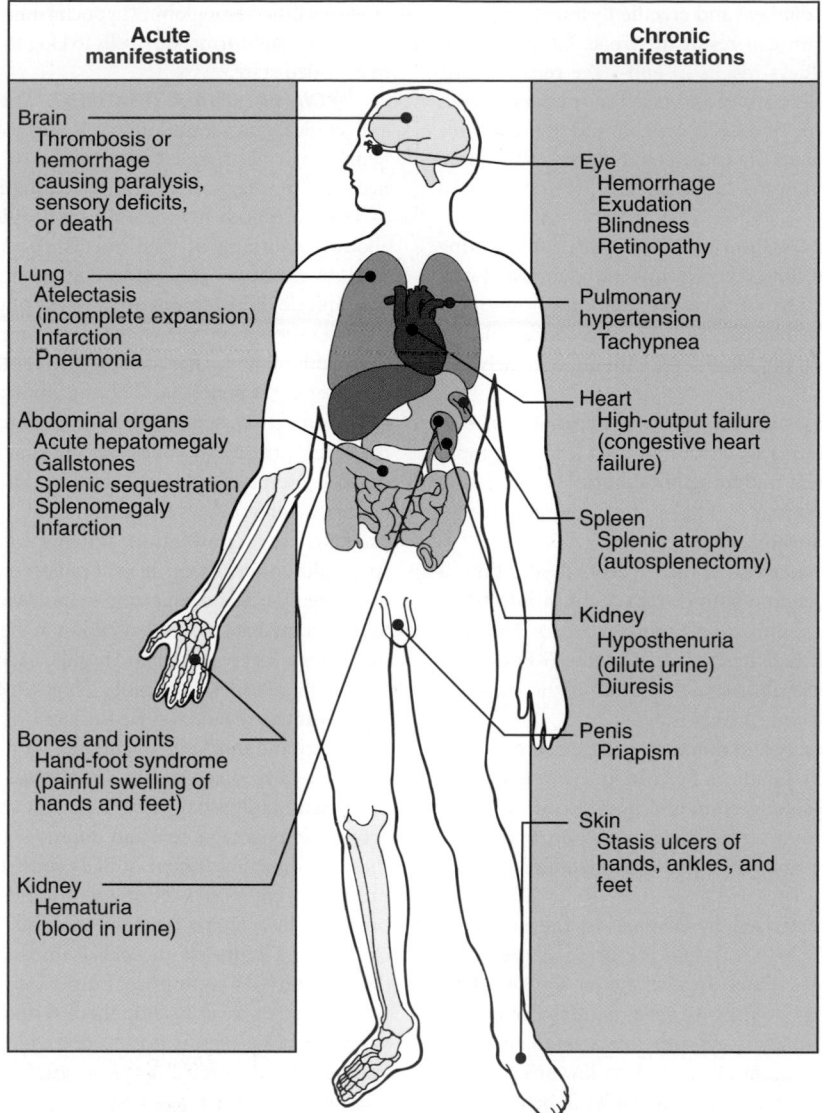

Acute manifestations

Brain
  Thrombosis or hemorrhage causing paralysis, sensory deficits, or death

Lung
  Atelectasis (incomplete expansion)
  Infarction
  Pneumonia

Abdominal organs
  Acute hepatomegaly
  Gallstones
  Splenic sequestration
  Splenomegaly
  Infarction

Bones and joints
  Hand-foot syndrome (painful swelling of hands and feet)

Kidney
  Hematuria (blood in urine)

Chronic manifestations

Eye
  Hemorrhage
  Exudation
  Blindness
  Retinopathy

Pulmonary hypertension
  Tachypnea

Heart
  High-output failure (congestive heart failure)

Spleen
  Splenic atrophy (autosplenectomy)

Kidney
  Hyposthenuria (dilute urine)
  Diuresis

Penis
  Priapism

Skin
  Stasis ulcers of hands, ankles, and feet

FIGURE 31.8 Clinical Manifestations of Sickle Cell Disease.

Once sickling begins, it tends to continue until the Po_2 returns to normal; then it ceases spontaneously. The extent, severity, and clinical manifestations of sickling depend to a great extent on the percentage of hemoglobin that is HbS. That is why homozygous inheritance of HbS produces the severest form of SCD—sickle cell anemia. Heterozygous inheritance of SCD results in less sickling because the individual's erythrocytes contain other forms of abnormal hemoglobin that, although defective, do not contribute to sickling to any great degree. Heterozygous inheritance (sickle cell trait), in which abnormal hemoglobin is inherited from one parent and normal hemoglobin from the other, rarely results in sickling because normal HbF and HbA do not contribute to sickling at all. Anemia persists because HbF does not live 120 days.

◆**CLINICAL MANIFESTATIONS.** There is much variation in the clinical manifestations of sickle cell disease. Some individuals have mild symptoms and others suffer from repeated vaso-occlusive crises.[7] Clinical manifestations of SCD may first be seen at 6 to 12 months of age as fetal hemoglobin is replaced by HbS. Two characteristics of SCD determine presentation: the first is its nature to be a chronic disease with acute exacerbations; the second is that it is a condition affecting RBCs that supply oxygen to all cells of the body. Therefore SCD can

affect any part of the body. When sickling occurs, the general manifestations of hemolytic anemia—pallor, fatigue, jaundice, and irritability—sometimes are accompanied by acute manifestations called *crises*. Extensive sickling can precipitate four types of crises: (1) vaso-occlusive crisis, (2) aplastic crisis, (3) sequestration crisis, or rarely (4) hyperhemolytic crisis. Sites of specific dysfunction are shown in Fig. 31.8.

Vaso-occlusive crises (pain crises) are events of hypoxic injury and infarction that can cause severe pain in affected areas. However, the specific cause of sensory pain lacks sufficient characterization.[38,39] The most common sites include bones, lungs, spleen, liver, brain, and penis. Painful bone crises are very common in children and are difficult to distinguish from acute osteomyelitis.[7] These bone alterations can manifest as painful swelling of the hands and feet (*hand-foot syndrome* or *dactylitis*).

A high-risk type of vaso-occlusive crisis involves the lungs known as acute chest syndrome. It typically presents with fever, cough, chest pain, and accumulations of lung infiltrates. The complications in the lungs create a worsening cycle of hypoxemia, sickling, and vaso-occlusion.[7] Acute chest syndrome is the cause of death in approximately 25% of all deaths in people with SCD.[40,41] *Priapism,* or prolonged erection of the penis, can lead to hypoxic damage and erectile dysfunction. Vaso-occlusion in vessels to the brain can result in stroke. Chronic vaso-occlusion in vessels to the kidneys results in end-stage renal disease. Vaso-occlusive crisis is extremely painful and may last for days or even weeks. The frequency of this type of crisis is variable and unpredictable because it may develop spontaneously or be precipitated by infection, exposure to cold, dehydration, low Po_2, acidosis (low pH), or localized hypoxemia.

Aplastic crisis, a transient cessation in RBC production resulting in acute anemia, occurs as a result of a viral infection, almost always infection with parvovirus B1. The virus causes temporary shutdown of RBC production in the bone marrow but hemolysis continues. The outcome is a sudden drop in hemoglobin level with an extremely low reticulocyte count.

In sequestration crisis, large amounts of blood become pooled in the spleen. Massive large amounts of sickle red cells lead to a rapid splenic enlargement, hypovolemia, and sometimes shock.[7] Sequestration crisis and acute chest syndrome may be fatal and can require prompt treatment with exchange transfusions.

Hyperhemolytic crisis, an accelerated rate of RBC destruction, is unusual but may occur in association with certain drugs or infections. It is characterized by anemia, jaundice, and reticulocytosis. The concomitant presence of G6PD deficiency (see Glucose-6-Phosphate Dehydrogenase Deficiency) contributes to hyperhemolytic episodes, especially when combined with infections.

A significant cause of morbidity and mortality is infection, especially for those with impaired splenic function. Splenic function is severely altered in children with splenic congestion and poor blood flow, and severe splenic damage in adults occurs from splenic infarction. In children, infections from *Pneumococcus pneumoniae* and *Haemophilus influenzae* are common.

Glomerular disease, characterized by damage to the glomeruli allowing protein and often RBCs to leak into the urine, is caused by sickling of RBCs in the kidneys. Extensive damage to the glomeruli results in nephropathy that may progress to renal failure. The earliest manifestation of SCD in the kidney is hyposthenuria, or the inability of the tubules of the kidneys to concentrate urine. Very low urine specific gravity occurs and in young children this often results in bed-wetting. Proteinuria also is an early manifestation of sickle nephropathy.

Cholecystitis, inflammation of the gallbladder that occurs when a gallstone blocks the cystic duct, can be caused by hemolysis resulting in an increase of bilirubin concentration, which in turn causes the formation of gallstones in the gallbladder. The presence of gallstones can cause right upper quadrant pain, nausea, vomiting, and an elevated white blood cell count and alkaline phosphatase level. Cholecystectomy may be required.

Sickle cell–hemoglobin C (HbC) disease is usually milder than sickle cell anemia. HbC results when lysine is substituted for glutamic acid in the amino acid chain. HbC is less soluble than HbA; however, it does not polymerize under conditions of decreased oxygen tension as does HbS. The main clinical problems are related to vaso-occlusive crises and are proposed to result from higher hematocrit values and viscosity. In older children, sickle cell retinopathy, renal necrosis, and aseptic necrosis of the femoral heads occur along with obstructive crises.

Sickle cell–thalassemia has the mildest clinical manifestations of all the SCDs. Individuals with sickle cell–thalassemia have mutations in each allele coding for hemoglobin. One mutation results in HbS formation and the other is associated with β-thalassemia and results in decreased production of hemoglobin. Even though most of the child's hemoglobin is HbS (60% to 90%), normal hemoglobins (HbA and HbF) also are present. The normal hemoglobins, particularly HbF, inhibit sickling. In addition, the erythrocytes tend to be small (microcytic) and to contain

relatively little hemoglobin (hypochromic). Their small size makes them less likely than normal-size cells to clog the microcirculation, even when in a sickled state.

◆**EVALUATION AND TREATMENT.** The parents' hematologic history and clinical manifestations may suggest that a child has SCD, but hematologic tests and the presence of irreversibly sickled cells are necessary for diagnosis. If the sickle solubility test confirms the presence of HbS in blood, hemoglobin electrophoresis provides information about the amount of HbS in erythrocytes. Prenatal diagnosis can be made by chorionic villus sampling as early as 8 to 10 weeks of gestation or amniotic fluid analysis at 15 weeks of gestation. Newborn screening for SCD should be performed according to state law.

Health maintenance as early interventions in populations identified by screening is beneficial.[28] Young children with SCA have a very high risk of infection, septicemia, and meningitis. The fatality is high and the risk is greatest in young people who lack immunity against pneumococcal serotype causing infection. These infections arise because of abnormal or absent splenic function.[28] A recent proposal has been presented as a prevention strategy to use prophylactic antibiotics (penicillin), vaccination against pneumococcus and other encapsulated microorganisms, and education to those with SCD, parents, and caregivers to seek immediate medical attention in the event of fever.[28] Other recommendations for treatment and health maintenance are available at https://www.nhlbi.nih/sites/www.nhlbi.nih.gov/filessickle-cell-disease-report.pdf.

Treatment advances since the late 1980s have significantly decreased morbidity and mortality in children with SCD. Aggressive management of fever, early diagnosis of *acute chest syndrome* (hypoxia, anemia, progressive multilobar pneumonia, fat emboli), RBC transfusions, and proper pain management can improve quality of life and prognosis for these children. Treatment of SCD consists of supportive care aimed at preventing consequences of anemia and avoiding crises. Crises can be prevented by avoiding fever, infection, acidosis, dehydration, constricting clothes, and exposure to cold. Immediate correction of acidosis and dehydration with appropriate intravenous fluids is imperative. Infections require aggressive antibiotic therapy and infections can be reduced by vaccination. Oxygen is not needed unless the child becomes hypoxic. Pain associated with SCD is very complex, requiring accurate assessment and multimodal management.[42]

A common treatment is hydroxyurea, an inhibitor of DNA synthesis. It increases HbF synthesis, which decreases the proportion of HbS. Transfusion or exchange transfusion also can achieve these changes. Genetic counseling and psychologic support are important for the child and family.

Thalassemias

The α- and β-thalassemias are inherited autosomal recessive disorders that cause an impaired synthesis of one of the two chains—α or β—of adult hemoglobin (HbA). The disorder was named thalassemia, which is derived from the Greek word for *sea*, because it was initially described in people with origins near the Mediterranean Sea. β-Thalassemia, in which synthesis of the β-globin chain is slowed or defective, is prevalent among Greeks, Italians, and some Arabs and Sephardic Jews. α-Thalassemia, in which the α chain is affected, is most common among Chinese, Vietnamese, Cambodians, and Laotians. Both α- and β-thalassemias are common among blacks. Anemia associated with thalassemia is microcytic-hypochromic hemolytic anemia.

◆**PATHOPHYSIOLOGY.** The β-thalassemias are classified into two types depending on the severity of symptoms: thalassemia major and thalassemia intermedia. Thalassemia major is more severe. The β-thalassemias are caused by mutations in the *HBB* gene that decrease the synthesis of β-globin chains. Thalassemia major (Cooley anemia) and thalassemia intermedia are inherited in an autosomal recessive pattern where both copies of the *HBB* gene in each cell have mutations. In a small percentage of families, the *HBB* gene mutation is inherited in an autosomal dominant manner.[43] The mutations are classified as (1) β^0 mutations or absent β-globin synthesis and (2) β^+ mutations with reduced amounts of β-globin synthesis. Genetic studies have identified more than 100 different causative mutations, and most are point (missense) mutations. Clinical classification of β-thalassemias is based on the severity of the anemia, which is dependent on the type of mutation (β^0 or β^+ allele) and gene dosage (homozygous or heterozygous).[7] β-Chain production is depressed in the heterozygous form, thalassemia minor (β^0 or β^+ allele); and anemia, if present, is mild; however, anemia is severe in the homozygous form, β-thalassemia major. β-Thalassemia major may lack HbA (β^0/β^0 genotype) or contain small amounts (β^+/β^+ or β^0/β^+ genotypes). The main type of hemoglobin is HbF and sometimes HbA$_2$ is high and often normal or low.[7] Depression of β-chain synthesis results in erythrocytes having a reduced amount of hemoglobin and accumulations of free α chains. The free α chains are unstable and easily precipitate in the cell (Fig. 31.9). Most erythroblasts that contain precipitates are destroyed by mononuclear phagocytes in the marrow, resulting in ineffective erythropoiesis and anemia. Some of the precipitate-carrying cells do mature and enter the bloodstream, but they are destroyed prematurely in the spleen, resulting in mild hemolytic anemia.

The α-thalassemias result from deletions involving the *HBA1* and *HBA2* genes. These genes provide instructions for making a protein called α-globin, a subunit of hemoglobin. The different types of α-thalassemia result from the loss of some or all of the alleles (two copies of the *HBA1* gene and two copies of the *HBA2* gene in each cell; for each gene, one allele is inherited from the father and the other from the mother). Characteristic features of α-thalassemia are anemia, weakness, fatigue, and other more severe complications (see Clinical Manifestations). Types of α-thalassemia include:

1. *Hb Bart syndrome* is the most severe form of α-thalassemia and is caused by the loss of all four α-globin alleles. In the fetus, hydrops fetalis is the most severe form of α-thalassemia caused by the deletion of all four α-globin genes. Excess γ-globin chains do have a high affinity for oxygen but deliver small quantities to tissue. Signs of fetal distress may become evident in the third trimester of pregnancy, and intrauterine transfusions may save the baby.

2. HbH disease is caused by a loss of three of the four α-globin alleles. In both Hb Bart syndrome and *HbH disease*, the decrease in α-globin prevents cells from making normal hemoglobin. Instead, cells produce abnormal forms of hemoglobin called *Bart* (Hb Bart) or *hemoglobin H* (HbH). These abnormal forms of hemoglobin do not carry oxygen effectively, which causes anemia and other related consequences.[44]

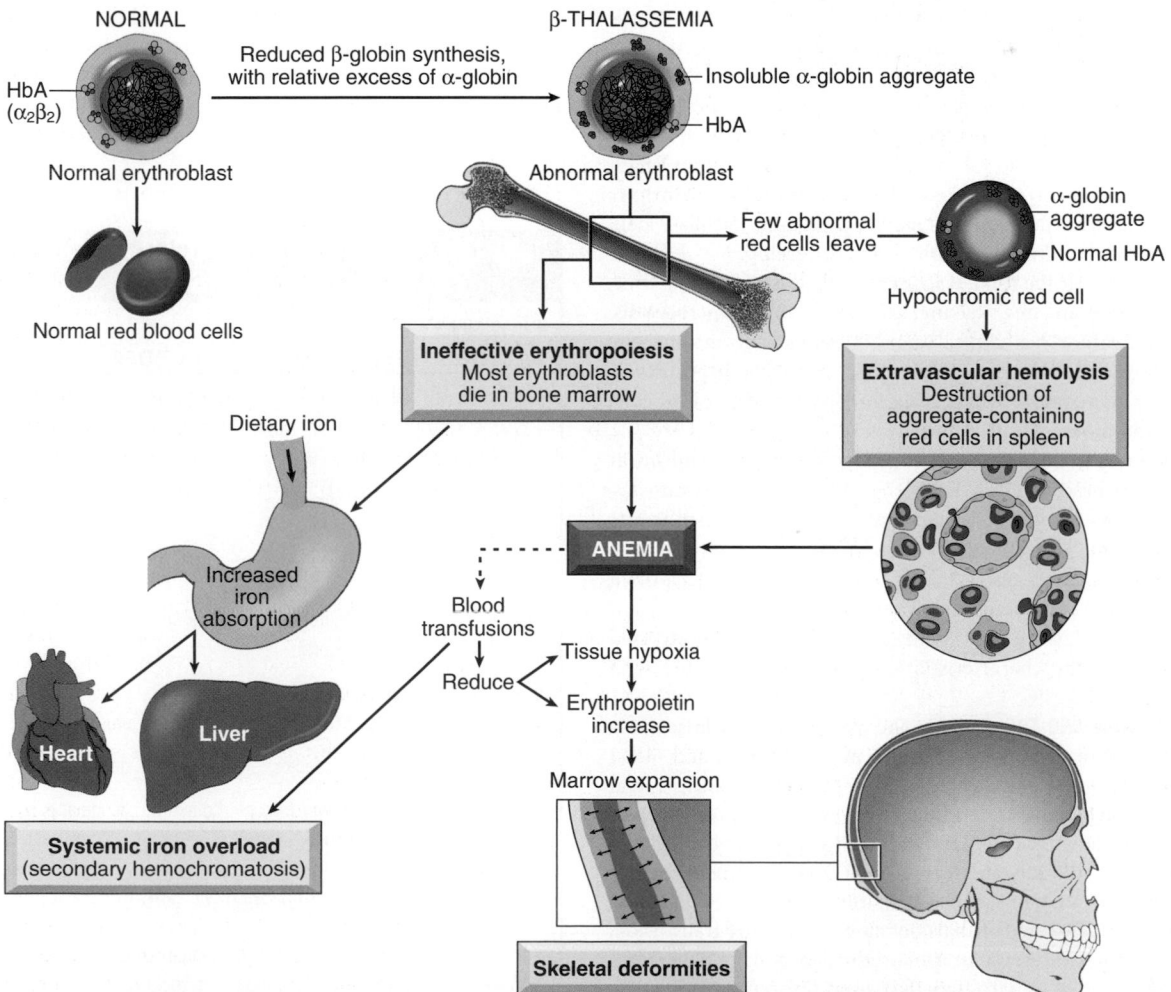

FIGURE 31.9 Pathogenesis of β-Thalassemia Major. The aggregates of unpaired α-globin chains are a hallmark of the disease. Blood transfusions can diminish the anemia but they add to the systemic iron overload. (From Kumar V et al: *Robbins and Cotran pathologic basis of disease,* ed 9, Philadelphia, 2015, Saunders.)

3. Two other variants of α-thalassemia are related to reduced amounts of α-globin. These variants still produce some normal hemoglobin and therefore cause few or no health problems.[44]

4. α-Thalassemia trait results from a loss of two of the four α-globin alleles. These individuals may have small, pale erythrocytes and mild anemia. A loss of one α-globin allele is found in α-thalassemia silent carriers, meaning these individuals have no related clinical manifestations.[44]

β-Thalassemia occurs more frequently than does α-thalassemia. Occasionally synthesis of γ- or δ-polypeptide chains is defective, resulting in γ- or δ-thalassemia. (Hemoglobin chains are described in Chapter 28.)

◆**CLINICAL MANIFESTATIONS.** β-Thalassemia minor causes mild to moderate microcytic-hypochromic hemolytic anemia. The degree of reticulocytosis depends on the severity of the anemia. Hemolysis of immature (and therefore fragile) erythrocytes may cause a slight elevation in serum iron and indirect bilirubin levels. Although persons with β-thalassemia minor may be asymptomatic, mild splenomegaly, bronze coloring of the skin, and hyperplasia of the bone marrow resulting in skeletal changes can occur.

Persons with β-thalassemia major may become quite ill with impaired physical growth and development. The severe anemia resulting from this condition can cause significant cardiovascular burden with high-output congestive heart failure. Historically, death results from cardiac failure by 5 or 6 years of age. Today, blood transfusions can increase life span by one to two decades, and death usually is caused by hemochromatosis (from transfusions).[45] (Hemosiderosis and hemochromatosis are described in Chapters 28 and 29.) Liver enlargement occurs as a result of progressive hemosiderosis, whereas enlargement of the spleen is caused by extramedullary hematopoiesis and increased destruction of RBCs. Skeletal changes include spinal impairment that starts in infancy and retards linear growth and subsequent upper and lower limb-length discrepancy. Bone marrow hyperplasia causes a characteristic deformity of the facial bones, as the nasal bridge, mandible, and maxilla widen. Osteopenia, osteochondrosis, or both also may develop.

People who inherit the mildest form of α-thalassemia, the α trait, usually are symptom free, having, at most, mild microcytosis. α-Thalassemia minor has clinical manifestations that are virtually identical to those of β-thalassemia minor: mild microcytic-hypochromic reticulocytosis, bone marrow hyperplasia, increased serum iron concentrations, and moderate splenomegaly.

α-Thalassemia major causes hydrops fetalis and fulminant intrauterine congestive heart failure. In addition to edema and massive ascites, the fetus has a grossly enlarged heart and liver. Most affected babies are stillborn or die shortly after birth. Diagnosis usually is made postmortem. Prenatal screening for this disorder can be performed by use of chorionic villus sampling. These cells can be analyzed, and a deoxyribonucleic acid (DNA) genetic map can be constructed and evaluated for the characteristic abnormalities associated with hydrops fetalis.

◆**EVALUATION AND TREATMENT.** The diagnosis of thalassemia is based on familial disease history, clinical manifestations, and blood tests. Laboratory tests reveal microcytic-hypochromic anemia and nucleated RBCs on peripheral blood smear, whereas hemoglobin analysis shows decreased amounts of HbA and increased amounts of hemoglobin F (HbF) after age 12 months, and severity of anemia. Treatment involves a regular transfusion program and chelation therapy to reduce transfusion iron overload. Milder forms of thalassemia rarely require transfusion, and these individuals are at risk for iron overload secondary to increased intestinal absorption of iron from ineffective erythropoiesis.[46] The only available definitive cure for thalassemia major is by allogeneic hematopoietic stem cell transplantation (HSCT) from a matched family or unrelated donor or cord blood transplantation from a related donor.[46]

Optimal clinical management may decrease the need for splenectomy. For less severe thalassemia (sometimes called *intermedia*), splenectomy may be done for those with the most affected symptoms, as well as sporadic red cell transfusions for some, folic acid supplementation, and iron chelation.[46]

Prenatal diagnosis is sometimes done and families are referred for genetic counseling. Molecular genetic testing of at-risk siblings should be offered to allow for early diagnosis and appropriate treatment. Women with thalassemia intermedia who have never received a blood transfusion or who received a minimal quantity of blood are at risk for severe alloimmune anemia if blood transfusions are required during pregnancy.[46]

DISORDERS OF COAGULATION AND PLATELETS

Inherited Hemorrhagic Disease
Hemophilias

Awareness of a serious bleeding disorder in males was documented nearly 2000 years ago in the Babylonian Talmud, which exempted those boys having male relatives prone to excessive bleeding from the rite of circumcision. In 1803 the first description of this disorder appeared in the medical literature, where it was noted to be X-linked and associated with joint bleeding and crippling.

Table 31.3 lists the coagulation factors. Until 1952 the term *hemophilia* was reserved for deficiency of factor VIII (antihemophilic factor). Since then two additional coagulation proteins, factor IX (plasma thromboplastin component [PTC]) and factor XI (plasma thromboplastin antecedent [PTA]), have been identified and their deficiency associated

TABLE 31.3	THE COAGULATION FACTORS	
CLOTTING FACTORS	**SYNONYM**	**DISORDER**
I	Fibrinogen	Congenital deficiency (afibrinogenemia) and dysfunction (dysfibrinogenemia)
II	Prothrombin	Congenital deficiency or dysfunction
V	Labile factor, proaccelerin	Congenital deficiency (parahemophilia)
VII	Stable factor or proconvertin	Congenital deficiency
VIII	Antihemophilic factor (AHF)	Congenital deficiency is hemophilia A (classic hemophilia)
IX	Christmas factor	Congenital deficiency is hemophilia B
X	Stuart-Power factor	Congenital deficiency
XI	Plasma thromboplastin antecedent	Congenital deficiency, sometimes referred to as hemophilia C
XII	Hageman factor	Congenital deficiency is *not* associated with clinical symptoms
XIII	Fibrin-stabilizing factor	Congenital deficiency

with similar clinical manifestations. Congenital deficiencies of these three plasma clotting factors—VIII, IX, XI—account for 90% to 95% of the hemorrhagic bleeding disorders collectively called *hemophilia*.

Types of Hemophilia. Hemophilia is a bleeding disorder with a wide range of clinical severity. The major types of hemophilia are hemophilia A (classic hemophilia or factor VIII deficiency) and hemophilia B (Christmas disease or factor IX deficiency). Hemophilia A is the most common hereditary disease associated with life-threatening bleeding, with an incidence of 1 in 4000 to 5000 male births and an incidence of hemophilia B of 1 in 20,000 newborn males worldwide.[47] Hemophilia A is caused by changes in the *F8* gene, and mutations in the *F9* gene cause hemophilia B. The *F8* gene provides instructions for making the protein called coagulation VIII. The *F9* gene produces coagulation factor IX.[47] These factors are important for blood clotting. Factor VIII is an essential cofactor for factor IX in the coagulation cascade. The alterations or deficiencies of the coagulation factors decrease the ability to form blood clots in response to injury. The decreased or ineffective blood clotting leads to continuous bleeding. The most severe types of hemophilia are derived from mutations that eliminate factor VIII or coagulation factor IX. Mutations that reduce but do not eliminate the activity of these proteins are responsible for mild and moderate hemophilia.[47] Hemophilia A and hemophilia B are inherited as an X-linked recessive pattern. The genes associated with the disorders are located on the X chromosome; in males one altered copy of the disorder causes the condition, which is why it affects mainly males (females are carriers) and very rarely homozygous females. In about 30% of individuals with no family history, their disease is caused by acquired new mutations.[7]

Hemophilias A and B occur with varying degrees of clinical severity, depending on concentrations of clotting factor VIII or IX in the blood. Severe hemophilia (concentration of clotting factors less than 1% of normal) is associated with spontaneous bleeding. In moderate hemophilia (1% to 5% of normal), bleeding usually occurs only after trauma; in the mild form (6% to 50% of normal), bleeding occurs only after severe trauma or surgery.

PATHOPHYSIOLOGY. Multiple types of genetic mutations are associated with hemophilias A and B with more than 2000 unique mutations identified for hemophilia A[48] and more than 1000 mutations described for hemophilia B.[49] The type of mutation also affects the phenotype of the disease. Mutations tend to be identical among affected members of a given family; however, mutations often differ across families.[50,51]

Inversions in introns 1 and 22 of the factor VIII gene are the most frequently observed mutations and account for the majority of severe cases of hemophilia A.[50] Point mutations, in which a single base in the DNA is inserted in the place of another base, are another type of mutation that causes hemophilia. Point mutations comprise the majority of unique mutations associated with hemophilia.[52] When a point mutation gives rise to a de novo stop codon (nonsense mutation), translation of the protein ceases and a shortened version of the protein is synthesized. Usually the protein is destroyed intracellularly and never reaches the plasma. This type of defect also is associated with severe hemophilia, that is, with coagulant activity levels below 1%. Point mutations resulting in the substitution of one amino acid for another can cause phenotypes of varying severity. The altered amino acid chain can destroy protein function, activation, or folding; inhibit intracellular processing; or cause protein clearance.[52]

Table 31.3 summarizes the types of coagulation disorders. Not all the disorders are discussed in this chapter because some are extremely rare (congenital dysfibrinogenemias) and others have no clinical significance. For example, Hageman factor deficiency is a condition with profound laboratory deficiency of factor XII yet is associated with no clinical defects in humans.

CLINICAL MANIFESTATIONS. Children with severe hemophilia manifest prolonged bleeding times at different ages. Many boys with hemophilia are circumcised without excessive bleeding. Normal hemostasis is achieved in these infants because clotting is activated through the extrinsic coagulation cascade, which does not involve factors VII, IX, or XI.

During the first year of life spontaneous bleeding often is minimal, but hematoma formation may result from immunizations and from firm holding (e.g., under the arms). Many children are diagnosed around the time they become mobile (i.e., crawling, pulling to stand) and become easily injured (i.e., increased bruising, swelling, redness at joints, mouth bleeding). By 3 to 4 years of age, 90% of children with hemophilia have had episodes of persistent bleeding from relatively minor traumatic lacerations (e.g., to the lip or tongue). These episodes are often the first clinical manifestations of hemophilia. Hemorrhage into the joints, elbows, knees, and ankles causes pain and limited joint mobility and predisposes the child to degenerative joint changes. Spontaneous hematuria and epistaxis are troublesome but minor complications. Oral bleeding can occur with dental surgery.

Recurrent bleeding—spontaneous and after minor trauma—is a lifelong problem. Many affected individuals experience cycles of spontaneous bleeding episodes. Intracranial bleeds; bleeding of internal organs; and bleeding into the tissues of the neck, chest, or abdomen are life-threatening. Delayed or suboptimal treatment of these bleeds may lead to permanent brain injury, loss of organ function, or death.

EVALUATION AND TREATMENT. Since hemophilia is most often an inherited disease, a positive family history may expedite a diagnosis of hemophilia. When a suspected carrier mother is expecting, genetic testing in utero through amniocentesis or chorionic villus sampling (CVS) may reveal a hemophilia diagnosis before birth. In the absence of a positive family history, when a bleeding disorder is suspected, personal bleed history, laboratory testing, family history, and physical assessment contribute to a thorough evaluation and accurate diagnosis. In general, those with hemophilia A or B will have a prolonged partial thromboplastin time (PTT) and the prothrombin time (PT) will be normal. An accurate diagnosis is made from factor VIII (hemophilia A) and factor IX (hemophilia B) levels.

The majority of children with hemophilia A (factor VIII deficiency) can be treated with recombinant factor VIII, and the majority of children with hemophilia B (factor IX deficiency) can be treated with recombinant factor IX. Recombinant factor is reconstituted in a small volume of diluent and administered by slow intravenous push, which raises the factor level almost immediately.

Primary prophylaxis consists of regular infusions of factor VIII or IX with the goal of preventing joint bleeding. It is usually given to children with severe hemophilia. A 5-year, multicenter trial, which has now become the standard of care,[53] found prophylaxis initiated in children between 6 and 30 months of age to be effective in the prevention of joint bleeding, structural joint damage, and frequency of bleeding in boys with factor VIII deficiency. Recent multisite trials have demonstrated the safety and efficacy of pegylated, recombinant factors VIII and IX. These pegylated products have extended half-lives and require less frequent dosing.[54,55]

von Willebrand Disease

von Willebrand disease results from an inherited trait with variable clinical manifestations and hematologic findings resulting from a deficiency or dysfunction in von Willebrand factor. von Willebrand factor binds factor VIII and platelets to the blood vessel wall as part of the clotting process. As a result, factor VIII activity is decreased in individuals with von Willebrand disease. Most cases of von Willebrand disease demonstrate an autosomal dominant pattern of inheritance;

however, some cases demonstrate an autosomal recessive or compound heterozygous pattern. The pattern of inheritance depends on the type of mutation that is present.[56]

Congenital Hypercoagulability and Thrombosis

Hereditary bleeding disorders, such as hemophilia, have been recognized and treated for centuries; however, the counterpart of these disorders, thrombophilia, has not been recognized until the past 50 years. The inherited thrombophilic conditions generally are caused by defects in the clotting factors that inhibit clot formation; thus the balance between bleeding and clotting is directed toward the clotting aspects of hemostasis. Although the majority of thrombotic events occurring in children, adolescents, and young adults are believed to be spontaneous, studies are investigating the role of mutations in multiple genes that may contribute to an increased risk of thrombosis. A recent study investigating genetic mutations in 115 adolescents and young adults presenting with thrombotic events identified single gene mutations in two-thirds of this sample, and some individuals had more than one mutation.[57] Ongoing studies are needed to further investigate the specific roles of these mutations.

Defects in specific proteins (C and S) and antithrombin (AT), as well as resistance to activated protein C (APC) and hyperhomocysteinemia, are the major recognized causes of inherited thrombophilia. Both proteins C and S are inhibitors of coagulation and depend on vitamin K for synthesis in the hepatocytes of the liver. Decreased levels of either of these proteins interfere with the normal homeostatic balance of procoagulant and anticoagulant activity at the endothelial level. Protein C and S deficiency states predispose affected individuals to thrombosis, especially venous thrombosis of the lower extremities.

Inheritance of protein C deficiency is autosomal dominant and results from mutations in the *PROC* gene. Its prevalence is approximately 0.2% to 0.4% in the general population. Genetic mutations may result in quantitative (type I) or qualitative (type II) deficiencies of protein C. *Type I deficiencies* involve a reduction in both biologic and immunologic activity of protein C. Type I is caused by deletion of the entire gene. *Type II deficiencies* are less common and result in decreased functional levels of protein C activity despite the presence of a normal level of protein C.[58]

Heterozygotes have protein C levels 50% to 60% of normal and may develop superficial thrombophlebitis, deep venous thrombosis, or pulmonary embolism in their late teens and early 20s. Homozygotes have less than 1% of normal levels of protein C and tend to develop thrombosis of the cutaneous vessels with large areas of skin necrosis. Arterial thrombosis is rare among individuals with protein C deficiency.

Neonatal purpura fulminans is a fatal syndrome found in neonates who are homozygous or double heterozygous for types I and II protein deficiency. Ecchymosis becomes apparent on the first day of life and develops around the head, trunk, and extremities and often is accompanied by cerebral thrombosis and infarction. The ecchymotic areas often coalesce, and ulceration and necrosis develop. Treatment includes administration of fresh frozen plasma (FFP) and heparinization, although the infant rarely survives.

Treatment for protein C deficiency depends on the clinical manifestations. Individuals who are asymptomatic may not require therapy unless a strong family history of thrombosis is present. Heparin is the treatment for acute episodes of thrombosis caused by protein C deficiency. Long-term therapy is required and consists of either oral warfarin sodium (Coumadin) or subcutaneous heparin. Supplemental protein C concentrates (human) also are available and have been approved for use in children.[59]

Protein S deficiency results from mutations in the *PROS1* gene and is similar to protein C deficiency. The inheritance pattern (autosomal dominant) also is similar. The severity of the clinical manifestations can vary, and many affected individuals never develop an abnormal blood clot.[58]

Protein S deficiency exists in three forms: type I, type II, and type III.[60] *Type I* deficiency is identified as a quantitative deficiency and manifests as low levels of total protein S antigen and free protein S antigen. *Type II* deficiency is identified as a qualitative deficiency with normal levels of free and total protein S antigen but reduced protein S activity. *Type III deficiency* results in low free protein S levels; however, the total plasma concentration of protein S is normal. Type III deficiency has not been established as a risk factor for venous or arterial thromboembolism.

Heterozygotes with a more severe deficiency demonstrate a strong tendency for deep venous thrombosis, with the first incidence often occurring before age 25 years. Other manifestations include superficial thrombophlebitis and pulmonary emboli. Although clots may occur spontaneously in individuals with protein S deficiency, risk factors, such as increasing age and immobility, can raise the risk of thrombus formation.

Homozygotes demonstrate severe manifestations of the condition and may develop a form of purpura fulminans in the neonatal period. The homozygous state also may lead to intrauterine death. Treatment with heparin, warfarin (Coumadin), and protein C concentrate is similar to that for protein C deficiency.

Antithrombin III (AT III) deficiency is inherited as an autosomal dominant condition—the heterozygous state is the most common. AT III deficiency results from mutations in the *SERPINC1* gene and exists in forms type I and type II. Type I is a quantitative deficiency of the AT III antigen resulting from decreased production. Type II is characterized by decreased functional activity; normal levels of AT III are present, however, activity is reduced.

Individuals with AT III deficiency are at risk for early development of venous thrombosis and pulmonary embolism. These events often occur in the middle to late teens, but can occur as early as 10 years of age. The deep veins of the lower extremities are usually involved, most commonly the iliofemoral vein. Other sites include the mesenteric veins, vena cava, renal veins, and retinal veins. Cerebral thromboses also have been described, and arterial thrombotic events are rare. In some cases thrombosis is precipitated by surgery, trauma, pregnancy, oral contraceptives, and infection.

The treatment of choice for AT III deficiency is heparin. Antiplatelet agents (e.g., aspirin, dipyridamole) may be used, as well as AT III concentrates.

Antibody-Mediated Hemorrhagic Disease

The antibody-mediated hemorrhagic diseases are a group of disorders caused by the immune response. Antibody-mediated destruction of platelets or antibody-mediated inflammatory reactions to allergens damage blood vessels and cause seepage into tissues. The thrombocytopenic purpuras may be intrinsic or idiopathic, or they may be transient phenomena transmitted from mother to fetus. The inflammatory, or "allergic," purpuras occur in response to allergens in the blood. All these disorders first appear during infancy or childhood.

Primary Immune Thrombocytopenia

Primary immune thrombocytopenia (ITP) (previously referred to as idiopathic thrombocytopenic purpura) is the most common of the thrombocytopenic purpuras of childhood. It is a disorder of platelet consumption in which antiplatelet autoantibodies bind to the plasma membranes of platelets, causing platelet sequestration and destruction by mononuclear phagocytes in the spleen and other lymphoid tissues at a rate that exceeds the ability of the bone marrow to produce them.

The destruction of platelets is triggered by drugs, infections, lymphomas, or an unknown cause.

An international working group of experts updated definitions and terminology for ITP in 2007. The goal of this effort was to reduce heterogeneity across studies and support standardization of reporting patient outcomes.[61] Key outcomes of this effort included distinguishing between primary and secondary ITP, defining the phases of the illness, and establishing criteria for evaluating the response to therapy. Specific phases include *newly diagnosed ITP*, within 3 months of diagnosis; *persistent ITP*, describing individuals with 3 to 12 months of diagnosis who have not achieved remission or complete response off therapy; *chronic ITP*, symptoms lasting longer than 12 months; and *severe ITP*, the presence of bleeding that requires treatment either at diagnosis or following initiation of treatment.

◆**PATHOPHYSIOLOGY.** The autoantibodies that produce the destruction are often of the IgG class and are usually against the platelet membrane glycoproteins (IIb–IIIa or Ib–IX). Approximately 70% of cases of ITP are preceded by a viral disease (e.g., cytomegalovirus [CMV], Epstein-Barr virus [EBV], HIV, parvovirus, or viral respiratory infection), suggesting that viral sensitization has occurred. The typical interval between infection and onset of purpura is 1 to 3 weeks.

◆**CLINICAL MANIFESTATIONS.** One to 3 weeks after a viral infection, bruising and a generalized petechial rash often occur with acute onset. Petechiae can develop into ecchymoses. Asymmetric bleeding is typical and is found most often on the legs and trunk. Hemorrhagic bullae of the gums, lips, and other mucous membranes may be prominent. Epistaxis (nosebleed) may be severe and difficult to control. Except for the signs of bleeding, the child appears well. The principal changes are found in the spleen, bone marrow, and blood.[7] The acute phase of the disease associated with spontaneous hemorrhages lasts 1 to 2 weeks, but thrombocytopenia often persists. Intracranial hemorrhage is the most serious complication of ITP, although the incidence is less than 1%. In some cases, the onset is more gradual and clinical manifestations consist of moderate bruising and scattered petechiae.

◆**EVALUATION AND TREATMENT.** Laboratory examination reveals an isolated low platelet count, and the few platelets observed on a peripheral blood smear are large in size, reflecting increased bone marrow production. The Ivy bleeding time is prolonged. Bone marrow aspiration is not recommended for children with typical features of ITP. The primary treatment for children with ITP is observation regardless of platelet count. When bleeding is present, primary treatment is with an infusion of intravenous immune globulin (IVIG) or a short course of corticosteroids only if thrombocytopenia is severe (suppresses immune attack).

Even without treatment the prognosis for children with ITP is excellent—75% recover completely within 3 months. After the initial acute phase, clinical manifestations typically subside. By 6 months after onset, 80% to 90% of affected children have regained normal platelet counts.[62] ITP that persists longer than 12 months in children is considered chronic and immunosuppressive therapies are utilized.[63,64]

Parents should be instructed to discourage activities that might cause trauma that could result in bleeding (e.g., contact sports, skateboarding, skiing, bicycle riding). Splenectomy should be reserved for chronic cases that fail to respond to nonsurgical intervention.

Autoimmune Neonatal Thrombocytopenias

Antibody-mediated thrombocytopenic purpura occurs in neonates in either autoimmune or alloimmune form. Both forms are characterized by the immunologic destruction of platelets by autoantibodies (IgG) against tissue-specific antigens expressed by the platelets (i.e., platelet-specific antigens).

Autoimmune neonatal thrombocytopenia was first noted in the early 1950s, when it was observed that mothers with ITP often delivered infants who were transiently thrombocytopenic. Neonatal thrombocytopenia was observed in approximately 50% of infants at risk and lasted an average of 1 month. As platelet counts returned to normal, a concomitant drop in the level of maternal antiplatelet antibody on the child's platelets occurred. The antibody is directed against antigens common to maternal and neonatal platelets. The prognosis generally is favorable and the frequency of intracranial hemorrhage is rare (1% to 3% of cases). Medical management of affected infants is to prevent the severe thrombocytopenia that can cause significant morbidity by administering intravenous immunoglobulins.

Neonatal alloimmune thrombocytopenic purpura (NATP) is less common, estimated to occur in 1 to 2 per 1000 live births. NATP is caused by maternal immunization against fetal paternally derived platelet-specific antigens (similar to rhesus [Rh] disease). The mother has a normal platelet count, whereas the fetus can be severely thrombocytopenic.

The diagnosis of NATP is confirmed by detection in the maternal serum of antibody that reacts with platelets from the infant and father but not with platelets from the mother. In approximately 75% to 85% of cases, NATP recurs in subsequent pregnancies. Purpura usually develops in the affected infant shortly after delivery, and intracranial, renal, and gastrointestinal hemorrhages are possible. The mortality rate from intracranial hemorrhage has been estimated at 10% to 15%. Management of the newborn with NATP includes an immediate cranial ultrasound because of the significant risk of intracranial hemorrhage. Severely thrombocytopenic newborns (<10,000/μL) or newborns with intracranial or visceral hemorrhages should receive a matched platelet transfusion (maternal or homozygous human platelet antigen 1b [HPA-1b] donor) as soon as possible. If maternal platelets are used, they must be processed to remove platelet alloantibodies. Newborn thrombocytopenia is difficult to predict because newborn platelet counts do not correlate with maternal platelet counts or antiplatelet antibody titers.[65]

Most of the life-threatening clinical manifestations of transient neonatal thrombocytopenia and NATP can be avoided through cesarean delivery. If the mother has antiplatelet disease, however, surgery can result in hemorrhage and serious maternal morbidity. Maternal morbidity resulting from NATP during pregnancy is low (less than 5%): the principal maternal risk is bleeding from surgical incisions during cesarean delivery. The incidence of transient thrombocytopenia in infants born to mothers with NATP is about 50%. If all deliveries were cesarean, half the mothers would undergo cesarean delivery unnecessarily. Conversely, if all deliveries were vaginal, half the infants—those with thrombocytopenia—would be at risk for intracranial bleeding. Therefore in the absence of any clear benefit to the neonate (given the low rate of intracranial hemorrhage in infants born to mothers with ITP), cesarean delivery should be reserved for the usual obstetric indications.

Autoimmune Vascular Purpura

Autoimmune vascular purpura (allergic purpura) is caused by antibody-mediated injury of blood vessel walls, typically arterioles and capillaries. The inflammatory reaction is to foreign proteins or chemicals in the blood (microorganisms, drugs, or other chemicals).

Autoimmune vascular purpura usually is seen in young children, with the incidence decreasing in adolescents and adults and occurring only rarely in older adults. The average age at onset is 5 years, with a slightly higher proportion of males affected. Purpura occurs as vessel integrity is disrupted by inflammatory processes, causing effusion of serosanguineous exudate to perivascular tissues.

Clinical manifestations include headache, anorexia, fever, abdominal pain, constipation, arthralgias and urticaria, and erythema that are located symmetrically on the proximal portions of the extremities, particularly on the legs and buttocks, and may be accompanied by itching or paresthesias. Abdominal pain results from hemorrhage into the bowel, which may lead to colic, nausea, and vomiting. These symptoms may precede the appearance of skin lesions. The pain usually is midabdominal but may radiate to other parts of the abdomen. Joint pain and tenderness may be present, but hemarthrosis does not occur. Periarticular swelling and edema of the hands and feet are common and may precede the onset of abdominal pain and purpura. Subacute glomerulonephritis occurs in some cases but usually is reversible.

The characteristic skin lesions (purpura and cutaneous manifestations of allergy), accompanied by a history of joint and abdominal pain, are suspicious for diagnosis. Laboratory test results often reveal no major abnormalities. Attacks may last several weeks and may recur at odd intervals and with changing manifestations with each episode. Treatment, if necessary, consists of symptom management.

NEOPLASTIC DISORDERS

Leukemia

Leukemia is cancer of the blood-forming tissues, such as the bone marrow, that most often produce abnormal white blood cells called *leukemic cells*. Once in the blood, leukemic cells can spread to other organs, such as the lymph nodes, spleen, and brain. Leukemia is the most common malignancy of children and adolescents. Of the varieties of acute childhood leukemia, 75% to 80% of leukemias in children are *acute lymphoblastic leukemia (ALL)* or *acute leukemia of ambiguous lineage*. The remaining 20% to 25% are classified as *acute myeloid leukemia (AML)* and *related neoplasms*. The related neoplasms include acute promyelocytic, myelomonocytic, and myelomonoblastic leukemias, as well as the very rare RBC leukemia erythroid leukemia.[66] Chronic leukemias are rare in children and account for fewer than 5% of cases. Leukemia accounts for 25% of cases of cancer in black children and 34% of cases of cancer in white children.

In the United States, 75% of all cases of ALL are diagnosed in individuals less than 20 years of age, and the peak incidence for childhood ALL is between 2 and 6 years of age.[67,68] A sharp peak in ALL incidence is reported among children aged 2 to 3 years (>90 cases per 1 million per year), and rates decrease to fewer than 30 cases per million by age 8 years. Since 1975, there has been a gradual increase in the incidence of ALL.[68] New leukemia cases have been rising on average 0.3% a year in the last 10 years.[69] ALL affects more white and Hispanic than black children and more males than females. The incidence of ALL also is higher in Western and industrialized nations.[67]

Types of Leukemia

A number of different classifications are used for the leukemias. First, acute leukemia is differentiated from chronic leukemia. Second, the cell line determines whether lymphoid cells or myeloid cells are involved. In acute leukemia this difference separates ALL from AML and vice versa. Within each of these categories, further subdivisions have been developed. (See Chapter 30 for a discussion of leukemias in adults.)

Cytogenic studies of leukemic cells are performed routinely at most major treatment centers during the diagnostic process. Abnormal morphologic characteristics, as well as abnormalities in the number of copies of chromosomes, are often found in leukemic cells. Hyperdiploidy (the presence of greater than the diploid [46] number of chromosomes) is associated with a good prognosis. Common translocations associated with ALL are TEL-AML1, MLL rearrangements, and BCR-ABL. TEL-AML1 is the most common abnormality (in 20% to 30% of cases) and occurs when the *TEL* gene on chromosome 12p13 fuses with the

AML1 gene on chromosome 21q22. TEL-AML1 is associated with a favorable outcome. MLL rearrangements are translocations between the *MLL* gene on chromosome 11q23 and other partner chromosomes. One of the most noted MLL rearrangements involves chromosome 4 as the partner chromosome t(4;11). This specific MLL rearrangement occurs most frequently among leukemia in infants less than 1 year of age and is associated with a poor prognosis despite intensive therapy.[70] A translocation involving the long arms of chromosomes 9 and 22, t(9;22)(q34;q11), also described as the Philadelphia chromosome, occurs in more than 95% of cases of chronic myeloid leukemia (CML) and in only 2% to 3% of cases of ALL.[66] The specific breakpoint varies in CML and ALL. The translocation results in the generation of the *BCR-ABL* fusion gene and the bcr-abl protein results in unregulated tyrosine kinase activity.

Classification of childhood leukemia has become a complex but essential process to determine treatment. Previous classification by the French-American-British Cooperative Group (FAB) was based primarily on the morphologic and biochemical system. A classification scheme developed by the World Health Organization (WHO) is based on a more comprehensive system that uses morphology, immunophenotyping, and cytogenic and clinical features.[66]

Flow cytometric immunophenotyping has made distinguishing between lymphoblastic and nonlymphoblastic leukemia much easier than in the past, when the degree of immaturity of the cell sometimes made such distinction difficult. Molecular cytogenetic techniques, such as fluorescence in situ hybridization (FISH), allow for further detection of specific genetic abnormalities associated with leukemia subtypes.

Immunologic classification has been used on identification of various surface markers. Categories of ALL have been identified on the basis of their presumed origin from thymic cells (T cells) and bursa-equivalent cells (B cells) of normal lymphocytes:

1. T-cell ALL—characterized by the presence of abnormal T lymphocytes and found more commonly in adolescent boys whose initial presentation often includes mediastinal masses, high white blood cell counts, and hepatosplenomegaly (15% to 20% of ALL)
2. Mature B-cell ALL—also called *Burkitt leukemia*; characterized by the presence of abnormal B lymphoblasts and associated with a poor prognosis (5% of ALL)
3. B-precursor ALL—characterized by the presence of pre-B lymphoblasts (80% to 85% of ALL); this category includes the pro-B (3% to 4%), early pre-B (60% to 70%), and pre-B (20% to 30%)
4. Acute leukemia of ambiguous lineage—includes acute undifferentiated leukemia and mixed phenotype acute leukemia (less than 5% of ALL)

◆ETIOLOGY. The cause of most childhood cancer is unknown. About 5% of all childhood cancers are caused by inherited mutations. Genetic mutations can occur during fetal development. Examples of genetic diseases that predispose a child to ALL include Down syndrome, neurofibromatosis, Fanconi anemia, Bloom syndrome, Li-Fraumeni syndrome, and ataxia-telangiectasia.[71] Genetic disorders associated with AML include Down syndrome, Fanconi anemia, neurofibromatosis type 1, Noonan syndrome, and Shwachman-Diamond syndrome. AML in children is sometimes associated with loss or deletion of chromosome 7 in the leukemia cells. AML can develop from preexisting myeloproliferative disorders that also are preleukemia syndromes (i.e., myelodysplastic syndrome). Epigenetic modifications, including DNA methylation, have been proposed as mediating events between environmental exposures and subsequent disease development.[72]

Many studies have shown that exposure to ionizing radiation (prenatal exposure to x-rays and postnatal exposure to high doses of radiation) can lead to the development of childhood leukemia.[71] There is recent concern about performing computed tomography (CT) scans in children because increased use combined with wide variability in radiation doses has resulted in many children receiving a high dose of radiation.[73] Studies of other possible environmental risk factors, including parental exposure to cancer-causing chemicals, prenatal exposure to pesticides, childhood exposure to common infectious agents, and environmental exposure to a nuclear power plant, have so far produced inconsistent results. Higher risks of cancer have not been seen in children of individuals treated for sporadic cancer (cancer not caused by an inherited mutation).[74,75]

The occurrence of leukemia in monozygotic twins is estimated as being as high as 25%. In 2006, the Office of the U.S. Surgeon General suggested evidence of a causal relationship between childhood leukemia, lymphoma, and brain tumors and prenatal or postnatal environmental tobacco smoke exposure.[76] A French case-control study failed to identify an association between maternal smoking and childhood leukemia; however, paternal preconception smoking was associated with an increased risk of both ALL and AML.[77] Likewise, an Italian case-control study demonstrated an association between paternal smoking and AML; however, an increased risk was not demonstrated for ALL. An association between maternal smoking and an increased risk of leukemia was not observed.[78,79] The pooled analysis of the Childhood Leukemia International Consortium (CLIC1974-2012) suggests an association between paternal smoking and childhood AML.[80] Exposure to both alcohol and cigarette smoke is associated with AML. Being Hispanic increases the risk of AML.[81]

Prenatal exposure to pesticides is hypothesized to increase the risk of childhood leukemia by resulting in oxidative stress leading to the generation of free radicals that induce breaks in the DNA of early hematopoietic stem cells.[82] Results of recent meta-analyses support associations between parental exposure to pesticides and other potential environmental toxins before or during pregnancy and subsequent development of childhood leukemia.[83,84]

Chemicals such as benzene have been associated with the development of AML in adults. A recent meta-analysis provides evidence of a possible association between benzene exposure and childhood leukemia.[85] Previous treatment with chemotherapy is a risk factor for developing ALL.[71]

Leukemic "clusters" that represent a greater number of leukemia cases occurring in a particular geographic location have raised speculation about environmental factors or infectious patterns of transmission. Careful follow-up, however, has failed to document the abnormal clustering.[86-88]

◆**PATHOPHYSIOLOGY.** Acute lymphoblastic leukemia (ALL) is composed of immature B (pre-B) or T (pre-T) cells called *lymphoblasts.* The bone marrow is dense with lymphoblasts, considered hypercellular, that replace the normal marrow and disrupt normal function. Many of the chromosomal abnormalities documented in ALL cause dysregulation of the expression and function of transcription factors required for normal B-cell and T-cell development.[7] The mutations can include both gain of function and loss of function that are required for normal development.

Acute myeloid leukemia (AML) is caused by acquired oncogenic mutations that impair differentiation, resulting in the accumulation of immature myeloid blasts in the marrow and other organs. Epigenetic alterations are frequent in AML and have a central role. The bone marrow crowding by blasts produces marrow failure and complications, including anemia, thrombocytopenia, and neutropenia. AML is very heterogeneous because myeloid cell differentiation is very complex. To be called *acute,* the bone marrow usually must include greater than 20% leukemic blasts.

◆**CLINICAL MANIFESTATIONS.** The onset may be abrupt or insidious, but the most common symptoms reflect the consequences of bone marrow failure: decreased levels of RBCs and platelets and changes in white blood cells. Pallor, fatigue, petechiae, purpura, bleeding, and fever

generally are present. Approximately 45% of children have a hemoglobin level less than 7 g/dL; in contrast to adults, children seem to demonstrate fewer symptoms. If acute blood loss occurs, however, characteristic symptoms of tachycardia, air hunger, restlessness, and thirst may be present. Epistaxis, excessive bruising, and hematuria may occur in children with severe thrombocytopenia. Three-quarters of children with ALL have platelet counts less than $100,000/mm^3$ at diagnosis, and 28% have platelet counts less than $20,000/mm^3$. Half of all children newly diagnosed with AML have platelet counts less than $50,000/mm^3$. Disseminated intravascular coagulation occurs more commonly with AML, particularly with promyelocytic leukemia. The granules in the leukemic promyelocytes likely possess thromboplastin activity.

Fever usually is present as a result of two causes: (1) infection associated with the decrease in functional neutrophils and (2) hypermetabolism associated with the ongoing rapid growth and destruction of leukemic cells. In most children with ALL, the total white blood count at diagnosis is less than $10,000/mm^3$, and with AML most present with white cell counts less than $50,000/mm^3$. In a few children, however, the peripheral white blood count at presentation may be greater than $100,000/mm^3$. White blood cell counts greater than $200,000/mm^3$ can cause leukostasis, an intravascular clumping of cells that results in infarction and hemorrhage, usually in the brain and lung. The three most important favorable prognostic factors are age at diagnosis (2 to 10 years), initial leukocyte count ($<50,000/mm^3$), and initial response to treatment.

Renal failure as a result of hyperuremia (high uric acid levels) can be associated with ALL, particularly at diagnosis or during active treatment. Uric acid levels rise as an end product of purine metabolism from cellular destruction. Because the major excretory pathway is through the kidney, urates can precipitate in renal tubules or ureters and can lead to oliguria and acute renal failure. Renal failure is preventable if uric acid levels are monitored and treatment is aimed at optimal hydration, alkalinization of urine to assist with the excretion of soluble urates, and blockage of further uric acid formation by administration of the drug allopurinol.

Extramedullary invasion with leukemic cells can occur in nearly all body tissue. Most children with ALL have some extramedullary involvement at diagnosis. Leukemic invasion of tissue other than bone marrow is believed to represent metastatic infiltration. Hepatosplenomegaly and lymphadenopathy, resulting from extramedullary hematopoiesis, occur in nearly half of children with ALL, but they are less common in children with AML.

The central nervous system (CNS) is a common site of infiltration of extramedullary leukemia, although less than 10% of children with ALL have CNS involvement at diagnosis. CNS infiltration manifests later in the course of the disease. Because successful chemotherapy prolongs the time of remission, the incidence of CNS involvement has increased. The most common symptoms of CNS involvement relate to increased intracranial pressure, causing early morning headaches, nausea, vomiting, irritability, and lethargy.

Gonadal involvement, with testicular and ovarian infiltration, has been demonstrated in postmortem examination in 57% and 35% of children, respectively. Clinical detection of gonadal involvement is much less frequent. The incidence of testicular involvement, like CNS involvement, has increased with lengthened duration of remission.

Leukemic infiltration into bones and joints is common in children. Reports of bone or joint pain actually lead to the diagnosis of leukemia in some children. In most children bone pain is characterized as migratory, vague, and without areas of swelling or inflammation. If joint pain is the primary symptom and some swelling is associated with the pain, however, misdiagnoses of rheumatoid arthritis may occur.

Other organs reported to be sites of leukemic invasion include the kidneys, heart, lungs, thymus, eyes, skin, and gastrointestinal tract. Of these, the kidneys, lungs, and gastrointestinal tract are the most frequently reported sites. Skin involvement is more common in AML than in ALL.

◆**EVALUATION AND TREATMENT.** The diagnosis of leukemia is made from blood tests and examination of peripheral blood smears. A bone marrow aspiration is usually performed to further characterize the leukemia. The blast cell is the hallmark of acute leukemia (see Fig. E 31.1 on Evolve). The blast cell is a relatively undifferentiated cell characterized by diffusely distributed nuclear chromatin, with one or more nucleoli and basophilic cytoplasm (see Fig. E 31.2 on Evolve).

Healthy children have less than 5% blast cells in the bone marrow and none in the peripheral blood. The bone marrow is categorized on the basis of blast percentage. In ALL the bone marrow often is replaced by 80% to 100% blast cells, with a reduction in normally developing RBCs and granulocytes. The marrow, which is considered hypercellular, is composed of a homogeneous population of cells. Occasionally, however, the marrow appears hypocellular, making the diagnosis difficult to differentiate from aplastic anemia. When this occurs, bone marrow biopsy or biopsy of extramedullary sites is necessary to confirm the diagnosis.

Remarkable success has occurred with treatment of ALL in children. Chemotherapy is the treatment of choice for acute leukemia. Radiation has special considerations for use. In ALL, identification of various risk groups has led to the development of different intensities of drug protocols. Thus treatment is tailored specifically for a particular risk group.

Treatment of the CNS, usually with intrathecal medication, is part of most pediatric acute leukemia protocols.[71,81] CNS irradiation is used only in selected cases of ALL. For children with AML, CNS irradiation is not necessary either as prophylaxis or for those presenting with cerebrospinal fluid leukemia that clears with intrathecal and systemic chemotherapy.[71]

Chronic myelogenous leukemia accounts for less than 5% of childhood leukemia. Biologically targeted therapies, specifically tyrosine kinase inhibitors, are becoming the mainstay of treatment, specifically for individuals with the BCR/ABL translocation.[89]

Lymphomas

Lymphomas are malignant proliferations that arise from discrete tissue masses.[7] These neoplasms involve some recognizable stage of lymphocyte B- or T-cell differentiation. Emerging is the understanding that some lymphomas occasionally have leukemic presentations and evolution to "leukemia" is not unusual during the progression of incurable "lymphomas." Therefore the terms merely reflect the usual tissue distribution.[7] Much controversy has surrounded the classifications of lymphoma and a consensus has been reached with the current World Health Organization (WHO) classification scheme found at www.cancer.gov/cancertopics/pdq/treatment/adult-non-hodgkins/HealthProfessional/page3. Non-Hodgkin lymphoma (NHL) and Hodgkin lymphoma (HL) constitute approximately 11% of all cases of childhood cancer. Approximately 2200 cases of lymphoma are diagnosed in children and adolescents less than 20 years of age in the United States annually.[67] Either group of diseases is rare before age 5 years, and the relative incidence increases throughout childhood and adolescence. NHL (including Burkitt lymphoma) occurs more often than HL in children. Boys are more likely to be diagnosed with a malignant lymphoma than are girls. The incidence of lymphoma is increased in children with congenital immunodeficiency syndromes such as Wiskott-Aldrich syndrome, severe combined immunodeficiency (SCID), X-linked lymphoproliferative disease, and ataxia-telangiectasia. An increased incidence of NHL also is associated with immunosuppression after solid organ and stem cell transplants, particularly T-cell–depleted stem

cell transplantation. The strongest association between viruses and the development of cancer in children has been the EBV, Burkitt lymphoma, and HL. Children with AIDS have an increased risk of developing NHL. However, with the use of highly active antiretroviral therapy in the developed world, the incidence of AIDS-related malignancies has declined dramatically.[90]

Non-Hodgkin Lymphoma

Non-Hodgkin lymphomas (NHLs) are neoplasms of immune cells. NHLs are diverse and include a large group of tumors; some are slow growing (indolent) and others are fast growing and aggressive. Almost without exception, childhood NHL becomes evident as a diffuse disease and can be further subdivided into three major types: (1) mature B-cell NHL (Burkitt and Burkitt-like lymphoma, Burkitt leukemia, and diffuse large B-cell lymphoma), (2) lymphoblastic lymphoma, and (3) anaplastic large cell lymphoma.[91] The common types of NHL in children are different than those in adults. The most common types of NHL in children are Burkitt lymphoma (40%), lymphoblastic lymphoma (25% to 30%), and large cell lymphoma (10%). Little data have been published on the etiology of childhood NHL. Known risk factors include Epstein-Barr virus (EBV) with most cases in the immunodeficient population, congenital and acquired immunodeficiency, and after a previous (subsequent to treatment) neoplasm (is rare in the child population).

◆**PATHOPHYSIOLOGY.** Burkitt lymphoma will be discussed as an example of pathogenesis of NHL in children. All forms of Burkitt lymphoma are associated with translocations of the MYC gene on chromosome 8 that lead to increased MYC protein levels.[7] MYC is a transcriptional regulator that increases the expression of genes required for aerobic glycolysis, called the *Warburg effect* (see Chapter 12). Most Burkitt lymphomas are latently infected with the Epstein-Barr virus (EBV).[7] EBV also is present in about 25% of HIV-associated tumors and 15% to 20% of sporadic cases.[7] There is increased evidence of NHL in children with congenital immunodeficiency syndromes, such as Wiskott-Aldrich syndrome, ataxia-telangiectasia, and Bloom syndrome.

◆**CLINICAL MANIFESTATIONS.** NHL has been found to arise from any lymphoid tissue. Signs and symptoms therefore are specific for the site involved. Some children have such widespread involvement that no original site can be determined. Because some childhood NHL is rapidly progressive, symptoms are typically present only a few weeks before diagnosis is made. Rapidly enlarging lymphoid tissue and painless lymphadenopathy are common in about one-third of children with abdominal sites of involvement, usually representing a gastrointestinal origin for the disease. Symptoms often include abdominal pain and vomiting, but a palpable mass is not always present. The other common site of childhood NHL is the chest region. Overall, associated signs of NHL include swelling of the lymph nodes in the neck, underarm, stomach, or groin; trouble swallowing; painless lump or swelling in a testicle; weight loss for unknown reason; night sweats; and possibly trouble breathing. Involvement of facial bones, particularly the jaw, is common in African Burkitt lymphoma.

◆**EVALUATION AND TREATMENT.** Diagnosis is made by physical examination and health history, followed by biopsy of disease sites, usually the involved lymph nodes, tonsils, bone marrow, spleen, liver, bowel, or skin. Burkitt lymphoma is very aggressive and responds well to treatment. Most children and young adults can be cured with intensive chemotherapy.

Hodgkin Lymphoma

Hodgkin lymphoma (HL) is a group of lymphoid neoplasms that, unlike NHL, arises in a single chain of lymph nodes and spreads first in a contiguous way to lymphoid tissue. NHL typically arises at extranodal

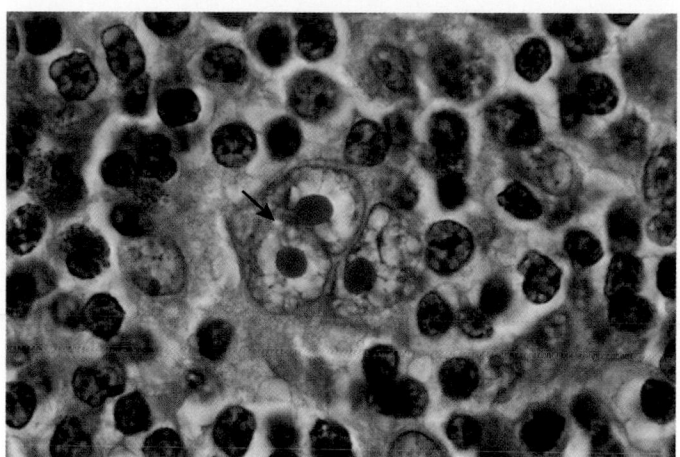

FIGURE 31.10 Diagnostic Reed-Sternberg Cell. A large multinucleated or multilobated cell with inclusion body–like nucleoli *(arrow)* surrounded by a halo of clear nucleoplasm. (From Damjanov I, Linder J: *Pathology: a color atlas*, St Louis, 2000, Mosby.)

sites and spreads in a noncontiguous or unpredictable manner. HL is characterized by the presence of Reed-Sternberg cells, which are large cells that come from the germinal center of B cells (Fig. 31.10). HL is a common type of cancer in young adults and adolescents but rare in childhood. The World Health Organization (WHO) has identified five types of HL: (1) nodular sclerosis, (2) mixed cellularity, (3) lymphocyte

rich, (4) lymphocyte depletion, and (5) lymphocyte predominance. Similar expression of Reed-Sternberg cells occurs in the first four types; therefore they are considered the *classic* types. In the lymphocyte predominance type, the Reed-Sternberg cell is distinctive but different than the others. Risk factors for HL include having EBV, being infected with HIV or other immunologic disorders (immunodeficiencies, autoimmune lymphoproliferative syndrome), having a personal history of mononucleosis, and having a parent or sibling with a personal history of HL.[92] HL accounts for 6% of all childhood cancers with a significant male-to-female dominance of 4:1 in young children. HL occurs infrequently among children younger than 2 years with relatively few cases observed before age 5 years. A gradual rise in incidence occurs through age 11 years, with a marked increase through adolescence that continues into the 30s.

Individuals typically have painless supraclavicular or cervical adenopathy. These nodes are firm and rubbery and may be sensitive to palpation if they have grown rapidly. At least two-thirds of individuals have mediastinal involvement that may cause symptoms ranging from a nonproductive cough to tracheal or bronchial compression leading to airway obstruction. Systemic symptoms may include fatigue, anorexia, weight loss, fever, drenching night sweats, and pruritus.

The Ann Arbor staging system considers extent and location of disease, as well as substage classifications that consider systemic symptoms (presence of fever of 38°C [100.4°F] for 3 consecutive days, drenching night sweats, or unexplained loss of 10% or more of body weight in the 6 months preceding diagnosis), extranodal manifestations, or bulky disease. Combination chemotherapy used with or without low-dose radiation has been shown to be an effective treatment, with long-term cure rates reported from 90% to 95%.[67]

SUMMARY REVIEW

Fetal and Neonatal Hematopoiesis

1. After 2 weeks of gestation, circulating erythrocytes play a major role in delivering oxygen to embryonal tissues.
2. Erythropoiesis in the liver and, to a lesser extent, in the spleen and lymph nodes reaches a peak at about 4 months of gestation.
3. By the fifth month of gestation, hematopoiesis begins to occur in the bone marrow, and by the time of delivery it is the only significant site of hematopoiesis.
4. Embryonal (Gower 1, Gower 2, and Portland) and fetal (HbF) hemoglobins are biochemically distinct from adult hemoglobin (HbA and HbA_2). They are composed of two α- and two γ-chains of polypeptides and have a greater affinity for oxygen.
5. Production of adult hemoglobin begins at approximately 16 to 20 weeks of gestation. Hemoglobin in the average term neonate is approximately 70% HbF, 29% HbA, and 1% HbA_2.

Postnatal Changes in the Blood

1. Blood cell counts tend to rise above adult levels at birth and then decline gradually throughout childhood.
2. The immediate postnatal rise in blood cell counts is the result of increased hematopoiesis during fetal life, trauma of birth, and cutting of the umbilical cord.
3. Polycythemia in the term neonate is the result of accelerated erythropoiesis during fetal life that is stimulated by the hypoxic intrauterine environment.
4. Erythrocyte values are age-dependent, and differences in values between males and females are apparent in adolescence.

5. The lymphocyte count is high at birth, and continues to rise in some healthy infants during the first year of life.
6. Platelet counts in full-term neonates are comparable to platelet counts in children and adults.

Disorders of Erythrocytes

1. Iron deficiency anemia (IDA) is the most common blood disorder of infancy and childhood; the highest incidence occurs between 6 months and 2 years of age.
2. Hemolytic disease of the fetus and newborn (HDFN) results from incompatibility between the maternal and the fetal blood, which may involve differences in Rh factors or blood type (ABO). Maternal antibodies enter the fetal circulation and cause hemolysis of fetal erythrocytes. Because the immature liver is unable to conjugate and excrete the excess bilirubin that results from the hemolysis, icterus neonatorum, or kernicterus, or both can develop.
3. Kernicterus, which may result from other causes of hyperbilirubinemia as well as HDFN, is the deposition of excess bilirubin in the brain.
4. Infections of the newborn, often acquired by the mother and transmitted to the infant, may result in hemolytic anemia; the mechanism is unclear.
5. Glucose-6-phosphate dehydrogenase (G6PD) deficiency is an inherited enzyme deficiency in erythrocytes that impairs the ability of RBCs to protect themselves against oxidative stress injuries that lead to hemolysis.
6. Hereditary spherocytosis is the most common of the hereditary hemolytic states in which there is no abnormality of hemoglobin.

SUMMARY REVIEW—cont'd

The basic defect is an undefined abnormality of the proteins or spectrins of the erythrocyte membrane in which affected cells are unduly permeable to sodium and acquire a characteristic structure.

7. Sickle cell disease (SCD) is an autosomal recessive condition resulting in defects in the β-globin units of the hemoglobin molecule. Conditions resulting in decreased oxygen tension result in polymerization of the abnormal hemoglobin, causing the RBC to take on the characteristic sickled shape. SCD is most common among Africans, blacks, and those of Mediterranean descent.

8. The thalassemias are a heterogeneous group of hereditary microcytic-hypochromic anemias of varying severity. The genetic defects cause an impaired synthesis of one of the two chains—α or β—of adult hemoglobin (HbA). The thalassemias are further classified based on the severity of the anemia, type of mutation present, and whether the individual is heterozygous or homozygous for the given mutation.

Disorders of Coagulation and Platelets

1. Hemophilias A and B are characterized by hereditary deficiencies in coagulation factors resulting in a decreased ability to form blood clots in response to injury. Because transmission is X-linked recessive, hemophilia occurs almost exclusively in males.

2. von Willebrand disease is an autosomal dominant condition characterized by prolonged bleeding, resulting from a deficiency or dysfunction in von Willebrand factor, which binds factor VIII and platelets to the blood vessel wall as part of the clotting process.

3. Hereditary disorders of congenital hypercoagulability and thrombosis include protein C deficiency, protein S deficiency, and antithrombin III deficiency. Genetic mutations may result in quantitative (type I) or qualitative (type II) deficiencies of the given clotting factor.

4. Immune thrombocytopenia (ITP), the most common of the childhood antibody-mediated hemorrhagic diseases, is a disorder of platelet consumption in which antiplatelet antibodies bind to the plasma membranes of platelets. This results in platelet sequestration and destruction by mononuclear phagocytes at a rate that exceeds the ability of the bone marrow to produce them.

5. Antibody-mediated neonatal thrombocytopenia can occur as either an autoimmune or an alloimmune disorder.

6. The autoimmune vascular purpuras (allergic purpuras) occur as an inflammatory reaction to foreign proteins or chemicals in the blood.

Neoplastic Disorders

1. Leukemia is the most common malignancy of childhood and adolescence, with a peak incidence in children between 2 and 6 years of age. More than 95% of childhood leukemia cases are acute leukemia.

2. Although the cause of childhood leukemia is not known, it is probably the result of multiple interactions between hereditary or genetic predisposition and environmental influences.

3. Acute lymphoblastic leukemia is a potentially curable disease, with more than 85% of cases cured.

4. The lymphomas of childhood are non-Hodgkin lymphoma and Hodgkin lymphoma.

5. Non-Hodgkin lymphoma is a diverse group of tumors. Factors that have been implicated in the development of non-Hodgkin lymphoma include defective host immunity, a viral agent, chronic immunostimulation, and genetic predisposition.

6. The risk of Hodgkin lymphoma is associated in part with infectious diseases, immune deficits, and genetic susceptibility.

7. The incidence of Hodgkin lymphoma increases during adolescence. Approximately 90% to 95% of individuals who develop Hodgkin lymphoma will be cured.

KEY TERMS

Acute chest syndrome, 1003
α-Globin, 1005
α-Thalassemia, 1005
α-Thalassemia major, 1006
α-Thalassemia minor, 1006
α trait, 1006
Antithrombin III (AT III) deficiency, 1008
Aplastic crisis, 1004
Autoimmune neonatal thrombocytopenia, 1009
Autoimmune vascular purpura (allergic purpura), 1009
β-Globin, 1000
β-Thalassemia, 1004
Blast cell, 1012
Cholecystitis, 1004
Embryonic hemoglobin (Gower 1, Gower 2, Portland), 993
Erythroblastosis fetalis, 998
Fetal hemoglobin (HbF), 993
Glomerular disease, 1004
Glucose-6-phosphate dehydrogenase (G6PD) deficiency, 999

Hemolytic disease of the fetus and newborn (HDFN), 996
Hemophilia A (classic hemophilia, factor VIII deficiency), 1007
Hemophilia B (Christmas disease, factor IX deficiency), 1007
Hereditary spherocytosis (HS), 1000
Hodgkin lymphoma (HL), 1012
Hydrops fetalis, 998
Hyperdiploidy, 1010
Hyperbilirubinemia, 998
Hyperhemolytic crisis, 1004
Icterus gravis neonatorum, 998
Icterus neonatorum (neonatal jaundice), 998
Immune thrombocytopenia (ITP; idiopathic thrombocytopenic purpura), 1008
Kernicterus, 998
Lymphoma, 1012
Microvascular occlusion, 1001
Neonatal alloimmune thrombocytopenic purpura (NATP), 1009
Neonatal purpura fulminans, 1008

Non-Hodgkin lymphoma (NHL), 1012
Philadelphia chromosome, 1010
Polymerization, 1001
Protein C deficiency, 1008
Protein S deficiency, 1008
Prothrombin time (PT), 1007
S1P level, 1001
Sequestration crisis, 1004
Sickle cell anemia (SCA, HbSS), 1001
Sickle cell disease (SCD), 1000
Sickle cell trait (HbAS), 1001
Spherocyte, 1000
Thalassemia, 1004
Thalassemia intermedia, 1004
Thalassemia major (Cooley anemia), 1004
Thrombophilia, 1008
Vaso-occlusive crisis (pain crisis), 1003
von Willebrand disease, 1007

REFERENCES

1. Christensen RD, et al: Reference intervals for reticulocyte parameters of infants during their first 90 days after birth. *J Perinatol* 36:61–66, 2016.
2. Nagaoka H: Immunization and infection change the number of recombination activating gene1 (Rag) expressing B cells in the periphery by altering immature lymphocyte production. *J Exp Med* 191:2113–2120, 2000.
3. Schmutz N, et al: Expected ranges for blood neutrophil concentrations of neonates: the Manroe and Mouzinho charts revisited. *J Perinatol* 28:275–281, 2008.
4. Lim EM, et al: Race-specific WBC and neutrophil count reference intervals. *Int J Lab Hematol* 32(6 Pt 2):590–597, 2010.

5. Aldrimer M, et al: Population-based pediatric reference intervals for hematology, iron and transferrin. *Scand J Clin Lab Invest* 73:253–261, 2013.

6. Christensen RD, et al: Reference ranges for blood concentrations of eosinophils and monocytes during the neonatal period defined from over 63,000 records in a multihospital health-care system. *J Perinatol* 30:540–545, 2010.

7. Kumar V, Abbas AK, Aster JC: *Robbins and Cotran pathologic basis of disease*, ed 9, Philadelphia, 2015, Elsevier Saunders.

8. Jo J, et al: Review article: role of cellular immunity in cow's milk allergy: pathogenesis, tolerance induction, and beyond. *Mediators Inflamm* 2014: 249784, 2014.

9. Paoletti G, Bogen DL, Ritchey AK: Severe iron-deficiency anemia still an issue in toddlers. *Clin Pediatr (Phila)* 53(14):1352–1358, 2014.

10. Baker RD, Greer FR, Committee on Nutrition American Academy of Pediatrics: Clinical report–diagnosis and prevention of iron deficiency and iron-deficiency anemia in infants and young children (0-3 years of age). *Pediatrics* 126: 1040–1150, 2010.

11. Suchdev PS, Pena-Rosas JP, De-Regil LM: Multiple micronutrient powders for home (point-of-use) fortification in pregnant women. *Cochrane Database Syst Rev* (6):CD011158, 2015.

12. Beutler E, et al: Polymorphisms and mutations of human TMPRSS6 in iron deficiency anemia. *Blood Cells Mol Dis* 44(1):16–21, 2010.

13. West AR, Oates PS: Mechanisms of heme iron absorption: current questions and controversies. *World J Gastroenterol* 14(26):4101–4110, 2008.

14. Gheibi SH, et al: Refractory iron deficiency anemia and *Helicobacter pylori* infection in pediatrics: a review. *Iran J Ped Hematol Oncol* 5(1):50–64, 2015.

15. Cancelo-Hidalgo MJ, et al: Tolerability of different oral iron supplements: a systematic review. *Curr Med Res Opin* 29(4):291–303, 2013.

16. Lopez A, et al: Iron deficiency anaemia. *Lancet* 387(10021):907–916, 2016.

17. Zipursky A, Bhutani VK: Impact of Rhesus disease on the global problem of bilirubin-induced neurologic dysfunction. *Semin Fetal Neonatal Med* 20(1):2–5, 2015.

18. Delaney M, Matthews DC: Hemolytic disease of the fetus and newborn: managing the mother, fetus, and newborn. *Hematology Am Soc Hematol Educ Program* 2015:146–151, 2015.

19. Qureshi H, et al: BCSH guideline for the use of anti-D immunoglobulin for the prevention of haemolytic disease of the fetus and newborn. *Transfus Med* 24(1):8–20, 2014.

20. Lamola AA, Russo M: Fluorescence excitation spectrum of bilirubin in blood: a model for the action spectrum for phototherapy of neonatal jaundice. *Photochem Photobiol* 90(2):294–296, 2014.

21. Lacroix J, Tucci M, DuPont-Thibodeau G: Red blood cell transfusion decision making in critically ill children. *Curr Opin Pediatr* 27(3):286–291, 2015.

22. Luzzatto L, Seneca E: G6PD deficiency: a classic example of pharmacogenetics with on-going clinical implications. *Br J Haematol* 164(4): 469–480, 2014.

23. Christensen RD, Yaish HM, Gallagher PG: A pediatrician's practical guide to diagnosing and treating hereditary spherocytosis in neonates. *Pediatrics* 135(6):1107–1114, 2015.

24. Forde DG, Cope A, Stone B: Acute parvovirus B19 infection in identical twins unmasking previously unidentified hereditary spherocytosis. *BMJ Case Rep* 2014.

25. Rice HE, et al: Clinical outcomes of splenectomy in children: report of the splenectomy in congenital hemolytic anemia registry. *Am J Hematol* 90(3): 187–192, 2015.

26. National Institutes of Health (NIH): *Sickle cell disease*, Bethesda, MD, 2017, U.S National Library of Medicine, U.S. Department of Health and Human Services.

27. American Society of Hematology (ASH): *ASH clinical practice guidelines*, Washington, DC, 2016, Author.

28. National Institutes of Health (NIH): *Evidence report evidence-based management of sickle cell disease*, Bethesda, MD, 2014, U.S. Department of Health and Human Services, National Institutes of Health, National Heart, Lung and Blood Institute.

29. Carden MA, et al: Normal saline is associated with increased sickle red cell stiffness and prolonged transit times in a microfluidic model of the capillary system. *Microcirculation* 2017 Jan 20. [Epub ahead of print.].

30. Dessap AM, et al: Environmental influences on daily emergency admissions in sickle-cell disease patients. *Medicine (Baltimore)* 93(29):e280, 2014.

31. Zhang Y, et al: Elevated spingosine-1-phosphate promotes sickling and sickle cell disease progression. *J Clin Invest* 124(6):2750–2761, 2014.

32. Pappu R, et al: Promotion of lymphocyte egress into blood and lymph by distinct sources of spingosine-1-phosphate. *Science* 316(5822): 295–298, 2007.

33. Darrow MC, et al: Visualizing red blood cell sickling and the effects of inhibition of sphingosine kinase 1 using soft X-ray tomography. *J Cell Sci* 129(18):3511–3517, 2016.

34. Voskou S, et al: Oxidative stress in β-thalassemia and sickle cell disease. *Redox Biol* 6:226–239, 2015.

35. Zhang D, et al: Neutrophils, platelets, and inflammatory pathways at the nexus of sickle cell disease. *Blood* 127(7):801–809, 2016.

36. Chang HY, et al: MD/DPD multiscale framework for predicting morphology and stresses of red blood cells in health and disease. *PLoS Comput Biol* 12(10):e1005173, 2016.

37. Lu X, et al: A microfluidic platform to study the effects of vascular architecture and oxygen gradients on sickle blood flow. *Microcirculation* 2017 Jan 27. [Epub ahead of print.].

38. Nogrady B: Neurobiology: life beyond the pain. *Nature* 515:S8–S9, 2014.

39. Wilkie DJ, et al: Patient-reported outcomes: descriptors of nociceptive and neuropathic pain and barriers to effective pain management in adult outpatients with sickle cell disease. *J Natl Med Assoc* 102(1):18–27, 2010.

40. Creary SE, Krishnamurti L: Prodromal illness before acute chest syndrome in pediatric patients with sickle cell disease. *J Pediatr Hematol Oncol* 36(6):480–483, 2014.

41. Novelli EM, Gladwin MT: Crises in sickle cell disease. *Chest* 149(4):1082–1093, 2016.

42. Kavanagh PL, et al: Improving the management of vaso-occlusive episodes in the pediatric emergency department. *Pediatrics* 136(4):e1016, 2015.

43. National Institutes of Health (NIH): *Genetics home reference beta thalassemia*, Bethesda, MD, 2017, U.S. Department of Health and Human Services, National Institutes of Health, National Library of Medicine.

44. National Institutes of Health (NIH): *Genetics home reference alpha thalassemia*, Bethesda, MD, 2017, U.S. Department of Health and Human Services, National Institutes of Health, National Library of Medicine.

45. Pennell DJ, et al: Cardiovascular function and treatment in β-thalassemia major: a consensus statement from the American Heart Association. *Circulation* 218:281–308, 2013.

46. Origa R: *GeneReviews [Internet]: beta-thalassemia NCBI resources.* Available at: University of Washington, Seattle, WA, 1993–2017.

47. National Institutes of Health (NIH): *Hemophilia*, Bethesda, MD, 2017, U.S Department of Health and Human Services, National Institutes of Health.

48. Rallapalli P, et al: *Factor VIII variant database.* Available at: http://www.factorviii-db.org/.

49. Rallapalli PM, et al: An interactive mutation database for human coagulation factor IX provides novel insights into the phenotypes and genetics of hemophilia B. *J Thromb Haemost* 11(7):1329–1340, 2013.

50. Konkle BA, Josephson NC, Nakaya Fletcher S: Hemophilia A, 2000 Sep 21 [updated 2014 Jun 5]. Pagon RA, et al, editors: *GeneReviews [Internet]*, Seattle, WA, 1993–2016, University of Washington.

51. Konkle BA, Josephson NC, Nakaya Fletcher S: Hemophilia B, 2000 Oct 2 [updated 2014 Jun 5]. Pagon RA, et al, editors: *GeneReviews [Internet]*, Seattle, WA, 1993–2016, University of Washington.

52. Swystun LL, James P: Using genetic diagnostics in hemophilia and von Willebrand disease. *Hematology Am Soc Hematol Educ Program* 2015:152–159, 2015.

53. Manco-Johnson MJ, et al: Prophylaxis versus episodic treatment to prevent joint disease in boys with severe hemophilia. *N Engl J Med* 357:535–544, 2007.

54. Konkle BA, et al: Pegylated, full-length, recombinant factor VIII for prophylactic and on-demand treatment of severe hemophilia A. *Blood* 126(9):1078–1085, 2015.

55. Santagostino E, et al: Long-acting recombinant coagulation factor IX albumin fusion protein (rIX-FP) in hemophilia B: results of a phase 3 trial. *Blood* 127(14):1761–1769, 2016.

56. Leebeek FW, Eikemboom JC: von Willebrand's disease. *N Engl J Med* 375(21):2067–2080, 2016.

57. Yokus O, et al: Risk factors for thrombophilia in young adults presenting with thrombosis. *Int J Hematol* 90(5):583–590, 2009.

58. U.S. National Library of Medicine: *Genetics home reference: protein C deficiency.* Available at: https://ghr.nlm.nih.gov/condition/protein-c-deficiency#.

59. Shah R, et al: Severe congenital protein C deficiency: practical aspects of management. *Pediatr Blood Cancer* 63(8):1488–1490, 2016.

60. Anderson JAM, Weitz JI: Hypercoagulable states. *Crit Care Clin* 27:933–952, 2011.

61. Rodeghiero F, et al: Standardization of terminology, definitions and outcome criteria in immune thrombocytopenic purpura of adults and children: report from an international working group. *Blood* 113:2386–2393, 2009.

62. Provan D, Newland AC: Current management of primary immune thrombocytopenia. *Adv Ther* 32:875–887, 2015.

63. Neunert C, et al: The American Society of Hematology 2011 evidence-based practice guideline for immune thrombocytopenia. *Blood* 117: 4190–4207, 2011.

64. Provan D, et al: International consensus report on the investigation and management of primary immune thrombocytopenia. *Blood* 115:168–186, 2010.

65. Cremer M, et al: Thrombocytopenia and platelet transfusion in the neonate. *Semin Fetal Neonatal Med* 21(1):10–18, 2016.

66. Arber DA, et al: The 2016 revision to the World Health Organization classification of myeloid neoplasms and acute leukemia. *Blood* 127(20): 2391–2405, 2016.

67. American Cancer Society (ACS): *Cancer facts and figures 2016*, Atlanta, 2016, Author.

68. Howlader N, et al, editors: *SEER cancer statistics review, 1975–2013*, Bethesda, MD, 2013, National Cancer Institute. Available at: http://seer.cancer.gov/csr/1975_2013/. Based on November 2015 SEER data submission, posted to the SEER web site April 2016.

69. Howlader N, et al, editors: *SEER cancer statistics review, 1975–2014*, Bethesda, MD, 2014, National Cancer Institute. Available at: https://seer.cancer.gov/csr/1975_2014/. Based on November 2016 SEER data submission, posted to the SEER web site, April 2017.

70. Guest EM, Stam RW: Updates in the biology and therapy for infant acute lymphoblastic leukemia. *Curr Opin Pediatr* 29(1):20–26, 2016.

71. National Cancer Institute (NCI): *Childhood acute lymphoblastic leukemia treatment (PDQ): health professional version*, Bethesda, MD, 2017, National Institutes of Health, National Cancer Center.

72. Timms JA, et al: DNA methylation as a potential mediator of environmental risks in the development of childhood acute lymphoblastic leukemia. *Epigenomics* 8(4):519–536, 2016.

73. Miglioretti DL, et al: The use of computed tomography in pediatrics and the associated radiation exposure and estimated cancer risk. *JAMA Pediatr* 167(8):700–707, 2013.

74. Hudson MM: Reproductive outcomes for survivors of childhood cancer. *Obstet Gynecol* 116(5): 1171–1183, 2010.

75. National Cancer Institute (NCI): *Cancer in children and adolescents*, Bethesda, MD, 2014, National Institutes of Health, National Cancer Institute.

76. Clapp RW, Howe GK, Jacobs MM: Environmental and occupational causes of cancer: a call to act on what we know. *Biomed Pharmacother* 61(10): 631–639, 2007.

77. Orsi L, et al: Parental smoking, maternal alcohol, coffee and tea consumption during pregnancy, and childhood acute leukemia: the ESTELLE study. *Cancer Causes Control* 26(7):1003–1017, 2015.

78. Farioli A, et al: Tobacco smoke and risk of childhood acute lymphoblastic leukemia: findings from the SETIL case-control study. *Cancer Causes Control* 25(6):683–692, 2014.

79. Mattioli S, et al: Tobacco smoke and risk of childhood acute non-lymphocytic leukemia: findings from the SETIL study. *PLoS ONE* 9(11): e111028, 2014.

80. Metayer C, et al: Parental tobacco smoking and acute myeloid leukemia: the Childhood Leukemia International Consortium. *Am J Epidemiol* 184(4): 261–573, 2016.

81. National Cancer Institute (NCI): *Childhood acute myeloid leukemia/other myeloid malignancies treatment (PDQ): patient version*, Bethesda, MD, 2016, National Institutes of Health, National Cancer Institute.

82. Hernandez AF, Menendez P: Linking pesticide exposure with pediatric leukemia: potential underlying mechanisms. *Int J Mol Sci* 17(4):461, 2016.

83. Turner MC, Wigle DT, Krewski D: Residential pesticides and childhood leukemia: a systematic review and meta-analysis. *Environ Health Perspect* 118(1):33–41, 2010.

84. Vinson F, et al: Exposure to pesticides and risk of childhood cancer: a meta-analysis of recent epidemiological studies. *Occup Environ Med* 68(9):694–702, 2011.

85. Carlos-Wallace FM, et al: Parental, in utero, and early-life exposure to benzene and the risk of childhood leukemia: a meta-analysis. *Am J Epidemiol* 183(1):1–14, 2016.

86. Kulkarni K, et al: Leukemia and lymphoma incidence in children in Alberta, Canada: a population-based 22-year retrospective study. *Pediatr Hematol Oncol* 28(8):649–660, 2011.

87. Laurier D, et al: Epidemiological studies of leukaemia in children and young adults around nuclear facilities: a critical review. *Radiat Prot Dosimetry* 132:182–190, 2008.

88. Wheeler DC: A comparison of spatial clustering and cluster detection techniques for childhood leukemia incidence in Ohio, 1996–2003. *Int J Health Geogr* 6:13, 2007.

89. National Cancer Institute (NCI): *Chronic myelogenous leukemia treatment (PDQ): health professional version*, Bethesda, MD, 2017, National Institutes of Health, National Cancer Institute.

90. Chiappini E, et al: Pediatric human immunodeficiency virus infection and cancer in the Highly Active Antiretroviral Treatment (HAART) era. *Cancer Lett* 347(1):38–45, 2014.

91. National Cancer Institute (NCI): *Childhood non-Hodgkin lymphoma treatment (PDQ)*, Bethesda, MD, 2015, National Institutes of Health, National Cancer Institute.

92. National Cancer Institute (NCI): *Childhood Hodgkin lymphoma treatment (PDQ): patient version*, Bethesda, MD, 2016, National Institutes of Health, National Cancer Institute.

Structure and Function of the Cardiovascular and Lymphatic Systems

Kathryn L. McCance, Susanna G. Cunningham

ⓔvolve WEBSITE

http://evolve.elsevier.com/McCance/
- Content Updates
- Chapter Summary Review
- Review Questions
- Case Studies
- Animations

CHAPTER OUTLINE

The functions of the circulatory system include delivery of oxygen, nutrients, hormones, cells of the immune system, and other substances to body tissues and removal of the waste products of cellular metabolism. Delivery and removal are achieved by an extensive array of tubing—the blood and lymphatic vessels—connected to a pump—the heart. The heart continuously pumps blood through the blood vessels in collaboration with other systems, particularly the nervous and endocrine systems, which are intrinsic regulators of the heart and blood vessels. Immune system cells, nutrients, and oxygen are supplied by the immune, digestive, and respiratory systems; gaseous wastes of cellular metabolism are blown off by the lungs; and other wastes are removed by the kidneys and digestive tract.

A critical component of the circulatory system is the vascular endothelium, which is considered by some to be a separate endocrine organ. The endothelium is a multifunctional tissue whose health is essential to normal vascular, immune, and hemostatic system function. Endothelial dysfunction is a critical factor in the pathogenesis of vascular and other diseases.

CIRCULATORY SYSTEM

The heart is comprised of two conjoined pumps moving blood through two separate circulatory systems; one to the lungs and one to all other parts of the body. Structures on the right side of the heart, or **right heart**, pump blood through the lungs. This system, termed the **pulmonary circulation**, is described in Chapter 35. The left side of the heart, or **left heart**, sends blood throughout the **systemic circulation**, which supplies all of the body except the lungs (Fig. 32.1). These two

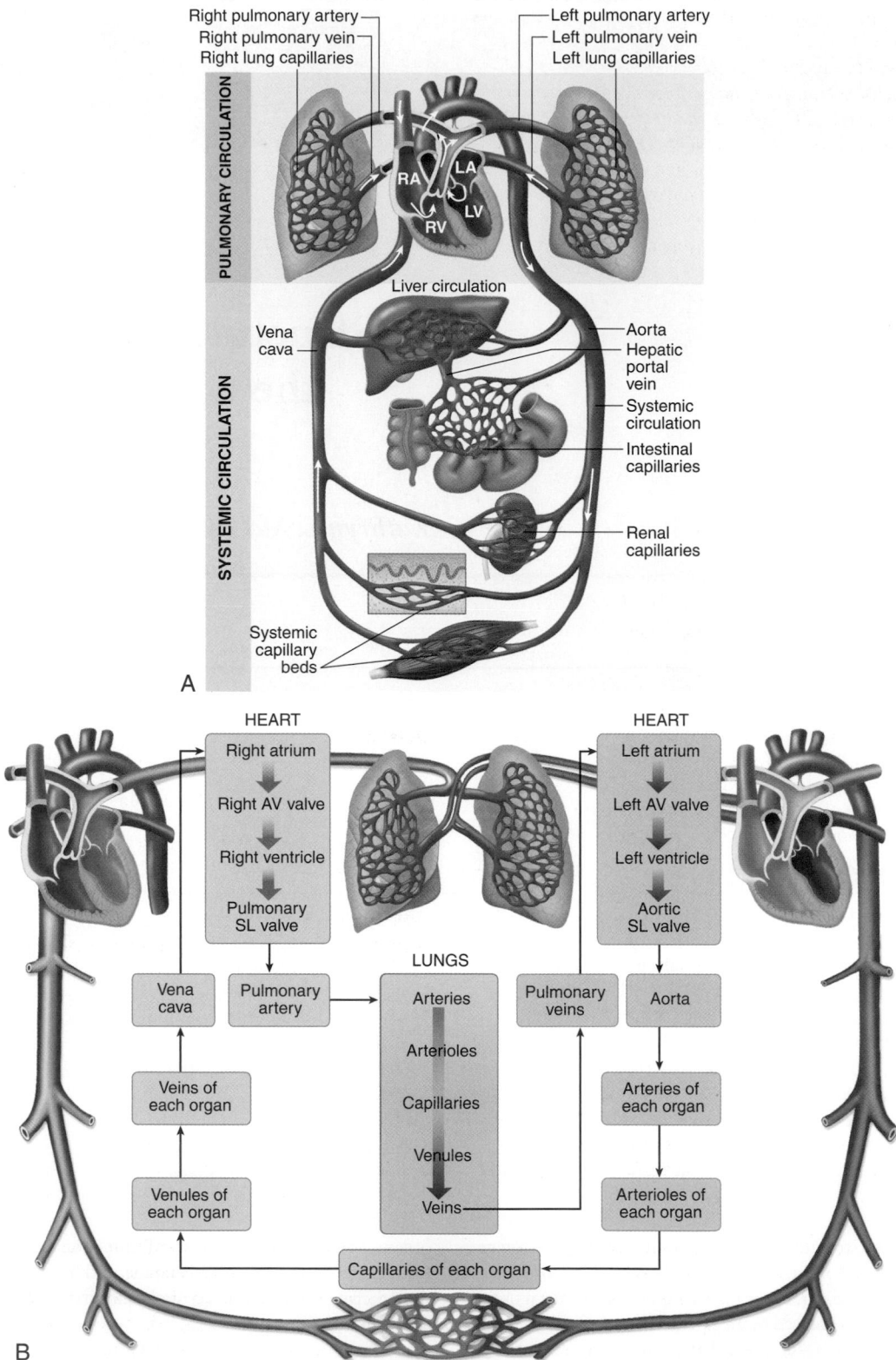

FIGURE 32.1 Diagram Showing Serially Connected Pulmonary and Systemic Circulatory Systems and How to Trace the Flow of Blood. **A,** Right heart chambers propel unoxygenated blood through the pulmonary circulation, and the left heart propels oxygenated blood through the systemic circulation. **B,** The direction of blood flow begins at the left ventricle of the heart; flows to the arteries, arterioles, capillaries of each body organ, venules, veins, right atrium, right ventricle, pulmonary artery, lung capillaries, pulmonary veins, and left atrium; and then returns to the left ventricle. *LA,* Left atrium; *LV,* left ventricle; *RA,* right atrium; *RV,* right ventricle; *SL,* semilunar. (**A** From Patton KT, Thibodeau GA, Douglas MM: *Essentials of anatomy & physiology,* St Louis, 2012, Mosby. **B** From Patton KT, Thibodeau GA: *The human body in health & disease,* ed 7, St Louis, 2018, Mosby.)

systems are serially connected so that the output of one pump becomes the input of the other.

Arteries carry blood from the heart to all parts of the body, where they branch into arterioles and even smaller vessels until they become a fine meshwork of capillaries. Capillaries allow the closest contact and exchange between the blood and the interstitial space, or interstitium—the environment in which the cells live. Venules and then veins then carry blood from capillaries back to the heart. Some of the plasma or liquid component of the blood passes through the walls of the capillaries into the interstitial space. This fluid, called *lymph,* is returned to the cardiovascular system by vessels of the lymphatic system. The lymphatic system is also a critical component of the immune system as described in Chapters 7 and 8.

THE HEART

The adult heart is about the size of a fist and weighs between 200 and 350 grams. It lies obliquely (diagonally) in the mediastinum, the area above the diaphragm and between the lungs. Heart structures can be categorized by function:

1. *Structural support of heart tissues and circulation of pulmonary and systemic blood through the heart.* This category includes the heart wall and fibrous skeleton, which enclose and support the heart and divide it into four chambers; the valves that direct flow through the chambers; and the great vessels that conduct blood to and from the heart.
2. *Maintenance of heart cells.* This category comprises vessels of the coronary circulation—the arteries and veins that serve the metabolic needs of all the heart cells—and the heart's lymphatic vessels.
3. *Stimulation and control of heart action.* Among these structures are the nerves and specialized muscle cells that direct the rhythmic contraction and relaxation of the heart muscles, propelling blood throughout the pulmonary and systemic circulatory systems.

Structures That Direct Circulation Through the Heart
Heart Wall

The heart wall has three layers—the epicardium, myocardium, and endocardium—and is enclosed in a double-walled membranous sac, the pericardium (Fig. 32.2). The pericardial sac has several functions: it prevents displacement of the heart during gravitational acceleration or deceleration, serves as a physical barrier that protects the heart against infection and inflammation from the lungs and pleural space, and contains pain receptors and mechanoreceptors that can cause changes in blood pressure and heart rate. The two layers of the pericardium, the *parietal* and *visceral* pericardia (see Fig. 32.2), are separated by a fluid-containing space called the pericardial cavity. The pericardial fluid (about 20 mL) is secreted by cells of the mesothelial layer of the pericardium and lubricates the membranes that line the pericardial cavity, allowing them to slide smoothly over one another with minimal friction as the heart beats. The amount and character of the pericardial fluid are altered if the pericardium is inflamed (see Chapter 33).

The outer layer of the heart, the epicardium, provides a smooth surface that allows the heart to contract and relax within the pericardium with a minimal amount of friction. The thickest layer of the heart wall, the myocardium, is composed of cardiac muscle and is anchored to the heart's fibrous skeleton. The heart muscle cells, cardiomyocytes, provide the contractile force needed to propel blood through the heart and into the pulmonary and systemic circulations. About 0.5% to 1% of cardiomyocytes are replaced annually; thus over a lifetime about one-half of these muscle cells are replaced.[1-3] The limited myocyte

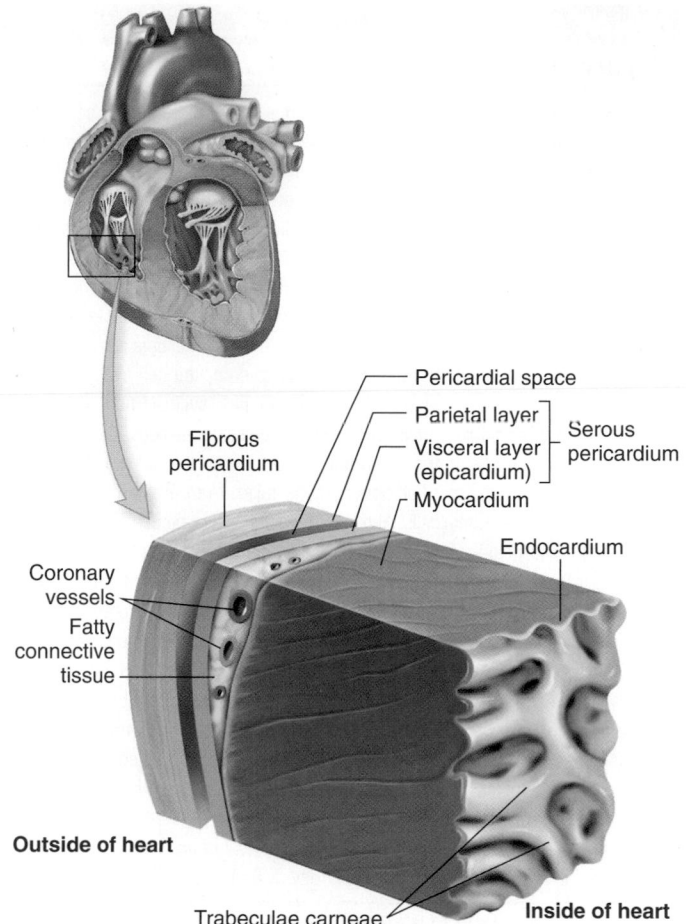

FIGURE 32.2 Wall of the Heart. The cutout section of the heart wall shows the outer fibrous pericardium and the parietal and visceral layers of the serous pericardium (with the pericardial space between them). Note that a layer of fatty connective tissue is located between the visceral layer of the serous pericardium (epicardium) and the myocardium. Note also that the endocardium covers beamlike projections of myocardial muscle tissue, called *trabeculae carneae.* (Modified from Patton KT, Thibodeau GA: *The human body in health & disease,* ed 7, St Louis, 2018, Mosby.)

turnover is insufficient for restoration of contractile function. The capacity to generate cardiomyocytes in the adult human heart has created great interest and investigation for potential cardiomyocyte replacement for persons with cardiac pathologies (see *What's New?* Myocardial Regeneration).

The thickness of the myocardium varies tremendously from one heart chamber to another. Thickness is related to the amount of resistance the muscle must overcome to pump blood from the different chambers. The internal lining of the myocardium is composed of connective tissue and a layer of squamous cells called the *endocardium* (see Fig. 32.2). The endocardial lining of the heart is continuous with the endothelium that lines all the arteries, veins, and capillaries of the body, creating a continuous, closed circulatory system.

Chambers of the Heart

The heart has four chambers: the right atrium, left atrium, right ventricle, and left ventricle. These chambers form two pumps in series: the right heart, a low-pressure system pumping blood through the lungs; and the left heart, a high-pressure system pumping blood through

WHAT'S NEW?

Myocardial Regeneration

Myocardial infarction causes the loss of some of the muscle cells needed to maintain cardiac output, thus increasing the risk of heart failure in survivors. Given that heart failure is a growing problem with a poor prognosis in both the United States and internationally, finding an effective therapy is a critical need.

To replace the approximately 1 billion cardiomyocytes that are estimated to be lost with a myocardial infarction, researchers have identified four possible approaches: (1) accelerating the rate of heart cell division, (2) inserting new cells into the heart, (3) stimulating the heart muscle precursor cells already in the heart, and (4) reprogramming other cells so that they will become cardiomyocyte precursor cells. To stimulate adult heart cells to enter the cell cycle and thus accelerate cell division, various signaling molecules, such as neuregulin and fibroblast growth factor 1, have been used with some success. Currently the most promising cell types that have been injected into the heart include cells from the bone marrow, cardiac-derived cells taken from myocardial biopsies, and human pluripotent stem cells. Although there are cardiac progenitor or precursor cells in the heart, their rate of division is not adequate to replace lost tissue after an infarction. Some of the methods being investigated to stimulate these cardiomyocytes or other progenitor cells in the heart include treatment with peptides that act as paracrines and some types of modified ribonucleic acids (RNAs) for vascular endothelial growth factor (VEGF). Reprogramming from one cell type into a pluripotent stem cell has been attempted with fibroblasts with some success. Each of these four approaches to replacing cardiomyocytes after injury comes with its own set of risks and challenges. Associated risks include increasing the chances for tumor development, damage to other organs, and myocardial scarring.

Portello and colleagues demonstrated that removal of up to 15% of the heart apex of the left ventricle of postnatal day 1 (P1) mice results in complete regeneration within 3 weeks without any measurable fibrosis and cardiac dysfunction. This response involved vigorous proliferating myocytes and gradual restoration of normal cardiac structure. Genetic studies confirmed that the majority of newly formed cardiomyocytes are derived from proliferation of preexisting cardiomyocytes. Using an injury model, investigators found the response similar to the resection model; however, the regenerative capacity was lost by postnatal day 7 (P7). By P7, injury results in typical cardiomyocyte hypertrophy and scar formation of the adult mammalian heart. Importantly, why does the loss of the regenerative capacity occur? The investigators hypothesized that oxidative damage might increase in cardiomyocytes postnatally and play a role in postnatal cell cycle arrest (i.e., stop proliferation). From their study, they found that oxidative base damage modification of DNA was undetectable at P1 but significantly increased at P7 and P14.

Overall, the factors that mediate increased mitochondrial reactive oxygen species (ROS) production and eventual oxidative damage are not well-known. Compared to the oxygenation state, energy metabolism of the embryonic and adult heart is quite distinct. During embryonic development, when cardiomyocytes rapidly proliferate, the relatively hypoxic embryonic heart utilizes anaerobic glycolysis as a main source of energy, whereas adult cardiomyocytes utilize the oxygen-dependent mitochondrial oxidative phosphorylation as an energy source. Therefore to further advance this field, it is necessary to study changes in oxygenation of cardiomyocytes. Eulalio and colleagues report, that in rodents, exogenous administration of selected microRNAs stimulates cardiomyocyte proliferation and promotes cardiac repair. Morrison and colleagues, studying a similar approach in large mammals (sheep), found some inconsistency and differences in sheep, potentially highlighting differences between species.

Data from Elhelaly WM et al: *Front Cell Dev Biol* 4:137, 2016; Eulalio A et al: *Nature* 492(7429):376–381, 2012; Fisher DJ, Heymann MA, Rudolph AM: *Am J Physiol* 238:H399–H405, 1980; Gerbin KA, Murray CE: *Cardiovasc Pathol* 24(3):133–140, 2015; Laflamme AM, Murry CE: *Nat Biotechnol* 23(7):845–856, 2005; Lin Z, Pu WT: *Sci Transl Med* 6(239):239rv1, 2014; Lopaschuk GD, Collins-Nakai RL, Itoi T: *Cardiovasc Res* 26,1172–1180, 1992; Morrison JL et al: *BMC Genomics* 16(1):541, 2015; Ounzain S, Pedrazzini T: *Trends Cardiovasc Med* 25(7):592–602, 2015; Porrello ER et al: *Science* 331(6020):1078–1080, 2011; Porrello ER et al: *Proc Natl Acad Sci U S A* 110(1):187–192, 2012.

the rest of the body. (Blood flow through these chambers is illustrated in Fig. 32.3.) The atria are smaller than the ventricles and have thinner walls. The ventricles have a thicker myocardial layer and make up much of the bulk of the heart. The wall of the right ventricle is about 4 to 5 mm thick, and that of the left ventricle, the most muscular chamber, is about 12 to 15 mm thick.[4] The ventricles are formed by a continuum of muscle fibers that originate from the fibrous skeleton at the base of the heart (chiefly around the aortic orifice).

The wall thickness of each cardiac chamber depends on the amount of pressure or resistance it must overcome to eject blood. The two atria have the thinnest walls because they are low-pressure chambers that serve as storage units and conduits for blood that is emptied into the ventricles. Normally, there is little resistance to flow from the atria to the ventricles. The ventricles, on the other hand, must propel blood all the way through the pulmonary or systemic circulation. The ventricular myocardium must be strong enough to pump against pressures in the pulmonary or systemic vessels. The mean pulmonary capillary pressure, the force the right ventricle must overcome, is only 15 mmHg whereas the mean arterial pressure, the force the left ventricle must overcome, is about 92 mmHg. Because the pressure is markedly higher in the systemic circulation, the wall of the left ventricle is several times thicker than that of the right ventricle.

The right ventricle is shaped like a crescent, or triangle, enabling it to function like a bellows and efficiently eject large volumes of blood

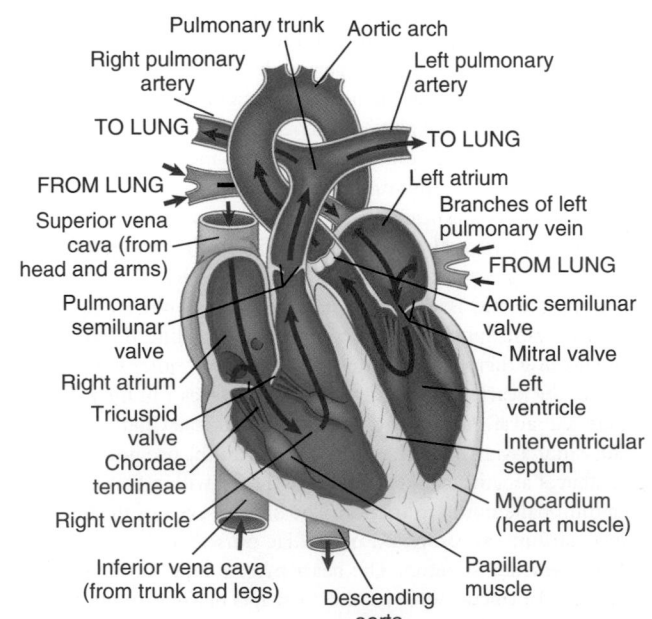

FIGURE 32.3 Structures That Direct Blood Flow Through the Heart. Arrows indicate path of blood flow through chambers, valves, and major vessels.

through the pulmonary semilunar valve into the low-pressure pulmonary system. The left ventricle is larger and bullet shaped, helping it to eject blood through the larger aortic semilunar valve into the high-pressure systemic circulation.

The ventricles are structurally more complex than the atria. Each ventricle contains muscle fibers that divide it roughly into an **inflow tract**, which receives blood from the atrium, and an **outflow tract**, which sends blood to the circulation (see Fig. 32.3).

Normally blood does not flow between the chambers of the right side of the heart and the chambers of the left side of the heart except in the fetus before delivery. The atria are separated by the interatrial septum and the ventricles by the interventricular septum. There is an opening between the right and left atria before birth called the *foramen ovale;* however, this opening closes shortly after birth in most individuals (see Chapter 34). The interventricular septum is an extension of the fibrous skeleton of the heart. Indentations of the endocardium form valves that separate the atria from the ventricles and the ventricles from the aorta and pulmonary arteries.

Fibrous Skeleton of the Heart

Four rings of dense fibrous connective tissue provide a firm anchorage for the attachments of the atrial and ventricular musculature, as well as the valvular tissue. The fibrous rings are adjacent and form a central, fibrous supporting structure collectively termed the *annuli fibrosi cordis*.

Valves of the Heart

One-way blood flow through the heart is ensured by the four heart valves as well as the pressure gradients that they maintain. During ventricular relaxation the two **atrioventricular valves** open and blood flows from the relatively higher pressure in the atria to the lower pressure in the relaxed ventricles. With increasing ventricular pressure these valves close and prevent backflow into the atria as the ventricles contract. The **semilunar valves** of the heart open when intraventricular pressure exceeds aortic and pulmonary pressures and blood flows out of the ventricles and into the systemic and pulmonary circulations, respectively. After ventricular contraction and ejection, intraventricular pressure decreases and the **pulmonic** and **aortic semilunar valves** close when the pressure in the vessels is greater than the pressure in the ventricles, thus preventing backflow into the right and left ventricles, respectively (Fig. 32.4; also see Fig. 32.3).

The atrioventricular (AV) (tricuspid and mitral) valve openings are composed of tissue flaps called *leaflets* or *cusps* that are attached at the upper end to one of the rings in the fibrous skeleton of the heart and at the lower end to papillary muscles by the **chordae tendineae** (see Fig. 32.3). The **papillary muscles** are extensions of the myocardium that help hold the cusps together and downward at the onset of ventricular contraction, thus preventing their backward expulsion, or **prolapse**, into the atria.

The right AV valve is called the **tricuspid valve** because it has three cusps. The tricuspid opening (orifice) has the largest diameter of all the heart valves. The left AV valve is a bicuspid (two cusps) valve called the **mitral valve**. The tricuspid and mitral valves function as a unit because the atria, fibrous rings, valvular tissue, chordae tendineae, papillary muscles, and ventricular walls are connected. Collectively, these six structures are known as the **mitral and tricuspid complex**. Damage to any one of the six components of this complex can significantly alter function and contribute to heart failure.

Blood leaves the right ventricle through the pulmonic semilunar valve, and it leaves the left ventricle through the aortic semilunar valve (see Figs. 32.3 and 32.4). Both the pulmonic and aortic semilunar valves have three cup-shaped cusps that arise from the fibrous skeleton. The pulmonic cusps are slightly thinner than the aortic cusps. The lower

edges of each cusp are suspended from the root of the pulmonary artery or aorta, with the upper valve edges freely projecting into the vessel lumen. When the ventricles contract, the cusps behave like one-way swinging doors. The force of the blood propels the cusps outward against the vessel wall. When the ventricles relax, blood fills the cusps and causes their free edges to meet in the middle of the vessel, closing the valve and preventing any backflow.

Great Vessels

Blood moves in and out of the heart through several large vessels (see Fig. 32.3). The right heart receives venous deoxygenated blood from the systemic circulation through the **superior vena cava** and the **inferior vena cava**, which enter the right atrium. Blood leaves the right ventricle and enters the pulmonary circulation through the pulmonary artery. The **pulmonary artery** divides into **right** and **left pulmonary arteries** to transport deoxygenated blood from the right heart to the right and left lungs. The pulmonary arteries branch further into the pulmonary capillary bed, where oxygen enters the blood and carbon dioxide leaves it as each gas moves from its higher to lower concentration gradient.

Four **pulmonary veins**, two from the right lung and two from the left lung, carry oxygenated blood from the lungs to the left side of the heart. The oxygenated blood moves through the left atrium and ventricle and out into the **aorta**, which delivers it to systemic vessels that supply the body.

Blood Flow During the Cardiac Cycle

The pumping action of the heart consists of contraction and relaxation of the heart muscle or myocardium. Each ventricular contraction and the relaxation that follows it constitute one **cardiac cycle**. (Blood flow through the heart during a single cardiac cycle is illustrated in Fig. 32.4.) During the period of relaxation, termed **diastole**, blood fills the ventricles. The ventricular contraction that follows, termed **systole**, propels the blood out of the ventricles and into the pulmonary and systemic circulations. Contraction of the left ventricle occurs slightly earlier than contraction of the right ventricle.

During ventricular systole, blood from the veins of the systemic circulation enters the thin-walled right atrium from the superior and inferior venae cavae (see Figs. 32.3 and 32.4). Venous blood from the coronary circulation enters the right atrium through the *coronary sinus*. The right atrium fills, which, along with the falling right ventricular pressures, allows the right AV (tricuspid) valve to open and fill the right ventricle during ventricular diastole (occasionally called *atrial systole*). The same sequence of events occurs a split second earlier in the left heart. The four pulmonary veins, two from the right lung and two from the left lung, carry blood from the pulmonary circulation to the left atrium. As the left atrium fills and left ventricular pressure falls, the mitral valve opens and blood flows into the left ventricle. Left atrial contraction, termed *atrial kick*, provides significant increases in the volume of blood entering the left ventricle at the end of diastole. Filling of the right and left ventricles occurs during one period of diastole. Five phases of the cardiac cycle can be identified (Figs. 32.5 and 32.6). As blood is pushed through the inflow and outflow tracts of the ventricles, it flows around the **crista supraventricularis**—the muscle that separates the inflow from the outflow tracts—and is mixed by passing through the strands of the **trabeculae carneae**.

Normal Intracardiac Pressures

Normal intracardiac pressures are shown in Table 32.1 and Fig. 32.7. Atrial pressure (see venous pulse in Fig. 32.5) curves are composed of the **a wave**, which is generated by atrial contraction, and the **v wave**, which is an early diastolic peak caused by filling of the atrium from the peripheral veins. A smaller pressure increase, the **c wave**, occurs

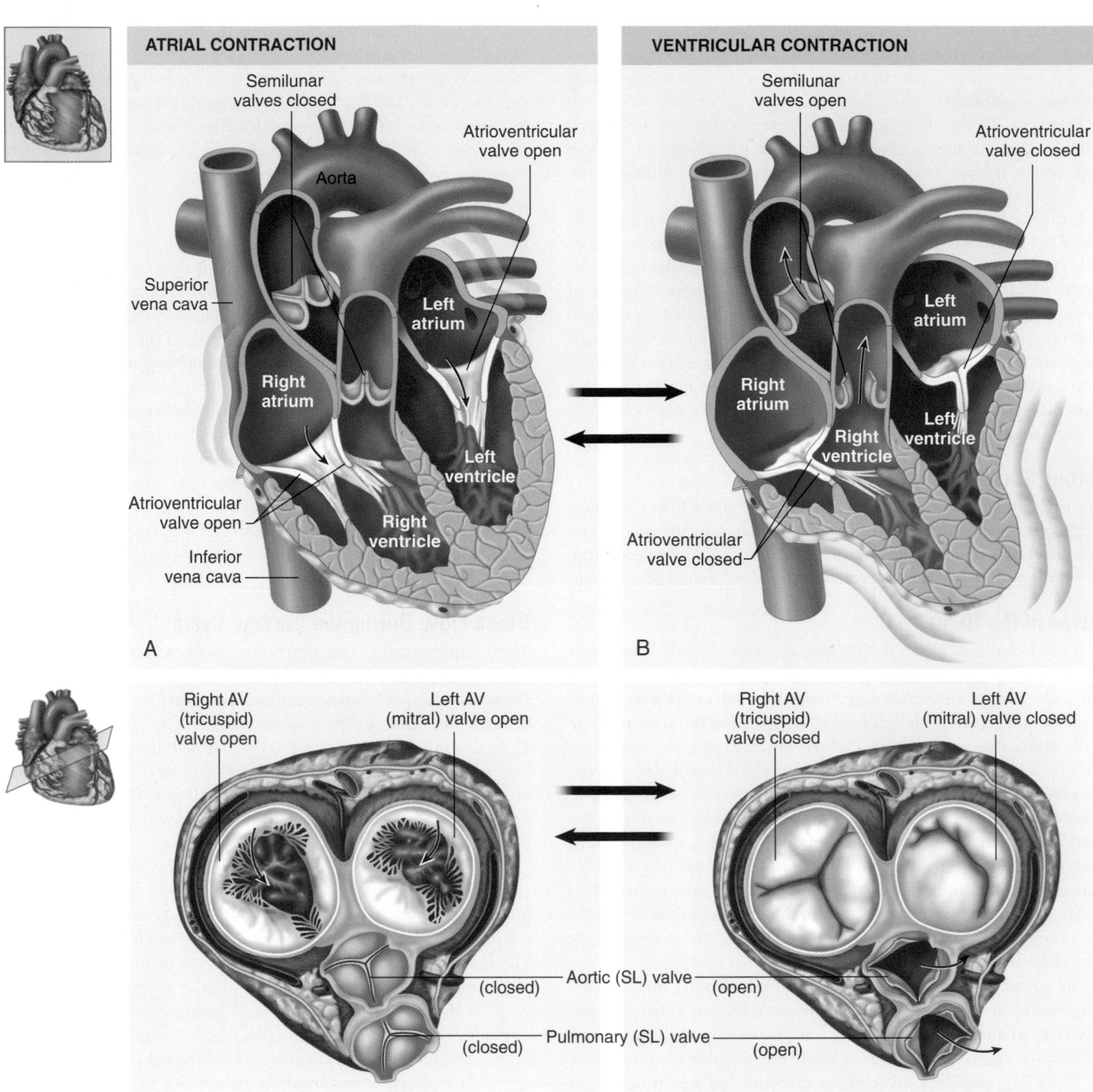

FIGURE 32.4 Chambers and Valves of the Heart. Chambers and valves of the heart. **A,** During atrial contraction cardiac muscle in the atrial wall contracts, forcing blood through the atrioventricular *(AV)* valves and into the ventricles. Bottom illustration shows superior view of all four valves, with semilunar *(SL)* valves closed and AV valves open. **B,** During ventricular contraction that follows, the AV valves close and the blood is forced out of the ventricles through the SL valves and into the arteries. Bottom illustration shows superior view of SL valves open and AV valves closed. (From Patton KT, Thibodeau GA: *The human body in health & disease,* ed 7, St Louis, 2018, Mosby.)

after the a wave in early systole and may represent bulging of the mitral valve into the left atrium during early systole. Two aspects of falling atrial pressure have also been named. The **x descent** follows the a wave and is produced by the descent of the tricuspid valve ring and by the ejection of blood from both ventricles. The **y descent** that follows the v wave reflects the rapid flow of blood from the great veins and right atrium into the right ventricle. Left ventricular pressures are illustrated by a peak systolic pressure and an end-diastolic pressure, which is the

ventricular pressure immediately before the onset of systole. The minimal left ventricular pressure occurs in early diastole.

Structures That Support Cardiac Metabolism: The Coronary Vessels

The myocardium and other heart structures are supplied with oxygen and nutrients by the coronary circulation, which is part of the systemic circulation. The **coronary arteries** originate just beyond the aortic

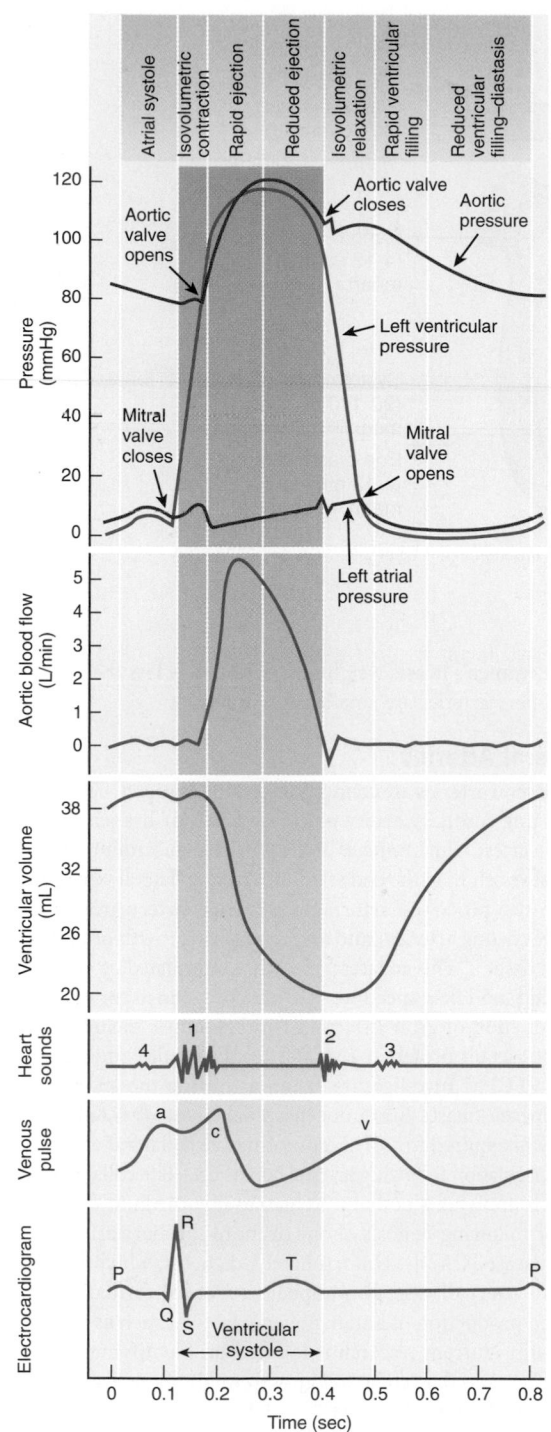

FIGURE 32.5 Composite Chart of Heart Function. This chart is a composite of several diagrams of heart function (blood pressure, blood flow, volume, heart sounds, venous pulse, and electrocardiogram [ECG]), all adjusted to the same time scale.

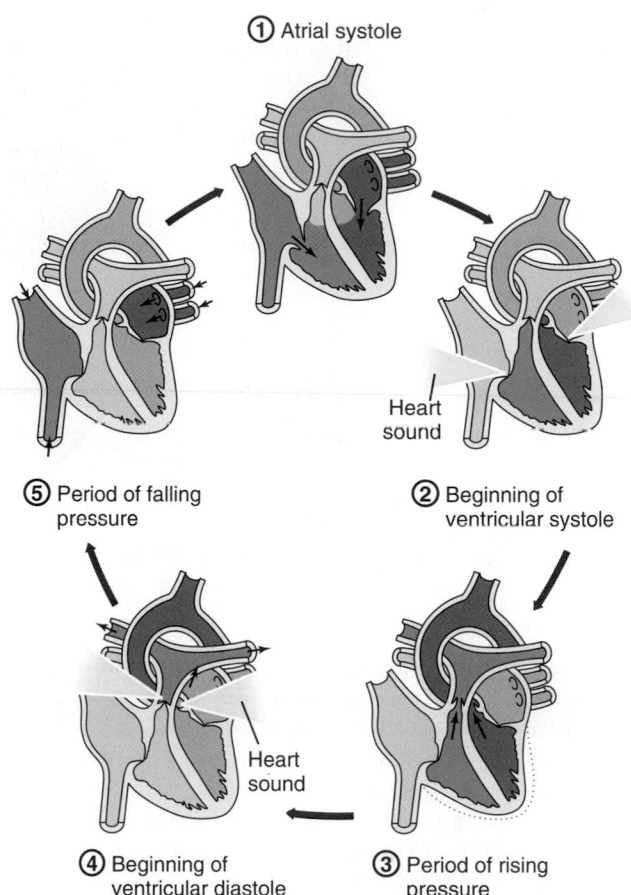

FIGURE 32.6 The Five Phases of the Cardiac Cycle. 1, Atrial systole: Atria contract, pushing blood through the open tricuspid and mitral valves into the ventricles. Semilunar valves are closed. **2,** Beginning of ventricular systole: Ventricles contract, increasing pressure within the ventricles. The tricuspid and mitral valves close, causing the first heart sound. **3,** Period of rising pressure: Semilunar valves open when pressure in the ventricle exceeds that in the arteries. Blood spurts into the aorta and pulmonary arteries. **4,** Beginning of ventricular diastole: Pressure in the relaxing ventricles drops below that in the arteries. Semilunar valves snap shut, causing the second heart sound. **5,** Period of falling pressure: Blood flows from veins into the relaxed atria. Tricuspid and mitral valves open when pressure in the ventricles falls below that in the atria. (Adapted from Solomon E: *Introduction to human anatomy and physiology,* ed 4, St Louis, 2016, Saunders.)

TABLE 32.1	NORMAL INTRACARDIAC PRESSURES	
	MEAN (mmHg)	**RANGE (mmHg)**
Right atrium	4	0–8
Right ventricle		
Systolic	24	15–28
End-diastolic	4	0–8
Left atrium	7	4–12
Left ventricle		
Systolic	130	90–140
End-diastolic	7	4–12

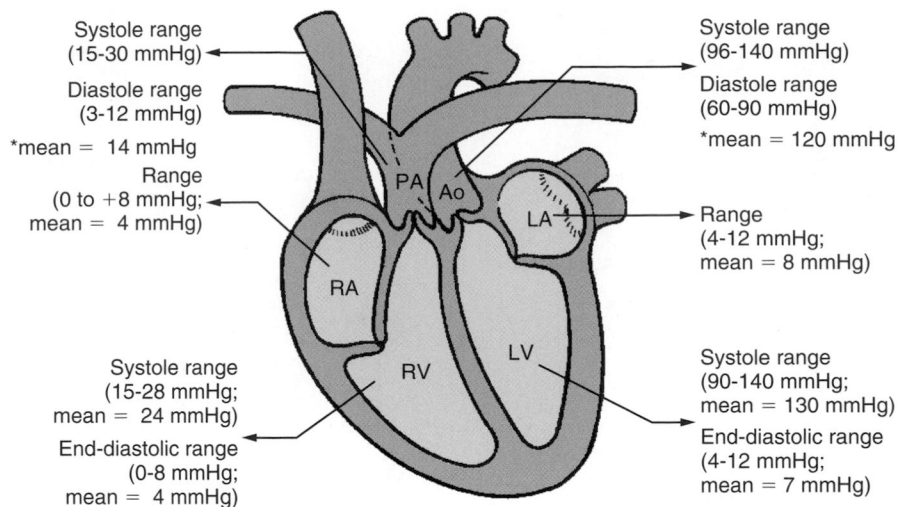

FIGURE 32.7 Normal Intracardiac Pressures. *Ao,* Aorta; *LA,* left atrium; *LV,* left ventricle; *PA,* pulmonary artery; *RA,* right atrium; *RV,* right ventricle. *Main mean pressure.

BOX 32.1   MAIN BRANCHES OF THE CORONARY ARTERIES

Left coronary artery. Arises from a single ostium behind the left cusp of the aortic semilunar valve; ranges from a few millimeters to a few centimeters long; passes between left arterial appendage and pulmonary artery and generally divides into two branches: the left anterior descending (LAD) artery and the circumflex artery; other branches are distributed diagonally across the free wall of the left ventricle.

Left anterior descending (LAD) artery (or anterior interventricular artery). Delivers blood to portions of the left and right ventricles and much of the interventricular septum; travels down the anterior surface of the interventricular septum toward the apex of the heart.

Circumflex artery. Travels in a groove *(coronary sulcus)* that separates the left atrium from the left ventricle and extends to the left border of the heart; supplies blood to the left atrium and the lateral wall of the left ventricle; often branches to posterior surfaces of the left atrium and left ventricle.

Right coronary artery. Originates from an ostium behind the right aortic cusp, travels from behind the pulmonary artery, and extends around the right heart to the heart's posterior surface, where it branches to the atrium and ventricle; three major branches are the conus (supplies blood to upper right ventricle), right marginal branch (supplies right ventricle to the apex), and posterior descending branch (lies in posterior interventricular sulcus and supplies smaller branches to both ventricles).

---

semilunar valve cusps and receive blood through openings in the aorta called the coronary ostia. The cardiac veins empty into the right atrium through another ostium, the opening of a large vein called the coronary sinus (Fig. 32.8). (Regulation of the coronary circulation is described in a later section.)

Coronary Arteries

The major coronary arteries are the right coronary artery (RCA) and the left coronary artery (LCA) (see Fig. 32.8). They traverse the epicardium, myocardium, and endocardium and branch to become arterioles and then capillaries. Their main branches are outlined in Box 32.1.

Because women's hearts weigh proportionately less than men's hearts, the coronary arteries are smaller in women.

Collateral Arteries

The collateral arteries are connections, or anastomoses, between branches of the same coronary artery or connections of branches of the right coronary artery with branches of the left. The epicardium contains more collateral vessels than the endocardium. New collateral vessels are formed through two processes: arteriogenesis (new artery growth branching from preexisting arteries) and angiogenesis (growth of new capillaries within a tissue).[5] This collateral growth is stimulated by shear stress, an increased blood flow speed near an area of stenosis, or narrowing, and the production of growth factors and cytokines, including monocyte chemoattractant protein-1 (MCP-1) and vascular endothelial growth factor (VEGF).[6] Investigators, using a murine model, show that the mixed lineage kinases-Jun amino-terminal kinases (MLK-JNK) signaling pathway is required for formation of native collateral arteries that can restore circulation following arterial occlusion.[7] The collateral circulation assists in supplying blood and oxygen to myocardium that has become ischemic following stenosis of one or more coronary arteries (coronary artery disease [CAD]). Unfortunately, diabetes, which predisposes to coronary artery disease, also impedes collateral formation because of increased production of antiangiogenic factors, such as endostatin and angiostatin. Current research is focused on identifying whether some factors that stimulate collateral growth might be useful treatments for myocardial ischemia.

Coronary Capillaries

The heart has an extensive capillary network. Blood travels from the arteries to the arterioles and then into the capillaries, where exchange of oxygen and other nutrients takes place.

Alterations of the cardiac muscles dramatically affect blood flow in the capillaries. For example, in ventricular hypertrophy (enlargement of the ventricular myocardium), the capillary network does not expand along with muscle fiber size. Therefore the same number of capillaries must now perfuse a larger area. This results in decreased exchange of oxygen and nutrients. At rest, the heart extracts 70% to 80% of the oxygen delivered to it and coronary blood flow is directly correlated with myocardial oxygen consumption.[8] Investigators are studying the microcirculation—capillaries and arterioles—and not just the main coronary arteries in congestive heart failure.[9]

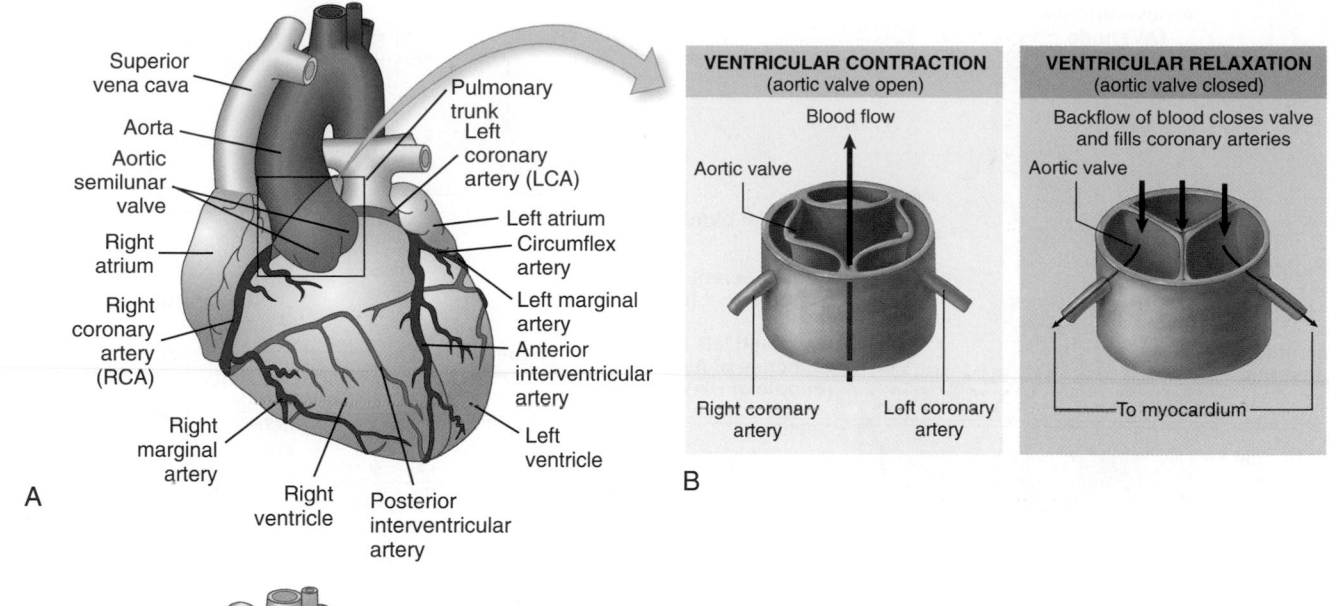

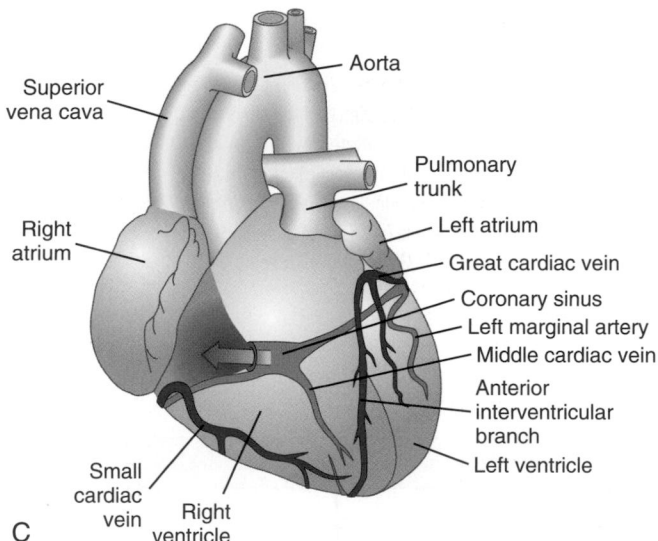

FIGURE 32.8 Coronary Circulation. A, Arteries. **B,** Coronary artery openings from the aorta. **C,** Veins. Both **(A)** and **(C)** are anterior views of the heart. Vessels near the anterior surface are more darkly colored than vessels of the posterior surface seen through the heart. **B,** Placement of the coronary artery opening behind the leaflets of the aortic valve allows the coronary arteries to fill during ventricular relaxation. (From Patton KT, Thibodeau GA: *The human body in health & disease,* ed 7, St Louis, 2018, Mosby.)

Coronary Veins and Lymphatic Vessels

After passing through the extensive capillary network, blood from the coronary arteries drains into the cardiac veins, which travel alongside the arteries. Most of the venous drainage of the heart occurs through veins in the visceral pericardium. The veins then feed into the great cardiac vein (see Fig. 32.8, *C*) and coronary sinus on the posterior surface of the heart, between the atria and ventricles, in the coronary sulcus.

The myocardium has an extensive system of lymphatic capillaries and collecting vessels within the layers of the myocardium and also in the valves. Impairment of cardiac lymphatic function has been hypothesized to impact cardiac conduction, protection from infection, and the development of myocardial fibrosis and atherosclerosis.[10]

Structures That Control Heart Action

People's lives depend on the continuous repetition of the cardiac cycle (systole and diastole) that occurs because of the transmission of electrical impulses, termed cardiac action potentials, through the myocardium (action potentials are described in Chapters 1 and 3). As an electrical impulse passes from cell to cell (fiber to fiber) in the myocardium, it stimulates an intracellular process that results in fiber shortening—that is, muscular contraction or systole. Between action potentials, the fibers relax and return to their resting length, causing diastole. The muscle fibers of the myocardium are electrically coupled so that action potentials pass from cell to cell very rapidly and efficiently. The myocardial structures that allow the action potentials to move so rapidly through the heart are the gap junctions in the intercalated disks. In the intercalated disks, the channel-forming proteins, called connexins, form pores in the gap junctions.[11] As a result of these structures plus the heart's conduction system, an action potential generated in one part of the myocardium passes very quickly throughout the heart, causing rapid, organized, sequential contraction of the atria and then the ventricles.

The myocardium contains its own pacemakers and conduction system—specialized cells that enable it to generate and transmit action potentials without input from the nervous system (Fig. 32.9). The pacemaker cells are concentrated at two sites in the myocardium called nodes, the sinoatrial (SA) node and the atrioventricular (AV) node. Although the heart is innervated by the autonomic nervous system (sympathetic and parasympathetic fibers), neural impulses are not needed to maintain the cardiac cycle. Thus the heart will beat in the absence of any nervous connection, one of the many factors that allow

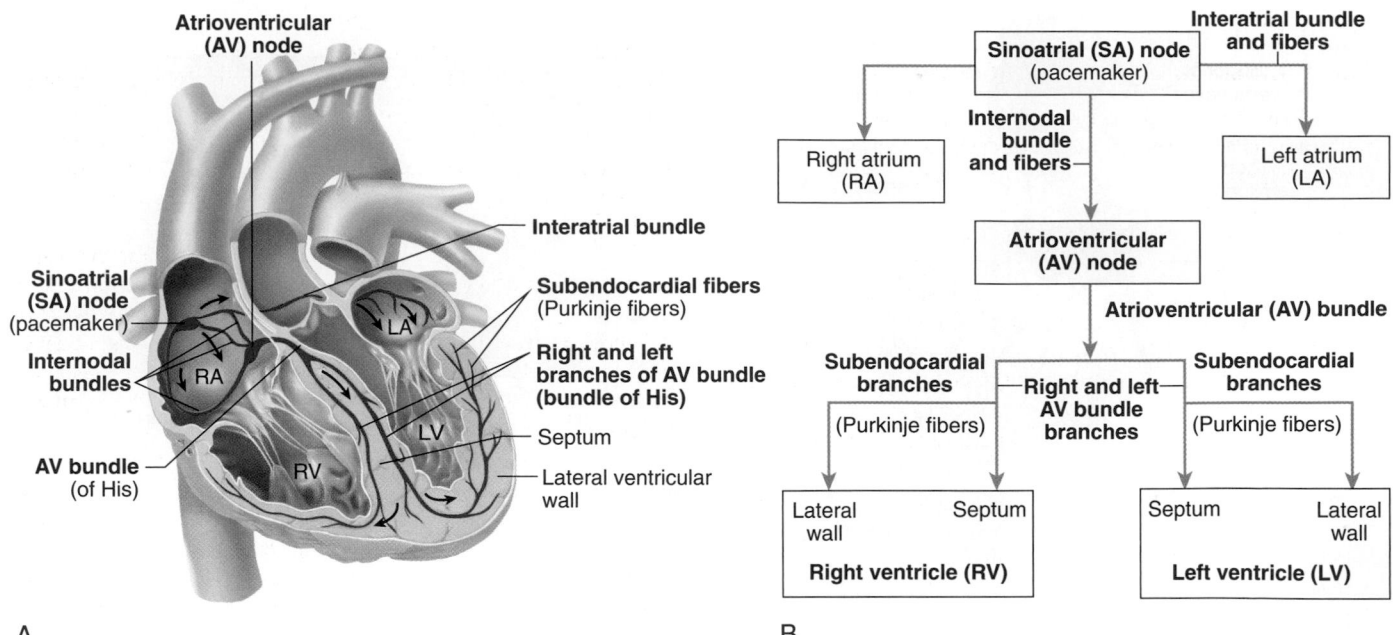

A

B

FIGURE 32.9 Conduction System of the Heart. Specialized cardiac muscle cells *(boldface type)* in the wall of the heart rapidly initiate or conduct an electrical impulse throughout the myocardium. Both the sketch of the conduction system **(A)** and the flowchart **(B)** show the origin and path of conduction. The signal is initiated by the SA node (pacemaker) and spreads to the rest of the right atrial myocardium directly, to the left atrial myocardium by way of a bundle of interatrial conducting fibers, and to the AV node by way of three internodal bundles. The AV node then initiates a signal that is conducted through the ventricular myocardium by way of the AV bundle (of His) and subendocardial branches (Purkinje fibers). (From Patton KT, Thibodeau GA: *The human body in health & disease,* ed 7, St Louis, 2018, Mosby.)

heart transplantation to be successful. The cardiac cycle is stimulated by the nodes of specialized cells and then adjusted to the physical needs of the body by the autonomic fibers. The sympathetic and parasympathetic nerves affect the speed of the cardiac cycle (**heart rate,** or beats per minute), the force of contraction, and the diameter of the coronary vessels (Fig. 32.10 and *What's New?* More Understanding on the Heart-Brain Axis). The sympathetic nervous system increases heart rate and conduction through the nodes, the parasympathetic nervous system slows heart rate and prolongs intranodal conduction time, and both systems cause coronary vasodilation.[12]

Heart action also is influenced by substances delivered to the myocardium in coronary blood. Nutrients and oxygen are needed for cellular survival and normal function, and hormones and biochemical substances, including medications, can affect the strength and duration of myocardial contraction and the degree and duration of myocardial relaxation. Normal or appropriate function depends on the availability of these substances, which is why coronary artery disease can seriously disrupt heart function.

The Conduction System

Electrical impulses normally arise in the sinoatrial (SA) node, the usual *pacemaker of the heart.* The SA node is located at the junction of the right atrium and superior vena cava, just above the tricuspid valve (see Fig. 32.9). The SA node sits only about 1 mm beneath the visceral pericardium, making it vulnerable to injury and disease, especially pericardial inflammation. The SA node is nourished by the sinus node artery, which passes through the center of the node. The SA node is heavily innervated by both sympathetic and parasympathetic nerve fibers.

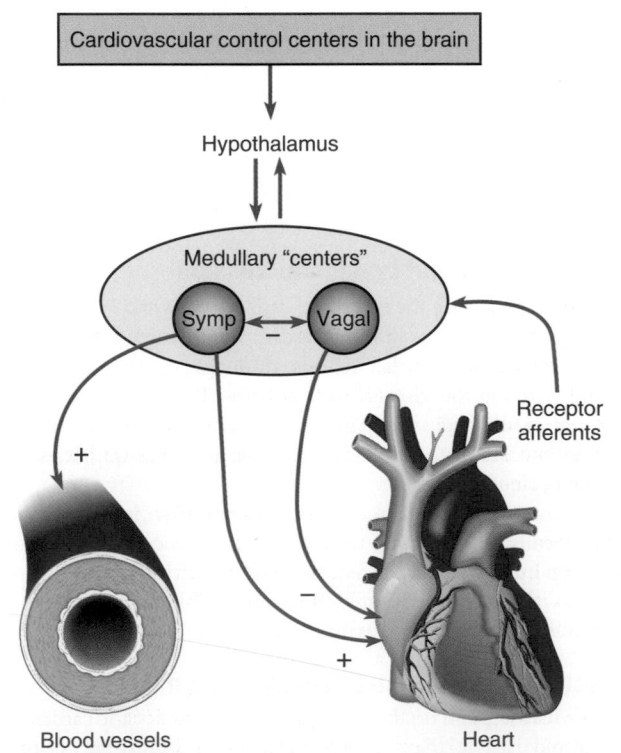

FIGURE 32.10 Autonomic Innervation of Cardiovascular System. +, Activation; −, inhibition; *Symp,* sympathetic.

More Understanding on the Heart-Brain Axis

Some of the effects of cardiovascular disease on the nervous system have been known for a long time; however, effects of neurologic disorders on the cardiovascular system are now expanding. Many pathologies of the nervous system can lead to several alterations in function and structure of the cardiovascular system including changes in the electrocardiogram (ECG), myocardial injury, cardiomyopathy, and cardiac death. The effects of neurologic injury on cardiac function and structure include electrocardiographic alterations, both benign and fatal after brain injury; and cardiac conduction disturbances from central nervous system (CNS) injury because of released enzymes that can alter automaticity, refractoriness, and repolarization. Neurologic injury and psychologic stressors (see Chapter 11) can affect cardiac structure by rapid (within minutes) development of subendocardial infarctions, calcification, and myofibrillar degeneration or *myocytolysis*. Paroxysmal sympathetic hyperactivity (PSH) can develop in pathologies of the autonomic nervous system (ANS), such as ischemia, inflammation, and trauma. The problems associated with PSH include aneurysmal subarachnoid hemorrhage (SAH), postcardiac arrest, cerebral ischemia, severe traumatic brain injury (TBI), and, less frequently, brain tumors. The prevalence of neuropsychiatric disorders including SAH, TBI, stroke, seizure, depression, and intense emotions, such as loss of a loved one, is related to stress-induced cardiomyopathy, especially in postmenopausal women. Emotional stressors are linked to sudden cardiac death (SCD), such as anger, fear, grief, and natural disasters. Neurologic injury can result in SCD by inducing fatal dysrhythmias, massive myocytolysis, and myocardial infarction. These changes are hypothesized as a result of catecholamines (see Chapter 11). More data are emerging related to the interaction between the nervous and cardiovascular systems. Dysfunction in one system may lead to changes in function in the other system.

Data from Tahsili-Fahadan P, Geocadin RG: *Circ Res* 120(3):559–572, 2017.

In the resting adult the SA node generates about 60 to 100 action potentials per minute depending on age and physical condition. Each action potential travels rapidly from cell to cell and through the atrial myocardium, onward to the atrioventricular node (AV node), as well as causing both atria to contract and begin systole. The AV node, located in the right atrial wall superior to the tricuspid valve and anterior to the ostium of the coronary sinus, conducts the action potentials onward to the ventricles. It is innervated by nerves from the autonomic parasympathetic ganglia that serve as receptors for the vagus nerve and cause slowing of impulse conduction through the AV node.

From the AV node, conducting fibers converge to form the bundle of His (atrioventricular bundle) within the posterior border of the interventricular septum. The bundle of His then gives rise to the right and left bundle branches. The right bundle branch (RBB) is thin and travels without much branching to the right ventricular apex. The thinness and relative lack of branches of the RBB make it susceptible to interruption of impulse conduction by damage to the endocardium. The left bundle branch (LBB) in some hearts divides into two branches, or fascicles. The left anterior bundle branch (LABB) passes the left anterior papillary muscle and the base of the left ventricle and crosses the aortic outflow tract. The LABB is susceptible to damage from the aortic valve or the left ventricle. The left posterior bundle branch (LPBB) travels posteriorly, crossing the left ventricular inflow tract to the base of the left posterior papillary muscle. This branch spreads diffusely through the posterior inferior left ventricular wall. Because of relatively nonturbulent blood flow through this portion of the left ventricle, the LBB is somewhat protected from injury caused by wear and tear.

Terminal branches of the RBB and LBB are the Purkinje fibers. They extend from the ventricular apexes to the fibrous rings and penetrate the heart wall to the outer myocardium. Portions of the interventricular septum of the ventricles are the first areas to be excited. Both the RBB and the LBB activate the septum. The rapid spread of the impulse to the ventricular apexes is accomplished from the extensive network of Purkinje fibers. Last to be activated are the basal and posterior portions of the ventricles.

Cardiac Excitation. From the SA node, the impulse that begins systole spreads throughout the right atrium at a conduction velocity of about 35 cm/sec.[12] Because impulses from the SA node arrive at the AV node very quickly, investigators have proposed that these nodes are connected by internodal pathways, called the *anterior, middle,* and *posterior internodal pathways.* However, the existence of these pathways is controversial; not all experts agree that they exist.[12]

The action potential is delayed in the region of the AV node, possibly because of electrophysiologic differences in the cells that comprise the AV region. Conduction velocity within the node is about 10 cm/sec, markedly slower than conduction through the atria.[12] The delay between atrial and ventricular excitation permits an additional boost to ventricular filling by atrial contraction (atrial kick). From the AV node the impulse travels from the AV bundle and through the bundle branches to the Purkinje fibers. Conduction velocities in the AV and Purkinje fibers are the most rapid in the heart.

Ventricular activation occurs sequentially in three phases: (1) septal activation, (2) apical activation, and (3) basal (upper) and posterior activation. The first areas of the ventricles to be excited are portions of the interventricular septum. The septum is activated from both the RBB and the LBB, although the impulse travels from left to right. The extensive network of Purkinje fibers promotes the rapid spread of the impulse to the ventricular apexes. Activation traverses the heart wall from the inside outward (from the endocardium to the epicardium; see Fig. 32.2). The basal and posterior portions of the ventricles are the last to be activated. Deactivation, which begins in diastole, occurs in the opposite direction, spreading from the outside inward (epicardium to endocardium). All areas of the ventricle recover at about the same time.

Propagation of Cardiac Action Potentials. Electrical activation of the muscle cells, termed depolarization, is caused by the movement of ions, including sodium, potassium, calcium, and chloride, across cardiac cell membranes. Deactivation, called repolarization, occurs the same way. (Movement of ions across cell membranes is described in Chapter 1; electrical activation of muscle cells is described in Chapter 44.)

Movement of ions into and out of the cell creates an electrical (voltage) difference across the cell membrane called the *membrane potential.* The resting membrane potential of myocardial cells is between −80 and −90 millivolts, whereas that of the SA node is between −50 and −60 millivolts and that of the AV node is between −60 and −70 millivolts.[12] During depolarization the inside of the cell becomes less negatively charged as positive ions move inside. In cardiac cells the difference between resting membrane potential (in millivolts) and the decreased negative charge caused by depolarization is the cardiac action potential. Table 32.2 summarizes the intracellular and extracellular ionic concentrations of cardiac muscle. The various phases of the cardiac action potential are related to changes in the permeability of the cell membrane to sodium, potassium, chloride, and calcium. Threshold is the point at which the cell membrane's selective permeability to these ions is temporarily disrupted, leading to depolarization. If the resting membrane potential becomes more negative as a result of a decrease in extracellular potassium concentration (hypokalemia), it is termed *hyperpolarization.*

TABLE 32.2 INTRACELLULAR AND EXTRACELLULAR ION CONCENTRATIONS IN THE MYOCARDIUM

ION	INTRACELLULAR CONCENTRATION	EXTRACELLULAR CONCENTRATION
Sodium (Na⁺)	15 mM	145 mM
Potassium (K⁺)	150 mM	4 mM
Chloride (Cl⁻)	5-30 mM	120 mM
Calcium (Ca⁺⁺)	10^{-7} M	2 mM

M, Moles; *mM,* millimoles per kilogram.
From Bonow RO et al, editors: *Braunwald's heart disease: a textbook of cardiovascular medicine,* ed 9, Philadelphia, 2012, Elsevier Saunders.

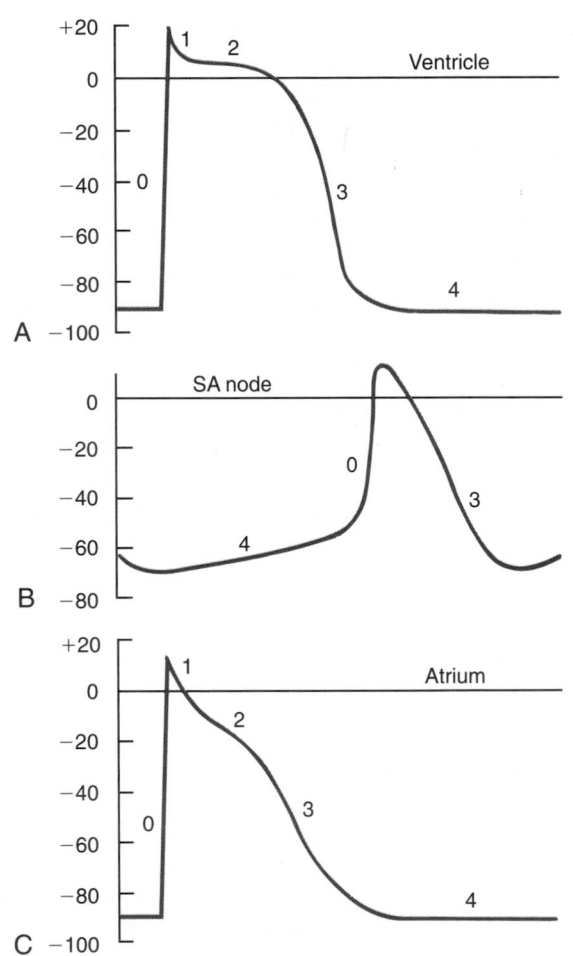

FIGURE 32.11 Cardiac Action Potentials. **A,** Ventricle. **B,** Sinoatrial *(SA)* node. **C,** Atrium. Sweep velocity in **B** is half that in **A** or **C.** (Modified from Koeppen BM, Stanton BA: *Berne and Levy physiology,* ed 6, Philadelphia, 2010, Mosby.)

Normal myocardial cell depolarization and repolarization occur in five phases numbered 0 through 4 (Fig. 32.11). Phase 0 consists of depolarization. This phase lasts 1 to 2 milliseconds (ms) and represents rapid sodium entry into the cell. Phase 1 is early repolarization, in which calcium slowly enters the cell. Phase 2, also called the *plateau,* is a continuation of repolarization, with slow entry of calcium and

sodium into the cell. Potassium is moved out of the cell during phase 3, with a return to resting membrane potential in phase 4.[12] The time between action potentials corresponds to diastole.

The phases of depolarization and repolarization occur somewhat differently in the SA and AV node cells, a difference that enables these cells to generate cardiac action potentials independently. The cells of the Purkinje fibers, atria, and ventricles begin with a negative resting membrane potential and proceed to a rapid upstroke, or depolarization (phase 0), a rapid early repolarization (phase 1), a plateau (phase 2), and a rapid later repolarization (phase 3) (see Fig. 32.11, *A* and *C*). The fast inward current of phase 0 is mediated by sodium ions flowing through "fast channels" in the cell membrane and causes the rapid upstroke of the action potential in Purkinje fibers, atria, and ventricles. In contrast, the cells of the SA and AV nodes begin with a less negative resting membrane potential, proceed to a slow upstroke (phase 0), and usually lack a plateau (phase 2) (see Fig. 32.11, *B*). The slow inward current, mediated by calcium through transient and long-lasting channels and sodium ions flowing through "slow channels" of the cell membrane, is responsible for the action potential of the SA node and the AV node. Hence, drugs that block calcium have profound effects on the slow inward current and can alter heart rate. Slow channel-blocking drugs, such as verapamil, are used to treat a variety of cardiovascular disorders.

A refractory period, during which no new cardiac action potential can be initiated by a stimulus, follows depolarization. This effective or absolute refractory period corresponds to the time needed for the reopening of channels that permit sodium and calcium influx (phase 0 through half of phase 3). A relative refractory period occurs near the end of repolarization, following the effective refractory period. During this time the membrane can be depolarized again but only by a greater than normal stimulus. Abnormal refractory periods as a result of disease can cause abnormal heart rhythms, or dysrhythmias, including ventricular fibrillation and cardiac arrest (see Chapter 33).

Normal Electrocardiogram. The genesis of the normal electrocardiogram is from electrical activity recorded by skin electrodes, that is, the sum of all cardiac action potentials (Fig. 32.12). The P wave represents atrial depolarization. The PR interval is a measure of time from the onset of atrial activation to the onset of ventricular activation; it normally ranges from 0.12 to 0.20 second. The PR interval represents the time necessary to travel from the sinus node through the atrium, AV node, and His-Purkinje system to activate ventricular myocardial cells. The QRS complex represents the sum of all ventricular muscle cell depolarizations. The configuration and amplitude of the QRS complex vary considerably among individuals. The duration is normally between 0.06 and 0.10 second. During the ST interval the entire ventricular myocardium is depolarized. The QT interval is sometimes called the *electrical systole* of the ventricles. It lasts about 0.4 second, but it varies inversely with the heart rate.

Automaticity. Automaticity, or the property of generating spontaneous depolarization to threshold, enables the SA and AV nodes to generate cardiac action potentials without any stimulus. Cells capable of spontaneous depolarization are called automatic cells. The automatic cells of the cardiac conduction system can stimulate the heart to beat even when the heart is transplanted and, thus, has no innervation. Spontaneous depolarization is possible in automatic cells because the membrane potential does not "rest" during phase 4. Instead, it slowly creeps toward threshold during the diastolic phase of the cardiac cycle. Because threshold is approached during diastole, phase 4 in automatic cells is called diastolic depolarization. The electrical impulse normally begins in the SA node because its cells depolarize more rapidly than other automatic cells.

Rhythmicity. Rhythmicity is the regular generation of an action potential by the heart's conduction system. The SA node sets the pace

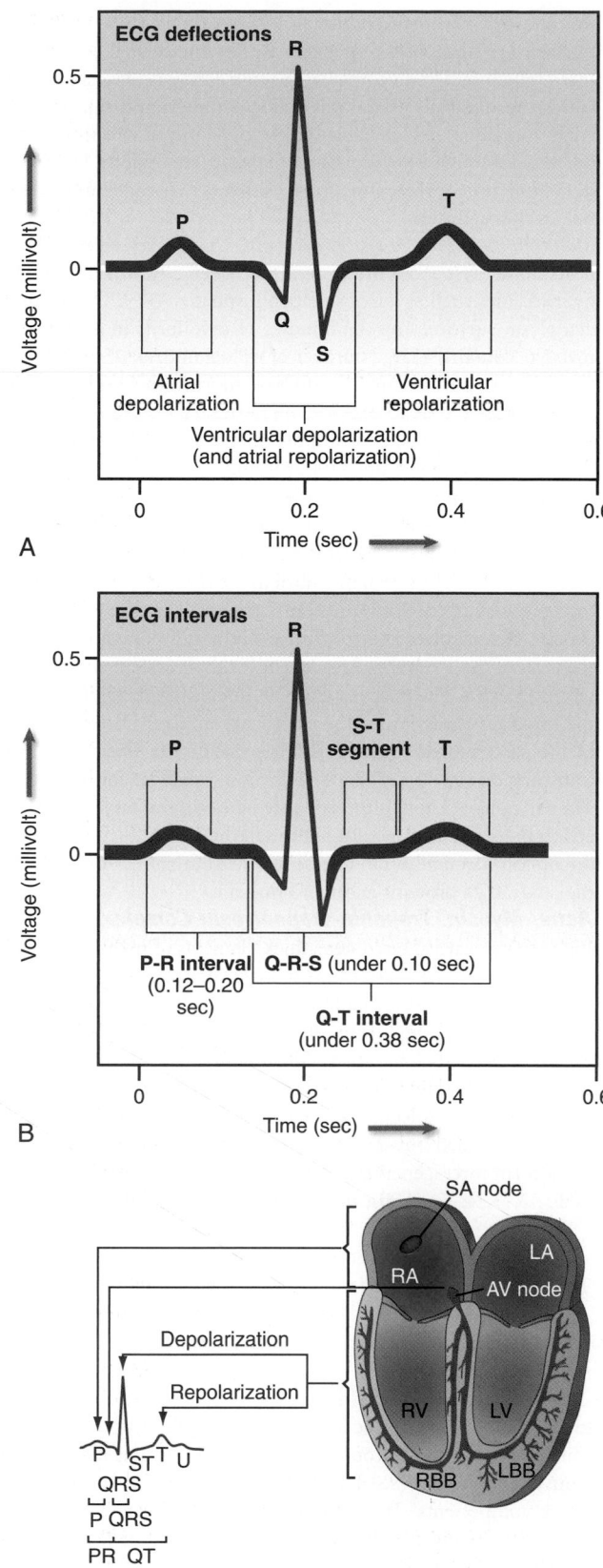

FIGURE 32.12 Electrocardiogram (ECG) and Cardiac Electrical Activity. **A,** Normal ECG. Depolarization and repolarization. **B,** ECG intervals among P, QRS, and T waves. **C,** Schematic representation of ECG and its relationship to cardiac electrical activity. *AV,* Atrioventricular; *LA,* left atrium; *LBB,* left bundle branch; *LV,* left ventricle; *RA,* right atrium; *RBB,* right bundle branch; *RV,* right ventricle; *SA node,* sinoatrial node.

because normally it has the fastest rate of depolarization. The SA node depolarizes spontaneously 60 to 100 times per minute. If the SA node is damaged, the AV node can become the heart's pacemaker at a rate of about 40 to 60 spontaneous depolarizations per minute. Eventually, however, conduction cells in the atria usually take over from the AV node. Purkinje fibers also are capable of spontaneous depolarization but at a slower rate. Therefore the Purkinje fibers only function as pacemakers when the SA and AV nodes are diseased or there is interruption to movement of electrical current through the heart.

Cardiac Innervation

Although the heart's nodes and conduction system generate cardiac action potentials independently, the autonomic nervous system influences the rate of impulse generation (firing), depolarization, and repolarization of the myocardium and the strength of atrial and ventricular contraction. Autonomic neural transmission produces changes in the heart and circulatory system faster than metabolic or humoral agents (see Fig. 32.10). Speed is important, for example, in stimulating the heart to increase its pumping action during times of stress and fear, the *fight-or-flight response*, or with increased physical activity. Although increased delivery of oxygen, glucose, hormones, and other blood-borne factors sustains increased cardiac activity, the rapid initiation of increased activity depends on the sympathetic and parasympathetic fibers of the autonomic nervous system. (The autonomic nervous system is described and illustrated in Chapter 15.)

Sympathetic and Parasympathetic Nerves. Sympathetic and parasympathetic nerve fibers innervate all parts of the atria and ventricles and the SA and AV nodes. In general, sympathetic stimulation increases electrical conductivity and the strength of myocardial contraction, and vagal parasympathetic nerve activity does the opposite, slowing the conduction of action potentials through the heart and reducing the strength of contraction. Therefore the sympathetic and parasympathetic nerves affect the speed of the cardiac cycle (heart rate, or beats per minute). The sympathetic nerves also influence the diameter of the coronary vessels (see Fig. 32.10) and overall myocardial performance. Stimulation of the SA node by the sympathetic nervous system rapidly increases heart rate. In addition, neurally released norepinephrine or circulating catecholamines interact with β-adrenergic receptors on the cardiac cell membranes. The final effect is an increased influx of Ca^{++}, which increases the contractile strength of the heart and increases the speed of electrical impulses through the heart muscle and the nodes.[13] Finally, increased sympathetic discharge dilates the coronary vessels by causing the release of vasodilating metabolites resulting from increased myocardial contraction.[14]

Efferent sympathetic fibers originate in the thoracic spinal cord and branch into the superior middle and inferior cardiac nerves. They join at the cardiac plexus, a neural junction located at the root of the aorta in front of the trachea. The efferent parasympathetic fibers originate in the medulla oblongata and travel by way of the vagus nerves to join the sympathetic nerves in the cardiac plexus.

Parasympathetic (vagal) activity causes the release of acetylcholine. Receptors for these neurotransmitters are found in the myocardium and coronary vessels of the heart. Acetylcholine decreases heart rate, slows conduction through the AV nodes, and reduces myocardial contraction strength.[12]

Adrenergic Receptor Function. Sympathetic neural stimulation of the myocardium and coronary vessels depends on the presence of G-protein–coupled adrenergic receptors, which bind specifically with neurotransmitters of the sympathetic nervous system. (Receptor physiology is discussed in Chapter 1.) The effects of sympathetic stimulation depend on whether (1) the α- or β-adrenergic receptors are most plentiful on cells of the effector tissue, (2) the neurotransmitter is norepinephrine or epinephrine, and (3) the extent to which the individual variations in receptor structure caused by single nucleotide polymorphisms (SNPs) influence receptor responsiveness.[15,16]

There are five types of adrenergic receptors: β_1, β_2, β_3, α_1, and α_2 (see Table 15.7). Each of the α-adrenergic receptors also has three subtypes, so some sources indicate that there are nine types of adrenergic receptors.[16,17] Overall, cardiovascular structures have more β- than α-receptors; therefore effects mediated by the β-receptors predominate. Norepinephrine is released by postsynaptic sympathetic nerve endings in the heart, whereas epinephrine is mainly released by the adrenal medulla and reaches the heart through the bloodstream.

The β_1-receptors are found mostly in the heart, specifically the conduction system (AV and SA nodes, Purkinje fibers) and the atrial and ventricular myocardium. The β_2-receptors are found in the heart and also on vascular smooth muscle. Stimulation of both the β_1- and β_2-receptors results in an increase in heart rate (chronotropy) and force of myocardial contraction (inotropy).[18] In addition, stimulation of the β_2-receptors results in vasodilation because of the location of the receptors on vascular smooth muscle. Overall β_1 and β_2 stimulation enables the heart to pump more blood and β_2 stimulation also increases coronary blood flow, and β_3-receptors are also found in the myocardium and coronary vessels. In the heart, stimulation of these receptors opposes the effects of β_1- and β_2-receptor stimulation and decreases myocardial contractility (negative inotropic effect).[18] Thus β_3-receptors may provide a "safety mechanism" to prevent overstimulation of the heart by the sympathetic nervous system.

Norepinephrine binding with α_1-receptors, all of which are post-synaptic in the systemic and coronary arteries, causes smooth muscle contraction and thus vasoconstriction. One of the three subtypes of α_2-receptors, α_{2a}, is located on the sympathetic ganglia and nerve terminals. The effect of norepinephrine on these receptors is to inhibit release of more norepinephrine, which promotes vasodilation, thus providing another safety mechanism to prevent excess blood pressure elevation.[18] Dysfunction of α- and β-adrenergic receptors can occur in many conditions (e.g., diabetes, hypertension) and has been implicated in the pathogenesis of many cardiac diseases, including heart failure, myocardial ischemia, and dysrhythmias.[15,16,18]

Myocardial Cells

Cardiomyocytes are composed of long, narrow fibers that contain bundles of longitudinally arranged myofibrils; a nucleus; mitochondria; an internal membrane system (the sarcoplasmic reticulum); cytoplasm (sarcoplasm); and a plasma membrane (the sarcolemma), which encloses the cell. Cardiac and skeletal muscle cells also have an "external" membrane system made up of transverse tubules (T tubules) formed by inward pouching of the sarcolemma. The sarcoplasmic reticulum forms a network of channels that surrounds the muscle fiber.

Myofibrils in both cardiac and skeletal fibers consist of alternating light and dark bands of protein, causing the fibers to appear striped, or striated. The dark and light bands of the myofibrils create repeating longitudinal units, called *sarcomeres*, which are between 1.6 and 2.2 μm long (Fig. 32.13, A). The length of these sarcomeres determines the limits of myocardial stretch at the end of diastole and subsequently the force of contraction during systole. Alterations in sarcomere size occur in both physiologic and pathologic myocardial hypertrophy.

There are differences between skeletal and cardiac muscle, which reflect cardiac function. Skeletal muscle cells tend to be arranged in parallel units throughout the length of the muscle, whereas cardiac cells are arranged in branching networks throughout the myocardium. Skeletal muscle cells have many nuclei, but cardiac fibers have only one nucleus. Other differences enable cardiac fibers to accomplish the following:
1. *Transmit action potentials quickly from cell to cell.* Electrical impulses are transmitted rapidly from cardiac fiber to cardiac fiber because

the network of fibers connects at intercalated disks, which are thickened portions of the sarcolemma. The intercalated disks contain three junctions: desmosomes or macula adherens; fascia adherens, which mechanically attach one cell to another; and gap junctions (tight junctions), which allow the electrical impulse to spread from cell to cell through a low-resistance pathway (see Chapter 1). Changes in the function of these junctional elements may cause an increased risk of dysrhythmias.[13]
2. *Maintain high levels of energy synthesis.* Unlike skeletal muscle, the heart cannot rest and is in constant need of energy, which is supplied by molecules such as adenosine triphosphate (ATP). Therefore the cytoplasm surrounding the bundles of myofibrils in each cardio-myocyte contains a large number of mitochondria (25% to 33% of cell volume). Cardiac muscle cells have more mitochondria than do skeletal muscle cells to provide the necessary respiratory enzymes for aerobic metabolism and supply quantities of ATP sufficient for the constant action of the myocardium.[19]
3. *Gain access to more ions, particularly sodium and potassium, in the extracellular environment.* Cardiac fibers contain more T tubules than do skeletal muscle fibers (Fig. 32.14). This increased closeness to the T tubules gives each myofibril in the myocardium faster access to molecules needed for the transmission of action potentials, a process that involves transport of sodium and potassium through the walls of the T tubules. Because the T tubule system is continuous with the extracellular space and the interstitial fluid, it facilitates the rapid transmission of the electrical impulses from the surface of the sarcolemma to the myofibrils inside the fiber. This rapid transmission activates all the myofibrils of one fiber simultaneously. The sarcoplasmic reticulum is located around the myofibrils. As an action potential is transmitted through the T tubules, it induces the sarcoplasmic reticulum to release its stored calcium, thus activating the contractile proteins actin and myosin.

Actin, Myosin, Troponin-Tropomyosin Complex, and Titin. Within each myocardial sarcomere, thick filaments of myosin constitute the central dark band called the anisotropic band, or A band (see Fig. 32.13, B). The myosin molecule resembles a golf club with two large bulbous heads protruding from one end of a straight shaft (Fig. 32.13, C). The bilobed heads contain an actin-binding site and a site of ATPase activity. A thick filament called *myosin microfilament* is composed of about 200 myosin molecules bundled together with outward-facing molecule heads called *cross-bridges* because with activation of contraction they will form force-generating bridges with exposed actin molecules (see Fig. 32.13, A, C). Actin molecules are part of the thin filaments (Fig. 32.15). The light bands, called isotropic bands, or I bands, of the sarcomere contain only actin molecules and no myosin (see Fig. 32.13, A). The thin filaments of actin extend from the Z line, a dense fibrous line that crosses the center of each I band. The area from one dark Z line to the next Z line defines one sarcomere. In the center of a sarcomere is the H zone, a somewhat less dense region. A thin, dark M line travels the center of the H zone. A single tropomyosin molecule (a relaxing protein) lies alongside seven actin molecules. Troponin, another relaxing protein, associates with the tropomyosin molecule, forming the troponin-tropomyosin complex (see Fig. 32.15). The troponin complex itself has three components. Troponin T aids in binding of the troponin complex to actin and tropomyosin; troponin I inhibits the ATPase of actomyosin; and troponin C contains binding sites for the calcium ions involved in contraction. Troponin T and I molecules are released into the bloodstream during myocardial injury. They are measured to evaluate if a myocardial infarction or other damage has occurred. Once troponin and tropomyosin cover the myosin-binding sites on actin, the cross-bridges release calcium and the myocardium relaxes. A giant elastic sarcomere protein (titin or connectin), which attaches myosin to the

FIGURE 32.13 Structure of a Sarcomere, Myofilaments, and Myosin. **A,** The sarcomere is the basic contractile unit of a muscle cell. The Z disk is the anchor for the contractile elements actin and myosin. Actin attaches directly to the Z disk, whereas myosin is attached to it by elastic titin filaments. The myosin filaments are connected to each other by M-protein at the M line. The A, H, and I bands refer to parts of the sarcomere as they were originally seen by light microscopy. **B,** Thin myofilaments and thick myofilament. **C,** Each myosin molecule is a coil of two chains wrapped around each other. At the end of each chain is a globular region, much like a golf club, called the *head.* Myosin molecules usually are combined into filaments, which are stalks of myosin from which the heads protrude at regular intervals.

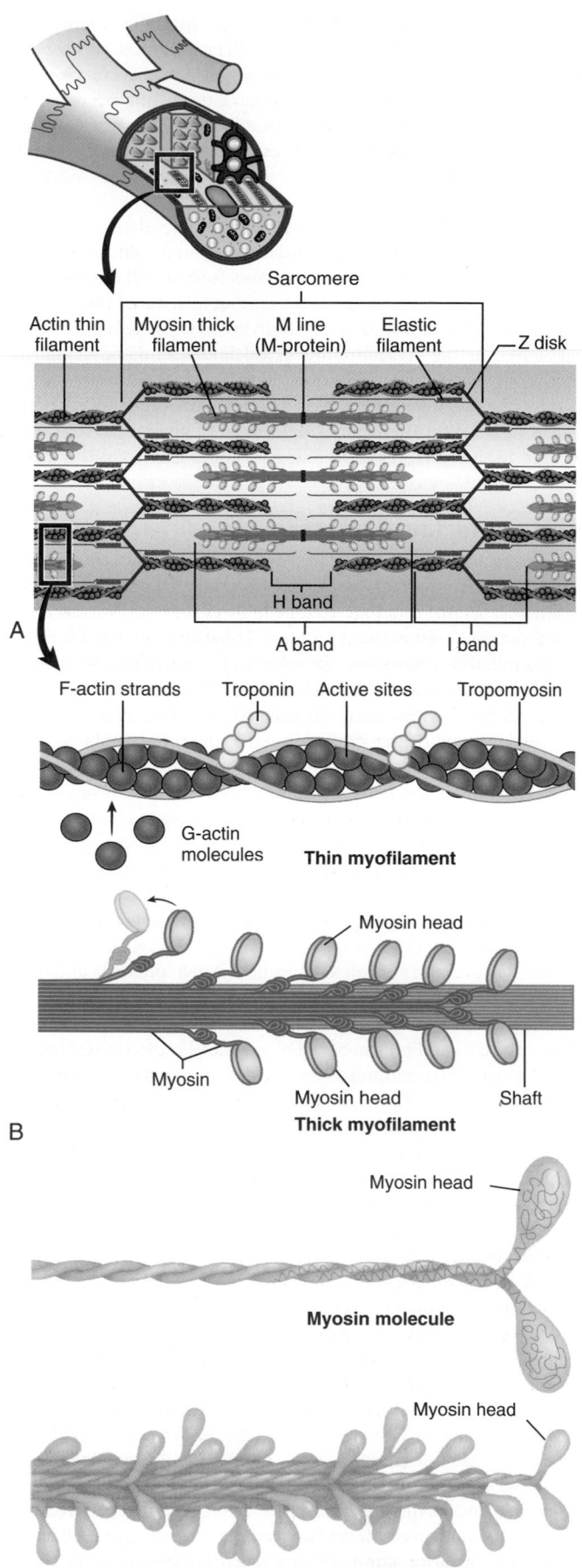

Z line, acts as a spring and influences myocardial stiffness.[19] Titin structure affects myocardial diastolic filling and has been found to play a role in heart failure.[20]

Myocardial Metabolism. Cardiomyocytes depend on the constant production of ATP, which is synthesized within the mitochondria mainly from glucose, fatty acids, and lactate. If the myocardium is underperfused because of coronary artery disease, anaerobic metabolism must be used as a source of energy (see Chapter 1). Energy produced by metabolic processes sustains muscle contraction and relaxation, electrical excitation, membrane transport, and synthesis of large molecules. Normally, the amount of ATP produced supplies sufficient energy to pump blood systemically.

Cardiac work often is expressed as myocardial oxygen consumption ($M\dot{V}O_2$), which is correlated with total cardiac energy requirements. $M\dot{V}O_2$ is determined by three major factors: (1) the amount of wall stress during systole, estimated by measuring the systolic blood pressure; (2) the duration of systolic wall tension, measured indirectly by the heart rate; and (3) the contractile state of the myocardium, which is not measured clinically.

The coronary arteries deliver oxygen (O_2) to the myocardium. From 70% to 75% of this O_2 is used immediately by cardiac muscle, leaving little O_2 in reserve. Therefore increased energy needs can be met only by increasing coronary blood flow. $M\dot{V}O_2$ can increase with exercise and decreases with hypotension and hypothermia. As myocardial metabolism and consumption of O_2 increases, the concentration of local vasoactive metabolic factors increases. Some of these, such as adenosine, nitric oxide, and prostaglandins, dilate coronary arterioles, thus increasing coronary blood flow.[21]

Myocardial Contraction and Relaxation

Myocardial contractility is a change in developed tension at a given resting fiber length, which is simply the ability of the heart muscle to shorten. At the molecular level, thin filaments of actin slide over thick filaments of myosin, called the cross-bridge cycle of muscle contraction. Anatomically, contraction occurs when the sarcomere shortens, causing adjacent Z lines to move closer together (Fig. 32.16). The width of the A band, which contains the thick myosin filaments, is unchanged whereas the I band becomes narrower as the overlap between the thick and thin filaments increases. The degree of shortening of the muscle fibers depends on how much the thin filaments overlap the thick filaments. Maximal contraction occurs when the sarcomere length is 2.2 mm. At 2.2 mm the number of cross-bridge attachments between actin and myosin is maximal.

Cross-Bridge Cycling. The globular head-end of the myosin contains a binding site for actin and a separate enzymatic site that catalyzes the breakdown of ATP to adenosine diphosphate (ADP) and inorganic phosphate (P_i) (see Fig. 32.16). This reaction releases the

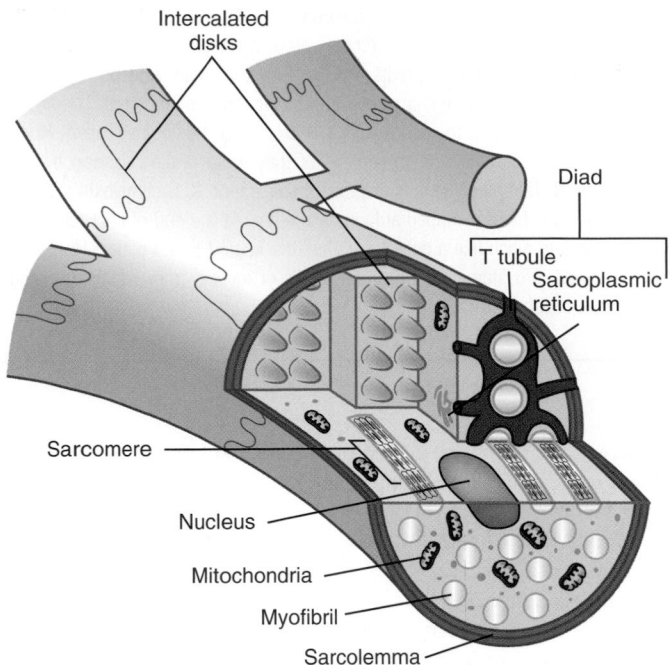

FIGURE 32.14 Cardiac Muscle Fiber. Unlike other types of muscle fibers, cardiac muscle fibers are typically branched with junctions, called *intercalated disks,* between adjacent myocytes. Like skeletal muscle cells, cardiac muscle cells contain sarcoplasmic reticula and T tubules, although these structures are not as highly organized as in skeletal muscle fibers.

chemical energy stored in ATP. Magnesium is required for the binding of ATP to the myosin site. The splitting of ATP occurs on the myosin molecule before it attaches to actin, but the ADP and inorganic phosphate released remain bound to the active site on myosin. The chemical energy released is transferred to myosin (m), producing a high-energy form of myosin (M):

$$M \bullet ATP \rightarrow M \bullet ADP + P_i$$

The binding of this high-energy myosin-actin form to a cross-bridge releases the energy stored in myosin (e.g., ADP and P_i), producing the force necessary for movement of the cross-bridge. With the attachment of actin to myosin at the cross-bridge, the myosin head molecule undergoes a position change, exerting traction on the rest of the myosin bridge, causing the thin filaments to slide past the thick filaments (see Fig. 32.16). During contraction each cross-bridge undergoes several cycles of attachment, movement, and dissociation from the thin filaments.[22]

Calcium and Excitation-Contraction Coupling. Excitation-contraction coupling is the process by which an action potential arriving at the plasma membrane of the muscle fiber triggers the cycle, leading to cross-bridge activity and contraction. Activation of this cycle depends on the availability of calcium, and the amount of force developed is regulated by how much the concentration of calcium ion increases within the cardiomyocytes.

Calcium is stored in the tubule system and the sarcoplasmic reticulum. It enters the myocardial cell from the interstitial fluid after electrical excitation, which increases the membrane permeability to calcium. Two types of calcium channels (L-type and T-type) are identified in cardiac tissues. The L-type, or long-lasting, channels are the predominant type of calcium channels and are the channels blocked by calcium channel–blocking drugs (verapamil, nifedipine, diltiazem).[19] The major effect

of these medications is to decrease the strength of cardiac contraction. The T-type, or transient, channels are much less abundant in the heart and are not blocked by currently available calcium channel–blocking drugs and are being investigated. Calcium entering the cell from the interstitial fluid triggers release of calcium from the storage sites within the sarcomere. Calcium from these sites diffuses toward the myofibrils, where it binds with troponin.

Myocardial Relaxation

Relaxation is as vital to optimal cardiac function as contraction, and calcium, troponin, and tropomyosin also facilitate relaxation. After contraction, free calcium ions are actively pumped out of the cell back into the interstitial fluid or taken up again by the sarcoplasmic reticulum and stored. As the concentration of calcium within the sarcomere subsequently falls, troponin releases its bound calcium. The tropomyosin complex blocks the active sites on the actin molecule, preventing cross-bridges with the myosin heads. Impairment of myocardial relaxation can lead to increased diastolic filling pressures and eventually heart failure.[23]

Factors Affecting Cardiac Output

Cardiac capability can be evaluated by measuring the cardiac output. Cardiac output is calculated by multiplying heart rate in beats per minute (beats/min) by stroke volume in liters per beat. Normal adult cardiac output at rest is about 5 L/min. The at-rest heart rate is about 70 beats/min with a normal stroke volume of about 70 mL.[14] With each heartbeat, the ventricles eject much of their blood volume; the amount ejected per beat is called the ejection fraction. The ejection fraction is calculated by dividing the stroke volume by the end-diastolic volume. The end-diastolic volume (EDV) of the normal ventricle is about 70 to 80 mL/m^2, and the normal ejection fraction of the resting heart measured with gated myocardial perfusion imaging was 66% ± 8% for women and 58% ± 8% for men.[24] The ejection fraction is increased by factors that increase contractility, for example, sympathetic nervous system activity. A decrease in ejection fraction may indicate ventricular failure. The effects of aging on cardiovascular function are summarized in Table 32.3.

Four factors affect cardiac output directly: preload, afterload, myocardial contractility, and heart rate (Fig. 32.17). Preload is the volume inside the ventricle at the end of diastole (ventricular end-diastolic volume [VEDV] and pressure [VEDP]). Preload is determined by two major factors: (1) the amount of venous blood returning to the ventricle during diastole and (2) the amount of blood left in the ventricle after systole (end-systolic volume). Blood volume and flow through the venous system and the atrioventricular valves determine *venous return.* The strength of ventricular contraction and the resistance to ventricular emptying determine *end-systolic volume.* Clinically, preload is estimated by measuring the central venous pressure (CVP) for the right side of the heart and the pulmonary artery wedge pressure for the left side. Normal values for these two estimates are 1–5 and 4–12 mmHg, respectively.[25] Heart failure can occur because of an increase in preload (VEDV), which causes a decline in stroke volume and also increases VEDP. Increased VEDP causes pressures to increase or "back up" into the pulmonary or systemic venous circulation, increasing plasma outflow through the vessel walls, causing pulmonary edema (see Chapter 36).

Left ventricular afterload is the resistance to ejection of blood from the left ventricle (see p. 1035). More simply, it is the load the muscle must move during contraction. An index of afterload is aortic systolic pressure. To understand the role of these factors in cardiac performance, it is first necessary to understand two physical laws that explain the mechanisms of heart action: the Frank-Starling law of the heart and Laplace's law.

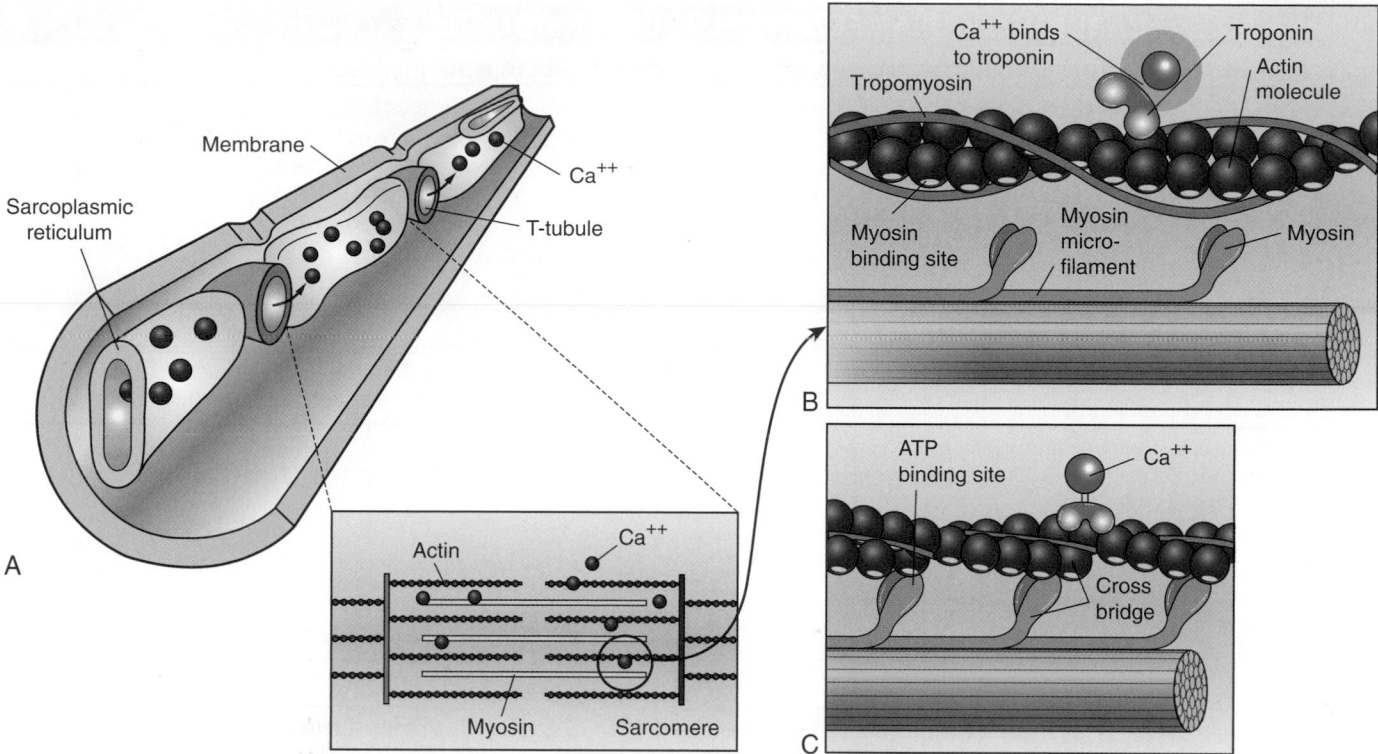

FIGURE 32.15 Myofilaments and Mechanisms of Muscle Contraction. A, Thin and thick myofilaments. In resting muscle, calcium ions are stored in the sarcoplasmic reticulum. When an action potential reaches the muscle cell, the T tubules carry the action potential deep into the sarcoplasm. The action potential causes the sarcoplasmic reticulum to release the store of calcium ions. **B,** In resting muscle the myosin-binding sites are covered by troponin and tropomyosin. The calcium ions released into the sarcoplasm as a result of the action potential bind to the troponin. This binding causes the tropomyosin and troponin to move out of the way of the myosin-binding sites, leaving the myosin heads free to bind to the actin microfilament. **C,** ATP is used as an energy molecule to the myosin cross-bridge. (Adapted from Raven PH, Johnson GB: *Understanding biology*, ed 3, Dubuque, IA, 1995, Brown.)

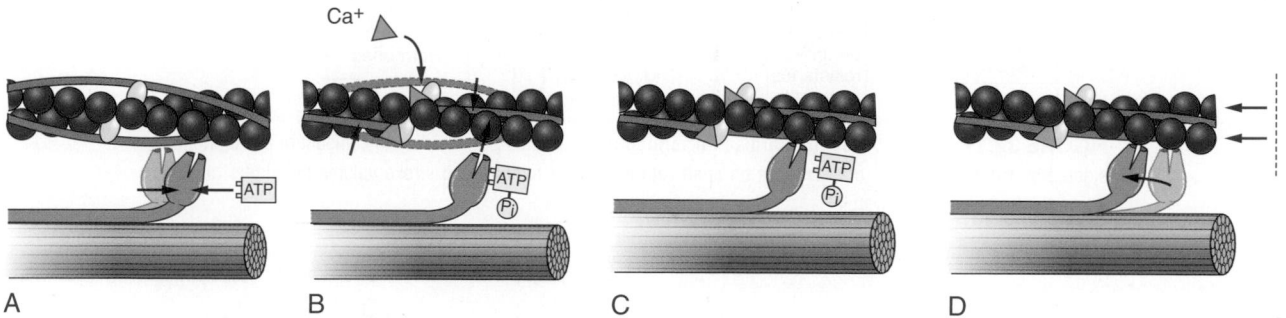

FIGURE 32.16 Cross-Bridge Theory of Muscle Contraction. A, Each myosin cross-bridge in the thick filament moves into a resting position after an adenosine triphosphate (ATP) molecule binds and transfers its energy. **B,** Calcium ions released from the sarcoplasmic reticulum bind to troponin in the thin filament, allowing tropomyosin to shift from its position blocking the active sites of actin molecules. **C,** Each myosin cross-bridge then binds to an active site on a thin filament, displacing the remnants of ATP hydrolysis—adenosine diphosphate (ADP) and inorganic phosphate (P_i). **D,** The release of stored energy from step **A** provides the force needed for each cross-bridge to move back to its original position, pulling actin along with it. Each cross-bridge will remain bound to actin until another ATP molecule binds to it and pulls it back into its resting position **(A).** (Adapted from Thibodeau GA, Patton KT: *Anatomy & physiology*, ed 4, St Louis, 1999, Mosby.)

Frank-Starling Law of the Heart

Cardiac muscle, like other muscle, increases its strength of contraction when it is stretched. This relationship was described in 1914 by a British physiologist, Ernest Starling, and was based on the earlier work of a German physiologist, Otto Frank. The Frank-Starling law of the heart, or the length-tension relationship of cardiac muscle, relates resting sarcomere length, expressed as the volume of blood in the heart at the end of diastole (end-diastolic volume), to tension generation, described as development of left ventricular pressure. Thus the volume of blood

TABLE 32.3	CARDIOVASCULAR FUNCTION IN OLDER ADULTS	
DETERMINANT	**RESTING CARDIAC PERFORMANCE**	**EXERCISE CARDIAC PERFORMANCE**
Cardiac index	Unchanged or slightly decreased in women only	Declines because of a decrease in heart rate and stroke volume
Heart rate	Slight decrease	Increases less than in younger people, possibly because of decreased cardiovascular response to catecholamines; overall slight decrease
Stroke volume	Slight increase	Slight increase
Ejection fraction	Unchanged	Increases less from rest to exercise in older people than in younger people
Afterload	Increased	Uncertain
End-diastolic volume	Unchanged	Unchanged
End-systolic volume	Unchanged	Higher in older people than in younger people
Contraction	Increased because of prolonged relaxation	Decreases with vigorous exercise*
Cardiac dilation	No change	Increases at end-diastole and end-systole
O_2 max	Not applicable	Declines because of a decline in skeletal muscle mass and increase in body fat

*As measured by end-systolic volume/systolic blood pressure (ESV/SBP), an index of contractility.
Data from Najjar SS, Gerstenblith G, Lakatta EG: Aging and the cardiovascular system. In Willerson JT et al, editors: *Cardiovascular medicine*, ed 3, London, 2007, Springer-Verlag.

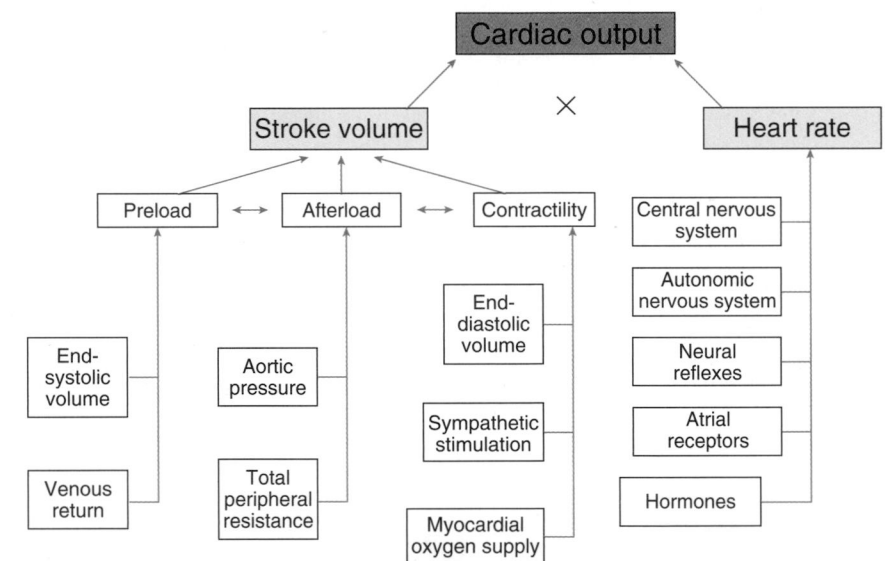

FIGURE 32.17 Factors Affecting Cardiac Performance. Cardiac output, which is the amount of blood (in liters) ejected by the heart per minute, depends on heart rate (beats per minute) and stroke volume (milliliters of blood ejected during ventricular systole).

in the heart at the end of diastole (the length of its muscle fibers) is directly related to the force of contraction during the next systole. Although the change in pressure is related to the volume of the ventricle and, consequently, to the length of the ventricular muscle fibers, preload (i.e., filling pressure) is commonly used as an index of ventricular volume. The length-tension mechanism is the main mechanism by which the normal right and left ventricles maintain equal minute outputs even though their stroke outputs may vary considerably during normal respiration. For example, changes in volume occur when an individual assumes a reclining position after being in a standing position; the volume of blood returning to the heart temporarily increases. The right ventricle stretches to accommodate this increase in volume and thereby increases its force of contraction. A larger stroke volume (i.e., the amount of blood ejected per beat) is pumped to the lungs, generating higher pressures. Pulmonary vascular pressure increases, causing a rise in the left ventricular filling pressure or preload. Left ventricular volume and

pressure increase. The left ventricle pumps a larger stroke volume, and arterial vascular pressure rises.

The mechanical function of the heart is characterized by a number of length-tension curves (Fig. 32.18). Factors that increase contractility (i.e., positive inotropic), such as sympathetic nerve stimulation, cause the heart to operate on a higher length-tension curve (curve *A* in Fig. 32.18). A higher tension or increase in ventricular stroke volume is generated without a necessary change in **left ventricular end-diastolic volume (LVEDV)** or fiber length. Heart failure (curve *C* in Fig. 32.18) is characterized by a lower length-tension curve (see Chapter 33). The Frank-Starling law of the heart may not apply to dilated or failing hearts because their fibers are already stretched beyond their optimal length. The failing heart responds to increased filling or stretch with a progressive decline in the force of contraction. Thus at the same left ventricular end-diastolic volume (LVEDV) as curves *A* and *B* (see Fig. 32.18), the force of contraction of stroke volume is decreased.

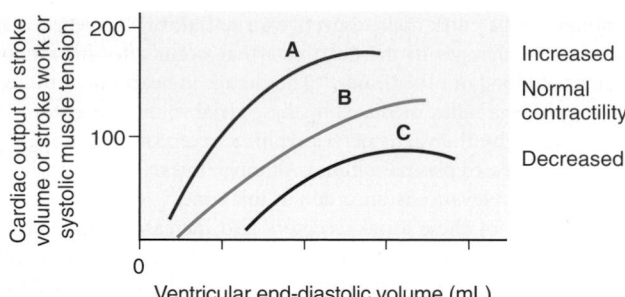

FIGURE 32.18 Frank-Starling Law of the Heart. Relationship between length and tension in the heart. End-diastolic volume determines end-diastolic length of ventricular muscle fibers and is proportional to tension generated during systole, as well as to cardiac output, stroke volume, and stroke work. A change in myocardial contractility causes the heart to perform on a different length-tension curve. (See text.) **A,** Increased contractility; **B,** normal contractility; **C,** heart failure or decreased contractility.

The cross-bridge arrangement with the sarcomere partially accounts for the length-tension mechanism of cardiac muscle. According to the Frank-Starling law, the longer the initial resting length of the cardiac muscle fiber (optimal length is between 2.2 and 2.4 mm), the greater the strength of contraction. At 2.2 mm an optimal number of active cross-bridges exist between actin and myosin. However, if the fibers are stretched beyond 2.2 to 2.4 mm, the force of contraction decreases because actin and myosin become partially disengaged, disrupting many of the cross-bridges. Excessive stretching, to about 3.65 mm, causes actin and myosin to become completely disengaged so that tension (force of contraction) drops to zero. The relationship between stretch and contraction can be compared with that of a rubber band. Up to a certain point, the more the rubber band is stretched the farther it will fly when one end is released; beyond that point, however, the rubber band will break but, of course, the myocardium does not actually break.

Laplace's Law

Laplace's law states that wall tension is related directly to the product of intraventricular pressure and internal radius and inversely related to the wall thickness as shown in the Laplace equation:

$$T = (p \times r)/\mu m$$

where T = wall tension, p = intraventricular pressure, r = internal radius of the sphere, and μm = wall thickness. In other words, the amount of tension generated in the ventricular wall (or any chamber or vessel) to produce a given intraventricular pressure depends on the size (radius and wall thickness) of the ventricle.

Laplace's law is useful for understanding aneurysm formation, distensibility in blood vessels, and the effects of ventricular dilation on myocardial contraction. Dilation is an important factor in heart failure (see Chapter 33). With a dilated ventricle, myocardial fibers in the wall must develop greater tension to produce a given pressure within the ventricle. The disadvantage of dilation is that the increased force, or tension, in the myocardial fibers required to develop a given pressure inside a dilated ventricle decreases the rate of fiber shortening, thereby decreasing the ability of the ventricle to eject blood.

Afterload

Ventricular afterload is the resistance to ejection of blood from the ventricle. Low aortic pressures (decreased afterload) enable the heart to contract more rapidly, whereas high aortic pressures (increased afterload) slow contraction and cause higher workloads against which

the heart must function to eject blood. Pressure in the ventricle must exceed aortic pressure before blood can be pumped out during systole. Increased aortic pressure is usually the result of increased systemic vascular resistance (SVR), also called total peripheral resistance (TPR). In individuals with hypertension, increased TPR means that afterload is chronically elevated, resulting in increased ventricular workload and hypertrophy of the myocardium. In some individuals, changes in afterload are the result of aortic valvular disease (see Fig. 32.17).

Myocardial Contractility

Stroke volume, or the volume of blood ejected per beat during systole, depends on the *force* of contraction, the myocardial contractility, or the degree of myocardial fiber shortening. Three major factors determine the force of contraction (see Fig. 32.17):

1. *Changes in the stretching of the ventricular myocardium caused by changes in VEDV (preload).* These changes were discussed earlier and an excessive increase in preload leads to decreased stroke volume.
2. *Alterations in the inotropic stimuli of the ventricles.* Inotropic agents affect contractility and include hormones, neurotransmitters, or medications. The sympathetic nervous system neurotransmitters, epinephrine and norepinephrine, are the most important endogenous positive inotropic agents. The most important negative inotropic agent is acetylcholine released from the vagus nerve. Many medications have positive or negative inotropic properties that can have significant effects on cardiac function. Cytokines released during sepsis, such as tumor necrosis factor-alpha (TNF-α) and interleukin-1β, are known to impair myocardial contractility.[26] Emerging is the understanding of mitochondrial dysfunction in sepsis and impaired myocardial function.[27]
3. *Adequacy of myocardial oxygen supply.* Both oxygen and carbon dioxide levels (tensions) in the coronary blood influence contractility. With oxygen saturation less than 50% (severe hypoxemia) myocardial contractility is decreased. Circulating catecholamines can increase contractility with moderate degrees of hypoxemia.[28]

Preload, afterload, and contractility all interact with one another to determine stroke volume and cardiac output. Changes in any one of these factors can result in deleterious effects on the others, resulting in heart failure (see Chapter 33).

Heart Rate

The SA node activity is the primary determinant of the heart rate. The control of heart rate includes activity of the CNS, autonomic nervous system, neural reflexes, atrial receptors, hormones (e.g., catecholamines [norepinephrine and epinephrine]), thyroid hormones, and growth hormones. Although these are principal factors, heart rate varies naturally with respiration, exercise, neuropsychologic factors (e.g., stressors, depression), cardiovascular disease, alcohol and drug consumption, air pollution, meditation, and others[29] (Figure E 32.1 [on Evolve]). This variability in heart rate is called heart rate variability (HRV); see Figure E 32.1(on Evolve) reveals physiologic, environmental, and psychologic elements linked with HRV.

In addition to HRV related to nervous system and hormonal factors, other factors include cardiovascular disease (CVD), depression, and proinflammatory cytokines, which can lead to immune dysfunction and inflammation.[29] Neurologic diseases linked with a HRV decrease include parkinsonian syndrome, spinocerebellar degeneration, Shy-Drager syndrome, multiple sclerosis, and Guillain-Barré syndrome. Temperature affects HRV; temperature decrease can induce bradycardia and temperature increase can increase heart rate. Estrogen levels correlated with HRV measures in healthy women and androgens have a parasympathetic effect (higher HPV with high testosterone levels).[29]Occupational settings can influence HRV, such as particulate matter, chemicals, electromagnetic fields (EMFs), vibrating tools, psychosocial environment, working time, fatigue, and others. A chronic exposure to these factors was linked to a decrease in HRV.[29] A high level of work stress also was associated with a low HRV.[29]

Heart rate varies naturally with respiration, the rate increasing with inspiration and decreasing with expiration. This normal alteration in rhythm pattern, called sinus arrhythmia, is caused by changes that occur within the chest cavity because of respiration. Inspiration results in stretch and an associated increase in firing of the SA node that increases heart rate. The stretch is reduced with expiration and the SA node firing rate slows, resulting in a decrease in heart rate.[30]

The average heart rate in healthy adults is about 70 beats/min. The average heart rate is typically greater in children. Heart rate diminishes by 10 to 20 beats/min during sleep and can accelerate to more than 100 beats/min during muscular activity or emotional excitement. In well-conditioned athletes the resting heart rate is about 50 to 60 beats/min. In highly trained or elite athletes, the resting heart rate can be less than 50 beats/min; these athletes have a greater stroke volume and lower peripheral resistance in active muscles than they had before training.

Cardiovascular Control Centers in the Brain.
The cardiovascular vasomotor control center is in the medulla and pons of the brainstem with additional areas in the hypothalamus, the cerebral cortex, and the thalamus. The hypothalamic centers regulate cardiovascular responses to changes in temperature; the cerebral cortex centers adjust cardiac reaction to a variety of emotional states; and the medullary control center regulates heart rate and blood pressure (see Fig. 32.10).

The nerve fibers from the cardiovascular control center synapse with the autonomic neurons that control the rate of firing of the SA node. As discussed earlier, sympathetic (adrenergic) stimulation increases heart rate. When the parasympathetic nerves to the heart are stimulated (primarily vagus nerve), the heart slows and the sympathetic nerves to the heart, arterioles, and veins are inhibited.

The resting heart rate in healthy individuals is primarily under the control of parasympathetic stimulation. While the individual is at rest, parasympathetic effects from the vagus nerves override sympathetic effects in the SA node. Interruption of the vagus nerves causes significant tachycardia (abnormally fast heart rate) because the inhibitory parasympathetic influence is lost.

Neural Reflexes.
The baroreceptor reflex is important in blood pressure control and is mediated by stretch receptors (baroreceptors or pressoreceptors) in the aortic arch and carotid arteries. (Because the receptors respond to mechanical factors, they are also called *aortic and carotid mechanoreceptors*.) When blood pressure falls, the baroreceptor reflex accelerates heart rate, increases myocardial contractility, and causes constriction of arterioles in the systemic circulation. These responses raise blood pressure back toward normal and are critical to maintaining adequate tissue perfusion. Aging is associated with dysfunction of the baroreceptor reflex (baroreflex) and can result in postural hypotension[31] (orthostatic hypotension, see Chapter 33).

The baroreflex also can reduce high blood pressure. The mechanoreceptors increase their rate of discharge when stretched by blood pressure elevations. Neural impulses are then transmitted over the glossopharyngeal nerve (ninth cranial nerve) from the carotid artery and through the vagus nerve from the aorta to the cardiovascular control centers in the medulla. These centers initiate an increase in parasympathetic activity and a decrease in sympathetic activity, causing blood vessels to dilate and heart rate to decrease. Responses to the baroreceptor reflex return the blood pressure to its previous level, which may or may not have been normal.

Atrial Receptors.
Mechanoreceptors that influence heart rate exist in both atria.[32] They are located where the veins, venae cavae, and pulmonary veins enter their respective atria. Bainbridge reflex is the name for the changes in the heart rate that occur after intravenous infusions of blood or other fluids.[33] The change in heart rate is thought to be caused by a reflex mediated by these atrial volume receptors that are innervated by the vagus nerves (volume receptors are thought to respond to increased plasma volume). Although this reflex can be elicited in humans, its relevance is uncertain at this time.[33]

Stimulation of these atrial receptors also increases urine volume, presumably because of a neurally mediated reduction in antidiuretic hormone. Peptides of the atrial natriuretic family also are released from atrial tissue in response to the increases in blood volume. These peptides have diuretic and natriuretic (salt excretion) properties, resulting in decreased blood volume and pressure. The atrial natriuretic peptides can relax vascular smooth muscle and oppose myocardial hypertrophy, leading to measurement of blood levels to evaluate clinical status and raising interest in their use as therapeutic agents.[34]

Hormones and Biochemicals.
Hormones and biochemicals affect the arteries, arterioles, venules, capillaries, and contractility of the myocardium. Norepinephrine increases heart rate, enhances myocardial contractility, and constricts blood vessels. Epinephrine dilates vessels of the liver and skeletal muscle and causes an increase in myocardial contractility. Some adrenocortical hormones, such as hydrocortisone, potentiate the effects of the catecholamines.

Thyroid hormone, specifically triiodothyronine, causes increases in both heart rate and contractility, resulting in an increase in cardiac output; it also decreases systemic vascular resistance. Triiodothyronine acts directly on the cardiac myocytes to cause gene transcription and cellular changes that result in more calcium release from the sarcoplasmic reticulum.[35] Awareness of these changes helps to understand the cardiovascular changes that occur with thyroid diseases. Growth hormone, working together with insulin-like growth factor 1 (IGF-1), also has been shown to increase myocardial contractility.[36] Decreases in levels of growth hormone or thyroid hormone may result in bradycardia, reduced cardiac output, and low blood pressure.

THE SYSTEMIC CIRCULATION

The arteries and veins of the systemic circulation are illustrated in Fig. 32.19. Oxygenated blood from the left side of the heart flows through the aorta and into the systemic arteries. These arteries branch into small arterioles that branch into the smallest vessels, the capillaries, where nutrient exchange between the blood and tissues occurs. Blood from the capillaries then enters tiny venules that join to form the larger veins, which return venous blood to the right heart. Peripheral vascular system is the term used to describe the part of the systemic circulation that supplies the skin and the extremities, particularly the legs and feet.

Structure of Blood Vessels

Blood vessel walls are composed of three layers: (1) the tunica intima (innermost or intimal layer); (2) the tunica media (middle or medial layer); and (3) the tunica externa or adventitia (outermost or external layer), which also contains nerves and lymphatic vessels. These layers are illustrated in Fig. 32.20. Blood vessel walls vary in thickness depending on the thickness or absence of one or more of these three layers. Cells of the larger vessels are nourished by the vasa vasorum, small vessels located in the tunica externa, and innervated by perivascular nerves. The vasa vasorum arises from the blood vessel itself or from other vessels nearby.

Adults are capable of growing new blood vessels through three processes, all of which are important in wound healing but also contribute to tumor growth. The three processes are angiogenesis, arteriogenesis, and vasculogenesis. Both angiogenesis and arteriogenesis occur by growth of new vessels that branch from existing vessels. Angiogenesis is branching of small vessels, such as capillaries, whereas arteriogenesis occurs by branching from larger vessels, such as arterioles. Vasculogenesis is a term that refers to the growth of vessels from progenitor or stemlike cells that originate in the bone marrow and other body tissues.[37]

Arterial Vessels

Arterial walls are composed of elastic connective tissue, fibrous connective tissue, and smooth muscle. There are two types of arteries: elastic and muscular. The elastic arteries have a very thick tunica media that contains more elastic fibers than smooth muscle fibers. Elastic arteries include the aorta and its major branches and the pulmonary trunk. Elasticity enables the vessel to absorb energy imparted to the blood by ventricular contraction and they stretch as blood is ejected from the heart during systole. During diastole, elasticity promotes recoil of the arteries, which is important for maintaining blood pressure within the vessels, and retransfers the energy from the elastic artery walls to the blood.

The muscular arteries are medium and small size arteries farther from the heart than the elastic arteries. They contain fewer elastic fibers and more muscle fibers than the elastic arteries and their function is to distribute blood to arterioles throughout the body. Because their smooth muscle can be stimulated to contract or relax, they play a role in controlling blood flow and in directing flow to the parts of the body with the highest need at any time. During exercise more blood is sent

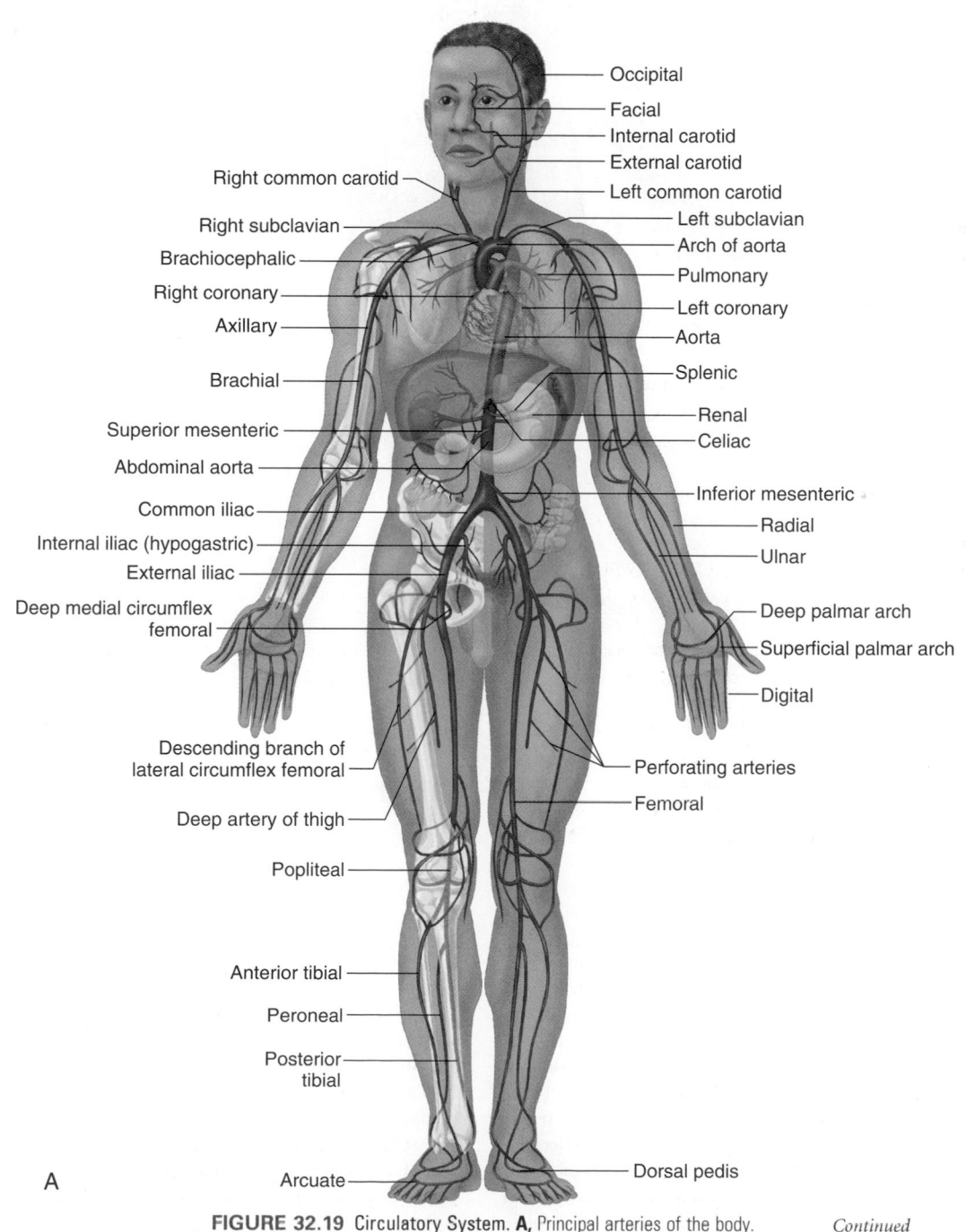

FIGURE 32.19 Circulatory System. **A,** Principal arteries of the body. *Continued*

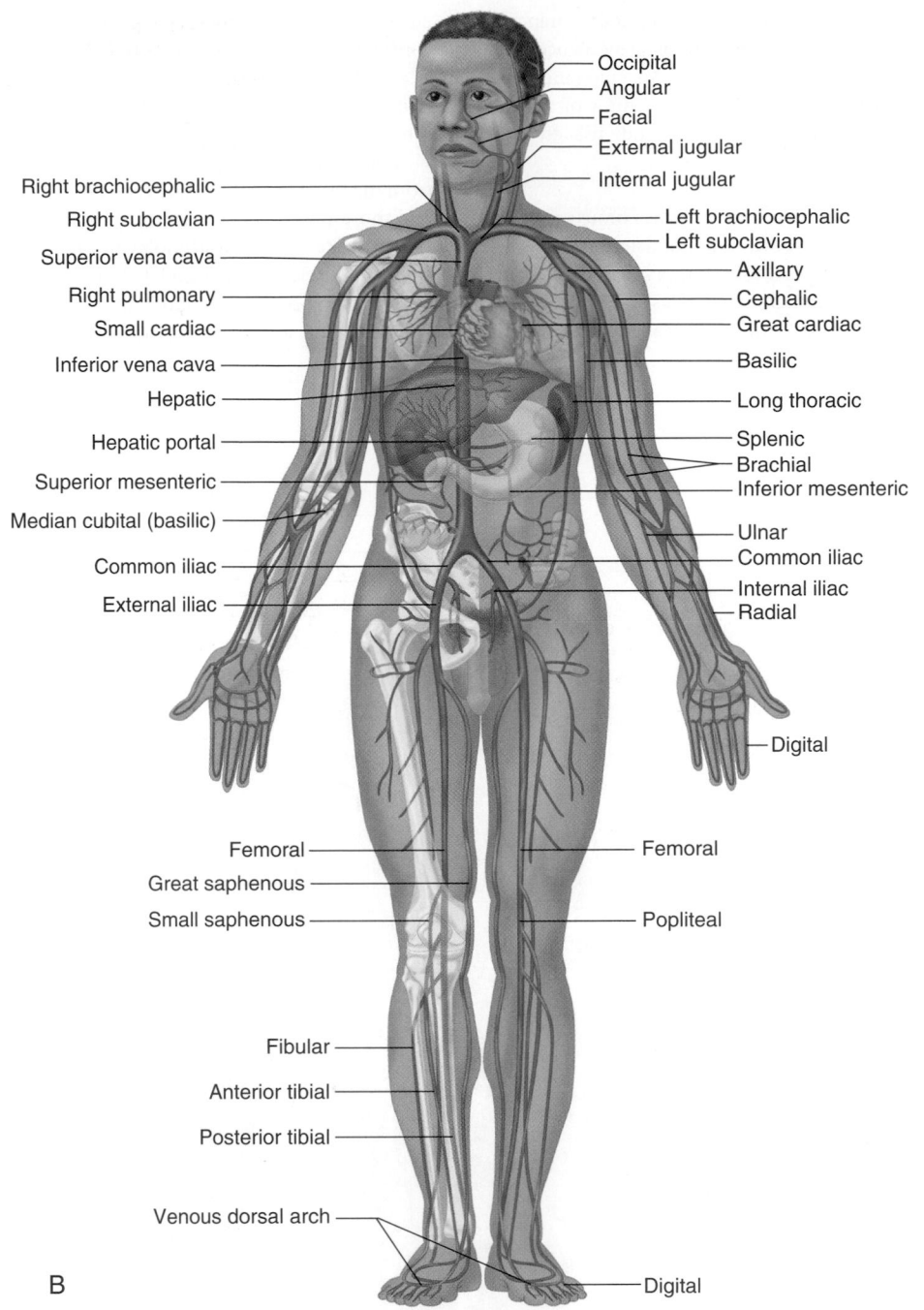

Occipital
Angular
Facial
External jugular
Internal jugular
Right brachiocephalic
Right subclavian
Superior vena cava
Right pulmonary
Small cardiac
Inferior vena cava
Hepatic
Hepatic portal
Superior mesenteric
Median cubital (basilic)
Common iliac
External iliac
Left brachiocephalic
Left subclavian
Axillary
Cephalic
Great cardiac
Basilic
Long thoracic
Splenic
Brachial
Inferior mesenteric
Ulnar
Common iliac
Internal iliac
Radial
Digital
Femoral
Great saphenous
Small saphenous
Femoral
Popliteal
Fibular
Anterior tibial
Posterior tibial
Venous dorsal arch
Digital

B

FIGURE 32.19, cont'd B, Principal veins of the body. (From Patton KT, Thibodeau GA: *The human body in health & disease,* ed 7, St Louis, 2018, Mosby.)

to the skeletal muscles, while after a meal more blood is directed to the gut and liver. Contraction narrows the vessel lumen (the internal cavity of the vessel), which diminishes flow through the vessel. This condition is termed vasoconstriction. When the smooth muscle layer relaxes, more blood flows through the vessel lumen, a state called vasodilation.

An artery becomes an arteriole at the point where the diameter of its lumen narrows to less than 0.5 mm. The arterioles are composed almost exclusively of smooth muscle, with little elastic tissue. Arterioles regulate the flow of blood into the capillaries by vasoconstriction, which retards the flow of blood into the capillaries, and vasodilation, which permits blood to enter the capillaries freely (Fig. 32.21). The thick, smooth muscle layer of the arterioles is a major determinant of the resistance blood encounters as it flows through the systemic circulation.

The capillary network is composed of connective channels called metarterioles, and "true" capillaries (see Fig. 32.21). Metarterioles have discontinuous smooth muscle cells in their tunica media whereas capillaries lack any smooth muscle cells. The capillaries branch from the metarterioles, meeting at a ring of smooth muscle called the precapillary sphincters. As the sphincters contract and relax, they regulate blood flow through the capillaries. Appropriately stimulated, the precapillary sphincters help maintain arterial pressure and regulate selective flow to vascular beds.

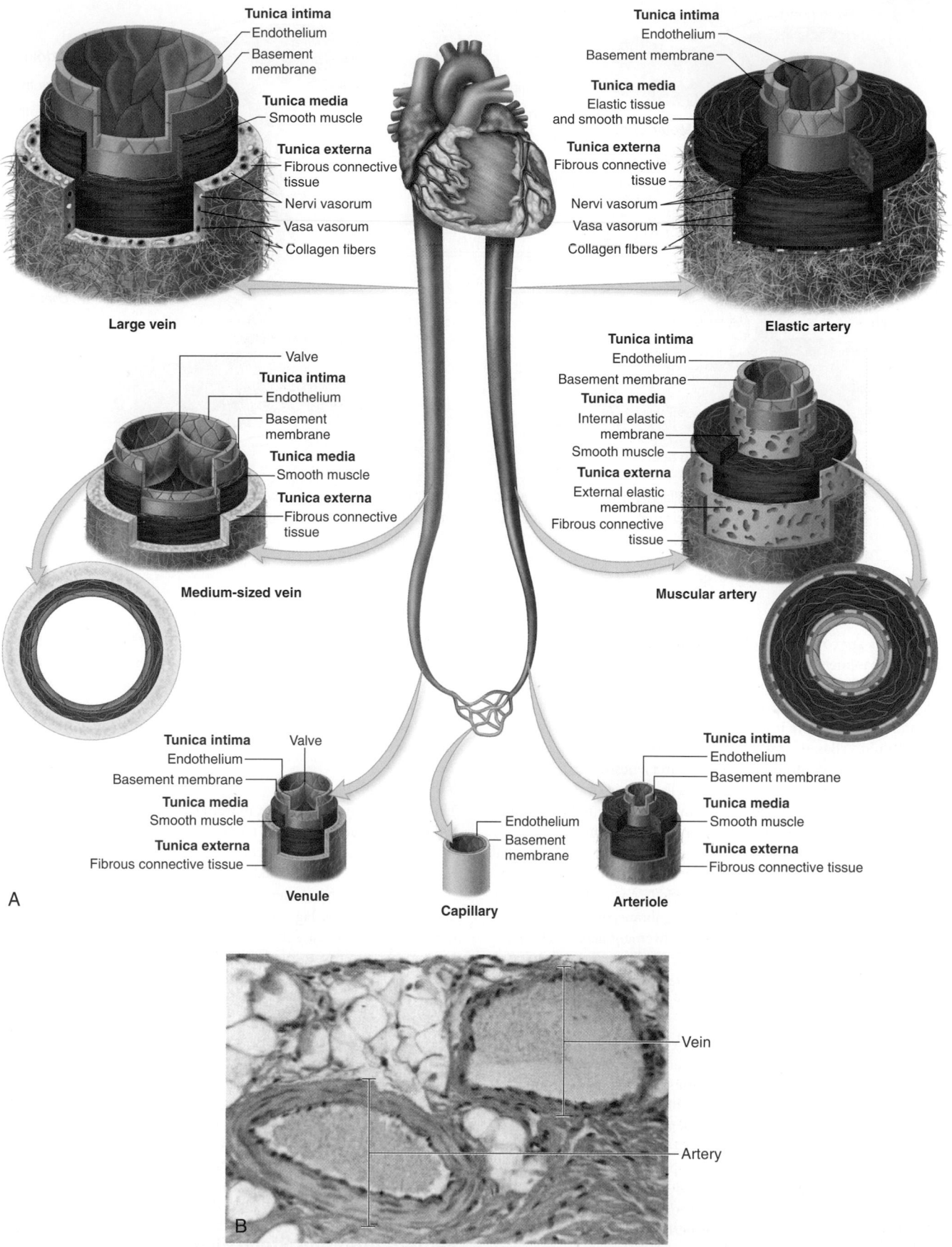

FIGURE 32.20 Structure of Blood Vessels, and an Artery and Vein. **A,** Structure of blood vessels. The tunica externa of the veins are color-coded blue and the arteries red. **B,** Artery and vein. Light micrograph of a cross section of similar-sized artery *(left)* and vein *(right)*. Notice the thick muscular wall of the artery as compared to the thin-walled vein. (From Patton KT, Thibodeau GA: *Anatomy & physiology,* ed 9, St Louis, 2016, Mosby.)

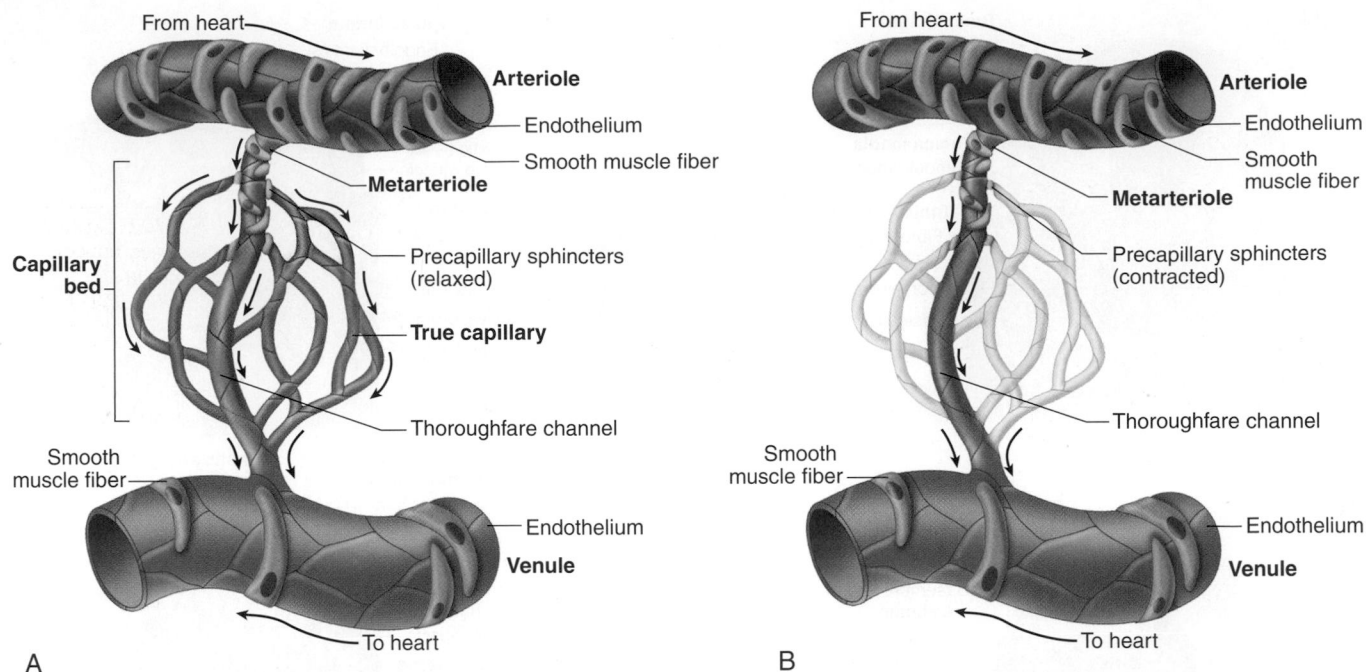

FIGURE 32.21 Capillary Wall and Microcirculation. Control of blood flow through a capillary network is regulated by the relative contraction of precapillary sphincters surrounding arterioles and metarterioles. **A,** Sphincters are relaxed, permitting blood flow to enter the capillary bed. **B,** With sphincters contracted, blood flows from the metarteriole directly into the thoroughfare channel, bypassing the capillary bed. (From Patton KT, Thibodeau GA: *Anatomy & physiology*, ed 9, St Louis, 2016, Mosby.)

Capillaries are composed solely of a layer of endothelial cells surrounded by a basement membrane. Their thin walls and unique structure make possible the rapid exchange of water, small (low-molecular-weight) soluble molecules, some larger molecules (such as albumin), and cells of the innate and adaptive immune system between the blood and the interstitial fluid.[38] Based on their structure, three types of capillaries have been described: continuous, sinusoid, and fenestrated. In the renal glomerulus, for example, the endothelial cells contain oval windows or pores termed fenestrations, which are covered by a thin diaphragm.[39] Sinusoid capillaries are found in the liver and bone marrow.

Substances pass between the capillary lumen and the interstitial fluid in several ways: (1) through junctions between endothelial cells, (2) through fenestrations in endothelial cells, (3) in vesicles moved by active transport across the endothelial cell membrane, or (4) by diffusion through the endothelial cell membrane. (Movement across cell membranes is described in Chapter 1.) A single capillary may be only 0.5 to 1 mm in length and 0.01 mm in diameter, but the capillaries are so numerous that their total surface area may be more than 600 m².

Endothelium

The vascular endothelium, or blood vessel lining, is important to several body functions and is considered by some to be a separate endocrine organ (Fig. 32.22). All tissues depend on blood supply and the blood supply depends on endothelial cells, which form the lining, or endothelium of the blood vessel (see Fig. 32.22). In addition to substance transport, the vascular endothelium has important roles in coagulation, antithrombogenesis, and fibrinolysis; immune system function; tissue growth and wound healing; and vasomotion, the contraction and relaxation of vessels. The endothelium performs these vital functions through synthesis and release of vasoactive chemicals (Table 32.4). Because of its varying roles, the actual structure of the endothelium may vary in different vascular beds. For example, within lymph nodes

the endothelial cells of specialized venules, called *high endothelial venules*, are uniquely structured to support the movement of lymphocytes from the blood into the lymph node.[40] Endothelial injury and dysfunction are central processes in many of the most common and serious cardiovascular disorders including hypertension and atherosclerosis (see Chapter 33).

Veins

The smallest venules downstream from the capillaries have an endothelial lining surrounded by fibrous tissue. The largest venules, those farthest from the capillaries, are surrounded by a few smooth muscle fibers comprising a thin tunica media.

Compared with arteries, veins are thin walled and fibrous with a larger diameter (see Fig. 32.20). A given vein is larger than the artery that lies within the same sheath. Veins are more numerous than arteries. In veins the tunica externa has less elastic tissue than that in arteries, so veins do not recoil after distention as quickly as arteries. Like arteries, veins receive nourishment from the tiny vasa vasorum. Some veins, typically in the legs, contain valves that regulate the one-way flow of blood toward the heart (Fig. 32.23). These valves are folds of the tunica intima and are structurally similar to the semilunar valves of the heart. Backflow in veins of the legs is stopped as the flaps of the valves fill with blood and block the vessel. The position of the valves also facilitates blood flow in the proper direction during venous compression. When a person stands up, contraction of the skeletal muscles of the legs compresses the deep veins of the legs and assists the flow of blood toward the heart. This important mechanism of venous return is called the *muscle pump* (see Fig. 32.23).

Factors Affecting Blood Flow

Blood flow, the amount of fluid moved per unit of time, is usually expressed as liters or milliliters per minute (L/min or mL/min). The

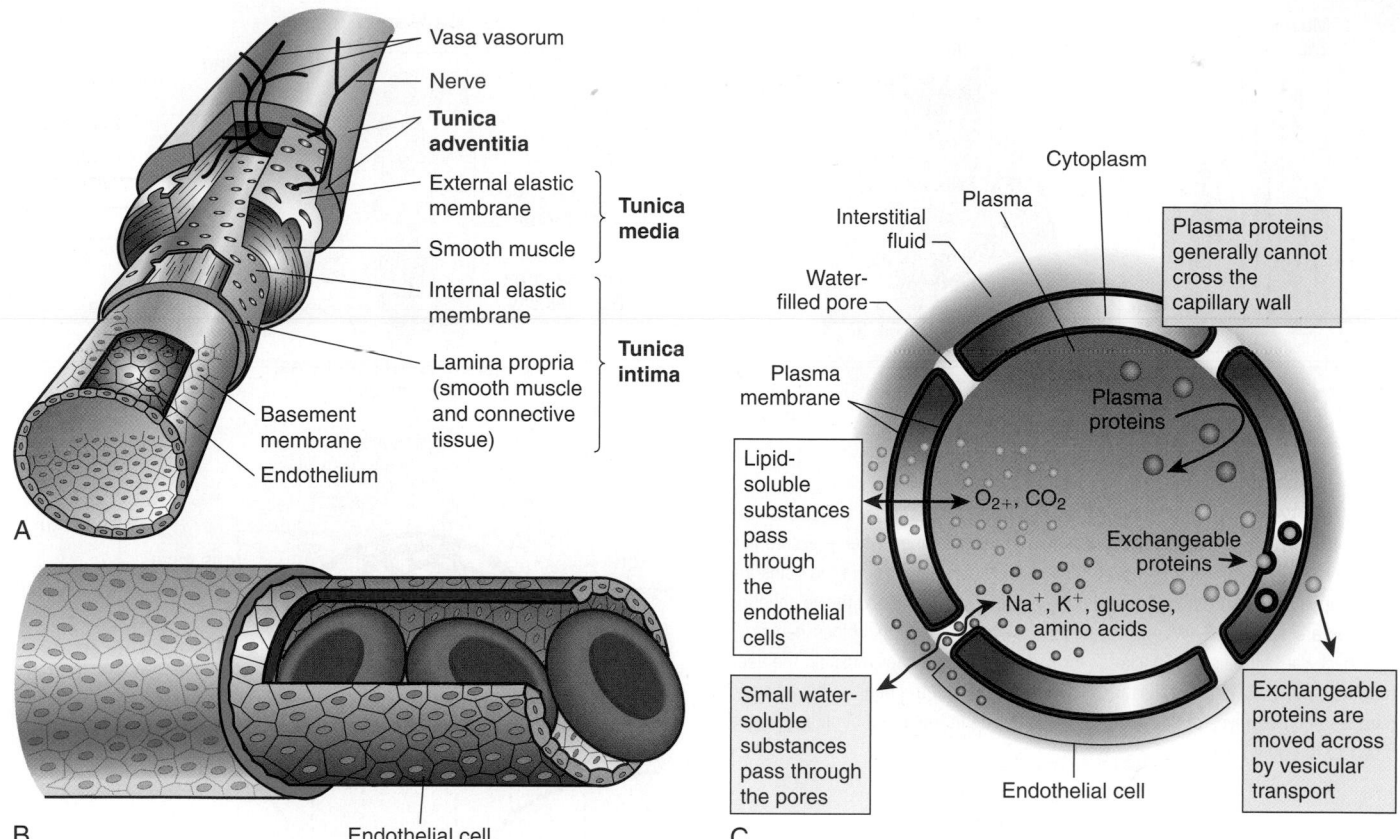

FIGURE 32.22 Endothelium. A, This schematic shows the endothelium in context with the entire blood vessel. Practically imperceptible, the endothelial cells arrange themselves as a fine lining that has numerous life support functions. **B,** The inset shows more clearly the endothelial cells. **C,** The endothelium supports numerous functions through synthesis and release of vasoactive fibers.

TABLE 32.4	FUNCTIONS OF THE ENDOTHELIUM
FUNCTION	**ACTIONS INVOLVED**
Filtration and permeability	Facilitates transport of large molecules via vesicular transport movement through intercellular junctions
	Facilitates transport of small molecules via movement of vesicles, through opening of tight junctions, and across cytoplasm
Vasomotion	Stimulates vascular relaxation through production of nitric oxide, prostacyclin, and other vasodilators
	Stimulates vascular constriction through production of endothelin-1 and of angiotensin II by the action of endothelial angiotensin-converting enzyme on angiotensin I
Hemostatic balance	Endothelial surface is normally antithrombotic and maintains a balance between pro- and anti-coagulant factors, as well as pro- and anti-fibrinolytic factors
	Anticoagulant factors include prostacyclin, nitric oxide, antithrombin, thrombomodulin, tissue factor pathway inhibitor, and heparins
	Procoagulant factors include tissue factor (factor VII), factor VIII, factor V, and plasminogen activator inhibitor-1 (PAI-1)
	Profibrinolytic factors are tissue- and urokinase-type plasminogen activating factor and plasminogen activator inhibitor-1 (PAI-1)
	Antifibrinolytic factor is tissue plasminogen activator
Inflammation/immunity	Expresses chemotactic agents and adhesion molecules that support white blood cells (including monocytes, neutrophils, and lymphocytes) moving into tissues
	Expresses receptors for oxidized lipoproteins, allowing them to enter vascular intima
Angiogenesis/vessel growth	Releases growth factors such as endothelin-1 and heparins for vascular smooth muscle cells
Lipid metabolism	Expresses receptors for lipoprotein lipase and low-density lipoproteins (LDLs)

From Griendling KK et al: Biology of the vessel wall. In Fuster et al, editors: *Hurst's the heart,* ed 13, Philadelphia, 2011, McGraw-Hill; Rajendran P et al: *Int J Biol Sci* 9(10):1057–1069, 2013.

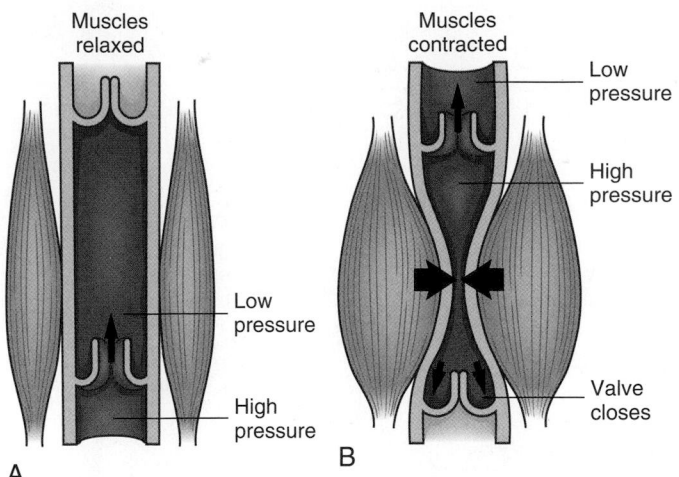

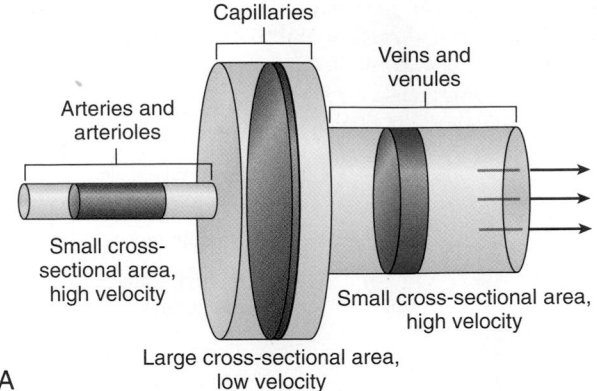

FIGURE 32.23 Venous Valves and the Muscle Pump. In veins, one-way valves aid circulation by preventing backflow of venous blood when pressure in a local area is low. **A,** Blood is moved toward the heart as valves in the veins are forced open by pressure from the volume of blood downstream and the neighboring muscles are relaxed. **B,** When pressure below the valve drops, blood begins to flow backward but fills the "pockets" formed by the valve flaps, pushing the flaps together and thus blocking further backward flow. Contraction in the adjacent muscles and the valves of the systemic veins assists in the return of unoxygenated blood to the right heart.

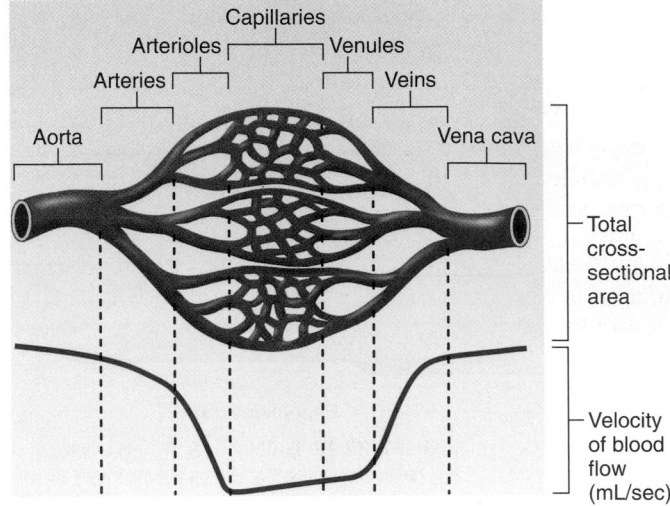

FIGURE 32.24 Relationship Between Cross-Sectional Area and Flow Rate of Blood. As can be seen in the simple diagram **(A)** and the blood vessel chart **(B)**, blood flows with great speed in the large arteries. However, branching of arterial vessels increases the total cross-sectional area of the arterioles and capillaries, reducing the flow rate. When capillaries merge into venules and venules merge into veins, the total cross-sectional area decreases, causing the flow rate to increase. (From Patton KT, Thibodeau GA: *Anatomy & physiology*, ed 9, St Louis, 2016, Mosby.)

most important factors that influence blood flow are pressure and resistance, followed by velocity, turbulent versus laminar flow, and compliance.

Pressure and Resistance

Pressure in a liquid system is the force exerted on the liquid per unit area and is expressed clinically as millimeters of mercury (mmHg), or torr (1 torr = 1 mmHg). Blood flow to a specific organ depends partly on the pressure difference between the arterial and venous vessels supplying that organ. Fluid moves from the arterial "side" of the capillaries, a region of greater pressure, to the venous side, a region of lesser pressure.

Resistance is the opposition to blood flow. Most opposition to blood flow results from the diameter and length of the blood vessels. Changes in blood flow through an organ result from changes in the vascular resistance within the organ because of increases or decreases in vessel diameter and the opening or closing of vascular channels. Resistance in a vessel is inversely related to blood flow; that is, increased resistance leads to decreased blood flow. Poiseuille's law indicates that resistance is directly related to tube length and fluid viscosity (blood viscosity) and inversely related to the radius of the tube to the fourth power (r^4). Blood flow is inversely related to resistance so that the greater the resistance in a vascular bed or tissue, the lower the blood flow. Resistance to flow cannot be measured directly but it can be calculated if the pressure difference and flow volumes are known. Resistance to blood flow in a single vessel is determined by the radius and length of the blood vessel and by the blood viscosity.

Clinically the most important factor determining resistance *in a single vessel* is the radius (diameter) of the vessel's lumen. Small changes in the lumen's radius lead to large changes in vascular resistance. Clinically, vasoconstriction will contribute to an increase in resistance whereas vasodilation will cause a decrease in resistance that may be reflected by a fall in blood pressure. Because vessel length is relatively constant and lumen size is quite variable, length is not as important as lumen size

in determining flow through a single vessel. Because viscosity is relatively constant, blood vessel radius is usually the key factor in determining total peripheral resistance. An exception to this rule is when red blood cell volume, measured as hematocrit, is elevated, which is relatively rare. Conditions with elevated hematocrits include a lack of body water, cyanotic congenital heart disease (see Chapter 34), or polycythemia (see Chapter 28) and can lead to increased cardiac work as a result of increased vascular resistance.

Resistance to flow through a *system of vessels*, or **total resistance**, depends not only on characteristics of individual vessels but also on whether the vessels are arranged in *series* (end-to-end) or in *parallel* (side-to-side) and on the total cross-sectional area of the system. Vessels arranged in parallel provide less resistance than vessels arranged in series. Blood flowing through the distributing arteries, beginning with branches off the aorta and ending at arterioles in the capillary bed, encounters more resistance than blood flowing through the capillary bed itself, where flow is distributed among many short, tiny branches arranged in parallel (Fig. 32.24). The total cross-sectional area of the arteriolar system is greater than that of the arterial system, yet the greater number of arterioles arranged in series leads to great resistance to flow in the arteriolar system. In contrast, the capillary system has a larger number of vessels arranged in parallel than the arteriolar system, and the total cross-sectional area is much greater; thus there is lower resistance overall through the capillary system. The resulting slow velocity of flow in each capillary is optimal for capillary-tissue exchange.

Velocity

Blood velocity, or *speed,* is the *distance* blood travels in a unit of time, usually centimeters per second (cm/sec). Blood velocity is directly related to blood flow (*amount* of blood moved per unit of time) and inversely related to the cross-sectional area of the vessel in which the blood is flowing (see Fig. 32.24). As blood moves from the aorta to the capillaries, the total cross-sectional area of the vessels increases and the velocity decreases.

Viscosity

Flow varies inversely with the viscosity—thick, sticky consistency of the fluid. Thick fluids move more slowly and cause greater resistance to flow than thin fluids—just think of honey as compared to water. The viscosity of blood depends on red cell content. The greater the percentage of red cells in the blood, the more viscous the blood. This relationship is expressed as the hematocrit—the ratio of the volume of more red blood cells to the volume of whole blood (see Chapter 28). A high hematocrit value reduces flow through the blood vessels, particularly the microcirculation (arterioles, capillaries, venules).

Laminar Versus Turbulent Flow

Flow through any tubular system can be either laminar or turbulent. Blood flow through the vessels, except where vessels split or branch, is mainly laminar. In laminar flow, concentric layers of molecules move "straight ahead." Each concentric layer flows at a different velocity (Fig. 32.25). The cohesive attraction between the fluid and the vessel wall prevents the molecules of blood that are in contact with the wall from moving. The next thin layer of blood is able to slide slowly past the stationary layer and so on until, at the center, the blood velocity is greatest. The centermost concentric layer of fluid is not slowed by friction against the vessel wall. Large vessels have room for a large center layer; therefore they have less resistance to flow and greater flow and velocity than smaller vessels.

Where flow is obstructed, the vessel turns, or blood flows over rough surfaces; it becomes turbulent with whorls or eddy currents that produce noise, causing a murmur to be heard on auscultation. Resistance increases with turbulence, which frequently occurs in areas with atherosclerotic plaques. Wall shear stress (WSS) is the complex interaction between the vessel wall's endothelial layer and blood hemodynamics. Much investigation is on the consequences of lower WSS and the promotion of plaque development distal to an induced stenosis.[41] Clarifying WSS and the perivascular changes with inflammation, macrophage activation, medial thinning, and plaque disruption is critical.

Vascular Compliance

Vascular compliance is the increase in volume a vessel is able to accommodate for a given increase in pressure. Compliance depends on the factors related to the nature of a vessel wall, such as the ratio of elastic fibers to muscle fibers in the vessel wall. Elastic arteries are more compliant than muscular arteries; the veins are more compliant than either type of artery because they have less smooth muscle. Because they are more compliant, veins serve as storage areas for the circulatory system.

Compliance determines a vessel's response to pressure changes. For example, with a very small increase in pressure, a large volume of blood

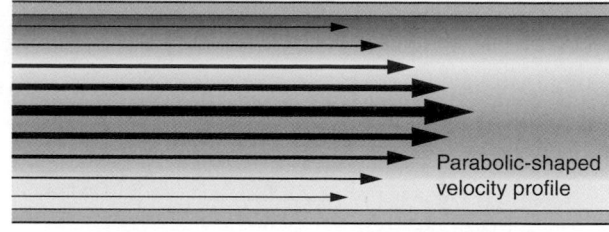

A

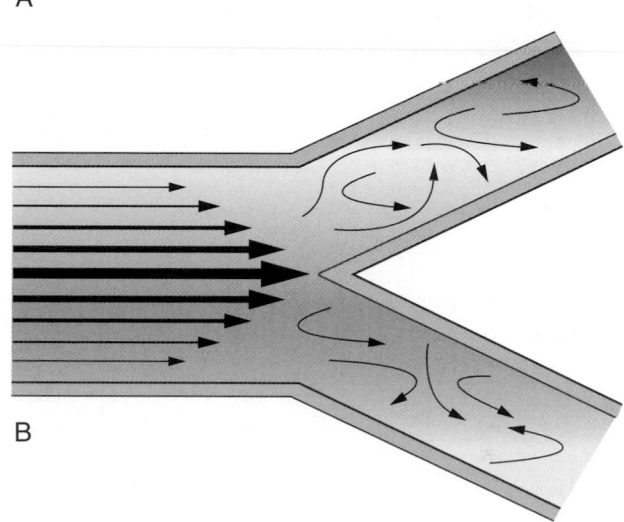

B

FIGURE 32.25 Laminar and Turbulent Flow. **A,** Laminar flow. Fluid flows in long smooth-walled tubes as if it is composed of a large number of concentric layers. **B,** Turbulent flow is caused by numerous small currents flowing crosswise or oblique to the long axis of the vessel, resulting in flowing whorls and eddy currents. (Adapted from Seeley RR, Stephens TD, Tate P: *Anatomy and physiology,* ed 3, St Louis, 1995, Mosby.)

can be accommodated by the venous system. In the less compliant arterial system, where smaller volumes and higher pressures are normal, small variations in pressure cause little or no change in the volume of blood within the arterial vessels.

Stiffness is the opposite of compliance. Several conditions and disorders can increase vascular stiffness, with the most common being aging and arteriosclerosis (see Chapter 33 and section on aging at the end of this chapter). Arteriosclerosis increases the rigidity or stiffness of arterial walls, which in turn increases peak arterial pressure at a given volume of blood.

Regulation of Blood Pressure
Arterial Pressure

Arterial pressure is determined by the cardiac output multiplied by the peripheral resistance (Fig. 32.26). The systolic blood pressure is the highest arterial blood pressure following ventricular contraction or systole. The diastolic blood pressure is the lowest arterial blood pressure that occurs during ventricular filling or diastole. The mean arterial pressure (MAP), which is the average pressure in the arteries throughout the cardiac cycle, depends on the elastic properties of the arterial walls and the mean volume of blood in the arterial system. MAP can be approximated from the measured values of the systolic (Ps) and diastolic (Pd) pressures as follows:

$$MAP = Pd + \frac{1}{3}(Ps - Pd)$$

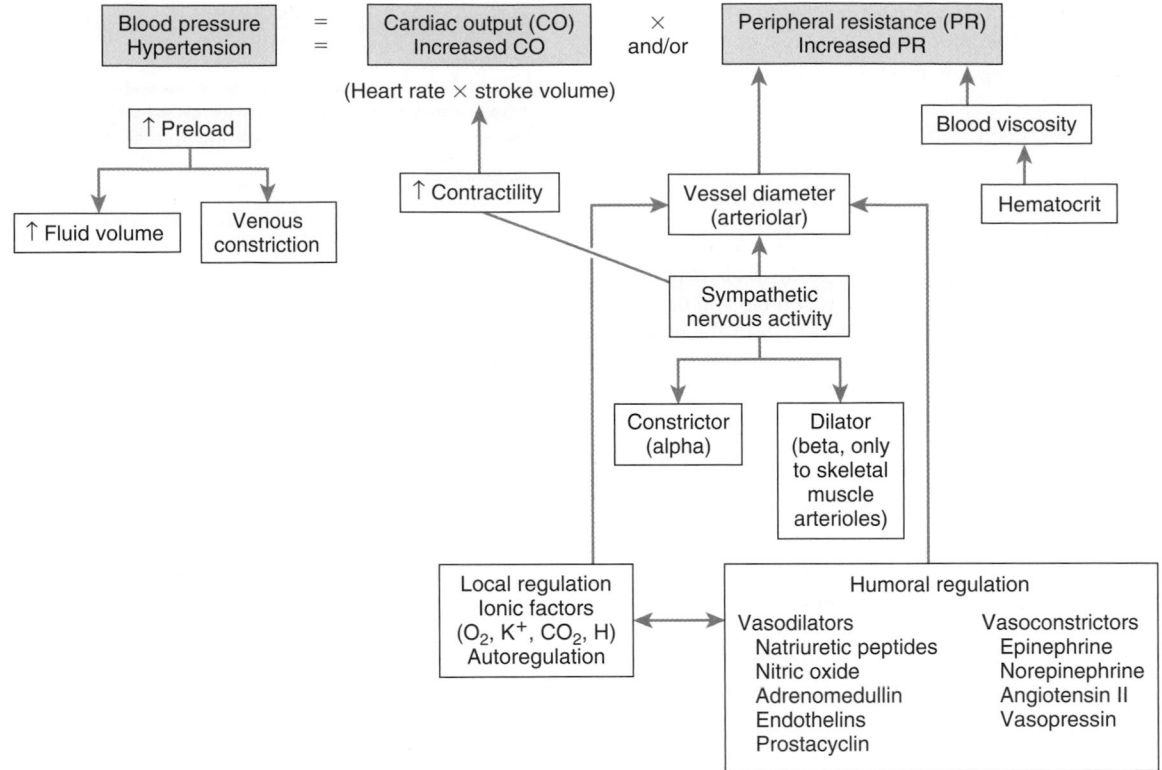

FIGURE 32.26 Factors Regulating Blood Pressure.

The normal range for the MAP is 70 to 110 mmHg.[42] The difference between the systolic pressure and diastolic pressure ($Ps - Pd$) is called the **pulse pressure** and typically is between 40 and 50 mmHg.[7] Pulse pressure is directly related to arterial wall stiffness and stroke volume.

During a wide range of physiologic conditions, including changes in body position, muscular activity, and circulating blood volume, arterial pressure is regulated within a fairly narrow range to maintain tissue **perfusion**, or blood supply to the capillary beds. The major factors and relationships that regulate arterial blood pressure are summarized in Fig. 32.26.

Effects of Cardiac Output

The cardiac output (minute volume) of the heart can be changed by alterations in heart rate, stroke volume (volume of blood ejected during each ventricular contraction), or both. An increase in cardiac output without a decrease in peripheral resistance will cause mean blood pressure and flow rate to increase. The higher arterial pressure increases blood flow through the arterioles. On the other hand, a decrease in the cardiac output causes an immediate drop in mean arterial blood pressure and flow rate (Table 32.5).

Effects of Total Peripheral Resistance and Blood Volume

Total resistance in the systemic circulation, often referred to as either *systemic vascular resistance (SVR)* or *total peripheral resistance (TPR)*, is primarily a function of the diameter of the arterioles. If cardiac output remains constant, arteriolar constriction raises mean arterial pressure by reducing the flow of blood into the capillaries and arteriolar dilation has the opposite effect. Reflex control of total cardiac output and peripheral resistance includes (1) sympathetic stimulation of heart, arterioles, and veins; and (2) parasympathetic stimulation of the heart (Fig. 32.27). The cardiovascular center in the medulla receives input

TABLE 32.5	**FACTORS THAT AFFECT MEAN ARTERIAL PRESSURE AND CAPILLARY FLOW**	
	MEAN ARTERIAL PRESSURE	**CAPILLARY FLOW**
Peripheral Resistance*		
Increased	Increased	Decreased
Decreased	Decreased	Increased
Heart Rate†		
Increased	Increased	Increased
Decreased	Decreased	Decreased
Stroke Volume‡		
Increased	Increased	Increased
Decreased	Decreased	Decreased

*Cardiac output maintained constant.
†Peripheral resistance and stroke volume constant.
‡Peripheral resistance and heart rate constant.
From Little RC: *Physiology of the heart and circulation,* ed 3, St Louis, 1985, Mosby.

from arterial baroreceptors and chemoreceptors throughout the vascular system and then modifies vagal and sympathetic output to control heart rate and contractility, plus vascular diameter. Vasoconstriction is regulated by an area of the brainstem that maintains a constant (tonic) output of norepinephrine from sympathetic fibers in the peripheral arterioles. This tonic activity is essential for maintenance of blood pressure.

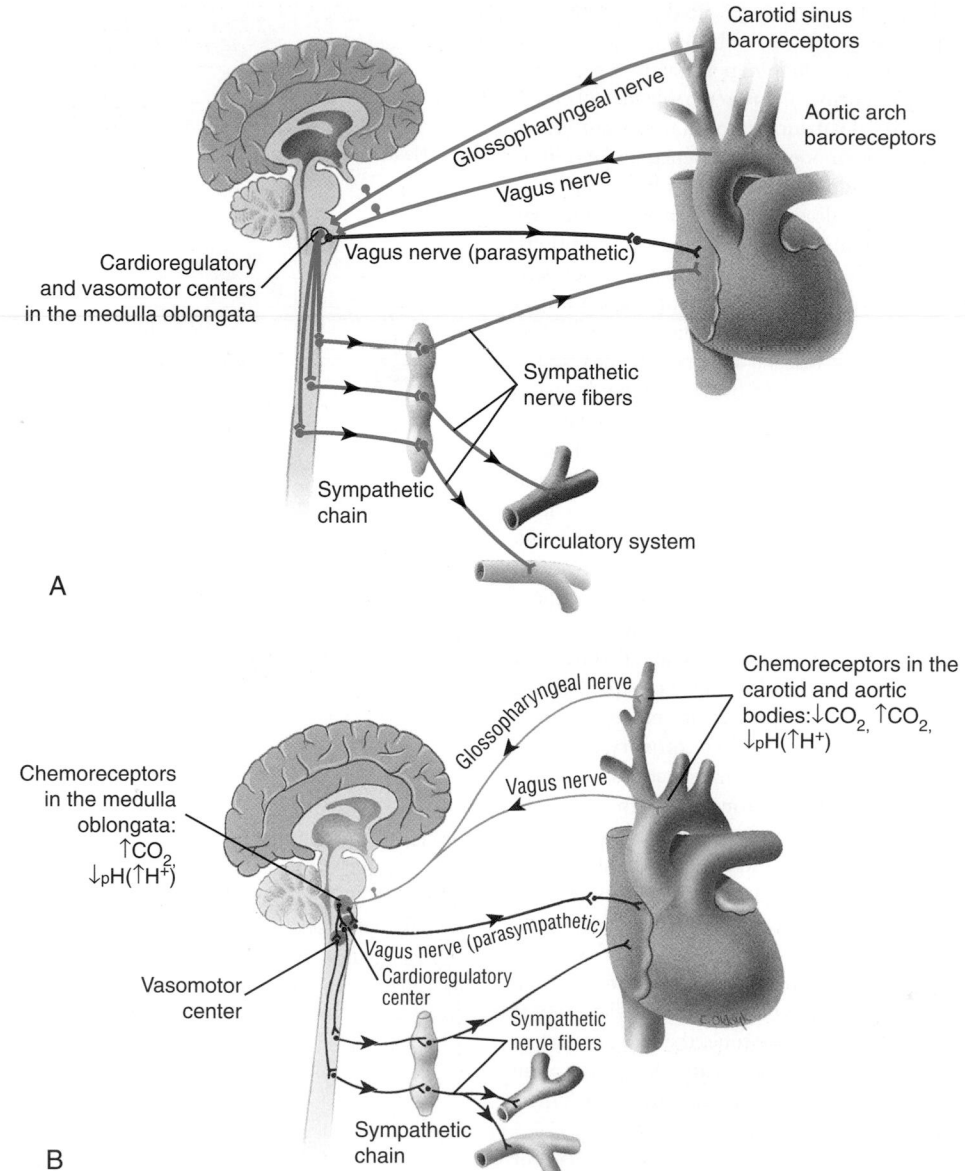

FIGURE 32.27 Baroreceptor and Chemoreceptor Reflex Control of Blood Pressure. A, Baroreceptor reflexes. Baroreceptors located in the carotid sinuses and aortic arch detect changes in blood pressure. Action potentials are conducted to the cardioregulatory and vasomotor centers. The heart rate can be decreased by the parasympathetic system; the heart rate and stroke volume can be increased by the sympathetic system. The sympathetic system also can constrict or dilate blood vessels. **B,** Chemoreceptor reflexes. Chemoreceptors located in the medulla oblongata and in the carotid and aortic bodies detect changes in levels of blood oxygen, carbon dioxide, or pH. Action potentials are conducted to the medulla oblongata. In response, the vasomotor center can cause vasoconstriction or dilation of blood vessels by the sympathetic system, and the cardioregulatory center can cause changes in the pumping activity of the heart through the parasympathetic and sympathetic systems. (From Seeley RR, Stephens TD, Tate P: *Anatomy & physiology,* ed 3, St Louis, 1995, Mosby.)

Baroreceptors. As discussed earlier, baroreceptors are stretch receptors located mainly in the aorta and the carotid sinus (see Fig. 32.27, *A*). They respond to changes in smooth muscle fiber length by altering their rate of discharge and supply sensory information to the cardiovascular center in the brainstem. When activated (stretched), the baroreceptors decrease cardiac output by lowering heart rate and stroke volume and peripheral resistance, and thus lower blood pressure.

Arterial Chemoreceptors. Specialized areas within the medulla oblongata and aortic and carotid arteries are sensitive to concentrations of arterial oxygen (Pao_2), arterial carbon dioxide ($Paco_2$), and arterial

hydrogen ions (pH) in the blood. Although these *chemoreceptors* are most important for respiratory control, they also transmit impulses to the medullary cardiovascular centers that regulate blood pressure. A decrease in arterial oxygen concentration (hypoxemia), an increase in arterial $Paco_2$ concentration, or to a lesser extent a decrease in arterial blood pH causes a reflexive increase (by a dominance of sympathetic impulses) in heart rate, stroke volume, and blood pressure.

Effects of Hormones. Hormones influence blood pressure regulation through their effects on vascular smooth muscle and blood volume. By constricting or dilating arterioles in organs, hormones can (1) increase or decrease the blood flow in response to the body's needs, (2) redistribute blood volume during hemorrhage or shock, and (3) regulate heat loss. The key vasoconstrictor hormones include angiotensin II, vasopressin (or antidiuretic hormone), epinephrine, and norepinephrine. The main vasodilator hormones are the atrial natriuretic hormones. Aldosterone, vasopressin, and the natriuretic hormones can influence stroke volume and thus blood pressure by causing fluid retention or loss.

A variety of other factors, including adipokines and insulin, may be related to the hypertension that occurs with chronic conditions, such as adiposity and diabetes mellitus; but these factors have not been clearly demonstrated to play a role in blood pressure regulation in healthy individuals.[43] Adiposity may increase cardiovascular disease (CVD) risk in part through effects on vascular stiffness.[44] Some research has suggested that the risk of cardiovascular disease and hypertension that often co-occurs with diabetes mellitus is more closely related to insulin resistance than to insulin levels.[45] Adrenomedullin (ADM) is a vasodilating peptide present in cardiovascular, pulmonary, renal, and other tissues. Because increases in ADM levels are associated with heart failure and myocardial infarction, ADM levels may be useful for risk categorization in people with these conditions.[46]

Vasoconstrictor Hormones. The vasoconstrictor hormones include epinephrine; norepinephrine; angiotensin II (Ang II), which is part of the renin-angiotensin-aldosterone system (RAAS); and vasopressin (also known as *antidiuretic hormone*). Epinephrine, the catecholamine hormone released from the adrenal medulla, causes vasoconstriction in most vascular beds except the coronary, liver, and skeletal muscle circulations. Norepinephrine mainly acts as a neurotransmitter; however, some also is released from the adrenal medulla. When released into the circulation, it is a more potent vasoconstrictor than epinephrine. Under normal circumstances, as vasoconstrictors—angiotensin II and vasopressin—are not thought to have a major role in blood pressure control. Vasopressin and aldosterone, however, affect blood pressure by increasing blood volume through their influence on fluid reabsorption in the kidney and by stimulating thirst. Vasopressin causes the reabsorption of water from tubular fluid in the distal tubule and collecting duct of the nephron. Aldosterone, the end product of the renin-angiotensin-aldosterone system, stimulates the reabsorption of sodium, chloride, and water from the same locations in the kidney (Fig. 32.28; also see Chapters 3 and 21).

Vasodilator Hormones. The natriuretic peptides (NPs) or hormones, including atrial natriuretic peptide (ANP), B-type natriuretic peptide (BNP), C-type natriuretic peptide (CNP), and urodilatin, function as both vasodilators and regulators of sodium and water excretion (natriuresis and diuresis). Increased pressure or diastolic volume in the heart stimulates the release of these peptide hormones. Increased levels of BNP predict increased risk of a poor outcome in heart failure, pulmonary embolism, valvular heart disease, and chronic coronary artery disease.[39]

Effects of Other Mediators. Several mediators produced by the vascular endothelium have been demonstrated to cause arteriolar vasodilation or vasoconstriction. Examples of vasodilating mediators include nitric oxide (NO), ADM, the endothelins, and prostacyclin. Nitric oxide (NO) is a soluble gas continuously synthesized from the amino acid L-arginine in endothelial cells by the calcium-calmodulin–dependent enzyme nitric oxide synthase (NOS).[47] NO has a wide range of biologic properties that maintain vascular homeostasis, including modulation of vascular dilator tone, regulation of local cell growth, and protection of the vessel from injurious consequences of platelets and cells circulating in blood (Fig. 32.29).

Therefore NO plays a crucial role in the normal endothelial function. An emerging list of conditions, including those commonly associated as risk factors for atherosclerosis such as hypertension, hypercholester-

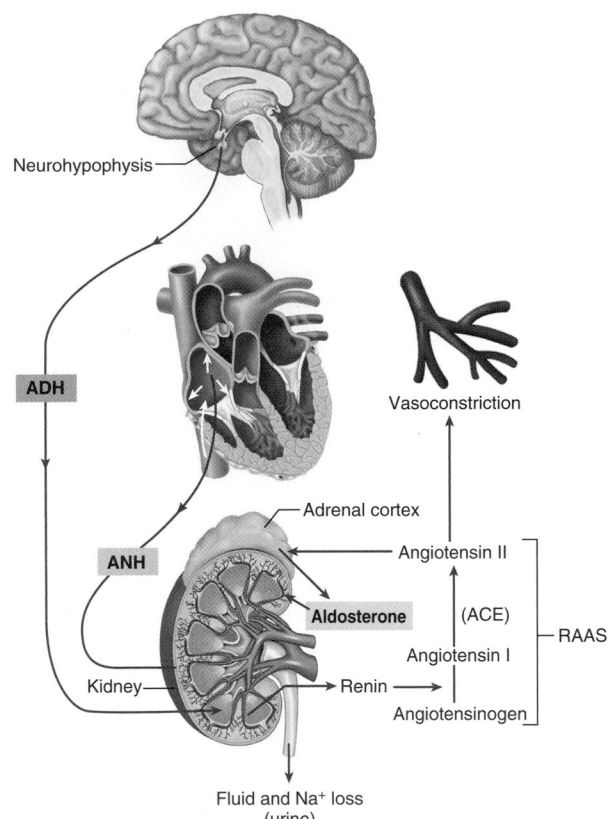

FIGURE 32.28 Three Mechanisms That Influence Total Plasma Volume. The antidiuretic hormone *(ADH)* mechanism and renin-angiotensin-aldosterone system *(RAAS)* tend to increase water, sodium, and chloride retention and thus increase total plasma volume. The atrial natriuretic hormone *(ANH)* mechanism antagonizes these mechanisms by promoting water, sodium, and chloride loss, thus promoting a decrease in total plasma volume. *ACE,* Angiotensin-converting enzyme. (From Patton KT, Thibodeau GA: *Anatomy & physiology,* ed 9, St Louis, 2016, Elsevier.)

olemia, smoking, diabetes mellitus, and heart failure, is associated with diminished release of nitric oxide into the arterial wall because of impaired synthesis or excessive oxidative degradation.[47] The decreased production of NO in these pathologic states causes serious problems in endothelial stability.

The velocity of blood movement within the arterioles causes shear stress at the vascular endothelial surface that in turn is the stimulus that causes the endothelial cells to produce these vasodilator substances. The flow-mediated dilation (FMD) test is used to evaluate endothelial function and to predict the risk of cardiovascular disease. A reduction in FMD is predictive of increased risk.[48]

ADM, a peptide with strong vasodilatory activity, is present in numerous tissues. It is a member of the calcitonin gene–related peptide family. Its exact role in adult human cardiovascular function and disease is unclear, but it has been found to have numerous cardiovascular effects, including a role in fetal cardiovascular system development and vasodilation

The *endothelins* are a family of three structurally similar peptides (ET-1, ET-2, and ET-3) and four receptors produced in cells in the vascular smooth muscle, the endothelium, the kidneys, and other organs. Because endothelin binding to the type A receptor causes vasodilation and natriuresis whereas binding to type B receptor causes the opposite

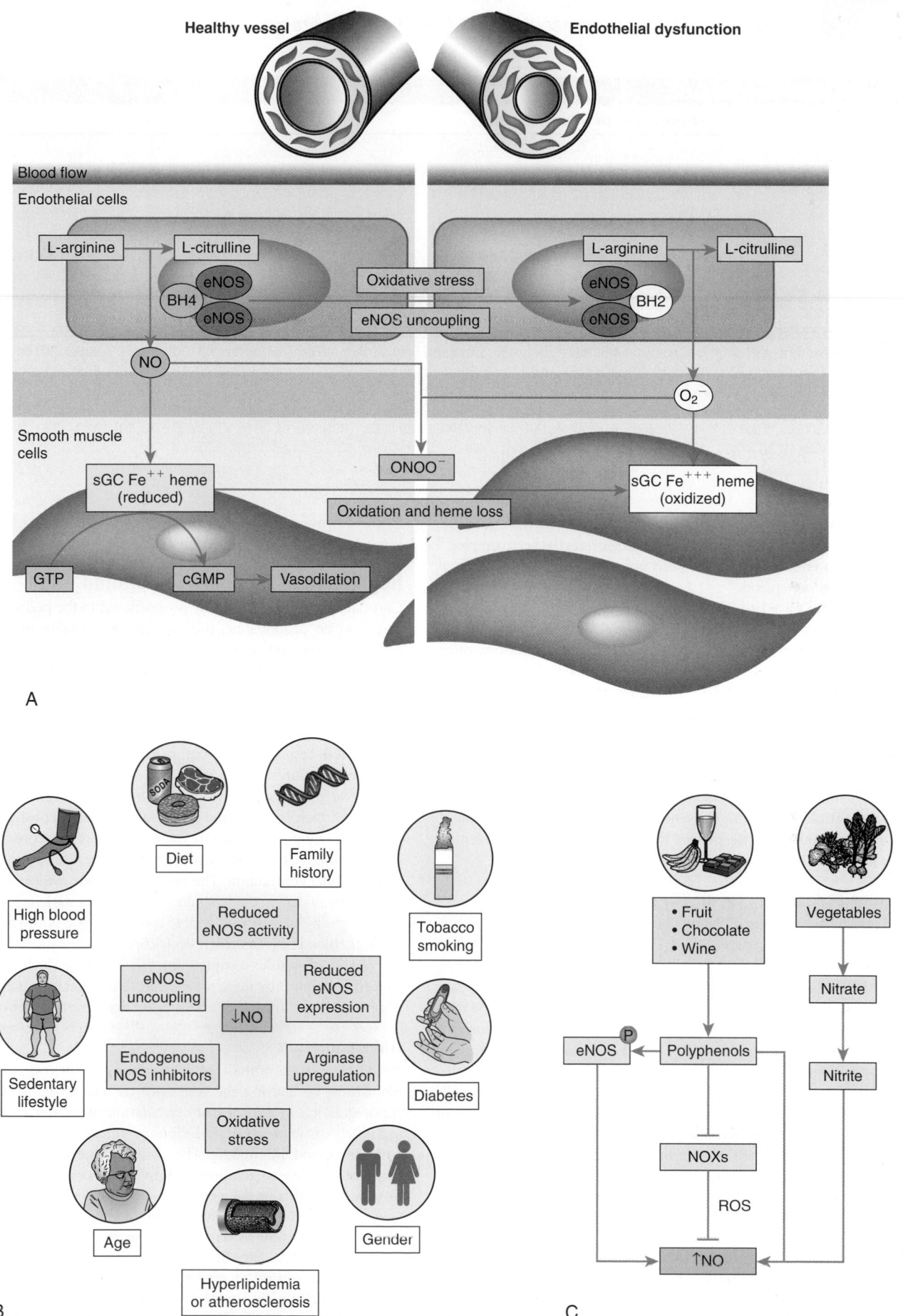

FIGURE 32.29 Importance of Nitric Oxide in Health and Disease and Lifestyle Factors Associated with Nitric Oxide Bioavailability. **A,** Nitric oxide in a healthy blood vessel and one with an altered or dysfunctional endothelium. **B,** Lifestyle factors associated with reduced bioavailability of nitric oxide. **C,** Dietary polyphenols can increase bioavailable nitric oxide. *BH4,* (6R) 5,6,7,8-tetrahydrobiopterin; *cGMP,* cyclic guanosine monophosphate; *eNOS,* endothelial nitric oxide synthase; *GTP,* guanosine triphosphate; *sGC,* soluble guanylate cyclase. (Adapted from Lundberg JO, Gladwin MT, Weitzberg E: *Nat Rev Drug Discov* 14:623–641, 2015.)

response—vasoconstriction plus sodium and water retention, the understanding of the physiologic and pathologic roles has been complex.[49] Inhibitors to endothelin-1 have been approved for the treatment of pulmonary hypertension.[50]

Prostacyclin is a vasodilator that is produced by the actions of cyclooxygenases (COX-1 and COX-2) on arachidonic acid. It also has the additional properties of opposing clot formation (antithrombotic), decreasing platelet activity, and inhibiting the release of growth factors from macrophages and the endothelial cells.[51] Nonsteroidal antiinflammatory drugs (NSAIDs) that inhibit these cyclooxygenases have been associated with cardiovascular disease risk in healthy people and in those with a known cardiovascular disease.[52,53]

Nattokinase (NK) activates multiple fibrinolytic and antithrombotic pathways simultaneously, either directly or indirectly (see *Nutrition & Disease*: Nattokinase for the Prevention of Thrombosis). In summary, NK intake could be an exceptional fibrinolytic/anticoagulant agent to reduce the risk of thrombosis in humans.

Venous Pressure

The main determinants of venous blood pressure are (1) the volume of fluid within the veins and (2) the compliance (distensibility) of the vessel walls. Typically, the venous system accommodates approximately 66% of the total blood volume with venous pressure averaging less than 10 mmHg. The systemic arteries accommodate about 11% of the total blood volume, with an average arterial pressure (blood pressure) of about 100 mmHg; the remainder of the blood volume is within the heart, capillaries, and pulmonary circulation.[42]

The sympathetic nervous system controls compliance. The walls of the veins are highly innervated by sympathetic fibers that control venous smooth muscle. Sympathetic innervation to the veins results in an increase in smooth muscle tone rather than vasoconstriction, which occurs in arteries. This increased smooth muscle tone stiffens the walls of the veins, reducing distensibility and increasing venous blood pressure, thus forcing more blood through the veins and into the right heart.

Two other mechanisms that increase venous pressure and venous return to the heart are (1) the skeletal muscle pump and (2) the respiratory pump. During skeletal muscle contraction the veins within the muscles are partially compressed, causing a decrease in venous capacity and increased return to the heart. The respiratory pump acts during inspiration, when the veins of the abdomen are partially compressed

by the downward movement of the diaphragm. Increased abdominal pressure moves blood toward the heart.

Regulation of Coronary Circulation

Coronary blood flow is directly proportional to the perfusion pressure and inversely proportional to the vascular resistance of the coronary bed. Coronary perfusion pressure is the difference between pressure in the aorta and pressure in the coronary vessels. Thus aortic pressure is the driving pressure that propels the perfusion of myocardial vessels. Vasodilation and vasoconstriction maintain coronary blood flow despite stresses imposed by the constant contraction and relaxation of the heart muscle and despite shifts (within a physiologic range) of coronary perfusion pressure.

Several unique anatomic factors influence coronary blood flow. Because of their location, the aortic valve cusps can obstruct coronary blood flow by pushing against the openings of the coronary arteries during systole. Also during systole, the coronary arteries are compressed by ventricular contraction. The resulting systolic compressive effect is particularly evident in the subendocardial layers of the left ventricular wall and can greatly increase resistance to coronary blood flow. Therefore most coronary blood flow in the left ventricle occurs during diastole. During the period of systolic compression, when flow is slowed or stopped, oxygen is supplied by myoglobin, a protein in heart muscle that binds oxygen during contraction and supplies oxygen to the myocardium.

Autoregulation

Autoregulation (automatic self-regulation) enables organs to regulate blood flow by altering the resistance (diameter) in their arterioles. Autoregulation in the coronary circulation maintains the blood flow at a nearly constant rate at perfusion pressures (mean arterial pressure) between 60 and 140 mmHg when other influencing factors are held constant. Thus autoregulation helps to ensure constant coronary blood flow despite shifts in the perfusion pressure within the stated range. Given that blood flow is directly related to pressure and inversely related to resistance, for flow to stay constant as pressure decreases, resistance also has to decrease; thus the mechanism(s) underlying autoregulation must relate to control of smooth muscle contraction in the arteriolar walls. Although the exact mechanisms underlying autoregulation are not known, research has indicated that factors influencing calcium release with the myocardium are involved and perhaps also the accumulation of vasodilatory products of metabolism, such as adenosine.[32,53]

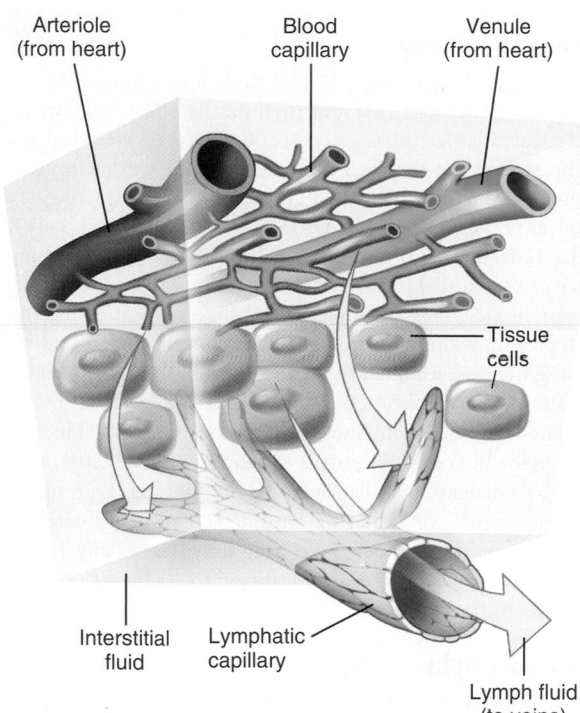

FIGURE 32.30 Role of the Lymphatic System in Fluid Balance. Fluid from plasma flowing through the capillaries moves into interstitial spaces. Although most of this interstitial fluid is either absorbed by tissue cells or reabsorbed by blood capillaries, some of the fluid tends to accumulate in the interstitial spaces. This lymph then diffuses into the lymphatic vessels that carry it to the lymph nodes and then into the systemic venous blood. Green is used to diagram the lymphatic vessels although the lymphatic vessels, particularly the smaller ones, are almost transparent. (Modified from Thibodeau GA, Patton KT: *Structure & function of the body,* ed 13, St Louis, 2008, Elsevier.)

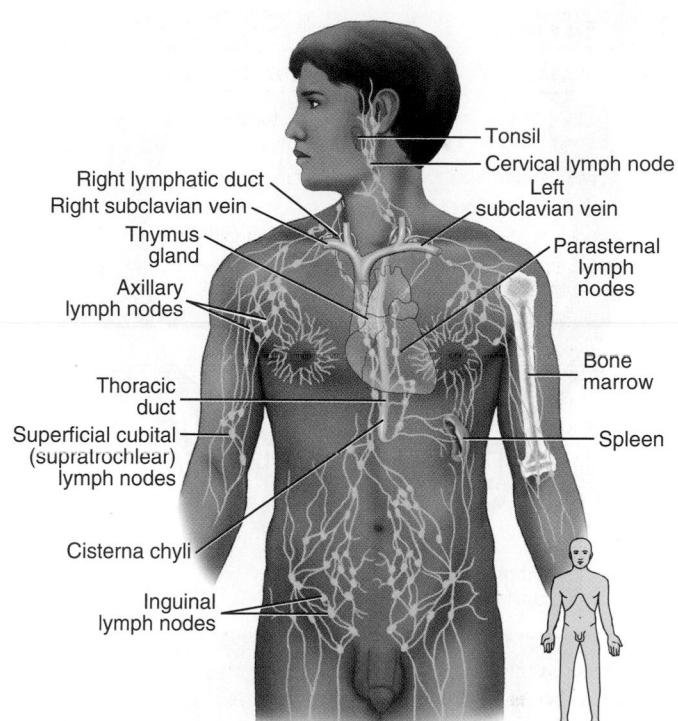

FIGURE 32.31 Principle Organs of the Lymphatic System. (From VanMeter KC, Hubert RJ: *Microbiology for the healthcare professional,* St Louis, 2010, Mosby.)

LYMPHATIC SYSTEM

The lymphatic system is a one-way network of lymphatic vessels and lymph nodes (Figs. 32.30 and 32.31) that is important for fluid balance, immune function, and transport of lipids, hormones, and cytokines. Every day about 3 liters of fluid filters out of venous capillaries in body tissues and is not reabsorbed. This fluid becomes the lymph that is carried by the lymphatic vessels to the chest where it enters the venous circulation. The lymphatic vessels run in the same sheaths with the arteries and veins. (Lymph nodes and lymphoid tissues are described in Chapters 7 and 28.) In this pumpless system a series of valves ensures one-way flow of the excess interstitial fluid (then called *lymph*) toward the heart. The lymphatic capillaries are closed at the distal ends (Fig. 32.32).

Lymph consists primarily of water and small amounts of dissolved proteins, mostly albumin, which are too large to be reabsorbed into the less permeable blood capillaries. Lymph also carries two types of cells—lymphocytes and antigen-presenting cells. The antigen-presenting cells are carried to the next lymph node in the system whereas lymphocytes traffic between lymph nodes. Once within the lymphatic system, lymph travels through lymphatic venules and veins that drain into one of two large ducts in the thorax—the right lymphatic duct and the thoracic duct. The right lymphatic duct drains lymph from the right arm and the right side of the head and thorax, whereas the larger thoracic duct receives lymph from the rest of the body (see Fig. 32.31). The right lymphatic duct and the thoracic duct drain lymph into the right and left subclavian veins, respectively.

Lymphatic veins are thin walled, like the veins of the cardiovascular system. In the larger lymphatic veins, endothelial flaps form valves similar to those in the blood-carrying veins (see Fig. 32.32). The valves permit lymph to flow in only one direction because lymphatic vessels are compressed intermittently by contraction of skeletal muscles, pulsatile expansion of an artery in the same sheath, and contraction of the smooth muscles in the walls of the lymphatic vessel.

As lymph is transported toward the heart, it is filtered through thousands of bean-shaped lymph nodes clustered along the lymphatic vessels (see Fig. 32.31). Lymph enters the nodes through several afferent lymphatic vessels, filters through the sinuses in the nodes, and leaves by way of efferent lymphatic vessels. Lymph flows slowly through a node, which facilitates the phagocytosis of foreign substances within the node by antigen-presenting cells and the entry of mature but naïve B and T lymphocytes, which then circulate through the body, moving from one lymph node to the next while waiting for a chance encounter with the antigen to which they are programmed to respond. (Phagocytosis is described in Chapter 7.)

TESTS OF CARDIOVASCULAR FUNCTION

Assessment of the individual with suspected cardiovascular disorders begins with a thorough history for determination of risk factors and symptoms. A careful physical examination looking for evidence of tissue ischemia, pulmonary congestion, and cardiac dysfunction is next. Blood samples are taken and sent for a variety of tests. For many individuals, these basic steps will be complemented with methods that measure heart and vascular function with greater specificity. Cardiac function can be evaluated using indicators calculated from pressures and flow rates in the heart and vessels. Table 32.6 defines the indicators most often used in the clinical setting. The normal values for several testing methods are different for men and women.[54,55] This textbook's inside back cover includes normal blood values for common laboratory tests.

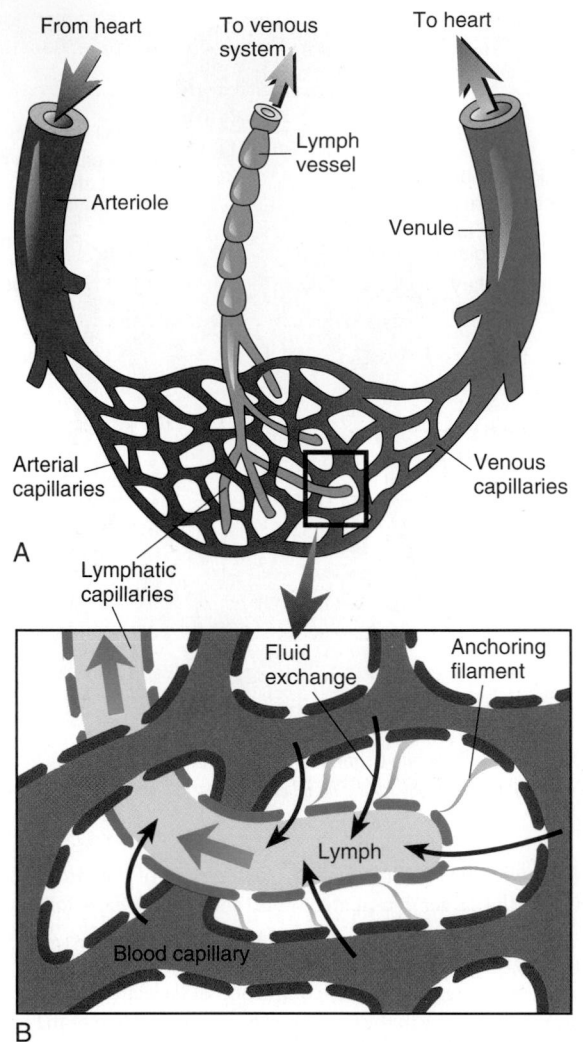

FIGURE 32.32 Lymphatic Capillaries. **A,** Schematic representation of lymphatic capillaries. **B,** Anatomic components of microcirculation.

Cardiac and Coronary Artery Evaluation

Many sophisticated tests are used to evaluate and diagnose cardiac or coronary artery diseases, and new ones are being tested each year. Some of the more commonly used modalities include chest x-ray, electrocardiography, echocardiography, stress testing, computed tomography (CT) and magnetic resonance imaging (MRI), technetium scanning, electrophysiology studies, and catheterization with angiography.

Chest Radiograph Examination

Chest x-rays allow for the examination of the size and contour of the heart and related structures. Evidence of chamber enlargement, pericardial disease, pulmonary edema, valvular calcification, ventricular hypertrophy, and pathology of the great vessels may be visualized. Chest x-ray also is useful to assess for appropriate placement of invasive cardiac conduction devices and for any complications caused by these devices (e.g., pneumothorax or hemothorax; see Chapter 36). A chest x-ray examination is a routine part of a cardiac examination. The most commonly obtained views are posteroanterior (PA) and lateral, with the individual standing upright and the lungs fully expanded. In those individuals confined to bed, an anteroposterior (AP) view may be obtained but is usually of lesser quality than the PA view.

Electrocardiography

Electrocardiography, typically a 12-lead electrocardiogram (ECG), gives information about heart rate and rhythm; the effects of activities of daily life, exercise, electrolytes, drugs, and disease on electrical activity in the heart; and the electrical orientation of the cardiac muscle. An ECG provides no direct information about the contractile state or mechanical performance of the heart.

Serial 12-lead ECGs are of primary importance in establishing the presence of myocardial ischemia and infarction or conduction defects and dysrhythmias. This examination has become part of the routine hospital preadmission/admission assessment, even when the admitting diagnosis is not cardiac in nature, because it establishes baseline information about the electrical function of the heart. Also, recent ECGs can be compared with ECGs obtained from the same individual in the past. Changes in the ECG over time assist in determining the cause, amount, or nature of changes in cardiac anatomy and physiology. Ambulatory electrocardiographic or Holter monitoring is used to evaluate rhythm changes that may occur in persons during activities of daily living. Cell phone technology also is rapidly advancing to enable ECG recording and relaying to healthcare providers.

Echocardiography

Echocardiography is the most effective and widely used noninvasive modality for evaluating the structures of the heart. Ultrasound beams reflected by cardiovascular structures produce shapes that can be visualized and allow for recognition of altered cardiac anatomy.[56] It is used to evaluate for suspected coronary artery disease, heart failure, valvular disease, infective endocarditis, cardiomyopathies, pericardial disease, prosthetic valve function, congenital heart disease, and aortic diseases. Through the use of M-mode, two- and three-dimensional techniques with Doppler and color flow imaging, accurate assessments of cardiac output, ejection fraction, and valvular function can be obtained.[56,57] Advances in technology now allow both intracardiac and transesophageal echocardiography for evaluation of the heart anatomy, although anesthesia is required for the transesophageal technique.[58]

Exercise or Stress Testing

Cardiac activity during exercise is examined during a stress test when an intervention is used to increase myocardial work. Stress testing elicits signs and symptoms of heart disease and coronary artery disease that may not appear at rest. Echocardiography or continuous 12-lead ECG and blood pressure measurements are obtained before, during, and after the study. Cardiac stress from exercise is usually induced by having the individual walk on a treadmill. Other, less frequently used forms of exercise include static exercise (hand ergometry or chemical stress), stair climbing (the Stairmaster's double two-step), arm ergometry, and bicycle ergometry. The individual exercises until the maximal heart rate for gender and age is reached or until other subjective or objective indicators of cardiac dysfunction or distress appear. Subjective indicators include chest pain, extreme fatigue, extreme dyspnea, leg pain, or the individual's request to stop the test. Objective criteria are ST-segment elevation or depression, SA node or atrial dysrhythmias, AV node dysrhythmias, ventricular dysrhythmias, elevated or decreased blood pressure, signs of cerebral hypoxia, and signs of circulatory insufficiency. One limitation of this test is that it cannot be used in persons whose capacity for exercise is limited.

Stress testing also may be used to evaluate either fitness for noncardiac surgery or progress in recovery after myocardial infarction or cardiac surgery. Graded exercise in individuals with low- to moderate-risk chest pain evaluated in an emergency department can be used as a prognostic

TABLE 32.6 INDICATORS OF CARDIAC FUNCTION

INDICATOR	DEFINITION*	COMMON CAUSE OF ABNORMALITY
Heart rate (HR)	Number of heartbeats (cardiac cycles) per minute Normal adult value: 70 beats/min	Ischemia, electrolyte disturbances, drug toxicity
Cardiac output (CO)	Amount of blood (in L) moved by the heart in 1 min Normal range: 4–8 L/min	Decrease indicates heart failure Increase indicates decreased systemic vascular resistance, common in sepsis
Cardiac index (CI)	Relationship between cardiac output and body surface area (BSA, in m²) Normal range: 2.8–4.2 L/min/m²	Decrease indicates heart failure Increase indicates decreased systemic vascular resistance, common in sepsis
Stroke volume (SV)	Amount of blood (in mL) ejected by the left ventricle during systole (i.e., per beat) Normal range: 60–100 mL/beat	Decrease indicates heart failure Increase indicates decreased systemic vascular resistance, common in sepsis
Stroke volume index (SVI)	Relationship between stroke volume and body surface area Normal range: 33–47 mL/beat/m²	Decrease indicates heart failure Increase indicates decreased systemic vascular resistance, common in sepsis
Oxygen consumption index ($\dot{V}O_2$)	Amount of oxygen (in mL) consumed per minute in relation to BSA	Decrease: sedation, anesthesia, hypothermia Increase: elevated temperature, sepsis, seizures
Stroke work index (SWI)	Amount of work (expressed as done) by the left or right ventricle per systole per square meter of BSA Normal value: 35 g/m²	Decreases within specific ranges indicate cardiogenic or hypovolemic shock (see Chapter 49) Increase: elevated systemic vascular resistance
Systemic mean arterial pressure (MAP)	Mean blood pressure (in mmHg) in the systemic arteries Normal range: 70–100 mmHg	Elevated: epinephrine release, diseases of arteries, primary hypertension Decreased: cardiac failure, decreased vascular resistance of sepsis
Pulmonary vascular resistance (PVR)	Relationship among cardiac output, preload, and afterload, expressed as units of force of resistance per second per centimeter of water Normal value: less than 250 dynes/sec/cm⁻⁵	Increased: acute respiratory distress syndrome (ARDS), pneumonia, primary pulmonary hypertension, congestive heart failure Decreased: late shock
Systemic vascular resistance (SVR)	Same definition as for PVR Normal range: 770–1500 dynes/sec/cm⁻⁵	Increased: epinephrine release Decreased: inflammatory response

*Values given are for adults at rest.

indicator of adverse cardiac events. When a differential diagnosis for chest pain has been difficult to determine, stress testing may help distinguish coronary artery insufficiency from other causes of pain. The risks associated with stress testing include dysrhythmias, myocardial infarction, and death. The risk is greater when the test is performed soon after an acute ischemic event.

Stress testing with ECG monitoring may not be sensitive enough to detect and localize areas of the myocardium at risk for ischemia and infarction. Currently, most stress testing includes the injection of a radiotracer that is absorbed by active heart cells. When the heart is scanned, during and after stress testing, areas where the radiotracer is not taken up by ischemic cells can be seen and those locations indicate areas of myocardial damage.

Single-Photon Emission Computed Tomography

Single-photon emission computed tomography (SPECT) is typically used to evaluate individuals for coronary artery disease and myocardial ischemia during stress testing. A radiotracer (usually thalium-201) is injected intravenously and is absorbed and retained for a while by healthy myocytes.[59] Photons are emitted from the radiotracer in the myocardium in proportion to perfusion of the tissue. A gamma camera visualizes the photons, and views are taken from 360 degrees by CT,

which digitizes the information and provides a three-dimensional view of myocardial perfusion. Data about where the myocardium absorbs the tracer normally, slowly, or not at all can be correlated with existing myocardial disease and can help quantify ischemic risk. A new development, high-speed SPECT, has the advantage of taking less time and, thereby, requiring less radiotracer, which decreases radiation exposure for the person being examined.[59]

Computed Tomography (CT) and Magnetic Resonance Imaging (MRI)

Computed tomography (CT) and magnetic resonance imaging (MRI) are used to evaluate cardiac anatomy and physiology. New techniques, including ECG gating (timing of data gathering to the cardiac cycle), electron beam CT, and spiral CT, have improved the ability of tomography to visualize cardiac structures. The high resolution of CT can provide information about calcification of coronary vessels and cardiac valves. Information about coronary artery calcification is being used to improve risk classification for coronary artery disease.[60] It also is a tool for evaluating large-vessel disease. Concerns and debate continue, however, about the radiation risks and use of variable protocols. The International Commission on Radiological Protection (ICRP) recently released a report on radiological protection in cardiology.[61]

MRI is based on the principle that the frequency of energy (resonant frequency) given up by a nucleus is exactly proportional to the surrounding magnetic field (see Chapter 15). The anatomy and physiology of the great blood vessels and myocardium are depicted in three dimensions with excellent resolution. Ventricular function can be evaluated using indexes of ventricular function, such as ejection fraction. Rapidly moving sequences (MRI) can determine regional wall motion and myocardial deformation. Flow direction and velocity also can be quantitatively determined. Stress testing also can be done with MRI using the drug dobutamine to increase the cardiac workload instead of exercise.[62]

Technetium Scanning

Radiopharmaceuticals labeled with [99m]technetium preparations, such as sestamibi, teboroxime, and tetrofosmin, are used to image the coronary arteries and myocardium. Technetium pyrophosphate ([99m]TcPYP) is injected intravenously into a resting individual during a "hot spot" imaging examination. Two hours after injection the distribution pattern of the radioactive solution is recorded by nuclear scan. During the 2-hour delay, the injected material will have been taken up by infarcted areas of the myocardium, particularly 1 to 3 days after the onset of symptoms. This type of scanning also is done with stress testing using exercise or dobutamine.[63] Study results are not definitive during the first 12 hours after an infarct.

Technetium scanning is used when (1) there is a conflicting history for myocardial infarction, (2) there are equivocal ECG abnormalities, or (3) an individual's cardiac enzymes have been elevated because of surgery or trauma. Ongoing research is determining any risks associated with radioactive substances.

Electrophysiology Studies

In-depth evaluation of electrical conduction within the heart can provide important information about the nature and causes of dysrhythmias, such as atrial and ventricular tachycardias and heart block. This evaluation is often referred to as *electrophysiologic mapping* of the myocardium. There are many types of electrophysiology studies that are specific to certain conduction disorders but they have the common goal of documenting abnormal conduction pathways. Furthermore, the techniques used may also allow for ablation of unwanted pathways or the appropriate placement of pacemakers and implantable defibrillators. Mapping can include the use of echocardiography and CT scanning.[64]

One example of an electrophysiology study is AV bundle electrocardiography. Two electrode-tipped catheters are inserted percutaneously into the femoral vein, floated up the inferior vena cava, and positioned in or near the right atrium during AV bundle (His bundle) electrocardiography. AV bundle electrocardiography can detect secondary sites of impulse generation (ectopic foci), as well as accessory pathways of conduction. Other conduction defects and the effects of drugs on conduction also can be illuminated. Risks related to this procedure can be grave and include dysrhythmias, death, vessel or heart perforation, clot or plaque embolization, and kidney failure.

Cardiac Catheterization and Angiography

One or both sides of the heart can be examined using cardiac catheterization. This invasive procedure requires the use of fluoroscopy and strict sterile techniques and takes place in a specially equipped catheterization laboratory. Local anesthetic is administered, and a catheter is introduced percutaneously into the vasculature and passed caudally into the atrium and ventricle. For a right-heart catheterization, the catheter is placed in either the jugular, subclavian, brachial, or femoral veins. The femoral artery is commonly used for a left-heart study. Once the catheter has been guided into the heart chambers, pressures are recorded, blood samples are obtained to examine oxygen content, and a contrast medium is injected to visualize chamber function and valve patency.

Cardiac catheterization provides a means to visualize the chambers of the heart continuously, although for a short time. A great deal of information can be obtained about heart structure and function. Pressures in each chamber and across heart valves can be precisely measured, along with timing of events in the cardiac cycle. Of particular value is the ability to compare the oxygen content of blood in each heart chamber. Risks for this procedure that have decreased over time include the development of dysrhythmias. Death can occur secondary to cardiac arrest after ventricular fibrillation.

Fluoroscopic visualization of the coronary arteries and left-heart structures using contrast dye is called coronary angiography or arteriography. Like cardiac catheterization, this study takes place in a catheterization laboratory using local anesthesia and a sterile field. A catheter is threaded into the left ventricle through the femoral artery. A ventriculogram generally is performed first. Contrast dye is injected into the apex of the ventricle, and the next few cardiac cycles are visualized and filmed. Like cardiac catheterization, coronary angiography is used to gain information about the structure and function of the ventricles and related valves. After the ventriculogram, catheters are introduced individually into the ostia of the coronary arteries. When the catheter is in position, a small volume of contrast dye is mechanically and rapidly injected into the artery and the results are visualized and filmed. Dye injection is repeated with the individual tilted at various angles to afford views of the artery other than the anteroposterior view.

The risks of for coronary angiography are similar to those of cardiac catheterization, with exceptions. As the blood supply to the cardiac muscle is briefly interrupted when dye is introduced into the coronary arteries, angina (chest pain) caused by ischemia (lack of oxygen) is much more common. Coronary artery spasms also can occur. Interrupted flow also causes decreased heart rate (bradycardia), as well as some tachydysrhythmias, hypotension, and ST-segment depression.

Systemic Vascular Evaluation

The systemic vascular system can be studied by a variety of techniques in order to evaluate for adequate flow rates, vascular obstruction, and structural defects. These techniques include Doppler ultrasonography, CT and MRI, venography, and arteriography.

Arterial Pressure Pulse Waveform Analysis

Pulsation, described by the flow of blood through an artery during the cardiac cycle, can be drawn as a waveform plotting pressure against time (Fig. 32.33). The waveform can be obtained noninvasively by placing a transducer on the skin over the carotid artery while the individual's

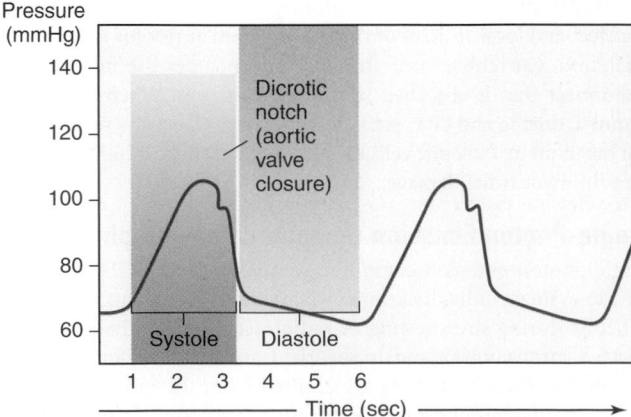

FIGURE 32.33 Arterial Pressure Pulse Waveforms.

head is turned slightly away from the transducer. The amplitude and shape of arterial waveforms can provide information about the elasticity of the arterial wall, or its inverse—the stiffness of the wall.

Doppler Ultrasonography Studies

A Doppler study is done using a microphone that amplifies and records the sounds made by blood flowing in peripheral vessels. The Doppler microphone is placed over the vessel to be studied, and sounds related to obstructions to flow, vessel wall mobility, and heart murmurs are transmitted through a lubricating gel to the microphone. The audio findings can be digitized into visual findings that can be analyzed for flow velocity and volume. These studies are useful in the evaluation for abnormalities of venous flow (e.g., deep venous thrombosis) and arterial flow (e.g., embolism). Ultrasound also is used to calculate the thickness of arterial walls, yielding a reading called *intimal-medial thickness*. Carotid intimal-medial thickness is used to assess for atherosclerosis.[65] Many people are familiar with ultrasound measurements because they are commonly used to assess fetal growth and development.

Computed Tomography and Magnetic Resonance Imaging

CT and MRI are used to evaluate the systemic circulation, providing information about the structure of the great vessels. Either can be used to evaluate for aneurysms and dissections of the thoracic or abdominal aorta. CT also is used to assess for vessel calcification and provide some insights into the risk for stroke and myocardial infarction through evaluation of the carotid and coronary vessels.

Venography and Arteriography

Radiopaque dye can be injected through intravenous or intraarterial catheters to allow for visualization of the internal structure, diameter, and patency of veins and arteries. Venography is performed primarily in the lower extremity to assess for the presence of thrombi in the large veins of the leg. Arteriography (angiography) can be used in almost any vascular system, including the great vessels and the pulmonary, coronary (see previously in this chapter), cerebral, mesenteric, renal, hepatic, and peripheral arteries. Risks include rupture, dissection, thrombosis, embolization, or organ infarction involving the arterial system being studied.

AGING AND THE CARDIOVASCULAR SYSTEM

Cardiovascular disease is the most common cause of morbidity and mortality in older adults in Western society and in much of the rest of the world.[66] In addition, age is a key driver of cardiovascular risk, which explains why it is the primary cause of death in persons older than age 65.[67] The most common cardiovascular disease condition is hypertension followed by coronary atherosclerosis for which hypertension is a risk factor.

It is challenging to determine the normal physiologic changes in cardiac function with aging because many pathologic changes are usually present and physical fitness is variable in older people as well. Studies of the effect of age on cardiovascular function must be rigorous in their

distinction between persons who are free of disease and those who have disease that may be evident only during testing. There is a wide range in the older population for nearly every cardiovascular variable. These variations are related to an increase in the prevalence of hypertension and coronary disease with advancing age; the growth in the segment of the population older than age 65; and major age-associated changes in lifestyle (e.g., fitness status).[67] The most relevant age-associated physiologic changes in cardiovascular performance include myocardial and blood vessel stiffening, changes in neurogenic control over vascular tone, increased occurrence of atrial fibrillation, and loss of exercise capacity plus left ventricular hypertrophy and fibrosis.[67,68] These changes pose considerable consequences with increased demand for flow, with changes in posture, or with disease.

Arterial stiffening occurs with aging even in the absence of clinical hypertension. It can, however, be an important contributor to systolic hypertension and its associated risks for cardiovascular events, dementia, and death. These changes result from alterations within the vascular media, including age-associated changes in cross-linking of collagen, an increase in the amount of collagen, deposition of calcium, and changes in the nature of elastin, the extracellular matrix, inflammatory molecules, endothelial cell function, and reactive oxygen species.[37] The increased arterial stiffness may not be related strictly to an age-associated change in vascular structure but may be caused by changes in baroreceptor activity. Baroreceptor activity may decrease with age, slowing physiologic adjustment to changes in blood pressure, and posture. In persons older than age 60, pulse pressure, which is directly influenced by arterial stiffness, is a better predictor of cardiovascular disease than either diastolic or systolic blood pressure.[69]

Left ventricular hypertrophy and fibrosis also are more common in the aging population, even in the absence of high blood pressure. As the arterial system becomes stiffer the ventricles must work harder to pump blood throughout the body, thus contributing to hypertrophy. Fibrosis, calcification, and increase in stiffness also impact valvular function, particularly the function of the atrioventricular valves. These changes make valvular disease a greater risk for the elderly, along with an increased risk of heart failure related to the left ventricular hypertrophy and stiffness.

The advent of genomic medicine and a deeper exploration of molecular changes with aging continue to enhance understanding of the myriad changes in people's bodies as they age.[67,68] The ongoing hope is that as understanding of the causative factors related to cardiovascular decline with aging improves, therapeutics that arrest or slow these changes may be developed.

Stress testing is used to uncover functional capacity losses that are not apparent at rest. In contrast to the subtle age effects on resting cardiac tests, more dramatic changes occur during exercise. Table 32.3 summarizes age-associated changes at rest and during exercise. Overall, long-term exercise conditioning in older individuals increases aerobic capacity and decreases arterial stiffness and left ventricular function so that cardiovascular diseases may be prevented or delayed in older adults. Although the risks and benefits of pharmacologic and invasive strategies must always be assessed carefully, many older adults can live longer and healthier lives if appropriate preventive and treatment regimens are offered, even quite late in life.

SUMMARY REVIEW

Circulatory System

1. The circulatory system is the body's transport system and a part of its communication system. It delivers oxygen, nutrients, hormones, blood cells, immune cells, and others throughout the

body and carries metabolic wastes to the kidneys and lungs for excretion.

2. The circulatory system consists of the heart, blood vessels, and the lymphatic vessels and is made up of two separate but conjoined,

serially connected pump systems: the pulmonary circulation and the systemic circulation, plus the lymphatics.

3. The low-pressure pulmonary circulation is driven by the right side of the heart. The function of the pulmonary circulation is to deliver blood to the lungs for oxygenation.

4. The higher pressure systemic circulation is driven by the left side of the heart, and its function is to move oxygenated blood to body tissues and to deliver waste products to the lungs, kidneys, and liver.

5. The lymphatic vessels collect fluids from the interstitium and return the fluids to the circulatory system. Another important function of the lymphatic system is the movement of lymphocytes and leukocytes between different components of the immune system.

The Heart

1. The heart consists of four chambers (two atria and two ventricles), four valves (two AV valves and two semilunar valves), a muscular wall, a fibrous skeleton, a conduction system, nerve fibers, systemic vessels (the coronary circulation), and openings where the great vessels enter the atria and ventricles.

2. The heart wall, which encloses the heart and divides it into chambers, is made up of three layers: the epicardium (outer layer), the myocardium (muscular layer), and the endocardium (inner lining). The heart is contained within the pericardium, a double-walled sac.

3. The myocardial layer of the two atria, which receive blood entering the heart, is thinner than the myocardial layer of the ventricles, which is stronger because it generates the pressure that causes the blood to circulate through the lungs or the systemic circulation.

4. The right and left sides of the heart are separated by portions of the heart wall called the *interatrial septum* and the *interventricular septum.*

5. Unoxygenated (venous) blood from the systemic circulation enters the right atrium through the superior and inferior venae cavae. From the right atrium the blood passes through the right AV (tricuspid) valve into the right ventricle. In the ventricle the blood flows from the inflow tract to the outflow tract and then through the pulmonic semilunar valve (pulmonary valve) into the pulmonary artery, which delivers it to the lungs for oxygenation.

6. Oxygenated blood from the lungs enters the left atrium through the four pulmonary veins (two from the left lung and two from the right lung). From the left atrium the blood passes through the left AV valve (mitral valve) into the left ventricle. In the ventricle the blood flows from the inflow tract to the outflow tract and then through the aortic semilunar valve (aortic valve) into the aorta, which delivers it to systemic arteries of the entire body.

7. The heart valves that ensure the one-way flow of blood from the atria to the ventricles are called the *atrioventricular valves.* The valves that ensure one-way flow from the ventricles to either the pulmonary artery or the aorta are called *semilunar valves.*

8. Oxygenated blood enters the coronary arteries through openings within the semilunar valves at the entrance to the aorta, and deoxygenated blood from the coronary veins enters the right atrium through the coronary sinus.

9. The pumping action of the heart consists of two phases: diastole, during which the myocardium relaxes and the chambers fill with blood; and systole, during which the myocardium contracts, forcing blood out of the ventricles. A cardiac cycle consists of one systolic contraction and the diastolic relaxation that follows it. Each cardiac cycle makes up one heartbeat.

10. The sinoatrial (SA) node generates electrical impulses, and the conduction system of the heart transmits these electrical impulses (cardiac action potentials) that stimulate systolic contraction. The autonomic nerves (sympathetic and parasympathetic fibers) can adjust heart rate and systolic force, but they do not stimulate the heart to beat.

11. Collateral arteries are connections between branches of the same coronary artery or connections of branches of the right coronary artery with branches of the left. New collateral vessels are formed through two processes: arteriogenesis and angiogenesis. This collateral growth is stimulated by shear stress, an increased blood flow speed near an area of stenosis, or narrowing, and the production of growth factors and cytokines.

12. The heart has an extensive capillary network.

13. The normal ECG is the sum of all cardiac action potentials. The P wave represents atrial depolarization; the QRS complex is the sum of all ventricular cell depolarizations. The ST interval occurs when the entire ventricular myocardium is depolarized.

14. Cardiac action potentials are generated by the SA node at the rate of between 60 and 100 impulses per minute. The impulses travel through the conduction system of the heart, stimulating myocardial contraction as they travel.

15. Cells of the cardiac conduction system possess the properties of automaticity and rhythmicity. Automatic cells return to threshold and depolarize rhythmically without an outside stimulus. The cells of the SA node depolarize faster than other automatic cells, making it the natural pacemaker of the heart. If the SA node is disabled, the next fastest pacemaker, the AV node, assumes control.

16. Each cardiac action potential travels from the SA node to the AV node to the bundle of His (AV bundle), through the bundle branches, and finally to the Purkinje fibers and the ventricular myocardium. There the impulse is stopped. It is prevented from reversing its path by the refractory period of cells that has just been polarized. The refractory period ensures that diastole (relaxation) will occur, thereby completing the cardiac cycle.

17. Adrenergic receptor number, type, and function govern autonomic (sympathetic) regulation of heart rate, contractile force, and dilation or constriction of coronary arteries. The presence of specific receptors (α_1, α_2, β_1, β_2, β_3) in the myocardium and coronary vessels determines the effects of the neurotransmitters norepinephrine and epinephrine.

18. Unique features that distinguish myocardial cells from skeletal cells enable myocardial cells to transmit action potentials faster (through intercalated disks), synthesize more ATP (because of a large number of mitochondria), and have readier access to ions in the interstitium (because of an abundance of transverse tubules). These combined differences enable the myocardium to work constantly, which is not required of skeletal muscle.

19. Cross-bridges between actin and myosin enable contraction to occur. Calcium and its interaction with the troponin complex facilitate the contraction process. With troponin release of calcium, myocardial relaxation begins.

20. Cardiac performance is affected by preload, afterload, heart rate, and myocardial contractility.

21. Preload, or pressure generated in the ventricles at the end of diastole, depends on the amount of blood in the ventricle. Afterload is the resistance to ejection of the blood from the ventricle. Afterload depends on pressure in the aorta.

22. Contractility is the potential for myocardial fiber shortening during systole. It is determined by the amount of stretch during

SUMMARY REVIEW—cont'd

diastole (i.e., preload) and by sympathetic stimulation of the ventricles.

23. The Frank-Starling law of the heart states that the myocardial stretch determines the force of myocardial contraction (the greater the stretch, the stronger the contraction).

24. Laplace's law states that the amount of contractile force generated within a chamber depends on the radius of the chamber and the thickness of its wall (the smaller the radius and the thicker the wall, the greater the force of contraction).

The Systemic Circulation

1. Blood flows from the left ventricle into the aorta and from the aorta into arteries that eventually branch into arterioles and capillaries, the smallest of the arterial vessels. Oxygen, nutrients, and other substances needed for cellular metabolism pass from the capillaries into the interstitium, where they are available for uptake by the cells. Capillaries also absorb products of cellular metabolism from the interstitium.

2. Venules, the smallest veins, receive capillary blood. From the venules the venous blood flows into larger and larger veins until it reaches the venae cavae, through which it enters the right atrium.

3. Vessel walls consist of three layers: the tunica intima (inner layer), the tunica media (middle layer), and the tunica externa (outer layer).

4. Layers of the vessel wall differ in thickness and composition from vessel to vessel, depending on the vessel's size and location within the circulatory system. In general, the tunica media of arteries close to the heart contains a greater proportion of elastic fibers because these arteries must be able to distend during systole and recoil during diastole. Distributing arteries farther from the heart contain a greater proportion of smooth muscle fibers because these arteries must be able to constrict and dilate to control blood pressure and volume within specific capillary beds.

5. Blood flow into the capillary beds is controlled by the contraction and relaxation of smooth muscle bands (precapillary sphincters) at junctions between metarterioles and capillaries. The endothelium is probably a source of prostaglandins that control vasomotion.

6. Blood flow through the veins is assisted by the contraction of skeletal muscles (the muscle pump), and backwards flow in the lower body is prevented by one-way valves, particularly in the deep veins of the legs.

7. Blood flow is affected by blood pressure; resistance to flow within the vessels; blood consistency (which affects velocity); anatomic features that may cause turbulent or laminar flow; and compliance (distensibility) of the vessels.

8. Poiseuille's law describes the relationship of blood flow, pressure, and resistance as the difference between pressure at the inflow end of the vessel and pressure at the outflow end divided by resistance within the vessel.

9. Resistance to blood flow depends on vessel length and radius and on the viscosity of the blood. The greater a vessel's length and the blood's viscosity and the narrower the radius of the vessel's lumen, the greater the resistance within the vessel.

10. Total peripheral resistance, or the resistance to flow within the entire systemic circulatory system, depends on the combined lengths and radii of all the vessels within the system and on whether the vessels are arranged in series (greater resistance) or in parallel (lesser resistance).

11. Blood flow is influenced also by neural stimulation (of vasoconstriction or vasodilation) and by autonomic features that cause turbu-

lence within the vascular lumen (e.g., protrusions from the vessel wall, twists and turns, bifurcations).

12. Arterial blood pressure is influenced and regulated by factors that affect cardiac output (heart rate and stroke volume), total resistance within the system, and blood volume.

13. Many hormones and other endothelial mediators alter vasomotion including epinephrine, norepinephrine, antidiuretic hormone, renin-angiotensin system, natriuretic peptides, adrenomedullin, nitric oxide, prostaglandins, and endothelium-derived relaxing factor.

14. Venous pressure is influenced by blood volume within the venous system and compliance of the venous walls.

15. Blood flow through the coronary circulation is governed not only by the same principles as flow through other vascular beds but also by two adaptations dictated by cardiac dynamics. First, blood flows into the coronary arteries during diastole rather than systole because during systole, the cusps of the aortic semilunar valve block the openings of the coronary arteries. Second, systolic contraction inhibits coronary artery flow by compressing the coronary arteries.

16. Autoregulation enables the coronary vessels to maintain optimal perfusion pressure despite systolic effects, and myoglobin in heart muscle stores oxygen for use during the systolic phase of the cardiac cycle.

Lymphatic System

1. The vessels of the lymphatic system run in the same sheaths as those of the arteries and veins.

2. Lymph (interstitial fluid plus cells of the immune system) is absorbed by lymphatic venules in the capillary beds and travels through ever larger lymphatic veins until it empties into the right lymphatic duct and the thoracic duct, which drain into the right and left subclavian veins, respectively.

3. As lymph travels toward the thoracic ducts, it passes through lymph nodes clustered around the lymphatic vessels. The lymph nodes are sites of immune function and are ideally placed to sample fluid and cells moving from the periphery into the central circulation.

Tests of Cardiovascular Function

1. The evaluation of an individual with known or suspected cardiovascular disease must include a careful history and physical examination including assessment of risk factors, symptoms, vital signs, level of consciousness, mucous membrane color, and cardiopulmonary functioning.

2. Important tests for cardiac disorders are ECG and Holter monitoring, which detect disturbances of impulse generation or conduction.

3. Stress tests elicit clinical manifestations of cardiovascular disease that might not be present at rest.

4. The sensitivity of stress testing is improved by the use of radiotracer imaging techniques such as SPECT.

5. Echocardiography detects structural and functional cardiac abnormalities over time.

6. Cardiac catheterization is used to measure the oxygen content and pressure of blood in the heart's chambers and to inject contrast media for x-ray examination of the size and shape of the chambers and valves. Injection of contrast medium into the coronary arteries (coronary angiography), on the other hand, permits visualization of the coronary circulation and every tissue perfused by the coronary arteries.

▮ SUMMARY REVIEW—cont'd

7. Evaluation of the systemic vascular system can include arterial pressure pulse waveform analysis, Doppler ultrasonography, venography, and arteriography.

Aging and the Cardiovascular System

1. Cardiovascular disease is the most common cause of morbidity and mortality in older adults in Western society and in much of the rest of the world. In addition, age is a key driver of cardiovascular risk, which explains why it is the primary cause of death in persons older than age 65.
2. The most common cardiovascular disease condition is hypertension followed by coronary atherosclerosis, for which hypertension is a risk factor.

3. It is challenging to determine the normal physiologic changes in cardiac function with aging because many pathologic changes are usually present and physical fitness is variable in older people as well.
4. The most relevant age-associated physiologic changes in cardiovascular performance include myocardial and blood vessel stiffening, changes in neurogenic control over vascular tone, increased occurrence of atrial fibrillation, and loss of exercise capacity plus left ventricular hypertrophy and fibrosis.
5. With active risk reduction, physical activity, and disease management, older adults can have markedly improved cardiovascular health.

▮ KEY TERMS

a wave, 1021
Actin, 1030
Adrenomedullin (ADM), 1046
Afferent lymphatic vessel, 1049
Afterload, 1032
Aldosterone, 1046
Angiogenesis, 1024
Angiotensin II (Ang II), 1046
Anisotropic band (A band), 1030
Aorta, 1021
Aortic semilunar valve, 1021
Arteriogenesis, 1024
Arteriole, 1036
Artery, 1036
Atrial natriuretic peptide (ANP), 1046
Atrioventricular (AV) node, 1027
Atrioventricular valve, 1021
Automatic cell, 1028
Automaticity, 1028
Autoregulation, 1048
B-type natriuretic peptide (BNP), 1046
Bainbridge reflex, 1036
Baroreceptor, 1053
Baroreceptor reflex, 1036
Blood velocity, 1043
Bundle branch, 1027
Bundle of His (atrioventricular bundle), 1027
C-type natriuretic peptide (CNP), 1046
c wave, 1021
Calcium channel–blocking drug, 1032
Capillary, 1040
Cardiac action potential, 1025
Cardiac catheterization, 1052
Cardiac cycle, 1021
Cardiac output, 1032
Cardiac plexus, 1029
Cardiac vein, 1024
Cardiomyocyte, 1019
Cardiovascular control center, 1036
Cardiovascular vasomotor control center, 1036
Chordae tendineae, 1021
Collateral artery, 1024
Conduction system, 1025
Connexin, 1025
Coronary angiography, 1052
Coronary artery, 1022
Coronary ostia, 1024
Coronary perfusion pressure, 1048
Coronary sinus, 1024
Crista supraventricularis, 1021
Cross-bridge cycle of muscle contraction, 1031
Depolarization, 1027

Diastole, 1021
Diastolic blood pressure, 1043
Diastolic depolarization, 1028
Efferent lymphatic vessel, 1049
Ejection fraction, 1032
Elastic artery, 1037
End-diastolic volume, 1033
Endocardium, 1019
Endothelial cell, 1040
Endothelium, 1040
Epinephrine, 1046
Excitation-contraction coupling, 1032
Fenestration, 1040
Frank-Starling law of the heart, 1033
Great cardiac vein, 1025
Heart rate, 1026, 1029
Heart rate variability (HRV), 1035
Hematocrit, 1043
Inferior vena cava, 1021
Inflow tract, 1021
Inotropic agent, 1035
Intercalated disk, 1030
Isotropic band (I band), 1030
Laminar flow, 1043
Left anterior bundle branch (LABB), 1027
Left atrium, 1019
Left bundle branch (LBB), 1027
Left coronary artery (LCA), 1024
Left heart, 1017
Left posterior bundle branch (LPBB), 1027
Left pulmonary artery, 1021
Left ventricle, 1019
Left ventricular end-diastolic volume (LVEDV), 1034
Lumen, 1038
Lymph, 1049
Lymphatic system, 1049
Lymphatic vein, 1049
Lymphatic venule, 1049
M line, 1030
Mean arterial pressure (MAP), 1043
Mediastinum, 1019
Metarteriole, 1038
Mitral and tricuspid complex, 1021
Mitral valve, 1021
Muscular artery, 1037
Myocardial contractility, 1031
Myocardial oxygen consumption ($M\dot{V}O_2$), 1031
Myocardium, 1019
Myoglobin, 1048
Myosin, 1030
Natriuretic peptide (NP), 1046

Nitric oxide (NO), 1046
Node, 1025
Norepinephrine, 1029
Outflow tract, 1021
P wave, 1028
Papillary muscle, 1021
Perfusion, 1044
Pericardial cavity, 1019
Pericardial fluid, 1019
Pericardial sac, 1019
Pericardium, 1019
Peripheral vascular system, 1036
Poiseuille's law, 1042
PR interval, 1028
Precapillary sphincter, 1038
Preload, 1032
Pressure, 1042
Prolapse, 1021
Pulmonary artery, 1021
Pulmonary circulation, 1017
Pulmonary vein, 1021
Pulmonic semilunar valve, 1021
Pulse pressure, 1044
Purkinje fiber, 1027
QRS complex, 1028
QT interval, 1028
Repolarization, 1027
Radius, 1042
Resistance, 1042
Rhythmicity, 1028
Right atrium, 1019
Right bundle branch (RBB), 1027
Right coronary artery (RCA), 1024
Right heart, 1017
Right lymphatic duct, 1049
Right pulmonary artery, 1021
Right ventricle, 1019
Semilunar valve, 1021
Shear stress, 1024
Sinoatrial (SA) node, 1026
Sinus arrhythmia, 1036
ST interval, 1028
Stenosis, 1024
Stroke volume, 1035
Superior vena cava, 1021
Systemic circulation, 1017
Systemic vascular resistance (SVR), 1035
Systole, 1021
Systolic blood pressure, 1043
Systolic compressive effect, 1048
Thoracic duct, 1049
Titin, 1030

KEY TERMS—cont'd

Total peripheral resistance (TPR), 1035
Total resistance, 1042
Trabeculae carneae, 1021
Tricuspid valve, 1021
Tropomyosin molecule, 1030
Troponin, 1030
Troponin C, 1030
Troponin I, 1030
Troponin T, 1030
Troponin-tropomyosin complex, 1030
Tunica externa (adventitia), 1036

Tunica intima, 1036
Tunica media, 1036
Turbulent, 1043
Urodilatin, 1046
v wave, 1021
Vasa vasorum, 1036
Vascular compliance, 1043
Vasculogenesis, 1037
Vasoconstriction, 1038
Vasoconstrictor hormone, 1046
Vasodilation, 1038

Vasomotion, 1040
Vasopressin, 1046
Vein, 1036
Venule, 1036
Visceral pericardium, 1025
Viscosity, 1043
Wall shear stress (WSS), 1043
x descent, 1022
y descent, 1022
Z line, 1030

REFERENCES

1. Bergmann O, et al: Evidence for cardiomyocyte renewal in humans. *Science* 324(5923):98–102, 2009.
2. Elhelaly WM, et al: Redox regulation of heart regeneration: an evolutionary tradeoff. *Front Cell Dev Biol* 4:137, 2016.
3. Nadal-Ginard B: Generation of new cardiomyocytes in the adult heart: prospects of myocardial regeneration as an alternative to cardiac transplantation. *Rev Esp Cardiol* 54:543–550, 2001.
4. Buja LM: Anatomy of the heart. In Willerson JT, et al, editors: *Cardiovascular medicine*, ed 3, London, 2007, Springer.
5. Faber JE, et al: A brief etymology of the collateral circulation. *Arterioscler Thromb Vasc Biol* 34:1854–1859, 2014.
6. Fung E, Helisch A: Macrophages in collateral arteriogenesis. *Front Physiol* 3:353, 2012.
7. Ramo K, et al: Suppression of ischemia in arterial occlusive disease by JNK-promoted native collateral artery development. *Elife* 5:2016.
8. Bache RJ: Coronary artery disease: regulation of coronary blood flow. In Willerson JT, et al, editors: *Cardiovascular medicine*, ed 3, London, 2007, Springer.
9. Chen J, et al: Abnormalities of capillary microarchitecture in a rat model of coronary ischemic congestive heart failure. *Am J Physiol Heart Circ Physiol* 308(8):H830–H840, 2015.
10. Loukas M, et al: The cardiac lymphatic system. *Clin Anat* 24(6):684–691, 2011.
11. Jansen JA, et al: Cardiac connexins and impulse propagation. *J Mol Cell Cardiol* 48(1):76–82, 2010.
12. Rubart M, Zipes DP: Genesis of cardiac arrhythmias: electrophysiologic considerations. In Bonow RO, et al, editors: *Braunwald's heart disease: a textbook of cardiovascular medicine*, ed 9, Philadelphia, 2012, Elsevier Saunders.
13. Rubart M, Zipes DP: Genesis of cardiac arrhythmias. In Mann DL, et al, editors: *Braunwald's heart disease: a textbook of cardiovascular medicine*, ed 10, Philadelphia, 2015, Saunders, p 33, 629–661.
14. Klabunde RE: *Cardiovascular physiology concepts*, ed 2, Baltimore, 2012, Lippincott Williams & Wilkins.
15. Opie LH, Hasenfuss G: Mechanisms of cardiac contraction and relaxation. In Bonow RO, et al, editors: *Braunwald's heart disease: a textbook of cardiovascular medicine*, ed 9, Philadelphia, 2012, Elsevier Saunders.
16. von Homeyer P, Schwinn DA: Pharmacogenomics of β-adrenergic physiology and response to β-blockade. *Anesth Analg* 113(6):1305–1318, 2011.
17. Harmar AJ, et al: IUPHAR-DB: the IUPHAR database of G protein-coupled receptors and ion channels. *Nucleic Acids Res* 37(Database issue):D680–D685, 2009.
18. Triposkiadis F, et al: The sympathetic nervous system in heart failure physiology, pathophysiology and clinical implication. *J Am Coll Cardiol* 54(19):1747–1762, 2009.
19. Opie LH, Bers DM: Mechanisms of cardiac contraction and relaxation. In Mann DL, et al, editors: *Braunwald's heart disease: a textbook of cardiovascular medicine*, ed 10, Philadelphia, 2015, Saunders, pp 429–453.
20. Linke WA, Hamdani N: Gigantic business: titin properties and function through thick and thin. *Circ Res* 114:1052–1068, 2014.
21. Deussen A, et al: Mechanisms of metabolic coronary flow regulation. *J Mol Cell Cardiol* 52(4):794–801, 2012.
22. Stehle R, Iorga B: Kinetics of cardiac sarcomeric processes and rate-limiting steps in contraction and relaxation. *J Mol Cell Cardiol* 48(5):843–850, 2010.
23. Sakata Y, et al: Left ventricular stiffening as therapeutic target for heart failure with preserved ejection fraction. *Circ J* 77(4):886–892, 2013.
24. Ababneh AA, et al: Normal limits for left ventricular ejection fraction and volumes estimated with gated myocardial perfusion imaging in patients with normal exercise test results: influence of tracer, gender, and acquisition camera. *J Nucl Cardiol* 7(6):661–668, 2000.
25. Davidson CJ, Bonow RO: Cardiac catheterization. In Mann DL, et al, editors: *Braunwald's heart disease: a textbook of cardiovascular medicine*, ed 10, Philadelphia, 2015, Saunders, pp 364–391.
26. Flynn A, et al: Sepsis-induced cardiomyopathy: a review of pathophysiologic mechanisms. *Heart Fail Rev* 15(6):605–611, 2010.
27. Cimolai MC, et al: Mitochondrial mechanisms in septic cardiomyopathy. *Int J Mol Sci* 16(8):17763–17778, 2015.
28. Goegel B, et al: Impact of acute normobaric hypoxia on regional and global myocardial function: a speckle tracking echocardiography study. *Int J Cardiovasc Imaging* 29(3):561–567, 2013.
29. Fatisson J, Oswald V, Lalonde F: Influence diagram of physiological and environmental factors affecting heart rate variability: an extended literature overview. *Heart Int* 11(1):e32–e40, 2016.
30. Larsen PD, et al: Respiratory sinus arrhythmia in conscious humans during spontaneous respiration. *Respir Physiol Neurobiol* 174(1-2):111–118, 2010.
31. Fisher JP: Carotid baroreflex control of arterial blood pressure at rest and during dynamic exercise in aging humans. *Am J Physiol Regul Integr Comp Physiol* 299(5):R1241–R1247, 2010.
32. Hoit BD, Walsh RA: Normal physiology of the cardiovascular system. In Fuster V, et al, editors: *Hurst's the heart*, ed 13, Philadelphia, 2011, McGraw-Hill.
33. Crystal GJ, Salem MR: The Bainbridge and the "reverse" Bainbridge reflexes: history, physiology, and clinical relevance. *Anesth Analg* 114(3):520–532, 2012.
34. Volpe M, et al: Natriuretic peptides in cardiovascular diseases: current use and perspectives. *Eur Heart J* 35(7):419–425, 2014.
35. Klein I, Ojamaa K: Thyroid hormone and the cardiovascular system. *N Engl J Med* 344(7):501–509, 2001.
36. Ren J, Samson WK, Sowers JR: Insulin-like growth factor I as a cardiac hormone: physiological and pathophysiological implications in heart disease. *J Mol Cell Cardiol* 31(11):2049–2061, 1999.
37. Lähteenvuo J, Rosenzweig A: Effects of aging on angiogenesis. *Circ Res* 110(9):1252–1263, 2012.
38. Mehta D, Malik AB: Signaling mechanisms regulating endothelial permeability. *Physiol Rev* 86(1):279–367, 2006.
39. Haraldsson B, Nyström J: The glomerular endothelium: new insights on function and structure. *Curr Opin Nephrol Hypertens* 21(3):258–263, 2012.
40. Girard J-P, Moussion C, Förster R: HEVs, lymphatics and homeostatic immune cell trafficking in lymph nodes. *Nat Rev Immunol* 12(11):762–773, 2012.
41. Millon A, et al: Low WSS induces intimal thickening, while large WSS variation and inflammation induce medial thinning, in an animal model of atherosclerosis. *PLoS ONE* 10(11):e0141880, 2015.
42. Patton KT, Thibodeau GA: *Anatomy & physiology online package*, ed 9, St Louis, 2016, Elsevier.
43. Kim DH, et al: Adiponectin levels and the risk of hypertension: a systematic review and meta-analysis. *Hypertension* 62(1):27–32, 2013.
44. Zachariah JP, et al: Circulating adipokines and vascular function: cross-sectional association in a community-based cohort. *Hypertension* 67(2):294–300, 2016.
45. Younk LM, et al: The cardiovascular effects of insulin. *Expert Opin Drug Saf* 13(7):955–966, 2014.
46. Yuyun MF, et al: Prognostic significance of adrenomedullin in patients with heart failure and with myocardial infarction. *Am J Cardiol* 115(7):986–991, 2015.
47. Tousoulis D, et al: The role of nitric oxide on endothelial function. *Curr Vasc Pharmacol* 10(1):4–18, 2012.
48. Stoner L, Sabatier MJ: Use of ultrasound for non-invasive assessment of flow-mediated dilation. *J Atheroscler Thromb* 19(5):407–421, 2012.
49. Kohan DE, et al: Regulation of blood pressure and salt homeostasis by endothelin. *Physiol Rev* 91(1):1–77, 2011.

50. Davenport AP, et al: Endothelin. *Pharmacol Rev* 68(2):357–418, 2016.

51. Griendling KK, et al: Biology of the vessel wall. In Fuster V, et al, editors: *Hurst's the heart*, ed 13, Philadelphia, 2011, McGraw-Hill.

52. Schjerning Olsen AM, et al: The impact of NSAID treatment on cardiovascular risk—insight from Danish observational data. *Basic Clin Pharmacol Toxicol* 115(2):179–184, 2014.

53. Singh BK, et al: Assessment of nonsteroidal anti-inflammatory drug-induced cardiotoxicity. *Expert Opin Drug Metab Toxicol* 10(2):143–156, 2014.

54. Lang RM, et al: Recommendations for chamber quantification: a report from the American Society of Echocardiography's Guidelines and Standards Committee and the Chamber quantification writing groups, developed in conjunction with the European Association of Echocardiography, a branch of the European Society of Cardiology. *J Am Soc Echo* 18(12):1440–1463, 2005.

55. Salton CJ, et al: Gender differences and normal left ventricular anatomy in an adult population free of hypertension. A cardiovascular magnetic resonance study of the Framingham heart study offspring cohort. *J Am Coll Cardiol* 39(6):1055–1060, 2002.

56. Connolly HM, Oh JK: Echocardiography. In Bonow RO, et al, editors: *Braunwald's heart disease: a textbook of cardiovascular medicine*, ed 9, Philadelphia, 2012, Elsevier Saunders.

57. Muraru D, et al: Mitral valve anatomy and function: new insights from three-dimensional echocardiography. *J Cardiovasc Med* 14(2):91–99, 2013.

58. Ali S, et al: Intracardiac echocardiography: clinical utility and application. *Echocardiography* 28(5):582–590, 2011.

59. Udelson JE, Dilsizian V, Bonow RO: Nuclear cardiology. In Bonow RO, et al, editors: *Braunwald's heart disease: a textbook of cardiovascular medicine*, ed 9, Philadelphia, 2012, Elsevier Saunders.

60. Polonsky TS, et al: Coronary artery calcium score and risk classification for coronary heart disease prediction. *JAMA* 303(16):1610–1616, 2010.

61. Cousins C, et al: ICRP publication 120: Radiological protection in cardiology. *Ann ICRP* 42(1):1–125, 2013.

62. Charoenpanichkit C, Hundley WG: The 20 year evolution of dobutamine stress cardiovascular magnetic resonance. *J Cardiovasc Magn Reson* 12:59, 2010.

63. McGhie AE, Gould KL, Willerson JT: Nuclear cardiology. In Willerson JT, et al, editors: *Cardiovascular medicine*, ed 3, London, 2007, Springer.

64. Joshi SB, et al: CT applications in electrophysiology. *Cardiol Clin* 27(4):619–631, 2009.

65. Darabian S, et al: The role of carotid intimal thickness testing and risk prediction for the development of coronary atherosclerosis. *Curr Atheroscler Rep* 15(3):306, 2013.

66. Lozano R, et al: Global and regional mortality from 235 causes of death for 20 age groups in 1990 and 2010: a systematic analysis for the Global Burden of Disease Study 2010. *Lancet* 380(9859):2095–2128, 2012.

67. North BJ, Sinclair DA: The intersection between aging and cardiovascular disease. *Circ Res* 110(8):1097–1108, 2012.

68. Dai D, et al: Cardiac aging: from molecular mechanisms to significance in human health and disease. *Antioxid Redox Signal* 16(12):1492–1526, 2012.

69. Franklin SS, et al: Does the relation of blood pressure to coronary heart disease risk change with aging? The Framingham Heart Study. *Circulation* 103(9):1245–1249, 2001.

Alterations of Cardiovascular Function

Valentina L. Brashers

⊖volve WEBSITE

http://evolve.elsevier.com/McCance/
- Content Updates
- Chapter Summary Review
- Review Questions
- Case Studies
- Animations

CHAPTER OUTLINE

Cardiovascular disease is the leading cause of death, in both the United States and worldwide.[1] Disorders of the veins, arteries, and heart wall comprise the scope of cardiovascular disease. Current understanding of the pathophysiology of cardiovascular disease is focused on genetic, neurohumoral, inflammatory, and metabolic mechanisms that underlie tissue and cellular alterations.

DISEASES OF THE VEINS

Varicose Veins and Chronic Venous Insufficiency

Chronic venous disease manifests along a continuum from asymptomatic telangiectasias to varicose veins to chronic vascular insufficiency. Telangiectasias are small, widened blood vessels visible in the skin. A varicose vein refers to a condition in which venous blood has pooled, producing distortion of the veins, leakage, increased intravascular hydrostatic pressure, and inflammation (Fig. 33.1). Varicose veins result from incompetent valves, venous obstruction, muscle pump dysfunction, or a combination of these conditions. The increase in venous hydrostatic pressure is associated with an increase in transforming growth factor

beta (TGF-β) and basic fibroblast growth factor (bfgf) in vessel walls resulting in permanent remodeling of the vessels. An altered ratio of prostacyclin to thromboxane A_2 with potential for clotting also occurs.[2] Risk factors for developing varicose veins include gender (women are at a much higher risk), pregnancy, increased weight, increased age, leg trauma, sitting or standing for long periods of time, and family history. Symptoms include visible distended veins; itching, burning, or throbbing around lower leg veins; and muscle cramping or pain in the lower legs.

Varicose veins can progress to chronic venous insufficiency (CVI), which is defined as persistent ambulatory lower extremity venous hypertension. Venous hypertension, circulatory stasis, and tissue hypoxia lead to an inflammatory reaction in vessels and tissue. These processes cause lower extremity edema, pain, skin changes (hyperpigmentation and lipodermatosclerosis), and necrosis (venous stasis ulcers)[3] (see Fig. 33.1). Infection can occur because poor circulation limits immune and inflammatory responses, especially as a complication of reparative surgery.

Treatment across the spectrum of chronic venous disease may include recommendations to lose weight and decrease time spent standing or

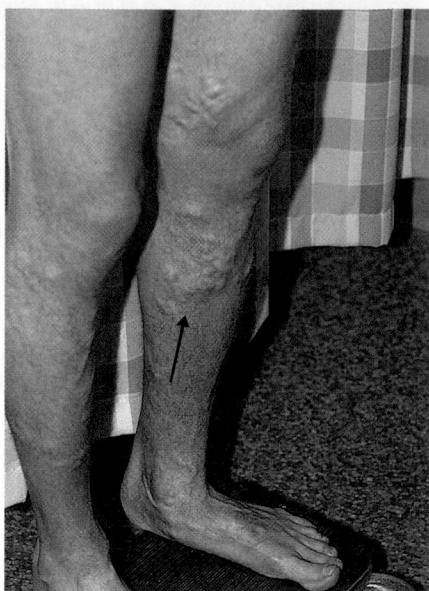

FIGURE 33.1 Varicose Veins of the Leg *(arrow)*. (Courtesy Dr. Magruder C. Donaldson, Brigham and Women's Hospital, Boston. From Kumar V et al: *Robbins basic pathology*, ed 8, Philadelphia, 2010, Saunders.)

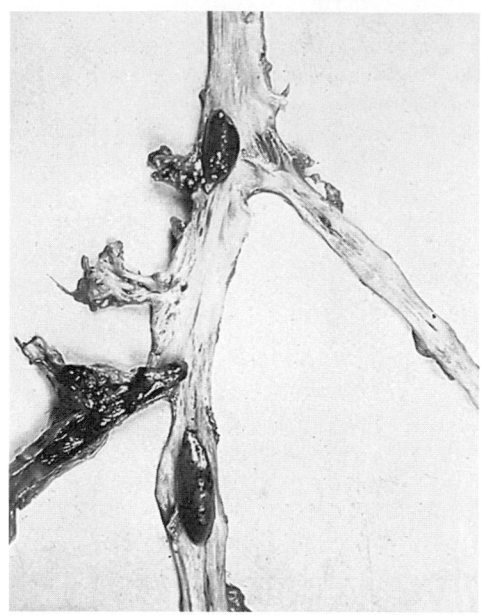

FIGURE 33.2 Multiple Venous Thrombi. (From Rosai J: *Ackerman's surgical pathology*, ed 8, vol 2, St Louis, 1996, Mosby.)

sitting, leg elevation, physical exercise, and use of compression stockings. If conservation treatment is not successful, endovenous ablation or foam sclerotherapy may be recommended. Both are associated with less pain and faster recovery compared to endovenous laser therapy and surgical stripping.[4]

Deep Venous Thrombosis

Venous thromboembolism (VTE) includes **deep venous thrombosis (DVT)** and pulmonary embolism (PE) (see Chapter 36). DVT is a blood clot that remains attached to a vessel wall, usually in a single side of a lower extremity (Fig. 33.2). A detached thrombus is a **thromboembolus**. Venous thrombi are more common than arterial thrombi because flow and pressure are lower in the veins than in the arteries. The American Heart Association (AHA) estimates that about 2 million people in the United States will have VTE annually with approximately 44,000 deaths.[5] Three factors (termed the triad of Virchow) promote venous thrombosis: (1) **venous stasis** (associated with immobility, obesity, prolonged leg dependency, age, congestive heart failure [CHF]), (2) **venous intimal damage** (related to trauma, venipuncture, IV medications), and (3) **hypercoagulable states** (from inherited disorders, smoking, malignancy, liver disease, pregnancy, oral contraceptives, hormone replacement, hyperhomocysteinemia, antiphospholipid syndrome).[6] Virtually everyone who is hospitalized is at significant risk for DVT, especially those with orthopedic trauma or surgery, spinal cord injury, age older than 60 years, and obstetric/gynecologic conditions. Individuals with malignancy (especially ovarian and pancreatic cancer), and women who are pregnant are also at significant risk. The most common heritable hypercoagulable states are abnormal factor V Leiden and prothrombin gene variant 20210A, both of which predispose patients to DVT.[6] Other less common causes are deficiencies of the endogenous anticoagulants protein C, protein S, and antithrombin.

Accumulation of clotting factors and platelets leads to thrombus formation in the vein, often near a venous valve. Inflammation around the thrombus promotes further platelet aggregation, and the thrombus grows proximally. Most thrombi eventually dissolve without treatment, but untreated DVT is associated with a high risk of **thromboembolization** of a part of the clot from the leg traveling to the lung resulting in a

pulmonary embolism[7] (see Chapter 36). In up to one-third of individuals with DVT, persistent venous outflow obstruction may lead to **post-thrombotic syndrome (PTS)** characterized by chronic, persistent pain; edema; and ulceration of the affected limb.[8]

Clinical manifestations of DVT are often absent. If a symptom is present, it is typically pain. Other signs of DVT include unilateral leg swelling, dilation of superficial veins, calf tenderness, and skin that is mottled or cyanotic. Because DVT is usually asymptomatic and difficult to detect clinically, prevention of DVT is a high priority. Prevention strategies are dependent upon the condition of the individual and prior history of DVT. In general, individuals should be mobilized as soon as possible after illness, injury, or surgery. Additional prophylactic treatment for individuals at low risk can include aspirin or pneumatic devices.[9] People at higher risk are treated prophylactically with low-molecular-weight heparin or, in some cases, direct thrombin inhibitors.

Diagnosis is made by combining measurement of serum D-dimer concentration plus lower extremity compression Doppler ultrasonography. D-dimer is an indirect measure of the presence of thrombosis that is very sensitive but is not specific. If the D-dimer is negative, DVT is ruled out. If it is positive, the diagnosis must be confirmed with ultrasonography. Because of its high rate of sensitivity and specificity, use of digital photoplethysmography is becoming more widespread.[10]

Management of deep venous thrombosis is based on the risk of extension of the clot or embolization. For low-risk individuals, serial imaging of the deep veins may be indicated. For individuals at high risk for clot extension or pulmonary embolism, anticoagulation with low-molecular-weight heparin is indicated.[11,12] Other options include direct thrombin inhibitors, such as fondaparinux, apixaban, argatroban, or dabigatran.[7,13] Catheter-directed thrombolytic therapy may be used to dissolve the clot more quickly and reduce the risk of postphlebitic syndrome, especially when a large clot is located in a proximal vein; however, bleeding risk is increased and many people have contraindications to the use of thrombolytics.[14] Pharmacomechanical treatment involves catheter-directed thrombolysis in combination with catheter-mediated removal of clots and can be used in selected individuals.[15] DVT has a high recurrence rate after discontinuation of anticoagulant therapy. In people with proximal DVT or pulmonary embolism, at least

3 months of therapy is indicated. Recent updated guidelines suggest that for long-term therapy of individuals with DVT without underlying cancer, direct thrombin inhibitors are recommended. For those with DVT and cancer, continued low-molecular-weight heparin is indicated.[16] If the individual is active and no identifiable underlying condition is discovered, aspirin therapy alone may be indicated.[9]

Superior Vena Cava Syndrome

Superior vena cava syndrome (SVCS) is a clinical manifestation of progressive compression of the superior vena cava (SVC) that leads to venous distention in the upper extremities and head. The leading causes of SVCS are nonsmall cell lung cancer, small cell lung cancer, and lymphoma. Nonmalignant causes of SVCS include thrombosis; infection, such as tuberculosis or histoplasmosis; mediastinal fibrosis; cystic fibrosis; and retrosternal goiter. Pacemaker wires, central venous catheters, and pulmonary artery catheters also can lead to SVCS.[17]

The SVC is a thin-walled and relatively low-pressure vessel that lies in the closed thoracic compartment; therefore tissue expansion can easily compress the SVC. The right main stem bronchus abuts the SVC so that cancers occurring in the bronchus may press on the vessel and obstruct venous return to the right atrium. Additionally, the SVC is surrounded by lymph nodes and lymph chains that commonly become involved in infection and thoracic cancers. If the onset of SVCS is slow, surrounding collateral vessels may enlarge in response to the increased pressure and symptoms may occur more gradually.

The most common clinical manifestations of SVCS include edema and venous distention in the face, neck, trunk, and upper extremities. More rarely, cyanosis may be observed. Individuals may complain of dyspnea, dysphagia, hoarseness, stridor, cough, and chest pain. Central nervous system (CNS) edema may cause malaise, headache, visual disturbances, vertigo, awareness or memory disorders, and impaired consciousness. The skin of the face and arms may become purple and taut, and capillary refill time can be prolonged. Respiratory distress may be present because of edema of bronchial structures or compression of the bronchus by a carcinoma.

Diagnosis is made by chest x-ray, Doppler ultrasound studies, computed tomography (CT), and contrast-enhanced magnetic resonance imaging (MRI). If laryngeal constriction or cerebral edema is present, emergency intervention may be required to address the underlying cause of SVCS. Similarly, if a rapidly growing malignancy is found, immediate treatment is indicated, including radiation or chemotherapy. With a slow-growing malignancy, stenting of the SVC may be considered for immediate symptom relief, followed by appropriate chemotherapy. For an infectious cause of SVCS, antibiotics are used. Fluid restriction, diuretics, supplemental oxygen, and elevation of the head also can provide symptomatic relief.[17]

DISEASES OF THE ARTERIES

Hypertension

Hypertension (HTN) is consistent elevation of systemic arterial blood pressure. Hypertension was defined in 2014 as a sustained systolic blood pressure (SBP) of 140 mmHg or greater or a diastolic blood pressure (DBP) of 90 mmHg or greater.[18] In 2017 hypertension was redefined as a SBP of 130 or greater or a DBP of 80 or greater (Table 33.1).[18a] Hypertension is the most common primary diagnosis in the United States— approximately one in three adults older than 20 years of age has hypertension; this increases to nearly two in three in those older than age 60. In individuals younger than age 45, the prevalence of hypertension is higher in men than in women; from ages 45 to 65 prevalence is the same in men and women; and after age 65 the prevalence of hypertension is greater in women than in men.[5] The prevalence of HTN is higher in

TABLE 33.1	CLASSIFICATION OF BLOOD PRESSURE FOR ADULTS*			
CATEGORY	**SYSTOLIC (mmHg)**		**DIASTOLIC (mmHg)**	
Normal	<120	*AND*	<80	
Elevated	120–129	*OR*	<80	
Hypertension				
Stage 1 hypertension	130–139	*OR*	80–89	
Stage 2 hypertension	≥140	*OR*	≥90	
Hypertensive crisis	>180	*AND/OR*	>120	

*Individuals with systolic blood pressure and diastolic blood pressure in two categories should be designated to the higher blood pressure category. Blood pressure indicates an average of more than two careful readings obtained on more than two occasions. Data from Whelton PK, Carey RM, Aronow WS, et al: *Hypertension.* 2017 Nov 13. doi: 10.1161/HYP.0000000000000065.

blacks and in those with diabetes. Those who fall into the prehypertension category (which includes between 25% and 37% of the U.S. population) are at risk for developing hypertension unless lifestyle modification and treatment are instituted. Some individuals have isolated systolic hypertension. **Isolated systolic hypertension (ISH)** is elevated systolic blood pressure accompanied by normal diastolic blood pressure (less than 90 mmHg). ISH is becoming more prevalent in all age groups and is strongly associated with cardiovascular and cerebrovascular events.[5]

Approximately 95% of cases of hypertension have no known cause and therefore are diagnosed as primary hypertension (also commonly called *essential hypertension*). Secondary hypertension accounts for 5% of cases and is associated with an underlying primary disorder, such as renal disease. Hypertension is a complex disorder that affects the entire cardiovascular system, and all types and stages of hypertension are associated with increased risk for target organ disease events, such as myocardial infarction (MI), kidney disease, and stroke.

Factors Associated with Primary Hypertension

A combination of genetic and environmental factors is thought to be responsible for the development of primary hypertension. Genetic predisposition to hypertension is polygenic, including polymorphisms associated with renal sodium excretion, insulin and insulin sensitivity, activity of the sympathetic nervous system (SNS) and renin-angiotensin-aldosterone system (RAAS), and cell membrane sodium or calcium transport.[19] Epigenetic links between environmental factors, such as diet, exercise, and smoking, with gene expression also are being defined.[20,21]

Risk factors associated with primary hypertension include age, ethnicity, family history of hypertension and genetic factors, lower education and socioeconomic status, tobacco use, psychosocial stressors, sleep apnea, and dietary factors (including dietary fats, higher sodium intake, lower potassium intake, and excessive alcohol intake).[5] Glucose intolerance (diabetes mellitus) and obesity also are significant risk factors. Many of these factors also are risk factors for other cardiovascular disorders. In fact, hypertension, dyslipidemia, and glucose intolerance are often found together in a condition called *metabolic syndrome* (see Chapter 22).

◆ **PATHOPHYSIOLOGY.** Hypertension is caused by increases in cardiac output, total peripheral resistance, or both. Cardiac output is increased by any condition that increases heart rate or stroke volume, whereas peripheral resistance is increased by any factor that increases blood viscosity or reduces vessel diameter (vasoconstriction). (The many factors affecting cardiac output and peripheral resistance are described in Chapter 32.)

Primary Hypertension

Primary hypertension is the result of a complicated interaction between genetics and the environment that increases vascular tone (increased peripheral resistance) and blood volume, thus causing sustained increases in blood pressure. Multiple pathophysiologic mechanisms mediate these effects including the sympathetic nervous system (SNS), the RAAS, and natriuretic peptides. Inflammation, endothelial dysfunction, obesity-related hormones, and insulin resistance also contribute to both increased peripheral resistance and increased blood volume. Increased vascular volume is related to a decrease in renal excretion of salt, often referred to as a shift in the **pressure-natriuresis relationship**. This means that for a given blood pressure, individuals with hypertension tend to secrete less salt in their urine. The pathophysiology of primary hypertension is summarized in Fig. 33.3.

The SNS contributes to the pathogenesis of hypertension in many people. In the healthy individual, the SNS contributes to the maintenance of adequate blood pressure and tissue perfusion by promoting cardiac contractility and heart rate (maintenance of adequate cardiac output) and by inducing arteriolar vasoconstriction (maintenance of adequate peripheral resistance). In individuals with hypertension, overactivity of the SNS can result from increased production of catecholamines (epinephrine and norepinephrine) or from increased receptor reactivity involving these neurotransmitters.[22] Increased SNS activity causes increased heart rate and systemic vasoconstriction, thus raising the blood pressure. Efferent sympathetic outflow stimulates renin release,

increases tubular sodium reabsorption, and reduces renal blood flow. Additional mechanisms of SNS-induced hypertension include structural changes in blood vessels (vascular remodeling), insulin resistance, increased renin and angiotensin levels, and procoagulant effects.[22] The SNS is implicated in the cardiovascular and renal complications of hypertension. Beta-blocking medications oppose the effects of the SNS and have been used for decades in the treatment of hypertension. However, because of their side effects, these medications are no longer considered first-line treatment. The role of the SNS in the pathogenesis of cardiovascular disease is summarized in Fig. 33.4.

In the healthy individual, the RAAS provides an important homeostatic mechanism for maintaining adequate blood pressure and therefore tissue perfusion (see Chapter 32). In hypertensive individuals, overactivity of the RAAS contributes to salt and water retention and increased vascular resistance. In the brain, angiotensin (ang) II enhances sympathetic neural outflow and alters the release of hormones that contribute to endothelial dysfunction, insulin resistance, dyslipidemia, and platelet aggregation.[23] Further, ang II mediates arteriolar remodeling, which is a structural change in the vessel wall that results in permanent increases in peripheral resistance[24] (see Figs. 33.5 and 32.28). Ang II is associated with end-organ effects of hypertension, including atherosclerosis, renal disease, and cardiac hypertrophy. Finally, aldosterone not only contributes to sodium retention by the kidney but also has other deleterious effects on the cardiovascular system.[24] Medications, such as angiotensin-converting enzyme (ACE) inhibitors and angiotensin-receptor blockers (ARBs), oppose the activity of the RAAS and are

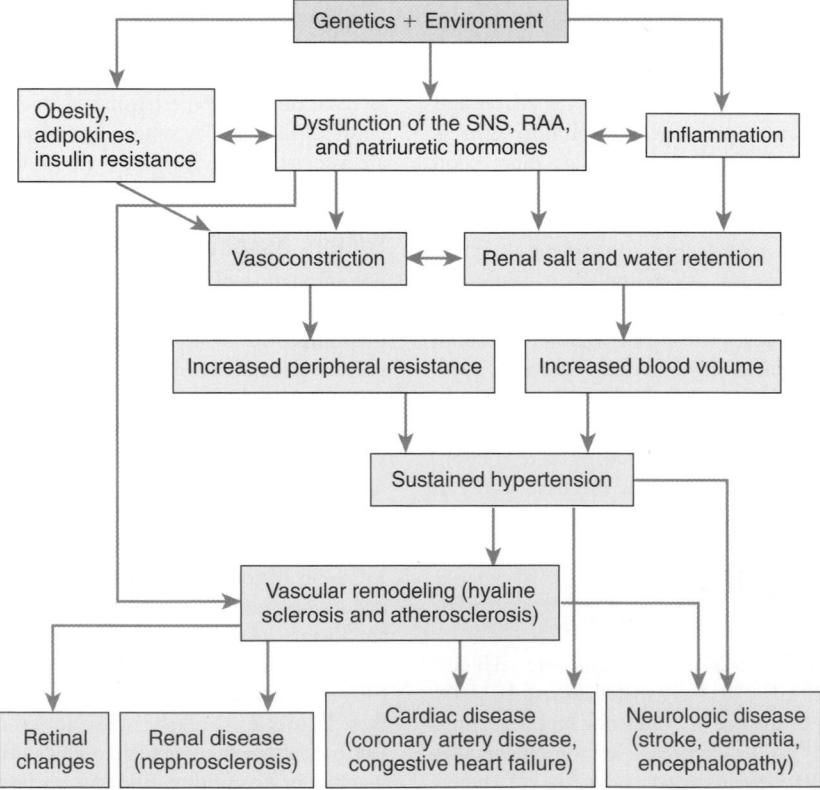

FIGURE 33.3 **Pathophysiology of Hypertension.** Numerous genetic vulnerabilities have been linked to hypertension and these, in combination with environmental risks, cause neurohumoral dysfunction (sympathetic nervous system *[SNS]*, renin-angiotensin-aldosterone *[RAA]* system, and natriuretic hormones) and promote inflammation and insulin resistance. Insulin resistance and neurohumoral dysfunction contribute to sustained systemic vasoconstriction and increased peripheral resistance. Inflammation contributes to renal dysfunction, which, in combination with the neurohumoral alterations, results in renal salt and water retention and increased blood volume. Increased peripheral resistance and increased blood volume are two primary causes of sustained hypertension.

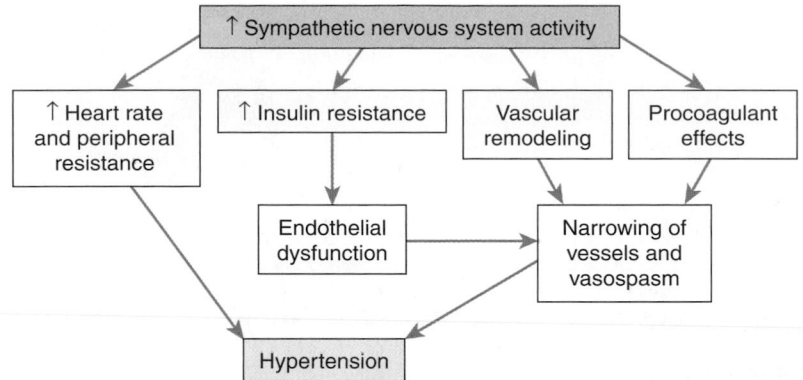

FIGURE 33.4 Role of the Sympathetic Nervous System in the Pathogenesis of Hypertension. Increased activity of the sympathetic nervous system (SNS) not only increases heart rate and peripheral resistance but also causes vascular remodeling with narrowing and vasospasm of arteries. The SNS contributes to insulin resistance, which is associated with endothelial dysfunction and decreased production of vasodilators, such as nitric oxide. The SNS also has procoagulant properties, making vascular spasm and thrombosis more likely. All of these factors contribute to sustained increases in blood pressure.

WHAT'S NEW?

The Renin-Angiotensin-Aldosterone System (RAAS) and Cardiovascular Disease

The RAAS has multiple effects on the cardiovascular system. There are four known RAA systems. The first and best known pathway includes the release of renin, the synthesis of angiotensin II (ang II) through angiotensin-converting enzyme (ACE), and stimulation of the AT1 receptor with secretion of aldosterone. Activation of the AT1 receptor causes systemic vasoconstriction and renal salt and water retention, and stimulates tissue growth and inflammation. AT1 activation also contributes to insulin resistance; remodeling of blood vessels, glomeruli, and the myocardium; atherogenesis and dysrhythmias; and decreased release of endothelial vasodilators and anticoagulants. Drugs that block this RAA pathway include ACE inhibitors, direct renin inhibitors, Ang II receptor blockers (ARBs), and aldosterone inhibitors. The second RAA pathway involves activation of a second ACE (ACE2) leading to the synthesis of angiotensin (1-7) from ang II. Ang (1-7) stimulates Mas receptors in the brain, blood vessels, heart, kidney, gut, pancreas, and inflammatory cells and has vasodilatory, antiproliferative, antifibrotic, and antithrombotic effects. These protective effects lead to lower blood pressure,
less vascular inflammation and clotting, improved insulin sensitivity, and decreased tissue remodeling and damage to target organ tissues. Research is underway to develop pharmacologic interventions, such as synthetic Mas agonists, Ang (1-7) formulations, and ACE2 activators that will stimulate these protective RAA pathways. More recently, additional RAA pathways have been identified. The third RAA system involves activation of the AT2 receptor by Ang II and by Ang III (derived from Ang II through the action of aminopeptidase). This pathway is up-regulated in brain, heart, and kidney injury and is antifibrotic, neuroprotective, and antiinflammatory but has no effect on blood pressure. AT2 agonists are being explored. Finally, the fourth RAA pathway is mediated by Ang IV which is derived from Ang III and activates the insulin-responsive aminopeptidase (IRAP) receptor. This pathway contributes to target organ damage in hypertension, and inhibitors of IRAP are under investigation. It may not be long before a fifth RAA pathway is described since a new homolog of ACE called ACE3 is now being identified in animal models.

Data from de Silva AR et al: *Eur J Clin Invest* 45:274–287, 2015; Mavtavelli LC, Siragy HM: *J Cardiovasc Pharm* 65:226–232, 2015; Oparil S, Schmieder, RE: *Circ Res* 116:1074–1095, 2015; Patel VB et al: *Circ Res* 118:1313–1326, 2016; Te Riet L et al: *Circ Res* 116(6):960–975, 2015; Romero CA, Orias M, Wier MR: *Nat Rev Endocrinol* 11:242–252, 2015; Santos RA: *Hypertension* 63:1138–1147, 2014; Yu CJ et al: *J Am Heart Assoc* 5(2):e002680, 2016; Zhang YH et al: *Inflamm Res* 64:253–260, 2015.

effective in reducing blood pressure and protecting against target organ damage, including the synthesis of angiotensins III and IV, which also are hypothesized to contribute to hypertension.[24] Another RAAS system has been identified that is proposed to be protective. This system uses ACE2 to create angiotensin (ang) 1-7, which reduces the blood pressure and has cardiovascular protective effects. Its discovery may lead to new and more effective medications.[24-26] Other RAAS pathways also have been described (see *What's New? The Renin-Angiotensin-Aldosterone System [RAAS] and Cardiovascular Disease*).

Populations with high dietary sodium intake have long been shown to have an increased incidence of hypertension.[27] Low levels of dietary potassium, calcium, and magnesium also are risk factors because sodium is retained without their intake. The natriuretic hormones modulate renal sodium (Na+) excretion and require adequate potassium, calcium, and magnesium to function properly. The natriuretic hormones include atrial natriuretic peptide (ANP), B-type natriuretic
peptide (BNP), C-type natriuretic peptide (CNP), and urodilatin. These hormones induce diuresis; enhancement of renal blood flow and glomerular filtration rate, systemic vasodilatation, and suppression of aldosterone; and inhibition of the SNS. Dysfunction of these hormones, along with alterations in the RAAS and the SNS, cause an increase in vascular tone and a shift in the pressure-natriuresis relationship. When there is inadequate natriuretic function, serum levels of the natriuretic peptides rise in an attempt to compensate. In hypertension, increased ANP and BNP levels are linked to an increased risk for ventricular hypertrophy, atherosclerosis, and heart failure.[28] Salt retention leads to water retention and increased blood volume, which contributes to an increase in blood pressure. Subtle renal injury results, with renal vasoconstriction and tissue ischemia. Tissue ischemia causes inflammation of the kidney and contributes to dysfunction of the glomeruli and tubules and promotes additional sodium retention. Increasing dietary intake of potassium, calcium, and magnesium can enhance

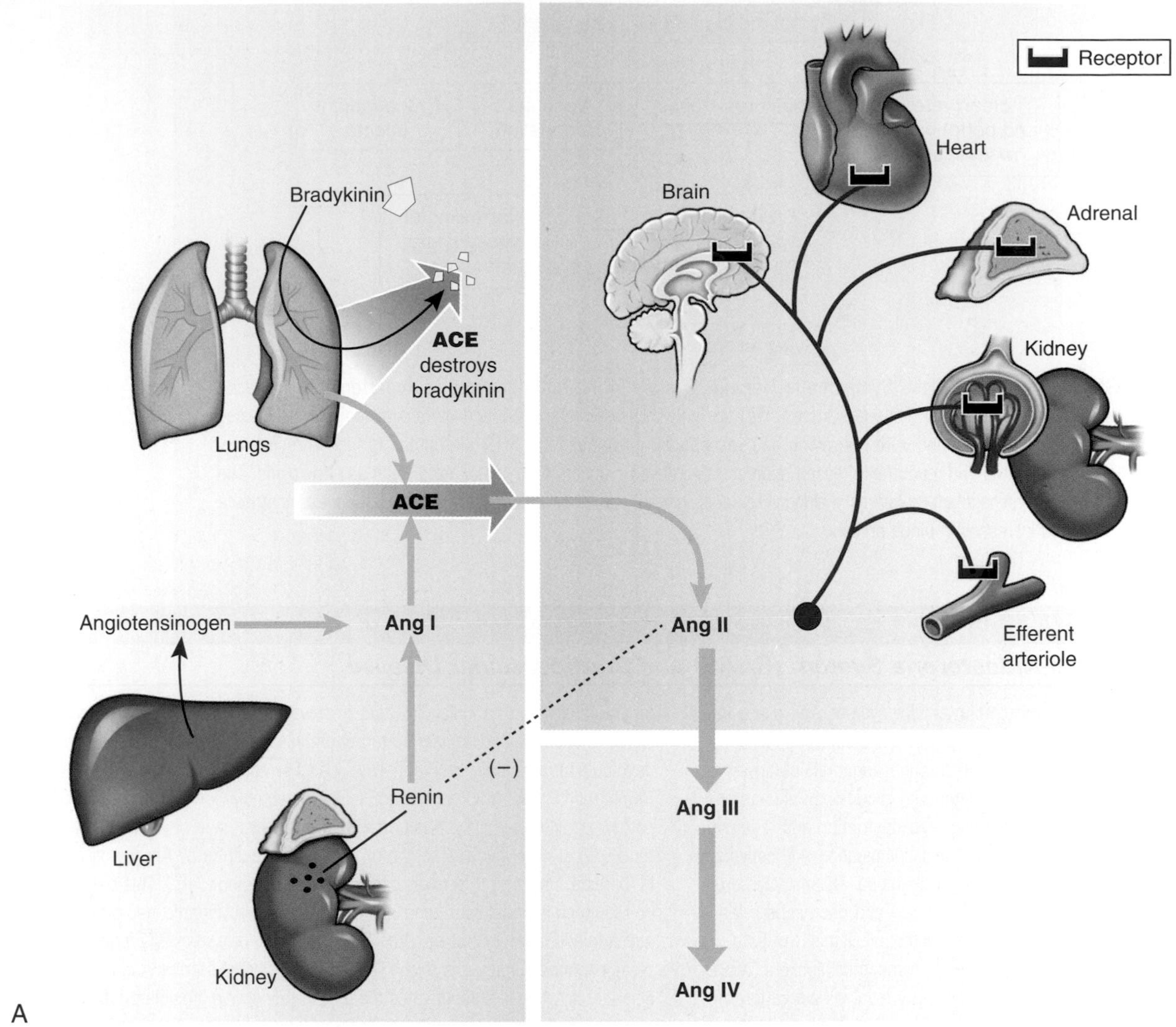

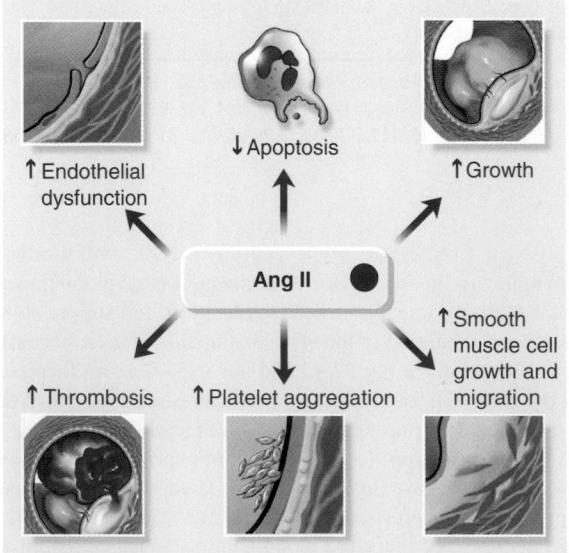

A

B

FIGURE 33.5 Angiotensins and the Organs Affected. A, The shaded blue area is the classical pathway of biosynthesis that generates the renin and angiotensin (ang) I. Ang is synthesized in the liver and is released into the blood where it is cleaved to form ang I by renin secreted by cells in the kidneys. Angiotensin-converting enzyme *(ACE)* in the lung catalyzes the formation of ang II from ang I, and destroys the potent vasodilator bradykinin. Further cleavage generates angs III and IV. The reddish shading shows the organs affected by ang II including the brain, heart, adrenals, kidney, and the kidney's efferent arterioles. The dashed line (on the left) shows the inhibition of renin by ang II. **B,** Summary of ang II effects on blood vessel structure and function leading to arteriosclerosis. (Redrawn from Goodfriend TL et al: *N Engl J Med* 334:2649–2654, 1996.)

natriuretic peptide function. New natriuretic peptide agonists are being studied.[29]

Inflammation also plays a role in the vascular dysfunction of hypertension. Endothelial injury and tissue ischemia result in the release of vasoactive inflammatory cytokines. Although many of these cytokines (e.g., histamine, prostaglandins) have vasodilatory actions in acute inflammatory injury, chronic inflammation contributes to vascular remodeling and smooth muscle contraction.[30] Endothelial injury and dysfunction in primary hypertension are further characterized by decreased production of vasodilators, such as nitric oxide, and increased production of vasoconstrictors, such as endothelin.[31]

Obesity is recognized as an important risk factor for hypertension in both adults and children and contributes to many of the neurohumoral, metabolic, renal, and cardiovascular processes that cause hypertension.[32] Obesity causes changes in what are called the *adipokines* (leptin, resistin, and adiponectin) and is associated with increased activity of the SNS and the RAAS.[33,34] Obesity is linked to inflammation, small artery remodeling, endothelial dysfunction, insulin resistance, and an increased risk for cardiovascular complications from hypertension.[35,36] The association between obesity and hypertension begins in adolescence and can have lifelong effects on health.

Finally, insulin resistance is common in hypertension, even in individuals without clinical diabetes. Insulin resistance is associated with endothelial injury and affects renal function, causing renal salt and water retention.[37] Insulin resistance is associated with overactivity of the SNS and the RAAS. It is interesting to note that in many individuals with diabetes treated with drugs that increase insulin sensitivity, blood pressure often declines, even in the absence of antihypertensive drugs. The interactions between obesity, hypertension, insulin resistance, and lipid disorders in the metabolic syndrome result in a high risk of cardiovascular disease.[38,39]

It is likely that primary hypertension is an interaction between many of these factors leading to sustained increases in blood volume and peripheral resistance. The role of these mechanisms in increasing blood volume in the pathophysiology of primary hypertension is summarized in Fig. 33.6.

Secondary Hypertension

Secondary hypertension is caused by an underlying disease process that raises peripheral vascular resistance or cardiac output. Examples include renal vascular or parenchymal disease, adrenocortical tumors, adrenomedullary tumors (pheochromocytoma), and drugs (oral contraceptives, corticosteroids, antihistamines). Blood pressure returns to normal if the cause is identified and removed before permanent structural changes occur.

Complicated Hypertension

Complicated hypertension is chronic hypertension that damages the walls of systemic blood vessels. Within the walls of arteries and arterioles, smooth muscle cells undergo hypertrophy and hyperplasia with associated fibrosis of the tunica intima and media in a process called *vascular remodeling* (Fig. 33.7). Endothelial dysfunction, ang II, catecholamines, insulin resistance, and inflammation contribute to this process. Once significant fibrosis has occurred, reduced blood flow and dysfunction of the organs perfused by these affected vessels are inevitable. Target organs include the kidney, brain, heart, extremities, and eyes (these effects are summarized in Table 33.2).

Cardiovascular complications include angina pectoris, left ventricular hypertrophy leading to CHF (left heart failure, congestive heart failure), coronary heart disease (CAD), MI, and sudden death. Myocardial hypertrophy is mediated by several neurohormonal substances, including the SNS and ang II.[40] Hypertrophy is characterized by changes in the

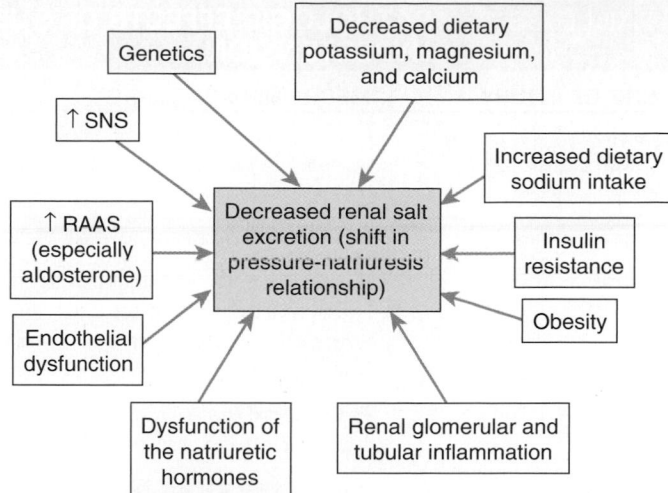

FIGURE 33.6 Shift in the Pressure-Natriuresis Relationship. Numerous factors have been implicated in the pathogenesis of sodium retention in individuals with hypertension. These factors cause less renal excretion of salt than would normally occur with increased blood pressure. This is called a *shift in the pressure-natriuresis relationship* and is believed to be a central process in the pathogenesis of primary hypertension. *RAAS,* Renin-angiotensin-aldosterone system; *SNS,* sympathetic nervous system.

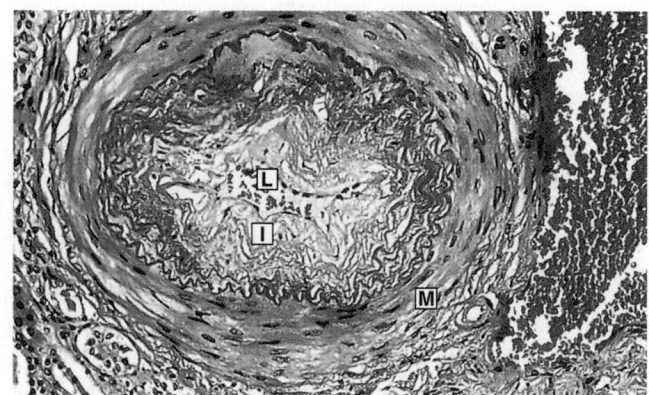

FIGURE 33.7 Dramatic Hypertension Change in Small Arterioles. Fibrous intimal proliferation *(I)* with reduction in lumen vessel caliber (radius) *(L)* and normal media *(M).* (From Stevens A, Lowe JS, Scott I: *Core pathology,* ed 3, London, 2009, Mosby.)

myocyte proteins, apoptosis of myocytes, and deposition of collagen in heart muscle, which causes it to become thickened, scarred, and less able to relax during diastole, leading to heart failure with preserved ejection fraction.[41] In addition, the increased size of the heart muscle increases demand for oxygen delivery over time, contractility of the heart is impaired, and the individual is at increased risk for systolic heart failure. Vascular complications include the formation, dissection, and rupture of aneurysms (outpouchings in vessel walls); intermittent claudication; and gangrene resulting from vessel occlusion. Renal complications are parenchymal damage, nephrosclerosis, renal arteriosclerosis, and renal insufficiency or failure. Microalbuminuria (small amounts of protein in the urine) is an early sign of impending renal dysfunction and significantly increased risk for cardiovascular events.[42]

Changes in the vascular beds can be estimated by viewing the arterioles of the retina. Complications specific to the retina include retinal vascular sclerosis, exudation, and hemorrhage. Cerebrovascular complications are

TABLE 33.2	PATHOLOGIC EFFECTS OF SUSTAINED, COMPLICATED PRIMARY HYPERTENSION	
SITE OF INJURY	**MECHANISM OF INJURY**	**POTENTIAL PATHOLOGIC EFFECT**
Heart Myocardium	Increased workload combined with diminished blood flow through coronary arteries	Left ventricular hypertrophy, myocardial ischemia, heart failure
Coronary arteries	Accelerated atherosclerosis (coronary artery disease)	Myocardial ischemia, myocardial infarction, sudden death
Kidneys	Reduced blood flow, increased arteriolar pressure, renin-angiotensin-aldosterone system (RAAS) and sympathetic nervous system (SNS) stimulation, and inflammation	Glomerulosclerosis and decreased glomerular filtration, end-stage renal disease
Brain	Reduced blood flow and oxygen supply; weakened vessel walls, accelerated atherosclerosis	Transient ischemic attacks, cerebral thrombosis, aneurysm, hemorrhage, acute brain infarction
Eyes (retinas)	Retinal vascular sclerosis, increased retinal artery pressures	Hypertensive retinopathy, retinal exudates and hemorrhages
Aorta	Weakened vessel wall	Dissecting aneurysm
Arteries of lower extremities	Reduced blood flow and high pressures in arterioles, accelerated atherosclerosis	Intermittent claudication, gangrene

similar to those of other arterial beds and include transient ischemia, stroke, cerebral thrombosis, aneurysm, and hemorrhage. Chronic hypertension also has been linked to cognitive decline with aging.[43,44]

Hypertensive crisis (or malignant hypertension) is rapidly progressive hypertension in which diastolic pressure is usually greater than 140 mmHg. It can occur as an uncommon complication of primary hypertension. Other causes include complications of pregnancy, cocaine or amphetamine use, reaction to certain medications, adrenal tumors, and alcohol withdrawal. High arterial pressure renders the cerebral arterioles incapable of regulating blood flow to the cerebral capillary beds. High hydrostatic pressures in the capillaries cause vascular fluid to exude into the interstitial space. If blood pressure is not reduced, cerebral edema and cerebral dysfunction (encephalopathy) increase until death occurs. Besides encephalopathy, hypertensive crisis can cause papilledema, cardiac failure, uremia, retinopathy, and cerebrovascular accident and is considered a medical emergency. Treatment must be initiated rapidly to avoid these serious complications.[45]

◆CLINICAL MANIFESTATIONS. The early stages of hypertension have no clinical manifestations other than elevated blood pressure; for this reason, hypertension is called a *silent disease*. Some hypertensive individuals never have signs, symptoms, or complications, whereas others become very ill, and hypertension can be a cause of death. Still other individuals have anatomic and physiologic damage caused by past hypertensive disease, despite current blood pressure measurements being within normal ranges. If elevated blood pressure is not detected and treated, it becomes established, setting the stage for the complications of hypertension that begin to appear during the fourth, fifth, and sixth decades of life.

Most clinical manifestations of hypertensive disease are caused by complications affecting the target organs. Evidence of heart disease, renal insufficiency, central nervous system dysfunction, impaired vision, impaired mobility, vascular occlusion, or edema can all be caused by sustained hypertension.

◆EVALUATION AND TREATMENT. A single elevated blood pressure reading does not mean that a person has hypertension. Diagnosis requires the measurement of blood pressure on at least two separate occasions averaging two readings at least 2 minutes apart, with the individual

seated, the arm supported at heart level, after 5 minutes rest, with no smoking or caffeine intake in the past 30 minutes. Some individuals benefit from 24-hour ambulatory blood pressure monitoring because of better correlation with end-organ damage and the ability to screen out "white coat hypertension" (elevated blood pressure that occurs only in a clinic setting) and "masked hypertension" (normal blood pressure in the clinic setting but elevated elsewhere).[46] Ambulatory measurement also detects those who fail to have a nocturnal decrease in blood pressure and who may be at higher cardiovascular risk. It is especially recommended for individuals with drug resistance, hypotensive symptoms with medications, episodic hypertension, and autonomic dysfunction.[47]

Evaluation of the hypertensive individual should include a complete medical history and assessment of lifestyle and other risk factors for hypertension and cardiovascular disease, as well as evidence of possible secondary causes of hypertension. Physical examination should include examination of the optic fundi; calculation of body mass index; auscultation for carotid, abdominal, and femoral bruits; examination of the heart and lungs; palpation of the abdomen; assessment of lower extremity pulses and edema; and neurologic examination. Diagnostic tests include complete blood count, urinalysis, biochemical blood profile (measures levels of plasma glucose, sodium, potassium, calcium, magnesium, creatinine, cholesterol, and triglycerides), and an electrocardiogram (ECG). Individuals who have elevated blood pressure are assumed to have primary hypertension unless their history, physical examination, or initial diagnostic screening indicates secondary hypertension. Once the diagnosis is made, a careful evaluation for other cardiovascular risk factors and for target organ damage should be done.

Treatment of primary hypertension depends on its severity. Fig. 33.8 illustrates an overview of the 2017 recommendations.[18a] Treatment begins with reducing or eliminating risk factors. Lifestyle modification can prevent hypertension from developing in those individuals who fall into the elevated category, may control the blood pressure in stage I hypertension, and can enhance the effects of drug treatment for those with more significant blood pressure elevation. Dietary modifications, such as the Dietary Approaches to Stop Hypertension (DASH) diet, are recommended[48] (also see *Nutrition & Disease*: Mediterranean Diet and

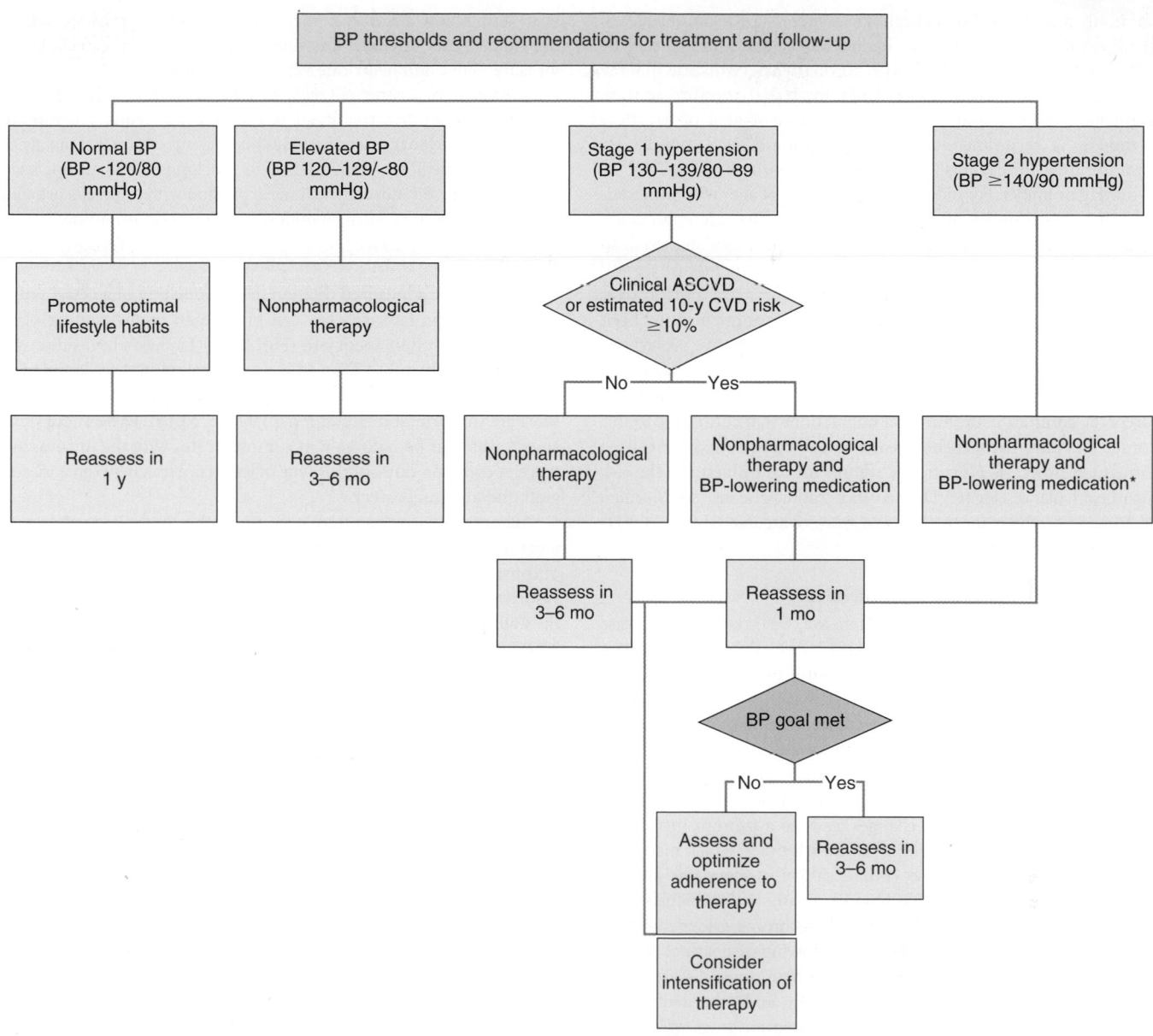

FIGURE 33.8 Blood Pressure Thresholds and Recommendations for Treatment and Follow-Up. Note: Patients with diabetes mellitus (DM) or chronic kidney disease (CKD) are automatically placed in the high-risk category. For initiation of renin-angiotensin system or diuretic therapy, assess blood tests for electrolytes and renal function 2 to 4 weeks after initiating therapy. *Consider initiation of pharmacological therapy for stage 2 hypertension with 2 antihypertensive agents of different classes. Patients with stage 2 hypertension and BP ≥160/100 mmHg should be promptly treated, carefully monitored, and subject to upward medication dose adjustment as necessary to control BP. Reassessment includes BP measurement, detection of orthostatic hypotension in selected patients (e.g., older or with postural symptoms), identification of white coat hypertension or a white coat effect, documentation of adherence, monitoring of the response to therapy, reinforcement of the importance of adherence, reinforcement of the importance of treatment, and assistance with treatment to achieve BP target. *ASCVD,* Atherosclerotic cardiovascular disease; *BP,* blood pressure; *CVD,* cardiovascular disease. Data from Whelton PK, Carey RM, Aronow WS, et al: ACC/AHA/AAPA/ABC/ACPM/AGS/APhA/ASH/ASPC/NMA/PCNA guideline for the prevention, detection, evaluation, and management of high blood pressure in adults: A report of the American College of Cardiology/American Heart Association Task Force on Clinical Practice Guidelines. *Hypertension.* 2017 Nov 13. doi: 10.1161/HYP.0000000000000065. [Epub ahead of print.]

Cardiovascular [CV] Disease and Recent Findings on Sugar). Physical training increases stroke volume, which has the effect of lowering heart rate and hence systolic blood pressure, and should consist of regular aerobic physical activity. Individuals are counseled to stop smoking to eliminate vasoconstrictor effects of nicotine.

Pharmacologic treatment of hypertension reduces the risk of end-organ damage and prevents major diseases, such as myocardial ischemia and stroke. Recent recommendations describe specific target blood pressure outcomes and medication choices for individuals based on age, ethnicity, and comorbidities, such as diabetes and renal disease.[18a]

Commonly recommended medications include thiazide diuretics, ACE inhibitors or ARBs, and calcium channel blockers. Additional considerations are necessary for those with coronary artery disease.[49] Some individuals require two or more drugs for blood pressure control. Treatment of hypertension with a SBP treatment goal of less than 130 mmHg is recommended for noninstitutionalized ambulatory community-dwelling adults (≥65 years of age) with an average SBP of 130 mmHg or higher. For older adults (≥65 years of age) with hypertension and a high burden of comorbidity and limited life expectancy, clinical judgment, patient preference, and a team-based approach to assess risk/benefit is reasonable for decisions regarding intensity of BP lowering and choice of antihypertensive drugs.[18a,50] Attempts to treat hypertension with techniques, such as renal denervation, have not been consistently successful to date; however, the use of invasive procedures for resistant hypertension continues to be explored.[51,52] Many new approaches to the treatment of hypertension are being explored that address the complex neurohumoral interactions that contribute to this disorder, and pharmacogenetic research is leading to more personalized treatment regimes.[53,54] Nutrition is significant for influencing the risk for cardiovascular disease (CVD) and other chronic diseases (see *Nutrition and Disease*: Mediterranean Diet and Cardiovascular Disease [CVD] and Recent Findings on Sugar).

Orthostatic (Postural) Hypotension

The term orthostatic (postural) hypotension (OH) refers to a decrease in systolic blood pressure of at least 20 mmHg or a decrease in diastolic blood pressure of at least 10 mmHg within 3 minutes of moving to a standing position.[55] Primary OH is often called *neurogenic* and is usually the result of neurologic disorders that affect autonomic function. Compensatory changes during standing normally increase sympathetic activity mediated through stretch receptors (baroreceptors) in the carotid sinus and the aortic arch (see Chapter 32). This reflex response to shifts in volume caused by postural changes leads to a prompt increase in heart rate and constriction of the systemic arterioles, which maintains a stable blood pressure. These compensatory mechanisms are not effective in maintaining a stable blood pressure in individuals with orthostatic hypotension. Primary OH is often chronic. Older adults are susceptible to this type of OH because of slowing of postural reflexes as part of the aging process. It also occurs in neurologic diseases, such as Parkinson disease, multiple system atrophy, and inherited neurologic disorders. Multiple system atrophy is a severe form of chronic autonomic failure in which there are multiple central nervous system degenerative changes, and Parkinson disease. Individuals with this disorder also may exhibit supine hypertension, altered drug sensitivity, hyperresponsiveness of blood pressure to hypo/hyperventilation, sleep apnea, and other neurologic disturbances.[56] Primary OH is a significant risk factor for falls and associated injury. It also is associated with an increased risk of death, coronary artery disease, heart failure, and stroke.[57]

Secondary OH is often acute and associated with (1) altered body chemistry, (2) drug action (e.g., antihypertensives or antidepressants), (3) prolonged immobility caused by illness, (4) starvation, (5) physical exhaustion, (6) any condition that produces volume depletion (e.g., massive diuresis, potassium or sodium depletion), and (7) any condition that results in venous pooling (e.g., pregnancy, extensive varicosities of the lower extremities). Other more chronic forms of secondary OH are seen with adrenal insufficiency, diabetes mellitus, cardiovascular diseases, and paraneoplastic syndromes.[57]

Orthostatic hypotension often is accompanied by dizziness, blurring or loss of vision, and syncope or fainting. To assess hypotensive episode frequency, severity, and correlation with symptoms, 24-hour blood pressure monitoring is recommended. Basic diagnostic tests include

ECG and blood electrolyte measurements. Other tests in selected individuals may include autonomic testing, serum catecholamine measurements, and heart rate variability testing.

Treatment for secondary OH is focused on correcting the underlying disorder. No curative treatment is available for primary orthostatic hypertension. Management includes liberalizing salt intake; raising the head of the bed; wearing thigh-high stockings; and administering erythropoietin, somatostatin, volume expansion with mineralocorticoids, and vasoconstrictors, such as midodrine and pyridostigmine.[56,57]

Aneurysm

An aneurysm is a localized dilation or outpouching of a vessel wall or cardiac chamber. Laplace's law can provide an understanding of the hemodynamics of an aneurysm (Fig. 33.9). (Laplace's law is discussed in detail in Chapter 32.) True aneurysms involve all three layers of the arterial wall and are best described as a weakening of the vessel wall. Most are fusiform and circumferential (Fig. 33.10). False aneurysm is an extravascular hematoma that communicates with the intravascular space. A common cause of this type of lesion is a leak between a vascular graft and a natural artery.

Aneurysms most commonly occur in the thoracic or abdominal aorta. The aorta is particularly susceptible to aneurysm formation because of constant stress on the vessel wall and the absence of penetrating vasa vasorum in the media layer (Fig. 33.11, *A*). Chronic inflammation of the wall of the aorta causes weakening of the intima and medial layers.[58] Arteriosclerosis and hypertension are found in more than half of all individuals with aneurysms. Chronic hypertension results in mechanical and shear forces that contribute to remodeling and weakening of the vessel wall. Atherosclerosis is a common cause of aneurysms because plaque formation erodes the vessel wall. From studies of abdominal aortic aneurysm (AAA) the main pathologic features include extracellular matrix remodeling, loss of vascular smooth muscle cells, and accumulation of inflammatory cells. The inflammatory process has a critical role in AAA influencing aortic wall remodeling, possibly as the result of *distinct* subsets of monocytes and macrophages.[59] Infections, such as syphilis, collagen disorders (such as Marfan syndrome), and traumatic injury to the chest or abdomen, also can cause aortic aneurysms. Genetic susceptibilities have been identified including gene polymorphisms for the production of growth factors, myosin, and proteases. Inflammation (with the production of toxic oxygen radicals) and changes in cytokines, such as TGF-β, activate matrix-degrading proteins and smooth muscle cell apoptosis, resulting in loss of medial elastic lamellae and thinning of the tunica media.[60]

Formation of a ventricular wall aneurysm most often occurs when intraventricular tension stretches noncontracting infarcted muscle (see Fig. 33.11, *B*). The stretching produces infarct expansion, a weak and thin layer of necrotic muscle, and fibrous tissue that bulges with each systole. With time the aneurysm becomes more fibrotic but continues to bulge with each systole, thus acting as a "reservoir" and reducing stroke volume.

Clinical manifestations depend on where the aneurysm is located. Aneurysms in the heart present with dysrhythmias, heart failure, and embolism of clots to the brain or other vital organs. Aortic aneurysms often are asymptomatic until they rupture, when they become painful. Symptoms of dysphagia (difficulty in swallowing) and dyspnea (breathlessness) are caused by the pressure of a thoracic aneurysm on surrounding organs. An abdominal aneurysm can impair flow to an extremity and cause symptoms of ischemia. Aneurysms that occur elsewhere in the body have variable symptoms and signs related to the size of the aneurysm and the potential for rupture and hemorrhage.

The diagnosis of an aneurysm is usually confirmed by ultrasonography, CT, MRI, or angiography.[61] The goals of medical treatment of

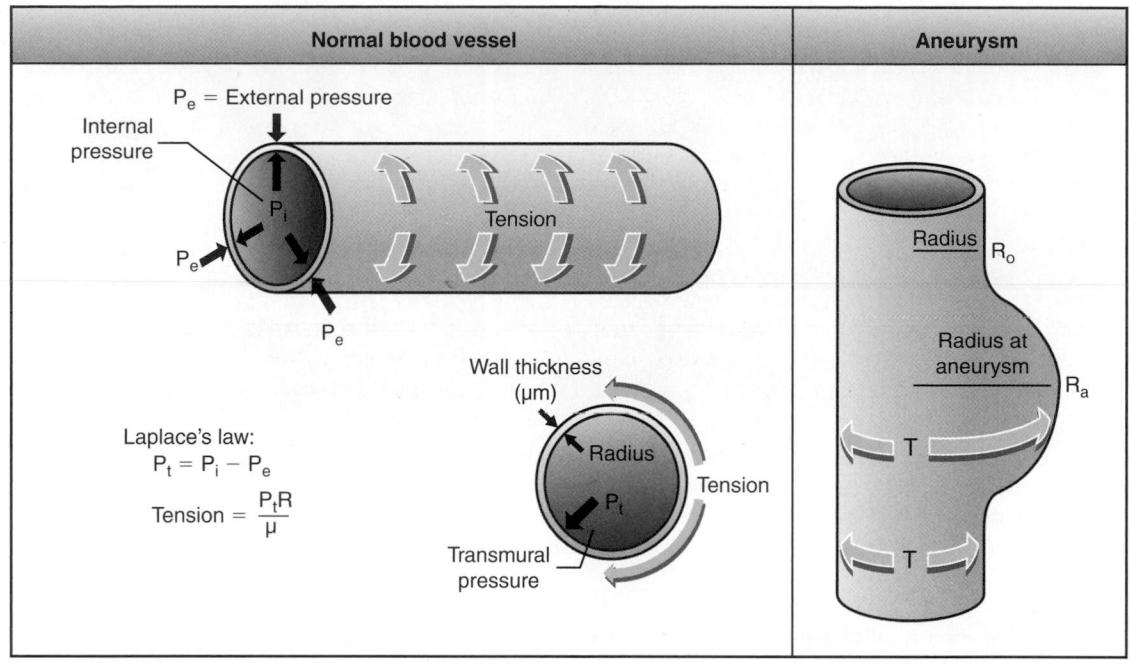

FIGURE 33.9 Pressure-Tension and Wall Thickness Relations in Blood Vessels or Cardiac Chambers (Laplace's Law).

Laplace's law:
$$P_t = P_i - P_e$$
$$\text{Tension} = \frac{P_t R}{\mu}$$

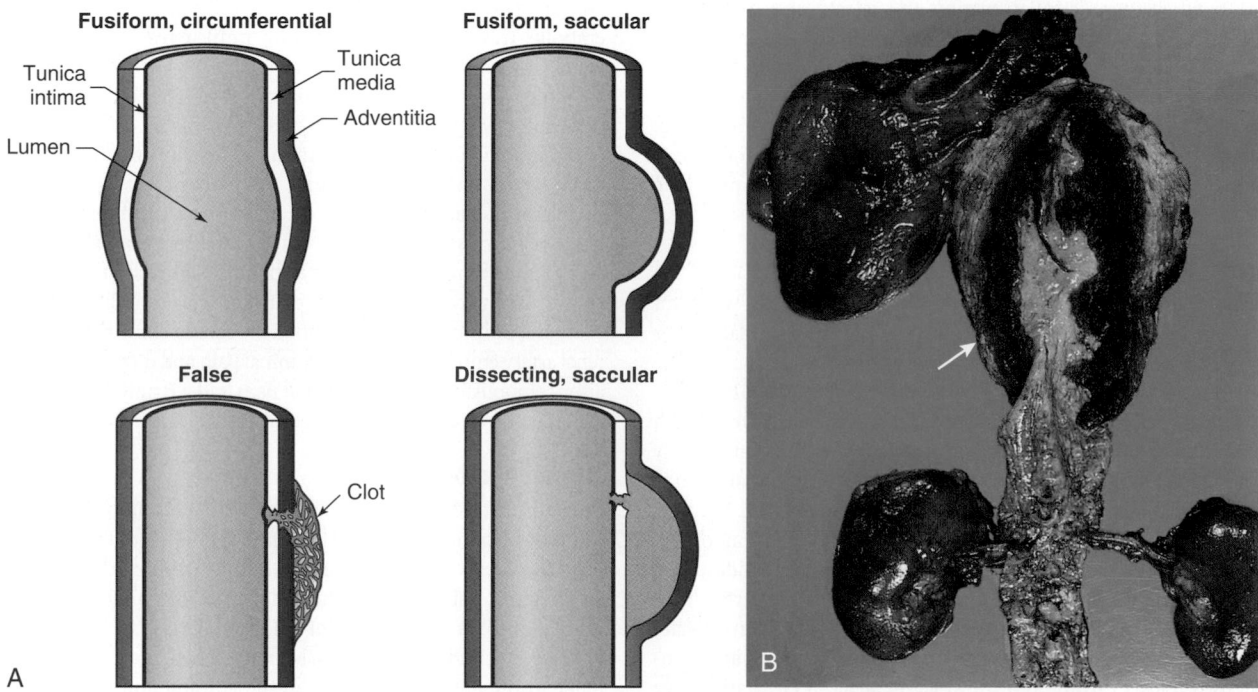

FIGURE 33.10 Longitudinal Sections Showing Types of Aneurysms. **A,** The fusiform circumferential and fusiform saccular aneurysms are true aneurysms, caused by weakening of the vessel wall. False and saccular aneurysms involve a break in the vessel wall, usually caused by trauma. **B,** Dissecting aneurysm of thoracic aorta *(arrow).* (**B** From Damjanov I, Linder J, editors: *Anderson's pathology,* ed 10, St Louis, 1996, Mosby.)

aneurysms are to maintain a low blood volume and low blood pressure to decrease mechanical forces thought to contribute to vessel wall dilation. Medical treatment is indicated for slow-growing aortic aneurysms, particularly in early stages, and includes smoking cessation, reducing blood pressure and blood volume, and administering β-adrenergic blockage medications. Aortic aneurysms can be complicated by the acute aortic syndromes that include vessel rupture and aortic dissection.[62] Rapidly expanding aneurysms are prone to rupture, and urgent surgical treatment often is indicated. New endovascular surgical techniques with placement of a stent make aneurysm repair possible even in those individuals with acute symptoms or complications.[63] **Aortic dissection** is a devastating complication that can involve any part of the aorta.

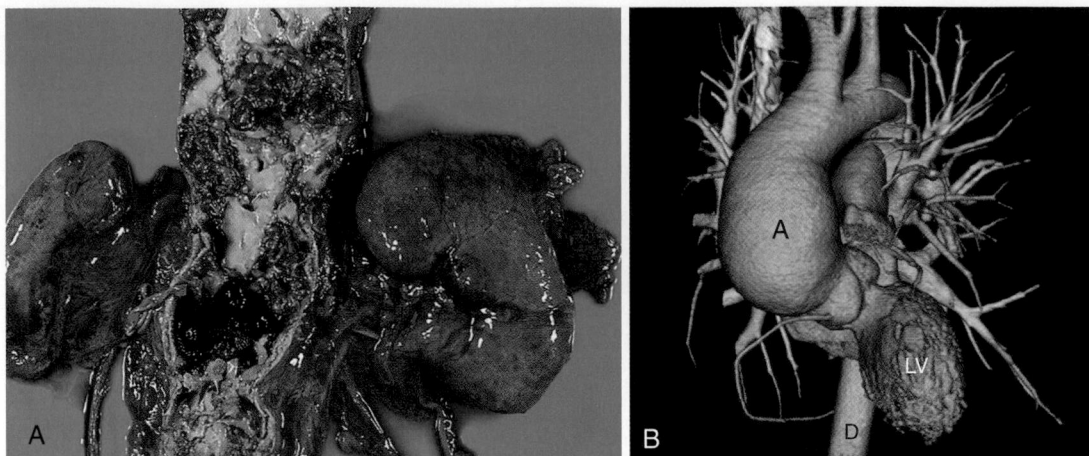

FIGURE 33.11 Aneurysms. **A,** Abdominal aortic atherosclerotic aneurysm. **B,** Thoracic aortic aneurysm. A three-dimensional CT scan shows the aneurysm. *A,* Ascending thoracic aorta; *D,* descending aorta; *LV,* left ventricle. (**A** From Damjanov I, Linder J, editors: *Anderson's pathology*, ed 10, St Louis, 1996, Mosby.)

Dissection of the ascending aorta is called *Type A,* and in any other part of the aorta it is called *Type B.* Dissection can disrupt flow through arterial branches, thus creating a surgical emergency. The risk is increased in individuals with hypertension, congenital heart disorders, atherosclerosis, and Marfan syndrome. Dissection of the layers of the arterial wall occurs when there is inflammation and release of enzymes that damage the vessel wall followed by a tear in the intima and blood that enter the wall of the artery (see Fig. 33.10). Individuals with acute aortic dissection complain of severe pain in the neck, jaw, chest, back, or abdomen; and diagnosis is made emergently with CT, echocardiography, or MRI. Although medical therapy may be indicated for Type B dissection, Type A is considered an emergency needing immediate surgical intervention.[64]

Arterial Thrombus Formation

As in venous thrombosis, arterial thrombi tend to develop wherever intravascular conditions promote activation of the coagulation, or clotting, cascade. In the arteries, activation of the coagulation cascade is most often caused by roughening of the tunica intima by atherosclerosis. Another important cause is anatomic changes of an artery (such as an aneurysm) that can stimulate thrombus formation, particularly if the change results in pooling of arterial blood. Thrombi also form on heart valves altered by calcification or bacterial vegetation. Valvular thrombi are associated most commonly with inflammation of the endocardium (endocarditis) and rheumatic heart disease. Widespread arterial thrombus formation can occur in shock, particularly shock resulting from septicemia. In septic shock, systemic inflammation activates the intrinsic and extrinsic pathways of coagulation, resulting in microvascular thrombosis throughout the systemic arterial circulation (see Chapters 29 and 49).

Arterial thrombi pose two potential threats to the circulation. First, the thrombus may grow large enough to occlude the artery, causing ischemia in tissue supplied by the artery. Second, the thrombus may dislodge, becoming a thromboembolus that travels through the vascular system until it occludes flow into a distal systemic vascular bed.

Diagnosis of arterial thrombi is usually accomplished through the use of Doppler ultrasonography and angiography. Pharmacologic treatment involves the administration of heparin, warfarin derivatives, thrombin inhibitors, or thrombolytics. A balloon-tipped catheter also can be used to remove or compress an arterial thrombus. Various combinations of drug and catheter therapies are sometimes used concurrently.

Embolism

Embolism is the obstruction of a vessel by an embolus—a bolus of matter that is circulating in the bloodstream. The embolus may consist of a dislodged thrombus; an air bubble; an aggregate of amniotic fluid; an aggregate of fat, bacteria, or cancer cells; or a foreign substance. An embolus travels in the bloodstream until it reaches a vessel through which it cannot fit. No matter how tiny it is, an embolus eventually will lodge in a systemic or pulmonary vessel. The source of the embolus determines whether the embolus will lodge in a vessel of the pulmonary or systemic circulation. Embolism causes ischemia or infarction in tissues distal to the obstruction. A limb that is ischemic because of arterial occlusion is characterized by an almost waxy whiteness of the skin because the vasculature is devoid of erythrocytes, and by numbness and pain resulting from neural ischemia. Embolism to a central organ causes organ dysfunction and pain and can be life threatening. For example, pulmonary artery embolism causes chest pain and dyspnea; renal artery embolism causes abdominal pain and oliguria; and mesenteric artery embolism causes abdominal pain and a paralytic, ischemic bowel. Embolism to a coronary or cerebral artery can result in MI or stroke.

Thromboembolism

Thromboembolism is a vascular obstruction resulting from a dislodged thrombus. Pulmonary emboli originate in the venous circulation (mostly from the deep veins of the legs) or in the right heart (also see Chapter 36). Arterial emboli most commonly originate from thrombi in the left heart that form as the result of MI, valvular disease, left heart failure, endocarditis, and dysrhythmias. More than half of these thromboemboli lodge in the lower extremities (in the femoral and popliteal arteries). Others lodge in the coronary arteries and the cerebral vasculature.

Air Embolism

Room air that enters the circulation through intravenous lines is a common cause of air embolism. Air also can be introduced into the bloodstream if trauma to the chest causes air from the lungs to enter the vascular space. For example, gunshot wounds and puncture wounds of the thorax sometimes introduce air emboli. Room air is about 70% nitrogen. Although nitrogen dissolves quickly in blood, large amounts of air cannot be dissolved rapidly enough to prevent the displacement of blood in the arterioles and capillary beds. Ischemia and necrosis occur when air totally blocks a vessel. Treatment for air embolism is supportive, including bed rest and supplemental oxygen, once the connection between the source of air and the vascular system is eliminated.

Amniotic Fluid Embolism

The great intraabdominal pressures generated during labor and delivery may force amniotic fluid into the mother's bloodstream through the highly vascular uterine wall. Amniotic fluid not only displaces blood, reducing oxygen, nutrient, and waste exchange, but also introduces antigens, cells, and protein aggregates that trigger inflammation, coagulation, and the immune response within the bloodstream. Capillary beds usually are affected by amniotic fluid emboli, especially the capillary beds of the lungs and kidneys. Treatment is supportive and may include dialysis, particularly after a cesarean delivery or hysterectomy.

Bacterial Embolism

Isolated bacteria in the bloodstream do not cause embolism, but aggregates of bacteria may be large enough to do so. The most common cause of bacterial embolism is infectious endocarditis, during which clumps of bacterial vegetations are dislodged from infected cardiac valves and ejected into the pulmonary or systemic circulation. A less common cause is erosion of an artery or vein by bacteria at a source of infection, such as an abscess. Treatment for bacterial embolism includes bed rest, supplemental oxygen, and antibiotics to eradicate the source of infection.

Fat Embolism

Trauma to the long bones is associated with fat embolism, particularly to the lungs. Two mechanisms have been proposed to account for the generation of fat emboli after skeletal trauma. The first is that trauma to the bones initiates defective fat metabolism, causing globules of fat to form in the blood. Platelets adhere to these globules until the conglomerate is large enough to lodge in a capillary bed. The second possible explanation is that globules of fat are released from fatty bone marrow exposed by fracture. Again, platelets adhere to the fat globules, and embolism occurs. Treatment for fat embolism consists of prompt immobilization of fractures and supportive measures that include administration of supplemental oxygen and steroids. Steroid administration may decrease the inflammation that occurs with vascular occlusion. Inflammation in the pulmonary bed is especially dangerous because it can cause acute respiratory distress syndrome (ARDS) (see Chapter 36).

Foreign Matter

Foreign matter can enter the bloodstream during trauma or through an intravenous or intraarterial line. Small particles, such as drug precipitates, small glass shards, or fibers from linen, are sometimes introduced unintentionally into a vessel through intravenous injections or manipulation of monitoring lines. Once in the blood, these small particles initiate the coagulation cascade. The thromboemboli that form around the particles are large enough to occlude a vessel and result in ischemia. Treatment is aimed at prevention of thrombus formation around the particle, dissolution of the particle, and supportive measures to alleviate ischemia. If the bolus of foreign matter is relatively large, it usually is removed surgically.

Peripheral Vascular Diseases
Thromboangiitis Obliterans (Buerger Disease)

Thromboangiitis obliterans (Buerger disease) is an idiopathic autoimmune condition strongly associated with smoking that is characterized by the formation of thrombi filled with inflammatory and immune cells that disrupt flow in the peripheral arteries.[65] Inflammatory cytokines

and toxic oxygen radicals contribute to accompanying vasospasm. Over time, these thrombi become organized and fibrotic and result in permanent occlusion and obliteration of portions of small- and medium-sized arteries in the feet and sometimes in the hands. Typically affected are the digital, tibial, and plantar arteries of the feet and the digital, palmar, and ulnar arteries of the hands.

The chief symptoms of thromboangiitis obliterans are pain and tenderness of the affected part. Clinical manifestations are caused by sluggish blood flow and include rubor (redness of the skin caused by dilated capillaries) and cyanosis (blueness of the skin caused by blood that remains in the capillaries after its oxygen has diffused into the interstitium). Chronic ischemia causes the skin to thin and become shiny and the nails to become thickened and malformed. In advanced disease, ischemia can cause gangrene, which may require amputation.

Diagnosis of thromboangiitis obliterans is made by identification of common features, such as age younger than 45 years, smoking history, and evidence of peripheral ischemia; and by exclusion of other causes of arterial insufficiency. The most important part of treatment is cessation of cigarette smoking. Vasodilators are prescribed to alleviate vasospasm, and the individual receives instruction in exercises that use gravity to improve blood flow. If vasospasm persists, sympathectomy may be performed. Newer therapies include immunomodulation, spinal cord stimulation, and bone marrow transplantation.[66]

Raynaud Phenomenon and Disease

Raynaud phenomenon and Raynaud disease are characterized by attacks of vasospasm in the small arteries and arterioles of the fingers and, less commonly, the toes. Although the clinical manifestations of the phenomenon and the disease are the same, their causes differ.

Raynaud disease (or primary Raynaud's) is a primary vasospastic disorder of unknown origin. It is estimated to affect nearly 5% of the general population and is associated with female gender, family history, smoking, manual occupation, migraine, and cardiovascular disease.[67] Blood vessels in affected individuals demonstrate endothelial dysfunction with an imbalance between endothelium-derived vasodilators (e.g., nitric oxide) and vasoconstrictors (e.g., endothelin-1). Platelet activation may play a role and vasospastic attacks triggered by brief exposure to cold or by emotional stress.

Raynaud phenomenon (or secondary Raynaud's) is secondary to systemic diseases, such as collagen vascular disease (e.g., scleroderma), chemotherapy, cocaine use, hypothyroidism, pulmonary hypertension, thoracic outlet syndrome, serum sickness, vasculitis, or malignancy. Vascular inflammation and vasospasm may reflect progression of the underlying disease.

The clinical manifestations of the vasospastic attacks of either disorder are pallor, numbness, and the sensation of cold in the digits. Attacks tend to be bilateral, and manifestations usually begin at the tips of the digits and progress to the proximal phalanges. Sluggish blood flow resulting in ischemia may cause the skin to appear cyanotic. Rubor follows as vasospasm ends and the capillaries become engorged with oxygenated blood. Rubor often is accompanied by throbbing and paresthesias. Skin color returns to normal after the attack, but frequent, prolonged attacks may cause the skin of the fingertips to thicken and the nails to become brittle. In severe, chronic Raynaud phenomenon or disease, ischemia eventually can cause ulceration and gangrene.

Once evident, the clinical manifestations confirm the diagnosis of Raynaud phenomenon; however, nailfold capillaroscopy is a more sensitive method of diagnosis and can improve management and follow-up of individuals with associated collagen-vascular disorders. The diagnostic criteria for Raynaud disease include not only the characteristic clinical manifestations described previously but also the absence of necrosis, no detectable underlying cause, normal digital photoplethysmography and pulse contour analysis, normal laboratory tests for inflammation, and negative tests for antinuclear factors.[68]

Treatment of Raynaud disease consists of avoidance of stimuli that trigger attacks (e.g., emotional stress, cold) and use of arm exercises, vasodilators, and biofeedback. Treatment for Raynaud phenomenon consists of removing the stimulus or treating the primary disease process. When Raynaud phenomenon is associated with malignancy, surgical removal of the tumor may resolve the ischemia. For Raynaud phenomenon not associated with malignancy, management includes arm exercises, vasodilators, sympathectomy, or botulinum toxin.[69]

Atherosclerosis

Atherosclerosis is a form of arteriosclerosis in which thickening and hardening of the vessel are caused by the accumulation of lipid-laden macrophages within the arterial wall, which leads to the formation of a lesion called a plaque. Atherosclerosis is not a single disease but rather a pathologic process that can affect vascular systems throughout the body, resulting in ischemic syndromes that can vary widely in their severity and clinical manifestations. It is the leading cause of coronary artery and cerebrovascular disease. (Atherosclerosis of the coronary arteries is described in the Coronary Artery Disease, Myocardial Ischemia, and Acute Coronary Syndrome section; atherosclerosis of the cerebral arteries is discussed in Chapter 18.)

◆**PATHOPHYSIOLOGY.** Atherosclerosis is a chronic inflammatory condition that results from the interaction of numerous pathophysiologic processes culminating in damage to arterial walls.[70] Pathologically, the lesions progress from endothelial injury and dysfunction to fatty streak fibrotic plaque to complicated lesions (Fig. 33.12).

Atherosclerosis begins with injury to the endothelial cells that line artery walls.[71] There are many possible causes of endothelial injury such as aging, smoking, hypertension, and diabetes. The risk factors for atherosclerosis are discussed in more detail in the following section on coronary artery disease. Injured endothelial cells become inflamed and cannot make normal amounts of antithrombotic and vasodilating cytokines. The adventitia also plays an important role through production of reactive oxygen species and activation of endothelial inflammation.[72] Low-density lipoprotein (LDL) penetrates into the subintima of arterial walls, where it is trapped by proteoglycans (Fig. 33.13). Inflammation, oxidative stress, and activation of macrophages cause the aggregated LDL to become oxidized. Hypertension, increased levels of LDL, oxidative stress, and activation of the renin-angiotensin-aldosterone system all contribute to an acceleration of this step in atherogenesis.[73] Inflammation and oxidized LDL cause endothelial cells to express adhesion molecules that bind monocytes and other inflammatory and immune cells. Monocytes penetrate the vessel wall becoming macrophages. Several types of receptors on these macrophages (toll-like receptors [TLRs] and LDL receptor-related protein [LRP]) enable detection and engulfment of the oxidized LDL.[74] These lipid-laden macrophages are now called *foam cells,* and when they accumulate in significant amounts, they form a lesion called a *fatty streak* and numerous inflammatory cytokines are released (e.g., tumor necrosis factor-alpha [TNF-α], interferons, interleukins, and C-reactive protein), as well as enzymes that further injure the vessel wall.[75] Growth factors also are released, including ang II, fibroblast growth factor, TGF-β, and platelet-derived growth factor, which stimulate smooth muscle cell proliferation in the affected vessel. These smooth muscle cells produce collagen and migrate over the fatty streak forming a fibrous plaque (see Fig. 33.12).[71] The fibrous plaque may calcify, protrude into the vessel lumen, and obstruct blood flow to distal tissues, especially during exercise, which may cause symptoms (e.g., angina or intermittent claudication).

Many plaques, however, are "unstable," meaning they are prone to rupture even before they affect blood flow and are clinically silent until they rupture. Plaque rupture occurs because of the inflammatory activation of proteinases (matrix metalloproteinases and cathepsins), apoptosis of cells within the plaque, and bleeding within the lesion (plaque hemorrhage).[76,77] Plaques that have ruptured are called complicated plaques (see Fig. 33.12). Once rupture occurs, exposure of underlying tissue results in platelet adhesion, initiation of the clotting cascade, and rapid thrombus formation that may suddenly occlude the affected vessel, resulting in ischemia and infarction. Aspirin or other antithrombotic agents are used to prevent this complication of atherosclerotic disease.

◆**CLINICAL MANIFESTATIONS.** Atherosclerosis presents with symptoms and signs that result from inadequate tissue perfusion because of obstruction of the vessels that supply them. Partial vessel obstruction may lead to transient ischemic events, often associated with exercise or stress. Once the lesion becomes complicated, increasing obstruction with superimposed thrombosis may result in tissue infarction. Obstruction of peripheral arteries can cause significant pain and disability. CAD caused by atherosclerosis is the major cause of myocardial ischemia and is one of the most important health issues in the United States. Atherosclerotic obstruction of the vessels supplying the brain is the major cause of stroke. Often more than one vessel is involved with this disease process; consequently, an individual may present with symptoms from several ischemic tissues at the same time, and disease in one area may indicate that the individual is at risk for ischemic complications elsewhere.

◆**EVALUATION AND TREATMENT.** In evaluating individuals for the presence of atherosclerosis, a complete health history (including risk factors and symptoms of ischemia) is essential. Physical examination may reveal arterial bruits and evidence of decreased blood flow to tissues. Laboratory tests include measurement of lipids, blood glucose, and high-sensitivity CRP (hs-CRP). Judicious use of x-ray films, electrocardiography, ultrasonography, nuclear scanning, CT, MRI, and angiography may be necessary to identify affected vessels, particularly coronary vessels.

Prevention of atherosclerosis encompasses a broad range of nonpharmacologic and pharmacologic approaches to reducing risk factors such as dyslipidemia, hypertension, diabetes, smoking, and obesity. (Management of atherosclerotic risk factors for coronary artery disease is discussed further in the Coronary Artery Disease, Myocardial Ischemia, and Acute Coronary Syndromes section.) Current management of atherosclerosis is focused on detecting and treating preclinical lesions with drugs aimed at stabilizing and reversing plaques before they rupture. Once a lesion obstructs blood flow, the primary goal in managing atherosclerosis is to restore adequate blood flow to the affected tissues. If an individual has presented with acute ischemia (e.g., MI, stroke), interventions are specific to the diseased area and are discussed further under those topics. In situations in which the disease process does not require immediate intervention, management focuses on reducing risk factors, removing the initial causes of vessel damage, and preventing lesion progression. This includes exercise, smoking cessation, and control of hypertension and diabetes when appropriate while reducing LDL cholesterol by diet or medications or both. (Management of atherosclerotic risk factors is discussed further in the Coronary Artery Disease, Myocardial Ischemia, and Acute Coronary Syndromes section.)

Peripheral Artery Disease

Peripheral artery disease (PAD) refers to atherosclerotic disease of arteries that perfuses the limbs, especially the lower extremities. PAD affects 10% to 15% of those who are 60 years of age or older, and

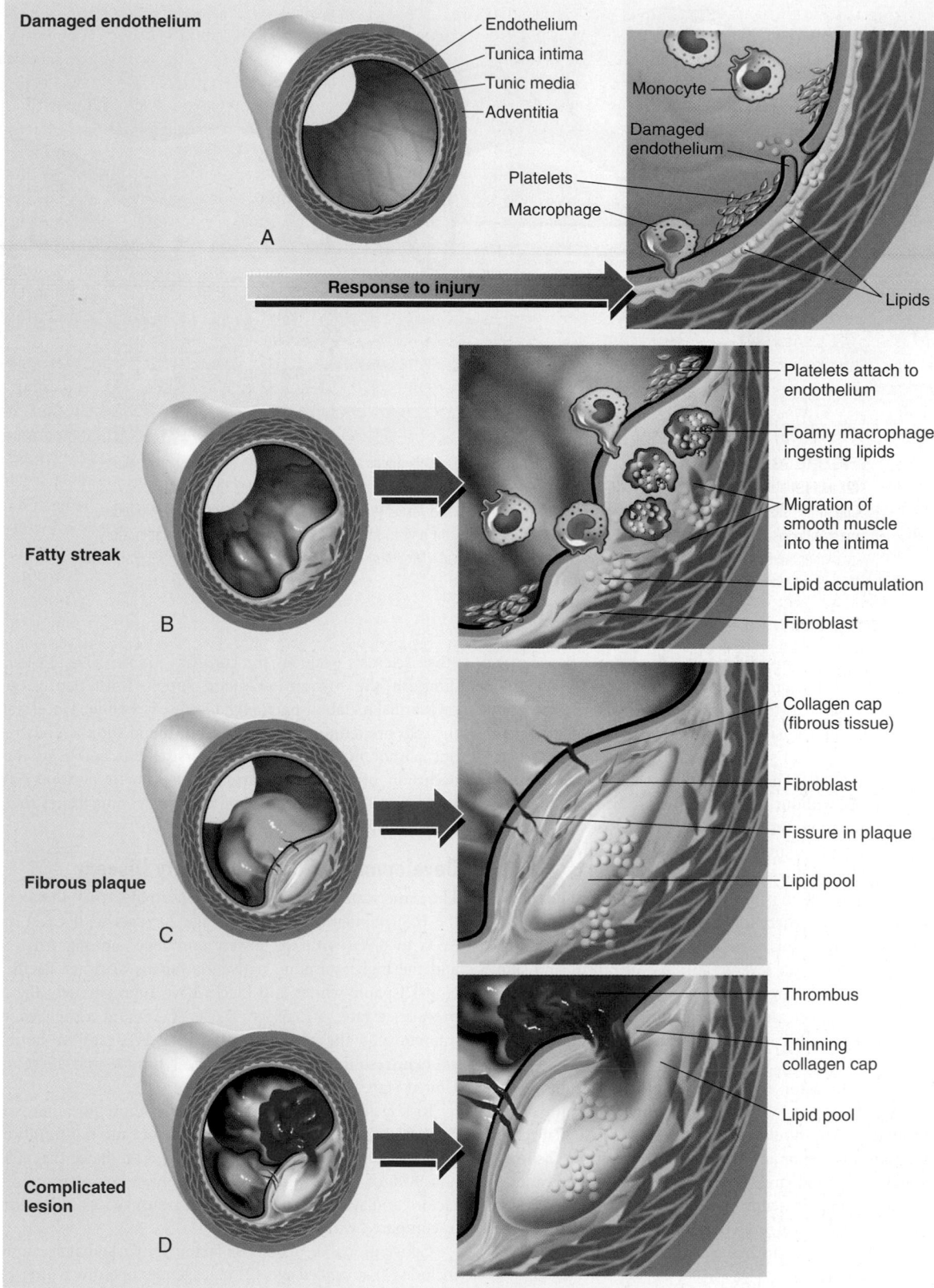

FIGURE 33.12 Progression of Atherosclerosis. A, Damaged endothelium. **B,** Fatty streak and lipid core formation. **C,** Fibrous plaque (raised plaques are visible: some are yellow; others are white). **D,** Complicated lesion (thrombus is red; collagen is blue).

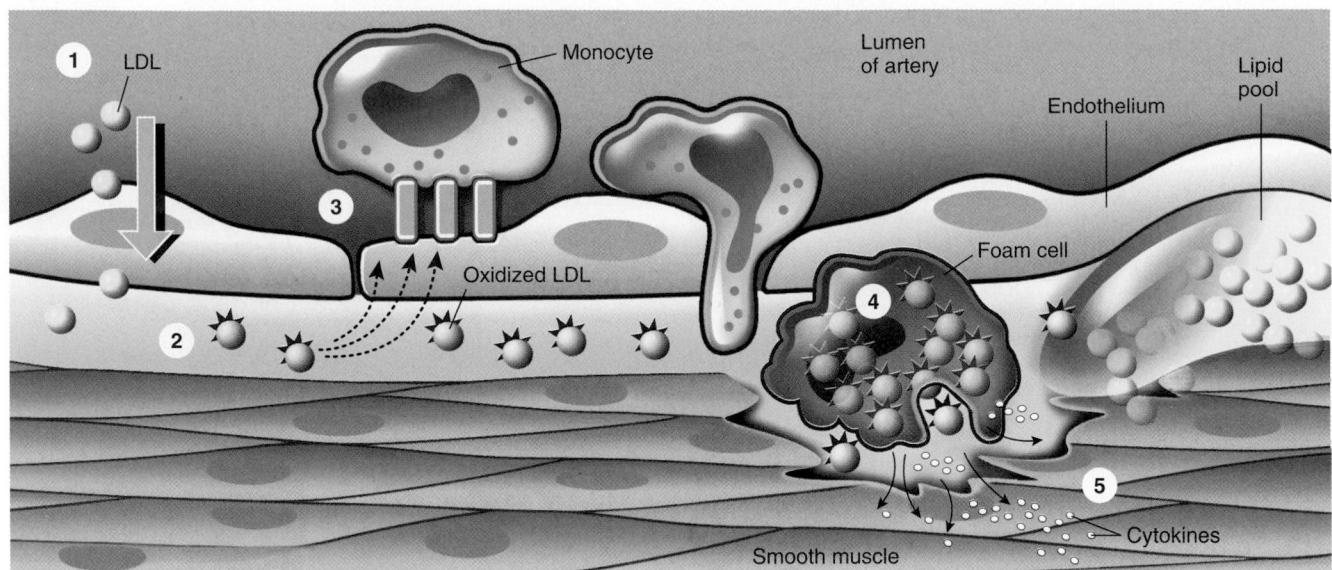

FIGURE 33.13 Low-Density Lipoprotein Oxidation. (1) LDL enters the arterial intima through an intact endothelium. **(2)** and **(3)** Inflammation and oxidized LDL cause endothelial cells to express adhesion molecules that bind monocytes and other inflammatory and immune cells. Monocytes penetrate the vessel wall, becoming macrophages. **(4)** Lipid-laden macrophages are called "foam cells." **(5)** Foam cells accumulate and form the fatty streak, and many inflammatory cytokines and enzymes are released that injure the vessel wall. (Modified from Crawford MH, DiMarco JP, Paulus WJ: *Cardiology*, ed 3, London, 2010, Mosby.)

is associated with significant morbidity and mortality.[5] Prevalence increases with age, and PAD disproportionately affects blacks. The risk factors for PAD are the same as those for atherosclerotic disease, and it is especially prevalent in individuals who smoke and those with diabetes. PAD is a significant predictor of systemic atherosclerotic disease such that those with documented PAD have nearly double the risk of coronary artery disease than those without PAD.

Lower-extremity ischemia, resulting from arterial obstruction in PAD, can be gradual or acute. In many individuals, gradually increasing obstruction to arterial blood flow to the legs caused by atherosclerosis in the iliofemoral vessels results in pain with ambulation called **intermittent claudication**; however, ischemia may not be painful and may go undetected for years. If a thrombus forms over the atherosclerotic lesion, perfusion can cease acutely with severe pain, loss of pulses, and skin color changes in the affected extremity.

Evaluation for PAD requires a careful history and physical examination that focuses on evidence of atherosclerotic disease (e.g., bruits), ankle-brachial index, and noninvasive Doppler measurement of blood flow. Treatment includes risk factor reduction (smoking cessation and treatment of diabetes, hypertension, and dyslipidemia) and antiplatelet therapy. Symptomatic PAD should be managed with vasodilators in combination with antiplatelet or antithrombotic medications (aspirin, cilostazol, ticlopidine, or clopidogrel), cholesterol-lowering medications, and exercise rehabilitation. If acute or refractory symptoms occur, emergent percutaneous or surgical revascularization may be indicated.[78,79] Newer treatment modalities that are being explored include autologous stem cell and gene therapies.[80,81]

Coronary Artery Disease, Myocardial Ischemia, and Acute Coronary Syndromes

CAD, myocardial ischemia, and MI form a pathophysiologic continuum that impairs the pumping ability of the heart by depriving the heart muscle of blood-borne oxygen and nutrients. The earliest lesions of the continuum are those of **coronary artery disease (CAD)** in which

atherosclerosis occludes the coronary arteries (Fig. 33.14). CAD can diminish the myocardial blood supply until deprivation impairs myocardial metabolism enough to cause **ischemia**, a local state in which the cells are temporarily deprived of blood supply. They remain alive but cannot function normally. Persistent ischemia or the complete occlusion of a coronary artery causes **acute coronary syndromes**. **Infarction** (irreversible myocardial injury) constitutes the often-fatal event known as a *heart attack*.

Development of Coronary Artery Disease

The American Heart Association estimates that the percentage of the U.S. population older than age 20 years with CAD ranges from 3.3% to 6.9% with the lowest prevalence among Asian Americans and the highest among native Hawaiians or other Pacific Islanders. Non-Hispanic whites and blacks have approximately the same CAD prevalence rates at 5.5% to 5.6%.[5] CAD and associated myocardial infarction is the number one cause of death in both men and women, resulting in a death every 1 minute and 20 seconds in the United States.

Risk factors for CAD are the same as those for atherosclerosis and can be categorized as conventional (major) and nontraditional (novel) and modifiable versus nonmodifiable. It is estimated that 65% of whites and 90% of blacks with CAD events have one or more of these risk factors, and avoidable death rates are nearly twice as high among blacks as compared with whites.[5]

Conventional or major risk factors for CAD that are nonmodifiable include (1) advanced age, (2) male gender or women after menopause, and (3) family history. Aging and menopause are associated with increased exposure to risk factors and poor endothelial healing. Family history may contribute to CAD through genetics and shared environmental exposure.[82] Many gene polymorphisms have been associated with CAD and its risk factors.[83]

Major modifiable conventional risks include (1) dyslipidemia, (2) hypertension, (3) cigarette smoking, (4) diabetes and insulin resistance,

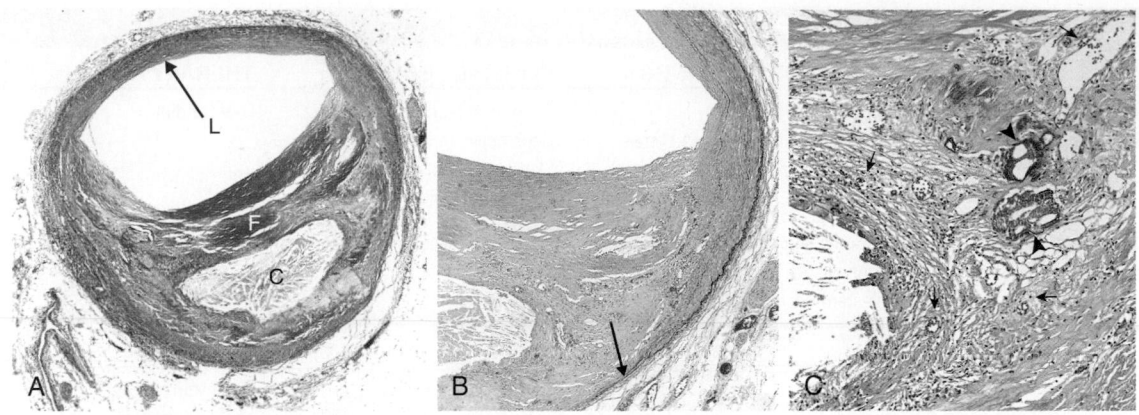

FIGURE 33.14 Histologic Features of Atheromatous Plaque in the Coronary Artery. **A,** Overall architecture demonstrating fibrous cap *(F)* and a central necrotic (largely lipid) core *(C)*. The lumen *(L)* has been moderately narrowed. Note that a segment of the wall is plaque free *(arrow)*, so that there is an eccentric lesion. In this section, collagen has been stained blue (Masson's trichrome stain). **B,** Higher power photograph of a section of the plaque shown in **(A),** stained for elastin *(black)*, demonstrating that the internal and external elastic membranes are destroyed and the media of the artery is thinned under the most advanced plaque *(arrow)*. **C,** Higher magnification photomicrograph at the junction of the fibrous cap and core, showing scattered inflammatory cells, calcification *(arrowhead)*, and neovascularization *(small arrows)*. (From Kumar V et al: *Robbins basic pathology*, ed 9, St Louis, 2007, Saunders.)

TABLE 33.3	CRITERIA FOR DYSLIPIDEMIA						
	OPTIMAL	NEAR OPTIMAL	DESIRABLE	LOW	BORDERLINE	HIGH	VERY HIGH
Total cholesterol			<200		200–239	≥240	
LDL	<100	100–129			130–159	160–189	≥190
Triglycerides			<150		150–199	200–499	≥500
HDL				<40		≥60	

HDL, High-density lipoprotein; *LDL,* low-density lipoprotein.
Data from Expert Panel on Detection, Evaluation, and Treatment of High Blood Cholesterol in Adults: *J Am Med Assoc* 285:2486–2497, 2001.

(5) obesity and sedentary lifestyle, and (6) an atherogenic diet. If individuals receive appropriate preventive care, modification of these factors can significantly reduce the risk for CAD.

Dyslipidemia. The link between CAD and abnormal plasma lipoprotein concentrations is well documented.[5] The term **lipoprotein** refers to lipids, phospholipids, cholesterol, and triglycerides bound to carrier proteins. Lipids (cholesterol in particular) are required by most cells for the manufacture and repair of plasma membranes. Cholesterol is also a necessary component for the manufacture of such essential substances as bile acids and steroid hormones. Although cholesterol can easily be obtained from dietary fat intake, most body cells also can manufacture cholesterol.

The cycle of lipid metabolism is complex. Dietary fat is packaged into particles known as **chylomicrons** in the small intestine that transport exogenous lipid from the intestine to the liver and peripheral cells. Chylomicrons are the least dense of the lipoproteins and primarily contain triglyceride. Some of the triglyceride may be removed and either stored by adipose tissue or used by muscle as an energy source. The chylomicron remnants, composed mainly of cholesterol, are taken up by the liver. A series of chemical reactions in the liver results in the production of several lipoproteins that vary in density and function. These include **very-low-density lipoproteins (VLDLs)**, primarily triglyceride and protein; **low-density lipoproteins (LDLs)**, mostly cholesterol and protein; and **high-density lipoproteins (HDLs)**, mainly phospholipids and protein.

Dyslipidemia (or **dyslipoproteinemia**) refers to abnormal concentrations of serum lipoproteins as defined by the *Third Report of the National Cholesterol Education Program* (Table 33.3).[84] It is estimated that nearly half of the U.S. population has some form of dyslipidemia.[5] These abnormalities are the result of a combination of genetic and dietary factors. Primary or familial dyslipoproteinemias result from genetic defects that cause abnormalities in lipid-metabolizing enzymes and abnormal cellular lipid receptors (Table 33.4). Secondary causes of dyslipidemia include several common systemic disorders, such as diabetes, hypothyroidism, pancreatitis, and renal nephrosis, as well as the use of some medications such as certain diuretics, beta-blockers, glucocorticoids, interferons, and antiretrovirals.

An increased serum concentration of LDL is an indicator of coronary risk; however, the relative risk of elevated LDL depends on the presence of other risk factors such as age, diabetes, and chronic kidney disease. Thus new guidelines from the American Heart Association and the American College of Cardiology focus on treating dyslipidemia in the context of other risk factors.[85] LDL is responsible for the delivery of cholesterol to the tissues. Serum levels of LDL are normally controlled by hepatic receptors that bind LDL and limit liver synthesis of this lipoprotein. High dietary intake of cholesterol and fats, often in combination with a genetic predisposition to accumulations of LDL in the serum (e.g., dysfunction of the hepatic LDL receptor), results in high levels of LDL in the bloodstream. LDL oxidation, migration into the vessel wall, and phagocytosis by macrophages are key steps

TABLE 33.4   FAMILIAL DYSLIPOPROTEINEMIAS

NAME	LABORATORY FINDINGS	CLINICAL FEATURES	THERAPY
Type I: exogenous hyperlipidemia; fat-induced hypertriglyceridemia	Cholesterol normal Triglycerides increased three times Chylomicrons increased	Abdominal pain Hepatosplenomegaly Skin and retinal lipid deposits Usual onset: childhood	Low-fat diet
Type IIa: hypercholesterolemia	Triglycerides normal LDL increased Cholesterol increased	Premature vascular disease Xanthomas of tendons and bony prominences Common Onset: all ages	Low-saturated-fat and low-cholesterol diet Cholestyramine[a] Colestipol[b] Lovastatin[c] Nicotinic acid[d] Neomycin[e] Intestinal bypass
Type IIb: combined hyperlipidemia; carbohydrate-induced hypertriglyceridemia	LDL, VLDL increased Cholesterol increased Triglycerides increased	Same as IIa	Same as IIa; *plus* carbohydrate restriction Clofibrate[f] Gemfibrozil[g] Lovastatin
Type III: dysbetalipoproteinemia	IDL or chylomicron remnants increased Cholesterol increased Triglycerides increased	Premature vascular disease Xanthomas of tendons and bony prominences Uncommon Onset: adulthood	Weight control Low-carbohydrate, low-saturated-fat, and low-cholesterol diet Alcohol restriction Clofibrate Gemfibrozil Lovastatin Nicotinic acid Estrogens[h] Intestinal bypass
Type IV: endogenous hyperlipidemia; carbohydrate-induced hypertriglyceridemia	Glucose intolerance Hyperuricemia Cholesterol normal or increased VLDL increased Triglycerides increased	Premature vascular disease Skin lipid deposits Obesity Hepatomegaly Common onset: adulthood	Weight control Low-carbohydrate diet Alcohol restriction Clofibrate Nicotinic acid Intestinal bypass
Type V: mixed hyperlipidemia; carbohydrate and fat-induced hypertriglyceridemia	Glucose intolerance Hyperuricemia Chylomicrons increased VLDL increased LDL increased Cholesterol increased Triglycerides increased three times	Abdominal pain Hepatosplenomegaly Skin lipid deposits Retinal lipid deposits Onset: childhood	Weight control Low-carbohydrate and low-fat diet Clofibrate Lovastatin Nicotinic acid Progesterone[i] Intestinal bypass

IDL, Intermediate-density lipoprotein; *LDL,* low-density lipoprotein; *VLDL,* very-low-density lipoprotein.

[a]*Cholestyramine* (Questran), anion exchange resin; binds bile acids; enhances cholesterol excretion.

[b]*Colestipol* (Colestid), same as cholestyramine.

[c]*Lovastatin,* 3-hydroxy-3-methylglutaryl coenzyme A (HMG-CoA) reductase inhibitor; decreases cholesterol synthesis in the liver.

[d]*Nicotinic acid* (niacin), decreases release of free fatty acids from adipose tissue; increases lipogenesis in liver; decreases glucagon release; most effective for type V disorder.

[e]*Neomycin,* experimental medication; questionable mode of action; decreases LDLs.

[f]*Clofibrate* (Atromid-S), decreases release of free fatty acids from adipose tissue; decreases hepatic secretion of VLDL and increases catabolism of VLDL.

[g]*Gemfibrozil* (Lopid), similar to clofibrate but increases HDLs more.

[h]*Estrogens,* decrease IDL levels in type III disorders; experimental.

[i]*Progesterone,* decreases plasma triglycerides in type V disorders; experimental.

in the pathogenesis of atherosclerosis (see Fig. 33.13). The term LDL actually describes several types of LDL molecules. Measurement of LDL subfractions allows for better prediction of coronary risk. For example, low density lioporotein-cholesterol (LDL-C) measurements allow for detection of the small dense LDL particles that are the most atherogenic, and apolipoprotein B (structural protein found in both LDL and VLDL) levels are a strong predictor of future coronary events.[86] Lowering serum levels of LDL can reduce the risk for CAD. For example, recent studies found that for every 1% reduction in LDL-C, there is a 1% reduction in coronary risk in both men and women.[87,88] Although

WHAT'S NEW?

New and Future Drugs for Treatment of Dyslipidemia

A new guideline for the treatment of blood cholesterol was released by the American College of Cardiology (ACC) and the American Heart Association (AHA) in 2014. This guideline linked decisions about treatment of dyslipidemia to the presence of other cardiovascular risks, such as diabetes. Statins have been shown to be effective in reducing low density lipoprotein (LDL) and overall cardiovascular risk but there continue to be considerable concerns about potential side effects of their use and their lack of effect on high density lipoprotein (HDL). The PCSK9 inhibitors are a new class of drugs that are now being used to treat increased LDL. These drugs prevent the breakdown of the LDL receptor, thus reduce hepatic synthesis of LDL. Early studies suggest that these drugs are safe and effective in lowering serum LDL levels in selected individuals. The FDA currently approves the use of two PCSK9 inhibitors (alirocumab and evolocumab) for individuals on maximally-tolerated statin therapy, who have familial hypercholesterolemia, or who have clinical coronary artery disease and require additional LDL lowering. Low levels of HDL also are a significant risk factor for cardiovascular disease. Unfortunately, most new drugs aimed at increasing HDL levels (e.g., cholesterol ester transfer protein [CETP] inhibitors) have been ineffective in reducing cardiovascular risk. Recent studies suggest that high density lipoprotein-cholesterol (HDL-C) is the most important HDL particle, and that this molecule becomes dysfunctional independent of serum levels in inflammatory conditions, such as atherosclerosis. Diet and exercise appear to improve HDL functionality. Assays to evaluate dysfunctional HDL and new drugs to improve HDL function are in development.

Data from Gadi R, Figueredo VM: *J Cardiovasc Med* 16(1):1–10, 2015; Leander K et al: *Circulation* 133:1230–1239, 2016; McKenney JM: *J Clin Lipidol* 9(2):170–186, 2015; Nofer JR: *Handb Exp Pharmacol* 224:229–256, 2015; Rosenson RS et al: *Nat Rev Cardiol* 13(1):48–60, 2016; Sattar N et al: *Lancet Diabetes Endocrinol* 4:403–410, 2016; Shapiro MD, Fazio S, Tavori H: *Curr Atheroscler Rep* 17(4):499, 2015; Siddiqi HK, Kiss D, Rader D: *Curr Opin Cardiol* 30(5):536–542, 2015; Waters DD, Hsue PY, Bangalore S: *J Am Med Assoc* 2315:1571–1572, 2016.

the 3-hydroxy-3-methyl-glutaryl-CoA reductase medications (statins) continue to be used for many people with elevated LDL levels and other risk factors for CAD,[85] new and future medications aimed at lowering LDL levels, such as the proprotein convertase subtilisin/kexin 9 (PCSK9) inhibitors, are being developed[89] (see *What's New?* New and Future Drugs for Treatment of Dyslipidemia).

Low levels of HDL cholesterol also are a strong indicator of coronary risk. HDL is responsible for "reverse cholesterol transport," which returns excess cholesterol from the tissues to the liver, where it binds to hepatic receptors (including the LDL receptor) and is processed and eliminated as bile or converted to cholesterol-containing steroids. HDL can remove excess cholesterol from the arterial wall through several pathways, including mediating the efflux of cholesterol from lipid-laden macrophages (foam cells) through the activation of adenosine triphosphate (ATP)–binding cassette transporter proteins (ABC proteins). Additional actions of HDL include protecting LDL from oxidation, preserving endothelial function, and also promoting antiinflammatory and antithrombotic effects.[90] As HDL cholesterol is transported, it progresses through three subtypes of HDL: pre-β HDL, HDL3, and HDL2. Apolipoprotein (ApoA-I) on the pre-β HDL binds cholesterol where it is converted to cholesteryl ester creating HDL3. HDL3 then increases in size to form HDL2, which is fully loaded with cholesterol. The smaller HDL3 molecule is the most protective in preventing atherosclerosis, and research continues to explore the best approach to increasing this

type of HDL. These various types of HDL exert both distinct and overlapping activities, which may be compromised by inflammatory conditions, obesity, and diabetes resulting in HDL dysfunction.[91,92] Drugs aimed at increasing HDL have not been effective to date, but new therapies are being explored that address HDL dysfunction (see *What's New?* New and Future Drugs for Treatment of Dyslipidemia).

Other lipoproteins associated with increased cardiovascular risk include elevated levels of serum VLDL (triglycerides) and increased lipoprotein(a). Triglycerides are associated with an increased risk for CAD, especially in combination with other risk factors such as diabetes. Because of this, the measurement of "non-HDL cholesterol" (LDL plus VLDL) is frequently used to assess cardiovascular risk rather than just LDL or HDL levels alone. **Lipoprotein(a) (Lp[a])** is a genetically determined molecular complex between LDL and a serum glycoprotein called *apoprotein(a)* that has been shown to be an important risk factor for coronary atherosclerosis, especially in women.[93]

Hypertension. Hypertension is responsible for a two- to threefold increased risk of atherosclerotic cardiovascular disease including MI.[5] It contributes to endothelial injury, a key step in atherogenesis and causes myocardial hypertrophy, which increases myocardial demand for coronary flow. The overactivity of the SNS and RAAS commonly found in hypertension also contributes to the genesis of coronary artery disease. Drugs that block the effects of the SNS and RAAS to treat hypertension have many positive effects on the vasculature.[94]

Cigarette Smoking. In the United States, approximately 17% of adults are active cigarette smokers, and direct and passive (environmental) smoking account for approximately one-third of all deaths related to CAD.[5] Smoking has a direct effect on endothelial cells and the generation of oxygen radicals that contribute to atherogenesis.[95] Nicotine stimulates the release of catecholamines (epinephrine and norepinephrine), which increases heart rate and causes peripheral vascular constriction. As a result blood pressure increases, as do cardiac workload and oxygen demand. Cigarette smoking is associated with an increase in LDL and a decrease in HDL levels, and contributes to vessel inflammation and thrombosis. The risk of CAD increases with heavy smoking and decreases when smoking is stopped.

Diabetes Mellitus. Diabetes mellitus and insulin resistance are extremely important risk factors for CAD.[5] Insulin resistance, hyperinsulinemia, and hyperglycemia have multiple effects on the cardiovascular system. These effects can include endothelial damage, thickening of the vessel wall, increased inflammation and leukocyte adhesion, increased thrombosis, glycation of vascular proteins, and decreased production of endothelial-derived vasodilators such as nitric oxide[96] (diabetes is discussed in Chapter 22). Diabetes is also associated with dyslipidemia, and aggressive management of this additional risk factor can significantly improve CAD risk in individuals with diabetes.[85]

Obesity and Sedentary Lifestyle. It is estimated that approximately one-third of children and two-thirds of adults in the United States are overweight or obese, resulting in a much increased risk for CAD and stroke. An estimated 47 million U.S. residents have a combination of obesity, dyslipidemia, and hypertension (called **metabolic syndrome**) (see Chapter 22), which is associated with an even higher risk for CAD events.[5] Obesity is caused by genetics, diet, and inadequate physical exercise. Abdominal obesity (also known as **android obesity**) has the strongest link with increased CAD risk and is related to insulin resistance, decreased HDL levels, increased blood pressure, and inflammation. Obesity is associated with changes in the adipokines (see the following) and is associated with the deposition of perivascular adipose tissue that contributes to atherogenesis.[97] A sedentary lifestyle not only increases the risk of obesity but also has an independent effect on increasing CAD risk. It is estimated that physical inactivity is responsible for approximately 12% of myocardial infarctions.[5] Physical activity and

NUTRITION & DISEASE

Mediterranean Diet and Cardiovascular (CV) Disease and Recent Findings on Sugar

The Mediterranean diet comprises a high intake of fruits, vegetables, legumes, whole-grain products, fish, and unsaturated fatty acids (especially olive oil), with low consumption of red meat, dairy products, and saturated fatty acids. Included in this dietary pattern is moderate consumption of alcohol (mostly wine, consumed with meals). However, investigators from a recent mendelian randomization study, including 59 epidemiologic studies, reported that the lowest risks for CV outcomes were in abstainers and that any amount of alcohol is associated with elevated blood pressure and body mass index (BMI).

The proportion of calories derived from carbohydrates has been associated with risk of diabetes and cardiovascular disease in observational studies and clinical trial. Some studies have shown that a diet higher in glycemic index (GI) is associated with higher levels of C-reactive protein, a marker of inflammation associated with risk for diabetes or cardiovascular disease. This observation has led to the hypothesis that inflammation may mediate the association of GI with cardiovascular disease. Ongoing studies are identifying these interactions. Investigators report that the oral glucose tolerance test does not represent the overall glycemic effects of dietary patterns that vary in both amount and type of carbohydrate. Glycated albumin and fructosamine, markers of 2- to 3-week cumulative exposure to blood glucose, may be especially suited for evaluating the effects of dietary carbohydrates on glycemia. Both glycated albumin and fructosamine are formed by glycation reactions, where glucose binds with intravascular proteins, including albumin, and are associated with risk of diabetes and cardiovascular disease events. Using an isocaloric feeding study (OmniCarb trial) in adults without diabetes, investigators found that reducing dietary carbohydrates lowered markers of 2- to 3-week glycemia (i.e., glycated albumin and fructosamine). Additionally, changes to GI had no effect on glycated albumin or fructosamine and neither reducing dietary carbohydrates or modifying glycemic index affected C-reactive protein. Overall, this study suggests that reducing carbohydrate content, rather than GI, is a better strategy for lowering glycemia in adults at risk for diabetes and, therefore, cardiovascular disease. The largest single food source of calories in the United States and Europe is sugar-sweetened soft drinks.

Data from Holmes MV et al: *BMJ* 349:g4164, 2014; Juraschek SP et al: *BMJ Open Diabetes Res Care* 4(1):e000276, 2016.

weight loss offer substantial reductions in risk for CAD.[98] There is emerging evidence that bariatric surgery procedures can provide sustained improvement in risk factors for cardiovascular disease such as hypertension, dyslipidemia, and diabetes.[5]

Atherogenic Diet. Diet plays a complex role in atherogenic risk. Diets high in salt, fats, trans fats, and carbohydrates have all been implicated. There are many recommendations regarding diet modification to reduce coronary risk; one of the most studied dietary patterns is the Mediterranean diet.[99] A recent randomized control trial in high-risk individuals suggested that following a Mediterranean diet over a 5-year period, compared with a control diet, was related to a 29% lower risk of CVD[100] (see *Nutrition & Disease:* Mediterranean Diet and Cardiovascular [CV] Disease and Recent Findings on Sugar).

Nontraditional Risk Factors. Nontraditional, or novel, risk factors for CAD include (1) increased serum markers for inflammation, ischemia, and thrombosis; (2) adipokines; (3) chronic kidney disease; (4) air pollution and ionizing radiation; (5) medications; (6) coronary artery calcification and carotid wall thickness; and (7) the microbiome. The amount of risk conferred by these relatively newly identified factors is still being explored.

Markers of Inflammation, Ischemia, and Thrombosis. Of the numerous markers of inflammation that have been linked to an increase in CAD risk, highly sensitive C-reactive protein (hs-CRP) has been explored in the greatest depth. hs-CRP is an acute phase reactant or protein mostly synthesized in the liver and is an indirect measure of atherosclerotic plaque-related inflammation and plaque progression.[101] Elevated levels of hs-CRP are associated with numerous other CAD risk factors including smoking, obesity, and diabetes and, while they have been found to be an independent risk factor for coronary disease, the risk is highest when there is an associated elevation in LDL-C.[102] Current recommendations suggest that hs-CRP should be used as a part of overall cardiovascular risk assessment in selected individuals.[103] Troponin I (TnI) is a serum protein whose measurement is used as a sensitive and specific diagnostic test to help identify myocardial ischemia during acute coronary syndromes. Highly sensitive TnI assays are used in individuals without a history of CAD to assess risk for future CHD events, mortality, and heart failure.[104] Markers of thrombosis associated with CAD include fibrinogen and protein C.

Adipokines. Adipokines are a group of hormones released from adipose cells. The two that are most studied are adiponectin and leptin. Increased serum leptin is primarily implicated because of its contributions to the complications of obesity, hypertension, and diabetes but it is also being implicated in autoimmunity and decreased endothelial angiogenesis.[105] Decreased adiponectin (hypoadiponectinemia) in obese individuals has been linked to a significant increase in cardiovascular risk. Antiatherogenic effects of adiponectin include antiinflammatory, insulin-sensitizing enhancement of nitric oxide generation, attenuation of reactive oxygen species production in endothelial cells, and reduced vascular smooth muscle cell proliferation.[106] A more recently described adipokine is resistin, which has been linked to inflammation, endothelial dysfunction, thrombosis, and smooth muscle cell dysfunction. Emerging evidence suggests that adipokine changes occurring in perivascular adipose cells may play a significant role in metabolic and vascular disorders.[107] Weight loss and exercise improve adipokine levels and are correlated with improved cardiovascular risk, and new therapies, such as peroxisome proliferator-activated receptor (PPAR) gamma agonists, upregulation of adiponectin receptors, and direct infusions of adiponectin, are being explored.[106]

Chronic Kidney Disease. People with chronic kidney disease (CKD) are at increased risk for CAD events, and risk increases as glomerular filtration rate declines. In CKD, dyslipidemia, endothelial dysfunction, vascular calcification, elevated levels of growth factors, and toxic oxygen radicals all contribute to atherogenesis and CAD.[108,109]

Air Pollution and Ionizing Radiation. Exposure to air pollution is strongly correlated with coronary risk. It is postulated that toxins in pollution contribute to macrophage activation, oxidation of LDL, autonomic imbalance, thrombosis, and inflammation of vessel walls.[110] Ionizing radiation is most often linked to cancer risk, but there is emerging evidence that even low doses of radiation may contribute to CAD.[111] A recent hypothesis is somatic mutations in hematopoietic cells contribute to the development of human atherosclerosis.[112]

Medications. An increase in CAD-related ischemic events can occur within weeks of beginning NSAID use.[113] The likelihood of MI or stroke is greatest among those with preexisting disease, and risk increases at higher doses and with longer duration of use. There also is evidence that NSAIDs decrease the effectiveness of aspirin in preventing clot formation on atherosclerotic plaques (see *What's New?* Nonsteroidal Antiinflammatory Drugs and Coronary Artery Disease). Antirejection drugs and protease inhibitors also increase the risk for CAD.

Coronary Artery Calcification and Carotid Artery Wall Thickness. Coronary risk related to changes in vessel walls can be assessed using various types of vascular imaging techniques. Coronary

WHAT'S NEW?

Nonsteroidal Antiinflammatory Drugs and Coronary Artery Disease

Nonsteroidal antiinflammatory drugs (NSAIDs) are some of the most widely used medications in the world, and approximately 13% of Americans take them regularly. The first NSAIDs linked to cardiovascular disease were the cyclooxygenase-2 (COX-2) inhibitors that were designed to protect the gastrointestinal tract from ulceration, but were found to increase the risk of acute coronary syndromes. Since then, all NSAIDs have been found to be linked to coronary risk, and no NSAID is considered "safe," especially in those with underlying coronary artery atherosclerosis. Pathophysiologically, all NSAIDs have effects on the mitochondria in myocytes, including generation of toxic reactive oxygen species through pathways, such as nicotinamide adenine dinucleotide phosphate (NADPH), cytochrome 450, and lipoxygenase. Furthermore, NSAIDs alter the thromboxane/prostacyclin balance contributing to platelet aggregation. More recently, they have been shown to block the anti-platelet effects of aspirin. Finally, NSAIDs may contribute to hypertension, heart failure, and chronic kidney disease which have significant associated cardiovascular complications. The FDA has added label warnings, and high-risk individuals are recommended to avoid their use when possible.

Data from Campbell CL, Moliterno DJ: *J Am Med Assoc* 313(8):801–802, 2015; Danelich IM et al: *Pharmacotherapy* 35(5):520–535, 2015; Ghosh R, Alajbegovic A, Gomes AV: *Oxid Med Cell Longev* 2015:536962, 2015; Schjerning Olsen AM et al: *J Am Med Assoc* 313(8):805–814, 2015; Yoemans ND: *BMC Med* 13:56–59, 2015.

artery calcification (CAC), as detected by CT scanning, carotid intima-media thickness test (CIMT), and ultrasonography, are two important imaging modalities in widespread use for determining coronary heart disease risk. CAC is likely to be the most useful of the current approaches to improving risk assessment among individuals found to be at intermediate risk after formal risk assessment.[103]

The Microbiome. The effects of diet and other lifestyle measures on the microbiome and CVD risk increasingly are being explored. These effects may be mediated through their impact on other risk factors, such as diabetes and autoimmunity, or through more direct effects on microbiota function. For example, hyperhomocysteinemia has been linked to cardiovascular risk, yet the addition of folate (which increases homocysteine breakdown) has not improved risk. It is now postulated that the microbiome may be an important modulator of lipid and homocysteine metabolism, as well as many other atherosclerotic risk factors.[114,115]

In coronary artery disease, atherosclerotic plaques that form in the coronary circulation can develop in two primary ways. **Stable plaques** gradually increase in size and may partially occlude the vessel lumina, thus limiting coronary flow and causing ischemia especially during exercise. **Unstable plaques** are prone to ulceration or rupture even if there has been no significant impairment of coronary blood flow before the event (see Fig. 33.19). When this ulceration or rupture occurs, underlying tissues of the vessel wall are exposed, resulting in platelet adhesion and thrombus formation. Thrombus formation can suddenly cut off blood supply to the heart muscle, resulting in acute myocardial ischemia, and if the vessel obstruction cannot be reversed rapidly, ischemia will progress to infarction.

Transient Myocardial Ischemia

As described previously, CAD can diminish the myocardial blood supply causing ischemia. The process of atherosclerotic plaque progression can be gradual, which usually results in transient myocardial ischemic syndromes when demand for blood supply exceeds supply, but perfusion is restored before there is permanent damage to the heart muscle. Ischemia also can occur with coronary vasospasm even in the absence of atherosclerosis. Transient myocardial ischemia can result in unstable angina, Prinzmetal angina, or silent ischemia.

PATHOPHYSIOLOGY. The coronary arteries normally supply blood flow sufficient to meet the demands of the myocardium because it labors under varying workloads. Oxygen extraction from these vessels occurs with maximal efficiency. If efficient exchange does not meet myocardial oxygen needs, healthy coronary arteries are able to dilate to increase the flow of oxygenated blood to the myocardium. Narrowing of a major coronary artery by more than 50% impairs blood flow sufficiently to hamper cellular metabolism under conditions of increased myocardial demand (see Fig. 33.14).

Myocardial ischemia develops if the supply of coronary blood cannot meet the demand of the myocardium for oxygen and nutrients. Imbalances between myocardial demand and coronary blood supply can result from a number of conditions. Common causes of increased myocardial demand for blood include tachycardia, exercise, hypertension (hypertrophy), and valvular disease. Myocardial ischemia also can result from other causes of decreased blood and oxygen delivery to the myocardium, such as coronary spasm, hypotension, dysrhythmias, decreased oxygen-carrying capacity of the blood (anemia, hypoxemia), and aortic valvular disease.

Myocardial cells become ischemic within 10 seconds of coronary occlusion. After several minutes the heart cells lose the ability to contract, and cardiac output decreases. Ischemia also causes conduction abnormalities that lead to changes in the electrocardiogram and may initiate dysrhythmias. Anaerobic processes take over, and lactic acid accumulates. Cardiac cells remain viable for approximately 20 minutes under ischemic conditions. If blood flow is restored, aerobic metabolism resumes, contractility is restored, and cellular repair begins. If the coronary artery occlusion persists beyond 20 minutes, MI occurs (Fig. 33.15).

CLINICAL MANIFESTATIONS. Individuals with reversible myocardial ischemia present clinically in several ways. Chronic atherosclerotic coronary obstruction usually results in recurrent predictable chest pain called stable angina. Abnormal vasospasm of coronary vessels results in unpredictable chest pain called Prinzmetal angina. Myocardial ischemia that does not cause detectable symptoms is called silent ischemia.

Stable Angina

Angina pectoris is chest pain caused by myocardial ischemia. Stable angina is caused by gradual luminal narrowing and hardening of the arterial walls, so that affected vessels cannot dilate in response to increased myocardial demand associated with physical exertion or emotional stress. With rest, blood flow is restored and no necrosis of myocardial cells results. Angina pectoris is typically experienced as transient substernal chest discomfort, ranging from a sensation of heaviness or pressure to moderately severe pain. Individuals often describe the sensation by clenching a fist over the left sternal border. The discomfort may be mistaken for indigestion. The pain is caused by the buildup of lactic acid or abnormal stretching of the ischemic myocardium that irritates myocardial nerve fibers. These afferent sympathetic fibers enter the spinal cord from levels C3 to T4, accounting for the variety of locations and radiation patterns of anginal pain. Pain may radiate to the neck, lower jaw, left arm, and left shoulder or occasionally to the back or down the right arm. Pallor, diaphoresis, and dyspnea may be associated with the pain. The pain is usually relieved by rest and nitrates.

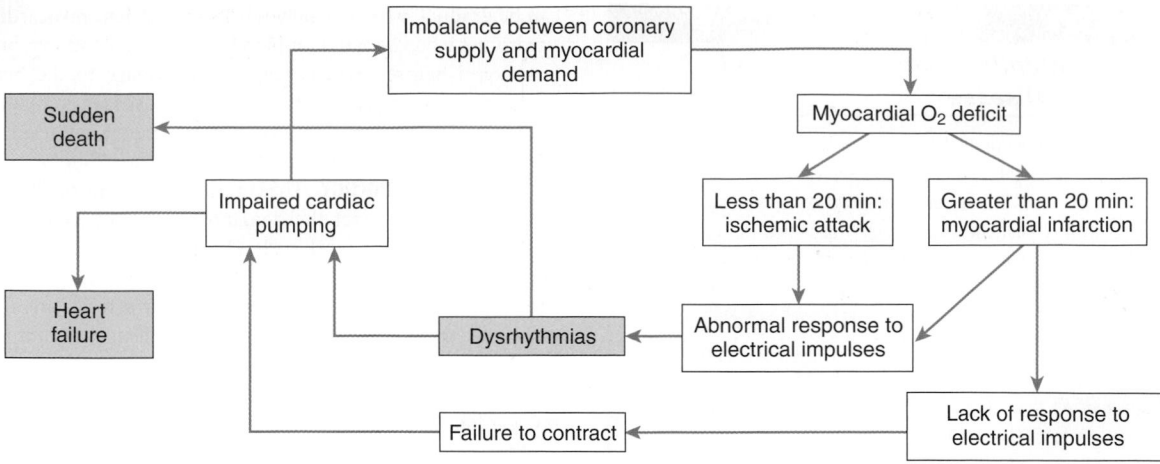

FIGURE 33.15 Cycle of Ischemic Events.

WHAT'S NEW?

Women and Microvascular Angina

Women with myocardial ischemia often have either no or atypical symptoms, such as palpitations, anxiety, weakness, and fatigue. Additionally, many women with angina are found to have cardiac ischemia, yet no evidence of obstructive coronary artery disease on cardiac catheterization. Evidence is accumulating that nearly half of women with myocardial ischemia suffer from coronary microvascular disease, a condition often called *microvascular angina (MVA)*. Small intramyocardial arterioles constrict in MVA causing ischemic pain that is less predictable than with typical epicardial coronary artery disease (CAD). The pathophysiology is complex and still being elucidated, but there is strong evidence that endothelial dysfunction, decreased endogenous vasodilators, inflammation, changes in adipokines, and platelet activation are contributing factors. The diagnosis of MVA may require catheterization during which there is assessment of the microcirculatory response to adenosine or acetylcholine and measurement of coronary and fractional flow reserve. New techniques include positron emission tomography (PET) scanning, cardiac magnetic resonance imaging (MRI), and transthoracic Doppler echocardiography. Managing MVA can be challenging, for example, women with this condition have less coronary microvascular dilation in response to nitrates than do those without MVA. Women with MVA often have traditional risk factors for CAD such as obesity, dyslipidemia, diabetes, and hypertension. Aggressive interventions to reduce modifiable risk factors are an important component of management, especially smoking cessation, exercise, and diabetes management. The combination of nonnitrate vasodilators, such as calcium channel blockers and angiotensin converting enzyme (ACE) inhibitors along with 3-hydroxy-3-glutaryl-coenzymeA (HMG-CoA) reductase inhibitors (statins), also has been shown to be effective in many women, and new drugs, such as Ranolazine and Ivabradine, have shown promise in the treatment of MVA. Other approaches include spinal cord stimulators, adenosine receptor blockade, and psychiatric intervention.

Data from Cattaneo M et al: Int J Cardiol 181:376–381, 2015; Celik T et al: *Int J Cardiol* 218:233–234, 2016; Lanza GA et al: *Circ J* 2016 May 27 [Epub ahead of print]; Marinescu MA et al: *JACC Cardiovasc Imaging* 8(2):210–220, 2015; Selthofer-Relatic K, Boxnjak I, Kibel A: *Cardiol Res Pract* 2016:8173816, 2016; Titterington JS, Hung OY, Wenger NK: *Future Cardiol* 11(2):229–242, 2015.

Myocardial ischemia in women may not present with typical angina. Common symptoms in women include atypical chest pain, palpitations, sense of unease, and severe fatigue. In addition, it is estimated that half of women with stable angina do not have obstructive coronary artery disease, but rather have *microvascular angina* that results from vasoconstriction of small coronary arterioles deep in the myocardium[116] (see *What's New? Women and Microvascular Angina*). Similarly, in individuals who have autonomic nervous system dysfunction, such as older adults or those with diabetes, angina may be mild, atypical, or even silent (see the following).

Prinzmetal Angina

Prinzmetal angina (also called *variant angina*) is chest pain attributable to transient ischemia of the myocardium that occurs unpredictably and almost exclusively at rest. This form of angina often occurs at night during rapid eye movement sleep and may have a cyclic pattern of occurrence. Pain is caused by vasospasm of one or more major coronary arteries with or without associated atherosclerosis. The angina may result from decreased vagal activity, hyperactivity of the sympathetic nervous system, and decreased nitric oxide activity. Other causes include altered calcium channel function in arterial smooth muscle and endothelial dysfunction with release of inflammatory mediators, such as serotonin, histamine, endothelin, or thromboxane.[117] The level of hs-CRP may be elevated in individuals with this form of angina. Prinzmetal angina is usually a benign condition, but can occasionally cause serious dysrhythmias especially if treatment is withdrawn; therefore calcium channel blockers or long-acting nitrates, or both, should be continued even if clinical remission is achieved. If the spasm persists long enough, infarction or serious dysrhythmias may occur.[118]

Silent Ischemia and Mental Stress (Induced Ischemia)

Myocardial ischemia does not always cause angina and may be associated only with nonspecific symptoms such as fatigue, dyspnea, or feeling of unease. Some individuals only have silent ischemia, whereas episodes of silent myocardial ischemia may occur in individuals who also experience angina. Global or regional abnormalities in left ventricular sympathetic afferent innervation have been implicated in diabetes mellitus, following surgical denervation during coronary artery bypass grafting

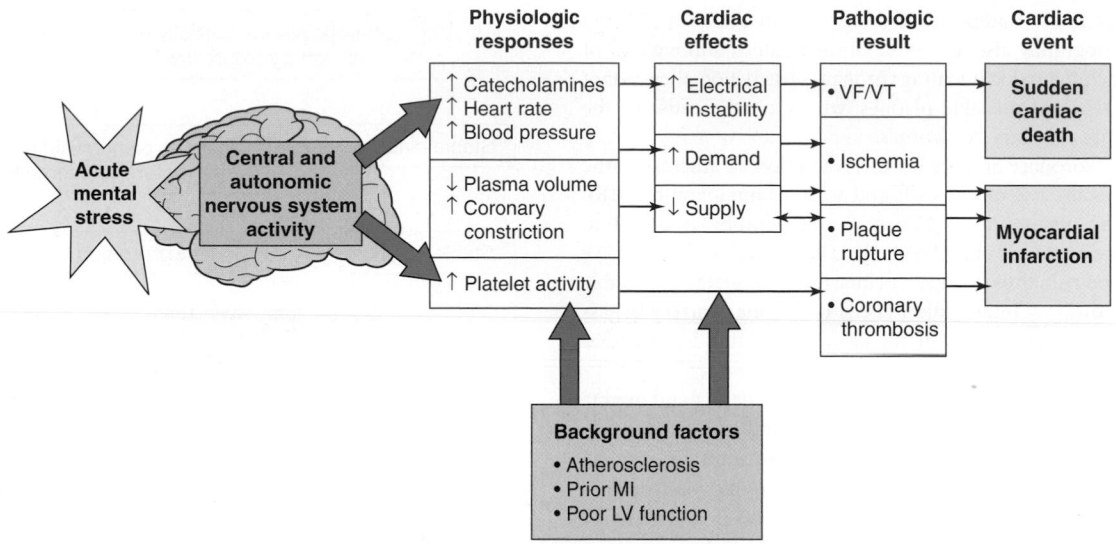

FIGURE 33.16 Pathophysiologic Model of Acute Stress Effects Triggering Cardiac Clinical Events. Acting via the central and autonomic nervous systems, stress can produce a cascade of physiologic responses that may lead to myocardial ischemia, potentially fatal dysrhythmia, plaque rupture, or coronary thrombosis. *LV,* Left ventricle; *MI,* myocardial infarction; *VF,* ventricular fibrillation; *VT,* ventricular tachycardia. (From Kranz DS et al: Mental stress as a trigger of myocardial ischemia and infarction. In Deedwania PC, Tofler GH, editors: *Triggers and timing of cardiac events,* ed 2, London, 1996, Saunders.)

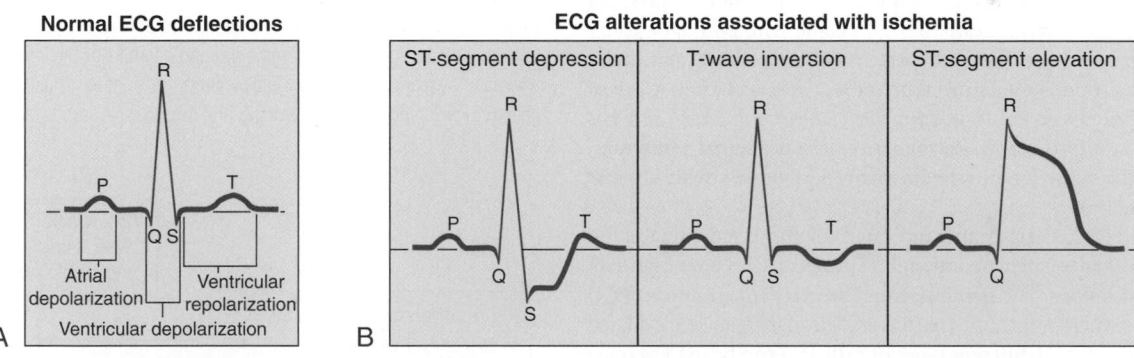

FIGURE 33.17 Electrocardiogram (ECG) and Ischemia. **A,** Normal ECG. **B,** Electrocardiographic alterations associated with ischemia.

(CABG) or cardiac transplantation, or following ischemic local nerve injury by MI. There also is evidence that individuals with silent ischemia produce less lactate than those with angina.[119] Silent ischemia also may occur in some individuals during mental stress and anger.[120] Mental stress results in the release of catecholamines and an increase in heart rate, blood pressure, and vascular resistance, as well as electrical instability (see Fig. 33.16). In addition, it has been linked to increased hs-CRP level, decreased activity of vasodilators such as nitric oxide, and a hypercoagulable state that may contribute to acute ischemic events.

◆ **EVALUATION AND TREATMENT.** Many individuals with reversible myocardial ischemia exhibit a normal physical examination between episodes. Physical examination of an individual experiencing myocardial ischemia may disclose tachycardia, extra heart sounds (gallops or murmurs), and pulmonary congestion indicating impaired left ventricular function. The presence of xanthelasmas (small fat deposits) around the eyelids or arcus senilis of the eyes (a yellow lipid ring around the cornea) suggests dyslipidemia and possible atherosclerosis. The presence of peripheral or carotid arterial bruits suggests probable atherosclerotic disease and increases the likelihood that CAD is present.

Electrocardiography is a critical tool for diagnosing myocardial ischemia. Because many individuals have normal ECGs in the absence of pain, diagnosis may require that electrocardiography be performed during an attack of angina. Transient ST-segment depression and T-wave inversion are characteristic signs of subendocardial ischemia frequently seen in angina. ST elevation, indicative of transmural ischemia, can be seen in individuals with Prinzmetal angina but is more common in infarction (Fig. 33.17). The ECG also can give some indication of which coronary artery is involved. Approximately 30% of individuals with angina have nondiagnostic ECG tracings and require other diagnostic studies.

Stress radionuclide imaging is indicated to detect ischemic changes in asymptomatic individuals with multiple risk factors for coronary disease, such as diabetes and dyslipidemia, and for older individuals who plan to start vigorous exercise. Stress testing is made more sensitive when radioisotope imaging is added to the ECG as an indicator of myocardial ischemia. Currently, the modality of choice for the diagnosis of myocardial ischemia is single-photon emission computed tomography (SPECT), which is effective at identifying ischemia and estimating risk for coronary events.[121] Radioisotope imaging with thallium-201 and stress echocardiography also are used. Unfortunately, although all of these tests are helpful in documenting coronary obstruction, they cannot detect the presence of unstable plaques, which are the cause of the majority of acute coronary syndromes.

Imaging the coronary arteries for the evaluation of atherosclerotic plaques involves the use of CT with and without angiography, MRI, or intravascular ultrasound.[122] Coronary angiography is useful in determining the anatomic extent of CAD. The procedure is expensive and carries some risk; thus it is used primarily to evaluate for possible percutaneous coronary intervention (PCI) or coronary artery bypass grafting (CABG) surgery for individuals whose noninvasive studies suggest severe disease.

The primary aims of therapy for myocardial ischemia and angina are to increase delivery of oxygen by improving coronary artery blood flow and to reduce myocardial oxygen consumption. Recommendations for appropriate diet, exercise, and risk reduction strategies have been widely distributed. Coronary blood flow is improved by reversing vasoconstriction, preventing clotting, and reducing plaque growth and rupture. Myocardial oxygen consumption is reduced by manipulation of blood pressure, heart rate, contractility, and left ventricular volume. Many different classes of drugs are available to manage stable angina, including nitrates, β-adrenergic receptor blockers, and calcium channel blockers.[123] Statins are indicated for primary prevention in high-risk individuals and for all those with known CAD.[85] Antithrombotics, such as aspirin or clopidogrel, reduce the risk of clot formation. Angiotensin-converting enzyme (ACE) inhibitors or ang II receptor blockers are indicated for all people with coronary artery disease who also have diabetes, hypertension, and/or left ventricular systolic dysfunction. Ranolazine represents a relatively new class of antianginal drugs known as *sodium ion channel inhibitors* and has been found to improve exercise tolerance, lessen anginal symptoms, and reduce the need for nitrates in many individuals with chronic stable angina.[124]

Coronary revascularization is indicated for those individuals who do not respond adequately to antianginal drugs or who have high-risk atherosclerotic lesions.[123,125] **Percutaneous coronary intervention (PCI)** is a procedure whereby stenotic (narrowed) coronary vessels are dilated with a catheter. Several different types of catheters can be used to open the blocked vessel. PCI is most often used to treat single-vessel disease, but it can be effective with multiple-vessel disease or restenosis of a coronary artery bypass graft in selected individuals. Restenosis of the artery is the major complication of the procedure; however, placement of a coronary stent can reduce this risk and antithrombotic treatment, such as aspirin, clopidogrel, or glycoprotein IIb/IIIa receptor antagonists, after stenting can improve outcomes. Severe CAD can be surgically treated by CABG, usually using the saphenous vein from the lower leg. In selected individuals, a modified CABG procedure called *minimally invasive direct coronary artery bypass (MIDCAB)* can be used with much less surgical morbidity and more rapid recovery. Investigational treatment for refractory angina includes gene and stem therapies for myocardial angiogenesis and spinal cord stimulation.[126,127]

Acute Coronary Syndromes

When there is sudden coronary obstruction caused by thrombus formation over a ruptured or ulcerated atherosclerotic plaque, acute coronary syndromes result (Fig. 33.18). The acute coronary syndromes (ACS) include unstable angina and myocardial infarction. **Unstable angina** is the result of reversible myocardial ischemia and is a harbinger of impending infarction. **Myocardial infarction (MI)** results when prolonged ischemia causes irreversible damage to the heart muscle. MI can be further subdivided into non–ST-elevation MI (non-STEMI) and

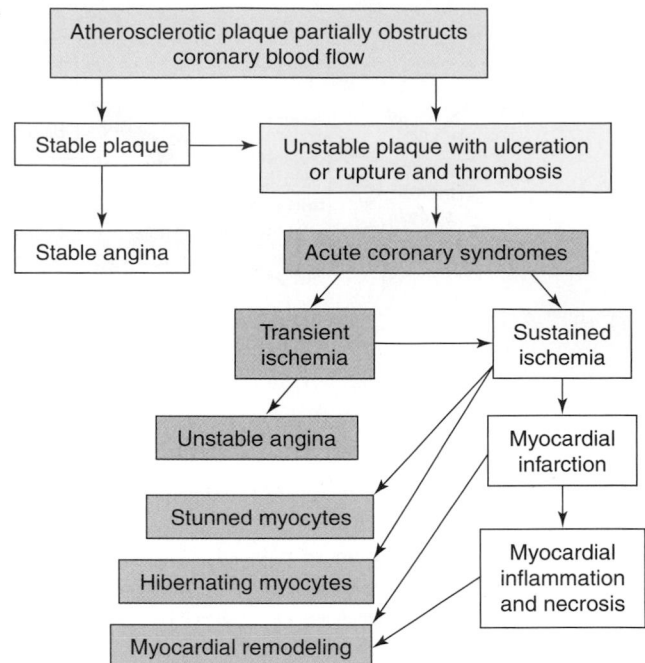

FIGURE 33.18 Pathophysiology of Acute Coronary Syndromes. The atherosclerotic process can lead to stable plaque formation and stable angina or can result in unstable plaques that are prone to rupture and thrombosis. Thrombus formation on a ruptured plaque that disperses in less than 20 minutes leads to transient ischemia and unstable angina. If the vessel obstruction is sustained, myocardial infarction with inflammation and necrosis of the myocardium result. In addition, myocardial infarction is associated with other structural and functional changes, including myocyte stunning and hibernation and myocardial remodeling.

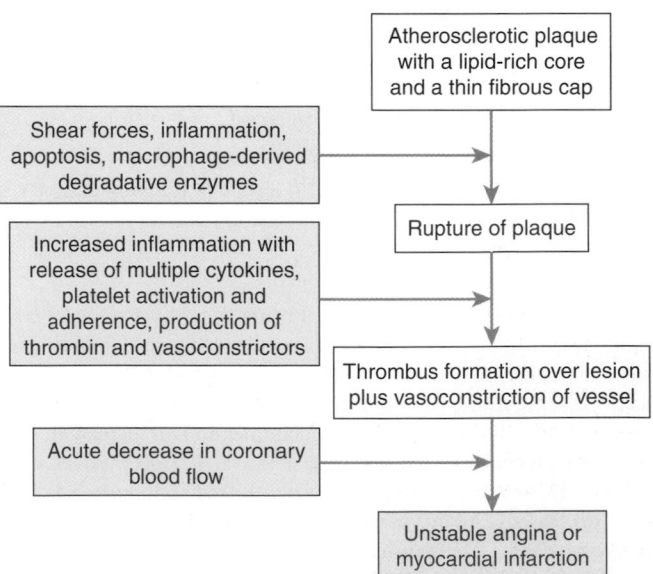

FIGURE 33.19 Pathogenesis of Unstable Plaques and Thrombus Formation.

ST-elevation MI (STEMI) (see the Pathophysiology section). Sudden cardiac death can occur as a result of any of the acute coronary syndromes.

An unstable atherosclerotic plaque is prone to rupture. It has a core that is especially rich in deposited oxidized LDL and a thin fibrous cap (Fig. 33.19). These unstable plaques may not extend into the lumen of

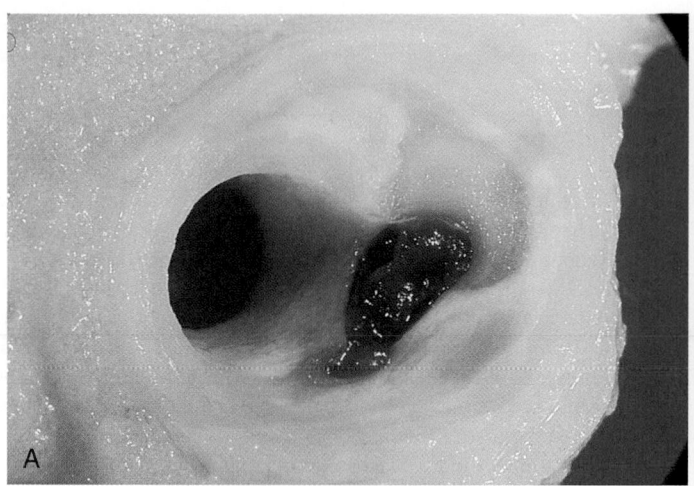
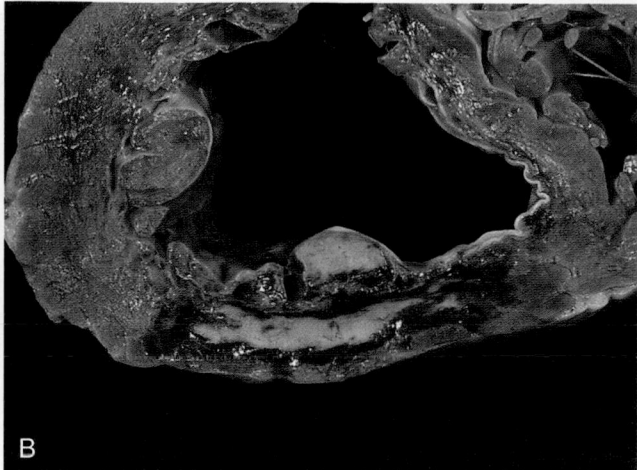

FIGURE 33.20 Plaque Disruption and Myocardial Infarction. **A,** Plaque disruption. The cap of the lipid-rich plaque has become torn with the formation of a thrombus, mostly inside the plaque. **B,** Myocardial infarction. This infarct is 6 days old. The center is yellow and necrotic with a hemorrhagic red rim. The responsible coronary artery occlusion is probably in the right coronary artery. The infarct is on the posterior wall. (From Damjanov I, Linder J, editors: *Anderson's pathology*, ed 10, St Louis, 1996, Mosby.)

the vessel and may be clinically silent until they rupture. Plaque disruption (ulceration or rupture) occurs because of shear forces, inflammation with release of multiple inflammatory mediators, secretion of macrophage-derived degradative enzymes, and apoptosis of cells at the edges of the lesions. Exposure of the plaque substrate activates the clotting cascade. In addition, platelet activation results in the release of coagulants and exposure of platelet glycoprotein IIb/IIIa surface receptors, resulting in further platelet aggregation and adherence. The resulting thrombus can form very quickly (Fig. 33.20, *A*). Vessel obstruction is further exacerbated by the release of vasoconstrictors, such as thromboxane A_2 and endothelin. The thrombus may break up before permanent myocyte damage has occurred (unstable angina) or it may cause prolonged ischemia with resultant MI (see Fig. 33.20, *B*). Diagnostic tests aimed at identifying unstable plaques before they rupture include intravascular ultrasound or MRI, angioscopy, and spectroscopy. Medications such as statins, ACE inhibitors, and beta-blockers can help stabilize plaques and prevent rupture.

Unstable Angina. Unstable angina is a form of acute coronary syndrome that results in reversible myocardial ischemia. It is important to recognize this syndrome because it signals that the atherosclerotic plaque has ruptured, and infarction may soon follow.

◆**PATHOPHYSIOLOGY.** Unstable angina occurs when fissuring or superficial erosion of the plaque leads to transient episodes of thrombotic vessel occlusion and vasoconstriction at the site of plaque damage. This thrombus is labile and occludes the vessel for no more than 10 to 20 minutes, with return of perfusion before significant myocardial necrosis occurs.

◆**CLINICAL MANIFESTATIONS.** Unstable angina presents as new-onset angina, angina that is occurring at rest, or angina that is increasing in severity or frequency (Box 33.1). Individuals may experience increased dyspnea, diaphoresis, and anxiety as the angina worsens.

◆**EVALUATION AND MANAGEMENT.** Physical examination may reveal evidence of ischemic myocardial dysfunction such as tachycardia or pulmonary congestion. The ECG most commonly reveals ST-segment depression and T-wave inversion during pain that resolves as the pain is relieved. The serum cardiac biomarkers (troponins, creatine phosphokinase-myocardial bound [CPK-MB]) remain normal. Manage-

---

BOX 33.1   THREE PRINCIPAL PRESENTATIONS OF UNSTABLE ANGINA

Rest angina*—angina occurring at rest and prolonged, usually >20 minutes

New-onset angina—new-onset angina of at least Canadian Cardiovascular Society (CCS) class III severity (CCS class III indicates "marked limitations of ordinary physical activity")

Increasing angina—previously diagnosed angina that has become distinctly more frequent, longer in duration, or lower in threshold (i.e., increased by ≥1 CCS class to at least CCS class III severity)

*Individuals with non–ST-elevation myocardial infarction (non-STEMI) usually present with angina at rest.
From Anderson J et al: *J Am Coll Cardiol* 50:e1–e157, 2007.
Originally adapted from Braunwald E: *Circulation* 80:410–414, 1989.

ment of unstable angina is the same as the management for non-STEMI and requires immediate hospitalization. Administration of nitrates, antithrombotics (aspirin, ticagrelor, and/or GP IIb/IIIa platelet receptor antagonists), and anticoagulants (heparin, low-molecular-weight heparin, or direct thrombin inhibitors, such as fondaparinux) is recommended. If the individual stabilizes, then continued anticoagulation plus beta-blockers and ACE inhibitors are indicated. If the patient is refractory to medical treatment, then emergent PCI is indicated.[128]

Myocardial Infarction

When coronary blood flow is interrupted for an extended period, myocyte necrosis occurs. This results in MI. Pathologically there are two major types of MI: subendocardial infarction and transmural infarction. Clinically, however, MI is categorized as STEMI or non-STEMI.

◆**PATHOPHYSIOLOGY.** Plaque progression, disruption, and subsequent clot formation are the same for myocardial infarction as they are for unstable angina (see Figs. 33.18, 33.19, and 33.20). In this case, however, the thrombus is less labile and occludes the vessel for a prolonged

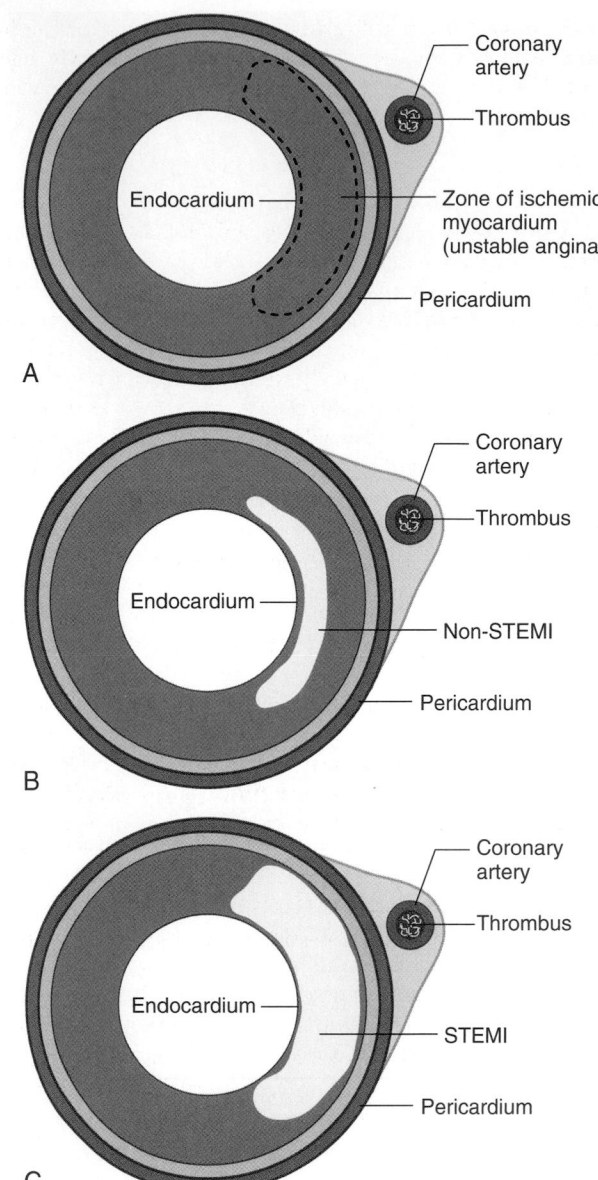

FIGURE 33.21 Unstable Angina, Non-STEMI, and STEMI. A, Unstable angina. Coronary thrombosis leads to myocardial ischemia. **B,** Non-ST-segment elevation myocardial infarction (Non-STEMI). Persistent coronary occlusion leads to infarction of the myocardium closest to the endocardium. **C,** ST-segment elevation myocardial infarction (STEMI). Continued coronary occlusion leads to transmural infarction extending from endocardium to pericardium.

period, such that myocardial ischemia progresses to myocyte necrosis and death (Fig. 33.21). The duration of ischemia determines the size and character of the infarction. If the thrombus breaks up before complete distal tissue necrosis has occurred, the infarction will involve only the myocardium directly beneath the endocardium (subendocardial MI). This infarction usually presents with ST depression and T-wave inversion and is termed non-STEMI. It is especially important to recognize this form of acute coronary syndrome because recurrent clot formation on the disrupted atherosclerotic plaque is likely to occur unless some intervention is undertaken as soon as possible. If the thrombus lodges permanently in the vessel, the infarction will extend through the myocardium all the way from endocardium to epicardium (transmural MI), resulting in severe cardiac dysfunction. Transmural infarction usually causes marked elevations in the ST segments on ECG, called

STEMI. Clinically it is important to identify those with STEMI because they are at highest risk for serious complications and require immediate intervention.

Cellular Injury

Cardiac cells can withstand ischemic conditions for about 20 minutes before cellular death takes place. After only 30 to 60 seconds of hypoxia, ECG changes are visible. Yet even if cells are metabolically altered and nonfunctional, they can remain viable if blood flow returns within 20 minutes. Reports suggest previous recurrent episodes of myocardial ischemia can result in myocyte adaptation to oxygen deprivation and preservation of myocardium. This process, termed ischemic preconditioning, results in changes in reactive oxygen species, calcium ions, adenosine, bradykinin, catecholamines, and opioids that exert protective effects on the myocardium.[129] Therapeutic ischemic preconditioning has been used in individuals undergoing elective CABG or valvular replacement and in individuals with STEMI before emergent PCI; however, more studies are needed to determine the best use of this modality.[130]

After 8 to 10 seconds of decreased blood flow, the affected myocardium becomes cyanotic and cooler. Myocardial oxygen reserves are used very quickly (within about 8 seconds) after complete cessation of coronary flow. Glycogen stores decrease as anaerobic metabolism begins. Unfortunately, glycolysis can supply only 65% to 70% of the total myocardial energy requirement and produces much less ATP than aerobic processes. Hydrogen ions and lactic acid accumulate. Because myocardial tissues have poor buffering capabilities and myocardial cells are very sensitive to low cellular pH, accumulation of these products further compromises the myocardium. Acidosis may make the myocardium more vulnerable to the damaging effects of lysosomal enzymes and may suppress impulse conduction and contractile function, thereby leading to heart failure.

Oxygen deprivation also is accompanied by electrolyte disturbances, specifically loss of potassium, calcium, and magnesium from cells. Myocardial cells deprived of necessary oxygen and nutrients lose contractility, thereby diminishing the heart's pumping ability. Ischemic myocardial cells release catecholamines (epinephrine and norepinephrine), predisposing the individual to serious imbalances of sympathetic and parasympathetic function, irregular heartbeats (dysrhythmia), and heart failure. Catecholamines mediate the release of glycogen, glucose, and stored fat from body cells. Therefore plasma concentrations of free fatty acids and glycerol rise within 1 hour after onset of acute MI. Excessive levels of free fatty acids can have a harmful detergent effect on cell membranes. Norepinephrine elevates blood glucose levels through stimulation of liver and skeletal muscle cells. It also suppresses pancreatic B-cell activity, which reduces insulin secretion and elevates blood glucose level further.

Ang II is released during myocardial ischemia and contributes to the pathogenesis of MI in several ways. First, it results in the systemic effects of peripheral vasoconstriction and fluid retention. These homeostatic responses are counterproductive in that they increase myocardial work and thus exacerbate the effects of the loss of myocyte contractility. Ang II is also released locally, where it is a growth factor for vascular smooth muscle cells, myocytes, and cardiac fibroblasts promoting catecholamine release and coronary artery spasm.

Ischemic injury can be exacerbated by what is termed reperfusion injury once blood flow is restored. This process involves the release of toxic oxygen radicals, calcium flux, and pH changes that cause a sustained opening of mitochondrial permeability transition pores (mPTPs) and contribute to resultant cellular death.[131] Infiltration of inflammatory cells contributes to tissue injury. Therapies aimed at reducing reperfusion injury are being explored, including targeted temperature management, use of adenosine or atrial natriuretic peptide, and ischemic postconditioning.[132,133]

Cellular Death

After about 20 minutes of myocardial ischemia, irreversible hypoxic injury causes cellular death and tissue necrosis. (Types of necrosis are described in Chapter 2.) Necrosis of myocardial tissue results in the release of intracellular enzymes, such as troponin, through the damaged cell membranes into the interstitial spaces. The lymphatics pick up the enzymes and transport them into the bloodstream, where they can be detected by serologic tests. Recent evidence has found that, along with necrosis, myocardial tissue is also destroyed by apoptosis and autophagy. An increased understanding of these processes in MI may lead to new therapies aimed at limiting infarct size.[134]

Structural and Functional Changes

As a result of an MI, structural and functional changes occur within cardiac tissue (Fig. 33.22). Gross tissue changes in the area of infarction may not become apparent for several hours, despite almost immediate onset (within 30 to 60 seconds) of ECG changes. The infarcted myocardium is surrounded by a zone of hypoxic injury, which may progress to necrosis, undergo remodeling (scarring), or return to normal.

Myocardial stunning is a temporary loss of contractile function that persists for hours to days after perfusion has been restored. This pathophysiologic state can occur both with MI and in individuals who suffer ischemia during cardiovascular procedures such as cardiac surgery. Stunning is caused by the alterations in electrolyte pumps, calcium homeostasis, and the release of toxic oxygen radicals. It is characterized by decreased contraction and conduction and can contribute to heart failure, shock, and dysrhythmias. Hibernating myocardium refers to tissue that is persistently ischemic and undergoes metabolic adaptation to prolong myocyte survival until perfusion can be restored. Restoring adequate perfusion to the myocardium with revascularization therapies can improve myocardial function; however, future therapies aimed specifically at maintaining myocyte viability are needed.[135] Myocardial remodeling is a process mediated by ang II, aldosterone, catecholamines, adenosine, oxidative stress, and inflammatory cytokines, which causes myocyte hypertrophy, scarring, and loss of contractile function in the areas of the heart distant from the site of infarction.

These changes can be limited and even reversed (reverse remodeling) through rapid restoration of coronary flow and the use of ACE inhibitors, beta-blockers, statins, sequential pacemakers, and ventricular assist devices after MI.

Repair

MI causes a severe inflammatory response that ends with wound repair (see Chapter 7). Repair consists of degradation of damaged cells, proliferation of fibroblasts, and synthesis of scar tissue. Many cell types, hormones, and nutrient substrates must be available for optimal healing to proceed. Within 24 hours, leukocytes infiltrate the necrotic area and proteolytic enzymes from scavenger neutrophils degrade necrotic tissue. A collagen matrix is deposited and is initially weak, mushy, and vulnerable to reinjury. Unfortunately it is at this time in the recovery period (10 to 14 days after infarction) that individuals feel more capable of increasing activities and thus may stress the newly formed scar tissue. After 6 weeks the necrotic area is completely replaced by scar tissue, which is strong but unable to contract and relax like healthy myocardial tissue.

The severity of functional impairment depends on the size of the lesion and the site of infarction. Functional changes can include (1) decreased cardiac contractility with abnormal wall motion, (2) altered left ventricular compliance, (3) decreased stroke volume, (4) decreased ejection fraction, (5) increased left ventricular end-diastolic pressure and volume, and (6) sinoatrial node malfunction. Life-threatening dysrhythmias and heart failure often follow myocardial infarction. With infarction, ventricular function is abnormal and the ejection fraction falls, resulting in increases in ventricular end-diastolic volume (VEDV). If the coronary obstruction involves the perfusion to the left ventricle, pulmonary venous congestion ensues; if the right ventricle is ischemic, increases in systemic venous pressures occur.

CLINICAL MANIFESTATIONS. The first symptom of acute MI is usually sudden, severe, chest pain. It is not possible to distinguish between angina and MI by symptoms alone, although the pain associated with MI tends to be more severe and prolonged. It may be described as heavy and crushing, such as an "elephant sitting on my chest." Radiation to the neck, jaw, back, shoulder, or left arm is common. Some individuals (especially older adults or those with diabetes) experience no pain, thereby having a "silent" infarction. Infarction often simulates a sensation of unrelenting indigestion. Nausea and vomiting may occur because

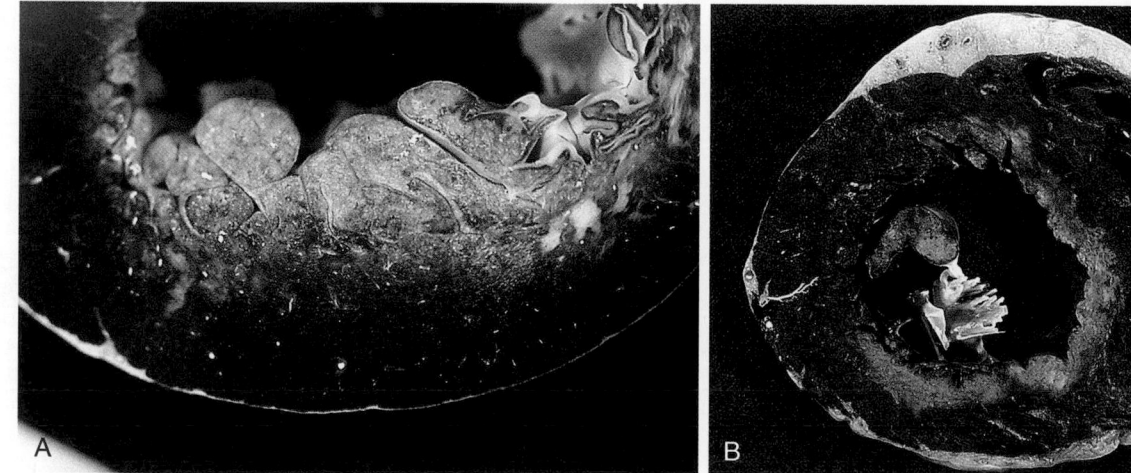

FIGURE 33.22 Myocardial Infarction. A, Local infarct confined to one region. **B,** Massive large infarct caused by occlusion of three coronary arteries. (From Damjanov I, Linder J, editors: *Anderson's pathology*, ed 10, St Louis, 1996, Mosby.)

of reflex stimulation of vomiting centers by pain fibers. Vasovagal reflexes from the area of the infarcted myocardium also may affect the gastrointestinal tract. Various cardiovascular changes are found on physical examination:

1. The sympathetic nervous system (SNS) is reflexively activated to compensate, resulting in a temporary increase in heart rate and blood pressure, although severe myocardial damage may cause hypotension despite elevated catecholamine activity.
2. Abnormal extra heart sounds reflect left ventricular dysfunction.
3. Cardiac murmurs may indicate acute valvular insufficiency.
4. Pulmonary findings of congestion including dullness to percussion and inspiratory crackles at the lung bases can occur if the individual develops heart failure.
5. Peripheral vasoconstriction may cause the skin to become cool and clammy.

◆**EVALUATION AND TREATMENT.** The diagnosis of acute MI is made on the basis of history, physical examination, ECG, and serial cardiac biomarker alterations (Box 33.2). It is important to note that nearly half of MIs are not preceded by any previous angina symptoms and up to one-third present with STEMI as the first symptomatic manifestation of coronary disease. MI can occur in various regions of the heart wall and may be described as anterior, inferior, posterior, lateral, subendocardial, or transmural depending on its location and extent of

tissue damage from infarction. Twelve-lead ECGs help localize the affected area through identification of changes in ST segments and T waves (Fig. 33.23). In STEMI, a characteristic Q wave often develops on ECG some hours later.

Cardiac troponin I (cTnI) is the most specific indicator of MI and should be obtained on admission to the emergency department. cTnI elevation is detectable 2 to 4 hours after onset of symptoms. Additional measurements within 6 to 9 hours and again at 12 to 24 hours are recommended if clinical suspicion is high and previous samples were negative. Troponin levels also can be used to estimate infarct size and therefore the likelihood of complications. Other biomarkers released by myocardial cells include CPK-MB and LDH. Additional laboratory data may reveal leukocytosis and elevated CRP, both of which indicate inflammation. The individual's blood glucose level is usually elevated and the glucose tolerance level may remain abnormal for several weeks. Individuals with acute coronary syndromes require admission to the hospital. The individual should be placed on supplemental oxygen and given an aspirin immediately (clopidogrel or prasugrel if intolerant to aspirin). Pain is treated with morphine sulfate, which also has vasodilatory effects on the coronaries. Continuous monitoring of cardiac rhythms and biomarker changes is essential because the first 24 hours after onset of symptoms is the time of highest risk for sudden death. Non-STEMI is treated in the same way as unstable angina including antithrombotics,

---

BOX 33.2   THE UNIVERSAL DEFINITION OF MYOCARDIAL INFARCTION

The term *myocardial infarction* should be used when there is evidence of myocardial necrosis in a clinical setting with myocardial ischemia. Under these conditions any one of the following criteria meets the diagnosis for myocardial infarction (MI):

- Detection of rise and/or fall of cardiac biomarkers (preferably cardiac troponin [cTn]) with at least one value above the 99th percentile of the upper reference limit (URL) together with evidence of myocardial ischemia with at least one of the following:
  Symptoms of ischemia
  New or presumed new significant ST-segment-T wave (ST-T) changes or new left bundle branch block (LBBB)
  Development of pathologic Q waves in the electrocardiogram (ECG)
  Imaging evidence of new loss of viable myocardium or new regional wall motion abnormality
  Identification of an intracoronary thrombus by angiography or autopsy
- Cardiac death with symptoms suggestive of myocardial ischemia and presumed new ischemic ECG changes or new LBBB, but death occurring before cardiac biomarkers were obtained, or before cardiac biomarker values would be increased.

- Percutaneous coronary intervention (PCI)–related MI is arbitrarily defined by an elevation of cTn values (>5 x 99th percentile URL) in patients with normal baseline values (≤99th percentile URL) or a rise of cTn values >20% of the baseline values are elevated and are stable or falling. In addition, either (i) symptoms suggestive of myocardial ischemia, (ii) new ischemic ECG changes, (iii) angiographic findings are consistent with a procedural complication, or (iv) imaging demonstration of new loss of viable myocardium or new regional wall motion abnormality are required.
- Stent thrombosis–associated MI when detected by coronary angiography or autopsy in the setting of myocardial ischemia and with a rise and/or fall of cardiac biomarker values with at least one value over the 99th percentile URL.
- Coronary artery bypass grafting (CABG)–related MI is arbitrarily defined by an elevation of cardiac biomarker values (>10 x 99th percentile URL) in patients with normal baseline cTn values (≤99th percentile URL).
  In addition, either (i) new pathologic Q waves or new LBBB, (ii) angiographically documented new graft or new native coronary artery occlusion, or (iii) imaging evidence of new loss of viable myocardium or new regional wall motion abnormality.

Data from Thygesen K, Alpert J, Jaffe, AS et al: *Circulation* 126:2020–2035, 2012.

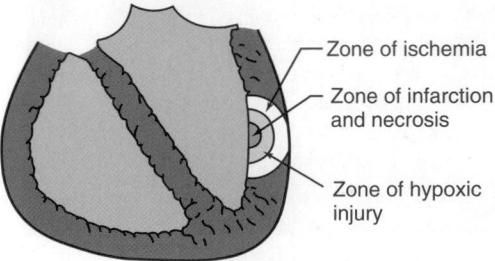

Normal	Ischemia	Injury	Infarction/necrosis

Zone of ischemia
Zone of infarction and necrosis
Zone of hypoxic injury

FIGURE 33.23 Electrocardiographic Alterations Associated with the Three Zones of Myocardial Infarction.

anticoagulation or PCI, or both.[128] STEMI is best managed with emergent PCI and antithrombotics.[136,137] Careful monitoring for dysrhythmias, heart failure, and shock is essential. Hyperglycemia is treated with insulin. Once the person is stabilized, further management includes ACE inhibitors, beta-blockers, and statins.

Bed rest, followed by gradual return to activities of daily living, reduces the myocardial oxygen demands of the compromised heart. Individuals not receiving thrombolytic or heparin infusion must receive deep venous thrombosis (DVT) prophylaxis as long as their activity is significantly limited. Stool softeners are given to eliminate the need for straining. Education on diet, caffeine, smoking cessation, exercise, and other aspects of risk factor reduction is crucial for secondary prevention of recurrent myocardial ischemia.

Approximately 1% to 2% of people initially diagnosed with STEMI do not have myocardial infarction, but rather have a stress-induced syndrome known as the *broken heart syndrome* or *Takotsubo cardiomyopathy*.[138] These individuals present with the acute onset of chest pain, ST elevation, and elevated troponins after emotional stress, but generally do not have coronary artery disease and must be managed differently (see *What's New? The Broken Heart Syndrome*).

◆**COMPLICATIONS.** The number and severity of postinfarction complications depend on the location and extent of necrosis, the individual's physiologic condition before the infarction, and the availability of swift therapeutic intervention.

Dysrhythmias (arrhythmias), which are disturbances of cardiac rhythm, are the most common complication of acute MI. Dysrhythmias can be caused by ischemia, hypoxia, autonomic nervous system (ANS) imbalances, lactic acidosis, electrolyte abnormalities, alterations of impulse conduction pathways or conduction defects, drug toxicity, or hemodynamic abnormalities. Dysrhythmias may originate from the atria, ventricles, nodal regions, or conduction tissues. The seriousness of dysrhythmias depends on the hemodynamic consequences. (Dysrhythmias are described in Tables 33.9 and 33.10.) Prophylactic use of antiarrhythmics, such as lidocaine and amiodarone, does not improve mortality; however, individuals at high risk should be considered for implantable cardioverter-defibrillators (ICDs).

Acute MI is accompanied by functional impairment of the myocardium. Many infarctions result in some degree of heart failure, which is characterized by pulmonary congestion, reduced myocardial contractility, and abnormal heart wall motion. Anterior infarction is associated with more severe left heart failure than is inferior infarction. If cardiac output is insufficient to maintain normal arterial pressure and to perfuse the kidneys and other organs adequately, cardiogenic shock develops. (Cardiogenic shock is discussed in Chapter 49.)

Inflammation of the pericardium (pericarditis) is a common complication of acute MI. Pericardial friction rubs often are noted 2 to 3 days after MI and are associated with anterior chest pain that worsens with respiratory effort. Specific treatment is not required; however, corticosteroids dramatically relieve symptoms.

Cardiac complications of MI can include rupture of heart structures and aneurysm formation. Tissue necrosis in or around the papillary muscles can cause rupture of these muscles or of the chordae tendineae. Weakening of the wall of the infarcted ventricle can cause ventricular aneurysm formation. Left ventricular aneurysm is a late complication of MI, occurring months or years after the acute event. The ventricle wall bulges with systole, resulting in impaired pump function and a significant risk for dysrhythmias. Although rare, rupture may occur when the tension becomes too great.

Thromboembolism is found during postmortem examinations of many individuals who have died of MI. Thromboemboli may disseminate from debris and clots that collect inside dilated aneurysmal sacs or from the infarcted endocardium and travel to the pulmonary or systemic vascular systems. Pulmonary emboli also may result from the breaking loose of deep venous thrombi of the legs in individuals who are confined to bed (see the Thromboembolism section and Chapter 36). Early mobilization and prophylactic anticoagulation therapy are essential to reduce the incidence of this complication.

Several factors contribute to the risk of death during acute infarction or reduce the chances of long-term survival, despite the best possible treatment. They are (1) the degree of left ventricular dysfunction, (2) the degree of left ventricular ischemia, (3) the potential for ventricular dysrhythmias, and (4) the individual's age.

WHAT'S NEW?

The Broken Heart Syndrome

Episodes of extreme mental stress, like the loss of a loved one, have been linked to sudden onset of myocardial ischemia, arrhythmias, heart failure, shock, and even death. This has been called the *broken heart syndrome*. This phenomenon, now called *Takotsubo cardiomyopathy*, was first described in Japan in 1990, where it was found to occur most often in postmenopausal women at times of acute stress. Since then it has been found to occur in women and men of all ages, and many other stressful triggers have been identified such as earthquakes, lightning strikes, noncardiac surgery, seizures, trauma, anesthesia, and alcohol withdrawal to name just a few. Although the manifestations are variable, it has been found that many individuals have weakening and ballooning of the left ventricular apex during systole that begins within minutes to hours after the stressful episode. Although the pathophysiology is still being explored, catecholamines play an important role in the pathogenesis causing coronary artery spasm, coronary microvascular abnormalities, direct myocardial damage, and neurogenic myocardial stunning. Intracellular calcium overload, oxidative stress, and estrogen deficiency also are implicated. Postmenopausal women may be especially vulnerable because of estrogen deficiency–mediated effects on the microvasculature. On myocardial biopsy, most people have inflammation without necrosis. People with Takotsubo cardiomyopathy present clinically with the same symptoms as acute ST-elevation myocardial infarction (STEMI), including chest pain, dyspnea, ST-segment elevation, and moderately elevated cardiac biomarkers, such as troponins and brain natriuretic peptide. Echocardiography and MRI are often used to make the diagnosis, along with cardiac catheterization in selected individuals. The American Heart Association Criteria for the diagnosis describe transient dyskinesis of the left ventricle in the absence of acute coronary artery disease, acute head trauma, myocarditis, or other forms of cardiomyopathy. Management usually includes aspirin, beta-blockers, angiotensin-converting enzyme inhibitors, and statins, although targeted emotional support and standard psychologic counseling have the greatest effect on recovery and reducing the risk for recurrence. An interprofessional team that includes a social worker, pastor, and mental health care providers has been found beneficial for those suffering from this cardiomyopathy. While many individuals recover without complication, recent population studies indicate that there is significant mortality with 30-day and 1-year mortality rates of 2.5% and 6.9%, respectively, in the United States.

Data from Akashi YJ, Nef HM, Lyon AR: *Nat Rev Cardiol* 12(7):387–397, 2015; Dastidar AG et al: *Heart Fail Rev* 20(4):415–421, 2015; Madias JE: *Int J Cardiol* 188:19-21, 2015; Peters S: *Int J Cardiol* 218:284, 2016; Stiermaier T, Thiele H, Eitel I: *JACC Heart Fail* 4(6):519–520, 2016; Yoshikawa T: *Int J Cardiol* 182.297–303, 2015.

DISORDERS OF THE HEART WALL

Disorders of the Pericardium

Pericardial disease is often a manifestation of another disorder, such as infection (bacterial, viral, fungal, rickettsial, parasitic); trauma or surgery; neoplasm; or a metabolic, immunologic, or vascular disorder (uremia, rheumatoid arthritis, systemic lupus erythematosus, periarteritis nodosa). The pericardial response to injury from these diverse causes may consist of acute pericarditis, pericardial effusion, or constrictive pericarditis.

Acute Pericarditis

Acute pericarditis is acute inflammation of the pericardium. The etiology of acute pericarditis is most often idiopathic (autoimmune) or caused by viral infection. Other causes include MI, trauma, neoplasm, surgery, uremia, bacterial infection (especially tuberculosis), connective tissue disease (especially systemic lupus erythematosus and rheumatoid arthritis), or radiation therapy. The pericardial membranes become inflamed and roughened, and a pericardial effusion may develop that can be serous, purulent, or fibrinous (Fig. 33.24). Possible sequelae of pericarditis include recurrent pericarditis, pericardial constriction, and cardiac tamponade.

Symptoms may follow several days of fever and usually begin with the sudden onset of severe, retrosternal chest pain that worsens with respiratory movements and when assuming a recumbent position. The pain may radiate to the back as a result of irritation of the phrenic nerve (innervates the trapezius muscles) as it traverses the pericardium. Individuals with acute pericarditis also report dysphagia, restlessness, irritability, anxiety, weakness, and malaise.

Physical examination often discloses low-grade fever (<38°C) and sinus tachycardia. A friction rub—a scratchy, grating sound—may be heard at the cardiac apex and left sternal border and is caused by the roughened pericardial membranes rubbing against each other. Friction rubs are not always present and may be intermittently heard and transient. Serum measures of inflammation, such as hs-CRP, are elevated. Electrocardiographic changes may reflect inflammatory processes through PR-segment depression and diffuse ST-segment elevation without Q waves, and they may remain abnormal for days or even weeks. Ultrasound, CT scanning, and MRI may be used as diagnostic modalities. Acute

pericarditis requires at least two of the following four criteria for diagnosis: (1) chest pain characteristic of pericarditis, (2) pericardial rub, (3) characteristic electrocardiographic (ECG) changes, and (4) new or worsening pericardial effusion.

Treatment for uncomplicated acute pericarditis relies on the use of antiinflammatory medications. Combined nonsteroidal antiinflammatory medications and colchicine (prevents fibrosis) is a highly effective regimen.[139] The level of hs-CRP in the blood should be followed to determine resolution before discontinuation of treatment. Additional analgesics may be given to relieve pain. Exploring the underlying cause is important. If pericardial effusion develops, aspirating the excessive fluid may be necessary.

Pericardial Effusion

Pericardial effusion, the accumulation of fluid in the pericardial cavity, can occur in all forms of pericarditis. Most are idiopathic (20%) but other causes, such as neoplasm and infection, must be considered. The fluid may be a transudate, such as the serous effusion that develops with left heart failure, overhydration, or hypoproteinemia. More often, however, the fluid is an exudate, which indicates pericardial inflammation like that seen with acute pericarditis, heart surgery, chemotherapeutic agents, infections, and autoimmune disorders, such as systemic lupus erythematosus. (Types of exudate are described in Chapter 7.) If the fluid is serosanguineous, the underlying cause is likely to be tuberculosis, neoplasm, uremia, or radiation. Effusions of frank blood are generally related to aneurysms, trauma, or coagulation defects. If chyle leaks from the thoracic duct, it may enter the pericardium and lead to cholesterol pericarditis.

Pericardial effusion may create sufficient pressure to cause cardiac compression, which is a serious condition known as tamponade. If an effusion develops gradually, the pericardium can stretch to accommodate large quantities of fluid without compressing the heart. If the fluid accumulates rapidly, however, even a small amount (50 to 100 mL) may cause serious tamponade. The danger is that pressure exerted by the pericardial fluid will eventually equal diastolic pressure within the heart chambers, which will interfere with right atrial filling during diastole. This causes increased venous pressure, systemic venous congestion, and signs and symptoms of right heart failure (distention of the jugular veins, edema, hepatomegaly). Decreased atrial filling leads to decreased ventricular filling, decreased stroke volume, and reduced cardiac output.

Individuals with cardiac tamponade most often present with dyspnea, tachycardia, jugular venous distention, cardiomegaly, and pulsus paradoxus. Pulsus paradoxus means that the arterial blood pressure during expiration exceeds the arterial pressure during inspiration by more than 10 mmHg. This clinical finding reflects impairment of diastolic filling of the left ventricle plus reduction of blood volume within all four cardiac chambers. Other clinical manifestations of pericardial effusion are distant or muffled heart sounds, poorly palpable apical pulse, dyspnea on exertion, and dull chest pain. A chest x-ray may disclose a "water-bottle" configuration of the cardiac silhouette. An echocardiogram can detect an effusion as small as 20 mL and is considered the most accurate and reliable method of diagnosis, although CT or MRI also are used.[140]

Treatment of pericardial effusion or tamponade generally consists of pericardiocentesis (aspiration of excessive pericardial fluid). Pericardiocentesis is diagnostic and therapeutic: the fluid is analyzed to identify the cause of the effusion, and its removal alone may bring dramatic relief from symptoms. Removal of large amounts of fluid may be associated with pericardial decompression syndrome, a potentially fatal condition complicated by pulmonary edema and cardiovascular shock.[141] Persistent pain may be treated with analgesics, antiinflammatory medications, or

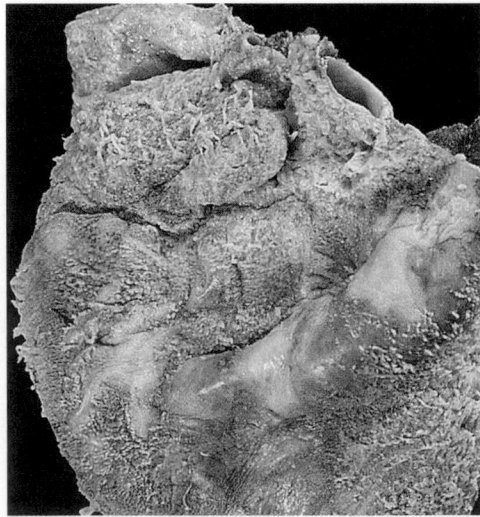

FIGURE 33.24 Acute Pericarditis. Note shaggy coat of fibers covering surface of heart. (From Damjanov I, Linder J: *Pathology: a color atlas*, St Louis, 2000, Mosby.)

steroids. Surgery may be required if the underlying cause of tamponade is trauma or aneurysm. If an effusion is neoplasm induced, sclerosing agents may be injected into the pericardial space. Recurrent pericardial effusions may require surgical creation of a pericardial "window" that allows for continual drainage and prevents tamponade.

Constrictive Pericarditis

Constrictive pericarditis, or restrictive pericarditis (chronic pericarditis), was once synonymous with tuberculosis. In the United States this form of pericardial disease is more often idiopathic or associated with radiation exposure, heart surgery (including transplantation), acute pericarditis, rheumatologic disease, trauma, or malignancy.[142] In constrictive pericarditis, fibrous scarring with occasional calcification of the pericardium causes the visceral and parietal pericardial layers to adhere, obliterating the pericardial cavity. The fibrotic lesions encase the heart in a rigid shell (Fig. 33.25). Like tamponade, constrictive pericarditis compresses the heart, which impairs ventricular relaxation during diastole, reduces ventricular filling, and eventually reduces cardiac output.

Because the onset of constrictive pericarditis is gradual, clinical manifestations develop slowly. Symptoms include exercise intolerance, dyspnea on exertion, fatigue, and anorexia. Approximately two-thirds of individuals present with heart failure.[142] Clinical assessment shows edema, jugular vein distention, and hepatic congestion. Restricted ventricular filling may cause a pericardial knock (early diastolic sound). ECG findings include T-wave inversions and atrial fibrillation. Chest x-ray often discloses prominent pulmonary vessels and calcification of the pericardium. CT, MRI, and transesophageal echocardiography (TEE) are used to detect pericardial thickening and constriction. Pericardial biopsy may be needed to determine the etiology.

Initial treatment for chronic constrictive pericarditis consists of dietary sodium restriction and diuretics. Management also may include use of antiinflammatory drugs and treatment of any underlying disorder. If these modalities are not successful, surgical excision of the restrictive pericardium (pericardiectomy) is indicated.[142]

Disorders of the Myocardium: The Cardiomyopathies

The cardiomyopathies are a diverse group of diseases that affect the myocardium. Most are the result of remodeling caused by the effect of the neurohumoral responses to ischemic heart disease or hypertension on the heart muscle. Cardiomyopathies also can be secondary to inherited disorders, infectious disease, exposure to toxins, systemic connective tissue disease, infiltrative and proliferative disorders, or nutritional deficiencies. Many cases of cardiomyopathy are idiopathic. The cardiomyopathies are categorized as dilated, hypertrophic, or restrictive depending on their tissue characteristics, genomics, and hemodynamic effects (Fig. 33.26 and Table 33.5). An individual may display characteristics of more than one type.

Dilated Cardiomyopathy

Dilated cardiomyopathy is usually the result of ischemic heart disease, valvular disease, diabetes, renal failure, alcohol or drug toxicity, hyperthyroidism, nutritional deficiencies (niacin, vitamin D, and selenium), or infection. Peripartum cardiomyopathy occurs in previously healthy women in the final month of pregnancy and up to 5 months after delivery and can lead to shock.[143] Dilated cardiomyopathy also can be associated with inherited disorders.[144,145] This form of cardiomyopathy is characterized by impaired systolic function leading to increases in

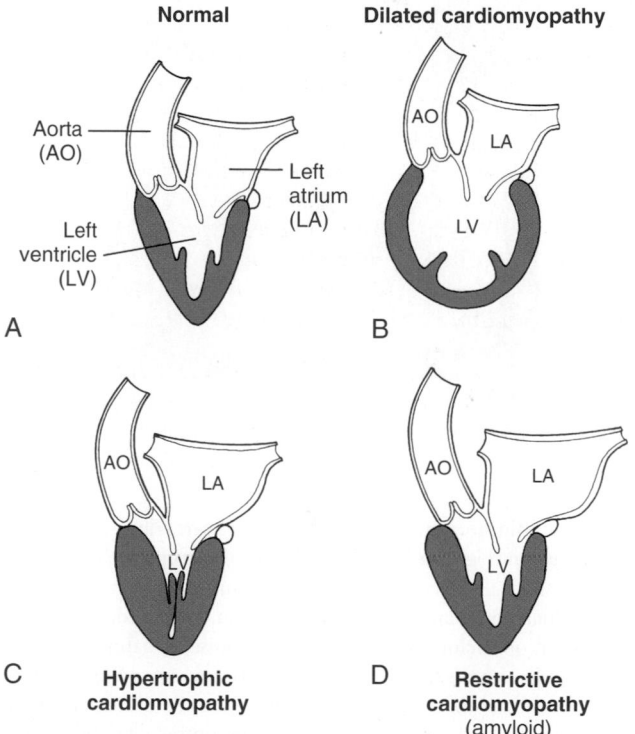

FIGURE 33.26 Diagram Showing Major Distinguishing Pathophysiologic Features of the Types of Cardiomyopathy. **A,** The normal heart. **B,** In the dilated type of cardiomyopathy, the heart has a globular shape, and the largest circumference of the left ventricle is not at its base but midway between apex and base. **C,** In the hypertrophic type of cardiomyopathy, the wall of the left ventricle is greatly thickened; the left ventricular cavity is small, but the left atrium may be dilated because of poor diastolic relaxation of the ventricle. **D,** In the restrictive type the left ventricular cavity is of normal size, but again, the left atrium is dilated because of the reduced diastolic compliance of the ventricle. (From Kissane JM, editor: *Anderson's pathology*, ed 9, St Louis, 1990, Mosby.)

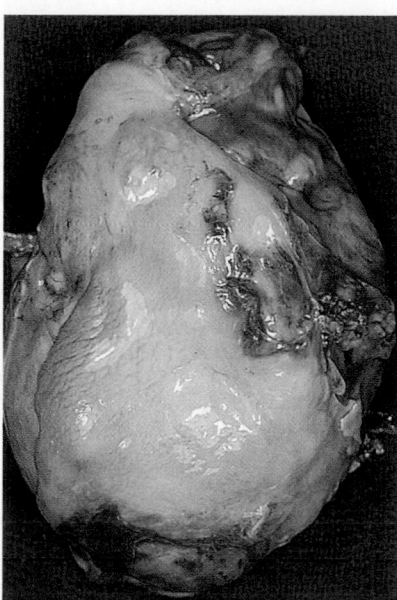

FIGURE 33.25 Constrictive Pericarditis. The fibrotic pericardium encases the heart in a rigid shell. (From Damjanov I, Linder J: *Pathology: a color atlas*, St Louis, 2000, Mosby.)

TABLE 33.5   PATHOPHYSIOLOGIC EFFECTS OF THE CARDIOMYOPATHIES

PATHOPHYSIOLOGY	TYPE OF CARDIOMYOPATHY		
	DILATED	HYPERTROPHIC	RESTRICTIVE
Associated conditions	Ischemic heart disease, alcoholism, pregnancy, infection, nutritional deficiency, exposure to toxins	Untreated hypertension and inherited defect of muscle growth and development	Infiltrative disease
Alterations of chamber volume	Volume increased	Volume decreased, particularly in left ventricle	Volume normal to decreased
Alterations of chamber compliance	Compliance increased	Compliance decreased, particularly in left ventricle	Compliance decreased, particularly in left ventricle
Alterations of myocardial contractility	Contractility decreased in left ventricle	Contractility normal	None
Dysrhythmias	Sinoatrial tachycardia; atrial and ventricular dysrhythmias	Atrial and ventricular dysrhythmias	Tachydysrhythmias
Eventual cardiovascular event	Left heart failure	Left heart failure	Right heart failure

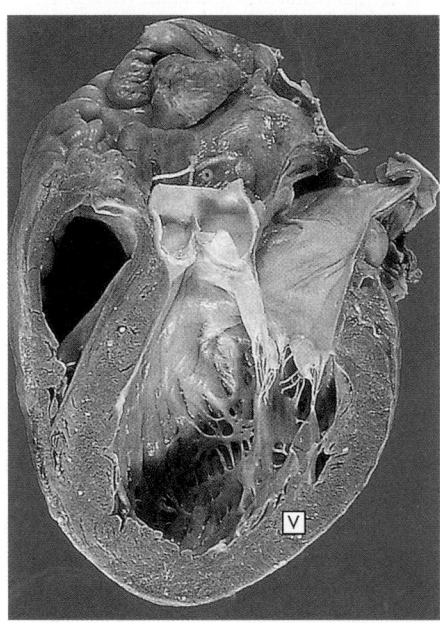

FIGURE 33.27 Dilated Cardiomyopathy. The dilated left ventricle has a thin wall *(V)*. (From Stevens A, Lowe JS, Scott I: *Core pathology*, ed 3, London, 2009, Mosby.)

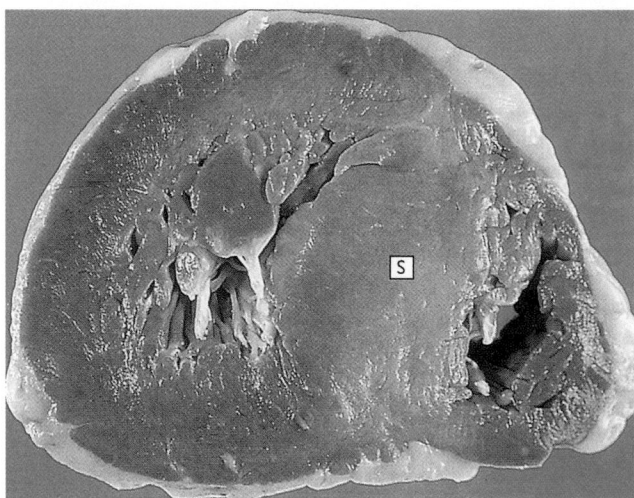

FIGURE 33.28 Hypertrophic Cardiomyopathy. There is marked left ventricular hypertrophy. This often affects the septum *(S)*. (From Stevens A, Lowe JS, Scott I: *Core pathology*, ed 3, London, 2009, Mosby.)

intracardiac volume, ventricular dilation, and heart failure with reduced ejection fraction (Fig. 33.27). Arrhythmias also are common. (Pathophysiologic effects of the cardiomyopathies are summarized in Table 33.5.)

Individuals complain of dyspnea, fatigue, and pedal edema. Findings on examination include a displaced apical pulse, S_3 gallop, peripheral edema, jugular venous distention, and pulmonary congestion. Diagnosis is confirmed by chest x-ray and echocardiogram, and management is focused on reducing blood volume, increasing contractility, and reversing the underlying disorder if possible.[146] Heart transplant is required in severe cases.

Hypertrophic Cardiomyopathy

Hypertrophic cardiomyopathy refers to two major categories of thickening of the myocardium: (1) hypertrophic obstructive cardiomyopathy (asymmetrical septal hypertrophic cardiomyopathy or idiopathic hypertrophic subaortic stenosis [IHSS]) and (2) hypertensive or valvular hypertrophic cardiomyopathy. These two categories are very different in their etiology, pathophysiology, and clinical presentation.

Hypertrophic obstructive cardiomyopathy is the most common inherited heart defect associated with left ventricular hypertrophy, occurring in 1 of 500 individuals through autosomal dominant inheritance.[147,148] It is characterized by thickening of the septal wall (Fig. 33.28), which may cause outflow obstruction to the left ventricle outflow tract. Additional changes include abnormalities of collagen deposition and altered contractile proteins in the myocytes. The thickening of the septum results in a hyperdynamic state, especially with exercise. Obstruction of left ventricular outflow can occur when heart rate is increased and intravascular volume is decreased. Individuals complain of angina, syncope, palpitations, and symptoms of MI and left heart failure. Sudden death may occur. Examination may reveal extra heart sounds and murmurs. Echocardiography and MRI are used to confirm the diagnosis and determine the best therapeutic approach.[149] Management includes beta-blockers to slow the heart rate, ACE inhibitors to reverse hypertrophic changes, and surgical resection or ablation of the hypertrophied myocardium.[148] Placement of an implantable cardioverter-defibrillator significantly decreases the risk of arrhythmia-related sudden death.[150]

Hypertensive or valvular hypertrophic cardiomyopathy occurs because of increased resistance to ventricular ejection; it is commonly seen in hypertension or in valvular stenosis (usually aortic). In this case, hypertrophy of the myocytes is an attempt to compensate for increased myocardial workload. Long-term dysfunction of the myocytes develops over time, with first diastolic dysfunction leading eventually to systolic dysfunction of the ventricle (see Heart Failure). Individuals with hypertrophic cardiomyopathy may be asymptomatic or may complain of angina, syncope, dyspnea on exertion, and palpitations. Examination may reveal extra heart sounds and murmurs. Echocardiography and cardiac catheterization can confirm the diagnosis.

Restrictive Cardiomyopathies

Restrictive cardiomyopathy is characterized by restrictive filling and reduced diastolic volume of either or both ventricles with normal or near-normal systolic function and wall thickness. It may occur idiopathically or as a cardiac manifestation of systemic diseases, such as scleroderma, amyloidosis, sarcoidosis, lymphoma, and hemochromatosis, or a number of inherited storage diseases. The myocardium becomes rigid and noncompliant, impeding ventricular filling and raising filling pressures during diastole. The overall clinical and hemodynamic picture mimics and may be confused with that of constrictive pericarditis.

The most common clinical manifestation of restrictive cardiomyopathy is right heart failure with systemic venous congestion. Cardiomegaly and dysrhythmias are common. A thorough evaluation for the underlying cause should be initiated (and may include myocardial biopsy). Treatment is aimed at the underlying cause; however, many individuals require placement of left ventricular assist devices (LVADs) followed by heart transplantation.[151]

Disorders of the Endocardium
Valvular Dysfunction

Disorders of the endocardium (the innermost lining of the heart wall) damage the heart valves, which are made up of endocardial tissue. Endocardial damage can be either congenital or acquired. Congenital valvular disease is discussed in Chapter 34. The acquired forms result from inflammatory, ischemic, traumatic, degenerative, or infectious alterations of valvular structure and function. Structural alterations of the heart valves result from remodeling changes in the valvular extracellular matrix and lead to stenosis, regurgitation, or both. Although all four heart valves may be affected, those of the left heart (mitral and aortic valves) are more commonly affected than those of the right heart (tricuspid and pulmonic valves).

In **valvular stenosis** the valve orifice is constricted and narrowed, impeding the forward flow of blood and increasing the workload of the cardiac chamber proximal to the diseased valve (Fig. 33.29). Intraventricular or atrial pressure increases in the chamber to overcome resistance to flow through the valve. Increased pressure causes the myocardium to work harder, causing myocardial hypertrophy. In **valvular regurgitation** (also called *insufficiency* or *incompetence*) the valve leaflets, or cusps, fail to shut completely, permitting blood flow to continue even when the valve is supposed to be closed (see Fig. 33.29). During systole or diastole some blood leaks back into the chamber proximal to the incompetent valve, producing a murmur on auscultation. Valvular regurgitation increases the volume of blood the heart must pump and increases the workload of the affected heart chamber. Increased volume leads to chamber dilation, and increased workload leads to hypertrophy.

Valvular dysfunction stimulates chamber dilation and/or myocardial hypertrophy, both of which are compensatory mechanisms intended to increase the pumping capability of the heart. Eventually, myocardial contractility is diminished, the ejection fraction is reduced, diastolic pressure increases, and the affected heart chamber fails from overload. Depending on the severity of the valvular dysfunction and the capacity of

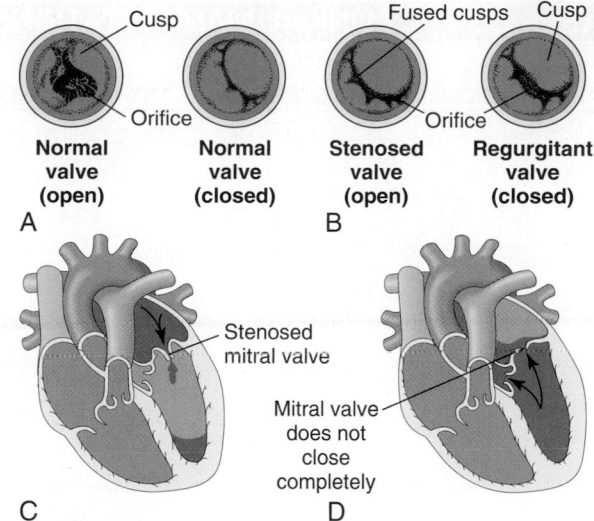

FIGURE 33.29 Valvular Stenosis and Regurgitation. **A,** Normal position of the valve leaflets, or cusps, when the valve is open and closed. **B,** Open position of a stenosed valve *(left)* and open position of a closed regurgitant valve *(right)*. **C,** Hemodynamic effect of mitral stenosis. The stenosed valve is unable to open sufficiently during left atrial systole, inhibiting left ventricular filling. **D,** Hemodynamic effect of mitral regurgitation. The mitral valve does not close completely during left ventricular systole, permitting blood to reenter the left atrium.

the heart to compensate, valvular alterations cause a range of symptoms and some degree of incapacitation (Table 33.6). In general, valvular disease is diagnosed by transthoracic echocardiography (TTE), which can be used to assess the severity of valvular obstruction or regurgitation before the onset of symptoms. CT or MRI may be indicated in certain settings. Valvular lesions are staged using four general categories: (1) at risk, (2) progressive, (3) asymptomatic severe, and (4) symptomatic severe, which determine the appropriate management. Management almost always includes careful medical management, valvular repair, or valve replacement followed by long-term anticoagulation therapy and prophylaxis for endocarditis as needed.[152] The purpose of valvular intervention is to improve symptoms and prolong survival, as well as to minimize complications such as asymptomatic irreversible ventricular dysfunction, pulmonary hypertension, stroke, and atrial fibrillation (AF).[152]

Stenosis

Aortic Stenosis. Aortic stenosis (AS) is the most common valvular abnormality, affecting approximately 5% of adults older than 75 years.[153] The three common causes are (1) calcific degeneration related to aging (aortic sclerosis), (2) congenital bicuspid valve, and (3) inflammatory damage caused by rheumatic heart disease (RHD). Aortic sclerosis affects up to 40% of those older than age 75 with about 2% per year progressing to hemodynamically significant AS, whereas congenital bicuspid aortic valve occurs in 0.5% to 0.8% of the population.[153] RHD is a less frequent cause of AS.

The pathophysiology of AS is complex and numerous gene abnormalities have been implicated, including polymorphisms of genes that code for LDL.[5] AS results from lipoprotein deposition in the valve tissue with chronic inflammation and leaflet calcification. Autoimmunity disorders in calcium transport, apoptosis of endocardial cells, and decreased nitric oxide synthesis have been implicated.[154,135] In AS from any cause, the orifice of the aortic semilunar valve narrows, causing diminished blood flow from the left ventricle into the aorta (Fig. 33.30). Outflow obstruction increases pressure within the left ventricle as it tries to eject blood through the narrowed opening. Left ventricular

TABLE 33.6   CLINICAL MANIFESTATIONS OF VALVULAR STENOSIS AND REGURGITATION

MANIFESTATION	AORTIC STENOSIS	MITRAL STENOSIS	AORTIC REGURGITATION	MITRAL REGURGITATION	TRICUSPID REGURGITATION
Most common cause	Congenital bicuspid valve, degenerative (calcification) changes with aging, rheumatic fever	Rheumatic heart disease	Infective endocarditis; aortic root disease (connective tissue diseases, Marfan syndrome); dilation of the aortic root due to hypertension and aging	Myxomatous degeneration (mitral valve prolapse)	Congenital
Cardiovascular outcome (untreated)	Left ventricular hypertrophy followed by left heart failure; decreased coronary blood flow with myocardial ischemia	Left atrial hypertrophy and dilation with fibrillation, followed by right ventricular failure	Left ventricular hypertrophy and dilation, followed by heart failure	Left atrial hypertrophy and dilation, followed by left heart failure	Right heart failure
Pulmonary effects	Pulmonary edema: dyspnea on exertion	Pulmonary edema: dyspnea on exertion, orthopnea, paroxysmal, nocturnal dyspnea, predisposition to respiratory infections, hemoptysis, pulmonary hypertension, and edema	Pulmonary edema with dyspnea on exertion	Pulmonary edema with dyspnea on exertion	Dyspnea
Central nervous system effects	Syncope, especially on exertion	Neural deficits only associated with emboli (e.g., hemiparesis)	Syncope	None	None
Pain	Angina pectoris	Atypical chest pain	Angina pectoris	Atypical chest pain	Palpitations
Heart sounds	Systolic murmur heard best at the right parasternal second intercostal space and radiating to the neck	Low rumbling diastolic murmur heard best at the apex and radiating to the axilla, accentuated first heart sound, opening snap	Diastolic murmur heard best at the right parasternal second intercostal space and radiating to the neck	Murmur throughout systole heard best at the apex and radiating to the axilla	Murmur throughout systole heard best at the left lower sternal border

Data from Braunwald E, editor: *Heart disease: a textbook of cardiovascular medicine,* ed 7, Philadelphia, 2005, Saunders; Carabello BA, Paulus WJ: Valvular heart disease. In Crawford MH, DiMarco JP, editors: *Cardiology,* London, 2001, Mosby-Wolfe.

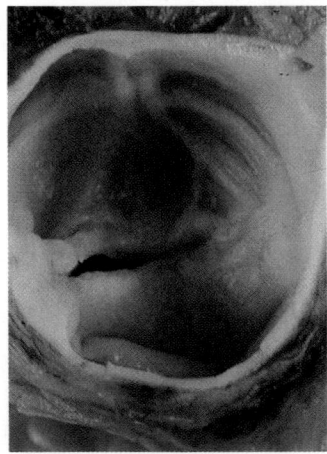

FIGURE 33.30 Aortic Stenosis. Mild stenosis in valve leaflets of a young adult. (From Damjanov I, Linder J: *Pathology: a color atlas,* St Louis, 2000, Mosby.)

hypertrophy develops to compensate for the increased workload.[156] Eventually hypertrophy increases myocardial oxygen demand that the coronary arteries may not be able to supply. If this occurs, ischemia may cause attacks of angina. Untreated aortic stenosis can lead to dysrhythmias, myocardial infarction, and heart failure.

Aortic stenosis tends to develop gradually. The classic manifestations of aortic stenosis are angina, syncope, and heart failure. Clinical manifestations include decreased stroke volume, reduced systolic blood pressure, and narrowed pulse pressure (difference between systolic and diastolic pressure). Heart rate is often slow, and pulses are faint. Resistance to flow through the stenotic valve gives rise to a crescendo-decrescendo systolic heart murmur heard best at the second intercostal space and may radiate to the neck. Echocardiography is used to follow valve orifice and cardiac functioning. Medical management with careful monitoring for complications, such as heart failure and myocardial ischemia, may be indicated for selected individuals. Surgical valve replacement with either a mechanical or a bioprosthetic valve is indicated for both symptomatic and asymptomatic individuals with severe stenosis.[152,154] Transcatheter aortic valve replacement (TAVR) is used increasingly to avoid major heart surgery in selected individuals.[157] The prognosis is poor once an individual becomes symptomatic from aortic stenosis.[154]

Mitral Stenosis. Mitral stenosis impairs the flow of blood from the left atrium to the left ventricle. Mitral stenosis is the most common form of rheumatic heart disease (see the Acute Rheumatic Fever and Rheumatic Heart Disease section). Autoimmune activation of lymphocytes and macrophages leads to inflammatory damage and subsequent scarring of the valve leaflets.[158] Scarring causes the leaflets to become fibrous and fused, and the chordae tendineae cordis becomes shortened (Fig. 33.31). Impedance to blood flow results in incomplete emptying

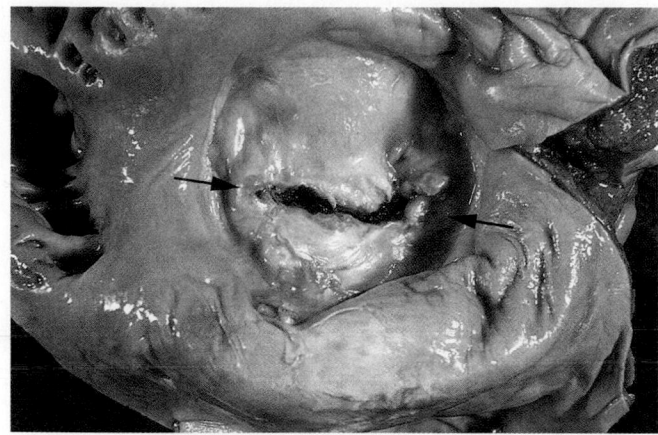

FIGURE 33.31 Mitral Stenosis with Classic "Fish Mouth" *(Arrows)* Orifice. (From Kumar V et al: *Robbins & Cotran pathologic basis of disease*, ed 9, St Louis, 2015, Elsevier.)

of the left atrium and elevated atrial pressure as the chamber tries to force blood through the stenotic valve. Continued increases in left atrial volume and pressure cause chamber dilation and hypertrophy and eventually result in pulmonary hypertension. The outcomes of untreated chronic mitral stenosis are pulmonary hypertension and right ventricular failure. The risk of developing atrial dysrhythmias (especially fibrillation) and dysrhythmia-induced thrombi is high.

Clinical manifestations depend on the size of the valvular orifice. As mitral stenosis progresses, symptoms of decreased cardiac output occur, especially during exertion. Blood flow through the stenotic valve gives rise to a rumbling decrescendo diastolic murmur heard best over the cardiac apex and radiating to the left axilla. If the mitral valve is forced open during diastole, it may make a sharp noise called an *opening snap*. The first heart sound (S_1) is often accentuated and somewhat delayed because of increased left atrial pressure. Other signs and symptoms, such as jugular venous distension and peripheral edema, result from pulmonary congestion and right heart failure. Atrial enlargement is demonstrated by chest x-rays and electrocardiography. Mitral stenosis can often be repaired with percutaneous balloon commissurotomy, but valve replacement may be required in advanced cases.[152] New minimally invasive procedures for mitral valve replacement are being explored, including percutaneous transcatheter techniques.[159]

Regurgitation

Aortic Regurgitation. Aortic regurgitation results from an inability of the aortic valve leaflets to close properly during ventricular diastole, resulting from abnormalities of the leaflets or the aortic root, or both. It can be primary, caused by congenital bicuspid valve disease or degeneration or secondary, caused by chronic hypertension, rheumatic heart disease, bacterial endocarditis, syphilis, connective tissue disorders (e.g., Marfan syndrome and ankylosing spondylitis), appetite-suppressing medications, trauma, or atherosclerosis. More than one-third of cases of aortic regurgitation are idiopathic. The hemodynamic repercussions depend on the size of the "leak." During systole, blood is ejected from the left ventricle into the aorta. During diastole, some of the ejected blood flows back into the left ventricle through the leaking valve. Volume overload occurs in the ventricle because it receives blood from the left atrium and the aorta during diastole. As the end-diastolic volume of the left ventricle increases, myocardial fibers stretch to accommodate the extra fluid. Compensatory dilation permits the left ventricle to increase its stroke volume and maintain cardiac output. Ventricular hypertrophy also occurs as an adaptation to the increased volume and

increased afterload created by the high stroke volume and resultant systolic hypertension. Ventricular dilation and hypertrophy eventually cease to compensate for aortic incompetence, and heart failure develops.

Clinical manifestations include widened pulse pressure resulting from increased stroke volume and diastolic backflow. Turbulence across the aortic valve produces a diastolic decrescendo murmur heard best in the second, third, or fourth intercostal spaces parasternally and may radiate to the neck. Large stroke volume and rapid runoff of blood from the aorta cause prominent carotid pulsations and bounding peripheral pulses (Corrigan pulse). Other symptoms are usually associated with heart failure that occurs when the ventricle can no longer pump adequately. Dysrhythmias and endocarditis are common complications of aortic regurgitation. The severity of regurgitation can be estimated by echocardiography, and surgical or transcatheter valve replacement may be delayed for many years through careful use of vasodilators and inotropic agents.[152,160]

Mitral Regurgitation. Mitral regurgitation occurs in approximately 1.7% of the U.S. population.[5] It can be primary because of mitral valve prolapse, rheumatic heart disease, infective endocarditis, MI, connective tissue diseases (Marfan syndrome), and dilated cardiomyopathy. It can also be secondary because of ischemic or nonischemic myocardial disease that damages the chordae tendineae or the mitral annulus.[152] Mitral regurgitation permits backflow of blood from the left ventricle into the left atrium during ventricular systole, giving rise to a loud pansystolic (throughout systole) murmur heard best at the apex that radiates into the back and axilla. The volume of backflow reentering the left atrium gradually increases, causing atrial dilation and associated atrial fibrillation. As the left atrium enlarges, the valve structures stretch and become deformed, leading to further backflow. The increased volume in the left atrium increases the volume that enters the ventricle; the left ventricle becomes dilated and hypertrophied to maintain adequate cardiac output. As mitral valve regurgitation progresses, left ventricular function may become impaired to the point of failure. Eventually, increased atrial pressure also causes pulmonary hypertension and failure of the right ventricle. Mitral incompetence is usually well tolerated—often for years—until ventricular failure occurs. Most clinical manifestations are caused by heart failure. The severity of regurgitation can be estimated by echocardiography, and surgical repair or valve replacement may become necessary.[152,161] In acute mitral regurgitation caused by MI, surgical repair or replacement must be done emergently.[162]

Tricuspid Regurgitation. Tricuspid regurgitation is more common than tricuspid stenosis and usually is associated with dilation and failure of the right ventricle secondary to pulmonary hypertension. Rheumatic heart disease and infective endocarditis are less common causes. Tricuspid valve incompetence leads to volume overload in the right atrium and ventricle, increased systemic venous blood pressure, and right heart failure. Pulmonic valve dysfunction can have the same consequences as tricuspid valve dysfunction.

Mitral Valve Prolapse Syndrome. Mitral valve prolapse syndrome is a condition in which the anterior and posterior cusps of the mitral valve billow upward (prolapse) into the atrium during systole (Fig. 33.32). To maintain competency, the mitral valve must be supported by what is called the *mitral valve complex*, which includes the annulus, leaflets, chordae tendineae, papillary muscles, and the left ventricular wall; dysfunction of any of these elements can lead to prolapse of the valve.[163] The most common cause of mitral valve prolapse is myxomatous degeneration of the leaflets in which the cusps are redundant, thickened, and scalloped because of changes in tissue proteoglycans, increased proteinases, and infiltration by myofibroblasts. The chordae tendineae may be elongated, permitting the valve cusps to stretch upward. Mitral

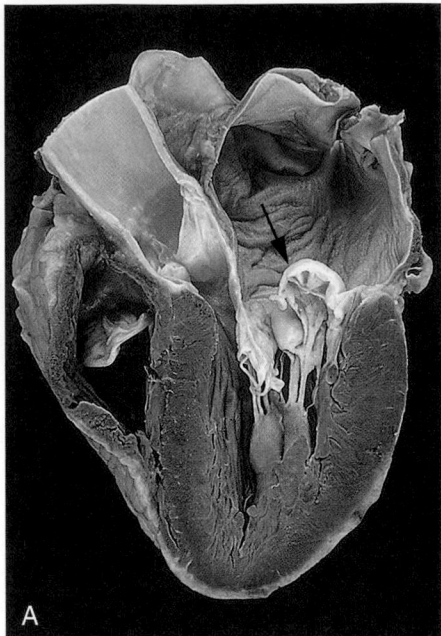
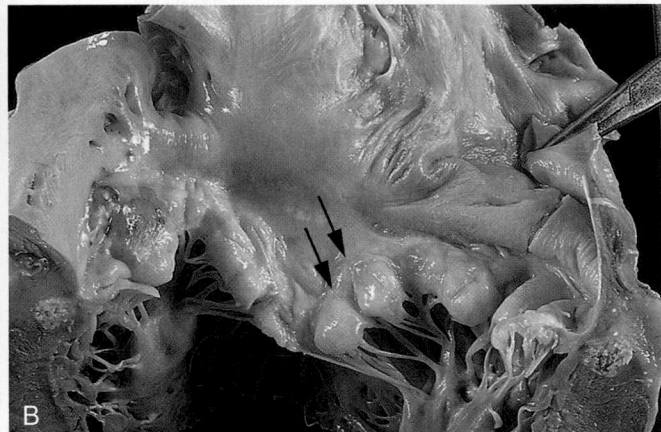

FIGURE 33.32 Mitral Valve Prolapse. **A,** Prolapsed mitral valve. Prolapse permits the valve leaflets to billow back *(arrow)* into the atrium during left ventricular systole. The billowing causes the leaflets to part slightly, permitting regurgitation into the atrium. **B,** Looking down into the mitral valve, the ballooning *(arrows)* of the leaflets is seen. (From Kumar V et al: *Robbins & Cotran pathologic basis of disease,* ed 9, St Louis, 2015, Mosby.)

regurgitation occurs if the ballooning valve permits blood to leak into the atrium.

Mitral valve prolapse (MVP) is the most common valve disorder in the United States, with a prevalence estimated at 3%. MVP tends to be most prevalent in young women. Genetic studies suggest several candidate genes that influence cardiac fibroblast and endothelial cell function.[164] Because mitral valve prolapse often is associated with other inherited connective tissue disorders (Marfan syndrome, Ehlers-Danlos syndrome, osteogenesis imperfecta), it is thought to result from a genetic or environmental disruption of valvular development during the fifth or sixth week of gestation. There may be a relationship between symptomatic mitral valve prolapse and hyperthyroidism.

Many cases of mitral valve prolapse are completely asymptomatic. Cardiac auscultation on routine physical examination may disclose a regurgitant murmur or midsystolic click in an otherwise healthy individual. Echocardiography may demonstrate the condition in the absence of auscultatory findings. Symptomatic mitral valve prolapse can cause palpitations related to dysrhythmias, tachycardia, lightheadedness, syncope, fatigue (especially in the morning), lethargy, weakness, dyspnea, chest tightness, hyperventilation, anxiety, depression, panic attacks, and atypical chest pain. Many symptoms are vague and puzzling and are unrelated to the degree of prolapse. Most individuals with mitral valve prolapse have an excellent prognosis, do not develop symptoms, and do not require any restriction in activity or medical management. Occasionally, beta-blockers are needed to alleviate syncope, severe chest pain, or palpitations. Surgical repair is only necessary if significant mitral regurgitation develops.

Acute Rheumatic Fever and Rheumatic Heart Disease

Rheumatic fever is a systemic, inflammatory disease caused by an immune and inflammatory response to infection by group A beta-hemolytic streptococci in genetically predisposed individuals.[165] In its acute form, rheumatic fever is a febrile illness that occurs approximately 2 to 3 weeks after infection and is characterized by inflammation of the joints, skin, nervous system, and heart. If untreated, rheumatic fever can cause scarring and deformity of cardiac structures resulting in rheumatic heart disease (RHD).

The incidence of acute rheumatic fever declined in the United States during the 1960s, 1970s, and early 1980s because of medical and socioeconomic improvements, as well as changes in the virulence of group A streptococci.[153] It occurs most often in children between 5 and 15 years of age. Appropriate antibiotic therapy given within the first 9 days of infection usually prevents rheumatic fever. Individuals who have experienced one attack of acute rheumatic fever are more susceptible to recurrent attacks.

PATHOPHYSIOLOGY. Acute rheumatic fever can develop *only* as a sequela to pharyngeal infection by group A beta-hemolytic streptococci. Streptococcal skin infections do not progress to acute rheumatic fever because the strains of the microorganism that infect the skin do not have the same antigenic molecules in their cell membranes as do those that cause pharyngitis and therefore do not elicit the same kind of immune response. Acute rheumatic fever is the result of an abnormal humoral and cell-mediated immune response to the M proteins on the microorganisms that cross-react with normal tissues (Fig. 33.33). Antibodies against streptococci bacterial antigens display cross-reactivity against laminin, a protein present in extracellular tissues around heart cells and in the valves. Cardiac myosin and vimentin are other target antigens.[153]

Autoimmunity and associated intense inflammation result in diffuse, proliferative, and exudative lesions in the connective tissues, especially in the heart, joints, and skin.[165] Repeated attacks of acute rheumatic fever cause chronic proliferative changes with resultant scarring, granulomas, and thromboses. Approximately 10% of cases of rheumatic fever develop RHD.[153] RHD begins as carditis, or inflammation of the

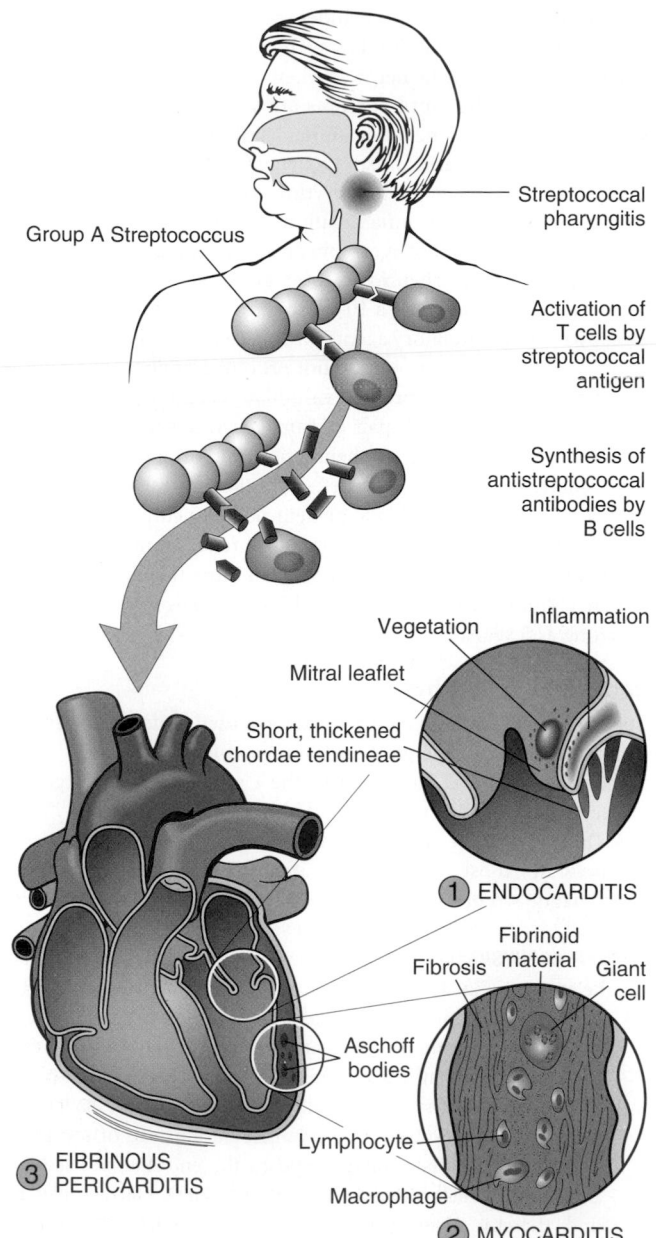

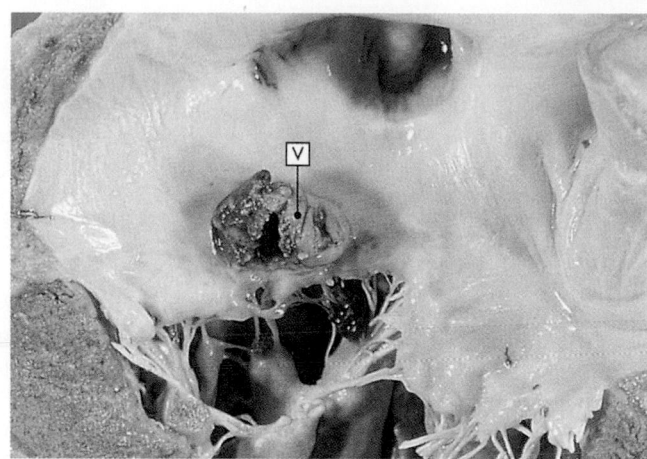

FIGURE 33.34 Valvular Vegetations in Mitral Stenosis. Mitral stenosis and clumps of vegetation *(V)* containing platelets and fibrin. Mitral leaflets are thickened and fused and have clumps of vegetation containing platelets and fibrin. (From Stevens A, Lowe JS, Scott I: *Core pathology,* ed 3, London, 2009, Mosby.)

FIGURE 33.33 Pathogenesis and Structural Alterations of Acute Rheumatic Heart Disease. Beginning usually with a sore throat, rheumatic fever can develop only as a sequela to pharyngeal infection by group A beta-hemolytic streptococcus. Suspected as a hypersensitivity reaction, it is proposed that antibodies directed against the M proteins of certain strains of streptococci cross-react with tissue glycoproteins in the heart, joints, and other tissues. The exact nature of cross-reacting antigens has been difficult to define, but it appears that the streptococcal infection causes an autoimmune response against self antigens. Inflammation is found in various sites including **(1)** endocardium, **(2)** myocardium, and **(3)** pericardium. The most distinctive inflammatory lesions within the heart are called *Aschoff bodies.* The chronic sequelae result from progressive fibrosis because of healing of the inflammatory lesions and the changes induced by valvular deformities. (From Damjanov I: *Pathology for the health professions,* ed 4, Philadelphia, 2012, Saunders.)

heart. Although rheumatic fever can cause carditis in all three layers of the heart wall (endocardium, myocardium, pericardium) (see Chapter 32, Fig. 32.2), the primary lesion usually involves the endocardium, which includes the heart valves. Endocardial inflammation causes swelling of the valve leaflets, with secondary erosion along the lines of leaflet

contact. Small beadlike clumps of vegetation containing platelets and fibrin are deposited on eroded valvular tissue and on the chordae tendineae (Fig. 33.34). The valves lose their elasticity, and the leaflets may adhere to each other. Scarring and shortening of the involved structures occur over time.

If inflammation penetrates the myocardium, localized fibrin deposits develop that are surrounded by areas of necrosis. These fibrinoid necrotic deposits are called *Aschoff bodies.* Pericardial inflammation is usually characterized by serofibrinous effusion within the pericardial cavity. Cardiomegaly and left heart failure may occur during episodes of untreated acute or recurrent rheumatic fever. Conduction defects and atrial fibrillation often are associated with rheumatic heart disease.

◆**CLINICAL MANIFESTATIONS.** The common symptoms of acute rheumatic fever are fever, lymphadenopathy, arthralgia, nausea, vomiting, epistaxis (nosebleed), abdominal pain, and tachycardia. The major clinical manifestations of acute rheumatic fever (carditis, acute migratory polyarthritis, subcutaneous nodules, chorea, and erythema marginatum) usually occur singly or in combination 1 to 5 weeks after streptococcal infection of the pharynx.

Carditis

Carditis occurs a few weeks after the initial infection in about 50% of patients with acute rheumatic fever with the mitral valve being the most affected structure.[165] Cardiac manifestations of acute rheumatic fever may be a previously undetected murmur caused by mitral or aortic valve dysfunction, chest pain, and pericardial rub caused by pericardial inflammation or unexplained cardiomegaly with heart failure.[166]

Polyarthritis

Acute migratory asymmetrical polyarthritis (inflammation of more than one joint) occurs in the majority of individuals with rheumatic fever, although a severe monoarthritis also is a presenting feature in high-risk populations.[165] Although all of the synovial joints may be involved, the large joints of the extremities are most often affected. Two or more joints are usually involved simultaneously or in succession, with each joint being symptomatic for approximately 2 to 3 days while the overall polyarthritis continues for up to 3 weeks. Exudative synovitis causes heat, redness, swelling, severe pain, and tenderness but no permanent disability.

Subcutaneous Nodules

Palpable subcutaneous nodes occur in less than 5% of cases of acute rheumatic fever.[165] They develop over bony prominences and along extensor tendons of elbows, wrists, knees, and ankles. They do not interfere with joint function and often go unnoticed.

Chorea

Sydenham chorea, or St. Vitus dance, is a disorder of the CNS characterized by sudden, aimless, irregular, involuntary movements. (Chorea is described in Chapter 17.) It affects up to 15% of people with rheumatic fever, and is the most common acquired chorea in children.[165] The chorea is self-limiting, although severe cases may require the use of dopamine receptor blockers and antiepileptic medications. It resolves within 1 to 6 months and has no permanent neural sequelae.

Erythema Marginatum

Erythema marginatum is an uncommon manifestation and presents as a distinctive truncal rash that often accompanies acute rheumatic fever. It consists of an annular erythema with the appearance of nonpruritic, pink, erythematous macules that spread outwards. The rash is transitory and may change in appearance within minutes or hours.

◆EVALUATION AND TREATMENT. The original Jones Criteria for the diagnosis of rheumatic fever have been updated by the American Heart Association[167] (Table 33.7). Supportive evidence for group A

beta-hemolytic streptococci includes positive throat cultures and measurement of serum antibodies against the hemolytic factor streptolysin O. Cultures may be negative when the rheumatic attack begins, however. Several other antibody tests are sensitive prognosticators of streptococcal infection, including antideoxyribonuclease B (anti-DNase B), antihyaluronidase, and antistreptozyme (ASTZ). Elevated measurements of white blood cell count, erythrocyte sedimentation rate, and C-reactive protein indicate inflammation. All three are usually increased at the time cardiac or joint symptoms begin to appear.

Therapy for acute rheumatic fever is aimed at eradicating the streptococcal infection using a 10-day regimen of antibiotics. NSAIDs are used as antiinflammatory agents for rheumatic carditis and arthritis and help relieve symptoms, but do not prevent complications. Serious carditis may require diuretics and vasodilators, and recovery can take up to 12 months. Surgical repair of damaged valves may be necessary in cases of chronic recurrent rheumatic fever or carditis. Persistent chorea requires psychosocial support, protection against falls and injury, and treatment with antiepileptic or neuroleptic medications. NSAIDs or paracetamol may provide symptomatic relief from arthralgias.[165] Because recurrent rheumatic fever occurs in more than half of affected children, continuous prophylactic antibiotic therapy may be necessary for as long as 5 years.

Infective Endocarditis

Infective endocarditis (IE) is a general term used to describe infection and inflammation of the endocardium, especially the cardiac valves. The incidence of IE is increasing in the United States, in large part because of the increase in the implantation of prosthetic valves[168] (Box 33.3). Bacteria are the most common cause of IE with *Staphylococcus aureus* the most common causative agent worldwide.[169] Other causes include streptococci, enterococci, viruses, fungi, rickettsia, and parasites.[168]

◆PATHOPHYSIOLOGY. The pathogenesis of IE requires at least three critical elements (Fig. 33.35):

1. Trauma, congenital heart disease, valvular heart disease, and the presence of prosthetic valves are the most common risk factors for endocardial damage that leads to IE. Turbulent blood caused by these abnormalities usually affects the atrial surface of atrioventricular valves or the ventricular surface of semilunar valves. Endocardial damage exposes the endothelial basement membrane, which contains a type of collagen that attracts platelets and thereby stimulates sterile thrombus formation on the membrane. This causes an inflammatory reaction (nonbacterial thrombotic endocarditis).

TABLE 33.7	MAJOR AND MINOR DIAGNOSTIC CRITERIA FOR ACUTE RHEUMATIC FEVER ACCORDING TO THE JONES CRITERIA
For all patient populations with evidence of preceding group A streptococcal infection: one major plus two minor manifestations	
MAJOR CRITERIA IN LOW-RISK POPULATIONS	**MAJOR CRITERIA IN MODERATE- AND HIGH-RISK POPULATIONS**
Carditis (clinical and/or subclinical)	Carditis (clinical and/or subclinical)
Arthritis (polyarthritis only)	Arthritis (monoarthritis or polyarthritis; polyarthralgia)
Chorea	Chorea
Erythema marginatum	Erythema marginatum
Subcutaneous nodules	Subcutaneous nodules
MINOR CRITERIA IN LOW-RISK POPULATIONS	**MINOR CRITERIA IN MODERATE- AND HIGH-RISK POPULATIONS**
Polyarthralgia	Monoarthralgia
Fever (≥38°C; 100.4°F)	Fever (≥38°C; 100.4°F)
ESR ≥60 mm/hr and/or CRP >3.0 mg/dL	ESR ≥30 mm/hr and/or CRP >3.0 mg/dL
Prolonged PR interval	Prolonged PR interval

CRP, C-reactive protein; ESR, erythrocyte sedimentation rate.
From Gewitz MH et al: *Circulation* 131:1806–1818, 2015.

BOX 33.3	RISK FACTORS FOR INFECTIVE ENDOCARDITIS

- Implantation of prosthetic heart valves
- Congenital lesions associated with highly turbulent flow (e.g., ventricular septal defect)
- Acquired valvular heart disease (especially mitral valve prolapse)
- Previous attack of infective endocarditis
- Intravenous drug use
- Long-term indwelling intravenous catheterization (e.g., for pressure monitoring, feeding, hemodialysis)
- Implantable cardiac pacemakers
- Heart transplant with defective valve

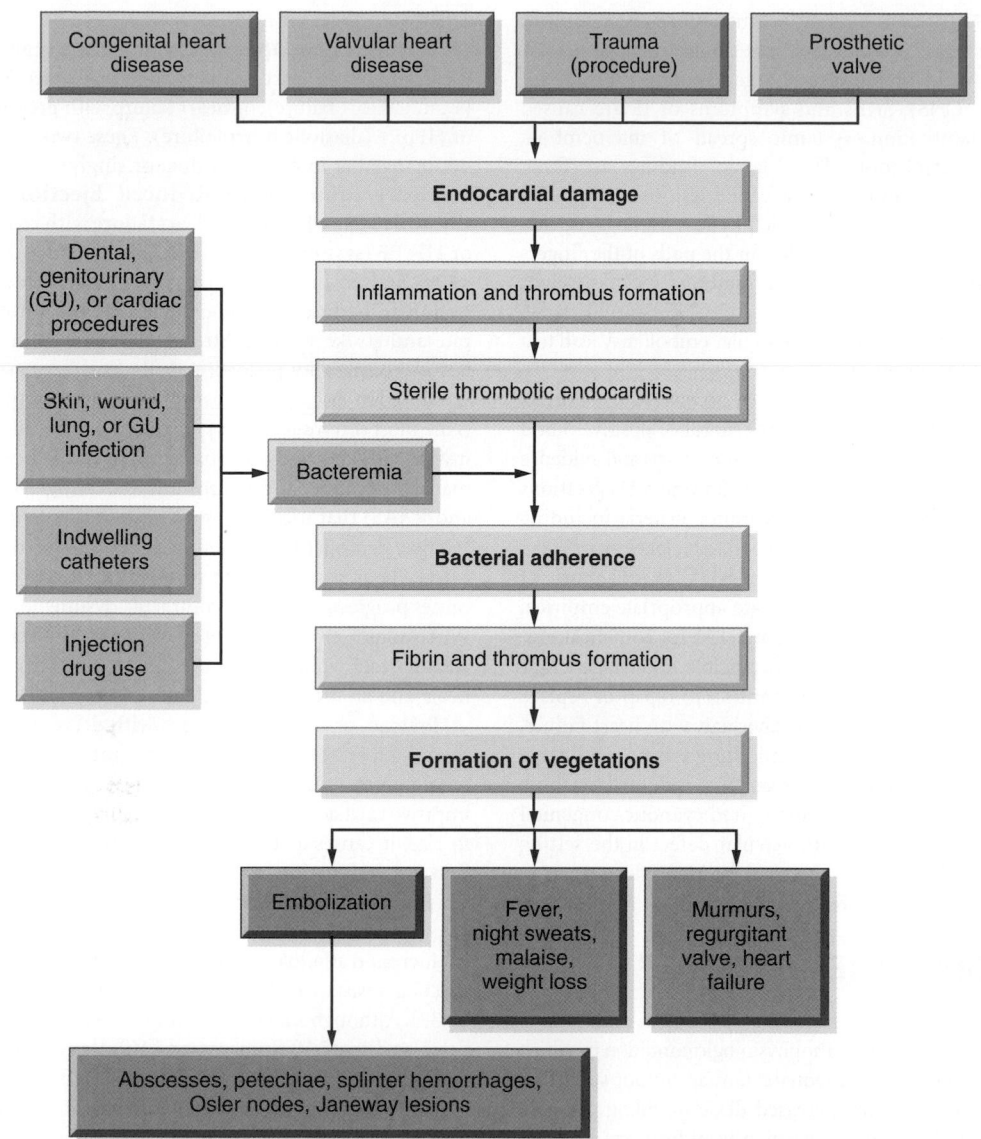

FIGURE 33.35 Pathogenesis of Infective Endocarditis.

2. Blood-borne microorganism adherence to the damaged endocardial surface. Bacteria may enter the bloodstream during injection drug use, trauma, dental procedures that involve manipulation of the gingiva, cardiac surgery, genitourinary procedures and indwelling catheters in the presence of infection, or gastrointestinal instrumentation, or may spread from uncomplicated upper respiratory tract or skin infections. Bacteria adhere to the damaged endocardium using adhesins.

3. Formation of infective endocardial vegetations (Fig. 33.36). Bacteria infiltrate the sterile thrombi and accelerate fibrin formation by activating the clotting cascade. These vegetative lesions can form anywhere on the endocardium but usually occur on heart valves and surrounding structures. Although endocardial tissue is constantly bathed in antibody-containing blood and is surrounded by scavenging monocytes and polymorphonuclear leukocytes, bacterial colonies are inaccessible to host defenses because they are embedded in the protective fibrin clots. Embolization from these vegetations can lead to abscesses and characteristic skin changes, such as petechiae, splinter hemorrhages, and Janeway lesions (nonpainful hemorrhagic lesions on the palms and soles).

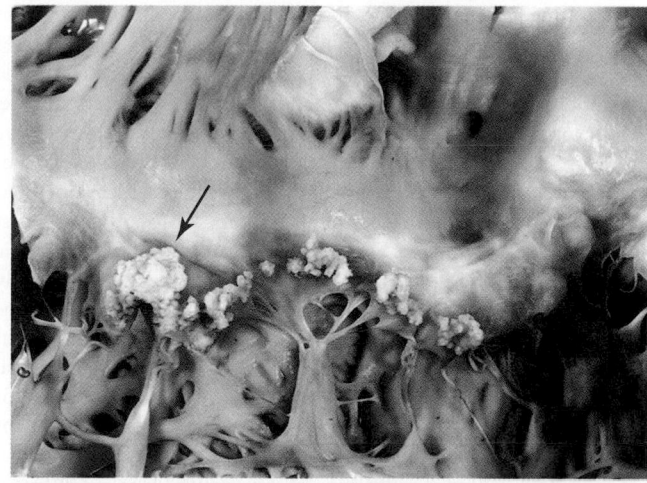

FIGURE 33.36 Bacterial Endocarditis of Mitral Valve. Lesion *(arrow)* in combination with old rheumatic valvulitis. (From Damjanov I, Linder J: *Pathology: a color atlas*, St Louis, 2000, Mosby.)

◆**CLINICAL MANIFESTATIONS.** IE may be acute, subacute, or chronic. It causes varying degrees of valvular dysfunction and may be associated with manifestations involving several organ systems (lungs, eyes, kidneys, bones, joints, CNS). Signs and symptoms of IE are caused by infection and inflammation, systemic spread of microemboli, and immune complex deposition. The "classic" findings are fever, new or changed cardiac murmur, and petechial lesions of the skin, conjunctiva, and oral mucosa. Characteristic physical findings include Osler nodes (painful erythematous nodules on the pads of the fingers and toes) and Janeway lesions. Other manifestations include weight loss, back pain, night sweats, and heart failure. CNS, splenic, renal, pulmonary peripheral arterial, coronary, and ocular emboli may lead to a wide variety of signs and symptoms.

◆**EVALUATION AND TREATMENT.** The widely accepted Duke criteria for the diagnosis of IE include the two major criteria of positive blood cultures (at least 2 positive cultures drawn >12 hours apart) and evidence for endocardial involvement (echocardiographic findings of vegetations and valvular dysfunction or damage), plus minor criteria including predisposing conditions, fever, evidence of emboli (e.g., Janeway lesions), and immunologic phenomena (e.g., Osler nodes).[169] The diagnosis of IE must be made as soon as possible to initiate appropriate empirical antibiotic therapy and to identify patients at high risk for complications. Antimicrobial therapy should begin as soon as possible, and it is generally continued for several weeks. Surgical intervention to repair or replace the valve may be required, especially in individuals with heart failure, abscess, infection with highly resistant microorganisms, and large vegetations.[169] Antibiotic prophylaxis to prevent IE is indicated for those with prosthetic valves, a history of IE, unrepaired cyanotic congenital heart disease, and heart transplant with valvular defect in the setting of gingival procedures or in the presence of documented acute gastrointestinal or genitourinary infection.[152]

MANIFESTATIONS OF HEART DISEASE

Heart Failure

Heart failure (HF) is defined as the pathophysiologic condition in which the heart is unable to generate an adequate cardiac output such that inadequate perfusion of tissues or increased diastolic filling pressure of the left ventricle, or both, occurs; consequently, pulmonary capillary pressures are increased. It is estimated that 5.7 million Americans ≥20 years of age have HF and it causes 1 in 9 deaths in the United States.[5] HF is a pressing, world-wide problem with millions of people experiencing worsening heart failure.[170] Ischemic heart disease and hypertension are the most important predisposing risk factors with 75% of HF cases occurring in individuals with hypertension. Other risk factors include age, smoking, obesity, diabetes, renal failure, valvular heart disease, cardiomyopathies, myocarditis, congenital heart disease, and excessive alcohol use. Numerous genetic polymorphisms have been linked to an increased risk for heart failure, including genes for cardiomyopathies, sarcomere proteins, and neurohumoral receptors.[144] Most causes of heart failure result in dysfunction of the left ventricle (systolic and diastolic heart failure). The right ventricle also may be dysfunctional, especially in pulmonary disease (right ventricular failure). Finally, some conditions cause inadequate perfusion despite normal or elevated cardiac output (high-output failure). A current area of investigation is mitochondrial dysfunction.[170] Mitochondrial abnormalities include impaired mitochondrial electron transport chain activity, increased formation of reactive oxygen species, altered metabolic substrate usage, abnormal mitochondrial dynamics, and altered ion hemostasis.[170] Abnormal mitochondrial energy production is involved in many symptoms found in individuals with heart failure and include skeletal muscle dysfunction and renal pathologies.[170]

Types

Left Heart Failure. Left heart failure (congestive heart failure) is categorized as heart failure with reduced ejection fraction, or HFrEF (systolic heart failure), or heart failure with preserved ejection fraction, or HFpEF (diastolic heart failure). These two types of heart failure can occur together in one individual or singly.

Heart Failure with Reduced Ejection Fraction (HFrEF) (Systolic Heart Failure). Heart failure with reduced ejection fraction, or HFrEF (systolic heart failure), is defined as an ejection fraction of <40% and an inability of the heart to generate an adequate cardiac output to perfuse vital tissues. Cardiac output depends on the heart rate and stroke volume. Stroke volume is influenced by three major factors: contractility, preload, and afterload (see Chapter 32). Contractility is reduced by diseases that disrupt myocyte activity. Myocardial infarction is the most common cause of decreased contractility; other causes include myocarditis and cardiomyopathies. These diseases contribute to inflammatory, immune, and neurohumoral changes (activation of the SNS and RAAS) that mediate a process called *ventricular remodeling*. Ventricular remodeling results in disruption of the normal myocardial extracellular structure with resultant dilation of the myocardium and causes progressive myocyte contractile dysfunction over time (Fig. 33.37). When contractility is decreased, stroke volume falls, and left ventricular end-diastolic volume (LVEDV) increases. This causes dilation of the heart and an increase in preload.

Preload, or LVEDV, increases with decreased contractility or when there is an excess of plasma volume (intravenous fluid administration, renal failure, mitral valvular disease). Increases in LVEDV can actually improve cardiac output up to a certain point, but as preload continues to rise, it causes a stretching of the myocardium that eventually can lead to dysfunction of the sarcomeres and decreased contractility. This relationship is described by the Frank-Starling law of the heart (see Fig. 32.18).

Increased afterload is most commonly a result of increased peripheral vascular resistance (PVR), such as that seen with hypertension (Fig. 33.38). Although much less common, it also can be the result of aortic valvular disease. With increased PVR, there is resistance to ventricular emptying and more workload for the left ventricle, which responds with hypertrophy of the myocardium. This process differs from the physiologic myocyte response to increased workload (exercise) in which the workload is intermittent rather than sustained, resulting in an increase in muscle mass but no distortion of the cardiac architecture. Sustained afterload leads to pathologic hypertrophy which is characterized by myocyte death, fibrosis, inflammation, and alterations in cardiac energetics and is mediated by ang II, catecholamines, and changes in intracellular signaling within the myocytes[171] (see Fig. 33.37). This pathologic increase in muscle mass results in an increase in oxygen and energy demand. When demand for energy is greater than the ability of these systems to supply the necessary ATP, contractility of the myocardium is compromised. An energy-starved state develops that further contributes to changes in the myocytes themselves and ventricular remodeling that significantly impairs contractility and therefore ventricular function. Remodeling also results in the deposition of collagen between the myocytes, which can disrupt the integrity of the muscle, decrease contractility, and make the ventricle more likely to dilate and fail.[172] Weakness of the cardiac muscle due to hypertension-induced hypertrophy is called *hypertensive hypertrophic cardiomyopathy*.[173,174]

As cardiac output falls, renal perfusion diminishes with activation of the RAAS, which acts to increase PVR and plasma volume, thus increasing afterload and preload further. In addition, baroreceptors in the central circulation detect the decrease in perfusion and stimulate the SNS to cause yet more vasoconstriction and to cause the hypothalamus to produce

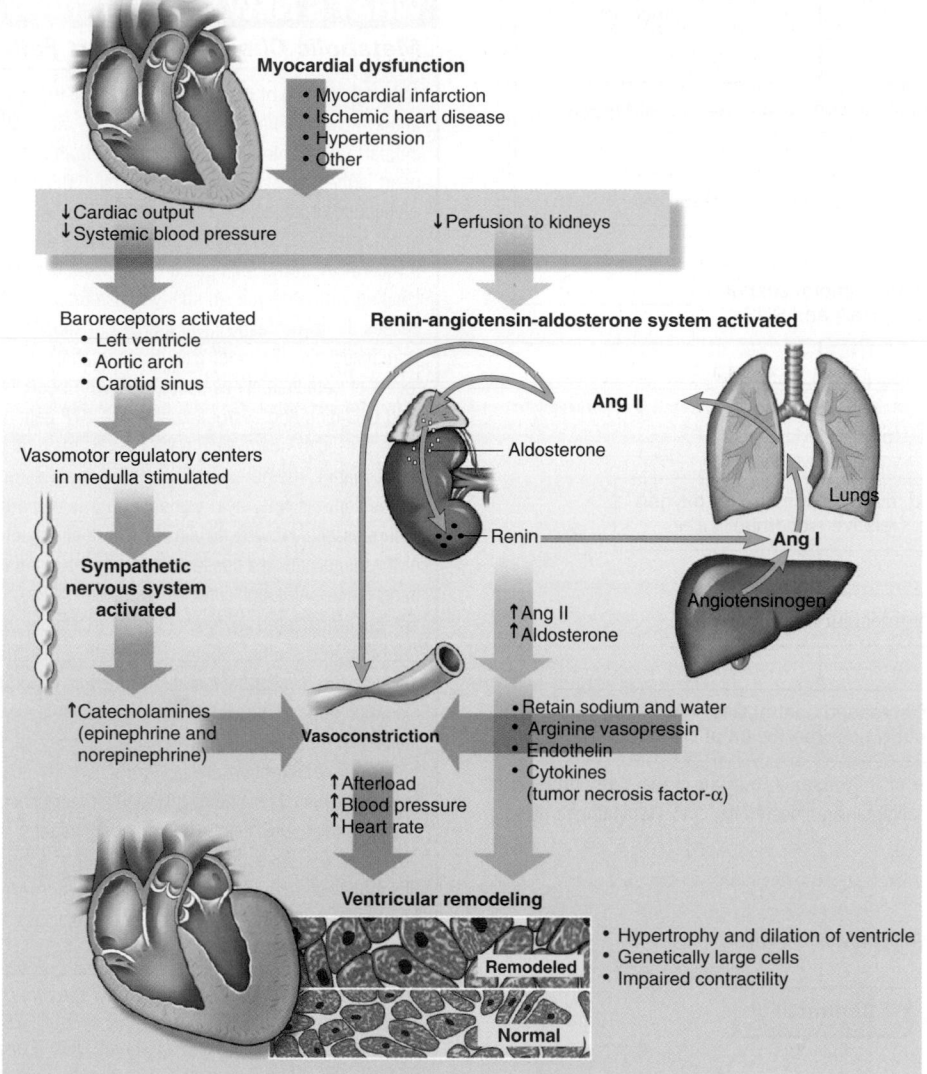

FIGURE 33.37 Pathophysiology of Ventricular Remodeling. Myocardial dysfunction activates the renin-angiotensin-aldosterone and sympathetic nervous systems, releasing neurohormones (angiotensin [ang] II, aldosterone, catecholamines, and cytokines). These neurohormones contribute to ventricular remodeling. (Redrawn from Carelock J, Clark AP: *Am J Nurs* 101[12]:27, 2001.)

antidiuretic hormone. This vicious cycle of decreasing contractility, increasing preload, and increasing afterload causes progressive worsening of left heart failure (Fig. 33.39).

In addition to these hemodynamic interactions, systolic congestive heart failure is characterized by a complex constellation of neurohumoral, inflammatory, and metabolic processes:

1. *Catecholamines.* Sympathetic nervous system activation initially compensates for a decrease in cardiac output by increasing heart rate and peripheral vascular resistance. However, catecholamines cause numerous deleterious effects on the myocardium, including direct toxicity to myocytes, induction of myocyte apoptosis, myocardial remodeling, downregulation of adrenergic receptors, facilitation of dysrhythmias, and potentiation of autoimmune effects on the heart muscle.

2. *RAAS*
   a. Angiotensin II (Ang II). Activation of the RAAS causes not only increases in preload and afterload, but also causes direct toxicity to the myocardium (see Fig. 33.37). Ang II mediates remodeling

of the ventricular wall, contributing to sarcomere death, loss of the normal collagen matrix, and interstitial fibrosis. This leads to decreased contractility, changes in myocardial compliance, and ventricular dilation.[175]

   b. Aldosterone. Aldosterone not only causes salt and water retention by the kidney but also contributes to myocardial fibrosis, autonomic dysfunction, and dysrhythmias. It also has been implicated in endothelial dysfunction and prothrombotic effects.

3. *Arginine vasopressin.* Arginine vasopressin is also known as *antidiuretic hormone* and causes both peripheral vasoconstriction and renal fluid retention. These actions exacerbate hyponatremia and edema in heart failure. The arginine vasopressin type 2 antagonist tolvaptan is indicated for the treatment of heart failure that is resistant to conventional diuretics.[176]

4. *Natriuretic peptides.* Atrial natriuretic peptides (ANPs) and B-type natriuretic peptides (BNPs) are increased and may have some protective effect by decreasing preload; however, their compensatory mechanisms are inadequate in heart failure.[177]

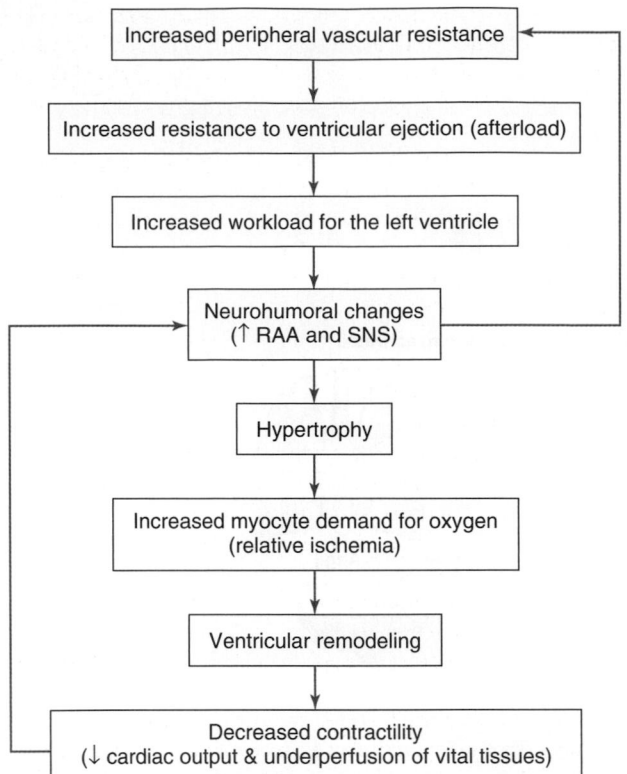

FIGURE 33.38 The Role of Increased Afterload in the Pathogenesis of Heart Failure. *RAA,* Renin-angiotensin-aldosterone, *SNS,* sympathetic nervous system.

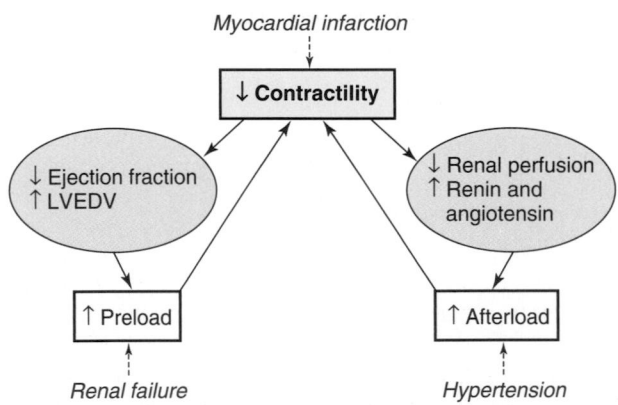

FIGURE 33.39 The Vicious Cycle of Systolic Heart Failure. Although the initial insult may be one of primary decreased contractility (e.g., myocardial infarction), increased preload (e.g., renal failure), or increased afterload (e.g., hypertension), all three factors play a role in the progression of left heart failure. *LVEDV,* Left ventricular end-diastolic volume.

5. *Inflammatory cytokines*
   a. Endothelial hormones. Endothelin is a potent vasoconstrictor and is associated with a poor prognosis in individuals with heart failure.
   b. TNF-α and IL-6. TNF-α is elevated in heart failure and contributes to myocardial hypertrophy and remodeling. It down-regulates the synthesis of the vasodilator nitric oxide (NO), induces myocyte apoptosis, and may contribute to weight loss and weakness in individuals with heart failure (cardiac cachexia). IL-6 also is

Data from Ahmad T et al: *J Am Coll Cardiol* 67:291–299, 2016; Czarnowska E et al: *PPAR Res* 2016:7508026, 2016; Horton JL et al: *JCI Insight* 1(2), 2016; Kim TT, Dyck JR: *Trends Endocrinol Metab* 26(1):40–48, 2015; Loudon BL et al: *Br J Pharmacol* 173(12):1911–1924, 2016; Rame JE: *J Am Coll Cardiol* 67:300–302, 2016.

elevated in individuals with severe heart failure and cardiogenic shock and may contribute to further deleterious immune activation.[178]

6. *Myocyte calcium transport.* Calcium transport into, out of, and within myocytes is critical to normal contractile function. Changes in calcium ion channels, intracellular transport mechanisms in the sarcoplasmic reticulum, and calcium cycling have all been implicated in decreased myocardial contractility and heart failure.[179]

7. *Insulin resistance and diabetes.* Insulin resistance is a likely contributor to, as well as complication of, heart failure.[180] Insulin resistance causes abnormal myocyte fatty acid metabolism and generation of ATP, which contributes to decreased myocardial contractility and remodeling (see *What's New?* Metabolic Changes in Heart Failure). Heart failure activates the SNS and RAAS, which contribute to insulin resistance. Diabetes contributes to heart failure through disturbed calcium metabolism, oxidative stress, changes in fatty acid and glucose metabolism, and mitochondrial dysfunction.[181] In addition, receptors on myocytes for damaging advanced glycation end-products (RAGE) (see Chapter 22) are up-regulated in injuries to the heart, including ischemia and reperfusion injury. Measurement of levels of RAGE in plasma or serum may correlate with the degree of heart failure.

Unfortunately, many of the new medications used to treat diabetes and insulin resistance have deleterious side effects on cardiac functioning, Newer agents, such as the sodium/glucose cotransporter 2 (SGLT2) inhibitors and the incretin-based drugs (see Chapter 22), are safer and may even reduce hospitalization and mortality from heart failure.[182,183]

The interaction of these metabolic, neurohumoral, and inflammatory processes results in a gradual decline in myocardial function. Pathologically, the heart muscle exhibits progressive changes in myocyte myofilaments, decreased contractility, myocyte apoptosis and necrosis, abnormal fibrin deposition in the ventricle wall, myocardial hypertrophy, and changes in the ventricular chamber geometry. Remodeling, endothelial dysfunction, venous congestion, and worsening renal function all contribute to the pathophysiology of acute heart failure.[175] These changes reduce myocardial function and cardiac output and lead to increased morbidity and mortality. These discoveries have led to the routine use of ACE inhibitors, aldosterone blockers, and beta-blockers in the management of heart failure, which has resulted in significant decreases in morbidity and mortality.[184]

◆**EVALUATION.** The clinical manifestations of HFrEF are the result of pulmonary vascular congestion and inadequate perfusion of the systemic circulation. Individuals experience dyspnea, orthopnea, cough of frothy sputum, fatigue, decreased urine output, and edema. Physical examination often reveals pulmonary edema (cyanosis, inspiratory crackles, pleural effusions), hypotension or hypertension, an S_3 gallop, and evidence of underlying CAD or hypertension. An ECG and serum troponin should be obtained to evaluate for acute ischemia. A chest x-ray should be obtained to assess heart size and evidence of pulmonary congestion, and echocardiography, to confirm decreased cardiac output and cardiomegaly.[184] Invasive catheterization to monitor hemodynamics or to document underlying coronary disease may be needed. Serum BNP levels should be measured to assist in diagnosing heart failure and to monitor its severity and response to treatment.[184] Other biomarkers that may aid in the diagnosis and management of heart failure include cardiac troponins and soluble suppression of tumorigenicity 2 (ST2).[185]

Management of HFrEF is aimed at interrupting the worsening cycle of decreasing contractility, increasing preload, and increasing afterload, as well as blocking the neurohormonal mediators of myocardial toxicity. The acute onset of left heart failure is often the result of acute myocardial ischemia and must be managed in conjunction with the underlying coronary disease. Oxygen, nitrates, and morphine administration improve myocardial oxygenation and help relieve coronary spasm while lowering preload through systemic venodilation. Diuretics reduce preload and are the mainstay of therapy. Intravenous inotropic drugs, such as dobutamine and milrinone, increase contractility and can help raise the blood pressure in hypotensive individuals. Calcium-sensitizing inotropic drugs (e.g., levosimendan) have shown promise for acute heart failure in selected individuals. ACE inhibitors (which reduce preload and afterload) and intravenous beta-blockers (which reduce myocardial demand) have been found to reduce mortality but must be used with caution in hypotensive individuals. Intravenous administration of nesiritide (recombinant BNP) also improves preload and contractility; however, results of this therapy have been mixed. Individuals with severe systolic failure because of myocardial ischemia may benefit from acute coronary bypass or PCI. Those with refractory hypotension may be supported with the intraaortic balloon pump (IABP) until they can be taken safely to the operating room; the IABP is positioned in the aorta just distal to the aortic valve and is inflated during diastole to improve coronary perfusion and deflated during systole to reduce afterload. Left ventricular assist devices (LVADs) also can be lifesaving.

Management of **chronic left heart failure** also relies on increasing contractility and reducing preload and afterload. In all patients with reduced ejection fraction, ACE inhibitors and beta-blockers are indicated to reduce mortality.[184] Salt restriction, loop diuretics, and aldosterone-blockers such as spironolactone and eplerenone are effective in reducing preload and improving outcomes. ACE inhibitors reduce preload and afterload and have been shown to significantly reduce mortality in chronic left heart failure. ARBs do not improve morbidity or mortality in individuals with heart failure and should be used only in those who do not tolerate ACE inhibitors. Renin inhibitors, such as aliskiren, can be effective in selected individuals.[186] Beta-blockers improve symptoms and increase survival. A new class of medications, called *neprilysin (NEP) inhibitors,* has been developed and, when combined with ARBs, can improve HF outcomes.[177] Pharmacogenetics may improve the individualization of therapies.[187] Anticoagulants and antithrombotics may be indicated in selected individuals, particularly those with intracardiac thrombi or atrial fibrillation. Although many individuals with left heart failure die suddenly from dysrhythmias, prophylactic administration of antidysrhythmics has not been shown to improve survival. In individuals with sustained ventricular tachycardia, amiodarone or ICDs are indicated. Cardiac resynchronization therapy is proving to be an important modality in selected individuals. Coronary bypass surgery or PCI may improve perfusion to ischemic myocardium (hibernating myocardium) and improve cardiac output. Other types of surgical intervention that improve ventricular geometry may be considered. Left ventricular assist devices have lengthened survival significantly for those with end-stage heart failure.[188] Heart transplant may be the only remaining option. Experimental therapies, including gene and stem cell therapies, are being explored[189,190] (see *What's New? Gene Therapy for Heart Failure*).

Heart Failure with Preserved Ejection Fraction (Diastolic Heart Failure)

Heart failure with preserved ejection fraction, or **HFpEF (diastolic heart failure)**, can occur singly or along with systolic heart failure. Isolated diastolic heart failure is defined as pulmonary congestion despite a normal stroke volume and cardiac output. It is the cause of approximately 50% of all cases of left heart failure and is more common in women.[191] The major causes of HFpEF include hypertension-induced myocardial hypertrophy and myocardial ischemia with resultant ventricular remodeling. Hypertrophy and ischemia cause a decreased ability of the myocytes to actively pump calcium from the cytosol, resulting in impaired relaxation. Other causes include aortic valvular disease, mitral valve disease, pericardial diseases, and cardiomyopathies.[192] Diabetes also increases the risk for diastolic dysfunction.[191]

Two areas of pathophysiologic changes in the ventricle have been identified in diastolic dysfunction: decreased compliance of the left ventricle and abnormal diastolic relaxation (lusitropy). Decreased ventricular compliance has been linked to changes in myocardial structure such as that seen with molecular alterations in collagen, which forms the extracellular matrix for myocytes. Another recently identified structural change is because of abnormalities in an intracellular protein component of the myocyte cytoskeleton called *titin*. Abnormal lusitropy is caused by changes in calcium transport from myocytes and may be related to the activity of sarcoplasmic reticulum–calcium adenosine triphosphatase (ATPase). Other pathophysiologic processes implicated include autonomic and endothelial dysfunction.[193] The resultant noncompliant and poorly lusitropic ventricle cannot accept filling with blood without significant resistance and an increase in wall tension. Thus HFpEF occurs because a normal LVEDV is associated with an increased LVEDP. The resultant increase in left atrial pressure is then reflected proximally into the pulmonary circulation and results in pulmonary edema. The increase in pressure is made worse when ventricular filling is rapid so symptoms worsen with tachycardia (e.g., with exercise).

Gene Therapy for Heart Failure

The effectiveness and safety of recent gene therapy trials for heart failure have led to an explosion of interest in innovative methods for restoring cardiac function. Multiple components of cardiac contractility have been identified as targets for gene therapy, including calcium channel cycling, beta adrenergic functioning, and cellular proliferation. The most studied of the potential gene targets include sarcoendoplasmic reticulum calcium ATPase (SERCA2a) and S100A1, which affect intracellular myocyte calcium handling. Another exciting target is adenylyl cyclase 6 (AC6), the enzyme catalyzing cyclic adenosine monophosphate (cAMP) formation and beta-adrenergic receptor function. Other targets include SDF1/CXCR4 complex, which promotes homing of stem cells to infarcted myocardium; microRNAs; and genes that code for critical neuro-humoral factors, including insulin-like growth factor-1 (IGF-1), growth hormone, and B-type natriuretic peptide. Viruses are the most widely used vectors for cardiovascular gene transfer, especially adeno-associated virus (AAV). These viruses exhibit fairly good cardiotropism, and various methods are being explored for delivering these gene vectors most efficiently to the myocardium, including antegrade or retrograde coronary infusion, intravenous infusion, direct myocardial injection, and pericardial injection. Intracoronary infusion of AAV with SERCA2a for individuals with severe heart failure significantly improved mortality and heart failure outcomes with positive effects and no reported safety concerns reported at 3 years. Unfortunately, a follow-up study by the same author provided less positive results. Most recently, a study reported that gene transfer of AC6 improved LV function and reduced hospitalizations for individuals with moderate to severe heart failure with preserved ejection fraction (HFrEF). Another avenue for gene therapy uses drugs to inhibit microRNAs that block essential gene expression and protein translation. It is clear that the future will reveal many new and potentially lifesaving gene therapies for those with intractable heart failure.

Data from Braunwald E: *Lancet* 385(9970):812-824, 2015; Donahue JK: *Lancet* 387(10024):1137-1139, 2016; Fish KM, Ishikawa K: *Dis Med* 19(105):285-291, 2015; Greenberg B: *J Cardiol* 66(3):195-200, 2015; Greenberg B et al: *Lancet* 387(10024):1178-1186, 2016; Hammond HK et al: *J Am Med Assoc Cardiol* 1(2):163-171, 2016.

Individuals with HFpEF most often present with dyspnea on exertion and fatigue. If diastolic dysfunction is severe, there may be evidence of pulmonary edema (inspiratory crackles on auscultation, pleural effusions). Pulmonary hypertension and right ventricular failure may develop. Late in diastole, atrial contraction with rapid ejection of blood into the noncompliant ventricle may give rise to an S_4 gallop. Electrocardiography often reveals evidence of left ventricular hypertrophy, and chest x-ray shows pulmonary congestion without cardiomegaly (Table 33.8). There also may be evidence of underlying coronary disease, hypertension, or valvular disease. Diagnosis is based on three factors: signs and symptoms of heart failure, normal left ventricular ejection fraction, and evidence of diastolic dysfunction. The diagnosis is initially made by echocardiography, which demonstrates poor ventricular filling, abnormal relaxation, hypertrophy, and/or left atrial enlargement with normal ejection fractions.[191] Management is aimed at improving ventricular relaxation and prolonging diastolic filling times to reduce diastolic pressure. Physical training (aerobic and weight training) improves endurance and quality of life. Nitrates, beta-blockers, ACE inhibitors, ARBs, and aldosterone blockers have been used with varying success, however current guidelines focus on treating hypertension, ischemia or valvular disease.[184,193] Outcomes for individuals with HFpEF can be as poor as those with systolic heart failure, and there has been little improvement in prognosis despite numerous new treatment trials.

TABLE 33.8	COMPARISON OF SYSTOLIC AND DIASTOLIC HEART FAILURE	
CHARACTERISTIC	**SYSTOLIC HEART FAILURE**	**DIASTOLIC HEART FAILURE**
Gender	Male > female	Female > male
Left ventricular ejection fraction	Decreased	Normal
Left ventricular chamber size	Increased	Decreased
Left ventricular hypertrophy on electrocardiogram	Possible	Probable
Chest radiography	Pulmonary congestion with cardiomegaly	Pulmonary congestion without cardiomegaly
Gallop	S_3	S_4

Adapted from Jessup M, Brozena S: *N Engl J Med* 348(20):2007–2018, 2003.

Right Heart Failure

Right heart failure is defined as the inability of the right ventricle to provide adequate blood flow into the pulmonary circulation at a normal central venous pressure. It most often results from severe left heart failure when the increased left ventricular filling pressure is reflected back into the pulmonary circulation. As pressure in the pulmonary circulation rises, the resistance to right ventricular emptying increases. The right ventricle hypertrophies in response to this increased workload, however it undergoes progressive diastolic and systolic deterioration and will dilate and fail. When this happens, pressure will rise in the systemic venous circulation, resulting in jugular venous distention, peripheral edema, and hepatosplenomegaly. Treatment relies on management of the left ventricular dysfunction as just outlined. When right heart failure occurs in the absence of left heart failure, it is caused most commonly by pulmonary hypertension resulting from diffuse hypoxic pulmonary disease, such as chronic obstructive pulmonary disease (COPD) and cystic fibrosis, or from primary pulmonary arterial hypertension (Fig. 33.40). The mechanisms for this type of right ventricular dysfunction (*cor pulmonale*) are discussed in Chapter 36. Finally, right heart failure can result from right ventricular MI, cardiomyopathies, and pulmonic valvular disease. Management relies on treating the underlying condition, managing intravascular volume, and assisting right ventricular contractility.[194] Vasodilators may improve outcomes in primary pulmonary arterial hypertension (see Chapter 36).

High-Output Failure

High-output failure is the inability of the heart to adequately supply the body with blood-borne nutrients, despite adequate blood volume and normal or elevated myocardial contractility. In high-output failure the heart increases its output but the body's metabolic needs are still not met. Common causes of high-output failure are anemia, septicemia, hyperthyroidism, and beriberi (Fig. 33.41).

Anemia decreases the oxygen-carrying capacity of the blood (see Chapter 29). Metabolic acidosis occurs as the body's cells switch to anaerobic metabolism (see Chapter 3). In response to metabolic acidosis, heart rate and stroke volume increase in an attempt to circulate blood faster. If anemia is severe, however, even maximum cardiac output does not supply the cells with enough oxygen for metabolism.

In septicemia, disturbed metabolism, bacterial toxins, and the inflammatory process cause systemic vasodilation and fever. Faced with a lowered systemic vascular resistance (SVR) and an elevated metabolic rate, cardiac output increases to maintain blood pressure and prevent metabolic acidosis. In overwhelming septicemia, however, the heart

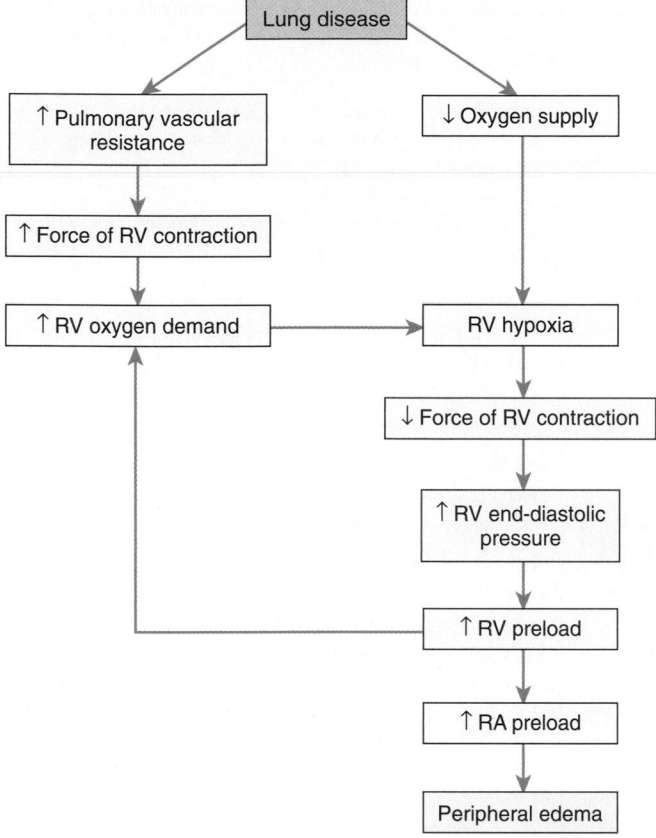

FIGURE 33.40 Right Heart Failure (Cor Pulmonale) Caused by Lung Disease. The presence of peripheral edema in cor pulmonale is caused by lung disease. *RA,* Right atrial; *RV,* right ventricular.

may not be able to raise its output enough to compensate for vasodilation (septic shock). Body tissues show signs of inadequate blood supply despite a very high cardiac output.

Hyperthyroidism accelerates cellular metabolism through the actions of elevated levels of thyroxine from the thyroid gland. This may occur chronically (thyrotoxicosis) or acutely (thyroid storm). Because the body's increased demand for oxygen threatens to cause metabolic acidosis, cardiac output increases. If blood levels of thyroxine are high and the metabolic response to thyroxine is vigorous, even an abnormally elevated cardiac output may be inadequate.[195]

In the United States, beriberi (thiamine deficiency) usually is caused by malnutrition secondary to chronic alcoholism. Beriberi actually causes a mixed type of heart failure. Thiamine deficiency impairs cellular metabolism in all tissues, including the myocardium. In the heart, impaired cardiac metabolism leads to insufficient contractile strength. In blood vessels, thiamine deficiency leads mainly to peripheral vasodilation, which decreases SVR. Heart failure ensues as decreased SVR triggers increased cardiac output, which the impaired myocardium is unable to deliver. The strain of demands for increased output in the face of impaired metabolism may deplete cardiac reserves until low-output failure begins.

Dysrhythmias

A dysrhythmia, or arrhythmia, is a disturbance of heart rhythm. Normal heart rhythms are generated by the SA node and travel through the heart's conduction system, causing the atrial and ventricular myocardium to contract and relax at a regular rate that is appropriate to maintain circulation at various levels of physical activity (see Chapter 32). Dysrhythmias range in severity from occasional "missed" or rapid beats to serious disturbances that impair the pumping ability of the heart, contributing to heart failure and death. Dysrhythmias can be caused by either an abnormal rate of impulse generation (Table 33.9) by the SA node or other pacemaker, or by the abnormal conduction of impulses (Table 33.10) through the heart's conduction system, including the myocardial cells themselves. The pathophysiology, diagnosis, and treatment of dysrhythmias are highly complicated. Atrial fibrillation provides an example of the many factors that must be considered (Box 33.4).

Text continued on p. 1108

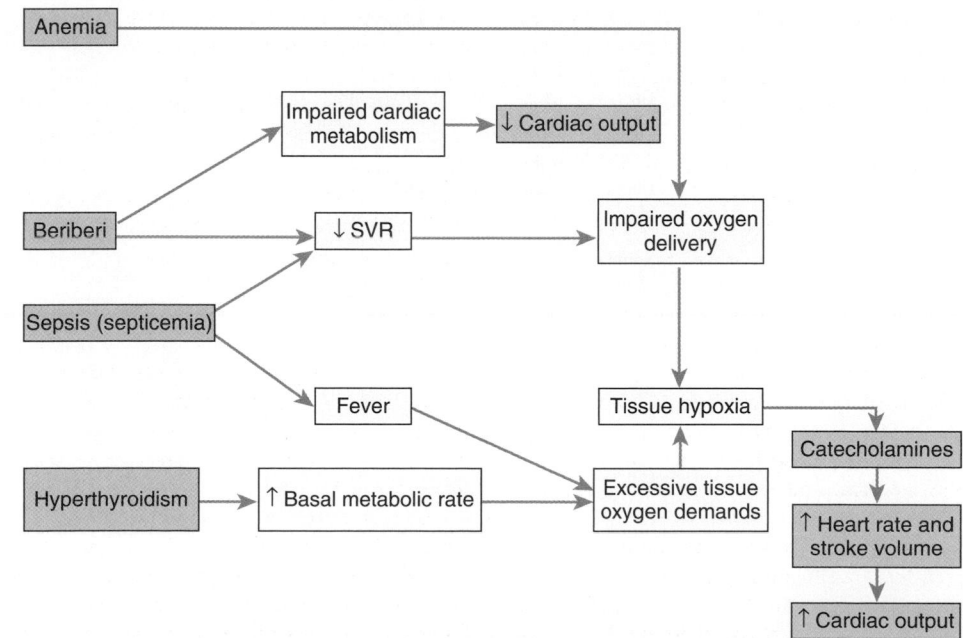

FIGURE 33.41 High-Output Failure. *SVR,* Systemic vascular resistance.

TABLE 33.9   DISORDERS OF IMPULSE FORMATION

TYPE	ELECTROCARDIOGRAM	EFFECT	PATHOPHYSIOLOGY	TREATMENT
Sinus bradycardia	P rate 60 or less PR interval normal QRS for each P	Increased preload Decreased mean arterial pressure	Hyperkalemia: slows depolarization Vagal hyperactivity: unknown Digoxin toxicity common Late hypoxia: lack of adenosine triphosphate (ATP)	If hypotensive, treat cause and support Follow with sympathomimetics, cardiotonics, and pacer Vagolytics
Simple sinus tachycardia	P rate 100-150 PR interval normal QRS for each P	Decreased filling times Decreased mean arterial pressure Increased myocardial demand	Catecholamines; rise in resting potential, calcium influx Fever: unknown Early failure and lung disease: hypoxic cell metabolism Hypercalcemia	Oxygen, bed rest Calcium channel blockers
Premature atrial contractions (PACs) or beats*	Early P waves that may have changed morphology PR interval normal QRS for each P	Occasional decreased filling time and mean arterial pressure	Electrolyte disturbances: decrease in all phases Hypoxia and elevated preload: cell membrane disturbances Hypercalcemia	Treat underlying cause Digoxin
Sinus dysrhythmias	Rate varies P-P regularly irregular, short with inspiration, long with exhalation PR interval normal QRS for each P	Variable filling times Variable mean arterial pressures Variable oxygen demand	Unknown Common in young children and young adults	None
Atrial tachycardia (includes premature atrial tachycardia if onset is abrupt)	P rate 151-250; morphology may differ from sinus PPR interval normal P:QRS ratio variable	Decreased filling time Decreased mean arterial pressure Increased myocardial demand	Same as PACs: leads to increased atrial automaticity, atrial reentry Digoxin toxicity: common	Control ventricular rate Digoxin, calcium channel blockers, vagus stimulation Pace to override
Atrial flutter*	P rate 251-300; morphology may vary from sinus P PR interval usually not observable P:QRS ratio variable	Decreased filling time Decreased mean arterial pressure	Same as atrial tachycardia Aging	Same as atrial tachycardia Synchronous cardioversion
Atrial fibrillation*	P rate >300 and usually not observable No PR interval QRS rate variable and rhythm irregular	Same as atrial flutter	Same as atrial tachycardia Aging	Same as atrial tachycardia
Idiojunctional rhythm	P absent or independent QRS normal, rate 41-59, regular	Decreased cardiac output from loss of atrial contribution to ventricular preload Decreased mean atrial pressure as a result of bradycardia	Atrial and sinus bradycardia, standstill, or block	Same as sinus bradycardia
Junctional bradycardia	P absent or independent QRS normal, rate 40 or less	Same as idiojunctional rhythm	Same as idiojunctional rhythm Vagal hyperactivity	Same as sinus bradycardia

TABLE 33.9	DISORDERS OF IMPULSE FORMATION—cont'd			
TYPE	**ELECTROCARDIOGRAM**	**EFFECT**	**PATHOPHYSIOLOGY**	**TREATMENT**
Premature junctional contractions (PJCs) or beats	Early beats without P waves QRS morphology normal	Decreased cardiac output from loss of atrial contribution to ventricular preload for that beat	Hyperkalemia (6-5.4 mEq/L) Hypercalcemia, hypoxia, and elevated preload (see PACs)	Same as PACs
Accelerated junctional rhythm	P absent or independent QRS morphology normal, rate 60-99	Decreased cardiac output from loss of atrial contribution to ventricular preload	Same as PJCs	Same as PACs
Junctional tachycardia	P absent or independent QRS morphology normal, rate 100 or more	Decreased cardiac output from loss of atrial contribution to ventricular preload Increased myocardial demand because of tachycardia	Same as PJCs	Same as PACs
Idioventricular rhythm[†]	P absent or independent QRS >0.11 and rate 20-39	Same as idiojunctional rhythm	Sinus, atrial, and junctional bradycardia, standstill, or block	Same as sinus bradycardia
Ventricular bradycardia[†]	P absent or independent QRS >0.11 and rate 60-21	Same as idiojunctional rhythm	Same as idiojunctional rhythm	Same as sinus bradycardia
Agonal rhythm/ electromechanical dissociation[†]	P absent or independent QRS >0.11 and rate 20 or less	Absent or barely present cardiac output and pulse Not compatible with life	Depolarization and contraction not coupled: electrical activity present with little or no mechanical activity Usually caused by profound hypoxia	Vigorous pharmacology aimed at restoring rate and force Usually ineffective May attempt to pace
Ventricular standstill or asystole[†]	P absent or independent QRS absent	No cardiac output Not compatible with life	Profound ischemia, hyperkalemia, acidosis	Same as agonal rhythm, including electrical defibrillation
Premature ventricular contractions (PVCs) or depolarizations*	Early beats with P waves QRS occasionally opposite in deflection from usual QRS	Same as PJCs	Same as PJCs, including aging and induction of anesthesia Impulse originates in cell outside normal conduction system and spreads through intercalated disks	Pharmacology to change thresholds, refractory periods; reduce myocardial demand, increase supply Removal of cause
Accelerated ventricular rhythm	P absent or independent QRS >0.11 and rate 41-99	Same as accelerated junctional rhythm	Same as PVCs	Same as PVCs
Ventricular tachycardia[†]	P absent or independent QRS >0.11 and rate 100 or more	Same as junctional tachycardia	Same as PVCs	Same as PVCs, including electrical cardioversion
Ventricular fibrillation[†]	P absent QRS >300 and usually not observable	Same as ventricular standstill	Same as PVCs Rapid infusion of potassium	Same as PVCs including electrical defibrillation

*Most common in adults.
[†]Life threatening in adults.

TABLE 33.10   DISORDERS OF IMPULSE CONDUCTION

TYPE	ELECTROCARDIOGRAM	EFFECT	PATHOPHYSIOLOGY	TREATMENT
Sinus block	Occasionally absent P, with loss of QRS for that beat	Occasional decrease in cardiac output. Increase in preload for the following beat	Local hypoxia, scarring of intraatrial conduction pathways, electrolyte imbalances. Increased atrial preload	Conservative. Usually do not progress in severity. Pharmacologic treatment includes vagolytics, sympathomimetics, pacing
First-degree block*	PR interval >0.2	None	Same as sinus block. Hyperkalemia (>7 mEq/L). Hypokalemia (<3.5 mEq/L). Formation of myocardial abscesses in endocarditis	Conservative. Discovery and correction of cause
Second-degree block, Mobitz I, or Wenckebach*	Progressive prolongation of PR interval until one QRS is dropped. Pattern of prolongation resumes	Same as sinus block	Hypokalemia (<3.5 mEq/L). Faulty cell metabolism in atrioventricular (AV) node. Severity increases as heart rate increases. Supports theory that AV node is fatiguing. Digoxin toxicity, beta-blockade. Coronary artery disease (CAD), myocardial infarction (MI), hypoxia, increased preload, valvular surgery and disease, diabetes	Same as sinus block
Second-degree block or Mobitz II	Same as sinus block	Same as sinus block	Hypokalemia (<3.5 mEq/L). Faulty cell metabolism below AV node. Antidysrhythmics, cyclic antidepressants. CAD, MI, hypoxia, increased preload, valvular surgery and disease, diabetes	More aggressively than Mobitz I because block can progress to type III. Pacemaker after pharmacologic treatment
Third-degree block†	P waves present and independent of QRS. No observed relationship between P and QRS. Always AV dissociation	Same as idiojunctional rhythm	Hypokalemia (<3.5 mEq/L). Faulty cell metabolism low in bundle of His. MI, especially inferior wall, as nodal artery interrupted; results in ischemia of AV node	Pharmacologic until pacemaker inserted. Temporary pacing if caused by inferior MI because ischemia usually resolves
Atrioventricular dissociation	P waves present and independent of QRS, but not always because of block (e.g., ventricular tachycardia). AV dissociation not always third-degree block	Decreased cardiac output from loss of atrial contribution to ventricular preload. Variable effect on myocardial demand, depending on ventricular rate	May result from third-degree block or accelerated junctional or ventricular rhythm, or be caused by sinus, atrial, and junctional bradycardias	Treat according to cause. Pacemaker or reducing rate of AV or ventricular discharge, or increasing rate of sinus or AV node discharge
Ventricular block	QRS >0.11. R-S-R' in V_1, V_2, V_5, V_6	None	Faulty cell metabolism in right and left bundle branches. RBBB more common than LBBB because of dual blood supply to left bundle branch. Congestive heart failure, mitral regurgitation, especially anterior MI, because of infarct of fascicles. Left anterior hemiblock more common than left posterior hemiblock, since posterior fascicles have dual blood supply	Isolated right bundle branch block (RBBB) or left bundle branch block (LBBB) or hemiblock not treated. If acute and/or associated with acute anterior MI, treated with permanent pacer and vigorous pharmacology
Aberrant conduction	QRS >0.11	None unless ventricular rate abnormalities present	Conduction of impulse through intercalated disks because conduction system transiently blocked because of hypoxia, electrolyte imbalances, digoxin toxicity, excessively rapid rates of discharge	Correct underlying cause

TABLE 33.10 DISORDERS OF IMPULSE CONDUCTION—cont'd

TYPE	ELECTROCARDIOGRAM	EFFECT	PATHOPHYSIOLOGY	TREATMENT
Preexcitation syndromes (Wolff-Parkinson-White and Lown-Ganong-Levine)	P present with QRS for each P PR interval >0.12 and QRS >0.11 because of presence of delta wave in PR interval	None	Congenital presence of accessory pathways (bundle of Kent and fiber of Mahaim) that conduct very rapidly and bypass the AV node, causing early ventricular depolarization in relation to atrial depolarization Prone (reason unknown) to tachycardias and atrial fibrillation that can result in very rapid ventricular rates	Aimed at lining up refractory periods of accessory pathway and AV node to prevent reentry May slow rate with pharmacology May surgically cut pathways

*Most common in adults.
†Life threatening in adults.

BOX 33.4 ATRIAL FIBRILLATION

Atrial fibrillation (AF) is the most common cardiac rhythm disorder. It occurs when electrical impulses in the heart become disorganized leading to a rapid and irregular heart rhythm. People with AF have a four- to fivefold increased risk of stroke and a two- to threefold increased risk of heart failure.

Mechanisms

Efficient pumping of blood by the heart relies on the coordinated activity of the atria and ventricles, which involves contraction of cardiomyocytes in response to membrane depolarization. Electrical impulses begin in the sinoatrial (SA) node and first propagate through the atria, then pass through atrioventricular (AV) node (which delays their transit) and enter the ventricles, causing sequential cardiomyocyte contraction. In AF, the electrical activity in the atria is rapid and irregular. As a result, there is no coordinated atrial contraction and, depending on the filtering effect of the SA node, the response of the ventricles can also be rapid and irregular. Although several explanations have been put forward for this disordered atrial activity, AF fundamentally involves atrial remodeling that generates ectopic foci or 'triggers'—additional sources of electrical impulses—and mechanisms that act to maintain inappropriate conduction within vulnerable 'substrates'.

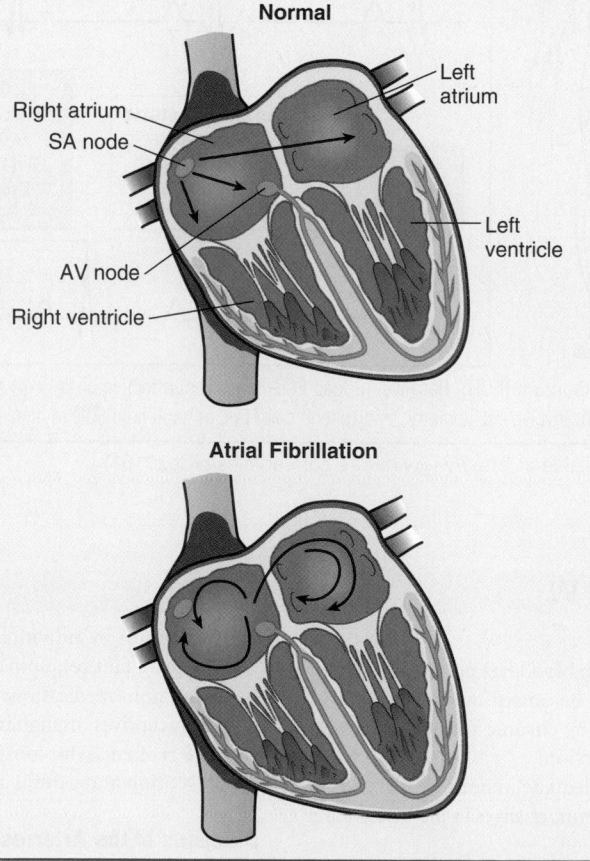

Normal

Right atrium
SA node
Left atrium
Left ventricle
AV node
Right ventricle

Atrial Fibrillation

Continued

BOX 33.4   ATRIAL FIBRILLATION—cont'd

Diagnosis

Symptoms of AF include palpitations, fatigue, dizziness, lightheadedness and dyspnea. They are nonspecific and are often not present. Diagnosis of AF is made by first checking a patient's pulse and then confirming it with a 12-lead electrocardiogram (ECG), which detects the electrical activity of the heart through electrodes placed on the skin. In AF, the space between the activation of the ventricles (QRS complexes) is "irregularly irregular" and there is often an absence of coordinated atrial contractions (P waves) prior to ventricular contraction.

Management

Treatment of AF involves strategies to achieve a normal heart rate, restore normal rhythm and reduce the risk of stroke, which is the most important priority for AF management. Rate-controlling drugs such as β-blockers usually act to modulate the activity of the SA and AV nodes. Rhythm control can be achieved either using antiarrhythmic drugs or the catheter-based introduction of lesions to ablate AF triggers and modify AF substrates. Finally, patients with AF commonly have comorbid conditions, the risk factors for which must also be appropriate addressed.

   NOTE: Ineffective blood pumping raises the likelihood of coagulation and thrombosis. As a result, patients with AF have an increased risk of stroke and often require oral anticoagulant therapy.

Epidemiology

Globally, in 2010 an estimated 20.9 million men and 12.6 million women had AF, and in developed countries AF is thought to be present in 3%-6% of those admitted to hospital with acute conditions. Risk factors for developing AF include conditions that have been found to promote atrial remodeling, such as heart failure, ischemic heart disease, hypertension, obesity, and obstructive sleep apnea. In addition, AF is associated with other classic cardiovascular disease risk factors such as diabetes, advanced age, male sex, alcohol consumption, and smoking. In developing countries, rheumatic heart disease often contributes to AF.

Outlook

Improved understanding of the mechanisms that trigger and maintain AF—such as changes in intracellular calcium ion handling, subtle alterations in atrial structure, and genetic factors—might lead to better strategies to prevent or treat the condition, whereas advances in catheter ablation will likely broaden the subset of patients who are eligible to undergo this procedure. In addition, although rates of stroke in patients in AF are declining owing to improved management, the identification of asymptomatic patients remains a challenge that might be addressed through new approaches to community-based screening.

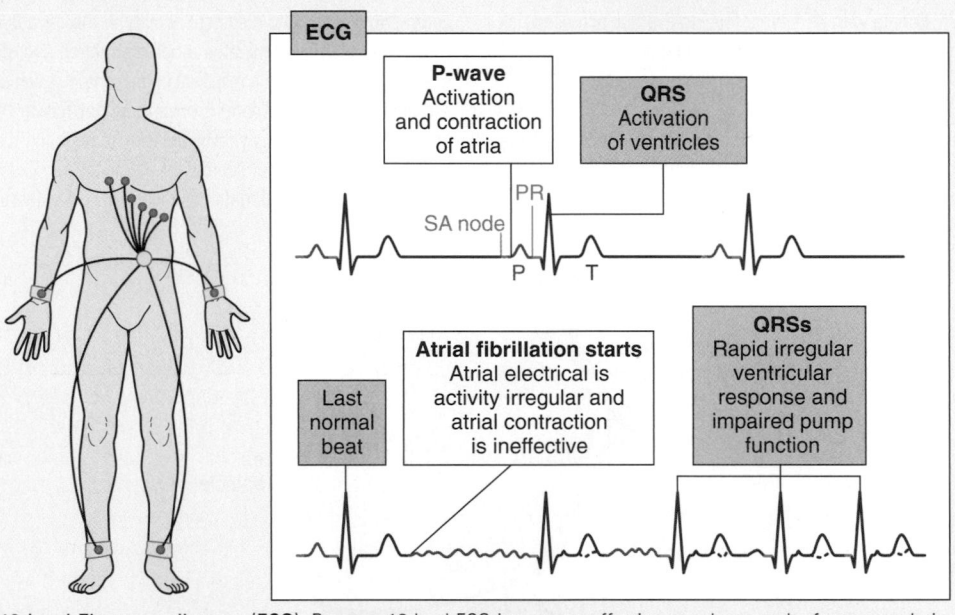

12-Lead Electrocardiogram (ECG). Because 12-lead ECG is not cost-effective on a large scale, future population screening for AF might involve oscillometry, smartphone cameras, or hand-held ECG rhythm strips.

Nat Rev Dis Primers 2:16017, 2016. Available at http://www.nature.com/articles/nrdp201617.

▌ S U M M A R Y   R E V I E W

Diseases of the Veins

1. Varicosities are areas of veins in which blood has pooled, usually in the saphenous veins. Varicosities may be caused by damaged valves as a result of trauma to the valve or by chronic venous distention involving gravity and venous constriction.
2. Chronic venous insufficiency is inadequate venous return over a long period that causes pathologic ischemic changes in the vasculature, skin, and supporting tissues.
3. Superior vena cava syndrome most often results from compression of the SVC by tumors.

4. DVT occurs in individuals who have venous stasis (immobility, age, left heart failure), spinal cord injury, vein wall damage (trauma, intravenous medications), or hypercoagulable states (pregnancy, oral contraceptives, malignancy, genetic coagulopathies).
5. DVT is often asymptomatic but may lead to fatal pulmonary emboli; prevention and careful assessment in individuals at risk are crucial.

Diseases of the Arteries

1. Hypertension is a sustained elevation of the systemic arterial blood pressure resulting from increases in cardiac output or total peripheral

SUMMARY REVIEW—cont'd

resistance, or both. Hypertension can be primary (without known cause) or secondary (caused by disease or drugs). Systolic hypertension is the most significant factor in causing target organ damage.

2. The risk factors for hypertension include a positive family history; male gender; advanced age; black race; obesity; high sodium intake; low potassium, calcium, and magnesium intake; diabetes mellitus; labile blood pressure; cigarette smoking; and heavy alcohol consumption.

3. Primary hypertension is the result of extremely complicated interactions of genetics and the environment mediated by a host of neurohumoral effects. These genes interact with diet, smoking, age, and the other risk factors to cause chronic changes in vasomotor tone and blood volume.

4. The most frequently cited theories of the pathogenesis of primary hypertension include overactivity of the SNS; overactivity of the RAAS; alterations in other neurohumoral mediators of blood volume and vasomotor tone such as ANP, BNP, and adrenomedullin; inflammation; a complex interaction involving insulin resistance and endothelial function; and obesity-related hormonal changes.

5. Clinical manifestations of hypertension result from damage of organs and tissues outside the vascular system. These include heart disease, renal disease, CNS problems, and retinal changes.

6. Hypertension is managed pharmacologically, using diuretics, adrenergic blockers, calcium channel blockers, ACE inhibitors, and Ang II receptor blockers. Nonpharmacologic methods include cessation of smoking, dietary modifications, and exercise.

7. Orthostatic hypotension is a drop in blood pressure that occurs on standing. The compensatory vasoconstriction response to standing is altered by a marked vasodilation and blood pooling in the muscle vasculature.

8. Orthostatic hypotension may be primary or secondary. The primary form is caused by neurologic changes that affect the autonomic reflexes that control blood pressure upon standing.

9. The clinical manifestations of orthostatic hypotension include fainting and may result in falls and significant injury.

10. An aneurysm is a localized dilation of a vessel wall to which the aorta is particularly susceptible.

11. A thrombus is a clot that remains attached to a vascular wall.

12. An embolus is a mobile aggregate of a variety of substances that occludes the vasculature. Sources of emboli include thrombi, air, amniotic fluid, bacteria, fat, and foreign matter.

13. The most common sources of arterial thrombotic emboli from the heart are mitral and aortic valvular disease and atrial fibrillation. Tissues affected include the lower extremities, the brain, and the heart.

14. Emboli to the central organs cause tissue death in lungs, kidneys, and mesentery.

15. The generation of air emboli requires a connection between the vascular compartment and a source of air. These emboli cause ischemia and necrosis when a vessel is totally blocked.

16. Amniotic fluid may be forced into the bloodstream and generate an embolus during the labor and delivery of pregnancy.

17. Aggregates of bacteria in the vasculature may be large enough to form an embolus.

18. Fat emboli are caused mainly by trauma to the long bones, either through defective fat metabolism after trauma or through the release of fat globules from bone marrow exposed by fracture.

19. The introduction of foreign matter into the vasculature can occur with trauma and also can occur in a hospital setting in which intravenous and intraarterial lines are being used.

20. Vasospastic disorders include thromboangiitis obliterans and Raynaud disease, involving arterioles of the extremities.

21. Atherosclerosis is a form of arteriosclerosis and is the leading cause of coronary artery and cerebrovascular disease.

22. Atherosclerosis is an inflammatory disease that begins with endothelial injury and progresses through several stages to become a fibrotic plaque.

23. Once a plaque has formed it can rupture, resulting in thrombosis and vasoconstriction that leads to obstruction of the lumen and inadequate perfusion of distal tissues.

24. PAD is atherosclerosis of arteries that perfuse the limbs, especially the lower extremities.

25. PAD is often asymptomatic but can present with intermittent claudication (pain in leg on walking). Treatment includes risk factor reduction and antiplatelet therapy.

26. CAD is occlusion of the coronary arteries and is most often the result of atherosclerotic lesions that limit the flow of blood to the heart.

27. Many risk factors contribute to the onset and escalation of CAD, including advanced age, gender, hypertension, dyslipidemia, diabetes mellitus, smoking, obesity, sedentary lifestyle, elevated hs-CRP, chronic kidney disease, and environmental exposures, such as air pollution and ionizing radiation.

28. CAD results in an imbalance between coronary supply of blood and myocardial demand for oxygen and nutrients such that reversible myocardial ischemia or irreversible infarction may result.

29. Reversible myocardial ischemia presents clinically in several ways. Chronic coronary obstruction results in recurrent predictable chest pain called *stable angina*. Abnormal vasospasm of coronary vessels results in unpredictable chest pain called *Prinzmetal angina*. Myocardial ischemia that does not cause detectable symptoms is called *silent ischemia*.

30. Stable angina is evaluated by noninvasive techniques of assessing coronary flow with or without exercise (stress ECG, thallium, or SPECT). Management may include lifestyle changes, vasodilators, antithrombotics, PCI, or CABG surgery.

31. When there is sudden coronary obstruction because of thrombosis formation over a ruptured atherosclerotic plaque, the acute coronary syndromes result. Unstable angina causes reversible myocardial ischemia and is a harbinger of impending infarction. MI results when prolonged ischemia causes irreversible damage to the heart muscle. Sudden cardiac death can occur in any of the acute coronary syndromes.

32. Unstable angina occurs because of transient episodes of thrombotic vessel occlusion and vasoconstriction at the site of plaque damage, with return of perfusion before significant myocardial necrosis occurs. This must be managed aggressively with antithrombotic agents to prevent MI.

33. When coronary blood flow is interrupted for an extended period, myocyte necrosis occurs; this is called *MI*. Pathologically, there are two major types of myocardial infarction: subendocardial infarction and transmural infarction. In addition to myocyte necrosis, other changes in the heart with MI include hibernating, stunning, and remodeling of the myocardium.

34. Acute coronary syndromes are assessed by measuring serum enzymes, such as troponins, as well as looking for characteristic changes in the ECG. Those individuals at highest risk for complications present with ST-segment elevations on the ECG (STEMI) and require immediate intervention. Smaller subendocardial infarctions are not associated with ST-segment elevations (non-STEMI) but

■ SUMMARY REVIEW—cont'd

suggest that additional myocardium is still at risk for recurrent ischemia and infarction. Management may include thrombolytic drugs, antithrombotic drugs, vasodilators, PCI, or immediate surgery.

35. Dysrhythmias, congestive heart failure, and sudden death are the most common complications of the acute coronary syndromes.

Disorders of the Heart Wall

1. Inflammation of the pericardium (pericarditis) may result from innumerable sources (infection, drug therapy, tumors). Pericarditis presents with symptoms that are physically troublesome, but in and of themselves they are not life threatening.

2. Fluid may collect within the pericardial sac (pericardial effusion). Cardiac function may be severely impaired if a large volume of fluid accumulates rapidly.

3. Cardiomyopathies are a diverse group of primary myocardial disorders that are poorly understood. The cardiomyopathies are categorized as dilated (congestive), restrictive (rigid and noncompliant), and hypertrophic (asymmetrical).

4. Hemodynamic integrity of the cardiovascular system depends to a great extent on properly functioning cardiac valves. Congenital or acquired disorders that structurally alter the valves result in stenosis or regurgitation, or both.

5. Characteristic heart sounds, cardiac murmurs, and systemic complaints assist in determining which valve is abnormal. If severely compromised function exists, a prosthetic heart valve may be surgically implanted to replace the faulty one.

6. Mitral valve prolapse is a common finding, especially in young women. Although not grossly abnormal, the mitral valve leaflets do not position themselves properly during systole. Mitral valve prolapse may be a completely asymptomatic condition or may progress to mitral regurgitation.

7. Rheumatic fever is an inflammatory disease that results from a delayed autoimmune response to a streptococcal infection. The disorder usually resolves without sequelae if treated early.

8. Untreated cases of rheumatic fever may progress to rheumatic heart disease, a potentially disabling cardiovascular disorder primarily affecting the heart valves.

9. Infective endocarditis is a general term for infection and inflammation of the endocardium, especially the cardiac valves. A wide range of conditions predisposes one to the development of this disorder. If infective endocarditis is left unchecked, severe valve abnormalities, chronic bacteremia, and systemic emboli may occur as vegetations break off the valve surface and travel through the bloodstream. Antibiotic therapy is essential to prevent serious complications.

Manifestations of Heart Disease

1. Heart failure is an inability of the heart to supply the metabolism with adequate circulatory volume and pressure.

2. Left heart failure can be categorized as heart failure with reduced ejection fraction (systolic) or heart failure with preserved ejection fraction (diastolic).

3. Heart failure with reduced ejection fraction is defined as an inability of the heart to generate an adequate cardiac output to perfuse vital tissue.

4. Cardiac output depends on the heart rate and stroke volume. Stroke volume is influenced by contractility, preload, and afterload. MI is the most common cause of decreased contractility. Myocardial ischemia results in ventricular remodeling that causes progressive myocyte contractile dysfunction over time.

5. Preload LVEDV is increased when there is decreased contractility or excess plasma volume.

6. Increased afterload is most commonly the result of increased peripheral vascular resistance. This increase in resistance decreases ventricular emptying and makes more workload for the left ventricle, resulting in hypertrophy and ventricular remodeling. The vicious cycle of decreasing contractility, increasing preload, and increasing afterload causes progressive worsening.

7. Neurohumoral mechanisms of congestive heart failure (CHF) include abnormalities in the SNS, RAAS, arginine vasopressin, natriuretic peptides, inflammatory cytokines, and myocyte metabolism.

8. The clinical manifestations of left heart failure are the result of pulmonary vascular congestion and inadequate systemic perfusion.

9. Management of left heart failure relies on increasing contractility and reducing preload and afterload.

10. Heart failure with preserved ejection fraction can occur singly or with systolic heart failure. The major causes of diastolic dysfunction include hypertension-induced myocardial hypertrophy and ischemia with resultant ventricular remodeling.

11. Right heart failure can result from left heart failure and/or diffuse hypoxic pulmonary disease, such as COPD, cystic fibrosis, and ARDS.

12. High output failure is the inability of the heart to adequately supply the body with blood-borne nutrients despite adequate volume and normal or elevated myocardial contractility. Common causes are anemia, septicemia, hyperthyroidism, and beriberi.

13. A dysrhythmia (arrhythmia) is a disturbance of heart rhythm. Dysrhythmias range in severity from occasional missed beats or rapid beats to disturbances that impair myocardial contractility and are life threatening.

14. Dysrhythmias can occur because of an abnormal rate of impulse generation or the abnormal conduction of impulses.

■ KEY TERMS

Acute coronary syndrome, 1074
Acute pericarditis, 1088
Android obesity, 1077
Aneurysm, 1068
Angina pectoris, 1079
Aortic dissection, 1069
Aortic regurgitation, 1093
Aortic stenosis (AS), 1091
Arcus senilis, 1081
Atherosclerosis, 1072
Cardiogenic shock, 1087
Cardiomyopathy, 1089

Carditis, 1094
Chronic left heart failure, 1101
Chronic venous insufficiency (CVI), 1059
Chylomicron, 1075
Complicated hypertension, 1065
Complicated plaque, 1072
Constrictive pericarditis (restrictive pericarditis, chronic pericarditis), 1089
Coronary artery disease (CAD), 1074
Deep venous thrombosis (DVT), 1060
Dilated cardiomyopathy, 1089
Dyslipidemia (dyslipoproteinemia), 1075

Dysrhythmia (arrhythmia), 1087
Embolism, 1070
Embolus, 1070
Erythema marginatum, 1096
False aneurysm, 1068
Heart failure (HF), 1098
Heart failure with preserved ejection fraction, or HFpEF (diastolic heart failure), 1101
Heart failure with reduced ejection fraction, or HFrEF (systolic heart failure), 1098
Hibernating myocardium, 1085
High-density lipoprotein (HDL), 1075

KEY TERMS—cont'd

Highly sensitive C-reactive protein (hs-CRP), 1078
High-output failure, 1102
Hypercoagulable state, 1060
Hypertension (HTN), 1061
Hypertensive crisis (malignant hypertension), 1066
Hypertrophic cardiomyopathy, 1090
Hypertrophic obstructive cardiomyopathy, 1090
Infarction, 1074
Infective endocarditis (IE), 1096
Intermittent claudication, 1074
Ischemia, 1074
Ischemic preconditioning, 1084
Isolated systolic hypertension (ISH), 1061
Left heart failure (congestive heart failure), 1098
Lipoprotein, 1075
Lipoprotein (a) (Lp[a]), 1077
Low-density lipoprotein (LDL), 1075
Metabolic syndrome, 1077
Mitral regurgitation, 1093
Mitral stenosis, 1092
Mitral valve prolapse syndrome, 1093
Myocardial infarction (MI), 1082

Myocardial remodeling, 1085
Myocardial stunning, 1085
non-STEMI, 1084
Orthostatic (postural) hypotension (OH), 1068
Percutaneous coronary intervention (PCI), 1082
Pericardial effusion, 1088
Pericarditis, 1087
Peripheral artery disease (PAD), 1072
Plaque, 1072
Post-thrombotic syndrome (PTS), 1060
Pressure-natriuresis relationship, 1062
Primary hypertension, 1062
Prinzmetal angina, 1079
Raynaud disease, 1071
Raynaud phenomenon, 1071
Reperfusion injury, 1084
Restrictive cardiomyopathy, 1091
Rheumatic fever, 1094
Rheumatic heart disease (RHD), 1094
Right heart failure, 1102
Secondary hypertension, 1065
Silent ischemia, 1079
Stable angina, 1079

Stable plaque, 1079
STEMI, 1084
Superior vena cava syndrome (SVCS), 1061
Sydenham chorea (St. Vitus dance), 1096
Tamponade, 1088
Thromboangiitis obliterans (Buerger disease), 1071
Thromboembolism, 1070
Thromboembolization, 1060
Thromboembolus, 1060
Tricuspid regurgitation, 1093
True aneurysm, 1068
Unstable angina, 1082
Unstable plaque, 1079
Valvular regurgitation, 1091
Valvular stenosis, 1091
Varicose vein, 1059
Venous intimal damage, 1060
Venous stasis, 1060
Venous stasis ulcer, 1059
Ventricular aneurysm, 1087
Ventricular remodeling, 1098
Very-low-density lipoprotein (VLDL), 1075
Xanthelasma, 1081

REFERENCES

1. World Health Organization (WHO): *Cardiovascular diseases (CVD) fact sheet*, 2016. Available at: http://www.who.int/mediacentre/factsheets/fs317/en/. (Accessed 22 February 2016).
2. Cronewett J, Johnson K: *Rutherford's vascular surgery*, St Louis, 2014, Elsevier.
3. Eberhardt R, Raffetto J: Chronic venous insufficiency. *Circulation* 130:333–346, 2014.
4. Lin F, et al: The management of varicose veins. *Int Surg* 100(1):185–189, 2015.
5. Mozaffarian D, et al: Heart disease and stroke statistics—2016 Update: a report from the American Heart Association. *Circulation* 133(4):e38–e360, 2016.
6. Coleman D, Obi A, Henke PK: Update in venous thromboembolism pathophysiology, diagnosis, and treatment for surgical patients. *Curr Prob Surg* 52(6):233–259, 2015.
7. Spandorfer J, Galanis T: In the clinic, deep venous thrombosis. *Ann Intern Med* 162(9):2015.
8. Kahn S, et al: Guidance for the prevention and treatment of the post-thrombotic syndrome. *J Thromb Thrombolysis* 41(1):144–153, 2016.
9. Mekaj YH, Daci FT, Mekai AY: New insights into the mechanisms of action of aspirin and its use in the prevention and treatment of arterial and venous thromboembolism. *Ther Clin Risk Manag* 11:1449–1456, 2015.
10. van der Hulle T, et al: Current standings in diagnostic management of acute venous thromboembolism: still rough around the edges. *Blood Rev* 30(1):21–26, 2016.
11. Kearon C, et al: Antithrombotic therapy for VTE disease: antithrombotic therapy and prevention of thrombosis, ed 9, American College of Chest Physicians evidence-based clinical practice guidelines. *Chest* 141(2 Suppl):e419S–e494S, 2012.
12. Lenchus JD, et al: In-hospital management and follow-up treatment of venous thromboembolism: focus on new and emerging treatments. *J Intensive Care Med* 32(5):299–311, 2017.
13. Hull RD, Gersh MH: The current landscape of treatment options for venous thromboembolism: a focus on novel oral anticoagulants. *Curr Med Res Opin* 31(2):197–210, 2015.

14. Du GC, Zhang MC, Zhao JC: Catheter-directed thrombolysis plus anticoagulation versus anticoagulation alone in the treatment of proximal deep vein thrombosis—a meta-analysis. *Vasa* 44(3):195–202, 2015.
15. Blackwood S, Dietzek AM: Pharmacomechanical thrombectomy: 2015 update. *Expert Rev Cardiovasc Ther* 14(4):463–475, 2015.
16. Kearon C, et al: Antithrombotic therapy for VTE disease: CHEST guideline and expert panel report. *Chest* 149(2):315–352, 2016.
17. Straka C, et al: Review of evolving etiologies, implications and treatment strategies for the superior vena cava syndrome. *Springerplus* 5:229, 2016.
18. James PA, et al: 2014 evidence-based guideline for the management of high blood pressure in adults. Report from the panel members appointed to the Eighth Joint National Committee (JNC 8). *J Am Med Assoc* 311(5):507–520, 2014.
18a. Whelton PK, Carey RM, Aronow WS, et al: 2017 ACC/AHA/AAPA/ABC/ACPM/AGS/APhA/ASH/ASPC/NMA/PCNA Guideline for the prevention, detection, evaluation, and management of high blood pressure in adults: a report of the American College of Cardiology/American Heart Association Task Force on Clinical Practice Guidelines. *Hypertension* 2017 Nov 13 doi: 10.1161/HYP.0000000000000065. [Epub ahead of print.]
19. Padmanabhan S, Caulfield M, Dominiczak AF: Genetic and molecular aspects of hypertension. *Circ Res* 116(6):937–959, 2015.
20. Friso S, et al: Epigenetics and arterial hypertension: the challenge of emerging evidence. *Transl Res* 165(1):154–165, 2015.
21. Morris BJ: Renin, genes, microRNAs, and renal mechanisms involved in hypertension. *Hypertension* 65(5):956–962, 2015.
22. Grassi G, Mark A, Esler M: The sympathetic nervous system alterations in human hypertension. *Circ Res* 116(6):976–990, 2015.
23. Young CN, Davisson RL: Angiotensin-II, the brain, and hypertension: an update. *Hypertension* 66(5):920–926, 2015.

24. Te Riet L, et al: Hypertension: renin-angiotensin-aldosterone system alterations. *Circ Res* 116(6):960–975, 2015.
25. Farag E, et al: An update of the role of renin angiotensin in cardiovascular homeostasis. *Anesth Analg* 120(2):275–292, 2015.
26. Santos RA: Angiotensin (1-7). *Hypertension* 63:1138–1147, 2014.
27. O'Donnell M, Mente A, Yusuf S: Sodium intake and cardiovascular health. *Circ Res* 116(6):1046–1057, 2015.
28. Patel P, Chen HH: Natriuretic peptides as a novel target in resistant hypertension. *Curr Hypertens Rep* 17(3):18, 2015.
29. Bavishi C, et al: Role of neprilysin inhibitor combinations in hypertension: insights from hypertension and heart failure trials. *Eur Heart J* 36(30):1967–1973, 2015.
30. McMaster WG, et al: Inflammation, immunity, and hypertensive end-organ damage. *Circ Res* 116(6):1022–1033, 2015.
31. Montezano AC, et al: Oxidative stress and human hypertension: vascular mechanisms, biomarkers, and novel therapies. *Can J Cardiol* 31(5):631–641, 2015.
32. Hall JE, et al: Obesity-induced hypertension: interaction of neurohumoral and renal mechanisms. *Circ Res* 116(6):991–1006, 2015.
33. Li YX, et al: Association of two well-defined polymorphisms in leptin and leptin receptor genes with hypertension and circulating leptin: a meta-analysis. *Arch Med Sci* 46(1):38–46, 2015.
34. Zachariah JP, et al: Circulating adipokines and vascular function: cross-sectional associations in a community-based cohort. *Hypertension* 67(2):294–300, 2016.
35. Sabbatini AR, et al: An update on the role of adipokines in arterial stiffness and hypertension. *J Hypertens* 33(3):435–444, 2015.
36. Soltani Z, et al: The impacts of obesity on the cardiovascular and renal systems: cascade of events and therapeutic approaches. *Curr Hypertens Rep* 17(2):7, 2015.
37. DeWitt D, Dugdale DC, Adam WR: Nonglycemic targets in diabetes. *Med Clin North Am* 99(1):187–200, 2015.

38. Rao A, Pandya V, Whaley-Connell A: Obesity and insulin resistance in resistant hypertension: implications for the kidney. *Adv Chronic Kidney Dis* 22(3):211–217, 2015.

39. Reisin E, Owen J: Treatment: special conditions. Metabolic syndrome: obesity and the hypertension connection. *J Am Soc Hypertens* 9(2):156–159, quiz 160, 2015.

40. Nadruz W: Myocardial remodeling in hypertension. *J Human Hypertens* 29(1):1–6, 2015.

41. Ishizu T, et al: Left ventricular strain and transmural distribution of structural remodeling in hypertensive heart disease. *Hypertension* 63(3):500–506, 2014.

42. Lioudaki E, et al: Microalbuminuria: a neglected cardiovascular risk factor in non-diabetic individuals? *Curr Pharm Des* 19(27):4964–4980, 2013.

43. Kokubo Y, Iwashima Y: Higher blood pressure as a risk factor for diseases other than stroke and ischemic heart disease. *Hypertension* 66(2):254–259, 2015.

44. Riba-Llena I, et al: High daytime and nighttime ambulatory pulse pressure predict poor cognitive function and mild cognitive impairment in hypertensive individuals. *J Cereb Blood Flow Metab* 36(1):253–263, 2016.

45. Muiesan ML, et al: An update on hypertensive emergencies and urgencies. *J Cardiovasc Med (Hagerstown)* 16(5):372–382, 2015.

46. Piper MA, et al: Diagnostic and predictive accuracy of blood pressure screening methods with consideration of rescreening intervals: a systematic review for the U.S. Preventive Services Task Force. *Ann Intern Med* 162(3):192–204, 2015.

47. Turner JR, Viera AJ, Shimbo D: Ambulatory blood pressure monitoring in clinical practice: a review. *Am J Med* 128(1):14–20, 2015.

48. Schwingshackl L, Hoffmann G: Diet quality as assessed by the healthy eating index, the alternate healthy eating index, the dietary approaches to stop hypertension score, and health outcomes: a systematic review and meta-analysis of cohort studies. *J Acad Nutr Diet* 115(5):780–800, e5, 2015.

49. Rosendorff C, et al: Treatment of hypertension in patients with coronary artery disease: a scientific statement from the American Heart Association, American College of Cardiology, and American Society of Hypertension. *Hypertension* 65:1372–1407, 2015.

50. Cushman WC, et al: SPRINT trial results: latest news in hypertension management. *Hypertension* 67(2):263–265, 2016.

51. Bhatt DL, et al: A controlled trial of renal denervation for resistant hypertension. *N Engl J Med* 370:1393–1401, 2014.

52. Laffin LJ, Bakris GL: Renal denervation for resistant hypertension and beyond. *Adv Chronic Kidney Dis* 22(2):133–139, 2015.

53. Cooper-DeHoff RM, Johnson JA: Hypertension pharmacogenomics: in search of personalized treatment approaches. *Nat Rev Nephrol* 12(2):110–122, 2016.

54. Oparil S, Schmieder RE: New approaches in the treatment of hypertension. *Circ Res* 116(6):1074–1095, 2015.

55. Ricci F, De Caterina R: Fedorowski A: Orthostatic hypotension: epidemiology, prognosis, and treatment. *J Am Coll Cardiol* 66(7):848–860, 2015.

56. Kanjwal K, et al: Orthostatic hypotension: definition, diagnosis and management. *J Cardiovasc Med* 16(2):75–81, 2015.

57. Ricci F, et al: Cardiovascular morbidity and mortality related to orthostatic hypotension: a meta-analysis of prospective observational studies. *Eur Heart J* 36(25):1609–1617, 2015.

58. Dale MA, Ruhlman MK, Baxter BT: Inflammatory cell phenotypes in AAAs: their role and potential as targets for therapy. *Arterioscler Thromb Vasc Biol* 35(8):1746–1755, 2015.

59. Raffort J, et al: Monocytes and macrophages in abdominal aortic aneurysm. *Nat Rev Cardiol* 14(8):457–471, 2017.

60. Andelfinger G, Loeys B, Dietz H: A decade of discovery in the genetic understanding of thoracic aortic disease. *Can J Cardiol* 32(1):13–25, 2016.

61. Mellnick VM, Heiken JP: The acute abdominal aorta. *Radiol Clin North Am* 53(6):1209–1224, 2015.

62. Ridge CA, Litmanovich DE: Acute aortic syndromes: current status. *J Thorac Imaging* 30(3):193–201, 2015.

63. Roselli EE, et al: Endovascular stent grafting for ascending aorta repair in high-risk patients. *J Thorac Cardiovasc Surg* 149(1):144–151, 2015.

64. Clough RE, Nienaber CA: Management of acute aortic syndrome. *Nat Rev Cardiol* 12:103–114, 2015.

65. Malecki R, et al: The pathogenesis and diagnosis of thromboangiitis obliterans: is it still a mystery? *Adv Clin Exp Med* 24(6):1085–1097, 2015.

66. Klein-Weigel PF, Richter JG: Thromboangiitis obliterans (Buerger's disease). *Vasa* 43(5):337–346, 2014.

67. Garner R, et al: Prevalence, risk factors and associations of primary Raynaud's phenomenon: systematic review and meta-analysis of observational studies. *BMJ Open* 5(3):e006389, 2015.

68. Linnemann B, Erbe M: Raynauds phenomenon—assessment and differential diagnoses. *Vasa* 44(3):166–177, 2015.

69. Merritt WH: Role and rationale for extended periarterial sympathectomy in the management of severe Raynaud syndrome: techniques and results. *Hand Clin* 31(1):101–120, 2015.

70. Viola J, Soehnlein O: Atherosclerosis—a matter of unresolved inflammation. *Sem Immunol* 27(3):184–193, 2015.

71. Tabas I, Garcia-Cardena G, Owens GK: Recent insights into the cellular biology of atherosclerosis. *J Cell Biol* 209(1):13–22, 2015.

72. Meijles DN, Pagano PJ: Nox and inflammation in the vascular adventitia. *Hypertension* 67:14–19, 2016.

73. Ivanovic B, Tadic M: Hypercholesterolemia and hypertension: two sides of the same coin. *Am J Cardiovasc Drugs* 15(6):403–414, 2015.

74. Seneviratne AN, Monaco C: Role of inflammatory cells and toll-like receptors in atherosclerosis. *Curr Vasc Pharmacol* 13(2):146–160, 2015.

75. Lu H, Daugherty A: Atherosclerosis. *Arterioscler Thromb Vasc Biol* 35(3):485–491, 2015.

76. Chistiakov DA, Orekhov AN, Bobryshev YV: Contribution of neovascularization and intraplaque haemorrhage to atherosclerotic plaque progression and instability. *Acta Physiol* 213(3):539–553, 2015.

77. Wang M, et al: Matrix metalloproteinases promote arterial remodeling in aging, hypertension, and atherosclerosis. *Hypertension* 65(4):698–703, 2015.

78. Abu Dabrh AM, et al: Bypass surgery versus endovascular interventions in severe or critical limb ischemia. *J Vasc Surg* 63(1):244–253, e11, 2016.

79. Vartanian SM, Conte MS: Surgical intervention for peripheral arterial disease. *Circ Res* 116(9):1614–1628, 2015.

80. Peeters Weem SM, et al: Bone marrow derived cell therapy in critical limb ischemia: a meta-analysis of randomized placebo controlled trials. *Eur J Vasc Endovasc Surg* 50(6):775–783, 2015.

81. Sanada F, et al: Gene therapy in peripheral artery disease. *Expert Opin Biol Ther* 15(3):381–390, 2015.

82. Rankinen T, et al: Are there genetic paths common to obesity, cardiovascular disease outcomes, and cardiovascular risk factors? *Circ Res* 116(5):909s–922s, 2015.

83. Björkegren JL, et al: Genome-wide significant loci: how important are they? Systems genetics to understand heritability of coronary artery disease and other common complex disorders. *J Am Coll Cardiol* 65(8):830–845, 2015.

84. Expert Panel on Detection: Evaluation and treatment of high blood cholesterol in adults: executive summary of the third report of the National Cholesterol Education Program (NCEP) Expert Panel on Detection, Evaluation, and Treatment of High Blood Cholesterol in Adults (Adult Treatment Panel III). *J Am Med Assoc* 285(19):2486–2497, 2001.

85. Stone NJ, et al: 2013ACC/AHA guideline on the treatment of blood cholesterol to reduce atherosclerotic cardiovascular risk in adults: a report of the American College of Cardiology/American Heart Association Task Force on practice guidelines. *J Am Coll Cardiol* 63(25 Pt B):3024–3025, 2014.

86. Rosenson RS, Hegele RA, Gotto AM, Jr: Integrated measure for atherogenic lipoproteins in the modern era: risk assessment based on apolipoprotein B. *J Am Coll Cardiol* 67(2):202–204, 2016.

87. Cholesterol Treatment Trialists' (CTT) Collaboration: Efficacy and safety of LDL-lowering therapy among men and women: meta-analysis of individual data from 174,000 participants in 27 randomised trials. *Lancet* 385:1397–1405, 2015.

88. Jarcho JA, Keaney JF, Jr: Proof that lower is better—LDL cholesterol and IMPROVE-IT. *N Engl J Med* 372:2448–2450, 2015.

89. Grundy SM: Dyslipidemia in 2015: advances in treatment of dyslipidemia. *Nat Rev Cardiol* 13:74–75, 2016.

90. Annema W, von Eckardstein A, Kovanen PT: HDL and atherothrombotic vascular disease. *Handb Exp Pharmacol* 224:369–403, 2015.

91. Constantinou C, et al: Advances in high-density lipoprotein physiology: surprises, overturns, and promises. *Am J Physiol Endocrinol Metab* 310(1):E1–E14, 2016.

92. Rosenson RS, et al: Dysfunctional HDL and atherosclerotic cardiovascular disease. *Nat Rev Cardiol* 13(1):48–60, 2016.

93. Mathur P, et al: Gender-related differences in atherosclerosis. *Cardiovasc Drugs Ther* 29(4):319–327, 2015.

94. Rosendorff C, et al: Treatment of hypertension in patients with coronary artery disease: a scientific statement from the American Heart Association, American College of Cardiology, and American Society of Hypertension. *Hypertension* 65(6):1372–1407, 2015.

95. Messner B, Bernhard D: Smoking and cardiovascular disease: mechanisms of endothelial dysfunction and early atherogenesis. *Arterioscler Thromb Vasc Biol* 34(3):509–515, 2014.

96. Eelen G, et al: Endothelial cell metabolism in normal and diseased vasculature. *Circ Res* 116(7):1231–1244, 2015.

97. Mazurek T, Opolski G: Pericoronary adipose tissue: a novel therapeutic target in obesity-related coronary atherosclerosis. *J Am Coll Nutr* 34(3):244–254, 2015.

98. Backshall J, et al: Physical activity in the management of patients with coronary artery disease: a review. *Cardiol Rev* 23(1):18–25, 2015.

99. Sala-Vila A, et al: Dietary α-linolenic acid, marine ω-3 fatty acids, and mortality in a population with high fish consumption: findings from the PREvención con DIeta MEDiterránea (PREDIMED) study. *J Am Heart Assoc* 5(1):2016.

100. Estruch R, et al: Primary prevention of cardiovascular disease with a Mediterranean diet. *N Engl J Med* 368:1279–1290, 2013.

101. Ammirati E, et al: Markers of inflammation associated with plaque progression and instability in patients with carotid atherosclerosis. *Mediators Inflamm* 2015:718329, 2015.

102. Lin GM, et al: Low-density lipoprotein cholesterol concentrations and association of high-sensitivity C-reactive protein concentrations with incident coronary heart disease in the multi-ethnic study of atherosclerosis. *Am J Epidemiol* 183(1):46–52, 2016.

103. Goff DC, et al: 2013 ACC/AHA guideline on the assessment of cardiovascular risk: a report of the American College of Cardiology/American Heart Association Task Force on practice guidelines. *Circulation* 129:549–573, 2014.

104. Iribarren C, et al: High-sensitive cardiac troponin-I and incident coronary heart disease among asymptomatic older adults. *Heart* 102(15):1177–1182, 2016.

105. Adya R, Tan BK, Randeva HS: Differential effects of leptin and adiponectin in endothelial angiogenesis. *J Diabetes Res* 2015:648239, 2015.

106. Hossain MM, Mukheem A, Kamarul T: The prevention and treatment of hypoadiponectinemia-associated human diseases by up-regulation of plasma adiponectin. *Life Sci* 135:55–67, 2015.

107. Carbone F, Mach F, Montecucco F: The role of adipocytokines in atherogenesis and atheroprogression. *Curr Drug Targets* 16(4):295–320, 2015.

108. Di Lullo L, et al: Chronic kidney disease and cardiovascular complications. *Heart Fail Rev* 20(3):259–272, 2015.

109. Gargiulo R, Suhail F, Lerma EV: Cardiovascular disease and chronic kidney disease. *Dis Mon* 61(9):403–413, 2015.

110. Franklin BA, Brook R, Arden Pope C, 3rd: Air pollution and cardiovascular disease. *Curr Prob Cardiol* 40(5):207–238, 2015.

111. Borghini A, et al: Ionizing radiation and atherosclerosis: current knowledge and future challenges. *Atherosclerosis* 230(1):40–47, 2013.

112. Jaiswal S, et al: Clonal hematopoiesis and risk of atherosclerotic cardiovascular disease. *N Engl J Med* 377(2):111–121, 2017.

113. Danelich IM, et al: Safety of nonsteroidal antiinflammatory drugs in patients with cardiovascular disease. *Pharmacotherapy* 35(5):520–535, 2015.

114. Clifford A, Hoffman GS: Evidence for a vascular microbiome and its role in vessel health and disease. *Curr Opin Rheumatol* 27(4):397–405, 2015.

115. Drosos I, Tavridou A, Kolios G: New aspects on the metabolic role of intestinal microbiota in the development of atherosclerosis. *Metabolism* 64(4):476–481, 2015.

116. Titterington JS, Hung OY, Wenger NK: Microvascular angina: an update on diagnosis and treatment. *Future Cardiol* 11(2):229–242, 2015.

117. Ong P, et al: Structural and functional coronary artery abnormalities in patients with vasospastic angina pectoris. *Circ J* 79(7):1431–1438, 2015.

118. Pasupathy S, et al: Systematic review of patients presenting with suspected myocardial infarction and nonobstructive coronary arteries. *Circulation* 131(10):861–870, 2015.

119. Abd El-Aziz TA, et al: A new metabolic mechanism for absence of pain in patients with silent myocardial ischemia. *Arch Med Res* 46(2):127–132, 2015.

120. Pimple P, et al: Association between anger and mental stress-induced myocardial ischemia. *Am Heart J* 169(1):115–121, 2015.

121. Petretta M, et al: Quantitative assessment of myocardial blood flow with SPECT. *Prog Cardiovasc Dis* 57(6):607–614, 2015.

122. Qayyum AA, Kastrup J: Measuring myocardial perfusion: the role of PET, MRI and CT. *Clin Radiol* 70(6):576–584, 2015.

123. Fihn SD, et al: 2014 ACC/AHA/AATS/PCNA/SCAI/STS focused update of the guideline for the diagnosis and management of patients with stable ischemic heart disease: a report of the American College of Cardiology/American Heart Association Task Force on practice guidelines, and the American Association for Thoracic Surgery, Preventive Cardiovascular Nurses Association, Society for Cardiovascular Angiography and Interventions, and Society of Thoracic Surgeons. *J Thorac Cardiovasc Surg* 149(3):e5–e23, 2015.

124. Ohman EM: Clinical Practice. Chronic stable angina. *N Eng J Med* 374(12):1167–1176, 2016.

125. Gada H, et al: Meta-analysis of trials on mortality after percutaneous coronary intervention compared with medical therapy in patients with stable coronary heart disease and objective evidence of myocardial ischemia. *Am J Cardiol* 115(9):1194–1199, 2015.

126. Hou L, et al: Stem cell-based therapies to promote angiogenesis in ischemic cardiovascular disease. *Am J Physiol Heart Circ Physiol* 310(4):H455–H465, 2016.

127. Tsigaridas N, et al: Spinal cord stimulation in refractory angina. A systematic review of randomized controlled trials. *Acta Cardiol* 70(2):233–243, 2015.

128. Amsterdam EA, et al: AHA/ACC guideline for the management of patients with non-ST-elevation acute coronary syndromes: a report of the American College of Cardiology/American Heart Association Task Force on practice guidelines. *Circulation* 130(25):2354–2394, 2014.

129. Heusch G: Molecular basis of cardioprotection: signal transduction in ischemic pre-, post-, and remote conditioning. *Circ Res* 116(4):674–699, 2015.

130. Williams TM, et al: Ischemic preconditioning-an unfulfilled promise. *Cardiovasc Revasc Med* 16(2):101–108, 2015.

131. Ong SB, et al: The mitochondrial permeability transition pore and its role in myocardial ischemia reperfusion injury. *J Mol Cell Cardiol* 78:23–34, 2015.

132. McAlindon E, et al: Infarct size reduction in acute myocardial infarction. *Heart* 101(2):155–160, 2015.

133. Touboul C, et al: Ischaemic postconditioning reduces infarct size: systematic review and meta-analysis of randomized controlled trials. *Arch Cardiovasc Dis* 108(1):39–49, 2015.

134. Ma S, et al: The role of the autophagy in myocardial ischemia/reperfusion injury. *Biochim Biophys Acta* 1852(2):271–276, 2015.

135. Holley CT, et al: Recovery of hibernating myocardium: what is the role of surgical revascularization? *J Card Surg* 30(2):224–231, 2015.

136. Levisman J, Price MJ: Update on the guidelines for the management of ST-elevation myocardial infarction. *Am J Cardiol* 115(5 Suppl):3A–9A, 2015.

137. O'Gara PT, et al: ACCF/AHA guideline for the management of ST-elevation myocardial infarction: a report of the American College of Cardiology Foundation/American Heart Association Task Force on practice guidelines. *Circulation* 127:e362–e425, 2013.

138. Akashi YJ, Nef HM, Lyon AR: Epidemiology and pathophysiology of Takotsubo syndrome. *Nat Rev Cardiol* 12(7):387–397, 2015.

139. Imazio M, Gaita F, LeWinter M: Evaluation and treatment of pericarditis: a systematic review. *J Am Med Assoc* 314(14):1498–1506, 2015.

140. Patel R, et al: Diagnostic performance of cardiac magnetic resonance imaging and echocardiography in evaluation of cardiac and paracardiac masses. *Am J Cardiol* 117(1):135–140, 2016.

141. Imazio M: Pericardial decompression syndrome: a rare but potentially fatal complication of pericardial drainage to be recognized and prevented. *Eur Heart J Acute Cardiovasc Care* 4(2):121–123, 2015.

142. Welch TD, Oh JK: Constrictive pericarditis: old disease, new approaches. *Curr Cardiol Rep* 17(4):20, 2015.

143. Scardovi AB, De Maria R, Ricci R: Acute peripartum cardiomyopathy rapidly evolving in cardiogenic shock. *Int J Cardiol* 189:255–256, 2015.

144. Skrzynia C, et al: Genetics and heart failure: a concise guide for the clinician. *Curr Cardiol Rev* 11(1):10–17, 2015.

145. Ware JS, et al: Shared genetic predisposition in peripartum and dilated cardiomyopathies. *N Engl J Med* 374(3):233–241, 2016.

146. Spinarova L, Spinar J: Pharmacotherapy of dilated cardiomyopathy. *Curr Pharm Des* 21(4):449–458, 2015.

147. Argulian E, Sherrid MV, Messerli FH: Misconceptions and facts about hypertrophic cardiomyopathy. *Am J Med* 129(2):148–152, 2016.

148. Hensley N, et al: Hypertrophic cardiomyopathy: a review. *Anesth Analg* 120(3):554–569, 2015.

149. Geske JB, Ommen SR: Role of imaging in evaluation of sudden cardiac death risk in hypertrophic cardiomyopathy. *Curr Opin Cardiol* 30(5):493–499, 2015.

150. Maron BJ, et al: What do patients with hypertrophic cardiomyopathy die from? *Am J Cardiol* 117(3):434–435, 2016.

151. Grupper A, et al: Role of ventricular assist therapy for patients with heart failure and restrictive physiology: improving outcomes for a lethal disease. *J Heart Lung Transplant* 34(8):1042–1049, 2015.

152. Nishimura RA, et al: 2014 AHA/ACC guideline for the management of patients with valvular heart disease: a report of the American College of Cardiology/American Heart Association Task Force on practice guidelines. *J Thorac Cardiovasc Surg* 148(1):e1–e132, 2014.

153. Coffey S, Cairns BJ, Iung B: The modern epidemiology of heart valve disease. *Heart* 102(1):75–85, 2016.

154. Bonow RO, et al: Management strategies and future challenges for aortic valve disease. *Lancet* 387(10025):1312–1323, 2016.

155. Mathieu P, Bouchareb R, Boulanger MC: Innate and adaptive immunity in calcific aortic valve disease. *J Immunol Res* 2015:851–945, 2015.

156. Rader F, et al: Left ventricular hypertrophy in valvular aortic stenosis: mechanisms and clinical implications. *Am J Med* 128(4):344–352, 2015.

157. Sarkar K, Sarkar M, Ussia GP: Current status of transcatheter aortic valve replacement. *Med Clin North Am* 99(4):805–833, 2015.

158. Breed ER, Binstadt BA: Autoimmune valvular carditis. *Curr Allergy Asthma Rep* 15(1):491, 2015.

159. Sorajja P, et al: Initial experience with commercial transcatheter mitral valve repair in the United States. *J Am Coll Cardiol* 67:1129–1140, 2016.

160. de Meester C, et al: Early surgical intervention versus watchful waiting and outcomes for asymptomatic severe aortic regurgitation. *J Thorac Cardiovasc Surg* 150(5):1100–1108, 2015.

161. Taramasso M, Maisano F: Valvular disease: functional mitral regurgitation: should all valves be replaced? *Nat Rev Cardiol* 13(2):65–66, 2016.

162. Goldstein D, et al: Two-year outcomes of surgical treatment of severe ischemic mitral regurgitation. *N Engl J Med* 374:344–353, 2016.

163. Watanabe N: The mitral valve complex: divine perfection. *Circ Cardiovasc Imaging* 9(1):2016.

164. Dina C, et al: Genetic association analyses highlight biological pathways underlying mitral valve prolapse. *Nat Genet* 47(10):1206–1211, 2015.

165. Webb RH, Grant C, Harnden A: Acute rheumatic fever. *BMJ* 351:h3443, 2015.

166. Bagnall EM, Ho MJ, McCormick IA: A 39-year-old man with recurrent rheumatic fever. *CMAJ* 187(1):50–54, 2015.

167. Gewitz MH, et al: Revision of the Jones criteria for the diagnosis of acute rheumatic fever in the era of Doppler echocardiography: a scientific statement from the American Heart Association. *Circulation* 131:1806–1818, 2015.

168. Pant S, et al: Trends in infective endocarditis incidence, microbiology, and valve replacement in the United States from 2000 to 2011. *J Am Coll Cardiol* 65(19):2070–2076, 2015.

169. Baddour LM, et al: AHA scientific statement: infective endocarditis in adults: diagnosis, antimicrobial therapy, and management of complications: a scientific statement for healthcare professionals from the American Heart Association. *Circulation* 132:1435–1486, 2015.

170. Brown DA, et al: Expert consensus document: mitochondrial function as a therapeutic target in heart failure. *Nat Rev Cardiol* 14:238–250, 2017.

171. Miao R: Regulator of G-protein signaling 10 negatively regulates cardiac remodeling by blocking mitogen-activated protein kinase-extracellular signal-regulated protein kinase 1/2 signaling. *Hypertension* 67(1):86–98, 2016.

172. Moon JC, Treibel TA, Schelbert EB: Myocardial fibrosis in hypertensive heart failure: does quality rather than quantity matter? *J Am Coll Cardiol* 67(3):261–263, 2016.

173. Ishizu T, et al: Left ventricular strain and transmural distribution of structural remodeling in hypertensive heart disease. *Hypertension* 63(3):500–506, 2014.

174. Nadruz W: Myocardial remodeling in hypertension. *J Human Hypertens* 29(1):1–6, 2015.

175. Mentz RJ, O'Connor CM: Pathophysiology and clinical evaluation of acute heart failure. *Nat Rev Cardiol* 13(1):28–35, 2016.

176. Izumi Y, Miura K, Iwao H: Therapeutic potential of vasopressin-receptor antagonists in heart failure. *J Pharmacol Sci* 124:1–6, 2014.

177. Volpe M, Carnovali M, Mastromarino V: The natriuretic peptides system in the pathophysiology of heart failure: from molecular basis to treatment. *Clin Sci* 130(2):57–77, 2016.

178. Mann DL: Innate immunity and the failing heart: the cytokine hypothesis revisited. *Circ Res* 116(7):1254–1268, 2015.

179. Hwang PM, Sykes BD: Targeting the sarcomere to correct muscle function. *Nat Rev Drug Discov* 14(5):313–328, 2015.

180. Kristensen SL, et al: Risk related to pre-diabetes mellitus and diabetes mellitus in heart failure with reduced ejection fraction: insights from prospective comparison of ARNI with ACEI to determine impact on global mortality and morbidity in heart failure trial. *Circ Heart Fail* 9(1):2016.

181. Dei Cas A, et al: Concomitant diabetes mellitus and heart failure. *Curr Prob Cardiol* 40(1):7–43, 2015.

182. Filion KB, et al: A multicenter observational study of incretin-based drugs and heart failure. *N Eng J Med* 374(12):1145–1154, 2016.

183. Kober L: Heart failure in 2015: better results from prevention than from additional treatment. *Nat Rev Cardiol* 13(2):75–77, 2016.

184. Writing Committee Members, et al: 2013 ACCF/AHA guideline for the management of heart failure: a report of the American College of Cardiology Foundation/American Heart Association Task Force on practice guidelines. *Circulation* 128(16):e240–e327, 2013.

185. Januzzi JL, Mebazaa A, Di Somma S: ST2 and prognosis in acutely decompensated heart failure: the international ST2 consensus panel. *Am J Cardiol* 115(7 Suppl):26B–31B, 2015.

186. McMurray JJ, et al: Aliskiren, enalapril, or aliskiren and enalapril in heart failure. *N Engl J Med* 374(16):1521–1532, 2016.

187. Oeser C: Pharmacogenetics: CRTR2 gene is associated with response to HF therapy. *Nat Rev Cardiol* 13(2):64, 2016.

188. Mancini D, Colombo PC: Left ventricular assist devices: a rapidly evolving alternative to transplant. *J Am Coll Cardiol* 65(23):2542–2555, 2015.

189. Braunwald E: The war against heart failure: the *Lancet* lecture. *Lancet* 385(9970):812–824, 2015.

190. Donahue JK: Cardiac gene therapy: a call for basic methods development. *Lancet* 387(10024):1137–1139, 2016.

191. Ferrari R, et al: Heart failure with preserved ejection fraction: uncertainties and dilemmas. *Eur J Heart Fail* 17(7):665–671, 2015.

192. Jumean MF, Konstam MA: Heart failure with preserved ejection fraction: what is in a name? *Cardiol Rev* 23(4):161–167, 2015.

193. Nanayakkara S, Kaye DM: Management of heart failure with preserved ejection fraction: a review. *Clin Ther* 37(10):2186–2198, 2015.

194. Kholdani CA, Fares WH: Management of right heart failure in the intensive care unit. *Clin Chest Med* 36(3):511–520, 2015.

195. McCulloch B: High-output heart failure caused by thyrotoxicosis and beriberi. *Crit Care Nurs Clin North Am* 27(4):499–510, 2015.

Alterations of Cardiovascular Function in Children

Nancy Pike, Jennifer K. Peterson

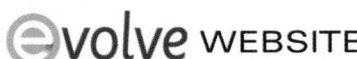

WEBSITE

http://evolve.elsevier.com/McCance/
- Content Updates
- Chapter Summary Review
- Review Questions
- Case Studies
- Animations

CHAPTER OUTLINE

Cardiovascular disease in children can be classified as congenital or acquired heart disease. Congenital heart disease is the most common. The diagnosis and management of congenital heart defects continue to improve with the use of fetal echocardiography, early interventional catheterization, and refined surgical repair or palliation. Acquired heart disease in children continues to present challenges to the practitioner; guidelines for diagnosis are available; standards of treatment and long-term follow-up are in progress.

DEVELOPMENT OF THE CARDIOVASCULAR SYSTEM
Developmental Anatomy
Embryology

Cardiogenesis begins at approximately 3 weeks' gestation; however, most cardiovascular development occurs between the fourth and seventh weeks.[1] The heart arises from the mesenchyme and begins development as an enlarged blood vessel with a large lumen and a muscular wall (Fig. 34.1, *A*). Initially, two lateral endocardial heart tubes fuse to form

a single structure (see Fig. 34.1, *B*). During the fifth week of gestation, the midsection of this tube begins to grow faster than its ends. This single heart tube elongates and rotates to the right (D-loop formation), creating a bulboventricular loop by approximately the 28th day[1] (see Fig. 34.1, *C*). Also at this time the first fetal heart contractions occur. At this stage the primitive heart structures include a common atrium; a common ventricle; the sinus venosus, which eventually evolves into the superior and inferior venae cavae; the bulbus cordis, which eventually evolves into the ventricular outflow tracts; and the truncus arteriosus, which eventually yields the main pulmonary artery (PA) and aorta (see Fig. 34.1, *D*). By the fourth week of gestation, cardiovascular septation, ventricular development, aortic arch evolution, and circulation begin.

Cardiac Septation

Separation first begins when collections of mesenchymal cells cause the endocardial lining of the heart to bulge into the internal lumen. These changes, known as endocardial cushions, are instrumental in closing the lower portion of the atrial septum, dividing the atrioventricular (AV) canals into the right and left AV orifices and forming the upper portion of the interventricular septum. Altered formation of the

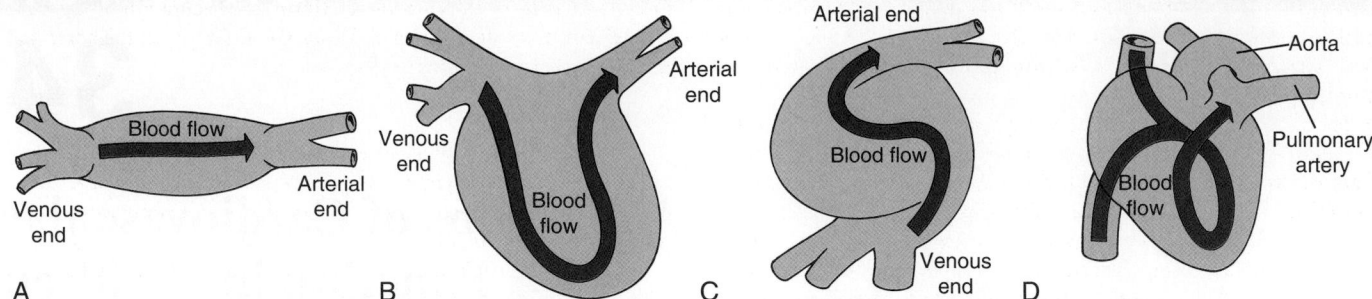

FIGURE 34.1 Embryologic Development of the Heart. **A,** The earliest heart structure consists of a muscular tube with a large lumen. About the fifth week of gestation, the tube, **B,** bulges and, **C,** twists until, **D,** the ends come together and fuse.

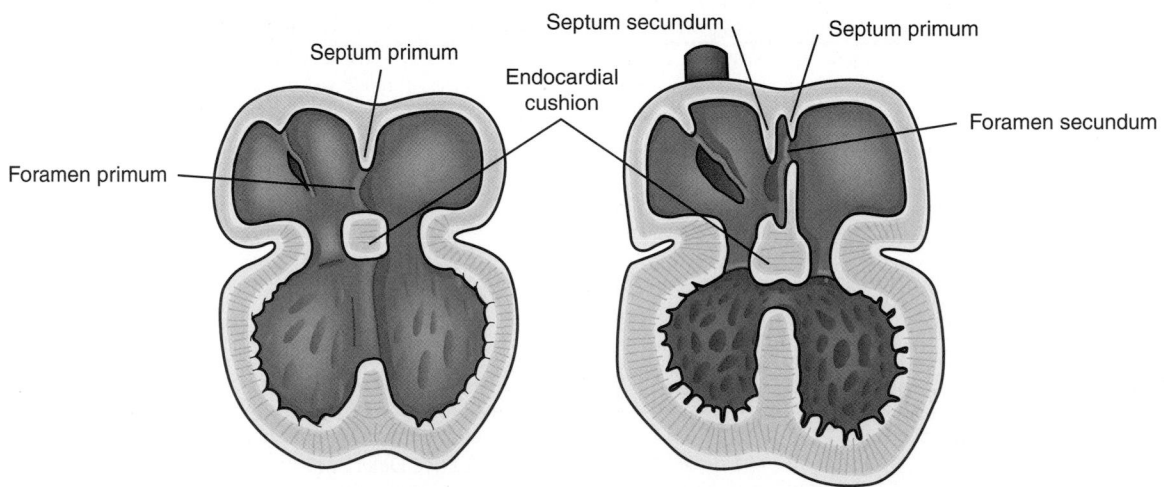

FIGURE 34.2 Development of the Cardiac Septa.

endocardial cushions can result in atrial septal defects (ASDs), inlet ventricular septal defects (VSDs), malformation of the AV valves, or a complete AV defect (also known as *atrioventricular septal defect*).[2]

Atrial septation begins when two thin membrane-like structures, known as the septum primum and the septum secundum, grow toward the area of the endocardial cushions (Fig. 34.2). The septum primum forms along the posterior wall of the common atrium and grows downward toward the center portion of the heart. The gap between the two structures, known as the ostium primum, normally closes by extensions from the endocardial cushions. At the time of closure, fenestrations or openings develop in the superior portion of the septum primum, creating the ostium secundum. Failure of the septum primum to fuse with the endocardial cushions results in an ostium primum defect in the atrial septum near the AV valve area.

The septum secundum is also a fenestrated, membrane-like structure located anteriorly that grows toward the endocardial cushions. During fetal development this structure does not completely fuse with the endocardial cushions to achieve complete atrial septal closure. The nonfused septum secundum and ostium secundum result in the formation of a flapped orifice known as the *foramen ovale,* which allows the right-to-left shunting necessary for fetal circulation. Altered development in any of these structures can lead to an ASD.

Ventricular septation develops when the muscular ridge located at the apex, endocardial tissue, and the bulbar ridges in the bulbus cordis fuse together (Fig. 34.3). Closure of the interventricular septum ensures communication between the right ventricle (RV) and the PA and between the left ventricle (LV) and the aorta. Further evolution of the endocardial

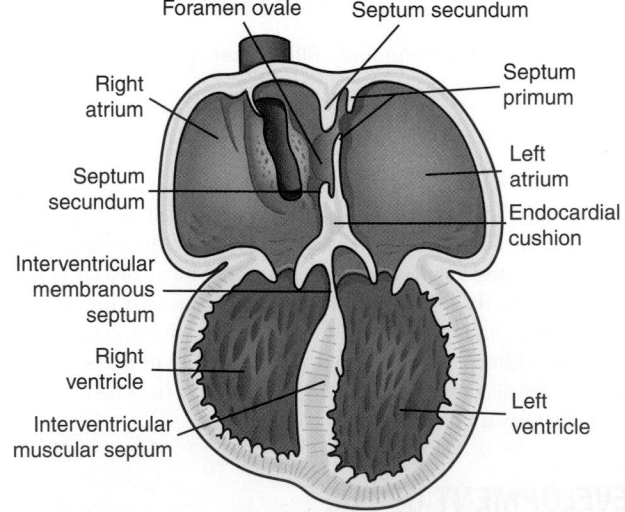

FIGURE 34.3 Septal Development of the Heart.

tissue gives rise to the membranous ventricular septum and the AV valves. The conal portion of the ventricular septum that separates the aorta from the PA forms from the bulbus cordis.

When the single primitive heart tube begins to form the D-loop, the venous and arterial poles of the heart are fixed, resulting in torsion within the anterosuperior region of the loop, known as the *truncus arteriosus.* This torsion creates a spiral ridgelike structure or septum within the truncus arteriosus that divides it into the PA and the aorta. The semilunar valves evolve from tubercles after this division is complete.

Before this division occurs, however, two large arteries form at the distal end of the truncus arteriosus. Over time they give rise to a series of arterial vessels, collectively called the *six aortic arches.* By the fifth week of gestation, the first two pairs disappear and the third eventually evolves into the common carotid artery, the external carotid artery, and part of the internal carotid artery. The fourth pair of aortic arches will form part of the true aortic arch and the proximal segment of the right subclavian artery. The fifth pair disappears; however, the sixth pair yields the proximal and branch pulmonary arteries within the lung parenchyma and the ductus arteriosus.

Swellings in the conal region at the base of the main trunk separate the right ventricular outflow (pulmonary outflow) tract from the left ventricular outflow (aortic outflow) tract. The conus also contributes to complete closure of the interventricular septum, and normal reabsorption of the subaortic conal region ensures rotation of the great arteries so that the aorta is positioned posterior and to the right of the PA.

Despite division of the truncus arteriosus and separation of the right and left outflow tracts, a communication exists between the aorta and the PA known as the *ductus arteriosus.*

Fetal Circulation

In order to deliver maximally oxygenated blood to the developing brain, fetal circulation differs from the adult pattern by the presence of alternate pathways known as *fetal shunts* (Fig. 34.4). Fetal shunts include the foramen ovale, ductus arteriosus, and ductus venosus. Fetal oxygenation occurs in the placenta instead of the fetal lungs. Therefore fetal lungs are not aerated despite the fetus making breathing motions.

In utero the fetus receives oxygenated blood and nutrients from the placenta through the umbilical vein. The blood travels to the liver, where a portion enters the portal and hepatic circulation; approximately half the flow is diverted away from the liver through the ductus venosus and into the inferior vena cava. Because the blood received from the inferior vena cava yields a higher pressure, blood entering the right atrium (RA) from the inferior vena cava is shunted through the foramen ovale and into the left atrium (LA) and is then pumped through the LV and into the aorta. Approximately two-thirds of the blood flows to

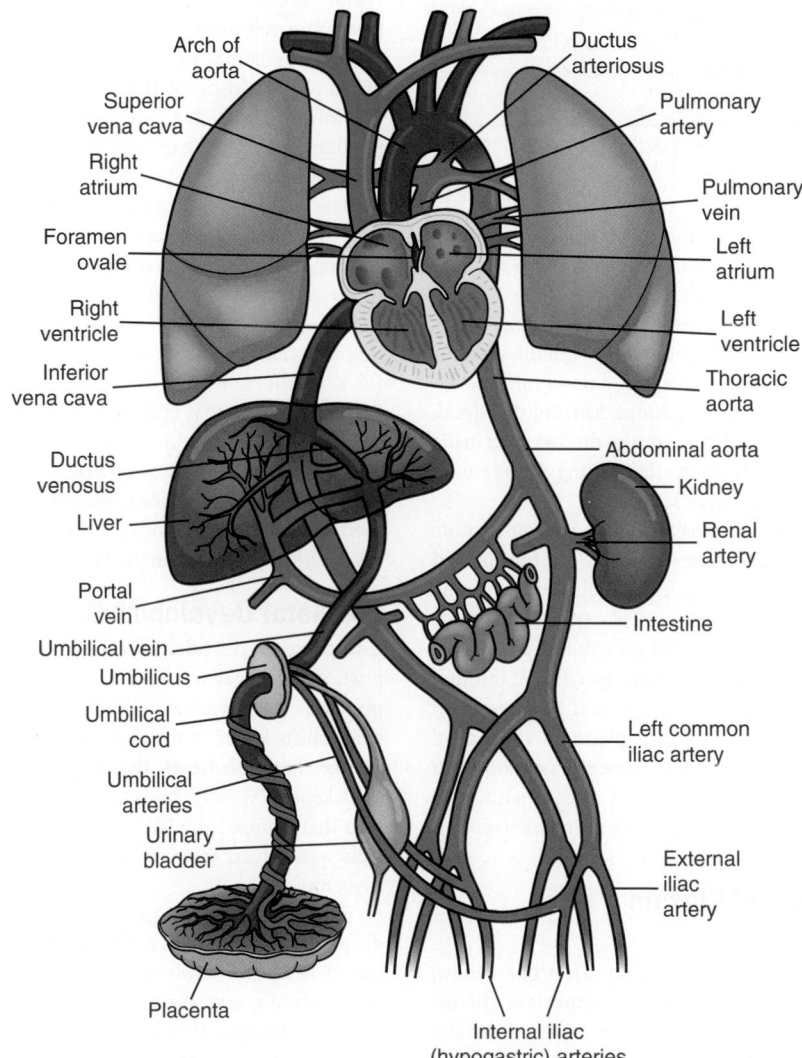

FIGURE 34.4 Fetal Circulation. Circulation of the fetus reflects the fact that oxygenation of fetal blood does not take place in the lungs, but rather in the placenta. Therefore the pulmonary circulatory system is essentially "bypassed." Instead of traveling from the right heart to the lungs, as occurs after birth, the majority of blood entering the right heart is shunted into systemic circulation through the ductus arteriosus.

Fetal Intervention for Complex Congenital Heart Disease

It is now possible to diagnose many types of CHD prenatally (as early as 16 to 18 weeks' gestation) through the use of fetal echocardiography. Fetal cardiac dysrhythmias are commonly treated by medication administration to the mother; the drugs are then transferred to the fetus through the placenta. Some types of CHD can progress in severity during fetal development—for example, severe aortic valve stenosis can sometimes progress to hypoplastic left heart syndrome (HLHS), because of reduced blood flow through the left ventricle. In some large centers, fetal balloon aortic valvuloplasty is available for some types of aortic valve stenosis. In this procedure, the apex of the fetal left ventricle is punctured with a needle placed through the mother's abdominal wall. A catheter can then be placed through the fetal aortic valve and a balloon inflated to dilate the valve. In HLHS, some fetuses have an intact or restrictive atrial septum, which can cause fetal lung damage or early death postnatally because of obstructed pulmonary venous return. Fetal intervention for intact atrial septum in HLHS involves direct puncture of the fetal heart through the mother's abdominal wall, and a catheter is then placed across the atrial septum to perform a balloon atrial septostomy. The intent of these procedures is to improve postnatal hemodynamic stability and potentially to allow a two-ventricle repair, rather than a single-ventricle treatment pathway. Although fetal intervention for severe CHD is in early stages of development, the potential to reduce CHD morbidity and mortality is great.

Data from Moon-Grady AJ, et al: *J Am Coll Cardiol* 66(4):388-399, 2015.

the head and upper extremities. The brain and coronary arteries receive the blood with the highest oxygen concentration, and the remaining blood flows into the descending aorta to perfuse distal organs.

Less-saturated blood, with an oxygen tension of 15 to 19 torr, returns from the upper body, head, neck, and arms and travels from the superior vena cava into the RA. A small portion of this blood flows into the RV and out the PA, entering the nonfunctioning lungs. Most of the blood, however, bypasses the lungs by flowing through the ductus arteriosus and into the descending aorta. Blood from the descending aorta returns to the placenta through two umbilical arteries.[1]

The nonaerated lungs and low oxygen tension induce vasoconstriction, creating high pulmonary vascular resistance (PVR). This is transmitted to the right side of the heart and the PAs. Conversely, fetal systemic resistance is low because of the large-volume placenta and ductus arteriosus. Therefore, because blood flow follows the path of least resistance, high PVR diverts most of the blood flow into the PA, through the ductus arteriosus, and into the aorta. From there it perfuses distal organs before traveling into the low-resistance placenta. Of clinical note, prenatal ultrasounds performed at 18 to 20 weeks' gestation can reveal up to 50% of all complex congenital heart disease with rates varying depending on provider training[3] (*What's New?* Fetal Intervention for Complex Congenital Heart Disease).

Transitional Circulation and Closure of Fetal Shunts

At birth a series of circulatory changes occur that affect blood flow, vascular resistance, and oxygen tension. The most important change that takes place in the circulation is the shift of gas exchange from the placenta to the lungs. In addition, alterations in pressure and volume of blood flowing through the heart chambers functionally close the ductus arteriosus, ductus venosus, and foramen ovale. A decrease of PVR and an increase of systemic vascular resistance (SVR) lead to changes in the size and shape of the heart chambers.

Clamping of the umbilical cord and expansion of the lungs at birth shift gas exchange from the placenta to the lungs. Removal of the low-resistance placenta from circulation also causes an immediate increase in SVR to about twice that before birth. Conversely, PVR decreases because of expansion of the lungs, which result from the infant's respirations and exposure to more oxygen-rich blood.

Once the umbilical cord is clamped, the umbilical arteries and vein, which comprise the cord, vasoconstrict and undergo fibrous changes. Therefore blood flow through the ductus venosus falls instantly; absence of fetal shunting through this vessel usually occurs within the first 7 days of life. Once the ductus venosus closes, its remnants form the ligamentum venosum, or round ligament of the liver.

Increased pulmonary venous return and decreased inferior vena cava return cause functional closure of the foramen ovale within the first month of life. In the fetus the foramen ovale is held open by the blood flow from the higher-pressure right side, reflecting the increased PVR, to the lower-pressure area on the left side of the heart, reflecting the decreased SVR. At birth the pressure gradients reverse (left atrial pressure exceeds right atrial pressure by a small degree), causing the valve flaps of the foramen ovale to close. Functional closure occurs by the adherence of these flaps to the atrial septum. Anatomic closure occurs within the first month of life after deposition of fibrin tissue and cell products permanently seals the flaps closed. Until this occurs, any condition that stimulates an increase in the right-sided pressures or causes dilation of the RA can reopen the foramen ovale. Conditions in which a patent foramen ovale (PFO) may continue past the first month of life include pulmonary hypertension, RV failure, and tricuspid atresia.

The ductus arteriosus closes more gradually. Increased oxygen saturation in the systemic arterial blood is thought to be the major stimulus causing vasoconstriction of the ductus arteriosus. In addition, a decrease in the amount of endogenous prostaglandins promoting dilation and the release of vasoactive substances stimulate further ductal closure. Vasoconstriction of the ductal medial smooth muscle shortens and thickens the intima of the ductal wall within 15 hours after birth. Permanent closure is complete several weeks after birth. Fibrous tissue adheres to the remaining structure, and the ductus arteriosus eventually evolves into the ligamentum arteriosum. Conditions that involve low arterial oxygen saturations, such as cyanotic heart disease, decreased medial muscle layer within the ductus, or increased levels of circulating vasodilating substances in the blood, may delay or prevent ductal closure.[4]

Postnatal Development

Compared to the adult, the infant's cardiopulmonary system is proportionally larger in relation to body surface area. The infant's heart points at a transverse angle, but as the lungs and heart mature, the heart shifts lower in the chest and is rotated at a more oblique angle. Unlike the adult heart, the newborn heart has RV dominance with a thickened RV wall. This is because of the high PVR during fetal circulation that exposed the RV to a high afterload, which in turn causes the right ventricular myocardial mass to become similar to the adult LV myocardium.

After birth the RV myocardium becomes less dominant as PVR drops. As SVR increases, the LV myocardium becomes thicker. By 1 month of age, the newborn's ventricles are approximately equal in weight. As the child grows, the heart size increases accordingly. The weight of the heart doubles during the first year of life and increases to six times that by 9 years of age.[4]

Postnatal changes involve a rise in arterial oxygen tension and an increase in alveolar oxygenation that stimulates vasodilation, resulting in a decrease in PVR. During the first 2 to 9 weeks of life, the inner medial linings of the small pulmonary arterioles become thinner in response to decreased pulmonary arterial pressure. This increased diameter of the pulmonary vessels, along with further development of the pulmonary bed in response to lung growth, results in a decrease in PVR. By 2 months of age, pulmonary resistance may approximate adult levels. During the neonatal period the pulmonary vascular bed remains hyperactive. Adverse conditions, such as alveolar hypoxia, acidosis, and hypothermia, may trigger pulmonary vasoconstriction and lead to pulmonary hypertension.

Postnatal Hemodynamics

As stated, SVR begins to rise once the placenta is removed from the circulation. Normal levels in the infant range from approximately 10 to 15 Wood units × body surface area (in square meters) and gradually increase to 15 to 30 Wood units × body surface area (in square meters) by childhood.[5] Likewise, the systolic pressure is low in the full-term newborn (approximately 39 to 59 mmHg), reflecting the low SVR. As the SVR increases, the LV becomes more developed and the systolic pressure rises steadily until it equals adult levels once the child reaches puberty.

The heart rate of the newborn ranges from 100 to 180 beats per minute, which gradually decreases as the child grows. Similarly, the newborn's cardiac output is high, which is a reflection of the fetal circulation described earlier. Oxygen consumption doubles at birth; to maintain adequate oxygen delivery, the cardiac output also remains high. These changes, however, cause minimal cardiac reserve in the newborn. Additional stressors could increase oxygen demands and result in acute deterioration. For example, stroke volume is fixed because of a decreased myocardial compliance; however, bradycardia may result in severely decreased cardiac output.[2] As the newborn grows, stroke volume steadily increases while the heart rate decreases, thus maintaining cardiac output.[2] By 2 months of age, oxygen consumption decreases by half.

Postnatal Circulation

Postnatal circulation allows the lungs to oxygenate the venous blood and allows fully saturated blood to be delivered to the systemic circulation. Desaturated blood returning from the superior vena cava, inferior vena cava, and coronary veins enters the RA and is pumped to the RV through the tricuspid valve. The RV then pumps the blood through the pulmonic valve to the PA; the blood flows to the lungs, where it is oxygenated. The oxygenated blood returns from the lungs through the pulmonary veins and enters the LA, which pumps blood to the LV through the mitral valve. The LV then pumps blood through the aortic valve and into the aorta. The coronary arteries receive the saturated blood along with delivery to the systemic circulation.

CONGENITAL HEART DEFECTS

Congenital heart disease (CHD) is the leading cause of death, excluding prematurity, during the first year of life[3] (Box 34.1). There are more than 35 documented types of congenital heart defects, and the frequency of occurrence in the United States continues to rise. Although researchers have not determined the reason for this increase, one explanation is that it may be the result of improved methods for early detection (*What's New?* Screening for Critical Congenital Heart Disease).

The underlying cause of CHD is known in only 10% of cases. Several factors place the fetus at risk for developing CHD, including prenatal, environmental, and genetic factors. Among the prenatal factors are maternal rubella, maternal insulin-dependent diabetes, maternal lupus, maternal alcohol or illicit drug use, maternal age (older than 40 years), maternal phenylketonuria, and maternal hypercalcemia (Table 34.1). The use of some drugs during pregnancy is associated with an above-average incidence of CHD. Examples of these drug teratogens include

---

BOX 34.1 ENDOCARDITIS RISK

Children with congenital heart disease are at risk for developing endocarditis. Although the risk is low, a transient bacteremia has been noted to follow dental and surgical procedures and instrumentation involving mucosal surfaces. A blood-borne pathogen can inhabit areas of the heart where there is high turbulence (such as an abnormal valve or vessel) or reside on artificial material (such as a valve or homograft). *Streptococcus viridans* (α-hemolytic streptococci) is the most commonly found pathogen following dental or oral procedures. *Enterococcus faecalis* (enterococci) is the most common bacterium found following genitourinary and gastrointestinal tract surgery or instrumentation. The American Heart Association has provided updated guidelines for the prevention of bacterial endocarditis. The type and dose of antibiotic prophylaxis recommended depend on the procedure and the cardiac classification of risk for endocarditis. Good dental hygiene with daily brushing and flossing is critically important along with regular dental check-ups.

Data from the American Heart Association. Available at: www.americanheart.org.

WHAT'S NEW?

Screening for Critical Congenital Heart Disease

Some newborn infants with severe congenital heart disease (CHD) may appear to be physically normal, without cyanosis or a significant heart murmur, but may become critically ill or even die when fetal shunts close, usually after discharge home. In 2011, the U.S. Department of Health and Human Services added pulse oximetry screening for critical congenital heart disease (CCHD) to the *Recommended Uniform Screening Panel* for all newborn infants. The requirement is a pulse oximeter recording from the right hand (preductal) and one foot (postductal) 24 hours after birth or prior to hospital discharge. A pulse oximeter reading less than 95% in either site or more than 3% difference between hand and foot means a positive (or failed) screen. If failed, the screen is repeated and if failed again, the infant should be evaluated and undergo a diagnostic echocardiogram prior to discharge. As of 2015, 43 states had enacted legislation, regulations, or hospital guidelines for CCHD screening. Studies are underway to evaluate the effect of this screening on CHD morbidity and mortality.

Data from Glidewell J, et al: *MMWR Morb Mortal Wkly Rep* 64(23):625-630, 2015.

---

anticonvulsants, angiotensin-converting enzyme (ACE) inhibitors, lithium, retinoic acid, and warfarin. The incidence of heart defects also has been found to be higher in stillbirths, spontaneous abortions, and low-birth-weight or small-for-gestational-age infants.[2] In general, the likelihood of unaffected parents having a child with CHD is about 1%. The risk of recurrence in a sibling is approximately 3%; however this may vary depending on the type of CHD (e.g., the risk may be up to 10% with hypoplastic left heart syndrome).[2]

Genetic factors also have been implicated in the development of CHD, although the mechanism of causation is often multifactorial. Recent progress, accelerated through the Human Genome Project, has resulted in the rapid identification of many genes causing CHD.[3]

◆ETIOLOGY. The etiology of most CHD is unknown. Early epidemiologic studies report a multifactorial influence to be the cause of up to 90% of cardiac anomalies.[2] Associated risk factors include maternal, gestational, and familial conditions. (Maternal risk factors are discussed in the previous section.) Exposure to teratogens in utero also may be a risk factor. Likewise, fetal exposure to active maternal infections, such as rubella, herpesvirus, coxsackievirus B5, and cytomegalovirus, may be a risk.

TABLE 34.1	ENVIRONMENTAL FACTORS ASSOCIATED WITH HEART DISEASE	

CAUSE	TYPE OF CONGENITAL HEART DEFECT
Infection	
Intrauterine	Patent ductus arteriosus (PDA), pulmonary stenosis (PS), coarctation of aorta (COA)
Systemic viral	PDA, PS, COA
Rubella	PDA, PS, COA
Coxsackie B5	Endocardial fibroelastosis
Herpesvirus Cytomegalovirus (HCMV)	Can infect endothelial cells and vascular endothelium
Radiation	Studies of cancer survivors reveal radiation can cause atherosclerosis; myocardial, endocardial, and pericardial disease; conduction disturbances; and endothelial vessel disease
Metabolic Disorders	
Diabetes	Ventricular septal defect (VSD), ventricular hypertrophy, cardiomegaly, transposition of the great vessels
Phenylketonuria (PKU)	COA, PDA
Hypercalcemia	Supravalvular aortic stenosis, PS; aortic hyperplasia
Drugs	
Alcohol	Tetralogy of Fallot (TOF), atrial septal defect (ASD), VSD
Lithium	Exact effect not known
Phenytoin	Embryonic dysrhythmia and valvular heart disease
Warfarin	ASD and PDA
Peripheral Conditions	
Increased maternal age	VSD, TOF (relationship unclear)
Antepartal bleeding	Various defects (relationship unclear)
Prematurity	PDA, VSD
High altitude	PDA, ASD (increased incidence)

TABLE 34.2	CONGENITAL HEART DISEASE IN SELECTED FETAL CHROMOSOMAL ABERRATIONS	

CONDITIONS	INCIDENCE OF CHD (%)	COMMON DEFECTS (IN DECREASING ORDER OF FREQUENCY)
5p (cri du chat syndrome)	25	VSD, PDA, ASD
Trisomy 13 syndrome	90	VSD, PDA, dextrocardia
Trisomy 18 syndrome	99	VSD, PDA, PS
Trisomy 21 (Down syndrome)	50	AVSD, VSD
Turner syndrome (XO)	35	COA, AS, ASD
Klinefelter variant (XXXXY)	15	PDA, ASD

AS, Aortic stenosis; *ASD,* atrial septal defect; *AVSD,* atrioventricular septal defect; *COA,* coarctation of the aorta; *PDA,* patent ductus arteriosus; *PS,* pulmonary stenosis; *VSD,* ventricular septal defect. From Park MK: *Pediatric cardiology for practitioners,* ed 6, St Louis, 2014, Mosby.

Classification of Congenital Heart Defects and Associated Conditions

There are more than 35 different types of congenital anomalies that can be classified into 4 categories based on blood flow pattern: (1) lesions increasing pulmonary blood flow; (2) lesions decreasing pulmonary blood flow; (3) obstructive lesions, in which right- or left-sided outflow tract obstructions curtail or prohibit blood flow out of the heart; and (4) mixing lesions, in which desaturated blood and saturated blood mix within the chambers or great arteries of the heart (Table 34.4). By classifying lesions in this way, the clinical manifestations, as well as associated sequelae, are more predictable.

Associated conditions and their clinical manifestations are lesion dependent. The two most common conditions associated with CHD are heart failure and hypoxemia. Lesions increasing pulmonary blood flow include defects that allow blood flow to shunt from the high-pressure left side to the lower-pressure right side, resulting in pulmonary congestion. Lesions that cause decreased pulmonary blood flow are generally complex and result in cyanosis. Obstructive lesions increase the pressure needed to eject the blood from the ventricles. The two types of obstructive lesions are right-sided lesions that may result in hypoxemia and cyanosis, and left-sided lesions that may result in HF. Mixing lesions are variable in their physiology and clinical manifestations.

Heart Failure

Heart failure (HF) is classified as an acquired condition. HF occurs when the heart is unable to maintain sufficient cardiac output to meet the metabolic demands of the body. HF can occur as the result of decreased myocardial function or excessive metabolic demands. The most common causes of HF in infancy and childhood are cardiomyopathy or the result of poor ventricular function. Table 34.5 lists the congenital heart defects that cause HF by age. Pulmonary overcirculation from large left-to-right shunts (mixing) is often called *congestive heart failure (CHF)* but is not usually associated with decreased cardiac output and failure to meet metabolic demands. However, the clinical manifestations are similar, such as failure to thrive (FTT), tachypnea, tachycardia, and respiratory tract infections.

◆**PATHOPHYSIOLOGY.** In general, the pathophysiologic mechanisms of HF in infants and children are very similar to those in adults. The

Chromosomal aberrations account for about 6% of all CHD (Table 34.2). Many genetic and hereditary diseases are associated with CHD, although the mechanism of causation is unknown (Table 34.3). As many as 50% of infants with trisomy 21 have a CHD, usually either an AV canal defect or a VSD. Noncardiac defects are noted in as many as 35% of infants with cardiac lesions. Prospective studies using chromosomal analysis have suggested that congenital cardiac malformations may be the result of a single gene defect.[3]

Because of improved screening methods, surgical interventions, and management, children with congenital heart defects are now surviving into adulthood and bearing children of their own. Studies report up to 15% incidence of CHD in offspring of a parent having a congenital heart lesion.[2] Subsequent siblings could have as high as a 50% chance of having a cardiac malformation.

TABLE 34.3	DISORDERS COEXISTENT WITH CONGENITAL OR ACQUIRED HEART DISEASE
DISORDER	**ASSOCIATED CARDIOVASCULAR DEFECT**
Connective Tissue Disorders	
Marfan syndrome	Aortic or mitral regurgitation, aortic aneurysm
Hurler syndrome (mucopolysaccharidosis type I)	Aortic or mitral regurgitation, pseudoatherosclerosis
Hunter syndrome (mucopolysaccharidosis type II)	Aortic or mitral regurgitation, pseudoatherosclerosis
Osteogenesis imperfecta	Incompetent aortic valve
Complex Syndromes	
Alagille syndrome	Peripheral pulmonary artery stenosis, complex cardiac defects
CHARGE syndrome	Tetralogy of Fallot (TOF), truncus arteriosus, interrupted aortic arch (IAA), vascular ring
DiGeorge syndrome	TOF, IAA, truncus arteriosus
Ellis–von Creveld syndrome	Defect or absence of atrial septum
Goldenhar syndrome	Ventricular septal defect (VSD), TOF
Holt-Oram syndrome	Atrial septal defect (ASD), VSD
Kartagener syndrome	Dextrocardia
Pierre Robin	VSD, patent ductus arteriosus (PDA)
Thrombocytopenia Absent Radius (TAR) syndrome	TOF, ASD, dextrocardia
Tuberous sclerosis	Cardiac rhabdomyoma
VATER syndrome	VSD, other defects
Velocardiofacial syndrome (VCFS)	TOF, truncus arteriosus, pulmonary atresia with VSD, IAA, VSD, D-transposition of the great arteries
Williams syndrome	Supravalvar aortic stenosis, pulmonary artery stenosis
Inborn Errors of Metabolism	
Pompe disease (glycogen storage disease II)	Cardiomegaly, left heart failure, supraventricular tachycardia
Homocystinuria	Thromboembolic episodes, pulmonic and aortic regurgitation

CHARGE, Coloboma, heart defects, atresia choanae, growth retardation, genital abnormalities, and ear abnormalitites; *VATER,* vertebral defects, anal atresia, cardiac defects, tracheo-esophageal fistula, renal anomalies.
Data from Park MK: *Pediatric cardiology for practitioners,* ed 6, St Louis, 2014, Mosby.

BOX 34.2	CLINICAL MANIFESTATIONS OF HEART FAILURE
IMPAIRED MYOCARDIAL FUNCTION	**PULMONARY CONGESTION**	**SYSTEMIC VENOUS CONGESTION**
Tachycardia	Tachypnea	Weight gain
Sweating (inappropriately)	Dyspnea	Hepatomegaly
Decreased urinary output	Retractions (infants)	Peripheral edema (rare)
Fatigue	Flaring nares	Ascites
Weakness	Exercise intolerance	Neck vein distention
Restlessness	Orthopnea	(rare in children)
Anorexia	Cough, hoarseness	
Pale, cool extremities	Cyanosis	
Weak peripheral pulses	Wheezing (rare)	
Decreased blood pressure	Grunting	
Gallop rhythm		
Cardiomegaly		

From Hockenberry MJ, Wilson D: *Wong's nursing care of infants and children,* ed 10, St Louis, 2015, Mosby.

results in retention of sodium and fluid by the kidneys, which in turn increases volume in the circulatory system.

These neurohumoral and hemodynamic changes create abnormal ventricular wall stress and cause the myocardium to hypertrophy. After excessive hypertrophy, the myocardial fibers begin to stretch to accommodate the increased volume. Hypertrophy and fiber stretch temporarily increase contractility and hence the force of ventricular contraction. However, these mechanisms eventually fail to maintain cardiac output as HF progresses. A review of the Frank-Starling law of the heart (see Chapter 32) is useful for an understanding of the cycle of compensation and decompensation that occurs in HF.

CLINICAL MANIFESTATIONS. Symptomatic HF in children has many causes. It is not usually necessary to determine if it is right- or left-sided HF. When assessing a child with HF, a combination of symptoms generally is present. Pulmonary overcirculation is the predominant cause associated with congenital defects.

HF in infants is manifested as poor feeding and sucking, often leading to failure to thrive (FTT). Dyspnea, tachypnea, and diaphoresis may be accompanied by retractions, grunting, and nasal flaring. Wheezing, coughing, and rales are rare even with significant HF. Common skin changes, such as pallor or mottling, are often present.

Hepatomegaly (enlargement of the liver) is atypically attributable to systemic venous congestion. In infants the normal liver is soft, sharp-edged, and palpable 1 to 2 cm below the costal margin. However, the absence of hepatomegaly does not rule out HF.

Periorbital edema and weight gain without caloric increase are uncommon manifestations of right ventricular failure in infants. Peripheral edema, which is a common finding in adults, is rare in infants and young children and more often signifies renal disease rather than cardiac disease. The clinical manifestations of HF are listed in Box 34.2.

EVALUATION AND TREATMENT. A thorough physical examination with an emphasis on cardiac and pulmonary findings often will reveal the degree of HF. Plotting the child's growth (height, weight, head circumference) is an important method for monitoring a child's health. Infants with HF and pulmonary overcirculation usually have low weight with normal length and head circumference. FTT is usually the result of increased metabolic expenditure relative to caloric intake. Increasing caloric density or nasogastric feeding, or both, may be necessary to optimize caloric intake to promote weight gain. An electrocardiogram

same compensatory mechanisms are activated in the face of inadequate cardiac output. An acute decrease in blood pressure stimulates stretch receptors and baroreceptors in the aorta and carotid arteries, which in turn stimulate the sympathetic nervous system. With the release of catecholamines and the stimulation of β receptors, heart rate and the force of myocardial contraction increase. Venous smooth muscle tone also increases, which increases return of venous blood to the heart. Sympathetic stimulation also decreases blood flow to the kidneys, skin, spleen, and extremities so that maximum flow to the brain, heart, and lungs can be maintained. Decreased blood flow to the kidneys causes the release of renin, angiotensin, and aldosterone. If chronic, this cycle

TABLE 34.4 CLASSIFICATION OF CONGENITAL HEART DEFECTS

CLASSIFICATION	SHUNT DIRECTION	PRESENTATION	SPECIFIC DEFECTS
Lesions increasing pulmonary blood flow	Left to right	Acyanotic congestive heart failure	Patent ductus arteriosus, atrial septal defect, ventricular septal defect, complete atrioventricular canal defect
Lesions decreasing pulmonary blood flow	Right to left	Cyanotic	Tetralogy of Fallot, tricuspid atresia
Obstructive lesions*	None	Low cardiac output Shock	Coarctation of the aorta, aortic stenosis, pulmonary stenosis
Mixed lesions†	Variable	Variable	Transposition of the great arteries, total anomalous pulmonary venous connection, truncus arteriosus, hypoplastic left heart syndrome*

*If patent ductus arteriosus closes, newborns with hypoplastic left heart syndrome, coarctation of the aorta, or critical aortic stenosis will present with shock. Newborns with aortic stenosis or pulmonary stenosis may have only mild symptoms depending on severity of stenosis.
†Transposition of the great arteries, truncus arteriosus, and hypoplastic left heart syndrome will present with cyanosis as patent ductus arteriosus starts to close. Total anomalous pulmonary venous connection usually presents with heart failure, but may present with severe hypoxemia if pulmonary venous return is obstructed.

TABLE 34.5 CONGENITAL HEART DEFECTS CAUSING HEART FAILURE

AGE	CONGENITAL HEART DEFECT
Time of birth	Hypoplastic left heart syndrome
	Volume overload caused by tricuspid regurgitation (rare)
	Arteriovenous fistula
Birth to 1 week	Hypoplastic left heart syndrome
	Aortic atresia
	Transposition of the great vessels with ventricular septal defect (VSD)
	Coarctation of the aorta
	Total anomalous pulmonary venous connection (TAPVC) with obstruction
	Patent ductus arteriosus (PDA) in premature infants
First 4 weeks	Coarctation of the aorta
	TAPVC
	Large left-to-right shunt caused by VSD, PDA in premature infants
	Tricuspid atresia
	Persistent truncus arteriosus with large left-to-right shunt
	All previously mentioned defects
4 to 6 weeks	Transposition of the great vessels with VSD
	Large left-to-right shunt caused by endocardial cushion defect
6 weeks to 6 months	VSD
6 months	Endocardial fibroelastosis

(ECG) should be performed to determine the presence of dysrhythmias or hypertrophy. A chest radiograph is useful in assessing the presence of cardiomegaly and signs of increased pulmonary circulation. However, echocardiography is the gold standard for definitive diagnosis of structural and functional cardiac disease.

Treatment is aimed at decreasing cardiac workload and increasing the efficiency of heart function. Medical management initially consists of diuretics, such as furosemide. Depending on the degree of HF, other diuretics can be used in combination with furosemide to counteract potassium losses. Agents that reduce afterload, such as ACE inhibitors, angiotensin receptor blockers, and beta-blockers, are used to further

manage severe HF. In severe cases of HF, anticoagulation and mechanical circulatory support may be indicated to support the failing myocardium.[6]

Hypoxemia

Heart defects that allow desaturated blood to enter the systemic system without passing through the lungs result in hypoxemia and cyanosis. Hypoxemia occurs when arterial oxygen tension is below normal and results in low oxygen arterial saturations and cellular function alteration. Cyanosis, a blue discoloration of the mucous membranes and nail beds, results from deoxygenated hemoglobin in a concentration of at least 5 g/dL of blood or from arterial saturations less than 85%.[2,5] Anemia may mask the signs of hypoxemia, whereas children who are polycythemic with a normal arterial saturation may appear cyanotic. Older children who have an unrepaired septal defect with a left-to-right shunt may become cyanotic because of pulmonary vascular changes secondary to increased pulmonary blood flow. Because of these progressive pulmonary vascular changes, PVR increases to exceed or equal SVR, resulting in a reversal of shunting known as Eisenmenger syndrome. Three types of defects cause hypoxemia and cyanosis:

1. Lesions that cause right ventricular outflow tract obstruction and shunting from the right side of the heart to the left side, as in tetralogy of Fallot (see Classification of Congenital Heart Defects and Associated Conditions section).
2. Defects involving the mixing of saturated and unsaturated blood within the heart chambers, as in a univentricular heart (also referred to as *single ventricle*)
3. Defects in children with transposition of the great arteries (see Classification of Congenital Heart Defects and Associated Conditions section), in which two parallel circulations exist and survival depends on the existence of a patent ductus arteriosus or septal defect

◆ **CLINICAL MANIFESTATIONS.** Infants with mild hypoxemia may show signs of cyanosis only occasionally when stressed; otherwise, they may exhibit near-normal age-projected growth and development. Infants with severe hypoxemia may display signs of feeding intolerance, poor weight gain, tachypnea, and dyspnea. Children with chronic hypoxemia are small for their age, may display cognitive and motor skill delays, experience shortness of breath with exertion, fatigue easily, and have exercise intolerance. Acute, severe hypoxemia will lead to tissue hypoxia, metabolic acidosis, hyperventilation, poor perfusion, and eventually shock.

In response to chronic hypoxemia, polycythemia occurs as the body generates additional red blood cells to increase the oxygen-carrying capacity of the blood. In some infants, however, microcytic anemia may result because of limited stores of iron. Polycythemia or hyperviscosity and the associated platelet dysfunction also place children at risk for thromboembolic events, especially infants with severe cyanosis and iron deficiency anemia. Children with right-to-left shunting are at risk for systemic embolic events, cerebrovascular accident (stroke), and brain abscess.[5] Clubbing of the nail beds occurs because of chronic tissue hypoxemia and polycythemia.

Defects Increasing Pulmonary Blood Flow

Cardiac lesions that increase pulmonary blood flow include defects that involve septal abnormalities or communications between the great arteries. These allow the shunting of blood from the high-pressure left side to the lower-pressure right side. Infants with left-to-right shunts are acyanotic and, depending on the degree of shunting, may develop signs and symptoms of HF. Children with significant left-to-right shunts left untreated are at risk for development of irreversible pulmonary hypertension.

Patent Ductus Arteriosus

The patent ductus arteriosus (PDA) is a vessel located between the junction of the main and left pulmonary arteries and the lesser curvature of the descending aorta, usually just distal to the left subclavian artery (Fig. 34.5, *A* and *B*). During fetal circulation the PDA allows blood to

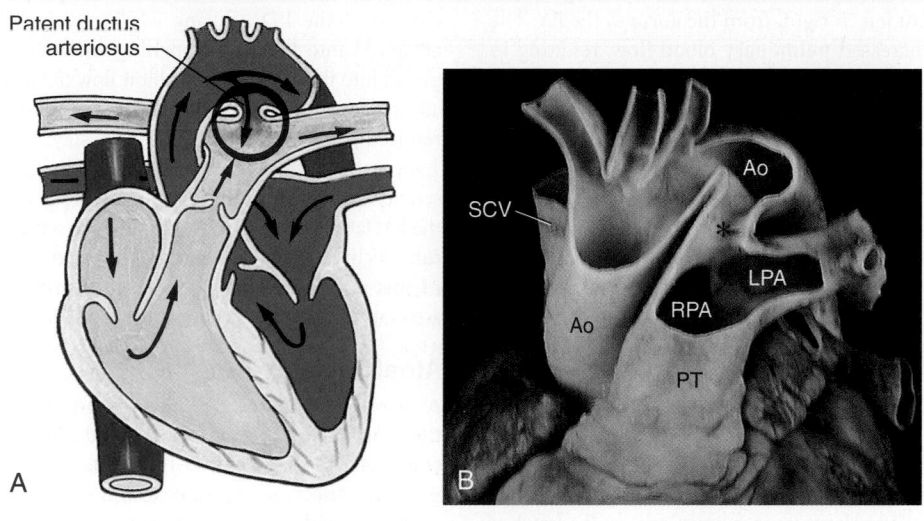

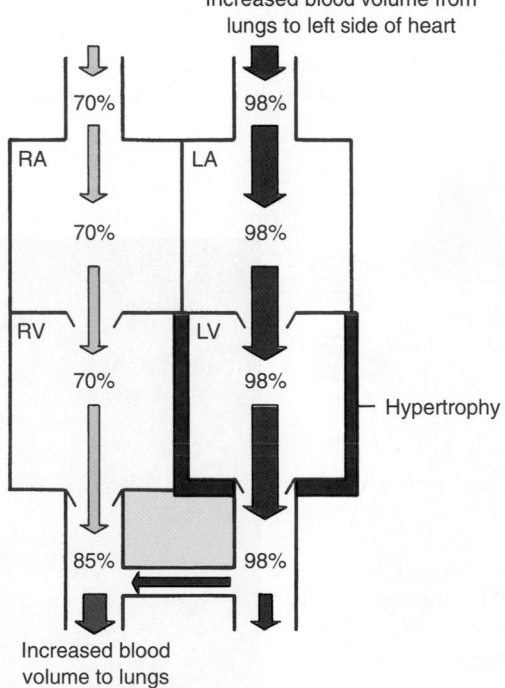

FIGURE 34.5 Patent Ductus Arteriosus (PDA). **A,** PDA with left-to-right shunt. **B,** PDA *(asterisk)* in an adult with pulmonary hypertension. **C,** Changes in oxygen saturation, left ventricular volume, and the myocardium caused by left-to-right shunt through a PDA. *Ao,* Aorta; *LA,* left atrium; *LPA,* left pulmonary artery; *LV,* left ventricle; *PT,* pulmonary trunk; *RA,* right atrium; *RPA,* right pulmonary artery; *RV,* right ventricle; *SCV,* subclavian vein. (**A** from Hockenberry MJ, Wilson D: *Wong's nursing care of infants and children,* ed 9, St Louis, 2011, Mosby; **B** from Damjanov I, Linder J, editors: *Anderson's pathology,* ed 10, St Louis, 1996, Mosby.)

shunt from the PA to the aorta. At birth, once the placenta is removed and the lungs are expanded, the PDA will start to constrict within the first hours of life. Closure of the PDA in full-term infants is usually noted in the first few weeks of life.[7] As an isolated defect, PDA occurs in 5% to 10% of all CHD, but the incidence of PDA is much higher in preterm infants because of high circulating levels of prostaglandins and immature pulmonary vascular smooth muscle.[2,8]

◆**PATHOPHYSIOLOGY.** Failure of the PDA to close results in persistent patency of the ductus arteriosus. The hemodynamic effects of PDA depend on the size of the lumen and the resistance in the pulmonary and systemic circulations. At birth the PVR and SVR are almost equal and are reflected in the PA and aorta, respectively; therefore shunting is minimal. However, as PVR falls, a reversal of fetal shunting occurs. Blood now begins to shunt left to right, from the aorta to the PA. The hemodynamic effect is increased pulmonary blood flow, resulting in increased pulmonary venous return to the LA and LV with increased workload on the left side of the heart (see Fig. 34.5, *C*). The increased workload is caused by increased pulmonary venous return to the LA and, potentially, an increase in right ventricular pressure if pulmonary vascular changes occur in response to the increased blood flow, leading to an increase in pulmonary vascular pressure.

◆**CLINICAL MANIFESTATIONS.** If PVR has fallen, infants with PDA will characteristically have a continuous-machinery type murmur heard best at the left upper sternal border throughout systole and diastole. If the PDA is significant, the infant also will have bounding pulses, an active precordium, a thrill upon palpation, and signs and symptoms of pulmonary overcirculation. Infants with a small PDA will usually remain asymptomatic.

◆**EVALUATION AND TREATMENT.** Chest radiograph will reveal cardiomegaly and increased pulmonary vascular markings. An ECG may demonstrate ventricular enlargement, particularly on the left, but in most cases it is within the normal range. Echocardiography and auscultation confirm the diagnosis based on the characteristic continuous-machinery type of murmur.

PDA closure in asymptomatic children with a murmur is recommended because of the risk of infective endocarditis or pulmonary overcirculation that may lead to pulmonary hypertension and eventually develop a right-to-left shunt.[9] Treatment of a small PDA in a child with the absence of a murmur or other cardiac conditions remains controversial.[9] Premature infants who develop respiratory distress are initially given indomethacin or ibuprofen (both prostaglandin inhibitors) to close the duct. If this is unsuccessful or contraindicated because of renal impairment, surgical ligation and division may be warranted.

Historically the most widely used method for PDA closure is surgical repair involving ligation and division of the ductus with extremely low surgical mortality. However, there continues to be some morbidity associated with the approach through a left thoracotomy incision.

Several other options for PDA closure are available depending on the size of the child and the PDA. Many specialists perform transcatheter closure of the PDA during cardiac catheterization. The catheter is advanced into the ductal opening whereby coils or other devices are placed into the lumen that prohibit flow through the ductus. The greatest advantages to this procedure are the avoidance of a thoracotomy incision, reduced pain, and a shorter hospital stay.

Another surgical option is closure through video-assisted thoracoscopic surgery. This procedure involves making three small incisions in the left lateral chest wall, through which a tube is inserted. Through the tube, a clip is then placed across the ductus to occlude it. An advantage of this procedure over open surgical procedures is that there is less associated morbidity because of the avoidance of a thoracotomy incision.[10]

Atrial Septal Defect

An **atrial septal defect (ASD)** is an abnormal communication between the atria (Fig. 34.6, *A* and *B*). Isolated ASD occurs in 5% to 10% of all congenital cardiac defects. The three major types are (1) an ostium primum defect, an opening found low in the septum that may be associated with AV valve abnormalities, especially mitral insufficiency; (2) an ostium secundum defect, an opening in the center of the septum (this is the most common type of atrial defect); and (3) a sinus venosus defect, an opening that occurs high up in the atrial septum near the superior vena cava and RA junction. This defect is often associated with partial anomalous pulmonary venous connection.

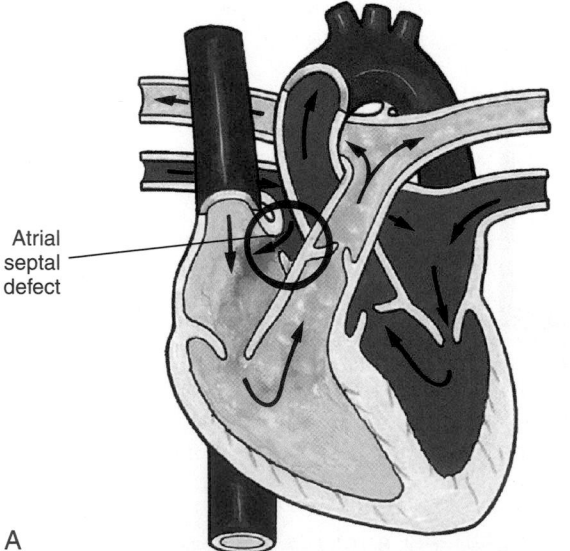

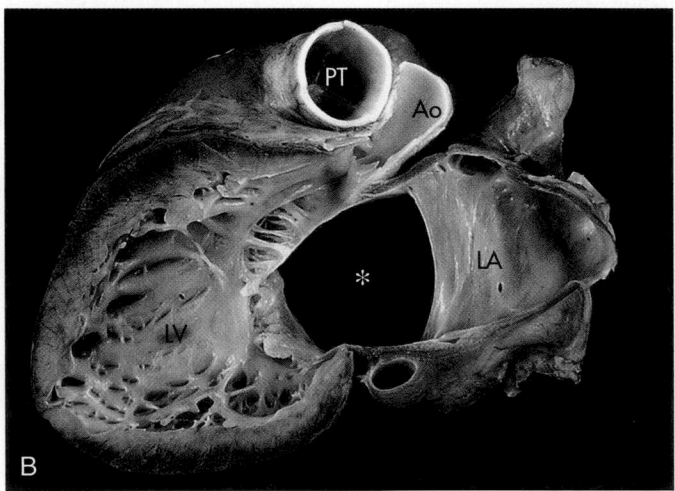

FIGURE 34.6 Atrial Septal Defect (ASD). A, Abnormal opening between the atria causing blood from the higher-pressure left atrium to flow into the lower-pressure right atrium. **B,** Complete ASD *(asterisk)* form in children. *Ao,* Aorta; *LA,* left atrium; *LV,* left ventricle; *PT,* pulmonary artery trunk. (**A** from Hockenberry MJ, Wilson D: *Wong's nursing care of infants and children,* ed 9, St Louis, 2011, Mosby; **B** from Damjanov I, Linder J, editors: *Anderson's Pathology,* ed 10, St Louis, 1996, Mosby.)

◆**PATHOPHYSIOLOGY.** Although the pressure difference between the two atria is minimal, the ASD allows blood to be shunted from left to right because of the slightly higher pressure of the left atrial chamber and lower PVR as compared with SVR. Right atrial and ventricular enlargement develops as a result of left-to-right shunting. Children with ASD are generally asymptomatic and rarely display signs of pulmonary overcirculation. Moderate to large ASDs allow an increase in pulmonary blood flow and, over time, pulmonary vascular changes can occur that may, although rarely, result in pulmonary hypertension.

◆**CLINICAL MANIFESTATIONS.** Because most children with ASD are asymptomatic, diagnosis usually is made during a routine physical examination by the auscultation of a crescendo-decrescendo systolic ejection murmur that reflects increased blood flow through the pulmonary valve. The location of the murmur is between the second and third intercostal spaces along the left sternal border. A wide fixed splitting of the second heart sound is also characteristic of ASD, reflecting volume overload to the RV, causing prolonged ejection time and delay of pulmonic valve closure.

◆**EVALUATION AND TREATMENT.** In most cases an echocardiogram is sufficient to confirm the diagnosis of an ASD. A chest radiograph may reveal cardiomegaly and increased pulmonary vascular markings in an asymptomatic child. An ECG may demonstrate right-axis deviation and diastolic overload of the RV manifested as right ventricular hypertrophy.[2]

ASDs are generally closed before school age. If left unrepaired, continued left-to-right shunting through the ASD may result in pulmonary hypertension and right ventricular hypertrophy, placing the child at risk for the development of HF, atrial dysrhythmias, or embolic events. Surgical closure involves a pericardial patch or suture closure of the defect, depending on the size of the opening. Repair can be done through a sternotomy or right anterior thoracotomy approach with the use of cardiopulmonary bypass. Some centers perform minimally invasive techniques for ASD repair in adults and children. Sinus venosus defects require a slightly different approach that consists of a synthetic or pericardial patch to close the opening and baffle the anomalous right pulmonary venous drainage to the LA. Surgical mortality and morbidity are extremely low.[7] Depending on the size and location of the ASD, a routinely used alternative to surgery is transcatheter closure performed in the catheterization laboratory using various septal occluder devices.[9] In the United States, the Amplatzer (AGA Medical Corporation) and Helex (Gore Medical) septal occluders are the only FDA-approved devices for transcatheter ASD closure. Advantages of transcatheter ASD closure include reduced pain, no surgical incision, and same day or overnight hospital stay. Potential complications include rare device embolization, which may require surgical retrieval, and rare device erosion.[9]

Ventricular Septal Defect

A ventricular septal defect (VSD) is an abnormal communication between the ventricles (Fig. 34.7, A). VSDs are the most common type of congenital heart lesion and account for 15% to 20% of all CHDs. The four types of VSDs are based on location in the septum. The perimembranous type, which occurs in the outflow tract of the LV immediately below the aortic valve, is the most common type, accounting for up to 80% of all VSDs that require treatment. Muscular VSDs, which occur low or anterior in the ventricular septum between the trabeculae (see Fig. 34.7, B) are most likely to close spontaneously and are difficult to close surgically because of their location low in the ventricular apex. Most muscular VSDs are hemodynamically insignificant and require no medical or surgical treatment. Supracristal VSDs (also called *outlet VSDs*) occur in the right ventricular outflow tract or infundibulum, below the pulmonary valve. AV canal or inlet VSDs occur posterior

and inferior to the membranous septum, beneath the septal cusp of the tricuspid valve, and inferior to the papillary muscles of the conus.

◆**PATHOPHYSIOLOGY.** The direction of shunting in a child with a VSD is from the high-pressure left side to the lower-pressure right side. The amount of shunting depends on the size of the defect and the degree of PVR. Small VSDs present increased resistance to shunting and limit blood flow through the defect; thus the degree of pulmonary vascular congestion and ventricular chamber enlargement is minimal (see Fig. 34.7, C).

After 1 to 2 weeks of life, when PVR has decreased, moderate-sized to large VSDs allow a large amount of shunting from left to right. The shunted blood flows directly out the RV outflow tract and into the PA rather than remain in the RV cavity (see Fig. 34.7, D). Therefore the main PA, LA, and LV all enlarge. LV hypertrophy occurs to effectively pump the additional volume. Pulmonary overcirculation accounts for the symptoms associated with a large VSD in most cases.

Over time the pulmonary bed also undergoes changes because of increased pulmonary blood flow caused by the left-to-right shunting. The smooth muscle layer in the arteriolar walls thickens, and proliferation of the intimal layer occurs. The effect of these changes is a decrease in the diameter of the pulmonary vessels, which increases the resistance to blood flow. If the PVR is severely increased, these changes eventually become irreversible, and PVR continues to rise. In some cases it exceeds SVR, causing the shunt through the VSD to reverse direction. Deoxygenated blood now flows into the systemic circulation, and cyanosis occurs, a phenomenon known as *Eisenmenger syndrome*.

◆**CLINICAL MANIFESTATIONS.** Clinical manifestations in children with VSDs depend on the age of the child, size of the defect, and level of PVR. Newborns with small VSDs are relatively asymptomatic. Initially no murmur is present because the newborn's high PVR causes equalization of the pressures between both ventricles. Once PVR has dropped, left-to-right shunting occurs, creating a murmur. Infants with large VSDs display symptoms of HF and poor weight gain. Adults who develop pulmonary hypertension as a result of unrepaired VSD will be cyanotic and have clubbing.

On physical examination a loud, harsh, holosystolic murmur and systolic thrill can be detected at the left lower sternal border. The intensity of the murmur reflects the pressure gradient across the VSD. An apical diastolic rumble may be present with a moderate to large defect, reflecting increased flow across the mitral valve.

◆**EVALUATION AND TREATMENT.** ECG and chest radiographs reflect the amount of shunting through the defect. The ECG of an individual with a small VSD may be normal, whereas the ECG of an individual with a large VSD may reveal biventricular hypertrophy and LA enlargement. Chest roentgenographic findings are significant for cardiomegaly and increased pulmonary vascular markings; again, the severity is directly related to the magnitude of shunting. An echocardiogram identifies the position, size, direction of shunting, and dimensions of the LA, LV, and RV chambers. It also can provide an estimate of PA and RV pressures. Cardiac catheterization may be performed to determine hemodynamics and, in some instances, the location of other defects and additional VSDs.

Many VSDs spontaneously close during the first year of life.[2] Infants with symptoms of HF and poor weight gain despite medical management should have their VSD corrected as soon as possible. Left-to-right shunting with a pulmonary flow/systemic flow (Q_p/Q_s) ratio of greater than 2:1 or evidence of elevated PVR are indications for closure. Closure of the VSD at this time is to prevent the development of pulmonary hypertension.

Placement of a PA band to decrease the amount of pulmonary blood flow was initially used as a palliative procedure but is now rarely used unless the presence of an additional lesion makes complete repair difficult.

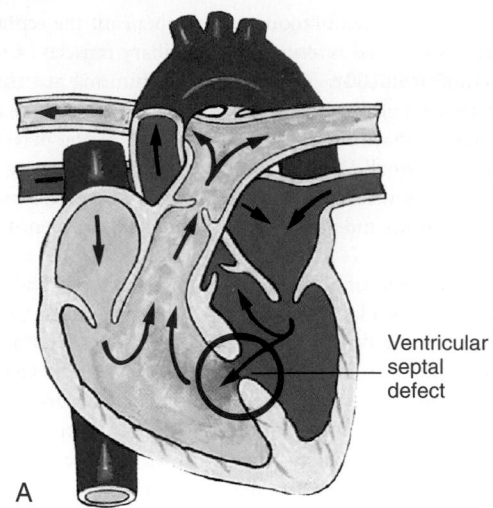

A

Ventricular septal defect

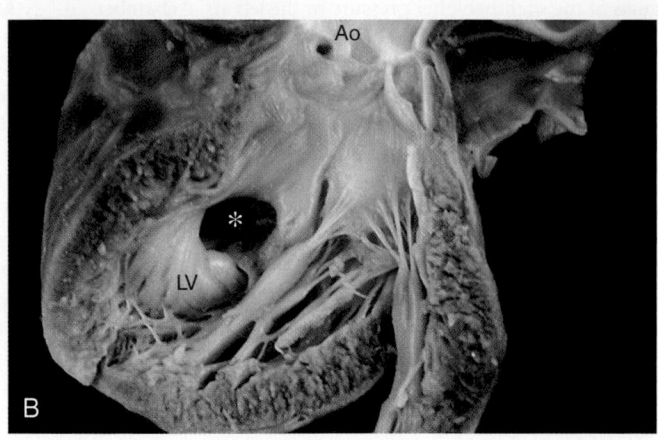

B

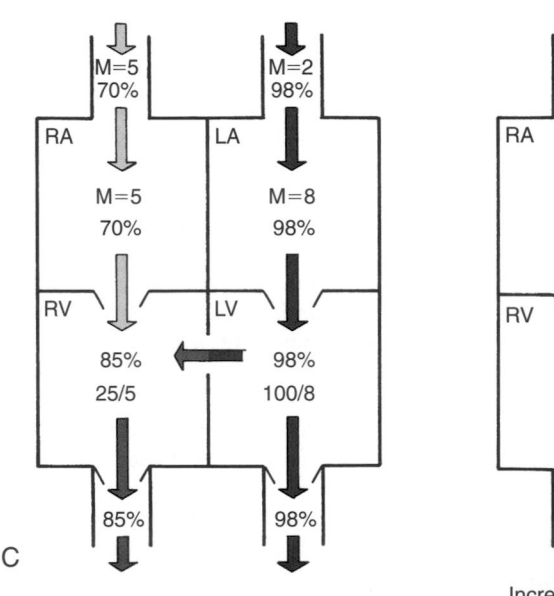

C

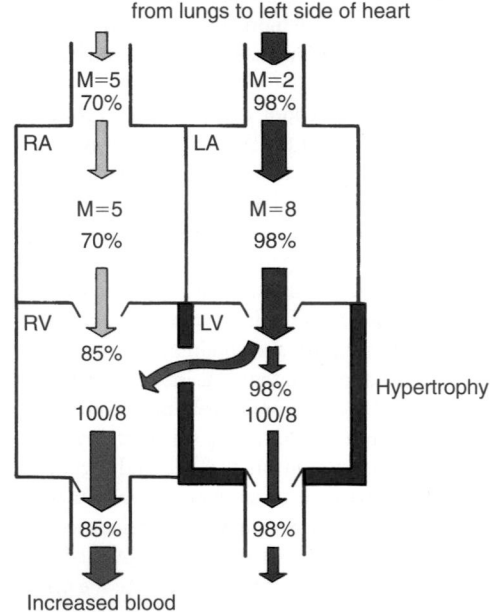

Increased blood volume
from lungs to left side of heart

Hypertrophy

Increased blood
volume to lungs

D

FIGURE 34.7 Ventricular Septal Defects (VSDs). **A,** VSD with left-to-right shunt. **B,** Muscular *(asterisk)* defect (opened left ventricle). **C,** Hemodynamics of a small VSD with left-to-right shunt. Mean *(M)* indicates mean of pressure; systolic/diastolic pressures are in mmHg; and percentages indicate oxygen saturation. **D,** Hemodynamics of a large VSD with left-to-right shunt. Like the shunting that occurs in preductal coarctation of the aorta, the shunting pictured here causes left ventricular overload and hypertrophy. *Ao,* Aorta; *LA,* left atrium; *LV,* left ventricle; *RA,* right atrium; *RV,* right ventricle. (**A** from Hockenberry MJ, Wilson D: *Wong's nursing care of infants and children,* ed 9, St Louis, 2011, Mosby; **B** from Damjanov I, Linder J, editors: *Anderson's pathology,* ed 10, St Louis, 1996, Mosby.)

Patch closure, using a synthetic material or pericardium, is accomplished through a sternotomy and with the use of cardiopulmonary bypass. A transatrial approach is preferable to a right ventriculotomy because of the increased incidence of conduction disturbances and impaired RV function associated with ventriculotomy. Contraindications for VSD closure include evidence of pulmonary hypertension or Eisenmenger syndrome.[2,7] Septal occluder devices for perimembranous VSD closure (performed in the cardiac catheterization laboratory) are not currently available in the United States but are under clinical evaluation in Europe.[9]

However, transcatheter muscular VSD devices are currently available for use depending on size and location of the defect.[9]

Atrioventricular Canal Defect

An atrioventricular canal (AVC) defect results from nonfusion of the endocardial cushions during fetal life, yielding abnormalities in both the atrial and ventricular septa and the AV valves (Fig. 34.8). This defect accounts for as many as 2% of all CHD, and approximately 70% of complete AVC defects occur in children with trisomy 21 (also referred

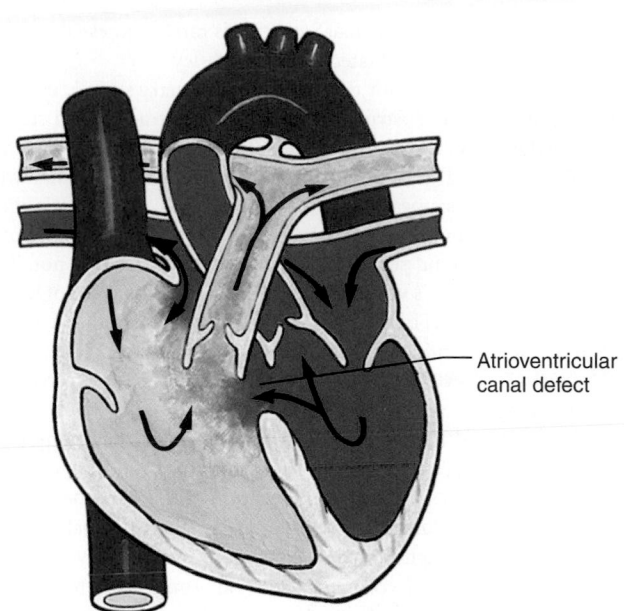

Atrioventricular
canal defect

FIGURE 34.8 Atrioventricular Canal Defect. (From Hockenberry MJ, Wilson D: *Wong's nursing care of infants and children*, ed 9, St Louis, 2011, Mosby.)

to as *Down syndrome*).[7] The three types of AVC defects are based on the cardiac components involved. Complete AVC (CAVC) defects consist of an inlet VSD, a primum type of ASD, and defects in both the mitral and tricuspid valves. Partial AVC (PAVC) defects consist of a primum type of ASD and a cleft in the septal or anterior leaflet of the mitral valve. Transitional AVC (TAVC) defects involve partial fusion of the endocardial cushions, resulting in variable AV valve abnormalities.[7]

◆**PATHOPHYSIOLOGY.** Hemodynamic abnormalities seen in AVC defects depend on the components of the lesion and the level of PVR. Shunting is minimal during the neonatal period when PVR is high. However, once PVR drops, left-to-right shunting occurs through the septal defects, resulting in increased pulmonary blood flow and HF.

PAVC defects mimic the hemodynamics of secundum ASD in which the left-to-right shunting through the primum ASD causes RA and RV dilation and increased pulmonary blood flow. The mitral regurgitation that occurs, caused by the cleft mitral valve, is usually hemodynamically insignificant.

CAVC defects reflect the hemodynamics of an ASD and a VSD, resulting in biatrial and biventricular enlargement. RA and RV volume overload occurs because of shunting through the primum ASD and tricuspid regurgitation. Likewise, LA and LV volume overload occurs because of shunting through the VSD, increased pulmonary venous return, and mitral regurgitation.

◆**CLINICAL MANIFESTATIONS.** Children with PAVC defects are generally asymptomatic. Findings on physical examination are similar to those of secundum ASD with the addition of a holosystolic, regurgitant murmur of mitral regurgitation at the apex. At 4 to 12 weeks of age, when PVR drops, children with CAVC defects usually begin to show symptoms of HF. Physical findings are similar to those found in individuals with VSDs with the addition of a holosystolic murmur radiating to the back and apex, reflecting mitral regurgitation. A mid-diastolic rumble at the left lower sternal border or apex reflects relative stenosis of the mitral or tricuspid valve from increased flow. Infants with CAVC may have signs of HF and frequent respiratory tract infections.

◆**EVALUATION AND TREATMENT.** The ECG generally demonstrates a superior left-axis deviation (−90 to −180 degrees), first-degree AV block, and RV hypertrophy or right bundle branch block. The ECG of

CAVC defects also may show LV hypertrophy. Chest radiograph shows cardiomegaly, increased pulmonary vascular markings, and a prominent main PA. Echocardiography allows visualization of the components of the defect, including continuity between the AV valves, their sizes, and chordal attachments. Cardiac catheterization is rarely indicated but may be performed to evaluate the reversibility of pulmonary vascular disease. Timing of surgical repair depends on the severity of symptoms, degree of shunting, and level of PVR. The trend is to perform complete repair between 3 and 6 months after birth to avoid the development of pulmonary vascular changes. Surgical repair is performed through a sternotomy, implementing a one- or two-patch repair to close the septal defects and repair the involved AV valves. Mortality is low unless the child is a newborn, has severe AV valve incompetence, or has univentricular anatomy (unbalanced AV canal).[11] Postoperative complications include heart block, dysrhythmias, or mitral regurgitation requiring further surgical intervention or valve replacement.[7,11]

Defects Decreasing Pulmonary Blood Flow

Defects decreasing pulmonary blood flow involve obstruction to pulmonary blood flow and septal communications. Because of RV outflow tract obstruction, right-sided pressures exceed left-sided pressures, resulting in right-to-left shunting. Children with these defects have hypoxemia and cyanosis.

Tetralogy of Fallot

Tetralogy of Fallot (TOF) consists of four defects: a large VSD that is high in the septum, an overriding aorta that straddles the VSD, pulmonary stenosis (PS), and RV hypertrophy (Fig. 34.9, *A*). It is the most common cyanotic congenital heart defect and accounts for 5% to 10% of all defects.[2]

◆**PATHOPHYSIOLOGY.** The pathophysiology associated with TOF varies widely, depending primarily on the degree of pulmonary stenosis, the size of the VSD, and the pulmonary and systemic resistance to flow. Because the VSD is usually large, pressures are equal in the RV and LV. Therefore the major determinant of shunt direction through the VSD is the difference between PVR and SVR (see Fig. 34.9, *B*). Infants who have little or no right-to-left shunting are acyanotic and are known as *pink tets*. They may have a net left-to-right shunt similar to a large VSD. If PVR is higher than SVR, the shunt is from right to left. Because many factors can alter the balance between PVR and SVR, shunt direction is not necessarily constant.

Pulmonary stenosis decreases blood flow to the lungs and, consequently, the amount of oxygenated blood that returns to the left heart. If blood also shunts from right to left through the VSD, deoxygenated blood mixes with the oxygenated blood returning from the lungs. The result is low oxygen saturation (hypoxemia) in the systemic circulation. The body attempts to compensate for chronic hypoxemia by producing more red blood cells (thereby causing polycythemia) and by increasing blood flow to the lungs through collateral bronchial vessels in long-standing cases.

◆**CLINICAL MANIFESTATIONS.** In cases with decreased pulmonary flow through the right ventricular outflow tract as long as the ductus arteriosus remains open, the newborn's pulmonary blood flow may be adequate. As the ductus closes, however, cyanosis becomes apparent. Chronic hypoxemia causes clubbing of the fingers and toes (see Chapter 36).

A rare manifestation of TOF is the sudden onset of dyspnea, cyanosis, and restlessness, sometimes called a *hypercyanotic spell* or a *tet spell*, that generally occurs with crying and exertion. The cause of these episodes is unknown, but it is theorized that the RV outflow tract goes into spasm or the systemic resistance drops suddenly. In either case the relative or actual increase in PVR increases the right-to-left shunt and

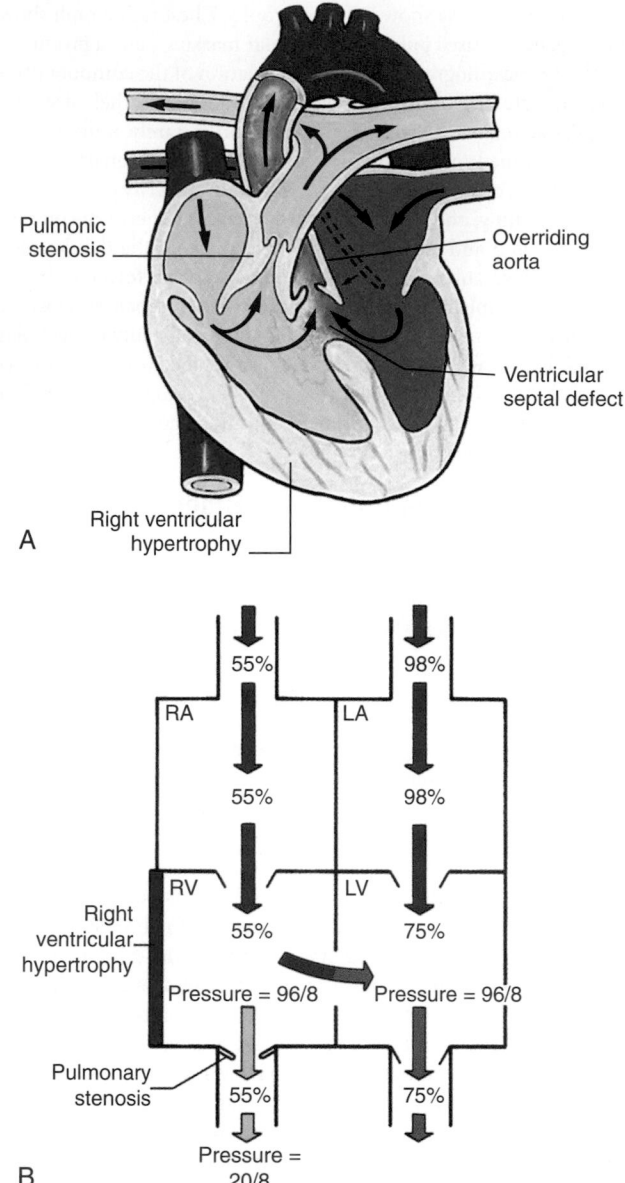

A

B

FIGURE 34.9 Tetralogy of Fallot. **A,** Anatomic defects in tetralogy of Fallot. **B,** Hemodynamics of tetralogy of Fallot with right-to-left shunt. *Ao,* Aorta; *LA,* left atrium; *LV,* left ventricle; *PT,* pulmonary artery trunk; *RA,* right atrium; *RV,* right ventricle. (**A** from Hockenberry MJ, Wilson D: *Wong's nursing care of infants and children,* ed 9, St Louis, 2011, Mosby.)

the cyanosis. Hypercyanotic spells are often the event that initiates surgical intervention. If the spells are frequent or do not terminate spontaneously, they are considered a medical-surgical emergency.[7]

Infants with TOF may have difficulty with feeding because the exertion required increases hypoxia, and therefore they experience slow growth and FTT. However, most infants with TOF grow normally.

Squatting is a spontaneous compensatory mechanism used by older children with unrepaired TOF to alleviate hypercyanotic spells. Squatting and its variants increase SVR while decreasing venous return to the heart from the inferior vena cava. The decrease of systemic venous return makes relatively more oxygenated blood available to the body. The increase of systemic resistance also reverses the shunt through the VSD to a left-to-right shunt, which has the effect of increasing pulmonary blood flow. Through both of these mechanisms, squatting temporarily

decreases the degree of hypoxemia. Squatting is rarely witnessed because most cases are surgically palliated in early infancy.

The typical heart murmur of TOF is a pulmonary systolic ejection murmur caused by the obstruction in the outflow tract, which creates turbulence during systole. More obstruction to flow (e.g., smaller orifice for the flow of blood) produces a louder murmur. This explains why the murmur often disappears during a hypoxic spell, when obstruction increases and pulmonary blood flow decreases to a minimal amount. The second heart sound seems to be single, but in fact it is not. The pulmonary component is very soft and delayed and usually is not heard, although it is present. The enlarged RV may cause the left side of the chest to be more prominent, and a "heave" also may be palpated.

◆**EVALUATION AND TREATMENT.** The ECG indicates RV hypertrophy. Chest radiographic examination shows that the heart is shaped like a boot (upturned apex because of a small main PA) and that pulmonary vascular markings are decreased. Echocardiograms and angiograms enable the clinician to see the size and position of the VSD, the stenotic pulmonary infundibulum or valve, the smaller-than-normal PA, and the overriding aorta. Diagnostic cardiac catheterization is rarely indicated, except to define unusual coronary artery anatomy crossing the RV outflow tract that may complicate surgical palliation.

The current practice is to repair acyanotic TOF before 1 year of age, and cyanotic TOF in early infancy. Staged procedures include the placement of a shunt from the subclavian or innominate artery to pulmonary artery known as the *modified Blalock-Taussig shunt* (using a prosthetic graft) or *classic Blalock-Taussig shunt* (using the native subclavian artery) to increase pulmonary blood flow. These shunts may cause PA distortion but may be necessary in a very small symptomatic child. Corrective repair involves patch closure of the VSD, resection of infundibular or valvular stenosis, and patch augmentation of the RV outflow tract that can extend across the pulmonary valve annulus (transannular patch). The procedure is done through a sternotomy incision while the child is on cardiopulmonary bypass. Operative mortality is low, and potential complications include dysrhythmias, low cardiac output because of RV dysfunction, and occasionally heart block. Many children require further surgery or transcatheter intervention to relieve recurrent pulmonary artery stenosis or treat severe pulmonary insufficiency.[12] More recently, a less invasive treatment for severe pulmonary insufficiency, depending on the size of the pulmonary outflow tract, is transcatheter pulmonary valve replacement performed in the catheterization laboratory.[9]

Tricuspid Atresia

Tricuspid atresia consists of an imperforate tricuspid valve, resulting in no communication between the RA and RV (Fig. 34.10). This defect accounts for 1% to 3% of congenital heart defects and is the third most common cyanotic heart defect. Tricuspid atresia is a combination of defects, including the imperforate tricuspid valve as well as a septal defect, hypoplastic or absent RV, enlarged mitral valve and LV, and varying degrees of pulmonic stenosis. Tricuspid atresia also may be associated with transposition of the great vessels. The most common type of tricuspid atresia involves a hypoplastic RA with decreased pulmonary blood flow, ASD, VSD, and normally related great vessels.[2]

◆**PATHOPHYSIOLOGY.** Systemic blood returns through the superior and inferior venae cavae to the RA. Venous return flows through the ASD into the LA, mixing with blood returning from the pulmonary circulation. The blood then enters the LV. Most of this blood passes into the systemic circulation through the aorta, but varying amounts flow through the VSD into the hypoplastic RV and to the lungs. Pulmonary circulation depends on the presence of a VSD and the presence of a functioning RV of reasonable capacity. If the RV is absent, the pulmonary valve is usually imperforate as well. If this is the case, a PDA

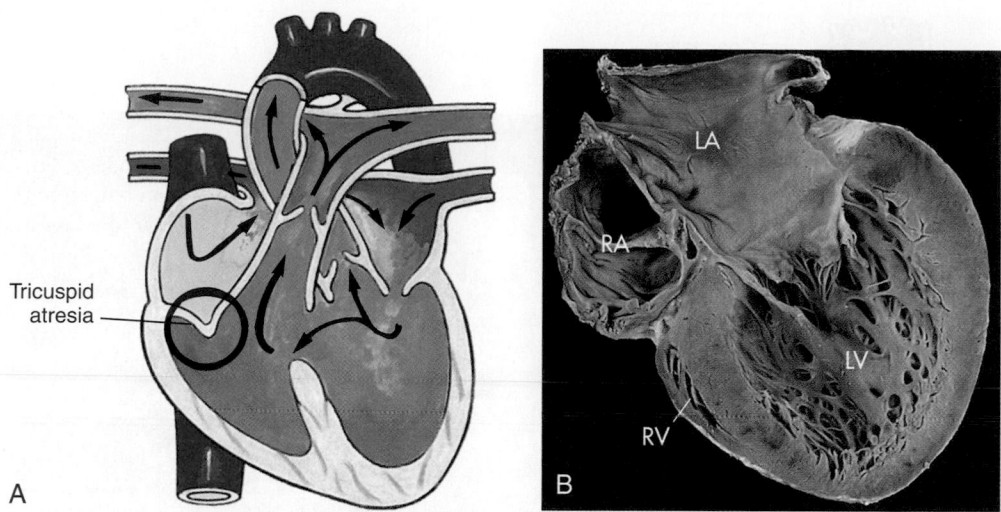

Tricuspid atresia

FIGURE 34.10 Tricuspid Atresia. **A,** No communication from the right atrium to the right ventricle. **B,** Tricuspid atresia with absent right atrioventricular connection with a hypoplastic right ventricle (four-chamber view). *LA,* Left atrium; *LV,* left ventricle; *RA,* right atrium; *RV,* right ventricle. (**A** from Hockenberry MJ, Wilson D: *Wong's nursing care of infants and children,* ed 9, St Louis, 2011, Mosby; **B** from Damjanov I, Linder J, editors: *Anderson's pathology,* ed 10, St Louis, 1996, Mosby.)

is necessary to ensure that some blood flows into the pulmonary circulation.[7]

Pulmonary circulation also depends on the relationship between PVR and SVR. As long as PVR is lower than SVR, blood flows through the VSD from left to right, feeding the pulmonary circulation. If PVR rises above SVR, pulmonary blood flow will be significantly diminished.

◆**CLINICAL MANIFESTATIONS.** Some degree of central cyanosis is common in tricuspid atresia, depending on the amount of pulmonary blood flow. Growth failure also is common. Children experience exertional dyspnea, tachypnea, and hypoxemia. Long-term effects of hypoxia are polycythemia and clubbing. These children also may display hypercyanotic spells. Hepatomegaly may be present if the ASD is restrictive or CHF occurs as a result of increased pulmonary blood flow.

The murmur heard with tricuspid atresia may have several components. The VSD causes a systolic regurgitant murmur; the murmur is likely to be softer and shorter as the VSD enlarges. A narrowly split second heart sound caused by decreased pulmonary blood flow may be present, or the second heart sound may be single if there is pulmonary atresia.

◆**EVALUATION AND TREATMENT.** Chest radiographic examination shows a heart size that is normal or slightly increased. ECG usually shows RA, LA, and LV hypertrophy with left-axis deviation. Echocardiography depicts left-to-right shunting at the ventricular level, inability of blood flow to enter the RV from the absent tricuspid opening, and the presence of associated defects.

Newborns with ductal dependent pulmonary blood flow are immediately given prostaglandins to maintain adequate pulmonary blood flow. Treatment is accomplished in stages. Initial surgical intervention involves the placement of a Blalock-Taussig shunt (or its modification). If the ASD is restrictive, a Rashkind procedure (balloon atrial septostomy) may be performed during catheterization or under echocardiographic guidance at the bedside. Children who experience increased pulmonary blood flow may require the placement of a PA band.

Further surgery is undertaken between 4 and 8 months of age, depending on the child's growth and degree of cyanosis. The second-stage procedure is the bidirectional Glenn shunt, in which the SVC is anastomosed to the PA. At that time, the PA may be ligated and the

Blalock-Taussig shunt is removed. The final separation of the pulmonary circulation to the systemic circulation is the modified Fontan procedure. In this stage, the inferior vena cava blood flow is routed to the PA using an intra- or extracardiac tube graft or baffle. The procedure is typically performed between 2 and 4 years of age. Surgical outcomes are best in the child with normal ventricular function, minimal systemic valve regurgitation, and low PVR. For children with borderline PVR, a fenestration (or opening) can be created in the baffle or graft to relieve high systemic pulmonary venous pressures if needed. Postoperative complications that increase hospital stay include pleural effusions, elevated pulmonary vascular resistance, and ventricular dysfunction.[12,13] Exercise tolerance is limited in many children following the Fontan procedure, but their general health is usually good.

Obstructive Defects

Obstructive defects are conditions in which anatomic stenosis (narrowing) in either the right or the left outflow tract obstructs blood flow and results in a pressure load on the affected ventricle. The gradient reflects the severity of the narrowing; the higher the gradient, the more obstruction to flow and the more afterload on the ventricle. Valvular stenosis refers to stenosis of the valve itself; subvalvular indicates that the obstruction is below the valve or in the ventricular outflow tract; and supravalvular is the area above the valve in the great artery. The obstructive defects include coarctation of the aorta, aortic stenosis, and pulmonary stenosis. Symptoms associated with the defect depend on the site and severity of stenosis.

Coarctation of the Aorta

Coarctation of the aorta (COA) is a narrowing of the lumen of the aorta that impedes blood flow. This defect accounts for 8% to 10% of all congenital heart defects. COA is almost always in a juxtaductal position, although it can occur anywhere between the origin of the aortic arch and the bifurcation of the aorta in the lower abdomen. About 50% to 80% of individuals with COA have a bicuspid aortic valve and also may have an associated VSD (Fig. 34.11).[2]

◆**PATHOPHYSIOLOGY.** COA may develop because of abnormal contractile ductal tissue that constricts at the time of ductal closure.

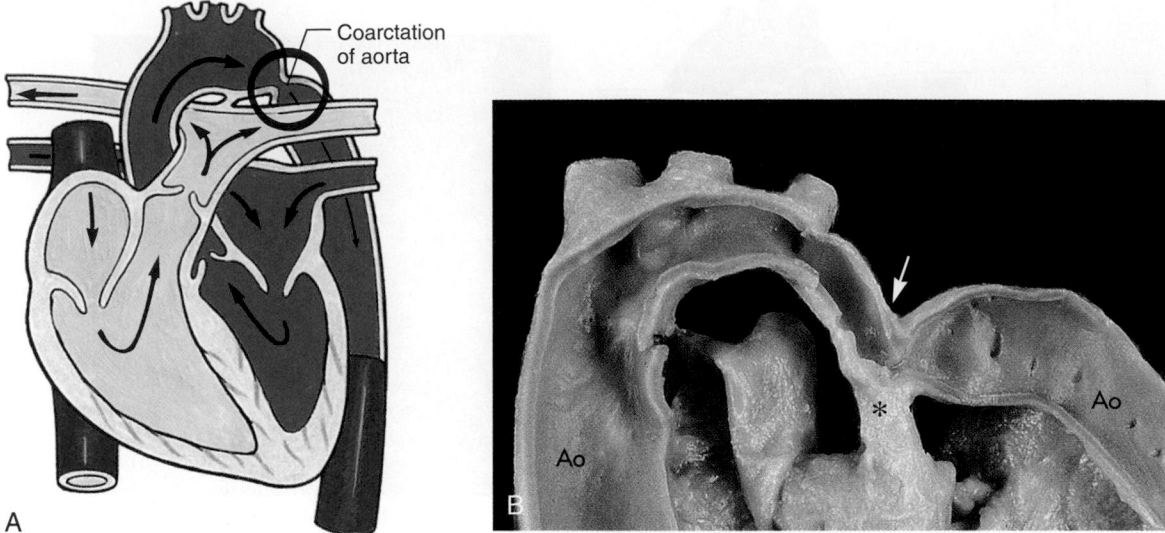

FIGURE 34.11 Postductal Coarctation of the Aorta. A, Postductal coarctation occurs distal to ("after") the insertion of the closed ductus arteriosus into the aortic arch. The coarctation consists of a flap of tissue that protrudes from the tunica media of the aortic wall. **B,** Coarctation of the aorta with typical indentation of the aortic wall *(arrow)* opposite the ductal arterial ligament *(asterisk)*. *Ao,* Aorta. (**A** from Hockenberry MJ, Wilson D: *Wong's essentials of pediatric nursing,* ed 10, St Louis, 2015, Mosby; **B** from Damjanov I, Linder J, editors: *Anderson's pathology,* ed 10, St Louis, 1996, Mosby.)

COA causes a condition in which there are higher pressures proximal to the site of stenosis and lower pressures distal to the site. In the neonate with a preductal COA, the RV acts as a systemic pump, sending unoxygenated blood through the ductus (right to left) into the descending aorta below the coarctation. As the PVR drops, blood will start to shunt left to right through the ductus, and symptoms of HF will appear (Fig. 34.12). In postductal COA the RV cannot pump enough blood through the ductus to the descending aorta because of pressure caused by the narrowed aorta. Systolic pressure increases in the ascending aorta and LV and decreases in the descending aorta beyond the COA (Fig. 34.13). In neonates with severe COA, adequate systemic blood flow may depend on the presence of a PDA to supply blood flow distal to the obstruction. In long-standing COA, collateral circulation, which involves small arteries arising from the subclavian arteries, joins intercostal arteries that flow into the descending aorta. These collateral vessels bypass the COA and supply blood to the lower extremities. The direction of shunting through the ductus, if present, depends on the pressure difference between the PA and aorta and the location of the ductus. When blood pressure is greater in the aorta than in the PA, blood flow through the ductus will be left to right toward the lungs, resulting in increased pulmonary venous return to the left side of the heart. This may place an additional strain on the LA and LV, leading to increased volume and workload. With time, prolonged LV hypertrophy will cause HF symptoms because of increased afterload and obstruction to flow caused by the coarctation.

CLINICAL MANIFESTATIONS. Clinical manifestations vary depending on the severity of the coarctation and age of presentation. In newborns the onset of symptoms depends on the timing of ductal closure after a fall in PVR, the location of the COA, and the presence of associated defects. The newborn usually presents with HF symptoms. Once the ductus closes, these infants will deteriorate rapidly from the development of hypotension, acidosis, and shock. Older children may not be diagnosed until hypertension is noted. Hypertension is noted in the upper extremities with decreased or absent pulses in the lower extremities. Children may have cool, mottled skin and occasionally leg cramps during exercise.

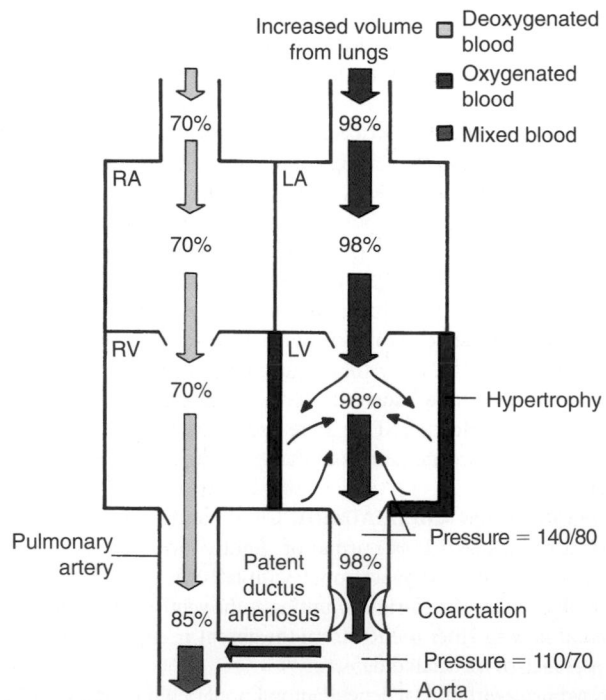

FIGURE 34.12 Hemodynamics of Preductal Coarctation of the Aorta with a Patent Ductus Arteriosus. The left-to-right shunt through the ductus arteriosus increases the volume of blood in the pulmonary circulation. Afterload *(small black arrows)* is increased in the left heart by increased return from the lungs and decreased ventricular outflow caused by the coarctation. The outcome is heart failure. *LA,* Left atrium; *LV,* left ventricle; *RA,* right atrium; *RV,* right ventricle.

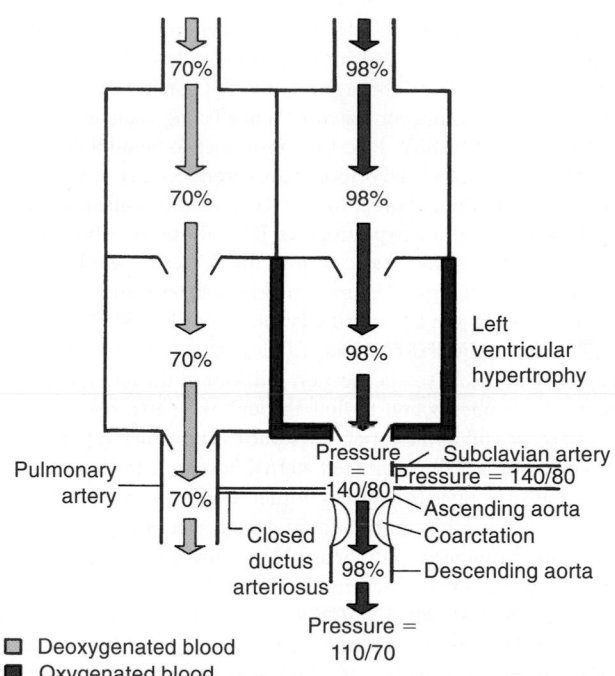

FIGURE 34.13 Hemodynamics of Postductal Coarctation of the Aorta. Blood pressure increases in the ascending aorta and subclavian artery and decreases in the descending aorta. These pressure changes eventually occur in the parts of the systemic circulation served by arteries that branch from the aorta before and after the coarctation.

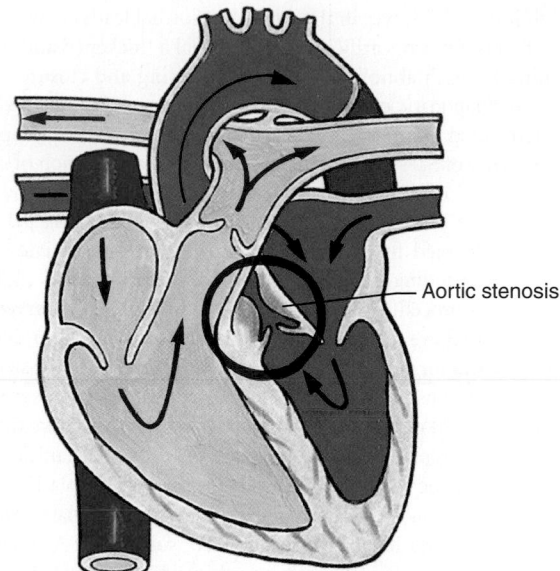

FIGURE 34.14 Aortic Stenosis. Narrowing of the aortic valve causing resistance to blood flow in the left ventricle, decreased cardiac output, left ventricular hypertrophy, and pulmonary congestion. (From Hockenberry MJ, Wilson D: *Wong's nursing care of infants and children,* ed 9, St Louis, 2011, Mosby.)

A systolic ejection murmur, heard best at the left interscapular area, is caused by rapid blood flow through the narrowed area.

◆ **EVALUATION AND TREATMENT.** A chest radiograph shows an enlarged heart with congested lung fields in newborns. Rib notching between the fourth and eighth ribs may be seen in children older than 5 years, reflecting erosion of the ribs as a result of enlarged collateral vessels from the ascending aorta to the descending aorta, bypassing the coarctation. An ECG may be normal or reveal LV hypertrophy. An echocardiogram will confirm the diagnosis and rule out other intracardiac defects. Cardiac catheterization and/or magnetic resonance imaging (MRI) is performed only if the echocardiogram is inconclusive.

The first step in treatment of the symptomatic infant is stabilization, which may require prostaglandin administration, mechanical ventilation, and inotropic support to maintain adequate cardiac output. Once this is achieved, surgical intervention is indicated. Surgical repair consists of a resection with end-to-end anastomosis of the arch segments, arch augmentation, or subclavian flap aortoplasty technique to enlarge the constricted area. Depending on the arch morphology (hypoplastic transverse arch), a modification of this procedure enlarges the aorta beyond the area of constriction.[12] Cardiopulmonary bypass may not be required in isolated COA, and approach can be through a left thoracotomy incision. However, COA repair may be a part of a more complex operation, and sternotomy incision with cardiopulmonary bypass may be required.

Operative mortality is relatively low. Postoperative complications include recoarctation and paradoxical postoperative hypertension. Residual permanent hypertension requiring continued medical therapy is related to age at repair; therefore surgical intervention is recommended at the time of diagnosis. Percutaneous balloon dilation angioplasty with or without stent implantation may be a less invasive option for treating native COA (greater than 6 months of age) or for reducing significant

residual COA in most children. However, aortic aneurysm formation and blood vessel injury from arterial access have been noted.[9,12,14]

Aortic Stenosis

Aortic stenosis (AS) is a narrowing of the aortic outflow tract (Fig. 34.14). The lesion accounts for up to 10% of all congenital heart defects.[2] Valvular stenosis is caused by malformation or fusion of the cusps. It is the most common type of AS, tends to be progressive, and, in rare cases, can lead to sudden death as a result of low cardiac output or myocardial ischemia. For children with mild AS, no exercise restrictions may be needed. For those with moderate AS, some exercise limitations may be advised. Severe AS is an indication for limiting exercise until the repair is accomplished. Less common forms of AS are subvalvular stenosis caused by a constricting fibrous ring below the valve and supravalvular stenosis that occurs above the valve.[7]

◆ **PATHOPHYSIOLOGY.** Obstruction to blood flowing out of the aorta causes an increased workload on the LV, resulting in left ventricle hypertrophy (LVH). LV failure may develop, leading to an increase in LA pressure and a backup in the system, eventually resulting in pulmonary vascular congestion and pulmonary arterial hypertension. LVH can decrease coronary artery perfusion, resulting in myocardial ischemia, and it can alter the LV papillary muscle, causing mitral insufficiency.

◆ **CLINICAL MANIFESTATIONS.** Most children with mild to moderate AS are asymptomatic. Signs of exercise intolerance may not appear until preadolescence. Syncopal episodes, epigastric pain, and exertional chest pain may occur in more severe forms of AS. A systolic ejection murmur at the right upper sternal border that transmits to the neck and left lower sternal border is produced by blood flow through the stenotic area. An ejection click may be heard with valvular AS. Severe forms of AS, especially critical AS in the newborn, result in shock and require immediate intervention.

◆ **EVALUATION AND TREATMENT.** Diagnosis may be made based on previous medical history and physical findings. Chest radiographic examination may reveal a dilated ascending aorta or LV enlargement. Increased pulmonary vascular markings may be seen in severe forms. In mild cases the ECG is normal. LVH with strain pattern (features of

LVH with inverted T waves in the lateral precordial leads) may be seen in severe forms. An echocardiogram may reveal a thickened and poorly functioning LV with abnormal structure, opening and closure of the aortic valve. Diagnostic cardiac catheterization is rarely indicated, but may be performed for intervention, such as balloon aortic valvuloplasty.

The presence of ST-segment changes on ECG, manifestation of severe HF, and evidence of discrete severe stenosis at the aortic outflow tract are indications for intervention. Balloon aortic valvuloplasty is a palliative procedure performed for valvular AS; however, it is associated with complications, including aortic insufficiency and dysrhythmia.[9] Children undergoing this procedure almost always require surgical intervention at some time to relieve recurrent narrowing or worsening regurgitation. Surgical treatment for valvular AS depends on the severity of the stenosis, previous interventions, and age of the child. Aortic valve commissurotomy or valvotomy may be performed as an initial procedure for severe valvular AS. Aortic valve replacement (Ross procedure or mechanical valve replacement) may be required if the valve is severely dysplastic.

Subvalvular AS and supravalvular AS require surgical repair involving excision of the area causing the constriction. For subvalvular AS involving a small LV outflow tract and aortic annulus, a Konno procedure may be required to enlarge the LV outflow tract and aortic annulus with a patch.[12,15] Severe supravalvar AS may require balloon angioplasty and stent placement or surgical enlargement with coronary reimplantation.

Pulmonary Stenosis

Pulmonary stenosis (PS) is the narrowing of the pulmonary outflow tract. This may be in the form of abnormal thickening of the valve leaflets or narrowing of the arterial (supravalvular) or ventricular (subvalvular) side of the valve (Fig. 34.15, A). Pulmonary atresia is the severe form of PS and involves complete fusion of the commissures and narrowing of the main PA, allowing no blood flow out of the RV to the PA. Pulmonary blood flow to the lungs is now dependent on a

PDA or from extra blood vessels (multiple aortopulmonary collaterals) that arise from the aorta and connect to the pulmonary arteries with decompression of the RV through an ASD/PFO or, in rare cases, a VSD for survival. PS accounts for 8% to 12% of all congenital heart defects.[2]

◆**PATHOPHYSIOLOGY.** PS creates resistance to blood flow from the RV to the PA. The narrowed orifice (valve) produces increased resistance (afterload) to ejection. In order for the RV to maintain adequate cardiac output, the myocardium hypertrophies. If the RV outflow tract obstruction is severe, blood may back up into the RA, causing dilation. This may result in reopening of the foramen ovale with resultant unoxygenated blood shunting to the LA, causing cyanosis (see Fig. 34.15, B).

◆**CLINICAL MANIFESTATIONS.** Clinical manifestations depend on the severity of PS. A systolic ejection murmur at the left upper sternal border reflects obstruction to flow through the narrowed pulmonary valve. In some children a variable systolic ejection click is present with valvular stenosis at the upper left sternal border. A thrill also may be palpated at the upper left sternal border. Children with moderate PS may have exertional dyspnea and fatigability because of the inability of the body to increase pulmonary blood flow to meet demands for increased cardiac output. Severe PS will produce cyanosis and HF.

◆**EVALUATION AND TREATMENT.** A chest radiograph shows a normal-size heart with a prominent main PA caused by poststenotic dilation. An ECG is usually normal but may reveal right-axis deviation and RV hypertrophy with moderate PS. Echocardiography confirms the diagnosis and detects associated defects. Cardiac catheterization, if performed for interventional purposes, further demonstrates PA anatomy.

Mild to moderate PS will not likely require intervention but should be observed closely. Most mild PS is not progressive. Treatment is indicated when a significant pressure gradient is detected across the RV outflow tract.

Critical (severe) PS must be addressed immediately. The treatment of choice is balloon angioplasty. This procedure is considered highly

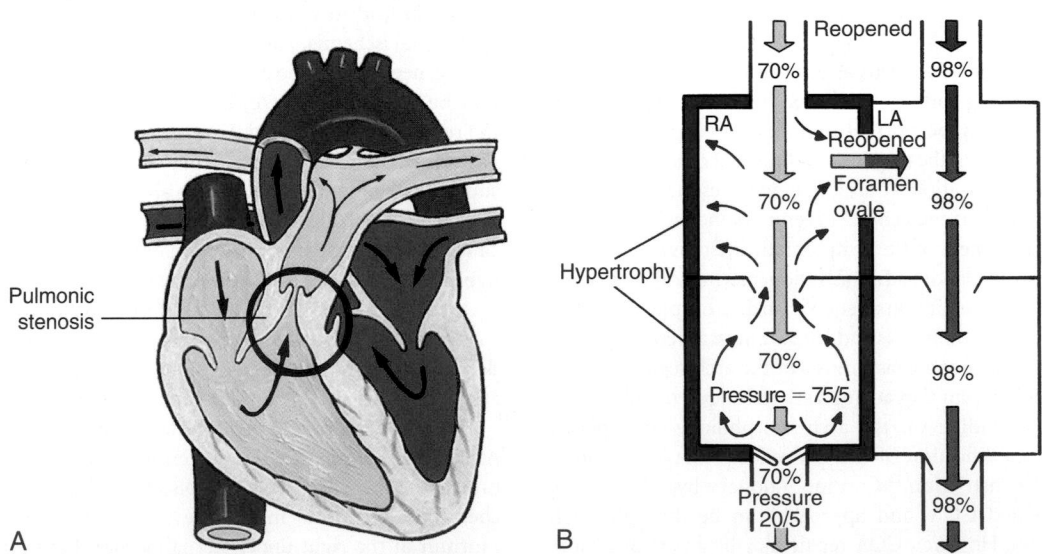

FIGURE 34.15 Pulmonary Stenosis. A, Obstruction of right ventricular outflow caused by pulmonary stenosis. Pressure on the ventricular side of the pulmonic semilunar valve (pulmonary valve) is much greater than that on the pulmonary arterial side. This difference disrupts the normal pressure gradient across the valve. Pulmonary stenosis increases ventricular afterload by decreasing blood flow through the valve, which causes ventricular hypertrophy. **B,** The backup of ventricular afterload into the right atrium reopens the foramen ovale. Venous blood then flows from the area of higher pressure (the right atrium) to the area of lower pressure (the left atrium), causing a right-to-left shunt. Cyanosis occurs if enough venous blood shunts from right to left to reduce oxygen saturation in the systemic circulation by 3% to 5%. *LA,* Left atrium; *RA,* right atrium. (**A** from Hockenberry MJ, Wilson D: *Wong's nursing care of infants and children,* ed 9, St Louis, 2011, Mosby.)

effective in decreasing the pressure gradient across the pulmonic valve and is noted to have few associated complications.[9] Surgical correction involves a pulmonary valvotomy incising the fused commissures.[2] Both valvotomy and balloon angioplasty may result in some pulmonary valve incompetence, and long-term follow-up may reveal the need for pulmonary valve replacement. Treatment for PA depends on the size of the native/branch pulmonary arteries and associated cardiac defects. Initial treatment may consist of an aortopulmonary shunt to supply stable blood flow to the lungs and later a second procedure to connect the RV to the PA.

Mixing Defects

Many complex defects are classified as mixing defects because of their dependence on the mixing of pulmonary and systemic circulations for survival during the postnatal period. This mixing results in desaturated systemic blood flow and cyanosis. Pulmonary congestion occurs because of preferential pulmonary blood flow because PVR is normally lower than SVR. Clinically each defect has varying degrees of cyanosis and HF depending on the various components of the lesion.

Transposition of the Great Arteries

Transposition of the great arteries (TGA) refers to a condition in which the aorta arises from the RV and the PA from the LV (Fig. 34.16, *A*). The result is two separate, parallel circuits in which unoxygenated blood circulates continuously through the systemic circulation and oxygenated blood circulates repeatedly through the pulmonary circulation. This condition is incompatible with extrauterine life unless a communication exists between the two circuits to provide the necessary oxygen to the body. Communication is accomplished by mixing of pulmonary and systemic circulations through a PDA, ASD, or VSD (see Fig. 34.16, *B*). Dextro-transposition of the great arteries (D-TGA) accounts for 5% to 7% of all congenital heart defects; *dextro* refers to the aorta remaining to the right of the PA.[2,7]

Two factors allow newborns with complete transposition to survive long enough to be treated. First, blood from the two closed systems can mix through the ductus arteriosus for a short time after birth if PVR remains high. Some mixing also may occur through the foramen ovale. If the child has a VSD, mixing occurs through that opening as well.

◆**PATHOPHYSIOLOGY.** It is not known precisely which embryologic events lead to transposition, but researchers have proposed that the fault lies in the development of conal tissue in the fibrous skeleton of the heart.[1] The conus is a segment of muscle that separates the AV (tricuspid and mitral) valves from the semilunar (aortic and pulmonic) valves. (The fibrous skeleton and heart valves are described and illustrated in Chapter 32; see Fig. 32.4.) The interventricular septum is intact in about 60% to 70% of cases of transposition; a VSD is present in the remaining 30% to 40%.[2,7] The following discussion is limited to the pathophysiology of transposition with an intact interventricular septum.

◆**CLINICAL MANIFESTATIONS.** The degree of mixing permitted by fetal structures determines the type and severity of clinical manifestations. Cyanosis may be mild shortly after birth and worsen during the first day because of functional closure of the ductus arteriosus. Low oxygen levels in the blood (hypoxemia) cause metabolic acidosis, tachycardia, and tachypnea. The presence of a PDA or large ASD allows for more mixing and results in only mild cyanosis, but the infant may develop HF.

The first heart sound is normal, and the second sound may be heard as a single sound even though both the aortic and pulmonic valves are functioning. The loud single S_2 may occur because transposition places the aortic valve closer to the chest wall than the pulmonic valve. No murmur is noted with transposition of the great arteries with an intact ventricular septum.

◆**EVALUATION AND TREATMENT.** On chest radiograph the heart has a characteristic shape—like an egg on its side—and pulmonary vascular markings are increased. The heart may be enlarged if the infant is a few weeks old and has a VSD. ECG findings reveal a right-axis deviation and some RV hypertrophy. Echocardiography confirms the diagnosis of transposition of the great arteries. Cardiac catheterization or bedside echocardiogram-guided balloon atrial septostomy may be needed for additional mixing in children with intact ventricular septum and severe hypoxemia.[9]

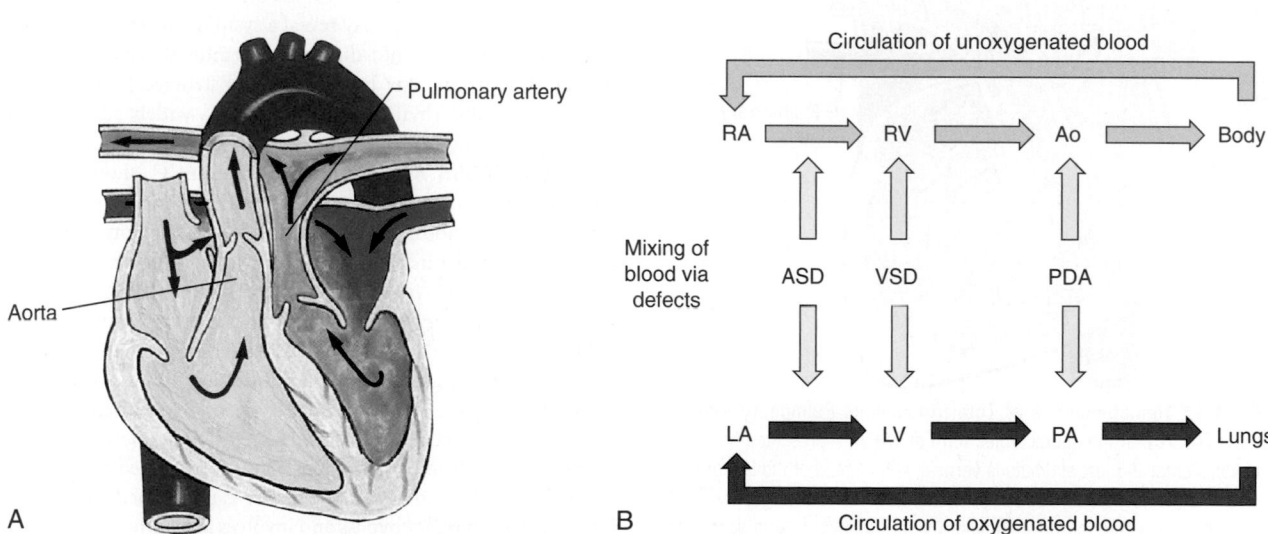

FIGURE 34.16 Hemodynamics in Transposition of the Great Arteries (TGA). **A,** Complete transposition of the great vessels with an intact interventricular septum. The aorta arises from the right ventricle and the pulmonary artery from the left. **B,** Oxygen saturation in the two parallel circuits. *Ao,* Aorta; *ASD,* atrial septal defect; *LA,* left atrium; *LV,* left ventricle; *PA,* pulmonary artery; *PDA,* patent ductus arteriosus; *RA,* right atrium; *RV,* right ventricle; *VSD,* ventricular septal defect. (**A** from Hockenberry MJ, Wilson D: *Wong's essentials of pediatric nursing,* ed 10, St Louis, 2015, Mosby.)

The most preferred type of surgical repair for D-TGA, performed in the first weeks of life, is the arterial switch procedure. The arterial switch involves transecting the great arteries and anastomosing the main pulmonary artery to the native proximal aorta and anastomosing the ascending AO to the native proximal PA. The coronary arteries are reimplanted with a *button* of tissue onto the new aortic outflow. Reimplantation of the coronary arteries is critical to survival, and they must be reattached without kinking or torsion. Potential complications include narrowing of the great artery anastomosis, neoaortic valve regurgitation, and coronary artery insufficiency. Long-term results for the arterial switch operation are usually good.[7]

The Rastelli procedure is used in children with transposition, VSD, and severe PS. This procedure involves closing the VSD with a baffle by rerouting LV blood through the VSD to the aorta. The pulmonary valve is closed, and an RV-to-PA prosthetic or homograft valve conduit is placed. This procedure requires prosthetic conduit replacement as the child grows and is associated with ventricular failure and dysrhythmias in the postoperative period.[7]

Total Anomalous Pulmonary Venous Connection

Total anomalous pulmonary venous connection (TAPVC), or total anomalous pulmonary venous return, occurs when the pulmonary veins abnormally connect to the right side of the heart either directly or through one or more systemic veins that drain into the RA (Fig. 34.17). An ASD also is generally present. This defect is extremely rare, accounting for only 1% of all congenital heart defects. The four types of TAPVC are based on the site of drainage. Supracardiac TAPVCs are the most common form (50%) and drain to the superior vena cava through the

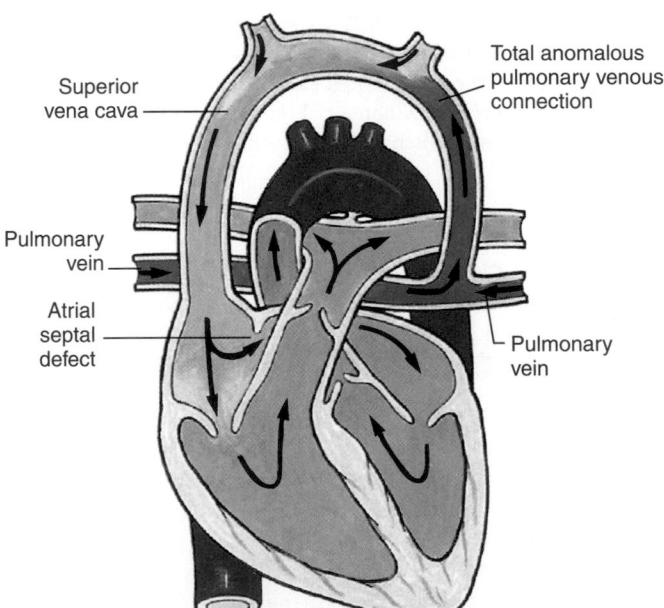

FIGURE 34.17 Hemodynamics of Total Anomalous Pulmonary Venous Connection (TAPVC). In the supracardiac form of TAPVC represented here, the pulmonary veins enter the left anomalous vertical vein instead of the left atrium. From the left anomalous vertical vein, the mixed blood from the lungs flows into the superior vena cava through an innominate vein (literally, a "vein without a name"). Oxygen saturation within the four heart chambers, the pulmonary artery, and the aorta is the same. Blood pressure in the right heart exceeds that in the left heart because the right heart is receiving blood from both the pulmonary and systemic circulatory systems. Abnormal vessels are shaded. (From Hockenberry MJ, Wilson D: *Wong's essentials of pediatric nursing*, ed 10, St Louis, 2015, Mosby.)

vertical or innominate vein. Cardiac TAPVCs (20%) drain directly into the RA or through the coronary sinus. Infracardiac TAPVCs (20%) traverse the diaphragm and drain into the portal or hepatic vein or the inferior vena cava. Mixed TAPVCs (10%) are a combination of the various types. Partial anomalous venous connection is a condition in which only one or two of the pulmonary veins, usually the right-sided veins, drain into the RA or one of its tributaries.[2]

◆**PATHOPHYSIOLOGY.** Physiologically TAPVC can be differentiated into two groups: nonobstructive and obstructive, depending on the absence or presence of obstruction to pulmonary venous drainage. The hemodynamics of the nonobstructive group involve the RA receiving the oxygenated blood that would normally flow into the LA. The amount of blood shunted into the LA vs. the volume entering the RV depends on the size of the ASD and compliance of the RV. Therefore if the ASD is restrictive and RV compliance approaches normal, more blood will enter the RV than the LA, resulting in RA and RV enlargement, as well as increased pulmonary blood flow. This causes increased pulmonary venous blood return and larger amounts of saturated blood in the RA. If the ASD is unrestrictive and the RV does not become thinner to increase compliance, the majority of mixed saturated blood is shunted from the higher-pressure RA to the LA.

The hemodynamics of obstructed TAPVC cause pulmonary venous hypertension because of resistance caused by the obstruction resulting in an elevation in pulmonary vascular and RV pressures. Pulmonary edema occurs from hydrostatic capillary pressure exceeding the osmotic pressure of the blood and eventually contributing to the development of HF. This group has a strong association with the infracardiac type of TAPVC and is a surgical emergency.

◆**CLINICAL MANIFESTATIONS.** The predominant clinical manifestation in infants with TAPVC is cyanosis caused by mixture of oxygenated and deoxygenated blood entering the systemic circulation. The degree of cyanosis is inversely related to the amount of pulmonary blood flow. Children with unobstructed TAPVC may be asymptomatic until PVR drops, at which time pulmonary blood flow will increase, resulting in signs of pulmonary overcirculation, particularly slow growth and frequent pulmonary infections, in addition to mild cyanosis. Obstructed TAPVC results in cyanosis and rapid deterioration necessitating immediate surgical correction, or death will occur.

Physical examination may reveal a systolic murmur at the left upper sternal border and a mid-diastolic murmur at the left lower sternal border. A murmur may be absent in obstructed TAPVC. A characteristic quadruple rhythm, consisting of S_1, widely split S_2, and S_3 or S_4, or a gallop rhythm also is present.

◆**EVALUATION AND TREATMENT.** The ECG shows a right-axis deviation, RV hypertrophy, and occasionally RA hypertrophy. The chest radiograph of unobstructed TAPVC reveals cardiomegaly, increased pulmonary vascular markings, and a snowman or figure-eight appearance in the supracardiac type. A chest roentgenogram of obstructed TAPVC shows a normal-size heart and a ground-glass appearance of the lung fields, reflecting pulmonary venous congestion or edema. The echocardiogram reveals the abnormal pulmonary venous connections.

Surgical repair varies with the type of TAPVC and whether the defect is obstructed or unobstructed. Obstructed lesions are repaired at the time of diagnosis, whereas the unobstructed type generally is repaired during infancy. The procedure is performed while the patient is on cardiopulmonary bypass and involves anastomosis of the common pulmonary vein to the LA and closing the ASD, as in the supracardiac and infracardiac types. Repair of the supracardiac type involves baffling the pulmonary venous drainage to the LA. This repair has the highest success rate because of the low technical difficulty, whereas infracardiac repair is associated with a high mortality and morbidity. Potential complications include reobstruction at the anastomosis site; atrial dysrhythmias, including sick sinus syndrome; PA hypertension; and LV dysfunction.[12]

Truncus Arteriosus

Truncus arteriosus is the failure of the large embryonic artery, the truncus arteriosus, to divide into the PA and the aorta. This results in a single vessel arising from both ventricles, providing blood flow to the pulmonary and systemic circulations (Fig. 34.18, A). This common trunk straddles the VSD (always present) and has a single valve with three or four leaflets, which may result in stenosis, regurgitation, or both. The incidence is 1% of all CHD and a right aortic arch is present 30% of the time. There are four types of truncus arteriosus. Type I is the most common and involves the main PA arising from the truncus and then dividing into the right and left PAs. Type II is less common and involves the PAs arising from the posterior aspect of the truncus. Type III is the least common and involves the PAs arising from the lateral aspect of the truncus. Type IV, also known as *pseudotruncus*, is now considered a severe form of TOF with the bronchial arteries arising from the descending aorta to supply the lungs.[2] Types 1 and II constitute 85% of cases, with types III and IV constituting the remaining 15%.

◆**PATHOPHYSIOLOGY.** Blood flow from the RV and LV is pumped into the main truncus, resulting in mixing of the pulmonary and systemic circulations (see Fig. 34.18, B). The differential flow out to either the pulmonary bed or the systemic circulation depends on the PVR and SVR. Generally, the PVR is less than the SVR, resulting in the majority of blood flow traveling to the lungs. This may be altered, however, because of PS, small pulmonary arteries, or increased PVR. Pulmonary vascular disease develops early with this defect because of increased pulmonary blood flow.

◆**CLINICAL MANIFESTATIONS.** Physical findings depend on the amount of pulmonary blood flow and the presence of other cardiac anomalies. If PS is present, a newborn will present with cyanosis, caused by already elevated PVR, but no HF. Conversely, if PS is not present,

the newborn initially will have mild to moderate cyanosis that worsens with activity. Once PVR drops, the pulmonary bed will receive preferential flow and the infant will have signs of HF. A harsh systolic regurgitant murmur is usually present along the left sternal border as a result of the VSD, and a systolic click at the apex and left upper sternal border may be present, reflecting opening of the truncal valve. An apical rumble with or without a gallop rhythm also may be present because of increased pulmonary blood flow. If truncal valve insufficiency exists, an early diastolic, high-pitched decrescendo murmur may be present.

◆**EVALUATION AND TREATMENT.** An ECG generally reveals biventricular hypertrophy and occasionally LA enlargement. A chest radiograph reveals cardiomegaly with biventricular and LA enlargement, as well as increased pulmonary vascular markings. When PS is present, the heart size is normal and the pulmonary vascular markings are decreased. Echocardiography determines the type of truncal defect, competency of the truncal valve, and differential blood flow.

Surgical repair in early infancy is recommended to prevent the sequelae of severe HF and pulmonary vascular disease. The definitive repair consists of a modified Rastelli procedure involving VSD patch closure to divert the blood flow from the LV outflow tract into the truncus. The pulmonary arteries are excised from the aorta and connected to the RV through a tissue homograft (cadaver conduit). Postoperative complications include HF, residual VSD, truncal valve (now the aorta) stenosis or insufficiency, dysrhythmias, and pulmonary hypertension. These children require additional procedures to replace the conduit as its size becomes inadequate in relation to growth or narrows because of calcification over time.[12]

Hypoplastic Left Heart Syndrome

Hypoplastic left heart syndrome (HLHS) refers to the abnormal development of the left-sided cardiac structures, resulting in obstruction to blood flow from the LV outflow tract. HLHS involves underdevelopment of the LV, aorta, and aortic arch, as well as mitral atresia or stenosis

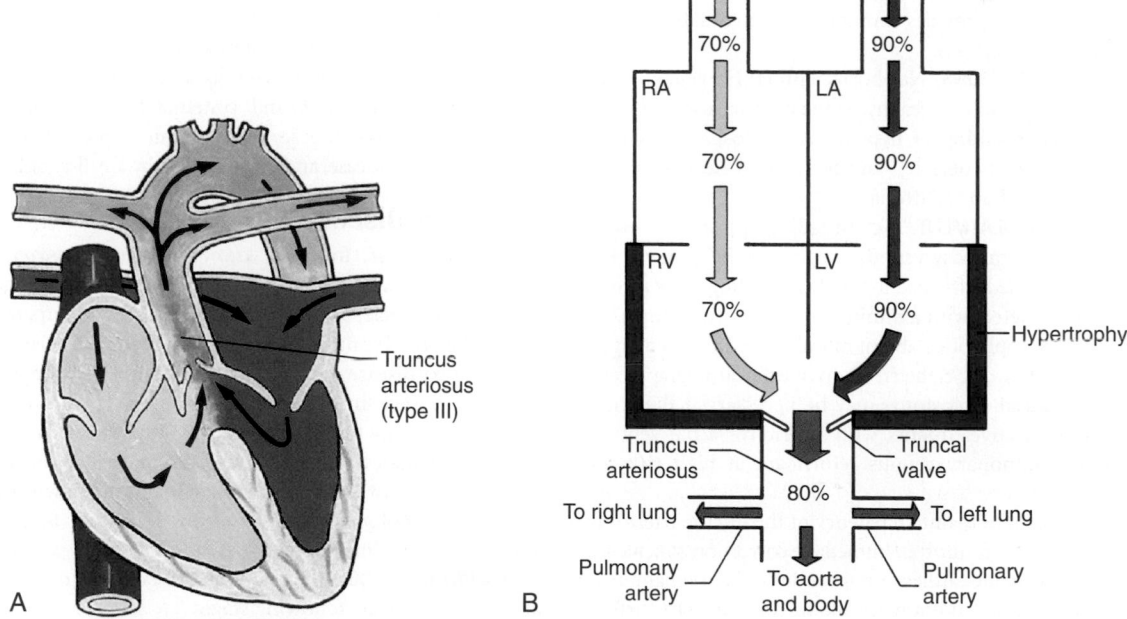

FIGURE 34.18 Truncus Arteriosus. A, Persistent truncus arteriosus. The truncus arteriosus fails to divide into the pulmonary artery and aorta, and the interventricular septum fails to close at the top. Blood from both ventricles mixes in the truncus arteriosus and then enters the pulmonary and systemic circuits. **B,** Alterations of hemodynamics and oxygen saturation by persistent truncus arteriosus. *LA,* Left atrium; *LV,* left ventricle; *RA,* right atrium; *RV,* right ventricle. (**A** from Hockenberry MJ, Wilson D: *Wong's essentials of pediatric nursing,* ed 10, St Louis, 2015, Mosby.)

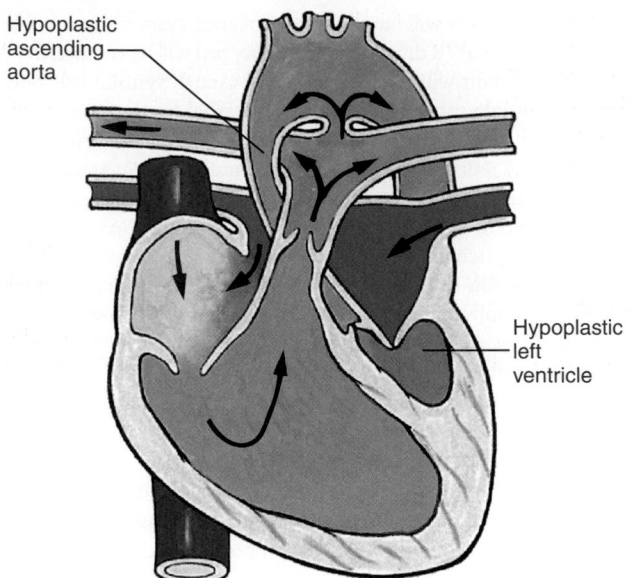

Hypoplastic ascending aorta

Hypoplastic left ventricle

FIGURE 34.19 Hypoplastic Left Heart Syndrome. (From Hockenberry MJ, Wilson D: *Wong's essentials of pediatric nursing,* ed 10, St Louis, 2015, Mosby.)

(Fig. 34.19). Therefore infants with HLHS must have a well-functioning RV and the presence of a PDA and atrial septal communication for survival. HLHS accounts for 5% of all congenital heart defects and is considered the most complex congenital defect.[7]

◆**PATHOPHYSIOLOGY.** Because of the high pressures caused by LV outflow tract obstruction, saturated blood enters the LA and mixes with desaturated blood in the RA through an atrial septal communication. Blood flow follows the normal pathways through the right side of the heart. Exiting the PA, the mixed-saturation blood flows through the ductus and to the descending aorta. The amount of blood flow that travels to the pulmonary and systemic circulations depends on vascular resistance in the respective systems. Retrograde blood flow through the hypoplastic ascending aorta provides coronary and cerebral blood flow if there is complete aortic atresia.

◆**CLINICAL MANIFESTATIONS.** Newborns with HLHS generally are born full-term and initially appear healthy. As the ductus closes, systemic perfusion is decreased resulting in hypoxemia, acidosis, and shock. Usually no heart murmur is detected and the second heart sound is loud and single because of aortic atresia.

◆**EVALUATION AND TREATMENT.** A chest radiograph shows cardiomegaly and increased pulmonary venous congestion. ECG shows RV hypertrophy and diminished left-sided forces. Echocardiography reveals the components of the defect with a diminutive LV cavity, hypoplastic aortic valve and arch, hypoplastic or absent mitral valve, and an enlarged RV cavity. Interventional cardiac catheterization or echocardiographically guided with balloon atrial septostomy may be necessary if the atrial communication is restrictive. Infants with restrictive atrial septum causing obstructive pulmonary venous return are at high risk for interventions.[7]

Prostaglandin infusion to maintain patency of the ductus arteriosus is essential for newborn infant survival. Immediate correction of acidosis, inotropic support for adequate cardiac output, and ventilatory manipulation to balance systemic and pulmonary blood flow prevent further deterioration and achieve stabilization.

Surgical intervention includes a three-stage approach that classically begins with the Norwood procedure. The Norwood procedure consists of an atrial septectomy, placement of a pulmonary-to-systemic artery shunt to maintain adequate pulmonary blood flow, creation of a permanent communication between the RV and aorta, and patch augmentation of the hypoplastic aorta. The Sano modification of the Norwood procedure uses a tube graft between the RV and PA to provide stable pulmonary blood flow rather than a pulmonary-to-systemic arterial shunt.[16] Postoperative complications include imbalance of systemic and pulmonary blood flow leading to inadequate cardiac output and persistent HF. Although the procedure is considered to be high risk, survival in most centers is now averaging greater than 80%.

Another option for high-risk infants with HLHS (those with significant comorbidities or prematurity) is the Hybrid Stage I palliation. This procedure involves placement of bilateral pulmonary artery bands to regulate PBF, stenting the ductus arteriosus to provide stable systemic blood flow, and a balloon atrial septostomy to allow unobstructed pulmonary venous return. This procedure can be done without the use of cardiopulmonary bypass and systemic heparinization. However, the second-stage bidirectional Glenn procedure will require the addition of an aortic arch augmentation as described in the original Norwood procedure.

The second stage is the bidirectional Glenn procedure, and the third stage is the modified Fontan procedure, which were described previously in the section Tricuspid Atresia. Long-term health problems following the Fontan procedure are related to reduced ventricular function and high central venous pressures.[13]

Few centers perform cardiac transplant as a primary treatment for HLHS because of the scarcity of neonatal donors. Disadvantages of neonatal transplantation include risk of rejection, long-term problems with chronic immunosuppression, and infection. Infants who are not candidates for staged procedures or transplantations are offered palliative care. Infants with HLHS have improved survival rates because of advances in surgical and medical technology. However, many infants and children with complex CHD have long-term neurodevelopmental disabilities.[7,17]

ACQUIRED CARDIOVASCULAR DISORDERS

Acquired heart diseases are those disease processes or abnormalities that occur after birth. They result from various causes, such as infection, genetic disorders, autoimmune processes in response to infection, environmental factors, or autoimmune diseases. Examples of acquired heart diseases include Kawasaki disease, myocarditis, rheumatic heart disease, cardiomyopathy, and systemic hypertension. This chapter discusses Kawasaki disease and systemic hypertension. Myocarditis, rheumatic heart disease, and cardiomyopathy are discussed in Chapter 33.

Kawasaki Disease

Kawasaki disease, formerly known as *mucocutaneous lymph node syndrome,* is an acute, self-limiting systemic vasculitis that may result in cardiac sequelae. Although Kawasaki disease occurs throughout the world, the greatest number of cases are reported in Japan.

Kawasaki disease is primarily a condition of young children: 80% of cases are seen in children younger than 5 years of age, with the incidence peaking in the toddler age group. Males are affected slightly more than females. Its peak incidence is in winter and spring.[18]

The etiology of Kawasaki disease remains unknown. Theories center on an immunologic response to an infectious, toxic, or antigenic substance (including superantigens).[2,7,18]

◆**PATHOPHYSIOLOGY.** Kawasaki disease progresses pathologically and clinically in the following stages:

Stage I (days 1 to 12): Small capillaries, arterioles, and venules become inflamed, as does the heart itself.
Stage II (days 13 to 25): Inflammation spreads to larger vessels, and aneurysms of the coronary arteries develop.

Stage III (days 26 to 40): Medium-size arteries begin the granulation process, causing coronary artery thickening; inflammation resolves in the microcirculation; and there is risk of thrombus formation.
Stage IV (day 41 and beyond): Vessels develop scarring, intimal thickening, calcification, and stenosis of coronary arteries.

◆CLINICAL MANIFESTATIONS. The clinical course of the disease progresses in three stages: acute, subacute, and convalescent. In the acute phase the child has fever, conjunctivitis, oral changes ("strawberry" tongue), rash, and lymphadenopathy and is often irritable. During this phase myocarditis in addition to the vasculitis may develop. The subacute phase begins when the fever ends and continues until the clinical signs have resolved. It is at this time that the child is most at risk for coronary artery aneurysm development. Desquamation of the palms and soles occurs at this time, as well as marked thrombocytosis. The convalescent phase is marked by the continued elevation of the erythrocyte sedimentation rate and platelet count. Arthritis still may be present. This phase continues until all laboratory values return to normal—usually about 6 to 8 weeks after onset.

◆EVALUATION AND TREATMENT. The diagnosis is based on the diagnostic criteria for Kawasaki disease, which state that the child must exhibit five of six criteria, including fever (Box 34.3). These children usually have leukocytosis, increased erythrocyte sedimentation rates, marked thrombocytosis, and elevated levels of liver enzymes. An echocardiogram is obtained at the time of diagnosis as a baseline to assess for coronary aneurysms or inflammation. Serial echocardiograms are obtained after treatment to assess for future development of coronary aneurysms.

The use of aspirin and intravenous immunoglobulin during the acute phase has decreased the mortality of Kawasaki disease and has reduced the incidence of coronary abnormalities from approximately 25% to 5% at 6 to 8 weeks after initiation of therapy. Most children recover completely from Kawasaki disease, including the regression of aneurysms. The most common, although rare, cardiovascular sequela is coronary artery aneurysms and resulting thrombosis or myocardial infarction. On average, studies have shown 30-year survival rates up to 90%; however, some children with giant aneurysms may require coronary artery bypass grafting (CABG).[18]

Systemic Hypertension

Hypertension (HTN) in children differs from adult HTN in etiology and presentation. Children diagnosed with HTN are often found to have some underlying disease, such as renal disease or COA (Box 34.4). In recent years an increased prevalence of primary HTN in older children has been noted. Research has shown that primary HTN in older children,

---

BOX 34.3   DIAGNOSTIC CRITERIA FOR KAWASAKI DISEASE

The child must exhibit five of the following six criteria, including fever:
1. Fever for 5 or more days (often diagnosed with shorter duration of fever if other symptoms are present)
2. Bilateral conjunctival infection without exudation
3. Changes in the oral mucous membranes, such as erythema, dryness, and fissuring of the lips; oropharyngeal reddening; or "strawberry tongue"
4. Changes in the extremities, such as peripheral edema, peripheral erythema, and desquamation of palms and soles, particularly periungual peeling
5. Polymorphous rash, often accentuated in the perineal area
6. Cervical lymphadenopathy (one lymph node >1.5 cm)

Modified from Hockenberry MJ, Wilson D: *Wong's nursing care of infants and children,* ed 10, St Louis, 2015, Mosby.

BOX 34.4   CONDITIONS ASSOCIATED WITH SECONDARY HYPERTENSION IN CHILDREN

Renal Disorders
Congenital defects
    Polycystic kidney, ectopic kidney, horseshoe kidney, etc.
    Obstructive anomalies
    Hydronephrosis
Renal tumor
    Wilms tumor
    Retrovascular tumor
Abnormalities of renal arteries
Renal vein thrombosis
Acquired disorders
    Glomerulonephritis—acute or chronic
    Pyelonephritis
    Nephritis associated with collagen disease

Cardiovascular Disease
Coarctation of the aorta
Arteriovenous fistulae
Patent ductus arteriosus
Aortic or mitral insufficiency

Metabolic and Endocrine Diseases
Adrenal tumors
    Adenoma
    Pheochromocytoma

Neuroblastoma
Cushing syndrome
Adrenogenital syndrome
Hyperthyroidism
Aldosteronism
Hypercalcemia
Diabetes mellitus

Neurologic Disorders
Space-occupying lesions of cranium (increased intracranial pressure)
    Tumors, cysts, hematoma
    Cerebral edema
    Encephalitis (including Guillain-Barré and Reye syndromes)

Miscellaneous Causes
Drugs (corticosteroids, oral contraceptives, pressor agents, amphetamines)
Burns
Genitourinary surgery
Trauma (e.g., stretching of femoral nerve with leg traction)
Insect bites (e.g., scorpion)
Intravascular overload (blood, fluid)
Hypernatremia
Toxemia of pregnancy
Heavy metal poisoning

From Hockenberry MJ, Wilson D: *Wong's essentials of pediatric nursing,* ed 10, St Louis, 2015, Mosby.

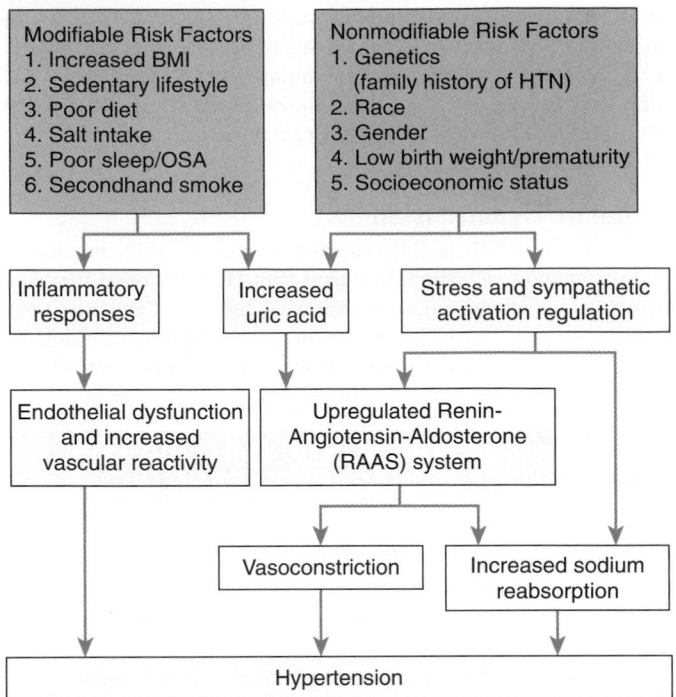

FIGURE 34.20 Mechanisms Believed to Influence Blood Pressure in Children. According to this model, a critical factor in the development of hypertension is obesity during childhood. Increased body mass, coupled with excessive sodium intake, can cause primary hypertension in children or set the stage for its development later in life. *BMI*, Body mass index; *HTN*, hypertension; *OSA*, obstructive sleep apnea.

TABLE 34.6 SUGGESTED NORMAL BP VALUES (mmHg) BY AUSCULTATORY METHOD (SYSTOLIC/DIASTOLIC K5)

AGE (YEARS)	MEAN BP LEVELS	90th PERCENTILE	95th PERCENTILE
6–7	104/55	114/73	117/78
8–9	106/58	117/76	120/82
10–11*	108/60	120/77	124/82
12–13*	112/62	124/78	128/83
14–15			
Boys	116/66	132/80	138/86
Girls	112/68	126/80	130/83
16–18			
Boys	121/70	136/82	140/86
Girls	110/68	125/81	127/84

*Values for ages 10 to 13 years have been extrapolated from these two studies using age-related increments from other studies.
BP, Blood pressure; *K5*, phase V of Korotkoff sound.
From Park MK: *Pediatric cardiology for practitioners*, ed 6, Philadelphia, 2014, Mosby; modified from Goldring D, et al: *J Pediatr* 91:884, 1977; Prineas RJ, et al: *Hypertension* 1(Suppl):18, 1980.

TABLE 34.7 NORMATIVE BP LEVELS (SYSTOLIC/DIASTOLIC [MEAN]) BY DINAMAP/MONITOR IN CHILDREN 5 YEARS OLD AND YOUNGER

AGE	MEAN BP LEVELS (mmHg)	90th PERCENTILE	95th PERCENTILE
1–3 days	64/41 (50)	75/49 (50)	78/52 (62)
1 month–2 years	95/58 (72)	106/68 (83)	110/71 (86)
2–5 years	101/57 (74)	112/66 (82)	115/68 (85)

BP, Blood pressure.
From Park MK: *Pediatric cardiology for practitioners*, ed 6, Philadelphia, 2014, Mosby; modified from Park MK, Menard SM: *Am J Dis Child* 143:860, 1989.

as well as other risk factors such as obesity, diabetes, and dyslipidemia, is related to the development of early atherosclerotic disease.[19]

Systemic hypertension in children is defined as systolic and diastolic blood pressure levels greater than the 95th percentile for age and sex on at least three occasions. The Fourth Task Force on Blood Pressure Control in Children uses height as an additional criterion to the blood pressure guide.[20,20a]

◆PATHOPHYSIOLOGY. Hypertension is classified as (1) primary (or essential) hypertension, in which a specific cause cannot be identified; or (2) secondary hypertension, in which a cause is secondary to another alteration such as renal disease or COA (see Box 34.4). In infants and children, the most common type of HTN is secondary HTN; this requires a thorough history and physical examination to identify the cause.[19] Primary HTN is more common in males than females, and among Hispanic and black children.[5]

The pathophysiology of primary HTN in children is not clearly understood but may result from complex interactions between modifiable risk factors, such as obesity and sedentary lifestyle, and nonmodifiable risk factors, such as genetics, race, and socioeconomic factors. These risk factors may result in inflammatory processes, activation of the sympathetic nervous system which leads to upregulation of the renin-angiotensin-aldosterone (RAAS) system, increased sodium reabsorption, and increased vascular reactivity with the end result leading to hypertension[21] (Fig. 34.20). New studies have shown an increased level of leptin, a hormone produced by adipose tissue, to be associated with HTN in obese children.[22]

◆CLINICAL MANIFESTATIONS. Most children with systemic HTN are asymptomatic. It is necessary that a thorough history (including family history of HTN and heart disease) and physical examination be obtained. The examination should include an accurate blood pressure measurement obtained on the right arm with the arm supported at the level of the heart; three separate measurements should be taken using a cuff of appropriate size (Tables 34.6 and 34.7).

Many factors influence blood pressure in children, including smoking, obesity, and sedentary lifestyles. However, obesity is one of the most important factors in the increasing prevalence of HTN in children.

◆EVALUATION AND TREATMENT. In children the history and physical examination should be directed at determining the etiology of HTN (Table 34.8). Blood pressure difference between upper and lower extremities and echocardiogram are performed to identify COA. If COA is found, surgical correction or balloon angioplasty with or without stent implantation is performed, depending on the child's age and severity of the coarctation. A complete blood count, serum chemistry levels, urinalysis, urine culture, lipid profile, and renal ultrasound are part of the routine evaluation for renal disease (Table 34.9).

Although the criteria for the diagnosis of hypertension are based on the use of a standard blood pressure cuff, some children have what is termed "white coat hypertension." Elevated blood pressure readings in these children occur only when measured in the clinic and may be

TABLE 34.8 MOST COMMON CAUSES OF CHRONIC SUSTAINED HYPERTENSION

AGE GROUP	CAUSES
Newborn	Renal artery thrombosis, renal artery stenosis, congenital renal malformation, COA, bronchopulmonary dysplasia
<6 years	Renal parenchymal disease, COA, renal artery stenosis
6–10 years	Renal artery stenosis, renal parenchymal disease, primary hypertension
>10 years	Primary hypertension, renal parenchymal disease

COA, Coarctation of the aorta.
From Park MK: *Pediatric cardiology for practitioners*, ed 6, Philadelphia, 2014, Mosby; adapted from Report of the Second Task Force on Blood Pressure Control in Children: *Pediatrics* 79:1, 1987.

WHAT'S NEW?

Ambulatory Blood Pressure Monitoring in Children

Ambulatory blood pressure monitoring (ABPM) records blood pressure over a 24-hour period. Its use in children was endorsed by the Fourth Report of the National High Blood Pressure Education Program Working Group on High Blood Pressure in Children primarily to help identify those children with "white coat hypertension." Paradoxically, some children have normal blood pressure readings in the clinic but are hypertensive during other parts of the day. This is called *masked hypertension* and also can be identified by ABPM. ABPM is useful in documenting what is called the *BP load*, which is the total amount of time the blood pressure (BP) is elevated above normal limits during a 24-hour period. By measuring BP load, ABPM may be able to identify those children who are at greatest risk for target organ damage. It can also help with management of children who suffer hypotensive episodes in response to pharmacologic therapy for their hypertension. Finally, ABPM facilitates medication changes in those with hypertension resistant to medication.

Data from Flynn JT et al: *Hypertension* 63(5):1116-1135, 2014.

caused by fear and anxiety. The use of ambulatory blood pressure monitoring (ABPM) records the blood pressure over a 24-hour period. In addition to identifying children with white coat hypertension, ABPM has been found to be useful in children with hypertension that is resistant to treatment (see Box 34.4 and *What's New?* Ambulatory Blood Pressure Monitoring in Children).[23,24]

If HTN is found to be essential, or primary, in nature, nonpharmacologic, lifestyle-based therapy is used initially. Moderate weight loss can decrease systolic and diastolic pressures in many children. Appropriate diet, regular physical activity, and avoidance of smoking have been shown to be effective in reducing blood pressure.[19]

Pharmacologic therapy is controversial in children with primary hypertension; however, when nonpharmacologic therapy fails, a staged approach with the use of ACE inhibitors, angiotensin receptor blockers (ARB), and calcium channel blockers is indicated. Effective treatment of HTN in children may reduce the incidence of long-term sequelae, such as left ventricular hypertrophy, renal failure, and cerebrovascular accident (CVA or stroke). The emphasis on preventive cardiology, especially for children, is significant because many investigators believe signs of atherosclerosis and other cardiovascular risk factors are present from childhood.[19]

TABLE 34.9 ROUTINE AND SPECIAL LABORATORY TESTS FOR HYPERTENSION

LABORATORY TEST	SIGNIFICANCE OF ABNORMAL RESULTS
Urinalysis, urine culture, blood urea nitrogen, creatinine, uric acid	Renal parenchymal disease
Serum electrolyte levels (hypokalemia)	Hyperaldosteronism (primary or secondary); Adrenogenital syndrome; Renin-producing tumors
ECG, chest x-ray studies, and possibly echocardiography	Cardiac cause of hypertension, also baseline function
Intravenous pyelogram (or ultrasonography, radionuclide studies, computed tomography, or magnetic resonance imaging of the kidneys)	Renal parenchymal disease; Renovascular hypertension; Tumors (neuroblastoma, Wilms tumor)
Plasma renin activity (peripheral)	High-renin hypertension (renovascular hypertension, renin-producing tumors, some Cushing syndrome, some essential hypertension); Low-renin hypertension (adrenogenital syndrome, primary hyperaldosteronism)
24-hour urine collection for 17-ketosteroids and 17-hydroxycorticosteroids	Cushing syndrome; Adrenogenital syndrome
24-hour urine collection for catecholamine levels and vanillylmandelic acid	Pheochromocytoma; Neuroblastoma
Aldosterone	Hyperaldosteronism (primary or secondary); Renovascular hypertension; Renin-producing tumors
Renal vein plasma renin activity	Unilateral renal parenchymal disease; Renovascular hypertension
Abdominal aortogram	Renovascular hypertension; Abdominal coarctation of the aorta; Unilateral renal parenchymal diseases; Pheochromocytoma
Intraarterial digital subtraction angiography	Renovascular hypertension

ECG, Electrocardiogram.
From Park MK: *Pediatric cardiology for practitioners*, ed 6, Philadelphia, 2014, Mosby.

Childhood Obesity

Childhood obesity is considered an epidemic not only in the United States but also in other countries.[25,26] The prevalence of obesity in children and young adults has remained fairly steady in the past two decades, with approximately 31.8% of children aged 2 to 19 years being overweight or obese, and 16.9% being obese.[25] Attention from U.S. federal and state initiatives has kept childhood obesity in the spotlight and, although obesity rates have not increased, obesity continues to be an important contributor to lifelong health problems. Percentile of body mass index (BMI) expressed as weight/height[2] (BMI-kg/m[2]) is used to identify overweight and obesity in children and adolescents. The Centers for Disease Control and Prevention (CDC), the supplier of national growth charts and prevalence data, classifies *overweight* as BMI from the 85th percentile to less than the 95th percentile for age, and *obese* as BMI at 95th percentile or greater for age.[27]

Causes of obesity in young children and adolescents are multivariable and multidimensional. Risk factors associated with developing childhood obesity include race, socioeconomic status, and lack of health insurance. Children of black and Hispanic race are at higher risk, as well as children with no insurance.[25,28] The presence of parental obesity also is associated with childhood obesity.[26] In addition, early childhood nutrition, level of physical activity, sleep disturbances, and engagement in sedentary activities, such as watching television and computer use, are associated with the development of overweight and obese children.[25,26,29,30]

Similar to obese adults, overweight and obese children are at risk for acquiring numerous other serious and potentially life-threatening illnesses, such as asthma, sleep apnea, HTN, type 2 diabetes, dyslipidemia, and cardiovascular disease.[7,28,31] Researchers also have reported a multitude of social and economic consequences in adolescents as a result of being overweight. Obese children have been reported to have increased anxiety and depression, as well as decreased self-esteem and quality of life and poorer school performance, and they are more likely to be the target of bullying compared to nonobese children.[28,31]

As in other acquired diseases, efforts should be focused on prevention (see *What's New? Guidelines on Reducing Cardiovascular Disease in Children*). The initial approach is a combined program of physical activity with nutritional improvements. Healthcare professionals play a vital role in recognizing the need for intervention, immediate referral, and support. Successful outcomes for most overweight and obese children require support, change in lifestyle at home, and involvement of family members. Researchers are involving school-based programs in preventing obesity in the young.[26,32,33]

WHAT'S NEW?

Guidelines on Reducing Cardiovascular Disease in Children

In 2011, the National Heart Lung and Blood Institute (NHLBI) released cardiovascular disease (CVD) guidelines for children and adolescents that are endorsed by the American Academy of Pediatrics (AAP) and American Heart Association (AHA) and are integrated into the *Bright Futures* guidelines on pediatric health maintenance. These universal lipid screening guidelines include (1) all children should undergo cholesterol screening once between ages 9 to 11 years and once between ages 17 to 21 years; (2) nonfasting total cholesterol and high-density lipoprotein (HDL) can be used for the initial lipid screening test; (3) clinicians may recommend low-fat or no-fat dairy at age 1 year for high-risk children; (4) for children who fail lifestyle changes and require lipid-lowering medications, pharmacologic treatment should be considered at age 10 years; and (5) once low-density lipoprotein (LDL) is optimized, high non-HDL cholesterol may be targeted for residual CVD risk reduction. However, the U.S. Preventive Services Task Force (USPSTF) evaluated the evidence to support such screening and issued a statement in 2016 that the current evidence is "insufficient" to assess the risk versus benefit of screening for lipid disorders in children and adolescents <20 years of age. The USPSTF statement has created controversy among leading experts in pediatric dyslipidemia. Although change in practice should be based on the highest level of evidence, randomized controlled trials (RCTs) are often lacking in the pediatric population. With the mounting evidence of early atherosclerosis development in children at high risk (obesity, hypertension, and type 2 diabetes) or with a genetic predisposition to dyslipidemia (e.g., familial hypercholesterolemia; more than 500,000 infants born each year), clinical decision making on whether to provide universal lipid screening to children and adolescents may need to be based on more than available evidence. All agree that future RCTs are needed to support universal lipid screening.

Data from U.S. Preventive Services Task Force (USPSTF): *JAMA* 316(6):625-633, 2016; Urbina EM, de Ferranti SD: *JAMA* 316(6):589-591, 2016; National Heart & Lung Institute Expert Panel: *Pediatrics* 128(5):S213-S256, 2011.

▪ SUMMARY REVIEW

Development of the Cardiovascular System

1. The heart arises from the mesenchyme and begins as an enlarged blood vessel with a large lumen and a muscular wall. By approximately the seventh week of gestation, all structures of the fetal heart and vascular system are present.

2. The endocardial cushions are instrumental in closing the atrial septum, dividing the AV canals into the right and left AV orifices, and closing the septum.

3. In the fetus the pulmonary and systemic circulatory systems are connected by the foramen ovale, an opening between the atria; by the ductus arteriosus, a fetal vessel that joins the PA to the aorta; and by the ductus venosus, a fetal vessel that connects the inferior vena cava to the umbilical vein.

4. Fetal circulation is different from postnatal circulation because of the presence of fetal shunts and altered metabolic needs of the various organs.

5. Fetal blood flow depends on resistance for its distribution through the body. Resistance in the pulmonary circulation is higher than resistance in the systemic circulation, so myocardial thickness is about the same in the right heart and the left heart.

6. After birth, SVR increases and PVR decreases.

7. PVR drops suddenly at birth because the lungs expand and the pulmonary vessels dilate. It continues to decrease gradually during the first 8 weeks after birth. Decreased PVR causes the right myocardium to become thinner.

8. SVR increases markedly at birth because severance of the umbilical cord removes the low-resistance placenta from the systemic circulation. Increased SVR causes the left myocardium to become dominant and thicken over time.

9. Changes in resistance cause disappearance of the fetal connections between the pulmonary and systemic circulatory systems. The foramen ovale closes functionally at birth and anatomically several months later; the ductus arteriosus closes functionally 15 hours after birth and anatomically within the first several weeks; and the ductus venosus closes within 1 week after birth.

10. At birth a series of circulatory changes occur that affect blood flow, vascular resistance, and oxygen tension. The most important change is the shift of gas exchange from the placenta to the lungs.

11. After birth, significant postnatal changes occur, including thinning of the right ventricular myocardium as the PVR drops. As the SVR increases, the left ventricular myocardium becomes thicker and more dominant as it is in the adult heart.

■ SUMMARY REVIEW—cont'd

Congenital Heart Defects

1. Most congenital cardiovascular defects have begun to develop by the fourth week of gestation, and most have many causes, both environmental and genetic.

2. Environmental risk factors associated with the incidence of CHD typically are maternal conditions. Among these are viral infections, diabetes, drug intake, alcohol intake, metabolic disorders, and advanced maternal age.

3. Genetic factors associated with CHD include, but are not limited to, trisomy 21 or Down syndrome, trisomy 13, trisomy 18, cri du chat syndrome, and Turner syndrome. It now appears, however, that most genetic mechanisms of causation are multifactorial.

4. Classification of CHDs is based on whether they (a) cause blood flow to the lungs to increase or decrease, (b) obstruct ventricular blood flow patterns, or (c) cause mixing of unoxygenated and oxygenated blood.

5. Symptoms of HF are usually the result of CHDs that increase blood volume and pressure in the pulmonary circulation, or myocardial failure. Clinical manifestations are almost the same as the manifestations of HF in adults, with the addition of FTT in children.

6. Cyanosis, a bluish discoloration of the skin, indicates that the tissues are not receiving fully adequate oxygenated blood. Cyanosis can be caused by defects that (a) reduce pulmonary blood flow; (b) overload the pulmonary circulation, causing pulmonary hypertension, pulmonary edema, and respiratory difficulty; and (c) cause large amounts of unoxygenated blood to shunt from the pulmonary to the systemic circulation.

7. Congenital heart defects that maintain or create direct communication between the pulmonary and systemic circulatory systems cause blood to shunt from one system to another, mixing oxygenated and unoxygenated blood and increasing blood volume and pressure on the receiving side of the shunt.

8. The direction of shunting through an abnormal communication depends on differences in pressure and resistance between the two systems. Flow is always from an area of high pressure to an area of low pressure. The resistance to flow determines the volume of the shunting.

9. Acyanotic CHDs that increase pulmonary blood flow consist of abnormal openings (PDA, ASD, VSD, AVC defect, or truncus arteriosus) that permit blood to shunt from left (systemic circulation) to right (pulmonary circulation). Cyanosis does not occur because the left-to-right shunt does not interfere with the flow of oxygenated blood through the systemic circulation.

10. If the abnormal communication between the left and right circuits is large, volume and pressure overload in the pulmonary circulation leads to HF.

11. In truncus arteriosus the main trunk fails to divide longitudinally into the aorta and PA. All blood from both ventricles enters the truncus, so that mixed blood is delivered by both circulatory systems, causing varying degrees of cyanosis and HF.

12. In CHDs that decrease pulmonary blood flow (TOF, tricuspid atresia), myocardial hypertrophy cannot compensate for restricted right ventricular outflow. Flow to the lungs decreases, and cyanosis is caused by mixing of systemic and pulmonary venous return.

13. Obstruction of ventricular outflow commonly is caused by PS, AS, COA, or interrupted aortic arch.

14. Despite obstruction, ventricular output remains normal for a long time because of compensatory ventricular hypertrophy stimulated by increased afterload and, in postductal COA, development of collateral circulation around the coarctation.

15. Complex CHDs that depend on mixing of the pulmonary and systemic circulations for survival during the postnatal period include TGA, HLHS, and TAPVC. This mixing results in desaturated systemic blood flow and cyanosis.

16. In TGA the circulatory systems are not connected serially or through a shunt, so that oxygenated blood remains permanently in the pulmonary circulation and unoxygenated blood remains in the systemic circulation. Survival depends on patency of the ductus arteriosus; in the absence of patency, surgical intervention is mandatory.

17. TAPVC is caused by abnormal pulmonary vein development and the lack of direct pulmonary venous return to the LA. All blood from the pulmonary and systemic circulations enters the RA. Mixed blood enters the LA through an ASD; it then flows into the systemic circulation and causes cyanosis.

18. Tricuspid atresia [left] and HLHS [right] are types of single-ventricle defects that commonly require three staged palliative surgical procedures.

19. Treatment for all hemodynamically severe CHDs is surgical or interventional palliation of the anomaly and management of cyanosis and HF.

Acquired Cardiovascular Disorders

1. The most common acquired cardiovascular disorders of childhood are Kawasaki disease, rheumatic heart disease (see Chapter 33), obesity, and HTN.

2. Kawasaki disease is an acute systemic vasculitis that may result in the development of coronary artery aneurysms and thrombosis.

3. Essential or primary HTN in children is the same as that in adults, except that it is more likely to be diagnosed at a younger age and most are at an asymptomatic stage. Most cases of secondary HTN in young children are because of an underlying cause, such as renal disease or COA.

4. Obesity in childhood is epidemic in the United States and other countries, but more recent data shows that obesity prevalence is not increasing.

5. Obese children are at risk for acquiring numerous other serious and potentially life-threatening illnesses, such as asthma, sleep apnea, HTN, type 2 diabetes mellitus, dyslipidemia, and cardiovascular disease.

■ KEY TERMS

Aortic stenosis (AS), 1131
Atrial septal defect (ASD), 1124
Atrial septation, 1116
Atrioventricular canal (AVC) defect, 1126
Bulbus cordis, 1116
Coarctation of the aorta (COA), 1129

Complete AVC (CAVC) defect, 1127
Conus, 1133
Cyanosis, 1122
Ductus arteriosus, 1118
Ductus venosus, 1117
Eisenmenger syndrome, 1122

Endocardial cushion, 1115
Foramen ovale, 1117
Heart failure (HF), 1120
Hypoplastic left heart syndrome (HLHS), 1135
Kawasaki disease, 1136
Ligamentum venosum, 1118

KEY TERMS—cont'd

Ostium primum, 1116
Ostium secundum, 1116
Partial AVC (PAVC) defect, 1127
Patent ductus arteriosus (PDA), 1123
Pulmonary atresia, 1132
Pulmonary stenosis (PS), 1132

Septum primum, 1116
Septum secundum, 1116
Systemic hypertension, 1138
Tetralogy of Fallot (TOF), 1127
Total anomalous pulmonary venous connection (TAPVC), 1134

Transitional AVC (TAVC) defect, 1127
Transposition of the great arteries (TGA), 1133
Tricuspid atresia, 1128
Truncus arteriosus, 1135
Ventricular septal defect (VSD), 1125
Ventricular septation, 1116

REFERENCES

1. Nakanishi T, et al, editors: *Etiology and morphogenesis of congenital heart disease: from gene function and cellular interaction to morphology*, Tokyo, 2016, Springer.
2. Park MK: *Pediatric cardiology for practitioners*, ed 6, St Louis, 2014, Mosby.
3. American Heart Association (AHA): Heart disease and stroke statistics, 2016 update. *Circulation* 133(4):e38–e360, 2016.
4. Wilson D, Hockenberry MJ: *Wong's clinical manual of pediatric nursing*, ed 10, St Louis, 2015, Mosby.
5. Hazinski MF: *Manual of pediatric critical care*, ed 3, St Louis, 2013, Mosby.
6. Stout KK, et al: Chronic heart failure in congenital heart disease: a scientific statement from the American Heart Association. *Circulation* 133: 770–801, 2016.
7. Allen HD: *Moss and Adam's heart disease in infants, children, and adolescents: including the fetus and young adult*, ed 9, Philadelphia, 2016, Wolters Kluwer Health/Lippincott Williams & Wilkins.
8. Benitz WE, et al: Patent ductus arteriosus in preterm infants. *Pediatrics* 137(1):e20153730, 2016.
9. Feltes TF, et al: Indications for cardiac catheterization and intervention in pediatric heart disease: a scientific statement from American Heart Association. *Circulation* 123(22):2607–2625, 2011.
10. Stankowski T, et al: Is thoracoscopic patent ductus arteriosus superior to conventional surgery? *Interact Cardiovasc Thorac Surg* 21(4):532–538, 2015.
11. St. Louis JD, et al: Contemporary outcomes of complete atrioventricular septal defect repair: analysis of the Society of Thoracic Surgeons congenital heart surgery database. *J Thorac Cardiovasc Surg* 148(6):2526–2531, 2014.
12. Mavroudis C, Backer CL, editors: *Pediatric cardiac surgery*, ed 4, St Louis, 2013, Wiley-Blackwell.
13. Pike NA, et al: Reduced pleural drainage, length of stay, and readmissions using a modified Fontan management protocol. *J Thorac Cardiovasc Surg* 150(3):481–487, 2015.
14. Forbes TJ, et al: Comparison of surgery, stent, or balloon angioplasty of native coarctation of the aorta: an observational study by the CCICS (Congenital Cardiovascular Interventional Study Consortium). *J Am Coll Cardiol* 58(25):2664–2674, 2011.
15. Nelson JS, et al: Long-term survival and reintervention after the Ross procedure across the pediatric age spectrum. *Ann Thorac Surg* 99:2086–2095, 2015.
16. Feinstein JA, et al: Hypoplastic left heart syndrome current considerations and expectations. *J Am Coll Cardiol* 59(Suppl 1):S1–S42, 2012.
17. Newburger JW, et al: Early developmental outcome in children with hypoplastic left heart syndrome and related anomalies: the single ventricle reconstruction trial. *Circulation* 125(17):2081–2091, 2012.
18. Newburger JW, Takahashi M, Burns JC: Kawasaki disease. *J Am Coll Cardiol* 67(14):1738–1749, 2016.
19. Rao G: Diagnosis, epidemiology, and management of hypertension in children. *Pediatrics* 138(2): e20153616, 2016.
20. National High Blood Pressure Education Program Working Group on High Blood Pressure in Children: The fourth report on the diagnosis, evaluation, and treatment of high blood pressure in children and adolescents. *Pediatrics* 114:555–576, 2004.
20a. Flynn JT, Kaelber DC, Baker-Smith CM, et al: Clinical practice guideline for screening and management of high blood pressure in children and adolescents. *Pediatrics* 140(3):e20171904, 2017.
21. Bucher BS, et al: Primary hypertension in childhood. *Curr Hypertens Rep* 15:444–452, 2013.
22. Becton LJ, Shatat IF, Flynn JT: Hypertension and obesity: epidemiology, mechanisms, and clinical approach. *Indian J Pediatr* 79(8):1056–1061, 2012.
23. Flynn JT, et al: Update: ambulatory blood pressure monitoring in children and adolescents: a scientific statement from the American Heart Association. *Hypertension* 63(5):1116–1135, 2014.
24. Lubrano R, et al: Impact of ambulatory blood pressure monitoring on the diagnosis of hypertension in children. *J Am Soc Hypertens* 9(10):780–785, 2015.
25. Ogden CL, et al: Prevalence of childhood and adult obesity in the United States, 2011-2012. *JAMA* 311(8):806–814, 2014.
26. Robertson W, Murphy M, Johnson R: Evidence base for the prevention and management of child obesity. *Paediatr Child Health* 26(5):212–218, 2015.
27. Centers for Disease Control and Prevention (CDC): *Defining childhood obesity*. Available at: https://www.cdc.gov/obesity/childhood/defining.html 2015.
28. Gurnani M, Birken C, Hamilton J: Childhood obesity: causes, consequences, and management. *Pediatr Clin North Am* 62(4):821–840, 2015.
29. Broussard JL, Van Cauter E: Disturbances of sleep and circadian rhythms: novel risk factors for obesity. *Curr Opin Endocrinol Diabetes Obes* 23(5): 353–359, 2016.
30. Li J, et al: Approaches to the prevention and management of childhood obesity: the role of social networks and the use of social media and related electronic technologies. *Circulation* 127(2):260–267, 2013.
31. Estrada E, et al: Children's Hospital Association consensus statements for comorbidities of childhood obesity. *Child Obes* 10(4):304–317, 2014.
32. Centers for Disease Control and Prevention (CDC): Guidelines for school health programs to promote lifelong healthy eating: Centers for Disease Control. *MMWR Recomm Rep* 45(RR-9):1–41, 2011.
33. Morano M, et al: A multicomponent, school-initiated, obesity intervention to promote healthy lifestyles in children. *Nutrition* 32: 1075–1080, 2016.

CHAPTER

35

Structure and Function of the Pulmonary System

Valentina L. Brashers

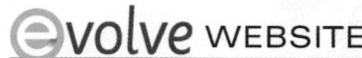

WEBSITE

CHAPTER OUTLINE

The primary function of the pulmonary system is the exchange of gases between the environmental air and the blood. There are three steps in this process: (1) ventilation, the movement of air into and out of the lungs; (2) diffusion, the movement of gases between air spaces in the lungs and the bloodstream; and (3) perfusion, the movement of blood into and out of the capillary beds of the lungs to body organs and tissues. The first two functions are carried out by the pulmonary system and the third by the cardiovascular system (see Chapter 32). Normally the pulmonary system functions efficiently under a variety of conditions and with little energy expenditure.

STRUCTURES OF THE PULMONARY SYSTEM

The pulmonary system includes two lungs and the upper and lower airways, and the blood vessels that serve them (Fig. 35.1); the chest wall, or thoracic cage; and the diaphragm. The lungs are divided into lobes: three in the right lung (upper, middle, lower) and two in the left lung (upper, lower). Each lobe is further divided into segments and lobules. The mediastinum is the space between the lungs and contains the heart, great vessels, and esophagus. A set of conducting airways, or bronchi, delivers air to each section of the lung. The lung tissue that surrounds the airways supports them, preventing their distortion or collapse as gas moves in and out during ventilation. The diaphragm is a dome-shaped muscle that separates the thoracic and abdominal cavities and is involved in ventilation.

The lungs are protected from a variety of exogenous contaminants by a series of mechanical and cellular defenses (Table 35.1). These defense mechanisms are so effective that in the healthy individual, contamination of the lung tissue itself, particularly by infectious agents, is rare.

Conducting Airways

The conducting airways provide a passage for the movement of air into and out of the gas-exchange structures of the lung. The nasopharynx, oropharynx, and related structures are called the *upper airway* (Fig. 35.2). These structures are lined with ciliated mucosa with a rich vascular supply that warms and humidifies inspired air and removes foreign

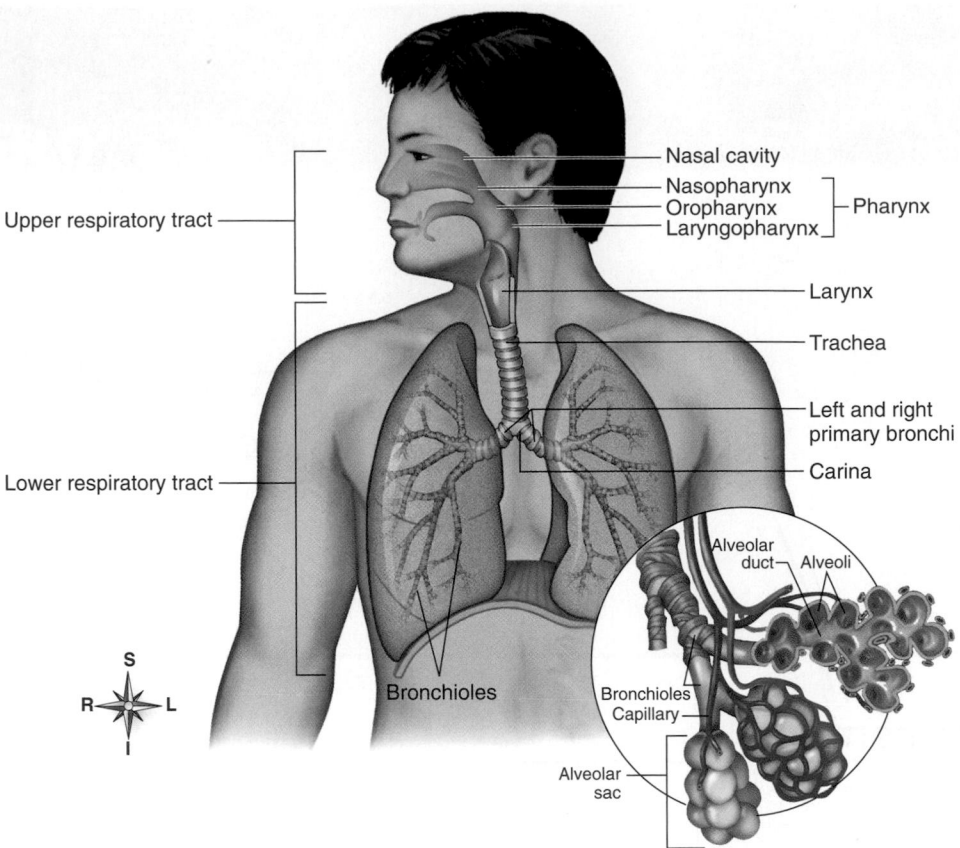

FIGURE 35.1 Structural Plan of the Respiratory System. The inset shows alveolar sacs where the interchange of oxygen and carbon dioxide takes place through the walls of the grapelike alveoli. Capillaries surround the alveoli. (From Patton KT, Thibodeau GA: *The human body in health & disease,* ed 7, St Louis, 2018, Mosby.)

TABLE 35.1   PULMONARY DEFENSE MECHANISMS

STRUCTURE OR SUBSTANCE	MECHANISM OF DEFENSE
Upper respiratory tract mucosa	Maintains constant temperature and humidification of gas entering the lungs; traps and removes foreign particles, some bacteria, and noxious gases from inspired air
Nasal hairs and turbinates	Trap and remove foreign particles, some bacteria, and noxious gases from inspired air
Branching airways	Disrupt laminar flow and enhance deposition of particles and pathogens on ciliated mucosa
Mucous blanket	Protects trachea and bronchi from injury; traps most foreign particles and bacteria that reach the lower airways
Innate immune proteins	Lysozyme, lactoferrin, defensins, collectins (surfactant protein A [SP-A] and surfactant protein D [SP-D]), and immunoglobulin A (IgA); recognize and promote killing of pathogens
Cilia	Propel mucous blanket and entrapped particles toward the oropharynx, where they can be swallowed or expectorated
Alveolar macrophages	Ingest and remove bacteria and other foreign material from alveoli by phagocytosis (see Chapter 7)
Surfactant	Enhances phagocytosis of pathogens and allergens in alveoli; down-regulates inflammatory responses
Irritant receptors in nares (nostrils)	Stimulation by chemical or mechanical irritants triggers sneeze reflex, which results in rapid removal of irritants from nasal passages
Irritant receptors in trachea and large airways	Stimulation by chemical or mechanical irritants triggers cough reflex, which results in removal of irritants from the trachea and large airways

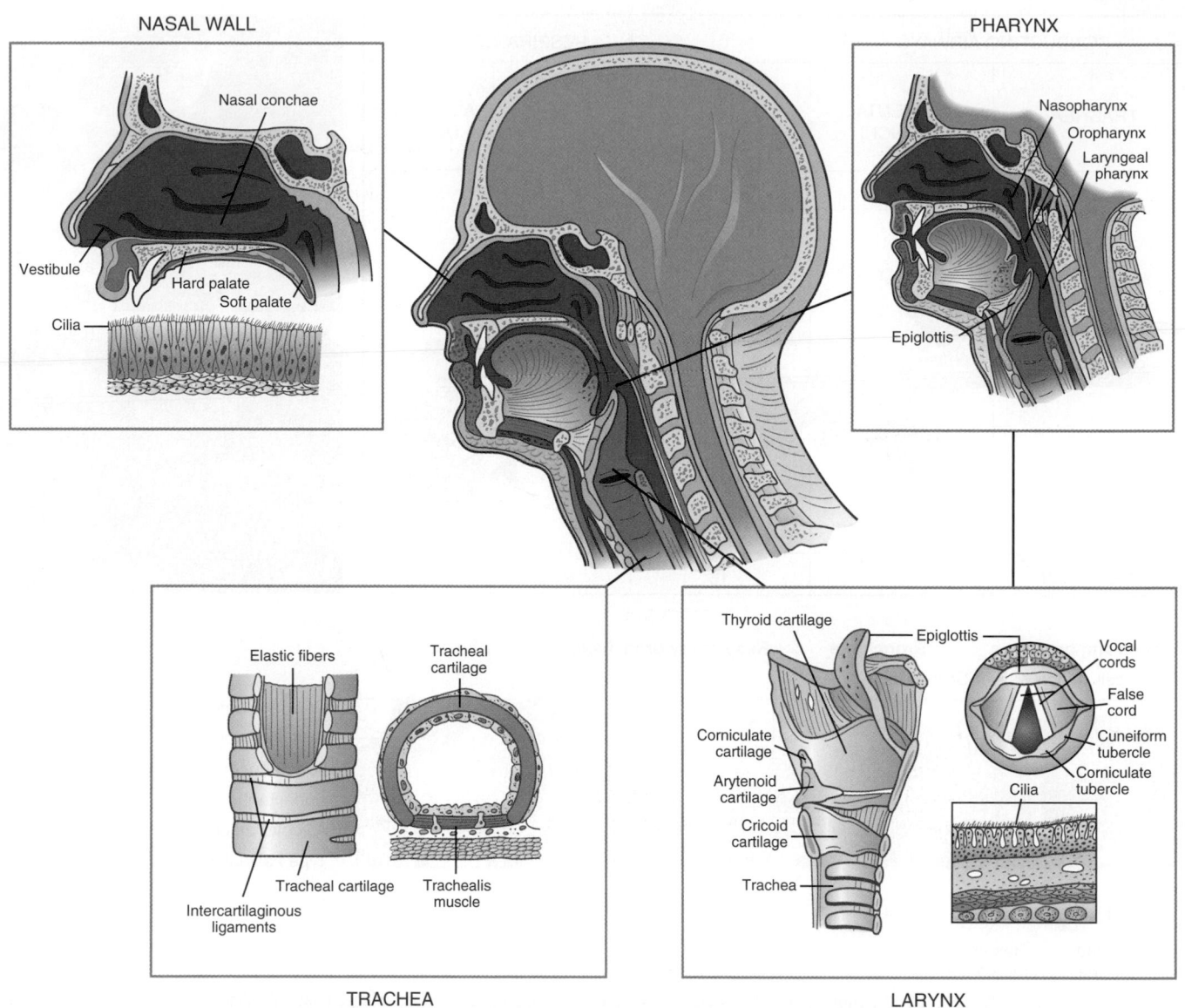

FIGURE 35.2 Structures of the Upper Airway. (Redrawn from Thompson JM et al: *Mosby's clinical nursing,* ed 5, St Louis, 2002, Mosby.)

particles from it as it passes into the lungs. The mouth and oropharynx provide for ventilation when the nose is obstructed or when increased flow is required, for example, during exercise. Filtering and humidifying are not as efficient with mouth breathing.

The larynx connects the upper and lower airways and consists of the endolarynx and its surrounding triangular-shaped bony and cartilaginous structures. The endolarynx is formed by two pairs of folds: the false vocal cords (supraglottis) and the true vocal cords. The slit-shaped space between the true cords forms the glottis (see Fig. 35.2). The vestibule is the space above the false vocal cords. The laryngeal box is formed by three large cartilages—the epiglottis, thyroid, and cricoid—and three smaller cartilages—the arytenoid, corniculate, and cuneiform—connected by ligaments. The supporting cartilages prevent collapse of the larynx during inspiration and swallowing. The internal laryngeal muscles control vocal cord length and tension, and the external laryngeal muscles move the larynx as a whole. Both sets of muscles are important to swallowing, respiration, and vocalization. The internal muscles contract

during swallowing to prevent aspiration into the trachea and contribute to voice pitch.[1]

The trachea, which is supported by U-shaped cartilage, connects the larynx to the bronchi, the conducting airways of the lungs. The trachea divides into the two main airways, or bronchi, at the carina (see Fig. 35.1). This area is very sensitive and when stimulated can cause coughing and airway narrowing. The left mainstem bronchus branches from the trachea at about a 45-degree angle. The right mainstem bronchus is slightly larger and more vertical than the left (branches at about a 20- to 30-degree angle from the trachea). Aspirated fluids or foreign particles thus tend to enter the right lung rather than the left. The right and left main bronchi enter the lungs at the hila, or "roots" of the lungs, along with the pulmonary blood and lymphatic vessels. From the hila the main bronchi branch into lobar bronchi and then to segmental and subsegmental bronchi, and finally end at the sixteenth division in the smallest of the conducting airways, the terminal bronchioles (Fig. 35.3). With these multiple divisions, the cross-sectional area of the airways

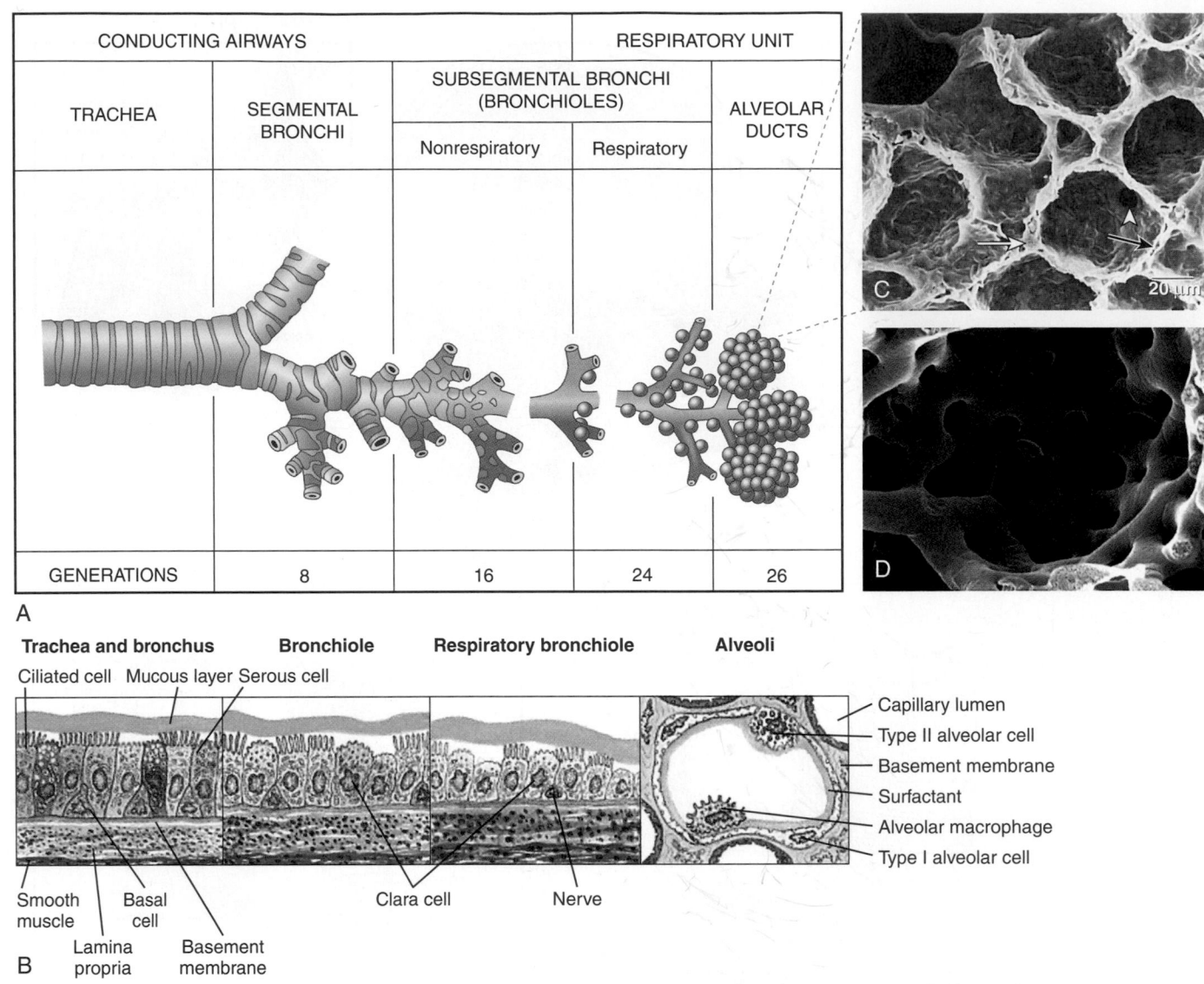

CONDUCTING AIRWAYS				RESPIRATORY UNIT
TRACHEA	SEGMENTAL BRONCHI	SUBSEGMENTAL BRONCHI (BRONCHIOLES)		ALVEOLAR DUCTS
		Nonrespiratory	Respiratory	
GENERATIONS	8	16	24	26

A

Trachea and bronchus   **Bronchiole**   **Respiratory bronchiole**   **Alveoli**

Ciliated cell   Mucous layer   Serous cell

Capillary lumen
Type II alveolar cell
Basement membrane
Surfactant
Alveolar macrophage
Type I alveolar cell

Smooth muscle   Basal cell   Clara cell   Nerve

B   Lamina propria   Basement membrane

FIGURE 35.3 Conducting Airways and Respiratory Unit. **A,** Structures of respiratory airways. **B,** Changes in bronchial wall with progressive branching. **C,** Electron micrograph of alveoli: long white arrow identifies type II alveolar cells (pneumocytes - secretes surfactant); short white arrowhead identifies pores of Kohn; red arrow identifies alveolar capillary. **D,** Plastic cast of pulmonary capillaries at high magnification. (**A** redrawn from Thompson JM et al: *Mosby's clinical nursing,* ed 5, St Louis, 2002, Mosby; **B** from Wilson SF, Thompson JM: *Respiratory disorders,* St Louis, 1990, Mosby; **C** from Mason RJ et al: *Murray and Nadel's textbook of respiratory medicine,* ed 5, Philadelphia, 2010, Saunders; **D** courtesy A. Churg, MD, and J. Wright, MD, Vancouver, Canada. From Leslie KO, Wick MR: *Practical pulmonary pathology: a diagnostic approach,* ed 2, Philadelphia, 2011, Saunders.)

increases to 20 times that of the trachea. This results in decreased velocity of airflow into the gas-exchange portion of the lung and allows for optimal gas diffusion.

The bronchial walls have three layers: an epithelial lining, a smooth muscle layer, and a connective tissue layer. In the large bronchi (up to approximately the tenth division), the connective tissue layer contains cartilage. The epithelial lining of the bronchi contains single-celled exocrine glands—the mucus-secreting goblet cells—and ciliated cells. High columnar pseudostratified epithelium lines the larger airways and becomes progressively thinner, changing to columnar cuboidal epithelium in the bronchioles and squamous epithelium in the alveoli (types of epithelia are reviewed in Chapter 1). The submucosal glands of the bronchial lining produce a mucous blanket that protects the bronchial epithelium. The ciliated epithelial cells rhythmically beat this mucous

blanket toward the trachea and pharynx, where it can be swallowed or expectorated by coughing. Toward the terminal bronchioles, ciliated cells and goblet cells become more sparse, and smooth muscle and connective tissue layers thin (see Fig. 35.3).

Gas-Exchange Airways

The conducting airways terminate in the respiratory (terminal) bronchioles, alveolar ducts, and alveoli (*sing.,* alveolus). These thin-walled structures participate in gas exchange, and the clusters of alveoli are sometimes called the acinus (see Fig. 35.3).

The bronchioles from the sixteenth through the twenty-third divisions contain increasing numbers of alveoli and are called *respiratory bronchioles.* The walls of the respiratory bronchioles are very thin, consisting of an epithelial layer devoid of cilia and goblet cells, very little smooth

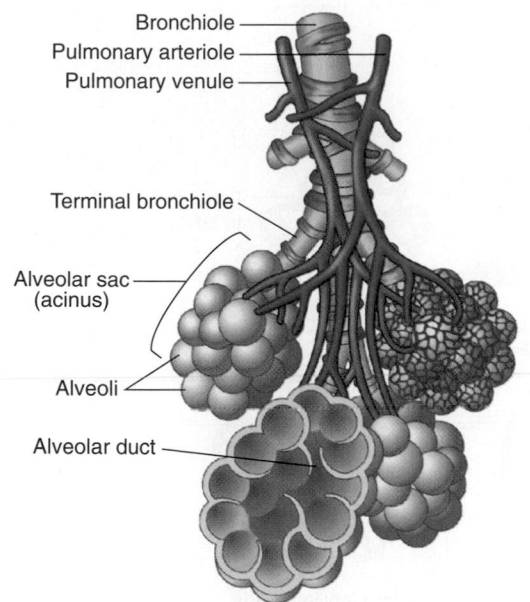

FIGURE 35.4 Alveoli. Bronchioles subdivide to form tiny tubes called *alveolar ducts* that end in clusters of alveoli called *alveolar sacs*. (From Patton KT, Thibodeau GA: *The human body in health & disease*, ed 7, St Louis, 2018, Mosby.)

muscle fiber, and a very thin and elastic connective tissue layer. These bronchioles end in **alveolar ducts**, which lead to alveolar sacs made up of numerous alveoli.

The **alveoli** are the primary gas-exchange units of the lung, where oxygen enters the blood and CO_2 is removed (Fig. 35.4). Tiny passages called *pores of Kohn* permit some air to pass through the septa from alveolus to alveolus, promoting collateral ventilation and even distribution of air among the alveoli. The lungs contain approximately 50 million alveoli at birth and about 480 million by adulthood.[2]

Lung epithelial cells provide a protective interface with the environment and are essential for adequate gas exchange, preventing entry of foreign agents, regulating ion and water transport, and maintaining mechanical stability of the alveoli. The alveolar septa consist of an epithelial layer and a thin, elastic basement membrane but no muscle layer (see Fig. 35.3). Two major types of epithelial cells (pneumocytes) appear in the alveolus. Type I alveolar cells provide structure, and type II alveolar cells secrete **surfactant**, a lipoprotein that coats the inner surface of the alveolus and facilitates its expansion during inspiration, which lowers alveolar surface tension at end-expiration, thereby preventing lung collapse (atelectasis). Surfactant proteins contribute to control of lung inflammation by decreasing release of proinflammatory mediators, preventing oxidative injury, and regulating the role of fibroblasts in airway remodeling. Surfactant proteins also are bacteriostatic and function as opsonins in presenting pathogens to alveolar macrophages.[3]

Macrophages are the most numerous immune cells present in the lung environment and provide innate immune defense of the airway from the bronchi to the alveoli. In the alveoli, *alveolar macrophages* provide protection by clearing surfactant from the lung and ingesting foreign material and pathogens that reach the alveolus, preparing these substances for removal through the lymphatics.[4] (Phagocytosis and the mononuclear phagocyte system are described in Chapters 7 and 8.) Surfactant and alveolar macrophages work together with the normal pulmonary microbiota to prevent lower lung infection. Changes in the pulmonary microbiome are associated with many pulmonary diseases (see *What's New? The Pulmonary Microbiome*).

WHAT'S NEW?

The Pulmonary Microbiome

Until recently, it was believed that the lower lungs were sterile. The first report of a healthy lung microbiome was published in 2010, and many more confirmatory articles have been published since then. The pulmonary microbiome is dynamic and is constantly influenced by the movement of air, mucus, and microbes in and out of the lung. The lung's natural defense mechanisms, such as the presence of bacteriostatic surfactant and active bronchial and alveolar macrophages, limit bacterial density along the mucosal surfaces, but those microorganisms that do survive provide important immunologic roles in preventing disease.[1] There is an interaction between the oral and gut mucosa and the pulmonary microbiome (gut-lung axis), and these relationships are just beginning to be understood in terms of causing and treating lung disease.[2]

A healthy pulmonary microbiome confers protection against many infectious and inflammatory conditions. Changes in lung microbiota have been associated with tobacco smoking, use of corticosteroids and antibiotics, and frequency of exacerbations in bronchiectasis, cystic fibrosis, asthma, and chronic obstructive pulmonary disease (COPD). Alterations in the pulmonary microbiome result in increased mortality in idiopathic pulmonary fibrosis and decreased responsiveness to corticosteroids in patients with asthma. Pulmonary changes include the presence of pathogenic species and alterations in the distribution and diversity of microbes normally found in healthy states.[3–5]

References

1. Man WH, de Steenhuijsen Piters WA, Bogaert D: The microbiota of the respiratory tract: gatekeeper to respiratory health. *Nat Rev Microbiol* 15(5):259–270, 2017.
2. Budden KF, et al: Emerging pathogenic links between microbiota and the gut-lung axis. *Nat Rev Microbiol* 15(1):55–63, 2017.
3. Dickson RP: The microbiome and critical illness. *Lancet Respir Med* 4:59–72, 2016.
4. Huang YJ, LiPuma JJ: The microbiome in cystic fibrosis. *Clin Chest Med* 37(1):59–67, 2016.
5. Yang X, et al: Does IL-17 respond to the disordered lung microbiome and contribute to the neutrophilic phenotype in asthma? *Mediators Inflamm* 2016:6470364, 2016.

Pulmonary and Bronchial Circulation

The **pulmonary circulation** provides an extensive surface area for gas exchange, delivers nutrients to lung tissues, acts as a blood reservoir for the left ventricle, and serves as a filtering system that removes clots, air, and other debris from the circulation (Fig. 35.5). The pulmonary vasculature is composed of three compartments connected in series: arteries, capillaries, and veins.

Although the entire cardiac output from the right ventricle goes into the lungs, the pulmonary circulation has a lower pressure and resistance than the systemic circulation. Pulmonary arteries are exposed to about one-fifth the pressure of the systemic circulation and have a much thinner muscle layer. (Systemic vessels are described in Chapter 32.) Mean pulmonary artery pressure is 18 mmHg; mean aortic pressure is 90 mmHg. About one-third of the pulmonary vessels are filled with blood (perfused) at any given time. More vessels become perfused when right ventricular cardiac output increases. Therefore, increased delivery of blood to the lungs does not normally increase mean pulmonary artery pressure. During exercise, pulmonary arterial pressure will normally increase, but not to more than 30 mmHg and is age and sex dependent.[5]

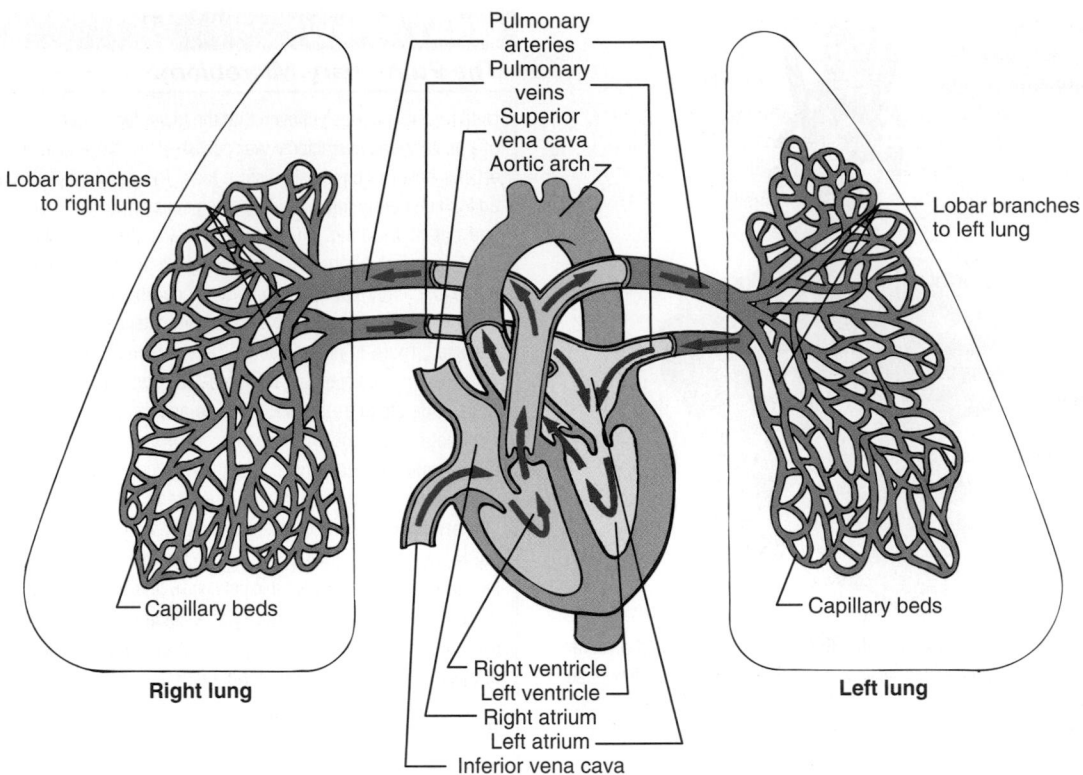

FIGURE 35.5 The Pulmonary Circulation. The right and left pulmonary veins and arteries and the branching capillaries are illustrated. Note the pulmonary artery carries venous blood, and the pulmonary vein carries arterial blood.

The **pulmonary artery** divides and enters the lung at the hilus, branching with each main bronchus, and with the bronchi at every division. Thus every bronchus and bronchiole has an accompanying artery or arteriole. The arterioles divide at the terminal bronchiole to form a network of **pulmonary capillaries** around the acinus. Capillary walls consist of an endothelial layer and a thin basement membrane, which often fuses with the basement membrane of the alveolar septum (see Fig. 35.3).

The shared alveolar and capillary walls compose the **alveolocapillary membrane**, a very thin membrane made up of the alveolar epithelium, the alveolar basement membrane, an interstitial space, the capillary basement membrane, and the capillary endothelium (Fig. 35.6). There is only about a 0.2-μm separation between blood in the capillary and gas in the alveolus.[6] Gas exchange occurs across the alveolocapillary membrane. These extremely thin alveolar walls are easily damaged and can leak plasma and blood into the alveolar space. With normal perfusion, approximately 100 mL of blood in the pulmonary capillary bed is spread very thinly over about 70 to 100 m² of alveolar surface area. Any disorder that thickens the membrane impairs gas exchange (e.g., fibrotic lung disease).

Each **pulmonary vein** drains several pulmonary capillaries. Unlike the pulmonary arteries, which follow the branching bronchi, pulmonary veins are dispersed randomly throughout the lungs and then leave the lung at the hila and enter the left atrium. They are similar to veins in the systemic circulation, but they have no valves.

The **bronchial circulation** is part of the systemic circulation and receives 1% of the cardiac output. The bronchial arteries supply blood to the trachea, bronchi and its branches, esophagus, visceral pleura, the vasa vasorum of the thoracic aorta, and the pulmonary arteries and to the nerves, pulmonary veins, and lymph nodes in the thorax.[7] Not all of the capillaries drain into their own venous system. Some empty into

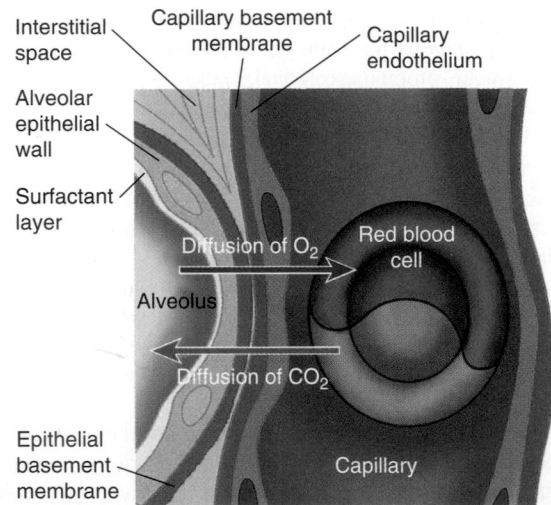

FIGURE 35.6 Cross Section Through an Alveolus Showing Histology of the Alveolar-Capillary Membrane (Respiratory Membrane). The dense network of capillaries forms an almost continuous sheet of blood in the alveolar walls, providing a very efficient arrangement for gas exchange. (Adapted from Montague SE, Watson R, Herbert R: *Physiology from nursing practice*, ed 3, London, 2005, Elsevier.)

the pulmonary vein and contribute to the normal venous admixture of oxygenated and deoxygenated blood or right-to-left shunt (right-to-left shunts are described in Chapter 36). The bronchial circulation does not participate in gas exchange.

Lung vasculature also includes deep and superficial **pulmonary lymphatic capillaries**. The deep lymphatic capillaries begin at the level of the terminal bronchioles. Fluid and alveolar macrophages migrate from the alveoli to the terminal bronchioles, where they enter the lymphatic system. The superficial lymphatic capillaries drain the membrane that surrounds the lungs. Both deep and superficial lymphatic vessels leave the lung at the hilum through a series of mediastinal lymph nodes. The lymphatic system plays an important role in keeping the lung free of fluid and providing immune defense.[8] (The lymphatic system is described in Chapter 32.)

Control of the Pulmonary Circulation

The caliber of pulmonary artery lumina decreases as smooth muscle in the arterial walls contracts. Contraction increases pulmonary artery pressure. Caliber increases as these muscles relax, decreasing blood pressure. Contraction (vasoconstriction) and relaxation (vasodilation) primarily occur in response to local humoral conditions, even though the pulmonary circulation is innervated by the autonomic nervous system (ANS), as is the systemic circulation.

The most important cause of pulmonary artery constriction is a low alveolar partial pressure of oxygen (P_{AO_2}). Vasoconstriction caused by alveolar and pulmonary venous hypoxia, often termed **hypoxic pulmonary vasoconstriction**, results from an increase in intracellular calcium levels in vascular smooth muscle cells in response to low oxygen concentration and the presence of charged oxygen molecules called *oxygen free radicals*. It can affect only one segment of the lung (i.e., one lobe that is obstructed, decreasing its P_{AO_2}) or the entire lung. If only one segment of the lung is involved, the arterioles to that segment constrict, shunting blood to other, well-ventilated portions of the lung. This reflex improves the lung's efficiency by better matching ventilation and perfusion. If all segments of the lung are affected, vasoconstriction occurs throughout the pulmonary vasculature, and pulmonary hypertension (elevated pulmonary artery pressure) can result. The pulmonary vasoconstriction caused by low P_{AO_2} values is reversible if the P_{AO_2} level is corrected. Chronic alveolar hypoxia can result in inflammation and structural remodeling in pulmonary arterioles, causing permanent pulmonary artery hypertension that eventually leads to right heart failure[9] (see *What's New? Update on Hypoxic Pulmonary Vasoconstriction*).

Acidemia also causes pulmonary artery constriction. If the acidemia is corrected, the vasoconstriction is reversed. (Respiratory acidosis and metabolic acidosis are described in Chapter 3.) An elevated Pa_{CO_2} value without a drop in pH does not cause pulmonary artery constriction. Other biochemical factors that affect the caliber of vessels in pulmonary circulation are histamine, prostaglandins, endothelin, serotonin, nitric oxide, and bradykinin.

Chest Wall and Pleura

The chest wall (skin, ribs, intercostal muscles) protects the lungs from injury. The intercostal muscles of the chest wall, in conjunction with the **diaphragm**, perform the muscular work of breathing. The **thoracic cavity** is contained by the chest wall and encases the lungs (Fig. 35.7). A serous membrane called the **pleura** adheres firmly to the lungs. It then folds over itself and attaches firmly to the chest wall. The membrane covering the lungs is the *visceral pleura;* that lining the thoracic cavity is the *parietal pleura*. The area between the two pleurae is called the **pleural space**, or **pleural cavity**. Normally only a thin layer of fluid secreted by the pleura (pleural fluid) fills the pleural space. About 18 mL of fluid is in the pleural space with a pH of about 7.6, a few cells, about 1 g/dL protein, and glucose and electrolyte concentrations that approximate those of the plasma. This lubricates the pleural surfaces, allowing the two layers to slide over each other without separating. Pressure in the pleural space is usually negative or subatmospheric (−4 to −10 mmHg).

Update on Hypoxic Pulmonary Vasoconstriction

Hypoxic pulmonary vasoconstriction is a physiologic response to changes in the environment and pulmonary pathologic conditions that affect alveolar oxygen content (P_{AO_2}). Decreases in P_{AO_2} to less than 12% of normal induce a locally controlled constriction of preacinar arteriolar smooth muscle and endothelial cells and therefore decrease blood flow through those vessels. When a pulmonary disorder is characterized by localized areas of acutely decreased alveolar oxygen content, vasoconstriction of the arterioles perfusing those areas is a positive compensatory mechanism that reduces shunt (wasted perfusion). However, in diffuse and chronic lung disorders (e.g., chronic obstructive pulmonary disease [COPD] or cystic fibrosis), widespread and persistent hypoxic pulmonary vasoconstriction creates resistance to pulmonary blood flow and raises the pressure in the pulmonary artery, causing a condition known as *secondary pulmonary artery hypertension*. Pulmonary hypertension can cause permanent arteriolar remodeling, and when it is severe enough to impede right ventricular ejection, it can lead to right heart failure, known as *cor pulmonale*. To prevent these complications, the processes involved in hypoxic pulmonary vasoconstriction are being studied intensely. The release of reactive oxygen species during hypoxia causes changes in smooth muscle cell membrane ion channels, particularly those for calcium and potassium. Calcium influx into the cell occurs through transient receptor potential (TRP) channels such as TRPV4 and TRPC6, causing vasoconstriction. Inhibitors of these channels are being studied for the treatment of secondary pulmonary artery hypertension. Other mechanisms that are being studied include microRNA dysregulation of potassium channels and alterations in tissue renin-angiotensin-aldosterone pathways. Of particular interest is the potential role of the cystic fibrosis transmembrane conductance regulator (CFTR) protein. This protein regulates sphingolipids in smooth muscle cell membranes and promotes hypoxic pulmonary vasoconstriction. Blockers of this protein are also being studied.

Data from Dunham-Snary KJ et al: *Chest* 151(1):181–192, 2017; Evans AM et al: *Adv Exp Med Biol* 860:89–99, 2015; Jernigan NL: *Exp Physiol* 100(2):111–120, 2015; Lai N, Lu W, Wang J: *Int J Clin Exp Pathol* 8(2):1081–1092, 2015; Sommer N et al: *Eur Respir J* 47:288–303, 2016; Tabeling C et al: *Proc Natl Acad Sci U S A* 112(13):E1614–1623, 2015.

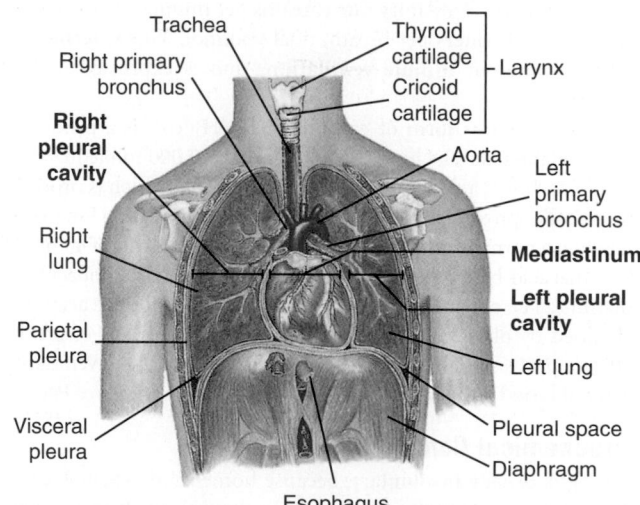

FIGURE 35.7 Thoracic (Chest) Cavity and Related Structures. The thoracic cavity is divided into three subdivisions (left and right pleural divisions and mediastinum) by a partition formed by a serous membrane called the *pleura*. (From Thibodeau GA, Patton KT: *Anatomy & physiology*, ed 3, St Louis, 1996, Mosby.)

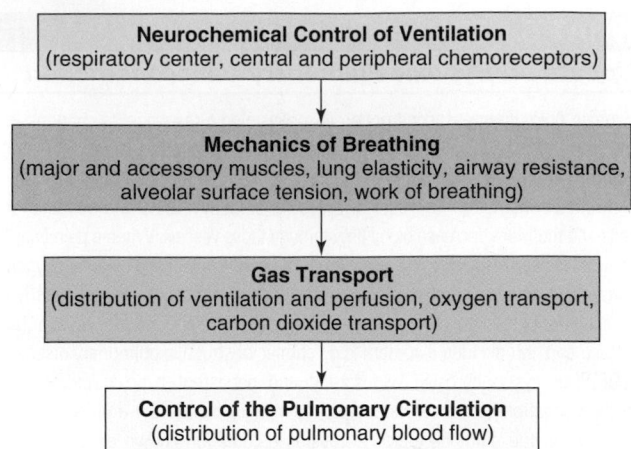

FIGURE 35.8 Functional Components of the Respiratory System. The central nervous system responds to neurochemical stimulation of ventilation and sends signals to the chest wall musculature. The response of the respiratory system to these impulses is influenced by several factors that affect the mechanisms of breathing and therefore affect the adequacy of ventilation. Gas transport between the alveoli and pulmonary capillary blood depends on a variety of physical and chemical activities. The control of the pulmonary circulation plays a role in the appropriate distribution of blood flow.

FUNCTIONS OF THE PULMONARY SYSTEM

The pulmonary system (1) ventilates the alveoli, (2) diffuses gases into and out of the blood, and (3) perfuses the lungs so that the organs and tissues of the body receive blood that is rich in oxygen and low in CO_2. Each component of the pulmonary system contributes to one or more of these functions (Fig. 35.8).

Ventilation

Ventilation is the mechanical movement of gas or air into and out of the lungs. Ventilation often is misnamed respiration, which is actually the exchange of O_2 and CO_2 during cellular metabolism. The ventilatory rate (or respiratory rate) is the number of times gas is inspired and expired per minute. The amount of effective ventilation is calculated by multiplying the ventilatory rate (breaths per minute) by the volume of air per breath (liters per breath, tidal volume). This is termed the minute volume (or minute ventilation) and is expressed in liters per minute.

CO_2, the gaseous form of carbonic acid (H_2CO_3), is a product of cellular metabolism. The lung eliminates about 10,000 milliequivalents (mEq) of carbonic acid per day in the form of CO_2, which is produced at the rate of approximately 200 mL/minute. CO_2 elimination is necessary to maintain a normal partial pressure of arterial CO_2 ($Paco_2$) of 40 mmHg and normal acid-base balance (see Chapter 3 for a discussion of acid-base regulation). The adequacy of alveolar ventilation *cannot* be accurately determined by observation of ventilatory rate, pattern, or effort. If a healthcare professional needs to determine the adequacy of ventilation, an arterial blood gas analysis must be performed to measure $Paco_2$.

Neurochemical Control of Ventilation

Breathing is usually involuntary, because homeostatic changes in the ventilatory rate and volume are adjusted automatically by the nervous system to maintain normal gas exchange. Voluntary breathing is necessary for talking, singing, laughing, and holding one's breath.

The respiratory center in the brainstem controls respiration by transmitting impulses to the respiratory muscles, causing them to contract and relax (Fig. 35.9). The medullary rhythmicity area is composed of interconnected groups of neurons located bilaterally in the brainstem: the dorsal respiratory group (DRG) and the ventral respiratory group (VRG).[10] The basic automatic rhythm of respiration is set by the VRG, a cluster of inspiratory nerve cells located in the medulla that sends efferent impulses to the diaphragm and inspiratory intercostal muscles. The DRG receives afferent impulses from peripheral chemoreceptors in the carotid and aortic bodies; from mechanical, neural, and chemical stimuli; and from receptors in the lungs, and it alters breathing patterns to restore normal blood gases. The pontine respiratory center and apneustic center, situated in the pons, do not generate primary rhythm, but rather act as modifiers of the rhythm established by the medullary rhythmicity area. Breathing can be modified by input from the cortex, the limbic system, and the hypothalamus, and the pattern of breathing can be influenced by emotion and by disease.

Chemoreceptors. Chemoreceptors monitor pH, $Paco_2$, and Pao_2. Central chemoreceptors monitor arterial blood indirectly by sensing changes in the pH of cerebrospinal fluid (CSF). They are located near the respiratory center and are sensitive to hydrogen ion concentration in brain interstitial fluid and the CSF (Chapter 3 describes the relationship between ions and the pH, or acid-base status, of body fluids). The pH, or concentration of hydrogen ions in the CSF, reflects arterial pH because CO_2 in arterial blood diffuses across the blood-brain barrier (the capillary wall separating blood from cells of the central nervous system) into the CSF until the partial pressure of CO_2 (Pco_2) is equal on both sides. CO_2 that has entered the CSF combines with H_2O to form carbonic acid, which subsequently dissociates into hydrogen ions that are capable of stimulating the central chemoreceptors. In this way $Paco_2$ regulates ventilation through its effect on the pH (hydrogen ion content) of the CSF.[11]

If alveolar ventilation is inadequate, $Paco_2$ increases. CO_2 diffuses across the blood-brain barrier until Pco_2 values in the blood and the CSF reach equilibrium. Because the central chemoreceptors sense the resulting decrease in pH (increase in hydrogen ion concentration), they stimulate the respiratory center to increase the depth and rate of ventilation. Increased ventilation causes the $Paco_2$ of arterial blood to decrease below that of the CSF, and CO_2 diffuses out of the CSF, returning its pH to normal.

The central chemoreceptors are sensitive to very small changes in the pH of CSF (equivalent to a 1 to 2 mmHg change in Pco_2) and are able to maintain a normal $Paco_2$ level under many different conditions, including strenuous exercise.[11] If inadequate ventilation, or hypoventilation, is a long-term condition (e.g., in chronic obstructive pulmonary disease), these receptors become insensitive to small changes in $Paco_2$ and regulate ventilation poorly. In addition, prolonged increases in $Paco_2$ result in renal compensation through bicarbonate retention. This bicarbonate gradually diffuses into the CSF, where it normalizes the pH and negates the effect on ventilatory drive.

The peripheral chemoreceptors are located in aortic bodies, the aortic arch, and carotid bodies at the bifurcation of the carotids, near the baroreceptors (see Chapter 32). They are somewhat sensitive to changes in $Paco_2$ and pH but are primarily sensitive to oxygen levels in arterial blood (Pao_2). As Pao_2 and pH decrease, peripheral chemoreceptors, particularly in the carotid bodies, send signals to the respiratory center to increase ventilation. However, the Pao_2 must drop well below normal (to approximately 60 mmHg) before the peripheral chemoreceptors have much influence on ventilation. If $Paco_2$ is elevated as well, ventilation increases much more than it would in response to either abnormality alone. The peripheral chemoreceptors become the major stimulus to ventilation when the central chemoreceptors are "reset" by chronic hypoventilation.[12]

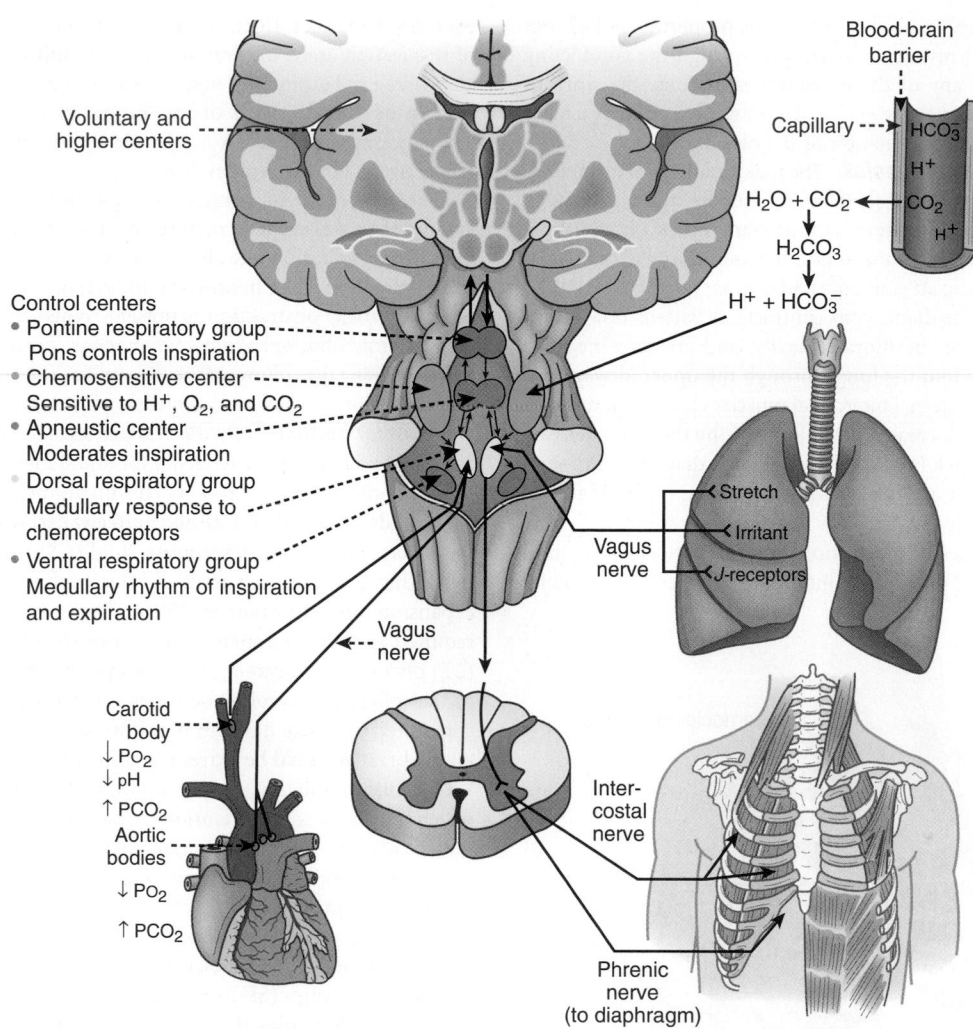

Control centers
- Pontine respiratory group
  Pons controls inspiration
- Chemosensitive center
  Sensitive to H^+, O_2, and CO_2
- Apneustic center
  Moderates inspiration
- Dorsal respiratory group
  Medullary response to chemoreceptors
- Ventral respiratory group
  Medullary rhythm of inspiration and expiration

Voluntary and higher centers

Blood-brain barrier

Capillary

HCO_3^-
H^+
CO_2
H^+

$H_2O + CO_2$

H_2CO_3

$H^+ + HCO_3^-$

Stretch
Irritant
J-receptors

Vagus nerve

Vagus nerve

Carotid body
↓ PO_2
↓ pH
↑ PCO_2
Aortic bodies
↓ PO_2
↑ PCO_2

Inter-costal nerve

Phrenic nerve (to diaphragm)

FIGURE 35.9 Neurochemical Respiratory Control System.

Lung Innervation. Three types of lung sensory receptors send impulses from the lungs to the dorsal respiratory group:

1. **Irritant receptors** (rapidly adapting receptors) are found in the epithelium of the conducting airways.[13] They are sensitive to noxious aerosols (vapors), gases, and particulate matter (e.g., inhaled dusts), which cause them to initiate the cough reflex. When stimulated, irritant receptors also cause bronchoconstriction and increased ventilatory rate. These receptors are located primarily in the proximal larger airways and are nearly absent in the distal airways; thus it is possible for secretions to accumulate in the distal respiratory tree without initiating cough.

2. **Stretch receptors** (slowly adapting receptors) are located in the smooth muscles of airways and are sensitive to increases in the size or volume of the lungs. They decrease ventilatory rate and volume when stimulated, an occurrence sometimes referred to as the *Hering-Breuer expiratory reflex*. This reflex is active in newborns and assists with ventilation.[14] In adults, this reflex is active only at high tidal volumes (such as with exercise and mechanical ventilation) and may play a role in protecting against excess lung inflation.

3. **Pulmonary C-fiber receptors** (previously known as *J-receptors juxtapulmonary capillary receptors*) are located near the capillaries in the alveolar septa and in other airway locations as nociceptors. They are sensitive to increased pulmonary capillary pressure,

which stimulates them to initiate rapid, shallow breathing; laryngeal constriction on expiration and mucus secretion; hypotension; and bradycardia. They may be associated with the sensation of dyspnea.[15]

The lung is innervated by the autonomic nervous system (ANS). Fibers of the sympathetic division of the ANS in the lung branch from the upper thoracic and cervical ganglia of the spinal cord. Fibers of the parasympathetic division of the ANS travel in the vagus nerve to the lung. (Structures and function of the ANS are discussed in detail in Chapter 15.) The parasympathetic and sympathetic divisions of the ANS control airway caliber (interior diameter of the airway lumen) by stimulating bronchial smooth muscle to contract or relax. The parasympathetic receptors cause smooth muscle to contract, whereas sympathetic receptors cause it to relax. Bronchial smooth muscle tone depends on equilibrium, that is, equal stimulation of contraction and relaxation. The parasympathetic division of the ANS is the main controller of airway caliber under normal conditions.[16] Constriction occurs if the irritant receptors in the airway epithelium are stimulated by irritants in inspired air, by inflammatory mediators (e.g., histamine, serotonin, prostaglandins), by many drugs, and by humoral substances.

Mechanics of Breathing

The mechanical aspects of inspiration and expiration are known collectively as the *mechanics of breathing* and involve (1) major and accessory muscles of inspiration and expiration, (2) elastic properties of the lungs and chest wall, and (3) resistance to airflow through the conducting airways. Alterations in any of these properties increase the work of breathing, and thus the metabolic energy that must be exerted to achieve adequate ventilation and oxygenation of the blood.

Major and Accessory Muscles. The major muscles of inspiration are the diaphragm and the external intercostal muscles (muscles between the ribs) (Fig. 35.10). The diaphragm is the primary muscle of ventilation, is dome-shaped, and separates the abdominal and thoracic cavities. It has multiple intrathoracic attachments and is innervated by the paired phrenic nerves. When the diaphragm contracts, it flattens downward, increasing the volume of the thoracic cavity, and creates a negative pressure that draws gas into the lungs through the upper airways and trachea. Contraction of external intercostal muscles elevates the anterior portion of the ribs. This increases the volume of the thoracic cavity by increasing its front-to-back (anteroposterior [AP]) diameter. Although the external intercostal muscles may contract during quiet breathing, inspiration at rest usually is assisted by the diaphragm only.

The accessory muscles of inspiration are the sternocleidomastoid and scalene muscles. Like the external intercostal muscles, these muscles enlarge the thorax by increasing its AP diameter. The accessory muscles of inspiration assist inspiration when the minute volume (volume of air inspired and expired per minute) is very high, such as during strenuous exercise or when the work of breathing is increased because of disease. The accessory muscles do not increase the volume of the thorax as efficiently as the diaphragm does.[17]

There are no major muscles of expiration because normal, relaxed expiration is passive and requires no muscular effort. The accessory muscles of expiration, the abdominal and internal intercostal muscles, assist expiration when minute volume is high, when the person coughs, or when airway obstruction is present. When the abdominal muscles contract, intraabdominal pressure increases, pushing up the diaphragm and decreasing the volume of the thorax. The internal intercostal muscles pull down the anterior ribs, decreasing the AP diameter of the thorax.

Alveolar Surface Tension. Surface tension occurs at any gas-liquid interface and refers to the tendency for liquid molecules that are exposed to air to adhere to one another. This phenomenon can be seen in the way liquids "bead" when splashed onto a waterproof surface, decreasing the surface area exposed to the air.

Within a sphere, such as an alveolus, surface tension tends to make expansion difficult. According to the law of Laplace, the pressure *(P)* required to inflate a sphere is equal to two times the surface tension *(2T)* divided by the radius *(r)* of the sphere, or $P = 2T/r$. As the radius of the sphere (or alveolus) becomes smaller, more and more pressure is required to inflate it. If the alveoli were lined with a water-like fluid, taking breaths would be extremely difficult.

Alveolar ventilation, or distention, is made possible by surfactant, which lowers the surface tension by coating the air-liquid interface in the alveoli (see Fig. 35.3). Surfactant, a lipoprotein (90% lipids and 10% protein) produced by type II alveolar cells, includes two groups of surfactant proteins (SPs). One group (SP-B and SP-C) consists of small hydrophobic molecules that have a detergent-like effect that separates the liquid molecules, thereby decreasing alveolar surface tension. The second group (SP-A and SP-D) consists of large hydrophilic molecules called collectins (pattern recognition molecules) that are capable of inhibiting foreign pathogens[3] (see Chapter 7).

Surfactant lines the alveolar side of the alveolocapillary membrane and, in effect, reverses the law of Laplace. As the radius of a surfactant-lined sphere (alveolus) becomes smaller, the surface tension *decreases,* and as the radius grows larger, the surface tension *increases.* This occurs because the surfactant molecules have much weaker intermolecular attraction than do liquid molecules. The surfactant molecules occupy most of the air-fluid interface and disrupt the intermolecular forces that tend to collapse the alveoli. Therefore, the alveoli are much easier to inflate at low lung volumes (i.e., after expiration) than at high volumes (i.e., after inspiration). The decrease in surface tension caused by surfactant also is responsible for keeping the alveoli free of fluid. If surfactant production is disrupted or surfactant is not produced in adequate quantities (e.g., as in premature infants), alveolar surface tension increases, causing alveolar collapse, decreased lung expansion, increased work of breathing, and severe gas-exchange abnormalities.

Elastic Properties of the Lung and Chest Wall. The lung and chest wall have elastic properties that permit expansion during inspiration and return to resting volume during expiration. The elasticity of the lungs is caused both by elastin fibers in the alveolar walls and in the surrounding small airways and pulmonary capillaries and by surface tension at the alveolar air-liquid interface. The elasticity of the chest wall is supported by the configuration of its bones and musculature.

Elastic recoil is the tendency of the lungs to return to the resting state after inspiration. Normal elastic recoil permits passive expiration, eliminating the need for major muscles of expiration. Passive elastic recoil may be insufficient during labored breathing (high minute volume),

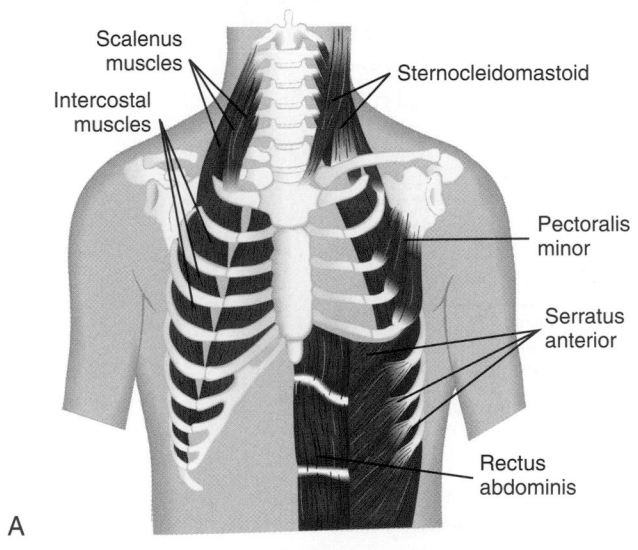

Scalenus muscles
Intercostal muscles
Sternocleidomastoid
Pectoralis minor
Serratus anterior
Rectus abdominis

A

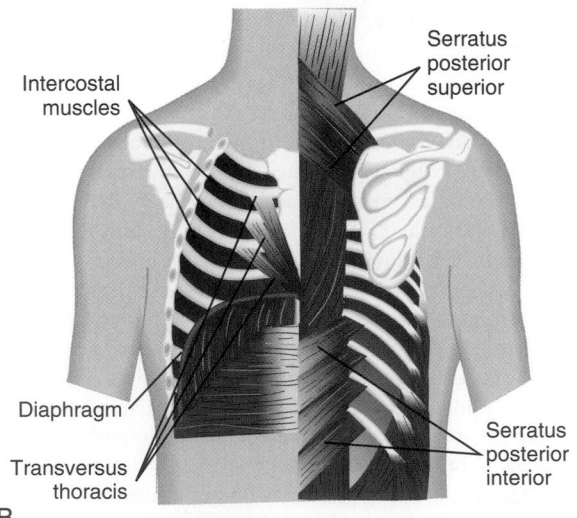

Intercostal muscles
Serratus posterior superior
Diaphragm
Transversus thoracis
Serratus posterior interior

B

FIGURE 35.10 Muscles of Ventilation. A, Anterior view. **B,** Posterior view. (Modified from Thompson JM et al: *Mosby's clinical nursing,* ed 5, St Louis, 2002, Mosby.)

in which case the accessory muscles of expiration may be needed. The accessory muscles also are used if disease compromises elastic recoil (e.g., in emphysema) or blocks the conducting airways.

Normal elastic recoil depends on the equilibrium between opposing forces of recoil in the lungs and chest wall. Under normal conditions the chest wall tends to recoil by expanding outward. When the sternum is split to open the thoracic cavity, the chest wall moves outward laterally. The tendency of the chest wall to recoil by expanding is balanced by the tendency of the lungs to recoil or collapse inward around the hila. This reaction is caused by elastic recoil and surface tension in the alveoli. The opposing forces of the chest wall and lungs create, in part, the small negative intrapleural pressure.

Balance between the outward recoil of the chest wall and the inward recoil of the lungs occurs at the resting level, at the end of expiration. During inspiration the diaphragm and intercostal muscles contract, air flows into the lungs, and the chest wall expands. Muscular effort is needed to overcome the resistance of the lungs to expansion. During expiration the muscles relax and the elastic recoil of the lungs causes the thorax to decrease in volume until, once again, balance between the chest wall and lung recoil forces is reached[18] (Fig. 35.11).

Compliance is the measure of lung and chest wall distensibility. It represents the relative ease with which these structures can be stretched. Compliance is therefore the reciprocal of elasticity. Compliance is determined by the alveolar surface tension and the elastic recoil of the lung and chest wall. It can be measured with the following formula:

$$C = \frac{\Delta V}{\Delta P}$$

where C = compliance in liters per centimeter of water, ΔV = volume change (usually tidal volume), and ΔP = pressure change (airway or pleural pressure) in centimeters of water.

Increased compliance indicates that the lungs or chest wall is abnormally easy to inflate and has lost some elastic recoil. A decrease in compliance indicates that the lungs or chest wall is abnormally stiff or difficult to inflate. Compliance increases with normal aging and with disorders such as emphysema; it decreases in individuals with acute respiratory distress syndrome, pneumonia, pulmonary edema, and fibrosis. (These disorders are described in Chapter 36.)

Airway Resistance. Airway resistance, which is similar to resistance to blood flow (described in Chapter 32), is determined by the length, radius, and cross-sectional area of the airways and by the density, viscosity, and velocity of the gas (Poiseuille's law). Resistance is computed by dividing change in pressure *(P)* by rate of flow *(F)*, or *R = P/F* (Ohm's law), and can easily be measured in the pulmonary function laboratory.[19] Airway resistance is normally very low. One-half to two-thirds of total airway resistance occur in the nose. The next

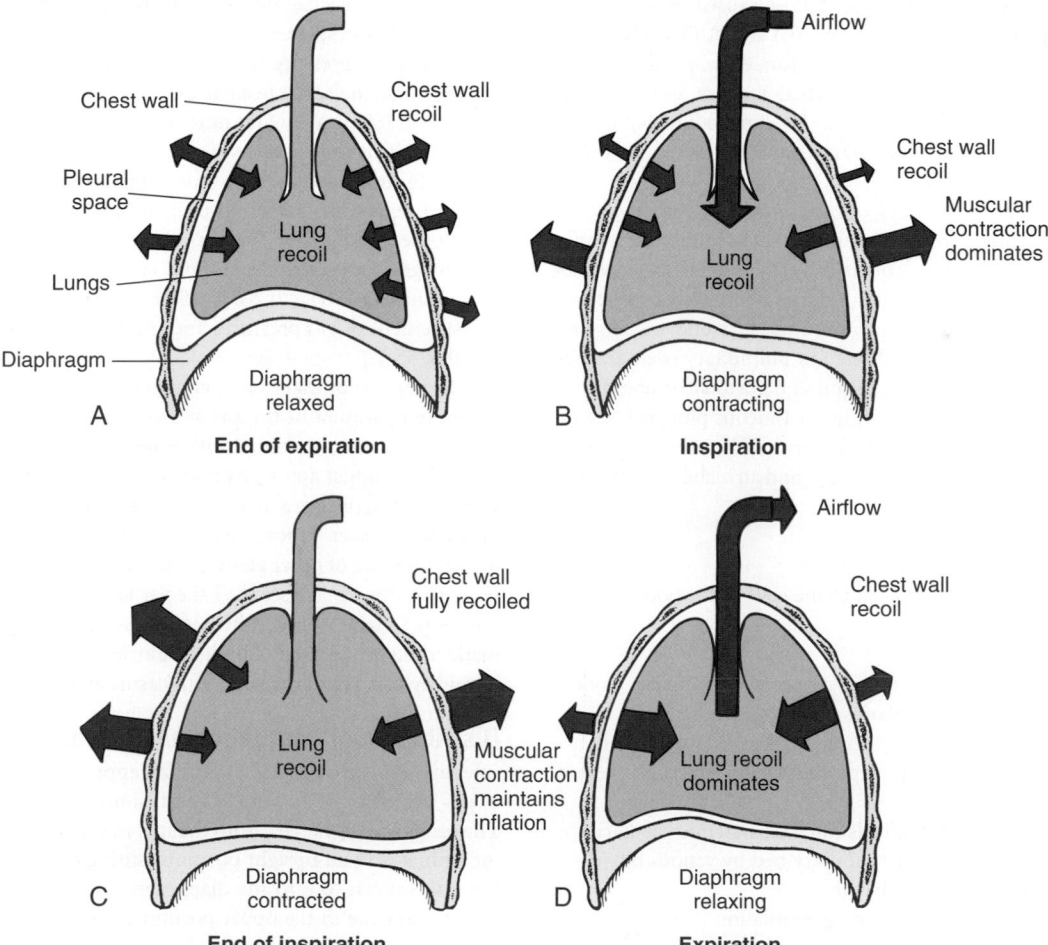

FIGURE 35.11 Interaction of Forces During Inspiration and Expiration. **A,** Outward recoil of the chest wall equals inward recoil of the lungs at the end of expiration. **B,** During inspiration, contraction of respiratory muscles, assisted by chest wall recoil, overcomes tendency of lungs to recoil. **C,** At the end of inspiration, respiratory muscle contraction maintains lung expansion. **D,** During expiration, respiratory muscles relax, allowing elastic recoil of the lungs to deflate the lungs.

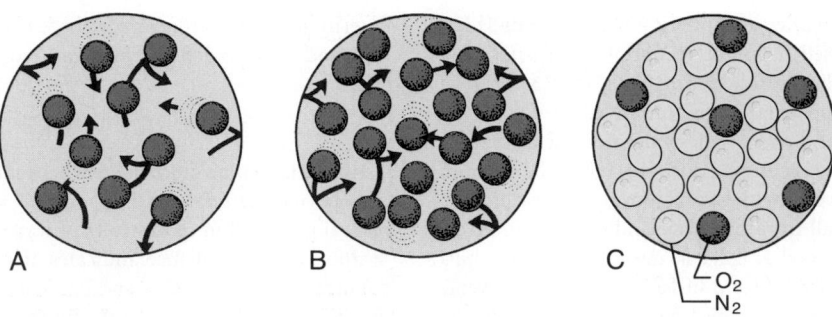

FIGURE 35.12 Relationship Between Number of Gas Molecules and Pressure Exerted by the Gas in an Enclosed Space. **A,** Theoretically, 10 molecules of the same gas exert a total pressure of 10 mmHg within the space. **B,** If the number of molecules is increased to 20, the total pressure is 20 mmHg. **C,** If there are different gases in the space, each gas exerts a partial pressure: here the partial pressure of nitrogen *(yellow)* is 18, the partial pressure of oxygen *(blue)* is 6, and the total pressure is 24 mmHg.

highest resistance is in the oropharynx and larynx. Airway resistance also is affected by the diameter of the airways, and there is very little resistance in the conducting airways of the lungs because of their large cross-sectional area. **Bronchodilation**, which decreases resistance to airflow, is caused by β_2-adrenergic receptor stimulation. **Bronchoconstriction**, which increases airway resistance, can be caused by stimulation of parasympathetic receptors in the bronchial smooth muscle and by numerous irritants and inflammatory mediators. Airway resistance also can be increased by edema of the bronchial mucosa and by airway obstructions such as mucus, tumors, or foreign bodies. Pulmonary function tests (PFTs) measure lung volumes and flow rates and can be used to diagnose lung disease.

Work of Breathing. The **work of breathing** is determined by the muscular effort (and therefore oxygen and energy) required for ventilation. The work of breathing is normally very low, but may increase considerably in disease states that disrupt the equilibrium between forces exerted by the lung and chest wall. More muscular effort is required when lung compliance is decreased (e.g., in pulmonary edema), chest wall compliance is decreased (e.g., in spinal deformity or obesity), or airways are obstructed by bronchospasm or mucous plugging (e.g., in asthma or bronchitis). An increase in the work of breathing can result in a marked increase in oxygen consumption and an inability to maintain adequate ventilation.

Gas Transport

Gas transport, the delivery of oxygen to the cells of the body, requires four steps:

1. Ventilation of the lungs
2. Diffusion of oxygen from the alveoli into the capillary blood
3. Perfusion of systemic capillaries with oxygenated blood
4. Diffusion of oxygen from systemic capillaries into the cells

The removal of CO_2 also has four steps and occurs in reverse order of oxygen delivery:

1. Diffusion of CO_2 from the cells into the systemic capillaries
2. Perfusion of the pulmonary capillary bed by venous blood
3. Diffusion of CO_2 into the alveoli
4. Removal of CO_2 from the lung by ventilation

If any step in gas transport is impaired by a respiratory or cardiovascular disorder, gas exchange at the cellular level is compromised.

Measurement of Gas Pressure

The properties of air, once it enters the body, are determined by interactions among gas molecules at a given temperature. The millions of gas molecules are moving randomly, colliding with each other and the wall of the space in which they are contained. These collisions exert pressure. If the same number of gas molecules is contained in a small and a large container, the pressure is greater in the small container because more collisions occur in the smaller space (Fig. 35.12). Heat increases the speed of the molecules, which increases the number of collisions and, therefore, the pressure.

Barometric pressure (P_B) (atmospheric pressure) is the pressure exerted by gas molecules in air at specific altitudes. At sea level, barometric pressure is 760 mmHg. This number is the sum of the pressure exerted by each gas in the air at sea level. The portion of the total pressure exerted by any individual gas is its **partial pressure** (see Fig. 35.12). At sea level the air is made up of oxygen (20.9%), nitrogen (78.1%), and a few other trace gases. The partial pressure of oxygen is equal to the percentage of oxygen in the air (20.9%) times the total P_B (760 mmHg), or 159 mmHg ($760 \times 0.209 = 158.84$ mmHg). (Symbols used in the measurement of gas pressures and pulmonary ventilation are defined in Table 35.2.)

The amount of water vapor contained in a gas mixture is determined by the temperature of the gas and is unrelated to P_B. Gas that enters the lungs becomes saturated with water vapor (humidified) as it passes through the upper airway. At body temperature (37°C [98.6°F]), water vapor exerts a pressure of 47 mmHg regardless of total P_B. The partial pressure of water vapor must be subtracted from the P_B before the partial pressure of other gases in the mixture can be determined. In air saturated with water at sea level, the partial pressure of oxygen is therefore $(760 - 47) \times 0.209 = 149$ mmHg. All pressure and volume measurements made in pulmonary function laboratories specify the temperature and humidity of a gas at the time of measurement.

Distribution of Ventilation and Perfusion

Effective gas exchange depends on an approximately even distribution of gas (ventilation) and blood (perfusion) in all portions of the lungs. The lungs are suspended from the hila in the thoracic cavity. When the individual is in an upright position (sitting or standing), gravity pulls the lungs down toward the diaphragm and creates a greater negative pleural pressure in the upper portions, or apexes of the lungs, than at the base. The alveoli in the apexes also contain a greater residual volume of gas and are larger and less numerous than those in the lower portions. Surface tension increases as the alveoli become larger. The combination of greater negative pleural pressure and higher surface tension in the larger alveoli in the apex of the lung makes them more difficult to inflate (less compliant, or less distensible) than the smaller alveoli in

TABLE 35.2	COMMON PULMONARY ABBREVIATIONS
SYMBOL*	**DEFINITION**
V	Volume or amount of gas
Q	Perfusion or blood flow
P	Pressure (usually partial pressure) of a gas
PiO_2	Partial pressure of inspired oxygen (varies with altitude)
PaO_2	Partial pressure of oxygen in arterial blood
PAO_2	Partial pressure of oxygen in alveolar blood
$PaCO_2$	Partial pressure of carbon dioxide in arterial blood
PH_2O	Partial pressure of water vapor
PN_2	Partial pressure of nitrogen
PvO_2	Partial pressure of oxygen in mixed venous or pulmonary artery blood
$P(A-a)O_2$	Difference between alveolar and arterial partial pressure of oxygen (A–a gradient)
P_B	Barometric or atmospheric pressure
SaO_2	Saturation of hemoglobin (in arterial blood) with oxygen
$S\overline{v}O_2$	Saturation of hemoglobin (in mixed venous blood)
V_A	Alveolar ventilation—effective total lung capacity
V_D	Dead-space ventilation
V_E	Minute capacity
V_T	Tidal volume or average breath
$\dot{V}/\dot{Q}$	Ratio of ventilation to perfusion
FiO_2	Fraction (percent) of inspired oxygen (0.21)
FRC	Functional residual capacity
FVC	Forced vital capacity
FEV_1	Forced expiratory volume in 1 second
ERV	Expiratory reserve volume
IRV	Inspiratory reserve volume
IC	Inspiratory capacity

*Subscripts identify the particular gas, volume, or pressure being discussed. An overhead dot, such as in $\dot{V}/\dot{Q}$, means measurement over time, usually 1 minute.
From Kacmarek RM, Stoller JK, Heuer AJ: *Egan's fundamentals of respiratory care*, ed 11, St Louis, 2017, Mosby.

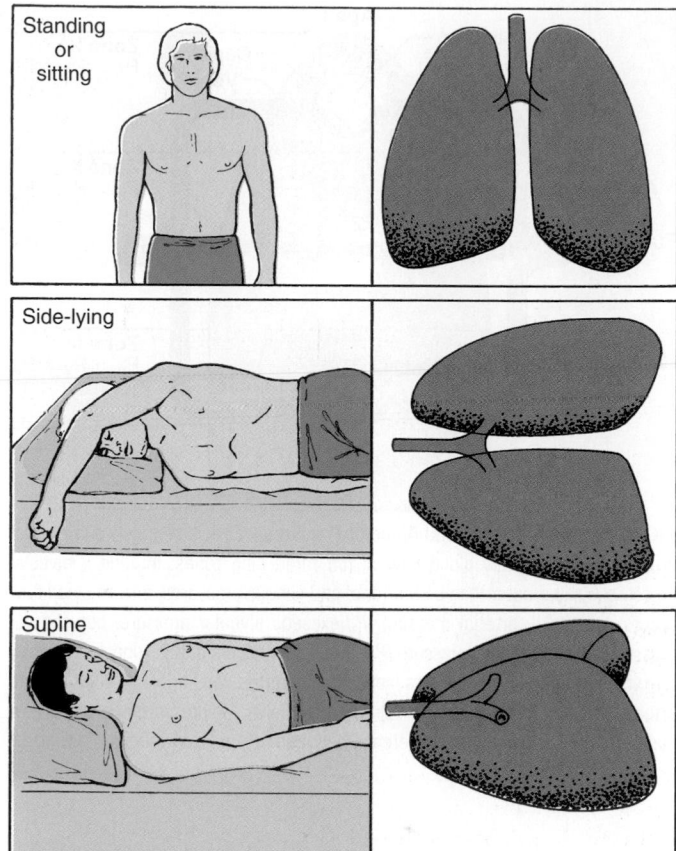

FIGURE 35.13 Pulmonary Blood Flow and Gravity. The greatest volume of pulmonary blood flow will normally occur in the gravity-dependent areas of the lungs. Body position has a significant effect on the distribution of pulmonary blood flow. Shaded areas represent gravity-dependent pulmonary blood flow.

the lower portions of the lung. Therefore, during ventilation most of the tidal volume is distributed to the bases of the lungs, where compliance is greater.

The heart pumps against gravity to perfuse the pulmonary circulation. As blood is pumped into the lung apexes of a sitting or standing individual, some blood pressure is dissipated in overcoming gravity. As a result, blood pressure at the apexes is lower than that at the bases. Because greater pressure causes greater perfusion, the bases of the lungs are better perfused than the apexes (Fig. 35.13). Thus ventilation and

perfusion are greatest in the same lung portions: the lower lobes. Ventilation and perfusion depend on body position. If a standing individual assumes a supine or side-lying position, the areas of the lungs that are then most dependent become the best ventilated and perfused.

Distribution of perfusion in the pulmonary circulation also is affected by alveolar pressure (gas pressure in the alveoli). The pulmonary capillary bed differs from the systemic capillary bed in that it is surrounded by gas-containing alveoli. If the gas pressure in the alveoli exceeds the blood pressure in the capillary, the capillary collapses and flow ceases. This occurs in portions of the lung where blood pressure is lowest and alveolar gas pressure is greatest, that is, the apex of the lung. The lungs are divided into three zones on the basis of the combination of factors affecting pulmonary blood flow. Alveolar pressure and the forces of gravity, arterial blood pressure, and venous blood pressure determine the distribution of perfusion (Fig. 35.14).

In zone I, alveolar pressure exceeds pulmonary arterial and venous pressures. The capillary bed collapses, and normal blood flow ceases. Zone I is a very small part of the lung at the apex. In zone II, alveolar pressure is greater than venous pressure, but not greater than arterial pressure. Blood flows through zone II, but it is impeded to a certain extent by alveolar pressure. Zone II is above the level of the left atrium. In zone III arterial and venous pressures are greater than alveolar pressure and blood flow is not affected by alveolar pressure. Zone III is in the base of the lung. Blood flow through the pulmonary capillary bed increases in regular increments from the apex to the base.

Although blood flow and ventilation are greater at the base of the lungs than at the apexes, they are not perfectly matched in any zone.

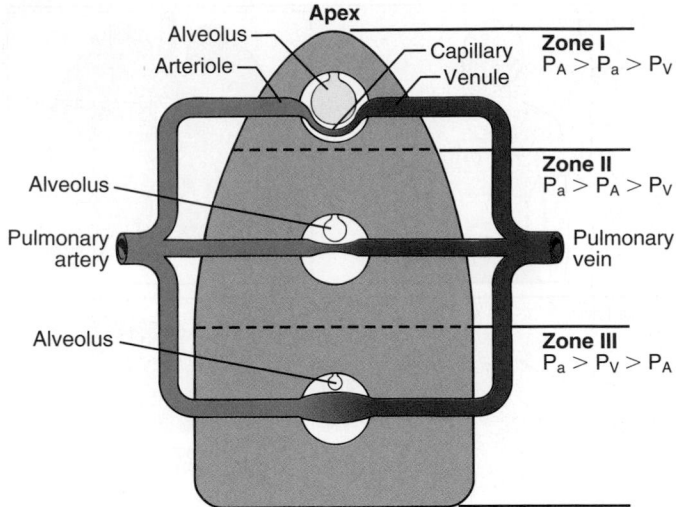

FIGURE 35.14 Gravity and Alveolar Pressures. Effects of gravity and alveolar pressure on pulmonary blood flow in the three lung zones. In zone I, alveolar pressure (P_A) is greater than both arterial and venous pressures, and no blood flow occurs. In zone II, arterial pressure (P_a) exceeds alveolar pressure, but alveolar pressure exceeds venous pressure (P_V). Blood flow occurs in this zone, but alveolar pressure compresses the venules (venous ends of the capillaries). In zone III, both arterial and venous pressures are greater than alveolar pressure and blood flow fluctuates, depending on the difference between arterial and venous pressures.

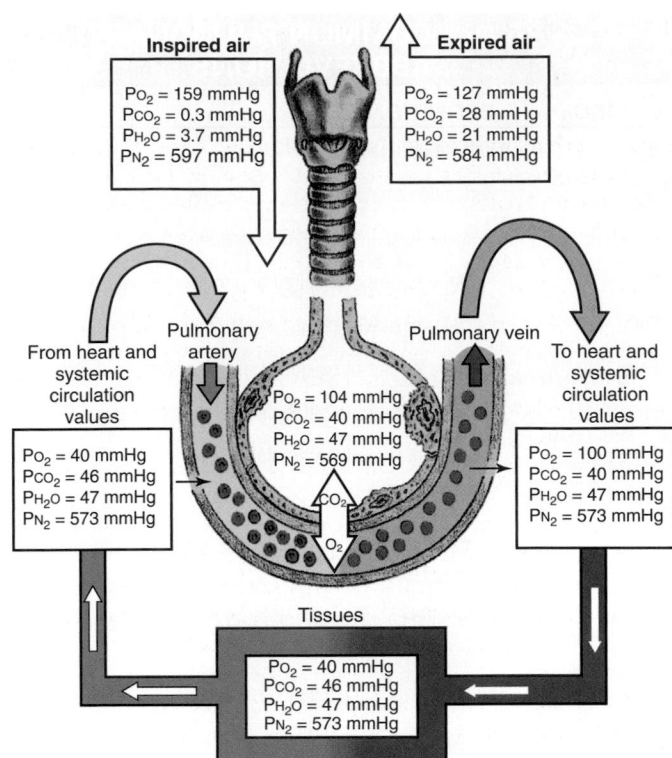

FIGURE 35.15 Partial Pressure of Respiratory Gases in Normal Respiration. These are average values. The values of Po_2, Pco_2, and Pn_2 fluctuate from breath to breath. CO_2, Carbon dioxide; O_2, oxygen; Pco_2, partial pressure of carbon dioxide; Ph_2o, partial pressure of water; Pn_2, partial pressure of nitrogen; Po_2, partial pressure of oxygen.

Perfusion exceeds ventilation in the bases, and ventilation exceeds perfusion in the apexes of the lung. The relationship between ventilation and perfusion is expressed as a ratio called the **ventilation-perfusion ratio**, or $\dot{V}/\dot{Q}$. The normal $\dot{V}/\dot{Q}$ ratio is 0.8. This is the amount by which perfusion exceeds ventilation under normal conditions.

Oxygen Transport

Approximately 1000 mL (1 L) of oxygen is transported to the cells of the body each minute. Oxygen is transported in the blood in two forms: a small amount dissolves in plasma, and the remainder binds to hemoglobin molecules. Without hemoglobin, oxygen would not reach the cells in amounts sufficient to maintain normal metabolic function. (Hemoglobin is discussed in detail in Chapter 28; cellular metabolism is discussed in Chapter 1.)

Diffusion Across the Alveolocapillary Membrane. The alveolocapillary membrane is the ideal medium for oxygen diffusion, because it has a large total surface area (70 to 100 m²) and is very thin (0.5 μm). In addition, the partial pressure of oxygen molecules (Po_2) is much greater in alveolar gas than in capillary blood, a condition that promotes rapid diffusion down the concentration gradient from the alveolus into the capillary.[20]

The amount of oxygen in the alveoli (Pao_2) depends on the amount of oxygen in the inspired air and on the amount of oxygen that remains in the alveoli and tracheobronchial tree (**physiologic dead space**) between breaths (i.e., the amount of oxygen that has not been consumed).[21] The Pao_2 can be estimated by using the alveolar gas equation:

$$Pao_2 = Pio_2 - Paco_2/0.8 \text{ (the respiratory quotient)}$$

where Pio_2 is the inspired partial pressure of oxygen and is calculated as:

$$Pio_2 = (\text{Barometric pressure} - 47\,\text{mmHg [vapor pressure of water]}) \times Fio_2(0.21)$$

The Pao_2 value is approximately 104 mmHg at sea level with relaxed breathing; therefore a pressure gradient of approximately 60 mmHg facilitates the diffusion of oxygen from the alveolus into the capillary (Fig. 35.15). Different values for Pao_2 can be calculated if there are changes in the inspired oxygen content or the $Paco_2$, which are common occurrences in clinical settings.

Blood remains in the pulmonary capillary for about 0.75 second, but only 0.25 second is required for oxygen concentration to equilibrate (equalize) across the alveolocapillary membrane. Therefore, oxygen has ample time to diffuse into the blood, even during increased cardiac output, which speeds blood flow, shortening the time the blood remains in the capillary.

Determinants of Arterial Oxygenation. As oxygen diffuses across the alveolocapillary membrane, it dissolves in the plasma, where it exerts pressure (the partial pressure of oxygen in arterial blood, or Pao_2). As the Pao_2 increases, oxygen moves from the plasma into the red blood cells (erythrocytes) and binds with hemoglobin molecules. Oxygen continues to bind with hemoglobin until the hemoglobin binding sites are filled or saturated. Oxygen then continues to diffuse across the alveolocapillary membrane until the Pao_2 and Pao_2 equilibrate, eliminating the pressure gradient across the alveolocapillary membrane. At this point diffusion ceases (see Fig. 35.15).

The majority (97%) of the oxygen that enters the blood is bound to hemoglobin. The remaining 3% stays in the plasma. The Pao_2 can be measured in the blood by obtaining an arterial blood gas measurement. The oxygen saturation (Sao_2) is the percentage of the available hemoglobin that is bound to oxygen and can be measured using a device called an *oximeter*. The total amount of oxygen carried in the blood is the **oxygen content** and is measured in milliliters per deciliter (1 dL =

100 mL) of blood. It is the combined value of the oxygen in oxygen-saturated hemoglobin and the oxygen dissolved in the blood.

To calculate the total arterial oxygen content, one must know (1) the hemoglobin concentration, or the amount of hemoglobin that is available to bind with oxygen (hemoglobin [Hb] in grams per deciliter); (2) the oxygen saturation, or the percentage of available hemoglobin that is bound to oxygen (Sao_2); and (3) the partial pressure of oxygen (Pao_2). The maximum amount of oxygen that can be transported by hemoglobin is 1.34 mL/g. The amount of oxygen that can be physically dissolved in blood is 0.003 mL/dL per mmHg. With the specific values known, the oxygen content of arterial blood can be calculated. To calculate the oxygen content of venous blood, the partial pressure of mixed venous blood (Pvo_2) and venous oxygen saturation (Svo_2) are substituted for the arterial values in the basic formula. Normal venous oxygen content is 15 to 16 mL/dL.

Because hemoglobin transports all but a small fraction of the oxygen carried in arterial blood, increases in hemoglobin concentration affect the oxygen content of the blood. Decreases in hemoglobin concentration below the normal value of about 15 mL/dL of blood reduce oxygen content. Increases in hemoglobin concentration may increase oxygen content, minimizing the effect of impaired gas exchange. In fact, increased hemoglobin concentration is a major compensatory mechanism in pulmonary diseases that impair gas exchange. For this reason, measurement of hemoglobin concentration is important in assessing individuals with pulmonary disease. If cardiovascular function is normal, the body's initial response to low oxygen content is to accelerate cardiac output. In individuals who also have cardiovascular disease, this compensatory mechanism is ineffective. An elevated Hb level can compensate for an inability to accelerate cardiac output, making increased hemoglobin concentration an even more important compensatory mechanism.

Oxyhemoglobin Association and Dissociation. Oxyhemoglobin (HbO_2) forms when hemoglobin molecules bind with oxygen. Binding occurs in the lungs and is called *oxyhemoglobin association* or *hemoglobin saturation with oxygen* (Sao_2). The reverse process, where oxygen is released from hemoglobin, occurs in the body tissues at the cellular level and is called *hemoglobin desaturation*. When hemoglobin saturation and desaturation are plotted on a graph, the result is a distinctive S-shaped curve known as the oxyhemoglobin dissociation curve (Fig. 35.16). For Pao_2 values less than 60 mmHg, oxygen is readily unloaded to peripheral tissues and hemoglobin's affinity for oxygen diminishes, reflecting the steep part of the curve. For Pao_2 values greater than 60 mmHg, the curve becomes relatively flat, reflecting the maximum saturation of hemoglobin with oxygen in the lungs.

Several factors can change the relationship between Pao_2 and Sao_2 and influence hemoglobin's affinity for oxygen (see Fig. 35.16). At a Pao_2 of 26.6 mmHg, hemoglobin is 50% saturated, known as P_{50}. An increase in the P_{50} value shifts the curve to the right, indicating hemoglobin's decreased affinity for oxygen or an increase in the ease with which oxyhemoglobin dissociates and oxygen moves into the cells. A larger partial pressure is necessary to maintain 50% oxygen saturation. A shift to the left depicts hemoglobin's increased affinity for oxygen, which promotes association in the lungs and inhibits dissociation in the tissues. A lower partial pressure is necessary to maintain 50% oxygen saturation.

The oxyhemoglobin dissociation curve is shifted to the right by acidosis (low pH) and hypercapnia (increased $Paco_2$). In the tissues, increased levels of CO_2 and hydrogen ions produced by metabolic activity decrease the affinity of hemoglobin for oxygen. Hyperthermia and increased levels of 2,3-diphosphoglycerate (2,3-DPG, a substance normally present in erythrocytes) also shift the curve to the right. The curve is shifted to the left by alkalosis (high pH), hypocapnia (decreased $Paco_2$), hypothermia, and decreased 2,3-DPG levels.

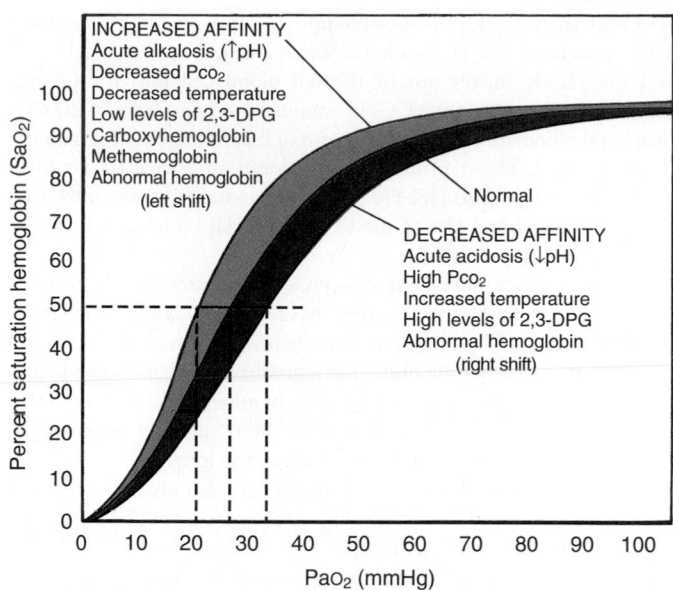

FIGURE 35.16 Oxyhemoglobin Dissociation Curve. The horizontal or flat segment of the curve at the top of the graph is the arterial or association portion, or that part of the curve where oxygen is bound to hemoglobin and occurs in the lungs. This portion of the curve is flat because partial pressure changes of oxygen between 60 and 100 mmHg do not significantly alter the percentage saturation of hemoglobin with oxygen and allow adequate hemoglobin saturation at a variety of altitudes. If the relationship between Sao_2 and Pao_2 was linear (in a downward sloping straight line) instead of flat between 60 and 100 mmHg, there would be inadequate saturation of hemoglobin with oxygen. The steep part of the oxyhemoglobin dissociation curve represents the rapid dissociation of oxygen from hemoglobin that occurs in the tissues. During this phase, there is rapid diffusion of oxygen from the blood into tissue cells. The P_{50} is the Pao_2 at which hemoglobin is 50% saturated, normally 26.6 mmHg. A lower than normal P_{50} represents increased affinity of hemoglobin for O_2; a high P_{50} is seen with decreased affinity. Note that variation from the normal is associated with decreased (low P_{50}) or increased (high P_{50}) availability of O_2 to tissues *(dashed lines)*. The shaded area shows the entire oxyhemoglobin dissociation curve under the same circumstances. *2,3-DPG,* 2,3-Diphosphoglycerate. (From Lane EE, Walker JF: *Clinical arterial blood gas analysis,* St Louis, 1987, Mosby.)

In the lungs, as CO_2 diffuses from the blood into the alveoli, the blood CO_2 level is reduced and the affinity of hemoglobin for oxygen is increased. The shift in the oxyhemoglobin dissociation curve caused by changes in CO_2 and hydrogen ion concentration in the blood is called the Bohr effect.

Carbon Dioxide Transport

Approximately 200 mL of CO_2 is produced by the tissues per minute at rest as a byproduct of cellular metabolism. This CO_2 equilibrates with carbonic acid (H_2CO_3) and must be eliminated continuously to prevent acidosis. The elimination of CO_2 by the lungs plays an important role in the regulation of acid-base balance (see Chapter 3).

CO_2 is carried in the blood in three ways: (1) dissolved in plasma, (2) transported as bicarbonate, and (3) combined with blood proteins to form carbamino compounds. As CO_2 diffuses out of the cells into the blood, it dissolves in the plasma. Approximately 10% of the total CO_2 in venous blood and 5% of the CO_2 in arterial blood are carried dissolved in the plasma. As CO_2 moves into the blood, it diffuses into the red blood cells. Within the red blood cells, CO_2, with the help of the enzyme carbonic anhydrase, combines with water to form carbonic acid and then quickly dissociates into H^+ and HCO_3^-. As carbonic acid dissociates, the H^+ binds to hemoglobin, where it is buffered, and the HCO_3^- moves out of the red blood cell into the plasma. Approximately 60% of the CO_2 in venous blood and 90% of the CO_2 in arterial blood are carried in the form of bicarbonate. The remainder combines with blood proteins, hemoglobin in particular, to form carbamino compounds (see Fig. 3.13). Approximately 30% of the CO_2 in venous blood and 5% of the CO_2 in arterial blood are carried as carbamino compounds.

CO_2 is 20 times more soluble than O_2 and diffuses quickly from the tissue cells into the blood. The amount of CO_2 that is able to enter the blood is enhanced by diffusion of oxygen out of the blood and into the cells. Reduced hemoglobin (hemoglobin that is dissociated from oxygen) is able to carry more CO_2 than hemoglobin that is saturated with O_2. Therefore, the drop in Sao_2 at the tissue level increases the ability of hemoglobin to carry CO_2 back to the lung.

The diffusion gradient for CO_2 in the lung is only approximately 6 mmHg (venous $Pvco_2 = 46$ mmHg; alveolar $Paco_2 = 40$ mmHg), yet CO_2 is so soluble in the alveolocapillary membrane that the CO_2 in the blood quickly diffuses into the alveoli, where it is removed from the lung with each expiration. Diffusion of CO_2 in the lung is so efficient that diffusion defects that cause hypoxemia (low oxygen content of the blood) do not cause hypercapnia (excessive CO_2 in the blood).

The diffusion of CO_2 out of the blood also is enhanced by oxygen binding with hemoglobin in the lung. As hemoglobin binds with O_2, the amount of CO_2 carried by the blood is decreased. Thus in the tissue capillaries, O_2 dissociation from hemoglobin facilitates the pickup of CO_2, and the binding of O_2 to hemoglobin in the lungs facilitates the release of CO_2 from the blood. This effect of oxygen on CO_2 transport is called the Haldane effect.

TESTS OF PULMONARY FUNCTION

Several laboratory tests aid in the diagnosis and evaluation of pulmonary system abnormalities. Most of them are easy to perform at hospitals and clinics. They provide valuable information about the possible cause of a respiratory abnormality and evaluate the progression or resolution of disease.[22] Spirometry measures the volume and flow of air inhaled and exhaled and is plotted against time (flow rate) during different breathing maneuvers. Several different types of spirometer are available. The procedure produces a spirogram, which is a record of the individual's ventilation in relation to time (Fig. 35.17). Clinically the most important spirometric tests are the forced vital capacity (FVC) and the forced expiratory volume in 1 second (FEV₁). (These tests and other important measurements are described in Table 35.3.) Spirometry enables clinicians to detect restrictive or obstructive deficits early in the course of disease. *Restrictive lung diseases* restrict the lungs' volume; the lungs are unable to expand normally, diminishing the amount of gas that can be inspired and reducing the FVC. *Obstructive lung diseases* affect gas flow; airflow into and out of the lungs is obstructed, reducing the FEV₁.

Lung capacities, such as vital capacity (sum of inspiratory reserve volume, tidal volume, and expiratory reserve volume) and total lung capacity (sum of the vital capacity and the residual capacity), are always the sum of two or more volumes. Norms for volumes and capacities are based on age, sex, and height and are referred to as *predicted values*. Differences from predicted or changes from baseline values are taken into account in diagnosing and assessing respiratory disorders.

Pulmonary diffusing capacity (transfer factor) is a measure of the rate of gas diffusion across the alveolocapillary membrane. Oxygen, or more commonly carbon monoxide, is used to measure diffusing capacity. Carbon monoxide has high affinity for hemoglobin and is not limited by pulmonary blood flow and therefore is an excellent measure of

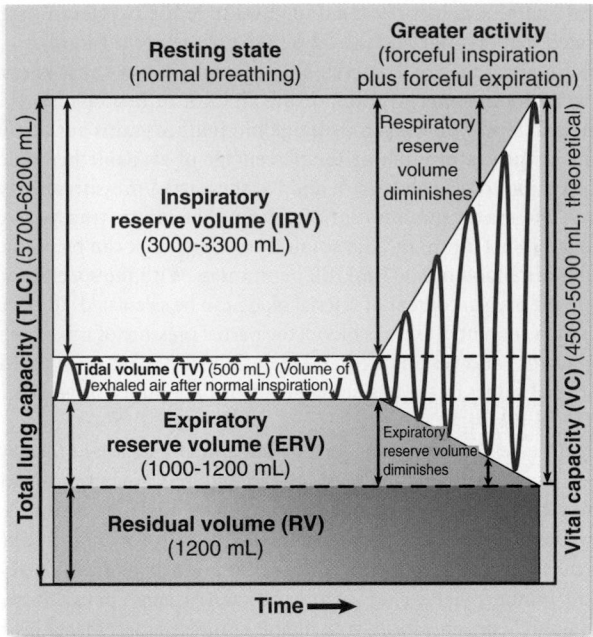

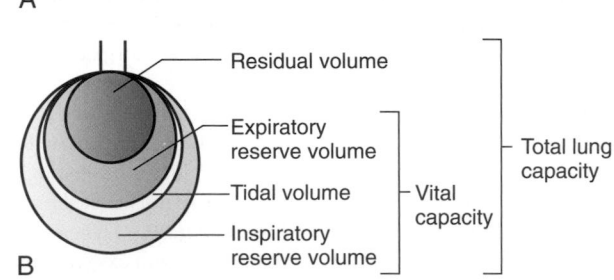

FIGURE 35.17 Pulmonary Ventilation and Lung Capacities. **A,** Spirogram. During normal, quiet respirations the atmosphere and lungs exchange about 500 mL of air (V_T). With a forcible inspiration, about 3300 mL more air can be inhaled *(IRV)*. After a normal inspiration and normal expiration, approximately 1000 mL more air can be forcibly expired *(ERV)*. Vital capacity is the amount of air that can be forcibly expired after a maximal inspiration and indicates, therefore, the largest amount of air that can enter and leave the lungs during respiration. Residual volume *(RV)* is the air that remains trapped in the alveoli. **B,** Lung capacities. (From Patton KT, Thibodeau GA: *The human body in health & disease,* ed 7, St Louis, 2018, Mosby.)

diffusion. The measurement is made by determining how much carbon monoxide is taken up by the blood and dividing this amount by the pressure gradient across the alveolocapillary membrane. Helium (an inert gas poorly soluble in alveolar blood and lung tissue) often is added to the gas mixture to obtain a simultaneous measurement of residual volume (RV), functional residual capacity (FRC), and total lung capacity (TLC). Individuals are asked to perform ventilatory maneuvers similar to those used in spirometry testing. A decreased diffusing capacity can be the result of an abnormal ventilation-perfusion ratio or an actual diffusion defect. For example, diffusing capacity is decreased in individuals with emphysema, where there is a decrease in the surface area of pulmonary capillaries available for gas exchange.

Oximetry is commonly performed for individuals with suggested or diagnosed pulmonary disease. It indirectly measures hemoglobin oxygen saturation and can suggest that the Pao_2 is low. However, it is prone to inaccurate measurements, particularly in individuals with poor peripheral circulation, and does not measure the $Paco_2$ or pH of the blood. Capnography measures the amount of CO_2 in expired air and thus estimates Paco2, but this test is also prone to inaccuracy. Arterial blood gas analysis is the direct measurement of the pH and gas concentrations in arterial blood and provides more accurate and complete information about an individual's gas exchange and acid-base status. Acidosis (low pH), alkalosis (high pH), ventilatory alterations, and decreased Pao2 can be diagnosed accurately only by arterial blood gas analysis. A blood gas report may be divided into an acid-base/ventilation portion and an oxygenation portion. (Normal values for arterial blood gases are given in Table 35.4; acid-base alterations are described in Chapter 3.) Oximetry can be used to monitor oxygen saturation once the arterial blood gas analysis has accurately measured the Pao2, but it does not measure Paco2 or pH.

Signs and symptoms of most respiratory abnormalities first appear when the system is stressed during exercise. Therefore, if pulmonary disease is suspected, the individual is evaluated at rest and during exercise. Evaluation during exercise usually entails spirometry and oximetry to monitor hemoglobin saturation. The exercise usually consists of riding a stationary bicycle or walking on a treadmill. Exercise testing enables clinicians to detect early changes in respiratory function and thus begin treatment. Exercise tests also are used in planning and evaluating exercise and rehabilitation programs.

Thoracic imaging techniques are among the most common examinations for diagnosis and detection of pulmonary disease and tumors and for evaluation of disease progression. Numerous techniques are available and include chest radiography, computed tomography (CT), magnetic resonance imaging (MRI), positron emission tomography, and ultrasonography. Pulmonary angiography is used for detection of pulmonary embolism and pulmonary arteriovenous malformations. Techniques may be combined for the best evaluation of pulmonary structure and function.

AGING AND THE PULMONARY SYSTEM

Most knowledge about pulmonary structure and function is based on norms for the middle-age years. Less is known about structure and function in the very young (see Chapter 37) and in older adults, but a few normal physiologic (developmental and degenerative) changes are known to occur from birth to old age. An understanding of these changes is needed to provide appropriate care and to differentiate between age-associated alterations and disease. Normal alterations in the pulmonary system include (1) loss of elastic recoil, (2) stiffening of the chest wall, (3) changes in gas exchange, and (4) increases in flow resistance. These changes, which affect lung volumes, are gradual and usually without adverse consequences in healthy individuals (Fig. 35.18). They are influenced by genetics, sociocultural factors, nutritional status, exercise, decreased immune function, respiratory disease, body size, sex, and race. Exposure to environmental toxins, such as some respiratory

TABLE 35.3 VALUES MEASURED BY SPIROMETRY

SYMBOL	VENTILATORY PROPERTY MEASURED
FVC	Forced vital capacity; maximum amount of gas that can be displaced from the lung during a forced expiration
FEV_1	Forced expiratory volume in 1 second; maximum amount of air that can be expired from the lung in 1 second
FEV_1/FVC	Percentage of maximum inspiration that is expired in 1 second; usually 80% of FVC
FEV_3	Forced expiratory volume in 3 seconds; maximum amount of gas that can be expired in 3 seconds
FEV_3/FVC	Percentage of FVC that is expired in 3 seconds; usually 95% of FVC
$FEF_{25-75\%}$	Forced expiratory flow rate during the middle 50% of expiration; sometimes reported as maximum midexpiratory flow rate (MMFR)
MVV	Maximum voluntary ventilation
PEF	Peak expiratory flow

TABLE 35.4 NORMAL RANGES FOR ARTERIAL AND MIXED VENOUS BLOOD GASES

MEASUREMENT	ARTERIAL BLOOD	MIXED VENOUS BLOOD*	CLINICAL NOTES
Acid-base status (pH)	7.35–7.45	7.33–7.43	Most important acid-base value; detects acidosis or alkalosis
Partial pressure of carbon dioxide (Pco_2)	35–45 mmHg	41–57 mmHg	Measures adequacy of ventilation and respiratory contribution of acid-base abnormality (respiratory acidosis)
Bicarbonate concentration (HCO_3^-)	22–26 mEq/L	24–28 mEq/L	Measures metabolic contribution to acid-base abnormality (metabolic acidosis); calculated from pH and Pco_2
Base excess (BE)	−2 to +2	0 to +4	Reflects deviation of bicarbonate concentration from normal
Partial pressure of oxygen (Po_2) (sea level)	80–100 mmHg	35–40 mmHg	Indicates driving pressure that causes oxyhemoglobin binding; varies with age and barometric pressure
Saturation of hemoglobin with oxygen (So_2)	96%–98%	70%–75%	Indicates abnormalities of oxyhemoglobin association and dissociation; may be measured directly or calculated from Pco_2, pH, and body temperature
Concentration of hemoglobin in the blood	15 g/dL	15 g/dL	Detects alterations of gas transport caused by anemia

*Mixed venous (pulmonary artery) blood is analyzed for critically ill individuals and those undergoing cardiac catheterization (it is not practical to withdraw samples except from a pulmonary artery catheter). Mixed venous blood gas analysis, in conjunction with arterial analysis, provides important information about the adequacy of cardiac output and tissue oxygenation.

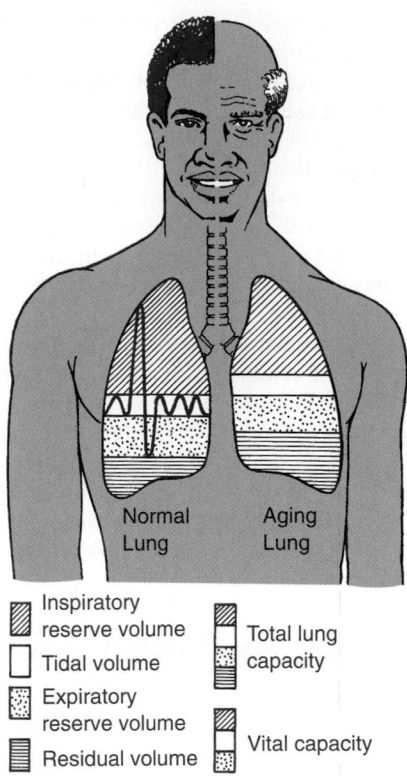

Inspiratory reserve volume

Tidal volume

Expiratory reserve volume

Residual volume

Total lung capacity

Vital capacity

FIGURE 35.18 Changes in Lung Volumes with Aging. In aging, vital capacity decreases and residual volume increases.

tract infections, tobacco smoke, air pollution, and occupational dusts, also contributes to decreased lung function with aging. These changes contribute to increased lung disease morbidity and mortality in older adults, including chronic obstructive lung disease, lung cancer, pulmonary fibrosis, and infection.[23]

During adulthood and as age advances, the alveoli tend to lose alveoli wall tissue and capillaries. This process increases alveolar size, diminishes the alveolar surface area available for gas diffusion, and decreases airway support provided by normal lung tissues. These changes are similar to those seen in emphysema and change the elastic properties of the lungs. Chest wall compliance decreases with age, because the ribs become ossified (less flexible) and the joints become stiffer. As a result the chest wall loses some of its ability to expand. In addition, respiratory muscle strength and endurance decrease by up to 20% by age 70. These mechanical changes in the lung and chest wall, along with structural changes in the alveoli, reduce the ventilatory capacity in older adults. Vital capacity decreases and residual volume increases; however, total lung capacity remains unchanged. These changes decrease ventilatory reserves and lead to decreased ventilation-perfusion ratios. With advancing age there is also increased immune dysregulation, asymptomatic low-grade inflammation ("inflamm-aging"), and increased risk of infection.[24]

Alterations in gas exchange are reflected by blood gas analysis. With advancing age, pH and $Paco_2$ levels do not change much, even though it has been documented that the chemoreceptors become less sensitive to gas partial pressures with age.[25] Older adults have a decreased compensatory response to hypercapnia and hypoxemia; however, the perception of dyspnea remains intact and is even enhanced. Pao_2 declines with age as a result of structural and mechanical changes, such as loss of alveolar surface area, thickening of plural septa, loss of lung elasticity, and increase in ventilation-perfusion mismatch. The maximum Pao_2 value in an older adult at sea level can be estimated by multiplying the person's age by 0.3 and subtracting the product from 100. For example, an 80-year-old individual would have an estimated maximum Pao_2 of 76 mmHg ($0.3 \times 80 = 24$; $100 - 24 = 76$).[26]

The decrease in Pao_2 and the diminished ventilatory reserve in an older adult lead to a decrease in exercise tolerance. Respiratory muscle strength and endurance decrease with age.[27] Furthermore, older adults are at greater risk for respiratory depression caused by medications. Changes in respiratory structure and function can vary considerably from person to person, however. Changes also are affected by activity and fitness earlier in life.[28]

SUMMARY REVIEW

Structures of the Pulmonary System

1. The pulmonary system consists of the two lungs, upper and lower airways, chest wall, diaphragm, and pulmonary and bronchial circulations.
2. Air is inspired and expired through the conducting airways, which include the nasopharynx, oropharynx, trachea, bronchi, and bronchioles to the sixteenth division.
3. Gas exchange occurs in structures beyond the sixteenth division: the respiratory bronchioles, alveolar ducts, and alveoli. Together these structures comprise the acinus.
4. The chief gas-exchange units of the lungs are the alveoli. The membrane that surrounds each alveolus and contains the pulmonary capillaries is called the *alveolocapillary membrane.*
5. The gas-exchange airways are served by the pulmonary circulation, a separate division of the circulatory system. The bronchi and other lung structures are served by a branch of the systemic circulation called the *bronchial circulation.*
6. The pulmonary circulation is innervated by the ANS, but vasodilation and vasoconstriction are controlled mainly by local and humoral factors, particularly arterial oxygenation and acid-base status.
7. Vasoconstriction of the pulmonary arterial system is caused by alveolar hypoxia, acidemia, and inflammatory mediators (histamine, serotonin, prostaglandins, and bradykinin).
8. The chest wall, which contains and protects the contents of the thoracic cavity, consists of the skin, ribs, and intercostal muscles, which lie between the ribs.
9. The chest wall is lined by a serous membrane called the *parietal pleura;* the lungs are encased in a separate membrane called the *visceral pleura.* The area where these two pleurae come into contact and slide over each another is called the *pleural space.*

Functions of the Pulmonary System

1. The pulmonary system enables oxygen to diffuse into the blood and CO_2 to diffuse out of the blood.
2. Ventilation is the process by which air flows into and out of the gas-exchange airways.
3. Ventilation is involuntary most of the time. It is controlled by the respiratory center in the brainstem and by the sympathetic and parasympathetic divisions of the ANS, which adjust airway caliber (by causing bronchial smooth muscle to contract or relax) and control the rate and depth of ventilation.

SUMMARY REVIEW—cont'd

4. Neuroreceptors in the lungs (lung receptors) monitor the mechanical aspects of ventilation. Irritant receptors sense the need to expel unwanted substances and stretch receptors sense lung volume (lung expansion), and J-receptors sense alveolar size.

5. Chemoreceptors in the circulatory system and brainstem sense the effectiveness of ventilation by monitoring the pH status of cerebrospinal fluid and the oxygen and carbon dioxide content of arterial blood (Pao_2 and $Paco_2$).

6. Successful ventilation involves the mechanics of breathing: the interaction of forces and counterforces involving the muscles of inspiration and expiration, alveolar surface tension, elastic properties of the lungs and chest wall, and resistance to airflow.

7. The major muscle of inspiration is the diaphragm. When the diaphragm contracts, it moves downward in the thoracic cavity, creating a vacuum that causes air to flow into the lungs. There are no major muscles in expiration. Normal elastic recoil permits passive expiration.

8. The alveoli produce surfactant, created by type II alveolar cells. Surfactant is a lipoprotein that lines the alveoli. Surfactant reduces alveolar surface tension and permits the alveoli to expand more easily with air intake.

9. Elastic recoil is the tendency of the lungs and chest wall to return to their resting states after inspiration. The elastic recoil forces of the lungs and chest wall are in opposition and pull on each other, creating the normally negative pressure of the pleural space.

10. Compliance is a measure of lung and chest wall distensibility during inspiration. Lung compliance is determined by the adequate production of surfactant and the elastic recoil of the lungs and chest wall.

11. Airway resistance is determined by the length, radius, and cross-sectional area of the airways and by the density, viscosity, and velocity of the gas. Airway resistance is normally very low because of the large cross-sectional area of the lungs.

12. The work of breathing is determined by the muscular effort (i.e., the energy required to achieve adequate oxygenation) necessary for ventilation.

13. Gas transport depends on ventilation of the alveoli, diffusion across the alveolocapillary membrane, perfusion of the pulmonary and systemic capillaries, and diffusion between systemic capillaries and tissue cells.

14. Efficient gas exchange depends on an even distribution of ventilation and perfusion within the lungs. Ventilation and perfusion are greatest in the bases of the lungs because the alveoli in the bases are more compliant, and perfusion is greater as a result of gravity.

15. Almost all of the oxygen that diffuses into pulmonary capillary blood is transported by hemoglobin, a protein contained within red blood cells. The remainder of the oxygen is transported dissolved in plasma.

16. Oxygen enters the body by diffusing down the concentration gradient, from high concentrations in the alveoli to lower concentrations in the capillaries. Diffusion ceases when alveolar and capillary oxygen pressures equilibrate.

17. Oxygen is loaded onto hemoglobin by the driving pressure exerted by Pao_2 in the plasma. As pressure decreases at tissue level, oxygen dissociates from hemoglobin and enters tissue cells by diffusion, again down the concentration gradient.

18. CO_2 is more soluble in plasma than oxygen is and diffuses readily from tissue cells into plasma. CO_2 returns to the lungs dissolved in plasma, transported as bicarbonate, or combined with blood proteins to form carbamino compounds (e.g., bound to hemoglobin).

Tests of Pulmonary Function

1. Spirometry measures the volume and flow rate of air during forced expiration.

2. The alveolar-arterial oxygen gradient is used to evaluate the cause of hypoxia.

3. Diffusing capacity is a measure of the gas diffusion rate at the alveolocapillary membrane.

4. Arterial blood gas analysis can be used to determine pH and oxygen and CO_2 concentrations.

5. Thoracic imaging techniques are used to detect pulmonary disease and tumors and to evaluate disease progression.

Aging and the Pulmonary System

1. Aging affects the mechanical aspects of ventilation by decreasing chest wall compliance and elastic recoil of the lungs. Changes in these elastic properties reduce ventilatory reserve.

2. Aging causes loss of alveolar wall tissue and alveolar enlargement, thus diminishing the surface area available for gas diffusion.

3. Aging can cause the Pao_2 level to decrease but does not affect the $Paco_2$ level.

4. Vital capacity decreases and residual volume increases with age; however, total lung capacity remains unchanged.

KEY TERMS

KEY TERMS—cont'd

REFERENCES

1. Bautista TG, Sun QJ, Pilowsky PM: The generation of pharyngeal phase of swallow and its coordination with breathing: interaction between the swallow and respiratory central pattern generators. *Prog Brain Res* 212:253–275, 2014.

2. Ochs MD, et al: The number of alveoli in the human lung. *Am J Respir Crit Care Med* 169:120–124, 2004.

3. Olmeda B, Martínez-Calle M, Pérez-Gil J: Pulmonary surfactant metabolism in the alveolar airspace: biogenesis, extracellular conversions, recycling. *Ann Anat* 209:78–92, 2017.

4. Byrne AJ, et al: Pulmonary macrophages: key players in the innate defence of the airways. *Thorax* 70(12):1189–1196, 2015.

5. Esfandiari S, et al: Pulmonary artery wedge pressure relative to exercise work rate in older men and women. *Med Sci Sports Exerc* 49(7):1297–1304, 2017.

6. West JB: Fragility of pulmonary capillaries. *J Appl Physiol* 115(1):1–15, 2013.

7. Walker CM, et al: Bronchial arteries: anatomy, function, hypertrophy, and anomalies. *Radiographics* 35(1):32–49, 2015.

8. Sozio F, et al: Morphometric analysis of intralobular, interlobular and pleural lymphatics in normal human lung. *J Anat* 220(4):396–404, 2012.

9. Lai N, Lu W, Wang J: Ca^{2+} and ion channels in hypoxia-mediated pulmonary hypertension. *Int J Clin Exp Pathol* 8(2):1081–1092, 2015.

10. Urfy MZ, Suarez JI: Breathing and the nervous system. *Handb Clin Neurol* 119:241–250, 2014.

11. Guyenet PG, Bayliss DA: Neural control of breathing and CO_2 homeostasis. *Neuron* 87(5):946–961, 2015.

12. Dempsey JA, Smith CA: Pathophysiology of human ventilatory control. *Eur Respir J* 44(2):495–512, 2014.

13. Taylor-Clark TE: Peripheral neural circuitry in cough. *Curr Opin Pharmacol* 22:9–17, 2015.

14. Landolfo F, et al: Hering-Breuer reflex, lung volume and position in prematurely born infants. *Pediatr Pulmonol* 43(8):767–771, 2008.

15. Anand A, et al: Dyspnea in Eisenmenger syndrome and its amelioration by sildenafil: role of J receptors. *Int J Cardiol* 174(3):574–578, 2014.

16. Mazzone SB, Undem BJ: Vagal afferent innervation of the airways in health and disease. *Physiol Rev* 96(3):975–1024, 2016.

17. De Troyer A, Boriek AM: Mechanics of the respiratory muscles. *Compr Physiol* 1(3):1273–1300, 2011.

18. Lumb AB: *Nunn's applied respiratory physiology*, ed 7, St Louis, 2010, Elsevier.

19. Kaminsky DA: What does airway resistance tell us about lung function? *Respir Care* 57(1):85–96, discussion 96–99, 2012.

20. Wagner PD: The physiological basis of pulmonary gas exchange: implications for clinical interpretation of arterial blood gases. *Eur Respir J* 45(1):227–243, 2015.

21. Robertson HT: Dead space: the physiology of wasted ventilation. *Eur Respir J* 45(6):1704–1716, 2015.

22. Gold WM, Doth LL: Pulmonary function testing. In *Murray & Nadel's textbook of respiratory medicine*, ed 6, Philadelphia, 2016, Saunders, pp 407–435.

23. Thannickal VJ, et al: Blue journal conference. Aging and susceptibility to lung disease. *Am J Respir Crit Care Med* 191(3):261–269, 2015.

24. Brandenberger C, Mühlfeld C: Mechanisms of lung aging. *Cell Tissue Res* 367(3):469–480, 2017.

25. Dyer C: The interaction of ageing and lung disease. *Chron Respir Dis* 9(1):63–67, 2012.

26. Hardie JA, et al: Reference values for arterial blood gases in the elderly. *Chest* 125(6):2053–2060, 2004.

27. Lowery EM, et al: The aging lung. *Clin Interv Aging* 8:1489–1496, 2013.

28. Kim J, Im JS, Choi YH: Objectively measured sedentary behavior and moderate-to-vigorous physical activity on the health-related quality of life in US adults: the National Health and Nutrition Examination Survey 2003–2006. *Qual Life Res* 25(6):1315–1326, 2017.

Alterations of Pulmonary Function

Valentina L. Brashers, Sue E. Huether

CHAPTER OUTLINE

Pulmonary disease is often classified as acute or chronic, obstructive or restrictive, and infectious or noninfectious. The symptoms and signs of lung disease, such as dyspnea and tachypnea, are common and associated not only with primary lung disorders but also with diseases of other organ systems, particularly the heart.

CLINICAL MANIFESTATIONS OF PULMONARY ALTERATIONS

Signs and Symptoms of Pulmonary Disease

Pulmonary disease is associated with many signs and symptoms and their specific characteristics often help in identifying the underlying disorder. The most common are dyspnea and cough. Others include abnormal sputum, hemoptysis, altered breathing patterns, hypoventilation and hyperventilation, cyanosis, clubbing of the digits, and chest pain.

Dyspnea

Dyspnea is a subjective experience of breathing discomfort and is the most common symptom of cardiac and respiratory diseases. It also can occur with pain, trauma, anxiety, and psychogenic disorders. The experience derives from interactions among multiple physiologic, psychologic, social, and environmental factors, and it may induce secondary physiologic and behavioral responses. The American Thoracic Society proposes that dyspnea evolves across three different constructs: sensory (intensity), affective (distress), and impact on daily activities.[1] It is comprised of qualitatively distinct sensations that vary in intensity. Individuals with dyspnea may complain of breathlessness, air hunger, shortness of breath, increased work of breathing, chest tightness, and preoccupation with breathing.

The severity of the experience of dyspnea may not directly correlate with the severity of the underlying disease. Either diffuse or focal disturbances of ventilation, gas exchange, or ventilation-perfusion relationships can cause dyspnea, as can increased work of breathing or diseases that damage lung tissue (lung parenchyma). Neurophysiologic mechanisms for dyspnea involve an impaired sense of effort where the perceived work of breathing is greater than the actual motor response generated. Stimulation of a variety of receptors can contribute to the sensation experience of dyspnea, including lower airway mechanoreceptors (the stretch receptors, irritant receptors, and C-fiber receptors [*J*-receptors]), upper airway receptors, and central and peripheral chemoreceptors that interact with the respiratory center and the sensory and motor cortex.[2] The more severe signs of dyspnea include flaring of the nostrils and use of accessory muscles of respiration. Retraction (pulling back) of the supracostal or intercostal spaces predominates in children. In dyspnea caused by parenchymal disease (e.g., pneumonia), retractions of tissue between the ribs (subcostal and intercostal retractions) are observed more often than supercostal retractions (retractions of tissues above the ribs), which predominate in upper airway obstruction. Retractions of any type are more commonly seen in children or in adults who are thin and have poorly developed thoracic musculature. Dyspnea can be quantified by the use of ordinal rating scales or visual analog scales.[3]

Dyspnea can occur transiently or can become chronic. Dyspnea first presents during exercise and is called **dyspnea on exertion**. **Orthopnea** is dyspnea that occurs during heart failure when an individual is recumbent, which causes the abdominal contents to exert pressure on the diaphragm and decreases the efficiency of the respiratory muscles. **Paroxysmal nocturnal dyspnea (PND)** occurs when individuals with pulmonary or cardiac disease awake at night gasping for air and must sit up or stand to relieve the dyspnea.

Cough

Cough is a protective reflex that helps clear the airways by an explosive expiration. Inhaled particles, accumulated mucus, inflammation, or the presence of a foreign body initiates the cough reflex by stimulating irritant receptors in the airway. There are few such receptors in the most distal bronchi and the alveoli; thus it is possible for significant amounts of secretions to accumulate in the distal respiratory tree without cough being initiated. Stimulation of cough receptors is transmitted centrally through the vagus nerve. The cough reflex consists of inspiration of air, closure of the glottis and vocal cords, contraction of the expiratory muscles, and reopening of the glottis, causing a sudden, forceful expiration that removes the offending matter. The effectiveness of the cough depends on the depth of the inspiration and the degree to which the airways narrow, increasing the velocity of expiratory gas flow. Somatosensory nerves innervating the chest wall, diaphragm, and abdominal musculature regulate cough patterning and sensitivity. Cough occurs frequently in healthy individuals, and those with an inability to cough effectively are at greater risk for pneumonia. Cough, the urge-to-cough sensation, and the cough motor response can be manipulated by distraction and cognitive states, such as anxiety, reflecting a voluntary component of cough.[4] Central modulation of the cough reflex can be influenced by opiates and serotonergic agents.[5]

Acute cough is cough that resolves within 2 to 3 weeks of the onset of illness or resolves with treatment of the underlying condition. It is most commonly the result of upper respiratory tract infections, allergic rhinitis, acute bronchitis, pneumonia, congestive heart failure, pulmonary embolus, or aspiration. **Chronic cough** is defined as cough that has persisted for more than 3 weeks, although some researchers have suggested that 7 or 8 weeks is a more appropriate timeframe because acute cough and bronchial hyperreactivity can be prolonged in some cases of viral infection. In persons who do not smoke, chronic cough is commonly caused by postnasal drainage syndrome, nonasthmatic eosinophilic bronchitis, asthma, gastroesophageal reflux disease, or heightened cough reflex sensitivity.[6] In those individuals who smoke, chronic bronchitis is the most common cause of chronic cough, although lung cancer must always be considered. Individuals taking angiotensin-converting enzyme inhibitors for hypertension may develop chronic cough that resolves with discontinuation of the drug.

Abnormal Sputum

Changes in the amount, consistency, color, and odor of **sputum** provide information about the progression of disease and the effectiveness of therapy. The gross and microscopic appearances of sputum enable the clinician to identify cellular debris or microorganisms that aid in diagnosis and choice of therapy.

Hemoptysis is the expectoration of blood or bloody secretions from the lower respiratory tract. This is sometimes confused with hematemesis, which is the vomiting of blood. Blood that is expectorated is usually bright red, has an alkaline pH, and is mixed with frothy sputum. Blood that is vomited is dark, has an acidic pH, and is mixed with food particles.

Hemoptysis usually indicates infection or inflammation that damages the bronchi (bronchitis, bronchiectasis) or the lung parenchyma (pneumonia, tuberculosis, lung abscess). Other causes include cancer and pulmonary infarction. The amount and duration of bleeding provide important clues about its source. Bronchoscopy, combined with chest imaging, is used to confirm the site of bleeding.[7]

Abnormal Breathing Patterns

Normal breathing (eupnea) is rhythmic and effortless. The ventilatory rate is 8 to 16 breaths per minute, and the tidal volume ranges from 400 to 800 mL. A short expiratory pause occurs with each breath, and the individual takes an occasional deeper breath or sigh. Sigh breaths, which help maintain normal lung function, are usually 1.5 to 2 times the normal tidal volume and occur approximately 10 to 12 times per hour.

The rate, depth, regularity, and effort of breathing undergo characteristic alterations in response to physiologic and pathophysiologic conditions. Patterns of breathing automatically adjust to minimize the work of respiratory muscles. Strenuous exercise or metabolic acidosis induces **Kussmaul respirations (hyperpnea)**. Kussmaul respirations are characterized by a slightly increased ventilatory rate, very large tidal volume, and no expiratory pause.

Labored breathing occurs whenever there is an increased work of breathing, especially if the airways are obstructed, as in chronic obstructive pulmonary disease (COPD). If the large airways are obstructed, a slowed ventilatory rate, increased effort, prolonged inspiration or expiration, and stridor (high-pitched sounds made during inspiration) or audible wheezing (whistling sounds on expiration) are typical. In small airway obstruction, like that seen in asthma and chronic obstructive pulmonary disease, a rapid ventilatory rate, small tidal volume, increased effort, prolonged expiration, and wheezing are often present. *Restricted breathing* is commonly caused by disorders such as pulmonary fibrosis that stiffen the lungs or chest wall and decrease compliance, resulting in small tidal volumes and rapid ventilatory rate (tachypnea).

Shock and severe cerebral hypoxia (insufficient oxygen in the brain) contribute to gasping respirations that consist of irregular, quick inspirations with an expiratory pause. Anxiety can cause sighing respirations that consist of irregular breathing characterized by frequent, deep sighing inspirations. **Cheyne-Stokes respirations** are characterized by alternating periods of deep and shallow breathing. Apnea lasting 15 to 60 seconds is followed by ventilations that increase in volume until a peak is reached, after which ventilation (tidal volume) decreases again to apnea. Cheyne-Stokes respirations result from any condition that slows the blood flow to the brainstem, which in turn slows impulses sending information to the respiratory centers of the brainstem. Neurologic impairment above the brainstem is also a contributing factor (see Table 17.4 and Fig. 17.1).

Hypoventilation and Hyperventilation

Hypoventilation is inadequate alveolar ventilation in relation to metabolic demands. Hypoventilation occurs when the minute volume (tidal volume × respiratory rate) is reduced. It is caused by alterations in pulmonary mechanics or in the neurologic control of breathing. When alveolar ventilation is normal, carbon dioxide (CO_2) is removed from the lungs at the same rate at which it is produced by cellular metabolism, and arterial CO_2 pressure ($Paco_2$) remains at normal levels (40 mmHg).

With hypoventilation, CO_2 removal lags behind CO_2 production and $Paco_2$ increases, causing hypercapnia ($Paco_2$ greater than 44 mmHg). (Table 35.1 contains the definition of gas partial pressure and other pulmonary abbreviations.) This results in an increase in hydrogen ion concentration in the blood, termed respiratory acidosis, which can affect the function of many tissues throughout the body.

Hypoventilation is often overlooked until it is severe because breathing pattern and ventilatory rate may appear normal, and changes in tidal volume can be difficult to detect clinically. Blood gas analysis (i.e., measurement of the $Paco_2$ level of arterial blood) or capnography (i.e., measurement of the CO_2 concentration in expired air) reveals the hypoventilation (hypercapnia). Pronounced hypoventilation can cause somnolence or disorientation and secondary hypoxemia because the accumulation of alveolar CO_2 displaces oxygen (see Hypercapnia under Conditions Caused by Pulmonary Disease or Injury).

Hyperventilation is alveolar ventilation that exceeds metabolic demands. The lungs remove CO_2 at a higher rate than it is produced by cellular metabolism, resulting in decreased $Paco_2$ or **hypocapnia** ($Paco_2$ less than 36 mmHg). Hypocapnia results in respiratory alkalosis that also can interfere with tissue function. Like hypoventilation, hyperventilation can be verified by arterial blood gas analysis or capnography. Hyperventilation commonly occurs with severe anxiety, acute head injury, and conditions that cause hypoxemia.

Cyanosis

Cyanosis is a bluish discoloration of the skin and mucous membranes caused by increasing amounts of desaturated or reduced hemoglobin (which is bluish) in the blood. It generally develops when 5 g of hemoglobin is desaturated, regardless of hemoglobin concentration.

Peripheral cyanosis (slow blood circulation in fingers and toes) is most often caused by poor circulation resulting from intense peripheral vasoconstriction, like that seen in Raynaud's disease, cold environments, or severe stress. Peripheral cyanosis is best seen in the nail beds. *Central cyanosis* is caused by decreased arterial oxygenation (low Pao_2) from pulmonary diseases or pulmonary or cardiac right-to-left shunts. Central cyanosis is best seen in buccal mucous membranes and lips.

Lack of cyanosis does not necessarily indicate that oxygenation is normal. In adults, cyanosis is not evident until severe hypoxemia is present and, therefore, is an insensitive indication of respiratory failure. Severe anemia (inadequate hemoglobin concentration) and carbon monoxide poisoning (in which hemoglobin binds with carbon monoxide instead of binding with oxygen) can result in inadequate oxygenation of tissues without causing cyanosis. Individuals with polycythemia (an abnormal increase in numbers of red blood cells), however, may have cyanosis when tissue oxygenation is adequate. Therefore the significance of cyanosis as a clinical finding must be interpreted in relation to the underlying pathophysiology. If cyanosis is observed, the Pao_2 level should be measured.

Clubbing

Clubbing is the selective bulbous enlargement of the end (distal segment) of a digit (finger or toe) (Fig. 36.1); its severity can be graded from 1 to 5 based on the extent of nail bed hypertrophy and the number of changes in the nails themselves. It is usually painless and develops gradually over weeks. Clubbing is commonly associated with diseases that disrupt the normal pulmonary circulation and cause chronic hypoxemia, such as bronchiectasis, cystic fibrosis, pulmonary fibrosis, lung abscess, and congenital heart disease. It is rarely reversible with treatment of the underlying pulmonary condition.

Although the pathogenesis of clubbing is unknown, the megakaryocyte hypothesis proposes that megakaryocytes and platelet clumps escape filtration in the pulmonary bed and enter the systemic circulation.

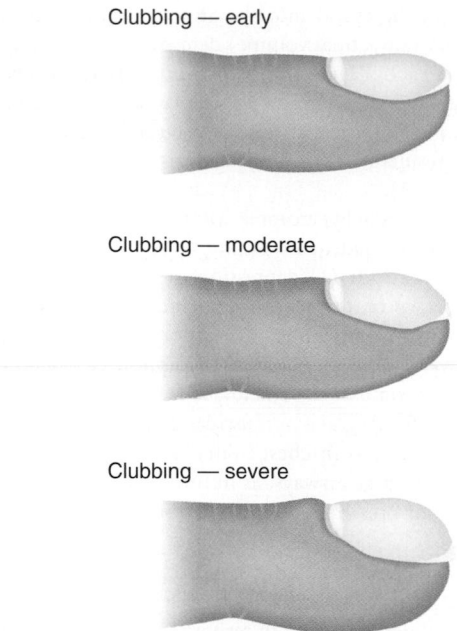

Clubbing — early

Clubbing — moderate

Clubbing — severe

FIGURE 36.1 Clubbing of Fingers Caused by Chronic Hypoxemia. (From Seidel HM et al: *Mosby's guide to physical examination,* ed 7, St Louis, 2011, Mosby.)

Platelets may then release platelet-derived growth factor at the nail bed, causing periosteal changes. *Secondary hypertrophic osteoarthropathy* can sometimes be seen in individuals with lung cancer even without hypoxemia because of the effects of inflammatory cytokines and growth factors.[8]

Pain

Pain caused by pulmonary disorders originates in the pleurae, airways, or chest wall.[9] Pleural pain is the most common pain caused by pulmonary disease and is usually sharp or stabbing in character. Infection and inflammation of the parietal pleura (pleuritis or pleurisy) cause pain when the pleurae stretch during inspiration. The pain is usually localized to a portion of the chest wall, where a unique breath sound called a *pleural friction rub* may be heard over the painful area. Laughing or coughing makes pleural pain worse.

Infection and inflammation either of the trachea or of the trachea and bronchi (tracheitis or tracheobronchitis, respectively) can cause central chest pain that is pronounced after coughing. Central chest pain can be difficult to differentiate from cardiac pain (see Chapter 33). High blood pressure in the pulmonary circulation (pulmonary hypertension) can cause pain during exercise that is often mistaken for cardiac pain (angina pectoris). Pleural pain is also common with pulmonary infarction (tissue death) caused by pulmonary embolism and emanates from the area around the infarction.

Pain in the chest wall is muscle pain or rib pain. The common causes of chest wall pain are rib fractures and excessive coughing, which make the muscles sore. Inflammation of the costochondral junction (costochondritis) also can cause chest wall pain. Chest wall pain can often be reproduced by pressing on the sternum or ribs.

Conditions Caused by Pulmonary Disease or Injury
Hypercapnia

Hypercapnia, or increased CO_2 concentration in the arterial blood (increased $Paco_2$), is caused by hypoventilation of the alveoli. CO_2 is easily diffused from the blood into the alveolar space; thus minute volume (respiratory rate × tidal volume) determines not only alveolar ventilation but also $Paco_2$. Hypoventilation is often overlooked because the breathing pattern and ventilatory rate may appear normal; it is important to obtain blood gas analysis to determine the severity of hypercapnia and resultant respiratory acidosis (acid-base balance is described in Chapter 3).

There are many causes of hypercapnia. Most are a result of a decreased drive to breathe or an inadequate ability to respond to ventilatory stimulation. Causes include (1) depression of the respiratory center by drugs; (2) diseases of the medulla, including infections of the central nervous system or trauma; (3) abnormalities of the spinal conducting pathways, as in spinal cord disruption or poliomyelitis; (4) diseases of the neuromuscular junction or of the respiratory muscles themselves, as in myasthenia gravis or muscular dystrophy; (5) abnormalities of the thoracic cage, as in chest injury or congenital deformity; (6) obstruction of the large airways, as in tumors or sleep apnea; and (7) increased work of breathing or increased physiologic dead space, as in emphysema.

Hypercapnia and the associated respiratory acidosis can result in several important clinical manifestations. Of greatest concern are electrolyte abnormalities that occur in response to the low pH that may cause dysrhythmias. Individuals also may have somnolence and even be in a coma because of changes in intracranial pressure associated with high levels of arterial carbon dioxide, which causes cerebral vasodilation. Alveolar hypoventilation with increased alveolar carbon dioxide concentration limits the amount of alveolar oxygen available for diffusion into the blood, leading to secondary hypoxemia.

Hypoxemia

Hypoxemia, or reduced oxygenation of arterial blood (reduced Pao_2), is caused by respiratory alterations, whereas hypoxia (ischemia), or reduced oxygenation of cells in tissues, may be caused by alterations of other systems as well. Cyanosis, hypoxemia, and hypoxia can exist independently of each other but they are interrelated.[10] For example, although hypoxemia can lead to tissue hypoxia, tissue hypoxia can result from other abnormalities, such as low cardiac output or cyanide poisoning.

Hypoxemia results from problems with one or more of the major mechanisms of oxygenation[11]:

1. Oxygen delivery to the alveoli
   a. Oxygen content of the inspired air (Fio_2)
   b. Ventilation of the alveoli
2. Diffusion of oxygen from the alveoli into the blood
   a. Balance between alveolar ventilation and perfusion ($\dot{V}/\dot{Q}$ mismatch)
   b. Diffusion of oxygen across the alveolocapillary membrane
3. Perfusion of pulmonary capillaries

Table 36.1 lists some of the common clinical causes of these problems.

The partial pressure of oxygen in the alveoli is called PAO_2 and is dependent on two factors. The first factor is amount of oxygen in inspired air and is expressed as the percentage or fraction of air that is composed of oxygen, called the Fio_2. The Fio_2 of air at sea level is approximately 21% or 0.21. Anything that decreases the Fio_2 (such as high altitude) decreases the PAO_2. A second factor is the amount of alveolar minute ventilation (tidal volume × respiratory rate). Hypoventilation results in an increase in $PACO_2$ and a decrease in PAO_2 such that there is less oxygen available in the alveoli for diffusion into the blood. This type of hypoxemia can be completely corrected if alveolar ventilation is improved by increases in the rate and depth of breathing. Examples of conditions in which hypoventilation causes hypoxemia include

TABLE 36.1	CAUSES OF HYPOXEMIA
MECHANISM	**COMMON CLINICAL CAUSES**
Decrease in inspired oxygen (decreased Fio_2)	High altitude Low oxygen content of gas mixture Enclosed breathing spaces (suffocation)
Hypoventilation of the alveoli	Lack of neurologic stimulation of the respiratory center (oversedation, drug overdose, neurologic damage) Defects in chest wall mechanics (neuromuscular disease, trauma, chest deformity, air trapping) Large airway obstruction (laryngospasm, foreign body aspiration, neoplasm) Increased work of breathing (emphysema, severe asthma)
Ventilation-perfusion mismatch	Asthma Chronic bronchitis Pneumonia Acute respiratory distress syndrome Atelectasis Pulmonary embolism
Alveolocapillary diffusion abnormality	Edema Fibrosis Emphysema
Decreased pulmonary capillary perfusion	Intracardiac defects Intrapulmonary arteriovenous malformations

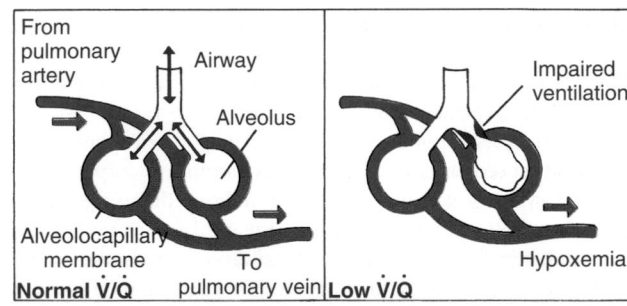

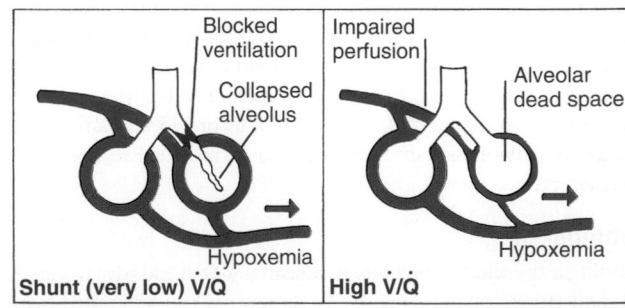

FIGURE 36.2 Ventilation-Perfusion Abnormalities. (Data from Glenny RW: *Adv Physiol Educ* 32[3]:192–195, 2008.)

unconsciousness; neurologic, muscular, or bone diseases that restrict chest expansion; and COPD.

Diffusion of oxygen from the alveoli into the blood is also dependent on two factors. The first is the balance between the amount of air getting into alveoli ($\dot{V}$) and the amount of blood perfusing the capillaries around the alveoli ($\dot{Q}$). An abnormal ventilation-perfusion ratio ($\dot{V}/\dot{Q}$) is the most common cause of hypoxemia (Fig. 36.2). In the healthy lung, alveolocapillary lung units receive almost equal amounts of ventilation and perfusion. The normal $\dot{V}/\dot{Q}$ is 0.8 to 0.9 because perfusion is somewhat greater than ventilation in the lung bases and because some blood is normally shunted to the bronchial circulation. $\dot{V}/\dot{Q}$ mismatch refers to an abnormal distribution of ventilation and perfusion. Hypoxemia can be caused by inadequate ventilation of well-perfused areas of the lung (low $\dot{V}/\dot{Q}$). Mismatching of this type, called shunting, occurs in atelectasis, in asthma as a result of bronchoconstriction, and in pulmonary edema and pneumonia when alveoli are filled with fluid. When blood passes through portions of the pulmonary capillary bed that receive no ventilation, right-to-left shunt occurs, resulting in decreased systemic PaO_2 and hypoxemia. Hypoxemia also can be caused by poor perfusion of well-ventilated portions of the lung (high $\dot{V}/\dot{Q}$), resulting in wasted ventilation. The most common cause of high $\dot{V}/\dot{Q}$ is a pulmonary embolus that impairs blood flow to a segment of the lung. An area where alveoli are ventilated but not perfused is termed alveolar dead space.

A second factor affecting diffusion of oxygen from the alveoli into the blood is the alveolocapillary barrier. Diffusion of oxygen through the alveolocapillary membrane is impaired if the alveolocapillary membrane is thickened or the surface area available for diffusion is decreased. Abnormal thickness, as occurs with edema (tissue swelling) and fibrosis (formation of fibrous lesions), increases the time required for diffusion across the alveolocapillary membrane. If diffusion is slowed enough, the oxygen in the alveolar gas (PAO_2) and capillary blood does not have time to equilibrate during the fraction of a second that blood remains in the capillary. Destruction of alveoli, such as that which occurs in emphysema, decreases the alveolocapillary membrane surface area available for diffusion. Hypercapnia is rarely produced by impaired diffusion, because carbon dioxide diffuses easily from capillary to alveolus even when oxygen diffusion is significantly impaired.

Hypoxemia also can result from blood flow bypassing the lungs. This can occur because of intracardiac defects that cause right-to-left shunting or because of intrapulmonary arteriovenous malformations. Administration of oxygen in these cases does not improve hypoxemia.

Hypoxemia is most often associated with a compensatory hyperventilation and resultant respiratory alkalosis (i.e., decreased $PaCO_2$ measurement and increased pH level). However, in individuals with associated ventilatory difficulties, hypoxemia may be complicated by hypercapnia and respiratory acidosis. Hypoxemia results in widespread tissue dysfunction and, when severe, can lead to organ infarction. In addition, hypoxic pulmonary vasoconstriction can contribute to increased pressures in the pulmonary artery (pulmonary artery hypertension) and lead to right-sided heart failure or *cor pulmonale* (see Cor Pulmonale under Pulmonary Vascular Disease). Clinical manifestations of acute hypoxemia may include cyanosis, confusion, tachycardia, edema, and decreased renal output.

Acute Respiratory Failure

Respiratory (lung) failure is defined as inadequate gas exchange, that is, hypoxemia in which PaO_2 is ≤50 mmHg or hypercapnia in which $PaCO_2$ is ≥50 mmHg with a pH ≤7.25.[12] Respiratory failure can result from direct injury to the lungs, airways, or chest wall or can occur indirectly as a result of disease or injury involving another body system, such as the brain, spinal cord, liver, or heart. It can occur in individuals who have an otherwise normal respiratory system or in those with underlying chronic pulmonary disease. Most pulmonary diseases can cause episodes of acute respiratory failure. If the respiratory failure is primarily hypercapnic, it is the result of inadequate alveolar ventilation (see Hypercapnia under Conditions Caused by Pulmonary Disease or Injury) and the individual must receive ventilatory support, such as

with a bag-valve mask, noninvasive positive pressure ventilation, or intubation and placement on mechanical ventilation. If the respiratory failure is primarily hypoxemic, it is the result of inadequate exchange of oxygen between the alveoli and the capillaries (see Hypoxemia under Conditions Caused by Pulmonary Disease or Injury) and the individual must receive supplemental oxygen therapy. Many individuals have a combined hypercapnic and hypoxemic respiratory failure and require both kinds of support.

Respiratory failure is an important potential complication of any major surgical procedure, especially those that involve the central nervous system, thorax, or upper abdomen. Persons who smoke are at risk, particularly if they have preexisting lung disease. Limited cardiac reserve, chronic renal failure, chronic hepatic disease, underlying lung disease, and infection also increase the tendency to develop postoperative respiratory failure. The most common postoperative pulmonary problems are atelectasis, pneumonia, pulmonary edema, and pulmonary emboli (these conditions are discussed later in this chapter).

Prevention of postoperative respiratory failure includes frequent turning and position changes, deep breathing exercises, incentive spirometry, avoidance of oversedation, and early ambulation to prevent atelectasis and accumulation of secretions. Incentive spirometry gives individuals immediate feedback about tidal volumes, which encourages them to breathe deeply. Supplemental oxygen is given for hypoxemia, and antibiotics are given as appropriate to treat infection. If respiratory failure develops, the individual may require conventional mechanical ventilation, high-frequency ventilation, or extracorporeal membrane oxygenation.[13]

DISORDERS OF THE CHEST WALL AND PLEURA
Disorders of the Chest Wall
Chest Wall Restriction

If the chest wall is deformed, traumatized, immobilized, or made heavy by fat, the work of breathing is increased and ventilation may be compromised because of a decrease in tidal volume. The degree of ventilatory impairment depends on the severity of the chest wall abnormality. Grossly obese individuals are often dyspneic on exertion or when recumbent. Individuals with severe kyphoscoliosis (bending and rotation of the spinal column with distortion of the thoracic cage) often present with dyspnea on exertion that can progress to respiratory failure. Obesity and kyphoscoliosis are risk factors for respiratory failure or infection in individuals admitted to a hospital for other problems, particularly those who require surgery. Other musculoskeletal abnormalities that can impair ventilation are ankylosing spondylitis and pectus excavatum (a deformity characterized by depression of the sternum) (see Chapters 45 and 46, respectively).

Impairment of respiratory muscle function caused by neuromuscular disease, such as poliomyelitis, muscular dystrophy, myasthenia gravis, and Guillain-Barré syndrome, also can restrict the chest wall or impair pulmonary function. Muscle weakness can result in hypoventilation and hypercapnia, inability to remove secretions, and hypoxemia.

Pain from chest wall injury, surgery, or disease can cause significant hypoventilation not only because of pain but also because of structural and mechanical changes that impair the ability of the chest to expand normally. Flail chest results from the fracture of several consecutive ribs in more than one place, or the fracture of the sternum and several consecutive ribs. These multiple fractures result in instability of a portion of the chest wall, causing paradoxical movement of the chest with breathing. During the negative intrathoracic pressure of inspiration, the unstable portion of the chest wall moves inward and during expiration it moves outward, impairing movement of gas in and out of the lungs (Fig. 36.3). Flail chest is usually associated with significant underlying

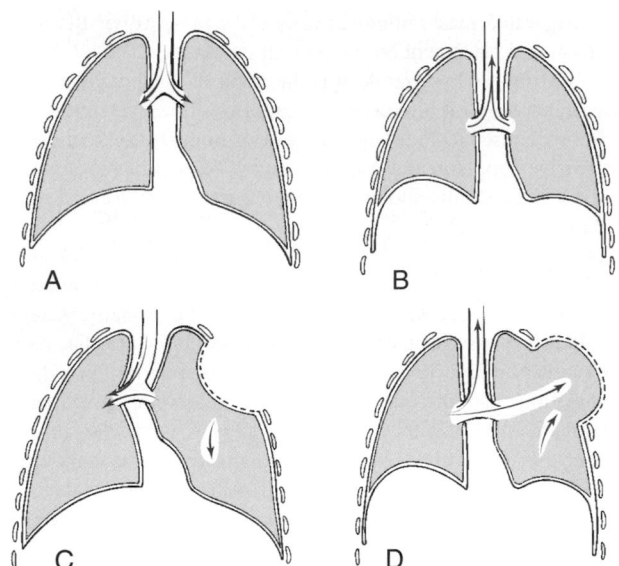

FIGURE 36.3 Flail Chest. Normal respiration: **A,** inspiration; **B,** expiration. Paradoxical motion: **C,** inspiration, area of lung underlying unstable chest wall sucks in on inspiration; **D,** expiration, unstable area balloons out. Note movement of mediastinum toward opposite lung during inspiration.

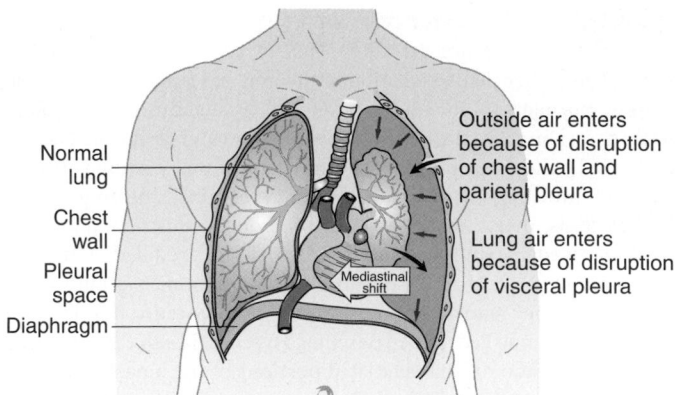

FIGURE 36.4 Tension Pneumothorax. Air in the pleural space causes the lung to collapse around the hilum and may shift the trachea and mediastinal contents (heart and great vessels) toward the other lung.

lung contusion. The clinical manifestations of flail chest are pain, dyspnea, unequal chest expansion, and hypoventilation. Treatment is internal fixation by controlled mechanical ventilation until the chest wall is stabilized.

Chest wall restriction results in decreased tidal volume. An increase in respiratory rate can temporarily compensate and restore minute ventilation, but many individuals will eventually progress to hypercapnic respiratory failure. Diagnosis of chest restriction is made by pulmonary function testing (reduction in forced vital capacity [FVC]), arterial blood gas measurement (hypercapnia), and radiographs. Treatment is aimed at any reversible underlying cause, but is otherwise supportive. In severe cases, mechanical ventilation may be indicated.

Pleural Abnormalities
Pneumothorax

Pneumothorax is the presence of air or gas in the pleural space caused by a rupture in the visceral pleura (which surrounds the lungs) or the parietal pleura and chest wall (see Chapter 35). As air is drawn into the pleural space during inspiration, it separates the visceral and parietal pleurae and destroys the negative pressure of the pleural space. This disrupts the state of equilibrium that normally exists between elastic recoil forces of the lung and chest wall. No longer held in check by the recoil forces of the chest wall, the lung fulfills its tendency to recoil by collapsing toward the hilum.

Primary (spontaneous) pneumothorax occurs unexpectedly in healthy individuals (usually men) between ages 20 and 40 years and is caused by the spontaneous rupture of blebs (blister-like formations) on the visceral pleura. Smoking is a risk factor.[14] Bleb rupture can occur during sleep, rest, or exercise. The ruptured bleb or blebs are usually located in the apexes of the lungs. The cause of bleb formation is not known, although more than 80% of these individuals have been found to have emphysema-like changes in their lungs even if they have no history of smoking or no known genetic disorder. Approximately 10% of affected individuals have a significant family history of primary pneumothorax that has been linked to autosomal dominant mutations in the *folliculin*

gene, which influences cell-to-cell adhesion and cell growth and causes cystic lung disease and kidney tumors (Birt-Hogg-Dubé syndrome).[15] Ruptured blebs damage the visceral pleura and create a conduit for air to travel from the lower airways into the pleural space (bronchopleural fistulae).

Secondary (traumatic) pneumothorax can be caused by chest trauma, such as a rib fracture, stab or bullet wounds, or a surgical procedure that tears the pleura; rupture of a bleb or bulla (larger vesicle) as occurs in COPD; or mechanical ventilation, particularly if it includes positive end-expiratory pressure (PEEP).[16] *Iatrogenic pneumothorax* is most commonly caused by transthoracic needle aspiration.[17]

Primary and secondary pneumothorax can present as either open or tension. In *open pneumothorax (communicating pneumothorax)*, air pressure in the pleural space equals barometric pressure because air that is drawn into the pleural space during inspiration (through the damaged chest wall and parietal pleura or through the lungs and damaged visceral pleura) is forced back out during expiration. In *tension pneumothorax*, however, the site of pleural rupture acts as a one-way valve, permitting air to enter on inspiration but preventing its escape by closing during expiration. As more and more air enters the pleural space, air pressure in the pneumothorax begins to exceed barometric pressure. Air pressure in the pleural space pushes against the already recoiled lung, causing compression atelectasis, and against the mediastinum, compressing and displacing the heart, great vessels, and trachea (Fig. 36.4). The pathophysiologic effects of tension pneumothorax are life-threatening.

Clinical manifestations of primary or secondary pneumothorax begin with sudden pleural pain, tachypnea, and dyspnea. Depending on the size of the pneumothorax, physical examination may reveal absent or decreased breath sounds and hyperresonance to percussion on the affected side. Tension pneumothorax may be complicated by severe hypoxemia, tracheal deviation away from the affected lung, and hypotension (low blood pressure). Deterioration occurs rapidly and immediate treatment is required. Diagnosis of pneumothorax is made with chest radiographs, ultrasound, and computed tomography (CT). Pneumothorax is treated by aspiration, usually with insertion of a chest tube that is attached to a water-seal drainage system with suction. After the pneumothorax is evacuated and the pleural rupture is healed, the chest tube is removed. For individuals with persistent air leaks, other interventions may be needed including thoracoscopic surgical techniques or pleurodesis (instillation of a caustic substance into the pleural space). Heimlich valves (one-way valves connected to the end of the chest drain) provide an option for home care in persistent spontaneous pneumothorax. Smoking cessation is strongly advised.[18]

TABLE 36.2	MECHANISMS OF PLEURAL EFFUSION	
TYPE OF FLUID/EFFUSION	**SOURCE OF ACCUMULATION***	**PRIMARY OR ASSOCIATED DISORDER**
Transudate (hydrothorax)	Watery fluid that diffuses out of capillaries beneath the pleurae (i.e., capillaries in lung or chest wall)	Cardiovascular disease that causes high blood pressure; liver or kidney disease that disrupts plasma protein production, causing hypoproteinemia (decreased oncotic pressure in the blood vessels)
Exudate	Fluid rich in proteins (leukocytes, plasma proteins of all kinds; see Chapter 7) that migrates out of capillaries	Infection, inflammation, or malignancy of the pleurae that stimulates mast cells to release biochemical mediators that increase capillary permeability
Empyema (pus)	Detritus of infection (microorganisms, leukocytes, cellular debris) dumped into the pleural space by blocked lymphatic vessels	Pulmonary infections, such as pneumonia; lung abscesses; infected wounds
Hemothorax (blood)	Hemorrhage into the pleural space	Traumatic injury, surgery, rupture, or malignancy that damages blood vessels
Chylothorax (chyle)	Chyle (milky fluid containing lymph and fat droplets) that is dumped by lymphatic vessels into the pleural space instead of passing from the gastrointestinal tract to the thoracic duct	Traumatic injury, infection, or disorder that disrupts lymphatic transport

*__NOTE:__ The principles of diffusion are discussed in Chapter 1; mechanisms that increase capillary permeability and cause exudation of cells and proteins are discussed in Chapter 7.

Pleural Effusion

Pleural effusion is the presence of fluid in the pleural space. The source of the fluid is usually from blood vessels or lymphatic vessels lying beneath either pleura, but occasionally an abscess or other lesion may drain into the pleural space. Pleural effusions that enter the pleural space from intact blood vessels can be transudative (watery) or exudative (proteinaceous) with fluid accumulating at a rate faster than it can be removed by the lymphatics. Other types of pleural effusion are characterized by the presence of pus (empyema), blood (hemothorax), or chyle (lymphatic fluid [chylothorax]). Mechanisms of pleural effusion are summarized in Table 36.2.

Transudative pleural effusions are often clear or slightly discolored and contain few cells and little protein. Examples are congestive heart failure, in which venous and left atrial pressures are increased, and liver or kidney disorders that cause hypoproteinemia. Hypoproteinemia decreases capillary oncotic pressure, which promotes diffusion of water out of the capillaries. (This mechanism is discussed in Chapter 3). *Exudative effusion* occurs in response to inflammation, infection, or malignancy and involves inflammatory processes that increase capillary permeability (see Chapter 7). When stimulated by biochemical mediators of inflammation, junctions in the capillary endothelium separate slightly, which enables leukocytes and plasma proteins to migrate out into affected tissues. Thus high concentrations of white blood cells and plasma proteins are evident in exudative effusion. Exudative effusions that occur in association with pneumonia are called *parapneumonic effusions*. These often resolve with treatment of the underlying infection but can progress to empyema (see following section).

Small collections of fluid may not affect lung function and remain undetected. Most will be removed by the lymphatic system once the underlying condition is resolved. Dyspnea, compression atelectasis with impaired ventilation, and pleural pain are common in larger effusions. Mediastinal shift and cardiovascular manifestations occur in a large, rapidly developing effusion. Physical examination reveals decreased breath sounds and dullness to percussion on the affected side. A pleural friction rub can be heard over areas of inflamed pleura.

Diagnosis is confirmed by chest imaging and thoracentesis (needle aspiration), which can determine the type of effusion and provide symptomatic relief. If the effusion is large, drainage usually requires the placement of a chest tube and surgical interventions may be needed to prevent recurrence of the effusion.[19]

Empyema

Empyema (infected pleural effusion) is the presence of pus in the pleural space and develops when the pulmonary lymphatics become blocked, leading to an outpouring of contaminated lymphatic fluid into the pleural space. Empyema progresses through three stages: (1) exudative stage, (2) fibrinopurulent stage, and (3) organizing stage with pleural peel formation. Empyema occurs most commonly in older adults and in children and usually develops as a complication of pneumonia, surgery, trauma, or bronchial obstruction from a tumor. Commonly documented infectious microorganisms include *Staphylococcus aureus*, *Escherichia coli*, anaerobic bacteria, and *Klebsiella pneumoniae*.

Individuals with empyema present clinically with cyanosis, fever, tachycardia (rapid heart rate), cough, and pleural pain. Breath sounds are decreased directly over the empyema. Diagnosis is made by chest radiographs, thoracentesis, and sputum culture. Treatment for empyema includes the administration of appropriate antimicrobials and drainage of the pleural space with a chest tube. In severe cases, ultrasound-guided pleural drainage, instillation of fibrinolytic agents, and/or injection of deoxyribonuclease (stimulates pleural fluid formation, reduces pleural fluid viscosity, and promotes resolution of systemic inflammation) into the pleural space may be needed to achieve adequate drainage. Surgical débridement may be required.[20]

PULMONARY DISORDERS

Restrictive Lung Disorders

Restrictive lung disorders are characterized by decreased compliance of the lung tissue. This means that it takes more effort to expand the lungs during inspiration, which increases the work of breathing. Individuals with lung restriction have dyspnea, an increased respiratory rate, and decreased tidal volume. Pulmonary function testing reveals a decrease in FVC. Restrictive lung diseases can cause $\dot{V}/\dot{Q}$ mismatch and affect the alveolocapillary membrane, which reduces the diffusion of oxygen from the alveoli into the blood and results in hypoxemia. Some of the most common restrictive lung diseases in adults are aspiration, atelectasis, bronchiectasis, bronchiolitis, pulmonary fibrosis, inhalational disorders, pneumoconiosis, allergic alveolitis, pulmonary edema, and acute respiratory distress syndrome. These disorders are characterized by activation of macrophages, polymorphonucleocytes, and lymphocytes with release of numerous inflammatory and immune cytokines.

Aspiration

Aspiration is the passage of fluid and solid particles into the lung. It tends to occur in individuals whose normal swallowing mechanism and cough reflex are impaired by a decreased level of consciousness or central nervous system abnormalities. Predisposing factors include altered level of consciousness caused by substance abuse, sedation, or anesthesia; seizure disorders; neuromuscular disorders that cause dysphagia; esophageal disorders, such as achalasia and esophageal strictures; and feeding through a nasogastric tube. Intubation of the trachea also is associated with aspiration. The right lung, particularly the right lower lobe, is more susceptible to aspiration than the left lung because the branching angle of the right mainstem bronchus is straighter than the branching angle of the left mainstem bronchus.

Aspiration of large food particles has serious consequences. Solid food particles can obstruct a bronchus, resulting in bronchial inflammation and collapse of airways distal to the obstruction. If the aspirated solid is not identified and removed by bronchoscopy, a chronic, local inflammation develops that may lead to recurrent infection and bronchiectasis (permanent dilation of the bronchus).

Aspiration of oral or pharyngeal secretions can lead to aspiration pneumonia. Intubation of the trachea also can cause aspiration and bacterial pneumonia. Aspiration of acidic gastric fluid with a pH of less than 2.5 may cause severe pneumonitis. Bronchial damage includes inflammation, loss of ciliary function, and bronchospasm. In the alveoli, acidic fluid damages the alveolocapillary membrane. This allows plasma and blood cells to move from capillaries into the alveoli, resulting in hemorrhagic pneumonitis. The lung becomes stiff and noncompliant as surfactant production is disrupted, leading to further edema and collapse. Infection is a common complication. Hypoventilation may develop as this process progresses, and systematic complications, such as hypotension, may occur.

Clinical manifestations of aspiration include the sudden onset of choking and intractable cough with or without vomiting, fever, dyspnea, and wheezing. Some individuals have no symptoms acutely; instead they have recurrent lung infections, chronic cough, or persistent wheezing over months and even years.

Preventive measures for individuals at risk are more effective than treatment of known aspiration. The most important preventive measures include the avoidance of fully recumbent positioning and excessive sedation, surveillance of enteral feeding, and use of promotility agents. Individuals being administered general anesthetics should not receive food or fluid for several hours before or after surgery. Antacids are sometimes given to individuals at risk for aspiration to keep the gastric pH greater than 2.5. Nasogastric tubes, which often are used to remove stomach contents and reduce the risk for aspiration, also can cause aspiration if fluid and particulate matter are regurgitated as the tube is being placed.

Treatment of aspiration, pneumonia, or pneumonitis includes supplemental oxygen and may require mechanical ventilation. Fluid intake may be restricted to decrease blood volume and minimize pulmonary edema. Corticosteroids may be administered during the first 72 hours after aspiration. Bacterial pneumonia that develops as a complication of aspiration pneumonitis must be treated with broad-spectrum antibiotics.[21]

Atelectasis

Atelectasis is the collapse of lung tissue. There are three types of atelectasis: compression, absorption, and surfactant impairment:

1. Compression atelectasis is caused by the external pressure exerted on lung tissue, such as occurs with tumors, or by fluid or air in the pleural space. Atelectasis at the base of the lungs can be caused by abdominal distention pressing on a portion of the lung, causing the alveoli to collapse.
2. Absorption atelectasis results from gradual absorption of air from obstructed or hypoventilated alveoli or from inhalation of concentrated oxygen or anesthetic agents.
3. Surfactant impairment results from decreased production or inactivation of surfactant, which is necessary to reduce surface tension in the alveoli and thus prevent lung collapse during expiration. Surfactant impairment can occur because of premature birth, acute respiratory distress syndrome, anesthesia, or mechanical ventilation.

Atelectasis tends to occur after surgery, especially in those who have been administered general anesthetics.[22] Postoperative individuals are often in pain, breathe shallowly, are reluctant to change position, and produce viscous secretions that tend to pool in dependent portions of the lung, particularly those who have surgical procedures involving the thorax or upper abdomen. Atelectasis increases pulmonary shunt, decreases compliance, and may lead to perioperative hypoxemia.

Clinical manifestations of atelectasis are similar to those of pulmonary infection: dyspnea, cough, fever, and leukocytosis. Prevention and treatment of postoperative atelectasis usually include deep breathing exercises (often with the aid of an incentive spirometer), frequent position changes, early ambulation, and pain management. Deep breathing is beneficial because it (1) promotes the ciliary clearance of secretions, (2) stabilizes the alveoli by redistributing surfactant, and (3) permits collateral ventilation of the alveoli through the pores of Kohn in the alveolar septa. The pores of Kohn, which open only during deep breathing, allow air to pass from well-ventilated alveoli to obstructed alveoli, minimizing their tendency to collapse and facilitating expectoration of the bronchial obstruction (Fig. 36.5).

Bronchiectasis

Bronchiectasis is persistent abnormal dilation of the bronchi. This disorder may result from a genetic predisposition or be caused by a defect in host defense. It usually occurs in conjunction with other respiratory conditions that are associated with chronic bronchial inflammation, such as obstruction of an airway with mucous plugs, atelectasis, aspiration of a foreign body, infection, cystic fibrosis, tuberculosis, congenital weakness of the bronchial wall, or immunocompromised status. Bronchiectasis is also associated with a number of systemic disorders such as rheumatologic disease, inflammatory bowel disease, and immunodeficiency syndromes (e.g., acquired immunodeficiency syndrome [AIDS]).[23] There may be no known cause. Recurrent infection and chronic inflammation of the bronchi leads to destruction of elastic and muscular components of their walls, bronchial lumen obstruction, traction from adjacent fibrosis, and permanent dilation.[24]

Bronchial dilation (Fig. 36.6) may be *cylindrical* (cylindrical bronchiectasis), with symmetrically dilated airways, as can be seen after pneumonia and is reversible; *saccular* (saccular bronchiectasis), in which the bronchi become large and balloon-like; or *varicose* (varicose bronchiectasis), in which constrictions and dilations deform the bronchi, creating a bulbous appearance. In both varicose and saccular bronchiectases, the smaller bronchial divisions are plugged with secretions or obliterated by fibrosis. Large anastomoses (connections) develop between the bronchial and pulmonary blood vessels, increasing blood flow through

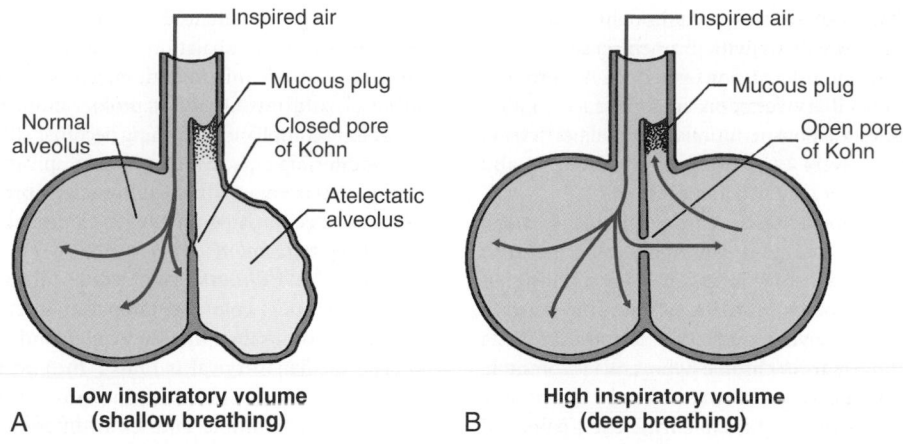

FIGURE 36.5 Pores of Kohn. **A,** Absorption atelectasis caused by lack of collateral ventilation through the pores of Kohn. **B,** Restoration of collateral ventilation during deep breathing.

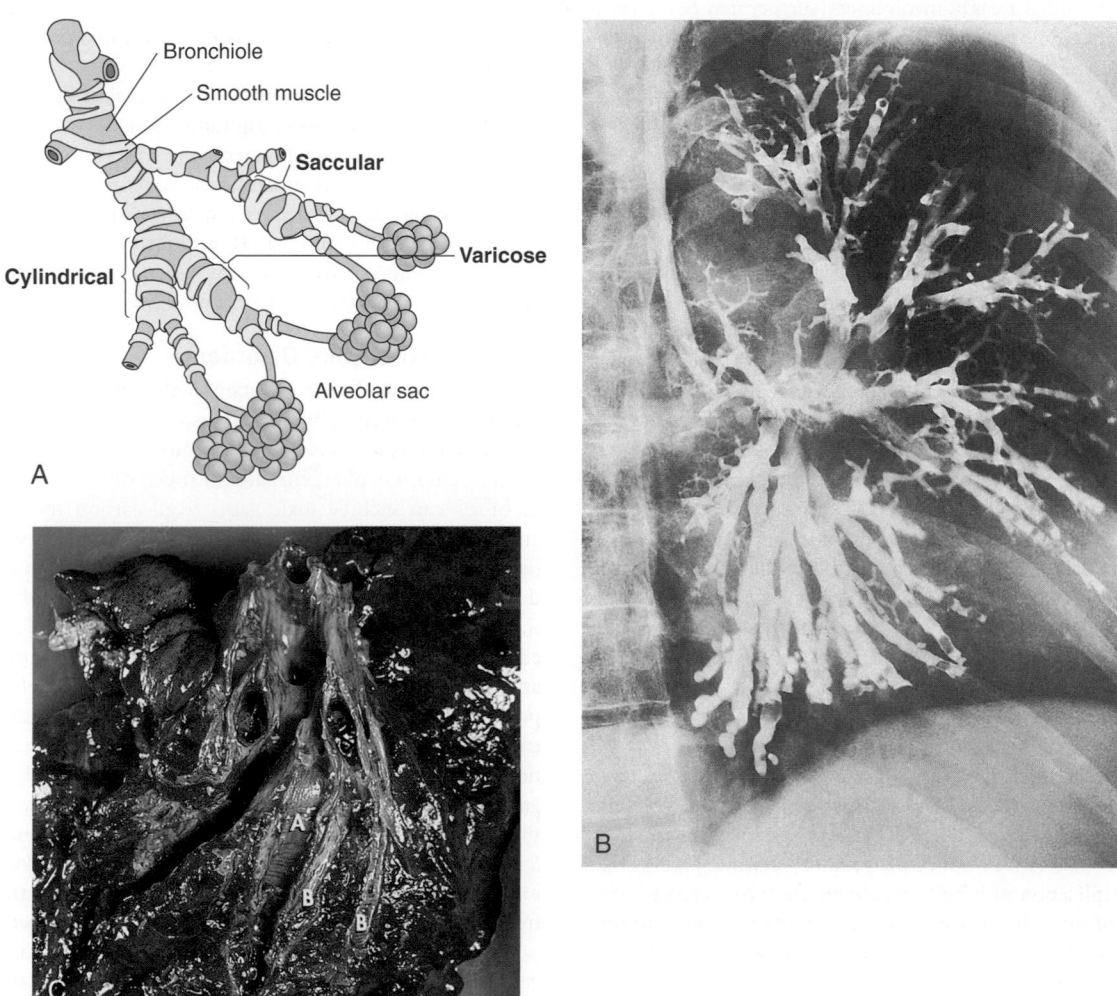

FIGURE 36.6 Bronchiectasis. **A,** Types of bronchiectasis. **B,** Left posterior oblique projection of a left bronchogram showing cylindrical bronchiectasis affecting the entire lower lobe except for the superior segment. Few side branches fill. The basal airways are crowded together, indicating volume loss of the lower lobe, a common feature in bronchiectasis. **C,** Cylindrical bronchiectasis. The dilated bronchi *(A)* and bronchioles *(B)* can be dissected almost to the pleural surface. (**B** from Hansell: *Imaging of diseases of the chest,* ed 5, St Louis, 2009, Mosby; **C** from Damjanov I, Linder J, editors: *Anderson's pathology,* ed 10, St Louis, 1996, Mosby.)

the bronchial circulation. These anastomoses are thought to cause the hemoptysis experienced by individuals with bronchiectasis. Airway damage leads to bronchospasm and colonization by bacteria that promote further lung damage, inhibit ciliary function, and produce copious amounts of purulent mucus. Ventilation-perfusion abnormalities develop and result in hypoxemia. In severe cases, minute ventilation is also compromised and the $Paco_2$ level may become elevated.

The primary symptom of bronchiectasis is chronic productive cough lasting for months or years. The disease is commonly associated with recurrent lower respiratory tract infections and expectoration of voluminous amounts of foul-smelling purulent sputum (measured in cups). If the individual is not receiving antibiotics, the sputum has a foul odor. Clubbing of the fingers from chronic hypoxemia is common. Hemoptysis can occur from mucosal inflammation and necrosis and, in some instances, can be massive. Dyspnea, pleuritic chest pain, and fatigue are common. Pulmonary function studies show decreases in FVC and expiratory flow rates. Hypoxemia eventually leads to cor pulmonale (see Cor Pulmonale under Pulmonary Vascular Disease). Diagnosis is usually confirmed by the use of high-resolution CT. Bronchiectasis is treated with antibiotics, bronchodilators, antiinflammatory drugs, chest physiotherapy, and supplemental oxygen. In selected individuals with localized areas of involvement, surgery may be indicated to remove the affected portion of the lung. Lung transplant is an option in advanced disease.[25]

Bronchiolitis

Bronchiolitis is diffuse inflammation of the small airways or bronchioles. It is most common in children (see Chapter 37). In adults it usually occurs with chronic bronchitis, but can occur in otherwise healthy individuals in association with an upper or lower airway viral infection (e.g., respiratory syncytial virus [RSV]) or with inhalation of toxic gases, or its etiology may be unknown.[26] Atelectasis or emphysematous destruction of the alveoli may develop distal to the inflammatory lesion. Bronchiolitis is usually diffuse. The resulting decrease in the ventilation-perfusion ratio results in hypoxemia. A decrease in minute ventilation with resulting carbon dioxide retention also may occur as lung restriction worsens.

Clinical manifestations include a rapid ventilatory rate; marked use of accessory muscles; low-grade fever; dry, nonproductive cough; and hyperinflated chest. If bronchiolitis is caused by an inhalation injury, pulmonary edema occurs rapidly. Respiratory distress with severe hypoxia frequently develops within 24 to 72 hours. Infiltrates can be seen on chest radiographs.[27] A decrease in the ventilation-perfusion ratio results in hypoxemia. Diagnosis is made by spirometry and bronchoscopy with biopsy. Bronchiolitis is treated with appropriate antibiotics, corticosteroids, immunosuppressive agents, and chest physical therapy (humidified air, coughing and deep breathing, postural drainage).

Bronchiolitis obliterans organizing pneumonia (BOOP) is a complication of bronchiolitis obliterans in which the alveoli and bronchioles become filled with plugs of connective tissue. Bronchiolitis obliterans syndrome (BOS) is an inflammatory, fibrotic process that occurs as a complication of lung transplantation. It is associated with persistent loss of lung allograft function 3 or more months following transplantation and has a high morbidity. Diagnosis is made by spirometry and bronchoscopy with biopsy. Treatment includes corticosteroids and other immunomodulatory agents.[28]

Pulmonary Fibrosis

Pulmonary fibrosis is an excessive amount of fibrous or connective tissue in the lung. Pulmonary fibrosis can be caused by formation of scar tissue after active pulmonary disease (e.g., acute respiratory distress syndrome, tuberculosis), in association with a variety of autoimmune

disorders (e.g., rheumatoid arthritis, progressive systemic sclerosis, sarcoidosis), or by inhalation of harmful substances (e.g., coal dust, asbestos). Chronic inflammation leads to fibrosis with alveolar epithelialization and myofibroblast proliferation. Fibrosis causes a marked loss of lung compliance. The lung becomes stiff and difficult to ventilate, and the diffusing capacity of the alveolocapillary membrane may decrease, causing hypoxemia. Diffuse pulmonary fibrosis has a poor prognosis. When no specific cause for the development of fibrosis is known, it is called *idiopathic pulmonary fibrosis.*

Idiopathic Pulmonary Fibrosis. Idiopathic pulmonary fibrosis (IPF) is the most common idiopathic interstitial lung disorder. It is more common in men than in women and most cases occur after age 60. The median survival is only 2 to 5 years after diagnosis. IPF is characterized by chronic inflammation, and recent studies suggest that it results from multiple injuries at different lung sites with aberrant alveolar wound healing, which probably occurs in response to the complex interaction of environmental insults and genetic, epigenetic, and metabolic factors.[29] Alveolar collapse and a fibroproliferative response result in thickening of the alveolocapillary membrane, causing decreased oxygen diffusion and hypoxemia. Progression of the disease results in decreased lung compliance, causing increased work of breathing, decreased tidal volume, and resultant hypoventilation with hypercapnia. Acute exacerbations of IPF can occur with rapid decompensation and a death rate as high as 50%.[30]

The primary symptom of IPF is increasing dyspnea on exertion. Examination shows diffuse inspiratory crackles, and diagnosis is confirmed by pulmonary function testing (decreased FVC), high-resolution CT, and lung biopsy. Treatment includes oxygen, corticosteroids, and cytotoxic drugs, although success rates are low and toxicities are high. Additional therapies may include antifibrotic drugs (N-acetylcysteine, pirfenidone, nintedanib), inhaled interferon, and anticoagulation therapy. Selected individuals may benefit from lung transplantation.[31,32]

Environmental Lung Disorders

Exposure to Toxic Gases. Inhalation of gaseous irritants can cause significant lung injury and respiratory dysfunction. Commonly encountered toxic gases include ammonia, hydrogen chloride, sulfur dioxide, chlorine, phosgene, and nitrogen dioxide. Inhalation injuries in burns can include toxic gases (e.g., carbon monoxide, cyanide, ammonia) from household or industrial combustants, heat, and smoke particles. Inhaled toxic particles can cause damage to the airway epithelium, cilia, and alveoli. There is increased secretion of mucus, promotion of inflammation, and development of mucosal and pulmonary edema with airway obstruction. Surfactant and other protective buffers and antioxidants are inactivated. The cellular effects of toxic gases and polluted air are described in Chapter 2. Acute toxic inhalation is frequently complicated by the development of bronchoconstriction, airway obstruction with fibrous mucus, microcirculatory coagulopathy, and impaired gas exchange. Initial symptoms include burning of the eyes, nose, and throat; coughing; chest tightness; and dyspnea. Hypoxemia is common. Secondary injury because of resuscitation, mechanical ventilation, and infection also can occur. Treatment includes supplemental oxygen, high frequency percussive ventilation, lung protective ventilation when possible, inhaled anticoagulants, bronchodilators, and support of the cardiovascular system. Inhaled beta agonists may help relieve bronchoconstriction. Most individuals respond quickly to therapy. Some, however, may improve initially and then deteriorate as a result of bronchiectasis or bronchiolitis.[33]

Prolonged exposure to high concentrations of supplemental oxygen at normal atmospheric pressure can result in a relatively rare iatrogenic condition known as oxygen toxicity. The basic underlying mechanism of injury is a severe inflammatory response mediated primarily by oxygen free radicals. The result is cellular necrosis or apoptosis with diffuse damage to alveolocapillary membranes, disruption of surfactant production, development of interstitial and alveolar edema, and decrease in compliance.[34] Treatment involves ventilatory support and reduction of inspired oxygen concentration to less than 60%, as soon as tolerated.

Pneumoconiosis. Pneumoconiosis represents any change in the lung caused by inhalation of inorganic dust particles, usually occurring in the workplace. As in all cases of environmentally acquired lung disease, the individual's history of exposure is important in determining the diagnosis. Pneumoconiosis often occurs after years of exposure to the offending dust with progressive fibrosis of lung tissue and an increased risk of lung cancer.

The dusts of silica, asbestos, and coal are the most common causes of pneumoconiosis. Others include talc, fiberglass, clays, mica, slate, cement, and metals (cadmium, beryllium, tungsten, cobalt, aluminum, iron, indium, and titanium dioxide nanoparticles). Deposition of these materials in the lungs causes the release of proinflammatory cytokines. This leads to chronic inflammation with scarring of the alveolocapillary membrane, resulting in pulmonary fibrosis and progressive pulmonary deterioration. Clinical manifestations with advancement of disease may include cough, sputum production, dyspnea, decreased lung volumes, and hypoxemia. In most cases, diagnosis is made by performing chest x-ray or CT and by obtaining careful occupational history. Treatment is usually symptomatic and palliative and focuses on preventing further exposure and promoting dust-free working conditions, along with pulmonary rehabilitation and management of associated hypoxemia and bronchospasm.

Silicosis is a type of pneumoconiosis resulting from the inhalation of free silica (silicon dioxide) and silica-containing compounds, which occurs in mining and in industries involved with the extraction and processing of ores, the preparation and use of sand, and the manufacture of pipe, building, and roofing materials. Silica exposure activates innate and adaptive immune mechanisms, and triggers inflammation with subsequent fibrosis.[35] Acute inflammation contributes to bronchospasm and wheezing. Release of proteolytic enzymes and toxic oxygen free radicals increases the risk for lung cancer. Exposed individuals may remain asymptomatic long after the nodules are visible on chest radiography. When clinical manifestations do appear, they include cough and dyspnea. There is no curative treatment for the disease, although corticosteroids may produce some improvement in the early, more acute stages. Screening for lung cancer should be included in the management plan.[36]

Coal worker pneumoconiosis (coal mine dust lung disease or anthracosis) is caused by coal dust deposits in the lung. Although coal dust itself is relatively well tolerated by the lung, it is frequently inhaled as a mixture of coal, silica, and quartz, which is strongly inflammatory and involves the small airways. Its mild form is asymptomatic, except for possible chronic bronchitis. Its advanced form manifests as severe pulmonary fibrosis. Individuals usually are seen with a productive cough and wheezing. Symptoms are more severe with advanced disease and mimic those of chronic bronchitis and emphysema. Diagnosis is made by obtaining a history of exposure and observing chest radiographs for characteristic signs. There is no specific treatment for coal worker pneumoconiosis. Individuals with the mild form of the disease usually have a favorable prognosis. Those with more complicated forms often develop marked cardiopulmonary dysfunction.[37]

Asbestos exposure affects not only factory workers but also individuals who live in areas of asbestos emission. Asbestos exposure can result in a type of pulmonary fibrosis called asbestosis, but can also cause lung cancer, mesothelioma (cancer of the pleura), or pleural plaques, especially in those also exposed to cigarette smoke.[38]

Asbestosis is caused by inhalation of hydrous silicates of various metals in fibrous form. Asbestos fibers cause inflammation and alveolitis. Activated macrophages release toxic oxygen free radicals and cause cellular apoptosis, leading to both fibrosis and malignancy. The most prominent clinical manifestations of asbestosis with fibrosis are dyspnea on exertion, a nonproductive cough, diffuse inspiratory crackles on examination, hypoxemia, and decreased lung volume. Progressive disease may take years and leads to respiratory failure and cardiac complications. Diagnosis is made by pulmonary function testing and low-dose CT. Therapy is supportive.

Hypersensitivity Pneumonitis. Hypersensitivity pneumonitis (extrinsic allergic alveolitis) is an allergic, inflammatory disease of the lungs caused by repeated inhalation of organic particles or fumes. Many allergens (antigens) can cause this disorder, including bacteria, fungi, and yeasts (moldy or contaminated hay, grain, compost, cork, or wood dust); mycobacteria (contaminated mists from standing water, showers, and hot tubs); animal proteins (bird droppings or feathers, animal pelts); and chemicals (fumes from paints, resins, and glues). A genetic predisposition may increase the risk for this disease. An autoimmune type III hypersensitivity response (see Chapter 9) is initiated by alveolar macrophages and results in immunoglobulin G (IgG) antibody production. Continued exposure results in a cellular immune type IV hypersensitivity response. The immune and inflammatory responses cause pneumonitis. Granuloma formation is common. Lung capacity and alveolocapillary diffusion are reduced.

Allergic alveolitis can be acute, subacute, or chronic. The acute form causes flulike symptoms with fever, cough, dyspnea, and chills a few hours after exposure that resolve without treatment in 1 to 3 days. With continued exposure, the disease becomes chronic and pulmonary fibrosis develops. Chronic allergic alveolitis causes cough, fever, fatigue, and weight loss and gradually progressive respiratory failure. Diagnosis is made by obtaining a history of allergen exposure and by performing serum testing for precipitating IgG antibodies, inhalation challenge, chest x-ray, high-resolution CT, bronchoscopy with bronchioalveolar lavage, and in rare cases lung biopsy. Treatment consists of avoidance of the offending agent, stopping smoking, and corticosteroid administration.[39]

Systemic Disorders and the Lungs

Several systemic diseases affect the airways, pleurae, or lung parenchyma, causing fibrosis, vasculitis, pulmonary hemorrhage, or granuloma formation. Clinical manifestations of lung involvement are usually nonspecific, and the diagnosis is based on involvement of other organs. There is usually no specific treatment, although corticosteroids often are used. Some of the systemic diseases affecting the lung are granulomatous disorders such as sarcoidosis, Wegener granulomatosis, lymphomatoid granulomatosis, and eosinophilic granuloma; connective tissue diseases such as rheumatoid arthritis, systemic lupus erythematosus, scleroderma, polymyositis or dermatomyositis, Sjögren syndrome, and polyarteritis nodosa; angioimmunoblastic or immunoblastic lymphadenopathy (a disease of the lymph nodes); cystic fibrosis (see Chapter 37); and Goodpasture syndrome (a pulmonary and renal disorder).

Pulmonary Edema

Pulmonary edema is excess water in the lung. The normal lung contains very little fluid and is kept dry by lymphatic drainage and a balance among capillary hydrostatic pressure, capillary oncotic pressure, and capillary permeability. In addition, surfactant lining the alveoli repels water, keeping fluid from entering the alveoli. Common predisposing factors for pulmonary edema include left-sided heart disease, causing increased pulmonary venous pressure; injury to pulmonary capillary endothelium, like that seen with adult respiratory distress syndrome

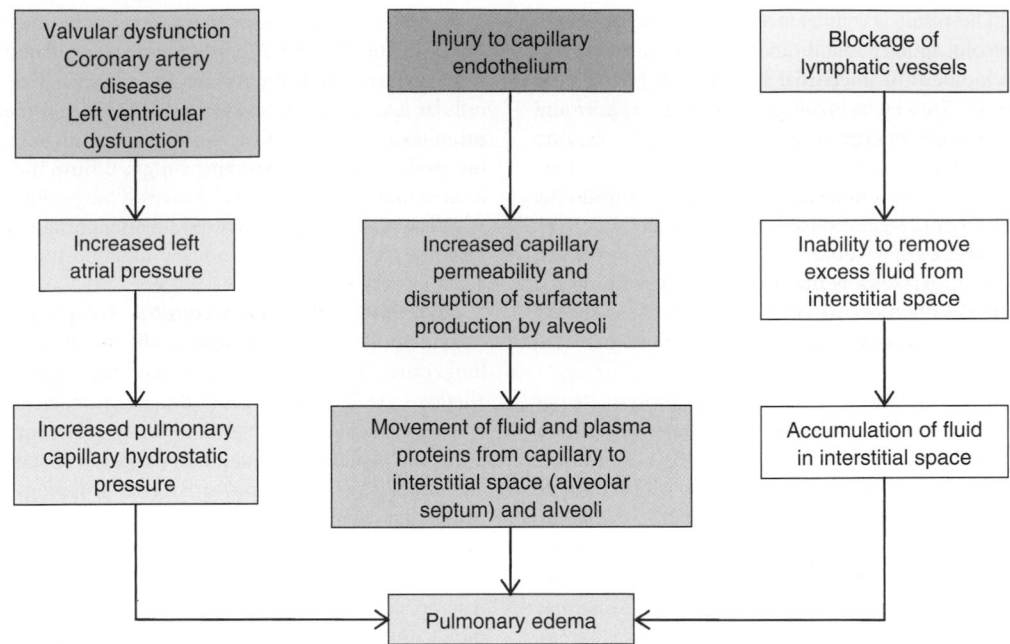

FIGURE 36.7 Pathogenesis of Pulmonary Edema.

(ARDS) and inhalation of toxic gases; and lymphatic obstruction. The pathogenesis of pulmonary edema is illustrated in Fig. 36.7. Other causes include rapid pulmonary reexpansion after upper airway obstruction and exposure to high altitude.

The most common cause of pulmonary edema is left-sided heart disease (see Chapter 33). When the left ventricle fails, filling pressures on the left side of the heart increase and cause a concomitant increase in pulmonary capillary hydrostatic pressure. When hydrostatic pressure exceeds oncotic pressure, fluid moves into the interstitium, or interstitial space (the space within the alveolar septum between the alveolus and capillary). Fluid moves to the lymphatic vessels and is then removed from the lung. When the flow of fluid out of the capillaries exceeds the lymphatic system's ability to remove it, alveolar flooding and pulmonary edema develop. Pulmonary edema usually begins to develop at a pulmonary capillary wedge pressure or left atrial pressure of 20 mmHg. If the capillary oncotic pressure is decreased for any reason (e.g., anemia, nephrotic syndrome, or liver disease), pulmonary edema develops at a lower hydrostatic pressure.

ARDS or inhalation of toxic gases causes injury to the alveolocapillary membrane. Capillary injury causes water and plasma proteins to leak out of the capillary and move into the interstitium. When plasma proteins move into the lung interstitium, they increase the interstitial oncotic pressure, which is usually very low. As the interstitial oncotic pressure begins to equal capillary oncotic pressure, water moves out of the capillary and into the lung. (Mechanisms of edema are discussed in Chapter 3.) Lymphatic drainage can be blocked by compression of lymphatic vessels caused by edema, tumors, and fibrotic tissue or by increased systemic venous pressure that elevates the hydrostatic pressure of the large pulmonary veins into which the pulmonary lymphatic system drains.

Postobstructive pulmonary edema ([POPE], negative pressure pulmonary edema, or reexpansion pulmonary edema) is a rare life-threatening complication that can occur after relief of upper airway obstruction (e.g., postextubation laryngospasm after anesthesia, epiglottitis, laryngeal tumor, or obstructive tonsils). Attempted inspiration against an occluded airway creates excessive intrathoracic negative pressure, causing increased venous return and blood flow to the right side of the heart and decreased outflow from the left side of the heart from the increased afterload.

This combination of events causes increased pulmonary blood volume and venous pressure and leads to pulmonary edema.[40]

High-altitude pulmonary edema (HAPE) can occur after arrival at altitudes usually more than 8000 to 10,000 feet and are related to a hypobaric hypoxic environment. The pathophysiology is not clearly known but hypoxic pulmonary vasoconstriction and increased pulmonary capillary permeability from increased pulmonary artery pressure are proposed mechanisms. The mechanisms are noncardiogenic and noninflammatory. Treatment includes moving to lower altitude and oxygen therapy. Drugs may be used for prevention.[41]

Clinical manifestations of pulmonary edema include dyspnea, hypoxemia, and increased work of breathing. Physical examination may reveal inspiratory crackles (rales), dullness to percussion over the lung bases, and evidence of ventricular dilation (S_3 gallop and cardiomegaly). In severe edema, pink and frothy sputum is expectorated, hypoxemia worsens, and hypoventilation with hypercapnia may develop.

The treatment of pulmonary edema depends on its cause. If the edema is caused by increased hydrostatic pressure resulting from heart failure, therapy is geared toward improving cardiac output and volume status with diuretics, vasodilators, and drugs that improve the contraction of the heart muscle. If edema is the result of increased capillary permeability resulting from injury, the treatment is focused on removing the offending agent and providing supportive therapy to maintain adequate oxygenation, ventilation, and circulation. POPE is treated with positive end-expiratory pressure ventilation. HAPE can be prevented with slow ascents, medications, and descent to lower altitudes when symptoms occur. Individuals with any type of pulmonary edema require supplemental oxygen. Mechanical ventilation may be needed if edema significantly impairs ventilation and oxygenation.

Acute Lung Injury/Acute Respiratory Distress Syndrome

Acute lung injury (ALI) and acute respiratory distress syndrome (ARDS) represent a spectrum of acute lung inflammation and diffuse alveolocapillary injury. ARDS is the most severe form and is defined as (1) the acute onset of bilateral infiltrates on chest radiograph not explained by cardiac failure or fluid overload and (2) a low ratio of the partial pressure of arterial oxygen to the fraction of inhaled oxygen.[42]

In the United States ARDS affects more than 190,000 people. Advances in therapy (particularly ventilator therapy) have decreased the overall death rate to approximately 35% to 46%, depending on severity of illness and comorbidities.[43] Older people and those who have severe infections or are immunocompromised continue to have a much higher mortality. The most common predisposing factors for ARDS are genetic factors, sepsis, and multiple trauma (especially when multiple transfusions are received). However, there are many other causes, including pneumonia, burns, aspiration, cardiopulmonary bypass surgery, pancreatitis, drug overdose, smoke or noxious gas inhalation, oxygen toxicity, radiation therapy, and disseminated intravascular coagulation.[44] Alcohol abuse and smoking are preventable environmental risk factors.[45]

◆ **PATHOPHYSIOLOGY.** ARDS can occur directly (aspiration of highly acidic gastric contents, inhalation of toxic gases, development of pneumonia) or indirectly, as from circulating proinflammatory mediators released in response to systemic disorders, such as sepsis, trauma, and multiple transfusions. All disorders causing ARDS cause acute immune cell–mediated injury to the alveolocapillary membrane producing massive inflammation, increased capillary permeability, and alveolar flooding with protein-rich fluid that overwhelms ion channels and lymphatic removal of fluid. Increasingly severe pulmonary edema (referred to as *noncardiogenic pulmonary edema*) develops with associated shunting, $\dot{V}/\dot{Q}$ mismatch, reduced lung compliance, and hypoxemia. ARDS progresses through three overlapping phases characterized by histologic changes in the lung: exudative (inflammatory), proliferative, and fibrotic (Figs. 36.8 and 36.9).[46]

Exudative (Inflammatory) Phase. Within 72 hours lung injury results in the release of inflammatory cytokines including interleukin-1β (IL-1β) and interleukin-6 (IL-6). This activates macrophages that release more proinflammatory cytokines, such as interleukin-8 (IL-8), tumor necrosis factor-alpha (TNF-α), surfactant protein-D (SPD), and mitochondrial DNA.[47,48] Neutrophils also are activated and release proteolytic enzymes, such as neutrophil elastase and metalloproteinases. Neutrophils release reactive oxygen species (superoxide radicals, hydrogen peroxide, hydroxyl radicals, singlet oxygen), nitric oxide, arachidonic acid metabolites (prostaglandins, thromboxanes, leukotrienes), and platelet-activating factor that damage the alveolocapillary membrane and increase capillary permeability. Fluid, protein, and cells are exuded into the interstitium and then into the alveoli, resulting in $\dot{V}/\dot{Q}$ mismatching.

Platelet and complement activation result in a hypercoagulable state with intravascular microthrombus formation and further damage to the lung capillary endothelium.[49] Furthermore, mediators released by platelets, neutrophils, and macrophages cause pulmonary vasoconstriction and microthrombus formation. Pulmonary hypertension occurs early in the course of the disease secondary to vasoconstriction.

Surfactant is inactivated, and its production by type II alveolar cells is impaired as alveoli and respiratory bronchioles fill with fluid or collapse. The intraalveolar hemorrhagic exudate becomes a cellular granulation tissue appearing as hyaline membranes and there is progressive hypoxemia. The lungs become less compliant, the work of breathing increases, ventilation of alveoli decreases, and hypercapnia develops.

Proliferative Phase. Within 1 to 3 weeks after the initial lung injury, there is resolution of the pulmonary edema and proliferation of fibroblasts, myofibroblasts, and type II pneumocytes with surfactant recovery. Type I pneumocyte differentiation with epithelial cell regeneration also occurs. This phase overlaps with the fibrotic phase.

Fibrotic Phase. About 2 to 3 weeks after the initial injury, remodeling (abnormal repair) and fibrosis occur. The fibrosis progressively obliterates the alveoli, respiratory bronchioles, and interstitium, leading to a decrease in functional residual capacity (FRC) and continuing $\dot{V}/\dot{Q}$ mismatch with severe right-to-left shunt and respiratory failure. Fibrosis of pulmonary capillaries contributes to pulmonary hypertension.

The same chemical mediators responsible for the alveolocapillary damage of ARDS often cause inflammation, endothelial damage, and capillary permeability throughout the body, resulting in the systemic inflammatory response syndrome (SIRS). SIRS then leads to multiple organ dysfunction syndrome (MODS). In fact, death may not be caused by respiratory failure alone, but by MODS associated with ARDS. (MODS is discussed in Chapter 49.)

◆ **CLINICAL MANIFESTATIONS.** The clinical manifestations of ARDS progress as follows:

Dyspnea and hypoxemia with poor response
to oxygen supplementation
↓
Hyperventilation and respiratory alkalosis
↓
Decreased tissue perfusion, metabolic acidosis,
and organ dysfunction
↓
Increased work of breathing, decreased tidal volume,
and hypoventilation
↓
Hypercapnia, respiratory acidosis, and worsening hypoxemia
↓
Decreased cardiac output, hypotension, and death

The new Berlin definition of ARDS provides categories of severity based on hypoxemia: mild (200 mmHg < Pao_2/Fio_2 ≤ 300 mmHg), moderate (100 mmHg < Pao_2/Fio_2 ≤ 200 mmHg), and severe (Pao_2/Fio_2 ≤ 100 mmHg) with bilateral infiltration on chest imaging which cannot be fully explained by cardiac failure or fluid overload.[50] Definitions for children are reviewed in Chapter 37.

Worsening hypoxemia and hypercapnia lead to respiratory failure. Decreased oxygen delivery to tissues results in metabolic acidosis and organ dysfunction (e.g., decreased urine output and a decline in cognitive functioning). Decreased cardiac output and hypotension may eventually lead to death.

◆ **EVALUATION AND TREATMENT.** Diagnosis is made on the basis of a history of lung injury, physical examination, analysis of arterial blood gases, and chest radiographs. Initial physical examination may show fine inspiratory crackles. Over the first 24 to 48 hours after injury, interstitial and alveolar infiltrates appear on chest radiographs. Serum biomarkers, such as TNF-α, brain natriuretic peptide (BNP), IL-6 and IL-8, and surfactant proteins, are being studied for ARDS prediction and treatment outcomes.[51]

Treatment strategies include early detection and management of contributing etiologies, supportive therapy to prevent progression of lung injury, and prevention of complications such as pneumonia and stress ulcer. There are no FDA-approved treatments for ARDS. Modes of protective ventilation are being used to reduce lung injury, including low tidal volume ventilation, noninvasive (through the mouth or nose, or both, with an external interface) positive-pressure ventilation, permissive hypercapnia, prone positioning, neuromuscular blockade (paralytics), and extracorporeal lung assistance. Some of these methods have shown reductions in death rates.[44,52]

Many studies are investigating new ways to prevent or treat ARDS. Prophylactic immunotherapy, antibodies against endotoxins, antioxidants, surfactant replacement therapy, nitric oxide inhalation, inhibition of various inflammatory mediators, gene therapy, and stem cells are among other possibilities being tested. Aspirin is currently being evaluated for treatment of sepsis-related ARDS.[53] The use of corticosteroids remains controversial but may be beneficial in persistent ARDS.[54] Some individuals who survive often have near-normal pulmonary function tests at 12

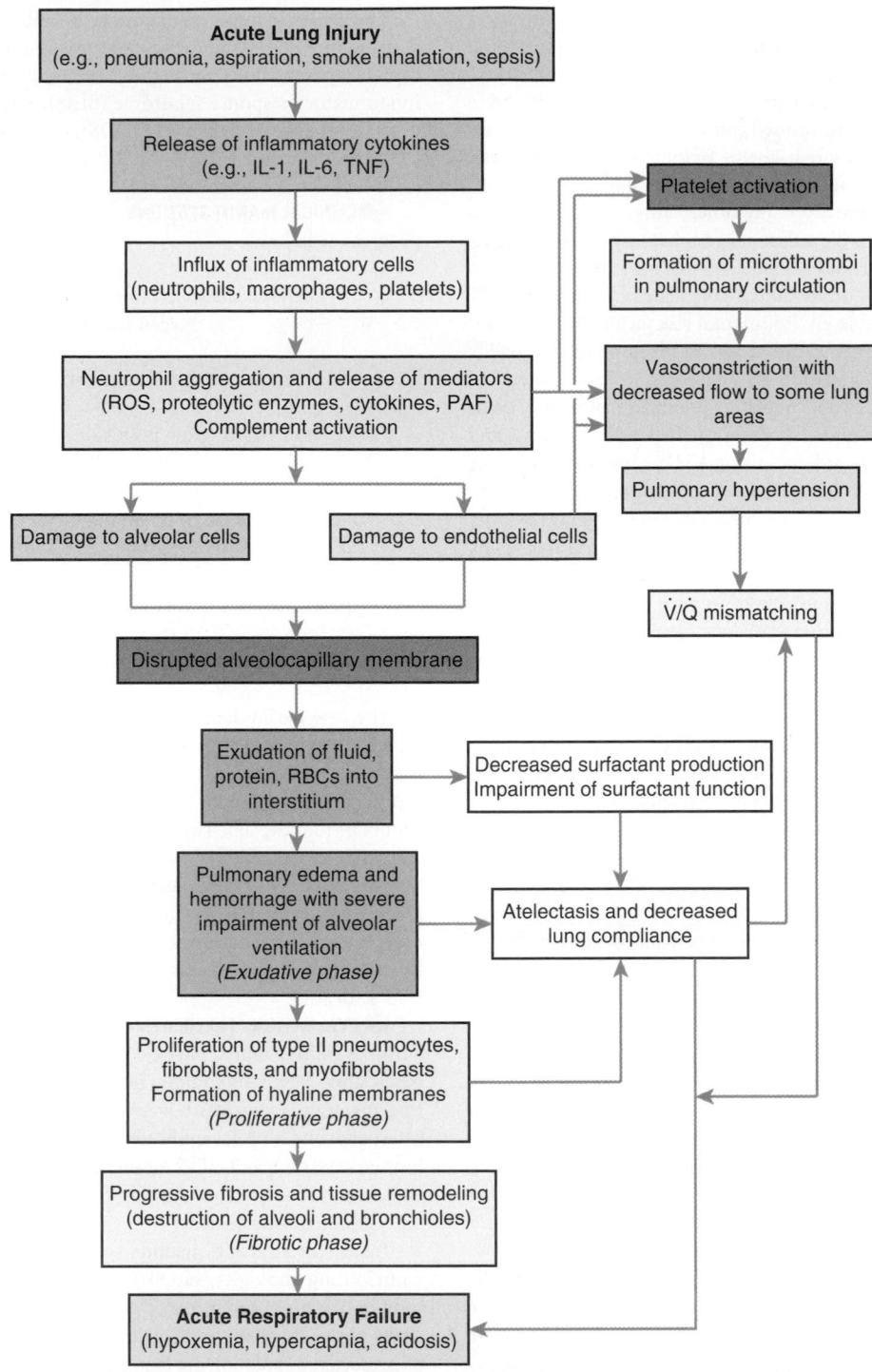

FIGURE 36.8 Pathogenesis of Acute Respiratory Distress Syndrome (ARDS). *IL-1,* Interleukin-1; *IL-6,* interleukin-6; *PAF,* platelet-activating factor; *RBCs,* red blood cells; *ROS,* reactive oxygen species; *TNF,* tumor necrosis factor.

months postrecovery, while others have persistent pulmonary dysfunction and poor quality of life associated with fibroproliferative changes in the lung, reduced exercise capacity, and long-term neurocognitive impairment.[55]

Obstructive Pulmonary Disease

Obstructive pulmonary disease is characterized by airway obstruction that is worse with expiration. More force (i.e., use of accessory muscles of expiration) or more time is required to expire a given volume of air,

and emptying of the lungs is slowed. These disorders are characterized by infiltration of the lung by inflammatory cells with the release of numerous cytokines that contribute to airway damage and mucus production. The unifying symptom of obstructive pulmonary disease is dyspnea and the unifying sign is wheezing. Individuals have an increased work of breathing, a mismatching of the ventilation-perfusion ratio, and a decreased forced expiratory volume in 1 second (FEV_1). The most common obstructive diseases are asthma and chronic obstructive pulmonary disease (COPD) (chronic bronchitis and emphysema).

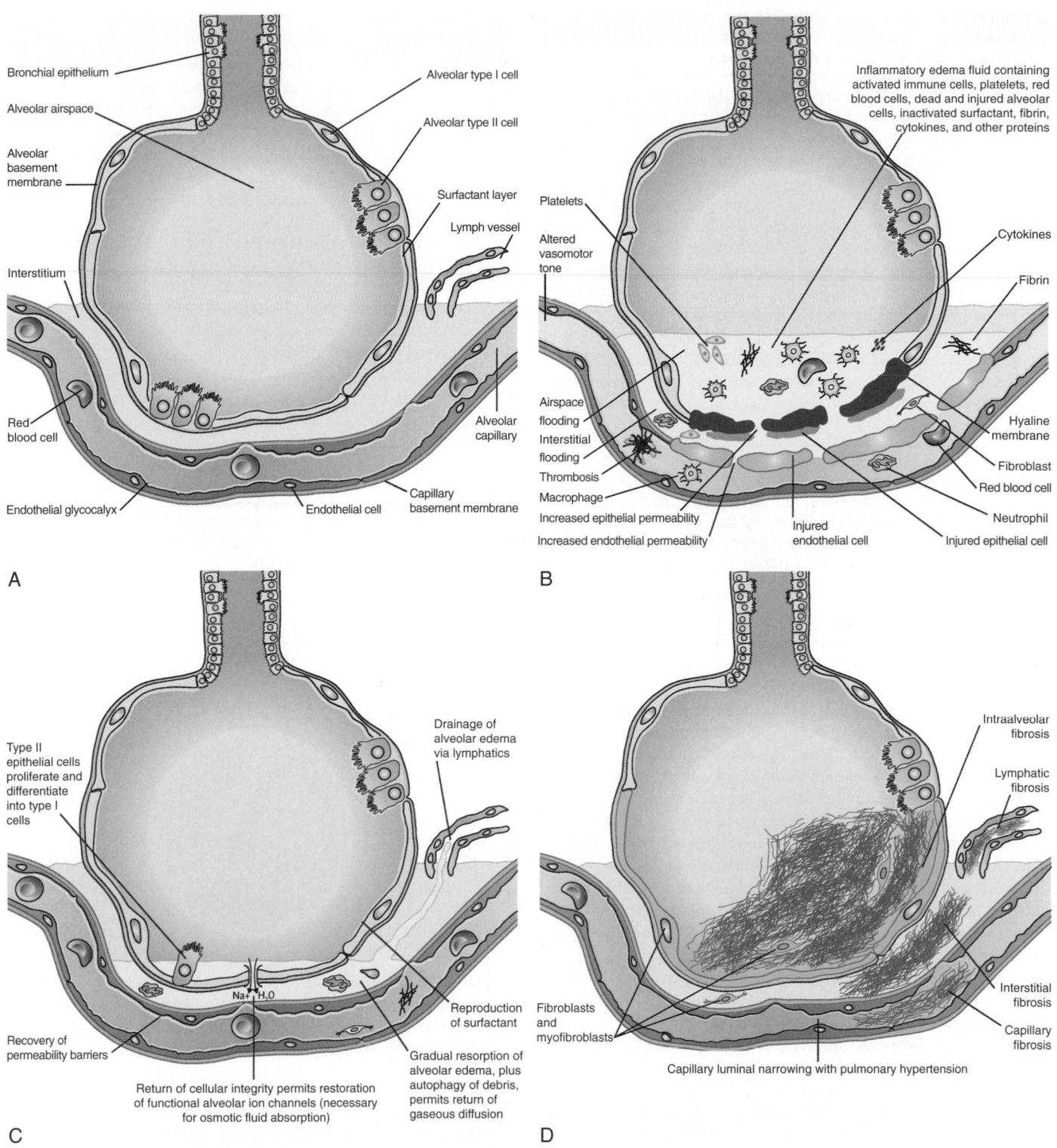

FIGURE 36.9 Acute Respiratory Distress Syndrome (ARDS). Cross-sectional views of alveoli in ARDS. A normal alveolus **(A)** plus the sequential exudative **(B)**, proliferative **(C)**, and fibrotic **(D)** phases in the pathogenesis of acute respiratory distress syndrome. (From Sweeney RM, McAuley DF: *Lancet* 388[10058]:2416–2430, 2016.)

Asthma

Asthma is a chronic inflammatory disorder of the bronchial mucosa that causes bronchial hyperresponsiveness, constriction of the airways, and variable airflow obstruction that is reversible. Asthma can develop at any age, with 6.3 million cases occurring among children (see Chapter 37)

and 17.7 million cases occurring among adults in the United States. The prevalence is increasing.[56] Death rates are highest for adult females, black persons, and adults older than 65.[57]

Asthma is a familial disorder and more than 100 genes have been identified that may play a role in the susceptibility, pathogenesis, and treatment response of asthma, including those that influence the

WHAT'S NEW?
Asthma and the Lung Microbiome

The term *microbiome* refers to the community of microorganisms that live in the human body. In the lung, the microbiome has been found to be essential to the development and maintenance of well-adapted immune and inflammatory responses to inhaled and ingested allergens, particles, and viruses. Asthma has been linked to changes in the lung microbiome (dysbiosis), particularly early in life. Of particular interest is the recent finding that airway colonization by large numbers of Proteobacteria, such as *Haemophilus influenzae* B and *Moraxella catarrhalis,* is more prevalent in individuals with asthma. Deleterious changes in the pulmonary microbiota have been associated with maternal and infant antibiotic use, maternal urinary tract infection, cesarean section mode of delivery, exposure to older siblings, vaccination, and changes in lifestyle and dietary habits. Newly developed sensitive methods for microbial detection have allowed researchers to more accurately explore in greater detail the relationship between the lung microbiome and pulmonary diseases. These studies will provide a foundation for developing new approaches for the prevention and treatment of asthma.

Data from Arrieta MC et al: *Sci Transl Med* 7(307):307ra152, 2015; Holt PG: *J Allergy Clin Immunol* 136(1):15–22, 2015; Huang YJ, Boushey HA: *J Allergy Clin Immunol* 135(1):25–30, 2015; Singanayagam A, Ritchie AI, Johnston SL: *Curr Opin Pulm Med* 23(1):41-47, 2017; Smits HH et al: *J Allergy Clin Immunol* 137(3):690–697, 2016; Wu P et al: *PLoS One* 11(3):e0151705, 2016.

BOX 36.1 ASTHMA AND IMMUNE CYTOKINES

IL-4: Activates B lymphocytes (plasma cells) and eosinophils
IL-5: Stimulates the activation, migration, and proliferation of eosinophils, which cause direct tissue injury and release of toxic neuropeptides that contribute to increased bronchial hyperresponsiveness, fibroblast proliferation, epithelial injury, and airway scarring
IL-8: Activates neutrophils that contribute to a more exaggerated inflammatory response
IL-9: Promotes mast cell proliferation and differentiation and increases production of IgE by B cells
IL-13: Impairs mucociliary clearance, enhances fibroblast secretion, indirectly increases number of eosinophils, and contributes to bronchoconstriction and airway remodeling
IL-17: Increases neutrophilic inflammation
IL-22: Stimulates airway epithelial cells and airway smooth muscle, and plays an important role in stimulating further innate and adaptive immune responses and bronchoconstriction
IL-25: Promotes airway remodeling
IL-33 Contributes to airway remodeling and promotes steroid-resistant asthma (see text)

Data from Erle DJ, Sheppard D: *J Cell Biol* 205(5):621–631, 2014; Farahani R et al: *Adv Biomed Res* 3:127, 2014; Lloyd CM, Saglani S: *Curr Opin Immunol* 34:52–58, 2015.

production of IL-4, IL-5, IL-13, IL-17, and IL-33; IgE; eosinophils; mast cells; adrenergic receptors; leukotrienes; nitric oxide; and transmembrane proteins in the endoplasmic reticulum.[58] Asthma phenotypes are observable characteristics not linked to a specific pathobiologic disease process. *Phenotypes* include eosinophilic asthma (allergic) versus neutrophilic asthma, recurrent respiratory tract viral infections, exercise-induced asthma, aspirin-sensitive asthma, age-at-onset asthma, or steroid nonresponsive asthma. Comorbidities associated with phenotypes include obesity, gastroesophageal reflux disease, allergic rhinitis, and vitamin D deficiency. *Endotypes* are subgroups that describe the specific underlying disease pathophysiology related to the observable phenotype (i.e., different clinical characteristics, histopathology, biomarkers including gene profiles, epidemiology, and treatment responses). An asthma endotype can encompass different phenotype clusters, and a specific phenotype may be present in several endotypes[59] (see Chapter 37, *What's New?* Asthma Phenotypes and Endotypes in Children).

Exposure to high levels of certain allergens during childhood increases the risk for asthma. Furthermore, decreased exposure to certain infectious organisms appears to create an immunologic imbalance that favors the development of allergy and asthma in some individuals. This complex relationship has been called the *hygiene hypothesis*[60] (see Asthma under Disorders of the Lower Airways in Chapter 37 for more detail). Recently, the relationship between the microbiome and asthma risk is shedding light on these complex interactions (see *What's New?* Asthma and the Lung Microbiome).

◆**PATHOPHYSIOLOGY.** Airway epithelial exposure to antigen initiates both an innate and an adaptive immune response in sensitized individuals (see Chapter 9).[61] Many cells and cellular elements contribute to the persistent inflammation of the bronchial mucosa and hyperresponsiveness of the airways, including dendritic cells (antigen-presenting macrophages), T helper 2 (Th2) lymphocytes, B lymphocytes, mast cells, neutrophils, eosinophils, and basophils. There is both an immediate (early asthmatic response) and a late (delayed) response.

The *early asthmatic response* is a phase of acute bronchoconstriction that reaches a maximum in the first 30 minutes and resolves within 1

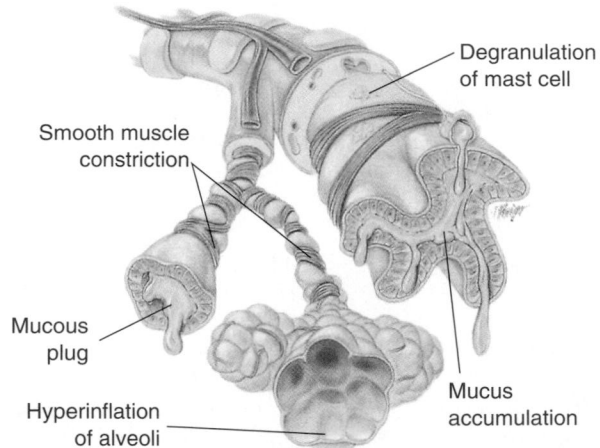

FIGURE 36.10 Bronchial Asthma. Thick mucus, mucosal edema, and smooth muscle spasm cause obstruction of small airways; breathing becomes labored and expiration is difficult. (Modified from Des Jardins T, Burton GG: *Clinical manifestations and assessment of respiratory disease,* ed 3, St Louis, 1995, Mosby.)

Labels in figure: Degranulation of mast cell; Smooth muscle constriction; Mucous plug; Hyperinflation of alveoli; Mucus accumulation

to 3 hours. During the early asthmatic response, antigen exposure to the bronchial mucosa activates dendritic cells to present the antigen to T helper cells (CD4+ T cells), which differentiate into Th2 cells releasing numerous inflammatory cytokines (Box 36.1). Together, these mediators activate inflammatory cells and cytokines, resulting in vasodilation, increased capillary permeability, mucosal edema, bronchial smooth muscle contraction (bronchospasm), and tenacious mucus secretion from mucosal goblet cells with narrowing of the airways and obstruction to airflow (Figs. 36.10, 36.11, and 36.12).

The *late asthmatic response* begins 4 to 8 hours after the early response with an increase in airway hyperresponsiveness.[62] Chemotactic recruitment of lymphocytes, eosinophils, neutrophils, basophils, and lymphocytes during the acute response causes a latent release of inflammatory

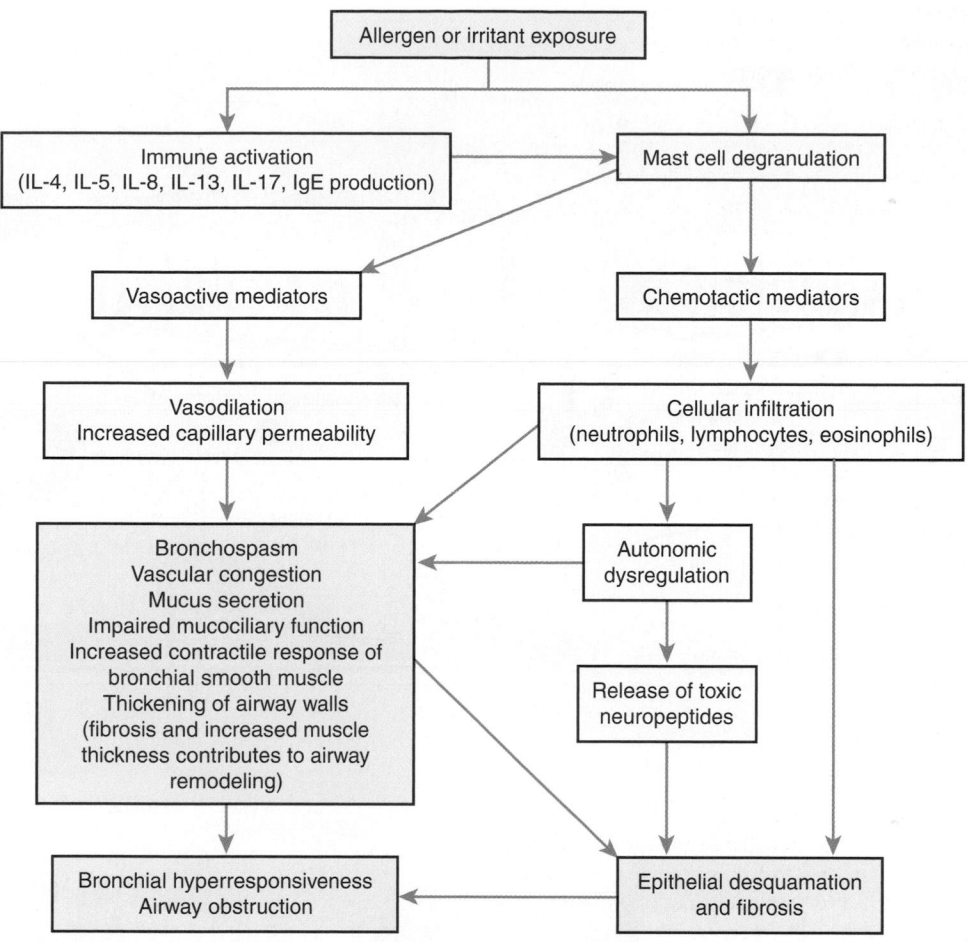

FIGURE 36.11 Pathophysiology of Asthma. Allergen or irritant exposure results in a cascade of inflammatory events leading to acute and chronic airway dysfunction. *IgE,* Immunoglobulin E; *IL,* interleukin.

mediators, and newly formed mediators (such as cysteinyl leukotrienes and prostaglandin D_2) cause bronchospasm, edema, and mucus secretion with obstruction to airflow. Eosinophil mediators cause direct tissue injury with fibroblast proliferation and airway scarring. Release of toxic neuropeptides (substance P, neurokinin A, and calcitonin gene–related peptide) contributes to increased bronchial hyperresponsiveness. Damage to ciliated epithelial cells contributes to impaired mucociliary function with accumulation of mucus and cellular debris forming plugs in the airways (increased synthesis of reactive nitrogen species [nitric oxide] contributes to oxidative injury and chronic inflammation).[63] A decrease in the number or function of T regulatory (Treg) cells also is associated with asthma.[64] Untreated inflammation can lead to long-term airway damage that is irreversible, known as *airway remodeling* (i.e., subepithelial fibrosis, smooth muscle and mucous gland hypertrophy).[65]

Airway obstruction increases resistance to airflow and decreases flow rates, especially expiratory flow. Impaired expiration causes air trapping, hyperinflation distal to obstructions, and increased work of breathing. Changes in resistance to airflow are not uniform throughout the lungs and the distribution of inspired air is uneven, with more air flowing to the less resistant portions. Continued air trapping increases intrapleural and alveolar gas pressures and causes decreased perfusion of the alveoli. Increased alveolar gas pressure, decreased ventilation, and decreased perfusion lead to variable and uneven ventilation-perfusion relationships within different lung segments. Hyperventilation is triggered by lung receptors responding to increased lung volume and obstruction. The result is early hypoxemia without CO_2 retention. Hypoxemia further

increases hyperventilation through stimulation of the respiratory center, causing the levels of $Paco_2$ to decrease and pH to increase (respiratory alkalosis). With progressive obstruction of expiratory airflow, air trapping becomes more severe and the lungs and thorax become hyperexpanded, putting the respiratory muscles at a mechanical disadvantage. This leads to a decrease in tidal volume with increasing CO_2 retention and respiratory acidosis. Respiratory acidosis signals respiratory failure.

◆ **CLINICAL MANIFESTATIONS.** Individuals with asthma are asymptomatic between attacks and pulmonary function tests are normal. No clinical symptoms are present during partial remission, but pulmonary function tests are abnormal. At the beginning of an attack, the individual experiences chest constriction, expiratory wheezing, dyspnea, nonproductive coughing, prolonged expiration, tachycardia, and tachypnea. Severe attacks involve the use of accessory muscles of respiration, and wheezing is heard during both inspiration and expiration. A **pulsus paradoxus** (decrease in systolic blood pressure during inspiration of more than 10 mmHg) may be noted. Peak flow measurements should be obtained. Because the severity of blood gas alterations is difficult to evaluate by clinical signs alone, arterial blood gas tensions should be measured if oxygen saturation falls below 90%. Usual findings are hypoxemia with an associated respiratory alkalosis. In the late asthmatic response, symptoms can be even more severe than during the initial attack.

If bronchospasm is not reversed by usual measures, the individual is considered to have severe bronchospasm or **status asthmaticus.** If status asthmaticus continues, hypoxemia worsens, expiratory flow rates decrease further, and effective ventilation decreases. Acidosis develops

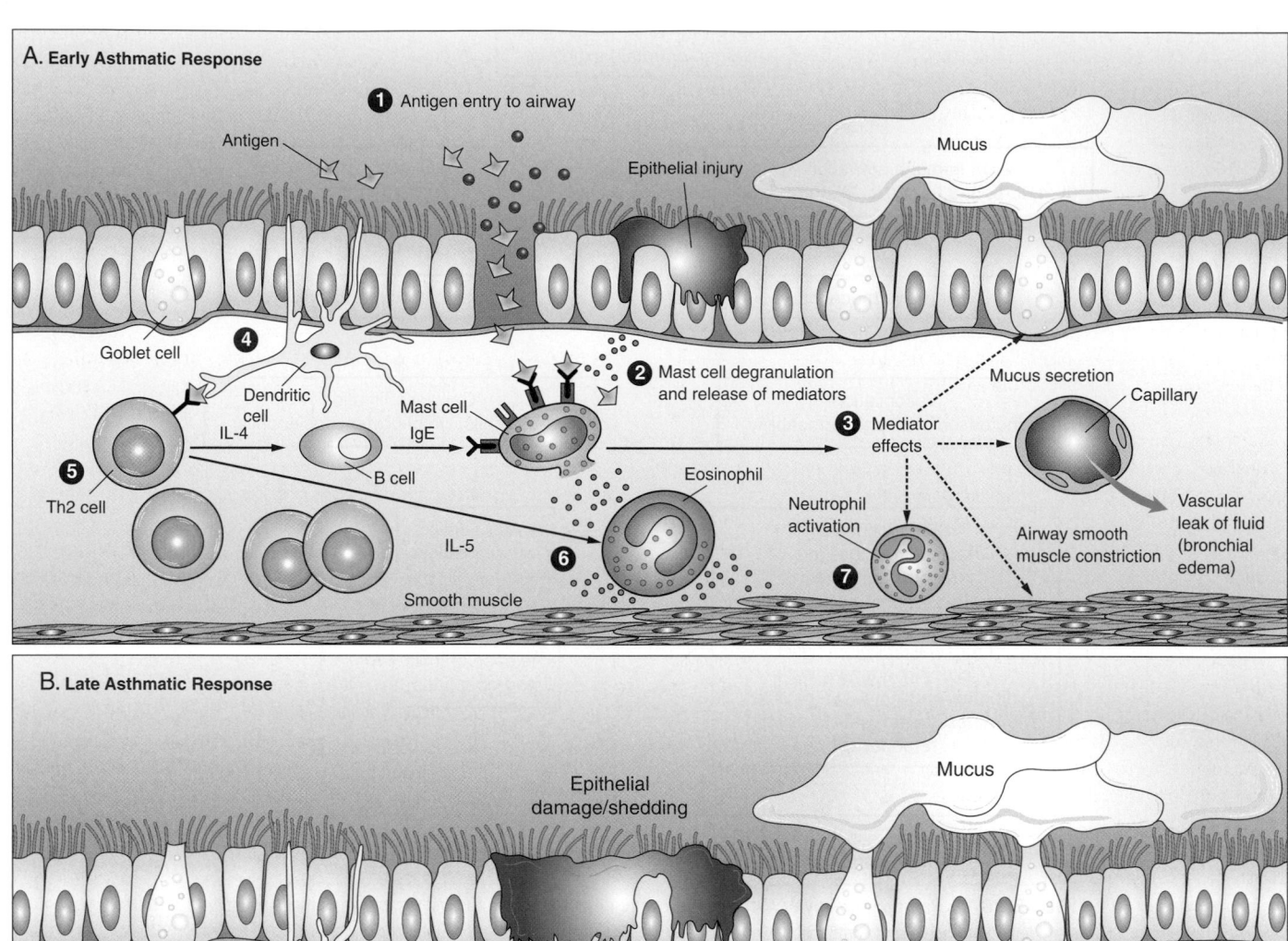

FIGURE 36.12 Early and Late Asthmatic Responses. **A,** *Early response:* Inhaled antigen **(1)** binds to mast cells covered with preformed immunoglobulin E (IgE). Mast cells degranulate **(2)** and release inflammatory mediators such as histamine, bradykinins, leukotrienes, prostaglandins, platelet-activating factor, and interleukins. Secreted mediators **(3)** induce active bronchospasm (airway smooth muscle constriction), edema from increased capillary permeability, and airway mucus secretion from goblet cells. At the same time, antigen is detected by **(4)** dendritic cells that process and present it to T-helper 2 (Th2) cells **(5),** which produce interleukin-4 *(IL-4)* and many other interleukins (see text). IL-4 promotes switching of B cells to favor IgE production. Th2 cells also produce IL-5 **(6),** which activates eosinophils. Many inflammatory cells, including neutrophils **(7),** also contribute to the inflammatory process. **B,** *Late response:* Areas of epithelial damage and shedding caused, at least in part, by toxicity of eosinophil products (major basic protein, eosinophilic cationic protein, eosinophil-derived neurotoxin, and eosinophil peroxidase). Many inflammatory cells are recruited by chemokines and upregulation of vascular cell adhesion molecules. Local T lymphocytes display a predominant Th2 cytokine profile. They produce IL-4 and IL-13, which promote switching of B cells to favor IgE production; and IL-3, IL-5, and granulocyte-macrophage colony–stimulating factor, which encourage eosinophil differentiation and survival. Inflammatory mediators also activate sensory nerves, further stimulating bronchoconstriction.

as the arterial $Paco_2$ value begins to rise. Asthma becomes life-threatening at this point if treatment does not reverse this process quickly. A silent chest (no audible air movement) and a $Paco_2$ value greater than 70 mmHg are ominous signs of impending death.

EVALUATION AND TREATMENT. The diagnosis of asthma is supported by a history of allergies and recurrent episodes of wheezing, dyspnea and cough, or exercise intolerance. Further evaluation includes spirometry, which may document reversible decreases in FEV_1 during an induced attack.

The evaluation of an acute asthma attack requires the rapid assessment of arterial blood gases and expiratory flow rates (using a peak flowmeter) and a search for underlying triggers, such as infection. Hypoxemia and respiratory alkalosis are expected early in the course of an acute attack. The development of hypercapnia with respiratory acidosis signals the need for mechanical ventilation. Management of the acute asthma attack requires immediate administration of oxygen and inhaled beta-agonist bronchodilators. In addition, inhaled corticosteroids should be administered early in the course of management.[66]

Careful monitoring of gas exchange and airway obstruction in response to therapy provides information necessary to determine whether hospitalization is necessary. Antibiotics are not indicated for acute asthma unless there is a documented bacterial infection.

Management of asthma includes the avoidance of allergens and irritants, control of symptoms, and prevention of exacerbations. Individuals with asthma tend to underestimate the severity of their asthma and extensive education is important, including use of a peak flowmeter and adherence to an action plan should symptoms worsen. In the mildest form of asthma (intermittent), short-acting beta-agonist inhalers are prescribed. For all categories of persistent asthma, antiinflammatory medications are essential, and inhaled corticosteroids are the mainstay of therapy. In individuals whose symptoms are not adequately controlled using inhaled corticosteroids, leukotriene antagonists can be considered. In more severe asthma, long-acting beta agonists can be used to control persistent bronchospasm; however, these agonists can actually worsen asthma in some individuals with certain genetic polymorphisms. Immunotherapy has been shown to be an important tool in reducing asthma exacerbations and can now be given sublingually. Monoclonal antibodies to IgE (omalizumab) have been found to be helpful as adjunctive therapy to inhaled corticosteroids.[67] The National Asthma Education and Prevention Program offers stepwise guidelines for the diagnosis and management of chronic asthma based on clinical severity, and they may be reviewed at http://www.nhlbi.nih.gov/guidelines/asthma/asthgdln.htm. More recent updates can be found at the Global Initiative for Asthma website (http://ginasthma.org/). Biomarkers and epigenetic markers are being evaluated to personalize treatment and reduce mortality.[68]

Chronic Obstructive Pulmonary Disease

Chronic obstructive pulmonary disease (COPD) is defined as a common, preventable disease characterized by airflow limitation that is not fully reversible and is usually progressive. COPD includes two primary phenotypes that frequently overlap each other. Chronic bronchitis is defined as hypersecretion of mucus and chronic productive cough that continues for at least 3 months of the year (usually the winter months) for at least 2 consecutive years. Emphysema is abnormal permanent enlargement of gas-exchange airways (acini) accompanied by destruction of alveolar walls without obvious fibrosis. Both phenotypes are associated with an enhanced chronic inflammatory response in the airways to noxious particles or gases. Exacerbations and comorbidities contribute to the overall severity of disease. COPD is the third leading cause of death in the United States with 2014 death rates at 44.3 per 100,000 men and at 35.6 per 100,000 women.[69]

Risk factors for COPD include tobacco smoke (cigarette, pipe, cigar, and environmental tobacco smoke), occupational dusts and chemicals (vapors, irritants, and fumes), indoor air pollution from biomass fuel used for cooking and heating (in poorly vented dwellings), and outdoor air pollution. Risks of lung disease with inhalation of marijuana are summarized in *What's New?* Inhalation of Marijuana and Lung Disease. The risk for COPD also is increased by factors that affect lung growth during gestation (smoking, antibiotic use, preterm birth, air pollution) and childhood (low birth weight, respiratory tract infections, obesity, childhood asthma).[70] Genetic and epigenetic susceptibilities have been identified, including polymorphisms of genes that code for tumor necrosis factor, surfactant, proteases, antiproteases, and acquired failure of DNA repair.[71] An inherited mutation in the α_1-antitrypsin gene results in the development of COPD (emphysema) at an early age, even in individuals who do not smoke.[72] The asthma-COPD overlap syndrome is a phenotype of chronic respiratory disease where there is an overlap of the clinical symptoms of asthma and COPD (see *What's New?* The Asthma-Chronic Obstructive Pulmonary Disease Overlap Syndrome).

PATHOPHYSIOLOGY. The pathologic changes of COPD occur in large central airways, small peripheral airways, and the lung parenchyma. In both chronic bronchitis and emphysema, chronic irritant exposure recruits neutrophils, macrophages, and lymphocytes to the lung, resulting in progressive damage from inflammation, oxidative stress, extracellular matrix proteolysis, and apoptotic and autophagic cell death.[73,74]

In chronic bronchitis, inspired irritants promote bronchial inflammation, causing bronchial edema, increases in the size and number of mucous glands and goblet cells in the airway epithelium, smooth muscle hypertrophy with fibrosis, and narrowing of airways. Hypersecretion of thick, tenacious mucus occurs and cannot be cleared because of impaired ciliary function (Fig. 36.13). The lung's defense mechanisms are therefore compromised, increasing susceptibility to pulmonary infection, which contributes to airway injury and ineffective repair. Frequent infectious exacerbations from bacterial colonization of damaged airways are complicated by bronchospasm with dyspnea and productive cough.[75] The pathogenesis of chronic bronchitis and emphysema is shown in Fig. 36.14. Initially chronic bronchitis affects only the larger bronchi, but eventually all airways are involved. The thick mucus and hypertrophied bronchial smooth muscle narrow the airways and lead to obstruction, particularly during expiration when the airways are

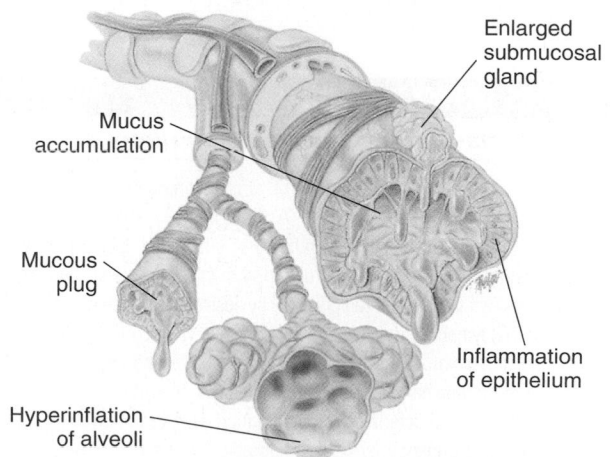

FIGURE 36.13 Chronic Bronchitis. Inflammation and thickening of mucous membrane with accumulation of mucus and pus leading to obstruction characterized by productive cough. (Modified from Des Jardins T, Burton GG: *Clinical manifestations and assessment of respiratory disease,* ed 3, St Louis, 1995, Mosby.)

WHAT'S NEW?
Inhalation of Marijuana and Lung Disease

Marijuana is the second most commonly smoked substance after tobacco. The recent legalization of marijuana *(Cannabis sativa)* in many states for recreational and medicinal use has raised questions about its health effects. To date, few investigations have explored the long-term lung effects of marijuana use and there is debate in the medical and scientific communities regarding its safety. Research has been limited because marijuana is an illegal drug according to federal law, although there has been some easing of restrictions on the study of cannabidiol for medical treatment (i.e., epilepsy, pain syndromes, and substance abuse disorders). *Cannabis* is a complex substance and contains 483 different compounds, including more than 80 cannabinoids.[1,2] Two cannabinoid receptors, CB1 and CB2, have been identified in humans and both are found in lung and bronchial tissue. Both endogenous and exogenous cannabinoids activate these receptors.[3] The general effect of cannabis on immune cells is to suppress immune function and inflammation, including immune cells in the lung. However, its overall impact on respiratory health remains unclear.

In some human studies, marijuana smoke has effects on the lungs similar to those caused by tobacco smoke, with large airway inflammation and symptoms of bronchitis, including increased cough and sputum production. Heavy marijuana smoking is associated with lung hyperinflation, increased forced vital capacity (FVC), upper lobe emphysematous changes, bronchial epithelial ciliary loss, and impairment of the phagocytic and bactericidal actions of alveolar macrophages. Despite these findings, evidence remains inconclusive regarding possible associated risks for asthma, chronic obstructive pulmonary disease (COPD), or lower respiratory tract infection.[4-7] Similarly, studies looking at the effects of marijuana on cancer risk also are inconclusive and contradictory. Epidemiologic studies regarding lung cancer development and smoking marijuana are inconsistent and not related to populations currently using marijuana legally. The carcinogenic effects of marijuana are unknown. Long-term heavy smoking of marijuana is associated with immuno-histopathologic changes, and epidemiologic evidence suggests a potential risk for developing lung cancer. However, in animal studies, cannabidiol has been shown to inhibit the progression of different types of cancer, including lung cancer.[8,9]

Marijuana is most commonly used by smoking, and the amount and depth of inhalation vary depending on the type of smoking device. Different varietals of marijuana, conditions of growth, stage of growth when harvested, and type of contaminants (such as pesticides, molds, and bacteria) affect the quality and number of active compounds contributing to the variability of their effects on the lungs and other tissues.[10] Furthermore, smokers of marijuana also may smoke tobacco, vape nicotine products, smoke cocaine, or use alcohol or other drugs,

making it difficult to discern the effects of marijuana on airway pathology. Together these factors make research on the lung effects of marijuana difficult. Thus the benefits and hazards of marijuana inhalation among the current population of users have yet to be determined. Collection of data relevant to the populations most likely to be exposed will require administration of pharmacologically approved preparations of marijuana in controlled trials. The Drug Enforcement Administration (DEA) has released new policies for supplying marijuana to medical researchers, thus advancing opportunities for investigation.[11]

References

1. Borgelt LM, et al: The pharmacologic and clinical effects of medical cannabis. *Pharmacotherapy* 33(2):195–209, 2013.
2. Elsohly MA, Slade D: Chemical constituents of marijuana: the complex mixture of natural cannabinoids. *Life Sci* 78(5):539–548, 2005.
3. Turcotte C, et al: Impact of cannabis, cannabinoids, and endocannabinoids in the lungs. *Front Pharmacol* 7:317, 2016.
4. Joshi M, Joshi A, Bartter T: Marijuana and lung diseases. *Curr Opin Pulm Med* 20(2):173–179, 2014.
5. Kempker JA, Honig EG, Martin GS: The effects of marijuana exposure on expiratory airflow. A study of adults who participated in the U.S. National Health and Nutrition Examination Study. *Ann Am Thorac Soc* 12(2):135–141, 2015.
6. Owen KP, Sutter ME, Albertson TE: Marijuana: respiratory tract effects. *Clin Rev Allergy Immunol* 46(1):65–81, 2014.
7. Tashkin DP: Effects of marijuana smoking on the lung. *Ann Am Thorac Soc* 10(3):239–247, 2013.
8. McAllister SD, Soroceanu L, Desprez PY: The antitumor activity of plant-derived non-psychoactive cannabinoids. *J Neuroimmune Pharmacol* 10(2):255–267, 2015.
9. Zhang LR, et al: Cannabis smoking and lung cancer risk: pooled analysis in the International Lung Cancer Consortium. *Int J Cancer* 136(4):894–903, 2015.
10. Biehl JR, Burnham EL: Cannabis smoking in 2015: a concern for lung health? *Chest* 148(3):596–606, 2015.
11. Drug Enforcement Administration, Department of Justice: Applications to become registered under the Controlled Substances Act to manufacture marijuana to supply researchers in the United States. Policy statement. *Fed Regist* 81(156):53846–53848, 2016.

WHAT'S NEW?
The Asthma-Chronic Obstructive Pulmonary Disease Overlap Syndrome

The asthma-COPD overlap syndrome (ACOS) is a condition in which a person has clinical features of both diseases. Asthma is an inflammatory disease of both the large and small airways with bouts of bronchial hyperresponsiveness, bronchoconstriction and airway obstruction with chest tightness, and coughing and wheezing. Asthma is mediated primarily by eosinophilic inflammation involving T-helper 2 (Th2) lymphocytes and is usually responsive to corticosteroid therapy. COPD is an inflammatory disease with primarily two phenotypes: (1) chronic bronchitis with inflammation and excessive mucus secretion in small airways and (2) emphysema characterized by inflammation with loss of alveolar structure. COPD is mediated primarily by neutrophils and CD8 lymphocytes (cytotoxic T

lymphocytes) with low Th2 activation and may be treated with macrolides, chemokine antagonists, monoclonal antibodies, or phosphodiesterase E4 inhibitors. Some individuals with asthma, particularly those who smoke, develop irreversible airway obstruction attributable to airway remodeling and clinically resemble individuals with COPD. Likewise, some individuals with COPD have eosinophilic inflammation and reversible airway obstruction and clinically resemble individuals with asthma. The overlap of these symptoms is described as ACOS and occurs later in life than in those with pure asthma. ACOS is more common in those with a history of smoking. Criteria have been developed for the diagnosis and targeted treatment of this syndrome.

Data from Barnes PJ: *J Allergy Clin Immunol* 136(3):531–545, 2015; Global Initiative for Asthma: *Diagnosis of disease of chronic airflow limitation, asthma COPD and asthma-COPD overlap syndrome (ACOS)*, 2015. Available at: http://www.msssi.gob.es/organizacion/sns/planCalidadSNS/pdf/GOLD_ACOS_2015.pdf; Nielsen M, Bårnes CB, Ulrik CS: *Int J Chron Obstruct Pulmon Dis* 10:1443–1454, 2015; Postma DS, Rabe KF: *N Engl J Med* 373(13):1241–1249, 2015; Slats A, Taube C: *Ther Adv Respir Dis* 10(1):57–71, 2016.

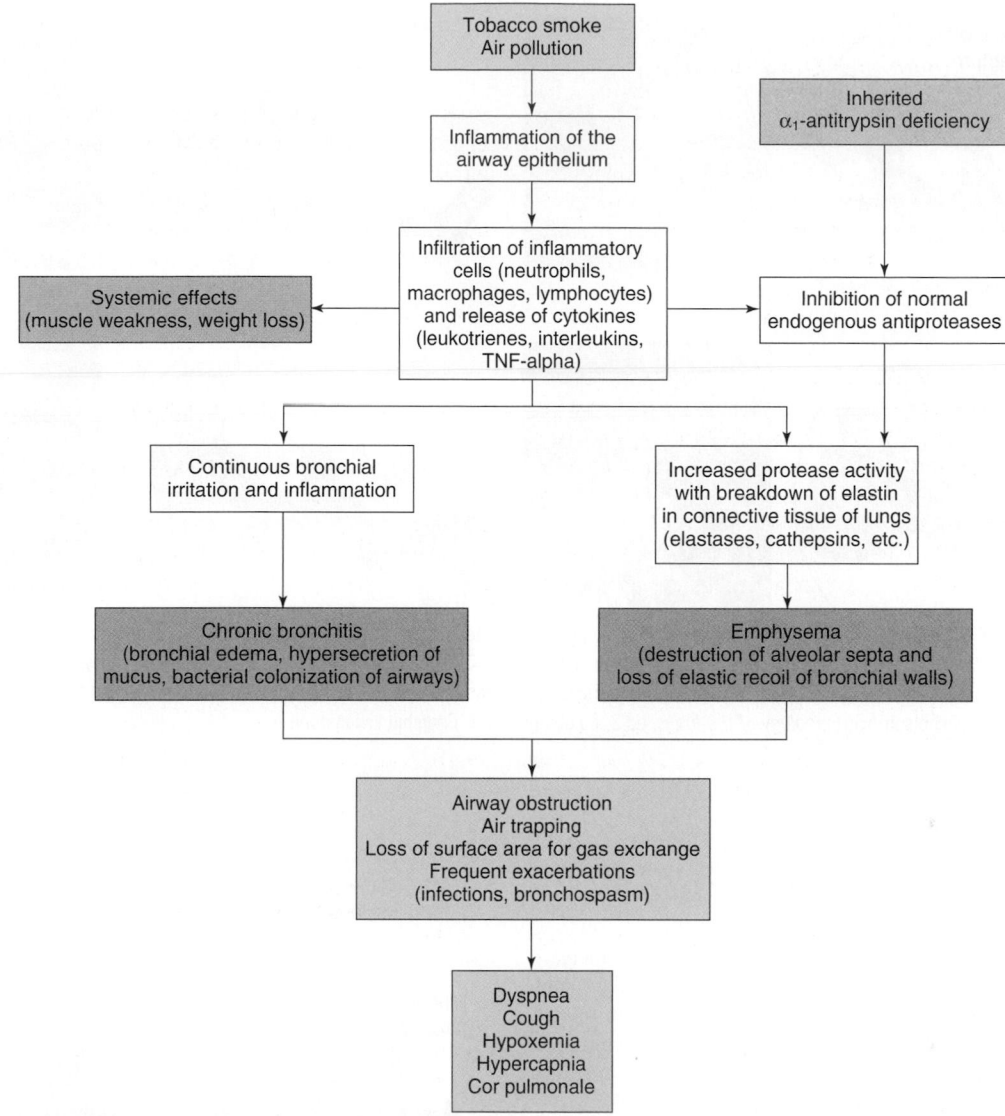

FIGURE 36.14 Pathogenesis of Chronic Bronchitis and Emphysema (Chronic Obstructive Pulmonary Disease [COPD]).

constricted. Obstruction also leads to ventilation-perfusion mismatch with hypoxemia.

Emphysema is characterized by destruction of alveoli through the breakdown of elastin within the septa caused by an imbalance between proteases and antiproteases, oxidative stress, and apoptosis of lung structural cells[76,77] (see Fig. 36.14). The number of neutrophils is increased in the airways of individuals with emphysema and they release elastase and proteases that cleave structural collagen and promote tissue breakdown, thus destroying bronchial and alveolar structures. Macrophages also are recruited to the lungs and enhance the release of pro-inflammatory mediators (i.e., tumor necrosis factor-alpha [TNF-α], IL-8, and chemokines). The role of T cells is less well described, but they may promote apoptosis and autophagic alveolar destruction.[78] Cellular apoptosis and early cellular senescence contribute to loss of alveolar cells and reduced surface area for gas exchange, and there is significant ventilation-perfusion ($\dot{V}/\dot{Q}$) mismatching and hypoxemia.

Emphysema can be centriacinar (centrilobular), paraseptal, or panacinar (panlobular); these variations can also occur in combination (Fig. 36.15) depending on the site of involvement. In **centriacinar (centrilobular) emphysema**, septal destruction occurs in the respiratory

bronchiolar walls and alveolar ducts in the center of the pulmonary lobule, usually in the upper lobes of the lung. The alveolar sac (alveoli distal to the respiratory bronchiole) remains intact. This type of emphysema tends to occur in smokers with chronic bronchitis. **Paraseptal emphysema** is similar to centriacinar emphysema but occurs adjacent to the pleura and septa of the pulmonary lobule and is associated with large bullae formation. **Panacinar emphysema** involves the alveolar and respiratory bronchiolar walls, resulting in global air space expansion with damage more randomly distributed and involving the lower lobes of the lung. It tends to occur in older adults and in those with α₁-antitrypsin deficiency.[79] Alveolar destruction also produces large air spaces within the lung parenchyma (bullae) and air spaces adjacent to pleurae (blebs).

Primary emphysema, which accounts for 1% to 3% of all cases of emphysema, is commonly linked to an autosomal recessive inherited deficiency of the enzyme α₁-antitrypsin.[80]

Normally, α₁-antitrypsin inhibits the action of many proteolytic enzymes; therefore individuals who have α₁-antitrypsin deficiency increase their likelihood of developing emphysema because proteolysis in lung tissues is not inhibited. Homozygous individuals have a 70%

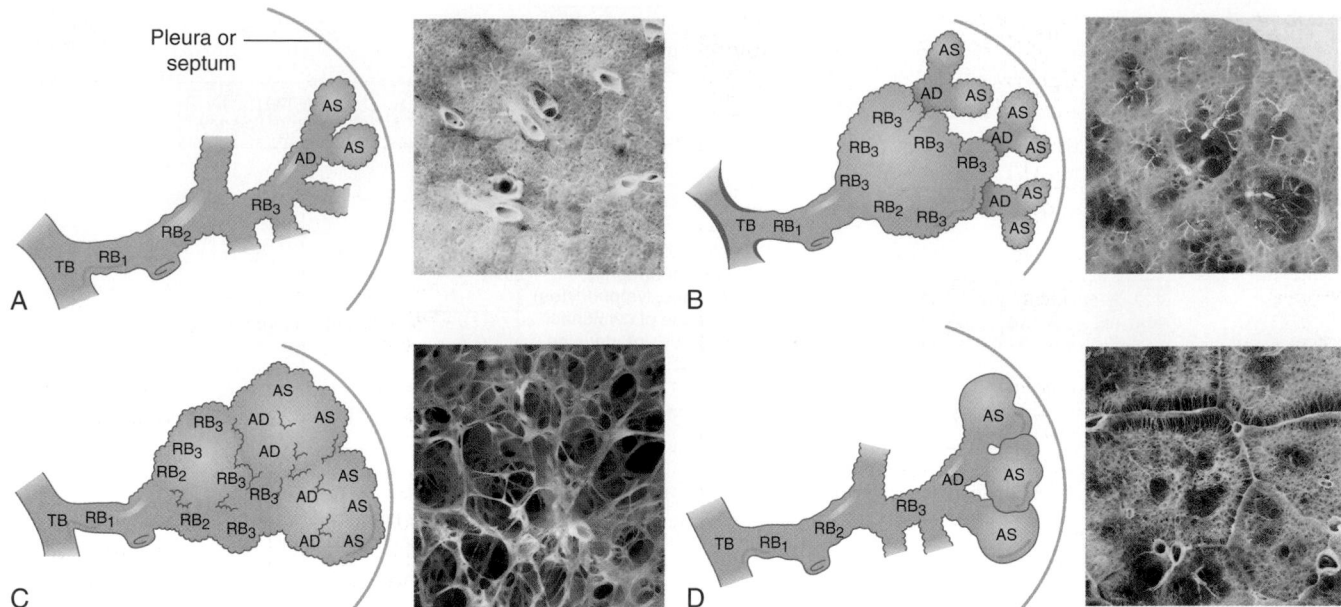

FIGURE 36.15 Types of Emphysema. Enlargement and destruction of alveolar walls with loss of elasticity and trapping of air. **A,** Normal lung. **B,** Centriacinar emphysema. **C,** Panacinar emphysema. **D,** Paraseptal emphysema. *AD,* Alveolar duct; *AS,* alveolar sac; *RB,* three orders of respiratory bronchioles; *TB,* terminal bronchiole. (From Corrin B, Nicholson AG: *Pathology of the lungs,* ed 3, Edinburgh, 2011, Churchill Livingstone.)

to 80% likelihood of developing lung disease. α_1-Antitrypsin deficiency is suggested in individuals who develop emphysema before 40 years of age and in those who do not smoke but still develop the disease.

Combined emphysema and idiopathic pulmonary fibrosis is increasingly recognized, particularly in heavy smokers with fibrosis predominant in the lower lobes and emphysema in the upper lobes. Symptoms are severe breathlessness and cough, and pulmonary hypertension is common. Specific pathogenic mechanisms are unknown. Diagnosis is confirmed with chest imaging and treatment is supportive.[81]

In COPD, expiration becomes difficult because of expiratory airway obstruction caused by accumulation of mucus, epithelial edema, and/or loss of elastic recoil and airway collapse. This reduces the volume of air that can be expired passively and air is trapped in the lungs (Fig. 36.16). **Air trapping** causes hyperexpansion of the chest, which puts the muscles of respiration at a mechanical disadvantage, resulting in increased work of breathing; consequently, many individuals will develop hypoventilation and hypercapnia. Persistent inflammation in the airways can result in hyperreactivity of the bronchi with bronchoconstriction, which may be partially reversible with bronchodilators. Chronic inflammation also can have significant systemic effects including weight loss, muscle weakness, and increased susceptibility to comorbidities, such as infection.

◆**CLINICAL MANIFESTATIONS.** Dyspnea on exertion that progresses to marked dyspnea, even at rest, is the most common symptom of COPD (see Table 36.3). In chronic bronchitis, individuals have a productive cough whereas in emphysema, cough is usually productive only during acute exacerbations. As COPD progresses, copious amounts of sputum are produced, accompanied by frequent pulmonary infections.[82] The individual with COPD is often thin, has tachypnea with prolonged expiration, and must use accessory muscles for ventilation. The anteroposterior diameter of the chest is increased (barrel chest), and the chest has a hyperresonant sound with percussion. To increase lung capacity, the individual often leans forward with arms extended and braced on

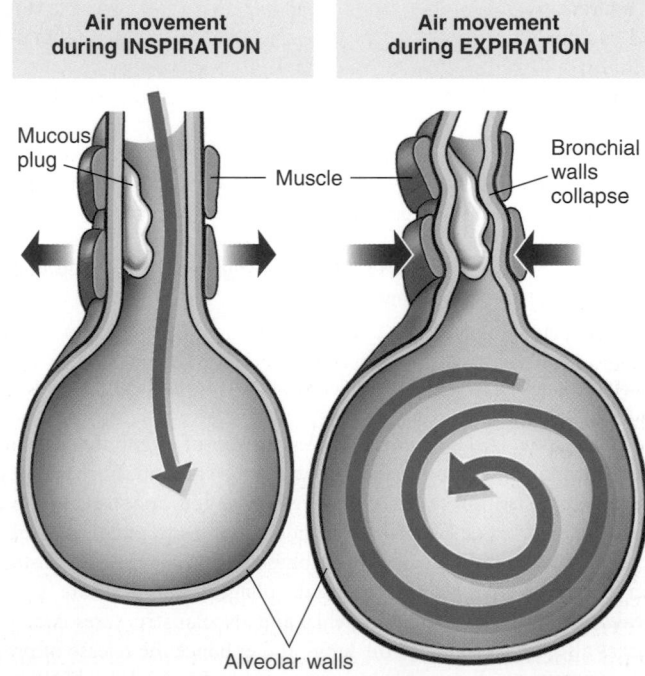

FIGURE 36.16 Mechanisms of Air Trapping in Chronic Obstructive Pulmonary Disease (COPD). Mucous plugs and narrowed airways cause air trapping and hyperinflation on expiration. During inspiration the airways are pulled open, allowing gas to flow past the obstruction. During expiration decreased elastic recoil of the bronchial walls results in collapse of the airways and prevents normal expiratory airflow.

TABLE 36.3   CLINICAL MANIFESTATIONS OF CHRONIC PULMONARY DISEASE

CLINICAL MANIFESTATIONS	CHRONIC BRONCHITIS	EMPHYSEMA
Productive cough	Classic sign	Late in course with infection
Dyspnea	Late in course	Common
Wheezing	Intermittent	Minimal
History of smoking	Common	Common
Barrel chest	Occasionally	Classic
Prolonged expiration	Always present	Always present
Cyanosis	Common	Uncommon
Chronic hypoventilation	Common	Late in course
Polycythemia	Common	Late in course
Cor pulmonale	Common	Late in course

BOX 36.2   PHARMACOLOGIC MANAGEMENT OF COPD

Short-acting anticholinergic (e.g., ipratropium)
Short-acting beta$_2$ agonist (e.g., levalbuterol)
Long-acting anticholinergic (e.g., tiotropium)
Long-acting beta$_2$ agonist (e.g., salmeterol)
Phosphodiesterase-4 inhibitor (e.g., roflumilast)
Inhaled corticosteroid (e.g., fluticasone)
Mucolytics and antioxidants (e.g., *N*-acetylcysteine)
Methylxanthine (e.g., theophylline)
Antibiotics (e.g., erythromycin)

Data from Global Initiative for Chronic Obstructive Lung Disease (GOLD): *Update 2016.* Available at: http://www.goldcopd.org/.

knees when sitting. In addition, people with COPD often exhale through pursed lips, a position that helps prevent expiratory airway collapse.

Airway obstruction results in decreased alveolar ventilation and hypercapnia and $\dot{V}/\dot{Q}$ mismatching with hypoxemia. Marked hypoxemia leads to polycythemia (overproduction of erythrocytes) and cyanosis. If not reversed, respiratory failure leads to pulmonary hypertension and eventually results in cor pulmonale (see Cor Pulmonale under Pulmonary Vascular Disease), which leads to severe disability or death. (Table 36.3 lists the common clinical manifestations of chronic bronchitis.)

◆**EVALUATION AND TREATMENT.** Diagnosis is based on history of symptoms, physical examination, chest imaging, pulmonary function tests, and blood gas analyses.[83] Pulmonary function testing reveals airway obstruction (decreased FEV_1) that is progressive and unresponsive to bronchodilators. Hypoxemia may first occur with exercise but gradually progresses to hypoxemia at rest. Hypercapnia develops as air trapping worsens and the work of breathing increases. Chest x-ray may reveal changes in thoracic diameter, distended lung fields, and flattening of the diaphragm. In individuals for whom chest x-ray and pulmonary function testing are not definitive for the diagnosis, high-resolution CT scanning is indicated.

Prevention of COPD is the best treatment because pathologic changes are not reversible. By the time an individual seeks medical care for symptoms, considerable airway damage is present. If the individual stops smoking, disease progression can be slowed. Influenza and pneumococcal vaccination should be kept up to date.

COPD is not reversible; therefore management is focused on symptom control (Box 36.2). Treatment is based on clinical stage as determined by the Global Strategy for the Diagnosis, Management and Prevention of COPD.[83] Bronchodilators (long-acting inhaled anticholinergics or long-acting inhaled beta agonists) and expectorants are prescribed to reduce dyspnea. Mucolytics, such as *N*-acetylcysteine, reduce cough and have been found to have antiinflammatory and antioxidant effects.[84] The addition of inhaled corticosteroids has been found to diminish the number of acute exacerbations, slow the rate of decline in quality of life, and reduce the rate of decline in FEV_1; however, their use must be weighed against the potential side effects (oropharyngeal candidiasis and hoarseness, risk of pneumonia). Phosphodiesterase-4 (PDE4)

inhibitors have been shown to reduce inflammation, cough, and sputum production. Chronic oral corticosteroids should be considered a last resort. During acute exacerbations (infection and bronchospasm), individuals require treatment with antibiotics and corticosteroids and may need mechanical ventilation. Macrolides are antiinflammatory and reduce neutrophil-elastase–induced mucous stasis in addition to their antibiotic properties.[85]

Chest physical therapy may be helpful and includes deep breathing and postural drainage. Teaching includes nutritional counseling, respiratory hygiene, recognition of the early signs of infection, and techniques that relieve dyspnea, such as pursed-lip breathing, all of which may be useful in the treatment of COPD in selected individuals[86] (see *Nutrition & Disease:* Chronic Obstructive Pulmonary Disease). Progressive pulmonary dysfunction with hypoxemia and hypercapnia may require long-term oxygen therapy and ventilation. Oxygen is titrated with care to individuals with severe hypoxemia and CO_2 retention. If titration of oxygen therapy cannot be achieved without significant hypercapnia, the individual's lungs must be mechanically ventilated.[87] In selected individuals with emphysema, lung volume reduction surgery, endoscopic techniques, or transplantation can be considered.[88] α_1-Antitrypsin augmentation may be indicated for primary emphysema.[89] In addition, many comorbidities accompany COPD and require monitoring and therapy, including bronchiectasis, cardiovascular disorders, metabolic diseases, bone disease, stroke, lung cancer, cachexia and muscle weakness, anemia, depression, and cognitive decline.

Respiratory Tract Infections

Respiratory tract infections are the most common cause of short-term disability in the United States. Most of these infections—the common cold, pharyngitis (sore throat), and laryngitis (inflammation of the larynx [voice box])—involve only the upper airways. Infections of the lower respiratory tract occur most often in the very young, the very old, or individuals with impaired immunity or underlying disease.

Acute Bronchitis

Acute bronchitis is acute infection or inflammation of the large airways or bronchi and is usually self-limiting. More than 90% of cases of acute bronchitis are caused by viruses.[90] Many of the clinical manifestations are similar to those of pneumonia (i.e., cough, fever, chills, malaise), but physical examination does not reveal signs of pulmonary consolidation and chest radiographs do not show infiltrates. Individuals with viral bronchitis usually have a nonproductive cough that occurs in paroxysms and is aggravated by cold, dry, or dusty air. However, purulent sputum may be produced with some viral infections. Chest pain often develops from the effort of coughing. Treatment consists of antitussive agents and beta₂ agonists for wheezing (especially in individuals with underlying asthma or COPD).[91]

Individuals with bacterial bronchitis have a productive cough, fever, and pain behind the sternum (breast bone) that is aggravated by coughing. It is rare in previously healthy adults except after viral infection, but is common in those with COPD. Bacterial bronchitis is treated with antitussive agents. Antibiotics have shown no difference in follow-up examinations compared with placebo, and potential side effects, antibiotic resistance, and cost need to be considered.[90,92]

NUTRITION & DISEASE
Chronic Obstructive Pulmonary Disease

Diet and nutrition have been linked to the development and progression of chronic obstructive pulmonary disease (COPD). For example, a high intake of omega-3 fatty acids has been linked to a decreased risk of COPD, whereas obesity and low levels of vitamin D are linked to an increased risk for COPD. Once the diagnosis of COPD has been established, and as the disease progresses, weight and muscle loss are common and are associated with reduced survival. The impact of poor nutrition on individuals with COPD is exacerbated by the fact that these individuals have increased work of breathing and elevated energy expenditure. Specifically, malnutrition (1) limits muscle strength and oxygen uptake, thus reducing exercise capacity; (2) decreases ventilatory capacity, contributing to hypercapnia; (3) limits surfactant production, negatively impacting lung function; (4) reduces cell-mediated immune responses, contributing to infection; and (5) decreases protein synthesis, contributing to widespread effects on cellular function. The goals of medical nutrition therapy are to maintain an acceptable and stable weight and supply adequate calories, minerals, vitamins, and antioxidants to promote optimal exercise capacity. However, dyspnea and fatigue, as well as the presence of inflammatory cytokines in COPD, impair appetite. Other nutrition impact symptoms (NISs) include dry mouth, stomachache, pain, and constipation or diarrhea. Consumption of high-energy foods, provision of oral nutritional support, promotion of frequent snacking that includes soft foods and beverages, and assistance with shopping and meal preparation can help overcome these barriers. Increasing omega-3 fatty acid supplementation and antioxidant intake may modulate the effects of systemic inflammation. Vitamin D and calcium supplementation is indicated to improve bone health. Serum phosphate levels also should be monitored to prevent hypophosphatemia, which can contribute to muscle weakness.

Data from Berthon BS, Wood LG: *Nutrients* 7(3):1618–1643, 2015; Liu Y et al: *Respir Med* 109(7):851–859, 2015; Mekal D et al: *Adv Exp Med Biol* 840:45–49, 2015; Norden J et al: *Eur J Clin Nutr* 69(2):256–261, 2015; Sanders KJ et al: *J Cachexia Sarcopenia Muscle* 7(1):5–22, 2016.

Pneumonia

Pneumonia is infection of the lower respiratory tract caused by bacteria, viruses, fungi, protozoa, or parasites. It is the eighth leading cause of death in the United States and is responsible for more disease and death than any other infection.[93] The incidence and mortality of pneumonia are highest in the elderly. Risk factors for pneumonia include advanced age; compromised immunity; underlying lung disease, particularly COPD; alcoholism; altered consciousness; chest trauma; impaired swallowing; smoking; endotracheal intubation; malnutrition; immobilization; underlying cardiac or liver disease; and residence in a nursing home.[94]

Pneumonia can be categorized as community-acquired (CAP), or healthcare-associated (HCAP), including hospital-acquired (HAP), or ventilator-associated (VAP). CAP is one of the most common reasons for hospitalization in the United States. HCAP is defined as occurring in individuals with recent hospitalization, residence in a nursing home or extended care facility, home infusion therapy, chronic dialysis, home wound care, nonambulatory status, and the use of tube feedings or gastric acid suppressive agents.[95] It is estimated that nearly one-third of all hospital admissions for pneumonia are now considered HCAP. HAP is the second most common nosocomial infection (urinary tract infection [UTI] most common), but has the greatest mortality (overall 20% to 50% mortality). VAP occurs in 9% to 27% of individuals who require intubation and mechanical ventilation.[96-98] The microorganisms that most commonly cause CAP are different from those infections that cause HCAP, HAP, and VAP (Box 36.3). In addition, the characteristics of the individual are important in determining which etiologic microorganism is likely; for example, immunocompromised persons tend to be susceptible to opportunistic infections that are uncommon in normal adults (see Box 36.3). Bacterial pneumonia can occur secondary to respiratory viral infection and is a cause of influenza deaths.[99] Mechanisms of viral and bacterial infection are reviewed in Chapter 10.

◆PATHOPHYSIOLOGY. Aspiration of oropharyngeal secretions is the most common route of lower respiratory tract infection; thus the nasopharynx and oropharynx constitute the first line of defense for most infectious agents. Another route of infection is through the inhalation of microorganisms that have been released into the air when an infected individual coughs, sneezes, or talks, or from aerosolized water, such as that from contaminated respiratory therapy equipment. This route of infection is most important in viral and mycobacterial pneumonias and in *Legionella* outbreaks. Endotracheal tubes become colonized with bacteria that form biofilms (protected colonies of bacteria that are resistant to host defenses and treatment with antibiotics) and can seed the lung with microorganisms, especially during endotracheal

BOX 36.3   ETIOLOGIC MICROORGANISMS FOR PNEUMONIA IN ADULTS

CAP	HCAP/HAP/VAP	IMMUNOCOMPROMISED INDIVIDUALS
Streptococcus pneumoniae	*Pseudomonas aeruginosa*	*Pneumocystis jiroveci* (formerly *P. carinii*)
Haemophilus influenzae	*Staphylococcus aureus* (including methicillin-resistant strains)	*Mycobacterium tuberculosis*
Staphylococcus aureus	*Klebsiella pneumoniae*	Atypical mycobacteria
Mycoplasma pneumoniae	*Enterobacter* species	Respiratory viruses
Chlamydia pneumoniae		Protozoa
Moraxella catarrhalis		Parasites
Legionella pneumophila		
Influenza		
Rhinovirus		
Coronavirus		

CAP, Community-acquired pneumonia; *HAP,* hospital-acquired pneumonia; *HCAP,* healthcare-associated pneumonia; *VAP,* ventilator-associated pneumonia.

suctioning.[100] Pneumonia also can occur when bacteria are spread to the lungs in the blood from bacteremia that can result from infection elsewhere in the body or from intravenous drug use.

In healthy individuals, pathogens that reach the lungs are expelled or controlled by mechanisms of self-defense (see Chapters 7, 8, and 10). If a microorganism overcomes the upper airway defense mechanisms, such as the cough reflex and mucociliary clearance, the next line of defense is the airway epithelial cell. Airway epithelial cells can recognize some pathogens directly (e.g., *Pseudomonas aeruginosa* and *Staphylococcus aureus*). However, the most important guardian cell of the lower respiratory tract is the alveolar macrophage, which recognizes pathogens through its pattern-recognition receptors (e.g., Toll-like receptors). Macrophages present infectious antigens to the adaptive immune system, activating T cells and B cells with the induction of cellular and humoral immunity. Release of TNF-α and IL-1 from macrophages and chemokines and chemotactic signals from mast cells and fibroblasts contributes to widespread inflammation in the lung with recruitment of neutrophils from the capillaries of the lungs into the alveoli.

Neutrophils are critical phagocytes that kill microbes through the formation of phagolysosomes filled with degradative enzymes, antimicrobial proteins, and toxic oxygen free radicals.[101] Neutrophils have also been found to extrude a meshwork of proteins called a *neutrophil extracellular trap (NET)* that can capture any bacteria that have not yet been phagocytosed. Unfortunately, many pathogens, such as the pneumococcus, can release a deoxyribonuclease (DNase) that cleaves the NET and thus escapes neutrophil defense.[102] The release of inflammatory mediators and immune complexes can damage bronchial, mucosal, and alveolocapillary membranes, causing the terminal bronchioles and acini to fill with infectious debris and exudate. In addition, some microorganisms release toxins from their cell walls that can cause further lung damage. Obstruction of bronchioles and accumulation of exudate in the acinus lead to V̇/Q̇ mismatching, hypoxemia, and dyspnea.

Pneumococcal Pneumonia. The pathogenesis of pneumococcal pneumonia (*Streptococcus pneumoniae*) is the most common cause of bacterial pneumonia and serves as a model for understanding other forms of bacterial pneumonia (Fig. 36.17). *S. pneumoniae* microorganisms initiate innate and adaptive immune responses (see Chapters 7 and 8). The immune response includes complement activation and the production of antibodies, which are crucial for opsonizing the encapsulated bacterium. Rapid lysis of pneumococcal bacteria (as occurs with antibiotic treatment) results in the release of intracellular bacterial proteins that can be toxic. The best known of these proteins is pneumolysin, which is cytotoxic to virtually every cell in the lung and is partially responsible for the worsening in clinical symptoms sometimes seen in individuals immediately after they begin antibiotic treatment.[103] Inflammatory cytokines and cells are released that cause alveolar edema. Edema creates a medium for the multiplication of bacteria and aids in the spread of infection into adjacent portions of the lung. The involved lobe undergoes consolidation, which alveoli fill with blood cells, fibrin, edematous fluid, and pneumococci, giving lung tissue a red appearance. This passes into the stage in which affected tissues become gray because of fibrin deposition over the pleural surfaces and the presence of fibrin and neutrophils in the consolidated alveoli, where phagocytosis is rapidly taking place. With resolution, increasing numbers of macrophages appear in the alveolar spaces, the neutrophils degenerate, and the fibrin threads and remaining bacteria are digested by macrophages and removed by lymphatic vessels. Usually infection is limited to one or two lobes.

Viral Pneumonia. Viral pneumonia is seasonal, usually mild and self-limiting, but it can set the stage for a secondary bacterial infection (especially by *S. aureus* and *Streptococcus pneumoniae*) by providing an ideal environment for bacterial growth and by damaging ciliated epithelial

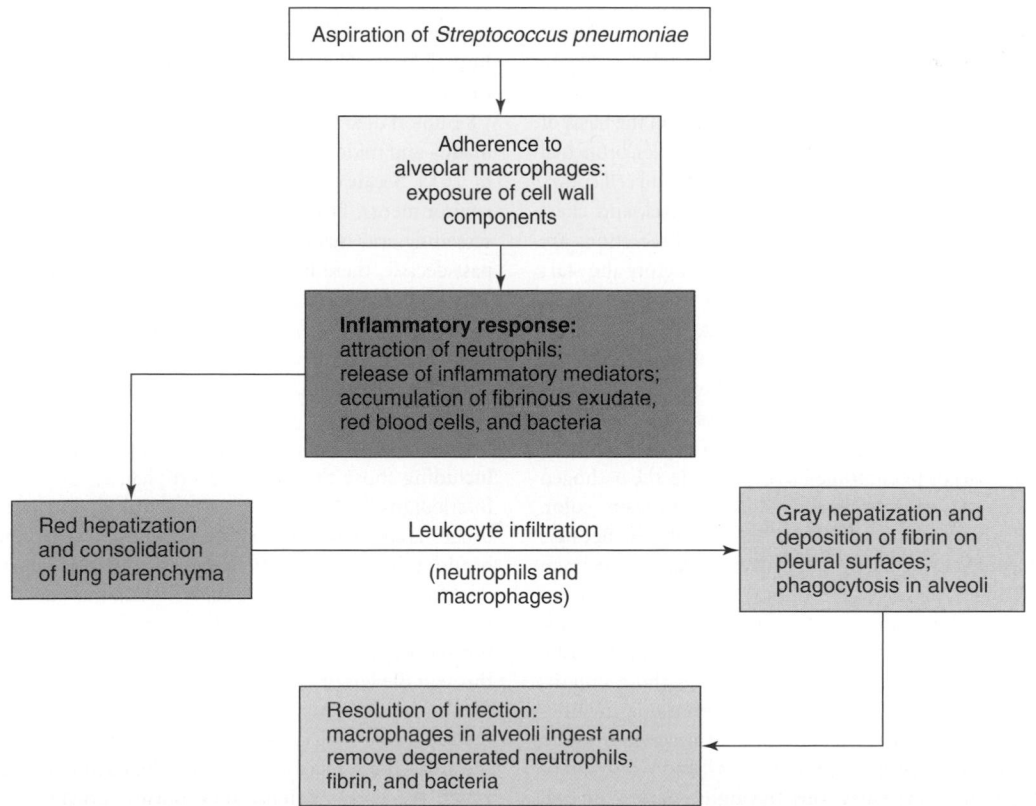

FIGURE 36.17 Pathophysiologic Course of Pneumococcal Pneumonia *(Streptococcus pneumoniae)*.

cells, which normally prevent pathogens from reaching the lower airways. Viral pneumonia can be a primary infection (e.g., influenza pneumonia) or a complication of another viral illness (e.g., chickenpox, measles). Influenza virus is the most common viral cause of pneumonia. Influenza viruses impair antibacterial defense mechanisms by increasing neutrophil apoptosis and neutrophil and monocyte dysfunction, depressing chemotaxis, and suppressing phagocytosis. The virus not only destroys the ciliated epithelial cells but also invades the goblet cells and bronchial mucous glands. Sloughing of destroyed bronchial epithelium occurs throughout the respiratory tract, preventing mucociliary clearance and promoting attachment of bacteria. Bronchial walls become edematous and infiltrated with leukocytes, and viruses can evade the protective effect of surfactant proteins in the alveoli.[104]

Some forms of viral pneumonia can progress to severe systemic illness and sepsis with many complications and a high morbidity and mortality. Severe viral pneumonia can include common types of influenza that can be fatal, especially in older adults.[105] Other severe viral infections are considered opportunistic infections, such as cytomegalovirus pneumonia in immunocompromised individuals. New or atypical forms of viral infection, such as swine influenza A (H1N1) virus, avian influenza A (H5N1 and H7N9) viruses, enterovirus D68 (EV-D68), and the coronavirus that causes severe acute respiratory syndrome (SARS), can affect previously healthy populations and pose a considerable threat for pandemics.[106,107]

◆**CLINICAL MANIFESTATIONS.** Most cases of pneumonia are preceded by an upper respiratory tract infection, which is usually viral. This is then followed by the onset of cough, dyspnea, and fever. The cough is often productive, but may be nonproductive, especially in viral pneumonia. Other symptoms include chills, malaise, and pleuritic chest pain. Physical examination may reveal signs of pulmonary consolidation, such as inspiratory crackles, increased tactile fremitus (palpable chest vibrations), egophony (a voice sound heard on auscultation as a prolonged "a" over consolidated lung tissue when a person says "e"), and whispered pectoriloquy (the sound of whispering heard on auscultation over consolidated lung tissue, which is abnormal). Individuals also may demonstrate symptoms and signs of underlying systemic disease or sepsis.

◆**EVALUATION AND TREATMENT.** Diagnosis is made on the basis of history, physical examination (tachypnea, tachycardia, crackles, bronchial breath sounds, and findings of pleural effusion), white blood cell count, measurement of procalcitonin or C-reactive protein level, and chest x-ray. Stains and cultures of blood and respiratory tract secretions are completed in more severe and hospitalized cases and before the start of antibiotic therapy. The white blood cell count is usually elevated, although it may be low if the individual is debilitated, is immunocompromised, or has overwhelming infection.[108] Serum procalcitonin or C-reactive protein levels can be used to help differentiate bacterial from viral infection in order to guide therapy. Chest imaging shows infiltrates that may involve a single lobe of the lung or may be more diffuse. Once the diagnosis of pneumonia has been made, the pathogen is identified by means of sputum characteristics (Gram stain, color, odor) and cultures or, if sputum is absent, blood cultures. Because many pathogens exist in the normal oropharyngeal flora, the specimen may be contaminated with pathogens from oral secretions. If sputum studies fail to identify the pathogen, the individual is immunocompromised, or the individual's condition worsens, further diagnostic studies may include molecular testing of blood or urine, thoracentesis, bronchoscopy, or lung biopsy.[109] Prevention of pneumonia includes prevention of aspiration, respiratory isolation of immunocompromised individuals, vaccination for appropriate populations, and reduction of ventilator-associated pulmonary infections through a variety of oral hygiene and endotracheal tube interventions.

The first step in the management of pneumonia is establishing adequate ventilation and oxygenation. Most individuals have hypoxemia and a respiratory alkalosis, although persons with underlying lung disease may require ventilation. Adequate hydration and good pulmonary hygiene (e.g., deep breathing, coughing, chest physical therapy) are also important. Severe pneumonia is a common cause of sepsis and septic shock (see Chapter 49) and requires intensive care.

Antibiotics should be given within 4 hours of presentation to treat bacterial pneumonia. When a specific microorganism is not identified, empirical antibiotics are chosen based on the likely causative microorganism and whether the individual has CAP, HCAP, HAP, or VAP.[110] The 2014 National Institute for Health and Care Excellence (NICE) guidelines recommend antibiotics only when the C-reactive protein level is greater than 20 mmol/L and positive clinical findings are evident.[111] Resistant strains of *Pneumococcus, Pseudomonas aeruginosa,* Enterobacteriaceae extended-spectrum β-lactamase (ESBL+), and methicillin-resistant *Staphylococcus aureus* (MRSA) are becoming more prevalent and require secondary antibiotics.[112] HCAP, HAP, and VAP require broad-spectrum empirical antibiotics, and sputum or blood cultures may indicate the need for additional therapies (e.g., antifungals).[113] Viral pneumonia is usually treated with supportive therapy alone (unless secondary bacterial infection is present); however, antivirals may be needed in severe cases. Infections with opportunistic microorganisms may be polymicrobial and require multiple drugs, including antifungals.

Tuberculosis

Tuberculosis (TB) is an infection caused by *Mycobacterium tuberculosis,* an acid-fast bacillus that usually affects the lungs, but may invade other body systems. TB is the leading cause of death from a curable infectious disease throughout the world. Since the 1992 peak resurgence in TB occurred (attributable to AIDS), the incidence of TB has declined every year and the death rate has declined by 67%. The highest number of reported cases is among foreign-born individuals, accounting for 67.9% of cases in the United States in 2016. The highest number of cases among racial and ethnic groups occurs among Asians and American Indian/Alaska Natives, Native Hawaiians and other Pacific Islanders.[114] In 2015 worldwide, 10.4 million people were diagnosed with TB and 1.8 million died from the disease, including 170,000 children primarily in low- and middle-income countries. One in three HIV deaths occurred in 2015 because of TB.[115] Crowded institutional settings or living environments, homelessness, substance abuse, and lack of access to screening and medical care contribute to the spread of TB. Over the past decade, there has been a rapid emergence of multidrug-resistant TB (MDR-TB) and extensively drug-resistant TB (XDR-TB) around the world (see *What's New?* Multidrug-Resistant and Extensively Drug-Resistant Tuberculosis).[116]

◆**PATHOPHYSIOLOGY.** TB is highly contagious and is transmitted from person-to-person by inhalation of airborne droplets. Host susceptibility to infection is influenced by host and parasite genetic polymorphisms, including those that affect macrophages, tumor necrosis factor, and interleukins.[117] In immunocompetent individuals, the microorganism usually is contained by the inflammatory and immune response systems, resulting in asymptomatic latent tuberculosis infection.[118]

After inhalation of *M. tuberculosis,* the bacilli lodge in the lung periphery, are phagocytized by resident macrophages, and cause nonspecific pneumonitis (lung inflammation). Some bacilli migrate through the lymphatics and become lodged in the lymph nodes, where they encounter lymphocytes and initiate the immune response. Inflammation in the lung causes neutrophils and macrophages to migrate to the area. These phagocytes engulf the bacilli and begin the process by which the body's defense mechanisms isolate the bacilli, preventing their spread. However, the bacterium is successful as a pathogen because

WHAT'S NEW?

Multidrug-Resistant and Extensively Drug-Resistant Tuberculosis

Multidrug-resistant tuberculosis (MDR-TB) refers to strains of *Mycobacterium tuberculosis* that are resistant to both isoniazid and rifampin. Extensively drug-resistant TB (XDR-TB) refers to strains that also are resistant to fluoroquinolones and at least one of three injectable second-line drugs (amikacin, kanamycin, or capreomycin). MDR-TB has been reported in hundreds of countries around the world, resulting in increased transmission and mortality. XDR-TB remains relatively rare, but concern is increasing, especially since the recognition of several cases of totally drug-resistant TB (TDR-TB). Mechanisms of drug resistance include mutations in ribonucleic acid (RNA) polymerase and the catalase peroxidase gene, especially in individuals exposed to inconsistent drug treatment (noncompliance) for TB infection. Other risk factors include prolonged hospitalization, HIV infection, and lack of directly observed therapy regimens or lack of consistently available drugs. The diagnosis of MDR-TB and XDR-TB combines culture and drug sensitivity testing with nucleic acid amplification assays that detect specific gene mutations associated with drug resistance. Second-line drugs for MDR-TB include aminoglycosides and fluoroquinolones. Drugs for XDR-TB include alanine analogs, thioamide drugs, salicylate antifolate, diarylquinoline, and oxazolidine; however, these drugs have significant side effects. The CDC reports that only 30% to 50% of people with XDR-TB can be successfully treated with these medications and the estimated cost of treatment exceeds $400,000. New medications are being explored in an attempt to improve success rates. One emerging approach is host-directed therapeutics, such as therapeutic vaccines and monoclonal antibodies, which seek to improve the immune response while reducing lung injury.

Data from Dheda K, Barry CE 3rd, Maartens G: *Lancet* 387(10024):1211–1226, 2016; Engstrom A: *Infect Dis (Lond)* 48(1):1–17, 2016; Wallis RS et al: *Lancet Infect Dis* 16(4):e34–e46, 2016; Wilson JW, Tsukayama DT: *Mayo Clinic Proc* 91(4):482–495, 2016; Yin J et al: *PLoS One* 11(3):e0150511, 2016.

it can survive within macrophages, resist lysosomal killing, multiply within the cell, and transit into a stage of dormancy rendering itself extremely resistant to host defense and drug treatment.[119] In defense, macrophages and lymphocytes release interferon, which inhibits the replication of the microorganisms and stimulates more macrophages to attack the bacterium. Apoptotic infected macrophages also can activate cytotoxic T cells (CD8). Neutrophils, lymphocytes, and macrophages seal off the colonies of bacilli, forming a granulomatous lesion called a *tubercle*. Infected tissues within the tubercle die, forming cheeselike material called *caseation necrosis*. (Necrosis is described in Chapter 2.) Collagenous scar tissue then grows around the tubercle, completing isolation of the bacilli. The immune response is complete after about 10 days, preventing further multiplication of the bacilli.

Once the bacilli are isolated in tubercles and immunity develops, TB may remain dormant for life. There is a range of tuberculosis infections that include individuals with effective immune responses that eradicate all viable bacilli; individuals who contain the infection but continue to maintain populations of bacilli that intermittently replicate in macrophages, granulomas, and other tissues as their immune system tries to control the bacilli; and individuals with no effective immunity, resulting in rapid progression to active disease. Liquefaction of the caseous center can occur, with extracellular bacterial growth and cavity formation. TB may spread through the blood and lymphatics and cause extrapulmonary disease. Coinfection with human immunodeficiency virus (HIV) is the single greatest risk factor for primary infection or reactivation of latent or controlled infection because the two diseases

(i.e., HIV and TB) potentiate each other, accelerating the decline of immune function.[120] Cancer, diabetes mellitus, immunosuppressive medications, poor nutritional status, renal failure, and other debilitating diseases can reactivate disease.[121,122]

◆**CLINICAL MANIFESTATIONS.** Latent TB infection is asymptomatic with no radiologic evidence of disease. Symptoms of active disease develop gradually and may not be noticed until the disease is advanced. However, symptoms can appear in immunosuppressed individuals within weeks of exposure to the bacillus. Common clinical manifestations include fatigue, weight loss, lethargy, anorexia (loss of appetite), a low-grade fever that usually occurs in the afternoon, and night sweats. (These are common signs and symptoms of all chronic infections.) A cough that produces purulent sputum develops slowly and becomes more frequent over several weeks or months. Dyspnea, chest pain, and hemoptysis also may occur as the disease progresses. Extrapulmonary TB disease is common in HIV-infected individuals and may cause neurologic deficits, meningitis symptoms, bone pain, and urinary symptoms.

◆**EVALUATION AND TREATMENT.** Screening for TB consists of obtaining a tuberculin skin test (TST; purified protein derivative [PPD]), immunoassays, and chest radiographs.[123] A positive tuberculin skin test indicates the need for yearly chest radiographs to detect active disease. The skin test does not differentiate between past, latent, or active forms of the disease. In addition, individuals who have received the TB vaccine with bacille Calmette-Guérin (BCG) will have a positive TST even if they have never had TB. Two immunoassays (enzyme-linked immunospot and quantitative blood interferon-gamma assay) are available. These newer tests are more sensitive and specific for the diagnosis of latent TB and are not confounded by previous BCG vaccination.

Sputum microscopy, culture, and indirect drug susceptibility testing (DST) remain the "gold standard" for diagnosing TB. When active pulmonary disease is present, sputum staining (using an acid-fast stain) and culture are positive for the tubercle bacillus. However, sputum culture can take up to 6 weeks to become positive. Current generation tuberculosis-specific nucleic acid amplification tests (NAATs) are important supplementary tests for the rapid direct detection of multidrug-resistant TB.[124] Chest radiographs of individuals with current or previous active disease demonstrate characteristic changes. Nodules, calcifications, cavities, and hilar enlargement (enlarged mediastinal lymph nodes) commonly are seen in the upper lobes. Screening and treatment of positive cases prevent transmission of the disease. Isolating individuals with active tuberculosis, limiting use of immunosuppressive medications, and treating underlying immunocompromising diseases, such as AIDS, are all critical steps.[125] Treatment consists of combinations of antibiotics (isoniazid, rifampin, pyrazinamide, and ethambutol) to control drug-sensitive disease or prevent reactivation of latent TB infection. The choice of drugs and the duration of treatment depend on the individual's health history, the likelihood of bacterial resistance to certain drugs, and the presence of active disease.[126]

The waxy coat of *M. tuberculosis* renders it impermeable to many common drugs. For drug-resistant bacilli, the recommended treatment is administration for an 18-month timeframe of a combination of at least four drugs to which the microorganism is susceptible, including injectable drugs, with intermittent review of drug effectiveness. New drugs and drug combinations, including drugs purposed for other infections, are being tested to overcome drug resistance, including immune modulators.[127] New vaccines are in clinical trials.[125]

Abscess Formation and Cavitation

An **abscess** is a circumscribed area of suppuration and destruction of lung parenchyma and is a type of liquefactive necrosis. Abscess formation follows **consolidation** of lung tissue, in which inflammation causes alveoli to fill with fluid, pus, and microorganisms. The development of a lung abscess may be acute (less than 6 weeks) or chronic (more than 6 weeks). Necrosis of consolidated tissue may progress proximally until it communicates with a bronchus. If this occurs, the abscess empties into the bronchus, leaving a cavity that has a radiographic appearance similar to that of a lesion of tuberculosis.

Pneumonia caused by aspiration or by exposure to *Klebsiella* or *Staphylococcus* is the most common cause of abscess formation. Aspiration abscess is usually associated with alcohol abuse, seizure disorders, general anesthesia, and swallowing disorders. Immunocompromised individuals also are at greater risk for lung abscesses and may be infected with opportunistic microorganisms, such as fungi and mycobacteria. The clinical manifestations of abscess formation are similar to those of pneumonitis: fever, cough, chills, excessive sputum production, and pleural pain. Abscess communication with a bronchus causes a severe cough, copious amounts of often foul-smelling sputum, and occasionally hemoptysis. Cavitation is the process of abscess emptying and cavity formation. Diagnosis is made by radiography.[128] Treatment includes the administration of appropriate antibiotics and chest physical therapy, including chest percussion and postural drainage. Bronchoscopy may be performed to drain the abscess.[129]

Pulmonary Vascular Disease

Blood flow through the lungs can be disrupted by a number of disorders that result in occlusion of the vessels, an increase in pulmonary vascular resistance, or destruction of the vascular bed. The consequences of altered pulmonary blood flow may be of little functional significance or can result in severe and life-threatening changes in ventilation-perfusion ratios. Major disorders that result from pulmonary vascular diseases include pulmonary embolism, pulmonary hypertension, and cor pulmonale.

Pulmonary Embolism

Pulmonary embolism (PE) is occlusion or partial occlusion of the pulmonary artery or its branches by an embolus. PE most commonly results from embolization of a clot from deep venous thrombosis (DVT) involving the lower leg (see Chapter 33). Other less common non-thrombotic emboli include tissue fragments, lipids (fats), a foreign body, an air bubble, or amniotic fluid (Fig. 36.18). Risk factors for PE include conditions and disorders that promote blood clotting as a result of *venous stasis* (immobilization, heart failure), *hypercoagulability* (inherited coagulation disorders, malignancy, hormone replacement, oral contracep-

tives, pregnancy), and *endothelial injury* to the cells that line the vessels (trauma, infection, caustic intravenous infusions). Increased risk for thrombosis associated with hemodynamic stasis, hypercoagulability, and endothelial injury is known as *triad of Virchow*[130] (see Chapter 33). Genetic risks include factor V Leiden mutation, antithrombin II deficiency, protein S deficiency, activated protein C deficiency, and prothrombin *20210* gene mutations. No matter its source, a blood clot becomes an embolus when all or part of it breaks away from the site of formation and begins to travel in the bloodstream. Thromboembolism is described further in Chapter 33.

◆**PATHOPHYSIOLOGY.** The effect of the embolus depends on the extent of pulmonary blood flow obstruction, the size of the affected vessels, the nature of the embolus, and the secondary effects. Pulmonary emboli can result in any of the following:

1. Embolus with infarction: an embolus that causes infarction (death) of a portion of lung tissue
2. Embolus without infarction: an embolus that does not cause permanent lung injury (perfusion of the affected lung segment is maintained by the bronchial circulation)
3. Massive occlusion: an embolus that occludes a major portion of the pulmonary circulation (i.e., main pulmonary artery embolus)
4. Multiple pulmonary emboli: multiple emboli that may be chronic or recurrent

As a result of the thrombus lodging in the pulmonary circulation, there is a release both of neurohumoral substances, such as serotonin, histamine, catecholamines, and angiotensin II, and of inflammatory mediators, such as endothelin, leukotrienes, thromboxanes, and toxic oxygen free radicals. This causes widespread vasoconstriction that further impedes blood flow to the lung. Hemodynamically, this results in increased pulmonary artery pressures (pulmonary hypertension) and can lead to right ventricular dilation and increased afterload.[131] Absent blood flow to a lung segment causes a ventilation-perfusion mismatch (increased dead space) and a decrease in surfactant production. The resulting atelectasis of the affected lung segments further contributes to hypoxemia. If the thrombus is large enough, infarction of lung tissue, dysrhythmias, decreased cardiac output, shock, and death are possible. The pathogenesis of pulmonary embolism is summarized in Fig. 36.19.

If the embolus does not cause infarction, the clot is dissolved by the fibrinolytic system (see Chapter 28) and pulmonary function returns to normal. If pulmonary infarction occurs, shrinking and scarring develop in the affected area of the lung.

◆**CLINICAL MANIFESTATIONS.** In most cases the clinical manifestations of PE are nonspecific; therefore evaluation of risk factors and predisposing factors is an important aspect of diagnosis. Consequently, the recognition of individuals at high risk for PE is crucial to assessing the clinical presentation. In suspected PE, assessment for DVT may indicate the presence of a lower extremity source for the thromboembolism. Calf pain and tenderness and also calf asymmetry (when documented with a tape measure) are some of the most important findings in DVT. Unfortunately, DVT is often asymptomatic and clinical examination has low sensitivity for the presence of a clot, especially in the thigh and pelvis. Therefore the lack of clinical indicators for DVT does not rule out the possibility for PE.

An individual with PE usually presents with the sudden onset of pleuritic chest pain, cough, dyspnea, tachypnea, tachycardia, and unexplained anxiety. Occasionally syncope (fainting) or hemoptysis occurs. With large emboli, a pleural friction rub, pleural effusion, fever, and leukocytosis may be noted. Recurrent pulmonary emboli occur in individuals with a history of previous emboli. Recurrent small emboli may not be detected until progressive incapacitation, precordial pain, anxiety, dyspnea, and right ventricular enlargement are exhibited. Massive occlusion causes severe pulmonary hypertension and shock.

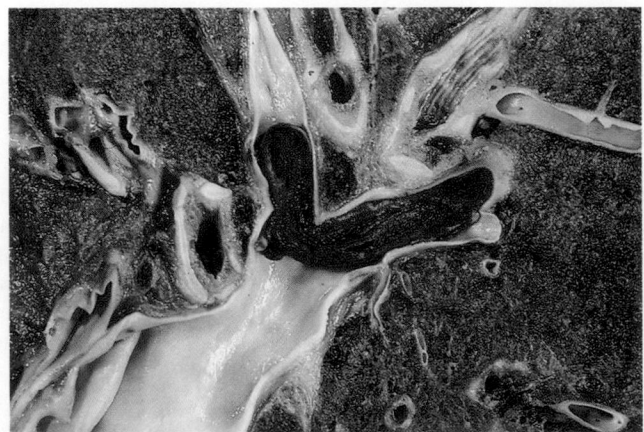

FIGURE 36.18 Pulmonary Embolus. The embolus extends into major branches of the pulmonary artery. (From Kumar V et al: *Robbins & Cotran pathologic basis of disease*, ed 8, Philadelphia, 2010, Saunders.)

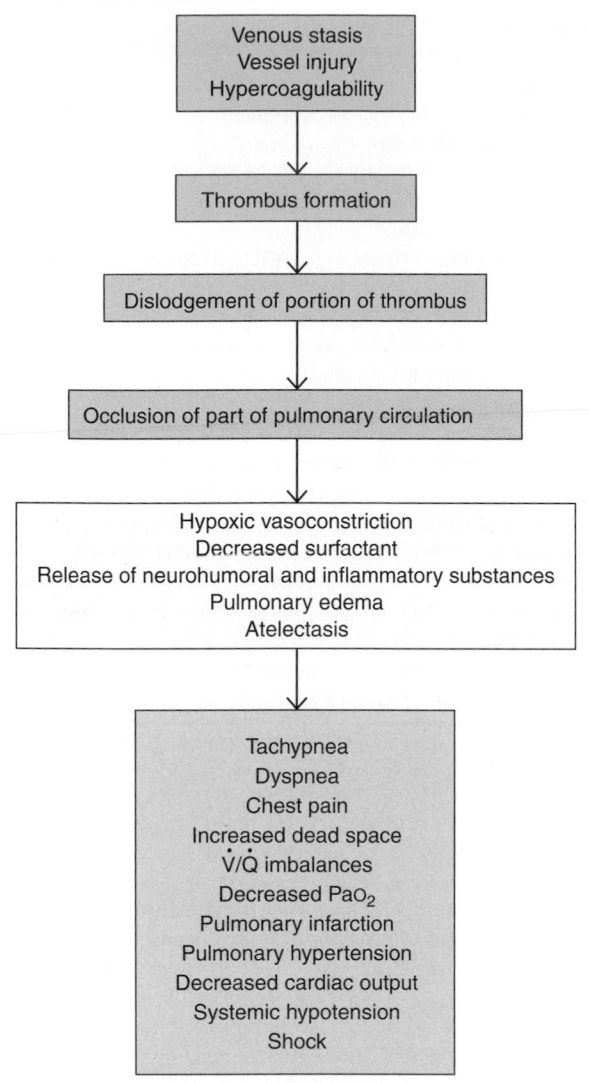

Venous stasis
Vessel injury
Hypercoagulability

↓

Thrombus formation

↓

Dislodgement of portion of thrombus

↓

Occlusion of part of pulmonary circulation

↓

Hypoxic vasoconstriction
Decreased surfactant
Release of neurohumoral and inflammatory substances
Pulmonary edema
Atelectasis

↓

Tachypnea
Dyspnea
Chest pain
Increased dead space
$\dot{V}/\dot{Q}$ imbalances
Decreased PaO_2
Pulmonary infarction
Pulmonary hypertension
Decreased cardiac output
Systemic hypotension
Shock

FIGURE 36.19 Pathogenesis of Massive Pulmonary Embolism Caused by a Thrombus (Pulmonary Thromboembolism).

EVALUATION AND TREATMENT. The evaluation of individuals suspected of having acute venous thromboembolism is based on the use of Clinical Decision Rules, such as the Well's score, which guide the sequence of diagnostic modalities based on pretest risk assessments.[132] Routine chest radiographs and pulmonary function tests are not definitive for pulmonary embolism in the first 24 hours. Oximetry and arterial blood gas analyses usually demonstrate hypoxemia. The ECG may show evidence of strain on the right side of the heart. The serum D-dimer level measures products of thrombus degradation (fibrinogen and fibrin) by the fibrinolytic system and, if normal, makes the presence of a PE highly unlikely. When D-dimer is positive, further evaluation may be conducted using single or multidetector spiral CT arteriography.[133] Magnetic resonance arteriography (MRA) is used in some centers. In rare cases, a pulmonary angiogram is necessary to confirm the diagnosis of PE. The measurement of elevated serum troponin I levels has been useful in stratifying the risk and severity of PE because it increases with right ventricular dysfunction and serious adverse events.[134] Diagnostic algorithms guide diagnosis and treatment.[131]

The ideal treatment of PE is prevention through risk factor recognition and elimination of predisposing factors. Venous stasis in hospitalized individuals is minimized by bed exercises, frequent position changes, early ambulation, and pneumatic calf compression. Most at-risk individuals also will receive prophylactic anticoagulation with low-molecular-weight heparin, warfarin, or fondaparinux. Oral anticoagulants that are not dependent on vitamin K levels, such as rivaroxaban, apixaban, and dabigatran, have been approved for the prevention and treatment of PE and DVT and do not require long-term anticoagulation monitoring.[135,136] Once venous thromboembolism has occurred, rapid assessment of hemodynamic stability and oxygenation is essential. Low-molecular-weight heparin, unfractionated heparin, fondaparinux, or one of the new anticoagulants not dependent on vitamin K levels are indicated for stable individuals.[131] In those with unstable hemodynamics, thrombolytic therapy, either intravenously provided or catheter directed, reduces mortality.[132] Oxygen and hemodynamic stabilization with fluids may be needed for life-threatening complications. Surgical embolectomy is indicated in massive PE. After stabilization, anticoagulation therapy is continued for several months. In individuals who have contraindications to anticoagulation therapy, the placement of a filter in the inferior vena cava can prevent emboli from reaching the lungs.[137,138]

Pulmonary Artery Hypertension

Pulmonary artery hypertension (PAH) is defined as a mean pulmonary artery pressure greater than 25 mmHg at rest (normal is 15 to 18 mmHg). Box 36.4 contains the World Health Organization (WHO) 2014 clinical categories for PAH. Left heart disease is the most common cause of PAH overall, and COPD is the most common lung disease associated with PAH. Idiopathic PAH is rare.

PATHOPHYSIOLOGY. Idiopathic PAH usually occurs in women between the ages of 20 and 40. It is characterized by endothelial dysfunction with overproduction of vasoconstrictors, such as thromboxane and endothelin-1, and decreased production of vasodilators, such as nitric oxide and prostacyclin-1.[139] Proinflammatory cytokines, abnormal calcium signaling (vasoconstriction), abnormal potassium channels (vasoconstriction), phosphodiesterases (modulate cellular proliferation), serotonin (vasoconstrictor), and adrenomedullin (vasodilator) also play a role in the pathogenesis of PAH. Release of growth factors causes proliferation of endothelial cells, smooth muscle cells, and fibroblasts, resulting in patchy intimal and medial hypertrophy, intimal fibrosis, abnormal angiogenesis, and in situ thrombosis in the small precapillary pulmonary arteries (resistance vessels). In individuals with *BMPR2* gene mutations (a member of the transforming growth factor-beta family), intracellular signaling abnormalities result in vascular proliferation. These processes result in *vascular remodeling* with luminal narrowing and abnormal vasoconstriction. The combined changes cause resistance to pulmonary artery blood flow, thus increasing the pressure in the pulmonary arteries.[140] As resistance and pressure increase, the workload of the right ventricle increases and subsequent right ventricular hypertrophy, followed by failure, may occur (cor pulmonale). Gas exchange is reduced with restriction in lung volumes. Eventually death results in most individuals with PAH. The pathogenesis of pulmonary artery hypertension and cor pulmonale, resulting from disease of the respiratory system or hypoxia, is shown in Fig. 36.20.

Pulmonary hypertension associated with hypoxia is a serious complication of many acute and chronic pulmonary disorders, such as COPD and hypoventilation associated with obesity. These conditions are complicated by hypoxic pulmonary vasoconstriction, which further increases pulmonary artery pressures.

CLINICAL MANIFESTATIONS. Pulmonary artery hypertension may not be detected until it is quite severe. The symptoms are often masked by underlying pulmonary or cardiovascular disease. The first indication of pulmonary hypertension is often an abnormality seen on a chest radiograph (enlarged pulmonary arteries and right heart border) or an electrocardiogram that shows right ventricular hypertrophy.

BOX 36.4   CLINICAL CLASSIFICATION OF PULMONARY HYPERTENSION*

1. Pulmonary artery hypertension (PAH)
   1.1 Idiopathic (IPAH) (rare)
   1.2 Heritable
      1.2.1 *BMPR2*
      1.2.2 *ALK1, endoglin* (with or without hereditary hemorrhagic telangiectasia), *SMAD9, CAV-1, KCNK3*
      1.2.3 Unknown
   1.3 Drug- and toxin-induced PAH
   1.4 Associated with PAH (APAH)
      1.4.1 Connective tissue disease
      1.4.2 HIV infection
      1.4.3 Portal hypertension
      1.4.4 Congenital heart disease
      1.4.5 Schistosomiasis
      1.4.6 Chronic hemolytic anemia
   1.5 Persistent pulmonary hypertension of the newborn
1′. Pulmonary veno-occlusive disease (PVOD) and/or pulmonary capillary hemangiomatosis (PCH)
1″. Persistent pulmonary hypertension of the newborn
2. Pulmonary hypertension caused by left-sided heart disease (most common)
   2.1 Left ventricular systolic dysfunction
   2.2 Left ventricular diastolic dysfunction
   2.3 Valvular disease
   2.4 Congenital/acquired left heart inflow/outflow tract obstruction and congenital cardiomyopathies
3. Pulmonary hypertension caused by lung diseases and/or hypoxia
   3.1 Chronic obstructive pulmonary disease
   3.2 Interstitial lung disease
   3.3 Other pulmonary diseases with mixed restrictive and obstructive pattern
   3.4 Sleep-disordered breathing
   3.5 Alveolar hypoventilation disorders
   3.6 Chronic exposure to high altitude
   3.7 Developmental abnormalities
4. Chronic thromboembolic pulmonary hypertension
5. Pulmonary hypertension with unclear multifactorial mechanisms
   5.1 Hematologic disorders: myeloproliferative disorders, splenectomy, chronic hemolytic anemia
   5.2 Systemic disorders: sarcoidosis, pulmonary Langerhans cell histiocytosis, lymphangioleiomyomatosis, neurofibromatosis, vasculitis
   5.3 Metabolic disorders: glycogen storage disease, Gaucher disease, thyroid disorders
   5.4 Others: tumoral obstruction, fibrosing mediastinitis, chronic renal failure on dialysis, segmental PH

*Pulmonary arterial hypertension (PAH) refers to group 1 PAH. Pulmonary hypertension (PH) refers to any of group 2 through group 5 PH, and also is used when referring to all five groups collectively.
HIV, Human immunodeficiency virus.
Data from Lau EM, Humbert M: *Can J Cardiol* 31(4):367–374, 2015.

Symptoms of fatigue, progressive shortness of breath with exertion, chest discomfort, tachypnea, palpitations, and cough are common. Examination may reveal peripheral edema, jugular venous distention, a right parasternal lift from an enlarged right ventricle, and splitting of the second heart sound with a loud pulmonic valve component as a result of forced closure of the pulmonic valve secondary to elevated pulmonary pressures.[139]

◆EVALUATION AND TREATMENT. Definitive diagnosis and accurate assessment of pulmonary artery pressure can be made only with right-sided heart catheterization. Common diagnostic modalities used to determine the cause include chest x-ray, echocardiography (to estimate right ventricular systolic pressures), and computed tomography. Other diagnostic studies to detect underlying causes of PAH can include arterial blood gas testing, liver function testing, HIV serology, electrocardiography, pulmonary function testing, polysomnography, and ventilation-perfusion scanning. The diagnosis of idiopathic PAH (IPAH) is made when all other causes of pulmonary hypertension have been eliminated. Disease severity is quantified using the New York Heart Association or WHO classification of functional status of patients with pulmonary artery hypertension.[141]

General therapies for PAH include administration of oxygen, diuretics, and anticoagulants and avoidance of contributing factors such as air travel, decongestant medications, nonsteroidal antiinflammatory medications, pregnancy, and tobacco use. Medications used in the treatment of PAH include prostacyclin analogs (epoprostenol, beraprost, iloprost), endothelin receptor antagonists (bosentan, ambrisentan), phosphodiesterase-5 inhibitors, and calcium channel blockers.[139,140] Those who fail medical therapy may be candidates for lung transplantation.

The most effective treatment for secondary pulmonary artery hypertension is treatment of the primary disorder. However, once pulmonary hypertension has persisted long enough for hypertrophy of the medial smooth muscle layer to develop (as it does with chronic hypoxemia), it is no longer reversible. Treatment relies on the use of supplemental oxygen to reverse hypoxic vasoconstriction.

Cor Pulmonale

Cor pulmonale is secondary to pulmonary artery hypertension and consists of right ventricular enlargement (hypertrophy, dilation, or both).[142]

◆PATHOPHYSIOLOGY. Cor pulmonale develops as pulmonary artery hypertension creates chronic pressure overload in the right ventricle. Pressure overload increases the work of the right ventricle, causes hypertrophy of the normally thin-walled heart muscle, and compromises right ventricular myocardial perfusion. The increased pressure decreases perfusion of the right coronary arteries, resulting in ischemia, decreased contractility, and right ventricular overload.[143] Acute hypoxemia, such as might occur with pneumonia, can exaggerate pulmonary hypertension and further stress the ventricle as well. Right ventricular filling pressures are normal until failure occurs. The right ventricle usually fails when pulmonary artery pressure equals systemic blood pressure.

◆CLINICAL MANIFESTATIONS. The clinical manifestations of cor pulmonale may be obscured by primary respiratory disease and appear only during exercise testing. The heart appears normal at rest, but with exercise, cardiac output falls. The electrocardiogram shows right ventricular hypertrophy. Chest pain is common. The pulmonary component of the second heart sound, which represents closure of the pulmonic valve, may be accentuated, and a pulmonic valve murmur also may be present. Tricuspid valve murmur may accompany the development of right ventricular failure. Increased pressure in the systemic venous circulation causes jugular venous distention, hepatosplenomegaly, and peripheral edema.

◆EVALUATION AND TREATMENT. Diagnosis is made on the basis of physical examination, radiographic imaging, and electrocardiogram or echocardiogram, or both. The goal of treatment for cor pulmonale is to decrease the workload of the right ventricle by lowering pulmonary artery pressure. Treatment is the same as that for pulmonary artery hypertension, and its success depends on reversal of the underlying lung disease.

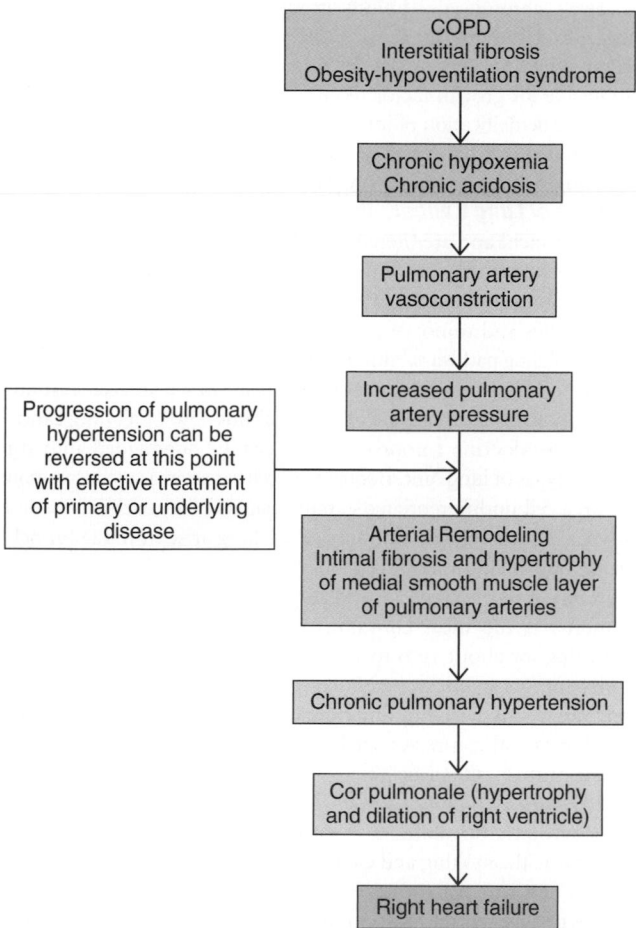

FIGURE 36.20 Pathogenesis of Pulmonary Hypertension and Cor Pulmonale Caused by Disease of the Respiratory System or Hypoxia. *COPD,* Chronic obstructive pulmonary disease.

Malignancies of the Respiratory Tract
Laryngeal Cancer

Laryngeal cancer represents less than 1% of all cancers in the United States. There were an estimated 13,360 new cases and 3660 deaths in 2017.[144] The highest incidence is in men between 50 and 75 years of age. The primary risk factor for laryngeal cancer is tobacco smoking; risk is further heightened with the combination of smoking and alcohol consumption. The human papillomavirus (HPV types 6 and 11) also has been linked to both benign and malignant disease of the larynx.[145]

◆**PATHOPHYSIOLOGY.** Carcinoma of the true vocal cords (glottis) is more common than that of the supraglottic structures (epiglottis, aryepiglottic folds, arytenoids, and false cords). Tumors of the subglottic area are rare. Squamous cell carcinoma is the most common cell type, although small cell carcinomas also occur (Fig. 36.21). Laryngeal dysplasia has a high risk of progressing to malignancy. Metastasis develops by spreading to the draining lymph nodes, and distant metastasis, usually to the lung, is rare.

◆**CLINICAL MANIFESTATIONS.** The presenting symptoms of laryngeal cancer include hoarseness, dyspnea, and cough. Progressive hoarseness is the most significant symptom and can result in voice loss. Dyspnea is rare in the case of supraglottic tumors, but can be severe in subglottic tumors. Cough occurs less commonly and may follow swallowing. Laryngeal pain or a sore throat is likely to be present with supraglottic lesions.

◆**EVALUATION AND TREATMENT.** Evaluation of the larynx includes external inspection and palpation of the larynx and the lymph nodes in the neck. Indirect laryngoscopy provides a stereoscopic view of the structure and movement of the larynx. A biopsy also can be obtained during this procedure. Direct laryngoscopy provides specific visualization of the tumor. Imaging procedures facilitate the identification of tumor boundaries and the degree of extension to surrounding tissue.

Combined chemotherapy and radiation therapy can result in cure in early-stage disease. Partial laryngectomies followed by combined chemotherapy and radiation therapy can result in local tumor control. For metastatic disease, combined chemotherapy and radiation therapy before surgery can reduce disease burden. Total laryngectomy is required when lesions are extensive and involve the cartilage. Swallowing and speech therapy after treatment can significantly improve recovery. Voice restoration after total laryngectomy includes instruction in esophageal speech, use of an electrolarynx, and tracheoesophageal puncture with

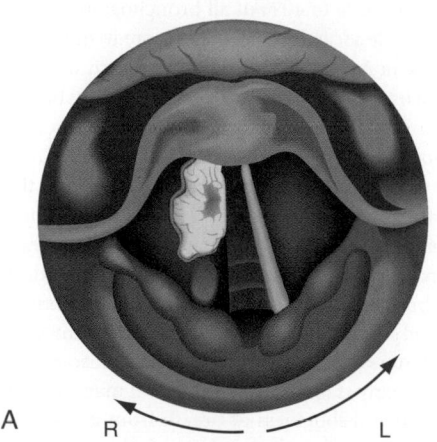
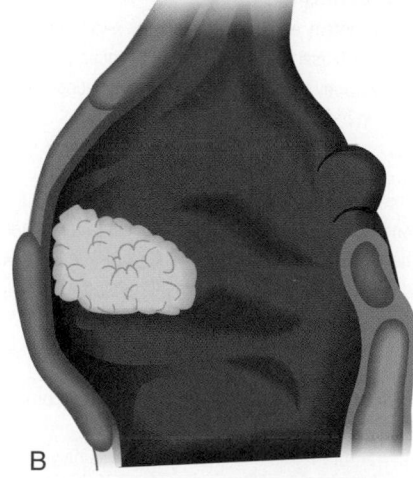

FIGURE 36.21 Laryngeal Cancer. **A,** Mirror view of carcinoma of right false cord partially hiding true cord. **B,** Lateral view. (From del Regato JA, Spjut HJ, Cox JD: *Ackerman and del Regato's cancer,* ed 2, St Louis, 1985, Mosby.)

voice prosthesis placement (the gold standard).[146] An artificial larynx is in development.[147]

Lung Cancer

Lung cancers (bronchogenic carcinomas) are tumors that arise from the epithelium of the respiratory tract. Other pulmonary tumors, including sarcomas, lymphomas, blastomas, and mesotheliomas (associated with asbestos exposure), occur less commonly. Lung cancer is the second most common cancer in the United States and the most common cause of cancer deaths. Important trends in lung cancer are summarized in Box 36.5.

The most common cause of lung cancer is tobacco smoking, and approximately 10% to 15% of active smokers will develop lung cancer.

BOX 36.5   IMPORTANT TRENDS FOR LUNG CANCER

Incidence
The incidence of lung cancer has been declining since the mid-1980s in men but only since the mid-2000s in women. There will be an estimated 222,500 new cases in 2017: 116,990 in men and 105,510 in women.

Mortality
Death rates have declined by 38% in men since 1990 and by 12% in women since 2002 because of the drop in smoking prevalence; however, lung cancer remains by far the greatest cancer killer in the United States. There will be an estimated 155,870 deaths in 2017: 84,590 in men and 71,280 in women.

Risk Factors
Cigarette smoking is the number one risk factor and accounts for 80% of lung cancer deaths in the United States. Environmental smoke exposure (exposure to someone else's cigarette smoke) increases the risk of lung cancer. Occupational risk factors include exposure to asbestos dust, arsenic, chromium, nickel, ionizing radiation, chloromethyl methyl ether, coal products, mustard gas, and vinyl chloride. Genetic susceptibility plays a role in the development of lung cancer.

Warning Signs
Warning signs include a persistent cough, sputum streaked with blood, chest pain, recurring attacks of pneumonia or bronchitis, weight loss, and hard nodes in the neck or axilla.

Early Detection and Prevention
Lung cancer is very difficult to detect early. Periodic chest x-ray films and sputum cytologic analysis are often used to screen for lung cancer; however, low-dose spiral computed tomography has been shown to reduce lung cancer mortality by 20% compared to standard chest x-ray in at-risk adults.

Treatment
Surgical resection of the entire tumor is the only treatment that results in cure; however, the disease is often too advanced by the time of diagnosis for surgery to be indicated. Radiation therapy and chemotherapy can be used as adjunctive or palliative treatment modalities. New treatments include gene therapy and immunotherapy.

Survival
Although the stage of cancer progression at the time of diagnosis greatly affects prognosis, the typical 1- and 5-year survival rates are 44% and 17%, respectively. The 5-year survival rate for small cell lung cancer is only 7%.

Data from American Cancer Society: *Cancer facts and figures 2017.* Available at: https://www.cancer.org/research/cancer-facts-statistics/all-cancer-facts-figures/cancer-facts-figures-2017.html.

Smokers with obstructive lung disease (low FEV_1 measurements) are at even greater risk. About 10% to 25% of lung cancers occur in persons who have never smoked, and it is estimated that 20% of lung cancer cases among never-smokers could be attributed to exposure to environmental tobacco smoke.[148] Environmental or occupational risk factors associated with lung cancer include exposure to benzopyrene, radon gas, metals (chromium, cadmium, arsenic), asbestos fibers, diesel exhaust, nitrogen and mustard gases, nickel, silica, vinyl chloride, and chloromethyl methyl ether. Genetic risks include polymorphisms of the genes responsible for growth factor receptors, angiogenesis, apoptosis, DNA repair, and detoxification of inhaled smoke.[149] Theories of carcinogenesis are discussed in Chapter 12. Currently there are no specific tools for predicting risk for or rate of progression of lung cancer.

Types of Lung Cancer. Primary lung cancers arise from cells that line the bronchi and are therefore called *bronchogenic carcinomas*. The development of lung cancer involves a multistep process of genetic, epigenetic, and environmental interactions resulting in the dysregulation of oncogenes and tumor-suppressor genes with activation of cancer-related signaling pathways. Although there are many types of lung cancer, they are divided into two major categories based on cell histology: nonsmall cell lung carcinoma (NSCLC, about 85% of all lung cancers) and neuroendocrine tumors. NSCLC can be subdivided into three common types of lung cancer: squamous cell carcinoma, adenocarcinoma, and large cell undifferentiated carcinoma, and they each have cellular subtypes. Neuroendocrine tumors of the lung arise from the bronchial mucosa and include small cell carcinoma, large cell neuroendocrine carcinoma, typical carcinoid, and atypical carcinoid tumors. Small cell carcinoma is the most common of these neuroendocrine tumors, accounting for about 10% to 15% of all lung cancers. Characteristics of these tumors are illustrated in Fig. 36.22 and described in Table 36.4. Many cancers that arise in other organs of the body metastasize to the lungs; however, these are not considered lung cancers and are categorized by their primary site of origin.

Nonsmall Cell Lung Cancer (NSCLC). Squamous cell carcinoma (SCC) accounts for about 30% of bronchogenic carcinomas and is associated with smoking and COPD. These tumors are typically located centrally near the hila and project into bronchi (Figs. 36.22, *A* and *B*). Because of this central location, nonproductive cough or hemoptysis is common. Pneumonia and atelectasis are often associated with squamous cell carcinoma. Chest pain is a late symptom associated with large tumors. These tumors are often fairly well localized and tend not to metastasize until late in the course of the disease.

Adenocarcinoma (tumor arising from glands) of the lung constitutes about 35% to 40% of all bronchogenic carcinomas (Figs. 36.22, *C* and *D*). Adenocarcinoma occurs more frequently in women, in nonsmokers, and in Asians. Environmental tobacco smoke, occupational carcinogens, viruses, hormones, and positive family history are associated with this tumor type.[150] *Epidermal growth factor receptor (EGFR)* mutations and *anaplastic lymphoma kinase (ALK)* gene rearrangements, as well as other tyrosine kinase inhibitors, are common in this type of lung cancer and are targets for therapy.[151] These tumors, which are usually smaller than 4 cm, more commonly arise in the peripheral regions of the pulmonary parenchyma. Pulmonary adenocarcinoma develops in a stepwise fashion through atypical adenomatous hyperplasia, adenocarcinoma in situ, and minimally invasive adenocarcinoma to invasive carcinoma. These tumors may be asymptomatic and discovered by routine chest x-ray in the early stages, or the individual may seek treatment for pleuritic chest pain and shortness of breath from pleural involvement by the tumor.

Included in the category of adenocarcinoma is bronchoalveolar cell carcinoma. These tumors arise from the terminal bronchioles and alveoli and are now being referred to as *adenocarcinoma in situ* or *minimally invasive adenocarcinoma.* They are slow-growing tumors with an

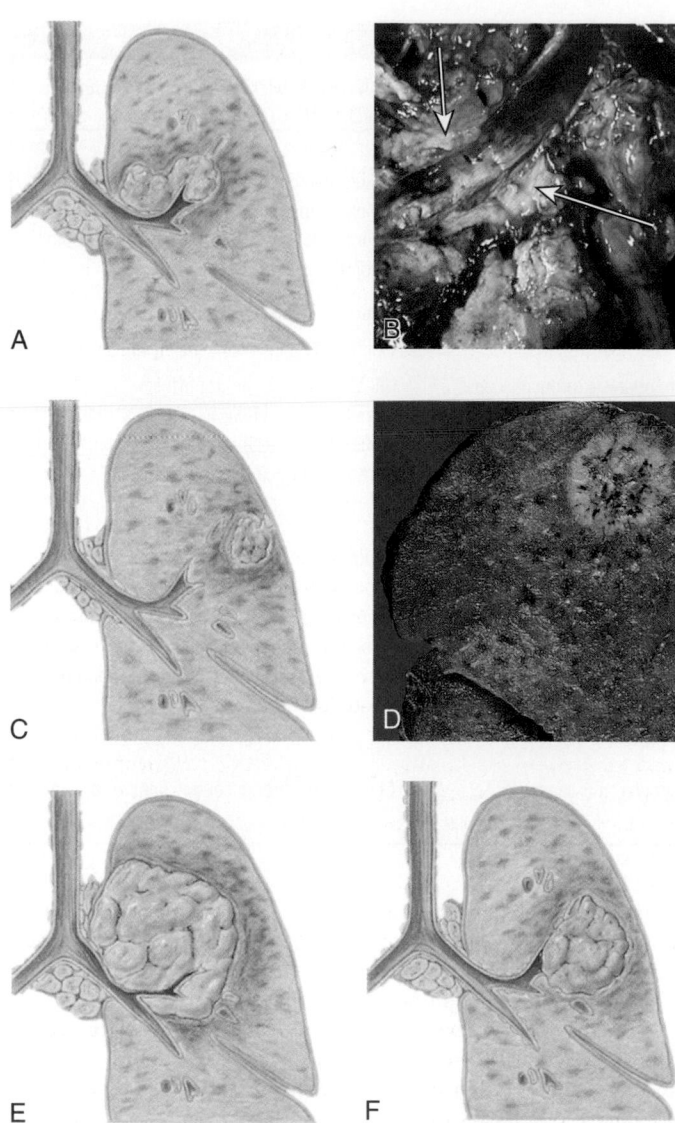

FIGURE 36.22 Lung Cancer. **A,** Squamous (epidermoid) cell carcinoma. **B,** Squamous cell carcinoma. This hilar tumor originates from the main bronchus. **C,** Adenocarcinoma. **D,** Peripheral adenocarcinoma. The tumor shows prominent black pigmentation, suggestive of having evolved in an anthracotic scar. **E,** Small cell (oat cell) carcinoma. **F,** Large cell carcinoma. (**A, C, E, F,** from Des Jardins T, Burton GG: *Clinical manifestations and assessment of respiratory disease,* ed 3, St Louis, 1995, Mosby. **B** and **D** from Damjanov I, Linder J, editors: *Anderson's pathology,* ed 10, St Louis, 1996, Mosby.)

unpredictable pattern of metastasis through the pulmonary arterial system and mediastinal lymph nodes.

Diagnosis of NSCLC requires cytologic analysis from biopsy, and treatment is based on histologic and molecular markers (e.g., EGFR tyrosine kinase inhibitors for adenocarcinoma) for a targeted approach to therapy. Surgical resection is possible in a high proportion of adenocarcinoma cases, but because metastasis occurs early (70% of lung cancers present in advanced stages), the 5-year survival rate remains less than 20%.[144] Clinical trials are in progress to develop immunotherapies/vaccines for NSCLC.[152]

Large cell carcinomas (undifferentiated) constitute about 10% to 15% of bronchogenic carcinomas (Fig. 36.22, *F*). These transformed epithelial cells have lost all evidence of differentiation. Recent studies have confirmed that these tumors arise from squamous, glandular, or

neuroendocrine precursor cells, and molecular analyses have made it possible to target some of these aggressive cancers for immunologic therapy.[153] These tumors commonly arise centrally and can grow to distort the trachea and cause widening of the carina.

Once metastasis has occurred, surgical therapy is limited to palliative procedures (comfort measures) designed to relieve obstructive pneumonitis or prevent recurrence of pleural effusion. Neither radiation therapy nor chemotherapy has been successful in increasing survival.

Neuroendocrine Lung Tumors. Small cell lung carcinomas (SCLCs) are the most common type of neuroendocrine lung tumors and constitute about 15% of lung cancers but cause 25% of lung cancer deaths. Most tumors arise from the central part of the lung (see Fig. 36.22, *E*). Cell sizes range from 6 to 8 μm. This cell type has the strongest correlation with tobacco smoking. Because these tumors show a rapid rate of growth and tend to metastasize early and widely, this type of carcinoma has the worst prognosis of all lung cancers. Survival time for untreated small cell carcinoma is about 8% at 5 years.

Small cell carcinoma arises from neuroendocrine cells that contain neurosecretory granules and exist throughout the tracheobronchial tree. Thus small cell carcinoma is often associated with tumor-derived hormone production. Hormone production is important to the clinician because resultant signs and symptoms called *paraneoplastic syndromes* (see Table 12.4) may be the first manifestations of the underlying cancer. Examples include hyponatremia (antidiuretic hormone), Cushing syndrome (adrenocorticotropic hormone), hypocalcemia (calcitonin), gynecomastia (gonadotropins), carcinoid syndrome (serotonin), and Lambert-Eaton myasthenic syndrome.[154]

Bronchial carcinoid tumors are rare, represent about 1% of all lung tumors, are not related to smoking, are slow growing, and have a low potential to metastasize. Carcinoid tumors can occur from childhood through older age. They arise more commonly in the main or segmental bronchi, are easily visualized bronchoscopically, and are found on routine chest radiographs. The tumor cells have dense granules containing neuroendocrine-like hormones, but they rarely produce endocrine symptoms. Fifty percent of individuals with bronchial carcinoid tumors are asymptomatic. Local surgical resection is curative if metastasis has not occurred; this can often be done by bronchoscopic resection. Histologic features determine typical and atypical characteristics and guide further treatment.[155]

Other Lung Cancers. Adenocystic tumors (cylindromas) and mucoepidermoid carcinomas are rare bronchial gland tumors. They arise predominantly in the trachea or large airways and cause obstruction. They can be malignant and metastasize early, although distal pulmonary metastases are usually slow growing. Thus it is not unusual for an individual to survive 10 to 15 years after diagnosis.

Mesotheliomas are rare tumors associated with asbestos exposure (80%) up to 40 years prior to diagnosis. Most tumors are aggressive malignant tumors arising from mesothelial cells that line the pleural cavities. A long latent interval between exposure to asbestos and the appearance of mesothelioma usually occurs, and the onset of symptoms may take 20 to 40 years. Clinical manifestations include dyspnea and chest pain that result from tumor-derived pleural fluid and invasion of the chest wall. Early detection is difficult because radiologic studies do not reveal the tumor at an early stage. Diagnosis is made by chest x-ray, CT scan, and thoracentesis with cytologic examination of the pleural fluid. Thoracoscopy also may be used for biopsy. Osteopontin and mesothelin are being explored as potential tumor markers for early diagnosis. Current management of malignant mesothelioma includes a combination of pleuropneumonectomy, chemotherapy, radiation, and hyperthermia. Molecular targeted approaches include vascular endothelial growth factor inhibition, monoclonal antibody immunotherapy, vaccination, and oncoviruses. Aspirin inhibition of asbestos-induced

TABLE 36.4   CHARACTERISTICS OF LUNG CANCERS

TUMOR TYPE	GROWTH RATE	METASTASIS	MEANS OF DIAGNOSIS	CLINICAL MANIFESTATIONS AND TREATMENT
Non–Small Cell Carcinoma				
Squamous cell carcinoma	Slow	Late; mostly to hilar lymph nodes	Biopsy, sputum analysis, bronchoscopy, electron microscopy, immunohistochemistry	Cough, hemoptysis, sputum production, airway obstruction, hypercalcemia; treated surgically, chemotherapy and radiation as adjunctive therapy
Adenocarcinoma	Moderate	Early; to lymph nodes, pleurae, bone, adrenal glands, and brain	Radiography, fiberoptic bronchoscopy, electron microscopy	Pleural effusion; treated surgically, chemotherapy as adjunctive therapy
Large cell carcinoma	Rapid	Early and widespread	Sputum analysis, bronchoscopy, electron microscopy (by exclusion of other cell types)	Chest wall pain, pleural effusion, cough, sputum production, hemoptysis, airway obstruction resulting in pneumonia; treated surgically
Neuroendocrine Tumors of the Lung				
Small cell carcinoma	Very rapid	Very early; to mediastinum, lymph nodes, brain, and bone marrow	Radiography, sputum analysis, bronchoscopy, electron microscopy, immunohistochemistry	Cough, chest pain, dyspnea, hemoptysis, localized wheezing, airway obstruction, signs and symptoms of excessive hormone secretion; treated by chemotherapy and ionizing radiation to thorax and central nervous system
Other Pulmonary Tumors				
Malignant pleural mesothelioma (MPM)	Rapid	Early; to lymph nodes, lungs, heart, and bone	Radiography, thoracentesis	Chest pain, chronic cough, signs of pleural effusion

inflammation may decrease or delay mesothelioma onset or growth, or both.[156]

◆**PATHOGENESIS.** Environmental carcinogens found in tobacco smoke and asbestos are associated with malignant transformations. Tobacco smoke contains as many as 30 lung carcinogens and is responsible for the vast majority of lung cancers. These carcinogens, along with inherited genetic predisposition to cancers and epigenetic mechanisms, result in tumor formation and the development of a microenvironment that promotes tumor progression.[157,158] Once lung cancer is initiated by these carcinogen-induced mutations, further tumor development is promoted by growth factors that alter cell growth and differentiation, and by cells and products of inflammation that promote immune suppression, neoangiogenesis and lymphangiogenesis, remodeling of extracellular matrix, invasion, and metastasis.[159] The bronchial mucosa suffers multiple carcinogenic "hits" because of repetitive exposure to tobacco smoke, and eventually epithelial cell changes begin to be visible on biopsy. These changes progress from metaplasia to carcinoma in situ to finally invasive carcinoma. Tumor progression includes invasion of surrounding tissues and, finally, metastasis to distant sites, including the brain, bone marrow, and liver.

◆**CLINICAL MANIFESTATIONS.** Table 36.4 summarizes the characteristic clinical manifestations according to tumor type. Symptoms are often nonspecific and are likely to be attributed by the individual to the effects of smoking. By the time manifestations are severe enough to motivate the individual to seek medical advice, the disease is usually advanced with signs and symptoms of metastatic disease (e.g., bone pain or alteration in liver function) or paraneoplastic syndromes (see Chapter 12).

◆**EVALUATION AND TREATMENT.** Diagnosing and treating lung cancer early in its development are crucial for long-term survival. Screening with a low-dose spiral CT scan promotes early detection and decreases the risk of dying from lung cancer by 20% in persons who are heavy smokers.[160] Diagnostic tests for the evaluation of lung cancer include sputum cytologic studies, chest imaging, virtual bronchoscopy, radial probe endobronchial ultrasound, electromagnetic navigational bronchoscopy, and biopsy. Biopsy determines the cell type. The evaluation of lymph nodes and other organ systems is used to determine the stage of the cancer. The histologic cell type, the genotype, and the stage of the disease are major factors that influence choice of therapy. The currently accepted system for the staging of NSCLC uses the TNM classification system in which T denotes the extent of the primary tumor, N indicates nodal involvement, and M describes the extent of metastasis (illustrated in Fig. 36.23). Staging for small cell carcinoma is divided into only two categories: limited disease (TNM stages I to III: 20% to 30%) and extensive disease (TNM stage IV: 70% to 80%).

For all types of early stage lung carcinoma, the preferred treatment is surgical resection. Once metastasis has taken place, total surgical resection is more difficult and survival rates dramatically decrease. NSCLC is less responsive to chemotherapy than is small cell carcinoma, but chemotherapy (e.g., platinum) and radiation are commonly used as adjuvant or palliative care. Targeted approaches based on histology and molecular markers guide the management of advanced stage NSCLC, and methodologies are being developed for all stages of the disease.[161] Small cell carcinoma is poorly differentiated and usually widely metastasized by the time of diagnosis. Palliative chemotherapy and radiation can initially improve survival, but mortality is high at 5 years primarily because of extreme genomic instability. Dose-intensified radiation radiofrequency ablation, microwave ablation, cryotherapy, and brachytherapy may be available as primary or palliative treatment for those for whom surgical removal is not an option. Antiangiogenic therapy, growth factor inhibitors, proapoptotic agents, epigenetic modulators, cancer stem cell targets, gene therapy, and immunotherapy continue to be evaluated for targeted treatment.[162] Prevention of lung cancer relies primarily on reduction of exposure to carcinogens. For most individuals this means smoking cessation.

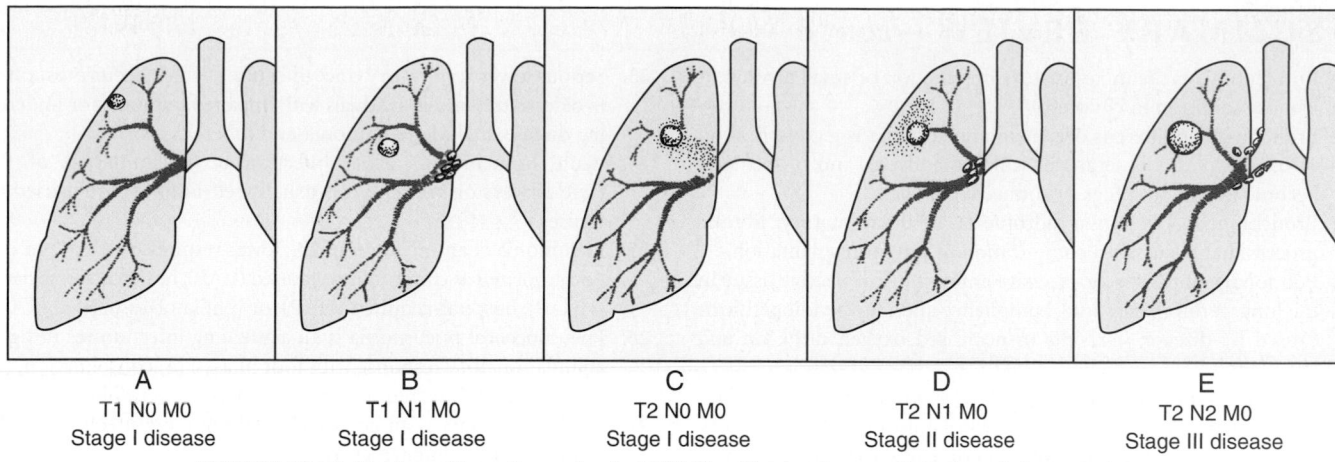

A	B	C	D	E
T1 N0 M0	T1 N1 M0	T2 N0 M0	T2 N1 M0	T2 N2 M0
Stage I disease	Stage I disease	Stage I disease	Stage II disease	Stage III disease

FIGURE 36.23 Staging of Lung Cancer by the TNM Classification System. A, B, Stage I disease includes tumors classified as T1, with or without metastasis to the lymph nodes in the ipsilateral hilar region. **C,** Also included in stage I are tumors classified as T2 but having no nodal or distant metastases. **D,** Stage II disease includes those tumors classified as T2, with metastasis only to the ipsilateral hilar lymph nodes. **E,** Stage III includes all tumors more extensive than T2 or any tumor with metastasis to the lymph nodes in the mediastinum or adjacent organs. Stage IV (not shown) involves spread to other organs.

SUMMARY REVIEW

Clinical Manifestations of Pulmonary Alterations

1. Dyspnea is a feeling of breathlessness and increased respiratory effort; it is associated with respiratory and cardiac diseases and causes distress. Orthopnea is dyspnea when a person is in the recumbent position and is associated with heart failure. Paroxysmal nocturnal dyspnea occurs at night and requires the person to sit or stand for relief.

2. Coughing is a protective reflex that expels secretions and irritants from the lower airways; the cough reflex is mediated by the vagus nerve.

3. Abnormal sputum is a change in the amount, consistency, color, and odor of sputum.

4. Hemoptysis is expectoration of bloody mucus that can be caused by bronchitis, TB, abscess, neoplasms, and other conditions that cause hemorrhage from damaged vessels.

5. Abnormal breathing patterns are adjustments made by the body to minimize the work of respiratory muscles. They include Kussmaul, obstructed, restricted, gasping, and/or Cheyne-Stokes respirations, and sighing.

6. Hypoventilation is decreased alveolar ventilation caused by airway obstruction, chest wall restriction, or altered neurologic control of breathing. Hypoventilation causes increased $Paco_2$.

7. Hyperventilation is increased alveolar ventilation produced by anxiety, head injury, or severe hypoxemia. Hyperventilation causes decreased $Paco_2$.

8. Cyanosis is a bluish discoloration of the skin caused by desaturation of hemoglobin, polycythemia, or peripheral vasoconstriction.

9. Clubbing of the fingertips is associated with diseases that disrupt the normal pulmonary circulation and cause chronic hypoxemia.

10. Chest pain can result from inflamed pleurae, the trachea, bronchi, or respiratory muscles.

11. Hypercapnia is increased $Paco_2$ caused by a decrease in minute volume (respiratory rate × tidal volume).

12. Hypoxemia is a reduced Pao_2 caused by (a) decreased oxygen content of inspired gas, (b) hypoventilation, (c) diffusion abnormality, (d) ventilation-perfusion mismatch, or (e) shunting.

13. Acute respiratory failure is caused by inadequate gas exchange or ventilation (Pao_2 ≤50 mmHg or $Paco_2$ ≥50 mmHg and pH ≥7.25).

Disorders of the Chest Wall and Pleura

1. If the chest wall is deformed, traumatized, immobilized, or made heavy by fat, the work of breathing is increased and ventilation is compromised by a decrease in tidal volume from compression of the lungs or impaired chest wall muscle function.

2. Flail chest results from rib or sternal fractures that disrupt the mechanics of breathing.

3. Pneumothorax is the accumulation of air in the pleural space. It can be caused by spontaneous rupture of weakened areas of the pleura or can be secondary to pleural damage caused by disease, trauma, or mechanical ventilation.

4. Tension pneumothorax is a life-threatening condition caused by trapping of air in the pleural space.

5. Pleural effusion is the accumulation of fluid in the pleural space, usually resulting from disorders that promote transudation or exudation from capillaries underlying the pleura but occasionally resulting from blockage or injury that causes lymphatic vessels to drain into the pleural space.

6. Empyema is the presence of pus in the pleural space (infected pleural effusion). The source of the pus is usually lymphatic drainage from sites of bacterial pneumonia.

Pulmonary Disorders

1. Aspiration is passage of fluid and solid particles into the lung, usually from impaired swallowing and coughing. It frequently results in pneumonitis and pulmonary infection.

2. Atelectasis is the collapse of alveoli resulting from compression of the lung tissue, absorption of gas from obstructed alveoli, or impairment of surfactant.

3. Bronchiectasis is abnormal dilation of the bronchi usually secondary to another pulmonary disorder, usually infection or chronic inflammation.

SUMMARY REVIEW—cont'd

4. Bronchiolitis is the inflammatory obstruction of small airways. It is most common in children.

5. Bronchiolitis obliterans organizing pneumonia is a complication of bronchiolitis obliterans in which the alveoli and bronchioles become filled with plugs of connective tissue.

6. Bronchiolitis obliterans syndrome is an inflammatory, fibrotic process that occurs as a complication of lung transplantation.

7. Pulmonary fibrosis is an excessive amount of connective tissue in the lung. It diminishes lung compliance and may be idiopathic or caused by disease; it results in decreased oxygen diffusion and hypoxemia.

8. Inhalation of noxious gases or prolonged exposure to high concentrations of oxygen can damage the bronchial mucosa or alveolocapillary membrane and cause inflammation or acute respiratory failure.

9. Pneumoconiosis is caused by inhalation of dust particles in the workplace, including coal dust (anthracosis), silica (silicosis), or asbestos. It causes chronic inflammation, pulmonary fibrosis, and susceptibility to lower airway infection and tumor formation.

10. Hypersensitivity pneumonitis (extrinsic allergic alveolitis) is an allergic or hypersensitivity reaction to many allergens.

11. Pulmonary edema is the presence of excess water in the lung caused by disturbances of capillary hydrostatic pressure, capillary oncotic pressure, or capillary permeability. A common cause is left-sided heart failure, which increases the hydrostatic pressure in the pulmonary circulation.

12. ALI/ARDS results from an acute, diffuse inflammatory injury to the alveolocapillary membrane and decreased surfactant production, which increases membrane permeability and causes pulmonary edema and atelectasis.

13. Obstructive pulmonary disease is characterized by airway obstruction that causes difficult expiration. Obstructive disease can be acute or chronic and includes asthma, chronic bronchitis, and emphysema.

14. Asthma is a chronic inflammatory disorder of the bronchial mucosa that causes bronchial hyperresponsiveness, mucosal edema, airway constriction, and variable obstruction to airflow that is reversible. Obstruction is caused by episodic airway epithelial exposure to antigen with attacks of bronchospasm, bronchial inflammation, mucosal edema, and increased production of mucus.

15. COPD is the coexistence of two primary phenotypes, chronic bronchitis and emphysema, which frequently overlap each other.

16. The asthma-COPD overlap syndrome is a phenotype of chronic respiratory disease where there is an overlap of the clinical symptoms of asthma and COPD.

17. Chronic bronchitis is chronic inflammation of the bronchi that causes airway obstruction resulting from bronchial smooth muscle hypertrophy, increases in the size and number of epithelial mucous glands and goblet cells, and increased production of thick, tenacious mucus.

18. Emphysema results from destruction of elastin in the alveolar septa and loss of passive elastic recoil, leading to airway collapse, obstruction to gas flow during expiration, and air trapping.

19. Emphysema in which septal deterioration is caused by α_1-antitrypsin deficiency or old age tends to be panacinar.

20. Emphysema in which septal deterioration results from smoking tends to be centriacinar.

21. Paraseptal emphysema is associated with large bullae formation.

22. Upper respiratory tract infections are the most common cause of short-term disability in the United States and include rhinitis (the common cold), pharyngitis, and laryngitis.

23. Serious lower respiratory tract infections, which occur most often in older adults and individuals with impaired immunity or underlying disease, include pneumonia and tuberculosis.

24. Acute bronchitis is acute infection or inflammation of the large airways or bronchi; it is usually self-limiting and caused by viruses.

25. Pneumonia is an infection of the lower respiratory tract and can be categorized as community-acquired (CAP), healthcare-associated (HCAP), hospital-acquired (HAP), or ventilator-associated (VAP).

26. Pneumococcal pneumonia is an acute lung infection resulting in an inflammatory response with four phases: (a) consolidation, (b) red hepatization, (c) gray hepatization, and (d) resolution.

27. Viral pneumonia is an acute, self-limiting lung infection usually caused by the influenza virus.

28. TB is a lung infection caused by *M. tuberculosis* (tubercle bacillus) and can also invade other organs. The bacterium is successful as a pathogen because it can survive within macrophages, resist lysosomal killing, multiply within the cell, and transit into a stage of dormancy rendering itself extremely resistant to host defense and drug treatment.

29. Bacilli may remain dormant within the tubercles for life; or if the immune system becomes compromised, they may cause recurrence of active disease.

30. Abscesses are circumscribed areas of destruction of lung parenchyma with suppuration usually resulting from aspiration pneumonia.

31. Acute bronchitis is acute infection or inflammation of the airways or bronchi usually caused by a virus.

32. Pulmonary vascular diseases are caused by embolism or hypertension in the pulmonary circulation.

33. PE is occlusion of a portion of the pulmonary vascular bed by a thrombus (most common), a tissue fragment, or an air bubble. Depending on its size and location, the embolus can cause hypoxic vasoconstriction, pulmonary edema, atelectasis, pulmonary hypertension, shock, and even death.

34. Pulmonary artery hypertension (pulmonary artery pressure) is defined as a mean pulmonary artery pressure greater than 25 mmHg at rest. It is caused by (a) elevated left ventricular pressure, (b) increased blood flow through the pulmonary circulation, (c) obliteration or obstruction of the vascular bed, or (d) active constriction of the vascular bed produced by hypoxemia or acidosis.

35. Cor pulmonale is right ventricular enlargement caused by chronic pulmonary hypertension. Cor pulmonale progresses to right ventricular failure if the pulmonary hypertension is not reversed.

36. Laryngeal cancer occurs primarily in men and represents less than 1% of all cancers. Squamous cell carcinoma of the true vocal cords is most common and manifests with a clinical symptom of progressive hoarseness.

37. Lung cancer, the most frequent cause of cancer death in the United States, is commonly caused by smoking of cigarettes or tobacco.

38. Cancer cell types include non–small cell lung cancer (squamous cell carcinoma, adenocarcinoma, large cell undifferentiated carcinoma) and neuroendocrine tumors (small cell carcinoma and bronchial carcinoid tumors). Other tumors include small cell (oat cell) carcinoma, bronchial adenoma, adenocystic tumors (cylindromas), mucoepidermoid carcinomas (bronchial tumors), and mesothelioma. Each type arises in a characteristic site or type of tissue, causes distinctive clinical manifestations, and differs in likelihood of metastasis and prognosis.

KEY TERMS

Abscess, 1189
Absorption atelectasis, 1170
Acute cough, 1164
Acute lung injury (ALI), 1174
Acute respiratory distress syndrome
  (ARDS), 1174
Adenocarcinoma, 1194
Adenocystic tumor (cylindroma), 1195
Air trapping, 1184
Alveolar dead space, 1167
Asbestos exposure, 1173
Asbestosis, 1173
Aspiration, 1170
Asthma, 1177
Atelectasis, 1170
Bronchial carcinoid tumor, 1195
Bronchiectasis, 1170
Bronchiolitis, 1172
Bronchiolitis obliterans organizing pneumonia
  (BOOP), 1172
Bronchiolitis obliterans syndrome (BOS), 1172
Cavitation, 1190
Centriacinar (centrilobular) emphysema, 1183
Cheyne-Stokes respiration, 1164
Chronic bronchitis, 1181
Chronic cough, 1164
Chronic obstructive pulmonary disease
  (COPD), 1181
Clubbing, 1165

Coal worker pneumoconiosis (coal mine lung disease,
  anthracosis), 1173
Compression atelectasis, 1170
Consolidation, 1189
Cor pulmonale, 1192
Cough, 1164
Cyanosis, 1165
Cylindrical bronchiectasis, 1170
Dyspnea, 1163
Dyspnea on exertion, 1164
Emphysema, 1181
Empyema (infected pleural effusion), 1169
Flail chest, 1167
Hemoptysis, 1164
Hypercapnia, 1165
Hypersensitivity pneumonitis (extrinsic allergic
  alveolitis), 1173
Hyperventilation, 1165
Hypocapnia, 1165
Hypoventilation, 1164
Hypoxemia, 1166
Hypoxia (ischemia), 1166
Idiopathic pulmonary fibrosis (IPF), 1172
Kussmaul respiration (hyperpnea), 1164
Large cell carcinoma (undifferentiated), 1195
Laryngeal cancer, 1193
Lung cancer, 1194
Mesothelioma, 1195
Mucoepidermoid carcinoma, 1195

Obstructive pulmonary disease, 1176
Orthopnea, 1164
Oxygen toxicity, 1172
Pain, 1165
Panacinar emphysema, 1183
Paraseptal emphysema, 1183
Paroxysmal nocturnal dyspnea (PND), 1164
Pleural effusion, 1169
Pneumoconiosis, 1173
Pneumonia, 1186
Pneumothorax, 1168
Pulmonary artery hypertension (PAH), 1191
Pulmonary edema, 1173
Pulmonary embolism (PE), 1190
Pulmonary fibrosis, 1172
Pulsus paradoxus, 1179
Respiratory (lung) failure, 1167
Saccular bronchiectasis, 1170
Shunting, 1167
Silicosis, 1173
Small cell lung carcinoma (SCLC), 1195
Sputum, 1164
Squamous cell carcinoma (SCC), 1194
Status asthmaticus, 1179
Surfactant impairment, 1170
TNM classification system, 1196
Tuberculosis (TB), 1188
Varicose bronchiectasis, 1170

REFERENCES

1. Parshall MB, et al: An official American Thoracic Society statement: update on the mechanisms, assessment, and management of dyspnea. *Am J Respir Crit Care Med* 185(4):435–452, 2012.
2. Laviolette L, Laveneziana P: A multidimensional and multidisciplinary approach. *Eur Respir J* 43(6):1750–1762, 2014.
3. Persichini R, et al: Diagnostic accuracy of respiratory distress observation scales as surrogates of dyspnea self-report in intensive care unit patients. *Anesthesiology* 123(4):830–837, 2015.
4. Ando A, Farrell MJ, Mazzone SB: Cough-related neural processing in the brain: a roadmap for cough dysfunction? *Neurosci Biobehav Rev* 47:457–468, 2014.
5. Canning BJ, et al: Anatomy and neurophysiology of cough: CHEST guideline and expert panel report. *Chest* 146(6):1633–1648, 2014.
6. Dicpinigaitis PV: Clinical perspective—cough: an unmet need. *Curr Opin Pharmacol* 22:24–28, 2015.
7. Larici AR, et al: Diagnosis and management of hemoptysis. *Diagn Interv Radiol* 20(4):299–309, 2014.
8. Owen CE: Cutaneous manifestations of lung cancer. *Semin Oncol* 43(3):366–369, 2016.
9. Brims FJ, Davies HE, Lee YC: Respiratory chest pain: diagnosis and treatment. *Med Clin North Am* 94(2):217–232, 2010.
10. Hiremath G, Kamat D: Diagnostic considerations in infants and children with cyanosis. *Pediatr Ann* 44(2):76–80, 2015.
11. Petersson J, Glenny RW: Gas exchange and ventilation-perfusion relationships in the lung. *Eur Respir J* 44(4):1023–1041, 2014.
12. Oana S, Mukherji J: Acute and chronic respiratory failure. *Handb Clin Neurol* 119:273–288, 2014.
13. Mulligan MS, Berfield KS, Abbaszadeh RV: Management of postoperative respiratory failure. *Thorac Surg Clin* 25(4):429–433, 2015.

14. Tschopp JM, et al: ERS task force statement: diagnosis and treatment of primary spontaneous pneumothorax. *Eur Respir J* 46(2):321–335, 2015.
15. Kennedy JC, Khabibullin D, Henske EP: Mechanisms of pulmonary cyst pathogenesis in Birt-Hogg-Dubé syndrome: the stretch hypothesis. *Semin Cell Dev Biol* 52:47–52, 2016.
16. Lin YC, et al: Pigtail catheter for the management of pneumothorax in mechanically ventilated patients. *Am J Emerg Med* 28(4):466–471, 2010.
17. Haynes D, Baumann MH: Management of pneumothorax. *Semin Respir Crit Care Med* 31(6):769–780, 2010.
18. Bintcliffe OJ, et al: Spontaneous pneumothorax: time to rethink management? *Lancet Respir Med* 3(7):578–588, 2015.
19. Bhatnagar R, Maskell N: The modern diagnosis and management of pleural effusions. *BMJ* 351: h4520, 2015.
20. Piccolo F, et al: Intrapleural tissue plasminogen activator and deoxyribonuclease therapy for pleural infection. *J Thorac Dis* 7(6):999–1008, 2015.
21. DiBardino DM, Wunderink RG: Aspiration pneumonia: a review of modern trends. *J Crit Care* 30(1):40–48, 2015.
22. Randtke MA, Andrews BP, Mach WJ: Pathophysiology and prevention of intraoperative atelectasis: a review of the literature. *J Perianesth Nurs* 30(6):516–527, 2015.
23. Calligaro GL, Gray DM: Lung function abnormalities in HIV-infected adults and children. *Respirology* 20(1):24–32, 2015.
24. Moulton BC, Barker AF: Pathogenesis of bronchiectasis. *Clin Chest Med* 33(2):211–217, 2012.
25. Rademacher J, et al: Lung transplantation for non-cystic fibrosis bronchiectasis. *Respir Med* 115:60–65, 2016.

26. Papiris SA, et al: Bronchiolitis: adopting a unifying definition and a comprehensive etiological classification. *Exp Rev Respir Med* 7(3):289–306, 2013.
27. Mosier MJ, et al: Predictive value of bronchoscopy in assessing the severity of inhalation injury. *J Burn Care Res* 33(1):65–73, 2012.
28. Meyer KC, et al: An international ISHLT/ATS/ERS clinical practice guideline: diagnosis and management of bronchiolitis obliterans syndrome. *Eur Respir J* 44(6):1479–1503, 2014.
29. Daccord C, Maher TM: Recent advances in understanding idiopathic pulmonary fibrosis. *F1000Res* 5:2016.
30. Song JW, et al: Acute exacerbation of idiopathic pulmonary fibrosis: incidence, risk factors and outcome. *Eur Respir J* 37(2):356–363, 2011.
31. Chauhan D, et al: Post-transplant survival in idiopathic pulmonary fibrosis patients concurrently listed for single and double lung transplantation. *J Heart Lung Transplant* 35(5): 657–660, 2016.
32. Fleetwood K, et al: Systematic review and network meta-analysis of idiopathic pulmonary fibrosis treatments. *J Manag Care Spec Pharm* 23(3-b Suppl):S5–S16, 2017.
33. Enkhbaatar P, et al: Pathophysiology, research challenges, and clinical management of smoke inhalation injury. *Lancet* 388(10052):1437–1446, 2016.
34. Thomson L, Paton J: Oxygen toxicity. *Paediatr Respir Rev* 15(2):120–123, 2014.
35. Luna-Gomes T, Santana PT, Coutinho-Silva R: Silica-induced inflammasome activation in macrophages: role of ATP and P2X7 receptor. *Immunobiology* 220(9):1101–1106, 2015.
36. Laney AS, Weissman DN: Respiratory diseases caused by coal mine dust. *J Occup Environ Med* 56(Suppl 10):S18–S22, 2014.

37. Go LH, et al: Lung disease and coal mining: what pulmonologists need to know. *Curr Opin Pulm Med* 22(2):170–178, 2016.

38. Markowitz S: Asbestos-related lung cancer and malignant mesothelioma of the pleura: selected current issues. *Semin Respir Crit Care Med* 36(3): 334–346, 2015.

39. Spagnolo P, et al: Hypersensitivity pneumonitis: a comprehensive review. *J Investig Allergol Clin Immunol* 25(4):237–250, 2015.

40. MacIver DH, Clark AL: The vital role of the right ventricle in the pathogenesis of acute pulmonary edema. *Am J Cardiol* 115(7):992–1000, 2015.

41. Luks AM, Swenson ER, Bärtsch P: Acute high-altitude sickness. *Eur Respir Rev* 26(143): 2017.

42. Ranieri VM, et al: Acute respiratory distress syndrome: the Berlin definition. *J Am Med Assoc* 307:2526–2533, 2012.

43. Bellani G, et al: Epidemiology, patterns of care, and mortality for patients with acute respiratory distress syndrome in intensive care units in 50 countries. *J Am Med Assoc* 315(8):788–800, 2016.

44. Przybysz TM, Heffner AC: Early treatment of severe acute respiratory distress syndrome. *Emerg Med Clin North Am* 34(1):1–14, 2016.

45. Moazed F, Calfee CS: Environmental risk factors for acute respiratory distress syndrome. *Clin Chest Med* 35(4):625–637, 2014.

46. Sweeney RM, McAuley DF: Acute respiratory distress syndrome. *Lancet* 388(10058):2416–2430, 2016.

47. Han S, Mallampalli RK: The acute respiratory distress syndrome: from mechanism to translation. *J Immunol* 194(3):855–860, 2015.

48. Mokra D, Kosutova P: Biomarkers in acute lung injury. *Respir Physiol Neurobiol* 209:52–58, 2015.

49. Yadav H, Kor DJ: Platelets in the pathogenesis of acute respiratory distress syndrome. *Am J Physiol Lung Cell Mol Physiol* 309(9):L915–L923, 2015.

50. ARDS Definition Task Force, Ranieri VM, et al: Acute respiratory distress syndrome: the Berlin definition. *JAMA* 307(23):2526–2533, 2012.

51. Baron RM, Levy BD: Recent advances in understanding and treating ARDS. *F1000Res* 5:2016.

52. Umbrello M, et al: Current concepts of ARDS: a narrative review. *Int J Mol Sci* 18(1):2016.

53. Toner P, McAuley DF, Shyamsundar M: Aspirin as a potential treatment in sepsis or acute respiratory distress syndrome. *Crit Care* 19:374, 2015.

54. Meduri GU, et al: Prolonged glucocorticoid treatment is associated with improved ARDS outcomes: analysis of individual patients' data from four randomized trials and trial-level meta-analysis of the updated literature. *Intensive Care Med* 42(5):829–840, 2016.

55. Chiumello D, et al: What's next after ARDS: long-term outcomes. *Respir Care* 61(5):689–699, 2016.

56. Centers for Disease Control and Prevention (CDC): *Most recent asthma data.* Last updated September 16, 2016. Available at: http://www.cdc .gov/asthma/most_recent_data.htm.

57. Akinbami LJ, et al: *Trends in asthma prevalence, health care use, and mortality in the United States, 2001–2010*, NCHS data brief, no. 94. Hyattsville, MD, 2012, National Center for Health Statistics. Available at: www.cdc.gov/nchs/data/databriefs/db94.htm. Page updated May 1, 2012; last reviewed November 6, 2015.

58. KleinJan A: Airway inflammation in asthma: key players beyond the Th2 pathway. *Curr Opin Pulm Med* 22(1):46–52, 2016.

59. Skloot GS: Asthma phenotypes and endotypes: a personalized approach to treatment. *Curr Opin Pulm Med* 22(1):3–9, 2016.

60. Liu AH: Revisiting the hygiene hypothesis for allergy and asthma. *J Allergy Clin Immunol* 136(4):860–865, 2015.

61. Holgate ST: Innate and adaptive immune responses in asthma. *Nat Med* 18(5):673–683, 2012.

62. Gauvreau GM, El-Gammal AI, O'Byrne PM: Allergen-induced airway responses. *Eur Respir J* 46(3):819–831, 2015.

63. Ghosh S, Erzurum SC: Modulation of asthma pathogenesis by nitric oxide pathways and therapeutic opportunities. *Drug Discov Today Dis Mech* 9(3-4):e89–e94, 2012.

64. Chapman TJ, Georas SN: Regulatory tone and mucosal immunity in asthma. *Int Immunopharmacol* 23(1):330–336, 2014.

65. Brightling CE, et al: Lung damage and airway remodelling in severe asthma. *Clin Exp Allergy* 42(5):638–649, 2012.

66. Castillo JR, Peters SP, Busse WW: Asthma exacerbations: pathogenesis, prevention, and treatment. *J Allergy Clin Immunol Pract* 5(4): 918–927, 2017.

67. Lin CH, Cheng SL: A review of omalizumab for the management of severe asthma. *Drug Des Devel Ther* 10:2369–2378, 2016.

68. Bagnasco D, et al: The path to personalized medicine in asthma. *Expert Rev Respir Med* 10(9):957–965, 2016.

69. Centers for Disease Control and Prevention (CDC): *Chronic obstructive pulmonary disease (COPD).* Last updated August 15, 2016. Available at: http://www.cdc.gov/copd/data.html.

70. Postma DS, Bush A, van den Berge M: Risk factors and early origins of chronic obstructive pulmonary disease. *Lancet* 385(9971):899–909, 2015.

71. Tzortzaki EG, et al: Immune and genetic mechanisms in COPD: possible targets for therapeutic interventions. *Curr Drug Targets* 14(2):141–148, 2013.

72. McElvaney NG: Diagnosing α1-antitrypsin deficiency: how to improve the current algorithm. *Eur Respir Rev* 24(135):52–57, 2015.

73. Kheradmand F, et al: Autoimmunity in chronic obstructive pulmonary disease: clinical and experimental evidence. *Exp Rev Clin Immunol* 8(3):285–292, 2012.

74. Tuder RM, Petrache I: Pathogenesis of chronic obstructive pulmonary disease. *J Clin Invest* 122(8):2749–2755, 2012.

75. Kim V, Criner GJ: Chronic bronchitis and chronic obstructive pulmonary disease. *Am J Respir Crit Care Med* 187(3):228–237, 2013.

76. Decramer M, Janssens W, Miravitlles M: Chronic obstructive pulmonary disease. *Lancet* 379(9823): 1341–1351, 2012.

77. Min T, et al: Critical role of proteostasis-imbalance in pathogenesis of COPD and severe emphysema. *J Mol Med* 89(6):577–593, 2011.

78. Bagdonas E, et al: Novel aspects of pathogenesis and regeneration mechanisms in COPD. *Int J Chron Obstruct Pulmon Dis* 10:995–1013, 2015.

79. Edwards RM, et al: Imaging of small airways and emphysema. *Clin Chest Med* 36(2):335–347, 2015.

80. Henao MP, Craig TJ: Understanding alpha-1 antitrypsin deficiency: a review with an allergist's outlook. *Allergy Asthma Proc* 38(2):98–107, 2017.

81. Mitchell PD, et al: Idiopathic pulmonary fibrosis with emphysema: evidence of synergy among emphysema and idiopathic pulmonary fibrosis in smokers. *Respir Care* 60(2):259–268, 2015.

82. Kim V, et al: The chronic bronchitic phenotype of COPD: an analysis of the COPD Gene Study. *Chest* 140(3):626–633, 2011.

83. Global Strategy for the Diagnosis, Management and Prevention of COPD: *Global initiative for chronic obstructive lung disease (GOLD)*, 2017. Available at: http://goldcopd.org.

84. Fowdar K, et al: The effect of N-acetylcysteine on exacerbations of chronic obstructive pulmonary disease: a meta-analysis and systematic review. *Heart Lung* 46(2):120–128, 2017.

85. Tarran R, et al: Nonantibiotic macrolides prevent human neutrophil elastase-induced mucus stasis and airway surface liquid volume depletion. *Am J Physiol Lung Cell Mol Physiol* 304(11):L746–L756, 2013.

86. Bettoncelli G, et al: The clinical and integrated management of COPD. *Sarcoidosis Vasc Diffuse Lung Dis* 31(Suppl 1):3–21, 2014.

87. Cousins JL, Wark PA, McDonald VM: Acute oxygen therapy: a review of prescribing and delivery practices. *Int J Chron Obstruct Pulmon Dis* 11:1067–1075, 2016.

88. Marchetti N, Criner GJ: Surgical approaches to treating emphysema: lung volume reduction surgery, bullectomy, and lung transplantation. *Semin Respir Crit Care Med* 36(4):592–608, 2015.

89. Strange C, Beiko T: Treatment of alpha-1 antitrypsin deficiency. *Semin Respir Crit Care Med* 36(4):470–477, 2015.

90. Harris AM, et al: Appropriate antibiotic use for acute respiratory tract infection in adults: advice for high-value care from the American College of Physicians and the Centers for Disease Control and Prevention. *Ann Intern Med* 164:425–434, 2016.

91. Tackett KL, Atkins A: Evidence-based acute bronchitis therapy. *J Pharm Pract* 25(6):586–590, 2012.

92. Smith SM, Smucny J, Fahey T: Antibiotics for acute bronchitis. *J Am Med Assoc* 312(24): 2678–2679, 2014.

93. Centers for Disease Control and Prevention (CDC): *Leading causes of death.* Last updated April 27, 2016. Available at: http://www.cdc.gov/nchs/fastats/leading-causes-of-death.htm.

94. Torres A, et al: Which individuals are at increased risk of pneumococcal disease and why? Impact of COPD, asthma, smoking, diabetes, and/or chronic heart disease on community-acquired pneumonia and invasive pneumococcal disease. *Thorax* 70(10):984–989, 2015.

95. American Thoracic Society, Infectious Diseases Society of America: Guidelines for the management of adults with hospital-acquired, ventilator-associated, and healthcare-associated pneumonia. *Am J Respir Crit Care Med* 171:388–416, 2005.

96. Ashraf M, Ostrosky-Zeichner L: Ventilator-associated pneumonia: a review. *Hosp Pract (Minneap)* 40(1):93, 2012.

97. Lobdell KW, Stamou S, Sanchez JA: Hospital-acquired infections. *Surg Clin North Am* 92(1):65–77, 2012.

98. Patterson CM, Loebinger MR: Community acquired pneumonia: assessment and treatment. *Clin Med* 12(3):283–286, 2012.

99. Lee KH, Gordon A, Foxman B: The role of respiratory viruses in the etiology of bacterial pneumonia: an ecological perspective. *Evol Med Public Health* 2016(1):95–109, 2016.

100. Loo CY, et al: Implications and emerging control strategies for ventilator-associated infections. *Expert Rev Anti Infect Ther* 13(3):379–393, 2015.

101. Pechous RD: With friends like these: the complex role of neutrophils in the progression of severe

pneumonia. *Front Cell Infect Microbiol* 7:160, 2017.

102. Storisteanu DM, et al: Evasion of neutrophil extracellular traps by respiratory pathogens. *Am J Respir Cell Mol Biol* 56(4):423–431, 2017.

103. Mitchell TJ, Dalziel CE: The biology of pneumolysin. *Subcell Biochem* 80:145–160, 2014.

104. Yoo JK, et al: Viral infection of the lung: host response and sequelae. *J Allergy Clin Immunol* 132(6):1263–1276, 2013.

105. Florescu DF, Kalil AC: The complex link between influenza and severe sepsis. *Virulence* 5(1):137–142, 2014.

106. Al-Hazmi A: Challenges presented by MERS corona virus, and SARS corona virus to health. *Saudi J Biol Sci* 23(4):507–511, 2016.

107. Messacar K, Abzug MJ, Dominguez SR: 2014 outbreak of enterovirus D68 in North America. *J Med Virol* 88(5):739–745, 2016.

108. Nair GB, Niederman MS: Community-acquired pneumonia: an unfinished battle. *Med Clin North Am* 95(6):1143–1161, 2011.

109. Prina E, Ranzani OT, Torres A: Community-acquired pneumonia. *Lancet* 386(9998):1097–1108, 2015.

110. Mandell LA, Wunderink RG, Anzueto A: Infectious Diseases Society of America/American Thoracic Society consensus guidelines on the management of community-acquired pneumonia in adults. *Clin Infect Dis* 44(Suppl 2):S27–S72, 2007.

111. Aabenhus R, et al: Biomarkers as point-of-care tests to guide prescription of antibiotics in patients with acute respiratory infections in primary care. *Cochrane Database Syst Rev* (11):CD010130, 2014.

112. Prina E, et al: Risk factors associated with potentially antibiotic-resistant pathogens in community-acquired pneumonia. *Ann Am Thorac Soc* 12(2):153–160, 2015.

113. Kalil AC, et al: Management of adults with hospital-acquired and ventilator-associated pneumonia: 2016 clinical practice guidelines by the Infectious Diseases Society of America and the American Thoracic Society. *Clin Infect Dis* 63(5):e61–e111, 2016.

114. Schmit KM, et al: Tuberculosis—United States, 2016. *MMWR Morb Mortal Wkly Rep* 66(11):289–294, 2017.

115. World Health Organization (WHO): *Tuberculosis fact sheet.* Available at: http://www.who.int/mediacentre/factsheets/fs104/en/. Reviewed March, 2017.

116. Wilson JW, Tsukayama DT: Extensively drug-resistant tuberculosis: principles of resistance, diagnosis, and management. *Mayo Clin Proc* 91(4):482–495, 2016.

117. Forrellad MA, et al: Virulence factors of the *Mycobacterium* tuberculosis complex. *Virulence* 4(1):3–66, 2013.

118. Haley CA: Treatment of latent tuberculosis infection. *Microbiol Spectr* 5(2):2017.

119. Sun J, et al: The tuberculosis necrotizing toxin kills macrophages by hydrolyzing NAD. *Nat Struct Mol Biol* 22(9):672–678, 2015.

120. Bruchfeld J, Correia-Neves M, Källenius G: Tuberculosis and HIV coinfection. *Cold Spring Harb Perspect Med* 5(7):a017871, 2015.

121. Lenaerts A, Barry CE, 3rd, Dartois V: Heterogeneity in tuberculosis pathology,

122. Noor KM, Shephard L, Bastian I: Molecular diagnostics for tuberculosis. *Pathology* 47(3):250–256, 2015.

123. U.S. Preventive Services Task Force: Screening for latent tuberculosis infection in adults; U.S. Preventive Services Task Force recommendation statement. *J Am Med Assoc* 316(9):962–969, 2016.

124. Leylabadlo HE, et al: Pulmonary tuberculosis diagnosis: where we are? *Tuberc Respir Dis (Seoul)* 79(3):134–142, 2016.

125. Rangaka MX, et al: Controlling the seedbeds of tuberculosis: diagnosis and treatment of tuberculosis infection. *Lancet* 386(10010):2344–2353, 2015.

126. Wallis RS, et al: Tuberculosis—advances in development of new drugs, treatment regimens, host-directed therapies, and biomarkers. *Lancet Infect Dis* 16(4):e34–e46, 2016.

127. Zumla A, et al: Potential of immunomodulatory agents as adjunct host-directed therapies for multidrug-resistant tuberculosis. *BMC Med* 14(1):89, 2016.

128. Mortensen KH, Babar JL, Balan A: Multidetector CT of pulmonary cavitation: filling in the holes. *Clin Radiol* 70(4):446–456, 2015.

129. Kuhajda I, et al: Lung abscess-etiology, diagnostic and treatment options. *Ann Transl Med* 3(13):183, 2015.

130. Wolberg AS, et al: Procoagulant activity in hemostasis and thrombosis: Virchow's triad revisited. *Anesth Analg* 114(2):275–285, 2012.

131. Konstantinides SV, et al: 2014 ESC guidelines on the diagnosis and management of acute pulmonary embolism. *Eur Heart J* 35(43):3033–3069, 3069a–3069k, 2014.

132. van der Hulle T, et al: Recent developments in the diagnosis and treatment of pulmonary embolism. *J Intern Med* 279(1):16–29, 2016.

133. Kubak MP, et al: Elevated d-dimer cut-off values for computed tomography pulmonary angiography-d-dimer correlates with location of embolism. *Ann Transl Med* 4(11):212, 2016.

134. Bajaj A, et al: Prognostic value of troponins in acute nonmassive pulmonary embolism: a meta-analysis. *Heart Lung* 44(4):327–334, 2015.

135. Konstantinides SV: Management of pulmonary embolism: an update. *J Am Coll Cardiol* 67(8):976–990, 2016.

136. Toth PP: Considerations for long-term anticoagulant therapy in patients with venous thromboembolism in the novel oral anticoagulant era. *Vasc Health Risk Manag* 12:23–34, 2016.

137. Davies MG, El-Sayed HF: Current status of clot removal for acute pulmonary embolism. *Ann Vasc Surg* 31:211–220, 2016.

138. Limbrey R, Howard L: Developments in the management and treatment of pulmonary embolism. *Eur Respir Rev* 24(137):484–497, 2015.

139. Ataya A, et al: Pulmonary arterial hypertension and associated conditions. *Dis Mon* 62(11):379–402, 2016.

140. McLaughlin VV, et al: Management of pulmonary arterial hypertension. *J Am Coll Cardiol* 65(18):1976–1997, 2015.

141. Simonneau G, et al: Updated clinical classification of pulmonary hypertension. *J Am Coll Cardiol* 62(SupplD):D34–D41, 2013.

142. Rich S: Right ventricular adaptation and maladaptation in chronic pulmonary arterial hypertension. *Cardiol Clin* 30(2):257–269, 2012.

143. Wilcox SR, Kabrhel C, Channick RN: Pulmonary hypertension and right ventricular failure in emergency medicine. *Ann Emerg Med* 66(6):619–628, 2015.

144. American Cancer Society (ACS): *Cancer facts & figures 2017*, Atlanta, 2017, Author. Available at: https://www.cancer.org/research/cancer-facts -statistics/all-cancer-facts-figures/cancer-facts -figures-2017.html.

145. Grce M, Mravak-Stipetić M: Human papillomavirus-associated diseases. *Clin Dermatol* 32(2):253–258, 2014.

146. Tang CG, Sinclair CF: Voice restoration after total laryngectomy. *Otolaryngol Clin North Am* 48(4):687–702, 2015.

147. Debry C, et al: Laryngeal replacement with an artificial larynx after total laryngectomy: the possibility of restoring larynx functionality in the future. *Head Neck* 36(11):1669–1673, 2014.

148. Schwartz AG, Cote ML: Epidemiology of lung cancer. *Adv Exp Med Biol* 893:21–41, 2016.

149. Sakashita S, Sakashita M, Sound Tsao M: Genes and pathology of non-small cell lung carcinoma. *Semin Oncol* 41(1):28–39, 2014.

150. Rivera GA, Wakelee H: Lung cancer in never smokers. *Adv Exp Med Biol* 893:43–57, 2016.

151. Bansal P, et al: Recent advances in targetable therapeutics in metastatic non-squamous NSCLC. *Front Oncol* 6:112, 2016.

152. Du L, Herbst RS, Morgensztern D: Immunotherapy in lung cancer. *Hematol Oncol Clin North Am* 31(1):131–141, 2017.

153. Rossi G, et al: Large cell carcinoma of the lung: clinically oriented classification integrating immunohistochemistry and molecular biology. *Virchows Archiv* 464(1):61–68, 2014.

154. Paraschiv B, et al: Paraneoplastic syndromes: the way to an early diagnosis of lung cancer. *Pneumologia* 64(2):14–19, 2015.

155. Anile M, et al: Bronchoplastic procedures for carcinoid tumors. *Thorac Surg Clin* 24(3):299–303, 2014.

156. Bononi A, et al: Latest developments in our understanding of the pathogenesis of mesothelioma and the design of targeted therapies. *Expert Rev Respir Med* 9(5):633–654, 2015.

157. Mittal V, et al: The microenvironment of lung cancer and therapeutic implications. *Adv Exp Med Biol* 890:75–110, 2016.

158. Sobus SL, Warren GW: The biologic effects of cigarette smoke on cancer cells. *Cancer* 120(23):3617–3626, 2014.

159. Orozco-Morales M, et al: Interplay between cellular and molecular inflammatory mediators in lung cancer. *Mediators Inflamm* 2016:3494608, 2016.

160. Nanavaty P, Alvarez MS, Alberts WM: Lung cancer screening: advantages, controversies, and applications. *Cancer Control* 21(1):9–14, 2014.

161. Gadgeel SM: Personalized therapy of non-small cell lung cancer (NSCLC). *Adv Exp Med Biol* 890:203–222, 2016.

162. Schneider BJ, Kalemkerian GP: Personalized therapy of small cell lung cancer. *Adv Exp Med Biol* 890:149–174, 2016.

Alterations of Pulmonary Function in Children

Valentina L. Brashers, Sue E. Huether

evolve WEBSITE

http://evolve.elsevier.com/McCance/
- Content Updates
- Chapter Summary Review
- Review Questions
- Case Studies
- Animations

CHAPTER OUTLINE

Alterations of respiratory function in children are influenced by age, development, gender, race, genes, and environmental conditions. Structural differences in infants and children render them less competent to tolerate conditions that cause increased work of breathing. Newborns, premature newborns in particular, are especially vulnerable to a variety of upper and lower airway infections caused by immaturity of the airways, circulation, chest wall, and the immune system. Access to health care and timeliness of immunizations influence the incidence and severity of pulmonary disorders.

STRUCTURE AND FUNCTION

A number of structural characteristics of the pulmonary system influence the way in which infants and children respond to respiratory disturbances. These include structural characteristics of the upper and lower respiratory tracts, chest wall and lung dynamics, metabolic requirements, immunologic immaturity, and physiologic control of respiration. Alterations in pulmonary blood flow that occur at birth are described in Chapter 35.

Upper Airway

All conducting airways (the portions of airway that do not participate in gas exchange) are present at birth and change only in size throughout childhood. Branching of the bronchial tree is in fact complete by the sixteenth week of fetal life.

Because infants and children naturally have smaller-diameter airways than adults, they suffer more obstruction for a given degree of mucosal edema or secretion accumulation. The relative sizes of tonsils, adenoids, and the epiglottis likewise are proportionately greater in the young child, and the presence of swelling can impose a significant site of obstruction. Infants up to 2 to 3 months of age are "obligatory nose breathers" and have difficulty inhaling through their mouths. Nasal congestion is therefore a serious threat to a young infant, especially during sleep.

Lower Airways and Lung Parenchyma

During fetal development the lung is transformed from a somewhat dense organ to one that is more delicately structured to facilitate air exchange. Beginning in the second trimester of pregnancy, there is loss of interstitial (mesenchymal) tissue with concomitant expansion of the future air spaces. Capillaries grow into the distal respiratory units that keep subdividing (alveolarization) to maximize the surface area for gas exchange. The number of alveoli continues to increase during the first 5 to 8 years of life, after which the alveoli increase in size and complexity. In addition to the structural development of the lung in utero, there is accompanying functional maturation during which specialized cell types, such as type II cells, manifest. (Fig. 37.1 contains a summary of alveolar development and stages of fetal lung development.)

Surfactant is a lipid-protein mixture that is produced by type II alveolar cells and is critical for maintaining alveolar expansion (thus allowing normal gas exchange, see Chapter 35). Surfactant is produced by 20 to 24 weeks' gestation and is secreted into the fetal airways by 30 weeks. Surfactant deficiency syndrome is often seen in premature infants and causes respiratory distress syndrome (RDS), previously known as *hyaline membrane disease*. The risk of acquisition of RDS escalates with increasing prematurity of the infant.

Chest Wall Dynamics

Chest wall compliance is high in infants, particularly premature infants. The cartilaginous structures of the thoracic cage are not yet well ossified (ossification continues to occur throughout childhood), and the chest wall is easily collapsible. During inspiration in the young child, air is drawn in by the downward movement of the diaphragm, but the resulting negative pressure causes the "soft" chest wall to be drawn *inward* (Fig. 37.2); this produces so-called *paradoxical breathing*, or *diaphragmatic breathing*. Paradoxical breathing is especially seen during rapid eye movement (REM) sleep of premature infants. With pulmonary compromise the accessory muscles are drawn inward, creating retraction of the intercostal and supraclavicular spaces (Fig. 37.3).

Resting lung volume, or functional residual capacity (FRC), represents the balance point between the natural elastic recoil of the lungs (to collapse) and the elastic recoil of the chest wall (to expand). In the face of an overly compliant chest wall, infants up to about 1 year of age are thought to maintain their FRC and avoid atelectasis by muscular "braking" of their expiration. This may occur either by active glottic narrowing or by increased activity of the inspiratory intercostal muscles.

Metabolic Characteristics

The basal metabolic rate of a child is greater than that of an adult, and thus oxygen consumption (Vo_2) is greater per unit of body weight. The Vo_2 of the child's normal work of breathing accounts for up to 25% of the total Vo_2. Respiratory distress increases the work of breathing and Vo_2 exponentially. Children have less muscle glycogen reserve, which limits the efficiency of accessory muscles, such that fatigue with lactic acidosis can occur quickly. Children also have a high proportion of extracellular fluid and therefore more quickly lose fluid and become dehydrated from fever, from environmental heat, or in association with tachypnea (which causes evaporation from the respiratory tract).

Immunologic Incompetence

Passive immunity with immunoglobulin G (IgG) is normally conveyed transplacentally from the mother to the fetus beginning at 20 weeks' gestation; thus IgG levels are lower in preterm than term infants. Breastfeeding allows transfer of secretory IgA, IgG, and IgM after birth. Because IgG has a half-life of approximately 21 days, the placentally transferred antibodies are depleted after just a few months. Infants are able to synthesize IgG, IgM, and IgA, and the levels of these immunoglobulins increase slowly with age. Cell-mediated immunity is also not fully developed in the neonate, which creates a situation of enhanced susceptibility to viral and fungal infections.

WHAT'S NEW?

Environmental Air Pollution and Childhood Respiratory Disease

Environmental exposures, such as tobacco smoke, air pollution (particulate matter, polycyclic aromatic hydrocarbons, and nitrogen dioxide), mold, respiratory viral infections, and medications, may contribute to pediatric pulmonary diseases, including increased asthma incidence and prevalence, risk of bronchitis and wheezing, susceptibility to infection, immune dysfunction, and deficits of lung growth and function. In the United States, 10.7% of pregnant mothers smoked during the last 3 months of pregnancy, which disturbs lung development in utero. Exposure to secondhand (environmental) tobacco smoke affects alveolar maturation during infancy and childhood. "Thirdhand smoke" results from tobacco chemicals that deposit on surfaces in the home. These tobacco products can react with chemicals in the environment, becoming even more toxic, and then can be inhaled or ingested by young children. In addition to smoke exposure, air pollution is increasingly recognized as a major contributor to pediatric pulmonary disease throughout the world. The impact of these exposures is mediated through changes in epigenetic controls on lung tissue genes and on immune cytokine synthesis and function. For example, both tobacco smoke and air pollution have been found to shift immune cytokine profiles toward allergy, increase airway inflammation, and increase expiratory airway obstruction, all of which are key components of asthma pathophysiology. Other epigenetic changes include increased airway fibroblast activation and disruption of normal respiratory center and peripheral chemoreceptor function. Clinicians, public health experts, and policy makers are expanding efforts to reduce prenatal, infant, and childhood exposure to these environmental risks.

Data from Chen Z et al: *J Thorac Dis* 7(1):46–58, 2015; Dick S et al: *BMJ Open* 4(11):e006554, 2014; Gibbs K, Collaco JM, McGrath-Morrow SA: *Chest* 149(2):552–561, 2016; Viera SE: *Int J Chron Obstruct Pulmon Dis* 10:1111–1121, 2015.

Physiologic Control of Respiration

Respiratory control in the neonate is immature compared to that in older children and adults, including respiratory responses to hypoxia and hypercapnia and an exaggerated apneic response to laryngeal stimulation. The mechanisms for this are not well understood but may reflect reduced activity of the peripheral chemoreceptors (in the carotid body) and nonadaptive responses or inhibitory influences on the respiratory center (in the brainstem). There is increased risk for apnea and hypoxia.[1] Congenital or acquired lesions of the central nervous system also may cause hypoventilation or apnea. Exposure to maternal smoking both during and after fetal development can have significant deleterious effects on lung development and subsequent susceptibility to pulmonary disorders. Exposure to environmental air pollution after birth also is associated with increased risk for childhood respiratory disease (see *What's New?* Environmental Air Pollution and Childhood Respiratory Disease).

DISORDERS OF THE UPPER AIRWAYS

Pulmonary dysfunction can be categorized into disorders of either the upper airway or the lower airway. Signs of acute respiratory failure are the same regardless of etiology. These include the following:

- Increased respiratory effort with retractions (see Fig. 37.3) or gasping (apnea in some conditions)
- Cyanosis or pallor
- Agitation
- Decreased level of consciousness

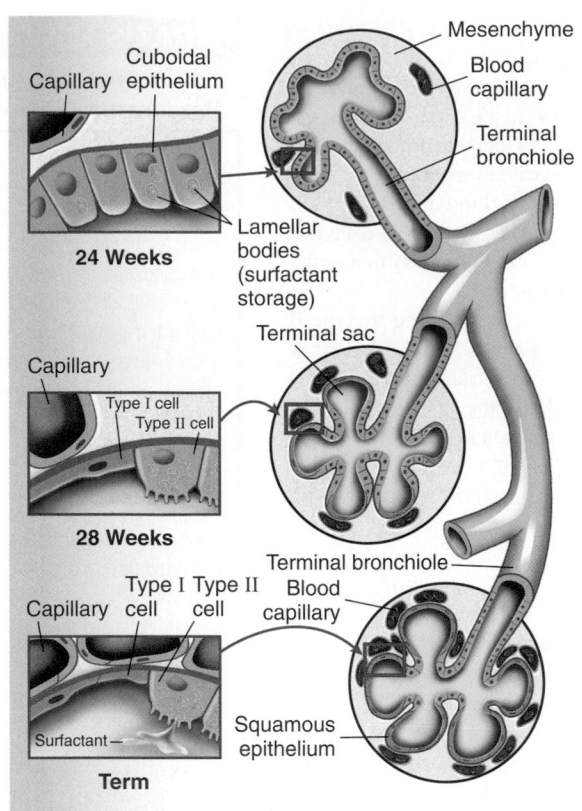

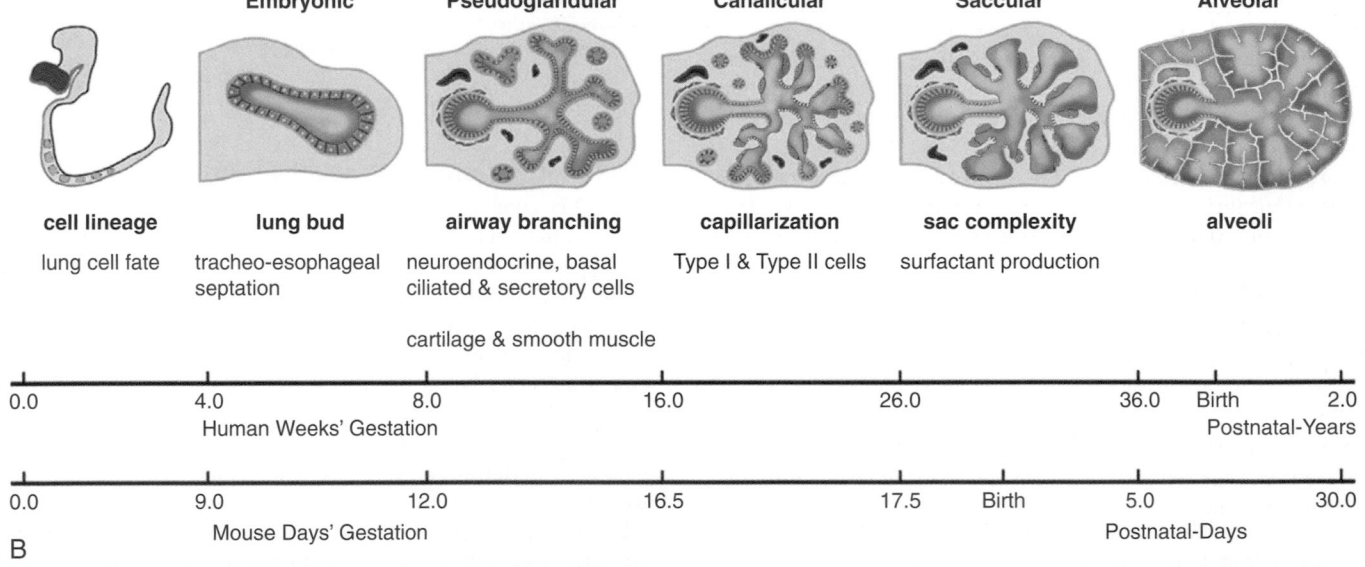

FIGURE 37.1 Prenatal Development of the Alveolar Unit and Stages of Lung Development. A, Epithelial cells differentiate into type II and type I cells. Mature type II cells are cuboidal, have apical microvilli, and contain lamellar bodies for surfactant storage and secretion. Type I cells are derived from type II cells and consist of flattened epithelium overlying capillaries, thus forming part of the desired thin air-blood barrier. During fetal development the pulmonary capillaries initially are randomly distributed in mesenchyme. They progressively arrange around the epithelial tubes and establish close contacts to the lining epithelium. Overall the volume of mesenchyme decreases and that of the potential air space increases. **B,** Stages of fetal lung development. (**B** adapted from Gleason CA, Devaskar S: *Avery's diseases of the newborn,* ed 9, Philadelphia, 2012, Saunders.)

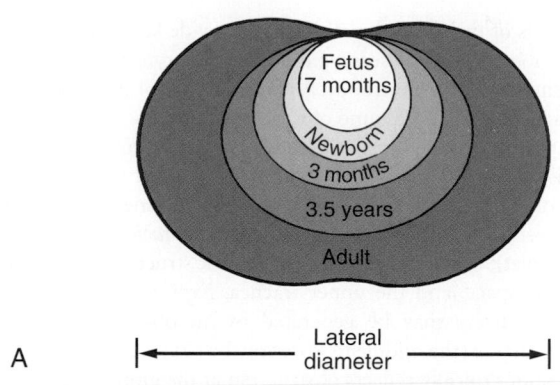

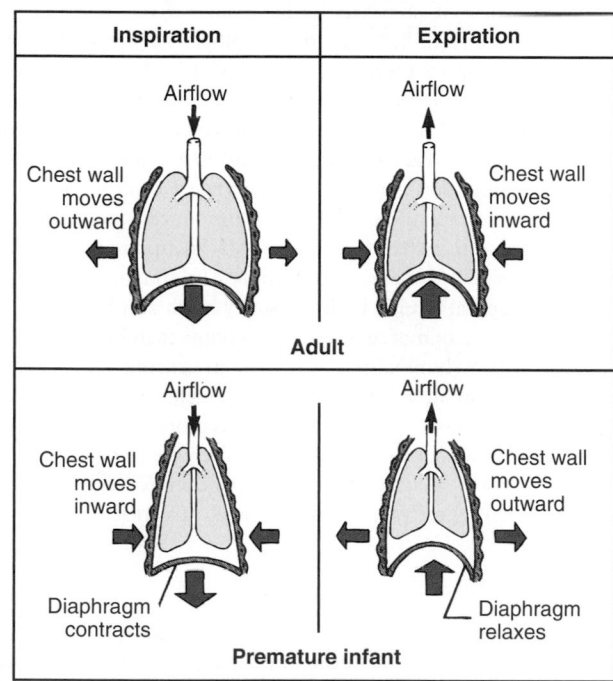

FIGURE 37.2 Developmental Differences in the Chest Wall and Lung Mechanics. **A,** Changes in chest wall shape with age. **B,** Differences in lung mechanics caused by differences in chest wall compliance (degree of rigidity) in premature infants and adults. (Arrows indicate direction of airflow, chest wall movement, and diaphragm movement.)

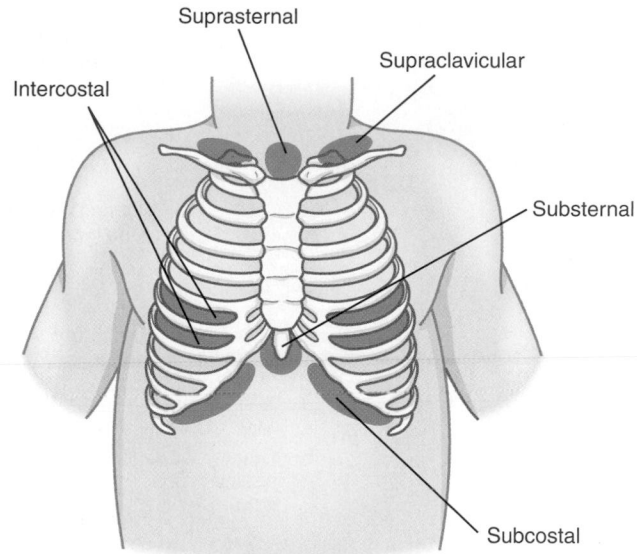

FIGURE 37.3 Areas of Chest Muscle Retraction.

BOX 37.1	**CAUSES OF UPPER AIRWAY OBSTRUCTION AND STRIDOR IN CHILDREN ACCORDING TO SITE OF OBSTRUCTION**

Nose and Pharynx	Vocal cord paralysis
Choanal atresia	Laryngotracheal stenosis
Lingual thyroid or thyroglossal cyst	Intubation trauma
Macroglossia	Foreign body
Micrognathia	Cystic hygroma
Hypertrophic tonsils/adenoids	Subglottic hemangioma
Retropharyngeal or peritonsillar abscess	Laryngeal papilloma
	Angioneurotic edema
	Laryngospasm (hypocalcemic tetany)
Larynx	Psychogenic stridor
Laryngomalacia	
Laryngeal web, cyst, or laryngocele	**Trachea**
Laryngotracheobronchitis (viral croup)	Tracheal stenosis
	Tracheomalacia
Acute spasmodic laryngitis (spasmodic croup)	Bacterial tracheitis
	External compression
Epiglottitis	

Data from Ida JB, Thompson DM: *Otolaryngol Clin North Am* 47(5):795–819, 2014; Mandal A, Kabra SK, Lodha R: *Indian J Pediatr* 82(8):737–744, 2015; Pfleger A, Eber E: *Paediatr Respir Rev* 18:64–72, 2016.

- Cardiovascular signs: tachycardia, mottled color, or bradycardia
- Physiologic compromise reflected by hemoglobin desaturation, hypoxemia, hypercarbia, and acidosis

Upper Airway Obstruction

The crucial issue in the upper airways is patency. The most common causes of *acute-onset* **upper airway obstruction (UAO)** in children are infections, foreign body aspiration, angioedema, obstructive sleep apnea, and trauma. *Chronic UAO* has many etiologies, including congenital malformations affecting the airway, cartilaginous weakness, vocal cord paralysis, and subglottic stenosis. Chronic upper airway symptoms should prompt referral to a pediatric pulmonologist or an otolaryngologist because specialized diagnostic studies may be needed. A summary of causes of pediatric UAO can be found in Box 37.1.

The site and nature of the obstruction are often discernible by assessing the noise or sounds associated with breathing, the quality of the voice or cry, and the presence of feeding difficulties (Fig. 37.4). This assessment often can be made without even touching the child. Likewise, the severity of the problem often can be judged by visual observation of signs, including retractions, nasal flaring, gasping or obstructed breaths, anxiety, restlessness, or need to maintain a specific head or body position. Agitation should be regarded as a likely sign of hypoxemia or obstruction. In acute UAO, increasing the child's anxiety by excessive physical examination can worsen the condition. The child should be kept as calm as possible. The clinician should never attempt a pharyngeal examination if there is any suspicion of epiglottitis or retropharyngeal abscess because this maneuver may precipitate acute obstruction of the airway.

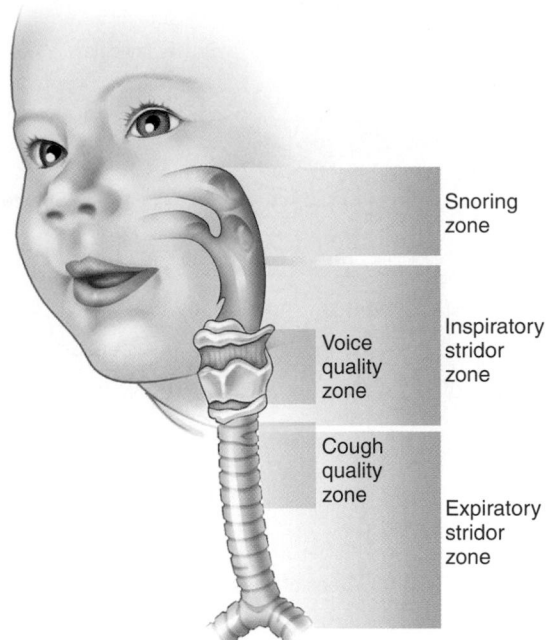

Snoring zone

Voice quality zone

Inspiratory stridor zone

Cough quality zone

Expiratory stridor zone

FIGURE 37.4 Listening Can Help Locate the Site of Airway Obstruction. A loud, gasping snore suggests enlarged tonsils or adenoids. Stridor during inspiration suggests the airway is compromised at the level of the supralaryngeal structures (epiglottis and arytenoid cartilages), vocal cords, and glottic region. With forced inspiration, intrathoracic pressure becomes quite negative and is less than atmospheric pressure, promoting collapse at or just above the site of obstruction. Expiratory stridor or central wheeze results from narrowing or collapse of the lower trachea or bronchi. During forced exhalation, rising pleural pressure may exceed intratracheal pressure. Airway noise during both inspiration and expiration often represents a fixed obstruction of the vocal cords or subglottic space. Hoarseness or a weak cry is a byproduct of obstruction at the vocal cords. If a cough is croupy or low pitched, suspect tracheal pathology. (Redrawn from Eavey RD: *Contemp Pediatr* 3[6]:78, 1986; used with permission; original illustration by Paul Singh-Roy.)

The sounds of the child's breathing can provide key clues (see Fig. 37.4). A sonorous, snoring noise is typical for nasopharyngeal obstruction, such as adenotonsillar hypertrophy. A common sign of pediatric UAO is *stridor*, a harsh, vibratory sound of variable pitch caused by turbulent flow through the partially obstructed airway.[2] A diagnostic approach to stridor is outlined in Fig. 37.5. Whether it is present in inspiration, expiration, or both reflects the site of the problem. In general, *inspiratory* stridor is generated with obstruction of the *extrathoracic* airway (above the thoracic inlet), which includes the supraglottic structures, the larynx, the subglottic space, and the upper trachea. *Expiratory* stridor or a monophonic wheeze may be generated by an obstruction in the *intrathoracic* airway (the middle to lower trachea and central bronchi). Biphasic stridor typically reflects obstruction at the glottis (e.g., vocal cord paralysis) itself or a *fixed* rather than a *dynamic* lesion in the subglottic space (e.g., hemangioma or subglottic stenosis). Biphasic noise may sometimes mean abnormalities of both the extrathoracic and intrathoracic trachea (long-segment stenosis or malacia).

Abnormalities of voice or cry (weak or hoarse) suggest problems at the larynx, such as vocal cord paralysis. Muffling of the voice, especially in an acute condition, suggests supralaryngeal obstruction, such as epiglottitis or retropharyngeal abscess. Pronounced cough may be an irritative symptom, such as that produced by an aspirated foreign body, or may be a sign of tracheal obstruction. The cough associated with croup or a tracheal foreign body is usually harsh and barking.

Airway obstruction occurs sooner in infants than in older children. Obviously, airway luminal size is smaller in accordance with smaller body size, but any decrease in luminal diameter will be much more significant. This is because airway resistance is proportional to the inverse of the *fourth* power of the radius; thus a decrease to half the original diameter increases resistance 16-fold. Furthermore, an infant's cartilaginous structures are more collapsible and thus are prone to creating or contributing to UAO.

Infections

Infections of the upper airway (Table 37.1) are common in children; some have the potential to cause life-threatening emergencies. Recognition and rapid evaluation of these problems are crucial pediatric care skills.

TABLE 37.1	COMPARISON OF UPPER AIRWAY INFECTIONS				
CONDITION	**AGE**	**ONSET**	**ETIOLOGY**	**PATHOPHYSIOLOGY**	**SYMPTOMS**
Acute laryngotracheo-bronchitis (croup)	6 mo–3 yr	Usually gradual	Viral (parainfluenza 1 and 3, influenza A, respiratory syncytial virus)	Inflammation from vocal cords to bronchial lumina	Harsh cough; stridor; low-grade fever; may have nasal discharge, conjunctivitis
Acute tracheitis	1–12 yr	Abrupt or following viral illness	*Staphylococcus aureus*/methicillin-resistant *S. aureus* (MRSA) *Haemophilus influenzae* type B Group A streptococci	Inflammation of upper trachea	High fever; toxic appearance; thick harsh cough; purulent secretions; may prefer head elevation
Epiglottitis	2–6 yr	Abrupt	*H. influenzae* type B (Hib) Group A streptococci	Inflammation of supraglottic structures	Severe sore throat; high fever; toxic appearance; muffled voice; may drool; sits erect and quietly
Retropharyngeal abscess	>6 yr	Gradual, 2–5 days; may follow oral trauma	*S. aureus*/MRSA *Streptococcus pyogenes* Anaerobes Group A beta-hemolytic streptococci Often polymicrobial	Abscess in posterior pharyngeal wall	Similar to epiglottitis
Peritonsillar abscess	>9 yr	May be abrupt	*S. pyogenes* *S. aureus*/MRSA	Abscess within or around tonsil	Similar to epiglottitis; may have trismus

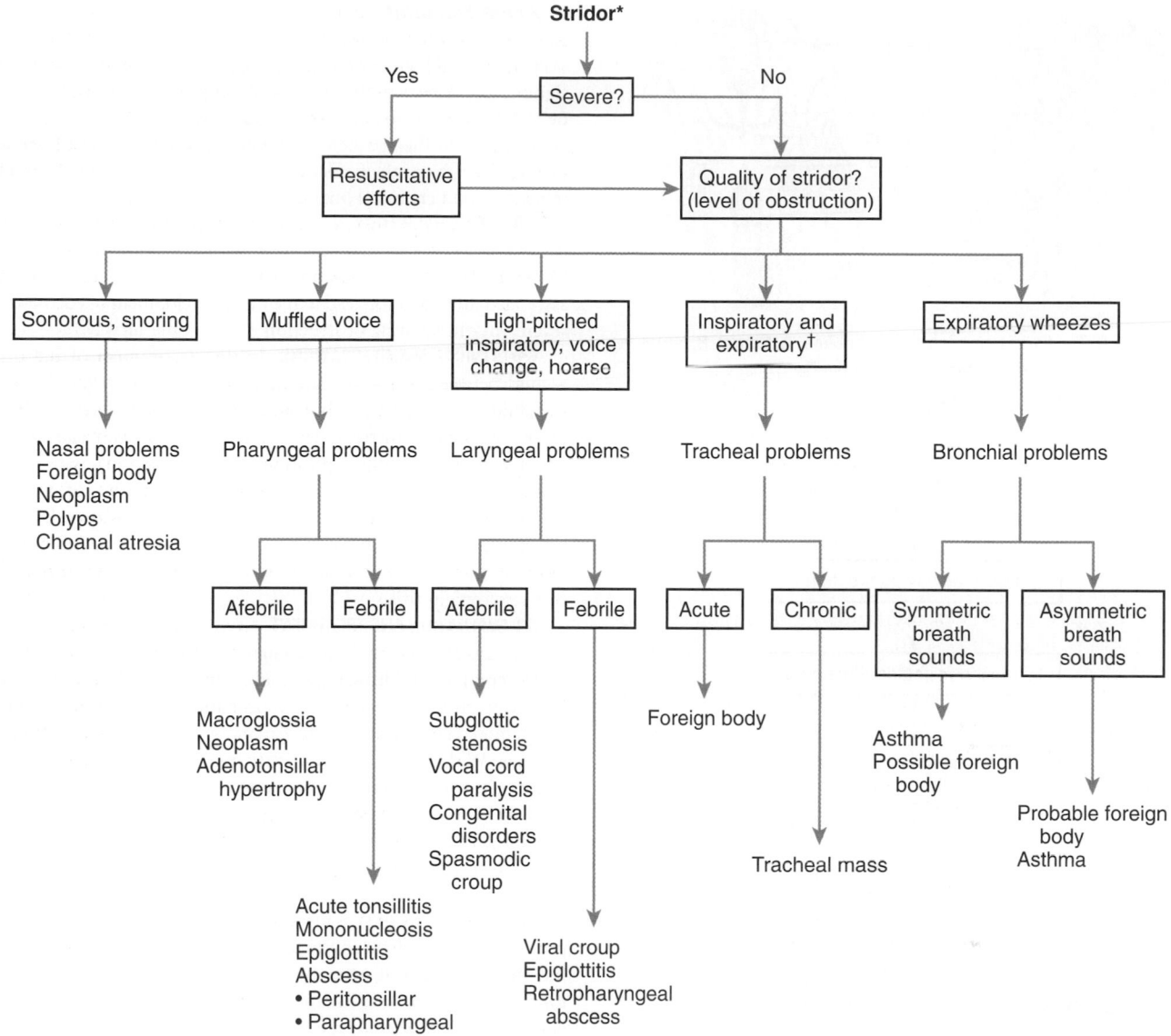

FIGURE 37.5 Diagnostic Approach to Stridor. *The age of the patient must be considered in making a specific diagnosis. †Laryngeal problems are frequently associated with inspiratory and expiratory stridor. (Adapted from Handler SD: Stridor. In Fleisher GR, Ludwig S, editors: *Textbook of pediatric emergency medicine*, Baltimore, 1993, Williams & Wilkins.)

Croup. Croup illnesses include viral croup (laryngotracheitis), recurrent croup (spasmodic croup), laryngotracheobronchitis, and laryngotracheobronchopneumonitis. Viral and recurrent croup are the most common. Diphtheria can be considered a croup illness but is now rare because of vaccinations. Croup illnesses are characterized by infection and obstruction of the upper airways.

Recurrent croup (spasmodic croup, also described as atypical croup) is two or more episodes of croup with symptoms similar to croup except it recurs without symptoms of respiratory tract infection. It often resolves as quickly as it develops and usually occurs in older children. The etiology is unknown but in some cases it is associated with an underlying congenital obstruction or airway narrowing (i.e., laryngomalacia or tracheomalacia). There also may be other associated illnesses such as gastroesophageal reflux disease or asthma.[3,4] Acute laryngotracheitis (croup) most commonly occurs in children from 6 months to 5 years of age, with peak incidence at about 2 years of age.[5]

◆**PATHOPHYSIOLOGY.** The pathophysiology of viral croup is caused primarily by subglottic edema from the infection. The mucous mem-branes of the larynx are tightly adherent to the underlying cartilage, whereas those of the subglottic space are looser and thus allow accumulation of mucosal and submucosal edema (Fig. 37.6). Furthermore, the cricoid cartilage is structurally the narrowest point of the airway, making edema in this area critical. As illustrated in Fig. 37.7, increased resistance to airflow leads to increased work of breathing, which generates more negative intrathoracic pressure, which in turn may exacerbate dynamic collapse of the upper airway.

◆**CLINICAL MANIFESTATIONS.** Typically there is a prodrome of rhinorrhea, sore throat, and low-grade fever for a few days. The child then develops the characteristic harsh (seal-like) barking cough, hoarse voice, and inspiratory stridor. Most cases are mild and resolve spontaneously after several more days. Occasionally, however, UAO becomes severe and requires urgent management.

◆**EVALUATION AND TREATMENT.** The degree of symptoms determines the level of treatment. Most children have a barking cough and viral symptoms and may need no specific treatment. However, the presence of stridor (especially at rest), retractions, or agitation suggests a sicker

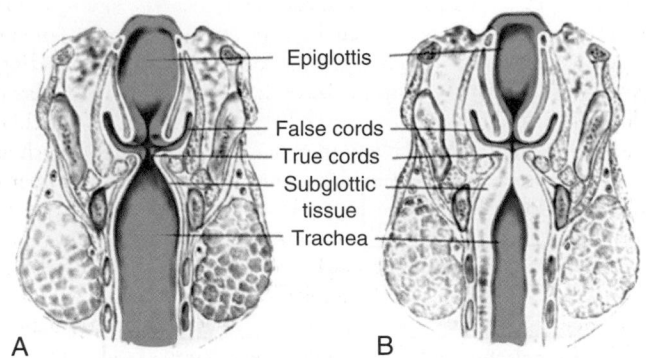

FIGURE 37.6 The Larynx and Subglottic Trachea. **A,** Normal. **B,** Narrowing and obstruction from edema caused by croup. (From Hockenberry MJ, Wilson D: *Wong's nursing care of infants and children,* ed 10, St Louis, 2015, Mosby.)

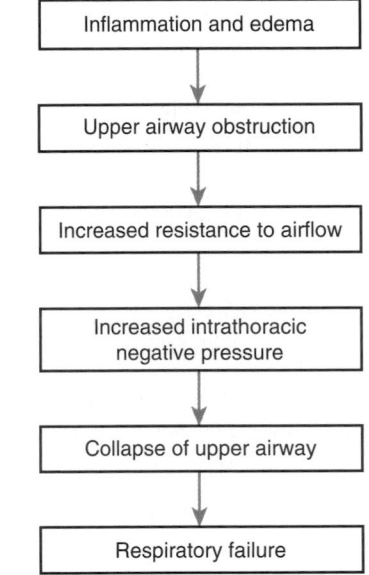

FIGURE 37.7 Upper Airway Obstruction with Croup.

child. The tool most often used for estimating croup severity is the Westley croup score, which provides a cumulative score for the degree of stridor, retractions, air entry, cyanosis, dyspnea, and level of consciousness in the child.[6]

The degree of seriousness of croup also is classified as mild, moderate, and severe. Most children with croup require no treatment. Inhalation of humidified air does not improve symptoms in mild to moderate croup. Glucocorticoids, either injected or oral (dexamethasone) or nebulized (budesonide), have been shown to improve symptoms within 6 hours. The use of nebulized racemic epinephrine improves outcomes with moderate to severe croup.[5,7] Epinephrine stimulates α- and β-adrenergic receptors and is thought to decrease airway secretions and mucosal edema. It is a temporizing measure until concomitantly given corticosteroids begin to take effect. Thus children who are given nebulized epinephrine should be closely observed for 2 to 3 hours to ensure that they will remain stable. Oxygen also should be administered. Heliox (helium/oxygen mixture of 80:20 or 70:30) may be used for severe cases of croup, although there is lack of scientific evidence to establish use in routine clinical practice.[8] In rare cases, croup and recurrent croup may require placement of an endotracheal tube. Children with recurrent croup require evaluation for anatomic abnormalities and the presence of associated diseases.[9]

Acute Epiglottitis. Historically, acute epiglottitis was caused by *Haemophilus influenzae* type B (Hib). Since the advent of Hib immunization, the overall incidence of acute epiglottitis in children has decreased significantly. However, up to 25% of epiglottitis cases are still caused by HiB.[10] Current pediatric cases usually represent vaccine failures or are caused by other pathogens. Infants less than 1 year of age are at greater risk.[11] Noninfectious causes include trauma from foreign body inhalation and chemical burns.

◆**PATHOPHYSIOLOGY.** The epiglottis arises from the posterior tongue base and covers the laryngeal inlet during swallowing. It has a rich blood and lymphatic circulation. Bacterial invasion of the mucosa and associated inflammation lead to the rapid development of edema causing severe, life-threatening obstruction of the upper airway.[12]

◆**CLINICAL MANIFESTATIONS.** In the classic form of the disease, a child between 2 and 6 years of age suddenly develops high fever, irritability, sore throat, a "hot potato voice," inspiratory stridor, and severe respiratory distress. The child appears ill and classically will adopt a forward-leaning position (tripod position) with drooling and dysphagia (inability to swallow). Examination of the throat may trigger laryngospasm and cause respiratory collapse. Death may occur in a few hours. Pneumonia, cervical lymph node inflammation, otitis, and, rarely, meningitis or septic arthritis may occur during the course of epiglottitis.

◆**EVALUATION AND TREATMENT.** Acute epiglottitis is a life-threatening emergency. The essentials are recognizing the presence of the disease, being careful not to disturb the child (which could worsen the obstruction), and securing the airway. Examination of the throat should not be attempted because it may trigger laryngospasm and cause respiratory collapse. With severe airway obstruction, the airway is secured with endotracheal intubation and anesthesia. Subsequent culture of the airway is obtained and intravenous broad-spectrum antibiotics are administered promptly. Therapy is reevaluated after culture results return. Corticosteroids also are generally used in treatment regimens.[13,14] Resolution with treatment is usually rapid. When Hib epiglottitis is diagnosed, the American Academy of Pediatrics (AAP) recommends that postexposure prophylaxis with rifampin be administered to household contacts of the infected child if they have not been fully vaccinated or are immunocompromised. Rifampin is given once daily for 4 days and eradicates *H. influenzae* type B in approximately 95% of carriers.[15]

Tonsillar Infections. Tonsillar infections (tonsillitis) are occasionally severe enough to cause UAO. As with other infections of the upper airway, the incidence of tonsillitis secondary to group A beta-hemolytic *Streptococci* (GABHS) and methicillin-resistant *Staphylococcus aureus* (MRSA) has risen in the past 15 years.[16] Significant swelling of the tonsils and pharynx occurs, and a tenacious membrane may cover the mucosa. UAO because of tonsillitis is a well-known complication of infectious mononucleosis, especially in a young child. The development of UAO in tonsillar infections requires the administration of appropriately selected antibiotics and the use of corticosteroids.[17] Some children with recurrent tonsillitis benefit from adenotonsillectomy. Tonsillitis may be complicated by formation of a tonsillar abscess, which can further contribute to airway obstruction. Peritonsillar abscess is usually unilateral and is most often a complication of acute tonsillitis.[18] The most common causative microorganism is GABHS. Symptoms in children include fever, sore throat, dysphagia, trismus, pooling of saliva, and muffled voice. Peritonsillar bulging (Fig. 37.8) and cervical adenopathy on the same side are usually visible. The abscess must be drained and the child given antibiotics. Death can occur from spontaneous abscess rupture with aspiration or airway obstruction.[19]

Bacterial Tracheitis. Bacterial tracheitis (pseudomembranous croup) is the most common, potentially life-threatening upper airway infection in children. It is most often caused by *S. aureus* (including

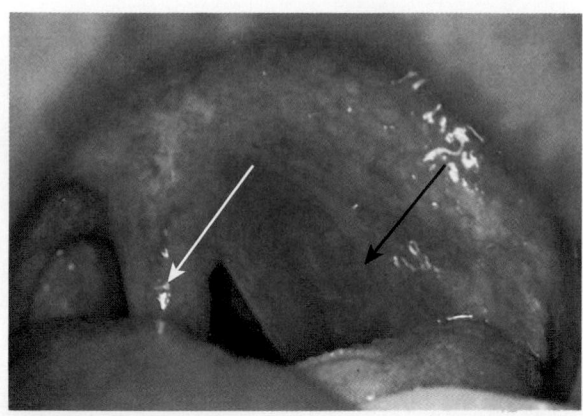

FIGURE 37.8 Peritonsillar Abscess. If the tonsils are inflamed and appear asymmetrical with unilateral palatal swelling *(black arrow)* and uvular deviation *(white arrow)*, a peritonsillar abscess should be suspected. (From Goldman L, Schafer AI: *Goldman's Cecil medicine,* ed 24, Philadelphia, 2012, Saunders.)

methicillin-resistant [MRSA] strains), *H. influenzae,* GABHS *(Streptococcus pyogenes),* or *Moraxella catarrhalis* virus. A fungus is more likely to be seen as the source of tracheitis in immunocompromised children.

The presence of airway edema and copious purulent secretions leads to airway obstruction that can be worsened by the formation of a tracheal pseudomembrane and mucosal sloughing. Increased morbidity can occur because of respiratory and cardiopulmonary arrest, respiratory failure, pneumonia, septic shock, toxic shock syndrome, acute respiratory distress syndrome (ARDS), and multiple organ dysfunction syndrome (MODS).[20] The onset of symptoms may be sudden or may be preceded by a preexisting viral upper respiratory tract infection or croup. The acute clinical presentation frequently includes tachypnea, stridor, hoarse voice, fever, cough, and/or increased secretions from the mouth and nose. There may be evidence of concurrent infections, such as sinusitis, otitis, pneumonia, or pharyngitis. Management requires the rapid administration of broad-spectrum intravenous antibiotics and endotracheal intubation in order to prevent airway obstruction.[21]

Retropharyngeal Abscess. Retropharyngeal abscess can be caused by aerobic, anaerobic, or polymicrobial infection. There has been an increase in GABHS strains associated with this condition, and the emergence of MRSA as the offending microorganism is increasingly noted.[22]

Retropharyngeal abscess usually occurs more commonly in children about 4 years of age and as a consequence of either nasopharyngeal infection or penetrating local injury.[23] Clinical signs include fever, dysphagia, drooling, stridor, respiratory distress, and neck pain. This condition requires emergency treatment with intravenous antibiotics targeted at the suspected microorganism, and sometimes incision and drainage.[24]

Aspiration of Foreign Bodies

Aspiration of foreign bodies into the airways is most common in children 1 to 4 years of age. More than 100,000 cases and 100 deaths occur each year.[25] Most objects are expelled by the cough reflex, but some objects may lodge in the larynx, trachea, or bronchi. Large objects (e.g., nuts, seeds, hard candy, a bite of hot dog, popcorn, grapes, beans, toy pieces, fragments of popped balloons, or coins) may occlude the airway and become life-threatening. Items of particular concern are batteries and multiple magnets. The aspiration event is often not witnessed or not recognized when it happens because the coughing, choking, wheezing, or gagging symptoms may resolve quickly. Foreign bodies lodged in the larynx or upper trachea cause cough, stridor, hoarseness or inability

to speak, decreased breath sounds, respiratory distress, and agitation or panic; the presentation is often dramatic and frightening.[26] Foreign bodies in the intrathoracic airways more commonly produce wheezing. Symptoms are determined by the size of the object and the site where it is located, as well as the child's age and size (see Fig. 37.4). If the child is acutely hypoxic and unable to move air, immediate action, such as sweeping the oral airway or performing abdominal thrusts (formerly called the *Heimlich maneuver*), may be required to prevent tragedy. Otherwise, bronchoscopic removal should be performed urgently. If an aspirated foreign body is small enough, it will be transferred to a bronchus before becoming lodged. If the foreign body is lodged in the airway for a notable period of time, local irritation, granulation, obstruction, and infection will ensue. Thus children may present with cough or wheezing, atelectasis, pneumonia, lung abscess, or blood-streaked sputum. Many objects are not radiopaque and will not be visible on a chest radiograph. Occasionally, air will accumulate distal to the obstruction if the object is causing a ball-valve effect. This effect can sometimes be documented by inspiratory and expiratory chest films (Fig. 37.9). These children are treated by prompt bronchoscopic removal of the object and administration of antibiotics as necessary. Children with an unexplained persistent cough and refractory parenchymal infiltrates also should be considered for unrecognized foreign body aspiration.[27]

Angioedema

Angioedema is a localized edema involving the deep, subcutaneous layers of skin or mucous membranes. Generally, angioedema causes facial swelling first, particularly around the eyes and lips, and may progress to airway swelling. Angioedema is usually secondary to mast cell–mediated allergic phenomena (e.g., allergy to peanuts, cow's milk, chicken eggs). Increased levels of bradykinin mediate this adverse effect by causing vasodilation, increased vascular permeability, and histamine release. An occasional cause of pediatric angioedema is use of angiotensin-converting enzyme inhibitors for treatment of hypertension or heart disease. If airway compromise is apparent, standard treatment includes epinephrine (subcutaneous), antihistamines, and corticosteroids.[28]

An inherited deficiency of the plasma protein C-1 inhibitor (C-1 INH) causes *hereditary angioneurotic edema (HAE),* a rare but serious problem in children. About 50% of cases occur during childhood.[29] The mean age of onset of initial symptoms is 8 to 19 years but it also may occur as early as the first year of life. This condition is characterized by nonallergic, recurring attacks of angioedema involving subcutaneous tissues (especially limbs, genitalia, and face); abdominal and pelvic viscera; and, much less often, the airway. Laryngeal attacks in these individuals may be life-threatening and do not respond reliably to standard measures for airway edema. Laboratory evaluation of complement and C-1 INH levels usually provides an accurate diagnosis.[30] The mortality of undiagnosed HAE can be as high as 50%. The mainstays of supportive care are airway monitoring, hydration, pain relief, and control of nausea. Treatments include concentrates of C-1 INH, ecallantide/kallikrein inhibitor, and icatibant/bradykinin receptor antagonist.[31,32]

Congenital Malformations

Congenital malformations can occur at multiple sites from the nasal openings to the subglottis. Anatomic or functional obstruction can cause severe respiratory distress.

Laryngomalacia and Tracheomalacia. Laryngomalacia results from abnormally soft laryngeal cartilages and is the most common cause of chronic stridor in infants. Boys are more likely than girls to present with symptoms. In laryngomalacia, the epiglottis or arytenoids, or both, fold inward with inspiration, partially covering the glottis (Fig. 37.10). The pathophysiology of these abnormalities is still not completely

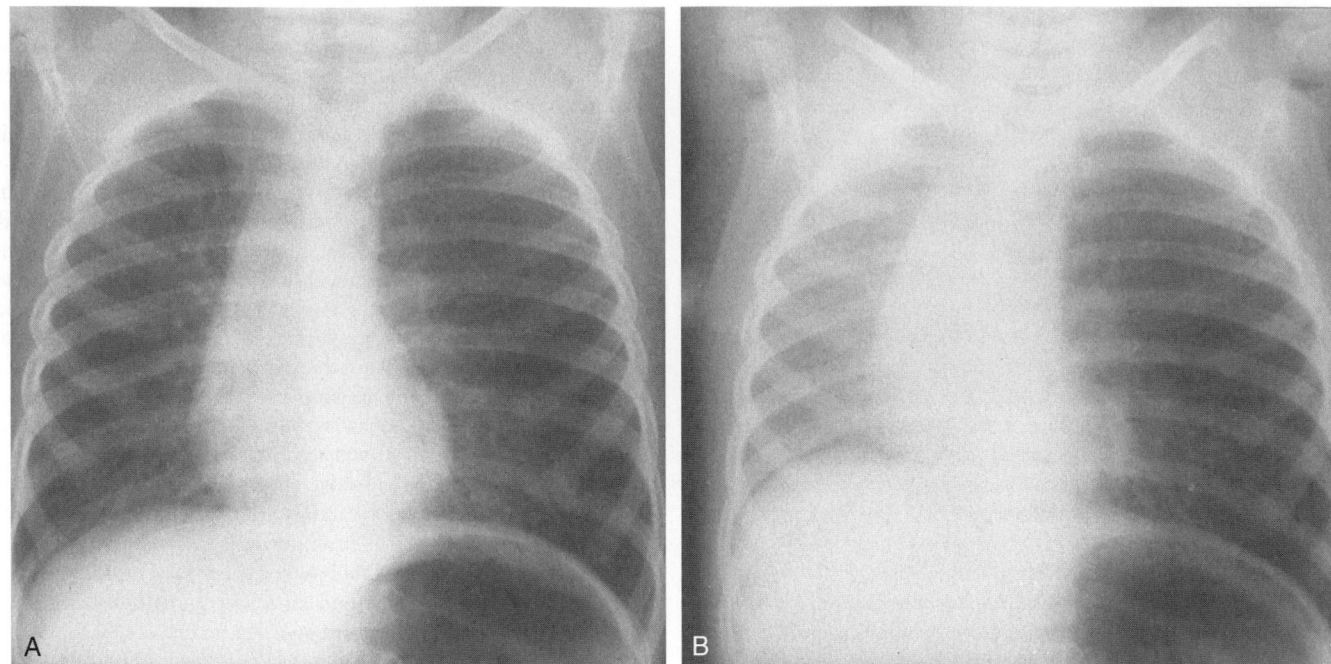

FIGURE 37.9 Foreign Body Aspiration. Anteroposterior inspiratory **(A)** and expiratory **(B)** chest radiographs. Air trapping in the left lung is caused by a peanut in the left mainstem bronchus. (From Taussig LM, Landau LI: *Pediatric respiratory medicine*, ed 2, St Louis, 2008, Mosby.)

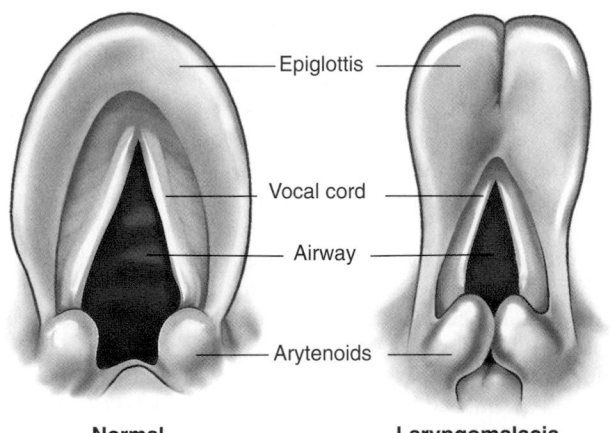

FIGURE 37.10 Laryngomalacia. In the normal larynx *(left)*, supralaryngeal structures maintain their upright orientation during inspiration. In contrast, in infants with laryngomalacia *(right)*, there is inward prolapse of the arytenoid masses, which include the prominent cuneiform tubercles and the arytenoid cartilages. The glottis becomes partially covered, and airflow is impeded. Sometimes the edges of the epiglottis curl inward, further exacerbating the obstruction. In expiration, these structures are "blown" aside passively.

understood. A neuromuscular hypothesis suggests there is immaturity or an abnormality of the sensorimotor integrative function of the brainstem, and peripheral reflexes are responsible for laryngeal tone and airway patency. Laryngeal nerve hypertrophy also has been documented.[33] Gastroesophageal reflux disease (GERD) and other comorbidities are associated with laryngomalacia.[34]

Typical signs of laryngomalacia include inspiratory stridor beginning in the first days or weeks of life that is accentuated with activity, and sometimes with positional changes (worse in supine or head-flexed positions). Feeding difficulties may be noted, but they are usually mild. Cry is normal. Laryngoscopy is used to confirm the diagnosis. Laryngomalacia is usually mild and improves spontaneously over the first year of life as the supralaryngeal cartilage structures stiffen; thus most cases are managed with watchful waiting. Supraglottoplasty is the surgery of choice for severe symptoms, including breathing and eating difficulties with weight loss or failure to thrive. A late-onset variant of this disease has been noted in the literature and should be suspected if the following occur: potential cause of feeding difficulties in toddlers, sleep apnea in children, and exercise intolerance in teenagers.[35,36]

In tracheomalacia, or tracheobronchomalacia, the tracheobronchial cartilages are flaccid and tend to collapse during the expiratory cycle, causing stridor. This may be classified as primary (idiopathic) or secondary. When malacia is caused by a secondary source, it is usually related to extrinsic compression of the trachea from a vascular malformation (congenital tracheomalacia). Tracheobronchomalacia involves the mainstem bronchi and presents clinically as a spectrum of respiratory illnesses that range from life-threatening conditions to chronic cough and wheeze conditions. In some cases symptoms may be more subtle than those associated with laryngomalacia. Low-pitched inspiratory stridor may be a sign of malacia of the upper trachea or a centrally located, single-pitch (monophonic) wheeze may be present in malacia of the middle to distal trachea. Tracheomalacia can be suspected clinically, usually by 2 to 3 months of age, and confirmed by bronchoscopy and imaging. Depending on the type and severity of the lesion, surgical approaches for repair may be indicated.[37]

Vocal Cord Paralysis. Vocal cord paralysis is second to laryngomalacia as a cause of stridor and is a relatively uncommon congenital disorder. The vocal cords should move apart to facilitate inspiration and move together to facilitate vocalization. Paralysis of one or both vocal cords may affect breathing, swallowing, and speech. The etiology of the congenital abnormality is unclear but may be caused by immaturity of the vagus nerve or brainstem, or both. Iatrogenic injury is frequently cited as the major secondary cause of vocal cord paralysis, such as surgical trauma to the recurrent laryngeal nerve during cardiac surgery. Other secondary causes include Arnold-Chiari malformation (the region of the brainstem in which the nucleus ambiguus acts as the "relay station" for laryngeal function), cerebral palsy, hydrocephalus, myelomeningocele, spina bifida, or hypoxia.[38] Other associations include infectious and neoplastic causes, trauma, and inflammatory conditions.[39] In older children and adolescents, exercise can result in inducible laryngeal obstruction (previously known as *vocal cord dysfunction [VCD]*).[40]

Clinical findings of vocal cord paralysis in children younger than 1 year include dysphonia, glottic incompetence, GERD, and stridor.[39] It sometimes resolves spontaneously (most often during the first year of life) or with correction of the underlying problem. Flexible laryngoscopy and chest x-ray are common evaluative tools that may help determine the cause. In some individuals, inducible laryngeal obstruction may be misdiagnosed as asthma.[41] Medical therapy may include the use of corticosteroids, proton pump inhibitors, and speech therapy. Recurrent pulmonary infections secondary to aspiration may occur and require treatment until the cords are repaired. Surgical treatment of unilateral vocal cord paralysis includes injection laryngoplasty, thyroplasty, and laryngeal reinnervation.[42] Tracheostomy may be used until the vocal cords are surgically repaired.

Subglottic Stenosis. Congenital subglottic stenosis is the third most common laryngeal anomaly and is defined as a subglottic airway diameter of less than 4 mm at the cricoid region (just below the vocal folds extending to the lower border of the cricoid cartilage) in a full-term infant, and less than 3 mm in a premature infant. Incomplete recanalization of the laryngotracheal tube during the third month of gestation results in this defect. The overall rate of symptomatic subglottic stenosis (stridor, intercostal retractions, and barking cough) in neonates is 0.2%.[43] Subglottic stenosis also is associated with eosinophilic esophagitis, Wegener granulomatosis, and neurofibromatosis.[44-46] Because of the rapid growth of the lumen of the trachea and cricoid cartilage in the first year (which triples in size), infants may outgrow the obstruction, particularly if it is mild or moderate. An endotracheal tube is placed in severe cases. Traumatic injury to the upper airway with development of secondary subglottic stenosis is a well-described complication of endotracheal intubation. Factors that contribute to secondary subglottic stenosis include utilization of long-term assisted ventilation, use of an endotracheal tube that is too large, excessive movement of the tube, and susceptibility of the individual. Neonates can tolerate long periods of endotracheal intubation and subglottic stenosis can be minimized by ensuring that the tube size allows a small air leak during inspiration (at a peak inspiratory force of approximately 25 mmHg) and that the tube is securely taped. Because of the rapid growth of the lumen of the trachea and cricoid cartilage in the first year (which triples in size), infants may outgrow the obstruction, particularly if mild or moderate. Serial balloon dilation can be effective. For severe subglottic stenosis, laryngotracheal reconstruction (LTR) along with cricotracheal resection and thyrotracheal anastomosis may be required.[47]

Other Congenital Malformations. Congenital malformations of the upper airways, trachea, and bronchial tree are rare and cause airway obstruction. Lesions include choanal atresia; laryngeal atresias, webs, cysts, clefts, and subglottic hemangiomas; and tracheal stenosis. Choanal atresia can be unilateral or bilateral and causes lack of patency of the nasal cavity within the nasopharynx. Bilateral choanal atresia can be life-threatening in newborns because they are obligate nasal breathers. Laryngeal atresias and webs are caused by failure of the larynx to recanalize during embryogenesis. Most of these disorders are in the area of the glottis with extension into the subglottis. Tracheal stenosis is a rare malformation characterized by inspiratory and expiratory stridor within the first few weeks of birth. It is usually associated with pulmonary, cardiovascular, and gastrointestinal malformations.[48] Structural abnormalities such as pectus excavatum or abnormalities involving the great vessels also can result in tracheal compression. For example, absent pulmonary valve syndrome dilates the pulmonary artery, which can compress the trachea and bronchi.[49] Tracheal or bronchial compression results in airway symptoms or feeding difficulties, or both, ranging from dysphagia, recurrent respiratory tract infections, wheezing, and stridor to acute respiratory distress or "dying spells." Many older children are first thought to have gastroesophageal reflux or asthma as the principal problem. Surgical management is usually required for these conditions, and some infants may require mechanical ventilation while awaiting surgery.[50]

Obstructive Sleep Apnea Syndrome

Obstructive sleep apnea syndrome (OSAS) is a form of sleep-disordered breathing (SDB) defined by partial or intermittent complete UAO during sleep with disruption of normal ventilation and sleep patterns. Childhood OSAS is common with an estimated prevalence of 2% to 3% of children 12 to 14 years of age, up to 13% of children ages 3 to 6 years, and about 60% of obese children.[51] Prevalence is estimated to be two to four times higher in vulnerable populations (blacks, Hispanics, and preterm infants) and there may be a family history of OSAS.[52] Possible influences early in life may include passive smoke inhalation, socioeconomic status, and snoring together with genetic modifiers that promote airway inflammation.

PATHOPHYSIOLOGY. The pathophysiology of childhood OSAS is likely to be multifactorial in origin, involving the central nervous, cardiovascular, metabolic, and immune systems. Airway narrowing and increased upper airway collapsibility are the common causes of OSAS. Obstruction of the upper airway during sleep results in cyclic episodes of increasing respiratory effort and changes in intrathoracic pressures with oxygen desaturation, hypercapnia, and arousal. The child goes back to sleep and the cycle repeats. Adenotonsillar hypertrophy, gastroesophageal reflux, obesity, and craniofacial anomalies are associated with airway narrowing. Infants are at risk because they have both anatomic and physiologic predispositions toward airway obstruction and gas-exchange abnormalities, including a superiorly placed larynx, increased chest wall compliance, ventilation-perfusion mismatching, and ventilatory control instability.

Reduced motor tone of the upper airways may be seen in neurologic disorders, such as cerebral palsy and Down syndrome. Upper airway inflammation and altered neurologic reflexes involving respiratory control of upper airway muscles are significant factors in reducing airway diameter. Allergy and asthma may contribute to inflammation, and children who have a history of a clinically significant episode of respiratory syncytial virus (RSV) bronchiolitis in infancy may exhibit altered neuroimmunomodulatory pathways toward inflammation in the upper airway. In obese children, current research links OSAS with airway inflammation and elevated levels of C-reactive protein, which also contribute to increased risk for cardiovascular and metabolic diseases.[53]

CLINICAL MANIFESTATIONS. Common manifestations of OSAS include snoring and failure to thrive in infants, labored breathing, restlessness, sweating during sleep (which can be continuous or intermittent), and sleepiness in children and adolescents. There may be episodes of increased respiratory effort but no audible airflow, often terminated by snorting, gasping, repositioning, or arousal. Affected children are often chronic mouth breathers and have large tonsils and adenoids. They also may exhibit nocturnal enuresis. Untreated OSAS can cause cardiovascular disease (particularly left ventricular hypertrophy and pulmonary hypertension) and insulin resistance as well as upper and lower respiratory tract infections. Cognitive and neurobehavioral impairment (e.g., inattention, hyperactivity, aggression, conduct problems, attention-deficit/hyperactivity disorder [ADHD]/emotional [mood]), impaired school performance, and poor quality of life are consequences of OSAS.[54]

◆EVALUATION AND TREATMENT. All parents should be asked if their child exhibits snoring and labored breathing, sweating, and restlessness during sleep, which may be continuous or intermittent. Screening tools and sleep questionnaires are helpful in evaluating the presence of SDB.[55] Imaging of the upper airway may be used to rule out adenoidal hypertrophy or upper airway narrowing. The most definitive evaluation ("gold standard") is the polysomnographic sleep study, which documents obstructed breathing and physiologic impairment and may be combined with nocturnal oximetry studies. If obstructive sleep apnea caused by tonsillar enlargement is documented or strongly suspected clinically, children are most often referred for tonsillectomy and adenoidectomy (T&A). For severely affected children who do not respond to T&A or who have different problems, such as obesity that cannot be rapidly remedied, use of continuous positive airway pressure (CPAP), antiinflammatory medications, dental treatments, or a high-flow nasal cannula as well as weight loss can be considered. Treatment is important to minimize associated morbidities.[56,57]

DISORDERS OF THE LOWER AIRWAYS

Lower airway disease is one of the leading causes of morbidity in the first year of life and continues to be an important component of other illnesses. Infants may have respiratory distress from immature lungs and surfactant deficiency, or from aspiration of amniotic fluid or meconium. Other disorders include congenital malformations, asthma, cystic fibrosis, infections, and acute respiratory distress syndrome (ARDS).

Surfactant Deficiency Disorder (Respiratory Distress Syndrome of the Newborn)

Surfactant deficiency disorder (SDD) (respiratory distress syndrome [RDS] of the newborn), previously known as **hyaline membrane disease (HMD)**, is a significant cause of neonatal morbidity and mortality. It occurs almost exclusively in premature infants, and the incidence has increased in the United States over the past two decades. Preterm births accounted for about 9.50% of all births in 2014 (about 8.0% for white mothers, about 13.23% for black mothers, and about 9.03% for Hispanic mothers).[58] The major predisposing factor is prematurity because the immature lung is not well structured for gas exchange and has not yet developed adequate surfactant production and secretion. SDD (RDS) occurs in 50% to 60% of infants born at 29 weeks' gestation and decreases significantly by 36 weeks. Infants of diabetic mothers and those with cesarean delivery (especially elective C-section) are more likely to develop SDD (RDS) because the labor-associated catecholamine and steroid surges do not occur, causing decreased pulmonary surfactant release.[59] It is more common in boys than girls, and in one cohort it was more common in black infants.[60,61] Death rates have declined significantly since the introduction of antenatal steroid therapy and postnatal surfactant therapy. The epidemiology, pathophysiology, and clinical presentation of SDD (RDS) are summarized in Box 37.2.

◆PATHOPHYSIOLOGY. SDD (RDS) is caused by surfactant deficiency. Surfactant lipoproteins have a detergent-like effect that separates the liquid molecules inside the alveoli, thereby decreasing alveolar surface tension. Without surfactant, alveoli collapse at the end of each exhalation, which decreases the alveolar surface area available for gas exchange.[62] Surfactant normally is not secreted by the alveolar cells until approximately 20 to 24 weeks' gestation (see Fig. 37.1). Premature infants also are born with underdeveloped and small alveoli that are difficult to inflate. Additionally, the alveoli have thick walls and an inadequate

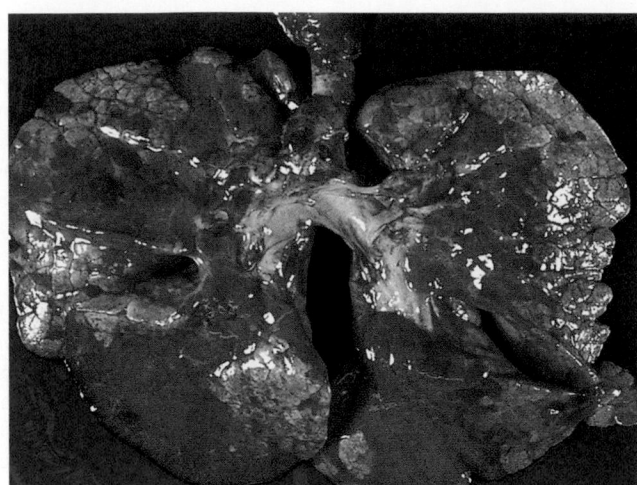

FIGURE 37.11 Patchy Atelectasis of Neonatal Lungs with Surfactant Deficiency Disorder (Respiratory Distress Syndrome). (From Damjanov I, Linder J, editors: *Anderson's pathology*, ed 10, St Louis, 1996, Mosby.)

capillary blood supply such that gas exchange is significantly impaired. The infant's chest wall is weak and highly compliant and, thus, the rib cage tends to collapse inward with respiratory effort. The net effect is *atelectasis* (Fig. 37.11), resulting in significant hypoxemia. Atelectasis is difficult for the neonate to overcome because it requires a significant negative inspiratory pressure to open the alveoli with each breath. The increased work of breathing and a decrease in tidal volume cause alveolar hypoventilation and hypercapnia. Hypoxia and hypercapnia cause pulmonary vasoconstriction and increase intrapulmonary resistance and shunting. This results in hypoperfusion of the lung and a decrease in effective pulmonary blood flow. Increased pulmonary vascular resistance may even cause a partial return to fetal circulation (see Chapter 35) with right-to-left shunting of blood through the ductus arteriosus and foramen ovale. Inadequate perfusion of tissues and hypoxemia contribute to metabolic acidosis.

Inadequate alveolar ventilation can be further complicated by increased pulmonary capillary permeability. Many premature infants with SDD (RDS) require positive pressure mechanical ventilation with high oxygen content, which damages the alveolar epithelium (e.g., barotrauma and oxygen toxicity). Together these conditions result in the leakage of plasma proteins into the alveoli and pulmonary edema. Fibrin deposits in the air spaces create the appearance of *hyaline membranes* for which the disorder was originally named. The plasma proteins leaked into the air space have the additional adverse effect of inactivating any surfactant that may be present. The pathogenesis of SDD (RDS) is summarized in Figs. 37.11 and 37.12.

◆CLINICAL MANIFESTATIONS. Signs of SDD (RDS) appear within minutes of birth and include tachypnea (respiratory rate more than 60 breaths per minute), expiratory grunting, intercostal and subcostal retractions, nasal flaring, and cyanosis. The natural course is characterized by progressive hypoxemia and dyspnea with severity progressing over the first hours after birth. Apnea and irregular respirations occur as the infant tires. The severity of the hypoxemia and the difficulty in providing adequate supplemental oxygenation result in the Vermont Oxford Network definition of RDS as a PaO_2 less than 50 mmHg in room air, central cyanosis in room air, or a need for supplemental oxygen to maintain a PaO_2 greater than 50 mmHg, as well as chest film appearance.[63] Typically, a chest radiograph shows diffuse, fine granular densities within the first 6 hours of life. This "ground glass" appearance is associated with alveolar flooding. In most cases the clinical

BOX 37.2   SURFACTANT DEFICIENCY DISORDER (RESPIRATORY DISTRESS SYNDROME OF THE NEWBORN)

Epidemiology
Worldwide
Prematurity predisposes
Cesarean section without labor predisposes
Perinatal asphyxia predisposes
Meconium aspiration predisposes
Male > female
White > black
Second-born twin at greater risk
PROM spares
IUGR spares
Advanced maternal age predisposes
Maternal stress spares
Maternal diabetes predisposes if less than 37 weeks
Maternal hemorrhage predisposes

Etiology
Surfactant deficiency
Probable inadequate hormonal (corticoid) stimulus in utero
DPL synthesis impaired and/or destruction increased
Autonomic dysfunction

Pathophysiology
Reduced lung compliance
Reduced FRC
Poor lung distensibility
Poor alveolar stability
Right-to-left shunts
Reduced effective pulmonary blood flow
If hypotensive and hypoxic, poor peripheral perfusion, poor renal perfusion, myocardial malfunction
Patent ductus arteriosus contributes

Clinical Signs
Onset near the time of birth
Tachypnea
Increased work of breathing:
    Nasal flaring
    Retractions of respiratory muscles

Expiratory grunt
Cyanosis
Systemic hypotension
Characteristic chest film
Course to death or improvement in 3 to 5 days
Fine inspiratory rales
Hypothermia
Peripheral edema
Pulmonary edema

Pathobiochemistry
Respiratory acidosis
Decreased saturated phospholipids
Low amniotic fluid L/S ratio
Low surfactant-associated proteins
Decreased total serum proteins
Decreased fibrinolysis
Low thyroxine levels

Pathology
Atelectasis
Injury to epithelial cells, edema
Membrane contains fibrin and cellular products
No tubular myelin
Osmiophilic lamellar bodies decreased early, increased later

Prevention
Prenatal glucocorticoids for more than 24 hours
Prevention of asphyxia
Surfactant replacement:
    Prophylactically—within 15 minutes after birth
    Early rescue—within 60 minutes after birth
    Established RDS—within 12 hours after birth
Continuous positive airway pressure
Lower tidal volumes

DPL, Dipalmitoyl lecithin; *FRC,* functional residual capacity; *IUGR,* intrauterine growth restriction; *L/S,* lecithin/sphingomyelin; *PROM,* prolonged rupture of membranes (>16 hours); *RDS,* surfactant deficiency disorder (respiratory distress syndrome).
Data from Jackson JC: Respiratory distress in the preterm infant. In Gleason CA, Devaskar SU, editors: *Avery's disease of the newborn,* ed 9, Philadelphia, 2011, Saunders; Jobe AH: Pathophysiology of respiratory distress syndrome. In Polin RA et al, editors: *Fetal and neonatal physiology,* ed 5, Philadelphia, 2017, Saunders.

manifestations reach a peak within 3 days, after which there is gradual improvement with appropriate treatment.

EVALUATION AND TREATMENT. Diagnosis is made on the basis of clinical manifestations, chest radiographs, and, if needed, analysis of amniotic fluid or tracheal aspirates to estimate lung maturity (lecithin/sphingomyelin ratio [L/S ratio]). The ultimate treatment for SDD (RDS) would be prevention of premature birth. There is extensive evidence that when there is risk of preterm labor, antenatal corticosteroid therapy given between 24 and 34 weeks' gestation reduces the incidence of SDD (RDS) and death. Repeated courses of corticosteroids may be safe in this setting.[64] Glucocorticoids induce a significant and rapid acceleration of lung maturation, particularly type 1 and type 2 pneumocytes, with stimulation of surfactant production and improved lung compliance

and gas exchange in the fetus. There is extensive evidence that maternal steroid therapy significantly reduces the incidence of SDD (RDS), bronchopulmonary dysplasia, central nervous system hemorrhage, and neonatal mortality. Efforts are in progress to determine the long-term effects on infant neurodevelopment with strategies to personalize dosage recommendations.[65] The American Congress of Obstetricians and Gynecologists recommends that administration of betamethasone may be considered in women with a singleton pregnancy between 34 0/7 and 36 6/7 weeks' gestation at imminent risk of preterm birth within 7 days.[66] Efforts are in progress to determine the long-term effects on infant development with personalization of dosage recommendations.[67]

Administration of exogenous surfactant (either synthetic or natural) is recommended as a prophylactic or preventive treatment for infants

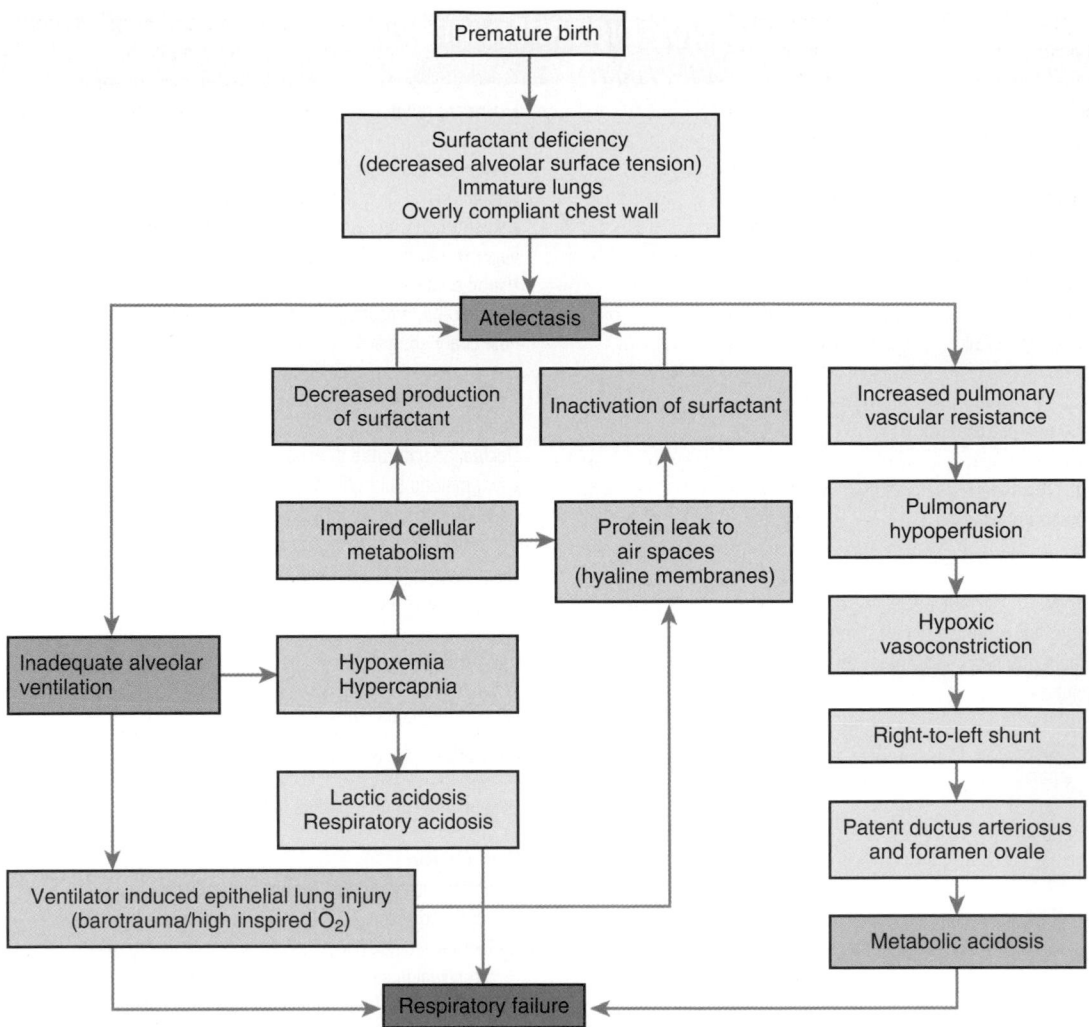

FIGURE 37.12 Pathogenesis of Surfactant Deficiency Disorder (Respiratory Distress Syndrome) of the Newborn.

weighing between 500 and 2000 g with prophylaxis beginning within 15 to 30 minutes of birth through a thin catheter (minimally invasive surfactant administration) or nebulizer or by nasal continuous positive airway pressure (CPAP) ventilation. Rescue surfactant therapy is given only to preterm infants with established SDD (RDS) and is most often administered within the first 12 hours after birth, when specified threshold criteria of severity of SDD (RDS) are met.[68] There is usually a dramatic improvement in oxygenation, as well as a decreased incidence of SDD (RDS) death, pneumothorax, and pulmonary interstitial emphysema. Surfactant therapy also can be considered complementary to antenatal glucocorticoids. The two therapies together appear to have an additive effect on improving lung function. Supplemental inositol also may promote maturation of surfactant and prevent adverse neonatal outcomes.[69]

Supportive care includes oxygen administration and mechanical ventilation. Mechanical ventilation can result in a proinflammatory state that may contribute to the development of chronic lung disease, such as bronchopulmonary dysplasia (BPD). Strategies that are lung protective, such as greater reliance on nasal continuous positive airway pressure (NCPAP) to prevent lung injury, permissive hypercapnia, lower oxygen saturation targets, modulation of tidal volume (V_T) settings, and use of high-frequency oscillation or jet ventilation, are being evaluated.[70,71] Mechanical ventilation with mixtures of oxygen and nitric oxide or helium may improve gas exchange and reduce airflow resistance and have improved outcomes.[72,73]

Most infants survive SDD (RDS) and, in many cases, recovery may be complete within 10 to 14 days. However, the incidence of subsequent chronic lung disease (i.e., bronchopulmonary dysplasia) is significant among very low birth weight infants.[74]

Bronchopulmonary Dysplasia

Bronchopulmonary dysplasia (BPD), also known as *chronic lung disease of prematurity*, is a chronic inflammatory lung disease associated with arrested pulmonary development and a need for supplemental oxygen. It is the major cause of pulmonary disease in infants and is associated with premature birth (usually before 28 weeks' gestation and birth weights less than 1500 g), SDD (RDS), perinatal supplemental oxygen, and positive pressure ventilation. Annually in the United States, approximately 10,000 to 15,000 infants are affected, including about 50% of infants weighing less than 1000 g. Up to 30% of very low and extremely low birth weight infants develop BPD.[75,76] The widespread use of antenatal glucocorticoids, postnatal surfactant, and NCPAP has lessened the incidence and severity of SDD (RDS) and thus also reduced the incidence of BPD. Surprisingly, some of the tiny infants who develop BPD have shown few or no clinical signs of SDD (RDS) at birth or have initially received only low levels of supplemental oxygen or ventilatory support for apnea. The presence of antenatal chorioamnionitis, preeclampsia, inflammation and postnatal sepsis, patent ductus arteriosus, hyperoxia and genetic susceptibility confers additive risk of developing BPD. Numerous biomarkers associated with immunity, inflammation, and oxidative stress also have been identified and are being used to develop risk factors and guidelines for diagnosis and treatment.[77]

BPD is a multisystem condition and is associated with developmental disorders in other systems, such as growth retardation, pulmonary hypertension, neurodevelopmental delays (e.g., cerebral palsy), hearing defects, and retinopathy of prematurity.[78]

◆**PATHOPHYSIOLOGY.** Lung immaturity and inflammation contribute to the development of BPD. In preterm infants born at less than 28 weeks' gestation, the fetal lung is in the *canalicular stage* of development (16 to 28 weeks), a critical period during which type II epithelial cells appear, capillaries grow into the future distal alveolar regions, and the interstitium begins to condense (see Fig. 37.1). Ultimately the alveoli must have a very thin interface between the air space and the capillary for appropriate gas exchange. The extensive network of alveoli develops by septation within the terminal respiratory unit, beginning in the *saccular stage,* starting at approximately 26 to 28 weeks. The alveoli are vulnerable to inflammation and impaired growth during this stage.

Before the widespread use of surfactant therapy, BPD was a disease characterized by airway injury, inflammation, and parenchymal fibrosis *(classic BPD).* Now, after the initiation of surfactant therapy, what is called *new BPD* is most often a form of arrested lung development with poor formation of the alveolar architecture. Alveoli are large and fewer in number, thereby presenting decreased surface area for gas exchange.

There is abnormal vascular endothelial growth factor that results in hypoplastic pulmonary capillary development and mild fibrosis accompanied by persistent inflammation contributing to ventilation-perfusion mismatch, pulmonary hypertension, and lasting pulmonary vascular disease.[79]

Levels of proinflammatory cytokines, such as tumor necrosis factor-alpha (TNF-α), interleukin-1β (IL-1β), interleukin 6 (IL-6), and interleukin 8 (IL-8), are all elevated in the amniotic fluid or tracheal aspirates, or both, of preterm infants who later develop BPD. Inflammation invites neutrophils and macrophages to release reactive oxygen species and proteolytic enzymes, initiating oxidative and immune injury. The predominant mediators of *new BPD* are profibrotic and angiogenic cytokines, which contribute to pulmonary hypertension.[80] Fig. 37.13 illustrates the pathophysiology of BPD.

◆**CLINICAL MANIFESTATIONS.** The clinical definition of BPD includes the need for supplemental oxygen at 36 weeks' postmenstrual age, which is also known as *gestational age* (the time elapsed between the first day of the last normal menstrual period and the day of birth) and for at least 28 days after birth. It also details graded severity dependent on required respiratory support at term (divided into mild, moderate, and severe based on oxygen requirements and ventilatory needs). Clinically, the infant exhibits hypoxemia caused by ventilation-perfusion mismatch and diffusion defects. Work of breathing is elevated, resulting in hypercapnia. The ability to feed may be impaired. Intermittent bronchospasm with wheezing, mucus plugging, and pulmonary hypertension characterizes the clinical course of the most severely affected babies. Of the most severely affected infants, dusky spells may occur with agitation, feeding, or gastroesophageal reflux. Infants with mild BPD may

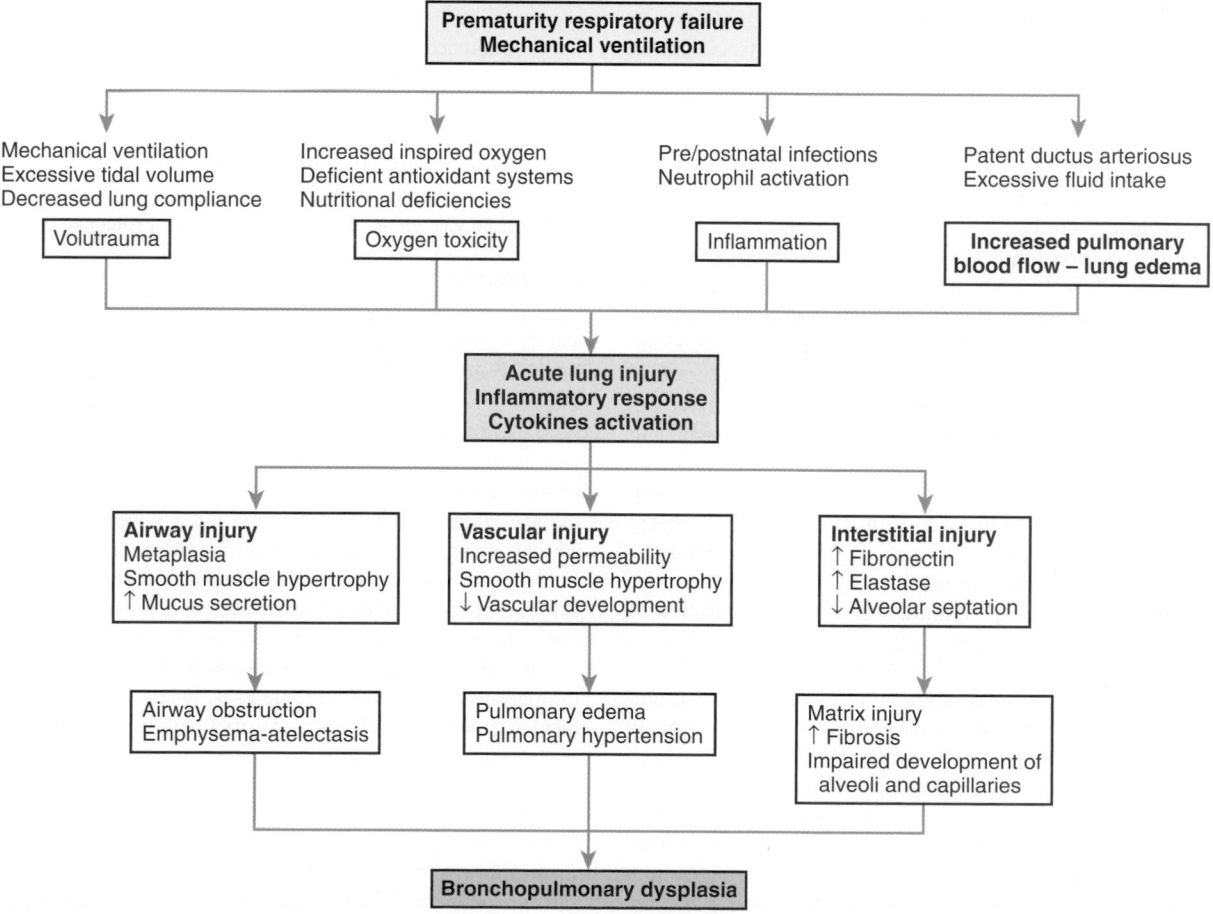

FIGURE 37.13 Pathophysiology of Bronchopulmonary Dysplasia (BPD).

demonstrate only mild tachypnea and difficulty handling respiratory tract infections.

◆**EVALUATION AND TREATMENT.** Infants with severe BPD require prolonged, assisted ventilation. Prevention of lung damage with non-invasive respiratory support (see Evaluation and Treatment section under Surfactant Deficiency Disorder [Respiratory Distress Syndrome of the Newborn]) or early nasal intermittent CPAP, or both, is used in clinical situations when permitted. When compared to mechanical ventilation, use of CPAP has resulted in fewer days of oxygen and ventilator requirement by reducing the amount of lung injury. Additionally, oxygen supplementation at lower than previously accepted values (89% to 94% saturations) is a means to reduce oxidant injury to the lungs and retinal vasculature. Diuretics are used to control pulmonary edema. Bronchodilators reduce airway resistance. Inhaled corticosteroids improve the rate of extubation and reduce the time that mechanical ventilation is required. Prophylactic caffeine citrate is used to prevent apnea and for neuroprotection. Supplementation with vitamin A provides antioxidant protection and stimulates lung growth and surfactant production.[81] New treatments are under consideration.[82] Careful nutritional and fluid and electrolyte support is routinely used and has resulted in improved outcomes.

Respiratory Tract Infections

Respiratory tract infections are common in children and are a frequent cause for emergency department visits and hospitalizations. Clinical presentation, age of the child, season of the year, and environmental exposures can often provide clues to the etiologic agent, even when the agent cannot be proven.

Bronchiolitis

Bronchiolitis is a common, viral-induced respiratory tract infection of the small airways that occurs almost exclusively in infants and young toddlers. There are distinct regional differences in the United States depending on geographic variation in the viral season. The most commonly associated pathogen is respiratory syncytial virus (RSV), but bronchiolitis also may be associated with rhinovirus (older children), adenovirus, influenza, parainfluenza virus (PIV), human metapneumovirus, and bocavirus. There are distinct regional differences in the United States depending on variation in the viral season based on geography. Healthy infants usually make a full recovery from RSV bronchiolitis, but infants who are premature (birth weight <2500 g) or who have underlying BPD, heart disease, or immune deficiency may have a much more severe or even deadly course. Their respiratory systems are immature, and maternal immunoglobulins do not protect against RSV infection.[83] Bronchiolitis has been linked to an increased risk for asthma later in childhood, particularly in those with a family history of asthma.[84]

◆**PATHOPHYSIOLOGY.** Viral infection causes inflammation and necrosis of the bronchial epithelium with destruction of ciliated epithelial cells. There is infiltration with lymphocytes around the bronchioles and a cell-mediated hypersensitivity to viral antigens with release of lymphokines causing inflammation, as well as activation of eosinophils, neutrophils, and monocytes. The submucosa becomes edematous, and cellular debris and fibrin form plugs within the bronchioles. Edema of the bronchiolar wall, accumulation of mucus and cellular debris, and possibly bronchospasm narrow or occlude many peripheral airways. Airway obstruction leads to atelectasis and uneven ventilation leads to ventilation-perfusion mismatch and hypoxemia. Airway narrowing causes obstruction of airflow that is worse with expiration. This leads to air trapping, hyperinflation, and an increase in FRC. Airway resistance and hyperinflation result in decreased lung compliance and increased work of breathing and may cause hypercapnia in severe cases.

◆**CLINICAL MANIFESTATIONS.** Symptoms usually begin with significant rhinorrhea followed by a tight, dry cough over the next several days, along with systemic signs of decreased appetite, lethargy, and fever. Infants may have tachypnea, expiratory wheezing, cough, rhinorrhea, mild fever, varying degrees of respiratory distress, and abnormal auscultatory findings of the chest. Wheezing is most common, but rales or rhonchi also may be present. Chest radiographs often show hyperexpanded lungs, patchy or peribronchial infiltrates, and atelectasis of the right upper lobe. With overexpansion of the lungs, the diaphragm is flattened, causing downward displacement of the liver and spleen. Abdominal distention results from air swallowing. Very young infants may present with severe apnea before lower respiratory tract symptoms appear, and these apneas frequently require mechanical ventilation.[83] Many children also may present with conjunctivitis or otitis media.

◆**EVALUATION AND TREATMENT.** Guidelines from the American Academy of Pediatrics are available for the evaluation, treatment, and prevention of bronchiolitis.[85] Diagnosis of bronchiolitis is made by review of history, signs, and symptoms (e.g., rhinitis, cough, wheezing, crackles, chest retractions and/or hyperinflation, tachypnea). Laboratory studies and radiologic or ultrasound examination are not routinely performed. Nasal washings/swabbings may be tested for specific viral agents, such as RSV. RSV swabs are positive in 70% of cases of bronchiolitis.

Treatment is determined by the severity of the disease and the age of the child. Most cases are mild and require no specific treatment, and affected children may be monitored as outpatients with supportive care. In more severe cases, supplemental oxygen with high-flow nasal cannula and increased hydration are commonly used. Nebulized 3% hypertonic saline has shown heterogenous outcomes. Continuous positive airway pressure (CPAP) increases positive end-expiratory pressure (PEEP) and warm humidified oxygen helps to overcome airway resistance.[86] Preventive treatment or prophylaxis with RSV-specific options includes immunotherapy with palivizumab an RSV-specific recombinant monoclonal antibody, although it is costly.[87] Other preventive measures include use of handwashing and alcohol-based decontamination, prevention of exposure to tobacco smoke, and promotion of infant breast-feeding. No licensed vaccine is currently available to protect against RSV.

Pneumonia

Pneumonia is infection and inflammation in the terminal airways and alveoli. Community-acquired pneumonia (CAP) is a major cause of morbidity and mortality in children, particularly in developing countries. The incidence of viral and bacterial pneumonia varies according to age, time of year, and geographic location. The most common agents are viruses, followed by bacteria and atypical microorganisms (e.g., mycoplasma); clinical symptoms often do not differentiate viral from bacterial or atypical pneumonia. Risk factors for developing CAP include age younger than 2 years, overcrowded living conditions, winter season, recent antibiotic treatment, attendance at daycare centers, and passive smoke exposure. Nutritional status, age, and underlying disease process influence morbidity and mortality related to CAP.

◆**PATHOPHYSIOLOGY AND CLINICAL MANIFESTATIONS.** Viral pneumonia is two to three times more likely in children than in adults, and incidence generally follows a seasonal pattern. Bacterial coinfections are common. The most common cause in infants and young children is respiratory syncytial virus (RSV). A number of other viruses are important, including parainfluenza, influenza, human rhinovirus, human metapneumovirus, adenoviruses, and *Mycoplasma pneumoniae*.[88] Acquisition of viruses is by direct contact, droplet transmission, or aerosol exposure. There is initial destruction of the ciliated epithelium of the distal airway with sloughing of cellular material. A mononuclear-predominant inflammatory response initially occurs in the interstitium and may later involve the alveoli. It is often difficult to determine whether the pneumonia is viral or bacterial early in the course of the disease. The clinical presentation of viral pneumonia often consists of cough and no fever, and the white blood count is often normal. In bacterial pneumonia, the degree of elevated temperature, absolute neutrophil counts, and percent of bands are consistently higher than in those cases of viral etiology.[89] Diagnosis of a viral etiology requires laboratory confirmation (immunofluorescence tests). Antiviral therapy may prevent development of influenza-associated CAP. Development of safe agents to treat and prevent viral pneumonias continues to be a priority, as is development of more effective vaccines.[90]

Bacterial pneumonia beyond the neonatal period is most commonly the result of infection with *Streptococcus pneumoniae*. It is the predominant bacteria isolated from bacterial CAP in children. Other causative microorganisms include *S. aureus* and atypical bacteria (e.g., *Mycoplasma pneumoniae*, *Chlamydia pneumoniae*) (Table 37.2). Childhood immunization with polyvariant pneumococcal conjugate vaccine is recommended to decrease the incidence of pneumococcal pneumonia in children younger than 2 years of age. *Haemophilus influenzae* pneumonia has become rare because of widespread immunization.[91]

Bacterial pneumonia usually begins with aspiration of one's own nasopharyngeal bacteria. A preceding viral infection sometimes sets the stage for bacterial infection by causing a damaged epithelium, reduced mucociliary clearance in the trachea and major bronchi, and a reduced immune response.[92] Once in the alveolar region, bacteria encounter local host defenses, such as antibodies, complement, phagocytes, and cytokines, that prepare bacteria for ingestion by alveolar macrophages.

Alveolar macrophages recognize bacteria with their surface receptors and phagocytose them. If these mechanisms fail, macrophages will release numerous inflammatory cytokines, neutrophils will be recruited, and an intense cytokine-mediated inflammation will ensue. Vascular engorgement, edema, and a fibrinopurulent exudate with tissue damage occur. Alveolar filling precludes gas exchange and, if extensive, can lead to respiratory failure. If sepsis occurs at the same time, shock and end-organ hypoperfusion will cause metabolic acidosis. Staphylococcal and group A streptococcal pneumonia can be particularly fulminant and necrotizing, with a high incidence of accompanying empyema, pneumatoceles, and sepsis. Empyema is associated with pneumococcal infections and antibiotic-resistant microorganisms.[93]

The clinical presentation of bacterial pneumonia, particularly pneumococcal, may include a preceding viral illness followed by fever with chills and rigors, shortness of breath, and an increasingly productive cough. Occasionally there is blood streaking of the sputum. Respiratory rate and oxygen saturation are important clinical indicators. Auscultation usually reveals such abnormalities as crackles or decreased breath sounds. Other less specific findings may include malaise, emesis, abdominal pain, and chest pain. Chest films will usually present with a lobar pattern in older children and adolescents but may appear patchier with a bronchopneumonic pattern in younger children.

Atypical pneumonia (*Mycoplasma pneumoniae*, *Chlamydophila pneumoniae*) is the most common cause of CAP for school-age children and young adults. *Chlamydophila pneumoniae* is clinically indistinguishable from and is typically grouped with *Mycoplasma* as "atypical pneumonia." Transmission is from person-to-person with a 2- to 3-week incubation period.

TABLE 37.2 COMMON TYPES OF PNEUMONIA IN CHILDREN

TYPE	CAUSAL AGENT	AGE	ONSET	SIGNS/SYMPTOMS	PATHOPHYSIOLOGY
Viral pneumonia	Respiratory syncytial virus (RSV), influenza (A and B), adenovirus, parainfluenza, human metapneumovirus (hMPV)	Infants for RSV All ages for others	Acute or gradual, winter and early spring	Mild to high fever, cough, rhinorrhea, malaise, rales, rhonchi, or wheezing; variable radiographic pattern	Edema, increased mucus, and interstitial pneumonia
Pneumococcal pneumonia	Pneumococci (*Streptococcus pneumoniae*)	1–4 yr	Acute, follows an upper respiratory tract infection, winter and early spring	High fever, productive cough, pleuritic pain, increased respiratory rate, decreased breath sounds in area of consolidation; lobar pattern or "round pneumonia" on radiograph	Inflammation of bronchial mucosa, alveolar exudate. *Early:* red hepatization with WBCs, RBCs, and fibrin consolidation. *Late:* gray hepatization with fibrin and neutrophils in alveoli. *Resolution:* many phagocytic macrophages
Staphylococcal pneumonia	*Staphylococcus aureus* Methicillin-resistant *S. aureus* (MRSA)	1 wk–2 yr	Acute, winter months	High fever, cough, respiratory distress, toxic appearance, sepsis, empyema, pneumatoceles are common; multilobar consolidation	Necrotizing patterns may occur in severe cases
Streptococcal pneumonia	Group A streptococci	All ages	Acute, any season	High fever, chills, respiratory distress, sepsis or shock; empyema, pneumatoceles	Tracheobronchitis, interstitial pneumonia with ulcers, exudate edema, and localized hemorrhage
Mycoplasma and *Chlamydophila* pneumonia	*M. pneumoniae* *C. pneumoniae*	School age and adolescents	Gradual	Low-grade fever; cough	Inflammation of bronchi with lymphocyte and chlamydia neutrophil recruitment

RBCs, Red blood cells; *WBCs,* white blood cells.

Mycoplasma is known to cause a wide spectrum of disease and has more extensive complications than previously recognized. Studies reveal that macrolide-resistant *Mycoplasma pneumoniae* is seen increasingly in infants and younger children.[94] Children experiencing recurrent respiratory tract infections often have been found to be infected with atypical bacteria.

Mycoplasma microorganisms lack cell walls but have a limiting membrane and a specialized tip for attaching to ciliated respiratory epithelial cells. Local sloughing of cells occurs. Peribronchial lymphocytic infiltration develops, along with neutrophil recruitment to the airway lumen. The pattern resembles bronchitis or bronchopneumonia.

Onset of symptoms is usually gradual, resembling a typical upper respiratory tract infection with low-grade fever and prominent cough. There may be accompanying wheezing, sore throat, myalgia, and headache. Cases are not usually clinically severe, and full recovery should be expected without complications. When complications do occur, they can include bronchopneumonia, parapneumonic effusions, and necrotizing pneumonitis.[93]

◆**EVALUATION AND TREATMENT.** Guidelines have been developed to improve and aid assessment and management of pediatric pneumonia.[95] Diagnosis of pneumonia is based on clinical and laboratory findings. The etiologic agent can sometimes be inferred from the age of the child and clinical scenario. Chest x-ray in bacterial pneumonia initially shows an alveolar infiltrate and later reveals a segmental or lobar disease. A viral infection is more likely to be associated with an interstitial pattern. Identifying etiologic pathogens can be very difficult in children, especially because there is often overlap between bacterial and viral pathogens. Biomarkers facilitate more rapid diagnosis, and procalcitonin is most specific to bacterial infection and can guide antibiotic therapy. The highly sensitive C-reactive protein (hs-CRP) is less specific and its level is elevated in both viral and bacterial infections.[96] Other laboratory tests that may be helpful include a white cell–granulocyte count or erythrocyte sedimentation rate (ESR) but do not indicate a specific etiology. Several microbiologic tests are available, such as polymerase chain reaction (PCR) and nucleic acid amplification tests (NAATs).

Some pneumonias may be treated on an outpatient basis; however, some children require oxygen supplementation and, occasionally, assisted ventilation. This is particularly true with infants who have a viral interstitial pneumonia like that caused by RSV. In addition, adequate hydration, nutrition, and supportive pulmonary therapy are required to reduce the duration and severity of illness. Many infants are markedly tachypneic and unable to coordinate their breathing with swallowing such that they may require enteral feeding. Aspiration is always a risk with infants in respiratory distress.

Appropriate antibiotic administration for bacterial pneumonias is dependent on age and severity assessment. Local patterns of drug resistance must be considered when choosing appropriate antibiotics. Pneumococcal and mycoplasmal pneumonias present some unique treatment obstacles and may need a multifaceted approach to care, including vaccine antigens and immunoadjuvant therapies.[97] Treatment of *Mycoplasma pneumoniae* with antibiotics is controversial.[98] Children should be vaccinated against influenza and pneumococcus.

Aspiration Pneumonitis

Aspiration pneumonitis is caused by a foreign substance, such as meconium, food, secretions (saliva or gastric secretions), or environmental compounds entering the lung and causing inflammation of lung tissue. The aspiration of meconium from amniotic fluid can occur at birth. Meconium contains bile salts and other constituents from the fetal intestinal tract that cause inflammation.[99] Neurologically compromised children or children with chronic lung disease may have chronic pulmonary aspiration (CPA), which can cause progressive lung

disease, bronchiectasis, and respiratory failure. This is the leading cause of death in children who are neurologically compromised because of failure of protective reflexes and difficulty swallowing.[100,101] Children undergoing sedation or administration of an anesthetic also may aspirate oral secretions contaminated with anaerobic bacteria or stomach contents.

The severity of lung injury after an aspiration incident is determined by the volume of material aspirated, the pH of the aspirated material, and the presence of pathogenic bacteria. Very low pH or very high pH causes a significant inflammatory response. With hydrocarbon ingestions, lung injury is determined by the volatility and viscosity of the aspirated substance. A low-viscosity substance, such as gasoline or lighter fluid, is the most toxic; high-viscosity hydrocarbons, such as petroleum jelly or mineral oil, are much less likely to cause a pneumonitis. Treatment for aspiration pneumonitis depends on the material aspirated but generally can include broad-spectrum antibiotics with failure to improve after 48 hours. Children with CPA and a large amount of upper respiratory tract secretions may benefit from salivary gland injection with botulinum toxin A (BTX-A) to suppress secretion.[102]

Bronchiolitis Obliterans

Bronchiolitis obliterans (BO) is fibrotic obstruction of the respiratory bronchioles and alveolar ducts secondary to intense inflammation. It is relatively rare in children. Two types are noted in the literature— proliferative and constrictive (obstructive)—with the latter being the more common form. BO most often occurs as a sequela of a severe viral pulmonary infection (e.g., adenovirus [most common], influenza, pertussis [whooping cough], or measles). Other cases may be secondary to parainfluenza, RSV, human immunodeficiency virus (HIV), or *M. pneumoniae* infection. It may occur after allograft transplantation (lung, heart-lung, and bone marrow) as a manifestation of graft-vs.-host disease. BO also is associated with collagen vascular disease, toxic fume inhalation, chronic hypersensitivity pneumonitis, Crohn disease, and Stevens-Johnson syndrome.[103,104] Cough, respiratory distress, and cyanosis initially occur, followed by a brief period of improvement. The progression of disease is then reflected by increasing tachypnea, sputum production, crackles, wheezing, increased anterior/posterior diameter, and hypoxemia.

There is no specific treatment for BO and, because it is so rare, there have been no randomized clinical trials. Therapeutic options include inhaled corticosteroids, bronchodilators, antibiotics (long-term azithromycin), and oxygen supplementation. Mechanical ventilation may contribute to the progression of the disease. Use of antiviral agents may be warranted in managing those with viral infection. For transplant recipients, augmentation of immunosuppressive therapies without increasing risk for infection and treatment with antiinflammatory agents are showing promise in reducing airway inflammation, thus improving pulmonary function.[105] Clinical progression can be quite variable depending on the predisposing condition. Some children experience partial recovery, whereas others follow a course of steady decline in lung function. Lung transplantation may be considered.[106]

Asthma

Asthma is a chronic inflammatory disease characterized by bronchial hyperreactivity and reversible airflow obstruction, usually in response to an allergen. It is the most prevalent chronic disease in childhood, affecting about 8.4% of U.S. children between birth and 17 years of age, and prevalence is increasing. Populations most affected include black and Puerto Rican children and those below 100% of poverty status.[107]

Childhood asthma and its severity result from a complex interaction between *genetic* susceptibility and *environmental* factors. Genetic studies have led to the identification of many candidate genes or chromosomal regions that are associated with asthma.[108] Included in the long list of asthma-associated genes are those that code for increased levels of immune and inflammatory mediators (e.g., IL-4, IL-5, IL-6, IL-13, IgE, and leukotrienes), adrenergic receptors, nitric oxide, and transmembrane proteins in the endoplasmic reticulum.[109] Various genotypes are associated with multiple phenotypes of asthma, including early-onset mild allergic asthma, asthma with severe exacerbations, later-onset asthma associated with obesity, atopic or nonatopic asthma, eosinophilic or noneosinophilic asthma, asthma associated with aspirin sensitivity or insensitivity, and asthma dependent or resistant to corticosteroids. Linking specific genes to specific asthma phenotypes is leading to targeted therapies and personalized approaches to asthma treatment[110] (see *What's New?* Asthma Phenotypes and Endotypes in Children).

Important environmental risk factors include early exposure to allergens (e.g., air pollution, dust mites, molds, cockroach antigen, and tobacco smoke), respiratory tract infections, gastroesophageal reflux, preterm birth, and childhood obesity. Additional confounding variables that affect disparity in asthma morbidity and therapy are social stress in the home (e.g., violence and depressed housing conditions), lack of health insurance, poor access to asthma specialists, inappropriate utilization of healthcare resources, and inadequate medical care.[111,112] Vitamin D insufficiency may be a risk factor for wheezing in children because vitamin D suppresses Th2-mediated allergic disease, suppresses inflammatory Th17 cells, inhibits IgE expression in B cells, is important for lung development, and suppresses infection.[113] Epigenetic mechanisms of asthma pathogenesis are being evaluated[114] (see *What's New?* Environmental Air Pollution and Childhood Respiratory Disease). Individual risk factors may overlap and vary in strength of association.[115] The *hygiene hypothesis* proposes that infants and children who are exposed to a highly hygienic environment, who receive vaccinations to prevent certain infections, or who are treated with antibiotics lack adequate exposure to common pathogens and therefore do not achieve balanced immune responses as they mature.[116] Consequently, this increases their risk for Th2-predominant allergic disease.[117] Early exposure to microbial products also may promote a microbiome that promotes Th1 immunity necessary to balance Th2 immune responses.[118]

PATHOPHYSIOLOGY. The pathophysiology of asthma in children is similar to that for adults and is described in Chapter 36; see Asthma under Obstructive Pulmonary Disease). Early-onset allergic asthma is initiated by a type I hypersensitivity reaction primarily mediated by Th2 lymphocytes whose cytokines activate mast cells and eosinophils, increase leukocyte synthesis, and enhance B-cell IgE production (see Figs. 36.10, 36.11, and 36.12). As in adults, inflammation, bronchospasm, and mucus production in the airways lead both to ventilation-perfusion mismatch with hypoxemia and to expiratory airway obstruction with air trapping and increased work of breathing. In young children, airway obstruction can be more severe because of the smaller diameter of their airways.

CLINICAL MANIFESTATIONS. Clinical manifestations of an acute asthma attack include coughing, wheezing, and shortness of breath. Expiratory wheezing is often described as high pitched and musical, along with prolongation of the expiratory phase of the respiratory cycle. Breath sounds may become faint when air movement is poor. The child may speak in clipped sentences or not at all because of dyspnea. Respiratory and heart rates are elevated. Nasal flaring and accessory muscle use are evident, with retractions in the substernal, subcostal, intercostal, suprasternal, or sternocleidomastoid areas. Infants may appear to be "head bobbing" because of sternocleidomastoid muscle use. Pulsus paradoxus (decrease in systolic blood pressure of more than 10 mmHg during inspiration) may be present. The child may appear anxious or diaphoretic, important signs of respiratory compromise. About 70% to 80% of acute wheezing episodes are associated with viral respiratory tract infections.[119] As a result, there may be signs of a preceding upper respiratory tract infection, such as rhinorrhea or low-grade fever. The most common of these is RSV in infants and toddlers younger than 2 years of age and rhinovirus in older children.

Findings in chronic asthma may include hyperinflation of the thorax (barrel chest) or pectus excavatum. Clubbing should not be seen in those with asthma and, if present, should trigger evaluation for other conditions, such as cystic fibrosis. Exercise intolerance may indicate underlying asthma.

EVALUATION AND TREATMENT. Currently, asthma cannot be prevented or cured, but it can be controlled. Asthma is often underdiagnosed and untreated, especially in preschool-age children because asthma symptoms overlap with other respiratory illness, such as bronchitis or upper respiratory tract infections. Diagnosis is based on episodes of wheezing, as well as a variety of risk factors including parental history of asthma, atopic dermatitis, sensitization to aeroallergens or foods, blood eosinophilia, increased IgE levels, or wheezing not associated with upper respiratory tract illnesses. The Modified Asthma Predictive Index (mAPI) can be used to help with asthma diagnosis and is

WHAT'S NEW?

Asthma Phenotypes and Endotypes in Children

The severity and clinical course of asthma in children can vary from mild and transient to severe and lifelong. Research is emerging that suggests genetically influenced differences in inflammatory and immune mechanisms may explain much of this variability. A phenotype is the observable characteristics (i.e., clinical manifestation, cell types, treatment response) of a disease without a link to a specific underlying pathology or pathophysiologic mechanism. Phenotypic heterogeneity in asthma includes the severity of airway obstruction, type of airway immune cells and inflammation, presence of airway remodeling, and response to medication. Inflammatory phenotypes include eosinophilic and neutrophilic asthma. The majority of asthmatic children have the well-described allergic (type I hypersensitivity) phenotype of asthma that is characterized by the presence of high levels of T helper2 (Th2) cytokines (interleukin [IL]-4, IL-5, and IL-13), synthesis of immunoglobulin E (IgE), and activation of eosinophils (therefore also called *eosinophilic asthma*), resulting in episodic bronchospasm that is responsive to inhaled bronchodilators and antiinflammatory medications, including corticosteroids. Children whose asthma phenotype is characterized by more severe symptoms and relative unresponsiveness to treatment with inhaled corticosteroids most often have *neutrophilic asthma*, or nonatopic asthma, in which the presence of Th1 cytokines and activation of large numbers of neutrophils appear to dominate lung injury. Neutrophilic asthma especially involves the cytokines tumor necrosis factor-alpha (TNF-α), interferon-gamma (IFN-γ), leukotriene B4 (LTB4), IL-17a, IL-6, and IL-8, and is corticosteroid resistant. *Endotypes* are subgroups that share an underlying disease pathobiology and explain the characteristic of the phenotype. At the molecular level, endotypes describe gene profiles of the airways that affect the development of airway remodeling and the response to treatment. For example, variation in candidate genes is associated with variability of response to leukotriene modifiers, glucocorticoids, inhaled corticosteroids, β2-adrenergic receptor agonists and anticholinergics, theophylline, mast cell stabilizers, and monoclonal antibodies to immunoglobulin E. Increased understanding of different asthma phenotypes and underlying endotypes is leading to drugs that target specific molecules and pathways that may provide significant improvements in personalized management of severe and drug-resistant asthma.

Data from Bostantzoglou C et al: *Breathe (Sheff)* 11(3):186–193, 2015; Desai M, Oppenheimer J: *Ann Allergy Asthma Immunol* 116(5):394–401, 2016; Landgraf-Rauf K, Anselm B, Schaub B: *Mol Cell Pediatr* 3(1):27, 2016; Panettieri RA Jr: *Immunol Allergy Clin North Am* 36(3):569–579, 2016.

recommended by the National Institutes of Health (NIH) guidelines.[120] Confirmation of the diagnosis of asthma relies on pulmonary function testing using spirometry, which can be accomplished only after the child is 5 to 6 years of age. Characteristic abnormalities of spirometry testing would be reduced expiratory flow rates that are reversible in response to an inhaled bronchodilator. For younger children, an empirical trial of asthma medications is commonly initiated. Many children with less severe asthma outgrow the disease by adulthood and may reflect a particular genetic phenotype of asthma.[121]

The goal of asthma therapy is to achieve long-term control by reduction in impairment and risk. Child and family education and appropriate allergen avoidance techniques should begin immediately. Care providers must periodically assess asthma control in children. Key features for assessment include nighttime awakenings, interference with normal activities, use of short-acting beta$_2$ agonists, pulmonary function testing, and exacerbations requiring corticosteroids. Peak flowmeters are often used to help guide treatment. Before therapy is augmented, care providers need to assess medication administration techniques, environmental controls, and comorbidities. Stepwise reduction in therapy can begin after the child's asthma has been well controlled for a minimum of 3 months.[120]

The pharmacologic treatment of asthma in children is essentially the same as that for adults and is initiated in a stepwise sequence based on asthma severity and response to treatment (see Chapter 36). Management of asthma medications in children is often difficult because there is commonly fluctuation in severity of symptoms.

Acute Lung Injury/Acute Respiratory Distress Syndrome

Acute respiratory distress syndrome (ARDS) occurs in children of all ages and is a dramatic, life-threatening condition resulting from a direct acute lung injury (ALI), such as pneumonia, aspiration, near drowning, or smoke inhalation; or from a systemic insult, such as sepsis or multiple trauma. ALI activates an inflammatory response that causes alveolocapillary injury and results in ARDS. ARDS accounts for approximately 10% of total admissions to pediatric intensive care units. Mortality in pediatric ARDS varies from 18% to 35%.[122]

PATHOPHYSIOLOGY. The pathophysiology of ARDS in children is the same as that described for adults in Chapter 36 (see Acute Lung Injury/Acute Respiratory Distress Syndrome in Chapter 36 and also see Fig. 36.8).

CLINICAL MANIFESTATIONS. The Pediatric Acute Lung Injury Consensus Conference[123] has developed a definition for pediatric ARDS (pARDS) that has some different elements than the definition for adults:

1. All pediatric age groups are affected from the neonatal period through adolescence. Perinatal causes of acute hypoxemia are excluded (i.e., lung disease related to prematurity, perinatal lung injury [meconium aspiration syndrome, pneumonia, and sepsis acquired during delivery], and congenital abnormalities [congenital diaphragmatic hernia or alveolar capillary dysplasia]).
2. Onset of hypoxemia and radiologic changes occur within 7 days after a known clinical insult.
3. Chest radiographs show new infiltrates (either unilateral or bilateral) consistent with parenchymal lung disease.
4. Children with left ventricular dysfunction presenting with acute-onset hypoxemia and new changes on chest radiographs not explained by left ventricular failure or fluid overload and who meet all other pARDS criteria are included in the definition.
5. The degree of hypoxemia used to define the severity of pARDS uses the oxygenation index (OI) (OI = mean airway pressure [M_{PAW}] × Fio_2/Pao_2) rather than the Pao_2/Fio_2 ratio (recommended in the Berlin consensus for adults). In the event that the Pao_2

is unavailable, the oxygen saturation index (OSI = MAP × $Fio_2/Sato_2$) can be used under the same conditions proposed for the OI.

Initially, hyperventilation occurs but CO_2 retention may ultimately develop because of inadequate functional air space, atelectasis, decreased pulmonary compliance, and respiratory muscle fatigue. The severity of the overall picture is modified by comorbid factors, such as the presence of sepsis or multisystem organ failure, and the development of complications, such as nosocomial pneumonia. More research is needed regarding the long-term outcomes of pediatric ARDS.[122]

EVALUATION AND TREATMENT. ARDS in older children and adolescents is similar to that in adults. However, infants have more compliant chest walls, lower hematocrit levels, higher baseline airway resistance, and lower functional residual capacity. The maturing lung may be at greater risk for ventilator-induced lung injury.[124] These factors have implications for management strategies that are different than those for older children and adolescents. Few randomized controlled trials have been completed to guide the clinical management of ALI/ARDS in infants and very young children.

Treatment of ARDS remains supportive in nature, including maintenance of fluid balance and nutrition. The goals of therapy are to maintain adequate tissue oxygenation, minimize acute lung injury, and avoid iatrogenic pulmonary complications. Most children with ARDS require mechanical ventilation and relatively high levels of positive end-expiratory pressure (PEEP) to promote alveolar ventilation and stabilization, and redistribution of alveolar edema fluid into the interstitium. Lung-protective ventilation strategies may include low tidal volumes, permissive hypercapnia, permissive hypoxemia to prevent oxygen toxicity, and airway pressure release ventilation. Use of corticosteroids in children with ARDS is controversial. One study reported fewer ventilator-free days and longer duration of ventilation in survivors.[125] Extracorporeal membrane oxygenation (ECMO) is used for reversible causes of pediatric ARDS and considers quality of life.[126]

Cystic Fibrosis

Cystic fibrosis (CF) is an autosomal recessive inherited disease that results from defective epithelial chloride ion transport. The CF gene is located on chromosome 7. More than 2000 different variants of this gene are known to produce CF.[127] They are divided into six classes with varying severity of disease expression. Classes 1 through 3 are associated with more severe disease and classes 4 through 6 with milder pulmonary disease (generally pancreatic sufficient). Mortality correlates respectively with the aforementioned classes, and therapy is currently being directed at specific gene classes.[128]

The incidence varies by race and is higher in whites.[129] Approximately 28,680 individuals in the United States and 70,000 worldwide manifest the disease. In the United States approximately 853 new cases of CF were diagnosed in 2015; the median age at diagnosis was 4 months and more than half of the CF population was age 18 years or older. The median predicted age at death was 30.1 years.[129,130]

PATHOPHYSIOLOGY. CF is a multiorgan disease that affects the airways, digestive tract, and reproductive organs (see Table 43.1). The *cystic fibrosis transmembrane conductance regulator (CFTCR) gene* mutation results in the abnormal expression of cystic fibrosis transmembrane conductance regulator (CFTCR) protein. There are many *CFTR* variants and they are grouped into six classes. The most common mutation is called *F508delCFTR*. The CFTCR protein is an activated chloride channel present on the surface of many types of epithelial cells, including those lining airways, bile ducts, the pancreas, sweat ducts, paranasal sinuses, and the vas deferens. The most important effects are on the lungs, and respiratory failure is almost always the cause of death. The typical features of CF lung disease are mucus plugging, chronic inflammation, and chronic infection of the small airways. The mucus plugging results from increased production of mucus from increased numbers and size of goblet cells, altered physicochemical properties of the mucus, and impaired mucociliary clearance. CF mucus is dehydrated and viscous because of defective chloride secretion and excess sodium absorption. The periciliary fluid layer is depleted in volume, impairing the mobility of the cilia and, thereby, allowing mucus to adhere to the airway epithelium along with bacteria and injurious byproducts from neutrophils. Neutrophils are present in great excess in the airways and release damaging oxidants and proteases (e.g., elastase) that cause direct damage to lung structural proteins, resulting in remodeling of the airway and, ultimately, development of bronchiectasis. Neutrophils promote inflammation and induce airway cells to produce interleukin-8 (IL-8), which attracts more neutrophils and stimulates mucus secretion, and destroys immunoglobulin G (IgG) and complement components important for opsonization and phagocytosis of pathogens.[131] Bacteria then form biofilms promoting chronic endobronchial infection. Progressive bronchiectasis becomes widespread. Parenchymal involvement occurs much later and includes microabscess formation, patchy consolidation and pneumonia, peribronchial fibrosis, and cyst formation (Fig. 37.14). The pathophysiology for these changes is outlined in Fig. 37.15. Airway obstruction and weakening of the airway wall can lead to the development of peripheral bullae, which may rupture and cause pneumothorax. Hemoptysis, sometimes life-threatening, may occur because of erosion of enlarged bronchial arteries that develop in response

to the inflammation associated with bronchiectasis. Over a long period of time, pulmonary vascular remodeling occurs because of localized hypoxia and arteriolar vasoconstriction; pulmonary hypertension and cor pulmonale may develop with end-stage disease.

◆CLINICAL MANIFESTATIONS. The most common manifestations involve the respiratory and gastrointestinal systems (see Chapter 43). Respiratory symptoms include persistent cough or wheeze, excessive sputum production, and recurrent or severe pneumonia. More subtle respiratory tract presentations of CF include chronic sinusitis and nasal polyps. Digital clubbing may appear quite early even in the absence of significant pulmonary impairment. Development of barrel chest or persistent crackles occurs much later in the course of the disease.

The overall severity of CF lung disease is highly variable. Even affected siblings may have disparate courses and different clinical phenotypes despite identical *CFTR* mutations, environment, and treatment strategy. The *CFTR* genotype is expressed differently in epithelial cells of different organs (airways, sinuses, gastrointestinal [GI] tract, pancreas, biliary system, sweat glands, and genitourinary system), and results in phenotypic variation in clinical manifestations with influences on disease progression and survival.[132]

◆EVALUATION AND TREATMENT. According to the Cystic Fibrosis Foundation, guidelines for the diagnosis of CF include one or more clinical features, history of CF in a sibling, or a positive newborn screen plus laboratory evidence of an abnormality in the *CFTR* gene or protein. The standard laboratory methods of diagnosis (screening) are the immunoreactive trypsinogen (IRT) blood test and the sweat chloride

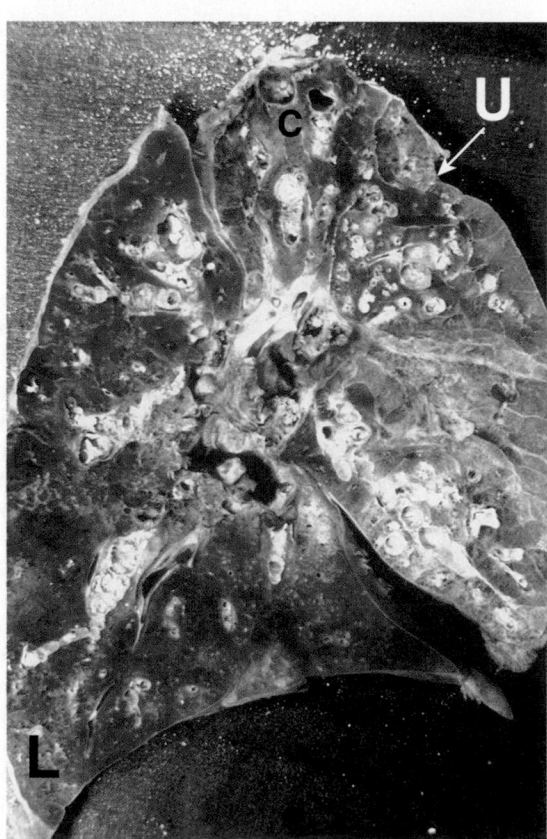

FIGURE 37.14 Pathology of the Lung in End-Stage Cystic Fibrosis. Key features are widespread mucus impaction of airways and bronchiectasis (especially in upper lobe, *U*), with hemorrhagic pneumonia in the lower lobe (*L*). Small cysts (*C*) are present at the apex of the lung. (From Kleinerman J, Vauthy P: *Pathology of the lung in cystic fibrosis,* Atlanta, 1976, Cystic Fibrosis Foundation.)

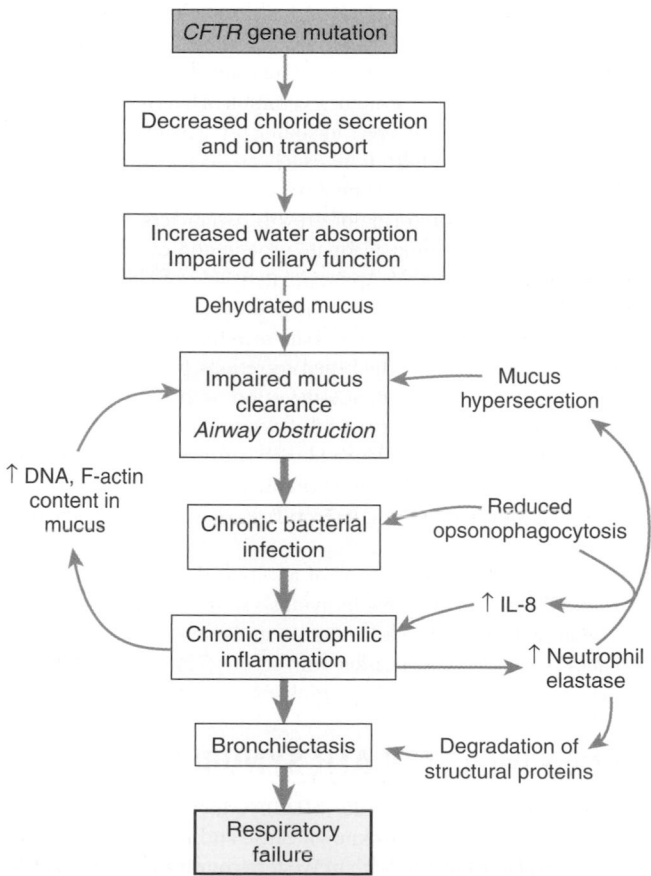

FIGURE 37.15 Pathogenesis of Cystic Fibrosis Lung Disease. *CFTR,* Cystic fibrosis transmembrane conductance regulator; *IL-8,* interleukin-8.

test, which reveal sweat chloride concentration in excess of 60 mEq/L. Alternative or supplemental methods include genotyping for *CFTR* mutations. Newborn screening for CF is universal in the United States.[133] Genetic counseling of CF gene carriers is important so they understand risk assessment in relation to disease.[134]

Treatment is primarily focused on pulmonary health and nutrition. Because the pulmonary decline in CF is slow and insidious, and because of the early onset of chronic inflammation and infection, treatment strategies begin immediately at diagnosis and are modified over time as disease progresses. Pulmonary therapies include techniques to promote mucus clearance, such as chest physical therapy and related mechanical devices (such as the high-frequency chest wall oscillation vest) and an assortment of hand-held positive expiratory pressure (PEP) devices. Aerosol therapy includes bronchodilators, dornase alfa, and hypertonic saline, which liquefy mucus.[133,135] Different classes of antibiotics and routes of administration (oral, inhaled, and intravenous) are used to treat different pathogens (e.g., *Pseudomonas aeruginosa, S. aureus, Burkholderia cepacia* nontuberculous mycobacteria) and to overcome antibiotic resistance.[136,137] Targeted therapy with oral *CFTR* modulators is available to treat specific *CFTR* mutation dysfunction. Ivacaftor has been approved in the United States, Canada, Australia, and the European Union for individuals 2 years of age and older for the *G551D CFTR* gating mutation. The corrector–potentiator pair lumacaftor–ivacaftor has been approved in the United States for individuals 12 years of age and older who are homozygous for the *CFTR* mutation *F508del* (34% of the U.S. CF population). The drugs are effective in the lung, GI tract, and sweat glands but are very expensive. Further research is in progress to target the other common genotypes.[138,139] Recombinant human growth hormone has been shown to improve lung function, height, and weight in children with severe CF.[140] Azithromycin, ibuprofen, and corticosteroids can reduce airway inflammation and improve lung function. New antiinflammatory drugs are under investigation.[141] Individuals with end-stage lung disease may consider lung transplantation.[142]

Nutritional problems are extremely common in CF, and poor nutrition is correlated with worse outcomes including progression of lung disease; onset of additional complications, such as decreased bone mineral density; and growth failure. Elements of aggressive nutritional support include meticulous monitoring of growth parameters, controlling fat malabsorption, maintaining adequate protein and caloric intake, and keeping overall health stable. Approximately 90% of children with CF have pancreatic insufficiency. This is the result of abnormal ion transport causing decreased fluid and bicarbonate secretion from the pancreatic acinar cells, which leads to thickened secretions plugging the smaller pancreatic ducts, and eventual autodigestion or atrophy of the acinar cells. Therefore, individuals must take exogenous pancreatic enzymes with meals and snacks in order to absorb nutrients and control malabsorptive symptoms (see *Nutrition & Disease:* Cystic Fibrosis [CF]).[143] Diabetes mellitus can develop as a secondary complication of pancreatic involvement.[144]

There is a growing contingent of adults with CF living into their forties and fifties. Care for these individuals shifts away from a pediatric focus because their care needs are unique and often extremely complex. Pregnancy also has become possible with advances in in vitro fertilization for men and women with fertility problems.[145]

SUDDEN INFANT DEATH SYNDROME

Sudden infant death syndrome (SIDS)/sudden unexpected infant death remains a disease of unknown cause and is the most common cause of unexplained infant death in Western countries.[146,147] It is defined as "sudden death of an infant under 1 year of age which remains unexplained after a thorough case investigation, including performance

---

NUTRITION & DISEASE
Cystic Fibrosis (CF)

Chronic inflammation, increased work of breathing, reduced nutrient absorption from pancreatic enzyme deficiency, and inadequate nutrient intake contribute to growth failure, poor clinical outcomes, and reduced life expectancy in CF. Adequate nutritional status is achieved when the weight-for-length value is greater than the 50th percentile in children younger than 2 years of age and the body mass index (BMI) is greater than the 50th percentile in children older than 2 years. Assessment of free fat mass assists evaluation of nutritional status. Energy requirements needed to meet normal growth and weight gain in children with CF necessitate a diet composed of 35% to 40% of calories from fat. Breast-feeding for the first 4 to 6 months has shown to be protective for the infant with CF, and then supplemental formula fortified with additional fat increases energy content. Oral pancreatic enzyme replacement is important in maintaining adequate nutritional status, particularly for fat absorption. The Food and Drug Administration now requires approval for the marketing of these products. Selection of dose and preparations is based on weight gain and individual response. High doses of lipase can be associated with fibrosing colonopathy, and new products are being tested in clinical trials. Fecal pancreatic elastase-1 is a common diagnostic test for evaluating pancreatic insufficiency. Yearly monitoring of fat-soluble vitamins (A, D, E, and K) is recommended with supplementation as needed. Vitamin D supplements are needed to maintain minimum serum concentrations at 30 ng/mL. Enteral feedings should be considered when weight gain and growth are inadequate. Current recommendations are to follow the Cystic Fibrosis Foundation nutrition care guidelines available at www.cff.org/treatments/CFCareGuidelines/Nutrition/. The management of CF-related diabetes mellitus is a particular challenge and occurs in up to 30% of CF individuals who are 18 years and older. Guidelines have been published by the American Diabetes Association. Nutritional guidelines and counseling are a necessary component of care for all individuals with CF.

Data from Lusman S, Sullivan J: *Pediatr Clin North Am* 63(4):661–678, 2016; Solomon M, Bozic M, Mascarenhas MR: *Clin Chest Med* 37(1):97–107, 2016; Wolfe SP, Collins C: *J Cyst Fibros* 16(4):436–438, 2017.

---

of a complete autopsy, examination of the death scene, and review of the clinical history."[148]

The incidence of SIDS is low during the first month of life but sharply increases in the second month of life, peaks at 2 to 4 months of age, and is unusual after 6 months of age. In 2014 about 3500 infants died a sudden unexpected death in the United States, of which 1500 were attributed to SIDS (44%). Other causes were accidental suffocation and strangulation in bed (25%) and unknown (31%). SIDS is more common among non-Hispanic blacks and American Indian/Alaskan Natives.[149] It almost always occurs during nighttime sleep, when infants are least likely to be observed. A seasonal variation has been noted, with higher frequencies during the winter months. This has been related to a higher rate of respiratory tract infection during those months, and such infections are often reported to have preceded the death. The sleeping room also may be overheated or the infant overwrapped.

Clinical risk groups are summarized in Box 37.3. About 75% of all SIDS victims have no known predisposing clinical risk factor. Epidemiologic studies have shown that SIDS rates decreased where massive public campaigns warned against prone sleeping for infants (e.g., the Back-to-Sleep Campaign).[150]

The etiology of SIDS remains unknown, but probably involves a combination of predisposing factors including a vulnerable infant in a critical developmental period for homeostatic control with altered

BOX 37.3   SUDDEN INFANT DEATH SYNDROME (SIDS)

- Prone and side-lying sleeping positions
- Sleeping on soft bedding
- Overheated sleeping environment
- Lower socioeconomic status
- Mothers younger than 20
- Mothers with less education
- Native American, Alaskan Native, Non-Hispanic blacks
- Low birth weight or growth-restricted infants
- Viral respiratory tract infection
- Male infants

- Preterm delivery
- Multiple gestations
- Sibling who died of SIDS
- Substance abuse during pregnancy (smoking, illicit drugs, alcohol)
- Exposure to tobacco smoke
- Lack of prenatal care
- Larger family size
- Polymorphism serotonin transporter gene (affects autonomic nervous system)

Data from Carlin RF, Moon RY: *JAMA Pediatr* 171(2):175-180, 2017; Jhun I et al: *Epidemiology* 2017 Jun 28 [Epub ahead of print]; Moon RY: *Pediatrics* 138(5), 2016.

cardiorespiratory, circulatory, and arousal characteristics, and environmental stressors (e.g., prone or side-resting position, soft bedding, or in utero or environmental tobacco exposure). There has been long-standing interest in hypotheses involving impaired autonomic regulation and failure of cardiovascular, ventilatory, and arousal responses.[151,152] Other theories involve immune dysregulation, airway inflammation, and responses to either bacterial pathogens from the nasopharynx or viral respiratory tract infections.[153] Finally, there is growing evidence that genetic factors may predispose certain individuals to SIDS. The most important risk factor genes include those involved in the regulation of the immune system and inflammation, cardiac function, and brainstem function.[152,154,155]

Currently, the best strategy to reduce SIDS and sudden unexpected infant death occurring during sleep is avoidance of risk factors as described by the American Academy of Pediatrics.[156] Breast-feeding has been identified as a specific risk reduction measure. Parents of infants with clinical risk should be taught cardiopulmonary resuscitation as a precaution. Some infants at risk for episodes of apnea and bradycardia may warrant cardiorespiratory monitoring after careful consideration of the individual situation.[157]

SUMMARY REVIEW

Structure and Function

1. The airways of infants and children are narrower than those of adults, thus making them more prone to obstruction.
2. Infants and young children continue to form new alveoli for several years after birth.
3. Surfactant production is an important marker of developmental maturity of the fetal lung and is secreted into the airways by 30 weeks' gestation.
4. The immature chest wall is soft and compliant, contributing to inefficient mechanisms of breathing.
5. Children have greater oxygen consumption than adults per unit of body weight.
6. Immune mechanisms are not fully developed at birth, making young infants more susceptible to infection.
7. Newborns have a blunted ventilatory response to hypoxia compared with older children and adults, increasing their risk for apnea and hypoxemia.
8. Neonatal exposure to air pollution increases the risk for respiratory disease.

Disorders of the Upper Airways

1. Physical examination can provide important clues in assessing the location and nature of UAO and stridor.
2. Upper airway infections can pose serious threats because of inflammatory edema and airway obstruction, including bacterial tracheitis, retropharyngeal abscess, and peritonsillar infections. Recognition and rapid evaluation are crucial.
3. Viral croup (laryngotracheobronchitis) is the most common cause of acute upper airway inflammatory obstruction in children ages 6 months to 5 years. Subglottic edema may be mild to severe. Parainfluenza is the most common cause.

4. Acute epiglottitis is a life-threatening emergency that is now rarely seen because of vaccination against *H. influenzae*, which had been the primary causative microorganism. Current cases usually represent vaccine failure or are caused by other bacteria, such as group A streptococci.
5. Tonsillar infections may be severe enough to cause UAO, and they are treated with appropriate antibiotics and corticosteroids. Complications can include tonsillar abscess.
6. Bacterial tracheitis causes airway edema and copious purulent secretions with UAO and requires administration of antibiotics and maintenance of the airway.
7. Retropharyngeal abscess is associated with nasopharyngeal infection or penetrating local injury and requires immediate antibiotic treatment.
8. Aspiration of a foreign body should be considered whenever there is a sudden onset of stridor, coughing, wheezing, or hoarseness. This usually occurs in children ages 1 to 3 years. Occasionally diagnosis is delayed and symptoms may be attributed to asthma, bronchitis, or pneumonia without recognition of the underlying cause.
9. Angioedema is a mast cell–mediated allergy to certain foods, causing edema of mucous membranes or subcutaneous layers of the skin; it can result in mucosal swelling and airway obstruction.
10. Chronic UAO may be manifested by stridor, abnormal cry, wheezing, or dyspnea. Causes of stridor in infants include laryngomalacia, tracheomalacia, subglottic stenosis, laryngeal atresias, tracheal stenosis, vocal cord paralysis, and vascular rings.
11. Obstructive sleep apnea syndrome usually occurs in older children rather than infants and is underdiagnosed. Typical symptoms are related to airway narrowing and include snoring, gasping, and restless sleep. OSAS is associated with airway narrowing and

SUMMARY REVIEW—cont'd

increased upper airway collapsibility. Adenotonsillar hypertrophy, gastroesophageal reflux, obesity, and craniofacial anomalies are common causes of OSAS.

Disorders of the Lower Airways

1. SDD (RDS) of the newborn usually occurs in premature infants who are born before surfactant production and alveolocapillary development are complete. Atelectasis and hypoventilation cause shunting, hypoxemia, and hypercapnia.
2. BPD is a chronic lung disease of infancy that is usually the consequence of acute respiratory disease in premature infants who required oxygen and positive pressure ventilatory support. Contributing factors include structural immaturity, inflammation, and disordered lung repair processes.
3. Bronchiolitis occurs in infants and toddlers, usually in the winter and early spring. It is caused by viruses, most commonly RSV. There is extensive edema, inflammation, and damage to the bronchiolar epithelium with airway obstruction and wheezing. Injection of monoclonal antibody against RSV or immunotherapy is recommended as a preventive measure for high-risk infants.
4. Childhood pneumonia is infection and inflammation in the terminal airways and alveoli usually caused by community-acquired viruses (most common), bacteria, or *Mycoplasma*. Lobar pneumonia is usually bacterial. Certain bacteria, such as *S. aureus* and group A streptococci, can cause particularly fulminant disease, as well as abscesses and empyema.
5. Aspiration pneumonitis can occur because of lung inflammation from entry of any foreign substance, including food, drink, or chemicals. Aspiration of oropharyngeal bacteria can occur because of loss of protective reflexes in neurologically impaired children, or during induction of anesthesia.
6. Bronchiolitis obliterans is fibrotic obstruction of the respiratory bronchioles and alveolar ducts usually secondary to severe respiratory viral infection or graft-versus-host disease after allograft transplantation. It is rare in children.
7. Asthma is a chronic inflammatory disease characterized by bronchial hyperreactivity and reversible airflow obstruction; it usually occurs in response to an allergen and has episodes of acute respiratory symptoms (cough, wheeze, dyspnea) and intermittent or chronic subacute symptoms. It is the most common chronic condition in children and results from genetic susceptibility and environmental factors with varying phenotypes. Environmental triggers cause inflammatory cell infiltration, mucosal edema, mucus plugging of airways, and epithelial damage with obstruction to airflow and long-term remodeling of airways.
8. ARDS is an acute life-threatening condition characterized by severe hypoxemia, poor lung compliance, atelectasis, and diffuse densities on chest radiographs. It can be triggered by direct acute lung injury (ALI), such as pneumonia, aspiration, near drowning, or smoke inhalation; or from a systemic insult, such as sepsis or multiple trauma. High-level ventilatory support is required, and mortality is significant.
9. CF is an autosomal recessive disease caused by the *cystic fibrosis transmembrane conductance regulator (CFTCR) gene* mutation. Defective chloride secretion and excess sodium absorption cause production of thick, tenacious mucus, plugging of airways, chronic pulmonary infection, and bronchiectasis related to airway epithelial chloride and sodium transport. The other major manifestations are digestive and nutritional, related to pancreatic insufficiency.

Sudden Infant Death Syndrome

1. SIDS is a diagnosis of exclusion after thorough investigation and autopsy following sudden death of an infant younger than 1 year of age. Usually the event occurs during nighttime sleep.
2. The cause is unknown. However, some known risk factors are avoidable, such as maternal smoking, prone sleeping, using soft bedding surfaces, and overheating of the infant. The incidence of SIDS has decreased significantly since public health campaigns have encouraged the supine sleeping position for babies.

KEY TERMS

Acute epiglottitis, 1208
Acute respiratory distress syndrome (ARDS), 1220
Angioedema, 1209
Aspiration of foreign body, 1209
Aspiration pneumonitis, 1218
Asthma, 1218
Atypical pneumonia (*Mycoplasma pneumoniae, Chlamydophila pneumoniae*), 1217
Bacterial pneumonia, 1217
Bacterial tracheitis (pseudomembranous croup), 1208
Bronchiolitis, 1216
Bronchiolitis obliterans (BO), 1218
Bronchopulmonary dysplasia (BPD), 1214

Choanal atresia, 1211
Community-acquired pneumonia (CAP), 1216
Cystic fibrosis (CF), 1220
Cystic fibrosis transmembrane conductance regulator (CFTCR) protein, 1220
Functional residual capacity (FRC), 1203
Hyaline membrane disease (HMD), 1212
Laryngeal atresia, 1211
Laryngomalacia, 1209
Laryngotracheitis (croup), 1207
Obstructive sleep apnea syndrome (OSAS), 1211
Peritonsillar abscess, 1208
Pneumonia, 1216
Recurrent croup, 1207

Retropharyngeal abscess, 1209
Stridor, 1206
Subglottic stenosis, 1211
Sudden infant death syndrome (SIDS)/sudden unexpected infant death, 1222
Surfactant, 1203
Surfactant deficiency disorder (SDD) (respiratory distress syndrome [RDS] of the newborn), 1212
Tonsillar abscess, 1208
Tracheal stenosis, 1211
Tracheomalacia (tracheobronchomalacia), 1210
Upper airway obstruction (UAO), 1205
Viral pneumonia, 1216

REFERENCES

1. Abu-Shaweesh JM: Maturation of respiratory reflex responses in the fetus and neonate. *Semin Neonatol* 9(3):169–180, 2004.
2. Ida JB, Thompson DM: Pediatric stridor. *Otolaryngol Clin North Am* 47(5):795–819, 2014.
3. Hiebert JC, Zhao YD, Willis EB: Bronchoscopy findings in recurrent croup: a systematic review and meta-analysis. *Int J Pediatr Otorhinolaryngol* 90:86–90, 2016.
4. Munson PD: Recurrent croup and persistent laryngomalacia: clinical resolution after supraglottoplasty. *Int J Pediatr Otorhinolaryngol* 84:94–96, 2016.
5. Zoorob R, Sidani M, Murray J: Croup: an overview. *Am Fam Physician* 83(9):1067–1073, 2011.
6. Westley CR, Cotton ED, Brooks JG: Nebulized racemic epinephrine by IPPB for the treatment of croup. *Am J Dis Child* 132:484–487, 1978.
7. Petrocheilou A, et al: Viral croup: diagnosis and a treatment algorithm. *Pediatr Pulmonol* 49(5):421–429, 2014.
8. Moraa I, et al: Heliox for croup in children. *Cochrane Database Syst Rev* (12):CD006822, 2013.

9. Greifer M, et al: Pediatric patients with chronic cough and recurrent croup: the case for a multidisciplinary approach. *Int J Pediatr Otorhinolaryngol* 79(5):749–752, 2015.

10. Westerhuis B, Bietz MG, Lindemann J: Acute epiglottitis in adults: an under-recognized and life-threatening condition. *S D Med* 66(8):309–311, 313, 2013.

11. Shah RK, Stocks C: Epiglottitis in the United States: national trends, variances, prognosis, and management. *Laryngoscope* 120(6):1256–1262, 2010.

12. Cirilli AR: Emergency evaluation and management of the sore throat. *Emerg Med Clin North Am* 31(2):501–515, 2013.

13. Abdallah C: Acute epiglottitis: trends, diagnosis and management. *Saudi J Anaesth* 6(3):279–281, 2012.

14. Lichtor JL, et al: Epiglottitis: it hasn't gone away. *Anesthesiology* 124(6):1404–1407, 2016.

15. Briere EC, et al: Prevention and control of *Haemophilus influenzae* type b disease: recommendations of the advisory committee on immunization practices (ACIP). *MMWR Recomm Rep* 63(RR-01):1–14, 2014.

16. Calò L, et al: Role of biofilms in chronic inflammatory diseases of the upper airways. *Adv Otorhinolaryngol* 72:93–96, 2011.

17. Stelter K: Tonsillitis and sore throat in children. *GMS Curr Top Otorhinolaryngol Head Neck Surg* 13:Doc07, 2014.

18. Bandarkar AN, et al: Tonsil ultrasound: technical approach and spectrum of pediatric peritonsillar infections. *Pediatr Radiol* 46(7):1059–1067, 2016.

19. Byard RW: Tonsillitis and sudden childhood death. *J Forensic Leg Med* 15(8):516–518, 2008.

20. Tak R, et al: Bacterial tracheitis and septic shock. *Pediatr Infect Dis J* 35(2):226–227, 2016.

21. Kuo CY, Parikh SR: Bacterial tracheitis. *Pediatr Rev* 35(11):497–499, 2014.

22. Abdel-Haq N, Quezada M, Asmar BI: Retropharyngeal abscess in children: the rising incidence of methicillin-resistant *Staphylococcus aureus*. *Pediatr Infect Dis J* 31(7):696–699, 2012.

23. Grisaru-Soen G, et al: Retropharyngeal and parapharyngeal abscess in children—epidemiology, clinical features and treatment. *Int J Pediatr Otorhinolaryngol* 74(9):1016–1020, 2010.

24. Hoffmann C, et al: Retropharyngeal infections in children. Treatment strategies and outcomes. *Int J Pediatr Otorhinolaryngol* 75(9):1099–1103, 2011.

25. Kim IA, et al: The national cost burden of bronchial foreign body aspiration in children. *Laryngoscope* 125(5):1221–1224, 2015.

26. Sink JR, et al: Predictors of foreign body aspiration in children. *Otolaryngol Head Neck Surg* 155(3):501–507, 2016.

27. Salih AM, Alfaki M, Alam-Elhuda DM: Airway foreign bodies: a critical review for a common pediatric emergency. *World J Emerg Med* 7(1):5–12, 2016.

28. Curtis RM, et al: ACE-1 angioedema: accurate clinical diagnosis may prevent epinephrine-induced harm. *West J Emerg Med* 17(3):283–299, 2016.

29. Farkas H: Pediatric hereditary angioedema due to C1-inhibitor deficiency. *Allergy Asthma Clin Immunol* 6(1):18, 2010.

30. Henao MP, et al: Diagnosis and screening of patients with hereditary angioedema in primary care. *Ther Clin Risk Manag* 12:701–711, 2016.

31. Guo C, Settipane RA: Clinical presentation, pathophysiology, diagnosis, and treatment of acquired and hereditary angioedema: exploring state-of-the-art therapies in RI. *R I Med J (2013)* 99(6):41–44, 2016.

32. Lumry W, et al: Safety and efficacy of C1 esterase inhibitor for acute attacks in children with hereditary angioedema. *Pediatr Allergy Immunol* 26(7):674–680, 2015.

33. Thorne MC, Garetz SL: Laryngomalacia: review and summary of current clinical practice in 2015. *Paediatr Respir Rev* 17:3–8, 2016.

34. Thompson DM: Laryngomalacia: factors that influence disease severity and outcomes of management. *Curr Opin Otolaryngol Head Neck Surg* 18(6):564–570, 2010.

35. Bedwell J, Zalzal G: Laryngomalacia. *Semin Pediatr Surg* 25(3):119–122, 2016.

36. Carter J, et al: International Pediatric ORL Group (IPOG) laryngomalacia consensus recommendations. *Int J Pediatr Otorhinolaryngol* 86:256–261, 2016.

37. Fraga JC, Jennings RW, Kim PC: Pediatric tracheomalacia. *Semin Pediatr Surg* 25(3):156–164, 2016.

38. Ada M, Isildak H, Saritzali G: Congenital vocal cord paralysis. *J Craniofac Surg* 21(1):273–274, 2010.

39. Ishman S, et al: Management of vocal paralysis: a comparison of adult and pediatric practices. *Otolaryngol Head Neck Surg* 135:590–594, 2006.

40. Olin JT, et al: Inducible laryngeal obstruction during exercise: moving beyond vocal cords with new insights. *Phys Sportsmed* 43(1):13–21, 2015.

41. Kennedy JL, Heymann PW, Platts-Mills TA: The role of allergy in severe asthma. *Clin Exp Allergy* 42(5):659–669, 2012.

42. Butskiy O, Mistry B, Chadha NK: Surgical interventions for pediatric unilateral vocal cord paralysis: a systematic review. *JAMA Otolaryngol Head Neck Surg* 141(7):654–660, 2015.

43. Sidman J, Jaguan A, Couser R: Tracheotomy and decannulation rates in a level 3 neonatal intensive care unit: a 12 year study. *Laryngoscope* 116:136–139, 2006.

44. Alvarez-Neri H, et al: Primary cricotracheal resection with thyrotracheal anastomosis for the treatment of severe subglottic stenosis in children and adolescents. *Ann Otol Rhinol Laryngol* 114(1 Pt 1):2–6, 2005.

45. Dauer EH, et al: Airway manifestations of pediatric eosinophilic esophagitis: a clinical and histopathologic report of an emerging association. *Ann Otol Rhinol Laryngol* 155(7):507–517, 2006.

46. Erickson VR, Hwang PH: Wegener's granulomatosis: current trends in diagnosis and management. *Curr Opin Otolaryngol Head Neck Surg* 15(3):170–176, 2007.

47. Jefferson ND, Cohen AP, Rutter MJ: Subglottic stenosis. *Semin Pediatr Surg* 25(3):138–143, 2016.

48. Koltai PJ: Pediatric tracheal stenosis. *Otolaryngol Clin North Am* 41(5):999–1021, 2008.

49. Martinez-Esteve Melnikova A, et al: Airway compression management in late-presenting absent pulmonary valve syndrome. *Cardiol Young* 25(2):295–300, 2015.

50. Kwong KM: Current updates on choanal atresia. *Front Pediatr* 3:52, 2015.

51. Bixler EO, et al: Sleep disordered breathing in children in a general population sample: prevalence and risk factors. *Sleep* 32(6):731–736, 2009.

52. Schwengel DA, Dalesio NM, Stierer TL: Pediatric obstructive sleep apnea. *Anesthesiol Clin* 32(1):237–261, 2014.

53. Dehlink E, Tan HL: Update on paediatric obstructive sleep apnoea. *J Thorac Dis* 8(2):224–235, 2016.

54. Blechner M, Williamson AA: Consequences of obstructive sleep apnea in children. *Curr Probl Pediatr Adolesc Health Care* 46(1):19–26, 2016.

55. Gozal D, Kheirandish-Gozal L, Kaditis AG: Home sleep testing for the diagnosis of pediatric obstructive sleep apnea: the times they are a changing …! *Curr Opin Pulm Med* 21(6):563–568, 2015.

56. Marcus CL, et al: Diagnosis and management of childhood obstructive sleep apnea syndrome. *Pediatrics* 130(3):e714–e755, 2012.

57. Tan HL, Kheirandish-Gozal L, Gozal D: Obstructive sleep apnea in children: update on the recognition, treatment and management of persistent disease. *Expert Rev Respir Med* 10(4):431–439, 2016.

58. Hamilton BE, et al: Births: final data for 2014. *Natl Vital Stat Rep* 64(12):1–64, 2015. Available at: http://www.cdc.gov/nchs/data/nvsr/nvsr64/nvsr64_12.pdf.

59. Raju TN: Developmental physiology of late and moderate prematurity. *Semin Fetal Neonatal Med* 17(3):126–131, 2012.

60. Colin A, McEvoy C, Castile R: Respiratory morbidity and lung function in preterm infants of 32 to 36 weeks' gestational age. *Pediatrics* 126:115–128, 2010.

61. Teune MJ, et al: A systematic review of severe morbidity in infants born late preterm. *Am J Obstet Gynecol* 205(4):374.e1–374.e9, 2011.

62. Pramanik AK, Rangaswamy N, Gates T: Neonatal respiratory distress: a practical approach to its diagnosis and management. *Pediatr Clin North Am* 62(2):453–469, 2015.

63. Sweet D, et al: European consensus guidelines on the management of neonatal respiratory distress syndrome. *J Perinat Med* 35:175–186, 2007.

64. Roberts D, et al: Antenatal corticosteroids for accelerating fetal lung maturation for women at risk of preterm birth. *Cochrane Database Syst Rev* (3):CD004454, 2017.

65. Carson R, et al: Effects of antenatal glucocorticoids on the developing brain. *Steroids* 114:25–32, 2016.

66. The American Congress of Obstetricians and Gynecologists: *Practice advisory: antenatal corticosteroid administration in the late preterm period.* Available at: http://www.acog.org/AboutACOG/News-Room/Practice-Advisories/Pracice-Advisory-Antenatal-Corticosteroid-Administration-in-the-Late-Preterm-Period.

67. Kamath-Rayne BD, et al: Antenatal corticosteroids beyond 34 weeks gestation: what do we do now? *Am J Obstet Gynecol* 215(4):423–430, 2016.

68. Polin RA, et al: Surfactant replacement therapy for preterm and term neonates with respiratory distress. *Pediatrics* 133(1):156–163, 2014.

69. Howlett A, Ohlsson A, Plakkal N: Inositol in preterm infants at risk for or having respiratory distress syndrome. *Cochrane Database Syst Rev* (2):CD000366, 2015.

70. Cools F, Offringa M, Askie LM: Elective high frequency oscillatory ventilation versus conventional ventilation for acute pulmonary dysfunction in preterm infants. *Cochrane Database Syst Rev* (3):CD000104, 2015.

71. Rojas-Reyes MX, Orrego-Rojas PA: Rescue high-frequency jet ventilation versus conventional ventilation for severe pulmonary dysfunction in preterm infants. *Cochrane Database Syst Rev* (10):CD000437, 2015.

72. Akter F, Coghlan G, de Mel A: Nitric oxide in paediatric respiratory disorders: novel interventions to address associated vascular phenomena? *Ther Adv Cardiovasc Dis* 10(4):256–270, 2016.

73. Long C, et al: Noninvasive ventilation with heliox for respiratory distress syndrome in preterm

infant: a systematic review and meta-analysis. *Can Respir J* 2016:9092871, 2016.

74. Gibson AM, Doyle LW: Respiratory outcomes for the tiniest or most immature infants. *Semin Fetal Neonatal Med* 19(2):105–111, 2014.

75. Hilgendorff A, et al: Chronic lung disease in the preterm infant. Lessons learned from animal models. *Am J Respir Cell Mol Biol* 50(2):233–245, 2014.

76. Jensen EA, Schmidt B: Epidemiology of bronchopulmonary dysplasia. *Birth Defects Res A Clin Mol Teratol* 100(3):145–157, 2014.

77. Rivera L, et al: Biomarkers for bronchopulmonary dysplasia in the preterm infant. *Front Pediatr* 4:33, 2016.

78. Groothuis JR, Makari D: Definition and outpatient management of the very low-birth-weight infant with bronchopulmonary dysplasia. *Adv Ther* 29(4):297–311, 2012.

79. Baker CD, Abman SH: Impaired pulmonary vascular development in bronchopulmonary dysplasia. *Neonatology* 107(4):344–351, 2015.

80. Balany J, Bhandari V: Understanding the impact of infection, inflammation, and their persistence in the pathogenesis of bronchopulmonary dysplasia. *Front Med (Lausanne)* 2:90, 2015.

81. Voynow JA: "New" bronchopulmonary dysplasia and chronic lung disease. *Paediatr Respir Rev* 2017 Jun 12. [Epub ahead of print].

82. Collins JJP, et al: The future of bronchopulmonary dysplasia: emerging pathophysiological concepts and potential new avenues of treatment. *Front Med (Lausanne)* 4:61, 2017.

83. Piedimonte G: RSV infections: state of the art. *Cleve Clin J Med* 82(11 Suppl 1):S13–S18, 2015.

84. Lu S, et al: Predictors of asthma following severe respiratory syncytial virus (RSV) bronchiolitis in early childhood. *Pediatr Pulmonol* 51(12):1382–1392, 2016.

85. Ralston SL, et al: Clinical practice guideline: the diagnosis, management, and prevention of bronchiolitis. *Pediatrics* 134(5):e1474–e1502, 2014. Available at: http://pediatrics.aappublications.org/content/134/5/e1474.

86. Florin TA, Plint AC, Zorc JJ: Viral bronchiolitis. *Lancet* 389(10065):211–224, 2017.

87. Rey-Jurado E, Kalergis AM: Immunological features of respiratory syncytial virus-caused pneumonia-implications for vaccine design. *Int J Mol Sci* 18(3):2017.

88. Jain S, et al: Community-acquired pneumonia requiring hospitalization among U.S. children. *N Engl J Med* 372(9):835–845, 2015.

89. Moreno L, et al: Development and validation of a clinical predication rule to distinguish bacterial from viral pneumonia in children. *Pediatr Pulmonol* 41:331–337, 2006.

90. Pavia AT: What is the role of respiratory viruses in community-acquired pneumonia? What is the best therapy for influenza and other viral causes of community-acquired pneumonia? *Infect Dis Clin North Am* 27(1):157–175, 2013.

91. Iroh Tam PY: Approach to common bacterial infections: community-acquired pneumonia. *Pediatr Clin North Am* 60(2):437–453, 2013.

92. Robinson KM, Kolls JK, Alcorn JF: The immunology of influenza virus-associated bacterial pneumonia. *Curr Opin Immunol* 34:59–67, 2015.

93. Loizzi M, et al: Pulmonary infections of surgical interest in childhood. *Thorac Surg Clin* 22(3):387–401, 2012.

94. Meyer Sauteur PM, van Rossum AM, Vink C: Mycoplasma pneumoniae in children: carriage, pathogenesis, and antibiotic resistance. *Curr Opin Infect Dis* 27(3):220–227, 2014.

95. Bradley JS, et al: The management of community acquired pneumonia in infants and children older than 3 months of age: clinical practice guidelines by the Pediatric Infectious Diseases Society and the Infectious Diseases Society of America. *Clin Infect Dis* 7:617–630, 2011.

96. Principi N, Esposito S: Biomarkers in pediatric community-acquired pneumonia. *Int J Mol Sci* 18(2):2017.

97. Mullholland S, et al: Antibiotics for community-acquired lower respiratory tract infections secondary to *Mycoplasma pneumoniae* in children. *Cochrane Database Syst Rev* (9):CD004875, 2012.

98. Gardiner SJ, Gavranich JB, Chang AB: Antibiotics for community-acquired lower respiratory tract infections secondary to *Mycoplasma pneumoniae* in children. *Cochrane Database Syst Rev* (1):CD004875, 2015.

99. Lindenskov PH, et al: Meconium aspiration syndrome: possible pathophysiological mechanisms and future potential therapies. *Neonatology* 107(3):225–230, 2015.

100. Boesch RP, et al: Advances in the diagnosis and management of chronic pulmonary aspiration in children. *Eur Respir J* 28:847–861, 2006.

101. Trinick R, et al: Reflux aspiration in children with neurodisability—a significant problem, but can we measure it? *J Pediatr Surg* 47(2):291–298, 2012.

102. Khan WU, et al: Botulinum toxin A for treatment of sialorrhea in children: an effective, minimally invasive approach. *Arch Otolaryngol Head Neck Surg* 137(4):339–344, 2011.

103. Kurland G, Michelson P: Bronchiolitis obliterans in children. *Pediatr Pulmonol* 39:193–208, 2005.

104. Fischer GB, et al: Post infectious bronchiolitis obliterans in children. *Paediatr Respir Rev* 11(4):233–239, 2010.

105. Snell GI, Paraskeva M, Westall GP: Managing bronchiolitis obliterans syndrome (BOS) and chronic lung allograft dysfunction (CLAD) in children: what does the future hold? *Paediatr Drugs* 15(4):281–289, 2013.

106. Yu J: Postinfectious bronchiolitis obliterans in children: lessons from bronchiolitis obliterans after lung transplantation and hematopoietic stem cell transplantation. *Korean J Pediatr* 58(12):459–465, 2015.

107. Centers for Disease Control and Prevention (CDC): *Most recent asthma data.* Available at: http://www.cdc.gov/asthma/most_recent_data.htm.

108. Thomsen SF: Genetics of asthma: an introduction for the clinician. *Eur Clin Respir J* 2, 2015.

109. Zissler UM, et al: Current and future biomarkers in allergic asthma. *Allergy* 71(4):475–494, 2016.

110. Sulaiman I, et al: Molecularly targeted therapies for asthma: current development, challenges and potential clinical translation. *Pulm Pharmacol Ther* 40:52–68, 2016.

111. Guibas GV, et al: Contributing factors to the development of childhood asthma: working toward risk minimization. *Expert Rev Clin Immunol* 11(6):721–735, 2015.

112. Milligan KL, Matsui E, Sharma H: Asthma in urban children: epidemiology, environmental risk factors, and the public health domain. *Curr Allergy Asthma Rep* 16(4):33, 2016.

113. Bantz SK, Zhu Z, Zheng T: The role of vitamin D in pediatric asthma. *Ann Pediatr Child Health* 3(1):2015.

114. DeVries A, Vercelli D: Epigenetic mechanisms in asthma. *Ann Am Thorac Soc* 13(Suppl 1):S48–S50, 2016.

115. Beasley R, Semprini A, Mitchell EA: Risk factors for asthma: is prevention possible? *Lancet* 386(9998):1075–1085, 2015.

116. Liu AH: Revisiting the hygiene hypothesis for allergy and asthma. *J Allergy Clin Immunol* 136(4):860–865, 2015.

117. Kuo CH, et al: Early life exposure to antibiotics and the risk of childhood allergic diseases: an update from the perspective of the hygiene hypothesis. *J Microbiol Immunol Infect* 46(5):320–329, 2013.

118. Panzer AR, Lynch SV: Influence and effect of the human microbiome in allergy and asthma. *Curr Opin Rheumatol* 27(4):373–380, 2015.

119. Garcia-Garcia ML, Calvo Rey C, Del Rosal Rabes T: Pediatric asthma and viral infection. *Arch Bronconeumol* 52(5):269–273, 2016.

120. Agency for Healthcare Quality and Research: National Guideline Clearing House and the Institute for Clinical Systems Improvement (ICSI): *Diagnosis and management of asthma.* Available at: http://www.guideline.gov/content.aspx?id=38255#Section420.

121. Brewczyński PZ, Brodziak A: Have recent investigations into remission from childhood asthma helped in understanding the pathogenesis of this disease? *Med Sci Monit* 21:570–575, 2015.

122. Yehya N, Thomas NJ: Relevant outcomes in pediatric acute respiratory distress syndrome studies. *Front Pediatr* 4:51, 2016.

123. The Pediatric Acute Lung Injury Consensus Conference Group: Pediatric acute respiratory distress syndrome: consensus recommendations from the Pediatric Acute Lung Injury Consensus Conference. *Pediatr Crit Care Med* 16(5):428–439, 2015.

124. Cheifetz IM: Pediatric acute respiratory distress syndrome. *Respir Care* 56(10):1589–1599, 2011.

125. Yehya N, et al: Corticosteroid exposure in pediatric acute respiratory distress syndrome. *Intensive Care Med* 41(9):1658–1666, 2015.

126. Dalton HJ, et al: Extracorporeal support in children with pediatric acute respiratory distress syndrome: proceedings from the Pediatric Acute Lung Injury Consensus Conference. *Pediatr Crit Care Med* 16(5 Suppl 1):S111–S117, 2015.

127. Cystic Fibrosis Center at the Hospital for Sick Children in Toronto: *Cystic fibrosis mutation database.* Available at: www.genet.sickkids.on.ca/cftr/StatisticsPage.html.

128. Egan ME: Genetics of cystic fibrosis: clinical implications. *Clin Chest Med* 37(1):9–16, 2016.

129. Spoonhower KA, Davis PB: Epidemiology of cystic fibrosis. *Clin Chest Med* 37(1):1–8, 2016.

130. Cystic Fibrosis Foundation: *Cystic fibrosis foundation patient registry 2015 annual data report,* Bethesda, MD, 2014, Author. Available at: https://www.cff.org/Our-Research/CF-Patient-Registry/2015-Patient-Registry-Annual-Data-Report.pdf.

131. López-Causapé C, et al: The problems of antibiotic resistance in cystic fibrosis and solutions. *Expert Rev Respir Med* 9(1):73–88, 2015.

132. Egan ME: Genetics of cystic fibrosis: clinical implications. *Clin Chest Med* 37(1):9–16, 2016.

133. Martiniano SL, et al: Advances in the diagnosis and treatment of cystic fibrosis. *Adv Pediatr* 61(1):225–243, 2014.

134. Dungan JS: Carrier screening for cystic fibrosis. *Obstet Gynecol Clin North Am* 37(1):47–59, 2010.

135. Rubin BK: Aerosol medications for treatment of mucus clearance disorders. *Respir Care* 60(6):825–829, discussion 830–832, 2015.

136. Chmiel JF, et al: Antibiotic management of lung infections in cystic fibrosis. I. The microbiome, methicillin-resistant *Staphylococcus aureus,*

gram-negative bacteria, and multiple infections. *Ann Am Thorac Soc* 11(7):1120–1129, 2014.

137. Chmiel JF, et al: Antibiotic management of lung infections in cystic fibrosis. II. Nontuberculous mycobacteria, anaerobic bacteria, and fungi. *Ann Am Thorac Soc* 11(8):1298–1306, 2014.

138. Corvol H, et al: Translating the genetics of cystic fibrosis to personalized medicine. *Transl Res* 168:40–49, 2016.

139. Mayer-Hamblett N, Boyle M, VanDevanter D: Advancing clinical development pathways for new CFTR modulators in cystic fibrosis. *Thorax* 71(5): 454–461, 2016.

140. Thaker V, et al: Recombinant growth hormone therapy for cystic fibrosis in children and young adults. *Cochrane Database Syst Rev* (5):CD008901, 2015.

141. Cantin AM, et al: Inflammation in cystic fibrosis lung disease: pathogenesis and therapy. *J Cyst Fibros* 14(4):419–430, 2015.

142. Lynch JP, 3rd, et al: Lung transplantation for cystic fibrosis: results, indications, complications, and controversies. *Semin Respir Crit Care Med* 36(2): 299–320, 2015.

143. Schindler T, Michel S, Wilson AW: Nutrition management of cystic fibrosis in the 21st century. *Nutr Clin Pract* 30(4):488–500, 2015.

144. Brennan AL, Beynon J: Clinical updates in cystic fibrosis-related diabetes. *Semin Respir Crit Care Med* 36(2):236–250, 2015.

145. Grigoriadis C, Tympa A, Theodoraki K: Cystic fibrosis and pregnancy: counseling, obstetrical management and perinatal outcome. *Invest Clin* 56(1):66–73, 2015.

146. American Academy of Pediatrics Task Force on Sudden Infant Death Syndrome: The changing concept of sudden infant death syndrome: diagnostic coding shifts, controversies regarding the sleeping environment, and new variables to consider in reducing risk. *Pediatrics* 116(5):1245, 2005.

147. Centers for Disease Control and Prevention: *Sudden infant death syndrome.* Updated October 1, 2012. Available at: www.cdc.gov/Features/SidsAwarenessMonth/.

148. Centers for Disease Control and Prevention (CDC): *Sudden unexpected infant death and sudden infant death syndrome.* Updated June 8, 2016. Available at: www.cdc.gov/sids/index.htm.

149. Centers for Disease Control and Prevention (CDC): *Sudden unexpected infant death and sudden infant death syndrome: data and statistics.* Updated February 8, 2016. Available at: http://www.cdc.gov.sids/data/htm.

150. Trachtenberg FL, et al: Risk factor changes for sudden infant death syndrome after initiation of Back-to-Sleep campaign. *Pediatrics* 129(4): 630–638, 2012.

151. Bergman NJ: Proposal for mechanisms of protection of supine sleep against sudden infant death syndrome: an integrated mechanism review. *Pediatr Res* 77:10–19, 2015.

152. Thach BT: Potential central nervous system involvement in sudden unexpected infant deaths and the sudden infant death syndrome. *Compr Physiol* 5(3):1061–1068, 2015.

153. Blackwell C, et al: Exploring the risk factors for sudden infant deaths and their role in inflammatory responses to infection. *Front Immunol* 6:44, 2015.

154. Ferrante L, Opdal SH: Sudden infant death syndrome and the genetics of inflammation. *Front Immunol* 6:63, 2015.

155. Hertz CL, et al: Genetic investigations of sudden unexpected deaths in infancy using next-generation sequencing of 100 genes associated with cardiac diseases. *Eur J Hum Genet* 24(6):817–822, 2016.

156. Task Force on Sudden Infant Death Syndrome: SIDS and other sleep-related infant deaths: updated 2016 recommendations for a safe infant sleeping environment. *Pediatrics* 138(5): e20162938, 2016. Available at: http://pediatrics.aappublications.org.ezproxy.lib.utah.edu/content/138/5.

157. Liu G, Molokhia E, Perkins A: Home apnea monitors—when to discontinue use. *J Fam Pract* 64(12):769–772, 2015.

CHAPTER

38

Structure and Function of the Renal and Urologic Systems

Sue E. Huether

evolve WEBSITE

http://evolve.elsevier.com/McCance/

- Content Updates
- Chapter Summary Review
- Review Questions
- Case Studies
- Animations

CHAPTER OUTLINE

The primary function of the kidney is to maintain a stable internal environment for optimal cell and tissue metabolism. The kidneys accomplish these life-sustaining tasks by balancing solute and water transport, excreting metabolic waste products, conserving nutrients, and regulating acids and bases. The kidney also has an endocrine function, secreting the hormones renin, erythropoietin, and 1,25-dihydroxy-vitamin D_3 for regulation of blood pressure, erythrocyte production, and calcium metabolism, respectively. The kidney also can synthesize glucose from amino acids, performing the process of gluconeogenesis (see *What's New? The Kidney and Glucose Regulation*). The formation of urine is achieved through the processes of glomerular filtration, tubular reabsorption, and secretion within the kidney. The bladder stores the urine that it receives from the kidney by way of the ureters. Urine is then removed from the body through the urethra.

STRUCTURES OF THE RENAL SYSTEM

Structures of the Kidney

The kidneys are paired organs located in the posterior region of the abdominal cavity behind the peritoneum (Fig. 38.1). They lie on either side of the vertebral column with their upper and lower poles extending from approximately the twelfth thoracic to the third lumbar vertebrae. The right kidney is slightly lower than the left and is displaced downward by the overlying liver. Each kidney is approximately 11 cm long, 5 to

The Kidney and Glucose Regulation

The human kidney contributes to the regulation of glucose concentration by making glucose through gluconeogenesis, by taking up glucose from the circulation, and by reabsorbing glucose from the glomerular filtrate. The human liver and kidneys release approximately equal amounts of glucose through gluconeogenesis in the postabsorptive state (4 to 12 hours after meal ingestion). Other tissues lack the enzyme necessary for gluconeogenesis (glucose-6-phosphatase) and cannot participate in gluconeogenesis. In the postprandial state (up to 4 hours after meal ingestion), although overall endogenous glucose release decreases substantially, renal gluconeogenesis accounts for 40% of glucose formed by gluconeogenesis.

About 180 grams of glucose are normally filtered each day by the kidneys. Almost all of this is actively reabsorbed by means of sodium-glucose cotransporter 2 (SGLT2), a transmembrane protein expressed in the luminal border of the proximal tubule. This ensures sufficient energy is available during fasting periods. When plasma glucose concentrations exceed a threshold, the SGLT2 becomes saturated and glucose appears in the urine. Individuals with diabetes mellitus have an increased transport maximum (Tm) for glucose from enhanced expression of SGLT2 and this contributes to hyperglycemia when there is poor glucose control. SGLT2 inhibitors are used for reducing hyperglycemia associated with diabetes mellitus.

Renal glucose release is stimulated by epinephrine and is inhibited by insulin. Insulin suppresses glucose release in both the liver and the kidney. The kidneys do not synthesize glycogen and, therefore, do not release glucose through glycogenolysis. In the postabsorptive state, the kidneys utilize about 10% of all glucose used by the body. When there is hypoglycemia, the liver initially releases glucose through glycogenolysis and then increases gluconeogenesis. The kidney also counter-regulates hypoglycemia through gluconeogenesis, which may explain in part why individuals with renal failure tend to develop hypoglycemia.

Data from Solini A: *Acta Diabetol* 53(6):863-870, 2016; Moen MF, et al: *Clin J Am Soc Nephrol* 4(6):1121-1127, 2009; White JR Jr: *Med Clin North Am* 2015 99(1):131-143, 2015.

6 cm wide, and 3 to 4 cm thick. A tightly adhering capsule (the renal capsule) surrounds each kidney, and the kidney then is embedded in a mass of fat. The capsule and fatty layer are covered with a double layer of renal fascia, composed of fibrous tissue that attaches the kidney to the posterior abdominal wall.

The cushion of fat and the position of the kidney between the abdominal organs and muscles of the back protect it from trauma. The hilum is a medial indentation in the kidney and is the location of the entry and exit for the renal blood vessels, nerves, lymphatic vessels, and ureter.

The structures of the kidney are summarized in Fig. 38.2. The outer layer of the kidney is called the cortex and contains all of the glomeruli, most of the proximal tubules, and some segments of the distal tubule. The medulla forms the inner part of the kidney and consists of regions called the pyramids. Renal columns are an extension of the cortex and lie between the pyramids and extend to the renal pelvis. The apexes of the pyramids project into minor calyces (cup-shaped cavities) that unite to form major calyces. The minor calyces receive urine from the collecting ducts through the renal papilla. The major calyces join to form the renal pelvis, which connects with the proximal end of the ureter. The walls of the calyces, pelvis, and ureter are lined with epithelial cells and contain smooth muscle cells that contract to move urine to the bladder. The structural unit of the kidney is the lobe. Each lobe is composed of a pyramid and the overlying cortex. On average, there are 14 lobes in each kidney.

Nephron

The nephron is the functional unit of the kidney. Each kidney contains approximately 1.2 million nephrons. The nephron is a tubular structure with subunits that include the renal corpuscle, proximal convoluted tubule, loop of Henle (nephron ansa), distal convoluted tubule, and collecting duct, all of which contribute to the formation of urine (Fig. 38.3). The different epithelial cells lining various segments of the tubule facilitate the special functions of reabsorption and secretion (Fig. 38.4).

The kidney has three kinds of nephrons: (1) superficial cortical nephrons (85% of all nephrons), which extend partially into the medulla; (2) midcortical nephrons with short or long loops; and (3) juxtamedullary nephrons, which lie close to and extend deep into

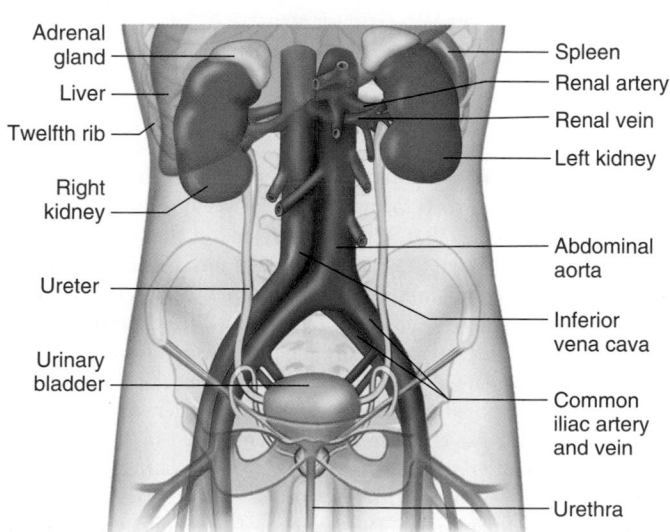

FIGURE 38.1 Organs of the Urinary System. (From Patton KT, Thibodeau GA: *The human body in health & disease*, ed 7, St Louis, 2018, Mosby.)

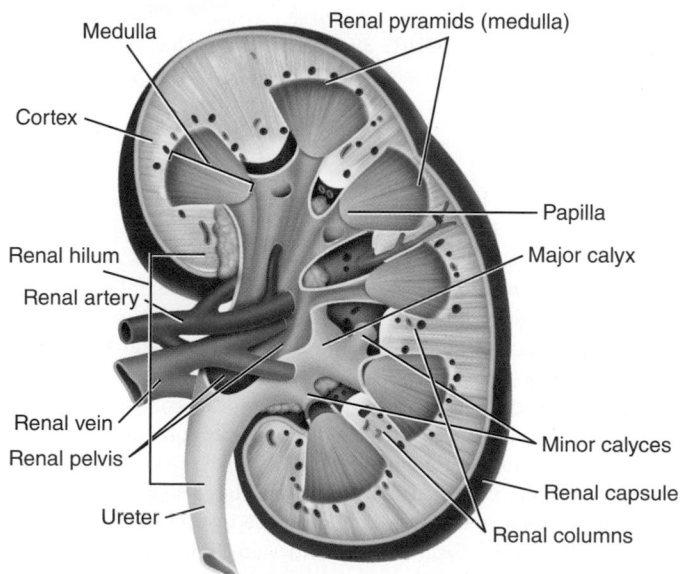

FIGURE 38.2 Kidney Structure. (From Solomon E: *Introduction to human anatomy and physiology*, ed 4, St Louis, 2016, Saunders.)

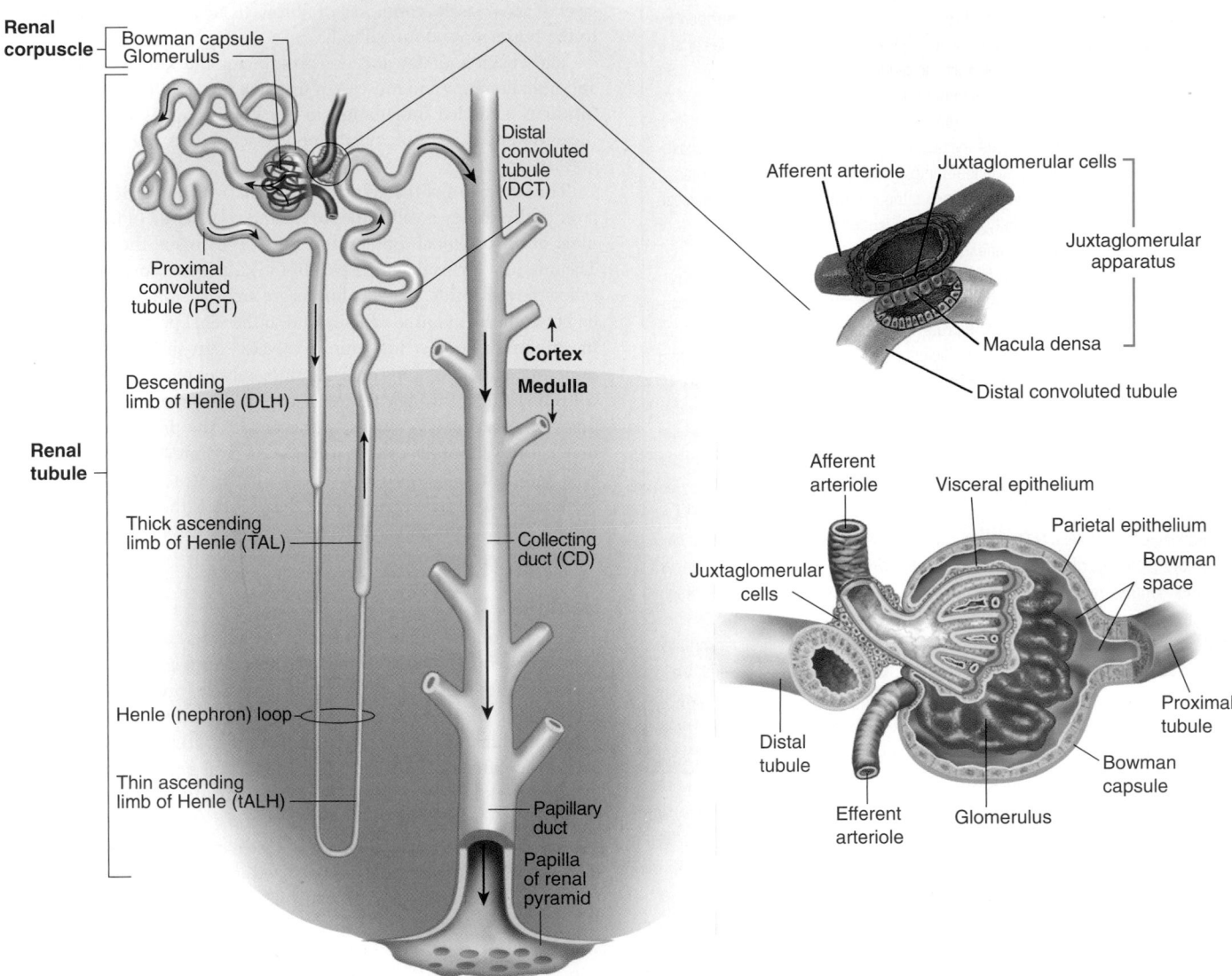

FIGURE 38.3 Components of the Nephron. (From Patton KT, Thibodeau GA, Douglass MM: *Essentials of anatomy & physiology*, St Louis, 2012, Mosby; Damjanov I: *Pathology for health professions*, ed 4, St Louis, 2012, Mosby.)

the medulla and are important for the concentration of urine (Fig. 38.5). The **glomerulus** (Fig. 38.6; see also Fig. 38.3) is a tuft of capillaries that loop into the circular Bowman capsule, like fingers pushed into bread dough. **Bowman capsule** is composed of a **visceral epithelium** (**visceral layer**) forming podocytes. The visceral epithelium is reflected back at the vascular pole to become the outer **parietal epithelium** (**parietal layer**) (see Fig. 38.3). **Mesangial cells** (shaped like smooth muscle cells) and the **mesangial matrix** (a type of connective tissue), secreted by mesangial cells, lie between and support the glomerular capillaries. Different mesangial cells contract like smooth muscle cells to regulate glomerular capillary blood flow. They also have phagocytic properties similar to monocytes and release inflammatory cytokines and growth factors.[1] Together, the glomerulus, Bowman capsule, and mesangial cells are called the **renal corpuscle**.

The **glomerular filtration membrane** filters blood components through its three layers: (1) an inner capillary endothelium; (2) a middle

glomerular basement membrane (GBM); and (3) an outer layer, the visceral epithelium, which forms the inner layer of Bowman capsule (Fig. 38.7; see also Fig. 38.6). The capillary endothelium is composed of cells in continuous contact with the basement membrane and contains pores. The pores are maintained by vascular epithelial growth factor (VEGF) produced by the visceral epithelium. The endothelial cells synthesize nitric oxide (a vasodilator) and endothelin-1 (a vasoconstrictor) that help regulate glomerular blood flow. The middle basement membrane is composed of a selectively permeable network of proteoglycans (type IV collagen) secreted and maintained by the epithelial cells.[2] The visceral epithelium is composed of specialized cells called **podocytes** from which pedicles (foot projections) radiate and adhere to the basement membrane. The pedicles of one podocyte interlock with the pedicles of adjacent podocytes, forming an elaborate network of intercellular clefts (**filtration slits** or **slit membranes**) (see Fig. 38.7) and modulate filtration. *Nephrin, podocin, CD2-associated protein,* and

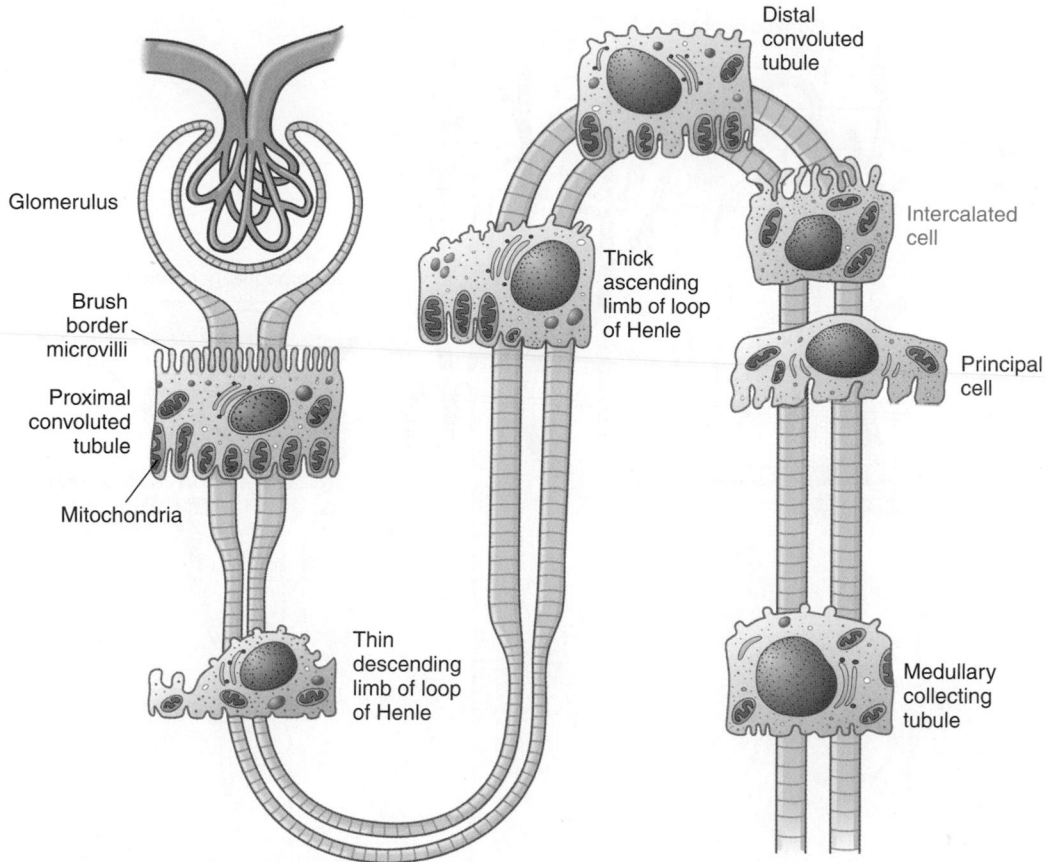

FIGURE 38.4 Epithelial Cells of the Various Segments of Nephron Tubules. The brush border and high number of mitochondria in the cells of the proximal convoluted tubule permit reabsorption of 60% of the glomerular filtrate. *Intercalated cells (blue text)* secrete either H^+ (reabsorb HCO_3^-) or HCO_3^- and reabsorb K^+. *Principal cells (magenta text)* reabsorb Na^+ and water and secrete K^+.

other transcellular protein molecules ensure proper function of the filtration slits and, when altered, cause glomerular disease.[3]

The space between the visceral and parietal epithelia is the Bowman space (urinary space), which is continuous with the lumen of the renal tubules. The endothelium, basement membrane, and podocytes are covered with protein molecules bearing anionic (negative) charges that retard the filtration of anionic proteins and prevent proteinuria. The glomerular filtration membrane separates the blood of the glomerular capillaries from the fluid in Bowman space and allows all components of the blood to be filtered, with the exception of blood cells and plasma proteins with a molecular weight greater than 70,000. The glomerular filtrate passes through the three layers of the glomerular membrane and forms the primary urine.

The glomerulus is supplied by the afferent arteriole and drained by the efferent arteriole. A group of specialized cells known as juxtaglomerular cells (renin-releasing cells) are located around the afferent arteriole where it enters the glomerulus (see Figs. 38.3 and 38.6). Between the afferent and efferent arterioles is the macula densa (sodium-sensing cells) of the distal convoluted tubule. Together the juxtaglomerular cells and macula densa cells form the juxtaglomerular apparatus (JGA) (see Fig. 38.6). Control of renal blood flow, glomerular filtration, and renin secretion occurs at this site.

The proximal convoluted tubule continues from the Bowman capsule and has an initial convoluted segment (pars convoluta) and then a straight segment (pars recta) that descends toward the medulla (see Fig. 38.3). The wall of the tubule consists of one layer of cuboidal epithelial cells with a surface layer of microvilli (a brush border) that

increases reabsorptive surface area. This is the only surface inside the nephron where the cells are covered with microvilli (see Fig. 38.4). The proximal convoluted tubule joins the hairpin-shaped loop of Henle. The loop is composed of a thin descending segment, a thin ascending segment, and a thick ascending segment. The thin descending segment is composed of squamous cells, has no active transport functions, and is highly permeable to water. The thin ascending segment is permeable to ions but not to water. The thick ascending segment actively transports ions into the interstitium and passes urine into the distal convoluted tubule (see Fig. 38.14). *Cortical nephrons* are more numerous and have glomeruli originating close to the surface of the cortex or in the midcortex. *Juxtamedullary nephrons* have glomeruli located deep in the cortex close to the medulla. The major structural difference between the two types of nephrons is the length of the loop of Henle. In cortical nephrons the loop is short and may not extend into the medulla. The loop of Henle for the juxtamedullary nephrons, however, may extend the whole length of the medulla (approximately 40 mm). Juxtamedullary nephrons represent about 12% of the total number of nephrons and are important for the concentration and dilution of urine.

The distal tubule has straight and convoluted segments. It extends from the macula densa to the collecting duct, a large tubule that descends down the cortex and through the renal pyramids of the inner and outer medullae, draining urine into the minor calyx. The distal tubule is composed of two epithelial cell types: principal cells that reabsorb sodium and water and secrete potassium, and intercalated cells that secrete hydrogen and reabsorb potassium (see Fig. 38.4).

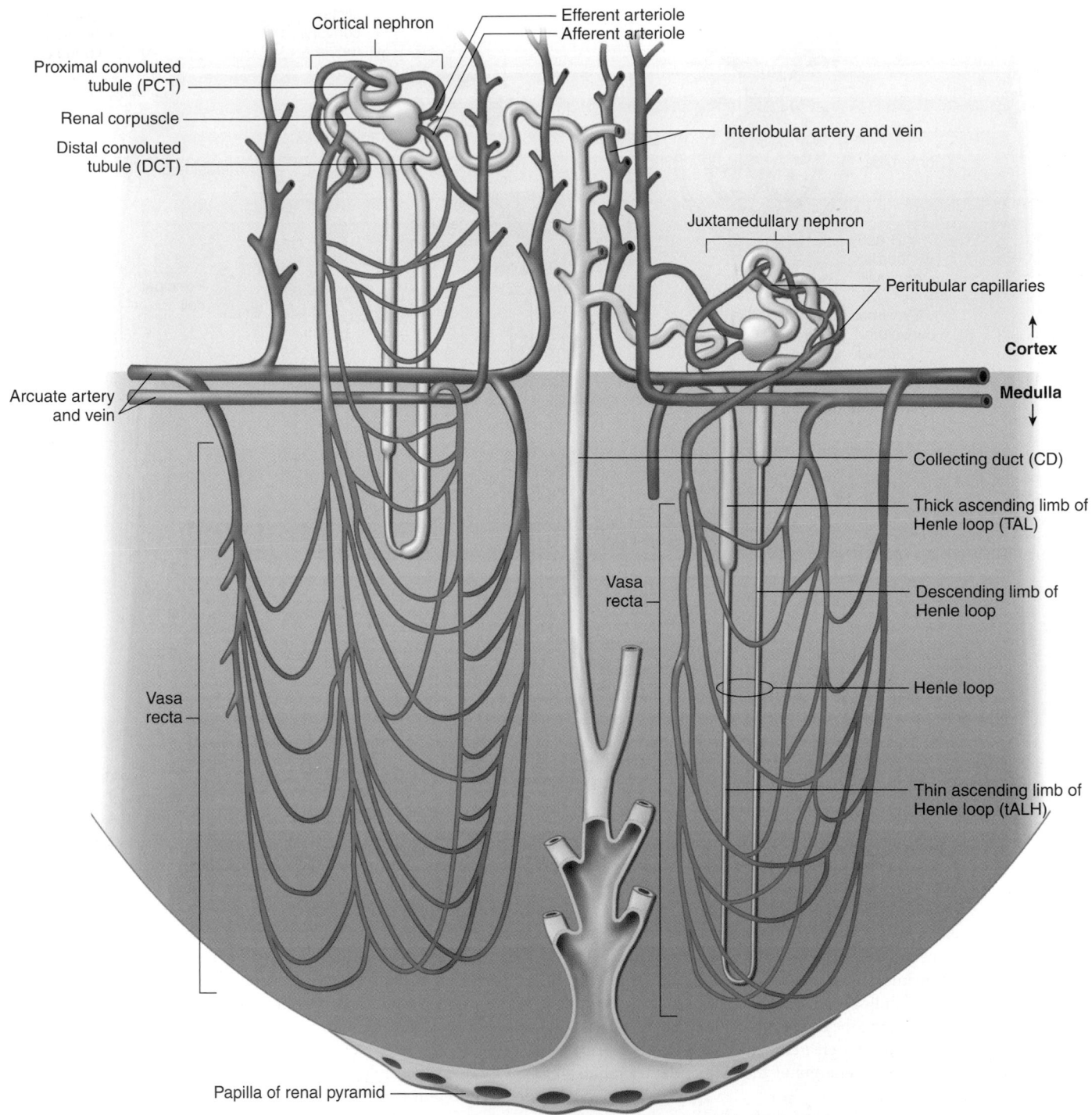

FIGURE 38.5 The Nephron Unit with Its Blood Vessels. Blood flows through nephron vessels as follows: interlobular artery, afferent arteriole, glomerulus, efferent arteriole, peritubular capillaries (around the tubules), venules, interlobular vein. (From Patton KT, Thibodeau GA, Douglass MM: *Essentials of anatomy & physiology*, St Louis, 2012, Mosby.)

Blood Vessels of the Kidney

The blood vessels of the kidney closely parallel nephron structure. The major vessels are as follows:

1. **Renal arteries** arise as the fifth branches of the abdominal aorta, divide into anterior and posterior branches at the renal hilum, and then subdivide into lobar arteries supplying blood to the lower, middle, and upper thirds of the kidney.

2. **Interlobar artery** subdivisions travel down renal columns and between pyramids and form afferent glomerular arteries (see Fig. 38.5).

3. **Arcuate arteries** consist of branches of interlobar arteries at the cortical-medullary junction; they arch over the base of the pyramids and run parallel to the surface.

4. **Glomerular capillaries** consist of four to eight vessels and are arranged in a fistlike structure; they arise from the **afferent arteriole** and

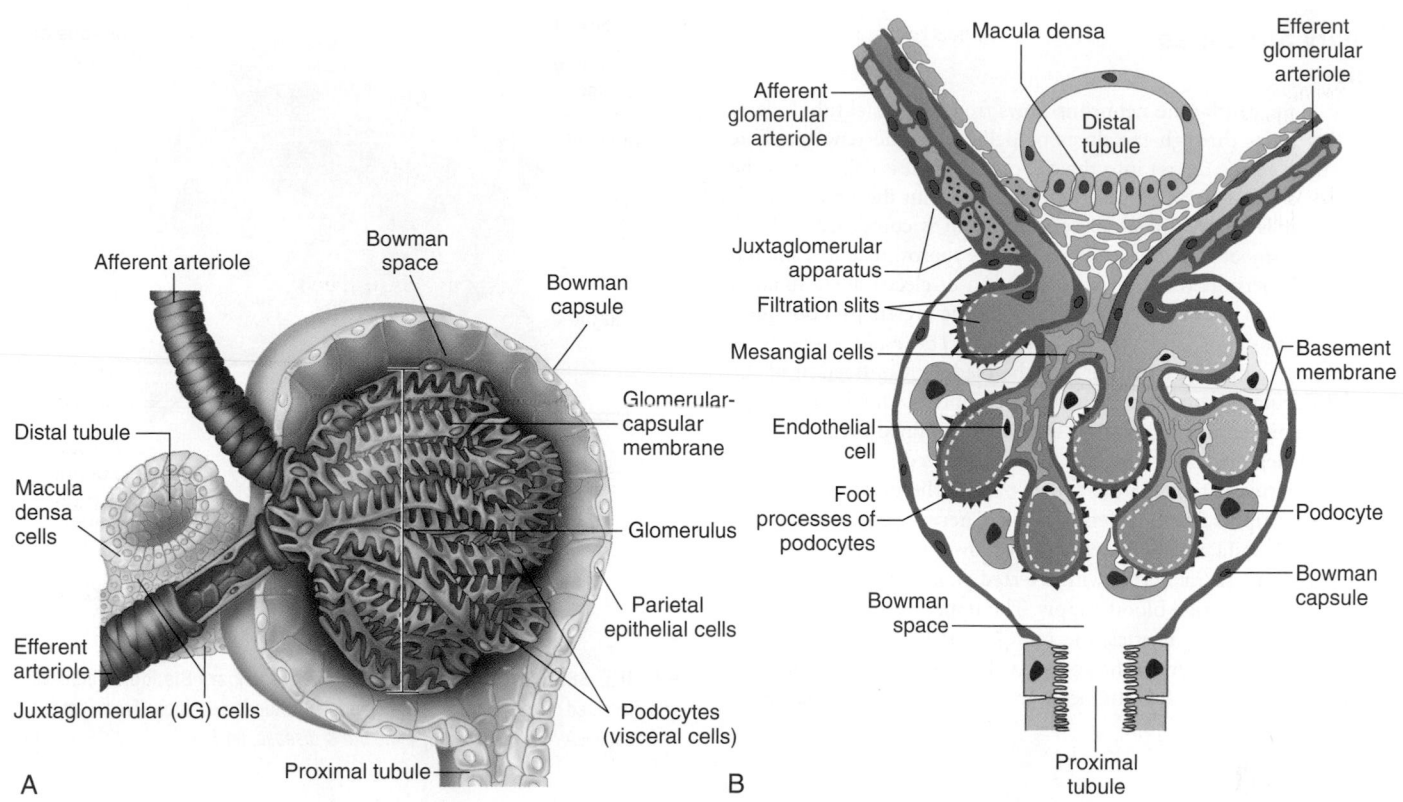

FIGURE 38.6 Anatomy of the Glomerulus and Juxtaglomerular Apparatus. **A,** Longitudinal cross section of glomerulus and juxtaglomerular apparatus. **B,** Longitudinal cross section illustrating detail of glomerular structures. (**B** from Goldman L, Schafer AI: *Goldman-Cecil medicine*, ed 25, Philadelphia, 2016, Elsevier.)

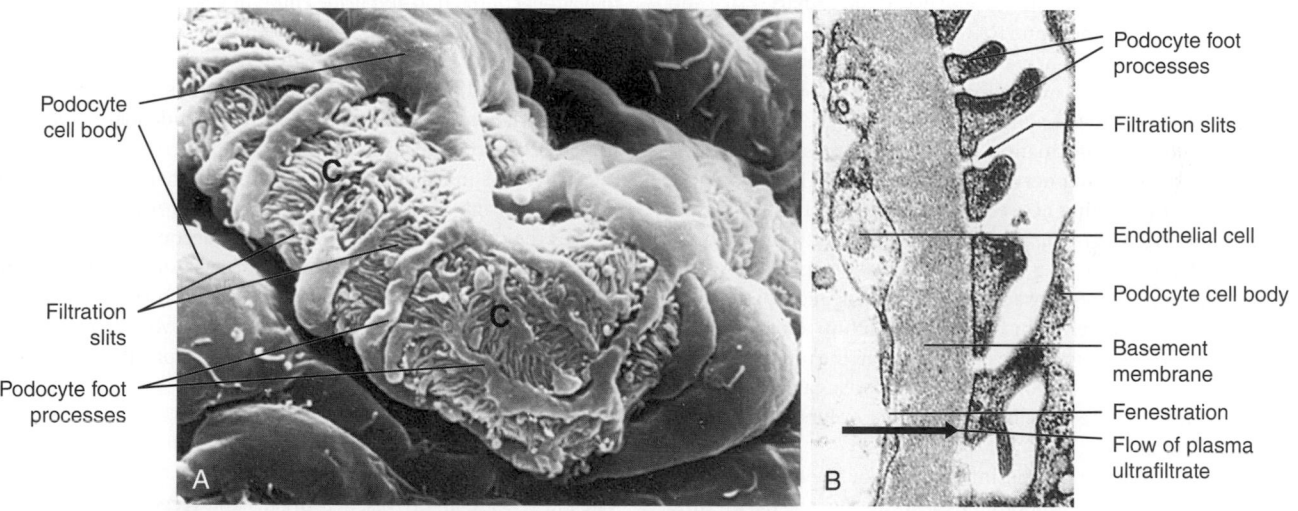

FIGURE 38.7 Glomerular Capillary. **A,** Scanning electron micrograph of normal glomerular capillary *(C)*. **B,** Glomerular capillary wall (filtration membrane) (×40,000). *Black arrow* indicates direction of urine flow. (From Kissane JM, editor: *Anderson's pathology*, ed 9, St Louis, 1990, Mosby.)

empty into the **efferent arteriole,** which carries blood to the peritubular capillaries. They are the major resistance vessels for regulating intrarenal blood flow (see under Autoregulation of Intrarenal Blood Flow).

5. **Peritubular capillaries** surround convoluted portions of the proximal and distal tubules and the loop of Henle; they are adapted for cortical and juxtamedullary nephrons.

6. **Vasa recta** is a network of capillaries that forms loops and closely follow the loops of Henle; it is the only blood supply to the medulla (important for formation of concentrated urine).

7. **Renal veins** follow the arterial path in reverse direction and have the same names as the corresponding arteries; they eventually empty into the inferior vena cava. The lymphatic vessels also tend to follow the distribution of the blood vessels.

Urinary Structures
Ureters

The urine formed by the nephrons flows from the distal tubules and collecting ducts through the ducts of Bellini and the **renal papillae** (projections of the ducts) into the calyces, where it is collected in the renal pelvis (see Fig. 38.2) and then funneled into the **ureters**. Each adult ureter is approximately 30 cm long and is composed of long, intertwining smooth muscle bundles. The close approximation of smooth muscle cells permits the direct transmission of electrical stimulation from one cell to another. The lower ends of the ureters pass obliquely through the posterior aspect of the bladder wall. The resulting downward peristaltic activity propels urine into the bladder. Contraction of the bladder during **micturition** (urination) compresses the lower end of the ureter, preventing reflux. Peristalsis is maintained even when the ureter is denervated, so ureters can be transplanted.

Sensory innervation for the upper part of the ureter arises from sympathetic inputs from the tenth thoracic nerve roots, with referred pain to the umbilicus. The innervation of lower segments arises from parasympathetic sacral nerves with referred pain to the vulva or penis. The ureters have a rich blood supply. The upper part of the ureter is supplied by the renal arteries, the middle part by the common iliac arteries and branches from the abdominal aorta and gonadal arteries, and the lower part mainly by branches from the internal iliac and vesical arteries.

Bladder and Urethra

The **bladder** is a bag composed of a basketweave of smooth muscle fibers that forms the **detrusor muscle** and its smooth lining of **uroepithelium (transitional epithelium)**. As the bladder fills with urine, it distends and the layers of uroepithelium within the lining slide past each other and become thinner as the volume of the bladder increases. The uroepithelium forms the interface between the urinary space and underlying vasculature and connective, nervous, and muscle tissue. Uroepithelium also lines the urinary tract from the renal pelvis to the urethra. The uroepithelium maintains an important barrier function to prevent movement of water and solutes between the urine and the blood. It communicates information about luminal pressure and urine composition to surrounding nerve and muscle cells.[4] The **trigone** is a smooth triangular area lying between the openings of the two ureters and the urethra (Fig. 38.8). The position of the bladder varies with age and sex. In infants and young children the bladder rises above the symphysis pubis, providing easy access for percutaneous aspiration. In adults it lies in the true pelvis, in front of the rectum and in front of the uterus in women. Inferiorly, the bladder sits on the prostate in men and on the anterior vagina in women. The bladder has a profuse blood supply, accounting for the bleeding that readily occurs with trauma, surgery, or inflammation.

The **urethra** extends from the inferior side of the bladder to the outside of the body. A ring of smooth muscle forms the **internal urethral sphincter** at the junction of the urethra and bladder. The **external urethral sphincter** is composed of striated skeletal muscle and is under voluntary control. The entire urethra is lined with mucus-secreting glands. The female urethra is short (3 to 4 cm). The male urethra is long (18 to 20 cm) and has three main segments: prostatic, membranous, and penile. The prostatic urethra is closest to the bladder. It passes through the prostate gland and contains the openings of the ejaculatory ducts. The membranous urethra is the segment that passes through the floor of the pelvis. The penile segment forms the remainder of the tube. The penile segment is surrounded by the corpus spongiosum erectile tissue and contains the openings of the bulbourethral glands.

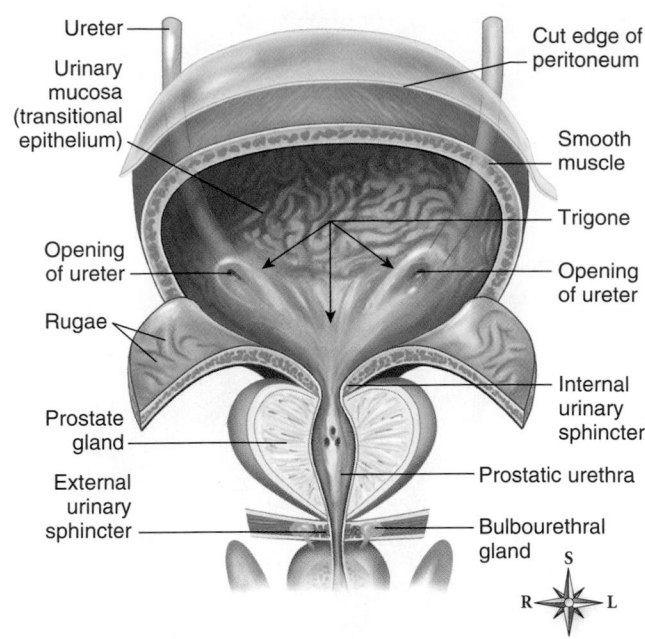

FIGURE 38.8 Structure and Location of the Urinary Bladder. Frontal view of a dissected urinary bladder (male) in a fully distended position. (From Patton KT, Thibodeau GA: *The human body in health & disease*, ed 7, St Louis, 2018, Mosby.)

The innervation of the bladder and internal urethral sphincter is supplied by parasympathetic fibers of the autonomic nervous system that arise from the sacral levels of the spinal cord (S2 to S4) and contribute to bladder contraction and urine emptying. Sympathetic fibers originate from T11-L2 and inhibit the bladder body and excite the lower bladder and proximal urethral sphincter to retain urine. Sensory fibers from the bladder and urethra may extend as high as the T6 portion of the spinal cord. Somatic motor neurons in the pudendal nerve innervate the striated external urethral sphincter. The reflex arc required for micturition is stimulated by mechanoreceptors that respond to stretching of tissue sensing bladder fullness and sending impulses to the sacral level of the spinal cord. When the bladder accumulates 250 to 300 mL of urine, the bladder contracts and the internal urethral sphincter relaxes through activation of the spinal reflex arc (known as the *micturition reflex*). At this time a person feels the urge to void. The reflex can be inhibited or facilitated by impulses coming from the brain, resulting in voluntary control of micturition.

RENAL BLOOD FLOW

The kidneys are highly vascular organs and receive about 20% to 25% of the cardiac output, which in adults is equivalent to 1000 to 1200 mL of blood per minute. With a normal hematocrit of 45%, about 600 to 700 mL of blood flowing through the kidney per minute is plasma. From the renal plasma flow (RPF), 20% (approximately 120 to 140 mL/min) is filtered at the glomerulus and passes into the Bowman capsule. The filtration of the plasma per unit of time is known as the **glomerular filtration rate (GFR)**, which is directly related to the perfusion pressure in the glomerular capillaries.

The remaining 80% (about 480 mL/min) of plasma flows through the efferent arterioles to the peritubular capillaries. The ratio of glomerular filtrate to RPF per minute (120/600 = 0.20) is called the *filtration fraction*. Normally all but 1 to 2 mL per minute of the glomerular filtrate

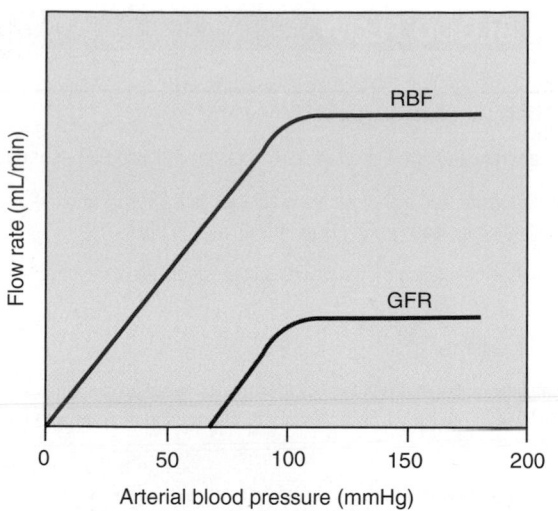

FIGURE 38.9 Autoregulation of Renal Blood Flow. Blood flow and glomerular filtration rate are stabilized with changes in mean arterial pressure between about 80 and 180 mmHg. *GFR*, Glomerular filtration rate; *RBF*, renal blood flow. (From Koeppen BM, Stanton BA: *Berne and Levy physiology* [updated], ed 6, St Louis, 2010, Mosby.)

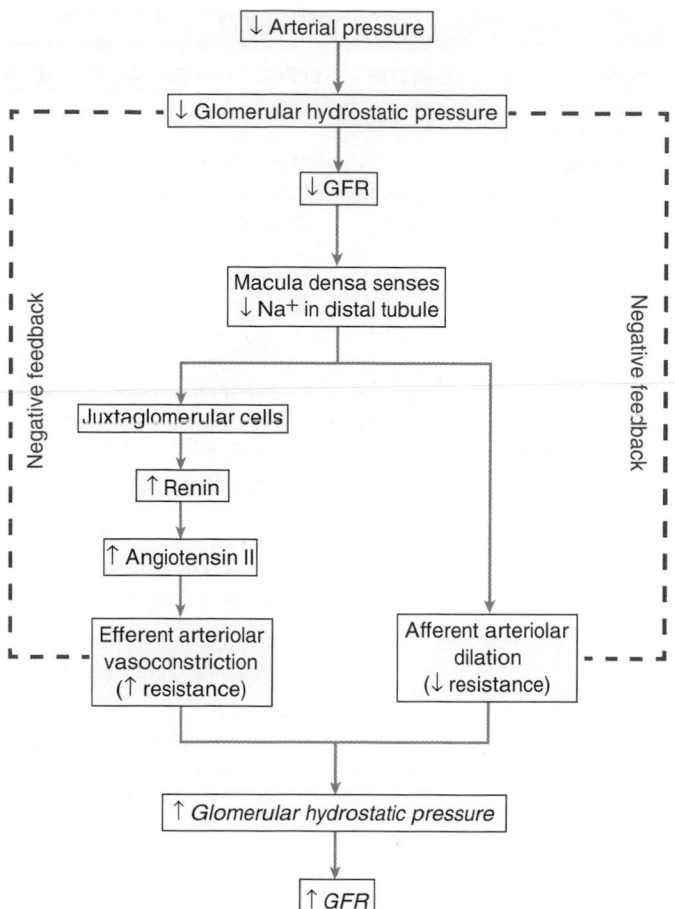

FIGURE 38.10 Tubuloglomerular Feedback. See text for details. *GFR*, Glomerular filtration rate.

is reabsorbed and returned to the circulation by the peritubular capillaries.

The GFR is directly related to renal blood flow (RBF), which is regulated by intrinsic autoregulatory mechanisms, neural regulation, and hormonal regulation. In general, blood flow to any organ is determined by the arteriovenous pressure differences across the vascular bed. If mean arterial pressure decreases or vascular resistance increases, RBF declines and urinary output decreases. Normal urinary output is about 30 mL/hour minimum in adults or 0.5 to 1.0 mL/kg/hr.

Autoregulation of Renal Blood Flow

In the kidney a local mechanism tends to keep the rate of glomerular perfusion and therefore the GFR fairly constant over a range of arterial pressures between 80 and 180 mmHg (Fig. 38.9). Changes in afferent arteriolar pressure and resistance occur in the same direction. Therefore, intrarenal blood flow and GFR are relatively constant independent of renal perfusion pressure, a relationship maintained by an intrinsic autoregulatory myogenic mechanism of contraction when blood vessels are stretched. The purpose of autoregulation of intrarenal blood flow is to keep RBF and GFR constant when there are increases or decreases in systemic blood pressure. Solute and water excretion, and thus blood volume, are regulated despite arterial pressure changes, and barotrauma is prevented in states of high systemic blood pressure.[5]

A second mechanism of autoregulation of RBF and GFR is tubuloglomerular feedback. Because the glomerular filtration rate in an individual nephron increases or decreases in relation to changing arterial pressure, the macula densa cells of the juxtaglomerular apparatus in the distal tubule sense the increasing or decreasing amounts of filtered sodium. When GFR and sodium concentration decrease, the macula densa cells stimulate afferent arteriolar vasodilation and increase GFR. At the same time, juxtaglomerular cells secrete renin which results in angiotensin II release causing vasoconstriction of the efferent arterioles increasing glomerular hydrostatic pressure and GFR. The opposite occurs with increases in GFR and sodium concentration at the macula densa (Fig. 38.10). This mechanism prevents large fluctuations in body water and sodium.[5]

Neural Regulation of Renal Blood Flow

The blood vessels of the kidney are innervated by sympathetic nerve fibers located primarily on afferent arterioles. When systemic arterial pressure decreases, increased renal sympathetic nerve activity is mediated reflexively through the carotid sinus and the baroreceptors of the aortic arch. The sympathetic nerves release catecholamines. This stimulates afferent renal arteriolar vasoconstriction and decreases RBF and GFR, increases renal tubular sodium and water reabsorption, and increases blood pressure. Decreased afferent renal sympathetic nerve activity produces the opposite effects. The integrated response regulates water and sodium balance. Renalase is a hormone released by the kidney and heart that may promote the metabolism of catecholamines and in this way participate in blood pressure regulation.[6] The sympathetic nervous system also participates in hormonal (i.e., angiotensin II) regulation of renal blood flow. There is no significant parasympathetic innervation. The innervation of the kidney arises primarily from the celiac ganglion and greater splanchnic nerve.

Hormones and Other Factors Regulating Renal Blood Flow

Hormones and other mediators can alter the resistance of the renal vasculature by stimulating vasodilation or vasoconstriction. A major hormonal regulator of renal blood flow is the renin-angiotensin-aldosterone system (RAAS), which can increase systemic arterial pressure

TABLE 38.1   HORMONES, MEDIATORS, AND RENAL BLOOD FLOW

HORMONE OR MEDIATOR	EFFECT ON RENAL BLOOD FLOW
Adenosine	Produced within kidney; causes vasoconstriction of afferent arteriole; decreases RBF and GFR
Angiotensin II	Produced systemically and within kidneys; constricts afferent and efferent arterioles; decreases RBF and GFR
Atrial and brain natriuretic peptides	Produced by atria and ventricles of the heart with hypertension and increased blood volume; cause vasodilation of afferent arteriole and vasoconstriction of efferent arteriole; modest increase in GFR with little change in RBF
Bradykinin	Produced in kidney from kininogen and causes vasodilation by release of nitric oxide and prostaglandins; increases RBF and GFR
Dopamine	Produced by the proximal tubule; increases RBF; inhibits renin secretion
Endothelin	Produced by renal vessel endothelial cells, mesangial cells, and distal tubule cells in response to bradykinin, angiotensin II, epinephrine, and stretch; most active with renal disease; profound vasoconstriction of afferent and efferent arterioles; decreases RBF and GFR
Histamine	Produced locally within the kidney; modulates RBF in basal state and during inflammation; increases RBF by decreasing afferent and efferent arteriolar resistance and does not decrease GFR
Nitric oxide	Produced by renal vessel endothelial cells with increased stretch and by stimulation of acetylcholine, histamine, bradykinin, ATP; increases vasodilation of afferent and efferent arterioles
Prostaglandins, PGI_2, PGE_2	Produced locally within kidney with decreased RBF; dampen vasoconstriction caused by sympathetic nerves and angiotensin II; prevent harmful vasoconstriction and renal ischemia
Urodilatin (a natriuretic peptide)	Produced by distal tubule and collecting duct when there is increased circulating volume and increased blood pressure; inhibits sodium and water reabsorption from medullary part of collecting duct, thereby producing diuresis

ATP, Adenosine triphosphate; *GFR*, glomerular filtration rate; *PGE2*, prostaglandin E2; *PGI2*, prostaglandin I2; *RBF*, renal blood flow.

and change RBF. Renin is an enzyme formed and stored in granular cells of the afferent arterioles of the JGA[7] (see Fig. 38.3). Renin release is triggered by decreased blood pressure in the afferent arterioles, decreased sodium chloride concentrations in the distal convoluted tubule, sympathetic nerve stimulation of β-adrenergic receptors on the juxtaglomerular cells, and release of prostaglandins.

When renin is released, it cleaves an α-globulin (angiotensinogen produced by liver hepatocytes) in the plasma to form angiotensin I, which is physiologically inactive. In the presence of angiotensin-converting enzyme (ACE) produced from the pulmonary and renal endothelium, angiotensin I is converted to angiotensin II. Angiotensin II stimulates secretion of aldosterone by the adrenal cortex, is a potent vasoconstrictor, and stimulates antidiuretic hormone secretion and thirst (see Chapter 3, Fig. 3.4; and Chapter 21, Fig. 21.20).

Numerous physiologic effects of the RAAS stabilize systemic blood pressure and preserve extracellular fluid volume during hypotension or hypovolemia. Actions include sodium reabsorption, potassium excretion, systemic vasoconstriction, sympathetic nerve stimulation, and thirst stimulation with increased drinking. The effects of aldosterone combine with those of antidiuretic hormone in regulating blood volume.

Natriuretic peptides are a group of peptide hormones, including atrial natriuretic peptide (ANP) secreted from myocardial cells in the atria and brain natriuretic peptide (BNP) secreted from myocardial cells in the cardiac ventricles. They are natural antagonists to the renin-angiotensin-aldosterone system. When the heart dilates during volume expansion or heart failure, ANP and BNP inhibit sodium and water absorption by kidney tubules, inhibit secretion of renin and aldosterone, vasodilate the afferent arterioles, and constrict the efferent arterioles. The result is increased urine formation, leading to decreased blood volume and blood pressure. C-type natriuretic peptide is secreted from vascular endothelium and in the nephron and causes vasodilation.[8]

Urodilatin is a renal natriuretic peptide secreted by the distal convoluted tubules and collecting ducts and causes vasodilation, increased renal blood flow, and diuretic effects. Other hormones and mediators that influence renal blood flow are summarized in Table 38.1.

KIDNEY FUNCTION

Nephron Function

The nephron can perform many functions simultaneously (Fig. 38.11) as follows:

1. Filters plasma at glomerulus.
2. Reabsorbs and secretes different substances along tubular structures.
3. Forms a filtrate of protein-free fluid (ultrafiltration).
4. Regulates the filtrate to maintain body fluid volume, electrolyte composition, and pH within narrow limits.

Glomerular filtration is the movement of fluid and solutes across the glomerular capillary membrane into the Bowman space. Tubular reabsorption is the movement of fluids and solutes from the tubular lumen to the peritubular capillary plasma. Tubular secretion is the transfer of substances from the plasma of the peritubular capillary to the tubular lumen. The transport mechanisms are active as well as passive. Excretion is the elimination of a substance in the final urine (Fig. 38.12).

Glomerular Filtration

The fluid filtered by the glomerular capillary filtration membrane and released into the proximal convoluted tubule is protein-free but contains electrolytes (such as sodium, chloride, and potassium) and organic molecules (such as creatinine, urea, and glucose) in the same concentrations as found in plasma. Like other capillary membranes, the glomerulus is freely permeable to water and relatively impermeable to

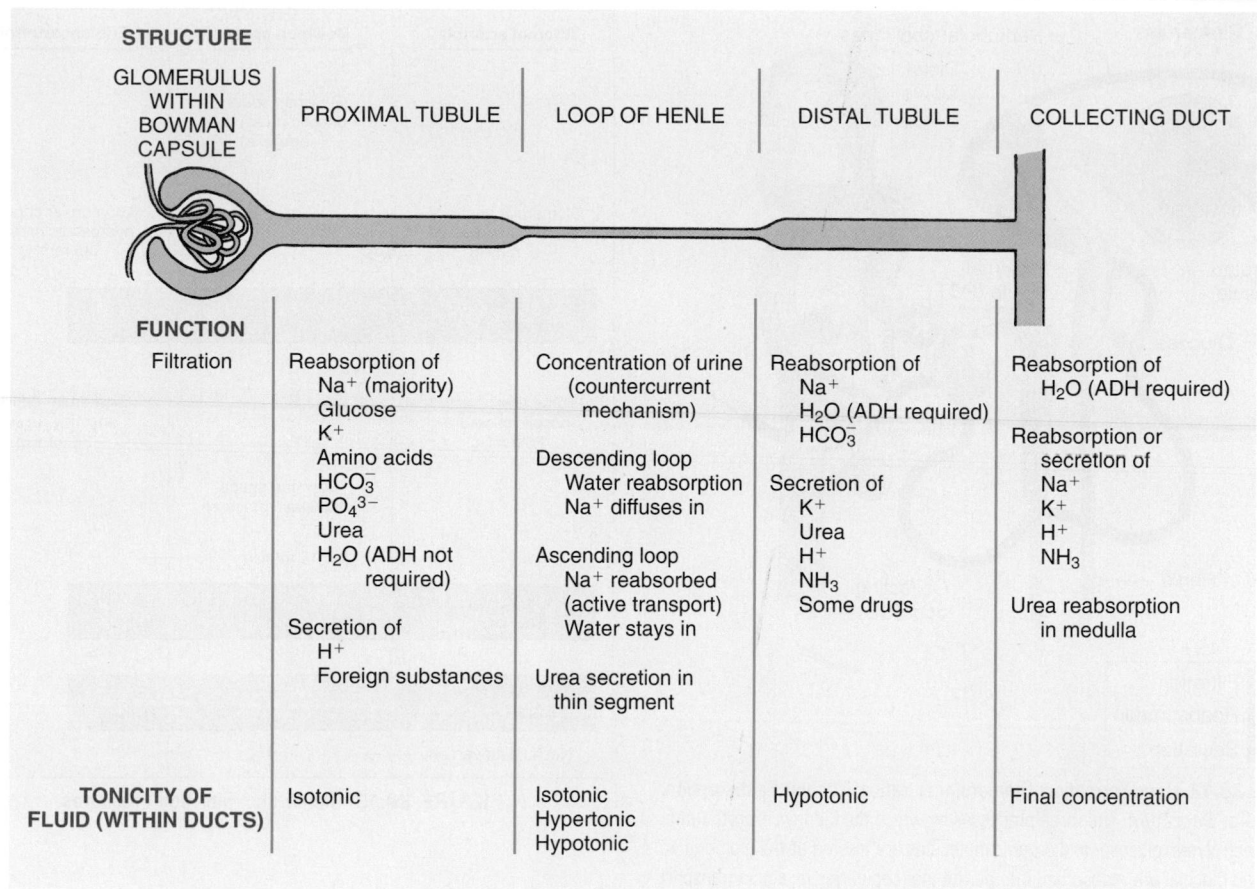

STRUCTURE				
GLOMERULUS WITHIN BOWMAN CAPSULE	PROXIMAL TUBULE	LOOP OF HENLE	DISTAL TUBULE	COLLECTING DUCT
FUNCTION				
Filtration	Reabsorption of Na$^+$ (majority) Glucose K$^+$ Amino acids HCO$_3^-$ PO$_4^{3-}$ Urea H$_2$O (ADH not required) Secretion of H$^+$ Foreign substances	Concentration of urine (countercurrent mechanism) Descending loop Water reabsorption Na$^+$ diffuses in Ascending loop Na$^+$ reabsorbed (active transport) Water stays in Urea secretion in thin segment	Reabsorption of Na$^+$ H$_2$O (ADH required) HCO$_3^-$ Secretion of K$^+$ Urea H$^+$ NH$_3$ Some drugs	Reabsorption of H$_2$O (ADH required) Reabsorption or secretion of Na$^+$ K$^+$ H$^+$ NH$_3$ Urea reabsorption in medulla
TONICITY OF FLUID (WITHIN DUCTS)	Isotonic	Isotonic Hypertonic Hypotonic	Hypotonic	Final concentration

FIGURE 38.11 Major Functions of Nephron Segments. *ADH,* Antidiuretic hormone. (Modified from Hockenberry MJ: *Wong's nursing care of infants and children,* ed 8, St Louis, 2007, Mosby.)

large colloids such as plasma proteins. The molecule's size and electrical charge are important factors, and the small size of the filtration slits in the glomerular epithelium restricts the passage of proteins and other macromolecules. The negative charge along the filtration membrane further impedes the passage of negatively charged macromolecules (because like forces repel each other). Positively charged macromolecules therefore permeate the membrane more readily than neutrally charged particles.

Capillary pressures also affect glomerular filtration. The hydrostatic pressure within the capillary is the major force for moving water and solutes across the filtration membrane into Bowman capsule. This pressure is determined by the systemic arterial pressure and the resistances to blood flow in the afferent and efferent arterioles. Two forces oppose the filtration effects of the glomerular capillary hydrostatic pressure (P_{GC}): (1) the hydrostatic pressure in Bowman space (P_{BC}), and (2) the effective oncotic pressure of the glomerular capillary blood (π_{GC}). Because the fluid in Bowman space normally contains only minute amounts of protein, it usually does not have an oncotic influence on the plasma of the glomerular capillary (Fig. 38.13).

The combined effect of forces favoring and forces opposing filtration determines the filtration pressure. The net filtration pressure (NFP) is the sum of forces favoring and opposing filtration and is expressed by the following equation:

$$NFP = (P_{GC} + \pi_{BC})(\text{forces favoring filtration}) - (P_{BC} + \pi_{GC})$$
$$(\text{forces opposing filtration})$$

The estimated values contributing to the forces of net filtration are presented in Fig. 38.13.

As the protein-free fluid is filtered into Bowman capsule, the plasma oncotic pressure increases and the hydrostatic pressure decreases. The increase in glomerular capillary oncotic pressure is great enough to reduce the net filtration pressure to zero at the efferent end of the capillary and to stop the filtration process effectively. The low hydrostatic pressure and increased oncotic pressure in the efferent arteriole then are transferred to the peritubular capillaries and facilitate reabsorption of fluid from the proximal convoluted tubules.

Filtration Rate. The total volume of fluid filtered by the glomeruli averages 180 L/day, or approximately 120 mL/min, a phenomenal amount considering the size of the kidneys. Because only 1 to 2 L of urine is excreted per day, 99% of the filtrate is reabsorbed into the peritubular capillaries and thus is returned to the blood. The factors determining the GFR are directly related to the pressures that favor or oppose filtration.

Obstruction to the outflow of urine (caused by strictures, stones, or tumors along the urinary tract) can cause a retrograde increase in pressure at Bowman capsule and a decrease in GFR. Low levels of plasma protein in the blood from severe malnutrition or liver disease result in a decrease in the effective oncotic pressure of the glomerular capillary blood (π_{GC}), which increases GFR. Excessive loss of protein-free fluid from vomiting, diarrhea, use of diuretics, or excessive sweating can increase glomerular capillary oncotic pressure and decrease the GFR. Renal disease also can cause changes in pressure relationships by

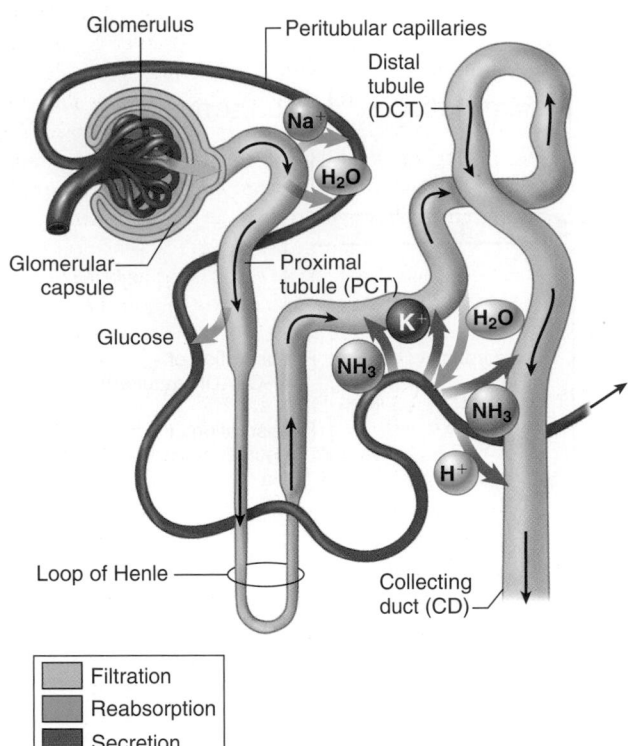

FIGURE 38.12 Urine Formation: Glomerular Filtration, Tubular Reabsorption, and Tubular Secretion. The three processes by which the kidneys excrete urine. Water, electrolytes, glucose, and organic molecules are filtered at the glomerulus. Sodium and glucose are reabsorbed into peritubular capillaries by active transport from the proximal convoluted tubules, and water reabsorption follows by osmosis. Sodium is reabsorbed by active transport from distal convoluted tubules; more sodium is conserved when aldosterone is secreted. Osmotic reabsorption of water from them occurs when antidiuretic hormone (ADH) is present. Secretion of ammonia (NH_3), hydrogen, and potassium occurs from peritubular capillaries into distal tubules by active transport. (From Patton KT, Thibodeau GA: *The human body in health & disease*, ed 7, St Louis, 2018, Mosby.)

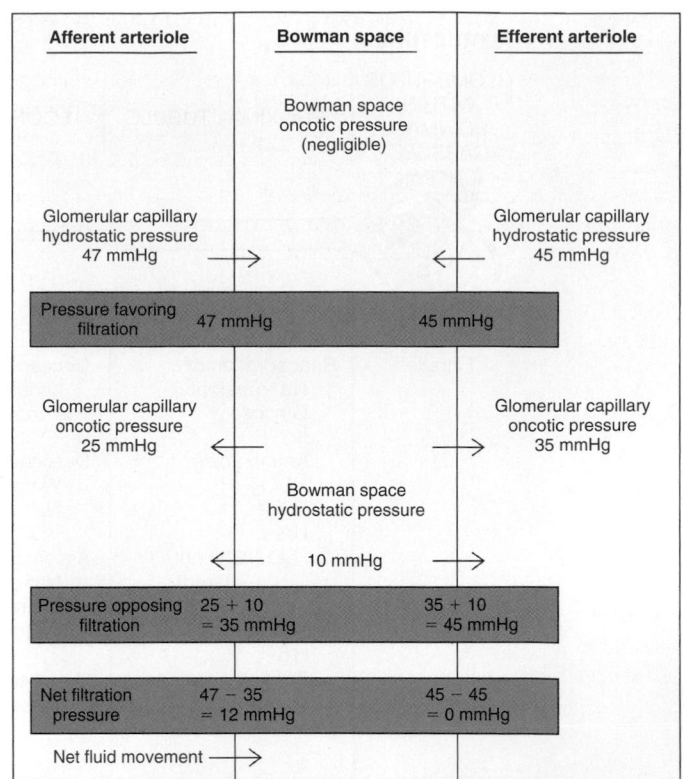

FIGURE 38.13 Glomerular Filtration Pressures.

altering capillary permeability and the surface area available for filtration (see Chapter 39).

Tubular Transport. At the end of the proximal convoluted tubule, approximately 60% to 70% of filtered sodium and water and about 50% of urea have been reabsorbed, along with 90% or more of potassium, glucose, bicarbonate, calcium, phosphate, amino acids, and uric acid. Chloride, water, and urea are reabsorbed passively but are linked to the active transport of sodium (a cotransport mechanism). For some molecules, active transport in the renal tubules is limited as carrier molecules become saturated, a phenomenon known as **transport maximum (Tm)**. For example, when the carrier molecules for glucose reabsorption in the proximal convoluted tubule become saturated (i.e., with the development of hyperglycemia and serum glucose values of 180 mg/dL or greater), the excess will be excreted in the urine.

Proximal Convoluted Tubule. Active reabsorption of sodium is the primary function of the proximal convoluted tubule. Water, most other electrolytes, and organic substances are cotransported with sodium. The osmotic force generated by active sodium transport promotes the passive diffusion of water out of the tubular lumen and into the peritubular capillaries. Passive transport of water is further enhanced by the elevated oncotic pressure of the blood in the peritubular capillaries,

which is created by the previous filtration of water at the glomerulus. The reabsorption of water leaves an increased concentration of urea within the tubular lumen, creating a gradient for its passive diffusion to the peritubular plasma. As the positively charged sodium ions leave the tubular lumen, negatively charged chloride ions passively follow to maintain electroneutrality. Because the inner membrane of the proximal tubular cell has a limited permeability to chloride, chloride reabsorption lags behind that of sodium.

Hydrogen ions are actively exchanged for sodium ions in the tubular lumen. The hydrogen ions (H^+) then combine with bicarbonate (HCO_3^-) in the tubular lumen to form carbonic acid (H_2CO_3).

Bicarbonate is completely filtered at the glomerulus, and approximately 90% is reabsorbed in the proximal tubule. In the tubular lumen, hydrogen and bicarbonate ions combine to form carbonic acid (H_2CO_3), which rapidly breaks down, or dissociates, to carbon dioxide (CO_2) and water (H_2O). CO_2 and H_2O then diffuse into the tubular cell, where carbonic anhydrase again catalyzes the CO_2 and H_2O to form HCO_3^- and H^+. The H^+ is secreted again and HCO_3^- combines with sodium and is transported to the peritubular capillary blood as $NaHCO_3$ (a sodium bicarbonate buffer). Bicarbonate is thus conserved, and the hydrogen is reabsorbed as water (see Fig. 3.14). Therefore, these ions normally do not contribute to the urinary excretion of acid or the addition of acid to the blood.

In addition to the proximal tubular secretion of hydrogen ions, secretory Tms exist for creatinine, other organic bases, and endogenous and exogenous organic acids, including *para*-aminohippurate (PAH) and penicillin (Box 38.1). These secretory mechanisms are important for eliminating drugs and other exogenous chemical products from the body, often after first conjugating them with sulfate and glucuronic acid in the liver. Many drugs and their metabolites are eliminated from the body in this way. When the renal tubules are damaged, metabolic byproducts and drugs may accumulate, causing toxic levels in the body.

Normally, 99% of the glomerular filtrate is reabsorbed. When the GFR spontaneously decreases or increases, the renal tubules and, primarily, the proximal tubules, automatically adjust their rate of reabsorption of sodium and water to balance the change in GFR. Thus a constant fraction of filtered sodium and water is reabsorbed from the proximal tubule. This prevents wide fluctuations in sodium and water excretion into the urine and maintains sodium and water balance and is known as **glomerulotubular balance (GTB)**. GTB and tubuloglomerular feedback (see Renal Blood Flow) together regulate sodium and water balance.

Loop of Henle and Distal Convoluted Tubule. Urine can be hypotonic, isotonic, or hypertonic. Urine concentration or dilution occurs principally in the loop of Henle, distal tubules, and collecting ducts. The structural features of the medullary hairpin loops allow the kidney to concentrate urine and conserve water for the body. The transition of the filtrate into the final urine reflects the concentrating ability of the loops. Final adjustments in urine composition are made by the distal tubule and collecting duct according to body needs.

Production of concentrated urine involves a **countercurrent exchange system**, in which fluid flows in opposite directions through the parallel tubes of the loop of Henle. A concentration gradient in the medulla causes fluid to be exchanged across the parallel pathways. The concentration gradient increases from the cortex to the tip of the medulla. The longer the loops of Henle, the greater their extension into the concentration gradient. The loops multiply the concentration gradient, and the vasa recta blood vessels act as a countercurrent exchanger for maintaining the gradient. The process is initiated in the thick ascending limb of the loop of Henle with the active transport of chloride and sodium out of the tubular lumen and into the medullary interstitium (Fig. 38.14). Because the lumen of the ascending limb is impermeable to water, water cannot follow the sodium chloride transport. This causes the ascending tubular fluid to become hypoosmotic and the medullary interstitium to become hyperosmotic. The descending limb of the loop, which receives fluid from the proximal tubule, is highly permeable to water, but it is the only place in the nephron that does not actively transport either sodium or chloride. Sodium and chloride may, however, diffuse into the descending tubule from the interstitium. The hyperosmotic medullary interstitium causes water to move out of the descending limb, and the remaining fluid in the descending tubule becomes increasingly concentrated while it flows toward the tip of the medulla. While the tubular fluid rounds the loop and enters the ascending limb, sodium and chloride are removed and water is retained. The fluid then becomes more and more dilute as it encounters the distal tubule.

BOX 38.1	SOME SUBSTANCES TRANSPORTED BY RENAL TUBULES	
REABSORPTION	**SECRETION**	
Albumin	Choline	
Ascorbate	Creatinine	
Fructose	Histamine	
	Dopamine	
	Catecholamines	
Galactose	Methyl guanidine	
Glucose	*para*-Aminohippurate	
Glutamate	Penicillin	
Phosphate	Steroid glucuronides	
Sulfate	Thiamine	
	Bile salts	
Xylose		

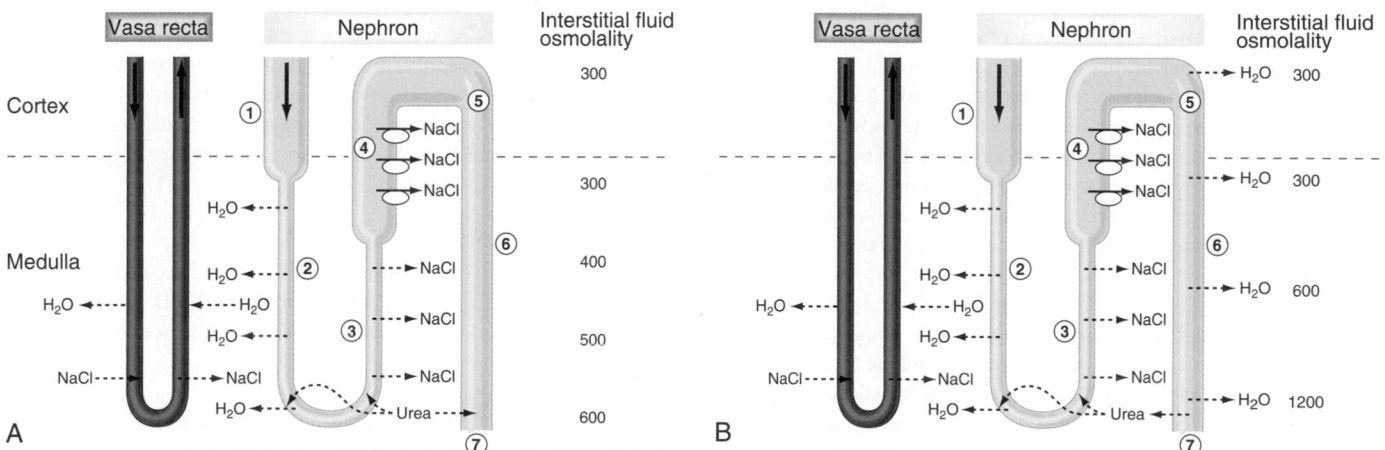

FIGURE 38.14 Countercurrent Mechanism for Diluting and Concentrating Urine. A, Urine dilution; **B,** urine concentration. **1,** Filtrate isotonic to plasma. **2,** Descending thin limb permeable to water. **3,** Ascending thin limb impermeable to water; permeable to ions. **4,** Ascending thick limb actively transports NaCl; impermeable to water and urea. **5,** Distal tubule actively resorbs NaCl; resorbs water in presence of ADH and adjusts the final concentration of the urine. **6,** Medullary CD actively resorbs NaCl, and slightly permeable to water and urea. **7,** Urine is dilute or concentrated depending on concentration of urea and other nonreabsorbed solutes (**NOTE:** Numbers under "Interstitial fluid osmolality" represent milliosmoles [mOsm/kg H₂O] of interstitial fluid.). See text for details. *ADH,* Antidiuretic hormone; *CD,* collecting duct, *NaCl,* sodium chloride, *H₂O,* water. (Adapted from: Koeppen BM, *Renal physiology,* ed 5, St Louis, 2013, Mosby.)

The slow rate of blood flow and the hairpin structure of the vasa recta blood vessels allow blood to flow through the medullary tissue without disturbing the osmotic gradient. When blood flows into the descending limb of the vasa recta, it encounters the increasing osmotic concentration gradient of the medullary interstitium. Water moves out and sodium and chloride diffuse into the descending vasa recta. The plasma becomes increasingly concentrated as it flows toward the tip of the medulla.

As blood flows away from the tip of the medulla and toward the cortex, the surrounding interstitial fluid becomes comparatively more dilute. Water then moves back into the vasa recta, and sodium and chloride diffuse out and the plasma again becomes more dilute. The net result is a preservation of the medullary osmotic gradient. If blood were to flow rapidly through the vasa recta, as occurs in some renal diseases, the medullary concentration gradient would be washed away and the ability to concentrate urine and conserve water would be lost. The efficiency of water conservation is related to the length of the loops of Henle: the longer the loops, the greater the ability to concentrate the urine.

Urea is the major constituent of urine along with water. The glomerulus freely filters urea, and tubular reabsorption depends on urine flow rate, with less reabsorption at higher flow rates. Approximately 50% of urea is excreted in the urine, and 50% is recycled within the kidney. This recycling contributes to the osmotic gradient within the medulla and is necessary for the concentration and dilution of urine (see Fig. 38.14). Because urea is an end product of protein metabolism, individuals with protein deprivation cannot maximally concentrate their urine.[9]

Another function of the loop of Henle is the production of uromodulin (also known as *Tamm-Horsfall protein [THP]*), the most abundant protein in human urine. This protein is produced in the thick ascending loop and binds to uropathogens to prevent urinary tract infection, protects the uroepithelium from injury, protects against kidney stone formation, and is associated with progression of kidney disease.[10]

The convoluted portion of the distal tubule is poorly permeable to water but readily absorbs ions and contributes to the dilution of the tubular fluid. The later, straight segment of the distal tubule and the collecting duct are permeable to water as controlled by antidiuretic hormone released from the posterior pituitary gland. Sodium is readily absorbed by the later segment of the distal tubule and collecting duct under the regulation of the hormone aldosterone (see Chapter 21). Potassium is actively secreted by principal cells and is reabsorbed in lesser amounts by intercalated cells in these segments. Potassium secretion is controlled by aldosterone and other factors related to the concentration of potassium in body fluids.

Hydrogen also is secreted by the distal tubule and combines with non-bicarbonate buffers (i.e., ammonium and phosphate) for the elimination of excess acids in the urine. The distal tubule thus contributes to the regulation of acid-base balance by excreting hydrogen ions into the urine and by adding new bicarbonate to the plasma (see Fig. 3.14). The mechanism is similar to the conservation of bicarbonate by the proximal tubule, except that the hydrogen ion is excreted in the urine. (The specific mechanisms of acid-base balance and acid excretion are described in Chapter 3.)

Urine Composition

Urine is normally clear yellow or amber in color. Cloudiness may indicate the presence of bacteria, cells, or high solute concentration. The pH ranges from 4.6 to 8.0, but it is normally acidic, providing protection against bacteria. Specific gravity ranges from 1.001 to 1.035. Normal urine does not contain glucose or blood cells and only occasionally contains traces of protein, usually in association with rigorous exercise.

Hormones and Nephron Function
Antidiuretic Hormone

The distal tubule in the cortex receives the hypoosmotic urine from the ascending limb of the loop of Henle. The concentration of the final urine is controlled by antidiuretic hormone (ADH), which is secreted from the posterior pituitary, or neurohypophysis. ADH increases water permeability in the last segment of the distal tubule and along the entire length of the collecting ducts, which pass through the inner and outer zones of the medulla. The water diffuses into the ascending limb of the vasa recta and returns to the systemic circulation. The excreted urine can have a high osmotic concentration, up to 1400 mOsm. The volume is normally reduced to about 1% of the amount that was filtered at the glomerulus.

Excess ADH secretion is therefore one cause of oliguria, or diminished excretion of urine, clinically defined as less than 400 mL/day or 30 mL/hr. The syndrome of inappropriate secretion of ADH occurs when the posterior pituitary hypersecretes ADH, resulting in excess water reabsorption and water excess in the plasma (see Chapters 3 and 22). Inadequate secretion of ADH results in diabetes insipidus, and causes the distal tubules and collecting ducts to become impermeable to water. Water remains in the tubular lumen and is excreted as a dilute and large volume of urine. (The mechanism for the regulation of ADH and plasma osmolality is described in Chapters 3 and 21.)

Natriuretic Peptides

The natriuretic peptides (urodilatin, ANP, and BNP) promote diuresis and were described under Hormones and Other Factors Regulating Renal Blood Flow.

Diuretics as a Factor in Urine Flow

A diuretic is any agent that enhances the flow of urine. Clinically, diuretics interfere with renal sodium reabsorption and reduce extracellular fluid volume. Diuretics are commonly used to treat hypertension and edema caused by heart failure, cirrhosis, and nephrotic syndrome.

Diuretics are divided into five general categories: (1) osmotic diuretics, (2) carbonic anhydrase inhibitors (inhibitors of urinary acidification), (3) inhibitors of loop sodium or chloride transport, (4) potassium sparing (i.e., aldosterone receptor antagonists), and (5) aquaretics. (The physiologic mechanism related to each category is summarized in Table 38.2.)

Renal Hormones

The kidneys activate or synthesize hormones that have systemic effects. These hormones include the active form of vitamin D, erythropoietin, renin-angiotensin-aldosterone, and natriuretic hormones.

Vitamin D

Vitamin D is a hormone that can be obtained in the diet or synthesized by the action of ultraviolet radiation (sun exposure) on cholesterol in the skin. These forms of vitamin D_3 (cholecalciferol) are inactive and require two hydroxylations to establish a metabolically active form. The first step occurs in the liver with hydroxylation at carbon-25 (calcifediol), and the second hydroxylation occurs at the first carbon position in the kidneys and is stimulated by parathyroid hormone. The end product is 1,25-dihydroxycholecalciferol, or 1,25-dihydroxy-vitamin D_3 (1,25-OH_2D_3) (calcitriol), the active form of vitamin D.

Calcitriol (1,25-dihydroxy-vitamin D_3) is necessary for the absorption of calcium and phosphate by the small intestine. A decreased plasma calcium level (less than 10 mg/dL) stimulates the secretion of parathyroid

TABLE 38.2	ACTION OF DIURETICS			
DIURETIC	**SITE OF ACTION**	**ACTION**		**SIDE EFFECTS**
Osmotic Diuretic				
Mannitol Glycerol Urea	Proximal tubule	Freely filtered but not reabsorbed; osmotically attracts water and diminishes sodium reabsorption		Hypokalemia, dehydration
Carbonic Anhydrase Inhibitors				
Acetazolamide	Proximal tubule	Inhibits carbonic anhydrase; blocks hydrogen ion secretion and reabsorption of sodium and bicarbonate		Hypokalemia, systemic acidosis, alkaline urine
Inhibitors of Sodium/Chloride Reabsorption (Loop Diuretics)				
Thiazides	Between end of ascending loop and beginning of distal tubule	Blocks sodium and chloride reabsorption; mildly suppresses carbonic anhydrase		Hypokalemia, metabolic alkalosis
Furosemide Ethacrynic acid Torsemide	Thick ascending limb of Henle loop	Blocks active transport of chloride, sodium, and potassium		Hypokalemia, uric acid retention
Bumetanide	Cortical vasodilation	Increased rate of urine formation		Hypokalemia, uric acid retention
Potassium Sparing				
Spironolactone Eplerenone	Distal tubule	Inhibits aldosterone, blocks sodium reabsorption, and results in potassium retention		Hyperkalemia, nausea, confusion, gynecomastia
Triamterene Amiloride	Distal tubule	Blocks sodium reabsorption and inhibits potassium excretion		Nausea, vomiting, headache, and amiloride granulocytopenia, skin rash
Aquaretics				
Vasopressin (V2 receptor) blockers (e.g., conivaptan)	Distal tubule and collecting ducts	Blocks action of antidiuretic hormone		Dehydration

hormone. Parathyroid hormone then stimulates a sequence of events that help restore plasma calcium level back toward normal including:

1. Calcium mobilization from bone
2. Synthesis of 1,25-dihydroxy-vitamin D_3
3. Absorption of calcium from the intestine
4. Increased renal calcium reabsorption
5. Decreased renal phosphate reabsorption

Serum phosphate concentration fluctuations also influence the renal hydroxylation of vitamin D. Decreased levels stimulate active 1,25-dihydroxy-vitamin D_3 formation, and increased levels inhibit formation. This results in compensatory changes in phosphate absorption from bone and the intestine. Individuals with renal disease have a deficiency of 1,25-dihydroxy-vitamin D_3 and manifest symptoms of disturbed calcium and phosphate balance (see Chapters 3 and 39).

Erythropoietin

Erythropoietin is produced by the fetal liver and the adult kidney and is essential for normal erythropoiesis. With decreased oxygen delivery in the kidneys, oxygen-sensing peritubular fibroblasts in the juxtamedullary cortex release erythropoietin, which stimulates the bone marrow to increase the rate of red blood cell production (see Chapter 28). Individuals with chronic renal failure develop anemia related to reduced erythropoietin secretion. Erythropoietin also affects the endothelium and promotes angiogenesis, mitogenesis, and antiapoptosis. It is also antiinflammatory, cytoprotective, and neurotrophic.[11]

TESTS OF RENAL FUNCTION

Renal Clearance

A number of specific renal functions can be measured by renal clearance. Renal clearance techniques determine how much of a substance can

be cleared from the blood by the kidneys per given unit of time. The application of this principle permits an indirect measure of GFR, tubular secretion, tubular reabsorption, and renal blood flow.

Clearance and Glomerular Filtration Rate

The GFR provides the best estimate of functioning renal tissue. Damage to the glomerular membrane or loss of nephrons leads to a corresponding decrease in GFR. The measurement of GFR requires use of a substance that has a stable plasma concentration, is not protein bound, is freely filtered at the glomerulus, does not influence GFR, and is not secreted, reabsorbed, or metabolized by the tubules and is easy to measure. *Inulin* (a fructose polysaccharide) is one substance that meets the criteria for measurement of GFR.

The kidney "clears" inulin from the plasma by filtering it at the glomerulus, reabsorbing nearly all of the fluid, and excreting the inulin left behind in the urine. The amount of inulin filtered is equal to the volume of plasma filtered (GFR) multiplied by the plasma concentration of inulin (P_{IN}). The amount of inulin in the urine is equal to a volume of urine per unit of time $\dot{V}$ (usually 24 hours) multiplied by the inulin concentration of urine (U_{IN}). Because all the inulin filtered is excreted in the urine,

$$GFR \times P_{IN} = U_{IN} \times \dot{V}$$

GFR can be calculated by rearranging the formula:

$$GFR\ (mL/min) = \frac{U_{IN} \times \dot{V}}{P_{IN}}$$

The accurate determination of **insulin clearance** requires constant infusion to maintain a stable plasma level. This is time consuming, inconvenient, and prone to error. Therefore, the clearance of *creatinine*, a natural substance produced by muscle and released into the blood at a relatively constant rate, is commonly used as an estimate clinically. It is freely filtered at the glomerulus and is not reabsorbed by the renal tubules, but a small amount is secreted by the renal tubules. Therefore, creatinine clearance overestimates the GFR but within tolerable limits. Creatinine clearance provides a good estimate of GFR because only one blood sample is required in addition to a 24-hour volume of urine. The GFR estimated by creatinine clearance is calculated as follows:

$$GFR\ (mL/min) = \frac{U_{CR} \times \dot{V}}{P_{CR}}$$

Cystatin C is a stable protein in serum filtered at the glomerulus and metabolized in the tubules. Serum levels of cystatin C also are a marker for estimating GFR, particularly for mild to moderate impaired renal function. A combined creatinine and cystatin C estimate of GFR was developed in 2012 and considers age, race, and gender.[12] Formulas are used to estimate GFR.[13] The Cockcroft and Gault creatinine-based formula is commonly used and considers age, body weight, and plasma creatinine (P_{cr}) values, and the National Kidney Foundation recommends the Modification of Diet in Renal Disease (MDRD) equation.[14] The Chronic Kidney Disease Epidemiology Collaboration (2009 CKD-EPI) equation has been developed as a more precise estimate of GFR than the MDRD and considers age, gender, and race.[15] In 2012, cystatin C and combined creatinine and cystatin C equations were developed. Calculators for estimates of GFR using these formulas are readily available on the Internet (see example at http://touchcalc.com/ip_epi_gfr/ip _ckd_epi). Normal values are 90 to 120 mL/min.

Plasma Creatinine Concentration

A chronic decline in GFR over weeks or months is reflected in the plasma creatinine (P_{CR}) concentration (normal value = 0.7 to 1.2 mg/dL). The P_{CR} concentration has a stable value when the GFR is stable because creatinine has a constant rate of production as a product of muscle metabolism. The amount filtered is approximately equal to the amount excreted. When the GFR declines, the P_{CR} increases proportionately. Thus the GFR and P_{CR} are inversely related. If the GFR were to decrease by 50%, the filtration and excretion of creatinine would be reduced by 50% and creatinine would accumulate in plasma to twice the normal value. Therefore, elevated P_{CR} values represent decreasing GFR. In the new steady state, however, the total amount of creatinine excreted in the urine would remain the same because of the proportionate decrease in GFR and increase in P_{CR}.

The application of this principle is simple and useful for monitoring progressive changes in renal function. The test is most valuable for monitoring the progress of chronic rather than acute renal disease because it takes 7 to 10 days for the plasma creatinine level to stabilize when GFR declines. Serial measures can be obtained over a long time and plotted as a curve of glomerular function. Normal P_{CR} value decreases with advanced age, since older adults experience a decrease in lean muscle mass. The P_{CR} value becomes elevated during trauma or breakdown of muscle tissue. In such instances the value is then not useful for estimating GFR.

Blood Urea Nitrogen

The concentration of urea nitrogen in the blood reflects glomerular filtration and urine-concentrating capacity. Because urea is filtered at the glomerulus, blood urea nitrogen (BUN) levels increase as glomerular filtration drops. Because urea is reabsorbed by the blood through the permeable tubules, the BUN value rises in states of dehydration and acute and chronic renal failure when passage of fluid through the tubules is slowed. BUN value also varies as a result of altered protein intake and protein catabolism and therefore is a poor measure of GFR. The normal range for BUN value in the adult is 10 to 20 mg/dL of blood.

Clearance and Renal Blood Flow

A clearance formula also can be used to estimate renal plasma flow (RPF) and RBF using a molecule called *para*-aminohippuric acid (PAH). Some PAH is filtered at the glomerulus, and most of the remainder is secreted into the tubules in one circulation through the kidney. If all the PAH were removed from the plasma during a single pass through the kidney, total RPF could be determined. Because the supporting and nonsecreting structures of the kidney receive 10% to 15% of effective renal blood flow (ERBF), clearance of PAH measures only what is known as the effective renal plasma flow (ERPF), which is 85% to 90% of the true renal plasma flow:

$$ERPF = \frac{U_{PAH} \times \dot{V}}{P_{PAH}}$$

where U_{PAH} = concentration of PAH in urine, and P_{PAH} = concentration of PAH in plasma.

The estimation of ERBF can then be calculated by considering the hematocrit in the following formula:

$$ERBF = \frac{ERPF}{1 - Hematocrit}$$
$$(1.0 - 0.45)$$

Evaluation of the biochemical components of the blood and urine provides valuable information regarding renal function.

Urinalysis

Urinalysis is a noninvasive and relatively inexpensive diagnostic procedure. The best results are obtained from a fresh, cleanly voided specimen because decay permits changes in the composition of urine. Urinalysis includes evaluation of color, turbidity, protein, pH, specific gravity, sediment, and supernatant.

Urine color is normally a clear, light yellow because of urochrome and other pigments. When formed substances (crystals, blood cells, or casts) are in the urine, it appears turbid. Protein in the urine creates marked foaming when shaken, and the foam is yellow or orange when the urine contains bile pigments. Urine does not normally contain protein or bile.

Urine pH normally ranges between 5 and 6.5, but it may vary from 4.5 to 8. Urine is more alkaline after eating and then becomes less alkaline before the next meal. Because sleep is accompanied by intermittent hypoventilation, urine is more acidic on awakening.

Specific gravity is an estimated measure of the solute concentration of the urine. The specific gravity of any solution is measured by comparing the weight of the solution with an equal volume of distilled water. Hence specific gravity is not a true measure of the number or concentration of particles, but it correlates well with osmolality and is a useful clinical tool. Specific gravity usually is measured with a hydrometer in a cylinder of urine; the normal value is 1.016 to 1.022. Dipstick evaluations may be falsely high when urine pH is less than 6 and falsely low when the pH is more than 7.

The final urine osmolality is primarily a function of ADH, which controls water reabsorption in the collecting ducts. If the kidney is unable to concentrate or dilute urine, given a stimulus, the cause is usually a malfunction of the renal tubules or inappropriate ADH secretion by the posterior pituitary gland. The state of hydration also affects the urine specific gravity, so hydration status should be evaluated before making a diagnosis. This determination is helpful for differentiating oliguria caused by intrinsic renal disease from hypovolemia as a result of dehydration.

Urine Sediment

The urine sediment is examined microscopically and may contain cells, casts, crystals, and bacteria. Epithelial cells may be seen in the microscopic field because they are shed naturally throughout the urinary tract.

Red Blood Cells. Normal urine contains few or no red blood cells. If a large number of red cells are present, this is known as hematuria, and the sediment may be red or brown. An alkaline or hypotonic urine causes lysis of red cells, however, so that the cells will not be seen. Urine then will be positive for hemoglobin, and the specific gravity will be elevated. Hematuria can occur with the administration of anticoagulants and with several renal diseases.

Casts. Casts (accumulations of cellular precipitates) originate in the renal tubules, from which they take their shape. They are cylindrical with distinct borders. All casts have a precipitated microprotein matrix and arise primarily from the ascending limb of the distal tubule. Red cell casts indicate bleeding into the tubules or escape of red blood cells through the glomerulus; white cell casts are associated with an inflammatory process. Epithelial cell casts indicate degeneration of the tubular lumen or necrosis of the renal tubules. The type of cast identified suggests the disease process occurring in the kidney.

Crystals. Numerous kinds of crystals can be observed in the urine. They may be composed of cystine, uric acid, calcium oxalate, or phosphate. They may not be initially observable, but as the urine cools, crystals will form. Crystals tend to form in a concentrated acidic or alkaline urine. Generally they are not clinically significant. Crystal formation is diagnostically significant, usually indicating inflammation, infection, or a metabolic disorder.

White Blood Cells. White blood cells (WBCs) in the urine (a condition termed pyuria) are indicative of urinary tract infection, particularly when bacteria are present. Glomerulonephritis and nephrotic syndrome also may demonstrate pyuria but usually in combination with proteinuria, red cells, and casts. The finding of WBC casts reflects a kidney infection because these casts are not formed in the bladder or prostate. If WBCs are present in the urine, a culture should be done for specific identification of bacteria and sensitivity of bacteria to antibiotics.

Other Measures

Dipsticks and reagent strips are available for detecting other substances in the urine, including glucose, bilirubin, urobilinogen, leukocyte esterase and nitrates, ketones, proteins, hemoglobin, and myoglobin.

AGING AND RENAL FUNCTION

Throughout life the kidney responds to an increased workload by compensatory hypertrophy. This hypertrophy is marked in individuals who have donated a kidney for transplant or have lost functioning nephrons from trauma or disease. The glomeruli increase in diameter, and the tubules enlarge effectively to maintain the regulatory functions of the kidney. Hypertrophy occurs more rapidly and with a larger size increase in younger individuals and in those with high protein intake.

Changes in the kidneys occur throughout life, resulting in a reduction in size and a linear decrease in renal blood flow and GFR; however, it is less pronounced in healthy individuals. Reference values for estimated GFR are available by age group.[16]

The number and size of nephrons decrease with aging, possibly related to oxidative stress, inflammation, and associated clinical conditions (e.g., hypertension and diabetes mellitus). The primary mechanism appears to be a change in the renal vasculature and perfusion patterns related to atherosclerosis that leads to a reduction in numbers of nephrons and nephrosclerosis. Tubular atrophy also occurs. The rate of nephron loss accelerates after 50 years of age. By about 75 years of age, the nephron population is reduced by 30% to 50% with loss of renal mass occurring primarily in the cortex.[17] Degenerative changes within nephrons also occur with aging. The glomerular capillaries become sclerotic, and remaining glomeruli become hypertrophic. The glomeruli may disappear completely. The arcuate and interlobular arteries become tortuous, contributing to ischemia. The loss of the glomerular tuft may cause a shunt between the afferent and efferent arterioles. Although loss of juxtaglomerular nephrons still allows the vasa recta to be perfused, the combination of events contributes to a reduced ability to excrete a concentrated urine.[18,19] Thus the specific gravity of the urine in older individuals tends to be on the low side of normal.

Tubular transport changes with aging, although under normal conditions the tubules function adequately. Adaptation to stressful conditions is more difficult. Glucose, bicarbonate, and sodium are not as efficiently reabsorbed, and hyperkalemia is more common because of decreased secretion. Response to acid or base loads is delayed and prolonged. Sudden or large changes in pH or fluid load may lead to serious imbalances with increased risk of hypervolemia or hypovolemia. Acute losses or chronic fluid deficits can lead to renal insufficiency in the older adult. Administration of drugs eliminated by renal processes may require dose modifications and more astute observations for toxic side effects. Contrast agents and nonsteroidal antiinflammatory drugs should be used with caution.

The Tm for glucose reabsorption decreases with age, contributing to a greater amount of glucose in the urine. This is an important consideration when glycosuria is used for screening or monitoring the process of diabetes mellitus in older adults. These changes occur independently of disease, however, indicating a normal process of aging. An age-related decline in renal activation of vitamin D decreases intestinal absorption of calcium, and older adults need more vitamin D to overcome diminishing renal function.[20] Previous or concurrent renal disease or urinary tract obstruction may amplify age-related changes in function.

Bladder symptoms are common among older adults and include frequency, urgency, and nocturia. Ischemic-induced neurogenic and myogenic changes in bladder structure and function may contribute to some symptoms as well as influences outside the urinary tract (i.e., cardiovascular disease, prostatic disease, uterine prolapse, stool impaction and hormonal changes). Changes in neurotransmission influence the micturition reflex and may lead to an overactive or underactive bladder.[21,22]

SUMMARY REVIEW

Structures of the Renal System

1. The primary functions of the kidney are to maintain fluid, electrolyte, acid-base, and blood pressure balance; excrete wastes; secrete the hormones renin and erythropoietin; and activate vitamin D.

2. The kidneys are paired structures lying in the retroperitoneal space between the twelfth thoracic and third lumbar vertebrae.

3. The kidney is composed of a capsule, an outer cortex containing the glomeruli, and an inner medulla containing the tubules and collecting ducts that drain into the calyces.

4. The calyces join to form the renal pelvis and are continuous with the upper end of the ureter.
5. The nephron is the urine-forming unit of the kidney and is composed of the glomerulus, proximal tubule, hairpin loops of Henle, distal tubule, and collecting duct.
6. The glomerulus contains loops of capillaries contained in the Bowman capsule. The capillary walls serve as a filtration membrane for the formation of the primary urine. The layers of the glomerular capillary include the endothelium, basement membrane, and epithelium. The epithelium is composed of podocytes that interlock to provide filtration slits. An anion charge across the filtration membrane restricts filtration of negatively charged molecules such as proteins.
7. Mesangial cells and matrix lie between and support the glomerular capillaries in the Bowman capsule.
8. Juxtaglomerular cells secrete renin and are located around the afferent arteriole. They are contiguous with the sodium-sensing macula densa cells of the distal convoluted tubule.
9. The Bowman capsule is the space between the visceral and parietal epithelium.
10. The proximal tubule is lined with microvilli to increase surface area and enhance reabsorption.
11. The hairpin-shaped loops of Henle selectively transport solutes and water, contributing to the hypertonic state of the medulla important for the concentration of urine.
12. The distal tubule adjusts acid-base balance by excreting acid into the urine and forming new bicarbonate ions.
13. The collecting duct contains principal cells that resorb sodium and water and excrete potassium and intercalated cells that secrete hydrogen or bicarbonate and potassium.
14. The ureters extend from the renal pelvis to the posterior wall of the bladder. Urine flows through the ureters by means of peristaltic contraction of the ureteral muscles.
15. The bladder is a bag composed of the detrusor and trigone muscles and innervated by branches of parasympathetic (contracts the bladder and relaxes the urethra), sympathetic (relaxes the bladder and contracts the proximal urethral sphincter), and somatic (striated urethral sphincter) pathways. When accumulation of urine reaches 250 to 300 mL, mechanoreceptors, which respond to stretching of tissue, stimulate the micturition reflex.

Renal Blood Flow

1. Renal blood flows at about 1000 to 1200 mL/min, or 20% to 25% of the cardiac output.
2. Blood flow through the glomerular capillaries is maintained at a constant rate in spite of a wide range of systemic arterial pressures (autoregulation).
3. The GFR is the filtration of plasma per unit of time and is directly related to the perfusion pressure of renal blood flow.
4. The renal blood vessels are innervated by the sympathetic noradrenergic nerves that regulate vasoconstriction.
5. Autoregulation of RBF and sympathetic neural regulation of vasoconstriction maintain a constant GFR.
6. Renin is an enzyme secreted from juxtaglomerular cells in the afferent arteriole; it causes the generation of angiotensin I, which is converted to angiotensin II by the action of ACE. Angiotensin II is a potent vasoconstrictor and also stimulates release of aldosterone from the adrenal cortex. Thus the renin-angiotensin-aldosterone system is a regulator of renal blood flow and blood pressure.

7. Natriuretic peptides from the myocardium antagonize the renin-angiotensin-aldosterone system and promote sodium chloride and water excretion.

Kidney Function

1. The major function of the nephron is urine formation, which involves the processes of glomerular filtration, tubular reabsorption, and tubular secretion and excretion.
2. Glomerular filtration is favored by capillary hydrostatic pressure and opposed by oncotic pressure in the capillary and hydrostatic pressure in the Bowman capsule. The balance of favoring and opposing filtration forces is the net filtration pressure (NFP).
3. The GFR is approximately 120 mL/min, and 99% of the filtrate is reabsorbed.
4. The proximal convoluted tubule reabsorbs about 60% to 70% of the filtered sodium and water and 90% of other electrolytes.
5. Because most molecules are reabsorbed by active transport, the carrier mechanism can become saturated at the Tm. Molecules not reabsorbed are excreted with the urine.
6. The distal tubules actively reabsorb sodium and water and secrete potassium and hydrogen for the regulation of fluid, electrolyte, and acid-base balance.
7. The concentration of the final urine is a function of the level of ADH that stimulates the distal tubules and collecting ducts to reabsorb water. The countercurrent exchange system of the long loops of Henle and their accompanying capillaries establishes a concentration gradient within the renal medulla to facilitate the reabsorption of water from the collecting duct.
8. The distal nephron regulates acid-base balance by excreting hydrogen ions and forming new bicarbonate.
9. The kidney secretes or activates a number of hormones that have systemic effects, including vitamin D_3 ($1,25-OH_2D_3$) which promotes calcium absorption in the gut, and erythropoietin, which stimulates erythropoiesis when there is hypoxia.

Tests of Renal Function

1. Tests that measure renal clearance indicate how much of a substance can be cleared from the blood by the kidneys per given amount of time.
2. Creatinine, a substance produced by muscle, is measured in plasma and urine to calculate a commonly used clinical estimate of GFR (creatinine clearance).
3. The plasma creatinine concentration, cystatin C plasma concentration, and BUN levels estimate glomerular function. Plasma creatinine and cystatin C are measured to monitor progressive renal dysfunction; BUN is an indicator of hydration status.
4. PAH clearance is used to determine renal plasma flow and blood flow.
5. Urinalysis involves evaluation of color, turbidity, protein, pH, specific gravity, sediment, and supernatant.
6. Presence of bacteria, red blood cells, white blood cells, casts, or crystals in the urine sediment may indicate a renal disorder.

Aging and Renal Function

1. As a person ages, a decrease occurs in the number and size of nephrons. Renal blood flow and glomerular filtration rate decline.
2. Tubular transport and reabsorption decrease with age. Response to acid-base changes and reabsorption of glucose are delayed. Drugs eliminated by the kidney can accumulate in the plasma, causing toxic reactions.
3. Neurogenic and myogenic changes in the bladder may lead to symptoms of urgency and frequency or urine retention.

KEY TERMS

Afferent arteriole, 1232
Angiotensin II, 1236
Antidiuretic hormone (ADH), 1240
Arcuate artery, 1232
Atrial natriuretic peptide (ANP), 1236
Autoregulation of intrarenal blood flow, 1235
Bladder, 1234
Blood urea nitrogen (BUN), 1242
Bowman capsule, 1230
Bowman space (urinary space), 1231
Brain natriuretic peptide (BNP), 1236
Calcitriol (1,25-dihydroxy-vitamin D_3), 1240
Cast, 1243
Collecting duct, 1231
Cortex, 1229
Countercurrent exchange system, 1239
Creatinine clearance, 1242
Crystal, 1243
C-type natriuretic peptide, 1236
Cystatin C, 1242
Detrusor muscle, 1234
Distal tubule, 1231
Diuretic, 1240
Effective renal blood flow (ERBF), 1242
Effective renal plasma flow (ERPF), 1242
Efferent arteriole, 1233
Excretion, 1236
External urethral sphincter, 1234
Filtration slit, 1230
Glomerular capillary, 1232
Glomerular filtration membrane, 1230

Glomerular filtration rate (GFR), 1234
Glomerulus, 1230
Glomerulotubular balance (GTB), 1239
Hematuria, 1243
Hilum, 1229
Insulin clearance, 1241
Intercalated cell, 1231
Interlobar artery, 1232
Internal urethral sphincter, 1234
Juxtaglomerular apparatus (JGA), 1231
Juxtaglomerular cell, 1231
Juxtamedullary nephron, 1229
Kidney, 1228
Loop of Henle, 1231
Macula densa, 1231
Major calyx, 1229
Medulla, 1229
Mesangial cell, 1230
Mesangial matrix, 1230
Micturition, 1234
Midcortical nephron, 1229
Minor calyx, 1229
Natriuretic peptide, 1236
Nephron, 1229
Net filtration pressure (NFP), 1237
Oliguria, 1240
Parietal epithelium (parietal layer), 1230
Peritubular capillary, 1233
Plasma creatinine (P_{CR}) concentration, 1242
Podocyte, 1230
Principal cell, 1231

Proximal convoluted tubule, 1231
Pyramid, 1229
Pyuria, 1243
Renal artery, 1232
Renalase, 1235
Renal capsule, 1229
Renal column, 1229
Renal corpuscle, 1230
Renal fascia, 1229
Renal papillae, 1234
Renal pelvis, 1229
Renal vein, 1233
Slit membrane, 1230
Specific gravity, 1242
Superficial cortical nephron, 1229
Transport maximum (Tm), 1238
Trigone, 1234
Tubular reabsorption, 1236
Tubular secretion, 1236
Tubuloglomerular feedback, 1235
Urea, 1240
Ureter, 1234
Urethra, 1234
Urinalysis, 1242
Urine color, 1242
Urine pH, 1242
Urodilatin, 1236
Uroepithelium (transitional epithelium), 1234
Vasa recta, 1233
Visceral epithelium (visceral layer), 1230
Vitamin D, 1240

REFERENCES

1. Abboud HE: Mesangial cell biology. *Exp Cell Res* 318(9):979–985, 2012.
2. Miner JH: The glomerular basement membrane. *Exp Cell Res* 318(9):973–978, 2012.
3. Garg P, Holzman LB: Podocytes: gaining a foothold. *Exp Cell Res* 318(9):955–963, 2012.
4. Merrill L, et al: Receptors, channels, and signalling in the urothelial sensory system in the bladder. *Nat Rev Urol* 13(4):193–204, 2016.
5. Carlström M, Wilcox CS, Arendshorst WJ: Renal autoregulation in health and disease. *Physiol Rev* 95(2):405–511, 2015.
6. Moran GR: The catalytic function of renalase: a decade of phantoms. *Biochim Biophys Acta* 1864(1):177–186, 2016.
7. Stefanska A, et al: Human kidney pericytes produce renin. *Kidney Int* 90(6):1251–1261, 2016.
8. Kobalava Z: SP 04-1 the role of natriuretic peptides in the pathogenesis of cardiovascular diseases. *J Hypertens* 34(Suppl 1):e377, 2016.
9. Weiner ID, Mitch WE, Sands JM: Urea and ammonia metabolism and the control of renal

nitrogen excretion. *Clin J Am Soc Nephrol* 10(8):1444–1458, 2015.
10. Scolari F, Izzi C, Ghiggeri GM: Uromodulin: from monogenic to multifactorial diseases. *Nephrol Dial Transplant* 30(8):1250–1256, 2015.
11. Nekoui A, Blaise G: Erythropoietin and nonhematopoietic effects. *Am J Med Sci* 353(1):76–81, 2017.
12. Stevens PE, et al: Evaluation and management of chronic kidney disease: synopsis of the kidney disease: improving global outcomes 2012 clinical practice guideline. *Ann Intern Med* 158(11):825–830, 2013.
13. Levey AS, et al: GFR estimation: from physiology to public health. *Am J Kidney Dis* 63(5):820–834, 2014.
14. Botev R, et al: Estimating glomerular filtration rate: Cockcroft-Gault and modification of diet in renal disease formulas compared to renal insulin clearance. *Clin J Am Soc Nephrol* 4(5):899–906, 2009.

15. Levey AS, et al: A new equation to estimate glomerular filtration rate. *Ann Intern Med* 150(9):604–612, 2009.
16. Hallan SI, et al: Age and association of kidney measures with mortality and end-stage renal disease. *J Am Med Assoc* 308(22):2349–2360, 2012.
17. O'Neill WC: Structure, not just function. *Kidney Int* 85(3):503–505, 2014.
18. Denic A, Glassock RJ, Rule AD: Structural and functional changes with the aging kidney. *Adv Chronic Kidney Dis* 23(1):19–28, 2016.
19. O'Sullivan ED, Hughes J, Ferenbach DA: Renal aging: causes and consequences. *J Am Soc Nephrol* 28(2):407–420, 2017.
20. Veldurthy V, et al: Vitamin D, calcium homeostasis and aging. *Bone Res* 4:16041, 2016.
21. Ranson RN, Saffrey MJ: Neurogenic mechanisms in bladder and bowel ageing. *Biogerontology* 16(2):265–284, 2015.
22. Vahabi B, et al: Can we define and characterize the aging lower urinary tract?-ICI-RS 2015. *Neurourol Urodyn* 36(4):854–858, 2015.

CHAPTER 39

Alterations of Renal and Urinary Tract Function

Sue E. Huether

evolve WEBSITE

http://evolve.elsevier.com/McCance/
- Content Updates
- Chapter Summary Review
- Review Questions
- Case Studies
- Animations

CHAPTER OUTLINE

Renal and urinary function can be affected by a variety of disorders. The most common type of urinary dysfunction is infection. Stones, tumors, or the associated inflammatory edema also can obstruct the urinary tract. Renal function can be impaired by disorders of the kidney itself or by many other systemic diseases and ultimately may result in acute kidney injury or chronic kidney disease. Because the kidney filters the blood, it is directly linked to every other organ system. Renal failure, whether acute or chronic, is a life-threatening condition.

URINARY TRACT OBSTRUCTION

Urinary tract obstruction is an interference with the flow of urine at any site along the urinary tract (Fig. 39.1). An obstruction may be anatomic or functional. The obstruction impedes urine flow, increases hydrostatic pressure and dilates structures proximal to the obstruction, increases risk for infection, and compromises renal function. Anatomic changes in the urinary system caused by obstruction are referred to as **obstructive uropathy**. The severity of an obstructive uropathy is

determined by (1) the location of the obstructive lesion, (2) the involvement of one or both upper urinary tracts (ureters and renal pelvis), (3) the completeness of the obstruction, (4) the duration of the obstruction, and (5) the nature of the obstructive lesion. Obstructions may be relieved or partially alleviated by correction of the obstruction, although permanent impairments occur if a complete or partial obstruction persists over weeks to months or longer.

Upper Urinary Tract Obstruction

Common causes of upper urinary tract obstruction include stricture or congenital compression of a calyx or the ureteropelvic or ureterovesical junction (e.g., stones [calculi]); ureteral compression from an aberrant vessel, tumor, or abdominal inflammation and scarring (retroperitoneal fibrosis); or ureteral blockage from stones or a malignancy of the renal pelvis or ureter.

Obstruction of the upper urinary tract causes increased hydrostatic pressure, dilation of the ureter, renal pelvis, calyces, and renal parenchyma proximal to the site of urinary blockage. The increased pressure is

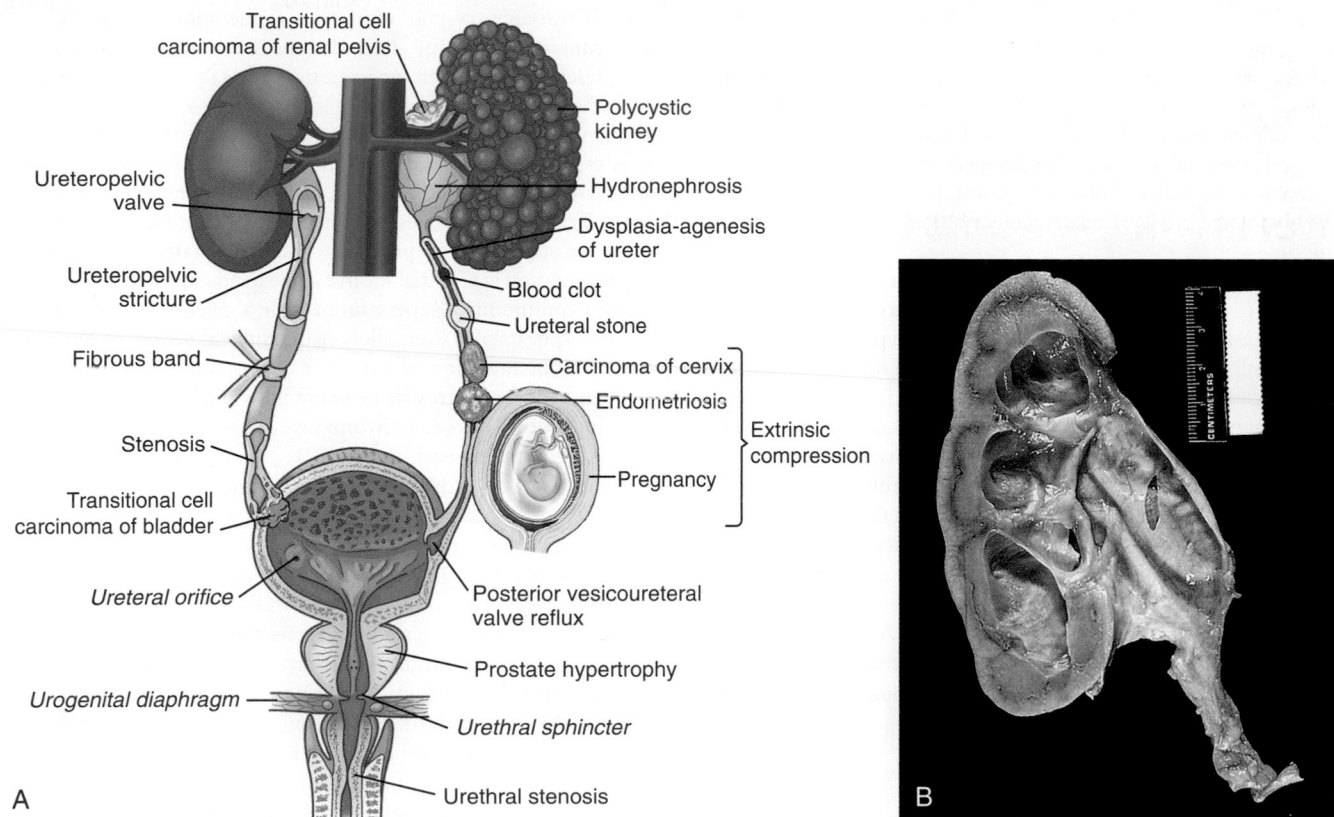

FIGURE 39.1 Urinary Tract Obstruction and Hydronephrosis. A, Causes of urinary tract obstruction. Terms in italics are normal structures. **B,** Hydronephrosis, marked dilation of renal pelvis and calyces with thinning of parenchyma. (**B** from Kumar V et al: *Robbins and Cotran pathologic basis of disease*, ed 9, Philadelphia, 2015, Saunders.)

transmitted to the glomerulus, which decreases glomerular blood flow and, ultimately, decreases glomerular filtration rate (GFR). Dilation of the ureter is referred to as **hydroureter** (accumulation of urine in the ureter), and dilation of the renal pelvis and calyces proximal to a blockage leads to **hydronephrosis** (enlargement of the renal pelvis and calyces) or **ureterohydronephrosis** (dilation of both the ureter and the pelvicaliceal system) (see Fig. 31.1, *B*). Dilation of the upper urinary tract is an early response to obstruction and includes smooth muscle hypertrophy and accumulation of urine above the level of blockage (urinary stasis/retention). Unless the obstruction is relieved, this dilation leads to enlargement with tubulointerstitial fibrosis and apoptosis affecting the renal nephrons and can lead to chronic kidney disease.

Tubulointerstitial fibrosis is the deposition of excessive amounts of extracellular matrix (collagen and other proteins) by activated fibroblasts with associated areas of tubular atrophy. Deposition of extracellular matrix is a normal process of kidney repair and maintenance, and the deposition of extracellular matrix is normally balanced by its breakdown under the influence of metalloproteinases. The dysregulated repair of tubulointerstitial fibrosis results from activation of multiple cytokines, and growth factors have been implicated in the process of tubulointerstitial fibrosis and irreversible loss of kidney function, including transforming growth factor-beta-1 (TGF-β1), angiotensin II, aldosterone, and various tumor necrosis factors.[1,2] **Apoptosis** is a normal process that the body uses to replace damaged or senescent cells with new ones (see Chapter 1), but the imbalance in growth factors provoked by obstruction leads to excess cellular destruction and death, ultimately resulting in loss of functioning nephrons and kidney damage.

Tubulointerstitial fibrosis and apoptosis result in detectable damage to the distal renal tubules within approximately 7 days. By 14 days, obstruction has adversely affected both distal and proximal aspects of the nephron. Within 28 days the glomeruli of the kidney have been damaged and the renal cortex and medulla are reduced in size (thinned). Distal tubular damage occurs initially and decreases the kidney's ability to concentrate urine, causing an increase in urine volume despite a decrease in GFR. The affected kidney is unable to conserve sodium, bicarbonate, and water or to excrete hydrogen or potassium, leading to metabolic acidosis and dehydration. The magnitude of this damage, and the kidney's ability to recover normal homeostatic function, is affected by the severity and duration of the obstruction. With complete obstruction, damage to the renal tubules and compression of the renal vasculature occur in a matter of hours, and irreversible damage occurs within 3 to 4 weeks. Nevertheless, even in the face of a complete obstruction, the human kidney may recover at least partial homeostatic function provided the blockage is removed within 56 to 69 days.[3] This recovery requires approximately 4 months. Partial obstruction, in the absence of renal infection, leads to subtler but ultimately permanent impairments including loss of the kidney's ability to concentrate urine, reabsorb bicarbonate, excrete ammonia, or regulate metabolic acid-base balance if the obstruction is not relieved. Complete bilateral obstruction causes anuria because the retrograde increase in tubular hydrostatic pressure completely opposes glomerular filtration.

The body is able to partially counteract the negative consequences of unilateral obstruction by a process called **compensatory hypertrophy** and **hyperfunction**.[4] The compensatory response is the result of compensatory growth that occurs under the influence of a hormone or hormones that have not yet been identified. Compensatory growth causes the contralateral (unobstructed) kidney to increase the size and function of individual glomeruli and tubules but not the total number of functioning nephrons. The ability of the body to engage in compensatory hypertrophy and hyperfunction diminishes with age, and the process is reversible when relief of obstruction results in recovery of function by the obstructed kidney. Unilateral obstruction may remain silent for a long time.

Relief of bilateral, partial urinary tract obstruction or complete obstruction of one kidney is usually followed by a brief period of diuresis (commonly called postobstructive diuresis).[5] It is a physiologic response and is typically mild, representing a restoration of fluid and electrolyte imbalance caused by the obstructive uropathy. Alterations in tubular transport and water reabsorption and volume expansion contribute to the diuresis. Occasionally relief of obstruction will cause rapid excretion of large volumes of water, sodium, or other electrolytes, resulting in a urine output of 10 L/day or more (minimal normal daily urine output is approximately 720 mL/day). Rapid postobstructive diuresis causes dehydration and fluid and electrolyte imbalances if not promptly corrected with fluid replacement. Risk factors for severe postobstructive diuresis include bilateral obstruction, impairment of one or both kidneys' ability to concentrate urine or reabsorb sodium *(nephrogenic diabetes insipidus)*, hypertension, edema and weight gain, congestive heart failure, and uremic encephalopathy.

Kidney Stones

Renal calculi (nephrolithiasis), or urinary stones (urolithiasis), are masses of crystals, protein, or other substances that are a common cause of urinary tract obstruction in adults. Calculi can be located in the kidneys, ureters, and urinary bladder. The prevalence of stones in the United States is approximately 8.8% (10.6% among men and 7.1% among women) and is increasing. The recurrence rate is approximately 30% to 40% at 10 and 15 years. The risk of urinary calculus formation is influenced by a number of factors, including age, sex, race, geographic location, seasonal factors, fluid intake, diet, occupation, genetic predisposition, and other conditions including urinary tract infection, hypertension, atherosclerosis, metabolic syndrome, obesity, and type 2 diabetes.[6] Most persons develop their first stone before age 50 years. Geographic location influences the risk of stone formation because of indirect factors, including average temperature, humidity, and rainfall and their influence on fluid intake and dietary patterns. Persons who regularly consume an adequate volume of water and those who are physically active are at reduced risk when compared with people who are inactive or consume lower volumes of water. Most kidney stones are unilateral and are a risk factor for chronic kidney disease and an increased risk for myocardial infarction.

Urinary calculi can be classified according to the primary minerals (salts) that make up the stones. The most common stone types include calcium oxalate or phosphate (70% to 85%), struvite (magnesium, ammonium, and phosphate) (1% to 5%), and uric acid (5% to 10%). Cystine stones are rare, less than 1%.[6] Less common stone elements include cystine, 2,8-dihydroxyadeninuria (a rare genetic disorder that increases risk of xanthine stones), triamterene (a diuretic), and indinavir (a protease inhibitor used in management of human immunodeficiency virus [HIV] infection). Urinary calculi also can be classified according to location and size. *Staghorn calculi* are large and fill the minor and major calyces. *Nonstaghorn calculi* are of variable size and are located in the calyces, in the renal pelvis, or at various sites along the ureter.

◆**PATHOPHYSIOLOGY.** Renal calculus formation is complex and related to (1) supersaturation of one or more salts in the urine, (2) precipitation of the salts from a liquid to a solid state (crystals), (3) growth through crystallization or agglomeration (sometimes called *aggregation*), and (4) the effect of stone inhibitors.[7] *Supersaturation* is the presence of a higher concentration of a salt within a fluid (in this case, the urine) than the volume is able to dissolve to maintain equilibrium. Human urine contains many positively and negatively charged ions capable of *precipitating* from solution and forming a variety of salts. The salts form crystals that are retained and grow into stones. *Crystallization* is the process by which crystals grow from a small *nucleus* to larger stones in the presence of supersaturated urine. Although supersaturation is essential for free stone formation, the urine need not remain continuously supersaturated for a calculus to grow once its nidus has precipitated from solution. Intermittent periods of supersaturation after the ingestion of a meal or during times of dehydration are sufficient for stone growth in many individuals. The apical papillae have interstitial sites where hydroxyapatite deposits, known as *Randall plaque*, become exposed and serve as sites for calcium oxalate stone formation. Calcium phosphate stone formation is rare and found at the end of the collecting ducts.[8] *Matrix* is an organic material (i.e., mucoprotein) in which the components of a kidney stone are embedded and form part of the stone and may protect the kidney from cellular injury.[9]

The pH of the urine also influences the risk of precipitation and calculus formation. An alkaline urinary pH (pH >7.0) significantly increases the risk of calcium phosphate stone formation, whereas acidic urine (pH <5.0) increases the risk of a uric acid stone. Cystine and xanthine precipitate more readily in acidic urine.

Stone or *crystal growth inhibiting substances,* including potassium citrate, uromodulin, pyrophosphate, and magnesium, are capable of crystal growth inhibition if they are not overwhelmed by the rate of supersaturation.[7] Thus they can reduce the risk of calcium phosphate or calcium oxalate precipitation in the urine and prevent subsequent stone formation.

Retention of *crystal particles* occurs primarily at the papillary collecting ducts. Although most crystals are flushed from the tract through antegrade urine flow, urinary stasis, anatomic abnormalities, or inflamed epithelium within the urinary tract may prevent prompt flushing of crystals from the system, thus increasing the risk of calculus formation.

The size of a stone determines the likelihood that it will pass through the urinary tract and be excreted through micturition. Stones smaller than 5 mm have about a 50% chance of spontaneous passage, whereas stones that are 1 cm have almost no chance of spontaneous passage.[10] Nevertheless, a person with ureteral dilation from the previous passage of a stone may be able to excrete larger stones when compared with a person experiencing an initial obstructing calculus.

Calcium stones (urolithiasis) account for 70% to 80% of all stones requiring treatment. Calcium oxalate accounts for about 80% of these stones and calcium phosphate about 5%. Both genetic and environmental factors may increase susceptibility. Most affected individuals have *idiopathic calcium oxalate urolithiasis (ICOU)*, a condition whose exact etiology has not yet been defined. Stones can form freely in supersaturated urine or detach from interstitial sites of formation (i.e., from Randall plaque). Hypercalciuria, hyperoxaluria, hyperuricosuria, hypocitraturia, mild renal tubular acidosis, crystal growth inhibitor deficiencies, and alkaline urine are associated with calcium stone formation. Hypercalciuria and hyperoxaluria are usually attributable to intestinal hyperabsorption and less commonly to a defect in renal calcium reabsorption. Hyperparathyroidism and bone demineralization associated with prolonged immobilization are also known to cause hypercalciuria.[8]

Struvite stones primarily contain magnesium ammonium phosphate as well as varying levels of matrix. Matrix forms in an alkaline urine and during infection with a urease-producing bacterial pathogen, such as a *Proteus, Klebsiella,* or *Pseudomonas.*[11] Struvite calculi may grow quite large and branch into a staghorn configuration (staghorn calculus) that approximates the pelvicaliceal collecting system. Women are at greater risk for struvite stones because they have an increased incidence of urinary tract infection.

Uric acid stones occur in persons who excrete excessive uric acid in the urine, such as those with gouty arthritis. Uric acid is primarily a product of biosynthesis of endogenous purines and is secondarily affected by consumption of purines (e.g., meat and beer) in the diet. A consistently acidic urine greatly increases this risk, including defective NH_4^+ excretion. Cystine and xanthine are amino acids that precipitate more readily in acidic urine.[12] *Cystinuria* and *xanthinuria* are genetic disorders of amino acid metabolism, and their excess in urine can cause cystinuric or xanthine stone formation in the presence of a low urine pH of 5.5 or less.

◆**CLINICAL MANIFESTATIONS.** Renal colic, described as moderate to severe pain often originating in the posterior hypochondrium (flank) and radiating to the groin, usually indicates obstruction of the renal pelvis or proximal ureter. Colic that radiates to the lateral flank or lower abdomen typically indicates obstruction in the midureter, and bothersome lower urinary tract symptoms (urgency, frequent voiding, urge incontinence) indicate obstruction of the lower ureter or ureterovesical junction. The pain can be severe and incapacitating and may be accompanied by nausea and vomiting. Gross (visible blood in the urine) or microscopic hematuria (three or more red blood cells per high power microscopic field) may be present.[10]

◆**EVALUATION AND TREATMENT.** The evaluation and diagnosis of urinary calculi are based on presenting symptoms and history combined with a focused physical assessment and imaging studies.[13] The history queries dietary habits; the age of the first stone episode; stone analysis; and presence of complicating factors, including recurrent urinary tract infection, hyperparathyroidism, or recent gastrointestinal or genitourinary surgery. Urinalysis (including pH) is obtained and a 24-hour urine is completed to identify calcium oxalate, calcium citrate, and other significant constituents. In addition, every effort is made to retrieve and analyze calculi that are passed spontaneously or retrieved through aggressive intervention. Additional tests are obtained in selected individuals, such as those with suspected hyperparathyroidism (elevated serum calcium levels) or cystine or uric acid stones, in order to diagnose and manage underlying metabolic disorders. Imaging of kidney stones includes plain abdominal radiography, ultrasound, intravenous pyelography, computed tomography, and magnetic resonance imaging.[14]

The goals of treatment are to manage acute pain, promote stone passage, reduce the size of stones already formed, and prevent new stone formation.[13] The components of treatment include (1) managing pain; (2) reducing the concentration of stone-forming substances by increasing urine flow rate with high fluid intake; (3) adjusting the pH of the urine (e.g., make it more alkaline with potassium citrate administration); (4) decreasing the amount of stone-forming substances in the urine by decreasing dietary intake or endogenous;[15] and (5) removing stones using percutaneous nephrolithotomy, ureteroscopy, or ultrasonic or laser lithotripsy to fragment stones for excretion in the urine. Obstructing kidney stones with a suspected proximal urinary tract infection are urologic emergencies requiring emergent decompression, stone removal, and antibiotics.[16] Prevention of recurrent stones includes increasing fluid intake to generate 2.5 L of urine per day; avoiding intake of colas and other soft drinks acidified with phosphoric acid; avoiding dietary oxalate (e.g., chocolate, beets, nuts, rhubarb, spinach, strawberries, tea, wheat bran); eating less animal protein; limiting sodium intake; and, for calcium stone prevention, maintaining a dietary calcium intake of 1000 to 1200 mg/day.[13,17]

Lower Urinary Tract Obstruction

Obstructive disorders of the lower urinary tract (LUT) are primarily related to storage of urine in the bladder or emptying of urine through the bladder outlet. The causes of the obstruction include neurogenic and anatomic alterations or, in some instances, a combination of both. Incontinence is a common symptom. Types of incontinence are reviewed in Table 39.1.

Neurogenic Bladder

Neurogenic bladder is a general term for bladder dysfunction caused by neurologic disorders and involves problems with urine storage or voiding. The types of dysfunction are related to the sites in the nervous system that control sensory and motor bladder function (Fig. 39.2). Lesions that develop in upper motor neurons of the brain and spinal cord result in dyssynergia (loss of coordinated neuromuscular contraction) and overactive or hyperreflexive bladder function. Lesions in the sacral area of the spinal cord or peripheral nerves result in underactive, hypotonic, or atonic (flaccid) bladder function, often with loss of bladder sensation.

Neurologic disorders that develop above the pontine micturition center result in detrusor hyperreflexia, also known as an *uninhibited* or *reflex bladder*. This is an upper motor neuron disorder in which the

TABLE 39.1	TYPES OF INCONTINENCE
TYPE	**DESCRIPTION**
Urge incontinence (most common in older adults)	Involuntary loss of urine associated with an abrupt and strong desire to void (urgency). Often associated with involuntary contractions of the detrusor (detrusor overactivity). When associated with a neurologic disorder, this is called *detrusor hyperreflexia.* When no neurologic disorder exists this is called *detrusor instability.* May be associated with decreased bladder wall compliance.
Stress incontinence (most common in women younger than 60 years and men who have had prostate surgery)	Involuntary loss of urine during coughing, sneezing, laughing, or other physical activity associated with increased abdominal pressure.
Overflow incontinence	Involuntary loss of urine with overdistention of the bladder.
	Associated with neurologic lesions below S1, polyneuropathies, and urethral obstruction (i.e., an enlarged prostate).
Mixed incontinence (most common in older women)	A combination of stress and urge incontinence.
Functional incontinence	Involuntary loss of urine caused by dementia or immobility.

Data from Agency for Healthcare Research and Quality: *Overview: urinary incontinence in adults, clinical practice guideline update,* Rockville, MD, 1996, Author. Available at: https://archive.ahrq.gov/clinic/uioverww.htm; MacLachlan LS, Rovner ES: *Adv Chronic Kidney Dis* 22(4):279-288, 2015.

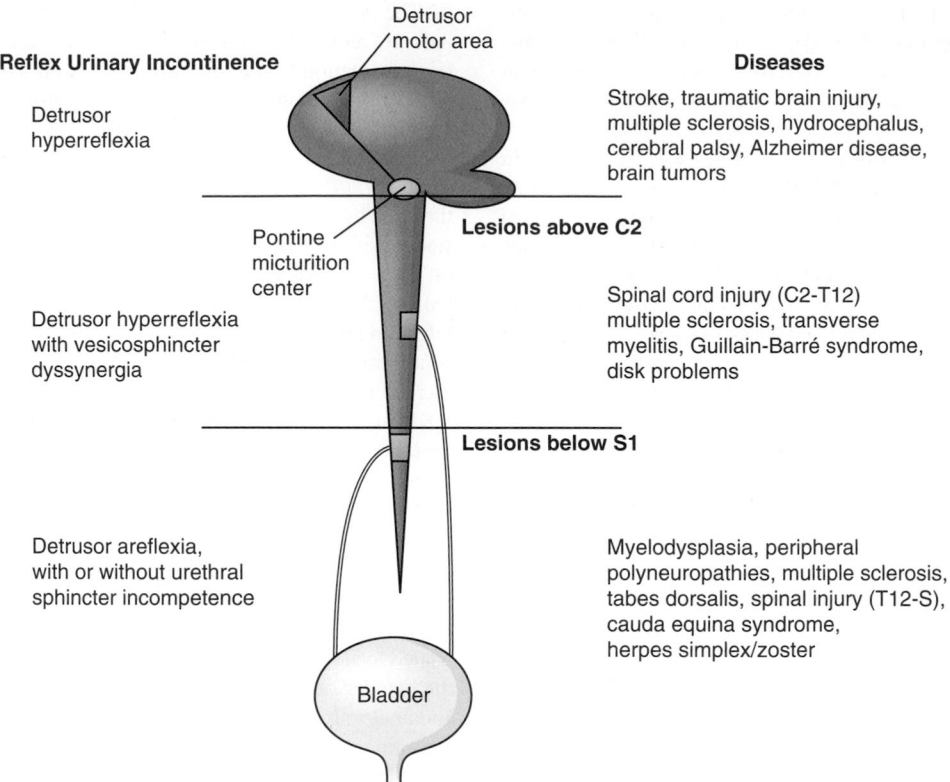

Reflex Urinary Incontinence

Detrusor
hyperreflexia

Detrusor
motor area

Pontine
micturition
center

Detrusor hyperreflexia
with vesicosphincter
dyssynergia

Detrusor areflexia,
with or without urethral
sphincter incompetence

Bladder

Diseases

Stroke, traumatic brain injury,
multiple sclerosis, hydrocephalus,
cerebral palsy, Alzheimer disease,
brain tumors

Lesions above C2

Spinal cord injury (C2-T12)
multiple sclerosis, transverse
myelitis, Guillain-Barré syndrome,
disk problems

Lesions below S1

Myelodysplasia, peripheral
polyneuropathies, multiple sclerosis,
tabes dorsalis, spinal injury (T12-S),
cauda equina syndrome,
herpes simplex/zoster

FIGURE 39.2 Causes of Neurogenic Bladder and Reflex Incontinence. (Adapted from Doughty DB, editor: *Urinary and fecal incontinence: current management concepts,* ed 3, Philadelphia, 2006, Mosby.)

bladder empties automatically when it becomes full and the external sphincter functions normally. Because the pontine micturition center remains intact, there is coordination between detrusor muscle contraction and the relaxation of the urethral sphincter. Stroke, traumatic brain injury, dementia, and brain tumors are examples of disorders that result in detrusor hyperreflexia. Symptoms include urine leakage and incontinence.

Neurologic lesions that occur below the pontine micturition center but above the sacral micturition center (between C2 and S1) are also upper motor neuron lesions and result in detrusor hyperreflexia with detrusor sphincter dyssynergia. There is loss of pontine coordination of detrusor muscle contraction and external sphincter relaxation, so both the bladder and the sphincter are contracting at the same time, causing a functional obstruction of the bladder outlet.[18] Spinal cord injury, multiple sclerosis, Guillain-Barré syndrome, and intervertebral disk problems are causes of this disorder. There is diminished bladder relaxation during storage with small urine volumes and high intravesicular (inside the bladder) pressures. This results in an overactive bladder syndrome (see later discussion) with symptoms of urgency, frequency, urge incontinence, and increased risk for urethral turbulence and urinary tract infection.

Lesions that involve the sacral micturition center (below S1; may also be termed *cauda equina syndrome*) or peripheral nerve lesions result in detrusor areflexia (acontractile detrusor), a lower motor neuron disorder. The result is an acontractile detrusor or atonic bladder with retention of urine and distention. If the sensory innervation of the bladder is intact, the full bladder will be sensed but the detrusor may not contract. This is an *underactive bladder syndrome* and may have symptoms of stress and overflow incontinence. Myelodysplasia, multiple sclerosis, tabes dorsalis, and peripheral polyneuropathies are associated with this disorder.

Because the bladder neck consists of circular smooth muscle with adrenergic innervation, overactive bladder (OAB) syndrome and detrusor sphincter dyssynergia may be managed by α-adrenergic blocking (antimuscarinic) medications or botulinum toxin A. Obstruction that is not adequately managed by pharmacotherapy may require bladder neck incision. Detrusor sphincter dyssynergia may be managed by intermittent catheterization in combination with higher dose antimuscarinic drugs to prevent overactive detrusor contractions and associated dyssynergia while ensuring regular, complete bladder evacuation through catheterization. Alternatively, men with dyssynergia may be managed by condom catheter containment, supplemented by an α-adrenergic blocking drug or transurethral sphincterotomy (surgical incision of the striated sphincter) in order to relieve obstruction. Low bladder wall compliance may be managed by antimuscarinic drugs and intermittent catheterization; however, more severe cases may require augmentation enterocystoplasty (enlargement of the low compliant bladder wall using a detubularized piece of small bowel), urinary diversion, or long-term indwelling catheterization.[18]

Overactive and Underactive Bladder Syndromes

Overactive bladder (OAB) syndrome is a chronic syndrome of detrusor overactivity in the absence of infection. It is estimated that 29.8 million adults over the age of 40 have bothersome OAB symptoms with a prevalence of 11% to 19%.[19] OAB is characterized by urgency with involuntary detrusor contractions during the bladder filling phase. The contraction may be spontaneous or provoked and associated with hyperexcitable nerves or involuntary reflexes. There is coordination between the contracting bladder and the external sphincter, but the detrusor is too weak to empty the bladder, resulting in urinary retention with overflow or stress incontinence. Overactive bladder is defined by the International Continence Society as a *symptom syndrome* of urgency, with or without urge incontinence and usually associated with frequency and nocturia.[20] Sexual dysfunction and bowel problems often accompany OAB. Diagnosis is usually made by evaluation of symptoms. Urodynamic evaluation confirms the diagnosis. Treatment options include lifestyle modifications, behavioral therapy, pharmacotherapy (e.g., antimuscarinics), neuromodulation therapy, and surgical interventions.[21] Adults are often reluctant to discuss this syndrome with their healthcare provider. When left untreated, OAB is costly, impairs health and quality of life, causes depression, and leads to social isolation. OAB is a risk for urinary tract infection and a risk for falls in older adults.

Underactive bladder (UAB) syndrome is defined by the International Continence Society (ICS) as bladder contraction of reduced strength and/or duration, resulting in prolonged bladder emptying or a failure to achieve complete bladder emptying, or both, within a normal time span.[20] Disruption of bladder innervation can occur with spinal cord injury, stroke, multiple sclerosis, Parkinson disease, and diabetic neuropathy. Aging can be a contributing factor. The symptoms may be indistinguishable from symptoms of lower urinary tract obstruction, including weak stream, intermittency, hesitancy, and straining to void. Urodynamic studies are required for evaluation. Treatment depends on the cause of the disorder and may include sacral neuromodulation, drugs that increase bladder contractility, and/or drugs that induce urethral relaxation.[22,23]

Anatomic Obstructions to Urine Flow

Anatomic causes of resistance to urine flow include urethral stricture, prostatic enlargement in men, pelvic organ prolapse in women, and tumor compression. Symptoms of lower urinary tract obstruction are more common in men and include (1) frequent daytime voiding (urination more than every 2 hours while awake); (2) nocturia (awakening more than once each night to urinate for adults younger than 65 years of age or more than twice for older adults); (3) bothersome urgency, often combined with hesitancy; (4) poor force of stream; (5) intermittency of urinary stream; and (6) feelings of incomplete bladder emptying despite micturition.

A urethral stricture is a narrowing of its lumen and occurs when infection, injury, or surgical manipulation produces a scar that reduces the caliber of the urethra. The vast majority of urethral strictures occur in men; they are less common in women. The severity of obstruction is influenced by its location within the urethra, its length, and the minimum caliber of urethral lumen within the stricture. Specifically, proximal urethral strictures cause more severe obstruction than do strictures of the distal urethra, longer strictures tend to be more obstructive, and the magnitude of blockage is in *reverse* proportion to the urethral caliber. Urethral stricture may be treated with urethral dilation. However, urethroplasty has become the first-line treatment of stricture disease, with long-term success for both men and women.[24,25]

Prostate enlargement is caused by acute inflammation, benign prostatic hyperplasia, or prostate cancer (see Chapter 26). Each of these disorders can cause encroachment on the urethra with obstruction to urine flow and the symptoms summarized previously. Prostate enlargement is managed by treating the underlying cause of the prostate enlargement with medication or surgery. Acute prostatitis is initially managed by broad-spectrum antibiotics until the results of a urine culture are obtained. Urinary retention may require transient placement of a suprapubic catheter. The management of benign prostatic hyperplasia and treatment options for prostate cancer are presented in Chapter 26.

Severe pelvic organ prolapse (POP) (see Chapter 25) in a woman causes bladder outlet obstruction when, most commonly, a cystocele (the downward protrusion of the bladder into the vagina) descends below the level of the urethral outlet. Rectoceles and prolapse of the uterus are additional causes of prolapse. Cystoceles (see Fig. 25.11) that

reach or protrude beyond the vaginal introitus create the greatest risk for obstruction, particularly if the bladder neck (in females the bladder neck and proximal urethra constitute the internal sphincter of the bladder) has been surgically repaired without simultaneous repair of the cystocele. In men the bladder may rarely herniate into the scrotum, causing a similar type of obstruction.

Mild POP can be treated effectively with pelvic floor muscle training.[26] A pessary (rubber or silicone device designed to compensate for vaginal wall prolapse) may be inserted to mechanically reverse severe pelvic organ (bladder, uterus, or rectum) prolapse. Depending on the device, the woman may be able to remove, cleanse, and replace the pessary, or it may be changed during a clinic visit. Intravaginal hormone replacement therapy may contribute to the long-term success of a pessary.[27] Alternatively, pelvic organ prolapse may be repaired surgically; the procedure may be combined with a urethral suspension to correct stress urinary incontinence or rectocele repair.[28]

Partial obstruction of the bladder outlet or urethra initially causes an increase in the force of detrusor contraction. If the blockage persists, afferent nerves within the bladder wall are adversely affected, leading to urinary urgency and, in some cases, overactive detrusor contractions (a myogenic cause of overactive bladder). When obstruction persists, there is an increased deposition of collagen within the smooth muscle bundles of the detrusor muscle *(trabeculation)*, possibly in an attempt to increase the force of its contraction strength. Ultimately, the bladder wall loses its ability to stretch and accommodate urine, a condition called low bladder wall compliance, and the detrusor loses its ability to contract efficiently. Low bladder wall compliance chronically elevates intravesicular pressure, greatly increasing the problems of hydroureter, hydronephrosis, and impaired renal function.

◆ EVALUATION OF LOWER URINARY TRACT DISORDERS. Although the history and physical examination are critical to the evaluation of lower urinary tract disorders, it must be remembered that no symptom or cluster of symptoms has been identified that accurately differentiates the various causes of these disorders. For example, symptoms such as urgency, urge incontinence, frequent urination, and nocturia may develop because of overactive bladder or either increased or decreased bladder outlet resistance. Reduced resistance is associated with the symptom of stress incontinence (incontinence with coughing or sneezing), and symptoms of increased resistance are similar to those of bladder outlet obstruction, including poor force of urinary stream, hesitancy, and feelings of incomplete bladder emptying.

Various diagnostic tests assist with evaluation.[29] A *cystometric test* uses a catheter and manometer to evaluate bladder urine volume and pressure in relation to involuntary bladder contraction (the leak point pressure) and the urge to void. The *postvoid residual urine* is measured by catheterization within 5 to 15 minutes of urination or through a bladder ultrasound machine that measures bladder height and width to provide an approximation of urine within the vesicle. This measurement may be combined with *uroflowmetry,* a graphic representation of the force of the urinary stream expressed as milliliters voided per second. Each of these measurements assesses the lower urinary tract's efficiency in evacuating urine through micturition but neither differentiates poor detrusor contraction strength from obstruction as a cause of urinary retention. Instead, *multichannel urodynamic testing* is used to identify obstruction, quantify its severity, and measure detrusor contraction strength (Fig. 39.3). *Video-urodynamic recordings* can also demonstrate overactive bladder and detrusor sphincter dyssynergia. An evaluation of renal function, including functional imaging studies and measurement of serum creatinine level, is completed particularly when obstruction is severe and associated with elevated residuals or urinary tract infection. *Electromyography* measures electrical activity in the bladder neck using surface or needle electrodes.

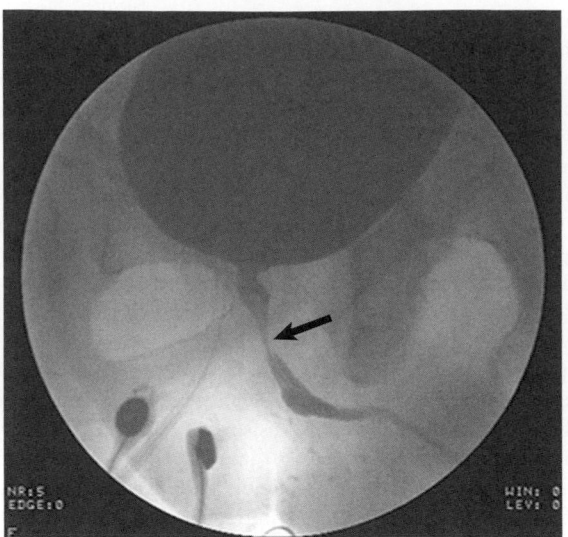

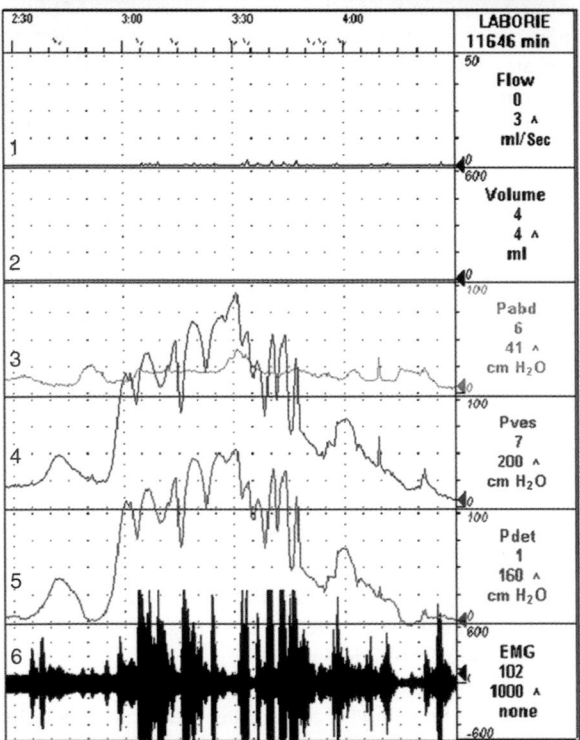

FIGURE 39.3 Neurogenic Detrusor Overactivity with Vesicosphincter. The arrow indicates narrowing of the striated sphincter consistent with electromyographic activity *(Line 6)* noted on the urodynamic tracing. Note the characteristic poor flow pattern *(Line 1)* with elevated voiding pressures *(Lines 4 and 5)* indicating obstruction. *Line 1* = Urine flow rate; *Line 2* = urine volume; *Line 3* = abdominal pressure *(Pabd)*; *Line 4* = intravesicular (inside bladder) pressure *(Pves)*; *Line 5* = detrusor muscle pressure *(Pdet)*; *Line 6* = bladder electromyogram *(EMG)*.

Tumors
Renal Tumors

Renal tumors account for about 62,700 (3.7%) of new cancer cases and 14,240 (2.4%) of deaths in 2016.[30] There are a number of different histologic subtypes of kidney tumors.[31] Renal adenomas (benign tumors) are uncommon but are increasing in number. The tumors are solid and encapsulated and are usually located near the cortex of the kidney. Because they can become malignant, they are usually surgically removed.

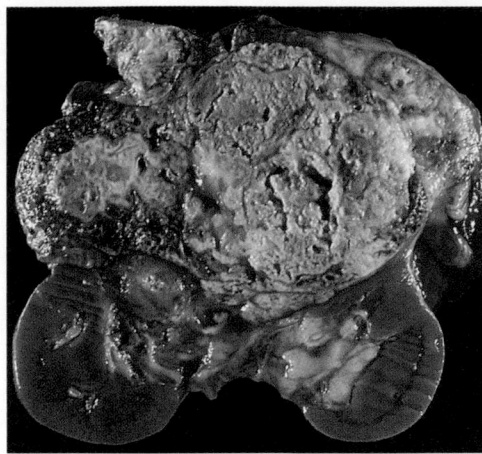

FIGURE 39.4 Renal Cell Carcinoma. Renal cell carcinomas usually are spheroidal masses composed of yellow tissue mottled with hemorrhage, necrosis, and fibrosis. (From Damjanov I, Linder J, editors: *Anderson's pathology*, ed 10, St Louis, 1996, Mosby.)

Renal cell carcinoma (RCC) is the most common renal neoplasm (approximately 80% of all renal neoplasms) (Fig. 39.4). Renal cell carcinoma usually occurs in men (1.5 times more often than in women) between 50 and 60 years of age, and the incidence is increasing. Blacks have a higher incidence and mortality. Risk factors include cigarette smoking, obesity, hypertension, nonsteroidal antiinflammatory drug use, advanced-stage chronic renal failure (CRF), and occupational exposure to trichloroethylene.[32] Several genes are associated with RCC. Five-year survival for stage I is about 80% and is about 8% for stage IV cancer (metastatic disease).[33]

PATHOPHYSIOLOGY. Renal cell carcinomas are adenocarcinomas and arise from tubular epithelium. The etiology is unknown. They are classified according to cell type and extent of metastasis. *Clear cell tumors,* the most common (80% of cases), are sporadic or hereditary dominated by mutations of the von Hippel-Lindau *(VHL)* gene located on chromosome 3p25. 3p mutations also can occur in sporadic tumors. They present a better prognosis than *non–clear cell renal cell carcinoma* (20%), which includes papillary (10%), chromophobe (5%), oncocytoma (3% to 4%), collecting duct tumors (1%), and unclassified (rare) tumors.[34] *Renal transitional cell carcinoma* is rare and primarily arises in the renal parenchyma and renal pelvis. Cortical tumors arise from proximal and distal convoluted tubular epithelium and have a growth pattern that pushes nonneoplastic nephrons to the periphery of the tumor. Medullary based tumors arise from the corticomedullary junction and typically invade the renal cortex. Renal pelvic tumors arise from the overlying urothelium with invasion through soft tissues and renal parenchyma, and retrograde growth up the collecting tubules.[35] Confinement within the renal capsule, together with treatment, is associated with a better survival rate. The tumors usually occur unilaterally (see Fig. 39.4). About 25% to 30% of individuals with RCC present with metastasis (stage IV) because they are highly vascular. The most common sites of distant metastasis are the lung, lymph nodes, liver, bone, thyroid, and central nervous system.[36]

CLINICAL MANIFESTATIONS. The classic clinical manifestations of renal tumors are hematuria, dull and aching flank pain, and palpable flank mass in thinner individuals. Systemic manifestations usually represent an advanced stage of disease and include weight loss, fatigue, intermittent fever from tumor cytokines, anemia from hematuria and lack of erythropoietin, polycythemia from tumor secretion of erythropoietin, hypertension from elevated renin levels, and alterations in liver function tests. All of these symptoms occur in less than 10% of cases. Further, they represent an advanced stage of disease, whereas earlier stages are often silent.

◆**EVALUATION AND TREATMENT.** Diagnosis is based on the clinical symptoms; ultrasound; plain x-ray films of the abdomen; intravenous pyelography; renal angiography; chest, abdominal and pelvic computed tomography; and magnetic resonance imaging. Biopsy provides identification of histologic cell types, molecular markers, and information for staging (Table 39.2). Treatment for localized disease is surgical removal of the affected kidney (radical nephrectomy) or partial nephron-sparing nephrectomy for smaller tumors. Use of high-dose interleukin-2 is limited by significant toxicity (hypotension requiring vasopressor support, oliguria, pulmonary congestion, arrhythmias, and neurologic toxicity). Agents targeting the vascular endothelial growth factor pathway and the mammalian target of rapamycin (mTOR) (axitinib) have shown efficacy in randomized clinical trials for treatment of metastatic disease. Tyrosine kinase inhibitors, sunitinib and pazopanib, have been effective in phase III clinical trials for first-line treatment of clear cell carcinoma with good prognosis. Bevacizumab or sorafenib, combined with interferon, are alternative options. Cabozantinib has been approved for advanced disease.[37] Non–clear cell renal cell carcinoma does not respond well to systemic therapy, and new treatment approaches are needed.[38] Techniques using stereotactic radiofrequency ablation, cryoablation,

and laparoscopy are effective for lower grade tumors.[39] Tumor obstruction is relieved by placement of ureteral catheters or nephrostomy tubes or by completion of urinary diversion procedures. Survival is related to tumor grade, tumor cell type, and extent of metastasis.

Bladder Tumors

Bladder tumors represent about 4.5% of all malignant tumors and are the fourth most common malignancy in white men over age 55 years. Approximately 76,960 people developed bladder cancer with 16,390 deaths (2.5% of all cancer deaths) in 2016. Risk factors include smoking; aromatic amines, such as benzidine and beta-naphthylamine; arsenic in drinking water; phenacetin; cyclophosphamide; and pioglitazone. *Schistosoma haematobium* is a risk factor in Asia and Africa.[30]

◆**PATHOGENESIS.** Urothelial (transitional cell) carcinoma is the most common bladder malignancy, appearing on the inner lining of the bladder. Oncogenes of the *ras* gene family and tumor-suppressor genes, including *TP53* mutations (more chemoresistant), and inactivation of *retinoblastoma gene (pRb)* are genomic subtypes of bladder cancer. Several other genes that are either deleted or amplified have been identified and contribute to tumorigenesis. Loss of heterozygosity at chromosome 9 has been found in all stages of urothelial cell carcinoma.[40,41]

The tumor is usually composed of uroepithelial cells (cells lining the bladder, ureters, urethra, and renal pelvis). They may have a papillary growth pattern (a tuftlike lesion attached to a stalk) or are flat with a velvety appearance (Fig. 39.5). Flat tumors (10% to 30% of bladder tumors) are not as common as papillary tumors and occur as carcinoma in situ or invasive carcinoma. Carcinoma in situ also can present with papillary tumors. High-grade papillary tumors have a complex papillary architecture and a high degree of nuclear atypia, with high risk of recurrence and metastasis.[42] Metastasis is usually to lymph nodes, liver, bones, lungs, and adrenal glands. Staging distinguishes between muscle invasive and nonmuscle invasive carcinoma and guides treatment and prognosis. Staging for bladder carcinoma is presented in Table 39.3. Secondary bladder cancer develops by invasion of cancer from bordering organs, such as cervical carcinoma in women or prostatic carcinoma in men.

◆**CLINICAL MANIFESTATIONS.** Gross painless microscopic hematuria is the common clinical manifestation of bladder cancer. Episodes of hematuria tend to recur, and they are often accompanied by other nonspecific lower urinary tract symptoms including daytime voiding frequency, dysuria, nocturia, urgency, and urge urinary incontinence. Flank pain may occur if tumor growth obstructs one or both ureterovesical junctions. Bothersome lower urinary tract symptoms are particularly intense in individuals with carcinoma in situ. Metastasis is the cause of death from bladder cancer, usually from high-grade muscle-invasive tumors.[43]

◆**EVALUATION AND TREATMENT.** Urinalysis for evidence of hematuria in the absence of infection provides a useful screening tool for high-risk patients. Urine cytology (pathologic analysis of sloughed cells within the urine) is completed in individuals with evidence of hematuria from unknown causes; cystoscopy or fluorescence cystoscopy with tissue biopsy can confirm the diagnosis. Transurethral resection of the tumor determines staging and guides treatment. Biologic markers for the diagnosis, prognosis, and treatment of bladder cancer are under investigation (e.g., tyrosine kinase receptors, epidermal growth factor and estrogen receptor pathways, cell-cycle regulators, chromatin remodeling, and immune mediators).[44]

Newer magnetic resonance techniques are helpful for local staging, and whole-body computed tomography detects metastasis. Transurethral resection or laser ablation, combined with intravesical chemotherapy (bacillus Calmette-Guerin [BCG]) or immunotherapy (according to guidelines), is effective for superficial tumors or carcinoma in situ.

TABLE 39.2	STAGING OF RENAL CELL CARCINOMA (TNM SYSTEM)
STAGE	**METASTASIS**
I	T1, N0, M0: The tumor is 7 cm across or smaller and is only in the kidney (T1). There is no spread to lymph nodes (N0) or distant organs (M0).
II	T2, N0, M0: The tumor is larger than 7 cm across but is still only in the kidney (T2). There is no spread to lymph nodes (N0) or distant organs (M0).
III	Either of the following:
	T3, N0, M0: The tumor is growing into a major vein (like the renal vein or the vena cava) or into tissue around the kidney, but it is not growing into the adrenal gland or beyond Gerota fascia (T3); there is no spread to lymph nodes (N0) or distant organs (M0).
	T1 to T3, N1, M0: The main tumor can be any size and may be outside the kidney, but it has not spread beyond Gerota fascia; the cancer has spread to nearby lymph nodes (N1) but has not spread to distant lymph nodes or other organs (M0).
IV	Either of the following:
	T4, any N, M0: The main tumor is growing beyond Gerota fascia and may be growing into the adrenal gland on top of the kidney (T4); it may or may not have spread to nearby lymph nodes (any N); it has not spread to distant lymph nodes or other organs (M0).
	Any T, Any N, M1: The main tumor can be any size and may have grown outside the kidney (any T); it may or may not have spread to nearby lymph nodes (any N); it has spread to distant lymph nodes and/or other organs (M1).

T, Tumor; *N,* node; *M,* metastasis.
From American Cancer Society: *Kidney cancer (adult)—renal cell carcinoma,* 2016. Available at: http://www.cancer.org/acs/groups/cid/documents/webcontent/003107-pdf.pdf.

Location of Tumors

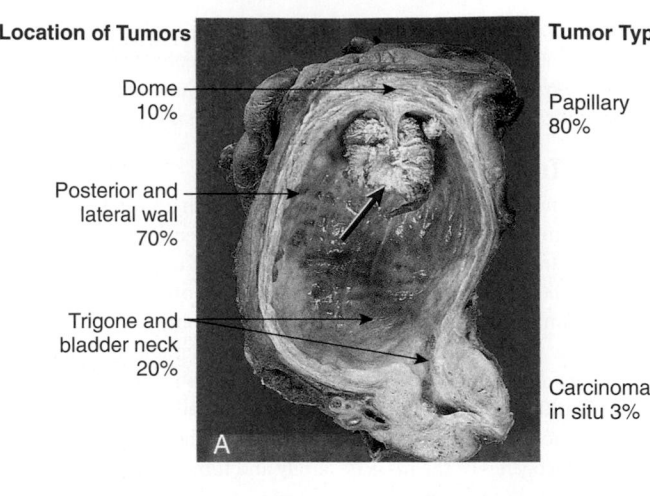

Tumor Type

Dome 10%

Papillary 80%

Posterior and lateral wall 70%

Trigone and bladder neck 20%

Carcinoma in situ 3%

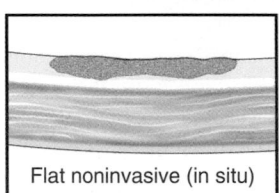

Flat noninvasive (in situ)

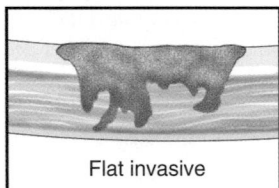

Flat invasive

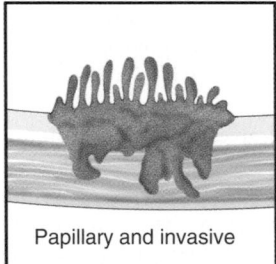

Papillary and invasive

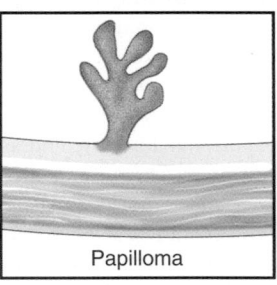

Papilloma

FIGURE 39.5 Carcinoma of the Bladder. A, Papillary transitional cell carcinoma arising in the dome of the bladder as a cauliflower-like lesion *(black arrow);* location and frequency of bladder tumor types noted. **B,** Bladder cancer with morphologic patterns of most common tumors. (**A** from Stevens A, Lowe J, Scott I, editors: *Core pathology,* ed 3, London, 2009, Mosby; **B** from Kissane JM, editor: *Anderson's pathology,* ed 9, St Louis, 1990, Mosby.)

TABLE 39.3	STAGING OF BLADDER CARCINOMA (TNM SYSTEM)
STAGE	**DESCRIPTION**
Primary Tumor	
T0	No primary tumor identified
Ta	Noninvasive papillary carcinoma—not in bladder muscle
Tis	Carcinoma in situ (CIS)
T1	Tumor invades connective tissue
T2	Tumor invades detrusor muscle
T3	Invasion of fatty tissue around bladder
T4	Tumor has invaded adjacent structures
Region of Lymph Nodes	
N0	No lymph node involvement
N1 to N3	Lymph node metastasis to pelvic or adjacent region
Distant Metastasis	
M0	No metastasis
M1	Distant metastasis

T, Tumor; *N,* node; *M,* metastasis.
Adapted from American Cancer Society: *Bladder cancer,* 2016. Available at: http://www.cancer.org/cancer/bladdercancer/detailedguide/bladder-cancer-staging.

Radical cystectomy with urinary diversion and adjuvant chemotherapy is required for locally invasive tumors, and short-course radiation therapy may be used to support palliative or adjuvant treatment for muscle-invasive tumors. Cisplatin-based combination chemotherapy is currently the first-line therapy for advanced-stage carcinoma. Targeted therapies are under investigation and include fibroblast, epidermal and endothelial growth factors, antiangiogenesis agents (bevacizumab), tyrosine kinase inhibitors (cabozantinib), and immune checkpoint inhibitors (drugs that overcome tumor resistance to immune attack).[45] Individuals with bladder cancer require lifelong surveillance, as there is a high recurrence rate.[46]

URINARY TRACT INFECTION

Causes of Urinary Tract Infection

A **urinary tract infection (UTI)** is an inflammation of the urinary epithelium usually caused by bacteria from gut flora. A UTI can occur anywhere along the urinary tract including the urethra, bladder, ureter, or kidney. At risk are premature newborns; prepubertal children; sexually active and pregnant women; women treated with antibiotics that disrupt

vaginal flora; spermicide users; estrogen-deficient postmenopausal women; individuals with indwelling catheters; and persons with diabetes mellitus, neurogenic bladder, or urinary tract obstruction (see *What's New?* Catheter-Associated Urinary Tract Infections [CAUTI]). Cystitis is more common in women because of the shorter urethra and the closeness of the urethra to the anus (increasing the possibility of bacterial contamination). Up to 50% of women may have a lower UTI at some time in their life.[47,48] *Uncomplicated UTIs* are generally mild and without complications, and they occur in individuals with a normal urinary tract. A *complicated (febrile) UTI* develops when there is an abnormality in the urinary system or a health problem that compromises host defenses, such as human immunodeficiency virus (HIV), renal transplant, diabetes, or spinal cord injury. UTI may occur alone or in association with pyelonephritis, prostatitis, or kidney stones. Up to 40% of cases of septic shock are caused by urosepsis that present in the emergency room.[48] *Recurrent UTI* is commonly defined as three or more UTIs within 12 months, or two or more occurrences within 6 months. It may occur as a *relapse* when there is a second UTI caused by the same pathogen within 2 weeks of the original treatment, or a *reinfection* that occurs more than 2 weeks after completion of treatment for the same or different pathogen. Mechanisms of UTI are summarized in Fig. 39.6.

Host Defense Mechanisms and Urinary Tract Infection

Host defense mechanisms maintain a sterile posterior urethra and bladder in a healthy individual. Even if bacteria manage to enter the bladder, these defense mechanisms prevent it from clinging to the walls of the bladder or ascending to the upper urinary tracts. Several factors normally combine to protect against UTI. Most bacteria are washed out of the urethra during micturition. The low pH and high osmolality of urea, the presence of uromodulin (Tamm-Horsfall protein, secreted by renal tubular cells in the distal loop of Henle), and secretions from the uroepithelium provide a bactericidal effect. The ureterovesical junction closes during bladder contraction, preventing reflux of urine to the ureters and kidneys. Periurethral mucus-secreting glands surround the

Bacterial factors

Capsular antigens
resist
phagocytosis

Hemolysin
damages
epithelium

Urease-positive
bacteria promote
infection (i.e., *Proteus*
and *Klebsiella*)

Adhesins: *Escherichia
coli* type I and P fimbriae
bind to uroepithelium

Host factors

Kidney stones

Diabetes
mellitus

Immunosuppression

Ureteral reflux

Pregnancy
Neurogenic bladder

P blood group
antigens

Prostatic hypertrophy

Short urethra in women
Indwelling catheters

E. coli contamination
from colon

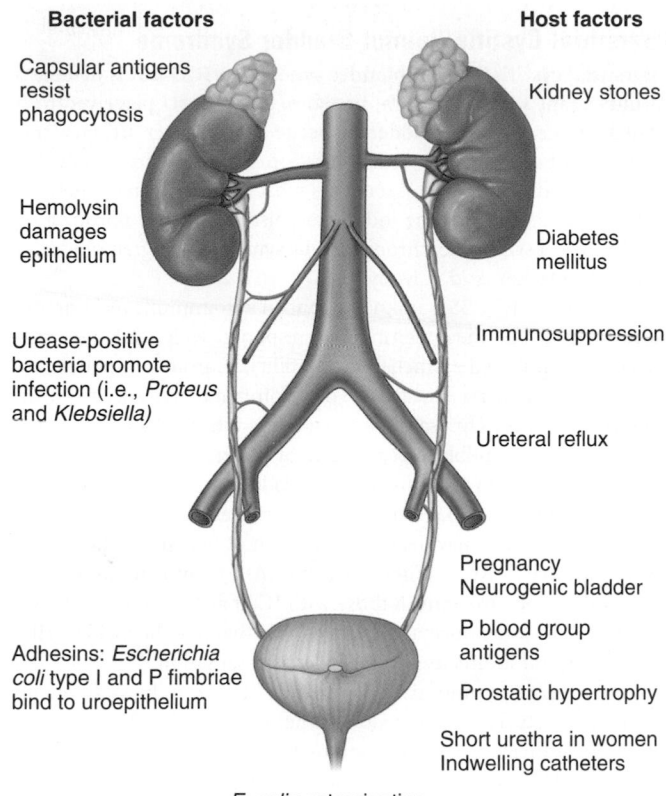

FIGURE 39.6 Mechanisms of Urinary Tract Infection.

distal two-thirds of the female urethra. Mucus from these glands traps bacteria before it can ascend from the proximal urethra to the bladder. In men, the length of the male urethra and secretions from the prostate and accessory periurethral glands combine to form a protective barrier against infection. In addition, the urethral sphincter mechanism acts as a mechanical barrier to bacterial ascent from the distal urethra.

Bacteria that successfully ascend the urethra face detection and destruction by components of the body's immune system, provided they come into contact with the bladder wall. Protective uroepithelial immune responses include Toll-like receptor (e.g., TLR4) recognition of pathogen-associated molecular patterns on the bacteria, neutrophil and macrophage recruitment, and phagocytosis. Susceptibility to infection also is influenced by genetic variation in the host immune response to bacterial virulence and by the virulence of the pathogen (see Chapter 10). Unfortunately, time is required for the immune system to respond to the potential threat, and this period may provide adequate time for bacteria or other pathogens to reproduce several times. The efficiency of the bladder's defenses is also influenced by the person's Lewis blood group. This taxonomy is based on recognition of inherited antigens associated with the ABO blood factors. Individuals with certain Lewis blood groups are more prone to UTIs because they secrete fewer antigens capable of resisting bacterial adherence by pilus formation.[49,50]

Most people are able to rapidly rid the urinary tract of invading bacteria, but some show evidence of bacteria in the urine that does not provoke an infection. This condition, called **asymptomatic bacteriuria**, does not harm urinary function or require intervention except in pregnant women or individuals experiencing urinary tract surgery.[51] A UTI occurs when a pathogen circumvents or overwhelms the host's defense mechanisms and rapidly reproduces.

Types of Urinary Tract Infection
Acute Cystitis

Acute cystitis is an inflammation of the bladder and the most common site of UTI. The morphologic appearance of the bladder through cystoscopy describes different types of cystitis. With mild inflammation, the mucosa is hyperemic (red). More advanced cases may show diffuse hemorrhage (termed *hemorrhagic cystitis*), pus formation, or suppurative exudates (termed *suppurative cystitis*) on the epithelial surface of the bladder. Prolonged infection may lead to sloughing of the bladder mucosa with ulcer formation (termed *ulcerative cystitis*). The most severe infections may cause necrosis of the bladder wall (termed *gangrenous cystitis*).

PATHOPHYSIOLOGY. Two factors account for the presence of a UTI: the efficiency of defense mechanisms within the host (individual) and the virulence of the pathogen (bacterium, fungus, or parasite). The most common infecting microorganisms are uropathic strains of *Escherichia coli* (80% to 85%), and the second most common is *Staphylococcus saprophyticus* (10%). Less common microorganisms include *Klebsiella, Proteus, Pseudomonas*, fungi, viruses, parasites, or tubercular bacilli. *Schistosoma haematobium* is the most common cause of parasitic invasion of the urinary tract on a global basis; it infects more than 200 million people and has a strong association with bladder cancer.[52]

Bacterial contamination of the normally sterile urine usually occurs by retrograde movement of uropathic gram-negative bacilli (usually *Escherichia coli*) from the gut into the urethra and bladder and then to the ureter and kidney. Strains of *E. coli* also produce *siderophores* for acquiring nutrient iron, are resistant to bactericidal effects of complement, and express toxins including *cytotoxin necrotizing factor-1* and *hemolysins*. Certain bacterial species also enhance their virulence by acting together to form a biofilm that enhances colonization and resists efficiency of innate host defense mechanisms and antimicrobial therapy, particularly in catheter-associated UTI. Uropathic strains of *E. coli* have *type-1 fimbriae* that bind to latex catheters and receptors on the uroepithelium. They resist flushing during normal micturition and have flagella that propel them upstream. These strains also have *P. fimbriae* (pyelonephritis-associated fimbriae) that bind to the uroepithelium of individuals with P blood group antigen and flagella that propel them upstream. Some women may be genetically susceptible to certain strains of *E. coli* attachment and may harbor pathogenic strains in their vaginal flora.[53] Fungal infections are comparatively uncommon. The most common pathogen is *Candida,* but multiple fungal species may colonize the urinary tract or urinary catheters and produce symptomatic UTIs, particularly in those who are immunosuppressed.[54] Hematogenous infections are uncommon and often preceded by septicemia. Infection initiates an inflammatory response and the symptoms of cystitis.

◆**CLINICAL MANIFESTATIONS.** Clinical manifestations of cystitis are related to the host inflammatory response and usually include frequency, urgency, dysuria (painful urination), and suprapubic and low back pain. The inflammatory edema in the bladder wall stimulates discharge of stretch receptors, initiating symptoms of bladder fullness with small volumes of urine and producing the urgency and frequency of urination associated with cystitis. Hematuria, cloudy and foul-smelling urine, and flank pain are more serious symptoms. Approximately 10% of individuals with bacteriuria have no symptoms,[55] and 30% of individuals with symptoms are abacteriuric. Older adults with cystitis may be asymptomatic or demonstrate confusion or vague abdominal discomfort. Older adults with recurrent UTI and other concurrent illness have a higher risk of morbidity and mortality.[56]

◆**EVALUATION AND TREATMENT.** Infections in symptomatic individuals are diagnosed by urine culture of specific microorganisms with counts of 10,000/mL or more from freshly voided urine. Urine dipstick that is positive for leukocyte esterase or nitrite reductase can be used for the diagnosis of uncomplicated UTI. Risk factors, such as a urinary tract obstruction, should be identified and treated. Evidence of bacteria from urine culture and antibiotic sensitivity warrants treatment with a microorganism-specific antibiotic. Acute uncomplicated cystitis in nonpregnant women can be diagnosed without an office visit or urine culture. If a urine culture and sensitivity are ordered, the urine specimen must be obtained before the initiation of any antibiotic therapy; 3 to 5 days of treatment is most common.[57] Complicated UTI requires 7 to 14 days of treatment. From 20% to 25% of women have relapsing infection within 7 to 10 days requiring prolonged antibiotic treatment. Follow-up urine cultures should be obtained 1 week after initiation of treatment and at monthly intervals for 3 months. Clinical symptoms are frequently relieved, but bacteriuria may still be present. Repeat cultures should be obtained every 3 to 4 months until 1 year after treatment for evaluation and treatment of recurrent infection. Recurrent UTI is effectively treated with short courses of antibiotics, but antibiotic resistance is an emerging problem.[58] Urosepsis and septic shock are medical emergencies that usually demand parenteral, broad-spectrum antibiotic therapy and may require hospitalization.[59] A UTI caused by schistosomiasis is treated with praziquantel.[60] Noninfectious cystitis is associated with radiation or chemotherapy treatment for pelvic and urogenital cancers and is treated symptomatically.[61]

Interstitial Cystitis/Painful Bladder Syndrome

Interstitial cystitis/painful bladder syndrome (IC/PBS) is defined as an unpleasant sensation (pain, pressure, discomfort) perceived to be related to the urinary bladder associated with lower urinary tract symptoms of more than 6 weeks' duration in the absence of infection or other identifiable causes.[62] It occurs most commonly in women ages 20 to 40 years of age. Some individuals also experience fibromyalgia, irritable bowel syndrome, chronic fatigue syndrome, Sjögren syndrome, chronic headaches, and vulvodynia

The cause of IC/PBS is unknown, but an autoimmune reaction may be responsible for the inflammatory response, which includes mast cell activation, altered epithelial permeability, neuroinflammation, and increased sensory nerve sensitivity. The inflammation is associated with a derangement of the glycosaminoglycan layer of the bladder mucosa that makes it more susceptible to penetration by bacteria and noxious urinary solutes. Inflammation and fibrosis of the bladder wall are accompanied by the presence of hemorrhagic ulcers (Hunner ulcers) in some individuals, and bladder volume may decrease as a result of fibrosis, particularly in older individuals.[63] Antiproliferative factor (APF), a protein expressed by the bladder uroepithelium in those with IC, may be a biomarker. APF appears to block the normal growth of cells that line the inside wall of the bladder and indirectly increases bladder sensation.[64]

Characteristic symptoms of IC include bladder fullness, frequency (including nocturia), small urine volume, and chronic pelvic pain with symptoms lasting longer than 6 months. Chronic pain and sleep deprivation can lead to depression. Diagnosis of IC requires a thorough history, physical examination and urinalysis, analysis of cystoscopic findings, and the exclusion of other diagnoses.[65] No single treatment is effective. Oral and intravesical therapies, sacral nerve stimulation, and onabotulinumtoxinA (Botox) are used for symptom relief. Surgery is used in refractory cases.[66] More research is needed to understand the pathogenesis and long-term treatment of this disease.

Acute Pyelonephritis

Pyelonephritis is an infection of one or both upper urinary tracts (ureter, renal pelvis, and kidney interstitium). Common causes are summarized in Table 39.4. Urinary obstruction and reflux of urine from the bladder (vesicoureteral reflux) are the most common underlying risk factors. Most cases occur in women.

◆**PATHOPHYSIOLOGY.** Microorganisms usually associated with acute pyelonephritis include *E. coli, Proteus,* and *Pseudomonas.* The latter two microorganisms are more commonly associated with infections after urethral instrumentation or urinary tract surgery. These microorganisms also split urea into ammonia, making alkaline urine that increases the risk of stone formation. The infection is probably spread by ascending uropathic microorganisms along the ureters. Dissemination also may occur by way of the bloodstream, and both kidneys are usually involved. The inflammatory process is usually focal and irregular, primarily affecting the pelvis, calyces, and medulla. The infection causes medullary infiltration of neutrophils with tubulointerstitial inflammation, renal edema, and purulent urine. In severe infections, localized abscesses may form in the medulla and extend to the cortex. Primarily affected are the renal tubules; the glomeruli usually are spared. Necrosis of renal papillae can develop. After the acute phase, healing occurs with deposition of scar tissue, fibrosis, and atrophy of affected tubules (Fig. 39.7).[67] Acute pyelonephritis rarely causes renal failure.[68]

◆**CLINICAL MANIFESTATIONS.** The onset of symptoms is usually acute, with fever, chills, and flank or groin pain. Symptoms characteristic of a UTI, including frequency, dysuria, and costovertebral tenderness, may precede systemic signs and symptoms. Older adults may have nonspecific symptoms, such as low-grade fever and malaise.

TABLE 39.4	**COMMON CAUSES OF PYELONEPHRITIS**
PREDISPOSING FACTORS	**PATHOLOGIC MECHANISMS**
Kidney stones	Obstruction and stasis of urine contributing to bacteriuria and hydronephrosis; irritation of epithelial lining with entrapment of bacteria
Vesicoureteral reflux	Chronic reflux of urine up the ureter and into kidney during micturition, contributing to bacterial infection
Pregnancy	Dilation and relaxation of ureter with hydroureter and hydronephrosis; partly caused by obstruction from enlarged uterus and partly from ureteral relaxation caused by higher progesterone levels
Neurogenic bladder	Neurologic impairment interfering with normal bladder and urethral sphincter contraction with residual urine and ascending infection
Instrumentation	Introduction of organisms into urethra and bladder by catheters and endoscopes introduced into the urinary tract for diagnostic purposes
Female sexual trauma	Movement of organisms from the urethra into the bladder with infection and retrograde spread to kidney

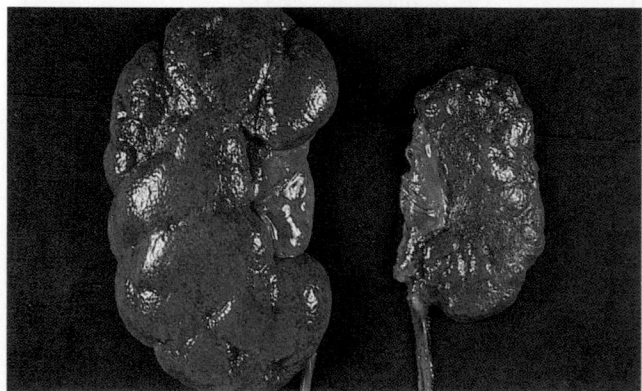

FIGURE 39.7 Pyelonephritis. *(Right)* Small, shrunken, irregularly scarred kidney of an individual with chronic pyelonephritis. *(Left)* Kidney is of normal size but also shows scarring on the upper pole. (From Damjanov I: *Pathology for the health professions,* ed 4, Philadelphia, 2012, Saunders.)

◆**EVALUATION AND TREATMENT.** Differentiating symptoms of cystitis from those of pyelonephritis by clinical assessment alone is difficult. The specific diagnosis is established by urine culture, urinalysis, and clinical signs and symptoms. White blood cell casts indicate pyelonephritis, but they are not always present in the urine. Complicated pyelonephritis requires blood cultures and urinary tract imaging.[69]

Uncomplicated acute pyelonephritis responds well to 2 to 3 weeks of microorganism-specific antibiotic therapy. Follow-up urine cultures are obtained at 1 and 4 weeks after treatment if symptoms recur. Antibiotic-resistant microorganisms or reinfection may occur in cases of urinary tract obstruction or reflux. Intravenous pyelography and voiding cystourethrography identify surgically correctable lesions.

Chronic Pyelonephritis

Chronic pyelonephritis is a persistent or recurrent infection of the kidney leading to scarring of the kidney. One or both kidneys may be involved. The specific cause of chronic pyelonephritis may be unknown (idiopathic) or associated with chronic UTIs, vesicoureteral reflux, renal stones, or obstructive uropathy. Recurrent infections from acute pyelonephritis may be associated with chronic pyelonephritis. Causes other than chronic pyelonephritis include drug toxicity from analgesics such as nonsteroidal antiinflammatory drugs, ischemia, irradiation, and immune-complex diseases.[70]

◆**PATHOPHYSIOLOGY.** Chronic urinary tract obstruction prevents elimination of bacteria and starts a process of progressive inflammation, alterations of the renal pelvis and calyces, destruction of the tubules, atrophy or dilation and diffuse scarring, and, finally, impaired urine-concentrating ability, leading to chronic kidney failure. The lesions of chronic pyelonephritis are sometimes termed *chronic interstitial nephritis* because the inflammation and fibrosis are located in the interstitial spaces between the tubules (see Fig. 39.7).

◆**CLINICAL MANIFESTATIONS.** The early symptoms of chronic pyelonephritis are often minimal and commonly include frequency, dysuria, and flank pain and may include hypertension. Progression of disease leads to renal failure, particularly in the presence of other risk factors (i.e., obstructive uropathy or diabetes mellitus). There is an inability to conserve sodium with loss of tubular function, and development of hyperkalemia and metabolic acidosis. Risk for dehydration must be considered if there is loss of the ability to concentrate the urine.

◆**EVALUATION AND TREATMENT.** Urinalysis, intravenous pyelography, and ultrasound are used diagnostically. Treatment is related to the underlying cause. Obstruction must be relieved. Antibiotics may be given, with prolonged antibiotic therapy for recurrent infection.

GLOMERULAR DISORDERS

Acute Glomerulonephritis

Acute glomerulonephritis is an inflammation of the glomerulus caused by *primary glomerular injury,* including immunologic responses, ischemia, free radicals, drugs, toxins, vascular disorders, and infection. *Secondary glomerular injury* is a consequence of systemic diseases, including diabetes mellitus, systemic lupus erythematosus, and, less commonly, congestive heart failure and HIV-related kidney disease. Glomerular disease is a significant cause of chronic kidney disease and end-stage renal failure worldwide.[71,72]

◆**PATHOPHYSIOLOGY.** Immune mechanisms are a major cause of injury for primary and secondary causes of glomerulonephritis (Fig. 39.8). The injury damages the glomerular capillary filtration membrane including the endothelium, basement membrane, and epithelium (podocytes). The most common types of immune injury are (1) deposition of circulating antigen-antibody immune complexes into the glomerulus (type III hypersensitivity); (2) reaction of antibodies in situ against planted antigens within the glomerulus (type II hypersensitivity, cytotoxic); (3) action of antibodies directed against the glomerular capillary wall (antiglomerular basement membrane antibodies), the least common and most severe form of immune injury (type II hypersensitivity); and (4) cell-mediated immune injury (type IV hypersensitivity) (Table 39.5). Nonimmune glomerular injury is related to ischemia, metabolic disorders (e.g., diabetes mellitus), toxin exposure, drugs, vascular disorders (e.g., vasculitis), and infection with direct injury to glomerular cells. Different causes of injury may result in more than one type of glomerular lesion; thus lesions are not necessarily disease specific (Table 39.6).

Immune injury is caused by activation of biochemical mediators of inflammation (i.e., complement and cytokines from leukocytes) and begins after the antigen-antibody complexes have deposited or formed in the glomerular capillary wall or mesangium. Complement can be

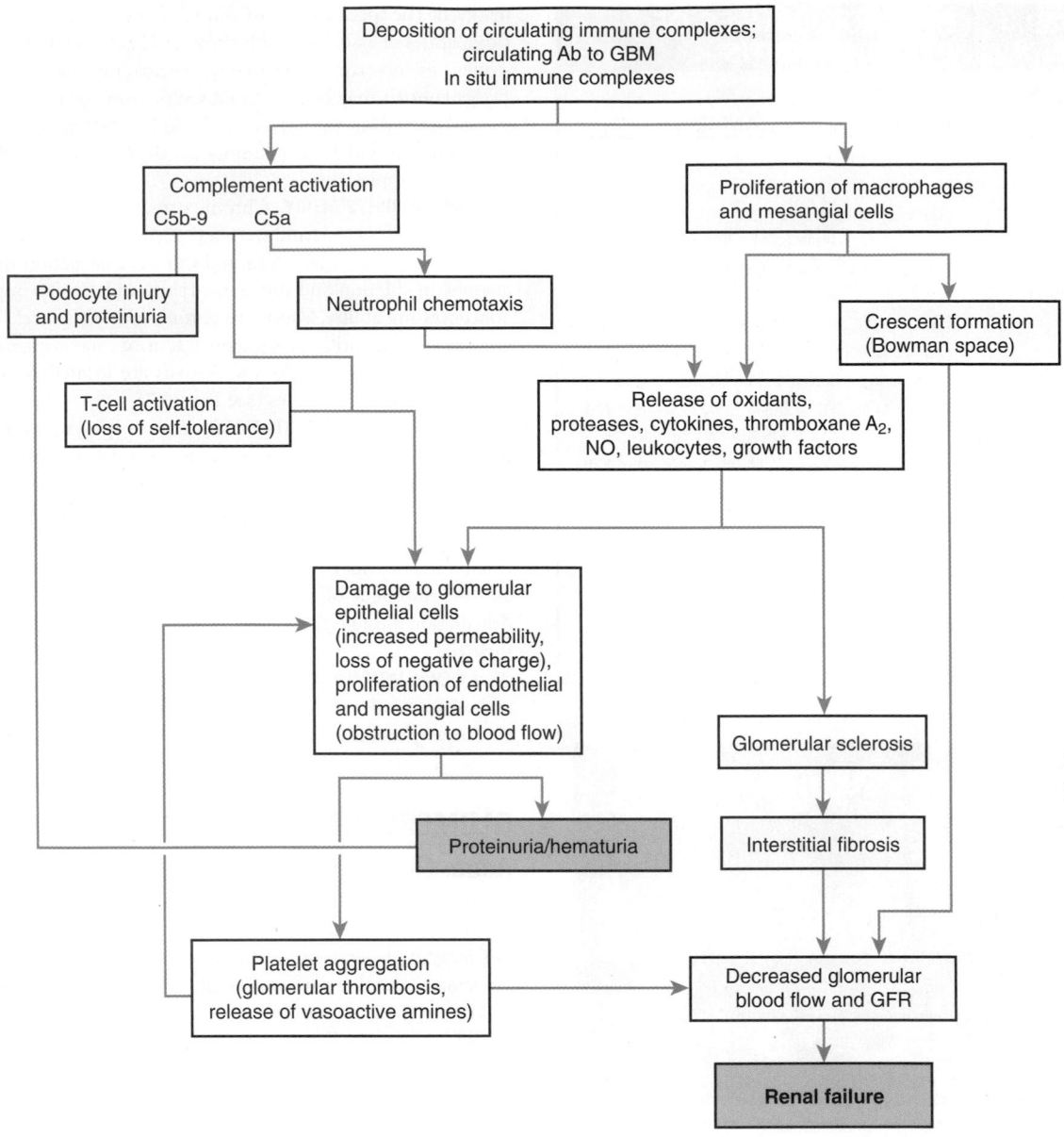

FIGURE 39.8 Mechanisms of Glomerular Injury. *Ab,* Antibody; *GBM,* glomerular basement membrane; *GFR,* glomerular filtration rate; *NO,* nitric oxide.

deposited with the antibodies, and activation can cause cell lysis or serve as a chemotactic stimulus for attraction of neutrophils, monocytes, and T lymphocytes. These phagocytes, along with activated platelets, further the inflammatory reaction by releasing mediators that injure the glomerular filtration membrane, including epithelial cells, glomerular basement membrane, and endothelial cells (podocytes and filtration slits).[73] The injury increases glomerular membrane permeability and reduces glomerular membrane surface area. There also may be swelling and proliferation of mesangial cells and expansion of the extracellular matrix in the Bowman space (Fig. 39.9), contributing to crescent formation (deposition of substances in the Bowman space, forming the shape of a crescent moon). The result is decreased glomerular blood flow, hypoxic injury, decreased driving hydrostatic pressure, decreased GFR, and increased serum creatinine levels.[74]

Loss of negative electrical charge across the glomerular filtration membrane and increase in filtration pore size enhance movement of proteins into the urine. Proteins are normally repelled because they

also have a negative charge. Red blood cells also escape if pore size is large enough. Proteinuria or hematuria, or both, develops. The severity of glomerular damage and decline in glomerular function is related to the size, number, and location (focal or diffuse) of cells injured; duration of exposure; and type of antigen-antibody complexes.

The mechanisms of acute glomerulonephritis are presented next, along with membranous glomerulonephritis, crescentic or rapidly progressive glomerulonephritis, mesangial proliferative glomerulonephritis, and membranous proliferative glomerulonephritis.[75] Immunoglobulin A (IgA) nephropathy is the binding of abnormal IgA to mesangial cells in the glomerulus resulting in injury and mesangial proliferation and presented in Chapter 40. Features of the types of glomerulonephritis are summarized in Table 39.7.

Focal segmental glomerulosclerosis is a scarring lesion that involves some but not all glomeruli (focal) and some but not all of the glomerular capillaries (segmental). The disease is characterized by primary podocyte injury related to gene alterations in podocyte structure (familial form)

TABLE 39.5 IMMUNOLOGIC PATHOGENESIS OF GLOMERULONEPHRITIS

GLOMERULAR INJURY	MECHANISM
Soluble immune-complex glomerulonephritis (90%)	Formation of antibodies stimulated by the presence of endogenous or exogenous antigens results in circulating soluble antigen-antibody complexes, which are deposited in glomerular capillaries, or the in situ formation of immune complexes to planted antigens or to structural components within the glomerulus; glomerular injury occurring with complement deposition and activation and release of immunologic substances that lyse cells and increase membrane permeability; immune deposits with a microscopic appearance that fluoresce in a *granular pattern* when stained with fluorescein and viewed under ultraviolet light; severity of glomerular injury related to the number of complexes formed; a type III hypersensitivity reaction; immunoglobulin A (IgA) nephropathy and poststreptococcal glomerulonephritis are examples
Antiglomerular basement membrane glomerulonephritis (5%)	Antibodies are formed and act directly against the glomerular basement membrane (type IV collagen); immune response that causes crescent formation and a *linear pattern* of immunofluorescence; generally associated with rapidly progressive renal failure such as Goodpasture syndrome (type II hypersensitivity reaction)
Alternative complement pathway	An immune mechanism associated with circulating autoantibodies and C3 complement and membranoproliferative glomerulonephritis
Cell-mediated immunity	A delayed hypersensitivity response that damages glomerulus; actual cellular mechanism not clearly understood but may involve cytokine secretion, activation of effector cells such as macrophages or by inducing autoantibodies or immune complexes; cytotoxic CD8+ T-cell responses and failure of regulatory T cells may represent two additional types of antirenal hypersensitivity (type IV hypersensitivity); often seen in rapidly progressive glomerulonephritis

Data from Foster MH: *Matrix Biol* 57-58:149-168, 2017; Nester CM, Smith RJ: *Semin Immunol* 28(3):241-249, 2016; Rodríguez-Iturbe B, Batsford S: *Kidney Int* 71(11):1094-1104, 2007.

TABLE 39.6 CLASSIFICATION OF GLOMERULAR LESIONS

LESION	DISTRIBUTION WHEN MANY GLOMERULI CONSIDERED
Diffuse	Relatively uniform involvement of most (>50%) or all glomeruli; most common form of glomerulonephritis
Focal	Changes in only some glomeruli (>50%), whereas others are normal

LESION	DISTRIBUTION WHEN SINGLE GLOMERULI CONSIDERED
Global	A lesion involving the entire glomerulus
Segmental-local	Changes in one part of the glomerulus with other parts unaffected

LESION	LESION CHARACTERISTICS
Mesangial	Deposits of immunoglobulins in the mesangial matrix; mesangial cell proliferation
Membranous	Thickening of the glomerular capillary wall with immune deposits (i.e., immunoglobulin G [IgG] and complement 3 [C3])
Proliferative	Increase in the number of glomerular cells: endothelial, epithelial, mesangial
Sclerotic	Glomerular scarring from previous glomerular injury
Crescentic	Accumulation of proliferating cells within Bowman space, making the appearance of a crescent
Interstitial fibrosis	Scarring between the glomerulus and the tubules

or a lesion that occurs secondarily in any type of chronic kidney disease (i.e., related to HIV or drugs). There are increases in mesangial matrix, loss of endothelial cells, and obliteration of capillary lumens by sclerosis and podocyte derangement. It is the most common cause of nephrotic syndrome in adults, compared to minimal change disease in children.[76]

Membranous nephropathy, also known as **membranous glomerulonephritis**, is one of the most common causes of acute glomerulonephritis, affects middle-aged and older adults, and is more common in men than women (sex ratio, 2:1). Primary membranous nephropathy is caused by subepithelial deposition of circulating antibodies or antibodies formed in situ to antigens located on glomerular podocytes. Assays are available to detect this antigen.[77] The antigen-antibody complexes activate C5b-C9 fragments of complement (the membrane attack complex) with injury and release of inflammatory mediators by mesangial and epithelial cells, resulting in increased membrane permeability, thickening of the glomerular membrane, and ultimately glomerular sclerosis. Secondary membranous nephropathy is associated with various disorders including infections (e.g., hepatitis B and C), systemic lupus erythematosus, some drugs (i.e., penicillamine), and some cancers. Proteinuria and nephrotic syndrome are the most common manifestations with risk for thromboembolism.[78] Alkylating agents plus corticosteroids or calcineurin inhibitors are used for treatment.

Rapidly progressive (crescentic) glomerulonephritis (RPGN), also known as *subacute* or *extracapillary glomerulonephritis*, is a rare disease and develops over days to weeks. The disease affects primarily adults in their 50s and 60s and may be idiopathic or associated with a proliferative glomerular disease (diffuse proliferation of extracapillary cells), such as lupus or poststreptococcal glomerulonephritis. Anti–glomerular basement membrane antibodies and anti-neutrophil cytoplasmic autoantibody (ANCA)-associated vasculitis are associated with glomerular injury and may be associated with pulmonary hemorrhage (Goodpasture syndrome). There is accumulation of T cells and macrophages with extensive proliferation of glomerular epithelial cells into the Bowman space. The accumulation of cells promotes crescent formation (the shape of the Bowman capsule). Heparin-binding epidermal growth factor–like growth factor (HB-EGF) released from glomerular epithelial cells is associated with the proliferation. Typically the glomerular injury is accompanied by a rapid decline in glomerular function, progressing to renal failure in a few weeks or months. Hematuria (nephritic syndrome) is common and may or may not be accompanied by proteinuria, edema, or hypertension (nephrotic syndrome). There are three types of RPGN distinguished by immunofluorescence and electron microscopic study of the renal biopsy. Types of RPGN are summarized in Table 39.7.[79]

RPGN has a relatively poor prognosis if not diagnosed and treated early. Anticoagulants may be of some benefit in reducing the fibrin component of crescent formation. Plasmapheresis is usually combined with corticosteroids and immunosuppression therapy. Dialysis or transplantation is required when failure is irreversible.[80]

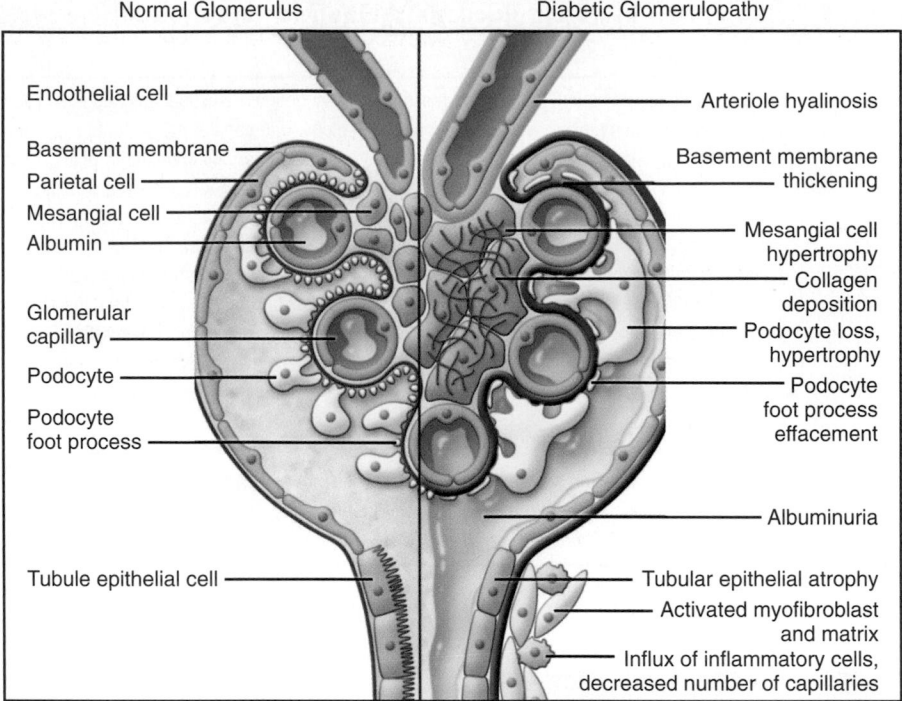

FIGURE 39.9 Diabetic Glomerulopathy. (Used with permission from Reidy K et al: *J Clin Invest* 124[6]:2333-2340, 2014.)

Mesangial proliferative glomerulonephritis is usually idiopathic and involves deposits of immune complex in the mesangium with mesangial cell proliferation. It can be associated with IgA nephropathy, lupus nephritis, or early diabetic nephropathy. Mesangial expansion reduces blood flow and alters filtration membrane permeability with development of hematuria, proteinuria, hypertension, and uremia (nephritic syndrome).

Membranoproliferative glomerulonephritis (MPGN) is an idiopathic pattern of glomerular injury that involves proliferation of mesangial cells and formation of crescents related to the deposition of complement (C3 component) and inflammatory injury. This disease is rare and can be associated with autoimmune diseases, infection such as hepatitis B and C, and monoclonal gammopathy. Hypocomplementemia is associated with all types of MPGN and they are differentiated by light microscopy. All three types stain positive for complement component C3 and are summarized in Table 39.7. Injury to the glomerular capillary wall in all types of MPGN can cause proteinuria, hematuria, nephrotic syndrome, and acute or chronic kidney failure.[81]

◆**CLINICAL MANIFESTATIONS.** The onset of glomerular disease may be sudden or insidious, and significant loss of nephron function can occur before symptoms develop. Acute glomerulonephritis may be silent, mild, moderate, or severe in symptom presentation; there are no specific clinical signs. Severe or progressive glomerular disease causes oliguria (urine output of 30 mL/hour or less), hypertension, and renal failure. Focal lesions tend to produce less severe clinical symptoms. Salt and water are reabsorbed, contributing to fluid volume expansion, edema, weight gain, and hypertension.

Two major symptoms of more severe glomerulonephritis are (1) proteinuria exceeding 3 g/day to 5 g/day with albumin (macroalbuminuria) as the major protein and (2) hematuria with red blood cell casts. Nephrotic syndrome is associated with gross proteinuria and lipid sediments (see the section on Nephrotic and Nephritic Syndromes). Nephritic syndrome is associated with red blood cells escaping through the glomerular membrane producing a smoky, brown-tinged urine;

red blood cell casts; and an accompanying proteinuria. Glomerular bleeding provides prolonged contact with the acidic urine and transforms hemoglobin to methemoglobin, which has a brownish color and no blood clots. In comparison, bleeding from sites lower in the urinary tract produces a pink- or red-colored urine. The urine sediment of chronic glomerular disease has waxy casts, granular casts, and less protein and blood than found in nephrotic or nephritic syndromes.

◆**EVALUATION AND TREATMENT.** The diagnosis of glomerular disease is confirmed by the progressive development of clinical manifestations and laboratory findings of abnormal urinalysis with proteinuria, red blood cells, white blood cells, and casts. Reduced GFR during glomerulonephritis is evidenced by elevated plasma urea, cystatin C, and creatinine concentrations, or by reduced renal creatinine clearance (see Chapter 38). Renal biopsy provides a specific determination of renal injury and type of pathologic condition. Patterns of antigen-antibody complex deposition or formation within the glomerular capillary filtration membrane have been established using light, electron, and immunofluorescent microscopy. Electron microscopy differentiates morphologic changes within the glomerular capillary wall (e.g., subendothelial and mesangial electron-dense deposits, increased mesangial matrix, mesangialization of capillary loops, and foot process fusion). Staining with fluorescein identifies complement and different antibodies (i.e., immunoglobulin G [IgG] or IgA) and their configurations when viewed under ultraviolet light with light microscopy (see Chapter 40, Fig. 40.5, *C*).

Management principles for treating glomerulonephritis are related to treating the primary cause; preventing or minimizing immune responses; and correcting accompanying problems, such as edema and hypertension. Specific treatment regimens are necessary for particular types of glomerulonephritis. Antibiotic therapy is essential for the management of underlying infections that may be contributing to ongoing antigen-antibody responses. Corticosteroids decrease antibody synthesis and suppress inflammatory responses. Cytotoxic agents (e.g., cyclophosphamide) may be used to suppress the immune response in

TABLE 39.7 FEATURES OF THE TYPES OF GLOMERULONEPHRITIS

TYPE AND CAUSE	HISTOPATHOPHYSIOLOGY
Associated with Nephritic Syndrome	
Acute postinfectious glomerulonephritis (PIGN) (e.g., group A beta-hemolytic streptococci [more common in children]; staphylococcus [more common in older adults])	Subepithelial deposits of IgG and complement complexes; infiltration of neutrophils and monocytes; proliferation of mesangial and epithelial cells with occlusion of glomerular capillary blood flow and decreased glomerular filtration; usually diffuse lesions
Rapidly progressive or crescentic glomerulonephritis (a clinical syndrome): *Type I:* Formation of IgG antibodies against pulmonary capillary and glomerular basement membrane (Goodpasture syndrome); activation of complement and neutrophils; more common in young men, causes pulmonary hemorrhage and renal failure *Type II:* Mesangial immune complex deposition (PIGN, SLE, IgA nephropathy) *Type III:* Pauci-immune, lack of anti-GBM antibodies or immune complexes; presence of serum antineutrophil cytoplasmic (ANC) antibodies associated with systemic vasculitides (usually idiopathic); nonspecific response to glomerular injury; can occur in any severe glomerular disease	Accumulation of fibrin, macrophages, and epithelial cell proliferation into the Bowman space forms crescents and occludes glomerular capillary blood flow, decreasing glomerular filtration; antiglomerular basement membrane antibodies lead to necrotizing, proliferative glomerulonephritis, and renal failure; diffuse lesions
Mesangial proliferative glomerulonephritis Can be associated with IgA nephropathy or lupus nephritis	Deposits of immune complexes in the mesangium with mesangial cell proliferation; results in decreased glomerular blood flow and glomerular filtration; leads to hematuria/proteinuria and nephrotic syndrome
Associated with Nephrotic Syndrome	
Minimal change nephropathy (lipoid nephrosis) Glomerular basement membrane appears normal Most common cause of nephrotic syndrome in children (see Chapter 40) Usually idiopathic	Glomeruli look normal under light microscopy; electron microscopy reveals uniform diffuse effacement of epithelial (podocyte) foot processes; loss of negative charge in basement membrane and increased permeability lead to severe proteinuria and nephrotic syndrome
Focal segmental glomerulosclerosis Usually idiopathic Can be associated with HIV infection, IgA nephropathy	Focal proliferation of endothelial and mesangial cells and glomerulosclerosis from hyaline deposits in segmental parts of the glomerular membrane; there is effacement (thinning or deletion) of epithelial podocytes, with a significant increase in pore size resulting in proteinuria and nephrotic syndrome; can progress to involve entire glomerulus and development of tubulointerstitial fibrosis
Membranous nephropathy (autoimmune response to unknown renal antigen) Usually idiopathic; can be associated with systemic diseases (i.e., hepatitis B virus, hepatitis C virus, systemic lupus erythematosus, solid malignant tumors)	Diffuse thickening of glomerular basement membrane and capillary wall from deposits of antibody, complement, and release of inflammatory cytokines; increased permeability with proteinuria and leading cause of nephrotic syndrome in white adults
Membranoproliferative glomerulonephritis (MPGN) Usually idiopathic; associated with hypocomplementemia *Type I:* Activation of classical complement pathway with nephrotic syndrome (hepatitides B and C, SLE) *Type II:* Activation of alternate complement pathway with hematuria (idiopathic); no circulating immune complexes *Type III:* Activation of alternative complement pathway with nephrotic syndrome; can be familial	Mesangial cell proliferation; thickening of basement membrane; subendothelial deposits of immune complex occlude glomerular capillary blood flow and decrease glomerular filtration; diffuse lesions
IgA Nephropathy (Berger Disease) Usually idiopathic (can be associated with cirrhosis and minimal change disease); elevated IgA plasma levels (also see Henoch-Schönlein purpura nephritis in Chapter 40)	Mesangial proliferation with deposition of IgA; release of inflammatory mediators with cellular proliferation; crescent formation, glomerulosclerosis, interstitial fibrosis, decreased GFR and hematuria; usually focal, some diffuse lesions

GBM, Glomerular basement membrane; *GFR,* glomerular filtration rate; *HIV,* human immunodeficiency virus; *IgA,* immunoglobulin A; *IgG,* immunoglobulin G; *SLE,* systemic lupus erythematosus.

corticosteroid-resistant cases. Anticoagulants may be useful for controlling fibrin crescent formation in rapidly progressive glomerulonephritis.

Chronic Glomerulonephritis

Chronic glomerulonephritis encompasses glomerular diseases with a progressive course leading to chronic kidney disease. There may be no history of renal disease before the diagnosis. Proteinuria and hypercholesterolemia have been associated with progressive glomerular and tubular injury.[82] The proposed mechanism is related to those observed in glomerulosclerosis and interstitial injury, such as hyperfiltration and inflammatory processes. The primary cause may be difficult to establish because advanced pathologic changes may obscure specific

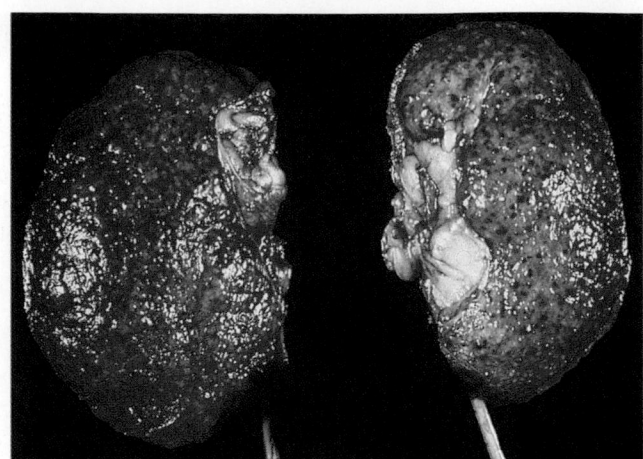

FIGURE 39.10 Chronic Glomerulonephritis. The kidneys appear small, are uniformly shrunken, and have a finely granular external surface. (From Damjanov I: *Pathology for the health professions*, ed 4, Philadelphia, 2012, Saunders.)

disease characteristics (Fig. 39.10). Renal insufficiency usually begins to develop after 10 to 20 years, followed by nephrotic syndrome and an accelerated progression to end-stage kidney failure. Symptom patterns vary depending on the underlying cause. Corticosteroids usually do not change the course of chronic glomerular disease, and dialysis or kidney transplantation ultimately may be needed. Diabetes mellitus and systemic lupus erythematosus are common secondary causes of chronic glomerular injury.

Diabetic nephropathy develops from metabolic (accumulation of advanced glycosylated end products), inflammatory (transforming growth factor-beta and protein kinase C), and macrovascular and microvascular complications related to chronic hyperglycemia (see Chapter 22). Changes in the glomerulus are characterized by podocyte injury, progressive thickening and fibrosis of the glomerular basement membrane, expansion of the mesangial matrix (diffuse diabetic glomerulosclerosis), and nodular glomerulosclerosis (Kimmelstiel-Wilson nodules; see Fig. 39.9) with proteinuria and progression to chronic renal failure. Decline in GFR can be independent of proteinuria.[83] Diabetic nephropathy is the most common cause of chronic kidney disease and end-stage renal failure for both type 1 and type 2 diabetes, although the incidence is declining.[84]

Lupus nephritis is an inflammatory complication of the chronic autoimmune syndrome systemic lupus erythematosus (see Chapter 9). The renal component of the disease may be caused by the formation of autoantibodies against double-stranded DNA and nucleosomes with glomerular deposition of the immune complexes. Immune complexes also may be formed in situ by binding to planted antigens of circulating autoantibodies. There is complement activation and a cascade of inflammatory events resulting in damage to the glomerular membrane with mesangial expansion (see Chapter 8).[85,86] Various glomerular lesion patterns are identifiable on biopsy, including membranous, mesangial, membranoproliferative, and diffuse proliferative glomerulonephritis; tubular fibrosis can also be present (see Table 39.6). Symptom presentation is variable depending on lesion involvement and can include proteinuria, microscopic hematuria, edema, and other signs of nephrotic syndrome. Disease progression may be silent or may progress to end-stage kidney failure over a period of years. Treatment includes the use of immunosuppressive agents and efforts to protect the kidney from secondary nonimmune consequences of acute injury.[87,88]

Nephrotic and Nephritic Syndromes

Nephrotic syndrome is the excretion of 3.5 g or more of protein in the urine per day, is characteristic of glomerular injury, and occurs when filtration of proteins exceeds tubular reabsorption. *Primary causes of nephrotic syndrome* include minimal change disease (lipoid nephrosis), membranous glomerulonephritis, and focal segmental glomerulosclerosis (see Table 39.7). *Secondary forms of nephrotic syndrome* occur in systemic diseases including diabetes mellitus, amyloidosis, systemic lupus erythematosus, and IgA vasculitis (i.e., Henoch-Schönlein purpura) (see Chapter 40). Nephrotic syndrome also is associated with certain drugs (e.g., nonsteroidal antiinflammatory drugs and penicillamine), infections, malignancies, and vascular disorders. Familial forms of nephrotic syndrome result from genetic defects that affect the function and composition of the glomerular capillary wall (i.e., alterations in basement membrane type IV collagen [Alport syndrome] and podocyte dysfunction).[89] It often signifies a more serious prognosis when present as a secondary complication. Nephrotic syndrome is more common in children than in adults and is more commonly idiopathic in adults.

Nephritic syndrome is hematuria and red blood cell casts in the urine. Proteinuria is usually less severe than in nephrotic syndrome and is related to infiltration of inflammatory cells in the mesangium driven by antigen deposition with damage to endothelial cells and escape of red blood cells and protein. It occurs with infection-related glomerulonephritis (i.e., hepatitis B and C and acute post-streptococcal glomerulonephritis), rapidly progressive crescentic glomerulonephritis, and lupus nephritis.[90]

◆**PATHOPHYSIOLOGY.** In nephrotic syndrome, disturbances in the glomerular basement membrane (GBM) and podocyte injury lead to loss of electrical negative charge and increased permeability (see Chapter 38). Loss of plasma proteins, particularly albumin and some immunoglobulins, occurs across the injured glomerular filtration membrane (Fig. 39.11). Loss of plasma proteins decreases plasma oncotic pressure, resulting in edema. The predominant cause of nephrotic syndrome is minimal-change nephropathy, which is common in children (see Chapter 40). Hypoalbuminemia results from urinary loss of albumin combined with a diminished synthesis of replacement albumin by the liver. Albumin is lost in the greatest quantity because of its high plasma concentration and low molecular weight. Decreased dietary intake of protein from anorexia or malnutrition or accompanying liver disease may also contribute to lower levels of plasma albumin. Loss of albumin stimulates lipoprotein synthesis by the liver and hyperlipidemia and can promote progression of glomerular disease. Loss of immunoglobulins may increase susceptibility to infections. Sodium retention is common. Hypercoagulation results from alterations in coagulation factors, fibrinolysis, and platelet function.[91,92]

◆**CLINICAL MANIFESTATIONS.** Many clinical manifestations of nephrotic and nephritic syndrome are related to loss of serum proteins (Table 39.8) and associated retention of sodium. They include edema, hypertension, hyperlipidemia, lipiduria, vitamin D deficiency, and hypothyroidism. Vitamin D deficiency is related to loss of serum transport proteins and decreased vitamin D activation by the kidney. Hyperlipidemia can promote atherosclerotic disease. Hypothyroidism can result from urinary loss of thyroid-binding protein and thyroxine, but there may be no symptoms. Hypercoagulability may lead to thromboembolic events.[93,94]

◆**EVALUATION AND TREATMENT.** Nephrotic syndrome is diagnosed when the protein level in a 24-hour urine collection is greater than 3.5 g. Serum albumin level decreases (to less than 3 g/dL), and concentrations of serum cholesterol, phospholipids, and triglycerides increase. Fat bodies may be present in the urine.

Nephrotic syndrome is commonly treated by consuming a moderate protein-restricted (i.e., 0.8 g/kg body weight/day), low-fat, and salt-restricted diet. Diuretics are used to control hypertension and eliminate fluid. Care must be taken to observe for hypovolemia and hypokalemia or potassium toxicity in the presence of renal insufficiency. Spironolactone may be combined with loop diuretics to suppress aldosterone activity to conserve potassium. Heparinoids are used for prophylactic anticoagulation. Glucocorticoids are used to control immune-mediated disease or may be combined with immunosuppressive drugs. Angiotensin-converting enzyme (ACE) inhibitors or angiotensin receptor blockers (ARBs) lower urine protein excretion and control blood pressure.[95,96]

The evaluation and treatment of nephritic syndrome are similar to those described for nephrotic syndrome. The course of glomerulonephritis is usually more severe with nephritic syndrome. High-dose corticosteroids and cyclophosphamide represent the standard therapy for rapidly progressive crescentic glomerulonephritis. The addition of plasma exchange (plasmapheresis) also may be helpful.[79]

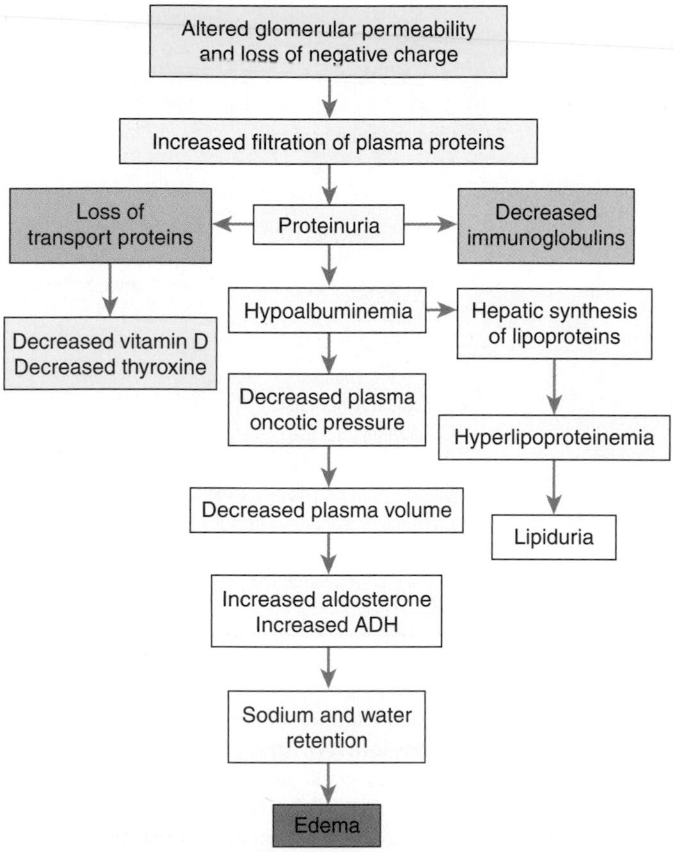

ACUTE KIDNEY INJURY

Classification of Kidney Dysfunction

Kidney injury may be acute and rapidly progressive (within hours), and the process may be reversible. Kidney injury also can be chronic, progressing to end-stage kidney failure over a period of months or years. The terms *renal insufficiency, renal failure, uremia,* and *azotemia* are associated with decreasing renal function but are not specific in relation to cause of kidney disease. Often they are used synonymously, although with some distinctions. Generally, renal insufficiency refers to a decline in renal function to about 25% of normal or a GFR of 25 to 30 mL/minute. Levels of serum creatinine and urea are mildly elevated. The term *acute kidney injury* is preferred to the term acute renal failure because it captures the diverse nature of this syndrome, ranging from minimal or subtle changes in renal function to complete renal failure requiring renal replacement therapy. Renal failure refers to significant loss of renal function. When less than 10% of renal function remains, this is termed end-stage kidney disease (ESKD). Specific criteria for acute renal dysfunction are discussed in the next section. Uremia (uremic syndrome) is a syndrome of renal failure and includes elevated blood urea and creatinine levels accompanied by fatigue, anorexia, nausea, vomiting, pruritus, and neurologic changes. Uremia represents numerous consequences related to renal failure, including retention of toxic wastes, deficiency states, electrolyte disorders, and immune activation promoting a proinflammatory state. Azotemia is characterized by increased serum urea levels and frequently increased creatinine levels (normal is 0.7 to 1.4 mg/dL). Renal insufficiency or renal failure causes azotemia. Both azotemia and uremia indicate an accumulation of nitrogenous waste products in the blood, a common characteristic that explains the overlap in definitions of terms.

FIGURE 39.11 Pathophysiology of Nephrotic Syndrome.

TABLE 39.8	**CLINICAL MANIFESTATIONS OF NEPHROTIC SYNDROME**	
MANIFESTATIONS	**CONTRIBUTING FACTORS**	**RESULT**
Proteinuria	Increased glomerular permeability, decreased proximal tubule reabsorption	Edema, increased susceptibility to infection from loss of immunoglobulins
Hypoalbuminemia	Increased urinary losses of protein	Edema
Edema	Hypoalbuminemia (decreased oncotic pressure, sodium and water retention, increased aldosterone and antidiuretic hormone [ADH] secretion), unresponsiveness to atrial natriuretic peptides	Soft, pitting, generalized edema
Hyperlipidemia	Decreased serum albumin; increased hepatic synthesis of very-low-density lipoproteins; increased cholesterol, phospholipids, triglycerides	Increased atherogenesis
Lipiduria	Sloughing of tubular cells containing fat (oval fat bodies); free fat from hyperlipidemia	Fat droplets that may float in urine
Decreased vitamin D	The globulin to which 1,25-dihydroxy-vitamin D_3 is attached for transport passes through the glomerulus and is lost in the urine	Decreased absorption of calcium from gut Risk for osteodystrophies
Hypothyroidism	Loss of thyroid-binding globulin and other thyroid hormone transport proteins in the urine	May have no symptoms; may have elevated thyroid-stimulating hormone

TABLE 39.9	STAGING OF ACUTE KIDNEY INJURY

STAGE	SERUM CREATININE
1	1.5–1.9 times baseline
	OR
	≥0.3 mg/dL (≥26.5 µmol/L) increase
2	2.0–2.9 times baseline
3	3.0 times baseline
	OR
	Increase in serum creatinine to ≥4.0 mg/dL (≥353.6 5 µmol/L)
	OR
	Initiation of renal replacement therapy OR in individuals <18 years, decrease in eGFR to <35 mL/min per 1.73 m^2

eGFR, Estimated glomerular filtration rate.
Data from: Kidney Disease: Improving Global Outcomes (KDIGO)
Acute Kidney Injury Work Group: *Kidney Inter Suppl* 2:1-138, 2012.
Available at: http://www.kdigo.org/clinical_practice_guidelines/AKI.php.

Acute Kidney Injury

Acute kidney injury (AKI) affects about 5% of hospitalized individuals with a higher percentage in intensive care units and has a mortality of 50% to 80%.[97] AKI is a sudden decline in kidney function with a decrease in glomerular filtration and urine output with an accumulation of nitrogenous waste products in the blood as demonstrated by an elevation in plasma creatinine and blood urea nitrogen levels. Staging criteria have been developed by the Kidney Disease: Improving Global Outcomes (KDIGO) Working Group to guide the diagnosis of acute renal injury (Table 39.9).

◆PATHOPHYSIOLOGY. AKI commonly results from extracellular volume depletion, decreased renal blood flow, or toxic/inflammatory injury to kidney cells that result in alterations in renal function that may be minimal or severe. Even small changes in renal function may be associated with significant morbidity and mortality. The etiologies of AKI can be described considering three categories of injury: (1) renal hypoperfusion (prerenal AKI); (2) disorders involving the renal parenchymal or interstitial tissue (intrarenal or intrinsic AKI); and (3) disorders associated with acute urinary tract obstruction (postrenal AKI) (Table 39.10). Most types of AKI are reversible if diagnosed and treated early.

Prerenal acute kidney injury is the most common cause of AKI and results from inadequate kidney perfusion. Poor perfusion can be caused by hypotension, hypovolemia associated with hemorrhage or fluid loss (e.g., burns), sepsis, inadequate cardiac output (e.g., myocardial infarct), multiple organ dysfunction, renal vasoconstriction (e.g., caused by nonsteroidal antiinflammatory drugs [NSAIDs] or radiocontrast agents), renal artery stenosis, or kidney edema that restricts arterial blood flow. During the early phases of hypoperfusion, protective autoregulatory mechanisms maintain GFR at a relatively constant level through afferent arteriolar dilation and efferent arteriolar vasoconstriction (mediated by angiotensin II). Tubuloglomerular feedback mechanisms also maintain GFR and distal tubular nephron flow (see Chapter 38). The GFR ultimately declines because of the decrease in filtration pressure. Sepsis/septic shock and cardiogenic shock following cardiac surgery are the most common causes of AKI in the critical care unit.[98,99] AKI may occur during chronic kidney failure if a sudden stress is imposed on already marginally functioning kidneys, hastening the progression to end-stage kidney disease. Failure to restore blood volume or blood pressure and oxygen delivery can cause cell injury and acute tubular necrosis and apoptosis or acute interstitial necrosis, a more severe form of AKI.

TABLE 39.10	CAUSES OF ACUTE KIDNEY INJURY

AREA OF DYSFUNCTION	POSSIBLE CAUSES
Prerenal	Hypovolemia
	Hemorrhagic blood loss (trauma, gastrointestinal bleeding, complications of childbirth)
	Loss of plasma volume (burns, peritonitis)
	Water and electrolyte losses (severe vomiting or diarrhea, intestinal obstruction, uncontrolled diabetes mellitus, inappropriate use of diuretics)
	Systemic hypotension or hypoperfusion
	Septic shock systemic inflammation
	Cardiac failure or shock
	Massive pulmonary embolism
	Stenosis or clamping of renal artery
	Increased intraabdominal pressure (abdominal compartment syndrome)
Intrarenal	Acute tubular necrosis (postischemic or nephrotoxic)
	Glomerulopathies
	Acute interstitial necrosis (tumors or toxins)
	Vascular damage
	Malignant hypertension, vasculitis
	Coagulation defects
	Renal artery/vein occlusion
	Bilateral acute pyelonephritis
Postrenal	Obstructive uropathies (usually bilateral—fibrosis)
	Ureteral destruction (edema, tumors, stones, clots)
	Bladder neck obstruction (enlarged prostate)
	Neurogenic bladder

Intrarenal (intrinsic) acute kidney injury (AKI) can result from ischemic acute tubular necrosis (ATN), nephrotoxic ATN (i.e., exposure to radiocontrast media or antibiotics), acute glomerulonephritis, vascular disease (malignant hypertension, disseminated intravascular coagulation, and renal vasculitis), allograft rejection, or interstitial disease (drug allergy, infection, tumor growth). ATN caused by ischemia is the most common cause of intrarenal AKI. It occurs most often after surgery and severe sepsis (40% to 50% of cases) but also is associated with obstetric complications and severe trauma, including severe burns. A combination of events and predisposing factors leads to the greatest risk for acute renal failure. The terms *acute tubular necrosis* and *acute kidney injury* are sometimes used interchangeably, but the conditions are not the same because acute kidney injury can occur without ATN. ATN is generally described as postischemic or nephrotoxic, or it can be a combination of both. Postischemic ATN involves persistent hypotension, hypoperfusion, and hypoxemia, producing ischemia and reduced levels of ATP and generating toxic oxygen free radicals with loss of antioxidant protection that causes cell swelling, injury, and necrosis. Activation of inflammatory cells (e.g., neutrophils, macrophages, and lymphocytes) and complement and release of inflammatory cytokines contribute to tubular injury. Transport of sodium and other molecules is disrupted with damage primarily to the proximal tubular epithelium and shedding of the brush border with the appearance of tubular granular casts in the urine. Ischemic necrosis tends to be patchy and may be distributed along any part of the nephron tubules. Injury is most severe in the outer medulla (the medulla has the highest oxygen extraction rate of all body tissues, ≈80%) with scattered necrosis in the cortex and loss of cells along the tubular epithelium.[100] Severe disease of the glomeruli

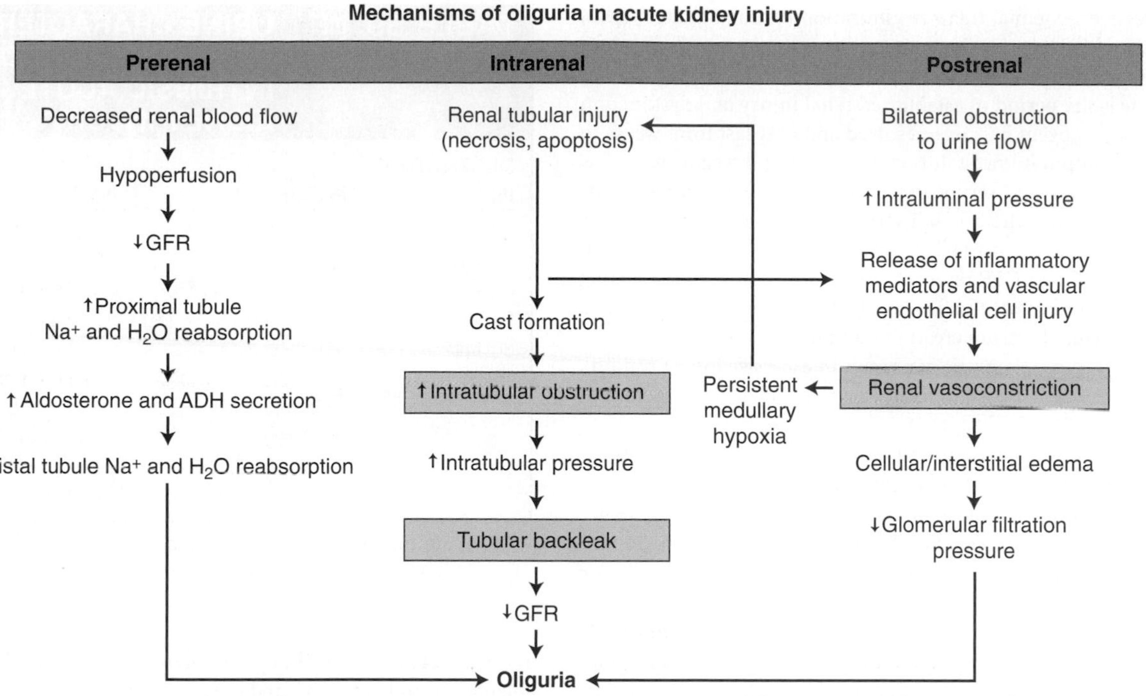

Mechanisms of oliguria in acute kidney injury

FIGURE 39.12 Acute Kidney Injury and Mechanisms of Oliguria. *ADH,* Antidiuretic hormone; *GFR,* glomerular filtration rate.

(i.e., acute or rapidly progressive glomerulonephritis) or renal microvascular disorders also can cause intrinsic kidney injury. Oliguria is common (urine output less than 30 mL/hour) with intrarenal AKI, but anuria is rare. Creatinine values in septic renal injury may not reflect renal injury because sepsis decreases production of creatinine without major alterations in body weight, hematocrit level, or amount of extracellular fluid. Creatinine level usually increases with decreased renal blood flow and decreased GFR. However, in sepsis-induced AKI, creatinine values can remain within normal ranges and may be related to alterations in intrarenal microcirculatory blood flow that are different from the kidney ischemia that develops related to systemic hypotension and hypoperfusion of nonseptic AKI. Sepsis-related tubular injury can occur in the absence of hypoperfusion and may be related to inflammation and changes in microcirculation and mitochondrial function.[99]

Nephrotoxic ATN can be produced by radiocontrast media and numerous antibiotics, particularly aminoglycosides (neomycin, gentamicin, tobramycin), because the drugs accumulate in the renal cortex. Other substances, such as carbon tetrachloride, heavy metals (mercury, arsenic), methoxyflurane anesthesia, or bacterial toxins, may promote renal failure. Endogenous substances toxic to renal tubules are excessive myoglobin (oxygen-transporting substance in muscles) and hemoglobin. Dehydration, advanced age, concurrent renal insufficiency, and diabetes mellitus tend to enhance nephrotoxicity. Necrosis and tubular cell apoptosis caused by nephrotoxins are usually uniform and limited to the proximal tubules. The high surface area of the brush border (microvilli) of the proximal tubular cells and the reabsorption properties of epithelial cells make them more vulnerable to toxic injury.

Postrenal acute kidney injury is rare and usually occurs with urinary tract obstruction that affects the kidneys bilaterally (e.g., bilateral ureteral obstruction, bladder outlet obstruction-prostatic hypertrophy, tumors or neurogenic bladder, and urethral obstruction). The obstruction causes an increase in intraluminal pressure upstream from the site of obstruction with a gradual decrease in GFR. A pattern of several hours of anuria with flank pain followed by polyuria is a characteristic finding. This type of AKI can occur after diagnostic catheterization of the ureters, a procedure that may cause edema with obstruction of the tubular lumen.

Oliguria (less than 400 mL of urine output per day) can occur in AKI, and three mechanisms have been proposed to account for the decrease in urine output. All three mechanisms probably contribute to oliguria in varying combinations and degrees throughout the course of the disease (Fig. 39.12). These mechanisms are as follows:[100,101]

1. *Alterations in renal blood flow.* In response to ischemia, blood flow is directed to the highly metabolic renal medulla. With continuing severe ischemia, tubular sodium chloride reabsorption fails and tubuloglomerular feedback at the macula densa activates the renin-angiotensis-aldosterone system (RAAS). There is an increased afferent arteriolar vasoconstriction and decreased GFR. Damaged endothelium and leukocyte activation activate coagulation and further impede microcirculatory blood flow, contributing to ischemia, reperfusion injury, and decreased GFR. Decreased GFR can be lifesaving; otherwise GFR would not change and death could result from continuing fluid loss during concurrent hypovolemia and hypotension. Autoregulation of blood flow also is impaired, contributing to decreased GFR.

2. *Tubular obstruction.* Necrosis of the tubules causes sloughing of cells, cast formation, and ischemic edema that result in tubular obstruction, which in turn causes a retrograde increase in pressure and reduces the GFR. Renal failure can occur within 24 hours.

3. *Tubular backleak.* Glomerular filtration remains normal, but tubular reabsorption or "leak" of filtrate is accelerated as a result of permeability caused by ischemia and increased tubular pressure from obstruction. Obstruction and backleak probably occur concurrently.

◆**CLINICAL MANIFESTATIONS.** The clinical progression of acute kidney injury, particularly acute tubular necrosis, occurs in phases: initiation phase, extension phase, maintenance phase, and recovery phase. The *initiation phase* is the phase of reduced perfusion or toxicity in which renal injury is evolving, usually lasting 24 to 36 hours. Prevention of injury is possible during this phase. During the *extension phase,* and with progressive ischemia, there is infiltration of inflammatory cells, mostly neutrophils; release of cytokines; inflammation; and cell injury contributing to tubular obstruction and backleak. The *maintenance* or *oliguric phase* is the period of established renal injury and dysfunction after the initiating event has been resolved and may last from weeks to months. Urine output is lowest during this phase, and serum creatinine, blood urea nitrogen, and serum potassium levels increase; metabolic acidosis develops; and there is salt and water overload. The *recovery phase* is the interval when renal injury is repaired and normal renal function is reestablished. GFR returns toward normal but the regenerating tubules cannot concentrate the filtrate. Diuresis is common during this phase, with a decline in serum creatinine and urea levels and an increase in creatinine clearance. Polyuria can result in excessive loss of sodium, potassium, and water. Fluid and electrolyte balance requires careful maintenance.

Oliguria begins within 1 day after a hypotensive event and lasts for 1 to 3 weeks, but it may regress in several hours or extend for several weeks, depending on the duration of ischemia or severity of toxic injury and the initiation of treatment. Anuria (urine output less than 50 mL/day) is uncommon in ATN, and 10% to 20% of cases have nonoliguric failure. Anuria involves both kidneys and suggests bilateral renal artery occlusion, obstructive uropathy, or acute cortical necrosis. **Nonoliguric renal failure** usually represents less severe injury and is associated with toxin exposure or drug toxicity. The renal tubules have impaired reabsorption and concentration and dilution function. The urine output may be greater than 2 L/day, but the blood urea nitrogen (BUN) and plasma creatinine concentrations increase.

Other early manifestations depend on the underlying cause of renal failure. Individuals who have experienced trauma or surgery or people in a catabolic state may have more rapid elevations in BUN level. They are prone to hyperkalemia and metabolic acidosis. Renal phosphate excretion is decreased, causing hyperphosphatemia. Fluid retention may cause edema. Symptoms of congestive heart failure develop in persons with cardiac disease. Nausea, vomiting, and fatigue accompany uremia and electrolyte imbalances. Wound healing is delayed, and the risk of infection, particularly pneumonia, is greater. Nonoliguric renal failure generally has a better prognosis because of fewer complications and regeneration of the tubular epithelium. Individuals with oliguria may require maintenance dialysis to attenuate symptoms of renal failure.

As renal function improves during the recovery phase, increase in urine volume (diuresis) is progressive. During the early diuretic phase the tubules are still recovering secretory and reabsorptive function. Sodium and potassium are lost in the urine, and the risk for hypokalemia is greater. Volume depletion may ensue, with fluid losses of 3 to 4 L/day. Fluid and electrolyte balance must be carefully monitored and excessive urinary losses replaced. Return to normal status may take 3 to 12 months. AKI is a risk factor for progression to end-stage kidney disease and other complications, such as cardiovascular events and stroke.[102,103]

◆ **EVALUATION AND TREATMENT.** The diagnosis of AKI is related to the cause of the disease. The history can help distinguish the different etiologies of AKI. Prerenal causes are associated with a history of blood volume depletion or other causes of poor kidney perfusion (e.g., shock, heart failure, renal artery thrombi). Intrinsic causes include exposure to nephrotoxins and infection. Postrenal causes are associated with obstructive uropathies (e.g., an enlarged prostate or stones). The diagnostic challenge is to differentiate prerenal acute renal injury from acute tubular necrosis. Urine composition may provide helpful diagnostic clues to changes in tubular function (Table 39.11).

The ratios of the BUN to plasma creatinine concentration and fractional excretion of sodium (the ratio of filtered sodium to excreted sodium) are helpful diagnostic indicators because the tests reflect renal

TABLE 39.11 URINE CHARACTERISTICS OF PRERENAL AND INTRINSIC ACUTE KIDNEY INJURY

DIAGNOSTIC INDEX	PRERENAL	ATN
Urine volume	<400 mL	<400 mL
Urine specificity	1.016–1.020	1.010–1.012
Urine osmolality	>500 mOsm	<300 mOsm
Urine sodium	<10 mEq/L	>30 mEq/L
BUN/plasma	>15:1	<15:1 creatinine
FE_{Na}	<1% (also seen in acute glomerulonephritis)	>1% (also seen in urinary tract obstruction and renal parenchymal disease)
Urine sediment	Usually no cells, some hyaline casts	Brown granular casts, epithelial cells

ATN, Acute tubular necrosis; *BUN,* blood urea nitrogen; *FE_{Na},* fractional excretion of sodium.

tubular reabsorption ability. In prerenal AKI, tubular function is maintained and salt, water, and urea are reabsorbed. With ATN, reabsorption and urinary concentration abilities are compromised. Other causes of renal failure also may exhibit similar clinical findings. *Cystatin C,* a serum protein constantly produced by nucleated cells, is freely filtered by the glomerulus, and its concentration can serve as a measure of GFR and may be useful for detecting early changes in glomerular filtration rate. Serial measurements of plasma creatinine concentration provide an index of renal function during the recovery phase. However, changes in serum creatinine level occur only if more than 50% of glomerular filtration is lost and are often delayed by more than 24 hours. Such diagnostic delays make the implementation of early therapy very difficult, contributing to disease progression and mortality. Advances are being made in the use of biomarkers that allow assessment of kidney injury and estimates of renal function[104] (see *What's New?* Biomarkers and Kidney Injury on Evolve.)

Prevention of AKI and maintenance of renal perfusion involve maintenance of fluid volume before and after surgery or diagnostic procedures or when nephrotoxic drugs or contrast agents are in use. There is no specific treatment for acute kidney injury, and it requires individualized therapy and monitoring. The primary goal of therapy, once AKI has occurred, is to maintain the individual's life until renal function has recovered. Management principles directly related to physiologic alterations generally include (1) correcting fluid and electrolyte disturbances, (2) managing blood pressure, (3) preventing and treating infections, (4) maintaining nutrition, and (5) remembering that certain drugs or their metabolites are not excreted and can be toxic. Fluid and electrolyte replacement must be carefully calculated with consideration of urine losses, insensible losses (up to 1000 mL/day), and production of endogenous water by oxidation (450 mL/day). Overhydration of individuals dilutes their plasma sodium concentration and can precipitate pulmonary, cerebral, myocardial, and liver edema, and other complications. Metabolic acidosis is treated when serum bicarbonate concentration less than 22 mEq/L.[105]

Hyperkalemia can be managed by restricting dietary sources of potassium, using non–potassium-sparing diuretics, or using cation ion exchange resins, which may be administered orally or rectally. These resins exchange potassium for another cation, such as sodium in the bowel, and the potassium is then excreted attached to the resin. With severe hyperkalemia (more than 6.5 mEq/L), dialysis may be required,

TABLE 39.12   STAGES OF CHRONIC KIDNEY DISEASE

STAGE	SEVERITY*	GFR (mL/min)	ALBUMINURIA (mg/24 hr urine)	PROGRESSION	SYMPTOMS
1	Kidney damage: normal or increased GFR	≥90	A1 <30	None apparent	Usually none Hypertension common
2	Kidney damage: mild ↓ GFR	60–89	Mildly increased	Increasing PTH Early bone disease Increasing plasma creatinine and urea	Subtle hypertension
3	Moderate: ↓ GFR	30–59	A2 30–300	Erythropoietin deficiency, anemia Increased plasma creatinine and urea	Mild hypertension
4	Severe: ↓ GFR	15–29	30–300 A3 >300	Increased triglycerides Metabolic acidosis Hyperkalemia Salt/water retention Increasing plasma creatinine and urea	Moderate hypertension Hyperphosphatemia Anemia
5	End-stage kidney disease; kidney failure	<15	30–300 A3 >300	Uremia	Severe hypertension Hyperphosphatemia Anemia

*Normal glomerular filtration rate in a 70-kg male is about 120 mL/min.
GFR, Glomerular filtration rate; *PTH*, parathyroid hormone.
Adapted from KDIGO 2012 clinical practice guideline for the evaluation and management of chronic kidney disease, *Kidney Int Suppl* 3(1):1-150, 2013. Available at: http://www.kdigo.org/clinical_practice_guidelines/pdf/CKD/KDIGO_2012_CKD_GL.pdf.

or potassium can be driven back temporarily into the cells by administering glucose and insulin or by infusing sodium bicarbonate or albuterol. Glucose metabolism causes potassium to move to the intracellular fluid, and insulin infusions therefore can be effective in shifting potassium from the extracellular to intracellular space, along with the transport of glucose, within 30 minutes. (Glucose metabolism is discussed in Chapter 1 and Chapter 21.) Using sodium bicarbonate to cause alkalemia also shifts potassium into cells in exchange for hydrogen ions but requires consideration of hypervolemia.[106] Careful monitoring of the electrocardiogram for peaking T waves is essential for individuals with hyperkalemia. Intravenous infusion of calcium is the most rapid method of treating cardiac effects of hyperkalemia. Calcium decreases the threshold potential and reduces the membrane excitability caused by hyperkalemia (see Chapter 3). Calcium should be used only in emergencies, however, because hypercalcemia also may cause cardiac arrest.

Azotemia is generally controlled and nutrition maintained with a low-protein, high-carbohydrate diet. Essential amino acid replacement can be given orally or parenterally. Adequate carbohydrate intake slows protein catabolism and helps prevent release of potassium from cellular breakdown. Because sepsis is a common serious and potentially fatal complication of renal failure, observation for signs of infection and early treatment with antibiotics are necessary. Drug dosage levels may require adjustment if they are metabolized or excreted by the kidneys. Recovery may take up to 1 year.

Continuous renal replacement therapy (CRRT [hemodialysis]) (mechanical removal of water, electrolytes, and toxins from the blood) is indicated for uncontrollable hyperkalemia or acidosis or severe fluid overload. CRRT is particularly promising in critically ill people with multiple organ dysfunction or sepsis. The timing and optimal dose-response relationships for CRRT are individually determined.[107]

CHRONIC KIDNEY DISEASE

Chronic kidney disease (CKD) is the progressive loss of renal function associated with systemic diseases such as hypertension, diabetes mellitus (most significant risk factor), hypertension, systemic lupus erythematosus, or intrinsic kidney disease, including acute kidney injury, chronic glomerulonephritis, chronic pyelonephritis, obstructive uropathies, or vascular disorders. The KDIGO guidelines define and stage CKD using estimates of GFR and albuminuria (Table 39.12). *Chronic kidney disease* is the preferred terminology and is referenced to declining GFR. The terms *renal insufficiency* and *chronic renal failure* are still often used to describe declining renal function, but they do not have the specificity of the stages recommended by KDIGO. CKD decreases filtration and tubular functions with consequences manifested throughout all organ systems.

◆**PATHOPHYSIOLOGY.** The kidneys have a remarkable ability to adapt to loss of nephron mass. Symptomatic changes result from increased levels of creatinine, urea, and potassium. Alterations in salt and water balance usually do not become apparent until renal function declines to less than 25% of normal when adaptive renal reserves have been exhausted.

Different theories have been proposed to account for the adaptation to loss of renal function. The *intact nephron hypothesis* proposes that loss of nephron mass with progressive kidney damage causes the surviving nephrons to sustain normal kidney function. These nephrons are capable of a compensatory hypertrophy and expansion or hyperfunction in their rates of filtration, reabsorption, and secretion and can maintain adaptive changes in solute and water regulation in the presence of overall declining GFR. Although the urine of an individual with chronic kidney failure may contain abnormal amounts of protein and red and white blood cells or casts, the major end products of excretion are similar to those of normally functioning kidneys until the advanced stages of renal failure, when there is a significant reduction of functioning nephrons. With severe or repeated injury, epithelial cells have an impaired proliferative response resulting in interstitial capillary loss and fibroblast proliferation. The progressive process of glomerulosclerosis and tubulointerstitial fibrosis contributes to end-stage kidney disease. The *particular location of kidney damage* also can influence loss of kidney function. For example, tubular interstitial diseases damage primarily

TABLE 39.13   FACTORS REPRESENTING PROGRESSION OF CHRONIC KIDNEY DISEASE

FACTOR	CHARACTERISTICS
Proteinuria	Glomerular hyperfiltration of protein contributes to tubular intestinal injury by accumulating in the interstitial space and promoting inflammation and progressive fibrosis.
Creatinine and urea clearance	In chronic renal failure, the GFR falls and the plasma creatinine concentration increases by a reciprocal amount; because there is no regulatory adjustment for creatinine, plasma levels continue to rise and serve as an index of changing glomerular function. As GFR declines, urea clearance increases. (**NOTE:** Urea is filtered and reabsorbed and varies with the state of hydration.)
Sodium and water balance	In chronic renal failure, sodium load delivered to nephrons exceeds normal, so excretion must increase; thus less is reabsorbed. Obligatory loss occurs, leading to sodium deficits and volume depletion. As GFR is reduced, ability to concentrate and dilute urine diminishes.
Phosphate and calcium balance	Changes in acid-base balance affect phosphate and calcium balance. The major disorders associated with chronic renal failure are reduced renal phosphate excretion, decreased renal synthesis of $1,25\text{-}(OH)_2\text{-vitamin }D_3$, and hypocalcemia. Hypocalcemia leads to secondary hyperparathyroidism, GFR falls, and progressive hyperphosphatemia, hypocalcemia, and dissolution of bone result.
Hematocrit	Lack of erythropoietin and anemia accompany chronic renal failure. Lethargy, dizziness, and low hematocrit are common.
Potassium balance	In chronic renal failure, tubular secretion of potassium increases until oliguria develops. Use of potassium-sparing diuretics also may precipitate elevated serum potassium levels. As disease progresses, total body potassium levels can rise to life-threatening levels and dialysis is required.
Acid-base balance	In early renal insufficiency, acid excretion and bicarbonate reabsorption are increased to maintain normal pH. Metabolic acidosis begins when GFR reaches 30% to 40%. Metabolic acidosis and hyperkalemia may be severe enough to require dialysis when end-stage renal failure develops.
Dyslipidemia	Chronic hyperlipidemia may induce glomerular and tubulointerstitial injury contributing to the progression of chronic kidney disease.

GFR, Glomerular filtration rate.

the tubular or medullary parts of the nephron, producing problems such as renal tubular acidosis, salt wasting, and difficulty diluting or concentrating the urine. When the damage is primarily vascular or glomerular, proteinuria, hematuria, and nephrotic syndrome are more prominent. A summary of factors involved in the progression of chronic kidney disease is outlined in Table 39.13 and Fig. 39.13.

The factors that contribute to the pathogenesis of CKD are complex and involve the interaction of many cells, cytokines, and structural alterations. Two factors that have consistently been recognized to advance renal disease are proteinuria and angiotensin II activity. Glomerular hyperfiltration and increased glomerular capillary permeability lead to proteinuria. Proteinuria contributes to tubulointerstitial injury by accumulating in the interstitial space and activating complement proteins and other mediators and cells, such as macrophages, that promote inflammation and progressive fibrosis.[108] Angiotensin II activity is elevated with progressive nephron injury. **Angiotensin II** promotes glomerular hypertension and hyperfiltration caused by efferent arteriolar vasoconstriction and also promotes systemic hypertension. The chronically high intraglomerular pressure increases glomerular capillary permeability, contributing to proteinuria. Angiotensin II also may promote the activity of inflammatory cells and growth factors that participate in tubulointerstitial fibrosis and scarring (see Fig. 39.13).[109]

◆**CLINICAL MANIFESTATIONS.** The clinical manifestations of chronic kidney disease are often described using the terms *azotemia* and *uremia*. Azotemia is manifested by increased levels of serum urea, serum creatinine, and other nitrogenous compounds related to decreasing kidney function. Uremia is a proinflammatory state with many systemic effects known as **uremic syndrome**[110] and is associated with the accumulation of urea and other nitrogenous compounds and toxins. Sources of toxins include the accumulation of end products of protein metabolism, alterations in fluid and electrolytes, metabolic acidosis, intestinal absorption of toxins produced by gut bacteria, and results of altered renal hormone synthesis (i.e., anemia, hyperphosphatemia, and hypocalcemia).

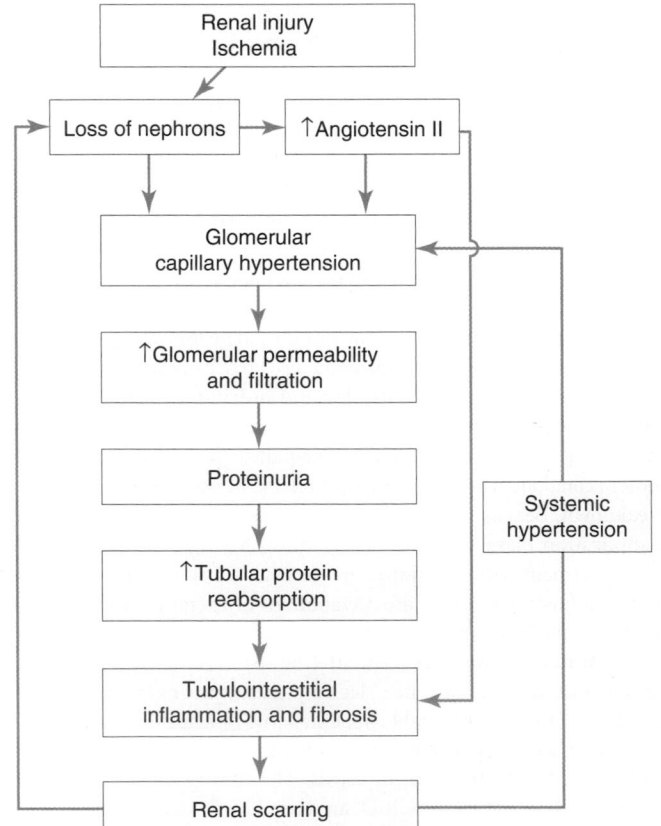

FIGURE 39.13 Mechanisms Related to the Progression of Chronic Kidney Disease.

TABLE 39.14   SYSTEMIC EFFECTS OF CHRONIC KIDNEY DISEASE AND UREMIA

SYSTEM	MANIFESTATIONS	MECHANISMS	TREATMENT
Skeletal	Spontaneous fractures and bone pain Deformities of long bones	Chronic kidney disease—mineral bone disorder: bone inflammation with fibrous degeneration related to hyperparathyroidism; bone resorption associated with vitamin D and calcium deficiency	Control of hyperphosphatemia to reduce hyperparathyroidism; administration of calcium and aluminum hydroxide antacids, which bind phosphate in the gut, together with a phosphate-restricted diet; vitamin D replacement; avoidance of magnesium antacids because of impaired magnesium excretion
Cardiopulmonary	Pulmonary edema, Kussmaul respirations	Fluid overload associated with pulmonary edema and metabolic acidosis leading to Kussmaul respirations	Angiotensin-converting enzyme (ACE) inhibitors; combination of propranolol, hydralazine, and minoxidil for those with high levels of renin; bilateral nephrectomy with dialysis or transplantation
Cardiovascular	Left ventricular hypertrophy, cardiomyopathy, and ischemic heart disease; hypertension, dysrhythmias, accelerated atherosclerosis; pericarditis with fever, chest pain, and pericardial friction rub	Extracellular volume expansion and hypersecretion of renin associated with hypertension; anemia increases cardiac workload; hyperlipidemia promotes atherosclerosis; toxins precipitate into pericardium	Volume reduction with diuretics that are not potassium sparing (to avoid hyperkalemia); lipid-lowering drugs; blood pressure–lowering strategies; dialysis
Neurologic	Encephalopathy (fatigue, loss of attention, difficulty with problem solving); peripheral neuropathy (pain and burning in the legs and feet, loss of vibration sense and deep tendon reflexes); loss of motor coordination, twitching, fasciculations, stupor, and coma with advanced uremia	Progressive accumulation of uremic toxins associated with end-stage renal disease Stroke or intracerebral hemorrhage associated with chronic dialysis	Dialysis or successful kidney transplantation
Endocrine	Restricted growth in children Higher incidence of goiter Osteomalacia	Elevated parathyroid hormone levels Decreased thyroid hormone	Endogenous recombinant human growth hormone; thyroid hormone replacement Same as skeletal above
Hematologic	Anemia, usually normochromic normocytic; platelet disorders with prolonged bleeding times	Reduced erythropoietin secretion and reduced red cell production; uremic toxins shorten red blood cell survival and alter platelet function	Dialysis; recombinant human erythropoietin (controversial) and iron supplementation; conjugated estrogens; DDAVP (1-deamino-[8-C-arginine] vasopressin); transfusion
Gastrointestinal	Anorexia, nausea, vomiting; mouth ulcers, stomatitis, urinous breath (uremic factor), hiccups, peptic ulcers, gastrointestinal bleeding, and pancreatitis associated with end-stage renal failure	Retention of metabolic acids and other metabolic waste products	Protein-restricted diet for relief of nausea and vomiting; Na+-based alkali or alkali-inducing food
Integumentary	Abnormal pigmentation and pruritus	Retention of urochromes, contributing to sallow, yellow color; high plasma calcium levels and neuropathy associated with pruritus	Dialysis with control of serum calcium and phosphate levels
Immunologic	Increased risk of infection that can cause death; increased risk of carcinoma	Suppression of cell-mediated immunity; reduction in number and function of lymphocytes, diminished phagocytosis	Routine dialysis
Reproductive	Sexual dysfunction: menorrhagia, amenorrhea, infertility, and decreased libido in women; decreased testosterone levels, infertility, and decreased libido in men	Dysfunction of ovaries and testes; presence of neuropathies	No specific treatment

Generally, the symptoms include hypertension, anorexia, nausea, vomiting, diarrhea or constipation, malnutrition and weight loss, pruritus, edema, anemia, and neurologic, cardiovascular disease, and skeletal changes. The many systemic manifestations associated with uremia are summarized in Table 39.14 and Fig. 39.14.

Creatinine, Urea Clearance, and Cystatin C

Creatinine is constantly released from muscle and excreted primarily by glomerular filtration. As the GFR declines in CKD, the serum creatinine (SCr) level increases by a reciprocal amount to maintain a constant rate of excretion (Fig. 39.15). Because no significant tubular adjustment occurs for creatinine (i.e., tubular secretion), the SCr levels continue to increase as the GFR decreases. Therefore measures of plasma creatinine can serve as an index of changing glomerular function. However, SCr as an estimate of GFR is limited when there is reduced muscle mass or fluid overload. Equations including cystatin C or combined with SCr provide a better index (see *What's New?* Biomarkers and Kidney Injury on Evolve). The clearance of *urea* follows a pattern similar to that of creatinine, but urea is filtered as well as reabsorbed and varies with the state of hydration; it is not a good index of GFR. However, as the GFR decreases, plasma urea concentration also increases.

Fluid and Electrolyte Balance

Fluid and electrolyte and acid-base balances are significantly disturbed with chronic kidney disease. A summary of electrolyte and acid-base balance alterations is presented in Table 39.15.

Levels of *sodium* must be regulated within narrow limits because sodium is the major extracellular solute. In CKD, sodium and water balance is maintained very close to normal until the development of stage 5 ESKD. This occurs because of the increased fractional excretion of sodium, particularly in the distal nephron, in relation to decreasing GFR. Hormones including aldosterone, prostaglandins, and natriuretic peptides also modulate sodium excretion, and their levels are elevated with progressive renal failure. Individual variation in the underlying pathology of CKD must be considered in the management of sodium intake or restriction. Sodium wasting may be present with tubulointerstitial causes of CKD, and there may also be extrarenal losses of sodium from vomiting, diarrhea, or fever. Sodium retention is more likely in ESKD, particularly in the presence of nephrotic syndrome or heart failure. Sodium retention contributes to hypertension, edema, heart

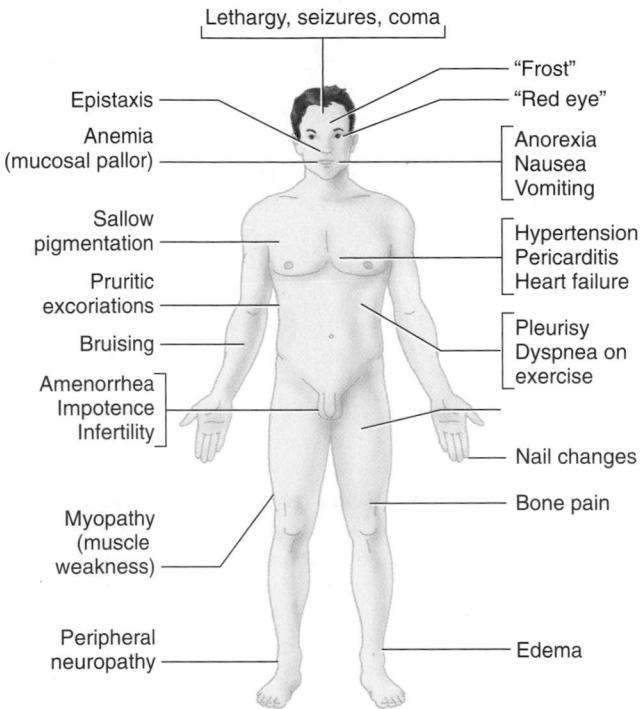

FIGURE 39.14 Common Signs and Symptoms of Kidney Dysfunction (See Text for Reference Site). (From Goldman L, Schafer AI: *Goldman-Cecil medicine*, ed 25, Philadelphia, 2016, Saunders; redrawn from Forbes CD, Jackson WF: *Color atlas and text of clinical medicine*, ed 3, London, 2003, Mosby.)

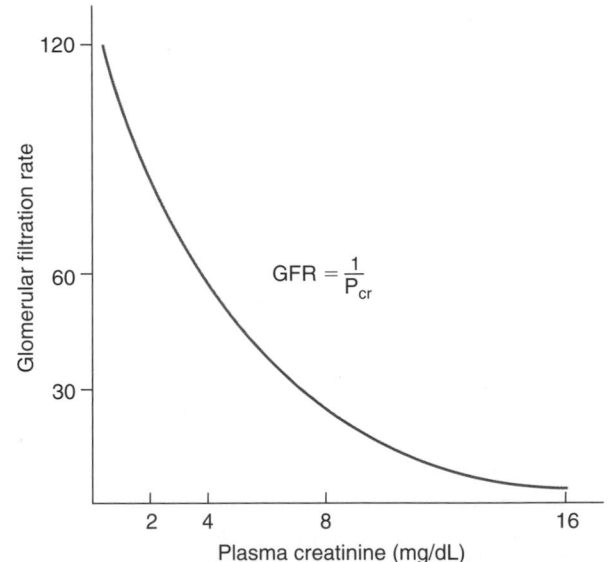

$$GFR = \frac{1}{P_{cr}}$$

FIGURE 39.15 Plasma Creatinine (P_{cr}) and Glomerular Filtration Rate (GFR).

TABLE 39.15	ELECTROLYTE AND ACID-BASE ALTERATIONS OF CHRONIC KIDNEY DISEASE
FACTOR	**CHARACTERISTICS**
Sodium and water balance	In chronic renal failure, sodium load delivered to nephrons exceeds normal, so excretion must increase; thus less is reabsorbed. Obligatory loss occurs, leading to sodium deficits and volume depletion. As GFR is reduced, ability to concentrate and dilute urine diminishes.
Phosphate and calcium balance	Changes in acid-base balance affect phosphate and calcium balance. The major disorders associated with chronic renal failure are reduced renal phosphate excretion, decreased renal synthesis of 1,25-$(OH)_2$-vitamin D_3 (calcitriol), and hypocalcemia. Hypocalcemia leads to secondary hyperparathyroidism, GFR falls, and progressive hyperphosphatemia, hypocalcemia, and dissolution of bone result.
Potassium balance	In chronic renal failure, tubular secretion of potassium increases until oliguria develops. Use of potassium-sparing diuretics also may precipitate elevated serum potassium levels. As disease progresses, total body potassium levels can rise to life-threatening levels and dialysis is required.
Acid-base balance	In early renal insufficiency, acid excretion and bicarbonate reabsorption are increased to maintain normal pH. Metabolic acidosis begins to develop when GFR decreases to 30% to 40% of normal. When end-stage renal failure develops, the metabolic acidosis may be severe enough to require dialysis.

GFR, Glomerular filtration rate.

failure, and mortality. Interdialytic water intake can cause volume overload and dilutional hyponatremia during dialysis. Management of salt and water balance requires individual assessment, and both hyponatremia and hypernatremia require management.[111,112]

The regulation of *water balance* and osmolality is normally achieved by urinary concentration mediated by antidiuretic hormone (ADH). As GFR is reduced, ability to concentrate and dilute the urine diminishes. In earlier stages of renal failure, this may be caused by osmotic diuresis produced by increased fractional excretion of solutes by the remaining nephrons or by a decreased tubular response to ADH. Individual nephrons can maintain water balance until severe renal failure occurs and GFR declines to 15% to 20% of normal with extensive loss of nephron and tubular function. At this stage the urinary concentration becomes fixed and approaches that of the plasma at 285 mOsm/L with a specific gravity of about 1.010.

Urinary excretion of *potassium* is related primarily to distal tubular secretion mediated by aldosterone and sodium-potassium adenosine triphosphatase (see Chapter 3). In renal failure there is increased tubular secretion that provides effective regulation until the onset of oliguria. With hyperkalemia, larger amounts of potassium can be eliminated through the bowel.[113]

Although nonoliguric patients can maintain potassium excretion with normal dietary intake, they are more prone to develop hyperkalemia with increased loading (i.e., use of salt substitutes). Use of potassium-sparing diuretics, such as spironolactone (Aldactone), volume depletion, acute infection, severe acidosis, or marked hyperglycemia also may precipitate elevated levels of serum potassium. With progression of disease to end-stage renal failure (ESRF), total body potassium can increase to life-threatening levels and must be controlled by dietary restriction, loop diuretics, cation exchange resins, and dialysis. Hyperkalemia also can be a side effect of ACE inhibitors or receptor blockers often used to prevent diabetic nephropathy. The new drug patiromer sorbitex calcium is FDA approved (exchanges calcium for potassium in the colon). Sodium zirconium cyclosilicate (traps potassium in the colon) is currently investigational. Both are effective in managing hyperkalemia.[114] Severe acute hyperkalemia is treated with intravenous 10% calcium gluconate or 10% calcium chloride, intravenous dextrose and insulin, and nebulized or intravenous salbutamol (sympathetic β_2 agonist, promotes Na^+-K^+-ATPase pump and intracellular movement of potassium). Renal replacement therapy may be required (support of renal function using hemodialysis or peritoneal dialysis).[115]

The intake of a normal diet produces 50 to 100 mEq of hydrogen per day. These ions are secreted from the renal tubules and excreted in the urine combined with phosphate and ammonia buffers (buffering is described in Chapter 3). *Metabolic acidosis* (Chapter 3) develops when GFR decreases to less than 20% to 25% of normal. The causes of acidosis

are primarily related to decreased hydrogen ion elimination and decreased bicarbonate reabsorption. With ESRF, metabolic acidosis may be severe enough to require alkali therapy and dialysis. Bicarbonate levels should be maintained at about 22 mEq/L.[116]

Calcium, Phosphate, and Bone

Bone and skeletal changes develop with alterations in calcium and phosphate metabolism (Table 39.16). These changes begin when the GFR decreases to 25% or less. *Hypocalcemia* is accelerated by impaired renal synthesis of 1,25-dihydroxy-vitamin D_3 (calcitriol) with decreased intestinal absorption of calcium. Renal phosphate excretion also decreases, and the increased serum phosphate binds calcium, further contributing to hypocalcemia. Acidosis also contributes to a negative calcium balance. Decreased serum calcium level stimulates parathyroid hormone secretion with mobilization of calcium from bone and may cause calcium levels to approach normal. The combined effect of *secondary hyperparathyroidism* and *vitamin D deficiency* can result in renal osteodystrophies (i.e., osteomalacia and osteitis fibrosa with increased risk for fractures)[117] (see Chapter 45) and vascular calcification, including coronary artery calcification.[118] Fractional excretion of magnesium increases as CKD progresses and also may contribute to cardiovascular complications.[119]

Protein, Carbohydrate, and Fat Metabolism

Protein, carbohydrate, and fat metabolism are altered in CKD. *Proteinuria* and a catabolic state contribute to a negative nitrogen balance. Levels of serum proteins diminish, including albumin, complement, and transferrin, and there is loss of muscle mass. Proteinuria may independently cause renal damage by promoting tubular inflammation and fibrosis.[108] The amount of proteinuria is also related to the extent of renal injury and predicts disease progression. Monitoring of proteinuria using the albumin-to-creatinine ratio can assist in staging chronic kidney disease.[120]

Hyperinsulinemia and glucose intolerance related to insulin resistance are common and may be related to alterations in adipokines that interfere with insulin action and oxidative stress that contributes to renal tubular and vascular injury in both nondiabetic and diabetic CKD.[121] Hyperparathyroidism also decreases insulin sensitivity and impairs glucose tolerance. High levels of adiponectin have been associated with increased mortality in progressive CKD.[122]

Dyslipidemia is common among individuals with CKD. There is a high ratio of low-density lipoprotein (LDL) to high-density lipoprotein (HDL), high levels of triglycerides, and accumulation of LDL particles with accelerated atherosclerosis and vascular calcification. Uremia causes a deficiency in lipoprotein lipase and decreased hepatic triglyceride lipase. Decreased lipolytic activity results in a reduction in HDL level. CKD also impairs the metabolism and protective effects of HDL.

TABLE 39.16 CALCIUM AND PHOSPHATE METABOLISM IN CHRONIC KIDNEY DISEASE

KIDNEY	PLASMA	BONE
Decreased renal production of vitamin D_3	Decreased calcium absorption from gut Decreased ionized calcium Increased PTH secretion (secondary hyperparathyroidism)	Decreased calcium deposition
Decreased phosphate excretion	Elevated phosphate Formation of $CaHPO_4$	Release of calcium and phosphate Osteitis fibrosa, osteomalacia, calcium deposits in soft tissue and vascular calcification (occurs when kidney fails to respond to PTH secretion because of loss of renal mass and calcium and phosphate continues to be absorbed from bone)

$CaHPO_4$, Calcium hydrogen phosphate; *PTH*, parathyroid hormone.

Apolipoprotein B concentration also is elevated, thereby accelerating atherogenesis.[123,124]

Cardiovascular System

Cardiovascular disease (see Chapter 33) is a major cause of morbidity and mortality in CKD. Proinflammatory mediators, oxidative stress, altered vitamin D metabolism, and metabolic derangements are significant contributors. Declining erythropoietin production causes anemia, which reduces oxygen delivery to the myocardium. Elevated renin level stimulates the secretion of aldosterone, increasing sodium and water reabsorption. *Hypertension* is the result of excess sodium and fluid volume. *Dyslipidemia* occurs early in CKD. Arterial wall thickness increases with decreased elastic fibers and increased extracellular matrix. Atheromatous plaque and arterial calcification contribute to loss of vessel elasticity and obstruction and are accelerated by the oxidative stress of CKD. Macrovascular disease is responsible for increased risk for ischemic heart disease, left ventricular hypertrophy, congestive heart failure, stroke, and peripheral vascular disease in individuals with uremia.[125] Endothelial cell dysfunction and calcium deposits lead to a loss of vessel elasticity and vascular calcification.[126] The resulting vascular disease increases the risk for *ischemic heart disease, left ventricular hypertrophy, congestive heart failure, stroke,* and *peripheral vascular disease* in individuals with uremia. *Pericarditis* can develop from inflammation caused by the presence of uremic toxins. Accumulation of fluid in the pericardial space can compromise ventricular filling and cardiac output.

Pulmonary System

Pulmonary edema results from fluid overload and congestive heart failure. *Dyspnea* is common in ESKD. Metabolic acidosis can cause Kussmaul respirations.

Hematologic System

Hematologic alterations include *normochromic normocytic anemia, impaired platelet function,* and *hypercoagulability.* Inadequate production of erythropoietin decreases red blood cell production and is the most significant factor in contributing to anemia. Chronic inflammation, iron deficiency, and decreased half-life of erythrocytes are also contributing factors. Anemia contributes to decreased tissue oxygenation and to progression of kidney disease. Low levels of hemoglobin and symptoms of anemia, such as lethargy, weakness, and dizziness, are common findings. Treatment of anemia includes erythropoiesis stimulating agents (i.e., recombinant human erythropoietin) and intravenous iron. The safety and cost benefit of new drug classes to stimulate erythropoiesis are under investigation.[127]

Disorders of hemostasis in CKD are primarily related to defective platelet aggregation, impaired adhesion of platelets to the vascular endothelium, and alterations in coagulation factors and the fibrinolytic pathway. The consequence is either (1) an increased bleeding tendency (more common with later stages of CKD) manifested by bruising, epistaxis and other mucosal bleeding, gastrointestinal bleeding, and cerebrovascular hemorrhage or (2) excessive formation of thrombi (i.e., deep vein thrombosis, pulmonary embolism and cardiovascular events), which is more common in earlier stages of CKD.[128]

Immune System

Immune system dysregulation with immune suppression, deficient response to vaccination, intestinal barrier dysfunction and dysbiosis, and increased risk for infection develop with CKD. Chemotaxis, phagocytosis, antibody production, and cell-mediated immune responses are suppressed.[129]

Malnutrition, metabolic acidosis, hyperglycemia, or effects of hemodialysis may amplify immunosuppression.

Neurologic System

Neurologic symptoms are common and progressive with CKD and are related to dysfunction of lower motor and sensory neurons associated with uremic toxicity, chronic hyperkalemic depolarization, and anemia. Neuromuscular irritation can cause hiccups, muscle cramps, and muscle twitching. In advanced stages of renal failure, symptoms may progress to seizures and coma. Peripheral neuropathies also develop with impaired sensations, decreased tendon reflexes, muscle weakness, and muscle atrophy, most commonly in the lower extremities. Symptoms may include headache, drowsiness, pain, sleep disorders, impaired concentration, memory loss, and impaired judgment (uremic encephalopathy). Diabetic neuropathy can occur concurrently. Renal replacement therapy or kidney transplant improves symptoms.[130]

Gastrointestinal System

Gastrointestinal complications are common in individuals with CKD. Uremic gastroenteritis can cause bleeding ulcer and significant blood loss. Nonspecific symptoms include anorexia, nausea, vomiting, and constipation or diarrhea. Uremic fetor is a form of bad breath caused by the breakdown of urea by salivary enzymes. Malnutrition is common.

Endocrine and Reproductive Systems

Endocrine and reproductive alterations develop with progression of CKD. Males and females have a decrease in the levels of circulating sex steroid hormones. Males often experience a reduction in testosterone levels and may be impotent. Oligospermia and germinal cell dysplasia can result in infertility. Females have reduced estrogen levels, amenorrhea, and difficulty with conception and maintaining a pregnancy to term. A decrease in libido occurs in both genders.[131] Renal replacement therapy and kidney transplantation improve sexual dysfunction. There are no guidelines related to sex hormone replacement therapy and end-stage kidney disease.[132]

Insulin resistance is common in uremia. Low-grade systemic inflammation, oxidative stress, vitamin D deficiency, and anemia may be contributing factors with increased risk for cardiovascular disease. As CKD progresses, the ability of the kidney to clear adiponectin and leptin and degrade insulin is reduced, and the half-life of insulin is prolonged. Individuals with diabetes mellitus and CKD need to carefully manage their insulin dosages. Low-protein diets and renal replacement therapy improve insulin sensitivity.[133]

CKD also causes alterations in thyroid hormone metabolism and low thyroid hormone levels and is known as *nonthyroidal illness syndrome (euthyroid sick syndrome)* and increases risk for cardiovascular disease. Low-grade inflammation and oxidative stress may be contributing factors. Uremia also reduces conversion of triiodothyronine (T_3) to tetraiodothyronine (T_4-thyroxine).[134]

Integumentary System

Skin changes are associated with other complications that develop with CKD. Anemia can cause pallor and bleeding into the skin and results in hematomas and ecchymosis. Retained urochromes manifest as a sallow skin color. Hyperparathyroidism and uremic skin residues, related to calcium and phosphorus levels and alterations in opioid receptors, are associated with irritation and pruritus with scratching, excoriation, increased risk for infection, impaired sleep, and depression.[135]

◆**EVALUATION AND TREATMENT.** Early screening and evaluation of CKD are based on risk factors, history, presenting signs and symptoms, and diagnostic testing. Prediction equations incorporating serum creatinine or cystatin C, or both, are used for estimating GFR. Markers of kidney damage include urine protein, particularly albumin, and examination of urine sediment. New biomarkers for predicting

End-Stage Kidney Disease (ESKD) and Protein-Energy Wasting

The malnutrition-inflammation complex syndrome or protein-energy wasting (decreased body storage of protein and energy) is a common condition associated with renal failure and loss of appetite and leads to accelerated atherosclerosis, cardiovascular disease, and increased mortality for individuals with ESKD. Elevated levels of leptin, ghrelin, adiponectin, and inflammatory cytokines, including interleukin-6, tumor necrosis factor-alpha, and interferon, suppress appetite and cause muscle proteolysis and decreased protein assimilation. Acidosis also acts synergistically with inflammatory cytokines and insulin resistance to promote mitochondrial dysfunction and protein catabolism. Reduced renal function, oxidative stress, decreased levels of antioxidants, infection and other comorbidities, exposure to dialysis tubing and membranes during hemodialysis, and back-filtration of contaminants during hemodialysis contribute to inflammation. Proteins and amino acids may be lost in the dialysate. The provision of supplemental formulations, including adequate calories and protein that includes amino acids, in the form of oral, enteral interdialytic, or enteral or parenteral intradialytic feeding helps a person to meet metabolic requirements. Dietary supplements of antioxidants, such as vitamins A and C, selenium, and carotenoids, are required. Low-protein, low-phosphorus, and low-sodium diets assist with reducing proteinuria, preventing hyperphosphatemia and secondary hyperparathyroidism, and lowering blood pressure, but diets must be individualized. Protein intake of plant origin may improve lipid profiles, provide fiber, and reduce phosphorus intake. Adequate nutritional support promotes renal recovery and may prevent consequences of muscle weakness and immune dysfunction.

Data from Akchurin OM, Kaskel F: *Blood Purif* 39(1-3):84-92, 2015; Carrero JJ, et al: *J Ren Nutr* 23(2):77-90, 2013; Ikizler TA: *Clin J Am Soc Nephrol* 8(12):2174-2182, 2013; Kalantar-Zadeh K, et al: *Semin Dial* 28(2):159-168, 2015; Sabatino A, et al: *Clin Nutr* 36(3):663-671, 2017.

progression of CKD are being evaluated (see *What's New?* Biomarkers and Kidney Injury on Evolve). Renal biopsy confirms the diagnosis.

Management involves dietary control, including management of protein intake, vitamin D supplementation, sodium and fluid maintenance, potassium restriction, adequate caloric intake, management of dyslipidemias, erythropoietin-stimulating agents (ESAs), and adjuvant iron therapy as needed[127,136] (see *Nutrition & Disease:* End-Stage Kidney Disease [ESKD] and Protein-Energy Wasting). Hyperphosphatemia is managed with a low phosphorus diet, phosphate binders, vitamin D replacement, calcimimetics, and parathyroidectomy while maintaining normal serum calcium levels. ESKD related to diabetic nephropathy can be significantly reduced with control of hyperglycemia, hypertension, hyperlipidemia, and albuminuria. ACE inhibitors or receptor blockers are often used to control systemic hypertension, decrease albuminuria, and provide renoprotection in the presence of diabetes mellitus and mild chronic kidney injury. They are under investigation for advanced CKD.[137]

Statins and fibrates are used to control hyperlipidemia (i.e., elevated low density lipoprotein cholesterol [LDL-C]).[138] Sodium glucose cotransporter 2 (SGLT2) inhibitors are being evaluated for nephroprotective actions and renal gluconeogenesis inhibition.[139] ESKD is treated with dialysis, supportive therapy, and renal transplantation.[140]

SUMMARY REVIEW

Urinary Tract Obstruction

1. Obstruction can occur anywhere in the urinary tract, and may be anatomic or functional, including kidney stones, tumors, an enlarged prostate gland, or strictures of the ureter or urethra. The most serious complications are hydronephrosis, hydroureter, ureterohydronephrosis, and infection caused by the accumulation of urine behind the obstruction.
2. Tubulointerstitial fibrosis and dysregulated apoptosis can result in progression to chronic kidney disease in untreated obstructive uropathy.
3. Compensatory hypertrophy and hyperfunction of the opposite kidney compensate for loss of function of the kidney with obstructive disease.
4. Relief of obstruction is usually followed by postobstructive diuresis and may cause fluid and electrolyte imbalance.
5. Kidney stones are caused by supersaturation of the urine with precipitation of stone-forming substances, changes in urine pH, or urinary tract infection. Most stones are unilateral.
6. The most common kidney stone is formed from calcium oxalate and most often causes obstruction by lodging in the ureter.
7. Obstructions of the bladder are a consequence of neurogenic or anatomic alteration of the bladder or both.
8. A neurogenic bladder is caused by a neural lesion that interrupts innervation of the bladder.
9. Upper motor neuron lesions above the pontine micturition center result in detrusor hyperreflexia and uninhibited or reflex bladder.
10. Upper motor neuron lesions between C2 and S1 result in overactive or hyperreflexive bladder function and detrusor sphincter dyssynergia (lack of coordinated neuromuscular contraction).
11. Lower motor neuron lesions below S1 result in detrusor areflexia with underactive, hypotonic, or atonic bladder function.
12. OAB syndrome is an uncontrollable or premature contraction of the bladder that results in urgency with or without incontinence, frequency, and nocturia.
13. Anatomic obstructions to urine flow include prostatic enlargement, urethral stricture, and pelvic organ prolapse in women.
14. Partial obstruction of the bladder can result in overactive bladder contractions with urgency. There is deposition of collagen in the bladder wall over time, resulting in decreased bladder wall compliance and ineffective detrusor muscle contraction.
15. Renal cell carcinoma is the most common renal neoplasm. The larger neoplasms tend to metastasize to the lung, liver, and bone.
16. Bladder tumors are commonly composed of transitional cells with a papillary appearance and a high rate of recurrence.

Urinary Tract Infection

1. UTIs are commonly caused by the retrograde movement of bacteria into the urethra and bladder. UTIs are uncomplicated when the urinary system is normal or complicated when there is a defect or abnormality.
2. Host defenses that protect against urinary tract infection include high osmolality and acidic pH of urine, mucus, uromodulin and

■ SUMMARY REVIEW—cont'd

other antimicrobial proteins that activate the immune response, sphincters that prevent reflux, and urine flow that washes out bacteria.

3. Virulent uropathogens have pili or fimbriae, or both, that promote binding to the uroepithelium and retrograde movement in the urinary tract. Formation of biofilms enhances colonization and resists host defenses and antimicrobial therapy.

4. Cystitis is an inflammation of the bladder commonly caused by bacteria and may be acute or chronic. Manifestations of frequency, urgency, and dysuria are caused by inflammation.

5. Interstitial cystitis/painful bladder syndrome may be an autoimmune injury with increased permeability of the glycosaminoglycan layer of the bladder mucosa.

6. Pyelonephritis is an acute or chronic inflammation of the renal pelvis often related to ascending infection and obstructive uropathies and may cause abscess formation and scarring with acute or chronic kidney injury.

Glomerular Disorders

1. Glomerular disorders are a group of related diseases of the glomerulus that can be primary and caused by immune injury, infection, ischemia, toxins or drugs, or vascular disorders or, secondarily, caused by systemic diseases.

2. Acute glomerulonephritis commonly results from inflammatory damage to the glomerulus as a consequence of immune reactions including deposition of circulating immune complexes, antibodies reacting in situ to planted antigens, antibodies directed against the glomerular basement membrane, and complement activation.

3. The urine sediment may contain large amounts of protein (nephrotic sediment) or have red and white blood cells and protein (nephritic sediment).

4. Acute postinfectious glomerulonephritis is commonly associated with immune complex deposition in the glomerulus or in situ formation.

5. Lupus nephritis is caused by the formation of autoantibodies against double-stranded DNA (dsDNA) and nucleosomes in the glomerulus, causing inflammation and injury.

6. IgA nephropathy is the binding of abnormal IgA to mesangial cells in the glomerulus resulting in injury and mesangial proliferation.

7. Focal segmental glomerulosclerosis is a scarring lesion that involves some but not all glomeruli (focal) and some but not all of the glomerular capillaries (segmental).

7. Membranous nephropathy is complement-mediated glomerular injury with increased glomerular permeability and glomerulosclerosis.

8. RPGN is associated with injury that results in the proliferation of glomerular capillary endothelial cells and a rapid loss of renal function.

9. Mesangial proliferative glomerulonephritis is usually idiopathic and involves deposits of immune complex in the mesangium with mesangial cell proliferation.

10. Membranoproliferative glomerulonephritis involves mesangial cell proliferation, complement deposition, and crescent formation.

11. Chronic glomerulonephritis is related to a variety of diseases that cause deterioration of the glomerulus and a progressive loss of renal function over a period of months to years, including diabetic nephropathy and lupus nephritis.

12. Diabetic nephropathy develops from metabolic, inflammatory, and microvascular complications associated with chronic hyperglycemia.

13. Lupus nephritis is caused by the formation of autoantibodies against dsDNA and nucleosomes in the glomerulus, causing inflammation and injury.

14. Nephrotic syndrome is the excretion of at least 3.5 g of protein (primarily albumin) in the urine per day primarily because of glomerular injury with increased capillary permeability and loss of membrane negative charge. The principal signs are hypoproteinemia, hyperlipidemia, and edema. The liver cannot produce enough protein to adequately compensate for urinary loss.

15. Nephritic syndrome is hematuria and red blood cell casts in the urine and less severe proteinuria.

Acute Kidney Injury

1. AKI is the sudden decline in kidney function with decreased glomerular filtration and an increase in serum creatinine, cystatin C, and BUN levels.

2. AKI is considered in three categories as prerenal, intrarenal, or postrenal and is usually accompanied by oliguria with elevated plasma BUN and plasma creatinine levels.

3. Prerenal acute renal failure is caused by decreased renal perfusion with a decreased GFR, ischemia, and tubular necrosis.

4. Intrarenal acute renal failure is associated with several systemic diseases or to drug toxicity but is commonly related to ATN.

5. Postrenal acute renal failure is associated with diseases that obstruct the flow of urine from the kidneys.

6. Oliguria is a urine output of less than 400 mL per day and can be caused by alterations in renal blood flow, tubular obstruction, or tubular fluid backleak, or by a combination of these events.

Chronic Kidney Disease

1. Chronic kidney disease is a progressive loss of renal function. Plasma creatinine levels gradually become elevated as GFR declines, sodium is lost in the urine, potassium is retained, acidosis develops, activation of vitamin D declines, calcium and phosphate metabolism are altered, and erythropoietin production is diminished.

2. Symptomatic changes usually do not become evident until renal function declines to less than 25%.

3. Glomerular hypertension, hyperfiltration, and tubulointerstitial inflammation and fibrosis contribute to the progression of chronic kidney disease. Proteinuria and angiotensin II promote the pathologic changes of chronic renal injury.

4. Uremic syndrome is a proinflammatory state with the accumulation of urea and other nitrogenous compounds as well as toxins and alterations in fluid, electrolyte, and acid-base balance that result from chronic kidney failure.

5. All organ systems are affected and contribute to disease symptoms.

■ KEY TERMS

Acute cystitis, 1255
Acute glomerulonephritis, 1257
Acute kidney injury (AKI), 1264
Acute renal failure, 1263
Acute tubular necrosis (ATN), 1264

Angiotensin II, 1268
Anuria, 1266
Apoptosis, 1247
Asymptomatic bacteriuria, 1255
Azotemia, 1263

Calcium metabolism, 1271
Calcium stone (urolithiasis), 1248
Chronic glomerulonephritis, 1261
Chronic kidney disease (CKD), 1267
Chronic pyelonephritis, 1257

■ KEY TERMS—cont'd

REFERENCES

1. Ding Y, Choi ME: Regulation of autophagy by TGF-β: emerging role in kidney fibrosis. *Semin Nephrol* 34(1):62–71, 2014.
2. Sulikowska B, et al: The role of interstitial changes in the progression of chronic kidney disease. *Postepy Hig Med Dosw (Online)* 69:830–837, 2015.
3. López-Novoa JM, et al: Common pathophysiological mechanisms of chronic kidney disease: therapeutic perspectives. *Pharmacol Ther* 128(1):61–81, 2010.
4. Helal I, et al: Glomerular hyperfiltration: definitions, mechanisms and clinical implications. *Nat Rev Nephrol* 8(5):293–300, 2012.
5. Halbgewachs C, Domes T: Postobstructive diuresis: pay close attention to urinary retention. *Can Fam Physician* 61(2):137–142, 2015.
6. Shoag J, et al: The new epidemiology of nephrolithiasis. *Adv Chronic Kidney Dis* 22(4):273–278, 2015.
7. Evan AP: Physiopathology and etiology of stone formation in the kidney and the urinary tract. *Pediatr Nephrol* 25(5):831–841, 2010.
8. Evan AP, et al: Mechanisms of human kidney stone formation. *Urolithiasis* 43(Suppl 1):19–32, 2015.
9. Narula S, et al: Kidney stone matrix proteins ameliorate calcium oxalate monohydrate induced apoptotic injury to renal epithelial cells. *Life Sci* 164:23–30, 2016.
10. Moran CP, Courtney AE: Managing acute and chronic renal stone disease. *Practitioner* 260(1790):17–20, 2-3, 2016.
11. Flannigan R, et al: Renal struvite stones—pathogenesis, microbiology, and management strategies. *Nat Rev Urol* 11(6):333–341, 2014.
12. Heilberg IP: Treatment of patients with uric acid stones. *Urolithiasis* 44(1):57–63, 2016.
13. Morgan MS, Pearle MS: Medical management of renal stones. *BMJ* 352:i52, 2016.
14. Brisbane W, Bailey MR, Sorensen MD: An overview of kidney stone imaging techniques. *Nat Rev Urol* 13(11):654–662, 2016.
15. Prezioso D, et al: Dietary treatment of urinary risk factors for renal stone formation. A review of CLU Working Group. *Arch Ital Urol Androl* 87(2):105–120, 2015.

16. Marien T, Miller NL: Treatment of the infected stone. *Urol Clin North Am* 42(4):459–472, 2015.
17. Qaseem A, et al: Dietary and pharmacologic management to prevent recurrent nephrolithiasis in adults: a clinical practice guideline from the American College of Physicians. *Ann Intern Med* 161:659–667, 2014.
18. Stoffel JT: Detrusor sphincter dyssynergia: a review of physiology, diagnosis, and treatment strategies. *Transl Androl Urol* 5(1):127–135, 2016.
19. Haab F: Chapter 1: The conditions of neurogenic detrusor overactivity and overactive bladder. *Neurourol Urodyn* 33(Suppl 3):S2–S5, 2014.
20. Abrams P, et al: The standardisation of terminology in lower urinary tract function: report from the Standardisation Subcommittee of the International Continence Society. *Urology* 61(1):37–49, 2003.
21. Nambiar A, Lucas M: Chapter 4: Guidelines for the diagnosis and treatment of overactive bladder (OAB) and neurogenic detrusor overactivity (NDO). *Neurourol Urodyn* 33(Suppl 3):S21–S25, 2014.
22. Aggarwal H, Zimmern PE: Underactive bladder. *Curr Urol Rep* 17(3):17, 2016.
23. Chuang YC, et al: Underactive bladder in older adults. *Clin Geriatr Med* 31(4):523–533, 2015.
24. Dugi DD, 3rd, Simhan J, Morey AF: Urethroplasty for stricture disease: contemporary techniques and outcomes. *Urology* 89:12–18, 2016.
25. Faiena I, Koprowski C, Tunuguntla H: Female urethral reconstruction. *J Urol* 195(3):557–567, 2016.
26. Lamin E, et al: Pelvic floor muscle training: underutilization in the USA. *Curr Urol Rep* 17(2):10, 2016.
27. Weber MA, et al: Local oestrogen for pelvic floor disorders: a systematic review. *PLoS ONE* 10(9):e0136265, 2015.
28. Hecht SL, Hedges JC: Diagnostic work-up of lower urinary tract symptoms. *Urol Clin North Am* 43(3):299–309, 2016.
29. Hecht SL, Hedges JC: Diagnostic work-up of lower urinary tract symptoms. *Urol Clin North Am* 43(3):299–309, 2016.
30. American Cancer Society (ACS): *Cancer facts & figures 2017*. Available at: http://www.cancer.org/

research/cancerfactsfigures/cancerfactsfigures/cancer-facts-figures-2013.
31. Delahunt B, Srigley JR: The evolving classification of renal cell neoplasia. *Semin Diagn Pathol* 32(2):90–102, 2015.
32. Navai N, Wood CG: Environmental and modifiable risk factors in renal cell carcinoma. *Urol Oncol* 30(2):220–224, 2012.
33. American Cancer Society (ACS): *Survival rates for kidney cancer by stage*. Available at: http://www.cancer.org/cancer/kidneycancer/detailedguide/kidney-cancer-adult-survival-rates#. (last revised 10 February 2016).
34. Valenca LB, et al: Non-clear cell renal cell carcinoma, part 1: histology. *Clin Adv Hematol Oncol* 13(5):308–313, 2015.
35. Hirsch MS, Signoretti S, Dal Cin P: Adult renal cell carcinoma: a review of established entities from morphology to molecular genetics. *Surg Pathol Clin* 8(4):587–621, 2015.
36. Brufau BP, et al: Metastatic renal cell carcinoma: radiologic findings and assessment of response to targeted antiangiogenic therapy by using multidetector CT. *Radiographics* 33(6):1691–1716, 2013.
37. Escudier B, et al: Renal cell carcinoma: ESMO clinical practice guidelines for diagnosis, treatment and follow-up. *Ann Oncol* 27(Suppl 5):v58–v68, 2016.
38. Vera-Badillo FE, et al: Systemic therapy for non-clear cell renal cell carcinomas: a systematic review and meta-analysis. *Eur Urol* 67(4):740–749, 2015.
39. Frey GT, Sella DM, Atwell TD: Image-guided renal intervention. *Radiol Clin North Am* 53(5):1005–1019, 2015.
40. Martin-Doyle W, Kwiatkowski DJ: Molecular biology of bladder cancer. *Hematol Oncol Clin North Am* 29(2):191–203, vii, 2015.
41. Volanis D, et al: Molecular mechanisms in urinary bladder carcinogenesis. *J BUON* 16(4):589–601, 2011.
42. Solomon JP, Hansel DE: Morphologic and molecular characteristics of bladder cancer. *Surg Pathol Clin* 8(4):663–676, 2015.
43. American Cancer Society (ACS): *Survival rates for bladder cancer*. Available at: http://www.cancer.org/

cancer/bladdercancer/detailedguide/bladder
-cancer-survival-rates. (Last revised 23 May 2016).

44. Netto GJ, Tafe LJ: Emerging bladder cancer biomarkers and targets of therapy. *Urol Clin North Am* 43(1):63–76, 2016.

45. Farina MS, Lundgren KT, Bellmunt J: Immunotherapy in urothelial cancer: recent results and future perspectives. *Drugs* 77(10):1077–1089, 2017.

46. Mbeutcha A, et al: Current status of urinary biomarkers for detection and surveillance of bladder cancer. *Urol Clin North Am* 43(1):47–62, 2016.

47. Dielubanza EJ, et al: Management of non-catheter-associated complicated urinary tract infection. *Infect Dis Clin North Am* 28(1):121–123, 2014.

48. Nicolle LE: Urinary tract infection. *Crit Care Clin* 29(3):699–715, 2013.

49. Abraham SN, Miao Y: The nature of immune responses to urinary tract infections. *Nat Rev Immunol* 15(10):655–663, 2015.

50. Hickling DR, Sun TT, Wu XR: Anatomy and physiology of the urinary tract: relation to host defense and microbial infection. *Microbiol Spectr* 3(4):2015.

51. Widmer M, et al: Duration of treatment for asymptomatic bacteriuria during pregnancy. *Cochrane Database Syst Rev* (11):CD000491, 2015.

52. Rinaldi G, et al: New research tools for urogenital schistosomiasis. *J Infect Dis* 211(6):861–869, 2015.

53. Stapleton AE: Urinary tract infection pathogenesis: host factors. *Infect Dis Clin North Am* 28(1):149–159, 2014.

54. Kauffman CA: Diagnosis and management of fungal urinary tract infection. *Infect Dis Clin North Am* 28(1):61–74, 2014.

55. Nielubowicz GR, Mobley HL: Host-pathogen interactions in urinary tract infection. *Nat Rev Urol* 7(8):430–441, 2010.

56. Detweiler K, Mayers D, Fletcher SG: Bacteriuria and urinary tract infections in the elderly. *Urol Clin North Am* 42(4):561–568, 2015.

57. Grigoryan L, et al: Diagnosis and management of urinary tract infections in the outpatient setting: a review. *J Am Med Assoc* 312(16):1677–1684, 2014.

58. Badalato G, Kaufmann M: *Adult UTI, American Urological Association.* Available at: https://www.auanet.org/education/adult-uti.cfm. (Amended July 2016).

59. Schneeberger C, Holleman F, Geerlings SE: Febrile urinary tract infections: pyelonephritis and urosepsis. *Curr Opin Infect Dis* 29(1):80–85, 2016.

60. Bamgbola OF: Urinary schistosomiasis. *Pediatr Nephrol* 29(11):2113–2120, 2014.

61. Zwaans BM, Chancellor MB, Lamb LE: Modeling and treatment of radiation cystitis. *Urology* 88:14–21, 2016.

62. Hanno P, Dmochowski R: Status of international consensus on interstitial cystitis/bladder pain syndrome/painful bladder syndrome: 2008 snapshot. *Neurourol Urodyn* 28(4):274–286, 2009.

63. Rais-Bahrami S, et al: Symptom profile variability of interstitial cystitis/painful bladder syndrome by age. *BJU Int* 109(9):1356–1359, 2012.

64. Grigorescu B, Powers K, Lazarou G: Update on urinary tract markers in interstitial cystitis/bladder pain syndrome. *Female Pelvic Med Reconstr Surg* 22(1):16–23, 2016.

65. Kim HJ: Update on the pathology and diagnosis of interstitial cystitis/bladder pain syndrome: a review. *Int Neurourol J* 20(1):13–17, 2016.

66. Cox A, et al: CUA guideline: diagnosis and treatment of interstitial cystitis/bladder pain syndrome. *Can Urol Assoc J* 10(5-6):E136–E155, 2016.

67. Fogo AB, et al: AJKD atlas of renal pathology: acute pyelonephritis. *Am J Kidney Dis* 68(4):e21–e22, 2016.

68. Hsiao CY, et al: Risk factors for development of acute kidney injury in patients with urinary tract infection. *PLoS ONE* 10(7):e0133835, 2015.

69. Colgan R, Williams M, Johnson JR: Diagnosis and treatment of acute pyelonephritis in women. *Am Fam Physician* 84(5):519–526, 2011.

70. Hou J, Herlitz LC: Renal infections. *Surg Pathol Clin* 7(3):389–408, 2014.

71. Barsoum RS: Glomerulonephritis in disadvantaged populations. *Clin Nephrol* 74(Suppl 1):S44–S50, 2010.

72. Segelmark M, Hellmark T: Autoimmune kidney diseases. *Autoimmun Rev* 9(5):A366–A371, 2010.

73. Kościelska-Kasprzak K, et al: The complement cascade and renal disease. *Arch Immunol Ther Exp (Warsz)* 62(1):47–57, 2014.

74. Hénique C, et al: Update on crescentic glomerulonephritism. *Semin Immunopathol* 36(4):479–490, 2014.

75. Floege J, Amann K: Primary glomerulonephritides. *Lancet* 387(10032):2036–2048, 2016.

76. Fogo AB: Causes and pathogenesis of focal segmental glomerulosclerosis. *Nat Rev Nephrol* 11(2):76–87, 2015.

77. Ronco P, Debiec H: Pathophysiological advances in membranous nephropathy: time for a shift in patient's care. *Lancet* 385(9981):1983–1992, 2015.

78. Ronco P, Debiec H: Membranous nephropathy: a fairy tale for immunopathologists, nephrologists and patients. *Mol Immunol* 68(1):57–62, 2015.

79. Moroni G, Ponticelli C: Rapidly progressive crescentic glomerulonephritis: early treatment is a must. *Autoimmun Rev* 13(7):723–729, 2014.

80. Silvariño R, Noboa O, Cervera R: Anti-glomerular basement membrane antibodies. *Isr Med Assoc J* 16(11):727–732, 2014.

81. Masani N, Jhaveri KD, Fishbane S: Update on membranoproliferative GN. *Clin J Am Soc Nephrol* 9(3):600–608, 2014.

82. Gyebi L, Soltani Z, Reisin E: Lipid nephrotoxicity: new concept for an old disease. *Curr Hypertens Rep* 14(2):177–181, 2012.

83. Toth-Manikowski S, Atta MG: Diabetic kidney disease: pathophysiology and therapeutic targets. *J Diabetes Res* 2015:697010, 2015.

84. Narres M, et al: The incidence of end-stage renal disease in the diabetic (compared to the non-diabetic) population: a systematic review. *PLoS ONE* 11(1):e0147329, 2016.

85. Podolska MJ, et al: Inflammatory etiopathogenesis of systemic lupus erythematosus: an update. *J Inflamm Res* 8:161–171, 2015.

86. Rekvig OP, et al: Future perspectives on pathogenesis of lupus nephritis: facts, problems, and potential causal therapy modalities. *Am J Pathol* 186(11):2772–2782, 2016.

87. Davidson A: What is damaging the kidney in lupus nephritis? *Nat Rev Rheumatol* 12(3):143–153, 2016.

88. Mok CC: Towards new avenues in the management of lupus glomerulonephritis. *Nat Rev Rheumatol* 12(4):221–234, 2016.

89. Hall G, Gbadegesin RA: Translating genetic findings in hereditary nephrotic syndrome: the missing loops. *Am J Physiol Renal Physiol* 309(1):F24–F28, 2015.

90. Dickinson BL: Unraveling the immunopathogenesis of glomerular disease. *Clin Immunol* 169:89–97, 2016.

91. Certikova-Chabova V, Tesar V: Recent insights into the pathogenesis of nephrotic syndrome. *Minerva Med* 104(3):333–347, 2013.

92. Timmermans SA, van Paassen P, Cohen Tervaert JW: Recent advances in the understanding of immune-mediated nephrotic syndrome: diagnostic and prognostic implications. *Expert Rev Clin Immunol* 11(4):489–500, 2015.

93. Chen G, Liu H, Liu F: A glimpse of the glomerular milieu: from endothelial cell to thrombotic disease in nephrotic syndrome. *Microvasc Res* 89:1–6, 2013.

94. Liebeskind DS: Nephrotic syndrome. *Handb Clin Neurol* 119:405–415, 2014.

95. Gibson KL, Glenn D, Ferris ME: Back to the future: therapies for idiopathic nephrotic syndrome. *Blood Purif* 39(1-3):105–109, 2015.

96. Tran TH, et al: Overview of current and alternative therapies for idiopathic membranous nephropathy. *Pharmacotherapy* 35(4):396–411, 2015.

97. Hofmann RM: Preventing harm during treatment of acute kidney injury: what do we really know? *Adv Chronic Kidney Dis* 19(3):142–148, 2012.

98. Bellomo R, et al: Acute kidney injury. *Lancet* 380(9843):756–766, 2012.

99. Shum HP, Yan WW, Chan TM: Recent knowledge on the pathophysiology of septic acute kidney injury: a narrative review. *J Crit Care* 31(1):82–89, 2016.

100. Glodowski SD, Wagener G: New insights into the mechanisms of acute kidney injury in the intensive care unit. *J Clin Anesth* 27(2):175–180, 2015.

101. Prowle JR, Bellomo R: Sepsis-associated acute kidney injury: macrohemodynamic and microhemodynamic alterations in the renal circulation. *Semin Nephrol* 35(1):64–74, 2015.

102. Doyle JF, Forni LG: Long-term follow-up of acute kidney injury. *Crit Care Clin* 31(4):763–772, 2015.

103. Horne KL, et al: Long term outcomes after acute kidney injury: lessons from the ARID Study. *Nephron* 131(2):102–106, 2015.

104. Kashani K, Cheungpasitporn W, Ronco C: Biomarkers of acute kidney injury: the pathway from discovery to clinical adoption. *Clin Chem Lab Med* 55(8):1074–1089, 2017.

105. Kraut JA, Madias NE: Metabolic acidosis of CKD: an update. *Am J Kidney Dis* 67(2):307–317, 2016.

106. Hewitt J, et al: Sodium bicarbonate supplements for treating acute kidney injury. *Cochrane Database Syst Rev* (6):CD009204, 2012.

107. Meersch M, et al: Timing of renal replacement therapy in critically ill patients with acute kidney injury. *Ann Transl Med* 4(18):360, 2016.

108. Zoja C, Abbate M, Remuzzi G: Progression of renal injury toward interstitial inflammation and glomerular sclerosis is dependent on abnormal protein filtration. *Nephrol Dial Transplant* 30(5):706–712, 2015.

109. Rutkowski B, Tylicki L: Nephroprotective action of renin-angiotensin-aldosterone system blockade in chronic kidney disease patients: the landscape after ALTITUDE and VA NEPHRON-D trails. *J Ren Nutr* 25(2):194–200, 2015.

110. Libetta C, et al: Oxidative stress and inflammation: implications in uremia and hemodialysis. *Clin Biochem* 44(14-15):1189–1198, 2011.

111. Combs S, Berl T: Dysnatremias in patients with kidney disease. *Am J Kidney Dis* 63(2):294–303, 2014.

112. Zhang R, et al: Hyponatremia in patients with chronic kidney disease. *Hemodial Int* 1(1):3–10, 2017.

113. Sorensen MV, et al: Colonic potassium handling. *Pflugers Arch* 459(5):645–656, 2010.

114. Schaefer JA, Gales MA: Potassium-binding agents to facilitate renin-angiotensin-aldosterone system

inhibitor therapy. *Ann Pharmacother* 50(6): 502–510, 2016.

115. Kovesdy CP: Management of hyperkalemia: an update for the internist. *Am J Med* 128(12): 1281–1287, 2015.

116. Kraut JA, Madias NE: Metabolic acidosis of CKD: an update. *Am J Kidney Dis* 67(2):307–317, 2016.

117. Babayev R, Nickolas TL: Bone disorders in chronic kidney disease: an update in diagnosis and management. *Semin Dial* 28(6):645–653, 2015.

118. Ritter CS, Slatopolsky E: Phosphate toxicity in CKD: the killer among us. *Clin J Am Soc Nephrol* 11(6):1088–1100, 2016.

119. Felsenfeld AJ, Levine BS, Rodriguez M: Pathophysiology of calcium, phosphorus, and magnesium dysregulation in chronic kidney disease. *Semin Dial* 28(6):564–577, 2015.

120. Vassalotti JA, et al: Practical approach to detection and management of chronic kidney disease for the primary care clinician. *Am J Med* 129(2): 153–162, 2016.

121. Ikee R, et al: Glucose metabolism, insulin resistance and renal pathology in non-diabetic chronic kidney disease. *Nephron Clin Pract* 108(2): c163–c168, 2008.

122. Sweiss N, Sharma K: Adiponectin effects on the kidney. *Best Pract Res Clin Endocrinol Metab* 28(1):71–79, 2014.

123. Reiss AB, et al: Cholesterol metabolism in CKD. *Am J Kidney Dis* 66(6):1071–1082, 2015.

124. Kon V, Yang H, Fazio S: Residual cardiovascular risk in chronic kidney disease: role of high-density lipoprotein. *Arch Med Res* 46(5):379–391, 2015.

125. Bhandari S: Risk factors and metabolic mechanisms in the pathogenesis of uraemic cardiac disease. *Front Biosci* 16:1364–1387, 2011.

126. Briet M, Burns KD: Chronic kidney disease and vascular remodelling: molecular mechanisms and clinical implications. *Clin Sci* 123(7):399–416, 2012.

127. Bonomini M, et al: New treatment approaches for the anemia of CKD. *Am J Kidney Dis* 67(1): 133–142, 2016.

128. Lutz J, et al: Haemostasis in chronic kidney disease. *Nephrol Dial Transplant* 29(1):29–40, 2014.

129. Kurts C, et al: The immune system and kidney disease: basic concepts and clinical implications. *Nat Rev Immunol* 13(10):738–753, 2013.

130. Baumgaertel MW, Kraemer M, Berlit P: Neurologic complications of acute and chronic renal disease. *Handb Clin Neurol* 119:383–393, 2014.

131. Nadeau-Fredette AC, et al: End-stage renal disease and pregnancy. *Adv Chronic Kidney Dis* 20(3): 246–252, 2013.

132. Holley JL, Schmidt RJ: Changes in fertility and hormone replacement therapy in kidney disease. *Adv Chronic Kidney Dis* 20(3):240–245, 2013.

133. Teta D: Insulin resistance as a therapeutic target for chronic kidney disease. *J Ren Nutr* 25(2): 226–229, 2015.

134. Dousdampanis P, et al: The thyroid and the kidney: a complex interplay in health and disease. *Int J Artif Organs* 37(1):1–12, 2014.

135. Combs SA, Teixeira JP, Germain MJ: Pruritus in kidney disease. *Semin Nephrol* 35(4):383–391, 2015.

136. Kowalski A, Krikorian A, Lerma EV: Dyslipidemia in chronic kidney disease. *Dis Mon* 61(9):396–402, 2015.

137. Bhandari S, et al: Multicentre randomized controlled trial of angiotensin-converting enzyme inhibitor/angiotensin receptor blocker withdrawal in advanced renal disease: the STOP-ACEi trial. *Nephrol Dial Transplant* 31(2):255–261, 2016.

138. Vaziri ND, Anzalone DA, Catini J: Statins in chronic kidney disease: when and when not to use them. *J Fam Pract* 65(8 Suppl):2016.

139. Novikov A, Vallon V: Sodium glucose cotransporter 2 inhibition in the diabetic kidney: an update. *Curr Opin Nephrol Hypertens* 25(1): 50–58, 2016.

140. Desai N, Rahman M: Nephrology update: end-stage renal disease and renal replacement therapy. *FP Essent* 444:23–29, 2016.

Alterations of Renal and Urinary Tract Function in Children

Patricia Ring, Sue E. Huether

evolve WEBSITE

CHAPTER OUTLINE

Renal and urinary disorders occur in children as well as adults. In childhood, however, the kidney and genitourinary structures are continuing to develop, so renal dysfunction may be associated with mechanisms and manifestations that are different from those in adults. In addition, some renal and urinary disorders are congenital and involve structural anomalies of the kidney and urinary drainage system.

STRUCTURE AND FUNCTION OF THE URINARY SYSTEM IN CHILDREN

Development of the Urinary System

The embryonic urinary system develops as three sets of sequentially replaced organs: the pronephros, mesonephros, and metanephros. The pronephros is a nonfunctional structure that arises at the level of the cervical and upper thoracic regions during the third fetal week and connects the primitive wolffian duct to the cloaca as the foundation for male sexual development (Fig. 40.1). The development of the mesonephros and metanephros is described in Fig. 40.1. The Wilms tumor 1 *(WT1)* gene plays an important role at all stages of kidney development and maintenance of kidney function.[1]

After glomeruli and tubules form, the tissues organize and progressively differentiate over approximately 30 days. Initial glomerular development is staggered, so there are glomeruli in various stages. In fact, a few of the first glomeruli that are formed degenerate and disappear during the later stages of fetal development. Progressive development continues into the ninth fetal month, when all metanephrogenic tissue then disappears.

As the embryo develops and the vertebral column straightens, the kidneys appear to ascend to the sacral area at about 6 weeks, to the third lumbar area by the third month, and to the first lumbar area at term. The kidneys rotate 90 degrees as they ascend so that renal tissue is lateral and the collecting system is medial.

While the kidneys mature, the *cloaca* becomes the urogenital sinus. It then differentiates into the vesicourethral canal, which forms the bladder and the upper urethra, and the urogenital sinus, which forms the main part of the urethra.

At birth the kidneys occupy a large portion of the posterior abdominal wall, and the ureters are proportionately shorter than those of an adult. All the nephrons are present at birth, and their number does not increase as the kidney grows and matures. The kidney reaches adult size by adolescence and, because of maturation of the tubular system, increases in weight fivefold from the time of birth.

Urine formation and excretion begin by the third month of gestation, contributing to the amniotic fluid. In infancy the bladder lies close to the abdominal wall, making urinary bladder aspiration for diagnostic purposes a relatively simple procedure. The bladder descends into the

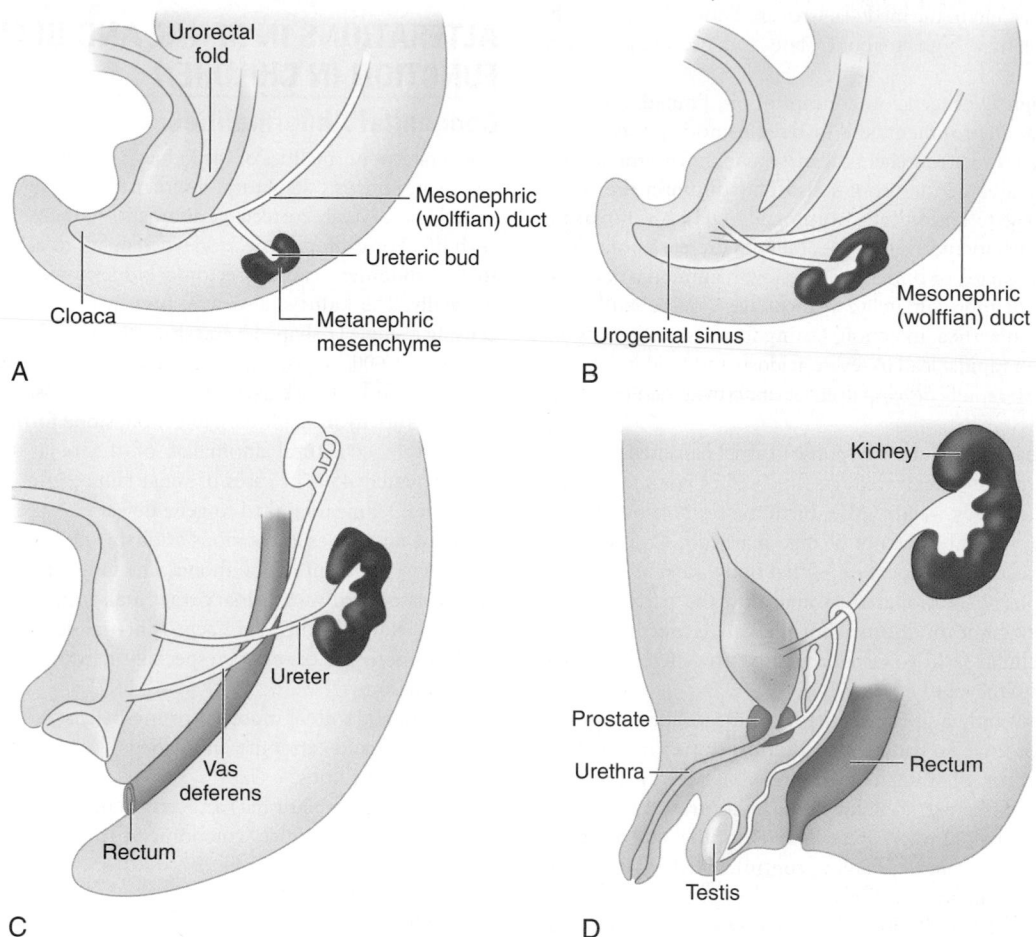

FIGURE 40.1 Embryonic Development of the Kidneys. The mesonephros begins development more caudally about the fourth fetal week and begins excretory function in the sixth week. Most of the mesonephros degenerates and disappears by the end of the embryonic period. The metanephros, the permanent kidney, arises distal to the bifurcation of the aorta and develops from two different sources: (1) the *ureteric bud* (metanephric duct) forms as an outgrowth of the mesonephric (wolffian) duct and grows dorsocranially and starts subdividing to become the collecting system for the kidneys by forming the ureter, renal pelvis, and calyces; by the fifth fetal month it will have progressively branched into the collecting ducts; and (2) the *metanephrogenic mesenchyme* sits atop the terminal branches of the collecting ducts and develops into primitive glomeruli and uriniferous tubules **(A)**. Genetic information from the metanephrogenic mesenchyme guides the development of the ureteric bud. Establishing the connection between the uriniferous tubules and the collecting ducts is a vital part of kidney development; errors in this stage can result in polycystic kidneys. As the embryo grows, the definitive kidneys migrate from the caudal position to the lumbar region and the ureters connect with the bladder **(B–D)**. In the 8-week male embryo, the wolffian duct begins to give rise to the epididymis, the seminal vesicles, and the caudal part of the vas deferens **(C)**. The external genitalia develop between 8 and 16 weeks, and testicular descent begins in month 7 of gestation **(D)**. (From Goldman L, Schafer AI: *Goldman's Cecil medicine,* ed 24, Philadelphia, 2012, Saunders.)

pelvis with growth, changing from a cylindrical organ to the adult pyramidal shape. Although small amounts of urine are found in the bladder at birth, the newborn may not void for 12 to 24 hours.

Immediately at birth the renal blood flow and glomerular filtration rate (GFR) increase because of a decrease in vascular resistance and the need to perform excretory functions no longer performed by the placenta. Renal vascular resistance remains higher in newborns and infants, however, which may be attributed to increased levels of circulating renin. The resistance progressively declines during the first year of development, with an increasing fraction of the cardiac output going to the kidney. The GFR continues to increase, achieving adult levels by 2 years of age.

Fluid and Electrolyte Balance in Children

Because the kidney develops from the center toward the periphery, renal distribution of blood flow during the newborn period is primarily to the renal medulla. The result is a preferential flow to the medullary nephrons, which have comparatively short loops at this stage of development. The combination of higher blood flow and shorter loops produces a more dilute urine up to 6 months of age—approximately 400 to 600 mOsm (compared with 800 to 1200 mOsm in adults) (see Chapter 3). The immature kidney is also less responsive to the actions of antidiuretic hormone (vasopressin)[2] (see Fig. 3.6). The dilute urine is accentuated by a low rate of urea excretion, which is necessary to establish the concentration gradient in the medulla. Urea excretion is low primarily because infants are in a high anabolic state and use their protein for growth.

Because of a high hydrogen ion concentration, limited ability to regulate the internal environment, and lowered osmotic pressure, the infant's renal system has a narrow chemical safety margin. The immaturity and smaller surface area of the tubules also may diminish the water reabsorption response to antidiuretic hormone (ADH). An immature tubular transport capacity means that the ability to excrete a potassium load, reabsorb bicarbonate, or buffer hydrogen with ammonia does not become efficient until approximately 2 years of age. Consequently, any disturbance such as diarrhea, infection, fasting for diagnostic tests, or improper feeding can rapidly lead to severe acidosis and fluid imbalance because the infant can rapidly develop over- or underhydration or edema (see Chapter 3).[3]

At birth infants have a natriuretic response to atrial natriuretic peptide and a normal contraction in extracellular fluid (ECF) volume with an accompanying loss of body weight. After birth the proportion of total body water to body weight does not change markedly. Considerable change occurs, however, in the location of that body water as the child matures (see Chapter 3). Compared to an adult, the percentage of extracellular fluid volume of the newborn infant is nearly double. Decrease in extracellular fluid volume occurs in two different periods of rapid growth—infancy and adolescence.

An infant has not only a greater content of extracellular fluid but also a greater rate of fluid exchange. The adult consumes and excretes approximately 2000 mL of water daily, representing 5% of the total body fluid or 14% of the extracellular fluid. In contrast, the infant's daily exchange of 600 to 700 mL represents 290% of the total or nearly 50% of the extracellular volume, making control of dehydration and overhydration more difficult.

The composition of body fluids differs slightly with age. The total electrolyte concentration in extracellular fluids is greater in the newborn than in the adult. The concentrations of sodium, chloride, phosphates, and organic acids are also greater. The concentration of bicarbonate ions is lower in the infant than in the older child, with a mild acidosis evidenced by a lowered pH. These variations, combined with a lowered plasma protein level, cause a reduced oncotic pressure of the vascular compartment and favor accumulation of fluid in the tissue spaces and an increased GFR. In the healthy child these differences remain for a few weeks or months. The premature infant and the normal newborn infant are usually in a state of well-compensated acidosis and potential edema.

ALTERATIONS IN RENAL AND BLADDER FUNCTION IN CHILDREN

Congenital Abnormalities

Congenital abnormalities of the kidney and urinary tract occur in about 1% of newborns.[4] Structural abnormalities range from minor, non-pathologic, or easily correctable anomalies to those that are incompatible with life. For example, the kidneys may fail to ascend from the pelvis to the abdomen, causing ectopic kidneys—which usually function normally. The kidneys also may fuse in the midline as they ascend, causing a single U-shaped horseshoe kidney, with an incidence rate of about 1 in 600 births.[5] Approximately one-third of individuals with horseshoe kidneys are asymptomatic. The most common associated problems are hydronephrosis, infection, stone formation, and tumors.[6] Collectively, structural anomalies of the renal system account for approximately 45% of cases of renal failure in children in developed countries. Many are linked to gene defects.[7]

Some anomalies are obvious at birth, whereas others remain silent or become apparent in childhood. The following structural anomalies can be associated with urinary tract malformations:[6,8]

- Low-set, malformed ears, sensorineural deafness
- Chromosomal disorders, especially trisomy 13 (Patau syndrome) and trisomy 18
- Absent abdominal muscles (prune-belly syndrome)
- Vertebral and extremity anomalies
- Imperforate anus
- Renal (nephroblastoma) and extrarenal tumors
- Ocular abnormalities (coloboma of the iris, congenital cataracts)
- Hepatic cysts or cirrhosis

Hypospadias

Hypospadias is a congenital condition in which the urethral meatus is located on the ventral side or undersurface of the penis. The meatus can be located anywhere on the glans (proximal hypospadias), the penile shaft, the base of the penis, the penoscrotal junction, or the perineum (distal hypospadias) (Fig. 40.2). Partial absence of the foreskin, inguinal hernia, and cryptorchidism (undescended testes; see Chapter 26) are associated with the anomaly. This is the most common anomaly of the penis. The incidence varies geographically ranging from 1.86 to 5 per 10,000 infant boys.[9] The etiology is multifactorial and related to disruptions in male hormones, including testosterone biosynthesis defects, steroid 5α-reductase type 2 mutations, genes associated with

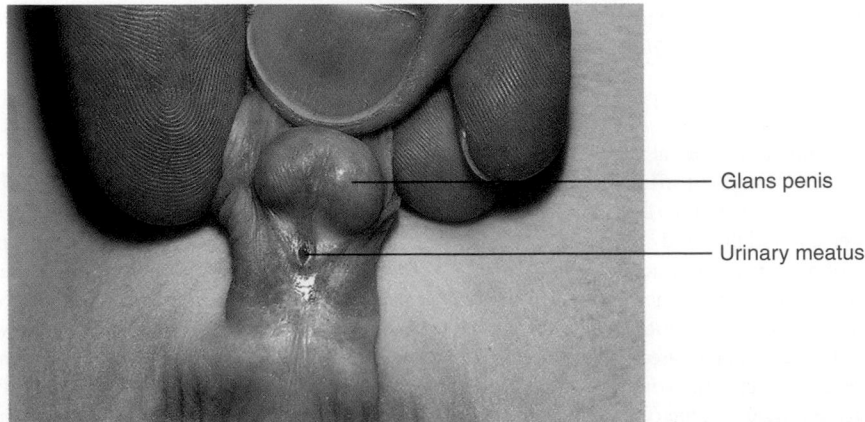

Glans penis

Urinary meatus

FIGURE 40.2 Hypospadias. (Courtesy H. Gil Rushton, MD, Children's National Medical Center, Washington, DC; from Hockenberry MJ, Wilson D: *Wong's nursing care of infants and children*, ed 10, St Louis, 2015, Mosby.)

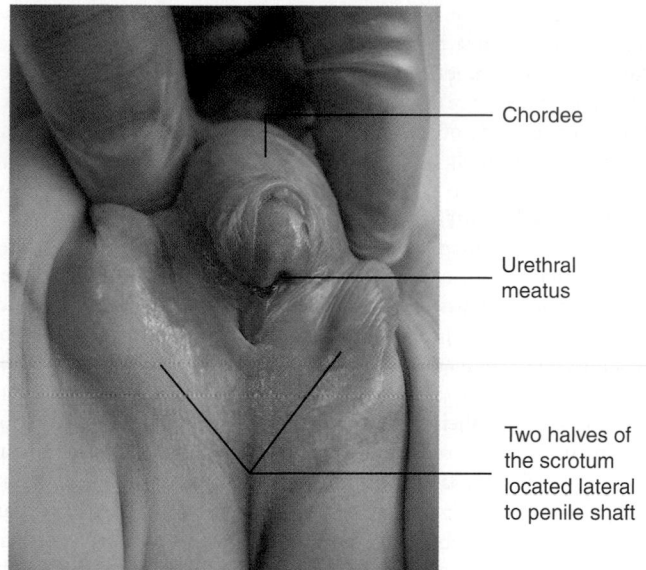

Chordee

Urethral meatus

Two halves of the scrotum located lateral to penile shaft

FIGURE 40.3 Perineal Hypospadias with Chordee and Partial Penoscrotal Transposition. (From Kliegman RM et al, editors: *Nelson textbook of pediatrics,* ed 19, Philadelphia, 2011, Saunders.)

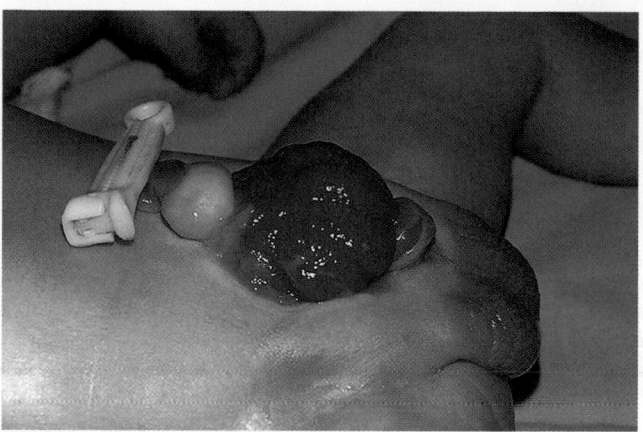

FIGURE 40.4 Exstrophy of Bladder. (Courtesy H. Gil Rushton, MD, Children's National Medical Center, Washington, DC; from Hockenberry MJ, Wilson D: *Wong's nursing care of infants and children,* ed 10, St Louis, 2015, Mosby.)

penile and urethral development, hormones administered for in vitro fertilization, advanced maternal age, and other environmental factors.[10] Chordee or penile torsion may accompany hypospadias. In *chordee* a shortage of skin on the ventral surface causes the penis to bend or to "bow" ventrally (Fig. 40.3). *Penile torsion* is a rotation, usually in a counterclockwise direction, of the penile shaft.[11]

The goals for corrective surgery on the child with hypospadias are (1) a straight penis when erect to facilitate sexual intercourse as an adult, (2) a uniform urethra of adequate caliber to prevent spraying during urinations, (3) a cosmetic appearance satisfactory to the individual, and (4) repair completed in as few procedures as possible. Improvements in microsurgical techniques have enhanced outcomes and decreased complications and the need for follow-up surgery. Surgery is usually performed between 6 and 12 months of age.[12]

Epispadias

Epispadias and exstrophy of the bladder are the same congenital defect but expressed to a different degree. The dorsal urethra is not fused in epispadias and has failed to form into a tube. In boys the urethral opening may be small and situated behind the glans (anterior epispadias), or a fissure may extend the entire length of the penis and into the bladder neck (posterior epispadias). In females a cleft along the ventral urethra usually extends to the bladder neck. The incidence of epispadias is about 9.25 per 100,000 in-hospital live births[13]; it is seen predominantly in males. Continence is determined in part by the location of the defect, with urinary incontinence rates of up to 75% in children with distal epispadias.[14] Treatment is surgical reconstruction.

Exstrophy of the Bladder

Exstrophy of the bladder is a rare extensive congenital anomaly of herniation of the bladder through the abdominal wall with failure of the abdominal muscles, pelvic ring, and pelvic floor musculature to fuse in the midline (Fig. 40.4). The posterior portion of the bladder mucosa is exposed and appears bright red. The prevalence of exstrophy of the bladder is about 1.7 in 100,000 live births.[13]

Exstrophy of the bladder is caused by intrauterine failure of the abdominal wall and the mesoderm of the anterior bladder to fuse. The clitoris in girls is divided into two halves with the urethra between them. The penis in boys is epispadias. Urine seeps onto the abdominal wall from the ureters, causing a constant odor of urine and excoriation of the surrounding skin. Because the exposed bladder mucosa becomes hyperemic and edematous, it bleeds easily and is painful. It should be covered with Silastic or a plastic dressing (e.g., kitchen plastic wrap) for protection from irritation while permitting urine drainage. The unrepaired exstrophic bladder is cosmetically unacceptable and prone to cancerous changes as soon as 1 year after birth. The rectus muscles below the umbilicus are separated, and the pubic rami (bony projections of the pubic bone) are not joined. In addition, the posterior aspect of the pelvis is externally rotated, which retroverts the acetabula and causes external rotation of the feet. This causes a waddling gait when the child first learns to walk. Most children learn to compensate, but surgical intervention may be required. Ideally the bladder and pubic defect should be closed before the infant is 72 hours old. Surgical reconstruction is usually performed within the first year, either as a complete primary repair or as staged procedures. Staged procedures may include bladder augmentation and bladder neck and epispadias repair.[15] Objectives of management include preservation of renal function, attainment of urinary control, prevention of infection, and improvement of sexual function and quality of life.

Cloacal exstrophy is the most rare and severe form of bladder exstrophy. The intestines, genitourinary tract, and spine may be involved, and reconstruction with restored urine and fecal control is difficult.

Ureteropelvic Junction Obstruction

Ureteropelvic junction (UPJ) obstruction is a blockage of the tapered point where the renal pelvis transitions into the ureter. Most cases are caused by intrinsic factors, such as a stricture or an aperistaltic ureteral segment, whereas extrinsic factors, such as crossing vessels, are rarely seen.[16] It is the most common cause of hydronephrosis in neonates.[17] Diagnosis is made by ultrasound. Open or endoscopic surgery to relieve the obstruction occurs if there is decline of renal drainage or function.[18] Secondary ureteropelvic junction obstruction is caused by kinking or extrinsic compression by an aberrant lower pole vessel.[19] Children with UPJ obstruction have an increased risk of vesicoureteral reflux.[20] UPJ obstruction can be associated with ureteral duplication, including complete ureteral duplication (abnormal growth of two ureters and ureteral orifices draining a single kidney) and incomplete duplication (bifurcation of the ureter terminates into one ureteral orifice and serves a single kidney). Obstruction of the distant ureter (**ureterovesical junction obstruction**) causes dilation of the entire ureter, renal pelvis, and calyceal system (megaureter). **Megaureter** can occur when a short acontractile segment of the ureter develops just above the ureterovesical junction or from ureteral reflux.[21] A **ureterocele** (cystic dilation of the intravesical ureter) impedes drainage from the associated kidney.

Bladder Outlet Obstruction

Congenital causes of bladder outlet obstruction are rare and include urethral valves, urethral polyps, and urethral atresia. A **urethral valve** is a thin membrane that occludes the urethral lumen and obstructs urinary outflow in males. It is the most common cause of congenital lower urinary tract obstruction and renal failure. Most valves occur in the posterior urethra (PUV), although a few arise from the embryologically distinct anterior urethra.[22] **Urethral polyps** arising from the prostatic urethra are rare. Symptoms of polyps may include hematuria; voiding issues, such as urinary retention or straining to void; and dilation of the upper tracts.[23] **Urethral atresia** is absence of the urethra and is rare. Congenital urethral valves or polyps can be diagnosed with prenatal ultrasound and treated with prenatal bladder shunting or with resection during the first days of life. Severe obstruction may impair renal embryogenesis and lead to renal failure.[24]

Hypoplastic or Dysplastic Kidneys

During embryologic development, the ureteric duct grows into the metanephric tissue, triggering the formation of the kidneys. If this growth does not occur, the kidney is absent—a condition called **renal aplasia**. A **hypoplastic kidney** is small with a decreased number of nephrons. These conditions may be unilateral or bilateral; the occurrence may be incidental or familial. Bilateral hypoplastic kidneys are a common cause of chronic renal failure in children. Segmental hypoplasia (the Ask-Upmark kidney) may be congenital or secondary to vesicoureteral reflux. Systemic hypertension is a common presentation.

Renal dysplasia usually results from abnormal differentiation of the renal tissues; for example, primitive glomeruli and tubules, cysts, and nonrenal tissue (such as cartilage) are found in the dysplastic kidney. Dysplasia may be secondary to antenatal obstruction of the urinary tract from ureteroceles, posterior urethral valves, or prune-belly syndrome.

Renal Agenesis

Renal agenesis (the absence of one or both kidneys) may be unilateral or bilateral and may occur randomly or be hereditary. It may be an isolated entity or associated with anomalies in other organs. *Unilateral renal agenesis* occurs in approximately 1 of 1000 live births in the United States. Males are more often affected, and it is usually the left kidney that is absent. The single kidney is often completely normal, so that the child can expect a normal, healthy life. The normal solitary kidney grows because of compensatory hypertrophy before and after birth. By the time the child is several years older, the volume of this kidney may approach twice the normal size. In some instances the single kidney is abnormally formed and associated with abnormalities of its collecting system.[25] Because the child has a decreased number of nephrons, there is a risk of "hyperfiltration injury," increasing the chance of developing proteinuria, hypertension, and chronic kidney disease.[26] Extrarenal congenital abnormalities of the urogenital, skeletal, cardiac, and other systems may coexist.[27] *Bilateral renal agenesis* (also called **Potter syndrome**) is a rare disorder incompatible with extrauterine life.[28] Approximately 75% of affected infants are male. Bilateral renal agenesis results from either an abnormal development of the normal progression from pronephros to mesonephros to metanephros or an isolated bilateral failure of development of the ureteral buds. The term *Potter syndrome*

refers to the association with a specific group of facial anomalies (wide-set eyes, parrot-beak nose, low-set ears, and receding chin). Oligohydramnios (low amount of amniotic fluid) leads to underdeveloped lungs. Affected infants rarely live more than 24 hours because of pulmonary insufficiency. Approximately 40% of affected infants are stillborn. Renal agenesis can be detected prenatally by ultrasound.

Polycystic Kidneys

Autosomal dominant polycystic kidney disease (ADPKD) is an inherited disorder that occurs in about 1 in 1000 live births in the United States. Mutations of two genes, *PKD-1* (chromosome 16) and *PKD-2* (chromosome 4), account for the disease most often presenting in late childhood or adulthood. The gene products (polycystins) regulate growth and differentiation of the tubular epithelium.[29] Defects in the formation of epithelial cells and their cilium result in cyst formation and obstruction accompanied by destruction of renal parenchyma, interstitial fibrosis, and loss of functional nephrons. Cysts may occur in other organs including the liver, seminal vesicles, and pancreas. Hypertension, heart valve defects, and cerebral and aortic aneurysms may develop.[30] Urinary tract infection, hematuria, and flank pain may occur. Diagnosis is usually confirmed by ultrasound. Individuals may live for decades before developing symptoms of renal disease, and not all progress to end-stage disease.[31] Tolvaptan (a competitive vasopressin receptor 2 antagonist) may slow progression of the condition.[32] **Autosomal recessive PKD (ARPKD)** with cystic changes in the kidney and liver is often first suspected on a prenatal ultrasound. Gene mutations in *PKHD1* result in reduced or absent function of fibrocystin which is required for tubulogenesis.[33] Renal replacement therapy is usually required during childhood or adolescence.[34]

Glomerular Disorders

The most common glomerular disorders in children are glomerulonephritis, nephrotic syndrome, and hemolytic uremic syndrome. Most glomerular diseases are acquired and immunologically mediated. The disease can be acute or chronic. The likelihood of developing renal failure depends on the specific condition. The most common glomerular disorders in children are presented next.

Glomerulonephritis

Acute glomerulonephritis includes a number of renal disorders in which inflammation of the glomeruli are secondary to an immune mechanism (Table 40.1). (The types of glomerulonephritis and their histologic characteristics can be reviewed in Chapter 39 and Table 39.7.) The symptoms usually include the sudden onset of hematuria with red blood cell casts and proteinuria, and can be accompanied by renal salt and water retention, edema, hypertension, and in severe cases azotemia (i.e., decreased glomerular filtration rate). Glomerulonephritis is the causative factor for 15% to 29% of end-stage renal disease in children.[35]

Acute Poststreptococcal Glomerulonephritis. Acute poststreptococcal glomerulonephritis (PSGN) is one of the most common immune complex–mediated renal diseases in children ages 5 to 15 years, and it is representative of acute glomerulonephritis. It most commonly occurs after a throat (pharyngitis) or skin (impetigo) infection with nephritogenic strains of group A beta-hemolytic streptococci, although other bacteria (e.g., *Staphylococcus*) and viruses also may be responsible. Occurrences have been observed after bacterial endocarditis, which may be associated with streptococcal or staphylococcal microorganisms, or after viral diseases, such as varicella and hepatitides B and C. Glomerulonephritis develops with the deposition of antigen-antibody complexes (immunoglobulin G [IgG] and C_3 complement) (see Chapter 8) in the glomerulus, or the antigen may be trapped within the glomerulus and

TABLE 40.1	PRIMARY GLOMERULONEPHRITIS IN CHILDREN
CLASSIFICATION	**FINDINGS**
Cause	Poststreptococcal infection
	Related to other bacterial or viral infection
	Unknown
Immunologic mechanism	Antigen-antibody complex deposition
	Planted antigens with immune complex formed in situ
	Formation of antiglomerular basement membrane antibodies (rare)
	No immunologic cause established
Histopathology	No lesion
	Diffuse, focal, or segmented
	Membranous, proliferative, or combination of types
	Lobular, exudative, necrotizing, and other types
	Chronic with glomerular proliferation
Clinical manifestations of disease	Acute glomerulonephritis
	Persistent (chronic) glomerulonephritis
	Idiopathic nephrotic syndrome

immune complexes formed in situ.[36] The exact mechanism of immune complex formation is unknown. The immune complexes initiate inflammation and glomerular injury. Immunofluorescence microscopy shows lumpy deposits of IgG and C_3 on the glomerular basement membrane (Fig. 40.5). The thickened glomerular membrane contributes to decreased GFR. Activated complement, inflammatory cytokines, oxidants, proteases, and growth factors attack epithelial cells, alter membrane permeability, and cause hematuria and proteinuria. Hypertension occurs primarily because of fluid retention.

Symptoms usually begin 1 to 2 weeks after an upper respiratory tract infection (more common during cold weather) and up to 6 weeks after skin infections, such as impetigo (more common during warm weather). The onset of symptoms in the child is abrupt, varying with disease severity. The urine is usually smoky brown or cola colored because of the presence of red blood cells. The child may complain of flank or midabdominal pain, irritability, general malaise, and fever. Acute hypertension may cause headache, vomiting, somnolence, and other central nervous system (CNS) manifestations, including seizures. Cardiovascular symptoms are related to circulatory overload and are compounded by hypertension. These include dyspnea, tachypnea, and an enlarged, tender liver. The most severely affected children develop acute renal failure with oliguria. The disease is usually mild and runs its course in 1 month, but urine abnormalities may be found up to 1 year after the onset. As many as half the children affected are asymptomatic.

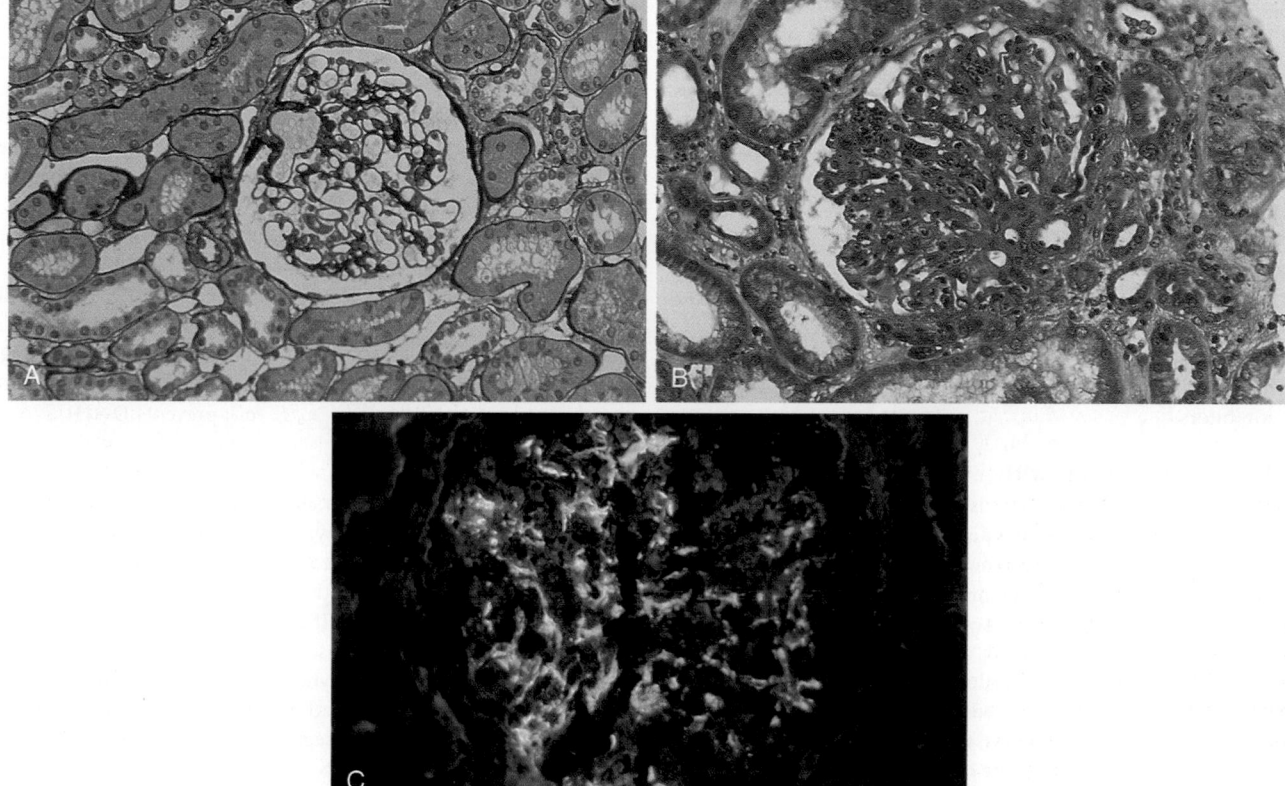

FIGURE 40.5 Glomerulonephritis. **A,** Normal glomerulus; note single-contoured walls, patent capillaries, inconspicuous mesangium, and degree of cellularity. (Periodic acid–methenamine silver stain.) **B,** Acute postinfectious glomerulonephritis. There is considerable increase in cellularity, mainly because of accumulation of numerous polymorphonuclear leukocytes in capillary lumina. Note numerous subepithelial hump-shaped fuchsinophilic deposits in many capillary walls. Protein precipitates (hyalinization) are in the arteriole. (Masson trichrome stain.) **C,** Postinfectious glomerulonephritis. Irregular mesangial and capillary wall immunostaining for C_3. (From Damjanov I, Linder J, editors: *Anderson's pathology*, ed 10, St Louis, 1996, Mosby.)

Fewer than 5% of children become oliguric or develop rapidly progressive glomerulonephritis, or progress to chronic glomerulonephritis. Prolonged proteinuria and abnormal GFR indicate an unfavorable prognosis. More than 95% recover completely. Fewer than 1% of children develop end-stage renal disease.[37]

Immunoglobulin A Nephropathy. Immunoglobulin A (IgA) nephropathy is the most common form of glomerulonephritis in children and young adults worldwide and occurs more often in males. The cause is unknown. It is characterized by deposition primarily of IgA and complement proteins in the mesangium of the glomerulus. Abnormal glycosylated IgA-1 (galactose-deficient IgA-1) is produced by the bone marrow. Glycan-specific IgA antibodies are formed against abnormal IgA-1, can activate complement, and bind to glomerular mesangial cells, stimulating them to proliferate, secrete extracellular matrix proteins, and release inflammatory cytokines and chemokines (interleukin-6, tumor necrosis factor-alpha, and transforming growth factor-beta 1) that cause injury. The immune response contributes to diffuse mesangioproliferative glomerular injury and glomerulosclerosis, which is usually reversible.[38] Children with this disease have recurrent gross hematuria concurrent with a respiratory tract infection (i.e., tonsillitis) or gastroenteritis. Most continue to have microscopic hematuria between the attacks of gross hematuria and have mild proteinuria. Treatment is supportive. Proteinuria, edema, and hypertension are more severe symptoms and must be treated to prevent future loss of kidney function. Some children recover completely, whereas 20% to 40% will eventually require dialysis and transplantation.[39] IgA nephropathy may recur following transplantation.

Henoch-Schönlein Purpura Nephritis. Henoch-Schönlein purpura (HSP) nephritis (anaphylactoid purpura) is an immune-mediated IgA vasculitis that affects glomerular blood vessels, causing inflammation and damage to the vessel wall. The disease also involves small vessels in the skin and gut. Classic symptoms of HSP include palpable purpura, arthritis, and abdominal pain. About 21% of children develop renal disease characterized by gross or microscopic hematuria with mild or no proteinuria,[40] usually within 4 weeks of disease onset. Kidney biopsy demonstrates IgA deposition in the mesangium.[41] The development of interstitial fibrosis and crescent formation from subepithelial immune deposits along the glomeruli increases the risk of chronic renal failure.[42] Most children recover with supportive care, although some progress to kidney failure. Severe symptoms require corticosteroids, other immunosuppressant drugs, or angiotensin-converting enzyme (ACE) inhibitors.[43]

Hemolytic Uremic Syndrome

Hemolytic uremic syndrome (HUS) is an acute disorder characterized by microangiopathic hemolytic anemia, thrombocytopenia, and renal impairment. It is the most common community-acquired cause of acute renal failure in young children. The disease occurs most frequently in infants and children younger than 4 years of age. The prognosis has improved dramatically in recent years, with more than 90% of children surviving and most regaining normal renal function.

◆**PATHOPHYSIOLOGY.** HUS has been associated with both bacterial and viral agents, as well as endotoxins, especially those from *Escherichia coli* 0157:H7 and recently *Escherichia coli* 0104:H4.[44] Potential sources of exposure include animals, unpasteurized beverages, and contaminated meat and vegetables. The disease also occurs with cancer and use of chemotherapeutic agents.[45] In HUS, verotoxin (Shiga toxin) from *E. coli* is absorbed from the intestines into the blood, binds to polymorphonuclear leukocytes, and is transported to the kidney, causing a cascade of effects, including lysis of glomerular capillary endothelial cells, separation of endothelial cells from the basement membrane, activation and aggregation of platelets, and activation of the coagulation cascade. The glomerular arterioles become swollen and occluded with platelets and fibrin clots. There is decreased glomerular filtration, and the damaged glomerular membrane results in hematuria and proteinuria. Oliguria with renal failure occurs in up to 50% of children. Narrowed vessels damage passing erythrocytes. These damaged red blood cells, identified as burr cells, helmet cells, and fragmented red blood cells, are removed by the spleen, causing acute hemolytic anemia. Fibrinolysis, the process of dissolution of a clot, acts on precipitated fibrin, causing the fibrin split products to appear in serum and urine. The platelet clustering within damaged vessels, combined with the damage and removal of platelets, produces thrombocytopenia. Fibrin-rich thrombi can be found throughout the microcirculation. Other tissues, including the brain, liver, heart, and intestines, are often involved.[46]

◆**CLINICAL MANIFESTATIONS.** Typical HUS is preceded by a prodromal gastrointestinal (GI) illness with diarrhea (usually caused by Shiga toxin–producing *E. coli*) and is known as *D+ HUS*. Atypical HUS (aHUS) is not associated with diarrhea and is known as *D– HUS*. Dysregulation of the alternative complement pathway is often noted.[47] Familial aHUS is rare and defined as the diagnosis of aHUS in at least two members of the same family at least 6 months apart.[48] The onset of D+ HUS occurs about 1 to 2 weeks after a GI illness with a symptom-free 1- to 5-day period. There is sudden onset of pallor, bruising or purpura, irritability, and oliguria. Slight fever, anorexia, vomiting, diarrhea (with the stool characteristically watery and blood stained—hemorrhagic diarrhea), abdominal pain, mild jaundice, and circulatory overload are accompanying symptoms. Seizures and lethargy indicate CNS involvement. Renal failure is apparent within 2 days to 2 weeks of onset. The renal failure causes metabolic acidosis, uremia, hyperkalemia, and often hypertension.

◆**EVALUATION AND TREATMENT.** Clinical evaluation includes history of preexisting illness, presenting symptoms, and urine and blood analysis. Antibiotics are not used in the initial treatment because they increase Shiga toxin release and increase the risk of HUS. Management consists of maintaining nutrition and hydration and controlling hypertension, hyperkalemia, and seizures. When renal failure occurs, dialysis is indicated. Blood transfusions with packed red blood cells are needed to maintain reasonable hemoglobin levels. Eculizumab, a C5 inhibitor, has been demonstrated to be efficacious in the treatment of aHUS.[49] Most children recover; however, some will develop hypertension, proteinuria, or renal insufficiency or failure. Death usually occurs from complications related to CNS, infectious, or myocardial causes.[50] Preventing Shiga toxin–producing bacterial infection (i.e., *E. coli*) prevents D+ HUS.

Nephrotic Syndrome

Nephrotic syndrome is a term used to describe a symptom complex characterized by proteinuria, hypoalbuminemia, hyperlipidemia, and edema. The syndrome is more common in children than adults. When no identifiable cause is found, the condition is termed primary (idiopathic) nephrotic syndrome. If it results from a systemic disease or other causes (e.g., drugs, toxins, diabetes mellitus, lupus nephritis) it is called secondary nephrotic syndrome. Primary nephrotic syndrome is usually described by histopathologic results (i.e., minimal change nephropathy [MCN], focal segmental glomerulosclerosis [FSGS], membranous nephropathy [MN], or membranoproliferative glomerulonephritis [MPGN]) (see Table 39.7). Secondary nephrotic syndrome has the same patterns of histopathology but is associated with an underlying cause.

Approximately 95% of cases of nephrotic syndrome in children occur in the absence of systemic or preexisting renal disease. Primary nephrotic syndrome is found predominantly in preschool children, with a peak incidence of onset between 2 and 3 years of age. Onset is rare after 8 years of age. Boys are affected more often than girls.

No prevalent racial or geographic distributions are evident. The incidence is approximately 2 to 3 per 100,000 children per year.[51]

◆PATHOPHYSIOLOGY. The cause of nephrotic syndrome in children is usually idiopathic and includes MCN (85%), FSGS (10%), and mesangial proliferative nephropathy (MPN) (5%)[52] (see Chapter 39, Table 39.7). Secondary nephrotic syndrome may develop during the course of several different renal or systemic diseases. The pathophysiology (see Fig. 39.11) and common clinical manifestations of nephrotic syndrome in adults are described in Chapter 39 (see Table 39.8) and are similar in children. The most common causes of nephrotic syndrome in children are presented here.

Minimal change nephropathy (MCN), also known as *lipoid nephrosis,* is the most common cause of nephrotic syndrome in children ages 2 to 6 years. A systemic immune mechanism is a likely cause of the disease, but the true etiology is unknown. The mechanism of increased glomerular permeability is unknown but is related, in part, to release of permeability factors from abnormal circulating T cells that injure the glomerular epithelial cells.[53] The glomeruli appear normal by light microscopy, and immunoglobulin deposition is usually absent. The only change is *fusion of epithelial cell podocyte foot processes.*[54] Loss of the electrical negative charge and increased permeability within the glomerular capillary wall lead to albuminuria. Hyperlipidemia leads to lipiduria and primarily results from increased hepatic lipid synthesis and decreased plasma lipid catabolism.

Focal segmental glomerulosclerosis (FSGS) is present in approximately 10% of children with nephrotic syndrome and is more common in blacks. The frequency of FSGS is increasing in children and adults.[55] The primary injury is effacement (thinning or deletion) of epithelial podocytes, with a significant increase in pore size leading to impairment of size selectivity and proteinuria. Progressive disease results in proliferation of endothelial and mesangial cells with occlusion and sclerosis of glomerular capillaries. The more severe the proteinuria, the more likely it is that end-stage renal disease will occur. FSGS is usually steroid resistant.[56]

Edema is the classic symptom of nephrotic syndrome. Factors theorized to contribute to edema formation include hypoalbuminemia (decreased plasma oncotic pressure) and sodium retention.[57] The movement of fluid from the vascular to the interstitial space can decrease blood volume, increase the activity of aldosterone and antidiuretic hormone (vasopressin), and decrease atrial natriuretic peptide concentration, all of which promote fluid retention.[58]

Hyperlipidemia occurs in inverse proportion to the decrease in plasma proteins, particularly albumin. There are high concentrations of triglycerides, low-density lipoprotein (LDL), and very-low-density lipoprotein (VLDL) cholesterol. High-density lipoprotein (HDL) cholesterol concentration is decreased. Hypoalbuminemia leads to a deficiency in the carrier protein for the transport of fatty acids, and they remain elevated in the serum. There is hepatic compensation for hypoalbuminemia with increased synthesis of lipoproteins to maintain plasma oncotic pressure. Hypoalbuminemia also leads to an increased hepatic stimulus for synthesis of LDL and VLDL cholesterol by the liver. Serum lipids may remain elevated from 1 to 3 months after remission of proteinuria.

Hypercoagulation with risk for arterial or venous thrombosis results from abnormalities in the coagulation pathways during nephrotic syndrome. Although rare, thrombosis can occur in the brain or lung. Family history and predisposing risk factors should be evaluated. Anticoagulants may be required.[59]

Congenital nephrotic syndrome—Finnish type is usually caused by an autosomal recessive mutation of the *NPHS1* gene that encodes an immunoglobulin-like protein, nephrin, at the podocyte slit membrane. Lack of nephrin causes heavy proteinuria. The disease usually manifests before 3 months of life. Treatment consists of intravenous albumin infusions, nutritional supplement, and bilateral nephrectomy followed by dialysis and kidney transplantation.[60]

◆CLINICAL MANIFESTATIONS. Onset of nephrotic syndrome is often insidious, with periorbital edema as the first sign. Periorbital edema is most noticeable in the morning but subsides during the day as fluid shifts to the abdomen and lower extremities (Fig. 40.6). Parents may notice diminished, frothy, or foamy urine output. When edema becomes pronounced, ascites, respiratory difficulty from pleural effusion, and labial or scrotal swelling may develop.

Edema of the intestinal mucosa may cause diarrhea, anorexia, and poor absorption. Edema often masks the malnutrition caused by malabsorption and protein loss. Because of protein deficiency, changes in the quality of hair indicate a malnourished state. Pallor, with shiny skin and prominent veins, may be present. Blood pressure is usually normal. The child has an increased susceptibility to infection, especially pneumonia, peritonitis, cellulitis, and septicemia. Irritability, fatigue, and lethargy are common. Infants born with congenital nephrotic syndrome have large fontanels and separated cranial sutures.

◆EVALUATION AND TREATMENT. The diagnosis of nephrotic syndrome is evident from the clinical presentation and findings of proteinuria, hyperlipidemia, and edema. Diagnostic tests, including kidney biopsy, may be required to determine whether the cause is an intrinsic renal disease or a consequence of systemic disease. The goals of treatment

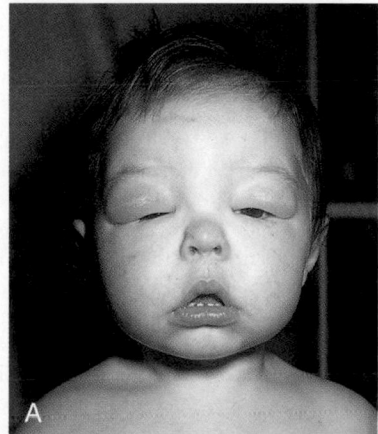
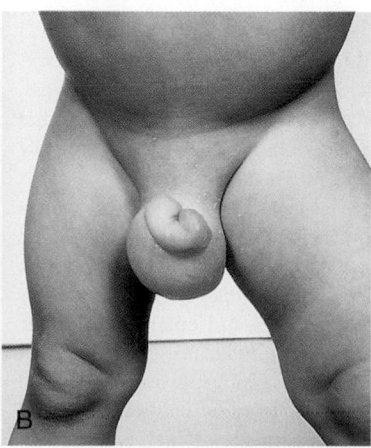

FIGURE 40.6 Nephrotic Syndrome. **A,** Facial edema. **B,** Gross edema of scrotum and legs with abdominal distention from ascites. (From Lissauer T, Clayden G: *Illustrated textbook of paediatrics,* ed 4, London, 2012, Mosby.)

TABLE 40.2   CORTICOSTEROID RESPONSE IN CHILDREN WITH NEPHROTIC SYNDROME

RESPONSE TO CORTICOSTEROID	OUTCOMES
Steroid sensitive	May have just one or recurrent episodes.
Steroid dependent or frequently relapsing	May require low-dose prednisone or treatment with other immunosuppressive agents to prevent recurrence
Steroid resistant	Treatment with immunosuppressive and nonimmunosuppressive medications; risk for development of end-stage kidney disease

Data from Hodson EM, et al: *Cochrane Database Syst Rev* 10:CD003594, 2016; Larkins N, et al: *Arch Dis Child* 101(4):404-408, 2016.

TABLE 40.3   PEDIATRIC-MODIFIED RIFLE (pRIFLE) CRITERIA

RISK CATEGORY	ESTIMATED CCL-GFR CRITERIA	URINE OUTPUT CRITERIA
Risk	eCCl decrease by 25%	<0.5 mL/kg/hr for 8 hr
Injury	eCCl decrease by 50%	<0.5 mL/kg/hr for 16 hr
Failure	eCCl decrease by 75% or eCCl <35 mL/min/1.73 m^2	<0.3 mL/kg/hr for 24 hr or anuric for 12 hr
Loss (of kidney function)	Persistent failure >4 weeks	
End-stage	End-stage renal disease (persistent failure >3 months)	

eCCl, Estimated creatinine clearance; *GFR,* glomerular filtration rate; *pRIFLE,* pediatric *r*isk, *i*njury, *f*ailure, *l*oss, and *e*nd-stage renal disease.
Data from Akcan-Arikan A et al: *Kidney Int* 71(10):1028-1035, 2007.

are to reduce the excretion of protein and to maintain protein-free urine. Prevention or treatment of infection, control of edema, establishment of a balanced nutritional state, and restoration of normal metabolic processes also are important in managing the disorder and avoiding adverse aspects of treatment. Basic management of nephrotic syndrome includes administering glucocorticosteroids (prednisone); adhering to a low-sodium, well-balanced diet; performing good skin care; and, if edema becomes problematic, administering diuretics (furosemide, metolazone).[61] ACE inhibitors inhibit formation of angiotensin II and aldosterone, resulting in decreased blood pressure and decreased renal sodium reabsorption. Nephrotic syndrome is often described by the response to steroid therapy (Table 40.2). **Steroid-sensitive nephrotic syndrome** results in remission with steroid therapy alone. **Steroid-resistant nephrotic syndrome** is the term for children who fail to respond to prednisone within 8 weeks. They may be treated with noncorticosteroid immunosuppressive agents (i.e., cyclophosphamide) or a combination of corticosteroids and noncorticosteroid immunosuppressives to prolong remission.[62] Intravenous rituximab, a monoclonal antibody, has been shown to induce and prolong remissions in some children with steroid-dependent or -resistant nephrotic syndrome.[63] Children with minimal change disease tend to have a very favorable prognosis, whereas those steroid-resistant nephrotic syndrome may develop end-stage kidney disease.[64]

Kidney Injury

Kidney injury is rare in children. The pathophysiology (see Fig. 39.12) and management are similar to those for kidney injury in adults. A modification of the RIFLE criteria (*R*, risk; *I*, injury; *F*, failure; *L*, loss; and *E*, end-stage kidney disease [ESKD]) that was proposed to standardize the definition of acute kidney injury in adults has been used in critically ill children (pRIFLE criteria)[65] (Table 40.3).

The most common causes of *prerenal acute kidney injury* are dehydration, hemorrhage, and sepsis. Glomerulonephritis, hemolytic uremic syndrome, and hypersensitivity reactions to drugs or infectious agents are the most common causes of *intrinsic acute kidney injury*. Obstructive uropathies, such as posterior urethral valves and obstruction of the ureteropelvic junction, are associated with *postrenal acute kidney injury*.

End-stage renal disease in children is commonly associated with congenital renal structural abnormalities. In older children the most common cause is a glomerulonephropathy.[66,67] Renal replacement modalities available for children with end-stage renal disease include peritoneal and hemodialysis and kidney transplant. The use of growth

hormone before and after transplant has contributed to normal growth and development.[68]

Nephroblastoma (Wilms tumor) is an embryonal tumor of the kidney arising from epigenetic and genetic changes that lead to abnormal proliferation of renal stem cells (metanephric blastema). The incidence of Wilms tumor remains constant in the United States, with approximately 500 children diagnosed each year. Most children are between 1 and 5 years of age when they are diagnosed. The peak incidence occurs between 2 and 3 years of age. Wilms tumor is slightly more common in females and in black than in white children and is less common in Asian children.[69]

Microscopically, Wilms tumor is composed of three cellular components: stromal, epithelial, and blastemic. This occurs because blastemic cells, which are primitive and undifferentiated, may have partially developed into epithelial or stromal tissue. With each of these three cellular components, varying stages of differentiation may be evident within the tumor.

◆PATHOGENESIS. Wilms tumor has sporadic and inherited origins. The sporadic form occurs in children with no known genetic predisposition. Inherited cases, which are relatively rare (1% to 2% of cases), are transmitted in an autosomal dominant fashion. A "two-hit" hypothesis for the development of Wilms tumor has been proposed wherein children who inherit a mutation in one allele of a tumor-suppression gene require just one more somatic mutation for a tumor to form[70] (see Fig. 20.16). This hypothesis may not apply to all Wilms tumors, however, because a number of genetic abnormalities have been identified in Wilms tumor. Wilms tumor–suppressor genes *WT1* and *WT2* are located on chromosome 11. Chromosomal abnormalities, including gains, losses, and rearrangements, are often present in Wilms tumors. Gains in chromosomes 1q, 2, 7q, 8, 12, and 13 and losses in chromosomes 1p, 7p, 16q, and 22q are among the most common findings, although multiple other chromosomal abnormalities also have been identified.[71] *WTX* is a tumor-suppressor gene located on the X chromosome. Approximately 10% of children who have Wilms tumor also have deletions or mutations of other genes and, therefore, have a number of congenital anomalies. These anomalies include aniridia (lack of an iris in the eye), hemihypertrophy (an asymmetry of the body), and genitourinary malformations (i.e., horseshoe kidneys, hypospadias, ureteral duplication, polycystic kidneys, or uterine abnormalities).[69] Children with congenital anomalies as well as Wilms tumor are more likely to have the inherited bilateral form of the disease.

◆CLINICAL MANIFESTATIONS. Most Wilms tumors (90%) present as an enlarging asymptomatic upper abdominal mass in a healthy,

TABLE 40.4	STAGING OF WILMS TUMOR (NEPHROBLASTOMA)
STAGE* (% OF TUMORS)	**TUMOR CHARACTERISTICS**
Stage I (40% to 45%)	Tumor limited to the kidney, completely resected
Stage II (20%)	Tumor ascending beyond the kidney or into vessels of renal sinus, but appearing to be totally resected
Stage III (20% to 25%)	Residual nonhematogenous tumor confined to the abdomen, positive lymph nodes in renal hila
Stage IV (10%)	Hematogenous metastases (e.g., lung, liver, bone, brain)
Stage V (5%)	Bilateral disease either at diagnosis or later, but need to stage each kidney

*NOTE: Staging system of the Third National Wilms Tumor Study Group (NWTS-3).
Data from American Cancer Society: *Wilms tumor.* Available at https://www.cancer.org/cancer/wilms-tumor/detection-diagnosis-staging/staging.html.

TABLE 40.5	NATIONAL WILMS TUMOR STUDY 4-YEAR SURVIVAL RATES	
TUMOR STAGE	**FAVORABLE HISTOLOGY**	**UNFAVORABLE HISTOLOGY (ANAPLASTIC WILMS TUMOR)**
I	99%	83%
II	98%	81%
III	94%	72%
IV	86%	38%
V	87%	55%

Last medical review: March 6, 2015; Last revised: February 16, 2016. From American Cancer Society: *Wilms tumor*, 2015. Available at https://www.cancer.org/cancer/wilms-tumor/detection-diagnosis-staging/survival-rates.html.

thriving child. Many tumors are discovered by the child's parent, who feels or notices an abdominal swelling, usually while dressing or bathing the child. Other presenting complaints include vague abdominal pain, hematuria, and fever. Hypertension may be present, likely because of excessive renin secretion by the tumor.[72]

◆ **EVALUATION AND TREATMENT.** On physical examination, the tumor feels firm, nontender, and smooth, and generally is a solitary mass of varying size confined to one side of the abdomen. Diagnostic imaging demonstrates a solid intrarenal mass.

Diagnosis is based on surgical biopsy. Additional laboratory and radiologic studies are used to evaluate the presence or absence of metastasis. The most common sites of metastasis are regional lymph nodes and the lungs and less commonly liver, brain, and bone.

Staging systems for Wilms tumor have been developed and serve as guides to treatment. The most widely accepted system in the United States was developed by the National Wilms Tumor Study Group (Table 40.4). The system is based on surgical findings and the extent of disease at diagnosis.[73] Children are further classified as either high or low risk according to favorable or unfavorable histologic presentation (anaplasia).

Primary treatment is usually (1) surgical exploration and resection followed by treatment based on histology, or (2) chemotherapy followed by surgical resection, which limits tumor spillage during surgery.[74] In bilateral disease, surgical intervention may include heminephrectomy of the less involved kidney and nephrectomy of the other. Radiation therapy may be used for children with higher stages of disease and metastases. Survival at 4 years is greater than 90% for localized disease and more than 85% for advanced disease with favorable histology (Table 40.5).[75] Congestive heart failure, renal failure, hypertension, and secondary malignancies occur more frequently in long-term survivors than in the general population.[76]

Bladder Disorders
Urinary Tract Infections

Urinary tract infection (UTI) is the colonization of a pathogen anywhere along the urinary tract (urethra, bladder, ureter, kidney) and occurs commonly in children. During the neonatal period, uncircumcised males and infants with congenital renal abnormalities are at increased risk.[77]

WHAT'S NEW?
Kidney Stones in Children

Nephrolithiasis in children is rare, although the incidence of calcium stones among children is increasing, particularly in adolescents. There are limited data available regarding the pathogenesis of kidney stones in children, but the mechanisms appear different compared to those in adults. Epidemiologic data indicate that nephrolithiasis is more common in boys during preadolescence and in girls during pubertal years. Proposed risk factors include diets high in salt, protein, or fructose, or low in water or calcium; and use of certain anti-seizure, diuretic, vitamin, or antibiotic medications. Kidney stones also can be associated with urinary tract malformations (reflux disease and megaureter). Calcium stones are the most common stone type (72% to 88%). Children who form stones often have supersaturation of urinary calcium, oxalate, or phosphate. The most common symptom presentations are pain and gross hematuria. Prevention and treatment are individualized, and any metabolic cause needs to be evaluated. Adequate fluid intake is the mainstay of treatment. Medications such as stone inhibitors (e.g., potassium citrate) or thiazide diuretics may be helpful for some children. Surgical methods include extracorporeal shock wave lithotripsy, ureteroscopy, and percutaneous nephrolithotomy.

Data from Hernandez JD, Ellison JS, Lendvay TS: *JAMA Pediatr* 169(10):964-970, 2015; Penido MG, Tavares Mde S: *World J Nephrol* 4(4):444-454, 2015; Sas DJ, et al: *Urolithiasis* 44(3):241-246, 2016.

Girls have a greater incidence after 1 year of age with an increasing incidence at adolescence. Sexually active female adolescents are at increased risk to have a UTI. Similar to adult women, susceptibility is increased when genetically controlled blood group antigens (P1 and Lewis blood group nonsecretor) are present on surface uroepithelial cells and act as receptors for bacterial attachment.[78] UTIs in females occur as a result of perineal bacteria, especially *E. coli*, ascending the urethra, which lies close to the anus.

The pathophysiology of UTIs in children is similar to that of adults (see Chapter 39). Although nephrolithiasis can be associated with UTI in adults, nephrolithiasis in children is rare, but is increasing in incidence (see *What's New?* Kidney Stones in Children). UTIs in children are often clinically categorized as first or recurrent infection. Individual susceptibility, bacterial virulence, anatomy (presence of reflux, obstruction, stasis, stones, or structural anomalies of the urinary tract), and genetics[79] affect the severity of the disease. The recurrence rate is approximately 20% to 30%.[80]

Cystitis, or infection of the bladder, results in mucosal inflammation and congestion. This causes detrusor muscle hyperactivity and a resulting decrease in the bladder capacity. It also can lead to transient reflux of urine up the ureters, sending bacteria all the way to the kidney, causing acute or chronic pyelonephritis and renal abscesses or scarring.

Symptoms of UTI in children are nonspecific, and differentiating whether an infection is in the bladder or kidneys is difficult based on symptoms alone. Infants usually develop fever, vomiting, diarrhea, or jaundice. Some children may present only with fever of undetermined origin, and others may present with urinary tract symptoms of frequency; urgency; enuresis or incontinence in a previously dry child; abdominal, flank, or back pain; foul-smelling urine; and sometimes hematuria. Acute pyelonephritis usually causes chills, fever, and flank or abdominal pain along with enlarged kidney(s) caused by edema. Chronic pyelonephritis may be asymptomatic.

Diagnosis of UTIs is by urine culture of a pathogen before antimicrobial treatment. An accompanying urinalysis can show pyuria, nitrites, and hematuria. The presence of casts in the urine can indicate pyelonephritis. Ultrasound, voiding cystourethrography (VCUG) or radionuclide cystography, or computed tomography (CT) scan may be necessary to rule out obstructions, abscesses, or reflux, particularly in young children who do not respond to antimicrobial therapy.

With treatment, UTI symptoms are usually relieved in 1 to 2 days, and the urine becomes sterile. A 2- to 4-day course of oral antibiotics is effective for an uncomplicated UTI.[81] Longer treatment may be required if the child has recurrent UTIs, has a complicated UTI including congenital abnormalities of the urinary tract, or is immunosuppressed. Imaging of children after a first UTI is controversial.[82] The age of the child and seriousness of the infection should be considered when making imaging decisions. Repeat urine cultures are not needed if a child has responded to treatment.[83] Management of constipation, promotion of adequate fluid intake, and elimination of dysfunctional voiding patterns are the cornerstones of minimizing the risk of recurrence.[84] Prophylactic antibiotics may be helpful for some children. Educating families about signs and symptoms of UTI allows for early identification and treatment. Surgical correction of vesicoureteral reflux or obstruction may be necessary.

Vesicoureteral Reflux

Vesicoureteral reflux (VUR) is the retrograde flow of bladder urine into the kidney and/or ureters. Reflux allows infected urine from the bladder to reach the kidneys. Reflux perpetuates infection by preventing complete emptying of the bladder as refluxed urine drains back into the bladder at the end of each void. In addition, reflux allows the maximal intravesical pressure to be transmitted to the renal calyces and pyramids. The combination of reflux and infection is an important cause of pyelonephritis, especially in children younger than 5 years.

Vesicoureteral reflux occurs more often in girls by a ratio of 10:1 and is less common in blacks. Its incidence is unknown because in the absence of urinary tract infections, VUR is often undiagnosed. Siblings of those affected have about a 27% to 51% chance of having reflux, and children with parents who had reflux have an almost 70% chance of reflux.[85] The shortness of the submucosal segment of the ureter during infancy and childhood renders the antireflux mechanism relatively inefficient and delicate. Thus reflux is seen commonly in association with infections during early childhood but rarely in older children and adults. (Among adults with UTIs, the incidence of reflux is approximately 5%.) Reflux may be unilateral or bilateral, and it can be classified or graded (Fig. 40.7) for comparative purposes:

Grade I—Reflux into a nondilated distal ureter
Grade II—Reflux into the upper collecting system without dilation
Grade III—Reflux into dilated ureter or blunting of calyceal fornices
Grade IV—Reflux into a grossly dilated ureter

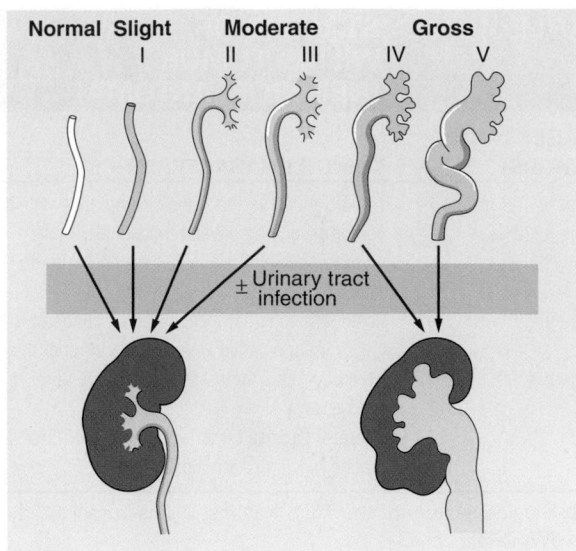

FIGURE 40.7 Grades of Reflux. (From Feehally J, Floege J, Johnson RJ: *Comprehensive clinical nephrology*, ed 3, Philadelphia, 2008, Mosby.)

Grade V—Massive reflux with ureteral dilation and tortuosity and effacement of the calyceal details; occurs almost exclusively in male infants[86]

◆**PATHOPHYSIOLOGY.** Primary reflux results from a congenitally abnormal or ectopic insertion of the ureter into the bladder (Fig. 40.8). Occasionally the condition is hereditary. Secondary reflux may be transient or persistent. It develops in association with infection, malformations of the ureterovesical (UV) junction, increased intravesical pressures, voiding disorders, or surgery on the UV junction. Urinary tract infection associated with VUR may lead to permanent renal scarring, particularly when there is pyelonephritis. The actual cause of renal cell damage and scarring is unknown, but contributing factors include inflammatory cytokines activated by bacterial virulence factors.[87]

◆**CLINICAL MANIFESTATIONS.** Children with reflux may be asymptomatic or may experience recurrent UTIs or unexplained fever, poor growth and development, irritability, and feeding problems. The family history may reveal VUR or urinary tract infections.

◆**EVALUATION AND TREATMENT.** Prompt treatment of UTIs in children with reflux is important to minimize the risk of renal scar development. Some infants with reflux already have renal scarring at birth.[88] In addition to the history of recurrent UTIs and other symptoms, imaging may be required for diagnosis and assessment of structural change, scarring, urinary tract function, and risk for future infection and renal damage. Identification and resolution of bowel and/or bladder dysfunction is imperative to decrease the risk of urinary tract infections and improve the rate of VUR resolution.[89] Spontaneous remission of grades I, II, and III reflux occurs in 50% to 80% of children. Approximately 20% of grades IV and V will resolve.[90] The use of prophylactic antibiotics for these children is controversial, with concerns regarding efficacy and the development of antibiotic resistance.[91] Recurrent infection or high-grade reflux are possible indications for surgical intervention or endoscopic injection of biomaterials into the bladder wall below the ureteral orifice. Surgical repair of reflux has been shown to decrease the incidence of pyelonephritis but does not decrease the risk of the development or progression of renal damage.[92] The value of screening asymptomatic siblings of children with vesicoureteral reflux is debatable. One current recommendation is to perform a renal ultrasound and consider a VCUG only in children with scarring or otherwise abnormal-appearing kidneys.[93]

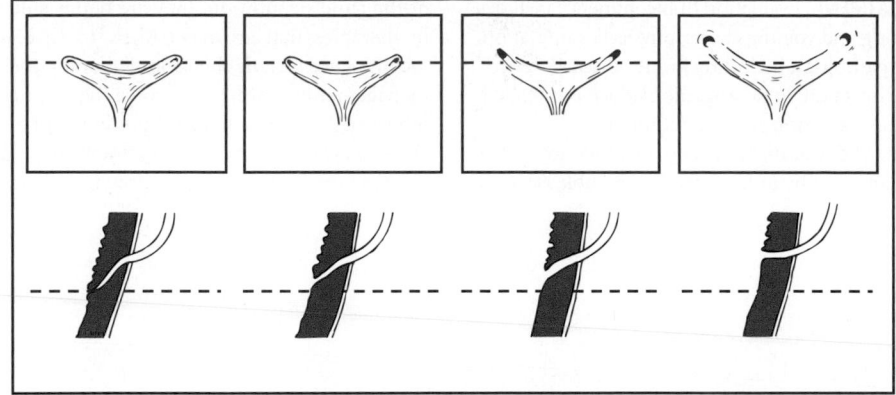

FIGURE 40.8 Normal and Abnormal Configuration of the Ureteral Orifices. *Left to right:* Progressive lateral displacement of the ureteral orifices and shortening of the intramural tunnels in the bladder. *Top row:* Endoscopic appearance. *Bottom row:* Sagittal view through the intramural ureter. (From Kliegman RM et al, editors: *Nelson textbook of pediatrics,* ed 19, Philadelphia, 2011, Saunders.)

Urinary Incontinence

Urinary incontinence refers to the involuntary passage of urine by a child who is beyond the age when voluntary bladder control should have been acquired. Bladder control is accomplished by most children before the age of 5 years, although this is largely influenced by cultural beliefs and parental toilet training practices. Nighttime wetting is called enuresis. Functional incontinence is urinary incontinence in which no structural or neurologic abnormality can be identified. The underlying mechanism may include disorders of both the storage and voiding phases of the bladder cycle. A child may have daytime incontinence or enuresis, or both.

The incidence of incontinence is difficult to determine because it is not a problem that parents readily share with others and because definitions vary according to cultural norms and family practices. The incidence of enuresis in children older than 5 years ranges from 15% to 20%. Boys are more enuretic than girls by a ratio of 2:1. Fewer than 2% of adults experience enuresis. Daytime incontinence occurs in up to 9% of early school-age children.[94]

◆**PATHOPHYSIOLOGY.** Multiple factors are likely responsible for incontinence. All or part of each one might be operating in a given child. A reasonable approach is to eliminate organic, behavioral, or physiologic causes before exploring the psychologic ones. Organic causes of incontinence account for 2% to 10% of cases. The causes include urinary tract infections; neurologic disturbances; congenital defects of the meatus, urethra, or bladder neck; allergies; constipation;[95] obesity;[96] or alteration in renal tubular ion and water transport related to prostaglandin secretion. Disorders that increase the normal output of urine, such as diabetes mellitus and diabetes insipidus, or disorders that impair the concentrating ability of the kidney must be considered in the evaluation of enuresis. Enuresis in children may be associated with a maturational lag. Studies have demonstrated that some children with enuresis have smaller functional bladder capacities than nonenuretic children.[97] Children who do not have the normal nocturnal elevation of vasopressin produce a higher volume of urine with a lower osmolality than controls.[98] A number of children experience bladder overactivity with elevated intravesical pressure and spikelike detrusor contractions during bladder filling. Incontinence often spontaneously disappears in children as they get older.

Genetic factors contribute to some types of incontinence. Multiple gene loci associated with enuresis have been identified. Bed-wetting occurs with high frequency among parents, siblings, and other near relatives of symptomatic children. These observations are further supported by a high concordance rate in enuretic monozygotic twins.[99]

Multiple studies have examined the role of sleep architecture in enuresis. Findings have ranged from elevated arousal thresholds[100] to increased light sleep with frequent cortical arousal without complete awakening.[101] Enuresis may be associated with obstructive sleep apnea. Inspiratory effort against a closed airway increases intrathoracic negative pressure, causing cardiac distention and release of atrial natriuretic hormone and decreased levels of vasopressin and renin-angiotensin-aldosterone complex.[102] A variety of psychosocial factors also have been postulated as explanations of enuresis. Enuresis has been associated with attention-deficit/hyperactivity disorders, anxiety disorders, depression, and oppositional defiant disorders.[103,104]

◆**CLINICAL MANIFESTATIONS.** Primary incontinence refers to a condition in which the child has never been continent. Secondary incontinence occurs when a child who has experienced a period of dryness of at least 6 months after toilet training becomes incontinent again. Secondary enuresis may be diurnal, nocturnal, or a combination of both. Types of incontinence are defined in Table 40.6.

TABLE 40.6 TYPES OF PEDIATRIC INCONTINENCE

TYPES OF INCONTINENCE	DEFINITION
Daytime voiding frequency	Decreased: three or fewer voids/day
	Increased: eight or more voids/day
Dysfunctional voiding	Habitual contraction of the urethral sphincter during voiding; intermittent urine flow, dribbling, hesitancy
Enuresis	Intermittent incontinence of urine while sleeping
Incontinence, intermittent	Leakage of urine in discrete episodes during the day and/or night
Incontinence, stress	Leakage of small amounts of urine with exertion or raised intraabdominal pressure
Urgency	Sudden, unexpected, immediate need to void
Overactive bladder	Child has urgency with or without frequency or incontinence
Underactive bladder	Decreased voiding frequency with use of raised intraabdominal pressure to void

Data from Nevéus T et al: *J Urol* 176(1):312-324, 2006.

◆**EVALUATION AND TREATMENT.** Evaluation of incontinence includes use of questionnaires, drinking and voiding charts, physical examination, and urinalysis. Underlying pathology, including kidney disease, vesicoureteral reflux, urinary tract infection, or neurogenic bladder, is excluded. Radiologic and urodynamic evaluation may be required.

Therapeutic management of day or night urinary incontinence begins with education. If the child and family understand the probable etiology of the child's condition, they are better able to choose and participate in therapies that are most likely to succeed. Treatment of daytime incontinence includes behavioral therapy, including timed voiding; fluid management; treatment of constipation, urinary tract infections, and other coexisting conditions if present; and medication (anticholinergic, alpha-blocker).[105] Enuresis treatment may also include enuresis alarms or other medications (desmopressin acetate tablets).[106]

▌ S U M M A R Y   R E V I E W

Structure and Function of the Urinary System in Children

1. The Wilms tumor 1 gene and *WNT* signaling are important for kidney development, growth, and differentiation.
2. The kidney develops from three sets of structures: the pronephros (nonfunctional by the end of the embryonic period), mesonephros (nonfunctional), and metanephros (the functional kidney).
3. All nephrons are present at full-term birth. The number does not increase with maturation, but they do increase in weight and function.
4. Urine formation begins by the third gestational month and contributes to the amniotic fluid.
5. Infants have a narrow chemical safety margin because of high hydrogen ion concentration, limited ability to regulate the internal environment, and lowered osmotic pressure.
6. Any disturbance, such as diarrhea, infection, fasting, or feeding alterations, can lead rapidly to severe acidosis and fluid imbalance in infants.
7. The composition of body fluids differs with age, thus making children more vulnerable to pathophysiologic changes.
8. Because the kidney develops from the medulla to the cortex, blood flow to the medullary nephrons is limited in infancy, and infants thus have limited urine-concentrating capacity.

Alterations in Renal and Bladder Function in Children

1. Congenital renal disorders affect about 1% of newborns. These disorders range in severity from minor, easily correctable anomalies to those incompatible with life.
2. Horseshoe kidney is a single U-shaped kidney that develops from fusion of the kidneys as they descend from the midline. The kidney may be asymptomatic or associated with hydronephrosis, stone formation, or infection.
3. Hypospadias is a congenital condition in which the urethral meatus is located on the undersurface of the penis; epispadias is a congenital condition in which the urethral opening is located on the dorsal surface of the penis.
4. Exstrophy of the bladder is a congenital malformation in which the pubic bones are separated, the lower portion of the abdominal wall and anterior wall of the bladder are missing, and the back wall of the bladder is everted through the opening.
5. Ureteropelvic junction obstruction is blockage where the renal pelvis joins the ureter and is often caused by smooth muscle or urothelial malformation or scarring that leads to hydronephrosis.
6. Bladder outlet obstruction is usually caused by urethral valves or polyps.
7. A dysplastic kidney is the result of abnormal differentiation of renal tissues. The hypoplastic kidney is a very small but otherwise normal kidney.

8. Renal agenesis is the failure of a kidney to grow or develop. The condition may be unilateral or bilateral and may occur as an isolated entity or in association with other disorders.
9. Polycystic kidney disease is an autosomal dominant or recessive disorder in which the renal tubule or epithelium proliferates; excessive fluid transport causes cyst formation and obstruction.
10. Glomerulonephritis is an inflammation of the glomeruli secondary to immune mechanisms characterized by hematuria, edema, and hypertension. Poststreptococcal glomerulonephritis may occur after infection, especially of the upper respiratory tract.
11. IgA nephropathy results from deposition of IgA immunoglobulins and other immune products in the mesangium of the glomerular capillaries. It is the most common type of childhood glomerulonephritis.
12. Henoch-Schönlein nephritis is an IgA nephropathy that affects glomerular blood vessels.
13. Hemolytic uremic syndrome is an acute disorder characterized by hemolytic anemia, acute renal failure, and thrombocytopenia and can be associated with *E. coli* verotoxin.
14. *Nephrotic syndrome* is a term used to describe a symptom complex characterized by proteinuria, hypoalbuminemia, hyperlipidemia, and edema. Metabolic, biochemical, or physiochemical disturbance in the glomerular basement membrane leads to increased permeability to protein. The most common form is minimal change nephropathy.
15. Acute or chronic renal injury is rare in children, and the most common cause is prerenal acute renal failure related to dehydration, sepsis, or hemorrhage.
16. Wilms tumor is an embryonal tumor of the kidney that usually presents between birth and 5 years of age as an inherited (1% to 2%) or sporadic form. The tumor can be successfully treated by surgery, with a combination of drugs, and sometimes with radiation therapy.
17. Urinary tract infections can result from general sepsis in the newborn but are usually caused by bacteria ascending the urethra in older children. The bladder alone is infected in cystitis. The infection ascends to the kidney or kidneys in pyelonephritis. Urinary tract anomalies may need surgical correction to prevent frequent recurrent infections.
18. Vesicoureteral reflux, which refers to the retrograde flow of bladder urine into the kidney and/or ureters, provides mechanisms for bladder and kidney infections in children. It can be unilateral or bilateral.
19. Urinary incontinence refers to the involuntary passage of urine beyond the age when normal continence should have occurred. This may occur during the day (incontinence) or night (enuresis). These disorders can have a variety of organic and psychologic causes.

KEY TERMS

REFERENCES

1. Wilm B, Muñoz-Chapuli R: The role of WT1 in embryonic development and normal organ homeostasis. *Methods Mol Biol* 1467:23–39, 2016.
2. Bonilla-Felix M: Development of water transport in the collecting duct. *Am J Physiol Renal Physiol* 287(6):F1093–F1101, 2004.
3. Quigley R: Developmental changes in renal function. *Curr Opin Pediatr* 24(12):184–190, 2012.
4. Caiulo VA, et al: Ultrasound mass screening for congenital anomalies of the kidney and urinary tract. *Pediatr Nephrol* 27(6):949–953, 2012.
5. Weizer AZ, et al: Determining the incidence of horseshoe kidney from radiographic data at a single institution. *J Urol* 170(5):1722–1726, 2003.
6. Je BK, Kim HK, Horn PS: Incidence and spectrum of renal complications and extrarenal diseases and syndromes in 380 children and young adults with horseshoe kidney. *AJR Am J Roentgenol* 205(6):1306–1314, 2015.
7. Vivante A, et al: Single-gene causes of congenital anomalies of the kidney and urinary tract (CAKUT) in humans. *Pediatr Nephrol* 29(4):695–704, 2014.
8. Akl K: The anomalies associated with congenital solitary functioning kidney in children. *Saudi J Kidney Dis Transpl* 22(1):67–71, 2011.
9. Springer A, van den Heijkant M, Baumann S: Worldwide prevalence of hypospadias. *J Pediatr Urol* 12(3):152, 2016.
10. Bouty A, et al: The genetic and environmental factors underlying hypospadias. *Sex Dev* 9(5):239–259, 2015.
11. Castagnetti M, et al: Benign penile skin anomalies in children: a primer for pediatricians. *World J Pediatr* 11(4):316–323, 2015.
12. No authors: Timing of elective surgery on the genitalia of male children with particular reference to the risks, benefits, and psychological effects of surgery and anesthesia. *Pediatrics* 97(4):590–594, 1996.
13. Lloyd JC, et al: Contemporary epidemiological trends in complex congenital genitourinary anomalies. *J Urol* 190(4 Suppl):1590–1595, 2013.
14. Frimberger D: Diagnosis and management of epispadias. *Semin Pediatr Surg* 20(2):85–90, 2011.
15. Inouye BM, et al: Modern management of the exstrophy-epispadias complex. *Surg Res Pract* 2014:587064, 2014.
16. Ellerkamp V, et al: Differences between intrinsic and extrinsic ureteropelvic junction obstruction related to crossing vessels: histology and functional analyses. *World J Urol* 34(4):577–583, 2016.
17. Sadeghi-Bojd S, et al: Postnatal evaluation and outcome of prenatal hydronephrosis. *Iran J Pediatr* 26(2):e3667, 2016.
18. Arora S, et al: Predictors for the need of surgery in antenatally detected hydronephrosis due to UPJ obstruction-a prospective multivariate analysis. *J Pediatr Urol* 11(5):248, 2015.
19. Delahunt B, Samarafunga H: Pathology of the renal pelvis and ureter. In Amin MB, et al, editors: *Urological pathology*, Philadelphia, 2014, Wolters Kluwer/Lippincott Williams & Wilkins, pp 261–294.
20. Hubertus J, et al: Children and adolescents with ureteropelvic junction obstruction: is an additional voiding cystourethrogram necessary? Results of a multicenter study. *World J Urol* 31(3):683–687, 2013.
21. Hodges SJ, et al: Megaureter. *ScientificWorldJournal* 10:603–612, 2012.
22. Farrugia MK: Fetal bladder outlet obstruction: embryopathology, in utero intervention and outcome. *J Pediatr Urol* 12(5):296–303, 2016.
23. Akbarzadeh A, Khorramirouz R, Kajbafzadeh AM: Congenital urethral polyps in children: report of 18 patients and review of literature. *J Pediatr Surg* 49(5):835–839, 2014.
24. Lopez Pereira P, et al: Long-term consequences of posterior urethral valves. *J Pediatr Urol* 9(5):590–596, 2013.
25. Calisti A, et al: The risk of associated urological abnormalities in children with pre- and postnatal occasional diagnosis of solitary, small or ectopic kidney: is a complete urological screening always necessary? *World J Urol* 26(3):281–284, 2008.
26. Westland R, et al: Clinical implications of the solitary functioning kidney. *Clin J Am Soc Nephrol* 9(5):978–986, 2014.
27. La Scola C, et al: Congenital solitary kidney in children: size matters. *J Urol* 196(4):1250–1256, 2016.
28. Stojanovic J, et al: Prevalence and 1 year outcome of severe congenital renal anomalies. *Arch Dis Child-Fetal* 96(Suppl 1):Fa18–Fa19, 2011.
29. Rangan GK, et al: Recent advances in autosomal-dominant polycystic kidney disease. *Intern Med J* 46(8):883–892, 2016.
30. Chapman AB, et al: Autosomal-dominant polycystic kidney disease (ADPKD): executive summary from a Kidney Disease: Improving Global Outcomes (KDIGO) Controversies Conference. *Kidney Int* 88(1):17–27, 2015.
31. Schrier RW, et al: Predictors of autosomal dominant polycystic kidney disease progression. *J Am Soc Nephrol* 25(11):2399–2418, 2014.
32. Mao Z, Chong J, Ong AC: Autosomal dominant polycystic kidney disease: recent advances in clinical management. *F1000Res* 5:2029, 2016.
33. Sweeney WE, Avner ED: Polycystic kidney disease, autosomal recessive, 2001 Jul 19 [updated 2016 Sep 15]. In Pagon RA, et al, editors: *GeneReviews*, Seattle, WA, 2016, University of Washington. Available at: http://www.ncbi.nlm.nih.gov/books/NBK1326/.
34. Patil A, et al: Chapter 2: childhood polycystic kidney disease. In Li X, editor: *Polycystic kidney disease [Internet]*, Brisbane AU, 2015, Codon Publications. Available at: http://www.ncbi.nlm.nih.gov/books/NBK373381/.
35. Ingelfinger JR, et al: World kidney day 2016 averting the legacy of kidney disease-focus on childhood. *Clin Nephrol* 85(2):63–69, 2016.
36. Couser WG: Pathogenesis and treatment of glomerulonephritis-an update. *J Bras Nefrol* 38(1):107–122, 2016.
37. VanDeVoorde RG, 3rd: Acute poststreptococcal glomerulonephritis: the most common acute glomerulonephritis. *Pediatr Rev* 36(1):2–12, 2015.
38. Fabiano RC, et al: Immunoglobulin A nephropathy: a pathophysiology view. *Inflamm Res* 65(10):757–770, 2016.
39. Lai KN, Leung JC, Tang SC: Recent advances in the understanding and management of IgA nephropathy. *F1000Res* 5:2016.
40. Chen JY, Mao JH: Henoch-Schönlein purpura nephritis in children: incidence, pathogenesis and management. *World J Pediatr* 11(1):29–34, 2015.
41. Kamath N, Rao S: Henoch-Schonlein purpura: an update. *Indian J Rheum* 7(Suppl 1):92–98, 2012.
42. Coppo R, Amore A: Henoch-Schoenlein purpura. In Avner E, et al, editors: *Pediatric nephrology*, ed 6, Berlin, 2009, Springer.
43. Davin JC, Coppo R: Henoch-Schönlein purpura nephritis in children. *Nat Rev Nephrol* 10(10):563–573, 2014.
44. Kemper MJ: Outbreak of hemolytic uremic syndrome caused by *E. coli* O104:H4 in Germany:

a pediatric perspective. *Pediatr Nephrol* 27(2): 161–164, 2012.

45. Scheiring J, Rosales A, Zimmerhackl LB: Today's understanding of the haemolytic uraemic syndrome. *Eur J Pediatr* 169(1):7–13, 2010.

46. Jenssen GR, et al: Clinical features, therapeutic interventions and long-term aspects of hemolytic-uremic syndrome in Norwegian children: a nationwide retrospective study from 1999-2008. *BMC Infect Dis* 16:285, 2016.

47. Durkan AM, et al: The long-term outcomes of atypical haemolytic uraemic syndrome: a national surveillance study. *Arch Dis Child* 101(4):387–391, 2016.

48. Bu F, et al: Familial atypical hemolytic uremic syndrome: a review of its genetic and clinical aspects. *Clin Dev Immunol* 2012:370426, 2012.

49. Karpman D, et al: Haemolytic uraemic syndrome. *J Intern Med* 281(2):123–148, 2017.

50. Mody RK, et al: Postdiarrheal hemolytic uremic syndrome in United States children: clinical spectrum and predictors of in-hospital death. *J Pediatr* 166(4):1022–1029, 2015.

51. Spencer JD, et al: Has the incidence of childhood steroid sensitive nephrotic syndrome changed? *Clin Nephrol* 78(2):112–115, 2012.

52. Gordillo R, Spitzer A: The nephrotic syndrome. *Pediatr Rev* 30(3):94–104, 2009.

53. Kim SH, et al: Pathogenesis of minimal change nephrotic syndrome: an immunological concept. *Korean J Pediatr* 59(5):205–211, 2016.

54. Ranganathan S: Pathology of podocytopathies causing nephrotic syndrome in children. *Front Pediatr* 4:32, 2016.

55. Woo K, et al: Global evolutionary trend of the prevalence of primary glomerulonephritis over the past three decades. *Nephron Clin Pract* 116(4): c337–c346, 2010.

56. Han KH, Kim SH: Recent advances in treatments of primary focal segmental glomerulosclerosis in children. *Biomed Res Int* 2016:3053706, 2016.

57. Teoh CW, Robinson LA, Noone D: Perspectives on edema in childhood nephrotic syndrome. *Am J Physiol Renal Physiol* 309(7):F575–F582, 2015.

58. Siddall EJ, Radhakrishnan J: The pathophysiology of edema formation in the nephrotic syndrome. *Kidney Int* 82(6):635–642, 2012.

59. Kerlin BA, Ayoob R, Smoyer WE: Epidemiology and pathophysiology of nephrotic syndrome-associated thromboembolic disease. *Clin J Am Soc Nephrol* 7(3):513–520, 2012.

60. Spahiu L, et al: Congenital nephrotic syndrome-Finish type. *Med Arch* 70(3):232–234, 2016.

61. Lombel RM, Gipson DS, Hodson EM: Kidney disease: improving global outcomes. Treatment of steroid-sensitive nephrotic syndrome: new guidelines from KDIGO. *Pediatr Nephrol* 28(3): 415–426, 2013.

62. Lombel RM, Hodson EM, Gipson DS: Kidney disease: improving global outcomes. Treatment of steroid-resistant nephrotic syndrome in children: new guidelines from KDIGO. *Pediatr Nephrol* 28(3):409–414, 2013.

63. Iijima K, Sako M, Nozu K: Rituximab for nephrotic syndrome in children. *Clin Exp Nephrol* 21(2):193–202, 2016.

64. Hjorten R, Anwar Z, Reidy KJ: Long-term outcomes of childhood onset nephrotic syndrome. *Front Pediatr* 4:53, 2016.

65. Akcan-Arikan A, et al: Modified RIFLE criteria in critically ill children with acute kidney injury. *Kidney Int* 71(10):1028–1035, 2007.

66. Harambat J, et al: Epidemiology of chronic kidney disease in children. *Pediatr Nephrol* 27(3):363–373, 2012.

67. Mong Hiep TT, et al: Clinical characteristics and outcomes of children with stage 3-5 chronic kidney disease. *Pediatr Nephrol* 25(5):935–940, 2010.

68. Rees L: Growth hormone therapy in children with CKD after more than two decades of practice. *Pediatr Nephrol* 31(9):1421–1435, 2016.

69. Ward E, et al: Childhood and adolescent cancer statistics, 2014. *CA Cancer J Clin* 64(2):83–103, 2014.

70. Knudson AG, Jr, Strong LC: Mutation and cancer: a model for Wilms' tumor of the kidney. *J Natl Cancer Inst* 48(2):313–324, 1972.

71. Szychot E, Apps J, Pritchard-Jones K: Wilms' tumor: biology, diagnosis and treatment. *Transl Pediatr* 3(1):12–24, 2014.

72. Davidoff AM: Wilms tumor. *Adv Pediatr* 59(1): 247–267, 2012.

73. Kieran K, Ehrlich PF: Current surgical standards of care in Wilms tumor. *Urol Oncol* 34(1):13–23, 2016.

74. Al-Hussain T, Ali A, Akhtar M: Wilms tumor: an update. *Adv Anat Pathol* 21(3):166–173, 2014.

75. Ali AN, et al: A Surveillance, Epidemiology and End Results (SEER) program comparison of adult and pediatric Wilms' tumor. *Cancer* 118(9): 2541–2551, 2012.

76. Lee JS, et al: Second malignant neoplasms among children, adolescents and young adults with Wilms tumor. *Pediatr Blood Cancer* 62(7): 1259–1264, 2015.

77. Beetz R: Evaluation and management of urinary tract infections in the neonate. *Curr Opin Pediatr* 24(2):205–211, 2012.

78. Khunda A, Elneil S: Recurrent urinary tract infections associated with gynecological disorders. *Curr Bladder Dysfunct Rep* 7(2):131–140, 2012.

79. Ambite I, et al: The genetics of urinary tract infections and the innate defense of the kidney and urinary tract. *J Pediatr Genet* 5(1):25–32, 2016.

80. Simões e Silva AC, Oliveira EA: Update on the approach of urinary tract infection in childhood. *J Pediatr (Rio J)* 91(6 Suppl 1):S2–S10, 2015.

81. Fitzgerald A, et al: Antibiotics for treating lower urinary tract infection in children. *Cochrane Database Syst Rev* (8):CD006857, 2012.

82. Riccabona M: Imaging in childhood urinary tract infection. *Radiol Med* 121(5):391–401, 2016.

83. Park KH, et al: The clinical usefulness of a repeat urine culture 48 hours after microbial treatment in anatomically normal and abnormal urinary tract infection. *J Korean Soc Pediatr Nephrol* 13(1): 49–55, 2009.

84. Shaikh N, et al: Recurrent urinary tract infections in children with bladder and bowel dysfunction. *Pediatrics* 137(1):1–7, 2016.

85. Hunziker M, Puri P: Familial vesicoureteral reflux and reflux related morbidity in relatives of index patients with high grade vesicoureteral reflux. *J Urol* 188(4 Suppl):1463–1466, 2012.

86. Lebowitz RL, et al: International system of radiographic grading of vesicoureteric reflux. International Reflux Study in Children. *Pediatr Radiol* 15(2):105–109, 1985.

87. Garcia-Roig ML, Kirsch AJ: Urinary tract infection in the setting of vesicoureteral reflux. *F1000Res* 5:2016.

88. Kangin M, et al: Significance of postnatal follow-up of infants with vesicoureteral reflux having antenatal hydronephrosis. *Iran J Pediatr* 20(4):427–434, 2010.

89. Johnston DL, et al: Contemporary management of vesicoureteral reflux. *Curr Treat Options Pediatr* 2(2):82–93, 2016.

90. Sung J, Skoog S: Surgical management of vesicoureteral reflux in children. *Pediatr Nephrol* 27(4):551–561, 2012.

91. Peters CA, et al: Summary of the AUA Guideline on Management of Primary Vesicoureteral Reflux in Children. *J Urol* 184(3):1134–1144, 2010.

92. Arslansoyu Çamlar S, et al: Antireflux surgery does not change ongoing renal functional deterioration. *Ren Fail* 38(3):348–351, 2016.

93. Skoog SJ, et al: Pediatric Vesicoureteral Reflux Guidelines Panel summary report: clinical practice guidelines for screening siblings of children with vesicoureteral reflux and neonates/infants with prenatal hydronephrosis. *J Urol* 184(3):1145–1151, 2010.

94. Buckley BS, Lapitan MC: Prevalence of urinary incontinence in men, women, and children-current evidence: findings of the Fourth International Consultation on Incontinence. *Urology* 76(2):265–271, 2010.

95. Veiga ML, et al: Constipation in children with isolated overactive bladders. *J Pediatr Urol* 9(6 Pt A):945–949, 2013.

96. Chang SJ, et al: Obese children at higher risk for having overactive bladder symptoms: a community-based study. *Neurourol Urodyn* 34(2):123–127, 2015.

97. Kim J: Diagnostic value of functional bladder capacity, urine osmolality, and daytime storage symptoms for severity of nocturnal enuresis. *Korean J Urol* 53(2):114–119, 2012.

98. Dossche L, et al: Circadian rhythm of glomerular filtration and solute handling related to nocturnal enuresis. *J Urol* 195(1):162–167, 2016.

99. von Gontard A, Heron J, Joinson C: Family history of nocturnal enuresis and urinary incontinence: results from a large epidemiological study. *J Urol* 185(6):2303–2306, 2011.

100. Gozmen S, Keskin S, Akil I: Enuresis nocturna and sleep quality. *Pediatr Nephrol* 23(2): 1293–1296, 2008.

101. Yeung CD, Diao M, Sreedhar B: Cortical arousal in children with severe enuresis. *N Engl J Med* 358(22):2414–2515, 2008.

102. Jeyakumar A, et al: The association between sleep-disordered breathing and enuresis in children. *Laryngoscope* 122(8):1873–1877, 2012.

103. von Gontard A: Equit M: Comorbidity of ADHD and incontinence in children. *Eur Child Adolesc Psychiatry* 24(2):127–140, 2015.

104. Yang T, et al: Correlation between symptoms of voiding dysfunction and attention deficit disorder with hyperactivity in children with lower urinary tract symptoms. *J Urol* 187(2):656–663, 2012.

105. Chang SJ, et al: Treatment of daytime urinary incontinence: a standardization document from the International Children's Continence Society. *Neurourol Urodyn* 36(1):43–50, 2017.

106. Bayne AP, Skoog SJ: Nocturnal enuresis: an approach to assessment and treatment. *Pediatr Rev* 35(8):327–334, quiz 335, 2014.

CHAPTER

41

Structure and Function of the Digestive System

Sue E. Huether

evolve WEBSITE

http://evolve.elsevier.com/McCance/
- Content Updates
- Chapter Summary Review
- Review Questions
- Case Studies
- Animations

CHAPTER OUTLINE

The digestive system consists of the gastrointestinal tract and accessory organs of digestion: the liver, gallbladder, and exocrine pancreas. The digestive system breaks down ingested food, prepares it for uptake by the body's cells, provides body water, and eliminates wastes. Food breakdown begins in the mouth with chewing and continues in the stomach, where food is churned and mixed with acid, mucus, and enzymes. From the stomach, the fluid and partially digested food pass into the small intestine, where bile and enzymes secreted by the liver, enzymes from the exocrine pancreas, and small intestinal epithelium break it down into absorbable components of proteins, carbohydrates, and fats. These nutrients pass through the small intestinal epithelium into underlying blood vessels and lymphatics that carry them to

the liver via the hepatic portal circulation for further processing and storage.

Ingested substances and secretions that are not absorbed in the small intestine pass into the large intestine, where fluid continues to be absorbed. Solid wastes pass into the rectum and are eliminated from the body through the anus.

Except for chewing, swallowing, and defecation of solid wastes, the activities of the digestive system are controlled by hormones and the autonomic nervous system. As ingested substances move through the gastrointestinal tract, they trigger the release of hormones that stimulate or inhibit (1) the muscular contractions (gastrointestinal motility) that mix and propel food from the esophagus to the anus, and (2) the timely secretion of substances that aid in digestion. The autonomic innervation, sympathetic and parasympathetic, is controlled by centers in the brain and by local stimuli that are mediated by neural plexuses of the enteric nervous system within the gastrointestinal walls.

THE GASTROINTESTINAL TRACT

The **gastrointestinal tract (alimentary canal)** consists of the mouth, esophagus, stomach, small intestine, large intestine, rectum, and anus (Fig. 41.1). It carries out the following digestive processes:

1. Ingestion of food
2. Propulsion of food and wastes from the mouth to the anus
3. Secretion of mucus, water, and enzymes
4. Mechanical digestion of food particles
5. Chemical digestion of food particles
6. Absorption of digested food
7. Elimination of waste products by defecation
8. Immune and microbial protection against infection

Histologically, the gastrointestinal tract consists of four layers. From the inside out, they are the mucosa, submucosa, muscularis, and serosa or adventitia (esophagus only). These concentric layers vary in thickness, and each layer has sublayers (Fig. 41.2). Neurons forming the **enteric nervous system** are located solely within the gastrointestinal tract and are controlled by local and autonomic nervous system stimuli. The enteric nervous system comprises three nerve plexuses located in different

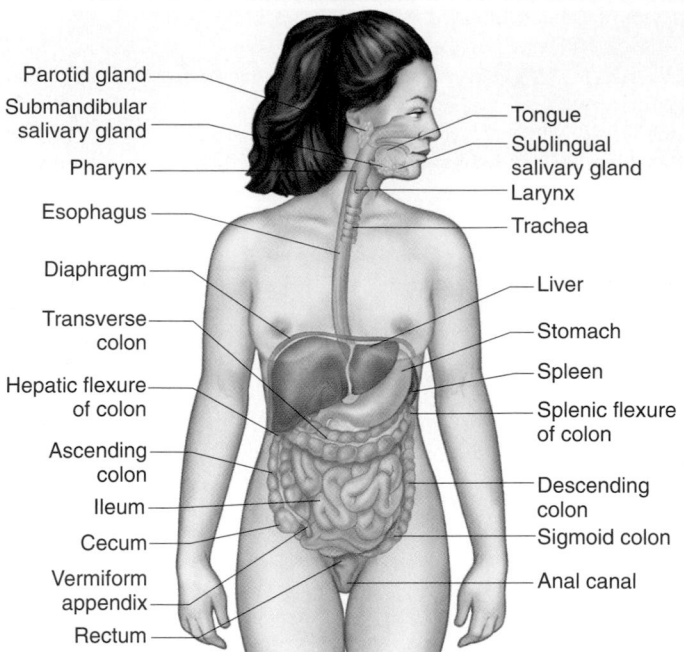

FIGURE 41.1 Structures of the Digestive System. (From Patton KT, Thibodeau GA: *The human body in health & disease*, ed 7, St Louis, 2018, Elsevier.)

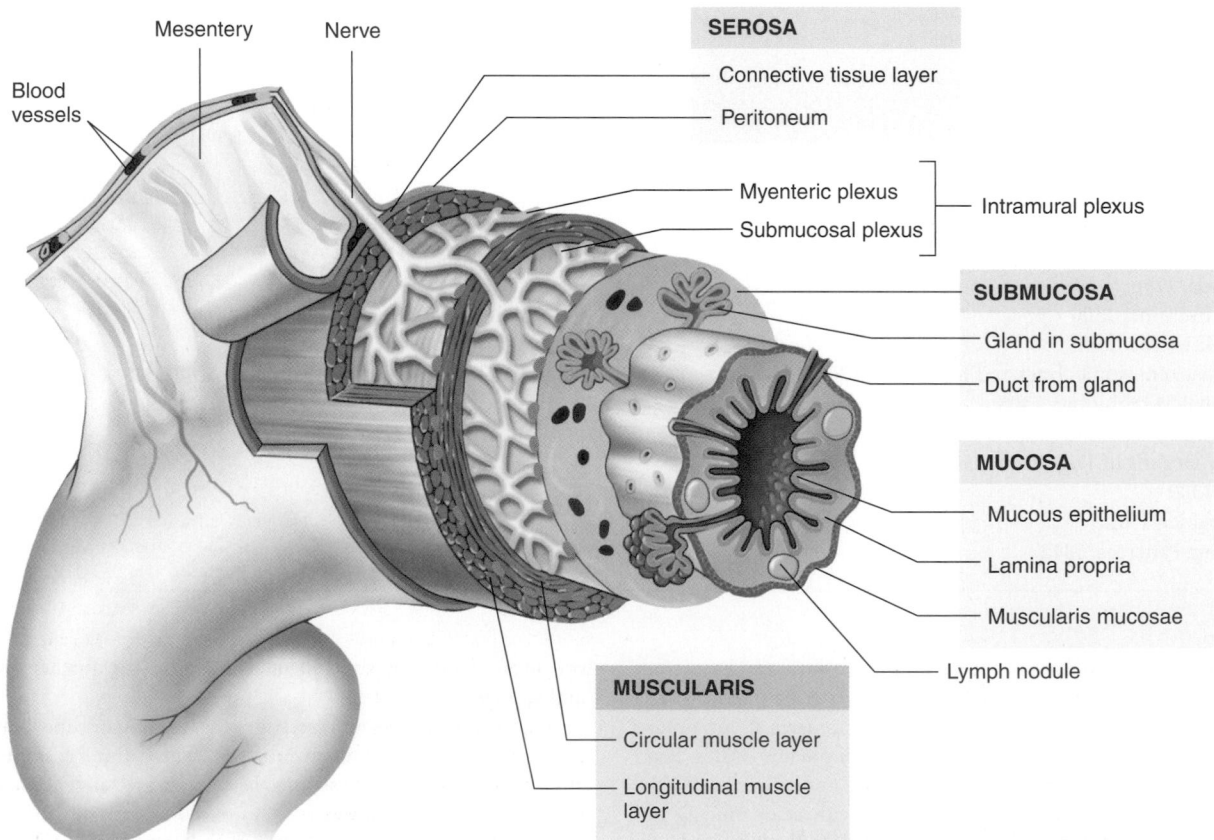

FIGURE 41.2 Wall of the Gastrointestinal (GI) Tract. The wall of the GI tract is made up of four layers with a network of nerves between the layers. Shown here is a generalized diagram of a segment of the GI tract. Note that the serosa is continuous with a fold of serous membrane called a *mesentery*. Note also that digestive glands may empty their products into the lumen of the GI tract by way of ducts. (From Patton KT, Thibodeau GA: *The human body in health & disease*, ed 7, St Louis, 2018, Elsevier.)

layers of the gastrointestinal walls. The submucosal plexus (Meissner plexus) is located in the muscularis mucosae, the myenteric plexus (Auerbach plexus) between the inner circular and outer longitudinal muscle layers in the muscularis, and the subserosal plexus just beneath the serosa. The enteric (intramural) plexus neurons regulate motility reflexes, blood flow, absorption, secretions, and immune response.

Mouth and Esophagus

The mouth is a site for the chewing and mixing of food with saliva. There are 32 permanent teeth in the adult mouth, and they are important for speech and mastication. As food particles become smaller and move around in the mouth, taste buds are continuously stimulated, adding to the satisfaction of eating. The tongue's surface and soft palate contains taste buds that contain taste receptors, that can distinguish salty, sour, bitter, savory (umami—taste of glutamate), and sweet tastes. Tastes and food odors, which stimulate the olfactory nerve, help initiate salivation and the secretion of gastric juice in the stomach. Efforts are in progress to identify the taste of fat and the relationship to food selection and diet.[1]

Salivation

The three pairs of salivary glands (the submandibular, sublingual, and parotid glands) (Fig. 41.3) secrete about 1 L of saliva per day. Saliva consists mostly of water that contains varying amounts of mucus, sodium, bicarbonate, chloride, potassium, and salivary α-amylase (ptyalin), an enzyme that initiates carbohydrate digestion in the mouth and stomach.

The sympathetic and parasympathetic divisions of the autonomic nervous system control salivation. Cholinergic parasympathetic fibers

stimulate the salivary glands, and atropine (an anticholinergic agent) inhibits salivation and makes the mouth dry. β-Adrenergic stimulation from sympathetic fibers also increases salivary secretion. The salivary glands are not regulated by hormones, although hormones are found in saliva (e.g., cortisol, testosterone, and estradiol).[2]

The composition of saliva depends on the rate of secretion. Aldosterone can decrease the rate of secretion by increasing an exchange of sodium for potassium. Sodium and water are conserved and potassium is excreted. The bicarbonate concentration of saliva sustains a pH of about 7.4, which neutralizes bacterial acids and prevents tooth decay. Saliva also contains mucin, immunoglobulin A (IgA), and other microbial substances that help prevent infection. Mucin provides lubrication. Exogenous fluoride (e.g., fluoride in drinking water) is absorbed and then secreted in the saliva, providing additional protection against tooth decay.

Swallowing

The esophagus is a hollow muscular tube approximately 25 cm long that conducts substances from the oropharynx to the stomach (see Fig. 41.1). Swallowed food is moved to the stomach by peristalsis, the coordinated sequential contraction and relaxation of outer longitudinal and inner circular layers of muscles. The pharynx and upper third of the esophagus contain striated muscle that is directly innervated by skeletal motor neurons that control swallowing. The middle third contains a mix of striated and smooth muscle, and the lower third is smooth muscle that is innervated by preganglionic cholinergic fibers from the vagus nerve. Peristalsis is stimulated when afferent fibers distributed along the length of the esophagus sense changes in wall tension caused by stretching as food passes. The greater the tension, the greater the intensity of esophageal contraction. Occasionally, intense contractions cause pain similar to "heartburn" or angina.

Each end of the esophagus is opened and closed by a sphincter. The upper esophageal sphincter (cricopharyngeal muscle) prevents entry of air into the esophagus during respiration. The lower esophageal sphincter (cardiac sphincter) prevents regurgitation from the stomach. The lower esophageal sphincter is located near the esophageal hiatus—the opening in the diaphragm where the esophagus ends at the stomach.

Swallowing is a complex event mediated by the trigeminal nucleus, nucleus tractus solitarius, and reticular formation of the brainstem and also involves other brain regions, including the insula/claustrum and cerebellum.

Swallowing occurs in two phases: the oropharyngeal (voluntary) phase and the esophageal (involuntary) phase. During the oral and pharyngeal phases of swallowing, food is segmented into a bolus by the tongue and forced posteriorly toward the pharynx as the tongue pushes upward against the hard palate. The superior constrictor muscle of the pharynx contracts, preventing movement of food into the nasopharynx. At the same time, respiration is inhibited and the epiglottis folds downward to prevent the bolus from entering the larynx and trachea. The movements of the tongue and pharyngeal constrictors propel the food into the esophagus in a series of coordinated events, taking less than 1 or 2 seconds.

During the esophageal phase of swallowing, the bolus is transported to the stomach by the coordinated sequential contraction and relaxation of outer longitudinal and inner circular layers of smooth muscle. The wave of relaxation reduces resistance and allows food to pass, after which the wave of contraction pushes food farther along. The terminal 1- to 2-cm portion of the musculature forms the lower esophageal sphincter, which relaxes just before the arrival of a peristaltic wave. The sphincter muscles return to their resting tone after the bolus of food passes into the stomach. The esophageal phase of swallowing takes 5 to 10 seconds, with the bolus moving 2 to 6 cm/second. Throughout

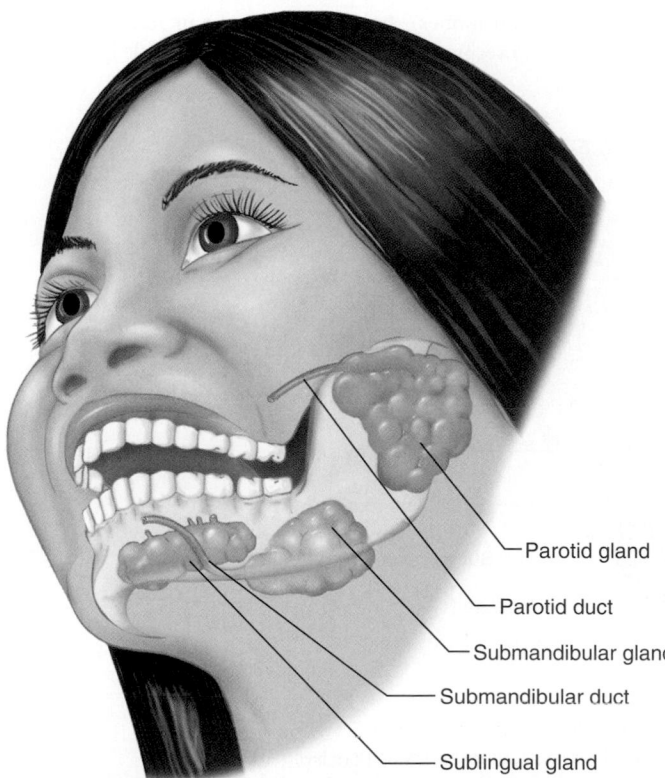

FIGURE 41.3 Salivary Glands. (From Patton KT, Thibodeau GA: *The human body in health & disease*, ed 7, St Louis, 2018, Elsevier.)

Parotid gland
Parotid duct
Submandibular gland
Submandibular duct
Sublingual gland

swallowing, the sphincters and esophagus work in concert with the peristaltic wave that moves food from the mouth to the stomach.

Peristalsis that immediately follows the oropharyngeal phase of swallowing is called primary peristalsis. If a bolus of food becomes stuck in the esophageal lumen, the distention of the esophageal wall stimulates secondary peristalsis, a wave of contraction and relaxation that is independent of voluntary swallowing. This is in response to stretch receptors that are stimulated by increased wall tension, causing an increase in impulses from the swallowing center of the brain.

The lower esophageal sphincter is normally constricted and serves as a barrier between the stomach and esophagus. The muscle tone of the lower sphincter changes with neural and hormonal stimulation and relaxes with swallowing. Cholinergic vagal stimulation and the digestive hormone gastrin increase sphincter tone. Nonadrenergic, noncholinergic vagal impulses relax the lower esophageal sphincter, as do the hormones progesterone, secretin, and glucagon.

Stomach

The stomach is a hollow muscular organ that stores food during eating, secretes digestive juices, mixes food with these juices, and propels partially digested food, called chyme, into the duodenum of the small intestine. The anatomy of the stomach is presented in Fig. 41.4. Its major anatomic boundaries are the lower esophageal sphincter, where food passes through the cardiac orifice at the gastroesophageal junction into the stomach, and the pyloric sphincter, which relaxes as food is propelled into the duodenum. Functional areas of the stomach are the fundus (upper portion), body (middle portion), and antrum (lower portion).

The stomach has three layers of smooth muscle: an outer, longitudinal layer; a middle, circular layer; and an inner, oblique layer (the most prominent) (see Fig. 41.4). These layers become progressively thicker in the body and antrum, where food is mixed, churned, and pushed into the duodenum. The circular layer is most prominent and the oblique layer is the least complete; the longitudinal layer is absent on the anterior and posterior surfaces. The glandular epithelium is discussed in the section on Gastric Secretion.

The stomach's blood supply comes from a branch of the celiac artery and is so abundant that nearly all arterial vessels must be occluded before ischemic changes occur in the stomach wall. A series of small veins (short gastric, left and right gastric, and left and right gastroomental) drain blood from the stomach toward the hepatic portal vein.[3]

Sympathetic and parasympathetic divisions of the autonomic nervous system innervate the stomach. Some of the autonomic nerves are extrinsic; that is, they originate in the central nervous system and are controlled by nerve centers in the brain. Extrinsic sympathetic fibers reach the stomach through the celiac plexus (solar plexus), whereas extrinsic parasympathetic fibers enter through the gastric branch of the vagus nerve. The myenteric (Auerbach) and submucosal (Meissner) plexuses are intrinsic and part of the enteric (intramural) nervous system. They originate within the stomach and respond to local stimuli.

Few substances are absorbed in the stomach. The stomach mucosa is impermeable to water, but the stomach can absorb alcohol and aspirin and other nonsteroidal antiinflammatory agents.

Gastric Motility

In its resting state the stomach is small and contains about 50 mL of fluid. There is minimal wall tension, and the muscle layers in the fundus contract very little. Swallowing causes the fundus to relax (receptive relaxation) to receive a bolus of food from the esophagus. Relaxation is coordinated by efferent, nonadrenergic, noncholinergic vagal fibers and is facilitated by gastrin and cholecystokinin, two polypeptide hormones secreted by the gastrointestinal mucosa. (The actions of digestive hormones and neurotransmitters are summarized in Table 41.1.) Food is stored in vertical or oblique layers as it arrives in the fundus, whereas fluids flow relatively quickly down to the antrum.

Gastric (stomach) motility increases with the initiation of peristaltic waves, which sweep over the body of the stomach toward the antrum. The rate of peristaltic contractions is approximately three per minute and is influenced by neural and hormonal activity. Gastrin, motilin (small intestine hormones), and the vagus nerve increase the rate of contraction by lowering the threshold potential of muscle fibers. (The

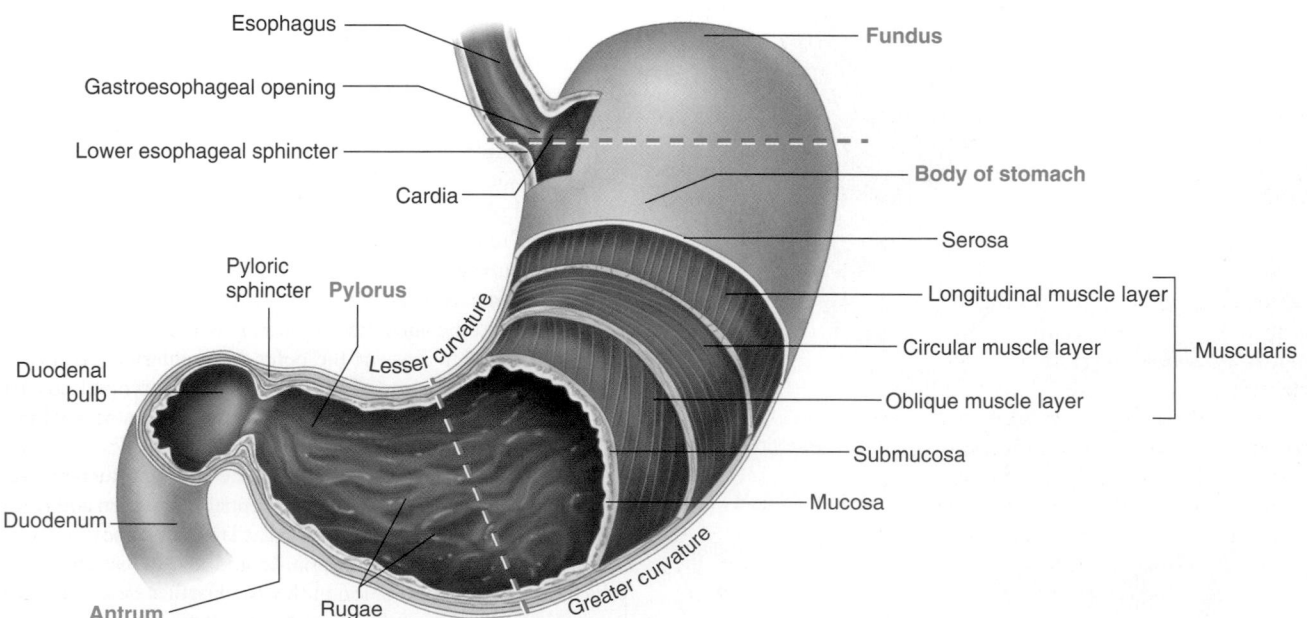

FIGURE 41.4 Stomach. A portion of the anterior wall has been cut away to reveal the muscle layers of the stomach wall. Note that the mucosa lining the stomach forms folds called *rugae*. The *dashed lines* distinguish the fundus, body, and antrum of the stomach. (From Patton KT, Thibodeau GA: *The human body in health & disease*, ed 7, St Louis, 2018, Elsevier.)

TABLE 41.1   **SELECTED HORMONES* AND NEUROTRANSMITTERS OF THE DIGESTIVE SYSTEM**

SOURCE	HORMONE/ NEUROTRANSMITTER	STIMULUS FOR SECRETION	ACTION
Mucosa of stomach	Gastrin	Presence of partially digested proteins in stomach	Stimulates gastric glands to secrete hydrochloric acid, pepsinogen, and histamine; growth of gastric mucosa
	Histamine	Gastrin	Stimulates acid secretion
	Somatostatin	Acid in stomach	Inhibits acid, pepsinogen, and histamine secretion and release of gastrin
	Acetylcholine	**Vagus and local nerves in stomach**	**Stimulates release of pepsinogen and acid secretion**
	Gastrin-releasing peptide (bombesin)	Vagus and local nerves in stomach	Stimulates gastrin and release of pepsinogen and acid secretion
	Ghrelin	High during fasting	Stimulates growth hormone secretion and hypothalamus to increase appetite
Mucosa of small intestine	Motilin	Presence of acid and fat in duodenum	Increases gastrointestinal motility
	Secretin	Presence of chyme (acid, partially digested proteins, fats) in duodenum	Stimulates pancreas to secrete alkaline pancreatic juice and liver to secrete bile; decreases gastrointestinal motility; inhibits gastrin and gastric acid secretion
	Serotonin (5-hydroxytryptamine)	**Intestinal distention; vagal stimulation; presence of acids, amino acids, or hypertonic fluids; released from enterochromaffin cells throughout intestine**	**Stimulates intestinal secretion, motility and sensation (i.e., pain and nausea), vasodilation; activates gut immune responses**
	Cholecystokinin	Presence of chyme (acid, partially digested proteins, fats) in duodenum	Stimulates gallbladder to eject bile and pancreas to secrete alkaline fluid; decreases gastric motility; constricts pyloric sphincter; inhibits gastrin
	Enteroglucagon	Intraluminal fats and carbohydrates	Weakly inhibits gastric and pancreatic secretion and enhances insulin release, lipolysis, ketogenesis, and glycogenolysis
	Gastric inhibitory peptide	Fat and glucose in small intestine	Inhibits gastric secretion and emptying; stimulates insulin release
	Peptide YY	Intraluminal fat and bile acids	Inhibits postprandial gastric acid and pancreatic secretion and delays gastric and small bowel emptying
	Pancreatic polypeptide	Protein, fat, and glucose in small intestine	Decreases pancreatic HCO_3^- and enzyme secretion
	Vasoactive intestinal peptide	Intestinal mucosa and muscle	Relaxes intestinal smooth muscle

*NOTE: The digestive hormones are not secreted into the gastrointestinal lumen but instead into the bloodstream, where they travel to target tissues. There are more than 30 peptide hormone genes expressed in the gastrointestinal tract and more than 100 hormonally active peptides. The green type indicates a neurotransmitter.
Modified from Johnson LR: *Gastrointestinal physiology*, ed 8, St Louis, 2014, Mosby. Data from Feldman M et al: *Sleisenger and Fordtran's gastrointestinal and liver disease*, ed 10, Philadelphia, 2015, Saunders.

neural and biochemical mechanisms of muscle contraction are described in Chapter 44.) Sympathetic activity and secretin (another small intestine hormone) are inhibitory and raise the threshold potential. The rate of peristalsis is mediated by pacemaker interstitial cells of Cajal that initiate a wave of depolarization (basic electrical rhythm), which moves from the upper part of the stomach to the pylorus.

Gastric mixing and subsequent emptying of gastric contents (chyme) from the stomach take several hours (3 to 6 hours depending on the composition and volume of food intake). Mixing occurs as food is propelled toward the antrum. As food approaches the pylorus, the velocity of the peristaltic wave increases, forcing the contents back toward the body of the stomach. This retropulsion effectively mixes food with digestive juices, and the oscillating motion breaks down large food particles. With each peristaltic wave a small portion of the chyme passes through the pylorus and into the duodenum. The pyloric sphincter is about 1.5 cm long and is always open about 2.0 mm. It opens wider

during antral contraction. Normally there is no regurgitation from the duodenum into the antrum.

The rate of gastric emptying (movement of gastric contents into the duodenum) depends on the volume, osmotic pressure, and chemical composition of the gastric contents. Larger volumes of food increase gastric pressure, peristalsis, and rate of emptying. Solids, fats, and nonisotonic solutions (i.e., hypertonic or hypotonic gastric tube feedings) delay gastric emptying. (Osmotic pressure and tonicity are described in Chapters 1 and 3.) Products of fat digestion, which are formed in the duodenum by the action of bile from the liver and enzymes from the pancreas, stimulate the secretion of cholecystokinin. This hormone inhibits food intake, reduces gastric motility, and decreases gastric emptying so that fats are not emptied into the duodenum at a rate that exceeds the rate of bile and enzyme secretion. Osmoreceptors in the wall of the duodenum are sensitive to the osmotic pressure of duodenal contents. The arrival of hypertonic or hypotonic gastric contents activates the osmoreceptors, which delays gastric emptying to facilitate formation of an isosmotic duodenal environment. The rate at which acid enters the duodenum also influences gastric emptying. Secretions from the pancreas, liver, and duodenal mucosa neutralize gastric hydrochloric acid in the duodenum. The rate of emptying is adjusted to the duodenum's ability to neutralize the incoming acidity. Peristaltic activity in the stomach is also affected by blood glucose levels. Low blood glucose levels stimulate the vagus nerve and gastric smooth muscles, increasing the rate of contraction and gastric emptying. Hyperglycemia delays gastric emptying.[4]

Gastric Secretion

The stomach produces large volumes of gastric secretions when stimulated by eating. Specialized cells located throughout the gastric mucosa produce mucus, acid, pepsinogen, enzymes, hormones, intrinsic factor, and gastroferrin. Intrinsic factor is necessary for the intestinal absorption of vitamin B_{12}, and gastroferrin facilitates small intestinal absorption of iron. The hormones are secreted into the blood and travel to target tissues in the bloodstream. The other gastric secretions are released directly into the stomach lumen under neural and hormonal regulation. Mucus covering the entire mucosa, intercellular tight junctions, bicarbonate secretion, and submucosal acid sensors form a protective barrier against acid and proteolytic enzymes, which otherwise would damage the gastric lining.[5]

In the fundus and body of the stomach the gastric glands of the mucosa are the primary secretory units (Fig. 41.5). Several of these glands (three to seven) empty into a common duct known as the gastric pit. The parietal cells (oxyntic cells) within the glands secrete hydrochloric acid, intrinsic factor, and gastroferrin. The chief cells within the glands secrete pepsinogen, an enzyme precursor that is readily converted to pepsin (a proteolytic enzyme) in the gastric fluid, and acidic lipase. The pyloric gland mucosa in the antrum synthesizes and releases the hormone gastrin from G cells. Enterochromaffin-like cells secrete histamine, and D cells secrete somatostatin.

The composition of gastric fluid depends on volume and flow rate (Fig. 41.6). Potassium level remains relatively constant, but its concentration is greater in gastric secretions than in plasma. The rate of secretion varies with the time of day: lower in the morning and higher in the afternoon and evening. Loss of gastric secretions through vomiting, drainage, or suction may decrease body stores of sodium, potassium, hydrogen, and chloride.

Acid. The major functions of gastric hydrochloric acid are to dissolve food fibers, act as a bactericide against swallowed microorganisms, and convert pepsinogen to pepsin. Gastric acid entering the duodenum facilitates the absorption of ferric iron. The production of acid by the parietal cells requires the transport of hydrogen and chloride from the parietal cells to the stomach lumen. Acid is formed in the parietal cells, primarily through the hydrolysis of water (Fig. 41.7). At a high rate of gastric secretion, bicarbonate moves into the plasma, producing an "alkaline tide" in the venous blood, which also may result in a more alkaline urine.

FIGURE 41.5 Gastric Pits and Gastric Glands. Gastric pits are depressions in the epithelial lining of the stomach. At the bottom of each pit is one or more tubular gastric glands. Chief cells produce the enzymes of gastric juice, and parietal cells produce stomach acid. (From Patton KT et al: *Essentials of anatomy & physiology,* St Louis, 2012, Mosby.)

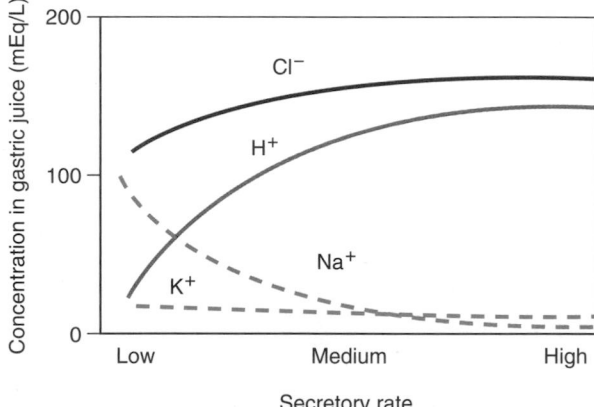

FIGURE 41.6 Relationship Between Secretory Rate and Electrolyte Composition of the Gastric Secretions. Sodium *(Na+)* concentration is lower in the gastric secretions than in the plasma, whereas hydrogen *(H+),* potassium *(K+),* and chloride *(Cl−)* concentrations are higher. Gastric secretions are close to isotonic. Secretory rate increases during the cephalic and gastric phases of digestion.

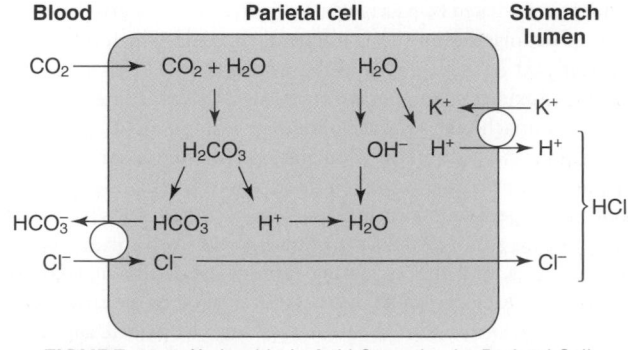

FIGURE 41.7 Hydrochloric Acid Secretion by Parietal Cell.

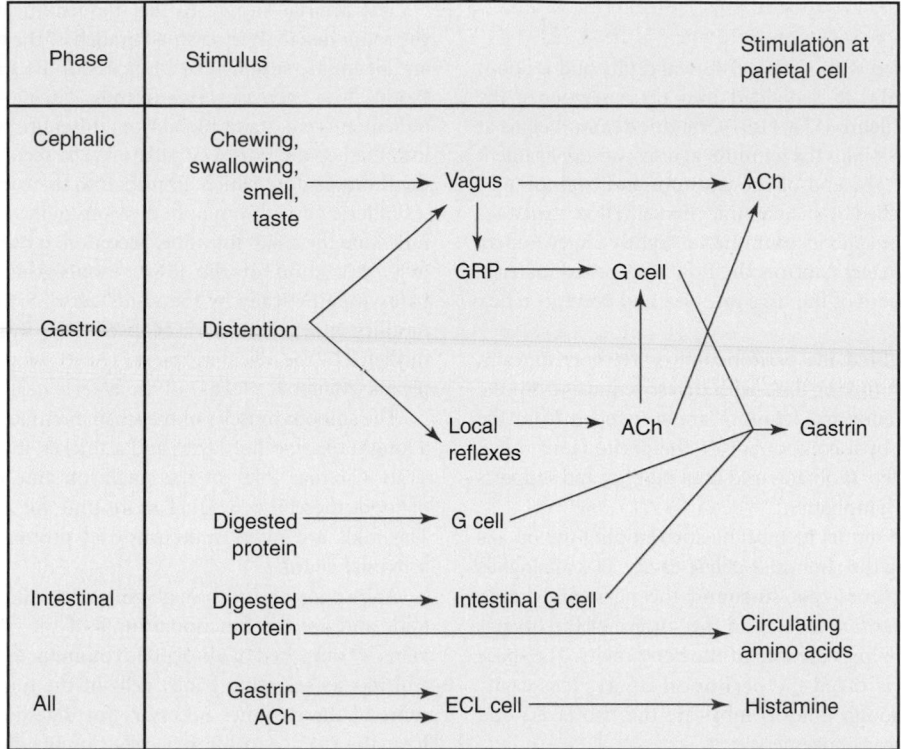

FIGURE 41.8 Mechanisms for Stimulating Acid Secretion. *ACh,* Acetylcholine; *ECL,* enterochromaffin-like cell; *GRP,* gastrin-releasing peptide. (From Johnson LR: *Gastrointestinal physiology,* ed 8, Philadelphia, 2014, Mosby.)

Acid secretion is stimulated by the vagus nerve, which releases acetylcholine and stimulates the secretion of gastrin; gastrin then stimulates the release of histamine from enterochromaffin-like cells in the gastric mucosa. Histamine stimulates acid secretion by activating histamine receptors (H2 receptors) on acid-secreting parietal cells. Caffeine, calcium, and ghrelin also stimulate acid secretion. Somatostatin, secretin, cholecystokinin, glucagon-like peptide-1, atrial natriuretic peptide, and prostaglandins inhibit acid secretion.[6]

Pepsin and Gastric Lipase. Acetylcholine, through vagal stimulation during the cephalic and gastric phases, is the strongest stimulation for pepsin secretion. The precursor pepsinogen is quickly converted to pepsin at a pH of 2. Acid also stimulates a local cholinergic reflex and stimulates chief cells to secrete pepsin. Gastrin and secretin are weaker pepsinogen secretagogues. Pepsin is a proteolytic enzyme that breaks down protein-forming polypeptides in the stomach. Once chyme has entered the duodenum, the alkaline environment of the duodenum inactivates pepsin. Gastric lipase is an acid lipase and does not require bile for activation like alkaline pancreatic and intestinal lipases and is active in an acid environment. It accounts for about 30% of fat digestion in adults and up to 50% percent of fat digestion in infants. It cleaves only one monoglyceride from triglyceride so is less efficient than alkaline lipase.

Mucus. The gastric mucosa is protected from the digestive actions of acid and pepsin by intercellular tight junctions, a coating of mucus called the mucosal barrier, and a rich gastric mucosal blood flow.[5] The quality and quantity of mucus and the tight junctions between epithelial cells make gastric mucosa relatively impermeable to acid. Prostaglandins and nitric oxide protect the mucosal barrier by stimulating the secretion of mucus and bicarbonate and by inhibiting the secretion of acid.

Intrinsic factor (IF), a mucoprotein produced by parietal cells, combines with vitamin B_{12} in the stomach. It is required for the absorption of vitamin B_{12} by the ileum. Atrophic gastritis and failure to absorb vitamin B_{12} result in pernicious anemia (see Chapter 29).

Phases of Gastric Secretion. The secretion of gastric juice is influenced by numerous stimuli that together facilitate the process of digestion. The phases of gastric secretion are the cephalic phase, gastric phase, and intestinal phase (Fig. 41.8).

Cephalic Phase. The anticipatory and sensory experiences of smelling, seeing, tasting, chewing, and swallowing food contribute to the cephalic phase of secretion. The cephalic phase of gastric secretion is mediated by the vagus nerve through the myenteric plexus. Insulin secretion by the endocrine pancreas, stimulated by hyperglycemia, also is a strong stimulus for gastric secretion and is mediated by the vagus nerve through sensors located in the hypothalamus. Maintenance of steady serum glucose levels suppresses the gastric response to insulin.

Gastric Phase. The gastric phase of secretion begins with the arrival of food in the stomach. Two major stimuli have a secretory effect: (1) distention of the stomach, and (2) the presence of digested protein. The vagus and enteric nerve plexuses are stimulated by distention and contribute to gastric secretion through a local reflex. Both neural reflexes are mediated by ACh and can be blocked by atropine. As digestion proceeds, products of protein break down, stimulating the release of more gastrin from G cells.

Intestinal Phase. The movement of chyme from the stomach into the duodenum initiates the intestinal phase of secretion. This phase represents a deceleration of the gastric secretory response; however, the presence of digested protein and amino acids in the duodenum continues to stimulate some gastric secretion.

Concurrently, in response to low duodenal pH and the presence of lipids, inhibitory vagal and enteric reflexes decrease gastric motility when chyme enters the duodenum. The release of secretin and cholecystokinin stimulates pancreatic secretions and inhibits gastric secretions.

Small Intestine

The small intestine is coiled within the peritoneal cavity and is about 5 to 6 m long. Functionally, it is divided into three segments: the duodenum, jejunum, and ileum (Fig. 41.9). The duodenum begins at the pylorus and ends where it joins the jejunum at a suspensory ligament called the *Treitz ligament*. The end of the jejunum and beginning of the ileum are not distinguished by an anatomic marker. These structures are not grossly different, but the jejunum has a slightly larger lumen. The ileocecal valve (sphincter) controls the flow of digested material from the ileum into the cecum of the large intestine and prevents reflux into the small intestine.

The duodenum lies behind the peritoneum, or retroperitoneally, and has an essential role in mixing food with digestive juices from the liver and pancreas. The ileum and jejunum are suspended from the posterior abdominal wall by a component of the peritoneum called the mesentery. The mesentery facilitates intestinal motility and supports blood vessels, nerves, and lymphatics.

The peritoneum is the serous membrane surrounding the organs of the abdomen and lining the abdominopelvic cavity. It is analogous to the pericardium and pleura that surround the heart and lungs, respectively. The *visceral peritoneum* lies on the surface of the organs, and the *parietal peritoneum* lines the wall of the body cavity. The space between these two layers is called the peritoneal cavity. This cavity normally contains just enough fluid to lubricate the two layers and prevent friction during organ movement.

The arterial supply to the duodenum arises primarily from the gastroduodenal artery, a small branch of the celiac artery. The jejunum and ileum are supplied by branches of the superior mesenteric artery. Blood flow increases significantly during digestion. The superior mesenteric vein drains blood from the entire small intestine and empties into the hepatic portal circulation. The regional lymphatics drain into the thoracic duct which empties into the subclavian vein.

Enteric nerves from both divisions of the autonomic nervous system innervate the small intestine. Secretion, motility, and intestinal reflexes (e.g., relaxation of the lower esophageal sphincter) are mediated parasympathetically by the vagus nerve. Sympathetic activity inhibits motility and produces vasoconstriction. Intrinsic reflexive activity is mediated by the myenteric plexus (Auerbach plexus) and the submucosal plexus (Meissner plexus) of the enteric nervous system.

The smooth muscles of the small intestine are arranged in two layers: a longitudinal, outer layer; and a thicker, inner circular layer (see Fig. 41.9). Circular folds of the small intestine mucosa slow the passage of food, thereby providing more time for digestion and absorption. The folds are most numerous and prominent in the jejunum and proximal ileum.

Absorption occurs through villi (*sing.*, *villus*), which cover the circular folds and are the functional units of the intestine (see Fig. 41.9). A villus is composed of absorptive columnar epithelial cells (enterocytes) and mucus-secreting goblet cells of the mucosa. Each villus secretes some of the enzymes necessary for digestion and absorbs nutrients. Near the surface, columnar cells closely adhere to each other at sites

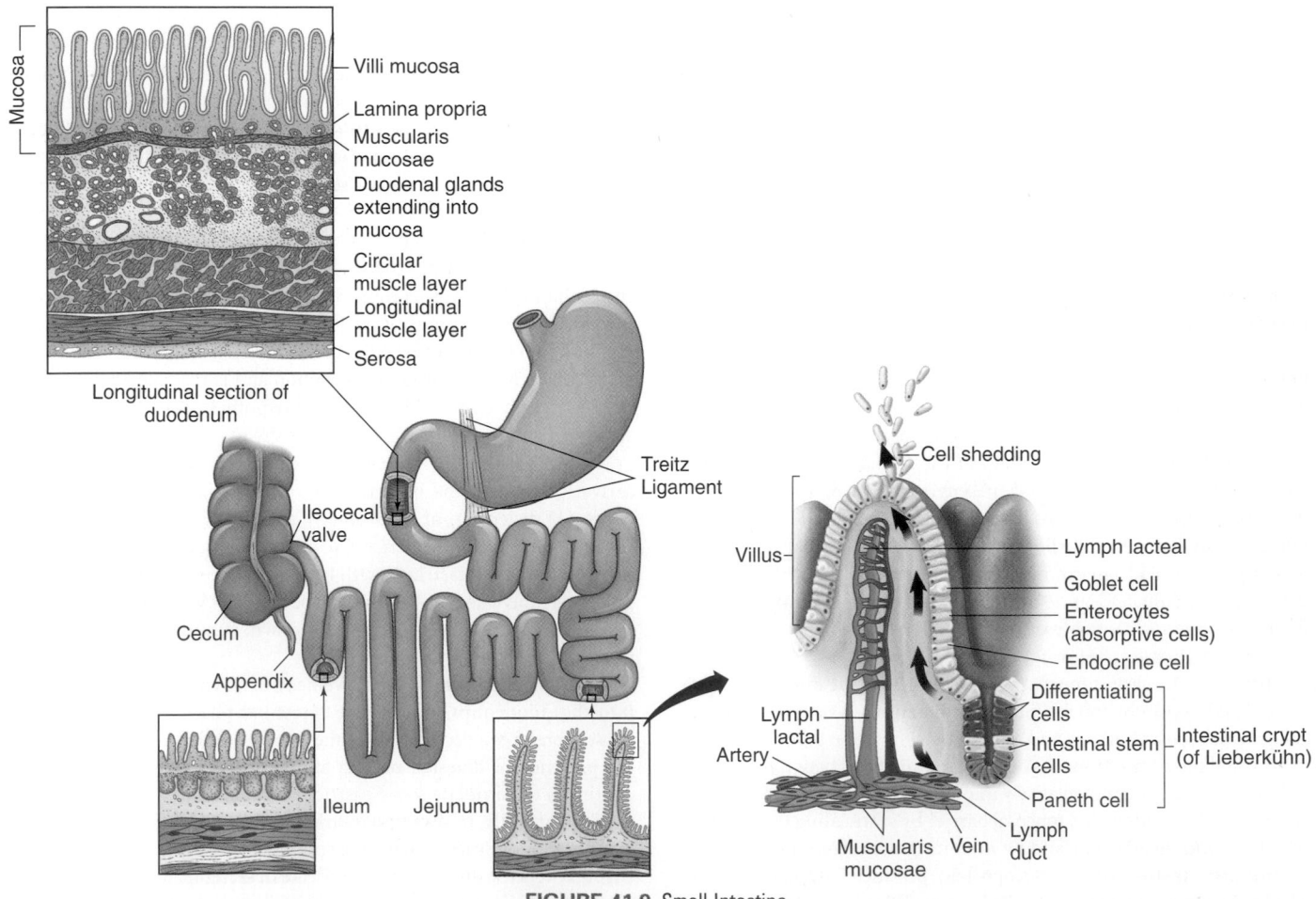

FIGURE 41.9 Small Intestine.

called *tight junctions.* Water and electrolytes are absorbed through these intercellular spaces. The surface of each columnar epithelial cell on the villus contains tiny projections called microvilli (see Fig. 41.9). Together the microvilli create a mucosal surface known as the brush border. The villi and microvilli greatly increase the surface area available for absorption. Coating the brush border is an "unstirred" layer of water that is important for the absorption of water-soluble substances, including emulsified micelles of fat. The lamina propria (a connective tissue layer of the mucous membrane) lies beneath the epithelial cells of the villi and contains lymphocytes and plasma cells, which produce immunoglobulins; and macrophages (see The Gastrointestinal Tract and Immunity section).

Central arterioles ascend within each villus and branch into a capillary array that extends around the base of the columnar cells and cascades down to the venules that lead to the hepatic portal circulation. The opposing ascending and descending blood flow provides a countercurrent exchange system for absorbed substances and blood gases. A central lacteal, or lymphatic capillary, is also contained within each villus and is important for the absorption and transport of fat molecules. Contents of the lacteals flow to regional nodes and channels that eventually drain into the thoracic duct[7] (see Fig. 41.9).

Between the bases of the villi are the crypts of Lieberkühn (intestinal glands), which extend to the submucosal layer. Undifferentiated cells arise from stem cells at the base of the crypt and move toward the tip of the villus, maturing to become columnar epithelial secretory cells (water, electrolytes, and enzymes) and goblet cells (mucus). After completing their migration to the tip of the villus, they function for a few days and then are shed into the intestinal lumen and digested. Discarded epithelial cells are an important source of endogenous protein. The entire epithelial population is replaced about every 4 to 7 days. Many factors can influence this process of cellular proliferation. Starvation, vitamin B_{12} deficiency, and cytotoxic drugs or irradiation suppresses cell division and shorten the villi. The decreased absorption that results can cause diarrhea and malnutrition. Nutrient intake and intestinal resection stimulate cell production.

Intestinal Digestion and Absorption

The process of intestinal digestion is initiated in the stomach by the actions of gastric hydrochloric acid and pepsin, which break down food fibers and proteins. The chyme that passes into the duodenum is a liquid that contains small particles of undigested food. Digestion continues in the proximal portion of the small intestine by the action of pancreatic enzymes, intestinal brush-border enzymes, and bile salts. Carbohydrates are broken down to monosaccharides and disaccharides in the proximal small intestine, proteins are degraded further to amino acids and peptides, and fats are emulsified and reduced to fatty acids (Box 41.1) and monoglycerides (Fig. 41.10). These nutrients, along with water, vitamins, and electrolytes, are absorbed across the intestinal mucosa and into the blood by active transport, diffusion, or facilitated diffusion. Products of carbohydrate and protein breakdown move into villus capillaries and then to the liver through the hepatic portal vein. Digested fats move into the lacteals and eventually reach the liver through the systemic circulation. Intestinal motility exposes nutrients to a large mucosal surface area by mixing chyme and moving it through the lumen. Different segments of the gastrointestinal tract absorb different nutrients. Digestion and absorption of all major nutrients occur in the small intestine. Sites of absorption are shown in Fig. 41.11.

Water and Electrolyte Transport by the Small Intestine.

The epithelial cell membranes of the small intestine are formed of lipids and therefore are hydrophobic, or tend to repel water. (The properties of cell membranes are described in Chapter 1.) Therefore water and electrolytes are transported in both directions (toward the capillary

BOX 41.1	SOURCES OF DIGESTIVE ENZYMES
Salivary Glands	Phospholipase A_2
Amylase	Cholesterol esterase–nonspecific
Lingual lipase	lipase
Stomach	**Small Intestine**
Pepsin	Enterokinase
Gastric lipase	Disaccharidases
	Maltase
Pancreas	Sucrase
Amylase	Lactase
Trypsin	α,α'-1 Trehalase
Chymotrypsin	Isomaltase
Carboxypeptidase	Peptidases
Elastase	Amino-oligopeptidase
Lipase-colipase	Dipeptidase

From Johnson LR: *Gastrointestinal physiology*, ed 8, St Louis, 2014, Mosby.

blood or toward the intestinal lumen) through the tight junctions and intercellular spaces rather than across cell membranes. Water diffuses passively across hydrostatic pressure and osmotic gradients established by the active transport of sodium and other substances. Approximately 85% to 90% of the water that enters the gastrointestinal tract each day is absorbed in the small intestine. The remaining water and electrolytes are absorbed at a constant rate in the large intestine. Sodium passes through the tight junctions and is actively transported across cell membranes. Sodium and glucose share a common active transport carrier (sodium-glucose ligand transporter1 [SGLT1]) so that sodium absorption is enhanced by glucose transport (Fig. 41.12). Potassium moves passively across the tight junctions with changes in the electrochemical gradient. Chloride is actively secreted throughout the large and small intestines.

Carbohydrates. Only monosaccharides (ribose, galactose, glucose, fructose) are absorbed by the intestinal mucosa; the complex carbohydrates (polysaccharides and oligosaccharides) must be hydrolyzed to their simplest form (see Fig. 41.10). The major disaccharides are sucrose (glucose-fructose), maltose (glucose-glucose), and lactose (glucose-galactose). Salivary and pancreatic amylases break down starches to oligosaccharides by splitting α-1,4-glucosidic linkages of long-chain molecules. Approximately half of starch hydrolysis occurs in the stomach and about half in the duodenum. In the small intestine, disaccharides are hydrolyzed by brush-border enzymes (sucrase, maltase, and lactase) to their respective monosaccharides.

The sugars are absorbed primarily in the duodenum and upper jejunum by facilitated diffusion mediated by glucose transporter proteins.[8] The monosaccharides pass through the unstirred layer by diffusion. At the cell membrane, glucose and galactose are actively transported with a sodium carrier (SGLT1) and fructose absorption is facilitated by glucose transporter 5 (GLUT5) and GLUT7. Transport of all three monosaccharides from the cytosol to the bloodstream is facilitated by GLUT2 (see Fig. 41.12). Insulin facilitates glucose transport into fat and muscle cells via glucose transporter 4 (GLUT4).

Insulin is not required for the intestinal absorption of glucose. Cellulose is a glucose polysaccharide found in plants. Humans lack enzymes to digest cellulose, and the undigested fiber contributes to stool volume and stimulates large intestine motility.

Proteins. Adults require 44 to 56 g of protein per day. Approximately 20 to 30 g of protein is derived endogenously from shed epithelial cells

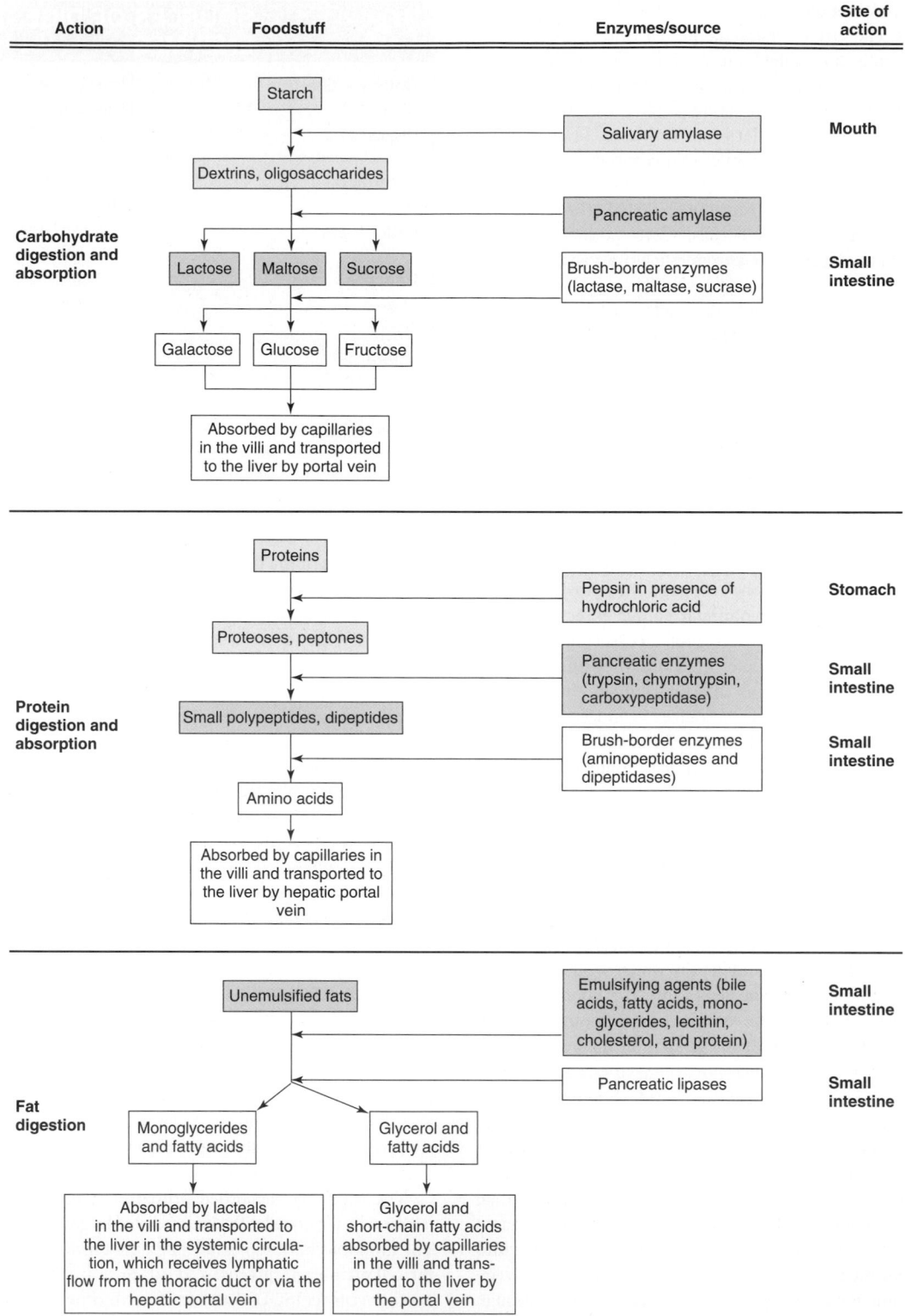

Action	Foodstuff	Enzymes/source	Site of action

Carbohydrate digestion and absorption

Starch → (Salivary amylase) — Mouth

Dextrins, oligosaccharides → (Pancreatic amylase) — Small intestine

Lactose, Maltose, Sucrose → Brush-border enzymes (lactase, maltase, sucrase)

Galactose, Glucose, Fructose

Absorbed by capillaries in the villi and transported to the liver by portal vein

Protein digestion and absorption

Proteins → Pepsin in presence of hydrochloric acid — Stomach

Proteoses, peptones → Pancreatic enzymes (trypsin, chymotrypsin, carboxypeptidase) — Small intestine

Small polypeptides, dipeptides → Brush-border enzymes (aminopeptidases and dipeptidases) — Small intestine

Amino acids

Absorbed by capillaries in the villi and transported to the liver by hepatic portal vein

Fat digestion

Unemulsified fats → Emulsifying agents (bile acids, fatty acids, mono-glycerides, lecithin, cholesterol, and protein) — Small intestine

→ Pancreatic lipases — Small intestine

Monoglycerides and fatty acids / Glycerol and fatty acids

Absorbed by lacteals in the villi and transported to the liver in the systemic circulation, which receives lymphatic flow from the thoracic duct or via the hepatic portal vein

Glycerol and short-chain fatty acids absorbed by capillaries in the villi and transported to the liver by the portal vein

FIGURE 41.10 Digestion and Absorption of Foodstuffs.

and small amounts of plasma proteins. Most ingested protein is absorbed; only 5% to 10% is eliminated in the stool.

The site of digestion of protein depends on the source of the protein. For example, casein from bovine milk precipitates in the stomach and is digested by gastric pepsin and acid, whereas the soluble proteins whey and soy pass rapidly through the stomach and are digested by pancreatic enzymes. Major protein hydrolysis is accomplished in the small intestine by the pancreatic enzymes trypsin, chymotrypsin, and carboxypeptidase (see Fig. 41.10). Trypsin and chymotrypsin (endopeptidase) hydrolyze the interior bonds of the large molecules, and carboxypeptidases cleave the end amino acids (exopeptidase). Hydrolysis of proteins is also carried out by the brush-border enzymes and enzymes

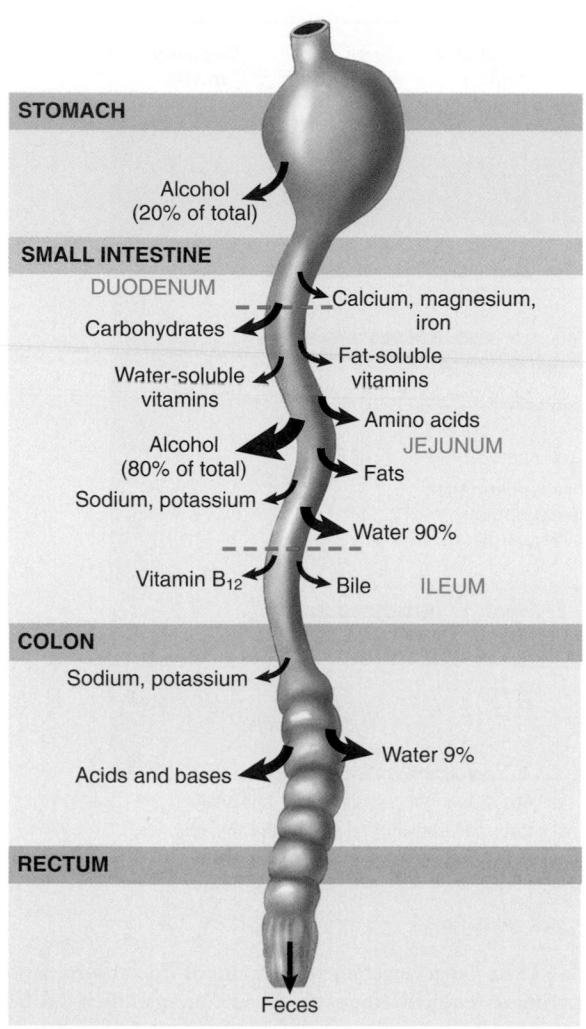

STOMACH

Alcohol
(20% of total)

SMALL INTESTINE

DUODENUM

Carbohydrates

Water-soluble
vitamins

Alcohol
(80% of total)

Sodium, potassium

Calcium, magnesium,
iron

Fat-soluble
vitamins

Amino acids

JEJUNUM

Fats

Water 90%

Vitamin B_{12}

Bile

ILEUM

COLON

Sodium, potassium

Water 9%

Acids and bases

RECTUM

Feces

FIGURE 41.11 Sites of Absorption of Major Nutrients.

in the epithelial cytosol (intracellular fluid). The brush-border enzymes hydrolyze the large oligopeptides (proteins composed of three to six amino acids) into smaller peptides, which can cross cell membranes. Enzymes in the cytosol then break them down to amino acids. Amino acids are actively transported from the cytosol into the bloodstream by a sodium-dependent carrier in the basolateral membrane. There also are free amino acids that can be absorbed directly from the intestinal lumen using a membrane transport protein. Like the sugars, proteins are absorbed primarily in the proximal area of the small intestine.

Fats. Approximately 90 to 100 g of fat is consumed daily by the average American. Fat is an important source of calories and is a primary structural component of cell membranes and organelles. Sources of dietary fat are reviewed in Box 41.2. Although triglycerides are the major dietary lipids, cholesterol, phospholipids, and fat-soluble vitamins also have nutritional importance. The digestion and absorption of fat occur in four phases: (1) emulsification and lipolysis, (2) micelle formation, (3) fat absorption, and (4) resynthesis of triglycerides and phospholipids.

The mechanical action of the stomach and small intestine disperses the triglyceride droplets into small particles. Emulsification is the process by which emulsifying agents (fatty acids, monoglycerides, lecithin, cholesterol, protein, bile salts) in the small intestinal lumen cover the small fat particles and prevent them from re-forming into fat droplets. Emulsified fat is then ready for lipolysis (lipid hydrolysis) by

lingual and gastric lipase (acid lipases), pancreatic lipase, phospholipase, and hydrolase (alkaline lipases). Lipase breaks down triglycerides to diglycerides, monoglycerides, free fatty acids, and glycerol (see Fig. 41.10). The action of alkaline lipases requires the presence of colipase, a pancreatic coenzyme that allows lipase to penetrate the triglyceride molecule. Phospholipase cleaves fatty acids from phospholipids, and cholesterol esterase breaks cholesterol esters into fatty acids and glycerol.

The products of lipid hydrolysis must be made water soluble if they are to be absorbed efficiently from the intestinal lumen. This is accomplished by the formation of water-soluble molecules known as micelles (Fig. 41.13). Micelles are formed of bile salts, the products of fat hydrolysis, fat-soluble vitamins, and cholesterol. The fats form the core of the micelle, and the polar bile salts form an outer shell, with the hydrophobic ("water-repelling") side facing the interior and the hydrophilic ("water-loving") side facing the aqueous (water-like) content of the intestinal lumen. Because the unstirred layer of the brush border is aqueous, the micelles readily diffuse through it. The micelles maintain the fat molecules in the dissolved or solubilized form, which allows them to move more rapidly from the micelle toward the absorbing surface of the intestinal epithelium. The fat products of the micelle then readily diffuse through the epithelial cell membrane, while the bile salts remain in the lumen and proceed to the ileum, where they are absorbed into the circulation and returned to the liver via the enterohepatic circulation (see Figs. 41.14 and 41.21). Almost all of the bile salts are recycled in this way.

When the fat products reach the inside of the epithelial cell, they are resynthesized into triglycerides and phospholipids. The triglycerides are covered with phospholipids, lipoproteins, and cholesterol to become particles called chylomicrons. The chylomicrons travel to the basolateral membrane of the columnar epithelial cells, where they are extruded

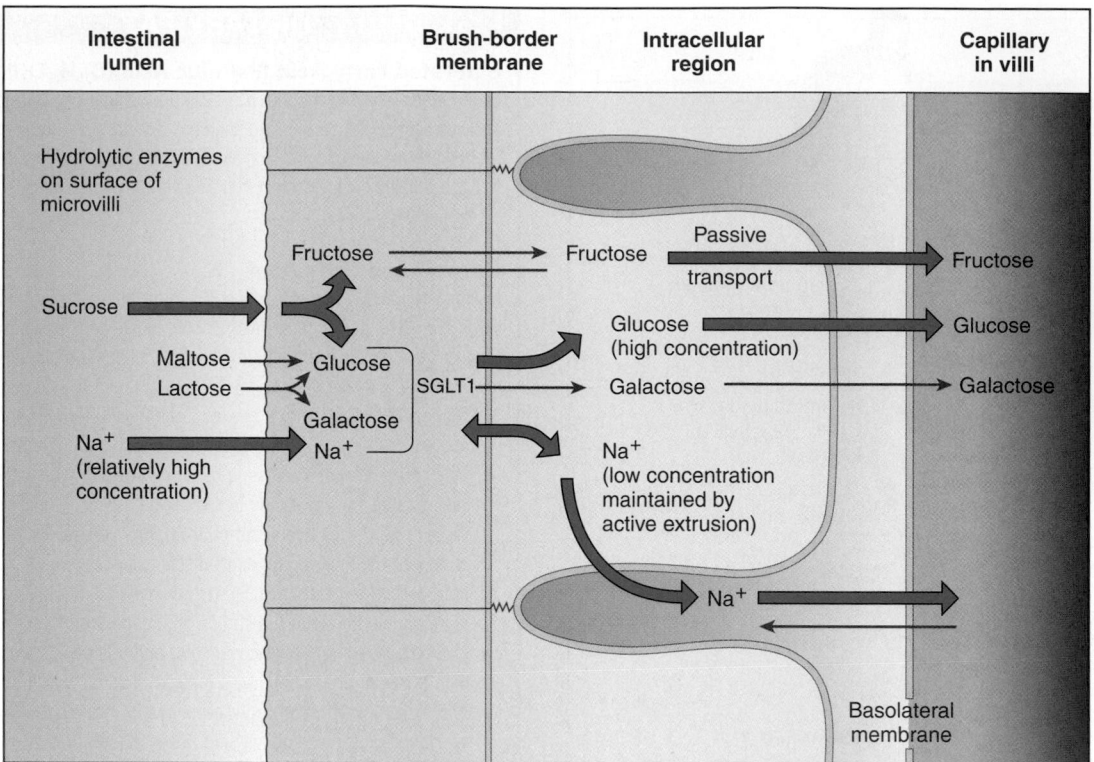

FIGURE 41.12 Monosaccharides and Sodium Transport. Schematic showing monosaccharides and sodium (Na+) transport through the small intestinal epithelium. Glucose, galactose, and sodium are transported into the epithelial cell by sodium-glucose ligand transporter 1 (SGLT1). See text for details regarding other glucose transporters.

into the intercellular spaces of the villus. From here they enter the lacteals and lymphatic channels and, eventually, the systemic circulation.

Minerals and Vitamins. The recommended intake of calcium ranges from 1000 to 1500 mg/day. Between 500 and 600 mg is secreted or shed into the lumen with desquamated epithelial cells. Not all of this calcium is absorbed. Daily absorption of calcium is approximately 600 mg. This amount increases with increased intake. When its concentration in the lumen is greater than 5 mmol/L, calcium is absorbed by passive diffusion. At concentrations less than 5 mmol/L, calcium is transported actively across cell membranes, bound to a carrier protein. The carrier formation requires the presence of the active form of vitamin D₃ (1,25-dihydroxy-vitamin D). The calcium-protein complex moves into the epithelial cell, where the calcium binds to proteins or other substances. Then these complexes move through the basolateral membrane to the interstitial fluid by diffusion or active transport. Calcium is absorbed throughout the small intestine, but primarily in the ileum. Increased serum calcium concentration inhibits parathyroid hormone, which in turn decreases the formation of vitamin D₃ by the kidney, thus regulating calcium absorption.

Increased demand for calcium results in increased uptake, as evidenced by the fact that calcium is absorbed more rapidly in children and pregnant or lactating women. Bile salts enhance calcium absorption indirectly by facilitating the absorption of vitamin D, which is fat soluble.

The recommended intake of magnesium for adults is 300 to 350 mg/day. Approximately 50% of it is absorbed by active transport or passive diffusion in the jejunum and ileum. Phosphate is also absorbed in the small intestine by passive diffusion and active transport.

The levels of iron in the body are regulated primarily by intestinal absorption and secretion. The average intake ranges from 15 to 30 mg/day. Of this amount, menstruating women absorb 1 to 1.5 mg and men

absorb 0.15 to 1 mg. Generally the amount of iron absorbed is equal to the amount required. Iron is absorbed more rapidly if a deficiency exists. A primary source of iron is heme from animal protein with a smaller amount of heme from recycling of senescent red blood cells. This iron is rapidly absorbed by the epithelial cells primarily in the proximal duodenum. Inorganic iron (e.g., iron in fruits, cereals, eggs, vegetables) is also readily absorbed. The presence of gastric acid and vitamin C in the duodenum reduces ferric iron to ferrous iron, which is the form more easily absorbed. Calcium phosphate and phospho-proteins (milk and antacids) in the intestinal lumen bind iron and reduce absorption. Tea also binds iron and inhibits absorption by forming iron tannate complexes.

Iron is bound to *intestinal transferrin* in the lumen and is absorbed and bound to the protein *ferritin* and to amino acid chelates in the cytosol of the enterocytes. Transport of iron across the basolateral membrane is determined by the amount of iron in the circulation. It is transported in the blood by *plasma transferrin,* a glycoprotein, and is carried to body tissues. When there is less need for iron, it remains in the enterocyte as ferritin and is carried into the lumen when the cell is sloughed from the end of the villus. Following hemorrhage, the intestinal cells require 3 days to increase their rate of iron absorption. This is because the need for iron is perceived by the precursor stem cells in the crypts of Lieberkühn, and they take 3 days to mature and migrate to the tips of the villi, where they absorb more iron. Hepcidin is a protein synthesized by the liver that inhibits apical uptake of iron by enterocytes and modulates iron trafficking.[9]

The absorption of vitamins is summarized in Table 41.2. Most of the water-soluble vitamins are absorbed passively or by sodium-dependent active transport. Most vitamin B₁₂ (cobalamin) is bound to intrinsic factor (making it resistant to digestion) and absorbed in the terminal

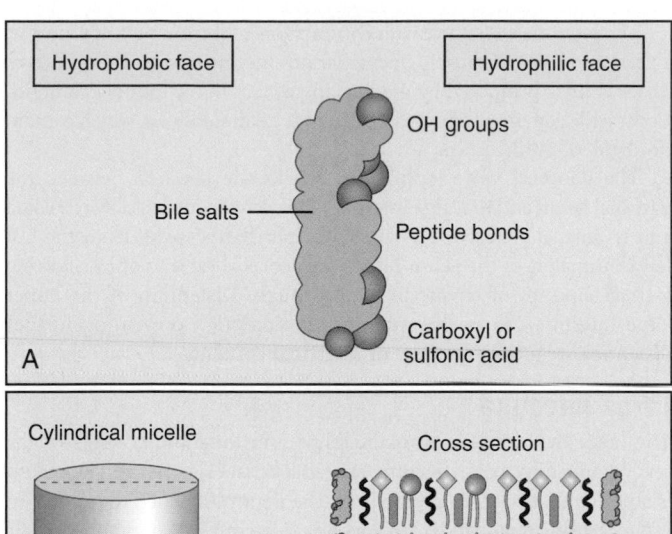

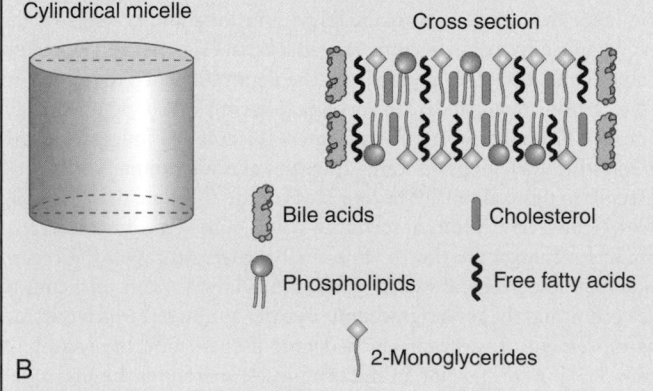

FIGURE 41.13 Structure of Bile Acid and Micelle. **A,** A bile salt molecule in solution. The molecule is amphipathic in that it has a hydrophilic face and a hydrophobic face. The amphipathic structure is key in the ability of the bile salts to emulsify lipids and form micelles. **B,** A model of the structure of a bile salt–lipid mixed micelle, an emulsified fat. (From Levy MN, Koeppen BM, Stanton BA: *Principles of physiology,* ed 4, St Louis, 2006, Mosby.)

TABLE 41.2   INTESTINAL ABSORPTION OF VITAMINS

VITAMIN	MECHANISMS OF ABSORPTION	SITE OF ABSORPTION
Fat-Soluble Vitamins	Micelle formation with bile salts; lipid diffusion	Ileum
A (retinal) D₃ (1,25-dihydroxy-vitamin D) E (α-tocopherol) K		
Water-Soluble Vitamins		
B₁ (thiamine)	Active transport (sodium dependent)	Duodenum and jejunum
B₂ (riboflavin)	Unknown	Duodenum and jejunum
Niacin (nicotinic acid)	Passive diffusion	Jejunum
C (ascorbic acid)	Passive diffusion; active transport (sodium dependent)	Ileum
Folic acid	Active transport (sodium dependent)	Jejunum
B₁₂ (cobalamin)	Active transport (intrinsic factor dependent)	Terminal ileum
B₆ (pyridoxine, pyridoxamine, pyridoxal phosphate)	Passive diffusion	Jejunum
Pantothenic acid	Passive diffusion	Duodenum and jejunum
Biotin	Unknown	Unknown

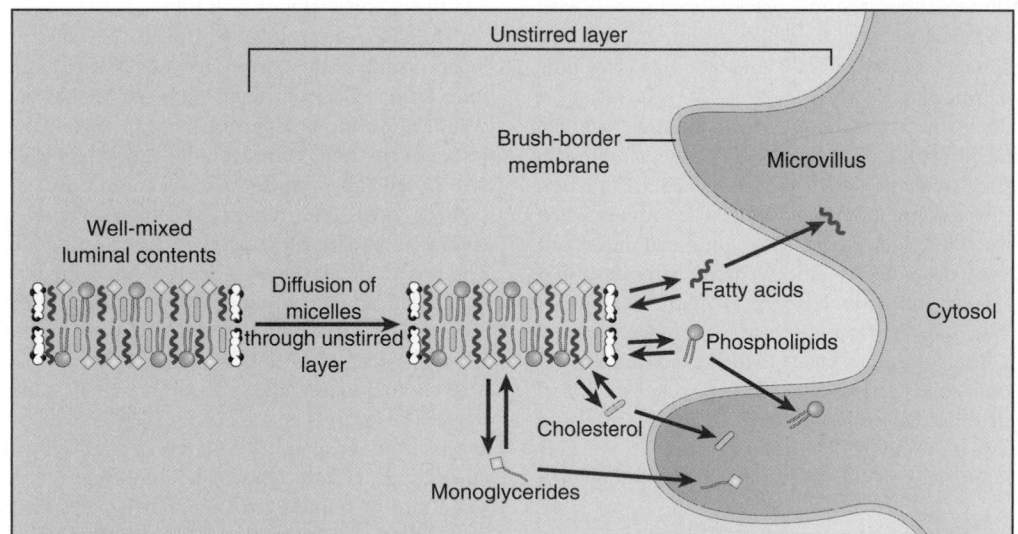

FIGURE 41.14 Lipid Absorption in the Small Intestine. Micelles of bile salts and products of lipid digestion diffuse through the unstirred layer and among the microvilli. As digestive products are absorbed from free solution by epithelial cells of the villi, more digestive products dissociate from the micelles. (From Levy MN, Koeppen BM, Stanton BA: *Principles of physiology,* ed 4, St Louis, 2006, Mosby.)

ileum, although a small amount of the vitamin is absorbed in its free (unbound) form.

Intestinal Motility

The movements of the small intestine facilitate digestion and absorption. Chyme leaving the stomach and entering the duodenum stimulates intestinal movements that help blend secretions from the liver, gallbladder, pancreas, and intestinal glands. A churning motion brings the luminal content into contact with the absorbing cells of the villi. Propulsive movements then advance the chyme toward the large intestine.

Intestinal motility is regulated by the enteric nervous system, vagal stimulation, and hormones (see Table 41.1). Two movements promote motility:

1. Haustral segmentation. Localized rhythmic contractions of circular smooth muscles divide and mix the chyme, enabling the chyme to have contact with digestive enzymes and the absorbent mucosal surface, and then propel it toward the large intestine.
2. Peristalsis. Waves of contraction along short segments of longitudinal smooth muscle allow time for digestion and absorption. The intestinal villi move with contractions of the muscularis mucosae, a thin layer of muscle separating the mucosa and submucosa, with absorption promoted by the swaying of the villi in the luminal contents.

Segmentation consists of localized rhythmic contractions of the circular smooth muscles and occurs more frequently than peristalsis. The contraction waves occur at different rates in different parts of the small intestine in segments of 1 to 4 cm. Frequency is greatest (12/minute) in the upper small intestine and least (8/minute) in the distal part of the ileum. Segmentation divides and mixes the chyme, bringing it into contact with the absorbent mucosal surface. It also helps to propel the chyme toward the large intestine. The frequency of the segmentation is regulated intrinsically by the frequency of the basic electrical rhythm, which arises in the myenteric plexus of longitudinal smooth muscle and is controlled by the interstitial cells of Cajal, the pacemaker cells of the gastrointestinal tract.[10] Although the basic rate of contraction is controlled intrinsically, the force of contraction can be enhanced extrinsically by vagal stimulation.

Intestinal peristalsis involves short segments (about 10 cm) of longitudinal smooth muscle and propels chyme through the intestine. The intestinal villi move with contractions of the muscularis mucosae, a thin layer of muscle separating the mucosa and submucosa, with absorption promoted by the swaying of the villi in the luminal contents. The wave of contraction moves slowly (1 to 2 cm/second) to allow time for digestion and absorption.

Neural reflexes along the length of the small intestine facilitate motility, digestion, and absorption. Through reflex action, receptors in one part of the intestine transmit signals that influence the function of another part. The ileogastric reflex inhibits gastric motility when the ileum becomes distended. This prevents the continued movement of chyme into an already distended intestine. The intestinointestinal reflex inhibits intestinal motility when one part of the intestine is overdistended or its mucosa is irritated. Both of these reflexes require extrinsic innervation. The gastroileal reflex, which is activated by an increase in gastric motility and secretion, stimulates an increase in ileal motility and relaxation of the ileocecal sphincter. This empties the ileum and prepares it to receive more chyme. The gastroileal reflex is probably regulated by the hormones gastrin and cholecystokinin or through the autonomic nerves.

During prolonged fasting or between meals, particularly overnight, slow waves sweep along the entire length of the intestinal tract from the stomach to the terminal ileum. This is known as the *interdigestive myoelectric complex,* and it appears to propel residual gastric and intestinal contents, including bacteria, into the colon.

The intestinal villi move with contractions of the muscularis mucosae, a very thin layer of muscle that separates the mucosa and submucosa. Absorption is promoted by the swaying of villi in the luminal contents. Contractile activity also helps to empty the central lacteals, which contain products of fat digestion.

The ileocecal valve (sphincter) marks the junction between the terminal ileum and the large intestine. This valve is intrinsically regulated and is normally closed. The arrival of peristaltic waves from the last few centimeters of the ileum causes the ileocecal valve to open, allowing a small amount of chyme to pass through. Distention of the upper large intestine causes the sphincter to constrict, preventing further distention or retrograde flow of intestinal contents.

Large Intestine

The large intestine is approximately 1.5 m long and consists of the cecum, appendix, colon, rectum, and anal canal (Fig. 41.15). The cecum is a pouch that receives chyme from the ileum. Attached to the cecum is the vermiform appendix, an appendage having little or no physiologic function. From the cecum, chyme enters the colon, a four-part length of intestine that loops upward, traverses the abdominal cavity, and descends to the anal canal. The four parts of the colon are the ascending colon, transverse colon, descending colon, and sigmoid colon. Two sphincters control the flow of intestinal contents through the cecum and colon: the ileocecal valve, which admits chyme from the ileum to the cecum, and the rectosigmoid (O'Beirne) sphincter, which controls the movement of wastes from the sigmoid colon into the rectum. A thick (2.5 to 3 cm) portion of smooth muscle surrounds the anal canal, forming the internal anal sphincter. Overlapping it distally is the striated skeletal muscle of the external anal sphincter.

In the cecum and colon the longitudinal muscle layer consists of three longitudinal bands called teniae coli (see Fig. 41.15). They are shorter than the colon, giving the colon its "gathered" appearance. The circular muscles of the colon separate the gathers into outpouchings called haustra (*sing.,* haustrum). The haustra become more or less prominent with the contractions and relaxations of the circular muscles. The mucosal surface of the colon has rugae (folds), particularly between the haustra, and Lieberkühn crypts but no villi. Columnar epithelial cells and mucus-secreting goblet cells form the mucosa throughout the large intestine. The columnar epithelium absorbs fluid and electrolytes, and the mucus-secreting cells lubricate the mucosa.

The enteric nervous system regulates motor and secretory activity independently of the extrinsic nervous system. Extrinsic parasympathetic innervation occurs through the vagus nerve and extends from the cecum up to the first part of the transverse colon. Vagal stimulation increases rhythmic contraction of the proximal colon. Extrinsic parasympathetic fibers reach the distal colon through the sacral parasympathetic splanchnic nerves. The internal anal sphincter is usually contracted, and its reflex response is to relax when the rectum is distended. The myenteric plexus provides the major innervation of the internal anal sphincter, but responds to sympathetic stimulation to maintain contraction and parasympathetic stimulation that facilitates relaxation when the rectum is full. Sympathetic innervation of this sphincter arises from the celiac and superior mesenteric ganglia and the sphincter nerve. The external anal sphincter is innervated by the pudendal nerve arising from sacral levels of the spinal cord. Sympathetic activity in the entire large intestine modulates intestinal reflexes, conveys somatic sensations of fullness and pain, participates in the defecation reflex, and constricts blood vessels. The blood supply of the large intestine and rectum is derived primarily from branches of the superior and inferior mesenteric artery.

The primary type of colonic movement is segmental. The circular muscles contract and relax at different sites, shuttling the intestinal

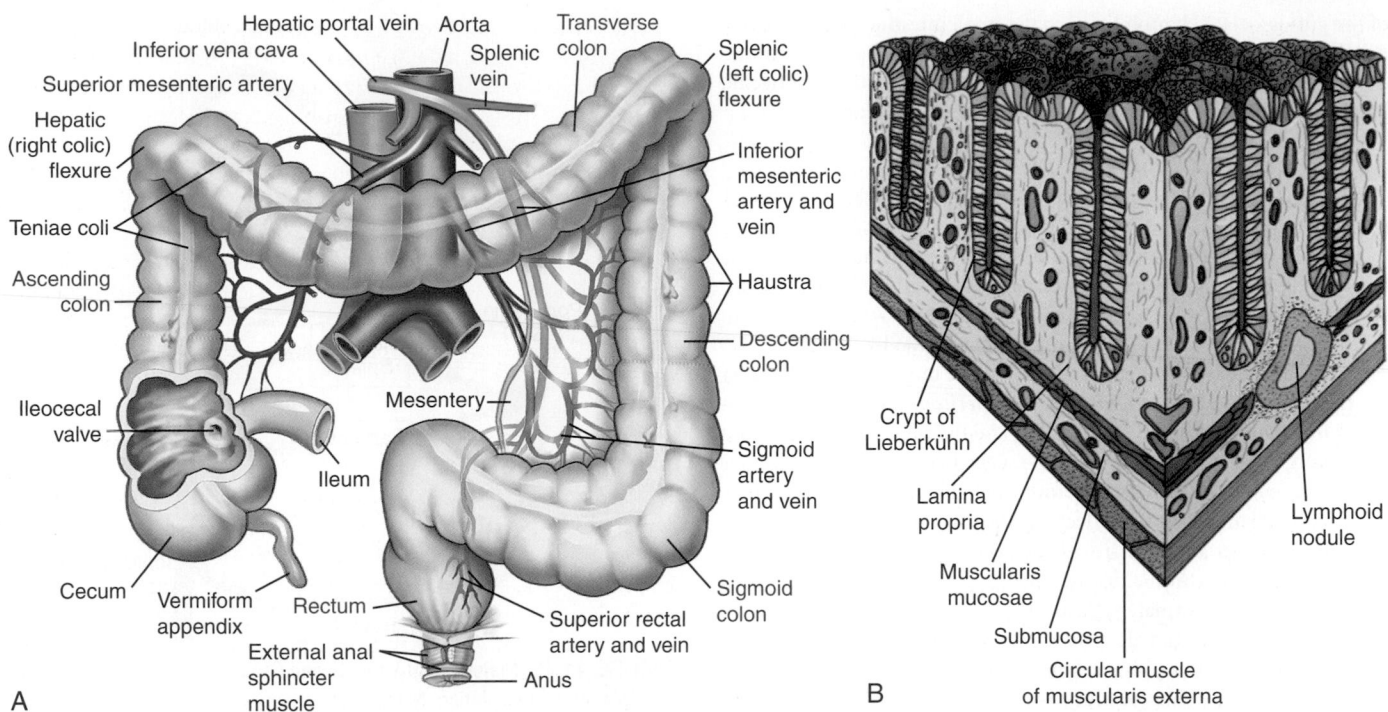

FIGURE 41.15 Large Intestine. **A,** Structure of the large intestine. **B,** Microscopic cross section illustrating cellular structures of the large intestine. The wall of the large intestine is lined with columnar epithelium, in contrast to the villi characteristic of the small intestine. The longitudinal layer of muscularis is reduced to become the teniae coli. (**A** modified from Patton KT, Thibodeau GA: *The human body in health & disease*, ed 7, St Louis 2018, Mosby; **B** from Gartner LP, Hiatt JL: *Color textbook of histology*, ed 3, Philadelphia, 2007, Saunders.)

contents back and forth between the contracting and relaxing haustra. The movements massage the intestinal contents, called the **fecal mass** at that point, and facilitate the absorption of water. Propulsive movement occurs with the proximal-to-distal contraction of several haustral units. **Peristaltic movements** also occur and promote the emptying of the colon. The **gastrocolic reflex** initiates propulsion in the entire colon, usually during or immediately after eating, when chyme enters from the ileum. The gastrocolic reflex causes the fecal mass to pass rapidly into the sigmoid colon and rectum, stimulating defecation. Gastrin may participate in stimulating this reflex. Epinephrine inhibits contractile activity as do exogenous opioids.

Approximately 500 to 700 mL of chyme flows from the ileum to the cecum per day. Most of the water is absorbed in the colon by diffusion and active transport. Aldosterone increases colon membrane permeability to sodium, thereby increasing both the diffusion of sodium into the cell and the active transport of sodium across the basolateral membrane to the interstitial fluid. (See Chapters 3, 21, and 38 for a discussion of aldosterone secretion.) This increases the cell-to-lumen diffusion gradient for potassium. Potassium moves outward, and chloride is absorbed with sodium as the complementary anion. Chloride also enters the cell in exchange for bicarbonate. The colon does not absorb monosaccharides and amino acids, but does absorb some short-chain free fatty acids produced by bacterial fermentation.

Absorption and epithelial transport occur in the cecum, ascending colon, transverse colon, and descending colon. By the time the fecal mass enters the sigmoid colon, the mass consists entirely of wastes and is called the **feces**, composed of food residue, unabsorbed gastrointestinal secretions, shed epithelial cells, and bacteria. The movement of feces into the sigmoid colon and rectum stimulates the **defecation reflex** (**rectosphincteric reflex**). The rectal wall stretches and the tonically constricted internal anal sphincter relaxes, creating the urge to defecate. The defecation reflex can be overridden voluntarily by contraction of the external anal sphincter and muscles of the pelvic floor. The rectal wall gradually relaxes, reducing tension, and the urge to defecate passes. Retrograde contraction of the rectum may displace the feces out of the rectal vault until a more convenient time for evacuation. Pain or fear of pain associated with defecation (e.g., rectal fissures or hemorrhoids) can inhibit the defecation reflex. The defecation reflex is regulated by parasympathetic cholinergic fibers. Voluntary inhibition or facilitation of defecation is mediated from cortical projections onto the medulla and down to sacral segments of the cord.

Squatting and sitting facilitate defecation because these positions straighten the angle between the rectum and anal canal and increase the efficiency of straining (increasing intraabdominal pressure). Intraabdominal pressure is increased by initiating the **Valsalva maneuver**—inhaling and forcing the diaphragm and chest muscles against the closed glottis to increase both intrathoracic and intraabdominal pressure which is transmitted to the rectum.

The Gastrointestinal Tract and Immunity

The gastrointestinal tract plays a major role in immune defenses by killing many microorganisms.[11] The mucosa of the intestine covers a large surface area, and mucosal secretions produce antibodies, particularly immunoglobulin A (IgA), and enzymes that provide defenses against pathogenic microorganisms. Small intestinal **Paneth cells**, located near the base of the crypts of Leiberkühn, produce defensins and other antimicrobial peptides and lysozymes important to mucosal immunity. Small intestinal **Peyer patches** (lymph nodes containing collections of lymphocytes, plasma cells, and macrophages) are most numerous in the ileum and produce antimicrobial peptides and IgA as a component of the gut-associated lymph tissue in the small intestine (see Fig. 40.15, *B*). Peyer patches are important for antigen processing and immune defense (see Fig. 8.3). Intestinal macrophages phagocytize pathogenic bacteria without releasing harmful inflammatory cytokines.[12]

Intestinal Microbiome

The bacterial flora vary greatly in their diversity and number throughout the normal gastrointestinal tract, with an increasing number of bacteria from the stomach to the distal colon. The intestinal tract is sterile at birth but becomes colonized with *Escherichia coli, Clostridium welchii,* and *Streptococcus* within a few hours. Within 3 to 4 weeks after birth, the normal flora are established and become stable by 2 years of age. There are hundreds of bacterial species, but the most common bacteria are from the genera *Bacteroides, Bifidobacterium, Eubacterium, Fusobacterium, Clostridium,* and *Lactobacillus,* and their diversity and number vary along the length of the intestine. Genetics, diet, environmental pollution, personal hygiene, vaccination, infection, antibiotics and other drugs, and radiation exposure affect the normal composition of bacterial flora. The number and diversity of bacteria change with aging and are influenced by diet, chronic disease, medications, and residential communities.[13] The intestinal bacteria do not have major digestive or absorptive functions but do play a role in metabolism of bile salts, estrogens, androgens, lipids, carbohydrates, various nitrogenous substances, and drugs. They produce antimicrobial peptides, hormones, neurotransmitters, antiinflammatory metabolites, vitamin K_2, and B vitamins; destroy toxins; prevent pathogen colonization; and alert the immune system to protect against infection. They are important to overall health, and when altered (dysbiosis) or translocated, they cause disease.[14] The normal flora do not have the virulence factors associated with pathogenic microorganisms, thus permitting immune tolerances.[15] The gastrointestinal microbiota also have regulatory influences on systemic innate and adaptive immune responses and inflammation, including expansion and activity of T-cell populations and systemic antiinflammatory signaling.[16,17]

Bacteria in the stomach are relatively sparse because of the secretion of hydrochloric acid that kills ingested pathogens or inhibits bacterial growth (with the exception of *Helicobacter pylori*). Bile acid secretion, intestinal motility, and antibody production suppress bacterial growth in the duodenum, and in the duodenum and jejunum there is a low concentration of aerobes (10^1 to 10^4/mL), primarily streptococci, lactobacilli, staphylococci, enterobacteria, and *Bacteroides*. Anaerobes are found distal to the ileocecal valve. They constitute about 95% of the fecal flora in the colon and contribute one-third of the solid bulk of feces.

Splanchnic Blood Flow

The splanchnic blood flow provides blood to the esophagus, stomach, small and large intestines, liver, gallbladder, pancreas, and spleen (Fig. 41.16). Blood flow is regulated by cardiac output and blood volume, the autonomic nervous system, hormones, and local autoregulatory blood flow mechanisms. The splanchnic circulation serves as an important reservoir of blood volume to maintain circulation to the heart and lungs when needed. The superior and inferior mesenteric arteries provide the blood supply to the large intestine (see Figs. 41.15 and 41.16).

ACCESSORY ORGANS OF DIGESTION

The liver, gallbladder, and exocrine pancreas all secrete substances necessary for the digestion of chyme. These secretions are delivered to the duodenum through the sphincter of Oddi at the major duodenal papilla (of Vater) (Fig. 41.17). The liver produces bile, which contains salts necessary for fat emulsification and absorption. Between meals

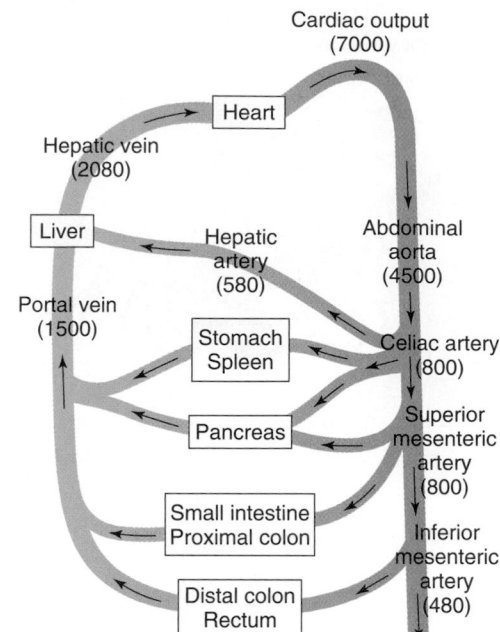

FIGURE 41.16 Major Blood Vessels and Organs Supplied with Blood in the Splanchnic Circulation. Numbers in parentheses reflect approximate blood flow values (mL/min) for each major vessel in an 80-kg normal, resting, adult human subject. Arrows indicate the direction of blood flow. (Modified from Johnson LR: *Gastrointestinal pathophysiology,* St Louis, 2001, Mosby.)

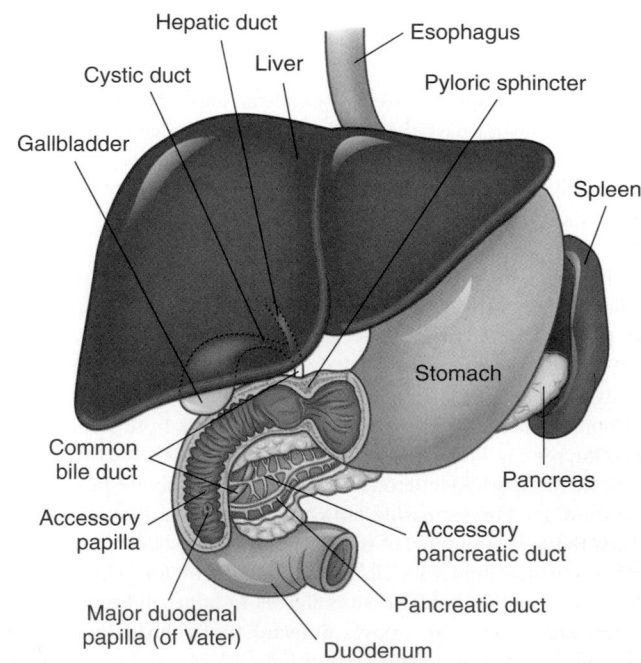

FIGURE 41.17 Locations of the Liver, Gallbladder, and Exocrine Pancreas, Which Are the Accessory Organs of Digestion.

bile is stored in the gallbladder. The exocrine pancreas produces enzymes needed for the complete digestion of carbohydrates, proteins, and fats. The exocrine pancreas also produces an alkaline fluid that neutralizes chyme, creating a duodenal pH that supports enzymatic action. The liver receives nutrients absorbed by the small intestine and metabolizes or synthesizes these nutrients into forms that can be absorbed by the

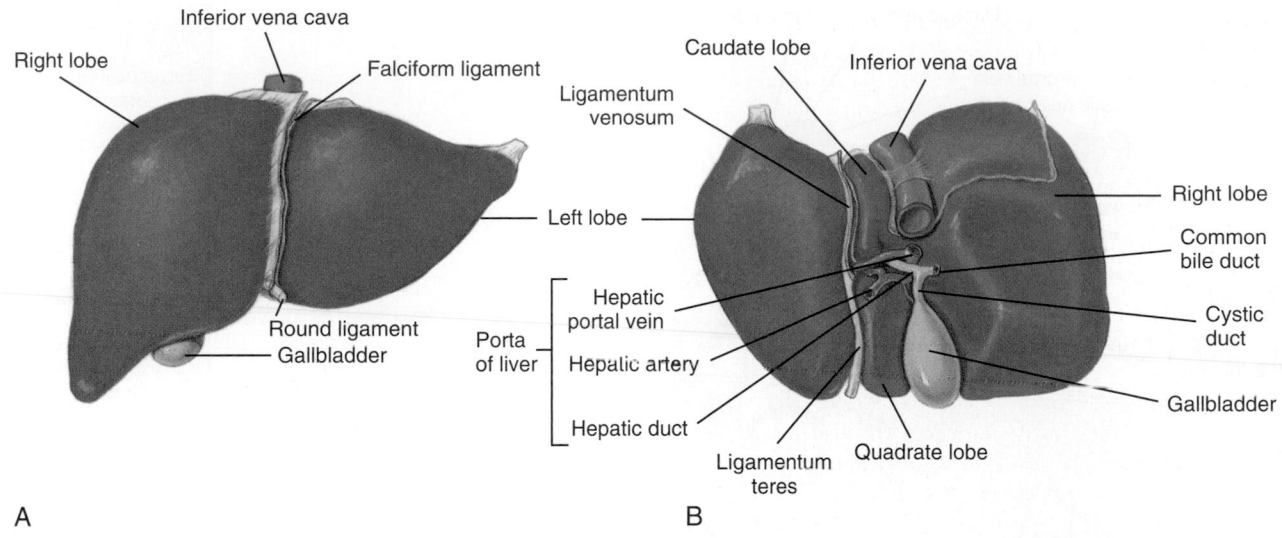

FIGURE 41.18 Gross Structure of the Liver. **A,** Anterior surface. **B,** Visceral surface. (From Applegate E: *The anatomy and physiology learning system*, ed 4, St Louis, 2011, Saunders.)

body's cells. It then releases the nutrients into the bloodstream or stores them for later use.

Liver

The liver, which weighs 1200 to 1600 g, is the largest solid organ in the body. It is located under the right diaphragm and is divided into right and left lobes. The larger, right lobe is divided further into the caudate and quadrate lobes (Fig. 41.18). The *falciform ligament* separates the right and left lobes and attaches the liver to the anterior abdominal wall. A fibrous cord called the *round ligament (ligamentum teres)* extends along the free edge of the falciform ligament. The round ligament is the remnant of the umbilical vein and extends from the umbilicus to the inferior surface of the liver. The *coronary ligament* branches from the falciform ligament and extends over the superior surface of the right and left lobes, binding the liver to the inferior surface of the diaphragm. The liver is covered by a fibroelastic capsule called the *Glisson capsule* which contains blood vessels, lymphatics, and nerves. When the liver is diseased or swollen, distention of the capsule causes pain because it is innervated by sensory neurons of the lower intercostal nerves.

The metabolic functions of the liver require a large amount of blood. The liver receives blood from both arterial and venous sources. The hepatic artery is formed by the confluence of superior mesenteric and splenic veins and receives blood from the inferior mesenteric, gastric, and cystic veins. It provides oxygenated blood to the liver at the rate of 400 to 500 mL/minute (about 25% of the cardiac output). The hepatic portal vein, which receives deoxygenated blood from the inferior and superior mesenteric veins and the splenic vein, delivers about 1000 to 1200 mL/minute of blood to the liver. The hepatic portal vein, which carries 70% of the blood to the liver, is rich in nutrients that have been absorbed from the intestinal tract (Fig. 41.19).

Within the liver lobes are multiple, smaller anatomic units called liver lobules (Fig. 41.20). The lobules are formed of cords or plates of hepatocytes, which are the functional cells of the liver. These cells are capable of regeneration; therefore damaged or resected liver tissue can regrow. Hepatocytes secrete electrolytes, lipids, lecithin, bile acids, and cholesterol into the canaliculi. Plasma proteins are also synthesized and released into the bloodstream. Lipocytes are star-shaped cells that store lipids, including vitamin A. Small capillaries, or sinusoids, are

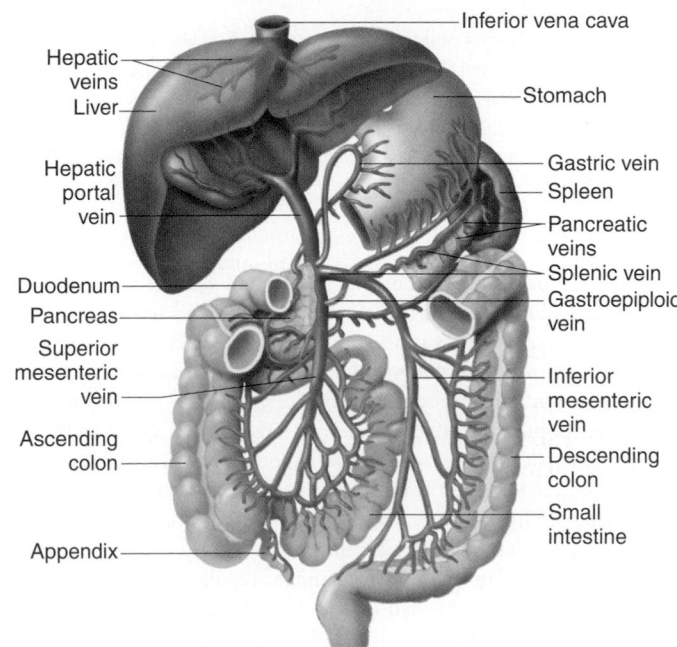

FIGURE 41.19 Hepatic Portal Circulation. In this unusual circulatory route, a vein is located between two capillary beds. The hepatic portal vein collects blood from capillaries in visceral structures located in the abdomen and empties into the liver for distribution to the hepatic capillaries. Hepatic veins return blood to the inferior vena cava. (Organs are not drawn to scale.) (From Patton KT, Thibodeau GA: *The human body in health & disease*, ed 7, St Louis, 2018, Elsevier.)

located between the plates of hepatocytes. They receive a mixture of venous and arterial blood from branches of the hepatic artery and hepatic portal vein. Blood from the sinusoids drains into a central vein in the middle of each liver lobule. Venous blood from all the lobules then flows into the hepatic vein, which empties into the inferior vena cava. The sinusoids of the liver lobules are lined with highly permeable endothelium. Their permeability enhances the transport of nutrients from the sinusoids into the hepatocytes, where they are metabolized.[18]

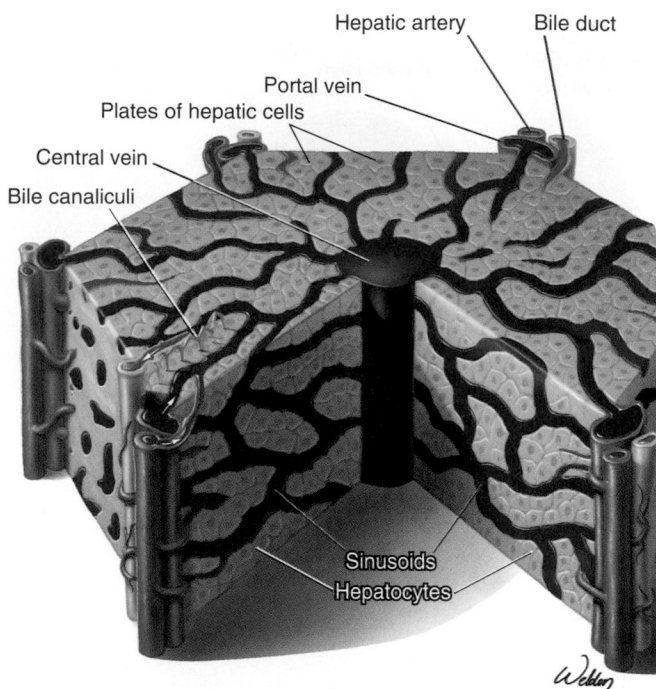

FIGURE 41.20 Diagrammatic Representation of a Liver Lobule. A central vein is located in the center of the lobule, with plates of hepatocytes disposed radially. Branches of the portal vein and hepatic artery are located on the periphery of the lobule, and blood from both vessels perfuses the sinusoids. Peripherally located bile ducts drain the bile canaliculi that run between the hepatocytes. (From Polin RA, et al: *Fetal and neonatal physiology*, ed 4, St Louis, 2011, Saunders.)

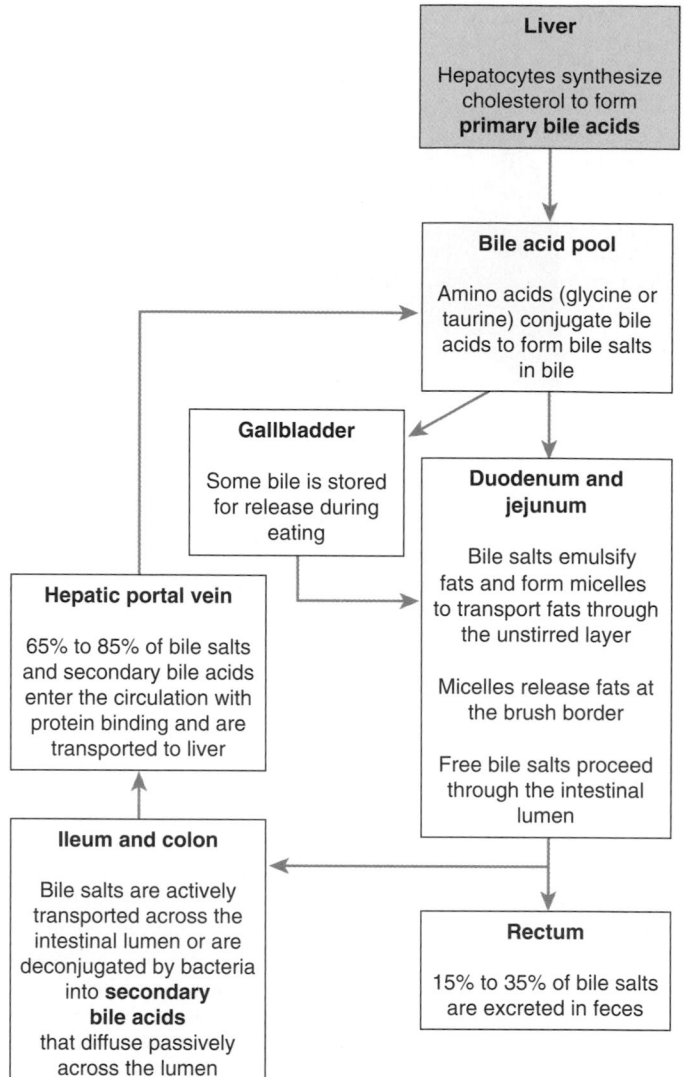

FIGURE 41.21 The Enterohepatic Circulation of Bile Salts.

Immune functions of the liver are carried out by various cells. Sinusoidal endothelial cells detect microbial infection through pattern recognition receptor activation and as antigen-presenting cells.[19] The sinusoids are lined with phagocytic **Kupffer cells** (macrophages), part of the mononuclear phagocyte system (see Chapters 7 and 28) and are the largest population of tissue macrophages in the body. They are found in the spaces between sinusoidal endothelial cells, are bactericidal, and are central to innate immunity. Kupffer cells also are important for healing of liver injury and for bilirubin production and lipid metabolism. **Stellate cells** are perisinusoidal cells and contain retinoids (vitamin A), are contractile in liver injury, regulate sinusoidal blood flow, can proliferate into myofibroblasts, participate in liver fibrosis, remove foreign substances from the blood, and trap bacteria. **Natural killer cells (pit cells)** also are found in the sinusoidal lumen; they produce interferon-γ and are important in tumor defense. Between the endothelial lining of the sinusoid and the hepatocyte is the **Disse space**, which drains interstitial fluid into the hepatic lymph system.

Secretion of Bile

The liver assists intestinal digestion by secreting 700 to 1200 mL of bile per day. **Bile** is an alkaline, bitter-tasting yellowish green fluid that contains bile salts (conjugated bile acids), cholesterol, bilirubin (a pigment), electrolytes, and water. It is formed by hepatocytes and secreted into the bile canaliculi, which are small channels adjacent to hepatocytes. **Bile salts** are required for the intestinal emulsification and absorption of fats. The **bile canaliculi** empty into hepatic bile ducts and eventually drain into the **common bile duct** (Fig. 41.21). The union of the common bile duct and pancreatic duct is at the papilla or **ampulla of Vater**, which empties into the duodenum through an opening called the **major duodenal papilla** and is surrounded by the **sphincter of Oddi**. Having

facilitated fat emulsification and absorption in the small intestine, most bile salts are actively absorbed in the terminal ileum and returned to the liver through the portal circulation for resecretion. The cycle of hepatic secretion, intestinal absorption, and hepatic resecretion of bile acids is termed the **enterohepatic circulation** (see Fig. 41.21).

Bile has two fractional components: the acid-dependent fraction and the acid-independent fraction. Hepatocytes secrete the **bile acid-dependent fraction** of the bile. This fraction consists of bile acids, cholesterol, lecithin (a phospholipid), and bilirubin (a bile pigment). The **bile acid-independent fraction** of the bile, which is secreted by the hepatocytes and epithelial cells of the bile canaliculi, is a bicarbonate-rich aqueous fluid that gives bile its alkaline pH.

Bile salts are conjugated in the liver from primary and secondary bile acids. The **primary bile acids** are cholic acid and chenodeoxycholic (chenic acid or chenodiol) acid. These acids are synthesized from cholesterol by the hepatocytes. The **secondary bile acids** are deoxycholic acid and lithocholic acid. These acids are formed in the small intestine by the action of intestinal bacteria, after which they are absorbed and flow to the liver (see Fig. 41.21). Both forms of bile acids are conjugated with amino acids (glycine or taurine) in the liver to form bile salts. Conjugation makes the bile acids more water soluble, thus restricting their diffusion from the duodenum and ileum. The primary and secondary bile acids together form the **bile acid pool**.

Some bile salts are deconjugated by intestinal bacteria to secondary bile acids. These acids diffuse passively into the portal blood from both small and large intestines. An increase in the plasma concentration of bile acids accelerates the uptake and resecretion of bile acids and salts by the hepatocytes. Bile secretion is called **choleresis**. A **choleretic agent** is a substance that stimulates the liver to secrete bile. One strong stimulus is a high concentration of bile salts. Other choleretics include secretin, which increases the rate of bile flow by promoting the secretion of bicarbonate from canaliculi and other intrahepatic bile ducts; cholecystokinin; and vagal stimulation.

Metabolism of Bilirubin

Bilirubin is a byproduct of destruction of aged red blood cells. It gives bile a greenish black color and produces the yellow tinge of jaundice. Aged red blood cells are taken up and destroyed by macrophages of the mononuclear phagocyte system, primarily in the spleen and liver. (In the liver these macrophages are Kupffer cells.) Within these cells, hemoglobin is separated into its component parts—heme and globin (Fig. 41.22). The globin component is further degraded into its constituent amino acids, which are recycled to form new protein. The heme moiety is converted to **biliverdin** by the enzymatic (heme oxygenase) cleavage of iron. The iron attaches to transferrin in the plasma and can be stored in the liver or used by the bone marrow to make new red blood cells. The biliverdin is enzymatically converted to bilirubin in the macrophage and then is released into the plasma. In the plasma, bilirubin binds to albumin and is known as **unconjugated bilirubin**, or free bilirubin, which is lipid soluble. Unconjugated bilirubin also has a role as an antioxidant and provides cytoprotection.[20]

In the liver, unconjugated bilirubin moves from plasma in the sinusoids into the hepatocyte. Within hepatocytes it joins with glucuronic acid to form **conjugated bilirubin**, which is water soluble. Conjugation transforms bilirubin from a lipid-soluble substance that can cross biologic membranes to a water-soluble substance that can be excreted in the bile. When conjugated bilirubin reaches the distal ileum and colon, it is deconjugated by bacteria and converted to **urobilinogen**. Urobilinogen is then reabsorbed in the intestines and transported to the kidney where it is excreted in the urine as urobilin, giving urine its yellow color. A small amount of urobilin is recirculated back into the liver and eliminated in feces as stercobilin, which contributes to the stool's brown pigmentation.

Vascular and Hematologic Functions

Because of its extensive vascular network, the liver can store a large volume of blood. The amount stored at any one time depends on pressure relationships in the arteries and veins. The liver also can release blood to maintain systemic circulatory volume in the event of hemorrhage.

The liver also has hemostatic functions. It synthesizes most of the clotting factors (see Chapters 7 and 28). Vitamin K_1 (phylloquinone, synthesized by plants and ingested in the diet) and vitamin K_2 (menaquinone, synthesized by intestinal bacteria) are fat-soluble vitamins essential for the synthesis of clotting factors (prothrombin and factors VII, IX, and X). Vitamin K_2 also activates matrix GLA protein (MGP), which inhibits the deposits of calcium in arterial walls.[21] Because bile salts are needed for absorption of fats, vitamin K absorption depends on adequate bile production in the liver. Impairment of vitamin K absorption diminishes production of clotting factors and increases risk of bleeding.

Metabolism of Nutrients

Fats. Ingested fat absorbed by lacteals in the intestinal villi enters the liver through the lymphatics, primarily as triglycerides. In the liver

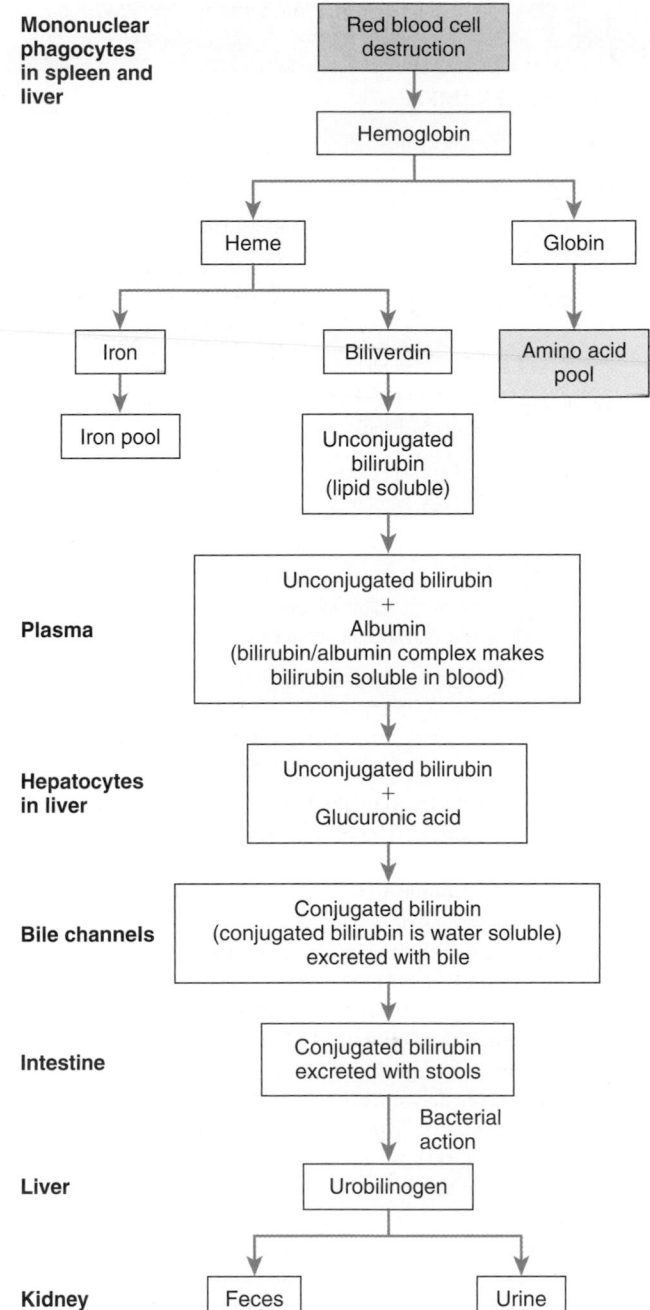

FIGURE 41.22 Bilirubin Metabolism. See text for further explanation.

the triglycerides can be hydrolyzed to glycerol and free fatty acids and used to produce metabolic energy adenosine triphosphate (ATP), or they can be released into the bloodstream bound to proteins (lipoproteins). The lipoproteins are carried by the blood to adipose cells for storage. The liver also synthesizes phospholipids and cholesterol, which are needed for the hepatic production of bile salts, steroid hormones, components of plasma membranes, and other special molecules.

Proteins. Protein synthesis requires the presence of all the essential amino acids (obtained only from food), as well as nonessential amino acids. Proteins perform many important functions in the body and are summarized in Table 41.3.

Within hepatocytes, amino acids are converted to carbohydrates by the removal of ammonia (NH_3), a process known as **deamination**. The

TABLE 41.3	PROTEIN FUNCTIONS IN THE BODY
ROLE	**EXAMPLE**
Contraction	Actin and myosin enable muscle contraction.
Energy	Proteins can be metabolized for energy.
Fluid balance	Albumin is a major source of plasma oncotic pressure.
Protection	Antibodies, complement, and C-reactive protein protect against infection and foreign substances. α_1-antitrypsin and α_1-antichymotrypsin inhibit proteolytic enzymes.
Regulation	Enzymes control chemical reactions; hormones regulate many physiologic processes.
Structure	Collagen fibers provide structural support to many parts of the body; keratin strengthens skin, hair, and nails.
Transport	Hemoglobin transports oxygen and carbon dioxide in the blood; plasma proteins serve as transport molecules; proteins in cell membranes control movement of materials into and out of cells.
Coagulation	Hemostasis is regulated by proteins that balance coagulation and anticoagulation (factors II, VII, IX and X).

ammonia is converted to urea by the liver and passes into the blood to be excreted by the kidneys. The plasma proteins, including albumins and α- and β- globulins (not gamma globulin, which is formed in lymph nodes and lymphoid tissue), are synthesized by the liver. The liver also synthesizes several nonessential amino acids and serum enzymes that become elevated with liver injury (and other diseases):

- Aspartate aminotransferase (AST) (previously called *serum glutamate-oxaloacetate transaminase [SGOT]):* also present in red blood cells and skeletal muscle; AST transfers an α-amino group between aspartate and glutamate.
- Alanine aminotransferase (ALT) (previously called *serum glutamate-pyruvate transaminase [SGPT]):* also present in small amounts in the kidneys, heart, skeletal muscle, and pancreas; ALT transfers an amino group from alanine to α-ketoglutarate to form pyruvate and glutamate.
- Lactate dehydrogenase (LDH): catalyzes the conversion of lactate to pyruvate; LDH is widely distributed throughout the body and different isoenzymes are found in different tissues.
- Alkaline phosphatase: removes phosphate groups, particularly in an alkaline environment.
- Gamma-glutamyltransferase: transfers the gamma-glutamyl moiety of glutathione to an acceptor to form glutamate and is a pro-oxidant.

Reference values for the listed enzymes can be reviewed in Table 41.6, later in this chapter, and are summarized on the inside back book cover.

Carbohydrates. The liver contributes to the stability of blood glucose levels by releasing glucose during states of hypoglycemia (low blood glucose levels) and taking up glucose during states of hyperglycemia (high blood glucose levels) and storing it as glycogen (glycogenesis) or converting it to fat. When all glycogen stores have been used, the liver can convert amino acids and glycerol to glucose.

Metabolic Detoxification

The liver alters exogenous and endogenous chemicals (e.g., drugs), foreign molecules, and hormones to make them less toxic or less biologically active. This process, called metabolic detoxification (biotransformation), diminishes intestinal or renal tubular reabsorption of potentially toxic substances and facilitates their intestinal and renal excretion. In this way alcohol, barbiturates, amphetamines, steroids, and hormones (including estrogens, aldosterone, antidiuretic hormone, and testosterone) are metabolized or detoxified, preventing excessive accumulation and adverse effects.

Although metabolic detoxification is usually protective, sometimes the end products of metabolic detoxification become toxins or active metabolites. Those of alcohol metabolism, for example, are acetaldehyde and hydrogen, which can damage hepatocytes. Acetaldehyde damages cellular mitochondria, and the excess hydrogen promotes fat accumulation, impairing the liver's ability to function (see Chapter 2).

Storage of Minerals and Vitamins

The liver stores certain vitamins and minerals, including iron and copper, in times of excessive intake and releases them in times of need. Iron is stored in the liver as ferritin, an iron-protein complex, and is released as needed for red blood cell production. The liver can store vitamins B_{12} and D for several months and vitamin A for several years. The liver also stores vitamins E and K. Iron is stored in the liver as ferritin, an iron-protein complex, and is released as needed for red blood cell production.

Gallbladder

The gallbladder is a saclike organ that lies on the inferior surface of the liver (see Figs. 41.18 and 41.23). Its primary function is to store and concentrate bile between meals. The wall of the gallbladder is composed of the mucous membrane, muscularis, and serosa. During the interdigestive period, bile flows from the liver through the right or left hepatic duct into the common bile duct and meets resistance at the closed sphincter of Oddi, which controls flow into the duodenum and prevents reflux of duodenal contents into the pancreatobiliary system. Bile then flows into the gallbladder through the cystic duct where it is concentrated and stored. The mucosa of the gallbladder wall readily absorbs water and electrolytes, leaving a high concentration of bile salts, bile pigments, and cholesterol. The gallbladder holds about 90 mL of bile.

Within 30 minutes after eating, the gallbladder begins to contract, forcing stored bile through the cystic duct and into the common bile duct. The sphincter of Oddi relaxes, and bile flows into the duodenum through the major duodenal papilla. During the cephalic and gastric phases of digestion (see the Phases of Gastric Secretion section), gallbladder contraction is mediated by cholinergic branches of the vagus nerve. Hormonal regulation of gallbladder contraction is derived primarily from the release of *cholecystokinin* secreted by the duodenal and jejunal mucosa in the presence of fat. Vasoactive intestinal peptide, pancreatic polypeptide, and sympathetic nerve stimulation relax the gallbladder.

Exocrine Pancreas

The pancreas is approximately 20 cm long, with its head tucked into the curve of the duodenum and its tail touching the spleen. The body of the pancreas lies deep in the abdomen, behind the stomach (see Fig. 41.17). The pancreas is unique in that it has endocrine as well as exocrine functions. The endocrine pancreas secretes insulin, glucagon, somatostatin, and pancreatic polypeptide (see Chapter 21).

The exocrine pancreas is composed of acinar cells that secrete enzymes and networks of ducts that secrete alkaline fluids with important digestive functions. The acinar cells are organized into spherical lobules (acini) around small secretory ducts (see Fig. 41.23). Secretions drain into a system of ducts that leads to the pancreatic duct (Wirsung duct),

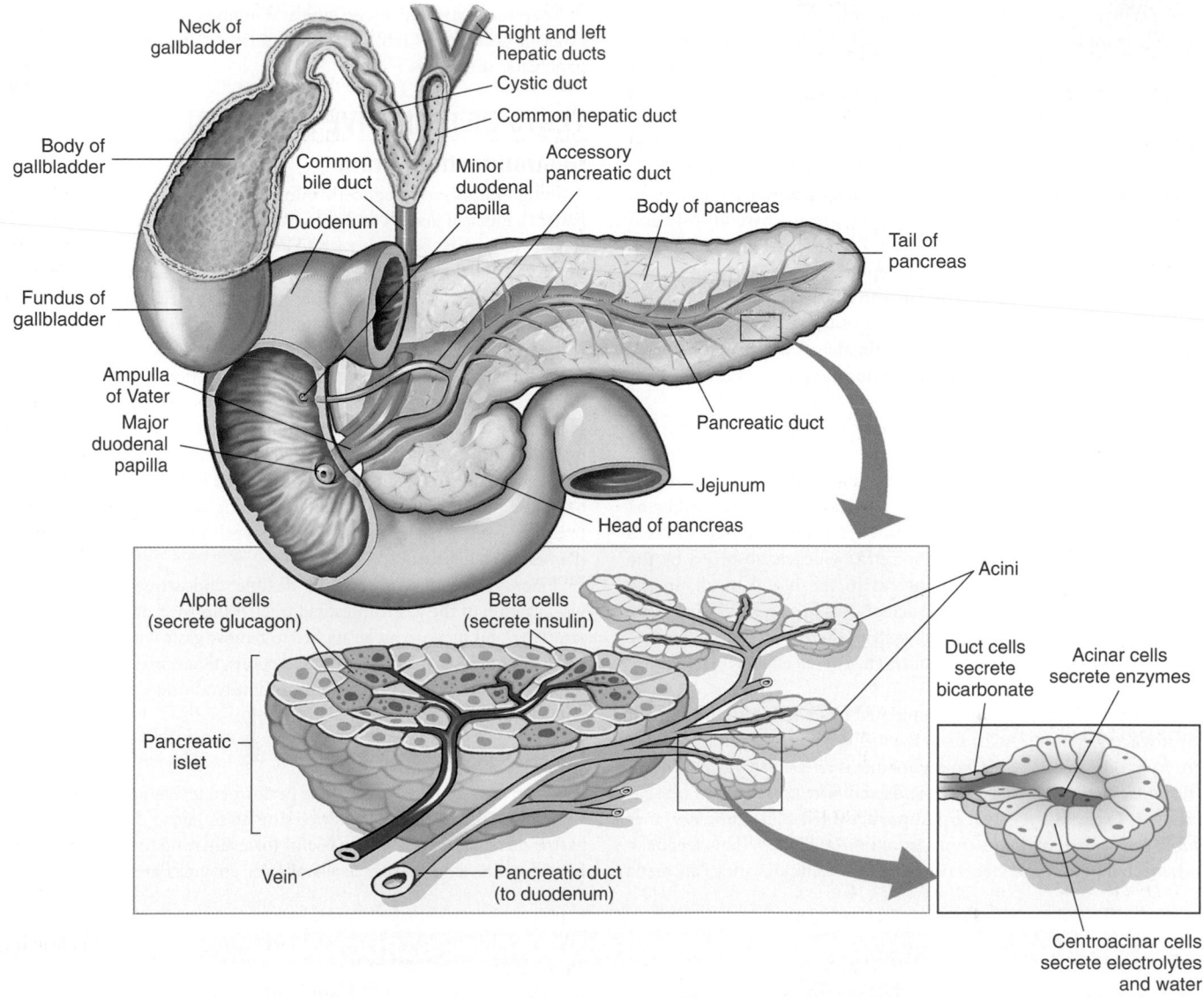

FIGURE 41.23 Associated Structures of the Gallbladder, Pancreas, and Pancreatic Acinar Cells and Duct. (Modified from Patton KT, Thibodeau GA: *Anatomy & physiology*, ed 6, St Louis, 2007, Mosby.)

which empties into the common bile duct at the ampulla of Vater and then through the duodenal papilla into the duodenum. In some individuals an accessory duct (the duct of Santorini) branches off the pancreatic duct and drains directly into the duodenum at an opening called the *minor duodenal papilla* (see Fig. 41.23).

Arterial blood is supplied to the pancreas by branches of the celiac and superior mesenteric arteries. Venous blood leaves the head of the pancreas through the tributaries to the hepatic portal vein, with the body and tail being drained through the splenic vein. All hormonal pancreatic secretions also pass through the hepatic portal vein into the liver.

Pancreatic innervation arises from parasympathetic neurons of the vagus nerve, which stimulate enzymatic and hormonal secretion. Sympathetic postganglionic fibers from the celiac and superior mesenteric plexuses innervate the blood vessels and cause vasoconstriction and inhibit pancreatic secretion.

The aqueous secretions of the exocrine pancreas are isotonic and contain potassium, sodium, bicarbonate, magnesium, calcium, and chloride. Sodium and potassium concentrations are about equal to those in the plasma. Pancreatic ductal cells secrete bicarbonate and the

concentration in pancreatic juice varies directly with the secretory flow rate. As bicarbonate secretion increases, chloride secretion decreases to maintain a constant anionic concentration. The highly alkaline pancreatic juice neutralizes the acidic chyme that enters the duodenum from the stomach and provides the alkaline medium needed for the actions of digestive enzymes and the intestinal absorption of fat.

In the pancreas, transport of water and electrolytes through the ductal epithelium involves active and passive mechanisms. The ductal cells actively transport hydrogen into the blood and bicarbonate into the duct lumen. Potassium and chloride are secreted by diffusion according to changes in electrochemical potential gradients. As the secretion flows down the duct, water is osmotically transported into the pancreatic juice until it becomes isosmotic. At low flow rates, bicarbonate is exchanged passively for chloride, but at higher flow rates there is less time for this exchange and bicarbonate concentration increases. Because eating stimulates the flow of pancreatic juice, the juice is most alkaline when it needs to be—during digestion.

The *pancreatic enzymes* hydrolyze proteins (proteases), carbohydrates (amylases), and fats (lipases). The proteolytic (protein-digesting) enzymes (proteases) include trypsin, chymotrypsin, carboxypeptidase, and elastase.

These enzymes are secreted in their inactive forms—that is, as trypsinogen, chymotrypsinogen, and procarboxypeptidase—to protect the pancreas from the digestive effects of its own enzymes. For further protection the pancreas produces **trypsin inhibitor**, which prevents the activation of proteolytic enzymes while they are in the pancreas. Once in the duodenum, the inactive forms (proenzymes) are activated by **enterokinase**, an enzyme secreted by the duodenal mucosa. Trypsinogen is the first proenzyme to be activated. Its conversion to trypsin stimulates the conversion of chymotrypsinogen to chymotrypsin and procarboxypeptidase to carboxypeptidase. Each of these enzymes cleaves specific peptide bonds to reduce polypeptides to smaller peptides.

Pancreatic α-amylase is secreted in active form and digests intestinal carbohydrate by cleaving interior α-1,4-glucosidic bonds to yield glucose and maltose at an optimum pH of approximately 6.9. **Pancreatic lipases** hydrolyze triglycerides, cholesterol, and phospholipids to free fatty acids in the intestine.

Secretion of the aqueous and enzymatic components of pancreatic juice is controlled by hormonal and vagal stimuli. *Secretin* stimulates the acinar and duct cells to secrete the bicarbonate-rich fluid that neutralizes chyme and prepares it for enzymatic digestion. As chyme enters the duodenum, its acidity (pH of 4.5 or less) stimulates the S cells of the duodenum to release secretin, which is absorbed by the intestine and delivered to the pancreas in the bloodstream. In the pancreas, secretin causes ductal and acinar cells to release alkaline fluid. Secretin also inhibits the actions of gastrin, thereby decreasing gastric hydrochloric acid secretion and motility. The overall effect is to neutralize the contents of the duodenum.

Enzymatic secretion follows, stimulated by **cholecystokinin**, which activates acetylcholine (ACh) from the vagus nerve and release of ACh from pancreatic stellate cells. Cholecystokinin is released in the duodenum in response to the essential amino acids and fatty acids already present in chyme. Once in the small intestine, activated pancreatic enzymes inhibit the release of more cholecystokinin and ACh. This feedback mechanism inhibits the secretion of more pancreatic enzymes. Pancreatic polypeptide is released after eating and inhibits postprandial pancreatic exocrine secretion. (Table 41.1 summarizes hormonal stimulation of pancreatic secretions.)

TESTS OF DIGESTIVE FUNCTION

Gastrointestinal Tract

Although important diagnostic information can be obtained from the patient's medical history and presenting symptoms, numerous disease-specific tests must be performed to evaluate the structure and function of the gastrointestinal tract. A description of selected studies is presented in Tables 41.4 and 41.5. Radiography and imaging techniques—including radionuclide, positron emission tomography (PET), magnetic resonance (MR), computed tomography (CT) scanning, and ultrasound—are procedures for evaluating structure and function. Plain radiographs using contrast media such as barium- or iodine-containing compounds can be used to outline the gastrointestinal lumen, biliary tree and pancreatic ducts, fistulae, and arteriovenous systems. CT scanning is particularly useful for diagnosis of intestinal lesions and pancreatic or hepatic tumors or cysts. Ultrasonic scanning is a safe, simple, and relatively inexpensive technique used to detect gallstones and intraabdominal masses, particularly abscesses.

Fiberoptic endoscopy, using flexible endoscopes, allows direct visualization of the gastrointestinal tract. A biopsy channel allows tissue sampling, and suction can be applied to remove gastrointestinal secretions or blood. Analysis of stool, gastric secretions, tissue, and plasma provides important clues to infection, malabsorption syndromes, ulcerative lesions, and tumor growth.

Liver

A variety of diagnostic tests can be performed to evaluate liver function (Table 41.6). Imaging techniques similar to those described for the gastrointestinal tract also are useful for evaluating liver structure and function. Elevated plasma levels of liver enzymes are associated with

TABLE 41.4 SELECTED STUDIES OF GASTROINTESTINAL STRUCTURE

TEST	DESCRIPTION	APPLICATION
Plain roentgenograms	Use of high-energy electromagnetic radiation to evaluate tissue structure by radiopacity or radiolucency	Visualization of the position, size, and structure of abdominal contents
Air or barium contrast roentgenograms	Introduction of radiopaque substances into the upper or lower gastrointestinal tract	Enhanced visualization of the contours, position, and size of the gastrointestinal tract to detect umbilical hernia, ulcers, diverticula, congenital anomalies, polyps, tumors, strictures, obstructions
Endoscopy Esophagoscopy (esophagus) Gastroscopy (stomach) Duodenoscopy (duodenum) Colonoscopy (large intestine) Sigmoidoscopy (sigmoid colon)	Passage of rigid or flexible (fiberoptic) endoscope into the gastrointestinal tract for visualization or biopsy	Visualization or biopsy of inflamed hernias, polyps, ulcers, strictures, varices, tumors, sites of bleeding, mucosal or neoplastic lesions and for culture of *Helicobacter pylori* from stomach
Ultrasound	Use of piezoelectric crystal to generate sound waves that are reflected from tissue interfaces to provide an image	Imaging of abdominal organs (gallbladder, liver, pancreas, spleen), masses, stones, abscesses, structural abnormalities
Computed tomography (CT)	Use of a computer to integrate differences in absorption of a large number of x-rays to produce a cross-sectional image; may be done with contrast agents	Imaging of gallbladder, liver, pancreas, spleen, cysts, hematomas, abscesses, stones, extrahepatic bile ducts, and portal vein
Magnetic resonance imaging	Projection of differences in magnetic properties of molecules within different cells and tissues, using the field of a large magnet	Same applications as CT scan; also can detect blood flow and vessel patency

TABLE 41.5 SELECTED TESTS OF GASTROINTESTINAL FUNCTION

TEST	NORMAL FINDINGS	CLINICAL SIGNIFICANCE OF ABNORMAL FINDINGS
Stool studies	Resident microorganisms: clostridia, enterococci, *Pseudomonas*, a few yeasts	Detection of *Salmonella typhi* (typhoid fever), *Shigella* (dysentery), *Vibrio cholerae* (cholera), *Yersinia* (enterocolitis), *Escherichia coli* (gastroenteritis), *Staphylococcus aureus* (food poisoning), *Clostridium botulinum* (food poisoning), *Clostridium perfringens* (food poisoning), *Aeromonas* (gastroenteritis)
	Fat: 2–6 g/24 hr	Steatorrhea (increased values) can result from intestinal malabsorption or pancreatic insufficiency
	Pus: none	Large amounts of pus are associated with chronic ulcerative colitis, abscesses, and anorectal fistula
	Occult blood: none (orthotolidine or guaiac test)	Positive tests associated with bleeding
	Ova and parasites: none	Detection of *Entamoeba histolytica* (amebiasis), *Giardia lamblia* (giardiasis), and worms
D-Xylose absorption	5-hr urinary excretion: 4.5 g/L Peak blood level: >30 mg/dL	Differentiation of pancreatic steatorrhea (normal D-xylose absorption) from intestinal steatorrhea (impaired D-xylose absorption)
Gastric acid stimulation	11–20 mEq/hr after stimulation	Detection of duodenal ulcers, Zollinger-Ellison syndrome (increased values), gastric atrophy, gastric carcinoma (decreased values)
Manometry (use of water-filled catheters connected to pressure transducers passed into the esophagus, stomach, colon, or rectum to evaluate contractility)	Values vary at different levels of the intestine	Inadequate swallowing, motility, sphincter function
Culture and sensitivity of duodenal contents	No pathogens	Detection of *Salmonella typhi* (typhoid fever)
Breath tests Glucose or D-xylose breath test Urea breath test Lactose breath test	 Negative for hydrogen or CO_2 Negative for isotopically labeled CO_2 Negative for exhaled hydrogen	 May indicate intestinal bacterial overgrowth Presence of *Helicobacter pylori* infection Lactose intolerance

many liver diseases because of the release of cytoplasmic enzymes into the circulation when there is damage to the hepatocyte. Of particular importance are elevations of aminotransferases and lactate dehydrogenase (LDH). Obstruction of bile canaliculi or ducts results in regurgitation of bile back into the hepatic sinusoids and into the circulation, manifesting with elevation of conjugated bilirubin levels. Prothrombin times (a measure of clotting tendency) are often prolonged with both hepatitis and chronic liver disease. In severe disease, other plasma proteins, such as albumin and globulins, may be diminished as a result of hepatocyte damage. Liver biopsies are often performed to evaluate the extent of liver involvement or degeneration with cirrhosis, hepatitis, or fatty liver disease.

Gallbladder

Evaluation of structural alterations in the gallbladder may be achieved by the use of various imaging techniques. Table 41.7 summarizes these techniques. Obstructive pathology of the bile ducts results in elevated values for both conjugated and total serum bilirubin, increased urine urobilinogen level, clay-colored stools, and development of jaundice. Fat absorption can be impaired and the prothrombin time prolonged if vitamin K is not absorbed. With inflammation of the gallbladder, the white cell count is elevated.

Exocrine Pancreas

Tests of pancreatic function are summarized in Table 41.8. Evaluation of serum lipase and urinary amylase provides particularly significant measures of pancreatic injury. Inflammation or obstruction of the

pancreas results in an early increase in serum amylase levels. Serum lipase level remains elevated after serum amylase has returned to normal levels and provides greater sensitivity with delayed presentation of pancreatitis. Elevation of urine amylase level also occurs later (after 48 hours) when serum amylase may have returned to normal levels. Urinary trypsinogen 2 (available as dipstick) is used to diagnose acute pancreatitis and is comparable to serum amylase and lipase.[22] Increased stool fat can reflect pancreatic insufficiency caused by decreased lipase secretion when biliary function is normal.

AGING AND THE GASTROINTESTINAL SYSTEM

Age-related change in gastrointestinal function is variable among individuals and is related to health status and disease treatments, genetics, and environmental factors.[23] Changes can begin to occur before 50 years of age. Tooth enamel and dentin wear down, making the teeth vulnerable to cavities. Teeth are lost, often as a result of periodontal (gum) disease, recession of the gums, osteoporotic bone changes, and more brittle roots that fracture easily. Taste buds decline in number, and the sense of smell diminishes. Together these losses decrease the sense of taste. These oral and sensory changes make eating less pleasurable and reduce appetite in very old adults. Food may not be chewed or lubricated sufficiently, making swallowing difficult. The esophagus develops decreased motility, and changes in the upper esophageal sphincter, history of stroke, and dementia may affect swallowing and contribute to gastroesophageal reflux.[24] Age also diminishes gastric

TABLE 41.6   COMMON LIVER FUNCTION TESTS

TEST	NORMAL VALUE	INTERPRETATION
Serum Enzymes		
Alkaline phosphatase	35–150 units/L	Increases with biliary obstruction and cholestatic hepatitis
Gamma-glutamyl transpeptidase	Male 12–38 units/L	Increases with biliary obstruction and cholestatic hepatitis
	Female 9–31 units/L	
Aspartate aminotransferase (previously serum glutamate-oxaloacetate transaminase)	Male 8–40 units/L Female 6–34 units/L	Increases with hepatocellular injury and injury in other tissues (e.g., skeletal and cardiac muscle)
Alanine aminotransferase (previously serum glutamate-pyruvate transaminase)	Male 10–40 units/L Female 9–32 units/L	Increases with hepatocellular injury and necrosis
Lactate dehydrogenase	110–220 units/L	Isoenzyme LD_5 is elevated with hypoxic and primary liver injury
5′-Nucleotidase	2–11 units/L	Increases with increase in alkaline phosphatase and cholestatic disorders
Bilirubin Metabolism		
Serum bilirubin		
Unconjugated (indirect)	0.1–1.0 mg/dL	Increases with hemolysis (lysis of red blood cells)
Conjugated (direct)	0.1–0.4 mg/dL	Increases with hepatocellular injury or obstruction
TOTAL	<1.0 mg/dL	Increases with biliary obstruction
Urine bilirubin	0	Increases with biliary obstruction
Urine urobilinogen	0–4 mg/24 hr	Increases with hemolysis or shunting of portal blood flow
Serum Proteins		
Albumin	3.5–5.5 g/dL	Reduced with hepatocellular injury
Globulin	2–4 g/dL	Increases with hepatitis
TOTAL	6–7 g/dL	
Albumin/globulin ratio	1.5:1 to 2.5:1	Ratio reverses with chronic hepatitis or other chronic liver disease
Transferrin	250–300 mcg/dL	Liver damage with decreased values, iron deficiency with increased values
Alpha fetoprotein	6–20 ng/mL	Elevated values in primary hepatocellular carcinoma
Blood-Clotting Functions		
Prothrombin time	10–13 sec or 90%–100% of control	Increases with chronic liver disease (cirrhosis) or vitamin K deficiency
Partial thromboplastin time	22–37 sec	Increases with severe liver disease or heparin therapy
Bromsulphthalein excretion	<6% retention in 45 min	Increased retention with hepatocellular injury

TABLE 41.7   DIAGNOSTIC EVALUATION OF THE GALLBLADDER

TEST	APPLICATION
Plain roentgenogram of the abdomen	Visualization of calcified gallstones
Oral cholecystogram (use of an oral contrast medium such as iopanoic acid, which is excreted with bile and concentrated in the gallbladder for visualization by radiography; may be administered as a double dose)	Visualization of gallstones; evaluation of filling and emptying of gallbladder
Intravenous cholangiography (use of intravenous contrast agents for visualization of gallbladder and bile ducts)	Diagnosis of acute gallbladder inflammation (cholecystitis) or disease of bile ducts
Cholecystography (ultrasound imaging of gallbladder and bile ducts including endoscopic ultrasound)	Preferred method for detecting gallstones; differentiation of hepatic disease from biliary obstruction; diagnosis of chronic cholecystitis
Cholescintigraphy (radioisotope imaging of gallbladder)	Diagnosis of cholecystitis in individuals allergic to iodine-containing contrast agents; diagnosis of cystic duct obstruction
Endoscopic retrograde cholangiography (instillation of contrast medium through cannulation of ampulla of Vater with a duodenoscope)	Differentiation of intrahepatic or extrahepatic obstructive jaundice Diagnosis of gallstones
Computed tomography	Diagnosis of biliary obstruction or malignancy when ultrasound is not successful
Magnetic resonance cholangiography	Diagnosis of complicated cholelithiasis or choledocholithiasis

TABLE 41.8 SELECTED TESTS OF PANCREATIC FUNCTION

TEST	NORMAL VALUE	CLINICAL SIGNIFICANCE
Serum amylase	25–125 units/mL	Elevated levels with pancreatic inflammation
Serum lipase	20–240 units/mL	Elevated levels with pancreatic inflammation (may be elevated with other conditions; differentiates with amylase isoenzyme study)
Urine amylase	35–260 Somogyi units/hr	Elevated levels with pancreatic inflammation
Secretin test	Volume 1.8 ml/kg/hr Bicarbonate concentration: >80 mEq/L Bicarbonate output: >10 mEq/L/30 sec	Decreased volume with pancreatic disease as secretin stimulates pancreatic secretion
Stool fat	2–5 g/24 hr	Measures fatty acids; decreased pancreatic lipase increases stool fat (malabsorption)
Fecal elastase	>200 μg/g of stool	Decreased in pancreatic insufficiency

motility, secretion, and blood flow with increased risk for mucosal injury. Acid content of gastric juice is related to gastric atrophy, which results in hypochlorhydria (insufficient hydrochloric acid), delayed gastric emptying, and compromise of the gastric mucosal barrier. Decreased production of intrinsic factor leads to inadequate small intestinal absorption of vitamin B_{12} and pernicious anemia.[25] Aging may be associated with a change in the composition of the intestinal microflora and a decline in pathogen-specific IgA with increased susceptibility to disease.[13,26] The ileal villi of the small intestine may become broader and shorter, perhaps because of a decrease in cell turnover. Degeneration and density of the enteric nervous system neurons can decrease intestinal absorption, motility, and blood flow, impairing nutrient absorption. Proteins, fats, minerals (including iron and calcium), and vitamins are absorbed more slowly and in lesser amounts, and absorption of carbohydrates is decreased. Intestinal transit time is delayed.

Constipation is often described as a condition of old age, but it is probably caused by lifestyle factors (e.g., diet, lack of fluid intake) rather than physiologic decline, although studies demonstrate there can be alterations in both enteric and external intestinal innervation.[27]

The rate of liver regeneration decreases with advancing age, but the volume of the liver can be maintained.[28] Liver blood flow and enzyme activity decrease with age and can influence the efficiency of drug and alcohol metabolism.[29] However, liver function test results often remain within relatively normal ranges. Alterations in liver function in older individuals are usually a sign of a pathologic condition. The pancreas undergoes structural changes, such as fibrosis, fatty acid deposits, and atrophy, and there is a decline in β-cell function.[30] Pancreatic secretion decreases, but there is usually no observable dysfunction.[31] Aging does not cause apparent changes in the structure and function of the gallbladder and bile ducts, but the incidence of gallstones increases.[32]

SUMMARY REVIEW

The Gastrointestinal Tract

1. The major functions of the gastrointestinal tract are the mechanical and chemical breakdown of food and the absorption of digested nutrients.
2. The gastrointestinal tract is a hollow tube that extends from the mouth to the anus.
3. The walls of the gastrointestinal tract have several layers: mucosa, muscularis mucosa, submucosa, muscularis (circular muscle and longitudinal muscle), and serosa (adventitia in the esophagus).
4. Except for swallowing and defecation, which are controlled voluntarily, the functions of the gastrointestinal tract are controlled by extrinsic autonomic nerves (vagus, parasympathetic splanchnic, and sympathetic nerves) and intrinsic autonomic nerves (enteric nervous system) and intestinal hormones.
5. Digestion begins in the mouth, with chewing and salivation. The digestive component of saliva is α-amylase, which initiates carbohydrate digestion.
6. The esophagus is a muscular tube that transports food from the mouth to the stomach. The muscularis in the upper part of the esophagus is striated muscle, and that in the lower part is smooth muscle.
7. Swallowing is controlled by the swallowing center in the reticular formation of the brain. The two phases of swallowing are the oropharyngeal phase (voluntary swallowing) and the esophageal phase (involuntary swallowing).
8. Food is propelled through the gastrointestinal tract by peristalsis: waves of sequential relaxations and contractions of the muscularis.
9. The lower esophageal sphincter opens to admit swallowed food into the stomach and then closes to prevent regurgitation of food back into the esophagus.
10. The stomach is a baglike structure that secretes digestive juices, mixes and stores food, and propels partially digested food (chyme) into the duodenum. The smooth muscles of the stomach include the outer longitudinal, middle circular, and internal oblique.
11. The vagus nerve stimulates gastric (stomach) secretion and motility.
12. The hormones gastrin and motilin stimulate gastric emptying; the hormones secretin and cholecystokinin delay gastric emptying.
13. Gastric glands in the fundus and body of the stomach secrete intrinsic factor, which is needed for vitamin B_{12} absorption, and hydrochloric acid, which dissolves food fibers, kills microorganisms, and activates the enzyme pepsin.
14. Chief cells in the stomach secrete pepsinogen, which is converted to pepsin in the acidic environment created by hydrochloric acid.
15. Acid secretion is stimulated by the vagus nerve, gastrin, and histamine and inhibited by sympathetic stimulation and cholecystokinin. Acetylcholine stimulates pepsin secretion.

16. Mucus is secreted throughout the stomach and protects the stomach wall from acid and digestive enzymes.

17. The three phases of acid secretion by the stomach are the cephalic phase (anticipation and swallowing), the gastric phase (food in the stomach), and the intestinal phase (chyme in the intestine).

18. The small intestine is 5 m long and has three segments: the duodenum, jejunum, and ileum. Digestion and absorption of all major nutrients and most ingested water occur in the small intestine.

19. The peritoneum is a double layer of membranous tissue. The visceral layer covers the abdominal organs, and the parietal layer extends along the abdominal wall.

20. Blood flow to the small intestine is primarily provided by the superior mesenteric artery.

21. The duodenum receives chyme from the stomach through the pyloric valve. The presence of chyme stimulates the liver and gallbladder to deliver bile and the pancreas to deliver digestive enzymes and alkaline secretions. Bile and enzymes flow through an opening guarded by the sphincter of Oddi.

22. Bile is produced by the liver and is necessary for fat digestion and absorption. Bile's alkalinity helps neutralize chyme, thereby creating a pH that enables the pancreatic enzymes to digest proteins, carbohydrates, and sugars.

23. Enzymes secreted by the small intestine (maltase, sucrase, lactase), pancreatic enzymes (proteases, amylase, and lipase), and bile salts act in the small intestine to digest proteins, carbohydrates, and fats.

24. Digested substances are absorbed across the intestinal wall and then transported to the liver through the hepatic portal vein, where they are metabolized further.

25. The ileocecal valve connects the small and large intestines and prevents reflux into the small intestine.

26. Villi are small finger-like projections that extend from the small intestinal mucosa and increase its absorptive surface area.

27. Carbohydrates, amino acids, and fats are absorbed primarily by the duodenum and jejunum; bile salts and vitamin B_{12} are absorbed by the ileum. Vitamin B_{12} absorption requires the presence of intrinsic factor.

28. Bile salts emulsify and hydrolyze fats and incorporate them into water-soluble micelles that transport them through the unstirred layer to the brush border of the intestinal mucosa. The fat content of the micelles readily diffuses through the epithelium into lacteals (lymphatic ducts) in the villi. From there fats flow into the lymphatics and into the systemic circulation, which delivers them to the liver.

29. Minerals and water-soluble vitamins are absorbed by active and passive transport throughout the small intestine.

30. Peristaltic movements created by longitudinal muscles propel the chyme along the intestinal tract, whereas contractions of the circular muscles (segmentation) mix the chyme and promote digestion.

31. The ileogastric reflex inhibits gastric motility when the ileum is distended.

32. The intestinointestinal reflex inhibits intestinal motility when one intestinal segment is overdistended.

33. The gastroileal reflex increases intestinal motility when gastric motility increases.

34. The large intestine consists of the cecum, appendix, colon (ascending, transverse, descending, and sigmoid), rectum, and anal canal.

35. The teniae coli are three bands of longitudinal muscle that extend the length of the colon.

36. Haustra are pouches of colon that are formed with alternating contraction and relaxation of the circular muscles.

37. The mucosa of the large intestine contains mucus-secreting cells and mucosal folds, but no villi.

38. The large intestine massages the fecal mass and absorbs water and electrolytes.

39. Distention of the ileum with chyme causes the gastrocolic reflex, or the mass propulsion of feces to the rectum.

40. Defecation is stimulated when the rectum is distended with feces. The conically contracted internal anal sphincter relaxes and, if the voluntarily regulated external sphincter relaxes, defecation occurs.

41. The largest numbers of intestinal bacteria are in the colon. They are anaerobes consisting of *Bacteroides,* clostridia, coliforms, and lactobacilli.

42. The intestinal tract is sterile at birth and becomes totally colonized within 3 to 4 weeks.

43. Endogenous infections of the gastrointestinal tract occur by excessive proliferation of bacteria, perforation of the intestine, or contamination from neighboring structures.

Accessory Organs of Digestion

1. The liver is the largest organ in the body. It has digestive, metabolic, hematologic, vascular, and immunologic functions.

2. The liver is divided into the right and left lobes and is supported by the falciform, round, and coronary ligaments.

3. Liver lobules consist of plates of hepatocytes, which are the functional cells of the liver.

4. The hepatic artery supplies blood to the liver. The hepatic portal vein, formed by the confluence of superior mesenteric and splenic veins, receives blood from the inferior mesenteric, gastric, and cystic veins.

5. Hepatocytes synthesize 700 to 1200 mL of bile per day and secrete it into the bile canaliculi, which are small channels between the hepatocytes. The bile canaliculi drain bile into the common bile duct and then into the duodenum through an opening called the *major duodenal papilla (sphincter of Oddi).*

6. Sinusoids are capillaries located between the plates of hepatocytes. Blood from the hepatic portal vein and hepatic artery flows through the sinusoids to a central vein in each lobule and then into the hepatic vein and inferior vena cava.

7. Kupffer cells, which are part of the mononuclear phagocyte system, line the sinusoids and destroy microorganisms in sinusoidal blood.

8. The primary bile acids are synthesized from cholesterol by the hepatocytes. The primary acids are then conjugated to form bile salts. The secondary bile acids are the product of bile salt deconjugation by bacteria in the intestinal lumen.

9. Most bile salts and acids are recycled. The absorption of bile salts and acids from the terminal ileum and their return to the liver are known as the *enterohepatic circulation of bile.*

10. Bilirubin is a pigment liberated by the lysis of aged red blood cells in the liver and spleen. Unconjugated bilirubin is fat soluble and can cross cell membranes. Unconjugated bilirubin is converted to water-soluble, conjugated bilirubin by hepatocytes and is secreted with bile.

11. Fats are synthesized by the liver from protein and carbohydrates and include glycerol, free fatty acids, phospholipids, and cholesterol. Fat absorbed by intestinal lacteals is primarily triglyceride, which is hydrolyzed to glycerol and free fatty acid.

■ SUMMARY REVIEW—cont'd

12. Protein synthesis by the liver requires all essential amino acids. The liver synthesizes albumin, globulin, and several serum enzymes and can convert amino acids to carbohydrates by removal of ammonia.

13. Carbohydrates can be released as glucose, stored as glycogen, or converted to fat.

14. The liver performs many metabolic functions including detoxification of exogenous and endogenous substances.

15. The gallbladder is a saclike organ located in the inferior surface of the liver. The gallbladder stores bile between meals and ejects it when chyme enters the duodenum.

16. Stimulated by cholecystokinin, the gallbladder contracts and forces bile through the cystic duct and into the common bile duct. The sphincter of Oddi relaxes, enabling bile to flow through the major duodenal papilla into the duodenum.

17. The pancreas is a gland located behind the stomach. The endocrine pancreas produces hormones (glucagon and insulin) that facilitate the formation and cellular uptake of glucose. The exocrine pancreas secretes an alkaline solution and the enzymes (trypsin, chymotrypsin, carboxypeptidase, α-amylase, lipase) that digest proteins, carbohydrates, and fats.

18. Secretin stimulates pancreatic secretion of alkaline fluid, and cholecystokinin and ACh stimulate secretion of enzymes. Pancreatic secretions originate in acini and ducts of the pancreas and empty into the duodenum through the common bile duct or an accessory duct that opens directly into the duodenum.

Tests of Digestive Function

1. Numerous diagnostic tests can evaluate structure and function (digestion, secretion, absorption) of the gastrointestinal tract. Radiographs and scans are most commonly used to evaluate structure, in addition to direct observation by endoscopy. Gastric and stool analysis and blood studies provide important information about digestion, absorption, and secretion.

2. Plasma chemistry levels and imaging procedures are commonly used to diagnose alterations in liver function. Of particular importance are the enzymes LDH, AST, and ALT. Plasma bilirubin levels reflect alterations in bilirubin and bile metabolism, and prothrombin times are prolonged in hepatitis and chronic liver disease.

3. Obstructive diseases of the gallbladder are evident by elevated serum bilirubin levels, elevated urine urobilinogen levels, and increased stool fat. The serum leukocyte levels become elevated with inflammation of the gallbladder.

4. The most significant indicators of pancreatic dysfunction are serum amylase and stool fat. Both values are increased with pathology of the pancreas.

Aging and the Gastrointestinal System

1. Advancing age is often associated with the loss or deterioration of teeth, diminished senses of taste and smell, and diminished salivary secretions, all of which may make eating difficult and reduce appetite.

2. Aging reduces gastric motility and secretions, particularly of hydrochloric acid. These changes slow gastric digestion and emptying.

3. Intestinal motility and absorption of carbohydrates, proteins, fats, and minerals decrease with age.

4. Efficiency of drug and alcohol metabolism decreases with age and can be related to decreased liver perfusion and decreased liver enzymes.

■ KEY TERMS

Alanine aminotransferase (ALT), 1312
Alkaline phosphatase, 1312
Ampulla of Vater, 1310
Antrum of stomach, 1296
Ascending colon, 1306
Aspartate aminotransferase (AST), 1312
Bile, 1310
Bile acid-dependent fraction, 1310
Bile acid-independent fraction, 1310
Bile acid pool, 1311
Bile canaliculi, 1310
Bile salt, 1310
Bilirubin, 1311
Biliverdin, 1311
Body of stomach, 1296
Brush border, 1301
Calcium, 1304
Carboxypeptidase, 1302
Cardiac orifice, 1296
Cecum, 1306
Cephalic phase of secretion, 1299
Chief cell, 1298
Cholecystokinin, 1314
Choleresis, 1311
Choleretic agent, 1311
Cholesterol esterase, 1303
Chylomicron, 1303
Chyme, 1296
Chymotrypsin, 1302
Colipase, 1303
Colon, 1306

Common bile duct, 1310
Conjugated bilirubin, 1311
Crypts of Lieberkühn, 1301
Cystic duct, 1312
D cell, 1298
Deamination, 1311
Defecation reflex (rectosphincteric reflex), 1307
Descending colon, 1306
Disse space, 1310
Duodenum, 1300
Emulsification, 1303
Enteric nervous system, 1294
Enterochromaffin-like cell, 1298
Enterohepatic circulation, 1310
Enterokinase, 1314
Esophageal phase of swallowing, 1295
Esophagus, 1295
Exocrine pancreas, 1312
External anal sphincter, 1306
Fat, 1303
Fecal mass, 1307
Feces, 1307
Fundus of stomach, 1296
G cell, 1298
Gallbladder, 1312
Gamma-glutamyltransferase, 1312
Gastric emptying, 1297
Gastric gland, 1298
Gastric hydrochloric acid, 1298
Gastric lipase, 1299
Gastric phase of secretion, 1299

Gastric pit, 1298
Gastrin, 1296
Gastrocolic reflex, 1307
Gastroileal reflex, 1306
Gastrointestinal tract (alimentary canal), 1294
Haustrum (*pl.*, haustra), 1306
Hepatic artery, 1309
Hepatic portal vein, 1309
Hepatic vein, 1309
Hepatocyte, 1309
Hepcidin, 1304
Histamine, 1298
Ileocecal valve (sphincter), 1300, 1306
Ileogastric reflex, 1306
Ileum, 1300
Internal anal sphincter, 1306
Intestinal peristalsis, 1306
Intestinal phase of secretion, 1299
Intestinointestinal reflex, 1306
Intrinsic factor (IF), 1299
Iron, 1304
Jejunum, 1300
Kupffer cell, 1310
Lactate dehydrogenase (LDH), 1312
Lacteal, 1301
Lamina propria, 1301
Large intestine, 1306
Lipase, 1303
Lipocyte, 1309
Lipolysis, 1303
Liver, 1309

■ KEY TERMS—cont'd

REFERENCES

1. Besnard P, Passilly-Degrace P, Khan NA: Taste of fat: a sixth taste modality? *Physiol Rev* 96(1): 151–176, 2016.

2. Gao W, Stalder T, Kirschbaum C: Quantitative analysis of estradiol and six other steroid hormones in human saliva using a high throughput liquid chromatography–tandem mass spectrometry assay. *Talanta* 143:353–358, 2015.

3. Granger DN, Holm L, Kvietys P: The gastrointestinal circulation: physiology and pathophysiology. *Compr Physiol* 5(3):1541–1583, 2015.

4. Marathe CS, et al: Relationships between gastric emptying, postprandial glycemia, and incretin hormones. *Diabetes Care* 36(5):1396–1405, 2013.

5. Yandrapu H, Sarosiek J: Protective factors of the gastric and duodenal mucosa: an overview. *Curr Gastroenterol Rep* 17(6):24, 2015.

6. Schubert ML: Functional anatomy and physiology of gastric secretion. *Curr Opin Gastroenterol* 31(6): 479–485, 2015.

7. Miller MJ, McDole JR, Newberry RD: Microanatomy of the intestinal lymphatic system. *Ann N Y Acad Sci* 1207(Suppl 1):E21–E28, 2010.

8. Muecker M, Thorens B: The SLC2 (GLUT) family of membrane transporters. *Mol Aspects Med* 34(2-3):121–138, 2013.

9. Schmidt PJ: Regulation of iron metabolism by hepcidin under conditions of inflammation. *J Biol Chem* 290(31):18975–18983, 2015.

10. Lammers WJ: Normal and abnormal electrical propagation in the small intestine. *Acta Physiol (Oxf)* 213(2):349–359, 2015.

11. Mowat AM, Agace WW: Regional specialization within the intestinal immune system. *Nat Rev Immunol* 14(10):667–685, 2014.

12. Schultze JL: Macrophage tolerance in the gut: it is in the epigenome! *Eur J Immunol* 46(8):1838–1841, 2016.

13. Vaiserman AM, Koliada AK, Marotta F: Gut microbiota: a player in aging and a target for anti-aging intervention. *Ageing Res Rev* 35:36–45, 2017.

14. Schippa S, Conte MP: Dysbiotic events in gut microbiota: impact on human health. *Nutrients* 6(12):5786–5805, 2014.

15. Khanna S, Tosh PK: A clinician's primer on the role of the microbiome in human health and disease. *Mayo Clin Proc* 89(1):107–114, 2014.

16. Denny JE, Powell WL, Schmidt NW: Local and long-distance calling: conversations between the gut microbiota and intra- and extra-gastrointestinal tract infections. *Front Cell Infect Microbiol* 6:41, 2016.

17. Samuelson DR, Welsh DA, Shellito JE: Regulation of lung immunity and host defense by the intestinal microbiota. *Front Microbiol* 6:1085, 2015.

18. Poisson J, et al: Liver sinusoidal endothelial cells: physiology and role in liver diseases. *J Hepatol* 66(1):212–227, 2016.

19. Knolle PA, Wohlleber D: Immunological functions of liver sinusoidal endothelial cells. *Cell Mol Immunol* 13(3):347–353, 2016.

20. Gazzin S, et al: A novel perspective on the biology of bilirubin in health and disease. *Trends Mol Med* 22(9):758–768, 2016.

21. Maresz K: Proper calcium use: vitamin K_2 as a promoter of bone and cardiovascular health. *Integr Med (Encinitas)* 14(1):34–39, 2015.

22. Huang W, et al: Prediction of the severity of acute pancreatitis on admission by urinary trypsinogen activation peptide: a meta-analysis. *World J Gastroenterol* 19(28):4607–4615, 2013.

23. Saffrey MJ: Aging of the mammalian gastrointestinal tract: a complex organ system. *Age (Dordr)* 36(3):9603, 2014.

24. Achem SR, DeVault KR: Gastroesophageal reflux disease and the elderly. *Gastroenterol Clin North Am* 43(1):147–160, 2014.

25. Patel KV: Epidemiology of anemia in older adults. *Semin Hematol* 45(4):210–217, 2008.

26. Sato S, Kiyono H, Fujihashi K: Mucosal immunosenescence in the gastrointestinal tract: a mini-review. *Gerontology* 61(4):336–342, 2015.

27. Keating C, Grundy D: Ageing and gastrointestinal sensory function. *Adv Exp Med Biol* 891:71–74, 2016.

28. Schmucker DL, Sanchez H: Liver regeneration and aging: a current perspective. *Curr Gerontol Geriatr Res* 2011:526379, 2011.

29. Tan JL, et al: Age-related changes in hepatic function: an update on implications for drug therapy. *Drugs Aging* 32(12):999–1008, 2015.

30. Barker CJ, et al: β-Cell Ca(2+) dynamics and function are compromised in aging. *Adv Biol Regul* 57:112–119, 2015.

31. Herzig KH, et al: Fecal pancreatic elastase-1 levels in older individuals without known gastrointestinal diseases or diabetes mellitus. *BMC Geriatr* 11:4, 2011.

32. Stinton LM, Shaffer EA: Epidemiology of gallbladder disease: cholelithiasis and cancer. *Gut Liver* 6(2):172–187, 2012.

Alterations of Digestive Function

Sue E. Huether

evolve WEBSITE

CHAPTER OUTLINE

Disorders of the gastrointestinal tract disrupt one or more of its functions. Structural and neural abnormalities can slow, obstruct, or accelerate the movement of intestinal content at any level of the gastrointestinal tract. Inflammatory and ulcerative conditions of the gastrointestinal wall disrupt secretion, motility, and absorption. Inflammation or obstruction of the liver, pancreas, or gallbladder can alter metabolism and result in local or systemic symptoms, or both. Many clinical manifestations of gastrointestinal tract disorders are nonspecific and can be caused by a variety of impairments. These manifestations are described in the following section.

DISORDERS OF THE GASTROINTESTINAL TRACT

Clinical Manifestations of Gastrointestinal Dysfunction

Anorexia

Anorexia is lack of a desire to eat despite physiologic stimuli that would normally produce hunger. Anorexia is a nonspecific symptom that is often associated with nausea, abdominal pain, diarrhea, psychologic distress, and aging. Side effects of drugs and disorders of other organ systems, including cancer, heart disease, and renal disease, are often accompanied by anorexia. Anorexia can lead to weight loss, sarcopenia, and functional decline and is often associated with cachexia.[1]

Vomiting

Vomiting is the forceful emptying of stomach and intestinal contents through the mouth. The vomiting center, called *area postrema*, lies in the medulla oblongata and includes the reticular formation, tractus solitarius nucleus, and the parabrachial nucleus. Stimulation of the vomiting center occurs directly by irritants or indirectly. Indirect stimulation includes the cerebral cortex and thalamus (anxiety and pain); the vestibular system through the eighth cranial nerve (motion sickness); several types of intestinal, vagal, or sympathetic input, including the presence of ipecac or copper salts in the duodenum; side effects of many drugs; distention of the stomach or duodenum; or torsion or trauma affecting the ovaries, testes, uterus, bladder, or kidney. Serotonin (5-hydroxytryptamine [5-HT]) stimulates the vomiting center and appears to be released from enterochromaffin cells in the intestinal wall, which activate vagal afferents leading to the chemoreceptor trigger zone (CTZ). Activation of the CTZ, which lies in the area postrema between the medulla and floor of the fourth ventricle, leads to vomiting by triggering receptors for substances such as dopamine (D_2), opioids, acetylcholine, substance P, serotonin (5-hydroxytryptamine type 3), and neurokinin-1. Serotonin and neurokinin-1 antagonists are effective antiemetics and have been used to treat nausea and vomiting associated with postoperative vomiting and cancer chemotherapy. Olanzapine is an antagonist to both serotonin and dopamine. Corticosteroids are usually given in combination with other therapies to prevent chemotherapy-induced nausea. Apomorphine, levodopa, and bromocriptine are dopamine D_2 agonists that cause nausea and vomiting. D_2 antagonists (metoclopramide, domperidone) are effective antiemetics.[2,3]

Nausea and retching usually precede vomiting, although they are distinct entities. Nausea is a subjective experience that is associated with various conditions, including visceral pain, labyrinthine stimulation (i.e., motion), and use of opiate medications. Specific neural pathways have not been identified for nausea. Hypersalivation and tachycardia are common associated symptoms. Retching is the muscular event of vomiting without the expulsion of vomitus.

Vomiting begins with deep inspiration. The glottis closes, the intrathoracic pressure falls, and the esophagus becomes distended. Simultaneously, the abdominal muscles contract, creating a pressure gradient from abdomen to thorax. The lower esophageal sphincter and body of the stomach relax, but the duodenum and antrum of the stomach spasm. The reverse peristalsis and pressure gradient force chyme from the stomach and duodenum up into the esophagus. Because the upper esophageal sphincter is closed, chyme does not enter the mouth. As the abdominal muscles relax, the contents of the esophagus drop back into the stomach. This process may be repeated several times before vomiting occurs. A diffuse sympathetic discharge causes the tachycardia, tachypnea, and sweating that accompany retching and vomiting. The parasympathetic system mediates copious salivation, increased gastric motility, and relaxation of the upper and lower esophageal sphincters.

With vomiting, the duodenum and antrum of the stomach produce retrograde peristalsis while the body of the stomach and the esophagus relax. When the stomach is full of gastric contents, the diaphragm is forced high into the thoracic cavity by strong contractions of the abdominal muscles. The higher intrathoracic pressure forces the upper esophageal sphincter to open, and chyme is expelled from the mouth. Then the stomach relaxes and the upper part of the esophagus contracts, forcing the remaining chyme back into the stomach. The lower esophageal sphincter then closes. The cycle is repeated if there is a volume of chyme remaining in the stomach.

Projectile vomiting is spontaneous vomiting that is not preceded by nausea or retching. It is caused by direct stimulation of the vomiting center by neurologic lesions (e.g., increased intracranial pressure, tumors, or aneurysms involving the brainstem [see Chapters 17 and 20]) or gastric outlet obstruction. The metabolic consequences of vomiting are fluid, electrolyte, and acid-base disturbances, including hyponatremia, hypokalemia, hypochloremia, and metabolic alkalosis (see Chapter 3).

Constipation

Constipation is difficult or infrequent defecation and is estimated to affect 2% to 28% of the population. Constipation must be individually defined because patterns of bowel evacuation differ greatly among individuals. Normal bowel habits range from two or three evacuations per day to one per week. Constipation is not significant until it causes health risks (e.g., severe abdominal distention or fecal impaction) or impairs quality of life.

◆**PATHOPHYSIOLOGY.** Constipation can occur as a primary or secondary condition. Primary constipation is generally classified into three categories. *Normal transit (functional) constipation* involves a normal rate of stool passage, but there is difficulty with stool evacuation. *Functional constipation* is most common and is associated with sedentary lifestyle, low-residue diet (the habitual consumption of highly refined foods), or low fluid intake, which decreases the volume and number of stools and can contribute to constipation. Lack of access to toilet facilities, consistent suppression of the urge to empty the bowel, and dehydration are other causes. *Slow-transit constipation* involves impaired colonic motor activity with infrequent bowel movements, straining to defecate, mild abdominal distention, and palpable stool in the sigmoid colon. *Pelvic floor dysfunction* (pelvic floor dyssynergia-anismus), or *outlet dysfunction*, is difficulty expelling stool because of failure of the pelvic floor muscles or anal sphincter to relax with defecation. Examples include pelvic floor dyssynergia, rectal fissures or fistula, strictures, or hemorrhoids.

Secondary constipation can be caused by diet, medications, or neurogenic disorders (e.g., stroke, Parkinson disease, spinal cord injury, multiple sclerosis, Hirschsprung disease) in which neurotransmitters or neural pathways are diseased or degenerated, resulting in delayed colon transit time. Antacids containing calcium carbonate or aluminum hydroxide; anticholinergics; iron; and bismuth tend to inhibit bowel motility. *Opioid-induced constipation* is caused by drugs that activate μ-opioid receptors in the gut. Endocrine or metabolic disorders associated with constipation include hypothyroidism, diabetes mellitus, hypokalemia, and hypercalcemia. Pelvic hiatal hernia (herniation of the bowel through the floor of the pelvis), diverticular disease, irritable bowel syndrome—constipation predominant, and pregnancy also are associated with constipation. Aging can result in constipation caused from changes in neurons in the myenteric plexus and decreased neurotransmitter function with decreased colon motility, use of medications, and comorbid medical conditions.[4] Many mechanical conditions can slow intestinal transit time. The abdominal muscles are normally used to create the intraabdominal pressure required to evacuate the rectum. Weakness or pain can interfere with the generation of adequate intraabdominal pressure. With the urge to defecate, the sphincter becomes hypertonic and the stool is not eliminated. Depression often impairs bowel evacuation, partly because depressed individuals tend to be sedentary and lack the motivation to eat a healthy diet. The problem is made worse if antidepressant drugs (e.g., anticholinergics) are used to treat the depression.

◆**CLINICAL MANIFESTATIONS.** Indicators of constipation include two of the following for at least 3 months: (1) straining with defecation at least 25% of the time, (2) lumpy or hard stools at least 25% of the time, (3) sensation of incomplete emptying at least 25% of the time, (4) manual maneuvers to facilitate stool evacuation for at least 25% of defecations, and (5) fewer than three bowel movements per week.[5] Changes in bowel evacuation patterns, such as less frequent defecation, smaller stool volume, hard stools, difficulty passing stools (straining), or a feeling of bowel fullness and discomfort or blood in the stools, require investigation. Fecal impaction (hard, dry stool retained in the rectum) is associated with rectal bleeding, abdominal or cramping pain, nausea and vomiting, weight loss, and episodes of diarrhea. Compression of capillary perfusion in the intestinal wall can lead to ischemia and necrosis.[6] Straining to evacuate stool may cause engorgement of the hemorrhoidal veins and hemorrhoidal disease or thrombosis with rectal pain, bleeding, and itching. Passage of hard stools can cause painful anal fissures.

◆**EVALUATION AND TREATMENT.** The history, current use of medications, physical examination, and stool diaries provide precise clues regarding the nature of constipation. Sudden-onset constipation can accompany the development of colorectal cancer and requires careful evaluation. The individual's description of frequency, stool consistency, associated pain, and presence of blood or whether evacuation was stimulated by enemas or cathartics (laxatives) is important. Cramping abdominal pain may be symptomatic of partial bowel obstruction. Palpation discloses colonic distention, masses, and tenderness. Blood may be caused by bleeding hemorrhoids or a neoplastic lesion of the colon.

Digital examinations of the rectum and anorectal manometry are performed to assess sphincter tone and detect anal lesions. Colonoscopy is performed with serious symptoms or for colon cancer screening. Colonic transit studies and imaging techniques can assist in identifying the etiology of constipation.

The treatment for constipation is to manage the underlying cause or disease for each individual. Management usually consists of bowel retraining, in which the individual establishes a satisfactory bowel evacuation routine without becoming preoccupied with bowel movements. Moderate exercise, increased fluid and fiber intake, bulking agents, stool softeners, and laxative agents (bisacodyl and senna) are useful and inexpensive for some individuals. Glycerine suppositories and enemas can be used to establish bowel routine, but they should not be used habitually. Biofeedback training maybe effective for dyssynergic defecation.[7] Drugs used to treat severe constipation include colonic secretagogues lubiprostone, linaclotide and plecanatide, and the 5-HT$_4$ agonist prucalopride. Peripherally acting μ-opioid receptor antagonists methylnaltrexone, naloxone, naloxegol, and alvimopan (for postoperative ileus) are used to treat opioid-induced constipation.[8]

Diarrhea

Diarrhea is the presence of loose, watery stools. Acute diarrhea is more than three loose stools developing within 24 hours and lasting less than 14 days. Persistent diarrhea lasts longer than 14 to 30 days and chronic diarrhea lasts longer than 30 days.[9,10] Diarrhea can have high rates of morbidity and mortality in children less than 5 years of age, particularly in developing countries (see Chapter 43) and in the elderly. Many factors determine stool volume and consistency, including the water content of the colon, diet, the presence of unabsorbed food, unabsorbable material, and intestinal secretions. Stool volume in the normal adult averages less than 200 g/day. Stool volume in children depends on age and size. An infant may pass up to 100 g/day. The adult intestine processes approximately 9 L of luminal contents per day; 2 L is ingested, and the remaining 7 L consists of intestinal secretions. Of this volume, 99% of the fluid is absorbed—90% (7 to 8 L) in the small intestine and 9% (1 to 2 L) in the colon. Normally, approximately 150 mL of water is excreted daily in the stool.

◆**PATHOPHYSIOLOGY.** Diarrhea in which the volume of feces is increased is called *large-volume diarrhea*. Large-volume diarrhea generally is caused by excessive amounts of water or secretions, or both, in the intestines. *Small-volume diarrhea*, in which the volume of feces is not increased, usually results from excessive intestinal motility.

The three major mechanisms of diarrhea are osmotic, secretory, and motility. (Specific mechanisms of diarrhea in children are described in Chapter 43.)

In osmotic diarrhea, a nonabsorbable substance in the intestine draws water into the lumen by osmosis and increases stool weight and volume, producing large-volume diarrhea. Large oral doses of poorly absorbed ions, such as magnesium, sulfate, and phosphate, can increase intraluminal osmotic pressure. Excessive ingestion of synthetic, non-absorbable sugars (e.g., sorbitol); introduction of full-strength tube feeding formulas; and dumping syndrome associated with gastric resection draw water into the intestinal lumen. Osmotic diarrhea disappears when ingestion of the osmotic substance stops. Malabsorption related to lactase deficiency, pancreatic enzyme or bile salt deficiency, small intestine bacterial overgrowth, or celiac disease also causes osmotic diarrhea.

Secretory diarrhea is a form of large-volume diarrhea caused by excessive mucosal secretion of chloride- or bicarbonate-rich fluid or inhibition of net sodium absorption. Infectious causes include viruses (e.g., rotavirus), bacterial enterotoxins (e.g., *Escherichia coli*, *Vibrio cholerae*, Shiga toxin), or exotoxins from overgrowth of *Clostridium difficile* following antibiotic therapy or small bowel bacterial overgrowth. These infections cause secretion of transmitters from enteroendocrine cells (e.g., 5-HT) and activation of afferent neurons that stimulate submucosal secretomotor neurons and altered sodium and chloride transport resulting in decreased water absorption. Neoplasms (such as gastrinoma or thyroid carcinoma) produce hormones that stimulate intestinal secretion causing diarrhea.

Small-volume diarrhea usually is caused by an inflammatory disorder of the intestine, such as ulcerative colitis, Crohn disease, or microscopic colitis. Inflammation of the colon causes smooth muscle contraction, cramping pain, urgency, and frequency. Small-volume diarrhea also can be caused by fecal impaction, a severe form of constipation. This diarrhea consists of secretions (mucus and fluid) produced by the colon to lubricate the impacted feces and move it toward the anal canal. These secretions flow around the impaction and cause low-volume, secretory diarrhea.

Motility diarrhea is caused by resection of the small intestine (short bowel syndrome), surgical bypass of an area of the intestine, fistula formation between loops of intestine, irritable bowel syndrome—diarrhea predominant, diabetic neuropathy, hyperthyroidism, and laxative abuse. Excessive motility decreases transit time, mucosal surface contact, and opportunities for fluid absorption, resulting in diarrhea.

◆**CLINICAL MANIFESTATIONS.** Diarrhea can be acute or chronic, depending on its cause. Systemic effects of prolonged diarrhea are dehydration, electrolyte imbalance (hyponatremia, hypokalemia), metabolic acidosis, and weight loss. Manifestations of acute bacterial or viral infection include fever, with or without vomiting or cramping pain. Most infectious diarrhea usually lasts less than 2 weeks. The exceptions are *Clostridium difficile*, *Aeromonas*, and *Yersinia enterocolitica*. Fever, cramping pain, and bloody stools accompany chronic diarrhea caused by inflammatory bowel disease or dysentery. Steatorrhea (fat in the stools), bloating, and diarrhea are common signs of malabsorption syndromes. Anal and perineal skin irritation can occur.

◆**EVALUATION AND TREATMENT.** A thorough history is taken to document the onset, frequency, and volume of stools. Exposure to contaminated food or water is indicated if the individual has traveled in foreign countries or areas where drinking water might be contaminated. Iatrogenic diarrhea is suggested if the individual has undergone abdominal radiation therapy, intestinal resection, or treatment with selected drugs (e.g., antibiotics, diuretics, antihypertensives, or laxatives). Physical examination helps the clinician to identify underlying systemic disease. Stool culture, polymerase chain reaction, examination of stool specimens for blood, microscopy for protozoal infections, abdominal roentgenograms, endoscopy, and intestinal biopsies provide more specific data.[11]

Treatment for diarrhea includes restoration of fluid and electrolyte balance, antimotility (e.g., loperamide [an opiate] or Lomotil [atropine]) and/or water-absorbent (e.g., attapulgite and polycarbophil) medications, and treatment of causal factors. Nutritional deficiencies need to be corrected in cases of chronic diarrhea or malabsorption. Natural bran and commercial preparations of psyllium are inexpensive and effective treatments for mild diarrhea. Probiotics can be useful for preventing and treating *Clostridium difficile*–associated diarrhea as an approach to restoring normal microflora in addition to antibiotic therapy.[12] Fecal transplantation can be used for cases that are resistant to conventional therapies, particularly *Clostridium difficile*–associated diarrhea.[13]

Abdominal Pain

Abdominal pain is the presenting symptom of a number of gastrointestinal (GI) diseases and can be acute or chronic. The pathophysiologic mechanisms are *mechanical, inflammatory,* or *ischemic.* Abdominal pain may be generalized to the abdomen or localized to a particular abdominal quadrant. The pain can be variably described as sharp, dull, or colicky. Generally, the abdominal organs are not sensitive to mechanical stimuli, such as cutting, tearing, or crushing. These organs are, however, sensitive to stretching and distention, which activate nerve endings in both hollow and solid structures. The onset of pain is associated with rapid distention; gradual distention causes little pain. Traction on the peritoneum caused by adhesions, distention of the common bile duct, or forceful peristalsis resulting from intestinal obstruction causes pain because of increased tension. Capsules that surround solid organs, such as the liver and gallbladder, contain pain fibers that are stimulated by stretching if these organs swell.

Biochemical mediators of the inflammatory response, such as histamine, bradykinin, and serotonin, stimulate pain nerve endings and produce abdominal pain. The edema and vascular congestion that accompany chemical, bacterial, or viral inflammation also cause painful stretching. Obstruction of blood flow from the distention of bowel obstruction or mesenteric vessel thrombosis produces the pain of ischemia, and increased concentrations of tissue metabolites stimulate pain receptors.

Abdominal pain can be parietal (somatic), visceral, or referred. Parietal pain arises from the parietal peritoneum. This pain is more localized and intense than visceral pain, which arises from the organs themselves. Nerve fibers from the parietal peritoneum are predominantly A-delta fibers and travel with somatic peripheral nerves to the spinal cord. The sensation of pain corresponds to skin dermatomes T6 and L1. Parietal pain lateralizes because, at any particular point, the parietal peritoneum is innervated from only one side of the nervous system.

Visceral pain arises from a stimulus (distention, inflammation, ischemia) acting on mechanical and chemical nociceptors of abdominal organs. Chronic low-grade inflammation can cause pain hypersensitivity with involvement of neurokinins, histamine, serotonin, proteases, and voltage-gated ion channels.[14] Pain is usually felt near the midline in the epigastrium, midabdomen, or lower abdomen because sensory afferents enter the spinal cord bilaterally and lack side specificity. Visceral pain, compared to somatic pain, is poorly localized, dull rather than sharp, and difficult to describe. Visceral pain is diffuse and vague because nerve endings in abdominal organs are predominantly unmyelinated C fibers, sparse, and multisegmented. Pain arising from the stomach, for example, is experienced as a sensation of fullness, cramping, or gnawing in the midepigastric area. Referred pain is visceral pain felt at some distance from a diseased or an affected organ. Referred pain is usually well localized and is felt in the skin dermatomes or deeper tissues because visceral afferent neurons and regional somatic neurons converge on second-order neurons at the same level of the spinal cord. Gallbladder pain is, for example, referred to the right shoulder or scapulae.[15,16]

Gastrointestinal Bleeding

Upper gastrointestinal (GI) bleeding is bleeding in the esophagus, stomach, or duodenum and is characterized by frank, bright red bleeding in emesis or dark, grainy digested blood ("coffee grounds") in stool. Upper GI bleeding is caused by bleeding esophageal or gastric varices, a Mallory-Weiss tear at the esophageal-gastric junction from severe retching, cancer, arteriovenous malformations, or peptic ulcers and is associated with various drugs (nonsteroidal antiinflammatory drugs [NSAIDs]), aspirin, selective serotonin reuptake inhibitors, and antiplatelet and anticoagulant medications.[17]

Lower gastrointestinal (GI) bleeding is bleeding from the jejunum or ileum of the small intestine, colon, or rectum and can be caused by polyps, inflammatory bowel disease, diverticular disease, cancer, mucosal vascular ectasias, or hemorrhoids.[18] Occult bleeding is usually caused by slow, chronic blood loss. It is not obvious and results in iron deficiency anemia as iron stores in the bone marrow are slowly depleted.

Physiologic response to gastrointestinal bleeding depends on the amount and rate of the loss (Fig. 42.1). Changes in blood pressure and heart rate are the best indicators of massive blood loss in the gastrointestinal tract. During the early stages of blood volume depletion, the peripheral arteries and arterioles constrict to maintain blood pressure and shunt blood to vital organs, including the brain. Blood losses of 1000 mL or more over a short time cause a decrease in blood pressure and a corresponding increase in heart rate. With losses of 1000 mL or more, the heart rate is greater than 100 beats/minute and systolic blood pressure is less than 100 mmHg. Signs of large-volume blood loss are postural hypotension (a drop in blood pressure that occurs with a change from the recumbent position to a sitting or upright position), lightheadedness, and loss of vision. Tachycardia develops as a compensatory response to maintain cardiac output and tissue perfusion. If blood loss continues, hypovolemic shock develops. Diminished blood flow to the kidneys causes decreased urine output and may lead to oliguria (low urine output), tubular necrosis, and renal failure. Ultimately, insufficient cerebral and coronary blood flow causes irreversible anoxia and death.

The presentation of GI bleeding is summarized in Table 42.1. Acute, severe GI bleeding is life threatening depending on the volume and rate of blood loss, associated disease, age, and effectiveness of treatment. The accumulation of blood in the gastrointestinal tract is irritating and increases peristalsis, causing vomiting (hematemesis) or diarrhea, or both. If bleeding is from the lower GI tract, the diarrhea is frankly bloody. Bleeding from the upper GI tract also can be rapid enough to produce bright red stools (hematochezia), but generally some digestion of the blood components will have occurred, producing melena, black or tarry stools that are sticky and have a characteristic foul odor. The digestion of blood proteins originating from massive upper GI bleeding is reflected by an increase in blood urea nitrogen (BUN) levels (see Fig. 42.1).

The hematocrit and hemoglobin values are not the best indicators of acute gastrointestinal bleeding because plasma and red cell volume are lost proportionately. As the plasma volume is replaced, the decreasing hematocrit and hemoglobin values begin to reflect the extent of blood

TABLE 42.1	PRESENTATIONS OF GASTROINTESTINAL BLEEDING
PRESENTATION	**DEFINITION**
Acute Bleeding	
Hematemesis	Bloody vomitus; either fresh, bright red blood or dark, grainy, digested blood with "coffee grounds" appearance
Melena	Black, sticky, tarry, foul-smelling stools caused by digestion of blood in the gastrointestinal tract
Hematochezia	Fresh, bright red blood passed from the rectum
Occult Bleeding	Trace amounts of blood in normal-appearing stools or gastric secretions; detectable with a guaiac test

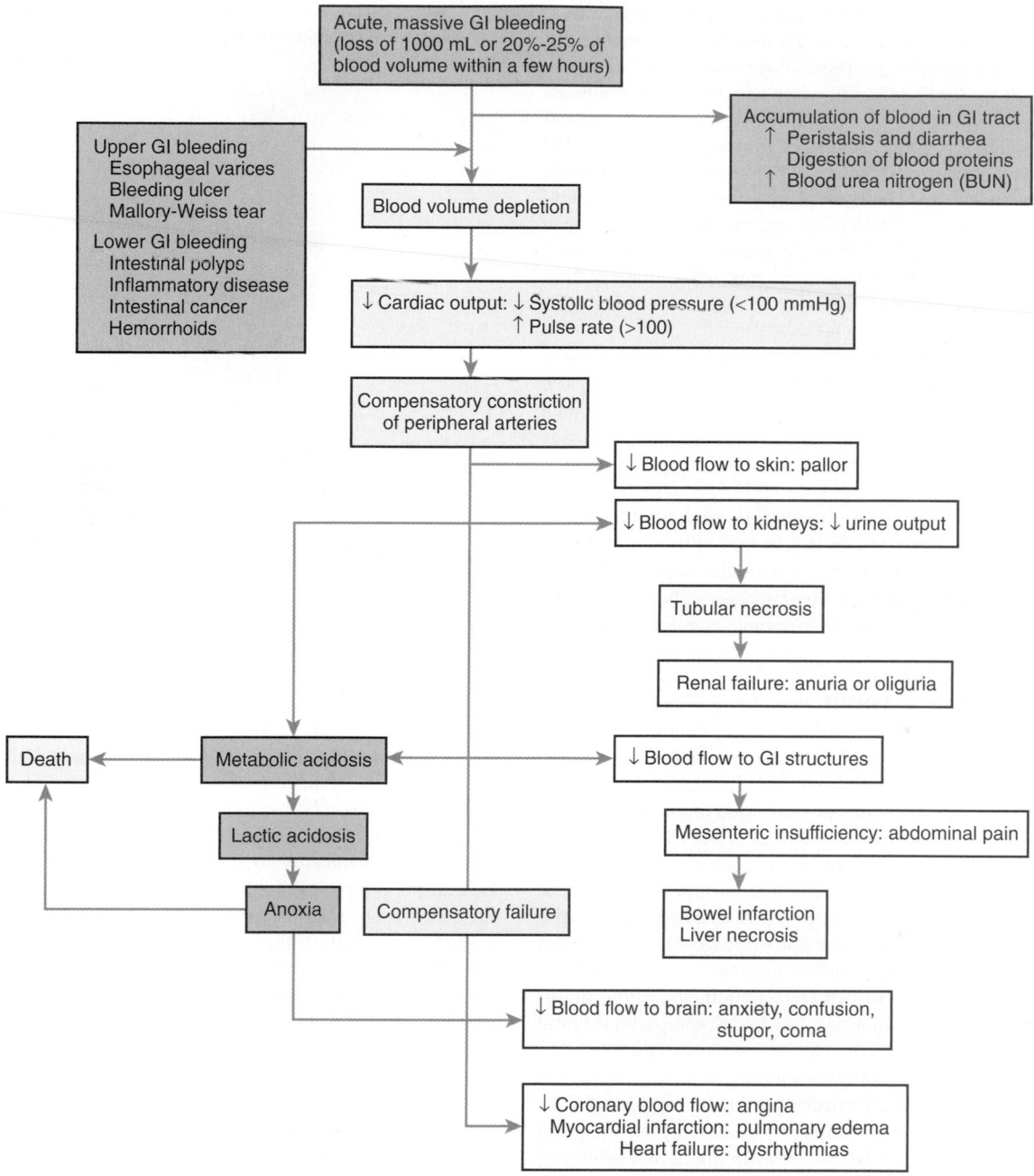

FIGURE 42.1 Pathophysiology of Gastrointestinal (GI) Bleeding.

loss. The interpretation of these values is modified to account for exogenous replacement of fluids and the hydration status of the tissues. Anemia associated with chronic GI bleeding is caused by iron depletion. Evaluation and treatment involve identifying and treating the source of the bleeding and replacing iron losses. Administration of blood products may be used for massive hemorrhage. Guidelines are available for the diagnosis and management of gastrointestinal bleeding.[19-21]

Disorders of Motility
Dysphagia

◆**PATHOPHYSIOLOGY.** Dysphagia is difficulty swallowing or perception of obstruction during swallowing. Dysphagia can be classified as oropharyngeal or substernal/esophageal, depending on the location of the sensation. It can result from mechanical obstruction of the esophagus

or a functional disorder that impairs esophageal motility. *Mechanical obstructions* can be intrinsic or extrinsic. Intrinsic obstructions originate in the wall of the esophageal lumen. Tumors, strictures, and diverticular herniations (outpouchings) are all causes of intrinsic mechanical obstruction. Extrinsic mechanical obstructions originate outside the esophageal lumen and narrow the esophagus by pressing inward on the esophageal wall. The most common cause of extrinsic mechanical obstruction is tumor.

Functional dysphagia is caused by neural or muscular disorders that interfere with voluntary swallowing or peristalsis. Disorders that affect the striated muscles of the upper esophagus interfere with the oropharyngeal (voluntary) phase of swallowing. Typical causes of functional dysphagia in the upper esophagus are dermatomyositis (a muscle disease) and neurologic impairments caused by stroke, multiple sclerosis, Parkinson disease, amyotrophic lateral sclerosis, or myasthenia gravis.[22]

Achalasia is a rare disorder related to loss of inhibitory neurons in the myenteric plexus with smooth muscle atrophy in the middle and lower portions of the esophagus. The etiology is unknown but may be related to a cell-mediated and antibody-mediated immune response against an unknown antigen in myenteric neurons. There is loss of inhibitory myenteric innervation, loss of esophageal peristalsis, and failure of lower esophageal sphincter (LES) relaxation, thus causing functional obstruction of the lower esophagus. Food accumulates above the obstruction, distends the esophagus, and causes dysphagia. Cough and aspiration can occur. As hydrostatic pressure increases, food is slowly forced past the obstruction into the stomach. Chronic inflammation from esophageal food retention can increase risk for esophageal cancer.

◆**CLINICAL MANIFESTATIONS.** Clinical manifestations of dysphagia vary according to the location of the obstruction. Distention and spasm of the esophageal muscles during eating or drinking may cause a mild or severe stabbing pain at the level of obstruction. Discomfort occurring 2 to 4 seconds after swallowing is associated with upper esophageal obstruction. Discomfort occurring 10 to 15 seconds after swallowing is more common in obstructions of the lower esophagus. If the cause of obstruction is a growing tumor, dysphagia begins with difficulty swallowing solids and advances to difficulty swallowing semisolids and liquids. Retrosternal pain, regurgitation of undigested food, unpleasant taste, vomiting, and weight loss are common manifestations of all types of dysphagia. Aspiration of esophageal contents can lead to chronic cough and pneumonia.

◆**EVALUATION AND TREATMENT.** Knowledge of the individual's history and clinical manifestations contributes significantly to a diagnosis of dysphagia. Videofluoroscopy and high-frequency ultrasound are used to visualize the contours of the esophagus and identify structural defects. High-resolution manometry with topography and intraluminal impedance monitoring documents motility disorders and the duration and amplitude of abnormal pressure changes associated with obstruction or loss of neural regulation. A video-modified barium swallow may be used for motility evaluation in oropharyngeal dysphagia. Esophageal endoscopy is performed to examine the esophageal mucosa, obtain biopsy specimens, or perform corrective surgery.[23]

The individual is taught to manage symptoms by eating slowly, eating small meals, taking fluid with meals, and sleeping with the head elevated to prevent regurgitation and aspiration. Oral medications may need to be formulated so they can be swallowed. Tube feedings may be required for some individuals, particularly following stroke. Definitive treatments include dilation or surgical myotomy of the lower esophageal sphincter (LES) or botulinum toxin injection if surgery or dilation is not an option.[24]

Gastroesophageal Reflux Disease

Gastroesophageal reflux disease (GERD) is the reflux of acid and pepsin or bile salts from the stomach to the esophagus that causes esophagitis. The prevalence of GERD is estimated at 18% to 27% in North America.[25] Risk factors for GERD include obesity, hiatal hernia, and drugs or chemicals that relax the LES (anticholinergics, nitrates, calcium channel blockers, nicotine). GERD may be a trigger for asthma, chronic cough, or sinusitis.[26] Gastroesophageal reflux that does not cause symptoms is known as *physiologic reflux*. In *nonerosive reflux disease (NERD)*, individuals have symptoms of reflux disease but no visible or minimal esophageal mucosal injury (functional heartburn).[27]

◆**PATHOPHYSIOLOGY.** Abnormalities in lower esophageal sphincter function, esophageal motility, and gastric motility or emptying can cause GERD. The resting tone of the LES tends to be lower than normal from either transient relaxation or weakness of the sphincter in those who develop GERD. Vomiting, coughing, lifting, bending, obesity, or

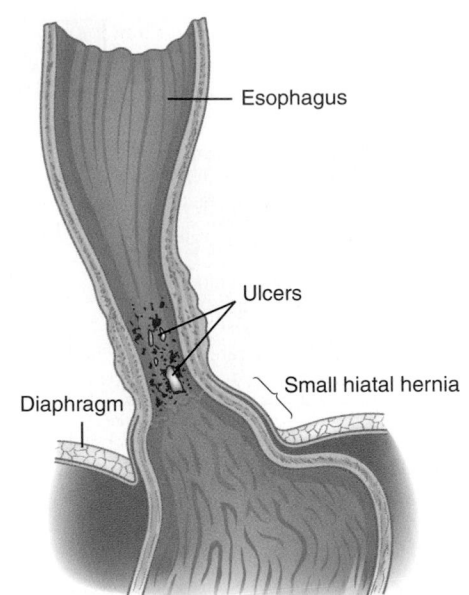

FIGURE 42.2 Esophagitis with Esophageal Ulcerations.

pregnancy increases abdominal pressure, contributing to the development of reflux esophagitis. Hiatal hernia can weaken the LES. Delayed gastric emptying contributes to reflux esophagitis by (1) lengthening the period during which reflux is possible and (2) increasing the acid content of chyme. Disorders that delay emptying include gastroparesis; gastric or duodenal ulcers, which can cause pyloric edema; and strictures that narrow the pylorus.[28]

The severity of the esophagitis depends on the composition of the gastric contents and esophageal mucosa exposure time. An acid pocket is an area of postprandial unbuffered gastric acid immediately distal to the gastroesophageal junction. It is enlarged in hiatal hernia and can contribute to GERD. If the gastric content is highly acidic or contains bile salts and pancreatic or intestinal enzymes, reflux esophagitis can be severe. In individuals with weak esophageal peristalsis, refluxed chyme remains in the esophagus longer than usual. This increases the amount of time the esophageal mucosa is exposed to acids, enzymes, and bile. The refluxate causes mucosal injury and inflammation with hyperemia, increased capillary permeability, edema, tissue fragility, erosions, and ulcerations (Fig. 42.2). Fibrosis and thickening may develop. Precancerous lesions (Barrett esophagus, see the Cancer of Gastrointestinal Tract section) with progression to adenocarcinoma can be a long-term consequence.

◆**CLINICAL MANIFESTATIONS.** The clinical manifestations of reflux esophagitis are related to mucosal injury from acid regurgitation and the frequency and duration of reflux events. Manifestations include heartburn, chronic cough, asthma attacks (Chapter 36), laryngitis, sinusitis, and upper abdominal pain within 1 hour of eating. The symptoms worsen if the individual lies down or if intraabdominal pressure increases (e.g., as a result of coughing, vomiting, or straining at stool). Symptoms may be present when no acid is in the esophagus. Edema, fibrosis (strictures), esophageal spasm, or decreased esophageal motility may result in dysphagia with weight loss. Alcohol or acid-containing foods, such as citrus fruits, can cause discomfort during swallowing.

◆**EVALUATION AND TREATMENT.** Diagnosis of GERD is based on the history and clinical manifestations. Esophageal endoscopy shows hyperemia, edema, erosion, and strictures. Dysplastic changes (Barrett esophagus) can be identified by tissue biopsy. Impedance/pH monitoring measures the movement of stomach contents upward into the esophagus and the acidity of the refluxate.

Proton pump inhibitors are the agents of choice for controlling symptoms and healing esophagitis. Other therapies include histamine-2 (H2) receptor antagonists, prokinetics, and antacids. Weight reduction, smoking cessation, elevation of the head of the bed 6 inches, and avoiding tight clothing also help to alleviate symptoms. Laparoscopic fundoplication is the most common surgical intervention when medical treatment fails.[29]

Eosinophilic esophagitis is a rare, idiopathic inflammatory disease of the esophagus characterized by esophageal infiltration of eosinophils associated with atopic disease, including asthma and food allergies. It occurs in adults and children. Dysphagia, food impaction, vomiting, and weight loss are common symptoms. Endoscopy with biopsy identifies the eosinophilic infiltration and differentiation from GERD. Treatment is symptomatic, including elimination diets and topical corticosteroids. Proton pump inhibitors are effective for many individuals.[30]

Hiatal Hernia

◆**PATHOPHYSIOLOGY.** Hiatal hernia is a type of diaphragmatic hernia with protrusion (herniation) of the upper part of the stomach through the diaphragm and into the thorax. There are four types: sliding (type I); paraesophageal (type II); and mixed (type III), which include elements of types I and II (Fig. 42.3). In type IV the entire stomach and other abdominal organs slide into the thorax.[31]

In type I, sliding hiatal hernia (the most common type, 90% to 95%), the proximal portion of the stomach moves into the thoracic

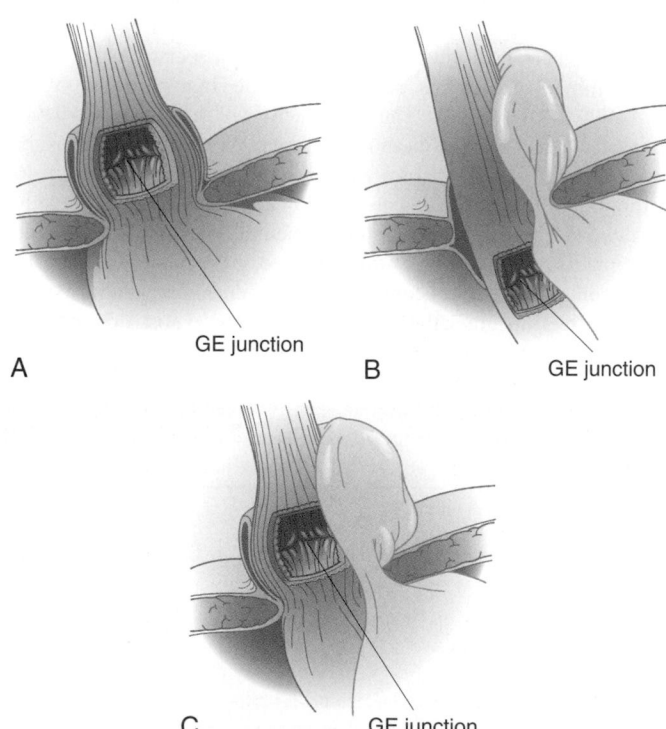

A

B

C

GE junction

FIGURE 42.3 Three Types of Hiatal Hernia. A, Type I—*sliding hernia.* The visceral peritoneum remains intact and restrains the size of the hernia in sliding hiatal hernia. **B,** Type II—*paraesophageal* or *rolling hernia.* The membrane becomes thinner or defective in paraesophageal hernia, allowing a true peritoneal sac to protrude into the posterior mediastinum where negative intrathoracic pressure causes it to enlarge. **C,** Type III—*mixed hernia. GE,* Gastroesophageal. **NOTE:** Type IV—complex paraesophageal hernia is not shown. (From Townsend CM et al: *Sabiston textbook of surgery,* ed 19, Philadelphia, 2012, Saunders.)

cavity through the esophageal hiatus, an opening in the diaphragm for the esophagus and vagus nerves. A congenitally short esophagus, fibrosis or excessive vagal nerve stimulation, or weakening of the diaphragmatic muscles at the gastroesophageal junction contributes to the hernia. While the individual is in the supine position, the lower esophagus and stomach are pulled into the thorax. Standing causes the organs to "slide" back into the abdomen. Sliding hiatal hernia is exacerbated by factors that increase intraabdominal pressure, such as coughing, bending, wearing tight clothing, ascites, obesity, or pregnancy. This type of hernia is associated with gastroesophageal reflux because the hernia diminishes the resting pressure of the LES. In pregnant women with sliding hiatal hernia, progesterone and estrogen may lower the resting pressure of the LES further.

In type II, paraesophageal hiatal hernia (rolling hiatal hernia), herniation of the greater curvature of the stomach is through a secondary opening in the diaphragm (see Fig. 42.3). A giant paraesophageal hiatal hernia develops when 30% to 60% of the stomach moves into the thorax. As the stomach protrudes through the opening into the thorax, it lies alongside the esophagus. The gastroesophageal junction remains below the diaphragm. With paraesophageal hernia, reflux is uncommon. The position of a portion of the stomach above the diaphragm, however, causes congestion of mucosal blood flow and can lead to gastritis and ulcer formation. A mechanical strangulation of the hernia is a major complication, and surgical correction is required. Strangulation occludes blood vessels and causes vascular engorgement, edema, ischemia, and hemorrhage.

Type III, mixed hiatal hernia, is a combination of both types I and II and tends to occur in conjunction with several other diseases, including gastroesophageal reflux, peptic ulcer, cholecystitis (gallbladder inflammation), cholelithiasis (gallstones), chronic pancreatitis, and diverticulosis. Type IV is an aggravated form of type III and includes herniation of other abdominal viscera.

◆**CLINICAL MANIFESTATIONS.** Hiatal hernias are often asymptomatic. Generally, a wide variety of symptoms develop later in life and are associated with other gastrointestinal disorders, primarily GERD. Manifestations of the various types of hiatal hernia are difficult to distinguish. Symptoms include heartburn, regurgitation, dysphagia, and epigastric pain. Ischemia from hernia strangulation causes acute, severe chest or epigastric pain, nausea, vomiting, and GI bleeding.

◆**EVALUATION AND TREATMENT.** Diagnostic procedures include chest x-ray with oral barium, endoscopy, high-resolution manometry, and reflux monitoring. A chest x-ray often will show the protrusion of the stomach into the thorax, indicating paraesophageal hiatal hernia.

Treatment for sliding hiatal hernia is usually conservative. The individual can diminish reflux by eating small, frequent meals and avoiding the recumbent position after eating. Abdominal supports and tight clothing are avoided, and weight control is recommended for obese individuals. Proton pump inhibitors alleviate reflux esophagitis. Histamine 2 receptor agonists and antacids are less effective. Drugs that relax the LES (anticholinergic, nitrates, calcium channel blockers) are contraindicated because they delay gastric emptying. Laparoscopic surgery (i.e., laparoscopic fundoplication) may be performed for paraesophageal hiatal hernia or if medical management fails to control symptoms.[32]

Gastroparesis is delayed gastric emptying in the absence of mechanical gastric outlet obstruction. It is most commonly associated with diabetes mellitus, surgical vagotomy, or fundoplication. It can be idiopathic. The pathophysiology is not well understood but involves abnormalities of the autonomic nervous system, smooth muscle cells, enteric neurons, and gastrointestinal hormones. Diabetic gastroparesis represents a form of neuropathy involving the vagus nerve and loss of interstitial cells of Cajal. Symptoms include nausea, vomiting, abdominal pain, postprandial fullness or bloating, and weight loss. Treatment options include dietary management; prokinetic drugs; and, in some cases, gastric electrical stimulation and/or pyloroplasty or surgical venting gastrostomy.[33]

Pyloric Obstruction

◆**PATHOPHYSIOLOGY.** Pyloric obstruction (gastric outlet obstruction) is the narrowing or blocking of the opening between the stomach and the duodenum. This condition can be congenital (i.e., infantile hypertrophic pyloric stenosis, see Chapter 43) or acquired. Acquired obstruction is caused by peptic ulcer disease or carcinoma near the pylorus. Duodenal ulcers are more likely than gastric ulcers to obstruct the pylorus. Ulceration causes obstruction resulting from inflammation, edema, spasm, fibrosis, or scarring. Tumors cause obstruction by growing into the pylorus.

◆**CLINICAL MANIFESTATIONS.** Early in the course of pyloric obstruction, the individual experiences vague epigastric fullness, which becomes more distressing after eating and later in the day. Nausea and epigastric pain may occur as the muscles of the stomach contract in attempts to force chyme past the obstruction. These symptoms disappear when the chyme finally moves into the duodenum. As obstruction progresses, anorexia develops, sometimes accompanied by weight loss. Severe obstruction causes gastric distention and atony (lack of muscle tone and gastric motility). Gastric distention stimulates gastric secretion, which increases the feeling of fullness. Rolling or jarring of the abdomen produces a sloshing sound called the *succussion splash*. At this stage, vomiting is a cardinal sign of obstruction. It is usually copious and occurs several hours after eating. The vomitus contains undigested food but no bile. Prolonged vomiting leads to dehydration, which is accompanied by a hypokalemic and hypochloremic metabolic alkalosis caused by the respective loss of gastric potassium and acid. Because food does not enter the intestine, stools are infrequent and small. Prolonged pyloric obstruction causes severe malnutrition and dehydration.

◆**EVALUATION AND TREATMENT.** Diagnosis is based on clinical manifestations, a history of peptic ulcer disease, and examination of residual gastric contents. Endoscopy is performed if gastric carcinoma is the suggested cause of pyloric obstruction.

Obstructions resulting from ulceration often resolve with conservative management. A large-bore nasogastric tube is used to aspirate stomach contents and relieve distention. Nasogastric suction is then maintained for 2 to 3 days to decompress the stomach and restore normal motility. Gastric secretions that contribute to inflammation and edema can be suppressed with proton pump inhibitors or histamine-2 (H2) receptor antagonists. Fluids and electrolytes (saline and potassium) are given intravenously to effect rehydration and correct hypochloremia, alkalosis, and hypokalemia (see Chapter 3). Severely malnourished individuals may require parenteral hyperalimentation (intravenous nutrition). Surgery or stenting may be required to treat gastric carcinoma or persistent obstruction caused by fibrosis and scarring.[34]

Intestinal Obstruction and Paralytic Ileus

Intestinal obstruction can be caused by any condition that prevents the normal flow of chyme through the intestinal lumen or failure of normal intestinal motility in the absence of an obstructing lesion (ileus) (Table 42.2). Obstructions can occur in either the small or the large intestine. The small intestine is more commonly obstructed because of its narrower lumen. Classifications of intestinal obstruction are summarized in Table 42.3. Intestinal obstruction is classified by cause as simple or functional. *Simple obstruction* is mechanical blockage of the lumen by a lesion, but blood flow is preserved. It is the most common type of intestinal obstruction. In a *strangulated obstruction*, blood flow is compromised, leading to intestinal ischemia and, if left untreated, necrosis and perforation. Paralytic ileus, or *functional obstruction*, is a failure of motility after intestinal or abdominal surgery, acute pancreatitis, or hypokalemia. Anesthetic agents, local inflammatory reactions, use of opioid analgesia, and hyperactivity of the sympathetic nervous system contribute to postoperative ileus.

Simple obstruction of the small intestine from fibrous adhesions is the most common type of intestinal obstruction. Acute obstructions usually have mechanical causes, such as adhesions or hernias (Fig. 42.4). Chronic or partial obstructions are more often associated with tumors or inflammatory disorders, particularly of the large intestine.[35]

◆**PATHOPHYSIOLOGY.** The consequences of intestinal obstruction are related to its onset and location, the length of intestinal tract proximal to the obstruction, and the presence and severity of ischemia. The major pathophysiologic alterations are presented in Fig. 42.5. Postoperative paralytic ileus results from inhibitory neural reflexes associated with inflammatory mediators, and the influence of exogenous (meperidine or morphine) and endogenous opioids (endorphins) that affect the entire GI tract, including the stomach.[36] Small bowel obstruction (SBO)

TABLE 42.2   COMMON CAUSES OF INTESTINAL OBSTRUCTION

CAUSE	PATHOPHYSIOLOGY
Herniation	Protrusion of the intestine through a weakness in the abdominal muscles or through the inguinal ring
Intussusception	Telescoping of one part of the intestine into another; this usually causes strangulation of the blood supply; more common in the ileocecal area in infants 10 to 15 months of age than in adults
Torsion (volvulus)	Twisting of the intestine on its mesenteric pedicle, with occlusion of the blood supply; often associated with fibrous adhesions in the small intestine; occurs most often in the large intestine in older adults
Diverticulosis	Inflamed saccular herniations (diverticula) of the mucosa and submucosa through the tunica muscularis of the colon; diverticula are interspersed between thick, circular, fibrous bands; most common in obese individuals older than 60 years
Tumor	Tumor growth into the intestinal lumen; adenocarcinoma of the colon and rectum is the most common tumoral obstruction; most common in individuals older than 60 years
Paralytic (adynamic) ileus	Loss of peristaltic motor activity in the intestine; associated with abdominal surgery, peritonitis, hypokalemia, ischemic bowel, spinal trauma, pneumonia, neuropathies, or myopathies; affects small and large intestines
Fibrous adhesions	Peritoneal irritation from surgery or trauma leads to formation of fibrin and adhesions that attach to intestine, omentum, or peritoneum and can cause traction and obstruction; most common in small intestine

TABLE 42.3 CLASSIFICATION OF INTESTINAL OBSTRUCTION

CRITERIA FOR CLASSIFICATION	DEFINITION
Onset	
Acute	Sudden onset; often caused by torsion, intussusception, or herniation
Chronic	Protracted onset; more commonly from tumor growth or progressive formation of strictures
Extent of Obstruction	
Partial	Incomplete obstruction of intestinal lumen
Complete	Complete obstruction of intestinal lumen
Location of Obstructing Lesion (Small Intestine or Colon)	
Intrinsic	Obstruction develops within intestinal lumen; examples: luminal edema or hemorrhage, foreign bodies (gallstones), tumors, intussusception, or intraluminal fibrosis
Extrinsic	Obstruction originates outside the intestine; examples: tumors, torsion, fibrosis, hernia
Effects on Intestinal Wall	
Simple	Luminal obstruction without impairment of blood supply
Strangulated	Luminal obstruction with occlusion of blood supply
Closed loop	Obstruction at each end of a segment of the intestine
Causal Factors	
Mechanical	Blockage of the intestinal lumen by intrinsic or extrinsic lesions; usually treated surgically
Functional (paralytic ileus)	Paralysis of the intestinal musculature as a result of accidental or surgical trauma, peritonitis, electrolyte imbalances, or spasmolytic agents; usually treated medically

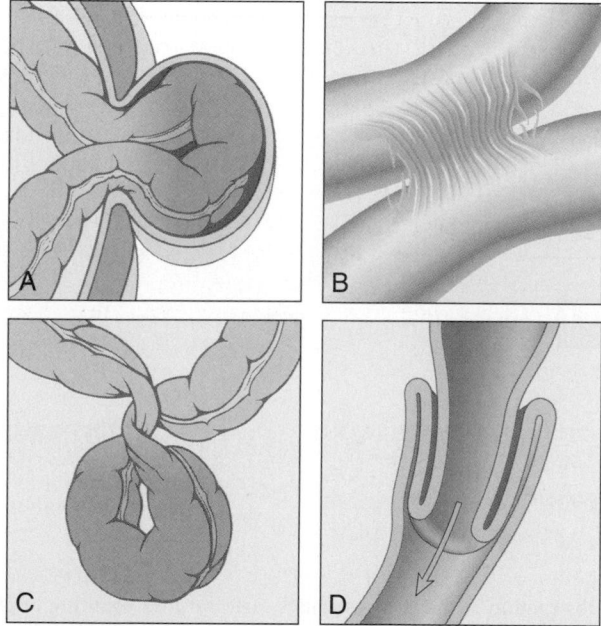

FIGURE 42.4 Intestinal Obstructions. A, Hernia. **B,** Constriction from adhesions. **C,** Volvulus. **D,** Intussusception. (From Kumar V, Abbas AK, Aster J: *Robbins basic pathology,* ed 9, Philadelphia, 2013, Saunders.)

is caused by postoperative adhesions (66%), tumors, Crohn disease, hernias, and intussusception. SBO leads to distention caused by impaired absorption and increased secretion with the accumulation of fluid and gas inside the lumen proximal to the obstruction. Distention decreases the intestines' ability to absorb water and electrolytes and increases the net secretion of these substances into the lumen. Gas from swallowed air, and to a lesser extent from bacterial overgrowth, contributes to the

distention. Distention begins almost immediately, as gases and fluids accumulate proximal to the obstruction. Within 24 hours, up to 8 L of fluid and electrolytes enters the lumen in the form of saliva, gastric juice, bile, pancreatic juice, and intestinal secretions. Distention initially increases peristalsis and then leads to decreased peristalsis and bacterial overgrowth. Copious vomiting or sequestration of fluids in the intestinal lumen prevents fluid reabsorption and produces severe fluid and electrolyte disturbances. Extracellular fluid volume and plasma volume decrease, causing dehydration. Hemoconcentration (decreased plasma volume) causes elevated hematocrit level, hypotension, and tachycardia. Severe dehydration leads to hypovolemic shock.

If the obstruction is at the pylorus or high in the small intestine, metabolic alkalosis develops initially as a result of excessive loss of hydrogen ions that normally would be reabsorbed from the gastric juice and vomiting. With prolonged obstruction or obstruction lower in the intestine, metabolic acidosis is more likely to occur because bicarbonate from pancreatic secretions and bile cannot be reabsorbed. Hypokalemia from vomiting and decreased potassium absorption can be extreme, promoting acidosis and atony of the intestinal wall. Metabolic acidosis also may be accentuated by ketosis, the result of declining carbohydrate stores caused by starvation. Lack of circulation permits the buildup of significant amounts of lactic acid, which worsen the metabolic acidosis. If pressure from the distention is severe enough, it occludes venous drainage and the arterial circulation, causing ischemia, necrosis, perforation, and peritonitis. Fever and leukocytosis are often associated with overgrowth of bacteria, ischemia, and bowel necrosis. Bacterial proliferation and translocation across the mucosa to the mesenteric lymph nodes or systemic circulation cause sepsis. The release of inflammatory mediators and toxins into the circulation causes multiple organ failure (see Chapter 49).

Large bowel obstruction is less common and often related to carcinoma. Diverticulitis, inflammatory bowel disease, volvulus, and other causes of obstruction are less common. **Acute colonic pseudo-obstruction (Ogilvie syndrome)** is a rare functional, massive dilation

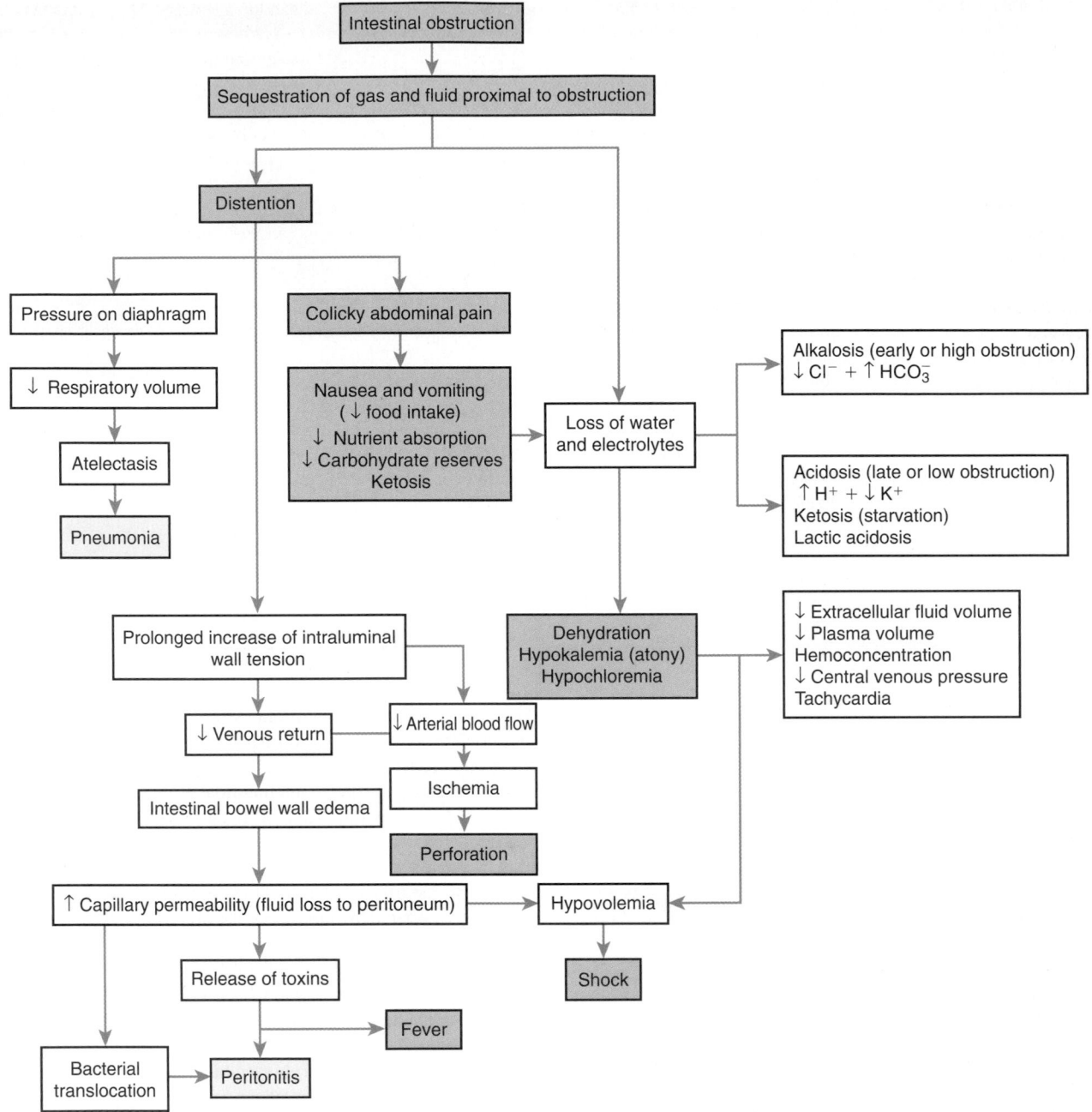

FIGURE 42.5 Pathophysiology of Intestinal Obstruction.

of the large bowel that is related to excessive sympathetic motor input or decreased parasympathetic motor input with absence of mechanical obstruction. It occurs primarily in people who are critically ill and immobilized older adults.[37]

◆**CLINICAL MANIFESTATIONS.** Signs and symptoms of *small intestine obstruction* include colicky pains caused by intestinal distention followed by nausea and vomiting. Pain intensifies for seconds or minutes as a peristaltic wave of muscle contraction meets the obstruction. Pain may be continuous with severe distention and then diminish in intensity. If ischemia occurs, the pain loses its colicky character, becoming more constant and severe. Sweating and tachycardia occur as a sympathetic nervous system response to hypotension. Fever, severe leukocytosis, abdominal distention, and rebound tenderness develop as ischemia progresses to necrosis, perforation, and peritonitis.

Obstruction at the pylorus causes early, profuse vomiting of clear gastric fluid. Obstruction in the proximal small intestine causes mild distention and vomiting of bile-stained fluid. Obstruction in the distal small intestine causes more pronounced distention because a greater length of intestine is proximal to the obstruction. In this case, vomiting may not occur or may occur later and contain fecal material. Partial obstruction can cause diarrhea or constipation, but complete obstruction usually causes constipation only. Complete obstruction increases the number of bowel sounds, which may be tinkly and accompanied by peristaltic rushes and crampy, abdominal pain. Signs of hypovolemia and metabolic acidosis may be observed as early as 24 hours after the occurrence of complete obstruction. Distention may be severe enough to push against the diaphragm and decrease lung volume. This can lead to atelectasis and pneumonia, particularly in debilitated individuals.

Large intestine obstruction usually presents with hypogastric pain and abdominal distention. Pain can vary from vague to excruciating, depending on the degree of ischemia and the development of peritonitis. Vomiting occurs late in the obstructive process. Small and large intestinal perforation presents the same with acute, persistent abdominal pain, nausea, vomiting, and fever.[38] *Acute colonic pseudo-obstruction* is characterized by abdominal distention, abdominal pain, and nausea and vomiting without any mechanical cause. Bowel sounds are usually present.

◆**EVALUATION AND TREATMENT.** Evaluation is based on clinical manifestations and imaging studies. Successful management requires early identification of the site and type of obstruction. Replacement of fluid and electrolytes and decompression of the lumen with gastric or intestinal suction are essential forms of therapy. Laparoscopic procedures can release adhesions. Immediate surgical intervention is required for strangulation and complete obstruction or perforation. Colonic stents may be placed for malignant obstruction. Neostigmine, a parasympathomimetic, is used for colonic pseudo-obstruction, and colonoscopic decompression may be required.[39] Management of intestinal perforation requires intravenous antibiotics, fluid resuscitation, and surgery related to the underlying cause of perforation.[38]

Gastritis

Gastritis is an inflammatory disorder of the gastric mucosa. It can be acute or chronic and can affect the corpus, fundus or antrum, or the entire mucosa (pangastritis).

Acute gastritis is caused by injury of the protective mucosal barrier by drugs, chemicals, or *Helicobacter pylori* infection (Fig. 42.6). Mucosal lesions can be superficial or deep erosions with or without hemorrhage. Nonsteroidal antiinflammatory drugs (NSAIDs [e.g., ibuprofen, naproxen, indomethacin, and aspirin]) inhibit the action of cyclooxygenase-1 (COX-1) and cause gastritis because they inhibit prostaglandin synthesis, which normally stimulates the secretion of mucus and suppresses inflammation. With the exception of aspirin, NSAIDs also cause gastric hypermotility, causing mucosal compression and injury. Alcohol, histamine, and metabolic disorders, such as uremia, are contributing factors. *H. pylori*–associated acute gastritis causes inflammation, increased gastric secretion in antral gastritis, decreased gastric section in fundal gastritis, pain, nausea, and vomiting (Box 42.1). Shock and hypotension can decrease mucosal blood flow contributing to acute gastritis.

The clinical manifestations of acute gastritis can include vague abdominal discomfort, epigastric tenderness, and bleeding. Healing usually occurs spontaneously within a few days. Discontinuing injurious drugs, using antacids, decreasing acid secretion with a histamine H2-receptor antagonist, or proton pump inhibitor also promote healing.

Chronic gastritis can occur at any age and involves chronic inflammation, mucosal atrophy, and epithelial metaplasia that progresses over years.[40] Chronic gastritis is usually classified as type A, or immune (fundal), or type B, nonimmune (antral) associated with *H. pylori*. When both types of chronic gastritis occur, it is known as *type AB*, or *pangastritis*, and the antrum is more severely involved. Type C gastritis is associated with reflux of bile and pancreatic secretions into the stomach, causing chemical injury.

BOX 42.1 **PATHOGENESIS OF *HELICOBACTER PYLORI*–RELATED DISEASE**

H. pylori is a gram-negative spiral bacterium with a flagellum and is a major cause of acute and chronic gastritis, peptic ulcer disease in the duodenum and stomach, gastric adenocarcinoma, and gastric mucosa–associated lymphoid tissue (MALT) in about 20% of infected individuals. *H. pylori* is transmitted through the fecal-oral route and is usually acquired in childhood. Infection is asymptomatic in about 70% of cases. In other cases, inflammation and immune responses promote mucosal ulcerations or prevent healing of injured tissue. Gene-environment interaction and different pathogenic strains of *H. pylori* increase risk for disease. Patterns of gastritis and disease progression vary by site of infection and strain of *H. pylori*. Pathogenic and virulence factors include the following:

1. An ability to colonize and adhere to gastric epithelial cells
2. The possession of flagella, which allows movement through the luminal mucous layer to a site of higher pH
3. A lipopolysaccharide membrane component evades immune protection and promotes inflammation
4. Secretion of urease that produces ammonia and carbon dioxide, resulting in a more alkaline environment
5. Release of vacuolating cytotoxin *(VacA)* that promotes bacterial survival and causes epithelial injury
6. The presence of cytotoxin-associated gene *(CagA)* strains that can escape normal immune responses and cause inflammation with release of inflammatory cytokines and reactive oxygen metabolites that damage mucosal epithelial cells and cause loss of the protective mucosal barrier; they also promote tumor development by degrading *tp53* tumor suppression
7. An ability of adherent strains to suppress acid secretion to improve their survival, particularly *CagA* and *VacA* strains
8. Recruitment and activation of neutrophils, macrophages, and mast cells with release of inflammatory cytokines (tumor necrosis factor-alpha [TNF-α], interleukin-1 [IL-1], IL-6, IL-8, IL-17, histamine) that promote cellular injury
9. Downregulation of antral somatostatin leading to increased gastrin, increased acid, impaired mucosal bicarbonate production, and increased mucosal exposure to acid and pepsin
10. Activation or inhibition of T- and B-cell immune responses that may contribute to mucosal injury
11. Release of cytokines and chemokines that promote gastric epithelial cell death (apoptosis) that can result in atrophy, ulcers or cell proliferation, and dysplasia or malignant growth

---

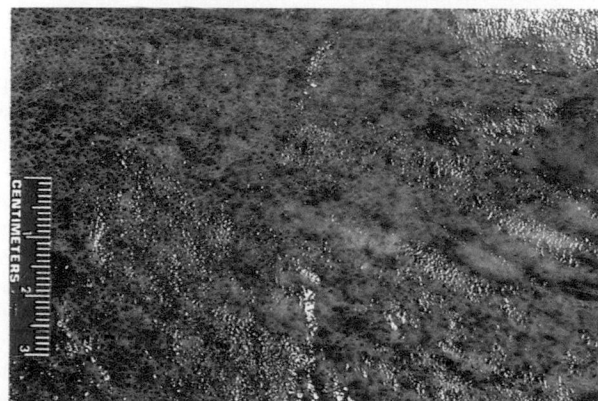

FIGURE 42.6 Acute Erosive Gastritis. Acute erosive gastritis is shown in the opened stomach. The mucosa appears hyperemic, and the foci of superficial ulceration are manifested as scattered, small, red areas termed *erosions*. (From Kumar V et al: *Pathologic basis of disease*, ed 7, Philadelphia, 2006, Saunders.)

Data from Amieva M, Peek RM Jr: *Gastroenterology* 150(1):64-78, 2016; Backert S et al: *Helicobacter* 21 Suppl 1:19-25, 2016; Li H et al: *Helicobacter* 21(6):445-461, 2016; Tohidpour A: *Microb Pathog* 93:44-55, 2016.

Chronic fundal gastritis, or type A, is the most rare and severe form of gastritis and is associated with loss of T-cell tolerance and development of autoantibodies against parietal cells or intrinsic factor, or both, with gastric H^+-K^+-ATPase protein as the causal antigen. The gastric mucosa degenerates extensively in the body and fundus of the stomach, leading to gastric atrophy. Loss of parietal cells leads to achlorhydria and loss of intrinsic factor. Pernicious anemia can develop from decreased vitamin B_{12} absorption (see Chapter 29). Because acid secretion is insufficient, the feedback mechanism that normally inhibits gastrin secretion is impaired, causing elevated plasma levels of gastrin. Chronic fundal gastritis occurs in association with other autoimmune diseases (e.g., rheumatoid arthritis, autoimmune thyroid disease, or type 1 diabetes mellitus) and is a risk factor for gastric carcinoma, particularly in individuals who develop pernicious anemia.

Type B chronic nonimmune (antral gastritis) generally involves the antrum only and is more common than fundal gastritis. Infection with *H. pylori* may trigger the immune response through molecular mimicry (a mechanism of autoimmune disease with similarities between foreign and self-antigens sufficient to result in cross-activation of autoreactive T or B cells)[41] or by causing mucosal injury and exposure of gastric H^+-K^+-ATPase protein.[42] Chronic use of alcohol, tobacco, and nonsteroidal antiinflammatory drugs are contributing factors. There are high levels of hydrochloric acid secretion with an increased risk of duodenal ulcers. *H. pylori* can also progress to autoimmune atrophic gastritis and involve the fundus, thus becoming pangastritis.[40]

Signs and symptoms of chronic gastritis often include vague symptoms such as anorexia, fullness, nausea, vomiting, and epigastric pain. Gastric bleeding may be the only clinical manifestation of gastritis. Gastroscopic examination and biopsy may show a long-standing inflammatory process and gastric atrophy in an individual with no history of abdominal distress. Gastric secretion analysis confirms achlorhydria and loss of intrinsic factor. Pernicious anemia can develop because intrinsic factor is less available to facilitate vitamin B_{12} absorption. There also may be iron deficiency. The presence of antiparietal cell antibody and elevated plasma ghrelin level are specific for atrophic gastritis. *H. pylori* infection is evidence for *H. pylori* chronic gastritis with infiltration of neutrophils and lymphocytes. Both invasive and noninvasive diagnostic tests are available. Surveillance for gastric carcinoma is recommended with chronic atrophic gastritis and *H. pylori* infection.[43]

Symptoms can usually be managed with consumption of smaller meals, including a soft, bland diet, and with avoidance of alcohol and NSAIDs. Combination antibiotics are used to eradicate *H. pylori*, and the emergence of antimicrobial resistance is a concern.[44] Vitamin B_{12} is administered to correct pernicious anemia (see Chapter 29).

Alkaline reflux gastritis is a stomach inflammation caused by reflux of bile and alkaline pancreatic secretions that contain proteolytic enzymes and disrupt the mucosal barrier in the remnant stomach. This form of gastritis occurs in 5% to 20% of individuals who have undergone gastrectomy, pyloroplasty, or pancreaticoduodenectomy. Clinical manifestations include nausea, bilious vomiting (vomiting in which the vomitus contains bile), and sustained epigastric pain that worsens after eating and is not relieved by antacids. Endoscopy shows a hemorrhagic and friable gastric mucosa. Antacids do not consistently improve symptoms. Avoidance of aspirin and alcohol may decrease gastric irritation, and a low-fat diet may limit bile secretion. Surgical correction may ultimately be required.[45]

Peptic Ulcer Disease

A **peptic ulcer** is a break, or ulceration, in the protective mucosal lining of the lower esophagus, stomach, or duodenum. The prevalence of peptic ulcer in 2011 in the United States was estimated at 15.5 million people.[46] Risk factors for peptic ulcer disease include genetic predisposi-

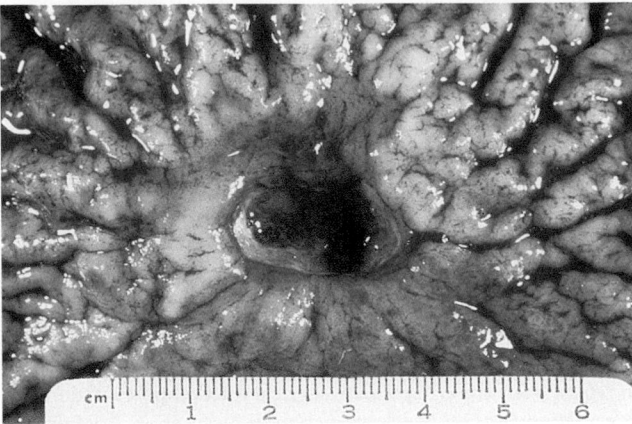

FIGURE 42.7 Chronic Peptic Ulcer. Gross photograph of a chronic peptic ulcer located in the lesser curvature, straddling the antrum and corpus of the stomach. (From Damjanov I, Linder J, editors: *Anderson's pathology*, ed 10, St Louis, 1996, Mosby.)

tion, *H. pylori* infection of the gastric mucosa (see Box 42.1), and habitual use of aspirin and NSAIDs. Additional factors include excessive use of alcohol, smoking, acute pancreatitis, chronic obstructive pulmonary disease, obesity, cirrhosis, age greater than 65 years, and socioeconomic status.[47,48] Psychologic stress contributes to risk for peptic ulcer disease but the exact mechanism of causation is not known.[49,50] Peptic ulcers also can be idiopathic or caused by gastrinoma.

Peptic ulcers can be single or multiple, acute or chronic, and superficial or deep. Superficial ulcerations are called *erosions* because they erode the mucosa but do not penetrate the muscularis mucosae (Fig. 42.7). True ulcers extend through the muscularis mucosae and damage blood vessels, causing hemorrhage or perforating the gastrointestinal wall.

Chronic use of NSAIDs suppresses mucosal prostaglandin synthesis, resulting in decreased bicarbonate secretion and mucin (a component of the gut barrier) production and increased secretion of hydrochloric acid. The interaction of NSAIDs and *H. pylori* can contribute to the pathogenesis of peptic ulcer. Disruption of the mucosa exposes submucosal areas to gastric secretions and autodigestion, causing erosion and ulceration.

Zollinger-Ellison syndrome is a rare syndrome also associated with peptic ulcers caused by a gastrin-secreting neuroendocrine tumor or multiple tumors (gastrinoma) of the pancreas or duodenum. Gastrin stimulates a proliferation of gastric parietal cells and chronic secretion of gastric acid. The resulting excess acid causes gastric and duodenal ulcers, gastroesophageal reflux with abdominal pain, and diarrhea. Diagnosis includes secretin- or calcium-stimulated measures of gastrin levels, gastric pH levels less than 2, and symptomatic evidence of peptic ulcer disease. Proton pump inhibitors reduce gastric acid secretion, and surgical removal of tumors limits metastasis.[51]

Duodenal Ulcers

Duodenal ulcers occur with greater frequency than other types of peptic ulcers and are commonly caused by *H. pylori* infection and NSAID use.[52] Idiopathic duodenal ulcers are rare and can be associated with altered mucosal defenses, rapid gastric emptying, elevated serum gastrin levels, or acid production stimulated by smoking.[53]

◆**PATHOPHYSIOLOGY.** Causative factors, singly or in combination, cause acid and pepsin concentrations in the duodenum to penetrate the mucosal barrier and lead to ulceration (Fig. 42.8). Acid in the duodenum facilitates *H. pylori* infection.

◆**CLINICAL MANIFESTATIONS.** The characteristic manifestation of a duodenal ulcer is chronic intermittent pain in the epigastric area. The

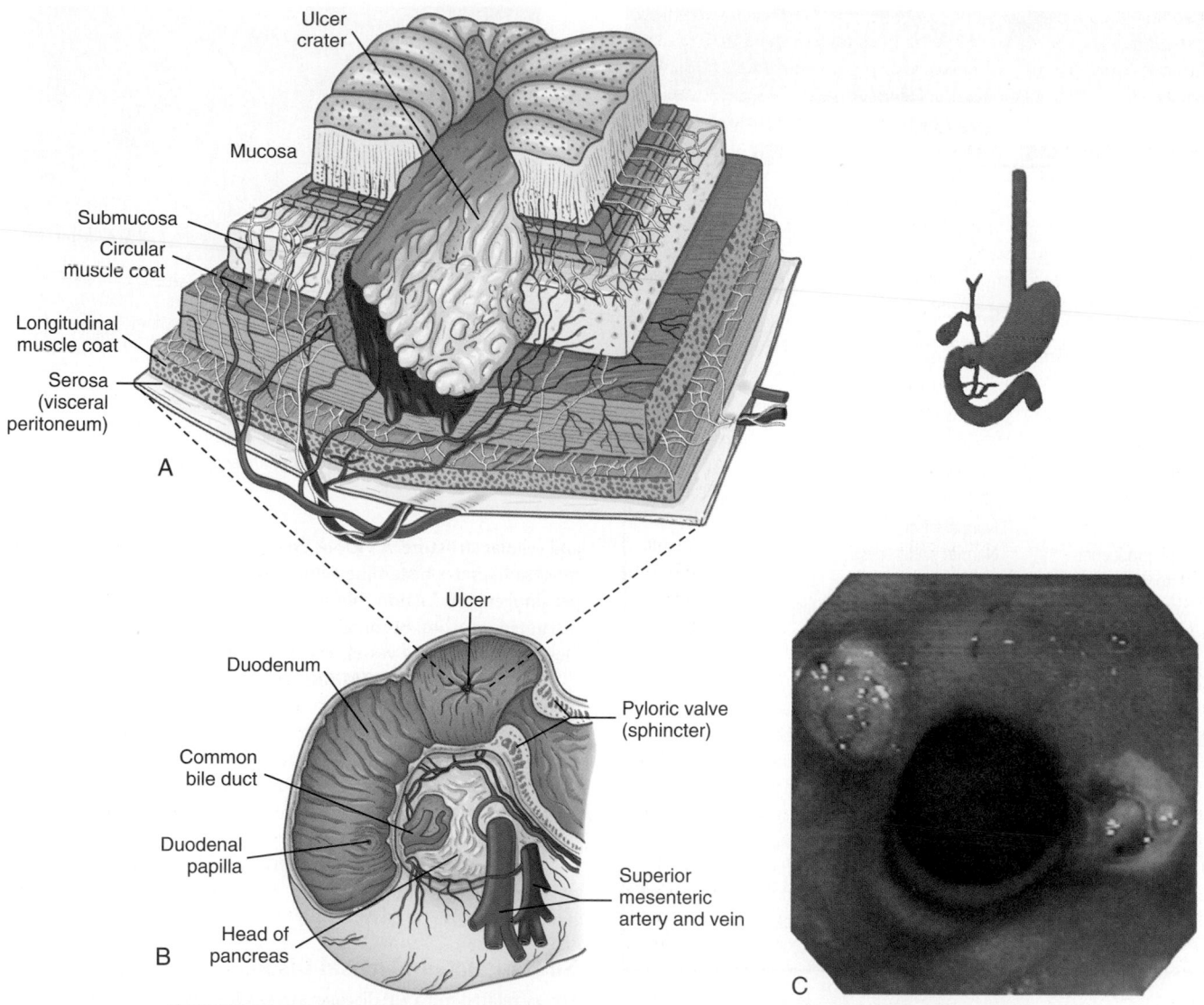

FIGURE 42.8 Duodenal Ulcer. A, A deep ulceration in the duodenal wall extending as a crater through the entire mucosa and into the muscle layers. **B,** Duodenal ulcer. **C,** Bilateral (kissing) duodenal ulcers in a person using nonsteroidal antiinflammatory drugs (NSAIDs). (**C** courtesy David Bjorkman, MD, Department of Gastroenterology, University of Utah School of Medicine, Salt Lake City, UT.)

pain begins 30 minutes to 2 hours after eating, when the stomach is empty. It is not unusual for pain to occur in the middle of the night and disappear by morning. The pain results from sensorineural stimulation by acid or muscle spasm, or both. Pain is relieved rapidly by ingestion of food or antacids, creating a typical "pain-food-relief" pattern. Some individuals with duodenal ulcer have no symptoms, particularly older adults; the first manifestation may be hemorrhage or perforation, particularly with a history of NSAID or anticoagulant use. Healing is accompanied by relief of pain. Constant, unremitting pain may be caused by complications, such as intestinal obstruction or perforation. Bleeding from duodenal ulcers causes hematemesis or melena. It is not clear why individuals infected with *H. pylori* duodenal ulcers are negatively associated with gastric cancer, but it may be related to heterogeneity of host and *H. pylori* genetic factors.[54]

◆**EVALUATION AND TREATMENT.** Several diagnostic approaches are used to differentiate duodenal ulcers from gastric ulcers or gastric carcinoma. Endoscopic evaluation allows visualization of lesions and biopsy. Radioimmune assays of gastrin levels are evaluated to identify

ulcers associated with gastric carcinomas. *H. pylori* is detected using the urea breath test, *H. pylori*–specific serum immunoglobulin G (IgG) and immunoglobulin A (IgA) antibodies, and measurement of *H. pylori* stool antigen levels. Findings from gastric biopsy detect *H. pylori* infection and confirm eradication after treatment. Polymerase chain reaction testing provides additional virulence and antibiotic sensitivity profiling.[55]

Management of duodenal ulcers is aimed at relieving the causes and effects of hyperacidity and preventing complications. Antacids neutralize gastric contents, elevate pH, inactivate pepsin, relieve pain, and are cytoprotective. Acid secretion can be suppressed with proton pump inhibitors or H2 receptor blockers. *H. pylori* is eradicated with combinations of antibiotics, although there is increasing drug resistance.[44] Probiotics may provide an added benefit.[56]

Ulcer-coating agents, such as sucralfate and colloidal bismuth, promote healing. Anticholinergic drugs may be used to inhibit gastric secretion, suppress gastric motility, and delay gastric emptying. Diet therapy includes a diet high in vitamin A, vitamin C, zinc, selenium, and fiber.[57] Surgical resection may be required for complications including

TABLE 42.4	CHARACTERISTICS OF GASTRIC AND DUODENAL ULCERS	
CHARACTERISTICS	**GASTRIC ULCER**	**DUODENAL ULCER**
Incidence		
Age at onset	50–70 years	20–50 years
Family history	Usually negative	Positive
Sex (prevalence)	Equal in women and men	Equal in women and men
Stress factors	Increased	Average
Ulcerogenic drugs	Normal use	Increased use
Cancer risk	Increased	Not increased
Pathophysiology		
Helicobacter pylori infection	Often present (60%–80%)	Often present (95%–100%)
Abnormal mucus	May be present	May be present
Parietal cell mass	Normal or decreased	Increased
Acid production	Normal or decreased	Increased
Serum gastrin	Increased	Normal
Serum pepsinogen	Normal	Increased
Associated gastritis	More common	Usually not present
Clinical Manifestations		
Pain	Located in upper abdomen	Located in upper abdomen
	Intermittent	Intermittent
	Pain-antacid-relief pattern	Pain-antacid or food-relief pattern
	Food-pain pattern	Nocturnal pain common
Clinical course	Chronic ulcer without pattern of remission and exacerbation	Pattern of remissions and exacerbations for years

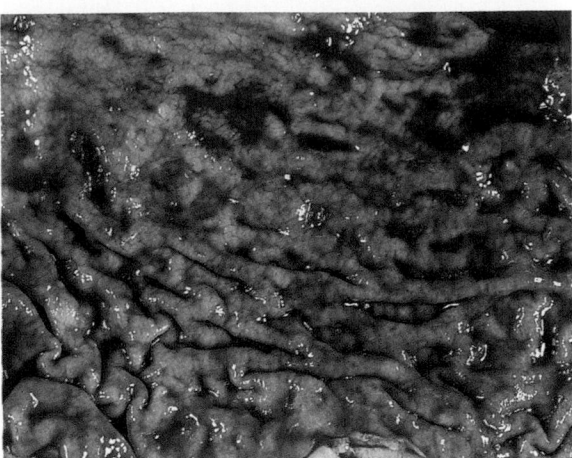

FIGURE 42.9 Macroscopic Appearance of Benign Gastric Ulcers. (From Damjanov I, Linder J, editors: *Anderson's pathology,* ed 10, St Louis, 1996, Mosby.)

bleeding, perforation, obstruction, or peritonitis. Development of a vaccine against *H. pylori* is progressing slowly.[58]

Gastric Ulcers

Gastric ulcers are ulcers of the stomach and usually occur between the ages of 55 and 65 years. They are less common than duodenal ulcers (Table 42.4 and Fig. 42.9).

◆**PATHOPHYSIOLOGY.** Gastric ulcers generally develop in the antral region, adjacent to the acid-secreting mucosa of the body (see Box 42.1). The primary defect is an abnormality that increases the mucosal barrier's permeability to hydrogen ions. Risk factors include *H. pylori* infection, duodenal reflux, and use of NSAIDs. Gastric secretion may be normal or less than normal, and there may be a decreased mass of parietal cells. Chronic autoimmune pangastritis is often associated with development of gastric ulcers and may precipitate ulcer formation by limiting the mucosa's ability to secrete a protective layer of mucus (Fig. 42.10).[41]

Duodenal reflux of bile is associated with gastric ulcer (alkaline reflux gastritis), and may occur after cholecystectomy, pyloroplasty, or gastrojejunostomy. The pyloric sphincter also may fail to respond to stimuli that normally increase resting tone, such as entry of acid, protein, and fat into the duodenum, allowing reflux of bile and pancreatic enzymes to damage the gastric mucosa. The damaged mucosal barrier permits hydrogen ions to diffuse into the mucosa, where they disrupt permeability

and cellular structure. A vicious cycle can be established as the damaged mucosa liberates histamine, which stimulates the increase of acid and pepsinogen production, blood flow, and capillary permeability. The disrupted mucosa becomes edematous and loses plasma proteins. Destruction of small vessels causes bleeding.

◆**CLINICAL MANIFESTATIONS.** The clinical manifestations of gastric ulcers are similar to those of duodenal ulcers (see Table 42.4). The pattern of pain, food, and relief is common, but the pain of gastric ulcers also occurs immediately after eating. Gastric ulcers also tend to be chronic rather than alternate between periods of remission and exacerbation and cause more anorexia, vomiting, and weight loss than duodenal ulcers.

◆**EVALUATION AND TREATMENT.** The evaluation and treatment of gastric ulcers are similar to the evaluation and treatment of duodenal ulcers.

Stress-Related Mucosal Disease

Stress-related mucosal disease (stress ulcer) is an acute form of erosive, inflammatory peptic ulcer that tends to accompany the physiologic stress of severe illness; multisystem organ failure; or major trauma, including severe burns or head injury. Usually, multiple sites of ulceration are distributed within the stomach or duodenum. Stress ulcers may be classified as ischemic ulcers or Cushing ulcers.

Ischemic ulcers develop within hours of an event—such as hemorrhage, multisystem trauma, severe burns, heart failure, or sepsis—that causes ischemia of the stomach and duodenal mucosa. Stress ulcers that develop as a result of burn injury are often called Curling ulcers. Cushing ulcer is a stress ulcer associated with severe head trauma or brain surgery. Decreased mucosal blood flow and hypersecretion of acid caused by overstimulation of the vagal nuclei damage the mucosal barrier, initiating the processes (see Fig. 42.10).

The primary clinical manifestation of stress-related mucosal disease is bleeding that occurs more readily with the presence of coagulopathy or mechanical ventilation. Other symptoms may not be present. The bleeding may be slight or, if a small vessel is perforated, amount to hundreds of milliliters. Prophylactic treatment regimens are used to prevent this disease.[59] Stress ulcers seldom become chronic.

Surgical Treatment of Ulcer

Advances in the medical treatment of peptic ulcer disease with proton pump inhibitors and eradication of *H. pylori,* as well as laparoscopic and endoscopic repair techniques, have significantly reduced the number

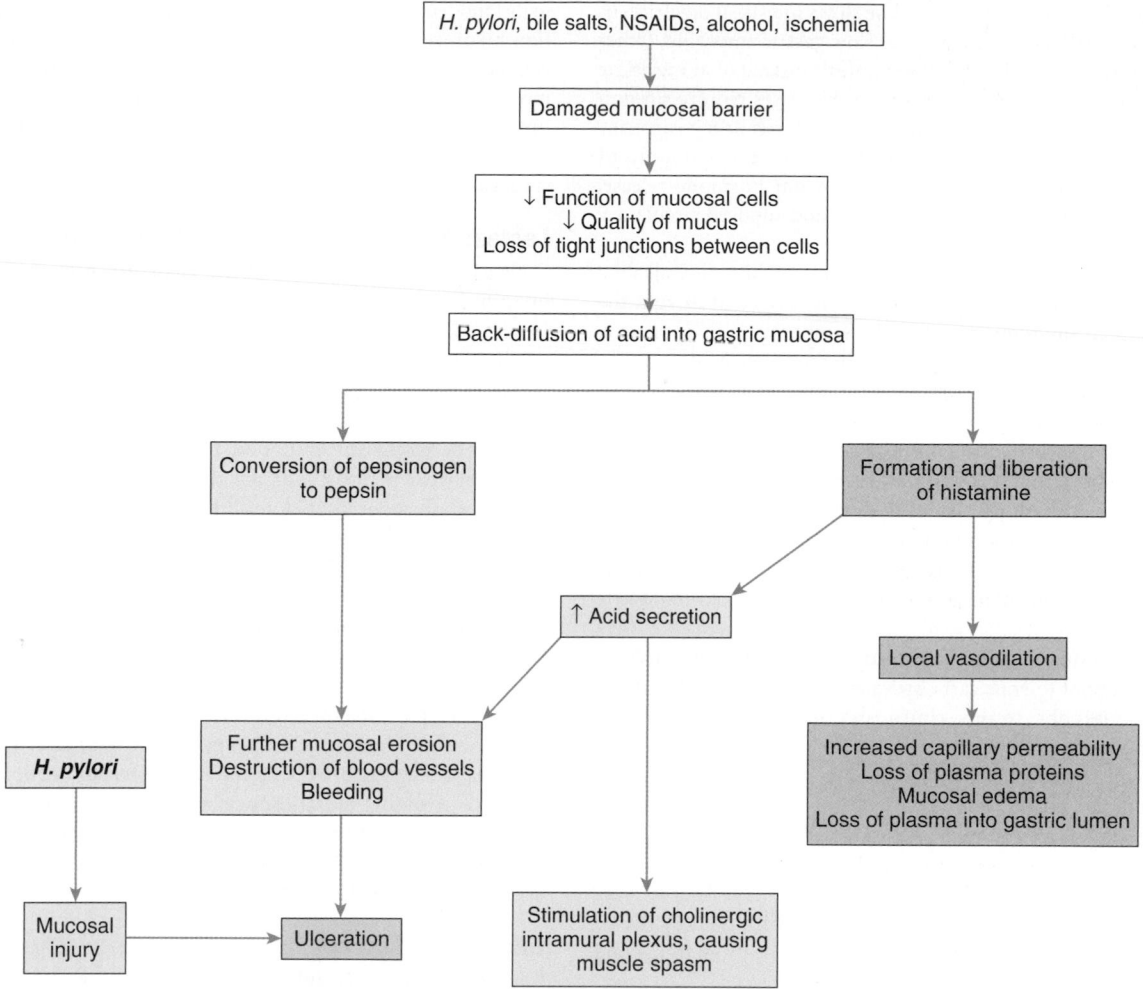

FIGURE 42.10 Pathophysiology of Gastric Ulcer Formation.

of cases requiring open surgery. The indications for ulcer surgery are recurrent or uncontrolled bleeding and complicated perforation of the stomach or duodenum. The primary objectives of surgical treatment are to reduce stimuli for acid secretion, decrease the number of acid-secreting cells in the stomach, and correct complications of ulcer disease.

Acute complications of gastrectomy or anastomosis, such as poor wound healing, abscess formation, or suture failure, are relatively uncommon except in the debilitated person. Chronic complications, however, occur more often and are likely to develop if a large portion of the stomach has been removed. These complications and their pathophysiologic mechanisms are described in the next section.

Postgastrectomy Syndromes

Postgastrectomy syndromes are a group of signs and symptoms that occur after gastric resection for the treatment of peptic ulcer, gastric carcinoma, or bariatric surgery for extreme obesity. They are caused by anatomic and functional changes in the stomach and upper small intestine.

Dumping syndrome is the rapid emptying of hypertonic chyme from the surgically created, residual stomach (the stomach component remaining after surgical resection following gastric or bariatric surgery) into the small intestine 10 to 20 minutes after eating (early dumping syndrome). It occurs with varying severity in 5% to 10% of individuals who have undergone partial gastrectomy, bariatric surgical procedures, or pyloroplasty.[60] It is not as common in individuals who have undergone

a Billroth II anastomosis (gastrojejunostomy) accompanied by vagotomy. Factors that promote *early dumping syndrome* include (1) loss of gastric capacity, (2) loss of emptying control when the pylorus is removed, and (3) loss of feedback control by the duodenum when it is removed. Rapid gastric emptying and creation of a nonphysiologic, high osmotic gradient within the small intestine cause a sudden shift of fluid from the vascular compartment to the intestinal lumen. Plasma volume decreases, causing vasomotor responses, such as increased pulse rate, hypotension, weakness, pallor, sweating, and dizziness. Rapid distention of the intestine produces a feeling of epigastric fullness, cramping pain, nausea, and vomiting. *Diarrhea* can accompany dumping syndrome or occur as a solitary symptom. Diarrhea can occur as frequent, persistent elimination of liquid stool or as intermittent, precipitous, and unpredictable elimination of a large volume of stool. Both types can be either mild or severe.

A less common form of dumping syndrome, *late dumping syndrome*, occurs 1 to 3 hours after eating. The symptoms include weakness, diaphoresis, and confusion. After a high-carbohydrate meal, individuals who have undergone gastrectomy may develop hypoglycemia, which causes the symptoms. The hypoglycemia is caused by an increase in insulin secretion stimulated by the hyperglycemia that follows eating. Other hormonal responses also may participate in the development of hypoglycemia.

Most cases of dumping syndrome respond well to dietary management. Frequent small meals that are high in protein and low in carbohydrates relieve symptoms. Acarbose slows intestinal digestion of carbohydrates, and somatostatin analogs slow gastric emptying. Other measures include drinking fluids between meals instead of at mealtime and reclining on the left side after eating. Some cases require surgical intervention, including reconstruction of the pylorus or a gastrojejunostomy. Octreotide reduces abdominal and vasomotor symptoms of dumping syndrome by inhibiting insulin and gut hormone release, slowing intestinal transit time, and inhibiting food-induced circulatory changes.[61]

Alkaline reflux gastritis is caused by reflux of bile and alkaline pancreatic secretions containing proteolytic enzymes that disrupt the mucosal barrier in the remnant stomach. Symptoms include nausea, bilious vomiting, and sustained epigastric pain that worsens after eating, is not relieved by antacids, and responds somewhat to avoidance of aspirin and alcohol.[62] Surgical correction may be required.

Afferent loop obstruction is a rare complication of Billroth II gastrojejunostomy. Symptoms include intermittent severe pain and epigastric fullness after eating as a result of volvulus, hernia, adhesion, or stenosis of the duodenal stump on the proximal side of the gastrojejunostomy; vomiting relieves symptoms; management includes low-fat diet, but decompression or surgery revision is required for complete obstruction.[63]

Weight loss is commonly caused by inadequate caloric intake because the individual cannot tolerate carbohydrates or a normal-size meal; the stomach is also less able to mix, churn, and break down food. In the case of bariatric surgery for extreme obesity, weight loss is the intended outcome, but nutrient deficiencies, including vitamins and minerals, must be supplemented.[64]

Anemia results from iron malabsorption caused by decreased acid secretion, lack of vitamin B_{12} or folate, and resection of the duodenum after a Billroth II gastrojejunostomy. Bone and mineral disorders are related to altered calcium absorption and metabolism with increased risk for fractures and deformity, and malabsorption of vitamins and nutrients, such as vitamin D.

Malabsorption Syndromes

Malabsorption syndromes interfere with nutrient absorption in the small intestine. Historically malabsorption disorders have been classified as maldigestion or malabsorption. Maldigestion is failure of the chemical processes of digestion that take place in the intestinal lumen or at the brush border of the intestinal mucosa of the small intestine. Malabsorption is the failure of the intestinal mucosa to absorb (transport) the digested nutrients. The two syndromes are often interrelated or occur together, making classification difficult. Generally, however, maldigestion is caused by deficiencies of enzymes, such as pancreatic lipase or intestinal lactase, which are necessary for digestion; inadequate secretion of bile salts; and inadequate reabsorption of bile in the ileum. Malabsorption is the result of mucosal disruption caused by gastric or intestinal resection, vascular disorders, or intestinal disease.

Pancreatic Exocrine Insufficiency

The pancreatic enzymes (lipase, amylase, trypsin, and chymotrypsin) are required for the digestion of proteins, carbohydrates, and fats. Pancreatic insufficiency is the deficient production of these enzymes by the pancreas. Causes of pancreatic insufficiency include chronic pancreatitis, pancreatic carcinoma, pancreatic resection, and cystic fibrosis. Significant damage to or loss of pancreatic tissue must occur before enzyme levels decrease sufficiently to cause maldigestion. Although pancreatic insufficiency causes poor digestion of all nutrients, fat maldigestion is the chief problem. Salivary amylase and enzymes secreted by the intestinal brush border assist in carbohydrate and protein digestion, but these enzymes do not digest fats. Absence of pancreatic bicarbonate in the duodenum and jejunum causes an acidic pH that worsens maldigestion by preventing activation of pancreatic enzymes that are present. A large amount of fat in the stool (steatorrhea) and weight loss are the most common signs of pancreatic insufficiency. Several pancreatic function tests are available.[65] Lipase supplementation, which may be in combination with antacids or antisecretory therapy, is usually successful.[66]

Lactase Deficiency (Lactose Intolerance)

Deficiency of disaccharidase at the villus brush border of the small intestine is caused by a genetic defect in which a single enzyme, usually lactase, is lacking. Lactase deficiency inhibits the breakdown of lactose (milk sugar) into monosaccharides and therefore prevents lactose digestion and absorption across the intestinal wall. Lactase deficiency is most common in blacks, Latinos, and Native Americans and usually does not develop until adulthood. Congenital lactase deficiency causes watery diarrhea in breast milk or lactose-containing formulas in infants. Lactase expression is lost before adulthood in adult-type lactose intolerance. Secondary (acquired) lactase deficiency can be caused by several diseases of the intestine, including celiac disease (see Chapter 43), enteritis, and bacterial overgrowth.[67]

The undigested lactose remains in the intestine, where bacterial fermentation causes formation of gases. Undigested lactose also increases the osmotic gradient in the intestine, causing irritation and osmotic diarrhea. Clinical manifestations of lactose consumption with lactase deficiency are bloating, crampy pain, diarrhea, and flatulence. The disorder is diagnosed by tests for lactose malabsorption and lactose tolerance. Avoiding milk products and adhering to a lactose-free diet relieve symptoms. Lactase enzyme replacement is an option. Maintaining an adequate calcium intake with restricted intake of milk products decreases risk of osteoporosis.[68]

Bile Salt Deficiency

Conjugated bile acids (bile salts) are necessary for the digestion and absorption of fats in the small intestine. Bile salts are conjugated in the bile that is synthesized from cholesterol and secreted from the liver. When bile enters the duodenum, the bile salts aggregate with fatty acids and monoglycerides to form micelles. Micelle formation makes fat molecules more soluble and allows them to pass through the unstirred layer at the brush border of the small intestinal villi (see Chapter 41). A minimum concentration of bile salts, termed the *critical micelle concentration,* is required to allow micelles to form. Therefore conditions that decrease the production or secretion of bile result in decreased micelle formation and fat malabsorption. These conditions include advanced liver disease, which decreases production of bile salts; obstruction of the common bile duct, which decreases flow of bile into the duodenum; intestinal stasis (lack of motility), which permits overgrowth of intestinal bacteria that deconjugate bile salts; and diseases or resection of the ileum, which prevent the reabsorption and recycling of bile salts (enterohepatic circulation).

Clinical manifestations of bile salt deficiency are related to poor intestinal absorption of fat and fat-soluble vitamins (A, D, E, and K). Increased fat in the stools (steatorrhea) leads to diarrhea and decreased plasma proteins. The losses of fat-soluble vitamins and their effects include the following:

1. Vitamin A deficiency results in night blindness.
2. Vitamin D deficiency results in decreased calcium absorption with bone demineralization (osteoporosis), bone pain, and fractures.
3. Vitamin K deficiency prolongs prothrombin time, leading to spontaneous development of purpura (bruising) and petechiae.
4. Vitamin E deficiency has uncertain effects but may cause testicular atrophy and neurologic defects in children.

The most effective treatment for fat-soluble vitamin deficiency is to increase the amount of medium-chain triglycerides in the diet, for example, by using coconut oil for cooking. Vitamins A, D, and K are given parenterally. Cholestyramine is used to treat steatorrhea related to ileal disease and failure of bile reabsorption.[69]

Inflammatory Bowel Disease

Ulcerative colitis and Crohn disease are chronic, relapsing idiopathic inflammatory bowel diseases (IBDs). The prevalence of IBD is about 3 million people in the United States.[70] The disease is more prevalent among white populations and Ashkenazi Jews. Risk factors and theories of causation include susceptibility genes, environmental factors, alterations in epithelial cell barrier functions, an altered immune response to intestinal microflora, and varying phenotypes.[71] Unknown environmental factors or infections are thought to alter the barrier function of the mucosal epithelium, promote loss of immune tolerance to normal intestinal antigens, and increase uptake of luminal antigens. There is possible loss of discrimination of potentially harmful pathogens from commensal microorganisms in the intestinal mucosa.[72] The loss of tolerance activates dendritic cells, triggering their transport to mesenteric lymph nodes, where they promote differentiation of naïve T cells to T helper1 (Th1), Th2, and Th17 cells, or T-regulatory cells. Production of proinflammatory cytokines and chemokines, including tumor necrosis factor, interleukins, toxic oxygen free radicals, and interferon-gamma (IFN-γ), damages the intestinal epithelium.[73] The risk of colon cancer increases significantly after 30 to 35 years of inflammatory bowel disease, particularly in untreated disease.[74] Future research is directed at an integration of these factors to refine understanding of disease cause and trajectory, particularly interactions between genetics, the microflora, mucosa, and immune responses.[75,76]

Ulcerative Colitis

Ulcerative colitis (UC) is a chronic inflammatory disease that causes ulceration of the colonic mucosa, most commonly in the rectum and sigmoid colon (Fig. 42.11). The lesions appear in susceptible individuals between 20 and 40 years of age. UC is less common in people who smoke, but smoking may not improve the natural history of ulcerative colitis.[77]

◆**PATHOPHYSIOLOGY.** The primary lesion of UC begins with inflammation at the base of the crypt of Lieberkühn. The disease involves the rectum (proctitis) and may extend proximally to the entire colon (pancolitis). The lesions are limited to the mucosa, are not transmural, and do not involve skip lesions. The inflammation involves infiltration and release of inflammatory cytokines from Th2-associated cytokines (i.e., IL-4 and IL-13) that activate neutrophils, lymphocytes, plasma cells, macrophages, eosinophils, and mast cells. Activated macrophages also contribute cytokines that cause fever and the acute phase response. The inflammation damages the epithelial mucosal barrier with leak of fluids into the gut.[78]

With milder inflammation, the mucosa is hyperemic and edematous and may appear dark red and velvety (Fig. 42.12). In more severe inflammation, the mucosa becomes hemorrhagic, and small erosions form and coalesce into ulcers. Abscess formation occurs in the crypts. Necrosis and ragged ulceration of the mucosa ensue with formation of granulation tissue. Edema and thickening of the muscularis mucosae may narrow the lumen of the involved colon. In chronic disease, inflammatory polyps (pseudopolyps) develop in the colon from rapidly regenerating epithelium.

◆**CLINICAL MANIFESTATIONS.** The course of UC consists of intermittent periods of remission and exacerbation. Clinical manifestations vary with the severity and extent of disease. Loss of the absorptive mucosal surface and decreased colonic transit time can cause large volumes of watery diarrhea. Mucosal destruction causes bleeding, cramping pain, and an urge to defecate. Frequent bloody diarrhea with passage of purulent mucus is common. Mild UC involves less mucosa and may be limited to proctitis, so that frequency of bowel movements, bleeding, and pain are minimal. Severe forms may involve the entire colon (pancolitis) and are characterized by fever, elevated pulse rate, frequent diarrhea (more than six movements per day), urgency, obviously bloody stools, continuous crampy pain, dehydration, weight loss, and anemia.[79] Complications include anal fissures, hemorrhoids, and perirectal abscess. Severe hemorrhage is rare, but chronic blood loss may precipitate

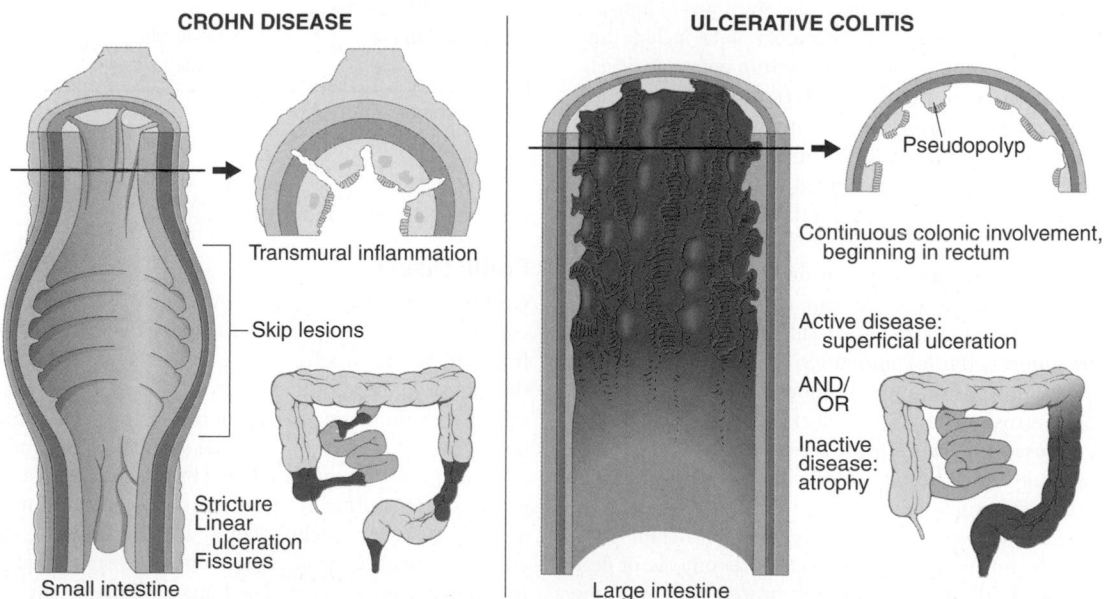

CROHN DISEASE

Transmural inflammation

Skip lesions

Stricture
Linear
ulceration
Fissures

Small intestine

ULCERATIVE COLITIS

Pseudopolyp

Continuous colonic involvement, beginning in rectum

Active disease: superficial ulceration

AND/ OR

Inactive disease: atrophy

Large intestine

FIGURE 42.11 Distribution Patterns of Crohn Disease and Ulcerative Colitis. Comparison of distribution patterns of Crohn disease and ulcerative colitis as well as different conformations of ulcers and wall thickenings. (From Kumar V et al: *Robbins basic pathology,* ed 8, St Louis, 2008, Mosby.)

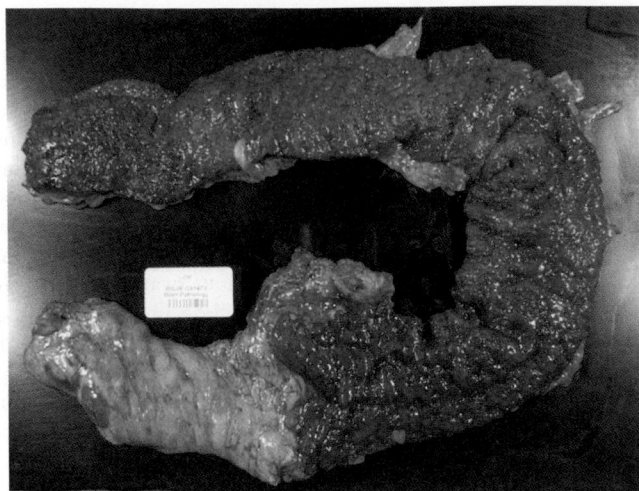

FIGURE 42.12 Acute Ulcerative Colitis. A gross specimen of subtotal ulcerative colitis showing diffuse continuous disease starting from the distal rectum and continuing up to the midportion of the ascending colon. (From Odze RD, Goldblum JR, editors: *Surgical pathology of the GI tract, liver, biliary tract, and pancreas*, ed 2, Philadelphia, 2009, Saunders.)

TABLE 42.5	FEATURES OF ULCERATIVE COLITIS AND CROHN DISEASE	
FEATURE	**ULCERATIVE COLITIS**	**CROHN DISEASE**
Risk Factors		
Age at onset	Any age; 10–40 years most common	Any age; 10–30 years most common
Family history	Less common	More common
Sex (prevalence)	Equal in women and men	About equal in women and men
Cancer risk	Increased	Increased
Pathophysiology		
Location of lesions	Colon and rectum, no "skip" lesions	All of GI tract: mouth to anus, "skip" lesions common
Inflammation and ulceration	Mucosal layer involved	Entire intestinal wall involved
Granulomas	Rare	Common
Friable mucosa	Common	Less common
Fistulae and abscesses	Rare	Common
Strictures and possible obstruction	Rare	Common
Clinical Manifestations		
Abdominal pain	Occasional	Common
Diarrhea	Common	Common
Bloody stools	Common	Less common
Abdominal mass	Rare	Common
Small intestinal malabsorption	Rare	Common
Steatorrhea	Rare	Common
Potential for malignancy	Common	Common
Antineutrophil cytoplasmic antibodies	Common	Rare
Anti–*Saccharomyces cerevisiae* antibodies	Rare	Common
Clinical Course	Remissions and exacerbations	Remissions and exacerbations

GI, Gastrointestinal.

hypotension and shock. Edema, strictures, or fibrosis can obstruct the colon. Perforation is an unusual but possible complication. The risk of colon cancer increases significantly after many years of ulcerative colitis.[80] Extraintestinal manifestations include cutaneous lesions (erythema nodosum and pyoderma gangrenosum), migratory polyarthritis and sacroiliitis, osteopenia and osteoporosis, mouth ulcers, episcleritis or anterior uveitis of the eye, and primary sclerosing cholangitis in the liver. Gallstones are common. Chronic inflammation causes alterations in coagulation and can cause life-threatening microthrombi, deep vein thrombosis, and other thromboembolic events.[81]

EVALUATION AND TREATMENT. Diagnosis of ulcerative colitis is based on the medical history, clinical manifestations, imaging procedures, and biopsy findings. Endoscopic evaluation shows an inflamed and hemorrhagic mucosa. Radiologic assessment may show loss of haustra, ulceration, and irregular mucosa. The laboratory data include low hemoglobin values, hypoalbuminemia, and low serum potassium levels. There are no specific serologic markers. Infectious causes are ruled out by stool culture. The symptoms of ulcerative colitis can be very similar to those of Crohn disease, making differential diagnosis challenging.[82] Chromoendoscopy is recommended over random biopsies in detecting dysplasia and colorectal cancer for those with long-standing disease.[83]

Treatment is individualized and depends on the severity of symptoms and the extent of mucosal involvement. Mild disease is treated with 5-aminosalicylic acid (mesalazine) or sulfasalazine followed by corticosteroids to suppress the inflammatory response and alleviate cramping pain. Azathioprine and immunomodulatory agents (cyclosporine and tumor necrosis factor [TNF] blocking agents) tacrolimus or vedolizumab are used for recurrent or serious disease.[84,85] Severe, unremitting disease can require hospital admission and administration of intravenous fluids. Extreme malnutrition may require intravenous hyperalimentation. Surgical approaches for severe UC include total proctocolectomy, with end ileostomy or ileorectal anastomosis, or ileal pouch anal anastomosis (IPAA), the preferred procedure.[86] *Pouchitis* is a complication of restorative proctocolectomy with ileal pouch anal anastomosis performed as surgical treatment for both UC and Crohn disease. Antibiotic treatment is usually successful.[87] New endoscopic imaging techniques are emerging to detect dysplasia and colorectal cancer with long-standing disease.[88]

Crohn Disease

Crohn disease (CD) (granulomatous colitis, ileocolitis, or regional enteritis) is an idiopathic inflammatory disorder that is distinguished from UC in that it affects any part of the gastrointestinal tract from the mouth to the anus and involves "skip lesions" with inflamed areas mixed with uninflamed areas, noncaseating granulomas, fistulas, and deep penetrating ulcers. The distal small intestine and proximal large colon are most commonly affected by the disease. In a small percentage of cases, CD is difficult to differentiate from ulcerative colitis (Table 42.5). Risk factors include family history, cigarette smoking, Jewish ethnicity, urban residency, age less than 40 years, a slight predominance in women, and an altered gut microbiome.[89] The *CARD15/NOD2* (nucleotide-binding-oligomerization-domain-containing protein 2) gene mutations have the strongest association with CD (35% to 45% of cases), although many other genes have been identified. The *CARD15/*

NOD2 genes code for a protein (a toll-like receptor; see Chapter 10) involved in the recognition of gram-negative and gram-positive bacterial wall fragments by intestinal epithelial cells. Their mutation may promote dysbiosis and reduced levels of defensins.[90] Th1-mediated inflammation with activation of TNF-α, IFN-γ, IL-12, and Th17-associated cytokines causes mucosal injury. Recruited leukocytes release proinflammatory substances, including prostaglandins, leukotrienes, proteases, reactive oxygen species, and nitric oxide, which cause further injury and inflammation.[73]

◆ **PATHOPHYSIOLOGY.** The inflammatory lesions begin in the intestinal submucosa and spread with discontinuous transmural involvement ("skip lesions"). The ascending colon and the transverse colon are the most common sites of the disease; however, both the large and small intestines may be involved, particularly the ileum. One side of the intestinal wall may be affected and not the other. Progression of the disease involves neutrophil infiltration of the crypts, resulting in abscess formation and crypt destruction. The ulcerations of CD produce longitudinal and transverse fissures that extend inflammation into lymphoid tissue. The typical lesion is a granuloma with cobblestone projections of inflamed tissue surrounded by areas of ulceration (Fig. 42.13). (Granulomas are described in Chapter 7.) Fistulae may form in the perianal area between loops of intestine or extend into the bladder, rectum, or vagina. Strictures may develop, promoting obstruction. Smoking increases the risk of relapse.[91]

◆ **CLINICAL MANIFESTATIONS.** Individuals with CD may have no specific symptoms other than an "irritable bowel" for several years. Symptoms vary according to the location of the disease but are similar to those for UC. Diarrhea is one of the most common symptoms and,

occasionally, rectal bleeding if the colon is involved. Other manifestations are related to the location and extent of intestinal involvement. Inflammation of the ileum, for example, causes tenderness in the lower right side of the abdomen, and the individual may be anemic as a result of malabsorption of vitamin B$_{12}$. There also may be deficiencies in folic acid, vitamin D absorption, and calcium leading to bone disease. Proteins may be lost, leading to hypoalbuminemia. Weight loss is common. Anal manifestations occur in about 30% of cases, including anal fissure, perianal abscess, and fistula. Individuals with CD of long duration also are at risk for intestinal adenocarcinoma. Extraintestinal manifestations include arthropathies, skin, oral, and ocular lesions and may be the presenting symptoms.[92]

◆ **EVALUATION AND TREATMENT.** The diagnosis and treatment of CD are similar to the diagnosis and treatment of ulcerative colitis. Imaging of the small intestine is used in the diagnosis of CD, including either a small bowel series or a capsule endoscopy (camera pill). There are no specific biomarkers or definitive treatments. Treatment includes corticosteroids, 5-aminosalicylates, and immunomodulatory agents (thiopurines and TNF-α–blocking agents). New biologic agents are under development.[93] Smoking cessation is a component of therapy. Surgery is generally performed to manage complications such as strictures, fistulae, abscesses, and perforation, or to relieve obstruction. When treatment involves surgical resection of small intestinal segments, complications related to short bowel syndrome can occur, including malabsorption, diarrhea, and nutritional deficiencies. Symptoms are related to the extent and location of resection. Cancer screening should be performed for long-standing disease.

Microscopic Colitis

Microscopic colitis is a relatively common cause of chronic, watery diarrhea. Risk factors include age 50 years or older, female sex, weight loss, absence of abdominal pain, use of proton pump inhibitors or nonsteroidal antiinflammatory drugs, celiac disease, and smoking. Although the mucosa appears normal, there are two histologic forms: lymphocytic and collagenous. Lymphocytic colitis shows more than 20 intraepithelial lymphocytes per 100 epithelial cells. Collagenous colitis is characterized by a thickened (10 to 20 μm) subepithelial collagen band, alteration of the vascular mucosal pattern, and mucosal nodularity. The cause is unknown.[94]

The symptoms of frequent, chronic, daily watery diarrhea are the same for both types and can be accompanied by abdominal pain and weight loss. Diagnosis is made by endoscopic biopsy. Antidiarrheal agents and budesonide (a local antiinflammatory steroid) are the best documented treatments. The disease is negatively associated with colorectal cancer.[95]

Irritable Bowel Syndrome

Irritable bowel syndrome (IBS) currently is considered a disorder of brain-gut interaction characterized by abdominal pain with altered bowel habits. The prevalence in North America is about 12% and is probably underestimated.[96] It is more common in women, with a higher prevalence in youth and middle age. Individuals with IBS are more likely to have anxiety and depression and reduced quality of life.[97]

◆ **PATHOPHYSIOLOGY.** There are no specific structural or biochemical alterations that have been currently identified as a cause of IBS, but there is increasing evidence to explain a multisystem interaction as a cause of the varying symptom presentations. They are summarized as follows:

1. *Visceral hypersensitivity or hyperalgesia*, particularly with distention of the rectum but also other areas of the gut. This occurs in about 30% to 40% of those with IBS. The cause is unknown; it may originate in the peripheral, enteric, or central nervous system. The mechanism

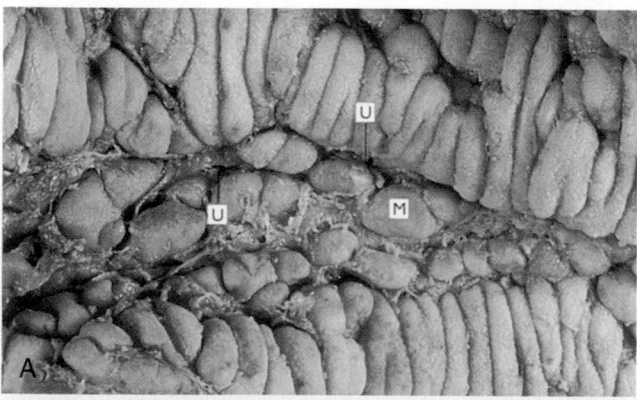

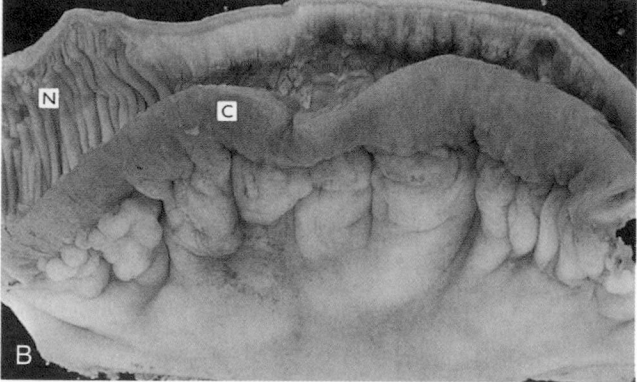

FIGURE 42.13   Crohn Disease. A, The mucosa in Crohn disease demonstrates a cobblestone pattern as a result of fissured ulcers *(U)* with intervening areas of edematous mucosa *(M).* **B,** Compared with normal small bowel wall *(N),* the Crohn segment *(C)* shows wall thickening that has caused a stenosis. (From Kumar V et al: *Pathologic basis of disease,* ed 7, Philadelphia, 2006, Saunders.)

may be related to pain and a dysregulation of the bidirectional "brain-gut axis" (alterations in gut or central nervous system processing of gut nociceptive information). Factors include genetic related changes in the function of serotonin-secreting cells of gut-brain pain modulation, alterations in gut microbiota metabolite production with activation of the gut immune system, increased visceral sensitivity, permeability, and altered motility and secretion.[98]

2. *Abnormal gastrointestinal permeability, motility, secretion, and sensitivity* are associated with IBS. Individuals with diarrhea-type IBS have more rapid colonic transit times and increased intestinal permeability. Those with bloating and constipation have delayed transit times and decreased intestinal permeability. The mechanisms may be related to dysregulation of the brain-gut axis or alterations in the function of gut neuroendocrine cells or dorsal root ganglion neurons. Enteroendocrine cells, mast cell proliferation, and activation with release of intrinsic and peripheral neuromediators, enzymes, and inflammatory mediators contribute to the symptoms of IBS. Sex hormones also may be a contributing factor.[99-101]

3. *Postinflammatory IBS* has been associated with intestinal infection (bacterial enteritis) and low-grade inflammation. Alterations in gut microbiota, immune activation in gut tissues, and changes in intestinal permeability with bidirectional neurohormonal communication between the gut and the brain have been proposed.[102]

4. *Alteration in gut microbiota (dysbiosis)* influences the sensory, motor, and immune systems of the gut and interacts with higher brain centers and may contribute to symptoms of IBS.[103] Small intestine overgrowth of normal gut bacteria may be associated with IBS symptoms in some cases.[104]

5. *Food allergy or food intolerance* is associated with IBS in some cases. Food antigens may activate the mucosal immune system, alter intestinal flora, or mediate hypersensitivity reactions and IBS symptoms. Allergic conditions, including rhinitis and asthma, have been associated with IBS.[105]

6. *Psychosocial factors (epigenetic factors)*, including early life trauma or abuse or chronic emotional stress, lead to alterations in neuroendocrine, neuroimmune, and autonomic nervous systems and gut microbiota; release of inflammatory mediators; and pain modulatory responses contributing to the symptoms of IBS.[106,107]

◆**CLINICAL MANIFESTATIONS.** IBS symptoms may be mild or debilitating. Clinical manifestations are characterized by lower abdominal pain and bloating. IBS can be subtyped as presented in Box 42.2 Individu-

---

BOX 42.2 **DIAGNOSTIC CRITERIA* FOR IRRITABLE BOWEL SYNDROME**

Rome IV Criteria

Recurrent abdominal pain, on average, at least 1 day per week in the last 3 months, associated with two or more of the following criteria:

1. Related to defecation
2. Associated with a change in frequency of stool
3. Associated with a change in form (appearance) of stool

IBS subtypes include:

IBS with predominant constipation (IBS-C)

IBS with predominant diarrhea (IBS-D)

IBS with mixed bowel habits (IBS-M)

IBS unclassified (IBS-U)

*Criteria fulfilled for the last 3 months with symptom onset at least 6 months before diagnosis.

IBS, Irritable bowel syndrome.

Adapted from Drossman DA: *Gastroenterology* 150(6):1262-1297, 2016; Lacey BE et al: *Gastroenterology* 150(6):1393-1407, 2016.

---

als also may describe fecal urgency and incomplete evacuation. Symptoms are usually relieved with defecation and usually do not interfere with sleep.

◆**EVALUATION AND TREATMENT.** The diagnosis of IBS is based on personal history of signs and symptoms, physical examination, and the exclusion of structural or biochemical causes of other diseases with symptoms similar to IBS (celiac disease, lactose intolerance, and inflammatory bowel disease). In the absence of "alarm symptoms," such as fever, weight loss, gastrointestinal bleeding, anemia, or abdominal mass, only limited diagnostic tests are needed (complete blood count and inflammatory markers [C-reactive protein or fecal calprotectin]). The individual may be evaluated for food allergies, lactose intolerance, parasites or bacterial growth, and thyroid disease. A colonoscopy may be completed if clinically indicated. The Rome IV criteria provide guidelines for diagnosing IBS and includes IBS subtypes (Box 42.2).[108]

There is no cure for IBS, and treatment is individualized based on predominant symptoms. Treatment may include laxatives, soluble dietary fiber, restriction of gluten and fermentable oligosaccharides, disaccharides, monosaccharides, polyols (FODMAPs), antidiarrheals, antispasmodics, pro-secretory drugs, visceral analgesics, low-dose antidepressants, serotonin agonists or antagonists (90% to 95% of the body's total serotonin is produced by intestinal enteroendocrine cells), and antibiotics. Alternative therapies including prebiotics (stimulate growth of healthy gut bacteria), probiotics, selected herbal treatments (e.g., peppermint oil), hypnosis, and psychotherapy are treatment options. Research continues to advance the understanding of the pathophysiology and specificity of treatment of this complex syndrome.[109]

Diverticular Disease of the Colon

Diverticula are herniations or saclike outpouchings of mucosa through the muscle layers of the colon wall. **Diverticulosis** is asymptomatic diverticular disease. **Diverticulitis** represents inflammation. The cause of diverticular disease is unknown. Approximately 300,000 hospital admissions per year are related to diverticular disease.[110] Predisposing factors include older age, genetic predisposition, obesity, smoking, diet, lack of physical activity, and medication use, such as aspirin and nonsteroidal antiinflammatory drugs. Lack of dietary fiber may or may not contribute to diverticular disease.[111] Altered intestinal microbiota, visceral hypersensitivity, and abnormal colonic motility also may be contributing factors.[112]

◆**PATHOPHYSIOLOGY.** Diverticula can occur anywhere in the gastrointestinal tract, with the most common sites in the left colon (prevalent in Western countries) and the right colon (prevalent in Asian countries). They rarely occur in the small intestine[113] and are associated with increased intracolonic pressure, abnormal neuromuscular function, and alterations in intestinal motility. The diverticula form at weak points in the colon wall, where arteries penetrate the tunica muscularis to nourish the mucosal layer. The colonic mucosa herniates through the smooth muscle layers (Fig. 42.14). A common associated finding is thickening of the circular and longitudinal (teniae coli) muscles surrounding the diverticula. Increased collagen and elastin deposition, not muscle hypertrophy, is associated with wall thickening and contributes to increased intraluminal pressure and herniation. Habitual consumption of a low-residue diet reduces fecal bulk, thus reducing the diameter of the colon. According to Laplace's law (see Chapter 32), wall pressure increases as the diameter of a cylindrical structure decreases. Therefore pressure within the narrow lumen can increase enough to cause local ischemia and rupture the diverticula. However, the exact cause of diverticula is uncertain.

◆**CLINICAL MANIFESTATIONS.** Symptoms of uncomplicated diverticular disease are usually vague or absent. Cramping pain of the lower abdomen can accompany constriction of the thickened colonic wall.

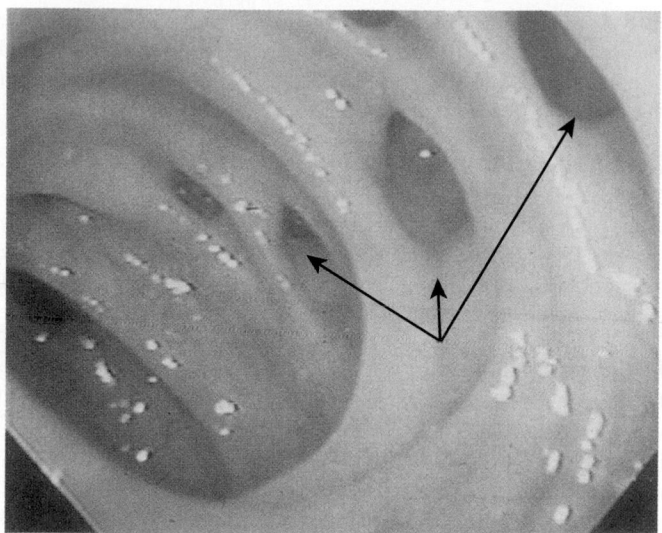

FIGURE 42.14 Diverticular Disease. In diverticular disease, the outpouches *(arrows)* of mucosa seen in the sigmoid colon appear as slitlike openings from the mucosal surface of the opened bowel. (From Townsend CM et al: *Sabiston textbook of surgery,* ed 19, Philadelphia 2012, Saunders.)

Diarrhea, constipation, distention, or flatulence may occur. If the diverticula become inflamed or abscesses form, the individual develops fever, leukocytosis (increased white blood cell count), and tenderness of the lower left quadrant.

◆**EVALUATION AND TREATMENT.** Diverticula are often discovered during diagnostic procedures performed for other problems. Ultrasound, sigmoidoscopy, or colonoscopy permits direct observation of the lesions. Abdominal computed tomography (CT) is used for complicated cases.

An increase of dietary fiber intake increases stool weight, lowers colonic pressures, improves transit times, and often relieves symptoms, although data are lacking (see *Nutrition & Disease:* Diverticular Disease and Diet). Uncomplicated diverticular disease is treated with bowel rest and analgesia. Antibiotics (i.e., rifaximin) and surgical resection are used to treat severe disease.[114] Radiographic, endoscopic, and laparoscopic procedures are implemented for more severe complications, including hemorrhage, bowel stenosis, obstruction, abscesses, fistulae, bowel perforation, and peritonitis.[115,116]

Appendicitis

Appendicitis is an inflammation of the vermiform appendix, which is a projection from the apex of the cecum. It is the most common surgical emergency of the abdomen, usually occurs between 10 years and 19 years of age (although it may develop at any age), and has an incidence in the United States of 7 to 10 per 10,000 persons.[117] Disease occurrence is higher in individuals with a family history of appendicitis.[118]

◆**PATHOPHYSIOLOGY.** The exact cause of appendicitis is controversial. Obstruction of the lumen with stool, tumors, or foreign bodies with consequent increased intraluminal pressure, ischemia, bacterial infection, and inflammation is the most common theory. The obstructed lumen does not allow drainage of the appendix, and as mucosal secretion continues, intraluminal pressure increases. The resultant increased pressure decreases mucosal blood flow, and the appendix becomes hypoxic. The mucosa ulcerates, promoting bacterial or other microbial invasion with further inflammation and edema. Inflammation may involve the distal or entire appendix. Gangrene develops from thrombosis of the luminal blood vessels, followed by perforation.[119] The appendix may harbor bacteria that contribute to the development of appendicitis.[120]

NUTRITION & DISEASE
Diverticular Disease and Diet

Daily consumption of fiber-enriched foods is being re-evaluated for the prevention of diverticula. A high-fiber diet increases fecal bulk, decreases transit time, lowers intracolonic pressures, and eases stool elimination. The recommendation for fiber has been 20 to 35 g/day. Some examples of high-fiber choices are whole wheat bread and other grain products, baked potato with skin, fresh fruit with skins, raw vegetables, beans, peas, legumes, wheat bran, and brown rice. Side effects may include flatulence, intestinal rumbling, cramps, and diarrhea and the possibility that frequent bowel movements promote a greater prevalence of diverticular disease. A gradual increase in dietary fiber over 1 or 2 months helps to avoid these problems. Other potential problems with an excessively high-fiber diet (greater than 40 to 45 g) might include a decrease in nutrient absorption because of the increased volume of intestinal contents, which in turn decreases the ability of the digestive enzymes to come into contact with the food. An increase of water intake (eight 8-ounce glasses) is important so intestinal blockage will not occur. For small children and older adults, a high-fiber diet increases the volume of food needed to meet energy requirements, and that increase may be difficult to obtain. Although some physicians recommend restricting nuts, seeds, and foods containing seeds such as berries, kiwi, and tomatoes that might lodge in the pouches, there is no evidence that this happens. If the diverticula become inflamed, a low-fiber, low-residue (no milk products), or elemental diet, or in complicated cases total parenteral nutrition (TPN), is required to prevent continued irritation of the inflamed tissue. Controlled clinical trials are needed to evaluate the effectiveness of high-fiber diets in preventing diverticular disease. The efficacy of probiotics in modifying gut microbiota and relieving symptoms of diverticular disease also requires more investigation.

Data from Carabotti M et al: *Nutrients* 9(2):2017; Lahner E et al: *J Gastrointest Liver Dis* 25(1):79-86, 2016; Mosadeghi S, Bhuket T, Stollman N: *Curr Opin Gastroenterol* 31(1):50-55, 2015.

◆**CLINICAL MANIFESTATIONS.** Epigastric or periumbilical pain is the typical symptom of an inflamed appendix. The pain may be vague at first, increasing in intensity over 3 to 4 hours. It may subside and then recur with a shift of location to the right lower quadrant with rebound tenderness. Right lower quadrant pain is associated with extension of the inflammation to the surrounding tissues. Nausea, vomiting, and anorexia follow the onset of pain, and fever is common. Diarrhea occurs in some individuals, particularly children; others have a sensation of constipation. Perforation, peritonitis, and abscess formation are the most serious complications of appendicitis.

◆**EVALUATION AND TREATMENT.** In addition to clinical manifestations, the clinician can usually locate the painful site with one finger. Rebound tenderness is usually referred to the right lower quadrant. There are no specific biomarkers. The white blood cell count ranges from 10,000 to 16,000 cells/mm³ with elevations in the levels of neutrophils and C-reactive protein. Abdominal ultrasound, CT scans, and MRI (particularly for pregnant women and children) assist with diagnostic accuracy and help rule out nonappendiceal disease. Clinical decision rules and risk scores can assist with diagnosis.[121] Antibiotics and appendectomy are the treatment for uncomplicated or perforated appendicitis. There is controversy regarding antibiotics first, then surgery.[122] Laparoscopic surgery provides quick recovery for uncomplicated appendicitis and provides an opportunity to discover malignancy. Nonoperative management is an option for some individuals.[123] Recovery is more complicated in cases of perforation or abscess formation and in individuals of older age.

Mesenteric Vascular Insufficiency

Mesenteric vascular insufficiency is rare with an incidence of about 2 to 3 cases per 100,000 persons. Mesenteric vascular insufficiency includes arterial, venous, occlusive, or nonocclusive etiologies. Three branches of the abdominal aorta supply the stomach and intestines: the celiac artery and the superior and inferior mesenteric arteries (see Fig. 42.15). The inferior mesenteric vein drains into the splenic vein. The superior mesenteric vein combines with the splenic vein to form the hepatic portal vein. Mesenteric venous thrombosis is the least common of the causes of mesenteric vascular insufficiency. Hypercoagulability, endothelial injury, malignancies, right-sided heart failure, and deep venous thrombosis are risk factors. Mesenteric venous thrombosis presents with nonspecific abdominal pain and is treated with anticoagulants.[124]

Acute mesenteric ischemia is more common in the elderly and results in a significant reduction in mucosal blood flow to the large and small intestines.[125] Preexisting morbidities include dissecting aortic aneurysms and arterial thrombi. Embolic obstruction is associated with atrial fibrillation, mitral valve disease, heart valve prostheses, or myocardial infarction. The superior mesenteric artery has a more direct line of flow from the aorta; therefore emboli enter it more readily than they enter the inferior branch, causing ischemia and necrosis of the small intestine. Ischemia and necrosis alter membrane permeability. Initially there is increased motility, nausea and vomiting, urgent bowel evacuation, and severe abdominal pain. Ischemia leads to decreased motility and distention. The damaged intestinal mucosa cannot produce enough mucus to protect itself from digestive enzymes. Mucosal alteration causes fluid to move from the blood vessels into the bowel wall and peritoneum. Fluid loss causes hypovolemia and further decreases in intestinal blood flow. As intestinal infarction progresses, shock, fever, bloody diarrhea, and leukocytosis develop. Bacteria invade the necrotic intestinal wall, causing gangrene and peritonitis.[126]

Chronic mesenteric ischemia is rare. It can develop secondary to atherosclerotic stenosis or occlusion (most common); secondary to congestive heart failure, acute myocardial infarction, dysrhythmias, hemorrhage, thrombus formation, or aortic aneurysm; or secondary to any condition that decreases arterial blood flow. Chronic occlusion is often accompanied by formation of collateral circulation. The collateral vessels may be able to nourish the resting intestine, but after eating, when the intestine requires more blood, the arterial supply may be insufficient. Ischemia develops, causing a cramping abdominal pain, called *abdominal angina,* a cardinal symptom. Some individuals suffer significant weight loss because they stop eating to control the pain. Progressive vascular obstruction eventually causes continuous abdominal pain and necrosis of the intestinal tissue and can precipitate acute mesenteric insufficiency.[127] Reperfusion injury related to reactive oxygen metabolites and inflammatory mediators contributes to tissue damage following revascularization.[128]

Diagnosis of acute and chronic mesenteric ischemia is based on clinical manifestations, laboratory findings, and imaging studies. A bruit often can be heard over a partially occluded artery. Treatment includes aggressive rehydration and the use of antibiotics, anticoagulation, vasodilators, and inhibitors of reperfusion injury. Surgery, including endovascular techniques, is required to remove necrotic tissue, repair sclerosed vessels, and revascularize affected tissue. Acute occlusion is a surgical emergency, and mortality is high (50% to 90%). Early diagnosis and aggressive treatment result in the best survival rates.[129,130]

DISORDERS OF THE ACCESSORY ORGANS OF DIGESTION

The accessory organs of digestion (liver, gallbladder, and pancreas) secrete substances necessary for digestion and, in the case of the liver, carry out metabolic functions needed to maintain life. Disorders of these organs include inflammatory disease, obstruction of ducts, and tumors. (Cancers of the digestive system are described at the end of this chapter.)

Common Complications of Liver Disorders

Of all the accessory organ disorders, acute or chronic liver disease leads to the most systemic, life-threatening complications. Complications of chronic liver disorders include portal hypertension, varices, splenomegaly, hepatopulmonary syndrome and portopulmonary syndrome, ascites, hepatic encephalopathy, jaundice, and hepatorenal syndrome.[131]

Portal Hypertension

Portal hypertension is abnormally high blood pressure in the portal venous system caused by resistance to portal blood flow. Pressure in this system is normally 3 to 5 mmHg; portal hypertension is the elevation of hepatic venous pressure above 5 mmHg.

◆ PATHOPHYSIOLOGY. Portal hypertension is caused by disorders that obstruct or impede blood flow through any component of the hepatic portal system. *Intrahepatic causes* result from vascular remodeling with intrahepatic shunts, thrombosis, inflammation, or fibrosis, as occurs in cirrhosis of the liver, viral hepatitis, or schistosomiasis (a parasitic infection). *Posthepatic causes* occur from hepatic vein thrombosis or cardiac disorders that impair the pumping ability of the right side of the heart (i.e., right-sided heart failure). This causes blood to back up and increases pressure in the portal system. The most common cause of portal hypertension is fibrosis and obstruction caused by cirrhosis of the liver. Thrombosis or narrowing of the hepatic portal vein is the major *prehepatic* cause. Long-term portal hypertension causes several pathophysiologic problems that are difficult to treat and can be fatal. These problems include varices, splenomegaly, hepatopulmonary syndrome, ascites, and hepatic encephalopathy.

Varices are distended, tortuous, collateral veins. Prolonged elevation of pressure in the hepatic portal vein causes collateral veins to open between the portal vein and systemic veins and their transformation into varices, particularly in the lower esophagus and stomach, but also over the abdominal wall (known as the *caput medusae [Medusa head]*), rectum (hemorrhoidal varices), or spleen (Fig. 42.15). Rupture of varices can cause life-threatening hemorrhage.

Splenomegaly is enlargement of the spleen. Portal hypertension contributes to congestive splenomegaly caused by increased pressure in the splenic vein, which branches from the portal vein. Thrombocytopenia from platelet sequestration is the most common symptom of congestive splenomegaly and can contribute to an increased bleeding tendency.[132] Splenomegaly also can be predictive of severity of esophageal varices.

Hepatopulmonary syndrome (HPS) (intrapulmonary vasodilation, intrapulmonary shunting, hypoxia), and portopulmonary hypertension (PPH) (pulmonary vasoconstriction and vascular remodeling) are respiratory complications of advanced liver disease and portal hypertension and occur in about 15% to 30% of cases. In HPS there is pulmonary vasodilation, probably because of increased nitric oxide synthesis, increased pulmonary venous congestion, and right-to-left shunting that induces hypoxemia. PPH is associated with vascular remodeling and pulmonary artery vasoconstriction. There are no specific clinical manifestations, although dyspnea, cyanosis, and digital clubbing may occur. Diagnosis is made by arterial blood gas analysis, contrast echocardiography, transthoracic echocardiography, and right heart catheterization. In portopulmonary hypertension, mean pulmonary artery pressure is greater than 25 mmHg at rest. There is no specific treatment for HPS. Treatment of PPH includes targeting the pulmonary arterial vasculature to reduce pulmonary hypertension with various medication

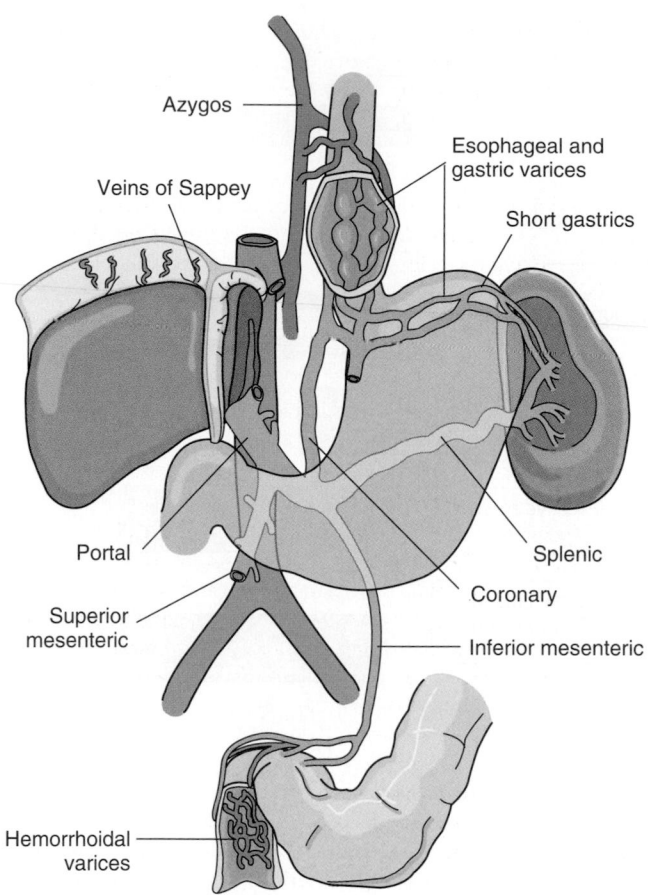

FIGURE 42.15 Varices Related to Portal Hypertension. Portal vein, its major tributaries, and the most important shunts (collateral veins) between the portal and caval systems. (From Monahan FD et al: *Phipps' medical-surgical nursing: concepts and clinical practice,* ed 8, St Louis, 2007, Mosby.)

options (endothelin receptor antagonists, phosphodiesterase type-5 inhibitors, and prostanoids). Liver transplant is required.[133]

◆**CLINICAL MANIFESTATIONS.** The most common clinical manifestation of portal hypertension is vomiting of blood from bleeding esophageal varices.[134] Bleeding is usually from varices that have developed slowly over a period of years. Slow, chronic bleeding from varices causes anemia or melena.

Acute rupture of esophageal varices causes hemorrhage and voluminous vomiting of dark blood. The ruptured varices are usually painless. Rupture is caused by a combination of erosion by gastric acid and elevated venous pressure. Mortality from ruptured esophageal varices ranges from 15% to 20%. Hemorrhoidal varices present as hematochezia and copious rectal bleeding. Recurrent bleeding of esophageal or gastric varices indicates a poor prognosis. Most individuals die within 1 year.

◆**EVALUATION AND TREATMENT.** Diagnosis of portal hypertension is often made at the time of variceal bleeding and confirmed by endoscopy and evaluation of portal venous pressure. Liver elastography (shear wave ultrasound or magnetic resonance imaging) provides a noninvasive measure of liver stiffness and extent of fibrosis.[135] Distended collateral veins may radiate over the abdomen, giving rise to caput medusae (Medusa head) from opening of the paraumbilical veins. The individual usually has a history of hepatitis or alcoholism.

Nonselective beta-blockers (that block both beta$_1$ [β$_1$] and beta$_2$ [β$_2$] receptors) can be effective in preventing variceal bleeding. Endoscopic vein ligation also is an option. Emergency management of bleeding

varices includes fluid resuscitation, red blood cell replacement, prophylactic antibiotics, vasoactive drugs (e.g., octreotide, somatostatin, terlipressin), endoscopic variceal band ligation, compression of the varices with an inflatable tube or balloon, and injection of a sclerosing agent. Surgical construction of a transjugular intrahepatic portosystemic shunt (TIPS) (anastomosis of the portal vein to the inferior vena cava) may decompress the varices, but this treatment can precipitate encephalopathy or liver failure resulting from reduced hepatic blood flow.[134] There is no definitive treatment for portal hypertension.

Ascites

Ascites is the accumulation of fluid in the peritoneal cavity and is a complication of portal hypertension. Ascites traps body fluid in the peritoneal cavity from which it cannot escape. The effect reduces the amount of fluid available for normal physiologic functions. Cirrhosis is the most common cause of ascites; ascites is the most common complication of cirrhosis. Other diseases associated with ascites include right heart failure, abdominal malignancies, nephrotic syndrome, and malnutrition. Twenty-five percent of individuals who develop ascites caused by cirrhosis die within 1 year. Continued heavy drinking of alcohol is associated with this mortality and is related to cirrhosis.

◆**PATHOPHYSIOLOGY.** Several factors contribute to the development of ascites, including portal hypertension, decreased synthesis of albumin by the liver, splanchnic arterial vasodilation, and renal sodium and water retention. The *overflow theory* proposes that portal hypertension and reduced serum albumin levels cause capillary hydrostatic pressure to exceed capillary osmotic pressure (see Chapter 3), pushing water into the peritoneal cavity (transudative effusion). Portal hypertension also increases capillary hydrostatic pressures in the intestinal wall, which causes fluid to "weep" into the peritoneal cavity. Reduced capillary oncotic pressure adds to the fluid shift. The *underfill theory* proposes an increase in hepatic sinusoidal hydrostatic pressure and decreased plasma oncotic pressure with weeping of lymph fluid from the surface of the liver. The resulting decrease in effective circulating plasma volume activates antidiuretic hormone release and the renin-angiotensin-aldosterone system, stimulating the kidney to retain water and sodium leading to intravascular volume overload. The *peripheral arterial vasodilation theory,* or *forward theory,* is a synthesis of the overflow and underfill theories and the most accepted theory. This theory proposes that circulating nitric oxide and carbon monoxide cause splanchnic vasodilation. The decrease in systemic vascular resistance overcomes compensatory cardiac output. Stimulation of baroreceptors activates renal sodium retention through activation of the renin-angiotensin-aldosterone system, increased sympathetic tone, secretion of antidiuretic hormones, and fluid retention. Combined portal hypertension and splanchnic vasodilation causes fluid transudation and lymph formation, producing ascites. Translocation of bacteria and release of endotoxin cause spontaneous peritonitis with an inflammatory response that increases mesenteric capillary permeability and fluid movement into the peritoneal cavity, promoting ascites. Fig. 42.16 summarizes the mechanisms by which cirrhosis of the liver causes ascites.

◆**CLINICAL MANIFESTATIONS.** The accumulation of ascitic fluid causes abdominal distention, increased abdominal girth, and weight gain (Fig. 42.17). Large volumes of fluid (10 to 20 L) displace the diaphragm and cause dyspnea by decreasing lung capacity. Respiratory rate increases, and the individual assumes a semi-Fowler position to relieve the dyspnea. Some peripheral edema is usually present. Dilutional hyponatremia is a consequence of excess fluid volume. Approximately 10% of individuals with ascites develop bacterial peritonitis, either spontaneously or as a result of paracentesis (needle aspiration of ascitic fluid). Peritonitis causes fever, chills, abdominal pain, decreased bowel sounds, and cloudy ascitic fluid.

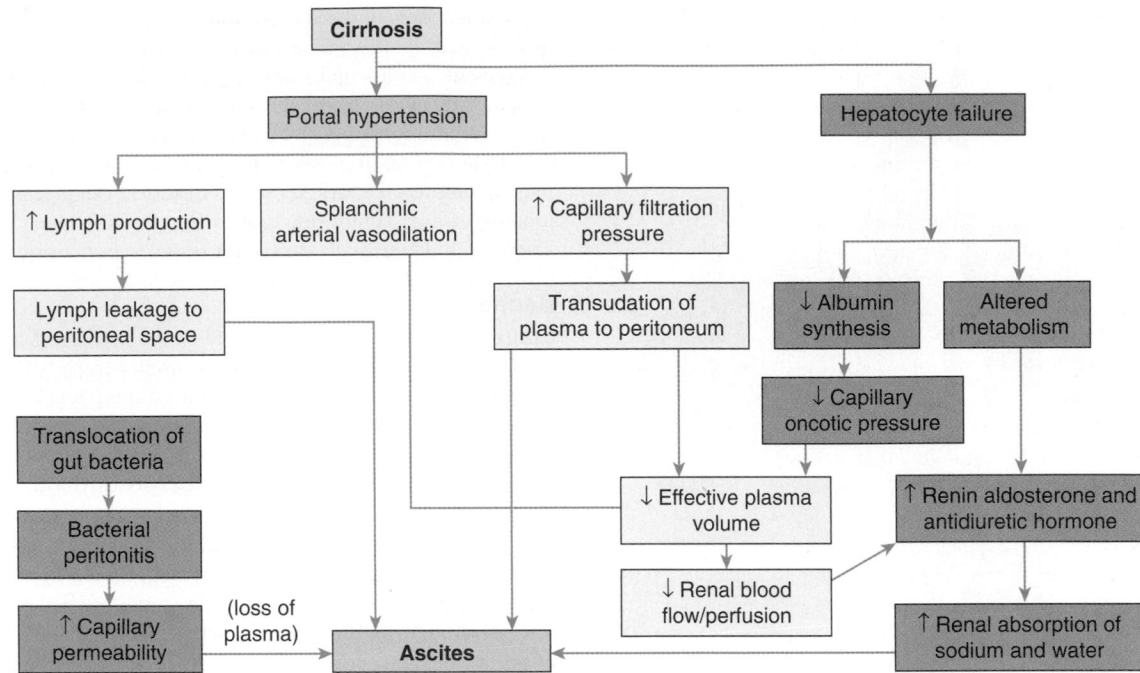

FIGURE 42.16 Mechanisms of Ascites Caused by Cirrhosis.

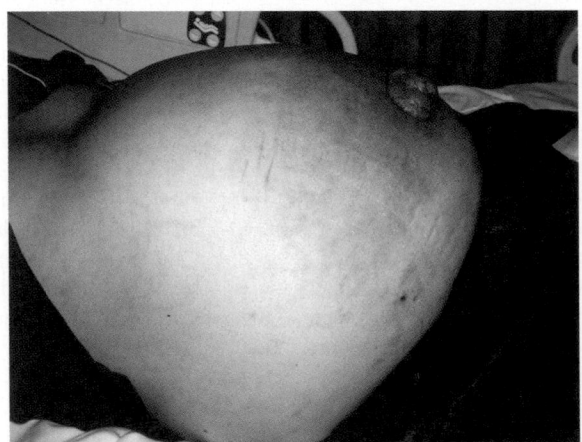

FIGURE 42.17 Massive Ascites in an Individual with Cirrhosis. Distended abdomen, dilated upper abdominal veins, and everted umbilicus are classic manifestations. (From Goldman L, Schafer AI: *Goldman's Cecil medicine,* ed 24, Philadelphia, 2012, Saunders.)

◆**EVALUATION AND TREATMENT.** Diagnosis of ascites is usually based on clinical manifestations and identification of liver disease. The serum-ascites albumin gradient (SAAG) from ascitic fluid analysis is the most specific diagnostic indicator for portal hypertension–related ascites. Chest and abdominal x-rays, ultrasonography, or CT scans are used to evaluate the cause and extent of the ascites and complications such as peritonitis. The goal of treatment is to relieve discomfort. If the restoration of liver function is possible (e.g., in ascites caused by viral hepatitis), the ascites diminishes spontaneously. In the meantime, dietary salt restriction and potassium-sparing diuretics (i.e., spironolactone, an aldosterone antagonist) can reduce ascites. Strong diuretics, such as furosemide or ethacrynic acid, may be used, and vasopressin receptor-2 antagonists are effective for dilutional hyponatremia. Albumin may be given. Serum electrolyte levels are monitored carefully because the individual is at risk for hyponatremia and hypokalemia.

Palliative measures include paracentesis to remove 1 or 2 L of ascitic fluid and relieve respiratory distress. This procedure can have serious complications, however. The removal of too much fluid too fast relieves pressure on blood vessels, causing arteriolar vasodilation, which carries the risk of hypotension, shock, or death. Despite repeated paracentesis, ascitic fluid reaccumulates in individuals with irreversible disease, drawing more albumin and electrolytes out of the vascular compartment. Paracentesis is also likely to cause peritonitis. Bacterial peritonitis is treated with antibiotics.[136] Other procedures include peritoneovenous shunt (peritoneal fluid into veins) and transjugular intrahepatic portosystemic shunt (TIPS) (bypass of blood flow from the portal venous branch to the hepatic venous branch). Individuals with ascites and portal hypertension have a poor prognosis, and liver transplant is the best treatment option.[137]

Hepatic Encephalopathy

Hepatic encephalopathy (portosystemic encephalopathy) is a complex neurologic syndrome characterized by impaired behavioral, cognitive, and motor function. The syndrome has three types and may develop rapidly during acute fulminant hepatitis (type A); after portosystemic bypass or shunting without liver disease (type B); or slowly during the course of cirrhosis, chronic liver disease, or portosystemic bypass (type C, which can be episodic, persistent, or covert).[138] Risk factors in the presence of advanced liver disease include gastrointestinal bleeding, increased dietary protein, electrolyte imbalance, and hypoxia.

◆**PATHOPHYSIOLOGY.** Hepatic encephalopathy results from a combination of biochemical alterations that affect neurotransmission.[139] Liver dysfunction and collateral vessels that shunt blood around the liver to the systemic circulation permit neurotoxins and other harmful substances absorbed from the gastrointestinal tract to accumulate and circulate freely to the brain. Substances include inflammatory cytokines, short-chain fatty acids, serotonin, tryptophan, and false neurotransmitters. The most hazardous substances are end products of intestinal protein digestion, particularly ammonia, which cannot be converted to urea by the diseased liver. The digestion of blood from leaking or ruptured varices adds to the amount of ammonia present in systemic blood, as does the action of ammonia-forming bacteria in the colon. Ammonia that reaches the brain is metabolized to glutamine, with osmotic disturbances and alterations in cerebral blood flow that interfere with neurotransmitters and cause astrocyte edema (cytotoxic edema) and oxidation. Permeability of the blood-brain barrier also may be increased (vasogenic edema), contributing to astrocytes swelling, brain edema, and intracranial hypertension. Excessive amounts of gamma-aminobutyric acid (GABA), an inhibitory neurotransmitter from benzodiazepine-like compounds from the intestinal flora, may contribute to reduced levels of consciousness. Infection, hemorrhage, inflammation, electrolyte imbalance, sedatives, and analgesics also can precipitate stupor and coma in the presence of liver disease

◆CLINICAL MANIFESTATIONS. Subtle changes in personality, memory loss, irritability, lethargy, and sleep disturbances are common initial manifestations of hepatic encephalopathy and can be covert (minimal hepatic encephalopathy). In acute liver failure, symptom onset can be rapid with confusion, disorientation to time and space, flapping tremor of the hands (asterixis), slow speech, bradykinesia, stupor, convulsions, and coma. Coma is usually a sign of severe liver dysfunction and ultimately results in death. Variceal bleeding and ascites may develop concurrently. Symptoms may be episodic, recurrent, or persistent.

◆EVALUATION AND TREATMENT. There is no specific diagnostic test for hepatic encephalopathy. Diagnosis is based on a history of liver disease, clinical manifestations, and psychometric testing. Electroen-cephalography and blood chemistry tests, including blood ammonia levels, provide supportive data. Tracking levels of serum ammonia assesses treatment effectiveness and liver function.

Correction of fluid and electrolyte imbalances and withdrawal of depressant drugs metabolized by the liver are the first steps in the treatment of hepatic encephalopathy. Cerebral edema can be managed with hypertonic saline, mannitol, or hypothermia. Dietary protein is maintained to prevent malnutrition, but at levels that reduce blood ammonia levels. Nonabsorbable disaccharides (e.g., lactulose) prevent ammonia absorption in the colon. Neomycin eliminates ammonia-producing intestinal bacteria but can be nephrotoxic. Glutaminase inhibitors reduce gut ammonia. Rifaximin decreases intestinal production of ammonia and is used for lactulose nonresponders. Extracorporeal liver support systems remove toxins from the blood and are an option for managing overt hepatic encephalopathy.[140]

Jaundice

Jaundice, or icterus, is a yellow or greenish pigmentation of the skin caused by hyperbilirubinemia (total plasma bilirubin concentrations greater than 2.5 to 3 mg/dL). Hyperbilirubinemia and jaundice can result from (1) extrahepatic (posthepatic) obstruction to bile flow (gallstones), (2) intrahepatic obstruction (hepatocellular disease such as cirrhosis or hepatitis), or (3) prehepatic excessive production of unconjugated bilirubin (i.e., excessive hemolysis of red blood cells)[141] (Fig. 42.18). Jaundice in newborns is caused by impaired bilirubin uptake and conjugation (see Chapter 43).

◆PATHOPHYSIOLOGY. Obstructive jaundice can result from extrahepatic or intrahepatic obstruction.[142] *Extrahepatic obstructive jaundice* develops if the common bile duct is occluded by a gallstone, tumor, or inflammation. Bilirubin conjugated by the hepatocytes cannot flow through the obstructed common bile duct into the duodenum. Therefore it accumulates in the liver and enters the bloodstream, causing hyperbilirubinemia and jaundice. *Intrahepatic obstructive jaundice* involves disturbances in hepatocyte function and obstruction of *bile canaliculi.*

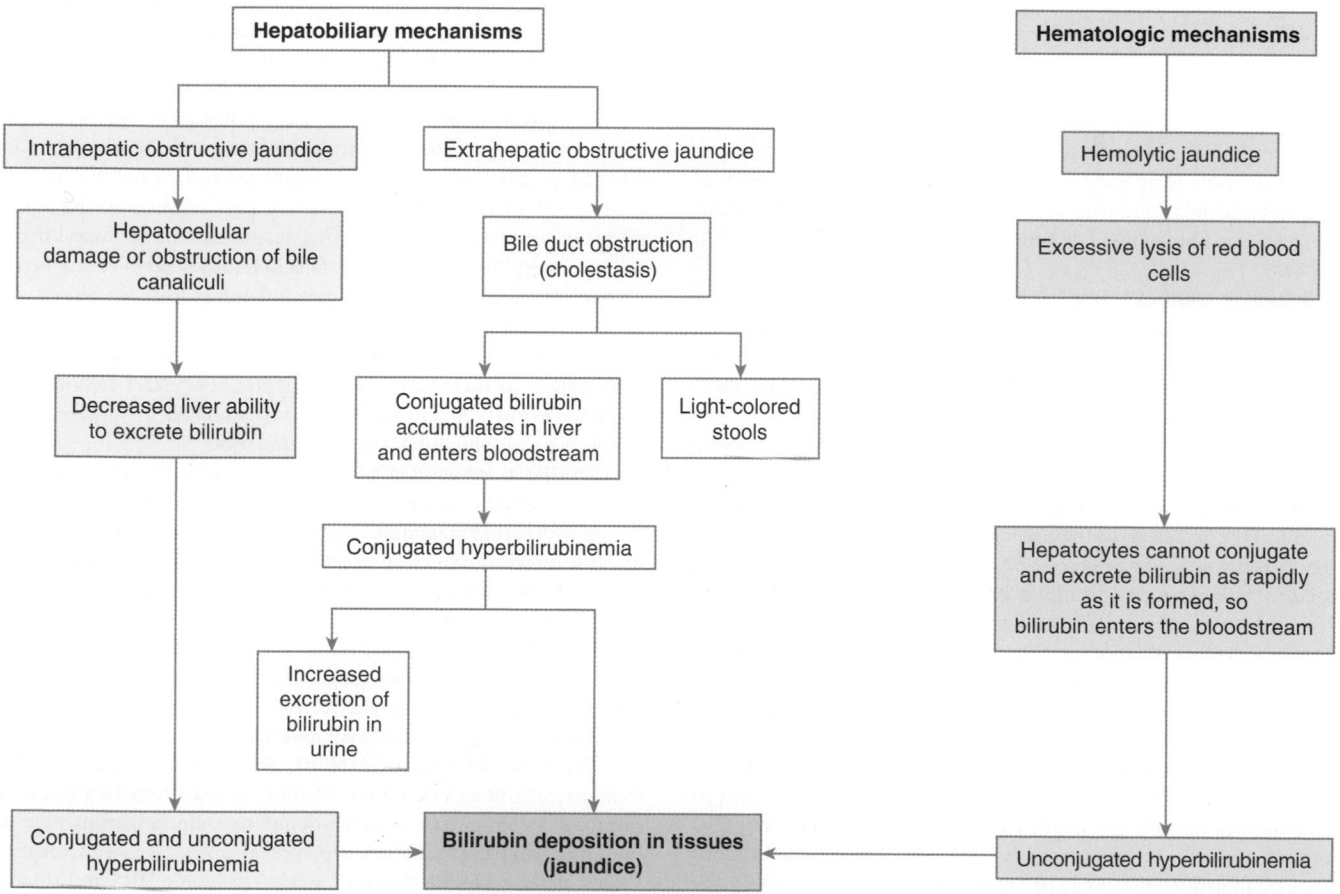

FIGURE 42.18 Mechanisms of Jaundice.

TABLE 42.6 THREE COMMON TYPES OF JAUNDICE

TYPE	MECHANISM	CAUSES
Hemolytic jaundice (predominantly unconjugated bilirubin)	Excessive destruction of erythrocytes	Membrane defect of erythrocytes Hemolytic anemias Immune reaction Severe infection Toxic substances in the circulation (e.g., snake venom) Transfusion of incompatible blood
Obstructive (cholestatic) jaundice (predominantly conjugated bilirubin)	Obstruction to passage of conjugated bilirubin from liver to intestine	Obstruction of bile duct by gallstones or tumor (extrahepatic obstructive jaundice) Obstruction of bile flow through the liver (intrahepatic obstructive jaundice) Drugs
Hepatocellular jaundice (both conjugated and unconjugated bilirubin)	Failure of liver cells (hepatocytes) to conjugate bilirubin and of bilirubin to pass from liver to intestine	Genetic defect of hepatocyte (decreased enzymes), such as occurs in premature infants (see Chapter 43) Hepatitis or biliary cirrhosis

The uptake, conjugation, and excretion of bilirubin can be affected with elevated levels of both conjugated and unconjugated bilirubin. Hepatocellular damage increases plasma concentrations of unconjugated bilirubin. The major disorder, however, is obstruction of bile canaliculi, which diminishes flow of conjugated bilirubin into the common bile duct with elevations in the plasma. In mild cases, some of the bile canaliculi open. Consequently, the amount of bilirubin in the intestinal tract may be only slightly decreased.

Excessive hemolysis (destruction) of red blood cells or absorption of hematoma causes hemolytic jaundice (prehepatic or nonobstructive jaundice). Increased unconjugated bilirubin is formed through metabolism of the heme component of destroyed red blood cells and exceeds the conjugation ability of the liver, causing blood levels of unconjugated bilirubin to rise. Decreased bilirubin uptake or conjugation also causes unconjugated hyperbilirubinemia, as occurs with reaction to some drugs (e.g., rifampin) and in genetic disorders such as Gilbert syndrome. Gilbert syndrome is an inherited autosomal dominant deficiency of glucuronyl transferase enzyme, which is required for the hepatic uptake of unconjugated bilirubin. The causes of jaundice are summarized in Table 42.6.

◆**CLINICAL MANIFESTATIONS.** The clinical manifestations of jaundice vary and are related to the underlying pathology. Conjugated bilirubin is water soluble and appears in the urine. Conjugated hyperbilirubinemia may cause the urine to darken several days before the onset of jaundice. The stools may be light colored or clay colored because they lack bile pigments. The stools also lack urobilinogen because bile is not available for conversion to urobilinogen. Extrahepatic biliary obstruction is associated with increased intestinal permeability and bacterial translocation and may contribute to the pathogenesis of sepsis.[143]

Fever, chills, and pain often accompany jaundice resulting from viral or bacterial inflammation of the liver (e.g., viral hepatitis). Manifestations of liver injury from any cause commonly include anorexia, malaise, and fatigue. Yellow discoloration may first occur in the sclera of the eye and then progress to the skin. Skin xanthomas (cholesterol deposits) and pruritus commonly accompany jaundice with an elevation of serum alkaline phosphatase level.

◆**EVALUATION AND TREATMENT.** Laboratory evaluation establishes whether the elevated level in plasma bilirubin is conjugated or unconjugated or both. The history, physical examination, and laboratory tests identify underlying disorders, such as alcoholism, exposure to hepatitis virus, or gallbladder disease. The treatment for jaundice consists of correcting the cause.

Hepatorenal Syndrome

Hepatorenal syndrome (HRS) is functional renal failure; it develops as a complication usually associated with alcoholic cirrhosis. The renal failure is not caused by primary renal disease or other extrinsic factors, but rather by arterial vasodilation of the splanchnic vasculature, reduced effective blood volume, and renal vasoconstriction in the presence of acute liver disease with advanced liver failure and portal hypertension.

◆**PATHOPHYSIOLOGY.** There are two types of HRS: type 1 and type 2. Type 1 involves rapid (within 2 weeks) progressive renal failure related to severe reduction in blood volume and decreased cardiac output secondary to massive gastrointestinal or variceal bleeding and hypotension caused by bleeding and splanchnic vasodilation. Type 2 is slower, is more stable, and is accompanied by refractory ascites.[144]

The decrease in blood volume and hypotension result in decreased renal perfusion, decreased glomerular filtration, and oliguria (see Chapter 39). In type 2 HRS, the ability to concentrate and dilute urine is usually maintained. Intrarenal vasoconstriction may result from the selective effects of vasoactive substances that accumulate in the blood because of liver failure. The diseased liver fails to remove excessive angiotensin, vasopressin, prostaglandins, and catecholamines from the blood, which travel to the kidneys and cause vasoconstriction. Vasoconstriction also may be a compensatory response to portal hypotension and vasodilation in the splanchnic circulation. The exact reason for the renal vasoconstriction is unknown but is related to vasoconstrictive mediators and sympathetic nerve stimulation.[144]

◆**CLINICAL MANIFESTATIONS.** The onset of hepatorenal manifestations may be acute or gradual. Type 1 HRS is a rapidly progressive renal failure with serum creatinine >2.5 mg/dL (>221 μmoL/L) or a decrease of 50% in creatinine clearance (<20 mL/min) in less than 2 weeks. Type 2 HRS is a more gradual renal failure with a serum creatinine of >1.5 mg/dL (>133 μmoL/L) with diuretic-resistant ascites.[145] Oliguria and complications of advanced liver disease, including jaundice, ascites, and gastrointestinal bleeding, are usually present. Systolic blood pressure is usually less than 100 mmHg. Nonspecific symptoms of hepatorenal syndrome include anorexia, weakness, and fatigue.

◆**EVALUATION AND TREATMENT.** Diagnosis of HRS is made by excluding all other causes of renal failure. Despite decreased glomerular filtration, serum potassium levels do not become dangerously elevated until the terminal stages of the hepatorenal syndrome. Serum creatinine values increase rapidly (within 2 weeks) in type 1 HRS and slowly or not at all in type 2 HRS. Urine osmolality is increased, but urine sodium concentrations are below normal (unlike acute tubular necrosis). Urine specific gravity is greater than 1.015. The prognosis for hepatorenal syndrome is usually poor and is related to liver function. Secondary problems, including fluid and electrolyte disorders, bleeding, infections, and encephalopathy, are vigorously treated. Treatments to increase renal perfusion include systemic vasoconstrictors (α-adrenergic agonists and octreotide) and albumin, which are effective in 50% of individuals with type 1 HRS. Vasoconstrictors also may be combined with TIPS as a bridge to liver transplant. Liver transplant reverses symptoms in most individuals, and it may be combined with kidney transplantation.[144]

Disorders of the Liver
Acute Liver Failure

Acute liver failure (fulminant liver failure) is a rare clinical syndrome (2000 cases in the United States annually)[146] resulting from severe impairment or necrosis of liver cells without preexisting liver disease or cirrhosis. Acetaminophen overdose is the leading cause of acute liver failure in the United States[147] (Box 42.3). Acute liver failure also can occur with concurrent liver disease (acute on chronic liver failure),[148] including complications of viral hepatitis, particularly hepatitis B virus (HBV) and hepatitis C virus (HCV) infection, and can be compounded by infection with the delta virus, as well as metabolic liver disorders. Edematous hepatocytes and patchy areas of necrosis and inflammatory cell infiltrates disrupt the parenchyma. The death of hepatocytes may be caused by viral or toxic injury or immunologic and inflammatory damage with necrosis or apoptosis.

Acute liver failure usually develops 6 to 8 weeks after the initial symptoms of viral hepatitis or a metabolic liver disorder (e.g., Wilson disease), or within 5 days to 8 weeks of acetaminophen overdose. Anorexia, vomiting, abdominal pain, and progressive jaundice are initial signs, followed by ascites and gastrointestinal bleeding. Hepatic encephalopathy is manifested as lethargy and altered motor functions. Coma is related to cerebral edema, ischemia, and brainstem herniation. Liver function tests show elevations in the levels of both conjugated and unconjugated serum bilirubin, serum transaminases, and blood ammonia. Prothrombin time is prolonged. Renal failure and pulmonary distress can occur.[149] Treatment of acute liver failure requires rapid evaluation and critical care. N-Acetylcysteine is used for acetaminophen poisoning; antiviral therapy appears to improve survival in cases of viral hepatitis; and lowering

---

BOX 42.3 ACETAMINOPHEN AND ACUTE LIVER FAILURE

Acetaminophen (paracetamol) toxicity from chronic use or intentional overdose is the leading cause of acute liver failure (46%) in the United States and Great Britain (40%-70%). Liver injury may occur with doses of 4 to 10 g/day, and hepatotoxicity with mitochondrial injury and hepatocyte necrosis should be suspected when doses exceed 4 g/day. The onset is sudden and unpredictable with abdominal pain and nausea developing between 12 and 24 hours followed by coagulopathy and encephalopathy within 72 to 96 hours. Elevated serum aminotransferase levels (may be up to 400 × normal) accompanied by hypo-prothrombinemia, lactic acidosis, and renal failure support a diagnosis of acute liver failure caused by acetaminophen. Complications of cerebral edema and infection are difficult to diagnose and treat and may lead to multiorgan failure, irreversible brain damage, and death. Early treatment (within 8 hours of overdose) with correct dosing with N-acetylcysteine provides a 66% chance of recovery, and there is 70% survival at 1 year after liver transplant.

Data from Jaeschke H: *Dig Dis* 33(4):464-471, 2015; Lee WM: *J Hepatol* 2017 Jul 29 [Epub ahead of print]; Yoon E, et al: *J Clin Transl Hepatol* 4(2):131-142, 2016.

---

blood ammonia levels may improve prognosis. Liver transplantation is lifesaving. Artificial liver support systems remove toxins and can be a bridge to transplant. Growth factors may promote hepatic regeneration, and stem cell therapy continues to be investigated.[150-152]

Autoimmune Hepatitis

Autoimmune hepatitis is a rare chronic, progressive, autoimmune inflammatory liver disease that affects genetically susceptible individuals, usually women and children. The cause is unknown, but certain infections and drugs are thought to trigger the autoimmune response. Autoreactive T cells trigger secretion of proinflammatory cytotoxic cytokines. Serologically, there are two types: type 1 with positivity for antinuclear and/or anti-smooth muscle antibody, and type 2 with anti-liver kidney microsomal type 1 antibody or anti-liver cytosol type 1 antibody. There is hypergammaglobulinemia and an elevation in aspartate and alanine aminotransferase. Biopsy confirms the diagnosis and shows lymphocytic infiltration with interface (parenchymal-connective tissue interface) hepatitis. There may be no symptoms or jaundice, fatigue, loss of appetite, amenorrhea, or acute liver failure. Most individuals respond to immunosuppressive drug therapy (e.g., corticosteroids or in combination with azathioprine) with remission within 24 months. Relapses are common with treatment withdrawal. About 10% of cases require liver transplant.[153]

Viral Hepatitis

Viral hepatitis is a relatively common systemic disease that affects primarily the liver. Different strains of viruses cause different types of hepatitis. The types and estimated incidence in the United States in 2014 were 2500 cases for hepatitis A virus (HAV), 19,200 cases for hepatitis B virus (HBV), an unknown number for hepatitis D virus (HDV) associated with HBV, 30,500 cases for hepatitis C virus (HCV), and an unknown number for hepatitis E virus (HEV). HVA, HVB, and HVC are the most common in the United States, and hepatitis C cases tripled from 2010 to 2015 with an estimate of 34,000 cases.[154,155] Characteristics of the various types of hepatitis are presented in Table 42.7.

Hepatitis A Virus (HAV). HAV is in the family Picornaviridae, is a *Hepatovirus,* and causes acute disease. HAV can be recovered from the feces, bile, and sera of infected individuals. The usual mode of transmission is the fecal-oral route (contaminated food or water), but the virus can be spread also by the transfusion of infected blood and men having sex with men.[156] Approximately 45% of adults in urban areas have HAV antibodies in their blood. The disease spreads readily in crowded, unsanitary conditions, usually through contaminated food or water. Person-to-person spread is more likely to occur in institutional care settings where there is contact between clients and caregivers who are not vaccinated.

The incubation period (the time between exposure and onset of symptoms) for HAV is 4 to 6 weeks (Fig. 42.19). Fecal shedding of the virus is greatest for 10 to 14 days before the onset of symptoms and during the first week of symptoms, and up to 3 months after onset of symptoms. The disease is most contagious during this time. Antibodies to HAV (anti-HAV) develop about 4 weeks after infection. The serum immunoglobulin M (IgM) concentration increases initially and is followed by an increase of serum IgG, whose levels remain elevated for several years after infection, creating immunity to the disease (see Chapters 7 and 8 for a description of immune functions). The administration of immunoglobulin before exposure or early in the incubation period can prevent hepatitis A. HAV vaccine and combined HAV and HBV vaccines are available and effective in preventing the disease and confer long-term immunity.[157] Transmission of HAV is prevented by handwashing and use of gloves when disposing fecal matter. Molecular procedures are available for direct surveillance of HAV in food and water.[158]

TABLE 42.7   CHARACTERISTICS OF VIRAL HEPATITIS

CHARACTERISTIC	HEPATITIS A	HEPATITIS B	HEPATITIS D	HEPATITIS C	HEPATITIS E
Size of virus	27–nm RNA virus	47–nm DNA virus	36–nm RNA virus, defective virus with HBsAg coat	30– to 60–nm RNA virus	32–nm RNA virus
Incubation phase	30 days	60–180 days	30–180 days; dependent on HBV for multiplication	35–72 days	15–60 days
Route of transmission	Fecal-oral, parenteral, sexual	Parenteral, sexual	Parenteral, fecal-oral, sexual	Parenteral	Fecal-oral
Onset	Acute with fever	Insidious	Insidious	Insidious	Acute
Carrier state	Negative	Positive	Positive	Positive	Negative
Severity	Mild	Severe; may be prolonged or chronic	Severe	Mild to severe	Severe in pregnant women
Chronic hepatitis	No	Yes	Yes	Yes	No
Age-group affected	Children and young adults	Any	Any	Any	Children and young adults
Prophylaxis	Hygiene, immune serum globulin, HAV vaccine	Hygiene, HBV vaccine	Hygiene, HBV vaccine	Hygiene, screening blood, interferon-alpha or combined with ribavirin; treatment also related to HCV genotype ± cirrhosis	Hygiene, safe water and meat

DNA, Deoxyribonucleic acid; *HAV,* hepatits A virus; *HBsAg,* hepatitis B surface antigen; *HBV,* hepatitis B virus; *HCV,* hepatitis C virus; *RNA,* ribonucleic acid.

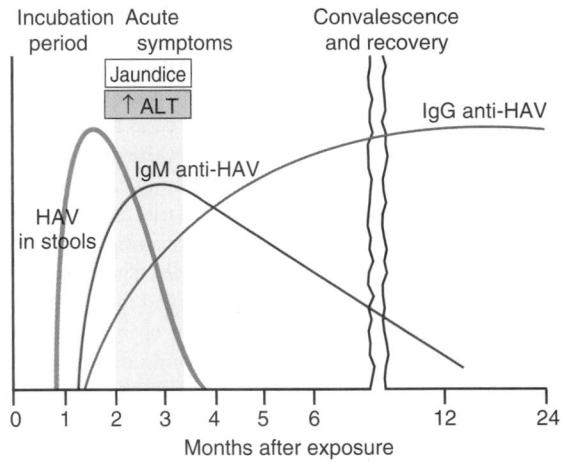

FIGURE 42.19 Course of Infection with the Hepatitis A Virus (HAV). *ALT,* Alanine transaminase; *IgG,* immunoglobulin G; *IgM,* immunoglobulin M.

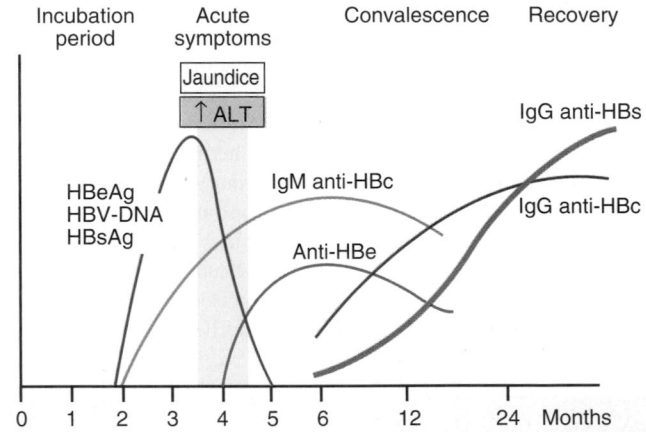

FIGURE 42.20 Course of Infection with the Hepatitis B Virus (HBV). *ALT,* Alanine transaminase; *anti-HBe,* antibody to HBeAg; *HBV-DNA,* hepatitis B virus deoxyribonucleic acid; *IgG,* immunoglobulin G; *IgM,* immunoglobulin M; *HBsAg,* hepatitis B surface antigen; *IgG anti-HBs,* antibody to HBsAg; *HBeAg,* hepatitis B e-antigen; *IgM anti-HBc,* antibody to hepatitis B core antigen.

Hepatitis B Virus (HBV). HBV is a parenterally and sexually transmitted hepadnavirus with eight genotypes (A through H) with many subgenotypes. The pathogenic characteristics are unknown. The genotypes vary by geographical region, disease progression, and treatment response.[159] People who are immunosuppressed; receive hemodialysis, multiple blood transfusions, or immunosuppressive drugs; have multiple sex partners; or share needles, syringes, or other drug equipment, as well as infants born to infected mothers, have a greater risk of exposure or less resistance to HBV. Coinfection with HCV, HDV, and HIV is common because these viruses share the same routes of transmission.

Mother-infant transmission of HBV occurs if the mother becomes infected during the third trimester of pregnancy. In women who are seropositive for both hepatitis B surface antigen (HBsAg) and hepatitis B e-antigen (HBeAg), vertical transmission is approximately 90%. Screening for HBV should occur for all pregnant women, and infants born to positive mothers should receive HBV vaccine and HBV immunoglobulin within 12 hours after birth.[160] Transmission among men having sex with men may be by oral or genital contact with bleeding lesions in the rectal mucosa. HBV is a major cause of chronic hepatitis, cirrhosis, and hepatocellular carcinoma.[161]

Three types of viral particles are involved in HBV infection. The larger (47 nm) Dane particle probably represents the intact HBV. The Dane particle has a double-layered outer coat and carries HBsAg, which was originally called the *Australia antigen.* HBsAg can be identified in the serum by radioimmunoassay. Hepatitis B core antigen (HBcAg) usually is not detected in the serum. The HBeAg is a derivative of HBcAg and is a marker of HBV replication. The HBV has an incubation period of 6 to 8 weeks. The initial serologic change is a transient increase in IgM levels. Levels of IgG antibodies to HBsAg rise more slowly and remain elevated for years (Fig. 42.20). *Chronic infection* develops in 15% to 30% of those with acute infection. HBV DNA and HBsAg measure viral load and the efficacy of drug treatment. Persistent liver cell injury, chronic low-grade inflammation, and deregulation of cellular growth control genes lead to increased risk for cirrhosis and liver failure and foster oncogenic transformation and hepatocellular carcinoma. Cancer risk is greater with HBV and HCV coinfection.[162]

Antiviral and immunomodulatory treatment for chronic hepatitis B includes monotherapy or combination therapy with nucleoside and nucleotide analogs (targets reverse transcriptase [e.g., entecavir, tenofovir]) and interferon (e.g., peginterferon). Drug resistance and disease recurrence develop because double-stranded HBV DNA is transformed in the nucleus to covalently closed circular DNA (cccDNA), the template necessary for viral RNA synthesis and replication of the virus. cccDNA remains in the hepatocytes after treatment and can be used as a marker of treatment effectiveness; HBV immune control is difficult to induce.[163,164] Vaccine prevents transmission of hepatitis B, the development of acute or chronic hepatitis B, and reduction of hepatocellular carcinoma, particularly in high-risk populations. Mutant strains can develop with escape from vaccine protection or diagnosis with HBsAg. Hepatitis B immunoglobulin provides postexposure prophylaxis against HBV after contact with blood or body fluids of individuals infected with hepatitis B. HBV vaccine or a combined vaccine for HAV and HBV provides protective immunity. New drugs that target different stages of the HBV life cycle and eradication of cccDNA and HBsAg, as well as vaccines that target different HBV proteins, are under investigation.[163,165]

Hepatitis C Virus (HCV). HCV (previously known as *non-A, non-B hepatitis*) is a parenterally transmitted flavivirus with 10 genotypes (A through J). Worldwide, a significant number of HCV cases involve intravenous drug users, who also have a high incidence of HIV infection.[166] HBV infection increases the risk for HCV infection. Approximately 80% of cases develop chronic liver disease.[167] HCV is diagnosed through detection of anti-HCV IgG. Persistent infection with recurring acute symptoms and elevated aminotransferase levels represents the clinical presentation. HCV is often undiagnosed as there may be no symptoms. Direct-acting antiviral drug therapy is available; it is genotype specific, depends on the presence or absence of cirrhosis, is oral, and is interferon free. Resistance to drug therapy is common, particularly when there is progression to chronic liver disease or selected viral genotypes.[168]

Progression of disease to cirrhosis is the most common cause of hepatocellular carcinoma in the United States and of liver transplant worldwide. Extrahepatic manifestations include cryoglobulinemia vasculitis and lymphoproliferative disorders.[169] Viral mutation, genetic diversity between genotypes, and reinfection after treatment have made vaccine development difficult, and there is no vaccine for HCV. The Centers for Disease Control and Prevention have recommended that all persons born from 1945 through 1965 be screened for HCV infection.[170] Individuals with HCV and cirrhosis or liver failure also should be screened for esophageal varices.[171]

Hepatitis D Virus (HDV). HDV is a defective, single-stranded RNA virus and occurs as a coinfection with hepatitis B. The delta virus depends on the viral coat of HBsAg molecules on HBV for its replication.[172] Hepatitis D has been shown to suppress replication of HBV. Parenteral drug users have a high incidence of HDV infection. HDV symptoms can be mild or severe with progression to fulminant liver failure. HDV is diagnosed by the presence of antibodies directed against HDAg (anti-HD) and HDV RNA in serum. Treatment for chronic HDV includes pegylated interferon alpha and is effective in about 25% of individuals. New treatments are in clinical development.[173]

Hepatitis E Virus (HEV). HEV is classified within the *Hepeviridae* family and is most common in Asian and African countries; human

genotypes vary by country. It is transmitted by the fecal-oral route, usually by way of contaminated water or uncooked meat. It is also found in developed countries and must be differentiated from drug-induced liver injury. Animal reservoirs of HEV with transmission to humans include domestic pigs, wild boars, deer, mongoose, and rabbits. It is more prevalent among adults and has the highest mortality in pregnant women and immunosuppressed individuals. Clinically, it can be asymptomatic and resemble HAV or progress to acute liver failure or chronic hepatitis. Extrahepatic manifestations include neurologic symptoms and impaired kidney function. Diagnosis is based on detection of anti-HEV IgM. Ribavirin and pegylated interferon are effective treatments. A vaccine for HEV has been approved in China but not in other countries.[174]

PATHOPHYSIOLOGY. The pathologic lesions of hepatitis are similar to those caused by other viral infection. Hepatic cell necrosis, scarring, Kupffer cell hyperplasia, and infiltration by mononuclear phagocytes occur with varying severity. Cellular injury is promoted by cell-mediated immune mechanisms (i.e., cytotoxic T cells, T regulatory cells, and natural killer cells).[175] Regeneration of hepatic cells begins within 48 hours of injury. The inflammatory process can damage and obstruct bile canaliculi, leading to cholestasis and obstructive jaundice. In milder cases the liver parenchyma is not damaged. Damage tends to be most severe in cases of hepatitis B and hepatitis C, as these viruses cause liver cell apoptosis. Hepatitis B is also associated with *acute liver failure,* a rare form of the disease that is characterized by massive hepatic necrosis. Mortality is high, but recovery can be complete.

CLINICAL MANIFESTATIONS. The clinical manifestations of the various types of viral hepatitis are very similar with nausea, malaise, abdominal pain, and jaundice. The spectrum of manifestations ranges from absence of symptoms to fulminating hepatitis, with rapid onset of liver failure and coma. Acute viral hepatitis causes abnormal liver function test results. The serum aminotransferase values, aspartate transaminase (AST) and alanine transaminase (ALT), are elevated, but their elevation may not be consistent with the extent of cellular damage. The clinical course of hepatitis usually consists of four phases: incubation, prodromal, icteric, and recovery phases. During the incubation phase, the virus is replicating and manifestations vary depending on the virus (see Table 42.7). There may be no symptoms, but there can be serologic and serum enzyme markers.

Prodromal Phase. The prodromal (preicteric) phase of hepatitis begins about 2 weeks after exposure and ends with the appearance of jaundice. Fatigue, anorexia, malaise, nausea, vomiting, headache, hyperalgia, cough, and low-grade fever are prodromal symptoms that precede the onset of jaundice. About 10% of individuals may develop extrahepatic symptoms including rash, arthralgias, and purpura. HBV and HCV may cause nephritis related to glomerular immune complex deposition.[176,177] Infection with HCV may have no symptoms. Right upper abdominal pain is common, and a weight loss of 2 to 4 kg is not unusual. The infection is highly transmissible during this phase.

Icteric Phase (Jaundice). The icteric phase begins about 1 to 2 weeks after the prodromal phase and lasts 2 to 6 weeks. Individuals who develop chronic HBV infection do not become jaundiced and may not be diagnosed.[178] Hepatocellular destruction and intrahepatic bile stasis cause jaundice (icterus). The urine may be dark and the stools clay colored before the onset of jaundice from conjugated hyperbilirubinemia. The icteric phase is the actual phase of illness. The liver is enlarged, smooth, and tender, and percussion over the liver causes pain. During the icteric phase, gastrointestinal and respiratory symptoms subside, but fatigue and abdominal pain may persist or become more severe. The stools may be lighter in color as a result of cholestasis. Serum bilirubin levels range from 5 to 10 mg/dL, with conjugated bilirubin fraction increasing. The jaundice may last 2 to 6 weeks or longer. Mild and transient itching often accompanies jaundice. The prothrombin time may be prolonged in individuals with more serious forms of the disease.

Recovery Phase. The posticteric or recovery phase begins with resolution of jaundice, about 6 to 8 weeks after exposure. Although the liver may still be enlarged and tender, symptoms diminish. In most cases, liver function test results return to normal within 2 to 12 weeks after the onset of jaundice.

Chronic hepatitis may begin at this point and is associated with HBV, HCV, and HDV infection. Chronic active hepatitis is the persistence of clinical manifestations and liver inflammation after the acute stages. Liver function tests remain abnormal for longer than 6 months, and HBsAg persists. Chronic, active HBV and HBC both predispose individuals to cirrhosis and primary hepatocellular carcinoma.[179] Chronic active hepatitis constitutes a carrier state, and HBV and HCV can be transmitted from mothers to infants.[180]

◆**EVALUATION AND TREATMENT.** Diagnosis and treatment were previously described for the different types of hepatitis viruses. Physical activity may be restricted. A low-fat, high-carbohydrate diet is beneficial if bile flow is obstructed.

There should be no direct contact with blood or body fluids of individuals with hepatitis B or hepatitis C. A combined vaccine for HAV and HBV is available. Hepatitis B immunoglobulin provides passive prophylactic immunity against HBV. Prophylaxis is recommended for healthcare workers, liver transplant recipients, and others who are at risk for contact with infected body fluids.[181]

Cirrhosis

Cirrhosis is an irreversible inflammatory, fibrotic liver disease and the eighth leading cause of death in the United States. Many disorders can cause cirrhosis and are summarized in Box 42.4. Alcohol abuse and HCV infection are the most common causes, and nonalcoholic steatohepatitis is an increasing cause. The process of cellular injury depends on the cause of cirrhosis; however, not all causes are clearly understood. Structural changes result from injury (alcoholism, viruses, steatosis, chemicals) and fibrosis. Fibrosis is a consequence of Kupffer cell (liver macrophages) activation with release of inflammatory mediators, reactive oxygen species, and growth factors and activation of fibrogenic hepatic stellate cells.[182] Chaotic fibrosis alters or obstructs biliary channels and

---

BOX 42.4   CAUSES OF CIRRHOSIS

Hepatitis virus—B and C (common)
Excessive alcohol intake (common)
Idiopathic (common)
Nonalcoholic fatty liver disease (NAFLD), also known as *nonalcoholic steatohepatitis (NASH)*
Autoimmune disorders
  Autoimmune hepatitis
  Primary biliary cirrhosis
  Primary sclerosing cholangitis
Hereditary metabolic disorder
  α_1-Antitrypsin deficiency
  Hemochromatosis
  Wilson disease
  Glycogen or lipid storage diseases
Prolonged exposure to chemicals (e.g., carbon tetrachloride, cleaning and industrial solvents, copper salts)
Hepatic venous outflow obstruction
  Budd-Chiari syndrome
  Right-sided heart failure

---

blood flow, producing jaundice and portal hypertension. New vascular channels form shunts, and blood from the portal vein bypasses the liver, contributing to portal hypertension, metabolic alterations, and toxin accumulation. The process of regeneration is disrupted by hypoxia, necrosis, atrophy, and (ultimately) liver failure. The formation of fibrous bands and regenerating nodules distorts the architecture of the liver parenchyma and gives the liver a cobbly appearance. The liver may be larger or smaller than normal and is usually firm or hard when palpated. Cirrhosis develops slowly over a period of years. Its severity and rate of progression depend on the cause. The complications of cirrhosis include jaundice, portal hypertension, ascites, hepatic encephalopathy, varices with gastrointestinal bleeding, hepatorenal syndrome, hepatopulmonary syndrome, and portopulmonary syndrome.[183]

If alcohol is involved, the rate of cell death and the severity of inflammation depend on the amount of alcohol present.[184] Removal of alcohol slows the progression of liver damage and enhances the process of regeneration.

Alcoholic Liver Disease. Abuse of any type of alcoholic beverage can cause alcoholic liver disease, and the severity of disease is related to the amount and duration of alcohol consumed and formation of acetaldehyde[184,185] (see Chapter 2 and Fig. 2.21). The spectrum of alcoholic liver disease includes steatosis, alcoholic hepatitis, and alcoholic cirrhosis (fibrosis). The incidence of alcoholic cirrhosis is greatest in middle-aged men; however, women develop more severe liver injury than men.[186] In the United States, mortality resulting from cirrhosis is highest among Hispanic white males and females; however, the death rates for all groups are declining.[187] Malnutrition may add to the risk of cirrhosis in alcohol abusers. Many alcoholics are malnourished, and the liver cannot regenerate without adequate nutrition.[188]

◆**PATHOPHYSIOLOGY.** Alcoholic fatty liver (steatosis) is the mildest form of alcoholic liver disease and is reversible with abstinence. It can be caused by chronic ingestion of relatively small amounts of alcohol (more than one alcoholic drink [14 grams of alcohol] per day for women and two alcoholic drinks [28 grams of alcohol] per day for men), may be asymptomatic, and is reversible with cessation of drinking.[189,190] Fat deposition (deposition of triglycerides) within the liver is caused primarily by increased lipogenesis and decreased fatty acid oxidation and fat metabolism by hepatocytes. Lipids mobilized from adipose tissue or dietary fat intake may contribute to fat accumulation.

Alcoholic hepatitis (steatohepatitis) is a precursor of cirrhosis characterized by inflammation; degeneration and necrosis of hepatocytes; infiltration of neutrophils, macrophages, and lymphocytes; immunologic alterations; and oxidative stress leading to lipid peroxidation. The injured hepatocytes contain Mallory bodies (hyaline endoplasmic reticulum), indicating the onset of fibrosis. Neutrophils infiltrate and surround degenerating hepatocytes. The mechanism of hepatocyte injury is not clearly understood, but inflammatory mediators, acetaldehyde, reactive oxygen and nitrogen species, and genetic factors are involved. Alcohol also increases gut permeability, and translocation of bacteria-derived lipopolysaccharide contributes to inflammation, oxidative stress, and the severity of alcoholic liver disease. Serum IgA level is often elevated in individuals with alcoholic hepatitis, and liver antigens and antibodies have been identified in persons with progressive alcoholic liver disease. The inflammation and necrosis caused by alcoholic hepatitis stimulate the fibrosis characteristic of the cirrhotic stage of disease. Treatment includes corticosteroids and/or pentoxifylline and alcohol abstinence supported by baclofen.[191]

Alcoholic cirrhosis is caused by the toxic effects of alcohol metabolism on the liver, immunologic alterations, oxidative stress from lipid peroxidation, and malnutrition. Alcoholic cirrhosis is more severe when associated with HCV. Although alcoholic cirrhosis is the most prevalent of the various types of cirrhosis, the occurrence of cirrhosis among persons with alcoholism is relatively low (approximately 35%). Alcohol is transformed to acetaldehyde. Excessive amounts of acetaldehyde are toxic, induce oxidative stress and lipid peroxidation, and disrupt cytoskeletal and membrane function. Acetaldehyde inhibits export of proteins from the liver, alters metabolism of vitamins and minerals, promotes liver fibrosis, and contributes to malnutrition. Mitochondrial function is impaired, decreasing oxidation of fatty acid. Enzyme and protein synthesis may be depressed or altered, and hormone and ammonia degradation is diminished. Alcohol also may stimulate the formation of autoantibodies specific to hepatic cells. Alcohol also increases gut permeability, and translocation of bacteria-derived endotoxin from the intestine contributes to progressive injury and inflammation. Cellular damage initiates an inflammatory response. Inflammatory cytokines, including TNF-α and IL-6, IL-8, and IL-18, and activation of complement are associated with alcoholic liver disease. Inflammation and necrosis result in excessive collagen formation. Transforming growth factor-beta (TGF-β) contributes to fibrosis and is produced in part by activated Kupffer cells. TGF-β activates hepatic stellate cells and transforms them to myofibroblasts, which produce excess collagen. Dense bands of fibrosis surround regenerative hepatocellular nodules. Fibrosis and scarring alter the structure of the liver and obstruct biliary and vascular channels, and hepatocytes lose their ability to regenerate.[192-194] There is increased risk for hepatocellular carcinoma. Examples of liver damage are shown in Fig. 42.21.

◆**CLINICAL MANIFESTATIONS.** Steatosis causes no specific symptoms or abnormal liver function test results. The liver is usually enlarged, however, and the individual has a history of continuous alcohol intake during the previous weeks or months. The clinical manifestations of alcoholic hepatitis can be mild or severe. Nonspecific symptoms include fatigue, weight loss, and anorexia. Manifestations of acute illness include nausea, anorexia, fever, abdominal pain, and jaundice. Toxic effects of alcohol also can cause gynecomastia, testicular atrophy, reduced libido, azoospermia, and decreased testosterone level in men. Cirrhosis is a multiple-system disease and causes hepatomegaly, splenomegaly, ascites, gastrointestinal hemorrhage, portal hypertension, hepatic encephalopathy, and esophageal varices. Anemia results from blood loss, malnutrition, and hypersplenism. Hepatorenal syndrome and portopulmonary syndrome are usually late complications. Risk for infection is greater, in part because of innate immune dysfunction. The presence of numerous and severe manifestations increases the risk of death. The clinical features of alcoholic cirrhosis depend on the duration of the disease and the severity of liver damage (Fig. 42.22).

◆**EVALUATION AND TREATMENT.** The diagnosis of alcoholic hepatitis is based on the individual's history and clinical manifestations. The results of liver function tests are abnormal, and serologic studies show elevated levels of serum enzymes (i.e., alanine aminotransferase, aspartate aminotransferase, and γ-glutamyltransferase) and bilirubin, and decreased serum albumin levels. Prolonged prothrombin time cannot easily be corrected with vitamin K therapy. Malnutrition is often present. Liver biopsy can confirm the diagnosis of cirrhosis, but biopsy is not necessary if clinical manifestations of cirrhosis are evident.[195]

There is no specific treatment for alcoholic liver disease, but many of the complications are treatable. Rest, a nutritious diet, corticosteroids, antioxidants, drugs that slow fibrosis, and management of complications such as ascites, gastrointestinal bleeding, anemia, infection, and encephalopathy slow disease progression.[183] Cessation of alcohol consumption slows the progression of liver damage, improves clinical symptoms, and prolongs life. Although the liver damage is irreversible, measures that halt the inflammation and destruction of liver cells and fibrosis prolong life. Guidelines are available to guide treatment and predict clinical outcome.[183] Liver transplant is the treatment for liver failure, and artificial liver support systems are being developed.[196]

Nonalcoholic Fatty Liver Disease and Nonalcoholic Steato-hepatitis. Nonalcoholic fatty liver disease (NAFLD) is infiltration of hepatocytes with fat, primarily in the form of triglycerides, but it occurs in the absence of alcohol intake. It is associated with polygenic susceptibility, obesity (including obese children), high levels of cholesterol and triglycerides, metabolic syndrome, type 2 diabetes mellitus, and alterations in the gut microbiome.[197] It is the most common chronic liver disease in the United States. Some individuals with NAFLD will develop nonalcoholic steatohepatitis (NASH), and the most severe forms of NASH progress to cirrhosis, end-stage liver disease, and an increased risk for hepatocellular carcinoma. NASH is difficult to distinguish from alcohol-induced liver disease and requires biopsy. NAFLD is usually asymptomatic and may remain undetected for years. Treatment includes lifestyle modification with diet and exercise. Pharmacotherapy with insulin sensitizers, vitamin E (antioxidant), and lipid-lowering drugs may be considered. Pioglitazone should be considered for those with NASH, especially those with fibrosis. Bariatric surgery may be an option. Liver transplant is the only option for liver failure.[198]

Biliary Cirrhosis. Biliary cirrhosis differs from alcoholic cirrhosis in that the damage and inflammation leading to cirrhosis begin in bile canaliculi and bile ducts, rather than in the hepatocytes. The two types of biliary cirrhosis are *primary* and *secondary*. Although both involve bile duct pathology, they differ with respect to cause, risk factors, and mechanisms of obstruction and inflammation.

Primary Biliary Cirrhosis. Primary biliary cirrhosis (PBC) is a chronic, autoimmune, cholestatic liver disease. It is caused by natural-killer T lymphocytes and highly specific antimitochondrial antibody

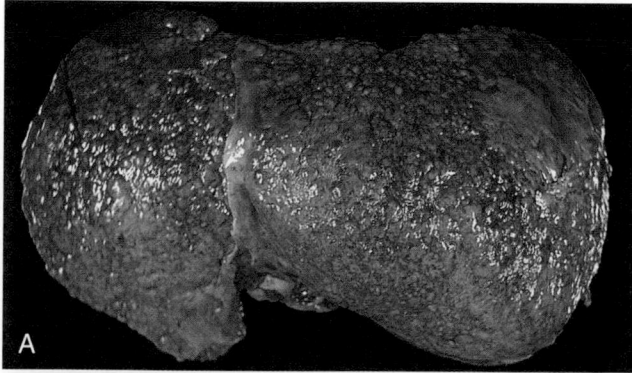
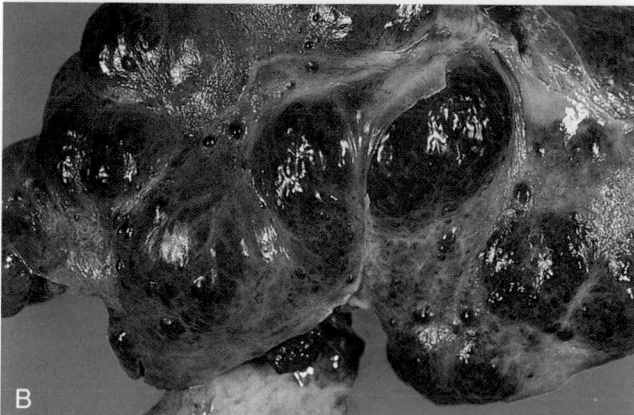

FIGURE 42.21 Cirrhosis. **A,** Micronodular cirrhosis. The nodular appearance develops from regeneration of hepatocytes projecting through fibrous bands of tissue. **B,** Macronodular cirrhosis. (From Damjanov I, Linder J, editors: *Anderson's pathology,* ed 10, St Louis, 1996, Mosby.)

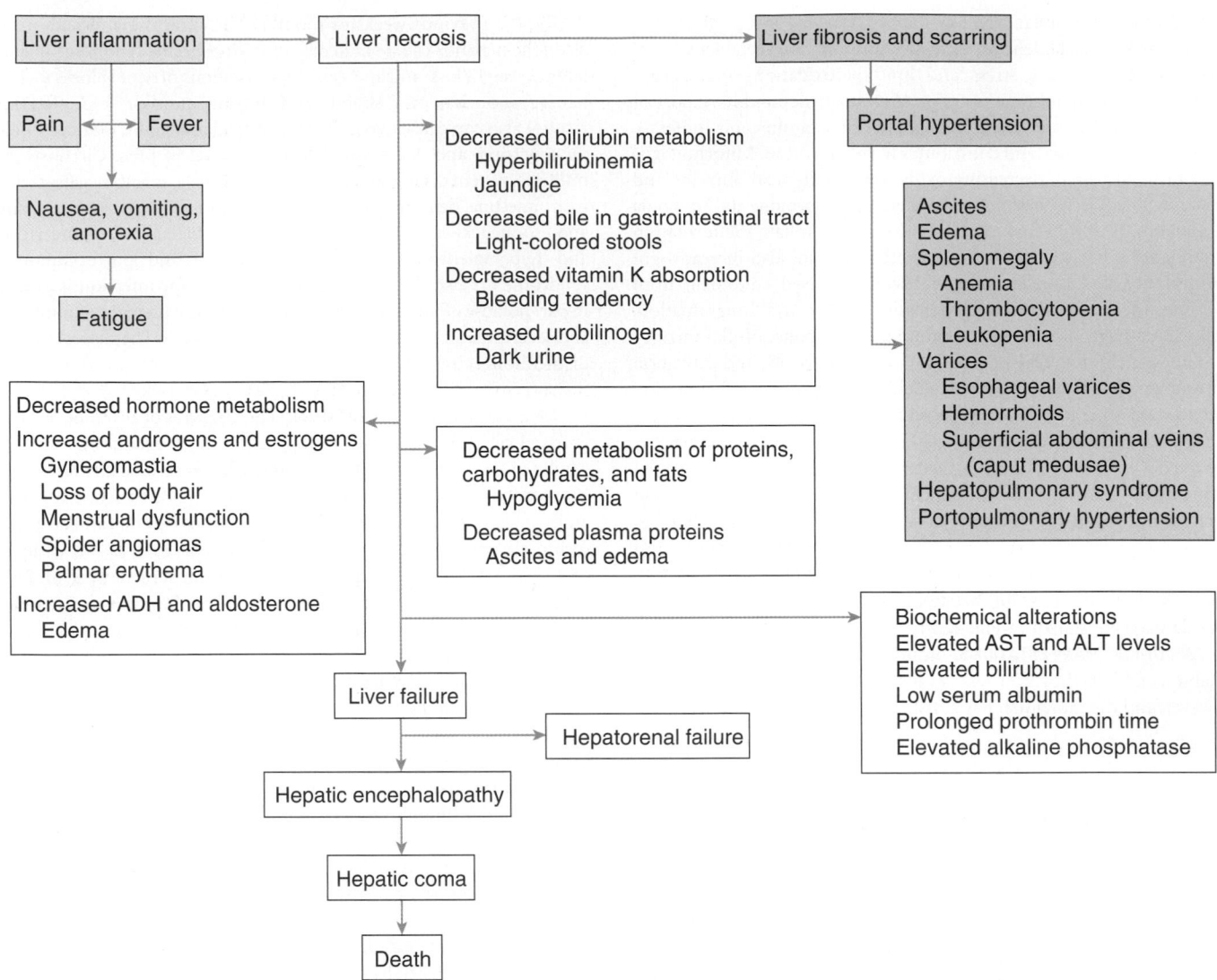

FIGURE 42.22 Clinical Manifestations of Cirrhosis. *ADH,* Antidiuretic hormone; *ALT,* alanine transaminase; *AST,* aspartate transaminase.

destruction of the small intrahepatic bile ducts. The disease is thought to be caused by superimposed environmental antigens (e.g., infectious agents) in genetically susceptible individuals, but the actual trigger of autoimmunity is unknown.[199] Women are affected more commonly (90%) than men. Symptoms rarely develop before the age of 30 years. Primary biliary cirrhosis often accompanies other autoimmune diseases.[200] PBC develops insidiously. Antimitochondrial antibody is the hallmark of the disease, and 30% to 50% of individuals have glycoprotein 210 antinuclear antibodies and anticentromere antibodies.[201] Pathogenesis includes inflammation, destruction, fibrosis, and obstruction of the intrahepatic bile ducts. Nodular regeneration, cirrhosis, and portal hypertension can develop during later stages of the disease.

Diagnosis is based on two of the following three criteria: (1) biochemical evidence of cholestatic liver disease of at least 6 months' duration, (2) antimitochondrial antibody (AMA) positivity, and (3) histologic features of PBC on liver biopsy. Serologic tests show elevated levels of alkaline phosphatase, γ-glutamyl transpeptidase and leucine aminopeptidase, hyperbilirubinemia, and hyperlipidemia with or without other clinical manifestations. Most individuals have a circulating IgG antimitochondrial antibody that is not found in other types of liver disease. Biopsy shows cholangitis and excludes other inflammatory liver

diseases. Evaluation involves ruling out biliary obstruction caused by gallstones, tumor, or inflammation of the common bile duct (i.e., secondary biliary cirrhosis).

Individuals with primary biliary cirrhosis may be asymptomatic or symptomatic at diagnosis and may have minimal disease or rapid progression to cirrhosis and liver failure. The earliest manifestations are pruritus, fatigue, and abdominal pain. Jaundice and light-colored stools are symptoms of advanced disease. These symptoms are caused by intrahepatic obstruction of bile flow. Steatorrhea and fat-soluble vitamin deficiencies are present in some cases. The malabsorption can lead to osteomalacia and osteoporosis. Cirrhosis, symptoms of portal hypertension, encephalopathy, and ultimately liver failure develop in untreated individuals.

Long-term treatment with ursodeoxycholic acid (UDCA) is highly effective. Bezafibrate may be effective for UDCA nonresponders. The distressing pruritus may be relieved by cholestyramine, which binds bile salts in the intestine. Use of rifampin has shown some success. Intramuscular injections of vitamins D and K alleviate the vitamin deficiency. The other symptoms of cirrhosis are managed as they develop. Liver transplant is the only option for those with progressive disease not responding to medical treatment.[202]

Secondary Biliary Cirrhosis. Secondary biliary cirrhosis develops when there is prolonged partial or complete obstruction of the common bile duct or its branches. The obstruction may be caused by gallstones, tumors, fibrotic strictures, or chronic pancreatitis. Biliary atresia and cystic fibrosis cause secondary biliary cirrhosis in children.

Chronic obstruction to bile flow increases pressure in the hepatic bile duct and results in the accumulation of bile in the centrilobular spaces. Necrotic areas develop and are followed by proliferation and inflammation of the portal ducts that result in edema and fibrosis. Pools of bile form when the portal ducts rupture into surrounding necrotic areas. Injury is accompanied by regeneration of hepatic cells with the development of finely nodular cirrhosis.

Clinical manifestations are similar to those of primary biliary cirrhosis, with jaundice and pruritus the most distressing symptoms. Right upper quadrant pain is common, and a low-grade fever may be present from bile duct inflammation (cholangitis).

Cholangiography provides the most definitive diagnosis. Laboratory tests usually show elevated conjugated bilirubin and alkaline phosphatase levels. Aminotransferase level increases if there is an accompanying cholangitis. Surgery or endoscopy relieves obstruction, prolongs survival, and diminishes or resolves symptoms. Continued obstruction leads to advanced cirrhosis and liver failure.

Sclerosing Cholangitis. Primary sclerosing cholangitis (PSC) is a rare, chronic inflammatory fibrotic disease of the hepatic bile ducts that leads to secondary biliary cirrhosis. The disease is immune-mediated, but the exact mechanism is unknown and does not respond to immunosuppressants. PSC is associated with proximal inflammatory bowel disease (75%) and primarily affects genetically susceptible young males. About 30% of cases occur in women. There is no effective sustaining medical or surgical therapy, and liver transplant is required for liver failure.[203] Secondary sclerosing cholangitis is associated with IgG4-related systemic disease, pyrogenic or ischemic cholangitis, eosinophilic cholangitis, or AIDS-related cholangitis.[204]

Disorders of the Gallbladder

Obstruction and inflammation are the most common disorders of the gallbladder. Obstruction is caused by gallstones (cholelithiasis), which are aggregates of substances in the bile. The gallstones may remain in the gallbladder or be ejected, with bile, into the cystic duct. Gallstones that become lodged in the cystic duct obstruct the flow of bile into and out of the gallbladder and cause inflammation. Gallstone formation is termed *cholelithiasis*. Inflammation of the gallbladder or cystic duct is known as *cholecystitis*.

Cholelithiasis (Gallstones)

Cholelithiasis is a prevalent disorder in developed countries, where the incidence is 15% in white adults and 60% to 70% in Native Americans. Risk factors include obesity; rapid weight loss in obese individuals; middle age; female sex; use of oral contraceptives; Native American ancestry; genetic predisposition; gallbladder, pancreatic, or ileal disease; low high density lipoprotein (HDL) cholesterol level and hypertriglyceridemia; and gene-environmental interactions.[205]

PATHOPHYSIOLOGY. Gallstones are formed from impaired metabolism of cholesterol, bilirubin, and bile acids. All gallstones contain cholesterol, unconjugated bilirubin, bilirubin calcium salts, fatty acids, calcium carbonates and phosphates, and mucin glycoproteins. Gallstones are of three types depending on chemical composition: *cholesterol* (70% cholesterol and the most common [70% to 80% of gallstones]); *pigmented* (black [hard] and brown [soft] with less than 30% cholesterol); and *mixed*. *Cholesterol gallstones* form in bile that is supersaturated with cholesterol produced by the liver and deficient in bile acids and phospholipids. Supersaturation sets the stage for cholesterol crystal formation,

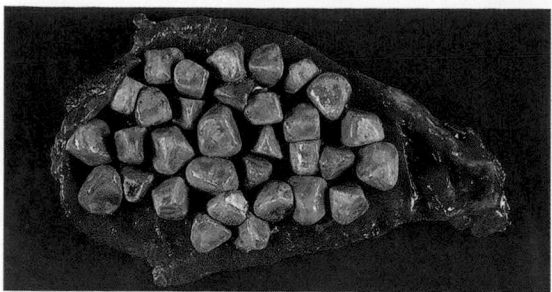

FIGURE 42.23 Resected Gallbladder Containing Mixed Gallstones. (From Kissane JM, editor: *Anderson's pathology*, ed 9, St Louis, 1990, Mosby.)

or the formation of "microstones." More crystals then aggregate on the microstones, which grow to form "macrostones." This process usually occurs in the gallbladder, which may have decreased motility and biliary stasis. The stones may lie dormant and silent or become lodged in the cystic or common duct, causing pain when the gallbladder contracts and cholecystitis. The stones can accumulate and fill the entire gallbladder (Fig. 42.23). *Pigmented brown gallstones* form from calcium bilirubinate and fatty acid soaps that bind with calcium, usually in common bile duct. They are associated with biliary stasis, bacterial infections, and biliary parasites. They are more common in East Asia. *Black gallstones* are rare and usually form in the gallbladder. They are associated with chronic liver disease and hemolytic disease and are composed of calcium bilirubinate with mucin glycoproteins.[206]

It is not known why the hepatocytes secrete bile that is supersaturated with cholesterol. Proposed mechanisms include (1) an enzymatic defect that increases the hepatocytes' synthesis of cholesterol; (2) diminished secretion of bile acids, which normally promote cholesterol solubility; (3) decreased resorption of bile salts from the ileum, which decrease the bile acid pool; (4) gallbladder smooth muscle hypomotility and stasis; (5) increased secretion of gallbladder mucin and biliary calcium; (6) genetic predisposition; and (7) some combination of these mechanisms. In obese individuals, the mechanism appears to involve cholesterol synthesis, whereas in nonobese individuals, it appears to involve decreased secretion of bile acids.[207]

CLINICAL MANIFESTATIONS. Cholelithiasis is often asymptomatic. Epigastric and right hypochondrium pain and intolerance to fatty foods are the cardinal manifestations of cholelithiasis. Vague symptoms include heartburn, flatulence, epigastric discomfort, pruritus, jaundice, and food intolerances, particularly to fats and cabbage. The pain (*biliary colic*) is most characteristic, occurs 30 minutes to several hours after eating a fatty meal, and is caused by the lodging of one or more gallstones in the cystic or common duct with obstruction and distention. It can be intermittent or steady and usually is located in the right upper quadrant and radiates to the mid-upper back. Jaundice indicates that the stone is located in the common bile duct. Abdominal tenderness and fever indicate cholecystitis. Complications can include pancreatitis from obstruction of the pancreatic duct.

EVALUATION AND TREATMENT. Diagnosis is based on the medical history, physical examination, and imaging evaluation. Imaging techniques include transabdominal ultrasound, endoscopic ultrasound, and magnetic resonance cholangiopancreatography.[208,209] Oral bile acids (ursodeoxycholic acid or chenodeoxycholic acid) may dissolve cholesterol stones, but the stones may recur when the drug is discontinued. Laparoscopic cholecystectomy is the preferred treatment for gallstones that cause obstruction or inflammation. Use of transluminal endoscopic surgery is advancing rapidly. Endoscopic retrograde cholangiopancreatography and sphincterotomy with stone retrieval are used for the treatment of bile duct stones. Large stones, or intrahepatic stones, may be managed with open surgery or lithotripsy.[210]

Cholecystitis

Cholecystitis can be acute or chronic. Both forms are almost always caused by the lodging of a gallstone in the cystic duct. Obstruction causes the gallbladder to become distended and inflamed. The pain is similar to that caused by gallstones. Pressure against the distended wall of the gallbladder decreases blood flow and can result in ischemia, necrosis, and perforation of the gallbladder. Fever, leukocytosis, rebound tenderness, and abdominal muscle guarding are common findings. Serum bilirubin and alkaline phosphatase levels may be elevated. Nevertheless, the acute abdominal pain of cholecystitis must be differentiated from the pain caused by other disorders, such as pancreatitis, intestinal vascular insufficiency, and acute pyelonephritis of the right kidney. Cholescintigraphy is the most sensitive imaging for cholecystitis. Ultrasound and magnetic resonance imaging have a substantial margin of error but can demonstrate nonspecific morphologic changes.[211]

Treatment includes pain control, replacement of fluid and electrolytes, and fasting. Antibiotics are often prescribed to manage bacterial infection in severe cases. Acute attacks usually require laparoscopic gallbladder resection (cholecystectomy). Obstruction also may lead to reflux of bile into the pancreatic duct, causing acute pancreatitis.[212,213]

Disorders of the Pancreas

Pancreatitis, or inflammation of the pancreas, is a relatively rare (about 15 cases per 100,000 people in the United States)[214] and potentially serious disorder. Incidence is about equal in men and women, is more common between 50 and 60 years of age, and is more likely to occur in blacks. Risk factors include obstructive biliary tract disease (particularly cholelithiasis), alcoholism, peptic ulcers, abdominal trauma, hyperlipidemia, smoking, certain drugs, and genetic factors (hereditary pancreatitis, cystic fibrosis). The cause is unknown in 15% to 25% of cases. Pancreatitis can be acute or chronic.

Acute Pancreatitis

Acute pancreatitis is usually a mild disease and resolves spontaneously, but about 20% of those with the disease develop a severe acute pancreatitis requiring hospitalization. Pancreatitis develops because of obstruction to the outflow of pancreatic digestive enzymes caused by bile duct or pancreatic duct obstruction (e.g., gallstones). Acute pancreatitis can also result from direct cellular injury from drugs or viral infection.[215]

◆ **PATHOPHYSIOLOGY.** In obstructive disease, the backup of pancreatic secretions or duodenal contents, or both, triggers activation and release of enzymes (activated trypsin activates chymotrypsin, lipase, and elastase) within the pancreatic acinar cells. The activated enzymes cause autodigestion (e.g., proteolysis, lipolysis) of pancreatic cells and tissues, resulting in inflammation and release of inflammatory cytokines. The autodigestion causes vascular damage, coagulative necrosis, fat necrosis (see Chapter 2), and formation of pseudocysts (walled-off collections of pancreatic secretions). Edema within the pancreatic capsule leads to ischemia and can contribute to necrosis. There also may be independent activation of inflammation within acinar cells contributing to the local and systemic responses occurring in acute pancreatitis.[216] In cases of alcohol abuse, the pancreatic acinar cell metabolizes ethanol with the generation of toxic metabolites that injure pancreatic acinar cells, causing release of activated enzymes. Chronic alcohol use also may cause formation of protein plugs in pancreatic ducts and spasm of the sphincter of Oddi, resulting in obstruction. The obstruction leads to intrapancreatic release of activated enzymes, autodigestion, inflammation, and pancreatitis.[217]

Systemic effects are associated with moderately severe and severe acute pancreatitis.[218] Proinflammatory cytokines (e.g., interleukin-6, TNF-α,

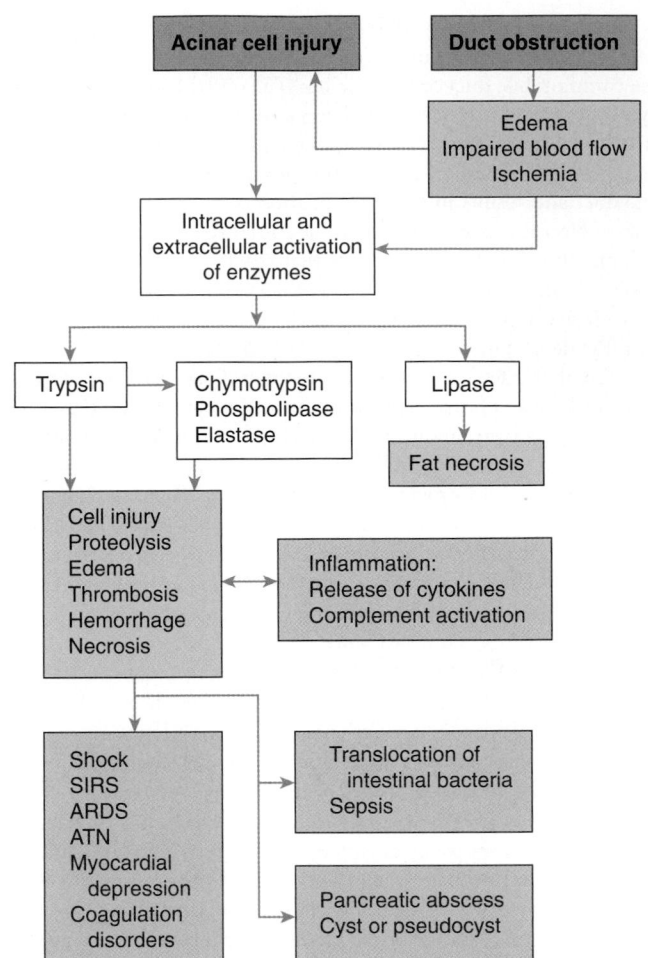

FIGURE 42.24 Pathophysiology of Acute Pancreatitis. *ARDS,* Acute respiratory distress syndrome; *ATN,* acute tubular necrosis; *SIRS,* systemic inflammatory response syndrome.

TGF-β, and platelet-activating factor) and vasoactive peptides are released into the bloodstream. There is activation of leukocytes, injury to vessel walls, and coagulation abnormalities with development of vasodilation, hypotension, and shock. Complications can include acute respiratory distress syndrome (ARDS), heart failure, renal failure, coagulopathies, intraabdominal hypertension, and the systemic inflammatory response syndrome (SIRS) (Chapter 49) (Figs. 42.24 and 42.25). Paralytic ileus and gastrointestinal bleeding can occur. Translocation of intestinal bacteria to the bloodstream causes peritonitis or sepsis. Recurrent inflammation activates pancreatic stellate cells, causing pancreatic fibrosis, strictures, and duct obstruction that lead to chronic pancreatitis.

◆ **CLINICAL MANIFESTATIONS.** The cardinal manifestation of acute pancreatitis is epigastric or midabdominal constant pain ranging from mild abdominal discomfort to severe, incapacitating pain. The pain may radiate to the back because of the retroperitoneal location of the pancreas. Pain is caused by (1) edema, which distends the pancreatic ducts and capsule; (2) chemical irritation and inflammation of the peritoneum; (3) irritation or obstruction of the biliary tract; and (4) inflammation of nerves. Fever and leukocytosis accompany the inflammatory response. Nausea and vomiting are caused by paralytic ileus secondary to the pancreatitis or peritonitis. Jaundice can occur from obstruction of the bile duct (e.g., a gallstone) or from pancreatic edema pressing on the duct. Abdominal distention accompanies bowel hypomotility or paralytic ileus and the accumulation of fluids in the

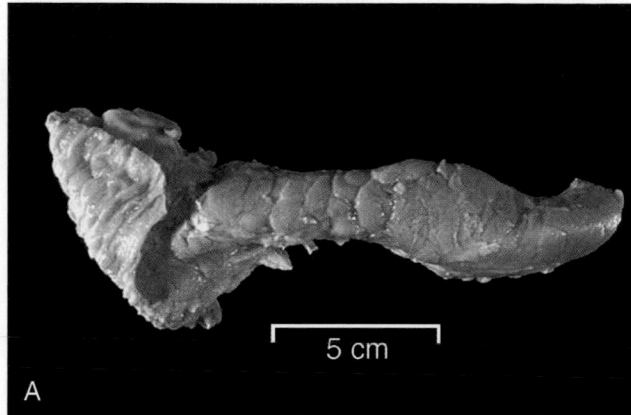
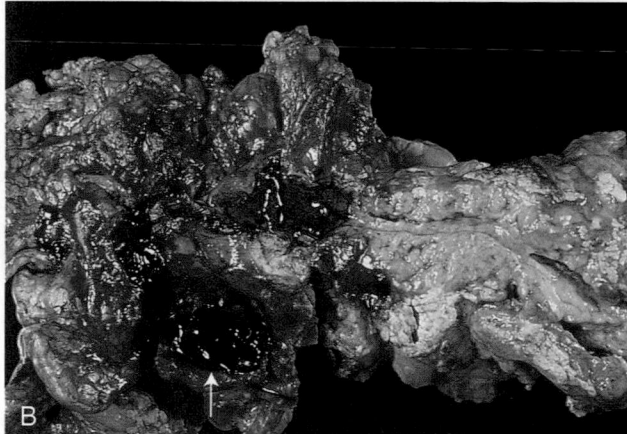

FIGURE 42.25 Acute Severe Pancreatitis with Hemorrhage. **A,** Normal pancreas. **B,** Acute hemorrhagic pancreatitis. The pancreas has hemorrhage, fat necrosis *(white patches),* and a pseudocyst filled with blood *(white arrow).* (**A** from Klatt EC, editor: *Robbins and Cotran atlas of pathology,* Philadelphia, 2006, Saunders. **B** from Damjanov I, Linder J, editors: *Pathology: a color atlas,* St Louis, 2000, Mosby.)

BOX 42.5   **ABDOMINAL COMPARTMENT SYNDROME**

Intraabdominal hypertension (IHA) and abdominal compartment syndrome (ACS) develop when there is abnormally high intraabdominal pressure associated with organ dysfunction. It occurs in 20% to 40% of intensive care unit patients. IHA and ACS are associated with abdominal injury, including trauma, ruptured aortic aneurysm, acute pancreatitis, sepsis, significant thermal injury, liver failure with ascites, massive fluid volume replacement with mechanical ventilation, and pregnancy. Increased intraabdominal pressure increases intrathoracic, intracardiac, and intracranial filling pressures and results in decreased cardiac output, decreased renal perfusion, atelectasis, pulmonary edema, oliguria, compromise of splanchnic and hepatic blood flow, and translocation of bacteria from the gut. The end consequence is multiple organ failure with high mortality.

Normally intraabdominal pressure is slightly greater than atmospheric pressure (5 to 7 mmHg, up to 12 mmHg). Organ dysfunction develops at pressures greater than 20 mmHg that last for more than 6 hours. ACS is difficult to detect from physical diagnosis alone. Automated serial or continuous monitoring of pressure inside the bladder provides a reliable estimate of intraabdominal pressure (greater than 12 mmHg being consistent with IHA and greater than 25 mmHg being consistent with ACS). Gastric monitoring is not always feasible, and inferior vena cava monitoring is more invasive. Treatment is tiered medical management and decompressive laparotomy, which may be performed at the bedside if the individual is too unstable to move. Paracentesis can be therapeutic in properly selected individuals. Elevating the head of the bed 20 degrees to 30 degrees is helpful for some individuals.

Data from Malbrain ML, Peeters Y, Wise R: *Crit Care* 20:67, 2016; Maluso P, Olson J, Sarani B: *Crit Care Clin* 32(2):213-222, 2016; Rogers WK, Garcia L: *Chest* 2017 Aug 2 [Epub ahead of print].

peritoneal and retroperitoneal cavities (ascites). Abdominal compartment syndrome is a potential life-threatening complication. Hypovolemia, hypotension, tachycardia, myocardial insufficiency, and shock occur because plasma volume is lost as inflammatory mediators released into the circulation increase vascular permeability and dilate vessels. Tachypnea and hypoxemia develop secondary to ascites, pulmonary edema, atelectasis, or pleural effusions. Hypovolemia can decrease renal blood flow sufficiently to impair renal function and can cause renal failure. Tetany may develop as a result of hypocalcemia when calcium is deposited in areas of fat necrosis or as a decreased response to parathormone. Transient hyperglycemia also can occur if glucagon is released from damaged alpha cells in the pancreatic islets. In severe acute pancreatitis, some individuals develop flank or periumbilical ecchymosis, a sign of poor prognosis. Multiple organ failure or SIRS accounts for most deaths of those with severe acute pancreatitis.

◆**EVALUATION AND TREATMENT.** Diagnosis is based on clinical findings, identification of associated disorders, laboratory studies, and imaging results (i.e., contrast-enhanced computed tomography, endoscopic ultrasound, or magnetic resonance cholangiopancreatography). Elevated serum amylase concentration is characteristic but is not diagnostic of severity or specificity of disease. Elevated serum lipase level is the primary diagnostic marker for acute pancreatitis. Both enzymes are elevated to at least three times their normal value. An elevated C-reactive protein is suggestive of severe disease.[219]

Acute pancreatitis is difficult to diagnose because several other disorders can cause similar clinical and laboratory findings (e.g., perforating duodenal ulcer, acute cholecystitis, and kidney stones). Intraabdominal pressure monitoring assesses risk for abdominal compartment syndrome[220] (Box 42.5). Scoring systems are available to predict disease severity.[221]

The goal of treatment is to stop the process of autodigestion and prevent systemic complications. Narcotics, nonsteroidal antiinflammatory drugs, and acetaminophen are used to relieve pain. Hemodynamic monitoring and parenteral fluids are essential to restore blood volume and prevent hypotension and shock, particularly in the first 24 hours. Nasogastric suction may not be necessary with mild pancreatitis but may help relieve pain and prevent paralytic ileus in individuals who are nauseated and vomiting. Feeding is usually initiated within 24 to 48 hours if ileus is not present. In severe acute pancreatitis, enteral nutrition with use of jejunal tube feeding is usually well tolerated and may decrease pancreatic enzyme secretion, prevent gut bacterial overgrowth, and maintain gut barrier function. Parenteral hyperalimentation should be initiated only when enteral feeding is not tolerated.[222] Drugs that decrease gastric acid production (e.g., H2 receptor antagonists) can decrease stimulation of the pancreas by secretin. Antibiotics are used if there is infection.[223] Necrotizing pancreatitis requires surgical debridement.[224]

Chronic Pancreatitis

Chronic pancreatitis is a process of progressive fibrotic destruction of the pancreas. Forms of the disease include chronic calcifying (most common), chronic obstructive, and steroid-responsive. Chronic alcohol abuse and smoking (nicotine induces oxidative stress in the pancreatic acinar cells) are the most common cause of chronic calcifying pancreatitis because repeated exacerbations of acute pancreatitis can lead to chronic changes. The disease is idiopathic in about 25% of cases.

Obstructive pancreatitis is associated with fibrosis and stricture from trauma endoscopic procedures, abdominal blunt trauma, gallstones, or tumors. In obstructive pancreatitis only the part of the pancreas distal to the obstruction is involved. Steroid-responsive disease is associated with autoimmune pancreatitis. *Autoimmune chronic pancreatitis* has two subtypes: type 1 (lymphoplasmacytic sclerosing pancreatitis) is a multisystem fibro-inflammatory syndrome known as *immunoglobulin G4- (IgG4-) related disease* that affects pancreatic ducts and veins and presents with painless obstructive jaundice; type 2 (idiopathic duct centric pancreatitis) involves a neutrophilic infiltrate in the pancreatic duct epithelium with duct obliteration and is pancreas specific. Both subtypes respond to corticosteroid therapy and immunomodulators.[225]

Toxic metabolites and chronic release of inflammatory cytokines contribute to the destruction of acinar cells and islets of Langerhans, fibrosis, strictures, calcification, ductal obstruction, ischemia, and pancreatic cysts. Pancreatic cysts can form, which are walled-off areas or pockets of pancreatic juice, necrotic debris, or blood within or adjacent to the pancreas.

Continuous intermittent abdominal pain is the classic symptom of all forms of chronic pancreatitis with the exception of type 1, steroid-sensitive pancreatitis. Pain is associated with increased intraductal pressure, increased tissue pressure, ischemia, neuritis, ongoing injury, and changes in central pain perception. Weight loss and, less commonly, steatorrhea, malnutrition, fat-soluble vitamin deficiency, and diabetes mellitus (known as *type 3C* to differentiate it from type 1 and type 2 diabetes mellitus) accompany disease progression. Treatment includes oral lipase and insulin. Preventing disease progression includes lifestyle modification to stop alcohol use and smoking. Pain management is complex, with use of analgesics, endoscopic therapy, nerve block, and surgical drainage of cysts or partial resection of the pancreas.[226] Chronic pancreatitis is a risk factor for pancreatic cancer.

CANCER OF THE DIGESTIVE SYSTEM

Table 42.8 contains information on the various gastrointestinal cancers by organ, percentage of death compared to all cancer deaths, risk factors, type of cell, and common manifestations. The biology of cancer is presented in Chapter 12.

Cancer of the Gastrointestinal Tract
Cancer of the Esophagus

Carcinoma of the esophagus is a rare disease with an estimated incidence of 16,940 new cases (13,360 males, 3580 females) and 15,690 deaths in 2017 in the United States.[227] Squamous cell carcinoma is more prevalent in China, Iran, South America, and South Africa, and in black men who use alcohol and smoke tobacco in the United States.[228] Squamous cell carcinoma is associated with smoking, chewing tobacco, or betel quid; alcohol, both intrinsic and extrinsic sources of the alcohol metabolite acetaldehyde; irritant drinks; food containing nitrosamines; achalasia; male sex; and older age. Squamous cell carcinomas are more common in the thoracic and cervical areas of the esophagus. Adenocarcinoma

	PERCENTAGE OF DEATHS			COMMON
ORGAN	**OF ALL CANCERS**	**RISKS**	**COMMON CELL TYPES**	**MANIFESTATIONS**
Esophagus	2.6	Malnutrition Alcohol Tobacco Chronic reflux	Squamous cell Adenocarcinoma	Chest pain Dysphagia
Stomach	1.8	Salty food Nitrates and nitrosamines Gastric atrophy	Adenocarcinoma Squamous cell	Anorexia Malaise Weight loss Upper abdominal pain Vomiting Occult blood
Colorectal	8.25	Polyps Ulcerative colitis Diverticulitis High–refined-carbohydrate, low-fiber, high-fat diet	Adenocarcinoma (left colon grows in ring; right colon grows as mass)	Pain Mass Anemia Bloody stool Obstruction Distention
Liver	4	Hepatitis B, C, and D viruses Cirrhosis Intestinal parasite Aflatoxin from moldy peanuts	Hepatomas Cholangiomas	Pain Anorexia Bloating Weight loss Portal hypertension Ascites, ± jaundice
Pancreas	7	Chronic pancreatitis Cigarette smoking Alcohol (?) Diabetic women	Adenocarcinoma (exocrine part of gland, ductal epithelium)	

TABLE 42.8   CANCER OF THE GUT, LIVER, AND PANCREAS

Data from American Cancer Society (ACS): *Cancer facts and figures, 2017,* Atlanta, 2016, American Cancer Society.

is more common in Western countries, accounts for about 58% of esophageal carcinoma cases in the United States, and is increasing. Adenocarcinoma is found in the distal one-third of the esophagus and is associated with risk factors that include reflux esophagitis, Barrett esophagus, abdominal obesity, drugs that decrease lower esophageal pressure, sliding hiatal hernia, and smoking. The *CagA*-positive strain of *H. pylori*, nonsteroidal antiinflammatory drugs, and statins may be a protection against esophageal adenocarcinoma.

◆**PATHOGENESIS.** The pathogenesis of esophageal adenocarcinoma is facilitated by chronic inflammation, intestinal metaplasia, and dysplasia (**Barrett esophagus** [columnar rather than squamous epithelium in the lower esophagus]) caused by gastroesophageal reflux. Long-term exposure to environmental irritants causes neoplastic transformation for both adenocarcinoma and squamous cell carcinoma (basal and squamous cell hyperplasia). Both genomic and epigenomic events are associated with esophageal cancers, and mutation of the *TP53* gene is an early event. Squamous cell carcinoma progresses from low-grade to high-grade intraepithelial neoplasia and, ultimately, to invasive carcinoma.[229]

◆**CLINICAL MANIFESTATIONS.** Early stages of esophageal carcinoma are asymptomatic. The two frequent symptoms of esophageal carcinoma are chest pain and dysphagia. The most common type of pain is heartburn (pyrosis). It is initiated by eating spicy or highly seasoned foods and assuming the recumbent position. Some individuals with esophageal cancer complain of a constant retrosternal pain that radiates to the back. Dysphagia (pain on swallowing), another common symptom, is usually pressure-like and may radiate posteriorly between the scapulae. Dysphagia usually progresses rapidly. Esophageal cancer metastasizes rapidly and, therefore, has a poor prognosis.

◆**EVALUATION AND TREATMENT.** Individuals who present with dysphagia undergo endoscopy so that specimens can be examined for neoplastic change and type of carcinoma. Endoscopic ultrasound and CT studies of the thorax are used for diagnosis and staging. Treatment of gastroesophageal reflux is essential for the prevention of Barrett esophagus. Esophageal carcinoma is treated with endoscopic radiofrequency mucosal ablation, cryotherapy, radiotherapy, resection, or combination therapy.[230]

Untreated esophageal cancer metastasizes rapidly and has a poor prognosis. At the time of diagnosis, 50% of esophageal cancers present with metastatic disease. The lymphatic vessels of the esophagus are continuous with vital mediastinal structures (trachea, heart, and great vessels) and drain to the celiac lymph nodes, making it impossible to remove all the lymph nodes with the tumor. Removal of the primary lesion and the local lymph nodes, however, can benefit the individual with esophageal cancer, and cure is likely if there is no metastasis.

Cancer of the Stomach

The incidence of gastric adenocarcinoma is estimated at 28,000 new cases (17,750 men and 10,250 women) and 10,960 deaths in the United States in 2017.[227] Most cases are adenocarcinoma. Squamous cell carcinoma is very rare and accounts for only 0.04% to 0.07% of all gastric carcinomas.[231] In countries such as Eastern Asia, Eastern Europe, and South America, the incidence of stomach cancer has remained consistently high.[232] Nonenvironmental risk factors include a family history of gastric adenocarcinoma; blood type (blood group A); type A atrophic gastritis; pernicious anemia, which is associated with atrophy of the gastric mucosa in the same locations where gastric tumors arise; and Epstein-Barr virus- (EBV-) associated gastric carcinoma in some individuals; however, the mechanism is unknown.[233,234]

The most important environmental risk factors in causing gastric cancer are:

1. Infection with *H. pylori* that carry selected virulence factors (i.e., *CagA* gene product cytotoxin-associated antigen A [80% of cases])

in genetically susceptible individuals. Only about 1% of individuals infected with *H. pylori* develop gastric cancer.[235,236] Infection with *H. pylori* and severe chronic gastritis change the mucosal cell proliferation pattern, destroy cell junctions, inhibit cell proliferation, and promote cell invasive ability, increasing the risk for gastric and duodenal carcinoma.[237-239] *H. pylori* also is causatively linked to **mucosa-associated lymphoid tissue (MALT) lymphoma** (a low-grade B-cell lymphoma) that can originate in the stomach.

2. Dietary factors, such as salt added to food, food additives (e.g., nitrates) in pickled or salted foods (e.g., bacon), and low intake of fruits and vegetables. Dietary salt enhances the conversion of nitrates to carcinogenic nitrosamines in the stomach. Salt is also caustic to the stomach and can cause chronic atrophic gastritis. Hypertonic salt solutions delay gastric emptying. Delayed emptying increases the time during which carcinogenic nitrosamines can exert their effects on the stomach mucosa. Nitrates interact with amino acids in the stomach to form nitrosamines. The conversion of these carcinogenic nitrosamines is enhanced at a low pH by iodides and thiocyanates. Nitrates are thought to be active only when converted to nitrites and to cause stomach cancer once atrophic gastritis has occurred.

3. Lifestyle factors, such as alcohol consumption and cigarette smoking. Alcohol is metabolized to the carcinogen acetaldehyde and decreases the production of prostaglandins that maintain gastric mucosal integrity. Smokers have a higher incidence of *H. pylori* infection.[240]

◆**PATHOGENESIS.** Environmental factors and genetic predisposition combine to cause injury, inflammation, and the progression to gastric adenocarcinoma. Epigenetic alterations (DNA methylation, histone methylation, and histone acetylation) and multiple genes are involved in gastric cancer, including oncogenes, tumor-suppressor genes, DNA repair genes, and cell cycle regulator genes. Genetics also can distinguish well-differentiated (intestinal) from undifferentiated (diffuse) gastric adenocarcinomas. About 1% to 3% of gastric cancers are familial.[241,242] Gastric adenocarcinoma usually begins in the glands of the stomach mucosa, commonly in the prepyloric antrum (Fig. 42.26). Atrophic gastritis progresses to intestinal metaplasia, dysplasia, and adenocarcinoma.

◆**CLINICAL MANIFESTATIONS.** The early stages of gastric cancer are generally asymptomatic or produce vague symptoms such as loss of appetite (especially for meat), malaise, and indigestion. Later manifestations include unexplained weight loss, upper abdominal pain, vomiting,

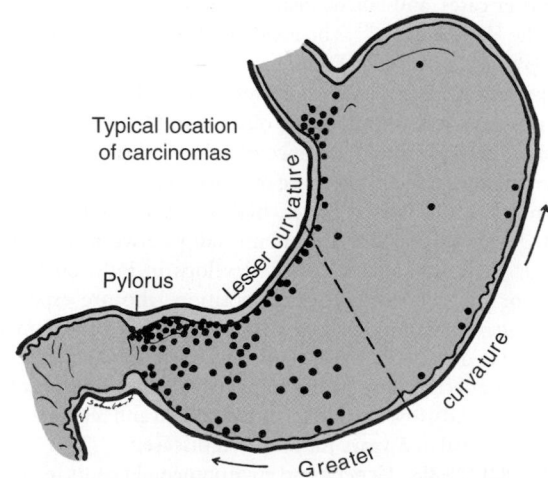

FIGURE 42.26 Typical Sites of Stomach Cancer. (From del Regato JA, Spjut HJ, Cox JD: *Cancer: diagnosis, treatment, and prognosis*, ed 2, St Louis, 1985, Mosby.)

change in bowel habits, and anemia caused by persistent occult bleeding. The prognosis is poor because symptoms usually do not occur until the tumor has penetrated the muscle layers of the stomach, spread to surrounding tissues, and entered the draining lymph nodes and veins, causing distant metastases. Generally the first manifestations of carcinoma are caused by distant metastases when the disease is already in an advanced stage.

◆**EVALUATION AND TREATMENT.** There are no specific biomarkers for gastric cancer. Micro RNAs, circulating tumor cells, and exhaled breath analysis are being evaluated as specific diagnostic and prognostic markers.[243] Most symptoms suggest a problem in the upper gastrointestinal tract, and a barium x-ray film shows the lesion. Direct endoscopic visualization and biopsy usually establish the diagnosis, or microscopic examination of exfoliated cells obtained by lavage during endoscopy.[244]

Screening and eradication of *H. pylori* infection are the best preventive approaches to gastric cancer. Vaccines to prevent *H. pylori* infection are under investigation and could eliminate a worldwide cause of gastric cancer death.[245] Surgery is the only curative treatment for early stages of disease. Staging is determined by pathologic findings after resection. Early diagnosis and chemotherapy combined with radiation improve postsurgical outcomes. Targeted therapy is being evaluated for molecular subtypes of gastric cancer. Abstinence from alcohol and smoking improves outcomes. Dietary modifications include high intake of fruits and vegetables, vitamin C, carotenoids, and fiber and reduced intake of salt, salted food, and red meat.[246]

Cancer of the Small Intestine

Small intestine carcinoma is rare and represents less than 3% of gastrointestinal cancers (10,190 estimated new cases and 1390 deaths in 2017).[227] Adenocarcinoma is the most common tumor type, followed by carcinoid tumors (neuroendocrine serotonin-producing tumors), sarcomas, and lymphomas. Carcinoma occurs more frequently in familial adenomatous polyposis and Crohn disease. Symptoms are nonspecific. Screening includes imaging and endoscopic surveillance. Urinary evaluation of 5-hydroxyindoloacetic acid can assist with diagnosis of carcinoid tumors. Treatment is surgical resection followed by tumor types specific treatment.[113,247]

Cancer of the Colon and Rectum

Colorectal cancer (CRC) is the third most common cause of cancer and cancer death with an estimated 95,520 new colon and 39,910 new rectal cancer cases, and 50,260 deaths (colon and rectal combined) in 2017 in the United States.[227] The incidence has been declining over the past several years because of successful screening programs, removal of polyps, and increased use of nonsteroidal antiinflammatory drugs. CRC tends to occur in individuals older than 50 years and is rare in children. Worldwide, the prevalence of colorectal cancer is highest in black populations, possibly because of a lack of access to screening and treatment.[248] In the United States, higher socioeconomic status was associated with lower incidence and mortality between 1998 and 2010 in a large Medicare cohort.[249] CRC develops in individuals with an acquired or inherited genetic predisposition who are exposed to a combination of environmental risk factors (Box 42.6). Lifestyle modifications related to diet, alcohol and tobacco use, exercise, and weight control are the most effective approaches to primary prevention of colorectal cancer. The 5- and 10-year survival rates are 65% and 58%, respectively, with 90% survival at 5 years for localized disease.[250]

◆**PATHOGENESIS.** Genetic and environmental factors (epigenetics) are associated with the development of CRC. CRC can develop through molecular pathways, gene mutations, and genomic instability (the cell cycle loses control of the gene mutation rate). Gene mutations may be

---

BOX 42.6 SELECTED RISK FACTORS AND COLORECTAL CANCER

Hereditary and Medical Factors
Family history of colorectal cancer
Familial adenomatous polyposis
Hereditary nonpolyposis colorectal cancer
Inflammatory bowel disease after 10 years
Type 2 diabetes mellitus

Modifiable Risk Factors
Smoking or chewing tobacco
Obesity
Physical inactivity
Moderate to heavy alcohol consumption
High consumption of processed meat
Red meat consumption (large variations among studies)
High-fat, low-fiber diet

Lower Risk
Diets high in cereal grains, vegetables, milk; fish; folic acid, calcium, and
     vitamin D; magnesium and selenium; and low in fat
Postmenopausal estrogen use
Physical activity
Use of NSAIDs

Other studies: Alexander DD, et al: *J Am Coll Nutr* 34(6):521-543, 2015; Le NT, et al: *Environ Health Perspect* 124(10):1529-1536, 2016. Data from American Cancer Society (ACS): *Cancer facts & figures 2017*, Atlanta, 2017, American Cancer Society. Available at: https://www.cancer.org/research/cancer-facts-statistics/all-cancer-facts-figures/cancer-facts-figures-2017.html.

---

inherited or acquired after birth (somatic mutations). Family history of CRC occurs in about 25% of cases, but only 5% to 6% of the 25% with a family history are related to highly penetrating gene mutations, mostly autosomal dominant. Familial adenomatous polyposis (FAP, 100% risk of developing CRC) and hereditary nonpolyposis colorectal cancer (HNPCC or Lynch syndrome, 40% risk of developing CRC) are examples of these types of cancers. The remainder of inherited CRCs are related to less penetrant genes, and environmental interactions increase risk. Most CRC is sporadic (nonhereditary or acquired), and the environment contributes to multiple somatic mutations. Chronic inflammatory bowel disease increases risk of CRC after 10 to 15 years of disease. Understanding the molecular events associated with CRC is allowing more targeted detection, diagnosis, and prognosis prediction, and more specific and personalized treatment approaches.[251] Most colorectal cancers arise from adenomatous polyps (Fig. 42.27), with the exception of HNPCC, which arises from apparently normal intestinal epithelial tissue. Other cancers are rare and include carcinoid (neuroendocrine) tumors, gastrointestinal stromal tumors, and lymphomas.

A polyp is a mass or finger-like projection arising from the intestinal mucosal epithelium. Most polyps are benign (nonneoplastic) and composed of normal glandular and stromal cells. Grossly, they are described as pedunculated or tubular (with a stalk) or sessile (flat, without a stalk) (Fig. 42.28). Neoplastic or cancerous polyps have progressed into adenocarcinomas. Histologically, they have different growth patterns and are classified as *tubular adenomas* with a stalk projecting from the intestinal wall (the most prevalent); *villous adenomas* with finger-like projections of the epithelium without stalks and tending to larger than 1 cm (more related to CRC); or *tubulovillous adenomas* with characteristics of both tubular and villous adenomas. *Serrated*

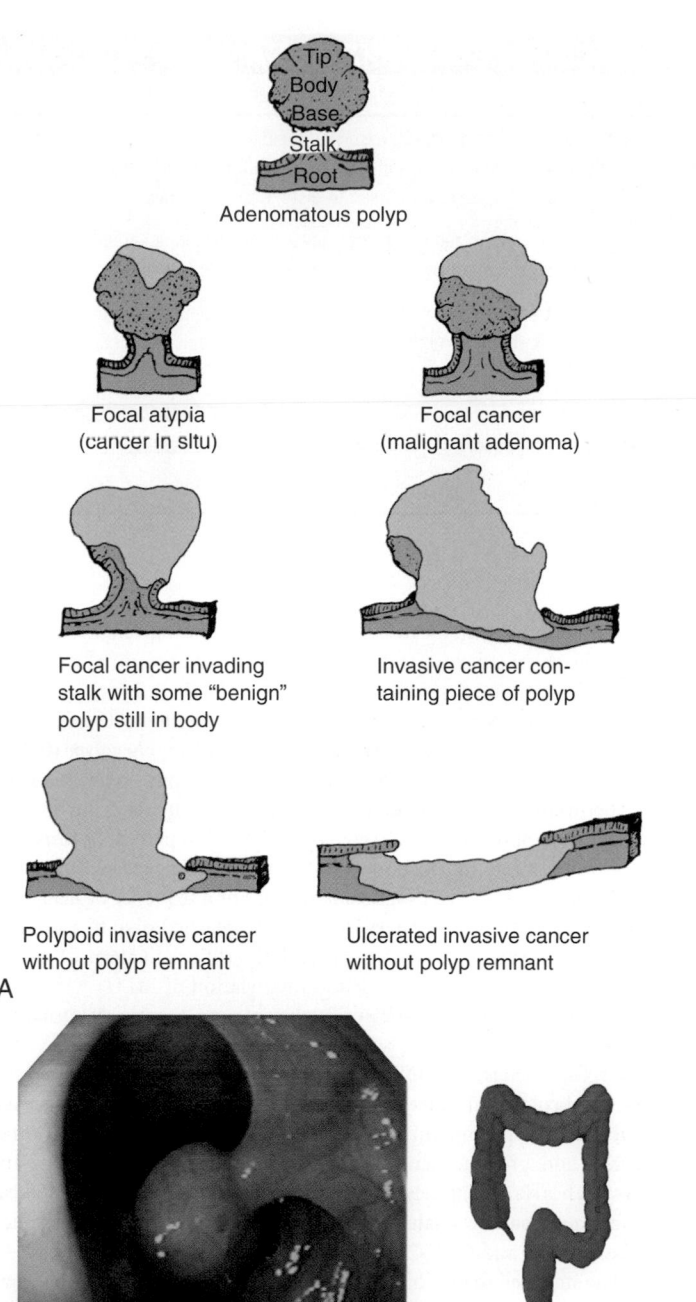

FIGURE 42.27 Development of Cancer of the Colon from Adenomatous Polyps. A, The tumor becomes invasive if it penetrates the muscularis mucosae and enters the submucosal layer. **B,** Endoscopic image of pedunculated polyp in descending colon. (**A** from del Regato JA, Spjut HJ, Cox JD: *Cancer: diagnosis, treatment, and prognosis,* ed 2, St Louis, 1985, Mosby. **B** courtesy David Bjorkman, MD, Department of Gastroenterology, University of Utah School of Medicine, Salt Lake City, UT.)

polyps are more rare, have a serrated (sawtooth appearance) of the crypt epithelium, and are larger and difficult to remove endoscopically. When polyps are larger than 2 cm, more numerous (greater than 20), and have a villous architecture, they have the most malignant potential. The adenomatous polyp forms in an area of epithelial cell hyperproliferation and crypt dysplasia. Once the adenoma traverses the muscularis mucosae,

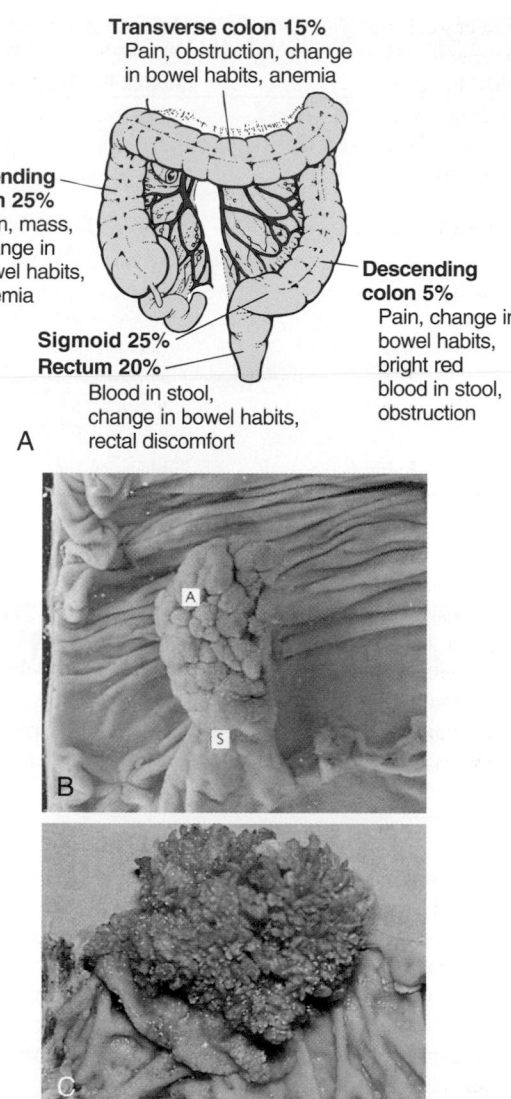

FIGURE 42.28 Signs and Symptoms of Colorectal Cancer by Location of Primary Lesion. A, Clinical manifestations are listed in order of frequency for each region (lymphatics of colon also shown). **B,** Tubular adenomas *(A)* are rounded lesions 0.5 to 2 cm in size that are generally red and sit on a stalk *(S)* of normal mucosa that has been dragged up by traction of the polyp in the bowel lumen. **C,** Villous adenomas are sessile (frondlike) lesions about 0.6 cm thick that occupy a broad area of mucosa generally 1 to 5 cm in diameter. (**B** and **C** from Stevens A, Lowe JS, Scott I: *Core pathology,* ed 3, London, 2009, Mosby.)

it becomes invasive and highly malignant. Adenomas can be detected early, however, and the submucosa may not be penetrated for several years. Thus screening colonoscopy with polypectomy is important when polyps are found. Table 42.9 gives other conditions commonly confused with colorectal cancer.

Progression from polyps to colon cancer involves a multistep cascade of genetic mutations that occur over 10 to 15 years (Box 42.7). Gene mutations include

1. loss of tumor-suppressor gene activity (genes that inhibit cell growth, e.g., *APC, TP53, SMAD4,* and *DCC*);
2. activation of proto-oncogenes (promote cell growth; e.g., *KRAS* [retrovirus-associated DNA sequence] and *BRAF*); and
3. abnormalities in DNA mismatch repair (MMR) genes (genes that fix errors in DNA replication and recombination, e.g., *TGF, EGFR, hMSH1, hMSH2,* and *hMSH6*).

TABLE 42.9   CONDITIONS COMMONLY CONFUSED WITH COLORECTAL CANCER

CONDITION	SIGNIFICANT CHARACTERISTICS
Diverticulitis	Left-sided pain similar to that of appendicitis; tender lower left quadrant; associated findings: nausea, vomiting, fever, obstruction, anorexia, and leukocytosis; mucosa is intact, and perforation, peritonitis, and abscesses occur more often than in cancer; ultrasound, CT scan, MRI, and proctosigmoidoscopy are used to distinguish from cancer
Ulcerative colitis	Younger people with chronic attacks of bloody diarrhea, crampy abdominal pain, fever, malnutrition, and dehydration; usually involves the left colon and rectum; endoscopy, barium enema, and biopsy performed for definitive diagnosis
Crohn disease (granulomatous colitis)	Generally involves the right colon; chronic diarrhea with abdominal cramps, fever, weight loss, and often a palpable abdominal mass; difficult at times to distinguish Crohn disease from ulcerative colitis; endoscopic examination and CT scan used to distinguish from cancer
Appendicitis	Vague abdominal symptoms, often with a tender or nontender mass in the lower right quadrant; associated symptoms: mild fever and leukocytosis; CT scan used to distinguish cancer of the cecum from appendiceal abscess
Thrombosed hemorrhoids	Examination shows a tender, swollen, bluish painful mass in the anus; individual has a history of hemorrhoids

CT, Computed tomography; *MRI,* magnetic resonance imaging.

BOX 42.7   COMMON GENES ASSOCIATED WITH COLORECTAL CANCER

APC (adenomatous polyposis coli): tumor suppressor; suppresses cell growth

TP53 (tumor protein 53): prevents gene mutations; a tumor suppressor gene

KRAS (V-Ki-ras2 Kirsten rat sarcoma viral oncogene homolog, proto-oncogene): promotes cell proliferation

BRAF (B-Raf proto-oncogene serine/threonine kinase): promotes cell proliferation

DCC (deleted in colon cancer): located at chromosome *18q*; tumor suppressor and apoptosis regulation

SMAD4 (Mothers against decapentaplegic homolog 4, proto-oncogene): promotes cell growth through TGF-β

TGF-β (transforming growth factor-beta): activates signaling pathways that facilitate tumor growth

EGFR (epidermal growth factor receptor): activates signaling pathways that facilitate tumor growth

COX-2 (cyclooxygenase-2): promotes cell growth and inflammation.

BAX: promotes apoptosis and normal cell life cycle

DNA: (mismatch repair genes [HNPCC/Lynch syndrome and some sporadic colorectal cancers]:
    hMLH1 (human mutator homolog 1)
    hMSH2 (human mutator S protein homolog 2)
    hMSH6 (human mutator S homolog 6)
    PMS2 (postmeiotic segregation increased 2)

LOH (loss of heterozygosity): loss of entire genome and surrounding chromosomal region

CRC is genetically unique for each individual; three molecular pathways of genomic instability have been recognized and can overlap in tumor development:

1. *Chromosomal instability* (CIN), or the tumor-suppressor pathway (adenoma-to-carcinoma sequence), is initiated by mutations in *APC/Wnt-β-catenin,* K-RAS, DCC, and tp53 and includes sporadic (50% to 70%) and the autosomal dominant inherited syndrome known as *familial adenomatous polyposis (FAP)* coli (100%). Tumors associated with CIN are primarily located on the left (descending) side in the distal colon.[252]

2. *Microsatellite instability* (MSI) pathway (15% of all CRCs) is associated with epigenetic methylation of DNA MMR genes and *APC* mutations.

These tumors are located in the right (ascending) colon proximal to the splenic flexure and are associated with autosomal dominant hereditary nonpolyposis colorectal cancer (HNPCC/Lynch syndrome [70%]) and sporadic epigenetic alterations (10% to 15%) of CRCs.[253]

3. *CpG (cytosine-phosphate-guanine) island methylator phenotype* (CIMP) pathway (about 15% to 20% of all CRCs) involves epigenetic DNA methylation of promoter CpG islands silencing genes involved in tumor suppression, cell cycle control, DNA repair, apoptosis, and invasion. It is found in about 30% to 40% of CRCs. Serrated adenomas are associated with a progression of steps or a sequence of malignant transformation that moves from a hyperplastic polyp to a serrated polyp to adenocarcinoma, particularly with activation of proto-oncogenes *KRAS* and *BRAF* and methylation of MLH1.[254,255]

Fig. 42.29 provides a summary of common genetic events in the development of CRC.

Cyclooxygenase-2 (COX-2) is variably expressed in right-sided and left-sided colorectal cancer. Platelets are activated with tissue damage, which induces proinflammatory mediators and activates expression of COX-2 and pro-oncogenic prostaglandin E2.[256] Use of aspirin and NSAIDs has shown efficacy in the prevention and treatment of colorectal cancer and may be related to suppression of platelet activation and inflammation and COX-2.[257]

The stem cell theory of CRC proposes that genetic mutations begin in crypt stem cells with strong oncogenicity. However, cells outside the stem cell zone can be cells of origin, so it is possible that other cells have the plasticity to revert to stemlike cells and acquire genetic mutations that initiate neoplasia.[258,259] The tumor microenvironment also influences the way mutations develop and progress in CRC. Factors include gut dysbiosis, chronic inflammation, and the cellular composition of the extracellular matrix, including fibroblasts and immune cells. Thus pathogenesis of CRC is promoted by the accumulation of genetic mutations within the context of tumor-promoting factors derived from adjacent tissue.[260]

Colorectal adenocarcinomas have a long preinvasive phase, and when they invade they tend to grow slowly over 10 to 15 years, with the exception of HNPCC/Lynch syndrome, which can progress more rapidly within 3 to 5 years. Because the lymphatic channels are located underneath the muscularis mucosae, the lesions must traverse this layer before metastasis can occur. Systemic lymphatic spread occurs along the aorta to the mesenteric and pancreatic lymph nodes. Liver metastasis follows invasion from the inferior mesenteric vein (left colon) or superior mesenteric vein (right colon), which drain into the portal circulation.

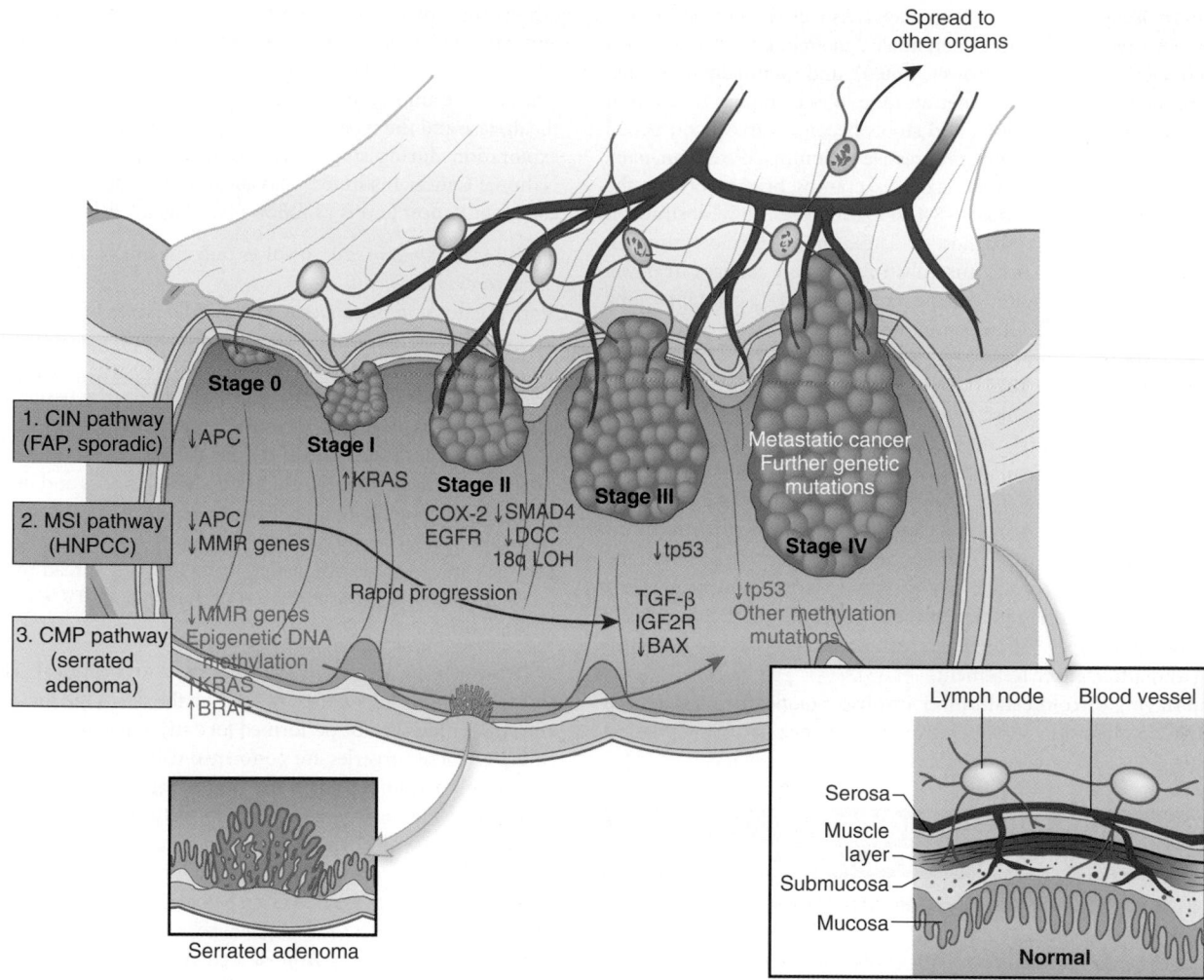

FIGURE 42.29 Multistage Development of Colonic Cancer. Colorectal carcinoma develops from the sequential progression of genetic abnormalities in different pathways. These pathways overlap in many tumors. **1,** Most colonic cancers arises in the chromosomal instability (CIN) pathway with imbalances in chromosomal numbers (aneuploidy) and loss of heterozygosity. Abnormalities in oncogenes and tumor-suppressor genes activate the pathways for CRC initiation and progression. Mutations in the *APC* gene are the earliest known event and inactivation of *APC* accelerates cell cycle progression. *K-ras* (proto-oncogene) overexpression leads to loss of other tumor-suppressor genes SMAD4, DCC, and *tp53* and transforms an adenoma into a metastatic carcinoma. *tp53* loss occurs in about 35% to 45% of colorectal carcinomas, and occurs less frequently in benign lesions. Growth factors COX-2 and EGFR promote tumor growth and angiogenesis in response to inflammatory cytokines and proto-oncogenes. **2,** The microsatellite instability *(MSI)* pathway involves the epigenetic mutation of DNA mismatch repair genes *(MMR)* that encode key molecules that repair DNA, resulting in replication errors and deactivation of proteins from other downstream mutations (*TGF-β, IGF2R, BAX*). **3,** The epigenetic pathway, CpG island methylator phenotype *(CIMP)*, involves early hypermethylation of DNA with gene silencing of *MMR* genes (i.e., *MLH1, MSH2, MSH6*). Proto-oncogenes *KRAS* and *BRAF* also are involved in this pathway. This pathway also can transform into the MSI pathway. **NOTE:** definitions for all abbreviations are listed in Box 42.7. (Adapted from National Institutes of Health: Advances in colorectal cancer research. Available at: https://www.nih.gov/research-training/advances-colorectal-cancer-research.)

Rectal carcinomas are defined as tumors occurring up to 15 cm from the anal opening. Most are adenocarcinomas and more rarely squamous cell or neuroendocrine tumors, sarcomas, and lymphomas. Tumors of the rectum can spread through the rectal wall to nearby structures: the prostate in men and the vagina in women. Penetration occurs more readily in the lower third of the rectum because it has no serosal covering. Systemic and pulmonary metastases occur through the hemorrhoidal plexus, which drains into the vena cava.[261]

◆**CLINICAL MANIFESTATIONS.** Polyps and early stage tumors usually do not have symptoms, making screening important for early detection.

Symptoms of colorectal cancer depend on the location, size, shape, and metastasis of the lesion. Tumors of the right and left colon evolve into two distinct types. On the right side the lesions are polypoid and extend along one wall of the cecum and ascending colon. These tumors may be silent, evolving to pain, with a palpable mass in the lower right quadrant, fatigue, dark red or mahogany-colored blood mixed with the stool, and anemia (see Fig. 42.28). These tumors can become large and bulky with necrosis and ulceration, contributing to persistent blood loss and anemia. Obstruction is unusual because the growth does not encircle the colon. These tumors are more common in women.[262]

Tumors of the left, or descending, colon are small, elevated, button-like masses. This type grows circumferentially, encircling the entire bowel wall (the left colon has a narrower lumen), and eventually ulcerating in the middle as the tumor penetrates the blood supply. Obstruction is common but occurs slowly, and stools become narrow and pencil shaped. Manifestations include progressive abdominal distention, pain, vomiting, constipation, need for laxatives, cramps, bright blood on the surface of the stool, and anemia. In 8% to 29% of cases, bowel obstruction is the primary symptom at diagnosis.[263] These tumors are more common in men. Rectal tumors also cause obstruction and changes in bowel habits, including constipation, diarrhea, and tenesmus (a constant feeling of needing to pass stool). Other symptoms can develop related to distant organ metastasis.

◆**EVALUATION AND TREATMENT.** Individuals with hereditary polyposis or a strong family history of CRC should begin screening at an early age (10 to 12 years) using colonoscopy and removal of polyps when they are found. Screening procedures for detection of nonhereditary CRC are summarized in Box 42.8. Specific, sensitive, and affordable molecular markers are being evaluated to assist with early diagnosis and evaluation of therapy. Chromoendoscopy (spraying dye onto the surface of the colon to make polyps more visible) and magnifying endoscopy help to differentiate between neoplastic and nonneoplastic colonic polyp subtypes.[264] Carcinoembryonic antigen (CEA) is evaluated during and after cancer treatment.

The staging of colorectal cancer involves preoperative testing and operative exploration. Preoperative testing begins with physical examination of the abdomen to detect liver enlargement and ascites and palpation of appropriate lymph nodes. Elevations in the level of CEA are often detected in the sera of individuals with colorectal carcinoma. The amount of CEA in the serum is a function of the stage of the disease and the type of tumor. Operative staging consists of careful exploration during surgery and biopsy of possible metastases. The National Cancer Institute[265] classification is widely used for staging of colorectal cancer and is as follows (see Fig. 42.29):

Stage 0 (carcinoma in situ): involves only the mucosal lining; also known as *carcinoma in situ*

Stage I: extension of cancer to the middle layers of the colon wall, no spread to lymph nodes; stage I colon cancer is sometimes called *Dukes A colon cancer*

Stage II: extension beyond the colon wall to nearby tissues around the colon or *rectum,* and/or through the *peritoneum*; stage II colon cancer is sometimes called *Dukes B colon cancer*

Stage III: spread beyond the colon into lymph nodes and nearby organs and/or through the *peritoneum*; stage III colon cancer is sometimes called *Dukes C colon cancer*

Stage IV: spread to nearby *lymph nodes* and has spread to other parts of the body, such as the *liver* or *lungs*; stage IV colon cancer is sometimes called *Dukes D colon cancer*

Treatment for cancer of the colon is always surgical. The location and amount of colon resected depend on the site of the cancer. Resection and anastomosis can be performed for early-stage tumors and is usually curative. These surgeries are performed using laparoscopic techniques or through abdominal incisions, and natural defecation is preserved. Growths in the lower portion of the rectum require removal of the entire rectum with formation of a permanent colostomy. Prognosis after surgery depends on the stage and location of the tumor.[266]

Radiation therapy is often given before surgery in the hope that it will shrink the tumor, alter the malignant cells, or both so that these cells will not survive after surgery. Adjuvant chemoradiotherapy is used to treat metastatic disease and cases with a high risk of recurrence. Monoclonal antibody therapy and other targeted therapies that are gene-specific may be added.[267] Vaccines for colon cancer are in clinical trials. Treatment of rectal cancer includes preoperative chemoradiotherapy, total mesorectal excision surgery, and adjuvant chemotherapy.

Anal carcinoma is rare (estimated 8200 cases and 1100 deaths in 2017).[227] The most common tumor type is squamous cell carcinoma, about 80%; other anal cancers are adenocarcinoma, lymphoma, or sarcoma. The most common risk factor is infection with human papillomavirus (93%) and less commonly anal involvement in Crohn disease. Squamous cell anal carcinoma is more common among the human immunodeficiency virus-infected population. Anal carcinomas are treated according to stage and include surgery and combined chemoradiation.[268,269]

Cancer of the Accessory Organs of Digestion
Cancer of the Liver

Cancer of the liver is a leading cause of cancer death worldwide and is highest in Eastern and Southeastern Asia.[270] The estimated number of new cases is 40,710, with 28,920 deaths in the United States in 2017. The overall 5-year survival rate is 18%.[227] In the United States, blacks and Hispanics are almost twice as likely to develop these cancers as whites.[271] In the United States, the incidence of primary hepatocellular carcinoma is increasing significantly as a result of chronic hepatitis C infection. Liver cancer is common in densely populated parts of Southeast Asia and sub-Saharan Africa, where hepatitis B virus infection is endemic.[227] Primary liver cancer is rare before the age of 40 years and

---

BOX 42.8 SCREENING FOR COLORECTAL CANCER

Beginning at age 50, both men and women should follow one of these testing schedules:

- Guaiac-based fecal occult blood test (gFOBT) with at least 50% sensitivity

  OR

- Fecal immunochemical test (FIT) with at least 50% sensitivity
- Yearly testing of spontaneously passed stool specimens

  Single stool testing during a clinician office visit is not recommended, nor are "throw in the toilet bowl" tests. In comparison with guaiac-based tests for the detection of occult blood, immunochemical tests are more patient-friendly and are likely to be equal or better in sensitivity and specificity. There is no justification for repeating gFOBT in response to an initial positive finding.

  OR

  Stool DNA test; every 3 years

  OR

  Flexible sigmoidoscopy (FSIG); every 5 years alone or consideration can be given to combining FSIG performed every 5 years with a highly sensitive gFOBT or FIT performed annually.

  OR

  Double-contrast barium enema; every 5 years

  OR

  Colonoscopy; every 10 years

  OR

  CT colonography, every 5 years

All positive tests (other than colonoscopy) should be followed up with colonoscopy.

Data from American Cancer Society (ACS): Recommendations for early detection of cancer in average risk asymptomatic people. In *Cancer facts & figures 2017*, p. 71, Atlanta GA, 2017, Author. Available at: https://www.cancer.org/research/cancer-facts-statistics/all-cancer-facts-figures/cancer-facts-figures-2017.html

most common after 60 years. Cancer in the liver is usually caused by metastatic spread from a primary site elsewhere in the body. Risk factors for primary liver cancer include the following:

1. Infection and inflammation associated with HBV, HCV, and HDV, particularly in conjunction with cirrhosis, acts either as a carcinogen or as a co-carcinogen in chronically infected hepatocytes[272]; primary liver cancer risks associated with HBV and HCV are decreasing with antiviral therapy and screening
2. Chronic alcoholic liver disease and nonalcoholic fatty liver disease that results in cirrhosis
3. Exposure to mycotoxins; the most significant mycotoxins are the aflatoxins, particularly those produced by *Aspergillus flavus,* a mold found on spoiled corn, peanuts, and grain; aflatoxins cause mutation of the *TP53* suppressor gene and activation of WNT signal transduction pathway
4. Long duration of heavy smoking (greater than 20 years)
5. Hepatic iron overload (hemochromatosis)
6. Obesity

◆**PATHOGENESIS.** Primary carcinomas of the liver are hepatocellular or cholangiocellular. **Hepatocellular carcinoma (hepatocarcinoma) (HCC)** develops in the hepatocytes and can be nodular (consisting of multiple, discrete nodules), massive (consisting of a large tumor mass having satellite nodules), or diffuse (consisting of very small nodules distributed throughout most of the liver). HCC is the type of primary liver cancer that is closely associated with cirrhosis (Fig. 42.30). Chronic hepatitis B and hepatitis C and cirrhosis give rise to HCC repetitive cellular proliferation that occurs in the inflamed liver in response to growth factor and cytokine stimulation and oxidative stress–induced DNA damage. Numerous genetic and epigenetic alterations, including activation of oncogenes, failure of tumor-suppressor genes, and signaling pathways, combine to promote carcinogenesis.[273] Because carcinoma of the liver invades the hepatic and portal veins, it often spreads to the heart and lungs. Other sites of metastases are the brain, kidney, and spleen.

Cholangiocellular carcinomas (cholangiocarcinoma) is rare (less than 1% of liver cancers), develops in the bile ducts, and occurs less often than hepatocellular carcinoma in the United States.[274] The disease predominates in men. Incidence demonstrates geographic variation and is common in Southeast Asia, where liver fluke infestation is prevalent. The mechanism by which fluke infestation causes cholangiocellular carcinoma is multifactorial and includes parasite secretions,

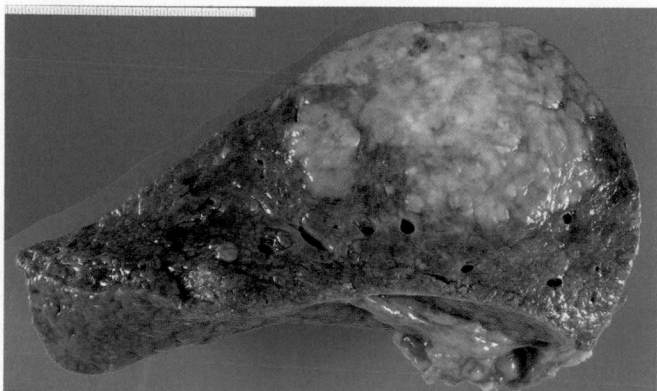

FIGURE 42.30 Primary Hepatocellular Carcinoma. Macroscopically, hepatocellular carcinomas may be single or multifocal. They usually develop in a liver already affected by cirrhosis as shown in this image. Tumor appears as the light-colored mass within the top part of the liver. (From Connolly AJ, et al, editors: *Autopsy pathology: a manual and atlas,* ed 3, Philadelphia, 2016, Saunders.)

immunopathology, and mechanical damage. Other risk factors include primary sclerosing cholangitis, hepatolithiasis, and choledochal cysts.[274] Intrahepatic cholangiocellular carcinoma also is associated with cirrhosis, HBV and HCV infection, obesity, and diabetes. However, most individuals diagnosed with cholangiocellular carcinoma do not have an identifiable risk factor except age. Cholangiocellular carcinoma can occur anywhere along the bile duct, both within and outside the liver, and usually is a solitary lesion. It is difficult to distinguish an invasion of cholangiocellular carcinoma from a metastatic adenocarcinoma except by neoplastic changes found in nearby ducts. A combined form of HCC is known as *combined (mixed) hepatocellular-cholangiocellular carcinoma.*

◆**CLINICAL MANIFESTATIONS.** HCC is usually asymptomatic. Manifestations can develop slowly or abruptly and include vague abdominal symptoms, such as nausea and vomiting; fullness or pressure; dull ache in the right hypochondrium; and weight loss. In individuals with cirrhosis, deepening jaundice or abrupt lack of appetite is a sign of hepatocellular carcinoma. Obstruction by the tumor can cause sudden worsening of portal hypertension and development of ascites. As the tumor enlarges, it causes pain. Cholangiocellular carcinoma more commonly presents insidiously as pain, loss of appetite, weight loss, and gradual onset of jaundice. Some carcinomas of the liver rupture spontaneously, causing hemorrhage. Others are discovered accidentally during laboratory evaluation, imaging, or surgery for other diseases or trauma.

◆**EVALUATION AND TREATMENT.** There is no specific test or biologic marker to guide diagnosis and treatment of HCC.[275]

Biopsy is not recommended because of the risk for tumor seeding. For HCC high-risk individuals, alpha fetoprotein associated with HBV (risk of high false-negative and false-positive results) and abdominal ultrasound are common screening tools. Additional serum markers are being evaluated.[276] Diagnosis is based on clinical manifestations, laboratory findings, imaging, biopsy findings, and exploratory laparotomy. In individuals without cirrhosis, liver scans can document filling defects. CT or ultrasonography is used to detect solid tumors, but neither can distinguish benign from malignant tumors. Serum levels of alkaline phosphatase, aspartate aminotransferase (AST), and alanine aminotransferase (ALT) are commonly elevated in individuals with HCC.

Staging of HCC is important for guiding treatment but does not accurately predict postoperative outcome. Surgical resection is possible with solitary tumors localized to a removable lobe of the liver and the absence of portal hypertension.

Radiofrequency (thermal) ablation has emerged as the most effective method for local tumor destruction.[277] Tyrosine kinase inhibitors (e.g., sorafenib) and monoclonal antibodies are improving survival; many new therapies are in clinical trials. Transarterial embolization, chemotherapy, and radiation are used for management of pain and to reduce tumor size.[278] Surgical resection or liver transplantation is the only alternative for cure; however, very early stage HCC is difficult to diagnose. Primary prevention of HCC is vaccination against HBV and antiviral therapy for HCV.

Cholangiocarcinoma causes duct obstruction. Most tumors are unresectable, and radiotherapy, chemotherapy, photodynamic therapy, and stenting can temporarily relieve the blockage.[279,280]

Cancer of the Gallbladder

Cancer of the gallbladder and biliary tract is a rare but lethal disease. The estimated number of new cases was 11,740 and 3830 deaths in 2017 in the United States.[227] It rarely occurs before age 40 and is most common between the ages of 50 and 60 years. Risk factors include gallstones, advancing age, female sex (2:1), anomalous pancreaticobiliary ductal junction, and obesity. Native populations in North and South America have greater risk of gallbladder cancer, and it is more common in Chile, Poland, India, Japan, and Israel.[281-284] Most cancerous tumors in the gallbladder are caused by metastasis.

◆**PATHOGENESIS.** Most primary cancers of the gallbladder are adenocarcinomas and, less commonly, squamous cell carcinomas. The pathogenesis is not clear. Chronic inflammation may trigger dysplasia and progression to metaplasia. The molecular mechanisms involve mutation of several genes, including tumor suppressor genes, oncogenes, and alterations in the extracellular matrix.[285] Infiltrative tumors are associated with gallstones, and invasion of the liver and lymph nodes occurs early. Spreading extends to the pancreas and retroperitoneal lymph nodes. Direct invasion of the stomach and the duodenum can cause pyloric obstruction. Infection often accompanies cancer of the gallbladder. Generalized peritonitis, gangrene, perforation, and liver abscesses are potential complications of infection.

◆**CLINICAL MANIFESTATIONS.** Early stages of gallbladder carcinoma are asymptomatic and the disease usually presents at an advanced stage. When symptoms develop, there is usually steady upper right quadrant pain for about 2 months, jaundice, and fever. Other symptoms mimic benign gallbladder disease, including diarrhea, belching, weakness, loss of appetite, weight loss, and vomiting. Obstructive jaundice can occur if an enlarging tumor presses on the extrahepatic ducts.

◆**EVALUATION AND TREATMENT.** Early diagnosis of gallbladder cancer is rare, and the disease may be found incidentally when removing gallstones. The disease is often in an early stage and resectable.[286] Therefore adults with gallstones, particularly older women, are evaluated for gallbladder carcinoma. Inflammatory disorders, such as cholangitis (bile duct inflammation) and peritonitis, often obscure an underlying malignancy. Diagnostic procedures include high resolution ultrasonography, CT, and MRI.[287]

Complete surgical resection of the gallbladder is the only effective treatment. Because advanced malignancies cannot be resected, gallbladders containing stones are removed as a preventive measure. Palliative chemotherapy or chemoradiation provides symptom improvement but does not improve survival. The prognosis of gallbladder cancer is extremely poor. Most individuals with advanced-stage disease die within 5 years.[288]

Cancer of the Pancreas

Pancreatic cancer represents about 2.6% of all new cancers. An estimated 53,670 new cases and 43,090 deaths occurred in 2017 in the United States.[227] The incidence of pancreatic cancer rises steadily with age. Men are affected more often than women, and blacks more often than whites.[227] Mortality is about 95% within 12 months and is related to lack of early diagnosis and ineffective treatment. Risk factors include use of tobacco (smoking and nonsmoking), heavy alcohol use, family history of pancreatic cancer, long-term type 2 diabetes mellitus, chronic pancreatitis, and non-O blood group. Obesity, with centralized fat distribution, is a risk factor, particularly in women, and is associated with decreased response to chemotherapy.[289,290]

◆**PATHOGENESIS.** Pancreatic cancer is a disease of inherited and multiple acquired mutations in cancer-related genes associated with chronic inflammation and growth factors.[291] A *K-ras* mutation (a proto-oncogene) is the most common and early genetic alteration; tumor-suppressor gene alterations also are found, including *TP53, CDKN2A, SMAD4, BRCA2,* and *PALB2.*[290,292]

Pancreatic cancer can arise from exocrine or endocrine cells. Most pancreatic tumors (95%) arise from metaplastic exocrine cells in the ducts and are called *ductal adenocarcinomas.* There is significant expansion of the extracellular matrix (stroma) from activation of pancreatic stellate cells, a type of fibroblast in the pancreas, which also promotes inflammation, angiogenesis, and tumor growth and contributes to therapeutic resistance.[293] Tumors arising in small ducts invade nearby

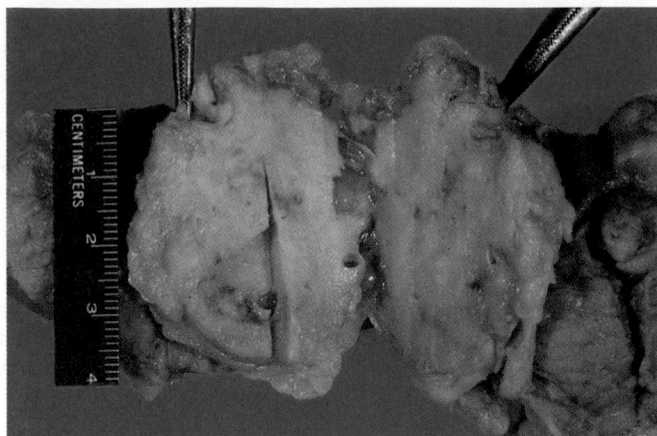

FIGURE 42.31 Pancreatic Carcinoma. Adenocarcinoma of the head of pancreas. Pancreatic adenocarcinoma may arise in the head (60%), body (15%), or tail (5%) of the pancreas; in 20% of cases there is involvement of more than one segment. (From Connolly AJ, et al: *Autopsy pathology: a manual and atlas,* ed 3, St Louis, 2016, Elsevier.)

glandular tissue, penetrate the covering of the pancreas, and extend into surrounding tissues. Tumors are staged using the TNM classification.

Ductal adenocarcinomas are the most common tumor and can occur in the head, body, or tail of the pancreas. Tumors of the head quickly spread to obstruct the common bile duct and portal vein (Fig. 42.31). These tumors can then infiltrate the superior mesenteric artery, the vena cava, and the aorta. Cancer cells that enter the blood vessels can form emboli. Tumors of the body and tail infiltrate the posterior abdominal wall. Lymphatic invasion occurs early and rapidly and involves local and regional lymph nodes. Venous invasion causes metastases to the liver. Tumor implants on the peritoneal surface can obstruct veins and promote development of ascites.

Ductal adenocarcinomas arising in the head of the pancreas cause biliary obstruction somewhat early in the disease. Individuals with such tumors survive slightly longer than those with cancer of the body and tail, presumably because they seek medical attention earlier.

Tumors of the endocrine pancreas are rare neoplasms of the islets of Langerhans known as *apudomas.* The first four letters in *apudoma* derive from *amine precursor uptake* and *decarboxylation.* The apudomas are so named because they contain neurosecretory granules. Endocrine neoplasms secrete abnormal amounts of hormones, such as insulin.

◆**CLINICAL MANIFESTATIONS.** Cancer of the body and tail of the pancreas is generally asymptomatic until there is intraductal obstruction or the tumor invades adjacent tissue. Alarm symptoms include lethargy, weight loss, abdominal pain, nausea and vomiting, bloating, dyspepsia, new-onset diabetes, changes in bowel habit, pruritus, lethargy, back pain, shoulder pain, and jaundice. Jaundice develops in most cases, usually caused by obstruction of the bile duct. Distant metastases are found in the cervical lymph nodes, the lungs, and the brain. Most individuals die of hepatic failure, malnutrition, or systemic complications.[294]

◆**EVALUATION AND TREATMENT.** Pancreatic cancer is usually diagnosed at an advanced stage after several years of silent tumor progression and has a poor prognosis. The most effective screening method for those at risk is endoscopic ultrasound because it detects small lesions and endoscopic ultrasonography-guided fine-needle aspiration for biopsy. Contrast CT scans or contrast MRI, or both, assist with diagnosis. *Autoimmune pancreatitis* is a rare, fibroinflammatory disorder of the pancreas that mimics radiologic and clinical symptoms (painless obstructive jaundice) of pancreatic cancer and must be differentiated from pancreatic cancer. Symptoms for this disease usually improve with steroid administration.[295] CA19-9 tumor antigen is a serum tumor biomarker useful for diagnosis and response to treatment of pancreatic cancer. The measurement of *K-ras* mutations has not been clinically beneficial.[296] The search for other biomarkers is continuing.[297] Laparotomy is used to establish a definitive diagnosis, evaluate the extent and resectability of disease, and determine whether palliative bypass surgery (i.e., cholecystojejunostomy and gastrojejunostomy) is needed. Laparoscopic and robotic approaches have been used in some centers.[298,299]

Individuals with small tumors and complete resection have the best possibility of cure (15% to 20% of cases), but 5-year survival is about 25% because of tumor recurrence. Pancreaticoduodenectomy (Whipple procedure) is the most common procedure performed to decompress duct obstruction. Some surgeons recommend a total pancreatectomy because cancer of the pancreas seldom consists of a single lesion. Islet cell autotransplantation minimizes the development of diabetes mellitus.[300] Neoadjuvant chemotherapy has shown encouraging long-term survival in borderline tumor resection. Evaluations are in progress for adjuvant radiation therapy. The dense stromal structure of the tumor impairs chemotherapeutic drug delivery and results in poor response to chemotherapy. Five classes of cytotoxic drugs (gemcitabine, fluoropyrimidines, oxaliplatin, irinotecan-nanoliposomal, or nanoparticle albumin-bound paclitaxel) are showing efficacy in disease treatment.[301] Chemoradiation therapy is used for advanced disease in some centers. Treatments with molecular targets are in clinical trials, including immune-modifying agents and vaccines, and combination agents.[302] Palliative care, including pain management and nutrition, is important.[303]

SUMMARY REVIEW

Disorders of the Gastrointestinal Tract

1. Anorexia (loss of appetite), vomiting, constipation, diarrhea, abdominal pain, and evidence of gastrointestinal bleeding are clinical manifestations of many disorders of the gastrointestinal tract.
2. Vomiting is the forceful emptying of the stomach effected by gastrointestinal contraction and reverse peristalsis of the esophagus. It is usually preceded by nausea and retching with the exception of projectile vomiting, which is associated with direct stimulation of the vomiting center in the brain.
3. Primary constipation is defined in three categories: functional, associated with low-residue, low-fluid diet; slow-transit, related to impaired colonic motor function; and pelvic floor dyssynergia-anismus. Secondary constipation results from a neurogenic disease, drugs that decrease intestinal motility, endocrine or metabolic disorders, or obstruction.
4. Diarrhea can be caused by excessive fluid drawn into the intestinal lumen by osmosis (osmotic diarrhea), excessive secretion of fluids by the intestinal mucosa (secretory diarrhea), or excessive gastrointestinal motility (motility diarrhea).
5. Abdominal pain is caused by stretching, inflammation, or ischemia and originates in the peritoneum (parietal pain) or in the organs themselves (visceral pain). Visceral pain is often referred to the back.
6. Gastrointestinal bleeding can occur in the upper or lower gastrointestinal tract. Obvious manifestations of gastrointestinal bleeding are hematemesis (vomiting of blood), melena (dark, tarry stools), and hematochezia (frank bleeding from the rectum). Occult bleeding can be detected only by testing stools or vomitus for the presence of blood.
7. Dysphagia is difficulty in swallowing or perception of obstruction during swallowing. It can be caused by a mechanical or functional obstruction of the esophagus. Functional obstruction is an impairment of esophageal motility.
8. Achalasia is a form of functional dysphagia caused by loss of esophageal innervation or relaxation of the lower esophageal sphincter.
9. Gastroesophageal reflux disease is the regurgitation of chyme from the stomach into the esophagus, causing esophagitis from repeated exposure to acids, enzymes, or bile salts in the regurgitated gastric contents.
10. Hiatal hernia is the protrusion of the upper part of the stomach through the hiatus (esophageal opening in the diaphragm) at the gastroesophageal junction. Hiatal hernia can be sliding, paraesophageal, or mixed.

11. Gastroparesis is delayed gastric emptying in the absence of mechanical gastric outlet obstruction.
12. Pyloric obstruction is the narrowing or blockage of the pylorus, which is the opening between the stomach and the duodenum. It can be caused by a congenital defect, inflammation and scarring secondary to a gastric ulcer, or tumor growth.
13. Intestinal obstruction can occur in the small or large intestine and prevents the normal movement of chyme through the intestinal tract. It is usually mechanical—that is, caused by torsion, herniation, or tumor. Functional obstruction is caused by paralytic ileus.
14. The most severe consequences of intestinal obstruction are fluid and electrolyte losses, hypovolemia, shock, intestinal necrosis, and perforation of the intestinal wall.
15. Gastritis is an acute or a chronic inflammation of the gastric mucosa.
16. Regurgitation of bile, use of antiinflammatory drugs or alcohol, *H. pylori* infection, and some systemic diseases are associated with gastritis.
17. Chronic fundal gastritis is rare and associated with autoantibodies to parietal cells and intrinsic factor, resulting in gastric atrophy and causing pernicious anemia.
18. Chronic antral gastritis is the most common gastritis and is associated with *H. pylori* and NSAIDs.
19. Alkaline reflux gastritis is stomach inflammation caused by the reflux of bile and pancreatic secretions from the duodenum into the stomach. These substances disrupt the mucosal barrier and cause inflammation.
20. A peptic ulcer is a circumscribed area of mucosal inflammation and ulceration caused by excessive secretion of gastric acid, disruption of the protective mucosal barrier, or both.
21. The three types of peptic ulcers are duodenal, gastric, and stress ulcers. Duodenal and gastric ulcers are associated with *H. pylori* infection and chronic use of NSAIDs.
22. Duodenal ulcers, the most common peptic ulcers, are associated with increased numbers of parietal (acid-secreting) cells in the stomach, elevated gastrin levels, and rapid gastric emptying. Pain occurs when the stomach is empty, and pain is relieved with food or antacids. Duodenal ulcers tend to heal spontaneously and recur frequently.
23. Gastric ulcers develop near parietal cells, generally in the antrum, and tend to become chronic. Gastric secretions may be normal or decreased, and pain may occur after eating.
24. Zollinger-Ellison syndrome is associated with a gastrinoma, chronic secretion of gastric acid, and gastric and duodenal ulcers.

■ SUMMARY REVIEW—cont'd

25. Stress ulcer (stress-related mucosal disease) is an acute form of peptic ulcer associated with severe illness or extensive trauma.

26. Ischemic stress ulcers develop suddenly after severe illness, systemic trauma, neural injury, or burns (Curling ulcer). Ulceration follows mucosal damage caused by ischemia (decreased blood flow to the gastric mucosa).

27. Cushing ulcer is a stress ulcer caused by head trauma. Ulceration follows hypersecretion of hydrochloric acid caused by overstimulation of the vagal nuclei.

28. Postgastrectomy syndromes are a group of signs and symptoms that occur after gastric resection for the treatment of peptic ulcer, gastric carcinoma, or bariatric surgery for extreme obesity.

29. Dumping syndrome causes malabsorption by the rapid emptying of hypertonic chyme from the surgically created residual stomach into the small intestine. It causes an osmotic shift of fluid from the vascular compartment to the intestinal lumen, which decreases plasma volume.

30. Malabsorption syndromes result in impaired digestion or absorption of nutrients.

31. Pancreatic insufficiency causes malabsorption associated with insufficient amounts of the enzymes that digest protein, carbohydrates, and fats into components that can be absorbed by the intestine.

32. Deficient lactase production in the brush border of the small intestine inhibits the breakdown of lactose. This prevents lactose absorption and causes osmotic diarrhea.

33. Bile salt deficiency causes fat malabsorption, including fat-soluble vitamins, and steatorrhea (fatty stools). Bile salt deficiency can result from inadequate secretion of bile, excessive bacterial deconjugation of bile, or impaired reabsorption of bile salts caused by ileal disease.

34. Ulcerative colitis is an inflammatory bowel disease that causes ulceration, abscess formation, and necrosis of the colonic and rectal mucosa. Cramping pain, bleeding, frequent diarrhea, dehydration, and weight loss accompany severe forms of the disease. A course of frequent remissions and exacerbations is common.

35. Crohn disease is similar to ulcerative colitis but it affects entire GI tract, including the large and small intestines. Ulceration tends to involve all layers of the lumen. "Skip lesion" fissures and granulomas are characteristic of Crohn disease. Abdominal tenderness, nonbloody diarrhea, and weight loss are the usual symptoms.

36. Microscopic colitis involves two histologic forms of the disease, lymphocytic and collagenous, with both resulting in frequent diarrhea.

37. Irritable bowel syndrome is a disorder of brain-gut interaction characterized by abdominal pain with altered bowel habits (diarrhea, constipation, or both).

38. Diverticula are outpouchings of colonic mucosa through the muscle layers of the colon wall. Diverticulosis is the presence of these outpouchings; diverticulitis is inflammation of the diverticula.

39. Appendicitis is caused by obstruction of the lumen and leads to increased pressure, ischemia, and inflammation of the appendix. Without surgical resection, inflammation may progress to gangrene, perforation, and peritonitis.

40. Vascular insufficiency in the intestine is associated most often with acute or chronic occlusion or obstruction of the mesenteric vessels or insufficient mesenteric arterial blood flow. The resulting ischemia and necrosis produce abdominal pain, fever, bloody diarrhea, hypovolemia, and shock.

Disorders of the Accessory Organs of Digestion

1. Portal hypertension, ascites, hepatic encephalopathy, jaundice, and hepatorenal syndrome are complications of many liver disorders.

2. Portal hypertension is an elevation of portal venous pressure to at least 10 mmHg. It is caused by increased resistance to venous flow in the portal vein and its tributaries, including the sinusoids and hepatic vein.

3. Portal hypertension is the most serious complication of liver disease because it can cause fatal complications, such as bleeding varices, ascites, hepatic encephalopathy, and renal failure.

4. Varices are distended, tortuous, collateral veins associated with portal hypertension.

5. Splenomegaly is an enlargement of the spleen resulting from increased splenic vein pressure caused by portal hypertension.

6. Hepatopulmonary syndrome is pulmonary hypertension related to the release of vasodilators that affect pulmonary arterioles and is associated with portal hypertension and severe liver disease.

7. Ascites is the accumulation and sequestration of fluid in the peritoneal cavity, often as a result of portal hypertension, decreased concentrations of plasma proteins, and sodium retention.

8. Hepatic encephalopathy (portosystemic encephalopathy) is impaired cerebral function caused by blood-borne toxins (particularly ammonia) not metabolized by the liver.

9. Jaundice (icterus) is a yellow or greenish pigmentation of the skin or sclera of the eyes caused by increases in plasma bilirubin concentration (hyperbilirubinemia).

10. Obstructive jaundice is caused by obstructed bile canaliculi (intrahepatic obstructive jaundice) or obstructed bile ducts outside the liver (extrahepatic obstructive jaundice). Bilirubin accumulates proximal to sites of obstruction, enters the bloodstream, and is deposited in the skin and other connective tissues.

11. Hemolytic jaundice is caused by destruction of red blood cells at a rate that exceeds the liver's ability to metabolize unconjugated bilirubin.

12. Hepatorenal syndrome is functional renal failure caused by advanced liver disease, particularly cirrhosis with portal hypertension. Renal failure is caused by a sudden decrease in blood flow to the kidneys, usually as a result of massive gastrointestinal hemorrhage or liver failure. Its chief clinical manifestation is oliguria.

13. Acute liver failure can be caused by toxic overdose of acetaminophen or complications of viral hepatitis.

14. Autoimmune hepatitis is T-cell mediated inflammatory liver disease with hypergammaglobulinemia, elevated transaminases, and absence of viral hepatitis.

15. Viral hepatitis is an infection of the liver caused by strains of the hepatitis virus. Modes of transmission are HAV and HEV, fecal-oral route; and HAV, HBV, HCV, HDV, and HEV, parenteral and sexual transmission. The hepatitis viruses can cause hepatic cell necrosis, Kupffer cell hyperplasia, and infiltration of liver tissue by mononuclear phagocytes. These changes obstruct bile flow and impair hepatocyte function.

16. The clinical manifestations of viral hepatitis depend on the stage of infection. Fever, malaise, anorexia, and liver enlargement and tenderness characterize the prodromal phase (stage 1). Jaundice and hyperbilirubinemia mark the icteric phase (stage 2). During the recovery phase (stage 3), symptoms resolve. Recovery takes several weeks.

17. Chronic active hepatitis can occur with HBV and HCV with predisposition to cirrhosis and hepatocellular carcinoma.

SUMMARY REVIEW—cont'd

18. Fulminant hepatitis is a complication of hepatitis B (with or without hepatitis D infection) or hepatitis C. It causes widespread hepatic necrosis and is often fatal.

19. Cirrhosis is an irreversible inflammatory disease of the liver that causes disorganization of lobular structure, fibrosis, and nodular regeneration. Bile obstruction causes jaundice. Vascular obstruction causes portal hypertension, shunting, and varices. Cirrhosis can result from hepatitis or exposure to toxins, such as acetaldehyde (a product of alcohol metabolism). The disease causes progressive irreversible liver damage, usually over a period of years.

20. Alcoholic liver disease results from formation of acetaldehyde impairing the hepatocytes' ability to oxidize fatty acids, synthesize enzymes and proteins, degrade hormones, and clear portal blood of ammonia and toxins. The disease is progressive and includes steatosis, steatohepatitis, and alcoholic cirrhosis.

21. Nonalcoholic fatty liver disease and nonalcoholic steatohepatitis is fat infiltration and inflammation of hepatocytes associated with obesity.

22. Primary biliary cirrhosis is an autoimmune disease with inflammatory destruction of intrahepatic bile ducts. Mitochondrial autoantibodies are found in this disease.

23. Secondary biliary cirrhosis develops from prolonged obstruction of bile flow (e.g., gallstones) with increased pressure in the hepatic bile ducts that causes pooling of bile and necrosis of tissue. Relief of obstruction alleviates symptoms of jaundice and pruritus. Continued obstruction causes cirrhosis and liver failure.

24. Primary sclerosing cholangitis is a fibrotic disease of medium- and large-sized bile ducts outside the liver.

25. Cholelithiasis (the formation of gallstones) is a result of bile aggregation of cholesterol crystals (cholesterol stones) or precipitates of unconjugated bilirubin (pigmented stones). Gallstones that fill the gallbladder or obstruct the cystic, or common, bile duct cause abdominal pain and jaundice.

26. Cholecystitis is an inflammation of the gallbladder. It is usually associated with obstruction of the cystic duct by gallstones.

27. Acute pancreatitis (pancreatic inflammation) is a serious but relatively rare disorder associated with biliary obstruction and alcoholism. Injury permits leakage of digestive enzymes into pancreatic tissue, where they become activated and begin the process of autodigestion, inflammation, and destruction of tissues. Release of pancreatic enzymes into the bloodstream or abdominal cavity causes damage to other organs.

28. Chronic pancreatitis results from structural or functional impairment of the pancreas usually related to alcoholism or recurrent acute pancreatitis. It causes recurrent abdominal pain and digestive disorders.

Cancer of the Digestive System

1. Cancer of the esophagus is rare and tends to occur in people older than 60 years. Alcohol and tobacco use, reflux esophagitis, radiation exposure, and nutritional deficiencies are associated with esophageal carcinoma. There are two types, squamous cell and adenocarcinoma.

2. Dysphagia and chest pain are the primary manifestations of esophageal cancer. Early treatment of tumors that have not spread into the mediastinum or lymph nodes results in a good prognosis.

3. Gastric carcinoma is associated with *H. pylori* (*CagA*), high salt intake, food preservatives (nitrates and nitrites), and atrophic gastritis.

4. Gastric cancers are commonly located in the prepyloric antrum. Clinical manifestations (weight loss, upper abdominal pain, vomiting, hematemesis, anemia) develop only after the tumor has penetrated the wall of the stomach.

5. Cancer of the colon and rectum (colorectal cancer) is the third most common type of cancer and cancer death in the United States. Small intestinal cancers are rare. Familial adenomatous polyposis coli and hereditary nonpolyposis colorectal cancer (HNPCC or Lynch syndrome) are inherited forms of colon cancer. Preexisting large and numerous polyps are highly associated with sporadic (acquired) adenocarcinoma of the colon.

6. Tumors of the right (ascending) colon are usually large and bulky; tumors of the left (descending, sigmoid) colon develop as small button-like masses. Manifestations of colon tumors include pain, bloody stools, and change in bowel habits.

7. Rectal carcinoma is located up to 15 cm from the opening of the anus. The tumor spreads transmurally to the vagina in women or to the prostate in men.

8. Metastatic invasion of the liver is more common than primary cancer of the liver.

9. Primary liver cancers are associated with chronic liver disease (cirrhosis and hepatitides B and C). Hepatocellular carcinomas arise from the hepatocytes, whereas cholangiocellular carcinomas arise from the bile ducts. Primary liver cancer spreads to the heart, lungs, brain, kidney, and spleen through the circulation.

10. Cancer of the gallbladder is relatively rare and tends to occur in women older than 50 years. Adenocarcinoma is most common. Because clinical manifestations occur late in the disease, metastases to lymph channels have usually occurred by the time of diagnosis, and the prognosis is poor.

11. Cancer of the pancreas represents about 2.6% of all cancers in the United States. Most tumors are adenocarcinomas that arise in the exocrine cells of ducts in the head, body, or tail of the pancreas. Symptoms may not be evident until the tumor has spread to surrounding tissues. Treatment is palliative, and mortality is nearly 100% for advanced tumors.

KEY TERMS

Achalasia, 1326
Acute colonic pseudo-obstruction (Ogilvie syndrome), 1329
Acute gastritis, 1331
Acute liver failure (fulminant liver failure), 1347
Acute mesenteric ischemia, 1342
Acute pancreatitis, 1354
Alcoholic cirrhosis, 1350
Alcoholic fatty liver (steatosis), 1350
Alcoholic hepatitis (steatohepatitis), 1350
Alkaline reflux gastritis, 1332

Anal carcinoma, 1362
Anorexia, 1321
Appendicitis, 1341
Ascites, 1343
Barrett esophagus, 1357
Biliary cirrhosis, 1351
Cholangiocellular carcinoma (cholangiocarcinoma), 1363
Cholecystitis, 1354
Cholelithiasis, 1353
Chronic active hepatitis, 1350

Chronic gastritis, 1331
Chronic mesenteric ischemia, 1342
Chronic pancreatitis, 1355
Cirrhosis, 1350
Constipation, 1322
Crohn disease (CD), 1338
Curling ulcer, 1334
Cushing ulcer, 1334
Diarrhea, 1323
Diverticula (*sing.*, diverticulum), 1340
Diverticulitis, 1340

KEY TERMS—cont'd

REFERENCES

1. Visvanathan R: Anorexia of aging. *Clin Geriatr Med* 31(3):417–427, 2015.
2. Natale JJ: Reviewing current and emerging antiemetics for chemotherapy-induced nausea and vomiting prophylaxis. *Hosp Pract* 43(4):226–234, 1995.
3. Navari RM: Treatment of breakthrough and refractory chemotherapy-induced nausea and vomiting. *Biomed Res Int* 2015:595894, 2015.
4. Vazquez Roque M, Bouras EP: Epidemiology and management of chronic constipation in elderly patients. *Clin Interv Aging* 10:919–930, 2015.
5. Lacy BE, Levenick JM, Crowell M: Chronic constipation: new diagnostic and treatment approaches. *Therap Adv Gastroenterol* 5(4):233–247, 2012.
6. Serrano Falcón B, et al: Fecal impaction: a systematic review of its medical complications. *BMC Geriatr* 16:4, 2016.
7. Chiarioni G, Bassotti G: Biofeedback therapy for constipation due to dyssynergic defecation: ready for prime time. *Tech Coloproctol* 19(6):331–332, 2015.
8. Wald A: Constipation: advances in diagnosis and treatment. *J Am Med Assoc* 315(2):185–891, 2016.
9. Guerrant RL, et al: Practice guidelines for the management of infectious diarrhea. *Clin Infect Dis* 32(3):331–351, 2001.
10. World Gastroenterology Organisation: *Acute diarrhea in adults and children: a global perspective*, February 2012. Available at: www.worldgastroenterology.org/assets/export/userfiles/Acute%20Diarrhea_long_FINAL_10604.pdf.
11. DuPont HL: Persistent diarrhea: a clinical review. *J Am Med Assoc* 315(24):2712–2723, 2016.
12. Spinler JK, Ross CL, Savidge TC: Probiotics as adjunctive therapy for preventing *Clostridium difficile* infection-What are we waiting for? *Anaerobe* 41:51–57, 2016.

13. Rao K, Safdar N: Fecal microbiota transplantation for the treatment of *Clostridium difficile* infection. *J Hosp Med* 11(1):56–61, 2016.
14. Basso L, Bourreille A, Dietrich G: Intestinal inflammation and pain management. *Curr Opin Pharmacol* 25:50–55, 2015.
15. Jänig W: [Neurobiology of visceral pain]. *Schmerz* 28(3):233–251, 2014.
16. Knowles CH, Aziz Q: Basic and clinical aspects of gastrointestinal pain. *Pain* 141(3):191–209, 2009.
17. Rahman SI, Saeian K: Nonvariceal upper gastrointestinal bleeding. *Crit Care Clin* 32(2):223–239, 2016.
18. Qayed E, Dagar G, Nanchal RS: Lower gastrointestinal hemorrhage. *Crit Care Clin* 32(2):241–254, 2016.
19. Kim BS, et al: Diagnosis of gastrointestinal bleeding: a practical guide for clinicians. *World J Gastrointest Pathophysiol* 5(4):467–478, 2014.
20. National Institute for Health and Clinical Excellence (NICE): *Clinical guideline no 141: acute upper gastrointestinal bleeding: management*, p 23, London, 2012, Author. Updated November 4, 2014. Available at: https://www.guideline.gov/summaries/summary/37563.
21. Strate LL, Gralnek IM: ACG clinical guideline: management of patients with acute lower gastrointestinal bleeding. *Am J Gastroenterol* 111(5):755, 2016.
22. Clavé P, Shaker R: Dysphagia: current reality and scope of the problem. *Nat Rev Gastroenterol Hepatol* 12(5):259–270, 2015.
23. Carucci LR, Turner MA: Dysphagia revisited: common and unusual causes. *Radiographics* 35(1):105–122, 2015.
24. Jansson-Knodell CL, Codipilly DC, Leggett CL: Making dysphagia easier to swallow: a review for the practicing clinician. *Mayo Clin Proc* 92(6):965–972, 2017.
25. Boeckxstaens G, et al: Symptomatic reflux disease: the present, the past and the future. *Gut* 63(7):1185–1193, 2014.

26. Naik RD, Vaezi MF: Extra-esophageal gastroesophageal reflux disease and asthma: understanding this interplay. *Expert Rev Gastroenterol Hepatol* 9(7):969–982, 2015.
27. Herregods TV, Bredenoord AJ, Smout AJ: Pathophysiology of gastroesophageal reflux disease: new understanding in a new era. *Neurogastroenterol Motil* 27(9):1202–1213, 2015.
28. Mikami DJ, Murayama KM: Physiology and pathogenesis of gastroesophageal reflux disease. *Surg Clin North Am* 95(3):515–525, 2015.
29. Patti MG: An evidence-based approach to the treatment of gastroesophageal reflux disease. *JAMA Surg* 151(1):73–78, 2016.
30. Blanchard C, et al: Eosinophilic esophagitis: unclear roles of IgE and eosinophils. *J Intern Med* 281(5):448–457, 2017.
31. Oleynikov D, Jolley JM: Paraesophageal hernia. *Surg Clin North Am* 95(3):555–565, 2015.
32. Roman S, Kahrilas PJ: The diagnosis and management of hiatus hernia. *BMJ* 349:g6154, 2014.
33. Tack J, Carbone F, Rotondo A: Gastroparesis. *Curr Opin Gastroenterol* 31(6):499–505, 2015.
34. Alonso-Lárraga JO, et al: Self-expanding metal stents versus antrectomy for the palliative treatment of obstructive adenocarcinoma of the gastric antrum. *Rev Esp Enferm Dig* 104(4):185–189, 2012.
35. Gore RM, et al: Bowel obstruction. *Radiol Clin North Am* 53(6):1225–1240, 2015.
36. Wehner S, et al: Immune mediators of postoperative ileus. *Langenbecks Arch Surg* 397(4):591–601, 2012.
37. Pereira P, et al: Ogilvie's syndrome-acute colonic pseudo-obstruction. *J Visc Surg* 152(2):99–105, 2015.
38. Brown CV: Small bowel and colon perforation. *Surg Clin North Am* 94(2):471–475, 2014.
39. Sawai RS: Management of colonic obstruction: a review. *Clin Colon Rectal Surg* 25(4):200–203, 2012.

40. Sipponen P, Maaroos HI: Chronic gastritis. *Scand J Gastroenterol* 50(6):657–667, 2015.

41. Toh BH: Diagnosis and classification of autoimmune gastritis. *Autoimmun Rev* 13(4-5):459–462, 2014.

42. Varbanova M, Frauenschläger K, Malfertheiner P: Chronic gastritis-an update. *Best Pract Res Clin Gastroenterol* 28(6):1031–1042, 2014.

43. Marqués-Lespier JM, González-Pons M, Cruz-Correa M: Current perspectives on gastric cancer. *Gastroenterol Clin North Am* 45(3):413–428, 2016.

44. Thung I, et al: Review article: the global emergence of *Helicobacter pylori* antibiotic resistance. *Aliment Pharmacol Ther* 43(4):514–533, 2016.

45. Tireli M: The results of the surgical treatment of alkaline reflux gastritis. *Hepatogastroenterology* 59(119):2352–2356, 2012.

46. Schiller JS, et al: *Summary health statistics for U.S. adults: National Health Interview Survey, 2011. Vital and Health Statistics, Series 10: data from the National Health Interview Survey*, Atlanta, 2011, Centers for Disease Control and Prevention. Available at: www.niddk.nih.gov/health-information/health-statistics/Pages/digestive-diseases-statistics-for-the-united-states.aspx#18.

47. Lee KM, et al: Association between acute pancreatitis and peptic ulcer disease. *World J Gastroenterol* 17(8):1058–1062, 2011.

48. Yeomans ND: The ulcer sleuths: the search for the cause of peptic ulcers. *J Gastroenterol Hepatol* 26(Suppl 1):35–41, 2011.

49. Levenstein S, et al: Psychological stress increases risk for peptic ulcer, regardless of *Helicobacter pylori* infection or use of nonsteroidal antiinflammatory drugs. *Clin Gastroenterol Hepatol* 13(3):498–506, 2015.

50. Overmier JB, Murison R: Restoring psychology's role in peptic ulcer. *Appl Psychol Health Well Being* 5(1):5–27, 2013.

51. Savarino V, et al: The appropriate use of proton pump inhibitors (PPIs): need for a reappraisal. *Eur J Intern Med* 37:19–24, 2017.

52. Talebi Bezmin Abadi A, Perez-Perez G: Role of dupA in virulence of *Helicobacter pylori*. *World J Gastroenterol* 22(46):10118–10123, 2016.

53. Gisbert JP, Cakvet X: Review article: *Helicobacter pylori*-negative duodenal ulcer disease. *Aliment Pharmacol Ther* 30(8):791–815, 2009.

54. Datta De D, Roychoudhury S: To be or not to be: the host genetic factor and beyond in *Helicobacter pylori* mediated gastro-duodenal diseases. *World J Gastroenterol* 21(10):2883–2895, 2015.

55. Atkinson NS, Braden B: *Helicobacter pylori* infection: diagnostic strategies in primary diagnosis and after therapy. *Dig Dis Sci* 61(1):19–24, 2016.

56. Boltin D: Probiotics in *Helicobacter pylori*-induced peptic ulcer disease. *Best Pract Res Clin Gastroenterol* 30(1):99–109, 2016.

57. Vomero ND, Colpo E: Nutritional care in peptic ulcer. *Arq Bras Cir Dig* 27(4):298–302, 2014.

58. Talebi Bezmin Abadi A: Vaccine against *Helicobacter pylori*: inevitable approach. *World J Gastroenterol* 22(11):3150–3157, 2016.

59. Bardou M, Quenot JP, Barkun A: Stress-related mucosal disease in the critically ill patient. *Nat Rev Gastroenterol Hepatol* 12(2):98–107, 2015.

60. Berg P, McCallum R: Dumping syndrome: a review of the current concepts of pathophysiology, diagnosis, and treatment. *Dig Dis Sci* 61(1):11–18, 2016.

61. Tack J, Deloose E: Complications of bariatric surgery: dumping syndrome, reflux and vitamin deficiencies. *Best Pract Res Clin Gastroenterol* 28(4):741–749, 2014.

62. Ersan Y, et al: Late results of patients undergoing remedial operations for alkaline reflux gastritis syndrome. *Acta Chir Belg* 109(3):364–370, 2009.

63. De Martino C, et al: Acute afferent loop obstruction treated by endoscopic decompression. Case report and review of literature. *Ann Ital Chir* 83(6):555–558, 2012.

64. Marcotte E, Chand B: Management and prevention of surgical and nutritional complications after bariatric surgery. *Surg Clin North Am* 96(4):843–856, 2016.

65. Laterza L, et al: Pancreatic function assessment. *Eur Rev Med Pharmacol Sci* 17(Suppl 2):65–71, 2013.

66. Trang T, Chan J, Graham DY: Pancreatic enzyme replacement therapy for pancreatic exocrine insufficiency in the 21(st) century. *World J Gastroenterol* 20(33):11467–11485, 2014.

67. Vandenplas Y: Lactose intolerance. *Asia Pac J Clin Nutr* 24(Suppl1):S9–S13, 2015.

68. Deng Y, et al: Lactose intolerance in adults: biological mechanism and dietary management. *Nutrients* 7(9):8020–8035, 2015.

69. Camilleri M: Advances in understanding of bile acid diarrhea. *Expert Rev Gastroenterol Hepatol* 8(1):49–61, 2014.

70. Dahlhamer JM, et al: Prevalence of inflammatory bowel disease among adults aged ≥18 years— United States, 2015. *MMWR Morb Mortal Wkly Rep*, 65:1166–1169, 2016.

71. Malik TA: Inflammatory bowel disease: historical perspective, epidemiology, and risk factors. *Surg Clin North Am* 95(6):1105–1122, 2015.

72. Ohkusa T, Koido S: Intestinal microbiota and ulcerative colitis. *J Infect Chemother* 21(11):761–768, 2015.

73. de Mattos BR, et al: Inflammatory bowel disease: an overview of immune mechanisms and biological treatments. *Mediators Inflamm* 2015:493012, 2015.

74. Beaugerie L, Itzkowitz SH: Cancers complicating inflammatory bowel disease. *N Engl J Med* 372(15):1441–1452, 2015.

75. de Lange KM, Barrett JC: Understanding inflammatory bowel disease via immunogenetics. *J Autoimmun* 64:91–100, 2015.

76. Hansen JJ: Immune responses to intestinal microbes in inflammatory bowel diseases. *Curr Allergy Asthma Rep* 15(10):61, 2015.

77. To N, Ford AC, Gracie DJ: Systematic review with meta-analysis: the effect of tobacco smoking on the natural history of ulcerative colitis. *Aliment Pharmacol Ther* 44(2):117–126, 2016.

78. Xu XR, et al: Dysregulation of mucosal immune response in pathogenesis of inflammatory bowel disease. *World J Gastroenterol* 20(12):3255–3264, 2014.

79. Conrad K, Roggenbuck D, Laass MW: Diagnosis and classification of ulcerative colitis. *Autoimmun Rev* 13(4-5):463–466, 2014.

80. Kinugasa T, Akagi Y: Status of colitis-associated cancer in ulcerative colitis. *World J Gastrointest Oncol* 8(4):351–357, 2016.

81. Marineață A, et al: Extra intestinal manifestations and complications in inflammatory bowel disease. *Rev Med Chir Soc Med Nat Iasi* 118(2):279–288, 2014.

82. Tontini GE, et al: Differential diagnosis in inflammatory bowel disease colitis: state of the art and future perspectives. *World J Gastroenterol* 21(1):21–46, 2015.

83. Sengupta N, Yee E, Feuerstein JD: Colorectal cancer screening in inflammatory bowel disease. *Dig Dis Sci* 61(4):980–989, 2016.

84. Bressler B, et al: Clinical practice guidelines for the medical management of nonhospitalized ulcerative colitis: the Toronto Consensus. *Gastroenterology* 148(5):1035–1058, 2015.

85. Petkau JM, Eksteen B: Selective biologics for ulcerative colitis and Crohn's disease-clinical utility of vedolizumab. *Biologics* 10:33–52, 2016.

86. Hindryckx P, Jairath V, D'Haens G: Acute severe ulcerative colitis: from pathophysiology to clinical management. *Nat Rev Gastroenterol Hepatol* 13(11):654–664, 2016.

87. Nitzan O, et al: Role of antibiotics for treatment of inflammatory bowel disease. *World J Gastroenterol* 22(3):1078–1087, 2016.

88. Knieling F, Waldner MJ: Light and sound-emerging imaging techniques for inflammatory bowel disease. *World J Gastroenterol* 22(25):5642–5654, 2016.

89. Feuerstein JD, Cheifetz AS: Crohn disease: epidemiology, diagnosis, and management. *Mayo Clin Proc* 92(7):1088–1103, 2017.

90. Lauro ML, Burch JM, Grimes CL: The effect of NOD2 on the microbiota in Crohn's disease. *Curr Opin Biotechnol* 40:97–102, 2016.

91. Martin TD, Chan SS, Hart AR: Environmental factors in the relapse and recurrence of inflammatory bowel disease: a review of the literature. *Dig Dis Sci* 60(5):1396–1405, 2015.

92. Colìa R, Corrado A, Cantatore FP: Rheumatologic and extraintestinal manifestations of inflammatory bowel diseases. *Ann Med* 48(8):577–585, 2016.

93. Ungar B, Kopylov U: Advances in the development of new biologics in inflammatory bowel disease. *Ann Gastroenterol* 29(3):243–248, 2016.

94. Pardi DS: Diagnosis and management of microscopic colitis. *Am J Gastroenterol* 112(1):78–85, 2017.

95. Ohlsson B: New insights and challenges in microscopic colitis. *Therap Adv Gastroenterol* 8(1):37–47, 2015.

96. Canavan C, et al: The epidemiology of irritable bowel syndrome. *Clin Epidemiol* 6:71–80, 2014.

97. Enck P, et al: Irritable bowel syndrome. *Nat Rev Dis Primers* 2:16014, 2016.

98. Deiteren A, et al: Irritable bowel syndrome and visceral hypersensitivity: risk factors and pathophysiological mechanisms. *Acta Gastroenterol Belg* 79(1):29–38, 2016.

99. Meleine M, Matricon J: Gender-related differences in irritable bowel syndrome: potential mechanisms of sex hormones. *World J Gastroenterol* 20(22):6725–6743, 2014.

100. Nasser Y, et al: Using human intestinal biopsies to study the pathogenesis of irritable bowel syndrome. *Neurogastroenterol Motil* 26(4):455–469, 2014.

101. Zhang L, Song J, Hou X: Mast cells and irritable bowel syndrome: from the bench to the bedside. *J Neurogastroenterol Motil* 22(2):181–192, 2016.

102. O'Malley D: Neuroimmune cross talk in the gut. Neuroendocrine and neuroimmune pathways contribute to the pathophysiology of irritable bowel syndrome. *Am J Physiol Gastrointest Liver Physiol* 311(5):G934–G941, 2016.

103. Eisenstein M: Microbiome: bacterial broadband. *Nature* 533(7603):S104–S106, 2016.

104. Ghoshal UC, Srivastava D: Irritable bowel syndrome and small intestinal bacterial overgrowth: meaningful association or unnecessary hype. *World J Gastroenterol* 20(10):2482–2491, 2014.

105. El-Salhy M, et al: Interaction between ingested nutrients and gut endocrine cells in patients with

irritable bowel syndrome (review). *Int J Mol Med* 34(2):363–371, 2014.

106. Fukudo S: Stress and visceral pain: focusing on irritable bowel syndrome. *Pain* 154(Suppl 1):S63–S70, 2013.

107. Konturek PC, Brzozowski T, Konturek SJ: Stress and the gut: pathophysiology, clinical consequences, diagnostic approach and treatment options. *J Physiol Pharmacol* 62(6):591–599, 2011.

108. Drossman DA: Functional gastrointestinal disorders: history, pathophysiology, clinical features and Rome IV. *Gastroenterology* 150: 1262–1279, 2016.

109. Morgan B: Drug development: a healthy pipeline. *Nature* 533(7603):S116–S117, 2016.

110. Tursi A: The role of colonoscopy in managing diverticular disease of the colon. *J Gastrointestin Liver Dis* 24(1):85–93, 2015.

111. Barroso AO, Quigley EM: Diverticula and diverticulitis: time for a reappraisal. *Gastroenterol Hepatol (N Y)* 11(10):680–688, 2015.

112. Scaioli E, et al: Pathophysiology and therapeutic strategies for symptomatic uncomplicated diverticular disease of the colon. *Dig Dis Sci* 61(3):673–683, 2016.

113. Aparicio T, et al: Small bowel adenocarcinoma: epidemiology, risk factors, diagnosis and treatment. *Dig Liver Dis* 46(2):97–104, 2014.

114. Feuerstein JD, Falchuk KR: Diverticulosis and diverticulitis. *Mayo Clin Proc* 2016(8):1094–1104, 2016.

115. Elisei W, Tursi A: Recent advances in the treatment of colonic diverticular disease and prevention of acute diverticulitis. *Ann Gastroenterol* 29(1):24–32, 2016.

116. Kaushik M, et al: Minimally invasive management of complicated diverticular disease: current status and review of literature. *Dig Dis Sci* 61(3): 663–672, 2016.

117. Buckius MT, et al: Changing epidemiology of acute appendicitis in the United States: study period 1993-2008. *J Surg Res* 175(2):185–190, 2012.

118. Ergul E: Heredity and familial tendency of acute appendicitis. *Scand J Surg* 96(4):290–292, 2007.

119. Bhangu A, et al: Acute appendicitis: modern understanding of pathogenesis, diagnosis, and management. *Lancet* 386(10000):1278–1287, 2015.

120. Rogers MB, et al: Acute appendicitis in children is associated with a local expansion of fusobacteria. *Clin Infect Dis* 63(1):71–78, 2016.

121. Leeuwenburgh MM, et al: A simple clinical decision rule to rule out appendicitis in patients with nondiagnostic ultrasound results. *Acad Emerg Med* 21(5):488–496, 2014.

122. Flum DR: Clinical practice. Acute appendicitis-appendectomy or the "antibiotics first" strategy. *N Engl J Med* 372(20):1937–1943, 2015.

123. Gandy RC, Wang F: Should the non-operative management of appendicitis be the new standard of care? *ANZ J Surg* 86(4):228–231, 2016.

124. Russell CE, Wadhera RK, Piazza G: Mesenteric venous thrombosis. *Circulation* 131(18): 1599–1603, 2015.

125. Kärkkäinen JM, Acosta S: Acute mesenteric ischemia (part I)—incidence, etiologies, and how to improve early diagnosis. *Best Pract Res Clin Gastroenterol* 31(1):15–25, 2017.

126. Dattani ND, Horvath R: Acute mesenteric ischemia. *CMAJ* 188(11):820, 2016.

127. Kärkkäinen JM: Acute mesenteric ischemia in elderly patients. *Expert Rev Gastroenterol Hepatol* 10(9):985–988, 2016.

128. Slone EA, Fleming SD: Membrane lipid interactions in intestinal ischemia/

reperfusion-induced injury. *Clin Immunol* 153(1):228–240, 2014.

129. Kärkkäinen JM, Acosta S: Acute mesenteric ischemia (part II)—vascular and endovascular surgical approaches. *Best Pract Res Clin Gastroenterol* 31(1):27–38, 2017.

130. Stephen E, et al: Acute mesenteric ischemia: the what, why, and when? *Indian J Vasc Endovasc Surg* 3:24–28, 2016.

131. Bloom S, Kemp W, Lubel J: Portal hypertension: pathophysiology, diagnosis and management. *Intern Med J* 45(1):16–26, 2015.

132. Møller S, et al: Extrahepatic complications to cirrhosis and portal hypertension: haemodynamic and homeostatic aspects. *World J Gastroenterol* 20(42):15499–15517, 2014.

133. Surani SR, Mendez Y, Anjum H, et al: Pulmonary complications of hepatic diseases. *World J Gastroenterol* 22(26):6008–6015, 2016.

134. Garcia-Tsao G, Bosch J: Varices and variceal hemorrhage in cirrhosis: a new view of an old problem. *Clin Gastroenterol Hepatol* 13(12): 2109–2117, 2015.

135. Chin JL, et al: Non-invasive markers of liver fibrosis: adjuncts or alternatives to liver biopsy? *Front Pharmacol* 7:159, 2016.

136. Sundaram V, Manne V, Al-Osaimi AM: Ascites and spontaneous bacterial peritonitis: recommendations from two United States centers. *Saudi J Gastroenterol* 20(5):279–287, 2014.

137. Pedersen JS, Bendtsen F, Møller S: Management of cirrhotic ascites. *Ther Adv Chronic Dis* 6(3): 124–137, 2015.

138. Tiberi O, et al: Diagnosing and treating hepatic encephalopathy. *Br J Hosp Med (Lond)* 76(11):646, 648-552, 654, 2015.

139. Patidar KR, Bajaj JS: Covert and overt hepatic encephalopathy: diagnosis and management. *Clin Gastroenterol Hepatol* 13(12):2048–2061, 2015.

140. Suraweera D, Sundaram V, Saab S: Evaluation and management of hepatic encephalopathy: current status and future directions. *Gut Liver* 10(4): 509–519, 2016.

141. Winger J, Michelfelder A: Diagnostic approach to the patient with jaundice. *Prim Care* 38(3): 469–482, viii, 2011.

142. Roche SP, Kobos R: Jaundice in the adult patient. *Am Fam Physician* 69(2):299–304, 2004.

143. Vaishnavi C: Translocation of gut flora and its role in sepsis. *Indian J Med Microbiol* 31(4):334–342, 2013.

144. Durand F, et al: Pathogenesis of hepatorenal syndrome: implications for therapy. *Am J Kidney Dis* 67(2):318–328, 2016.

145. Egerod Israelsen M, Gluud LL, Krag A: Acute kidney injury and hepatorenal syndrome in cirrhosis. *J Gastroenterol Hepatol* 30(2):236–243, 2015.

146. Lee WM: Acute liver failure. *Semin Respir Crit Care Med* 33(1):36–45, 2012.

147. Blieden M, et al: A perspective on the epidemiology of acetaminophen exposure and toxicity in the United States. *Expert Rev Clin Pharmacol* 7(3):341–348, 2014.

148. Moreau R, et al: Acute-on-chronic liver failure: recent concepts. *J Clin Exp Hepatol* 5(1):81–85, 2015.

149. Shalimar, Acharya SK: Management in acute liver failure. *J Clin Exp Hepatol* 5(Suppl 1):S104–S115, 2015.

150. Karvellas CJ, Subramanian RM: Current evidence for extracorporeal liver support systems in acute liver failure and acute-on-chronic liver failure. *Crit Care Clin* 32(3):439–451, 2016.

151. Sarin SK, Choudhury A: Acute-on-chronic liver failure: terminology, mechanisms and

management. *Nat Rev Gastroenterol Hepatol* 13(3):131–149, 2016.

152. Tolosa L, Pareja E, Gómez-Lechón MJ: Clinical application of pluripotent stem cells: an alternative cell-based therapy for treating liver diseases? *Transplantation* 100(12):2548–2557, 2016.

153. Liberal R, et al: Cutting edge issues in autoimmune hepatitis. *J Autoimmun* 75:6–19, 2016.

154. Campbell CA, et al: State HCV incidence and policies related to HCV preventive and treatment services for persons who inject drugs—United States, 2015-2016. *MMWR Morb Mortal Wkly Rep* 66(18):465–469, 2017.

155. Centers for Disease Control and Prevention (CDC): *Surveillance for viral hepatitis-United States, 2014.* Last updated June 22, 2016. Available at: http://www.cdc.gov/hepatitis/statistics/ 2014surveillance/commentary.htm#summary.

156. Vaughan G, et al: Hepatitis A virus: host interactions, molecular epidemiology and evolution. *Infect Genet Evol* 21:227–243, 2014.

157. Irving GJ, et al: Hepatitis A immunisation in persons not previously exposed to hepatitis A. *Cochrane Database Syst Rev* (7):CD009051, 2012.

158. Butot S, Zuber S, Baert L: Sample preparation prior to molecular amplification: complexities and opportunities. *Curr Opin Virol* 4:66–70, 2014.

159. Sunbul M: Hepatitis B virus genotypes: global distribution and clinical importance. *World J Gastroenterol* 20(18):5427–5434, 2014.

160. Society for Maternal-Fetal Medicine (SMFM), et al: #38: Hepatitis B in pregnancy screening, treatment, and prevention of vertical transmission. *Am J Obstet Gynecol* 214(1):6–14, 2016.

161. Kuo A, Gish R: Chronic hepatitis B infection. *Clin Liver Dis* 16(2):347–369, 2012.

162. Schinzari V, Barnaba V, Piconese S: Chronic hepatitis B virus and hepatitis C virus infections and cancer: synergy between viral and host factors. *Clin Microbiol Infect* 21(11):969–974, 2015.

163. Brahmania M, et al: New therapeutic agents for chronic hepatitis B. *Lancet Infect Dis* 16(2): e10–e21, 2016.

164. Ringelhan M, et al: The direct and indirect roles of HBV in liver cancer: prospective markers for HCC screening and potential therapeutic targets. *J Pathol* 235(2):355–367, 2015.

165. Michel ML, et al: Therapeutic vaccines in treating chronic hepatitis B: the end of the beginning or the beginning of the end? *Med Microbiol Immunol* 204(1):121–129, 2015.

166. Peters L, Klein MB: Epidemiology of hepatitis C virus in HIV-infected patients. *Curr Opin HIV AIDS* 10(5):297–302, 2015.

167. Tarr AW, Urbanowicz RA, Ball JK: The role of humoral innate immunity in hepatitis C virus infection. *Viruses* 4(1):1–27, 2012.

168. Pawlotsky JM: Hepatitis C virus resistance to direct-acting antiviral drugs in interferon-free regimens. *Gastroenterology* 151(1):70–86, 2016.

169. Tang L, Marcell L, Kottilil S: Systemic manifestations of hepatitis C infection. *Infect Agent Cancer* 11:29, 2016.

170. Smith BD, et al: Recommendations for the identification of chronic hepatitis C virus infection among persons born during 1945-1965. *MMWR Recomm Rep* 61(RR-4):1–32, 2012.

171. Belousova V, Abd-Rabou AA, Mousa SA: Recent advances and future directions in the management of hepatitis C infections. *Pharmacol Ther* 145:92–102, 2015.

172. Taylor JM: Hepatitis D virus replication. *Cold Spring Harb Perspect Med* 5(11):2015.

173. Elazar M, Koh C, Glenn JS: Hepatitis delta infection—current and new treatment options. *Best Pract Res Clin Gastroenterol* 31(3):321–327, 2017.

174. Lhomme S, et al: Hepatitis E pathogenesis. *Viruses* 8(8):2016.

175. Tian Z, Chen Y, Gao B: Natural killer cells in liver disease. *Hepatology* 57(4):1654–1662, 2013.

176. Elewa U, et al: Treatment of hepatitis B virus-associated nephropathy. *Nephron Clin Pract* 119(1):c41–c49, 2011.

177. Morales JM, Kamar N, Rostaing L: Hepatitis C and renal disease: epidemiology, diagnosis, pathogenesis and therapy. *Contrib Nephrol* 176:10–23, 2012.

178. Shiffman ML: Management of acute hepatitis B. *Clin Liver Dis* 14(1):75–91, 2010.

179. Lin J, et al: Virus-related liver cirrhosis: molecular basis and therapeutic options. *World J Gastroenterol* 20(21):6457–6469, 2014.

180. Dunkelberg JC, et al: Hepatitis B and C in pregnancy: a review and recommendations for care. *J Perinatol* 34(12):882–891, 2014.

181. Aspinall EJ, et al: Hepatitis B prevention, diagnosis, treatment and care: a review. *Occup Med (Lond)* 61(8):531–540, 2011.

182. Zhang CY, et al: Liver fibrosis and hepatic stellate cells: etiology, pathological hallmarks and therapeutic targets. *World J Gastroenterol* 22(48):10512–10522, 2016.

183. Ge PS, Runyon BA: Treatment of patients with cirrhosis. *N Engl J Med* 375(8):767–777, 2016.

184. Hill DB, Kugelmas M: Alcoholic liver disease: treatment strategies for the potentially reversible stages. *Postgrad Med* 103(4):261, 267, 1998.

185. Dunn W, Shah VH: Pathogenesis of alcoholic liver disease. *Clin Liver Dis* 20(3):445–456, 2016.

186. Eagon PK: Alcoholic liver injury: influence of gender and hormones. *World J Gastroenterol* 16(11):1377–1384, 2010.

187. Yoon Y-H, Yi H: *Surveillance report #93: liver cirrhosis mortality in the United States, 1970-2009*, Arlington, VA, 2012, U.S. Department of Health and Human Services. Available at: http://pubs.niaaa.nih.gov/publications/Surveillance93/Cirr09.htm.

188. Louvet A, Mathurin P: Alcoholic liver disease: mechanisms of injury and targeted treatment. *Nat Rev Gastroenterol Hepatol* 12(4):231–242, 2015.

189. Division of Population Health, National Center for Chronic Disease Prevention and Health Promotion: *Alcohol and public health*, Atlanta, GA, 2012, Centers for Disease Control and Prevention.

190. Völzke H: Multicausality in fatty liver disease: is there a rationale to distinguish between alcoholic and non-alcoholic origin? *World J Gastroenterol* 18(27):3492–3501, 2012.

191. Farooq MO, Bataller R: Pathogenesis and management of alcoholic liver disease. *Dig Dis* 34(4):347–355, 2016.

192. Alpert L, Hart J: The pathology of alcoholic liver disease. *Clin Liver Dis* 20(3):473–489, 2016.

193. Chayanupatkul M, Liangpunsakul S: Alcoholic hepatitis: a comprehensive review of pathogenesis and treatment. *World J Gastroenterol* 20(20):6279–6286, 2014.

194. Fujii H, Kawada N: Fibrogenesis in alcoholic liver disease. *World J Gastroenterol* 20(25):8048–8054, 2014.

195. Childers RE, Ahn J: Diagnosis of alcoholic liver disease: key foundations and new developments. *Clin Liver Dis* 20(3):457–471, 2016.

196. Koyama Y, et al: New developments on the treatment of liver fibrosis. *Dig Dis* 34(5):589–596, 2016.

197. Yu J, et al: The pathogenesis of nonalcoholic fatty liver disease: interplay between diet, gut microbiota, and genetic background. *Gastroenterol Res Pract* 2016:2862173, 2016.

198. Neuschwander-Tetri BA: Non-alcoholic fatty liver disease. *BMC Med* 15(1):45, 2017.

199. Webb GJ, Siminovitch KA, Hirschfield GM: The immunogenetics of primary biliary cirrhosis: a comprehensive review. *J Autoimmun* 64:42–52, 2015.

200. Carey EJ, Ali AH, Lindor KD: Primary biliary cirrhosis. *Lancet* 386(10003):1565–1575, 2015.

201. Nakamura M: Clinical significance of autoantibodies in primary biliary cirrhosis. *Semin Liver Dis* 34(3):334–340, 2014.

202. Purohit T, Cappell MS: Primary biliary cirrhosis: pathophysiology, clinical presentation and therapy. *World J Hepatol* 7(7):926–941, 2015.

203. Goode EC, Rushbrook SM: A review of the medical treatment of primary sclerosing cholangitis in the 21st century. *Ther Adv Chronic Dis* 7(1):68–85, 2016.

204. Seo N, et al: Sclerosing cholangitis: clinicopathologic features, imaging spectrum, and systemic approach to differential diagnosis. *Korean J Radiol* 17(1):25–38, 2016.

205. Stinton LM, Shaffer EA: Epidemiology of gallbladder disease: cholelithiasis and cancer. *Gut Liver* 6(2):172–187, 2012.

206. Goral V: Gallstone etiopathogenesis, lith and mucin genes and new treatment approaches. *Asian Pac J Cancer Prev* 17(2):467–471, 2016.

207. Bonfrate L, et al: Obesity and the risk and prognosis of gallstone disease and pancreatitis. *Best Pract Res Clin Gastroenterol* 28(4):623–635, 2014.

208. European Association for the Study of the Liver (EASL): EASL clinical practice guidelines on the prevention, diagnosis and treatment of gallstones. *J Hepatol* 65(1):146–181, 2016. Available at: easloffice@easloffice.eu.

209. National Guideline Clearinghouse: *Gallstones*, October 2014. Available at: https://www.guideline.gov/summaries/summary/49014/gallstone-disease.

210. Cremer A, Arvanitakis M: Diagnosis and management of bile stone disease and its complications. *Minerva Gastroenterol Dietol* 62(1):103–129, 2016.

211. Katabathina VS, Zafar AM, Suri R: Clinical presentation, imaging, and management of acute cholecystitis. *Tech Vasc Interv Radiol* 18(4):256–265, 2015.

212. Knab LM, et al: Cholecystitis. *Surg Clin North Am* 94(2):455–470, 2014.

213. Koti RS, Davidson CJ, Davidson BR: Surgical management of acute cholecystitis. *Langenbecks Arch Surg* 400(4):403–419, 2015.

214. Yadav D, Lowenfels AB: The epidemiology of pancreatitis and pancreatic cancer. *Gastroenterology* 144(6):1252–1261, 2013.

215. Hung WY, Abreu Lanfranco O: Contemporary review of drug-induced pancreatitis: a different perspective. *World J Gastrointest Pathophysiol* 5(4):405–415, 2014.

216. Sah RP, et al: New insights into the pathogenesis of pancreatitis. *Curr Opin Gastroenterol* 29(5):523–530, 2013.

217. Feng YC, et al: Study on acute recent stage pancreatitis. *World J Gastroenterol* 20(43):16138–16145, 2014.

218. Banks PA, et al: Classification of acute pancreatitis-2012: revision of the Atlanta classification and definitions by international consensus. *Gut* 62(1):102–111, 2013.

219. Greenberg JA, et al: Clinical practice guideline: management of acute pancreatitis. *Can J Surg* 59(2):128–140, 2015.

220. van Brunschot S, et al: Abdominal compartment syndrome in acute pancreatitis: a systematic review. *Pancreas* 43(5):665–674, 2014.

221. Kuo DC, et al: Acute pancreatitis: what's the score? *J Emerg Med* 48(6):762–770, 2015.

222. Oláh A, Romics L, Jr: Enteral nutrition in acute pancreatitis: a review of the current evidence. *World J Gastroenterol* 20(43):16123–16131, 2014.

223. Bakker OJ, et al: Treatment options for acute pancreatitis. *Nat Rev Gastroenterol Hepatol* 11(8):462–469, 2014.

224. Kokosis G, Perez A, Pappas TN: Surgical management of necrotizing pancreatitis: an overview. *World J Gastroenterol* 20(43):16106–16112, 2014.

225. Majumder S, Takahashi N, Chari ST: Autoimmune pancreatitis. *Dig Dis Sci* 62(7):1762–1769, 2017.

226. Majumder S, Chari ST: Chronic pancreatitis. *Lancet* 387(10031):1957–1966, 2016.

227. American Cancer Society (ACS): *Cancer facts and figures, 2016*. Available at: http://www.cancer.org/research/cancerfactsstatistics/cancerfactsfigures2016/.

228. Prabhu A, et al: The race-specific incidence of esophageal squamous cell carcinoma in individuals with exposure to tobacco and alcohol. *Am J Gastroenterol* 111(12):1718–1725, 2016.

229. Chung CS, Lee YC, Wu MS: Prevention strategies for esophageal cancer: perspectives of the East vs. West. *Best Pract Res Clin Gastroenterol* 29(6):869–883, 2015.

230. Best LM, Mughal M, Gurusamy KS: Non-surgical versus surgical treatment for oesophageal cancer. *Cochrane Database Syst Rev* (3):CD011498, 2016.

231. Segura S, et al: Primary squamous cell carcinoma of the stomach: a case report and review of the literature. *Conn Med* 80(4):209–212, 2016.

232. Nagini S: Carcinoma of the stomach: a review of epidemiology, pathogenesis, molecular genetics and chemoprevention. *World J Gastrointest Oncol* 4(7):156–169, 2012.

233. Chen XZ, et al: Epstein-Barr virus infection and gastric cancer: a systematic review. *Medicine (Baltimore)* 94(20):e792, 2015.

234. Vannella L, Lahner E, Annibale B: Risk for gastric neoplasias in patients with chronic atrophic gastritis: a critical reappraisal. *World J Gastroenterol* 18(12):1279–1285, 2012.

235. Anderl F, Gerhard M: Helicobacter pylori vaccination: is there a path to protection? *World J Gastroenterol* 20(34):11939–11949, 2014.

236. Wang MY, Liu XF, Gao XZ: *Helicobacter pylori* virulence factors in development of gastric carcinoma. *Future Microbiol* 10(9):1505–1516, 2015.

237. Bornschein J, et al: Gastric cancer: clinical aspects, epidemiology and molecular background. *Helicobacter* 16(Suppl 1):45–52, 2011.

238. Compare D, Rocco A, Nardone G: Risk factors in gastric cancer. *Eur Rev Med Pharmacol Sci* 14(4):302–308, 2010.

239. Wang P, et al: Effects of *Helicobacter pylori* on biological characteristics of gastric epithelial cells. *Histol Histopathol* 27(8):1079–1091, 2012.

240. Salaspuro M: Interactions of alcohol and tobacco in gastrointestinal cancer. *J Gastroenterol Hepatol* 27(Suppl 2):135–139, 2012.

241. Colvin H, et al: Hereditary gastric cancer syndromes. *Surg Oncol Clin N Am* 24(4):765–777, 2015.

242. Tan P, Yeoh KG: Genetics and molecular pathogenesis of gastric adenocarcinoma. *Gastroenterology* 149(5):1153–1162, 2015.

243. Wan QS, Zhang KH: Noninvasive detection of gastric cancer. *Tumour Biol* 37(9):11633–11643, 2016.

244. Yoon H, Kim N: Diagnosis and management of high risk group for gastric cancer. *Gut Liver* 9(1):5–17, 2015.

245. Blanchard TG, Czinn SJ: Current status and prospects for a *Helicobacter pylori* vaccine. *Gastroenterol Clin North Am* 44(3):677–689, 2015.

246. Yan L: The journey of personalizing gastric cancer treatment. *Chin J Cancer* 35(1):84, 2016.

247. Reynolds I, Healy P, McNamara DA: Malignant tumours of the small intestine. *Surgeon* 12(5):263–270, 2014.

248. Tammana VS, Laiyemo AO: Colorectal cancer disparities: issues, controversies and solutions. *World J Gastroenterol* 20(4):869–876, 2014.

249. Liang PS, et al: Temporal trends in geographic and sociodemographic disparities in colorectal cancer among Medicare patients 1973-2010. *J Rural Health* 2016 Aug 31. [Epub ahead of print].

250. American Cancer Society (ACS): *Can colorectal cancer be prevented?* Last revised March 1, 2017. Available at: https://www.cancer.org/cancer/colon-rectal-cancer/causes-risks-prevention/prevention.html.

251. Palma S, et al: From molecular biology to clinical trials: toward personalized colorectal cancer therapy. *Clin Colorectal Cancer* 15(2):104–115, 2016.

252. Szylberg Ł, et al: Large bowel genetic background and inflammatory processes in carcinogenesis—systematic review. *Adv Clin Exp Med* 24(4):555–563, 2015.

253. Kawakami H, Zaanan A, Sinicrope FA: Microsatellite instability testing and its role in the management of colorectal cancer. *Curr Treat Options Oncol* 16(7):30, 2015.

254. Dickinson BT, et al: Molecular markers for colorectal cancer screening. *Gut* 64(9):1485–1494, 2015.

255. Yang HM, et al: Molecular and histologic considerations in the assessment of serrated polyps. *Arch Pathol Lab Med* 139(6):730–741, 2015.

256. Guillem-Llobat P, et al: Platelets, cyclooxygenases, and colon cancer. *Semin Oncol* 41(3):385–396, 2014.

257. Burn J, Sheth H: The role of aspirin in preventing colorectal cancer. *Br Med Bull* 119(1):17–24, 2016.

258. Huels DJ, Sansom OJ: Stem vs non-stem cell origin of colorectal cancer. *Br J Cancer* 113(1):1–5, 2015.

259. Lamprecht S, Fich A: The cancer cells-of-origin in the gastrointestinal tract: progenitors revisited. *Carcinogenesis* 36(8):811–816, 2015.

260. Huang C, et al: Analysis of different components in the peritumoral tissue microenvironment of colorectal cancer: a potential prospect in tumorigenesis. *Mol Med Rep* 14(3):2555–2565, 2016.

261. Gaertner WB, et al: Rectal cancer: an evidence-based update for primary care providers. *World J Gastroenterol* 1(25):7659–7671, 2015.

262. Kim SE, et al: Sex- and gender-specific disparities in colorectal cancer risk. *World J Gastroenterol* 21(17):5167–5175, 2015.

263. De Salvo GL, et al: Curative surgery for obstruction from primary left colorectal carcinoma: primary or staged resection? *Cochrane Database Syst Rev* (2):CD002101, 2004.

264. Rath T, Neumann H, et al: High-definition endoscopy with digital chromoendoscopy for histologic prediction of distal colorectal polyps. *BMC Gastroenterol* 15:145, 2015.

265. National Cancer Institute (NCI): *Stage information for colon cancer in colon cancer treatment (PDQ®)-health professional version.* Updated August 12, 2016. Available at: http://www.cancer.gov/types/colorectal/hp/colon-treatment-pdq#cit/section_3.1.

266. National Cancer Institute (NCI): *Colon cancer treatment (PDQ®)-health professional version.* Updated August 12, 2016. Available at: https://www.cancer.gov/types/colorectal/hp/colon-treatment-pdq#section/_45.

267. Ohhara Y, et al: Role of targeted therapy in metastatic colorectal cancer. *World J Gastrointest Oncol* 8(9):642–655, 2016.

268. Ghosn M, et al: Anal cancer treatment: current status and future perspectives. *World J Gastroenterol* 21(8):2294–2302, 2015.

269. National Cancer Institute (NCI): *Rectal cancer treatment (PDQ®)-health professional version.* Updated August 12, 2016. Available at: https://www.cancer.gov/types/colorectal/hp/rectal-treatment-pdq#section/_43.

270. Choo SP, et al: Comparison of hepatocellular carcinoma in Eastern versus Western populations. *Cancer* 122(22):3430–3446, 2016.

271. National Cancer Institute (NCI): *A snapshot of liver and bile duct cancers.* Available at: www.cancer.gov/researchandfunding/snapshots/liverandbileduct.

272. Arzumanyan A, Reis HM, Feitelson MA: Pathogenic mechanisms in HBV- and HCV-associated hepatocellular carcinoma. *Nat Rev Cancer* 13(2):123–135, 2013.

273. Li L, Wang H: Heterogeneity of liver cancer and personalized therapy. *Cancer Lett* 379(2):191–197, 2016.

274. Blechacz B: Cholangiocarcinoma: current knowledge and new developments. *Gut Liver* 11(1):13–26, 2017.

275. Bruix J, Reig M, Sherman M: Evidence-based diagnosis, staging, and treatment of patients with hepatocellular carcinoma. *Gastroenterology* 150(4):835–853, 2016.

276. Kulik LM, Chokechanachaisakul A: Evaluation and management of hepatocellular carcinoma. *Clin Liver Dis* 19(1):23–43, 2015.

277. Ziemlewicz TJ, et al: Hepatic tumor ablation. *Surg Clin North Am* 96(2):315–339, 2016.

278. Raza A, Sood GK: Hepatocellular carcinoma review: current treatment, and evidence-based medicine. *World J Gastroenterol* 20(15):4115–4127, 2014.

279. Simo KA, et al: Multimodality treatment of intrahepatic cholangiocarcinoma: a review. *J Surg Oncol* 113(1):62–83, 2016.

280. Smith I, Kahaleh M: Biliary tumor ablation with photodynamic therapy and radiofrequency ablation. *Gastrointest Endosc Clin N Am* 25(4):793–804, 2015.

281. Dutta U: Gallbladder cancer: can newer insights improve the outcome? *J Gastroenterol Hepatol* 27(4):642–653, 2012.

282. Lowenfels AB, et al: Epidemiology of gallbladder cancer. *Hepatogastroenterology* 46(27):1529, 1999.

283. Pandy M: Risk factors for gallbladder cancer: a reappraisal. *Eur J Cancer Prev* 12(1):15–24, 2003.

284. Wang F, Wang B, Qiao L: Association between obesity and gallbladder cancer. *Front Biosci* 17:2550–2558, 2012.

285. Espinoza JA, et al: The inflammatory inception of gallbladder cancer. *Biochim Biophys Acta* 1865(2):245–254, 2016.

286. Ahn Y, et al: Incidental gallbladder cancer after routine cholecystectomy: when should we suspect it preoperatively and what are predictors of patient survival? *Ann Surg Treat Res* 90(3):131–138, 2016.

287. Kim SW, et al: Gallbladder carcinoma: causes of misdiagnosis at CT. *Clin Radiol* 71(1):e96–e109, 2016.

288. American Cancer Society (ACS): *Survival statistics for gallbladder cancer by stage.* Last revised 2/10/16. Available at: http://www.cancer.org/cancer/gallbladdercancer/detailedguide/gallbladder-survival-rates.

289. Arslan AA, et al: Anthropometric measures, body mass index, and pancreatic cancer: a pooled analysis from the Pancreatic Cancer Cohort Consortium (PanScan). *Arch Intern Med* 170:791–802, 2010.

290. Yeo TP: Demographics, epidemiology, and inheritance of pancreatic ductal adenocarcinoma. *Semin Oncol* 42(1):8–18, 2015.

291. Momi N, et al: Discovering the route from inflammation to pancreatic cancer. *Minerva Gastroenterol Dietol* 58(4):283–297, 2012.

292. Amundadottir LT: Pancreatic cancer genetics. *Int J Biol Sci* 12(3):314–325, 2016.

293. Birtolo C, et al: Phosphatidylinositol 3-kinase: a link between inflammation and pancreatic cancer. *Pancreas* 45(1):21–31, 2016.

294. Kamisawa T, et al: Pancreatic cancer. *Lancet* 388(10039):73–85, 2016.

295. Hart PA, Zen Y, Chari ST: Recent advances in autoimmune pancreatitis. *Gastroenterology* 149(1):39–51, 2015.

296. Bournet B, et al: Targeting KRAS for diagnosis, prognosis, and treatment of pancreatic cancer: hopes and realities. *Eur J Cancer* 54:75–83, 2016.

297. Chang JC, Kundranda M: Novel diagnostic and predictive biomarkers in pancreatic adenocarcinoma. *Int J Mol Sci* 18(3):2017.

298. de Rooij T, et al: Laparoscopic pancreatic surgery for benign and malignant disease. *Nat Rev Gastroenterol Hepatol* 13(4):227–238, 2016.

299. Riviere D, et al: Laparoscopic versus open distal pancreatectomy for pancreatic cancer. *Cochrane Database Syst Rev* (4):CD011391, 2016.

300. Arce KM, et al: Total pancreatectomy and islet cell autotransplantation: definitive treatment for chronic pancreatitis. *Cleve Clin J Med* 83:435–442, 2016.

301. Conroy T, et al: Current standards and new innovative approaches for treatment of pancreatic cancer. *Eur J Cancer* 57:10–22, 2016.

302. Javle M, Golan T, Maitra A: Changing the course of pancreatic cancer-focus on recent translational advances. *Cancer Treat Rev* 44:17–25, 2016.

303. Perone JA, Riall TS, Olino K: Palliative care for pancreatic and periampullary cancer. *Surg Clin North Am* 96(6):1415–1430, 2016.

Alterations of Digestive Function in Children

Sara J. Fidanza, Sharon Sables-Baus

evolve WEBSITE

http://evolve.elsevier.com/McCance/
- Content Updates
- Chapter Summary Review
- Review Questions
- Case Studies
- Animations

CHAPTER OUTLINE

Disorders of the gastrointestinal tract, liver, and pancreas in children include congenital anomalies with structural and functional alterations, enzyme deficiencies, and infections. These disorders lead to impairment of motility, digestion, nutrition, and normal growth and development.

DISORDERS OF THE GASTROINTESTINAL TRACT

Congenital Impairment of Motility
Cleft Lip and Cleft Palate

Cleft lip (CL) and cleft palate (CLP) are embryonic developmental anomalies of the first branchial arch (Fig. 43.1). The incidence of CL with or without CLP is estimated at 1 in 940 live births and the incidence of CLP without CL is estimated at 1 in 1574 live births in the United States between 2004 and 2006.[1] Incidence is lower in black populations and higher in Asian populations.[2] Cleft lip, with or without cleft palate, is more common in males and isolated cleft palate is more common in females. Both anomalies can be unilateral or bilateral, partial or complete, and may also be associated with other malformations. *Nonsyndromic (isolated) CLP* is a malformation with an incomplete separation between nasal and oral cavities without any associated anomaly (70% of cases). Syndromic CLP is associated with other malformations (e.g., Crouzon syndrome [craniofacial dysostosis], Treacher Collins syndrome [mandibulofacial dysostosis], hemifacial microsomia).[3]

In most cases, cleft lip and cleft palate are caused by multiple gene-environmental interactions, including maternal deficiency of B vitamins (B_6, folic acid, and B_{12}), maternal smoking and alcohol intake, steroid or statin use, maternal hyperhomocysteinemia, and maternal diabetes mellitus as well as many gene mutations.[4] (This phenomenon, called *multifactorial inheritance*, is discussed in Chapter 5.) Together these factors reduce the amount of neural crest mesenchyme that migrates into the area that will develop into the face of the embryo.[5]

PATHOPHYSIOLOGY. Cleft lip is caused by the incomplete fusion of the nasomedial and intermaxillary processes beginning during the fourth week of embryonic development, a period of rapid fetal growth. The cleft causes structures of the face and mouth to develop without the normal restraints of encircling lip muscles. The facial cleft may affect not only the lip but also the external nose, the nasal cartilages, the nasal septum, and the alveolar processes (bony ridge of the maxilla that contains the tooth sockets). The cleft is usually just beneath the center of one nostril. The defect may occur bilaterally and may be

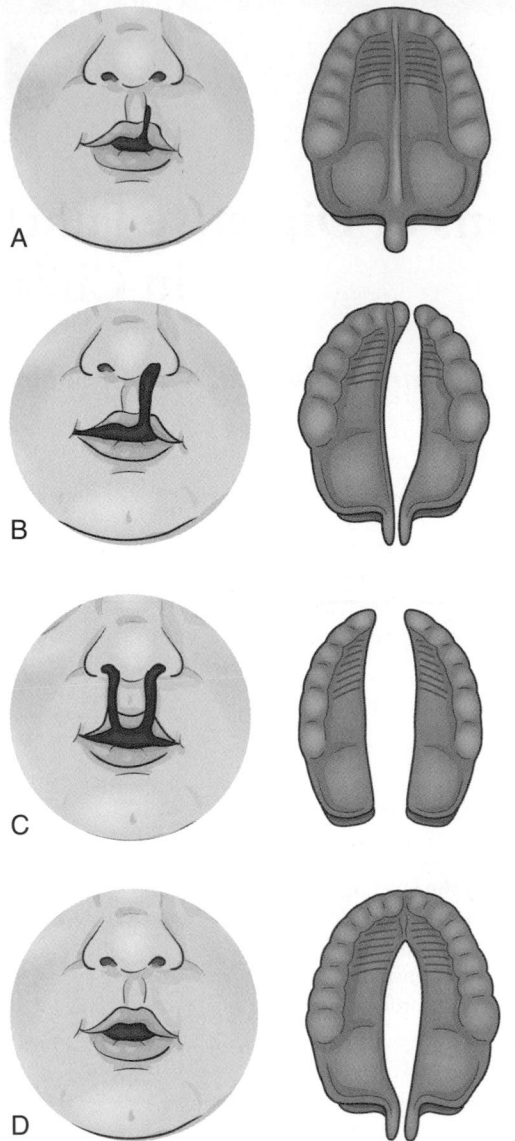

FIGURE 43.1 Variations in Clefts of the Lip and Palate. **A,** Notch in vermilion border. **B,** Unilateral cleft lip and palate. **C,** Bilateral cleft lip and cleft palate. **D,** Cleft palate.

symmetrical or asymmetrical. The cleft can range in severity from a slight indentation of the lip to a fissure that extends to the nostril, causing a sagging and flattening of the nose. The failure of lip fusion by 35 days' gestation may impair closure of the palatal shelves. The more complete the cleft lip, the greater the chance that teeth in the line of the cleft will be missing or malformed.

Cleft palate is often associated with cleft lip but may occur without it. Cleft palate results from the failure of the primary palatal shelves, or processes, to fuse during the third month of gestation. The fissure may affect only the uvula and soft palate, or it may extend forward to the nostril and involve the hard palate and the maxillary alveolar ridge. It may be unilateral or bilateral, with the cleft occupying the midline posteriorly and as far forward as the alveolar process, where it deviates to the involved side. Clefts involving the palate only are usually but not necessarily in the midline. In some cases the vomer process and nasal septum are partly or completely undeveloped. When these facial bones are involved, the nasal cavity may freely communicate with the oral cavity. Teeth in the cleft palate area may be missing or deformed.[6]

◆**CLINICAL MANIFESTATIONS.** Clefts of the lip or palate, or both, are immediately recognizable disruptions of normal facial structure. Feeding difficulty is the most significant clinical manifestation because of the oronasal communication and the inability to generate negative pressure needed for normal sucking.[7] There also may be swallowing difficulty.

◆**EVALUATION AND TREATMENT.** Prenatal diagnosis is made by ultrasound, and postnatal imaging confirms the extent of bone deformity. Soft tissue alterations are evaluated by history and physical examination. The nature and extent of the cleft, the infant's condition, and the method of surgical correction proposed determine the course of treatment. Surgical correction is planned at about the third to sixth month and may be performed in stages and may include preoperative nasal alveolar molding.[8] There are limited long-term outcome studies.[9]

Feeding the infant with cleft lip usually presents no difficulty if the cleft lip is simple and the palate intact. A baby with a complete cleft palate requires consultation with a feeding and swallowing specialist to ensure adequate and safe nutritional intake. Bottles with nipples specialized for feeding an infant with a cleft palate are required. Breast-feeding may be possible for some infants.[7] An orthodontic prosthesis for the roof of the mouth may facilitate sucking for some infants. Parental education and support is required for the long-term care of children with cleft palate. Longitudinal monitoring requires a cleft/orofacial multidisciplinary team including a plastic surgeon, speech therapist, orthodontist, and nurse.[10] The child should be evaluated for hearing loss.

Esophageal Malformations

The estimated incidence of congenital malformations of the esophagus is 1 in 3500 live births.[11] Other congenital malformations are present in up to 50% of cases. Esophageal atresia (EA) is the most common, where the esophagus ends in a blind pouch. EA is usually accompanied by a fistula between the esophagus and the trachea (tracheoesophageal fistula [EA/TEF]). Either defect can occur alone (Fig. 43.2). Environmental risk factors include maternal exposure to methimazole, exogenous sex hormones, infectious diseases, alcohol, or cigarette smoke; maternal diabetes; advanced maternal age; and maternal employment in agriculture.[12] There is a high frequency of anomalies and syndromes associated with esophageal atresias.[13] Two syndromes in particular are associated with esophageal atresia[14]:

- VACTERL (*V*ertebral anomalies, *A*nal atresia, *C*ardiac malformations, *T*racheoesophageal fistula, *E*sophageal atresia, *R*enal anomalies and *r*adial aplasia, and *L*imb anomalies)
- CHARGE (*C*oloboma, *H*eart defects, *A*tresia of the choanae, *R*etardation of mental and/or physical development, *G*enital hypoplasia, and *E*ar abnormalities)

◆**PATHOPHYSIOLOGY.** The pathogenesis of esophageal abnormalities is unknown, but postviral, infectious, environmental, and genetic factors have been suggested.[15] Defective growth of endodermal cells and impaired embryonic foregut development of the trachea and esophagus[16] lead to atresia.[16]

◆**CLINICAL MANIFESTATIONS.** Antenatal diagnosis of EA/TEF increases with the findings of polyhydramnios (excessive amniotic fluid) on ultrasound.[17] Swallowed amniotic fluid is usually absorbed into the placental circulation; therefore if the fetus cannot swallow, amniotic fluid accumulates in the uterus. EA will be diagnosed at birth on the basis of drooling, inability to swallow secretions or choking with feeding, respiratory distress, and inability to pass an orogastric tube. Confirmation is established by a radiopaque catheter, which determines the location of the atresia on x-ray. If a fistula connects the trachea with the distal esophagus, the abdomen fills with air and becomes distended, possibly interfering with breathing (see Fig. 43.2, *C* to *E*). Intermittent cyanosis may result.

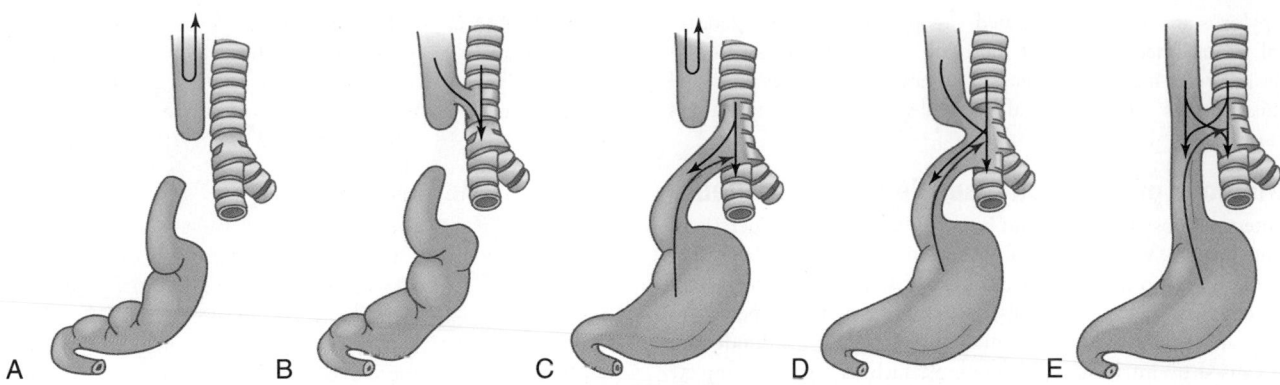

FIGURE 43.2 Five Types of Esophageal Atresia and Tracheoesophageal Fistulae. A, Simple esophageal atresia. Proximal esophagus and distal esophagus end in blind pouches, and there is no tracheal communication. Nothing enters the stomach; regurgitated food and fluid may enter the lungs. **B,** Proximal and distal esophageal segments end in blind pouches, and a fistula connects the proximal esophagus to the trachea. Nothing enters the stomach; food and fluid enter the lungs. **C,** Proximal esophagus ends in a blind pouch, and a fistula connects the trachea to the distal esophagus. Air enters the stomach; regurgitated gastric secretions enter the lungs through the fistula. **D,** Fistula connects proximal and distal esophageal segments to the trachea. Air, food, and fluid enter the stomach and the lungs. **E,** Simple tracheoesophageal fistula between otherwise normal esophagus and trachea. Air, food, and fluid enter the stomach and the lungs from the mouth through the fistula; and regurgitated gastric secretions enter the lungs through the fistula. Between 85% and 90% of esophageal anomalies are type C; 6% to 8% are type A; 3% to 5% are type E; and less than 1% are type B or D. **NOTE:** Type F, esophageal stenosis, is not shown.

Pulmonary complications are compounded by reflux of air and gastric secretions into the tracheobronchial tree through the fistula, causing severe chemical irritation. Infants with esophageal atresia but no fistulae have scaphoid (boat-shaped), gasless abdomens. In infants with fistulae but without atresia (see Fig. 43.2, *E*), the usual symptoms are recurrent aspiration, pneumonia, and atelectasis that remains unexpressed for days or even months. Late complications of esophageal atresia or tracheal esophageal fistula include stricture, reflux, dysphagia, chronic cough, and dyspnea on exertion.[18]

◆**EVALUATION AND TREATMENT.** Infants presenting with esophageal atresia are evaluated with ultrasound, echocardiogram, and vertebral and limb radiographs. Following diagnosis, a tube should be placed into the upper pouch and continuous suction should be applied to decrease the risk of aspiration. The head of the bed should be elevated slightly to assist drainage of the upper pouch. The infant should not be fed orally. Surgical repair is completed in the majority of cases and may be done in stages.[19] The overall survival rate for infants with esophageal defects is 95%.[20]

Infantile Hypertrophic Pyloric Stenosis

Infantile hypertrophic pyloric stenosis (IHPS) is the most common cause of intestinal obstruction in infancy. It is an acquired narrowing and distal obstruction of the pylorus and a common cause of postprandial vomiting. Its presentation most commonly occurs in the first few weeks or months of life.[21] The incidence of pyloric stenosis is approximately 2 to 5 in 1000 live births for males and 1 in 1000 live births for females.[22]

The causes of IHPS are multifactorial and may include environmental and hereditary factors. Potential etiologic factors include deficiency of nitric oxide synthase containing neurons, abnormal innervation of the myenteric plexus, the presence of infantile hypergastrinemia, and exposure to macrolide antibiotics. Whites are affected more often than blacks or Asians, and full-term infants are affected more often than premature infants. The cause is unknown but increased gastrin secretion by the mother in the last trimester of pregnancy raises the likelihood of pyloric stenosis in the infant. The overproduction of gastric secretions

in the infant may be caused by stress-related factors in the mother. Exogenous administration of prostaglandin E is associated with an increased incidence of pyloric stenosis. There is an increased incidence of pyloric stenosis in those children who have a family member with pyloric stenosis, suggesting a genetic predisposition.[23]

◆**PATHOPHYSIOLOGY.** Individual muscle fibers thicken, particularly the circular and longitudinal muscular layers of the pylorus, so the entire pyloric sphincter becomes enlarged and inflexible.[23] The mucosal lining of the pyloric opening is folded and the lumen is narrowed by the encroaching muscle. Because of the extra peristaltic effort necessary to force the gastric contents through the narrow pylorus, the muscle layers of the stomach may become hypertrophied as well.

◆**CLINICAL MANIFESTATIONS.** Between 2 and 3 weeks after birth, an infant who has fed well and gained weight begins forceful, nonbilious vomiting immediately after feeding.[24,25] The infant then demands to be refed. Constipation occurs because little food reaches the intestine.

In severe untreated cases, increased gastric peristalsis and vomiting lead to severe fluid and electrolyte imbalances (hypokalemic, hypochloremic metabolic alkalosis), malnutrition, and weight loss that can be fatal within 4 to 6 weeks. Infants with pyloric stenosis are irritable because of hunger, and they may have esophageal discomfort caused by repeated vomiting and esophagitis. The vomitus may be blood streaked because of rupture of gastric and esophageal vessels.

◆**EVALUATION AND TREATMENT.** Diagnosis is based on the history and clinical manifestations, such as nonbilious vomiting or regurgitation, which often is described as projectile, after which the infant is still hungry. The force and timing of the vomiting can help distinguish IHPS from gastroesophageal reflux, for which episodes of vomiting are not forceful and occur 10 minutes or more after feeding. The hypertrophied pylorus is palpable as a firm, small, movable mass, approximately the size of an olive, and is felt in the right upper quadrant in 70% to 90% of infants with pyloric stenosis. A visible gastric peristaltic wave after eating is observed in some infants. Ultrasound will show the hypertrophied pyloric muscles and narrowed pyloric channel.

The standard treatment for hypertrophic pyloric stenosis is corrective surgery, specifically a laparoscopic pyloromyotomy, in which the muscles of the pylorus are split and separated. Preoperative and postoperative medical management to correct fluid and electrolyte imbalance has been the key to the high success rate and low complication rates associated with this surgery.[26] Children usually can tolerate feeding several hours after surgery.[26]

Obstructions of the Duodenum, Jejunum, and Ileum

High intestinal obstruction should be considered whenever persistent vomiting occurs. With duodenal obstruction there will be upper abdominal distention, visible peristaltic waves, a decrease in the size and frequency of meconium stools, progressive weight loss, persistent vomiting, and dehydration. Congenital obstruction of the duodenum can be caused by intrinsic malformations, such as atresia (complete blockage), stenosis (partial obstruction or narrowing), or external pressure by a choledochal cyst or annular pancreas, and occurs in 2.5 to 10 per 100,000 live births.[27] Duodenal atresia is the third most common atresia of the gastrointestinal tract and is the failure of canalization during embryonic development because of an ischemic event or genetic factors. Duodenal obstruction may be partial or complete and is usually located at or near the major duodenal papilla. The classic "double bubble" sign is seen on imaging of the abdomen and represents duodenal obstruction. The larger, proximal "bubble" is air in a dilated stomach. The more distal, smaller "bubble" is air in a dilated proximal duodenum. There is usually little or no air in the bowel distal to the obstruction. Double bubble also may be seen on prenatal ultrasounds. An annular pancreas—a defect in which the head of the pancreas surrounds part of the duodenum—can obstruct the duodenum. Congenital obstructions of the jejunum and ileum can be attributable to atresia, stenosis, meconium ileus, megacolon (Hirschsprung disease), intussusception, Meckel diverticulum, intestinal duplication, or strangulated hernia. In ileal or jejunal atresia, the intestine ends blindly, proximal and distal to an interruption in its continuity, with or without a gap in the mesentery. Stenosis (narrowing of the lumen) causes dilation proximal to the obstruction and luminal collapse distal to it.

Intestinal Malrotation

Intestinal malrotation is the most common congenital anomaly of the small intestine. It has an estimated incidence of about 0.5%. Associated abnormalities are common and include duodenal, jejunal, or biliary atresia; pancreatic malformations; and heart defects.[28]

◆**PATHOPHYSIOLOGY.** In malrotation, the small intestine lacks a normal posterior fixation because it has only a rudimentary attachment near the origin of the superior mesenteric artery (Fig. 43.3). When rotation does not occur, the colon remains in the upper right quadrant where an abnormal membrane or band called a periduodenal band (Ladd band) may press on and obstruct the duodenum (Fig. 43.3, D). The mobile loops of intestine can twist upon themselves (volvulus) from the duodenojejunal junction to the middle of the transverse colon. The twisting can partly or completely occlude the superior mesenteric artery, causing infarction and necrosis of the entire midgut.

◆**CLINICAL MANIFESTATIONS.** Most cases of malrotation-associated volvulus and infarction develop during the neonatal period (90% of cases involve children younger than 1 year). Some develop during childhood or even adulthood.[29] Classic symptoms in infants are intermittent or persistent bile-stained vomiting after feeding and epigastric distention as the stomach and duodenum are dilated. Dehydration and electrolyte imbalance may occur rapidly with vomiting. Fever usually ensues with pain and scanty stools. Diarrhea and bloody stools are associated with progressive volvulus, vascular compression, and infarction of the intestine. Intermittent or partial volvulus may be seen in older children and adults. It may be asymptomatic or cause minor abdominal discomfort and be discovered during unrelated abdominal surgery.[30]

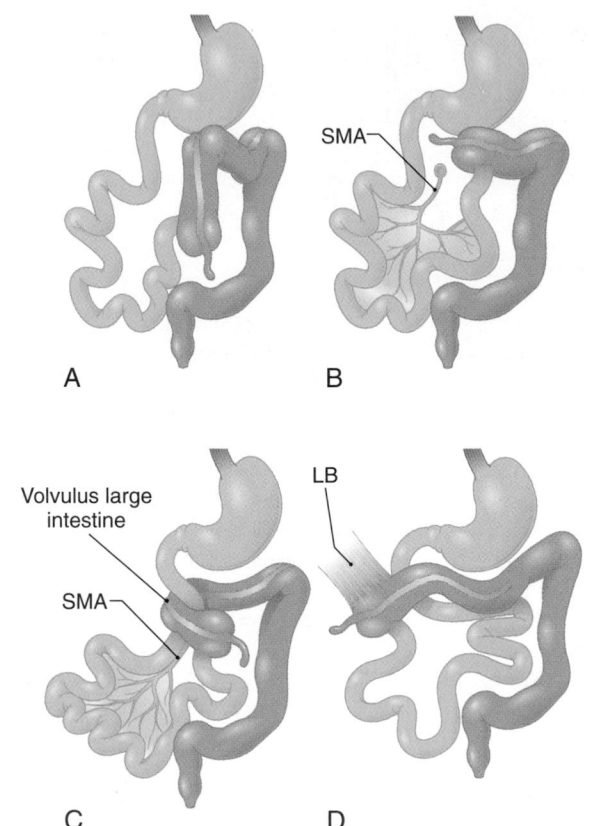

FIGURE 43.3 Variations of Intestinal Malrotation. **A,** Nonrotation. **B,** Incomplete rotation. **C,** Midgut volvulus with duodenal obstruction and obstruction of superior mesenteric artery blood flow. **D,** Incomplete rotation with Ladd bands extending from the lateral and posterior abdominal wall to the subhepatic cecum. *LB,* Ladd band; *SMA,* superior mesenteric artery. (From Gilbert-Barness E et al: *Potter's pathology of the fetus, infant and child,* ed 2, Philadelphia, 2007, Mosby.)

◆**EVALUATION AND TREATMENT.** Diagnosis of malrotation with volvulus and infarction is based on clinical manifestations, upper gastrointestinal contrast imaging, and explorative laparoscopy. Treatment includes laparoscopic or open Ladd procedure to reduce the volvulus.[31] Necrotic bowel is resected and a primary anastomosis performed. An enterostomy may be created. Most children have a good outcome; however, there is risk for adhesion-related bowel obstruction in about 15% of cases and its long-term sequelae.[32]

Meckel Diverticulum

Diverticula are small outpouches, or sacs, that have formed and pushed outward through weak spots of the intestinal wall. Meckel diverticulum is a true diverticulum in that it contains all layers of the intestinal wall and is a remnant of the embryonic yolk sac. It is the most prevalent congenital abnormality of the small bowel and is usually located in the distal ileum. Ectopic gastric mucosal cells are contained in the diverticuli and may cause peptic ulcer and painless bleeding or mimic colonic diverticulitis. Often referred to as *the rules of 2s,* a Meckel diverticulum occurs in approximately 2% of the general population, is typically located within 2 feet of the ileocecal valve (on the antimesenteric border of the ileum), is an average 2 inches in length, and its clinical symptomatology often occurs before 2 years of age. Meckel diverticulum develops when there is failure to obliterate the omphalomesenteric duct, which normally leaves a fibrous band that connects the small intestine to the umbilicus during the first months of fetal development. Ectopic gastric mucosal cells are contained in the diverticuli and may cause peptic ulcer. Although most Meckel diverticuli are asymptomatic, the most common symptom is painless rectal bleeding. Intestinal obstruction, intussusception, and volvulus occur more commonly in adults. Diagnosis is made by symptom presentation and imaging studies. Radionucleotide scintigraphy shows the gastric mucosal cells in the diverticuli. Treatment in those with symptoms is surgical resection.[33]

Hirschsprung Disease

Hirschsprung disease, congenital aganglionic megacolon, is a functional obstruction of the colon. It is the most common cause of colon obstruction, accounting for about one-third of all gastrointestinal obstructions in infants. The incidence is approximately 1 in 5000 live births with an increased incidence in males, siblings of children with Hirschsprung disease, and children with Down syndrome or other congenital malformations.[34] Familial occurrence is 5% to 20%. The exact cause is unknown but multiple interacting factors, including gene mutations and epigenetic mechanisms, have been described.[35]

◆**PATHOPHYSIOLOGY.** Hirschsprung disease is a congenital malformation resulting from failure of neural crest cells to migrate into the gastrointestinal (GI) tract. There is an absence of parasympathetic nervous system intrinsic ganglion cells in the submucosal and myenteric plexuses (Meissner and Auerbach plexuses) along variable lengths of the colon, and there may be skipped segments. Lacking neural stimulation, the muscle layers of the colon wall fail to propel feces through the colon, leading to functional obstruction. In 80% of cases the aganglionic segment is limited to the rectosigmoid region (short-segment Hirschsprung disease); in about 5% of cases the entire colon lacks ganglion cells and the ileum may be involved. The abnormally innervated colon impairs fecal movements, causing the proximal colon to become distended, hence the term *megacolon* (Fig. 43.4). In rare cases the entire bowel can be involved, known as *total intestinal Hirschsprung disease*.

◆**CLINICAL MANIFESTATIONS.** The infant typically becomes symptomatic during the first 24 to 72 hours after birth with delayed passage of meconium. Mild to severe constipation is the usual manifestation of Hirschsprung disease with poor feeding, poor weight gain, and progressive abdominal distention. However, diarrhea may be the first sign because only water can travel around the impacted feces. With

"ultrashort-segment" Hirschsprung disease, mild constipation is generally the only symptom. These children may not be diagnosed until adulthood.

The most serious complication in the neonatal period is Hirschsprung-associated enterocolitis (HAEC) and it can occur both preoperatively and postoperatively. The intestinal inflammation is related to fecal impaction, alterations in intestinal microbiota, impaired mucosal barrier function, and innate immunity with bacterial translocation.[36,37] Bowel dilation stretches and partly occludes the encircling blood and lymphatic vessels, causing edema, ischemia, infarction of the mucosa, and significant outflow of fluid into the bowel lumen. Copious liquid stools result. Infarction and destruction of the mucosa enable enteric microorganisms to penetrate the bowel wall. Frequently, gram-negative sepsis occurs, accompanied by fever and vomiting. Severe and rapid fluid and electrolyte changes may take place, causing hypovolemic or septic shock or death.

◆**EVALUATION AND TREATMENT.** Radiocontrast enema and anorectal manometry are screening tools for the diagnosis of Hirschsprung disease. The definitive diagnosis is made by rectal biopsy showing an absence of ganglion cells in the submucosa of the colon. Surgery is the definitive treatment in all cases of Hirschsprung disease with resection of the aganglionic segment and anastomosis of the proximal bowel to the anus, known as a *"pull-through" procedure*. Laparoscopic or open approaches may be used.[38] In general, the prognosis of Hirschsprung disease is satisfactory for children who undergo surgical treatment. Bowel training may be prolonged; however, most children achieve bowel continence before puberty whereas others have long-term constipation or fecal incontinence.[39,40]

Idiopathic Intestinal Pseudo-Obstruction

Idiopathic intestinal pseudo-obstruction is a rare condition characterized by repetitive episodes or continuous symptoms of intestinal obstruction without an obstructing lesion and can occur at any age. Alterations or atrophy of enteric nerves and/or muscles, or of the interstitial cells of Cajal, prevents normal contractions of the intestines and prevents the movement of food, fluid, and air through the intestines. It may have an acute or chronic onset and can be a cause of intestinal failure.[41]

Distal Intestinal Obstruction Syndrome

Distal intestinal obstruction syndrome (DIOS), formerly called *meconium ileus equivalent,* is the partial or complete obstruction of the colon of the terminal ileum by abnormally viscous intestinal contents, particularly after episodes of dehydration or lack of pancreatic enzymes. It is characterized by complete or incomplete intestinal obstruction of viscid fecal accumulation in the terminal ileum and proximal colon and affects approximately 7.4% of children and adults with cystic fibrosis.[42]

Anorectal Malformations

Anorectal malformations (ARMs) represent a spectrum of rare anomalies of the anus and rectum, including anorectal stenosis, imperforate anus, anorectal atresia, and rectal atresia (Fig. 43.5). Persistent cloaca is the most severe type of anorectal malformation and occurs primarily in girls. The rectum, urethra, and vagina fail to develop separately; instead, they drain through a single, common channel onto the perineum.[43] Approximately 40% of infants with anorectal malformations have other developmental anomalies (i.e., Down syndrome, Hirschsprung disease and duodenal atresia, neurogenic bladder, and spinal malformations).[44,45] ARMs occur in approximately 1 in 2500 to 1 in 5000 newborns.[46] The cause is unknown but may be associated with altered expression of the sonic hedgehog *(SHH)* gene, which is involved in anorectal development.[47]

Most ARMs are identified in routine physical examination during the neonatal period. Ultrasound and magnetic resonance imaging (MRI) can assist prenatal diagnosis. Types of imperforate anus include the

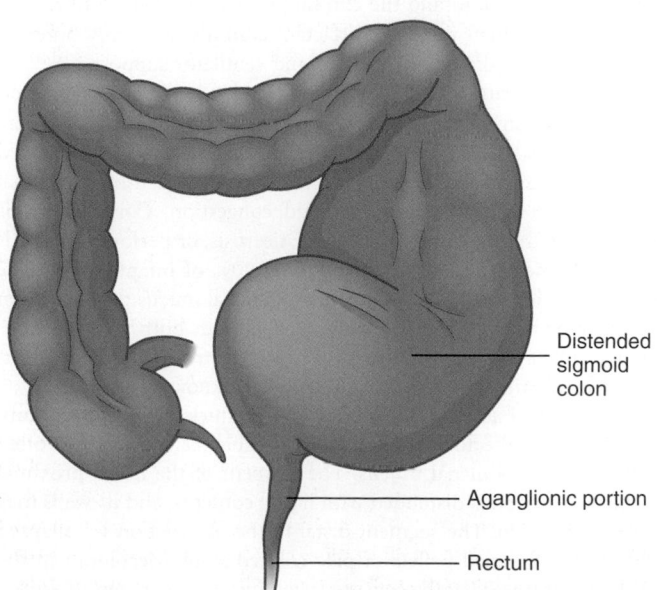

Distended sigmoid colon

Aganglionic portion

Rectum

FIGURE 43.4 Congenital Aganglionic Megacolon (Hirschsprung Disease).

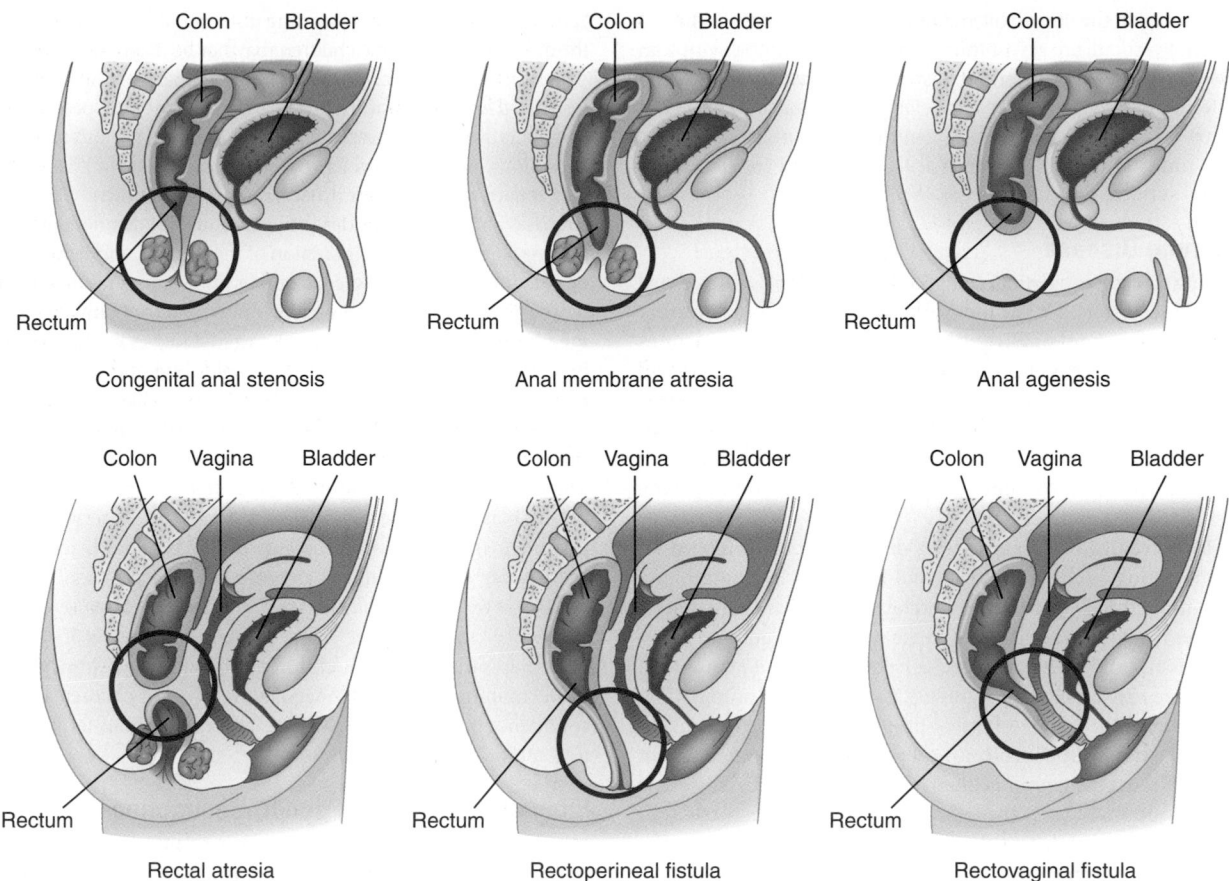

Colon Bladder

Rectum

Congenital anal stenosis

Colon Bladder

Rectum

Anal membrane atresia

Colon Bladder

Rectum

Anal agenesis

Colon Vagina Bladder

Rectum

Rectal atresia

Colon Vagina Bladder

Rectum

Rectoperineal fistula

Colon Vagina Bladder

Rectum

Rectovaginal fistula

FIGURE 43.5 Anorectal Stenosis and Imperforate Anus.

following: the anal opening may be narrow or misplaced; a membrane (covering) may be present over the anal opening; the rectum may not connect to the anus; the rectum may connect to part of the urinary tract or to the reproductive system through an opening called a *fistula*; or the anal opening may not be present. Treatment recommendations depend on the type of imperforate anus, the presence and type of associated abnormalities, and the child's overall health status. Anal stenosis can be treated by dilation. Infants with an imperforate anus and other anorectal malformations require surgical correction. Children with lower lesions and those with an intact sacrum and normal sacral vertebrae and spinal cord have better functional outcomes.[48]

Meconium Syndromes

Meconium is a substance that fills the entire intestine before birth. It is a dark greenish, odorless mass of desquamated cells, mucus, free fatty acids, pancreatic phospholipases, and bile that accumulates in the bowel of a fetus and is typically discharged during the first 12 to 48 hours after birth. Meconium plug syndrome, also termed *functional immaturity of the colon*, is a benign cause of bowel obstruction and a transient disorder of the newborn colon. It is more common in premature infants and characterized by delayed passage of meconium during the first 24 to 48 hours after birth with dilation of the intestine. Meconium plug syndrome is a diagnosis of exclusion. Contrast enema usually excludes congenital small bowel obstruction and rare colon abnormalities, such as atresia or duplication. The main differential consideration is Hirschsprung disease, which is eventually diagnosed in approximately 10% to 30% of children with apparent meconium plug syndrome.[49]

Meconium aspiration syndrome occurs following intestinal peristalsis, meconium release, and contamination of amniotic fluid associated with fetal hypoxia. Gasping respirations cause aspiration of the contaminated amniotic fluid deep into the fetal lung. Infants present with respiratory distress with expiratory airway obstruction, air trapping, surfactant inactivation, atelectasis, and chemical pneumonitis. Meconium aspiration also predisposes to infection and the development of persistent pulmonary hypertension of the newborn with shunting through the patent ductus arteriosus and foramen ovale.[50] The presence of meconium-stained amniotic fluid and the clinical presentation help confirm the diagnosis. Treatment includes surfactant administration (by bolus or lavage), oxygen, inhaled nitric oxide, and ventilator support.[51]

Meconium ileus (MI) is intestinal obstruction in the neonatal period caused by meconium formed in utero that is abnormally sticky. There are two forms of MI: simple and complex. In simple MI, thickened meconium accumulates and obstructs the ileum causing proximal dilatation, bowel wall thickening, and congestion. Complex MI is associated with bowel atresia, volvulus, necrosis, or perforation and is a surgical emergency. MI occurs in up to 20% of infants with cystic fibrosis, and is thought to result from abnormal mucus production in the intestine or impaired pancreatic enzymes, or both.[52] In the cases *not* associated with cystic fibrosis, genes other than *CFTR* mutations have been identified.[53] The cause usually is unknown.

The terminal ileum in MI is plugged with thick, viscous meconium resulting from the formation of an insoluble, calcium-glycoprotein compound in abnormal mucus. The segment of the ileum proximal to the obstruction is distended with liquid contents, and its walls may be hypertrophied. The segment distal to the obstruction is collapsed and filled with small pellets of pale-colored stool. Meconium in the obstructed segment has the consistency of thick syrup or glue. Peristalsis fails to propel this viscous material through the ileum, so it becomes impacted. Volvulus, atresia, or perforation of the bowel occurs in complicated MI.

Abdominal distention usually develops during the first few days after birth. The infant does not pass meconium and begins to vomit within hours or days of birth. Infants with cystic fibrosis may have signs of pulmonary involvement, such as tachypnea, intercostal retractions, and grunting respirations. The distended abdomen shows patterns of dilated intestinal loops that feel doughlike when palpated. Some of the loops contain scattered, firm, movable masses. Despite hyperactive peristalsis, the rectal ampulla is empty.

All women of reproductive age should be offered preconception and prenatal cystic fibrosis (CF) carrier screening (see Chapter 37). Prenatal diagnosis of MI can be made by ultrasound or MRI.[54] The treatment of choice for cases not complicated by volvulus or perforation is a hyperosmolar enema (e.g., meglumine diatrizoate [Gastrografin]) performed under fluoroscopy. A warm saline enema containing 4% *N*-acetylcysteine may be given to help complete the evacuation. Surgical management includes tube enterostomy (a percutaneous drain), open enterostomy, or resection to remove the meconium mass. Survival of infants with meconium ileus is improving, with survival rates approaching 100%.[52] Mortality increases if the obstruction is complicated by peritonitis.

Acquired Impairment of Motility
Gastroesophageal Reflux Disease

Gastroesophageal reflux (GER) is the passage of gastric contents into the esophagus independent of swallowing. GER is normal and non-pathologic in healthy infants and may be asymptomatic or exhibited by regurgitation and vomiting because of relaxation or incompetence of the lower esophageal sphincter. In newborns, gastroesophageal reflux or regurgitation is normal (physiologic reflux) because neuromuscular control of the gastroesophageal sphincter is not fully developed. The frequency of reflux is highest in premature infants and decreases during the first 6 to 12 months of life. Children usually outgrow their reflux. Gastroesophageal reflux disease (GERD) is different from GER and occurs when it is the cause of troublesome symptoms or complications, or both, described as esophageal or extraesophageal in nature. Children at greatest risk for complicated GERD are those with prematurity, neurologic impairment, esophageal atresia, obesity, hiatal hernia, achalasia, chronic lung diseases, and certain genetic disorders, including cystic fibrosis.

◆**PATHOPHYSIOLOGY.** GERD is influenced by genetic, environmental, anatomic, hormonal, and neurogenic factors. Although transient lower esophageal sphincter relaxations (TLESRs) are the most common pathophysiologic cause of GER, inadequate adaptation of sphincter tone to changes in abdominal pressure also may be implicated. Factors that maintain lower esophageal sphincter integrity in children include the location of the gastroesophageal junction in a high-pressure zone within the abdomen, mucosal gathering within the sphincter, and the angle at which the esophagus is inserted into the stomach. Reflux persists if any one of these pressure-maintaining factors is altered. Other mediators of GER are esophageal peristalsis or clearance, mucosal resistance that mediates the noxiousness of the refluxate, and delayed gastric emptying. Reflux of acidic gastric contents results in inflammation of the esophageal epithelium (esophagitis) and stimulation of the vomiting reflex.

Eosinophilic esophagitis is differentiated from GERD (see Chapter 42) and can occur in children. It is thought to be an allergic esophageal disease involving reactions to food antigens. A mast cell, eosinophil, and T lymphocyte infiltrate are associated with inflammation of the entire esophagus that is nonresponsive to acid-suppression therapy. Eosinophilic inflammation may lead to *progressive subepithelial fibrosis* with esophageal strictures, narrowing, and dysphagia.[55] Dysphagia, food impaction, and vomiting are common symptoms and other atopic diseases, such as asthma and eczema, may be present. Treatment includes elimination of aggravating foods and administration of oral corticosteroids.[56]

◆**CLINICAL MANIFESTATIONS.** The clinical manifestations of GERD include excessive regurgitation or vomiting; food refusal/anorexia; unexplained crying, choking, or gagging; sleep disturbance; dysphagia; and abdominal or epigastric pain, or both.[57] Esophageal complications of GER can be significant, such as esophagitis, hemorrhage, stricture, Barrett esophagus (metaplasia; see Chapter 42) and, rarely, adenocarcinoma. Extraesophageal symptoms include cough and wheezing, laryngitis, pharyngitis, dental erosions, sinusitis, recurrent otitis media, and Sandifer syndrome (a neurologic disorder).[58] This constellation of symptoms is often indistinguishable from those of cow's milk protein allergy, which may coexist with or overlap GERD.

◆**EVALUATION AND TREATMENT.** The clinical manifestations are often adequate to confirm a diagnosis of GERD. However, irritability, crying, feeding refusal, and regurgitation can be common problems in infants and not specific to GERD. Esophageal pH monitoring with or without impedance using a 24-hour pH probe and endoscopy with biopsy are used for diagnosis when there are unusual symptoms or treatment failure. Mild GER resolves without treatment usually within 12 months. Techniques for managing infant reflux include small, frequent feedings; prolonged feeding duration and slower flow rate; frequent burping and position changes; and thickened feedings.[59,60] Lifestyle changes for children and adolescents include weight loss, smoking cessation, sleeping position changes, and avoidance of caffeine, chocolate, alcohol, and spicy foods.

Medications are used to treat erosive esophagitis, including gastric acid suppression therapy with proton pump inhibitors (e.g., esomeprazole) and prokinetic agents (e.g., bethanechol).[61] Routine use of medications requires caution because of adverse side effects.[62] If no improvement is seen with medical management or if the child has life-threatening events with reflux, an antireflux surgical procedure, including gastropexy and fundoplication, is performed. A fundoplication re-creates a valve by wrapping the fundus of the stomach around the lower esophagus and can be completed using laparoscopic techniques.[63]

Intussusception

Intussusception is the telescoping of a proximal segment of intestine into a distal segment, causing an obstruction. It is the most common cause of small bowel obstruction in children with rates of hospitalization at about 4.0 to 5.5 per 10,000 children yearly in the United States.[64] Most cases occur between 5 and 7 months of age with seasonal peaks between fall and winter. Intussusception is more common in males and can be idiopathic, can be associated with lead points (polyps or tumors, Meckel diverticulum, intestinal adhesions) or cystic fibrosis, or can develop immediately after abdominal surgery. The health benefits of rotavirus vaccination far exceed the risk of intussusception.[64]

◆**PATHOPHYSIOLOGY.** In intussusception, the ileum commonly telescopes into the cecum and part of the ascending colon by collapsing through the ileocecal valve (ileocolic intussusception), although it can occur anywhere from the duodenum to the rectum. The proximal portion of the intestine (the intussusceptum) collapses into the distal portion (intussuscipiens) in the direction of peristaltic flow (Fig. 43.6). The intussusceptum then drags its mesentery into the enveloping lumen, causing an intussusception. Initially, the mesentery is constricted, obstructing venous return. Compression of the mesenteric vessels between the two layers of intestinal wall and at the U-shaped angle at either end of the intussusceptum leads within hours to venous stasis, engorgement, edema, exudation, and further vascular compression. The tension of the mesentery on the intussusceptum tends to arch the bowel in a curve with its center at the mesenteric root. Edema and compression obstruct

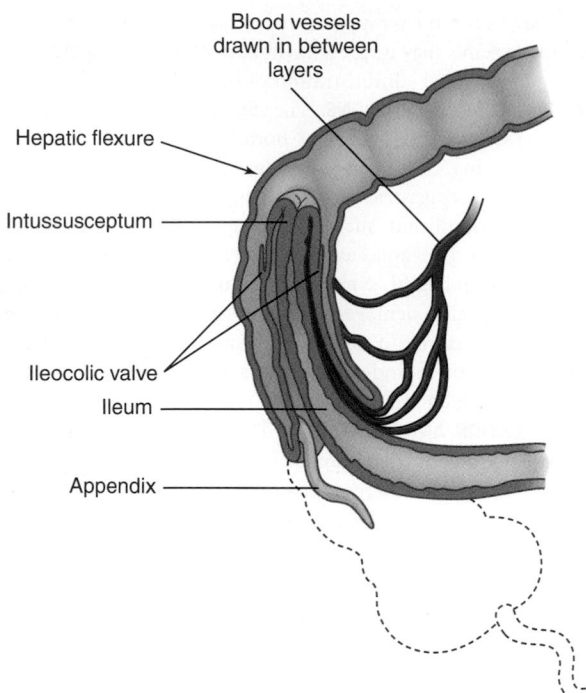

Blood vessels
drawn in between
layers

Hepatic flexure

Intussusceptum

Ileocolic valve

Ileum

Appendix

FIGURE 43.6 Ileocolic Intussusception.

the flow of chyme through the intestine. Unless the intussusception is treated, bleeding, necrosis, and bowel perforation ensue.

◆**CLINICAL MANIFESTATIONS.** The classic symptoms of intussusception include colicky abdominal pain, irritability, knees drawn to the chest, abdominal mass, vomiting, and bloody (currant-jelly) stools. A single normal stool may be passed, evacuating the colon distal to the apex of the intussusception. All of these symptoms may not occur and intussusception has been discovered incidentally by computed tomography (CT) or magnetic resonance imaging (MRI) scan for other indications.

◆**EVALUATION AND TREATMENT.** Diagnosis is based on clinical manifestations and onset of symptoms. Ultrasound of the abdomen and radiographic imaging studies are commonly completed for diagnosis.[65] For large bowel intussusception, an enema reduction is usually effective and avoids the progression to ischemia and perforation. Surgical reduction is done on children who fail or, in rare cases, have perforation.[66] Untreated intussusception in infants is nearly always fatal. Most infants recover if the intussusception is reduced within 24 hours. Spontaneous reduction of intussusception may occur in symptomatic or asymptomatic children.[67]

Appendicitis

Appendicitis is common in children between the ages of 10 and 11 years.[68] The mechanisms of disease, symptoms, and treatment are similar to those for adults and can be reviewed in Chapter 42.

Impairment of Digestion, Absorption, and Nutrition
Cystic Fibrosis

Cystic fibrosis (CF) is an autosomal recessive disease of the exocrine glands that involves multiple organ systems but primarily the gastrointestinal and respiratory systems. Prognosis is mainly determined by the degree of pulmonary involvement, with death caused by a combination of respiratory failure and cor pulmonale. This section focuses on gastrointestinal complications of CF (Chapter 37 discusses epidemiology and pulmonary involvement).

◆**PATHOPHYSIOLOGY.** The gastrointestinal presentation of CF is caused by a dysfunction of the CF transmembrane regulator (CFTR) protein, which is located on epithelial membranes and regulates chloride and sodium ion channels. It is found throughout the airways, sweat glands, digestive tract, pancreas, hepatobiliary system, and reproductive system (also called *mucoviscidosis* or *fibrocystic disease of the pancreas*). The hallmark pathophysiologic triad of CF includes obstruction, infection, and inflammation that are evident throughout the gastrointestinal tract and within the airways. The full spectrum of involvement is summarized in Table 43.1.

Dysfunction of the CFTR protein results in altered sodium, chloride, and potassium resorption, all of which remain external to the surface of the epithelial membrane with reduced clearance from tubular structures lined by affected epithelia. Maldigestion of proteins, carbohydrates, fats, and fat-soluble vitamins occurs because mucus obstruction of the pancreatic ducts blocks the flow of pancreatic enzymes, causing intestinal malabsorption and degenerative and fibrotic changes in the pancreas and gastrointestinal tract. Diabetes mellitus commonly develops as CFTR protein mutation results in dysregulation of beta-cell insulin secretion.[69]

◆**CLINICAL MANIFESTATIONS.** Clinical manifestations are presented in Table 43.1. Gastrointestinal symptoms often precede pulmonary manifestations. Approximately 85% of those with CF present early in life with pancreatic insufficiency (PI). PI is the cause of nutrient malabsorption and failure to thrive (FTT) in children with CF. Steatorrhea and abdominal distention are common symptoms with potential sequelae that include distal intestinal obstruction syndrome (DIOS) (see the Obstructions of the Duodenum, Jejunum, and Ileum section), fibrotic colonopathy, intussusception, and focal biliary cirrhosis. Children who are pancreatic sufficient (PS) are at greater risk of developing pancreatitis in addition to many other gastrointestinal complications, including gastrointestinal cancers and hepatobiliary abnormalities, which may lead to pancreatic transplant or death.[70,71]

◆**EVALUATION AND TREATMENT.** All states in the United States screen newborns for cystic fibrosis using a blood test to detect immunoreactive trypsinogen. Genetic screening and the sweat test are required for diagnosis. To determine the extent of pancreatic function, 72-hour fecal fat measurements are used, which are not easily obtained. Therefore the most common measurement of fat malabsorption is the level of fecal elastase. A serum test for trypsinogen level also can be used to detect pancreatic insufficiency in children older than 8 years of age.

The goal of treatment for PI is to reduce malabsorption of nutrients and improve growth. Most children with CF take pancreatic enzyme replacement therapy (PERT) for the rest of their lives. PERT is administered before or with every meal, snack, or enteral feeding supplementation. High doses of PERT are associated with DIOS; therefore minimal effective doses are indicated. High-caloric, high-protein diets with frequent snacks and vitamin supplements are used to treat malnutrition. Enteral supplements are used as needed.[72] Nutritional status and growth should be carefully monitored, and growth hormone may be included with nutritional supplements.[73]

Celiac Disease (CD)

Celiac disease (CD also known as *celiac sprue* or *gluten-sensitive enteropathy*), is an autoimmune disease that damages the small intestinal villous epithelium when there is ingestion of gluten (gliadin), which is commonly found in the wheat, rye, barley, and oats of cereal grains. CD is a multiorgan disease with a strong genetic predisposition associated with human leukocyte antigen DQ2 (HLA-DQ2) and HLA-DQ8. The disease has a prevalence of about 1% worldwide although evidence suggests only 10% to 15% of the population have been diagnosed and treated.[74] Nonceliac gluten sensitivity (GS) should not be confused

TABLE 43.1	PATHOPHYSIOLOGY, CLINICAL MANIFESTATIONS, AND COMPLICATIONS OF CYSTIC FIBROSIS		
ORGAN INVOLVED	**SECRETORY DYSFUNCTION**	**CLINICAL MANIFESTATIONS**	**COMPLICATIONS**
Sweat glands	Elevated concentrations of sodium and chloride in sweat	Hyponatremia; hypochloremia	Heat prostration; shock
Esophagus	None	Gastroesophageal reflux	Risk for aspiration events
Intestine			
Newborn	Viscid meconium	Meconium ileus with intestinal obstruction	Meconium peritonitis
Older child and adult	Inspissated (dried out) mucofecal masses (intestinal sludging)	Partial intestinal obstruction with severe cramping pains	Gastroesophageal reflux Volvulus (obstruction), intussusception (prolapse) Distal intestinal obstruction syndrome
Pancreas (enzyme deficiency)	Inspissation and precipitation of pancreatic secretions, causing obstruction of pancreatic ducts	Absence of pancreatic enzymes, causing malabsorption of food; fatty, bulky stools Decreased vitamins A, D, E, and K absorption Growth failure	Hypoproteinemia; iron deficiency anemia; malnutrition Recurrent pancreatitis, pancreatic cysts Vitamins A, D, E, and K deficiency and rectal prolapse Decreased bone density and risk of fractures in adolescents and adults
	Insulin deficiency	Glucose intolerance	Diabetes mellitus
Liver	Inspissation and precipitation of bile in biliary system	Focal biliary cirrhosis; shrunken, "hobnail" liver	Portal hypertension with esophageal varices, hematemesis and hypersplenism Hepatic steatosis Focal biliary cirrhosis Steatorrhea from lack of bile salts
Salivary glands	Inspissation and precipitation of secretions in small ducts of submaxillary and sublingual salivary glands	Mild patchy fibrosis of salivary glands	None
Paranasal structures	Viscid mucus	Retention of mucus; clouding seen on sinus roentgenograms	Mucopyoceles (pus accumulations) with nasal deformity or orbital cavity extension
Nose	Nasal polyps	Obstruction of nasal airflow	None
Lungs	Viscid mucus in bronchioles and bronchi	Obstruction of bronchioles causing bronchiolectasis, bronchiectasis, and chronic lung infection	Hemoptysis; pneumothorax; cor pulmonale; atelectasis; chronic bacterial infection; respiratory failure
Reproductive tract			
Male	Viscid genital tract secretions during embryologic development, causing failure of formation of normal vas deferens	Delayed puberty Sterility	None
Female	Distention of endocervical epithelial cells with cytoplasmic mucin	Delayed puberty Decreased fertility	Polypoid cervicitis (cervical inflammation) while taking oral contraceptives

Data from Assis DN, Freedman SD: *Clin Chest Med* 37(1):109–118, 2016; Lavelle LP et al: *Radiographics* 35(3):680–695, 2015; Leeuwen L, Fitzgerald DA, Gaskin KJ: *Paediatr Respir Rev* 15(1):69–74, 2014; Marcdante KJ, Kliegman RM, editors: *Nelson essentials of pediatrics,* ed 7, Philadephia, 2014, Saunders; Stalvey MS, Clines GA: *Curr Opin Endocrinol Diabetes Obes* 20(6):547–552, 2013.

with CD. Although it presents similarly after the ingestion of gluten. The individual does not have positive autoantibodies or classic intestinal villous atrophy but instead has variable HLA status with similar symptoms as CD. The cause is unknown and there is not a biologic marker for the disease.[75] IgE-mediated wheat allergy is a gluten-related disorder with gastrointestinal manifestation in younger children (vomiting and/or diarrhea) and dermatitis and wheezing in older children.[76]

The pathogenesis of CD is complex and involves genetic and both cellular and humoral immunologic factors. Environmental factors include early infections, gut microbiota in infants, feeding patterns, and timing and amount of gluten. CD presents with greater frequency in children with type 1 diabetes mellitus, autoimmune thyroid or liver disease, Down syndrome, Turner syndrome, Williams syndrome, selective immunoglobulin A (IgA) deficiency, Addison disease, and first-degree relatives with CD. Individuals with CD are also at greater risk for non-Hodgkin's lymphoma and rarely, small intestinal adenocarcinoma.[77]

◆**PATHOPHYSIOLOGY.** The major pathophysiologic characteristic is an HLA-DQ2- or HLA-DQ8-induced CD4+ T-cell–mediated autoimmune injury to the small intestinal epithelial cells of genetically susceptible individuals. There are increased numbers of intraepithelial lymphocytes, atrophy and flattening of villi, crypt hyperplasia in the upper small intestine, and malabsorption of most nutrients in the presence of cereal gluten, particularly wheat, rye, and barley (Figs. 43.7 and 43.8). The levels of transglutaminase 2 IgA (TG2) and endomysial IgA autoantibodies closely correlate with the acute phase of the disease in the presence of gluten.[78] The atrophy is caused by accelerated shedding of epithelial cells from the villi. To compensate for this loss, epithelial cell production increases, causing hypertrophy of the crypts

of Lieberkühn. Increased cell production is not sufficient to keep pace with cell loss, and the cells are not mature enough to sustain absorptive functions. The microvilli and brush border disappear, leaving patches of bald mucosa. The loss of mucosal surface area and brush-border enzymes leads to severe malabsorption. The pathologic process is most pronounced in the duodenum and jejunum. The ileum may be spared. The severity of disease correlates with the length of the small intestinal mucosa involved.[79]

Damage to the mucosa of the duodenum and jejunum exacerbates malabsorption. The secretion of intestinal hormones, such as secretin

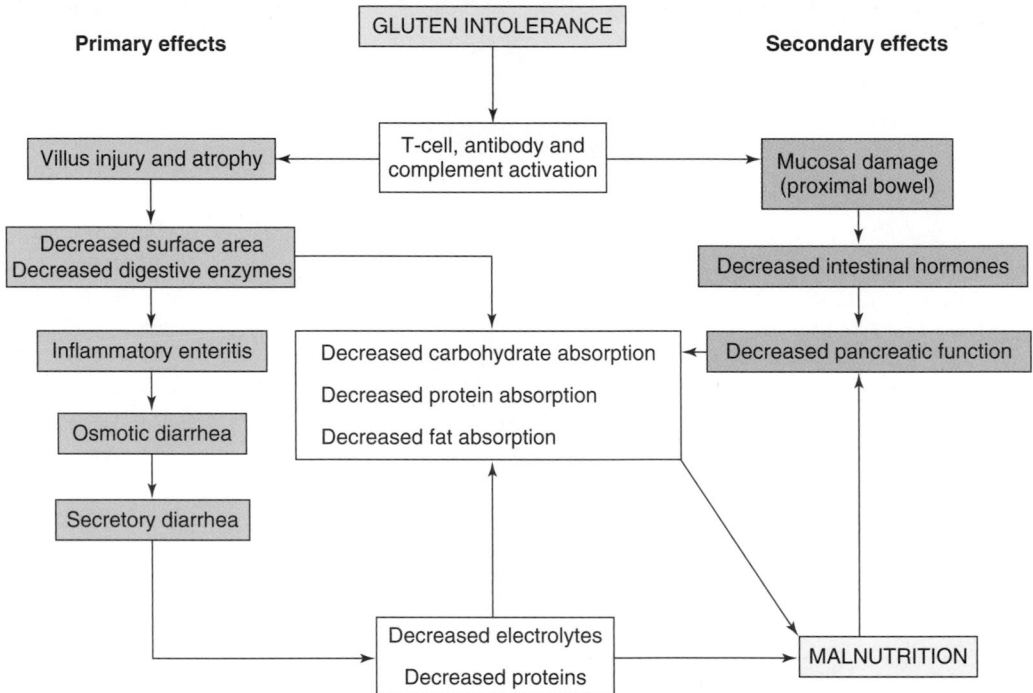

FIGURE 43.7 Pathophysiology of Gluten-Sensitive Enteropathy.

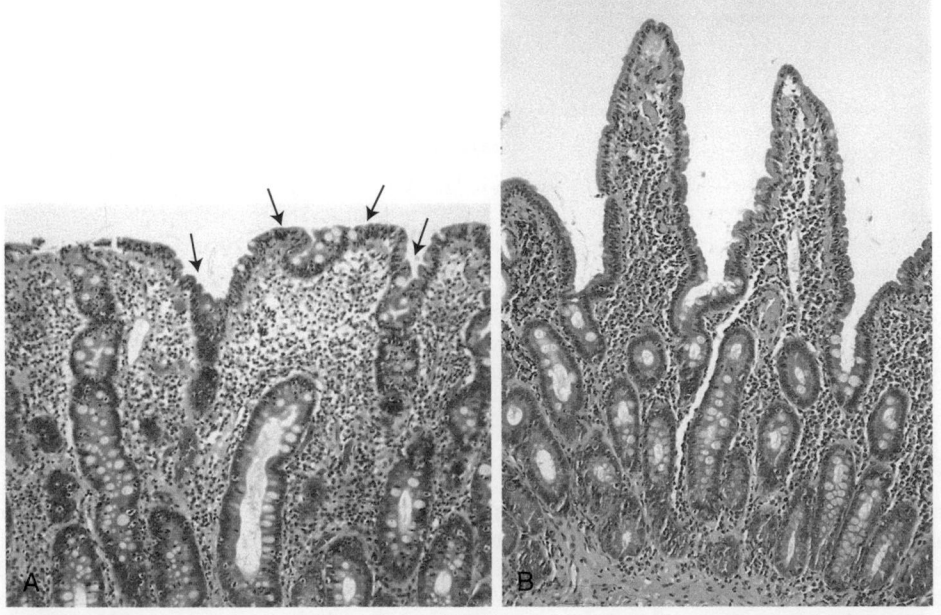

FIGURE 43.8 Gluten-Sensitive Enteropathy. **A,** Atrophy of villi and elongation of crypts that result in reduced surface area, loss of digestive enzymes, and malabsorption *(arrows).* **B,** Recovery of normal villous structure after 6 months of gluten-free diet. (From Damjanov I, Linder J: *Pathology: a color atlas,* St Louis, 2000, Mosby.)

and cholecystokinin, may be diminished. Consequently, secretion of pancreatic enzymes and expulsion of bile from the gallbladder are reduced, contributing to malabsorption. Destruction of mucosal cells causes inflammation, and water and electrolytes are secreted, leading to watery diarrhea. Potassium loss leads to muscle weakness. Magnesium and calcium malabsorption can cause seizures or tetany. Unabsorbed fatty acids combine with calcium, and secondary hyperparathyroidism increases phosphorus excretion, resulting in bone reabsorption. Calcium is no longer available to bind oxalate in the intestine and is absorbed, which causes hyperoxaluria. Gallbladder function may be abnormal, and bile salt conjugation may decrease.

Fat malabsorption in the jejunum is the major cause of steatorrhea (fatty stools). Deficiencies of fat-soluble vitamins are common in children with CD. Vitamin K malabsorption leads to hypoprothrombinemia. In one-third of cases, iron and folic acid malabsorption is manifested as cheilosis; anemia; and a smooth, red tongue. Vitamin B_{12} absorption is impaired in those with extensive ileal disease. Because the absorption of folate and iron is greatest in the proximal small intestine, deficiencies of these substances are common.

◆**CLINICAL MANIFESTATIONS.** The onset of clinical manifestations of CD depends on the age of the infant when gluten-containing substances are added to the diet. In 50% of affected children, onset occurs by 18 months of age; it is not uncommon to be diagnosed later in life. Severity of symptoms can vary tremendously, and children older than 3 years of age can present with mild to severe gastrointestinal symptoms or no symptoms.

Abdominal pain, abdominal distention, and diarrhea are early signs in most infants accompanied by failure to thrive and anemia. The stools are pale, bulky, greasy, and foul smelling, and may contain oil droplets. Three to five such movements occur daily. As early as 3 or 4 months of age, growth failure, anorexia, and constipation can begin. Some children present with constipation. Vomiting and abdominal pain are prominent in infants but unusual in older children. Anorexia is prevalent. The classic physical manifestations of organic failure to thrive, such as abdominal protuberance, wasted buttocks and limbs, and hypotonia, occur in less than 50% of infants with gluten-sensitive enteropathy. Growth is usually diminished.

Extraintestinal manifestations of malabsorption, such as rickets, tetany, frank or occult bleeding, or anemia, may be obvious. Some children urinate more at night. The tongue is smooth and red, and the child may bruise and bleed easily. Hypomagnesemia and hypocalcemia cause irritability, tremor, convulsions, tetany, bone pain, osteomalacia, and dental abnormalities. If vitamin D deficiency is prolonged, rickets and clubbing of the terminal phalanges are likely. Dermatitis herpetiformis is a cutaneous manifestation of itchy blister formation that presents with a symmetrical distribution on the extensor surfaces of the elbows (90%), knees (30%), shoulders, midline of the back, or buttocks. The sacral region, scalp, nuchal area, face, and groin also may be involved. Eighty-six percent of older children have fingerprint changes (ridge atrophy). In older children, delayed puberty and infertility may be a manifestation of otherwise subtle gluten-sensitive enteropathy. There is an increased incidence of malignant disease, particularly T-cell lymphoma, in individuals who have refractory celiac disease (failure to heal after 6 to 12 months of a strict gluten-free diet).[80]

◆**EVALUATION AND TREATMENT.** Diagnosis includes confirmation of clinical findings with serologic measurements of antiendomysial and antitransglutaminase IgA antibodies and HLA-DQ2 or HLA-DQ8 (human leukocyte antigen class II haplotypes that regulate immunity). Duodenal biopsy detects the classic mucosal changes caused by gluten-sensitive enteropathy and confirms the diagnosis. The initial biopsy may be followed by a second intestinal biopsy to demonstrate regeneration of intestinal villi after treatment with a gluten-free diet. Later age diagnosis

is associated with younger age gluten avoidance. Many children with celiac disease remain undiagnosed.[81,82]

Treatment consists of lifelong adherence to a gluten-free diet (GFD), which includes elimination of wheat, rye, barley, and malt. Lactose (milk sugar) intolerance may be present because of damage to the villi; therefore lactose is excluded from the diet but should be resumed after treatment. Infants are routinely given fat-soluble vitamins, iron, and folic acid supplements to treat deficiencies. Breast-feeding at the time of gluten introduction in the diet delays the appearance of celiac disease. Most children have complete remission of symptoms with clearing of serologic markers and an excellent prognosis. Refractory CD is resistant to treatment with a gluten-free diet and is rare. Steroids or immunosuppressants may be required for treatment.[80]

Malnutrition

Pediatric malnutrition is an imbalance between nutrient requirements and intake that results in energy, protein, and micronutrient deficits that negatively impact growth and development. Malnutrition also involves impaired absorption and altered nutrient utilization. Kwashiorkor and marasmus (all forms of inadequate nutrient intake) are the two most common types of malnutrition in children. Collectively, they are known as protein-energy malnutrition (PEM). PEM describes the effects of malnutrition but not the etiology or interactions that contribute to nutrient depletion.

Both Kwashiorkor and marasmus are states of severe long-term starvation and are the result of widespread nutritional deficiencies among children in developing countries and economically destitute populations, particularly when associated with human immunodeficiency virus (HIV) infection.[83] Kwashiorkor refers to edematous malnutrition and usually occurs in infants or children from 1 to 4 years of age who have been weaned from breast milk to a high-starch, protein-deficient diet. The death rate of kwashiorkor is higher than that for marasmus.

Marasmus can occur at any age but it is common in children younger than 1 year. In marasmus, starvation is attributable to lack of protein and carbohydrates, and in neglected children it can have a psychogenic basis. In developing countries and impoverished populations, early weaning of breast-fed infants to overdiluted commercial formulas is a risk factor for marasmus.

Although PEM is common in developing countries, it is underestimated in hospitalized children. A new paradigm used to define pediatric malnutrition includes the concepts of etiology (illness or environmental), identification of pathogenesis and chronicity, associations with inflammation, and resulting impact on functional outcomes.[84]

PEM is a known complication of chronic diseases, such as chronic fever; infectious diseases like tuberculosis; malignancy; digestive and malabsorption disorders; cardiac, pulmonary, renal, and neurologic diseases; burns or hypermetabolic states; anorexia and bulimia; and psychogenic illness. Treatments, such as radiation therapy and chemotherapy, also can contribute to malnutrition. PEM contributes to hospital-acquired conditions (HACs), longer time on mechanical ventilation, increased hospital length of stay, and increased morbidity and mortality.[85]

◆**PATHOPHYSIOLOGY.** The pathogenesis of kwashiorkor is uncertain but includes inadequate dietary protein, leaky gut syndrome (compromised gut barrier), and intestinal inflammation. The lack of sufficient plasma proteins results in generalized edema with a substantial loss of potassium. The liver swells with stored fat because no hepatic proteins are synthesized to form and release lipoproteins. Pancreatic atrophy and fibrosis may be present. Kwashiorkor also causes malabsorption, reduced bone density, and impaired renal function. If the condition is not reversed, the prognosis is very poor.

The metabolic response in marasmus is different, allowing sustained protein and lipid supply during periods of decreased dietary intake. Metabolic processes, including liver function, are preserved, but growth is severely retarded. Caloric intake is too low to support protein synthesis for growth or the storage of fat. Muscle and fat wasting occur, and anemia is common and can be severe.

Recent studies are now implicating alterations in gut microbiota in the pathophysiology of malnutrition.[86] Children with malnutrition show stunting of gut microbiota maturation, which may delay normal development of the gut, depress intestinal immune function, and promote inflammation and infection. Healthy gut bacteria also produce short-chain fatty acids, B vitamins, and vitamin K, and promote the absorption of minerals important for maintaining intestinal epithelium.[87]

◆**CLINICAL MANIFESTATIONS.** Children with kwashiorkor have marked generalized edema, dermatoses, hypopigmented hair, distended abdomen, hepatomegaly, and almost normal weight for age (because of edema). Children with marasmus demonstrate greater wasting of protein and fat stores yet have improved survival. Marasmus is characterized by muscle wasting, fatty liver and hepatomegaly, diarrhea, dermatosis, low hemoglobin level, and infection. There is loss of subcutaneous fat and an absence of edema. Both conditions lead to delays in physical, behavioral, and cognitive development and academic performance. Lastly, micronutrient deficiencies, especially with zinc, selenium, iron, and antioxidant vitamins, can lead to immune deficiency and infections. Severe vitamin A deficiency commonly results in blindness.[88]

◆**EVALUATION AND TREATMENT.** Evaluation of PEM is based on nutritional history and clinical manifestations, including anthropometric measurements. Laboratory monitoring is used to assess for macro- and micronutrient deficiencies, aminotransaminase alterations, and refeeding response. The provision of deficient nutrients will resolve clinical symptoms in 4 to 6 weeks. Use of antibiotics has been shown to improve recovery of PEM and decrease mortality.[89] Developmental sequelae of PEM may be irreversible; therefore early intervention is recommended. Nutritional rehabilitation with appropriate environmental stimulation for infants and young children resolves or improves cerebral shrinkage, physical growth, and psychomotor development. Advances are being made in the preparation of ready-to-use therapeutic food for both home- and community-based malnutrition management.[90] Breast-feeding needs to be encouraged and some infants and children require intensive inpatient treatment.[91] High morbidity and mortality occur in some regions of the world.

Failure to Thrive or Growth Faltering

Failure to thrive (FTT), or growth faltering, is a physical sign demonstrating that a child is receiving inadequate nutrition for optimal growth and development. It is manifested as a deceleration in weight gain, a low weight/height ratio, a low weight/height/head circumference ratio, or a low body mass index (BMI). FTT is a common problem and can present at any time in childhood. Approximately 80% of children present with FTT before 18 months of age.[92]

◆**PATHOPHYSIOLOGY.** Currently, there is a move away from describing FTT as organic versus nonorganic; instead, it is considered a multifactorial condition that includes biologic, psychosocial, and environmental contributions that are illness related or nonillness related (Box 43.1). An underlying medical condition is never found in more than 80% of cases of FTT. Categories of FTT include inadequate caloric intake, inadequate caloric absorption, or excessive caloric expenditure. Infants and children are at risk for FTT if their parents or primary caregivers are unable to provide nurturance.

◆**CLINICAL MANIFESTATIONS.** Clinical manifestations of FTT are delayed growth accompanied by manifestations of malnutrition or an underlying disease (e.g., diarrhea or infectious disease, or both).

BOX 43.1   FACTORS ASSOCIATED WITH FAILURE TO THRIVE OR GROWTH FALTERING

Poverty: food insecurity related to lack of money
Premature birth; low birth weight
Inadequate caloric intake or caloric absorption: infant feeding problems, underlying chronic disease, chronic infection, or malabsorption syndromes
Incorrect preparation of formula (too diluted, too concentrated)
Mechanical feeding difficulties (oromotor dysfunction, congenital anomalies, central nervous system disorders)
Unsuitable feeding habits (food fads, excessive juice)
Behavior problems affecting eating
Disturbed parent-child relationship; parental stress, parental lack of knowledge; child neglect

Data from Krishna A et al: *Glob Health Action* 8:26523, 2015; Kyle UG et al: *Nutr Clin Pract* 30(2):227–238, 2015; Mehta NM et al: *JPEN J Parenter Enteral Nutr* 37(4):460–481, 2013.

Symptoms include delayed growth; pallid or dry, cracked skin and sparse hair; poorly developed musculature; decreased subcutaneous fat; swollen abdomen with malabsorption, diarrhea, or anorexia; and signs of vitamin deficiencies, such as rickets. Social or emotional manifestations include reduced energy level, reduced responsiveness and interaction with the environment, social isolation, spasticity or rigidity when held or touched, inability to make eye contact or smile, refusal to eat, and rejection of foods.[93]

◆**EVALUATION AND TREATMENT.** FTT is suggested if a child falls below the third percentile on the growth curve or shows stagnation in length or weight measurements. Underlying medical conditions are evaluated. If illness is ruled out, a thorough review of psychosocial, emotional, and environmental components of care is necessary. Screening tools are available to assist with evaluation of nutrition status and to guide therapy, particularly in hospitalized children.[94]

Treatment of FTT includes treating an underlying illness if found, increasing volume or caloric density of formula, increasing frequency of breast-feeding (if found to be insufficient), structuring meals and snacks, and adding high-calorie foods and additives. Eliminating fruit juice, soda, or excessive milk also will improve appetite and absorption of nutrients. Medications are used to stimulate appetite. Nutrient deficiencies are supplemented. If unable to gain weight, an oral enteral supplement may be added to the diet or a nasogastric or gastrostomy tube can be used to supplement oral intake.

If the cause is not medical, management then involves the immediate total care of the child and measures to address (1) the psychosocial and emotional problems of the caregivers and (2) parent-child interactions. Counseling, parental modeling, and long-term family support are sometimes required.[95] Hospital admission and evaluation is recommended if the diagnosis is unclear or the child is in nutritional or emotional jeopardy. Eating patterns, food preferences, caloric intake, and family interactions can be assessed and treatment plans implemented during the hospital stay.

Necrotizing Enterocolitis

Necrotizing enterocolitis (NEC) is an acquired disease associated with an ischemic, inflammatory condition that causes bowel necrosis and perforation, and infant death if untreated. NEC is not a specific diagnosis but a constellation of signs and symptoms with several proposed etiologies. It is the most common severe neonatal gastrointestinal emergency that predominantly affects the smallest and most premature infants. Approximately 11% of infants born weighing less than 1500 g will develop NEC; of those, about 30% will not survive.[96] Isolated or focal intestinal perforation is sometimes confused with NEC and generally is not accompanied by an inflammatory component or by diffuse necrosis.[97] The risk of NEC decreases as the gastrointestinal tract matures.

◆**PATHOPHYSIOLOGY.** The exact etiology of NEC is unclear. Factors contributing to the development of NEC include infections, abnormal bacterial colonization, intestinal ischemia, immature immune responses, increases in proinflammatory mediators, immature intestinal motility, altered microcirculatory blood flow and barrier function, perinatal stress, effects of medications and formula feeding, and genetic predisposition.[97] The immature mucosal barrier delays digestion and motility is slower, allowing for the accumulation of noxious substances that damage the intestine, increase permeability, and increase risk for infection. Translocation of intestinal bacteria and other substances contributes to injury, inflammation, development of systemic inflammatory disease, and multiple organ failure and death. Immature intestinal innate immunity and an unfavorable balance between normal and pathogenic bacteria promote intestinal inflammation and release of proinflammatory mediators.[98] Accumulation of gas in the intestine can cause pressure that decreases blood flow, and an imbalance between vasodilator and vasoconstrictor inputs in the immature gut may lead to vasoconstriction, promoting ischemia and oxidative stress, reperfusion injury, necrosis, and perforation. Injury to Paneth cells located in the intestinal crypts has also been proposed.[99] The terminal ileum and proximal colon are most often involved.[100,101]

◆**CLINICAL MANIFESTATIONS.** Manifestations of NEC appear suddenly and usually within weeks of premature birth and sooner for term neonates. Signs and symptoms of "classic" NEC include feeding intolerance, abdominal distention and bloody stools after 8 to 10 days of age, septicemia with elevated white blood cell count, and falling platelet levels. Unstable temperature, bradycardia, and apnea are nonspecific signs. In late preterm infants, NEC is more likely to be associated with other predisposing factors, such as low Apgar scores, chorioamnionitis, exchange transfusions, prolonged rupture of membranes, congenital heart defects, and neural tube defects.

◆**EVALUATION AND TREATMENT.** Diagnosis is based on clinical manifestations, laboratory results, and plain films of the abdomen. Symptoms usually progress rapidly, often within hours, from subtle signs to abdominal discoloration, intestinal perforation, and peritonitis or even death. Abdominal radiographs show pneumoperitoneum, pneumatosis intestinalis (gas in the bowel wall), or unchanging "rigid" loops of small bowel. Systemic hypotension requires intensive medical support or bowel resection, or both. Efforts are in progress to identify predictive biologic markers for early diagnosis including urinary intestinal fatty acid–binding protein; a marker for intestinal cell wall integrity damage; and fecal calprotectin, a marker for intestinal inflammation.[102]

Preventive strategies include awareness of risk factors, encouragement of breast milk feeding, preferential feeding of human milk, judicious fluid management to prevent vascular fluid overload, and confirmation of patent ductus arteriosus (see Chapter 34). Additional treatments include avoidance of H2-receptor antagonists, administration of amino acids (i.e., arginine and glutamine supplements) to support intestinal epithelial cell growth, and utilization of enteral probiotics to support normal gut bacteria.[103,104] The rapid onset of symptoms makes primary prevention difficult.

Treatments include cessation of feeding, implementation of gastric suction to decompress the intestines, maintenance of fluid and electrolyte balance, and administration of antibiotics to control sepsis. Surgical resection is the treatment of choice for perforation, and peritoneal drainage may be used as an adjunct to laparotomy. Overall mortality is high, particularly for infants who have surgery.[96]

Diarrhea

Diarrhea is an increase in the water content, volume, or frequency of stools and can be acute or chronic. Diarrhea is usually defined as three or more watery or loose stools in 24 hours.[105] Children with acute gastroenteritis often remain mildly symptomatic for up to 4 weeks; therefore diarrhea that persists longer than 4 weeks is considered chronic. Diarrhea is a common gastrointestinal problem during infancy and early childhood, and infectious diarrhea is the leading cause of death in young children, particularly among preterm infants and in developing countries.[106] Severe, acute infectious diarrhea occurs one to three times during the first 3 years of life. Most episodes are self-limiting and resolve within 72 hours.

The pathophysiologic mechanisms of diarrhea in children are similar to those described for adults: osmotic, secretory, intestinal dysmotility, or inflammatory (see Chapter 42). Prolonged diarrhea is more dangerous in infants and children because they have much smaller fluid reserves and more rapid peristalsis and metabolism than adults. Therefore dehydration can develop rapidly if any disturbance increases fluid secretion into the gastrointestinal lumen (secretory diarrhea), draws fluid into the lumen by osmosis (osmotic diarrhea), reduces intestinal transit time with luminal fluid retention (intestinal dysmotility), or causes inflammation that results in malabsorption and increased luminal osmotic load from nutrients, fluid, and blood, which may increase gut motility (inflammatory diarrhea).[107]

Diarrhea in Infants and Children

There are numerous causes of diarrhea in infants and young children, including viral, bacterial, and systemic infections; malabsorption syndromes; autoimmune disorders; congenital malformations; and genetic disorders. Acute infection is a common cause of childhood diarrhea worldwide.[106]

Acute infectious diarrhea in infants and young children is usually associated with acute viral or bacterial gastroenteritis, and contaminated food or water is often the source of infection. Viral causes of diarrhea include rotaviruses, noroviruses, and adenoviruses. Rotavirus is the most common cause in young children and is associated with a higher death rate in low-income countries. Rotavirus invades enterocytes of the intestinal mucosa and releases an enterotoxin that damages these cells. Damage decreases viable absorptive surface area, causing an imbalance of secretion and absorption, and increases motility, resulting in diarrhea and dehydration. Recovery from mucosal damage may take several weeks. Rotavirus is transmitted by the fecal-oral route among humans.

Numerous bacteria or parasites can contaminate food or water and cause diarrhea. Specific bacteria can be identified using molecular analysis or stool culture. Bacterial causes of diarrhea have geographical variation and include *Cryptosporidium*, *Shigella* spp., and heat-stable toxin-producing enterotoxigenic *Escherichia coli* (ST-ETEC), *Vibrio cholerae*, *Campylobacter jejuni*, adenovirus 40/41, and *Aeromonas* spp.[108] *Clostridium difficile* is often associated with previous antibiotic therapy.

Infectious diarrhea has a rapid onset, with watery stools sometimes mixed with blood, abdominal cramping, fever, vomiting, and weight loss. Severe dehydration, acidosis, and shock can occur quickly from diarrhea and vomiting. Hemolytic uremic syndrome and renal failure can develop when diarrhea is associated with *Shigella* toxin and *Escherichia coli* infection (see Chapter 40). Other causes of acute diarrhea in the older child include antibiotic therapy, appendicitis, chemotherapy, inflammatory bowel disease, parasitic infestation, parenteral infections, and ingestion of toxic substances.

Treatment of diarrhea requires evaluation of cause by taking the individual's history, testing the stool for common pathogens, and performing laboratory analysis. Treatment of underlying illness is warranted when identified. Other treatments include hydration, electrolyte replacement, nutrition maintenance, and antibiotics if a pathogen is found. Antispasmodics may relieve abdominal cramping, and probiotics can reduce duration and improve morbidity and mortality.[109] Intravenous solutions are used only when oral solutions are not tolerated. Prevention includes clean water, environmental sanitation, and good hygiene. Licensed vaccines are available for rotavirus, cholera, and typhoid fever[110,111] (see *What's New?* Pediatric Inflammatory Bowel Disease).

Primary Lactose Intolerance. Lactose intolerance (lactose malabsorption) is the inability to digest lactose (milk sugar) and is caused by inadequate production or impaired activity of the enzyme lactase. It is a common cause of diarrhea in children, particularly nonwhite children younger than 7 years of age. The congenital form is a rare autosomal recessive disorder that manifests at birth. The malabsorption of lactose results in osmotic diarrhea accompanied by abdominal pain, bloating, and flatulence. Fluids move by osmosis from the vascular compartment into the intestinal lumen. The undigested sugar is processed by the colonic bacteria, and intestinal gas and short-chain fatty acids are produced.[112] Systemic manifestations include skin disease, rheumatologic complaints, chronic fatigue, and failure to thrive.

Diagnosis can be made by eliminating dietary lactose or by performing hydrogen lactose breath testing or an oral lactose tolerance test.[113] Treatment consists of reducing milk consumption or supplementing the diet with oral lactase. Some children can tolerate lactose in fermented forms, such as cheese and yogurt, or by adding soy food. Utilization of a diet low in fermentable oligo-, di-, and monosaccharides and polyols (FODMAPs) or administration of probiotics to alter intestinal flora has been found to be effective in children with lactose-intolerant irritable bowel syndrome who have persistent symptoms. Other sources of dietary calcium or supplements need to be provided if dairy products are eliminated.

DISORDERS OF THE LIVER
Disorders of Biliary Metabolism and Transport
Neonatal Jaundice

Jaundice (icterus) is a yellow pigmentation of the skin caused by an increased level of bilirubin in the bloodstream (i.e., total serum bilirubin [TSB] level that exceeds the 95th percentile for the infant's age in hours or is greater than 20 mg/dL, except in the low birth weight population). Jaundice usually becomes clinically apparent when the serum bilirubin concentration is greater than 2 mg/dL (34 μmol/L). Physiologic jaundice (hyperbilirubinemia) of the newborn is usually a transient, benign icterus that occurs during the first week of life in otherwise healthy full-term infants. It is caused by mild unconjugated (indirect-reacting) hyperbilirubinemia. Pathologic jaundice appears within 24 hours after birth with total serum bilirubin level greater than 20 mg/dL or an indirect bilirubin level greater than 15 mg/dL. Risk factors include fetal-maternal blood type incompatibility (ABO and Rh incompatibility), prematurity, exclusive breast-feeding, maternal age greater than or equal to 25 years, an infant of male gender, delayed meconium passage, and excessive birth trauma such as bruising or cephalohematomas.[114] Prediction tools for hyperbilirubinemia are available to reduce risk associated with early hospital discharge (within 48 hours) when hyperbilirubinemia may not yet be evident.

PATHOPHYSIOLOGY. Pathologic jaundice results from the complex interaction of factors that cause (1) increased bilirubin production (e.g., hemolysis), (2) impaired hepatic uptake or excretion of unconjugated bilirubin, and (3) delayed maturation of liver conjugating mechanisms. The most common cause is hemolytic disease of the newborn, also known as erythroblastosis fetalis[115] (ABO blood incompatibility; see Chapters 9 and 31), and all pregnant women should be tested for ABO and Rh incompatibility. Unconjugated bilirubin (indirect bilirubin) is lipid soluble and bound to albumin in the blood, and in the free form readily crosses the blood-brain barrier in infants. Bilirubin encephalopathy (kernicterus) is caused by the deposition of toxic, unconjugated bilirubin in brain cells and usually does not occur in healthy full-term infants. An elevated level of conjugated bilirubin is a sign of underlying disease (e.g., neonatal cholestasis). A late, acute rising indirect bilirubin level also may be a manifestation of glucose-6-phosphate dehydrogenase (an enzyme important in red blood cell metabolism) deficiency, a hereditary X-linked genetic defect.[115]

◆**CLINICAL MANIFESTATIONS.** Physiologic jaundice develops during the second or third day after birth and usually subsides in 1 to 2 weeks in full-term infants and in 2 to 4 weeks in premature infants. After this, increasing bilirubin values and persistent jaundice indicate pathologic hyperbilirubinemia. Manifestations include yellowing skin, dark urine, light-colored stools, and weight loss. Premature infants with respiratory distress, acidosis, or sepsis are at greater risk for kernicterus and the development of bilirubin-induced neurologic dysfunction (BIND) (e.g., neuromotor signs, hyperexcitable neonatal reflexes, and speech and hearing impairment).[116]

◆**EVALUATION AND TREATMENT.** Jaundice is detected by clinical assessment. Both total and direct (conjugated) bilirubin levels are monitored, and the bilirubin/albumin ratio is being evaluated as a corollary to unbound serum bilirubin level for predicting neurotoxicity, particularly in premature infants.[117] Transcutaneous bilirubin monitoring is readily available.[118] Pathologic jaundice should be suspected with serum bilirubin values that increase greater than 5 mg/dL per day, persistent jaundice (more than 7 to 10 days in the full-term infant), or conjugated bilirubin values greater than 2 mg/dL. Other causes of jaundice must be eliminated to confirm physiologic jaundice.

Treatment depends on the degree of hyperbilirubinemia. Physiologic jaundice is usually treated by phototherapy (ultraviolet light) with good eye protection; several techniques are available. Phototherapy produces isomers of bilirubin that are water soluble, can be more rapidly excreted in the stools and urine, and do not cross the blood-brain barrier. Pathologic jaundice requires high-intensity phototherapy, exchange transfusion, and treatment of the underlying cause.[119] Treatment with tin-mesoporphyrin (a heme oxygenase inhibitor) is useful in severe hyperbilirubinemia.[120]

Biliary Atresia

Biliary atresia (BA) is a rare congenital malformation characterized by the absence or obstruction of extrahepatic bile ducts, resulting in neonatal cholestasis. The etiology of duct injury is not clear but is thought to be related to either an embryonic (or congenital) abnormality or an acquired anomaly (e.g., perinatal viral-induced progressive inflammation with innate autoimmune destruction in genetically susceptible individuals). There is phenotypic variation in the timing of disease onset (embryonic or perinatal—80% of cases) and the association with other anomalies. The disease expression is a continuum in which the principal process is one of bile duct destruction. The atresia of the bile ducts is associated with inflammation, fibrosis, loss of epithelial cells, and obstruction of the bile canaliculi. Progressive obstruction leads to cholestasis and secondary biliary cirrhosis (see Chapter 42), portal hypertension, and liver failure, which can develop within a few weeks after birth. Liver failure can lead to death within 2 years without surgical intervention.[121]

Jaundice is the primary clinical manifestation of BA along with hepatomegaly and acholic (clay-colored) stools. Fat absorption is impaired because of the lack of bile salts. Abdominal distention caused by hepatomegaly and ascites may cause anorexia and FFT. Fat-soluble vitamin (A, D, E, K) deficiencies require supplementation. Manifestations of cirrhosis and liver failure include ascites, hypoalbuminemia, hypercoagulation, pruritus, esophageal varices, and gastrointestinal bleeding that may lead to death.

Early diagnosis of BA is essential with the best outcome occurring when diagnosed and treated in the first 30 to 45 days of life. Late diagnosis of BA does not respond well to current surgical treatment. Diagnosis of BA is based on clinical manifestations, abnormal liver function tests, liver biopsy results, and intraoperative cholangiogram. Serum aminotransaminase and alkaline phosphatase levels are elevated and conjugated (direct) serum bilirubin levels increase progressively.

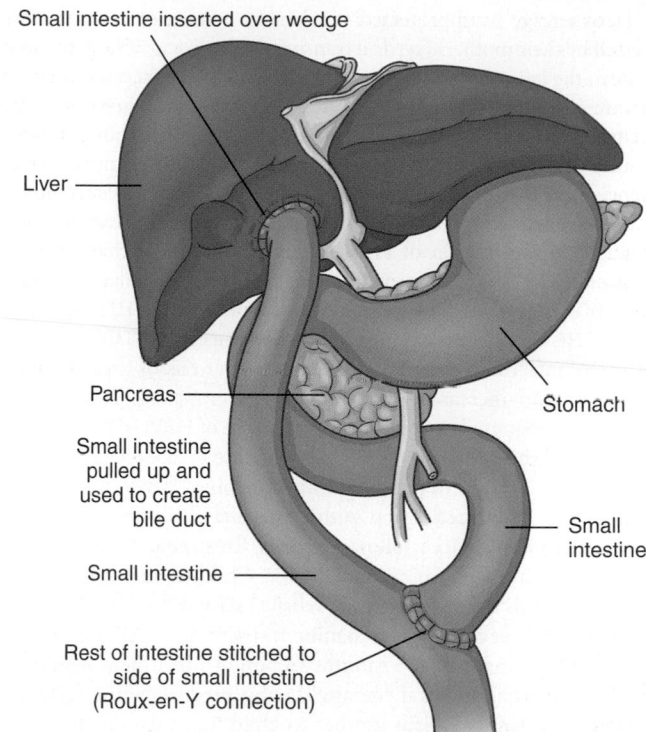

FIGURE 43.9 Kasai Procedure. Surgical correction for extrahepatic biliary atresia. The jejunal segment between the liver and the bowel may be externalized, creating a double-barrel portoenterostomy.

Surgical intervention removes the atretic biliary remnants and creates a Roux-en-Y intestinal conduit for bile drainage, also known as the *Kasai hepatoportoenterostomy* (Fig. 43.9). Even with initial restoration of bile flow, however, obliteration of intrahepatic bile ducts can continue and cirrhosis results. Liver transplantation is performed for 80% of children with BA and is the only long-term therapeutic option.[122]

Inflammatory Disorders
Hepatitis

Details related to viral hepatitis are presented in Chapter 42, including differentiation of types of viruses (see Table 42.7).

Hepatitis A. Approximately one-third to one-half of the reported cases of hepatitis A virus (HAV) occur in children, particularly children of nursery school age.[123] Outbreaks tend to occur in daycare centers with large numbers of children who are not toilet trained and with staff members who practice poor handwashing techniques. Vertical transmission from mother to newborn or from a transfusion is rare. HAV replicates in the liver and is excreted through the biliary system into the stool. HAV in young children is usually mild and asymptomatic but may include nausea, vomiting, and diarrhea. Older children have jaundice and elevated serum aminotransferase levels. Almost all children recover from hepatitis A without residual liver damage. Relapse HAV occurs in 3% to 20% of individuals. Vaccination programs for children 1 year and older have successfully reduced the incidence of HAV in the United States by 95%.[124]

Hepatitis B. Risk factors for hepatitis B virus (HBV) include infants of mothers who are chronic hepatitis B surface antigen (HBsAg) carriers, children from families that immigrated to the United States or are adopted from endemic areas, children who have been infected by HBsAg-positive household contacts, and children who abuse parenteral drugs or engage in unprotected sex. Ninety percent of newborns are infected by their mothers (vertical transmission); 25% to 50% of children between the ages of 1 and 5 years who are acutely infected will develop chronic infection, and 25% will develop cirrhosis or hepatocellular carcinoma.[125] Chronic hepatitis may develop more often in young children because of their immature immune systems. The most serious consequence of HBV infection is fulminant hepatitis, which occurs in 1% of cases. Hepatitis D virus (HDV) infection depends on active infection with HBV. Exacerbation of HBV is more common in children with superinfected HDV. There is evidence that the risk of fulminant hepatitis is higher in individuals with combined infections of HBV, HDV, hepatitis C virus (HCV), or human immunodeficiency virus (HIV) than in those with HBV infection alone. There also is a higher risk of hepatocellular carcinoma and increased mortality in this group. Aggressive HBV vaccination programs have reduced the incidence of HBV; HDV reduction has mirrored this response and there is decreased risk of hepatocellular carcinoma.[126] To prevent perinatal transmission of HBV, immunoprophylaxis and HBV vaccination within the first 12 hours of birth are recommended with close follow-up visits. Treatment is conservative and antivirals are used for chronic disease. Children ages 2 to 17 years who are hepatitis B surface antigen (HBsAg) seropositive for more than 6 months with elevated serum alanine transaminase (ALT) and HBV DNA levels for more than 3 months respond to treatment with antivirals.[127] Maternal antiviral therapy during pregnancy and lactation reduces the hepatitis B virus mother-to-child transmission rate.[128]

Hepatitis C. Hepatitis C virus (HCV) in children is most commonly transmitted vertically and is enhanced with maternal coinfection with HIV. Risk factors for vertical transmission include internal fetal monitoring, prolonged rupture of membranes, and fetal anoxia. HCV transmission also can occur through exposure to infected blood or contaminated materials (as in injection drug use or tattooing and body piercing) and, less commonly, following sexual encounters with HCV-infected partners. Transmission from blood transfusions has become a negligible risk with universal HCV screening of blood. With vertical transmission, spontaneous resolution of HCV is high, up to 40%; otherwise, the disease is usually mild in children and cirrhosis is rare. Treatment is genotype specific with high sustained viral response in children treated with pegylated interferon (Peg-IFN) + ribavirin with HCV genotypes 2 or 3 and about 45% to 55% in those infected with genotypes 1 or 4. Efforts are in progress to develop affordable direct-acting antiviral treatments with fewer adverse drug-related events.[129] Maternal antiviral therapy reduces vertical transmission. There is currently no vaccination available for hepatitis C and only those children with persistently elevated serum aminotransferase levels or progressive liver disease are treated with antiviral drugs.

Chronic Hepatitis. HBV and HCV are the main causes of chronic hepatitis in children. Manifestations of chronic hepatitis include malaise, anorexia, fever, gastrointestinal bleeding, hepatomegaly, edema, and transient joint pain. Often there are no symptoms. Serum alanine aminotransferase and bilirubin levels are elevated. There may be evidence of impairment of synthetic functions of the liver: prolonged prothrombin time, thrombocytopenia, and hypoalbuminemia. Diagnosis is based on the clinical manifestations and liver biopsy. There is no curative therapy for chronic HBV or HCV; hence children are treated with antiviral drugs and should continue to be monitored. About 3% develop cirrhosis or hepatocellular carcinoma before adulthood.[130] Liver transplant may ultimately be required for chronic hepatitis.[131]

There also is an autoimmune form of chronic hepatitis, known as *autoimmune hepatitis (AIH)* or *autoimmune primary sclerosing cholangitis (PSC)*, with unknown etiology. The pathogenic mechanism is thought to be immunologic, environmental, or genetic in nature. PSC is associated with a diagnosis of inflammatory bowel disease (IBD). Advances are being made in identifying serologic markers to guide diagnosis and treatment.[132] Elevations in the levels of aminotransferases, autoantibodies, and immunoglobulin G (IgG) are seen in both AIH and PSC. AIH is more common in female children, and both are treated with prednisone and/or immunosuppressive therapy; about 50% to 80% will achieve remission and long-term survival.[133]

Cirrhosis

Cirrhosis is fibrotic scarring of the liver in response to inflammation and tissue damage, resulting in obstruction to the flow of blood and bile (see Chapter 42). Most forms of chronic liver diseases in children can progress to cirrhosis, but they seldom do. The complications of cirrhosis in children are the same as those in adults: portal hypertension, the opening of collateral vessels between the portal and systemic veins, and varices. In addition, children with cirrhosis experience growth failure caused by nutritional deficits and developmental delay, particularly in gross motor function because of ascites and weakness. The cause of cirrhosis may influence its severity and course. Some types of cirrhosis can be stabilized if the cause is identified and treated early. The risk of cirrhosis is increased in obese children with nonalcoholic fatty liver disease (see *What's New?* Childhood Obesity and Nonalcoholic Fatty Liver Disease).

Portal Hypertension

Portal hypertension is increased pressure in the portal venous system and a major cause of morbidity and mortality in children with liver disease. There are two basic causes of portal hypertension in children: (1) increased resistance to blood flow within the portal system, and (2) increased volume of portal blood flow. The second cause is rare in children and is not discussed here. Increased resistance to flow can occur anywhere in the portal circulatory system. Portal hypertension

---

WHAT'S NEW?

Childhood Obesity and Nonalcoholic Fatty Liver Disease

Nonalcoholic fatty liver disease (NAFLD) is the most common cause of chronic liver disease in children and is associated with obesity, insulin resistance, genetic predisposition, ethnicity, the gut microbiome, and environmental factors (diet and lack of exercise). NAFLD is associated with dyslipidemia, hypertension, and early cardiac dysfunction in children. The rise in childhood obesity worldwide is contributing to the increasing prevalence of NAFLD. The disease usually presents in prepubertal children and is predominant in males and in children of Hispanic origin. Diagnosis is made by exclusion of other causes of the disease, usually by 12 to 13 years of age in the United States. Liver biopsy is required for definitive diagnosis of nonalcoholic steatohepatitis (NASH). Compared to adults, there are differences in the extent of fat, inflammation, and fibrosis in children and there is no standard scoring system. There is no consensus regarding treatment. Exercise and slow, consistent weight loss with a low glycemic index diet have been shown to be more effective than a low-fat diet in lowering body weight. Pharmacologic agents are being evaluated to control insulin resistance and prevent progression of liver disease and cirrhosis. Omega-3 fatty acids, probiotics, and vitamin E may delay disease progression. Research is in progress to define the pathophysiology of NAFLD, measures that can help prevent this disease, and also noninvasive diagnostic procedures.

Data from Clemente MG et al: *World J Gastroenterol* 22(36):8078-8093, 2016; Selvakumar PKC et al: *Pediatr Clin North Am* 64(3):659-675, 2017; Temple JL et al: *Int J Mol Sci* 17(6):E947, 2016.

can accompany cirrhosis, intraabdominal infections, portal vein thrombosis, congenital anomalies of the portal vein, and congenital hepatic fibrosis.

Types of Portal Hypertension

Extrahepatic Portal Hypertension. Extrahepatic (prehepatic) portal venous obstruction causes 50% to 70% of extrahepatic portal hypertension in children. No specific cause can be found in approximately two-thirds of these children. Obstruction is almost always in the portal vein and is usually caused by thrombosis as a complication of abdominal trauma, pancreatitis, abdominal infections, and some systemic disorders; however, these causes are rare. Umbilical infection with or without a history of catheterization of the umbilical vein may be a cause in neonates. It also has been associated with neonatal dehydration, inflammatory bowel disease, and hypercoagulable states, such as protein C and protein S deficiencies.[134] Life-threatening bleeding and coagulation disorders can occur. Mesoportal bypass (anastomosis of the mesenteric vein to the portal vein) restores normal physiologic portal flow to the liver and corrects portal hypertension.[135]

Intrahepatic Portal Hypertension. Liver fibrosis is the primary cause of intrahepatic portal hypertension. The fibrosis can lead to cirrhosis with increased resistance to portal blood flow by constricting and reducing the compliance of hepatic sinusoids. Chronic hepatitis, biliary atresia, nonalcoholic fatty liver disease, and congenital hepatic fibrosis are causes of liver fibrosis in children.

The clinical manifestations of portal hypertension are (1) splenomegaly, (2) upper gastrointestinal tract bleeding, (3) ascites, (4) hepatopulmonary syndrome, (5) hepatorenal syndrome, and (6) hepatic encephalopathy (see Chapter 42).

The objectives of the clinical investigation are to (1) locate the site of the venous block and (2) identify the disease responsible for the portal hypertension. Thorough physical examination; laboratory evaluation of liver function, white blood count, and platelet count; ultrasonographic imaging (e.g., sonoelastography); endoscopic evaluation; and

biopsy may be included in the diagnostic evaluation. Treatment in children is the same as that in adults (see Chapter 42). The outcome of portal hypertension depends almost entirely on its cause. Children with extrahepatic disease are expected to recover with little morbidity. For children with intrahepatic disease, the prognosis varies.

Metabolic Disorders

More than 5000 genetically determined metabolic pathways have been identified in liver tissue. The earliest possible identification of metabolic disorders is essential because (1) early treatment may prevent permanent damage to vital organs, such as the liver or brain; (2) precise genetic counseling may be possible with prenatal diagnosis; and (3) complications can be minimized, even if cure is not possible. Galactosemia,[136] fructosemia, and Wilson disease are rare treatable metabolic disorders that have hepatic clinical manifestations. These disorders are summarized in Table 43.2; Wilson disease is summarized here.

Wilson Disease

Wilson disease (hepatolenticular degeneration) is an autosomal recessive defect of copper metabolism related to loss of *ATP7B* gene expression that causes toxic amounts of copper to accumulate in the liver, brain, kidneys, and corneas. *ATP7B* is localized on chromosome 13 and encodes copper-transporting P-type adenosinetriphosphatase (ATPase) membrane-spanning protein. It is highly expressed in the liver, kidney, and placenta and is expressed in lower levels in the brain, heart, muscle, and pancreas. This defect in the uptake and excretion of copper by hepatocytes is an important cause of progressive liver disease in children and young adults. Wilson disease is very rare, with an incidence of 1 in 30,000 to 1 in 100,000 live births worldwide. About 1 in 90 persons are carriers.[137]

◆**PATHOPHYSIOLOGY.** Two major abnormalities in copper metabolism have been identified: (1) diminished biliary excretion of copper and (2) failure to insert copper into ceruloplasmin (a glycoprotein that transports copper in the blood). A positive copper balance is present

TABLE 43.2 GALACTOSEMIA, FRUCTOSEMIA, AND WILSON DISEASE

	GALACTOSEMIA	FRUCTOSEMIA	WILSON DISEASE
Mechanism of disease	Deficiency of galactose and phosphate, uridyl transferase An autosomal recessive trait Cannot convert galactose to glucose Toxic accumulation of galactose in body tissues, liver, and brain	Deficiency of fructose-1-phosphate aldolase An autosomal recessive trait Cannot metabolize fructose, sucrose, or honey; occurs when breast milk is replaced with cow's milk Toxic accumulation of fructose in body tissues	Autosomal recessive: *ATP7B* gene mutation on chromosome 13 Defect in copper excretion by liver Impaired transport of copper in blood caused by diminished transport protein (ceruloplasmin) Toxic accumulations of copper in liver, brain, kidney, corneas
Clinical manifestations	High levels of blood galactose Vomiting Hypoglycemia May have failure to thrive Symptoms of cirrhosis at 2 to 6 months—jaundice Intellectual disability if not treated Cataracts if not treated	High levels of blood fructose Vomiting Hypoglycemia May have failure to thrive Hepatomegaly Jaundice Seizures	Intention tremors Indistinct speech Dystonia Greenish yellow rings in cornea Hepatomegaly Jaundice Anorexia Renal tubular defects
Evaluation	Presence of reducing substances in urine when infant is receiving lactose	Detailed dietary history Liver or intestinal mucosa biopsy	Low plasma ceruloplasmin
Treatment	Galactose-free diet	Fructose-, sucrose-, honey-free diet Vitamin C supplementation	Chelation therapy to remove copper from body Decreased dietary intake of copper Liver transplant

from birth in children with Wilson disease, despite increased excretion of copper in the urine. Copper toxicity with accumulation in the liver and brain is the major abnormality. Excesses of copper generate free radicals that disrupt cellular organelles, deoxyribonucleic acid (DNA), microtubules, enzymes, and proteins. Copper overload is related to impaired biliary excretion of copper and may be related to failure of hepatocyte lysosomes to eliminate copper by exocytosis.[138]

Early in the disease, intestinal absorption of copper is normal, as is hepatic clearance of albumin-bound absorbed copper. As copper-binding proteins in the liver become saturated, hepatic uptake of copper diminishes, with elevated serum copper levels and biochemical and clinical evidence of liver damage caused by copper accumulation. In later stages of the disease, copper accumulates in extrahepatic tissues, including the eyes, brain, and kidneys.

When cerebral copper-binding proteins become saturated, a characteristic pattern of brain damage develops, particularly in the basal ganglia. Neural effects include intention tremor, unsteady gait, dystonia, and behavioral changes. Manifestations of renal tubular injury usually appear simultaneously. The uptake of copper by red blood cells is thought to cause hemolytic anemia, a condition sometimes seen early in the clinical course of Wilson disease.

◆**CLINICAL MANIFESTATIONS.** The clinical manifestations of Wilson disease may begin as young as 4 years of age, when control mechanisms responsible for copper homeostasis and biliary excretion should have matured. The classic clinical presentation of Wilson disease is a triad of neuromuscular abnormalities, intention tremors, dysarthria (indistinct speech), and dystonia (disordered muscular tonicity): (1) Kayser-Fleischer rings (accumulation of copper in the limbus of the cornea, causing a greenish yellow ring), (2) cirrhosis associated with elevated serum copper levels, and (3) low ceruloplasmin levels.[139] Initial symptoms vary from malaise and abdominal pain to jaundice. Changes in mental and motor performance may develop at age 6 years or into adult life. The earliest signs of liver involvement include enlargement of the liver and spleen, jaundice, and anorexia. Edema and ascites may develop suddenly, or gastrointestinal hemorrhage may be the initial sign of the disease. Occasionally Wilson disease begins with a hemolytic crisis caused by the toxic effects of copper on the red blood cells. Cirrhosis develops in all untreated cases. Copper deposition in the kidneys causes a proximal renal tubular defect that results in losses of glucose, amino acids, phosphate, and uric acid in the urine and renal tubular acidosis. All untreated individuals will develop behavioral or psychiatric disorders.

◆**EVALUATION AND TREATMENT.** Because Wilson disease is rare and has broad clinical manifestations, it may not be diagnosed until older childhood or adulthood. Laboratory tests detect a serum ceruloplasmin concentration less than 30 mg/dL. Serum copper values may be normal or high, and urine copper values are elevated. Liver biopsy confirms structural changes and measures copper concentrations. *ATP7B* gene sequencing can avoid the need for liver biopsy.[140] The goal of therapy is to decrease copper accumulation by decreasing dietary copper intake and intestinal copper absorption, and increasing renal excretion of copper. Medical treatments include D-penicillamine and trientine (copper chelating agents), and zinc and ammonium tetrathiomolybdate (reduces intestinal copper absorption).[141] Liver transplantation is the only therapy for Wilson disease, and gene therapy and hepatocyte cell transplantation are being investigated.[137]

SUMMARY REVIEW

Disorders of the Gastrointestinal Tract

1. Most alterations of digestive function in children are caused by congenital anomalies of the intestinal tract; disorders of digestion, absorption, or nutrition; or liver disease.

2. Cleft lip and cleft palate may occur separately or together, and both defects are associated with multiple gene-environmental interactions and deficiency of B vitamins. The fissure may affect the uvula, soft palate, hard palate, nostril, and maxillary alveolar ridge.

3. *Nonsyndromic (isolated) CLP* is the most common malformation with an incomplete separation between nasal and oral cavities without any associated anomaly.

4. Esophageal atresia, a condition in which the esophagus ends in a blind pouch, may occur with or without tracheoesophageal fistula, a connection between the esophagus and the trachea. As the infant swallows oral secretions or ingests milk, the pouch fills, causing either drooling or aspiration into the lungs.

5. Infantile hypertrophic pyloric stenosis, an obstruction of the pyloric outlet caused by hypertrophy and hyperplasia of circular muscles in the pyloric sphincter, is more common in male infants and may require surgical correction.

6. Intestinal malrotation occurs with failure of the colon to rotate during fetal development, and an obstructing band or volvulus (twisting of the bowel on itself) may partly or completely occlude the gastrointestinal tract and its blood vessels.

7. Meckel diverticulum is an outpouching of all layers of the small intestine caused by failure of the fibrous band that connects the small intestine to the umbilicus.

8. Hirschsprung disease (aganglionic megacolon) is caused by an absence of enteric ganglia and malformation of the parasympathetic nervous system in a segment of the colon, resulting in inadequate colon motility and functional obstruction.

9. Idiopathic intestinal pseudo-obstruction is repetitive episodes or continuous symptoms of intestinal obstruction without an obstructing lesion and may be associated with atrophy of enteric nerves and/or muscles.

10. DIOS, formerly called *meconium ileus equivalent,* can occur when intestinal contents become abnormally thick and obstruct the intestinal lumen. CF, pancreatic enzyme deficiency, and dehydration are common causes.

11. Duodenal, jejunal, and ileal obstructions can be caused by meconium ileus, atresia, peritoneal bands, or acquired obstructive disorders.

12. Malformations of the anus and rectum range from mild congenital stenosis of the anus to complex deformities, all of which are classified as imperforate anus.

13. Meconium aspiration syndrome is a type of newborn respiratory distress caused by fetal inspiration of meconium-contaminated amniotic fluid associated with fetal hypoxic distress and in utero gasping respirations.

14. Meconium ileus is a condition in the newborn in which intestinal secretions and amniotic waste products produce a thick tarry plug that obstructs the intestine, usually from lack of fetal digestive enzymes. From 10% to 15% of neonates with CF have meconium ileus as neonates.

15. GERD is caused by the relaxation or incompetence of the lower esophageal sphincter. Infants are susceptible to reflux because the

SUMMARY REVIEW—cont'd

sphincter is not fully mature, their diet consists of liquids, and they are seldom in an upright position.

16. Eosinophilic esophagitis involves an eosinophilic inflammation of the esophagus with dysphagia and vomiting that can be associated with asthma and eczema.

17. The most common cause of acquired intestinal obstruction in infants is intussusception, a condition in which one portion of the bowel telescopes or invaginates into another. It occurs most commonly in the area of the ileocecal junction.

18. CF is an inherited disease caused by a dysfunction of the CF transmembrane regulator (CFTR) protein with a pathophysiologic triad that includes pancreatic enzyme deficiency (which causes maldigestion), overproduction of mucus in the respiratory tract, and abnormally elevated sodium and chloride concentrations in sweat.

19. Celiac disease is an immune-mediated lifelong disease with a genetic predisposition characterized by the loss of mature villous epithelium in the presence of a gluten-containing diet. It results in malabsorption and growth failure. Nonceliac gluten sensitivity is wheat allergy without the autoantibodies associated with celiac disease.

20. Severe acute malnutrition is a group of disorders resulting from a severe dietary deficiency of proteins (kwashiorkor), carbohydrates, or both (marasmus). Starvation causes stunted mental and physical development. Kwashiorkor occurs most often in toddlers who have stopped breast-feeding and subsist on a high-carbohydrate diet.

21. Failure to thrive or growth faltering is inadequate physical growth of a child associated with multifactorial conditions that include biologic, psychosocial, and environmental contributions resulting in delayed growth and malnutrition.

22. Necrotizing enterocolitis is a disorder in neonates, particularly low birth weight or premature infants, thought to result from stress and anoxia of an immature bowel wall and immature intestinal innate immunity. Bacteria invade the mucosa and can cause colitis, necrosis, intestinal perforation, sepsis, and death.

23. Acute diarrhea in infants and children is often caused by infection from contaminated food and/or water and can rapidly cause dehydration and electrolyte imbalances because fluid reserves are relatively small. The most common cause of acute diarrhea in children is bacterial or viral enterocolitis.

24. Chronic diarrhea (diarrhea persisting longer than 4 weeks) can be caused by a wide variety of underlying conditions and often leads to growth failure and delayed development.

25. Lactose malabsorption and intolerance causes diarrhea when failure to produce lactase results in osmotic diarrhea with ingestion of lactose-containing dairy products.

Disorders of the Liver

1. Physiologic jaundice of the newborn is caused by mild hyperbilirubinemia that subsides in 1 to 2 weeks. Pathologic jaundice is caused by severe hyperbilirubinemia and can cause brain damage (kernicterus).

2. Biliary atresia is a congenital malformation of the bile ducts that obstructs bile flow. Atresia causes jaundice, biliary cirrhosis, portal hypertension, and liver failure. Biliary atresia is the most common reason for liver transplantation in children.

3. Acute hepatitis has the same clinical course in children and adults but children have milder cases of the disease. Hepatitis A is the most common form of childhood hepatitis and is spread by contact with contaminated stool and poor handwashing.

4. Young children more readily develop chronic HBV or HCV hepatitis because of their immature immune system. HBV and HCV can be acquired by maternal vertical transmission in newborns or by parenteral (i.e., use of shared needles) transmission in older children.

5. Cirrhosis is fibrotic scarring of the liver and is rare in children but can develop from most forms of chronic liver disease.

6. Portal hypertension in children usually is caused by extrahepatic obstruction. Thrombosis of the portal vein is the most common cause of portal hypertension in children and splenomegaly is the most common sign.

7. The three most common metabolic disorders that cause liver damage in children are galactosemia, fructosemia, and Wilson disease. All are rare, are inherited as genetic traits, and permit the accumulation of toxins in the liver.

8. Wilson disease causes defective copper uptake and metabolism. Copper that is not excreted accumulates in the liver, brain, kidney, and corneal cells. Damage from accumulated copper is gradual; the disease is usually not diagnosed before age 4 or 5 years.

KEY TERMS

Anorectal malformation (ARM), 1377
Biliary atresia (BA), 1387
Celiac disease (CD; celiac sprue or gluten-sensitive enteropathy), 1380
Cirrhosis, 1388
Cleft lip, 1373
Cleft palate, 1374
Cystic fibrosis, 1380
Dermatitis herpetiformis, 1383
Diarrhea, 1385
Distal intestinal obstruction syndrome (DIOS), 1377
Eosinophilic esophagitis, 1379
Esophageal atresia (EA), 1374
Extrahepatic (prehepatic) portal venous obstruction, 1389
Failure to thrive (FTT; growth faltering), 1384
Gastroesophageal reflux (GER), 1379

Gastroesophageal reflux disease (GERD), 1379
Glucose-6-phosphate dehydrogenase deficiency, 1386
Hepatitis A virus (HAV), 1387
Hepatitis B surface antigen (HBsAg), 1387
Hepatitis B virus (HBV), 1387
Hepatitis C virus (HCV), 1388
Hepatitis D virus (HDV), 1388
Hirschsprung disease (congenital aganglionic megacolon), 1377
Imperforate anus, 1377
Infantile hypertrophic pyloric stenosis (IHPS), 1375
Intestinal malrotation, 1376
Intrahepatic portal hypertension, 1389
Intussusception, 1379
Jaundice (icterus), 1386
Kernicterus, 1386

Kwashiorkor, 1383
Lactose intolerance (lactose malabsorption), 1386
Marasmus, 1383
Meckel diverticulum, 1376
Meconium, 1378
Meconium aspiration syndrome, 1378
Meconium ileus (MI), 1378
Meconium plug syndrome, 1378
Necrotizing enterocolitis (NEC), 1384
Nonceliac gluten sensitivity (GS), 1380
Pathologic jaundice, 1386
Periduodenal band (Ladd band), 1376
Physiologic jaundice (hyperbilirubinemia) of the newborn, 1386
Portal hypertension, 1388
Protein-energy malnutrition (PEM), 1383
Tracheoesophageal fistula (EA/TEF), 1374
Wilson disease, 1389

REFERENCES

1. Centers for Disease Control and Prevention (CDC): *Birth defects: data and statistics.* Last updated February 29, 2016. Available at: http://www.cdc.gov/ncbddd/birthdefects/data.html.

2. Cooper ME, Tatay JS, Marazita ML: Asian oral-facial cleft birth prevalence. *Cleft Palate Craniofac J* 43(5):580–589, 2006.

3. Drew SJ: Clefting syndromes. *Atlas Oral Maxillofac Surg Clin North Am* 22(2):175–181, 2014.

4. Twigg SR, Wilkie AO: New insights into craniofacial malformations. *Hum Mol Genet* 24(R1):R50–R59, 2015.

5. Mossey PA, et al: Cleft lip and palate. *Lancet* 374(9703):1773–1785, 2009.

6. Qureshi WA, Beiraghi S, Leon-Salazar V: Dental anomalies associated with unilateral and bilateral cleft lip and palate. *J Dent Child (Chic)* 79(2):69–73, 2012.

7. Goswami M, Jangra B, Bhushan U: Management of feeding problem in a patient with cleft lip/palate. *Int J Clin Pediatr Dent* 9(2):143–145, 2016.

8. Bhuskute AA, Tollefson TT: Cleft lip repair, nasoalveolar molding, and primary cleft rhinoplasty. *Facial Plast Surg Clin North Am* 24(4):453–466, 2016.

9. Shaye D: Update on outcomes research for cleft lip and palate. *Curr Opin Otolaryngol Head Neck Surg* 22(4):255–259, 2014.

10. Sitzman TJ, et al: Measuring outcomes in cleft lip and palate treatment. *Clin Plast Surg* 41(2):311–319, 2014.

11. Pedersen RN, et al: Oesophageal atresia: prevalence, prenatal diagnosis and associated anomalies in 23 European regions. *Arch Dis Child* 97(3):227–232, 2012.

12. de Jong EM, et al: Etiology of esophageal atresia and tracheoesophageal fistula: "mind the gap." *Curr Gastroenterol Rep* 12(3):215–222, 2010.

13. Holland AJ, Fitzgerald DA: Oesophageal atresia and tracheo-oesophageal fistula: current management strategies and complications. *Paediatr Respir Rev* 11(2):100–106, quiz 106–107, 2010.

14. Solomon BD, et al: An approach to the identification of anomalies and etiologies in neonates with identified or suspected VACTERL (vertebral defects, anal atresia, tracheo-esophageal fistula with esophageal atresia, cardiac anomalies, renal anomalies, and limb anomalies). *J Pediatr* 164(3):451–457, 2014.

15. Jacobs IJ, Ku WY, Que J: Genetic and cellular mechanisms regulating anterior foregut and esophageal development. *Dev Biol* 369(1):54–64, 2012.

16. El-Gohary Y, Gittes GK, Tovar JA: Congenital anomalies of the esophagus. *Semin Pediatr Surg* 19(3):186–193, 2010.

17. Langer JC, et al: Prenatal diagnosis of esophageal atresia using sonography and magnetic resonance imaging. *J Pediatr Surg* 36(5):804–807, 2001.

18. Gottrand M, et al: Motility, digestive and nutritional problems in esophageal atresia. *Paediatr Respir Rev* 19:28–33, 2016.

19. Teague WJ, Karpelowsky J: Surgical management of oesophageal atresia. *Paediatr Respir Rev* 19:10–15, 2016.

20. Alberti D, et al: Esophageal atresia: pre and post-operative management. *J Matern Fetal Neonatal Med* 24(Suppl 1):4–6, 2011.

21. Hernanz-Schulman M: Infantile hypertrophic pyloric stenosis. *Radiology* 227(2):319–331, 2003.

22. Krogh C, et al: Pre- and perinatal risk factors for pyloric stenosis and their influence on the male predominance. *Am J Epidemiol* 176(1):24–31, 2012.

23. Pandya S, Heiss K: Pyloric stenosis in pediatric surgery: an evidence-based review. *Surg Clin North Am* 92(3):527–539, 2012.

24. Askew N: An overview of infantile hypertrophic pyloric stenosis. *Paediatr Nurs* 22(8):27–30, 2010.

25. Peters B, et al: Advances in infantile hypertrophic pyloric stenosis. *Expert Rev Gastroenterol Hepatol* 8(5):533–541, 2014.

26. Ranells JD, Carver JD, Kirby RS: Infantile hypertrophic pyloric stenosis: epidemiology, genetics, and clinical update. *Adv Pediatr* 58(1):195–206, 2011.

27. Kliegman RM, et al: *Nelson textbook of pediatrics,* ed 19, Philadelphia, 2011, Saunders.

28. Langer JC: Intestinal rotation abnormalities and midgut volvulus. *Surg Clin North Am* 97(1):147–159, 2017.

29. Nehra D, Goldstein AM: Intestinal malrotation: varied clinical presentation from infancy through adulthood. *Surgery* 149(3):386–393, 2011.

30. Graziano K, et al: Asymptomatic malrotation: diagnosis and surgical management: an American Pediatric Surgical Association outcomes and evidence based practice committee systematic review. *J Pediatr Surg* 50(10):1783–1790, 2015.

31. Ooms N, et al: Laparoscopic treatment of intestinal malrotation in children. *Eur J Pediatr Surg* 26(4):376–381, 2016.

32. El-Gohary Y, Alagtal M, Gillick J: Long-term complications following operative intervention for intestinal malrotation: a 10-year review. *Pediatr Surg Int* 26(2):203–206, 2010.

33. Kotha VK, et al: Radiologist's perspective for the Meckel's diverticulum and its complications. *Br J Radiol* 87(1037):20130743, 2014.

34. Travassos D, van Herwaarden-Lindeboom M, van der Zee DC: Hirschsprung's disease in children with Down syndrome: a comparative study. *Eur J Pediatr Surg* 21(4):220–223, 2011.

35. Torroglosa A, et al: Epigenetics in ENS development and Hirschsprung disease. *Dev Biol* 417(2):209–216, 2016.

36. Gosain A, Brinkman AS: Hirschsprung's associated enterocolitis. *Curr Opin Pediatr* 27(3):364–369, 2015.

37. Jiao CL, Chen XY, Feng JX: Novel insights into the pathogenesis of Hirschsprung's-associated enterocolitis. *Chin Med J* 129(12):1491–1497, 2016.

38. Zhang S, et al: Comparison of laparoscopic-assisted operations and laparotomy operations for the treatment of Hirschsprung disease: evidence from a meta-analysis. *Medicine (Baltimore)* 94(39):e1632, 2015.

39. Chumpitazi BP, Nurko S: Defecation disorders in children after surgery for Hirschsprung disease. *J Pediatr Gastroenterol Nutr* 53(1):75–79, 2011.

40. More K, et al: Growth and developmental outcomes of infants with Hirschsprung disease presenting in the neonatal period: a retrospective study. *J Pediatr* 165(1):73–77, 2014.

41. Gfroerer S, Rolle U: Pediatric intestinal motility disorders. *World J Gastroenterol* 21(33):9683–9687, 2015.

42. Lavie M, et al: Long-term follow-up of distal intestinal obstruction syndrome in cystic fibrosis. *World J Gastroenterol* 21(1):318–325, 2015.

43. VanderBrink BA, Reddy PP: Early urologic considerations in patients with persistent cloaca. *Semin Pediatr Surg* 25(2):82–89, 2016.

44. Levitt MA, Pena A: Anorectal malformations. *Orphanet J Rare Dis* 2:33, 2007.

45. Marcelis C, de Blaauw I, Brunner H: Chromosomal anomalies in the etiology of anorectal malformations: a review. *Am J Med Genet A* 155A(11):2692–2704, 2011.

46. Forrester MB, Merz RD: Risk of selected birth defects with prenatal illicit drug use, Hawaii, 1986–2002. *J Toxicol Environ Health A* 70:7–18, 2007.

47. Huang Y, et al: Hypermethylation of SHH in the pathogenesis of congenital anorectal malformations. *J Pediatr Surg* 49(9):1400–1404, 2014.

48. Arnoldi R, et al: Anorectal malformations with good prognosis: variables affecting the functional outcome. *J Pediatr Surg* 49(8):1232–1236, 2014.

49. Cuenca AG, et al: "Pulling the plug"— management of meconium plug syndrome in neonates. *J Surg Res* 175(2):e43–e46, 2012.

50. Glen J, Kinsella JP: Pathophysiology of meconium aspiration syndrome. In Polin RA, et al, editors: *Fetal and neonatal physiology,* ed 5, Philadelphia, 2017, Elsevier, pp 1619–1624.

51. Vain NE, Batton DG: Meconium "aspiration" (or respiratory distress associated with meconium-stained amniotic fluid?). *Semin Fetal Neonatal Med* 22(4):214–219, 2017.

52. Carlyle BE, Borowitz DS, Glick PL: A review of pathophysiology and management of fetuses and neonates with meconium ileus for the pediatric surgeon. *J Pediatr Surg* 47(4):772–781, 2012.

53. Romi H, et al: Meconium ileus caused by mutations in GUCY2C, encoding the CFTR-activating guanylate cyclase 2C. *Am J Hum Genet* 90(5):893–899, 2010.

54. Furey EA, Bailey AA, Twickler DM: Fetal MR imaging of gastrointestinal abnormalities. *Radiographics* 36(3):904–917, 2016.

55. Moawad FJ, et al: Eosinophilic esophagitis: current perspectives from diagnosis to management. *Ann N Y Acad Sci* 1380(1):204–217, 2016.

56. Ruffner MA, Spergel JM: Eosinophilic esophagitis in children. *Curr Allergy Asthma Rep* 17(8):54, 2017.

57. Davies I, et al: Gastro-oesophageal reflux disease in children: NICE guidance. *BMJ* 350:g7703, 2015.

58. Sherman PM, et al: A global, evidence-based consensus on the definition of gastroesophageal reflux disease in the pediatric population. *Am J Gastroenterol* 104(5):1278–1295, 2009.

59. Baird DC, Harker DJ, Karmes AS: Diagnosis and treatment of gastroesophageal reflux in infants and children. *Am Fam Physician* 92(8):705–714, 2015.

60. Dupont C, Vandenplas Y, SONAR Study Group: Efficacy and tolerance of a new anti-regurgitation formula. *Pediatr Gastroenterol Hepatol Nutr* 19(2):104–109, 2016.

61. Lightdale JR, Gremse DA, Section on gastroenterology, hepatology, and nutrition: gastroesophageal reflux: management guidance for the pediatrician. *Pediatrics* 131(5):e1684–e1695, 2013.

62. Cohen S, Bueno de Mesquita M, Mimouni FB: Adverse effects reported in the use of gastroesophageal reflux disease treatments in children: a 10 years literature review. *Br J Clin Pharmacol* 80(2):200–208, 2015.

63. Wakeman DS, Wilson NA, Warner BW: Current status of surgical management of gastroesophageal reflux in children. *Curr Opin Pediatr* 28(3): 356–362, 2016.

64. Tate JE, et al: Intussusception rates before and after the introduction of rotavirus vaccine. *Pediatrics* 138(3):2016.

65. Ntoulia A, et al: Failed intussusception reduction in children: correlation between radiologic, surgical, and pathologic findings. *AJR Am J Roentgenol* 207(2):424–433, 2016.

66. Apelt N, Featherstone N, Giuliani S: Laparoscopic treatment of intussusception in children: a systematic review. *J Pediatr Surg* 48(8):1789–1793, 2013.

67. Parikh M, et al: Does all small bowel intussusception need exploration? *Afr J Paediatr Surg* 7(1):30–32, 2010.

68. Pepper VK, et al: Diagnosis and management of pediatric appendicitis, intussusception, and Meckel diverticulum. *Surg Clin North Am* 92(3): 505–526, vii, 2012.

69. Barrio R: Management of endocrine disease: cystic fibrosis-related diabetes: novel pathogenic insights opening new therapeutic avenues. *Eur J Endocrinol* 172(4):R131–R141, 2015.

70. Borowitz D, Gelfond D: Intestinal complications of cystic fibrosis. *Curr Opin Pulm Med* 19(6): 676–680, 2013.

71. Kelly T, Buxbaum J: Gastrointestinal manifestations of cystic fibrosis. *Dig Dis Sci* 60(7):1903–1913, 2015.

72. Schindler T, Michel S, Wilson AW: Nutrition management of cystic fibrosis in the 21st century. *Nutr Clin Pract* 30(4):488–500, 2015.

73. Thaker V, et al: Recombinant growth hormone therapy for cystic fibrosis in children and young adults. *Cochrane Database Syst Rev* (5):CD008901, 2015.

74. Guandalini S, Assiri A: Celiac disease: a review. *JAMA Pediatr* 168(3):272–278, 2014.

75. Watkins RD, Zawahir S: Celiac disease and nonceliac gluten sensitivity. *Pediatr Clin North Am* 64(3):563–576, 2017.

76. Czaja-Bulsa G, Bulsa M: What do we know now about IgE-mediated wheat allergy in children? *Nutients* 9(1):2017.

77. Shannahan S, Leffler DA: Diagnosis and updates in celiac disease. *Gastrointest Endosc Clin N Am* 27(1):79–92, 2017.

78. Husby S, Murray JA: Diagnosing coeliac disease and the potential for serological markers. *Nat Rev Gastroenterol Hepatol* 11(11):655–663, 2014.

79. Parzanese I, et al: Celiac disease: from pathophysiology to treatment. *World J Gastrointest Pathophysiol* 8(2):27–38, 2017.

80. Rishi AR, Rubio-Tapia A, Murray JA: Refractory celiac disease. *Expert Rev Gastroenterol Hepatol* 10(4):537–546, 2016.

81. Murch S: Recent advances in celiac disease. *Indian J Pediatr* 83(12-13):1428–1435, 2016.

82. Tanpowpong P, et al: Age-related patterns in clinical presentations and gluten-related issues among children and adolescents with celiac disease. *Clin Transl Gastroenterol* 3:e9, 2012.

83. Jesson J, Leroy V: Challenges of malnutrition care among HIV-infected children on antiretroviral treatment in Africa. *Med Mal Infect* 45(5): 149–156, 2015.

84. Garrett WS: Kwashiorkor and the gut microbiota. *N Engl J Med* 368(18):1746–1747, 2013.

85. Prieto MB, Cid JL: Malnutrition in the critically ill child: the importance of enteral nutrition. *Int J Environ Res Public Health* 8(11):4353–4366, 2011.

86. Million M, Diallo A, Raoult D: Gut microbiota and malnutrition. *Microb Pathog* 106:127–138, 2017.

87. Kane AV, Dinh DM, Ward HD: Childhood malnutrition and the intestinal microbiome malnutrition and the microbiome. *Pediatric Res* 77(0):256–262, 2015.

88. Wiseman EM, Bar-El Dadon S, Reifen R: The vicious cycle of vitamin A deficiency: a review. *Crit Rev Food Sci Nutr* 57(17):3703–3714, 2017.

89. Kismul H, et al: Diet and kwashiorkor: a prospective study from rural DR Congo. *Peer J* 2:e350, 2014.

90. Bahwere P, et al: Cereals and pulse-based ready-to-use therapeutic food as an alternative to the standard milk- and peanut paste-based formulation for treating severe acute malnutrition: a noninferiority, individually randomized controlled efficacy clinical trial. *Am J Clin Nutr* 103(4):1145–1161, 2016.

91. Vygen SB, et al: Treatment of severe acute malnutrition in infants aged <6 months in Niger. *J Pediatr* 162(3):515–521, 2013.

92. Cole SZ, Lanham JS: Failure to thrive: an update. *Am Fam Physician* 83(7):829–834, 2011.

93. Jaffe AC: Failure to thrive: current clinical concepts. *Pediatr Rev* 32(3):100–107, 2011.

94. Joosten KF, Hulst JM: Nutritional screening tools for hospitalized children: methodological considerations. *Clin Nutr* 33(1):1–5, 2014.

95. Black MM, et al: Early intervention and recovery among children with failure to thrive: follow-up at age 8. *Pediatrics* 120(1):59–69, 2007.

96. Cho SX, et al: The immunological landscape in necrotising enterocolitis. *Expert Rev Mol Med* 18:e12, 2016.

97. Terrin G, Scipione A, De Curtis M: Update in pathogenesis and prospective in treatment of necrotizing enterocolitis. *Biomed Res Int* 2014: 543765, 2014.

98. Tanner SM, et al: Pathogenesis of necrotizing enterocolitis: modeling the innate immune response. *Am J Pathol* 185(1):4–16, 2015.

99. McElroy SJ, Underwood MA, Sherman MP: Paneth cells and necrotizing enterocolitis: a novel hypothesis for disease pathogenesis. *Neonatology* 1:10–20, 2013.

100. Lee JH: An update on necrotizing enterocolitis: pathogenesis and preventive strategies. *Korean J Pediatr* 54(9):368–372, 2011.

101. Patel BK, Shah JS: Necrotizing enterocolitis in very low birth weight infants: a systemic review. *ISRN Gastroenterol* 2012:562594, 2012.

102. Frost BL, et al: New medical and surgical insights into neonatal necrotizing enterocolitis: a review. *JAMA Pediatr* 171(1):83–88, 2017.

103. Gephart SM, Wetzel C, Krisman B: Prevention and early recognition of necrotizing enterocolitis, a tale of two tools: eNEC and GutCheck. *Adv Neonatal Care* 14(3):201–210, 2014.

104. Zhou P, et al: The role of immunonutrients in the prevention of necrotizing enterocolitis in preterm very low birth weight infants. *Nutrients* 7(9): 7256–7270, 2015.

105. Churgay CA, Aftab Z: Gastroenteritis in children: part 1. Diagnosis. *Am Fam Physician* 85(11): 1059–1062, 2012.

106. Fischer-Walker CL, et al: Global burden of childhood pneumonia and diarrhea. *Lancet* 381(9875):1405–1416, 2013.

107. Zella GC, Israel EJ: Chronic diarrhea in children. *Pediatr Rev* 33(5):207–217, 2012.

108. Leung DT, Chisti MJ, Pavia AT: Prevention and control of childhood pneumonia and diarrhea. *Pediatr Clin North Am* 63(1):67–79, 2016.

109. Bernaola Aponte G, et al: Probiotics for treating persistent diarrhoea in children. *Cochrane Database Syst Rev* (8):CD007401, 2013.

110. Wang CM, Chen SC, Chen KT: Current status of rotavirus vaccines. *World J Pediatr* 11(4):300–308, 2015.

111. Venkatesan MM, Van de Verg LL: Combination vaccines against diarrheal diseases. *Hum Vaccin Immunother* 11(6):1434–1448, 2015.

112. Amiri M, et al: The diverse forms of lactose intolerance and the putative linkage to several cancers. *Nutrients* 7(9):7209–7230, 2015.

113. Berni Canani R, et al: Diagnosing and treating intolerance to carbohydrates in children. *Nutrients* 8(3):157, 2016.

114. Watson RI.: Hyperbilirubinemia. *Crit Care Nurs Clin North Am* 21(1):97–120, 2009.

115. Wong RJ, Stevenson DK: Neonatal hemolysis and risk of bilirubin-induced neurologic dysfunction. *Semin Fetal Neonatal Med* 20(1):26–30, 2015.

116. Bhutani VK, Johnson-Hamerman L: The clinical syndrome of bilirubin-induced neurologic dysfunction. *Semin Fetal Neonatal Med* 20(1): 6–13, 2015.

117. Hulzebos CV, Dijk PH: Bilirubin-albumin binding, bilirubin/albumin ratios, and free bilirubin levels: where do we stand? *Semin Perinatol* 38(7):412–421, 2014.

118. Engle WD, Jackson GL, Engle NG: Transcutaneous bilirubinometry. *Semin Perinatol* 38(7):438–451, 2014.

119. American Academy of Pediatrics: Management of hyperbilirubinemia in the newborn infant 35 or more weeks of gestation. *Pediatrics* 114(1): 297–316, 2004. Available at: http://aappolicy .aappublications.org/cgi/content/full/ pediatrics;114/1/297.

120. Bhutani VK, et al: Clinical trial of tin mesoporphyrin to prevent neonatal hyperbilirubinemia. *J Perinatol* 36(7):533–539, 2016.

121. Asai A, Miethke A, Bezerra JA: Pathogenesis of biliary atresia: defining biology to understand clinical phenotypes. *Nat Rev Gastroenterol Hepatol* 12(6):342–352, 2015.

122. Zagory JA, Nguyen MV, Wang KS: Recent advances in the pathogenesis and management of biliary atresia. *Curr Opin Pediatr* 27(3):389–394, 2015.

123. Degertekin B, Lok AS: Update on viral hepatitis: 2008. *Curr Opin Gastroenterol* 25(3):180–185, 2009.

124. Centers for Disease Control and Prevention (CDC): *Viral hepatitis–hepatitis A information, overview and statistics, last updated July 13, 2016.* Available at: http://www.cdc.gov/hepatitis/HAV/ HAVfaq.htm#general.

125. Gill US, Kennedy PT: Chronic hepatitis B virus in young adults: the need for new approaches to management. *Expert Rev Anti Infect Ther* 12(9): 1045–1053, 2014.

126. Kao JH: Hepatitis B vaccination and prevention of hepatocellular carcinoma. *Best Pract Res Clin Gastroenterol* 29(6):907–917, 2015.

127. Jonas MM, et al: Antiviral therapy in management of chronic hepatitis B viral infection in children: a systematic review and meta-analysis. *Hepatology* 63(1):307–318, 2016.

128. Komatsu H, Inui A: Hepatitis B virus infection in children. *Expert Rev Anti Infect Ther* 13(4): 427–450, 2015.

129. Granot E, Sokal EM: Hepatitis C virus in children: deferring treatment in expectation of direct-acting antiviral agents. *Isr Med Assoc J* 17(11):707–711, 2015.

130. El-Shabrawi M, Hassanin F: Treatment of hepatitis B and C in children. *Minerva Pediatr* 66(5): 473–489, 2014.

131. Su TH, Kao JH: Improving clinical outcomes of chronic hepatitis B virus infection. *Expert Rev Gastroenterol Hepatol* 9(2):141–154, 2015.

132. Czaja AJ: Transitioning from idiopathic to explainable autoimmune hepatitis. *Dig Dis Sci* 60(10):2881–2900, 2015.

133. Zhu JY, Han Y: Autoimmune hepatitis: unveiling faces. *J Dig Dis* 16(9):483–488, 2015.

134. Behrman RE, Kliegman R, Jenson HB: *Nelson textbook of pediatrics*, ed 18, Philadelphia, 2007, Saunders.

135. McKiernan P, Abdel-Hady M: Advances in the management of childhood portal hypertension. *Expert Rev Gastroenterol Hepatol* 9(5):575–583, 2015.

136. Berry GT: Galactosemia and amenorrhea in the adolescent. *Ann N Y Acad Sci* 1135:112–117, 2008.

137. Wu F, et al: Wilson's disease: a comprehensive review of the molecular mechanisms. *Int J Mol Sci* 16(3):6419–6431, 2015.

138. Rosencrantz R, Schilsky M: Wilson disease: pathogenesis and clinical considerations in diagnosis and treatment. *Semin Liver Dis* 31(3): 245–259, 2011.

139. Kanwar P, Kowdley KV: Metal storage disorders: Wilson disease and hemochromatosis. *Med Clin North Am* 98(1):87–102, 2014.

140. Poon KS, Tan KM, Koay ES: Targeted next-generation sequencing of the ATP7B gene for molecular diagnosis of Wilson disease. *Clin Biochem* 49(1-2):166–171, 2016.

141. Purchase R: The treatment of Wilson's disease, a rare genetic disorder of copper metabolism. *Sci Prog* 96(Pt 1):19–32, 2013.

CHAPTER

44

Structure and Function of the Musculoskeletal System

Geri C. Reeves, Leslie W. Hopkins, Benjamin A. Smallheer

evolve WEBSITE

http://evolve.elsevier.com/McCance/

- Content Updates
- Chapter Summary Review
- Review Questions
- Case Studies
- Animations

CHAPTER OUTLINE

The way an individual functions in daily life, moves, or manipulates objects physically depends on the integrity of the musculoskeletal system. The musculoskeletal system actually consists of the following two systems: (1) the skeleton composed of bones and joints and (2) soft tissues (skeletal muscles, tendons, and ligaments). Each of the systems contributes to mobility. The skeleton supports the body and provides leverage to the skeletal muscles so that movement of various parts of the body is possible. Contraction of the skeletal muscles and bending or rotation at the joints facilitate movement of the various body parts.

STRUCTURE AND FUNCTION OF BONES

Bones give form to the body, support tissues, and permit movement by providing points of attachment for muscles. Many bones meet in movable joints that determine the type and extent of movement possible. Bones also protect many of the body's vital organs. For example, the bones of the skull, thorax, and pelvis are hard exterior shields that protect the brain, heart, lungs, and reproductive and urinary organs.

Bone marrow is one of the sources of mesenchymal stem cells (MSCs) (Fig. 44.1). These nonhematopoietic stem cells consist of a small proportion of the stromal cell population in the bone marrow, and can generate bone cells, cartilage cells, and fat cells that support the formation of blood and fibrous connective tissue. Within certain bones, the marrow cavities also serve as a storage site for the hematopoietic stem cells that form both blood and immune cells. In adults, blood cells originate exclusively in the marrow cavities of the skull, vertebrae, ribs, sternum, shoulders, and pelvis. Bones also have a crucial role in mineral homeostasis (storing minerals [i.e., calcium, phosphate, carbonate, magnesium]) that is essential for the performance of many delicate cellular mechanisms, have a role in hormone homeostasis, and assist in maintaining normal immunologic function.

Elements of Bone Tissue

Mature bone is a rigid yet flexible connective tissue consisting of cells, fibers, a homogeneous gelatinous medium termed ground substance, and large amounts of crystallized minerals, mainly calcium, that give bone its rigidity. Ground substance consists of proteoglycans and hyaluronic acid secreted by chondroblasts. The structural elements of bone are summarized in Table 44.1.

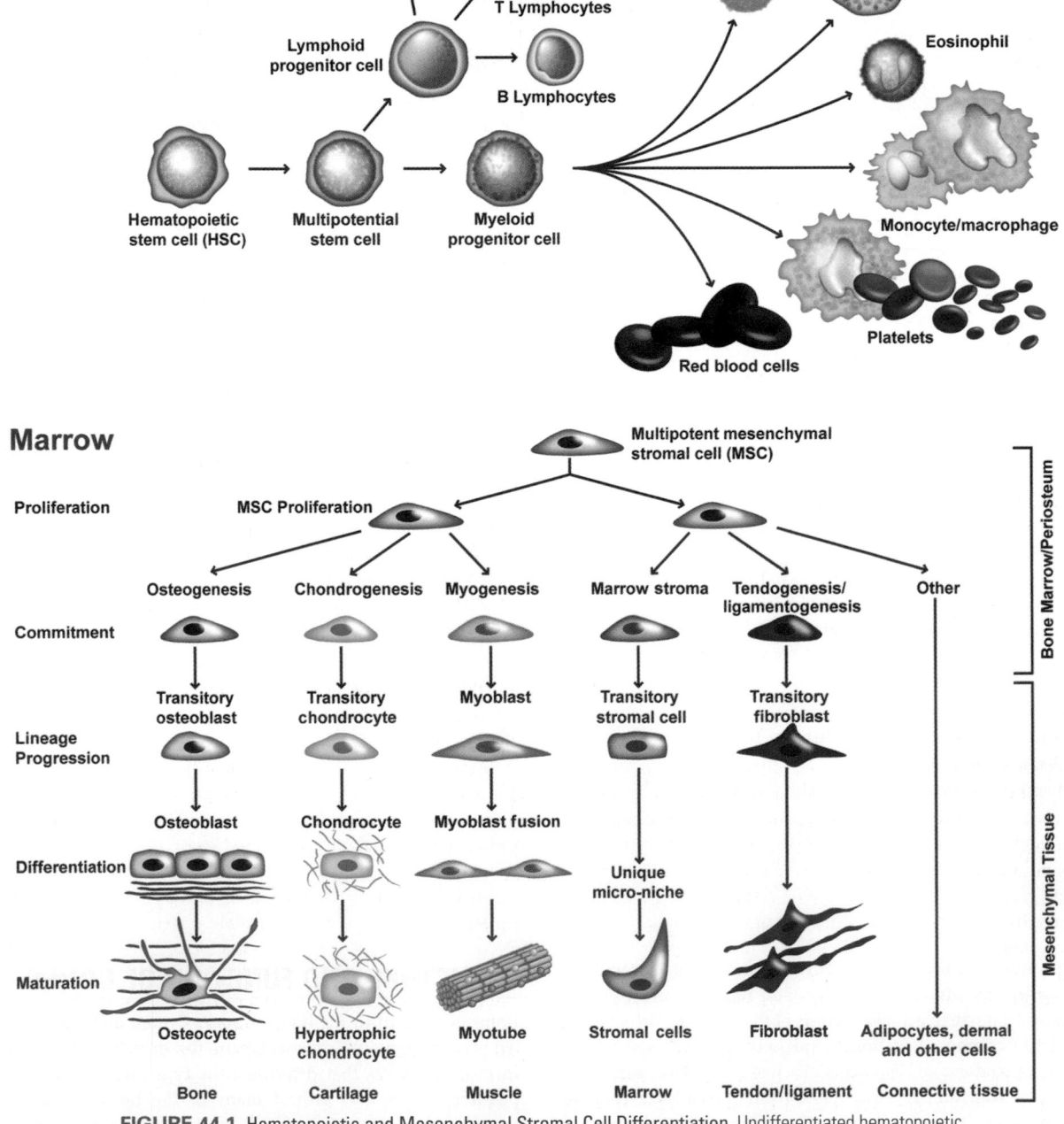

FIGURE 44.1 Hematopoietic and Mesenchymal Stromal Cell Differentiation. Undifferentiated hematopoietic and mesenchymal multipotential cells give rise to a variety of cell types with distinct functions. *NK*, Natural killer cell. (Adapted from abcam.com.)

TABLE 44.1	STRUCTURAL ELEMENTS OF BONE
STRUCTURAL ELEMENT	**FUNCTION**
Bone Cells	
Osteoblasts	Synthesize collagen and proteoglycans; stimulate bone formation and are also involved in some osteoclast resorptive activity
Osteocytes	Maintain bone matrix; act as mechanoreceptors; influence osteoblasts and osteoclasts
Osteoclasts	Resorb bone; major role in mineral homeostasis
Bone Matrix	
Collagen fibers	Lend support and tensile strength
Proteoglycans	Control transport of ionized materials through matrix
Bone morphogenic proteins (BMPs)*	Induce cartilage, bone, tendon, and ligament formation and repair
Glycoproteins	
Sialoprotein	Promotes calcification
Osteocalcin	Inhibits calcium phosphate precipitation; promotes bone resorption
Laminin	Stabilizes basement membranes in bones
Osteonectin	Binds calcium in bones
Albumin	Transports essential elements to matrix; maintains osmotic pressure of bone fluid
α-Glycoprotein	Promotes calcification
Minerals (elements)	Crystallize to lend rigidity and compressive strength
Calcium	Regulates vitamin D and thereby promotes mineralization
Phosphate	Balance of organic and inorganic phosphate required for proper bone mineralization; regulates vitamin D
Alkaline phosphatase	Promotes mineralization
Vitamins	
Vitamin D	Assists with differentiation, mineralization of osteoblasts
Vitamin K	Increases bone calcification; reduces serum osteocalcin level

*See Table 44.2 for BMP functions.

TABLE 44.2	BONE MORPHOGENIC PROTEINS (BMPs) AND THEIR KNOWN FUNCTIONS
BMP	**KNOWN FUNCTION**
BMP1	Involved in cartilage development; is actually a metalloprotease; key role in extracellular matrix (ECM) formation
BMP2	Induces bone and cartilage formation, osteoblast differentiation, bone healing
BMP3 (osteogenin)	Induces bone formation
BMP4	Regulates formation of teeth, limbs, and bone
BMP5	Involved in cartilage development
BMP6	Found in osteoblasts; helps maintain adult joint integrity; accelerates bone repair
BMP7	Has major role in osteoblast differentiation, chondrocyte formation, fracture healing; important in renal development and repair
BMP8a	Involved in bone and cartilage development; up-regulated in fracture nonunion
BMP9	Induces osteogenesis in mature osteoblasts
BMP10	Plays role in development of the heart
BMP12 (cartilage-derived morphogenic protein-3; CDMP-3)	Involved in tendon and ligament formation
BMP13	Involved in cartilage development; tendon and ligament repair
BMP14	Assists in bone and tendon healing; cartilage formation

Data from Caetano-Lopes J, Canhão H, Fonseca JE: *Arthritis Res Ther* 9(Suppl 1):S1, 2007; Hojo H et al: *J Bone Miner Metab* 28(5):489–502, 2010; Fajardo M, Liu C-J, Egol K: *Clin Orthop Relat Res* 467(12):3071–3078, 2009; Li Y et al: *Zhong Nan Da Xue Xue Bao Yi Xue Ban* 37(1):1–5, 2012.

Bone cells enable bone to grow, repair itself, change shape, and continuously synthesize new bone tissue and resorb (dissolve or digest) old tissue. The fibers in bone are made of collagen, which gives bone its tensile strength (the ability to hold itself together). Ground substance acts as a medium for the diffusion of nutrients, oxygen, metabolic wastes, biochemicals, and minerals between bone tissue and blood vessels.

Bone formation begins during embryonic development when mesenchymal stem cells begin differentiating into either chondrocytes or preosteoblasts. Endochondral ossification and intramembranous ossification are the two major mechanisms responsible for normal bone development.

Endochondral ossification occurs when mesenchymal (mesenchyme, or loose tissue found during embryonic development) stem cells begin differentiating into chondrocytes (see Fig. 44.1), which in turn develop a mineralized cartilage scaffold that allows formation of osteoblasts. Long bones and most other bone elements are formed this way. Intramembranous ossification is responsible for the development of skull

and flat bones.[1,2] With intramembranous ossification, mesenchymal stem cells differentiate into a preosteoblast line that forms osteoblasts without any cartilage framework.[2,3]

Multiple factors influence normal bone formation, maintenance, and remodeling. Bone morphogenic proteins (BMPs) are members of the transforming growth factor-beta (TGF-β) superfamily, and BMPs play a major role in bone formation.[3] This group is primarily responsible for initiation, differentiation, and commitment of precursor cells into osteoblasts. TGF-β signals are transmitted across the plasma membrane, combine with certain proteins that act as transcription factors (Smads), and then form specific receptors known as *R-Smads*.[3] These receptors, in turn, initiate intracellular signaling, interact with other transcription factors, and regulate other factors that are important in osteoblast formation, function, and maintenance.[3] Crosstalk between signaling pathways (including TGF-β, BMPs, fibroblast growth factors [FGFs], Wnt, Notch, MAPK, and Indian Hedgehog) is critical in regulating osteoblasts.

BMPs have multiple crucial functions in the skeletal system. BMP activities are regulated at different molecular levels. Table 44.2 summarizes the role of several important BMPs.

Wnt genes belong to a large family of protein-signaling factors that are required for the development of body systems, including the musculoskeletal system. They play a significant role in forming bone, developing bone mass, remodeling bone, and healing fractures. Wnt signaling regulates production and differentiation of osteoblasts and osteoclasts, and affects bone mass and density, joint formation, fracture repair, bone remodeling, and some bone diseases. Other important elements responsible for bone formation and homeostasis are presented in Table 44.3.

In mature bone the formation of new tissue begins with the production of an organic matrix by the bone cells. This bone matrix consists of ground substances, collagen, and other proteins (see Table 44.1) that take part in bone formation and maintenance.

The next step in bone formation is calcification, when minerals are deposited and crystallize. Minerals bind tightly to collagen fibers, producing tensile and compressional strength in bone, and withstand pressure and weightbearing.

Bone Cells

Bone contains three types of cells: osteoblasts, osteocytes, and osteoclasts (Fig. 44.2). Osteoblasts are the bone-forming cells, whose primary function is to lay down new bone. Once this function is complete, osteoblasts become osteocytes that are embedded in bone. Comprising 90% to 95% of bone cells, osteocytes develop dendritic processes that extend either to the bone surface or to the bone's vascular space.[4] Osteocytes help maintain bone by signaling osteoblasts and osteoclasts to form and resorb bone.[5] Osteoclasts are the major bone-resorbing cells responsible for remodeling.

Osteoblasts. Osteoblasts originate from mesenchymal stem cells (MSCs). Bone formation is initiated by osteoblasts. Mature osteoblasts produce inorganic calcium phosphate, which is converted to hydroxyapatite, and an organic matrix that is comprised mainly of type I collagen.[6] Once this process is complete, osteoblasts deposit new bone in response to the bone resorbed by osteoclasts.[6] Osteoblasts and osteocytes control osteoclast differentiation and bone resorption by producing receptor activator of nuclear factor κβ ligand (RANKL) and osteoprotegerin. Osteoclasts trigger an osteoblastic response to couple bone formation to bone resorption during bone remodeling.[7] The net result is continuous renewal of the skeletal system. Bone modeling and bone remodeling are the processes that allow the skeleton to adapt to environmental challenges and to regulate mineral metabolism.[7] Osteoblasts cause the formation of new bone and the orderly mineralization of bone matrix by concentrating some of the plasma proteins (growth factors) found in the bone matrix and by facilitating the deposit and exchange of calcium and other ions at the site. Enzymes, signaling proteins, and growth factors, including bone morphogenic proteins (BMPs) and other members of the transforming growth factor-beta (TGF-β) superfamily, are critical components of bone formation, maintenance, and remodeling (Table 44.4).

Osteoblasts are active on the outer surface of bones, where they form a single layer of cells. They are responsive to parathyroid hormone (PTH) and produce a protein called *osteocalcin* when stimulated by 1,25-dihydroxy-vitamin D_3.[8] Osteoblasts initiate the formation of new bone by their synthesis of osteoid (nonmineralized bone matrix). The mechanism of osteoblast stimulation is reported to be the production of so-called coupling factors generated during the resorption process. Osteoblasts alter levels of RANKL and osteoprotegerin (OPG); the balance of these two cytokines determines overall osteoclast formation[9] (see Fig. 45.11). As new bone is formed, it is shaped and remodeled through TGF-β, as well as other plasma proteins (growth factors) found in the bone marrow (see Table 44.4).

Osteocytes. Osteocytes, the most abundant cells in bone, are transformed osteoblasts that become trapped or surrounded in osteoid as it hardens because of minerals that enter during ossification (see Fig. 44.2, *B*). It is the final differentiation stage for an osteoblast. The osteocyte is within a space in the hardened bone matrix called a lacuna. Within the mineralized matrix, osteocytes are interconnected by a network of dendritic cytoplasmic processes through tunnels known as *canaliculi*.[1,4] These canaliculi radiate from each lacuna and contain cell processes from the resident osteocyte, thereby enabling it to form gap junctions with adjacent osteocytes.[10] Within this microenvironment, osteocytes detect mechanical forces and help to control calcium and phosphate levels.[1]

One of the osteocyte's primary functions is to act as a mechanoreceptor, responding to changes in weightbearing or other stressors ("loading") on bone. Lying within the lacunae are the osteocyte's primary cilia,

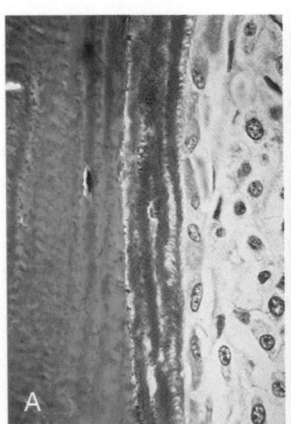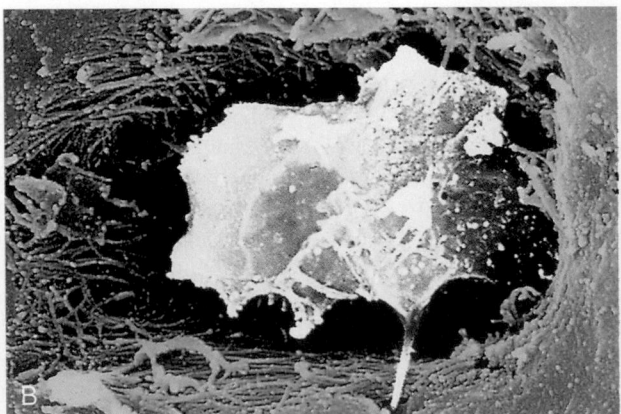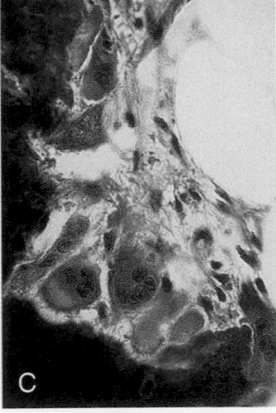

FIGURE 44.2 Bone Cells. **A,** Osteoblasts are responsible for the production of collagenous and noncollagenous proteins that compose osteoid. Active osteoblasts are aligned on the osteoid. Note the eccentrically located nuclei. **B,** Osteocyte. Scanning electron micrograph showing an osteocyte within a lacuna. The cell is surrounded by collagen fibers and mineralized bone. **C,** Osteoclasts actively resorb mineralized tissue. The scalloped surface in which the multinucleated osteoclasts rest is termed the *Howship lacuna.* (**A** and **C** from Damjanov I, Linder J, editors: *Anderson's pathology,* ed 10, St Louis, 1996, Mosby. **B** from Erlandsen S, Magney J: *Color atlas of histology,* St Louis, 1992, Mosby.)

TABLE 44.3 SELECTED FACTORS AFFECTING BONE FORMATION AND HOMEOSTASIS

FACTOR	FUNCTION
Transforming growth factor-beta (TGF-β)	Superfamily of polypeptides; regulates bone formation, many other cellular processes though signaling
Platelet-derived growth factor (PDGF)	Increases number of osteoblasts
Fibroblast growth factor-2 (FGF-2)	FGF-2 increases osteoblast population, but not function; inhibits alkaline phosphatase activity, osteocalcin, type I collagen, and osteopontin
Insulin-like growth factor (IGF)	
IGF-1	Increases peak bone mass during adolescence; decreases osteoblast apoptosis; maintains bone matrix
IGF-2	Increases BMP-9–induced endochondral ossification
Smad proteins	Mediate the signaling cascade of transforming growth factor-beta (TGF-β), especially in embryonic bone development; play a role in crosstalk between BMP/TGF-β and Wnt signaling pathways
Bone morphogenic proteins (BMPs)	Members of transforming growth factor-beta (TGF-β) superfamily of polypeptides; have many functions outside skeletal system; stimulate endochondral bone and cartilage formation and function, promote osteoblast maturation; augment bone remodeling by affecting both osteoblasts and osteoclasts
Tumor necrosis factors (TNFs)	Superfamily of cytokines; play major role in regulating bone metabolism, especially osteoclast function
Osteoprotegerin (OPG)	Inhibits bone remodeling/resorption; produced by several cells, including osteoblasts; is a decoy receptor for RANKL (binds to RANKL, inhibiting RANK/RANKL interactions, suppressing osteoclast formation and bone resorption)
Receptor activator of nuclear factor κβ (RANK)	Stimulates differentiation of osteoclast precursors; activates mature osteoclasts
Bone morphogenic protein antagonists	Prevent BMP signaling
Noggin	Binds BMP-2 and BMP-4, reducing osteoblast function
Gremlin	Multiple effects in and out of skeletal system, but also binds BMP-2, -4, and -7; may play a role in development of osteoporosis
Twisted gastrulation	Acts as either a BMP agonist or an antagonist
Activin (a BMP-related protein)	Affects both osteoblasts and osteoclasts; may promote bone formation and fracture healing; expressed by both osteoblasts and chondrocytes; helps regulate bone mass
Inhibin	Dominant over activin and BMPs; helps regulate bone mass and strength by affecting formation of osteoblasts and osteoclasts
Leptin	Plays role in bone formation and resorption
Wnt (a signaling pathway)	Important in differentiating osteoblasts and bone formation; has overlapping effects with BMPs; helps regulate bone formation and remodeling
Wnt antagonists	
Dickkopf family (Dkk)	Disrupts Wnt signaling, leading to reduced bone mass
Sclerostin	Protein secreted by osteocytes, osteoblasts, and osteoclasts; binds to BMP-6 and BMP-7; interferes with Wnt signaling pathway, inhibiting bone formation by osteoblasts
Transcription Factors	
Nuclear factor of activated κβ cells (NF-κβ)	Affects embryonic osteoclastogenesis; plays a role in certain osteoclast, osteoblast, and chondroblast functions
Matrix metalloproteinases (MMPs)	
Family of endopeptidases (enzymes) that includes collagenases, gelatinases, stromelysins, matrilysins	Help maintain equilibrium of extracellular matrix (ECM); break down almost all components of ECM
A disintegrin and metalloproteinase (ADAM)	Proteolytic enzymes; also have cell-signaling functions, usually linked to cell membrane
A disintegrin and metalloproteinase with thrombospondin motifs (ADAMTS)	Similar to ADAMs but are secreted into circulation, are found around cells; various subgroups affect multiple tissues
Cysteine Protease	
Cathepsin	K-expressed by osteoclasts; assists in bone remodeling by cleaving proteins, such as collagen type I, collagen type II, and osteonectin
Mmp Inhibitors	
Tetracyclines (especially doxycycline), bisphosphonates	Block enzymatic function of MMPs
Tissue inhibitors of metalloproteinases (TIMPs)	Balance effect of MMPs in maintaining ECM equilibrium

From Boyce GC, Zhenqiang, Zing L: *Ann N Y Acad Sci* 1192:367–375, 2010; Canalis E: *J Cell Biol* 108(4):769–777, 2009; Kim Y-S et al: *J Korean Med Sci* 25:985–991, 2010; Moester MJ et al: *Calcif Tissue Int* 87(2):99–107, 2010; Nicks KN et al: *Mol Cell Endocrinol* 310(1–2):11–20, 2009; Pasternak B, Aspenberg P: *Acta Orthopaedica* 80(6):693–703, 2009; Stewart A, Guan H, Yang K: *J Cell Physiol* 223(3):658–666, 2010; Tat SK et al: *Keio Med J* 58(1):29–40, 2009.

TABLE 44.4   EFFECTS OF SELECTED CYTOKINES (GROWTH FACTORS) ON SKELETAL TISSUES (BONE OR CARTILAGE)

CYTOKINE (GROWTH FACTOR)	BONE		CARTILAGE	
	FORMATION	RESORPTION	FORMATION	RESORPTION
Transforming growth factor-beta	+, −	+, −	+, −	−
Transforming growth factor-alpha or epidermal growth factor	+, −	+	+	0
Insulin-like growth factor	−	?	−	0
Fibroblast growth factor	+, −	?	−	0
Platelet-derived growth factor	0	+	?	?
Colony-stimulating factors	?	?	−	−
Interferon-gamma	−	?	−	+
Tumor necrosis factor	−	+	+, −	+
Interleukins-1, -3, and -6	−	+	?	?

+, −, Both stimulatory and inhibitory properties on the specific cell listed; *0*, no effects presently known; *?*, possible effects on the cell listed.

which are likely the primary mechanoreceptors in bone.[11,12] Once changes, such as mechanical stress, hormonal imbalance, loading, or unloading, in bone are detected by the osteocyte's mechanoreceptors, multiple molecular signals are produced and the process of bone remodeling begins.[6,13] Osteocytes communicate with other bone cells and instruct both osteoblasts and osteoclasts about when and where to form and resorb bone; concentrate nutrients in the matrix; regulate bone mass and minerals (especially calcium and phosphorus); and secrete other proteins, such as sclerostin and fibroblast growth factor-23 (FGF-23), that influence mineral metabolism.[4,14-16] Sclerostin inhibits osteoblasts, thus reducing bone formation. Additionally, osteocytes seem to function as endocrine receptors in regulating bone metabolism and are prime target cells of parathyroid hormone (PTH).[16-18] Through exchanges between these cells, hormone catalysts, and minerals, optimal levels of calcium, phosphorus, and other minerals are maintained in blood plasma. (Remodeling is described under Maintenance of Bone Integrity.)

Osteoclasts. Derived from the hematopoietic monocyte-macrophage lineage, osteoclasts are terminally differentiated multinucleated bone cells and are responsible for bone resorption.[1] Osteoclasts migrate over bone surfaces to resorption areas that have been prepared and stripped of osteoid by enzymes, such as collagenases produced by osteoblasts in the presence of parathyroid hormone (PTH), which are necessary for the resorptive process. Osteoclasts travel over the prepared bone surfaces, creating irregular, scalloped cavities, known as *Howship lacunae* or *resorption lacunae*, as they resorb bone areas and then acidify hydroxyapatite in order to dissolve it.[19]

A specific area of the cell membrane adjacent to the bone surface forms deep and irregular foldings. These foldings, known as the **ruffled border**, greatly increase the surface areas of cells under their scalloped or ruffled borders. Osteoclasts resorb bone by secretion of hydrochloric acid, acid proteases (such as cathepsin K), and matrix metalloproteinases (MMPs) that help digest collagen, along with the action of cytokines (see Table 44.3). Osteoclasts also resorb bone through the action of lysosomes (digestive vacuoles) filled with hydrolytic enzymes in their mitochondria.[19]

Osteoclasts bind to the bone surface through attachments called **podosomes**, which are footlike structures that cluster together along a sealing membrane that forms a "belt" containing multiple proteins, enzymes, and integrin receptors.[19-20] Once resorption is complete, the osteoclasts retract and loosen from the bone surface under the ruffled border through the action of calcitonin. Calcitonin binds to receptor areas of the osteoclasts' cell membranes to effectively loosen the osteoclasts from the bone surfaces. Once resorption is completed, osteoclasts disappear by the process of degeneration either by reverting to the form of

their parent cells or by undergoing cell movements away from the site, in which the osteoclast becomes an inactive or resting osteoclast.

In addition to resorption of bone, osteoclasts assist the endocrine and renal systems in maintaining appropriate serum calcium and phosphorus levels. Osteoclasts also appear to have a role in the body's immune response.[19]

The OPG/RANKL/RANK System. Osteoprotegerin (OPG) is a glycoprotein belonging to the tumor necrosis factor superfamily and inhibits bone remodeling/resorption by inhibiting osteoclast formation. Numerous cells, including osteoblasts and osteocytes, produce it. OPG is key in the interaction between osteoblasts and osteoclasts.[21] Osteoblasts and osteoclasts cooperate (a term called *coupling*) to maintain normal bone homeostasis. RANKL is an essential cytokine needed for the formation and activation of osteoclasts. RANKL increases bone loss. OPG decreases bone loss because when it is activated it promotes bone formation. When RANKL binds to its receptor RANK on osteoclast precursor cells, it triggers their proliferation and increases bone resorption. OPG, secreted by osteoblasts and B lymphocytes, serves as a decoy by binding to RANK, preventing RANKL binding to RANK and thereby preventing bone resorption.[22] Therefore the overall balance between RANKL and OPG determines the amount of bone loss and is regulated by cytokines and hormones.[23]

Alterations of the RANKL/RANK/OPG system can lead to dysregulation and pathologic conditions, including primary osteoporosis, immune-mediated bone diseases, malignant bone disorders, and inherited skeletal diseases. It is worth noting that dimethyl sulfoxide (DMSO), an FDA-approved organosulfur solvent, is reported to have osteoclast-inhibiting properties.[24] In a recent study, data showed that 1% DMSO significantly inhibited RANKL-induced osteoclastogenesis.[24] Specifically, DMSO inhibited both differentiation and function of osteoclasts. This is an important finding because it presents the potential use of DMSO for treatment of bone diseases related to increased osteoclast proliferation, such as osteoporosis.[24] One study demonstrated that daily injections of DMSO inhibited estrogen deficiency–induced osteopenia in rats by inhibiting the function of osteoclasts.[25]

Bone Matrix

Bone matrix is made of the extracellular elements of bone tissue. Bone matrix is composed of an organic component known as *osteoid* (35%) and a mineral component (65%). Osteoid is comprised of predominantly type I collagen with small amounts of glycosaminoglycans and other proteins[1] (Box 44.1).

The major inorganic components are the calcium and phosphate minerals. Other parts of the bone matrix are the proteins,

---

BOX 44.1   **PROTEINS OF BONE MATRIX**

Osteoblast-Derived Proteins
Type I collagen
Calcium-binding proteins
  Osteonectin, bone sialoprotein
Cell adhesion proteins
  Osteopontin, fibronectin, thrombospondin
Cytokines
  IGF-2, TGF-β, PDGF
Proteins involved in mineralization
  Osteocalcin

Proteins Concentrated from Serum
Albumin
β_2-Microglobulin

From Kumar V, Abbas AK, Aster JCF: *Robbins & Cotran pathologic basis of disease,* ed 9, Philadelphia, 2015, Elsevier Sanders.

TABLE 44.5   **TYPES OF COLLAGEN IN MUSCULOSKELETAL TISSUES**

TYPE OF COLLAGEN	DISTRIBUTION IN MUSCULOSKELETAL TISSUES
I	Bone, tendon, ligament, intervertebral disk, muscle*
II	Cartilage, intervertebral disk
III	Skin, muscle, often with type I
IV	Basement cell membrane, muscle
V	Codistributed with type I muscle, most interstitial tissues
VI	Ubiquitous, muscle
IX	Codistributed with type II muscle
X	Cartilage growth plate
XI	Cartilage, muscle
XII	Codistributed with type I and type III muscle
XIII	Molecule has not been isolated in connective tissues to date
XIV	Codistributed with type I muscle
XV	Muscle; contains heparin sulfate proteoglycans (HSPGs)
XVII	Muscle; contains HSPGs

*Refers specifically to skeletal muscle.

---

carbohydrate-protein complexes, and ground substances. Water comprises 5% to 8% of the matrix.

Collagen Fibers. Collagen fibers make up the bulk of bone matrix. They are formed as follows:

1. Osteoblasts synthesize and secrete type I collagen and osteocalcin.
2. Collagen molecules assemble into three thin chains (alpha chains) to form fibrils.
3. Fibrils organize into the staggered pattern, with each fibril overlapping its nearest neighbor by about one-fourth its length; this creates gaps into which mineral crystals are deposited.
4. After mineral deposition, fibrils interlink and twist to form ropelike fibers.
5. The fibers then join to form the framework that gives bone its tensile and supportive strength.

Collagen is the most abundant macromolecule in the body, accounting for approximately one-third of all protein and providing the structural framework for nearly all tissues. Collagen is one of the extracellular components, along with proteoglycans and noncollagenous matrix proteins, of articular cartilage. To date, more than 20 types of collagen have been identified, though all their functions are not yet known. Cartilage-specific collagens include types II (the principal component), VI, IX, X, and XI. Type IX collagen is thought to be the "glue" that holds together the type II collagen scaffold of articular cartilage, helps maintain the structural integrity of cartilage, and resists tensile forces on joint cartilage. Type XI regulates the fibril diameter of type II cartilage. Degradation of type IX collagen by proteolytic enzymes has been seen in the early stages of osteoarthritis and rheumatoid arthritis. Researchers have proposed that this degradation, or "unplugging," may be the mechanism for the degenerative changes seen in osteoarthritic and rheumatoid cartilage. Table 44.5 gives the musculoskeletal distribution of other types of collagen.

Proteoglycans. Proteoglycans are large complexes of numerous polysaccharides attached to a common protein core. They strengthen bone by forming compression-resistant networks between the collagen fibrils. Proteoglycans also control the transport and distribution of electrically charged particles (ions), particularly calcium, through the bone matrix, thereby playing a role in bone calcium deposition and calcification.

Glycoproteins. Glycoproteins are carbohydrate-protein complexes of bone. Glycoproteins control the collagen interactions that lead to fibril formation. They also may play a role in calcification.

Some of the glycoproteins in bone matrix include bone sialoprotein, osteocalcin, osteonectin, laminin, albumin, and α-glycoprotein. Other proteins found in bone matrix are the compounds currently called bone morphogenic proteins (BMPs) (see Table 44.2). Sialoprotein (osteopontin) comprises about 8% of the noncollagenous matrix of bone and easily binds with calcium.

Osteocalcin is also a calcium-binding protein that binds preferentially to calcium that has already crystallized. The roles of osteocalcin may be to inhibit calcium phosphate precipitation and to play a part in bone resorption by recruiting osteoclasts.

Osteonectin is a bone-specific protein that binds selectively to both hydroxyapatite and collagen in the bone matrix. Laminin is an abundant bone matrix protein in humans that stabilizes basement membranes in bones and is important in neurite and axon growth.

Bone albumin is identical to serum albumin. In calcified matrix, bone albumin is permanently fixed to bone mineral crystals and remains so until the bone is resorbed. Bone albumin transports essential elements such as hormones, ions, and other metabolites to and from the bone cells and maintains the osmotic pressure of bone fluid (fluid surrounding mineral crystals and osteoblasts).

Bone Minerals

After collagen synthesis and fiber formation, the final step in bone formation is mineralization. Mineralization has two distinct phases: (1) formation of hydroxyapatite crystals within matrix vesicles that bud from the surface membrane of chondrocytes, osteoblasts, and odontoblasts; and (2) proliferation or accretion of hydroxyapatite into the extracellular matrix and its deposition between collagen fibrils.[26]

Table 44.6 lists the sequence in which calcium and phosphate form amorphous (fluid) calcium phosphate compounds that are converted, in stages, to solid hexagonal crystals of hydroxyapatite (HAP). As the calcium and phosphorous concentrations increase in the bone matrix, the first precipitate to form is dicalcium phosphate dihydrate (DCPD). Once DCPD precipitation begins, the remaining phases of bone crystal formation proceed until insoluble HAP is produced, with approximately 80% to 90% of the HAP being incorporated into the collagen fibers.

TABLE 44.6	SEQUENCE OF CALCIUM AND PHOSPHATE COMPOUND FORMATION AND CRYSTALLIZATION*	
FORMULA	**NAME**	**ABBREVIATION**
$Ca(HPO_4) \times 2H_2O$	Dicalcium phosphate dehydrate	DCPD
$Ca_4H(PO_4)_3$	Octacalcium phosphate	OCP
$Ca_9(PO_4)_6$ (var.)	Amorphous calcium phosphate	ACP
$Ca_3(PO_4)_2$	Tricalcium phosphate	TCP
$Ca_5(PO_4)_3OH$	Hydroxyapatite	HAP

*NOTE: Compounds are listed in order in which precipitation and crystal formation occur.

Amorphous calcium phosphate is distributed throughout the bone matrix.

Types of Bone Tissue

Bone is composed of two types of bony (osseous) tissue: compact bone (cortical bone) and spongy bone (cancellous bone) (Fig. 44.3). Compact bone constitutes approximately 85% of the skeleton; spongy bone comprises the remaining 15%. Both types of bone tissue contain the same structural elements, and, with a few exceptions, both compact tissue and spongy tissue are present in every bone. The major difference between the two types of tissue is the organization of the elements.

Compact bone is highly organized, solid, and extremely strong. The basic structural unit in compact bone is the haversian system (Fig. 44.4). Each haversian system is made up of the following:

1. A central canal called the haversian canal
2. Concentric layers of bone matrix called lamellae
3. Tiny spaces (lacunae) between the lamellae
4. Bone cells (osteocytes) within the lacunae
5. Small channels or canals called canaliculi

Each haversian system is a separate cylindrical entity that looks like a set of concentric rings. In the center of the haversian system is the haversian canal that runs through the long axis of bone and contains one or two blood vessels and nerve fibers. The blood vessels in the canal communicate with blood vessels in the periosteum (surface cover) and marrow cavity to transport nutrients and wastes to and from the osteocytes contained within the lacunae. Surrounding each haversian canal are the concentric lamellae. Between the lamellae are the lacunae, each of which contains one osteocyte. The lacunae are connected to each other and to the haversian canal by the canaliculi, which run parallel to the horizontal axis of the bone. Each canaliculus encloses a small extension (cytoplasmic process) from the osteocyte contained in the lacuna. The canaliculi transport both nourishment and molecular signals into the lacunae, a mechanism essential for osteocyte survival.

Spongy bone is less complex and lacks haversian systems. In spongy bone the lamellae are not arranged in concentric layers but in plates or bars termed trabeculae that branch and unite with one another to form an irregular meshwork. The pattern of the meshwork is determined by the direction of stress on the particular bone. The spaces between the trabeculae are filled with red bone marrow. The osteocyte-containing lacunae are distributed between the trabeculae and interconnected by canaliculi. Capillaries pass through the marrow to nourish the osteocytes.

All bones are covered with a double-layered connective tissue called the periosteum. The outer layer of the periosteum contains blood vessels and nerves, some of which penetrate to the inner structures of the bone through channels called *Volkmann canals* (see Fig. 44.4). The inner

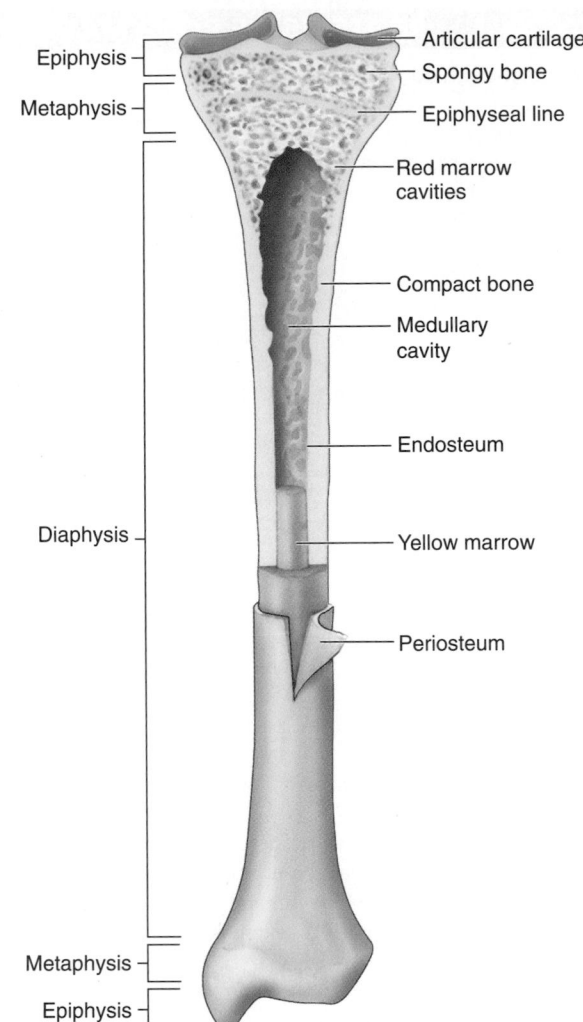

FIGURE 44.3 Cross Section of Bone. Longitudinal section of long bone (tibia) showing cancellous and compact bone. (From Patton KT, Thibodeau GA: *The human body in health & disease*, ed 7, St Louis, 2018, Mosby.)

layer of the periosteum is anchored to the bone by collagenous fibers (Sharpey fibers) that penetrate the bone. Sharpey fibers also help hold or attach tendons and ligaments to the periosteum of bones.[27]

Characteristics of Bone

The human skeleton consists of 206 bones that constitute the axial skeleton and the appendicular skeleton (Fig. 44.5). The axial skeleton consists of 80 bones that make up the skull, vertebral column, and thorax. The appendicular skeleton consists of 126 bones that make up the upper and lower extremities, the shoulder girdle (pectoral girdle), and the pelvic girdle (os coxae). The skeleton contributes about 14% of the weight of the adult body.

Bones can be classified by shape as long, flat, short (cuboidal), or irregular. Long bones are longer than they are wide and consist of a narrow tubular midportion (diaphysis) that merges into a broader neck (metaphysis) and a broad end (epiphysis) (see Fig. 44.3).

The diaphysis consists of a shaft of thick, rigid compact bone that can tolerate bending forces. Contained within the diaphysis is the elongated marrow (medullary) cavity. The marrow cavity of the diaphysis contains primarily fatty tissue, which is referred to as *yellow marrow*. The yellow marrow assists red bone marrow in hematopoiesis only during times of stress. The yellow marrow cavity of the diaphysis is

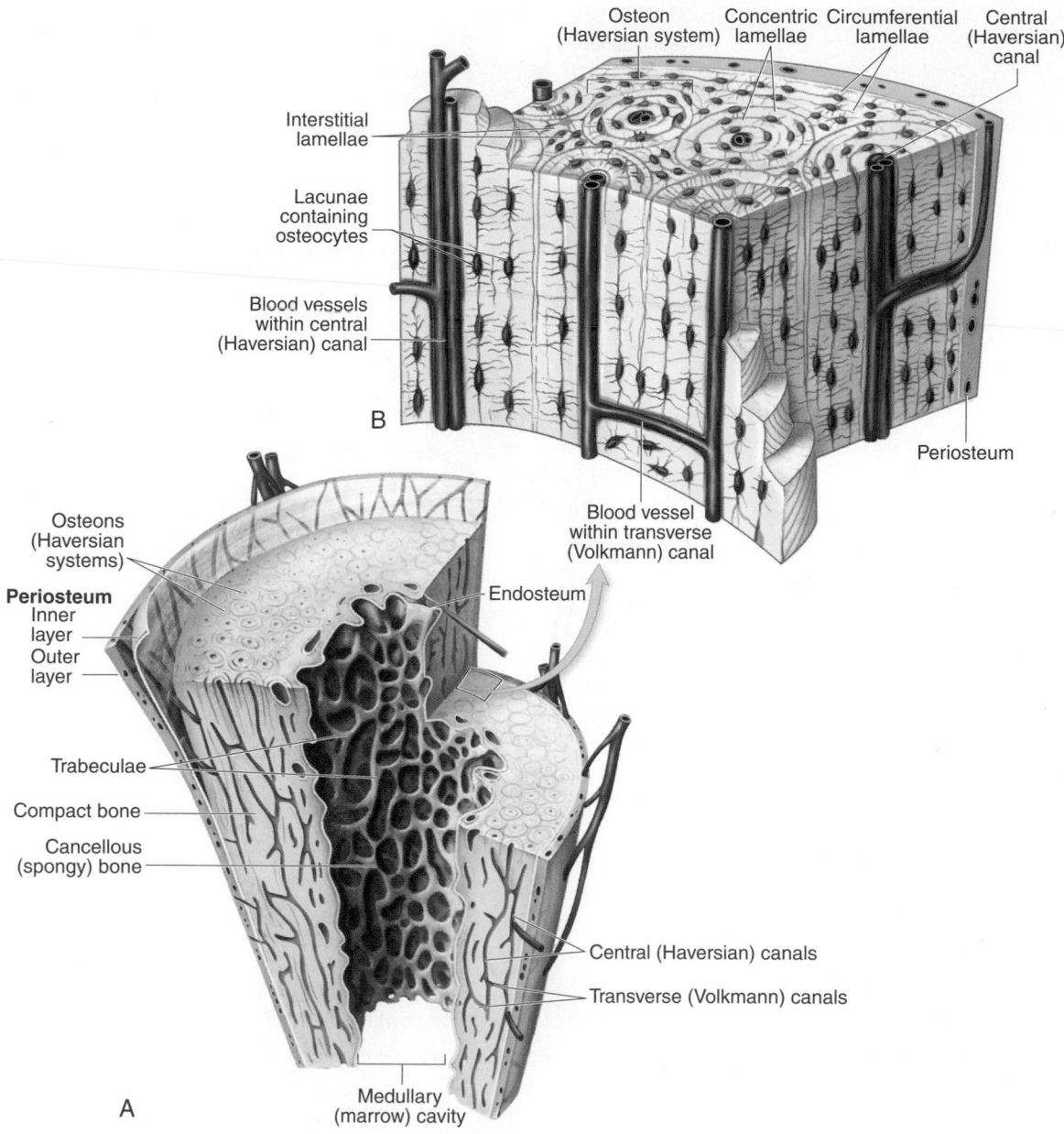

FIGURE 44.4 Structure of Compact and Spongy Bone. **A,** Longitudinal section of a long bone showing cancellous and compact bone. **B,** A magnified view of compact bone. (From Patton KT, Thibodeau GA: *Anatomy & physiology*, ed 9, St Louis, 2016, Mosby.)

continuous with marrow cavities in the spongy bone of the metaphysis and diaphysis. The marrow contained within the epiphysis is red because it contains primarily blood-forming tissue (see Chapter 28). A layer of connective tissue, the endosteum, lines the outer surfaces of both types of marrow cavity.

The broadness of the epiphysis allows weightbearing to be distributed over a wide area. The epiphysis is made up of spongy bone covered by a very thin layer of compact bone. In a child the epiphysis is separated from the metaphysis by a cartilaginous growth plate, the epiphyseal plate. After puberty the epiphyseal plate calcifies and the epiphysis and metaphysis merge. By adulthood the line of demarcation between the epiphysis and metaphysis is undetectable.

In flat bones, such as the ribs or scapulae, two plates of compact bone are roughly parallel to each other. Between the compact bone plates is a layer of spongy bone. Short bones (cuboidal bones), such

as the bones of the wrist or ankle, are often cuboidal in shape. They consist of spongy bone covered by a thin layer of compact bone.

Irregular bones, such as the vertebrae, mandible, or other facial bones, have various shapes that include thin and thick segments. The thin part of an irregular bone consists of two plates of compact bone with spongy bone between the plates. The thick part consists of spongy bone surrounded by a layer of compact bone.

Maintenance of Bone Integrity
Remodeling

The integrity of bone is maintained by bone remodeling, a three-phase process in which existing bone is resorbed and new bone is laid down to replace it. Osteoclasts and osteoblasts work together as a basic multicellular unit (BMU) to remove old bone by osteoclast activity

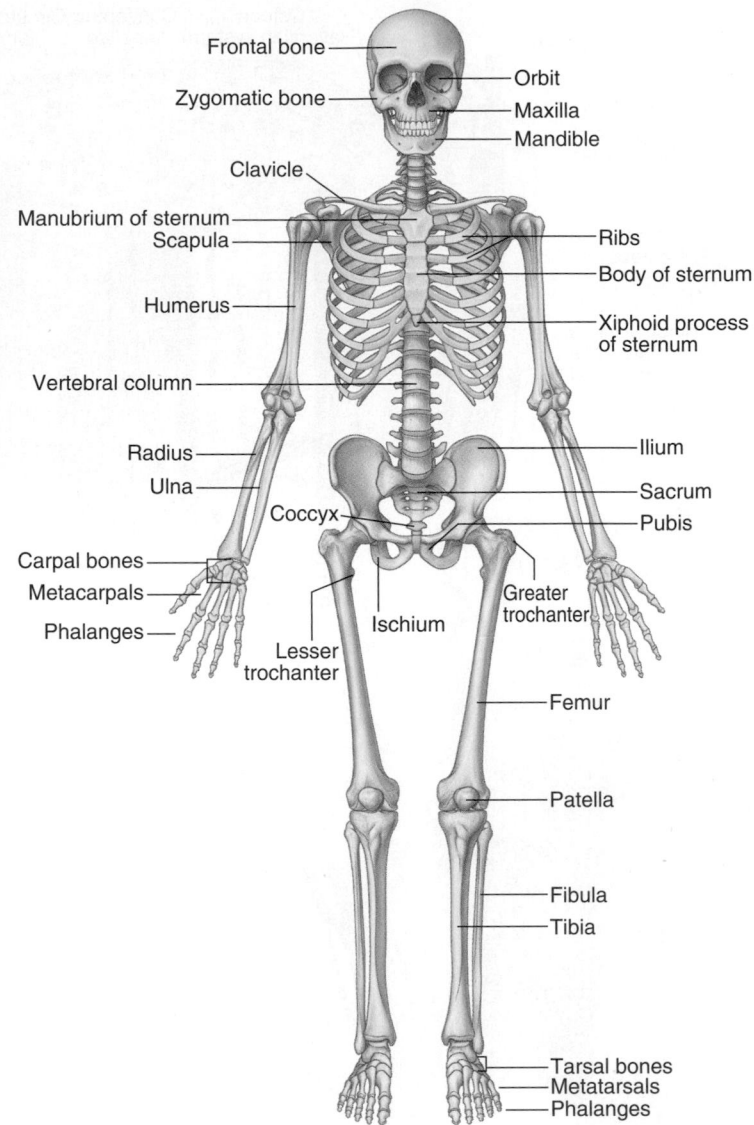

FIGURE 44.5 Anterior View of Skeleton. (From Drake R et al: *Gray's atlas of anatomy,* ed 2, Philadelphia, 2015, Churchill Livingstone.)

and to deposit new bone by osteoblast activity.[6] The basic multicellular units are made up of bone precursor cells that differentiate into osteoclasts and osteoblasts. Precursor cells are located on the free surfaces of bones and along the vascular channels (especially the marrow cavities).

In phase 1 (activation) of the remodeling cycle, a stimulus (e.g., hormone, drug, vitamin, physical stressor) activates programmed osteocyte cell death (apoptosis). The distribution of these apoptotic osteocytes provides the osteoclasts with information about where to begin resorbing damaged bone. In phase 2 (resorption), the osteoclasts form a "cutting cone," which gradually resorbs bone, leaving behind an elongated cavity termed a *resorption cavity*. Osteoclasts attach to the bone matrix by actin microfilaments and multiple other proteins that form footlike structures called *podosomes*. Once attached, the osteoclasts' integrin receptors anchor their microfilaments to the extracellular matrix, thus providing receptor pathways between the osteocyte and bone matrix. Lysosomal enzymes produced by osteoclasts "digest" bone; the osteoclasts then release the degraded bone products into the vascular system.[19]

In phase 3 (formation), new bone formation begins as osteoblasts lining the walls of the resorption cavity express osteoid and alkaline phosphatase, forming sites for calcium and phosphorus deposition. New bone is formed as the osteoid mineralizes. Successive layers (lamellae) in compact bone are laid down until the resorption cavity is reduced to a narrow haversian canal around a blood vessel. In this way, old haversian systems are destroyed and new haversian systems are formed. New trabeculae are formed in spongy bone. The formation phase takes 4 to 6 months in humans.[28]

Repair

The remodeling process can repair microscopic bone injuries, but gross injuries, such as fractures and surgical wounds (osteotomies), heal by the same stages as soft tissue injuries, except that new bone, instead of scar tissue, is the final result (see Chapter 7). In bone the stages of wound healing are as follows:

1. *Hematoma formation:* This process occurs if vessels have been damaged, causing hemorrhage. Fibrin and platelets within the hematoma form a meshwork that is the initial framework for healing with the help of hematopoietic growth factors such as platelet-derived growth factor and TGF-β (see Table 44.3).

2. *Procallus formation:* Fibroblasts, capillary buds, and osteoblasts move into the wound to produce granulation tissue called **procallus**. Cartilage is formed as a precursor of bone, and types I, II, and III collagen are formed. Enzymes and growth factors, such as insulin and insulin-like growth factors, plus bone morphogenic protein and osteogenin, aid in this stage of healing.

3. *Callus formation:* Osteoblasts in the procallus form membranous or **woven bone (callus)**. Enzymes increase the phosphate content and permit the phosphate to join with calcium to be deposited as mineral to harden the callus.

4. *Replacement:* Basic multicellular units of the callus are replaced with lamellar bone or trabecular bone (Fig. 44.6).

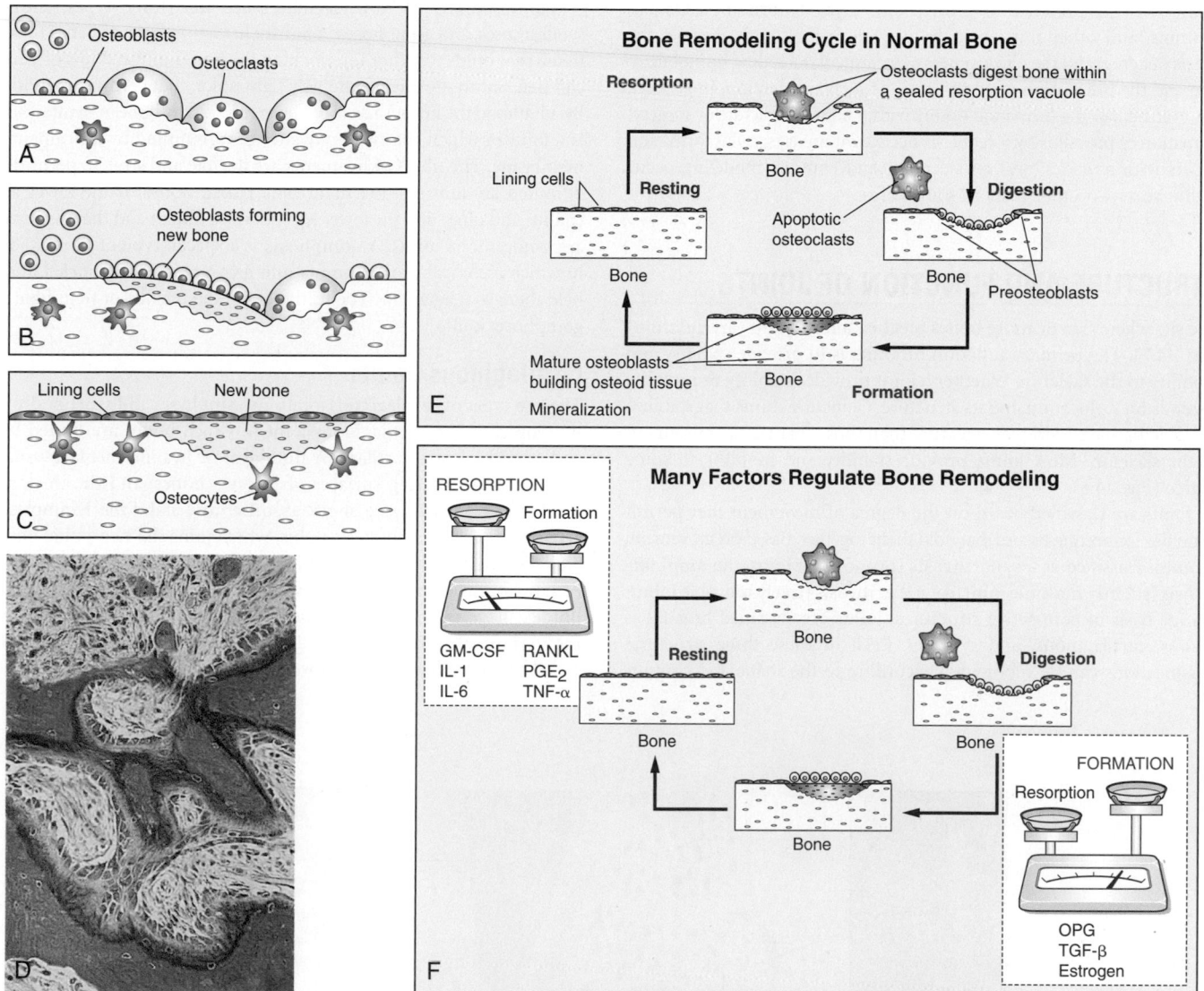

FIGURE 44.6 Bone Remodeling. All bone cells participate in bone remodeling. In the remodeling sequence bone sections are removed by bone-resorbing cells (osteoclasts) and replaced with a new section laid down by bone-forming cells (osteoblasts). Bone remodeling is necessary because it allows the skeleton to respond to mechanical loading, maintains quality control (repair and prevent microdamage), and allows the skeleton to release growth factors and minerals (calcium and phosphate) stored in bone matrix to the circulation. The cells work in response to signals generated in the environment (see **F**). Only the osteoclastic cells mediate the first phase of remodeling. They are activated, scoop out bone (**A**), and resorb it; then the work of the osteoblasts begins (**B**). They form new bone that replaces bone removed by the resorption process (**C**). The sequence takes 4 to 6 months. **D,** Micrograph of active bone remodeling seen in the settings of primary or secondary hyperparathyroidism. Note the active osteoblasts surmounted on red-stained osteoid. Marrow fibrosis is present. **E,** Bone remodeling cycle in normal bone (**F**). Numerous signaling factors are necessary for remodeling. Factors most important for resorption include granulocyte-macrophage colony–stimulating factor *(GM-CSF)*, interleukins-1 and -6 *(IL-1* and *IL-6)*, receptor activator for nuclear factor κβ ligand *(RANKL)*, prostaglandin E_2 *(PGE$_2$)*, and tumor necrosis factor-alpha *(TNF-α)*. Important factors for bone formation include osteoprotegerin *(OPG)*, transforming growth factor-beta *(TGF-β)*, and estrogen. (Adapted from Nucleus Medical Art. **D** from Damjananov I, Linder J, editors: *Anderson's pathology,* ed 10, St Louis, 1996, Mosby.)

5. *Remodeling:* The periosteal and endosteal surfaces of the bone are remodeled to the size and shape of the bone before injury. Synthesis of other types of collagen recedes in favor of type I, which is the collagen found in bone. This final stage of healing, or remodeling, is vital because bone that has not been remodeled does not have good mechanical properties for weightbearing and mobility.

The speed with which bone heals depends on the severity of the bone disruption; the type and amount of bone tissue that must be replaced (spongy bone heals faster); the blood supply and oxygen content at the site; the presence of growth and thyroid hormones, insulin, vitamins, and other nutrients; the presence of systemic disease; the effects of aging; and the effectiveness of treatment, including immobilization and the prevention of complications such as infection. In general, however, hematoma formation occurs within hours of fracture or surgery; formation of procallus by osteoblasts occurs within days; callus formation occurs within weeks; and replacement and contour modeling occur within years—up to 4 years in some cases.

STRUCTURE AND FUNCTION OF JOINTS

The site where two or more bones meet is called a joint (articulation) (Fig. 44.7). The primary function of joints is to provide stability and mobility to the skeleton. Whether a joint provides stability or mobility depends on its location and its structure. Generally, joints that stabilize the skeleton have a simpler structure than those that enable movement of the skeleton. Most joints provide stability and mobility to some degree (Fig. 44.8).

Joints are classified based on the degree of movement they permit or on the connecting tissues that hold them together. Based on movement, a joint is classified as a synarthrosis (immovable joint), an amphiarthrosis (slightly movable joint), or a diarthrosis (freely movable joint). On the basis of connective structures, joints are classified broadly as fibrous, cartilaginous, and synovial. Each of these three structural classifications can be subdivided according to the shape and contour of the articulating surfaces (ends) of the bones and the type of motion the joint permits.

Fibrous Joints

A joint in which bone is united directly to bone by fibrous connective tissue is called a fibrous joint. Generally, fibrous joints are synarthroses (immovable), but many fibrous joints allow some movement. The degree of movement depends on the distance between the bones and the flexibility of the fibrous connective tissue.

Fibrous joints are further subdivided into three types: sutures, syndesmoses, and gomphoses. A suture has a thin layer of dense fibrous tissue that binds together interlocking flat bones in the skulls of young children. Sutures form an extremely tight union that permits no motion. By adulthood the fibrous tissue has been replaced by bone. A syndesmosis is a joint in which the two bony surfaces are united by a ligament or membrane. The fibers of ligaments are flexible and stretch, permitting a limited amount of movement. The paired bones of the lower arm (radius and ulna) and the lower leg (tibia and fibula) and their ligaments are syndesmotic joints. A gomphosis is a special type of fibrous joint in which a conical projection fits into a complementary socket and is held there by a ligament. The teeth held in the maxilla or mandible are gomphosis joints.

Cartilaginous Joints

The two types of cartilaginous joints are symphyses and synchondroses. A symphysis is a cartilaginous joint in which bones are united by a pad or disk of fibrocartilage. A thin layer of hyaline cartilage usually covers the articulating surfaces of the two bones, and the thick pad of fibrocartilage acts as a shock absorber and stabilizer. Examples of symphyses are the symphysis pubis, which joins the two pubic bones, and the intervertebral disks, which join the bodies of the vertebrae. A synchondrosis is a joint in which hyaline cartilage, rather than fibrocartilage, connects the two bones. The joints between the ribs and the sternum are synchondroses. The hyaline cartilage of these joints is called *costal cartilage*. Slight movement at the synchondroses between

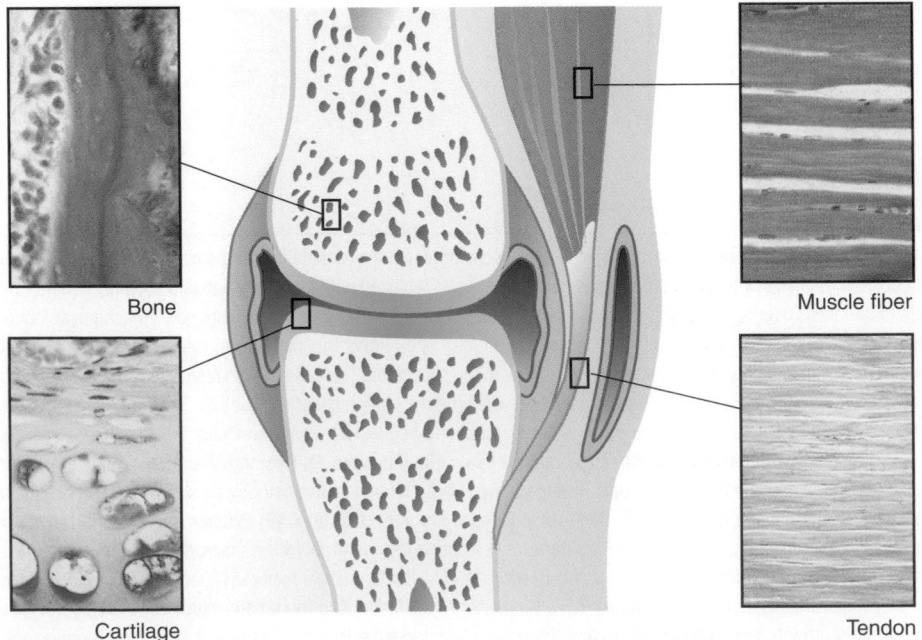

Bone

Muscle fiber

Cartilage

Tendon

FIGURE 44.7 Main Tissues of a Joint. (Micrographs from Erlandsen SL, Magney JE: *Color atlas of histology,* St Louis, 1992, Mosby.)

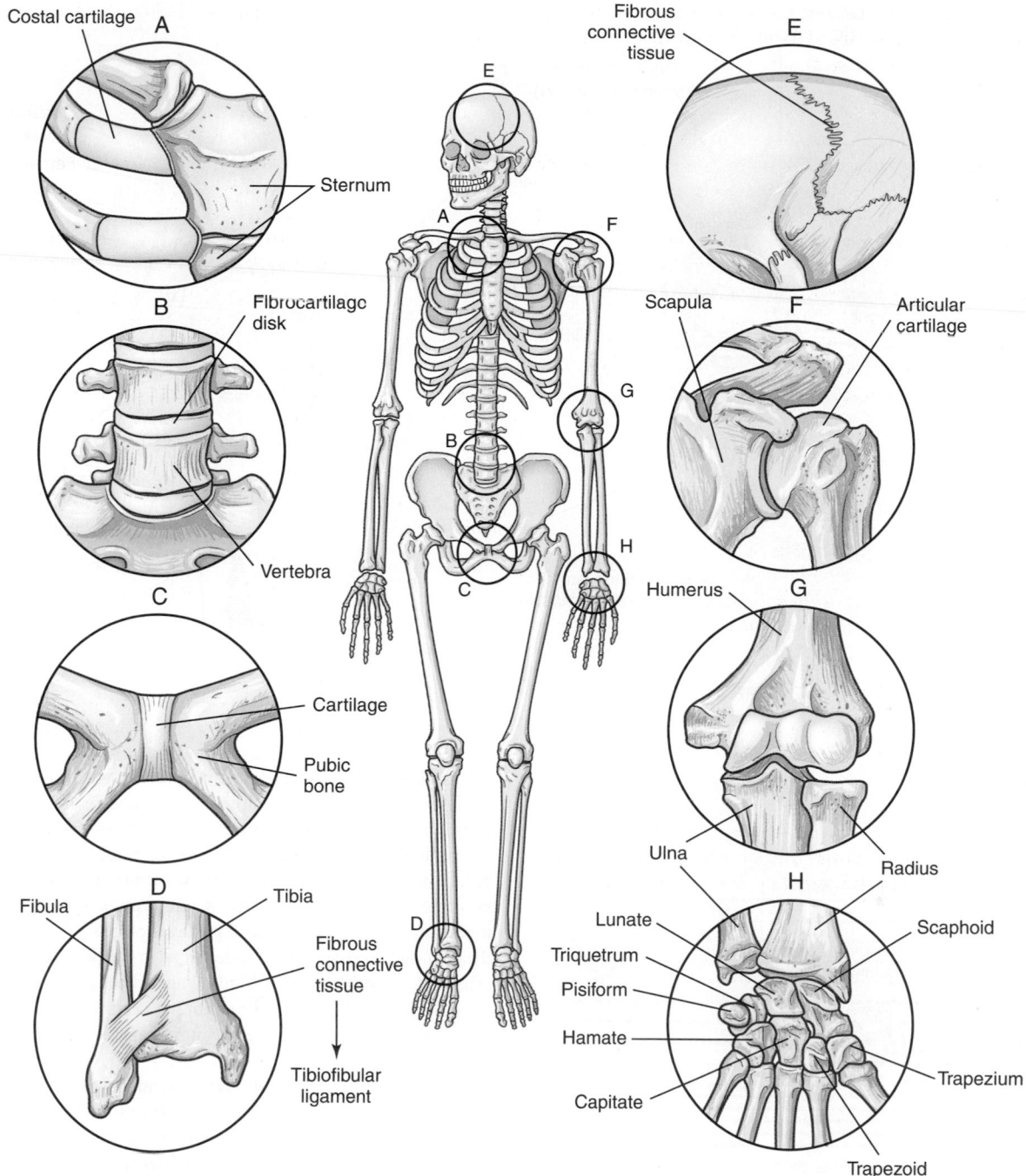

FIGURE 44.8 Types of Joints. Cartilaginous (amphiarthrodial) joints, which are slightly movable, include **(A)** a synchondrosis that attaches ribs to costal cartilage; **(B)** a symphysis that connects vertebrae; and **(C)** the symphysis that connects the two pubic bones. Fibrous (synarthrodial) joints, which are immovable, include **(D)** the syndesmosis between the tibia and fibula; **(E)** sutures that connect the skull bones; and the gomphosis (not shown), which holds teeth in their sockets. The synovial joints include **(F)** the spheroid type at the shoulder; **(G)** the hinge type at the elbow; and **(H)** the gliding joints of the hand.

the ribs and the sternum allows the chest to move outward and upward during breathing.

Synovial Joints
Structure

Synovial joints (diarthroses) are the most movable and the most complex joints in the body (Fig. 44.9). A synovial joint consists of the following parts:

1. A fibrous joint capsule (articular capsule)
2. A synovial membrane that lines the inner surface of the joint capsule
3. A joint cavity (synovial cavity), a space formed by the capsule
4. Synovial fluid, which fills the joint cavity and lubricates the joint surface
5. Articular cartilage, which covers and pads the articulating bony surfaces

Joint Capsule. The fibrous joint capsule (articular capsule) is connective tissue that covers the ends of the bones where they meet in

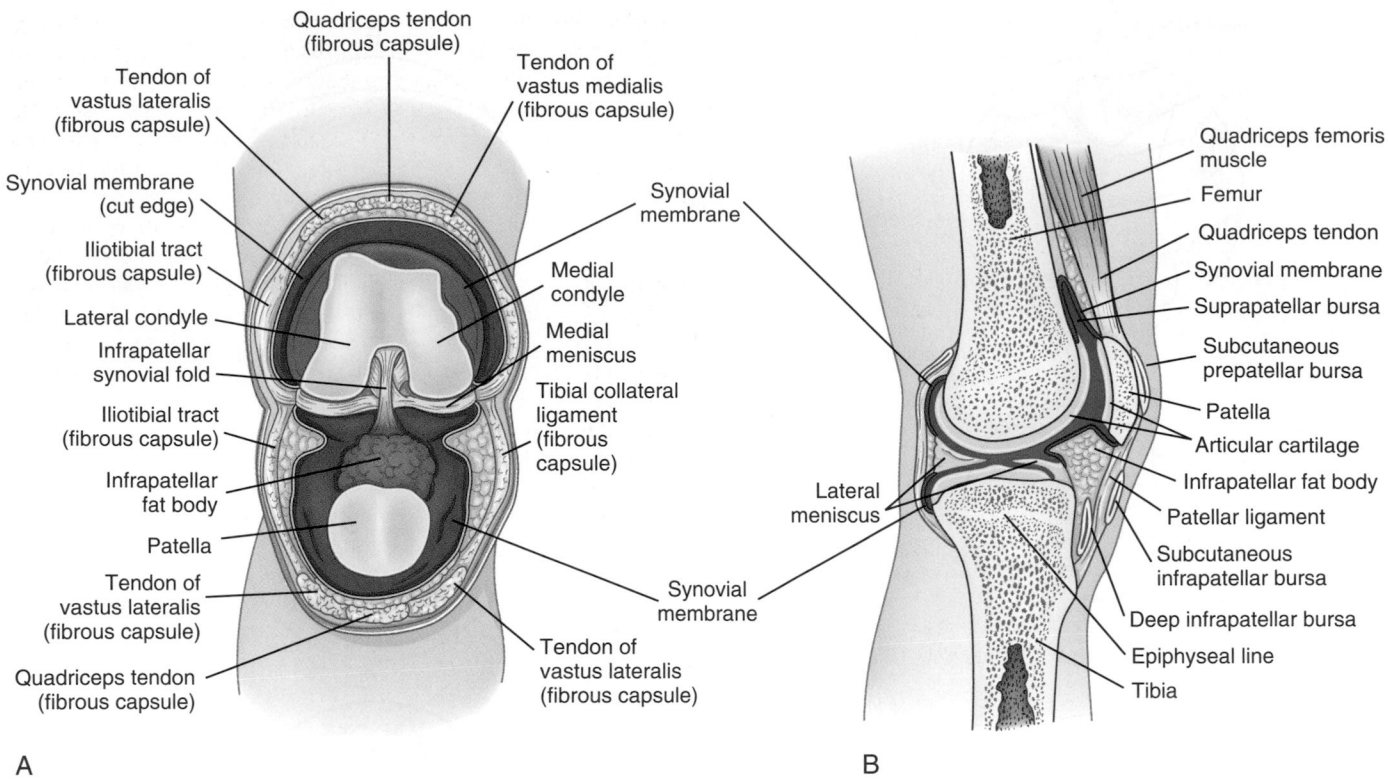

FIGURE 44.9 Knee Joint (Synovial Joint). **A,** Frontal view. **B,** Lateral view.

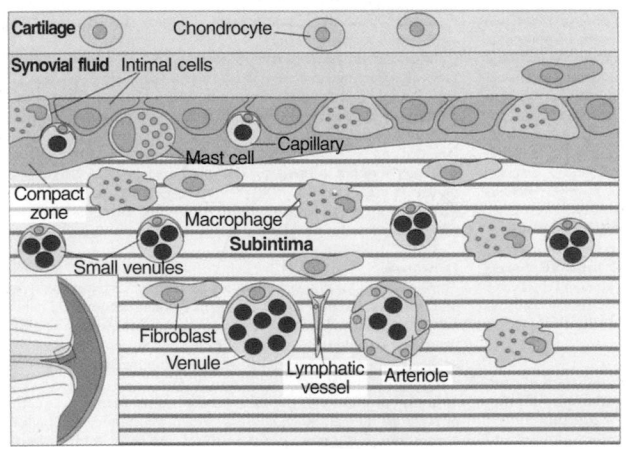

FIGURE 44.10 Synovium. Note the delicate synovial lining resting on a fibroadipose subintimal lining rich in capillaries, lymphatics, and nerve endings. (Modified from Hochberg MC et al: *Rheumatology*, ed 4, Philadelphia, 2008, Mosby.)

the joint. Sharpey fibers firmly attach the proximal and distal capsules to the periosteum and ligaments and tendons, which also reinforce the capsule. The joint capsule consists of parallel, interlacing bundles of dense, white fibrous tissue. It is richly supplied with nerves, blood vessels, and lymphatic vessels. The nerves in and around the joint capsule are sensitive to the rate and direction of motion, compression, tension, vibration, and pain.

Synovial Membrane. The synovial membrane (synovium) is the smooth, delicate inner lining of the joint capsule (Fig. 44.10). It lines the nonarticular portion of the synovial joint and any ligaments or tendons that traverse the joint cavity. It is made up of two layers—a

vascular layer (subintima) and a thin cellular layer (intima). The vascular subintima merges with the fibrous joint capsule and is composed of loose fibrous connective tissue, elastin fibers, fat cells, fibroblasts, macrophages, and mast cells. The intima consists of rows of synovial cells embedded in a fiber-free intercellular matrix. The intima contains two types of synovial cells: type A and type B. Type A synovial cells ingest and remove bacteria and particles of debris by phagocytosis in the joint cavity. (Phagocytosis is described in Chapter 7.) Type B synovial cells secrete hyaluronate, a binding agent that gives synovial fluid its viscous quality. The synovial membrane is richly supplied with blood and lymphatic vessels; therefore it is capable of rapid repair and regeneration.

Joint Cavity. The joint cavity (synovial cavity) is an enclosed fluid-filled space between the articulating surfaces of the two bones. This small cavity, often called the *joint space,* enables the two bones to move "against" one another. The synovial cavity is surrounded by the synovial membrane and filled with a clear, viscous, slick fluid called the *synovial fluid.*

Synovial Fluid. Synovial fluid is superfiltrated plasma from blood vessels in the synovial membrane. Synovial fluid lubricates the joint surfaces, nourishes the pad of the articular cartilage that covers the ends of the bones, and contains free-floating synovial cells and various leukocytes that phagocytize joint debris and microorganisms. Loss of synovial fluid leads to rapid deterioration of articular cartilage.

Articular Cartilage. Articular cartilage is a layer of hyaline cartilage that covers the end of each bone (Fig. 44.11). It ranges from 2 to 5 mm thick, depending on the size of the joint, the fit of the two bone ends, and the amount of weight and shearing force the joint normally withstands. Cartilage strength and its biologic properties are due to an extensive network of cross-linked collagen fibers. Fig. 44.12 illustrates how collagen cross-links from cartilage. The function of articular cartilage is to reduce friction in the joint and to distribute the forces of

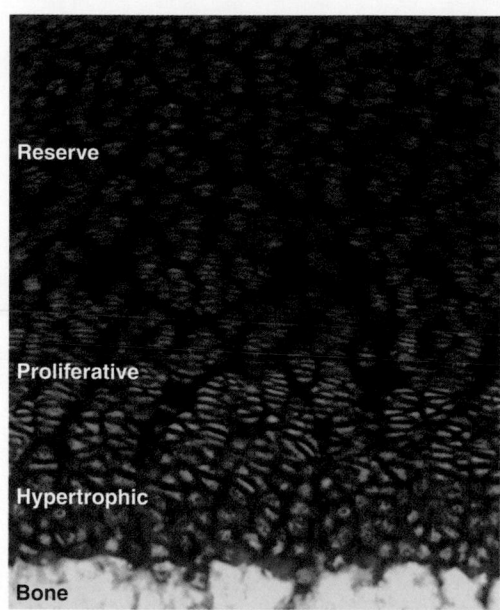

FIGURE 44.11 Collagen Zones. The three collagen zones (reserve, proliferative, and hypertrophic) are distinctly shown in a growth plate. (From Hjorten R et al: *Bone* 41[4]:535, 2007.)

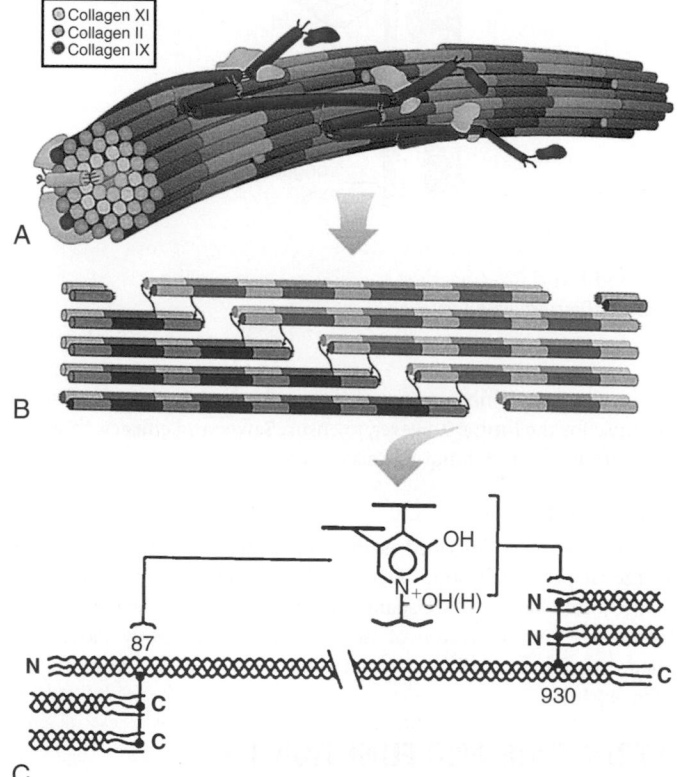

FIGURE 44.12 Heterotypic Collagen Fibril. Hierarchical depiction of heterotypic collagen fibril, emphasizing the internal axial relationships required for mature cross-link formation. **A,** Three-dimensional concept of the type II/IX/XI heterotypic fibril of developing cartilage matrix. **B,** Detail illustrating required nearest neighbor axial relationships for trifunctional intermolecular cross-links to form in collagens of cartilage, bone, and other high-tensile strength tissue matrices. The exact three-dimensional spatial pattern of cross-linking bonds is still unclear for any tissue. **C,** Detail of the axial stagger of individual collagen molecules required for pyridinoline cross-linking. (From Eyre DA, Weiss MA, Wu JJ: *Methods* 4[1]:65, 2008.)

weightbearing. Articular cartilage is composed of chondrocytes (cartilage cells) (making up about 2% of the tissue) and an intercellular matrix made up of collagen (making up about 10% to 30% of weight), protein polysaccharides (making up 5% to 10% of weight), and water. The water content ranges from 60% to almost 80% of the net weight of the cartilage, and individual molecules rapidly enter or exit the articular cartilage to contribute to the resiliency of the tissue.

The intercellular matrix is produced by the chondrocytes, which synthesize and extrude collagen that, like the collagen produced by bone cells, is distributed throughout the cartilage in a highly organized system of fibers. Collagen fibers in cartilage are made up of many fine fibrils that, like bone fibrils, are assembled in an orderly fashion that makes them resistant to physical, metabolic, or chemical breakdown. The main differences between bone collagen and cartilage collagen are the amino acid content of the α chains and the composition of the fibrils. Bone collagen fibrils are made up of two type I chains and one type II chain. Approximately 90% of the cartilage collagen fibrils are made up of three identical type II chains, with the remaining 10% consisting of types V, VI, IX, X, and XI.

At the surface of articular cartilage, the collagen fibers run parallel to the joint surface and are closely compacted into a dense, protective mat. (Loss of this dense, compacted configuration at the surface subjects the underlying fibers to splitting and thinning, in which case the cartilage is unable to tolerate weightbearing.) In the middle layer (the proliferative zone) of the cartilage, the fibers are arranged tangential to the surface, which allows them to deform and absorb some of the force of weightbearing (see Fig. 44.11). In the bottom layer (the hypertrophic zone) of the cartilage, the fibers are perpendicular to the joint surface, allowing them to resist shear forces, and are embedded in a calcified layer of cartilage called the tidemark. The tidemark anchors the collagen fibers to the underlying (subchondral) bone and represents the zone between calcified and noncalcified cartilage. Collagen fibers are important components of the cartilage matrix because they account for approximately 60% of the dry weight and because they (1) anchor the cartilage securely to underlying bone, (2) provide a taut framework for the cartilage, (3) control the loss of fluid from the cartilage, and (4) prevent the escape of protein polysaccharides (proteoglycans) from the cartilage.

The proteoglycans are macromolecules consisting of proteins, carbohydrates (glycosaminoglycans), and hyaluronic acid. One subgroup of proteoglycans, known as *heparin sulfate proteoglycans (HSPGs)*, binds to many proteins involved in musculoskeletal development and homeostasis, including FGF, BMPs, Wnts, chemokines, interleukins, and extracellular matrix (ECM) proteins.[29,30] The glycosaminoglycans (keratin sulfate and chondroitin sulfate) are attached to the protein core, and several protein cores (with their attached glycosaminoglycans) are bound to a hyaluronic acid chain by a special protein called link protein. The proteoglycans give articular cartilage its stiff quality and regulate the movement of synovial fluid through the cartilage. Without proteoglycans, normal weightbearing would rapidly and completely press all the synovial fluid out of the cartilage. Proteoglycans act as a pump, permitting enough fluid to be pressed out to ensure that a fluid film is always present on the surface of the cartilage, even after hours of weightbearing. The pumping action of proteoglycans also draws synovial fluid back into the cartilage after a weightbearing load is released. Mobility and weightbearing are necessary for the pumping action of proteoglycans to occur. Nonuse of a joint quickly reduces the pumping action, which changes the composition of the matrix and interferes with the nutrition of the chondrocytes.

Normal articular cartilage has no blood vessels, lymph vessels, or nerves. Therefore it is insensitive to pain and regenerates slowly and minimally after injury.[31,32] Regeneration occurs primarily at sites where the articular cartilage meets the synovial membrane, where blood vessels

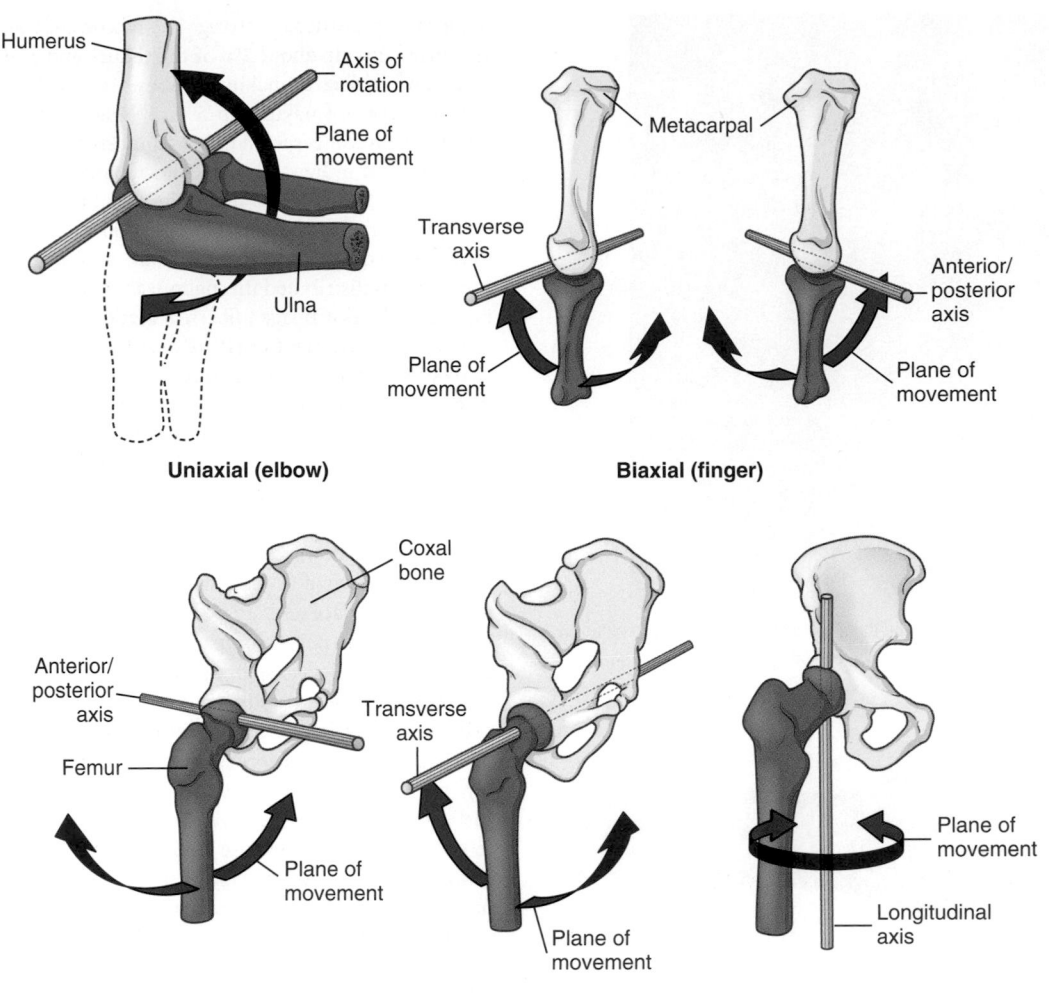

FIGURE 44.13 Movements of Synovial (Diarthrodial) Joints.

and nutrients are available. In general, it has been difficult to enhance cartilage repair, but that may be changing.

Progress in Rebuilding Cartilage. Although much research is needed, recent evidence suggests that mesenchymal stem cell therapies may be a potential solution to rebuilding articular cartilage.[33] Multipotent adult stem cells are largely available and accessible. It is theorized that bone marrow mesenchymal stem cells secrete proliferative and regenerative factors in the lesion site of articular cartilage (AC), thereby retarding osteoarthritis progression and promoting AC regeneration locally by trophic effects.[33-35]

Gene therapy (GT) also represents a novel approach to managing joint degradation. The principle of gene therapy is the overexpression of desired gene products. Gene therapy can support articular cartilage generation by targeting different genes involved in different cellular processes, such as inhibiting inflammatory and catabolic pathways, stimulating anabolic pathways, or preventing cell senescence and apoptosis.[33] Candidate transgene studies are currently in the exploratory phases, generally using animal models. Candidate transgenes with antiinflammatory action include interleukin-1 (IL-1) receptor antagonist and soluble tumor necrosis factor (sTNF). Gene therapy strategies also may target the catabolic effect of matrix metalloproteinases by the delivery of tissue inhibitor of metalloproteinase.[33,36-38]

The overexpression of growth factors has been shown to enhance matrix formation. TGF-β, in particular, was reported to aid cartilage

regeneration and enhance meniscal tissue healing in vitro.[33] GT shows promise for the future; however, to ensure safety and efficacy, thorough evaluation of the technique is necessary.

Movement

Synovial joints are described as uniaxial, biaxial, or multiaxial according to the shapes of the bone ends and the type of movement occurring at the joint (Fig. 44.13). Usually one of the bones is stable and serves as an axis for the motion of the other bone. The body movements made possible by various synovial joints are either circular or angular (Fig. 44.14).

STRUCTURE AND FUNCTION OF SKELETAL MUSCLES

Skeletal muscles arise from mesodermal progenitor cells; the most numerous are the somites. Actual formation of skeletal muscle is a complex process controlled by multiple signaling factors. A critical component of successful embryonic muscle formation (myogenesis) is protein kinase, an enzyme that adds phosphate groups to substrate proteins, thereby directing cell processes.[39] In muscle, these factors direct formation of myoblasts. Once myoblasts are formed, they fuse with other myoblasts and form myotubes, eventually developing into muscle fibers. At birth, the muscle fibers have completed development from

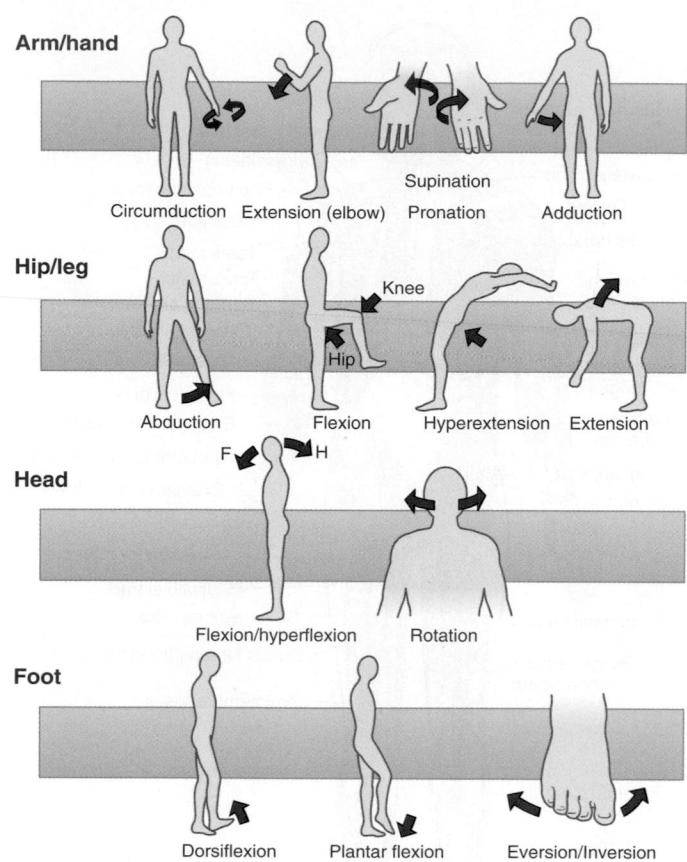

Arm/hand

Circumduction   Extension (elbow)   Supination / Pronation   Adduction

Hip/leg

Knee / Hip

Abduction   Flexion   Hyperextension   Extension

Head

F   H

Flexion/hyperflexion   Rotation

Foot

Dorsiflexion   Plantar flexion   Eversion/Inversion

FIGURE 44.14 Body Movements Provided by Synovial (Diarthrodial) Joints.

myoblasts. Final muscle type is determined by transcription factors that regulate both pre- and postnatal muscle development.[40]

All voluntary muscles are derived from the mesodermal layer of the embryo. Genetic transcription factors, most notably myoblast determination protein (MyoD), induce skeletal muscle differentiation. Myoblasts are the main cells responsible for muscle growth and regeneration. Myoblasts are termed *satellite cells* when in a dormant state and are crucial in muscle growth, maintenance, repair, and regeneration. Once muscle is injured, satellite cells become activated and increase the number of transcriptional factors necessary to form myoblasts and assist in repair.

Skeletal muscles are made up of millions of individual fibers that by the processes of contraction and relaxation do the work necessary to complete movements as varied as a ballerina's pirouette or an artist's deft stroke (Fig. 44.15). Muscle constitutes 40% of adults' body weight and 50% of children's body weight. Muscle is 75% water, 20% protein, and 5% organic and inorganic compounds; 32% of all protein stores for energy and metabolism is contained in muscle.

Whole Muscle

There are more than 350 named muscles; almost all are paired. The body's muscles vary dramatically; they range from 2 to 60 cm in length and are shaped according to function.[41] Fusiform muscles are elongated muscles shaped like straps and can run from one joint to another. Pennate muscles are broad, flat, and slightly fan shaped, with fibers running obliquely to the muscle's long axis. The multipennate deltoid muscle, which flexes and extends the arm, is a good example of a muscle shaped according to its function.

Each skeletal muscle is a separate organ encased in a three-part connective tissue framework called fascia. The layers of connective

tissue protect the muscle fibers, attach the muscle to bony prominences, and provide a structure for a network of nerve fibers, blood vessels, and lymphatic channels.

The outermost layer, the epimysium, is located on the surface of the muscle and tapers at each end to form the tendon (Fig. 44.16). Tendons allow a short muscle to exert power on a distant joint, whereas a thick muscle interferes with joint mobility. The next layer, the perimysium, further subdivides the muscle fibers into bundles of connective tissue, or fascicles. The endomysium surrounds the muscle fascicles, the smallest unit of muscle fibers visible without a microscope. The ligaments, tendons, and fascia are made up of connective tissue that also serves to buffer the limbs from the effects of sudden strains or changes in speed. The rapid recovery necessary for strenuous exercise is supported by the elastic property of muscle and its connective tissue.

Skeletal muscle is described, almost interchangeably, as voluntary, striated, or extrafusal. "Voluntary" indicates that the muscle is controlled directly by the central nervous system. "Striated" describes the striated, or striped, pattern of skeletal muscle viewed under a light microscope. The striations result from the organization of the muscle fibers into the contractile units called *sarcomeres*. "Extrafusal" distinguishes the skeletal muscle fibers from other contractile fibers located within the sensory organs of the muscle.

Other components that are visible on gross inspection of the whole muscle include the motor and sensory nerve fibers. These function together with the muscle, innervating portions of it and providing the electrical impulses needed for motor function.

Motor Unit

From the anterior horn cell of the spinal cord, the axons of motor nerves branch out to innervate a specific group of muscle fibers. Each anterior horn cell, its axon (part of a lower motor neuron; see Chapter 15), and the muscle fibers innervated by it are called a motor unit (Fig. 44.17). The motor units are composed of lower motor neurons, which extend to skeletal muscles. Often termed the *functional unit* of the neuromuscular system, the motor unit behaves as a single entity and contracts as a whole when it receives an electrical impulse.

The whole muscle may be controlled by several motor nerve axons. These branch out to innervate many motor units within the muscle. The whole muscle then may consist of many motor units. The number of motor units per individual muscle varies greatly. In the calf, for example, 1 motor axon will innervate approximately 2000 muscle fibers, out of a total of 1,200,000 muscle fibers. This is a high innervation ratio of muscle fibers to axons, and it contrasts markedly with the low innervation ratio in the laryngeal muscles, where two or three muscle fibers constitute each motor unit, and the innervation ratio can be of great functional significance. The greater the innervation ratio of a particular organ, the greater its endurance. Higher innervation ratios prevent fatigue, and lower innervation ratios allow for precision of movement.

Sensory Receptors. Although muscles function as effector organs, they also contain sensory receptors and are involved in sending different signals to the central nervous system. Among these are the muscle spindles and Golgi tendon organs. Spindles are mechanoreceptors that lie parallel to muscle fibers and respond to muscle stretching. Golgi tendon organs are dendrites that terminate and branch to tendons near the neuromuscular junction. Motor and sensory neurons secrete a proteoglycan called *neuregulin (NRG)* that increases the number of acetylcholine receptors and helps in the formation of muscle spindle fibers. Muscle spindles, Golgi tendon organs, and free nerve endings provide a means of reporting changes in length, tension, velocity, and tone in the muscle. This system of afferent signals is responsible for the muscle stretch response and maintenance of normal muscle tone.

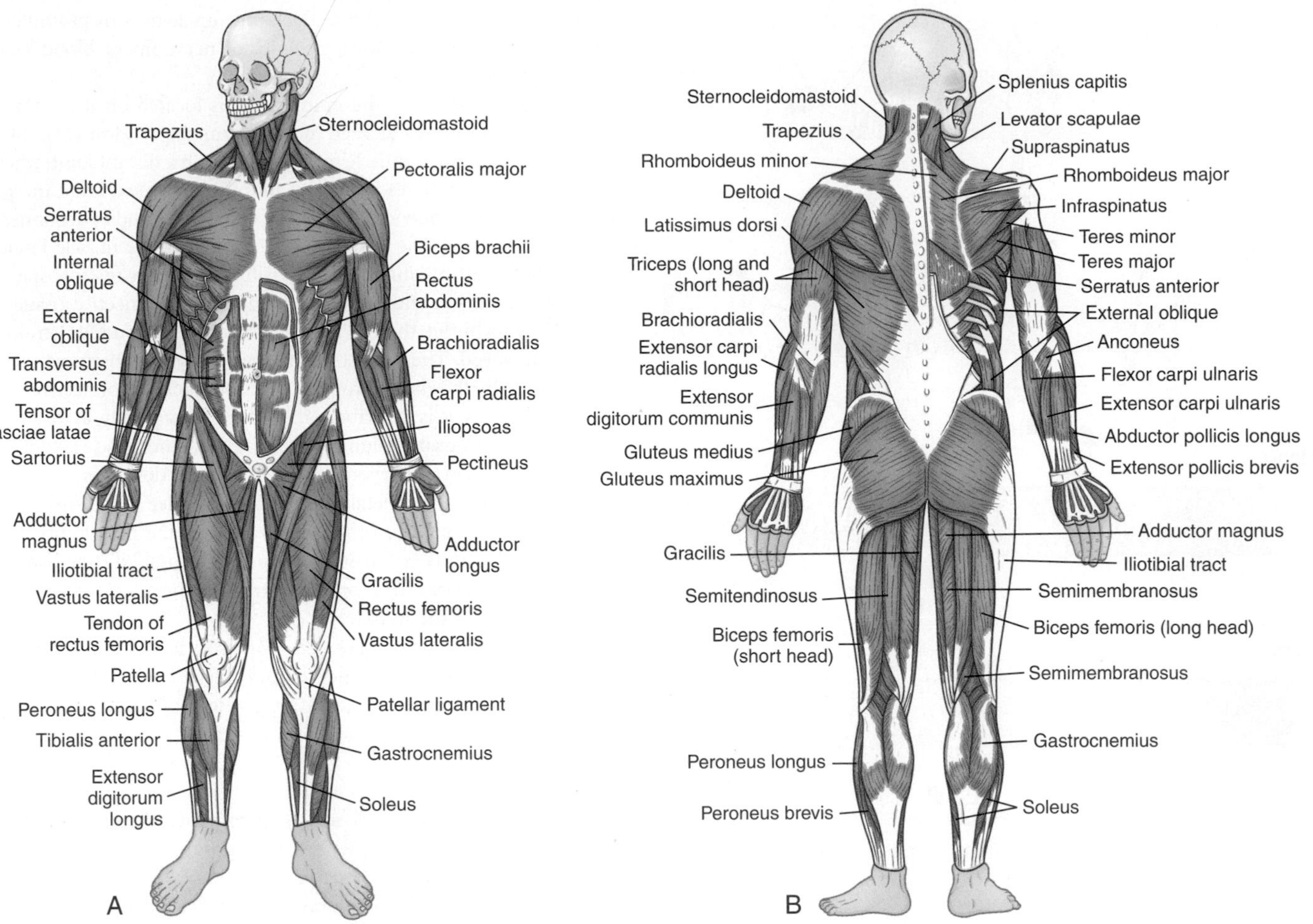

Anterior view labels (A):

Trapezius
Sternocleidomastoid
Deltoid
Serratus anterior
Internal oblique
External oblique
Transversus abdominis
Tensor of fasciae latae
Sartorius
Adductor magnus
Iliotibial tract
Vastus lateralis
Tendon of rectus femoris
Patella
Peroneus longus
Tibialis anterior
Extensor digitorum longus

Pectoralis major
Biceps brachii
Rectus abdominis
Brachioradialis
Flexor carpi radialis
Iliopsoas
Pectineus
Adductor longus
Gracilis
Rectus femoris
Vastus lateralis
Patellar ligament
Gastrocnemius
Soleus

A

Posterior view labels (B):

Sternocleidomastoid
Trapezius
Rhomboideus minor
Deltoid
Latissimus dorsi
Triceps (long and short head)
Brachioradialis
Extensor carpi radialis longus
Extensor digitorum communis
Gluteus medius
Gluteus maximus
Gracilis
Semitendinosus
Biceps femoris (short head)
Peroneus longus
Peroneus brevis

Splenius capitis
Levator scapulae
Supraspinatus
Rhomboideus major
Infraspinatus
Teres minor
Teres major
Serratus anterior
External oblique
Anconeus
Flexor carpi ulnaris
Extensor carpi ulnaris
Abductor pollicis longus
Extensor pollicis brevis
Adductor magnus
Iliotibial tract
Semimembranosus
Biceps femoris (long head)
Semimembranosus
Gastrocnemius
Soleus

B

FIGURE 44.15 Skeletal Muscles of the Body. **A,** Anterior view. **B,** Posterior view.

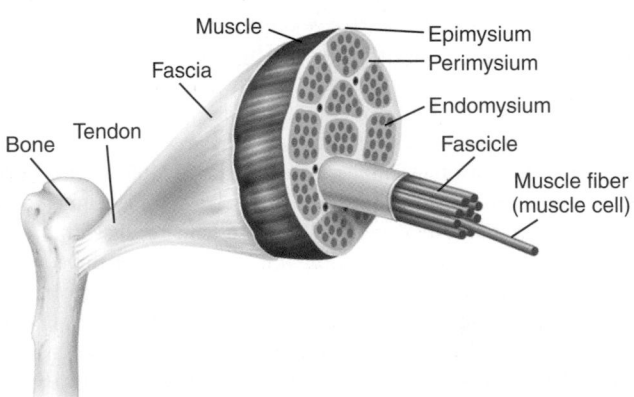

Labels: Muscle, Fascia, Tendon, Bone, Epimysium, Perimysium, Endomysium, Fascicle, Muscle fiber (muscle cell)

FIGURE 44.16 Cross Section of Skeletal Muscle Showing Muscle Fibers and Their Coverings. (Thibodeau GA, Patton KT: *Anatomy & physiology*, ed 5, St Louis, 2003, Mosby.)

Muscle Fibers. Each **muscle fiber** is a single **muscle cell**. This long cell is cylindrical and surrounded by a membrane capable of excitation and impulse propagation. The muscle fiber contains bundles of **myofibrils**, the fiber's functional subunits, in a parallel arrangement along the longitudinal axis of the muscle (Fig. 44.18). At birth the muscle fibers have completed development from precursor cells called **myoblasts**. All voluntary muscles are derived from the mesodermal layer of the embryo.

The type of peripheral nerve influences the muscle fiber and motor unit considerably; that is, the type of muscle fiber in the motor unit is determined by whether the motor nerve is fast or slow. Type II fibers, also called *white fast-motor fibers,* are innervated by relatively large type II alpha motor neurons with fast conduction velocities. These fibers rely on a short-term anaerobic glycolytic system for rapid energy transfer, whereas type I fibers depend on aerobic oxidative metabolism. Histo-chemical stains are now routinely used to describe the structure of muscle fibers and contractile elements of muscle biopsy specimens. White muscle (**type II fibers**) stains dark with the enzyme stain adenosinetriphosphatase (ATPase) at a pH of 9.4. Red muscle (**type I fibers**) appears lightly stained.

The overlap of muscle fibers that appear with staining gives the checkerboard appearance of muscle biopsy specimens and provides an equal distribution of fiber types throughout the muscle. This overlap also helps compensate for muscle fiber loss and fatigue of individual motor units during activity. In spite of this, some muscles contain proportionally more of one fiber type than another. The postural muscles have more type I fibers, allowing them the high resistance to fatigue that is necessary to maintain the same position for extended periods. Ocular muscles have more type II muscle fibers, allowing them to respond rapidly to visual changes. (Table 44.7 describes the specific characteristics of type I and type II fibers.)

The number of muscle fibers varies according to location. Large muscles, such as the gastrocnemius, have more fibers (1,200,000) than smaller muscles, such as the lumbrical muscles in the hand (10,000). The diameter of muscle fibers also varies. The closely packed polygons

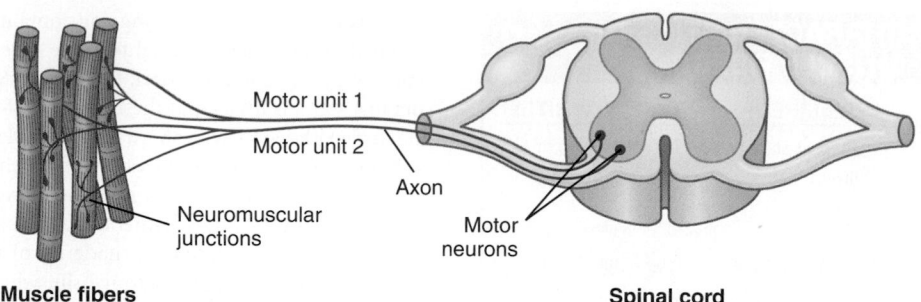

FIGURE 44.17 Motor Units of a Muscle. Each motor unit consists of a somatic motor neuron and all the muscle fibers (cells) supplied by the neuron and its axon branches.

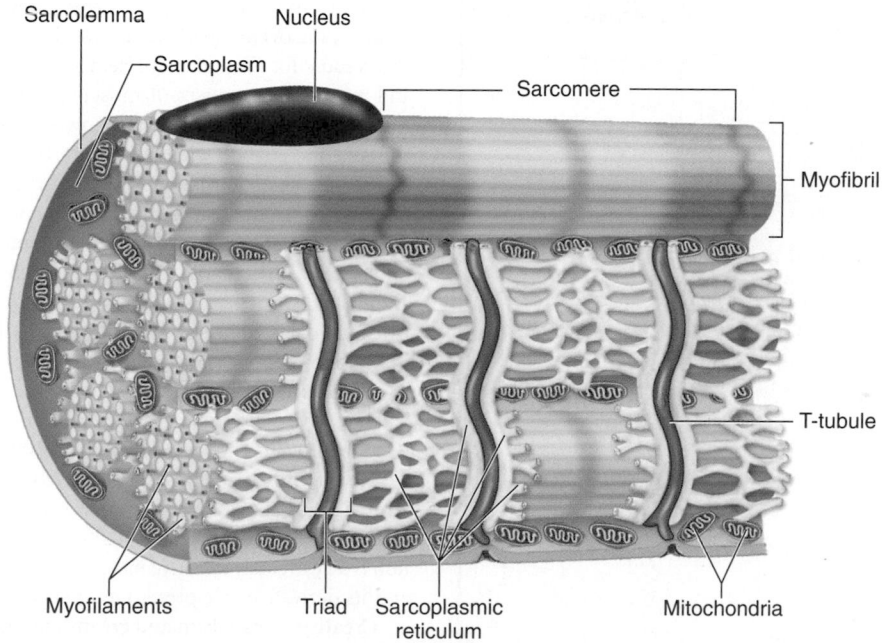

FIGURE 44.18 Myofibrils of a Skeletal Muscle Fiber (Cell) and Overall Organization of Skeletal Muscle. (Patton KT, Thibodeau GA: *Anatomy & physiology*, ed 9, St Louis, 2016, Mosby.)

are small (10 to 20 μm) until puberty, when they attain the normal adult diameter of 40 to 80 μm. Women usually have smaller-diameter fibers than men. Small muscles, such as the ocular muscles, are 15 μm in diameter; larger, more proximal muscles are 40 μm in diameter. Both fiber size and muscle length have functional significance. Studies have shown that larger fiber diameter is associated with generation of greater forces. Fiber diameter can be increased by activities that cause hypertrophied muscle, such as exercise or occupational overuse.

The major components of the muscle fiber include the muscle membrane, myofibrils, sarcotubular system, sarcoplasm, and mitochondria (Fig. 44.18). The **muscle membrane** is a two-part membrane. It includes the **sarcolemma**, which contains the plasma membrane of the muscle cell, and the cell's **basement membrane**. The sarcolemma is 7.5 μm thick and is capable of propagating electrical impulses to initiate contraction. At the motor nerve end plate, where the nerve impulse is transmitted, the sarcolemma forms the highly convoluted synaptic cleft. The sarcolemma is comprised of lipid molecules and protein systems. The protein systems perform special functions, such as transport of nutrients and synthesis of proteins. They also provide the sodium-potassium pump and include the cell's cholinergic receptor. The basement membrane is 50 μm thick and is composed primarily of proteins and polysaccharides. It serves as the cell's microskeleton and maintains the

shape of the muscle cell. The basement membrane also may function in some way to restrict further diffusion of electrolytes once they have crossed the sarcolemma.

The **sarcoplasm** is the cytoplasm of the muscle cell and contains the intracellular components that are common to all cells (see Chapter 1). The sarcoplasm is an aqueous substance that provides a matrix that surrounds the myofibrils. It contains numerous enzymes and proteins that are responsible for the cell's energy production, protein synthesis, and oxygen storage. The mitochondria house enzyme systems for energy production, particularly those that regulate such processes as the citric acid cycle and adenosine triphosphate (ATP) formation. Many other structures are present in the sarcoplasm. The ribosomes are composed primarily of ribonucleic acid (RNA) and participate in the process of protein synthesis. The cell nucleus, satellite cells, glycogen granules, and lipid droplets are suspended in the sarcoplasmic matrix. Blood vessels, nerve endings, muscle spindles, and Golgi tendon organs are also directly located within this structure.

Unique to the muscle is the **sarcotubular system**, a network that includes the transverse tubules and the sarcoplasmic reticulum, which crosses the interior of the cell. The **sarcoplasmic reticulum** is made in the same manner as the endoplasmic reticulum in other cells. In the muscle cells the sarcoplasmic reticulum is involved in calcium transport,

TABLE 44.7	CHARACTERISTICS OF MUSCLE FIBERS	
CHARACTERISTIC	**TYPE I (RED)**	**TYPE II (WHITE)**
Anatomic location	Deep axial portion of surface muscle	Surface portion of surface muscle
Contraction speed	Slow	Fast
Motor neuron type	Type I, small alpha	Type II, large alpha
Firing frequency	Low, long duration	Rapid, short duration
Resistance to fatigue	High	Low
Myoglobin	High	Low
Capillary supply	Profuse	Intermediate to sparse
Metabolism	Oxidative	Glycolysis
Mitochondria	Many	Few
Enzymes	Lactate dehydrogenase, types 1 to 3	Lactate dehydrogenase, types 4 and 5
Creatine kinase	Cardiac type	Fast, skeletal
Example (most muscles are mixed)	Greater proportion of slow-contracting fibers in soleus	Greater proportion of fast-contracting fibers in laryngeal and ocular muscles
Glycogen content	Low	High
Intensity of contraction	Low	High
Aerobic metabolic capacity	High	Low
Fiber diameter	Small	Large
Myosin-adenosinetriphosphatase (ATPase) activity	Low	High

From Spence AP, Mason EE: *Human anatomy and physiology*, ed 4, St Paul, MN, 1992, West Publishing.

which initiates muscle contraction at the sarcomere, a portion of the myofibril. The sarcoplasmic reticulum is composed of tubules that run parallel to the myofibrils. The longitudinal tubules are termed sarcotubules. The transverse tubules, which are closely associated with the sarcotubules, run across the sarcoplasm and communicate with the extracellular space. Together, the tubules of this membrane system allow for intracellular calcium uptake, regulation, and release during muscle contraction, and for the storage of calcium during muscle relaxation.

Myofibrils. Myofibrils, the most abundant subcellular muscle components, are the functional units of muscle contraction. Each myofibril contains sarcomeres, which, in turn, consist of repeating protein filaments[42] (see Fig. 44.18). Sarcomeres are chiefly composed of the proteins actin, myosin, titin, and nebulin. The sarcomere is responsible for converting chemical energy into movement.

On cross section they are irregular polygons with a mean diameter of less than 1 μm. Each myofibril is composed of serially repeating sarcomeres, separated by Z lines that give the muscle its striped, cross-striated appearance. Each sarcomere has a dark A band and is flanked by two light I bands (Fig. 44.19). Titin functions as a molecular spring that plays a significant role in determining muscle stiffness and elasticity.[43]

The A band is 1.5 to 1.6 μm long and contains thick myosin filaments. Included in the A band is a lighter zone called the *H band,* and in the center of the H band is the dark M band, or M line. The I band, which contains actin, is divided at the midpoint of each sarcomere by the Z line. Its length varies with the start of muscle contraction.

Myofibrils are composed of myofilaments. Each myofilament is structured in a closely packed hexagonal arrangement, with two thin filaments for every thick filament. The thick filament, along with C protein and M line protein, is made up of myosin. Myosin has two subunits, heavy and light meromyosin, which resemble twisted golf club shafts. The thin filaments are twisted double strands made up of actin, troponin, and tropomyosin (see Chapter 32 and Fig. 32.15).

Muscle Proteins. Table 44.8 summarizes muscle protein distribution, location, and possible functional significance. The contractile and regulatory functions of actin, myosin, and the troponin-tropomyosin complex (associated with actin) are the most commonly known. They also account for most of the protein found in the myofibril. The structural and regulatory processes of muscle proteins are less well understood. Alpha actin and beta actin are known to link the filaments. M protein contains the enzyme creatine kinase (CK). Creatine is released when muscle cells are damaged, making the serum creatine value an important measurement of pathologic conditions of muscles.

The most abundant proteins, actin and myosin, are also found in other cells, particularly motile cells such as platelets. The complete amino acid sequences of actin and myosin have been identified. Noteworthy is the presence of the amino acid 3-methylhistidine, found only in the thin filament, actin; 85% to 90% of 3-methylhistidine is found in skeletal muscle. The amino acids lysine and histidine, in addition to leucine, have been used to study protein synthesis by means of stable isotope infusion and muscle biopsy analysis.

Nonprotein Constituents of Muscle. Nitrogen, creatine, creatinine, phosphocreatine, purines, uric acid, and amino acids serve in the complex process of muscle metabolism. Phosphocreatine concentration is an extremely sensitive indicator of muscle fiber activity.[44] Glycogen and its derivatives are present as energy sources.

Creatine metabolism and creatinine metabolism have been used to measure muscle mass. Plasma creatine is taken up by muscle and converted into the high-energy phosphate compound *phosphocreatine* by the enzyme creatine kinase. Creatinine is formed in muscle from creatine at a constant rate of 2% per day. Creatine excretion is increased in muscle wasting. This change reflects the reduction in total body creatine stores and loss of muscle mass.

Inorganic compounds, anions (phosphate, chloride), and cations (calcium, magnesium, sodium, potassium) are important in regulating protein synthesis, muscle contraction, enzyme systems, and membrane stabilization. Intracellular calcium levels influence the force and duration of muscle contraction. Total body potassium (TBK) level, measured by the K_{40} method, has been used to measure muscle mass, also called *lean body mass.* TBK levels reflect changes in muscle mass seen during growth, malnutrition, and muscle wasting.

Components of Muscle Function

The ultimate function of muscle is to accomplish work. Although variously expressed in such measures as foot-pounds or kilogram-meters, work usually refers to the amount of energy liberated or force exerted over a distance (work = force × distance). Muscles usually contract or tense while doing work. Muscle contraction occurs on the molecular level and leads to the observable phenomenon of muscle movement.

Muscle Contraction at the Molecular Level

Muscle contraction is a four-step process: excitation, coupling, contraction, and relaxation. The initial contraction process is the

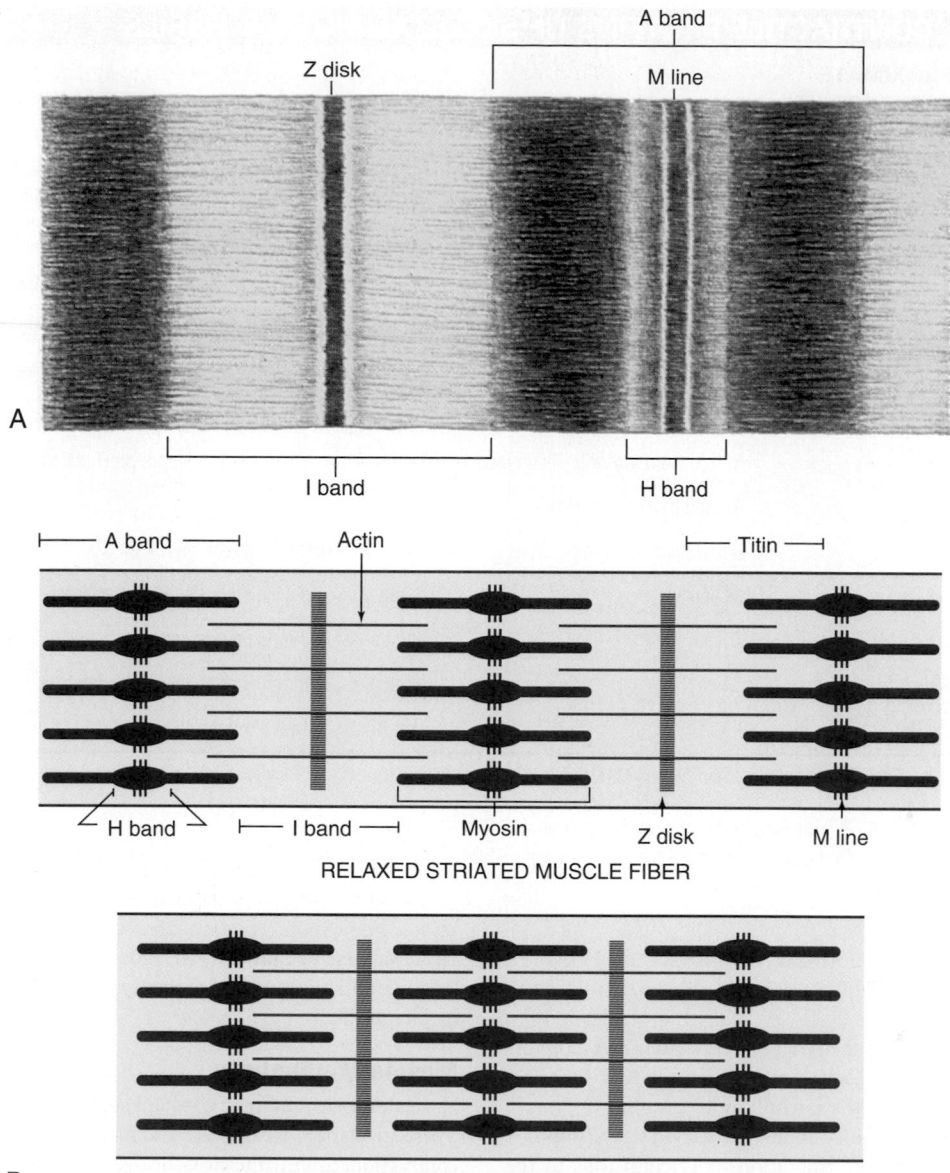

FIGURE 44.19 Muscle Fibers. A, The Z disks define the end of an individual sarcomere. The M line (which lies within the H band) is made of cross-connecting elements of the cytoskeleton. **B,** Actin is the primary protein of the I band (thin filament). Nebulin (not shown) also extends along the I band and contains binding sites for actin and myosin. Myosin (thick filament) extends through the A band. Titin extends from the Z disk to the M line, binding with myosin; strong titin anchoring within the I band is necessary for proper muscle function. During contraction, the I bands and H bands shorten, moving the Z disks closer together. (**A** modified from Thompson JM et al: *Mosby's clinical nursing,* ed 5, St Louis, 2002, Mosby.)

excitation-contraction coupling (ECC) series, which involves the electrical properties of all cells and the movement of ions across the plasma membrane (see Chapter 1). At rest an electrical charge of −90 mV is continually maintained across the muscle sarcolemma. This resting potential, generated by the separation of positive and negative charges on either side of the membrane, creates an electrochemical equilibrium caused by the selective permeability of the sarcolemma to electrolytes in the intracellular and extracellular fluids, particularly potassium and sodium.

Specific intracellular receptors within the skeletal muscle sarcoplasmic reticulum, called ryanodine receptors (RyRs), are the primary ion

channels that control calcium release. RyRs are the largest known ion channels, allowing for rapid movement of calcium. Three RyRs have been identified: RyR1 is predominantly found in skeletal muscle; RyR2 is found mostly in cardiac muscle; and RyR3 is in the diaphragm, smooth muscle, and brain.[45-47]

Excitation, the first step of muscle contraction, begins with the spread of an action potential from the nerve terminal to the neuromuscular junction. The rapid depolarization of the membrane initiates an electrical impulse in the muscle fiber membrane called the muscle fiber action potential. As the action potential advances along the sarcolemmal membrane, it spreads to the transverse tubules (T-tubules).

TABLE 44.8 CONTRACTILE PROTEINS OF SKELETAL MUSCLE FIBRILS

NAME	APPROXIMATE PERCENTAGE OF MYOFIBRILLAR PROTEIN	LOCATION	FUNCTION
Myosin	55	A band (thick filament)	Contraction; hydrolyzes ATP and develops tension
Actin	20	I band (thin filament)	Contraction; activates myosin ATPase and interacts with myosin
Troponin	7	Thin filament	Regulatory protein; in presence of Ca^{++}, promotes actin-myosin activation
Tropomyosin	5–7	Thin filament	Regulatory and structural function; links filaments, controls filament length
Alpha (α) actin	10	Z band	Regulatory and structural function; links filaments, controls filament length
Beta (β) actin	2	Z band	Regulatory and structural function; links filaments, controls filament length
M protein	2	M line (center of thick filaments)	Regulatory and structural function; provides enzyme creatine kinase
C protein	2	A band (thick filaments)	Possible structural role
Titin	Unknown	Z line (thick filament)	Interconnects thin filaments in Z line
Creatine kinase	Unknown	M line	Catalyzes the phosphorylation of ADP to form ATP
Desmin	Unknown	Z line	Interconnects thin filaments in Z line
Filamin*	Unknown	Z line	Interconnects thin filaments in Z line; stabilizes membrane
Nebulin*	Unknown	Z line	Determines filament length

*Data from Ma K, Wang K: *Fed Eur Biochem Soc Lett* 532(3):273–278, 2002; Sampson LJ, Leyland ML, Dart D: *J Biol Chem* 278(43):41988–41997, 2003.
ADP, Adenosine diphosphate; *ATP,* adenosine triphosphate; *ATPase,* adenosinetriphosphatase.
Modified from Simon SR, editor: *Orthopaedic basic science,* Chicago, 1994, American Academy of Orthopaedic Surgeons.

(The velocity of conduction is much slower in muscle fibers than in myelinated nerve fibers—only 3 to 5 m/second compared with 54 to 90 m/second in nerve fibers.)

The generated action potential then triggers voltage-sensitive receptors in the T-tubule wall; in turn, these receptors open the RyR channels, causing release of calcium from the sarcoplasmic reticulum.[45]

Following depolarization of the T-tubules, the second stage, **coupling,** occurs. This stage consists of the migration of calcium ions to the myofilaments. Calcium affects troponin and tropomyosin, muscle proteins that bind with actin when the muscle is at rest. In the presence of calcium, however, both of these proteins are attracted to calcium ions, leaving the actin free to bind with myosin.

Contraction begins as the calcium ions combine with troponin, a reaction that overcomes the inhibitory function of the troponin-tropomyosin system. The thin filament *actin* then slides toward the thick filament *myosin.* The two ends of the myofibril shorten after contraction when the myosin heads attach to the actin molecules, forming a cross-bridge that constitutes an actin-myosin complex. ATP, located on the actin-myosin complex, is released when the cross-bridges attach. This is the **sliding filament theory** and was first described by A. F. Huxley in the 1950s; however, it is now called the **cross-bridge theory** because of the formation of the actin-myosin cross-bridges. The process is so named because the actin actually slides onto the myosin, causing the sarcomere to shorten. The useful distance of contraction of a skeletal muscle is approximately 25% to 35% of the muscle's length. When actin and myosin filaments have maximal interactions, the muscle generates maximal force.[41]

The last step, **relaxation,** begins as the sarcoplasmic reticulum absorbs the calcium molecules, removing them from interaction with troponin. Calcium is pumped back into the sarcoplasmic reticulum by means of an active transport process. The cross-bridges detach, and the sarcomere lengthens. (The cross-bridge theory of muscle contraction is discussed in Chapter 32.)

Muscle Metabolism

Skeletal muscle requires a constant supply of ATP and phosphocreatine. These substances are necessary to fuel the complex processes of muscle contraction, driving the cross-bridges of actin and myosin together and transporting calcium from the sarcoplasmic reticulum to the myofibril. Other internal processes of the muscular system that require ATP include protein synthesis, which replenishes muscle constituents and accommodates growth and repair. The rate of protein synthesis is related to hormone levels (particularly insulin), amino acid substrates, and overall nutritional status. At rest the rate of ATP formation by oxidation of glucose or acetoacetate is sufficient to maintain internal processes, given normal nutritional status. During activity the need for ATP increases 100-fold. The metabolic pathways for muscle activity in Table 44.9 show reactions to the immediate need for increased ATP caused by contraction. Activity lasting longer than 5 seconds expends the available stored ATP and phosphocreatine.

Stored glycogen and blood glucose are converted anaerobically to sustain brief activity without increasing the demand for oxygen. Anaerobic glycolysis is much less efficient than aerobic glycolysis, using six to eight times more glycogen to produce the same amount of ATP. With increased activity, such as intense exercise, or ischemia, an increase in the level of lactic acid occurs because of the breakdown of glycogen, thus causing a shift in muscle pH (see Table 44.9). This short-term mechanism "buys time" by allowing ATP formation in spite of inadequate energy stores or oxygen supply. When the anaerobic threshold is reached and more oxygen is required, physiologic changes occur, including an increase in

TABLE 44.9 ENERGY SOURCES FOR MUSCULAR ACTIVITY

SOURCES	REACTIONS
Short-term (anaerobic) sources	Adenosine triphosphate (ATP) → Adenosine diphosphate (ADP) + Inorganic phosphate (Pi) + Energy
	Phosphocreatine + ADP ⇌ Creatine + ATP
	Glycogen/glucose + Pi + ADP → Lactate + ATP
Long-term (aerobic) sources	Glycogen/glucose + ADP + Pi + O_2 → H_2O + CO_2 + ATP
	Free fatty acids + ADP + Pi + O_2 → H_2O + CO_2 + ATP
	Creatine kinase catalyzes the reversible reaction of ATP to ADP: Creatine phosphate + ADP $\xrightleftharpoons[]{\text{Creatine kinase}}$ Creatine + ATP

From Spence AP, Mason EE: *Human anatomy and physiology*, ed 4, St Paul, MN, 1992, West Publishing.

lactic acid concentration and increases in oxygen consumption, heart rate, respiratory rate, and muscle blood flow.

Strenuous exercise requires oxygen, which activates the aerobic glycogen pathway for ATP formation. During maximal exercise, free fatty acid mobilization and the aerobic glycogen pathways provide ATP over an extended time. These pathways require oxygen to maintain maximal activity and return the muscle to the resting state. Maximal exercise increases oxygen uptake 15 to 30 times over the resting state.[48] When this system becomes exhausted or unable to respond to the need for ATP, fatigue and weakness finally force the muscle to reduce activity, with a resultant buildup of lactic acid in muscle fibers.

The ability to sustain maximal muscular activity leads to the accumulation of oxygen debt. Oxygen debt is the amount of oxygen needed to convert the buildup of lactic acid to glucose and replenish ATP and phosphocreatine stores. For example, after running at maximal speed for 10 seconds, the average person has consumed 1 L of oxygen. At rest, oxygen consumption for the same period is approximately 40 mL. As the person recovers, the measured oxygen debt is 4 L greater than the amount used during activity.

Oxygen consumption is measured to calculate the metabolic cost of activity in normal and diseased muscle. It is an indirect measure of energy expenditure, along with timed tests of activity, heart rate, and respiratory quotient (ratio of carbon dioxide to expired oxygen consumed). Energy expenditure is measured directly by heat production because heat is released whenever work is accomplished.

Another factor that changes energy requirements is muscle fiber type. Type II fibers rely on anaerobic glycolytic metabolism and fatigue readily. Type I fibers can resist fatigue for longer periods because of their capacity for oxidative metabolism.

Muscle Mechanics

Muscle contraction cannot be viewed in isolation. Several factors determine how force is transmitted from the cross-bridges on individual muscle fibers to accomplish whole-muscle contraction. First, when a motor unit responds to a single nerve stimulus, it develops a phasic contraction, also called *twitch*. Because the motor unit contracts in an "all or nothing" manner, the contraction that is generated will be a maximal contraction. The central nervous system smoothly grades the force generated by "recruiting" additional motor units and varying the discharge frequency of each active motor unit. This adding of motor units within the muscle is called repetitive discharge.

Recruitment and repetitive discharge of motor units allow the muscle to activate the number of motor units needed to generate the desired force. The total force developed is the sum of the force generated by each motor unit. As the strength, speed, and duration of stimuli increase, the summation of contractions reaches a critical frequency called tetanus. When tetanus is reached, no further increase in force can be achieved.

Other variables, such as fiber type, innervation ratio, muscle temperature, and muscle shape, influence the efficiency of muscular contraction. The two muscle fiber types differ in their responses to electrical activity. Tetanus and duration of phasic contractions, which take microseconds to accomplish, are achieved more rapidly in type II than in type I muscle fibers. Low-innervation ratios promote control and coordination, whereas high ratios promote strength and endurance. Muscles work best at normal body temperature (37°C [98.6°F]). Finally, muscles with a large cross-sectional area, such as the fan-shaped pennate muscles, develop greater contractile forces than smaller-diameter muscles. The initial length of a muscle and the range of shortening that occur when the muscle contracts also determine the forces it can generate. The long fusiform muscles have a greater range of shortening and can contract up to 57% of their resting length. A certain amount of elongation is necessary to generate sufficient tension and muscular force. The elongation that occurs during the swing of a golf club or tennis racquet is an example of how stretch improves contractile force.

Types of Muscle Contraction

During isometric contraction (static or holding contraction), the muscle maintains constant length as tension is increased. Isometric contraction occurs, for example, when the arm or leg is pushed against an immovable object. The muscle contracts, but the limb does not move.

During dynamic contraction, formerly known as *isotonic contraction*, the muscle maintains a constant tension as it moves. The terms "eccentric" for lengthening and "concentric" for shortening are technically inaccurate descriptions of muscle movement; the respective terms "lengthening" and "shortening" are more precise. Positive work is accomplished during shortening, and energy is released to exert force or lift a weight. In contrast, during lengthening the muscle lengthens and absorbs energy. Negative work is accomplished on the muscle by the load. Lengthening requires less energy to accomplish and may result in the development of pain and stiffness after unaccustomed exercise.

Movement of Muscle Groups

Muscles do not act alone but rather in groups, often under automatic control. When a muscle contracts it acts as a "prime mover," or agonist, and its reciprocal muscle, or antagonist, relaxes. This is easily tested by holding the right arm in the horizontal position in front of the body and then bending the elbow while feeling the upper arm, biceps in the front and the triceps in the back, with the other hand. The biceps is firm, and the triceps is soft. As the arm is extended, the muscles change. When the elbow is completely extended, the biceps is soft and the triceps firm. Completing this movement causes the agonist and antagonist to change automatically; only the movement is commanded, not the alternate contraction and relaxation of the specific muscle groups.

Other associated actions may be seen during walking; as the foot leaves the ground, the paravertebral and gluteal muscles on the opposite side of the body contract to maintain balance. One notices the loss of the associated muscle's action when paralysis offsets this process and decreases balance. If a person is paralyzed, difficulty in maintaining balance is noticeable.

TESTS OF MUSCULOSKELETAL FUNCTION

Tests of Bone Function

Diagnostic procedures to evaluate bone function include gait analysis, measurement of serum calcium and phosphorus levels, and imaging studies. Most imaging techniques provide morphologic rather than functional information about bone. Plain radiographs (x-rays) remain the standard initial imaging tool for bone evaluation because bone absorbs x-ray beams better than soft tissue. Computed tomography (CT) provides multiple images that are then processed into single (two-dimensional) or multiple images taken around a single axis to form (three-dimensional) pictures. Dual-energy computed tomography (DECT) utilizes x-ray beams at two different energy levels to determine different chemical compositions of tissues, thereby expanding CT imaging to include soft tissues, bone marrow, and crystals.[49] Advances in CT technology allow for detailed visualization of bone microstructure.[50]

Magnetic resonance imaging (MRI) provides detailed anatomic information and is useful for evaluating primary or metastatic bone lesions, infection, marrow edema, bony erosions, osteonecrosis, fractures, and other pathologic changes of bone. Magnetic resonance arthrography (MRa) involves injection of a contrast agent into the area of interest but allows better visualization of small abnormalities. Detailed functional imaging of bone can be attained with positron emission tomography (PET) scanning. A relatively new technology, MRI-PET combines MRI with functional imaging of molecular events seen with PET.

Nuclear medicine studies also provide imaging about metabolic activity in bone and soft tissue. After a small amount of radioactive tracer is injected, a special camera is used to identify bone absorption of the tracer. Bone scanning is very sensitive, but not specific about the cause of increased metabolic activity.

Dual-photon absorptiometry (DXA) is often used to measure the density of bones in the extremities and the fracture risk of vertebral bodies, femoral neck, and distal radius. Dual-photon absorptiometry allows the soft tissue components to be subtracted. New technology promises more accurate evaluation of bone.

Serum bone-specific alkaline phosphatase (BAP) is a marker of bone formation. Bone resorption is evaluated with urinary and serum measurements of cross-linked N-terminal telopeptides (NTx), a product of osteoclast bone resorption. NTx is specific for bone because the cross-links assessed are characteristic of bone collagen alone. Urine NTx is a more sensitive and specific biochemical marker of bone resorption than serum NTx.[51,52]

Tests of Joint Function

Procedures used to diagnose joint function include arthrography, arthroscopy, magnetic resonance imaging, and synovial fluid analysis. Arthrography (the injection of dye into the joint) is particularly useful to diagnose tears in the fibrocartilage of the knee (meniscus) and the rotator cuff of the shoulder. Arthroscopy is the direct visualization of a joint through an arthroscope. Magnetic resonance imaging (MRI) produces images of body tissues through the use of electromagnetic (radio) waves that alter the atoms (hydrogen ions) in the nuclei of cells being examined. When the polarized radio waves are stopped, the nuclear atoms return to their original positions, emitting energy as signals as they move back. The signals produce visible images for examination and diagnosis. MRI produces excellent contrast of soft tissues for evaluation of musculoskeletal conditions. Magnetic resonance arthroscopy (MRa) is injection of contrast into a joint, followed by MRI evaluation.

Analysis of synovial fluid may reveal inflammatory, septic, and noninflammatory joint diseases, which cause characteristic changes in the color, clarity, viscosity, and cellular elements of the fluid. The presence of blood in the joint fluid (hemarthrosis) usually indicates joint trauma. Normal synovial fluid is sterile, so the presence of bacteria in the fluid always indicates disease. Cell fragments and fibrous tissue in the fluid are the result of inflammation or wear-and-tear on the articular surfaces.

Tests of Muscular Function

When the individual's history and physical examination disclose abnormalities, such as weakness, atrophy, muscle tenderness, cramps, and stiffness, specific tests of muscle function are in order. One of the most useful tests is the serum creatine kinase (CK) concentration. CK is found in large quantities in the muscle fibers, and when these fibers are diseased or damaged, CK leaks into the serum. Myoglobin is also detectable in the urine after acute muscle damage caused by crush injury, ischemic disorders, extreme exertion, and some inherited diseases.

Because the muscle membrane tissue is excitable and carries an electrical charge, its capacity to function can be assessed by electromyography. Using sensitive needle electrodes, the electromyogram (EMG) records the summation of action potentials of the muscle fibers in each motor unit. The EMG is often compared with the electrocardiogram (ECG), but the activity recorded on the EMG is on a much smaller scale. The amplitude of the ECG is measured in volts, the duration of impulse is recorded in seconds, and both are recorded as the heart rate (e.g., 80 V/60 seconds). EMG amplitude is recorded in millivolts and the duration is measured in milliseconds, with a frequency of about 5 to 50 action potentials per second. Motor unit potentials are measured to determine rate of firing, duration, and amplitude. Abnormalities in EMG and nerve conduction velocities help differentiate muscle diseases (myopathy) from peripheral nerve (neuropathy) and neuromuscular junction disorders. The muscle biopsy (using histologic, histochemical, and electron microscopic studies) is used to further define the presence of myopathic and neuropathic disorders, many of which can be diagnosed only by muscle biopsy. Complex myography, a relatively new technique, allows a noninvasive way to gather information on the mechanical characteristics of muscle.

A new area of evaluation is genetics. Recent advances in molecular genetics, deoxyribonucleic acid (DNA) libraries, genetic probes, and gene localization techniques have enhanced the knowledge of neuromuscular diseases, including types of muscular dystrophy, Charcot-Marie-Tooth disease, and familial amyotrophic lateral sclerosis.

AGING AND THE MUSCULOSKELETAL SYSTEM

Aging of Bones

Aging is accompanied by the loss of bone tissue. Bones become less stiff, less strong, and more brittle with aging. The bone remodeling cycle takes longer to complete, and the rate of mineralization also decelerates. Studies have shown that an individual's bone mass at the end of the growth period helps determine the significance of bone loss as the person ages. With aging, women experience loss of bone density, accelerated by rapid bone loss during early menopause from increased osteoclastic bone resorption, fewer osteocytes, and decreased numbers of osteoblasts.[53] By age 70 years, susceptible women have, on average, lost 50% of their peripheral cortical bone mass.[1] Bone mass loss to this extent can lead to deformity, pain, stiffness, and high risk for fractures. Men also experience bone mass loss but at later ages and much slower rates than women. Also, peak bone mass in men is higher than that in women. Therefore bone loss in men causes less risk of disability than for women.[54] In general, age-related bone loss is caused by genetics, hormonal factors (decreased estrogen and estradiol levels), decreased bone formation, vitamin and mineral deficiencies (vitamin D, magnesium, and calcium), underlying conditions (malignancy, autoimmune diseases, hyperthyroidism), and lifestyle choices (physical inactivity, smoking, certain medications, and alcohol intake). Men's peak bone mass is related to race, heredity, hormonal factors (testosterone and estradiol levels), physical activity, and calcium intake during childhood.[55] Height also is lost with aging because of intervertebral disk degeneration and, sometimes, osteoporotic spinal fractures.

Bone mass can be gained in healthy young women up to the third decade through physical activity and intake of dietary calcium and magnesium. In postmenopausal women, aerobic exercises and strength training in particular have proven to be effective in improving and maintaining bone mass during the aging process.[56,57] In addition to the positive effects of exercise on bone mineral density (BMD), exercise has been shown to improve balance, coordination, muscle strength, lean body mass, and mobility, all of which may decrease the incidence of falls.[58,59]

Aging of Joints

With aging, cartilage becomes more rigid, fragile, and susceptible to fraying because of increased cross-linking of collagen and elastin, decreased water content in the cartilage ground substance, and decreased concentrations of glycosaminoglycans. Changes in collagen result in cartilage calcification and muscle stiffness. Decreased range of motion of the joint is related to the changes in ligaments and muscles. Bones in joints develop evidence of osteoporosis with fewer trabeculae and thinner, less dense bones, making them prone to fractures. Intervertebral disk spaces decrease in height.

Aging of Muscles

The function of skeletal muscle depends on many factors that are affected by aging, including the nervous, vascular, and endocrine systems. Mitochondrial dysfunction within cells contributes to oxidative stress and results in increased bone resorption and apoptosis of muscle cells.[60,61] In the young child, development of muscle tissue is highly dependent on continuing neurodevelopmental maturation. Muscle function remains trainable even into advanced age. Muscle diseases have a definite association with specific age groups. Muscular dystrophies occur in children, and muscle disabilities related to rheumatic diseases usually occur in advancing age.

Age-related loss in skeletal muscle is referred to as sarcopenia and is a direct cause of the age-related decrease in muscle strength. By 50 years of age, approximately 10% of muscle area is lost.[62] Parallel to sarcopenia, muscle strength declines by 15% per decade in the sixties and seventies and doubles to 30% after 80 years of age.[62] As the body ages, muscle bulk and strength decline slowly, beginning as early as age 50, with loss of about 1% per year thereafter. Muscle strength declines faster than muscle mass.[61] Type II fibers decrease to a greater extent than the slower-acting type I fibers. Loss of satellite cells appears to play a major role in the development of sarcopenia. Although muscle's regenerative function remains largely intact, satellite cell numbers are decreased.[63] Reduced RNA synthesis, loss of mitochondrial volume, shortening of telomeres, and reduction in the size of motor units contribute to sarcopenia. As much as 30% to 40% of skeletal muscle mass and strength may be lost from the third to ninth decades.

Maximal oxygen intake decreases with age. Reduced basal metabolic rate and decreased lean body mass are also seen in the older adult population.

■ SUMMARY REVIEW

Structure and Function of Bones

1. Bones provide support and protection for the body's tissues and organs and are important sources of minerals and blood cells.
2. Bone formation begins during embryonic development with the differentiation of mesenchymal cells into either chondrocytes or preosteoblasts. Bone minerals then either crystallize on a cartilage framework or become bone-forming cells without cartilage.
3. Bone tissue is continuously being resorbed and synthesized by bone-remodeling units of osteoclasts and osteoblasts.
4. RANKL induces osteoclast activation and bone resorption. OPG, a protein, binds to a protein called *OPG ligand*. This attachment serves as a decoy receptor for RANKL and blocks osteoclast activity, thus decreasing bone resorption. The balance between RANKL and OPG determines the quality of bone.
5. Bones in the body are made up of compact bone tissue and spongy bone tissue. Compact bone is highly organized into haversian systems that consist of concentric layers of crystallized matrix surrounding a central canal that contains blood vessels and nerves. Dispersed throughout the concentric layers of crystallized matrix are small spaces containing osteocytes. Smaller canals, called *canaliculi,* interconnect the osteocyte-containing spaces. The crystallized matrix in spongy bone is arranged in bars or plates. Spaces containing osteocytes are dispersed between the bars or plates and interconnected by canaliculi.
6. BMPs are part of the TGF-β superfamily and are involved in multiple crucial functions in the skeletal system.

7. There are 206 bones in the body, divided into the axial skeleton and the appendicular skeleton. Bones are classified by shape as long, short, flat, or irregular. Long bones have a broad end (epiphysis), broad neck (metaphysis), and narrow midportion (diaphysis) that contains the medullary cavity.
8. Bone injuries are repaired in stages. Hematoma formation provides the fibrin framework for formation and organization of granulation tissue. Granulation tissue provides a cartilage model for the formation and crystallization of bone matrix. Remodeling restores the original shape and size to the injured bone.

Structure and Function of Joints

1. A joint is the site of attachment of two or more bones. Joints provide stability and mobility to the skeleton.
2. Joints are classified as synarthroses, amphiarthroses, or diarthroses, depending on the degree of movement they allow. Joints also can be classified by the type of connecting tissue holding them together. Fibrous joints are connected by dense fibrous tissue, ligaments, or membranes. Cartilaginous joints are connected by fibrocartilage or hyaline cartilage. Synovial joints are connected by a fibrous joint capsule. Within the capsule is a small fluid-filled space. The fluid in the space nourishes the articular cartilage that covers the ends of the bones meeting in the synovial joint.
3. Articular cartilage is a highly organized system of collagen fibers and proteoglycans. The fibers firmly anchor the cartilage to the

SUMMARY REVIEW—cont'd

bone, and the proteoglycans control the loss of fluid from the cartilage.

4. Joints help move bones and muscle.

Structure and Function of Skeletal Muscles

1. Skeletal muscle is the largest organ in the body and is made up of millions of individual fibers.

2. Whole muscles vary in size (2 to 60 cm in length) and shape (fusiform and pennate). Each skeletal muscle is encased in a three-part connective tissue framework. The fundamental concept of muscle function is the *motor unit*, defined as all muscle fibers innervated by a single motor nerve.

3. Muscle fibers contain bundles of myofibrils arranged in parallel along the longitudinal axis and include the muscle membrane, myofibrils, sarcotubular system, aqueous sarcoplasm, and mitochondria. There are two types of muscle fibers, type I and type II, determined by motor nerve innervation.

4. Myofibrils and myofilaments contain the major muscle proteins actin and myosin, which interact to form cross-bridges during muscle contraction. The nonprotein muscle constituents provide an energy source for contraction and regulate protein synthesis, enzyme systems, and membrane stabilization.

5. Muscle contraction includes excitation, coupling, contraction, and relaxation.

6. Muscle strength is graded by the "all or nothing" phenomenon and recruitment. Speed of contraction is affected by several factors: muscle fiber type, temperature, stretch, and weight of the load.

7. The two types of muscle contraction are isometric and isotonic. Muscle shortening occurs during contraction but can be seen also during pathologic and physiologic contracture.

8. Actin and myosin filaments form cross-bridges that cause the sarcomere to shorten, a process now known as the *cross-bridge theory of muscle contraction*.

9. Skeletal muscle requires a constant supply of ATP and phosphocreatine to fuel muscle contraction and for growth and repair. ATP

and phosphocreatine can be generated aerobically or anaerobically. Phosphocreatine concentration is an extremely sensitive indicator of muscle fiber activity.

10. Several factors determine how force is transmitted from the actin-myosin cross-bridges on individual muscle fibers to accomplish whole-muscle contraction. When a motor unit responds to a single nerve stimulus, it develops a phasic contraction. The central nervous system smoothly grades the force generated by "recruiting" additional motor units and varying the discharge frequency of each active motor unit.

Tests of Musculoskeletal Function

1. Procedures used to evaluate bone function include analysis of gait, evaluation of urinary bone resorption markers, measurement of serum calcium and phosphorus levels and serum bone-specific alkaline phosphatase (BAP) level, x-ray films, angiography, bone scanning, and MRI.

2. Procedures used to evaluate joint function include arthrography, arthroscopy, MRI, and synovial fluid analysis.

3. Serum creatine kinase concentration is useful in detecting muscle damage. Electromyography is used to assess the muscle membrane's capacity to function. Genetic evaluation is useful in detecting, diagnosing, and developing specific treatment for certain inheritable muscle diseases such as muscular dystrophy.

Aging and the Musculoskeletal System

1. Muscle bulk and strength slowly decline with aging, although not to a pathologic degree. The bone remodeling cycle takes longer to complete, and the rate of mineralization slows.

2. Exercise in older adults improves muscle strength, helps increase bone mineral density, and improves balance, coordination, lean body mass, and mobility.

3. Age-related loss in skeletal muscle is referred to as *sarcopenia*. Loss of satellite cells appears to play a major role in the development of sarcopenia.

KEY TERMS

Actin, 1414
Agonist, 1417
Amphiarthrosis (slightly movable joint), 1406
Antagonist, 1417
Appendicular skeleton, 1402
Arthrography, 1418
Arthroscopy, 1418
Articular cartilage, 1408
Axial skeleton, 1402
Basement membrane, 1413
Basic multicellular unit (BMU), 1403
Bone albumin, 1401
Bone fluid, 1401
Bone matrix, 1398
Bone morphogenic protein (BMP), 1401
Calcification, 1398
Canaliculus (*pl.,* canaliculi), 1402
Chondrocyte, 1409
Collagen fiber, 1401
Compact bone (cortical bone), 1402
Contraction, 1416
Coupling, 1416
Creatine, 1414
Creatine kinase, 1414
Cross-bridge theory, 1416

Diaphysis, 1402
Diarthrosis (freely movable joint), 1406
Electromyogram (EMG), 1418
Endochondral ossification, 1397
Endomysium, 1411
Endosteum, 1403
Epimysium, 1411
Epiphysis, 1402
Excitation, 1415
Fascia, 1411
Fascicle, 1411
Fibril, 1401
Fibrous joint, 1406
Flat bone, 1403
Fusiform muscle, 1411
Glycoprotein, 1401
Glycosaminoglycan, 1409
Golgi tendon organ, 1411
Gomphosis, 1406
Ground substance, 1396
Growth plate (epiphyseal plate), 1403
Haversian canal, 1402
Haversian system, 1402
Hyaluronate, 1408
Hydroxyapatite (HAP), 1401

Intima, 1408
Intramembranous ossification, 1397
Irregular bone, 1403
Isometric contraction (static or holding contraction), 1417
Joint (articulation), 1406
Joint capsule (articular capsule), 1407
Joint cavity (synovial cavity), 1408
Lacuna, 1398
Lamellae, 1402
Laminin, 1401
Link protein, 1409
Long bone, 1402
Magnetic resonance imaging (MRI), 1418
Mesenchymal stem cell (MSC), 1396
Mesenchyme, 1397
Metaphysis, 1402
Motor unit, 1411
Muscle cell, 1412
Muscle fiber, 1412
Muscle fiber action potential, 1415
Muscle membrane, 1413
Myoblast, 1412
Myofibril, 1412
Myosin, 1414

KEY TERMS—cont'd

REFERENCES

1. Kumar V, Abbas AK, Aster JCF: *Robbins & Cotran pathologic basis of disease,* ed 9, Philadelphia, 2015, Elsevier Sanders.
2. van de Peppel J, van Leeuwen JP: Vitamin D and gene networks in human osteoblasts. *Front Physiol* 5:137, 2014.
3. Beederman M, et al: BMP signalling in mesenchymal stem cell differentiation and bone formation. *J Biomed Sci Eng* 6(8A):32–52, 2013.
4. Bonewald LF: The amazing osteocyte. *J Bone Miner Res* 26(2):229–238, 2012.
5. Bellido T: Osteocyte-driven bone remodelling. *Calcif Tissue Int* 94(1):25–34, 2014.
6. Hambli R: Connecting mechanics and bone remodelling process: an integrated finite element modelling. *Front Bioeng Biotechnol* 2:6, 2014.
7. Zanotti E, Canalis S: Notch signaling and the skeleton. *Endocr Rev* 37(3):223–253, 2016.
8. van der Meijen K, et al: Primary human osteoblasts in response to 25-hydroxyvitamin D3. *PLoS ONE* 9(10):e110283, 2014.
9. Zaudi M, et al: Osteoclastogenesis, bone resorption, and osteoclast-based therapeutics. *J Bone Miner Res* 18(4):599–609, 2003.
10. Alberts B, et al, editors: *Molecular biology of the cell,* ed 6, New York, 2015, Garland Science Taylor & Francis Group.
11. Nguyen AM, Jacobs CR: Emerging role of primary cilia as a mechanoreceptor in osteocytes. *Bone* 54(2):196–204, 2013.
12. Schaffler MB, Kennedy OD: Osteocyte signaling in bone. *Curr Osteoporos Rep* 19(2):118–125, 2012.
13. Xiong J, O'Brien CA: Osteocyte RANKL: new insights into control of bone remodeling. *J Bone Miner Res* 27:499–505, 2012.
14. Chen G, Deng C, Li Y-P: TGF-β and BMP signaling in osteoblast differentiation and bone formation. *Int J Biol Sci* 8:272–288, 2012.
15. Kennedy OD, Schaffler MB: The roles of osteocyte signaling in bone. *J Am Acad Orthop Surg* 20(10):670–671, 2012.
16. Quarles LD: Skeletal secretion of FGF-23 regulates phosphate and vitamin D metabolism. *Nat Rev Endocrinol* 8(5):276–286, 2012.
17. Bellido T, Saini V, Pajevic PD: Effects of PTH on osteocyte function. *Bone* 12:1245–1248, 2012.
18. Schaffler MB, Kennedy OD: Osteocyte signaling in bone. *Curr Osteoporos Rep* 10(2):118–125, 2012.

19. Cappariello A, et al: The great beauty of the osteoclast. *Arch Biochem Biophys* 561:13–21, 2014.
20. Luenburg C, et al: Involvement of actin polymerization in podosomes dynamics. *J Cell Sci* 125:1666–1672, 2012.
21. Yasuda H: Historically significant events in the discovery of RANK/RANKL/OPG. *World J Orthop* 4:186–197, 2013.
22. Manilay JO, Zouali M: Tight relationships between B lymphocytes and the skeletal system. *Trends Mol Med* 20:405–412, 2014.
23. Weitzman MN: The role of inflammatory cytokines, the RANKL/OPG axis and the immunoskeletal interface in physiological bone turnover and osteoporosis. *Scientifica (Cairo)* 2013:125705, 2013.
24. Yang C, et al: Inhibition of differentiation and function of osteoclasts by dimethyl sulfoxide (DMSO). *Cell Tissue Res* 362:577–585, 2015.
25. Tamjidipoor A, Tavafi M, Ahmadvand H: Effect of dimethyl sulfoxide on inhibition of post-ovariectomy osteopenia in rats. *Connect Tissue Res* 45:426–431, 2013.
26. Orimo H: The mechanism of mineralization and the role of alkaline phosphatase in health and disease. *J Nippon Med Sch* 77(1):4–12, 2010.
27. Thompson JC, editor: *Netter's concise orthopaedic anatomy,* ed 2, Philadelphia, 2010, Saunders.
28. Del Fattore A, Teti A, Rucci N: Bone cells and the mechanisms of bone remodeling. *Front Biosci (Elite Ed)* 4:2302–2321, 2012.
29. Bishop JR, Schuksz M, Esko JD: Heparan sulphate proteoglycans fine-tune mammalian physiology. *Nature* 446(7139):1030–1037, 2007.
30. Lortat-Jacob H, et al: Transglutaminase-2 intra-action with heparin. *J Biol Chem* 287(22):18005–18017, 2012.
31. Kock A, van Donkelaar CC, Ito K: Tissue engineering of functional articular cartilage: the current status. *Cell Tissue Res* 347(3):613–627, 2012.
32. Pesesse L, Sanchez C, Henrotin Y: Osteochondral plate angiogenesis: a new treatment target in osteoarthritis. *Joint Bone Spine* 78(2):144–149, 2011.
33. Ondresik M, et al: Management of knee osteoarthritis. Current status and future trends. *Biotechnol Bioeng* 114(4):717–739, 2017.

34. Wakitani S, et al: Safety of autologous bone marrow-derived mesenchymal stem cell transplantation for cartilage repair in 41 patients and 45 joints followed for up to 11 years and 5 months. *J Tissue Eng Regen Med* 5(2):146–150, 2011.
35. Wu L, et al: Trophic effects of mesenchymal stem cells in chondrocyte co-cultures are independent of culture conditions and cell sources. *Tissue Eng Part A* 18:1542–1551, 2012.
36. Casagrande D, Stains JP, Murthi AM: Identification of shoulder osteoarthritis biomarkers: comparison between shoulders with and without osteoarthritis. *J Shoulder Elbow Surg* 24:382–390, 2015.
37. Yang CC, Lin CY, Wang HS, et al: Matrix metalloproteases and tissue inhibitors of metalloproteinases in medial plica and pannus-like tissue contribute to knee osteoarthritis progression. *PLoS ONE* 8:1–11, 2013.
38. Zhang FY, et al: Effect of osteopontin on TIMP-1 and TIMP-2 mRNA in chondrocytes of human osteoarthritis in vitro. *Exp Ther Med* 8:391–394, 2014.
39. Knight JD, Kothary R: The myogenic kinome: protein kinases critical to mammalian skeletal myogenesis. *Skelet Muscle* 1:29–46, 2011.
40. Braun T, Gautel M: Transcriptional mechanisms regulating skeletal muscle differentiation, growth and homeostasis. *Nat Rev Mol Cell Biol* 12:349–361, 2011.
41. Lieber RL, Ward SR: Skeletal muscle design to meet functional demands. *Philos Trans R Soc Lond B Biol Sci* 366(1570):1466–1476, 2011.
42. Myhre JL, Pilgrim DB: At the start of the sarcomere: a previously unrecognized role for myosin chaperones and associated proteins during early myofibrillogenesis. *Biochem Res Int* 2012:712315, 2012.
43. Hsin J, et al: Molecular origin of hierarchical elasticity of titin: simulation, experiment, and theory. *Annu Rev Biophys* 40:187–203, 2011.
44. Sargeant AJ: Structural and functional determinants of human muscle power. *Exp Physiol* 92(2):323, 2007.
45. Capes EM, Loaiza R, Valdivia HH: Ryanodine receptors. *Skelet Muscle* 1(1):18, 2011.
46. Hamilton SL, Serysheva II: Ryanodine receptor structure: progress and challenges. *J Biol Chem* 284(7):4047–4051, 2009.

47. Lanner JT: Ryanodine receptor physiology and its role in disease. *Adv Exp Med Biol* 1(74):217–234, 2012.

48. Richardson RS: Oxygen transport and utilization: an integration of the muscle systems. *Adv Physiol Educ* 27(1-4):183–191, 2003.

49. Nicolaou S, et al: Dual-energy CT: a promising new technique for assessment of the musculoskeletal system. *AJR Am J Roentgenol* 199(Suppl 5):S78–S86, 2012.

50. Ito M: Recent progress in bone imaging for osteoporosis research. *J Bone Miner Metab* 29:131–140, 2011.

51. Abe Y, Ishikawa H, Fukao A: Higher efficacy of urinary bone resorption marker measurements in assessing response to treatment for osteoporosis in postmenopausal women. *Tohoku J Exp Med* 214(1):51, 2008.

52. Ulrich-Vinther M, et al: Articular cartilage biology. *J Am Acad Orthop Surg* 11(6):421–430, 2003.

53. Almeida M, O'Brien CA: Basic biology of skeletal aging: role of stress response pathways. *J Gerontol A Biol Sci Med Sci* 68(10):1197–1208, 2013.

54. Zanatta M, et al: Runx-2 gene expression is associated with age-related changes of bone mineral density in the healthy young-adult population. *J Bone Miner Metab* 30(6):706–714, 2012.

55. Adler RA: Osteoporosis in men: insights for the clinician. *Ther Adv Musculoskelet Dis* 3(4):191–200, 2011.

56. Gombos GC, et al: Direct effects of physical training on markers of bone metabolism and serum sclerostin concentrations in older adults with low bone mass. *BMC Musculoskelet Disord* 17:254, 2016.

57. Kemmler W, von Stengel S, Kohn M: Exercise frequency and bone mineral density development in exercising postmenopausal osteopenic women. Is there a critical dose of exercise for affecting bone? Results of the Erlangen Fitness and Osteoporosis Prevention Study. *Bone* 89:1–6, 2016.

58. Bergmann P, et al: Loading and skeletal development and maintenance. *J Osteoporos* 2011:786752, 2011.

59. Body JJ, et al: Non-pharmacological management of osteoporosis: a consensus of the Belgian Bone Club. *Osteoporos Int* 22:2769–2788, 2011.

60. Karasik D, Cohen-Zinder M: The genetic pleiotropy of musculoskeletal aging. *Front Physiol* 3:303, 2012.

61. Peterson CM, Johannsen DL, Ravussin E: Skeletal mitochondria and aging: a review. *J Aging Res* 2012:194821, 2012.

62. Kim CH, et al: The effect of aging on relationships between lean body mass and VO2max in rowers. *PLoS ONE* 11(8):e160275, 2016.

63. Shadrach JL, Wagers AJ: Stem cells for skeletal muscle repair. *Philos Trans R Soc Lond B Biol Sci* 366(1575):2297–2306, 2011.

Alterations of Musculoskeletal Function

⊖volve WEBSITE

http://evolve.elsevier.com/McCance/
- Content Updates
- Chapter Summary Review
- Review Questions
- Case Studies
- Animations

CHAPTER OUTLINE

The musculoskeletal system is comprised of the bones, muscles, cartilage, tendons, ligaments, and other connective tissues. This system provides structure, support, stability, and movement to the body. Injuries to the musculoskeletal system include fractures (traumatic and nontraumatic), dislocations, sprains, and strains. Additionally, alterations in bones, joints, and muscles may be caused by metabolic disorders, infections, inflammatory or noninflammatory diseases, or tumors. The most common disease affecting bones is osteoporosis and the incidence increases with age.[1]

MUSCULOSKELETAL INJURIES

Trauma has been termed "the neglected disease of modern society."[2] Unintentional traumatic injuries are the number one cause of death for people ages 1 to 44.[3] Fractures are most commonly caused by falls, car accidents, and athletic injuries. For those who survive traumatic injuries, the impact is significant. Injury affects their families, and impacts society because of related loss or limitation of daily activities and mobility, pain, and a decreased quality of life. Significant direct care costs are

associated with diagnosis and treatment; indirect care costs are related to time away from work, loss of employment, and decreased productivity. Several national organizations in the United States are collaborating to develop a centralized national resource for injury prevention.[4]

Skeletal Trauma
Fractures

A fracture is a break in the continuity of a bone. A break occurs when force is applied that exceeds the tensile or compressive strength of the bone. Fracture incidence varies depending on the bone involved, age, and gender. The highest incidence of fractures occurs in young males ages 15 to 24 and in adults 65 years and older. Rates of hip and wrist fractures tended to be higher in women. An estimated 158 million hip fractures occurred worldwide in 2015; this number is expected to increase to 316 million by 2040.[5]

Classification. Fractures are classified as complete or incomplete and open or closed (Fig. 45.1). In a complete fracture, the integrity of the bone is broken into two pieces, whereas in an incomplete fracture

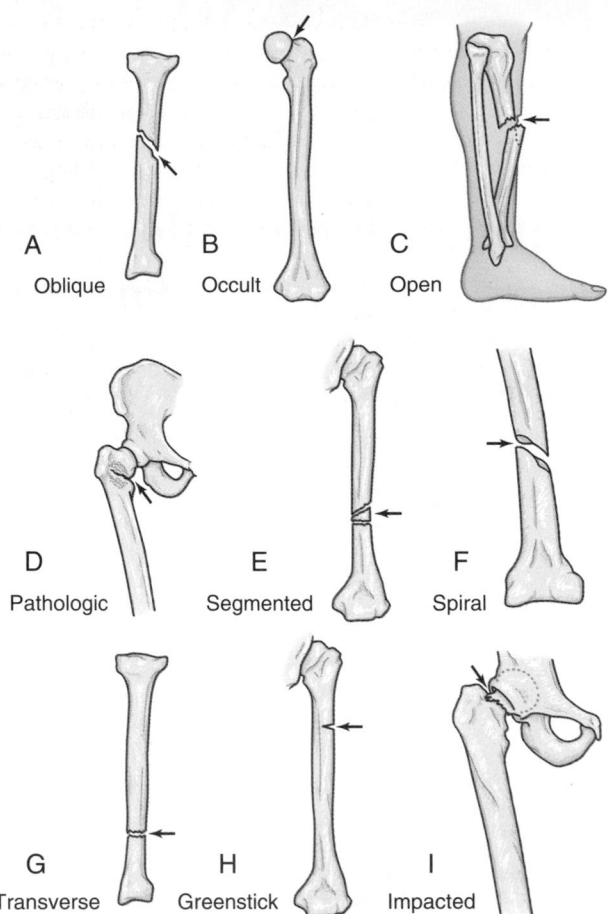

A, Oblique
B, Occult
C, Open
D, Pathologic
E, Segmented
F, Spiral
G, Transverse
H, Greenstick
I, Impacted

FIGURE 45.1 Examples of Types of Bone Fractures. **A,** *Oblique:* fracture at oblique angle across both cortices. *Cause:* direct or indirect energy, with angulation and some compression. **B,** *Occult:* fracture that is hidden or not readily discernible. *Cause:* minor force or energy. **C,** *Open:* skin broken over fracture; possible soft tissue trauma. *Cause:* moderate to severe energy that is continuous and exceeds tissue tolerances. **D,** *Pathologic:* transverse, oblique, or spiral fracture of bone weakened by tumor pressure or presence. *Cause:* minor energy or force, which may be direct or indirect. **E,** *Segmented:* fracture with two or more pieces or segments. *Cause:* direct or indirect moderate to severe force. **F,** *Spiral:* fracture that curves around cortices and may become displaced by twist. *Cause:* direct or indirect twisting energy or force with distal part held or unable to move. **G,** *Transverse:* horizontal break through bone. *Cause:* direct or indirect energy toward bone. **H,** *Greenstick:* break in only one cortex of bone. *Cause:* minor direct or indirect energy. **I,** *Impacted:* fracture with one end wedged into opposite end of inside fractured fragment. *Cause:* compressive axial energy or force directly to distal fragment. (Redrawn from Mourad L: Musculoskeletal system. In Thompson JM et al, editors: *Mosby's clinical nursing,* ed 7, St Louis, 2002, Mosby.)

TABLE 45.1	TYPES OF FRACTURES
TYPE	**DEFINITION**
Typical Complete Fractures	
Closed fracture	Skin overlying the bone is intact
Open fracture	Communicating wound between bone and skin
Comminuted fracture	Multiple bone fragments
Linear fracture	Fracture line parallel to long axis of bone
Oblique fracture	Fracture line at an angle to long axis of bone
Spiral fracture	Fracture line encircling bone (as in a spiral staircase)
Transverse fracture	Fracture line perpendicular to long axis of bone
Impacted	Fracture fragments are pushed into each other
Pathologic	Fracture occurs at a point in the bone weakened by disease (e.g., bones with tumors or osteoporosis)
Avulsion	A fragment of bone connected to a ligament or tendon breaks off from the main bone
Compression	Fracture is wedged or squeezed together on one side of bone
Displaced	Fracture with one, both, or all fragments out of normal alignment
Extracapsular	Fragment is close to the joint but remains outside the joint capsule
Intracapsular	Fragment extends into or is within the joint capsule
Fragility	Fracture caused by low-level trauma
Typical Incomplete Fractures	
Greenstick fracture	Break on one cortex of bone with splintering of inner bone surface (commonly occurs in children and older adults)
Torus fracture	Buckling of cortex
Bowing fracture	Bending of the bone
Stress fracture	Microfracture
Transchondral fracture	Separation of cartilaginous joint surface (articular cartilage) from main shaft of bone

the bone is damaged but still in one piece. Complete or incomplete fractures are further classified as open or closed. An **open fracture,** formerly referred to as a *compound fracture,* is characterized by a concurrent break in the skin in the area of the fracture. A **closed fracture,** formerly referred to as a *simple fracture,* has no break in the surrounding skin. Fractures are classified according to the direction of the fracture line. A **linear fracture** runs parallel to the long axis of the bone. An **oblique fracture** is a slanted fracture of the shaft of the bone. A **spiral fracture** encircles the bone, and a **transverse fracture** occurs straight across the bone. A fracture in which a bone breaks into more than two fragments is termed a **comminuted fracture.**

The three main types of incomplete fractures are greenstick, buckle or torus, and bowing. A **greenstick fracture** perforates one cortex and splinters the spongy bone and is relatively unstable. The term *greenstick* is derived from the damage sustained by a young tree branch (a green stick) when it is bent sharply. The outer surface of the bone (or tree branch) is disrupted, but the inner surface remains intact. Greenstick fractures typically occur in the metaphysis or diaphysis of the tibia, radius, and ulna. In a buckle or **torus fracture,** the cortex of the bone buckles but does not break, thus making it a relatively stable fracture. **Bowing fractures** usually occur when longitudinal force is applied to bone. This type of fracture is common in children and usually involves the paired radius-ulna or fibula-tibia. A complete diaphyseal fracture occurs in one bone of the pair, which disperses the stress sufficiently to prevent a complete fracture of the second bone, which bows. Treatment of a bowing fracture is difficult because the bowed bone interferes with the reduction of the fractured bone. In addition, a bowing fracture resists correction (reduction) because the force necessary to reduce it must be equal to the force that caused the initial injury. A fracture that results from a trauma that would not normally cause a fracture (a low-level trauma) is termed a **fragility fracture.** Fragility fractures are often a sequela of osteoporosis. Types of fractures are summarized in Table 45.1.

Fractures may be further classified by cause as pathologic, stress, or transchondral fracture. A **pathologic fracture** is a break at the site of a preexisting abnormality (such as a tumor), usually by force that would not fracture a healthy bone. Any disease process that weakens a bone (especially the cortex) predisposes the bone to pathologic fracture. This type of fracture is most commonly associated with tumors, infections, osteoporosis, and other metabolic bone disorders.

A **stress fracture** is caused by the cumulative effects of repeated forces over time, such as occurs during athletics. Fatigue and insufficiency fractures are subtypes of stress fractures. **Fatigue fractures** are caused by abnormal stress or torque applied to a bone with normal ability to deform and recover (e.g., joggers, dancers, military recruits). **Insufficiency fractures** include fragility fractures of osteoporosis and osteomalacia, and occur in bones lacking normal ability to deform and recover (i.e., normal weightbearing or activity fractures the bone).

A **transchondral fracture** consists of fragmentation and separation of a portion of the articular cartilage that covers the end of a bone at a joint. (Joint structures are defined in Chapter 44.) The fragments may consist of cartilage alone or cartilage and bone. Typical sites of transchondral fractures are the distal femur, the ankle, the kneecap, the elbow, and the wrist. Transchondral fractures are most prevalent in adolescents.

◆**PATHOPHYSIOLOGY.** When a bone is broken the periosteum and blood vessels in the cortex, marrow, and surrounding soft tissues are disrupted. Bleeding occurs from the damaged ends of the bone and from the neighboring soft tissue. A hematoma forms within the medullary canal, between the fractured ends of the bone, and beneath the periosteum. Bone tissue immediately adjacent to the fracture dies. This necrotic tissue and any debris in the fracture area stimulate an intense inflammatory response characterized by vasodilation, exudation of plasma and leukocytes, and infiltration by inflammatory leukocytes and mast cells. Cytokines, including transforming growth factor-beta (TGF-β), platelet-derived growth factor (PDGF), prostaglandins, and other factors that promote healing, are released. Within 48 hours after the injury, vascular tissue invades the fracture area from the surrounding soft tissue and marrow cavity, and blood flow to the entire bone is increased. Osteoblasts and osteoclasts (or bone-forming cells) in the periosteum, endosteum, and marrow are activated to produce subperiosteal procallus along the outer surface of the shaft and over the broken ends of the bone (Fig. 45.2). Healing generally occurs in three overlapping

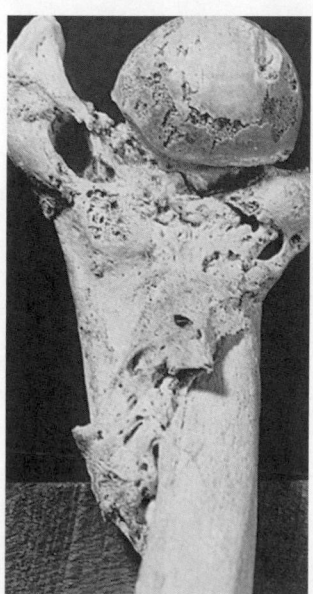

FIGURE 45.2 Exuberant Callus Formation Following Fracture. (From Rosai J: *Ackerman's surgical pathology*, ed 8, St Louis, 1996, Mosby.)

phases. The initial inflammatory phase of healing lasts 3 to 4 days. During the next few days, the repair phase begins and capillary ingrowth, together with mononuclear cells and fibroblasts, begins the transformation of a hematoma into granulation tissue. Next, osteoblasts within the procallus synthesize collagen and matrix, which becomes mineralized to form callus. As the repair process continues, remodeling occurs, during which unnecessary callus is resorbed and trabeculae are formed along lines of stress; at the end of this stage, bone can withstand normal stresses. The last phase, remodeling, lasts for months to years. Except for the liver, bone is unique among all body tissues in that after a fracture it will heal with normal, not scar, tissue.

◆**CLINICAL MANIFESTATIONS.** Clinical manifestations of a fracture can vary according to the type of fracture, site of the fracture, and associated soft tissue injury. In general, the signs and symptoms of a fracture include impaired function, unnatural alignment (deformity), swelling, muscle spasm, tenderness, pain, and impaired sensation. The position of the bone segments is determined by the pull of attached muscles, gravity, and the direction and magnitude of the force that caused the fracture. One or both segments of the fractured bone may be rotated inward or outward on the bone's long axis (rotation), misaligned at an angle (angulation), or slide over the other segment (overriding) or out of normal position (displaced).

Fractures are usually caused by trauma and immediate, often severe pain at the site of injury occurs. Subsequent pain is produced by muscle spasm, overriding of the fracture segments, or damage to adjacent soft tissues. Numbness also is common and caused by swelling, pinching, or severing of a nerve caused by the trauma or bone fragments. Pathologic fractures can cause angular deformity, painless swelling, or generalized bone pain. Stress fractures usually occur in weightbearing bones. Stress fracture symptoms can vary, but the most common is pain. The pain of a stress fracture is often gradual in onset and can be relieved with rest. Other symptoms of stress fractures include local tenderness and soft tissue swelling. Transchondral fractures may be entirely asymptomatic or painful during movement. Range of motion in the joint is limited and movement may evoke crepitation, a crunching sensation felt when bones rub against each other.

◆**EVALUATION AND TREATMENT.** Treatment of a displaced fracture involves manipulating the bone to realign bone fragments (reduction) to the correct anatomic position and holding the fragments in place (immobilization) so bone healing can occur. Many fractures heal without manipulation and require only adequate immobilization. Several methods of manipulation are available to reduce a fracture that will not heal with simple immobilization, including closed manipulation, traction, and open reduction. Maligned fractures require the most aggressive treatment of all types of fractures.

Fractures can be reduced by closed manipulation if the skin is not opened and the bone is able to be moved or manipulated into place. Appropriate use of closed manipulation occurs when the contour of the bone is well aligned and the alignment can be maintained with immobilization.

Traction is another option used to accomplish or maintain reduction of a fracture. When bone fragments are displaced (not in their anatomic position), weights are used to apply firm, steady traction (pull) and countertraction to the long axis of the bone. Traction stretches and fatigues muscles that pull the bone fragments out of place, allowing the distal fragment to align with the proximal fragment. Traction can be applied to the skin (skin traction), directly to the involved bone, or distal to the involved bone (skeletal traction). Skin traction is used when only a few pounds of pulling force are needed to realign the fragments or when the traction will be used for only a brief time, such as before surgery or for a few days before applying a cast. In skeletal traction, a pin or wire is drilled through the bone below the fracture site, and a traction bow, rope, and weights are attached to the pin or wire to apply tension by providing the pulling force needed to overcome the muscle spasm and helping realign the fracture fragments.

Open reduction is a surgical procedure that exposes the fracture site; the fragments are brought into alignment under direct visualization. Some form of hardware, such as a screw, plate, nail, or wire, is used to maintain the reduction (internal fixation). External fixation is a procedure used to reduce and immobilize significantly displaced open fractures. Pins are placed in the bone proximal and distal to the break and then stabilized by an external frame of clamps and rods (Fig. 45.3). Bone grafts also are used to repair fractures and filling voids in the bone. These grafts are from the injured individual (autograph), a cadaver (allograph), or a bone substitute (ceramic composites, bioactive cement).

Improper reduction or immobilization of a fractured bone may result in nonunion, delayed union, or malunion. Nonunion is failure of the bone ends to grow together (Fig. 45.4). The gap between the broken ends of the bone fills with dense fibrous and fibrocartilaginous tissue instead of new bone. Occasionally, the fibrous tissue contains a fluid-filled space that resembles a joint, termed a *false joint,* or *pseudarthrosis.* Delayed union is union that does not occur until approximately 8 to 9 months after a fracture. Malunion is the healing of a bone in a nonanatomic position. Treatment of delayed union and nonunion includes use of various modalities designed to stimulate new bone formation. Physical modalities, such as implantable or external electric current devices, electromagnetic field generations, and low-density ultrasound, have been effective in stimulating bone formation.[6] Stem cells and gene therapy also show promise in promoting formation of new bone.[7,8] Large defects in bone can be filled with bone graft or synthetic materials, such as calcium phosphate cement.

Dislocation and Subluxation

Dislocation and subluxation are caused by trauma, but also can be caused by ligamentous laxity, nerve injury, rheumatoid disease, or genetic problems. Dislocation is the temporary displacement of a bone from its normal position in a joint. If a dislocation does not involve a fracture, it is a simple dislocation; if there is an associated fracture, it becomes a complex dislocation. If the contact between the two joint surfaces is only partially lost, the injury is called a subluxation.

Dislocation and subluxation are most common in persons younger than 20 years and are generally associated with fractures. Dislocation and subluxation, however, may result from congenital or acquired disorders that cause (1) muscular imbalance, as occurs with congenital hip dislocation or neurologic disorders; (2) incongruities in the articulating surfaces of the bones, such as with rheumatoid arthritis (see Classic Inflammatory Joint Disease); or (3) joint instability.

Most often dislocated or subluxated are the joints of the shoulder, elbow, wrist, finger, hip, and knee (Fig. 45.5). The shoulder's glenohumeral joint is a relatively unstable joint because the articular surface of the glenoid cavity is only one-third as large as the surface of the humeral head. As a result, the glenohumeral joint is often injured. Physical trauma to the shoulder can cause anterior, posterior, superior, or inferior dislocation. Anterior dislocation is the most common and is usually the result of an indirect force that places the shoulder in extreme external rotation.

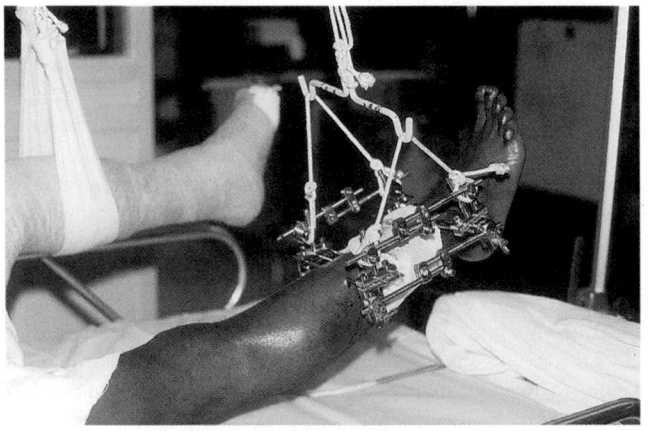

FIGURE 45.3 Example of an External Fixation Device on the Right Leg. The left leg is in a splint.

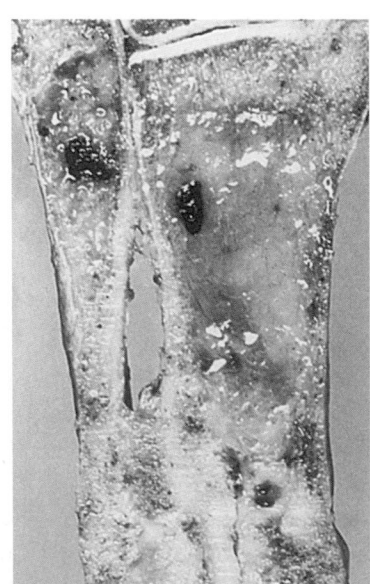

FIGURE 45.4 Nonunion of Old Fracture of Tibia and Fibula in a 53-Year-Old Man. Multiple fractures had occurred in 2 years previously and necessitated bone grafting. (From Rosai J: *Ackerman's surgical pathology,* ed 8, St Louis, 1996, Mosby.)

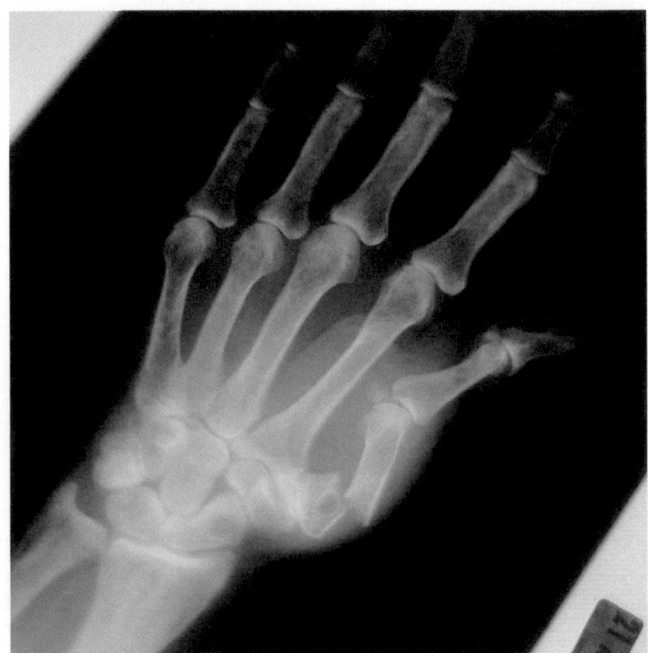

FIGURE 45.5 Displaced Fracture. An x-ray showing a displaced fracture of the base of the first metacarpal, also known as a *Bennett fracture.*

Posterior dislocations usually occur because of trauma. A superior dislocation is rare and usually the result of an extreme forward and upward force on an adducted arm. Inferior displacement is seen in persons with neurologic injuries of the brachial plexus and is believed to be caused by stretching of the supporting muscles or by joint effusion.

Traumatic dislocation of the elbow joint is common in the immature skeleton. In adults, however, an elbow dislocation is usually associated with a fracture of the ulna or head of the radius. Posterior dislocations occur when the individual falls on an outstretched hand with the elbow extended. Anterior dislocations are usually the result of a direct blow to the flexed elbow.

Traumatic dislocation of the wrist usually involves the distal ulna and carpal bones. Any one of the eight carpal bones can be dislocated after an injury. The most common cause is a fall on the hyperextended hand.

Dislocation in the hand usually involves the metacarpophalangeal and interphalangeal joints. Dislocation of the metacarpophalangeal joint is often the result of a fall on the outstretched hand that forces the joint into hyperextension. Dislocation of the interphalangeal joint occurs because of injury to the fingers in a hyperextended position.

Considerable trauma is needed to dislocate the hip. Anterior hip dislocation is rather rare and caused by forced abduction, for example, when an individual lands on the feet from a high fall. Posterior dislocation of the hip can occur in an automobile accident in which the flexed knee strikes the dashboard.

The knee is a relatively unstable joint that depends heavily on the soft tissue structures around it for support. Because the knee is an unstable weightbearing joint exposed to many different types of motion (flexion, extension, rotation), it is one of the most commonly injured joints. A knee dislocation can be anterior, posterior, lateral, medial, or rotary. It is often the result of a hyperextension injury that occurs during sports activities.

◆**PATHOPHYSIOLOGY.** Dislocations and subluxations are often accompanied by fracture because stress is placed on areas of bone not normally subjected to stress. In addition, as the bone separates from the joint, it may bruise or tear adjacent nerves, blood vessels, ligaments, supporting structures, and soft tissue. Dislocation of the shoulder may damage the shoulder capsule and the axillary nerve. Damage to the axillary nerve causes anesthesia in the sensory distribution of the nerve and paralysis of the deltoid muscle. Torn periosteum, ligaments, and muscle frequently accompany elbow dislocations. Bleeding from the damaged periosteum and muscle puts pressure on adjacent arteries that stops circulation to and from the forearm and hand. If the pressure is not promptly relieved, ischemic paralysis develops. Dislocations of the hand often result in permanent disability because of damage to the tendons and intricate mechanisms that allow smooth gliding in the joints. In the hip, avascular necrosis of the femoral head is a complication seen with dislocations. Knee dislocation usually tears both the collateral and the cruciate ligaments.

◆**CLINICAL MANIFESTATIONS.** Signs and symptoms of dislocations or subluxations include pain, swelling, limitation of motion, and joint deformity. Pain is caused by effusion of inflammatory exudate into the joint or associated tendon and injury to the ligament. Joint deformity is caused by muscle contractions that exert pull on the dislocated or subluxated joint or fluid within the joint. Limitation of motion may be a result of effusion into the joint or the displacement of bones.

Tenderness and deformity are prominent in dislocations of the fingers. Unusual muscle pull and pain often result in abnormal posturing of the fingers; for example, the fingers or thumb may be abnormally flexed. A dislocated elbow is often held in a flexed position, and the joint resists active or passive movement. Pain is the key symptom of shoulder injuries.

Attempts to lift the arm aggravate the pain. In most shoulder dislocations, the ability to elevate the arm is minimal and the individual supports the injured arm with the opposite hand. Pain and an abnormal gait or limp or inability to bear full weight usually accompanies traumatic dislocation of the hip. The pain is constant and severe and is felt in the inguinal region or thigh. The thigh and leg may assume a position of inward rotation, adduction, or flexion and appear shortened. In a rare anterior dislocation, the limb is not shortened and the joint is fixed in abduction, outward rotation, and flexion.

◆**EVALUATION AND TREATMENT.** Evaluation of dislocations and subluxations is based on clinical manifestations and roentgenograms. Treatment consists of reduction and immobilization for 2 to 6 weeks and exercises to maintain normal range of motion in the joint. Depending on the joint, healing is usually complete within months to years.

Support Structure Trauma
Sprains and Strains of Tendons and Ligaments

Tendon and ligament injuries can accompany fractures and dislocations. A tendon is fibrous connective tissue that attaches skeletal muscle to bone. A ligament is a band of fibrous connective tissue that connects bones where they meet at a joint. Tendons and ligaments support the bones and joints and either facilitate or limit motion. Tendons and ligaments can be torn, ruptured, or completely separated from bone at their points of attachment.

A tear in a tendon is known as a strain. Major trauma can tear or rupture a tendon at any site in the body. Most often injured are the tendons of the hands and feet, the knee (patellar), the upper arm (biceps and triceps), the thigh (quadriceps), the ankle, and the heel (Achilles). Lifting excessive weight with the arms can cause traumatic rupture of the biceps tendon. Rupture of the Achilles tendon occurs when forced dorsiflexion is applied to the foot when it is in plantar flexion. Spontaneous tendon ruptures can occur in individuals receiving local corticosteroid injections or fluoroquinolones and in persons with rheumatoid arthritis or systemic lupus erythematosus.

Ligament tears are known as sprains. Ligament tears and ruptures can occur at any joint, but are most common in the wrist, ankle, elbow, and knee joints. A complete separation of a tendon or ligament from its bony attachment site is known as an avulsion. An avulsion is the result of abnormal stress on the ligament or tendon and is commonly seen in young athletes, especially sprinters, hurdlers, and runners.

Strains and sprains are classified as first degree (least severe), second degree, and third degree (most severe).

◆**PATHOPHYSIOLOGY.** When a tendon or ligament is torn, an extensive inflammatory cascade process begins. Inflammatory mediators include cytokines, nitric oxide, prostaglandins, and lipoxins. An inflammatory exudate develops between the torn ends. Later, granulation tissue containing macrophages, fibroblasts, and capillary buds grows inward from the surrounding soft tissue and cartilage to begin the repair process. Within 3 to 4 days after the injury, collagen formation begins. At first, collagen formation is random and disorganized. As the collagen fibers interweave and connect with preexisting tendon fibers, they organize parallel to the lines of stress. Eventually, vascular fibrous tissue fuses the new and surrounding tissues into a single mass. As reorganization takes place, the healing tendon or ligament separates from the surrounding soft tissue. Usually, a healing tendon or ligament lacks sufficient strength to withstand strong pull for 4 to 5 weeks after the injury. If strong muscle pull does occur during this time, the tendon or ligament ends may separate again, which causes the tendon or ligament to heal in a lengthened shape with an excessive amount of scar tissue that renders the tendon or ligament functionless. Scar remodeling may take months to years before it is complete.[9]

◆**CLINICAL MANIFESTATIONS.** Tendon and ligament injuries are painful and cause functional limitation. These injuries are usually accompanied by soft tissue swelling, changes in tendon or ligament contour, and dislocation or subluxation of bones. The pain is generally sharp and localized, and tenderness persists over the distribution of the tendon or ligament. Painful joint swelling usually can be seen in finger and elbow sprains. Flexion deformities of the fingers and thumb occur in injuries to the extensor tendons. Crepitus may accompany tendon injury in the wrist. Tendon or ligament pain in the elbow is accentuated by flexion, supination, and extension of the elbow or by extension of the wrist. Lifting small objects requires extension of the wrist and therefore aggravates the pain. Tendon injuries in the upper arm cause weakness when the individual tries to flex the forearm. Pain is often the key symptom of shoulder injuries with pain radiating to the deltoid muscle or extending down the arm and is aggravated by attempts to actively raise the arms. Depending on the ligament or tendon involved, injuries to the knee may produce pronounced immobility, absence of lateral movement, instability when walking down stairs, flexion deformity, crepitus, or an upward or downward shift of the patella.

◆**EVALUATION AND TREATMENT.** Evaluation is based on clinical manifestations, stress radiography, arthroscopy, or arthrography. When possible, treatment consists of protection of the involved structures (splinting), promotion of early motion, and rehabilitation. Surgical intervention that sutures the tendon or ligament ends in close approximation may be necessary to treat complete rupture. If this is not possible because of the extent of damage, tendon or ligament grafting may be necessary. Prolonged rehabilitation exercises help ensure that the individual regains nearly normal functions.

Tendinopathy and Bursitis

Trauma and overuse injuries can cause painful degradation of collagen fibers (**tendinosis**), inflammation of tendons (**tendinitis**), or inflammation in bursal sacs (**bursitis**). The term *tendinopathy* includes tendinitis, tendinosis, and paratendinitis. Studies have shown that vascular ingrowth in tendinopathy (neovascularization) is accompanied with nerve ingrowth, facilitating pain transmission in Achilles and patellar tendinopathies.[10] Other causes of tendinopathy include crystal deposits, postural misalignment, and hypermobility in a joint. Table 45.2 summarizes classes of tendinopathies.

Epicondylitis is inflammation of a tendon where it attaches to a bone (at its origin). Most tendon pathology, however, is caused by tissue degeneration rather than inflammation.[11] Epicondylar areas of the humerus, radius, or ulna and the area around the knee are most often involved. **Lateral epicondylopathy**, commonly called **tennis elbow**, is

the result of tissue degeneration or irritation of the extensor carpi radialis brevis tendon at its origin. **Medial epicondylopathy**, referred to as **golfer's elbow**, is a degenerative process of the pronator teres, flexor carpi radialis, and palmaris longus tendons at the medial humeral condyle (Fig. 45.6). Epicondylopathy is also related to smoking, obesity, and work activities that involve forceful or repetitive cyclic flexion and extension of the elbow, or cyclic pronation, supination, extension, and flexion of the wrist that generates loads to the elbow and forearm region.

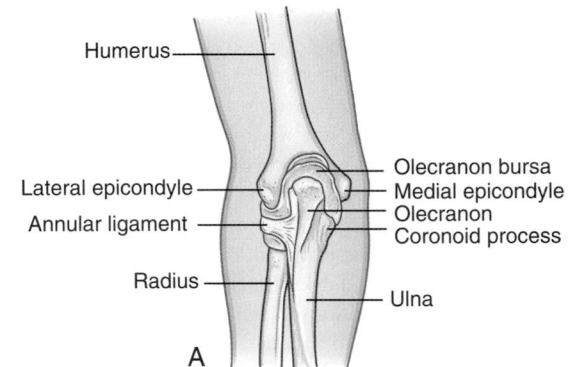

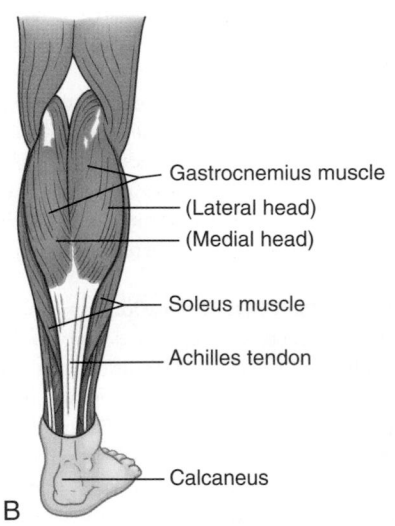

FIGURE 45.6 Tendinitis and Epicondylitis. **A,** Medial or lateral epicondyles of humerus, site of epicondylitis. **B,** Achilles tendon, site of commonly occurring tendinitis.

TABLE 45.2	**HISTOPATHOLOGIC CLASSIFICATION OF TENDON DISORDERS**	
PATHOLOGIC DIAGNOSIS	**MACROSCOPIC PATHOLOGY**	**HISTOPATHOLOGIC FINDINGS**
Tendinosis	Intratendinous degeneration (commonly due to aging, microtrauma, muscular compromise)	Collagen disorientation, disorganization, and fiber separation by an increase in mucoid ground substance, increased preponderance of cells and vascular spaces with or without neovascularization and focal necrosis or calcification
Tendinitis	Symptomatic degeneration of the tendon with vascular disruption and inflammatory repair response	Degenerative changes as noted above with superimposed evidence of tear, including fibroblastic and myofibroblastic proliferation, hemorrhage, and organizing granulation tissue
Paratenonitis	"Inflammation" of the outer layer of the tendon (paratenon) alone, whether or not the paratenon is lined by synovium	Mucoid degeneration if the areolar tissue is seen; a scattered mild mononuclear infiltrate with or without focal fibrin deposition and fibrinous exudate
Paratenonitis with tendinosis	Paratenonitis associated with intratendinous degeneration	Degenerative changes as noted in tendinosis with mucoid degeneration with or without fibrous and scattered inflammatory cells in the paratenon alveolar tissue

From Maffulli N, Wong J, Almekinders LC: *Clin Sports Med* 22(4):675–692, 2003.

Bursae are small sacs lined with synovial membrane and filled with synovial fluid; they are located between tendons, muscles, and bony prominences. Their primary function is to separate, lubricate, and cushion these structures. When irritated or injured, these sacs become inflamed and swell. Because most bursae lie outside joints, joint movement is rarely compromised with bursitis. Acute bursitis occurs primarily in the middle years and is often caused by trauma; repetitive irritation can cause chronic bursitis. Septic bursitis is caused by wound infection or bacterial infection of the skin overlying the bursae. Bursitis commonly occurs in the shoulder, hip, knee, and elbow.

◆**PATHOPHYSIOLOGY.** In tendinitis, inflammatory fluid accumulates, causing swelling of the tendon and its enclosing sheath. Inflammatory changes cause thickening of the sheath, which limits movements and causes pain. Microtears cause bleeding, edema, and pain in the involved tendons or surrounding structures. At times, after repeated inflammations, calcium may be deposited in the tendon origin area, causing a calcific tendinitis.

The typical bursitis is an inflammation that is reactive to overuse or excessive pressure. The inflamed bursal sac becomes engorged, and the inflammation can spread to adjacent tissues (Fig. 45.7). The inflammation may decrease with rest, heat, and aspiration of the fluid. (Inflammation is discussed in Chapter 7.)

◆**CLINICAL MANIFESTATIONS.** Tendinopathy may be asymptomatic, but generally there is localized pain that worsens with active more than passive motion. With symptomatic tendinopathy, the pain is localized over the involved tendon and movement in the affected joint is limited. In bursitis, onset of pain may be gradual or sudden, but movement of the joint itself is normal. Shoulder bursitis impairs arm abduction because of pain and swelling of the bursa. Bursitis in the knee produces pain when climbing stairs, and crossing the legs is painful in bursitis of the hip. Lying on the side of an inflamed trochanteric bursa is also very painful. Table

45.3 summarizes common sites of bursitis. Signs of infectious bursitis may include the presence of a puncture site, prior corticosteroid injection, severe inflammation, or an adjacent source of infection.

◆**EVALUATION AND TREATMENT.** Evaluation of tendinopathy, epicondylopathy, and bursitis is based on clinical manifestations, physical examination, arthroscopy, arthrography, ultrasound, and possibly magnetic resonance imaging (MRI). Treatment includes administration of systemic analgesics, application of ice or heat, or local injection of an anesthetic and a corticosteroid to reduce inflammation. Bursitis may require aspiration to drain excess fluid. Physical therapy to prevent loss of function begins after acute symptoms subside.

Muscle Strains

Mild injury such as muscle strain is usually seen after traumatic or sports injuries. *Muscle strain* is a general term for local muscle damage. It is often the result of sudden, forced motion causing the muscle to become stretched beyond normal capacity. Strains often involve the tendon as well. Muscles are ruptured more often than tendons in young people; the opposite is true in older adults. Muscle strain may be chronic when the muscle is repeatedly stretched beyond its usual capacity. There is evidence of tissue disruption with subsequent signs of muscle regeneration and connective tissue repair when a biopsy is performed. Hemorrhage into the surrounding tissue and signs of inflammation also may be present. Knife and gunshot wounds also cause traumatic rupture. Regardless of the cause of trauma, muscle cells usually can regenerate. Regeneration may take up to 6 weeks, and the affected muscle should be protected during this time. Types of muscle strain, together with their manifestations and treatment, are summarized in Table 45.4.

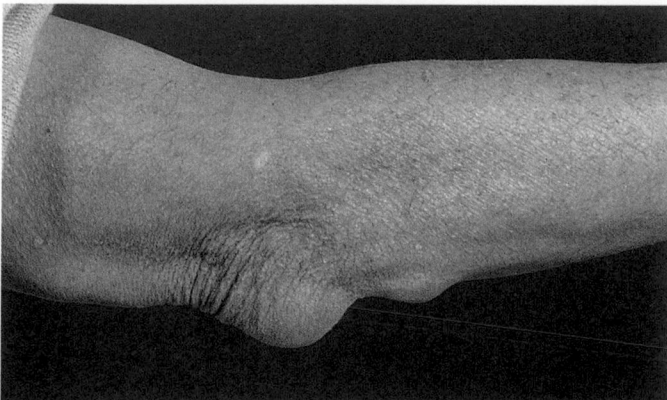

FIGURE 45.7 Olecranon Bursa. A case of olecranon bursitis in a patient with rheumatoid arthritis. A rheumatoid nodule is also shown. (From Hochberg MC et al: *Rheumatology*, ed 6, Philadelphia, 2015, Elsevier.)

TABLE 45.3	COMMON SITES AND CAUSES OF BURSITIS
SITE	**COMMON CAUSES**
Shoulder (subacromial)	Repetitive overhead activities
Elbow (olecranon)	Rheumatoid arthritis (RA), gout, tuberculosis, leaning on elbow
Hip (greater trochanter)	Acute trauma, chronic stress
Ischial (weaver's bottom)	Overuse (runner, ballet dancers), lumbosacral disease, RA, osteoarthritis (OA)
Knee	
Prepatellar (housemaid knee)	Trauma, frequent kneeling, infection
Pes anserine (medial knee)	Obesity, long-distance runner, OA, type 2 diabetes
Heel (calcaneal)	Poorly fitting footwear, Achilles tendinitis

TABLE 45.4	MUSCLE STRAIN	
TYPE	**MANIFESTATIONS**	**TREATMENT**
First degree (e.g., bench press in untrained athlete)	Muscle overstretched, painful	Ice should be applied 5 or 6 times in the first 24–48 hr; complete rest for up to 2 weeks, followed by weightbearing 3 times per week and range of motion daily
Second degree (e.g., any muscle strain with bruising and pain)	Muscle intact with some tearing pain, mild bruising; fascia is intact	Treatment similar to that for first-degree strains, with added mild analgesia; cryokinetics (a treatment system of alternating applications of cold with progressive exercise)
Third degree (e.g., traumatic injury)	Caused by tearing of fascia; muscle rupture palpable, bleeding present	Surgery to approximate ruptured edges; immobilization and rest for 6 weeks, followed by an individualized rehabilitation regimen of strengthening exercises

A late complication of localized muscle injury is abnormal bone formation in soft tissue, often called myositis ossificans or heterotopic ossification (HO). Its exact pathophysiology remains unknown, but the basic problem seems to be the inability of mesenchymal cells to differentiate into osteoblastic stem cells and the improper development of fibroblasts into bone-forming cells. Though uncommon, HO is associated with burns, joint surgery, and trauma to the musculoskeletal system or central nervous system. HO may involve muscle or tendons, ligaments, or bones near a muscle.[12] Examples include "rider's bone," in which the adductor muscle of the thigh of equestrians becomes calcified, as well as in football players after muscle injury to thigh muscles; and "drill bone," in which the same complication is seen in the deltoid and pectoral muscles of fencers and infantry soldiers.

Rhabdomyolysis

Once used interchangeably with the term *myoglobinuria*, rhabdomyolysis is the rapid breakdown of muscle that causes the release of intracellular contents, including protein pigment myoglobin, into the extracellular space and bloodstream. Physical interruptions in the sarcolemmal membrane, called *delta lesions*, suggest that the sarcolemmal membrane is the route through which muscle constituents are released. Myoglobinuria, first described in victims of crush injuries in London during World War II, refers to the presence of the muscle protein myoglobin in the urine. More recently, myoglobinuria has been reported in individuals found unresponsive and immobile for long periods, such as drug and alcohol overdoses.

◆**PATHOPHYSIOLOGY.** Rhabdomyolysis is sometimes incorrectly used interchangeably with *crush injury* (a description of injuries resulting from crushing of a body part), *compartment syndrome* (the consequences of increased intracompartmental pressures of a muscle), or *crush syndrome* (the pathophysiologic events caused by rhabdomyolysis, primarily involving the kidneys and coagulation syndrome).[13] Although relatively rare, rhabdomyolysis has many causes (Box 45.1) and can result in serious complications, including hyperkalemia (because of the release of intracellular potassium into the circulation), metabolic acidosis (from liberation of intracellular phosphorus and sulfate), acute renal failure (myoglobin precipitates in the tubules, obstructing flow through the nephron and producing injury), and even disseminated intravascular coagulation (DIC) (likely caused by activation of the clotting cascade by sarcolemma damage and release of intracellular components from the damaged muscles). Even the weight of a limp extremity can generate enough pressure to produce muscle ischemia (Fig. 45.8).

Malignant hyperthermia (MH) is a potentially life-threatening hereditary disorder of skeletal muscle ryanodine receptors (RyR1), allowing large quantities of calcium to be released from the sarcoplasmic reticulum (SR) after exposure to certain volatile anesthetics. The sustained elevation of calcium concentration allows excessive stimulation of aerobic and anaerobic glycolytic metabolism, causing a hypermetabolic state resulting in respiratory and metabolic acidosis, muscle rigidity, altered cell permeability, and hyperkalemia.[14] Dantrolene, a skeletal muscle relaxant, inhibits calcium release from the SR and is used to reverse the effects of MH.

Compartment syndromes occur when blood flow to the affected area is compromised because of increased venous pressure, leading to decreased arterial inflow, ischemia, and edema. Emergency treatment may be required to save an affected limb. Classic symptoms of compartment syndrome are (1) pain out of proportion to the injury, (2) paresthesia, (3) pallor, (4) pulselessness (uncommon), and (5)

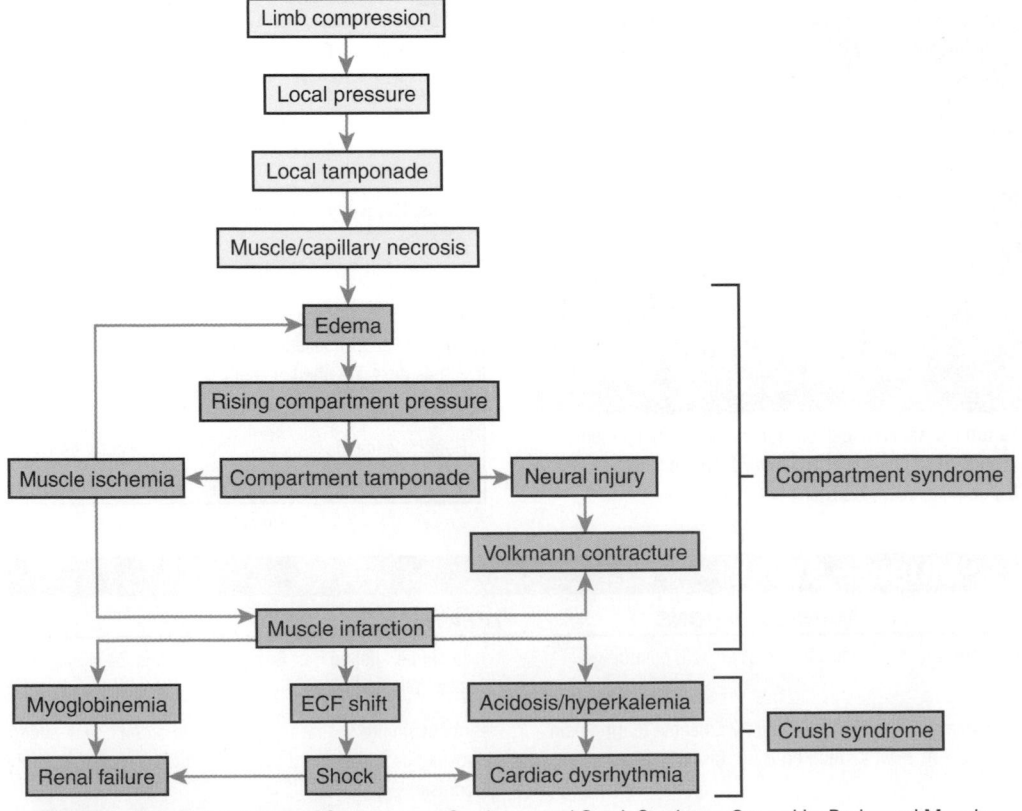

FIGURE 45.8 Pathogenesis of Compartment Syndrome and Crush Syndrome Caused by Prolonged Muscle Compression. *ECF*, Extracellular fluid.

BOX 45.1 SELECTED CAUSES OF RHABDOMYOLYSIS

Medications and Toxic Substances That Increase the Risk of Rhabdomyolysis
Direct Myotoxicity
HMG-CoA reductase inhibitors (statins), especially in combination with fibrate-derived lipid-lowering agents such as niacin (nicotinic acid; Nicolar)
Cyclosporine (Sandimmune)
Itraconazole (Sporanox)
Erythromycin
Colchicine
Zidovudine (Retrovir)
Corticosteroids

Other Medications and Toxins
Amphetamines
Anesthetic and paralytic agents (halothane, propofol, succinylcholine—malignant hyperthermia syndrome)
Antihistamines (diphenhydramine, doxylamine)
Anti-hyperlipidemic agents (statins, clofibrate, bezafibrate)
Antipsychotics and antidepressants (amitriptyline, doxepin, fluoxetine, haloperidol, lithium, protriptyline, perphenazine, promethazine, chlorpromazine, trifluoperazine)
Caffeine
Cocaine
HIV integrase inhibitor (raltegravir)
Hypnotics and sedatives (benzodiazepines, barbiturates)
Heroin
LSD
Methamphetamine
Methadone
Methylenedioxymethamphetamine (MDMA; "ecstasy")
Miscellaneous medications (amphotericin B, azathioprine, ε-aminocaproic acid, quinidine, penicillamine, salicylates, theophylline, terbutaline, thiazides, vasopressin)
Phencyclidine
Protease inhibitors

Indirect Muscle Damage
Alcohol
Central nervous system depressants
Cocaine
Amphetamines
Ecstasy (MDMA)
LSD
Neuromuscular-blocking agents

Traumatic, Heat-Related, Ischemic, and Exertional Causes
Traumatic Causes
Direct trauma
Lightning strike
Immobilization
Extensive third-degree burn
Crush injury

Heat-Related Causes
Heat stroke
Malignant hyperthermia
Neuroleptic malignant syndrome

Ischemic Causes
Ischemic limb injury

Exertional Causes
Marathon running
Physical overexertion in untrained athletes
Pathologic muscle exertion
Severe dystonia
Tetanus
Status epilepticus
Delirium tremens
Heat dissipation impairment
Physical overexertion in persons with sickle cell disease

Genetic Causes
Lipid Metabolism
Carnitine palmitoyltransferase deficiency
Carnitine deficiency
Short-chain and long-chain acetyl-coenzyme A dehydrogenase deficiency

Carbohydrate Metabolism
Myophosphorylase deficiency (McArdle disease)
Phosphorylase kinase deficiency
Phosphofructokinase deficiency
Phosphoglycerate mutase deficiency
Lactate dehydrogenase deficiency (characteristic elevation of creatine kinase level with normal lactate dehydrogenase level)

Purine Metabolism
Myoadenylate deaminase deficiency
Duchenne muscular dystrophy

Infectious, Inflammatory, Metabolic, and Endocrinologic Causes
Infectious Causes
Viruses: influenza virus B, parainfluenza virus, adenovirus, coxsackievirus, echovirus, herpes simplex virus, cytomegalovirus, Epstein-Barr virus, human immunodeficiency virus
Bacteria: *Streptococcus, Salmonella, Legionella, Staphylococcus,* and *Listeria* species

Inflammatory Causes
Polymyositis
Dermatomyositis
Capillary leak syndrome
Snake bites (mostly in South America, Asia, and Africa)

Metabolic and Endocrinologic Causes
Electrolyte imbalances: hyponatremia, hypernatremia, hypokalemia, hypophosphatemia, hypocalcemia
Hypothyroidism
Thyrotoxicosis
Diabetic ketoacidosis
Nonketotic hyperosmolar syndrome

Herbal Supplements
Red yeast rice (*Monascus purpureus*)
Compounds containing ma huang, guarana, and garcinia cambogia
Ephedra-based compounds, especially weight-loss supplements

HMG-CoA, 3-Hydroxy-3-methylglutaryl coenzyme A; *LSD,* lysergic acid diethylamide; *MDMA,* 3,4-methylenedioxymethamphetamine.
Data from Acharya S et al: *Ann Indian Acad Neurol* 13(3):221–222, 2010; Cervelin G, Comelli I, Lippe G: *Clin Chem Lab Med* 48(6):749–756, 2010; Croce F et al: *Int J STD AIDS* 21(11):783–785, 2010; Halpern P et al: *Hum Exp Toxicol* 29(5):259–266, 2010; Mammen AL, Amato AA: *Curr Opin Rheumatol* 22(6):644–650, 2010; Sauret JM, Narinides G, Wang GK: *Am Fam Physician* 65(3):907, 2002.

paralysis (a late finding). Of these symptoms, pain is the most sensitive clinical sign.[15]

When clinical evaluation is inconclusive, the rising compartment pressure can be directly measured by inserting a wick catheter, needle, or slit catheter into the muscle. Immediate fasciotomy and débridement are advocated for reducing elevated intracompartmental pressures.[15] Those frequently affected are the compartments of the leg, the volar compartment of the hand, the abdomen, and the gluteal compartments.

◆ **CLINICAL MANIFESTATIONS.** A *classic triad* of muscle pain, weakness, and dark urine is considered typical of rhabdomyolysis, but those affected may have no complaint of pain or muscle weakness.[13] Abnormally dark urine caused by myoglobinuria may be the first and only symptom. The renal threshold for myoglobin is low (approximately 0.5 mg/dL of urine), so only 200 g of muscle needs to be damaged to cause visible changes in the urine. Myoglobin is rapidly cleared and levels may return to normal within 24 hours of injury. Along with the release of myoglobin, creatine kinase (CK) and other serum enzymes are released in massive quantities. The efflux of proteins and enzymes also includes loss of potassium, phosphate, nucleotides, creatinine, and creatine. Serum hypocalcemia is seen early in the course of myoglobinuria and is followed by late hypercalcemia.

◆ **EVALUATION AND TREATMENT.** The most important and clinically useful measurement in rhabdomyolysis is serum creatine kinase (CK) level. With normal CK serum levels of 5 to 25 units/L for women and 5 to 35 units/L for men, a level five times the upper limit of normal (about 1000 units/L) is used to identify rhabdomyolysis. Once CK levels exceed 5000 units/L, acute renal failure is likely. A recent study evaluated the ultrasonographic appearance of rhabdomyolysis in damaged muscle from earthquake victims and found abnormalities in muscle texture and subcutaneous tissue, as well as areas of liquid in the damaged tissue.[16]

Maintaining adequate urinary flow and prevention of kidney failure are goals of treatment. Rapid intravenous hydration maintains adequate kidney flow. Other issues, such as hyperkalemia, may require temporary hemodialysis. Other treatments, such as using mannitol to cause an osmotic diuresis or bicarbonate to alkalinize the urine, have not been shown to consistently improve outcomes.

DISORDERS OF BONES

Metabolic Bone Diseases

Metabolic bone disease is characterized by abnormal bone structure that is caused by altered or inadequate biochemical reactions resulting in disorders of bone strength. Abnormalities include genetic, mineral, vitamin, hormone, and structural abnormalities.

Osteoporosis

Osteoporosis, or porous bone, is the most common bone disease in humans. It is characterized by low bone mineral density (BMD), impaired structural integrity of the bone, decreased bone strength, and the risk of fracture. Those with the lowest BMD are at most risk of fracture.[17] There are two types of osteoporosis: *primary* or *idiopathic osteoporosis*, which is the most common; and secondary osteoporosis. *Secondary osteoporosis* is caused by other conditions, including endocrine diseases (hormone imbalances, diabetes, hyperparathyroidism, hyperthyroidism), medications (such as heparin, corticosteroids, phenytoin, barbiturates, lithium), and other substances (including tobacco and ethanol). Other conditions (including rheumatoid disease, human immunodeficiency virus [HIV], malignancies, malabsorption syndromes, liver or kidney disease) also increase the risk for developing osteoporosis (Box 45.2). Cortical bone becomes more porous and thinner, making bone weaker

BOX 45.2	RISK FACTORS FOR OSTEOPOROSIS
Genetic	**Lifestyle**
Family history of osteoporosis	Sedentary
White/Asian race	Smoker
Increased age	Alcohol consumption (excessive)
Female gender	
	Concurrent
Anthropometric	Hyperparathyroidism
Small stature	
Fair or pale skinned	**Illness and Trauma**
Thin build	Renal insufficiency, hypocalciuria
	Rheumatoid arthritis
Hormonal and Metabolic	Spinal cord injury
Early menopause (natural or surgical)	Systemic lupus erythematosus
Late menarche	**Liver Disease**
Nulliparity	Marrow disease (myeloma,
Obesity	mastocytosis, thalassemia)
Hypogonadism	
Gaucher disease	**Drugs**
Cushing syndrome	Corticosteroids
Weight below healthy range	Dilantin
Acidosis	Gonadotropin-releasing hormone agonists
	Loop diuretics
Dietary	Methotrexate
Low dietary calcium and vitamin D	Thyroid
Low endogenous magnesium	Heparin
Excessive protein*	Cyclosporine
Excessive sodium intake	Depo-medroxyprogesterone acetate
High caffeine intake	Retinoids
Anorexia	
Malabsorption	

*Low levels of protein intake also have been reported.

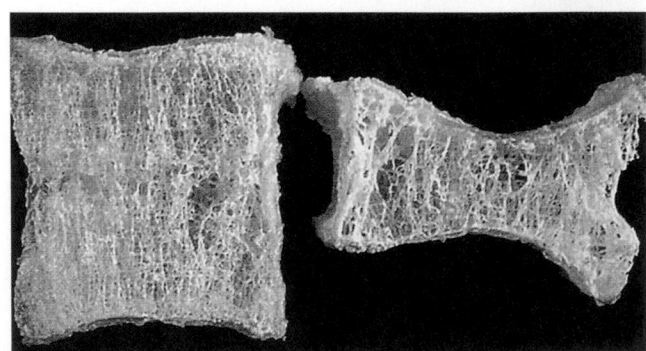

FIGURE 45.9 Vertebral Body. Osteoporotic vertebra *(right)* shortened by compression fractures compared with normal vertebral body *(left)*. Note that the osteoporotic vertebra has characteristic loss of horizontal trabeculae and thickened vertebral trabeculae. (From Kumar V et al: *Robbins & Cotran pathologic basis of disease*, ed 9, Philadelphia, 2015, Saunders.)

and prone to fractures (Fig. 45.9). The World Health Organization (WHO) has defined osteoporosis on the basis of bone density:
1. Normal bone mass is greater than 833 mg/cm^2.
2. Osteopenia, or decreased bone mass, is 833 to 648 mg/cm^2.
3. Osteoporosis is bone mass less than 648 mg/cm^2.

Osteoporosis is a complex, multifactorial chronic disease that often progresses silently for decades until fractures occur. It is the most common disease that affects bone. It is not necessarily a consequence of the aging process because some older adults retain strong, relatively dense bones. In osteoporosis, old bone is being reabsorbed faster than new bone is being made, causing the bones to lose density, becoming thinner and more porous. A progressive loss of bone mass may continue until the skeleton is no longer strong enough to support itself. Eventually, bones can fracture spontaneously. As bone becomes more fragile, fractures occur from falls or bumps that would not previously have caused fracture.

Severe or established osteoporosis is identified when there has been a fragility fracture. The disease can be (1) generalized, involving major portions of the axial skeleton, or (2) regional, involving one segment of the appendicular skeleton.

Throughout a lifetime, old bone is removed (resorption) and new bone is added (formation) to the skeleton. During childhood and teenage years, new bone is added faster than old bone is removed. Consequently, bones become larger, heavier, and denser. Bone formation continues at a pace faster than resorption until peak bone mass, or maximum bone density and strength, is reached, around age 30, after which bone resorption slowly exceeds bone formation. In women, bone loss begins before menopause, and is most rapid in the first years after menopause but persists throughout the postmenopausal years. Osteoporosis is most common in women at a rate of one in two women.[18] Men also are at risk, with an estimated one in four men experiencing an osteoporosis-related fracture at some point in one's lifetime.[18] In adults older than age 50, the prevalence of osteoporosis at either the spine or the femoral neck by age ranges from 3% to 10% in men and from 7% to 35% in women. One study showed that in men the prevalence of osteoporosis did not increase with age until age 80 years and older, but in women it increased for each decade after age 50 years.[19]

Approximately 52 million people in the United States are affected by osteoporosis or low bone density.[20] The major risks for persons with osteoporosis are fractures. Men lose bone density with aging; but because they begin with a higher bone density, they reach osteoporotic levels at an older age than do women.[21] In 2011 the United States Preventive Services Task Force (USPSTF) issued a recommendation that women age 65 and older be routinely screened for osteoporosis.[22] Hip fractures, in particular, can have devastating effects on an individual's life. In addition to direct medical costs, studies have shown decreased quality of life as well as excess loss of life-years for those experiencing hip or osteoporotic fractures.[23,24]

Vertebral fractures are the most common osteoporotic fracture but may be asymptomatic. Even if the fracture does not cause pain, vertebral fractures can cause deformity, reduced pulmonary function, and loss of height. The degree of compression necessary to define a vertebral fracture has not been standardized.

Osteoporosis affects all races and both sexes. Recent data from the National Health and Nutrition Examination Survey (NHANES) showed that Mexican-Americans had higher risk for osteoporosis, whereas non-Hispanic black persons had lower risk of osteopenia or osteoporosis at the lumbar spine or femoral neck.[19] Multiple genetic factors also influence development of osteoporosis.[25]

Whites are more susceptible than other races to osteoporosis caused by loss of bone density with age. Blacks have only about half the fractures found in whites, probably related to their higher peak bone mass, but black women remain at a high risk because of factors such as decreased dietary calcium intake, a high percentage of lactose intolerance, and increased prevalence of diseases, such as sickle cell disease and lupus, that increase the risk of developing osteoporosis.[26] Both black women and black men have generally been undertreated for osteoporosis.[26] Decreased bone strength with aging is partly due to lower bone mass, but other factors such as deterioration of type I collagen likely contribute to increased fracture risk.[27]

Measuring bone mineral density (BMD) by using dual x-ray absorptiometry (DXA) continues to be the most common method of estimating bone mass. Bone quality relates not just to bone mass (as measured by bone density) but also to the microarchitecture of the bone. Other variables include crystal size and shape, brittleness, vitality of the bone cells, structure of the bone proteins, water volume, integrity of the trabecular network, vascular supply, and the ability to repair tiny cracks.[28]

Because bone density relates to *quantity* of bone, bone *quality* is not accurately identified by bone density testing. Therefore bone density testing may or may not accurately identify individuals with increased fracture risk. An online tool called Fracture Risk Assessment (FRAX) (Fig. 45.10) incorporates clinical risk factors with BMD at the femoral

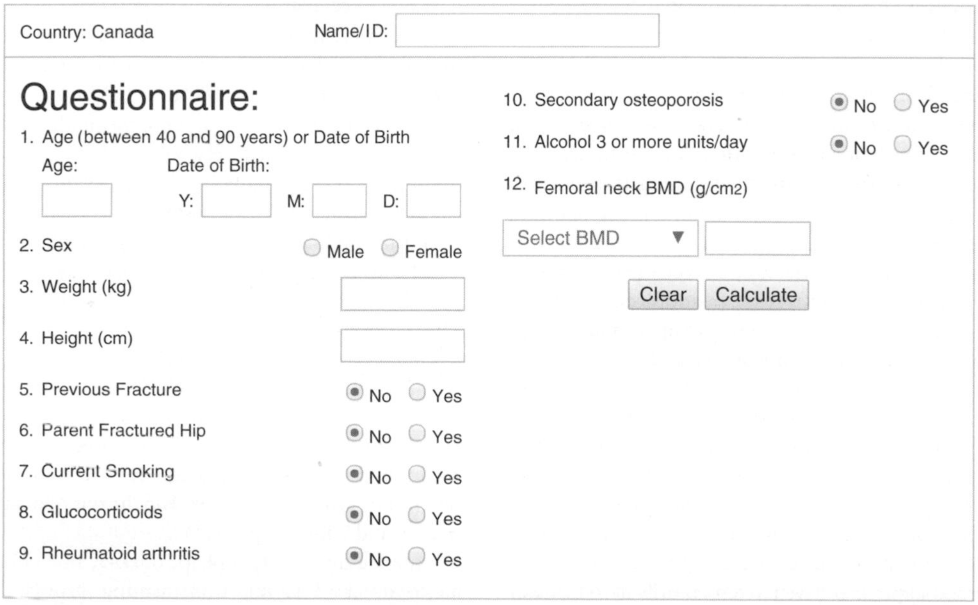

FIGURE 45.10 Fracture Risk Assessment Tool: FRAX. (Available at: http://www.shef.ac.uk/FRAX/tool.aspx ?country=19.)

neck to predict an individual's 10-year probability of fracture. This tool is available at http://www.shef.ac.uk/FRAX.

Postmenopausal osteoporosis occurs in middle-aged and older women. It can occur because of estrogen deficiency as well as estrogen-independent age-related mechanisms (e.g., secondary causes such as hyperparathyroidism and decreased mechanical stimulation). Recent studies indicate that increased oxidative stress (OS) and increased intracellular reactive oxygen species (ROS) play a significant role in the development of age-related bone loss, as well as other age-related changes in the body.[28] Hormonal deficiency also can increase with stress, excessive exercise, and low body weight. Postmenopausal changes include a substantial increase in bone turnover—that is, an imbalance between the remodeling activity of osteoclasts and osteoblasts. Increased formation and longevity of osteoclasts result in increased bone resorption and is associated with a cascade of proinflammatory cytokines. Increased cytokine activation, especially tumor necrosis factor (TNF), can occur with declining estrogen levels.[28] In addition, estrogen helps protect against the effects of OS and osteoclast apoptosis. Biologically, these processes involve the receptor activator of nuclear factor $\kappa\beta$ ligand (RANKL), transcription factors such as Forkhead proteins, the Wnt and osteoprotegerin (OPG) signaling pathways (see the following Pathophysiology section), and insulin-like growth factor (IGF). Other causes may include a combination of inadequate dietary calcium intake and lack of vitamin D, possibly decreased magnesium level, lack of exercise, low body mass, and family history. IGF is known to help in fracture healing and collagen synthesis and improves conditions for bone mineralization. IGF levels significantly decline by age 60.

The levels of sex hormones, especially estradiol (estrogen) and testosterone, are significant in premenopausal bone maintenance; however, when estrogen levels drop after menopause, it appears that circulating androgens become significant effectors on bone metabolism. In clinical studies of women, data have suggested that serum androgens influence bone density in pre-, peri-, and postmenopausal women. Androgens (i.e., testosterone and dihydrotestosterone) have long been recognized to stimulate bone formation. Other risk factors are identified in Box 45.2.

Poor nutrition and insufficient intake or malabsorption of dietary minerals, particularly calcium, are factors in the development of osteoporosis. Calcium absorption from the intestine decreases with age, and studies of individuals with osteoporosis show that their calcium intake is lower than that of age-matched controls. Deficiencies of vitamins, particularly vitamins C, D, E, and K, also contribute to bone loss.[29]

Skeletal homeostasis depends on a very narrow range of plasma calcium and phosphate concentrations, which are maintained by the endocrine system.[30] Therefore endocrine dysfunction ultimately can cause metabolic bone disease. In addition to declining levels of sex steroids, the hormones most commonly associated with osteoporosis are parathyroid hormone, cortisol, thyroid hormone, and growth hormone. Excessive intakes of caffeine, alcohol, and nicotine along with low body fat have been considered risk factors. In addition, significant differences in the levels of trace elements (zinc, copper, manganese) were noted in the bones and hair of unaffected individuals compared with those with osteoporosis. The development of selective estrogen receptor modulators (SERMs) for the treatment of postmenopausal osteoporosis increases bone formation and builds more muscle mass. In theory, selectively affecting bone, muscle mass, and other desired sites, while not affecting lipid or estrogen levels or blood pressure, side effects can be controlled but since the direct effects of SERMs on bone are not yet known, this remains a clinical challenge.[31]

Secondary osteoporosis sometimes develops temporarily in individuals receiving large doses of heparin, perhaps because heparin promotes bone resorption by decreasing collagen synthesis or by increasing collagen breakdown. Osteoporosis caused by heparin therapy usually resolves when therapy ceases. Treatment with other medications may lead to the development of osteoporosis, such as the use of glucocorticoid treatment for many chronic disease processes. Other medications that increase the risk of osteoporosis include lithium, methotrexate, anticonvulsants, cyclophosphamide, and cyclosporine.

One secondary cause, transient osteoporosis of the hip, is associated with the third trimester of pregnancy or the immediate postpartum period. However, most transient osteoporosis is a typically self-limiting syndrome affecting the lower extremity joints of middle-aged men. The etiology is unknown, and although most cases spontaneously resolve, some occurrences of bone demineralization may be related to osteonecrosis.[32]

Regional osteoporosis—osteoporosis confined to a region or segment of the appendicular skeleton—usually has a known cause. Transient regional osteoporosis has no known etiology, is characterized by bone marrow edema, and can cause severe pain. The lower extremity is most often affected, but other areas also may be involved.[33] Fortunately, it is usually self-limited. It tends to occur in middle-aged men and women in their late second or third trimester of pregnancy.[33] It is characterized by bone marrow edema, seen on magnetic resonance imaging (MRI), and areas of localized bone demineralization are seen on plain radiographs. Treatment is primarily symptomatic and the condition usually resolves spontaneously over 3 to 6 months, with no long-term adverse effects.

Classic regional osteoporosis is associated with disuse or immobilization of a limb because of fractures, motor paralysis, or bone or joint inflammation (see Fig. 45.14). A negative calcium balance develops early and continues throughout the period of immobilization. After 8 weeks of immobilization, significant osteoporosis is present, although it may develop earlier in persons younger than 20 years or older than 50 years. A uniform distribution of osteoporosis also has been observed in astronauts and in individuals treated with air suspension therapy as a result of weightlessness and lack of mechanical strain.

PATHOPHYSIOLOGY. Whatever the cause, osteoporosis develops when the remodeling cycle—the process of bone resorption and bone formation—is disrupted, leading to an imbalance in the coupling process. The explosion of new information in the field of bone biology has led to new understanding of the roles of hormones, growth and signaling factors, and cellular biology in osteoporosis. Although hormonal influences remain important in maintaining bone health, genetic factors and the role of oxidative stress are receiving increased attention as critical determinants of bone homeostasis.[25,28] Reactive oxygen species (ROSs) are normal byproducts of aerobic metabolism, and although they can cause cell damage, at levels below which they cause oxidative stress (OS), ROSs serve as signaling molecules for many cell types, including osteocytes, osteoblasts, and osteoclasts. When excess ROSs accumulate, OS occurs and can result in loss of bone mass and bone strength.[28]

The osteoclast differentiation pathway is directed by a series of processes that include proliferation, differentiation, fusion, and activation. These processes are controlled by hormones, cytokines, and paracrine stromal-cell microenvironment interactions. Thus the intercellular communication in bone and the key molecular regulators are necessary for bone homeostasis. Certain transcription factors, known as *Forkhead box (FoxO)*, help protect against the effects of OS by preventing excess accumulation of ROS and regulating certain genes that affect DNA repair and cell life span. FoxOs help remove damaged and abnormal cells by inducing apoptosis.[28]

Interleukins (IL-1, IL-4, IL-6, IL-7, IL-11, IL-17), tumor necrosis factor-alpha (TNF-α), transforming growth factor-beta (TGF-β), prostaglandin E_2, and hormones interact to control osteoclasts[34] (Fig. 45.11). Normal bone homeostasis is dependent on the balance between

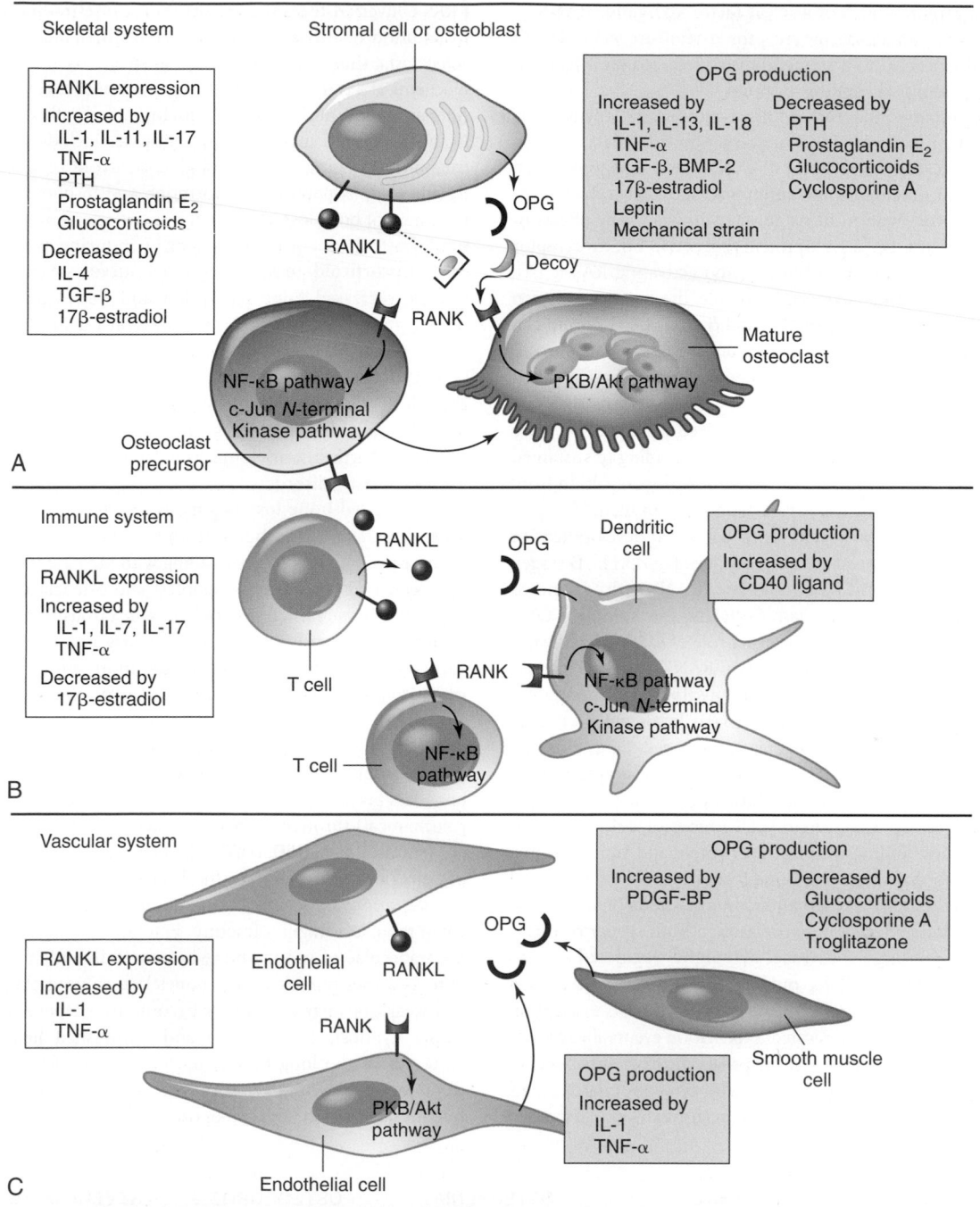

FIGURE 45.11 OPG/RANKL/RANK System. Receptor activator of nuclear factor κβ ligand (*RANKL*, which is a cytokine and part of the tumor necrosis factor *[TNF]* family) and osteoprotegerin (*OPG*, which is a glycoprotein receptor antagonist) are modulated by various cytokines, hormones, drugs, and mechanical strains *(see inserts)*. **A,** In bone, RANKL is expressed by both stromal cells and osteoblasts. RANKL stimulates the receptor RANK on osteoclast precursor cells and mature osteoclasts, and activates intracellular signaling pathways to promote osteoclast differentiation and activation and cytoskeletal reorganization and survival *(PKB/Akt pathway)* that increase resorption and bone loss. OPG, secreted by stromal cells and osteoblasts, acts as a "decoy" receptor and blocks RANKL binding to and activation of RANK. **B,** In the immune system, RANKL is expressed and secreted by T cells. T-cell–derived RANKL also can activate RANK on osteoclasts, T cells, and dendritic cells (antigen-presenting cells), which enhances bone loss that occurs in inflammatory bone diseases such as rheumatoid arthritis. Dendritic cells may regulate these processes by secreting OPG. **C,** In the vascular system, endothelial cells express RANKL and the RANK receptor. RANKL/RANK interactions contribute to endothelial and smooth muscle cells and can block RANKL binding. The physiologic significance of the OPG/RANKL/RANK system in endothelial and smooth muscle cells is being studied. *BMP-2,* Bone morphogenic protein 2; *IL,* interleukin; *PDGF-BP,* platelet-derived growth factor-beta polypeptide; *PTH,* parathyroid hormone; *TGF-α,* tumor necrosis factor-alpha; *TGF-β,* transforming growth factor-beta. (Adapted from Hofbauer LC, Schoppet M: *JAMA* 292[4]:490–495, 2004.)

the cytokine **receptor activator of nuclear factor κβ ligand (RANKL)**, its receptor **RANK**, and its decoy receptor **osteoprotegerin (OPG)**; understanding this has led to a tremendously increased knowledge of osteoclast biology and pathogenesis of bone loss.[35]

RANKL, a member of the TNF family, is expressed by osteoblasts and their immature precursors and is necessary for osteoclast development. RANKL activates the receptor RANK, which is expressed on osteoclasts and their precursors and suppresses apoptosis, which leads to activation and prolongation of osteoclast survival.[36] The effects of RANKL are blocked by OPG, a glycoprotein that acts as a decoy receptor for RANKL that prevents it from binding and activating RANK (see Fig. 45.11). Cytokines and hormones regulate the balance between RANKL and OPG. Alterations of the RANKL/RANK/OPG system can lead to dysregulation and pathologic conditions including osteoporosis, immune-mediated bone diseases, malignant bone disorders, and inherited skeletal diseases (see Fig. 45.11).

Postmenopausal osteoporosis is characterized by increased bone resorption relative to the rate of bone formation, leading to sustained bone loss resulting from estrogen deficiency. Bone loss resulting from estrogen deficiency also contributes to osteoporosis in men.[37,38]

Increased bone resorption results from enhanced development of osteoclasts and decreased osteoclast apoptosis (see Fig. 45.11). Estrogen stimulates OPG secretion and down-regulates RANKL; drugs known as *selective estrogen response modifiers (SERMs)* also stimulate OPG production. In estrogen deficiency, the exact role of OPG is less clear.[34] Postmenopausal women express higher levels of RANKL on bone marrow stromal cells, T cells, and B cells than premenopausal women. Importantly, RANKL expression is increased when estrogen levels are decreased, leading to increased formation of osteoclasts while reducing osteoclast apoptosis.[21] Other factors, such as sclerostin (SOST), a glycoprotein secreted by osteocytes, are powerful inhibitors of osteoblast formation by binding to low-density lipoprotein (LDL) receptor–related protein 5 (LRP5) and prevent binding with frizzled protein and Wnt signaling, important factors in osteoblast and bone formation.[34]

Sex steroids (e.g., estrogens) exert antiapoptotic effects on osteoblasts but exert proapoptotic effects on osteoclasts; in both scenarios this is accomplished by activating the **extracellular signal regulated kinases (ERKs)**. Estrogen activates ERKs outside the nucleus; ERKs then accumulate in the nucleus and activate downstream transcription factors.[39] This confusing and complicated information eventually revealed that the important determinant of whether proapoptosis or antiapoptosis was exhibited was the *length of time* that the phosphorylated ERKs remained in the nucleus. Prolonged nuclear accumulation of activated ERKs converted the antiapoptotic effect of estradiol to proapoptotic. In addition to ERKs, RANKL promotes the antiapoptotic effects on osteoclasts, thus increasing their life span.[40] Wnt signaling induces a biochemical series of events that increases osteoblast and bone formation. Alterations in Wnt signaling account for critical pathophysiologic changes in most acquired metabolic bone diseases including postmenopausal osteoporosis, aging effects, and glucocorticoid (i.e., cortisone) excess. Agents such as parathyroid hormone and bisphosphonates, used for treatment of bone loss, exert their positive effects by altering the formation of osteoblasts or osteoclasts or by inducing osteoclast apoptosis.

Glucocorticoid- (e.g., cortisone-) induced osteoporosis is characterized by increased bone resorption and decreased bone formation. Glucocorticoids increase RANKL expression and inhibit OPG production by osteoblasts (see Fig. 45.11). The use of immunosuppressive drugs (e.g., cyclosporine A) to reduce rejection of transplanted organs also alters the OPG/RANKL/RANK system and can lead to posttransplantation osteoporosis. Other conditions affected by OPG/RANKL/RANK include rheumatoid arthritis, myeloma, vascular diseases, and skeletal metastases from neoplastic disorders.

Age-related bone loss begins in the third to fourth decade. The cause remains unclear, but it is known that decreased serum growth hormone (GH) and IGF levels along with increased binding of RANKL and decreased OPG affect osteoblast and osteoclast function. Loss of trabecular bone in men proceeds in a linear fashion, with thinning of trabecular bone rather than complete loss as is noted in women (Fig. 45.12). Men have approximately 30% more bone mass than women, which may be a factor in their later involvement with osteoporosis (Fig. 45.13). Androgens promote osteoprotegerin production, thus inhibiting the osteoclastic effect of RANKL.[41] Reduction in physical activity in older persons also may be a major factor in the degree of bone loss because preservation of bone mass depends on skeletal stress (mechanical) through muscle contraction and weightbearing.[34]

◆**CLINICAL MANIFESTATIONS.** The specific clinical manifestations of osteoporosis depend on the bones involved. The most common manifestation, however, is bone deformity. Pain tends to occur only when there is a fragility fracture. Fractures are likely to occur because the trabeculae of spongy bone become thin and sparse and compact bone becomes porous. As the bones lose volume, they become brittle and weak and may collapse or become misshapen. Vertebral collapse causes kyphosis (hunchback) and diminished height (Fig. 45.14). Fractures of the long bones (particularly the femur and humerus), distal radius, ribs, and vertebrae are most common. The most serious fractures associated with osteoporosis are hip fractures because of their

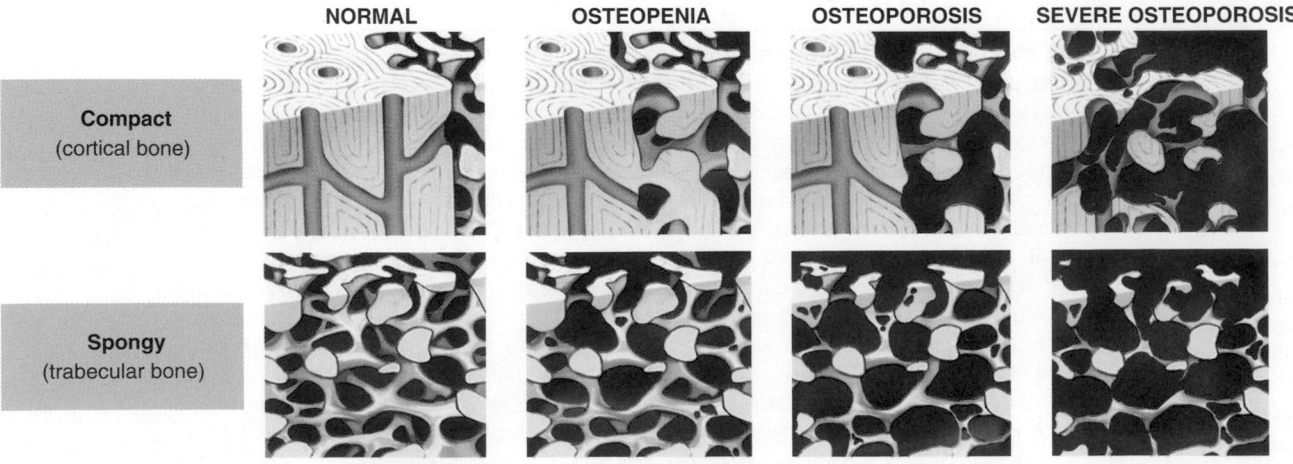

FIGURE 45.12 Osteoporosis in Cortical and Trabecular Bone.

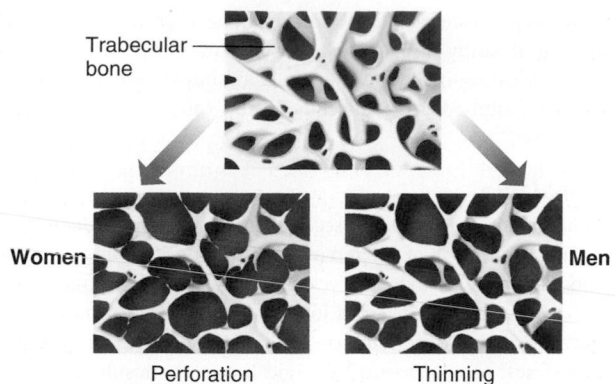

Trabecular bone

Women

Men

Perforation

Thinning

FIGURE 45.13 Mechanism of Loss of Trabecular Bone in Women and Trabecular Thinning in Men. Bone thinning predominates in men because of reduced bone formation. Loss of connectivity and complete trabecular loss predominate in women.

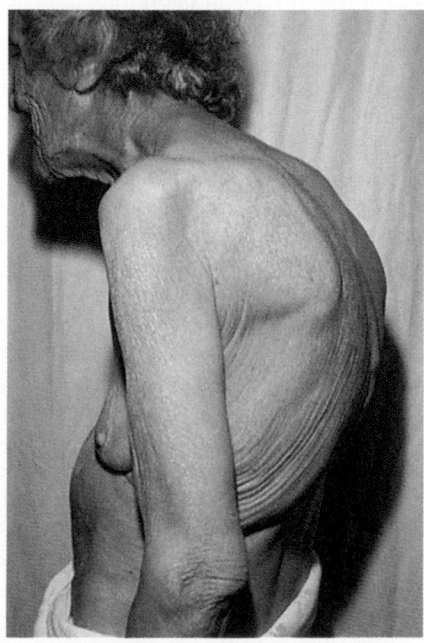

FIGURE 45.14 Kyphosis. This older adult woman's condition was caused by a combination of spinal osteoporotic vertebral collapse and chronic degenerative changes in the vertebral column. (From Kamal A, Brocklehurst JC: *Color atlas of geriatric medicine*, ed 2, St Louis, 1992, Mosby.)

TABLE 45.5	T-SCORE CLASSIFICATION*
T-SCORE	**CLASSIFICATION**
T ≥ −1.0	Normal bone density
T between −1.0 and −2.5	Osteopenia or low bone density
T ≤ −2.5	Osteoporosis

*The World Health Organization's T-score classification scale for the diagnosis of osteoporosis. *T*, T-score.
Data from National Osteoporosis Foundation: *Clinician's guide to prevention and treatment of osteoporosis*, Washington, DC, 2017, Author.

for diagnosis. Unfortunately, DXA does not provide information about bone strength or fracture risk.

Bone density is based on the number of standard deviations that differ from the mean bone mineral density of a young-adult reference population (a T-score) (Table 45.5). Osteopenia is categorized as a bone density score between 1.5 and 2.5 standard deviations below normal. A T-score of 2.5 or more standard deviations below normal bone density is considered osteoporosis. Severe or established osteoporosis is identified when there has been a fragility fracture associated with low bone density. The disease can be generalized as involving major portions of the axial skeleton or regional loss that involves one segment of the appendicular skeleton.[43]

Because fractures are the primary complication of osteoporosis, the World Health Organization (WHO) has developed an assessment tool to estimate an individual's 10-year risk of fracture. The WHO's Fracture Risk Assessment (FRAX) is a downloadable computer-drive questionnaire that has been developed for use in Europe, North America, Asia, and Australia. Once completed, the imbedded algorithms predict the 10-year probability of hip, spine, forearm, or shoulder fractures. This tool can be downloaded from http://www.shef.ac.uk/FRAX (see Fig. 45.10). Other evaluation procedures include tests for levels of serum calcium, phosphorus, and alkaline phosphatase as well as protein electrophoresis. Body calcium levels also can be measured by neuron activation analysis, a procedure involving use of radioactive calcium-49, whose gamma activity can be measured with a whole-body counter.

Though prevention of osteoporosis is paramount, treatment is more common and is focused on preventing fractures and maintaining optimal bone function. The role of calcium intake to prevent and treat osteoporosis is controversial. It is well accepted that oral calcium intake sufficient to maintain normal calcium balance is necessary during adolescence to ensure development of peak bone mass, and that calcium-deficient diets can aggravate bone loss associated with menopause and aging. Although recommendations have been established for young women of 1000 mg of calcium daily (particularly from dietary sources) and for postmenopausal women of 1500 mg daily (with vitamin D), it has been difficult to translate these recommendations into clear-cut clinical outcomes (see *Nutrition & Disease:* Postmenopausal Women Should Not Take Calcium and Vitamin D to Prevent Fractures). A significant relationship has been observed between an individual's lifetime history of calcium intake and peak bone mineral density. Diets with higher fruit and vegetable intake seem to correlate with higher BMD.[44] Other nutrients that appear to have a positive impact on bone health include magnesium, vitamin K_2, and docosahexaenoic acid or DHA (from purified fish oil).[45]

Magnesium (Mg^{++}), another mineral important for skeletal development, is an essential mineral in many biochemical and physiologic functions, including activation of enzymes, involvement in adenosine triphosphate (ATP) synthesis and protein synthesis, regulation of membrane channels, and contraction of muscle. Mg^{++} is important to

resultant chronic pain, disability, diminished quality of life, and premature death. Fracture of the neck of the femur (intertrochanteric fracture) tends to occur in older adult women with osteoporosis.[42] Fatal complications of fractures include fat or pulmonary embolism, hemorrhage, and shock. Approximately 20% of persons with a hip fracture die as a result of surgical complications.

EVALUATION AND TREATMENT. Generally, osteoporosis is detected radiographically as increased radiolucency of bone. By the time abnormalities are detected by x-ray examination, as much as 25% to 30% of bone tissue may have been lost.

Types of radiologic examinations include single- or dual-photon absorptiometry (SXA, DXA) and computed tomography (CT) scans. Because osteoporosis is asymptomatic unless a fracture occurs, diagnosis is often delayed. At present, DXA is the current examination of choice

NUTRITION & DISEASE

Postmenopausal Women Should Not Take Calcium and Vitamin D to Prevent Fractures

The beneficial effects of vitamin D on fracture risk are attributed to two explanations: (1) the decrease in bone loss in older adults, and (2) the increase in muscle strength and balance mediated through vitamin D receptors in muscle tissue. Vitamin D alone, however, does not appear to reduce fracture risk. In fact, the U.S. Preventive Services Task Force (USPSTF) has made the recommendation that postmenopausal women should not take supplementary calcium (1000 mg or less) and vitamin D (400 international units or less) because, at these doses, it appears that they do not prevent primary fracture risk and pose a small increased risk for renal stones. The USPSTF also concluded there is not enough evidence either supporting or opposing the use of higher doses of calcium and vitamin D for men or premenopausal women.

Data from Moyer V: *Ann Intern Med* Feb 2013 (online).

bone quality because it helps control hydroxyapatite crystal growth and thereby prevents formation of brittle bones. It seems reasonable that Mg^{++} is required for normal calcium (Ca^{++}) absorption because severe Mg^{++} deficiency results in hypocalcemia.

Regular, moderate weightbearing exercise can slow the rate of bone loss and, in some cases, reverse demineralization because the mechanical stress of exercise stimulates bone formation. It is important to reduce the risk of falls and enhance bone quality. Therefore an exercise program to enhance muscle strength is advised. Important new findings suggest that estrogen may prevent excessive bone loss before and after menopause by limiting osteoclast life span through promotion of apoptosis.

SERMs are being used to provide the positive effects of estrogen on bone but minimize estrogen's negative effect on breast and endometrial tissues. As a result, in addition to reducing vertebral fractures, SERMs reduce risk of estrogen receptor breast cancer and improve lipid profiles.[46] Raloxifene and tamoxifen are examples of SERMs.

Bisphosphonates are a class of inorganic pyrophosphate derivatives that bind bone mineral and improve osteoblast and osteocyte survival while promoting osteoclast apoptosis, thus slowing the bone remodeling process.[47] Nitrogen-containing bisphosphonates are highly effective in reducing both vertebral and nonvertebral osteoporotic fractures; because of this, bisphosphonates are the mainstay of osteoporosis treatment. Side effects include alterations in TGF-β signaling that may cause osteonecrosis of the jaw.[47] There also is a small risk of atypical femoral fractures, atrial fibrillation, and possibly esophageal cancer associated with bisphosphonates.[48-51] The optimal length of treatment with bisphosphonates has not yet been determined.[52]

One of the most promising treatments for osteoporosis is denosumab, a monoclonal antibody that binds the cytokine receptor activator of nuclear factor-κβ ligand (RANKL). RANKL inhibition blocks the maturation, function, and survival of osteoclasts, thus reducing bone resorption.[53]

Teriparatide, also called *PTH 1–34*, is a biosynthetic form of parathormone and contains the first 34 amino acids of parathyroid hormone; PTH 1–84 is a recombinant PTH that contains all 84 amino acids of naturally occurring PTH. Both work by stimulating osteoblasts when administered intermittently.[54] Given by subcutaneous injection, PTH reduces vertebral fractures but use is limited to a period of 24 months because of the risk of developing osteosarcoma. A recent large meta-analysis of osteoporosis treatment found improved BMD and reduced fractures with bisphosphonates, SERMs, and denosumab, though each regimen has potential adverse effects.[55] Restoration of a balanced RANKL/OPG ratio (see Chapter 44) or inhibition of RANK responsiveness is known to prevent osteoclast activation and bone resorption. Anti-RANKL therapy significantly reduces bone resorption. Other biologic agents under investigation include cathepsin K inhibitors, antisclerostin, and anti-dickkopf antibodies that affect the Wnt/β-catenin signaling pathway in osteoblasts.[56]

Osteomalacia

Osteomalacia is a metabolic disease characterized by inadequate and delayed mineralization of osteoid in mature compact and spongy bone. In osteomalacia the remodeling cycle proceeds normally through osteoid formation, but mineral calcification (hydroxyapatite formation) does not occur. Bone volume remains unchanged, but the replaced bone consists of soft osteoid instead of rigid bone. The result is abnormal bone matrix mineralization. Rickets is similar to osteomalacia in pathogenesis, but it occurs in the growing bones of children, whereas osteomalacia occurs in adult bone. Chronically low serum phosphate levels can be caused by tumors resulting in osteomalacia.[57] Fibroblast growth factor-23 (FGF-23) plays a significant role in maintaining normal serum phosphate levels. Primarily produced by osteocytes, FGF-23 functions to inhibit reabsorption of phosphate in the renal proximal tubule.[58] (Rickets is described in Chapter 46.)

Osteomalacia and rickets are rare in the United States and parts of Europe but are significant health problems in Great Britain, Ethiopia, Pakistan, Iran, and India. In the United States these diseases occur in older adults, in premature infants of very low birth weight, and in individuals adhering to rigid macrobiotic vegetarian diets. Breast-fed black infants who do not receive vitamin D supplementation have been shown to be at risk for developing nutritional rickets.[59,60]

Many factors contribute to the development of osteomalacia, but the most important is a deficiency of vitamin D. The major causes of vitamin D deficiency are diets deficient in vitamin D, decreased endogenous production of vitamin D, intestinal malabsorption of vitamin D, renal tubular diseases, and anticonvulsant therapy. Classic vitamin D deficiency is rare in the United States because of the addition of synthetic vitamin D to dairy products and bread. Still, disorders of the small bowel, kidneys, hepatobiliary system, and pancreas do cause vitamin D deficiency in the United States. In malabsorptive disease of the small bowel, vitamin D and calcium absorption are decreased, so vitamin D is lost in feces. Liver disease interferes with the metabolism of vitamin D to its more active form, and diseases of the pancreas and biliary system cause a deficiency of bile salts, which are necessary for normal intestinal absorption of vitamin D.

The mechanism by which anticonvulsant drug therapy results in decreased bone mineral density is not completely understood, but appears to be from direct impact on bone or effects on other regulators of bone metabolism such as calcium, vitamin D, and parathyroid hormone.[61] The anticonvulsants phenobarbital and phenytoin interfere with calcium absorption and increase degradation of vitamin D metabolism in the liver through activation of the cytochrome P-450 pathway.[62]

◆**PATHOPHYSIOLOGY.** Crystallization of minerals in osteoid requires adequate concentrations of calcium and phosphate. When the concentrations are too low, crystallization, and hence ossification, does not proceed normally.

Vitamin D deficiency disrupts mineralization because vitamin D normally regulates and enhances the absorption of calcium ions from the intestine. A lack of vitamin D causes the plasma calcium concentrations to fall. Low plasma calcium levels stimulate increased synthesis and secretion of parathyroid hormone (PTH). Although the increase in the level of circulating PTH raises the plasma calcium concentration, it also stimulates increased renal clearance of phosphate. When the concentration of phosphate in the bone decreases below a critical level, mineralization cannot proceed normally.

Abnormalities occur in spongy as well as compact bone. Trabeculae in spongy bone become thinner and fewer, whereas haversian systems in compact bone develop large channels and become irregular. Because osteoid continues to be produced but not mineralized, abnormal quantities of osteoid accumulate, coating the trabeculae and the linings of the haversian canals. Excessive osteoid also can accumulate in areas beneath the periosteum. The excess of osteoid leads to gross deformities of the long bones, spine, pelvis, and skull.

◆**CLINICAL MANIFESTATIONS.** Osteomalacia causes varying degrees of diffuse skeletal pain and tenderness. Bone pain is typically between joints, rather than within them.[59] Pain is noted particularly in the hips, and the individual may be hesitant to walk. Muscular weakness, particularly of the proximal muscles, is common and may contribute to a waddling gait. Facial deformities and bowed knees, or "knock-knees," may be present. Bone fractures and vertebral collapse occur with minimal trauma. Low back pain may be an early complaint, but pain also may involve ribs, feet, other areas of the vertebral column, and other sites. Uremia may be present in renal osteodystrophy.

◆**EVALUATION AND TREATMENT.** Laboratory data may include elevated blood urea nitrogen (BUN) and creatinine levels, normal or low serum calcium levels, and a serum inorganic phosphate level that is usually higher than 5.5 mg. Alkaline phosphatase and PTH levels are usually elevated. Radiographic findings show pseudofractures and radiolucent bands perpendicular to the surface of involved bones. Bone biopsy is useful in determining bone structure and remodeling.[63] Diagnosis of certain types of osteomalacia is becoming easier because of the ability to measure an individual's serum FGF-23 level. Elevated FGF-23 levels are common in X-linked hypophosphatemic and tumor-induced osteomalacia.[64]

Treatment of osteomalacia includes the following:
1. Adjusting serum calcium and phosphorous levels to normal
2. Suppressing secondary hyperthyroidism
3. Chelating bone aluminum if needed
4. Administering calcium carbonate to decrease hyperphosphatemia
5. Adding dietary supplements of vitamin D
6. Performing renal dialysis
7. Considering renal transplant for renal osteodystrophy

Paget Disease

Paget disease of bone (PDB or osteitis deformans) is a state of increased metabolic activity in bone characterized by abnormal and excessive bone resorption and formation (remodeling). Genetic manipulations involving the RANK–NF-κβ signaling pathways are significant in the development of Paget disease, resulting in increased osteoclast activity.[65] Chronic accelerated remodeling eventually enlarges and softens the affected bones. Classic PDB arises as a consequence of disorderly bone resorption and formation.

PDB most often affects the axial skeleton, especially the vertebrae, skull, sacrum, sternum, pelvis, and femur. The disease process may occur in one or more bones without causing significant clinical manifestations.

The disease is seldom found before age 40 years, but its incidence almost doubles each decade from age 50. It affects men more than women in a proportion of 1.8:1. Because it is often symptomless and can be diagnosed only by invasive procedures, few epidemiologic data are available. Autopsy data from England and Germany indicate that approximately 3% to 4% of persons older than 40 years have Paget disease. It is most prevalent in Australia, Great Britain, New Zealand, and the United States.

The cause of PDB is unknown; however, studies have implicated both genetic and environmental factors. About 10% to 30% of individuals with PDB have mutations of a specific gene, sequestosome-1. Even viral etiologies have been proposed.[65]

◆**PATHOPHYSIOLOGY.** Paget disease begins with excessive resorption of spongy bone and deposition of disorganized bone. The trabeculae diminish, and bone marrow is replaced by extremely vascular fibrous tissue. The resorption phase of Paget disease is followed by the formation of abnormal new bone at an accelerated rate. The collagen fibers are disorganized, and glycoprotein levels in the matrix decrease. Mineralization may extend into the bone marrow. Bone formation is excessive around partially resorbed trabeculae, causing them to thicken and enlarge. Eventually, Paget disease progresses to an inactive phase, in which abnormal remodeling is minimal or absent. Osteoclasts of individuals with Paget disease have increased responses to RANKL.[65]

◆**CLINICAL MANIFESTATIONS.** In the skull, abnormal remodeling is first evident in the frontal or occipital regions, and then encroaches on the outer and inner surfaces of the entire skull. The skull thickens and assumes an asymmetrical shape (Fig. 45.15). Thickened segments of the skull may compress areas of the brain, producing altered mentality and dementia. Impingement of new bone on cranial nerves causes sensory abnormalities, impaired motor function, deafness, atrophy of the optic nerve, and obstruction of the lacrimal duct. Headache is commonly noted.

Extensive alterations of the facial bones are rare except in the jaw, where sclerosis and thickening of the maxilla and mandible displace teeth and produce malocclusion. In long bones, resorption begins in the subchondral regions of the epiphysis and extends into the metaphysis and diaphysis. Warmth over the affected area, bone and joint pain, and bone deformity may occur. Occasionally, Paget disease affects both ends of a long bone. In the femur, PDB produces an exaggerated lateral curvature. In the tibia, anterior curvature is also exaggerated. Stress fractures are common in the lower extremities.

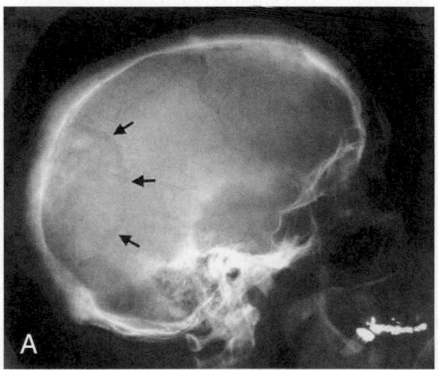
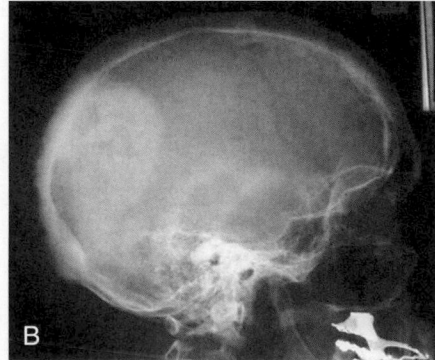

FIGURE 45.15 Paget disease of the skull. A, Active Paget disease of the skull, with marked cortical thickening and an area of osteoporosis circumscripta *(arrows).* **B,** The same individual several years later (after bisphosphonate treatment), with the lytic lesion largely replaced by sclerotic bone. (From Walsh JP: *Med J Aust* 181[5]:263, 2004.)

Clinical manifestations of PDB in the vertebral column depend on the level of involvement and are caused by compression of adjacent structures. In the cervical spine, cord compression can lead to spastic quadriplegia. Approximately 1% of persons with PDB develop osteogenic sarcoma. Paget-related sarcoma has a poor prognosis.

◆**EVALUATION AND TREATMENT.** Evaluation of PDB is made on the basis of radiographic findings of irregular bone trabeculae with a thickened and disorganized pattern. A typical V-shaped lesion in long bones and rounded areas of thinning bone in the skull are often seen on plain x-ray. Bone scanning can more readily detect early disease as well as extent of PDB through increased uptake of bone radionuclides. Serum total alkaline phosphatase and urinary hydroxyproline levels are elevated.[66]

Most individuals require no treatment because the disease is localized and does not cause symptoms. Treatment during active disease is for pain relief, prevention of deformity, or fracture. Bisphosphonates (alendronate, risedronate, and pamidronate) and calcitonin (salmon and human) are the mainstays of treatment. Surgery is indicated if there are neurologic complications or severe bony deformities.

Infectious Bone Disease: Osteomyelitis

Osteomyelitis is a bone infection most often caused by bacteria; however, fungi, mycobacteria, parasites, and viruses also can infect bone (Fig. 45.16). Exogenous osteomyelitis is an infection that enters from outside the body, for example, through open fractures, penetrating wounds, or surgical procedures. In exogenous osteomyelitis, infection spreads from soft tissues into adjacent bone. Endogenous osteomyelitis is caused by pathogens carried in the blood from sites of infection elsewhere in the body. In hematogenous osteomyelitis, infection spreads from bone to adjacent soft tissues. Hematogenous osteomyelitis is commonly found in infants, children, and older adults. (Osteomyelitis in children is discussed in Chapter 46.) In infants, incidence rates among males and females are approximately equal. In children and older adults, however, males are most commonly affected. Osteomyelitis is a common complication of sickle cell anemia and low oxygen tension.

Staphylococcus aureus (including methicillin-resistant *Staphylococcus aureus* [MRSA]) is the primary cause of hematogenous osteomyelitis.[67] Other microorganisms include group B streptococci, *Haemophilus influenzae*, *Salmonella*, and gram-negative bacteria. Group B streptococci and *H. influenzae* tend to infect young children; *Salmonella* infection is associated with sickle cell anemia; and gram-negative infections are most common in older adults and individuals with impaired immunity. Mycobacterial and fungal infections occur in immunocompromised individuals.

Cutaneous, sinus, ear, and dental infections are the primary sources of bacteria in hematogenous bone infections. Soft tissue infections,

disorders of the gastrointestinal tract, infections of the genitourinary system, and respiratory tract infections are also sources of bacterial contamination. In addition, infections contracted after total joint replacement surgeries can be causes of osteomyelitis. The vulnerability of a specific bone depends on the anatomy of its vascular supply. In adults, hematogenous osteomyelitis is more common in the spine, pelvis, and small bones.

Microorganisms reach the vertebrae through arteries, veins, or lymphatic vessels. The spread of infection from pelvic organs to the vertebrae is well documented. Vaginal, uterine, ovarian, bladder, and intestinal infections can lead to iliac or sacral osteomyelitis.

Exogenous osteomyelitis can be caused by human bites or fist blows to the mouth. Superficial animal or human bites inoculate local soft tissue with bacteria that later spread to underlying bone. Deep bites can introduce microorganisms directly onto bone. The most common infecting organism in human bites is *S. aureus*. In animal bites the most common infecting organism is *Pasteurella multocida*, which is part of the normal mouth flora of cats and dogs.

Direct contamination of bones with bacteria also can occur in open fractures or dislocations with an overlying skin wound. Intervertebral disk surgery and operative procedures involving implantation of large foreign objects, such as metallic plates or artificial joints, are associated with exogenous osteomyelitis. Local injections and venous punctures are significant causes of exogenous osteomyelitis. Exogenous osteomyelitis of the arm and hand bones tends to occur in drug abusers. *S. aureus* is the most common pathogen. In general, persons who are chronically ill, have diabetes or alcoholism, or are receiving large doses of corticosteroids or immunosuppressive drugs are particularly susceptible to exogenous osteomyelitis or recurring episodes of this disease.

◆**PATHOPHYSIOLOGY.** Regardless of the source of the pathogen, the pathologic features of bone infection are similar to those in any other body tissue (see Chapter 10). First, the invading pathogen provokes an intense inflammatory response. Inflammation in bone is characterized by vascular engorgement, edema, leukocyte activity, small blood vessel thrombosis, and abscess formation.[68] Once inflammation is initiated, the small terminal vessels thrombose and exudate seals the bone's canaliculi. Inflammatory exudate extends into the metaphysis and the marrow cavity and through small metaphyseal openings into the cortex. In children, exudate that reaches the outer surface of the cortex forms abscesses that lift the periosteum off underlying bone. Lifting of the periosteum disrupts blood vessels that enter bone through the periosteum, which deprives underlying bone of its blood supply; this leads to necrosis and death of the area of bone infected, producing sequestrum, an area of devitalized bone (see Fig. 45.16). Lifting of the periosteum also stimulates an intense osteoblastic response. Osteoblasts lay down new bone that can partially or completely surround the infected bone. This

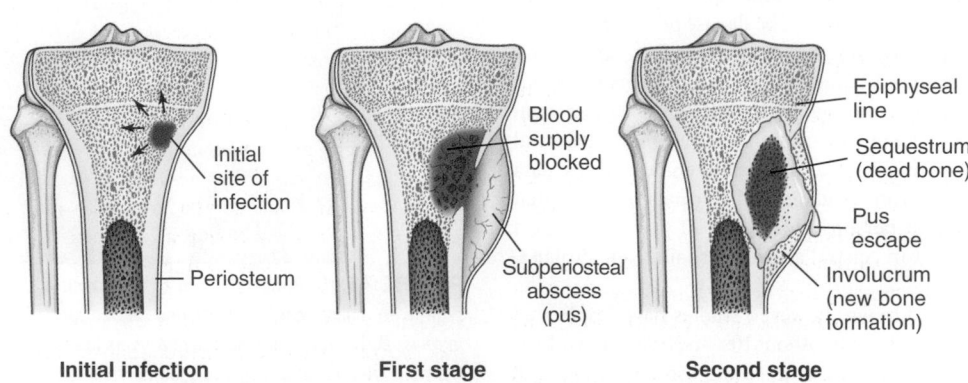

Initial infection   **First stage**   **Second stage**

FIGURE 45.16 Osteomyelitis Showing Sequestration and Involucrum.

layer of new bone surrounding the infected bone is called an involucrum. Openings in the involucrum allow the exudate to escape into surrounding soft tissue and ultimately through the skin by way of sinus tracts. Involucrum in adults is rare because the periosteum is firmly attached to the cortex and resists displacement. Instead, infection disrupts and weakens the cortex, which predisposes the bone to pathologic fracture.

◆**CLINICAL MANIFESTATIONS.** Clinical manifestations of osteomyelitis vary with the age of the individual, site of involvement, initiating event, infecting organism, and whether the infection is acute, subacute, or chronic. Acute osteomyelitis causes an abrupt onset of inflammation. If an acute infection is not completely eliminated, the disease may become subacute or chronic. In subacute osteomyelitis, signs and symptoms are usually vague. In the chronic stage, infection is indolent or silent between exacerbations. The microorganisms persist in small abscesses or fragments of necrotic bone and produce occasional flare-ups of acute osteomyelitis. The progression from acute to subacute osteo-myelitis may be the result of inadequate or inappropriate therapy or the development of drug-resistant microorganisms.

In the adult, hematogenous osteomyelitis has an insidious onset. The symptoms are usually vague and include fever, malaise, anorexia, and weight loss. Recent infection (urinary, respiratory, skin) or instru-mentation (catheterization, cystoscopy, myelography, diskography) usually precedes onset of symptoms.

Back pain is the primary symptom in vertebral osteomyelitis. Pain may be intermittent or constant, aggravated by motion, and throbbing at rest. It may radiate in a radicular distribution and is commonly accompanied by spinal tenderness and rigidity. Hip contracture can occur in the presence of soft tissue inflammation as a result of irritation of the psoas muscle.[69]

Signs and symptoms of sacroiliac osteomyelitis are generally severe and include local pain, tenderness, and a limp. The pain may radiate to the buttock or the abdomen.

Single or multiple abscesses (Brodie abscesses) characterize subacute or chronic osteomyelitis. Brodie abscesses are painless, circumscribed lesions 1 to 4 cm in diameter, usually in the ends of long bones, and surrounded by dense ossified bone matrix. The abscesses are thought to develop when the infectious microorganism has become less virulent or the individual's immune system is resisting the infection somewhat successfully.

In exogenous osteomyelitis, signs and symptoms of soft tissue infection predominate. Inflammatory exudate in the soft tissues disrupts muscles and supporting structures and forms abscesses. Low-grade fever, lymphadenopathy, local pain, and swelling usually occur within days of contamination by a puncture wound. Osteomyelitis in the hand causes exquisite tenderness over the course of tendon sheaths. The fingers are usually in a semiflexed position, and extension usually causes severe pain. Palmar swelling or symmetrical swelling of the fingers may be present.

◆**EVALUATION AND TREATMENT.** Laboratory data show an elevated white cell count. Radiographic studies include radionuclide bone scan-ning, CT, and MRI. MRI is especially useful in detecting early bone changes associated with infection.[70]

Infectious bone disease is expensive and difficult to treat and often culminates in extensive physical disability. The following factors con-tribute to the difficulty in treating bone infection:

1. Bone contains multiple microscopic channels that are impermeable to the cells and biochemicals of the body's natural defenses. Once bacteria gain access to these channels, they are able to proliferate unimpeded.
2. The microcirculation of bone is highly vulnerable to damage and destruction by bacterial toxins. Vessel damage causes local

thrombosis (blockage) of the small vessels, which leads to ischemic necrosis (death) of bone.
3. Bone cells have a limited capacity to replace bone destroyed by infections. Initially, osteoclasts are stimulated by infection to resorb bone, which opens up isolated bone channels so that cells of the inflammatory and immune system can gain access to the infected bone. At the same time, however, resorption weakens the structural integrity of the bone. New bone formation usually lags behind resorption, and the haversian systems in the new bone are incomplete.

Treatment of osteomyelitis includes surgical débridement with bone biopsy and culture before or as soon after initiating antibiotics as possible. Initial antibiotic therapy should be intravenous. Chronic conditions may require surgical removal of the inflammatory exudate followed by continuous wound irrigation with antibiotic solutions in addition to systemic treatment with antibiotics. Hyperbaric oxygen therapy of 100% oxygen, given at 2 atmospheres of pressure for 2 hours' duration per day for 30 treatments, is also beneficial for chronic refractory osteomyelitis. Implanted hardware may require removal to more thoroughly treat an infected joint.

Bone Tumors

Primary bone cancer is a rare but metastatic disease that commonly affects bone. Many different types of tumors involve the skeleton. Based on the tissue of origin, bone tumors are classified as osteogenic, chondrogenic, collagenic, or myelogenic. Each of the four types arises from one of the four stem cells that are ultimately derived from the primitive mesoderm (Fig. 45.17). In addition, bone tumors may be classified as being of histiocytic, notochordal, lipogenic, and neurogenic origins (Box 45.3).

The mesoderm contributes the primitive fibroblast and reticulum cells. The fibroblast is the progenitor of the osteoblast and the chon-droblast. Each cell synthesizes a specific type of intercellular ground substance, and the type of ground substance produced by the cell generally characterizes the tumor derived from the cell. For example, osteogenic tumors usually contain cells that have the appearance of osteoblasts and produce an intercellular substance that can be recognized as osteoid. Chondrogenic tumors contain chondroblasts and produce an intercellular substance similar to chondroid (cartilage). Collagenic tumors contain fibrous tissue cells and produce an intercellular substance similar to the type of collagen found in fibrous connective tissue.

Tumors also are classified as benign or malignant. The criteria used to identify tumor cells as malignant are (1) an increased nuclear/cytoplasmic ratio, (2) an irregular nuclear border, (3) an excess of chromatin, (4) a prominent nucleolus, and (5) an increase in the number of cells undergoing mitosis. However, many young, rapidly growing, normal cells and cells subjected to inflammation and change in their blood supply also exhibit many of these same characteristics. (Tumor biology is described in Chapter 12.)

Epidemiology

The incidence of bone tumors varies with age. Osteosarcoma is the most common primary malignant bone tumor in children and young adults.[71] Adolescents have the highest incidence of bone tumors, and adults between 30 and 35 years of age have the lowest incidence. After age 35, the incidence slowly increases until, at age 60, it equals the incidence in adolescents, primarily related to metastatic tumors.

Patterns of Bone Destruction

The general pathologic features of bone tumors include bone destruction, erosion or expansion of the cortex, and periosteal response to changes in underlying bone. The least amount of pathologic damage occurs

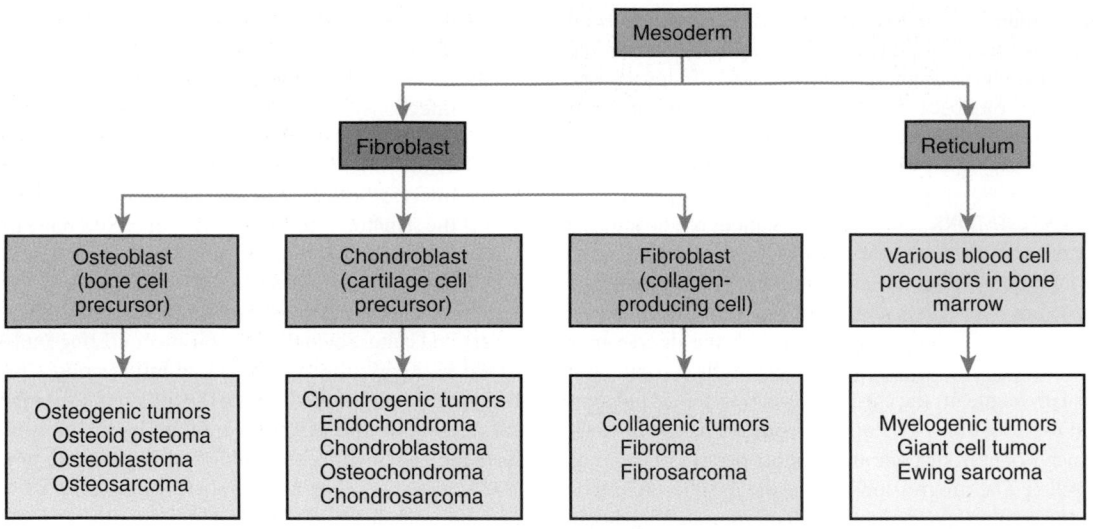

FIGURE 45.17 Derivation of Bone Tumors.

BOX 45.3 WORLD HEALTH ORGANIZATION CLASSIFICATION OF BONE TUMORS

Cartilage Tumors
Chondrosarcoma (M)
Chondroma (B)
Osteochondroma (B; but may become malignant)
Chondroblastoma (B)

Osteogenic Tumors
Osteoblastoma (B)
Osteoid osteoma (B)
Osteosarcoma (M)

Fibrogenic Tumors (Often Produce Collagen; Do Not Have a Mineralizing Matrix)
Fibrosarcoma (M)

Fibrohistiocytic Tumors (Comprised of Fibroblasts)
Benign fibrous histiocytoma (B)
Malignant fibrous histiocytoma (M)

Ewing Sarcoma
Ewing sarcoma (M)

Hematopoietic Tumors
Plasma cell myeloma (M)
Malignant lymphoma (M)

Giant Cell Tumor
Giant cell tumor (B, but can grow aggressively)
Malignancy in giant cell tumor (M; very rare tumor)

Smooth Muscle Tumors
Leiomyoma (B)
Leiomyosarcoma (M)

Miscellaneous Tumors
Adamantinoma (M; almost exclusively found in tibia)
Metastatic malignancy (M; most common skeletal malignancy)

Miscellaneous Lesions
Aneurysmal bone cyst (B)
Simple cyst (B)
Fibrous dysplasia (B; rarely can become malignant)
Osteofibrous dysplasia (B)
Langerhans cell histiocytosis (B, but can aggressively grow)
Chest wall hamartoma (B; is excessive growth of mesenchymal tissue [mostly cartilage])

Joint Lesions
Synovial chondromatosis (B; rarely becomes M)

B, Benign lesion; *M,* malignant lesion.
Data from Dorfman HD et al: WHO classification of tumours of the bone: introduction. In Christopher EM et al, editors: *World Health Organization classification of tumors, International Agency for Research on Cancer (IARC) pathology and genetics of tumours of soft tissue and bone,* Lyon, France, 2002, IARC Press, p 226.

---

with benign bone tumors that push against neighboring tissue. Because they usually have a symmetrical, controlled growth pattern, benign bone tumors tend to compress and displace neighboring normal bone tissue, which weakens the bone's structure until it is incapable of withstanding the stress of ordinary use, leading to pathologic fracture. Other tumors invade and destroy adjacent normal bone tissue by producing substances that promote resorption by increasing osteoclast activity or by interfering with a bone's blood supply. Three patterns of bone destruction by bone tumors have been identified: (1) the geographic

pattern, (2) the moth-eaten pattern, and (3) the permeative pattern (Table 45.6).

Tumors that erode the cortex of the bone usually stimulate a periosteal response, that is, new bone formation at the interface between the surface of the bone and the periosteum. Slow erosion of the cortex usually stimulates a uniform periosteal response. Additional layers of bone are added to the exterior surface of the bone to buttress the cortex. Eventually the additional layers expand the bone's contour. Aggressive penetration of the cortex usually elevates the periosteum and stimulates

TABLE 45.6 PATTERNS OF BONE DESTRUCTION BY BONE TUMORS

TYPE OF DESTRUCTION	PATTERN SEEN
Geographic	Well-defined margins separated from surrounding normal bone; well-defined lytic area in affected bone
Moth-eaten	Less-defined margin not easily separated from normal bone; areas of partially destroyed bone adjacent to completely lytic areas
Permeative	Poorly demarcated margins; abnormal lytic bone merges imperceptibly with surrounding normal bone

TABLE 45.7 THE ENNEKING SURGICAL STAGING SYSTEM FOR MALIGNANT BONE TUMORS

STAGE	GRADE	SITE (T)	METASTASIS (M)
IA	Low (G_1)	Intracompartmental (T_1)	None (M_0)
IB	Low (G_1)	Extracompartmental (T_2)	None (M_0)
IIA	High (G_2)	Intracompartmental (T_1)	None (M_0)
IIB	High (G_2)	Extracompartmental (T_2)	None (M_0)
IIIA	Low (G_1)	Intracompartmental or extracompartmental (T_1 or T_2)	Regional or distant (M_1)
IIIB	High (G_2)	Intracompartmental or extracompartmental (T_1 or T_2)	Regional or distant (M_1)

Data from National Comprehensive Cancer Network: *Recent updates to NCCN clinical practice guidelines in oncology: bone cancer, Version 1,* Fort Washington, PA, 2013, Author.

erratic patterns of new bone formation. Examples of erratic patterns include concentric layers of new bone; a sunburst pattern, in which delicate rays of new bone radiate toward the periosteum from a single focus on the underlying surface; and rays of new bone that grow perpendicularly, creating a brush or bristle pattern.

Diagnosis

Malignant bone tumors account for less than 0.2% of all cancers.[71] A tumor must be identified early to allow survival of the individual and the preservation of the affected limb. However, individuals often have only vague symptoms that may be attributed to minor trauma, degenerative changes, or inflammatory conditions. In addition, other conditions may obscure the diagnosis.

Thorough diagnostic studies are needed to determine the exact type and extent of bone tumor present, which also helps determine the optimal treatment regimen. Staging of any bone tumor is critical to determine future treatment and results. The American Joint Committee on Cancer (AJCC) staging system (also known as the *Enneking* or *TNM staging system*) is the most commonly used arrangement (Table 45.7). This system classifies tumors according to grade (G), tumor site (T), and metastasis (M). Benign tumors are given a numeric value of zero, whereas malignant tumors are low grade (G_1) or high grade (G_2).

Serum alkaline phosphatase levels are elevated in bone lytic tumors, and they are significantly elevated in osteosarcoma and Ewing sarcoma. Radiologic studies include plain radiologic film, technetium-99 bone scan, CT scan, and MRI, which has become the examination of choice for the local staging of bone tumors, especially the staging of peripheral osteosarcomas (see Table 45.6). MRI is also used to monitor the response of osteosarcomas to radiation or chemotherapy and to detect recurrent disease. A CT scan can evaluate involvement of osteosarcoma in flat bones when the tumor is not well-defined on a plain film, can assist in differentiating the tumor, and can locate pulmonary metastases. Radionucleotide bone scans show an increased uptake at the tumor site. Before any surgical procedure, placement of bone biopsy is critical.[72]

Additional diagnostic studies performed for specific bone tumors include a complete blood count and erythrocyte sedimentation rate (to rule out infection, myeloma, or Ewing sarcoma) and measurement of serum levels of calcium and phosphorus to detect hypercalcemia. Serum glucose levels may be elevated in chondrosarcoma. Acid phosphatase level may be moderately elevated in bone metastases, multiple myeloma, and advanced Paget disease. Serum protein electrophoresis and immunoelectrophoresis are done to rule out multiple myeloma. Fine-needle biopsy is done, usually at the time of surgery, to determine the exact tumor type.

Types

A very large number of lesions are classified as bone tumors. The bone tumors most representative of the four derivative types (see Fig. 45.17)—osteogenic, chondrogenic, collagenic, and myelogenic tumors—are described here.

Osteogenic Tumors: Osteosarcoma. Osteogenic (bone-forming) tumors are characterized by the formation of bone or osteoid tissue with a sarcomatous tissue. The tissue can have the appearance of compact or spongy bone. The most common malignant primary bone tumor is osteosarcoma. Osteosarcomas account for 38% of bone tumors. The male/female ratio is 3:2, and osteosarcoma occurs predominantly in adolescents and young adults; 60% of osteosarcomas occur in persons younger than 20 years. A secondary peak incidence for osteosarcoma occurs in the 60 and older age group, primarily in individuals with a history of radiation therapy several years previously for pelvic or other malignancies (Fig. 45.18).

An osteosarcoma is a malignant bone-forming tumor. It is aggressive and most often found in bone marrow; it has a moth-eaten pattern of bone destruction. The borders of the tumor are indistinct and merge into adjacent normal bone. Osteosarcomas always contain osteoid and callus (osteoblastic sarcoma) produced by anaplastic stromal cells, which are atypical, abnormal cells not seen in normal developing bone; they are neither normal nor embryonal. The osteosarcoma also may contain chondroid (cartilage) (chondroblastic sarcoma) and fibrinoid tissue (fibroblastic sarcoma) that may form the bulk of the tumor. The osteoid is deposited in thick masses or "streamers" between the trabeculae of callus, which infiltrate the normal compact bone, destroy it, and replace it with dense callus and masses of osteoid. Demonstrating the presence of osteoid aids in the diagnosis of osteosarcoma. Bone tissue produced by osteosarcomas never matures to compact bone.

Ninety percent of osteosarcomas are located in the metaphyses of long bones, especially the distal femur and proximal tibia, with 50% around the knee area. The tumor typically breaks through the cortex, lifts the periosteum, and forms a soft tissue mass that is *not* covered by a smooth shell of new bone. Lifting of the periosteum stimulates bizarre patterns of new bone formation called a *periosteal reaction.* Distinct osteosarcomas occur on the surface of long bones, called *parosteal, periosteal,* or *high-grade surface osteosarcomas;* dedifferentiated parosteal and central osteosarcomas also occur.

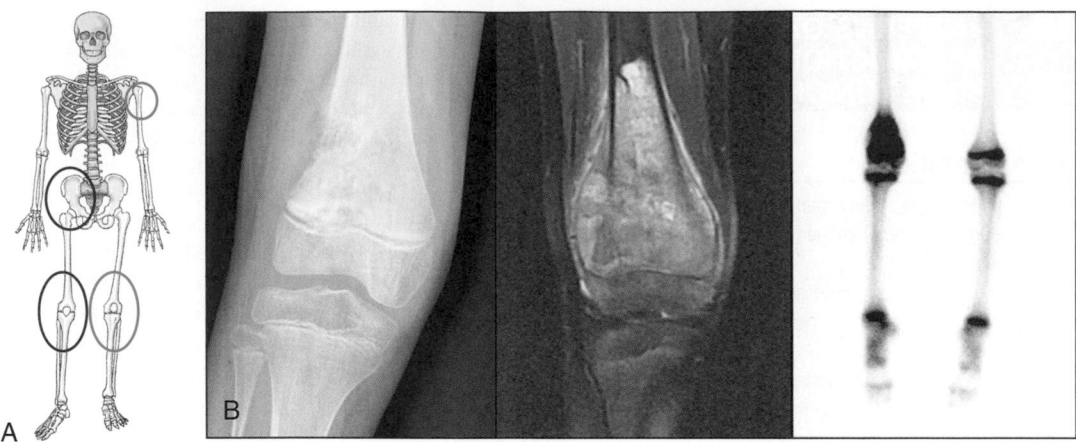

FIGURE 45.18 Osteosarcoma. **A,** Common locations of Ewing sarcoma and osteosarcoma. *Blue,* osteosarcoma; *red,* Ewing sarcoma. **B,** Comparison of plain radiograph, MRI, and nuclear bone scan appearances of osteosarcoma of the distal femur. Note destruction of the bone cortex and soft tissue component. (**A** adapted from Bontrager KL, Lampignanno JP, editors: *Textbook of radiographic positioning and related anatomy,* St Louis, 2013, Elsevier. **B** from HaDuong JH et al: *Pediatr Clin N Am* 62:179–200, 2015.)

The most common initial symptoms are pain and swelling. Initially the pain is slight and intermittent, but within a short time it increases in severity and duration. Pain is usually worse at night and gradually requires medication. Systemic symptoms are uncommon. Usually a coincidental history of trauma is noted. Occasionally the individual may have a pathologic fracture.

Systemic chemotherapy and surgery are the treatments of choice, with the location of the tumor and its size, malignancy grade, and evidence of metastasis dictating the type and extent of surgery. Preoperative chemotherapy has greatly increased the number of individuals qualifying for limb salvage surgery. Limb salvaging procedures have been made possible by advances in reconstructive techniques and endoprosthetics. Limb salvage ultimately may be successful in as many as 80% of persons. Individuals must have achieved most of their bone growth to be candidates for limb salvage procedures, which are preferred to amputation. Skeletally immature individuals may have a limb salvage operation, referred to as a *rotationplasty,* in which the major portions of the thigh, the tumor, and contaminated knee are resected while preserving the nerve supply (sciatic) to the leg and foot. The proximal tibia is internally fixed to the stump of the proximal femur after it has been rotated 180 degrees. The foot is positioned at a desired spot or direction, allowing the ankle joint to function as a knee joint with the foot supplying the traditional role of the tibial stump in a below-knee amputation.

If an amputation is done, individuals are monitored closely with chest roentgenograms and CT. Pulmonary metastases are surgically resected, and chemotherapy is now a common therapy given both before and after surgery, using combinations of chemotherapeutic agents. Promising agents under investigation include monoclonal antibodies, hormone antagonists, gene therapy, and other biologic agents that may dramatically improve survival.[73,74]

Chondrogenic Tumors: Chondrosarcoma. Chondrogenic (cartilage-forming) tumors produce cartilage or chondroid, a primitive cartilage or cartilage-like substance. The most common chondrogenic tumor is chondrosarcoma, accounting for 20% of bone tumors.

Chondrosarcoma, the second most common primary malignant bone tumor, is a tumor of middle-age and older adults; incidence peaks in the sixth decade of life.[75] The tumor is found more commonly in men than in women. Preexisting chondral lesions, such as osteochon-

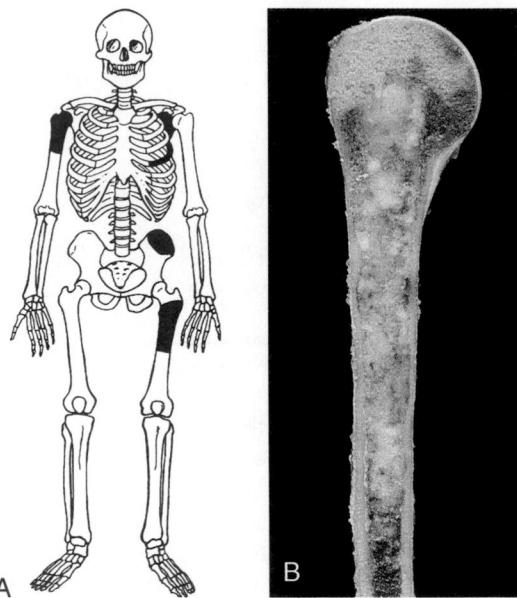

FIGURE 45.19 Chondrosarcoma. **A,** Common locations of chondrosarcoma. **B,** Chondrosarcoma of humerus. (From Damjanov I, Linder J, editors: *Anderson's pathology,* ed 10, St Louis, 1996, Mosby.)

dromas, can give rise to secondary chondrosarcoma, which, generally, has a fairly good prognosis.[76]

A chondrosarcoma is a large ill-defined malignant tumor that infiltrates trabeculae in spongy bone. It produces cartilage-forming cells but there is no ossification, as in normal endochondral bone formation.[77] It occurs most often in the metaphysis or diaphysis of long bones, especially the femur, and in the bones of the pelvis (Fig. 45.19). The tumor contains large lobules of hyaline cartilage that are separated by bands of fibrous tissue and anaplastic cells. Chondrosarcomas typically implant in surrounding tissue ("seeding").

Symptoms associated with chondrosarcoma have an insidious onset. Local swelling and pain are the usual symptoms that cause a person to seek treatment. At first the pain is dull and intermittent, and then gradually intensifies and becomes constant. It may awaken the person at night.

Diagnostic studies include radiographs, which must be reviewed carefully for an accurate diagnosis. Biopsy is done at the time of surgery. (If biopsy is done before scheduled surgical incision, seeding of tumor cells could occur.) Sufficient tumor material must be obtained to facilitate an accurate diagnosis.

Wide surgical excision is generally regarded as the treatment of choice because chemotherapy and radiation seem to have little effect.[77] Many surgically treated individuals demonstrate recurrences, however, so amputation is becoming one treatment of choice. Therefore individuals with tumors located in the limbs have a better prognosis than those with pelvic lesions.

Collagenic Tumors: Fibrosarcoma. Collagenic (collagen-forming) tumors produce fibrous connective tissue. The most typical collagenic tumor is the fibrosarcoma.

Fibrosarcomas come from fibroblasts that originate from mesenchymal stem cells and represent 4% of primary malignant bone tumors, with a broad age distribution. They may occur at any age but are most common in adults between 30 and 50 years of age. Fibrosarcoma also may be a secondary complication of radiation therapy, Paget disease, and long-standing osteomyelitis; secondary fibrosarcoma tends to be more aggressive, with poorer outcome.

Fibrosarcoma is a solitary tumor that most often affects the metaphyseal region of the femur or tibia. The tumor is composed of a firm fibrous mass of tissue that contains collagen, malignant fibroblasts, and occasional osteoclast-like giant cells.

The tumor begins in the marrow cavity of the bone and infiltrates the trabeculae. It demonstrates a permeative growth pattern, destroys the cortex, and extends into the soft tissue. Metastasis to the lung is common.

Symptoms associated with the tumor have an insidious onset, which delays diagnosis. Pain and swelling, the usual symptoms that cause the individual to seek treatment, usually indicate that the tumor has broken through the cortex. Local tenderness, the presence of a palpable mass, and limitation of motion also may be present. A pathologic fracture in the affected bone is often the reason for seeking medical help. Diagnostic studies include radiographs and MRI.

Radical surgery and amputation are the treatments of choice for fibrosarcoma. Radiation therapy is generally considered ineffective treatment for this tumor.

Myelogenic Tumors. Myelogenic tumors originate from various bone marrow cells. Two types of myelogenic tumors are giant cell tumor and myeloma. Myeloma is discussed in Chapter 30.

Giant Cell Tumor. Giant cell tumor is the sixth most common of the primary bone tumors, accounting for 4% to 5% of bone tumors. Giant cell tumors have a wide age distribution; however, they are rare in persons younger than 10 years or older than 70 years. Most giant cell tumors are found in persons between 20 and 40 years of age. Unlike most other bone tumors, giant cell tumors affect females more often than males.[78]

Giant cell tumors are generally benign, solitary, circumscribed tumors that cause extensive bone resorption because of their osteoclastic origin (Fig. 45.20). There is a high rate of recurrence but metastasis is rare. The tumor is rich in osteoclast-like giant cells and anaplastic stromal cells. It also may contain osteoid, callus, and collagen. Overexpression of several genes, including osteoprotegerin ligand (OPGL), occurs in giant cell tumors. The giant cell tumor is typically located in the center of the epiphysis in the femur, tibia, radius, or humerus. The tumor has a slow, relentless growth rate and is usually contained within the original contour of the affected bone. Tumors are often associated with pathologic fractures because of aggressive bone resorption.[79] It may, however, extend

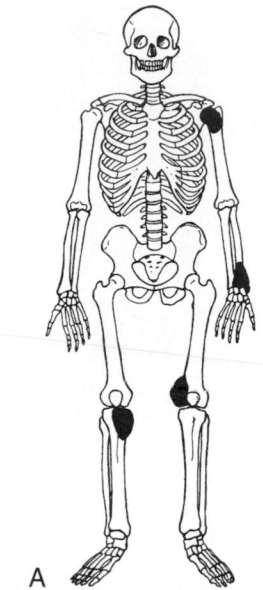

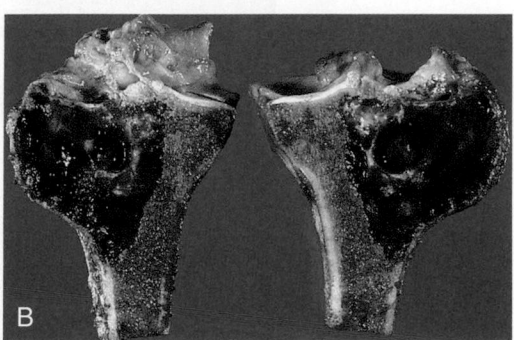

FIGURE 45.20 Giant Cell Tumor of Bone. **A,** Common skeletal locations. **B,** Gross picture of cell tumor of bone (epimetaphysis). (From Damjanov I, Linder J, editors: *Anderson's pathology*, ed 10, St Louis, 1996, Mosby.)

into the articular cartilage. When the tumor extends, it is usually covered by periosteum or periosteal bone growth.

The most common symptoms associated with giant cell tumor are pain, local swelling, and limitation of movement. Diagnostic studies include radiographs, CT, and MRI. Cryosurgery and resection of the tumor with the use of adjuvant polymethylmethacrylate (PMMA) for bone grafts decrease recurrence and are more successful treatments than curettage and radiation.[80] Amputation may be necessary but is not common.

DISORDERS OF JOINTS

The American College of Rheumatology (ACR) recognizes a growing body of evidence identifying and classifying joint diseases called arthropathies. The two major categories of these disorders include noninflammatory joint disease and inflammatory joint disease. Current detection methods, through diagnostic imaging and serum and synovial fluid analysis, allow for a clearer delineation between the inflammatory and noninflammatory pathways once poorly understood.

Osteoarthritis

Osteoarthritis (OA) is the most common form of joint disease and leading cause of disability in middle-aged and older populations.[81] In

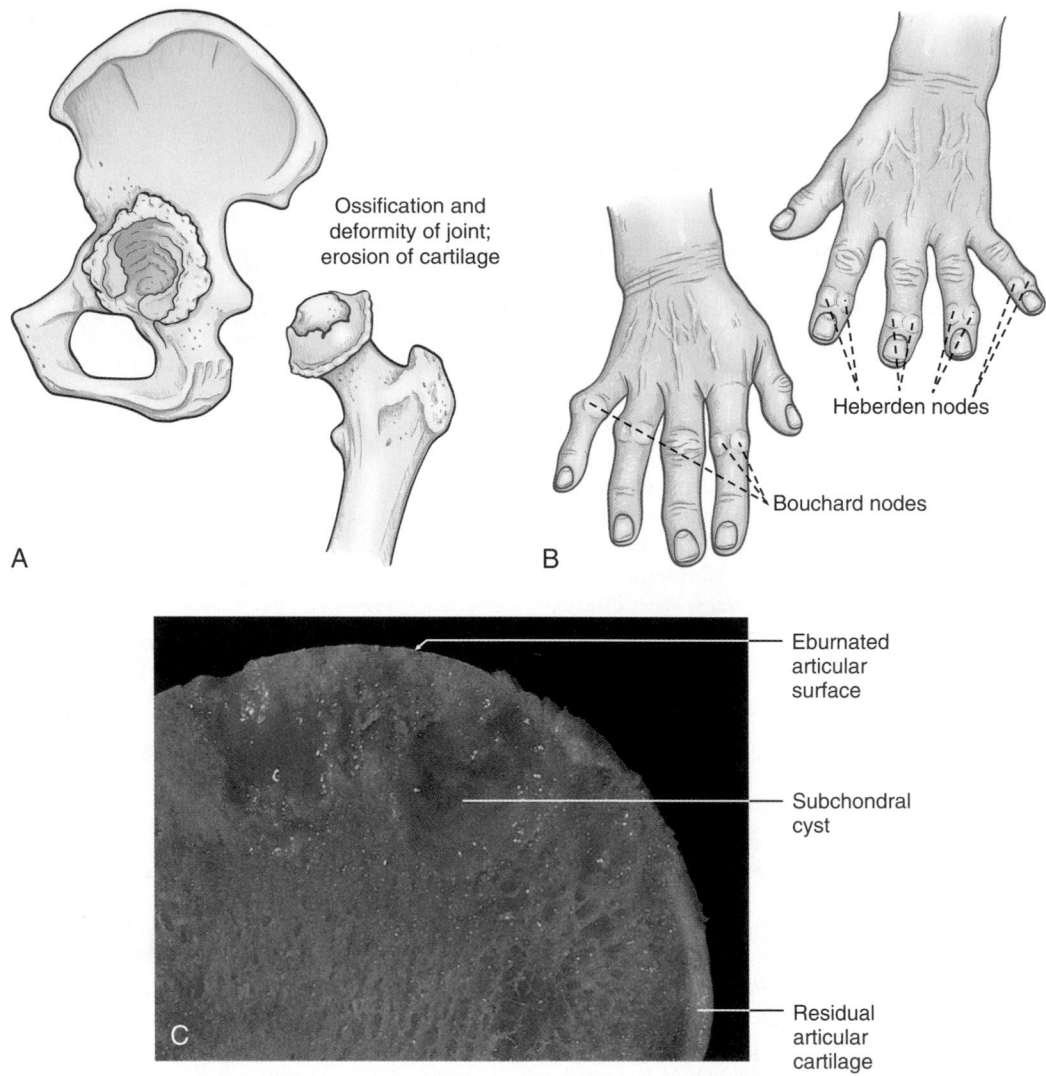

Ossification and deformity of joint; erosion of cartilage

A

B

Heberden nodes

Bouchard nodes

Eburnated articular surface

Subchondral cyst

Residual articular cartilage

C

FIGURE 45.21 Osteoarthritis (OA). **A,** Cartilage and degeneration of the hip joint resulting from osteoarthritis. **B,** Heberden nodes and Bouchard nodes. **C,** Severe osteoarthritis with small islands of residual articular cartilage next to exposed subchondral bone. (**C** from Kumar V et al: *Robbins & Cotran pathologic basis of disease*, ed 9, Philadelphia, 2015, Saunders.)

the United States, OA affects about 27 million people.[82] OA is characterized by local areas of loss and damage of articular cartilage, new bone formation of joint margins (osteophytosis), subchondral bone changes, variable degrees of mild synovitis, and thickening of the joint capsule (Fig. 45.21). Currently, there is no single specific cause of OA; historically it has been viewed as a mechanical problem and emerging is the evidence of molecular events interacting with mechanical issues.[81] OA has been commonly classified as noninflammatory joint disease. However, more recent discoveries have identified the presence of numerous cytokines, chemokines, prostaglandins, and apoptotic molecules within the disease process.[83-85] The ensuing low-grade inflammation, calcification of articular cartilage, and interaction between transcription factors, cytokines, growth factors, matrix molecules, and enzymes affect development and progression of OA. This chemical cascade outlines how the process of cartilaginous destruction begins long before osteoarthritic changes can be detected through the use of MRI, arthroscopy, or traditional x-ray films.

OA often occurs without a known precipitating cause (insidious) with aging, known as *idiopathic* or *primary osteoarthritis*. This

progression is usually noted in a few joints but can be generalized.[86] OA is not a common outcome in younger people with predisposing events, such as injury (e.g., trauma, strains, dislocations, fractures), long-term mechanical stress (e.g., athletics, ballet dancing, repetitive physical tasks, and obesity), or chronic disease (e.g., diabetes, ochronosis, and hemochromatosis). Certain medications can stimulate collagen-digesting enzyme activity in the synovial membrane (e.g., colchicine, indomethacin, and steroids). With these conditions, the disease is noted as secondary osteoarthritis.[86] The incidence of OA increases with age and is more common in women than in men older than age 50. The prevalence in individuals younger than age 45 is uncommon and generally does not exceed 20% in the elderly.[87] OA is generally distributed throughout the peripheral and central joints of the body (hips, hands, knees, and spine). The most commonly affected joints include the hips, knees, lower lumbar and cervical vertebrae, proximal and distal interphalangeal joints of the fingers, first carpometacarpal joints, and first tarsometatarsal joints. The distribution of OA seems affected by gender; the hands and knees are more commonly affected in women whereas

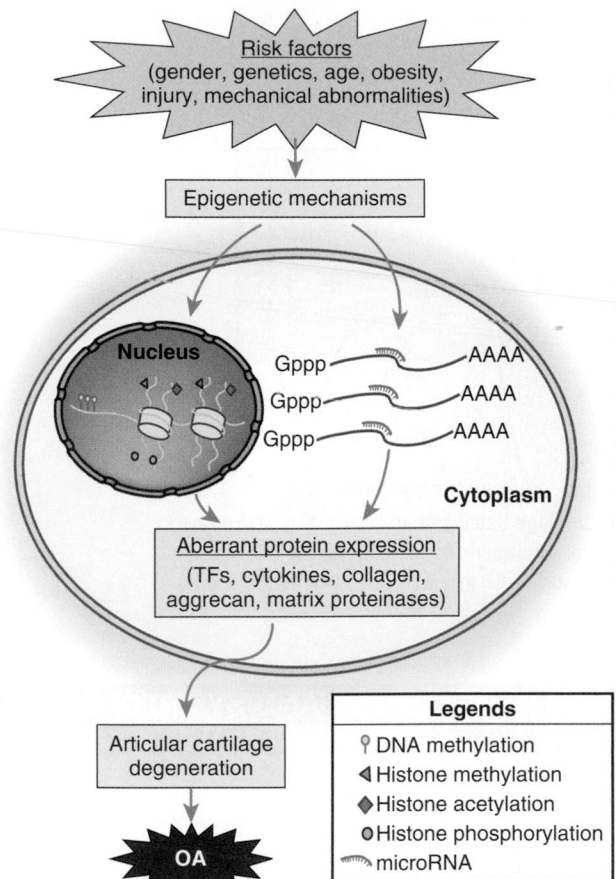

FIGURE 45.22 Working Model Epigenetic Changes in the Pathophysiology of OA. From the proposed effects of risk factors, chondrocytes experience epigenetic events of DNA methylation and histone modifications that occur in the nucleus and miRNAs, which function in the cytoplasm. Overall, these factors result in aberrant expression of transcription factors (TFs), cytokines, collagen, aggrecan, and matrix proteinases. Altered expression of these factors may disrupt the fine balance of anabolic and catabolic activity and affect cartilage homeostasis, resulting in articular cartilage degradation and the development of OA. (Adapted from Zhang M, Wang J: *Genes Dis* 2[1]:69–75, 2015.)

the hips are more affected in men.[86] Advancing disease reveals narrowing of the joint space because of cartilage loss, bone spurs (osteophytes), and often changes in the subchondral bone.

PATHOPHYSIOLOGY. Genome-wide studies show that OA is genetically heterogeneous, and recent advances in epigenetic studies also have indicated the importance of gene expression in the development of OA.[81] The primary pathogenesis in OA is degeneration and then eventual loss and disordered repair of articular cartilage. The chondrocytes of the articular cartilage become damaged early in the disease process because of atypical load bearing as well as both genetic/epigenetic and biochemical factors (Fig. 45.22). These changes lead to increased remodeling of the articular cartilage and a loss of the smooth, frictionless joint.[88,89] Visually, the articular cartilage loses its glistening appearance, becoming yellow-gray or brownish gray. As the disease progresses, surface areas of the articular cartilage flake off and deeper layers develop longitudinal fissures (fibrillation). The cartilage becomes thin and may be absent over some areas, leaving the underlying subchondral bone unprotected. Consequently, the unprotected subchondral bone becomes sclerotic. Cysts sometimes develop within the subchondral bone and communicate with the longitudinal fissures in the cartilage. Pressure

builds in the cysts until the cystic contents are forced into the synovial cavity, breaking through the articular cartilage on the way. As the articular cartilage erodes, cartilage-coated osteophytes may grow outward from the underlying bone and alter the bone contours and joint anatomy. These spurlike bony projections enlarge until small pieces, called *joint mice*, break off into the synovial cavity. If osteophyte fragments irritate the synovial membrane, synovitis and joint effusion result. The joint capsule also becomes thickened and at times adheres to the deformed underlying bone, which may contribute to the limitation of movement (see Fig. 45.21).

Articular cartilage is lost through a cascade of cytokine, biochemical, and growth factor pathways.[90] Enzymatic processes, particularly those involving collagenase, break down the macromolecules of proteoglycans, glycosaminoglycans, and collagen into large, diffusible fragments. The fragments are then taken up by the chondrocytes and digested by the cell's own lysosomal enzymes. (Processes of cellular uptake and lysosomal digestion are described in Chapter 1.) The loss of proteoglycans from articular cartilage is a hallmark of the osteoarthritic process.

Enzymatic destruction of articular cartilage begins in the matrix, with destruction of proteoglycans and collagen fibers. Stromelysin and collagenase enzymes affect proteoglycans by interfering with assembly of the proteoglycan subunit or the proteoglycan aggregate (see Chapter 44); levels of these enzymes are markedly elevated in OA. Changes in the conformation of proteoglycans disrupt the regulation of water and synovial fluid movement into and out of the cartilage. It is the distribution and active redistribution of this water and synovial fluid that evenly disperse the joint load across the cartilage.[88] Without the regulatory action of the proteoglycan pump, cartilage absorbs too much fluid and becomes less able to withstand the stresses of weightbearing.

With aging, the proteoglycan content is decreased and the water content in cartilage can be increased by as much as 8%, affecting the strength of the cartilage. Persons with OA, even those with fairly extensive cartilage destruction, have elevated levels of proteoglycans or fragments of proteoglycans in their synovial fluid, perhaps indicative of a more pronounced reparative phase. Inflammatory cytokines (IL-1β, IL-6, and TNF-α), apoptotic molecules (COX-2, nitric oxide [NO], prostaglandin E_2 [PGE$_2$]), and prostaglandins play a major role in cartilage degradation in part through induction of nitric oxide synthase (iNOS) and increased nitric oxide (NO) generation.[83] (Chapter 8 contains a discussion of cytokines.) These chemical mediators release and activate proteolytic and collagenolytic enzymes (e.g., chemokines and metalloproteinases), causing an imbalance of cell responses to growth factor activity. Chondrocyte apoptosis is increased in OA cartilage, along with increased deposition of calcium phosphate crystals. These deposits are attributed to the disequilibrium between inorganic phosphates and mineralization inhibitors.[91] Nitric oxide stimulates apoptosis in chondrocytes. The resultant cartilage destruction initiates the IL-1β and TNF-α pathways of inflammation.

Genetic deficiencies of inhibitors of calcification also may contribute to a proliferative calcification cascade of the articular cartilage (Fig. 45.23). Recent epigenetic discoveries continue to outline the role of microRNAs in cartilage development and homeostasis. MicroRNAs provide an inhibitor effect on other cartilage-degrading enzymes, such as MMP13 and ADAMTS4.[92] When deficits of these microRNA exist, destruction of the fibrils that give articular cartilage its tensile strength accelerates and exposes the chondrocytes to continued mechanical stress and enzymatic attack.

CLINICAL MANIFESTATIONS. Asymptomatic articular surface changes are common after age 40, although clinical manifestations of OA typically appear during the fifth or sixth decade of life. Pain and stiffness in one or more weightbearing or load-bearing joints are often the first symptoms of the disease. Examination typically reveals

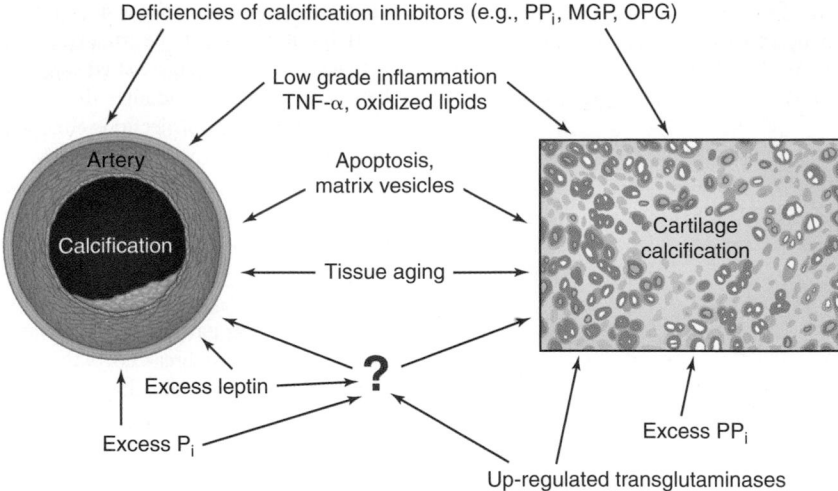

FIGURE 45.23 Possible Mechanisms Driving Artery and Cartilage Calcification. All specified factors have been demonstrated to promote calcification in either arteries and/or cartilage (see text). *MGP,* Matrix GLA-protein; *OPG,* osteoprotegerin; *Pi,* inorganic phosphate; *PPi,* inorganic pyrophosphate. (From Rutsch F, Terkeltaub R: *Joint Bone Spine* 72:110–118, 2005.)

involvement of peripheral and central joints (see earlier discussion). Joint pain related to overuse is typically relieved by rest.

Pain and stiffness are the predominant symptoms of OA; other symptoms include swelling, tenderness, or enlargement/deformity of joints[93] (Box 45.4). Symptoms are usually aggravated by weightbearing or use of the joint and relieved through resting, supporting, bracing, or splinting the joint. Referred pain also may be experienced. Osteoarthritis of the lumbosacral spine, for example, may mimic sciatica, causing severe pain in the back of the thigh along the course of the sciatic nerve. OA in the lower cervical spine may cause brachial neuralgia aggravated by movement of the neck. Additionally, osteoarthritic conditions in the hip cause pain that may be referred to the lower thigh and knee area.

The mechanism of joint pain perception is complex. Cartilage lacks innervation; therefore the sensation of pain is not experienced from cartilaginous damage alone. There is little correlation between the radiologic appearance of OA and the perception of pain.[88,94] Subchondral bone injury, ligamentous injury, weightbearing stress, and inflammation contribute to the sources of joint pain in OA. Articular distention and stretching of the fibrous joint capsule, which has an abundant nerve supply, significantly contribute to the sensation of pain. Finally, inflammation of the joint capsule leads to remodeling and a fibrous contraction of the capsule, causing the joint to become stiff and painful with movement[95,96] (Fig. 45.24).

Joint stiffness is generally defined as difficulty in initiating joint movement, immobility, or a loss of range of motion. The extent of cartilage degeneration, along with joint capsule remodeling and fibrous contraction, also contributes to a limitation in range of motion. Stiffness is typically worse in the morning as joint movement begins but dissipates within 30 minutes of continued movement. Enlargement and bulging of joint contour, commonly described as swelling, are actually attributed to thickening of the subchondral bone from the proliferation of osteophytes around the margins of the joint and hypertrophy of the joint capsule.[96] These types of joint deformities in the fingers are termed Heberden and Bouchard nodes.

Swelling may also occur in response to tissue injury. Such injuries initiate the inflammatory cascade of cytokines and chemokines, resulting in capillary permeability and interstitial fluid collection.[96] If inflammatory exudate or blood enters the joint cavity, the total volume of synovial

---

BOX 45.4   SIGNS AND SYMPTOMS OF OSTEOARTHRITIS

Hand
Pain on range of motion
Hypertrophic changes at distal and proximal interphalangeal joints (Heberden nodes and Bouchard nodes)
Tenderness over carpometacarpal joint of thumb

Shoulder
Pain on range of motion
Limitation of range of motion, especially external rotation
Crepitus on range of motion

Knee
Pain on range of motion
Joint effusion
Crepitus on range of motion
Presence of popliteal cyst (Baker cyst)
Lateral instability
Valgus or varus deformity

Hip
Pain on range of motion
Pain in buttock
Limitation of range of motion, especially internal rotation

Foot
Pain on ambulation, especially at first metatarsophalangeal joint
Limited range of motion of first metatarsophalangeal joint, hallux rigidus
Hallux valgus deformity

Spine
Pain on range of motion
Limitation of range of motion
Lower extremity sensory loss, reflex loss, motor weakness caused by nerve root impingement
Pseudoclaudication caused by spinal stenosis

Data from Sinusas K: *Am Fam Physician* 85(1):49–56, 2012.

fluid will be increased. This condition, termed joint effusion, is attributed to (1) the presence of osteophyte fragments in the synovial cavity, (2) drainage of cysts from diseased subchondral bone, or (3) acute trauma to joint structures, resulting in hemorrhage and inflammatory exudation into the synovial cavity.

Abnormal knee alignment also has been shown to increase the incidence and progression of OA.[97] Both varus or valgus disorders of the knee of more than 5 degrees have been associated with increased

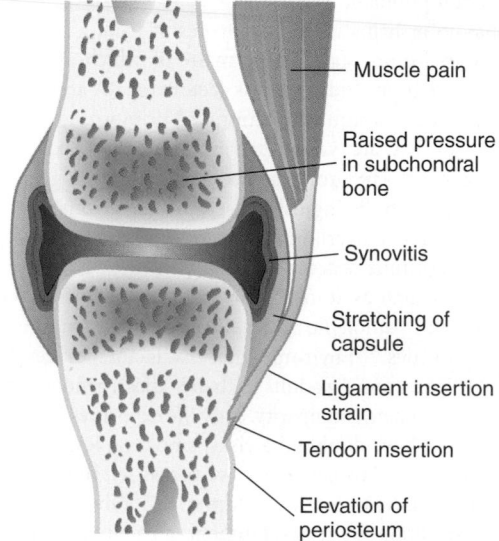

Muscle pain

Raised pressure in subchondral bone

Synovitis

Stretching of capsule

Ligament insertion strain

Tendon insertion

Elevation of periosteum

FIGURE 45.24 Possible Causes of Pain in Osteoarthritis.

risk of development and progression of OA. Although the use of biomechanical devices, such as foot wedges or alignment braces, has been shown to decrease pain, the reduction of disease progression has yet to be supported.[98]

◆**EVALUATION AND TREATMENT.** Evaluation consists of individual subjective reports, clinical assessment, and radiologic studies, which may include CT scan, arthroscopy, and MRI. Treatment is often determined by the severity of symptoms of pain and immobility. Possible treatment regimens span conservative to surgical, as well as nonpharmacologic to pharmacologic. Complementary and alternative therapies also may be considered.

Lifestyle modification, particularly exercise and weight reduction, is a core management approach. Use of supportive devices is recommended, such as a cane, walker, braces, or other devices to decrease weightbearing.[98-101] Physical therapy is an important management strategy for OA. Losing weight reduces pain-associated inflammation, and weight loss combined with physical activity has a greater benefit.[102] Dietary recommendations include increasing intake of long-chain *n*-3 fatty acids, preferably by eating oily fish twice a week; aiming for a safe level of sun exposure; eating rich vitamin D dietary sources or taking vitamin D supplements (≤25 μg/day); and increasing vitamin K intake by eating green, leafy vegetables.[102] Pharmacologic therapy may include the use of analgesic and antiinflammatory drug therapies. The combination of glucosamine and chondroitin may be effective. Other alternative and complementary therapies include the use of magnetic bracelets, therapeutic ultrasound,[103] balneotherapy, and acupuncture.[93,104]

Surgical intervention may be used to improve joint movement. However, emerging evidence, based on systematic reviews[105] (see *What's New?* Evidence Against the Use of Arthroscopy for Nearly All Patients with Degenerative Knee Disease), cautions against the use of arthroscopy

WHAT'S NEW?

Evidence Against the Use of Arthroscopy for Nearly All Patients with Degenerative Knee Disease

An international expert panel provided recommendations on the role of arthroscopic surgery in degenerative disease. These recommendations were based on a recent randomized trial of patients with a degenerative medial meniscus tear; the panel found that knee arthroscopy was no better than exercise therapy alone for these patients.[1] This study adds to the growing evidence that the benefits of arthroscopy may not outweigh the burdens and risks.[2,3] The panel made a strong recommendation against arthroscopy for degenerative knee disease.[4] This recommendation applies to patients with or without imaging evidence of osteoarthritis, mechanical symptoms, or sudden symptom onset. Here, the term degenerative knee disease included patients with knee pain, particularly if they are >35 years old, with or without imaging evidence of osteoarthritis, meniscal tears, locking, clicking, or other mechanical symptoms. However, degenerative knee disease did not include patients with persistent locked knee, patients with acute or subacute onset of symptoms, or patients with major knee trauma and acute onset of joint swelling (such as hemarthrosis).[4] The international panel included orthopedic surgeons, a rheumatologist, physiotherapists, a general practitioner, general internists, epidemiologists, methodologists, and patients who had experienced degenerative knee disease. Characteristics of patients and trials included in this systemic review were as follows: 13 trials were examined; 12 of 13 trials were free of industry funding; 1668 patients were followed (median age 54.8 years); symptom duration was 3 months (12 months median, 52 months maximum); percent of women studied was 49.2; mean BMI was 27; no patients were involved in designing or conducting trials. In addition, 12 observational studies for complications (>1.8 million patients) were reviewed. In general, it takes 2 to 6 weeks to recover from arthroscopy. Patients may experience pain, swelling, and limited function. Most patients cannot bear full weight on the leg

(i.e., they may need crutches) in the first week after surgery, and physical activity and driving are limited during the recovery period. Degenerative knee disease is a chronic condition and symptoms fluctuate. Pain, on average, tends to improve with time after seeing a physician[5,6] and delaying knee replacement is encouraged when possible.[7]

References

1. Kise NJ, et al: Exercise therapy versus arthroscopic partial meniscectomy for degenerative meniscal tear in middle aged patients: randomised controlled trial with two-year follow-up. *BMJ* 354:i3740, 2016.
2. Khan M, et al: Arthroscopic surgery for degenerative tears of the meniscus: a systematic review and meta-analysis. *CMAJ* 186(14):1057–1064, 2014.
3. Thorlund JB, et al: Arthroscopic surgery for degenerative knee: systematic review and meta-analysis of benefits and harms. *BMJ* 350:h2747, 2015.
4. Siemieniuk RAC, et al: Arthroscopic surgery for degenerative knee arthritis and meniscal tear: a clinical guideline. *BJM* 357:j1982, 2017.
5. Brignardello-Peterson R, et al: Knee arthroscopy versus conservative management in patients with degenerative knee disease: a systematic review. *BMJ Open* 7(5):e016114, 2017.
6. de Roolij M, et al: Prognosis of pain and physical functioning in patients with knee osteoarthritis: a systematic review and meta-analysis. *Arthritis Care Res (Hoboken)* 68(4):481–492, 2016.
7. McGrory B, et al: American Academy of Orthopaedic Surgeons evidence-based clinical practice guideline on surgical management of osteoarthritis. *J Bone Joint Surg Am* 98(8):688–692, 2016.

in nearly all persons with degenerative knee disease. This recommendation was triggered by a randomized trial that found, among persons with a degenerative medial meniscus tear, knee arthroscopy was no better than exercise.[106] More aggressive surgical procedures involve creating a new joint with artificial implants.[107]

Classic Inflammatory Joint Disease

Inflammatory joint disease, commonly referred to as *arthritis*, is characterized by damage or destruction in the synovial membrane or articular cartilage and by systemic signs of inflammation (fever, leukocytosis, malaise, anorexia, hyperfibrinogenemia).

Inflammatory joint disease can be infectious or noninfectious. In infectious inflammatory joint disease, inflammation is caused by invasion of the joint by bacteria, mycoplasmas, viruses, fungi, or protozoa. These microorganisms can invade the joint through a number of ports of entry, such as a traumatic wound, surgical incision, or contaminated needle. Additionally, these pathogens can be delivered by the bloodstream from sites of entry through the body's mucous membranes, as well as infections elsewhere in the body, such as in bones, heart valves, or blood vessels.[108] In noninfectious inflammatory joint diseases such as gout, inflammation is caused by an immune response to the deposition of crystals of monosodium urate in and around the joint. Immune and hypersensitivity reactions occur in conditions such as rheumatoid arthritis, psoriatic arthritis, and ankylosing spondylitis.

Rheumatoid Arthritis

Rheumatoid arthritis (RA) is a chronic, systemic inflammatory autoimmune disease that may involve many tissues and organs but particularly affects the joints. RA involves synovial inflammation, joint swelling, and ankylosis and destruction of articular cartilage. The first joint tissue to be affected is the synovial membrane, which lines the joint cavity (see Chapter 44 and Fig. 44.9). Multiple immunoregulatory cytokines and inflammatory enzymes, such as interleukins, B cells, and collagenase, contribute to the development of an exaggerated immune response resulting in leukocyte infiltration into the synovium.[109] This leads to the development of synovitis and eventual joint damage. Inflammation may spread to the articular cartilage, fibrous joint capsule, and surrounding ligaments and tendons, causing pain, joint deformity, and loss of function (Fig. 45.25). The joints most commonly affected are in the fingers, feet, wrists, elbows, ankles, and knees. Other joints,

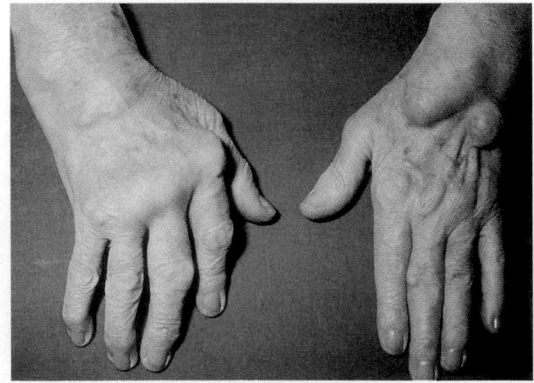

FIGURE 45.25 Rheumatoid Arthritis of the Hand. Note swelling from chronic synovitis of metacarpophalangeal joints, marked ulnar drift, subcutaneous nodules, and subluxation of metacarpophalangeal joints with extension of proximal interphalangeal joints and flexion of distal joints. Note also deformed position of thumb. (From Walker BR et al: *Davidson's principles and practice of medicine,* ed 22, London, 2014, Churchill Livingstone.)

such as shoulders, hips, and cervical spine, also may be involved as well as the tissues of the lungs, heart, kidneys, and skin. In addition to joint inflammation and tissue damage, RA can cause fever, malaise, rash, lymph node or spleen enlargement, and Raynaud phenomenon (transient lack of circulation to the fingertips and toes).

Internationally, the prevalence of rheumatoid arthritis ranges from 0.4% to 1.3%. The incidence of RA increases with age and peaks at ages 65 to 74 years, with women having a greater lifetime risk than men (4% vs. 3%).[110] However, over the past five decades the incidence and prevalence of RA have decreased in developed countries to approximately 1% of the adult population.[111,112]

Rheumatoid arthritis is thought to result from a combination of genetic and environmental factors, many of which are unknown.[113] Many genes have been studied as risk factors for RA and most of these genes are involved in immune function.[113] The most significant genetic risk factors for RA are variations in HLA genes, particularly the HLA-DRB1 gene.[113] The proteins produced from HLA genes assist the immune system with distinguishing self proteins from proteins made by invaders such as bacteria and viruses. Investigation of epigenetic factors, such as histone deacetylases, can confer the effects of environmental triggers, such as smoking or diet (e.g., n-3 fatty acids, or in combination with γ-linolenic acid [GLA]), or treatment on expression levels of target genes.[114] Environmental risk factors for developing RA include age (highest among adults in their sixties), gender (two to three times higher in women), nulliparity, early life exposures (children whose mothers smoked have double the risk), smoking, low socioeconomic status, and obesity.[115] Women who have breast-fed their infants have a decreased risk of developing RA. Additionally, individuals who have a genetic predisposition to the development of rheumatoid arthritis have an increased risk when they smoke or subject themselves to other forms of repeated bronchial stress or infectious agents, such as Epstein-Barr virus, cytomegalovirus, *Proteus* species, and *Escherichia coli.*[116]

PATHOPHYSIOLOGY. The pathologic events are mediated by antibodies against self antigens and inflammatory cytokines, especially CD4+ T cells that promote inflammation. Acting together, T cells produce cytokines that stimulate other inflammatory cells and promote tissue injury.[86] The most significant cytokines include interferon-gamma (IFN-γ) (activates macrophages and synovial cells), IL-17 (stimulates neutrophils and monocytes), TNF and IL-1 (stimulate synovial cells to secrete proteases that damage hyaline cartilage), and RANKL (activates bone resorption and erosion).[86]

During inflammation, arginine (an α-amino acid) can be enzymatically modified into another α-amino acid, citrulline. This process (citrullination) changes the structure and function of the protein. Other proteins, like fibrin and vimentin, can become citrullinated during cell death and tissue inflammation.[117] In turn, the citrullinated proteins may act as antigens.[118,119]

The inflammatory cytokines convert the synovium into a thick, abnormal layer of granulation tissue known as **pannus** (see Figs. 45.27 and 45.28, *A*). The pannus acts *like* a locally invasive tumor.[116,120,121] Macrophages, components of pannus (Fig. 45.26), stimulate the release of IL-1, platelet-derived growth factor (PDGF), and fibronectin. The pathogenesis of rheumatoid arthritis is summarized in Fig. 45.26.

The ensuing inflammatory and immune process instigates the migration of several types of leukocytes out of the circulation and into the synovial membrane, resulting in a damaging effect on the synovial membrane. The phagocytes of inflammation (neutrophils and macrophages) ingest the immune complexes and, in the process of doing so, release powerful enzymes that degrade synovial tissue and articular cartilage (Fig. 45.27). The immune system's B and T lymphocytes also are activated.[116] With long-term or intensive exposure to the antigen, normal antibodies (immunoglobulins [Igs]) become autoantibodies

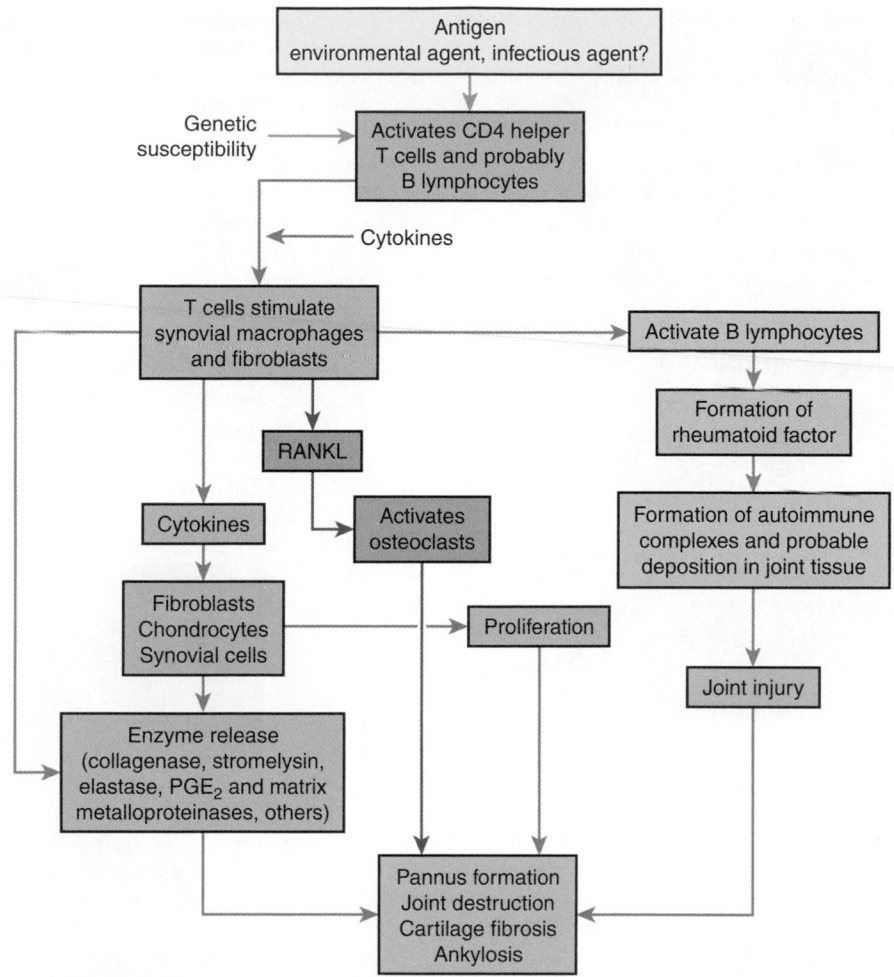

FIGURE 45.26 Emerging Model of Pathogenesis of Rheumatoid Arthritis. Rheumatoid arthritis is an autoimmune disease of a genetically susceptible host triggered by an unknown antigenic agent. Chronic autoimmune reaction with activation of CD4+ helper T cells and possibly other lymphocytes and the local release of inflammatory cytokines and mediators eventually destroy the joint. T cells stimulate cells in the joint to produce cytokines that are key mediators of synovial damage. Apparently immune complex deposition also plays a role. Tumor necrosis factor *(TNF)* and interleukin-1 *(IL-1)*, as well as some other cytokines, stimulate synovial cells to proliferate and produce other mediators of inflammation, such as prostaglandin E$_2$ *(PGE$_2$)*, matrix metalloproteinases, and enzymes, which all contribute to destruction of cartilage. Activated T cells and synovial fibroblasts also produce receptor activator of nuclear factor κβ ligand *(RANKL)*, which activates the osteoclasts and promotes bone destruction. Pannus is a mass of synovium and synovial stroma with inflammatory cells, granulation tissue, and fibroblasts that grows over the articular surface and causes its destruction.

and attack host tissues (self antigens). Because they are usually present in individuals with rheumatoid arthritis, the altered antibodies are termed **rheumatoid factors (RFs)**. RFs usually consist of two classes of immunoglobulin antibodies (antibodies for IgM and IgG) but occasionally involve antibodies for IgA. Their main antigenic targets are portions of the immunoglobulin molecules. RFs bind with their target self antigens in blood and synovial membrane, forming immune complexes (antigen-antibody complexes) (see Chapter 8).

The B lymphocytes are stimulated to produce more RFs, and the T lymphocytes eventually cause release of enzymes that amplify and perpetuate the inflammatory response. Cartilage destruction is mediated by collagenase, which activates the synoviocytes to invade the synovium and cartilaginous matrix.[118,122] In addition, RANKL is expressed by various cells in the synovium and induces osteoclast maturation and activation, thus producing increased bone resorption (also see Chapter 44).

Along with the swelling and damage to the synovial membrane caused by leukocyte infiltration, the synovial membrane undergoes hyperplastic thickening as its cells proliferate and become abnormally large. As synovial inflammation progresses to involve its blood vessels, small venules become occluded by the hypertrophied endothelial cells, fibrin, platelets, and inflammatory cells, which decrease vascular flow to the synovial tissue. Compromised circulation, coupled with increased metabolic needs because of hypertrophy and hyperplasia, causes hypoxia and metabolic acidosis. Acidosis stimulates the release of hydrolytic enzymes from synovial cells into the surrounding tissue, initiating erosion of the articular cartilage and inflammation in the supporting ligaments and tendons. Inflammation causes hemorrhage, coagulation, and fibrin deposition on the synovial membrane, in the intracellular matrix, and in the synovial fluid[116,118] (Fig. 45.28).

◆**CLINICAL MANIFESTATIONS.** The onset of RA is usually insidious, although as many as 15% of cases have an acute onset. RA begins with

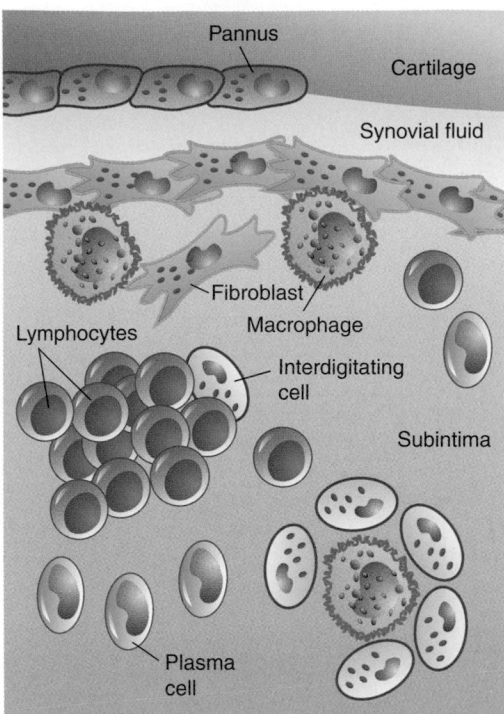

FIGURE 45.27 Synovitis. Inflamed synovium showing typical arrangements of macrophages and fibroblastic cells.

general systemic manifestations of inflammation, including fever, fatigue, weakness, anorexia, weight loss, and generalized aching and stiffness. Local manifestations appear gradually over weeks or months. The joints typically become painful, tender, and stiff. Pain early in the disease is caused by pressure from swelling; later it is caused by sclerosis of subchondral bone and new bone formation. Stiffness usually lasts for about 1 hour after arising in the morning and may be caused by synovitis. Initially the most commonly involved joints are the metacarpophalangeal (MCP), proximal interphalangeal (PIP), and wrists, with later involvement of larger weightbearing joints.

Widespread and symmetrical joint swelling is caused by increasing amounts of inflammatory exudate (leukocytes, plasma, plasma proteins) in the synovial membrane, hyperplasia of inflamed tissues, and formation of new bone. On palpation, the swollen joint feels warm and the synovial membrane feels "boggy." The skin over the joint may have a ruddy or cyanotic hue and may look thin and shiny.

An inflamed joint may lose some of its mobility; even mild synovitis can lead to loss of range of motion. Extension becomes limited and is eventually lost if flexion contractures form. Chronic synovitis weakens ligamentous structures, leading to deformities of the fingers, toes, and limbs, including ulnar deviation of the hands, boutonnière and swan-neck deformities of the finger joints, plantar subluxation of the metatarsal heads of the foot, and hallux valgus (angulation of the great toe toward the other toes). Flexion contractures of the knees and hips are also common.[123]

Joint deformities cause the physical limitations experienced by persons with RA. Loss of joint motion is quickly followed by secondary atrophy of the surrounding muscles. With secondary muscle atrophy the joint becomes unstable, which further aggravates joint pathology.

Two complications of chronic RA are caused by an excessive amount of inflammatory exudate in the synovial cavity. One complication is the formation of cysts in the articular cartilage or subchondral bone. Occasionally these cysts communicate with the skin surface (usually

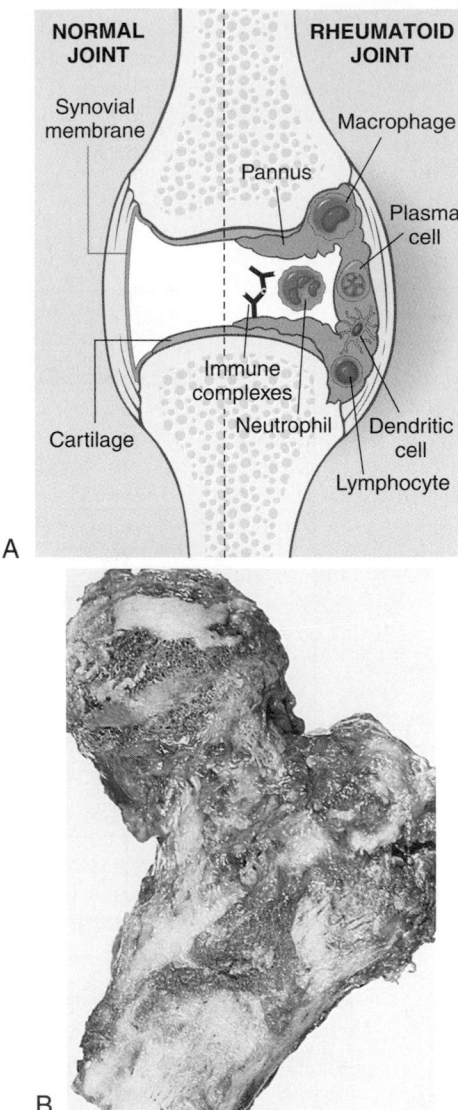

FIGURE 45.28 Rheumatoid Arthritis. **A,** Schematic view of the joint lesion. **B,** Advanced rheumatoid arthritis involving femur. There is prominent proliferation of synovium and almost complete destruction of overlying articular cartilage. (**A** modified from Feldmann M: *Nat Rev Immunol* 2:364, 2002; **B** from Rosai J: *Ackerman's surgical pathology,* ed 10, Philadelphia, 2011, Mosby.)

the sole of the foot) and begin to drain, causing a fistula. The second complication is rupture of a cyst or of the synovial joint itself, usually caused by strenuous physical activity that places excessive pressure on the joint. Both of these complications contribute to the formation of bone erosion and worsened outcomes for the individual with RA.[124]

Extrasynovial **rheumatoid nodules**, or swellings, are observed in areas of pressure or trauma in up to 30% of individuals with RA. Each nodule is an aggregate of inflammatory cells surrounding a central core of fibrinoid and cellular debris. T lymphocytes are the predominant leukocytes in the nodule; B lymphocytes, plasma cells, and phagocytes are found around the periphery. Nodules are found most often in subcutaneous tissue over the extensor surfaces of elbows and fingers. Less common sites are the scalp, back, feet, hands, buttocks, and knees.

Rheumatoid nodules also may invade the skin, cardiac valves, pericardium, pleura, lung parenchyma, and spleen.[125] These nodules are identical to those encountered in some individuals with rheumatic fever and are characterized by central tissue necrosis surrounded by proliferating connective tissue. Also noted are large numbers of lymphocytes and occasional plasma cells. Acute glaucoma may result, with nodules forming on the sclera. Pulmonary involvement may result in diffuse pleuritis or multiple intraparenchymal nodules. Together, the occurrence of pulmonary nodules and pneumoconiosis (chronic inflammation of the lungs from inhalation of dust) creates Caplan syndrome.[126] Diffuse pulmonary fibrosis may occur because of immunologically mediated immune complex deposition.

Rheumatoid nodules within the heart may cause valvular deformities, particularly of the aortic valve leaflets. Pericardial effusion or other pericardial problems occur in almost 50% of individuals with RA.[127] Lymphadenopathy of the nodes close to the affected joints may develop. Rheumatoid nodules within the spleen result in splenomegaly. Involvement of any blood vessel can result in the development of necrotizing vasculitis.[128] Thromboses of such involved vessels may give rise to myocardial infarctions, cerebrovascular occlusions, mesenteric infarction, kidney damage, and vascular insufficiency in the hands and fingers (Raynaud phenomenon). Vascular changes are noted primarily in

individuals receiving corticosteroid therapy; thus there is some concern that the therapy may play a role in initiating these lesions. Changes in skeletal muscle are often noted in the form of nonspecific atrophy secondary to joint dysfunction.

◆**EVALUATION AND TREATMENT.** In 2010 the American College of Rheumatology (ACR) and the European League Against Rheumatism (EULAR) revised their classification criteria to better identify early stages of RA.[129] Box 45.5 summarizes the criteria for diagnosing RA. These criteria are dependent upon a combination of physical examination and serologic evaluation of rheumatoid factor (RF) or the much more specific serum marker anti–citrullinated protein antibody (ACPA). These serum markers can be present for years to decades before synovial or radiographic changes become apparent.[117,129-131] Early, aggressive treatment of RA can decrease the systemic impact of RA, leading to a decreased development of disability and joint destruction.

Early treatment of RA begins with disease-modifying antirheumatic drugs (DMARDs) such as methotrexate (MTX), azathioprine, sulfasalazine, hydroxychloroquine, leflunomide, and cyclosporine. MTX remains the first line of treatment. More recently, targeted treatment of RA has

---

BOX 45.5   THE 2010 AMERICAN COLLEGE OF RHEUMATOLOGY/EUROPEAN LEAGUE AGAINST RHEUMATISM CLASSIFICATION CRITERIA FOR RHEUMATOID ARTHRITIS

Target population (Who should be tested?) includes individuals:
1. who have at least one joint with definite clinical synovitis (swelling)*
2. who have synovitis not better explained by another disease[†]

Classification criteria for RA (score-based algorithm: add scores of categories A–D; a score ≥6/10 is needed for definite classification of RA)

CLINICAL FINDING	SCORE
A. Joint Involvement[‡]	
1 large joint[§]	0
2–10 large joints	1
1–3 small joints (with or without involvement of large joints)[¶]	2
4–10 small joints (with or without involvement of large joints)	3
>10 joints (at least 1 small joint)[#]	5

CLINICAL FINDING	SCORE
B. Serology (At Least One Test Result Is Needed for Classification)**	
Negative RF *and* negative ACPA	0
Low-positive RF *or* low-positive ACPA	2
High-positive RF *or* high-positive ACPA	3
C. Acute-phase Reactants (At Least One Test Result Is Needed for Classification)[††]	
Normal CRP *and* normal ESR	0
Abnormal CRP *or* abnormal ESR	1
D. Duration of Symptoms[‡‡]	
<6 weeks	0
≥6 weeks	1

*The criteria are aimed at classification of newly presenting patients. In addition, patients with erosive disease typical of rheumatoid arthritis (RA) and with a history compatible with prior fulfillment of the 2010 criteria should be classified as having RA. Patients with longstanding disease, including those whose disease is inactive (with or without treatment) and who (based on retrospectively available data) have previously fulfilled the 2010 criteria, should be classified as having RA.

[†]Differential diagnoses vary among patients with different presentations, but may include conditions such as systemic lupus erythematosus, psoriatic arthritis, and gout. If it is unclear about the relevant differential diagnoses to consider, an expert rheumatologist should be consulted.

[‡]Joint involvement refers to any swollen or tender joint in examination, which may be confirmed by imaging evidence of synovitis. Distal interphalangeal joints, first metacarpophalangeal joints, and first metatarsophalangeal joints are excluded from assessment. Categories of joint distribution are classified according to the location and number of involved joints, with placement into the highest category possible based on the pattern of joint involvement.

[§]"Large joints" refer to shoulders, elbows, hips, knees, and ankles.

[¶]"Small joints" refer to the metacarpophalangeal joints, proximal interphalangeal joints, second through fifth metatarsophalangeal joints, thumb interphalangeal joints, and wrists.

[#]In this category, at least one of the involved joints must be a small joint; the others can include any combination of large and additional small joints, as well as other joints not specifically listed elsewhere (e.g., temporomandibular, acromioclavicular, sternoclavicular).

**Negative refers to international unit values that are less than or equal to the upper limit of normal (ULN) for the laboratory and assay; low-positive refers to international unit values that are >3 times the ULN for the laboratory and assay. Where rheumatoid factor (RF) information is only available as positive or negative, a positive result should be scored as low-positive for RA. *ACPA,* Anti–citrullinated protein antibody.

[††]Normal/abnormal is determined by local laboratory standards.

[‡‡]Duration of symptoms refers to patient self-report of the duration of signs and symptoms of synovitis (e.g., pain, swelling, tenderness) of joints that are clinically involved at the time of assessment, regardless of treatment status.

CRP, C-Reactive protein; *ESR,* erythrocyte sedimentation rate.

Data from Aletaha D: *Arthritis Rheum* 62(9):2574, 2010.

involved use of agents aimed at interrupting the pathogenesis of the disease. Known as *biological DMARDs (bDMARDs)*, these medications affect specific processes in the development of RA and include tumor necrosis factor (TNF) inhibitors, such as etanercept, adalimumab, and infliximab, golimumab, and certolizumab. Other agents interfere with cytokine function (anakinra inhibits IL-1 function; tocilizumab targets IL-6), inhibit T-cell activation (abatacept), or deplete B cells (rituximab).

Other treatments and therapies include nonsteroidal antiinflammatory drugs (NSAIDs), glucocorticoids, intraarticular steroid injections, physical and occupational therapy with therapeutic exercise, and use of assistive devices. Surgery is used to treat deformities or mechanical deficiencies of joints and can include synovectomy or joint replacement.

Ankylosing Spondylitis

Ankylosing spondylitis (AS) is the most common of a group of inflammatory arthropathies known as *spondyloarthropathies.* It is a chronic inflammatory joint disease characterized by stiffening and fusion (ankylosis) of the spine and sacroiliac joints.

◆**PATHOPHYSIOLOGY.** The exact cause of AS continues to be unknown; however, a high association with the histocompatibility antigen human leukocyte antigen (HLA-B27) has been known for decades. A misfolding of HLA-B27 occurs in the endoplasmic reticulum (ER) and, as a result, the misfolded proteins accumulate. This results in a stress response of the ER and increased production of interleukin-23 (IL-23), a potent cytokine that may also act on T-helper 17 cells, promoting their survival.[132,133]

The prevalence of AS globally is predicted to be between 0.1% and 1.4% with greater incidence in North American and European countries.[134] Worldwide, the disease also has shown a greater prevalence in men, three times as often as women. In women, AS may affect the peripheral joints of the appendicular skeleton rather than the axial skeleton, progress less rapidly, and cause less dramatic spinal changes. Many individuals with AS remain undiagnosed. Primary AS usually develops in late adolescence or young adulthood, with peak incidence at about 20 years of age. Secondary AS affects older age groups and is often associated with other inflammatory diseases (e.g., psoriatic arthropathy, inflammatory bowel disease, Reiter syndrome).

◆**CLINICAL MANIFESTATIONS.** The most common signs and symptoms of early AS are low back pain and stiffness. Typically, the individual with primary disease develops low back pain during the early twenties. The pain is at first insidious but progressively becomes persistent. It is often worse after prolonged rest and is alleviated by physical activity. Early morning stiffness usually accompanies the low back pain, and the individual typically has difficulty sitting up or twisting the spine. Forward flexion, rotation, and lateral flexion of the spine are restricted and painful. Early pain and resultant loss of motion are caused by the underlying inflammation and reflex muscle spasm rather than by soft tissue or bony fusion.

As the disease progresses, the normal convex curve of the lower spine (lumbar lordosis) diminishes and concavity of the upper spine (kyphosis) increases. The individual becomes increasingly stooped. The thoracic spine becomes rounded, the head and neck are held forward on the shoulders, and the hips are flexed (Fig. 45.29).

Inflammation in the tendon insertions of the many costosternal and costovertebral muscles can cause pleuritic chest pain and restricted chest movement. The pain is usually worse on inspiration. Movement in the diaphragm is normal and full. Pressure on the anterior chest wall over the sternum, ribs, and costal cartilages may cause tenderness. Tenderness over the pelvic brim may cause discomfort at night and interfere with sleep because turning onto the iliac crests causes pain. Tenderness over the ischial tuberosities may make sitting on hard seats

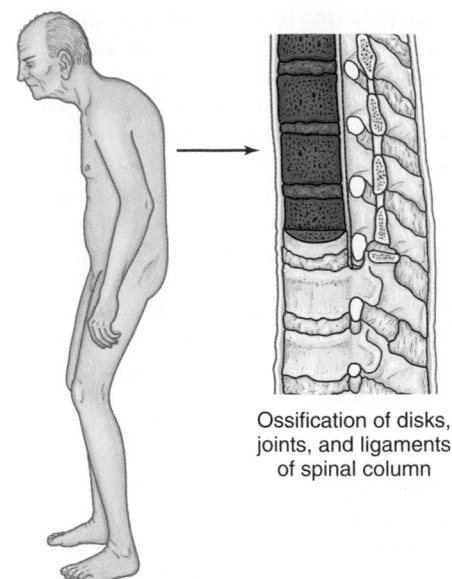

Ossification of disks, joints, and ligaments of spinal column

FIGURE 45.29 Ankylosing Spondylitis. Characteristic posture and primary pathologic sites of inflammation and resulting damage.

unbearable. Tenderness in the heels may contribute to a limp or the cautious placement of the feet during walking.

Pain in the sacroiliac joint in men is often the first clinical manifestation, while initial symptoms typically present as knee pain in women.[133,135] Along with low back pain, many individuals have peripheral joint involvement, uveitis, fibrotic changes in the lungs, cardiomegaly, aortic incompetence, amyloidosis, and Achilles tendinitis. Symptoms may include fatigue, weight loss, low-grade fever, hypochromic anemia, and an increased erythrocyte sedimentation rate.

◆**EVALUATION AND TREATMENT.** Diagnosis of AS is made on the basis of both clinical and radiologic findings. Low back pain and stiffness lasting more than 3 months that improves with exercise but is not relieved by rest, limited spine range of motion (ROM) in both frontal and sagittal planes, and limited chest expansion relative to normal values for age and gender are the classic clinical criteria. Radiologic changes at the sacroiliac joint are graded according to severity of abnormality; abnormalities include sclerosis, widening, narrowing, or ankylosis.[136] With traditional radiographic imaging, a delay exists between the onset of joint damage and radiographic identification. Laboratory tests, including serum analysis for the presence of the histocompatibility antigen HLA-B27, elevated erythrocyte sedimentation rate (ESR) (normal is 0 to 9 mm/hour in males, 0 to 2 mm/hour in females), and elevated alkaline phosphatase levels, can be used to help monitor the course of the disease.

Treatment of individuals with AS consists of a multidisciplinary approach: physical therapy to maintain skeletal mobility and prevent the natural progression of contractures, support groups to help individuals cope with the disease process, nonsteroidal antiinflammatory drugs (NSAIDs) to suppress some of the pain and stiffness and to facilitate exercise, and corticosteroid injections to help reduce inflammation in joints.[137] Surgical interventions also have been shown to help in decreasing severe disabling deformity.

Gout

Gout is an inflammatory response to excessive quantities of uric acid in the blood (hyperuricemia) and in other body fluids, including synovial fluid. These elevated levels lead to the formation of monosodium urate (MSU) crystals in and around joints.[138] When the uric acid concentration is >6.8 mg/dL in fluids, it crystallizes and forms insoluble precipitates of MSU that are deposited in connective tissues throughout the body. Crystallization in synovial fluid triggers TNF-α, causing the release of chemokines and interleukins. The result of crystallization in synovial fluid is acute, painful inflammation of the joint. This inflammatory response triggers macrophages. When macrophages phagocytize MSU crystals, they form a protein scaffold known as an *inflammasome*. Inflammasomes then convert inactive interleukins of IL-1β and IL-18 into their active forms.[139,140] Prolonged accumulation results in joint damage, a condition known as **gouty arthritis**. With time, crystal deposition in subcutaneous tissues causes the formation of small, white nodules, or **tophi**, that are visible through the skin. Hyperuricemia and tophi deposits are significantly associated with joint damage; however, associations also exist with hypertension, heart disease, diabetes mellitus type 2, kidney disease, and metabolic syndrome and increased death rates.[141-143]

Although hyperuricemia is essential for the development of gout, it is not the only factor. Other factors include age (rare before 30 years), genetic predisposition (X-linked alteration of the enzyme hypoxanthine-guanine phosphoribosyltransferase [HGPRT]), excessive alcohol consumption, obesity, certain drugs (especially thiazides), and lead toxicity. Dietary intake of purine-rich foods, such as organ meats, pork, some fish, and beer, also has been shown to contribute to the incidence of gout. Additionally, evidence exists identifying the contributory nature of foods high in fructose and sugar-sweetened soft drinks. Conversely, dairy products, coffee, and vitamin C have been shown to have a protective effect against gout.[138]

In classic gouty arthritis, monosodium urate crystals form and cause joint inflammation. **Pseudogout** mimics gout; however, it is caused by the formation and deposition of calcium pyrophosphate dihydrate (CPPD) crystals. Calcium pyrophosphate dihydrate crystals predominantly deposit in joint cartilage and intervertebral disks.[144] The effect of either crystal is the same—the onset of a cytokine-mediated acute inflammatory response (see Chapter 7).

Gout is rare in children and premenopausal women and is uncommon in males younger than 30 years. Gout is more common in men and is thought to occur at a 3:1 ratio compared to women. Onset in men often peaks between the ages of 40 and 50 years. Onset of gout in females tends to occur at a later age since it is rarely seen in premenopausal women.[144,145] Additionally, a greater correlation exists in women with coexisting diseases, such as hypertension and renal insufficiency.[145] The plasma urate concentration is an important determinant of the risk of developing gout (Table 45.8). The risk of developing gouty arthritis is similar in males and females for particular urate concentrations.

Uric acid (UA) is a byproduct of protein metabolism that normally assists with removal of nitrogen waste from the body. At lower levels,

UA is an important antioxidant but at higher levels it acts as a pro-oxidant where it increases levels of free radicals and causes other inflammatory changes.[146] When ionized, uric acid can form salts with various cations but 98% of extracellular uric acid is in the form of monosodium urate (uric acid salt). At any time, the proportion of uric acid or urate is pH dependent, so the ratio of these two forms varies considerably in urine (Fig. 45.30).

The solubility of urate and uric acid is critical to the development of crystals. Urate is more soluble in plasma, synovial fluid, and urine than in aqueous solutions; the solubility in urine rises dramatically as the pH increases to more than 4. There is little change, however, in the solubility of urate within the normal pH range that exists in the plasma, synovial fluid, and other tissues. Decreasing temperatures cause both urate and uric acid solubility to fall. The pathways of production of uric acid are shown in Fig. 45.31.

◆**PATHOPHYSIOLOGY.** The pathophysiology of gout is closely linked to purine metabolism and kidney function. At the cellular level, purines are synthesized to purine nucleotides, which are used in the synthesis of nucleic acids, adenosine triphosphate, cyclic adenosine monophosphate (cAMP), and cyclic guanosine monophosphate (cGMP). Uric acid is a breakdown product of purine nucleotides (uric acid synthesis and elimination are illustrated in Fig. 45.32).[141] Individuals with gout may have an accelerated rate of purine synthesis accompanied by an overproduction of uric acid. Other individuals break down purine nucleotides at an accelerated rate, also resulting in an overproduction of uric acid. A deficiency of the enzyme HGPRT (see earlier) can lead to an increased production of uric acid. A complete absence of HGPRT is uncommon but can occur in the X-linked Lesch-Nyhan syndrome, with males at risk for hyperuricemia, neurologic alterations, and sometimes gouty arthritis. The majority of individuals with gout, however, have an unknown metabolic defect, which is referred to as **primary gout**. When the etiology is known, it is referred to as **secondary gout**.

Most uric acid is eliminated from the body through the kidneys. Urate is filtered at the glomerulus and undergoes reabsorption and

TABLE 45.8	MEAN URATE CONCENTRATIONS BY AGE AND GENDER	
CHARACTERISTIC	**MEAN URATE LEVELS (mg/dL)**
Prepuberty	3.5
Males (at puberty)	Steep rise to 5.2
Females (puberty to premenopause)	Slow rise to ≅4
Females (after menopause)	4.7
Hyperuricemia	
Men	7
Women	6

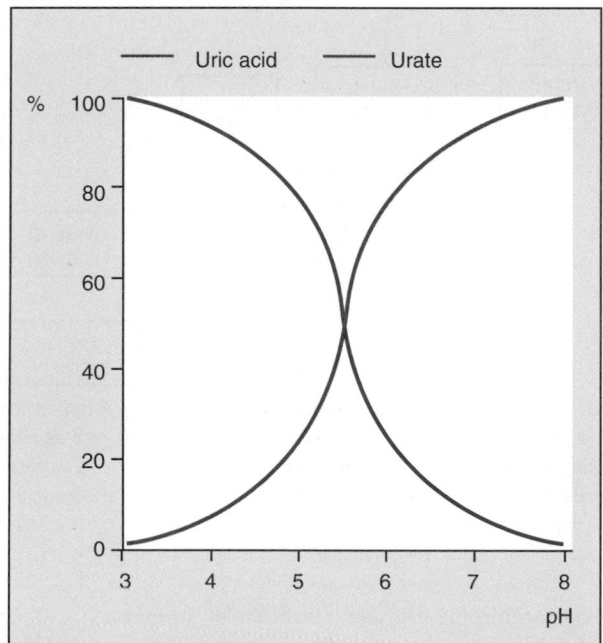

FIGURE 45.30 Effect of pH on Uric Acid and Urate Equilibrium. At pH 5.7, equal amounts of uric acid and urate are present in the solution. (Redrawn from Klippel JH, Dieppe PA, editors: *Rheumatology,* ed 2, London, 1998, Mosby-Wolfe.)

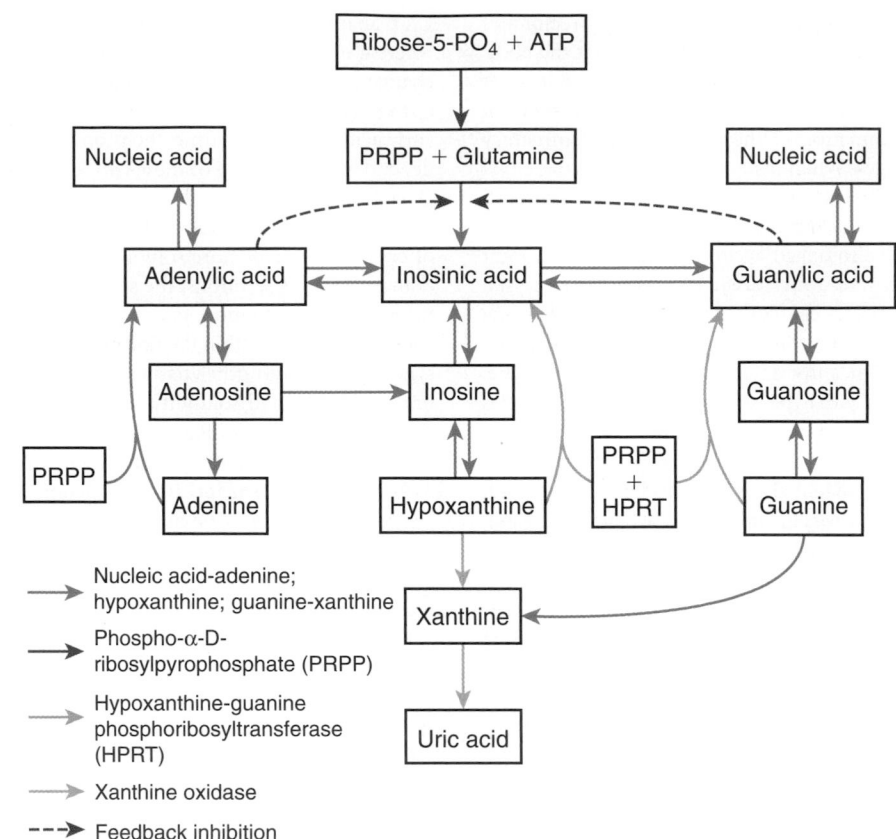

FIGURE 45.31 Production of Uric Acid. The major pathways involved in purine nucleotide synthesis. (Redrawn from Klippel JH, Dieppe PA, editors: *Rheumatology,* ed 2, London, 1998, Mosby-Wolfe.)

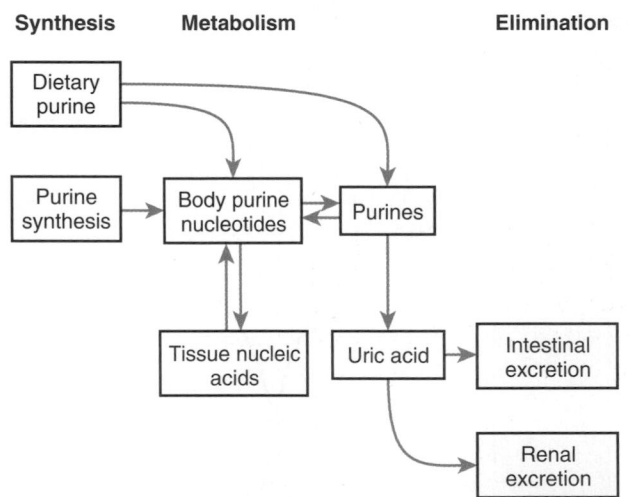

FIGURE 45.32 Uric Acid Synthesis and Elimination. Uric acid is derived from ingested purines or synthesized from ingested foods, as well as recycled following cell breakdown. Uric acid is then eliminated through the kidneys and gastrointestinal tract. (Redrawn from Klippel JH, Dieppe PA, editors: *Rheumatology,* ed 2, London, 1998, Mosby-Wolfe.)

excretion within the proximal renal tubules. In primary gout, urate excretion by the kidneys is sluggish; this may be the result of a decrease in glomerular filtration of urate or acceleration in urate reabsorption. In addition, MSU crystals deposited in renal tubules can cause acute nephropathy.[141] (Kidney function is described in Chapter 38.)

Monosodium urate crystals can stimulate and perpetuate the inflammatory response (Fig. 45.33). The presence of MSU crystals triggers the acute inflammatory response. Initiation of the complement system activates cytokines and interleukins, which draw neutrophils out of the circulation to begin phagocytizing the crystals.

A variety of inflammatory mediators are released during the crystal/cell response, of which IL-1β appears to be of prime importance. Other factors including chemotactic factors, lysosomal enzymes, eicosanoids, prostaglandin E_2 (PGE_2), reactive oxygen species, and collagenase also are released[141] (see Fig. 45.33, *A*). Some of these mediators stimulate the influx of neutrophils, monocytes, and lymphocytes. (Acute inflammation and phagocytosis are described in Chapter 7.)

Within the joint fluid, urate crystals react particularly with neutrophils and monocytes. Tissue damage begins to occur, principally when the neutrophils release the contents of their phagolysosomes (see Fig. 45.33, *B*). These contents also perpetuate inflammation. At an early phase of an acute gouty attack, synovial microtophi have been demonstrated. As the process continues, numerous microtophi may be present on the synovial membrane (see Fig. 45.33, *C*).

◆**CLINICAL MANIFESTATIONS.** Gout is manifested by (1) an increase in serum urate concentration (hyperuricemia); (2) recurrent attacks of monoarticular arthritis (inflammation of a single joint); (3) deposits of monosodium urate monohydrate (tophi) in and around the joints; (4) renal disease involving glomerular, tubular, and interstitial tissues and blood vessels; and (5) the formation of renal stones. These manifestations appear in three clinical stages:

1. **Asymptomatic hyperuricemia:** The serum urate level is elevated but arthritic symptoms, tophi, and renal stones are not present; may persist throughout life.

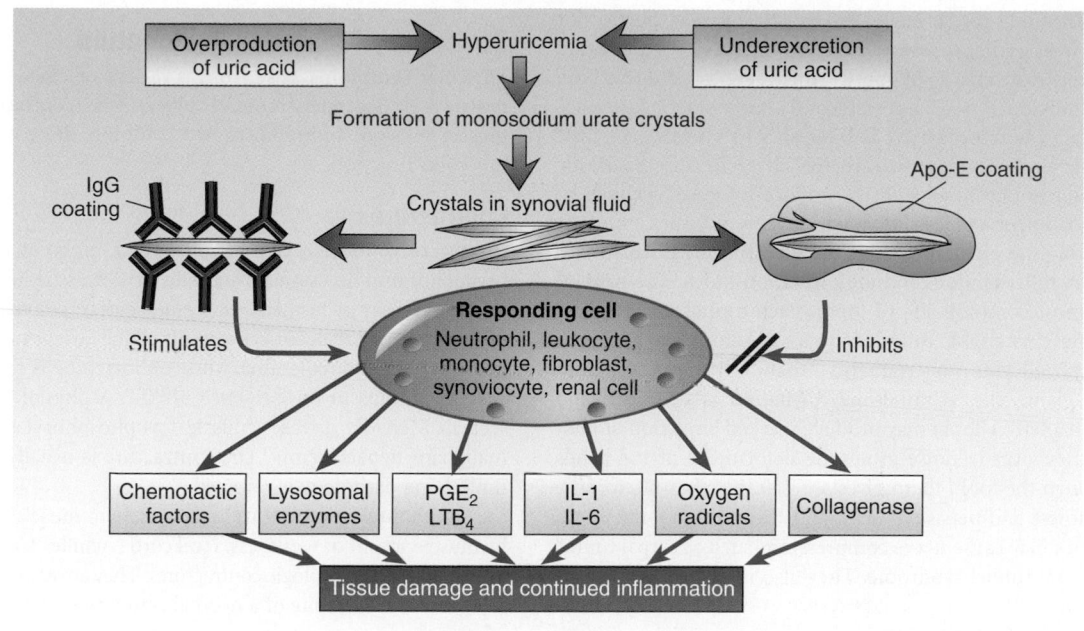

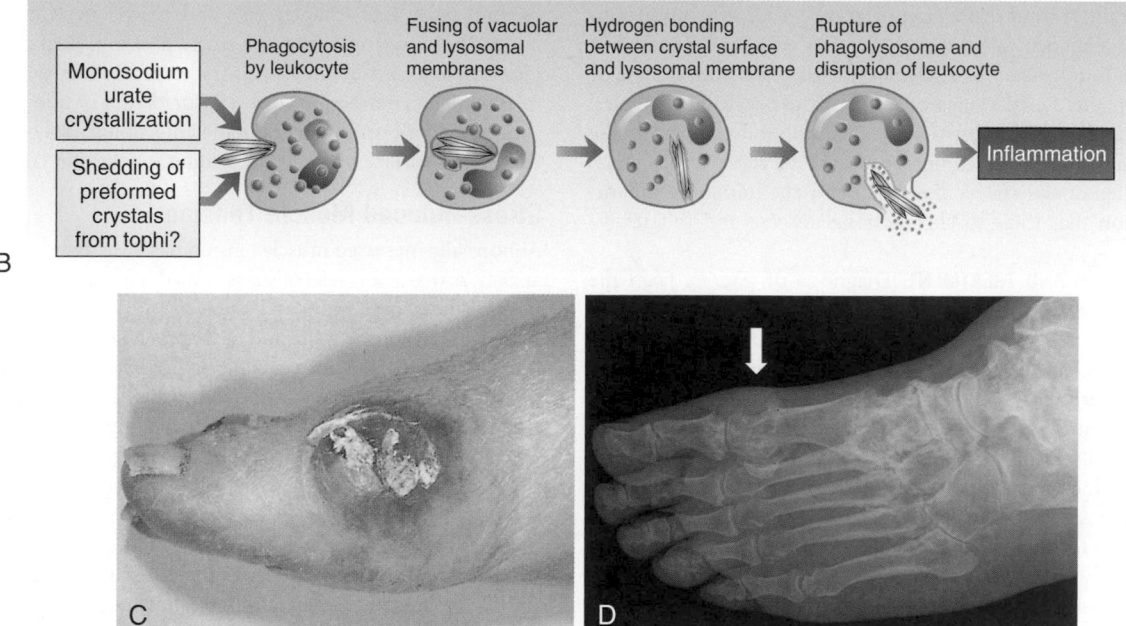

FIGURE 45.33 Pathogenesis of Acute Gouty Arthritis. **A,** Depending on the urate crystal coating, a variety of cells may be stimulated to produce a wide range of inflammatory mediators. **B,** Sequence of events in the production of inflammatory response to urate crystals. **C,** Gouty tophus on right foot. **D,** Bone destruction of first metatarsal because of gout. *Apo-E,* Apolipoprotein E; *IgG,* immunoglobulin G; *IL,* interleukin; *LTB₄,* leukotriene B₄; *PGE₂,* prostaglandin E. (**C** from Dieppe P et al: *Arthritis and rheumatism in practice,* London, 1991, Gower. **D** from Chhana A, Dalbeth N: *Rheum Dis Clin North Am* 40[2]:291–309, 2014.)

2. **Acute gouty arthritis:** Attacks develop with increased serum urate concentrations; tends to occur with sudden or sustained increases of hyperuricemia but also can be triggered by trauma, drugs, and alcohol.

3. **Tophaceous gout:** The third and chronic stage of disease; can begin as early as 3 years or as late as 40 years after the initial attack of gouty arthritis. Progressive inability to excrete uric acid expands the urate pool until urate crystal deposits (tophi) appear in cartilage, synovial membranes, tendons, and soft tissue.

Attacks of gouty arthritis occur abruptly, usually in a peripheral joint. The primary symptom is severe pain. Approximately 50% of the initial attacks occur in the metatarsophalangeal joint of the great toe. The other 50% involve the heel, ankle, and instep of the foot; knee; wrist; or elbow. The pain is usually noticed at night. Within a few hours the affected joint becomes hot, red, and extremely tender and may be slightly swollen. Lymphangitis and systemic signs of inflammation (leukocytosis, fever, elevated sedimentation rate) occasionally are present. Untreated, mild attacks usually subside in several hours but may persist for 1 or 2 days. Severe attacks may persist for several days or weeks. After recovery, the symptoms resolve completely. Intervals between acute attacks of gouty arthritis are called *intercritical periods*. Some individuals never have a second attack; others experience subsequent attacks within days to as long as 5 to 10 years after the first episode. Tophaceous deposits are the characteristic diagnostic lesions of chronic gout. These deposits produce irregular swellings of the fingers, hands, knees, and feet. Tophi within the soft tissue commonly form lumps along the ulnar surface of the forearm, the tibial surface of the leg, the Achilles tendon, and the olecranon bursa. The helix of the ear is the most common site of tophi. Each tophus consists of a deposit of urate crystals, surrounded by a granuloma made up of mononuclear phagocytes (macrophages) that have developed into epithelial and giant cells. (Granuloma formation is described and illustrated in Chapter 7.) Tophi may produce marked limitation of joint movement and eventually cause grotesque deformities of the hands and feet. Although the tophi themselves are painless, they often cause progressive stiffness and persistent aching of the affected joint. Tophi in the extremities may cause nerve compressions such as carpal tunnel syndrome or tarsal tunnel syndrome. They also may erode and drain through the skin.

Renal stones are 1000 times more prevalent in individuals with primary gout than in the general population. The stones can vary in size from a grain of sand to the size of gravel. A large accumulation can produce a staghorn calculus. Renal stones may be comprised of purse monosodium urate, but also may consist of calcium oxalate or calcium phosphate. Renal stones can form in the collecting tubules, pelvis, or ureters, causing obstruction, dilation, and atrophy of the more proximal tubules and leading eventually to acute renal failure. Stones deposited directly in renal interstitial tissue initiate an inflammatory reaction that leads to chronic renal disease and progressive renal failure.

◆**EVALUATION AND TREATMENT.** Diagnosis of gout is from the individual's history and physical examination; also included may be blood tests, possible joint aspiration, and the use of diagnostic imaging.[147,148] The goals of gout treatment are to terminate the acute gouty attack as promptly as possible; decrease serum uric acid levels; avoid recurring attacks; prevent or reverse complications associated with urate deposits in the joints, soft tissues, and kidneys; and prevent formation of kidney stones.[149] Numerous drugs are used to prevent or abort attacks of arthritis. Nonpharmacologic treatment includes the application of ice to relieve pain and inflammation of the joint. Weight-bearing on the involved joint is avoided until the acute attack subsides. Reducing body weight, avoiding alcohol, and changing dietary practices may reduce recurrent gouty episodes.[140]

DISORDERS OF SKELETAL MUSCLE

Weakness and fatigue are common symptoms of disorders of the skeletal muscles. In many cases, neural, traumatic, and psychogenic causes provide an adequate explanation for the failure to generate force (weakness) or sustain force (fatigue) seen in myopathies. The pathophysiologic mechanisms in some of the metabolic and inflammatory muscle diseases have been explored, but the cause of many of the myopathies remains obscure. Recognition and improved understanding of ryanodine receptor (RyR1) function have allowed identification of therapeutic targets in treating central core disease (CCD). The term *CCD* refers to the mitochondrial lack of oxidative enzyme activity in the central cytoplasmic area of the muscle caused by a genetic abnormality on chromosome 19. Complex interactions between muscles and nerves affect muscular function as well. Only inherited and acquired disorders of skeletal muscles are discussed here.

Secondary Muscular Dysfunction

Muscular symptoms arise from a variety of causes unrelated to the muscle itself. Secondary muscular phenomena (contracture, stress-related muscle tension, immobility) are common disorders that influence muscular function.

Contractures

Contractures are the lack of full passive range of motion of a joint because of muscle, connective tissue, or soft tissue limitations.[150] These limitations may be termed either *pathologic* or *physiologic*. A *physiologic muscle contracture* occurs as a result of the absence of a muscle action potential in the sarcolemma. Muscle shortening is caused by failure of calcium pumps in the presence of ATP. A physiologic contracture is seen in McArdle disease (muscle myophosphorylase deficiency) and malignant hyperthermia. The contracture is usually temporary if the underlying pathology is reversed.

A pathologic contracture is a permanent muscle shortening caused by muscle spasm or weakness. Heel cord (Achilles tendon) contractures are examples of pathologic contractures. They are associated with plentiful ATP and occur in spite of a normal action potential. Most occurrences of pathologic contractures are seen in neuromuscular disorders such as Charcot-Marie-Tooth disease, amyotrophic lateral sclerosis (ALS), cerebral palsy (see Chapter 46), and central nervous system (CNS) injury. Prolonged splinting in a single position, such as an elbow, also may lead to a contracture.[151] Contractures also may develop secondary to scar tissue contraction in the flexor tissues of a joint, for example, contracture of burned tissues in the antecubital area of the forearm or the palmar surface of the hand leading to a flexion contracture.[152]

Stress-Induced Muscle Tension

Abnormally increased muscle tension has been associated with chronic anxiety, as well as a variety of stress-related muscular symptoms, including neck stiffness, back pain, and headache.[153] Abnormalities in the CNS, reticular activating system, and autonomic nervous system (ANS) have been implicated. The underlying pathophysiology may be related to the fact that as a muscle contracts, the muscle spindle is activated. This gamma-feedback system produces a series of impulses that are transmitted to the brain by the sensitive 1A afferent fibers. Unconscious tension is thought to increase the activity of the reticular activating system as well. This causes increased firing of the efferent loop of the gamma fibers and produces further muscle contraction, which increases muscle tension. ANS function that regulates increased blood flow to the muscle during sympathetic activity may be related to increased muscle contraction tension.

Various forms of treatment have been used to reduce the muscle tension associated with stress. Progressive relaxation training, yoga, meditation, and biofeedback are examples of stress reduction therapies.

Fibromyalgia

Fibromyalgia (FM) is a chronic musculoskeletal syndrome characterized by widespread joint and muscle pain, fatigue, and tender points. The absence of systemic or localized inflammation and the presence of increased sensitivity to touch (i.e., tender points), fatigue/nonrestorative sleep, and anxiety and depression are common. Individuals with FM report diffuse tenderness in all body regions and an increased sensitivity to numerous types of stimuli, including heat, cold, and electrical stimuli. Other research also identifies sensitivity to light and sound.[154] New research suggests the possible link between an inflammatory process and the development of FM.[155-157] In the past, a common misdiagnosis has been chronic fatigue syndrome and there is overlap of symptoms between these two conditions. From 80% to 90% of individuals affected

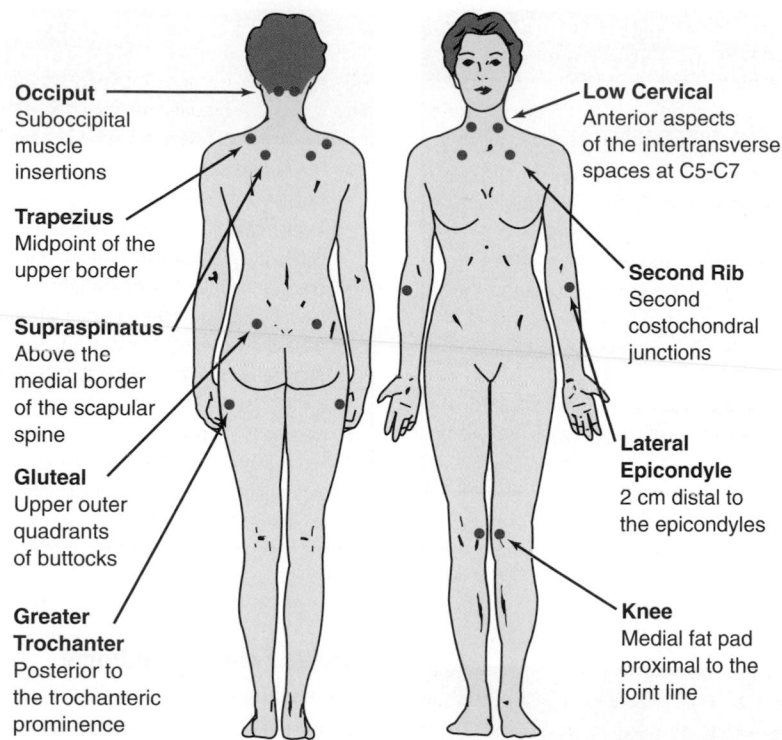

Occiput
Suboccipital muscle insertions

Trapezius
Midpoint of the upper border

Supraspinatus
Above the medial border of the scapular spine

Gluteal
Upper outer quadrants of buttocks

Greater Trochanter
Posterior to the trochanteric prominence

Low Cervical
Anterior aspects of the intertransverse spaces at C5-C7

Second Rib
Second costochondral junctions

Lateral Epicondyle
2 cm distal to the epicondyles

Knee
Medial fat pad proximal to the joint line

FIGURE 45.34 Location of Specific Tender Points for Diagnostic Classification of Fibromyalgia. (Redrawn from Freundlich B, Leventhal L: The fibromyalgia syndrome. In Schumacher HR Jr, Klippel JH, Koopman WJ, editors: *Primer on the rheumatic diseases,* ed 11, Atlanta, 1997, Arthritis Foundation. Copyright ©1997. Reprinted with permission of the Arthritis Foundation.)

are women, and the peak age is 30 to 50 years. Although the incidence is unknown, the prevalence is reported to be 2% to almost 6% and increases with age.[158] The American College of Rheumatology has identified new criteria for the diagnosis of FM. A tender point evaluation is no longer required; instead, the use of a widespread pain index (WPI) and symptom severity inventory (SSI) is recommended.[159] For the WPI evaluation, the individual also is asked to identify body regions where pain has been experienced during the last 1-week time period (Fig. 45.34). For the SSI evaluation, the individual is then asked to rank specific symptoms of fatigue, waking unrefreshed, cognitive symptoms, and somatic symptoms on a scale of 0 to 3. A diagnosis of FM is then determined on the basis of both the WPI score and the SSI score.[158,159] For example, a WPI of at least 7 and SSI of at least 5; or a WPI of 3 to 6 and SSI of at least 9.

Although the etiology of FM is unknown, it is thought to involve both genetic susceptibility and environmental exposure that triggers alterations in gene expression (epigenetics).[160] Current hypotheses for the etiology of FM include numerous interacting factors: psychologic, genetic/epigenetic, neurobiologic, and environmental.[160] Despite much debate on the classification and pathophysiology of FM, it is now recognized as a disorder.[160]

◆**PATHOPHYSIOLOGY.** FM has unclear pathophysiology. Genetic factors are increasingly being suggested as important in developing FM. Aggregation of fibromyalgia within families and other coexisting conditions, such as irritable bowel syndrome, chronic fatigue, and mood disorders, suggest a major role for neuroendocrine and stress-response alterations (see Chapter 11). Studies of genetic factors have implicated alterations in genes affecting serotonin, catecholamines, and dopamine—all of these substances are involved in the stress response and sensory processing.[161,162] In spite of these studies, the role of genetic factors in FM has not yet been fully identified. Studies have suggested a link between stress/stressors (such as infection including Lyme disease, psychosocial stress, sleep abnormalities, immune dysfunction, physical or emotional trauma) and FM.[154] These relationships continue to be researched.

Functional magnetic resonance imaging (fMRI) and positron emission tomography (PET) scans of the brains of persons with FM have shown activity in different areas of the brain than in healthy individuals when exposed to painful stimuli.[163] Individuals with fibromyalgia have lowered mechanical and thermal pain thresholds, high pain ratings for provoking stimuli, and altered temporal summation of pain stimuli. Functional abnormalities within the CNS are shown in Fig. 45.34. Other pathophysiologic evidence includes hypothalamic-pituitary-adrenal (HPA) axis alterations that demonstrate abnormal response to pain.[164] Recent investigations suggest cytokines are involved in the pathogenesis of FM.[157] Corticotropin-releasing hormone (CRH) and locus ceruleus–norepinephrine (LC/NE), their peripheral effectors, and the hypothalamic-pituitary-adrenal axis are the main components of the stress system. Impaired functioning of the HPA axis and LC/NE system may be associated with fibromyalgia.[154]

◆**CLINICAL MANIFESTATIONS.** The prominent symptom of fibromyalgia is diffuse, chronic pain. As discussed previously, the American College of Rheumatology has identified new criteria for the diagnosis of FM that expand to include other nonpain symptoms.[165] A tender point evaluation is no longer required. Instead, the use of a widespread pain index (WPI) and symptom severity inventory (SSI) is recommended. Pain often begins in one location, especially the neck and shoulders, but then becomes more generalized. Fatigue is most notable when arising from sleep and during the midafternoon. Headaches, symptoms of irritable bowel syndrome, and excess sensitivity to cold (Raynaud-like) are reported in 50% of individuals.

TABLE 45.9   DIFFERENTIAL DIAGNOSIS OF FIBROMYALGIA

DIFFERENTIAL DIAGNOSIS	HELPFUL DIFFERENTIAL FEATURES
Rheumatoid arthritis*	Synovitis, serologic tests, elevated erythrocyte sedimentation rate (ESR)
Systemic lupus erythematosus	Dermatitis, serositis (renal, central erythematosus,* nervous system, etc.)
Polymyalgia rheumatica*	Elevated ESR, older adults, response to corticosteroids
Myositis	Increased muscle enzymes, weakness more than pain
Hypothyroidism*	Abnormal thyroid function tests
Neuropathies	Clinical and electrophysiologic evidence of neuropathy

*Fibromyalgia may also more commonly coexist with these conditions.
Data from Klippel JH, Dieppe PA, editors: *Rheumatology*, ed 2, London, 1998, Mosby-Wolfe.

TABLE 45.10   CONCOMITANT CONDITIONS WITH FIBROMYALGIA

CONCOMITANT CONDITION	RELATIONSHIP TO FIBROMYALGIA
Depression	Present in 25%–60% of fibromyalgia cases
Irritable bowel syndrome	Present in 50%–80% of fibromyalgia cases
Migraine	Present in 50% of fibromyalgia cases
Chronic fatigue syndrome (CFS)	70% of CFS cases meet criteria for fibromyalgia
Myofascial pain	May be a localized form of fibromyalgia

Data from Klippel JH, Dieppe PA, editors: *Rheumatology*, ed 2, London, 1998, Mosby-Wolfe.

Almost 25% of individuals seek psychologic support for depression. Anxiety, particularly in regard to their diagnosis and future, is almost universal. Again, the only reliable finding on examination is the presence of multiple tender points.

◆EVALUATION AND TREATMENT. Because the manifestations of chronic, generalized pain and fatigue are present in many musculoskeletal (e.g., rheumatic) disorders, these disorders should be considered in the diagnosis of fibromyalgia (Tables 45.9 and 45.10). The WPI and SSI are then used for diagnostic and evaluation purposes.

No single regimen of medication has proved successful for fibromyalgia. Current recommendations outline a combination of both pharmacologic and nonpharmacologic therapies.[158] Stress reduction, sleep, and exercise remain central lifestyle modifications for individuals living with FM. Medications that improve sleep may be helpful as well as vitamin D supplementation. Antiinflammatories have been used despite the fact there is no evidence of tissue inflammation, but these medications have not been effective. Certain CNS-active medications, most notably pregabalin, were better than placebo in controlled trials.[166] Other medications, designed to augment the activity of neurotransmitters and the endogenous opioid system, also have been shown to provide symptom relief.[158] The most effective approach is a combination of modalities, including education, medication, exercise, and cognitive-behavioral therapy.[167-169] Box 45.6 lists some of these modalities.

BOX 45.6   EDUCATION AND REASSURANCE FOR INDIVIDUALS WITH FIBROMYALGIA

- Stress that the illness is real, not imagined.
- Explain that fibromyalgia is not a deforming or deteriorating condition.
- Explain that fibromyalgia is neither life-threatening nor markedly debilitating, although it is an irritating presence.
- Discuss the role of sleep disturbances and the relationship of neurohormones to pain, fatigue, abnormal sleep, and mood.
- Reassure individual that although the cause is unknown, some information is known about the physiologic changes responsible for the symptoms.
- Use muscle "spasms" and perhaps low muscle blood flow to lay the groundwork for exercise recommendations.
- Assist individual to use aerobic exercise to reduce stress and increase rapid eye movement (REM) sleep.

Chronic Fatigue Syndrome

Chronic fatigue syndrome (CFS), also known as myalgic encephalomyelitis (ME), is a debilitating and complex disorder characterized by profound fatigue, musculoskeletal pain, cognitive impairment, unrefreshing sleep, impaired neurologic energy production, and immune impairments. Additionally, individuals may experience sore throat, headache, and tender lymph nodes. These symptoms, however, occur without a clear pathophysiologic explanation.[170] Without a clear etiology, diagnosis of CFS is often a diagnosis of exclusion. Current research is investigating the potential impact of the immune and adrenal systems, as well as genetics and biopsychosocial involvement.[171] As a result, CFS/ME is believed to be less of a musculoskeletal disorder and more related to hypersensitivity of the central nervous system, a condition also known as *central sensitization*. Although individuals with CFS have widespread pain and fatigue, they do not have the tender points associated with fibromyalgia.[172]

◆PATHOPHYSIOLOGY. The exact etiology and pathophysiology of CFS remain unknown. Therefore recent International Consensus Criteria have recommended use of the term myalgic encephalomyelitis (ME) rather than chronic fatigue syndrome, because ME indicates an underlying pathophysiology.[173] Studies are currently investigating the possible involvement of skeletal muscle abnormalities, mitochondrial dysfunction, abnormal cytokine regulation, and dysfunction of the hypothalamic-pituitary-adrenal (HPA) axis.[174,175] In support of this, functional MRI (fMRI) has shown lower blood perfusion to the brainstem in individuals affected by CFS.[172] Other researchers have shown apparent central nervous system abnormalities, immunologic dysregulation, and higher-than-normal levels of proinflammatory cytokines. Certain points in skeletal muscle may be affected by oxidative stress reactions (see Chapter 2), accounting for the muscle pain and fatigue associated with CFS; however, other research implicates central sensitization of the CNS.[176]

◆CLINICAL MANIFESTATIONS. Unrestful sleep is a hallmark of CFS. Defining symptoms include debilitating fatigue made worse by physical or mental exercise (postexertional fatigue), muscle pain, noninflammatory joint pain, headaches, flulike symptoms, and memory or concentration problems.[171] Other common symptoms include bloating, morning joint stiffness, chest or jaw pain, chills and night sweats, visual disturbances, sore throat, and tender axillary or cervical lymph nodes. Symptoms and their consequences can be severe.

◆**EVALUATION AND TREATMENT.** Diagnosis of CFS is often delayed or missed because there is no biologic marker or specific laboratory test for CFS, many CFS symptoms are shared with other illnesses, individuals with CFS do not necessarily appear sick, and symptoms typically have a variable course. Currently, the CDC recommends considering a diagnosis of CFS if the following two criteria are met[177]:

1. Unexplained, persistent fatigue is not due to ongoing exertion, is not substantially relieved by rest, is of new onset (not lifelong), and results in a significant reduction of previous levels of activity.
2. Four or more of the following symptoms are present for 6 months or more:

   Impaired memory or concentration
   Postexertional malaise (extreme, prolonged exhaustion and exacerbation of symptoms following physical or mental exertion)
   Unrefreshing sleep
   Muscle pain
   Multijoint pain without swelling or redness (adults)
   Headaches of a new type or severity
   Sore throat that is frequent or recurring
   Tender cervical or axillary lymph nodes

Treatment of CFS should focus on symptom management, especially management of sleep disturbances, depression, and pain.[171] Consideration of the person's individual needs also must be made, and involves consideration of psychosocial factors as well as symptomatic and supportive care. Acknowledging the validity of the person's symptoms is important. Collaborative decision making between the individual and healthcare provider with regard to treatment, professional counseling, medication, diet, and activity helps CFS sufferers deal with the limitations imposed by the disease. Alternative therapies such as acupuncture, massage, and therapeutic touch can relieve anxiety.

Disuse Atrophy

Disuse atrophy describes the pathologic reduction in normal size of muscle fibers from an accelerated degradation of myofibrillar proteins. This may be associated with the normal aging process (sarcopenia), as well as following periods of prolonged immobilization and low mechanical load, such as from inactivity during bed rest, trauma (casting), local nerve damage, and space flight.[178] Disease-induced atrophy also is seen in debilitating conditions, such as cancer, acquired immunodeficiency syndrome (AIDS), renal failure, congestive heart failure, chronic obstructive pulmonary disease, and burns.[179] Studies have shown the effects of muscular deconditioning associated with lack of physical activity have been seen in as few as 5 days after immobility.[180] Oxidative stress from lack of muscle activity causes decreased protein synthesis and increased proteolysis, leading to muscle atrophy.[181] The normal individual on bed rest loses muscle strength from baseline levels at a rate of 3% per day. Bed rest also is associated with cardiovascular, skeletal, and other organ system changes.

The most effective restorative measure for disuse atrophy is to reapply mechanical load to the muscle group. Resistance exercise, stretching, and electrical stimulation have been shown to reduce the extent of atrophy in individuals who are immobilized or on bed rest.[179] Measures to prevent atrophy include adequate nutrition, frequent forceful isometric muscle contractions, and passive lengthening exercises. If reuse is not restored within 1 year, regeneration of muscle fibers becomes impaired.

Muscle Membrane Abnormalities

Two defects of the muscle membrane (plasma membrane of the muscle fiber) have been linked to clinical syndromes: the hyperexcitable membrane seen in the myotonic disorders and the intermittently unresponsive membrane seen in periodic paralyses. Although these are infrequent disorders, research into the pathologic processes has led to an improved understanding of the cell membrane channelopathies.

Skeletal Muscle Channelopathies

Skeletal muscle channelopathies can be divided into two primary groups: those presenting with myotonia (nondystrophic myotonias) and those associated with episodes of weakness (periodic paralysis). In **myotonic channelopathies**, muscle relaxation is delayed after voluntary contractions, such as handgrip or eye closure, leading to a disabling muscle stiffness and/or weakness. Periodic paralysis is an autosomal dominant disorder in which depolarization of the sarcolemma is severe enough that the muscle cannot be "fired" again, resulting in paralysis or even myotonia.[182]

Myotonia can be reproduced by removing extracellular chloride, thus reducing chloride conductance across the plasma membrane. The delicate balance in which sodium diffuses into the intracellular fluid, potassium diffuses out of the intracellular fluid, and chloride is in flux is thus interrupted. Because the normal diffusion processes (described in Chapter 3) stabilize the membrane, the shift in chloride ions is thought to increase membrane excitability. The chloride abnormality may explain the resting membrane hyperexcitability, but it does not explain the delayed relaxation present in myotonia and has not been detected in human myotonia.

Myotonia is seen in several disorders: myotonia congenita, paramyotonia congenita, myotonic muscular dystrophy, and some forms of periodic paralysis. Most are inherited disorders and are mild in symptomatology, with the exception of myotonic muscular dystrophy (see Chapter 46). Myotonia is treated by drugs that reduce muscle fiber excitability, such as sodium channel blocking agents (mexiletine, procainamide) and phenytoin.[183]

Central core disease (CCD) is another inherited channelopathy that involves mutations in ryanodine receptors (RyR1) and affects calcium channels. In CCD, RyR1 channels are defective and either too much or too little calcium is released from the cell's sarcoplasmic reticulum, resulting in symmetrical proximal muscle weakness. This weakness, however, is typically not progressive in nature.[184] Classified as a neuromuscular disorder, CCD typically manifests during infancy as decreased muscle tone, delayed motor development, muscle weakness (particularly around the hip girdle), and other skeletal deformities, such as scoliosis.[185] Thought to be the most common congenital myopathy, the pathology of CCD relates to the lack of "cores" within skeletal myofibers that do not contain mitochondria and their oxidative enzymes. Therefore definitive diagnosis is made through muscle biopsy.[184]

Periodic Paralysis

Periodic paralysis (PP) encompasses a group of muscle diseases caused by the inheritance of an autosomal dominant mutation of skeletal muscle sodium, calcium, or potassium channels.[186,187] During an attack of PP the muscle membrane is unresponsive to neural stimuli and the resting membrane potential is reduced from −90 to −45 mV. Periodic paralysis can be either hyper- or hypokalemic. As the name implies, PP is usually transient.

The paralysis, which leaves the individual flaccid and weak, typically only affects the skeletal muscles and not the respiratory muscles. The weakness is accompanied by a change in serum potassium level, although in most individuals the change is negligible unless a secondary underlying condition affecting potassium distribution coexists.[188] For this reason, cardiac dysrhythmias, although not common, have been present during attacks.

Hypokalemic periodic paralysis is most often triggered by thyrotoxicosis caused by alterations in potassium ion channels that are regulated by triiodothyronine (T_3).[188,189] (The effect of potassium on the resting membrane potential is discussed in Chapter 3.) Glucose and insulin infusions and oral potassium loading are used as provocative tests; oral and intravenous potassium can relieve acute attacks. Treatment includes potassium-sparing diuretics and a high-salt diet. Acetazolamide, dichlorphenamide, and a low-salt diet are useful for long-term therapy. Hyperkalemic periodic paralysis is caused by an *SNC4A* genetic mutation affecting sodium channels and can be precipitated by several factors including pregnancy, alcohol, illness, exercise, and increased potassium intake.[190] Attacks are usually less severe than the hypokalemic form. Treatment includes small carbohydrate-rich meals, light exercise, and intravenous calcium gluconate.[191]

Metabolic Muscle Diseases

Metabolic muscle diseases are a collection of disorders caused by a genetic mutation impacting a muscle's metabolism. Disorders in muscle metabolism can be caused by endocrine abnormalities or by diseases of energy metabolism, such as glycogen storage disease, enzyme deficiencies, and abnormalities in lipid metabolism and mitochondrial function.

Endocrine Disorders

Often the systemic effects of hormonal imbalance overshadow the individual's muscular symptoms. For example, individuals with thyrotoxicosis may have signs of proximal weakness, paresis of the extraocular muscles (exhibited as exophthalmic ophthalmoplegia), or hypokalemic periodic paralysis, as discussed earlier in the previous section. Hypothyroidism is often associated with a decrease in muscle mass and strength, with weak, flabby skeletal muscles and sluggish movements.

Thyroid hormone is believed to regulate muscle protein synthesis and electrolyte balance. Changes in muscle protein synthesis and electrolyte balance may therefore explain the alterations in muscle mass and contractility seen in endocrine disorders. The muscle symptoms subside with appropriate treatment of the primary hormonal disorder.

Other endocrine disorders affecting the musculoskeletal system include Dent disease (a syndrome that causes bone deformities); rickets or osteomalacia (softening of the bone because of deficiencies in vitamin D and calcium); and osteopetrosis (also known as *Albers-Schönberg disease*) caused by failure of osteoclasts to resorb bone, which thereby results in increased bone mass while causing increased bone fragility, growth abnormalities, and bone marrow failure in infants as bone marrow is replaced by bony masses.[192] Familial hypomagnesemia is an autosomal recessive disease that primarily affects the renal system, causing hypomagnesemia and secondary hypocalcemia, and can result in tetany and convulsions.[193]

Diseases of Energy Metabolism

Muscle relies on carbohydrates, such as glycogen and lipids (free fatty acids), for energy. When stored glycogen or lipids cannot be used because of a lack of the enzyme necessary to convert energy for contraction, the individual experiences cramps, fatigue, and exercise intolerance. Disorders of muscle metabolism can be self-limiting, such as is seen in McArdle disease and some lipid disorders, or can cause widespread irreparable muscle destruction, as in acid maltase deficiency.

McArdle Disease. McArdle disease, or glycogen myophosphorylase deficiency, is an autosomal recessive disease and was the first myopathy in which a single enzyme defect was identified (Fig. 45.35). Individuals with McArdle disease lack muscle phosphorylase, which is responsible for the breakdown of glycogen in muscle.[194] Normally after the body uses the short-term ATP and phosphocreatine stores, intramuscular lactic acid accumulates as glycogen is used (see Chapter 44). The individual with McArdle disease is not able to break down muscle glycogen stores or produce lactic acid.[195]

The altered energy production manifests itself in exercise intolerance, fatigue, and painful muscle cramps. When exercise is carried to an extreme, painful muscle contracture and myoglobinuria develop.[196] Some individuals describe a "second wind" phenomenon, in which exercise tolerance increases if they slow their pace once the initial sensation of fatigue commences. This is caused by the use of free fatty acids as a secondary source of energy.[195] As the disease progresses, some individuals have pronounced muscle weakness and wasting. Other organs are not involved because the absence of phosphorylase is limited to muscle. Generally, individuals with McArdle disease learn to adapt their daily routine to avoid muscle symptoms. Usually the diagnosis of McArdle disease is made by the histochemical evaluation of myophosphorylase activity in frozen sections. There is no staining of myofibrils in affected individuals.

Acid Maltase Deficiency. Acid maltase deficiency is an uncommon, autosomal recessive disorder affecting glycogen storage from an accumulation of glycogen in the lysosomes of muscle and other tissue cells.[197] The usual pathways of glycogen degradation are preserved. However, deficiency of α-glucosidase (GAA) enzyme is responsible for the abnormality in glycogen metabolism.

The infantile form, Pompe disease, is often recognized shortly after birth because of the presence of hypotonia, respiratory weakness, dysreflexia, and physiologic abnormalities such as cardiomegaly, an

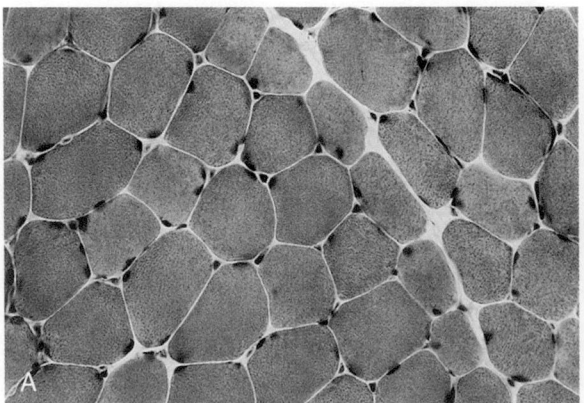
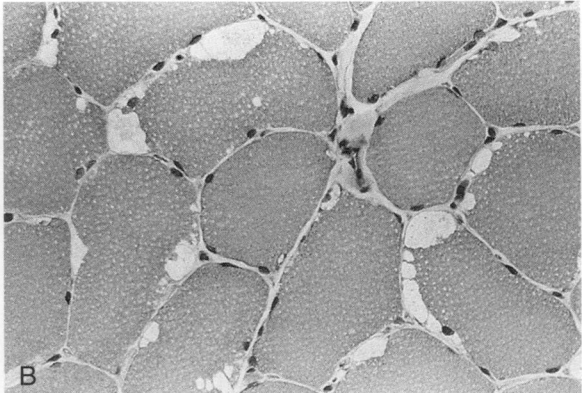

FIGURE 45.35 McArdle Disease. **A,** Normal muscle fibers. **B,** Muscle fibers of McArdle disease. Note the enlarged *(white)* peripheral vacuoles. (From Damjanov I, Linder J, editors: *Anderson's pathology,* ed 10, St Louis, 1996, Mosby.)

enlarged tongue, and hepatomegaly.[198] The adult form tends to be less severe than the infantile form. Hypertrophy of these tissues is thought to be the result of glycogen deposition. Diagnosis of Pompe disease can be made through the evaluation of GAA activity in blood or through muscle biopsy.[199] Previously, children with Pompe disease often died of cardiac or respiratory failure before age 2; now enzyme replacement therapy (ERT) with recombinant human acid α-glucosidase and physical therapy has shown a significant improvement in symptom presentation.[200,201]

Myoadenylate Deaminase Deficiency. Myoadenylate deaminase deficiency (MDD), also referred to as *adenosine monophosphate deaminase deficiency,* is a fairly common, autosomal recessive, enzyme deficiency that causes changes in skeletal muscles and is associated with exercise intolerance accompanied by muscle pain and cramps, although the majority of individuals are asymptomatic.[202,203] Because these individuals lack myoadenylate deaminase, they have a poor capacity for sustained energy production. Myoadenylate deaminase is the catalytic enzyme that forms phosphocreatine and ATP during exercise through a metabolic pathway that binds the purine and phosphate molecules that constitute ATP. Persons with MDD differ from those with McArdle disease in that during the ischemic exercise test, lactate production is normal when ATP and phosphocreatine are synthesized. Symptoms range from minimal complaints to exercise-induced muscle pain, to rhabdomyolysis.[204] Currently, there are limited reports of successful treatments. Avoidance of rigorous exercise is generally recommended.[203]

Lipid Deficiencies. Inherited disorders of lipid metabolism are uncommon but account for severe changes in muscle metabolism. The lipid content of muscle cells consists of free fatty acids, which are oxidized in the mitochondria. These acids require carnitine and the enzyme carnitine palmitoyltransferase (CPT) to transport long-chain fatty acids to the mitochondria. Individuals with CPT deficiency often have mild muscular symptoms but can experience bouts of renal failure caused by rhabdomyolysis. Individuals with a deficiency of carnitine alone have progressive muscle weakness and can experience sudden exacerbations.[205]

Measuring the CPT and carnitine content in muscle aids in the diagnosis. Cells in the muscle biopsy show vacuoles and lipid deposits. Treatments with riboflavin, medium-chain triglycerides, oral carnitine, prednisone, and propranolol are proposed.[206]

Inflammatory Muscle Diseases: Myositis
Viral, Bacterial, and Parasitic Myositis

Viral, bacterial, and parasitic infections of varying severity are known to produce inflammatory changes in skeletal muscle, a group of conditions collectively described by the term myositis. In tuberculosis and sarcoidosis, chronic inflammatory changes and granulomas are found in muscle, as well as in other affected tissues. In trichinellosis, *Trichinella* larvae reside in infected muscles of infected animals, such as pigs, horses, and other wildlife, such as cougars and black bears.[207] After ingestion, the parasites migrate to the intestinal mucosa and from there to the lymphatic and circulatory systems. Initial symptoms occur 1 to 2 days following consumption of infected meat and present as gastrointestinal distress (nausea, diarrhea, vomiting, abdominal pain). The more traditional trichinellosis symptoms generally occur from 2 to 8 weeks after ingestion and include muscle pain and stiffness, fever, rash, itching, and headaches.[207] Treatment includes administration of corticosteroids, such as prednisone, and antiparasitic agents, such as albendazole. Mebendazole also may be used, though it is not available in the United States.[208] Toxoplasmosis, a common parasitic infection, is also associated with a generalized polymyositis that responds rapidly to therapy.

In the tropics, more prevalent disorders include bacterial infections with *Staphylococcus aureus* and parasites such as cysticercus, the larva

of the tapeworm *Taenia solium.* Viral infections can be associated with an acute myositis. Muscle pain, tenderness, signs of inflammation, and elevation of creatine kinase (CK) level are common manifestations of viral myositis. The self-limiting symptoms of muscle aches and pains during a bout of influenza may actually be a subacute form of viral myopathy.

Polymyositis, Dermatomyositis, and Inclusion-Body Myositis

Idiopathic inflammatory myopathies (IIMs) are a group of autoimmune diseases that typically target skeletal muscles, though cutaneous manifestations have been documented in 50% to 60% of individuals.[209] IIMs are characterized by symmetrical proximal muscle weakness (hip and neck flexors, and shoulder girdle) and myalgia that develops over weeks to months. The four principle types are polymyositis (PM), dermatomyositis (DM), necrotizing myopathy (NM), and inclusion-body myositis (IBM).[210] The incidence of IIM appears to be increasing, but this may simply reflect improved diagnosis. With an incidence of 5 to 22 per 100,000, it is more prevalent in nonwhite women older than age 50.

PATHOPHYSIOLOGY. Polymyositis and dermatomyositis are characterized by inflammation of connective tissue and muscle fibers. Polymyositis is mediated by T cells, whereas dermatomyositis is humorally mediated.[211] CD8+ T cells and macrophages are typically found in PM-affected muscles. Fig. 45.36 shows the distribution of CD4+ and CD8+ lymphocytes in myositis. Innate and adaptive immune responses are activated in these myopathies, including myositis-specific antibodies and cytokines.[212] Inflammatory cells, including T cells, macrophages, and plasma cells, surround, displace, and even invade muscle fibers in

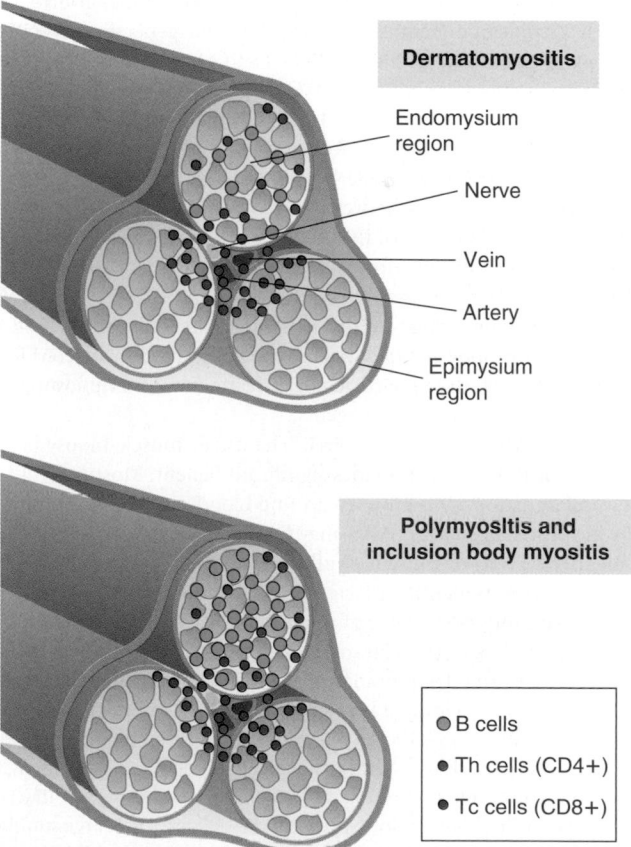

FIGURE 45.36 Distribution of CD4+ and CD8+ Lymphocytes in Different Types of Myositis. Dermatomyositis shows perivascular and CD4+ T cells (helper T cells). Polymyositis shows mostly CD8+ T cells (cytotoxic T cells).

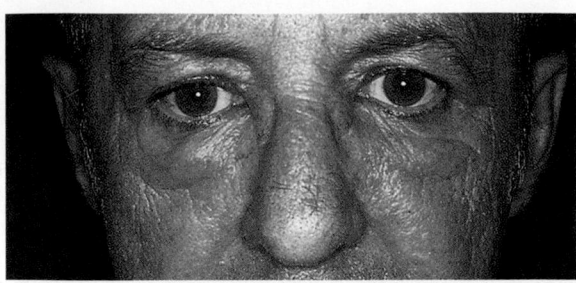

FIGURE 45.37 Dermatomyositis. Heliotrope (violaceous) discoloration around the eyes and periorbital edema. (From Habif TP: *Clinical dermatology*, ed 3, St Louis, 1996, Mosby.)

PM. Perimysial and perivascular sites are selectively enriched in B cells and helper T cells in those with DM.

◆**CLINICAL MANIFESTATIONS.** The acute symptoms include many of those seen in any inflammatory process: malaise, fever, muscle swelling, pain and tenderness, lethargy, and listlessness. In adults, weakness of the shoulder and pelvic girdle muscles is a primary manifestation of PM. Both PM and DM often are associated with symmetrical proximal muscle weakness and initially can be confused with other myopathies. A thorough evaluation is required to exclude other disorders. Clinical features common to both are dysphagia, reduced esophageal motility, vasculitis, Raynaud phenomenon, cardiomyopathy, and interstitial pulmonary fibrosis. Some individuals have other coexisting collagen vascular disorders, such as RA, systemic lupus erythematosus (SLE), and progressive systemic sclerosis (formerly called *scleroderma*).

Although PM and DM have similar histories of onset, DM includes cutaneous manifestations. The two most classic signs of skin involvement are (1) a heliotrope (reddish purple) rash that generally covers the eyelids and periorbital area (Fig. 45.37), and often includes the chest; and (2) erythematous, scaly lesions (Gottron lesions) that cover joints, such as the knees and elbows.[212] DM is slightly more common in children and older adults, with onset before age 15 or after age 50. The adult with DM occasionally has underlying malignancies.[213]

Additional differences between PM and DM exist. Muscle biopsy and histopathologic studies of IBM show degenerative changes of muscle, accumulation of multiple proteins within muscle fibers, and evidence of endoplasmic reticular stress with misfolding of proteins.[214,215] Clinically, IBM may show weakness of the wrist and finger flexors as well as asymmetrical atrophy and quadriceps weakness. Additionally, IBM does not respond to standard pharmacologic treatment of immunosuppressants and immune-modifying agents.[216]

◆**EVALUATION AND TREATMENT.** The use of muscle biopsy in the diagnosis of PM or DM provides significant benefit. Most individuals show inflammatory cells grouped around blood vessels and atrophy of cells in muscle fascicles.[213] MRI may be used concomitantly not only to identify regions of muscular inflammation and edema suitable for biopsy but also to identify affected muscles not otherwise recognized on clinical examination. Levels of creatine kinase (CK) and other muscle enzymes, including aspartate transaminase (AST), lactate dehydrogenase (LDH), and alanine transaminase (ALT), and the sedimentation rate are often extremely elevated in both disorders. The presence of serum antinuclear antibodies (ANAs) also may be helpful in diagnosing DM. Electromyography (EMG) shows a typical "myopathic" pattern, with short, low-amplitude polyphasic potentials, as well as signs of marked muscle irritability. This is done through the delivery of a large number of low-amplitude action potentials of brief duration in which signs of muscle irritability and myopathic changes are identified.[213]

Treatment primarily includes pharmacologic immunosuppression, although the evidence surrounding the effectiveness of this treatment is not robust. The use of pulsed intravenous glucocorticoids is followed by a 4-week oral regimen, concluding with a tapering of medication. High-dose intravenous immunoglobulin administration is sometimes used during active disease. Successful treatment with intravenous immunoglobulin (IVIg), azathioprine, methotrexate, mycophenolate mofetil, and cyclosporine has been reported.[213,217]

Myopathy

Myopathy is the term applied to a primary muscle disorder. Many pathologic processes affect muscles and cause loss of functional muscle cells. Myopathies affect muscle strength, tone, and bulk. Primary muscle disease is invariably associated with marked weakness. The distribution of the weakness in myopathy is usually symmetrical and proximal, although occasionally the weakness is predominantly distal, such as in myotonic dystrophy. The weakness is associated with mild fatigue. Tone is decreased, as are the tendon reflexes. Atrophy may be present. Some myopathies are associated with muscle hypertrophy as in cretinism and the familial progressive muscular dystrophies of childhood, in which hypertrophied muscles are rubbery and weak. Fasciculations are not present with myopathy because no denervation is present. No sensory changes are found. (Specific neurologic-associated myopathies are discussed in Chapter 17.)

Toxic Myopathies

A number of agents, including corticosteroids, chloroquine, alcohol, phenytoin, azathioprine, organophosphates, and reverse transcriptase inhibitors, have been shown to cause toxic myopathy. Other contributing agents may include lipid-lowering agents, and opioids, such as heroin.

Alcohol specifically has been attributed to myopathies since the mid-nineteenth century and is associated with approximately 50% of skeletal muscle myopathies.[218,219] Alcoholic toxic myopathies may have either an acute or a chronic presentation.[220] The mechanisms by which alcohol affects the muscle include increasing the rate of proteolysis and amino acid oxidation and causing impaired cellular metabolism, gene dysregulation, and premature initiation of apoptosis.[218]

Acute alcoholic myopathy can range from benign cramps and pain resolving in a matter of hours to severe weakness and markedly increased CK level associated with myoglobinuria and renal failure. Individuals are prone to repeated attacks following recovery. The first-line treatment remains abstinence from alcohol and improved nutrition.[218] An individual with chronic alcoholic myopathy often has a coexisting peripheral neuropathy that complicates the diagnosis.

Repeated intramuscular injections have been associated also with changes in muscle fibers. Local necrosis of muscle fiber and elevated CK concentration have been reported after intramuscular injections of certain cephalosporins, lidocaine, diazepam, and digoxin; these effects were not produced with injections of saline. When drugs are injected over long periods, a chronic focal myopathy develops. Proliferation of connective tissue both in the muscle fiber and in the overlying skin and subcutaneous tissue has been reported. Over time, segments of the muscles, particularly the deltoid and quadriceps, are converted into fibrotic bands. Pathophysiologic mechanisms for these changes include repeated needle trauma and infection, along with the nonphysiologic acidity and alkalinity of the injected material. Box 45.7 lists some of the causes of toxic myopathy.

Muscle Tumors
Rhabdomyoma

Rhabdomyoma is an extremely rare benign tumor of striated muscle that generally occurs in the tongue, neck muscles, larynx, uvula, nasal cavity, axilla, vulva, and heart. These tumors are usually treated by

BOX 45.7 AGENTS THAT CAN CAUSE TOXIC MYOPATHY

Drug-Induced

Alcohol

Amiodarone (and others that inhibit CYP3A4 when combined with simvastatin)

Amphotericin B

Azathioprine

AZT (zidovudine)

Chloroquine

Clofibrate

Cocaine

Colchicine

Ethanol

Ipecac (withdrawn from U.S. markets)

3,4-Methylenedioxymethamphetamine (MDMA, "ecstasy")

Pentachlorophenol (PCP)

Statins

Steroids (especially with prolonged high doses; doses >25 mg/day; fluorinated steroids)

Endocrine Disorders

Adrenal disorders (Addison disease, Cushing disease)

Hyperparathyroidism

Hyperthyroidism (creatine kinase may be normal)

Hypothyroidism (creatine kinase may be mildly elevated)

Infectious disorders

Coxsackie A and B viruses

Human immunodeficiency virus (HIV)

Influenza

Lyme disease

Staphylococcus aureus muscle infection (frequent cause of pyomyositis)

Toxoplasmosis

Trichinosis

Miscellaneous

Licorice

Certain edible wild mushrooms

Lead poisoning

Organophosphates

Red yeast rice

European migratory quail (quail eat toxic hemlock, hellebore seeds)

Any medication that alters serum concentrations of sodium, potassium, calcium, phosphorus, or magnesium

Data from Kuncl RW: *Curr Opin Neurol* 22(5):506–515, 2009; Valiyil R, Christopher-Stine L: *Curr Rheumatol Rep* 12(3):213–220, 2010.

surgical excision and do not recur. When malignant, these tumors are referred to as *rhabdomyosarcomas*.

Rhabdomyosarcoma

A rare malignant tumor of striated muscle is called rhabdomyosarcoma, which is a subgroup of sarcoma. It is the most common soft tissue sarcoma in children and adolescents, constituting 50% of all soft tissue sarcomas and 10% of all malignant tumors in children. These tumors are highly malignant, with rapid metastasis. They are located in the muscle tissue of the head, neck, and genitourinary tract in 75% of cases. The remaining 25% of these tumors are located in the trunk, extremities, and urinary tract.[221-223]

Three types of rhabdomyosarcoma are differentiated on pathologic section: pleomorphic, embryonal, and alveolar. The pleomorphic, or spindle cell, type is considered to be one of the most highly malignant tumors of the extremities seen in adulthood, but has a better outcome in children.[221] Embryonal tumors are most commonly seen in childhood and appear on biopsy to be shaped like a tadpole or tennis racquet. Alveolar-type tumors, which appear lattice-like, resemble alveolar lung tissue and have the poorest outcome.[224]

The diagnosis and staging of rhabdomyosarcoma are made by history, physical examination, serologic testing, CT, and MRI. Diagnosis is confirmed by incisional biopsy with surgical resection and by examination of the specimen by a pathologist.[221] On electron microscopy the tissue demonstrates myofilaments and Z-band material; CT scan helps define the tissue borders. Staging is based on the site of origin, residual disease, lymph node involvement, and distant metastases.[221] This information allows a diagnosis of rhabdomyosarcoma (RMS) to be classified into one of the following four different groups: group I, completely resected without lymph node involvement; group II, localized disease with or without complete resection, or microscopic residual disease with or without lymph node involvement; group III, localized gross residual disease; and group IV, distant metastases.[225] This staging is then helpful in determining prognosis and treatment.

Treatment consists of a combination of surgical excision, systemic chemotherapy, and adjuvant radiation therapy. Overall survival of childhood rhabdomyosarcoma has improved over the past decades but adult survival remains poor (see Chapter 46).

Other Tumors

Metastatic muscle tumors are rare in spite of the extensive vascular supply of skeletal muscles. It is suggested that local pH or metabolic changes discourage metastatic involvement from other tumors. When adjacent carcinomas do cause muscle damage, it is usually related to the compression of tissue and resultant muscle atrophy.

SUMMARY REVIEW

Musculoskeletal Injuries

1. The most common skeletal injury is a fracture. A bone can be completely or incompletely fractured. A closed fracture leaves the skin intact. An open fracture has an overlying skin wound. The direction of the fracture line can be linear, oblique, spiral, or transverse. Greenstick, torus, and bowing fractures are examples of incomplete fractures that occur in children. Stress fractures occur in normal or abnormal bone that is subjected to repeated stress. Fatigue fractures occur in normal bone subjected to abnormal stress. Normal weightbearing can cause an insufficiency fracture in abnormal bone.

2. Dislocation is complete loss of contact between the surfaces of two bones. Subluxation is partial loss of contact between two bones. As a bone separates from a joint, it may damage adjacent nerves, blood vessels, ligaments, tendons, and muscle.

3. Tendon tears are called *strains*, and ligament tears are called *sprains*. A complete separation of a tendon or ligament from its attachment is called an *avulsion*.

4. Epicondylopathy is degeneration of a tendon where it attaches to a bone. Bursitis is inflammation of the bursae (small sacs lined with synovial membrane and filled with synovial fluid). Bursitis can be inflammatory, septic, or hemorrhagic.

5. Muscle strain can range from mild injury to severe damage that can result in loss of muscle function.

6. Rhabdomyolysis can be a life-threatening complication of severe muscle trauma wherein muscle cell contents are released into the circulation. It may result in myoglobinuria, the presence of myoglobin in the urine, and is often associated with acute renal failure.

Disorders of Bones

1. Metabolic bone diseases are characterized by abnormal bone structure. In osteoporosis bone tissue is normally mineralized, but the density or mass of bone is reduced because the bone remodeling cycle is disrupted. Osteoporosis is a complex, multifactorial, chronic disease that often progresses silently for decades until fractures occur. It is the most common bone disease. Multiple factors are involved including alteration in the OPG/RANKL/RANK system.

2. Postmenopausal osteoporosis occurs in middle-aged and older women and is caused by increased osteoclast activity (probably caused by changes in osteoprotegerin), decreased IGF levels, a combination of inadequate dietary calcium intake and lack of vitamin D, possibly decreased levels of magnesium, lack of exercise, decreased levels of estrogen, and family history.

3. Glucocorticoids increase RANKL expression and inhibit OPG production by osteoblasts, thus leading to lower bone density.

4. Osteomalacia is a metabolic bone disease characterized by inadequate bone mineralization.

5. Excessive and abnormal bone remodeling occurs in Paget disease. Sporadic Paget disease involves overexpression of RANKL.

6. Osteomyelitis is a bone infection caused most often by bacteria (e.g., *S. aureus*) that can enter bone from outside the body (exogenous osteomyelitis) or from infection sites within the body (hematogenous osteomyelitis).

7. Bone tumors originate from bone cells, cartilage cells, fibrous tissue cells, or vascular marrow cells. Each cell produces a specific type of ground substance that is used to classify the tumor as osteogenic (bone cell), chondrogenic (cartilage cell), collagenic (fibrous tissue cell), or myelogenic (vascular marrow cell). Malignant bone tumors are large, aggressively destroy surrounding bone, invade surrounding tissue, and initiate independent growth outside the site of origin. Benign bone tumors are less destructive, limit their growth to the anatomic confines of the bone, and have a well-demarcated border.

Disorders of Joints

1. Noninflammatory joint disease is differentiated from inflammatory joint disease by the absence of synovial membrane inflammation, the absence of systemic signs and symptoms, and the presence of normal synovial fluid.

2. OA is an inflammatory joint disease and is characterized by the degeneration and loss of articular cartilage, sclerosis of underlying bone, and formation of bone spurs (osteophytes).

3. RA is an inflammatory joint disease characterized by inflammatory destruction of the synovial membrane, articular cartilage, joint capsule, and surrounding ligaments and tendons. RA involves an aberrant immune response and the transformed antibodies are called *rheumatoid factors*. The OPG/RANKL/RANK system is also involved. Rheumatoid nodules may also invade the skin, lung, and spleen and involve small and large arteries. RA is a systemic disease that affects the heart, lungs, kidneys, and skin, as well as the joints.

4. AS is a chronic inflammatory joint disease characterized by stiffening and fusion of the spine and sacroiliac joints. Recent data show that synovitis and bone marrow inflammation, rather than solely the connective tissue between tendon or ligament and bone (enthesis) involvement, explain the alteration in sacroiliac joints.

5. Gout is a metabolic disorder associated with high levels of uric acid in the blood and body fluids. Uric acid crystallizes in the connective tissue of a joint, where it initiates inflammatory destruction of the joint.

Disorders of Skeletal Muscle

1. A pathologic contracture is permanent muscle shortening caused by muscle spasticity, as seen in CNS injury or severe muscle weakness.

2. Stress-induced muscle tension is presumably caused by increased activity in the reticular activating system and gamma loop in the muscle fiber. Progressive relaxation training and biofeedback have been advocated to reduce muscle tension.

3. Fibromyalgia is a chronic musculoskeletal syndrome characterized by diffuse pain and tender points. Current research indicates that muscle is the end organ responsible for the pain and fatigue of the disease. Comorbidities (e.g., irritable bowel syndrome, mood disorders, and chronic fatigue) suggest a major role for neuroendocrine and stress-response alterations.

4. Chronic fatigue syndrome (CFS) is a debilitating and complex disorder with profound fatigue not improved by bed rest. The cause of CFS is hypothesized to include central nervous system alterations, immunologic disruptions, and chronic proinflammatory cytokines.

5. Atrophy of muscle fibers and overall diminished size of the muscle are seen after prolonged inactivity. Isometric contractions and passive lengthening exercises decrease atrophy to some degree in immobilized persons.

6. Hyperexcitable membranes cause the physical and electrical phenomenon of myotonia. The disorder is treated with drugs that reduce fiber excitability. Periodic paralysis is caused by an unresponsive muscle membrane and is accompanied by changes in the level of serum potassium. The biochemical defect is possibly related to changes in the muscle membrane and sarcoplasmic reticulum.

7. Metabolic muscle diseases are caused by endocrine disorders, glycogen storage disease, enzyme deficiencies, and abnormal lipid function. The muscle depends on a complex system of carbohydrates and fats converted by enzymes to produce energy for the muscle cell. Abnormalities in these pathways can inhibit function or cause damage to the muscle fiber. These illnesses are rare, yet they account for significant functional abnormalities.

8. Viral, bacterial, and parasitic infections of muscles produce the characteristic clinical and pathologic changes associated with inflammation. These are usually treatable and self-limiting disorders.

9. Polymyositis (generalized muscle inflammation) and dermatomyositis (polymyositis accompanied with skin rash) are characterized by inflammation of connective tissue and muscle fibers, and muscle fiber necrosis. Cell-mediated and humoral immune factors have been implicated. Treatment with immunosuppressive agents is effective in many cases.

10. Primary disorders with weakness and atrophy are known as *myopathies.*

11. The most common toxic myopathy is caused by alcohol abuse. Direct toxic effects of alcohol-producing necrosis of muscle fibers and nutritional deficiency have been identified. The most effective treatment is abstinence and improved nutrition. The toxic effects

SUMMARY REVIEW—cont'd

of many drugs on muscle fibers cause local trauma to the muscle fibers from direct effects of the needle, secondary infection, and changes caused by nonphysiologic acidity and alkalinity in the fibers.

12. Sarcomas of muscle tissue are rare. Rhabdomyosarcoma has a uniformly poor prognosis because of an aggressive invasion and early, widespread dissemination. The usual treatment includes surgical excision, radiation therapy, and systemic chemotherapy.

KEY TERMS

Acid maltase deficiency, 1462
Acute gouty arthritis, 1457
Age-related bone loss, 1436
Ankylosing spondylitis (AS), 1454
Arthropathy, 1445
Asymptomatic hyperuricemia, 1456
Avulsion, 1427
Bouchard node, 1448
Bowing fracture, 1424
Bursae, 1429
Bursitis, 1428
Caplan syndrome, 1453
Central core disease (CCD), 1461
Chondrogenic (cartilage-forming) tumor, 1444
Chondroid, 1444
Chondrosarcoma, 1444
Chronic fatigue syndrome (CFS; myalgic encephalomyelitis [ME]), 1460
Closed fracture, 1424
Collagenic (collagen-forming) tumor, 1445
Comminuted fracture, 1424
Complete fracture, 1423
Contracture, 1458
Delayed union, 1426
Dislocation, 1426
Disuse atrophy, 1461
Epicondylitis, 1428
Extracellular signal regulated kinases (ERKs), 1436
Fatigue fracture, 1425
Fibromyalgia (FM), 1458
Fibrosarcoma, 1445
Fracture, 1423
Fragility fracture, 1424
Glucocorticoid (cortisone) induced osteoporosis, 1436
Gout, 1454
Gouty arthritis, 1455
Greenstick fracture, 1424

Heberden node, 1448
Heterotopic ossification (HO), 1430
Hyperbaric oxygen therapy, 1441
Hyperkalemic periodic paralysis, 1462
Hypokalemic periodic paralysis, 1461
Idiopathic inflammatory myopathy (IIM), 1463
Incomplete fracture, 1423
Inflammatory joint disease, 1450
Insufficiency fracture, 1425
Involucrum, 1441
Joint effusion, 1449
Joint stiffness, 1448
Lateral epicondylopathy (tennis elbow), 1428
Ligament, 1427
Linear fracture, 1424
Malunion, 1426
McArdle disease, 1462
Medial epicondylopathy (golfer's elbow), 1428
Muscle strain, 1429
Myelogenic tumor, 1445
Myoadenylate deaminase deficiency (MDD), 1463
Myopathy, 1464
Myositis, 1463
Myositis ossificans, 1430
Myotonic channelopathy, 1461
Noninflammatory joint disease, 1446
Nonunion, 1426
Oblique fracture, 1424
Open fracture, 1424
Osteoarthritis (OA), 1445
Osteogenic (bone-forming) tumor, 1443
Osteomalacia, 1438
Osteomyelitis, 1440
Osteopenia, 1432
Osteophyte, 1447
Osteoporosis, 1432
Osteoprotegerin (OPG), 1436
Osteosarcoma, 1443

Paget disease of bone (PDB; osteitis deformans), 1439
Pannus, 1450
Pathologic contracture, 1458
Pathologic fracture, 1424
Peak bone mass, 1433
Periodic paralysis (PP), 1461
Pompe disease, 1462
Postmenopausal osteoporosis, 1434
Primary gout, 1455
Primary osteoarthritis, 1446
Pseudogout, 1455
RANK, 1436
Receptor activator of nuclear factor κβ ligand (RANKL), 1436
Regional osteoporosis, 1434
Rhabdomyolysis, 1430
Rhabdomyosarcoma, 1465
Rheumatoid arthritis (RA), 1450
Rheumatoid factor (RF), 1451
Rheumatoid nodule, 1452
Secondary gout, 1455
Secondary osteoarthritis, 1446
Sequestrum, 1440
Spiral fracture, 1424
Sprain, 1427
Strain, 1427
Stress fracture, 1425
Subluxation, 1426
Tendinitis, 1428
Tendinosis, 1428
Tendon, 1427
Tophaceous gout, 1457
Tophus (pl., tophi), 1455
Torus fracture, 1424
Toxic myopathy, 1464
Transchondral fracture, 1425
Transverse fracture, 1424

REFERENCES

1. Centers for Disease Control and Prevention (CDC): Osteoarthritis fact sheet. Last updated 2 Feb 2017. Available at: http://www.cdc.gov/arthritis/basics/osteoarthritis.htm.
2. Committee on Trauma, Division of Medical Sciences, National Academy of Sciences (US), National Research Council: Accidental death and disability: the neglected disease of modern society, 1966. Washington, DC, National Academy of Sciences, National Research Council. Available at: http://www.ncbi.nlm.nih.gov/books/NBK222962/.
3. Centers for Disease Control and Prevention (CDC), Injury Center: Key injury and violence data, 2016. Available at: http://www.cdc.gov/injury/wisqars/overview/key_data.html.
4. American College of Surgeons/Injury Prevention and Control (ACS/IPC): Resources for the optimal care of the injured patient, 2017. Chicago, Il.,

Committee on Trauma. Available at: https://www.facs.org/quality%20programs/trauma/ipc.
5. Einhorn TA, Gerstenfeld LC: Fracture healing: mechanisms and interventions. Nat Rev Rheumatol 11:45–54, 2015.
6. Assiotis A, Sachinis NP, Chalidis BE: Pulsed electromagnetic fields for the treatment of tibial delayed unions and nonunions. A prospective clinical study and review of the literature. J Orthop Surg Res 7:24, 2012.
7. Shenaq DS, et al: Mesenchymal progenitor cells and their orthopedic applications: forging a path towards clinical trials. Stem Cells Int 2010:519028, 2010.
8. Virk MS, et al: "Same day" ex-vivo regional gene therapy: a novel strategy to enhance bone repair. Mol Ther 5:960–968, 2011.
9. Millar NL, Murrell GAC, McInnes IB: Inflammatory mechanisms in

tendinopathy-towards translation. Nat Rev Rheumatol 13:110–122, 2017.
10. Knobloch K: The role of tendon microcirculation in Achilles and patellar tendinopathy. J Orthop Surg Res 3:18, 2008.
11. Weinreb JH, et al: Tendon structure, disease, and imaging. J Muscles Ligaments Tendons 1(4):66–73, 2014.
12. Baird EO, Kang QK: Prophylaxis of heterotopic ossification–an updated review. J Orthop Surg Res 4:12, 2009.
13. Cervellin G, Comelli I, Lippi G: Rhabdomyolysis: historical background, clinical, diagnostic, and therapeutic features. Clin Chem Lab Med 48(6): 749–756, 2010.
14. Kollmann-Camaiora A, et al: Clinical protocol for the management of malignant hyperthermia. Rev Esp Anestesiol Reanim 64(1):32–40, 2017.

15. Murdock M, Murdock MM: Compartment syndrome: a review of the literature. *Clin Podiatr Med Surg* 29(2):301–310, 2012.

16. Su B-H, et al: Ultrasonic appearance of rhabdomyolysis in patients with crush injury in the Wenchuan earthquake. *Chin Med J* 122(16): 1872–1876, 2009.

17. Cosman F, et al: Clinician's guide to prevention and treatment of osteoporosis. *Osteoporos Int* 25(10):2359–2381, 2014.

18. National Osteoporosis Foundation: *Clinician's guide to prevention and treatment of osteoporosis*, Arlington, VA, 2017, Author.

19. Looker AC, et al: *Osteoporosis or low bone mass at the femur neck or lumbar spine in older adults: United States, 2005–2008*, 2012. Washington, DC, National Center for Health Statistics.

20. Crandall CJ, et al: *Treatment to prevent fractures in men and women with low bone density or osteoporosis: update of a 2007 report*, 2012. Rockville, MD, Agency for Healthcare Research and Quality.

21. Clarke BL, Khosla S: Physiology of bone loss. *Radiol Clin North Am* 48(3):483–495, 2010.

22. Nordin C: Screening for osteoporosis: U.S. Preventive Services Task Force recommendation statement. *Ann Intern Med* 155(4):276–277, 2011.

23. Adachi JD, et al: Impact of prevalent fractures on quality of life: baseline results from the global longitudinal study of osteoporosis in women. *Mayo Clin Proc* 85(9):806–813, 2010.

24. Vestergaard P, Rejnmark L, Mosekilde L: Loss of life years after a hip fracture: effects of age and sex. *Acta Orthop* 80(5):525–530, 2009.

25. Estrada K, et al: Genome-wide meta-analysis identifies 56 bone mineral density loci and reveals 14 loci associated with risk of fracture. *Nat Genet* 44(5):491–501, 2012.

26. National Institute of Arthritis and Musculoskeletal and Skin Diseases: *Osteoporosis and African American women*, Washington, DC, 2015, Author.

27. Manolagas SC, Parfitt AM: What old means to bone. *Trends Endocrinol Metab* 21(6):369–374, 2010.

28. Manolagas SC: From estrogen-centric to aging and oxidative stress: a revised perspective of the pathogenesis of osteoporosis. *Endocr Rev* 31(3): 266–300, 2010.

29. Nieves JW: Skeletal effects of nutrients and nutraceuticals, beyond calcium and vitamin D. *Osteoporos Int* 24(3):771–786, 2012.

30. Bonjour JP: Calcium and phosphate: a duet of ions playing for bone health. *J Am Coll Nutr* 30(5 Suppl 1):438S–448S, 2011.

31. Nanes MS, Kallen CB: Osteoporosis. *Semin Nucl Med* 44(6):439–450, 2014.

32. Mahadevan S, Kumaravel V, Bharath R: Calcium and bone disorders in pregnancy. *Indian J Endocrinol Metab* 16(3):358–363, 2012.

33. Klontzas ME, et al: MR imaging of transient osteoporosis of the hip: an update on 155 hip joints. *Eur J Radiol* 84(3):431–436, 2015.

34. Demontiero O, Vidal C, Duque G: Aging and bone loss: new insights for the clinician. *Ther Adv Musculoskel Dis* 4(2):61–76, 2012.

35. Trouvin A-P, Goëb V: Receptor activator of nuclear factor-κB ligand and osteoprotegerin: maintaining the balance to prevent bone loss. *Clin Interven Aging* 5:345–354, 2010.

36. Silva I, Branco JA: Rank/Rankl/opg: literature review. *Acta Rheumatol Port* 36(3):209–218, 2011.

37. Chin KY, Ima-Nirwana S: Sex steroids and bone health status in men. *Int J Endocrinol* 2012:208719, 2012.

38. Oury F: A crosstalk between bone and gonads. *Ann N Y Acad Sci* 1260:1–7, 2012.

39. Plotkin LI, et al: Bisphosphonates and estrogens inhibit osteocyte apoptosis via distinct molecular mechanisms downstream of extracellular signal-regulated kinase activation. *J Biol Chem* 280(8):7317–7325, 2005.

40. Cicek M, et al: TGF-β inducible early gene 1 regulates osteoclast differentiation and survival by mediating the NFATc1, AKT, and MEK/ERK signaling pathways. *PLoS ONE* 6(3):e17522, 2011.

41. Ciangherotti L, Branidi ML: Muscle-bone interactions: basic and clinical aspects. *Endocrine* 45(2):165–177, 2014.

42. Tanner DA, et al: Hip fractures in men and women change differently with age. *BMC Geriatr* 10:12, 2010.

43. World Health Organization (WHO): *WHO Scientific Group on the assessment of osteoporosis at primary health care level, summary meeting report*, Geneva, 2007, Author.

44. Nieves JW: Skeletal effects of nutrients and nutraceuticals, beyond calcium and vitamin D. *Osteoporos Int* 24(3):771–786, 2013.

45. Genius SJ, Bouchard T: Combination micronutrients for bone (COMB) study: bone density after micronutrient intervention. *J Environ Public Health* Jan 15 2012. [Published online.].

46. An K-C: Selective estrogen receptor modulators. *Asian Spine J* 10(4):787–791, 2016.

47. Fung PPL, et al: Time to onset of bisphosphonate-related osteonecrosis of the jaws: a multicenter retrospective cohort study. *Oral Disease* 23(4): 477–483, 2017.

48. Alshahrani F, Kendler D: Femoral fractures in osteoporotic patients on bisphosphonates: a case report. *J Clin Densitom* 15(3):380–384, 2012.

49. Kennel KA, Drake MT: Adverse effects of bisphosphonates: implications for osteoporosis management. *Mayo Clin Proc* 84(7):632–639, 2009.

50. McClung M, et al: Bisphosphonate therapy for osteoporosis: benefits, risks and drug holiday. *Am J Med* 126(1):13–20, 2013.

51. Salari P, Abdollahi M: Long term bisphosphonate use in osteoporotic patients: a step forward, two steps back. *J Pharm Sci* 15(2):305–317, 2012.

52. Black DM, et al: Continuing bisphosphonate treatment for osteoporosis—for whom and for how long? *N Engl J Med* 366(22):2015–2053, 2012.

53. Hanley DA, et al: Denosumab: mechanism of action and clinical outcomes. *Int J Clin Pract* 66(12):1139–1146, 2012.

54. Vescini F, Grimaldi F: PTH 1–84: bone rebuilding as a target for the therapy of severe osteoporosis. *Clin Cases Miner Bone Metab* 9(1):31–36, 2012.

55. Crandall CJ, et al: *Treatment to prevent fractures in men and women with low bone density or osteoporosis: update of a 2007 report [Internet], comparative effectiveness reviews, no. 53*, 2012. Rockville, MD, Agency for Healthcare Research and Quality.

56. Lim V, Clarke BL: New therapeutic targets for osteoporosis: beyond denosumab. *Maturitas* 73(3):269–272, 2012.

57. Penido MG, Alon US: Phosphate homeostasis and its role in bone health. *Pediatr Nephrol* 27(11): 2039–2048, 2012.

58. Fukumoto S: FGF23-FGF receptor/klotho pathway as a new drug target for disorders of bone and mineral metabolism. *Calcif Tissue Int* 98(4): 334–340, 2016.

59. Thacher TD, Clarke BL: Vitamin D deficiency. *Mayo Clin Proc* 86(1):50–60, 2011.

60. Unuvar T, Buyukgebiz A: Nutritional rickets and vitamin D deficiency in infants, children and adolescents. *Pediatr Endocrinol Rev* 7(3):283–291, 2011.

61. Jain SK, et al: Unusual presentation of altered bone metabolism with long-term antiepileptic therapy: pathological fracture of neck of femur due to brown tumor at calcar. *Musculoskelet Surg* 95(3):265–268, 2011.

62. Jones AN, Hansen KE: Recognizing the musculoskeletal manifestations of vitamin D deficiency. *J Musculoskelet Med* 26(10):389–396, 2009.

63. Kulak CA, Dempster DW: Bone histomorphometry: a concise review for endocrinologists and clinicians. *Arq Bras Endocrinol Metabol* 54(2):87–98, 2010.

64. Bergwitz C, Jüppner H: Phosphate sensing. *Adv Chronic Kidney Dis* 18(2):132–144, 2011.

65. Tan A, Ralston SH: Paget's disease of bone. *QJM* 107(11):865–869, 2014.

66. Michou L, Brown JP: Emerging strategies and therapies for treatment of Paget's disease of bone. *Drug Design Develop Ther* 5:225–239, 2011.

67. Harik NS, Smeltzer MS: Management of acute hematogenous osteomyelitis in children. *Expert Rev Anti Infect Ther* 8(2):175–181, 2010.

68. Calhoun JH, Manring MM, Shirtliff M: Osteomyelitis of the long bones. *Semin Plast Surg* 23(2):59–72, 2009.

69. Hernigou P, et al: Septic arthritis in adults with sickle cell disease often is associated with osteomyelitis or osteonecrosis. *Clin Orthop Relat Res* 468:1676–1681, 2010.

70. Kapoor A, et al: Magnetic resonance imaging for diagnosing foot osteomyelitis: a meta-analysis. *Arch Intern Med* 167(2):125, 2007.

71. Brown HK, Tellez-Gabriel M, Heymann D: Cancer stem cells in osteosarcoma. *Cancer Lett* 386(1): 189–195, 2017.

72. National Comprehensive Cancer Network (NCCN): *Recent updates to NCCN clinical practice guidelines in oncology: bone cancer*, Fort Washington, PA, 2017, Author.

73. Buddingh EP, et al: Intact interferon signaling in peripheral blood leukocytes of high-grade osteosarcoma patients. *Cancer Immunol Immunother* 61(6):941–947, 2012.

74. Sadikovic B, et al: Expression analysis of genes associated with human osteosarcoma tumors shows correlation of RUNX2 overexpression with poor response to chemotherapy. *BMC Cancer* 10:202, 2010.

75. Wesolowski R, Budd GT: Use of chemotherapy for patients with bone and soft-tissue sarcomas. *Clev Clin J Med* 77(Suppl 1):S23–S26, 2010.

76. Lin PP, Moussallem CD, Deavers MT: Secondary chondrosarcoma. *J Am Acad Orthop Surg* 18(10): 608–615, 2010.

77. Onishi AC, Hincker AM, Lee FY: Surmounting chemotherapy and radioresistance in chondrosarcoma: molecular mechanisms and therapeutic targets. *Sarcoma* 2011:381654, 2011.

78. Karpik M: Giant cell tumor (tumor gigantocellularis, osteoclastoma)—epidemiology, diagnosis, treatment. *Orthop Traumatol Rehabil* 12(3):207–215, 2010.

79. Cowan RW, Singh G: Giant cell tumor of bone: a basic science perspective. *Bone* 52(1):238–246, 2013.

80. Kivioja AH, et al: Cement is recommended in intralesional surgery of giant cell tumors: a Scandinavian Sarcoma Group study of 294 patients followed for a median time of 5 years. *Acta Orthop* 9(2):86, 2008.

81. Zhang M, Wang J: Epigenetics and osteoarthritis. *Genes Dis* 2(1):69–75, 2015.

82. Murphy L, Helmick CG: The impact of osteoarthritis in the United States: a

population-health perspective. *Am J Nurs* 112(3 Suppl 1):S13–S19, 2012.

83. Rigoglou S, Papavassiliou AG: The NF-B signaling pathway in osteoarthritis. *Int J Biochem Cell Biol* 45(1):2580–2584, 2013.

84. Scanzello C, Goldring S: The role of synovitis in osteoarthritis pathogenesis. *Bone* 51:249–257, 2012.

85. Scanzello C, et al: Synoval inflammation in patients undergoing arthroscopic meniscectomy: molecular characterization and relationship to symptoms. *Arthritis Rheum* 63:391–400, 2011.

86. Kumar V, Abbas AK, Aster JCF: *Robbins & Cotran pathologic basis of disease*, ed 9, Philadelphia, 2015, Elsevier Sanders.

87. Cooper C, Javaid M, Arden N: Epidemiology of osteoarthritis. In *Atlas of osteoarthritis*, New York, 2014, Springer Healthcare. doi:10.1007/978-1-910315-16-3_2.

88. Amoako AO, Pujalte GG: Osteoarthritis in young, active, and athletic individuals. *Clin Med Insights Arthritis Musculoskelet Disord* 7:27–32, 2014.

89. Vincent K, et al: The pathophysiology of osteoarthritis: a mechanical perspective of the knee joint. *PM R* 4(Suppl 5):S3–S9, 2012.

90. van der Kraan PM: Age-related alterations in TGE beta signaling as a causal factor of cartilage degeneration in osteoarthritis. *Biomed Mater Eng* 24(Suppl 1):75–80, 2014.

91. Clement T, et al: Identification of new microRNAs targeting genes regulating the Pi/PPi balance in chondrocytes. *Biomed Mater Eng* 24(Suppl 1):3–16, 2014.

92. Trzeciak T, Czarny-Ratajczak M: MicroRNAs: important epigenetic regulators in osteoarthritis. *Curr Genomics* 15(6):481–484, 2014.

93. Sinusas K: Osteoarthritis: diagnosis and treatment. *Am Fam Physician* 85(1):49–56, 2012.

94. Schiphof D, et al: Factors for pain in patients with different grades of knee osteoarthritis. *Arthritis Care Res (Hoboken)* 65(5):695–702, 2013.

95. Bijlsma B, Berenbaum F, Lafeber F: Osteoarthritis: an update with relevance to clinical practice. *Lancet* 377(9783):2115–2126, 2011.

96. Loeser R, et al: Osteoarthritis: a disease of the joint as an organ. *Arthritis Rheum* 64(6):1697–1707, 2011.

97. Sharma L, et al: The role of varus and valgus alignment in the initial development of knee cartilage damage by MRI: the MOST study. *Ann Rheum Dis* 72(2):235–240, 2013.

98. Jones R, et al: A comparison of the biomechanical effects of valgus knee braces and lateral wedged insoles in patients with knee osteoarthritis. *Gait Posture* 37(3):368–372, 2013.

99. Frasen M, et al: Exercise for osteoarthritis of the knee. *Cochran Database Syst Rev* (1):CD004376, 2015.

100. Koonce R, Bravman J: Obesity and osteoarthritis: more than just wear and tear. *J Am Acad Orthop Surg* 21(3):161–169, 2013.

101. Messier S, et al: Effects of intensive diet and exercise on knee joint loads, inflammation, and clinical outcomes among overweight and obese adults with knee osteoarthritis: the IDEA randomized clinical trial. *JAMA* 310(12):1263–1273, 2013.

102. Rayman MP: Diet, nutrition, and osteoarthritis. *BMC Musculoskelet Disord* 16(Suppl 1):S7, 2015.

103. Rutjes AWS, et al: Therapeutic ultrasound for osteoarthritis of the knee or hip. *Cochrane Database Syst Rev* 20 (1):CD003132, 2010.

104. Alaaeddine N, et al: Use of complementary and alternative therapy among patients with rheumatoid arthritis and osteoarthritis. *J Clin Nurs* 21(21-22):3198–3204, 2012.

105. Siemieniuk RAC, et al: Arthroscopic surgery for degenerative knee arthritis and meniscal tear: a clinical guideline. *BMJ* 357:j1982, 2017.

106. Kise NJ, et al: Exercise therapy versus arthroscopic partial meniscectomy for degenerative meniscal tear in middle aged patients: randomized controlled trail with two-year follow-up. *BMJ* 354:i3740, 2016.

107. Gomoll A, et al: Surgical treatment for early osteoarthritis. Part II: allografts and concurrent procedures. *Knee Surg Sports Traumatol Arthrosc* 20(3):468–486, 2012.

108. Schmidtt S: *Infectious arthritis (septic arthritis)*. Available at: http://www.merckmanuals.com/home/bone,-joint,-and-muscle-disorders/bone-and-joint-infections/infectious-arthritis.

109. You S, et al: Identification of key regulators for the migration and invasion of rheumatoid synoviocytes through a systems approach. *Proc Natl Acad Sci USA* 111(1):550–555, 2015.

110. Center for Disease Control and Prevention (CDC): *Rheumatoid arthritis fact sheet (2016)*. Available at: https://www.cdc.gov/arthritis/basics/rheumatoid-arthritis.html.

111. Gibofsky A: Epidemiology, pathophysiology, and diagnosis of rheumatoid arthritis: a synopsis. *Am J Manag Care* 20(Suppl 7):S128–S135, 2014.

112. Eyre S, et al: High-density genetic mapping identifies new susceptibility loci for rheumatoid arthritis. *Nat Genet* 44(12):1336–1340, 2012.

113. National Institutes of Health (NIH): *Rheumatoid arthritis: genetics home reference*, 2017. Bethesda, MD, U.S. Department of Health and Human Services, National Institutes of Health.

114. Klein K, Gay S: Epigenetics in rheumatoid arthritis. *Curr Opin Rheumatol* 27(1):76–82, 2015.

115. Centers for Disease Control and Prevention (CDC): *Rheumatoid arthritis fact sheet*, 2017. Atlanta, GA, Centers for Disease Control and Prevention, National Center for Chronic Disease Prevention and Health Promotion, U.S. Department of Health and Human Services.

116. McInnes IB, Schett G: The pathogenesis of rheumatoid arthritis. *N Engl J Med* 365(23):2205–2219, 2011.

117. Song YW, Kang EH: Autoantibodies in rheumatoid arthritis: rheumatoid factors and anticitrullinated protein antibodies. *Q J Med* 103(3):139–146, 2010.

118. Cooles F, Isaacs JD: Pathophysiology of rheumatoid arthritis. *Curr Opin Rheumatol* 23(3):233–240, 2011.

119. Valesini G, et al: Citrullination and autoimmunity. *Autoimmun Rev* 14(6):490–497, 2015.

120. Bartok B, Firestein GS: Fibroblast-like synoviocytes: key effector cells in rheumatoid arthritis. *Immunol Rev* 233(1):233–255, 2010.

121. Laragione T, Shah A, Gulko PS: The vitamin D receptor regulates rheumatoid arthritis synovial fibroblast invasion and morphology. *Mol Med* 18(1):194–200, 2012.

122. Sabeh F, Fox D, Weiss SJ: Membrane-type I matrix metalloproteinase-dependent regulation of rheumatoid arthritis synoviocytes function. *J Immunol* 184:6396–6406, 2010.

123. Longo UG, Petrillo S, Denaro V: Current concepts in the management of rheumatoid hand. *Int J Rheumatol* 2015:648073, 2015.

124. Schett G, Gravallcse E: Bone erosion in rheumatoid arthritis: mechanisms, diagnosis and treatment. *Nat Rev Rheumatol* 8(11):656–664, 2012.

125. Turesson C: Extra-articular rheumatoid arthritis. *Curr Opin Rheumatol* 25(3):360–366, 2013.

126. Kelly CA: Rheumatoid arthritis: classical rheumatoid lung disease. *Baillieres Clin Rheumatol* 7(1):1–16, 1993.

127. Marijon E, et al: Rheumatic heart disease. *Lancet* 379(9819):953–964, 2012.

128. Ntatsaki E, et al: Systemic rheumatoid vasculitis in the era of modern immunosuppressive therapy. *Rheumatology (Oxford)* 53(1):145–152, 2014.

129. Aletaha D, et al: 2010 Rheumatism classification criteria for rheumatoid arthritis: an American College of Rheumatology/European League Against Rheumatism collaborative initiative. *Arthritis Rheum* 62(9):2569–2581, 2010.

130. Goronzy JJ, Weyand CM: Developments in the scientific understanding of rheumatoid arthritis. *Arthritis Res Ther* 11(5):249, 2009.

131. Pruijn GJ, Wiik A, van Venrooij WJ: The use of citrullinated peptides and proteins for the diagnosis of rheumatoid arthritis. *Arthritis Res Ther* 12(1):203, 2010.

132. Colbert RA, et al: From HLA-B27 to spondyloarthritis: a journey through the ER. *Immunol Rev* 233(1):181–202, 2010.

133. Colbert RA, Tran TM, Layh-Schmitt G: HLA-B27 misfolding and ankylosing spondylitis. *Mol Immunol* 57(1):44–51, 2014.

134. Dean LE, et al: Global prevalence of ankylosing spondylitis. *Rheumatology* 53(4):650–657, 2014.

135. Roussou E, Sultana S: Early spondyloarthritis in multiracial society: differences between gender, race, and disease subgroups with regard to first symptom at presentation, main problem that the disease is causing to patients, and employment status. *Rheumatol Int* 32(6):1597–1604, 2012.

136. Braun J, et al: 2010 update of the ASAS/EULAR recommendations for the management of ankylosing spondylitis. *Ann Rheum Dis* 70(6):896–904, 2011.

137. Sari I, Öztürk MA, Akkoç N: Treatment of ankylosing spondylitis. *Turk J Med Sci* 45(2):416–430, 2015.

138. Roddy E, Choi HK: Epidemiology of gout. *Rheum Dis Clin North Am* 40(2):155–175, 2014.

139. Crittenden DB, Pillinger MH: The year in gout 2010-2011. *Bull NYU Hosp Joint Dis* 69(3):257–263, 2011.

140. Gonzales EB: An update on the pathology and clinical management of gouty arthritis. *Clin Rheumatol* 31:13–21, 2012.

141. Jin M, et al: Uric acid, hyperuricemia and vascular diseases. *Front Biosci (Landmark Ed)* 17:656, 2012.

142. Perez-Ruiz F, et al: Tophaceous gout and high level of hyperuricaemia are both associated with increased risk of mortality in patients with gout. *Ann Rheum Dis* 73(1):177–182, 2014.

143. Sriranganathan MK, et al: Interventions for tophi in gout: a Cochrane systematic literature review. *J Rheumatol Suppl* 92:63–69, 2014.

144. Busso N, Ea HK: The mechanisms of inflammation in gout and pseudogout (CPP-induced arthritis). *Reumatismo* 63(4):230–237, 2011.

145. Hueskes BA, et al: Use of diuretics and the risk of gouty arthritis: a systematic review. *Semin Arthritis Rheum* 41(6):879–889, 2012.

146. Álvarez-Lario B, Macarrón-Vicente J: Is there anything good in uric acid? *QJM* 104(12):1015–1024, 2011.

147. Girish G, Glazebrook KN, Jacobson JA: Advanced imaging in gout. *Am J Roentgenol* 201(3):515–525, 2013.

148. Perez-Ruiz F, Herrero-Beites AM: Evaluation and treatment of gout as a chronic disease. *Adv Ther* 29(11):935–946, 2012.

149. Sivera F, et al: Multinational evidence-based recommendations for the diagnosis and

management of gout: integrating systematic literature review and expert opinion of a broad panel of rheumatologists in the 3e initiative. *Ann Rheum Dis* 73(2):328–335, 2013.

150. Skalsky AJ, McDonald CM: Prevention and management of limb contractures in neuromuscular diseases. *Phys Med Rehab Clin N Am* 23(3):675–687, 2012.

151. Olsen BS: Treatment of the stiff elbow joint. *Orthop Trauma* 26(6):397–404, 2012.

152. Saaiq M, Zaib S, Ahmad S: The menace of post-burn contractures: a developing country's perspective. *Ann Burns Fire Disasters* 25(3): 152–158, 2012.

153. Larsman P, Kadefors R, Sandsjö L: Psychosocial work conditions, perceived stress, perceived muscular tension, and neck/shoulder symptoms among medical secretaries. *Int Arch Occup Environ Hlth* 86(1):57–63, 2013.

154. Schmidt-Wilcke T, Clauw DJ: Fibromyalgia: from pathophysiology to therapy. *Nat Rev Rheumatol* 7(9):518–527, 2011.

155. Pernambuco AP, et al: Increased levels of IL-17A in patients with fibromyalgia. *Clin Exp Rheumatol* 31(6 Suppl 79):S60–S63, 2013.

156. Rodriguez-Pintó I, et al: Fibromyalgia and cytokines. *Immunol Lett* 161(2):200–203, 2014.

157. Sturgill J, McGee E, Menzies V: Unique cytokine signature in the plasma of patients with fibromyalgia. *J Immunol Res* 2014:938576, 2014.

158. Clauw DJ: Fibromyalgia: a clinical review. *JAMA* 311(15):1547–1555, 2014.

159. Jahan F, et al: Fibromyalgia syndrome: an overview of pathophysiology, diagnosis and management. *Oman Med J* 27(3):192–195, 2012.

160. Park D-J, et al: Exploring genetic susceptibility to fibromyalgia. *Chonnam Med J* 51(2):58–65, 2015.

161. Arnold LM, et al: The fibromyalgia family study: a genome-wide linkage scan study. *Arthritis Rheum* 65(4):1122–1128, 2013.

162. Diatchenko L, et al: The phenotypic and genetic signatures of common musculoskeletal pain conditions. *Nat Rev Rheumatol* 9(6):340–350, 2013.

163. Cagnie B, et al: Central sensitization in fibromyalgia? A systematic review on structural and functional brain MRI. *Semin Arthritis Rheum* 44(1):68–75, 2014.

164. Harbeck B, et al: High prevalence of fibromyalgia-associated symptoms in patients with hypothalamic-pituitary disorders. *Clin Exp Rheumatol* 31(6 Suppl 79):S16–S21, 2012.

165. Wolfe F, et al: Fibromyalgia criteria and severity scales for clinical and epidemiological studies: a modification of the ACR Preliminary Diagnostic Criteria for Fibromyalgia. *J Rheumatol* 38(6): 1113–1122, 2011.

166. Smith MT, Moore BJ: Pregabalin for the treatment of fibromyalgia. *Expert Opin Pharmacother* 13(10): 1527–1533, 2012.

167. Bidonde J, et al: Aquatic exercise training for fibromyalgia. *Cochrane Database Syst Rev* (10): 2014.

168. Bidonde J, et al: Exercise for adults with fibromyalgia: an umbrella systematic review with synthesis of best evidence. *Curr Rheumatol Rev* 10(1):45–79, 2014.

169. O'Connor SR, et al: Walking exercise for chronic musculoskeletal pain: systematic review and meta-analysis. *Arch Phys Med Rehabil* 96(4): 724–734, 2015.

170. Bansal AS, et al: Chronic fatigue syndrome, the immune system and viral infection. *Brain Behav Immun* 26(1):24–31, 2012.

171. Yancey JR, Thomas SM: Chronic fatigue syndrome: diagnosis and treatment. *Am Fam Physician* 86(8):741–746, 2012.

172. Nijs J, et al: Pain in patients with chronic fatigue syndrome: time for specific pain treatment? *Pain Physician* 15(5):E677–E686, 2012.

173. Carruthers BM, et al: Myalgic encephalomyelitis: international consensus criteria. *J Intern Med* 270:327–338, 2011.

174. Booth NE, Myhill S, McLaren-Howard J: Mitochondrial dysfunction and the pathophysiology of myalgic encephalomyelitis/chronic fatigue syndrome. *Int J Clin Exp Med* 5(3):208–220, 2012.

175. Romano GF, et al: Fibromyalgia and chronic fatigue: the underlying biology and related theoretical issues. *Adv Psychosom Med* 34:61–77, 2015.

176. Medow MS, et al: Modulation of the axon-reflex response to local heat by reactive oxygen species (ROS) in subjects with chronic fatigue syndrome. *J Appl Physiol* 114(1):45–51, 2013.

177. Centers for Disease Control and Prevention (CDC): *Chronic fatigue syndrome*. Available at: http://www.cdc.gov/cfs/diagnosis/index.html.

178. Suetta C, et al: Aging affects the transcriptional regulation of human skeletal muscle disuse atrophy. *PLoS ONE* 7(12):e51238, 2012.

179. Brooks NE, Myburgh KH: Skeletal muscle wasting with disuse atrophy is multi-dimensional: the response and interaction of myonuclei, satellite cells and signaling pathways. *Front Physiol* 5:99, 2014.

180. Dirks ML, et al: Neuromuscular electrical stimulation prevents muscle disuse atrophy during leg immobilization in humans. *Acta Physiol (Oxf)* 210(3):628–641, 2014.

181. Calvani R, et al: Mitochondrial pathways in sarcopenia of aging and disuse muscle atrophy. *Biol Chem* 394(3):393–414, 2013.

182. Burge JA, Hanna MG: Novel insights into the pathomechanisms of skeletal muscle channelopathies. *Curr Neurol Neurosci Rep* 12(1):62–69, 2012.

183. Statland JM, et al: Mexiletine for symptoms and signs of myotonia in nondystrophic myotonia: a randomized controlled trial. *JAMA* 308(13): 1357–1365, 2012.

184. Malicdan MC, Nishino I: Central core disease. In Pagon RA, Adam MP, Bird TD, editors: *GeneReviews*, Seattle, WA, 2014, University of Washington. Available at: https://www.ncbi.nlm.nih.gov/books/NBK1391/.

185. Lanner JT: Ryanodine receptor physiology and its role in disease. *Adv Exp Med Biol* 740:217–234, 2012.

186. Francis DG, et al: Leaky sodium channels from voltage sensor mutations in periodic paralysis, but not paramyotonia. *Neurology* 76(19):1635–1641, 2011.

187. Tricarico D, Camerino DC: Recent advances in the pathogenesis and drug action in periodic paralyses and related channelopathies. *Front Pharmacol* 2:8, 2011.

188. Falhammar H, Thorén M, Calissendorff J: Thyrotoxic periodic paralysis: clinical and molecular aspects. *Endocrine* 43(2):274–284, 2013.

189. Lin SH, Huang CL: Mechanism of thyrotoxic periodic paralysis. *J Am Soc Nephrol* 23(6): 985–988, 2012.

190. Weber F, Jurkat-Rott K, Lehmann-Horn F: Hyperkalemic periodic paralysis. In Pagon RA, et al, editors: *GeneReviews*, Seattle, WA, 2016, University of Washington. Available at: https://www.ncbi.nlm.nih.gov/books/NBK1496/?report=printable.

191. Charles G, et al: Characterization of hyperkalemic periodic paralysis: a survey of genetically diagnosed individuals. *J Neurol* 260(10): 2606–2613, 2013.

192. Sobacchi C, et al: Osteopetrosis: genetics, treatment and new insights into osteoclast function. *Nat Rev Endocrinol* 9(9):522–536, 2013.

193. Guran T, et al: Clinical and molecular characterization of Turkish patients with familial hypomagnesaemia: novel mutations in TRPM6 and CLDN16 genes. *Nephrol Dial Transplant* 27(2):667–673, 2012.

194. Bollig G: McArdle's disease (glycogen storage disease type V) and anesthesia–a case report and review of the literature. *Paediatr Anesth* 23(9): 817–823, 2013.

195. Lucia A, et al: The 'McArdle paradox': exercise is a good advice for the exercise intolerant. *Br J Sports Med* 47(12):728–789, 2012.

196. Gurgel-Giannetti J, et al: Clinical and molecular characterization of McArdle's disease in Brazilian patients. *Neuromolecular Med* 15(3):470–475, 2013.

197. Zaidman CM, et al: Qualitative and quantitative skeletal muscle ultrasound in late-onset acid maltase deficiency. *Muscle Nerve* 44(3):418–423, 2011.

198. Toscano A, Schoser B: Enzyme replacement therapy in late-onset Pompe disease: a systematic literature review. *J Neurol* 260(4):951–959, 2013.

199. Werneck LC, et al: Muscle biopsy in Pompe disease. *Arq Neuropsiquiatr* 71(5):284–289, 2013.

200. Angelini C, Semplicini C: Enzyme replacement therapy for Pompe disease. *Curr Neurol Neurosci Rep* 12(1):70–75, 2012.

201. Kishnani PS, Beckemeyer AA, Mendelsohn NJ: The new era of Pompe disease: advances in the detection, understanding of the phenotypic spectrum, pathophysiology, and management. *Am J Med Genet C Semin Med Genet* 160(1):1–7, 2012.

202. Hayes LD, Houston FE, Baker JS: Genetic predictors of adenosine monophosphate deaminase deficiency. *J Sports Med Doping Stud* 3(124):2161–2673, 2013.

203. Jinnah HA, Sabina RL, Van Den Berghe G: Metabolic disorders of purine metabolism affecting the nervous system. *Handb Clin Neurol* 113:1827, 2013.

204. Landau ME, et al: Exertional rhabdomyolysis: a clinical review with a focus on genetic influences. *J Clin Neuromuscul Dis* 13(3):122–136, 2012.

205. Van Der Vusse GJ, Reneman RS: Lipid metabolism in muscle. In *Comprehensive physiology supplement 29: handbook of physiology, exercise: regulation and integration of multiple systems*, New York, 2011, Wiley., pp 952–994. doi:10.1002/cphy.cp120121.

206. Liang WC, Nishino I: State of the art in muscle lipid diseases. *Acta Myol* 29(2):351–356, 2010.

207. Center for Disease Control and Prevention (CDC): *Parasites – trichinellosis (also known as trichinosis): epidemiology and risk factors*, 2012. Available at: https://www.cdc.gov/parasites/trichinellosis/epi.html.

208. Bruschi F, Dupouy-Camet J: Trichinellosis. In Bruschi F, editor: *Helminth infections and their impact on global public health*, Wien Heidelberg, New York, Dordrecht, London, 2014, Springer, pp 229–273.

209. Callen JP: Cutaneous manifestations of dermatomyositis and their management. *Curr Rheumatol Rep* 12(3):192–197, 2010. 2010.

210. Dimachkie MM, Barohn RJ: Idiopathic inflammatory myopathies. *Semin Neurol* 32(3): 227–236, 2012.

211. Raychaudhuri SP, Mitra A: Polymyositis and dermatomyositis: disease spectrum and classification. *Indian J Dermatol* 57(5):366–370, 2012.

212. Vincze M, Danko K: Idiopathic inflammatory myopathies. *Best Pract Res Clin Rheumatol* 26(1): 25–45, 2012.

213. Carstens PO, Schmidt J: Diagnosis, pathogenesis and treatment of myositis: recent advances. *Clin Exp Immunol* 175(3):349–358, 2014.

214. Dimachkie MM, Barohn RJ: Inclusion body myositis. *Neurol Clin* 32(3):629–646, 2014.

215. Schmidt J, Dalakas MC: Inclusion body myositis: from immunopathology and degenerative mechanisms to treatment perspectives. *Expert Rev Clin Immunol* 9(11):1125–1133, 2013.

216. Mastaglia FL, Needham M: Inclusion body myositis: a review of clinical and genetic aspects, diagnostic criteria and therapeutic approaches. *J Clin Neurosci* 22(1):6–13, 2015.

217. Schiopu E, et al: Predictors of survival in a cohort of patients with polymyositis and dermatomyositis: effect of corticosteroids, methotrexate and azathioprine. *Arthritis Res Ther* 14(1):R22, 2012.

218. Molina PE, et al: Alcohol abuse: critical pathophysiological processes and contribution to disease burden. *Physiology (Bethesda)* 29(3): 203–215, 2014.

219. Pasnoor M, Barohn RJ: Dimachkie MM: Toxic myopathies. *Neurol Clin* 32(3):647–670, 2014.

220. Wijnia JW, et al: Is vitamin D deficiency a confounder in alcoholic skeletal muscle myopathy? *Alcohol Clin Exp Res* 37(Suppl 1):E209–E215, 2013.

221. Carroll SJ, Nodit L: Spindle cell rhabdomyosarcoma: a brief diagnostic review and differential diagnosis. *Arch Pathol Lab Med* 137(8):1155–1158, 2013.

222. Damor A, et al: Congenital rhabdomyosarcoma: a rare axillary presentation. *Int J Biomed Adv Res* 3(3):212–214, 2012.

223. Zanola A, et al: Rhabdomyosarcomas: an overview on the experimental animal models. *J Cell Mol Med* 16(7):1377–1391, 2012.

224. Gosiengfiao Y, Reichek J, Walterhouse D: What is new in rhabdomyosarcoma management in children? *Paediat Drugs* 14(6):389–400, 2012.

225. Raney RB, et al: Rhabdomyosarcoma and undifferentiated sarcoma in the first two decades of life: a selective review of intergroup rhabdomyosarcoma study group experience and rationale for Intergroup Rhabdomyosarcoma Study V. *J Pediatr Hematol Oncol* 23(4):215–220, 2001.

Alterations of Musculoskeletal Function in Children

Marcella R. Woiczik, McCall G. McDaniel, Russel J. Butterfield

evolve WEBSITE

CHAPTER OUTLINE

Musculoskeletal alterations in children are very common. They may be congenital, such as clubfoot; hereditary, such as muscular dystrophy; or acquired, such as Legg-Calvé-Perthes disease. Some of these disorders are acute, and the child will recover completely; other disorders are chronic or, in some cases, terminal. An understanding of the pathophysiology of these alterations will aid in providing the best care possible for these children.

MUSCULOSKELETAL DEVELOPMENT IN CHILDREN

Bone Formation

Bone formation, which begins at about the sixth week of gestation, involves two phases: (1) the delivery of bone cell precursors to sites of bone formation and (2) the aggregation of these cells at primary centers of ossification, where they mature and begin to secrete osteoid (see Chapter 44). Some of the bone cell precursors are present in fetal connective tissues, whereas others migrate in blood to sites of bone formation after blood vessels have grown into the tissue.

Cellular aggregation and maturation occur in two types of fetal tissue, depending on which bones are being formed. The cranium, facial bones, clavicles, and parts of the jawbone (classically called *flatbones*) arise from a fetal membrane termed the *mesenchyme*. Bones that develop on or within the mesenchyme grow by the process of intramembranous formation of bone. As the mesenchyme becomes vascularized, the immature bone cells aggregate and mature into osteoblasts, which form the centers of ossification and create solid bone or osteoid.

Endochondral formation of bone is the development of new bone from cartilage (Fig. 46.1). First, mesenchymal tissue forms a cartilage anlage, which defines the shape of the bone. This is usually found by 6 weeks' gestation. Blood vessel invasion to inside the anlage brings osteoprogenitor cells leading to primary centers of calcification by 8 weeks. Endochondral bone formation begins in the outer layer of the cartilage model, which consists of a layer of dense connective tissue called perichondrium. The perichondrium contains cells that develop into osteoblasts, forming a collar of bone, termed the periosteal collar, around the cartilage model. Cartilage enclosed within the periosteal collar degenerates, and capillaries from outside the perichondrium

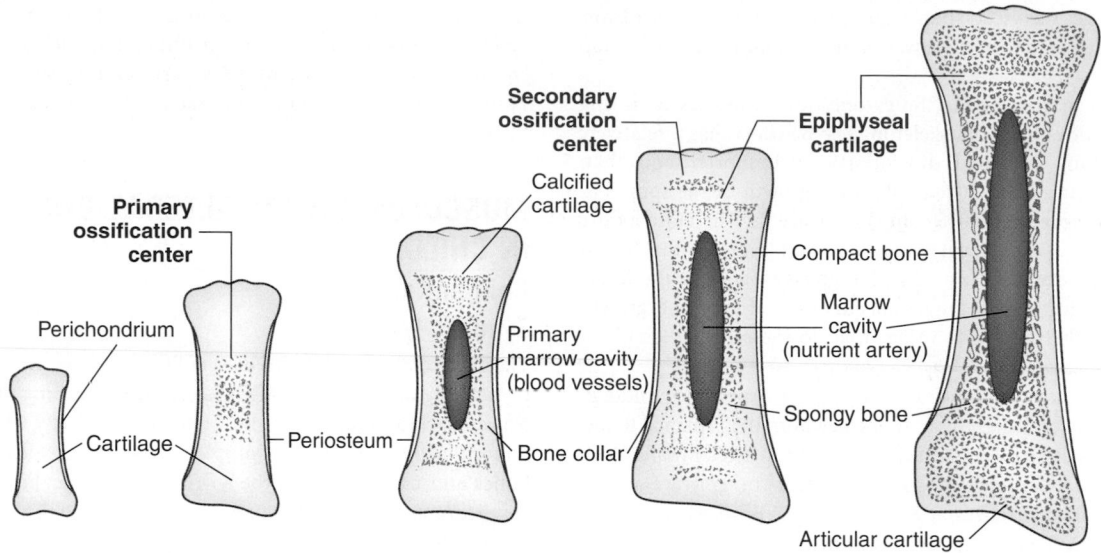

FIGURE 46.1 Stages of Endochondral Bone Formation and Centers of Ossification in Long Bone.

invade the degenerating cartilage cells, carrying with them osteoblast precursors from the inner layer of the perichondrium and osteoclast precursors from the blood itself.

Endochondral bone formation progresses at the primary center of ossification in the middle of the cartilage model and extends toward either end of the developing bone. At the same time, the periosteal collar thickens and becomes wider toward the epiphyses. By the end of gestation secondary centers of ossification (i.e., the epiphyseal centers) begin to lay down bone at both ends of the cartilage model. Here, too, cartilage within the periosteal collar degenerates, and blood vessels grow inward, delivering bone cell precursors. Once the osteoblasts begin to secrete osteoid, ossification spreads from the secondary centers in all directions until all the cartilage within the model is replaced by bone.

Two regions of cartilage remain at the ends of long bones: (1) articular cartilage over the free ends of the bone, and (2) the physeal plate, a layer of cartilage between the metaphysis and epiphysis. (These structures are described and illustrated in Chapter 44; see Fig. 44.3). The physeal plate retains the ability to form and calcify new cartilage and deposit bone until the skeleton matures approximately 1 year after sexual maturity (11 to 15 years of age in females, 15 to 18 in males).

Bone Growth

Until adult stature is reached, growth in the length of long bones occurs at the physeal plate through endochondral ossification. Cartilage cells at the epiphyseal side of the physeal plate multiply and enlarge. As rapidly as new cartilage cells form, cartilage cells at the metaphyseal side of the plate are destroyed and replaced by bone.

In the shaft of new bone, where growth is relatively slow, the bone produced by accretion is compact and dense. The compact bone is thickest where it has to withstand the maximal stresses, which generally occur in the middle of the shaft.

The two physes of the long bone often have varying activity rates. For example, the distal physis in the femur contributes 80% of the overall length, whereas the proximal physis at the hip contributes only 20%. The more active of the two has more power to remodel deformity but also can be more sensitive to injury. The architecture of the physis also dictates its sensitivity to injury. The distal femur, for example, has an undulating pattern that increases its resistance to sheer force; when injured, however, growth disturbance is highly likely. On the other hand,

the distal radius, which contributes 80% of overall radial length, is a flat, smooth physis that is far more resistant to traumatic injury.

Growth in the diameter of bone occurs by deposition of new bone on an existing bone surface. Bone matrix is laid down by osteoblasts on the periosteal surface and subsequently becomes calcified. At the same time, bone resorption occurs on the endosteal surface. Endosteal resorption increases the diameter of the medullary cavity, which contains marrow and spongy bone.

Many factors affect the development, physiology, and rate of growth of the epiphyseal plate. Growth hormone must be secreted by the pituitary gland at a constant rate to stimulate the growth plate consistently. Other known factors affecting growth include peptide regulatory factors (e.g., fibroblast growth factor [FGF]); changes in cell-to-cell interactions through cell adhesion molecules (CAMs) and cell junctions; and complex interactions or changes in the extracellular matrix (ECM), nutrition, general health, and other hormones (e.g., thyroid hormone, adrenal and gonadal androgens, estrogens). When these factors are poorly controlled, skeletal dysplasias, such as achondroplasia, can occur.

Even after physeal closure at skeletal maturity, bone is constantly being destroyed and re-formed (see Chapter 44). This is a rapid process in young children, allowing them to heal bone injury more quickly than adults. By adulthood, however, bone turnover, or remodeling, occurs at a relatively slow rate. Peak bone mass is achieved by the middle to late twenties and slowly decreases throughout life; therefore ensuring appropriate intake of calcium and phosphorus, performing weightbearing exercises, and minimizing caffeine intake are especially important for a young female if she is to avoid osteoporosis in later life. Recently, the importance of vitamin D levels also has been emphasized. In one study, nearly 70% of American children had low levels of vitamin D.[1] The actual percentages of children and adults with low levels of vitamin is debated. Children with vitamin D insufficiency have a higher incidence of fracture[2] and also may be at greater risk for sustaining more severe fractures.[3]

Skeletal Development

The axial skeleton changes shape with growth. (The axial skeleton and appendicular skeleton are described and illustrated in Chapter 44; see Fig. 44.5.) In a newborn the entire spine is concave anteriorly, or kyphosed. In the first 3 months of life, with the infant's ability to control the head, the upper (cervical) spine begins to arch, or become lordotic. The normal lordotic curve of the lower (lumbar) spine begins to develop with sitting.

The appendicular skeleton (the extremities) grows faster during childhood than does the axial skeleton. The newborn has a relatively large head and long spine with disproportionately shorter limbs than an adult. By 1 year of age, 50% of the total growth of the spine has occurred and is more than 70% complete by age 8.[4] Therefore failure of the spine to grow (e.g., spinal fusion) does not limit eventual height as much as the premature fusion of the growth plates of the lower extremities. In children with congenital curvature of the spine, growth tends to worsen the deformity rather than to increase the length of the spine.

Besides getting longer, growing bones of the extremities undergo changes in rotation and alignment. In the newborn the proximal femur is rotated forward up to 40 degrees and the tibia is rotated inward. With growth the femur assumes its normal alignment (by 12 years of age) and tibial rotation neutralizes at 8 years of age.[5] Bowlegs and knock knees can be normal at certain stages of growth. At birth the newborn's legs are bowed because of stresses in utero. Genu varum (bowleg) reaches a peak by 30 months of age, whereas genu valgum (knock knee) maximizes by 5 to 6 years of age. If genu varum or genu valgum persists past these ages, a pathologic process rather than a physiologic phase may be present. Pathologic causes of genu varum are Blount disease, rickets, skeletal dysplasias (such as achondroplastic dwarfism), traumatic injury, and musculoskeletal infection. Genu valgum also may persist in children with a skeletal dysplasia, benign musculoskeletal tumors (multiple hereditary exostoses), osteogenesis imperfecta, or following a traumatic injury or infection. A genetic predisposition to genu valgum also may be evident.

Muscle Growth

The composition and size of muscles vary with age. In the fetus, muscle tissue contains a large amount of water and much intercellular matrix. After birth, both are reduced considerably as the muscle fibers (cells) enlarge by accumulating cytoplasm. Little information is available about the numbers of fibers in a given muscle at various ages, but the total mass of muscle in the body can be estimated from the amount of creatinine excreted in the urine, because the conversion of creatine to creatinine takes place only in muscle (see Chapter 44). Between birth and maturity the number of muscle nuclei in the body increases 14 times in boys and 10 times in girls. Muscle fibers reach their maximal size in girls at approximately 10 years of age and in boys by 14 years. Growth in length occurs at the ends of muscles, and the increase in length is accompanied by an increase in number of nuclei in the fibers. Muscle fibers increase in diameter as the fibrils become more numerous. The fibrils themselves do not increase in diameter. Connective tissue components of muscle grow where the tendon and muscle meet.

A potent stimulus to the growth of a muscle is the separation of its attachments as the skeleton grows. The length of a muscle fiber is the direct consequence of its intended range of movement. The stimulus for the formation of a tendon is probably the pull of the muscle rudiment on undifferentiated connective tissue. If the normal opponents of a muscle are paralyzed, the muscle fails to grow properly and can result in contracture of a joint.

Muscle growth during adolescence is a major factor in weight gain. Gender differences in muscle size and weight are minor in childhood but become considerable with the onset of puberty.

In the infant, muscle accounts for approximately 25% of total body weight, compared with 40% in the adult. In the adult, approximately 55% of muscle weight is in the lower limb muscles, whereas in the infant the majority of the weight is axial musculature. The respiratory

and facial muscles are well developed at birth so that the infant can perform the vital functions of breathing and sucking. Other muscle groups, such as the pelvic muscles, take several years to develop fully. Throughout life the weight of the skeletal muscles can be increased by exercise.

MUSCULOSKELETAL ALTERATIONS IN CHILDREN

Congenital Defects

Syndactyly

The most common congenital defect of the upper extremity is syndactyly, or webbing of the fingers (Fig. 46.2). Simple webbing involves the soft tissue envelope alone and is best released surgically when the child is 6 months to 1 year of age. Complex syndactyly involves fusion of the bones and nails as well as the soft tissues; it may be associated with absence or anomaly of bony or neurovascular units. The primary goal in surgical correction of these defects is to achieve maximal function and appearance. Ideally, corrective surgery is deferred until the child is 1 to 2 years old and completed before the child enters school. Vestigial tabs, such as an extra digit, however, are best removed during the immediate neonatal period. Anomalies on the radial aspect of the arm, such as a foreshortened or absent radius, are often associated with abnormalities of blood, heart, or kidneys. Lateral or ulnar-sided defects are less often associated with systemic anomalies and are extremely rare.

Developmental Dysplasia of the Hip

Developmental dysplasia of the hip (DDH), formerly known as *congenital dislocation of the hip,* is an abnormality in the development of the proximal femur, acetabulum, or both (Fig. 46.3). Although most often present at birth, it may occur at any time in the newborn or infant period.

The incidence of true dislocation of the hip or a dislocatable hip is 1 in 1000 live births. Some degree of instability of the hip is present in approximately 10 per 1000 live births. The left hip is affected in 60% of cases, whereas the right hip alone is affected only 20% of the time. Bilateral DDH occurs 20% of the time.

Risk factors for DDH include family history, female gender (6:1), metatarsus adductus (20%), torticollis (10%), oligohydramnios, first pregnancy, and breech presentation. First pregnancies and oligohydramnios (deficient volume of amniotic fluid) are thought to limit fetal movement, and breech presentation not only limits movement but also places the hips in a position of flexion and adduction, which creates a

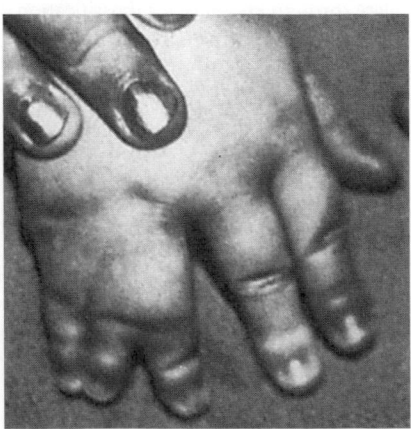

FIGURE 46.2 Syndactyly with Polydactyly.

more shallow socket, or acetabulum. Although only 2% of births have breech history, as many as 40% of infants with DDH had a breech birth. Maternal hormones that reportedly increase joint laxity also have an effect on DDH, although the exact mechanism is unknown. DDH also is more common in whites and those cultures that swaddle infants with the hips in extension and adduction. It is almost unknown in African cultures where infants are carried, with legs abducted, on the back.

◆**PATHOPHYSIOLOGY.** The hip can be described as subluxated (partial contact only), dislocated (no contact between femoral head and acetabulum), and acetabular dysplasia (the femoral head is located properly but the acetabulum is shallow or underdeveloped) (Fig. 46.4). The

subluxated hip maintains contact with the acetabulum but is not well seated within the hip joint. The acetabulum is often dysplastic (or shallow) although the femur is often normal. The dislocatable hip is sometimes located but can be dislocated easily. The dislocated hip has no contact between the femoral head and the acetabulum. Some degree of acetabular dysplasia is present in almost all cases. Typically, the acetabulum is shallow or sloping rather than cup shaped.

By approximately 10 weeks' gestation, the femur, acetabulum, and hip joint capsule are well developed. It appears that most hip dysplasia develops within the second and third trimesters and is often the result of positioning factors (i.e., breech positioning). There also can be a genetic component, although this is still poorly understood. In addition, 2% of DDH cases are teratologic or caused by a systemic syndrome, such as arthrogryposis or spina bifida, in which muscle contracture or imbalance leads to DDH.

If DDH is left untreated in the growing child, secondary changes occur. If the hip remains subluxated or dislocated, the acetabulum becomes increasingly shallow and the soft tissues shorten around the proximal femur. Subluxation leads to early osteoarthritis (OA), and it is now estimated that at least 60% of all OA of the hip is related to DDH. If the hip is dislocated, the bone acetabulum fills with soft tissue and a false acetabulum forms where the femoral head contacts the iliac crest. An apparent limb length inequity and hip muscle weakness occur, leading to a waddling gait. Back pain and hip pain develop in adulthood. Adult reconstruction of a dislocated hip, even with an artificial hip, is very difficult.[6]

◆**CLINICAL MANIFESTATIONS.** The clinical manifestations of DDH vary with the severity of the condition and the age of the child. Signs and symptoms that should be noted include the following:

1. Asymmetry of gluteal or thigh folds
2. Limb length discrepancy (Galeazzi sign)
3. Limitation of hip abduction
4. Positive Barlow maneuver (hip reduced, but dislocatable) (Fig. 46.5, *A*)
5. Positive Ortolani sign (hip dislocated, but reducible) (Fig. 46.5, *B*)
6. Positive Trendelenburg gait (waddling)
7. Pain (very late)

The child also should be examined for other anomalies, such as torticollis or metatarsus adductus, which can be associated with DDH.

◆**EVALUATION AND TREATMENT.** In the newborn period clinical examination is the most important diagnostic tool. Real-time ultrasound, in which the hip is examined while the ultrasound is performed, also

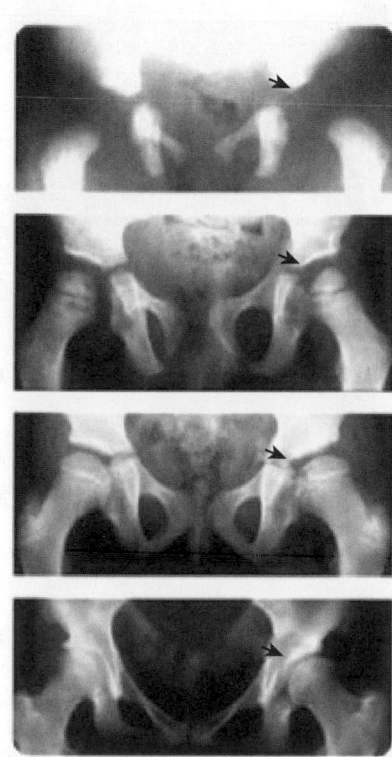

FIGURE 46.3 Hip Dysplasia in Children. Developmental dysplasia of the hip (DDH) with residual acetabular dysplasia *(red arrows)*. Radiographs at birth, 3, 10, and 19 years (top to bottom) show persisting dysplasia.

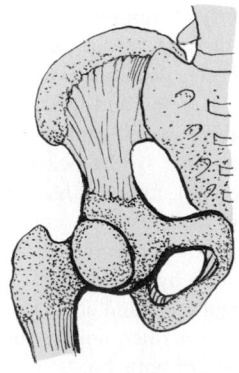 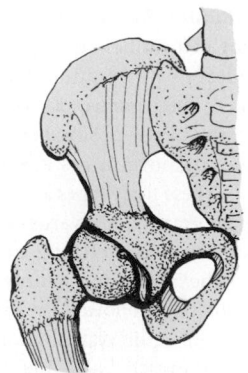 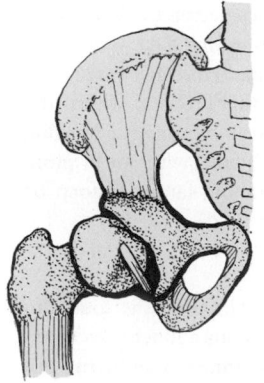 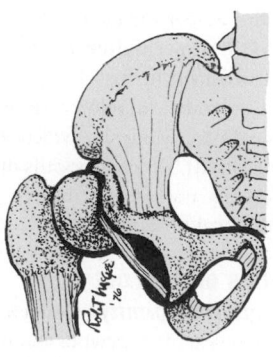

Normal   Dysplasia   Subluxation   Dislocation

FIGURE 46.4 Configuration and Relationship of Structures in Developmental Dysplasia of the Hip. (From Hockenberry MJ, Wilson D: *Wong's nursing care of infants and children,* ed 10, St Louis, 2015, Mosby.)

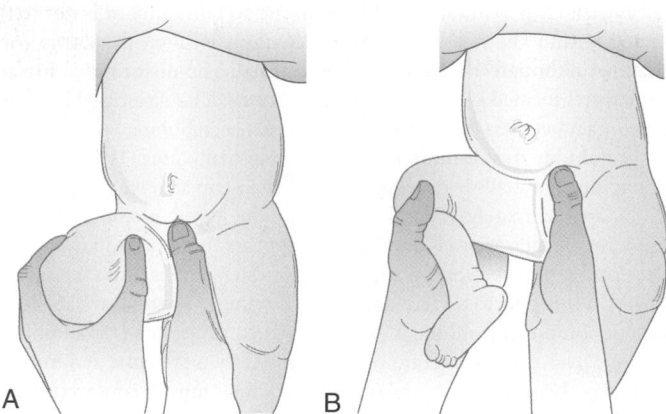

FIGURE 46.5 Congenital Dislocation of the Hip. **A,** Barlow maneuver. With one hand pressing the symphysis in front and the sacral spine in back, lateral pressure is applied to the thigh with the thumb of the other hand while pressure is applied with the palm to the knee on the side being examined. The hip that has been flexed to 90 degrees is then adducted. A positive sign is a sensation of abnormal movement, indicating dislocation of the femoral head from the acetabulum. The hands are reversed for examining the other hip. This sign and Ortolani sign may be found only in the first weeks of life. **B,** Ortolani maneuver. Sign of jerking into correct position. After the Barlow maneuver **(A),** the hip should be abducted to about 80 degrees while the femur is lifted anteriorly with the fingers along the thigh. A positive sign is a sensation of a jerk or snap with reduction into the joint socket. (Adapted from Specht EE: *Am Fam Physician* 9:88–96, 1974.)

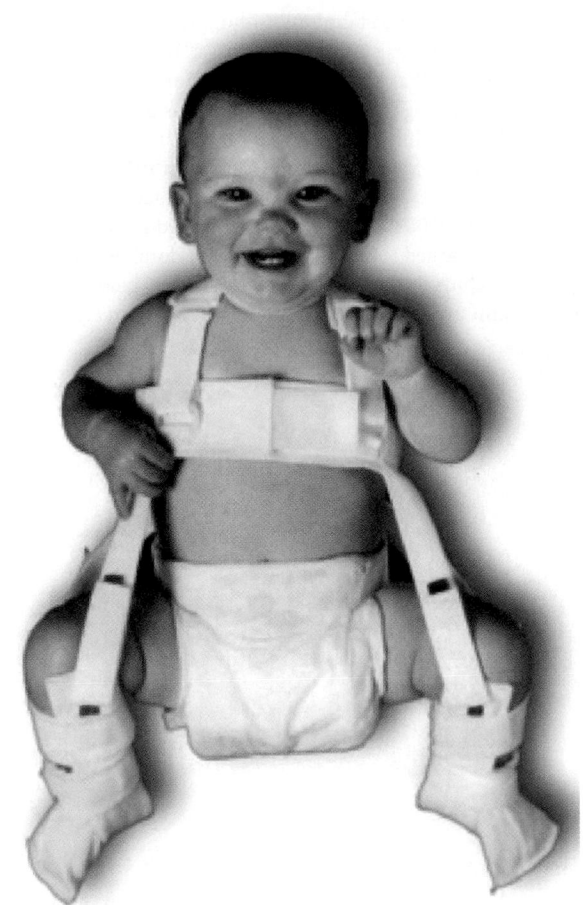

FIGURE 46.6 Pavlik Harness for Bilateral Hip Dislocation. (From Wheaton Brace Co.)

is extremely valuable in the newborn period, especially in high-risk infants. The use of ultrasound allows visualization of the cartilaginous structures of the hip (the femoral head and the outer lip of the acetabulum), which are not seen on plain roentgenogram. Radiographs are used after age 6 months when the ossific nucleus of the femoral head appears.[7]

Treatment depends on the age of the child, severity of dysplasia, and duration of dysplasia. The earlier that treatment is begun, the better the result. In children less than 4 to 6 months of age, a Pavlik harness can brace the hip in abduction and flexion, and the acetabulum will remodel as the femoral head rests centered in the socket (Fig. 46.6). With this treatment, up to 98% of children will have an excellent result. A "closed" reduction (without opening the joint) followed by spica or body casting for up to 3 months can be done in children up to 12 months of age. After 12 months, surgical intervention—including opening the joint and cutting and realigning the femur and/or acetabulum—may be required. The percentage of good outcomes decreases as the child ages. Up to 70% of children treated surgically for DDH after age 3 develop early osteoarthritis.[8] Early intervention before age 1 is critical for a good outcome; therefore vigilance for this problem within the first year is essential. Moderate evidence supports performing an imaging study (ultrasound) before 6 months of age in infants with one or more of the following risk factors: breech presentation, family history, or history of clinical instability.[9]

Deformities of the Foot

Congenital Deformity. Congenital foot deformity is found in approximately 4% of all newborns, and metatarsus adductus accounts for 75% of these deformities (Table 46.1). Metatarsus adductus is a forefoot adduction deformity associated with a normal, plantigrade hindfoot and is believed to be secondary to intrauterine positioning. It is associated with developmental dysplasia of the hip in 20% of cases; consequently, the hips of these infants must be carefully evaluated.

Metatarsus adductus is usually classified by two criteria: flexibility (passively correctable vs. rigid) and degree of deformity. The degree of deformity (mild, moderate, severe) is ascertained by the heel bisection line. A mild deformity is one in which the heel bisection line passes medial to the third toe; moderate, through the third or fourth toes; and severe, lateral to the fourth toe. Serial casts during the first 6 months of life are suggested for moderate to severe deformities and those deformities that appear less flexible. By 6 years of age, 87% of children usually correct *spontaneously*, and 95% by 15 years of age. Even in those children with some residual deformity, functional symptoms are rare.

Clubfoot: Equinovarus Deformity. Clubfoot describes a range of foot deformities in which the foot turns inward and downward. Technically called equinovarus, the heel is positioned varus (inwardly deviated) and equinus (plantar flexed) (Figs. 46.7 and 46.8). The clubfoot deformity can be positional (correctable passively), idiopathic, or teratologic equinovarus (as a result of another syndrome, such as spina bifida). These three types are discussed in the following sections. Overall, the positional equinovarus deformity lends itself to rapid correction by conservative stretching exercises or by application of a few serial casts. The idiopathic variety is treated by weekly cast correction/manipulation, followed by Achilles tenotomy and abduction bracing. Teratologic equinovarus deformities more often require surgical correction or muscle-balancing procedures, or both; however, initial serial casting may achieve correction of the foot deformity albeit with a higher risk of recurrence.

Positional Equinovarus. Positional equinovarus is a deformity in which an infant's foot is in equinovarus position but does have

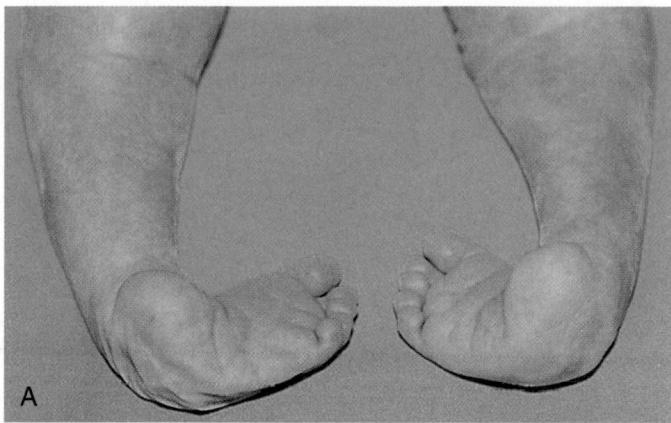

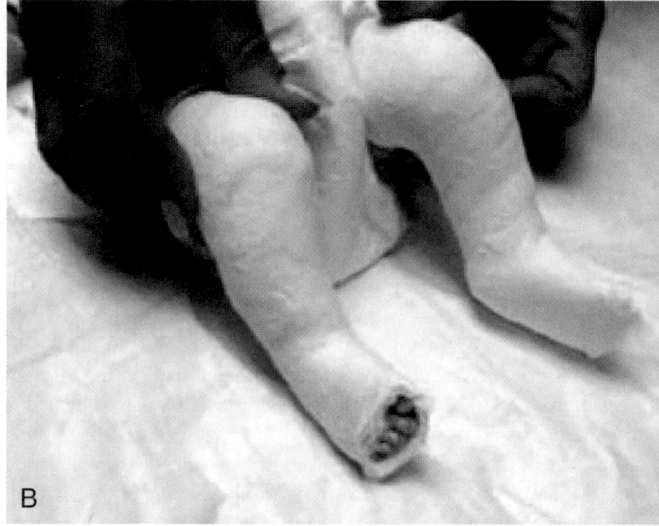

FIGURE 46.7 Bilateral Clubfoot. **A,** Infant with bilateral congenital talipes equinovarus. **B,** Ponseti casting. (**A** courtesy Dr. A.E. Chudley, Section of Genetics and Metabolism, Department of Pediatrics and Child Health, Children's Hospital and University of Manitoba, Winnipeg, Manitoba, Canada. In Moore KL et al: *The developing human,* ed 10, Philadelphia, 2016, Saunders.)

TABLE 46.1	TERMS USED TO DESCRIBE FOOT ABNORMALITIES
TERM	**DEFINITION**
Position	
Abduction	Lateral deviation away from the midline of the body
Adduction	Lateral deviation toward the midline of the body
Eversion	Twisting of the foot outward along its long axis
Inversion	Twisting of the foot inward along its long axis
Dorsiflexion	Bending the foot upward and backward
Plantar flexion	Bending the foot downward and forward
Abnormality	
Talipes	Congenital abnormality of the foot (clubfoot)
Pes	Acquired deformity of the foot
Varus	Inversion and adduction of the heel and forefoot
Valgus	Eversion and abduction of the heel and forefoot
Equinus	Plantar flexion of the foot in which the heel is lower than the toes
Calcaneus	Dorsiflexion of the foot in which the heel is lower than the toes
Planus	Flattening of the medial longitudinal arch of the foot (flatfoot)
Cavus	Elevation of the medial longitudinal arch of the foot (high arch)
Equinovarus	Coexistent equinus and varus deformities
Calcaneovarus	Coexistent calcaneus and varus deformities
Equinovalgus	Coexistent equinus and valgus deformities
Calcaneovalgus	Coexistent calcaneus and valgus deformities

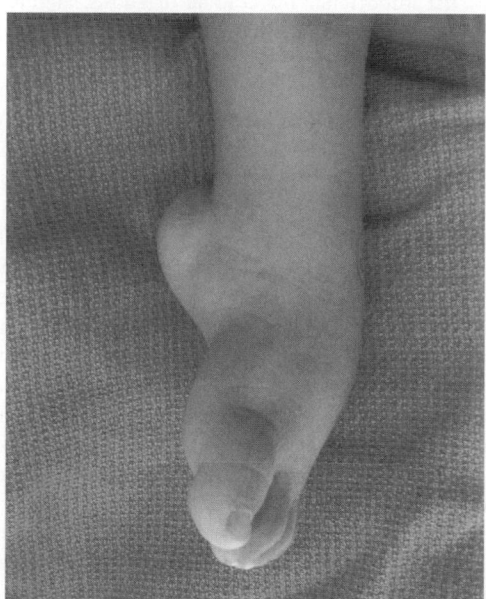

FIGURE 46.8 Idiopathic Clubfoot. Idiopathic clubfoot displaying forefoot adduction (toward midline of body) and supination (upturning) and hindfoot equinus (pointed downward). Note skin creases along arch and back of heal.

flexibility without deep creases at the posterior ankle or midfoot. The Achilles tendon is still flexible. The foot can be passively brought to a plantigrade position and is amenable to stretching and casting. In general, conservative therapy corrects this foot without the need for surgical intervention or lengthy bracing.

Idiopathic Congenital Equinovarus. The etiology of idiopathic equinovarus (clubfoot) is unknown. In one human fetal study, all clubfeet were associated with identifiable anterior horn cell changes in L5 and S1. Muscle biopsies of both the anterior tibialis long flexors and the peroneus brevis muscles in clubfoot reveal that at least 50% of cases show a decreased number of muscle fibers and/or abnormal fiber histology. The soleus often has an increase in type 1 fibers, whereas the peroneus brevis has a fiber type disproportion. The more abnormal the histopathology, the more severe the deformity, and the greater the chance of recurrent deformity after treatment. The genetic component is unclear and studies are ongoing.

Idiopathic equinovarus occurs in approximately 0.3 to 7.8 per 1000 newborns, with males being affected twice as often as females. Historically, these deformities were treated by posteromedial release, a surgical procedure that lengthened all tight structures and opened the capsule of all tight joints in the foot. However, since 1998 the casting technique developed by Ignacio Ponseti (see Fig. 46.7, *B*) has been used; the

technique involves six to eight above-knee casts, left on for 5 to 7 days each, followed by a percutaneous tendo achilles lengthening procedure performed with local anesthesia. The child then uses special braces at night until 3 to 4 years of age. Noncompliance with braces leads to increased recurrence and need for additional casting or surgery. Nearly

BOX 46.1   PONSETI CASTING

Ponseti casting implements toe-to-groin casts changed weekly for 6 weeks. Casting begins as early as possible after birth and culminates in a percutaneous tendo achilles lengthening in the clinic, followed by a final cast worn for 3 weeks. In recalcitrant cases, a full surgical posteromedial release (PMR) still may be required. The need for PMR in idiopathic clubfoot has decreased from 90% to less than 20% of infants when this casting technique is used. Long-term results, presumably because of less scarring and more long-term flexibility, are better with Ponseti casting than with the PMR method.

30% of children may need an anterior tibialis transfer around age 3.[10] Studies comparing operative posteromedial release with Ponseti techniques show better long-term results with the less invasive Ponseti method[11] (Box 46.1).

Teratologic Equinovarus. The most common cause of teratologic equinovarus is either neuromuscular (such as spina bifida) or syndromic (such as arthrogryposis or osteochondrodysplasia [e.g., diastrophic dwarfism]). The teratologic clubfoot, unlike the idiopathic type, more often fails to be corrected with Ponseti casting and may require operative intervention. The surgery is often more extensive than that for an idiopathic clubfoot, and revision surgery is also more common (see Box 46.1).

Pes Planus (Flatfoot) Deformity. Pes planus (flatfoot) commonly raises parental concern. Despite medical evidence to the contrary, it can be very difficult to convince families that a flexible flatfoot is often as functional as one with a "normal" arch. The majority of babies are born with flat (or "fat") feet, with the arch becoming more apparent with age. The relatively benign natural history, however, should not overshadow the importance of accurate diagnosis. Significant ankle valgus, vertical talus, tarsal coalition, and skewfoot must be accurately differentiated from flexible pes planus.

Flexible flatfoot deformity appears to be familial, with occasional association of generalized ligamentous laxity. Careful evaluation of possible occult Achilles contracture is done by holding the hindfoot in varus position and dorsiflexing the ankle. Achilles contracture can signify a more severe flatfoot variant. The flexibility of the hindfoot is evaluated by having the child stand on his or her toes facing away from the examiner. In flexible pes planus, the hindfoot swings into a varus position as the planter fascia tightens in toe raise. In rigid pes planus, the hindfoot stays in valgus and the child has more difficulty going up onto tip-toe.

Surgical or orthotic treatment of *asymptomatic* flexible pes planus is unnecessary. Custom orthotics, Helfet heel cups, and corrective orthopedic shoes have no influence over the natural history (clinically or radiographically) of flat feet. Adult studies on army recruits have shown that soldiers with flat feet perform just as well as their counterparts without "fallen" arches.

There is a small subset of children with painful, flexible flat feet. For these children careful attention to the possibility of Achilles contracture or tarsal coalition (congenital union of the hindfoot bones) must be made. This group of children is best treated with inexpensive shoe inserts and then expectantly watched. If pain continues into adolescence, requiring more aggressive treatment, calcaneal lengthening will correct the pes planus without decreasing hindfoot motion. In rigid flat feet, a computed tomographic (CT) scan often will reveal a coalition, a bony or cartilaginous connection between the bones—if painful, this can be resected. Heel cord contractures can be surgically lengthened if stretching alone is inadequate. All surgery carries risk; if a foot is flat but nonpainful, treatment is not required. The painless flatfoot should be viewed as a variation of normal feet.

Abnormal Density or Modeling of the Skeleton
Osteogenesis Imperfecta

Osteogenesis imperfecta (OI) (brittle bone disease) is a collagen-related bone dysplasia. Collagen is the main component of bone and blood vessels. The disorder was first described in 1840 as a syndrome in newborns that consisted of osteoporosis with fractures and skeletal deformities. The Sillence classification is based on both models of inheritance and clinical findings (Table 46.2), and has been useful to describe the most common types of OI. Newer classifications also exist and are based on the mode of inheritance, identifying the defective gene, protein, or mechanism[12] (Table 46.3).

In the most severe form of this disorder, the child is usually stillborn or dies soon after birth, although some survive into childhood. OI in its more severe forms is evident at birth because fractures and deformity have occurred in utero. The less severe forms may not become evident until the child begins to walk. Some children with this milder form then experience numerous fractures that can be mistaken for nonaccidental trauma until the diagnosis is made. The prevalence rate of the most common form is about 1 in 30,000. Inheritance is usually autosomal dominant but can be autosomal recessive. At least four syndromes have been identified that have various clinical manifestations and prognoses (see Table 46.2).

◆**PATHOPHYSIOLOGY.** The major errors in OI lie in the synthesis of collagen, a triple helix with two matching α chains and one β chain. Collagen is present in bone, cartilage, eye tissue, skin, and the vascular system. The severity of the OI phenotype and the related anomalies of the eye, dentition, or vascular system are all dependent on the severity of the genetic anomaly and the part of the triple helix that is affected.[13] (Genes are discussed in Chapter 4.)

A number of metabolic abnormalities are associated with OI. Some individuals have increased serum thyroxine levels, suggesting hyperthyroidism. This is consistent with the findings of increased sweating, heat intolerance, increased body temperature, a resting tachycardia, and tachypnea. Studies of leukocyte metabolism suggest an uncoupling of oxidative phosphorylation. Reports of alterations of platelet function with defects in adhesion and clot retraction also exist.

◆**CLINICAL MANIFESTATIONS.** The classic clinical manifestations of OI are osteoporosis and increased rate of fractures, possible bony deformation, triangular facies, possible vascular weakness (i.e., aortic aneurysm), possible blue sclerae, and poor dentition. The Sillence classification designated types I through IV on the basis of severity. The most severe, types II and III, are comparable to *osteogenesis imperfecta congenita*. These two types are characterized by autosomal recessive inheritance and early onset of manifestations. Both can cause stillbirth or severe neonatal deformity and a short life expectancy. Less severe are types I and IV, which are comparable to *osteogenesis imperfecta tarda*. Type I is slightly more common than types II and III, and type IV is quite rare. Types I and IV are inherited as autosomal dominant traits and vary in age of onset from birth to adulthood. Type IV, especially when the sclerae are white, is the least deforming type and is often confused with nonaccidental trauma (child abuse).

◆**EVALUATION AND TREATMENT.** Evaluation of OI is based primarily on clinical manifestations. Serum alkaline phosphatase level is elevated in all forms of the disease. OI can be diagnosed prenatally by ultrasound or chorionic villi sampling. Quantitative analysis of cultured skin fibroblast collagen by electrophoresis shows a decreased quantity of collagen in 95% of individuals.

Type II OI is often terminal in the perinatal period, and therefore little is known about appropriate treatment for the few children who survive. For other types of OI, careful positioning and handling of the newborn help prevent fractures. Beyond the neonatal period, various

TABLE 46.2 SILLENCE CLASSIFICATION OF OSTEOGENESIS IMPERFECTA SYNDROMES

TYPE	TRANSMISSION	MAIN BIOCHEMICAL DEFECT	ORTHOPEDIC	MISCELLANEOUS
IA	AD	Decreased production of type I collagen	Mild to moderate bone fragility, osteoporosis, normal stature	Blue sclera, hearing loss, easy bruising, dentinogenesis imperfecta absent
IB	AD		Short stature	More severe in IA with dentinogenesis imperfecta
II	AD, AR, and mosaic	Substitutions of glycyl residue in X1 or X2 chains in triple helix	Multiple intrauterine fractures, extreme bone fragility	Usually lethal in perinatal period, delayed ossification of skull, intrauterine growth restriction
IIA			Long bones broad, crumpled; ribs broad with continuous beading	
IIB			Long bones broad, crumpled; ribs discontinuous or beading	
IIC			Long bones thin, fractured; ribs thin, beaded	
IID			Severely osteoporotic with generally well-formed skeleton; normal-shaped vertebrae and pelvis	
III	AD and AR	Abnormal type I collagen	Progressive deforming phenotype, severe bone fragility with fractures	Hearing loss, short stature, blue sclerae becoming less blue with age, shortened life expectancy, dentinogenesis imperfecta, relative macrocephaly with triangular facies
IVA	AD	Shortened pro-α (I) chains	Mild to moderate bone fragility, osteoporosis, bowing of long bones, scoliosis	Light sclerae, normal hearing, normal dentition, dentinogenesis imperfecta absent
IVB	AD			Dentinogenesis imperfecta present

AD, Autosomal dominant; *AR*, autosomal recessive.
Reproduced with permission from Vaccaro AR, editor: *Orthopaedic knowledge update 8*, Rosemont, IL, 2005, American Academy of Orthopaedic Surgeons, p 248.

TABLE 46.3 OSTEOGENESIS IMPERFECTA (OI) TYPES CAUSED BY DEFECTS IN GENES AND THE COLLAGEN-RELATED PROTEINS THAT THEY ENCODE

	OI TYPE	DEFECTIVE GENE	DEFECTIVE PROTEIN	DEFECTIVE MECHANISM	
Autosomal dominant	I	*COL1A1*	α1(I) collagen	Collagen quantity	85%–90% of OI case types
	II	*COL1A1* or *COL1A2*	α1(I)/ α2(I) collagen	Collagen structure	I–IV
	III	*COL1A1* or *COL1A2*	α1(I)/ α2(I) collagen		
	IV	*COL1A1* or *COL1A2*	α1(I)/ α2(I) collagen		
	V	*IFITM5*	BRIL	Matrix mineralization	10%–15% of OI cases
Autosomal recessive	VI	*SERPINF1*	PEDF	Collagen 3-hydroxylation	10%–15% of OI case types VI
	VII	*CRTAP*	CRTAP		to unclassified
	VIII	*LEPRE1*	P3H1		
	IX	*PPIB*	CyPB		
	X	*SERPINH1*	HSP47	Collagen chaperoning	
	XI	*FKBP10*	FKBP65	Telopeptide hydroxylation	
	XII	*BMP1*	BMP1/mTLD	Collagen processing	
	Unclassified	*SP7/OSX*	SP7/OSTERIX	Osteoblast development	
		WNT1	WNT1		
		TMEM38B	TRIC-B		
		CREB3L1	OASIS		

Data from Marini J et al: *Curr Opin Pediatr* 26(4):500–506, 2014.

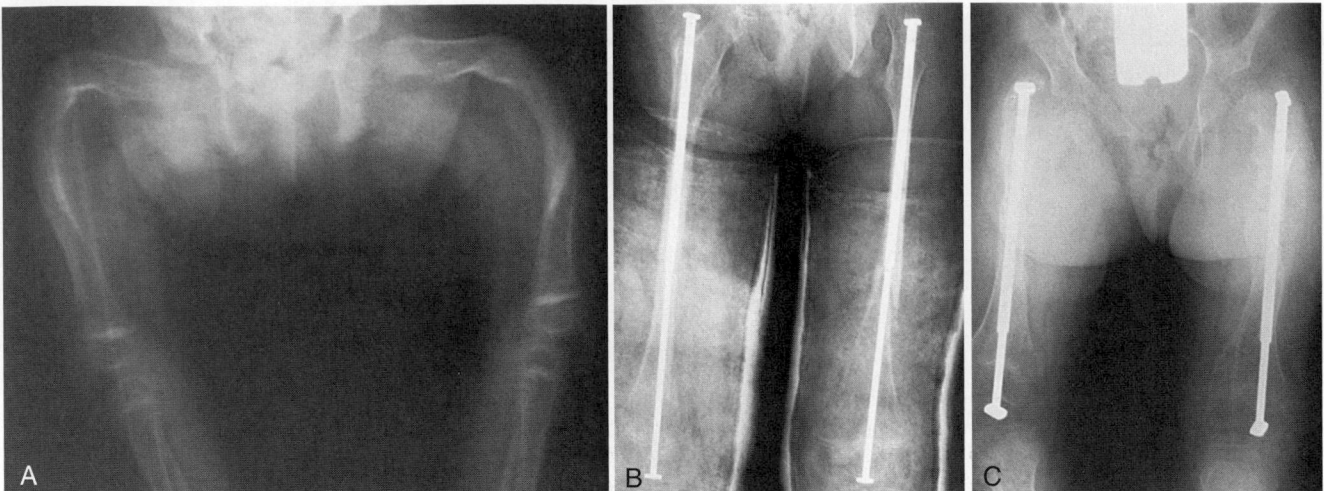

FIGURE 46.9 Osteogenesis Imperfecta Treated with Osteotomies and Telescoping Medullary Rods. **A,** Severe deformity of both femurs. **B,** Same individual after multiple osteotomies with telescoping medullary rod fixation. **C,** Same individual 4 years later demonstrating growth of femurs, no recurrence of deformity, and elongation of rods. (Plaster casts are in place for immobilization of tibial osteotomies.) (From Crenshaw AH, editor: *Campbell's operative orthopaedics,* ed 8, vol 3, St Louis, 1992, Mosby.)

orthopedic measures are applied, such as prompt splinting of fractures and correction of deformities arising from the progressive bowing or bending of the skeleton by intramedullary rodding of the bones (Fig. 46.9). Newer, telescoping rods, which grow with the child, have been shown to reduce the reoperative rate by 30%.[14] Scoliosis is present in up to 50% of Sillence III cases and often requires surgery. A multicenter study of a bisphosphonate therapy showed promising results in type III OI, with marked improvements of bone density (up to 30%). Chronic bone pain and fatigue also are thought to be lessened with routine bisphosphonate therapy. Despite these results, there is concern that the healing of fractures and surgical intervention can be more difficult. More study is needed to address the efficacy and safety of these types of drugs. Genetic counseling for affected families should aim at primary prevention.

Rickets

Rickets is a disorder in which growing bone fails to become mineralized (ossified), resulting in "soft" bones and skeletal deformity (Fig. 46.10). Rickets results from either insufficient vitamin D, insensitivity to vitamin D, wasting of vitamin D by the kidney, or inability to absorb vitamin D and calcium in the gut. The most common form is X-linked hypophosphatemic rickets in industrialized nations. In addition to the severe form of metabolic rickets, dietary and lifestyle changes in the United States have led to widespread vitamin D deficiency in children.[15] Although unprotected exposure to ultraviolet rays is not suggested, children still need 15 to 20 minutes per week of true sun exposure to activate vitamin D, the mineral necessary for absorption and metabolism of calcium and phosphate. In one recent study, up to 90% of *normal* American children had a low vitamin D level, especially children of color. This can lead to early fracture or slow bone healing after fracture.[16]

Severe metabolic rickets in the immature skeleton leads to short stature and bowing of the limbs with broad, irregular growth plates. The rows of cells in the growth plate that are intended to ossify fail to do so as they reach the metaphysis since calcification is impeded.

Children with rickets are often listless and irritable. They have hypotonia and muscle weakness and may be unable to walk without support. Abnormal parietal flattening and frontal bossing occur in the skull. The calvaria become soft, and the sutures may widen. Cartilaginous

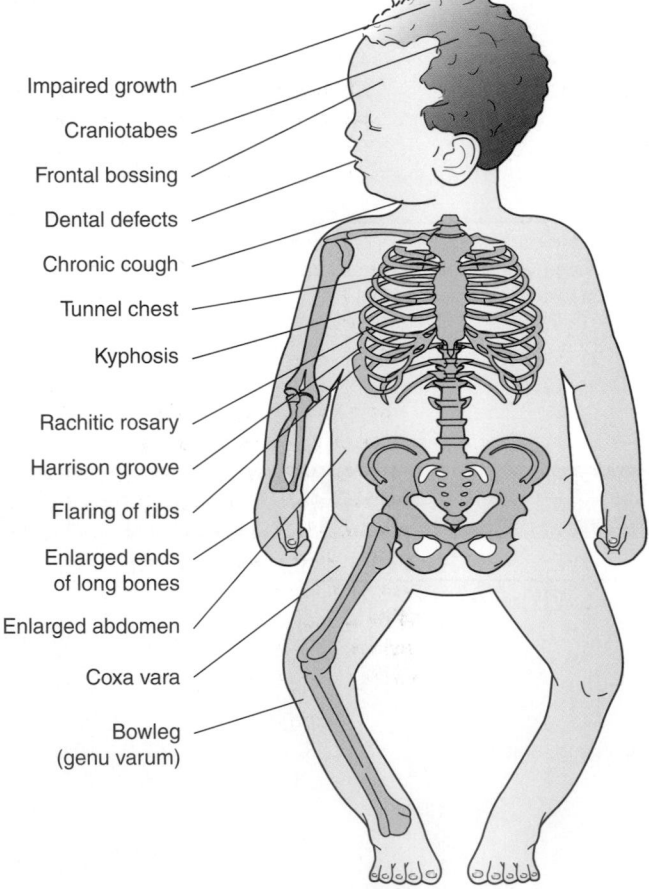

Impaired growth
Craniotabes
Frontal bossing
Dental defects
Chronic cough
Tunnel chest
Kyphosis
Rachitic rosary
Harrison groove
Flaring of ribs
Enlarged ends of long bones
Enlarged abdomen
Coxa vara
Bowleg (genu varum)

FIGURE 46.10 Rickets.

attachments of the ribs become prominent, and the long bones of the extremities (tibia, femur, radius, ulna) may be bowed. Growth is restricted, and fractures are common.

Like osteogenesis imperfecta, surgical treatment of bony deformity can be required. However, medical management of calcium, phosphorous, and vitamin D levels must be optimized before surgical intervention. In addition to medical management, children may benefit from guided growth techniques to correct persistent deformity (Fig. 46.11).

Scoliosis

Scoliosis is a rotational curvature of the spine most obvious in the anteroposterior plane (Fig. 46.12). It can be classified as nonstructural or structural. Nonstructural scoliosis results from a cause other than the spine itself, such as posture, leg length discrepancy, or pain. Structural scoliosis is curvature of the spine associated with vertebral rotation. Nonstructural scoliosis can become structural if the underlying cause is not found and treated.

Structural scoliosis can be caused by a great variety of conditions. It can result from congenital skeletal abnormalities (15%), neuromuscular diseases (15%), trauma, extraspinal contractures, bone infections that involve the vertebrae, metabolic bone disorders (e.g., rickets, osteoporosis, osteogenesis imperfecta), joint disease, and tumors. Most cases of structural scoliosis, however, have no known cause, although genetic factors are suggested. Structural scoliosis with no known cause, termed idiopathic scoliosis, accounts for at least 70% of cases.

Idiopathic scoliosis is classified as infantile, juvenile, or adolescent, depending on the child's age at the time of onset. In infantile scoliosis, also known as *early onset scoliosis*, spinal curvature develops during the first 3 years of life; in juvenile scoliosis, curvature develops between the skeletal age of 4 years and the onset of adolescence; and in adolescent scoliosis, it develops after the skeletal age of 10. Adolescent idiopathic scoliosis is the most common. Scoliosis in its milder forms occurs equally in boys and girls; however, girls are 10 times more likely than boys to develop curves greater than 30 degrees.

◆PATHOPHYSIOLOGY. It has been hypothesized that in individuals with adolescent scoliosis, there is an abnormality of the central nervous system involving the balance mechanism (reticular system) in the midbrain. A genetic component is also suggested because 30% occur within families.

Experimentally it also has been shown that individuals with adolescent idiopathic scoliosis have an abnormality in the function of the posterior columns of the spinal cord. This results in abnormal proprioception and is not evident clinically except in the presence of scoliosis. The exact cause of scoliosis, however, remains elusive.[17]

The earliest pathologic changes, which are probably secondary changes, occur in the soft tissues. The muscles, ligaments, and other

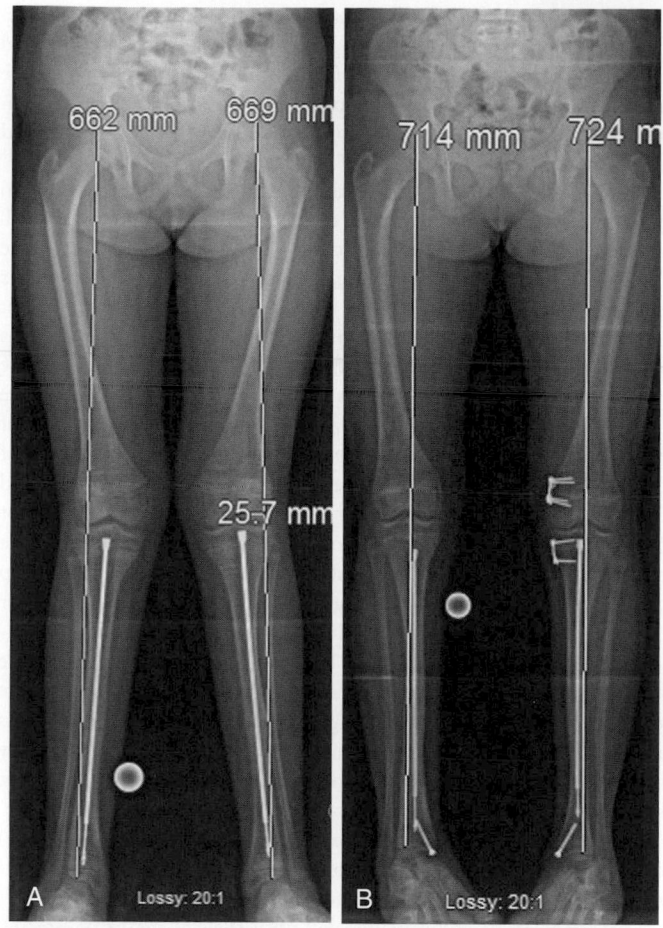

FIGURE 46.11 Guided Growth Technique. **A,** Right genu valgum and bilateral ankle valgus deformity in a 10-year-old female with osteogenesis imperfecta. **B,** Corrected left genu valgum and ankle valgus with guided growth technique. (Used with permission from M. Woiczik personal patient collection, images taken from 2012 and 2013.)

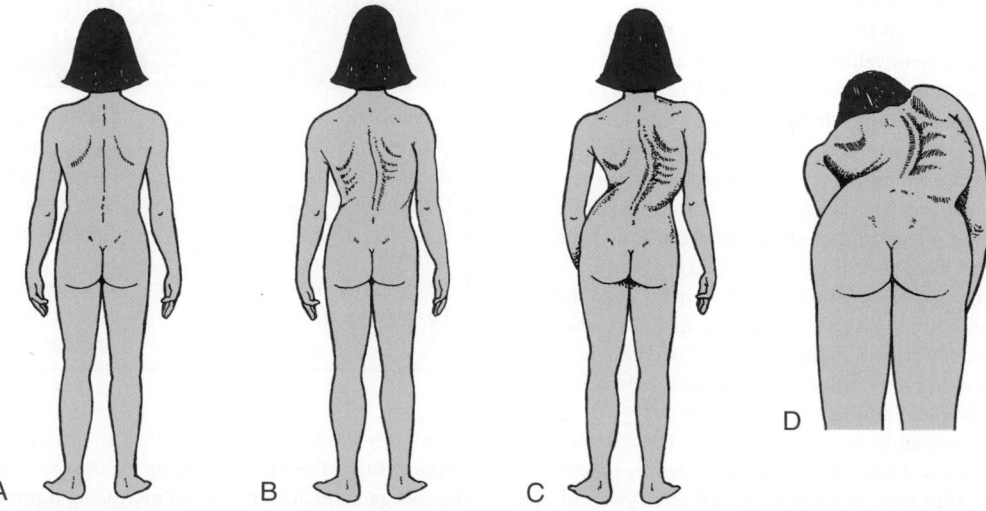

FIGURE 46.12 Scoliosis in Children. Normal spinal alignment and abnormal spinal curvatures associated with scoliosis. **A,** Normal. **B,** Mild. **C,** Severe. **D,** Rotation and curvature of scoliosis.

soft tissues become shortened on the concave side of the curve. Vertebral deformity occurs as asymmetrical forces are applied to the epiphyseal center of the ossification by shortened and tight soft tissues on the concave side of the curve. True curves involve not only bending but also twisting of the torso, leading to the "rib hump" seen when the child bends forward.

The curves increase most rapidly during periods of rapid skeletal growth. If the curve is less than 40 degrees at skeletal maturity, the risk of progression is quite small. In curves greater than 50 degrees, the spine is biomechanically unstable, and the curve usually progresses even after the cessation of growth. Curves in the thoracic spine greater than 80 degrees result in decreased pulmonary function, whereas the most common complication of large curves in the lumbar spine is back pain.

◆**CLINICAL MANIFESTATIONS.** The clinical manifestations of nonstructural scoliosis are mild spinal curvature with prominence of one hip or rounded shoulders. The curvature disappears with forward flexion of the spine, lying down, or traction of the head. Treatment for nonstructural scoliosis is correction of the underlying disorder. The clinical manifestations of structural scoliosis include asymmetry of hip height, asymmetry of shoulder height, shoulder and scapular (shoulder blade) prominence, and rib prominence.

◆**EVALUATION AND TREATMENT.** Spinal curvature is usually visible or palpable, and muscles on one side of the lower back (the convex side) may be prominent or bulging. Most cases of idiopathic scoliosis are noticed during school screening programs. In girls the deformity may be noticed because clothing does not "hang" properly on the body. Diagnosis is made by roentgenographic examinations.

Brace treatment is indicated for children with curves of 25 to 40 degrees who have at least 2 years of growth remaining.[18] A rigid, low-profile thoracolumbar brace is used in most cases. Low-profile braces are worn for 18 to 23 hours per day until skeletal maturity. Bracing will only prevent progression of the curve; it will not correct the curvature. Bracing is not effective in large curves or in skeletally mature individuals; the most effective time for bracing is in growing prepubescents with a small curve.[19] Extensive chiropractic manipulations and electrical stimulation have not been shown to change natural history. Surgical treatment using spinal fusion with instrumentation is recommended for curves greater than 40 to 50 degrees. If surgery is indicated, it is better performed during the adolescent years while there is greater flexibility of the curves and less risk of complications.

Bone Infection: Osteomyelitis

Osteomyelitis is an infection of the bone. Occurring twice as often in males as females, acute osteomyelitis may affect infants and children of any age, but it occurs most often between 3 and 12 years of age.

Bacteria enter the bone through the bloodstream and lodge in the medullary cavity, where a rich phagocytic mechanism often prevents most of the bacteria from establishing an infectious state. In some cases, however, the bacteria may lodge at the end of the venous loops beneath the epiphyseal plate, and infection then develops because there are no phagocytic cells present to remove the bacteria[20-22] (Fig. 46.13).

The microorganism responsible for osteomyelitis varies and is related to the age of the child (Box 46.2). Osteomyelitis in the newborn is caused primarily by *Staphylococcus aureus*. Group B streptococcus and *Escherichia coli* infections are responsible for some cases, especially those of multiple bone involvement and in high-risk infants.[22]

S. aureus is the responsible microorganism in 80% to 90% of osteomyelitis cases in older children. *Haemophilus influenzae*, a previously common cause of osteomyelitis in children less than 5 years of age, has become rare with the improvements in immunization. However, cases of methicillin-resistant *Staphylococcus aureus* (MRSA) have risen

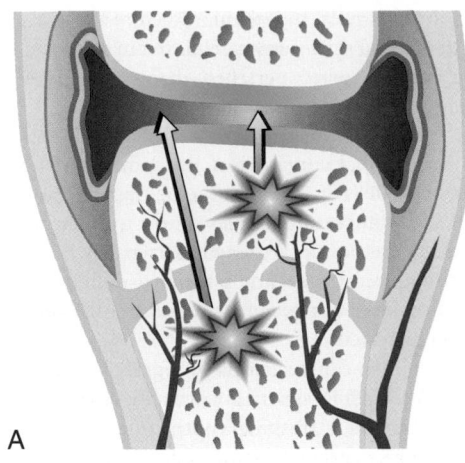

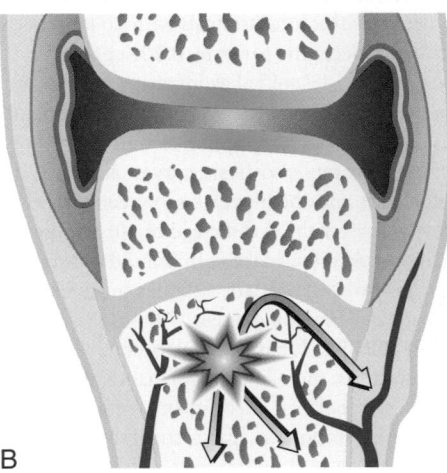

FIGURE 46.13 Pathogenesis of Acute Osteomyelitis Differs with Age. **A,** In infants younger than 1 year the epiphysis is nourished by penetrating arteries through the physis, allowing development of the condition within the epiphysis. **B,** In children up to 15 years of age the infection is restricted to below the physis because of interruption of the vessels.

BOX 46.2   CAUSATIVE MICROORGANISMS OF OSTEOMYELITIS ACCORDING TO AGE

Newborns
Staphylococcus aureus
Group B *Streptococcus*
Gram-negative enteric rods

Infants
S. aureus (MRSA 70, MRSA 30)
Haemophilus influenzae

Older Children
Staphylococcus aureus
Pseudomonas
Salmonella
Neisseria gonorrhoeae

Adolescents and Adults
Pseudomonas
Mycobacterium tuberculosis

alarmingly in the past 5 years. Once an infrequent cause of childhood osteomyelitis, MRSA now causes up to 30% of new cases.[23] Gram-negative microorganisms account for an increasing number of infections of the vertebrae,[24,25] whereas *Salmonella* infections are associated with sickle cell disease.

Factors that predispose an individual to the development of osteomyelitis include impetigo, furunculosis, infected lesions of varicella (chickenpox), infected burns, cerebral abscesses, immunization with bacille Calmette-Guérin (BCG) vaccine, prolonged intravenous or central parenteral alimentation, drug addiction, and direct trauma to the area adjacent to the site of osteomyelitis.

◆**PATHOPHYSIOLOGY.** Osteomyelitis usually begins as a bloody abscess in the metaphysis of the bone. The abscess ruptures under the periosteum and spreads along the bone shaft or into the bone marrow cavity if untreated. Infection rarely spreads down the medullary cavity of the bone but rather first gains entrance to the subperiosteal space in the metaphysis. The bone cortex in this area is porous, allowing easier entry for the bacteria than the shaft of the bone.[26] Because of the accumulation of debris caused by the infection, the periosteum may separate and form a shell of new bone around the infected portion of the shaft. Because the periosteum is separated from an adequate blood supply, sections of the bone die; these pieces of dead bone are called sequestra. The periosteum that maintains a blood supply generates new bone and is responsible for the appearance of the periosteal new bone, or involucrum. The presence of the sequestra and involucrum indicates that the disease is highly aggressive or established.

In cases in which the infection in the metaphysis occurs near the joint, the accumulating pus (bacteria, white blood cells, fluid) creates increasing pressure that may cause a rupture into the joint cavity. If rupture into the joint occurs, the pus causes inflammation and a condition called secondary septic arthritis.[24] Studies show that up to 40% of children will have adjacent joint involvement with osteomyelitis. The most common joint to be affected is the knee. Osteomyelitis is most commonly caused by bacteria that reach the metaphysis through the bloodstream but may occur through secondary inoculation of microorganisms caused by trauma or contagious spread of infection from cellulitis in adjacent soft tissue.

Osteomyelitis in infants is often associated with septic arthritis because the infant's bone has blood vessels that perforate the growth plate. Because of the unique nature of the blood supply to an infant's bones, the occurrence of osteomyelitis and septic arthritis in combination is higher than 50%. Normal anatomic variations in infants allow infection to spread directly to the epiphysis, which causes both joint disease and permanent injury to the growth plate. Multiple sites of osteomyelitis are also common in children younger than 2 years of age. Other areas of osteomyelitis and possibly septic arthritis must be evaluated through a bone scan of the entire skeleton.[27]

Children are susceptible to joint involvement for several reasons (Fig. 46.14). In the immature infant, there is no epiphyseal plate or an ossific nucleus at the end of the bone and the cartilage precursor of bone is penetrated by vascular channels. In these infants the infection begins in the vulnerable cartilage precursor of the end bone itself and results in rapid destruction of the joint and arrested growth of the bone. For this reason early detection and treatment of osteomyelitis are crucial if the infant's joint is to be saved from destruction. As the child matures and the epiphyseal, or growth, plate forms, a temporary barrier is established against infection because the arterioles end beneath the epiphyseal plate.[26]

In children older than 2 years, the epiphyseal plate prevents the spread of a metaphyseal abscess into the epiphysis and the cortex of the metaphysis is thicker. These anatomic differences increase the likelihood that the metaphyseal abscess will extend into the diaphysis, and the blood supply of the bone will be disrupted. The periosteum is also more difficult to perforate in older children; this may lead to a larger subperiosteal abscess that could endanger the periosteal blood supply as well. This process results in extensive sequestrum formation and chronic osteomyelitis.[26]

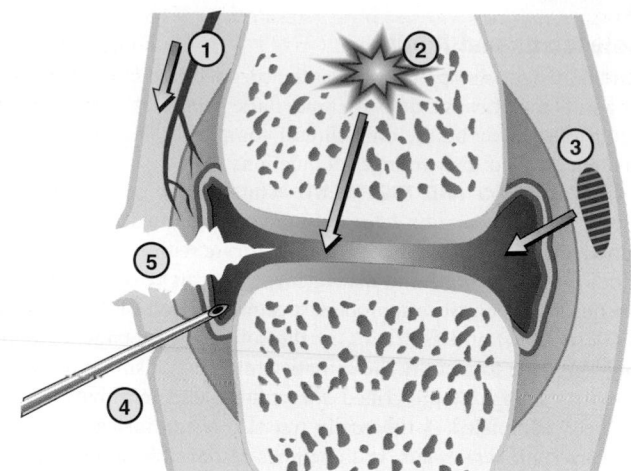

FIGURE 46.14 Routes of Infection to the Joint. **(1)** The hematogenous route; **(2)** dissemination from osteomyelitis; **(3)** spread from an adjacent soft tissue infection; **(4)** diagnostic or therapeutic measures; **(5)** penetrating damage by puncture of cutting.

Osteomyelitis is much less common after the physeal plates are closed, except in the vertebral body. Infection may develop in any part of a bone, and abscesses spread slowly. Destruction of the cortex in a localized area may result in a pathologic fracture.[24,25]

Spread of infection to contiguous joints is related to the child's age. Metaphyseal infection may spread to contiguous joints if the fibrous joint capsule includes the metaphysis and epiphysis. This special situation exists at the hip joint, distal femur, proximal humerus and radius, and lateral ankle. Careful clinical vigilance helps protect children with osteomyelitis from suffering permanent joint injury. Unlike bone, the articular cartilage of joints is unable to repair itself after injury from infection.[27]

◆**CLINICAL MANIFESTATIONS.** The clinical manifestations of osteomyelitis are age dependent and are related to the differing vascular patterns found in the skeletal system at various ages. Three distinct groups may be identified: (1) infants younger than 1 year, (2) children from 1 year of age to puberty, and (3) adolescents after cessation of bone growth and adults.

Infants

Osteomyelitis may be an acute illness characterized by fever and failure to move the affected limb (pseudoparalysis). Infantile osteomyelitis is characterized by involvement of multiple sites within the same bone or in multiple bones. If untreated, involvement of the adjacent growth plate can result in growth arrest.

Children

Osteomyelitis in children between the ages of 1 year and puberty is characterized by fever and systemic signs of toxicity. The illness is sometimes subacute, with the child complaining of swelling, fever, tenderness, and decreasing ability to bear weight on or move the affected area. Onset can be abrupt. Osteomyelitis during childhood most often affects the long bones but also may be found in the pelvis and spine. Clinical manifestations are usually accompanied by elevated white blood cell counts and elevated erythrocyte sedimentation rates. When the level of C-reactive protein (CRP) is elevated, it is a sensitive sign of osteomyelitis and can rapidly decrease with appropriate treatment. Evidence of infection using roentgenograms can be delayed but bone scan is positive within 48 hours.

Adolescents and Adults

In addition to the sites previously mentioned, osteomyelitis in adolescents and adults may involve the vertebrae. Back pain, with a duration of several weeks, may be the only clinical complaint. This age group is less often affected than younger populations.

◆**EVALUATION AND TREATMENT.** White blood cell counts and erythrocyte sedimentation rates are sometimes elevated, but this is not a consistent finding. Monitoring of erythrocyte sedimentation rates is an indication of response to management but can be delayed. CRP is more quickly responsive to appropriate treatment. Blood cultures (positive in 30% to 40%) and aspiration of the soft tissue or bone, or both, should be done to identify the causative microorganism. Appropriate antibiotics should be prescribed *after* culture and sensitivity studies have been completed. A tuberculin test also is administered because *Mycobacterium tuberculosis* is sometimes responsible and has had a slight resurgence in incidence. Bone scans can be quite helpful with diagnosis and in children younger than 1 year are absolutely required to define whether multiple sites are involved.

Treatment includes intravenous (IV) antibiotics or, in highly reliable children and families, a combination of IV and oral antibiotics for 6 weeks. Drainage and margination of bone are required if changes are present on radiographs signifying abscess. Immobilization may help with pain control. If a joint is also infected (termed *septic arthritis*), the situation becomes a *surgical emergency;* surgery on the affected joint can help prevent damage to the articular cartilage by lysozymes released from the involved neutrophils.

Death is rare, but serious sequelae may occur. The course of the disease and prognosis depend on the age of the child, the rapidity with which the diagnosis is established, the initiation of early treatment, and maintenance of treatment for an adequate time. The most serious complications are growth arrest, osseous necrosis, and recurrence. Recurrence with presently available antibiotic regimens is less than 10%.

Rheumatologic Disorders

The rheumatic diseases are a group of diverse conditions having in common the inflammation of connective tissues. They include juvenile idiopathic arthritis (JIA, formerly known as *juvenile rheumatoid arthritis*), systemic lupus erythematosus, dermatomyositis, and progressive systemic sclerosis (formerly called *scleroderma*). The incidence of these disorders in children is estimated in Table 46.4.

Juvenile idiopathic arthritis (JIA) is the most common rheumatologic disorder in childhood. Like adult-onset rheumatoid arthritis (RA), JIA is a syndrome that is often accompanied by systemic manifestations (see Chapter 45). Approximately 5% of all cases of RA begin in childhood. An estimated 250,000 children in the United States have JIA.

The basic pathophysiology of JIA is the same as that of adult RA; however, the clinical manifestations of JIA may differ. Unlike adult RA, which begins insidiously with systemic signs of inflammation and generalized aches, JIA has three distinct modes of onset: arthritis in fewer than five joints (pauciarticular arthritis), arthritis in more than five joints (polyarticular arthritis), and systemic or Still disease. JIA differs from the adult form in the following respects[28,29]:

1. Predominantly the large joints are affected.
2. Subluxation and ankylosis of the cervical spine are common if the disease progresses.
3. Joint pain may not be severe, as in the adult type.
4. Serologic tests often detect antinuclear antibody (ANA).
5. Chronic uveitis is common, especially if ANA positive.
6. Serologic tests seldom detect rheumatoid factor.
7. Rheumatoid nodules are not limited to subcutaneous tissue but are found in the heart, lungs, eyes, and other organs.
8. Cyclic citrullinated peptide antibody is often positive.

Many children with pauciarticular arthritis who are seronegative for ANA will resolve their symptoms over time. However, with systemic onset (Still disease) or seropositivity, JIA may progress to true adult RA. Treatment is supportive and aims to control inflammation and minimize deformity. The emergence of new treatments, including use of biologics and targeting of key cytokines and other inflammatory mediators, has dramatically improved the prognosis for children with JIA.[30]

Avascular Diseases of the Bone: Osteochondrosis

The avascular diseases of the bone, collectively termed osteochondroses, are caused by insufficient blood supply to growing bones. Disturbances of blood supply to primary and secondary centers of ossification during periods of rapid bone growth result in a variety of skeletal abnormalities.

The cause of the osteochondroses remains obscure. In the past, infection, nutritional deficiencies, and hormonal imbalances were blamed, but these causes have been largely disproved. Currently, vascular impairment and trauma, coupled with an underlying developmental or genetic predisposition, have been identified as probable causes of osteo-chondroses. The most common osteochondroses are Osgood-Schlatter disease (tibial tubercle), Sinding-Larsen-Johansson syndrome (distal patellar pole), Panner disease (radial head), Kohler disease (the navicular bone of the foot), and Sever disease (calcaneus). All are associated with activity-related pain of the affected region that improves with rest. All are more common in boys than girls and in athletes more than nonathletes.

The osteochondroses involve areas of significant tensile or compressing stress that undergo partial osseous necrosis, progressive bony weakness, and then microfracture. Most of these are associated with trauma and overuse and improve with rest. Use of antiinflammatories, modification of activities, and even immobilization of the affected area are used during active stages of the disease. Reparative correction by revascularization is the rule, although this may be a lengthy process.

Legg-Calvé-Perthes Disease

Legg-Calvé-Perthes (LCP) disease, commonly called *Perthes disease,* is classically thought to be an osteochondrosis like those previously described. This self-limited disease of the hip is presumably produced by recurrent interruption of the blood supply to the femoral head. The

TABLE 46.4	INCIDENCE OF CONNECTIVE TISSUE DISEASES IN CHILDREN				
DISEASE	ANNUAL RATE/10⁵	GENDER RATIO (FEMALE/MALE)	RACE RATIO (WHITE/BLACK)	PEAK AGE GROUP AT RISK (yr)	CHILDHOOD ONSET (%)
Rheumatoid arthritis	40	3:1	Equal	Increases with age (20–50)	5
Systemic lupus erythematosus	6	8:1	1:4	15–45	18
Dermatomyositis	0.8	2:1	1:3	45–65	20
Progressive systemic sclerosis	0.4	3:1	Equal	Increases with age (30–50)	3
Polyarteritis	0.2	1:3	Equal	Middle adulthood	Rare

Data from Hollingworth P. In Klippel JH, Dieppe PA, editors: *Rheumatology*, St Louis, 1994, Mosby.

ossification center first becomes necrotic and collapses and then is gradually remodeled by live bone.

LCP disease is relatively common (1 in 5000 children), usually occurring in children between 3 and 10 years of age, with a peak incidence at 6 years. It is more common in boys than in girls by a ratio of about 5:1. The condition is bilateral in approximately 10% of affected children; however, bilateral cases are temporally separated. If LCP disease appears at identical stages and the femoral heads show matched radiographic involvement, then another diagnosis, such as an epiphyseal dysplasia, should be considered.

The cause of decreased blood supply to the head of the femur is unknown. Several theories have been proposed, including trauma, infection, and protein C and S deficiencies, which cause a hypercoagulable state or vascular anomalies.[31] A plausible theory is that acute synovitis (infection of the synovial membrane) and increased hydrostatic pressure in the hip joint compress blood vessels that supply the femoral head.

Constitutional factors definitely play a role. Skeletal maturation is delayed an average of 2 years in children with LCP disease, and affected children are between 2.5 and 7 cm shorter than unaffected children of the same age. Familial occurrence is 30% to 40%. The disease is rare in blacks, and it is frequent in children of Japanese and central European ancestry.

◆**PATHOPHYSIOLOGY.** LCP disease runs its natural course in 2 to 5 years. In the initial stage the soft tissues of the hip (synovial membrane and joint capsule) are swollen, edematous, and hyperemic, often with fluid present in the joint (Fig. 46.15). The joint space widens, and the joint capsule bulges. The first stage lasts only a few weeks. In the second stage, called *fragmentation,* the entire epiphysis or the anterior half of the epiphysis of the femoral head loses blood supply and the metaphyseal bone at the junction of the femoral neck and capital epiphyseal plate is softened because of decalcification. Soon granulation tissue (procallus) and blood vessels invade the dead bone. This stage lasts several months to 1 year.

The third (or regenerative healing) stage ordinarily lasts 2 to 3 years. The dead femoral head is replaced by procallus, and new bone is laid down. Collapse and flattening of the femoral head occur, and the femoral neck becomes short and wide (see Fig. 46.15).

In the fourth (or healed) stage, remodeling takes place and the newly formed bone is organized into a live spongy bone. Children less than 6 years of age at onset have more time to remodel the damage LCP has caused and have the best outcome. Recent multicenter studies, using the Herring "lateral pillar" classification,[32] have shown that hips younger than 6 years with *no* involvement of the lateral femoral head (type A) do better than those with involvement of the lateral femoral head. Those children with complete collapse of the lateral femoral head (type C) have the worst prognosis. Long-term studies of type C hips show that 70% to 90% progress to osteoarthritis by 40 years of age.[33]

◆**CLINICAL MANIFESTATIONS.** Injury or trauma precedes the onset of clinical manifestations in approximately one-third of children with LCP disease. Onset of symptoms is insidious unless trauma aggravates the disease process. The pain often is referred to the knee and can lead to misdiagnosis as a knee injury. The inner thigh and groin also can be painful. In some children, pain may be absent or minimal. If pain is present, it is usually aggravated by activity and relieved by rest.

The typical physical findings include spasm on inward rotation of the hip and a limitation of internal rotation flexion and abduction. If the child is walking, an abnormal gait, termed a *Trendelenburg gait* or *abductor lurch,* is apparent. The child dips the trunk toward the affected side with stance to compensate for weak abductor musculature. If the hip pain or limp has been present for a prolonged period, muscles of the hip and thigh atrophy. A limb length inequity may be present if the proximal femoral physis is involved.

◆**EVALUATION AND TREATMENT.** Diagnosis is confirmed by radiographic examination. Principles of treatment are *containment* (keeping the ball completely in the socket) and *motion* to maintain the articular cartilage. In the past, children were treated with bed rest and a variety of braces. Most children can be managed with antiinflammatory medications and crutches for episodes of synovitis and with activity modification (avoidance of jumping activities that place increased stress on the hip) during the active phase of the disease. Serial roentgenograms monitor the progress of the disease and ensure that the hip remains congruent. Surgery may be necessary if the femoral head becomes subluxated or incongruent with the acetabulum before the reparative process. The ball must be congruent to take on the shape of the socket as remodeling occurs. Newer treatments, such as intraarticular injection of bisphosphonates (that reduce the function of osteoclasts), are being studied.[34]

Factors affecting the outcome of LCP disease are the age of the child at onset, the extent of necrosis, and the congruence of the joint at skeletal maturity. Recent studies have shown that girls, despite earlier skeletal maturity, do as well as boys. Outcome is 70% satisfactory with Herring stage A; for Herring stages B and C or age greater than 8 years, outcome is guarded. Present prospective studies are evaluating more aggressive early treatment (i.e., osteotomy of the femur or pelvis) on the more involved hips to change long-term outcome.

Osgood-Schlatter Disease

Osgood-Schlatter disease consists of tendinitis of the anterior patellar tendon, within which the patella (kneecap) is embedded, and associated osteochondrosis of the tubercle of the tibia. Osgood-Schlatter disease occurs most often in preadolescents and adolescents who participate in sports. The incidence is higher in boys than in girls, many of whom have increased outward tibial torsion compared to controls.[35]

◆**PATHOPHYSIOLOGY.** The severity of the lesion varies from mild tendinitis to a complete separation of the anterior extension of the tibial epiphysis, which is the part of the epiphysis that contributes to growth of the tibial tubercle. The underlying pathologic alterations also vary. The mildest form of Osgood-Schlatter disease causes ischemic (avascular) necrosis in the region of the bony tibial tubercle, with

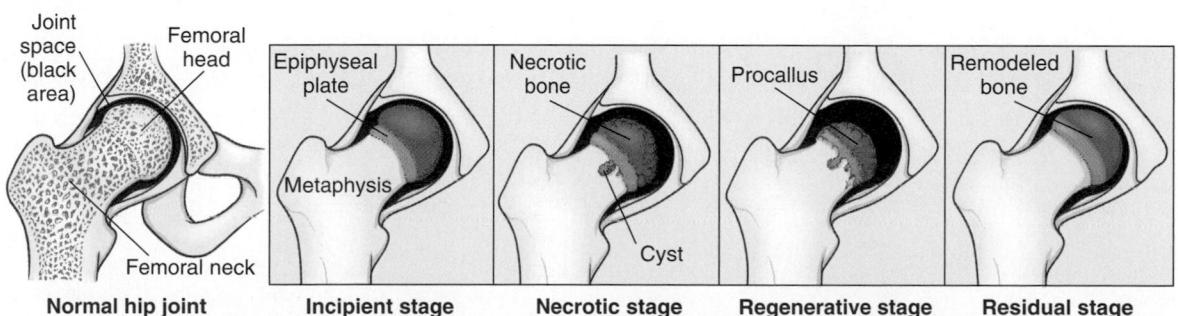

FIGURE 46.15 Stages of Legg-Calvé-Perthes Disease, a Form of Osteochondrosis.

hypertrophic cartilage formation during the stages of repair. In more severe cases the abnormality involves a true epiphyseal separation of the tibial tubercle.

◆**CLINICAL MANIFESTATIONS.** The child experiences pain and swelling in the region of the patellar tendon and tibial tubercle, which becomes prominent and is tender to direct pressure. The pain is most severe after physical activity that involves vigorous quadriceps contraction or direct local trauma to the tibial tubercle area. Often the child experiences sudden acute discomfort referable to the affected region. Sudden onset of pain can represent a pathologic fracture through an area of ischemic necrosis.

◆**EVALUATION AND TREATMENT.** Diagnosis is confirmed by roentgenographic examination. The goal of treatment for Osgood-Schlatter disease is to decrease the stress at the tubercle. Often a period of 4 to 8 weeks of restriction from strenuous physical activity is sufficient. If pain relief is not achieved, a cast or brace is required to immobilize the knee, a situation that is particularly difficult if the condition is bilateral.

Gradual resumption of activity is permitted after 8 weeks, but return to unrestricted athletic participation requires an additional 8 weeks to allow for revascularization, healing, and ossification of the tibial tubercle. All types of osteochondroses resolve once skeletal maturity is reached.

Cerebral Palsy

Cerebral palsy (CP) is a general term that refers to nonprogressive disorders of movement and posture resulting from injury or malformation of the developing central nervous system. The resulting disability may be mild, manifesting as a stiff (spastic) gait, or severe, in which the child is in a wheelchair and needs lifelong help eating, ambulating, and communicating. Comorbid conditions, such as intellectual disability, seizures, scoliosis, and hearing or vision loss, are common, especially in children with more severe forms. The overall incidence is 3% to 5%; this number has stayed approximately the same although changes in prenatal and newborn care have been associated with shifts in the etiologies of CP.[36,37]

◆**EVALUATION AND TREATMENT.** The diagnosis of CP is often made after failure to meet gross motor milestones at predicted ages. In some infants, diagnosis is made at birth or in the first months of life because the child has an underlying diagnosis, such as a major brain malformation, that is known to be associated with CP.[38] Classic patterns of motor involvement include hemiplegia, involving only one side of the body; diplegia, involving only the lower extremities; and quadriplegia, involving all four extremities. In addition to physical therapy, children with CP should receive speech/language therapy with trials of augmentative communication devices so that underlying cognitive abilities, which may not be apparent because of motor problems, are given a chance to manifest.

Treatment of CP is multifaceted and focused on maximizing functional abilities. Physical and occupational treatments, use of orthotics, spasticity reduction (by selected dorsal rhizotomy, oral, or intrathecal baclofen injections), botulinum-A (Botox) toxin injections, and surgery are commonly used approaches. In many centers, a multispecialty approach at "CP clinics" occurs so that a family may, within one clinic visit, see neurology, pediatrics, orthotics, orthopedic surgery, and rehabilitation clinicians.

Children with CP should be carefully followed and given all possible opportunities to flourish. Although CP is a static disorder, progressive deformity because of increased muscle tone can occur. Monitoring these children as they grow with a multispecialty approach is essential to their optimal outcome.

Neuromuscular Disorders

The neuromuscular disorders are a group of inherited disorders that cause progressive muscle fiber loss leading to weakness, mostly of the voluntary muscles. Duchenne muscular dystrophy (DMD) and spinal muscular atrophy (SMA) are the most prevalent of the muscle diseases in childhood (Table 46.5). Neuromuscular disorders cause significant disability in affected children resulting in lifelong neurologic,

TABLE 46.5   MAJOR NEUROMUSCULAR DISORDERS IN CHILDREN

DISEASE	MODE OF INHERITANCE	AGE AT CLINICAL ONSET	USUAL DISTRIBUTION	RATE OF PROGRESSION	INTELLECTUAL DISABILITY	DISTINGUISHING FINDINGS
Duchenne muscular dystrophy (DMD)	X-linked recessive	About 3 years	Hips and shoulders, quadriceps femoris, gastrocnemius (pseudohypertrophy)	Rapid	Frequent	Elevated serum enzymes (CPK, LDH, SGOT, aldolase)
Spinal muscular atrophy (SMA)	Autosomal recessive	Variable depending on subtype (infant to childhood)	Proximal greater than distal, especially involving hip and shoulder girdles	Rapid	Absent	Tongue fasciculation, tremor
Facioscapulohumeral dystrophy	Autosomal dominant	In first or second decade	Shoulder girdle, neck, face, pelvic girdle (late)	Moderate	Occasional	Several distinct muscle pathologic findings
Limb girdle (LG) dystrophy	Poorly defined or recessive	Variable	Pelvic and shoulder girdles	Variable	Variable	Collection of several diseases
Myotonic dystrophy (MyD)	Autosomal dominant	Variable—birth to fifth decade	Distal extensor muscle, eyelids, face, neck, hands, pharynx	Slow, related to age at clinical onset, faster with younger patients	Frequent	Percussion myotonia, cataracts, diabetic glucose tolerance test despite increased insulin, testicular atrophy, decreased IgG

orthopedic, and pulmonary complications necessitating complex, multispecialty care.

Although historically the classification of neuromuscular disorders was based on age of onset, rate of progression, distribution of muscular involvement, findings from muscle biopsy, and patterns of inheritance, increasingly genetic testing is used for diagnosis and classification. Current paradigms follow the traditional approach with respect to the clinical history, physical examination, and family history to narrow the differential diagnosis to one or a few disorders that can then be tested directly with a genetic test. For common disorders with distinctive phenotypes, such as DMD, myotonic dystrophy, facioscapulohumeral dystrophy (FSHD), and SMA, genetic testing has become a first-line test based on clinical history and examination (Fig. 46.16).

Duchenne Muscular Dystrophy

In 1868 the French neurologist G.B.A. Duchenne described boys with progressive weakness associated with large calf muscles, said to be **pseudohypertrophic**, because they consisted of fat and connective tissue rather than muscle. Duchenne muscular dystrophy (DMD) is the most common of the muscular dystrophies, affecting approximately 1 in 3500 male births.[39] DMD occurs primarily in boys because of an X-linked inheritance.

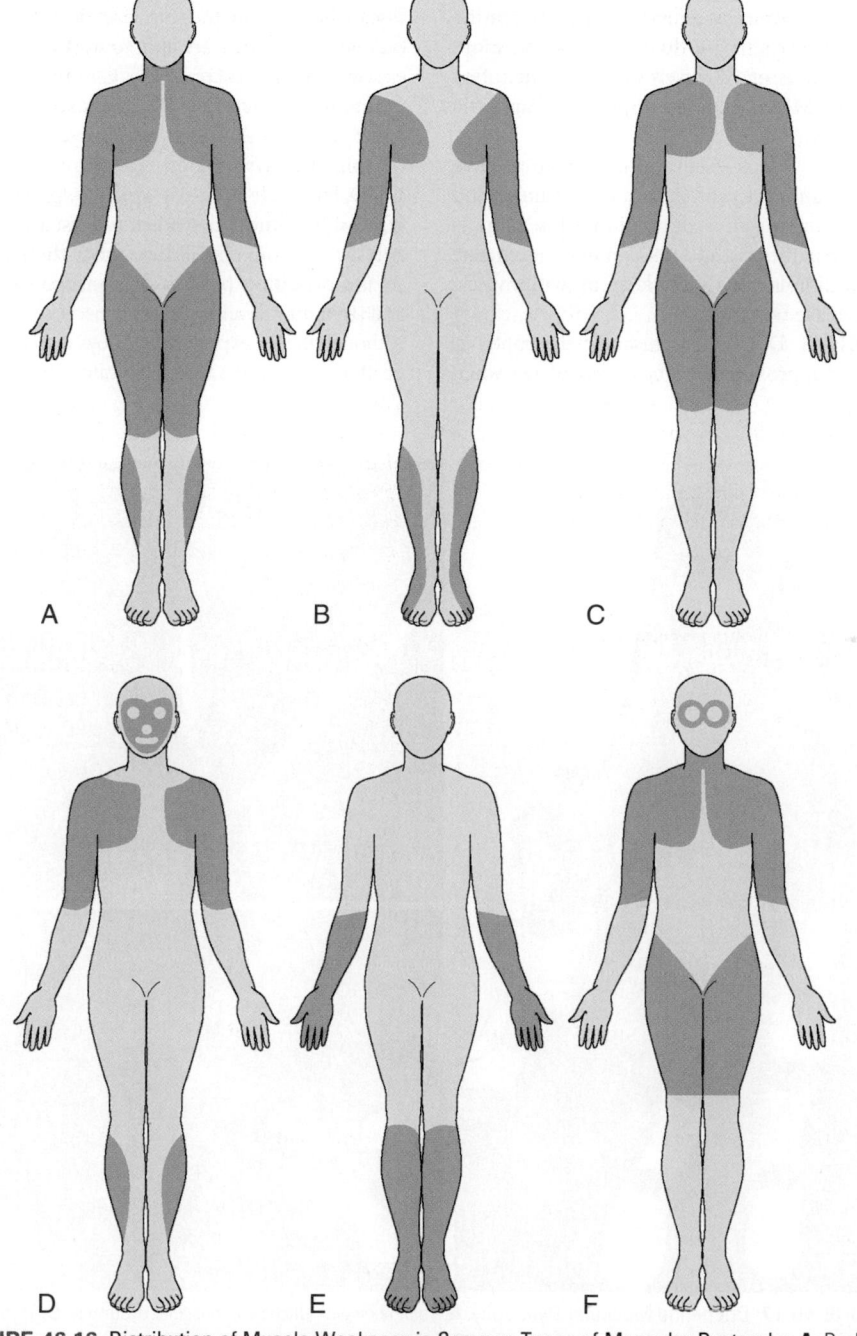

FIGURE 46.16 Distribution of Muscle Weakness in Common Types of Muscular Dystrophy. A, Duchenne muscular dystrophy. **B,** Emery-Dreifuss muscular dystrophy. **C,** Limb girdle. **D,** Facioscapulohumeral. **E,** Distal. **F,** Oculopharyngeal. (From Emery-Dreifuss AE: *Lancet* 359[9307]:687–695, 2002.)

◆**PATHOPHYSIOLOGY.** Duchenne muscular dystrophy (DMD) is caused by deletion of one or more exons of the *DMD* gene on the X chromosome or, more rarely, by a nonsense mutation resulting in premature termination of translation.[40] *DMD* is the largest gene in the human genome and encodes **dystrophin,** a large, membrane-stabilizing protein.

Dystrophin is present in normal muscle cells and absent in DMD. Milder mutations with residual dystrophin expression result in **Becker muscular dystrophy,** a milder syndrome. Dystrophin mediates anchorage of the actin cytoskeleton of skeletal muscle fibers to the basement membrane through a membrane glycoprotein complex. The lack of dystrophin results in poorly anchored fibers that are torn apart under the repeated stress of contraction. Free calcium then enters the muscle cells, causing cell death and fiber necrosis[41] (Fig. 46.17). Disruption of the cell membrane allows escape of creatine kinase (CK), increasing serum levels to 100 to 1000 times or more its normal level. Marked elevations of CK levels are easily identified in children suspected to have DMD and are an important diagnostic screen.

As muscle degenerates, there is increased endomysial connective tissue and fat; loss of striations; and concomitant hyaline, granular, and fatty degeneration of fibers. Disorganization of tendinous insertions is associated with fat accumulation in these areas. Although fibers regenerate in the younger child, regeneration is not able to keep up with muscle cell death, resulting in progressive weakness.

◆**CLINICAL MANIFESTATIONS.** Duchenne muscular dystrophy is usually identified in children at approximately 3 to 4 years of age, when the parents first notice gait abnormalities, including toe walking, difficulty getting up from the ground, and frequent falls.[42]

Muscular weakness begins in the pelvic girdle, causing a "waddling" gait. Hypertrophy of the calf muscles is apparent in 80% of cases. The method of rising from the floor by "climbing up the legs" (Gower sign) is characteristic and is caused by weakness of the lumbar and gluteal muscles. The foot assumes an equinovarus position (see Fig. 46.7), and the child tends to walk on the toes because of weakness of the anterior tibial and peroneal muscles. Within 3 to 5 years, muscles of the shoulder girdle become involved.

Progressive weakness results in loss of ambulation between 12 and 15 years of age. Subsequent progression includes slowly progressive respiratory insufficiency, cardiomyopathy, and orthopedic complications including scoliosis. Treatment with oral corticosteroids early in the disease has become the standard of care and has dramatically improved outcomes. Children are able to walk an additional 2 to 5 years and life expectancy has increased.[43] Complications, such as compromised pulmonary function and kyphoscoliosis ("humped" upper spine combined with scoliosis), are delayed.

Cognitive dysfunction is a common and often overlooked aspect of DMD. Full-scale IQ is 85, which is significantly lower than the average IQ of 100, although studies suggest this decrease may be caused by specific learning disabilities rather than a true decreased intelligence. As the condition progresses, constipation and incontinence of urine and stool may develop, possibly because of smooth muscle involvement. Although the life expectancy of boys with Duchenne continues to increase, death usually occurs from respiratory tract infection and a compromised

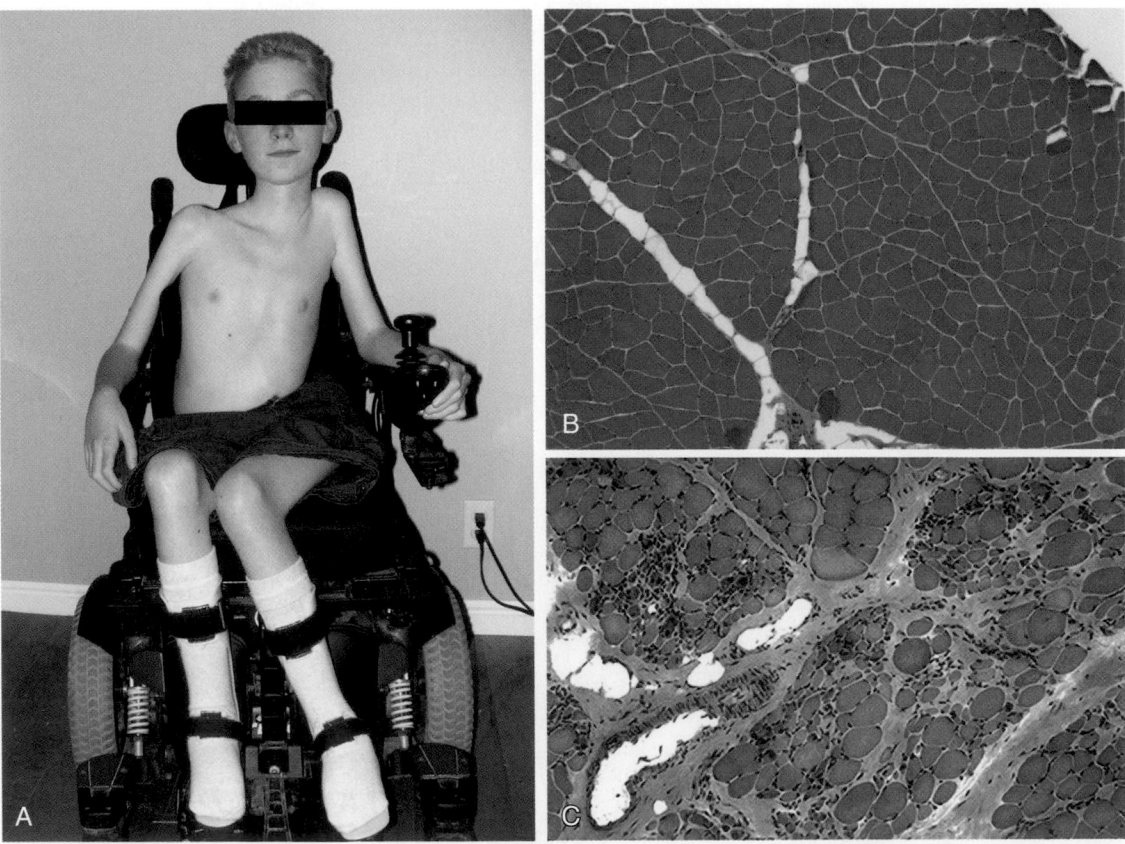

FIGURE 46.17 Duchenne Muscular Dystrophy. **A,** Young boy with Duchenne muscular dystrophy. **B,** Transverse section of gastrocnemius muscle from a healthy boy. **C,** Transverse section of gastrocnemius muscle from a boy with Duchenne muscular dystrophy. Normal muscle fiber is replaced with fat and connective tissue. (From Jorde LB, Carey JC, Bamshad MJ: *Medical genetics,* ed 5, Philadelphia, 2016, Mosby.)

respiratory system, with the majority living into their middle twenties. Some individuals who have chosen ventilatory support live a decade or more longer. With increased survival, cardiac complications are becoming an important contributor to mortality.

◆**EVALUATION AND TREATMENT.** Diagnosis is confirmed by genetic testing, which is informative in 95% of cases. Levels of serum enzymes, especially CK, are increased 100 to 1000 times normal, even during infancy and before the onset of weakness.

Genetic counseling is recommended for all families who have children with DMD. About one-third of the time, the mutation in a boy with DMD is sporadic; that is, the boy is the first person in the family to develop the mutation causing DMD. With X-linked inheritance, male siblings of an affected child have a 50% chance of being affected and female siblings have a 50% chance of being carriers. Prenatal diagnosis is now possible and female carriers can be identified, especially if there is a known genetic defect in another family member. However, a negative carrier test cannot exclude the female being a carrier since the female's germ cells (her eggs) may be of two different types: one with Duchenne and one without (mosaicism). Various strategies to develop gene modification or gene replacement are currently in development for children with DMD.[44] An exon-skipping approach to gene modification was recently accepted as the first FDA-approved treatment for DMD.

Children with DMD require a multidisciplinary approach to care, including attention to heart and breathing problems, weight loss/gain, constipation, rehabilitative/developmental problems, psychosocial needs, neurologic issues, and orthopedic problems (Fig. 46.18). Maintaining function in unaffected muscle groups for as long as possible is the primary goal of treatment. Although activity fosters maintenance of muscle function, strenuous exercise may hasten the breakdown of muscle fibers.

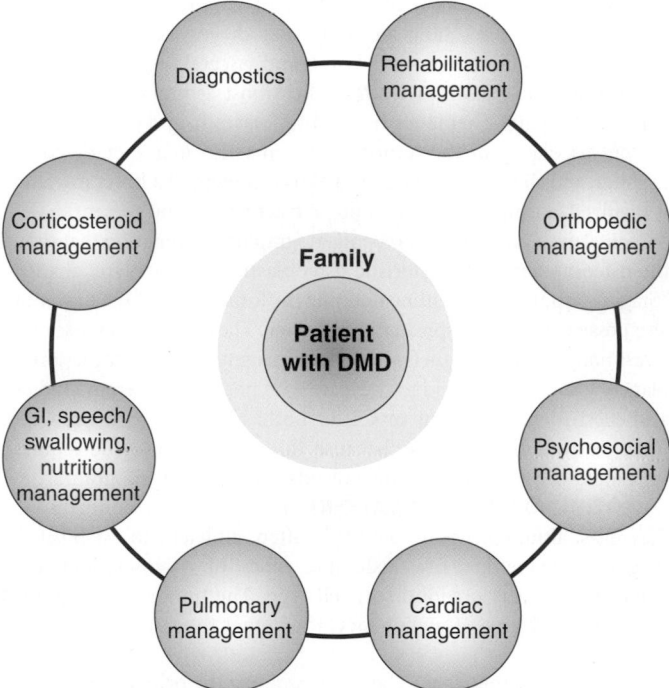

FIGURE 46.18 Multisystem Approach for Evaluation and Treatment of Duchenne Muscular Dystrophy. *DMD,* Duchenne muscular dystrophy; *GI,* gastrointestinal. (Adapted from Bushby K: Diagnosis and management of Duchenne muscular dystrophy part 1: diagnosis and pharmacological and psychosocial management, 2009; Bushby K: Diagnosis and management of Duchenne muscular dystrophy part 2: implementation of multidisciplinary care, 2009. Available at www.thelancet.com/neurology. Published online November 30, 2009.)

Range-of-motion exercises, bracing, and surgical release of contracture deformities are used to maintain normal function as long as possible. To prolong respiratory function or walking ability, or both, surgery for scoliosis is suggested when curves reach greater than 20 degrees.

Spinal Muscular Atrophy

Spinal muscular atrophy (SMA) is a common, autosomal recessive disorder characterized by degeneration of motor neurons in the spinal cord leading to progressive muscle atrophy. Children have progressive weakness and loss of motor skills. Clues to diagnosis include tongue fasciculation and a bell-shaped chest in the most severely affected infants, and tremor and quadriceps atrophy in older children. Genetically, SMA is caused by a mutation in the *SMN1* gene. About 1 in 40 individuals carries the common mutation in the *SMN1* gene, making it one of the most common recessive disorders, affecting approximately 1 in 6000 individuals.[45,46] The severity of SMA is variable. Type 1 SMA is the most common and is seen in infants with profound weakness from the first months of life. These children never achieve independent sitting, have significant respiratory compromise, and rarely survive the second year. Children with type 2 SMA achieve sitting independently but never walk. These children have significant disability, including profound weakness, but can survive into adulthood. Type 3 SMA is more variable in severity and includes children who can walk at least 10 meters independently. Treatment is supportive and, like DMD, requires multidisciplinary specialty care. The new drug nusinersen (Spinraza), an antisense oligonucleotide, has been approved for treatment.[47] Genetic replacement and gene modification therapies are rapidly evolving, and may have a significant impact on survival and progression in coming years.

Facioscapulohumeral Muscular Dystrophy

Facioscapulohumeral muscular dystrophy (FSHD) is a mild form of progressive, autosomal dominant muscular dystrophy. Age at onset varies from early childhood to adulthood, and the disease affects males and females equally. As the name implies, clinical manifestations begin with weakness and atrophy of facial and shoulder girdle (scapulohumeral) muscles. The illness progresses slowly. Inability to close the eyes completely may be noted from early childhood. The face is expressionless, and pouting of the lips makes whistling impossible. The first symptoms usually include drooping of the shoulders with difficulty in raising the arms above the head. Onset of weakness in the lower limbs often is delayed for 20 to 30 years, and pseudohypertrophy of muscles is rare. Contractures and skeletal deformities develop less often and are less prominent than in DMD. FSHD is rare compared to the other dystrophies in that it often manifests asymmetrically.

Treatment includes supportive physiotherapy to prevent contractures and prolong ambulation. Lightweight plastic ankle-foot orthoses (AFOs) for footdrop are extremely helpful. Shoulder pain is often present and figure-of-eight bracing or surgery to stabilize the shoulder is sometimes advised.

Musculoskeletal Tumors in Children
Bone Tumors

Bone tumors are uncommon childhood tumors and comprise less than 5% of all childhood malignancies. Of the malignant tumors, osteosarcoma and Ewing sarcoma are the most common. Fortunately, the majority of pediatric tumors are benign, most commonly nonossifying fibroma, osteochondroma, simple bone cyst, aneurysmal bone cyst, osteoid osteoma, and fibrous dysplasia.

Benign Bone Tumors
Nonossifying Fibroma. Nonossifying fibromas are sharply demarcated, cortically based lesions of fibrocytes that have replaced

normal bone. These fibromas constitute about 50% of benign bone tumors. Most fibrous cortical defects are metaphyseal and resolve spontaneously or are obliterated by reparative ossification or remodeling. In some cases, however, the nonossifying fibroma persists and proliferates, affecting the structural integrity of the bone.

Nonossifying fibromas are usually asymptomatic and found incidentally on radiographs. In the 1950s, when fluoride was added to drinking water, random skeletal surveys were done on hundreds of children. Nonossifying fibromas were discovered in 20% to 30% of children and were distributed in nearly every bone of the body.

Nonossifying fibroma is not treated until it occupies more than 50% of the diameter of the bone or extends more than 3 to 4 cm into the cortex. When the tumor grows to this size, a pathologic fracture may occur, and curettage and bone grafting of the defect is undertaken. Quantitative CT scans help define a large lesion clearly and are used for preoperative planning.

Osteochondroma. Osteochondroma (or exostosis) is a very common benign tumor that results in a bony protuberance of bone growing near the growth plate. They can occur as a solitary lesion or as an inherited syndrome of hereditary multiple exostoses (HMEs). Osteochondromas are covered with a cartilage cap that, very rarely, can degenerate into malignant chondrosarcoma. Osteochondromas can occur on any bone and mature while a child is growing. They are the most commonly removed bony tumor.

Hereditary multiple exostosis (HME) occurs in about 1 of every 50,000 live births and results in multiple osteochondroma. It is autosomal dominant and caused by inactivation of *EXT1* and *EXT2* mutations on chromosomes 8 and 11, respectively. Multiple surgeries are common in affected individuals because the lesions lead to angulation of the bones, pain from pressure on nerves or tendons, and growth abnormalities. The malignant transformation rate is higher, reaching 5%. All affected children should be screened with a spinal MRI to discover if the cord is at risk of injury by spinal exostosis. Involvement of the spine in children with multiple hereditary exostoses is common.[48]

Simple Bone Cyst. Simple bone cysts (SBCs) are cystic lesions of the central region of the metaphyseal area in children. With growth these lesions may appear within the diaphysis. Affected children are usually asymptomatic until pathologic fracture or incidental discovery occurs. Lesions often heal after a fracture, but large lesions may require treatment. A large prospective, randomized study compared steroid injection (the classic treatment for these lesions) with bone marrow injection for treatment. Both treatment modalities were found to have comparable healing rates if the pseudolining of the lesion was scraped from the cyst wall.[49] Very large lesions in weightbearing areas may require internal fixation and bone grafting.

Aneurysmal Bone Cyst. Aneurysmal bone cysts (ABCs) are typically eccentric, metaphyseal lesions that occur in a slightly older population than SBCs. The etiology remains controversial; many consider ABC a lesion secondary to another process, such as giant cell tumor. This lesion must be differentiated from malignant telangiectatic osteosarcoma; thus biopsy is necessary. Recent findings of genetic aberration in chromosome band 17p13 suggest a neoplastic basis for ABC.[50] Once diagnosed, curettage with complete removal of the "pseudolining" must be done with chemical cautery or electrocautery to minimize recurrence. Bone graft is placed in the defect. Even with modern techniques, recurrence can be as high as 21%.[51]

Osteoid Osteoma. Osteoid osteoma, or the larger counterpart osteoblastoma, presents as painful lesions of the diaphysis or metadiaphysis of long bones. Involvement of the posterior elements of the spine—with resultant "splinting" scoliosis—can occur. Night pain is common, as is relief from symptoms with nonsteroidal antiinflammatory drugs (NSAIDs), because these tumors release prostaglandins. When

pain is too extreme to be controlled medically, resection of the "nidus," or central portion, of the lesion is uniformly successful. CT guidance to the lesion is often used and, if possible, CT-guided laser ablation can be done. When present in the spine, surgical resection must be used because the heat of laser ablation can injure the spinal cord.

Fibrous Dysplasia. Fibrous dysplasia (FD) is a disease that causes thinning of the bone or formation of growths or lesions that can occur in one bone (monostotic) or in multiple bones (polyostotic). Albright syndrome is a triad of polyostotic FD, precocious puberty, and cutaneous pigmentation. Although any bone can be affected, the long bones, ribs, and skull are the most common. A radiographic "ground glass" appearance is present primarily in the metaphyseal or metadiaphyseal areas. Deformity can be marked and necessitate operative intervention. When Albright syndrome is present, endocrine abnormalities also must be addressed.

Malignant Bone Tumors

Osteosarcoma. Osteosarcoma is the most common malignant bone tumor that occurs during childhood; it originates from bone-producing mesenchymal cells. It accounts for 60% of all malignant bone tumors and strikes between the ages of 10 and 18.

Molecular analysis has demonstrated deletion of genetic material on the long arm of chromosome 13, leading to the identification of a tumor-suppressor gene as part of the mechanism for tumor development. The oncogene *src* also has been associated with osteosarcoma.

◆**PATHOPHYSIOLOGY.** Osteosarcoma occurs mainly in the metaphyses of long bones. Most tumors arise in bones involved with the knee joint at the distal end of the femur or proximal end of the tibia. As a tumor of mesenchymal cells, osteosarcoma makes osteoid tissue.

Osteosarcoma is a bulky tumor that extends beyond the bone into the soft tissues. It may encircle the bone and destroy the trabeculae of the diseased bone. Osteosarcoma disseminates through the bloodstream, usually to the lung. As many as 25% of children diagnosed with osteosarcoma exhibit lung metastases at diagnosis. Other sites of metastatic spread include other bones and visceral organs.

◆**CLINICAL MANIFESTATIONS.** The most common presenting complaint is pain. There may be swelling, warmth, and redness caused by the vascularity of the tumor. Symptoms also may include cough, dyspnea, and chest pain if lung metastasis is present. If a lower extremity is involved, a limp or even pathologic fracture may be present.

Initial evaluation includes roentgenographic examination that shows the osteosarcoma's characteristic osteoblastic and osteolytic changes. "Staging" studies to determine not only the local extent of the tumor but also possible metastatic spread must be done. These include bone scan (to assess bony spread), magnetic resonance imaging (MRI) of the lesion (to plan surgical resection and to compare with postchemotherapy studies), and chest roentgenograms or CT, or both. The chest roentgenogram must be done *before* biopsy because the general anesthetic required for biopsy can give false-positive results on the roentgenogram.

◆**EVALUATION AND TREATMENT.** Tissue biopsy confirms the diagnosis, although needle biopsy is often sufficient to establish the diagnosis. There are five histologic types of osteosarcoma, each determined by the predominant cell type. The tumor is then graded according to degree of malignancy; the higher the number, the worse the prognosis.

Surgery and multiagent chemotherapy are the primary treatments for osteosarcoma. Radiation is occasionally used. The 5-year survival rate with modern protocols is 70% to 80%.[52]

Chemotherapy is used preoperatively to shrink the size of the tumor and minimize metastatic growth. Following chemotherapy, the child is given a short "rest period" to regain strength for surgery. Following adjunctive chemotherapy, the majority of children undergo "limb salvage" rather than amputation procedures. The long-term survival rate of children treated with limb salvage and chemotherapy is now nearly equal to amputation in 5- and 10-year survival.[53]

Ewing Sarcoma. Ewing sarcoma is a malignant round cell tumor of bone and soft tissue that has a poor prognosis. It is the second most common and most lethal malignant bone tumor that can occur during childhood. The peak incidence is 10 to 20 years. Like osteosarcoma, Ewing sarcoma is slightly more common in males than females and is linked with periods of rapid bone growth. The incidence of Ewing sarcoma is less than 2% in blacks.[54]

◆**PATHOPHYSIOLOGY.** Ewing sarcoma commonly occurs in the diaphysis of long bones or in flat bones. The most common sites include the pelvis, femur, and tibia (Fig. 46.19). The femur is involved in most cases, with the pelvis being the second most common site. It can occur in any bone.

Arising from bone marrow, Ewing sarcoma can break through the cortex of the bone to form a soft tissue mass. It does not form bone, but abundant reactive bone may be present in an attempt to contain this quickly growing lesion. Metastasis occurs early and is usually apparent at diagnosis or within 1 year. The most common sites are the lung, other bones, lymph nodes, bone marrow, liver, spleen, and central nervous system, although invasion of any organ is possible.

◆**CLINICAL MANIFESTATIONS.** Like osteosarcoma, the most common complaint is pain. A soft tissue mass is often present. Additional symptoms may include fever, malaise, and anorexia. Known as *the great imitator,* Ewing sarcoma can appear radiographically identical to infection or even benign lesions such as Langerhans cell granulomatosis. Any pervasive diaphyseal or rib lesion must be regarded with a high index of suspicion.

◆**EVALUATION AND TREATMENT.** In addition to plain roentgenogram, CT and MRI are needed to help establish the diagnosis and extent of the tumor. Bone scan, chest roentgenogram, chest CT scan, and bone marrow biopsy also are used to detect metastases.[55] No specific laboratory test is diagnostic; however, the sedimentation rate will be elevated and lactic dehydrogenase (LDH) level often is elevated. An elevated LDH level is a poor prognostic sign. Biopsy is used to conclusively establish the diagnosis. The identification of an 11:22 chromosomal translocation within the tumor cells confirms the diagnosis of Ewing sarcoma.

The use of multidrug chemotherapy has improved survival rates. Treatment protocols call for preoperative chemotherapy followed by radiation or surgical resection or both, with continuation of chemotherapy for 12 to 18 months afterward. Surgical resection is essential.

Historically, Ewing sarcoma had a dismal prognosis with 5-year survival rates no better than 5% to 10%. Combinations of aggressive radiation, chemotherapy, and surgical resection have improved the survival rate for extremity disease to 65% to 75%.[56] Disease of the trunk or pelvis continues to have a 5-year survival of only 40%. The major predictor of prognosis appears to be the location of the primary tumor and the presence of metastases at diagnosis.

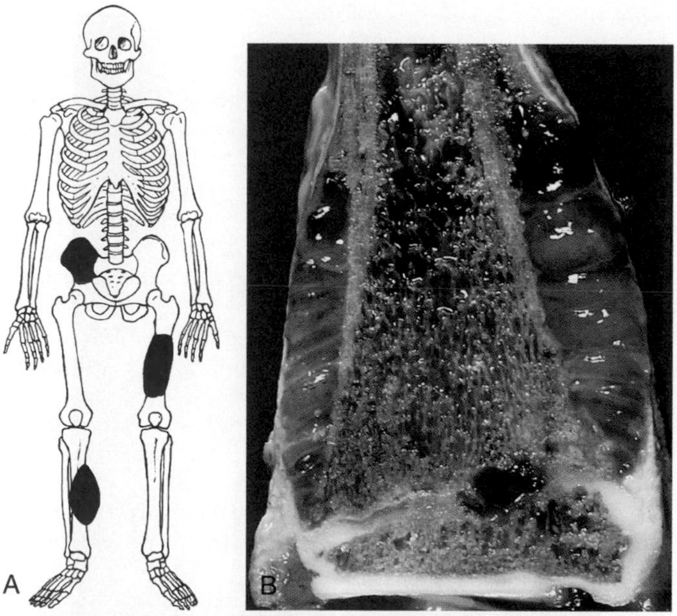

Muscle Tumors

Most soft tissue tumors in children are benign. Only two malignant soft tissue tumors occur with any frequency—rhabdomyosarcoma in the younger child and synovial cell sarcoma in the teenager. Both of these occur rarely. The annual incidence is 8 cases per million for white children and 7.7 per million for black children. About 230 U.S. children are diagnosed with a soft tissue tumor each year. Soft tissue tumors originate from the primitive mesenchymal cells that normally give rise to muscle, tendons, blood vessels, lymphatic structures, fibrous and connective tissue, and bursa and fascia. Table 46.6 identifies the classification of soft tissue tumors according to origin. All malignant soft tissue tumors are characterized as highly aggressive tumors that invade surrounding structures and metastasize early.

Rhabdomyosarcoma (RMS) is the most common soft tissue sarcoma of childhood and accounts for more than 50% of soft tissue tumors but less than 3% of all childhood cancers. RMS arises from embryonal rhabdomyoblasts that normally differentiate into mature striated muscle.

RMS can develop anywhere striated muscle is located. The primary locations and percentage range of incidence are the head and neck (including the orbit), 36% to 61%; the trunk, 8% to 33%; the extremities, 14% to 24%; and the genitourinary tract, 10% to 17%. Two age ranges (2 to 6 years and 15 to 19 years) are associated with RMS. More than two-thirds of children with RMS are diagnosed by 10 years of age, and RMS is slightly more common in males than females.

Recent studies demonstrate an association between *TP53* (a tumor-suppressor gene) mutations and sporadic rhabdomyosarcoma.[57] Three oncogenes (*src, ras,* and *c-myb*) have been associated with this tumor.[58]

◆**PATHOPHYSIOLOGY.** RMS generally appears as a firm, fleshy, grayish white mass. RMS has various appearances, depending on the phase of differentiation of the rhabdomyoblast. The cells may be round, spindle shaped, tadpole shaped, or multinucleated giant cells.

FIGURE 46.19 Ewing Sarcoma. **A,** Most common anatomic sites. **B,** Close-up view of Ewing sarcoma of the distal end of the tibia. Tumor extends into the soft tissue. (From Damjanov I, Linder J, editors: *Anderson's pathology,* ed 10, St Louis, 1996, Mosby.)

TABLE 46.6	CLASSIFICATION OF TUMORS BY ORIGIN	
TISSUE	**TUMOR**
Muscle	
Striated	Rhabdomyosarcoma
Smooth	Leiomyosarcoma
Adipose	Liposarcoma
Fibrous	Fibrosarcoma
Synovial mesothelium	Synovial sarcoma
Lymphatic structures	Lymphangiosarcoma
Blood vessels	Hemangiopericytoma
Nerve sheath	Neurogenic sarcoma

At least 20% of children with RMS have metastatic disease at diagnosis. The preferred sites of metastases include the lungs, lymph nodes, bone marrow, liver, brain, and bone. Another 30% have disease that is unresectable, although not widely spread.

◆**CLINICAL MANIFESTATIONS.** The signs and symptoms of RMS depend on the anatomic location of the primary tumor and the presence of symptomatic metastases. The tumors are usually painless, and early detection of RMS is facilitated by the presence of a palpable or visible mass. Deep-seated tumors may cause functional impairment but can be silent until they are very large. The clinical manifestations of RMS are outlined in Table 46.7.

◆**EVALUATION AND TREATMENT.** Diagnostic studies during the pretreatment phase are used to determine the extent of the primary tumor and metastases. Specific diagnostic studies depend on the primary site, but a combination of radiographic, nuclear, and CT scanning or MRI technology and blood studies is used. A biopsy of the primary tumor is necessary to confirm the diagnosis.

RMS is treated by a combination of surgery, radiation, and chemotherapy. Complete surgical resection combined with multiagent chemotherapy has increased the overall survival rate to 70%. If surgical resection leads to serious disfigurement or functional disability (e.g., enucleation for orbital tumors or cystectomy for bladder tumors), chemotherapy and radiation serve as the primary treatment, and surgery is avoided or minimized.

The primary prognostic factor in RMS is the degree of residual disease after surgical resection. Children with localized disease (stages I and II) have long-term survival rates of 70% to 80%. With widespread disease, long-term survival rates drop to 20%. Orbital tumors have an overall favorable prognosis, probably because of the lack of lymphatics in the area and early physical signs of disease.

NONACCIDENTAL TRAUMA

Abuse is estimated to occur in more than 1.5 million U.S. children per year. The maltreatment may be psychologic, sexual, or physical. Of children who suffer physical abuse, 30% are initially seen by an orthopedist. Accurate and appropriate referrals to child protection services are not only legally mandated but also essential for the well-being of the child; an abused child who returns unmonitored to an abusive situation has a 15% chance of mortality.

Children who are not yet ambulatory and present with a long bone fracture have a greater than 75% chance of that fracture being caused by nonaccidental trauma. "Corner" metaphyseal fractures, caused by a twisting force, are *nearly pathognomonic* of abuse but occur only 25% of the time (Fig. 46.20). Fractures at multiple stages of healing are also suggestive; however, osteogenesis imperfecta must be ruled out. The most common presentation is a transverse tibial fracture.[59] After walking age, only 2% of long bone fractures are the result of nonaccidental trauma.[60]

◆**EVALUATION AND TREATMENT** If suspected, nonaccidental trauma necessitates early consultation with child protective services. The child should undergo skeletal radiographic survey, especially if less than 2 years of age, and have a complete physical examination to evaluate for patterned bruising, burns, or multiple soft tissue injuries. Ophthalmologic

TABLE 46.7	CLINICAL MANIFESTATIONS OF RHABDOMYOSARCOMA
LOCATION	**MANIFESTATION**
Head and Neck	
Orbit	Ptosis
	Exophthalmos
	Proptosis
Paranasal sinuses	Nasal obstruction
	Epistaxis
	Swelling
	Chronic sinusitis
Nasopharynx	Hypernasal speech
	Nasal discharge
	Visible polypoid mass
Oropharyngeal	Dysphagia
	Painful mastication
Middle ear	Chronic serous otitis media
	Discharge from affected ear
	Facial nerve palsy
	Conduction hearing loss
	Visible polypoid mass
Extremities	
All locations	Deep-seated, fixed palpable mass
Retroperitoneal	
All locations	Usually asymptomatic
	May have vague abdominal pain
	Bowel or genitourinary obstruction (late)
	Possible palpable mass
Genitourinary	
Vaginal	Abnormal vaginal bleeding
	Protruding polypoid mass
Prostate	Urinary tract obstruction
Bladder	Urinary retention
	Straining to void
	Hematuria
Paratesticular	Mass in scrotum that may be painful

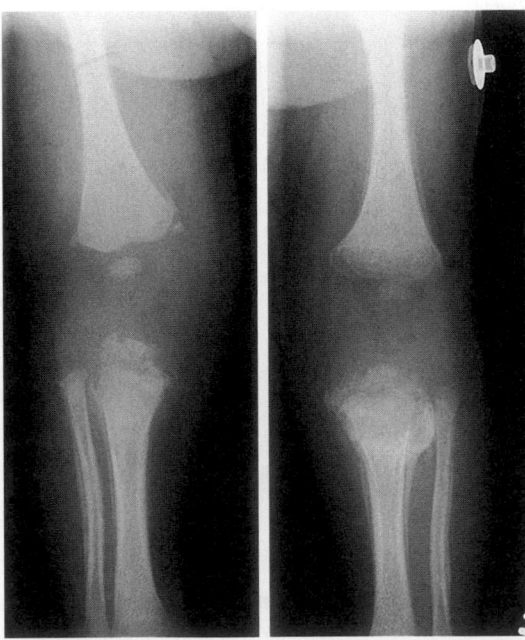

FIGURE 46.20 Corner Fracture. Bilateral knee radiograph showing healing corner fractures of bilateral proximal tibias and distal femurs. Note the varying amount of callus formation signifying fractures at different stages of healing.

examination and brain CT should be used to evaluate for retinal or brain hemorrhage caused by shaking. A thorough history must be obtained for all identified injuries. Bone scan can be helpful in diagnosing subtle injuries, especially rib fractures. Posterior rib fractures are especially likely to be caused by abuse. It is important to remember that social isolation can lead to increased likelihood of abuse, but no social stratum is immune.

A nonjudgmental attitude on the part of the treating healthcare provider is essential. The child and family involved in nonaccidental trauma are delicate and require not only physical but also emotional care. Social workers need to be involved early to ensure appropriate medical care to the child. Fortunately, fractures heal quickly in young children; neurologic injury and social disease, however, are much more difficult to cure.

SUMMARY REVIEW

Musculoskeletal Development in Children

1. Skeletal growth and development consists of two phases: (a) delivery of bone cell precursors to sites of bone formation and (b) the aggregation of these cells at primary centers of ossification where they mature to secrete osteoid.
2. Ossification takes place in two centers in long bones: (a) the primary center, or the diaphysis (the long, central portion of the bone); and (b) the secondary center, or the epiphysis (the end portions of the bone).
3. Peak bone mass is achieved by the middle to late twenties.
4. By 1 year of age 50% of the total growth of the spine has occurred, and most children have achieved 50% of their adult height by 2 years of age.
5. The appendicular skeleton (extremities) grows faster during childhood than does the axial skeleton.
6. Muscle fibers reach their maximal size in females at 10 years of age and at 14 years of age in males.

Musculoskeletal Alterations in Children

1. The most common congenital defect of the upper extremities is syndactyly (webbing of the fingers).
2. Developmental dysplasia of the hip (DDH) is an abnormality in the development of the femoral head, acetabulum, or both. It is a serious and disabling condition in children if not diagnosed and treated early, preferably in infancy.
3. Clubfoot (equinovarus) is a common deformity in which the foot is twisted out of its normal shape or position. Clubfoot can be positional, idiopathic, or teratologic.
4. Congenital muscle disorders (myopathies) include absence of muscles, hypoplasia, hyperplasia, and faulty intrinsic development.
5. Osteogenesis imperfecta (brittle bone disease) is a genetic disorder of collagen that affects primarily bones and results in fractures of many bones.
6. Rickets is a condition caused by deficiencies in vitamin D, calcium, and usually phosphorus that is characterized by the failure of bones to become mineralized (ossified) and results in skeletal deformity.
7. Scoliosis is a lateral curvature of the spinal column that can be caused by congenital malformations of the spine, neuromuscular disease, trauma, extraspinal contractures, bone infections, metabolic bone disorders, joint disease, and tumors.
8. Osteomyelitis is a local or generalized bacterial infection of bone and bone marrow. Bacteria are usually introduced by direct extension from a nearby infection, through the bloodstream, or by trauma. Septic arthritis (bacteria within the joint) may be associated with osteomyelitis and is a surgical emergency.
9. Juvenile idiopathic arthritis is an inflammatory joint disorder characterized by pain and swelling. Large joints are most commonly affected.
10. Avascular diseases of the bone are collectively referred to as *osteochondroses* and are caused by an insufficient blood supply to growing bones.
11. Legg-Calvé-Perthes disease is one of the most common osteochondroses. This disorder is characterized by epiphyseal necrosis or degeneration of the head of the femur followed by regeneration or recalcification.
12. Osgood-Schlatter disease is characterized by inflammation or partial separation of the tibial tubercle caused by chronic irritation, usually as a result of overuse of the quadriceps muscles. The condition is seen primarily in muscular, athletic adolescent males.
13. The muscular dystrophies are a group of genetically transmitted diseases characterized by progressive atrophy of symmetrical groups of skeletal muscles without evidence of involvement or degeneration of neural tissue. There is an insidious loss of strength in all forms of the disorder with increasing disability and deformity.
14. The two most common forms of benign bone tumors include nonossifying fibroma and osteochondroma. Other benign bone tumors include simple bone cysts, aneurysmal bone cysts, osteoid osteoma, and fibrous dysplasia.
15. The two main types of malignant childhood bone tumors are osteosarcoma and Ewing sarcoma.
16. Osteosarcoma, the most common malignant childhood bone tumor, originates in bone-producing mesenchymal cells and is most often located in the distal end of the femur or proximal end of the tibia.
17. Most childhood osteosarcoma tumors occur between the ages of 10 and 18 years.
18. Ewing sarcoma originates from cells within the bone marrow space and is located most often in the midshaft of long bones, in ribs, or in flat bones.
19. Ewing sarcoma is more common in males and is diagnosed most often between the ages of 5 and 15 years.
20. Pain is the usual presenting symptom for either osteosarcoma or Ewing sarcoma.
21. The primary treatments for osteosarcoma are surgery and chemotherapy. The primary treatment for Ewing sarcoma is a combination of chemotherapy, radiation, and surgery.
22. The most common type of childhood soft tissue tumor is rhabdomyosarcoma.
23. Rhabdomyosarcoma originates from embryonal rhabdomyoblasts that normally differentiate into mature striated muscle.
24. Clinical manifestations of rhabdomyosarcoma depend on the anatomic location; superficial tumors exhibit a painless palpable mass, whereas deep-seated tumors cause functional impairment.
25. Rhabdomyosarcoma is treated with a combination of surgery, radiation, and chemotherapy.

SUMMARY REVIEW—cont'd

Nonaccidental Trauma

1. Nonaccidental trauma must be considered with any long bone injury in a preambulatory child.
2. Evidence of soft tissue injury, corner fractures, and fractures at different stages of healing is extremely helpful in making a diagnosis of nonaccidental trauma.
3. When nonaccidental trauma is suspected, a child must be evaluated radiographically for other fractures, head trauma, and retinal hemorrhage.
4. All social strata are at risk for nonaccidental trauma.
5. The healthcare provider is legally responsible to report suspected nonaccidental trauma.

KEY TERMS

Acetabular dysplasia, 1475
Albright syndrome, 1490
Aneurysmal bone cyst (ABC), 1490
Becker muscular dystrophy, 1488
Cartilage anlage, 1472
Cerebral palsy (CP), 1486
Clubfoot, 1476
"Corner" metaphyseal fracture, 1492
Developmental dysplasia of the hip (DDH), 1474
Dislocatable hip, 1475
Duchenne muscular dystrophy (DMD), 1488
Dystrophin, 1488
Endochondral formation of bone, 1472
Equinovarus, 1476
Ewing sarcoma, 1491
Facioscapulohumeral muscular dystrophy (FSHD), 1489
Fibrous dysplasia (FD), 1490
Genu valgum (knock knee), 1474
Genu varum (bowleg), 1474

Hereditary multiple exostosis (HME), 1490
Idiopathic equinovarus, 1477
Idiopathic scoliosis, 1481
Intramembranous formation of bone, 1472
Involucrum, 1483
Juvenile idiopathic arthritis (JIA), 1484
Kyphosed, 1473
Legg-Calvé-Perthes (LCP) disease, 1484
Lordotic, 1474
Metatarsus adductus, 1476
Neuromuscular disorder, 1486
Nonossifying fibroma, 1489
Nonstructural scoliosis, 1481
Osgood-Schlatter disease, 1485
Osteochondroma (exostosis), 1490
Osteochondrosis, 1484
Osteogenesis imperfecta (OI) (brittle bone disease), 1478
Osteoid osteoma, 1490
Osteomyelitis, 1482

Osteosarcoma, 1490
Perichondrium, 1472
Periosteal collar, 1472
Pes planus (flatfoot), 1478
Positional equinovarus, 1476
Primary centers of ossification, 1472
Pseudohypertrophic, 1487
Rhabdomyosarcoma (RMS), 1491
Rickets, 1480
Scoliosis, 1481
Secondary center of ossification, 1473
Secondary septic arthritis, 1483
Sequestrum (pl., sequestra), 1483
Simple bone cyst (SBC), 1490
Spinal muscular atrophy (SMA), 1489
Structural scoliosis, 1481
Subluxated hip, 1475
Syndactyly, 1474
Teratologic equinovarus, 1478
Vestigial tab, 1474

REFERENCES

1. Misra M, et al: Vitamin D deficiency in children and its management: review of current knowledge and recommendations. *Pediatrics* 122(2):398–417, 2007.
2. Thompson R, et al: Vitamin D insufficiency and fracture risk in urban children. *J Pediatr Orthop* 37(6):368–373, 2017.
3. Minkowitz B, et al: Low vitamin D levels are associated with need for surgical correction of pediatric fractures. *J Pediatr Orthop* 37(1):23–29, 2017.
4. Simkin P: The musculoskeletal system. In Klippel JH, Dieppe PA, editors: *Rheumatology*, ed 2, London, 1998, Mosby-Wolfe.
5. Sankar WN, Laird CT, Baldwin KD: Hip range of motion in children: What is the norm? *J Pediatr Orthop* 32(4):399–405, 2012.
6. Weinstein SL: Congenital hip dislocation: long range problems, residual signs, and symptoms after successful treatments. *Clin Orthop Relat Res* Aug(281):69–74, 1992.
7. Weintroub S, Grill F: Ultrasonography in developmental dysplasia of the hip. *J Bone Joint Surg Am* 82A(7):1004–1018, 2000.
8. Holman J, et al: Long term follow-up of open reduction surgery for DDH. *J Pediatr Orthop* 32(2):121–124, 2012.
9. Mulpuri K, et al: Detection and nonoperative management of pediatric developmental dysplasia of the hip in infants up to six months of age. *J Bone Joint Surg Am* 97:1717–1718, 2015.
10. Ippolito E, et al: Long-term comparative results in patients with congenital clubfoot treated with two different protocols. *Arch Gynecol Obstet* 268(4):331–332, 2003.
11. Zionts LE, et al: Treatment of idiopathic clubfoot: experience with the Mitchell-Ponseti brace. *J Pediatr Orthop* 32(7):706–713, 2012.
12. Marini J, et al: Osteogenesis imperfect due to mutations in non-collagenous genes: lessons in the biology of bone formation. *Curr Opin Pediatr* 26(4):500–506, 2014.
13. Zaleske DJ, Doppelt SH, Mankin HJ: Endocrine abnormalities of the immature skeleton. In Lovell WW, Winter RB, editors: *Pediatric orthopedics*, ed 2, Philadelphia, 1986, Lippincott.
14. Zeitlin L, Fassier F, Glorieux FH: Modern approach to children with osteogenesis imperfecta. *J Pediatr Orthop B* 12(2):77–87, 2003.
15. Wharton B, Bishop N: Rickets. *Lancet* 362(9393):1389–1400, 2003.
16. Parry J, Sullivan E, Scott AC: Vitamin D sufficiency screening in preoperative pediatric orthopaedic patients. *J Pediatr Orthop* 31(3):331–333, 2011.
17. Barrack R, et al: Vibratory hypersensitivity in idiopathic sclerosis. *J Pediatr Orthop* 8(4):389, 1988.
18. Weinstein SL, et al: Effects of bracing in adolescents with idiopathic scoliosis. *N Engl J Med* 369(16):1512–1521, 2013.
19. Vijermans V, et al: Factors determining the final outcome of treatment of idiopathic scoliosis with the Boston brace: a longitudinal study. *J Pediatr Orthop B* 13(3):143–149, 2004.
20. Caksen H, et al: Septic arthritis in childhood. *Pediatr Int* 42(5):534, 2000.
21. Gillespie WJ, et al: Aspects of the microbe:host relationship in staphylococcal hematogenous osteomyelitis. *Orthopedics* 10(3):475, 1987.
22. Hedström SA, Lidgren L: Septic arthritis and osteomyelitis. In Klippel JH, Dieppe PA, editors: *Rheumatology*, ed 2, London, 1998, Mosby-Wolfe.
23. Stanitski C: Changes in pediatric acute hematogenous osteomyelitis management. *J Pediatr Orthop* 24(4):444–445, 2004.
24. Przybylski GJ, Sharan AD: Single-stage autogenous bone grafting and internal fixation in the surgical management of pyogenic discitis and vertebral osteomyelitis. *J Neurosurg* 94(Suppl 1):1, 2001.
25. Ray NJ, Basset RL: Pyogenic vertebral osteomyelitis. *Orthopedics* 8(4):504, 1985.
26. Mader JT, et al: The host and skeletal infection: classification and pathogenesis of acute bacterial bone and joint sepsis. *Baillieres Best Pract Res Clin Rheumatol* 13(1):1, 1999.
27. Perlman M, et al: The incidence of joint involvement of adjacent osteomyelitis in pediatric patients. *J Pediatr Orthop* 20(1):40, 2000.
28. Cassidy JT: *Textbook of pediatric rheumatology*, New York, 1982, Wiley & Sons.
29. Hollingworth P: Juvenile chronic arthritis. In Klippel JH, Dieppe PA, editors: *Rheumatology*, ed 2, London, 1998, Mosby-Wolfe.
30. Stoll ML, Cron RQ: Treatment of juvenile idiopathic arthritis: a revolution in care. *Pediatr Rheumatol Online J* 12:13, 2014.
31. Glueck CJ, et al: Association of antithrombotic factor deficiencies and hypofibrinolysis with Legg-Perthes disease. *J Bone Joint Surg Am* 78(1):3–13, 1996.
32. Herring JA, et al: The lateral pillar classification of Legg-Calvé-Perthes disease. *J Pediatr Orthop* 12(2):143–150, 1992.

33. Schoenecker PL, et al: Legg-Perthes disease in children under 6 years old. *Orthop Rev* 22:201, 1993.

34. Little DG, et al: Potential for bisphosphonate treatment in Legg-Calve-Perthes disease. *J Pediatr Orthop* 31(Suppl 2):S182–S188, 2011.

35. Gigante A, et al: What is the best treatment for Osgood-Schlatter disease? *J Fam Pract* 53(2):153–156, 2004.

36. Himmelmann K, et al: The changing panorama of cerebral palsy in Sweden. IX. Prevalence and origin in the birth-year period 1995-1998. *Acta Paediatr* 94(3):287–294, 2005.

37. Hagberg B, et al: The changing panorama of cerebral palsy in Sweden. V. The birth year period 1979-82. *Acta Paediatr Scand* 78(2):283–290, 1989.

38. Swanson MW, et al: Identification of neurodevelopmental abnormality at 4 and 8 months by the movement assessment of infants. *Dev Med Child Neurol* 34(4):321–337, 1992.

39. Mah JK, et al: A systematic review and meta-analysis on the epidemiology of Duchenne and Becker muscular dystrophy. *Neuromuscul Disord* 24(6):482–491, 2014.

40. Aartsma-Rus A, Ginjaar IB, Bushby K: The importance of genetic diagnosis for Duchenne muscular dystrophy. *J Med Genet* 53(3):145–451, 2016.

41. Stevens A, Lowe J: *Pathology*, London, 1995, Mosby-Wolfe.

42. Ciafaloni E, et al: Delayed diagnosis in Duchenne muscular dystrophy: data from the Muscular Dystrophy Surveillance, Tracking, and Research Network (MD STARnet). *J Pediatr* 155(3):380–385, 2009.

43. Moxley RT, 3rd, et al: Change in natural history of Duchenne muscular dystrophy with long-term corticosteroid treatment: implications for management. *J Child Neurol* 25(9):1116–1120, 2010.

44. Wein N, Alfano L, Flanigan KM: Genetics and emerging treatments for Duchenne and Becker muscular dystrophy. *Pediatr Clin North Am* 62(3):723–742, 2015.

45. Ogino S, et al: Genetic risk assessment in carrier testing for spinal muscular atrophy. *Am J Med Genet* 110:301–307, 2002.

46. Prior TW, et al: Newborn and carrier screening for spinal muscular atrophy. *Am J Med Genet A* 152A:1605–1607, 2010.

47. Corey DR: Nusinersen, an antisense oligonucleotide drug for spinal muscular atropy. *Nat Neurosci* 20(4):497–499, 2017.

48. Roach JW, Klatt JW, Faulkner ND: Involvement of the spine in patients with multiple hereditary exostoses. *J Bone Joint Surg Am* 91(8):1942–1948, 2009.

49. Wright JG, et al: A randomized clinical trial comparing intralesional bone marrow and steroid injections for simple bone cysts. *J Bone Joint Surg Am* 90:722–730, 2008.

50. Oliveira AM, et al: Aneurismal bone cyst variant translocations upregulate USP6. *Oncogene* 24(21):3410–3426, 2005.

51. Dorman JP, et al: Surgical treatment and recurrence rate of aneurismal bone cysts in children. *Clin Orthop* 421:205–211, 2004.

52. Glasser DB, et al: Survival, prognosis, and therapeutic response in osteogenic sarcoma: the Memorial Hospital experience. *Cancer* 69(3):698–708, 1992.

53. Bielack SS, et al: Prognostic factors in high-grade osteochondromas of the extremity and trunk: an analysis of 1702 patients treated on neoadjuvant cooperative osteosarcoma study group protocols. *J Clin Oncol* 20(3):776–790, 2002.

54. Ayala AG, Ro JY, Raymond AK: Bone tumors. In Damjanov I, Linder J, editors: *Anderson's pathology*, ed 10, St Louis, 1996, Mosby.

55. Carvajal RL, Meyers P: Ewing's sarcoma and primitive neuroectodermal family of tumors. *Hematol Oncol Clin North Am* 19(3):501–525, vi–vii, 2005.

56. Ruymann FB, Grovas AC: Progress in the diagnosis and treatment of rhabdomyosarcoma and related soft tissue sarcomas. *Cancer Invest* 18(3):223, 2000.

57. Lugo-Vicente H: Molecular biology and genetics affecting pediatric solid tumors. *Bol Asoc Med P R* 92(4-8):72–82, 2000.

58. Israel MA: Molecular and cellular biology in pediatric malignancies. In Pizzo PA, editor: *Principles and practice of pediatric oncology*, Philadelphia, 1989, Lippincott.

59. King J, et al: Analysis of 429 fractures in 189 battered children. *J Pediatr Orthop* 8(5):585–589, 1988.

60. Thomas SA, et al: Long-bone fracture in young children: distinguishing accidental injuries from child abuse. *Pediatrics* 88(3):471–476, 1991.

CHAPTER

47

Structure, Function, and Disorders of the Integument

Sue Ann McCann, Sue E. Huether

evolve WEBSITE

http://evolve.elsevier.com/McCance/
- Content Updates
- Chapter Summary Review
- Review Questions
- Case Studies
- Animations

CHAPTER OUTLINE

The skin covers the entire body and is the body's largest organ, accounting for approximately 20% of the body's weight. Combined with the accessory structures of hair, nails, and glands, it forms the *integumentary system*. The primary function of the skin is to protect the body from the environment by serving as a barrier against microorganisms, ultraviolet (UV) radiation, loss of body fluids, and the stress of mechanical forces. The skin regulates body temperature within a very narrow range and is involved in immune surveillance and the activation of vitamin D. Touch and pressure receptors provide important protective functions and pleasurable sensations. The commensal (normal) microorganisms of the skin (skin microbiota) protect against pathologic bacteria.

STRUCTURE AND FUNCTION OF THE SKIN

Layers of the Skin

The skin is formed of three major layers: (1) a superficial or outer layer of epidermis; (2) a deeper layer of dermis; and (3) the subcutaneous layer (hypodermis), the lowest lying layer of connective tissue that contains macrophages, fibroblasts, fat cells, nerves, fine muscles, blood vessels, lymphatics, and hair follicle roots (Fig. 47.1). Each skin layer contains cells that represent progressive stages of skin cell differentiation and function as the skin grows. These are summarized in Table 47.1.

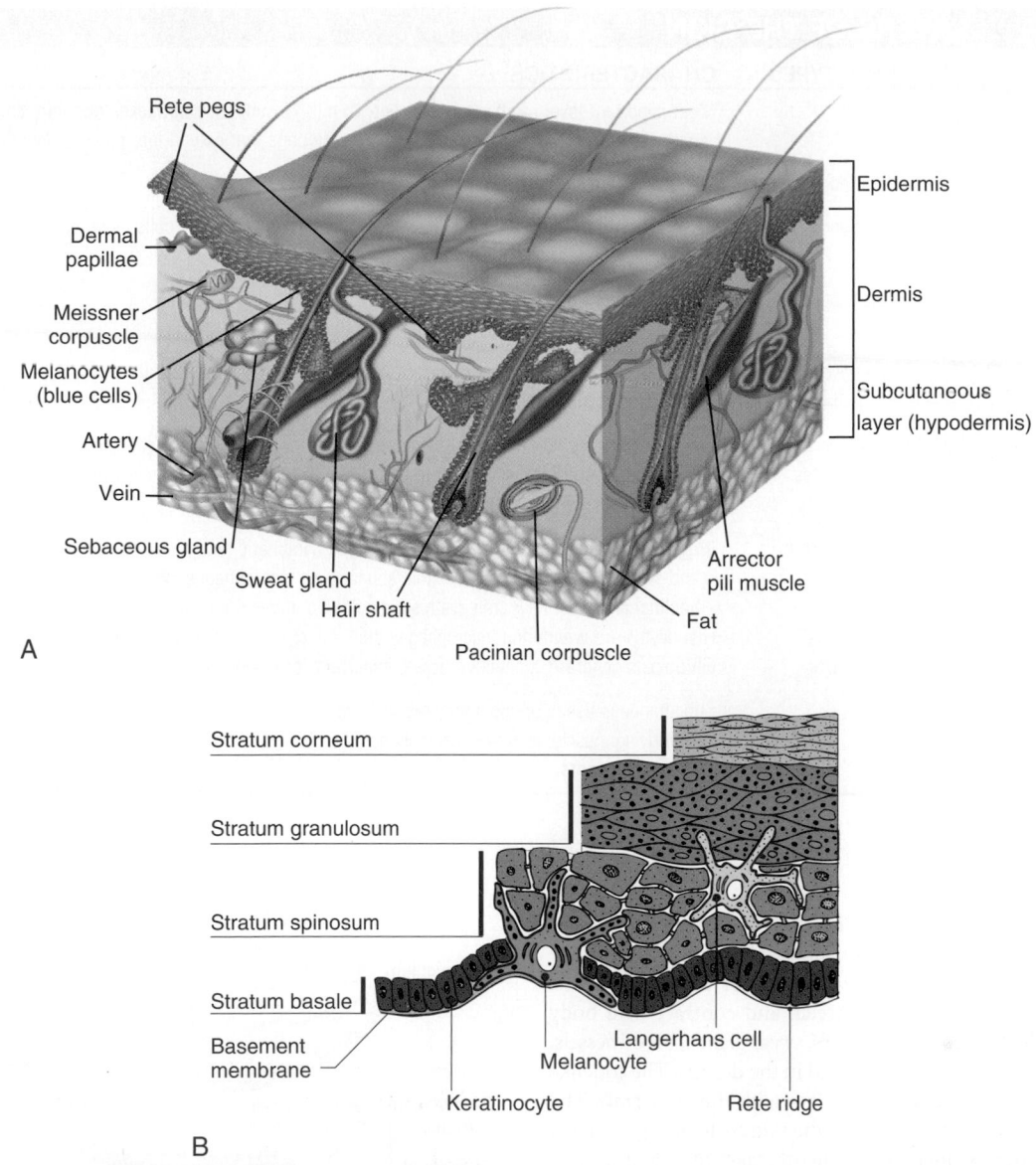

FIGURE 47.1 Structure of the Skin. **A,** Cross section showing major skin structures. **B,** Layers of the epidermis. (**A** from Kumar V et al: *Robbins & Cotran pathologic basis of disease,* ed 9, St Louis, 2015, Saunders; **B** from Gawkrodger D, Ardern-Jones MR: *Dermatology,* ed 5, Philadelphia, 2012, Churchill Livingstone.)

Epidermis

The epidermis is a defensive barrier that continually renews itself by shedding the superficial layer of stratum corneum. It is formed primarily of keratinocytes embedded in a lipid matrix. These cells are named for the substances they produce. Keratinocytes produce keratin, a sclero-protein that provides protection from mechanical stress. Keratin is the main constituent of skin, hair, and nail cells. The thickness of the epidermis varies from 0.05 mm on the eyelids to 1.5 mm on the palms of the hands and soles of the feet and averages about 0.12 mm. New cells (keratinocytes) formed in the basal layer (stratum basale) move upward and differentiate, forming the spinous layer (stratum spinosum). Together they form the germinative layer (stratum germinativum) and ensure continual renewal of the skin. The cells enlarge and then become flattened, stacked, and cornified (stratum corneum) as they ascend to the skin surface. Cornification, or keratinization, prevents

dehydration of deeper skin layers and loss of body water. The average turnover of the epidermis is about 30 days.

The epidermis has three additional types of cells that facilitate its functional characteristics: melanocytes, Langerhans cells, and Merkel cells. The melanocytes are usually located near the base of the epidermis. They synthesize and secrete the pigment melanin with exposure to UV light in response to melanocyte-stimulating hormone (MSH). Melanin in the epidermis provides a shield against UV radiation and determines skin color. Vitiligo is thought to be an autoimmune-related loss of melanocytes resulting in the depigmentation of patches of skin (see "Patch" in Table 47.3). Langerhans cells migrate to the epidermis from the bone marrow. Langerhans cells (a type of dendritic cell) and dermal dendritic cells initiate an immune response by presenting processed antigen to T cells, thus providing a defense against environmental antigens.[1] Merkel cells are associated with touch receptors and function as slowly adapting mechanoreceptors when stimulated by deformation of the epidermis.

TABLE 47.1   LAYERS OF THE SKIN

LAYER	CELL TYPES	CHARACTERISTICS
Epidermis		Most important layer of skin; normally very thin (0.12 mm) but can thicken and form corns or calluses with constant pressure or friction; includes rete pegs that extend into papillary layer of dermis
Stratum corneum	Keratinocytes	Tough superficial sheets of cornified cells
Stratum lucidum	Keratinocytes	Clear layers of cells containing eleidin, which becomes keratin as cells move up to the corneum layer; found only in palmoplantar skin
Stratum granulosum	Keratinocytes	Lose their nuclei Keratohyalin gives a granular appearance to this layer
Stratum spinosum	Keratinocytes Langerhans cells	Polygonal-shaped with spinous processes projecting between adjacent keratinocytes Cells with dendritic processes and immune function
Stratum basale (germinativum)	Keratinocytes Melanocytes Merkel cells	Basal layer where keratinocytes divide and move upward to replace cells shed from the surface Originate in neural crest and migrate to stratum basale and produce melanin Light touch mechanoreceptors
Dermis Papillary layer (thin) Reticular layer (thick)	Macrophages Mast cells Histiocytes Fibroblasts	Irregular connective tissue layer with rich blood, lymphatic, and nerve supply; contains sensory receptors and sweat glands (apocrine, eccrine, sebaceous); macrophages (phagocytic and important for wound healing) and mast cells (release histamine) have immune functions (see Chapter 7) Histiocytes are wandering macrophages that collect pigments and inflammatory debris Fibroblasts generate connective tissue; important for wound healing
Subcutaneous **(Hypodermis)**		Subcutaneous tissue or superficial fascia of varying thickness that connects the overlying dermis to underlying muscle; contains macrophages, fibroblasts, fat cells, nerves, blood vessels, lymphatics, and hair follicle roots

Dermis

The **dermis** is 1 to 4 mm thick and is composed of three types of connective tissue: (1) collagen, (2) elastin and reticulin, and (3) a gel-like ground substance. The haphazard arrangement of connective tissue allows the skin to be mobile and to stretch and contract with body movement. Hair follicles, sebaceous glands, sweat glands, blood vessels, lymphatic vessels, and nerves are contained in the dermis. The conelike projections of the papillary dermis interface with the epidermis. The papillae provide texture to the surface of the skin by forming *rete pegs*.

The cells of the dermis include fibroblasts, mast cells, and macrophages. Fibroblasts secrete the connective tissue matrix and collagen. Mast cells release histamine and play a role in hypersensitivity reactions in the skin. Macrophages are phagocytic and participate in immune responses. Histiocytes are macrophages that reside in loose connective tissue and phagocytize pigments and the debris of inflammation.

Subcutaneous Layer

The third layer of the skin is subcutaneous tissue (**hypodermis**) and consists of adipose tissue. The lobules are separated by fibrous walls (septa) of collagen and large blood vessels. Dermal collagen is continuous with the collagen found in the subcutaneous tissue.

Dermal Appendages

The **dermal appendages** include the nails, hair, sebaceous glands, and the eccrine and apocrine sweat glands. The **nails** are protective keratinized plates composed of six structural units: (1) the proximal nail fold, (2) the eponychium (cuticle), (3) the matrix from which the nail grows and its nail root, (4) the hyponychium (nail bed), (5) the nail plate, and (6) the paronychium (lateral nail fold) (Fig. 47.2). Nail growth is continuous throughout life at a rate of 1 mm or less per day.

Hair follicles and sebaceous glands are integrated units (see Fig. 47.1). Hair color, density, grain, and pattern of distribution have

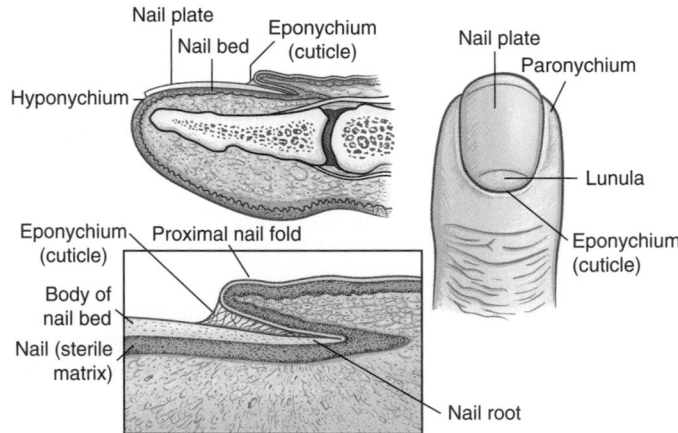

FIGURE 47.2 Structures of the Nail. (Redrawn from Thompson JM et al: *Mosby's clinical nursing,* ed 5, St Louis, 2002, Mosby.)

considerable variability and depend on age, gender, and race. **Hair follicles** arise from the matrix (or bulb) located deep in the dermis. They extend from the dermis at an angle and have an arrector pili muscle attached near the mid-dermis that straightens the follicle when contracted, causing the hair to stand up. Hair growth begins in the bulb, with cellular differentiation of stem cells occurring as the hair progresses up the follicle. Hair is fully hardened, or cornified, by the time it emerges at the skin surface. Hair growth is cyclic, with periods of growth and rest that vary over different body surfaces. Hair color is determined by melanin-secreting follicular melanocytes.

The **sebaceous glands** open onto the surface of the skin through a canal. They are found in greatest numbers on the face, chest, and back;

modified glands are found on the eyelids, lips, nipple, glans penis, and prepuce. Sebaceous glands secrete sebum, composed primarily of lipids, that oils the skin and hair and prevents drying. Growth of sebaceous glands is stimulated by androgens, and their enlargement is one of the early signs of puberty.

The eccrine sweat glands are distributed over the body, with the greatest numbers in the palms of the hands, soles of the feet, and forehead. These secretions are important in thermoregulation and cooling of the body through evaporation. The apocrine sweat glands, located in the axillae, scalp, face, abdomen, and genital area, are fewer in number and have very limited proven function.

Blood Supply and Innervation

The blood supply to the skin is limited to the papillary capillaries, or plexus, of the dermis. These capillary loops arise from a subpapillary plexus that is supplied by a deeper horizontal cutaneous arterial plexus. Branches from the deep plexus supply hair follicles and sweat glands. A subpapillary network of veins drains the capillary loops. Arteriovenous anastomoses in the dermis facilitate the regulation of body temperature. Heat loss can be regulated by varying blood flow through the skin by opening and closing the arteriovenous anastomoses in conjunction with evaporative heat loss of sweat. The sympathetic nervous system regulates vasoconstriction and vasodilation of hair-bearing skin through α-adrenergic receptors. Non–hair-bearing skin (glabrous skin) of the palms, soles, and lips is innervated solely by sympathetic vasoconstrictors with passive vasodilation.[2] The lymphatic vessels arise in the papillary dermis and drain into larger subcutaneous trunks, removing cells, proteins, and immunologic mediators.

AGING AND SKIN INTEGRITY

Many age-associated changes in the skin are generalized and readily observable. Genetics and cumulative environmental factors, including UV radiation from sun exposure (photoaging), inflammatory responses, tobacco smoke, and gravity, contribute to cutaneous changes with aging. Structurally the skin becomes thinner, less elastic, drier, and wrinkled with a change in pigmentation. There is loss of adipose tissue volume, particularly in the face. The cellular alterations contributing to the changes include a flattening of the dermoepidermal junction with a shortening and decrease in the number of capillary loops. There are fewer melanocytes, resulting in decreased protection against UV radiation. A significant decrease in the number of Langerhans cells reduces the skin's immune response with aging. The thickness of the dermis also decreases, with loss of extracellular matrix and elastic fibers, and accounts for the translucent, paper-thin quality of the skin. Loss of the rete pegs gives the skin a smooth, shiny appearance.

As the skin microcirculation ages, there is decreased vascular compliance and loss of vasoreactive responses with decreases in skin blood flow. Temperature regulation is compromised in older adults, with an increased risk for heat stroke and hypothermia. Loss of cutaneous vasomotion and subcutaneous fat, reduced vascularity, and decreased eccrine sweat production are contributing factors.[3] The decreased vasculature and lymphatic drainage contribute to loss of barrier protection, and the atrophy of eccrine, apocrine, and sebaceous glands promotes dry skin. Loss of elastin fibers is associated with wrinkling. Collagen fibers become fragmented, and fibroblasts decrease in number, resulting in a decreased ability of the skin to stretch and regain shape. Decreased cell proliferation, diminished blood supply, and depressed immune responses can delay wound healing in aging skin.[4] Changes in hair color and distribution also occur. Graying is caused by loss of melanocytes from hair bulbs, and thinning occurs from loss of stem cells and a gradual decline in the number of hair follicles and growth of finer hair.[5]

Epidermal cells change shape, and the barrier function of the stratum corneum is reduced. There is increased permeability and decreased clearance of toxic oxidative substances from the dermis that are formed from exposure to environmental toxins and UV radiation.[6] Pressure and touch receptors and free nerve endings decrease in number and reduce sensory perception.

Tests of Skin Function

Initial diagnostic evaluations of skin disorders are completed by gathering historical information, performing a physical examination, and observing the distribution and characteristics of the presenting lesions. Additional diagnostic studies are summarized in Table 47.2.

Clinical Manifestations of Skin Dysfunction
Lesions

Lesions of the skin are readily observable and easily assessed for distribution and structure. Identification of the morphologic structure, including a differentiation between the primary and secondary lesions, and the general appearance of the skin is critical. The physical examination, in combination with a thorough health history, is essential to identify the underlying pathophysiology. Table 47.3 describes and illustrates the primary lesions of the skin, and Table 47.4 describes and illustrates the secondary lesions of the skin. Special skin lesions are described in Table 47.5.

Pressure Injury. Pressure injury is localized damage to the skin that results from unrelieved pressure, shearing forces, friction, and moisture. Pressure that consistently interrupts arterial and venous blood flow to and from the skin or deeper tissue is the most significant cause.[7] The term *decubitus injury* refers to a pressure injury that results when an individual lies or sits in one position for a long time. Mucosal membrane pressure injury is related to injury caused from use of medical devices, such as endotracheal tubes. Risk factors for pressure injuries are summarized in Box 47.1.

Pressure injuries usually develop over bony prominences, such as the sacrum, heels, ischia, and greater trochanters. Continuous pressure on tissue between the bony prominence and a resistant outside surface distorts capillaries and occludes the blood flow and oxygen supply. Individuals with darkly pigmented skin are at greater risk for developing pressure injuries because early signs of skin damage may not be clearly visible.[8] Pressure injury also can occur in soft tissues from unrelieved pressure, for example, from nasal cannulas or endotracheal tubes. If the pressure is relieved within a few hours, a brief period of reactive hyperemia (redness) occurs and there may be no lasting tissue damage. If the pressure continues unrelieved, the endothelial cells lining the capillaries become disrupted with platelet aggregation, forming microthrombi that block blood flow and cause anoxic necrosis of surrounding tissues (see Fig. 47.3). Shearing and friction are mechanical forces moving parallel to the skin (dragging) and can extend to the bony skeleton, causing detachment and injury of tissues. Several scales are available for predicting pressure injury risk; the Braden Scale is one of those most frequently used.[9,10] Pressure injury staging is illustrated at http://www.npuap.org/resources/educational-and-clinical-resources/npuap-pressure-injury-stages/. One classification of stages or grades is summarized as follows[11]:

1. Nonblanchable erythema of intact skin usually over bony prominence; darkly pigmented skin may not have visible blanching
2. Partial-thickness skin loss with exposed dermis (erosion or intact or ruptured blistering) involving epidermis or dermis presenting as a shallow open ulcer with a red-pink wound bed, without slough. Deeper tissues are not visible.
3. Full-thickness skin loss involving damage or necrosis of subcutaneous tissue that may extend to, but not through, underlying fascia. Adipose

TABLE 47.2   SUMMARY OF SKIN DIAGNOSTIC PROCEDURES

TEST	PURPOSE
Dermoscopy	Magnified illumination of the skin using a liquid medium and transparent plate to examine skin lesions
Reflectance confocal microscopy	High-resolution assessment of cellular details and microstructures of the skin for evaluation of skin cancer
Skin biopsy	Histologic examination of tissue to determine differential diagnosis of cellular structure (i.e., benign growths vs. carcinoma, chronic infections, blistering diseases, and vasculitis)
Microscopic immunofluorescence	Identification of antibodies, immunoglobulins, and complement components for diseases such as pemphigus, vasculitis, and discoid lupus erythematosus using fluorescent light on slide-mounted biopsy specimens
Gram stain	Differentiation of gram-positive from gram-negative bacteria according to stain absorption
Culture	Identification of chronic bacterial and fungal infections by incubating skin specimens in culture media
Wood lamp examination	Examination of skin or hair to identify fungus that fluoresces bright yellow-green under ultraviolet light
Patch and scratch tests	Application of suspected allergens to skin by patch or scratch for evaluation of immune system responses to known allergens and evaluation of cell-mediated immune function (*Candida albicans*, skin fungus, chemicals, aeroallergens, and foods)
Skin scrapings	Application of potassium hydroxide and low heat to skin scrapings on a glass slide to identify dermatophytes and *C. albicans*
Side lighting	Indirect lighting of the skin using light to the side of the lesions to evaluate patterns of depression and elevation of skin lesions
Diascopy	Use of glass or clear plastic pressed on the skin to differentiate erythema caused by dilated capillaries (blanching) from extravasation of blood (no blanching)
Tzanck smear	A microscopic examination of cellular material from skin lesions to help diagnose vesicular diseases, including herpes simplex virus and varicella-zoster virus

BOX 47.1   PRESSURE INJURY RISK FACTORS

Prolonged Pressure/Immobilization

Lying in bed or sitting in chair or wheelchair without changing position or relieving pressure over an extended period

- Lying for hours on hard x-ray and operating tables
- Neurologic disorders (coma, spinal cord injuries, peripheral neuropathy, cognitive impairment, or cerebrovascular disease)
- Fractures or contractures
- Debilitation: elderly persons in hospitals and nursing homes
- Pain
- Sedation

Shearing forces

- Turning by dragging on coarse bed sheets

Disease/Tissue Factors

Thin or fragile skin
Impaired perfusion; ischemia

Fecal or urinary incontinence; prolonged exposure to moisture
Malnutrition, dehydration
Chronic diseases accompanied by anemia, edema, renal failure, malnutrition, peripheral vascular disease, or sepsis
Previous history of pressure ulcers

Additional Risk Factors for the Critically Ill

Norepinephrine infusion
Acute Physiology and Chronic Health Evaluation (APACHE II) score
Anemia
Age greater than 40 years
Multiple organ system disease or comorbid complications
Length of hospital stay
Use of ventilators or extracorporeal membranous oxygenation support

Data from Coleman S et al: *Int J Nurs Stud* 50(7):974-1003, 2013; Dealey C et al: *Int Wound J* 12(3):309-312, 2015; Edsberg LE et al: *J Wound Ostomy Continence Nurs* 41(4):313-334, 2014.

tissue visible in the ulcer, granulation tissue and rolled wound edges are often present.

4. Full-thickness skin and tissue loss with exposure of muscle, bone, or supporting structures (tendons or joint capsules); can include undermining and tunneling

5. Unstageable pressure injury with obscured full-thickness skin and tissue loss. Full-thickness skin and tissue loss in which the extent of tissue damage within the ulcer cannot be confirmed because it is obscured by slough or eschar.

6. Deep tissue pressure injury with persistent nonblanchable skin. Deep red, maroon, or purple discoloration of intact skin or epidermal separation revealing a dark wound bed or blood-filled blister caused by underlying soft tissue damage from pressure or shear forces, or both, at the bone-muscle interface.

Superficial damage results in a layer of dead tissue that appears as an abrasion, blister, erosion, or nonblanchable red/darkened skin or as a reddish-blue-purple discoloration when there is deeper tissue damage. Superficial injuries are more common on the sacrum as a result of shearing or friction forces. Deep injuries develop closer to the bone as a result of tissue distortion and vascular occlusion from pressure that is perpendicular to the tissue (over the heels, trochanter, and ischia). Bacteria colonize the dead tissue, and infection is usually localized and

TABLE 47.3 PRIMARY SKIN LESIONS

Macule[a]

A flat, circumscribed area that is a change in the color of the skin; less than 1 cm in diameter

Examples: Freckles, flat moles (nevi), petechiae, measles, scarlet fever

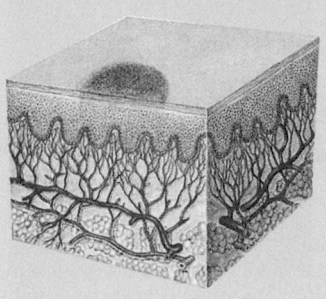 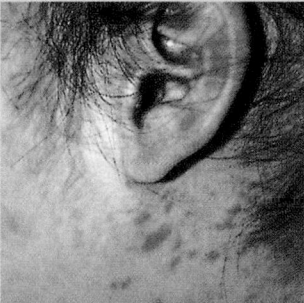

A, Macules

Papule[b]

An elevated, firm, circumscribed area less than 1 cm in diameter

Examples: Wart (verruca), elevated moles, lichen planus, fibroma, insect bite

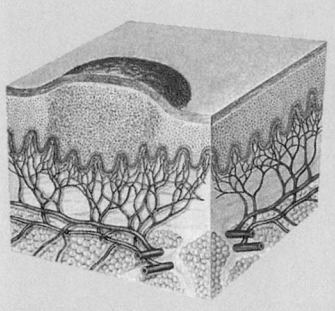 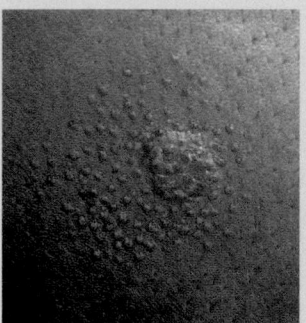

B, Lichen planus

Patch[c]

A flat, nonpalpable, irregular-shaped macule more than 1 cm in diameter

Examples: Vitiligo, port-wine stains, mongolian spots, café-au-lait spots

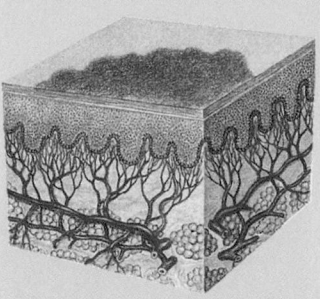 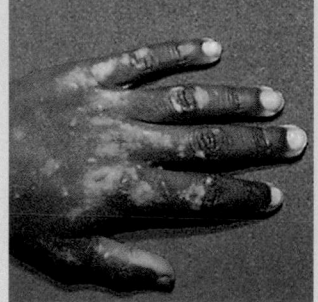

C, Vitiligo

Plaque[d]

Elevated, firm, and rough lesion with flat top surface greater than 1 cm in diameter

Examples: Psoriasis, seborrheic and actinic keratoses

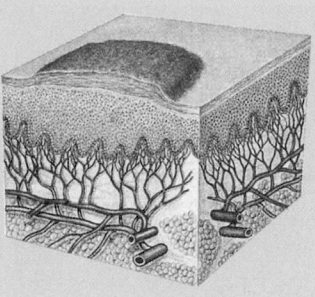 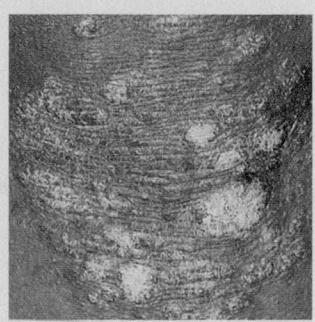

D, Plaque

Wheal[e]

Elevated, irregular-shaped area of cutaneous edema; solid, transient; variable diameter

Examples: Insect bites, urticaria, allergic reaction

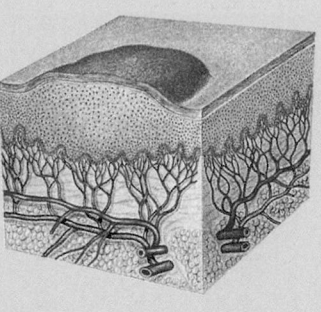 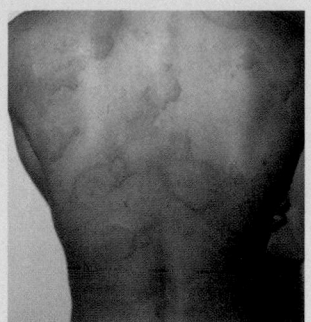

E, Wheal

Nodule[f]

Elevated, firm, circumscribed lesion; deeper in dermis than a papule; 1–2 cm in diameter

Examples: Erythema nodosum, lipomas

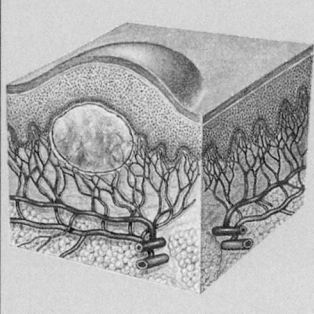 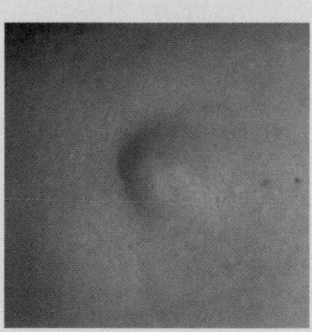

F, Lipoma

Continued

TABLE 47.3 PRIMARY SKIN LESIONS—cont'd

Tumor[f]
Elevated, solid lesion; may be clearly demarcated; deeper in dermis; greater than 2 cm in diameter
Examples: Neoplasms, benign tumor, lipoma, neurofibroma, hemangioma

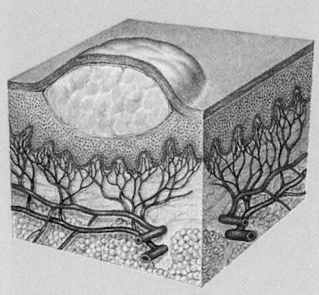
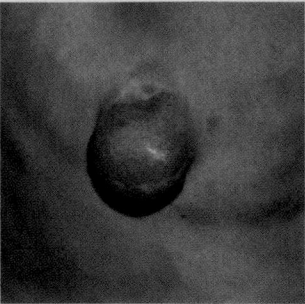

G, Neurofibroma

Vesicle[g]
Elevated, circumscribed, superficial, does not extend into dermis; filled with serous fluid; less than 1 cm in diameter
Examples: Varicella (chickenpox), herpes zoster (shingles), herpes simplex

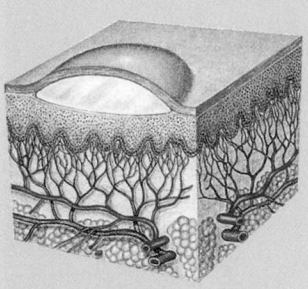
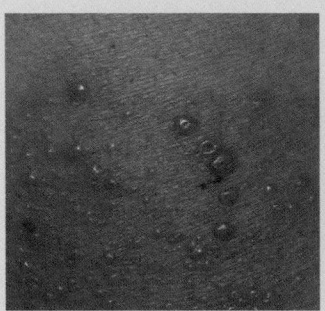

H, Vesicles

Bulla[h]
Vesicle greater than 1 cm in diameter
Examples: Blister, pemphigus vulgaris

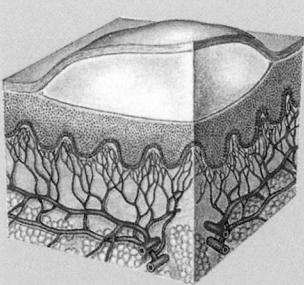
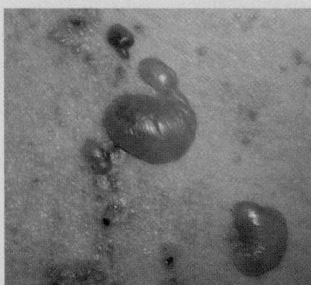

I, Bullae

Pustule[c]
Elevated, superficial lesion; similar to a vesicle but filled with purulent fluid
Examples: Impetigo, acne

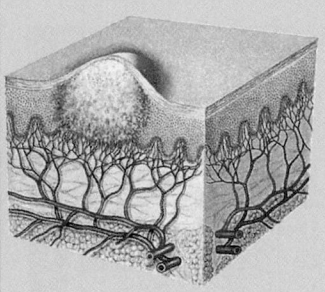
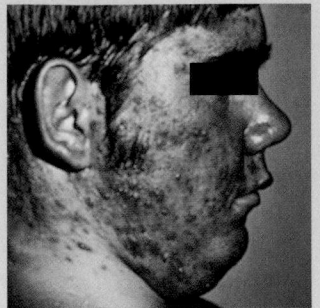

J, Acne

Cyst[c]
Elevated, circumscribed, encapsulated lesion; in dermis or subcutaneous layer; filled with liquid or semisolid material
Examples: Sebaceous cyst, cystic acne

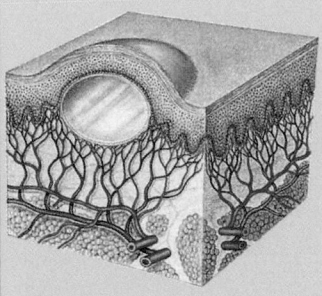
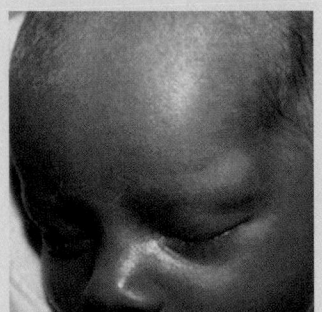

K, Sebaceous cyst

Telangiectasia[e]
Fine (0.5–1.0 mm), irregular red lines produced by capillary dilation; can be associated with acne rosacea (face), venous hypertension (spider veins in legs), systemic sclerosis, or developmental abnormalities (port-wine birthmarks)
Example: Telangiectasia in rosacea

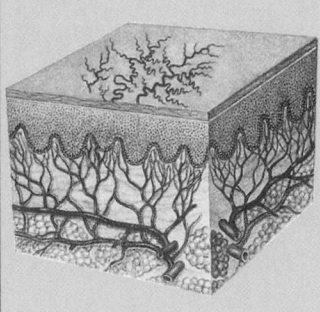
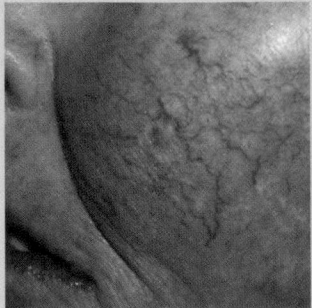

L, Telangiectasia

[a]Farrar WE et al: *Infectious diseases,* ed 2, London, 1992, Gower.
[b]James WD, Berger T, Elston DMD: *Andrews' diseases of the skin,* ed 11, Philadelphia, 2011, Saunders.
[c]Weston WL, Lane AT: *Color textbook of pediatric dermatology,* ed 3, Philadelphia, 2002, Mosby.
[d]Habif TP: *Clinical dermatology: a color guide to diagnosis and therapy,* ed 5, Philadelphia, 2010, Mosby.
[e]Bolognia JL, Jorizzo JL, Schaffer JV: *Dermatology,* ed 3, Philadelphia, 2012, Saunders.
[f]Weston WL, Lane AT, Morelli JG: *Color textbook of pediatric dermatology,* ed 4, Philadelphia, 2007, Mosby.
[g]Black MM et al: *Obstetric and gynecologic dermatology,* ed 3, Philadelphia, 2008, Mosby.
[h]Marks JG, Miller JJ: *Lookingbill & Marks' principles of dermatology,* ed 4, London, 2006, Saunders.

TABLE 47.4 SECONDARY SKIN LESIONS

Scale[a]

Heaped-up, keratinized cells; flaky skin; irregular-shape; thick or thin; dry or oily; variation in size

Examples: Flaking of skin with seborrheic dermatitis following scarlet fever, or flaking of skin following a drug reaction; dry skin

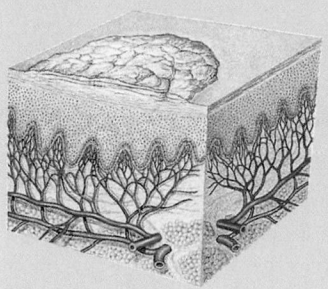 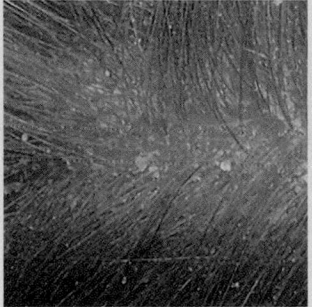

A, Fine scaling

Lichenification[b]

Rough, thickened epidermis secondary to persistent rubbing, itching, or skin irritation; often involves flexor surface of extremity

Example: Chronic dermatitis

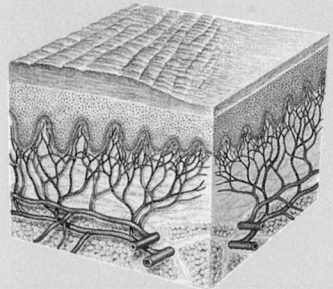 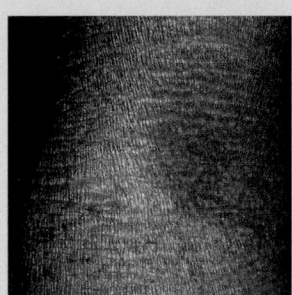

B, Atopic dermatitis of arm

Keloid[c]

Irregular-shaped, elevated, progressively enlarging scar; grows beyond the boundaries of the wound; caused by excessive collagen formation during healing

Example: Keloid formation following surgery

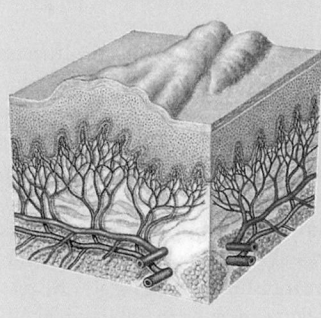 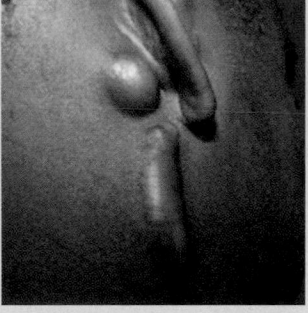

C, Keloid

Scar[d]

Thin to thick fibrous tissue that replaces normal skin following injury or laceration to the dermis

Examples: Healed wound or surgical incision

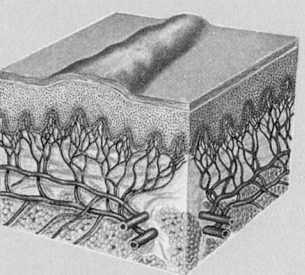 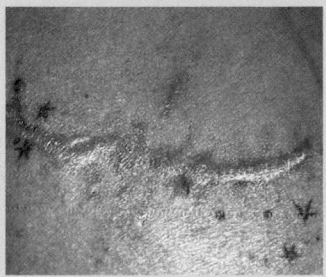

D, Hypertrophic scar

Excoriation[c]

Loss of the epidermis; linear, hollowed-out, crusted area

Examples: Abrasion or scratch, scabies

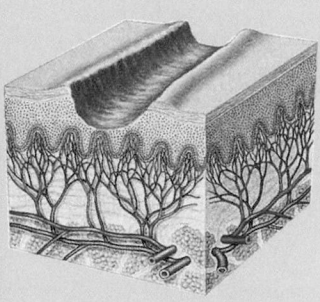 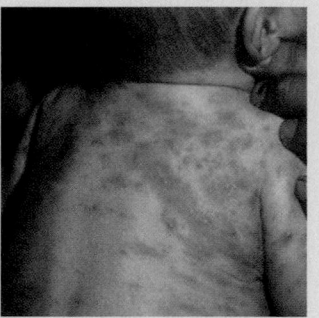

E, Scabies

Fissure[c]

Linear crack or break from the epidermis to the dermis; may be moist or dry

Examples: Athlete's foot, cracks at the corner of the mouth, anal fissure, dermatitis

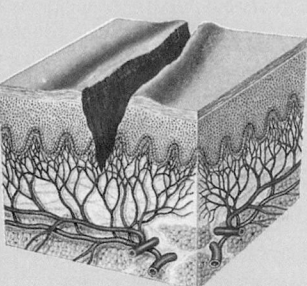 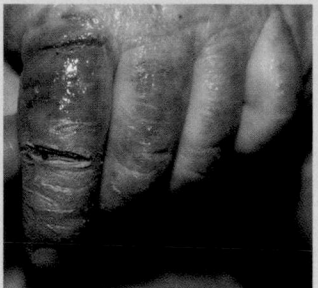

F, Fissures from infected dermatitis

Continued

TABLE 47.4   SECONDARY SKIN LESIONS—cont'd

Erosion[e]
Loss of part of the epidermis; depressed, moist, glistening; follows rupture of a vesicle or bulla or chemical injury
Example: Chemical injury

Atrophy[g]
Thinning of the skin surface and loss of skin markings
Examples: Aged skin, striae

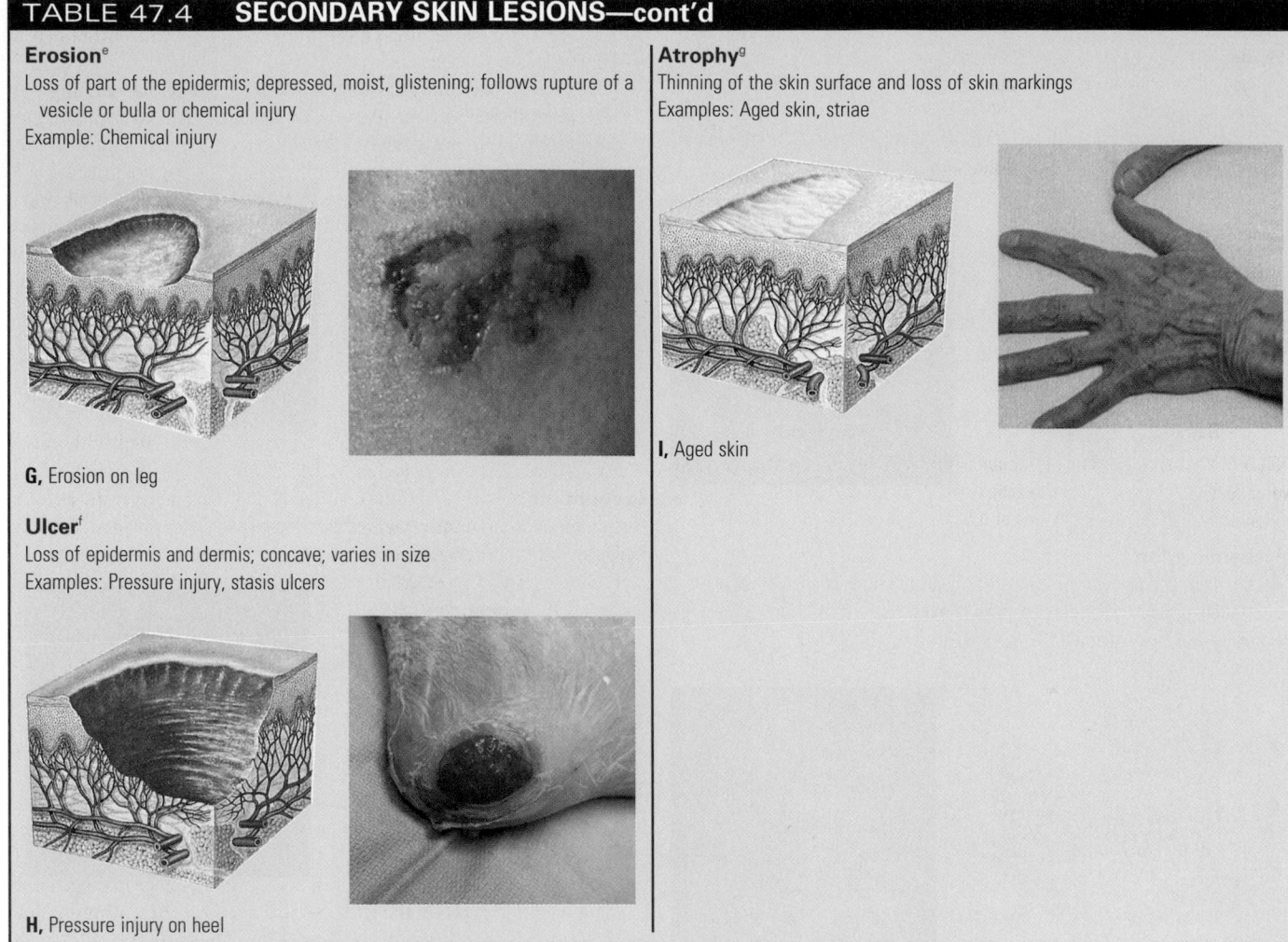

G, Erosion on leg

I, Aged skin

Ulcer[f]
Loss of epidermis and dermis; concave; varies in size
Examples: Pressure injury, stasis ulcers

H, Pressure injury on heel

[a]Baran R, Dawber RR, Levene GM: *Color atlas of the hair, scalp, and nails,* St Louis, 1991, Mosby.
[b]James WD, Berger T, Elston DMD: *Andrews' diseases of the skin,* ed 11, Philadelphia, 2011, Saunders.
[c]Weston WL, Lane AT, Morelli JG: *Color textbook of pediatric dermatology,* ed 4, Philadelphia, 2007, Mosby.
[d]Nouri K, Leal-Khouri S: *Techniques in dermatologic surgery,* Philadelphia, 2003, Mosby.
[e]Bolognia JL, Jorizzo JL, Schaffer JV: *Dermatology,* ed 3, Philadelphia, 2012, Saunders.
[f]Robinson JK et al: *Surgery of the skin,* ed 3, Philadelphia, 2015, Mosby.
[g]Seidel HM et al: *Mosby's guide to physical examination,* ed 8, St Louis, 2015, Mosby.

TABLE 47.5   SPECIAL SKIN LESIONS

TYPE	CLINICAL MANIFESTATIONS
Comedone	A plug of sebaceous and keratin material lodged in the opening of a hair follicle; an open comedone has a dilated orifice (blackhead), and a closed comedone has a narrow opening (whitehead)
Burrow	A narrow, raised, irregular channel caused by a parasite
Petechiae	A circumscribed area of blood less than 0.5 cm in diameter
Purpura	A circumscribed area of blood greater than 0.5 cm in diameter

self-limiting. Proteolytic enzymes from bacteria and macrophages dissolve necrotic tissues and cause a foul-smelling discharge that resembles, but is not, pus. The necrotic tissue initiates an inflammatory response with potential pain, fever, and leukocytosis. If the ulceration is large, toxicity and pain lead to a host of possible complications, including loss of appetite, debility, local/systemic infections, and renal insufficiency (Fig. 47.3).

The primary goal for those at risk for pressure injury is prevention and early detection. Prevention strategies include education of caregivers; frequent skin assessment with repositioning and turning; use of prophylactic dressings to high-risk bony prominences; promotion of movement; implementation of pressure reduction (repositioning and use of specialty beds/supportive surfaces) and pressure removal (positioning interval); and elimination of excessive moisture and drainage. Adequate nutrition, oxygenation, and fluid balance must be maintained.[12]

Superficial injuries should be covered with flat, moisture-retaining dressings (e.g., hydrogel dressings) that cannot wrinkle and cause increased pressure or friction; multiple options are available. Successful healing requires continued adequate relief of pressure; débridement of dead tissue; opening of deep pockets for drainage; and repair of damaged tissue by construction of skin flaps for large, deep ulcers. Negative-pressure wound healing is used in the treatment of advanced-stage pressure injuries, but clinical trials are lacking.[13] Infection requires

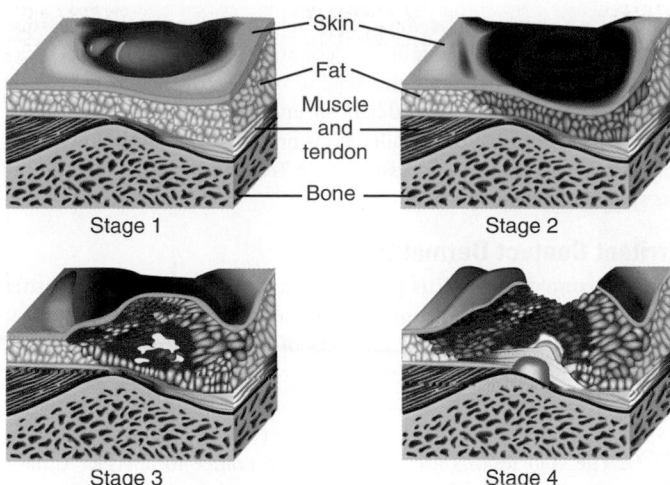

FIGURE 47.3 Progression of Decubitus Pressure Injury. Sustained pressure over a bony prominence compresses the tissue and reduces blood flow, resulting in progressive ischemia and necrosis of tissue.

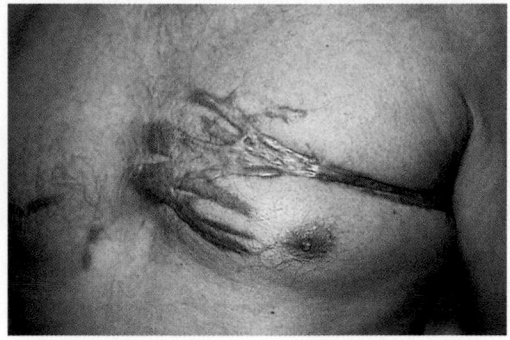

FIGURE 47.4 Keloid. (Courtesy Department of Dermatology, School of Medicine, University of Utah.)

treatment with topical and/or systemic agents, but there are no clear guidelines.[14] Pain must be controlled. Randomized controlled trials are needed to determine the best methods for treating pressure injuries.

Keloids and Hypertrophic Scars. Keloids are rounded, firm, elevated scars with irregular clawlike margins that extend beyond the original site of injury. They are most common in darkly pigmented skin types and generally appear weeks to months after a stable scar has formed. Keloids have excessive deposition of fibroblast-derived extracellular matrix proteins, particularly types I and III collagen with persistent inflammation and fibrosis. The fibroblasts have high metabolic and mitotic rates. Keloids first appear as pink or red, firm, well-defined rubbery plaques that persist for several months after trauma. Later, uncontrolled overgrowth causes extension beyond the site of the original wound, and the tumor becomes smoother, irregularly shaped, hyperpigmented, and harder with clawlike prolongations (Fig. 47.4).

Hypertrophic scars are elevated erythematous fibrous lesions that do not expand beyond the border of injury and primarily contain type III collagen. Hypertrophic scars appear within 3 to 4 months and usually regress within 1 year. Both lesions are caused by abnormal wound healing with excessive fibroblast activity and collagen formation and loss of control of normal tissue repair and regeneration.[15] Genetic susceptibility is likely.

Excessive or poorly aligned tension on a wound, introduction of foreign material into the skin, infection, and certain types of trauma (e.g., burns) are provocative factors. The parts of the body at risk include

the shoulders, back, chin, ears, and lower legs. Individuals 10 to 30 years of age develop lesions much more commonly than do children before puberty or older adults.

Keloids are the most extreme example of cutaneous scarring and the most difficult to treat. Preventive measures such as avoidance of unnecessary elective surgeries, recognition of familial tendency, and early detection are of paramount importance. Management of keloids and hypertrophic scars includes pressure therapy, topical and intralesional corticosteroids, intralesional interferon, bleomycin and 5-fluorouracil (5-FU), cryotherapy, radiotherapy, surgical/laser procedures, silicone gel sheeting, onion extract–containing preparations, and other therapies directed at collagen synthesis.[16,17] The calcium antagonist verapamil is an emerging treatment. There remains a need for research to improve prevention strategies and treatment outcomes.

Pruritus

Pruritus, or itching, is a common symptom associated with many primary skin disorders, such as eczema, psoriasis, or lice infestations, or it can be a manifestation of systemic disease (e.g., xerosis, chronic renal failure, cholestatic liver disease, thyroid disorders, iron deficiency, neuropathies, or malignancy) or the use of opiate drugs. It may be acute (e.g., mosquito bite) or chronic (neuropathic itch), localized or generalized, and migratory.

Multiple stimuli can produce itching, and there is interaction between itch and pain sensations. Peripheral pruritogenic (itch) mediators include histamine, neuropeptides, serotonin, prostaglandins, bradykinin, substance P, opioids, acetylcholine, interleukins 2 and 31, proteinases (trypsin and papain), and nerve growth factor. Small unmyelinated type C nerve fibers transmit itch sensations, and specific spinal pathways carry itch sensations through the spinal cord to the brain. These nerve fibers also may interact with dermal eosinophils, lymphocytes, and mast cells.[18]

Central nervous system mechanisms also can modulate itching, which is less perceptible when the mind is distracted by other stimuli. How the central nervous system influences the itch sensation is unclear. *Neuropathic itch* (itch without pruritogenic stimuli) is related to pathology along an afferent pathway (i.e., postherpetic neuropathy).[19] *Psychogenic itch* is associated with psychologic disorders (e.g., depression and obsessive-compulsive disorder).[20]

Chronic itching is an unpleasant sensation that may or may not be relieved by scratching—often done so intensely that trauma to the skin occurs, resulting in infection, skin thickening (lichenification), and scarring. Both central and peripheral sensitization occurs.[18] Management of itching is challenging and depends on the cause; the primary condition must be treated. Both topical and systemic therapies are used.[21]

DISORDERS OF THE SKIN

Disruptions in skin integrity may be precipitated by trauma, abnormal cellular function, infection and inflammation, and systemic diseases. Many skin disorders are benign and self-limiting, whereas others are severe and life threatening.

Inflammatory Disorders

The most common inflammatory disorders of the skin are eczema and dermatitis. Eczema and dermatitis are general terms that describe a particular type of inflammatory response in the skin and can be used interchangeably. Eczematous disorders are generally characterized by pruritus, lesions with indistinct borders, and epidermal changes. These lesions either can appear as erythema, papules, or scales and can present in an acute, subacute, or chronic phase. Edema, serous discharge, and crusting occur with continued irritation and scratching. In chronic eczema the skin becomes thickened, leathery, and hyperpigmented from recurrent irritation and scratching. The location of eczema is related to the underlying cause. Eczematous inflammations need to be differentiated from other dermatoses, particularly psoriasis.

Allergic Contact Dermatitis

Allergic contact dermatitis is a common form of T-cell-mediated or delayed hypersensitivity (type IV). (See Chapter 9 for various types of allergic responses.) The response is a consequence of alterations in skin barrier function with reaction to irritants/allergens; release of cytokines, chemokines, and cytotoxins from keratinocytes; dendritic cells (Langerhans cells); and natural killer cells and neuronal responses, such as pruritus. Genetic susceptibility involves several genes, and specific mutations are not clearly known.[22] Allergens (e.g., microorganisms, chemicals, foreign proteins, drugs, metals, latex) can form the sensitizing antigen; contact with poison ivy is a common example (Fig. 47.5). When the allergen comes into contact with the skin, the allergen is bound to a carrier protein, forming a hapten-specific sensitizing antigen. Langerhans cells process the antigen and carry it to T cells in the draining lymph nodes. T cells then become sensitized to the antigen, releasing cytokines and chemokines leading to leukocyte infiltration and antigen-specific inflammation.[23] Latex allergy can be either a type IV hypersensitivity reaction to chemicals used in latex rubber processing or a type I immediate hypersensitivity reaction with immunoglobulin E (IgE) antibodies formed in response to latex rubber protein.[24]

In delayed hypersensitivity, several hours pass before an immunologic response is apparent. The T cells play an important role because they differentiate and secrete lymphokines that affect skin macrophage (Langerhans cells) movement and aggregation, coagulation, and other inflammatory responses (see Chapter 9). Sensitization usually develops with first exposure to the antigen, and symptoms of dermatitis occur with reexposure.

The manifestations of allergic contact dermatitis include erythema and swelling with pruritic vesicular lesions in the areas of allergen contact. The pattern of distribution provides clues to the source of the antigen (e.g., hands exposed to chemical solutions or boundaries from rings and bracelets). Chronic atopic dermatitis (AD) results in lichenification, fissuring, thickening, and scaling of the skin. Patch tests with specific antigens assist with diagnosis and differentiation from other dermatoses. Removal of the allergen is necessary for resolution of the inflammatory response and tissue repair. Treatment may require topical or systemic steroids.[25]

Irritant Contact Dermatitis

Irritant contact dermatitis is a nonspecific, inflammatory dermatitis caused by activation of the innate immune system by proinflammatory properties of chemicals. The intensity of the inflammation is related to the concentration of the irritant, exposure time, disruption of the skin barrier, and age.[26] Irritation can occur from almost anything, especially if the epidermal barrier is compromised in any way (Box 47.2). The skin lesions are similar in appearance to allergic contact dermatitis. Removing the source of irritation and using topical agents (i.e., corticosteroids and petroleum-based emollients) and nonirritating soaps constitute effective treatment.

Atopic Dermatitis

Atopic dermatitis (atopic eczema) is more common in infancy and childhood; however, some individuals are affected throughout life (see Chapter 48 for details).

BOX 47.2	SUBSTANCES KNOWN TO CAUSE CONTACT DERMATITIS*

Alkalis
    Soaps
    Detergents
    Ammonia preparations
    Lye
    Drainpipe cleaners
    Toilet bowl cleaners
    Oven cleaners
Acids
Metal salts
    Cyanides of calcium, copper, mercury, nickel, silver, zinc
    Chlorides of calcium and zinc
Bromine, chlorine, iodine, fluorine
Insecticides
Herbicides
Dusts of lime, zinc, arsenic
Dyes and fragrances
Wood dust from teak, cinchona bark, quinine, pyrethrum
Tobacco dust from cigars
Topical antibiotics
Explosive powders
Hydrocarbons
    Crude petroleum, lubricating oil, cutting oil
    Paraffins, mineral oils
    Asphalt, other tar products
Soot, peat
Preservatives
    Formaldehyde-releasing and nonformaldehyde-releasing

*For chemicals that cause occupational allergic contact dermatitis, see National Library of Medicine: *Haz-map Table 1: Chemicals that cause occupational allergic contact dermatitis*, Bethesda, MD, last updated April 2013. Available at: www.hax-map.com/allergic.htm.

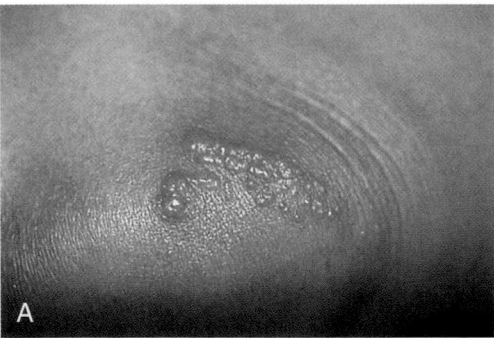
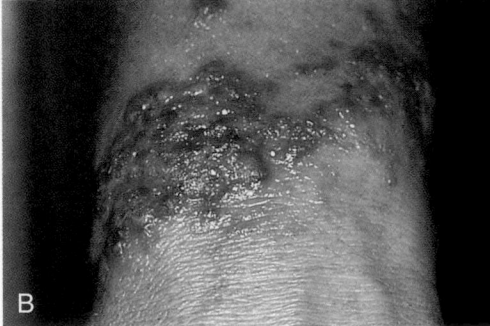

FIGURE 47.5 Poison Ivy. A, Poison ivy on knee. **B,** Poison ivy dermatitis. (Courtesy Department of Dermatology, School of Medicine, University of Utah.)

Stasis Dermatitis

Stasis dermatitis usually occurs on the legs as a result of venous stasis and edema. The disorder is associated with varicosities (incompetent venous valves), phlebitis, and vascular trauma (see Chapter 33). Pooling of venous blood traps leukocytes that may release proteolytic enzymes. Increased venous pressure widens interendothelial pores with deposition of red blood cells, fibrin, and other macromolecules, making them unavailable for repair and promoting inflammation.[27] Edema evolves to erythema and pruritus with progression to scaling, petechiae, and hyperpigmentation. Progressive lesions become ulcerated (stasis ulcers), particularly around the ankles and tibia (Fig. 47.6).

Treatment includes elevating the legs as often as possible, refraining from wearing tight clothes around the legs, compression stockings, and avoiding standing for long periods. Defined infections are treated with antibiotics. Chronic lesions with ulceration are treated with moist dressings, external compression/dressings, and vein ablation surgery.[28]

Seborrheic Dermatitis

Seborrheic dermatitis is a common chronic inflammation of the skin involving the scalp, eyebrows, eyelids, ear canals, nasolabial folds, axillae, chest, and back (Fig. 47.7). In infants it is known as *cradle cap*. Proposed theories include genetic predisposition, phospholipases from *Malassezia* yeasts, immunosuppression, and epidermal hyperproliferation. *Malassezia* infection causes inflammation with stratum corneum hyperproliferation (scaling) and incomplete corneocyte differentiation. Alteration in the stratum corneum barrier allows water to more readily leave the skin.[29]

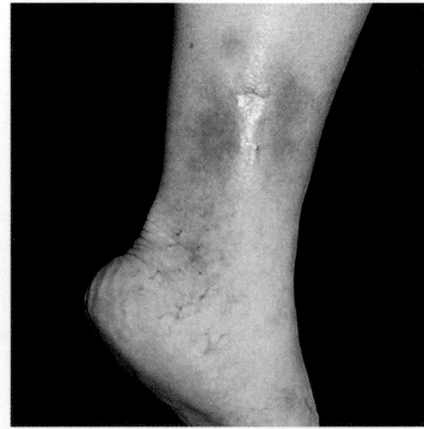

FIGURE 47.6 Stasis Ulcer. (Courtesy Department of Dermatology, School of Medicine, University of Utah.)

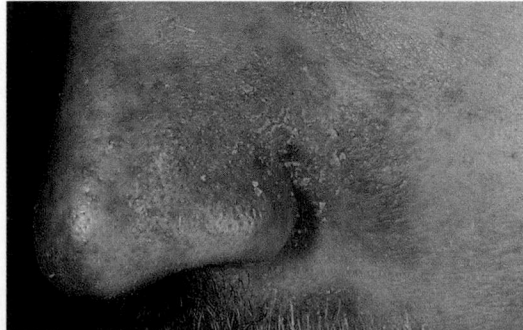

FIGURE 47.7 Seborrheic Dermatitis. (Courtesy Department of Dermatology, School of Medicine, University of Utah.)

Lesions develop from infancy to old age, with periods of remission and exacerbation. The lesions appear as greasy, scaly, white, or yellowish inflammatory plaques in sebaceous areas with mild pruritus. Topical agents are first-line therapy and include antifungal agents (ketoconazole), keratolytics (coal tar shampoo), and antiinflammatory agents (short-term use of corticosteroids).[30]

Papulosquamous Disorders

Psoriasis, pityriasis rosea, and lichen planus are inflammatory disorders characterized by papules, scales, plaques, and erythema. Collectively they are described as papulosquamous disorders.

Psoriasis

Psoriasis is a chronic, relapsing, proliferative, inflammatory disorder that involves the skin, scalp, and nails and can occur at any age. Psoriasis affects about 1% to 11% of the world population and is more common in countries north of the equator.[31] The onset is generally established by 40 years of age. A family history of psoriasis is estimated at 60% to 90% of cases. The genetic mechanisms are complex and involve skin barrier function and innate and adaptive immunity.[32] The onset of psoriasis later in life is less familial and more secondary to comorbidities, such as obesity, smoking, hypertension, and diabetes.

Triggers of psoriasis include physical injury (which causes Koebner phenomenon [new plaque formation]), infections (particularly streptococcal), and medications (e.g., β-blockers, lithium). The inflammatory cascade of psoriasis involves the complex interactions between macrophages, fibroblasts, dendritic cells, natural killer cells, T helper cells, and regulatory T cells. Psoriasis is a T helper (Th) cell-mediated autoimmune disease. The interleukin (IL)-23/T helper (Th) 17 cell axis plays an important role in the pathogenesis of psoriasis. Inflammatory cytokines involved include tumor necrosis factor-alpha (TNF-α), interferon-gamma (IFN-γ), and numerous interleukins derived from activated T cells, B cells, dendritic cells, and macrophages.[33] These inflammatory markers are the target for several therapeutic drugs known as the *biologics* (biotherapy or immunotherapy).[34]

Both the dermis and epidermis are thickened because of keratinocyte hyperproliferation, altered keratinocyte differentiation, and expanded dermal vasculature. The turnover time for shedding the epidermis is decreased to 3 to 4 days from the normal 26 to 30 days with many more germinative cells and an increase in transit time of cells through the dermis. Cell maturation and keratinization are bypassed, and the epidermis thickens and plaques form. The loosely cohesive keratin gives the lesion a silvery, scaly appearance. Capillary dilation and increased vascularization occur from release of angiogenic factors, such as vascular endothelial growth factor (VEGF), and accommodate the increased cell metabolism and causes erythema. The disease can be mild, moderate, or severe depending on the size, distribution, inflammation, and type of lesion. Psoriasis is marked by remissions and exacerbations.[35]

The types of psoriasis include plaque (psoriasis vulgaris), inverse, guttate, pustular, and erythrodermic. Plaque psoriasis is the most common and affects 80% to 90% of individuals with psoriasis. Early-onset psoriasis is an inflammatory lesion with epidermal hyperproliferation, the presence of activated T lymphocytes and numerous cytokines including IL-1, IL-6, IL-17, IL-22, TNF-α, and IFN-γ.[33] The typical lesion of plaque psoriasis is a well-demarcated, thick, silvery, scaly, erythematous plaque surrounded by normal skin that can appear anywhere on the body (Fig. 47.8). Small erythematous papules enlarge and coalesce into larger inflammatory lesions more commonly on the face, scalp, trunk, elbows, and knees and at sites of trauma (Koebner phenomenon). Inverse psoriasis is rare and involves lesions that develop in skinfolds (i.e., axilla or groin). Often misdiagnosed as a fungal infection, they are large, smooth, dry, and deep red.[36]

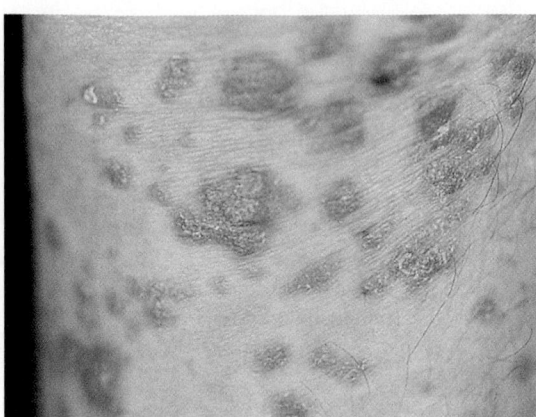

FIGURE 47.8 Psoriasis. Typical oval plaques with well-defined borders and silvery scale. (Courtesy Department of Dermatology, School of Medicine, University of Utah.)

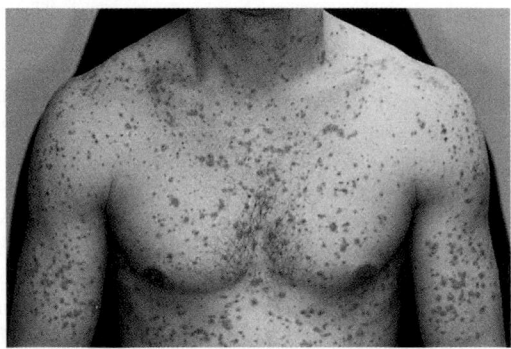

FIGURE 47.9 Guttate Psoriasis After Streptococcal Infection. Numerous uniformly small lesions may abruptly occur after streptococcal pharyngitis. (Courtesy Department of Dermatology, School of Medicine, University of Utah.)

In guttate psoriasis, small papules (1 to 10 mm) appear suddenly on the trunk and extremities (Fig. 47.9). The lesions may appear a few weeks after a streptococcal respiratory tract infection and are more common in children. Guttate psoriasis may resolve spontaneously in weeks or months. Pustular psoriasis appears as blisters of noninfectious pus (collections of neutrophils) that develop over areas of plaque psoriasis and represents a flare of disease with involvement of IL-1α, IL-1β, IL-36, TNF-α, and IFN-α.[33] Erythrodermic (exfoliative) psoriasis is characterized by widespread red, scaling lesions that cover a large body surface area (BSA) and is often accompanied by itching or pain associated with constitutional symptoms (fever, chills, fatigue) and skin infections.

Psoriatic arthritis (PsA) is associated with the proinflammatory cytokines that cause psoriatic skin lesions, particularly the IL-23/Th17 axis and TNF-α.[37] There are several phenotypes including asymmetric arthritis of the major joints, enthesitis (inflammation of ligaments and tendons), dactylitis (involvement of finger and toes), and nail disease. Psoriatic arthritis mutilans involves pronounced bone destruction, and there is greater risk of cardiovascular disease with PsA. Psoriatic nail disease can occur in all psoriasis subtypes with pitting, onycholysis, subungual hyperkeratosis, and nail plate dystrophy. Psoriasis also is a risk factor for a number of comorbidities, including uveitis; inflammatory bowel disease; metabolic syndrome, including hypertension insulin resistance, dyslipidemias, and abdominal obesity; depression and anxiety; chronic obstructive pulmonary disease; and increased risk for atherosclerosis and cardiovascular disease that is independent of traditional risk factors for these diseases.[38]

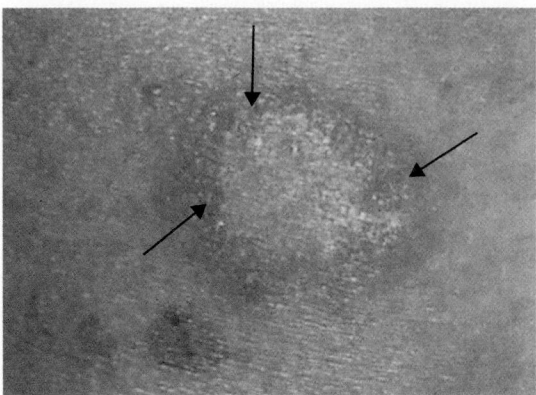

FIGURE 47.10 Pityriasis Rosea Herald Patch. A collarette pattern has formed around the margins. (Courtesy Department of Dermatology, School of Medicine, University of Utah.)

Treatment is individualized and related to maintaining skin moisture, reducing epidermal cell turnover and pruritus, and promoting immunomodulation. Mild lesions are usually treated with emollients (maintains skin moisture), keratolytic agents (removes scale), corticosteroids (suppresses inflammation), and vitamin D analogs (reduces epidermal proliferation). Narrow band phototherapy, cyclosporine, methotrexate, acitretin, or biologics such as TNF-α antagonists and drugs that target the IL-23/IL-17 axis are reserved for moderate to severe forms of disease. New drugs are under investigation for safety, efficacy, and cost.[34,39]

Pityriasis Rosea

Pityriasis rosea is a self-limiting inflammatory disorder that occurs more often in children and young adults. The cause is thought to be a herpes-like virus (e.g., human herpesvirus 6 [HHV-6] and HHV-7).[40] Pityriasis rosea begins as a single lesion known as a herald patch (Fig. 47.10) that is circular, demarcated, and salmon-pink; is approximately 3 to 10 cm in diameter; and is usually located on the trunk. Early lesions are macular and papular, followed by lesions that develop within 14 to 21 days and extend over the trunk and upper part of the extremities and, rarely, on the face. The small erythematous rose-colored papules expand into characteristic oval lesions that are bilateral and symmetrically distributed. There may be few or hundreds of lesions. The pattern of distribution follows the skin lines around the trunk and resembles a drooping pine tree. Scales slough from the margin of the lesions, forming a collarette pattern. Itching is the most common symptom. Occasional headache, fatigue, or sore throat may precede the development of the lesions.

The diagnosis of pityriasis rosea follows the clinical appearance of the lesion. Secondary syphilis, psoriasis, drug eruption, nummular eczema, and seborrheic dermatitis are among the differential diagnosis considerations. The disorder is usually self-limiting and resolves in a few months with symptomatic treatment for pruritus or cosmetic concerns. UV light (with some risk for hyperpigmentation), antihistamines, or topical corticosteroids may be used to control itching. Erythromycin and acyclovir also may be used for treatment. When diagnosed during pregnancy, there is increased risk for miscarriage or premature delivery from viral infection, and antiviral therapy should be considered.[41]

Lichen Planus

Lichen planus (LP) is a benign, autoimmune inflammatory disorder of the skin and mucous membranes with multiple clinical variations. The age of onset is usually between 30 and 70 years. The stimulating antigen is unknown, but T cells, adhesion molecules, inflammatory

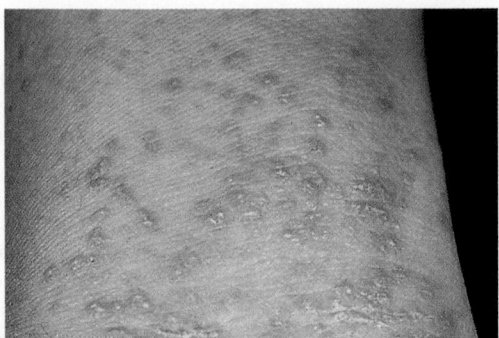

FIGURE 47.11 Hypertrophic Lichen Planus on Arms. (Courtesy Department of Dermatology, School of Medicine, University of Utah.)

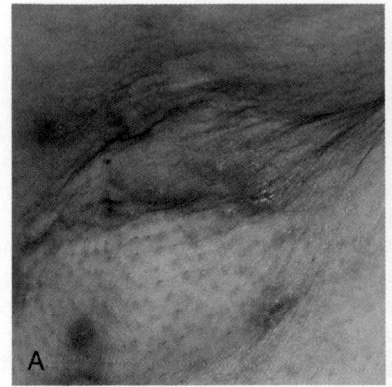 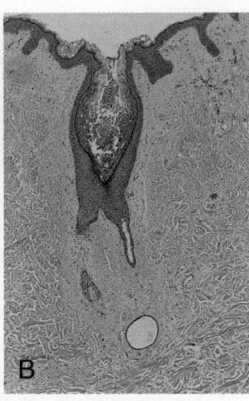

FIGURE 47.12 Hidradenitis Suppurativa. **A,** Characteristic painful pustules and draining sinus tracts. **B,** Histology shows follicular plugging and connection to a dilated apocrine duct. (**A** courtesy Kalman Watsky, MD; from Bolognia JL, Jorizzo JL, Schaffer JV, editors: *Dermatology*, ed 3, Philadelphia, 2012, Saunders. **B** from Bolognia JL, Jorizzo JL, Rapini RP, editors: *Dermatology*, ed 2, Philadelphia, 2008, Saunders.)

cytokines, perforin, and antigen-presenting cells are involved. The infiltrate of T cells mediates immunoreactivity against basal layer keratinocytes, which have altered surface antigens and adhesion molecules. LP is also linked to hepatitis C virus. The disorder begins with nonscaling, purple-colored, flat-topped, polygonal pruritic papules 2 to 4 mm in size, usually located on the wrists, ankles, lower legs, and genitalia (Fig. 47.11). New lesions are pale pink and evolve into a dark violet. Persistent lesions may be thickened and red, forming hypertrophic lichen planus.[42] Oral lesions (oral lichen planus) appear as lacy white rings that must be differentiated from leukoplakia or oral candidiasis, and they may be precancerous lesions in about 1% of cases.[43] Fine white lines, known as *Wickham striae*, can be seen throughout the oral lesions on magnification. These lesions also can develop on the penis and vulvovaginal area. Oral lesions do not commonly ulcerate, but if present are painful and require treatment. Chronic ulcerated lesions become malignant in 1% of individuals with the disease. Thinning and splitting of nails are common, and all or part of the nail may be shed.

Pruritus is the most distressing symptom. The lesions are self-limiting and may last for months or years, with an average duration of 6 to 18 months. Postinflammatory hyperpigmentation is a common consequence of the lesion. Approximately 20% of individuals have a recurrence. Diagnosis is made by the clinical appearance and histopathology of the lesion. Treatment is individualized and includes topical, intralesional, or systemic corticosteroids (second line for resistant LP) and systemic acitretin and narrow-band ultraviolet light therapy. Antihistamines are given for itching, and short-term use of topical or systemic glucocorticoids may control inflammation. Mucous membrane lesions are treated with potent topical steroids, topical retinoids or immunomodulators (or both), and systemic glucocorticoids.[44]

Acne Vulgaris

Acne vulgaris is an inflammatory disorder of the pilosebaceous follicle (the sebaceous gland contiguous with a hair follicle). It occurs most commonly during adolescence. Details of this disorder are presented in Chapter 48.

Hidradenitis Suppurativa (Inverse Acne)

Hidradenitis suppurativa is a chronic, inflammatory, recurring scarring disease of the pilosebaceous follicular ducts involving areas of skin where there are folds, hair follicles, and apocrine (sweat) glands (i.e., axillary, inguinal, inframammary, genital, buttocks, and perineal areas of the body) (Fig. 47.12). The incidence is unknown but is estimated at 1% to 4% of the population and is more common in females. The pathogenesis of the disease is complex and includes a combination of genetic, hormonal, immune, and environmental factors. Aggravating factors include smoking (the most significant factor, as nicotine activates

keratinocytes, fibroblasts, and immunocytes), tight clothing, heat and perspiration, obesity, and stress.[45] An aberrant response to commensal follicular bacteria results in inflammatory cytokine production with follicular hyperkeratosis and occlusion of the pilosebaceous unit causing perifolliculitis, abscess formation, sinus tracts, and scarring. The sweat glands are not primarily involved.[46] The lesions present as deep, firm, painful subcutaneous nodules that track and rupture horizontally under the skin. They are differentiated from "boils" (carbuncles) because boils extend vertically and discharge onto the skin.

Diagnosis can be difficult, delaying effective treatment. Treatment can include administering systemic medications, performing incision and drainage of nodules, obtaining a culture of the exudate, and giving antibiotics (combination of clindamycin and rifampicin) with concern about the presence of methicillin-resistant *Staphylococcus aureus* (MRSA), topical or intralesional corticosteroids, and retinoids. Biologics (i.e., infliximab or adalimumab) are options when other treatments fail.[47] Lesions often require surgical excision and skin grafting. Complete, spontaneous resolution is rare, and there is risk for squamous cell carcinoma. Deterrence includes avoiding heat and perspiration, losing weight if obese, wearing loose clothing, refraining from shaving affected areas, stopping smoking, and using zinc gluconate supplements to reduce inflammation. The disease can recur for years with negative effects on quality of life. Clinical trials are needed to identify the best treatment options.[48]

Acne Rosacea

Acne rosacea is a chronic inflammatory skin disease with varied presentations and extent of involvement that develops primarily in middle-age adults. There are four subtypes of lesions that can occur singly or in combination: erythematotelangiectatic, papulopustular, phymatous, and ocular. The cause is unknown. There is a familial tendency, and several genes have been identified. Neurovascular dysregulation, infection, and factors that trigger altered innate and adaptive immune response are involved (i.e., chronic sun exposure and damage, heat, drinking alcohol or hot beverages, hormonal fluctuations, *Demodex folliculorum* [mites] colonization, and mental stress).[49] The most common lesions are erythema and edema, papules, pustules, and telangiectasia occurring most commonly on the forehead, nose, cheeks, and chin (Fig. 47.13). Neurovascular dysregulation is associated with flushing, a burning sensation, and vasodilation. Alterations in epidermal barrier function and activation of T and B cells promote inflammation and the production of angiogenic factors and fibrogenic cytokines (i.e., transforming growth factor-β1 [TGF-β1]), promoting formation of telangiectasias, fibrosis, and cutaneous thickening.[50] Sebaceous hypertrophy, fibrosis, and telangiectasia may be severe enough to produce an irreversible bulbous appearance of the nose, known as *rhinophyma*. Facial application of fluorinated topical steroids may increase the severity of telangiectasias. Disorders of the eye often accompany rosacea, particularly conjunctivitis and, more rarely, keratitis which can result in visual impairment.[51]

Photoprotection, such as sunscreens or protective clothing, is essential along with avoidance of other triggers. Both topical (metronidazole, azelaic acid, low-dose isotretinoin, and ivermectin) and oral drugs (doxycycline, tetracycline, and an α2 receptor agonist) may be effective as well as treatment using pulsed lasers.[52] Surgical excision of excessive tissue may be required for rhinophyma.

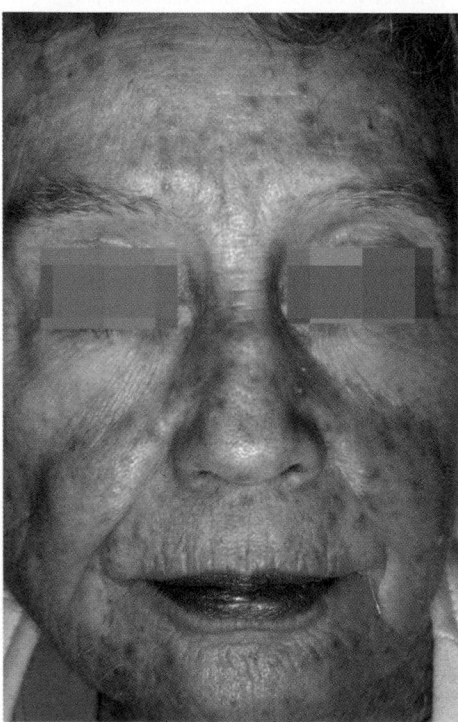

FIGURE 47.13 Rosacea. Pustules and erythema occur on the forehead, cheeks, and nose. (From Habif TP: *Clinical dermatology*, ed 6, Philadelphia, 2016, Saunders.)

Lupus Erythematosus

Lupus erythematosus is a systemic inflammatory, autoimmune disease with cutaneous manifestations (see Chapter 9). Cutaneous (or discoid) lupus erythematosus (CLE) is limited to the skin and often progresses to systemic lupus erythematosus (SLE) (70% to 80% of cases)[53] (Fig. 47.14).

Cutaneous Lupus Erythematosus. Cutaneous lupus erythematosus (CLE) usually occurs in genetically susceptible adults, particularly women in their late 30s or early 40s, but people of any age can be affected. Environmental triggers can initiate the inflammatory response, including infections, hormones (estrogen and prolactin), UV radiation, and exposure to drugs and chemicals. There are three subtypes of CLE with specific manifestations of the disease: acute, subacute, and chronic. The lesions may be single or multiple and of various sizes. Often the lesions are located on light-exposed areas of the skin, and photosensitivity is common. The face is the most common site of lesion involvement. The characteristic manifestations of the different categories of CLE are summarized in Table 47.6.

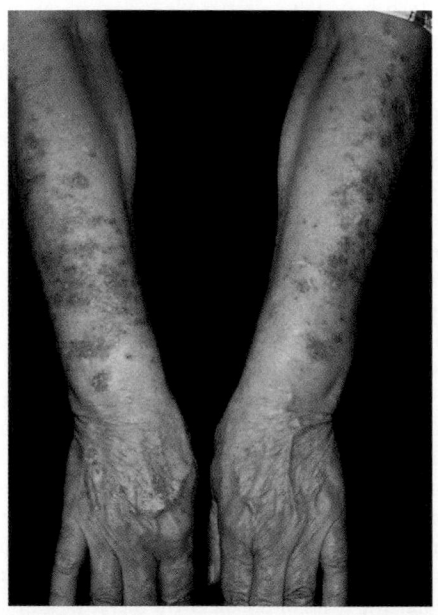

FIGURE 47.14 Subacute Cutaneous Lupus (Discoid Lupus Erythematosus). (Courtesy Department of Dermatology, School of Medicine, University of Utah.)

TABLE 47.6	CATEGORIES AND MANIFESTATIONS OF CUTANEOUS LUPUS ERYTHEMATOSUS	
CATEGORY OF CLE	**CLINICAL MANIFESTATIONS**	
Acute		
Localized	Butterfly pattern of erythema over bridge of nose and malar areas of face (malar rash); may have fine surface scales and underlying edema; scalp areas may develop alopecia; lasts for hours to days	
Generalized	Diffuse or papular erythema of face, upper trunk, or extremities; develops quickly and lasts hours to days	
Subacute	Erythematous macules and papules that evolve into *papulosquamous* or *annular* plaques developing on sun-exposed areas of the upper body (V area of neck, upper chest, back, shoulders, extensor surface of arms and hands); can be associated with reaction to drugs; may be accompanied by mild systemic disease	
Chronic	Classic cutaneous (discoid) lupus erythematosus is the most common form; lesions are red to purple macules or papules with a superficial brownish scale; scale can penetrate hair follicle leaving a carpet-tack appearance when removed; may have residual scarring, dermal atrophy hypopigmentation, alopecia, and telangiectasia; Raynaud phenomenon occurs in some individuals	

CLE, Cutaneous lupus erythematosus.
Data from Hejazi EZ, Werth VP: *Am J Clin Dermatol* 17(2):135-146, 2016; Tull TJ et al: *Br J Hosp Med (Lond)* 76(11):C162-C165, 2015.

The cause is unknown but thought to be related to genetic and environmental factors and an altered immune response to an unknown antigen or response to UVB wavelengths with the development of self-reactive T and B cells, decreased number of regulatory T cells, and increased levels of proinflammatory cytokines. Autoantibodies and immune complexes cause tissue damage and inflammation.[54]

Diagnosis of CLE is made from the presenting symptoms, biopsy of skin lesions with direct immunofluorescence, as well as histologic results. Skin biopsy with immunofluorescent observation reveals lumpy deposits of immunoglobulins, including IgM, IgG, and C3. The Revised Cutaneous Lupus Erythematosus Disease Area and Severity Index (CLASI) can be used to assess disease severity.[55]

Individuals with CLE must use sunscreen and sun protection because direct sun exposure initiates or exacerbates lesions. Treatment options include topical steroids, calcineurin inhibitors, and antimalarial drugs (e.g., hydroxychloroquine sulfate). These medications must be used with caution to prevent serious side effects.[53] Immunotherapy is being evaluated for treatment of CLE.[56]

Vesiculobullous Disorders

Vesiculobullous skin diseases share a common characteristic of vesicle, or blister, formation. Two such diseases are pemphigus and erythema multiforme.

Pemphigus

Pemphigus (meaning to blister or bubble) is a group of rare autoimmune blistering diseases of the skin and oral mucous membranes. It is caused when circulating immunoglobulin G (IgG) autoantibodies and C3 complement bind to the desmoglein adhesion molecules, resulting in the destruction of cell-to-cell adhesion (acantholysis) at the desmosomal cell junction in the suprabasal layer of the epidermis with fluid accumulation and the resulting symptom of blister formation.[57] Pemphigus can occur in all age groups but is more prevalent between 40 and 50 years of age. There is a genetic predisposition as well as environmental influences (viral infections, drug-induced, dietary intake), physical effects (such as radiation or surgery), and endogenous (emotional or hormonal stressors). Pemphigus presents in varying forms, often with painful, superficial erosions prone to infection:

- Pemphigus vulgaris is the most common form. Oral lesions precede the onset of skin blistering, which is more prominent on the face, scalp, and axilla. The blisters rupture easily because of the thin, fragile overlying portion of epidermis, resulting in painful erosions.
- Pemphigus vegetans is a rare variant of pemphigus vulgaris with large blisters that progress to hypertrophic granulomas with tissue erosion and pustules (vegetating plaques). They usually occur in tissue folds.
- Pemphigus foliaceus is a milder form of the disease and involves acantholysis at the subcorneal level with blistering, erosions, scaling, crusting, and erythema usually of the face and chest. Oral mucous membranes are rarely involved.
- Pemphigus erythematosus is a subset of pemphigus foliaceus often associated with systemic lupus erythematosus with positive antinuclear antibodies. The lesions are generally less widely distributed.
- Paraneoplastic pemphigus is the most severe form of pemphigus and is associated with lymphoproliferative neoplasms. Internal organs, including lungs, thyroid, kidney, smooth muscle, and the gastrointestinal tract, also are involved, leading to the term *paraneoplastic autoimmune multiorgan syndrome*. In contrast to pemphigus vulgaris, the lesions develop from inflammatory papules or macules rather than normal skin.
- IgA pemphigus is the most benign form of pemphigus characterized by tissue-bound and circulating IgA antibodies targeting desmosomal

or nondesmosomal cell surface components in the basement membrane of the epidermis. Acantholysis is not as severe as that in pemphigus vulgaris, but there is still blister formation.
- Pemphigus herpetiformis is a very rare form of pemphigus that resembles dermatitis herpetiformis (blistering lesions that have the appearance of herpes lesions) but with immunologic and histologic findings consistent with those of pemphigus.

The diagnosis of pemphigus is made from the clinical manifestations and histologic findings of autoantibodies in the epidermis or mucosal epithelium.[58] Immunofluorescence demonstrates the presence of antibodies at the site of blister formation. The clinical course of the disease may range from rapidly fatal to relatively benign. The primary treatment for pemphigus is systemic corticosteroids in combination with adjuvant immunosuppressants and, in difficult cases, adjuvant protein A immunoadsorption intravenous immunoglobulins, plasmapheresis, and anti-CD20 monoclonal antibody therapy. Newer methods of treatment and a clearer understanding of the pathogenesis have improved the prognosis and decreased mortality.[59]

Bullous Pemphigoid

Bullous pemphigoid (BP) is a more benign autoimmune disease than pemphigus vulgaris, with blistering of the basement membrane of the skin, not the cell junctions. Autoantibodies (IgG and IgE) to transmembrane collagen protein (collagen XVII/ BP 180) have been found. There are numerous triggers, including drugs and skin trauma. The autoantibodies activate complement with inflammatory infiltration of neutrophils, eosinophils, and lymphocytes. Loss of dermal-epidermal adhesion is caused by inflammatory cytokines.[60] The lesions of pemphigoid begin with localized erythema or as pruritic plaques that extend and become edematous. The plaques turn reddish purple by 2 to 3 weeks, with vesicles and bullae emerging on the surface (Fig. 47.15). Oral lesions can occur. The bullae do not extend with pressure. The blisters rupture within 1 week and heal rapidly. BP occurs more commonly after 60 years of age.

Diagnostic criteria include age more than 70 years, absence of atrophic scars, mucosal involvement and bullous lesions of the head and neck, and results of skin biopsy and immunofluorescent examination. The presence of subepidermal blistering and eosinophils distinguishes pemphigoid from pemphigus. Treatment usually includes antihistamines for itching and topical (i.e., clobetasol propionate) or systemic corticosteroids. Adjuvant immunosuppressive drugs may be prescribed. Relapse may occur with discontinuation of treatment.[61]

Erythema Multiforme

Erythema multiforme (EM) minor is a syndrome characterized by inflammation of the skin with minimal or no mucous membrane

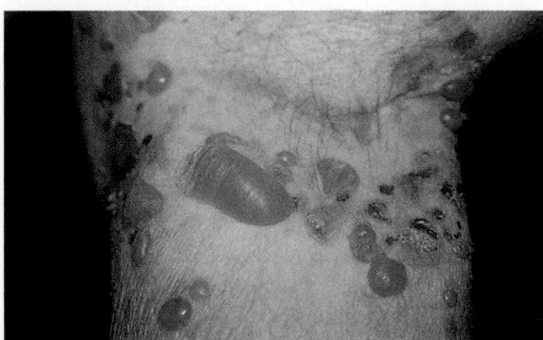

FIGURE 47.15 Bullous Pemphigoid. Generalized eruption with blisters arising from an edematous, erythematous annular base. (Courtesy Department of Dermatology, School of Medicine, University of Utah.)

involvement and no systemic symptoms. *Erythema multiforme major* has moderate to severe mucosal involvement and some systemic symptoms (fever, weakness, and arthralgia). EM is often associated with a T-cell-mediated type IV hypersensitivity reaction to a microorganism, particularly a viral infection (e.g., herpes simplex virus, Epstein-Barr virus) or more rarely histoplasmosis and *Mycoplasma pneumoniae*, that targets small blood vessels in the skin or mucosa. It is rarely related to drug reactions.[62] The incidence of EM is not well defined and can occur at any age, but is more common in children and young adults. Immune complex formation and deposition of complement (C3), IgM, and fibrinogen around the superficial dermal blood vessels, basement membrane, and keratinocytes are common histology findings. Edema develops in the superficial dermis, leading to the formation of vesicles and bullae. Both EM minor and major have characteristic "bull's-eye" or "target" lesions that occur on the skin surface with a central dusky region surrounded by concentric rings or alternating edema and inflammation commonly over the extensor surfaces of the limbs. The lesions usually occur suddenly in groups over 2 to 3 weeks. Urticarial plaques, 1 to 2 cm in diameter, can develop without the target lesion. EM major (vesiculobullous form) includes mucous membrane lesions and erythematous plaques. Single or multiple vesicles or bullae may arise on a part of the plaque, accompanied by pruritus and burning. EM is self-limiting; lesions heal within 3 to 4 weeks and rarely recur.[63,64] For extensive involvement, systemic steroids may be indicated along with supportive care for mucositis and skin erosions, or daily viral suppression for recurrent infectious etiology[65] (Fig. 47.16).

Stevens-Johnson Syndrome and Toxic Epidermal Necrolysis

Stevens-Johnson syndrome (SJS) and toxic epidermal necrolysis (TEN) are the same disease with a continuum of symptoms based on clinical presentation and symptom severity. They are rare, distinct from EM, and are usually associated with severe cutaneous drug reactions and extensive keratinocyte cell death characterized by extensive bullous epidermal detachment, mucositis, and other organ involvement. SJS involves <10% of the BSA and is milder than TEN. TEN involves >30% of BSA. SJS/TEN overlap is BSA involvement between 10% and 30%.[66] Lesions appear 3 to 10 days after drug introduction. Cytotoxic T lymphocytes (CTLs) in a human leukocyte antigen (HLA)-restricted fashion mediate the immune mechanism related to drug reactions. Genetic markers have been identified for these reactions and are used to guide prevention and therapy.[67]

Prodromal symptoms of TEN include fever, headache, malaise, sore throat, and cough in approximately one-third of cases. Blisters and bullae form and large areas of necrotic epidermis may be shed, leaving open, weeping, painful areas of underlying skin. Mucosal involvement may be extensive and involve the mouth, air passages, esophagus, urethra,

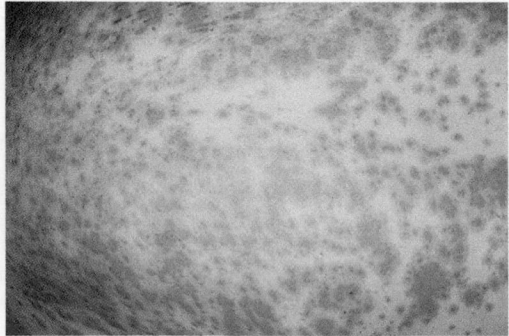

FIGURE 47.16 Erythema Multiforme Caused by Doxepin. (Courtesy Department of Dermatology, School of Medicine, University of Utah.)

and conjunctiva. Blindness can result from corneal ulcerations. Difficulty with eating, breathing, and urinating may develop with severe manifestations. The SJS/TEN overlap also can affect the gastrointestinal, genitourinary, and respiratory systems. The mortality rate for these conditions is as high as 40% and usually related to infection or multiple organ failure, or both.

Medical/medication history preceding the development of lesions and a skin biopsy are required to establish the diagnosis and differentiate the reaction from staphylococcal scalded-skin syndrome (SSSS). A severity of illness score for toxic epidermal necrolysis (SCORTEN) syndrome guides treatment and predicts mortality.[68] Any ongoing drug therapy should be withdrawn or reevaluated and underlying infections treated. Treatment is individualized according to severity and, in severe cases, requires the care of a burn unit.[66]

Fluid and electrolyte balance should be monitored in severe forms of these diseases, and mucous membranes must be carefully managed with a bland diet, warm saline eyewashes, topical anesthetics, or corticosteroids to maintain comfort and prevent infection. Use of systemic steroids is controversial. Cutaneous blisters can be treated with wet compresses of Burow solution. Ophthalmic, kidney, and lung involvement requires special care. Resolution occurs in 8 to 10 days, usually without scarring. Mucosal lesions may take 6 weeks to heal.[63]

Infections

Cutaneous infections are common forms of skin disease. They generally remain localized; however, serious, potentially life-threatening complications can develop with systemic involvement. The types of skin infection include bacterial, viral, and fungal. The commensal (normal) flora of the skin often provides protection against pathogens that cause skin infections, including *Staphylococcus* and *Streptococcus*.

Bacterial Infections

Most bacterial infections of the skin are caused by local invasion of pathogens. Coagulase-positive *Staphylococcus aureus* and, less often, beta-hemolytic *Streptococci* are the common causative microorganisms. Community-acquired methicillin-resistant *Staphylococcus aureus* (CA-MRSA) is also a cause of serious skin infection, particularly skin abscesses (Box 47.3).

Folliculitis. Folliculitis is an inflammation of the hair follicle and can be infectious, caused by bacteria, viruses, fungi, or a noninfectious, caused by trauma or plugging of the follicle. *S. aureus* is a common causative microorganism. The infection develops from proliferation of the microorganism around the opening of the follicle and then spreads into the follicle. Inflammation is caused by the release of chemotactic factors and enzymes from the bacteria. The lesions appear as pustules and papules with a surrounding area of erythema. The pus is sterile in noninfectious folliculitis. Lesions are most prominent on the scalp and extremities and rarely cause systemic symptoms. Prolonged skin moisture, occlusive clothing, topical agents, skin trauma (e.g., shaving facial hair), and poor hygiene are associated contributing factors to the development of folliculitis. Cleaning with soap and water and topical application of antibiotics are effective forms of treatment.[69]

Furuncles and Carbuncles. Furuncles, or "boils," are inflammations of the hair follicles. They may develop from a preceding folliculitis that spreads through the follicular wall into the surrounding dermis. The invading microorganism is usually *S. aureus,* including CA-MRSA. The infecting strain may spread to the skin from the anterior nares. Any skin area with hair can be infected, and one or several lesions may be present. The precipitating events are similar to those for folliculitis. The initial lesion is a deep, firm, red, painful nodule 1 to 5 cm in diameter (Fig. 47.17). Within a few days the initial erythematous nodule changes to a large fluctuant and tender cystic nodule that may be

BOX 47.3   COMMUNITY-ACQUIRED METHICILLIN-RESISTANT *STAPHYLOCOCCUS AUREUS*

Community-acquired methicillin-resistant *Staphylococcus aureus* (CA-MRSA) is a serious skin and soft tissue infection that includes abscesses, cellulitis, and necrotizing fasciitis and can serve as a source for bloodstream infections. Infections are documented among healthy individuals who have no known risk factors, that is, no recent hospitalization, surgical procedures, or prolonged antibiotic treatment. Outbreaks have been documented among athletic teams, among prisoners, in daycare centers, and in homeless shelters. CA-MRSA strains are epidemiologically and clonally different from hospital- or nursing home–acquired MRSA, although CA-MRSA onset in hospitals is emerging. The most common tests involve genotyping for the staphylococcal chromosomal cassette *mec* (SCC*mec*) type IV that encodes resistance to methicillin and Panton-Valentine leukocidin, and other genes that encode virulence toxins. The USA300-0114 strain has been epidemic in the United States and is difficult to treat because of the development of biofilm formation. It also has caused life-threatening pneumonia, osteomyelitis, and septic arthritis and is spreading internationally. CA-MRSAs are more sensitive to antibiotic treatment, and there is a wider choice of antibiotic treatment options for CA-MRSA compared with hospital-acquired MRSA. CA-MRSA is usually susceptible to a variety of oral non–beta-lactam antibiotics, including trimethoprim-sulfamethoxazole, clindamycin, tetracyclines, and linezolid. Parenteral therapy with vancomycin or daptomycin also can be considered. Ceftaroline has been effective for both skin and systemic infections. Dalbavancin, oritavancin, and tedizolid are options for drug-resistant strains. Mupirocin may be used to clear MRSA from nasal secretions if cultures show contamination in the nose. New drugs are under investigation. Preventive measures include practicing good hand hygiene, applying antiseptics and covering cuts and abrasions, using antibacterial soaps for showers after contact sports, avoiding sharing towels and razors, and frequently washing towels. Development of a vaccine is a priority for prevention.

Data from Gleghorn K, Grimshaw E, Kelly EK: *Skin Therapy Lett* 20(5):7-9, 2015; Gupta AK, Lyons DC, Rosen T: *Int J Dermatol* 54(11):1226-1232, 2015; Kale P, Dhawan B: *Indian J Med Microbiol* 34(3):275-285, 2016; Olaniyi R et al: *Curr Top Microbiol Immunol* 2016 Oct 16 [Epub ahead of print].

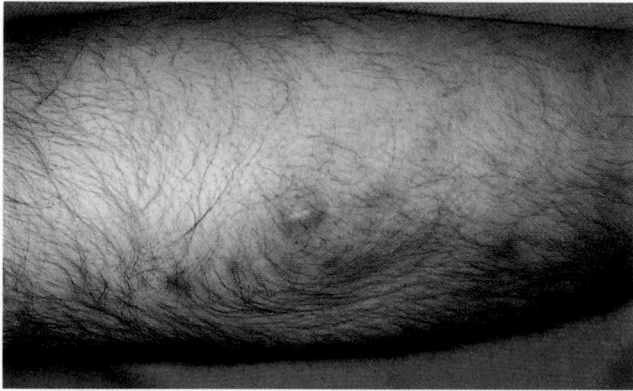

FIGURE 47.17 Furuncle on the Forearm. (Courtesy Department of Dermatology, School of Medicine, University of Utah.)

accompanied by cellulitis. No systemic symptoms are present, and the lesion may drain large amounts of pus and necrotic tissue.

A **carbuncle** is a collection of infected hair follicles and usually occurs on the back of the neck, upper back, and lateral thighs. The lesion begins in the subcutaneous tissue and lower dermis as a firm mass that evolves into an erythematous, painful, swollen mass that drains through many openings. Abscesses may develop. Chills, fever, and malaise are systemic symptoms that can occur during the early stages of lesion development.

Furuncles and carbuncles are treated with warm compresses to provide comfort and promote localization and spontaneous drainage. Abscess formation requires incision and drainage, and recurrent infections, extensive lesions, or those associated with cellulitis or systemic symptoms are treated with systemic antibiotics.

Cellulitis. **Cellulitis** is an infection of the dermis and subcutaneous tissue usually caused by *Staphylococcus*, CA-MRSA, or group B streptococci. Cellulitis can occur as an extension of a skin wound, of an ulcer, or from furuncles or carbuncles. It can be associated with chronic venous insufficiency and stasis dermatitis. Risk factors include diabetes mellitus, edema, peripheral vascular disease, tinea pedis, insect bites, and immune suppression. The infected area is erythematous, warm, swollen, and painful and can extend to lymph nodes and the blood. Initial systemic treatment with antibiotics should cover both *Staphylococci* and *Streptococci*, and Burow soaks can be used to relieve pain. Corticosteroids are used for adjuvant therapy.[70]

Cellulitis must be differentiated from necrotizing fasciitis. Necrotizing fasciitis (also known as *flesh-eating disease*) is a rare, rapidly spreading infection. It is commonly caused by *Streptococcus pyogenes* which resists phagocytosis and releases toxins. Infection starts in the fascia, muscles, and subcutaneous fat with subsequent necrosis of the overlying skin and can progress to sepsis and death without early diagnosis and treatment. Risk factors include older age; chronic disease, such as cirrhosis, diabetes mellitus, or chronic renal failure; immunosuppression; and malnutrition. Treatment requires antibiotics and often surgical débridement.[71]

Erysipelas. **Erysipelas** is an acute superficial infection of the upper dermis (a superficial form of cellulitis) most often caused by *Streptococcus pyogenes*, beta-hemolytic streptococci, and *S. aureus*. The face, ears, and lower legs are common sites of involvement, and the site of initial infection may not be identified. Chills, fever, and malaise precede the onset of lesions by 4 hours to 20 days. The initial lesions appear as firm, red spots that enlarge and coalesce to form a clearly circumscribed, advancing edge, bright red, hot lesion with a raised border. Vesicles may appear over the lesion and at the border, producing a bullous form of the disease. Pruritus, burning, and tenderness accompany the development of the lesion. Cold compresses provide symptomatic relief, and systemic antibiotics are required to arrest the infection.[72]

Impetigo. **Impetigo** is a superficial infection of the skin caused by coagulase-positive *S. aureus* or alpha-hemolytic streptococci. The disease does occur in adults but is more common in children (see Chapter 48).

Lyme Disease. **Lyme disease** is a multisystem inflammatory disease caused by the spirochete *Borrelia burgdorferi* transmitted by *Ixodes* tick bites and is the most frequently reported vector-borne illness. The highest incidence is among children. The microorganism is difficult to culture; escapes immune defenses through antigenic variation; blocks complement-mediated killing; impedes release of antimicrobial peptides, leukocyte chemotaxis, and antimicrobial killing; and hides in tissue. It spreads to other tissues by entering capillary beds.

Symptoms of the disease occur in three stages, although 50% of infected individuals are symptom free. *Localized infection* occurs soon after the bite (within 3 to 32 days) with erythema migrans and a bull's-eye rash (commonly appearing at the site of tick attachment) with or without fever, fatigue, malaise, myalgias, and arthralgias. Erythema migrans is a T-cell-mediated response. Within days to weeks after the onset of the illness, there is *disseminated infection* with secondary erythema migrans, usually with myalgias, arthralgias, and, more rarely, meningitis, neuritis, or carditis. *Post Lyme disease syndrome* or *chronic Lyme disease* can continue for years with arthritis, encephalopathy, polyneuropathy, or heart failure.[73]

The diagnosis of Lyme disease is based on the clinical presentation and history of tick bite, if known. Serologic tests may be used to confirm the diagnosis, although there is a delay in antibody response and the test may be negative during the first 3 weeks after infection. Antibiotics (e.g., oral doxycycline [not used in children younger than 8 years or in pregnant or breast-feeding women], amoxicillin, or cefuroxime) are used for treatment, with longer treatment required for arthritis or active neurologic disease. Reinfection can occur. There currently is not a vaccine for Lyme disease.[74]

Viral Infections

Herpes Simplex Virus. Skin infections with herpes simplex virus (HSV) are commonly caused by two types: HSV-1 and HSV-2. Either type can occur in different parts of the body, including oral and genital locations.[75] Their differences are distinguished by laboratory tests. HSV-1, transmitted by contact with infected saliva, is generally associated with oral infections (cold sore or fever blister) or infection of the cornea (herpes keratitis), mouth (gingivostomatitis), and orolabia (lips/labialis), but it also can cause genital herpes. With initial (primary) infection, the virus infects epithelial cells, embeds in sensory nerve endings, and moves by retrograde axonal transport to the dorsal root ganglion, where the virus develops lifelong latency. The incubation period ranges from 2 to 14 days. During the secondary phase, the lesions occur at the same site from reactivation of the virus. The virus travels down the peripheral nerve to the site of the original infection, where it is shed. Exposure to ultraviolet light, skin irritation, fever, fatigue, menses, or stress may cause reactivation.

The lesions for HSV-1 appear as a rash or clusters of inflamed and painful vesicles (e.g., within the mouth, over the tongue, on the lips, within and/or around the nose) (Fig. 47.18). Increased sensitivity, paresthesias, and mild burning often occur before onset of the lesions. The vesicles rupture, forming a crust. Lesions may last from 2 to 6 weeks. Treatment is symptomatic and includes topical antiviral agents; lesions usually resolve within 2 weeks. Oral antivirals may be indicated at the time of acute infection or through daily suppressive dosing to prevent acute infections.

Genital infections are more commonly caused by HSV-2. The virus is spread by skin-to-skin mucous membrane contact during viral shedding. Risk of infection is high in immunosuppressed persons or in persons who have sexual contact with infected individuals and increases risk for human immunodeficiency virus (HIV) infection.[76] Vertical transmission from mother to neonate is associated with significant neonatal neurologic morbidity and mortality. The primary infection is asymptomatic. With recurrent exposure, the lesions begin as small vesicles that progress to ulceration within 3 to 4 days with pain, itching, and weeping. Treatment is symptomatic and includes topical or oral antiviral agents or daily antiviral suppression for recurrent episodes. Progress is being made with prophylactic vaccines.[77]

Herpes Zoster and Varicella. Herpes zoster (shingles) and herpes varicella (chickenpox, see Chapter 48) are caused by the same herpes virus—varicella-zoster virus (VZV). VZV occurs as a primary infection followed years later by activation of the virus when immunity declines to cause herpes zoster (shingles). During this time the virus remains latent in trigeminal and dorsal (sensory) root ganglia.[78]

Herpes zoster has initial symptoms of pain and paresthesia localized to the affected dermatome (the cutaneous area innervated by a single spinal nerve; see Chapter 15), followed by vesicular eruptions along a facial, cervical, or thoracic lumbar dermatome (Fig. 47.19). Lesions do not usually cross the midline. Local symptoms are alleviated with compresses, calamine lotion, or baking soda. Persistent pain may last for weeks or months and is a debilitating complication, particularly in older adults, and requires treatment. Approximately 15% to 20% of individuals experience postherpetic neuralgias, particularly those older than age 60. There is no cure for herpes zoster. Antiviral drugs are useful if used within the first 72 hours. Tricyclic antidepressants and analgesics are helpful treatments. The varicella vaccine is safe and effective in both children and adults, particularly those older than age 60. In children, the vaccine is given to prevent chickenpox and in adults, particularly the elderly, the vaccine is given to prevent herpes zoster (shingles).[79]

Warts. Warts (verrucae) are benign lesions of the skin caused by the many different types of human papillomavirus (HPV) that infect the stratified epithelium of skin and mucous membranes. Specific viruses are associated with specific kinds and locations of lesions. The lesions can occur anywhere, are flat, round, or fusiform and elevated with a rough, grayish surface. Warts are transmitted by touch. *Common warts* (verrucae vulgaris) occur most often in children and are usually on the fingers (Fig. 47.20). Plantar warts are usually located at pressure points on the bottom of the feet.

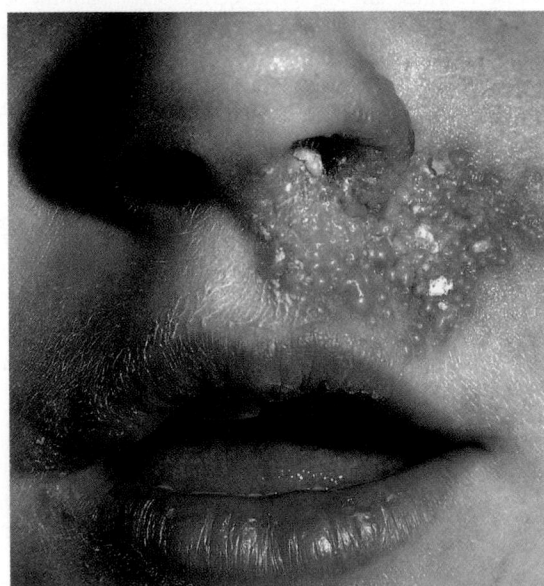

FIGURE 47.18 Herpes Simplex. Typical presentation with tense vesicles involving the nasal mucosa and extending onto the skin. (From Habif TP: *Clinical dermatology: a color guide to diagnosis and therapy,* ed 4, Philadelphia, 2004, Mosby.)

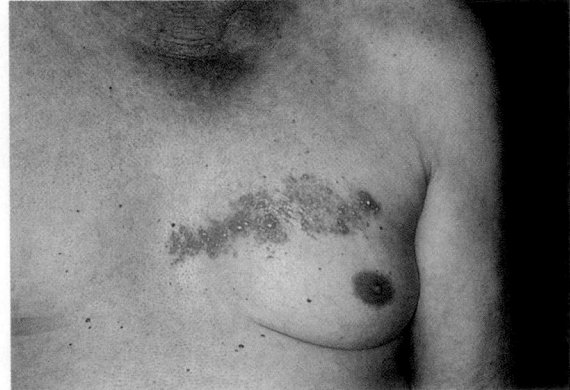

FIGURE 47.19 Herpes Zoster. Diffuse involvement of a dermatome. (Courtesy Department of Dermatology, School of Medicine, University of Utah.)

Diagnosis of warts is by visualization. Treatment considers age of the individual and size and location of the lesion. Warts can be removed by freezing with liquid nitrogen, electrocauterization, vaporization with lasers, application of keratolytics, or application of irritants and corrosives such as salicylic acid, formaldehyde, interferons, or podophyllum.[80]

Recalcitrant warts may benefit from application of topicals such as imiquimod 5% cream (immunomodulatory) or 5-fluorouracil, by intralesional injections of bleomycin or *Candida* (immunoreactive antigen), or by more aggressive surgical procedures.[81] Many warts resolve spontaneously but often recur.

Condylomata acuminata (venereal warts) are highly contagious and sexually transmitted. The cauliflower-like lesions occur in moist areas along the glans of the penis, vulva, and anus (see Chapter 27). Oncogenic HPV (e.g., types 16 and 18) is a primary cause of cervical and other types of cancer (see Chapter 25).

Fungal Infections

The fungi causing superficial skin infections are called *dermatophytes,* and they thrive on keratin (stratum corneum, hair, nails). Fungal disorders are known as *mycoses;* when caused by dermatophytes, the mycoses are termed *tinea* (dermatophytosis or ringworm).

Tinea Infections. Tinea infections are classified according to their location on the body. Tinea pedis is shown in Fig. 47.21, and the most common sites are summarized in Table 47.7. (Chapter 48 contains a discussion of fungal infections in children.)

Tinea is diagnosed by culture, microscopic examination of skin scrapings prepared with potassium hydroxide wet mount, or observation of the skin with a UV light (Wood lamp). Cultures establish the particular type of fungus and are necessary for hair and nail infections. Fungi have characteristic spores and filaments known as hyphae that are more prominent when prepared in potassium hydroxide. The spores fluoresce blue-green when exposed to UV light. Treatment is related to the type of fungi and includes both topical and systemic antifungal medications.[82]

Candidiasis. Candidiasis is caused by the yeastlike fungus *Candida albicans* and normally can be found on mucous membranes, on the skin, in the gastrointestinal tract, and in the vagina. *C. albicans* can, under certain circumstances, change from a commensal (normal) microorganism to a pathogen (invasive candidiasis), particularly in the critically ill and those who are immunosuppressed.[83]

Factors that predispose to infection include (1) a local environment of moisture, warmth, maceration, or occlusion; (2) the systemic administration of antibiotics; (3) pregnancy; (4) diabetes mellitus; (5) Cushing disease; (6) debilitated states; (7) infants younger than 6 months as a result of decreased immune reactivity; (8) immunosuppression;

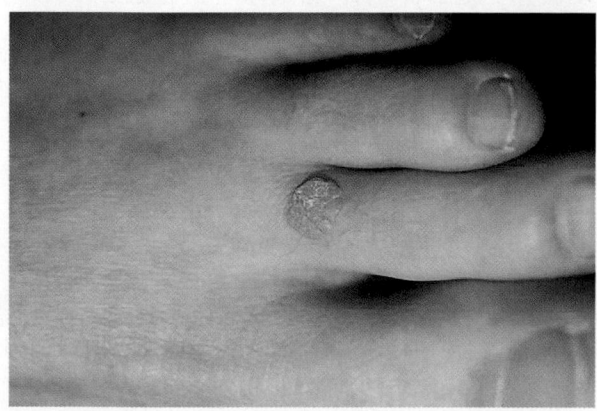

FIGURE 47.20 Verruca Vulgaris. (Courtesy Department of Dermatology, School of Medicine, University of Utah.)

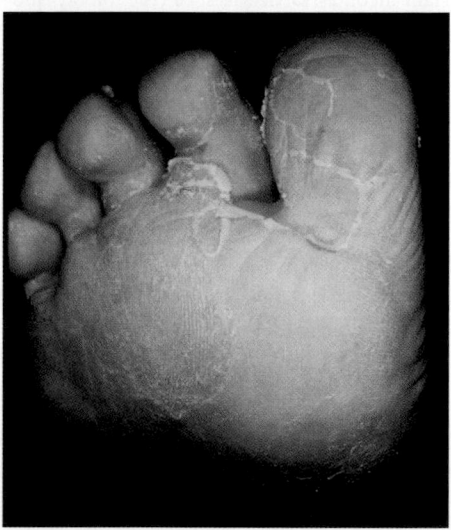

FIGURE 47.21 Tinea Pedis. Inflammation has extended from the web area onto the dorsum of the foot. (Courtesy Department of Dermatology, School of Medicine, University of Utah.)

TABLE 47.7	COMMON SITES OF TINEA INFECTIONS
SITE	**CLINICAL MANIFESTATIONS**
Tinea capitis (scalp)	Scaly, pruritic scalp with bald areas; hair breaks easily
Tinea corporis (skin areas, excluding scalp, face, hands, feet, groin)	Circular, clearly circumscribed, mildly erythematous scaly patches with a slightly elevated ringlike border; some forms are dry and macular, and other forms are moist and vesicular
Tinea cruris (groin, also known as *jock itch*)	Small erythematous and scaling vesicular patches with a well-defined border that spreads over the inner and upper surfaces of the thighs; occurs with heat and high humidity
Tinea pedis (foot, also known as *athlete's foot*)	Occurs between the toes and may spread to the soles of the feet, nails, and skin of toes; slight scaling, macerated painful skin, occasionally with fissures and vesiculation
Tinea manus (hand)	Dry, scaly, erythematous lesions, or moist vesicular lesions that begin with clusters of intensely itching, clear vesicles; often associated with fungal infection of the feet
Tinea unguium or onychomycosis (nails)	A superficial or deep inflammation of the nail that develops yellow-brown accumulations of brittle keratin over all or portions of the nail

TABLE 47.8	SITES OF CANDIDIASIS		
SITE	**RISK FACTORS**	**CLINICAL MANIFESTATIONS**	**TREATMENT**
Vagina (vulvovaginitis)	Heat, moisture, occlusive clothing Pregnancy Systemic antibiotic therapy Diabetes mellitus Sexual intercourse with infected male	Vaginal itching; white, watery, or creamy discharge Red and swollen vaginal and labial membranes with erosions Lesions may spread to anus and groin	Miconazole cream Clotrimazole tablets or cream Nystatin tablets Ketoconazole cream Loose cotton clothing
Penis (balanitis)	Uncircumcised Sexual intercourse with infected female	Pinpoint, red, tender papules and pustules on glans and shaft of penis	Any of creams listed above Topical steroids for severe inflammation
Mouth	Diabetes mellitus Immunosuppressive therapy Inhaled steroids	Red, swollen, painful tongue and oral mucous membranes Localized erosions and plaques appear with chronic infection	Nystatin oral suspension Clotrimazole troches Ketoconazole Fluconazole
Skinfolds	Heat and moisture Diabetes mellitus Immunosuppressive therapy	Pruritic red rash progressing to vesicles and papules that enlarge and rupture	Topical antifungals (e.g., clotrimazole, econazole, ciclopirox, miconazole, ketoconazole, nystatin)

and (9) certain neoplastic diseases of the blood and monocyte-macrophage system. The commensal bacteria on the skin, mainly cocci, inhibit proliferation of *C. albicans*. Cell-mediated immunity plays a major role in the defense against monilial infections. *C. albicans* can activate the complement system by the alternative pathway and produce small abscesses. Candidiasis affects only the outer layers of mucous membranes and skin and occurs in the mouth, vagina, uncircumcised penis, nail folds, interdigital areas, and large skinfolds (inframammary area, intertriginous area, perianal region, and abdominal creases). Table 47.8 lists selected sites of candidiasis. *C. albicans* is highly adaptable in the human host environment, thus promoting its infection and colonization[84] (see Chapter 10, Box 10.3).

The initial lesion is a thin-walled pustule that extends under the stratum corneum with an inflammatory base that may burn or itch. The accumulation of inflammatory cells and scale produces a whitish-yellow curdlike substance over the infected area. The lesion ceases to spread when it reaches dry skin. Topical antifungal medication is most commonly used for treatment.[85]

Vascular Disorders

Vascular abnormalities are commonly associated with skin diseases; they may be congenital or may involve vascular responses to local or systemic vasoactive substances. Blood vessels may increase in number, dilate, constrict, or become obliterated by disease processes.[86]

Cutaneous Vasculitis

Vasculitis (angiitis) is an inflammation of the blood vessel wall that can result in bleeding aneurysm formation, or occlusion with ischemia or infection of surrounding tissue. The extensive vascular bed in the skin results in vasculitic syndromes that may be localized and self-limiting or generalized with multiorgan involvement. The initiating site may be the blood, the vessel wall, or adjacent tissue. Small vessels are usually affected.

Cutaneous vasculitis develops from the deposit of immune complexes in small blood vessels as a toxic response to drugs (phenothiazines, barbiturates, sulfonamides) or allergens, or streptococcal or viral infection, or as a component of systemic vasculitic syndromes. The deposits activate complement, which is chemotactic for neutrophils and other mediators of inflammation that disrupt adhesion molecules and the vessel wall.[87]

The disorder is also known as *cutaneous small vessel vasculitis* or *cutaneous leukocytoclastic angiitis* (from the presence of leukocytes [i.e.,

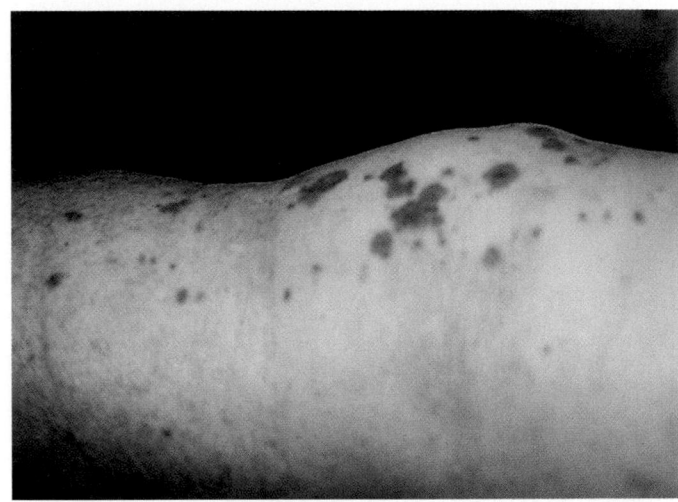

FIGURE 47.22 Vasculitis of the Leg. (Courtesy Department of Dermatology, School of Medicine, University of Utah.)

neutrophils] in and around vessel walls). The extremities are the chief sites affected primarily the lower legs and feet. The lesion may initially present with burning, itching, and pain. The pattern of skin involvement includes palpable purpuras (from the leakage of blood from damaged vessels) that may progress to hemorrhagic bullae with necrosis and ulceration from occlusion of the vessel (Fig. 47.22). Lesions appear in clusters and persist for 1 to 4 weeks. The disease may be self-limiting and occur as a single episode. Biopsy and direct immunofluorescence confirm the diagnosis. A systemic form (cutaneous systemic vasculitis) can involve other organs, including the kidneys, lungs, and gastrointestinal tract (e.g., Wegener granulomatosis).

Identifying the primary disease or removing the antigen (chemical, drug, or source of infection) is the first step of treatment. Supportive treatment and topical steroids can relieve pruritus and burning. Systemic therapy and immunosuppressants are used when symptoms are severe.[87]

Urticaria

Urticaria (hives) is a circumscribed area of raised erythema and edema of the superficial dermis. Urticarial lesions are most commonly associated with type I hypersensitivity reactions to drugs (e.g., penicillin, aspirin),

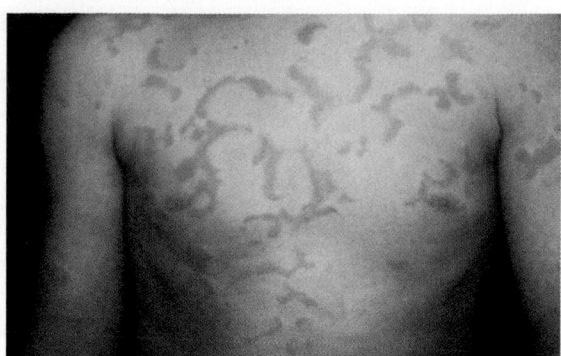

FIGURE 47.23 Urticaria. (Courtesy Department of Dermatology, School of Medicine, University of Utah.)

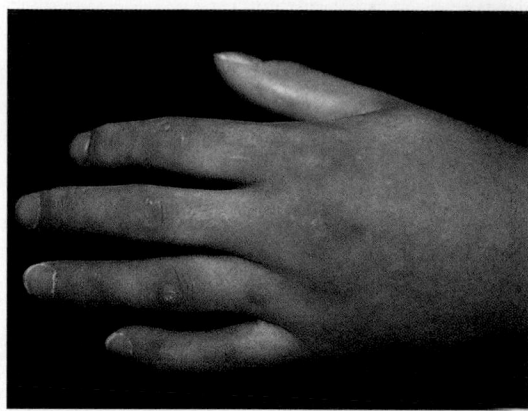

FIGURE 47.24 Scleroderma. Note inflammation and shiny skin. (Courtesy Department of Dermatology, School of Medicine, University of Utah.)

certain foods (e.g., strawberries, shellfish, food dyes), systemic diseases (e.g., intestinal parasites, lupus erythematosus), or physical agents (e.g., heat, cold). They may occur with angioedema (edema of the dermis and subcutaneous tissue). The lesions are mediated by IgE-stimulated release of histamine, bradykinin, or kallikrein from mast cells or basophils, or both, which causes the endothelial cells of skin blood vessels to contract, increasing their permeability. IgG antibody directed against the IgE receptor and other inflammatory and vasodilatory substances, such as serotonin, leukotrienes, prostaglandins, and kinins, also may be mediators of urticaria. The leakage of fluid from vessels appears as wheals, welts, or hives that may be distributed over the entire body (Fig. 47.23). Most lesions resolve spontaneously within 24 hours, but new lesions may appear and a life-threatening reaction can occur. All possible causes should be removed. Antihistamines (H1 antagonists) usually reduce hives and provide relief of itching. Corticosteroids and β-adrenergic agonists may be required for severe attacks. Chronic urticaria (recurrent wheals for more than 6 weeks) is either idiopathic or autoimmune in origin, rarely because of allergy, and involves inappropriate activation of mast cells. Angioedema (welts or swelling deeper within the skin or mucous membranes) is associated with both groups and more commonly affects the eyes and mouth.[88]

Scleroderma

There are two categories of scleroderma. Localized scleroderma or morphea is usually benign and self-limiting and is confined to the skin and/or underlying tissues. Systemic sclerosis is characterized by cutaneous sclerosis with visceral involvement.

Localized scleroderma (morphea) means sclerosis of the skin and underlying tissue. The disease is rare, more common in females, and the cause is unknown. Genetic predisposition, autoimmunity, and an immune reaction to a toxic substance are possible initiating mechanisms of the disease. T helper cells (Th1 and Th17) and their cytokines are associated with fibroblast proliferation and fibrosis. Several autoantibodies also have been identified, including antinuclear antibody (ANA), antihistone antibody (AHA), and single-stranded DNA antibody (ss-DNA Ab).[89] Impaired regulation of collagen gene expression by fibroblasts probably underlies the persistent fibrosis. There are subtypes of localized scleroderma, but all involve thickening of the skin. Localized scleroderma is differentiated from the systemic form of the disease by the absence of the following: sclerodactyly, Raynaud phenomenon, abnormalities of the nail bed capillaries, or internal organ involvement.[90]

Systemic scleroderma (SSc) involves the connective tissues of the skin and many organs, including the kidneys, gastrointestinal tract, and lungs. Fibrosis occurs in the papillary and reticular dermis and in the subcutaneous tissue and deep fascia. There are massive deposits of type

> **BOX 47.4** **CLINICAL FEATURES OF SYSTEMIC SCLERODERMA**
>
> Raynaud phenomenon—episodes of arteriolar vasoconstriction or spasm in response to cold or stress, often a sentinel sign of disease
> Skin thickening of the fingers of both hands
> Sclerodactyly—tightening of skin over the fingers and toes leading to tapering of the digits with scarring and tissue atrophy
> Abnormal nail fold capillaries
> Telangiectasias—dilation of capillaries causing small weblike (0.5 cm) red marks on skin surface
> Pulmonary arterial hypertension and/or interstitial lung disease
> Esophageal changes—swallowing difficulty related to acid reflux and increased esophageal fibrosis
> Pericardial or myocardial disease
> Arthralgias
> Kidney disease

Data from Desbois AC, Cacoub P: *Autoimmun Rev* 15(5):417-426, 2016.

I collagen with progressive fibrosis accompanied by inflammatory reactions, as well as vascular changes in the capillary network with a decrease in the number of capillary loops, dilation of the remaining capillaries, formation of perivascular infiltrates, and development of occlusion and ischemia.

The cutaneous lesions are most often on the face and hands, the neck, and the upper chest, although the entire skin can be involved. The skin is hard, hypopigmented, taut, shiny, and tightly attached to the underlying tissue. The tightness of the facial skin projects an immobile, masklike appearance and the mouth may not open completely. The nose may assume a beaklike appearance. The hands are shiny and sometimes red and edematous (Fig. 47.24). The fingers become tapered and flexed, often with contractures, depressed scars, and loss of fingertips from atrophy. Progression to body organs can occur, and death is caused by subsequent respiratory failure, renal failure, cardiac dysrhythmias, or esophageal or intestinal obstruction or perforation. The clinical features of systemic scleroderma are summarized in Box 47.4.

Suitable clothing and a warm environment are essential to protecting the hands. Trauma and smoking should be avoided. Treatment is individualized and based on organ involvement and progression of the disease. Immunosuppressive medications, ultraviolet light treatment, and targeted therapies are prescribed.[91]

Benign Tumors

Most benign tumors of the skin are associated with aging. Benign tumors include seborrheic keratosis, keratoacanthoma, actinic keratosis, and moles.

Seborrheic Keratosis

Seborrheic keratosis is a benign proliferation of cutaneous basal cells that produces smooth or warty elevated lesions. The pathogenesis is unknown. These tumors are usually seen in older people and occur as multiple lesions on the chest, back, and face. The color varies from tan to waxy yellow, flesh colored, or dark brown-black. Lesion size varies from a few millimeters to several centimeters, and they are often oval and greasy appearing with a hyperkeratotic scale (Fig. 47.25). Both cryotherapy with liquid nitrogen and electrocautery are effective treatments, and the lesions usually slough 2 to 3 weeks after treatment.

Keratoacanthoma

A keratoacanthoma is a benign self-limiting tumor of squamous cell differentiation arising from hair follicles. It usually occurs on sun-damaged skin of older adults and smokers; the incidence is high in males. The most commonly affected sites are the face, back of the hands, forearms, neck, and legs (Fig. 47.26). The lesion develops over a period of 1 to 2 months and has a histologic course resembling a well-differentiated squamous cell carcinoma as follows:

Proliferative stage: Lesion develops as a rapidly growing, dome-shaped nodule with a central crust.

Mature stage: Lesion fills with whitish keratin and requires differentiation from squamous cell carcinoma.

Involution stage: Occurs over a 3- to 4-month period with regression of the lesion.

Although the lesions resolve spontaneously, treatment is the optimal approach. They can be removed by curettage or excision to improve cosmetic appearance and reduce the risk of evolution to squamous cell carcinoma. Intralesional 5-FU, bleomycin, interferon, or methotrexate also have been effective.[92]

Actinic Keratosis

Actinic keratosis (solar keratosis) is a common premalignant lesion composed of aberrant proliferations of epidermal keratinocytes caused by prolonged exposure to UV radiation. The prevalence is highest in individuals with unprotected light-colored skin. Actinic keratosis is rare in black skin. The lesions appear as rough or scaly, poorly defined pink to reddish or reddish brown papules that are felt more than seen (Fig. 47.27) and are considered an early in situ squamous cell carcinoma. Surrounding areas may have telangiectasia. Dermoscopy and biopsy aid evaluation. Treatment options include ablative and photodynamic therapy, laser surgery, and topical therapies, such as 5-FU, diclofenac, imiquimod cream, and ingenol mebutate. The lesions should continue to be evaluated for progressive squamous cell carcinoma. Protection from the sun with clothing or a sunblock to prevent lesions from developing elsewhere is advised.[93]

Nevi

Nevi (moles) are benign pigmented or nonpigmented lesions (Fig. 47.28) that form from melanocytes beginning at ages 3 to 5 years. Melanocytic nevus, formed from melanocytes, may be congenital or acquired and small (less than 1 cm) or large (greater than 20 cm). Larger congenital melanocytic nevus may be removed to reduce risk of cutaneous malignant melanoma.[94] During the early stages of development, the cells accumulate at the junction of the dermis and epidermis (junctional nevi) and are macular lesions. Over time the cells move deeper into the dermis and the nevi become nodular and symmetric without irregular borders (compound nevi). Nevi may appear on any part of the skin, and vary in size, occur singly or in groups and may undergo transition to malignant melanomas. Nevi repeatedly traumatized, irritated by clothing, or considered too large may be excised. Multiple and changing moles require regular evaluation.

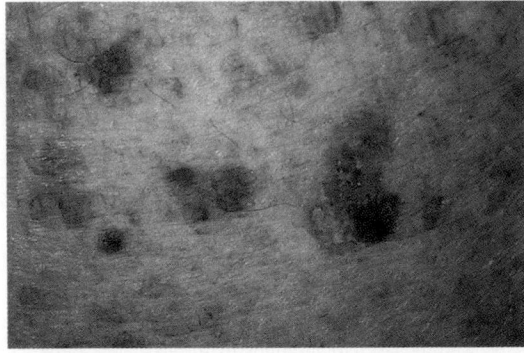

FIGURE 47.25 Seborrheic Keratosis. Typical lesion that is broad, flat, and comparatively smooth surfaced. (Courtesy Department of Dermatology, School of Medicine, University of Utah.)

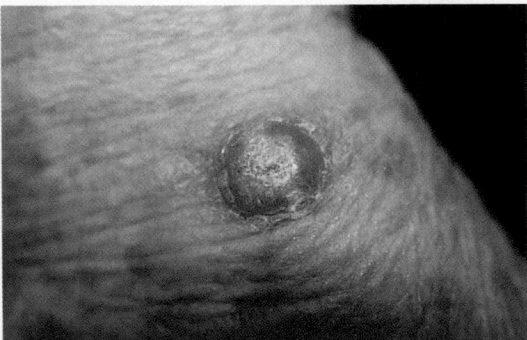

FIGURE 47.26 Keratoacanthoma. Classic presentation of a fully developed tumor. Round, smooth, dome-shaped mass with a central keratin-filled crater. (Courtesy Department of Dermatology, School of Medicine, University of Utah.)

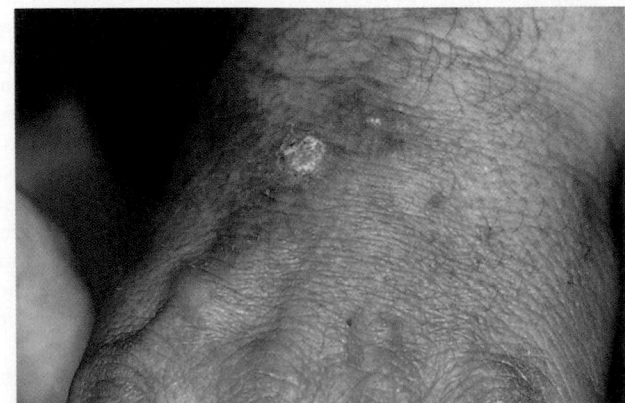

FIGURE 47.27 Actinic Keratosis. (Courtesy Department of Dermatology, School of Medicine, University of Utah.)

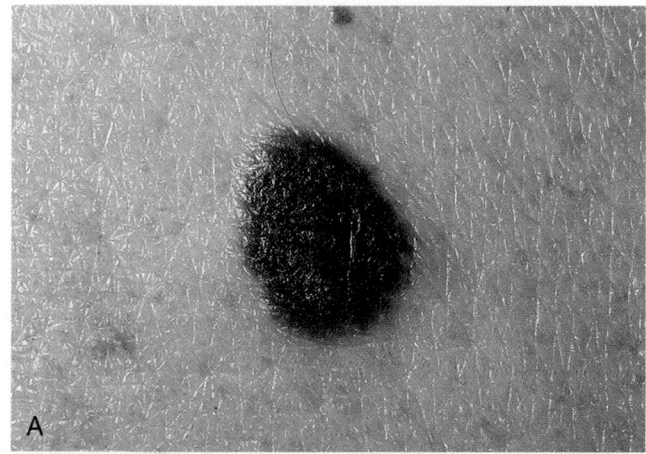

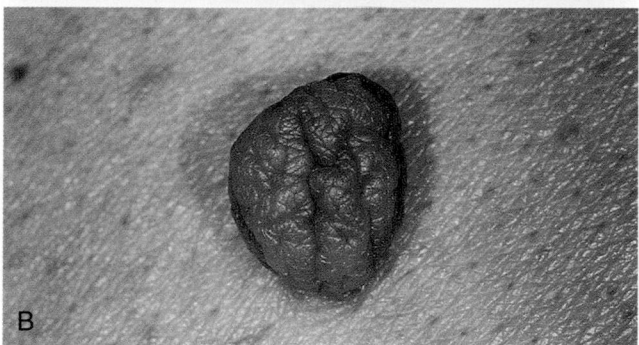

FIGURE 47.28 Nevi. **A,** Junction nevus: slightly raised, dark, and uniform. **B,** Dermal nevus: pedunculated with a soft, flabby, wrinkled surface. (From Habif TP: *Clinical dermatology: a color guide to diagnosis and therapy,* ed 5, Philadelphia, 2010, Mosby.)

Skin Cancer

Cutaneous basal cell carcinoma and squamous cell carcinoma (collectively known as *nonmelanoma skin cancers*) are the most prevalent forms of cancer. Malignant melanoma is the most serious and the most common cause of death from skin cancer. Important trends related to skin cancer are presented in Box 47.5.

Chronic ultraviolet (UV) radiation causes most skin cancers. Lesions are most common on the face, neck, hands, and other areas exposed to intense sunlight. Protection from the sun and avoidance of tanning beds, particularly during childhood, significantly reduces the risk of skin cancer in later years. Genetic mutations in oncogenes and tumor-suppressor genes (see Chapter 12) are associated with skin cancers. This leads to loss of keratinocyte repair functions and apoptosis resistance of DNA-damaged cells. Dark-skinned persons and those avoiding sunlight are significantly less likely to develop these malignant tumors. In dark-skinned persons, basal cells contain the pigment melanin, a protective factor against sun exposure.

Basal Cell Carcinoma

Basal cell carcinoma (BCC) of the skin is the most common cancer in the world, making it the most common skin cancer by default. Risk factors for BCC include chronic ultraviolet light exposure, radiation exposure, severe actinic damage, fair skin, radiation therapy, chronic arsenic exposure, long-term immunosuppression, and older age.[95]

BCC is a surface epithelial tumor of the skin originating from undifferentiated basal or stem cells. BCC arises from mutation in the *TP53* tumor-suppressor gene, leading to loss of keratinocyte repair functions and apoptosis resistance of DNA-damaged cells. Other

---

BOX 47.5   IMPORTANT TRENDS FOR SKIN CANCER

Incidence

More than 5.4 million nonmelanoma skin cancers in 2012 with likely underreporting because of lack of a nonmelanoma skin cancer registry; and an estimated 87,110 cases of melanoma in 2017

Greater in women younger than age 40 years; greater in men after age 40 years; 40 times more prevalent in whites than in blacks; increases steadily with age; increasing among young individuals with chronic exposure to artificial UV radiation

Majority of cases are highly curable basal or squamous cell cancers, and the most serious is malignant melanoma; it represents 4% of all skin cancer cases but causes about 79% of all skin cancer deaths

Mortality

Total estimated deaths in 2017 were 9730 from melanoma and approximately 3860 from other nonepithelial types of skin cancer

Risk Factors

Excessive exposure to ultraviolet radiation from the sun

Exposure to artificial UV radiation, particularly in ages less than 25 years

Fair complexion, blue eyes, blonde hair

Occupational exposure to coal tar, pitch, creosote, arsenic compounds, and radium

Exposure to human papillomavirus and human immunodeficiency virus

Immunosuppression

Family history of skin cancer

Skin cancer is negligible in blacks because of heavy skin pigmentation

Warning Signals

Any change on the skin, especially a change in the size or color of a mole or other darkly pigmented growth or spot

Prevention and Early Detection

Avoidance of artificial UV radiation and sun when ultraviolet light is strongest (e.g., 10 AM to 3 PM); use of protective clothing and sunscreen preparations, especially those containing ingredients such as *para*-aminobenzoic acid (PABA); prevention for all types of skin cancer should begin in childhood

Routine visual screening for skin cancer may be a benefit for those at highest risk

Survival

For basal cell and squamous cell cancers, cure is highly likely with early detection and treatment; malignant melanoma metastasizes quickly, accounting for a lower 5-year survival rate

Data from American Cancer Society: *Cancer facts and figures 2017,* Atlanta, 2017, Author; Brunssen A et al: *J Am Acad Dermatol* 76(1):129-139, 2017.

---

oncogenic pathways include inhibition of the *PTCH* gene with overexpression in the Sonic Hedgehog signaling pathway (codes for smoothened protein important for cell growth and differentiation).[96]

BCCs have numerous subtypes, including superficial, nodular, pigmented, morpheaform (sclerosing), and combinations of each. Thus they can have very different clinical presentations from superficial erythematous papules; to thick, pigmented nodules resembling melanomas; to erosive, necrotic, and ulcerating lesions (Fig. 47.29); and autosomal dominant basal cell nevus syndrome (early onset with

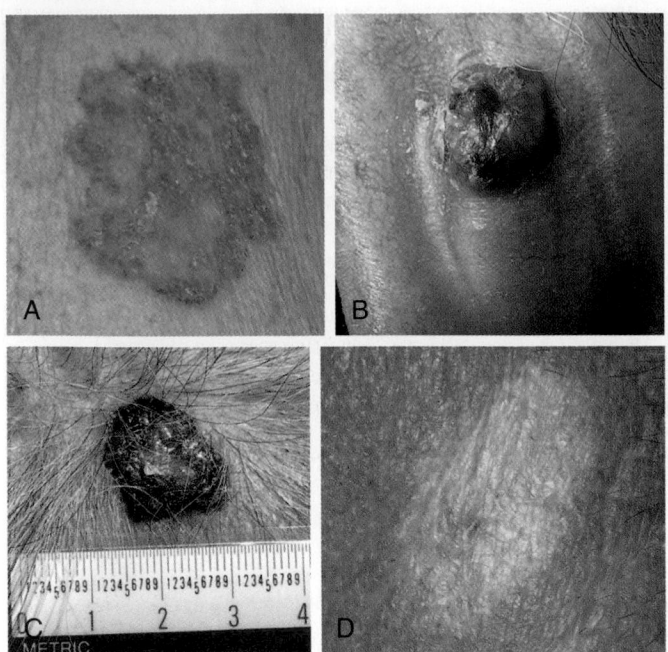

FIGURE 47.29 Types of Basal Cell Carcinoma. **A,** Superficial. **B,** Nodular. **C,** Pigmented. **D,** Morpheaform-recurrent tumor. (**A** and **D** from Bolognia JL, Jorizzo JL, Schaffer JV: *Dermatology,* ed 3, Philadelphia, 2012, Saunders; **B** and **C** from James WD, Berger TG, Elston DM: *Andrews' diseases of the skin: clinical dermatology,* ed 11, Philadelphia, 2011, Saunders.)

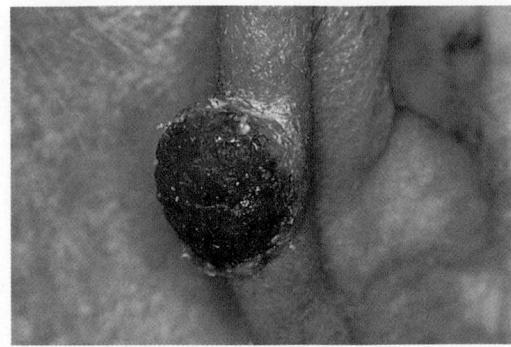

FIGURE 47.30 Squamous Cell Carcinoma. The sun-exposed ear is a common site for squamous cell carcinoma. (Courtesy Department of Dermatology, School of Medicine, University of Utah.)

numerous lesions). The lesion often begins as a nodule (greater than 5 mm across) that is pearly or ivory in appearance and slightly elevated above the skin surface with small blood vessels on the surface (telangiectasias). The tumors grow upward and laterally or downward to the dermal-epidermal junction. They usually have depressed centers and rolled borders. As the lesion grows, it often ulcerates, develops crusting, and becomes firm to the touch.

Treatment includes complete surgical excision (micrographic surgery with histologic analysis), radiotherapy, curettage, cryotherapy, photodynamic therapy, and topical applications of imiquimod or 5-fluorouracil. If left untreated, basal cell lesions invade surrounding tissues and, over months or years, destroy tissue (i.e., nose, eyelid, or ear). These are known as *locally advanced basal cell carcinomas (laBCC)*. Metastatic spread is rare because these tumors do not invade blood or lymph vessels. In laBCC or inoperable tumors, the Smoothened receptor in the Sonic Hedgehog pathway can be inhibited by use of vismodegib.[97]

Cutaneous Squamous Cell Carcinoma

Squamous cell carcinoma (SCC) is a tumor of the epidermis with uncontrolled growth of keratinocytes and the second most common human cancer. Two types are characterized: in situ (Bowen disease [BD]) and invasive. Ultraviolet radiation exposure causes SCC, and actinic keratosis is a precursor lesion. Other risk factors include genetic predisposition; chronic arsenic exposure; chronic, nonhealing wounds; radiation exposure; immunosuppression; and light-colored skin. Areas affected are the head and neck (75%) and the hands (15%), with 10% of squamous cell carcinomas occurring elsewhere on the body. UV exposure causes SCC, particularly mutation of the *TP53* gene and other oncogenic signals. It is unclear how UV light produces alterations in DNA, DNA repair, and resistance to apoptosis.[98]

In situ SCC is usually confined to the epidermis (intraepidermal) but may extend into the dermis. Bowen disease is a dysplasia of the epidermis or carcinoma in situ found on unexposed areas of the body, such as the glans penis (erythroplasia of Queyrat). The lesions are flat, reddish, scaly patches. These lesions may enlarge to more than 1 cm in diameter, rarely invading surrounding tissue, very rarely metastasize, and are associated with human papillomavirus. Other cellular components in the skin (e.g., sweat glands, hair follicles) can give rise to SCC, but these cancers are relatively uncommon. Invasive SCC can arise from premalignant lesions of the skin. It rarely arises from normal-appearing skin or de novo. Invasive SCC grows more rapidly than basal cell carcinomas, penetrates the basement membrane between epidermis and dermis, and can spread to regional lymph nodes with metastasis. These tumors are firm and increase in elevation and diameter. The surface may be granular and bleed easily (Fig. 47.30).[96]

SCC is the most common cause of lip cancer and is prevalent in older white men, with about 3000 new cases per year.[99] The lower lip is the most common site. Long-term environmental exposure results in dryness, chapping, hyperkeratosis, and predisposition to malignancy. Immunosuppression, pipe smoking, and chronic alcoholism increase the risk for lip cancer. The most common lesion is termed *exophytic* and usually develops in the outer part of the lip along the vermilion border. The lip becomes thickened and evolves to an ulcerated center with a raised border (Fig. 47.31). These lesions have an irregular surface, follow cracks in the lip, and tend to extend toward the inner surface.

Treatment includes cryotherapy, 5-FU, and photodynamic therapy for small, low-risk, superficial SCC and complete microsurgical excision with histologic analysis and radiotherapy with consideration of adjuvant chemotherapy for advanced disease.[100]

Cutaneous Melanoma

Cutaneous melanoma is a malignant tumor of the skin originating from the transformation of melanocytes, the cells that synthesize the pigment melanin and arise from the neural crest. Melanoma is the most serious skin cancer with an estimated 87,110 new cases and 9730 deaths in the United States in 2017.[99] Noncutaneous melanoma is rare but is most common in the uvea of the eye and in mucous membranes.[101] The incidence of melanoma is increasing in the United States and worldwide. There is uncertainty regarding how much of the increase is attributable to greater melanoma screening activities, potential detection bias, or overdiagnosis.[102] However, discovering melanoma at an early stage increases 5-year survival.[103] Risk factors include personal or family history, or both; solar and artificial ultraviolet light exposure; immunosuppression; fair hair; light skin with repeated sunburns; freckles; younger females and older males; geographic location; past pesticide exposure; and three or more clinically atypical (dysplastic) melanocytic

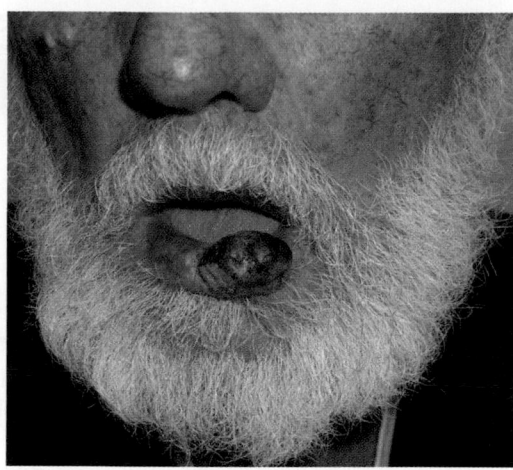

FIGURE 47.31 Lip Cancer. Biopsy confirmed squamous cell carcinoma. Lip vermilion shows diffuse actinic keratosis. (From Bagheri SC et al: *Current therapy in oral and maxillofacial surgery,* Philadelphia, 2012, Saunders.)

TABLE 47.9	CLASSIFICATION OF NEVI
NEVI	**COMMON CHARACTERISTICS**
Junctional nevus	Flat, well circumscribed, vary in size up to 2 cm, dark color, hairs may be present; originate in basal layer of epidermis and can eventually reach the cutaneous surface; rarely develop into a melanoma
Compound nevus	Most common in adolescents; the majority of pigmented lesions are in children; rarely develops into melanoma; usually 1 cm in size; hairs may be present; surface is elevated and smooth
Intradermal nevus	Small (less than 1 cm) with regular edges and bristle-like hairs; color ranges from skin tone to light brown; has a slight likelihood of developing into a melanoma

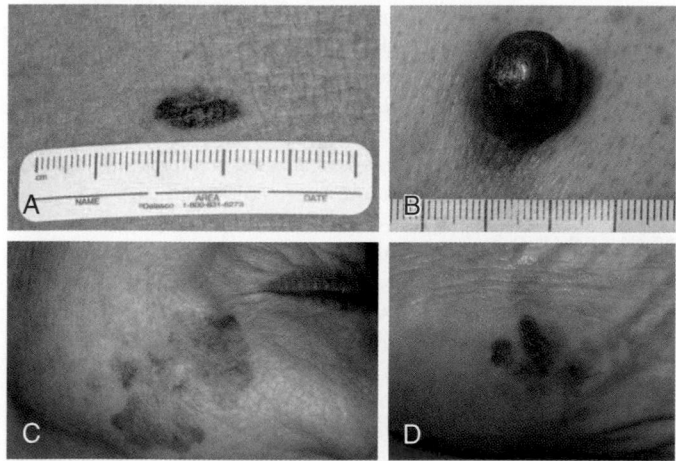

FIGURE 47.32 Malignant Melanoma. A, Superficial spreading melanoma. **B,** Nodular melanoma. **C,** Lentigo malignant melanoma. **D,** Acral lentiginous melanoma on plantar surface of foot. (From Bolognia JL et al: *Dermatology essentials,* Philadelphia, 2014, Saunders.)

nevi.[104] Multiple melanocytic nevi are associated with nonchronic sun-damage melanomas and *BRAF* mutations and occur more commonly on the trunk and extremities. Melanoma is the most common cancer in white women 25 to 29 years old.[105]

Cutaneous melanomas arise as a result of chronic sun exposure or pathways associated with melanocytic nevi (nonchronic sun exposure) resulting in malignant degeneration of melanocytes located either along the basal layer of the epidermis or in a benign melanocytic nevus. They grow vertically, eventually penetrate the endothelium of capillaries, and enter the bloodstream and lymphatics allowing them to form distant metastases. The clinical types of cutaneous melanoma are based on their histologic growth patterns. Melanomas in situ are in a radial growth phase and include *superficial spreading melanoma* (SSM), the most common with radial growth preceding vertical growth; *lentigo malignant melanoma* (LMM), frequently found in the elderly and confused with age spots and an aggressive vertically growing tumor; and *acral lentiginous melanoma* (ALM) (Fig. 47.32). It is rare and aggressive and occurs on

non—hair-bearing surfaces (i.e., palms of the hands and soles of the feet) and in mucous membranes more commonly in black and Asian people.[106] *Primary nodular melanomas* (PNMs) are in a vertical growth phase and are more aggressive. Rare and difficult to diagnose subtypes include desmoplastic melanoma, which resembles a scar, and amelanotic (nonpigmented) melanoma tumors.[107]

The pathogenesis of malignant melanoma is complex. There is an accumulation of genetic mutations that activate oncogenes, inactivate tumor suppressor genes, and impair DNA repair genes. Most familial melanomas are associated with cyclin-dependent kinase 4 gene *(CDK4)* and cyclin-dependent kinase inhibitor 2A gene *(p16/CDKN2A)* located on chromosome 9p21. The *CDKN2A* gene encodes two potent tumor-suppressor proteins (p16 and p14^{ARF}) that are cell-cycle inhibitors. Both *CDNKN2A* and *CDK4* are highly penetrant susceptibility genes and result in melanomas.[108] A number of proto-oncogenes have been identified, including *BRAF* point mutations (the most common) and *NRAS,* and genes involved in the regulation of mitogen-activated protein kinase *(MAPK)* and other signaling pathways (RAS [N/H/K], NF1, and Triple-WT). Melanomas have a high mutation rate stimulated by UVR, making gene sequencing difficult.

The relationship between nevi (see Fig. 47.28) and melanoma makes it important for the clinician to understand the various neval forms (Table 47.9). Most nevi never become suspicious; however, suspicious nevi should be evaluated and removed. Indications for biopsy include changes in color and size; irregular notched margin; itching, bleeding or oozing; nodularity; scab formation; ulceration; or an unusual pattern of presentation. The ABCDE rule is used as a guide: **A**symmetry, **B**order irregularity, **C**olor variation, **D**iameter larger than 6 mm, and **E**levation, which includes raised appearance or rapid enlargement.[109] Clinical characteristics are summarized in Table 47.10.

Surveillance strategies include clinician-based total body skin examination, total body photography, dermoscopy that may be combined with confocal microscopy, and individual-based self-skin examination.[110] Staging of melanoma is determined using tumor, node, metastasis (TNM) criteria established by the American Joint Committee on Cancer and is summarized in Box 47.6.

Prognostic factors include the thickness of the lesion, mitotic index, immunohistochemical assessment, ulceration, and metastasis (e.g., number of lymph nodes or viscera involved). Efforts are in progress to refine the morphologic classifications by adding subgroups that include molecular markers for proto-oncogene mutations and specific signaling pathways.[111] Early detection of cutaneous melanomas can have a major

TABLE 47.10   CLINICAL CHARACTERISTICS OF SUBTYPES OF CUTANEOUS MELANOMA

CHARACTERISTIC	DESCRIPTION
Lentigo Malignant Melanoma	
Frequency	5% to 15% of cutaneous melanomas
Age at diagnosis	50 to 80 years old, mean age 65 years
Primary location	Head, neck, dorsum of hands (sun-exposed areas)
Pigmentation according to thickness	
<1.5 mm (levels I and II)	Tan and brown
>1.5 mm (level III)	Tan, brown, and blue-black
>1.5 mm (levels IV and V)	Nodule formation
Superficial Spreading Melanomas	
Frequency	50% to 75% of cutaneous melanomas
Age at diagnosis	20 to 60 years old
Primary location	Legs of females; upper back of both genders
Pigmentation according to thickness	
<1.5 mm (levels I and II)	Tan and brown
>1.5 mm (level III)	Tan, brown, and blue-black
>1.5 mm (levels IV and V)	Nodule formation
Acral-Lentiginous Melanoma	
Frequency	5% to 8% in whites; 30% to 75% in blacks, Hispanics, Asians
Age at diagnosis	20 to 60 years old, male more common
Primary location	Palms, soles of feet, mucous membranes
Pigmentation at any thickness	Blue-black irregular macules, papules, or nodules
Primary Nodular Melanoma (Usually Invasive at Diagnosis)	
Frequency	15% to 35% of cutaneous melanomas
Age at diagnosis	20 to 60 years old, mean age 53 years
Primary location	Trunk, head, or neck
Pigmentation according to thickness	
>1.5 mm (level III)	Small nodule (any hue)
>1.5 mm (levels IV and V)	Large nodule (any hue)

Data from Johnston RB: *Weedon's skin pathology essentials*, ed 2, Elsevier, 2017; Longo C, Pellacani G: *Dermatol Clin* 34(4):411-419, 2016.

BOX 47.6   TUMOR, NODE, METASTASIS (TNM) STAGING CRITERIA FOR MELANOMA

Stage 0: carcinoma in situ (TisN0M0)
Stage I A/B: includes lesions up to 2 mm with no nodal or distant metastases (T1aN0M0, T1bN0M0, T2aN0M0).
Stage II A/B/C: includes larger lesions, greater than 2 mm without positive nodes or distant metastases (T2bN0M0, T3aN0M0, T3bN0M0, T4aN0M0, T4bN0M0).
Stage III: includes lesions of any size with positive lymph nodes (TxN1M0, TxN2M0, TxN3M0).
Stage IV: includes lesions of any size with distant metastases (TxNxM1).

Data from Piris A, Lobo AC, Duncan LM: *Dermatol Clin* 30(4):581-592, v, 2012.

metastases. There also is significant morbidity associated with residual lymphedema.[112] Survival rate for advanced disease is very low.

Radiation therapy, chemotherapy, and immunotherapy inhibiting the *MAPK* pathway and *BRAF* mutations and MEK inhibition are used to treat metastatic disease and have demonstrated long-term improvement in disease outcome. Promising new immunotherapies are used for advanced disease, including checkpoint inhibitors, programmed cell death protein 1 (PD-1) receptor antibody, anti-CTLA4 antibody, and targeted therapy including *BRAF* and/or MEK inhibition, C-kit gene inhibitors of tyrosine kinases, and platelet-derived growth factor.[113] Vaccines, cell therapy, and biomarkers to assess treatment effectiveness are under continuing investigation.

Merkel Cell Carcinoma

Merkel cell (a skin mechanoreceptor) carcinoma is a very rare aggressive cutaneous carcinoma usually localized to the head and neck. Risk factors include ultraviolet radiation, immunosuppression, age older than 50 years, male gender, and Merkel cell polyomavirus infection. The lesions appear as nodules or skin-colored or purple dome-shaped papules or plaques. Treatment includes wide excision and adjuvant radiotherapy. Targeted therapies are being evaluated. Mortality is high for metastatic lesions.[114,115]

Kaposi Sarcoma

Kaposi sarcoma (KS) is a vascular malignancy associated with immunodeficiency states and occurs among transplant recipients taking immunosuppressive drugs. Genetic and environmental cofactors determine disease progression. Human herpesvirus type 8 (HHV8) is found in all lesions of KS. Four forms of the disease have been described: classic (more benign), epidemic (rapidly progressive and associated with AIDS), African endemic, and iatrogenic (associated with immunosuppressant treatment including organ transplant).[116,117]

The endothelial cell is thought to be the progenitor of KS with inflammation and angioproliferation.[118] The lesions emerge as purplish brown macules and develop into plaques and nodules. They tend to be multifocal rather than spreading by metastasis. The lesions initially appear over the lower extremities in the classic form (Fig. 47.33). The rapidly progressive form associated with AIDS tends to spread symmetrically over the upper body, particularly the face and oral mucosa. The lesions are often pruritic and painful. About 75% of individuals with epidemic KS have involvement of lymph nodes, particularly in the lung and gastrointestinal tract. Organ involvement is much less common in the classic form. The rapidly progressive form has a poor prognosis and shorter survival rates than the classic form. (See Chapter 10 for a further discussion on AIDS.)

effect on achieving a surgical cure and decreasing mortality from metastatic disease.

Prevention of melanoma includes avoidance of UV radiation exposure through use of protective clothing and sunscreens, and avoidance of artificial UV radiation exposure. Treatment of melanoma with no evidence of metastatic disease involves wide surgical excision of the primary lesion site. A lymph node biopsy of the peripherally draining lymph node (sentinel node) is warranted for lesions greater than 1 mm deep and if positive, regional lymphadenectomy is performed. Lesions on the extremities have the best surgical prognosis. Immediate complete lymph-node dissection increases the rate of regional disease control and provides prognostic information but does not increase melanoma-specific survival among individuals with melanoma and sentinel-node

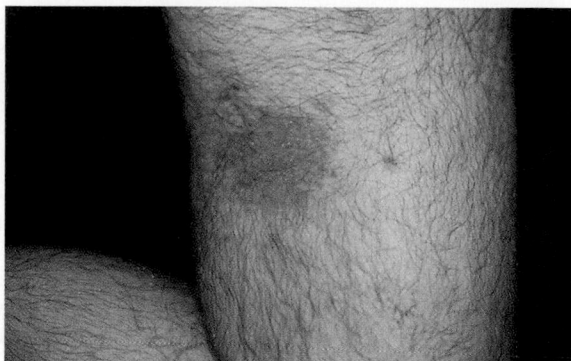

FIGURE 47.33 Kaposi Sarcoma. The purple lesion commonly seen on the skin. (Courtesy Department of Dermatology, School of Medicine, University of Utah.)

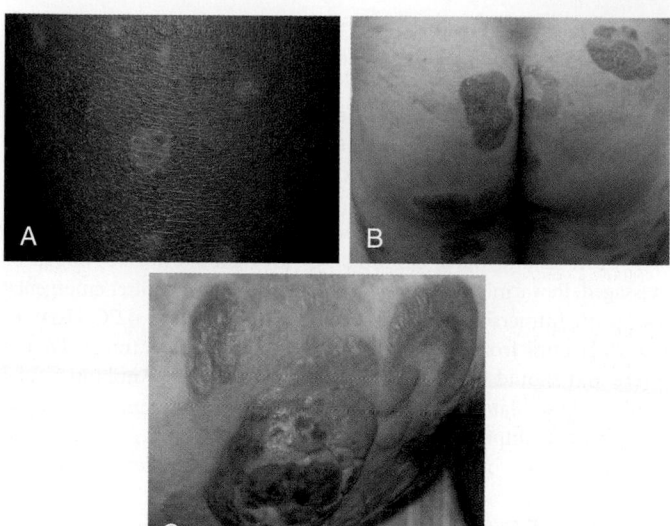

FIGURE 47.34 Mycosis Fungoides. **A,** Hypopigmented patches of mycosis fungoides. **B,** Plaques of mycosis fungoides. **C,** Tumors of mycosis fungoides combined with patches. (Courtesy of Ellen Korn, M.D. In James WD, Berger TG, Elston DM: *Andrews' diseases of the skin: clinical dermatology,* ed 11, Philadelphia, 2011, Saunders.)

Diagnosis is by medical history, physical examination, and skin biopsy with a high index of suspicion for those with immunodeficiency. Chest imaging reveals lesions in the lungs, and endoscopy is completed if there is suspicion of gastrointestinal involvement. Local lesions can be excised. Multiple disseminated lesions may be treated with a combination of α-interferon, radiotherapy, and cytotoxic drugs. Antiangiogenic agents are being tested. Individuals receiving highly active antiretroviral therapy (HAART) have a markedly reduced incidence of KS.[117]

Primary Cutaneous Lymphomas

Primary cutaneous lymphomas are cutaneous T-cell and B-cell lymphomas that are present in the skin without evidence of extracutaneous disease at the time of diagnosis (see Chapter 30 for classification and general pathophysiology of lymphomas). Cutaneous lymphomas are rare but are the second most common site of extranodal non-Hodgkin lymphoma. The incidence rate is about 14/100,000, and their cause is unknown.[119] Cutaneous lymphomas are more common in men and generally present after age 50 years; 75% of cases are T-cell lymphomas and 25% are B-cell lymphomas.

Cutaneous lymphomas develop from clonal expansion of B cells; T-helper cells; and, rarely, T-suppressor cells. The most common is cutaneous T-cell lymphoma (about 75%), and mycosis fungoides is the most prominent subtype. Sézary syndrome (a leukemic variant of T-cell lymphoma) and primary cutaneous CD30-positive lymphoproliferations (less than 10% of cases) are the most aggressive. Mycosis fungoides can present as focal or widespread erythematous patches or plaques, follicular papules, comedone-like lesions, and tumors (Fig. 47.34). Lesions are pruritic and cause considerable distress and debilitation. There may be patches of alopecia. The lesions progress over a period of months or years. Involvement of other organs can occur in advanced stages of the disease.

The differential diagnosis of the different types of cutaneous lymphomas is based on clinical manifestations, skin biopsy, and histologic appearance, immunologic and cytogenetic features, and response to appropriate treatment.[120] Treatment is based on staging of the disease following consensus-based guidelines that include a range of topical and systemic therapies, such as antiinflammatory, immunomodulatory, and biologic agents; histone deacetylase inhibitors; rexinoids; phototherapy; and chemotherapeutics. Radiotherapy has historically been the most common successful therapy. Stem cell transplant is the only cure for cutaneous T-cell lymphoma.[121,122]

Cold Injury

Exposure to extreme cold includes a spectrum of injuries[123]:

1. *Frostnip*—mild and completely reversible injury characterized by skin pallor and numbness

2. *Chilblains*—more serious injury than frostnip, violaceous skin color with plaques or nodules, pain, and pruritus but no ice crystal formation; chronic vasculitis can develop and is usually located on the face, anterior lower leg, hands, and feet

3. *Frostbite*—tissues freeze and form ice crystals at temperatures less than −2°C (28°F), progressing from distal to proximal; is potentially reversible

4. *Flash freeze*—rapid cooling with intracellular ice crystals associated with contact with cold metals or volatile liquids

The most common areas affected are fingers, toes, ears, nose, and cheeks, and skin damage can range from mild to severe. Initially, the body responds with alternating cycles of vasoconstriction and vasodilation—the "hunting reflex." The mechanism of injury is complex but is related to direct cold injury to cells, indirect injury, cell death from extracellular and intracellular ice crystal formation, impaired circulation with anoxia because of thrombosis in the exposed area, and reperfusion injury. Mild frostbite causes pallor and pain followed by redness and discomfort during rewarming with no tissue damage. Frozen skin becomes white or yellowish and has a waxy texture. There is numbness and no sensation of pain. Frostbite injury is related to direct cold injury to cells, indirect injury from ice crystal formation, and endothelial cell damage. During rewarming, there is progressive microvascular thrombosis followed by reperfusion injury with release of inflammatory mediators (including thromboxanes, prostaglandins, bradykinins, and histamines) and with impaired circulation and anoxia to the exposed area. Cyanosis and mottling develop followed by redness, edema, and burning pain on rewarming in more severe cases. Edema can cause capillary compression and vascular stasis.

Within 24 to 48 hours, vesicles and bullae appear and resolve into crusts that eventually slough off, leaving thin, newly formed skin. The most severe cases result in gangrene with loss of the affected part. Frostbite may be classified by depth of injury after rewarming as follows[124]:

First degree: superficial, characterized by a numb central white area surrounded by erythema and edema and including partial skin freezing without blistering

Second degree: full-thickness skin freezing with blistering surrounded by edema and hyperemia

Third degree: deep, characterized by full-thickness skin and subcutaneous freezing with tissue necrosis and hemorrhagic vesicles and blisters

Fourth degree: deep tissue freezing with full-thickness necrosis and gangrene with a line of demarcation.

Immediate treatment of frostbite is to cover affected areas with other body surfaces and warm clothing. The area should not be rubbed or massaged. Rewarming for severe frostbite should occur after emergency transport. Immersion in a warm water bath (40° to 42°C [104° to 107.6°F]) until frozen tissue is thawed is the best treatment. Pain is severe and should be treated with potent analgesics. Antibiotics may be given. Vasodilators, thrombolytics, hyperbaric oxygen, and sympathectomy may improve healing responses. Débridement or amputation of necrotic tissue occurs when there is a clear line of demarcation.[125]

DISORDERS OF THE HAIR

Alopecia

Alopecia means loss of hair from the head or body. Hair loss occurs when there is disruption in the growth phase of the hair follicle. Hair loss can be associated with systemic disorders such as hypothyroidism and iron deficiency, chemotherapy for cancer, malnutrition, compulsive hair pulling (trichotillomania), traction on hair from braiding and ponytails, use of hair treatment chemicals, hormonal alterations, and immune reactions.[126]

Androcentric Alopecia

Androcentric alopecia is localized hair loss and occurs in about 80% of men and about 50% of women with alopecia. It is not a disease but rather a variation in the androgen receptor *(AR)* gene that clusters in families. The mechanism of inheritance is unknown. Within the distribution of hair over the scalp, androgen-sensitive hair follicles are on top and androgen-insensitive follicles are on the sides and back. In genetically predisposed men, the androgen-sensitive follicles are transformed into vellus follicles. The normal hair is shed and replaced by fine, light, short hair. Male-pattern baldness begins with frontotemporal recession and progresses to loss of hair over the top of the scalp. Minoxidil may be used to stimulate hair growth, and finasteride may decrease the effect of androgens on hair follicles. Affected individuals may choose to wear wigs or have hair transplants.[127]

Female-Pattern Alopecia

Women in their 20s and 30s (6% to 12%) and women older than 70 years (55%) experience thinning and loss of hair over the central, frontal, and parietal scalp regions. Often there is a family history and an earlier presentation. Hair follicles are miniaturized and less functional with a reduction in hair density. Many of these women have elevated levels of serum adrenal androgen dehydroepiandrosterone sulfate (DHEAS), and treatment with antiandrogens can be effective. Lower levels of estrogen can also decrease hair growth after menopause. Minoxidil and light therapy or combinations of therapy may be used and work best when started early. Finasteride is no more effective than placebo.[128] In rare instances, a male-pattern baldness develops. Laboratory evaluation of serum androgenic hormones shows elevations, and some women have decreased hair loss when treated with daily doses of spironolactone.[129]

Alopecia Areata

Alopecia areata is an autoimmune T-cell-mediated chronic inflammatory disease directed at hair follicles that results in hair loss.[130] Hair loss occurs in multiple areas of the scalp. The eyebrows, eyelashes, beard, and other areas of the body can be involved. The cause is unknown, but stressful events, cell-mediated immune factors, and genetic susceptibility are linked to hair loss. Other autoimmune diseases, such as Addison disease, thyroid disease, and lupus erythematosus, also are associated in some individuals with alopecia areata.

The affected areas have round or oval areas of hair loss that may coalesce. The skin is smooth or may have short shafts of poorly developed hair that breaks at the surface. Regrowth occurs within 1 to 3 months, but hair loss may recur at the same site. Permanent regrowth of hair usually occurs. Total loss of hair (alopecia totalis) occurs in some young people; the long-term prognosis for total hair regrowth is poor. Diagnosis is made by observation of the pattern of hair loss. Biopsy may show a lymphocytic infiltrate around the follicle. There are several treatments for alopecia areata including watchful waiting, topical and intralesional corticosteroids, light therapy, minoxidil, and topical immunotherapy.[131]

Hirsutism

Hirsutism is the abnormal growth and distribution of hair on the face, body, and pubic area in a male pattern that occurs in about 5% to 10% of women. There is also frontotemporal hair recession. These areas of hair growth are androgen sensitive. Variations of hair growth in women are great, and a male pattern can be normal. Women who develop hirsutism may be secreting hormones associated with ovarian or adrenal disease, and they should be evaluated for polycystic ovaries, adrenal hyperplasia, or adrenal tumors. If no hormonal pathologic conditions exist, undesirable hair can be removed mechanically, by electrolysis, or with lasers. Endocrine therapy to suppress androgens may be considered.[132]

DISORDERS OF THE NAIL

Paronychia

Paronychia is an acute or chronic infection of the cuticle. One or more fingers or toes may be involved. Individuals whose hands are frequently exposed to moisture are at greatest risk. The most common causative microorganisms are *Staphylococcus* or *Streptococcus,* and occasionally *Candida.* Acute paronychia is manifested by the rapid onset of painful inflammation of the cuticle, usually after minor trauma. The skin around the nail becomes more edematous and painful with progressive infection. Pus may be expressed from the proximal nail fold, and an abscess may develop, requiring incision and drainage (I&D) for pain relief. The nail plate is usually not affected, although it can become discolored with ridges. Chronic paronychia develops slowly, with tenderness and swelling around the proximal or lateral nail folds. Treatment includes prevention by keeping the hands dry and avoidance of predisposing factors such as trauma through cuticle manipulation or excessive manicures. Oral antifungals are not effective because they do not penetrate the affected tissues. Several topical agents are available.[133]

Onychomycosis

Onychomycosis is a fungal or dermatophyte infection of the nail unit. The most common pattern is a nail plate that turns yellow or white (infection develops from the dorsal surface) and becomes elevated as a result of the accumulation of hyperkeratotic debris within the plate. Fungal infections of the nail are differentiated from psoriasis, lichen planus, and trauma by culture and microscopy and the absence of pitting on the nail surface, which is characteristic of psoriasis. Treatment is difficult because topical or systemic antifungal agents do not penetrate the nail plate readily. Two topical agents, efinaconazole and tavaborole, have been approved and are applied for 12 months. Terbinafine is an effective systemic antifungal drug. Surgical excision of the nail may be required. Education is essential to preventing recurrence.[133]

SUMMARY REVIEW

Structure and Function of the Skin

1. The skin is the largest organ of the body and equals about 20% of body weight.
2. The skin has three layers: the dermis, epidermis, and subcutaneous layer.
3. Keratinocytes produce keratin to form the superficial layer of the epidermis. The underlying epidermis contains a basal and a spinous layer with melanocytes, Langerhans cells, and Merkel cells.
4. The dermis is composed of connective tissue elements, hair follicles, sweat glands, sebaceous glands, blood vessels, nerves, and lymphatic vessels.
5. The subcutaneous layer contains macrophages, fibroblasts, fat cells, nerves, fine muscles, blood vessels, lymphatics, and hair follicle roots.
6. The dermal appendages include the nails, hair, sebaceous glands, and the eccrine and apocrine sweat glands.
7. The papillary capillaries provide the major blood supply to the skin, arising from deeper arterial plexuses. The sympathetic nervous system regulates skin blood flow.
8. Heat loss and heat conservation are regulated by arteriovenous anastomoses that lead to the papillary capillaries.
9. Older skin is thinner and drier with less collagen; it has fewer capillary loops and fewer changes in pigmentation.
10. Loss of melanocytes and hair follicles leads to gray and thinner hair.
11. The skin of older adults is more permeable; there is decreased sweating and loss of thermal regulation and decreased protective functions.
12. Pressure injuries develop from continuous pressure and shearing forces that occlude capillary blood flow with resulting ischemia and necrosis. Areas at greatest risk are pressure points over bony prominences, such as the greater trochanter, sacrum, ischia, and heels. Immobilized individuals with fractures and neurologic deficits are most likely to develop pressure injuries.
13. Keloids are scars that extend beyond the border of injury and result from abnormal fibroblast activity and excess collagen formation and fibrosis. Hypertrophic scars are elevated erythematous fibrous lesions that do not expand beyond the border of injury.
14. Pruritus (itching) is associated with many skin disorders. Itch mediators, peripheral unmyelinated polymodal C nerve fibers, and central processes contribute to itching. Scratching can cause skin trauma, infection, and scarring.

Disorders of the Skin

1. Allergic contact dermatitis is a form of delayed hypersensitivity that develops with alterations in skin barrier function and sensitization to allergens, such as microorganisms, metals, chemicals, or poison ivy.
2. Irritant contact dermatitis develops as an inflammatory response to prolonged exposure to chemicals, such as acids or soaps.
3. Atopic dermatitis or atopic eczema is associated with a family history of allergies, hay fever, elevated IgE levels, and increased histamine sensitivity; it is more common in children.
4. Stasis dermatitis occurs on the legs and results from venous stasis and edema.
5. Seborrheic dermatitis involves scaly, yellowish, inflammatory plaques of the scalp, eyebrows, eyelids, ear canals, chest, axillae, and back and may be associated with *Malassezia* yeasts, immunosuppression, and epidermal hyperproliferation.

6. Papulosquamous disorders are characterized by papules, scales, plaques, and erythema.
7. Psoriasis is a chronic autoimmune T-cell-mediated inflammatory skin disease with thickening of the epidermis and dermis characterized by scaly, erythematous pruritic plaques. The forms of psoriasis are plaque, inverse, guttate, pustular, and erythrodermic. Systemic complications can accompany the disease, including arthritis, nail disease, and cardiovascular disease.
8. Pityriasis rosea is a self-limiting disease associated with herpes type viruses and characterized by oval lesions with scales around the edges (herald patch) located along skin lines of the trunk.
9. Lichen planus is a papular violet-colored autoimmune inflammatory lesion involving T cells and inflammatory cytokines manifested by severe pruritus and can involve both skin and mucous membrane lesions.
10. Acne vulgaris is an inflammation of the pilosebaceous follicles with hypertrophy of sebaceous glands and telangiectasia, particularly of the nose.
11. Hidradenitis suppurativa, a chronic, inflammatory, recurring scarring disease of the pilosebaceous follicular ducts involves areas of skin where there are folds, hair follicles, and apocrine (sweat) glands and is related to immune and environmental factors.
12. Acne rosacea is inflammation with erythema, edema, papules, pustules, and telangiectasia that develops on the middle third of the face with hypertrophy and inflammation of the sebaceous glands that may be the result of infection or immune-mediated inflammation.
13. Cutaneous lupus erythematosus is an inflammatory autoimmune disease that affects only the skin. The inflammatory lesions usually occur in sun-exposed areas with a butterfly distribution over the nose and cheeks.
14. Pemphigus is a chronic, autoimmune, blistering disease that begins in the mouth or on the scalp and spreads to other parts of the body, often with a fatal outcome. The forms of pemphigus include pemphigus vulgaris (most common), pemphigus foliaceus, paraneoplastic pemphigus, IgA pemphigus, and pemphigus herpetiformis.
15. Bullous pemphigoid is a benign autoimmune blistering disease that resolves rapidly.
16. Erythema multiforme minor is an acute inflammation of the skin without involvement of mucous membranes. Erythema multiforme major involves acute inflammation of the skin with mucosal involvement. The lesions of erythema multiforme appear target-like with alternating rings of edema and inflammation; it is most often associated with HSV or other infections and rarely with drug reactions.
17. Stevens-Johnson syndrome (SJS), toxic epidermal necrolysis (TEN), and SJS/TEN overlap syndrome are the same disease with progressively more extensive blistering caused by keratinocyte cell death characterized by extensive bullous epidermal detachment, mucositis, and other organ involvement mediated by a cytotoxic T-cell drug reaction.
18. Folliculitis is a bacterial infection of the hair follicle.
19. A furuncle is an infection of the hair follicle that extends to the surrounding tissue.
20. A carbuncle is a collection of infected hair follicles that forms a draining abscess.
21. Cellulitis is a diffuse infection of the dermis and subcutaneous tissue usually caused by *Staphylococcus,* CA-MRSA, or group B streptococci.

SUMMARY REVIEW—cont'd

22. Erysipelas is a superficial streptococcal infection of the skin commonly affecting the face, ears, and lower legs.

23. Impetigo may have a bullous or an ulcerative form, is caused by *Staphylococcus* or *Streptococcus,* and is more common in children.

24. HSV-1 causes cold sores but can infect the cornea, mouth, and labia. HSV-2 causes genital lesions and is usually spread by sexual contact.

25. Herpes zoster and varicella (chickenpox) are both caused by the same herpesvirus, with herpes zoster manifesting years after the initial infection.

26. Warts (verrucae) are benign, rough, elevated lesions caused by papillomavirus. Venereal warts (condylomata acuminata) are spread by sexual contact.

27. Tinea skin infections (fungal infections) can occur anywhere on the body and are classified by location (i.e., tinea pedis, tinea corporis, tinea capitis).

28. Candidiasis is a yeastlike fungal infection caused by *C. albicans* occurring on skin, on mucous membranes, and in the gastrointestinal tract.

29. Cutaneous vasculitis is an immune-mediated inflammation of small skin blood vessels with purpura, ischemia, and necrosis resulting from disruption of the vessel wall.

30. Urticarial lesions are associated with type I hypersensitivity responses and appear as wheals, welts, or hives.

31. Scleroderma is an immune-mediated sclerosis of the skin that may be localized to the skin or systemic and affect muscle, bone, and other body organs that involves T helper cells, cytokines, and autoantibodies.

32. Seborrheic keratosis is a proliferation of squamous cells that produce elevated, smooth, or warty lesions of varying size, usually in sun-damaged skin. They are most common among older adults.

33. Keratoacanthoma arises from hair follicles on sun-exposed areas. There are three stages of development that result in a dome-shaped, crusty lesion filled with keratin that resolves in 3 to 4 months.

34. Actinic (solar) keratosis is a pigmented scaly lesion that develops in sun-exposed individuals with fair skin. The lesion may become malignant in the form of squamous cell carcinoma.

35. Nevi arise from melanocytes and may be pigmented or fleshy pink. They occur singly or in groups and may undergo transition to malignant melanoma.

36. Basal cell carcinoma is the most common skin cancer and occurs most often on sun-exposed areas with different subtypes and morphologic presentations.

37. Squamous cell carcinoma is a tumor of the epidermis with uncontrolled growth of keratinocytes associated with sun exposure and can be localized (in situ) or invasive.

38. Cutaneous melanoma is a malignant tumor that arises from melanocytes. If it is not excised early, metastasis occurs through the lymph nodes. Cutaneous melanomas arise in chronic sun-exposed skin or from melanocytic nevi.

39. KS is an endothelial cell vascular malignancy associated with immunodeficiency states and herpesvirus 8.

40. Cutaneous lymphomas are cutaneous T-cell and B-cell lymphomas that present in the skin but may develop disease in extracutaneous sites.

41. Frostbite usually occurs on cheeks and digits, causing direct injury to cells and impaired circulation.

Disorders of the Hair

1. Androcentric alopecia is an inherited form of irreversible baldness with hair loss in the central scalp and recession of the temporofrontal hairline that occurs in both men and women.

2. Female-pattern alopecia is a thinning of the central hair of the scalp beginning in women at 20 to 30 years of age and is often associated with elevated levels of serum adrenal androgen dehydroepiandrosterone sulfate.

3. Alopecia areata is patchy loss of hair associated with an autoimmune process and triggered by stress or metabolic diseases; it is usually reversible.

4. Hirsutism is a male pattern of hair growth in women that may be normal or the result of excessive secretion of androgenic hormones.

Disorders of the Nail

1. Paronychia is an inflammation of the cuticle that can be acute or chronic and is usually caused by staphylococci or streptococci.

2. Onychomycosis is a fungal infection of the nail plate.

KEY TERMS

Acne rosacea, 1509
Acne vulgaris, 1509
Actinic keratosis, 1518
Allergic contact dermatitis, 1506
Alopecia, 1524
Alopecia areata, 1524
Androcentric alopecia, 1524
Apocrine sweat gland, 1499
Atopic dermatitis (atopic eczema), 1506
Basal cell carcinoma (BCC), 1519
Basal layer (stratum basale), 1497
Bullous pemphigoid (BP), 1511
Candidiasis, 1515
Carbuncle, 1513
Cellulitis, 1513
Condylomata acuminata, 1515
Cutaneous lupus erythematosus (CLE), 1510
Cutaneous melanoma, 1520
Cutaneous vasculitis, 1516
Dermal appendage, 1498

Dermis, 1498
Dermatitis, 1505
Eccrine sweat gland, 1499
Eczema, 1505
Epidermis, 1497
Erysipelas, 1513
Erythema multiforme (EM) minor, 1511
Erythrodermic (exfoliative) psoriasis, 1508
Folliculitis, 1512
Furuncle, 1512
Germinative layer (stratum germinativum), 1497
Guttate psoriasis, 1508
Hair follicle, 1498
Herald patch, 1508
Herpes simplex virus (HSV), 1514
Herpes varicella, 1514
Herpes zoster, 1514
Hidradenitis suppurativa, 1509
Hirsutism, 1524
Human papillomavirus (HPV), 1514

Hypertrophic scar, 1505
Hyphae, 1515
Hypodermis, 1498
IgA pemphigus, 1511
Impetigo, 1513
Inverse psoriasis, 1507
Irritant contact dermatitis, 1506
Kaposi sarcoma (KS), 1522
Keloid, 1505
Keratin, 1497
Keratinocyte, 1497
Keratoacanthoma, 1518
Langerhans cell, 1497
Lichen planus (LP), 1508
Localized scleroderma (morphea), 1517
Lupus erythematosus, 1510
Lyme disease, 1513
Melanocyte, 1497
Merkel cell, 1497
Mycosis fungoides, 1523

REFERENCES

1. Chopin M, Nutt SL: Establishing and maintaining the Langerhans cell network. *Semin Cell Dev Biol* 41:23–29, 2015.
2. Tansey EA, Johnson CD: Recent advances in thermoregulation. *Adv Physiol Educ* 39(3):139–148, 2015.
3. Bentov I, Reed MJ: The effect of aging on the cutaneous microvasculature. *Microvasc Res* 100:25–31, 2015.
4. Thomas DR, Burkemper NM: Aging skin and wound healing. *Clin Geriatr Med* 29(2):xi–xx, 2013.
5. Goodier M, Hordinsky M: Normal and aging hair biology and structure 'aging and hair'. *Curr Probl Dermatol* 47:1–9, 2015.
6. Rinnerthaler M, et al: Oxidative stress in aging human skin. *Biomolecules* 5(2):545–589, 2015.
7. Anders J, et al: Decubitus ulcers: pathophysiology and primary prevention. *Dtsch Arztebl Int* 107(21):371–381, 2010.
8. Clark M: Skin assessment in dark pigmented skin: a challenge in pressure ulcer prevention. *Nurs Times* 106(30):16–17, 2010.
9. Cox J: Predictive power of the Braden scale for pressure sore risk in adult critical care patients: a comprehensive review. *J Wound Ostomy Continence Nurs* 39(6):613–621, 2012.
10. Mortenson WB, Miller WC: SCIRE Research Team: a review of scales for assessing the risk of developing a pressure ulcer in individuals with SCI. *Spinal Cord* 46(3):168–175, 2008.
11. National Pressure Ulcer Advisory Panel: *Pressure ulcer stages revised by NPUAP*, 2016. Available at: http://www.npuap.org/resources/educational-and-clinical-resources/npuap-pressure-injury-stages/.
12. Tayyib N, Coyer F: Effectiveness of pressure ulcer prevention strategies for adult patients in intensive care units: a systematic review. *Worldviews Evid Based Nurs* 13(6):432–444, 2016.
13. Dumville JC, et al: Negative pressure wound therapy for treating pressure ulcers. *Cochrane Database Syst Rev* (5):CD011334, 2015.
14. Norman G, et al: Antibiotics and antiseptics for pressure ulcers. *Cochrane Database Syst Rev* (4):CD011586, 2016.
15. Jumper N, Paus R, Bayat A: Functional histopathology of keloid disease. *Histol Histopathol* 30(9):1033–1057, 2015.
16. Rabello FB, Souza CD, Farina Júnior JA: Update on hypertrophic scar treatment. *Clinics (Sao Paulo)* 69(8):565–573, 2014.
17. Verhiel S, et al: Mechanism of action, efficacy, and adverse events of calcium antagonists in hypertrophic scars and keloids: a systematic review. *Dermatol Surg* 41(12):1343–1350, 2015.

18. Hassan I, Haji ML: Understanding itch: an update on mediators and mechanisms of pruritus. *Indian J Dermatol Venereol Leprol* 80(2):106–114, 2014.
19. Dhand A, Aminoff MJ: The neurology of itch. *Brain* 137(Pt 2):313–322, 2014.
20. Potenzieri C, Undem BJ: Basic mechanisms of itch. *Clin Exp Allergy* 42(1):8–19, 2012.
21. Pereira MP, Ständer S: Chronic pruritus: current and emerging treatment options. *Drugs* 77(9):999–1007, 2017.
22. Friedmann PS, Sanchez-Elsner T, Schnuch A: Genetic factors in susceptibility to contact sensitivity. *Contact Dermatitis* 72(5):263–274, 2015.
23. Honda T, Kabashima K: Novel concept of iSALT (inducible skin-associated lymphoid tissue) in the elicitation of allergic contact dermatitis. *Proc Jpn Acad Ser B Phys Biol Sci* 92(1):20–28, 2016.
24. Chełmińska M, et al: Differentiating of cross-reactions in patients with latex allergy with the use of ISAC test. *Postepy Dermatol Alergol* 33(2):120–127, 2016.
25. Bernstein DI: Contact dermatitis for the practicing allergist. *J Allergy Clin Immunol Pract* 3(5):652–658, 2015.
26. Ale IS, Maibach HI: Irritant contact dermatitis. *Rev Environ Health* 29(3):195–206, 2014.
27. Raffetto JD, Marston WA: Venous ulcer: what is new? *Plast Reconstr Surg* 127(Suppl 1):279S–288S, 2011.
28. Alavi A, et al: What's new: management of venous leg ulcers: treating venous leg ulcers. *J Am Acad Dermatol* 74(4):643–664, 2016.
29. Dessinioti C, Katsambas A: Seborrheic dermatitis: etiology, risk factors, and treatments: facts and controversies. *Clin Dermatol* 31(4):343–351, 2013.
30. Gupta AK, Versteeg SG: Topical treatment of facial seborrheic dermatitis: a systematic review. *Am J Clin Dermatol* 18(2):193–213, 2017.
31. Michalek IM, Loring B, John SM: A systematic review of worldwide epidemiology of psoriasis. *J Eur Acad Dermatol Venereol* 31(2):206–212, 2017.
32. Mahil SK, Capon F, Barker JN: Genetics of psoriasis. *Dermatol Clin* 33(1):1–11, 2015.
33. Hedrich CM: Shaping the spectrum-from autoinflammation to autoimmunity. *Clin Immunol* 165:21–28, 2016.
34. Mahil SK, Capon F, Barker JN: Update on psoriasis immunopathogenesis and targeted immunotherapy. *Semin Immunopathol* 38(1):11–27, 2016.
35. Boehncke WH: Etiology and pathogenesis of psoriasis. *Rheum Dis Clin North Am* 41(4):665–675, 2015.
36. Milavec-Puretić V, et al: Drug induced psoriasis. *Acta Dermatovenerol Croat* 19(1):39–42, 2011.

37. Barnas JL, Ritchlin CT: Etiology and pathogenesis of psoriatic arthritis. *Rheum Dis Clin North Am* 41(4):643–663, 2015.
38. Takeshita J, et al: Psoriasis and comorbid diseases: implications for management. *J Am Acad Dermatol* 76(3):393–403, 2017.
39. Stein Gold LF: Topical therapies for psoriasis: improving management strategies and patient adherence. *Semin Cutan Med Surg* 35(2 Suppl 2):S36–S44, 2016.
40. Ayanlowo O, Akinkugbe A, Olumide Y: The pityriasis rosea calendar: a 7 year review of seasonal variation, age and sex distribution. *Nig Q J Hosp Med* 20(1):29–31, 2010.
41. Chuh A, et al: A position statement on the management of patients with pityriasis rosea. *J Eur Acad Dermatol Venereol* 30(10):1670–1681, 2016.
42. Gorouhi F, Davari P, Fazel N: Cutaneous and mucosal lichen planus: a comprehensive review of clinical subtypes, risk factors, diagnosis, and prognosis. *ScientificWorldJournal* 2014:742826, 2014.
43. Greenberg MS: AAOM Clinical Practice Statement: subject: oral lichen planus and oral cancer. *Oral Surg Oral Med Oral Pathol Oral Radiol* 122(4):440–441, 2016.
44. Atzmony L, et al: Treatments for cutaneous lichen planus: a systematic review and meta-analysis. *Am J Clin Dermatol* 17(1):11–22, 2016.
45. Kelly G, Prens EP: Inflammatory mechanisms in hidradenitis suppurativa. *Dermatol Clin* 34(1):51–58, 2016.
46. Prens E, Deckers I: Pathophysiology of hidradenitis suppurativa: an update. *J Am Acad Dermatol* 73(5 Suppl 1):S8–S11, 2015.
47. Deckers IE, Prens EP: An update on medical treatment options for hidradenitis suppurativa. *Drugs* 76(2):215–229, 2016.
48. Woodruff CM, Charlie AM, Leslie KS: Hidradenitis suppurativa: a guide for the practicing physician. *Mayo Clin Proc* 90(12):1679–1693, 2015.
49. Holmes AD, Steinhoff M: Integrative concepts of rosacea pathophysiology, clinical presentation and new therapeutics. *Exp Dermatol* 26(8):659–667, 2017.
50. Woo YR, et al: Rosacea: molecular mechanisms and management of a chronic cutaneous inflammatory condition. *Int J Mol Sci* 17(9):2016.
51. Vieira AC, Mannis MJ: Ocular rosacea: common and commonly missed. *J Am Acad Dermatol* 69(6 Suppl 1):S36–S41, 2013.
52. van Zuuren EJ, et al: Interventions for rosacea. *Cochrane Database Syst Rev* (4):CD003262, 2015.

53. Kuhn A, Landmann A: The classification and diagnosis of cutaneous lupus erythematosus. *J Autoimmun* 48-49:14–19, 2014.

54. Kirchhof MG, Dutz JP: The immunopathology of cutaneous lupus erythematosus. *Rheum Dis Clin North Am* 40(3):455–474, 2014.

55. Kuhn A, et al: Revised cutaneous lupus erythematosus disease area and severity index (RCLASI): a modified outcome instrument for cutaneous lupus erythematosus. *Br J Dermatol* 163(1):83–92, 2010.

56. Presto JK, Hejazi EZ, Werth VP: Biological therapies in the treatment of cutaneous lupus erythematosus. *Lupus* 26(2):115–118, 2016.

57. Kasperkiewicz M, et al: Pemphigus. *Nat Rev Dis Primers* 3:17026, 2017.

58. Baum S, et al: Diagnosis and classification of autoimmune blistering diseases. *Autoimmun Rev* 13(4-5):482–489, 2014.

59. Gregoriou S, et al: Management of pemphigus vulgaris: challenges and solutions. *Clin Cosmet Investig Dermatol* 8:521–527, 2015.

60. Ujiie H: IgE autoantibodies in bullous pemphigoid: supporting role, or leading player? *J Dermatol Sci* 78(1):5–10, 2015.

61. Zhao CY, Murrell DF: Advances in understanding and managing bullous pemphigoid. *F1000Res* 4: 2015.

62. Tomasini C, et al: From erythema multiforme to toxic epidermal necrolysis. Same spectrum or different diseases? *G Ital Dermatol Venereol* 149(2): 243–261, 2014.

63. Kohanim S, et al: Stevens-Johnson syndrome/toxic epidermal necrolysis-a comprehensive review and guide to therapy. I. Systemic disease. *Ocul Surf* 14(1):2–19, 2016.

64. Samim F, et al: Erythema multiforme: a review of epidemiology, pathogenesis, clinical features, and treatment. *Dent Clin North Am* 57(4):583–596, 2013.

65. Chan M, Goldman RD: Erythema multiforme in children: the steroid debate. *Can Fam Physician* 59(6):635–636, 2013.

66. Dodiuk-Gad RP, et al: Stevens-Johnson syndrome and toxic epidermal necrolysis: an update. *Am J Clin Dermatol* 16(6):475–493, 2015.

67. Darlenski R, Kazandjieva J, Tsankov N: Systemic drug reactions with skin involvement: Stevens-Johnson syndrome, toxic epidermal necrolysis, and DRESS. *Clin Dermatol* 33(5): 538–541, 2015.

68. Schwartz RA, McDonough PH, Lee BW: Toxic epidermal necrolysis: part II. prognosis, sequelae, diagnosis, differential diagnosis, prevention, and treatment. *J Am Acad Dermatol* 69(2):187.e1– 187.e16, 2013.

69. Sardana K: Follicular disorders of the face. *Clin Dermatol* 32(6):839–872, 2014.

70. Raff AB, Kroshinsky D: Cellulitis: a review. *JAMA* 316(3):325–337, 2016.

71. Sun X, Xie T: Management of necrotizing fasciitis and its surgical aspects. *Int J Low Extrem Wounds* 14(4):328–334, 2015.

72. Ibrahim F, Khan T, Pujalte GG: Bacterial skin infections. *Prim Care* 42(4):485–499, 2015.

73. Lantos PM: Chronic Lyme disease. *Infect Dis Clin North Am* 29(2):325–340, 2015.

74. Sanchez JL: Clinical manifestations and treatment of Lyme disease. *Clin Lab Med* 35(4):765–778, 2015.

75. Ramdass P, Mullick S, Farber HF: Viral skin diseases. *Prim Care* 42(4):517–567, 2015.

76. Desai DV, Kulkarni SS: Herpes simplex virus: the interplay between HSV, host, and HIV-1. *Viral Immunol* 28(10):546–555, 2015.

77. Stanfield B, Kousoulas KG: Herpes simplex vaccines: prospects of live-attenuated HSV vaccines to combat genital and ocular infections. *Curr Clin Microbiol Rep* 2(3):125–136, 2015.

78. Dayan RR, Peleg R: Herpes zoster—typical and atypical presentations. *Postgrad Med* 129(6): 567–571, 2017.

79. Gagliardi AM, et al: Vaccines for preventing herpes zoster in older adults. *Cochrane Database Syst Rev* (3):CD008858, 2016.

80. Bruggink SC, et al: Monochloroacetic acid application is an effective alternative to cryotherapy for common and plantar warts in primary care: a randomized controlled trial. *J Invest Dermatol* 135(5):1262–1267, 2015.

81. Leung L: Recalcitrant nongenital warts. *Aust Fam Physician* 40(1-2):40–42, 2011.

82. Kaushik N, Pujalte GG, Reese ST: Superficial fungal infections. *Prim Care* 42(4):501–516, 2015.

83. Hani U, et al: Candidiasis: a fungal infection-current challenges and progress in prevention and treatment. *Infect Disord Drug Targets* 15(1):42–52, 2015.

84. Polke M, Hube B, Jacobsen ID: Candida survival strategies. *Adv Appl Microbiol* 91:139–235, 2015.

85. Zeichner JA: New topical therapeutic options in the management of superficial fungal infections. *J Drugs Dermatol* 14(10 Suppl):s35–s41, 2015.

86. Gru AA, Salavaggione AL: Vasculopathic and vasculitic dermatoses. *Semin Diagn Pathol* 34(3): 285–300, 2017.

87. Micheletti RG, Werth VP: Small vessel vasculitis of the skin. *Rheum Dis Clin North Am* 41(1):21–32, 2015.

88. Schaefer P: Acute and chronic urticaria: evaluation and treatment. *Am Fam Physician* 95(11):717–724, 2017.

89. Kurzinski K, Torok KS: Cytokine profiles in localized scleroderma and relationship to clinical features. *Cytokine* 55(2):157–164, 2011.

90. Bielsa Marsol I: Update on the classification and treatment of localized scleroderma. *Actas Dermosifiliogr* 104(8):654–666, 2013.

91. Elhai M, et al: Systemic sclerosis: recent insights. *Joint Bone Spine* 82(3):148–153, 2015.

92. Chitwood K, Etzkorn J, Cohen G: Topical and intralesional treatment of nonmelanoma skin cancer: efficacy and cost comparisons. *Dermatol Surg* 39(9):1306–1316, 2013.

93. Dirschka T, et al: Real-world approach to actinic keratosis management: practical treatment algorithm for office-based dermatology. *J Dermatolog Treat* 28(5):431–442, 2017.

94. Schaffer JV: Update on melanocytic nevi in children. *Clin Dermatol* 33(3):368–386, 2015.

95. Marzuka AG, Book SE: Basal cell carcinoma: pathogenesis, epidemiology, clinical features, diagnosis, histopathology, and management. *Yale J Biol Med* 88(2):167–179, 2015.

96. Feller L, et al: Basal cell carcinoma, squamous cell carcinoma and melanoma of the head and face. *Head Face Med* 12:11, 2016.

97. Gandhi SA, Kampp J: Skin cancer epidemiology, detection, and management. *Med Clin North Am* 99(6):1323–1335, 2015.

98. Emmert S, et al: Molecular biology of basal and squamous cell carcinomas. *Adv Exp Med Biol* 810:234–252, 2014.

99. American Cancer Society (ACS): *Cancer facts & figures 2017*, Atlanta, 2017, Author.

100. Kauvar AN, et al: Consensus for nonmelanoma skin cancer treatment, part II: squamous cell carcinoma, including a cost analysis of treatment methods. *Dermatol Surg* 41(11):1214–1240, 2015.

101. Kibbi N, Kluger H, Choi JN: Melanoma: clinical presentations. *Cancer Treat Res* 167:107–129, 2016.

102. US Preventive Services Task Force, et al: Screening for skin cancer: US Preventive Services Task Force recommendation statement. *JAMA* 316(4): 429–435, 2016.

103. Glazer AM, et al: Analysis of trends in US melanoma incidence and mortality. *JAMA Dermatol* 153(2):225–226, 2016.

104. Azoury SC, Lange JR: Epidemiology, risk factors, prevention, and early detection of melanoma. *Surg Clin North Am* 94(5):945–962, 2014.

105. Little EG, Eide MJ: Update on the current state of melanoma incidence. *Dermatol Clin* 30(3): 355–361, 2012.

106. Paluncic J, et al: Roads to melanoma: key pathways and emerging players in melanoma progression and oncogenic signaling. *Biochim Biophys Acta* 1863(4):770–784, 2016.

107. Elder DE: Pathology of melanoma. *Surg Oncol Clin N Am* 24(2):229–237, 2015.

108. Ransohoff KJ, et al: Familial skin cancer syndromes: increased melanoma risk. *J Am Acad Dermatol* 74(3):423–434, 2016.

109. American Academy of Dermatology Ad Hoc Task Force for the ABCDEs of Melanoma, et al: early detection of melanoma: reviewing the ABCDEs. *J Am Acad Dermatol* 72(4):717–723, 2015.

110. Kwak J, et al: Volatile biomarkers from human melanoma cells. *J Chromatogr B* 932:90–96, 2013.

111. Wick MR: Cutaneous melanoma: a current overview. *Semin Diagn Pathol* 33(4):225–241, 2016.

112. Faries MB, et al: Completion dissection or observation for sentinel-node metastasis in melanoma. *N Engl J Med* 376(23):2211–2222, 2017.

113. Wick MR, Gru AA: Metastatic melanoma: pathologic characterization, current treatment, and complications of therapy. *Semin Diagn Pathol* 33(4):204–218, 2016.

114. Brummer GC, Bowen AR, Bowen GM: Merkel cell carcinoma: current issues regarding diagnosis, management, and emerging treatment strategies. *Am J Clin Dermatol* 17(1):49–62, 2016.

115. Saini AT, Miles BA: Merkel cell carcinoma of the head and neck: pathogenesis, current and emerging treatment options. *Onco Targets Ther* 8:2157–2167, 2015.

116. Dezube BJ, Sullivan R, Koon HB: Emerging targets and novel strategies in the treatment of AIDS-related Kaposi's sarcoma: bidirectional translations science. *J Cell Physiol* 209(3):659–662, 2006.

117. Ruocco E, et al: Kaposi's sarcoma: etiology and pathogenesis, inducing factors, causal associations, and treatments: facts and controversies. *Clin Dermatol* 31(4):413–422, 2013.

118. Schulz TF, Cesarman E: Kaposi sarcoma-associated herpesvirus: mechanisms of oncogenesis. *Curr Opin Virol* 14:116–128, 2015.

119. Bradford PT, et al: Cutaneous lymphoma incidence patterns in the United States: a population based study of 3884 cases. *Blood* 113:5064–5073, 2009.

120. Olsen EA: Evaluation, diagnosis, and staging of cutaneous lymphoma. *Dermatol Clin* 33(4): 643–654, 2015.

121. DeSimone JA, et al: Recent advances in primary cutaneous T-cell lymphoma. *Curr Opin Oncol* 27(2):128–133, 2015.

122. Lima M: Cutaneous primary B-cell lymphomas: from diagnosis to treatment. *An Bras Dermatol* 90(5):687–706, 2015.

123. Mohr WJ, Jenabzadeh K, Ahrenholz DH: Cold injury. *Hand Clin* 25(4):481–496, 2009.

124. Petrone P, et al: Management of accidental hypothermia and cold injury. *Curr Probl Surg* 51(10):417–431, 2014.

125. Handford C, et al: Frostbite: a practical approach to hospital management. *Extrem Physiol Med* 3:7, 2014.

126. Qi J, Garza LA: An overview of alopecias. *Cold Spring Harb Perspect Med* 4(3):a013615, 2014.

127. Varothai S, Bergfeld WF: Androgenetic alopecia: an evidence-based treatment update. *Am J Clin Dermatol* 15(3):217–230, 2014.

128. van Zuuren EJ, Fedorowicz Z, Schoones J: Interventions for female pattern hair loss. *Cochrane Database Syst Rev* (5):CD007628, 2016.

129. Ramos PM, Miot HA: Female pattern hair loss: a clinical and pathophysiological review. *An Bras Dermatol* 90(4):529–543, 2015.

130. Spano F, Donovan JC: Alopecia areata: part 1: pathogenesis, diagnosis, and prognosis. *Can Fam Physician* 61(9):751–755, 2015.

131. Perera E, Yip L, Sinclair R: Alopecia areata. *Curr Probl Dermatol* 47:67–75, 2015.

132. Somani N, Turvy D: Hirsutism: an evidence-based treatment update. *Am J Clin Dermatol* 15(3):247–266, 2014.

133. Iorizzo M: Tips to treat the 5 most common nail disorders: brittle nails, onycholysis, paronychia, psoriasis, onychomycosis. *Dermatol Clin* 33(2):175–183, 2015.

Alterations of the Integument in Children

Noreen Heer Nicol, Sue E. Huether

CHAPTER OUTLINE

Skin diseases in children may be minor or severe, localized or generalized, and may have different causative mechanisms and different patterns of distribution than those found in adults, although there may be similarities. Some skin diseases resolve spontaneously and require no treatment. Diagnosis is commonly made from the history, appearance, and distribution of the lesion or lesions. Common skin diseases of childhood are presented here.

ACNE VULGARIS

Acne vulgaris is the most common skin disease and affects 85% of the population between the ages of 12 and 25 years. Onset is occurring at a younger age and may be associated with earlier onset of puberty in the United States. Acne tends to occur in families, and genetic susceptibility may determine an individual's susceptibility and severity of disease.[1] The incidence of acne is the same in both sexes, although severe disease affects males more often. Acne develops at distinctive pilosebaceous units, known as *sebaceous follicles*. Located primarily on the face and upper parts of the chest and back, these follicles have many large sebaceous glands, a small vellus hair (very short, nonpigmented, and very thin hair), and a dilated follicular canal that is visible as a pore on the skin surface. Acne lesions are associated with obstruction of the follicle and may be noninflammatory or inflammatory. In noninflammatory acne, the comedones are open (blackheads) and closed (whiteheads), with the accumulated material causing obstruction and distention of the follicle and thinning of follicular canal walls. Inflammatory acne (cystic) develops in closed comedones when the follicular wall ruptures, expelling sebum into the surrounding dermis and initiating inflammation. Pustules form when the inflammation is close to the surface, and papules and cystic nodules can develop when the inflammation is deeper, causing mild to severe scarring (Fig. 48.1). Both noninflammatory and inflammatory lesions may exist in the same individual.

The principal factors contributing to acne are (1) follicular proliferation of *Propionibacterium acnes* (a gram-positive anaerobic bacterium), (2) hyperkeratinization of follicular epithelium, (3) excessive sebum production, and (4) inflammation and rupture of a follicle from accumulated debris and bacteria within the follicle (see Fig. 48.1).

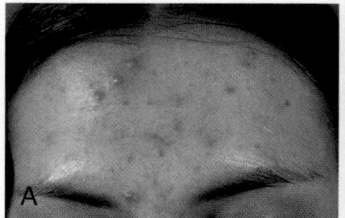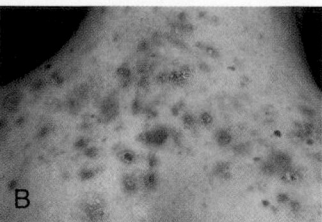

FIGURE 48.1 Inflammatory Acne. **A,** Inflammatory pustules and papules. **B,** Multiple erythematous papules, pustules, and cysts are present, and several have become confluent. (From Kliegman RM et al, editors: *Nelson textbook of pediatrics,* ed 19, Philadelphia, 2011, Saunders.)

P. acnes shifts from being symbiotic to pathogenic and from being noninflammatory to inflammatory. The causal mechanism is unknown.[2] Androgens (dihydrotestosterone and testosterone) synthesized in increasing amounts during puberty boost the size and productivity of the sebaceous glands that promote *P. acnes. P. acnes* produces extracellular porphyrins and proinflammatory molecules, including chemotactic factors and lipolytic and proteolytic enzymes. The hydrolytic action of the enzymes converts triglycerides into free fatty acids (FFAs). FFAs activate toll-like receptors, T-cell–associated and Th17-associated inflammation, and edema that results in pus formation and breakdown of the follicle wall. Chemotactic substances attract polymorphonuclear leukocytes with release of proinflammatory cytokines.[3] Increased sebum production feeds bacterial growth. Acne also is associated with polycystic ovarian syndrome, congenital adrenal hyperplasia, and various endocrine tumors as a result of higher circulating levels of androgens.

The treatment of acne should be individualized according to severity. Combinations of a topical retinoid, benzoyl peroxide, and antimicrobial agents are preferred. Retinoids target all four principal factors contributing to acne: comedogenesis, *P. acnes*, inflammation, and sebum production. Benzoyl peroxide and topical antibiotics target comedogenesis, *P. acnes*, and inflammation.[4] Combined oral contraceptives are of benefit in both inflammatory and noninflammatory acne.[5] Use of systemic therapies, including oral antibiotics, sex hormones, corticosteroids, and isotretinoin (requires pregnancy prevention), may be limited by side effects. Acne surgery, including comedo extraction, intralesional steroids, and cryosurgery, is useful in selected individuals. Severe scarring may be treated with dermabrasion, lasers, and resurfacing techniques. Evidence suggests that high–glycemic-index diets may be associated with acne, but given current data, no specific dietary changes are recommended in the management of acne.[4] Psychologic support is important because acne negatively affects quality of life, self-esteem, and mood in adolescents and is associated with an increased risk of anxiety, depression, and suicidal ideation.[5] Special consideration must be given to treatment for those with darker skin, because they have greater risk for hyperpigmentation and keloidal scarring. Research is continuing on the development of new drugs, vaccines, and other immunotherapies to prevent *P. acnes* infection.[6]

Acne conglobata is a highly inflammatory form of severe acne with communicating cysts and abscesses beneath the skin that can cause scarring. Remissions tend to occur during the summer, perhaps from more exposure to sunlight. This type of acne requires the use of systemic and combination therapies to prevent drug resistance.

DERMATITIS

Atopic Dermatitis

Atopic dermatitis (AD), also known as *atopic eczema,* is the most common cause of eczema in children. The prevalence is approximately 25% of children and 2% to 3% of adults.[7] Onset is usually from 2 to

6 months of age, and most cases occur within the first 5 years of life. More than half of individuals with AD develop asthma and allergies later in life.[8] Positive skin tests to a variety of common food and inhalant allergens are seen in approximately 80% of individuals.

The cause of this chronic, relapsing form of pruritic eczema is not clearly understood but involves an interplay of genetic predisposition, altered skin barrier function associated with filaggrin gene missense mutations (proteins that bind keratin in the epidermis and protect hydration), claudin (tight junction proteins), reduced ceramide (a stratum corneum lipid) levels, altered innate immunity, and altered immune responses to allergens, irritants, and microbes.[9] There is debate as to whether the pathophysiology favors an "inside-out" explanation with immunologic dysregulation leading to epidermal barrier abnormality, or an "outside-in" explanation with primary barrier dysfunction as the cause of the immunologic perturbations.[10] Regardless of the debate, both are involved, and barrier repair is required. In AD, memory T cells in the blood express cutaneous lymphocyte antigen (CLA), which leads to the homing of lymphocytes to the skin. Inflammation is associated with activation of a Th2 phenotype with a switch to Th1 cells in the chronic phase of the disease. There is release of numerous cytokines, chemokines, interferon-gamma (IFN-γ), and granulocyte-macrophage colony-stimulating factor (GM-CSF). Activation of mast cells, eosinophils, macrophages, and IgE-mediated autoreactivity to epidermal proteins contribute to the inflammation.[11]

Deficiency in filaggrin protein leads to a defect of the epidermal barrier that causes transepidermal water loss and allows easy penetration of pathogens and allergens through the skin and a systemic hyperactive immune response.[12] Keratinocytes are deficient in their ability to express toll-like antimicrobial peptides (see Chapter 7) and may predispose such individuals to skin colonization and infection with *Staphylococcus aureus,* viruses, and fungi. Alterations in the skin microbiome may promote colonization with pathogenic microorganisms.[13]

AD has a constellation of clinical features that include frequent exacerbations, severe pruritus, and a characteristic appearance with redness, edema, and scaling (Fig. 48.2). The skin becomes increasingly dry, sensitive, itchy, and easily irritated because the barrier function is impaired. Microscopic epidermal cracks that allow water to be expelled and irritants, allergens, and microbes to enter further inflammation, drying, and cracking. Itching is the hallmark of atopic dermatitis, and rubbing and scratching to relieve the itch are responsible for many of the clinical skin changes of AD. Histamine level is elevated in AD lesions but is not considered a major pruritogen because blockage of H1 and H2 receptors alone is ineffective at relieving itch.

In young children, the rash appears primarily on the face, scalp, trunk, and extensor surfaces of the arms and legs. In older children and adults, the rash tends to be found on the neck, antecubital and popliteal fossae, and hands and feet. Lichenification (thickening of the epidermis from constant scratching) is more common in adults with chronic eczema. The irritation and itching interfere with sleep and cause irritability.

There are no specific laboratory features of AD that can be used for diagnostic and treatment purposes. Most affected individuals show increased serum levels of immunoglobulin E (IgE), interleukin-4 and interleukin-13, eosinophils, and positive skin tests to a variety of common food and inhalant allergens. Management of individuals with AD includes accurate diagnosis and comprehensive evaluation of triggers and response to treatment; management of confounding factors, including sleep disruption; and education of individuals and caregivers. Avoidance of triggers and promotion of skin hydration, including emollients and cleansing with mild or nonsoap cleansers, are key to good therapy. Bleach baths may be helpful for recurrent infection. For acute treatment and frequent flares, antiinflammatory

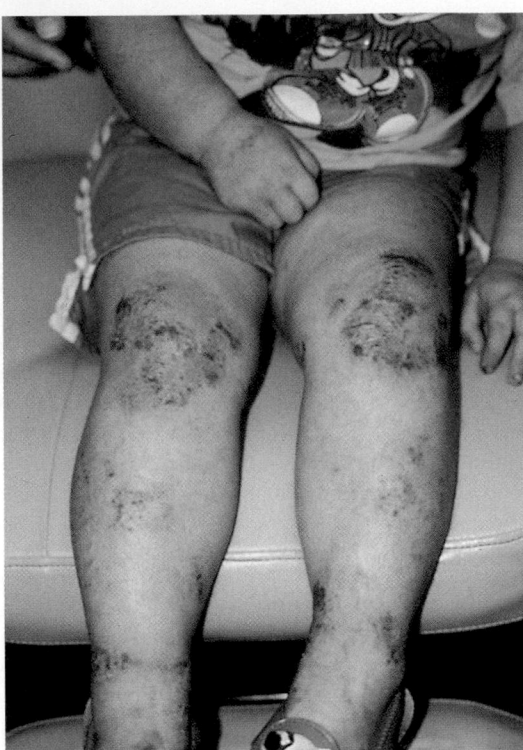

FIGURE 48.2 Atopic Dermatitis. Characteristic lesions with crusting from irritation and scratching over knees and around ankles. (Courtesy Department of Dermatology, School of Medicine, University of Utah.)

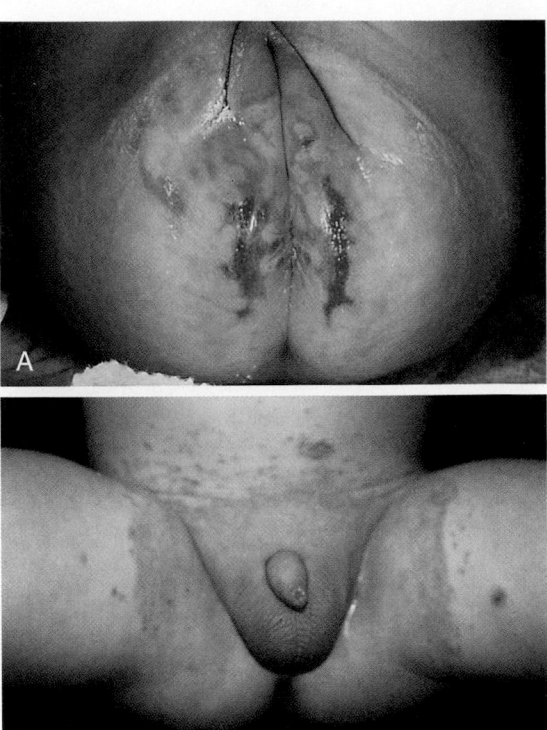

FIGURE 48.3 Diaper Dermatitis. **A,** Diaper dermatitis with erosions. **B,** Diaper dermatitis with *Candida albicans* secondary infection. (Courtesy Department of Dermatology, School of Medicine, University of Utah.)

agents, such as topical corticosteroids and calcineurin inhibitors, are necessary.[14] Wet wrap therapy is used for severe eczema.[15]

Although temporarily effective, systemic steroids (oral or parenteral) should generally be avoided in adults and children with AD because the potential short- and long-term adverse effects largely outweigh the benefits. Systemic therapy includes immunomodulators, the use of sedating antihistamines, antibiotics, and phototherapy. Research is in progress to develop molecule-specific targets to produce long-term disease remission.[16]

Diaper Dermatitis

Diaper dermatitis is a form of irritant contact dermatitis initiated by a combination of factors that include prolonged exposure to and irritation by urine ammonia and feces, maceration, and friction by wet diapers or use of airtight plastic diaper covers. The lesions vary from mild erythema to erythematous papular lesions. Diaper dermatitis is often secondarily infected with *Candida albicans*. Candidal (monilial) diaper dermatitis is usually very erythematous, with sharp margination and pustulovesicular satellite lesions affecting the lower aspect of the abdomen, genitalia, buttock, and upper portion of the thigh[17] (Fig. 48.3). Disposable diaper designs have decreased the incidence of diaper dermatitis in infants.[18]

Treatment involves frequent diaper changes to keep the area clean and dry or regular exposure of the perineal area to air, use of super-absorbent diapers, and topical protection with a product containing petrolatum or zinc oxide, or both. Topical antifungal medication is used to treat *C. albicans* when present.

INFECTIONS OF THE SKIN

Infectious diseases caused by bacteria, viruses, and fungi constitute the major forms of skin disease. Breaks in the skin integrity, particularly those that inoculate pathogens into the dermis and epidermis, may cause or exacerbate infections. Most infections tend to occur superficially; however, systemic signs and symptoms develop occasionally and can be life-threatening in immunosuppressed children.

Bacterial Infections
Impetigo Contagiosum

Impetigo is a common bacterial skin infection in infants and children 2 to 5 years of age. *Staphylococcus aureus* (*S. aureus*) and, less commonly, *Streptococcus pyogenes* cause impetigo. The mode of transmission is by both direct and indirect contact. The disease is more common in midsummer to late summer, with a higher incidence in hot, humid climates. Impetigo is particularly infectious among people living in crowded conditions with poor sanitary facilities or in settings such as daycare facilities. It affects children in good health, but conditions such as anemia and malnutrition are predisposing factors.

Bacterial invasion occurs through minor breaks in the cutaneous surface or as a secondary infection of a preexisting dermatosis or infestation. The staphylococci produce bacterial toxins called *exfoliative toxins (ETs)* that cause a disruption in desmosomal adhesion molecules with blister formation. There are two types of impetigo: nonbullous and, more rarely, bullous (caused only by *S. aureus*) where blisters enlarge or coalesce to form bullae (Box 48.1). Both forms of impetigo begin as vesicles with a thin vesicular roof composed of stratum corneum that ruptures to form a honey-colored crust (Fig. 48.4). The lesions are often located on the face, around the nose and mouth, but the hands and other exposed areas also are involved. The lesions must be differentiated from herpes simplex lesions (see Fig. 47.18). Impetigo is clinically characterized by crusted erosions or ulcers that may arise as a primary infection or as a secondary infection of a preexisting dermatosis or infestation.

BOX 48.1   IMPETIGO

Vesicular Impetigo

- Contagious, acute, superficial, vesiculopustular, and most common form
- Caused by group A *Streptococcus pyogenes* (alone or with *Staphylococcus aureus*)
- Spread by direct physical contact with other infected individuals or through insect bites
- Presents as small vesicles with a honey-colored serum; yellow to white-brown crusts form as vesicles rupture and extend radially
- Untreated lesions last for weeks and cover large area
- Regional lymphadenitis common
- Most significant complication is acute glomerulonephritis
- Treatment is aggressive in light of this complication

Bullous Impetigo

- Caused by *Staphylococcus aureus*
- Bacterial toxin produced (exfoliative toxin [ET]) causes disruption in cellular adhesion with blister formation
- Occurs in neonates
- Highly contagious
- Source is family member with pustule or asymptomatic carrier with pathogen in anterior nares, perineal region, or fingernails
- Transmitted by contact with individual or contaminated equipment
- Presents with vesicles that enlarge or coalesce to form superficial bullae, few localized lesions, or many lesions scattered over the skin surface; as bullae rupture, thin, flat, honey-colored crust appears (hallmark of impetigo)
- Lesions found on face around the nose and mouth; hands and other exposed areas also susceptible

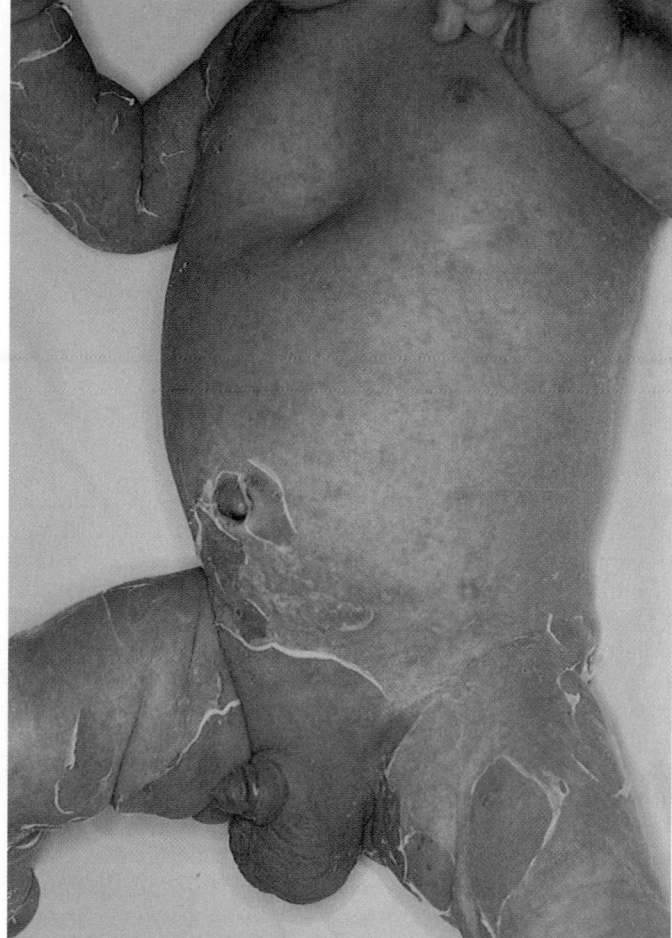

FIGURE 48.5 Staphylococcal Scalded-Skin Syndrome (SSSS). The skin lesions, showing desquamation and wrinkling of the skin margins, appeared 1 day after drainage of a staphylococcal abscess. (From Kliegman RM et al: *Nelson textbook of pediatrics,* ed 19, St Louis, 2011, Saunders.)

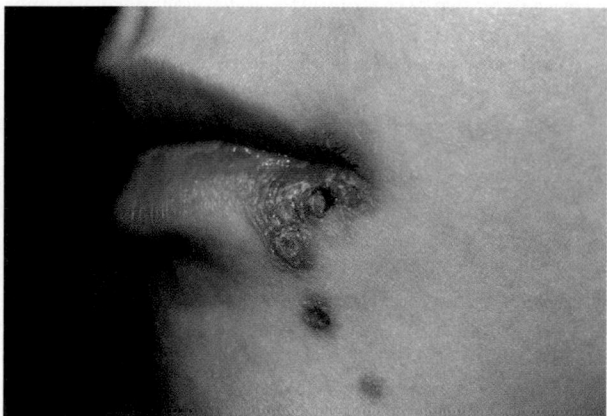

FIGURE 48.4 Impetigo. Multiple crusted and oozing lesions of impetigo. (From Kliegman RM et al: *Nelson textbook of pediatrics,* ed 19, Philadelphia, 2011, Saunders.)

Staphylococcal Scalded-Skin Syndrome

Staphylococcal scalded-skin syndrome (SSSS) is the most serious staphylococcal infection that affects the skin and usually is seen in infants and children younger than 5 years of age. SSSS is caused by virulent group II staphylococci that produce an exfoliative toxin. The toxin attacks desmoglein and adhesion molecules and causes a separation of the skin just below the granular layer of the epidermis. The toxins are usually produced at body sites other than the skin and arrive at the epidermis through the circulatory system. Staphylococci typically are not found in the skin lesions themselves. Adults have circulating antistaphylococcal antibodies and are better able to metabolize and excrete the toxin. Neonates are at the highest risk because of their lack of immunity and no prior exposure to the toxin.[21] A source of the infection in neonates may be from healthcare workers who are nasal carriers of the microorganism. This reinforces the need for good infection control practices for all neonates.[22]

The clinical symptoms begin with fever, malaise, rhinorrhea, and irritability followed by generalized erythema with exquisite tenderness of the skin. There may be an associated impetigo, but the infection often begins in the throat or chest. The erythema spreads from the face and trunk to cover the entire body except the palms, soles, and mucous membranes. Within 24 to 48 hours, blisters and bullae may develop, giving the child the appearance of being scalded (Fig. 48.5). The pain

Treatment of choice for both types of impetigo is topical mupirocin and fusidic acid for uncomplicated lesions. For extensive or complicated impetigo, systemic antibiotics may be warranted, but β-lactam antibiotics should be avoided if methicillin-resistant *S. aureus* (MRSA) is suspected. Prompt treatment avoids complications, such as glomerulonephritis, necrotizing fasciitis, and septic shock syndrome.[19] Using good handwashing techniques and isolating the infected child's washcloth, towels, drinking glass, and linen are important for prevention.[20]

is severe and requires analgesics. Fluid loss from ruptured blisters and water evaporation from denuded areas may cause dehydration and loss of body heat. Perioral and nasolabial crusting and fissures develop. In severe cases the skin of the entire body may slough. When secondary infection can be prevented, healing of the involved skin occurs in 10 to 14 days, usually without scarring.

Before medical intervention is initiated, culture and histologic or exfoliative cytology must be performed to differentiate SSSS from Stevens-Johnson syndrome and toxic epidermal necrolysis, which are associated with drug reactions. When the infection is confirmed, treatment with oral or intravenous antibiotics is begun. Topical antibiotics are ineffective. Fluid balance must be maintained. The skin should be treated the same as that with a severe burn—with meticulous aseptic technique. Skin substitutes may be used for adjuvant therapy. Special care is required in serious cases and when the lips and eyelids are involved.

Fungal Infections

Fungal disorders are known as *mycoses* and, when caused by dermatophytes (fungi that thrive on keratin), the mycoses are termed *tinea* (dermatophytosis or ringworm). The different types of tinea are classified according to their location on the body. Dermatophytes of the genus *Epidermophyton* are the major cause of superficial fungal infections in children. These dermatophytes invade the stratum corneum and not the remainder of the epidermis or dermis. The inflammatory response is a cell-mediated immune response.[23]

Tinea pedis (a chronic, superficial fungal infection of the skin of the foot) occurs in children but is rare. Scaling disorders of the toes and feet in prepubertal children are usually eczema.

Tinea capitis (scalp ringworm), a fungal infection of the scalp, is the most common fungal infection of childhood. It rarely affects infants and is seen in children between 2 and 10 years of age. The primary microorganism responsible for this infection is *Trichophyton tonsurans* (*T. tonsurans*); however, *Microsporum canis* (*M. canis)* also is a pathogenic microorganism in this infection and is found on cats, dogs, and certain rodents. Humans are a terminal host for *M. canis.* Children who handle such animals are possible hosts. Direct transmission between humans does not occur; however, there is direct human transmission of *T. tonsurans,* particularly in crowded areas, the most prevalent environment of the fungus.[24] The prevalence of asymptomatic carriers among household contacts of a child with active *T. tonsurans* disease is high.

The lesions are often circular and manifested by broken hairs 1 to 3 mm above the scalp, leaving a partial area of alopecia from 1 to 5 cm in diameter (Fig. 48.6). A slight erythema and scaling with raised borders can be observed. Diagnosis is best confirmed by potassium hydroxide

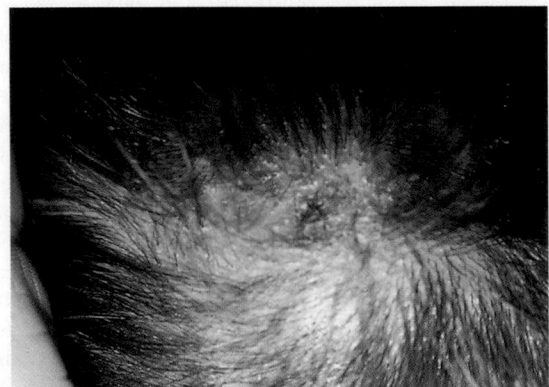

FIGURE 48.6 Tinea Capitis. (Courtesy Department of Dermatology, School of Medicine, University of Utah.)

(KOH) examination, and fungal culture. Use of Wood light examination has become unpopular because there are a number of dermatophytes that fluoresce under an ultraviolet light. Tinea capitis always requires systemic treatment because topical antifungal agents do not penetrate the hair follicle. Several oral antifungal agents, particularly griseofulvin, are available for treatment. Terbinafine, itraconazole, and fluconazole are effective alternatives.[25]

Tinea corporis (ringworm) is a common superficial dermatophyte infection in children. The microorganisms most commonly responsible for this disease are *M. canis* and *Trichophyton mentagrophytes.* As in tinea capitis, contact with kittens and puppies is a common source of the disorder. Tinea corporis preferentially affects the nonhairy parts of the face, trunk, and limbs. Lesions are often erythematous, round or oval scaling patches that spread peripherally with clearing in the center, creating the ring appearance, which is why this disease is commonly referred to as *ringworm.* The lesions are distributed asymmetrically, and multiple lesions (when present) overlap. Transmission occurs by direct contact with an infected lesion and through indirect contact with personal items used by the infected person. Potassium hydroxide examination of the scale from the border of the lesions confirms the diagnosis for most lesions. Most lesions respond well to applications of appropriate topical antifungal medications.[26]

Thrush

Thrush is the term used to describe the presence of *Candida albicans* (*C. albicans*) in the mucous membranes of the mouth of infants. It occurs less commonly in adults; however, infected adults are usually immune compromised. *C. albicans* penetrates the epidermal barrier more easily than other microorganisms because of its keratolytic proteases and other enzymes. It attracts neutrophils to skin sites of invasion but evades neutrophil killing.[27] Thrush is characterized by the formation of white plaques or spots in the mouth that lead to shallow ulcers caused by keratolytic proteases from the microorganism. The tongue may have a dense, white covering. The underlying mucous membrane is red and tender and may bleed when the plaques are removed. The disease is often accompanied by fever and gastrointestinal irritation. The infection commonly spreads to the groin, buttocks, and other parts of the body. Diagnosis is by clinical evaluation but may include direct microscopy.[28]

Treatment may be difficult and may include oral antifungal washes, such as nystatin oral suspension. Simultaneous treatment of a *Candida* nipple infection or vaginitis in the mother is helpful in reducing the *C. albicans* surface colonization of the infant. Feeding bottles and nipples should be sterilized to prevent reinfection.[29]

Viral Infections

Viral infections of the skin in children are caused by poxvirus, papovavirus, and herpesvirus. The most common infections are described here.

Molluscum Contagiosum

Molluscum contagiosum is a common, highly contagious poxvirus infection of the skin epidermis and occasionally conjunctiva that affects school-aged children and sexually active young adults. The disease can be more severe or prolonged in individuals with atopic dermatitis and a variety of immunodeficient states, including acquired immunodeficiency syndrome (AIDS). It is transmitted by skin-to-skin contact (e.g., contact sports), autoinoculation, and fomites, such as clothing, wash devices, and towels, when there is a break in the skin. The poxvirus induces epidermal cell proliferation and blocks immune responses that would control the virus. The epidermis grows down into the dermis to form saccules containing clusters of virus. The characteristic molluscum body

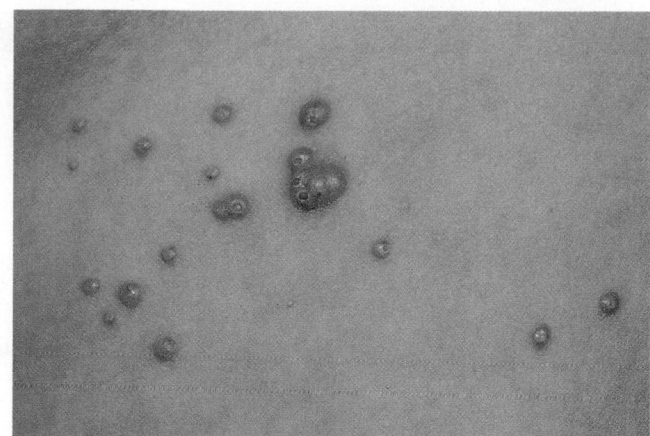

FIGURE 48.7 Molluscum Contagiosum. Waxy pink globules with umbilicated centers. (From Habif TP: *Clinical dermatology: a color guide to diagnosis and therapy*, ed 6, St Louis, 2016, Mosby.)

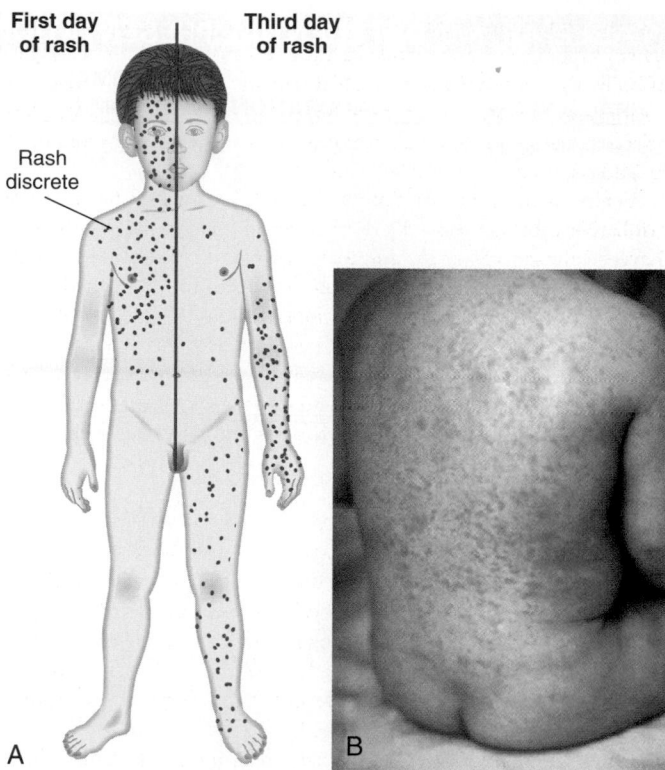

FIGURE 48.8 Rubella (3-Day Measles). **A,** Typical distribution of full-blown maculopapular rash with tendency to coalesce. **B,** Rash of rubella. (From Centers for Disease Control and Prevention: Public Health Image Library, Figure #712. Available at: https://phil.cdc.gov/phil/quicksearch.asp. Accessed November 18, 2016.)

is composed of mature, immature, and incomplete viruses and cellular debris. The lesions of molluscum are discrete, slightly umbilicated, dome-shaped, waxy or pearl-like papules 1 to 5 mm in diameter that appear anywhere on the skin or conjunctiva. The skin distribution in children is mainly on the trunk, face, and extremities (Fig. 48.7). The pubic, genital, and perineal areas are favored in adults. Usually no inflammation surrounds molluscum lesions unless they are traumatized or secondary infection occurs. Scarring may occur with healing.[30]

The best diagnostic procedures are (1) visual inspection using dermoscopy that may be combined with reflectance confocal microscopy, (2) staining smears of the expressed molluscum body, (3) examining a biopsy, (4) inoculating a molluscum suspension into cell cultures to demonstrate the cytotoxic reactions, and (5) polymerase chain reaction amplification of parts of the molluscum contagiosum virus genome.[30] Most lesions are self-limiting and clear in 6 to 9 months if not manipulated. However, because children often do manipulate these lesions, spontaneous involution may take 2 to 4 years without therapy.

Treatment options include immunomodulatory and antiviral therapy and destructive procedures (cryotherapy, curettage, or laser ablation); however, no treatment is universally effective. Cantharidin, a compound secreted by the blister beetle, is the most commonly used therapeutic, and it is thought to kill the virus and trigger an antiviral immune response.[31] Treatment is recommended for genital molluscum to prevent sexual transmission and autoinoculation. Destructive therapy is poorly tolerated by children. Measures to prevent spread of infection must be taken, and recurrences are common.[32]

Rubella (German or 3-Day Measles)

Rubella is a common communicable disease of children and young adults caused by a ribonucleic acid (RNA) virus that enters the bloodstream through the respiratory route. This disease is mild in most children. The incubation period ranges from 14 to 21 days. Prodromal symptoms are few but may include enlarged cervical and postauricular lymph nodes, low-grade fever, headache, sore throat, runny nose, and cough. A faint pink-to-red, coalescing maculopapular rash develops on the face, with spread to the trunk and extremities, sparing the palms of the hands and soles of the feet, 1 to 4 days after the onset of initial symptoms (Fig. 48.8). The rash is thought to be the result of virus dissemination to the skin. The rash subsides after 2 to 3 days, usually without complications. Children are generally not contagious after development of the rash. Differential presentations of viral diseases producing rashes are given in Table 48.1.

Vaccination for rubella is usually combined with vaccines for mumps and measles (rubeola) (MMR). The Centers for Disease Control and Prevention vaccine recommendations are available at http://www.cdc.gov/vaccines/schedules/index.html. Measles are known to occur in previously immunized children.[33] Rubella has almost been eliminated in the United States because of vaccination campaigns. However, challenges to maintain elimination include large outbreaks of measles in highly traveled developed countries, frequent international travel, and clusters of U.S. residents who remain unvaccinated because of personal belief exemptions.[34] Rubella virus is a candidate for global eradication, as humans are the only known host.

Although the MMR vaccine may rarely be associated with adverse neurologic events (e.g., seizures because of fever, deafness), studies conclude that MMR immunization does not cause autism.[35,36] However, findings in congenital rubella syndrome (which can occur when pregnant women contract the rubella virus during the first trimester of pregnancy) share an overlap of findings in autism, including deafness, congenital heart disease, hyperactivity, spasticity, and increased risk for type 1 diabetes as young adults. Some sources have proposed that rubella is a vaccine-preventable cause of autism.[37,38] The benefits of vaccination exceed the lack of vaccination, which leads to significant morbidity and mortality, with pneumonia, croup, and encephalitis being causes of death worldwide.[39]

Women of childbearing age are immunized if their rubella hemagglutination-inhibition titer is low. Pregnancy should be avoided for 3 months after vaccination because the attenuated virus in the vaccine may remain for this period. However, accidental receipt of MMR vaccination is not known to cause maternal or fetal complications, or both.[40] Pregnant women who have rubella early in the first trimester

TABLE 48.1	DIFFERENTIAL PRESENTATION OF VIRAL DISEASES PRODUCING RASHES			
VIRAL DISEASE	INCUBATION	PRODROMAL SYMPTOMS	DURATION/ CHARACTERISTICS	CLINICAL SYMPTOMS
Rubella (German measles; rubivirus)	14–21 days	1–2 days Mild fever Malaise Respiratory symptoms	1–3 days Pink-red maculopapular rash Face and trunk	Enlarged and tender occipital and periauricular nodes
Rubeola (measles; paramyxovirus)	7–12 days	2–5 days Fever Cough Respiratory symptoms	3–5 days Purple-red to brown maculopapular papules Face, trunk, extremities	Koplik spots 1–3 days before rash Rash develops when fever subsides
Roseola (exanthema subitum; human herpesvirus 6 and 7)	5–15 days	2–5 days High fever	1–3 days Pink-red macular papules Neck and trunk	
Varicella (chickenpox; herpes zoster virus)	11–20 days	1–2 days Low-grade fever Cough May be asymptomatic	Red papules, vesicles, pustules in clusters	Eruption of new lesions for 4–5 days Occasional ulcerative lesion in the mouth
Hand, foot, and mouth disease (coxsackie A virus)	4–6 days	Fever, sore throat, anorexia	3–7 days Gray thick-walled vesicles 3–6 mm in diameter on a red or noninflamed base, commonly on palms and soles and sides of feet, and mouth mucosa	None or fever, diarrhea, sore throat

may have a fetal death or a fetus that develops congenital defects (congenital rubella syndrome).[38]

There is no specific treatment for rubella. Recovery is spontaneous, although lymph nodes may remain enlarged for weeks. Supportive therapy includes rest, fluids, and use of a vaporizer. In rare cases a mild encephalitis or peripheral neuritis may follow rubella.

Rubeola (Red Measles)

Rubeola is a highly contagious, acute viral disease of children. It is transmitted by direct contact with droplets from infected persons and is caused by an RNA-containing paramyxovirus with an incubation period of 7 to 12 days, during which there are no symptoms. The virus enters the respiratory tract and attaches to dendritic cells and alveolar macrophages, amplifies in local lymphatic tissue, and progresses to systemic disease.[41] Prodromal symptoms include high fever (up to 40.5°C [104.9°F]), malaise, enlarged lymph nodes, runny nose, conjunctivitis, and "barking" cough. Within 3 to 4 days, an erythematous maculopapular rash develops over the head and spreads distally over the trunk, extremities, hands, and feet. Early lesions blanch with pressure, followed by a brownish hue that does not blanch as the rash fades. Characteristic pinpoint white spots surrounded by an erythematous ring develop over the buccal mucosa and are known as *Koplik spots*. These spots precede the rash by 1 to 2 days and are usually missed because they appear so early. The rash then subsides within 3 to 5 days.

Complications associated with measles may be caused by the primary infection or a secondary bacterial infection. Measles encephalitis occurs in about 1 of 800 cases, and most children recover completely. Only a small minority develop permanent brain damage or die. Bacterial complications include otitis media and pneumonia, usually caused by group A hemolytic streptococcus, *Haemophilus influenzae*, or *S. aureus* infection.

Measles is prevented by vaccination although suboptimal vaccine delivery in developing countries and vaccination refusal have prevented

eradication. Postexposure prophylaxis with antivirals is a strategy for complementing vaccination and preventing viral transmission.[42] There is no specific treatment for measles, and supportive therapy is the same as for rubella. Antibiotic therapy is initiated if secondary bacterial infections develop.

Roseola (Exanthema Subitum or 6th Disease)

Roseola is caused by human herpesviruses 6 or 7 in infants between 6 months and 2 years of age, but it can be seen in children as old as 4 years. The incubation period is 5 to 15 days, followed by the sudden onset of fever (38.9° to 40.5°C [102° to 104.5°F]) that lasts 3 to 5 days. After the fever an erythematous, nonpruritic macular rash that lasts about 24 to 48 hours develops, primarily over the trunk, neck, and arms. Children usually feel well, eat normally, and have few other symptoms. Usually no treatment is required and there are no complications.[43]

Chickenpox and Herpes Zoster

Chickenpox (varicella) and herpes zoster (shingles) are both produced by the varicella-zoster virus (VZV). VZV is a complex deoxyribonucleic acid (DNA) virus of the herpes group. The incubation period is 10 to 27 days, averaging 14 days. Vesicular lesions occur in the epidermis as infection occurs within keratinocytes. An inflammatory infiltrate is often present. Vesicles eventually rupture, followed by crust formation or the development of transient ulcers on mucous membranes. Varicella occurs in people not previously exposed to VZV, whereas herpes zoster (shingles) occurs in individuals who had varicella in the past. The virus enters the dorsal root ganglia and remains latent (see Chapter 47 and Fig. 47.19). Since the introduction of live attenuated VZV vaccine in 1995, there has been a significant reduction in varicella incidence and its associated complications.[44]

Chickenpox (Varicella). Chickenpox is a disease of early childhood, with 90% of children contracting the disease during the first decade of life. It is a highly contagious virus that is spread by close

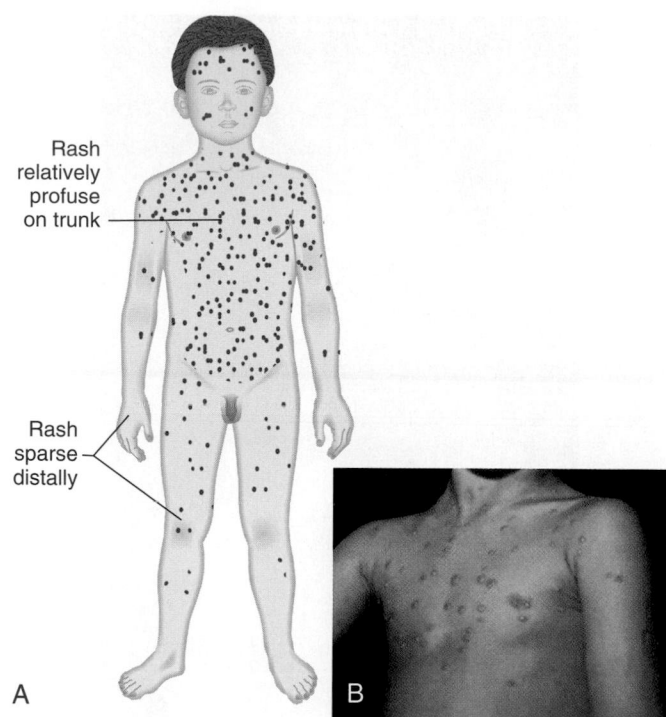

Rash relatively profuse on trunk

Rash sparse distally

A

B

FIGURE 48.9 Chickenpox. **A,** Pattern of generalized, polymorphous eruption. **B,** Chickenpox lesions on fifth day of illness. (From Centers for Disease Control and Prevention: Image Bank, Figure #2882. Available at: https://phil.cdc.gov/phil/quicksearch.asp. Accessed November 18, 2016.)

person-to-person contact and airborne droplets. Introduction of an infected person into a household results in a 90% possibility of susceptible persons in the household developing the disease within the incubation period—usually 14 days. Children are contagious for at least 1 day before development of the rash. Transmission of the virus may occur until approximately 5 to 6 days after the onset of the first skin lesions in healthy children. In immunocompromised children the virus is recoverable for a longer period, but these children must be considered contagious for at least 7 to 10 days. Healthy children who develop chickenpox have no prodromal symptoms. The first sign of illness may be itching or the appearance of vesicles, usually on the trunk, scalp, or face. The rash later spreads to the extremities. Characteristically, lesions can be seen in various stages of maturation with macules, papules, and vesicles present in a particular area at the same time (Fig. 48.9). The vesicular lesions are superficial and can be easily ruptured. New lesions will erupt for 4 to 5 days, until there are approximately 100 to 300 in different stages of development. The vesicles become crusted, with only the crust remaining. Occasionally a vesicle may appear on the palm later in the disease. Although uncommon, ulcerative lesions are sometimes seen in the mouth and, less commonly, on the conjunctiva and pharynx. Fever usually lasts 2 to 3 days and ranges from 38.5° to 40°C [101.3° to 104°F]).

Complications are rare in children but more common in adults. They can include transient hematuria (from rupture of vesicles in the bladder), epistaxis, laryngeal edema, and varicella pneumonia. One case of chickenpox produces almost complete immunity against a second attack. Rarely, the fetus may be malformed (congenital varicella syndrome) if chickenpox develops in the mother in the first trimester of pregnancy. Infants whose mothers have chickenpox at any stage of pregnancy have a higher risk of developing herpes zoster during the

first few years of life. Administration of maternal varicella-zoster immunoglobulin before rash development, with or without antiviral medication, can modify the progression of the disease.[45]

Uncomplicated chickenpox requires no specific therapy. Baths, wet dressings, and oral antihistamines are occasionally helpful to relieve itching and to prevent secondary infection as a result of scratching. Oral antistaphylococcal drugs should be given if secondary bacterial infection is present. Zoster immune globulin may be administered to immunodeficient individuals if given within 72 hours after exposure to chickenpox. Prophylactic acyclovir may be valuable in immunosuppressed or other select groups of children.[46] The varicella vaccine protects against both varicella and herpes zoster. However, wild-type (vaccine-resistant) viruses are a continuing threat.[47]

Hand, Foot, and Mouth Disease. Hand, foot, and mouth disease (HFMD) is a contagious viral disease primarily of infants and young children. It is commonly caused by the coxsackievirus A16 (CV-A16) and the enterovirus 71 (EV-A71), although coxsackievirus A6 and coxsackievirus A10 have been associated with sporadic cases. The infection manifests fever, vesicular ulcerous lesions in the mouth, and vesicular rashes on the hands, feet, and buttocks. A small number of children may experience severe complications, such as meningitis, encephalitis, acute flaccid paralysis, and neurorespiratory syndrome. The disease is self-limiting with supportive care. Research is in progress to develop a preventive vaccine.[48,49]

Herpes Zoster. Although herpes zoster (shingles) occurs mainly in adults, approximately 5% of cases are in children younger than 15 years. The pathophysiology and treatment are reviewed in Chapter 47.

Smallpox

Smallpox (variola) is a highly contagious and deadly but preventable disease caused by poxvirus variolae. Smallpox was eradicated worldwide in 1977. Routine vaccination in the United States was discontinued in 1972, and a new vaccine, ACAM2000, has been produced for the U.S. Strategic National Stockpile. Information is available from the Food and Drug Administration at www.fda.gov/biologicsbloodvaccines/vaccines/approvedproducts/ucm180810.htm.

INSECT BITES AND PARASITES

Insect bites and infestations are common causes of skin disorders in children and adults. Skin damage occurs by various mechanisms, including trauma of bites and stings, allergic reactions, transmission of disease, injection of substances that cause local or systemic reactions, and inflammatory reactions from retained mouthparts. Scabies and pediculosis are the most common parasitic skin infections. Lyme disease is a tick-bite–associated illness and is discussed in Chapter 47.

Scabies

Scabies is a contagious disease caused by the itch mite, *Sarcoptes scabiei* (Fig. 48.10, *A*), which can colonize the human epidermis.[50] Scabies is a common skin infection in tropical settings and affects large numbers of people, particularly children. It is transmitted by personal contact and by infected clothing and linens. Scabies is often epidemic in areas of overcrowded housing, in areas with poor sanitation, or in long-term care institutions. The scabies mite has adapted mechanisms to overcome host defenses, including complement inhibitors.[51] Immunocompromised individuals are at greater risk. Scabies can facilitate *Streptococcus pyogenes* and *Staphylococcus aureus* skin infection. Infestation is initiated by a female mite that tunnels into the stratum corneum, depositing eggs and creating a burrow several millimeters to 1 cm long. Over a 3-week period, the eggs mature into adult mites, which sometimes can be recognized as tiny dots at the end of intact burrows.

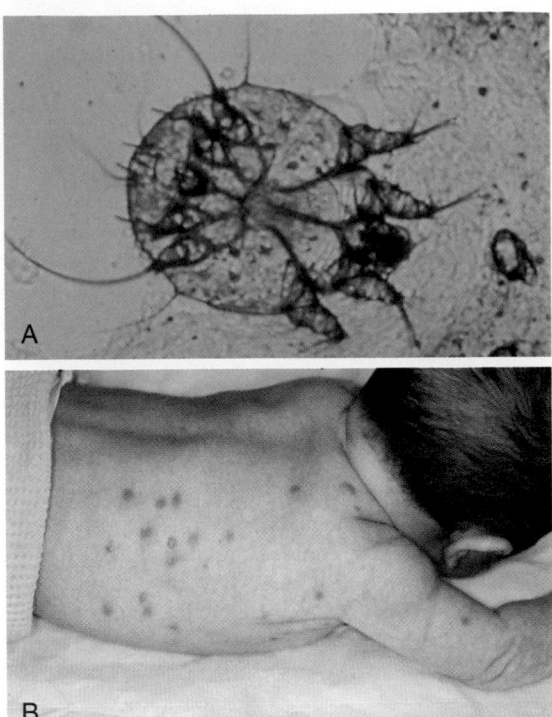

FIGURE 48.10 Scabies. A, Scabies mite, as seen clinically when removed from its burrow. **B,** Characteristic scabies bites. (Courtesy Department of Dermatology, School of Medicine, University of Utah.)

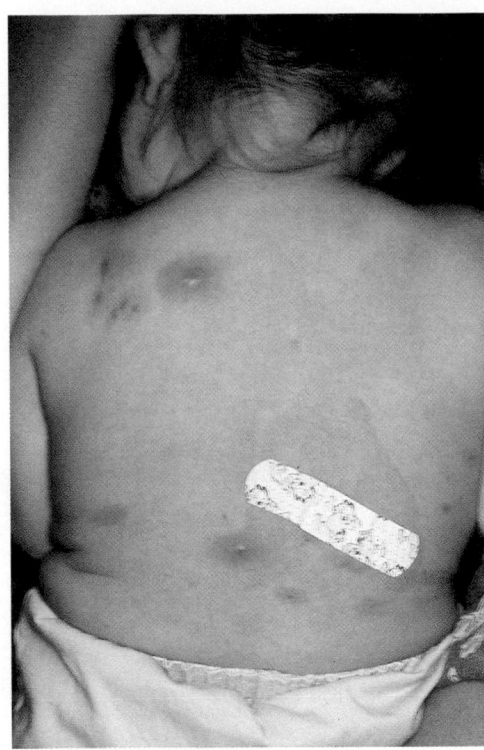

FIGURE 48.11 Flea Bites. Flea bite producing an urticarial wheal with central puncture. (Courtesy Department of Pediatrics, Division of Allergy and Immunology, National Jewish Health.)

The primary lesions are burrows 2 to 15 mm in length, papules, and vesicular lesions with severe itching that worsens at night. Two or three bites (commonly referred to as *breakfast, lunch, and dinner*) usually appear in a line on exposed areas of the skin. Pruritus is related to a type IV sensitivity reaction to the mite and its saliva, eggs, and feces. Consequently, the first symptoms appear 3 to 5 weeks after primary infestation and 1 to 2 days after reinfestation. In older children and adults, the lesions occur in the webs of fingers, axillae, and creases of the arms and wrists; along the belt line; and around the nipples, genitalia, and lower buttocks. Infants and young children have a different pattern of distribution, with involvement of the palms, soles, head, back, neck, and face (see Fig. 48.10, *B*). Secondary infections and crusting develop from scratching and eczematous changes.

Diagnosis of scabies is made by observation of the tunnels and burrows and by scraping of the skin with microscopic examination of the mite or its eggs or feces. Treatment involves the application of a scabicide or oral ivermectin, which is curative. Even with elimination of all viable scabies microorganisms, pruritus may persist for 10 days or longer. All clothing and linens should be washed and dried in hot cycles or dry-cleaned.

Pediculosis (Lice Infestation)

The three known types of human lice are (1) the head louse *(Pediculus capitis, most common)*, (2) the body louse *(Pediculus corporis)*, and (3) the crab or pubic louse *(Phthirus pubis)*.[50] They are highly contagious parasites that survive by sucking blood. The female louse has a 1-month life span and produces about 7 to 10 eggs (nits) per day, and mates and reproduces every 3 to 4 weeks. The mouthparts are shaped for piercing and sucking and attach to the skin while feeding. When piercing the skin, the louse secretes a toxic saliva; the mechanical trauma and toxin produce a pruritic dermatitis. Head and body lice are acquired directly by personal contact or indirectly by sharing combs, brushes, towels, or

contact with infested clothes, toys, furniture, carpets, or bedding. Crab lice are spread by body contact, such as contact with an infected adult. Other common sources of transmission include sharing clothing or headphones.

Pruritus is the major symptom of lice infestation. In head lice infestation the ova attach to hairs above the ears and in the occipital region. The primary lesion of the body louse is a pinpoint red macule, papule, or wheal with a hemorrhagic puncture site. The primary lesion often is not seen because it is masked by excoriations, wheals, and crusts. The crab louse is found on pubic hairs but also may involve other body hair such as eyelashes, mustache, beard, and axillae. Young children particularly may become infected with crab lice on their eyebrows or eyelashes.

The live louse, 2 to 3 mm long, is rarely observed, although the ova, or nits, can be observed as oval, yellowish pinpoint specks fastened to a hair shaft. The ova fluoresce under an ultraviolet light (Wood lamp) and can be best observed with a microscope. Infestations can be treated with a topical pediculicide (i.e., permethrin) or oral ivermectin. Head and pubic lice can be treated with wet combing every 3 days for 2 weeks to remove all nits, but it is less effective. All clothes, towels, bedding, combs, and brushes should be washed and dried in hot air or boiled, or the clothes should be ironed. Individuals who have personal contact also should be treated.

Fleas

Fleas are wingless, jumping insects that feed on blood. Young children are very susceptible to flea bites; the most common are the bites of cat, dog, and human fleas *(Pulex irritans)*.[52] Bites occur in clusters along the arms and legs or where clothing fits tightly. The bite produces an urticarial wheal with a central hemorrhagic puncture (Fig. 48.11). Flea bites can transmit plague, tularemia, and cat-scratch disease (caused by the bacterium *Bartonella henselae*). Treatment includes spraying

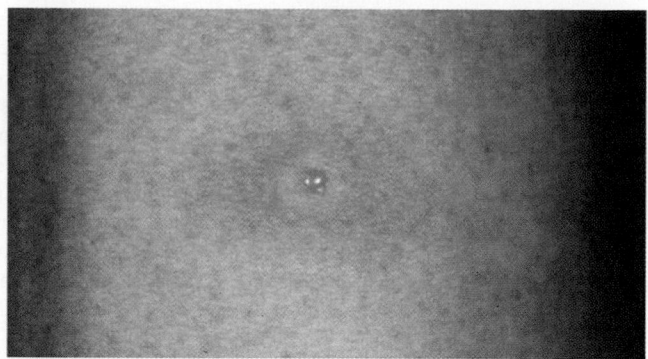

FIGURE 48.12 Bullous Bedbug Bites. (Courtesy Department of Dermatology, School of Medicine, University of Utah.)

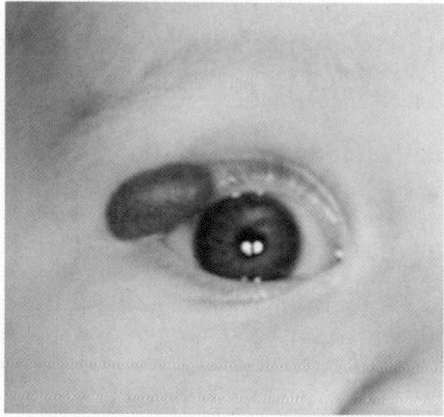

FIGURE 48.13 Strawberry Hemangioma. (Courtesy Department of Dermatology, School of Medicine, University of Utah.)

carpets, crevices, and furniture with malathion or lindane powder. Infected animals should be treated, and clothes and bedding should be washed in hot water.

Bedbugs

Bedbugs *(Cimex lectularius)* are blood-sucking parasites that live in the crevices and cracks of floors, walls, and furniture and in bedding or furniture stuffing. They are 3 to 5 mm long and reddish brown. Bedbugs are nocturnal, emerging to feed in darkness by attaching to the skin to suck blood, and are attracted by warmth and carbon dioxide. Feeding occurs for 5 to 15 minutes; then the bedbug leaves. It will move long distances to search for food and can travel from house to house.

Immunologic reactions to bedbug saliva vary, but bites typically yield erythematous and pruritic papules. The face and distal extremities, areas uncovered by sleeping clothes or blankets, are preferentially involved. If the host has not been previously sensitized, the only symptom is a red macule that develops into a nodule, lasting up to 14 days. In sensitized children and adults, pruritic wheals, papules, and vesicles may form (Fig. 48.12) and, rarely, anemia and angioedema. Most lesions respond to antihistamines or corticosteroids. Secondary infections require antibiotic treatment. Bedbugs are eliminated by inspecting and cleaning or disposing of bedding, mattresses, furniture, and other contaminated items, and by using applications of approved insecticides, usually by a professional.[53]

CUTANEOUS HEMANGIOMAS AND VASCULAR MALFORMATIONS

Cutaneous vascular anomalies are frequent tumors of early infancy and can be categorized as either vascular tumors (hemangiomas) or vascular malformations.[54]

Cutaneous Hemangiomas

Cutaneous hemangiomas are benign tumors that form from the rapid growth of vascular endothelial cells, which results in formation of extra blood vessels. Hemangiomas can be superficial or deep. *Superficial hemangiomas* are known as *infantile (capillary)* or *strawberry hemangiomas*. Deep lesions are known as *cavernous* or *congenital hemangiomas*. The etiology may be related to embolization of fetal placental endothelial cells with placental trauma or loss of placental angiogenic inhibitor of placental and maternal origin. Superficial hemangiomas are associated with endothelial glucose transporter 1 (GLUT1). There is proliferation of mast cells that are thought to promote the angiogenesis. Infiltration of fat cells, fibrosis, and the rich vascular network give the lesions a firm, rubbery feel. Females are affected more often than males.

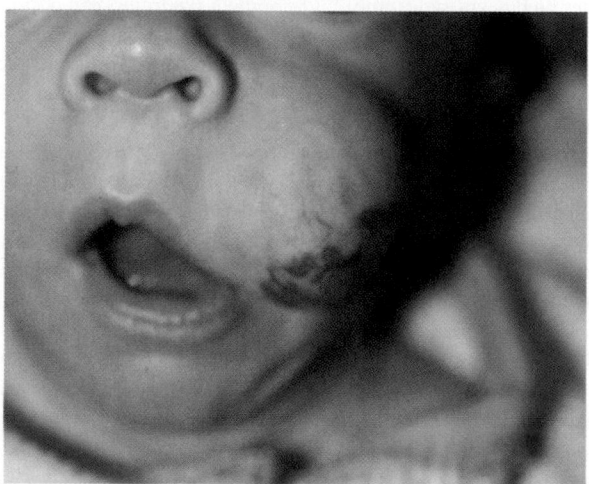

FIGURE 48.14 Cavernous Hemangioma. (Courtesy Department of Dermatology, School of Medicine, University of Utah.)

About 30% of hemangiomas are apparent at birth, but usually emerge during the first few weeks after birth. They grow rapidly during the first few years of life and become bright red and elevated with minute capillary projections that give them a strawberry appearance. Only one lesion is usually present and is located on the head and neck area or trunk (Fig. 48.13). After the initial growth, the lesion grows at the same rate as the child and then starts to involute at 12 to 16 months of age. Approximately 90% of strawberry hemangiomas involute by 5 to 9 years of age, usually without scarring. Most superficial hemangiomas require no treatment. Hemangiomas located over the eye, ear, nose, mouth, urethra, or anus may require treatment because they interfere with function and have a higher risk for infection or injury.

Cavernous hemangiomas are a rare variant of superficial hemangiomas and are GLUT1-negative. They are a fully grown solitary lesion present at birth and primarily located on the head, neck, or limbs. They appear as a spongy purplish mass of tissue with more mature and larger vessels within the lesion (Fig. 48.14). There are two groups of cavernous hemangiomas: rapidly involuting and noninvoluting. Rapidly involuting cavernous hemangiomas disappear by 12 months to 14 months of age, leaving an area of thin skin. Noninvoluting cavernous hemangiomas do not undergo involution.

Rapidly progressing hemangiomas are treated with a beta-blocker (e.g., propranolol),[55] which should be considered a first-line agent, with regression occurring within 2 weeks. Other therapies include systemic or intralesional steroids. Cryosurgery, laser surgery, sclerotherapy, and embolization are alterative treatment options. Interferons, vincristine, cyclophosphamide, and radiotherapy can suppress angiogenesis.[54]

Cutaneous Vascular Malformations

Cutaneous vascular malformations are rare congenital anomalies of blood vessels present at birth but may not be apparent for several years. They grow proportionately with the child and never regress.[54] The malformations occur equally among males and females. Occasionally they expand rapidly, particularly during the hormonal changes of puberty or pregnancy and in association with trauma. Vascular malformations are classified as low flow or high flow. *Low-flow malformations* involve capillaries, veins, and lymphatics. *High-flow malformations* are arteriovenous malformations. In addition to locations within the skin they may involve the gastrointestinal tract, bone, facial capillary malformation, skin, vascular malformation of the eye, and vascular malformation of the brain (Maffucci syndrome, Sturge-Weber syndrome, or blue rubber bleb nevus syndrome).[56] *Overgrowth syndromes* can occur with either high- or low-flow malformations, with overgrowth of the underlying structures (i.e., legs, arms, facial bones). The most common vascular malformation is nevus flammeus (port-wine stain) and salmon patches (stork bite, angel kiss).

Port-wine (nevus flammeus) stains are low-flow congenital malformations of the dermal capillaries. The lesions are flat and their color ranges from pink to dark reddish purple. They are present at birth or within a few days after birth and do not fade with age. Involvement of the face and other body surfaces is common, and the lesions may be large. Sturge-Weber syndrome is a port-wine stain distributed along the ophthalmic branch of the trigeminal nerve and is associated with the leptomeninges of the brain and choroid, glaucoma, seizures, stroke, and intellectual disability. These capillary malformations are associated with a mutation in the *GNAQ* gene (guanine nucleotide-binding protein G, q polypeptide). The lesions are flat, and their color ranges from pink to dark reddish purple. They are present at birth or within a few days after birth and do not fade with age. Involvement of the face and other body surfaces is common, and the lesions may be large (Fig. 48.15).

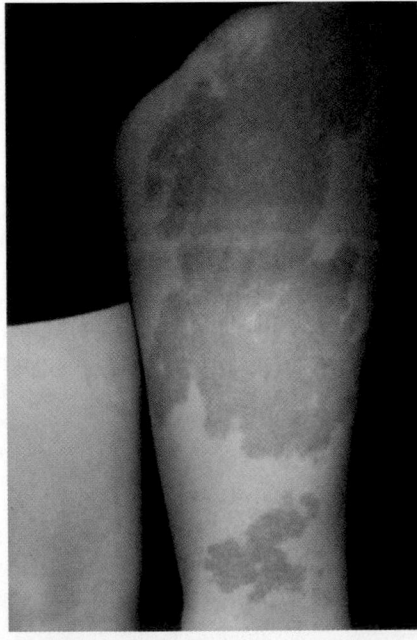

FIGURE 48.15 Capillary Malformation in a Child. (Courtesy Department of Dermatology, School of Medicine, University of Utah.)

During adolescence and later adult years, the port-wine stain may become papular and cavernous. The pulsed dye laser is the treatment of choice to successfully lighten the color and flatten the more nodular and cavernous lesions.[54] Waterproof cosmetics may be used to cover the lesions.

Salmon patches (nevus simplex) are macular pink lesions present at birth and located on the nape of the neck, forehead, upper eyelids, or nasolabial fold. They are a more superficial variant of nevus flammeus and one of the most common congenital malformations in the skin. The pink color results from distended dermal capillaries, and 95% of patches fade by 1 to 3 years of age. Those located at the nape of the neck may persist for a lifetime, but generally do not present a cosmetic problem.

OTHER SKIN DISORDERS

Miliaria

Miliaria is a dermatosis commonly seen in infants and is characterized by a vesicular eruption after prolonged exposure to perspiration, with subsequent obstruction of the eccrine ducts. There are two forms of miliaria: miliaria crystallina and miliaria rubra. In *miliaria crystallina*, ductal rupture occurs within the stratum corneum and appears as 1- to 2-mm clear vesicles without erythema. They rupture within 24 to 48 hours and leave a white scale. In miliaria rubra, the ductal rupture occurs in the lower epidermis, with inflammatory cells attracted to the site of the rupture. *Miliaria rubra (prickly heat)* is characterized by 2- to 4-mm discrete erythematous papules or papulovesicles (Fig. 48.16). Both forms resolve spontaneously, but may become secondarily infected, requiring treatment with systemic antibiotics. The key to management is avoidance of excessive heat and humidity, which cause sweating. Light clothing, cool baths, and air conditioning assist in keeping the skin surface dry and cool.

Erythema Toxicum Neonatorum

Erythema toxicum neonatorum (toxic erythema of the newborn) is a benign, erythematous accumulation of macules, papules, or pustules that appears at birth or 3 to 4 days after birth. The lesions first appear as a blotchy, macular erythematous rash. The macules vary from 1 mm to 1 cm. When papules or pustules develop, they are light yellow or white and 1 to 3 mm in diameter. There may be few or several hundred lesions, and any surface of the body can be affected, with the exception of the palms and soles, where there are no pilosebaceous follicles. The cause of the lesion is unknown, but it may be related to an innate immune response to the first commensal microflora with release of mast cell mediators. Eosinophils are abundant in the lesions.[57] It is self-limiting and resolves spontaneously within a few weeks of birth. No treatment is required.

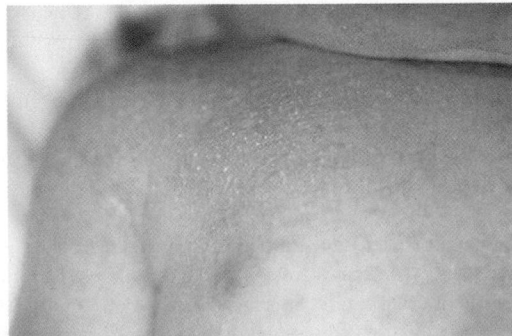

FIGURE 48.16 Miliaria Rubra. Note discrete erythematous papules or papulovesicles. (Courtesy Department of Dermatology, School of Medicine, University of Utah.)

SUMMARY REVIEW

Acne Vulgaris

1. Acne vulgaris is the most common skin disease, affecting 85% of the population between the ages of 12 and 25 years.
2. Acne is characterized by noninflammatory and inflammatory lesions related to follicular hyperkeratinization, excessive sebum production, plugging of sebaceous glands, and *P. acnes* colonization. Acne conglobata is a severe form of acne with communicating cysts and abscesses. The cause is unknown.

Dermatitis

1. Atopic dermatitis is associated with complex immunologic responses, a family history of asthma and hay fever, and deficient filaggrin protein resulting in altered skin barrier function. Red, scaly lesions commonly occur on the face, cheeks, and flexor surfaces of the extremities in infants and young children.
2. Diaper dermatitis is a type of irritant contact dermatitis initiated by a combination of factors that include prolonged exposure to urine and feces; frequently the infant becomes infected secondarily with *Candida albicans*.

Infections of the Skin

1. Impetigo is a contagious bacterial disease caused by *Staphylococcus aureus* (*S. aureus*) and, less commonly, *Streptococcus pyogenes* that occurs in two forms: bullous and vesicular (contagious). The toxins from the bacteria produce a weeping lesion with a honey-colored crust.
2. SSSS is a group II staphylococcal skin infection that produces an exfoliative toxin and occurs more commonly in young children with low titers of antistaphylococcal antibody. Painful blisters and bullae form over large areas of the skin, requiring systemic antibiotics for treatment.
3. Dermatophytes of the genus *Epidermophyton* invade the stratum corneum and are the major cause of superficial fungal (tinea) infections in children.
4. Tinea capitis (infection of the scalp) and tinea corporis (infection of the body) are fungal infections caused by dermatophytes.
5. *C. albicans* infection is a superficial fungal infection of the mouth (thrush).
6. Molluscum contagiosum is a poxvirus of the skin that produces pale papular lesions filled with viral and cellular debris.
7. Rubella (also known as *German* or *3-day measles*) is a communicable disease characterized by fever, sore throat, enlarged cervical and postauricular nodes, and a generalized maculopapular rash that lasts 1 to 4 days.
8. Rubeola is a highly contagious disease of children. Symptoms include high fever, enlarged lymph nodes, conjunctivitis, and a red rash that begins on the head and spreads to the trunk and extremities and lasts 3 to 5 days. Bacterial and viral complications may accompany rubeola.
9. Roseola is a benign disease of infants with a sudden onset of fever that lasts 3 to 5 days, followed by a rash that lasts 24 hours.
10. Chickenpox (varicella) is a highly contagious disease caused by VZV. Vesicular lesions occur on the skin and mucous membranes. Individuals are contagious from 1 day before the development of the rash until about 6 days after the rash develops.
11. Herpes zoster (shingles) is a viral eruption of vesicles on the skin along the distribution of a sensory nerve caused by latent activation of VZV. Children with immune suppression develop more serious complications.
12. Hand, foot, and mouth disease is a contagious disease caused by coxsackievirus A16 (CV-A16) and enterovirus 71 (EV-A71) with vesicular lesions in the mouth and on the hands, feet, and buttocks.
13. Smallpox (variola) is a highly contagious, deadly disease that has been eradicated worldwide by vaccination.

Insect Bites and Parasites

1. Scabies is an itching lesion caused by the itch mite that burrows into the skin, forming papules and vesicles. The mite is very contagious and is transmitted by direct contact.
2. Pediculosis (lice infestation) is caused by blood-sucking parasites that secrete a toxic saliva and damage the skin to produce a pruritic dermatitis. Lice are spread by direct contact and are recognized by the ova, or nits, that attach to the shaft of body hairs.
3. Flea bites produce a pruritic wheal with a central puncture site and occur as clusters in areas of tight-fitting clothing.
4. Bedbugs are blood-sucking parasites that live in cracks of floors, furniture, or bedding and feed at night. They produce pruritic wheals and nodules.

Cutaneous Hemangiomas and Vascular Malformations

1. Hemangiomas are benign vascular tumors that emerge at birth and resolve spontaneously through the childhood years. Strawberry hemangiomas (distinct, raised vascular lesions) are more superficial, and cavernous hemangiomas, with larger and more mature vessels, are deeper lesions.
2. Vascular malformations are congenital anomalies of blood vessels. Low-flow malformations involve capillaries, veins, and lymphatics; high-flow malformations involve arteries.
3. Nevus flammeus (port-wine stain) is a deeper congenital malformation of the dermal capillaries, and salmon patches are more superficial vascular malformations.

Other Skin Disorders

1. Miliaria is characterized by small pruritic papules or vesicles that result from prolonged exposure to perspiration and subsequent obstruction of the eccrine ducts in infants.
2. Erythema toxicum neonatorum is a benign, erythematous accumulation of macules, papules, and pustules that appear at birth or 3 to 4 days after birth and then spontaneously resolve within a few weeks.

KEY TERMS

Acne conglobata, 1531
Acne vulgaris, 1530
Atopic dermatitis (AD), 1531
Bedbug, 1539
Cavernous hemangioma, 1539
Chickenpox, 1536

Cutaneous hemangioma, 1539
Cutaneous vascular malformation, 1540
Diaper dermatitis, 1532
Erythema toxicum neonatorum, 1540
Flea bite, 1538
Hand, foot, and mouth disease (HFMD), 1537

Impetigo, 1532
Inflammatory acne, 1530
Miliaria, 1540
Molluscum contagiosum, 1534
Noninflammatory acne, 1530
Port-wine (nevus flammeus) stain, 1540

KEY TERMS—cont'd

REFERENCES

1. Bhate K, Williams HC: Epidemiology of acne vulgaris. *Br J Dermatol* 168(3):474–485, 2013.
2. Eichenfield LF, et al: Evolving perspectives on the etiology and pathogenesis of acne vulgaris. *J Drugs Dermatol* 14(3):263–272, 2015.
3. Kistowska M, et al: Propionibacterium acnes promotes Th17 and Th17/Th1 responses in acne patients. *J Invest Dermatol* 135(1):110–118, 2015.
4. Zaenglein AL, et al: Guidelines of care for the management of acne vulgaris. *J Am Acad Dermatol* 74(5):945–973, 2016.
5. Bhate K, Williams HC: What's new in acne? An analysis of systematic reviews published in 2011-2012. *Clin Exp Dermatol* 39(3):273–277, 2014.
6. Liu PF, et al: Propionibacterium acnes in the pathogenesis and immunotherapy of acne vulgaris. *Curr Drug Metab* 16(4):245–254, 2015.
7. Eichenfield LF, et al: Guidelines of care for the management of atopic dermatitis: section 1. Diagnosis and assessment of atopic dermatitis. *J Am Acad Dermatol* 70(2):338–351, 2014.
8. Thomsen SF: Epidemiology and natural history of atopic diseases. *Eur Clin Respir J* 2, 2015.
9. Kim JE, et al: Molecular mechanisms of cutaneous inflammatory disorder: atopic dermatitis. *Int J Mol Sci* 17(8):2016.
10. Wolf R, Wolf D: Abnormal epidermal barrier in the pathogenesis of atopic dermatitis. *Clin Dermatol* 30(3):329–334, 2012.
11. Navarrete-Dechent C, et al: Humoral and cellular autoreactivity to epidermal proteins in atopic dermatitis. *Arch Immunol Ther Exp (Warsz)* 64(6):435–442, 2016.
12. Cabanillas B, Novak N: Atopic dermatitis and filaggrin. *Curr Opin Immunol* 42:1–8, 2016.
13. Williams MR, Gallo RL: The role of the skin microbiome in atopic dermatitis. *Curr Allergy Asthma Rep* 15(11):65, 2015.
14. Eichenfield LF, et al: Current guidelines for the evaluation and management of atopic dermatitis: a comparison of the Joint Task Force Practice Parameter and American Academy of Dermatology guidelines. *J Allergy Clin Immunol* 139(4S):S49–S57, 2017.
15. Nicol NH, Boguniewicz M: Wet wrap therapy in moderate to severe atopic dermatitis. *Immunol Allergy Clin North Am* 37(1):123–139, 2017.
16. Eichenfield LF, et al: Translating atopic dermatitis management guidelines into practice for primary care providers. *Pediatrics* 136(3):554–565, 2015.
17. Bonifaz A, et al: Superficial mycoses associated with diaper dermatitis. *Mycopathologia* 181(9-10):671–679, 2016.
18. Dey S, et al: Modern diaper performance: construction, materials, and safety review. *Int J Dermatol* 55(Suppl 1):18–20, 2016.
19. Hartman-Adams H, Banvard C, Juckett G: Impetigo: diagnosis and treatment. *Am Fam Physician* 90(4):229–235, 2014.
20. May P, et al: Protocol for the systematic review of the prevention, treatment and public health management of impetigo, scabies and fungal skin infections in resource-limited settings. *Syst Rev* 5(1):162, 2016.
21. Mishra AK, Yadav P, Mishra A: A systemic review on staphylococcal scalded skin syndrome (SSSS): a rare and critical disease of neonates. *Open Microbiol J* 10:150–159, 2016.
22. Paranthaman K, et al: Nosocomial outbreak of staphylococcal scalded skin syndrome in neonates in England, December 2012 to March 2013. *Euro Surveill* 19(33):2014.
23. Sahoo AK, Mahajan R: Management of tinea corporis, tinea cruris, and tinea pedis: a comprehensive review. *Indian Dermatol Online J* 7(2):77–86, 2016.
24. Abdel-Rahman SM, et al: The prevalence of infections with *Trichophyton tonsurans* in schoolchildren: the CAPITIS study. *Pediatrics* 125(5):966–973, 2010.
25. John AM, Schwartz RA, Janniger CK: The kerion: an angry tinea capitis. *Int J Dermatol* 2016, doi:10.1111/ijd.13423. Oct 1, [Epub ahead of print].
26. Kaushik N, Pujalte GG, Reese ST: Superficial fungal infections. *Prim Care* 42(4):501–516, 2015.
27. Xie Z, et al: *Candida albicans* biofilms do not trigger reactive oxygen species and evade neutrophil killing. *J Infect Dis* 206(12):1936–1945, 2012.
28. Marty M, et al: Direct microscopy: a useful tool to diagnose oral candidiasis in children and adolescents. *Mycopathologia* 180(5-6):373–377, 2015.
29. Silk H: Diseases of the mouth. *Prim Care* 41(1):75–90, 2014.
30. Shisler JL: Immune evasion strategies of molluscum contagiosum virus. *Adv Virus Res* 92:201–252, 2015.
31. Moye V, et al: Beetle juice: a guide for the use of cantharidin in the treatment of molluscum contagiosum. *Dermatol Ther* 26(6):445–451, 2013.
32. Chen X, Anstey AV, Bugert JJ: Molluscum contagiosum virus infection. *Lancet Infect Dis* 13(10):877–888, 2013.
33. Parker Fiebelkorn A, et al: Measles in the United States during the postelimination era. *J Infect Dis* 202(10):1520–1528, 2010.
34. Reef SE, et al: Evidence used to support the achievement and maintenance of elimination of rubella and congenital rubella syndrome in the United States. *J Infect Dis* 204(Suppl 2):S593–S597, 2011.
35. Jain A, et al: Autism occurrence by MMR vaccine status among US children with older siblings with and without autism. *JAMA* 313(15):1534–1540, 2015.
36. Maglione MA, et al: Safety of vaccines used for routine immunization of U.S. children: a systematic review. *Pediatrics* 134(2):325–337, 2014.
37. Hutton J: Does rubella cause autism: a 2015 reappraisal? *Front Hum Neurosci* 10:25, 2016.
38. Lambert N, et al: Rubella. *Lancet* 385(9984):2297–2307, 2015.
39. Di Pasquale A, et al: Vaccine safety evaluation: practical aspects in assessing benefits and risks. *Vaccine* 34(52):6672–6680, 2016.
40. White SJ, et al: Measles, mumps, and rubella. *Clin Obstet Gynecol* 55(2):550–559, 2012.
41. de Vries RD, et al: The pathogenesis of measles. *Curr Opin Virol* 2(3):248–255, 2012.
42. Plattet P, et al: Measles virus fusion protein: structure, function and inhibition. *Viruses* 8(4):112, 2016.
43. Stone RC, Micali GA, Schwartz RA: Roseola infantum and its causal human herpesviruses. *Int J Dermatol* 53(4):397–403, 2014.
44. Schmader K: Herpes zoster. *Clin Geriatr Med* 32(3):539–553, 2016.
45. Bapat P, Koren G: The role of VariZIG in pregnancy. *Expert Rev Vaccines* 12(11):1243–1248, 2013.
46. Smedegaard LM, et al: Varicella vaccination of children with leukemia without interruption of maintenance therapy: a Danish experience. *Pediatr Infect Dis J* 35(11):e348–e352, 2016.
47. Ibraheem M, et al: Fatal wild-type varicella-zoster virus encephalitis without a rash in a vaccinated child. *Pediatr Infect Dis J* 32(2):183–185, 2013.
48. Aswathyraj S, et al: Hand, foot and mouth disease (HFMD): emerging epidemiology and the need for a vaccine strategy. *Med Microbiol Immunol* 205(5):397–407, 2016.
49. Nassef C, Ziemer C, Morrell DS: Hand-foot-and-mouth disease: a new look at a classic viral rash. *Curr Opin Pediatr* 27(4):486–491, 2015.
50. Dadabhoy I, Butts JF: Parasitic skin infections for primary care physicians. *Prim Care* 42(4):661–675, 2015.
51. Swe PM, et al: Parasitic scabies mites and associated bacteria joining forces against host complement defense. *Parasite Immunol* 36(11):585–593, 2014.
52. Juckett G: Arthropod bites. *Am Fam Physician* 88(12):841–847, 2013.
53. Vasievich MP, Villarreal JD, Tomecki KJ: Got the travel bug? A review of common infections, infestations, bites, and stings among returning travelers. *Am J Clin Dermatol* 17(5):451–462, 2016.
54. Slaughter KA, Chen T, Williams E, 3rd: Vascular lesions. *Facial Plast Surg Clin North Am* 24(4):559–571, 2016.
55. Raphael MF, et al: Treatment of infantile hemangiomas: therapeutic options in regard to side effects and adverse events-a review of the literature. *Expert Opin Drug Saf* 15(2):199–214, 2016.
56. Ballieux F, Boon LM, Vikkula M: Blue bleb rubber nevus syndrome. *Handb Clin Neurol* 132:223–230, 2015.
57. Ghosh S: Neonatal pustular dermatosis: an overview. *Indian J Dermatol* 60(2):211, 2015.

CHAPTER

49

Shock, Multiple Organ Dysfunction Syndrome, and Burns in Adults

Linda L. Martin, Dennis J. Cheek, Stephen E. Morris

⊖volve WEBSITE

http://evolve.elsevier.com/McCance/
- Content Updates
- Chapter Summary Review
- Review Questions
- Case Studies
- Animations

CHAPTER OUTLINE

Shock occurs when the circulatory system fails to perfuse tissues, cells, and organs adequately, resulting in widespread impairment of cellular metabolism and tissue function. **Tissue perfusion** is defined as the adequacy of blood flow through the small vessels to maintain tissue function.[1] Inadequate tissue perfusion occurs when there is decreased delivery of blood, oxygen, and nutrients to cells and tissues and increased oxygen consumption, such as from a decrease in cardiac output, a reduction in blood volume or hemoglobin level, or a significant reduction in blood pressure. Thus inadequate tissue perfusion can result in shock regardless of cause or type. Multiple etiologies exist for shock, but shock from any cause will progress to organ failure and death unless physiologic mechanisms reverse the process or clinical intervention succeeds in stopping the progression. Untreated, shock overwhelms the body's compensatory mechanisms and results in organ dysfunction that may progress to multisystem organ failure.

Multiple organ dysfunction syndrome (MODS) is progressive and involves the failure of two or more organ systems after a severe illness or injury. The disease process is initiated and perpetuated by uncontrolled systemic inflammatory and stress responses and is characterized by a hypermetabolic and hyperdynamic state that persists as organ dysfunction develops. For many years the syndrome was referred to as *multiple organ failure* or *multiple systems organ failure*. Gradually it was recognized that the term *organ dysfunction* more accurately describes the syndrome as a process of physiologic deterioration.

Major burns result in extensive immediate tissue injury and thus are a form of trauma with wide-reaching effects on all organ systems. The cause of injury may be thermal contact, flame, chemical agents, or electrical agents; each cause requires a different approach in diagnosis and treatment. Closely associated with thermal burns is smoke inhalation injury, which accounts for about 25% of all burn unit admissions. As a multiorgan problem, thermal injuries can have an overwhelming effect on survival of the burned individual. Regardless of the cause of burns, the result is a final common pathway of physiologic response dependent on the extent of burn surface involvement and the depth of tissue destruction.

SHOCK

Shock can be classified by type, principal pathophysiologic process, or clinical manifestations. Classification by type is perhaps the most useful

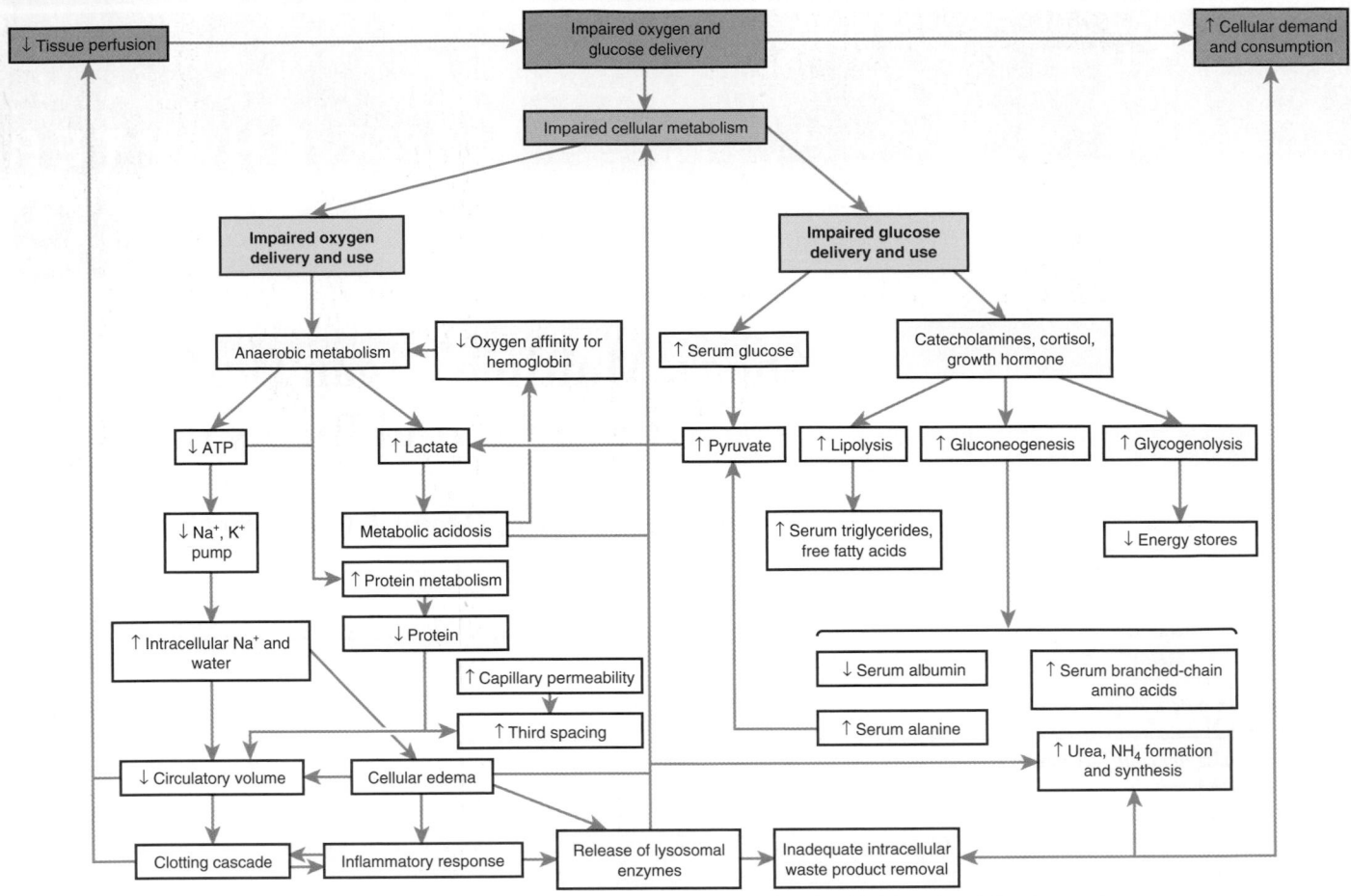

FIGURE 49.1 Impairment of Cellular Metabolism by Shock. *ATP,* Adenosine triphosphate.

because it suggests the cause and pathophysiologic process of the underlying disorder, which must be treated to prevent the irreversible cellular alterations and impairment of cellular metabolism. **Shock** is classified as cardiogenic (caused by heart failure); neurogenic or vasogenic (caused by alterations in vascular smooth muscle tone); anaphylactic (caused by hypersensitivity); septic (caused by infection); or hypovolemic (caused by insufficient intravascular fluid volume).

Cellular Alterations and Impairment of Cellular Metabolism

The body consists of many organs, tissues, and cells that may function or malfunction at different stages of metabolic impairment. The common pathway in all types of shock is impairment of cellular metabolism, attributable to decreased delivery of oxygen and nutrients, frequently coupled with an increased demand and consumption of oxygen and nutrients and a decreased removal of cellular waste products.[2] In septic shock, for example, a deficiency in cellular metabolism and the buildup of lactic acid often precede the decreased tissue perfusion. Fig. 49.1 illustrates the pathophysiology of shock at the cellular level.

Impairment of Oxygen Delivery, Increased Oxygen Consumption, and Volume Changes

Normal tissue perfusion allows for the delivery of more oxygen to the capillary beds and cells than is consumed at the cellular level. In all types of shock, the cells do not receive adequate amounts of oxygen because of decreased delivery or increased cellular consumption, or both, and therefore are unable to use oxygen normally (see Fig. 49.1).

In cardiogenic shock, cardiac output, either stroke volume or heart rate, is too low to deliver adequate oxygen to the cell. In hypovolemic shock, oxygen delivery is impaired by inadequate numbers of red blood cells or hemoglobin (which carries oxygen) and insufficient blood volume. In neurogenic, anaphylactic, and septic shock, systemic vascular resistance (SVR) becomes very low because of vasodilation, resulting in inadequate perfusion pressure in the capillaries. Thus the pressure needed to drive oxygen and nutrients across cell membranes is inadequate. In septic shock, hypoxia is worsened both by increased inflammatory responses (such as fever), which raise the cell's oxygen demands and consumption rate, and by direct toxic and inflammatory chemical disruption of cellular metabolism, which impairs the cell's ability to use oxygen. In particular, each molecule of hemoglobin is normally capable of carrying four molecules of oxygen but it delivers only one molecule of oxygen at the capillary bed for delivery to the cells; however, as tissue perfusion decreases and oxygen needs increase, two molecules of oxygen will be extracted to meet needs. When this compensatory mechanism is exhausted, cellular demand becomes abnormally greater than delivery. Without oxygen, the cells shift from aerobic to anaerobic metabolism, resulting in lactic acid production at the cellular level.

Both positive compensatory mechanisms, such as lysosomal enzyme and cytokine release, and negative compensatory mechanisms, such as anaerobic metabolism and decreased intravascular volume in any shock state, further impair oxygen delivery and use. Concurrently in the inflammatory state of sepsis, diffusion across capillary membranes is slowed because blood flow in the capillary beds becomes sluggish as a result of decreased fluid volume and increased blood viscosity.

Sluggish capillary flow decreases tissue perfusion, which may result in microvascular clot formation, and activation of the clotting cascade may begin (see Chapter 28). Microemboli formation and platelet aggregation account for common complications of shock caused by blocked tissue perfusion to end organs, such as the kidneys (causing acute tubular necrosis) or the lungs (causing acute respiratory distress syndrome [ARDS]). Disseminated intravascular coagulation (DIC) may be activated by the inflammatory response along with clotting cascade abnormalities.[3]

Anaerobic metabolism results in disruption of electrolyte and lysosomal enzymatic processes, thus changing the normal ionic and osmotic levels in cells governed by the physical law of diffusion. Diffusion of nutrients and wastes into and out of the cell takes longer, and cellular metabolism is further altered. Anaerobic metabolism is a less efficient method of extracting energy from carbon bonds, and the cell begins to use adenosine triphosphate (ATP) faster than it can be replaced. Without ATP the cell loses its ability to maintain an electrochemical gradient across its selectively permeable membrane. Specifically, the cell cannot operate the sodium-potassium pump. Sodium and chloride accumulate inside the cell and potassium exits the cell. Cells of the nervous system and myocardium are profoundly and immediately affected. The resting potentials of these cells are reduced, and the action potentials decrease in amplitude (see Chapter 1). Myocardial depressant factor is released, which decreases the contractility of the heart. A variety of clinical manifestations of impaired central nervous system and myocardial function results. As sodium moves into the cell, water follows. Throughout the body, the water drawn from the interstitium into the cells is "replaced" by water that is in turn drawn out of the vascular space, often called "third spacing" of fluid. This results in further decreases in circulatory volume. Within the cells, water causes cellular edema that disrupts cellular membranes, releasing lysosomal enzymes that injure the cells internally and then leak into the interstitium.

In addition to decreasing ATP stores, anaerobic metabolism affects the pH of the cell, and metabolic acidosis develops, which is indirectly measured by increasing lactate levels in the blood. A compensatory mechanism is initiated that enables cardiac and skeletal muscles to use lactic acid as a fuel source, but only for a limited time. The decreasing pH of the cell that is functioning under anaerobic conditions has serious consequences. Enzymes necessary for cellular function dissociate under acidic conditions. Enzyme dissociation stops cell function, repair, and division. As lactic acid is released systemically, blood pH drops, reducing the oxygen-carrying capacity of the blood (see Chapter 2), and the heart's ability to pump. Therefore less oxygen is delivered to the cells and further hypoxia results in metabolic acidosis, which triggers more lysosomal enzyme release caused by disruption of lysosomal membrane integrity. Lysosomal enzymes released during shock injure the cell that released them and injure adjacent cells. By damaging the mechanisms of surrounding cells, lysosomal enzymes extend areas of impaired metabolism and cellular injury.

Intravascular fluid loss into the intracellular and interstitial spaces, described as "third spacing" earlier, is amplified when serum albumin and other plasma proteins are consumed for fuel, which results in decreased intravascular osmotic pressure, shift of fluid to the interstitial or extracellular spaces, and decreased circulatory volume, which can cause a relative hypovolemic state. Decreased intravascular volume causes decreased cardiac output in septic, neurogenic, and anaphylactic shock states, but it is the decreased mechanical ability to eject volume from the heart pump that reduces cardiac output in cardiogenic shock. In individuals with anaphylactic, neurogenic, or septic shock and an already dilated vasculature, hypotension worsens as a result of decreased circulatory volume. New data on additional mechanisms for hypotension (vasodilation) are illustrated in Fig. 49.7.

Impairment of Glucose Delivery and Use

Impaired glucose use can be caused by either impaired glucose delivery or impaired glucose uptake by the cells (see Fig. 49.1). The reasons for inadequate glucose delivery are the same as those enumerated for inadequate oxygen delivery. In addition, in septic and anaphylactic shock, glucose metabolism and consumption may be increased or disrupted because of fever or bacteria, and glucose uptake can be prevented by the presence of vasoactive toxins, endotoxins, histamine, and kinins.

Some of the compensatory mechanisms activated by shock contribute to decreased glucose uptake and use by the cells. High serum levels of cortisol, growth hormone, and catecholamines account for hyperglycemia and insulin resistance, tachycardia, increased SVR, and increased cardiac contractility. Cells shift to glycogenolysis, gluconeogenesis, and lipolysis to generate fuel for survival (see Chapter 1). Except in the liver, kidneys, and muscles, the body's cells have extremely limited stores of glycogen. In fact, total body stores can fuel the metabolism for only about 10 hours. The depletion of fat and glycogen stores is not itself a cause of organ failure, but the energy costs of glycogenolysis and lipolysis are considerable and contribute to the cellular failure.

Impairment of Protein Metabolism and Depletion of Protein Stores

The depletion of protein is, however, a cause of organ failure. When gluconeogenesis causes proteins to be used for fuel, these proteins are no longer available to maintain cellular structure, function, repair, and replication. The breakdown of protein occurs in starvation states, hyperdynamic metabolic states, and septic shock. Under anaerobic metabolism, protein breakdown liberates alanine, which is converted to pyruvate. Pyruvic acid is changed into lactic acid, leading to an increased affinity for oxygen to bind to hemoglobin with resultant hypoxia and metabolic acidosis.

As proteins are metabolized anaerobically, ammonia and urea are produced. Ammonia is toxic to living cells. Uremia develops, and uric acid further disrupts cellular metabolism. Proteins are broken down preferentially. Serum albumin and other plasma proteins are consumed for fuel first. Serum protein consumption decreases capillary osmotic pressure and contributes to the development of interstitial edema, creating another negative compensatory outcome that decreases circulatory volume. In septic shock, plasma protein breakdown includes breakdown of immunoglobulins, thereby impairing immune system function when it is most needed.

Muscle wasting caused by protein breakdown weakens skeletal and cardiac muscle. Skeletal muscle wasting impairs the muscles that facilitate breathing. Muscle wasting therefore alters the actions of both heart and lungs. The delivery of oxygen and glucose to the cells is directly reduced, as is the removal of metabolic waste products, such as the formation of carbon dioxide and lactic acid, causing metabolic acidosis with resultant inability of muscles, organs, and tissues to function mechanically and electrically.

The metabolic wastes that accumulate in the cell and interstitial spaces are toxic to the cells and further disrupt cellular function and membrane integrity.

Types of Shock, Clinical Manifestations, and Treatment

Each type of shock (cardiogenic, hypovolemic, neurogenic, anaphylactic, septic) involves numerous clinical manifestations, signs, and symptoms that also may characterize other conditions, making diagnosis difficult. If there are overlapping shock states that occur simultaneously, the clear clinical manifestations confuse the diagnosis. An individual's history, risks, and situation are correlated with the specificity of the shock state suspected or anticipated. For example, clinical manifestations common in septic shock are fever, high heart rate, high respiratory rate, or elevations in immune responses, such as increased levels of white blood cells. Elevated circulating blood glucose level, cyanosis, mottling, decreased urine output, and decreases in blood pressure with altered mental status may be present in any shock state. Subjective complaints often are nonspecific and general, such as chief complaints of weakness, malaise, or shortness of breath.

The initial management for shock is to discover, diagnose, and correct or remove the underlying cause. Although this seems a simple tenet, it is one that is not always remembered. Thus treatment for cardiogenic shock begins with diagnosis and treatment of heart failure or at least enhancement of cardiac output. In hypovolemic shock, hemorrhage and other causes of fluid loss must be stopped and replaced. In neurogenic shock, as a result of spinal cord trauma, stabilization of the spine and surrounding tissue is an initial approach, followed by treatment to counteract the vasodilatory effect and decreased blood pressure related to the parasympathetic control below the level of spinal cord injury. For anaphylactic shock, antigens must be identified, removed, or neutralized. Management for septic shock begins with identification and eradication of the infective agent, with blood cultures followed by administration of antimicrobials and fluids.

Simultaneous to correcting the underlying cause or condition, treatment is directed at targeting improvement of microcirculatory tissue perfusion.[3] Optimizing oxygenation is an absolute necessity in all shock states. The goal has a dual purpose to both optimize oxygen delivery and reduce oxygen consumption. Intravenous fluid or blood products are administered to expand intravascular volume and thereby improve tissue perfusion by increasing blood pressure, hemoglobin level, and cardiac output, except in cases of cardiogenic shock, which requires diuresis to reduce preload, so that the pump is not overloaded, or augmentation therapies to increase cardiac output. Effective glucose level control in various shock states has been shown to improve outcomes. Hyperglycemia, caused by insulin resistance in the liver and muscle, is a common finding in the critically ill. This is most likely an adaptive response providing glucose for the brain, cell nourishment and production, and wound healing; it also causes the increase in circulating corticosteroids produced in the stress response. The extent of appropriate glucose level control has been evaluated in recent years, leading to more aggressive treatment with continuous, titrating insulin infusions to maintain blood glucose levels closer to normal, thus promoting normal cellular function and healing.[4]

Once cellular and organ dysfunction and physiologic derangement are established, risk of morbidity and mortality increases in all shock states. Prevention and early treatment offer the best prognosis.

Cardiogenic Shock

Cardiogenic shock results from the inability of the heart to pump adequate blood to tissues and end organs. Cardiogenic shock is a state of inadequate systemic tissue perfusion, despite adequate left ventricular filling pressure and intravascular volume. It is caused by extensive myocardial damage and appears to be aggravated by a systemic inflammatory response. The result is hypotension with metabolic acidosis and often has a fatal outcome; however, medical treatment and hypothermia in the treatment of post–cardiac arrest states have been shown to improve outcomes.[5,6] Overall, hospital mortality because of cardiogenic shock has decreased from approximately 90% in the 1970s to a recent estimate of 50%.[7]

Pathologic conditions that reduce contractility, cause pump failure, impair diastolic filling, or cause obstruction can lead to cardiogenic shock. Decreased contractility and pump failure can result from (1) acute myocardial infarction (AMI), cardiomyopathy, sepsis, myocarditis,

pericarditis, aneurysm, dysrhythmias, contusion, metabolic abnormalities, and papillary muscle rupture; (2) impaired diastolic filling related to dysrhythmias; and (3) obstruction attributable to pulmonary embolism, cardiac tamponade, valvular disorders, tumors, and wall rupture or defects.[8] Dysrhythmias or conditions related to post–cardiopulmonary resuscitation reduce cardiac function and output, and may be associated with any of the previous pathologies mentioned.

As cardiac output decreases, compensatory adaptive responses are activated, such as the renin-angiotensin, neurohormonal, and sympathetic nervous systems, that lead to fluid retention, systemic vasoconstriction, and tachycardia.[9] Activation of the inflammatory response (resulting in expression of inducible nitric oxide synthase), activation of inflammatory cytokines, and activation of the complement system appear to play an important role in the pathogenesis and outcome of cardiogenic shock.[10] Increases in contractility, heart rate, and blood pressure are maintained in mild shock states through vasoconstriction in response to catecholamine release from the adrenals. Vasoconstriction increases vascular resistance to normalize blood pressure and improves cardiac performance by returning more blood volume and increasing perfusion to the heart; however, this increases myocardial demand and consumption of oxygen and nutrients by the heart. Increasing myocardial requirements burden the already failing heart, which can no longer pump an adequate volume of blood with sufficient force to perfuse the tissues. Thus increased coronary, tissue, and cellular ischemia further deteriorates myocardial function and shock.

Morbidity and mortality caused by cardiogenic shock is reduced by use of percutaneous intravascular interventions to open coronary arteries; intraaortic balloon counterpulsation (intraaortic balloon pump [IABP]), cardiosupportive drug regimens, and mild hypothermia, which has been shown to increase contractility while decreasing oxygen demand and metabolism, also have shown improved outcomes.[10-12] Following myocardial infarction, reperfusion and revascularization can be achieved with treatment modalities that include fibrinolytic therapies (medications that disintegrate the coronary thrombus) and percutaneous interventions (balloon angioplasty, stent placement, and thrombectomies). Surgery (coronary artery bypass, ventriculoplasty, or heart transplant) is also utilized to open the coronary vessels during an acute myocardial infarction or to replace irreparable heart muscle. Cardiosupportive drug and fluid regimens are initiated to maintain adequate blood pressure and essential fluid and electrolyte balance, and to optimize coronary perfusion to the myocardium. Mechanical assist devices, specifically intraaortic balloon pumps and percutaneous or ventricular assist devices (VADs), are used to support cardiac output temporarily until the individual improves or transplantation is possible.[11] Implantable VADs, pacemakers, or internal defibrillator devices are sometimes used as permanent treatment for those who survive cardiogenic shock. Continuous hemodynamic monitoring should be employed to evaluate vascular volume and pressures, optimize fluid levels, and monitor drug administration with the goal of improving cardiac output and tissue perfusion.[13]

The clinical manifestations of cardiogenic shock are caused by inadequate perfusion to the heart and end organs (Fig. 49.2). Subjective complaints of chest pain, dyspnea, and faintness, along with feelings of impending doom, are often revealed. Classic observable signs and symptoms of tachycardia, tachypnea, hypotension, jugular venous distention, dysrhythmia, and low measured cardiac output are hallmarks. Cyanosis; skin mottling; rapid, faint, or irregular pulses; low urine output; and occasional peripheral edema are additional signs and symptoms of end-organ hypoperfusion. Myocardial dysfunction from fluid overload may result in extra heart sounds, pulmonary edema, hypoxemia, and elevated end-organ laboratory values. The amount of brain natriuretic peptide, produced when the heart stretches in relation

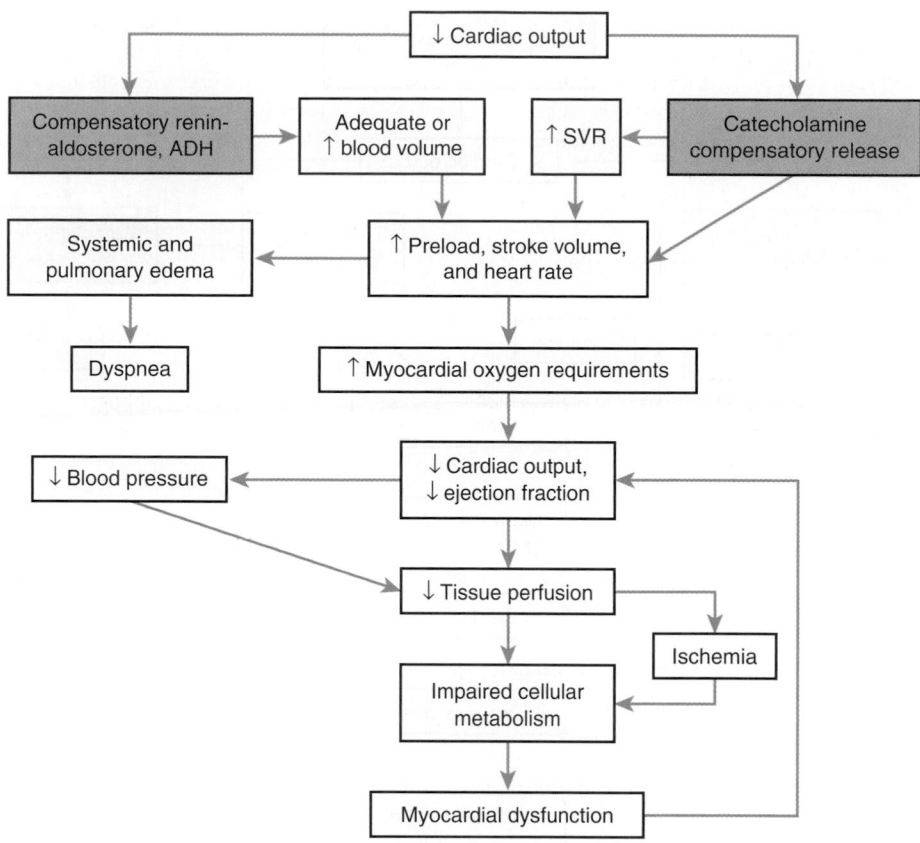

FIGURE 49.2 Cardiogenic Shock. Shock becomes life-threatening when compensatory mechanisms *(orange boxes)* cause increased myocardial oxygen requirements. *ADH,* Antidiuretic hormone; *SVR,* systemic vascular resistance.

to increased volume with decreased cardiac output, is increased to help the diuresis of fluid volume excess.[9] Pulmonary edema increases as volume accumulates and expands from the heart into the lungs as evidenced by audible crackles and wheezes, as well as abnormal vascular congestion on chest radiography. Metabolic abnormalities involving electrolyte imbalances, metabolic acidosis, and elevated levels of inflammatory markers may result from or concur with the cardiac cascade of shock.

Hypovolemic Shock

Hypovolemic shock is caused by loss of whole blood (hemorrhage), plasma (burns), or interstitial fluid (diaphoresis, diabetes mellitus, diabetes insipidus, emesis, or diuresis) in large amounts. Loss of whole blood or plasma causes hypovolemia directly. Loss of interstitial fluid causes an indirect "relative" hypovolemia by promoting diffusion of plasma from the intravascular to the extravascular space. Hypovolemic shock begins to develop when intravascular volume has decreased by about 15%.

Hypovolemia is offset initially by compensatory mechanisms (Fig. 49.3). Heart rate and vasoconstriction increase as a result of catecholamine release by the adrenals. This boosts cardiac output and tissue perfusion pressures. Compelled by a decrease in capillary hydrostatic pressures, interstitial fluid moves into the vascular compartment. The liver and spleen add to blood volume by disgorging stored red blood cells and plasma. In the kidneys, renin (through several intermediaries) stimulates aldosterone release and the retention of sodium (and hence water), whereas antidiuretic hormone (ADH, or vasopressin) from the posterior pituitary gland increases water retention. Data on the compensation

of ADH, however, show that as shock worsens, ADH in plasma decreases. Eventually, hypovolemic shock results in extreme vasoconstriction and increased systemic vascular resistance (SVR) and afterload in order to improve blood pressure and perfusion to core organs.

These compensatory mechanisms are, however, finite. If the initial fluid or blood loss is great or if loss continues, compensation fails, resulting in decreased tissue perfusion. Nutrient delivery to the cells is impaired, and cellular metabolism fails. Mortality from traumatic hemorrhagic shock ranges from 10% to 31%. Prompt control of hemorrhage is the treatment of choice. Fluid replacement is also important, but the type of fluid to be used and the rate of replacement are controversial.[14,15] The clinical manifestations of hypovolemic shock include high SVR, pallor and cool extremities, increased thirst, oliguria, low systemic and pulmonary preloads, and rapid heart rate.

Neurogenic Shock

Neurogenic shock, also called **vasogenic shock,** refers to a widespread and massive vasodilation that results from an imbalance between parasympathetic and sympathetic stimulation of vascular smooth muscle (see Chapter 33). Occasionally, parasympathetic overstimulation or sympathetic understimulation persists, causing vasodilation and low blood pressure for an extended period. Extreme, persistent vasodilation leads to neurogenic shock (Fig. 49.4). Neurogenic shock creates a "relative hypovolemia." Blood volume has not changed, but the amount of space containing the blood has increased, causing the SVR to decrease drastically as a result of vasodilation. Thus pressure in the vessels is inadequate to drive oxygen and nutrients across capillary membranes and delivery to the cells is impaired, thus leading to impaired cellular metabolism.

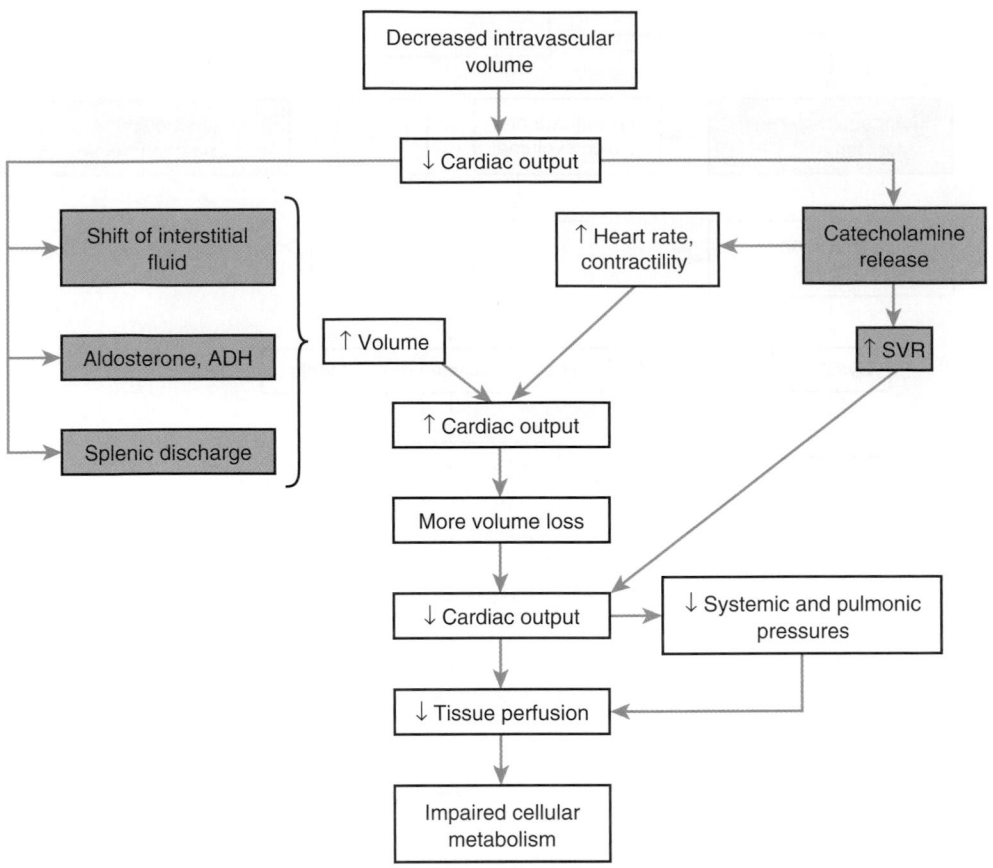

FIGURE 49.3 Hypovolemic Shock. This type of shock becomes life-threatening when compensatory mechanisms *(orange boxes)* are overwhelmed by continued loss of intravascular volume. *ADH,* Antidiuretic hormone; *SVR,* systemic vascular resistance.

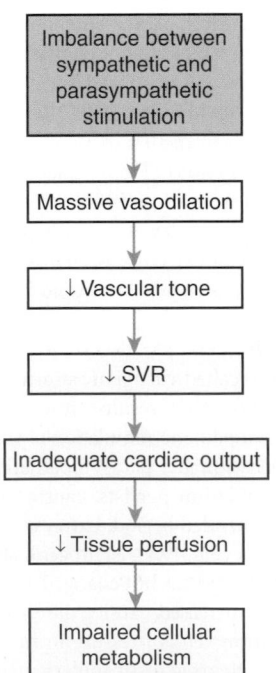

FIGURE 49.4 Neurogenic Shock. *SVR,* Systemic vascular resistance.

Neurogenic shock can be caused by any factor that stimulates parasympathetic activity or inhibits sympathetic activity of vascular smooth muscle. (Parasympathetic stimulation automatically inhibits sympathetic activity and vice versa; see Chapter 33.) Normally, sympathetic stimulation maintains muscle tone. If sympathetic stimulation is interrupted or inhibited, vasodilation occurs. Therefore trauma to the spinal cord or medulla, conditions that interrupt the supply of oxygen to the medulla, or conditions that deprive the medulla of glucose (e.g., insulin reactions) can cause neurogenic shock by interrupting sympathetic activity. Depressive drugs, anesthetic agents, and severe emotional stress and pain are other causes of neurogenic shock.

The clinical hallmark of neurogenic shock is a very low SVR, along with other indicators of excessive parasympathetic activity. Bradycardia is the most obvious manifestation, especially in the early stages. Bradycardia may cease when compensatory mechanisms, particularly an increase in sympathetic system activity, have been initiated. The ejection fraction remains high, indicating a healthy myocardium, whereas central venous pressure decreases as the veins dilate. Neurogenic shock causes fainting if blood pressure decreases to the point that cerebral metabolism is not sufficient to support consciousness. Most episodes of fainting are *not* shock, however; rarely do such episodes progress to shock. By allowing the blood pressure to equalize from head to toe as the individual becomes prone, fainting can actually prevent shock.

Anaphylactic Shock

Anaphylactic shock is the outcome of a widespread hypersensitivity to an allergen that triggers a reaction known as *anaphylaxis.* (An allergen

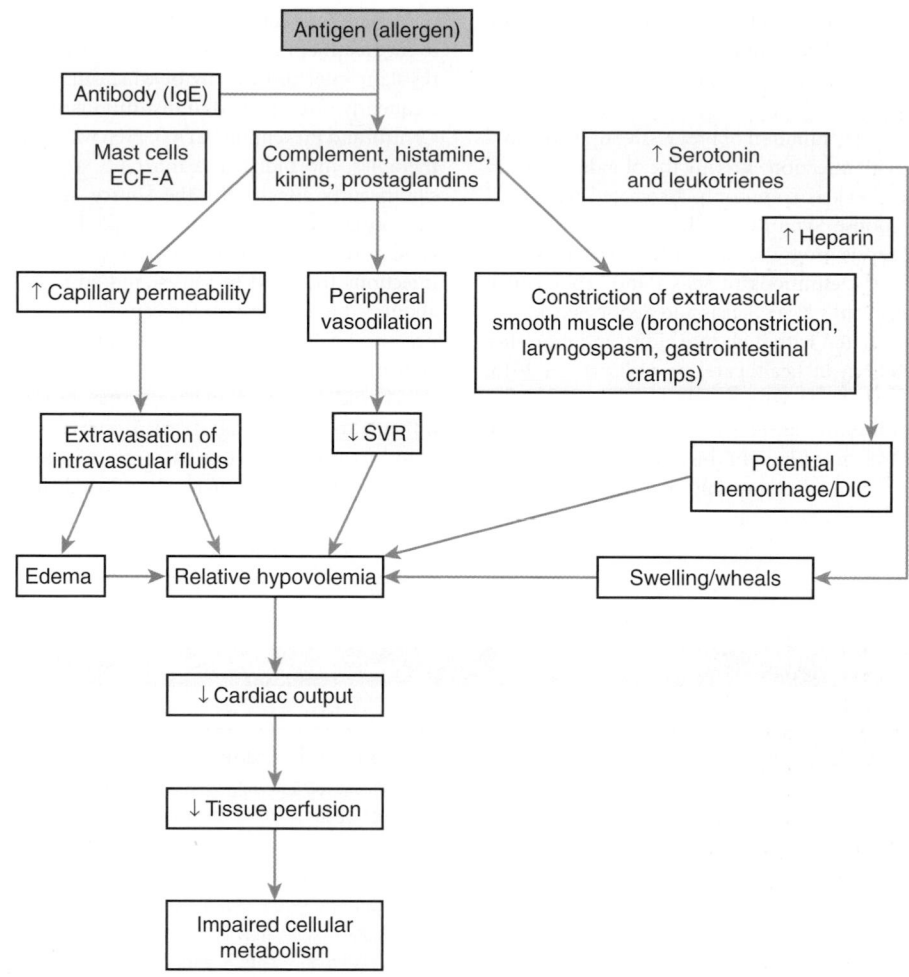

FIGURE 49.5 Anaphylactic Shock. *DIC,* Disseminated intravascular coagulation; *ECF-A,* eosinophil chemotactic factor of anaphylaxis; *IgE,* immunoglobulin E; *SVR,* systemic vascular resistance.

is an antigen to which an individual is hypersensitive; see Chapters 7, 8, and 9 for discussions of immunity, inflammation, and hypersensitivity.) Immunologic causes are related to the inflammatory and vasodilatory effects triggered by a pathologic allergic reaction to an antigen. Production of mast cells, immunoglobulin E (IgE), and low-affinity IgE receptor (FceRI) is induced by cellular response to the antigen and contributes to the induction of clinical manifestations and anaphylactic severity.[16] *Anaphylactoid* type reactions, which are nonimmunologic in origin, can be related to cold weather, exercise, and contaminants in medications.[17] Physiologic alterations related to the inflammatory and immune response, similar to neurogenic shock, are massive; vasodilation, peripheral pooling, and relative hypovolemia lead to decreased tissue perfusion and impaired cellular metabolism (Fig. 49.5). Anaphylactic shock is often severe and has immediate symptoms, including an itchy rash, throat swelling, and low blood pressure, related to the massive vasodilation and systemic inflammation that may progress to death in minutes if emergency treatment is not rendered.

Some allergens known to cause hypersensitivity reactions are foods, insect and snake venoms, pollens, medications, and latex. Once in the body, the allergen or antigen causes immune inflammatory responses that range from mild to life-threatening or fatal.[18] Vascular effects of this response include vasodilation and increased vascular permeability, resulting in peripheral pooling and tissue edema. Extravascular effects include constriction of extravascular smooth muscle, such as the smooth muscle found in the walls of airways (e.g., the larynx and bronchioles;

see Chapter 36), which may cause the extreme bronchoconstriction commonly associated with asthma and other severe allergic reactions.

Symptoms often affect multiple organ systems, including gastrointestinal (e.g., nausea, abdominal pain, vomiting, diarrhea), cutaneous (e.g., erythema, pruritus, urticaria, or angioedema), respiratory (e.g., shortness of breath, cough, rhinorrhea, tightening of throat, difficulty swallowing, wheezing), cardiovascular (e.g., diaphoresis, pallor, hypotension), or hematologic (e.g., fever, hemolysis). Other ominous clinical manifestations of anaphylactic shock may be anxiety, confusion, or impaired mentation. A precipitous decrease in blood pressure may account for altered mental status and may result in oliguria. Treatment begins with removal of the antigen (if possible). Epinephrine is administered to decrease mast cell and basophil degranulation, cause vasoconstriction, and reverse airway constriction.[19] Volume expanders (e.g., lactated Ringer solution) are given intravenously to reverse the relative hypovolemia, and antihistamines and corticosteroids are given to stop the inflammatory reaction.

In response to the need for improved anaphylaxis diagnosis and treatment, the World Allergy Organization (WAO) formulated global guidelines in 2011 for assessment and management of anaphylaxis.[19] These guidelines were further updated in 2012 to include recommendations for validation of the clinical criteria for diagnosis, use of epinephrine, development of in vitro tests to distinguish clinical risk from asymptomatic sensitization, and immune modulation to prevent anaphylaxis.[17] Currently, the emphasis on management of severe cases of anaphylaxis is shifting toward identification of triggers, determination of genetic predispositions, and prevention of recurrence.

Septic Shock

Septic shock is the endpoint of a continuum of progressive dysfunction.[20] The disease process begins with infection entering the bloodstream and causing bacteremia. Septic shock is commonly associated with both systemic inflammatory response syndrome (SIRS) and sepsis with multiorgan dysfunction. If sepsis progresses in severity to septic shock, multiorgan failure is evident. Definitions of sepsis and septic shock were updated in 2016[21] (see *What's New?* Sepsis and Septic Shock; also see Table 49.1). Sepsis is associated with high morbidity and mortality and accounted for $23.7 billion in healthcare expenditures in 2013, with rough mortality rates of 20% to 70%.[22]

Septic shock is most commonly caused by gram-negative bacteria, gram-positive bacteria, viruses, and fungi. In the intensive care setting, research suggests that the six most commonly identified infections associated with sepsis are pneumonia, bloodstream, intravascular catheter, intraabdominal, urosepsis, and surgical wounds, some of which are nosocomial.[23]

Advances in antibiotic therapy and broad-spectrum use of antibiotics in the treatment of sepsis have led to a significant increase in antibiotic-resistant infections, many of which may be hospital-acquired but are frequently not reported to institutions such as the Centers for Disease Control and Prevention (CDC). Even when properly treated with available therapies, morbidity and mortality are extremely high. Prognosis is significantly affected by the source and virulence of the infectious microorganism, which has prompted the expansion of efforts by the CDC and its partners to describe the epidemiology of sepsis, prevent infections that lead to sepsis, and educate clinicians and individuals about reducing the risk for sepsis.[24] Sepsis outcomes depend on the person's health before infection and the degree of organ dysfunction after infection.[25]

The nidus of infection in sepsis may be readily discernible or extremely difficult to locate (Fig. 49.6). Bacteria, viruses, and fungi enter the bloodstream to produce bacteremia in one of two ways: (1) directly from the site of infection or (2) indirectly from toxic substances released by the bacteria directly into the bloodstream. These toxic substances, which act as triggering molecules in the septic syndrome, include endotoxins released by gram-negative microorganisms, lipoteichoic

WHAT'S NEW?

Sepsis and Septic Shock

During the 2016 Third International Consensus Definitions for Sepsis and Septic Shock (Sepsis-3), experts eliminated the use of systemic inflammatory response syndrome (SIRS) criteria from the definition of sepsis and removed 'Severe Sepsis' from the previous definitions because of the fact that all sepsis should be considered severe. Meta-analysis of multiple studies and review of hospitalization records suggest that the use of SIRS criteria in diagnosing sepsis resulted in unnecessary admissions to the ICU and false-positive diagnosis of sepsis. Basically, both infectious and noninfectious pathologies may present with SIRS. SIRS criteria include (1) temperature >38°C (100.4°F) or <36°C (96.8°F); (2) heart rate >90 beats/min; (3) respiratory rate >20 breaths/min or $PaCO_2$ <32 mmHg; and (4) WBC >12,000/mm³, <4000/mm³, or >10% bands. When SIRS criteria are used as a screening tool, individuals exhibiting two of the four SIRS criteria met the previous consensus definition of sepsis. These criteria are still utilized in the clinical setting to assist in identifying potential infections leading to sepsis, but a source of infection and stratification of persons at high risk for infection—such as those who are immunocompromised; those who are very young or very old; those with invasive procedures, wounds, traumatic injury, or histories of chronic disease; or those suspected of respiratory tract, urinary tract, skin, or gastrointestinal sources of infection—should be considered before the diagnosis and workup for sepsis. Diagnosis codes, definitions, and core measurements for SIRS, sepsis, and severe sepsis identified by the Centers for Medicare and Medicaid Services (CMS) still apply in clinical settings for both children and adults. Latent, low systolic blood pressures (<90 mmHg), along with the use of organ dysfunction identifying tools such as LODS, SOFA, and qSOFA, are recommended for use in defining sepsis under the new 2016 consensus definition (see Table 49.1).

Improved early goal-directed therapies (EGDTs) to treat sepsis and the education of healthcare providers, as recommended by the Surviving Sepsis Campaign and others, have been adopted since 2002 and have been shown to reduce mortality in severe sepsis and shock. Research is now directed at the early identification

of pathogens and biomarkers indicative of organ dysfunction and the development of prognostic tools to identify types of infections. Using molecular assays designed to detect bacteria in the bloodstream is being studied, but molecular assays have not yet replaced the gold standard of obtaining blood cultures. Identifying and targeting metabolites of infection and biomarkers that consistently identify end-organ risk before clinical manifestations, such as TIMP-2 and IGFBP-7 in acute kidney injury, may become useful in differentiating the type of infection. Using less broad-spectrum antimicrobials with implementation of novel antimicrobial strategies—such as identification of antimicrobial gene resistance, bacterial biofilms, and bacterial gene resistance and employment of antimicrobial stewardship programs (ASPs) in hospitals, clinics, and communities—has been shown to assist in detecting and directing treatment toward the current epidemiology of microbial resistance and reduction of antimicrobial resistance (AMR).

Prevention and risk stratification for septicemia pose major challenges in the management, treatment, and clinical improvement of morbidity and mortality. Infection prevention strategies (e.g., vaccination, reduction of transmission of pathogens in healthcare environments, and appropriate management of chronic diseases) are likely to have a substantial impact on reducing sepsis. A recent large retrospective cohort study reported the increased risk of sepsis from the use of a short-term oral corticosteroid. The study reported that during the study time period the use of an oral corticosteroid for short-term treatment increased the person's risk for adverse effects, such as sepsis, venous thromboembolism, and fractures. The investigators postulated that the increased risk for these adverse effects was dependent upon the dose of the oral corticosteroid. The CDC, in partnership with organizations representing clinicians, patients, and other stakeholders, is launching a comprehensive campaign to demonstrate that prevention of infections that cause sepsis, surveillance of sepsis incidence, and early recognition of sepsis are integral to overall safety.

ICU, Intensive care unit; *IGFBP-7,* insulin-like growth factor-binding protein 7; *LODS,* logistic organ dysfunction score; *SOFA,* sequential organ failure assessment; *TIMP-2,* tissue inhibitor of metalloprotinase-2; *WBC,* white blood cell.
Data from Centers for Medicare and Medicaid Services (CMS): *Draft ICD-10-CM/PCS MS-DRGv28 definitions manual,* available at: https://www.cms.gov/icd10manual/fullcode_cms/P0324.html, retrieved September 28, 2016; Karanika S et al: *Antimicrob Agents Chemother* 60(8):4840–4852, 2016; Kashini K et al: *Crit Care* 17(R25), 2013; Marston HD et al: *JAMA* 316(11):1193–1204, 2016; Neugebauer S et al: *Crit Care Med* 44(9):1649–1662, 2016; Nguyen HB et al: *Crit Care* 20:1–16, 2016; Riedel S, Carroll KC: *Clin Chest Med* 37(2):191–207, 2016; Seymour C et al: *JAMA* 315(8):762–774, 2016; Shannon A et al: *MMWR Morb Mortal Wkly Rep* 65(33):864–869, 2016; Singer M et al: *JAMA* 315(8):801–810, 2016; Waljee AK et al: *BMJ* 357:1415–1422, 2017; Yende S, Iwashyna TJ, Angus DC: *Trends Mol Med* 20(4):234–238, 2014.

TABLE 49.1   DEFINITIONS OF SEPTIC SHOCK COMPONENTS

TERM	BASIC DEFINITION	COMMENTS
Infection	A pathologic process that results from an invasion of a normal part of the body by pathogenic or potentially pathogenic microorganisms	Suspicion of infection necessitates immediate identification of possible pathogens, bacteria, fungi, or viruses with blood culture(s). Without benefit of microbiologic confirmation, clinical judgment should be used to identify signs, symptoms, and risk stratification of potential infection to promote early identification. SIRS criteria may still be used to screen for infection (see *What's New?* Sepsis and Septic Shock).
Bacteremia	Presence of viable bacteria in the blood	Insufficient to make a diagnosis of sepsis, especially in the absence of organ dysfunction.
Organ dysfunction	Abnormality or impairment of normal organ function, with or without direct insult or damage to the organ	Indirect insult of organ perfusion is caused by the septic cascade and hypoperfusion. Organ dysfunction can be represented by an increase in the Sequential Organ Failure Assessment (SOFA) score by 2 points or more when evaluating 6 organ systems.

Evidence of 2 of 3 quickSOFA (qSOFA) criteria: respiratory rate of 22/min or greater; altered mentation, Glasgow Coma Scale <15 (new/worsening from baseline); or systolic blood pressure of 100 mmHg or less is considered positive for organ dysfunction.

The quickSOFA (qSOFA) is not as predictive as the full SOFA score in the intensive care setting; however, it is superior to SOFA when applied to individuals outside the intensive care unit. |
| Sepsis | Life-threatening organ dysfunction caused by a dysregulated host response to infection | Common organ systems showing dysfunction are the respiratory, hematologic, cardiac, renal, hepatic, and central nervous systems.

Additional clinical signs, symptoms, biomarkers, and variables that may be used to identify inflammation, inadequate tissue perfusion, and organ dysfunction:

1. General variables
   a. Fever >38°C (100.4°F) or hypothermia <36°C (96.8°F)
   b. Tachycardia, heart rate >90 beats/min
   c. Tachypnea
   d. Progressive deterioration of mental status
   e. Altered mental status
   f. Significant edema or positive fluid balance (>20 mL/kg over 24 hr)
   g. Hyperglycemia (blood glucose >140 mg/dL) in the absence of diabetes
2. Inflammatory variables
   a. Leukocytosis or leukopenia (WBC >12,000/mm^3, <4000/mm^3, or >10% bands)
   b. CRP >2 SD above the normal value
   c. PCT >2 SD above the normal value
3. Hemodynamic variables
   a. Arterial hypotension (SBP <90 mmHg; MAP <70 mmHg, or an SBP decrease >40 mmHg)
   b. S$\bar{v}o_2$ >70%
   c. Cardiac index >3.5 L/min
4. Organ dysfunction variables
   a. Arterial hypoxemia (Pao$_2$/Fio$_2$ <300 mmHg)
   b. Acute oliguria (urine output <0.5 mL/kg/hr or 45 mL for at least 2 hr)
   c. Creatinine increase >0.5 mg/dL
   d. Coagulation abnormalities (INR >1.5 or PTT >60 seconds)
   e. Ileus
   f. Thrombocytopenia (platelet count <100,000/m^3)
   g. Hyperbilirubinemia (plasma total bilirubin >4 mg/dL or 70 mmol/L)
5. Tissue perfusion variables
   a. Hyperlactatemia (>1 mmol/L)
   b. Decreased capillary refill or mottling |
| Septic shock | A subset of sepsis in which particularly profound circulatory, cellular, and metabolic abnormalities are associated with a greater risk of mortality than with sepsis alone | Clinically identified by a vasopressor requirement to maintain a mean arterial pressure of 65 mmHg or greater and serum lactate level greater than 2 mmol/L (>18 mg/dL) in the absence of hypovolemia. |

CRP, Plasma C-reactive protein; *INR,* international normalized ratio; *MAP,* mean arterial pressure; *Pao$_2$/Fio$_2$,* partial pressure of oxygen in arterial blood/fraction of inspired oxygen; *PCT,* plasma procalcitonin; *PTT,* partial thromboplastin time; *SBP,* systolic blood pressure; *SD,* standard deviation; *SIRS,* systemic inflammatory response syndrome; *S$\bar{v}o_2$,* saturation of hemoglobin with oxygen; *Temp,* core temperature; *WBC,* white blood cell(s).

Data from Dellinger RP et al: *Crit Care Med* 41(2):580–637, 2013; Levy MM et al: *Crit Care Med* 312:1250, 2003; Opal SM: *Scand J Infect Dis* 35:529, 2003; Seymour C: *JAMA* 315(8):762–774, 2016; Shankar-Hari M et al: *JAMA* 315(8):775–787, 2016; Singer M et al: *JAMA* 315(8):801–810, 2016.

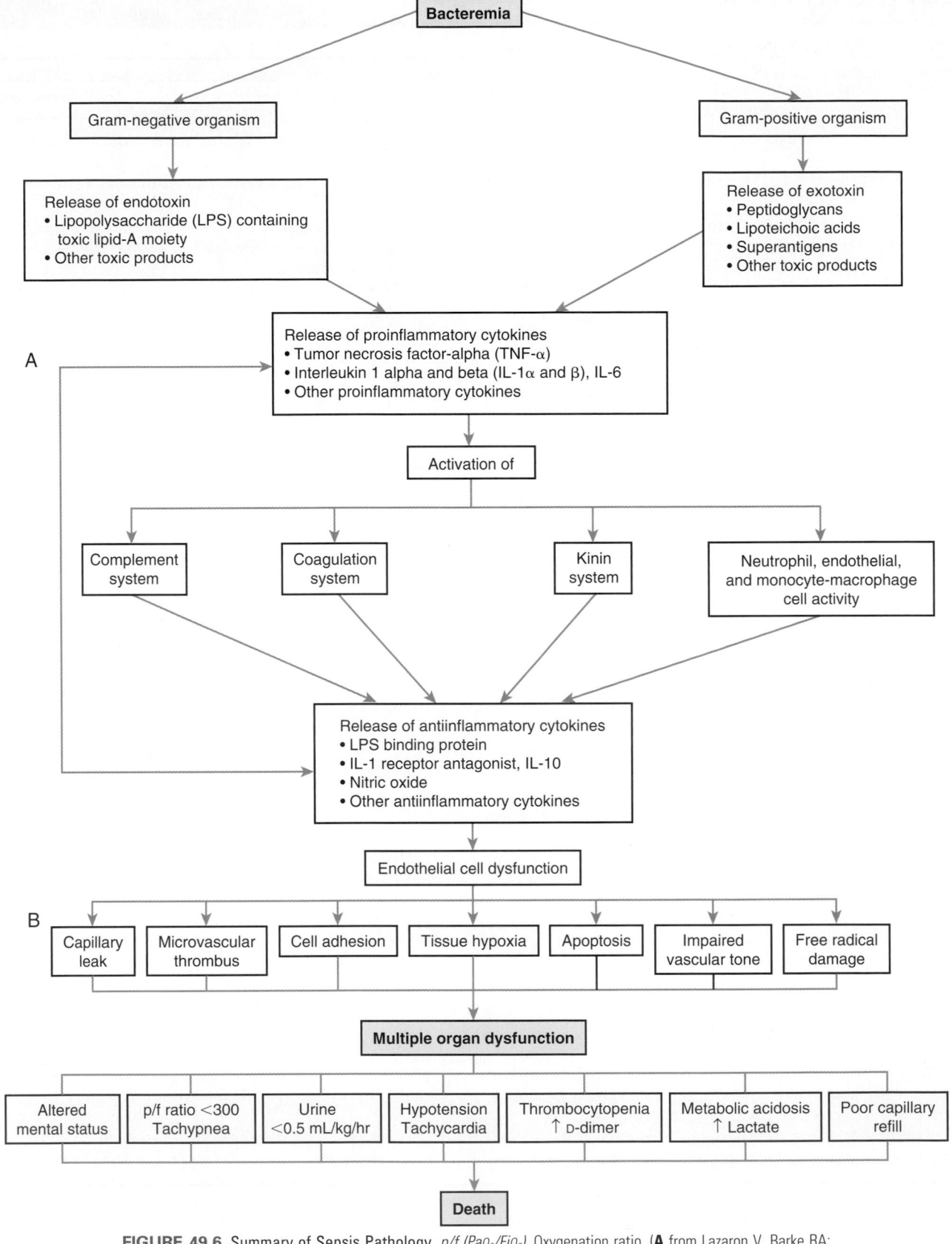

FIGURE 49.6 Summary of Sepsis Pathology. *p/f (PaO$_2$/FiO$_2$)*, Oxygenation ratio. (**A** from Lazaron V, Barke RA: *Urol Clin North Am* 26[4]:687, 1999. **B** copyright 2003, Eli Lilly and Company. All rights reserved. Reprinted with permission from Eli Lilly and Company.)

acids and peptidoglycan released by gram-positive microorganisms, and superantigens.[26]

The triggering molecules cause the host to initiate a proinflammatory response. Proinflammatory cells that are released include polymorphonuclear leukocytes, macrophages, monocytes, and platelets. The proinflammatory mediators released include the following: cytokines (interleukins [IL-1, IL-2, IL-6, IL-8, and IL-15], tumor necrosis factor-alpha [TNF-α], and granulocyte cell–stimulating factor); complement and complement cascade activation factors; kinins; arachidonic acid metabolites (prostaglandins, prostacyclin, leukotrienes, and thromboxane); soluble adhesion molecules; platelet-activating factor; endorphins; vasoactive neuropeptides; histamine; serotonin; monocyte chemoattractant proteins 1 and 2; proteolytic enzymes (e.g., elastase and lysosomal enzymes); protein kinase; tyrosine kinase; CD14; toxic oxygen metabolites (e.g., superoxide, hydroxyl radical, hydrogen peroxide, peroxynitrite); neopterin; and clotting cascade activation factors.[3,27,28] Proinflammatory cytokines enhance tissue factors, which initiate coagulation. Diminished thrombomodulin (cell surface glycoprotein of endothelial cells) inhibits the conversion of protein C and activated protein C. A compensatory antiinflammatory response syndrome is presumed to follow this response.[3,27,28] Antiinflammatory mediators released include lipopolysaccharide-binding protein; IL-1 receptor antagonist; soluble CD14; type 2 IL-1 receptor; leukotriene B$_4$ receptor antagonist; IL-4, IL-10, and IL-13; soluble tumor necrosis factor receptor; transforming growth factor-beta (TGF-β); epinephrine; and nitric oxide.[3,27,28] Presumably the end result is a mixed antagonistic response syndrome as proinflammatory and antiinflammatory mediators respond, intensify, and lead the host into MODS.

Clinical manifestations of septic shock are persistent low arterial pressure, low tissue perfusion, low SVR from vasodilation, and an alteration in oxygen extraction by all cells (see Comments column in Table 49.1). Two main mechanisms contribute to lactic acid accumulation in sepsis: tissue hypoxia and epinephrine-induced stimulation of aerobic glycolysis.[29] Low-flow states of prolonged shock causing tissue hypoxia with lactic acidosis increase nitric oxide synthesis, activate ATP-sensitive and calcium-regulated potassium channels (K$_{ATP}$ and K$_{Ca}$, respectively) in vascular smooth muscle (see Chapter 33), and lead to depletion of ADH (vasopressin) (Fig. 49.7). Tachypnea is a compensatory mechanism to increase oxygen. Tachycardia, in the initial stages of sepsis, supports cardiac output to remain normal or become elevated, although myocardial contractility is reduced. Sustained tachycardia is deleterious to improving cardiac output, especially when underlying comorbid states of heart disease exist. Temperature instability, ranging from hyperthermia to hypothermia, may indicate deterioration of the immune response, or may partially be caused by latent vasoconstriction or a vasopressor drug effect. Effects on other organ systems may result in deranged renal function, gastrointestinal mucosa changes, and ischemia that lead to translocation of bacteria from the gut, jaundice related to liver dysfunction, and clotting abnormalities that cause microemboli formation. Although deterioration of mental status and tachypnea are attributable to the low tissue perfusion described, complications such as stroke and acute respiratory distress syndrome (ARDS) often contribute to the distribution of these microemboli lodging in the microcirculation of the end organs, such as the brain, splanchnic organs, and pulmonary vascular system.

In 2001 the Surviving Sepsis Campaign established guidelines promoting early detection of high-risk illness and rapid implementation of early goal-directed therapy (EGDT) in the treatment of sepsis or septic shock. They described guidelines, or bundles of action, that should be implemented within both 3-hour and 6-hour timeframes, and these measures are increasingly being implemented by hospitals worldwide.[30-32] The EGDT protocol to be implemented within 3 hours of presenting

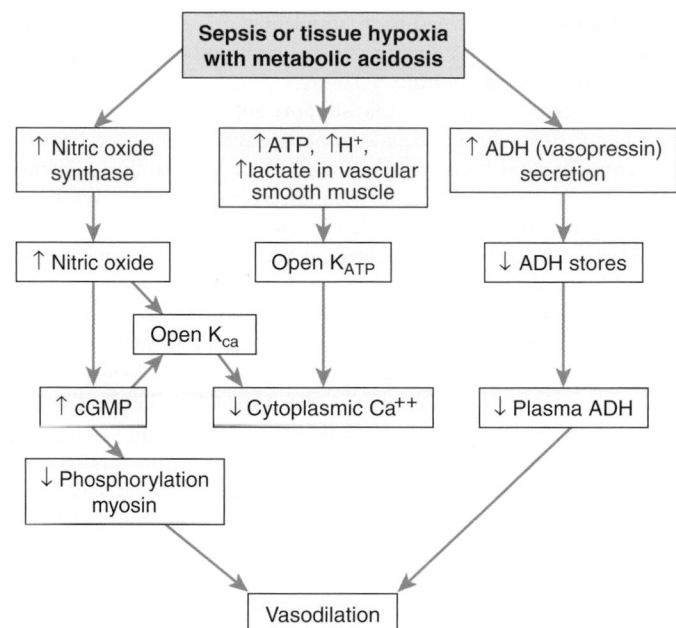

FIGURE 49.7 Mechanisms of Vasodilation in Shock. Vasodilatory shock is caused by the inappropriate activation of vasodilatory mechanisms and the failure of constrictor mechanisms. Unregulated nitric oxide, by regulating guanylate cyclase and generating cyclic guanosine monophosphate *(cGMP)*, causes dephosphorylation of myosin and, thus, vasodilation. Nitric oxide synthesis and metabolic acidosis activate the potassium channels (K$_{ATP}$ and K$_{Ca}$) in the plasma membrane of vascular smooth muscle. The resulting hyperpolarization (see Chapter 3) of the membrane presents the calcium that mediates norepinephrine-induced and angiotensin II–induced vasoconstriction from entering the cell. Therefore hypotension and vasodilation stubbornly persist despite high plasma levels of these hormones. In contrast, and unexpectedly, the plasma level of antidiuretic hormone *(ADH)* (vasopressin) is low despite the presence of hypotension. The early, massive release of ADH may result in future depletion.

with defined sepsis or septic shock is the following: (1) measure lactate level, (2) obtain blood cultures before administration of antibiotics, (3) administer broad-spectrum antibiotics, and (4) administer fluid challenge of 30 mL/kg crystalloid for hypotension or a lactate level ≤4 mmol/L. The EGDT protocol to be implemented within 6 hours of presentation is as follows: (5) administer vasopressors for hypotension that does not respond to initial fluid resuscitation to maintain a mean arterial pressure (MAP) ≥65 mmHg; (6) in the event of persistent hypotension (MAP <65 mmHg) after initial fluid administration or if the lactate level was ≤4 mmol/L, reassess volume status (central venous pressure [CVP]) and tissue perfusion (S$\bar{v}$O$_2$ or Sc$\bar{v}$O$_2$) and ensure adequate urine output; and (7) remeasure lactate level.[30-34] Specifically, fluid resuscitation should be goal directed to maintain the following values: CVP, 8 to 12 mmHg (or 12 to 15 mmHg when the person is being mechanically ventilated); urine output, 0.5 mL/kg/hour; mixed venous saturation (S$\bar{v}$O$_2$), 65%; and 70% venous pressure.

In addition, specific anatomic sites of infection with source identification should be determined so that appropriate antibiotics can be prescribed and control measures can be implemented that eliminate or reduce the spread of infection.[33,35] Fungal assays, including 1,3-β-D-glucan assay and mannan and anti-mannan antibody assays, are recommended to identify suspected fungal infection.[36] Normal saline, at least 1 L or 30 mL/kg body weight, is the initial fluid of choice and hetastarches with molecular weights >200 daltons are not recommended. Adequate and incremental fluid resuscitation is a prerequisite and should be continued to achieve perfusion; supplementation with vasopressors is recommended if the endpoints of tissue perfusion (CVP and normalized lactate levels) are not met.[30]

Pharmacologic hemodynamic support and adjunctive therapy to maintain tissue perfusion include vasoactive agents. Norepinephrine is now considered the initial vasopressor of choice.[30] Dopamine, epinephrine, phenylephrine, and vasopressin are alternatives; however, these are less preferred because of potential tachycardia, dysrhythmias, or reduction in splanchnic blood flow. Dobutamine, an inotropic agent, should be used if myocardial dysfunction is present or hypotension remains after intravascular volume and blood pressure are achieved. Similarly, intravenous corticosteroids are suggested in septic shock to help replace intrinsic loss of cortisol, but only when blood pressure remains unresponsive to volume.[33] Other supportive therapies in the treatment of severe sepsis include blood product administration to maintain hemoglobin levels between 7 and 9 g/dL, maintenance of targeted tidal volume (6 mL/kg) when mechanically ventilated with plateau pressure less than 30 cm H_2O, utilization of sedation and analgesic protocols when needed, and avoidance of neuromuscular blockers if possible. Glucose concentration is to be maintained at less than 140 mg/dL. If renal dialysis is required, intermittent hemodialysis and continuous venovenous hemofiltration are considered equivalent. Bicarbonate therapy is contraindicated for the purpose of treating hypoperfusion lactic acidemia, unless the pH is <7.15. Use of deep vein thrombosis prophylaxis, such as low-dose unfractionated heparin or low-molecular-weight heparin, or mechanical compression prophylaxis of heparin, is contraindicated. Stress ulcer prophylaxis with H2-receptor antagonists or proton pump inhibitors is indicated. Digestive tract decontamination and selective oropharyngeal decontamination are recommended in the prevention of ventilator-acquired pneumonia.[30,36] It is important to discuss advance directives with the individual and family.[33] Seeking to decrease use of antibiotics in the critically ill, and thereby prevent resistance to antibiotics, is an important strategy in treating infection. Research suggests that monitoring serial procalcitonin (PCT) levels, a precursor hormone to calcitonin, may be used to shorten antibiotic use in the treatment of respiratory tract infections.[37] Elevated procalcitonin (PCT) level indicates a nonspecific proinflammatory response seen in bacterial infection. PCT levels should not be used as an indicator to start antibiotics; however, if levels are monitored sequentially at the start of empirical antibiotics and then drop, discontinuation may be clinically indicated. However, no significant reduction in antibiotic treatment using a procalcitonin algorithm has been proven.[37-39] C-reactive protein (CRP) is an acute phase reactant protein produced by the liver, mainly in response to interleukin-6 produced by inflammation of any type. CRP is most sensitive to acute phase reactants; consequently, its level rises rapidly during inflammation. Similarly to PCT, CRP is nonspecific to types of inflammation, but may be used to trend severity of infection and response to treatment, especially in occult and resistant infections, such as osteomyelitis.

MULTIPLE ORGAN DYSFUNCTION SYNDROME

Multiple organ dysfunction syndrome (MODS) is the progressive dysfunction of two or more organ systems resulting from an uncontrolled inflammatory response to a severe illness or injury. The organ dysfunction can progress to organ failure and death. MODS occurs during severe sepsis. In 2016, an international consensus conference developed an updated set of definitions for sepsis and related disorders (see Table 49.1). MODS is the end stage of a variety of injuries that terminate in a severe, generalized inflammatory response.

MODS was first recognized as a distinct clinical syndrome in the early 1970s[40-42] when advances in resuscitation and support technologies

allowed many individuals to survive life-threatening illness or trauma only to die of complications of their disease. Today MODS remains a leading cause of mortality in surgical intensive care units (ICUs). Mortality for individuals with MODS increases progressively from 54% with two failing organ systems to 100% with five failing organ systems. Moreover, mortality has not improved much over the past 15 to 20 years.[43,44]

Although sepsis and septic shock are the most common causes, MODS can be initiated by any severe injury or disease process that activates a massive systemic inflammatory response by the host. Documented clinical infection is not necessary for its development. Other common triggers are severe trauma, major surgery, burns, circulatory shock, acute pancreatitis, acute renal failure, ARDS, blood transfusion, heat stroke, liver failure, mesenteric ischemia, propofol infusion syndrome, persistent inflammatory foci, disseminated intravascular coagulation (DIC), and tissue necrosis (Box 49.1). MODS is the major cause of death following septic shock, trauma, burn injuries, and ARDS. People at greatest risk for developing MODS are older adults and persons with significant tissue injury or preexisting disease.[21] The SOFA system (see Table 49.1), a clinically useful sepsis staging system, stratifies individuals with disease by baseline risk of adverse outcomes and potential to respond to therapy.[21]

◆ **PATHOPHYSIOLOGY.** In primary MODS, the organ injury is directly associated with a specific insult, most often ischemia or impaired perfusion from an episode of shock or trauma, thermal injury, soft tissue necrosis, or invasive infection.[45] This decreased perfusion is local (in the injured organs themselves) and generalized. The generalized hypoperfusion in primary MODS usually cannot be detected clinically. As a result of the insult, a stress response is initiated and stress hormones, catecholamines in particular, are released. The inflammatory and stress responses are not as evident because they are in secondary MODS. In primary MODS during the inflammatory response, presumably neutrophils and macrophages are "primed" by cytokines.[45] Any second insult, such as additional tissue injury, infection, or organ ischemia, may then activate the primed cells to produce an exaggerated response of secondary MODS[45,46] (Fig. 49.8).

BOX 49.1	OTHER COMMON TRIGGERS OF MODS
Severe trauma	Heat stroke
Major surgery	Liver failure
Burns	Mesenteric ischemia
Circulatory shock	Propofol infusion syndrome
Acute pancreatitis	Persistent inflammatory foci
Acute renal failure	Necrotic tissue
Acute respiratory distress syndrome	Disseminated intravascular
Blood transfusion	coagulation (DIC)

Data from Abboud D, Daher R, Boujaoude J: *World J Gastroenterol* 14(35):5361–5370, 2008; Abukauskiené D et al: *Medicina (Kaunas)* 44(7):536–540, 2008; Beger HG, Rau BM: *World J Gastroenterol* 13(38):5043–5051, 2007; Bouchama A, Knochel JP: *N Engl J Med* 346:1978–1988, 2002; Broessner G et al: *Crit Care* 9(5):R498–R501, 2006; Carnovale A et al: *J Pancreas (Online)* 6(5):438–444, 2005; Ciesla DJ et al: *Arch Surg* 140(5):432–440, 2005; Gando S: *Crit Care Med* 38(2):S35–S42, 2010; Kam PCA, Cardone D: *Anesthesia* 62(10):690–701, 2007; Oeckler RA, Hubmayr RD: *Eur Respir J* 30(6):1216–1226, 2007; Shaheen MA, Akhtar AJ: *J Nat Med Assoc* 99(12):1402–1406, 2007; Varghese GM et al: *Emerg Med J* 22:185–187, 2005; Vincent JL, Nelson DR, Williams MD: *Crit Care Med* 39(5):1050–1055, 2011; Zaccheo MM, Bucher DH: *Crit Care Nurse* 28(3):18–26, 2008.

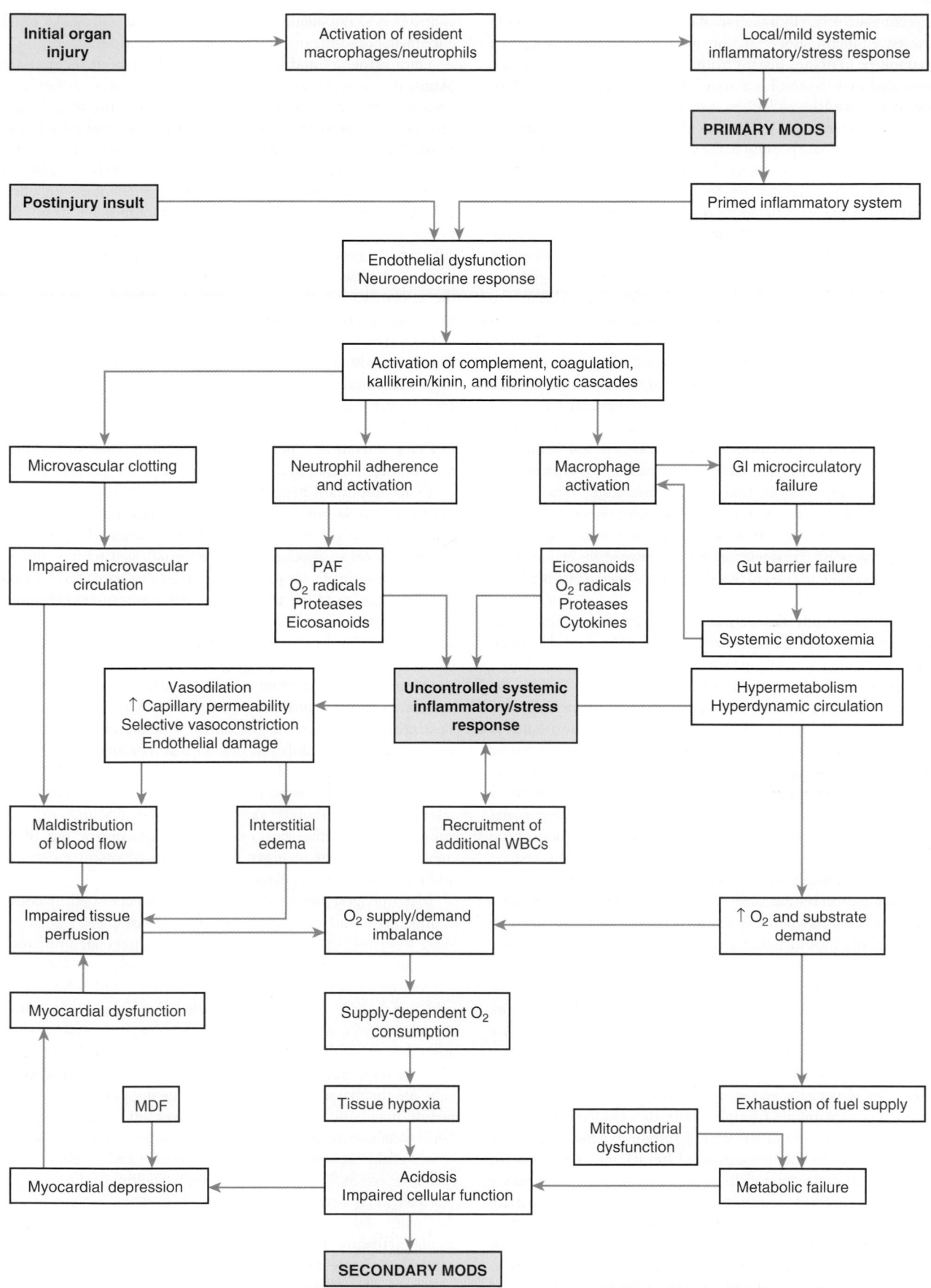

FIGURE 49.8 Pathogenesis of Multiple Organ Dysfunction Syndrome. *GI,* Gastrointestinal; *MDF,* myocardial depressant factor; *MODS,* multiple organ dysfunction syndrome; *PAF,* platelet-activating factor; *WBCs,* white blood cells.

The progressive organ dysfunction of secondary MODS is the result of an excessive inflammatory reaction, after a latent period following the initial injury, in organs distant from the site of the original injury. It is postulated that the resulting organ trauma is caused by the host response to a second insult rather than being a direct result of the primary injury. The second insult is often mild but produces an immense disproportionate response because of the previous priming of leukocytes. The interaction of injured organs then leads to a self-perpetuating inflammation.

Secondary MODS is initiated by the delayed postinjury insult as primed macrophages release a barrage of mediators, particularly the cytokines TNF and IL-1. These mediators damage the endothelium throughout the body. If a gram-negative bacterial infection is present, endotoxin released from the bacteria also causes severe damage to endothelial cells. Normal endothelial cells have little interaction with leukocytes, but when stimulated by TNF, IL-1, IL-6, or endotoxin, they change to a proinflammatory state and express adhesion molecules that mediate adhesion of neutrophils. The adhered neutrophils then migrate through the endothelium, aggregate in the area of damaged tissue, and amplify the inflammation.[3] The activated endothelial cells increase production and release of nitric oxide (endothelium), a potent vasodilator, that is considered an important factor in the blood flow changes and loss of vascular tone noted in systemic inflammation.[47] The injured endothelium also becomes much more permeable, allowing fluid and protein to leak into the interstitial spaces. An important function of normal endothelium is anticoagulation. When damaged, the endothelium loses much of its ability to prevent blood clotting, allowing microvascular thrombi to develop.

The postinjury insult also activates the neuroendocrine system, resulting in a second, more extensive stress response. The normal function of the stress response is to maintain basal and stress-related homeostasis[48]; however, homeostasis cannot be maintained in MODS. In fact, the endocrine response becomes excessive and injurious. There is an early increase in the levels of circulating catecholamines that contributes to many of the clinical manifestations of MODS, such as tachycardia, hypermetabolism, and increased oxygen consumption. Cortisol, glucagon, insulin, human growth hormone, ADH (which may become depleted), and endorphin levels also are increased. Many of these hormones contribute to the extreme catabolic state of MODS, and endorphins, which are vasodilators, decrease SVR. The sympathetic nervous system, to compensate for complications resulting from the injury (e.g., fluid loss, hypotension), also is stimulated. The stimulation persists throughout the period of critical illness.[48] The stress response can be amplified by a number of factors, including pain, anxiety, psychosis, and hyperthermia. (The stress response is discussed in detail in Chapter 11.)

Because of endothelial cell dysfunction and the release of mediators, four major plasma cascades are activated: complement, kallikrein-kinin, coagulation, and fibrinolytic.[49,50] Complement components, particularly the anaphylatoxins C3a and C5a, cause vasodilation by stimulating release of histamine from mast cells. They also have strong chemotactic properties. C5a, especially, causes adhesion and the activation and degranulation of neutrophils. Complement is thought to be a powerful trigger for the exaggerated inflammatory response. Activation of the kinin system results in the production of bradykinin, a very potent vasodilator known to decrease SVR. Coagulation mechanisms also are activated and, because tissue injury and endothelial dysfunction are extensive, microvascular thrombosis occurs throughout the body, resulting in impaired microvascular circulation and organ ischemia. Concurrently, fibrinolytic mechanisms are activated. The tendency toward clotting, however, is greater, resulting in a net procoagulant state that can lead to the development of DIC. The overall effect of the activation of the plasma cascades is a hyperinflammatory and hypercoagulant state that contributes to vasodilation, vasopermeability, cardiovascular instability, endothelial dysfunction, and clotting abnormalities.[45,50,51]

Once cytokines and other mediators have been released and the plasma enzyme cascades have been activated, a massive systemic inflammatory response develops. It involves several types of inflammatory cells, particularly neutrophils, macrophages, and mast cells. These cells, having been primed by their response to the initial organ injury, now pour large amounts of chemical mediators into tissues and into the systemic circulation. Neutrophils have tremendous inflammatory potential. The accumulation of activated neutrophils in organs is thought to play a key role in the pathogenesis of MODS.[52] When neutrophils adhere to the endothelium, they undergo a "respiratory burst" (oxidative burst) and release oxygen free radicals. The respiratory burst occurs as the activated neutrophil experiences a sudden increase in oxidative metabolism, producing large quantities of highly toxic oxygen free radicals. These reactive oxygen species (ROS) cause oxidative stress. The primary ROS produced are superoxide, hydrogen peroxide (H_2O_2), hydroxyl radical (OH^-), and singlet oxygen (O). Oxygen free radicals are extremely damaging to vascular endothelium and tissue cells, attacking deoxyribonucleic acid (DNA), cross-linking membrane structures, and inducing membrane peroxidation reactions that disorganize cell membranes and lead to tissue necrosis[3] (also see Chapter 2).

Other important mediators released by neutrophils are proteases, particularly collagenase and elastase. Proteases directly damage endothelium and neighboring cells, resulting in increased capillary permeability and organ damage. When activated, neutrophils also release platelet-activating factor (PAF), a mediator that damages endothelium, stimulates clot formation, and activates increasing numbers of phagocytes. Finally, neutrophils release arachidonic acid metabolites (eicosanoids) as a result of lipid peroxidation of their cell membranes. Of the arachidonic acid metabolites (prostaglandins, thromboxanes, leukotrienes), two are particularly important in the pathogenesis of organ hypoperfusion: prostacyclin (PGI_2) and thromboxane A_2 (TXA_2). TXA_2 is a powerful vasoconstrictor, and PGI_2 is a potent vasodilator. When released in varying amounts in different organ beds, they are largely responsible for the maldistribution of blood flow characteristic of MODS. In total, neutrophils produce at least 50 to 60 toxins.[53,54] Collectively, products released by neutrophils cause endothelial dysfunction, systemic vasodilation, selective vasoconstriction (vasoconstriction of certain organ beds or parts of organ beds), increased vascular permeability, and microvascular coagulation.

Macrophages, present in most tissues, are activated by endotoxin, complement, and monocyte chemotactic substances.[55] Macrophages share a key role in the development of the unregulated inflammation of secondary MODS with the neutrophils. Like neutrophils, they produce oxygen free radicals, proteases, cytokines, nitric oxide, and arachidonic acid metabolites. It has been reported that excessive or prolonged stimulation of macrophages leads to the overproduction of cytokines and nitric oxide that initiate the cycle of harmful effects in MODS.[3,55] TNF and IL-1, which share many of the same functions and act synergistically, are the major cytokines that mediate inflammation.[55,56] TNF has potent metabolic effects, including fever, anorexia, hyperglycemia, hypermetabolism, and weight loss. It activates neutrophils, damages endothelial cells, and potentiates hypotension and shock. IL-1 also has metabolic effects, inducing fever, hypermetabolism, and muscle wasting. Normally, TNF activates cytokines, the coagulation system, fibrinolysis, and neutrophils. With the exception of neutrophil activation, IL-1 causes similar activation in individuals with cancer.[53] In the pathogenesis of MODS, the cytokines are linked to all cellular, hemodynamic, and metabolic alterations.

The gastrointestinal mucosa is particularly vulnerable to inflammatory mediators released by macrophages and neutrophils. Under normal circumstances the gut mucosa serves as a barrier to prevent bacteria from the gastrointestinal tract from entering the systemic circulation. Damage to the mucosa results in microcirculatory failure of the gut and consequent loss of the gut barrier function. The loss of intestinal barrier function leads to the systemic spread of bacteria or endotoxin, or both, from the gut (systemic endotoxemia). This phenomenon is called *translocation of bacteria*. The idea that the gut acts as a reservoir of bacteria and endotoxin that can initiate or perpetuate the development of MODS is known as the **gut hypothesis**. The gut hypothesis provides a possible explanation for the fact that an infectious focus is not always found in individuals with MODS. Although this hypothesis has been substantiated by animal studies and has much support, the evidence from human studies is inconclusive.[57,58]

The numerous inflammatory processes operating in MODS cause maldistribution of blood flow and hypermetabolism. **Maldistribution of blood flow** refers to the uneven distribution of flow to various organs and between the large vessels and capillary beds of the body. It is caused by generalized vasodilation, increased capillary permeability, selective vasoconstriction, endothelial dysfunction, and impaired microvascular circulation. It is a major factor in the pathophysiology of MODS.[50] The alterations in blood flow—which can occur at the cellular, organ, or regional level—lead to impaired tissue perfusion and a decreased supply of oxygen to the cells. The organs most severely affected by hypoperfusion are the lungs, splanchnic bed, liver, and kidneys. Despite supernormal systemic blood flow, oxygen delivery to the tissues decreases. Several factors contribute to the problem. First, blood is shunted past selected regional capillary beds. Shunting, caused by loss of autoregulation in some organs, may be an early indicator of progression of sepsis into MODS.[59] This occurs because inflammatory mediators, particularly TXA$_2$, override the normal vascular control mechanisms to cause selective vasoconstriction and because injured endothelial cells are unable to respond to normal vasodilator mediators. Second, interstitial edema, resulting from microvascular permeability, contributes to decreased oxygen delivery to cells by increasing the distance oxygen must travel to reach the cells. Third, capillary obstruction occurs because of the formation of microvascular thrombi and the aggregation of leukocytes.[3,55]

Hypermetabolism, with accompanying alterations in carbohydrate, fat, and lipid metabolism, is initially a compensatory measure to meet the body's increased demands for energy. Eventually, however, hypermetabolism becomes detrimental, placing enormous demands on the heart. Hypermetabolism is the result of (1) the neuroendocrine response to stress with the release of catecholamines and cortisol, and (2) the action of TNF and IL-1. With increased metabolism the calorie requirements are markedly increased,[43] and the cardiac output increases to 1.5 to 2 times normal.[60,61] The alterations in metabolism affect all aspects of substrate use. Most important is the catabolism of protein, primarily of skeletal muscle and visceral organs. The extreme catabolism of protein can rapidly deplete lean body mass. Hyperglycemia occurs as gluconeogenesis by the liver increases and glucose use by the cells decreases. Fatty acids are mobilized from adipose tissue. The net result of the hypermetabolism is depletion of oxygen and fuel supplies.

Myocardial depression also accompanies MODS. The cause remains unclear, but possible explanations are the effects of myocardial depressant factor (MDF), TNF, and IL-1 on cardiac contractility; alterations in α-adrenergic receptors in the heart; and hypoxia of the myocardium.[62]

The decreased oxygen delivery to the cells (resulting from the maldistribution of blood flow) and the increased oxygen needs of the cells (resulting from hypermetabolism) combine to create an imbalance in oxygen supply and demand. This imbalance is critical in the pathogenesis of MODS because it results in a pathologic condition known as **supply-dependent oxygen consumption**. Ordinarily the amount of oxygen consumed by the cells depends only on the needs of the cells

because there is an adequate reserve of oxygen that can be delivered if required. In MODS, however, the reserve has been exhausted and the amount of oxygen consumed becomes dependent on the amount the circulation is able to deliver. Because the amount is inadequate in MODS, the tissues become hypoxic. Compounding the hypoxic damage to cells is a phenomenon called *reperfusion injury* (see Chapter 2). Much of the organ damage in MODS occurs with the reestablishment of blood flow after a period of ischemia. During the ischemic episode, energy stores and ATP are depleted and the enzyme *xanthine dehydrogenase* is converted to *xanthine oxidase*. With reperfusion of the ischemic tissue, oxygen free radicals are formed from oxygen by the action of xanthine oxidase, and they attack the already damaged tissues. Consequently, although reperfusion is necessary to restore oxygen supply to ischemic organs, it can increase the extent of injury. Therefore because of supply-dependent oxygen consumption and reperfusion injury, tissues become increasingly hypoxic. The result is cellular acidosis, impaired cellular function, and ultimately multiple organ failure.

CLINICAL MANIFESTATIONS. In MODS, the organs that show clinical manifestations of failure are not always the organs involved as part of the initial injury, and there is usually a lag time between the initial insult and the development of systemic organ failure. The development of primary MODS is difficult to monitor, but there is a well-established general pattern in the clinical development of secondary MODS.[45] Following the inciting event and aggressive resuscitation of an individual for approximately 24 hours, the individual develops low-grade fever, tachycardia, tachypnea, dyspnea, altered mental status, and a general hyperdynamic and hypermetabolic state (Box 49.2). Following this, the lungs begin to fail and ARDS may appear within 24 to 72 hours (see discussion of ARDS in Chapter 36). Between days 7 and 10, the hypermetabolic and hyperdynamic state intensifies; bacteremia with enteric organisms is common; and signs of hepatic, intestinal, and renal failure develop. During days 14 to 21, renal failure and liver failure become more severe. Hematologic failure and myocardial failure are usually later manifestations. Encephalopathy, characterized by mental status changes ranging from confusion to deep coma, may occur at any time. This sequence can evolve rapidly, with death occurring between 14 and 21 days later, or it can evolve over weeks. Individuals can recover from either the slowly or the rapidly evolving course.

The clinical manifestations of failure of individual organs in MODS are caused by inflammatory mediator damage, tissue hypoxia, and hypermetabolism. Respiratory failure progresses early to ARDS and is characterized by tachypnea, pulmonary edema with crackles and diminished breath sounds, use of accessory muscles, and hypoxemia. Liver failure, although early in its development, is not clinically detectable until the later stages of MODS, when jaundice, abdominal distention, liver tenderness, muscle wasting, and hepatic encephalopathy appear. All aspects of metabolism, substance detoxification, and immune response are impaired. Albumin and clotting factor synthesis decreases, protein wastes accumulate, and liver tissue macrophages (Kupffer cells) no longer function effectively.

The gastrointestinal system is very sensitive to ischemic and inflammatory injury. Clinical manifestations of bowel involvement are hemorrhage, ileus, stress ulcers, malabsorption, diarrhea or constipation, vomiting, anorexia, abdominal pain, and pancreatitis. Intolerance to enteral feeding may develop. Adding to damage caused by injury to the bowel is bacterial translocation into the bloodstream resulting from the loss of the gut barrier function. The overwhelmed liver is unable to clear the bacteria from the systemic circulation. Thus regardless of whether infection or some other injury was the precipitating cause of MODS, once intestinal bacteria enter the systemic circulation, it is likely that sepsis will be a problem. Renal failure develops at about the same time and is marked by progressive oliguria, azotemia, and

BOX 49.2   CLINICAL MANIFESTATIONS OF ORGAN DYSFUNCTION

Pulmonary
- Acute respiratory distress syndrome (ARDS) pattern of respiratory failure (dyspnea, patchy infiltrates, refractory hypoxemia, respiratory acidosis, abnormal O_2 indices)
- Pulmonary hypertension

Gastrointestinal
- Abdominal distention and ascites
- Intolerance to enteral feedings
- Paralytic ileus
- Upper and lower gastrointestinal bleeding (guaiac-positive stools)
- Diarrhea
- Ischemic colitis
- Mucosal ulceration
- Decreased bowel sounds
- Bacterial overgrowth in stool

Liver
- Increased serum bilirubin level (hyperbilirubinemia)
- Increased liver enzyme levels (serum aspartate transaminase [SAST], serum alanine aminotransferase [SALT], lactic dehydrogenase [LDH], alkaline phosphatase)
- Increased serum ammonia level
- Decreased serum transferrin level
- Jaundice
- Hepatomegaly

Gallbladder
- Right upper quadrant tenderness or pain
- Abdominal distention
- Unexplained fever
- Decreased bowel sounds

Metabolic/Nutritional
- Decreased lean body mass
- Muscle wasting
- Severe weight loss
- Negative nitrogen balance
- Hyperglycemia
- Hypertriglyceridemia

- Increased serum lactate levels
- Decreased serum albumin, serum transferrin, prealbumin, retinol-binding protein

Renal
- Increased serum creatinine level and blood urea nitrogen
- Oliguria, anuria, or polyuria consistent with prerenal azotemia or acute tubular necrosis
- Urinary indices consistent with prerenal azotemia or acute tubular necrosis

Cardiovascular
Hyperdynamic
- Decreased pulmonary capillary wedge pressure
- Decreased systemic vascular resistance
- Decreased right atrial pressure
- Decreased left ventricular stroke work index
- Increased oxygen consumption
- Increased cardiac output, cardiac index, heart rate

Hypodynamic
- Increased systemic vascular resistance
- Increased right atrial pressure
- Increased left ventricular stroke work index
- Decreased oxygen delivery and consumption
- Decreased cardiac output and cardiac index

Central Nervous System
- Lethargy
- Altered level of consciousness
- Fever
- Hepatic encephalopathy

Coagulation and Hematologic
- Thrombocytopenia
- Disseminated intravascular coagulation

Immune
- Infection
- Decreased lymphocyte count
- Anergy

Data from Thelan LA et al: *Critical care nursing: diagnosis and management,* ed 6, St Louis, 2010, Mosby.

edema. If renal shutdown is severe, anuria, hyperkalemia, and metabolic acidosis occur.

The first manifestations of cardiac failure are similar to those of septic shock: tachycardia, bounding pulse, increased cardiac output, fall in SVR, hypotension, warm skin, and supraventricular dysrhythmias. In the terminal stages, profound hypotension and ventricular dysrhythmias may develop. Changes in central nervous system function may be noted. Ischemia and inflammation are responsible for the changes, which include apprehension, confusion, disorientation, restlessness, agitation, headache, decreased cognitive ability and memory, and decreased level of consciousness. When ischemia is severe, seizures and coma can occur.

◆**EVALUATION AND TREATMENT.** Because there is no specific therapy for MODS, early detection or prevention is extremely important so that supportive measures are initiated instantly.[44] Frequent assessment of the clinical status of individuals at known risk is essential. Unfortu-

nately, there is no way to determine with certainty when an organ is failing. Indicators of organ dysfunction are presented in Table 49.1.

Several systems for scoring severity of illness also have been developed. Commonly used systems are the **Acute Physiology and Chronic Health Evaluation II and III (APACHE II and APACHE III)**, the logistic organ dysfunction score (LODS), the sequential organ failure assessment (SOFA), the MODS score, and the predisposition, infection (or insult), response, and organ dysfunction (PIRO) staging system.[63] Once organ failure develops, monitoring of laboratory values and hemodynamic parameters is necessary to assess the degree of clinical impairment.

The therapeutic management of MODS consists of prevention and support. Prevention of the syndrome is essential! First, if possible, the initial source of inflammation must be eliminated or controlled. Next, a second insult must be avoided. It is paramount to remove any potential site of infection by débriding necrotic tissue, draining abscesses, reducing the number of invasive procedures performed, and removing hematomas.

Nosocomial infections from contaminated lines and catheters are of concern and must be prevented. Nosocomial infection rates of 15% to 25% have been reported in critically ill individuals.[64] Early reduction of long-bone fractures and surgical repair of injured tissues also are important preventive measures.

The goals of therapy are to control infection, provide adequate tissue oxygenation, restore intravascular volume, and support the function of individual organs.[34,65-67] After the initial injury has been aggressively treated and sources of infection have been removed, antibiotics usually are administered. The choice of agents is based on the individual's disease process, but the regimen is usually a combination of antibiotics that covers both gram-negative and gram-positive organisms.

Because oxygen is not stored in the tissues, it must be continuously delivered. Maintaining an arterial oxygen saturation of 88% to 92% is recommended,[34,65-67] and hemoglobin levels should be kept greater than 9 g/dL.[34,65-67] Mixed venous oxygen saturation greater than or equal to 70% is recommended. Blood transfusions may be necessary to ensure an adequate hemoglobin level. To deliver oxygen to the organs in the face of profound systemic vasodilation, fluid volume must be restored. Therefore aggressive fluid therapy is initiated early. Usually large volumes of isotonic crystalloid solutions are administered, although colloids (often albumin) also may be added to maintain adequate preload and circulation volume.[34,65-67]

Finally, support for individual organ systems must be provided. Respiratory failure is treated with mechanical ventilation with low tidal volumes, high oxygen concentrations, and positive end-expiratory pressures (PEEPs).[68] To provide adequate nutrition and metabolic support, the failing gastrointestinal system is supported with enteral feedings. It is now well recognized that enteral feedings help preserve gut microbial barrier function, and thus are preferred to parenteral feedings.[69] However, if the individual is unable to tolerate the amount of enteral feeding required to meet the enormous metabolic demands, hyperalimentation may be added. Ideally the feeding formula is carefully calculated to meet the individual's nutritional requirements. Glucose level control (140 to 180 mg/dL) is recommended.[69] Once renal failure is established, dialysis or continuous hemofiltration may be required to maintain fluid and electrolyte balance. To support the failing cardiovascular system, inotropic drugs, such as low-dose dopamine and dobutamine, or vasopressors, such as norepinephrine, may be required to maximize cardiac contractility and maintain cardiac output. Although steroids have antiinflammatory effects, their use is controversial because they have been shown to be effective in adults with septic shock. Obtaining an adrenocorticotropic hormone (ACTH) level is not recommended. Deep vein thrombosis prophylaxis also is important.[45]

Scientific knowledge gained about MODS and inflammatory mediators has led to many investigational therapies. Novel molecular approaches targeting a variety of interdependent mediators of MODS are being investigated.[45]

BURNS

Major thermal injury is a source of massive tissue injury and destruction that has wide-reaching effects on virtually all organ systems. Burn is a generic term used to describe cutaneous injury caused by thermal, chemical, or electrical environmental causes. In addition to cutaneous injury, burns are often associated with smoke inhalation injury or other traumatic injuries that aggravate the local and systemic problems of burns. Pulmonary injury, both primary and secondary, is common in this population and often requires ventilator support. The use of tracheostomy has been examined in these populations.[70-73] This model of multisystem injury provides an opportunity to examine the interaction of shock, inflammation, and immunocompromise in a clinical setting.

Epidemiology and Etiology

The incidence of burns in the United States dropped from 4.2 per 100,000 during the years 1961 through 1964 to 1.5 per 100,000 during the period 1993 through 1996.[74] Burns and fire-related injuries requiring medical treatment are now estimated to be about 486,000 annually in the United States.[75] Deaths consequent to these injuries decreased more than 50%, from 9000 in 1971[76] to 3275 annually.[75] This clinical progress is the result of several factors, such as ongoing research in burn physiology and burn care,[77] a nationally increased focus on fire safety and burn prevention, the establishment of regional burn centers, the use of smoke detectors, regulation of consumer product safety, and occupational safety mandates. A decrease in hospitalization is a result of a shift to outpatient care and improved prehospital and emergency treatment, as well as an improvement in burn assessment and delivery of care.[78] This may reduce medical transport and treatment costs. Worldwide interest in telemedicine has blossomed over the past decade.[79,80] These advances in care are changing measures of healthcare value from burn survival to functional outcomes in burn survivors.[81,82]

The causes of burn injury may be thermal or nonthermal, such as chemical, electrical, or radioactive. Thermal burns may result from thermal contact, flame, or scald. Adherent materials (e.g., asphalt, tar, or plastic) may likewise produce a serious contact burn. Chemical injuries are a result of contact with substances that are directly toxic to the skin or the lining of the respiratory or alimentary tract. Such chemicals are often acidic, alkali, or organic agents, termed vesicants, that cause blistering of the epithelial surfaces. Electrical burns may be the result of the conduction of electrical current through the body with heating of tissue or flash over the body surface associated with an electrical discharge. Quality of life can be affected but life quality may exceed normal population averages with proper intervention.[83]

Burn Wound Depth

The classification of burn wound depth is usually based on the physical appearance and the symptoms associated with the affected skin. The definitive diagnosis is determined by the histologic depth of tissue necrosis. Such historic evaluation, unfortunately, necessitates a skin biopsy. Because of the invasive nature of biopsy, clinical depth assessment is used and the ultimate fate of the wound determines final diagnosis. Recent advances in laser Doppler technology have resulted in extensive exploration of noninvasive means for burn wound depth assessment.[84-96]

First-degree burns are a partial-thickness injury involving only the epidermis without injury to the underlying dermal or subcutaneous tissue (Table 49.2). The skin maintains water vapor and bacterial barrier functions. Many sunburns are first-degree injuries caused by exposure of the skin to ultraviolet radiation from the sun. Initially there is local pain and erythema, but no blisters appear until after about 24 hours. An extensive first-degree burn may cause systemic responses such as chills, headache, localized edema, and nausea or vomiting. No treatment of extensive first-degree burns is required unless the person is elderly or an infant, in which case severe nausea and vomiting may lead to inadequate fluid intake and dehydration. Therapy consists of intravenous hydration until the nausea and vomiting subside 24 to 72 hours after burn injury. Comfort measures for previously healthy children or adults with extensive first-degree burns consist of aspirin for adults or acetaminophen for children every 4 hours in age-appropriate doses and frequent application of a water-soluble lotion. First-degree burns heal in 3 to 5 days without scarring.

Second-degree burns describe two categories of burn depth with markedly different characteristics. Both of these are partial-thickness injuries, but they evoke vastly different responses. The hallmark of superficial partial-thickness injury is the appearance of thin-walled,

TABLE 49.2	DEPTH OF BURN INJURY			
	FIRST DEGREE	**SECOND DEGREE**		**THIRD DEGREE**
CHARACTERISTIC		**SUPERFICIAL PARTIAL THICKNESS**	**DEEP PARTIAL THICKNESS**	**FULL THICKNESS**
Morphology	Destruction of epidermis only	Destruction of epidermis and some dermis	Destruction of epidermis and dermis, leaving only skin appendages	Destruction of epidermis, dermis, and underlying subcutaneous tissue
Skin function	Intact	Absent	Absent	Absent
Tactile and pain sensors	Intact	Intact	Intact but diminished	Absent
Blisters	Present only after first 24 hr	Present within minutes, thin walled and fluid filled	May appear as fluid-filled blisters; often is layer of flat, dehydrated "tissue paper" that lifts off in sheets	Blisters rare; usually is a layer of flat, dehydrated "tissue paper" that lifts off easily
Appearance of wound after initial débridement	Skin peels at 24–48 hr, normal or slightly red underneath	Red to pale ivory, moist surface	Mottled with areas of waxy white, dry surface	White, cherry red, or black; may contain visible thrombosed veins; dry, hard leathery surface
Healing time	3–5 days	21–28 days	30 days to many months	Will not heal; may close from edges as secondary healing if wound is small
Scarring	None	May be present; low incidence influenced by genetic predisposition	Highest incidence because of slow healing rate promoting scar tissue development; also influenced by genetic predisposition	Skin graft; scarring minimized by early excision and grafting; influenced by genetic predisposition

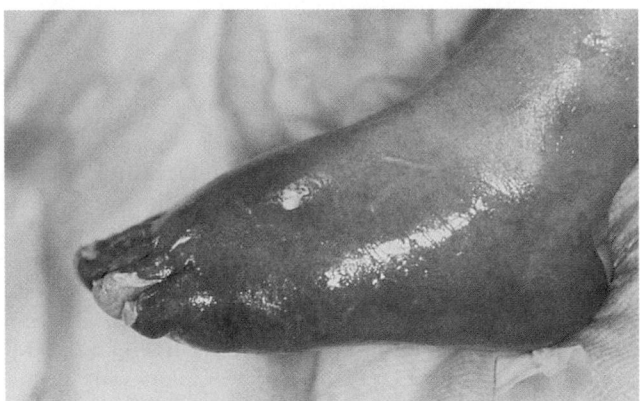

FIGURE 49.9 Superficial Partial-Thickness Injury. Scald injury following débridement of overlying blister and nonadherent epithelium. (Courtesy University of Utah Burn Center.)

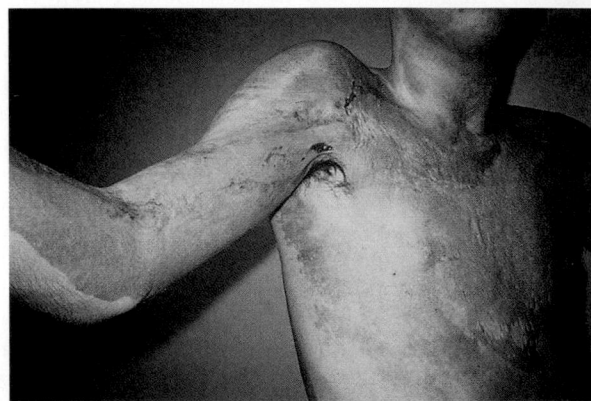

FIGURE 49.10 Axillary Burn Scar Contracture. Note the blanching of the anterior axillary fold and small ulceration, both indicating the diminished range of motion. (Courtesy University of Utah Burn Center.)

fluid-filled blisters that develop within just a few minutes after injury. Another dominant characteristic of superficial injury is pain. As blisters break or are removed, nerve endings are exposed to air (Fig. 49.9). Tactile and pain sensors remain intact throughout healing, with each wound care procedure causing substantial pain. Wounds heal in 3 to 4 weeks if the individual is adequately nourished and no complications develop (Fig. 49.10). Scar formation is unusual with this injury. The amount of scarring that develops is a genetically determined trait and is not predictable during the early course of treatment.

Deep partial-thickness burns involve the entire dermis, sparing skin appendages such as hair follicles and sweat glands (see Table 49.2). The burn often looks waxy white and is surrounded by margins of superficial partial-thickness injury. The injury is often clinically indistinguishable from a full-thickness injury (Fig. 49.11), but by 7 to 10

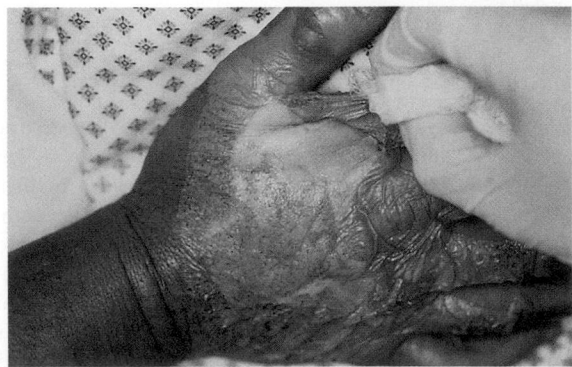

FIGURE 49.11 Deep Partial-Thickness Wound. Note pale appearance and minimal exudate. (Courtesy University of Utah Burn Center.)

days after burn injury, skin buds and hair will appear from hair follicles, indicating that skin appendages remain. These wounds take weeks to heal, and current therapy consists of surgical removal of the burn wound (excision) followed by application of the person's own unburned skin from another body area (autograft). Wounds that heal slowly produce more scar tissue and continue to be a potential source of infection until closed. In the presence of relative surgical contraindications, such as cardiopulmonary failure, deep partial-thickness wounds are not surgically treated but are allowed to heal primarily. The fate of partial-thickness burns can be affected by treatment, such as topical antibiotics, or by the condition of biologic membranes.[97] The ultimate healing of deep partial-thickness burns commonly results in hypertrophic scarring with poor functional and cosmetic results.

Third-degree burns, or **full-thickness injuries**, involve destruction of the entire epidermis, dermis, and often the underlying subcutaneous tissue (see Table 49.2). On occasion, all underlying subcutaneous tissue is destroyed and muscle or bone may be involved. Full-thickness wounds often appear relatively innocuous when their color is white and the delineation between normal and burned skin is not accompanied by a marked color change. Elasticity of the dermis is absent, leaving the wound dry and leathery in appearance and texture (Fig. 49.12). As marked edema develops, distal circulation may be compromised in areas of circumferential burns. **Escharotomies** (cutting through burned skin) are performed to release underlying pressure. Full-thickness burns are painless because all nerve endings have been destroyed by the injury.

The extent of the **total body surface area (TBSA)** burn is estimated using either the "rule of nines" (Fig. 49.13) or the Lund and Browder chart (Fig. 49.14). Areas of partial-thickness and full-thickness injury are marked on the diagram in Fig. 49.14. First-degree burns are not included in the TBSA estimate. The surface area of the palm, including palmar finger surface, averages 1% of the body surface area over a wide range of ages; thus it can be used to estimate burn areas of irregular size and shape.[98]

Severity of burn injury is a combination of many factors, including age, medical history, extent and depth of injury, and body area involved. The American Burn Association has defined criteria to assist healthcare professionals in identifying individuals who require care at a specialized burn center (Box 49.3). The multidisciplinary burn center is recommended for those persons who are at high risk for morbidity, mortality, or permanent functional loss.

◆**PATHOPHYSIOLOGY AND CLINICAL MANIFESTATIONS.** Burn injury results in dramatic changes in many physiologic functions of the body within the first few hours after the event. The effect of burn depends on two factors: first, the extent of body surface involved; and second, the depth of cutaneous injury. Body surface burn extent is described

by the percentage of TBSA injured. Burns exceeding 20% of TBSA in most adults are considered to be major burn injuries and are associated with massive evaporative water losses and flux of large amounts of fluid and electrolytes in the tissues, manifested as generalized edema and circulatory hypovolemia. Depth of cutaneous injury has been categorized

---

BOX 49.3   BURN CENTER REFERRAL CRITERIA

A burn center may treat adults or children, or both. Burn injuries that should be referred to a center include the following:

1. Partial-thickness burns greater than 10% total body surface area (TBSA).
2. Burns that involve the face, hands, feet, genitalia, perineum, or major joints.
3. Third-degree burns in any age group.
4. Electrical burns, including lightning injury.
5. Chemical burns.
6. Inhalation injury.
7. Burn injury in individuals with preexisting medical disorders that could complicate management, prolong recovery, or affect mortality.
8. Burns and concomitant trauma (such as fractures) in which the burn injury poses the greatest risk of morbidity or mortality. If the trauma poses the greater immediate risk, the individual's condition may be stabilized initially in a trauma center before being transferred to a burn center. Physician judgment will be necessary in such situations and should be in concert with the regional medical control plan and triage protocols.
9. Burns in children; children with burns should be transferred to a burn center verified to treat children. In the absence of a regional pediatric burn center, an adult burn center may serve as a second option for the management of pediatric burns.
10. Burn injury in individuals who will require special social, emotional, or rehabilitative intervention.

From *Resources for optimal care of the injured patient*, Chicago, IL, 2014, Committee on Trauma, American College of Surgeons.

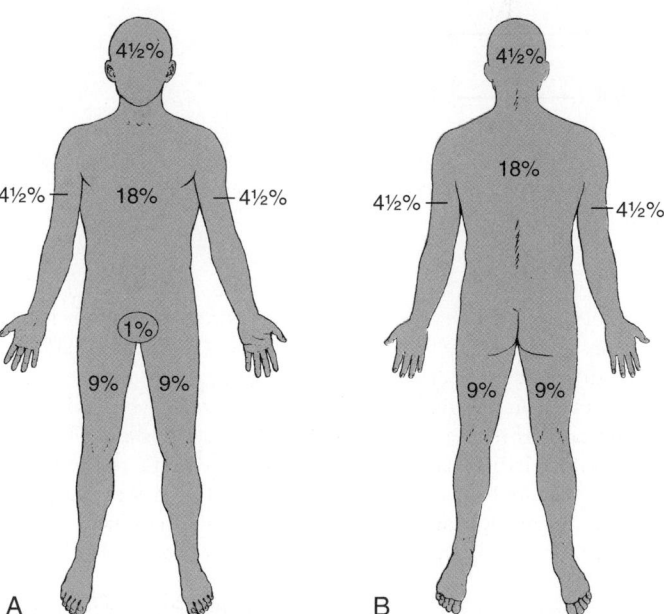

FIGURE 49.13 Rule of Nines. A commonly used assessment tool with estimates of the percentages (in multiples of 9) of the total body surface area burned. **A,** Adults (anterior view). **B,** Adults (posterior view).

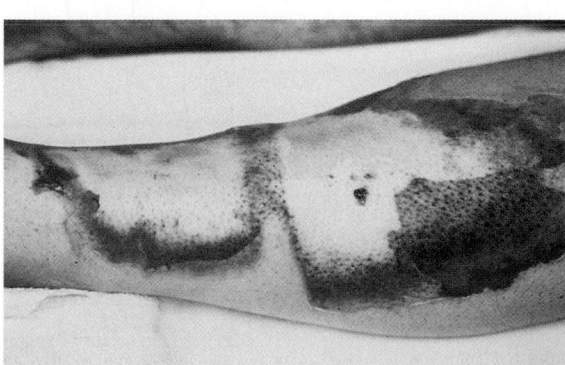

FIGURE 49.12 Full-Thickness Thermal Injury. The wound is dry and insensate. (Courtesy University of Utah Burn Center.)

Area	Birth 1 yr.	1-4 yr.	5-9 yr.	10-14 yr.	15 yr.	Adult	2°	3°	Total	Donor Areas
Head	19	17	13	11	9	7				
Neck	2	2	2	2	2	2				
Ant. Trunk	13	13	13	13	13	13				
Post. Trunk	13	13	13	13	13	13				
R. Buttock	2$\frac{1}{2}$	2$\frac{1}{2}$	2$\frac{1}{2}$	2$\frac{1}{2}$	2$\frac{1}{2}$	2$\frac{1}{2}$				
L. Buttock	2$\frac{1}{2}$	2$\frac{1}{2}$	2$\frac{1}{2}$	2$\frac{1}{2}$	2$\frac{1}{2}$	2$\frac{1}{2}$				
Genitalia	1	1	1	1	1	1				
R. U. Arm	4	4	4	4	4	4				
L. U. Arm	4	4	4	4	4	4				
R. L. Arm	3	3	3	3	3	3				
L. L. Arm	3	3	3	3	3	3				
R. Hand	2$\frac{1}{2}$	2$\frac{1}{2}$	2$\frac{1}{2}$	2$\frac{1}{2}$	2$\frac{1}{2}$	2$\frac{1}{2}$				
L. Hand	2$\frac{1}{2}$	2$\frac{1}{2}$	2$\frac{1}{2}$	2$\frac{1}{2}$	2$\frac{1}{2}$	2$\frac{1}{2}$				
R. Thigh	5$\frac{1}{2}$	6$\frac{1}{2}$	8	8$\frac{1}{2}$	9	9$\frac{1}{2}$				
L. Thigh	5$\frac{1}{2}$	6$\frac{1}{2}$	8	8$\frac{1}{2}$	9	9$\frac{1}{2}$				
R. Leg	5	5	5$\frac{1}{2}$	6	6$\frac{1}{2}$	7				
L. Leg	5	5	5$\frac{1}{2}$	6	6$\frac{1}{2}$	7				
R. Foot	3$\frac{1}{2}$	3$\frac{1}{2}$	3$\frac{1}{2}$	3$\frac{1}{2}$	3$\frac{1}{2}$	3$\frac{1}{2}$				
L. Foot	3$\frac{1}{2}$	3$\frac{1}{2}$	3$\frac{1}{2}$	3$\frac{1}{2}$	3$\frac{1}{2}$	3$\frac{1}{2}$				
						TOTAL				

Cause of Burn _____

Date of Burn _____

Time of Burn _____

Age _____

Sex _____

Weight _____

BURN DIAGRAM

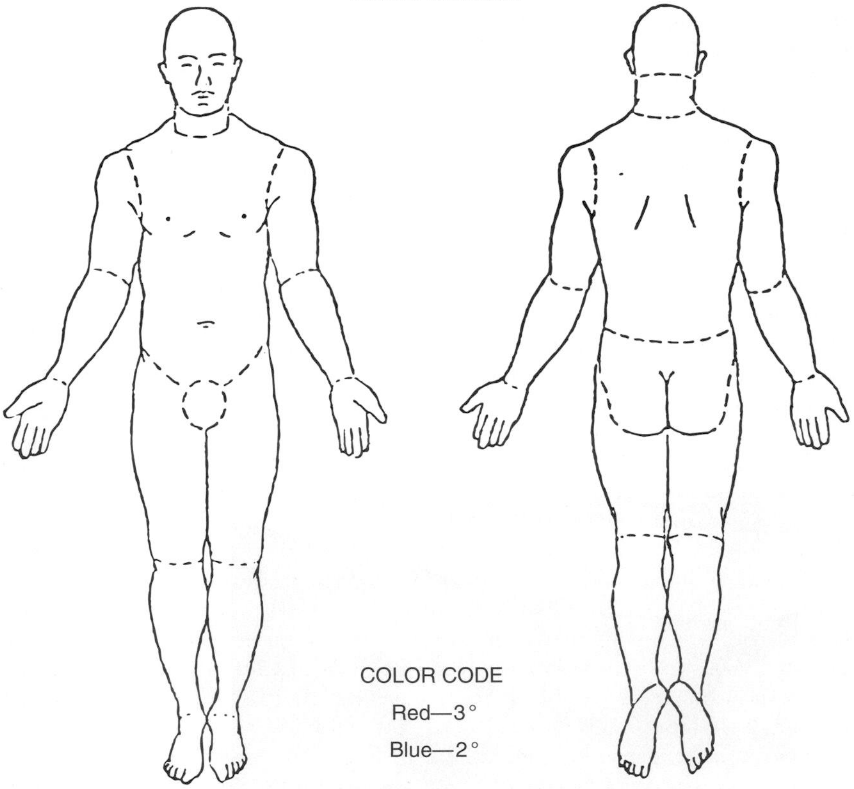

COLOR CODE

Red—3°

Blue—2°

FIGURE 49.14 Lund and Browder Chart. Regional differences in body surface area are calculated based on age. (Courtesy University of Utah Burn Center.)

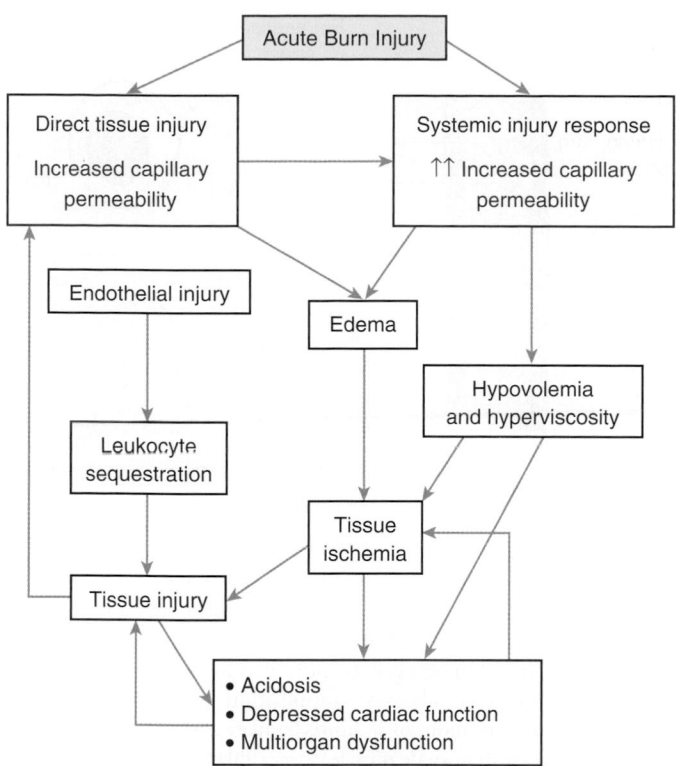

FIGURE 49.15 Immediate Cellular and Immunologic Alterations of Burn Shock.

TABLE 49.3	ELECTROLYTE CONTENT OF RINGER LACTATE SOLUTION AND EXTRACELLULAR FLUID	
ELECTROLYTE	**EXTRACELLULAR FLUID* (mEq/L)**	**LACTATED RINGER SOLUTION[†] (mEq/L)**
Sodium	135–145	130
Potassium	3.2–4.5	4
Chloride	95–105	109
Lactate (bicarbonate)	24–28	28

*Normal values may vary slightly between laboratories.
[†]Plus 80–100 mL of free water per liter.

in many ways but always depends on the severity of injury of epidermal and dermal elements of the skin and whether the alteration is a permanent or reversible injury.

With a major burn injury, a systemic pathophysiology ensues that requires therapeutic intervention to sustain life. The immediate (acute) physiologic consequences of a major burn injury center around the profound, life-threatening hypovolemic shock that occurs in conjunction with cellular and immunologic disruption within a few hours of injury (Fig. 49.15). **Burn shock** is a phenomenon consisting of both a hypovolemic cardiovascular component and a cellular component.

Hypovolemia associated with burn shock results from massive fluid losses from the circulating blood volume. The losses are caused by an increase in capillary permeability that persists for approximately 24 hours after burn injury. **Fluid resuscitation** is the administration of intravenous fluids, such as lactated Ringer solution, given in an effort to restore the circulating blood volume during the period of increasing capillary permeability. In addition to hypovolemia, most other organ systems are affected. Cardiac contractility is diminished during the initial 24-hour resuscitation period with shunting of blood away from the liver, kidney, and gut. This is often termed the *ebb phase* of the response to trauma and can be seen with other severe injuries. Normal blood volume does not result in restoration of normal cardiac output because of a phenomenon known as *myocardial depression*. The decrease in perfusion of viscera results in a decrease in their function. This may be an explanation for decreased gut barrier function seen in thermal injury.[99] Other mechanisms include hypoxia and inflammation with histologic damage of intestinal mucosa.[100]

There also is evidence that cellular metabolism is disrupted when the burn wound is created, resulting in altered cell membrane permeability and loss of normal electrolyte homeostasis. This cellular defect may be the pathophysiologic process responsible for the genesis of burn shock. There are numerous circulating factors in burn serum that may

play a role in these cellular processes. Although the cardiovascular and systemic responses are intricately interwoven into the cellular response, these responses are presented here as discrete entities for purposes of description.

Cardiovascular and Systemic Response to Burn Injury

The clinical manifestations of burn shock are the result of more than simple loss of extracellular fluid at the burn wound site. Hypovolemia and numerous local mediators in the burn wound,[101] as well as systemic signals, result in alteration of cellular function throughout the body. The restoration of normal intravascular volume with either saline solutions or colloid materials (e.g., albumin, blood, or dextrans) does not reverse changes such as increases in pulmonary vascular resistance or myocardial contractility.[102-104] This is reflected in cardiac output with precipitous decreases that often result in inadequate perfusion of most tissues at the capillary level, which is the hallmark of burn shock. Fluid infusion, likewise, does not return cardiac output to preburn levels.[105,106] These findings led to the postulation of a specific myocardial depressant factor (MDF).[102,107,108] Other causes also have been suggested, such as reactive oxygen free radicals that attack cell membranes and other subcellular organelles as a result of first ischemia and then reperfusion of tissues during burn shock and resuscitation.[109] A third factor may be the level of nitric oxide after burn injury, which could have a direct myocardial depressant effect.[110,111] The relationship of nitric oxide and myocardial function is not yet totally clear. Gamelli and colleagues[112] found nitric oxide production to be significantly depressed in burned individuals who did not survive their injuries. They postulated that nitric oxide may scavenge reactive oxygen free radicals and protect tissues from oxidative injury.

Regardless of the contribution of these mechanisms, fluid resuscitation eventually results in improved outcome of the massively burned person. This resuscitation involves infusion of intravenous fluid at a rate faster than the loss of circulatory vascular volume for a period of about 24 hours from the time of burn injury, and may require up to 30 L in a major burn. Resuscitation from burn shock can be accomplished using any of a number of infusion protocols. The most frequently used protocol is the Parkland formula.[113] Lactated Ringer solution is used because it closely approximates extracellular fluid, the repository of fluid leaving the circulatory system during this phase of extensive edema formation (Table 49.3). The use of electrolyte-free fluids, such as D_5W, results in life-threatening hypovolemia and hyponatremia. Resuscitation with hypertonic saline has been used in some centers but is reserved for special circumstances; its use can result in adverse outcomes.[114]

The massive edema associated with burn shock is inevitable with fluid resuscitation, and failure to administer resuscitation fluid results

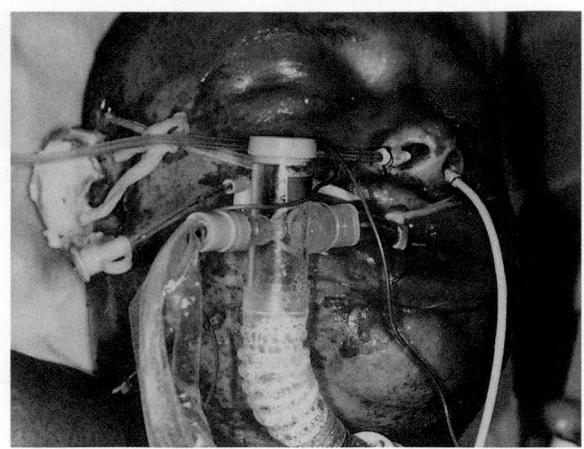

FIGURE 49.16 Edema Related to Burn Injury. Superficial facial burns can result in marked swelling, requiring prompt endotracheal intubation to maintain the airway. (Courtesy University of Utah Burn Center.)

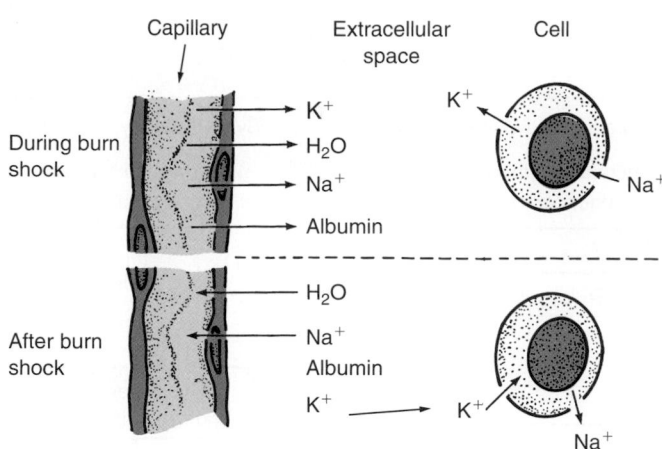

FIGURE 49.17 Direction of Fluid and Electrolyte Shifts Associated with Burn Shock. (Courtesy University of Utah Burn Center.)

in irreversible hypovolemic shock and death. The edema occurs in unburned as well as burned areas (Fig. 49.16). This often leads to mechanical airway obstruction, necessitation of tracheal intubation, and increased severity of the interstitial pulmonary edema associated with inhalation injury.

The most reliable criterion for adequate resuscitation of burn shock is urine output. The individual is in hypovolemic shock and will, as a compensatory mechanism, decrease or stop urine output in an effort to preserve circulation volume. The adult receiving sufficient intravenous fluids will excrete urine amounting to 30 to 50 mL/hour; children will produce 1 mL/kg/hour. If the individual does not have adequate urine output, it often indicates inadequate fluid resuscitation. The massive amount of intravenous fluid required by burned individuals during the shock phase is often intimidating to the person unfamiliar with burns. One common concern is that massive fluid administration will result in pulmonary edema. It should be remembered that the individual is in hypovolemic shock and that fluid is lost dramatically during the resuscitation period through third spacing, exudation, and evaporation.

The endpoint of burn shock is defined as the state in which the individual is able to maintain adequate urine output for 2 hours with the intravenous fluid administration rate equal to the individual's calculated maintenance rate. As burn shock ends, fluid administered remains in the circulating volume and is reflected as an increase in urine output. The mechanism whereby capillary integrity is restored is unknown but usually occurs about 24 hours after burn injury (Fig. 49.17). After the individual has reached the endpoint of burn shock, the term used to describe the vascular status of the individual is **capillary seal**. In individuals with large burns, colloid-containing fluids may be given to help maintain oncotic pressure during the resuscitation phase and afterward to enhance the mobilization of interstitial fluid and diuresis.[115] Efforts to decrease burn edema and fluid resuscitation volumes can involve the use of hypertonic fluid resuscitation as well.[116]

Cellular Response to Burn Injury

In addition to capillary endothelial permeability changes resulting in vascular fluid losses, transmembrane potential changes occur in cells not directly damaged by heat. The normal potential of −90 mV decreases to nearly −70 mV, with an increase in the levels of intracellular sodium and water. Such membrane potential changes may be caused by a circulating shock factor.[117] Apoptosis is central to the cellular responses to burn injury.[118] Other changes can be categorized as (1) a metabolic response to the burn injury or (2) an immunologic response to the burn injury.

Metabolic Response. The metabolic changes after a burn injury were described in 1967 by Welt and associates as "sick cell syndrome."[119] This was considered to be a cell membrane transport defect related to an alteration in the steady-state composition characterized by high intracellular concentrations of sodium. Trunkey and colleagues[120] found a marked decrease in primate muscle extracellular water and an increase in intracellular sodium and water during hypovolemic shock. In addition, other researchers demonstrated an associated decrease in resting membrane potential, a decrease in amplitude of the action potential, and a prolongation of the repolarization and depolarization times in association with a decreased intracellular potassium concentration.[121,122] The cellular dysfunction of burn injury extends beyond the transmembrane potential disruption and the sodium-potassium pump impairment to include a loss of intracellular magnesium and phosphate[123] and elevated serum lactic acid dehydrogenase (LDH) levels.[124] Thus impairment of basic cellular function may be the underlying cause of the diminished membrane potentials. The data suggest a decrease in the efficiency of the pump. The failure of rapid intravascular volume repletion to restore membrane potential completely suggests other pathways for cellular metabolic derangement.[125]

Metabolic reactions to the stress of a major burn injury involve the response of the sympathetic nervous system and other homeostatic regulators. Catecholamines are found in elevated amounts in both the serum and urine of burned individuals. Cortisol, glucagon, and insulin levels are elevated, with a corresponding increase in gluconeogenesis, lipolysis, and proteolysis. Changes in lipid metabolism are reflected as an elevation in the level of plasma free fatty acids (FFAs) and a decrease in the levels of plasma cholesterol and phospholipids.[126] Herndon and colleagues[127] found that the use of propranolol, a nonselective beta₁- and beta₂-blocker, could attenuate symptoms of the hypermetabolic response, including a decrease in heart rate and lipolysis. Glucose and lactate kinetics are altered after burn injury. Although tissue hypoxia produces lactic acidosis, its persistence in the presence of adequate tissue perfusion suggests an increased rate of glycogenolysis.[128] A small study conducted by Akcay and colleagues[129] showed that growth hormone levels are diminished in major burn injuries and appear to improve survival but more clearly affect wound healing.[130]

Burn injury induces a hypermetabolic state that persists until wound closure. Wilmore and colleagues[131] described the hypermetabolic state of 20 burned individuals as unrelated to ambient temperatures, with persistent elevation of core body temperatures. The metabolic rate increased with burn size in a curvilinear relationship, with oxygen consumption

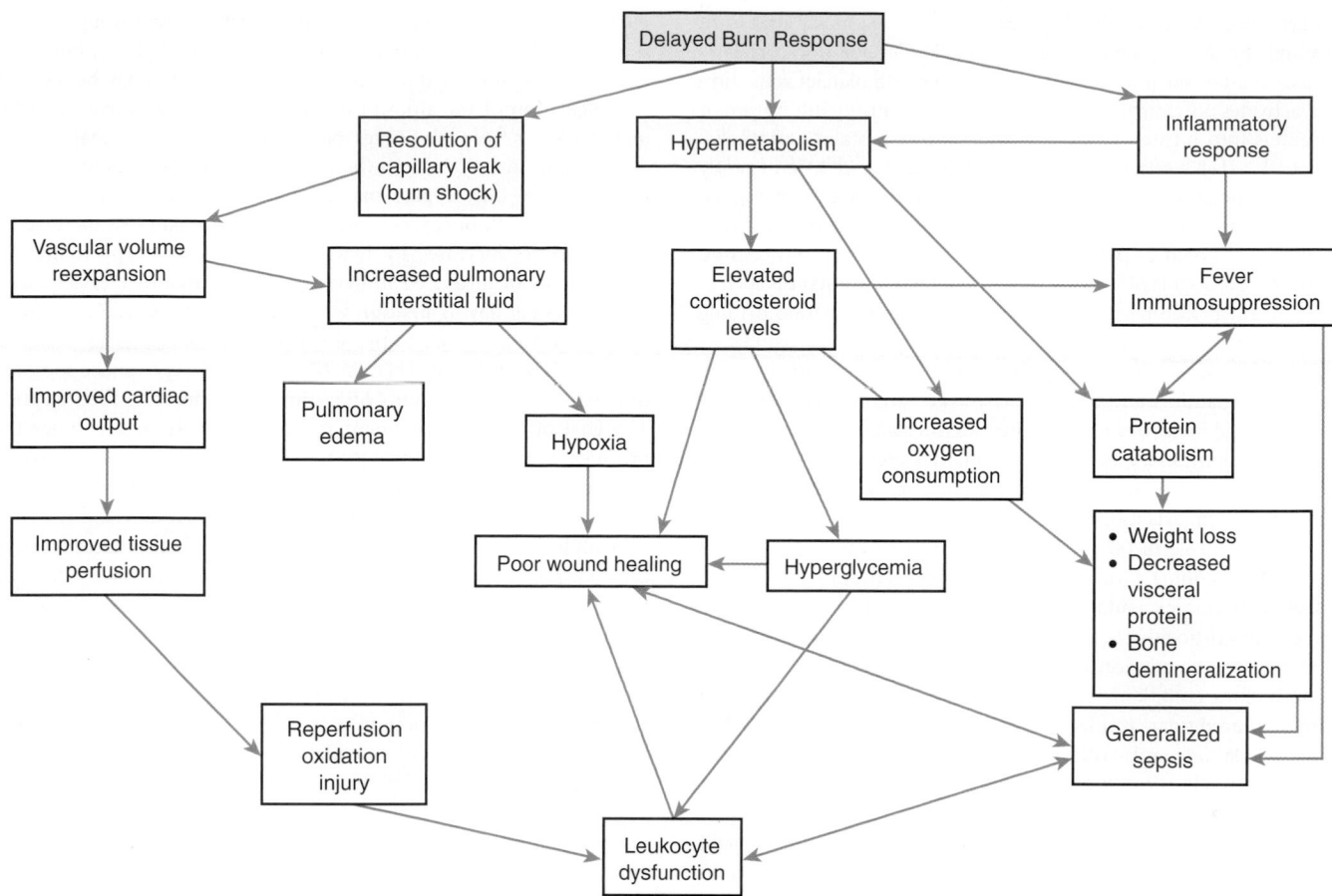

FIGURE 49.18 Physiologic Alterations in Inflammatory Burn Injury Response.

rarely exceeding two times basal levels. Evaporative water loss and surface cooling are not the primary stimulus for the hypermetabolic state; rather, the hypermetabolism is related to an increase and resetting of the thermal regulatory set point. A core body temperature of 38.5°C (101.3°F) is typical. A reflex arc mobilizes neural or hormonal afferent stimuli to the hypothalamus, producing a catecholamine response clinically manifested as hypermetabolism, hyperthermia, and hyperglycemia.

Evidence also exists that the burn wound itself directly mediates the response to injury at both the local and systemic levels. Cytokines, oxygen free radicals, chemotactic substances, and eicosanoids contribute to the systemic inflammatory response and hypermetabolic state. The inflammatory response to the wound level is magnified into a generalized systemic inflammatory response that is often deleterious.[132-134] Vasodilation, increased capillary permeability, and edema occur to facilitate healing of the local area. The distribution of the peripheral circulation after burn injury transports heat and glucose preferentially to the wound. The energy cost of these reparative and transport processes is reflected in the increased metabolism and hyperdynamic circulation.

The extensive evaporative water loss that occurs in burn tissue is a heat-consuming process, and the energy of evaporation is provided by increased visceral heat production. The signal for the response is unknown because individuals whose wounds have been denervated continue to have a **posttraumatic hypermetabolic response**. Hypothalamic function alterations result in the elevation of human growth hormone (hGH) serum levels in the presence of hyperglycemia, a finding opposite that in normal states.[131] Further, the hypermetabolic rate is not decreased during rest, sleep, or warmth.

Evidence of hepatic response to burn injury is characterized by alterations in the clotting factors.[135] A hypercoagulable state develops as manifested by an elevated plasma fibrinogen concentration in the presence of shortened prothrombin time (PT) and activated partial thromboplastin time (PTT).[136]

In summary, extensive burn injury initiates the most marked alterations in body metabolism associated with any illness (Fig. 49.18). Much of the work explaining this response has been conducted by Wilmore,[137,138] who reported that the persistent tachycardia, hyperpnea, hyperpyrexia, and marked body wasting seen in burn injury reflect heightened metabolic activity and accelerated body catabolism. The development of decreased bone density can last long after discharge from the hospital.[139] These systemic alterations occur as a result of the cutaneous inflammatory process and are thought to facilitate wound repair. The neural component of this alteration is in response to a sympathetic reaction that releases catecholamines in large amounts.

Immunologic Response. The immunologic response to burn injury is immediate, prolonged, and severe. The result in individuals surviving burn shock is immunosuppression with increased susceptibility to potentially fatal systemic burn wound sepsis.

Several cytokines have been identified in the immediate postburn period. Interkeukin-1 (IL-1) is detected in the serum of burned individuals. The level of IL-1 correlates inversely with burn survival; low levels may be associated with a higher mortality.[140] Fatal burn injury has often shown decreased levels of IL-2, which may result in decreased T helper 1 (Th1) lymphocytes. Th1 cells produce IL-2, interferon-gamma, and TNF, which help to initiate cellular immunity and immunoglobulin G (IgG) production. IL-4 is elevated after burn injuries and causes a shift in the T-helper cell production from Th1 to Th2 lymphocytes. Th2 cells secrete IL-4, which promotes further conversion of nonspecific Th cells to Th2 cells. Th2 cells also produce other cytokines and antibodies.[141] IL-6 levels increase quickly after burn injury and remain elevated for several weeks. The level of IL-6 correlates with the extent of burn injury.[142] IL-6, together with platelet activation factor, activates polymorphonuclear neutrophils, causing infiltration of neutrophils into burned tissue and adhesion to vascular endothelial surfaces.[143,144] IL-8 levels are elevated after burn injury with significantly greater elevations in individuals with a TBSA burn of 40% or higher. IL-8 activity may play a role in the strong and persistent activation of neutrophils noted in people with large burns.[145] Burn blister fluid contains large amounts of IL-6 and IL-8 in addition to substances such as epidermal growth factor, platelet-derived growth factor, and transforming growth factor.[146]

Macrophages, platelets, neutrophils, and vascular endothelial cells release prostaglandins and leukotrienes, which are the byproducts of arachidonic acid metabolism. These chemical mediators cause peripheral vasodilation, pulmonary vasoconstriction, increased capillary permeability, and local tissue ischemia in the burn wound.

A host of chemicals found in burn plasma in altered concentrations also may play a role in burn shock. These include vasoactive amines (histamine, serotonin), products of complement activation (C3a, C5a), prostaglandins, kinins, endotoxin, and metabolic hormones (catecholamines, glucocorticoids). A decrease in complement components C3a and C5a in the circulation after burn injury suggests a nonspecific activation of the complement system.[147] Activation of the complement system in injured tissue results in an inflammatory response caused by release of histamine and serotonin by C3a and C5a, because histamine and serotonin alter capillary permeability and participate in the mechanism of burn shock along with kinin polypeptides and other chemical mediators. Prostaglandins function in the inflammatory process by regulating the metabolism of cells of inflammation (see Chapter 7).

Burn shock can induce changes in the integrity of the intestinal wall, facilitating bacterial translocation and endotoxemia.[148] Bacterial translocation from the gut may be a mechanism of infection leading to septic shock after burn injury and other major trauma.[149] Circulating endotoxin is correlated with the development of MODS and death after major burn injury.[150]

White blood cells are also altered at this time, when their need to inhibit sepsis is vital. Natural resistance to infection in burn wounds is a function of the nonspecific immune system; that is, resistance to microorganisms that infect wounds rests almost solely on the ability of phagocytic cells (i.e., granulocytes, macrophages) to leave the bloodstream, migrate to the site of infection, and ingest and kill microorganisms.[151] Normally opsonins render bacteria susceptible to phagocytosis, but the burn injury triggers a consumptive opsoninopathy. Burn serum contains an inhibitor of C3 conversion that leads to decreased opsonization and polymorphonuclear (PMN) dysfunction.[152,153]

Individuals with altered immunocompetence before burn injury are at additional risk for complications. Opportunistic infections, such as fungal sepsis, can increase a hospital stay and intensive care unit (ICU) costs.[154] Included in this group are individuals at the extremes of age and those with cardiac disease, malnutrition, immunodeficiency disease, and a history of alcohol or drug abuse.[155,156] Additional risk factors include diabetes mellitus and pulmonary or renal dysfunction.

Evaporative Water Loss

One of the major purposes of intact skin is to serve as a barrier to evaporative water loss (EWL) from the body. With major burn injury, this ability of the skin to regulate evaporative water loss is totally disrupted. In a classic 1962 study, Moncrief and Mason[157] attempted to determine the magnitude of such a loss and determined that daily evaporative water loss was in the range of 20 times normal in the early phase of injury, with gradual decreases as wound closure is achieved.

Further studies indicated that insensible water loss through burned skin is not from evaporation of water from sweat glands but rather from water vapor formed within the body and lost through the skin.[158,159]

Calculation of the amount of fluid lost by evaporative water loss includes losses from all sources. Normally the skin is the major source of insensible loss (75%) and the lungs are minor sources (25%), with a total loss of only approximately 600 to 800 mL/day. This changes dramatically with burns, because not only does skin loss increase but also lung loss increases by hypermetabolism and hyperventilation, especially in an intubated individual. Total evaporative losses exceed many liters per day in an adult with large burn wounds. Replacement of the loss is mandatory to prevent volume deficit.

◆**EVALUATION AND TREATMENT.** Burn recovery can be long and difficult, with complications often the rule rather than the exception. The goal of burn management is wound closure in a manner that promotes survival. Scar formation with contractures is often a consequence of healing in deep partial-thickness and full-thickness burns (Fig. 49.19; see also Fig. 49.10). Assessment of tissue viability can be difficult in complex extremity injury; pyrophosphate nuclear scanning can assist in evaluation.[160] Early intervention may have effects on tissue survival as is evident in the zone of stasis and application of cerium nitrate.[161] The advancement in survival and outcome can be as simple as using antibiotic catheters to reduce catheter-associated bloodstream infections[162] or improving glycemic management during ICU treatment.[163] Advances in care systems have shown the value of advanced practice nurses in a collaborative role in the burn ICU and emergency departments.[164]

The three essential elements of survival of major burn injury are (1) meticulous wound management, (2) adequate fluids and nutrition, and (3) early surgical excision and grafting. Current therapy for deep partial- and full-thickness burn injury includes surgical removal of the burn tissue (excision) followed by grafting of the person's unburned skin (autograft) onto the excised wound. Techniques of early wound care, such as the use of amniotic membrane,[165] may well affect the nature of burn scarring. Satisfactory wound closure with cultured epithelial autograft (Fig. 49.20) has been inconsistent and costly.[166,167] Early enthusiasm for synthetic dermal replacement has been tempered by a high rate of dermal graft loss and slow epidermal engraftment.[168,169] Such advancements in skin replacement technology include sheets of acellular dermal matrix that can be used with thin, meshed autografts or cultured epithelial autografts.[170,171] This concept also is being used on the donor site, and glycosaminoglycan hydrogels may supplement donor site wound dressings, and even topical gene therapy or stem cell applications.[172-174] Scar reduction or prevention is a challenging problem

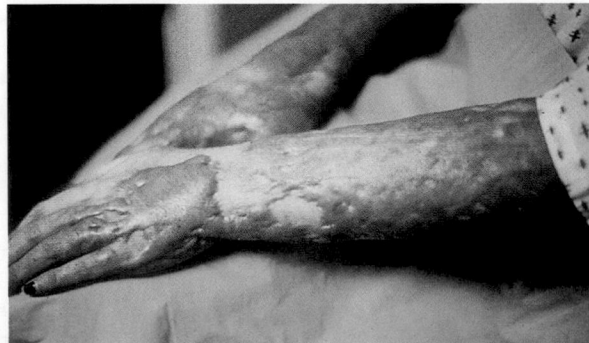

FIGURE 49.19 Hypertrophic Scarring. Deep partial-thickness thermal injury can result in extensive hypertrophic scarring. (Courtesy University of Utah Burn Center.)

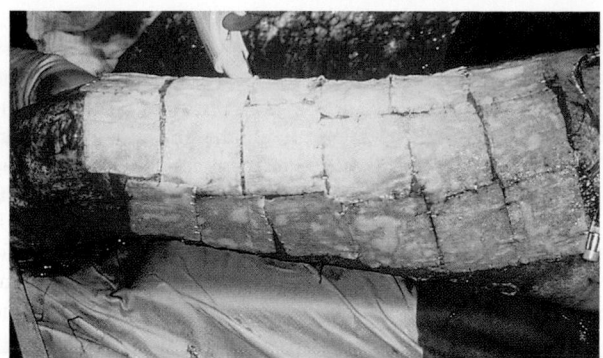

FIGURE 49.20 Application of Cultured Epithelial Autografts. The thin sheets of keratinocytes are attached to gauze backing to allow application onto the clean, excised thigh. (Courtesy University of Utah Burn Center.)

that is being addressed with pulsed-dye laser treatment.[175] Current research also is directed toward therapies to modulate hypermetabolic and inflammatory responses. Nutritional therapy is focused on early enteral feeding to reduce the potential of gut-mediated sepsis. Ongoing clinical trials using anabolic agents (e.g., recombinant human growth hormone) and pharmacologic agents that modulate inflammatory and endocrine mediators (e.g., ibuprofen, propranolol) show promise in the treatment of severe burn injuries.[113] Altered body image is a significant hurdle to those with facial burns. A framework for aiding individuals can often be useful for those reintegrating into the community.[176] Burn pain is almost always acute, and treatment strategies usually differ from strategies for chronic pain. The understanding and management of burn pain is key to recovery.[177,178] In addition to opioid-based agents, newer treatment approaches may include antianxiety agents, hypnosis, and relaxation techniques,[179] as well as virtual reality systems.[82,180]

SUMMARY REVIEW

Shock

1. Shock occurs when the cardiovascular system fails to perfuse tissue, cells, and organs adequately, causing a widespread impairment of cellular metabolism and tissue function. It is a downward physiologic spiral that, if not reversed, can lead to MODS.
2. Types of shock are cardiogenic, hypovolemic, neurogenic or vasogenic, anaphylactic, and septic.
3. The final common pathway in all types of shock is impaired cellular metabolism with cells switching from aerobic to anaerobic metabolism. Energy stores drop, and cellular mechanisms relative to membrane permeability, action potentials, and lysozyme release fail.
4. Anaerobic metabolism results in activation of the inflammatory response, decrease in circulatory volume, and decrease in pH.
5. Impaired cellular metabolism results in cellular inability to use glucose because of impaired glucose delivery or impaired glucose intake, resulting in a shift of glycogenolysis, gluconeogenesis, and lipolysis for fuel generation.
6. Glycogenolysis is affected for up to 10 hours. Gluconeogenesis results in the use of proteins necessary for structure, function, repair, and replication that leads to more impaired cellular metabolism. Lipolysis is ineffective because of a lack of transport serum proteins.
7. Gluconeogenesis contributes to lactic acid, uric acid, and ammonia buildup; interstitial edema; and impairment of the immune system, as well as general muscle weakness leading to decreased respiratory function and cardiac output.
8. Cardiogenic shock results from persistent hypotension and tissue hypoperfusion caused by cardiac dysfunction in the presence of adequate intravascular volume and left ventricular filling pressure.
9. Hypovolemic shock is caused by loss of whole blood, plasma, or interstitial fluid in large amounts. The use of compensatory mechanisms may be vigorous, but tissue perfusion ultimately decreases and results in impaired cellular metabolism.
10. Neurogenic (vasogenic) shock results from massive vasodilation that occurs from an imbalance between parasympathetic and sympathetic stimulation of vascular smooth muscle. It causes a relative hypovolemia (even though cardiac output may be high), and results in impaired cellular metabolism.
11. Anaphylactic shock is the outcome of a widespread hypersensitivity to an allergen that triggers anaphylaxis. The inflammatory response

is triggered, and massive vasodilation with fluid shift into the interstitium follows. The relative hypovolemia leads to impaired cellular metabolism.
12. Septic shock begins with impaired cellular metabolism caused by uncontrolled septicemia. The infecting agent triggers the inflammatory and immune responses. It is part of a continuum known as *SIRS*. Mortality for septic shock is very high.

Multiple Organ Dysfunction Syndrome

1. MODS is the progressive dysfunction of two or more organ systems resulting from a systemic inflammatory response after a severe illness or injury. The inflammatory response can be triggered by sepsis, necrotic tissue, trauma, burns, ARDS, acute pancreatitis, major surgery, circulatory shock, DIC, acute renal failure, blood transfusion, heat stroke, liver failure, mesenteric ischemia, propofol infusion syndrome, persistent inflammatory foci, and other severe injuries.
2. Primary MODS is the immediate local or mild systemic response to the triggering event or illness. It primes the inflammatory system.
3. Secondary MODS is the uncontrollable, excessive systemic inflammatory response that develops after a latent period and results in organ dysfunction.
4. People at greatest risk for developing MODS are older adults, those with significant tissue injury or preexisting disease, and those in whom resuscitation from the initiating illness or injury has been delayed or inadequate.
5. MODS is a leading cause of mortality in surgical intensive care units (ICUs). Mortality for individuals with MODS increases progressively from 54% with two failing organ systems to 100% with five failing organ systems.
6. Multiple organ dysfunction involves the stress response; release of complement, coagulation, and kinin proteins; changes in the vascular endothelium; and numerous inflammatory processes mediated by substances released by activated neutrophils and macrophages. The accumulation of activated neutrophils in organs is thought to play a key role in the pathogenesis of MODS, as well as macrophages.
7. The consequences of the release of inflammatory mediators in MODS are vasodilation, increased vasopermeability, and selective vasoconstriction resulting in maldistribution of blood flow; hypermetabolism; myocardial depression; and hypoxic injury to cells. Cellular hypoxia and acidosis impair cellular metabolism, leading to organ dysfunction.

SUMMARY REVIEW—cont'd

8. Clinical manifestations of the development of MODS are general during the first 24 hours: low-grade fever, tachycardia, tachypnea, dyspnea, and altered mental status. Over the next several days, beginning with the lungs, individual organ systems show signs of failure.

9. Because there is no specific therapy for MODS, early detection is extremely important so that supportive measures can be initiated as soon as possible.

10. At present the therapeutic management of MODS consists of prevention or removal of triggering mechanisms and support of individual organs. Recent scientific knowledge about inflammatory mediators has led to many promising future therapies for MODS.

Burns

1. Burns are classified according to depth and extent of injury.

2. First-degree burns involve the superficial skin without loss of protective function.

3. Second-degree burns are superficial (blister formation) or superficial involving partial skin thickness with a waxy white appearance and no involvement of dermal appendages.

4. Third-degree burns involve full skin thickness and often underlying tissues. They are painless and can be life-threatening as a result of hypovolemic shock and metabolic and immunologic responses.

5. The TBSA burned is estimated using either the rule of nines or the Lund and Browder chart.

6. Hypovolemia associated with burn shock is caused by increased capillary permeability with massive fluid losses from blood volume.

7. Altered cell membrane permeability and loss of electrolyte homeostasis contribute to burn shock.

8. Cardiac contractility is decreased during the first 24 hours with shunting of blood away from the liver, kidney, and gut.

9. Fluid resuscitation, such as with lactated Ringer solution, involves infusion of fluid at a rate faster than the loss of circulating volume.

10. The most reliable criterion for adequate resuscitation of burn shock is urine output.

11. *Capillary seal* is the term used to indicate the end of burn shock.

12. Transmembrane potentials are altered in cells not directly damaged by heat, with impairment of the sodium-potassium pump and loss of magnesium and phosphate.

13. The stress of a major burn activates the sympathetic nervous system with release of catecholamines, cortisol, glucagon, and insulin.

14. Burn injury produces a hypermetabolic state that persists until wound closure and is related to a higher thermal regulatory set point.

15. The local inflammatory response at the burn site releases cytokines, oxygen free radicals, chemotactic factors, and eicosanoids, which lead to a systemic inflammatory response and contribute to hypermetabolism.

16. A posttraumatic hypermetabolic response is associated with increased visceral heat production.

17. Alterations in clotting factors produce a hypercoagulable state following major burns.

18. The immune response following a burn is immediate, prolonged, and severe.

19. Numerous alterations in inflammatory cytokines are evident in the immediate burn period, affecting cellular immunity, antibody production, and attraction of neutrophils and contributing to the vasodilation and increased capillary permeability associated with burn shock.

20. White blood cells are altered, and there is decreased opsonization and phagocytosis, contributing to the development of sepsis.

21. Changes in intestinal wall integrity lead to translocation of bacteria, endotoxemia, and septic shock.

22. Loss of intact skin with a major burn results in significant evaporative water loss contributing to hypovolemia.

23. Treatment of major burns involves meticulous wound management, adequate fluids and nutrition, early surgical excision and grafting, modulation of the hypermetabolic state, and pain management.

KEY TERMS

Acute Physiology and Chronic Health Evaluation II and III (APACHE II and APACHE III), 1558
Anaphylactic shock, 1548
Burn, 1559
Burn shock, 1563
Burn wound depth, 1559
Capillary seal, 1564
Cardiogenic shock, 1546
Deep partial-thickness burn, 1560
Escharotomy, 1561
First-degree burn, 1559
Fluid resuscitation, 1563

Full-thickness injury, 1561
Gut hypothesis, 1557
Hypermetabolism, 1557
Hypovolemic shock, 1547
Maldistribution of blood flow, 1557
Multiple organ dysfunction syndrome (MODS), 1554
Myocardial depression, 1557
Neurogenic shock (vasogenic shock), 1547
Nonthermal injury, 1559
Partial-thickness injury, 1559
Posttraumatic hypermetabolic response, 1565
Primary MODS, 1554

Secondary MODS, 1556
Second-degree burn, 1559
Septic shock, 1550
Shock, 1544
Superficial partial-thickness injury, 1559
Supply-dependent oxygen consumption, 1557
Thermal injury, 1559
Third-degree burn, 1561
Tissue perfusion, 1543
Total body surface area (TBSA), 1561
Vesicant, 1559

REFERENCES

1. *Mosby's dictionary of medicine: nursing and health professions*, ed 10, St Louis, 2017, Elsevier.

2. Bonanno FG: Shock—a reappraisal: the holistic approach. *J Emerg Trauma Shock* 5(2):167–177, 2012.

3. Edul VS, Dubin A, Ince C: The microcirculation as a therapeutic target in the treatment of sepsis and shock. *Semin Respir Crit Care Med* 32(5):558–568, 2011.

4. Schmeltz LR: Management of inpatient hyperglycemia. *Lab Med* 42(7):427–434, 2011.

5. Topalian S, Ginsberg F, Parrillo J: Cardiogenic shock. *Crit Care Med* 36(1):S66–S77, 2008.

6. van der Pals J: Hypothermia in cardiogenic shock. *Crit Care* 16(Suppl 2):A21, 2012.

7. Babaev A, et al: Trends in management and outcomes of patients with acute myocardial infarction complicated by cardiogenic shock. *JAMA* 294(4):448–454, 2005.

8. Jackson C, Boenau IB: How to recognize cardiogenic shock. *Emerg Med* 39(10):11–19, 2007.

9. Omland T: Advances in congestive heart failure management in the intensive care unit: B-type natriuretic peptides in evaluation of acute heart failure. *Crit Care Med* 36(1):S17–S27, 2008.

10. Fox JT, Gowda RM, Khan IA: Cardiogenic shock: basics and clinical considerations. *Int J Cardiol* 123(3):221, 2008.

11. Myat A, et al: The intra-aortic balloon pump in high-risk percutaneous coronary intervention. *Interv Cardiol* 4(2):211–234, 2012.

12. Polderman KH: Mechanisms of action, physiological effects, and complications of hypothermia. *Crit Care Med* 37:S186–S202, 2009.

13. Hochman J, et al: Early revascularization and long-term survival in cardiogenic shock complicating acute myocardial infarction. *JAMA* 295(21):2511–2515, 2006.

14. Holmes CL, Walley KR: The evaluation and management of shock. *Clin Chest Med* 24(4):775–789, 2003.

15. Russell J: Vasopressin versus norepinephrine infusion in patients with septic shock. *N Engl J Med* 358(9):877–887, 2008.

16. Hogan SP, et al: Food induced anaphylaxis: mast cells as modulators of anaphylactic severity. *Semin Immunopathol* 34(5):643–653, 2012.

17. Simons FE, et al: 2012 update: World Allergy Organization Guidelines for the assessment and management of anaphylaxis. *Curr Opin Allergy Clin Immunol* 12(4):389–399, 2012.

18. Danoff TM, Borish L: Case fatality and population mortality associated with anaphylaxis in the United States. *J Allergy Clin Immunol* 133(4):1075–1083, 2014.

19. Simons FE, et al: World Allergy Organization anaphylaxis guidelines: summary. *J Allergy Clin Immunol* 127(3):587–593, e22, 2011.

20. Levy MM, et al: 2001 SCCM/ESICM/ACCP/ATS/SIS International Sepsis Definition Conference. *Crit Care Med* 31(4):1250–1256, 2003.

21. Singer M, et al: The Third International Consensus Definitions for Sepsis and Septic Shock (Sepsis-3). *JAMA* 315(8):801–810, 2016.

22. Torio CM, Moore BJ: *National inpatient hospital costs: the most expensive conditions by payer, 2013*, HCUP statistical brief no. 204. Rockville, MD, 2016, Agency for Healthcare Research and Quality.

23. Calandra T, Cohen J: The international sepsis forum consensus conference on definitions of infection in the intensive care unit. *Crit Care Med* 33(7):1538–1548, 2005.

24. Novosad SA, et al: Epidemiology of sepsis: prevalence of health care factors and opportunities for prevention. *MMWR Morb Mortal Wkly Rep* 65(33):864–869, 2016.

25. Greenberg JA, et al: Sequential organ failure assessment score modified for recent infection in patients with hematologic malignant tumors and severe sepsis. *Am J Crit Care* 25(5):409–417, 2016.

26. Albrecht SJ, et al: Reemergence of gram-negative health care-associated bloodstream infections. *Arch Intern Med* 166(12):1289–1294, 2006.

27. Kleinpell RM, Graves BT, Ackerman MH: Incidence, pathogenesis, and management of sepsis: an overview. *AACN Adv Crit Care* 17(4):385–393, 2006.

28. Papathanassoglou ED, et al: Association of proinflammatory molecules with apoptotic markers and survival in critically ill multiple organ dysfunction patients. *Biol Res Nurs* 5(2):129–141, 2003.

29. Kraut JA, Madias NE: Lactic acidosis: current treatments and future directions. *Am J Kidney Dis* 68(3):473–482, 2016.

30. Nguyen HB, et al: Early goal-directed therapy in severe sepsis and septic shock: insights and comparisons to ProCESS, ProMISe, and ARISE. *Crit Care* 20(160):1–16, 2016.

31. Levy MM, et al: Surviving Sepsis Campaign: association between performance metrics and outcomes in a 7.5 year study. *Intensive Care Med* 40:1623–1633, 2014.

32. Cannon CM, et al: The GENESIS Project (GENeralized Early Sepsis Intervention Strategies): a multicenter quality improvement collaborative. *J Intensive Care Med* 28(6):355–368, 2013.

33. Dellinger R, et al: Surviving Sepsis Campaign: international guidelines for management of severe sepsis and septic shock: 2012. *Crit Care Med* 41(2):580–637, 2013.

34. Rivers E, et al: Early goal-directed therapy in the treatment of severe sepsis and septic shock. *N Engl J Med* 345:1368–1377, 2001.

35. Wilson J, Bion J: *Surviving Sepsis Campaign: guidelines for management of severe sepsis and septic shock*. Available at: www.survivingsepsis.org.

36. Friswell AC: Surviving Sepsis Campaign previews updated guidelines for 2012. *Pulmon Rev* 17(5):1–5, 2012.

37. Kopterides P, et al: Procalcitonin-guided algorithms of antibiotic therapy in the intensive care unit: a systematic review and meta-analysis of randomized controlled trials. *Crit Care Med* 38(11):2229–2241, 2010.

38. Shehabi Y, et al: Procalcitonin algorithm in critically ill adults with undifferentiated infection or suspected sepsis. A randomized controlled trial. *Am J Respir Crit Care Med* 190(10):1102–1110, 2014.

39. Layios N, et al: Procalcitonin usefulness for the initiation of antibiotic treatment in intensive care unit patients. *Crit Care Med* 40(8):2304–2309, 2012.

40. Baue AE: Multiple, progressive or sequential system failure: a syndrome for the 70's. *Arch Surg* 110(7):779–781, 1975.

41. Tilney NL, Bailey GL, Morgan AP: Sequential system failure after rupture of abdominal aortic aneurysm: an unsolved problem in postoperative care. *Ann Surg* 178(2):117–122, 1973.

42. Skillman JJ, et al: Respiratory failure, hypotension, sepsis, and jaundice. A clinical syndrome associated with lethal hemorrhage from acute stress ulceration of the stomach. *Am J Surg* 117(4):523–530, 1969.

43. Awad SS: State-of-the-art therapy for severe sepsis and multisystem organ dysfunction. *Am J Surg* 186(Suppl):23S–30S, 2003.

44. Sauaia A, et al: Validation of postinjury multiple organ failure scores. *Shock* 31(5):438–447, 2009.

45. Osterbur K, et al: Multiple organ dysfunction in humans and animals. *J Vet Intern* 28(4):1141–1151, 2014.

46. Abraham E, Singer M: Mechanism of sepsis-induced organ dysfunction. *Crit Care Med* 35(10):2408–2416, 2007.

47. Shapiro NI, et al: The association of endothelial cell signaling, severity of illness, and organ dysfunction in sepsis. *Crit Care* 14(5):R182–R192, 2010.

48. Van den Berghe G: The 2016 ESPEN Sir David Cuthbertson lecture: interfering with neuroendocrine and metabolic responses to critical illness: from acute to long-term consequences. *Clin Nutr* 36(2):348–354, 2017.

49. Aird WC: The role of the endothelium in severe sepsis & MODS. *Blood* 101:3756–3777, 2003.

50. Fry DE: Sepsis, systemic inflammatory response, and multiple organ dysfunction: the mystery continues. *Am Surg* 78(1):1–8, 2012.

51. van Meurs M, et al: Early organ-specific endothelial activation during hemorrhagic shock and resuscitation. *Shock* 29(2):291–299, 2008.

52. Souto FO, et al: Essential role of CCR2 in neutrophil tissue infiltration and multiple organ dysfunction in sepsis. *Am J Respir Crit Care Med* 183(2):234–242, 2011.

53. Kimura F, et al: Immunosuppression following surgical and traumatic injury. *Surg Today* 40(9):793–808, 2010.

54. Baue AE: Mediators or markers of injury, inflammation, and infection (harbingers of doom or predictors of disaster) and biologic puzzles or ambiguities. *Arch Surg* 142(1):89–93, 2007.

55. Cohen HE, Mosser DM: Extrinsic and intrinsic control of macrophage inflammatory responses. *J Leukoc Biol* 94(5):913–919, 2013.

56. Opal SM, van der Poll T: Endothelial barrier dysfunction in septic shock. *J Intern Med* 277(3):277–293, 2015.

57. Deitch EA: Gut-origin sepsis: evolution of a concept. *Surgeon* 10(6):350–356, 2012.

58. Silvestri L, et al: Impact of selective decontamination of the digestive tract on multiple organ dysfunction syndrome: systematic review of randomized controlled trials. *Crit Care Med* 38(5):1370–1376, 2010.

59. Gando S: Microvascular thrombosis and multiple organ dysfunction syndrome. *Crit Care Med* 38(2):S35–S42, 2010.

60. Schmidt H, et al: Autonomic dysfunction predicts both 1- and 2-month mortality in middle-aged patients with multiple organ dysfunction syndrome. *Crit Care Med* 36(3):967–970, 2008.

61. Schmidt H, et al: Relation of impaired interorgan communication and parasympathetic activity in chronic heart failure and multiple-organ dysfunction syndrome. *J Crit Care* 29(3):367–373, 2014.

62. Fernandes CJ, Jr, de Assuncao MSC: Myocardial dysfunction in sepsis: a large, unsolved puzzle. *Crit Care Res Pract* 2012:896430, 2012.

63. MacDonald SPJ, et al: Comparison of PIRO, SOFA and MEDS scores for predicting mortality in emergency department patients with severs sepsis and septic shock. *Acad Emerg Med* 21(11):1257–1263, 2014.

64. Leistner R, et al: Costs and prolonged length of stay of central venous catheter-associated bloodstream infections (CVC BSI): a matched prospective cohort study. *Infection* 42(1):31–36, 2014.

65. Levy MM: Early goal-directed therapy: what do we do now? *Crit Care* 18(6):705, 2014.

66. Jaehne AK, Salem D, Garces JD: Early goal-directed therapy in the treatment of sepsis: the times have changed but not the therapy and benefit to patients. *Intensive Care Med* 41(9):1728–1729, 2015.

67. Nguyen HB, et al: Early goal-directed therapy in severe sepsis and septic shock: insights and comparisons to ProCESS, ProMISe and ARISE. *Crit Care* 20(1):160–176, 2016.

68. Thompson BT, Bernard GR: ARDS network (NHLBI) studies-successes and challenges in the ARDS clinical research. *Crit Care Clin* 27(3):459–468, 2011.

69. Taylor BE, et al: Guidelines for the provision and assessment of nutrition support therapy in the adult critically ill patient: Society of Critical Care Medicine (SCCM) and American Society for Parenteral and Enteral Nutrition (A.S.P.E.N). *Crit Care Med* 44(2):390–438, 2016.

70. Aggarwal S, Smailes S, Dziewulski P: Tracheostomy in burns patients revisited. *Burns* 35(7):962–966, 2009.

71. Caruso DM, et al: Rationale for 'early' percutaneous dilatational tracheostomy in patients with burn injuries. *J Burn Care Rehabil* 18(5):424–428, 1997.

72. Clayton N, Kennedy P, Maitz P: The severe burns patient with tracheostomy: implications for management of dysphagia, dysphonia and laryngotracheal pathology. *Burns* 36(6):850–855, 2010.

73. Saffle JR, Morris SE, Edelman L: Early tracheostomy does not improve outcome in burn patients. *J Burn Care Rehabil* 23(6):431–438, 2002.

74. Clark DE, Dainiak CN, Reeder S: Decreasing incidence of burn injury in a rural state. *Inj Prev* 6(4):259–262, 2000.

75. American Burn Association: *Burn incidence and treatment in the U.S.: 2016 fact sheet*, Chicago, IL, 2016, Author. Available at: www.ameriburn.org/rsources_factsheet.php.

76. Brigham PA, McLoughlin E: Burn incidence and medical care use in the United States: estimates, trends, and data sources. *J Burn Care Rehabil* 17(2):95–107, 1996.

77. Sen S, Greenhalgh D, Palmieri T: Review of burn research for the year 2010. *J Burn Care Res* 33(5):577–586, 2012.

78. Saffle JR, Edelman L, Morris SE: Regional air transport of burn patients: a case for telemedicine? *J Trauma* 57(1):57–64, 2004.

79. Syed-Abdul S, et al: Telemedicine utilization to support the management of the burns treatment involving patient pathways in both developed and developing countries: a case study. *J Burn Care Res* 33(4):e207–e212, 2012.

80. Wallace DL, et al: A systematic review of the evidence for telemedicine in burn care: with a UK perspective. *Burns* 38(4):465–480, 2012.

81. Falder S, et al: Core outcomes for adult burn survivors: a clinical overview. *Burns* 35(5):618–641, 2009.

82. Mackey SP, et al: Return to work after burns: a qualitative research study. *Burns* 35(3):338–342, 2009.

83. Cochran A, et al: Self-reported quality of life after electrical and thermal injury. *J Burn Care Rehabil* 25(1):61–66, 2004.

84. Altintas MA, et al: Differentiation of superficial-partial vs. deep-partial thickness burn injuries in vivo by confocal-laser-scanning microscopy. *Burns* 35(1):80–86, 2009.

85. Braue EH, Jr, et al: Noninvasive methods for determining lesion depth from vesicant exposure. *J Burn Care Res* 28(2):275–285, 2007.

86. Chiu T, Burd A: Laboratory assessment of burn depth. *Plast Reconstr Surg* 119(2):751–752, 2007.

87. Cross KM, et al: Clinical utilization of near-infrared spectroscopy devices for burn depth. *Wound Repair Regen* 15(3):332–340, 2007.

88. Devgan L, et al: Modalities for the assessment of burn wound depth. *J Burns Wounds* 5:e2, 2006.

89. Hoeksema H, et al: Accuracy of early burn depth assessment by laser Doppler imaging on different days post burn. *Burns* 35(1):36–45, 2009.

90. Kassira W, Namias N: Outpatient management of pediatric burns. *J Craniofac Surg* 19(4):1007–1009, 2008.

91. Mandal A: Burn wound depth assessment—is laser Doppler imaging the best measurement tool available? *Int Wound J* 3(2):138–143, 2006.

92. McGill DJ, et al: Assessment of burn depth: a prospective, blinded comparison of laser Doppler imaging and videomicroscopy. *Burns* 33(7):833–842, 2007.

93. Monstrey S, et al: Assessment of burn depth and burn wound healing potential. *Burns* 34(6):761–769, 2008.

94. Ng D, et al: The use of laser Doppler imaging for burn depth assessment after application of flammacerium. *Burns* 33(3):396–397, 2007.

95. Renkielska A, et al: Burn depths evaluation based on active dynamic IR thermal imaging—a preliminary study. *Burns* 32(7):867–875, 2006.

96. Tehrani H, et al: Spectrophotometric intracutaneous analysis: a novel imaging technique in the assessment of acute burn depth. *Ann Plast Surg* 61(4):437–440, 2008.

97. Hosseini SN, et al: Xenoderm versus 1% silver sulfadiazine in partial-thickness burns. *Asian J Surg* 32(4):234–239, 2009.

98. Sheridan RL, et al: Planimetry study of the percent of body surface represented by the hand and palm: sizing irregular burns is more accurately done with the palm. *J Burn Care Rehabil* 16(6):605–606, 1995.

99. Morris SE, Navaratnam N, Herndon DN: A comparison of effects of thermal injury and smoke inhalation on bacterial translocation. *J Trauma* 30(6):639–643, 1990.

100. Chen C, et al: Myosin light chain kinase mediates intestinal barrier disruption following burn injury. *PLoS ONE* 7(4):e34946, 2012.

101. Arturson G: Forty years in burns research—the postburn inflammatory response. *Burns* 26(7):599–604, 2000.

102. Baxter CR, Cook WA, Shires GT: Serum myocardial depressant factor of burn shock. *Surg Forum* 17:1–2, 1966.

103. Demling RH, Will JA, Belzer FO: Effect of major thermal injury on the pulmonary microcirculation. *Surgery* 83(6):746–751, 1978.

104. Horton JW, et al: Calcium antagonists improve cardiac mechanical performance after thermal trauma. *J Surg Res* 87(1):39–50, 1999.

105. Aikawa N, Martyn JA, Burke JF: Pulmonary artery catheterization and thermodilution cardiac output determination in the management of critically burned patients. *Am J Surg* 135(6):811–817, 1978.

106. Dobson EL, Warner GF: Factors concerned in the early stages of thermal shock. *Circ Res* 5(1):69–74, 1957.

107. Lefer AM, Martin J: Origin of myocardial depressant factor in shock. *Am J Physiol* 218(5):1423–1442, 1970.

108. Rosenthal SR, Hawley PL, Hakim AA: Purified burn toxic factor and its competition. *Surgery* 71(4):527–536, 1972.

109. Horton JW, Burton KP, White DJ: The role of toxic oxygen metabolites in a young model of thermal injury. *J Trauma* 39(3):563–569, 1995.

110. Onuoha G, Alpar K, Jones I: Vasoactive intestinal peptide and nitric oxide in the acute phase following burns and trauma. *Burns* 27(1):17–21, 2001.

111. Ungureanu-Longrois D, et al: Myocardial contractile dysfunction in the systemic inflammatory response syndrome: role of a cytokine-inducible nitric oxide synthase in cardiac myocytes. *J Mol Cell Cardiol* 27(1):155–167, 1995.

112. Gamelli RL, et al: Burn-induced nitric oxide release in humans. *J Trauma* 39(5):869–877, discussion 77–78, 1995.

113. Baxter CR: Fluid volume and electrolyte changes of the early postburn period. *Clin Plast Surg* 1(4):693–703, 1974.

114. Huang PP, et al: Hypertonic sodium resuscitation is associated with renal failure and death. *Ann Surg* 221(5):543–554, 1995.

115. Herndon DN, Spies M: Modern burn care. *Semin Pediatr Surg* 10(1):28–31, 2001.

116. Belba MK, Petrela EY, Belba GP: Comparison of hypertonic vs isotonic fluids during resuscitation of severely burned patients. *Am J Emerg Med* 27(9):1091–1096, 2009.

117. Evans JA, Darlington DN, Gann DS: A circulating factor(s) mediates cell depolarization in hemorrhagic shock. *Ann Surg* 213(6):549–556, 1991.

118. Duan H, et al: Effect of burn injury on apoptosis and expression of apoptosis-related genes/proteins in skeletal muscles of rats. *Apoptosis* 14(1):52–65, 2009.

119. Welt LG: Membrane transport defect: the sick cell. *Trans Assoc Am Physicians* 80:217–226, 1967.

120. Trunkey DD, et al: The effect of hemorrhagic shock on intracellular muscle action potentials in the primate. *Surgery* 74(2):241–250, 1973.

121. Cunningham JN, Jr, Shires GT, Wagner Y: Changes in intracellular sodium and potassium content of red blood cells in trauma and shock. *Am J Surg* 122(5):650–654, 1971.

122. Rosenthal SR, Tabor H: Electrolyte changes and chemotherapy in experimental burn and traumatic shock and hemorrhage. *Arch Surg* 51:244, 1945.

123. Turinsky J, Gonnerman WA, Loose LD: Impaired mineral metabolism in postburn muscle. *J Trauma* 21(6):417–423, 1981.

124. Deets DK, Glaviano VV: Plasma and cardiac lactic dehydrogenase activity in burn shock. *Proc Soc Exp Biol Med* 142(2):412–416, 1973.

125. Button B: Evidence of circulating membrane depolarization factor(s) in hemorrhagic shock. *Shock* 1(Suppl):15, 1994.

126. Okamoto R, Glaviano VV: Pindok M: Myocardial lipases and catecholamines in burn shock. *Proc Soc Exp Biol Med* 137(1):347–353, 1971.

127. Herndon DN, et al: Long-term propranolol use in severely burned pediatric patients: a randomized controlled study. *Ann Surg* 256(3):402–411, 2012.

128. Wilmore DW, Aulick HL, Goodwin CW: Glucose metabolism following severe injury. *Acta Chir Scand Suppl* 498:43–47, 1980.

129. Akcay MN, et al: The effect of growth hormone on 24-h urinary creatinine levels in burned patients. *Burns* 27(1):42–45, 2001.

130. Ikezu T, et al: A unique mechanism of desensitization to lipolysis mediated by beta(3)-adrenoceptor in rats with thermal injury. *Am J Physiol* 277(2 Pt 1):E316–E324, 1999.

131. Wilmore DW, et al: Alterations in hypothalamic function following thermal injury. *J Trauma* 15(8):697–703, 1975.

132. Gump FE, Price JB, Jr, Kinney JM: Blood flow and oxygen consumption in patients with severe burns. *Surg Gynecol Obstet* 130(1):23–28, 1970.

133. Wilmore DW, et al: Influence of the burn wound on local and systemic responses to injury. *Ann Surg* 186(4):444–458, 1977.

134. Wilmore DW, et al: Effect of injury and infection on visceral metabolism and circulation. *Ann Surg* 192(4):491–504, 1980.

135. Holder IA, Neely AN: Hageman factor dependent activation and its relationship to lethal *Pseudomonas aeruginosa* burn wound infections. *Agents Actions Suppl* 38(Pt 3):329–342, 1992.

136. McManus WF, Eurenius K, Pruitt BA, Jr: Disseminated intravascular coagulation in burned patients. *J Trauma* 13(5):416–422, 1973.

137. Wilmore DW, editor: *The metabolic management of the critically ill*, ed 2, New York, 1990, Plenum.

138. Wilmore DW, Aulick LH: Metabolic changes in burned patients. *Surg Clin North Am* 58(6):1173–1187, 1978.

139. Edelman LS, et al: Sustained bone mineral density changes after burn injury. *J Surg Res* 114(2):172–178, 2003.

140. Wright K, et al: Burn-activated neutrophils and tumor necrosis factor-alpha alter endothelial cell actin cytoskeleton and enhance monolayer permeability. *Surgery* 128(2):259–265, 2000.

141. Goebel A, et al: Injury induces deficient interleukin-12 production, but interleukin-12 therapy after injury restores resistance to infection. *Ann Surg* 231(2):253–261, 2000.

142. Nishiura T, et al: Gene expression and cytokine and enzyme activation in the liver after a burn injury. *J Burn Care Rehabil* 21(2):135–141, 2000.

143. Biffl WL, et al: Interleukin-6 delays neutrophil apoptosis via a mechanism involving platelet-activating factor. *J Trauma* 40(4):575–578, 1996.

144. Choi M, et al: Preventing the infiltration of leukocytes by monoclonal antibody blocks the development of progressive ischemia in rat burns. *Plast Reconstr Surg* 96(5):1177–1185, 1995.

145. Iocono JA, et al: Interleukin-8 levels and activity in delayed-healing human thermal wounds. *Wound Repair Regen* 8(3):216–225, 2000.

146. Ortega MR, Ganz T, Milner SM: Human beta defensin is absent in burn blister fluid. *Burns* 26(8):724–726, 2000.

147. Heideman M, Kaijser B, Gelin LE: Complement activation and hematologic, hemodynamic, and respiratory reactions early after soft-tissue injury. *J Trauma* 18(10):696–700, 1978.

148. Grzybowski J, et al: Antidietary antigen antibodies in the sera of patients with burns as a potential marker of gut mucosa integrity failure. *J Burn Care Rehabil* 13(2 Pt 1):194–197, 1992.

149. Deitch EA, Berg R: Bacterial translocation from the gut: a mechanism of infection. *J Burn Care Rehabil* 8(6):475–482, 1987.

150. Yao YM, et al: The association of circulating endotoxaemia with the development of multiple organ failure in burned patients. *Burns* 21(4):255–258, 1995.

151. Benhaim P, Hunt TK: Natural resistance to infection: leukocyte functions. *J Burn Care Rehabil* 13(2 Pt 2):287–292, 1992.

152. Alexander JW, et al: Consumptive opsoninopathy: possible pathogenesis in lethal and opportunistic infections. *Ann Surg* 184(6):672–678, 1976.

153. Bjornson AB, Altemeier WA, Bjornson HS: Changes in humoral components of host defense following burn trauma. *Ann Surg* 186(1):88–96, 1977.

154. Cochran A, et al: Systemic *Candida* infection in burn patients: a case-control study of management patterns and outcomes. *Surg Infect (Larchmt)* 3(4):367–374, 2002.

155. Goff DR, et al: Cardiac disease and the patient with burns. *J Burn Care Rehabil* 11(4):305–307, 1990.

156. McGill V, et al: The impact of substance use on mortality and morbidity from thermal injury. *J Trauma* 38(6):931–934, 1995.

157. Moncrief JA, Mason AD, Jr: Water vapor loss in the burned patient. *Surg Forum* 13:38–41, 1962.

158. Moncrief JA: Burns. In Schwartz SI, editor: *Principles of surgery*, ed 2, New York, 1974, McGraw-Hill.

159. Roe CF, Kinney JM: Water and heat exchange on third-degree burns. *Surgery* 56:212–220, 1964.

160. Affleck DG, et al: Assessment of tissue viability in complex extremity injuries: utility of the pyrophosphate nuclear scan. *J Trauma* 50(2):263–269, 2001.

161. Eski M, et al: Cerium nitrate treatment prevents progressive tissue necrosis in the zone of stasis following burns. *Burn* 38(2):283–289, 2012.

162. Weber JM, et al: Incidence of catheter-associated bloodstream infection after introduction of minocycline and rifampin antimicrobial-coated catheters in a pediatric burn population. *J Burn Care Res* 33(4):539–543, 2012.

163. Lee J, et al: Computerized insulin infusion programs are safe and effective in the burn intensive care unit. *J Burn Care Res* 33(3):e114–e119, 2012.

164. Zaletel CL: Factors affecting fluid resuscitation in the burn patient: the collaborative role of the APN. *Adv Emerg Nurs J* 31(4):309–320, 2009.

165. Fraser JF, et al: A randomized controlled trial of amniotic membrane in the treatment of a standardized burn injury in the merino lamb. *Burns* 35(7):998–1003, 2009.

166. Ronfard V, et al: Long-term regeneration of human epidermis on third degree burns transplanted with autologous cultured epithelium grown on a fibrin matrix. *Transplantation* 70(11):1588–1598, 2000.

167. Williamson JS, et al: Cultured epithelial autograft: five years of clinical experience with twenty-eight patients. *J Trauma* 39(2):309–319, 1995.

168. Fitton AR, Drew P, Dickson WA: The use of a bilaminate artificial skin substitute (Integra) in acute resurfacing of burns: an early experience. *Br J Plast Surg* 54(3):208–212, 2001.

169. Peck MD, et al: A trial of the effectiveness of artificial dermis in the treatment of patients with burns greater than 45% total body surface area. *J Trauma* 52(5):971–978, 2002.

170. Carsin H, et al: Cultured epithelial autografts in extensive burn coverage of severely traumatized patients: a five year single-center experience with 30 patients. *Burns* 26(4):379–387, 2000.

171. Wainwright D, et al: Clinical evaluation of an acellular allograft dermal matrix in full-thickness burns. *J Burn Care Rehabil* 17(2):124–136, 1996.

172. Branski LK, et al: A review of gene and stem cell therapy in cutaneous wound healing. *Burns* 35(2):171–180, 2009.

173. Curinga G, et al: Comments on "platelet-rich plasma in burns. *Burns* 36(6):944–945, 2010.

174. Pallua N, Wolter T, Markowicz M: Platelet-rich plasma in burns. *Burns* 36(1):4–8, 2010.

175. Liew SH, Murison M, Dickson WA: Prophylactic treatment of deep dermal burn scar to prevent hypertrophic scarring using the pulsed dye laser: a preliminary study. *Ann Plast Surg* 49(5):472–475, 2002.

176. Sainsbury DC: Body image and facial burns. *Adv Skin Wound Care* 22(1):39–44, 2009.

177. Connor-Ballard PA: Understanding and managing burn pain: part 1. *Am J Nurs* 109(4):48–56, 2009.

178. Connor-Ballard PA: Understanding and managing burn pain: part 2. *Am J Nurs* 109(5):54–62, 2009.

179. Jellish WS, et al: Effect of topical local anesthetic application to skin harvest sites for pain management in burn patients undergoing skin-grafting procedures. *Ann Surg* 229(1):115–120, 1999.

180. Konstantatos AH, et al: Predicting the effectiveness of virtual reality relaxation on pain and anxiety when added to PCA morphine in patients having burn dressings changes. *Burns* 35(4):491–499, 2009.

Shock, Multiple Organ Dysfunction Syndrome, and Burns in Children

Mary Fran Hazinski, Mary A. Mondozzi,
Rose A. Urdiales Baker

evolve WEBSITE

CHAPTER OUTLINE

This chapter reviews shock, multiple organ dysfunction syndrome, and burns in children. It focuses on the assessment and care of children but also notes many of the differences between these conditions in children and adults.

SHOCK AND MULTIPLE ORGAN DYSFUNCTION SYNDROME

Shock is a condition of acute and progressive circulatory dysfunction that results in inadequate delivery of oxygen and nutrients to the tissues. Shock in children most often results from severe dehydration, hemorrhage, progressive heart failure, or sepsis. It may also complicate the care of the child with congenital heart disease, pulmonary hypertension (cor pulmonale), drug toxicity, electrolyte or acid-base imbalance, dysrhythmias, obstruction to blood flow (e.g., pulmonary embolus, cardiac tamponade), or multiple organ failure.

In children, shock is present when there are signs of poor systemic perfusion, regardless of the blood pressure—shock may be present with normal, high, or low blood pressure. When the systolic blood pressure is adequate for age, but there are signs of inadequate tissue perfusion, the child is in compensated shock. In this child, although the systolic blood pressure may be normal, the diastolic or mean arterial pressure is typically low. When systolic hypotension is associated with inadequate tissue perfusion, the child is in hypotensive (formerly called *decompensated*) shock.[1-3]

Shock causes tissue ischemia (inadequate blood flow) and hypoxia (inadequate oxygen delivery) that leads to acidosis and cell dysfunction. Oxygen delivery may be inadequate because arterial oxygen content or cardiac output is low, or because there are increased tissue oxygen requirements or impaired cellular use of oxygen. Ischemia and hypoxia are primary insults to cells. Restoration of adequate blood flow and oxygen delivery may trigger the development of *reperfusion injury*, a secondary problem characterized by an exaggerated inflammatory response that may produce cellular death and organ failure.

Multiple organ dysfunction syndrome (MODS) is the concurrent failure of at least two organs resulting from a single cause,[4] most often from a systemic inflammatory response syndrome (SIRS), associated with acute insults such as sepsis or trauma. MODS also can complicate chronic diseases, such as cancer and congenital heart disease (CHD), as well as more acute insults including drowning, acute respiratory distress syndrome (ARDS), liver failure, pancreatitis, or cardiac arrest. Finally, MODS can result from treatments such as chemotherapy, surgical correction of CHD, or organ transplantation.[2,5-9] Children with chronic diseases have both an increased risk of and increased mortality from MODS.

MODS may be either primary or secondary. Primary MODS is directly attributable to an insult and typically occurs soon (3 to 7 days) after the insult. Secondary MODS typically occurs later and may be associated with more sequential development of organ dysfunction. New or progressive MODS (NPMODS) is a recently defined problem that can develop with severe sepsis. It is defined as a dysfunction of one or fewer organs on day 1 of sepsis recognition with subsequent development of two or more concurrent organ failures at any time during treatment.[4,9,10]

Types of Shock

Shock is categorized by type as follows:[2,3]

1. *Hypovolemic shock:* caused by inadequate intravascular volume relative to the vascular space
2. *Cardiogenic shock:* results from impairment of myocardial function
3. *Distributive shock* (including septic, anaphylactic, and neurogenic): results from inappropriate distribution of blood flow, increased capillary permeability, and myocardial dysfunction (e.g., septic or anaphylactic shock) or central nervous system injury (e.g., neurogenic or spinal shock)
4. *Obstructive shock:* caused by a mechanical obstruction to blood flow into and through the heart and great vessels (e.g., cardiac tamponade, pulmonary embolus, obstructive congenital heart lesions such as critical aortic stenosis) resulting in low cardiac output

An etiologic classification of shock is helpful because it suggests the initial therapy required. However, the etiologic classification is an oversimplification because any child with late or progressive shock is likely to demonstrate widespread cardiovascular dysfunction that may include inappropriate intravascular volume relative to the vascular space, poor myocardial function, and maldistribution of blood flow. Severe shock of any kind may be followed by complications such as reperfusion injury, MODS, or NPMODS.[4] Children with septic shock demonstrate elements of hypovolemic and cardiogenic shock in addition to the complications of infection and maldistribution of blood flow. Thus healthcare providers must assess and support all aspects of cardiovascular function and oxygen delivery during the treatment of any form of shock.

Clinical Manifestations of Shock

Signs of shock in children may initially be subtle, thus detection of shock and evaluation of response to therapy typically requires careful, repeated assessments over time. Inadequate cardiac output causes signs of inadequate blood flow to some tissue beds and evidence of organ system dysfunction (Box 50.1). Critical parameters to evaluate include assessment of consciousness, breathing, and color. This initial assessment is described in the Pediatric Advanced Life Support course.[3] Through this assessment the provider determines if the child "looks good" (appears stable, in no acute distress) or "looks bad" (in need of immediate intervention).[11] More detailed assessment will reveal evidence of inadequate organ function resulting from inadequate organ perfusion.

The child's level of *consciousness* and *responsiveness* often provide valuable information about the severity of illness. The healthy infant should orient to faces, make eye contact, and track bright objects across a visual field. The healthy toddler is reluctant to be separated from parents or examined by strangers, and the healthy child is alert and responds to questions. By comparison, the critically ill infant or child is often extremely irritable; lethargy indicates severe deterioration in the child's level of consciousness. A decreased response to painful stimulus is abnormal and usually indicates severe cardiorespiratory or neurologic compromise.[3,11]

The infant or child normally breathes without evidence of distress or increased effort, such as retractions or nasal flaring. An extremely rapid respiratory rate (tachypnea), increased depth of respirations (hyperpnea), or evidence of increased respiratory effort (e.g., retractions, grunting) may indicate the presence of heart failure or shock. The development of apnea or inadequate respiratory rate or effort generally indicates deterioration and need for immediate support of airway, oxygenation, and ventilation.

BOX 50.1 CLINICAL MANIFESTATIONS OF SHOCK IN NEWBORNS, INFANTS, AND CHILDREN

Signs of Shock in Infants and Children

- Change in responsiveness (initial irritability followed by lethargy)
- Tachypnea
- Mottled color, pallor (distributive shock may be associated with flushed skin)
- Tachycardia
- Cool skin, prolonged capillary refill (distributive shock may cause "flash" [instantaneous] refill)
- Diminished intensity of peripheral pulses (may also vary in intensity)
- Metabolic (lactic) acidosis (serum lactate >4 mmol/L is typically well above normal for arterial or venous blood)
- Decreased central venous oxygen saturation (more than 25% to 30% below arterial oxygen saturation)
- LATE: Hypotension, bradycardia

Nonspecific Signs of Distress in Newborns

- Jitteriness or lethargy with decreased tone
- Change in oxygen requirements
- Apnea
- Bradycardia or decreased heart rate variability
- Temperature instability, hypothermia
- Glucose instability, hypoglycemia
- Feeding intolerance (e.g., increased residual volume)

If perfusion is adequate and the ambient temperature is warm, the child's *color* will be consistent over the surface of the skin, and lips, nailbeds, and mucous membranes will be pink. Children who are in a cold environment, those who have undergone hypothermic surgery or a procedure in a cold room, and children in shock often demonstrate mottling (a marbled or "blotchy" appearance to the skin).[2,3,11] Pallor also may be observed when perfusion is poor (Fig. 50.1). Children with sepsis occasionally demonstrate flushed, bright red (plethoric) skin.[2,3,11]

If perfusion is adequate and the ambient temperature is warm, the child's capillary refill is normally brisk (<2 seconds). Prolonged capillary refill (>2 seconds) may indicate a compromise in systemic perfusion (see Fig. 50.1, *B*) and the development of shock.[2,3,11] Septic shock is associated with vasodilation that may result in instantaneous (flush) capillary refill, rather than delayed capillary refill. Evaluation of capillary refill time is subjective, and gradual changes may be difficult to detect.[12]

The child's *vital signs* must be evaluated in light of the child's clinical condition. Normal vital signs are not always appropriate for the seriously ill or injured child[11] (Box 50.2 and Table 50.1).

The child's heart rate should be appropriate for age and clinical condition. The child in shock is often tachycardic. The tachycardia may be primary (i.e., associated with a tachydysrhythmia) or secondary to stress (i.e., sinus tachycardia). If the heart rate is extremely rapid, especially in the child with decreased myocardial function, tachycardia may be the cause rather than the symptom of shock. In general, if the ventricular rate exceeds 200 to 220/min in the infant or 160 to 180 beats/min in the child, ventricular diastolic filling time and coronary artery perfusion time are significantly reduced and stroke volume falls. Cardiac output can then fall, leading to signs of heart failure or shock. Once supraventricular or ventricular tachycardia produces signs of shock, urgent treatment is required.[13,14]

Bradycardia, an abnormally low heart rate, can cause a fall in cardiac output or it can be a symptom of deterioration. In children, a fall in heart rate typically produces a commensurate fall in cardiac output.[15]

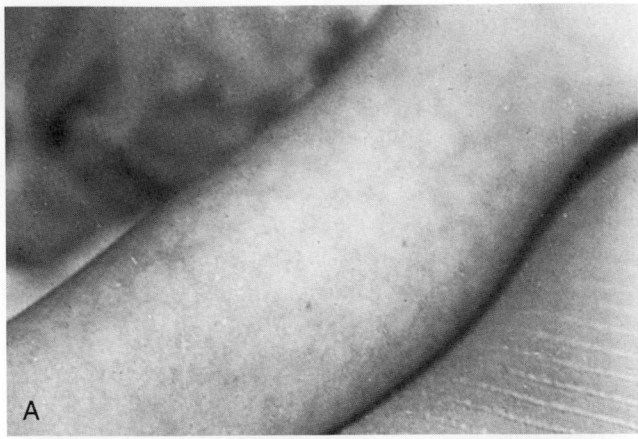
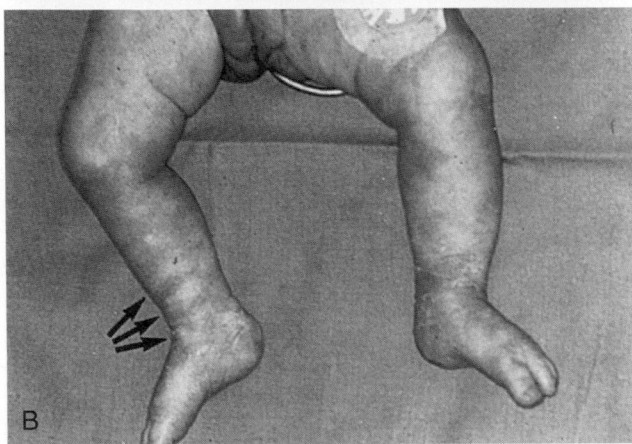

FIGURE 50.1 Mottling of Skin Caused by Poor Systemic Perfusion. **A,** Mottling of skin color often indicates inadequate tissue oxygenation; this may result from hypoxemia or poor systemic perfusion. This child developed myocardial dysfunction and signs of cardiogenic shock. **B,** Mottled skin color is often associated with other signs of compromise of skin perfusion, including delayed capillary refill. The skin over this infant's right ankle was blanched using three fingers (*arrows*), and the skin failed to perfuse for more than 5 seconds. This infant suffered from septic shock. (From Hazinski MF: Cardiovascular disorders. In Hazinski MF, editor: *Nursing care of the critically ill child,* ed 2, St Louis, 1992, Mosby.)

The most common cause of bradycardia in young children is hypoxia.[3,13] If the infant or child develops bradycardia with poor perfusion, the provider must immediately assess and support the child's airway, oxygenation, and ventilation, and be prepared to initiate chest compressions if the heart rate and systemic perfusion do not improve.[3,13]

Bradycardia often indicates impending cardiovascular collapse and is the most common terminal cardiac rhythm observed in children.[3,11,14] In neonates, especially preterm neonates, a *lack of heart rate variability* is a nonspecific sign of compromise, such as sepsis.[16]

The child's stroke volume may be altered by conditions affecting ventricular preload, compliance, contractility, and afterload (Table 50.2). Providers must evaluate and optimize each of these variables in the treatment of shock (see Chapter 49).

The child's *blood pressure* must be appropriate for age and clinical condition. Shock may be present despite a systolic blood pressure within the normal range for age. When hypovolemic or cardiogenic shock is present, compensatory vasoconstriction may initially maintain the systolic blood pressure, although the mean and diastolic arterial pressures may fall. The development of systolic hypotension in the child with hypovolemic or cardiogenic shock indicates severe shock, and rapid deterioration may follow. In septic shock, by comparison, mild systolic hypotension

| BOX 50.2 | ESTIMATING BLOOD PRESSURE IN CHILDREN 1 TO 10 YEARS OF AGE |

BOX 50.2 ESTIMATING BLOOD PRESSURE IN CHILDREN 1 TO 10 YEARS OF AGE

Typical systolic BP for 1–10 years of age: The typical "normal" (i.e., median, or 50th percentile) systolic blood pressure for a child 1 to 10 years of age of normal height may be estimated by adding 90 mmHg to twice the child's age in years (90 mmHg + [2 × age in years]); this corresponds to the 50th percentile systolic blood pressure for the child's age.

Hypotensive systolic BP for 1–10 years of age: A systolic pressure less than 70 mmHg plus twice the child's age in years (<70 mmHg + [2 × age in years]) is considered hypotensive for children 1 to 10 years of age because this blood pressure corresponds to the 5th percentile systolic blood pressure for age (i.e., only 5% of normal, healthy children of average height demonstrate a systolic blood pressure lower than that number).

Hypotensive mean arterial pressure for 1–10 years of age: A mean arterial pressure less than 40 mmHg + (1.5 × age in years) is consistent with hypotension because this mean arterial pressure corresponds to the 5th percentile mean arterial pressure in children of average height.

Data from Chameides L et al: Systemic approach to the seriously ill or injured child. In Samson RA et al, editors: *Pediatric advanced life support provider manual,* Dallas, 2016, American Heart Association; Hacque IU, Zaritsky AL: *Pediatr Crit Care* 8:138-144, 2007.

may develop early in the clinical course. In all children, the development of systolic hypotension or a fall in mean arterial pressure indicates hypotensive shock, and urgent treatment is needed.[2,3,11]

The central venous pressure (CVP) is normally 0 to 5 mmHg. The pulmonary artery wedge pressure (PAWP, also called *pulmonary artery occlusion pressure* [*PAOP*]) is normally 5 to 8 mmHg or less, although pulmonary artery catheters are now rarely used in children. Inadequate CVP or PAWP may indicate hypovolemia, whereas high measurements typically result from heart failure or cardiogenic shock. Note that in the absence of tricuspid valve disease, tension pneumothorax, or influence from positive pressure ventilation, the CVP reflects the right ventricular end-diastolic pressure (RVEDP). The RVEDP may differ substantially from the left ventricular end-diastolic pressure.

A central venous catheter is useful to evaluate CVP and provides a route for rapid volume administration. In addition, a CVP catheter in the superior vena cava (SVC) enables evaluation of the central venous oxygen saturation ($ScvO_2$). The $ScvO_2$ is used as a surrogate for the mixed venous oxygen saturation (which would require a sampling of blood from the pulmonary artery). If cardiac output is adequate and oxygen consumption is normal, the $ScvO_2$ will be no more than 25% to 30% below the arterial oxygen saturation. A fall in $ScvO_2$ can indicate a fall in oxygen delivery (caused by decreased arterial oxygen content or decreased cardiac output, or both), an uncompensated rise in oxygen consumption, or both.[2]

Near-infrared spectroscopy (NIRS) transmits near-infrared light through muscle, bone, tissue, and skin and captures reflected light to calculate tissue oxygen saturation. Adhesive NIRS sensors are placed on the forehead (cerebral) and over the abdomen (somatic) to evaluate changes in regional oxygenation and blood flow. The cerebral regional tissue oxygen saturation (cerebral rSO_2) is typically >50% and the somatic regional tissue oxygen saturation (somatic rSO_2) is typically 10% to 15% higher or >60% to >75%. A low or falling rSO_2 may indicate a fall in cardiac output and systemic perfusion, and rSO_2 may fall more quickly than the arterial oxygen saturation.[2,17]

Shock compromises renal perfusion, so despite adequate fluid intake, urine volume decreases, typically falling to less than 2 mL/kg per hour

TABLE 50.1 NORMAL PEDIATRIC VITAL SIGNS

HEART RATES

AGE	AWAKE HEART RATE (PER MIN)	SLEEPING HEART RATE (PER MIN)	RESPIRATORY RATE* (BREATHS PER MIN)
Newborn	100–205	90–160	30–60
Infant (6 mo)	100–180	90–160	30–53
Toddler	98–140	80–120	27–37
Preschooler	80–120	65–100	20–28
School-age child	75–118	58 90	18–25
Adolescent	60–100	50–90	12–20

BLOOD PRESSURES

AGE	SYSTOLIC BLOOD PRESSURE (mmHg)[†]	DIASTOLIC BLOOD PRESSURE (mmHg)[†]	MEAN ARTERIAL PRESSURE (mmHg)[‡]	SYSTOLIC HYPOTENSION (mmHg)[§]
Birth (12 hr, <1000 g)	39–59	16–36	28–42[¶]	<40–50
Birth (12 hr, 3-kg weight)	60–76	31–45	48–57	<50
Newborn (96 hr)	67–84	35–53	45–60	<60
Infant (1–12 mo)	72–104	37–56	50–62	<70
Toddler (1–2 yr)	86–106	42–63	49–62	<70 + (2 × age in years)
Preschool (3–5 yr)	89–112	46–72	58–69	<70 + (2 × age in years)
School-age child (6–9 yr)	97–115	57–76	66–72	<70 + (2 × age in years)
Preadolescent (10–12 yr)	102–120	61–80	71–79	<90
Adolescent (13–15 yr)	110–131	64–83	73–84	<90

NOTE: Always consider patient's normal range and clinical condition. Heart and respiratory rates normally increase with fever or stress.
From Hazinski MF: Children are different. In Hazinski MF, editor: *Nursing care of the critically ill child*, ed 3, St Louis, 2013, Mosby.
*Respiratory rates from Fleming S et al: *Lancet* 377:1011–1018, 2011.
[†]Systolic and diastolic blood pressure ranges assume 50th percentile for height for children 1 year and older, and are consistent with the Pediatric Advanced Life Support course (Chameides L et al: *Pediatric advanced life support provider manual*, Dallas, 2011, American Heart Association).
[‡]Mean arterial pressures (Diastolic pressure + [Difference between systolic and diastolic pressures ÷ 3]) for 1 year and older, assuming 50th percentile for height.
[§]Threshold for hypotension in children 1 to 10 years old from Pediatric Advanced Life Support course (Chameides L et al: *Pediatric advanced life support provider manual*, Dallas, 2011, American Heart Association).
[¶]Approximately equal to postconception age in weeks (may add 5 mmHg).
Blood pressure ranges from the following sources: Gemelli M et al: *Eur J Pediatr* 149:318–320, 1990; Versmold H et al: *Pediatrics* 67:107, 1981; Haque IU, Zaritsky AL: *Pediatr Crit Care* 8:138–144, 2007; National Heart, Lung and Blood Institute: *Fourth report on the diagnosis, evaluation, and treatment of high blood pressure in children and adolescents*, Bethesda, MD, 2004, National Heart, Lung and Blood Institute. Available at: www.nhlbi.nih.gov/guidelines/hypertension/child.tbl.htm.

in infants, less than 1 mL/kg per hour in children, and less than 0.5 mL/kg hour in adolescents. Liver enzymes may be elevated if hepatic perfusion is reduced. The development of metabolic acidosis and a rise in serum lactate to greater than 4 mg/dL indicate that blood flow to some tissues is inadequate to support aerobic metabolism.

Infants have high glucose needs and low glycogen stores that may be rapidly depleted during stress. For this reason, *hypoglycemia* (glucose ≤60 mg/dL) may be observed in seriously ill or injured infants and may be associated with cardiovascular or neurologic deterioration.[3,18] Severe physiologic stress, such as cardiac surgery, shock, sepsis, MODS, or NPMODS can produce *critical illness hyperglycemia* (CIH), a transient glucose concentration >150 mg/dL. CIH has been documented in adults and children. It is produced by a relative insulin-resistant state associated with high levels of endogenous catecholamines and hydrocortisone

secretion, with resultant gluconeogenesis and glycogenolysis. Glucose uptake by the liver is increased while glucose uptake by peripheral tissues is decreased. Inflammatory mediators can contribute to the relative insulin resistance.[2,18,19] In children, the serum glucose is often elevated in the first 12 to 18 hours after initial insult (such as injury, shock, sepsis or MODS development, or cardiac surgery), then falls to normal ranges. Although CIH is associated with poor survival in critically ill children,[20,21] it is not clear if the hyperglycemia is the cause or the marker of poor outcomes.[19]

Hypovolemic Shock

Hypovolemic shock, the most common type of shock in children, is caused by a reduction in the intravascular volume relative to the vascular space. Dehydration and trauma are the most common causes of

TABLE 50.2	FACTORS AFFECTING CARDIOVASCULAR PERFORMANCE IN CHILDREN
FACTOR	**COMMENTS**
Heart rate	Major factor affecting cardiac output in children. Normally more rapid in children than in adults. Because the *stroke volume* is smaller than in adults, the *cardiac output* of the child is more closely related to heart rate than to stroke volume. *Tachycardia* is expected in the seriously ill or injured child. The most common cause of *bradycardia* in young children is hypoxia; bradycardia is an ominous sign if present in association with poor perfusion. Urgent treatment is required once bradycardia or supraventricular or ventricular tachycardia produces signs of shock.
Stroke volume	Averages 1.5 mL/kg; affected by conditions altering ventricular preload, compliance, contractility, and afterload.
Ventricular end-diastolic pressure (VEDP)	Optimal pressure for children in shock is unknown. Aggressive fluid administration is linked to improved survival in children with *septic* shock.
Ventricular compliance or distensibility	Can be affected by congenital heart defects such as atrial septal defects (ASDs) and complex congenital heart defects. If compliance is low, such as in newborns and infants, volume administration may increase VEDP. Hypoplastic ventricles are often noncompliant. Hypertrophied ventricles, present in children with severe pulmonary stenosis or aortic stenosis, may become fibrotic and noncompliant. Increased compliance may be present in early septic shock.
Contractility	Contractility probably similar in normal newborns, infants, children, and adults. Newborn myocardium does have fewer contractile proteins and higher water content than adult myocardium, but the clinical significance of this is probably minimal.
Afterload	Newborn myocardium *can* adapt to mild, nonacute increases in afterload. Afterload may be increased in children with systemic vasoconstriction or pulmonary hypertension (constrictors include alveolar hypoxia, acidosis, hypothermia, and alveolar distention). Some uncorrected congenital heart defects may increase afterload. Coarctation of the aorta and aortic stenosis increase left ventricular afterload. Pulmonary stenosis increases right ventricular afterload. Afterload may be decreased in septic shock.
Oxygen delivery and consumption	Highest per kilogram body weight during the neonatal period and infancy. The young child requires a higher cardiac output and oxygen delivery per kilogram than the adult. Increased oxygen consumption occurs in critically ill newborns exposed to cold because they cannot shiver to generate heat. Other causes of increased oxygen consumption in children and infants include fever, sepsis, trauma, pain, and seizures.

hypovolemic shock in children. A relative hypovolemia may result from vasodilation and a redistribution of blood volume or from increased capillary permeability.

When hypovolemia is mild or moderate, such as with 5% to 10% dehydration or mild hemorrhage, compensatory adrenergic vasoconstriction redistributes blood from the skin, the mesenteric (gut), and renal circulations to maintain blood flow to the heart and brain. The blood pressure is typically adequate with mild hypovolemic shock. Hypotension is a sign of severe, decompensated hypovolemic shock and may not develop unless intravascular volume loss is rapid or severe.[2,3]

Relative hypovolemia may be caused by a decrease in the intravascular volume relative to the vascular space. This may be associated with the vasodilation of sepsis, anaphylaxis, or neurogenic shock (see following text) or with β_2-adrenergic drug toxicity. A relative hypovolemia also may be caused by increased capillary permeability with a redistribution of intravascular volume, such as with burns, anaphylaxis, or sepsis. The translocation of extravascular fluid to a location that is neither intravascular nor intracellular, as in edema, is termed "third spacing" of fluids.[18]

Compensatory Responses. Significant dehydration, hypovolemia, and low cardiac output stimulate adrenergic and renal compensatory mechanisms characterized by the "fight-or-flight" response. These include tachycardia and redistribution of blood from the skin, gut, and kidney to the brain and heart. Reduced renal perfusion stimulates the renin-angiotensin-aldosterone system, resulting in renal sodium and water retention. Decreased atrial stretch stimulates the secretion of antidiuretic hormone (ADH, also known as *arginine vasopressin* [*AVP*]) and produces free water retention by the kidneys.[2] These mechanisms are similar in adults and children and may help restore or maintain intravascular volume over time. Neonatal and young infant kidneys, however, are incapable of excreting concentrated urine, so these

compensatory mechanisms are relatively ineffective during the first weeks of life.[18]

Compensatory mechanisms cannot be maintained indefinitely. Systemic vasoconstriction increases left ventricular afterload and myocardial oxygen consumption and may produce tissue ischemia. Prolonged tachycardia may impair subendocardial blood flow and increase myocardial oxygen consumption; both may ultimately contribute to myocardial ischemia.[2] Extreme tachypnea increases oxygen demand and reduces effective ventilation. A severe compromise in blood flow and systemic perfusion contributes to cerebral, renal, or hepatic ischemia and possible organ failure.

◆**CLINICAL MANIFESTATIONS.** The child with hypovolemic shock demonstrates signs of inadequate blood flow to some tissue beds and some evidence of organ system dysfunction (see Box 50.1). The infant or child may be irritable or lethargic. Respirations will be rapid and may be labored if shock is severe or associated with myocardial failure. The skin will be mottled, although pallor also may be observed. A prolonged capillary refill time (>2 seconds) is consistent with the development of shock.[2,3,11,22]

The child in hypovolemic shock is often tachycardic. Bradycardia in the child with shock indicates impending cardiovascular collapse, and is the most common terminal cardiac rhythm observed in children.[2,3,14] When hypovolemic shock is present, compensatory vasoconstriction may initially maintain the systolic blood pressure, although the mean arterial pressure may fall. The development of systolic hypotension often indicates severe shock, and rapid deterioration may follow. The CVP is less than 5 to 8 mmHg, unless heart failure or pulmonary hypertension is present.

Hypovolemic shock compromises renal perfusion, so urine volume decreases despite adequate fluid intake. Liver enzymes may be elevated if hepatic perfusion is reduced. The development of metabolic acidosis

TABLE 50.3   DEHYDRATION AND HYPOVOLEMIA

TYPE OF DEHYDRATION	CLINICAL INDICATORS
Isotonic dehydration	Fluid output exceeds intake. Loss of free water is proportional to loss of sodium, so serum sodium concentration remains normal. Fluid loss is from intravascular and extravascular compartments. Compromises peripheral perfusion when the young child has lost approximately 10% (100 mL/kg) of body weight. Compromises systemic perfusion in the adolescent with acute fluid loss equivalent to 5% to 6% of body weight.
	Can produce hypotension (decompensated shock) when the young child has lost about 15% (150 mL/kg) of body weight. Can produce hypotension in the adolescent with a fluid loss equivalent to about 7% to 9% of body weight because body water constitutes a smaller percentage of body weight in older children and adults than in young children.
Hypotonic/hyponatremic dehydration	Associated with a proportionately greater loss of sodium than free water; thus the serum sodium falls. Resultant acute fall in serum osmolality produces an acute extravascular fluid shift and further loss of extravascular volume. Fluid loss in hypotonic dehydration is primarily from the intravascular compartment; thus a compromise in systemic perfusion will be observed after even small quantities of fluid loss.
	Poor peripheral perfusion can develop in a child with a fluid loss equivalent to about 5% (50 mL/kg) of body weight. Adolescents with hyponatremic dehydration may demonstrate a compromise in peripheral perfusion with a fluid loss equivalent to approximately 3% of body weight.
	Hypotension often is observed when fluid loss is equal to approximately 10% (100 mL/kg) of body weight. Hypotension in an adolescent is observed when the fluid loss equals approximately 5% to 6% of body weight.
Hypertonic/hypernatremic dehydration	Free water deficit is proportionately greater than the deficit of sodium, so serum sodium concentration rises, increasing serum osmolality and producing an intravascular shift of free water. For this reason the child with hypernatremic dehydration is likely to maintain intravascular volume and systemic perfusion until relatively large quantities of fluid are lost.
	Compromise in systemic perfusion is not likely to be observed in the *child* with hypernatremic dehydration until *severe* dehydration is present with a fluid loss equivalent to about 10% of body weight (or 5% to 6% of body weight in the adolescent).
	Hypotension may not be observed until the fluid loss approximates 15% or more of body weight (7% to 9% or more of body weight in the adolescent).
	Hypotension in the child with hypertonic/hypernatremic dehydration indicates a substantial fluid deficit. However, the deficit must be replaced carefully to correct shock and avoid rapid lowering of serum sodium concentrations.

Data in part from Roberts KE: *Pediatr Rev* 22:380–386, 2001; Roberts KE: Fluid, electrolyte and endocrine problems. In Hazinski MF, editor: *Nursing care of the critically ill child*, ed 3, St Louis, 2013, Mosby.

and a rise in serum lactate indicate that blood flow to some tissues is inadequate to support aerobic metabolism.

Hypoglycemia (glucose ≤60 mg/dL) may be observed in seriously ill or injured infants, especially if intake has been compromised, and may be associated with cardiovascular or neurologic deterioration. *Hyperglycemia* (>150 mg/dL) may develop in critically ill or injured children.

Clinically significant dehydration is associated with weight loss (Table 50.3). Fluid intake and output records (or reports from parents or primary caretakers) reveal a history of inadequate fluid intake or excessive fluid losses. The child with significant dehydration demonstrates dry mucous membranes, a sunken fontanel (in infants), and poor skin turgor[18] (Table 50.4). Moderate isotonic dehydration produces signs of peripheral circulatory compromise, and severe isotonic dehydration will produce hypotension. The blood urea nitrogen (BUN) and urine specific gravity are usually elevated. The serum sodium concentration and osmolality are affected by the type and severity of dehydration present. Hypotension typically develops with greater than 10% isotonic or hypotonic dehydration in the infant or child, or greater than 6% to 7% dehydration in the adolescent.[18]

Hemorrhage is another potential cause of hypovolemic shock. To appreciate the significance of any blood lost or drawn for laboratory analysis, the total blood loss should be considered as a percentage of the child's circulating blood volume (Table 50.5).

Tachycardia, peripheral vasoconstriction, and altered level of consciousness may be the only early signs of hemorrhage in the child with trauma (Table 50.6). Acute blood loss (hemorrhage) may not cause hypotension until an estimated 25% to 30% of intravascular volume is lost (i.e., an acute intravascular or blood loss of 16 to 24 mL/kg).[22-24] Once hypotension develops in the child with hemorrhage, cardiovascular collapse is imminent, and immediate, rapid intravascular volume expansion is required. Surgical intervention may be needed.

Redistribution of blood volume associated with systemic vasodilation, high capillary pressure or transudative fluid losses, or capillary leak may produce a relative hypovolemia and signs of poor systemic perfusion in the absence of evidence of absolute volume loss. For example, children with end-stage hepatic failure may demonstrate a relative hypovolemia associated with ascites and hepatorenal syndrome. Maldistribution of blood flow with distributive shock (e.g., with septic shock, neurogenic shock, or severe burns) also will produce signs of relative hypovolemia because intravascular volume is inadequate relative to the vascular space.

Cardiogenic Shock

Cardiogenic shock is present when impaired myocardial function compromises cardiac output. This form of shock is observed:
1. Following cardiovascular surgery or with inflammatory disease of the heart, such as cardiomyopathy and myocarditis
2. With drug toxicity or severe electrolyte or acid-base imbalances
3. As a complication of any form of shock, and early in septic shock

Compensatory Responses. In the early stages of cardiogenic shock, adrenergic compensatory mechanisms produce tachycardia, peripheral vasoconstriction, and constriction of the splanchnic arteries to divert blood flow from the skin, gut, and kidneys to maintain flow to the heart and brain.[2,3,22] These compensatory mechanisms may initially be sufficient to maintain the systolic blood pressure and effective coronary and cerebral blood flow. However, tachycardia and systemic arterial constriction increase myocardial oxygen consumption. In addition, reduction in gut and kidney blood flow may produce hepatic, mesenteric, or renal ischemia or failure. Decreased renal perfusion

TABLE 50.4	SEVERITY OF (ISOTONIC) DEHYDRATION BASED ON CLINICAL EXAMINATION*		
CLINICAL PARAMETERS	**MILD**	**MODERATE**	**SEVERE**
Approximate body weight loss			
Infant	5% (50 mL/kg)	10% (100 mL/kg)	15% (150 mL/kg)
Adolescent	3% (30 mL/kg)	5%–6% (50–60 mL/kg)	7%–9% (70–90 mL/kg)
General appearance	Alert, restless, thirsty	Lethargic, postural dizziness	Limp, coma, cold and cyanotic extremities
Radial pulse	Full	Thready, weak, rapid	Feeble, not palpable
Respiration	Normal	Deep	Deep, rapid
Skin elasticity	Pinch retracts immediately	Pinch retracts slowly	Pinch retracts very slowly (>2 seconds)
Eyes	Normal	Sunken	Very sunken
Tears	Present	Diminished	Absent
Mucous membranes	Moist	Dry	Very dry (parched)
Urine output	Normal	↓	↓ or absent
Capillary refill time	<2 seconds	>2 seconds	Prolonged
Heart rate	Varies with age	Varies with age	Varies with age
Blood pressure	Normal	Normal	Reduced

*The interpretation of the assessments must be appropriately modified for age and type of dehydration (hypotonic or hypertonic).
Modified from Perkin RM et al: Shock, cardiac arrest and resuscitation. In Hazinski MF, editor: *Nursing care of the critically ill child,* ed 3, St Louis, 2013, Mosby.

TABLE 50.5	ESTIMATION OF PEDIATRIC CIRCULATING BLOOD VOLUME	
AGE OF CHILD	**BLOOD VOLUME (mL/kg body weight)**	
Newborn	80–85	
Infant	75–80	
Child	70–75	
Adolescent	65–70	

From Hazinski MF: Children are different. In Hazinski MF, editor: *Nursing care of the critically ill child,* ed 3, St Louis, 2013, Mosby.

stimulates the renin-angiotensin-aldosterone system, as described for hypovolemic shock.

A fall in the mean arterial pressure or pulse pressure reduces stimulation of the baroreceptors in the carotid sinuses and aortic arch. This reduced baroreceptor activity removes inhibition from the vasomotor center in the medulla, resulting in increased adrenergic stimulation.[2] If myocardial dysfunction progresses, cardiac output and blood pressure ultimately fall. Myocardial ischemia then exacerbates myocardial dysfunction, and multisystem organ failure may result from persistent or severe organ ischemia.

◆**CLINICAL MANIFESTATIONS.** The child with cardiogenic shock demonstrates signs of inadequate systemic perfusion despite evidence of adequate intravascular volume or even relative hypervolemia. This form of shock is generally associated with low cardiac output. The child's extremities are cool to touch (the extremities will cool peripherally to proximally), with delayed capillary refill despite a warm, ambient temperature.[3,11,22] The skin may be mottled (see Fig. 50.1). If myocardial function is severely compromised, peripheral pulses may be diminished in intensity (dampened) or they may vary in intensity (pulsus alternans).

Evidence of systemic venous congestion, including high central venous pressure, hepatomegaly, and periorbital edema, is typically present in cardiogenic shock, particularly if right ventricular failure is involved. Evidence of pulmonary edema may be identified on a chest radiograph or clinical assessment (including signs of respiratory distress, reduced lung compliance during hand ventilation, or frothy pink sputum suctioned from the endotracheal tube) if left ventricular failure is present. The cardiac silhouette is usually enlarged on the chest radiograph, unless concurrent hypovolemia is present.

A low cardiac output may be documented by invasive or noninvasive devices. The $ScvO_2$ will be more than 25% to 30% below the arterial oxygen saturation.

Signs of low cardiac output and cardiogenic shock can be similar to signs of cardiac tamponade. Although some classic signs, including muffled heart tones or pulsus paradoxus, may be observed with tamponade, these signs may be difficult to appreciate if cardiac output and blood pressure are severely compromised. Therefore, if cardiogenic shock is suspected in a child after cardiovascular surgery or in any child at risk for the development of pericardial effusion, tamponade should be ruled out through an echocardiogram.

In infants following surgery for congenital heart disease, a low cardiac output syndrome score (LCOSS) can be calculated by assigning one point each for tachycardia (>20% higher than postinduction heart rate in operating room), oliguria (<1 mL/kg/hr), toe temperature less than 30°C (86°F), need for volume administration of >30 mL/kg/day, decreased near infrared spectrometry (NIRS) measurements (cerebral NIRS <50% and renal NIRS <75% of arterial saturation), arterial lactate >2 mmol/L, and need for vasoactive/inotropes beyond milrinone at 0.5 µg/kg per minute. The score is assessed at ICU admission, 8, 12, and 24 hours postoperatively. Morbidity and resource utilization can be significantly higher among infants with peak LCOSS ≥4 and those with a cumulative LCOSS ≥7.[25]

Distributive/Septic Shock

With distributive (septic, anaphylactic, and neurogenic) shock, vasodilation and increased capillary permeability are typically present

TABLE 50.6	CLASSIFICATION OF PEDIATRIC HEMORRHAGIC SHOCK IN TRAUMA PATIENTS BASED ON CLINICAL EVALUATION		
SYSTEM	MILD HEMORRHAGE, COMPENSATED SHOCK, SIMPLE HYPOVOLEMIA (<30%)	MODERATE HEMORRHAGE, DECOMPENSATED SHOCK, MARKED HYPOVOLEMIA (30%–45%)	SEVERE HEMORRHAGE, CARDIOPULMONARY FAILURE, PROFOUND HYPOVOLEMIA (>45%)
Cardiovascular	Tachycardia	Moderate tachycardia	Severe tachycardia
	Weak peripheral pulses, strong central pulses	Thready peripheral pulses, weak central pulses	Absent peripheral pulses, thready central pulses
	Low to normal blood pressure (systolic BP >70 mmHg + [2 × (age in years)])	Frank hypotension (systolic BP <70 mmHg + [2 × (age in years)])	Profound hypotension (systolic BP <50 mmHg)
	Mild acidosis	Moderate acidosis	Severe acidosis
Respiratory	Mild tachypnea	Moderate tachypnea	Severe tachypnea
Central nervous system	Irritable, confused	Agitated or lethargic	Obtunded, comatose
Skin	Cool extremities, mottling	Cool extremities, pallor	Cool extremities, cyanosis
	Poor capillary refill (72 sec)	Delayed capillary refill (72 sec)	Prolonged (>5 sec) capillary refill
Kidneys	Mild oliguria, increased specific gravity	Marked oliguria, increased blood urea nitrogen (BUN)	Anuria

From Soud T, Pieper P, Hazinski MF: Pediatric trauma. In Hazinski MF, editor: *Nursing care of the critically ill child*, ed 2, St Louis, 1992, Mosby.

and blood flow is unregulated throughout the skin and organ systems, so a normal cardiac output is likely to be inadequate to maintain sufficient perfusion of all tissue beds. Neurogenic shock is a form of hypovolemic and vasogenic (maldistributive) shock. It is caused by a loss of vasomotor tone after severe head or spinal cord injury. Massive vasodilation and loss of sympathomimetic tone result in a relative hypovolemia and hypotension. The loss of sympathetic tone prevents compensatory tachycardia.

Sepsis and its complications result from activation of biochemical and physiologic cascades that lead to the formation or activation of cytokines and other mediators that produce vasodilation, increased capillary permeability, maldistribution of blood flow, and cardiovascular and cellular dysfunction.[2] Sepsis and its complications may result in MODS or NPMODS and are leading causes of death in noncoronary intensive care units. In 2005 in the United States, there were more than 75,000 pediatric hospitalizations involving severe sepsis, with an overall mortality of 8.9% to 24%.[26]

Hartman and colleagues'[26] hospital data from seven states provide the most detailed information regarding causes of pediatric sepsis in the United States. In 2013, this group reported data through 2005. In this series, an infecting microorganism was identified in less than 40% of infants and children with severe sepsis.[26] The most common sites of identified infection were respiratory tract (roughly 50%) and bacteremia (about 20%).[26] In a more recent series from the Children's Hospital Association of nearly 50,000 children with pediatric severe sepsis from 2004 to 2012,[27] approximately two-thirds of children with severe sepsis had chronic disease. Among these children, bloodstream (67.8%) infections were most common, with a high incidence of respiratory (57.2%) sites of infection. Genitourinary infections were identified in one-fifth, with device infection, cardiovascular infection, and abdominal infections as additional sources.

An international series characterizing children with septic shock has been published by the Pediatric Acute Lung Injury and the Sepsis Investigators Network.[28] In this series, an infectious microorganism was identified in 65% of children with respiratory (40%) and bloodstream (19%) infections, the most frequent sources.

The microorganisms that cause sepsis vary according to age, immune function, and location. In the two large pediatric series from the United States, the most commonly reported infecting microorganisms were staphylococcus, streptococcus, and fungal infections, with fewer gram-negative and viral infections.[26,27] Fungal infections were much more common among children with cancer. When viral infections were documented, concomitant bacterial infections were nearly always present.[26] In the international series of children with severe sepsis, gram-negative (28%) and gram-positive (27%) microorganisms are identified approximately equally, followed by viruses (21%) and fungi (21%).[28]

Prevention of hospital-acquired infections can substantially reduce the risk of infection, sepsis, and its complications.[29] Clinicians must be aware of the common pathogens in various populations.

Factors associated with risk for the development of sepsis include extremes of age (risk highest among infants, young children, and older adults);[2,26,27] chronic diseases; invasive catheters, surgical incisions, or wounds or burns; immunocompromise; and long-term antibiotic therapy.[27,30] As noted earlier in data from children's hospitals, two-thirds of children with severe sepsis had a chronic disease.[27]

It is now clear that genetic characteristics of the child, as well as the invading microorganisms, alter the outcome of infections, sepsis, and septic shock.[31,32] Certainly, infectious diseases, such as meningococcal disease, can vary widely in invasiveness and severity of clinical consequences.[33]

Both proinflammatory and antiinflammatory cytokines serve essential protective functions in fighting infection and modulating the immune response. Sepsis is caused by the effects of the invading microorganism and its toxins, and most effects that contribute to septic shock result from a disruption in the balance between *proinflammatory* mediators (including tumor necrosis factor-alpha [TNF-α], interleukin [IL]-1, IL-6, and IL-8; platelet-activating factor; arachidonic acid metabolites; nitric oxide; and many kinins) and *antiinflammatory* mediators (IL-4, IL-10, IL-11, and IL-13; transforming growth factor-beta; colony-stimulating factors; soluble tumor necrosis factor receptor; IL-1 receptor antagonist; and activated protein C).[2] Extremely high levels of proinflammatory mediators, such as TNF, nitric oxide, and platelet-activating factor, can become destructive, even when they eradicate the triggering microorganism.[7,31]

High proinflammatory cytokine levels have been implicated in the development of sepsis-induced disseminated intravascular coagulation, pulmonary injury, and microcirculatory disruptions, similar to those observed with burns, severe trauma, shock reperfusion syndromes, postcardiac arrest, and MODS.[31] Tumor necrosis factor levels have been directly related to mortality in newborns and children with meningitis and sepsis,[2] and interleukin-8 levels have been shown to be reliable predictors of pediatric sepsis mortality.[32]

An increase in nitric oxide concentration contributes to vasodilation, hypotension, and decreased myocardial function that develop during adult sepsis. However, infants with sepsis often demonstrate pulmonary vasoconstriction from shock-induced acidosis and hypoxia and may benefit from administration of inhaled nitric oxide or other vasodilators.[34]

During sepsis, the endothelium becomes a secretory organ, changing from the normal profibrinolytic and anticoagulant state to an antifibrinolytic and precoagulant one.[34] This change can lead to the development of microthrombi in some areas of the microcirculation, further contributing to maldistribution of blood flow. Mediators that regulate coagulation pathways have been implicated in the sepsis process.[34] Activated protein C normally curtails the inflammatory process once the invading microorganism is destroyed, and a deficiency in activated protein C is a marker for severe sepsis in all ages.[35] Although administration of activated protein C improved survival in one study of adults with severe sepsis,[36] subsequent adult studies failed to replicate this result.[37] A study in children was halted because the activated protein C produced excessive bleeding complications.[34,37]

C-reactive protein (CRP) binds to both bacteria and macrophages and activates the complement system. The complement system is a series of proteins that helps macrophages eliminate (opsonize) invading microorganisms; these proteins also participate in the clotting cascade.

CRP concentration normally rises with infection and falls when the infection is adequately treated with antibiotics, so it is a useful component to monitor response to infection. Ferritin is released when macrophages are activated in response to sepsis, injury, and inflammation. In a small sample of children with severe sepsis, mortality was highest (46.5%) among those with both a CRP ≥4.08 mg/dL and a ferritin ≥1980 ng/mL, and lowest (0%) among those with a CRP and ferritin below these thresholds.[38]

There is clear interaction among catecholamines, adrenoreceptors, and glucocorticoids contributing to critical illness hyperglycemia. Endogenous glucocorticoids decrease activation of proinflammatory mediators, and the proinflammatory mediators contribute to a relative insulin resistance. The glucocorticoids modulate vasomotor tone by enhancing cardiovascular and vasomotor response to catecholamines.[39]

Critically ill children may have absolute or relative adrenal insufficiency, caused by adrenal hemorrhage, decreased renal perfusion, inhibition of corticosteroid production by TNF, or actual adrenal disease, with inadequate adrenal stress response or decreased response to circulating glucocorticoids.[40,41] When sepsis is present and the child fails to respond to initial fluid therapy and vasoactive support, providers should rule out adrenal insufficiency and consider hydrocortisone administration.[42]

◆ CLINICAL MANIFESTATIONS

Signs of Septic Shock. Sepsis and its complications produce a cascade of physiologic and biochemical changes. The clinical progression of sepsis in children was defined in 2005 by an international consensus panel[5] (Box 50.3). These definitions are still used today, but they have

---

BOX 50.3   INTERNATIONAL CONSENSUS DEFINITIONS OF SYSTEMIC INFLAMMATORY RESPONSE SYNDROME, SEPSIS, SEVERE SEPSIS, AND SEPTIC SHOCK IN CHILDREN

Systemic Inflammatory Response Syndrome (SIRS)

The presence of at least two of the following alteration criteria, one of which must be abnormal temperature or leukocyte count:

- ALTERATION IN TEMPERATURE: Core body temperature of >38.5°C (101.3°F) or <36°C (96.8°F)
- ALTERATION IN HEART RATE:
  - Tachycardia in the absence of external stimulus, chronic drugs, or painful stimuli, defined as follows:
    - Newborn to 1 year: >180 beats/min
    - 2–5 years: >140 beats/min
    - 6–12 years: >130 beats/min
    - 13 to <18 years: >110 beats/min
  - Otherwise unexplained persistent elevation over a 0.5- to 4-hour time period
  - For children younger than 1 yr: bradycardia, in the absence of external vagal stimulus, β-blocker drugs, or congenital heart disease, defined by one of the following rates:
    - Newborn to 1 month: <100 beats/min
    - 1 month to 1 year: <90 beats/min
    - Otherwise unexplained persistent depression over a 30-minute time period
- ALTERATION IN RESPIRATORY RATE:
  - Mean respiratory rate >95th percentile normal for age, defined as follows:
    - Newborn to 1 week: >50 beats/min
    - 1 week to 1 month: >40 beats/min
    - 1 month to 1 year: >34 beats/min
    - 2–5 years: >22 beats/min

- 6–12 years: >18 beats/min
- 13 to <18 years: >14 beats/min
- Mechanical ventilation for an acute process not related to underlying neuromuscular disease or the receipt of general anesthesia
- ALTERATION IN WHITE BLOOD CELL COUNT:
  - Leukocyte count elevated or depressed for age (not secondary to chemotherapy-induced leukopenia) or >10% immature neutrophils

Infection (one of the following):

- A suspected or proven (by positive culture, tissue stain, or polymerase chain reaction test) infection caused by any pathogen
- A clinical syndrome associated with a high probability of infection

NOTE: Evidence of infection includes positive findings on clinical examination, imaging, or laboratory tests (e.g., white blood cells in a normally sterile body fluid, perforated viscus, chest radiograph consistent with pneumonia, petechial or purpuric rash, purpura fulminans)

Sepsis

- SIRS in the presence of or as a result of suspected or proven infection

Severe Sepsis

- Sepsis plus one of the following:
  - Cardiovascular organ dysfunction
  - Acute respiratory distress syndrome
  - Two or more other organ dysfunctions (organ dysfunctions are defined in Box 50.4)

Septic Shock

- Sepsis and cardiovascular organ dysfunction as defined in Box 50.4

Data from Perkin RM et al: Shock, cardiac arrest and resuscitation. In Hazinski MF, editor: *Nursing care of the critically ill child* ed 3, St Louis, 2013, Mosby; Modified from Goldstein B et al: *Pediatr Crit Care Med* 6:2-8, 2005.

not been validated in newborns and are found in only about half of newborns with culture-positive sepsis.[16]

Systemic inflammatory response syndrome (SIRS) represents a nonspecific response to a variety of insults, including trauma, burns, pancreatitis, or infection. SIRS is present when the child demonstrates two or more of the following as an acute change from baseline: change in temperature, specifically fever (greater than 38.5°C [101.3°F]) or hypothermia (less than 36°C [96.8°F]), change in heart rate (tachypnea or, in infants, bradycardia), change in respiratory rate (or need for mechanical ventilation), or change in white blood cell (WBC) count (including leukocytes, leukopenia, or an increase in the percentage of immature or band forms of WBCs).[5] These clinical signs must be interpreted in light of the child's baseline organ and system function.

Sepsis is a systemic response to infection. It is present when manifestations of SIRS are observed in conjunction with suspected infection. Positive cultures are not necessary for the diagnosis, but suspicion of infection is required.[5]

Septic newborns are more likely to demonstrate a decrease in heart rate variability rather than overt tachycardia or bradycardia. Fever is uncommon in newborns, and hypothermia may relate more to inadequate temperature support rather than hypothermia. Finally, no complete blood count (CBC) variable has been shown to reliably identify septic newborns.[16]

Severe sepsis is present when the child with sepsis (SIRS + suspected infection) develops cardiovascular or pulmonary dysfunction, or if the child has sepsis and evidence of two or more other organ dysfunctions (Box 50.4).[5] The dysfunctional organ should be separate from the site of suspected infection and not explained by effects of drug therapy or other acute effects.[5] This important distinction helps separate signs of severe sepsis from signs of simple pneumonia with respiratory failure.

Septic shock is present when the septic child develops cardiovascular dysfunction characterized by hypotension despite adequate fluid resuscitation or by the need for vasopressors to maintain blood pressure.[5] Because children may develop hypotension only late in the course of shock, septic shock is present if the child develops signs of poor perfusion despite adequate fluid resuscitation. When the child with sepsis develops hypotension *plus* signs of poor perfusion, hypotensive septic shock is present, and mortality may be as high as 14% to 24%.[27,28,42]

The adult Sepsis-3 guidelines simplified the criteria to identify sepsis and recommend evaluation for infection-related organ failure for adults with tachypnea, abnormal mentation, or hypotension.[43] Simplified consensus pediatric criteria have not yet been published, but several have been proposed. Kissoon, Orr, and Carcillo[44] suggested a simplified triad of fever, tachycardia, and vasodilation as diagnostic for pediatric sepsis, with septic shock likely when an altered level of consciousness is added to this triad. Carcillo and colleagues[34,44] have also distilled the international consensus definitions of septic shock to include suspected infection with hypo- or hyperthermia and clinical signs of inadequate perfusion. These signs of inadequate perfusion include any of the following: decreased level of conscious or change in mental status; prolonged (>2 seconds) capillary refill; abnormal pulses (either diminished or bounding with wide pulse pressure); mottled, cool extremities; or decreased urine output. Hypotension is not required for the diagnosis but, if present, is confirmatory.[34,44]

Infants and children with septic shock may have a high, normal, or low cardiac output. Preterm newborns may maintain cardiac output

---

BOX 50.4 CRITERIA FOR ORGAN DYSFUNCTION IN CHILDREN WITH SEVERE SEPSIS OR SEPTIC SHOCK

Cardiovascular

Despite administration of isotonic intravenous fluid boluses of more than 40 mL/kg in 1 hour, is described by the characteristics in one or more of the following:

- Decrease in blood pressure (BP) (hypotension) to <5th percentile for age, estimated for children 1–10 years of age as follows:
  - Mean arterial pressure: <40 mmHg + (1.5 × age in years)
  - Systolic BP <70 mmHg + (2 × age in years)
- Need for vasoactive drug to maintain BP in normal range (dopamine >5 μg/kg/min; or dobutamine, epinephrine, or norepinephrine at any dose)
- Two of the following:
  - Unexplained metabolic acidosis: base deficit more severe than −5 mEq/L
  - Increased arterial lactate >2 times upper limit of normal
  - Oliguria: urine output <0.5 mL/kg/hr
  - Prolonged capillary refill: >5 seconds
  - Core to peripheral temperature gap >3°C (37.4°F)

Respiratory (one of the following)*

- $PaCO_2/FiO_2$ <300 in absence of cyanotic heart disease or preexisting lung disease

- $PaCO_2$ >65 torr or 20 mmHg over baseline $PaCO_2$
- Proven need† or >50% inspired oxygen to maintain saturation >92%
- Need for nonelective invasive or noninvasive mechanical ventilation‡

Neurologic (either of the following)

- Glasgow Coma Scale score ≤11
- Acute change in mental status with a decrease in Glasgow score ≥3 points from abnormal baseline

Hematologic (one of the following)

- Platelet count <80,000/mm³
- A decline of 50% in platelet count from highest value recorded over the past 3 days (for chronic hematology/oncology)
- International normalized ratio >2

Renal

- Serum creatinine ≥twofold upper limit of normal for age or twofold increase in baseline creatinine

Hepatic (either of the following)

- Total bilirubin ≥4 mg/dL (not applicable for newborn)
- ALT twofold upper limit of normal for age

*Acute respiratory distress syndrome must include a PaO_2/FiO_2 ratio <200 mmHg, bilateral infiltrates, acute onset, and no evidence of left heart failure. Acute lung injury is defined identically except the PaO_2/FiO_2 ratio must be <300 mmHg.
†Proven need assumes oxygen requirement was tested by decreasing flow with subsequent increase in flow if required.
‡In postoperative patients, this requirement can be met if the patient has developed an acute inflammatory or infectious process in the lungs that prevents them from being extubated.
ALT, Alanine transaminase.
From Perkin RM et al: Shock, cardiac arrest and resuscitation. In Hazinski MF, editor: *Nursing care of the critically ill child,* ed 3, St Louis, 2013, Mosby. Modified from Goldstein B et al: *Pediatr Crit Care Med* 6:2-8, 2005.

but demonstrate severe vasodilation.[45] Unlike adults, who typically present with vasodilation, hypotension, and normal or high cardiac output, approximately half of children with septic shock present with severe peripheral vasoconstriction, high systemic vascular resistance, and low cardiac output.[34,44] Among children with CHD, sepsis is most likely to produce a decrease in cardiac output and perfusion and, postoperatively, is more likely to lead to the development of MODS.[30]

The terms *warm* and *cold septic shock* are imprecise terms and should be used only in conjunction with other descriptions of systemic perfusion and cardiovascular function. **Warm shock** is typically associated with peripheral vasodilation, warm skin with flash capillary refill, bounding pulses, and wide pulse pressure. **Cold shock** is typically associated with peripheral vasoconstriction, cold skin with prolonged capillary refill, and decreased peripheral pulses; these characteristics are present in almost half of children who present with septic shock.[34] Cardiac output may be low, normal, or high regardless of skin temperature, perfusion, and pulses; these characteristics alone will not identify the cardiovascular support required.

Kissoon, Orr, and Carcillo[44] described a *shock index* calculated by dividing the heart rate by the systolic blood pressure in children with septic shock. This shock index is 2.4 or higher with untreated or inadequately treated septic shock but falls (e.g., to 1.75 or less) with effective treatment of septic shock. Two studies have supported the usefulness of this shock index in pediatric care. In one, among children 1 to 3 years of age and over 12 years of age, higher early shock index was associated with higher mortality.[46] In a retrospective application, shock index was significantly higher at the time of presentation and 6 hours after presentation among nonsurvivors than survivors of septic shock.[47] More data are needed regarding the sensitivity and specificity of this shock index.

Signs of Neurogenic Shock. Signs of neurogenic shock in the child with a recent, severe spinal cord injury include warm skin and hypotension with a low diastolic blood pressure. Signs of poor systemic perfusion also are observed (see Clinical Manifestations of Shock), although loss of sympathetic nervous system tone prevents the typical tachycardic response.

Obstructive Shock

Obstructive shock is inadequate cardiac output caused by an impediment to blood flow to or from the heart into the pulmonary or systemic circulation. Causes of obstructive shock in children include congenital heart defects (such as critical aortic stenosis and those with ductal-dependent pulmonary or systemic blood flow), tension pneumothorax, and pulmonary embolus. Obstruction to blood flow results in low cardiac output and circulatory collapse, typically with signs of peripheral vasoconstriction as adrenergic stimulation diverts blood flow from the skin, gut, and kidney to the heart and brain. Signs of systemic or pulmonary venous obstruction are observed.

Additional clinical manifestations of obstructive shock are based on the cause of the obstruction. For example, the newborn with ductal-dependent pulmonary blood flow develops profound hypoxemia when the ductus arteriosus begins to constrict. If a newborn has ductal-dependent systemic blood flow, systemic pulses become faint or absent, extremities become cold and pale, and signs of pulmonary venous congestion can develop when the ductus arteriosus begins to close. Tension pneumothorax produces signs of systemic venous obstruction and congestion, decreased breath sounds and chest expansion on the side of the pneumothorax, and shift of the mediastinum to the contralateral chest. Significant hypoxemia is present. When cardiac tamponade is the cause of the obstruction, signs of systemic or pulmonary edema, or both, develop with low cardiac output. Additional signs can include muffled heart sounds and pulsus paradoxus. When pulmonary embolus

is the cause of the obstruction, hypoxemia, severe respiratory distress (or shortness of breath), and signs of right ventricular failure are observed.[2,22]

Reperfusion and Inflammatory Injury

Reperfusion (reoxygenation) injury is cell damage caused by the restoration of blood flow and oxygen delivery to cells that have been exposed to injurious but nonlethal hypoxic conditions.[48] Ischemia causes changes in transmembrane permeability to sodium and calcium, and damage to intracellular organelles.[49] This damage triggers a proinflammatory and procoagulant response that can be very similar to that caused by septic shock (described previously).

Restoration of oxygen delivery to extremely ischemic tissues produces highly reactive oxygen intermediates (e.g., free oxygen radicals and superoxide) that damage cell membranes, denature proteins, and disrupt chromosomes (see Chapter 2).[49] The amount of free oxygen radical produced is directly related to the severity and duration of the ischemic period. The reperfusion process is most likely to affect endothelial cells of the microvasculature, compromising organ perfusion after shock resuscitation.[48,49]

An ischemic insult activates white blood cells, priming monocytes and macrophages and contributing to the release of inflammatory mediators or cytokines, including TNF, IL-1, IL-6, IL-8, and platelet-activating factor. These cytokines in turn contribute to vasodilation, increased capillary permeability, and altered platelet function. The ultimate result is a maldistribution of blood flow and a compromise in organ perfusion.[48,49] The role of these mediators is summarized in Table 8.4. Chapter 49 includes a more comprehensive discussion of MODS.

Signs of organ dysfunction include but are not limited to lactic acidosis, oliguria, and an acute alteration in level of consciousness (e.g., decrease in Glasgow Coma Scale score of 1 point or more); hypoxemia, hypotension, poor capillary refill, or shock plus signs of coagulopathy; respiratory, renal, or hepatic dysfunction; or neurologic dysfunction. Critical illness hyperglycemia also may be present. Gut injury and inflammation may enable translocation of gram-negative bacteria or endotoxin into the bloodstream and may contribute to gastrointestinal bleeding.[6] Box 50.4 contains information on other potential signs of organ system failure in children.

Several predictive and descriptive scoring systems are available to characterize the severity of illness in critically ill children with organ dysfunction. Outcome scores include the Pediatric Logistic Organ Dysfunction (PELOD) scoring system[50] and the Pediatric Multiple Organ Dysfunction Score (P-MODS).[50-52] These scoring systems may be useful as prognostic indicators when they are applied for several days. Important differences exist between neonates and children in terms of mortality associated with specific organ failures and with specific PELOD scores.[51]

Treatment of Shock and Reperfusion Injury

The goals of treatment of shock are maximization of oxygen delivery and minimization of oxygen demand. The airway, oxygenation, ventilation, and perfusion must be supported. Reduction of oxygen demand requires treatment of fever and pain. In addition, the child should be kept warm, and shivering should be prevented. Blood components and, perhaps, intravenous fluids should be warmed before administration to young infants and children with hypothermia. Fear and pain increase oxygen consumption, so care must be taken to reassure the child and treat pain as indicated.

To evaluate and support airway patency and ventilation, position the child in a manner that supports a patent airway, and assess airway and ventilation. Provide humidified supplementary oxygen as needed at up to 10 to 15 L/min by nonrebreathing mask or bag-valve mask

BOX 50.5   MOST COMMON PEDIATRIC DYSRHYTHMIAS

Heart (QRS) Rate Too Slow for Clinical Condition
QRS Duration (Width) Normal
Sinus bradycardia
Junctional rhythm
Heart block

QRS Duration (Width) Prolonged
Supraventricular tachycardia (SVT) with aberrant ventricular conduction
Ventricular rhythm
Heart block

Heart (QRS) Rate too Fast for Clinical Condition
QRS Duration (Width) Normal
Sinus tachycardia
SVT

QRS Duration (Width) Prolonged
SVT with aberrant ventricular conduction
Ventricular tachycardia

Collapse (Pulseless) Rhythms
Electromechanical dissociation
Ventricular tachycardia
Ventricular fibrillation
Asystole

ventilation. Advanced airway placement is indicated *before* respiratory deterioration or arrest complicates shock management. Monitor oxygenation continuously through pulse oximetry.

The child's heart rate must be adequate to support effective cardiac output and systemic perfusion. The most common pediatric dysrhythmias are listed in Box 50.5. Treat bradydysrhythmias and extreme tachydysrhythmias promptly. Pharmacologic therapy, pacing, or synchronized direct current (DC) cardioversion may be required.

The rhythms associated with loss of pulses ("arrest" rhythms) include asystole, electromechanical dissociation (EMD), pulseless ventricular tachycardia, and ventricular fibrillation. Regardless of electrocardiogram (ECG) findings, provide cardiopulmonary resuscitation, including cardiac compression, when pulses are lost or if, despite support of adequate oxygenation and ventilation, the child demonstrates a heart rate less than 60 beats/min with poor perfusion.

Unless shock is mild or responds immediately to volume therapy, insertion of a central venous (monitoring) catheter is advisable. Several multilumen catheters are available in pediatric sizes that enable simultaneous monitoring of central venous pressure and administration of fluids. Continuous or intermittent monitoring of the ScvO$_2$ will enable evaluation of the balance between the child's oxygen delivery and oxygen consumption. If cardiac output is adequate, the ScvO$_2$ will be no more than 25% to 30% lower than the arterial oxygen saturation. A larger arterial venous oxygen saturation difference suggests inadequate oxygen delivery (caused by inadequate arterial oxygen content or inadequate cardiac output or both) or excessive oxygen demand.[2]

Monitoring of the regional tissue oxygen saturation with NIRS is useful to identify episodes of perfusion compromise and to monitor response to therapy. The cerebral rSO$_2$ should exceed 50% and the somatic rSO$_2$ should be 10% to 15% higher, or >60% to >75%.

All sources of fluid intake and output should be monitored and recorded hourly or more frequently if needed. Urine output and specific gravity reflect the child's response to fluid therapy. A urinary catheter should be inserted if shock is present unless the child has sustained pelvic trauma or a urethral tear is suspected.

An intraarterial catheter is needed if shock persists. This enables reliable, continuous evaluation of arterial pressure. Noninvasive oscillometric blood pressure–monitoring devices may not accurately measure low or rapidly falling blood pressures and may *overestimate* the blood pressure,[53] particularly in trauma patients.[54]

The child's serum glucose concentration should be monitored using rapid bedside testing. Hypoglycemia requires glucose administration; continuous infusion is preferred to repeated intermittent bolus therapy. When hyperglycemia develops, it is unclear if treatment with insulin administration is warranted. A single study of tight glycemic control in critically ill children, most (75%) recruited following cardiovascular surgery, documented improved survival and shorter length of stay with maintenance of serum glucose at fasting glucose levels,[55] although frequent episodes of hypoglycemia were noted. However, a recent large, pediatric multicenter prospective randomized trial of tight glycemic control (to a serum glucose of 80 to 110 mg/dL) versus control to a higher glucose concentration (150 to 180 mg/dL) found no benefit to tight glycemic control. In addition, tight glycemic control was associated with higher rates of healthcare-associated infection and episodes of hypoglycemia.[56]

Electrolyte imbalances depress myocardial function and must be corrected when shock is present. Alterations in serum potassium concentration may affect myocardial contractility and conduction. However, children are far less sensitive than adults to minor changes in serum potassium concentration. Hypokalemia may result from inadequate potassium administration during volume therapy or from excessive potassium losses caused by drug therapy (e.g., furosemide). The serum potassium concentration falls in the presence of alkalosis; this represents an intracellular shift of potassium and is corrected when the pH is normalized. Treat true hypokalemia with an infusion of potassium chloride at a dose equivalent to 0.5 to 1 mEq/kg administered over several hours.[18]

Hyperkalemia may result from excessive potassium administration, reduced potassium excretion (e.g., in renal failure), or massive cell lysis (e.g., tumor lysis syndrome). Serum potassium concentration also rises when acidosis develops; the rise in serum potassium is caused by a shift of potassium from the intracellular to the vascular space (i.e., exchanged for vascular H$^+$) and falls when the serum pH is corrected.[18]

Providers must monitor both ionized and total calcium concentration and treat documented hypocalcemia. Note that the ionized serum calcium falls with alkalosis and rises with acidosis. Serum ionized calcium concentration is often low (less than 4.5 mEq/L) in children with septic shock.[18]

When conventional shock management fails, mechanical support such as with extracorporeal membrane oxygenation should be considered.[17] The child requires treatment at a center with appropriate pediatric critical care expertise.

Treatment of Hypovolemic Shock

Specific treatment of hypovolemic shock is volume resuscitation. Volume resuscitation is designed to restore intravascular volume relative to the vascular space and to optimize ventricular preload. The specific fluid selected and route of administration are determined by the child's clinical condition. In general, isotonic **crystalloids** (isotonic salt-containing solutions, such as normal saline or lactated Ringer solution) or **colloids** (protein-containing fluids, such as albumin or blood) are administered in boluses of 20 mL/kg (or 10 mL/kg of packed red blood cells) given over 5 to 20 minutes for hypovolemic and septic shock. If myocardial dysfunction is present, smaller fluid boluses (5 to 10 mL/kg) are administered over about 10 to 20 minutes. Hypotonic fluids should not be administered.[2,48,49,57] After each bolus, it is important to reassess systemic perfusion and administer additional fluids if indicated. Providers should halt bolus fluid administration immediately if the child develops new or worsening hepatomegaly, respiratory distress, or rales.

During treatment of shock caused by dehydration, providers must avoid acute or severe alterations in the serum sodium concentration.[2,18,57] Acute changes in serum sodium alter the serum osmolality and result in fluid shifts into and out of the vascular spaces. Such fluid shifts can be associated with neurologic complications including seizures, cerebral edema, and intracranial hemorrhage.[18]

Administration of blood or blood component therapy may be needed to treat hemorrhage. A "normal" hematocrit does not rule out the possibility of hemorrhage in the injured patient; the hematocrit typically falls in a person who has sustained whole blood loss after the blood loss is replaced with crystalloids or colloids. When blood loss is significant, 10 mL/kg boluses of packed red blood cells (PRBCs) are administered as needed to maintain hemoglobin and hematocrit.[23,24,57]

The optimal hemoglobin threshold for transfusion in critically ill children is unknown. In a multicenter trial of critically ill children, a hemoglobin red-cell transfusion threshold of 7 g/dL decreased transfusion requirements without increasing adverse outcomes.[58] However, that study excluded premature infants and children with severe hypoxemia, hemodynamic instability, active blood loss, and cyanotic heart disease. A more recent publication from the same researchers[59] recommends higher transfusion thresholds (9 to 12 g/dL or higher) for children with cardiac or respiratory disease, with the highest thresholds for children with cyanotic congenital heart disease and those with hemodynamic instability.

Transfusion for the child with chronic anemia and shock must be accomplished slowly to prevent further deterioration in myocardial function. A PRBC administration rate averaging 3 to 5 mL/kg hour over several hours may be well tolerated, particularly if it is preceded and followed by administration of diuretics.[60] If severe anemia is associated with severe hypervolemia and myocardial dysfunction, an exchange transfusion may be required. If a coagulopathy is present, administer specific blood component therapy necessary to prevent or treat hemorrhage.

Treatment of Cardiogenic Shock

Treatment targeting cardiogenic shock requires titration of fluid boluses as needed to optimize cardiac preload. These boluses of 5 mL/kg to 10 mL/kg of isotonic crystalloid are delivered over 10 to 20 minutes and should be stopped immediately if the child develops new or worsening hepatomegaly, respiratory distress, or rales. Vasoactive drugs are needed to improve myocardial function and vasodilators or vasoconstrictors may be needed to support systemic perfusion. Table 50.7 summarizes drug therapy for children in shock.

Treatment of Septic Shock

The child with septic shock has significant hypovolemia and maldistribution of blood flow. Treatment required within the first hour after the identification of septic shock includes administration of antibiotics, bolus fluid administration, and, if signs of shock persist despite bolus fluid administration, initiation and titration of vasoactive drugs, including inotropes and vasopressors or vasodilators.[42,57] Therapeutic goals include restoring systemic perfusion and blood pressure, normalizing heart rate and capillary refill, maintaining the $ScvO_2$ ≥70%, and maintaining high cardiac index (3.3 to 6 L/min/m² body surface area [BSA]), and high oxygen delivery (more than 200 mL/min/m²) BSA.[42,44,57,61,62]

In a small but seminal study of children with septic shock,[61] Carcillo, Davis, and Zaritsky[61] showed that rapid fluid resuscitation (more than

40 mL/kg administered within the first hour of therapy and more than 200 mL/kg administered during the first 8 hours of therapy) was associated with significantly higher survival than less aggressive fluid resuscitation. Bolus fluid administration should be halted if the child develops new or worsening respiratory distress, rales, or hepatomegaly.[42,57]

The 2015 Pediatric Advanced Life Support Guidelines[63] cautioned that in resource-limited settings (i.e., with limited critical care resources such as inotropic and mechanical ventilator support), fluid administration should proceed with caution in children with severe febrile illness. In such children, bolus fluid administration may be associated with higher mortality.

Implementation of the consensus recommendations for hemodynamic support of children with septic shock is reportedly associated with decreased mortality (from 35% to 40% mortality to 2% to 8% mortality).[42,44] In fact, for every hour of delay in the restoration of normal blood pressure for age and restoration of capillary refill less than 3 seconds, child mortality doubled.[34,42,44]

The ultimate goal of treatment of septic shock is to support adequate systemic oxygen delivery (reflected by $ScvO_2$ ≥70%) and organ perfusion and function. This requires careful titration of fluid administration, inotropic support, and vasoconstrictors or vasodilators to maximize systemic oxygen delivery and organ perfusion and function.

When inadequate systemic perfusion persists in the child with septic shock, the child likely needs additional fluid administration and titration of vasoactive drug therapy. Vasoactive drugs include milrinone, epinephrine, and/or norepinephrine. In a randomized prospective trial in children with septic shock, the use of epinephrine was associated with higher survival (14% vs. 7%) than the use of dopamine.[64]

Providers must be prepared to support organs and body systems that fail. Early use of renal replacement therapies aids in hemodynamic support and maintenance of appropriate intravascular volume.[2,42]

An algorithm for the treatment of septic shock, based on the recommendations of the American College of Critical Care Medicine and the Pediatric Advanced Life Support course, is presented in Fig. 50.2.

Treatment of Neurogenic Shock

Treatment of neurogenic shock includes positioning to enhance venous return, bolus fluid therapy as needed to support cardiac output, and administration of vasopressors to treat fluid-refractory hypotension. Supplementary warming or cooling is likely to be needed to support normothermia.[57]

Treatment of Obstructive Shock

Treatment of obstructive shock focuses on restoration of systemic oxygenation and perfusion, and elimination of the obstruction to flow. To support systemic oxygenation and perfusion, providers must establish and maintain an adequate airway and support oxygenation and ventilation. Diagnostic studies are limited to those essential to establishment of the diagnosis. Elimination of the cause of obstruction may require administration of prostaglandin E_1 (to reopen a constricted ductus arteriosus in newborns with ductal-dependent congenital heart disease), interventional cardiac catheterization for treatment of other defects causing obstruction, needle decompression of a tension pneumothorax or cardiac tamponade, and fibrinolytic therapy and fibrinolytics (and possible embolectomy) for treatment of massive pulmonary embolus.[2,57]

If cardiac tamponade is present, bolus fluid administration may improve cardiac output while preparations are made for pericardiocentesis. However, this should not delay definitive therapy.

Treatment of Reperfusion Injury

The best available model of reperfusion injury is the person who survives cardiac arrest. "Bundled" post–cardiac arrest care, including meticulous

TABLE 50.7   PEDIATRIC VASOACTIVE DRUGS FOR THE TREATMENT OF SHOCK*

DOSE	EFFECTS	CAUTIONS
Sympathomimetics		
Dobutamine: 2–20 µg/min	Selective β-adrenergic effects, increases cardiac contractility and also increases heart rate (this latter effect is variable); β_2 effects produce peripheral vasodilation; no dopaminergic or α-adrenergic effects	Extreme tachyarrhythmias have been reported, particularly in infants; hypotension may develop; may produce pulmonary vasoconstriction
Dopamine: 1–5 µg/kg/min	Dopaminergic effects predominate, including increase in glomerular filtration rate and urine volume	Can produce extreme tachyarrhythmias; can result in increase in pulmonary artery pressure; inhibits thyroid-stimulating hormone and aldosterone secretion
Dopamine: 2–10 µg/kg/min	Dopaminergic effects persist and β_1 effects are seen, especially an increase in heart rate	As Dopamine 1–5
Dopamine: 8–20 µg/kg/min	α-Adrenergic effects dominate	As Dopamine 1–5
Epinephrine: 0.05–0.15 µg/kg/min	Endogenous catecholamine, which produces α, β_1, and β_2 adrenergic effects; at low doses, β_1 effects dominate	Will increase myocardial work and oxygen consumption at any dose; splanchnic constriction will occur at even low doses
Epinephrine: 0.2–0.3 µg/kg/min	α-Adrenergic (vasoconstrictive) effects dominate	As Epinephrine 0.05–0.15
Isoproterenol: 0.05–0.1 µg/kg/min	β-Adrenergic effects; β_1 effects may result in rapid increase in heart rate; β_2 effects may produce peripheral vasodilation and also may effectively treat bronchoconstriction	Monitor for tachyarrhythmias, hypotension; will increase myocardial oxygen consumption
Norepinephrine: 0.05–1 µg/kg/min	Endogenous catecholamine with α- and β-adrenergic effects; produces potent peripheral and renal vasoconstriction; can increase blood pressure	May cause tachyarrhythmias, increased myocardial work, and increased oxygen consumption; may result in hepatic and mesenteric ischemia
Vasopressin		
Vasopressin: 0.2 to 2 milliunits/kg/min (0.0002 to 0.002 unit/kg/min)	Antidiuretic hormone analog that acts on vasopressin receptors; produces peripheral and splanchnic vasoconstriction; also used to treat GI hemorrhage for this reason	May cause hypertension, bradycardia
Phosphodiesterase Inhibitors and Inodilators		
Milrinone: loading dose, 0.05 mg/kg (50 µg/kg) over 10–60 min; infusion, 0.25–0.75 µg/kg/min	Nonadrenergic inotropic agent that produces phosphodiesterase inhibition and increase in intracellular cyclic adenosine monophosphate (cAMP); intracellular calcium uptake also is delayed; these effects result in improved cardiac contractility and vasodilation	Monitor for arrhythmias (especially accelerated junctional rhythm, junctional tachycardia, and ventricular ectopy); may produce hypotension (especially if patient is hypovolemic), liver and GI dysfunction, thrombocytopenia, and abdominal pain; experience in children is limited and recent Reduce dose when renal dysfunction present
Vasodilators		
Nitroglycerin: 0.25–0.5 µg/kg/min; increase as tolerated to maximum 10 µg/kg/min (adolescents, 5 µg/min; Note **not** per kg/min)	Arterial and venodilator	Is absorbed by polyvinyl chloride tubing; use special infusion set
Nitroprusside: 0.3–0.5 µg/kg/min; titrate up to 8 µg/kg/min (max. infusion dose: 8–10 µg/kg/min)	Arterial and venodilator	Light sensitive; use special infusion set or cover tubing when infusion slow; may produce thiocyanate and cyanide toxicity, particularly for higher doses or prolonged infusion

*Infusion rate = mL/hr = Weight (kg) × Dose (µg/kg per min) × 60 min/hr ÷ concentration (µg/mL).

GI, Gastrointestinal.

Modified from Perkin RM et al: Shock, cardiac arrest and resuscitation. In Hazinski MF, editor: *Nursing care of the critically ill child*, ed 3, p 120, St Louis, 2013, Mosby.

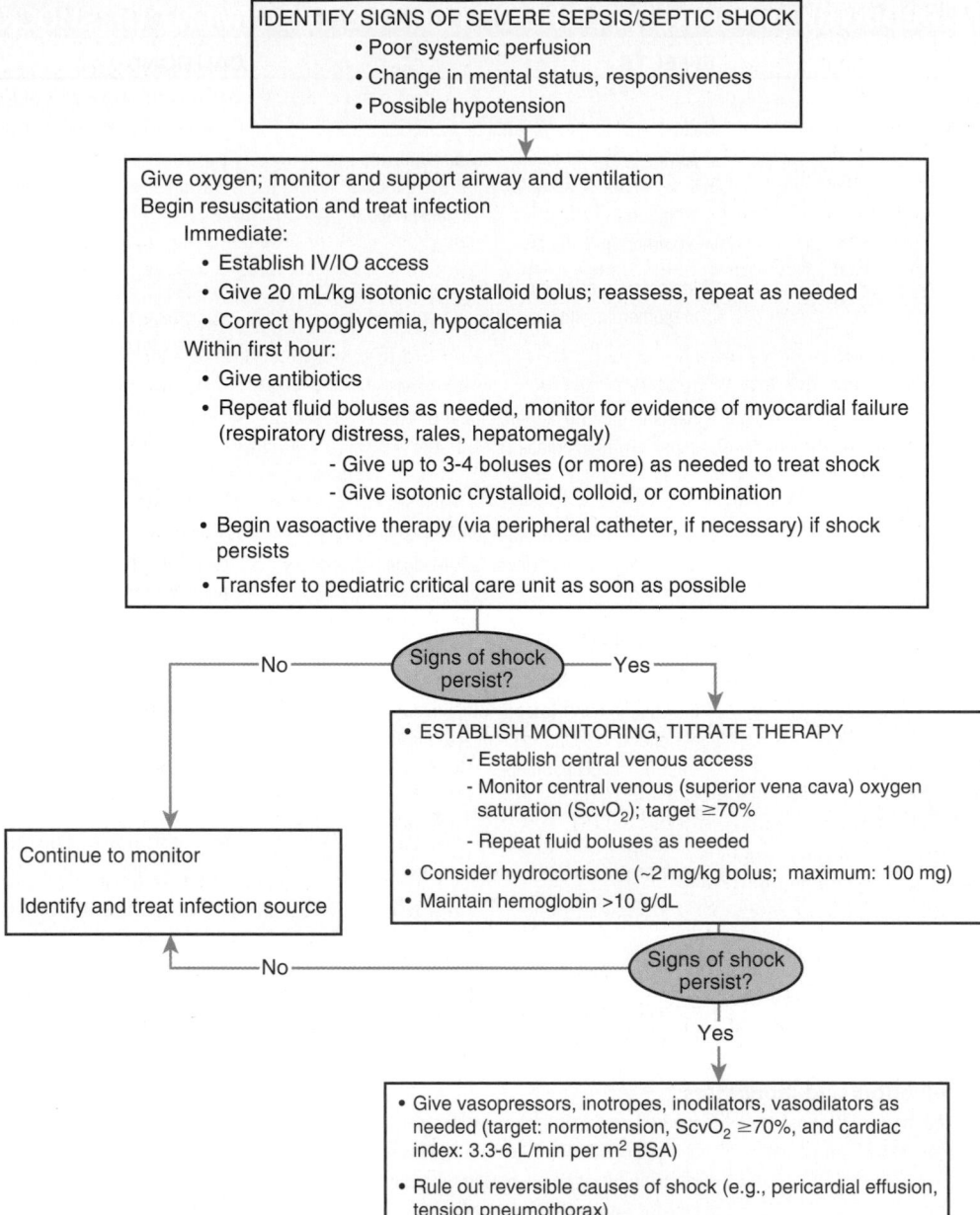

FIGURE 50.2 Hemodynamic Support in Pediatric Septic Shock. *BSA,* Body surface area; *IO,* intake/output; *IV,* intravenous. (From Perkin RM et al: Shock, cardiac arrest and resuscitation. In Hazinski MF, editor: *Nursing care of the critically ill child,* ed 3, p 126, St Louis, 2013, Mosby; data from Brierley J et al: *Crit Care Med* 37:666-688, 2009.)

targeted temperature management, as well as protocol-based support of cardiorespiratory function and function of other organ systems, has been shown to substantially increase neurologically intact survival to hospital discharge in adults who survive cardiac arrest[65]; such a "bundled" approach is now pursued with children. This care typically requires transfer of the child to a medical center with appropriate pediatric critical care expertise.[2,66]

Fever typically develops following resuscitation from cardiac arrest and is associated with unfavorable neurologic outcome.[67] Therapeutic hypothermia suppresses proinflammatory mediators and may enhance antiinflammatory mediators.[68,69] Mild to moderate induced hypothermia (to 32° to 34°C [89.6° to 93.2°F]) was associated with increased survival

in neurologic outcome in neonates with hypoxic-ischemic encephalopathy[70] and in comatose, hemodynamically stable adults following resuscitation from cardiac arrest.[71] However, the control groups in these neonatal and adult hypothermia studies were febrile, so that may have lowered survival in the control group. Three recent large, multicentered randomized clinical trials comparing strict maintenance of normothermia (36°C [96.8°F]) to moderate therapeutic hypothermia [33°C [91.4°F]) demonstrated no benefit to the use of cooling in adults[72] or children with out-of-hospital cardiac arrest[73] or in-hospital cardiac arrest.[74]

Support of airway, oxygenation, and ventilation includes oxygen administration and intubation and support of ventilation to maintain arterial oxygen saturation at 94% to 99% and avoid hypoxemia. Of course, if cyanotic heart disease is present, the arterial oxygen saturation is typically maintained at 65% to 75%. Support of ventilation is titrated to maintain a $PaCO_2$ within the child's normal range.

Continuous monitoring of blood pressure is indicated. Hypotension during post–cardiac arrest care can contribute to worse neurologic outcome, so it must be promptly detected and aggressively treated. Titration of inotropic and vasoactive drugs is typically required (see Table 50.7), and bolus fluid administration may be needed. Additional treatment of shock has been summarized earlier in this chapter. If the child remains hemodynamically unstable with conventional management of shock, mechanical support of circulation should be considered in the appropriate setting.

Prevention of secondary neurologic insult requires targeted temperature management with strict maintenance of normothermia and prevention or aggressive treatment of fever. In addition to support of airway, ventilation, and circulation, careful maintenance of fluid and electrolyte balance is imperative. If renal failure develops, early use of renal replacement therapies is indicated. If seizures develop, they must be managed aggressively.[66]

Emerging Therapies for Shock and Sepsis

Prevention of shock is important. Prevention of trauma (injury prevention) and treatment of dehydration can eliminate the two leading causes of hypovolemic shock in children. The incidence of septic shock from hospital-acquired infections, such as ventilator-associated pneumonia or catheter-related bloodstream infections, is decreasing with the use of quality improvement approaches.[29]

Advances in shock therapy show promise for continued improvement in treatment. First, there is a better understanding of resuscitation goals with an appreciation of the need to target high, rather than normal, cardiac output and oxygen delivery during resuscitation.

Trauma resuscitation also has become more targeted in adults and children. In the prehospital setting, prehospital fluid resuscitation is reserved for children with signs of shock. If penetrating trauma is associated with hypovolemic shock, the child requires urgent transport and surgical intervention, rather than attempts to aggressively treat the shock at the site of injury.

Because massive transfusions can produce immunologic and coagulation complications, the surgical approach to trauma has changed to include staged surgical repair of significant injuries (e.g., liver and bowel injuries). The initial surgery is performed to stabilize the child, and, if needed, subsequent procedures repair the injury. This multistage approach, based on battlefield experiences, reduces the volume of blood products administered and has been linked with reduced morbidity and mortality.[24]

Major advances have been made in understanding the pathophysiology of septic shock and MODS in children. These advances are beginning to be applied to the clinical setting.[75] Patterns of alterations in biomarkers of sepsis—so-called biomarker signatures—may enable identification of high-risk children requiring more careful monitoring and early intervention. In addition, if alterations in concentrations of biomarkers can be identified at the time they occur, modulation of biomarker activity may be possible using strategies such as receptor antagonists.

It soon may be possible to tailor sepsis and other critical therapies through the use of genetic profiling of the microorganism[33] and of the child.[32,75] Prospective identification of genetic markers for risk of sepsis and responsiveness to therapy may enable individual tailoring of surveillance and interventions to maximize survival and minimize risks from those therapies that are unlikely to be effective.

Finally, several devices are available that enable noninvasive or minimally invasive calculation of cardiac output and index, stroke volume, and circulating blood volume in children.[2] As providers gain experience with the use of such devices and more published data are available about their reliability in children, there will be more tools to confirm clinical assessment and monitor response to therapy.

BURNS

Management of pediatric burn injuries requires an understanding of the differences that exist in this population related to etiology of injury, growth and development, physiology, and clinical course. In 1988 the American Burn Association established criteria to guide transfer of a patient to a specialized burn center. These criteria remain a standard in burn care and are based on complex management issues related to treatment of acute burns and the long-term rehabilitation needs of children.[76]

Burn injuries in children often are preventable and often are the result of curiosity, inability to escape the burning agent, inadequate supervision, or nonaccidental burn trauma. Scald injuries (i.e., hot water, grease, other) are most common among young children, whereas flame burns are more prevalent among older children.[77] A child exposed to hot tap water at 60°C (140°F) for 5 seconds will sustain a third-degree burn.[78]

A child's skin is thinner and thus more susceptible to injury than an adult's. The extent of injury is determined by the temperature of the burning agent and the duration of exposure. Because very young children may be unable to escape the heat source, the depth of the injury is likely to be greater. The kitchen tends to be a common site for burn injury and often involves pulling over dishes or appliances containing hot liquids. These are common burn injury sources for children 2 years of age and younger.

Children 3 to 8 years of age are most often injured by flame during fire play. Lighters and matches ignite clothing and cause house fires. Young children may run when clothing ignites and increase the severity of injury. Approximately 50% of all deaths in burned children are caused by inhalation injury.[79] Escape from a burning residence or motor vehicle is often delayed because young children cannot cognitively comprehend the circumstances or physically remove themselves from the danger. Flame burns involving flammable liquids, especially gasoline, are more common in older children.

Although flame and scald burns account for the majority of thermal injuries in children, electrical burns result from direct contact with high- or low-voltage current. Most commonly these injuries occur as a result of risk-taking behavior on the part of young males. Trauma from contact with electrical energy results from the passage of current through vital organs, muscle compartments, and nerve or vascular pathways. Very young children are at risk for injury from chewing on electrical cords or inserting objects into electrical outlets (Fig. 50.3). Lightning strikes also account for some electrical burns. Chemical burns occur most often in an industrial setting for the adult. At home, children may be burned by swallowing corrosive agents. The type of causative agent has important implications for the evaluation, treatment, and prognosis of the child.

Although child abuse can occur at any age, young children are particularly vulnerable to serious injury. Approximately 8% to 12% of all forms of abuse cases in the United States are caused by burning.[80] Burns that may suggest nonaccidental trauma include (1) patterned burns, (2) classic forced immersion burn pattern with sharp stocking or glove demarcation and sparing of flexed protected areas, (3) splash/spill burn patterns not consistent with history or developmental level, and (4) cigarette burns.[81] Abuse is suggested with (1) incompatible history and physical examination; (2) incompatible burn and developmental level; (3) bilateral or mirror image burns; (4) localized burns

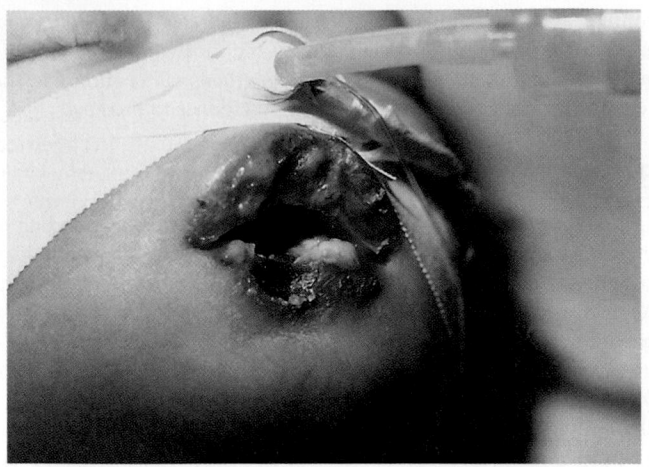

FIGURE 50.3 Commissure Burn Resulting from Biting an Electrical Wire.

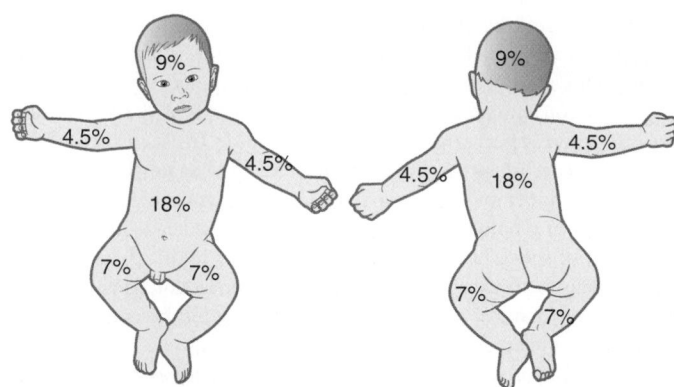

FIGURE 50.5 Rule of Nines for Pediatric Burns (Adapted from American Burn Association: *Pediatric burn injuries. Advanced burn life support provider manual 2016 update*, Chicago, 2016, American Burn Association.)

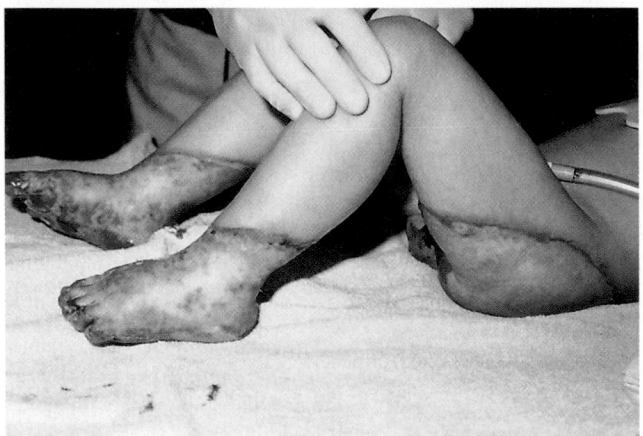

FIGURE 50.4 Burn Pattern Typically Seen After Forced Immersion in Hot Water.

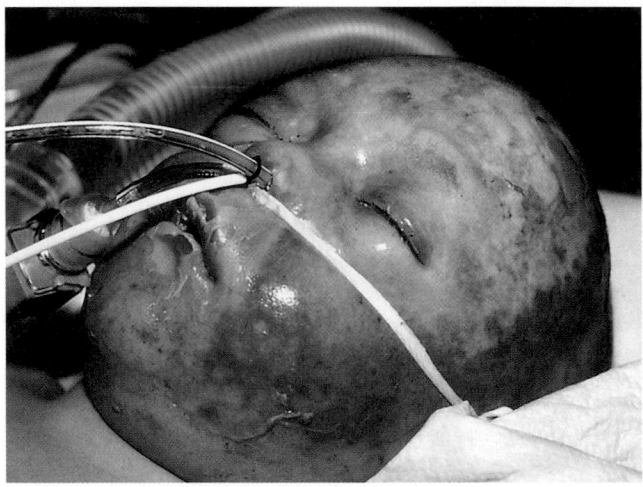

FIGURE 50.6 Areas of Indeterminate Depth of Injury in a Young Child.

to genitals, buttocks, and perineum (especially at toilet-training stage); (5) evidence of excessive delay in seeking treatment; and (6) presence of other forms of injury.[82] Forced immersion in hot water typically presents with deep symmetric injuries lacking any evidence of splash wounds (Fig. 50.4). By contrast, a pull-down splash burn usually has a triangular pattern with immediate skin contact reflected as the area of greatest burn injury. The burn injury then forms an arrow pointing downward. Contact burns also may be intentionally inflicted by contact with cigarettes or other hot objects, such as curling irons. Young children may inadvertently grasp a hot object. However, the pattern of injury will be confined to the palm. Burns to the dorsum of the hand are viewed with suspicion.[82,83] The provider must rule out diseases or conditions that mimic burn injury, such as diaper dermatitis, scalded skin syndrome, or impetigo, when assessing for abuse.

Severity of Injury

The severity of burn injury is assessed based on the percentage of the total body surface area (TBSA) involved. Use of the standard Rule of Nines results in inaccurate calculation of the percentage of TBSA involved in children. Although the infant's trunk and arms are of roughly the same proportion as the adult's, the head and neck make up 18% of TBSA and each lower extremity is 14% of TBSA. A modified Rule of Nines deducts 1% from the head and adds 0.5% to each leg for each year of life after 2 years[78] (Fig. 50.5). Various charts are available that

assign body proportions to children of different ages. These are generally used in pediatric burn facilities and accurately compute the extent of burn injury.

Because burn trauma represents a three-dimensional wound, the severity of injury is assessed also in relation to the **depth of injury**. The etiology of the burn and the duration of contact with the burning agent are important considerations in determining the depth of injury. In general, the more intense the heat source and longer the contact, the deeper the resulting injury; however, infant skin is extremely fragile and more likely to sustain a deeper burn. This makes the estimation of the depth of burn difficult in very young children, especially following scald injuries (Fig. 50.6). Intentionally inflicted burns tend to be more severe because contact with the burning agent is prolonged. Electrical injuries also may mask the extent of damage on initial assessment. Visible tissue damage may appear minimal despite severe injury to underlying structures.

Another important factor in assessing the severity of injury is the victim's age. Children younger than 2 years have a significantly higher risk for associated morbidity and mortality after sustaining a burn injury. They have not achieved maturity of the immune system and are at increased risk for infection and sepsis. In addition, very young children are intolerant of rapid fluid shifts and demonstrate immature renal function, which negatively affects their ability to retain sodium and water (see Shock).

The areas of the body injured are another consideration when assessing the severity of the burn. Burns of the hands, feet, and perineum and across joints carry the potential for scar formation and contracture that may interfere with function as well as growth and development. Specialized care is required to preserve maximal function. In addition, burns to the face and neck may result in airway compromise as well as deformity caused by damage to delicate cartilage of the nose and ears.

Concomitant injuries may be suggested by the circumstances of the burn and should always be investigated; for example, initially burns do not bleed. Bloody drainage suggests another source of trauma. Fractures may result from jumping from a window to escape a house fire. Electrical injuries and motor vehicle accidents often result in associated trauma. Any suspicion of nonaccidental burns should alert the burn team to assess for other injuries.

♦PATHOPHYSIOLOGY, CLINICAL MANIFESTATIONS, AND TREATMENT. Major burn trauma involves all body systems, and the consequences of injury include shock, infection, hypermetabolism, organ failure, and functional limitations. These effects can be magnified in the pediatric population as a result of physiologic immaturity and age-related variation in treatment modalities. Along with recognition of changes in the pathophysiology with a burn injury, clinical manifestations are apparent in all organ systems. Although the cutaneous trauma is the initiator of the chain of responses, it is important to consider all of the likely consequences of the injury. An awareness of the changing patterns of convalescence and the development of complications assists in the identification and early treatment of potential sequelae.

Integument

The local response manifested in the area of trauma includes cellular destruction and damage. Progressive injury caused by dermal ischemia may result from ineffective initial management, especially inadequate or delayed resuscitation. An increase in the permeability and hydrostatic pressure of the capillaries results in the loss of fluid, proteins, and electrolytes into the interstitial spaces. A diminishing intravascular oncotic pressure further enhances these losses and results in edema formation. Marked edema can result, not only in the area of injury but also in unburned areas. Loss of substantial areas of skin has immediate and profound physiologic effects. Direct and evaporative fluid losses are seen immediately.[84] Although these losses are maximal in the immediate postburn period, they persist until wound closure.

Circulatory alterations also occur in the area of injury. Reduced blood flow and capillary stasis result from hemoconcentration, the release of thromboplastin and clot-activating factors from heat-damaged cells, reduced cardiac output, and edema formation. Circulation in the area of partial-thickness wounds ceases for 24 to 48 hours after injury, after which it is usually restored. Vascular supply in the area of full-thickness injuries is completely occluded and is not restored until granulation tissue forms or the wound is surgically repaired. The dry, leathery eschar provides an ideal environment for bacterial growth. Infection, trauma, or applying ice to the burn area may convert a partial-thickness injury to a full-thickness one, especially in young children, who have thinner, more delicate skin.

Vitamin D, an essential factor for proper formation of bone during growth and development, is an important nutrient in children to facilitate intestinal absorption of calcium. Even though vitamin D plays no direct role in burn wound healing, a deficiency of this vitamin has been associated with adverse effects on the skeletal system, as well as on the immune system, which can lead to an increased risk of infection. Vitamin D production may be compromised in burned children, demonstrated by a high incidence of low serum vitamin D levels. Burn-wound scarring and lack of sunlight may limit cutaneous vitamin D biosynthesis.[85]

Cardiovascular System

The marked reduction in cardiac output immediately following injury is accompanied by an initial increase in systemic vascular resistance. As fluid is lost into the interstitial spaces, a further reduction in cardiac output occurs, accompanied by vasodilation. Because the infant maintains cardiac output by increasing heart rate preferentially to stroke volume, extremely elevated heart rates result in a decreased filling time and a further reduction in cardiac output.[86] Adequate resuscitation returns cardiac output to normal levels in approximately 24 to 36 hours. Without fluid replacement, cardiac output continues to decrease and results in organ failure and death.

The inefficient and labile peripheral circulation of the infant further complicates management of the burn shock phase of treatment. The rapid fluid shift to the interstitial space and drying of the eschar result in compromised circulation and a resultant tourniquet effect in the extremities. Blood vessels and nerves become entrapped because the fascia cannot expand to accommodate the massive edema. Release of pressure is required to restore blood flow and preserve nerve function (Fig. 50.7).

A higher risk of chest constriction and impairment of respiratory excursion may result because of the increased pliability of the rib cage, especially in very young children. Excessive fluid volume and burns to the chest or abdomen decrease compliance and can contribute to a serious complication (increased intraabdominal pressure) that may have an underestimated incidence in burned individuals. Although children with increased intraabdominal pressure readings tended to be younger, larger TBSA injuries and full-thickness components were significantly associated with elevated pressures and can result in tissue ischemia.[87] Increased intraabdominal pressure has the potential to impair hemodynamics, renal function, hepatic malperfusion, and pulmonary dysfunction. Despite maintaining cardiac output with fluid replacement, renal function remains impaired in the presence of increased intraabdominal pressure. Intraabdominal pressure, as a stressor, can stimulate the neuroendocrine system and elicit stress reactions directed at neutralizing the initial insult of the burn. Increases in the production and release of catecholamines, glucocorticoids, and beta-endorphins support the clinical finding of profoundly altered cardiovascular, pulmonary, and renal function.[88]

Pulmonary System

The clinical manifestations of burn injury related to the pulmonary system include a variety of complications ranging from inhalation injury,

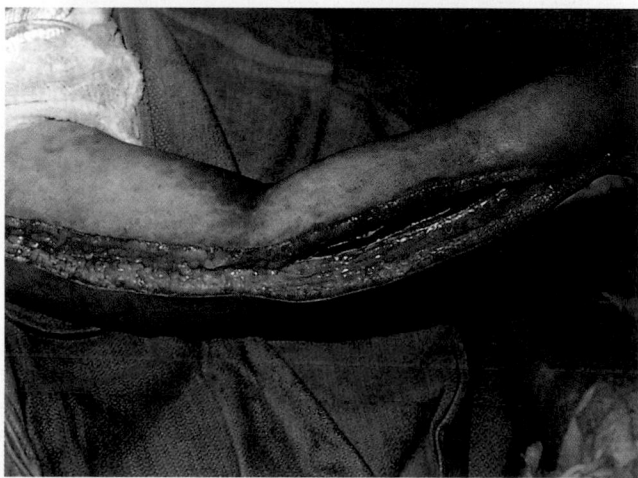

FIGURE 50.7 Escharotomy/Fasciotomy in a Severely Burned Arm.

pulmonary edema, and respiratory failure to aspiration of gastric contents and pneumonia. Inhalation injury has a negative, prolonged effect on pulmonary function that is associated with and remains a major determinant of increased morbidity and mortality.[89]

Anatomic differences in the pediatric airway affect the response to pulmonary complications, as well as therapeutic interventions. The infant airway is positioned anteriorly, making visualization of the cords more difficult. The difficult visualization is further compounded by the relatively large tongue and slanting vocal cords. A small degree of edema results in greatly increased work of breathing in the child (Fig. 50.8). These considerations are particularly important during the resuscitation phase when progressive edema threatens to obstruct the airway. Significant edema results in impairment of respiratory function unless an artificial airway is inserted (Fig. 50.9). Malposition of an endotracheal tube may result in inadvertent extubation, intubation of the bronchi, and atelectasis. Because of the relatively short length of the infant trachea, alterations of the position of the head and neck can affect tube position despite maintenance of the tube position at the teeth.[90-92]

Infants compensate for pulmonary compromise by increasing the respiratory rate. However, because the child possesses fewer type I muscle

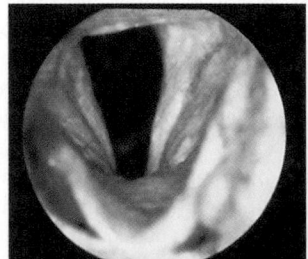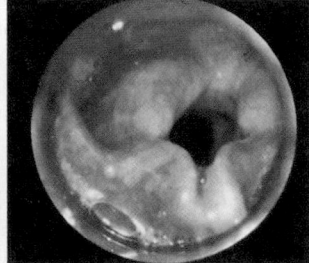

FIGURE 50.8 Airways. Adult airway *(left)*; smaller pediatric airway *(right)*.

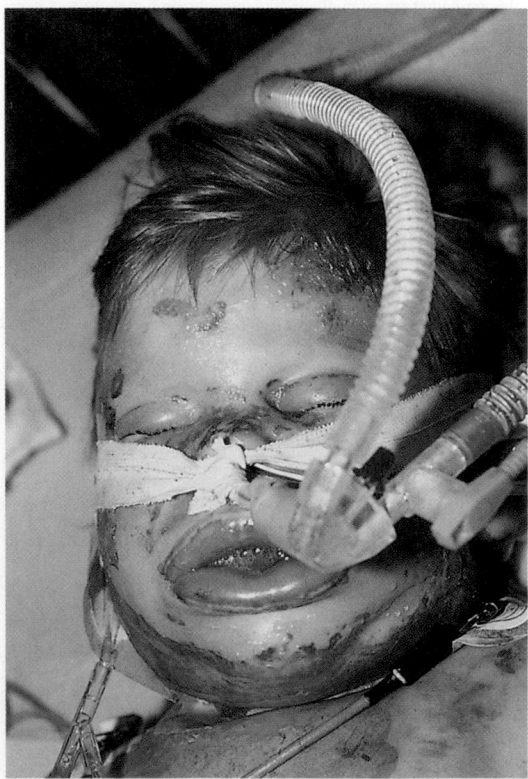

FIGURE 50.9 Severe Facial Edema During Burn Shock.

fibers, fatigue related to the increased work of breathing results in more rapid desaturation than in adults. The soft cartilage of the pediatric airway is prone to collapse in the presence of partial obstruction. Children with burns are at increased risk for these events because of underlying respiratory disease or injury.

Mechanical ventilation of severe inhalation injury is a dynamic and complex task.[93] Therapeutic interventions required for maintenance of pulmonary function have been implicated in postextubation stridor and barotrauma. Evidence suggests that barotrauma from mechanical ventilation may be minimized by protocols based on permissive hypercapnia. In addition, high-frequency oscillatory ventilation (HFOV) in severe pediatric burn patients provides significant, early, and sustained improvement in oxygenation. When HFOV is begun early in burn care, barotrauma is significantly reduced.[94] There also are studies among the pediatric population with inhalation injury that compare high tidal volume (HTV) ventilation versus low tidal volume (LTV) ventilation. Results conclude that those on HTV spent fewer days on the ventilator, had an increase in maximum peak inspiratory pressures, and had less incidence of atelectasis. One should be cautious, however, as HTV ventilation has been associated with a higher incidence of pneumothorax.[89]

The consequences of metabolic and physiologic changes occurring during the acute phase of injury remain apparent during convalescence. Severe burns result in a decrease in pulmonary function from restrictive and obstructive pulmonary disease evidenced by a reduction in pulmonary volumes and maximum voluntary ventilation lasting up to 8 years. At times, chest wall scarring in children caused by burns severely limits thoracic cage excursion.

Burn Shock

The pathophysiologic responses of burn injury result in **hypovolemia** and extracellular sodium depletion in the burn-injured individual. Manifestations for adults are discussed in Chapter 49. Hypotension is a late sign of shock in the child. A complete circulatory assessment, including heart rate and peripheral parameters, is a more reliable measure. Urine output is a reflection of end-organ perfusion and is therefore the most accurate monitor of adequate fluid resuscitation. A urine output of 30 to 50 mL/hr in adults and 1 mL/kg/hr in children weighing less than 30 kg are the suggested endpoints associated with many resuscitation formulas. Fluid is titrated to maintain the output within the parameters.[78]

The fluid of choice for burn shock resuscitation should approximate the fluid lost from the circulating volume, for example, lactated Ringer solution. Children require fluid resuscitation for smaller burns than do adults as a result of their limited physiologic reserves. The child's relatively greater ratio of body surface area to weight results in increased evaporative water losses and proportionately more fluid during resuscitation. Although **colloid replacement** during burn shock resuscitation remains controversial, colloids may be required in the very young child who fails to respond to fluid replacement.[95] A component for **maintenance fluid** *must* be included in the calculation of fluid needs during resuscitation. Maintenance fluids represent the body requirements in the absence of burn injury.

Successful resuscitation depends on establishment of intravenous access. Although this is usually accomplished by peripheral or central venous cannulation, circulatory collapse may preclude timely administration of fluid replacement. Cannulation of veins in the pediatric population is further complicated by small vessels and increased subcutaneous fat. Children are good candidates for **intraosseous cannulation** when traditional venous access techniques fail. Blood, drugs, and fluids are readily absorbed by red marrow that drains into medullary venous channels and thus to the systemic circulation. This technique is most effective in children younger than 5 years, because red marrow is steadily replaced by yellow marrow in the limbs, making infusion more difficult, hence decreasing the infusion rate.[96] Complications are minimal with proper care and removal as soon as other access is available.

Fluid Resuscitation

Fluid resuscitation is generally required for children after thermal injuries in excess of 10% to 15% of the TBSA. Fluid is administered to compensate for fluid and electrolytes extravasating into the interstitial spaces. This replacement restores circulating volume, improves perfusion, and alleviates organ dysfunction associated with impaired circulation.

Various protocols have been proposed as guidelines for fluid administration. It is important to remember that any regimen serves merely as a guideline and will require adjustment based on the individual response of each child. Because the linear relationship between weight and surface area does not exist in children (surface area varies to weight as a two-thirds function), use of adult formulas results in under- or over-resuscitation.[97] A commonly used protocol is a modification of the Parkland formula. Children also tend to require relatively more fluids than adults because they have higher evaporative losses because of their body surface area-to-weight ratio. Evaporative fluid loss can be a significant contributor to hypovolemia in the burned child. This evaporative fluid loss continues until the burn wounds are closed. As in adults, inhalation injury also continues until burn wounds are closed. And as in adults, inhalation injury increases the magnitude of total body surface area injury; therefore children with burn injuries require more fluids.[95]

Research suggests that in the acute phase of the burn injury children receive far more fluid resuscitation than calculated by the modified Parkland formula guidelines. This can lead to a syndrome termed *fluid creep*.[98] Onset maybe caused by higher fluid limits and increased use of opiates resulting in an increased abdominal pressure. The method to control fluid creep includes strict adherence to the modified Parkland formula. In children who have developed increased abdominal pressure, decompressive laparotomy may resolve the increased intraabdominal pressure.[95]

Renal System

Loss of circulating volume into the interstitial spaces results in reduced renal blood flow and decreased glomerular filtration. An important measure of the adequacy of volume replacement is urine excretion. Sufficient volume replacement maintains urine output during resuscitation. Approximately 36 hours after injury, edema fluid begins to mobilize and output increases.

Children younger than 2 years of age lack the ability to concentrate urine because of the immaturity of the renal system and are, therefore, at increased risk for dehydration. In addition, the child has a relatively larger TBSA in relation to weight than the adult. Combined with limited physiologic reserves, increased fluid requirements are necessary for children during burn shock resuscitation and to compensate for evaporative water losses.[97]

Evidence of pigment in the urine results from the hemolysis of red blood cells. This is especially common after extensive electrical injuries and destroyed muscle from deep thermal injury. The release of myoglobin may occlude the kidney tubules and result in renal failure.

Gastrointestinal System

The gastrointestinal (GI) system plays an important role in the pathophysiology of burns. Alterations in blood flow result in decreased perfusion to the GI tract. Ischemia may cause erosion and necrosis of GI tissue. The GI response to a burn injury often includes mucosal atrophy, changes in digestive absorption, and increased intestinal permeability. Depending on the proportion of burn size, atrophy of the GI tract

mucosa can occur immediately after injury. The atrophy results in gut barrier dysfunction leading to increased bacterial translocation and ultimately sepsis.[99]

Paralytic ileus occurs often after major burn injuries. Although digestion ceases in the stomach and the large bowel, the small intestine maintains motility and absorptive capacity. Intestinal motility returns as fluid losses are replaced unless irreversible necrosis of the bowel has occurred as a result of insufficient perfusion.

Immune Function

Burn trauma—induced immunosuppression results in increased susceptibility to infection and sepsis. Although the exact mechanisms responsible for this immunosuppression remain obscure, it is clear that complex interactions of the hypermetabolic response, nutritional support, bacterial translocation, and defects in both innate and acquired immune function are involved (Fig. 50.10). In addition, young children are at increased risk for microbial invasion caused by an immature immune system and limited antibody production.

Deitch reported that wound- or gut-derived endotoxemia may be one of the mediators of the hypermetabolic response observed after thermal injury, and this finding remains undisputed.[100] When bacteria translocate from the gut or from the burn wound, endotoxin may affect immunologic response as inflammatory mediators are released. A further complication in the activation of inflammatory mediators is the release of toxic metabolites, such as oxygen free radicals.[101]

Circulating immunoglobulins may be affected by several factors, including age and the severity of injury.[102] Therapeutic interventions

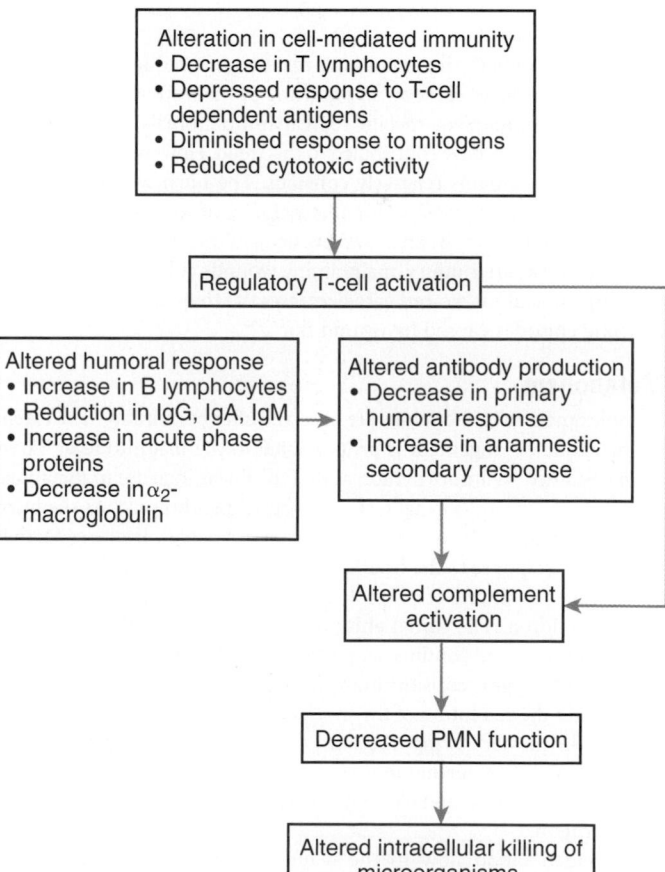

FIGURE 50.10 Altered Immune Function After Thermal Injury. Cell-mediated immunity, antibody production, humoral response. *PMN*, Polymorphonuclear leukocyte.

such as multiple transfusions, surgical procedures, and antibiotic and anesthetic administration also introduce elements that confound the evaluation of immunosuppressive effects. The immune system is activated systemically after a large burn injury with extensive tissue necrosis and may become ineffective or even self-destructive. Infections in burns may result in the loss of some components of innate immune function.[103]

An additional aspect of the immunopathologic consequence of a burn is the role of immunomodulatory cytokines that are suggested to regulate innate regulatory lymphocytes. The systemic inflammatory response increases proinflammatory cytokine production by the peripheral blood mononuclear cells.[104] In children with moderate to severe burn injury, cytokines have been found to increase inflammation by enhancing catabolism and hypermetabolism. In this immunomodulatory process, the proinflammatory function of cytokines enhances protection from sepsis, and the antiinflammatory function supports anabolism (i.e., tissue repair).[105]

Infection

Whereas shock and pulmonary compromise present the most immediate threat after burn trauma, local and systemic infections become the primary complication during healing. The burn wound initially is relatively free of pathogens; however, dead, avascular tissue and wound exudate provide a fertile environment for bacterial growth. Colonization of the wound is apparent by the fifth postburn day. Gram-positive microorganisms are usually recovered from cultures first, followed by opportunistic gram-negative bacteria. The impaired vascular supply to burned tissue enhances the proliferation of pathogenic microorganisms. Bacterial invasion results in thrombosis and a further impairment of circulation sufficient to convert a partial-thickness injury to a full-thickness wound.

Improvements in treatment have resulted in a reduction in wound infection. Aggressive excision and grafting of the wounds, the development of microorganism-specific topical antimicrobials, and improved nutritional support have contributed to this trend. However, the incidence of septicemia remains relatively constant. The burn wound serves as the site of primary invasion for the majority of instances of local or generalized infection. Because the burned child is immunosuppressed for many weeks after injury, maintaining wounds at low contamination levels by meticulous wound care decreases the frequency and duration of septic episodes caused by wound flora.[106]

Metabolism

Complex metabolic alterations are observed after burn injury. The extent of metabolic derangement is proportional to the magnitude of TBSA burn sustained. Wilmore demonstrated the linear increase in metabolic rate up to $2\frac{1}{2}$ times normal resting energy expenditure.[107] As the burn injury approaches 50% TBSA, a plateau is reached, limiting further physiologic response to the trauma or other challenges such as infection.

A biphasic pattern of physiologic response is evident in thermally injured children. The initial ebb phase occurs during the immediate postburn period and continues for 3 to 5 days. This phase is characterized by reduced oxygen consumption, impaired circulation, and cellular shock. After the resolution of the shock and the restoration of circulating volume, the metabolic response shifts to a catabolic (flow) phase (Table 50.8). A state of hypermetabolism ensues, characterized by increased oxygen consumption and elevation of catecholamines, glucocorticoids, and glucagon.

Increased blood flow to the wound supplies additional glucose necessary for tissue repair. Insulin levels are usually normal or even elevated but are inappropriately low in relation to glucagon. Catecholamines and glucocorticoids act as antagonists to insulin. This effect combined with a tissue resistance to insulin stimulates glycogenolysis

TABLE 50.8 METABOLIC ALTERATIONS FOLLOWING INJURY

RESPONSE	DOMINANT FACTORS	CLINICAL FINDINGS
Ebb Response	Loss of plasma volume Shock Low plasma insulin levels	Hyperglycemia Decreased oxygen consumption Depressed resting energy expenditure Decreased blood pressure Cardiac output below normal Decreased body temperature
Flow Response		
Acute phase	Elevated catecholamines Elevated glucagons Elevated glucocorticoids Normal or elevated insulin levels High glucagon/insulin ratio	Catabolic Hyperglycemia Increased respiratory rate Increased oxygen consumption Increased body temperature Redistribution of polyvalent cations such as zinc and iron Mobilization of metabolic reserves Increased urinary excretion of nitrogen, sulfur, magnesium, phosphorus, potassium Accelerated gluconeogenesis
Adaptive phase	Stress hormone response subsiding	Anabolic Normoglycemia Energy turnover diminished Convalescence

From Gottschlich M, Alexander JW, Bower RH. In Rombeau JL, Caldwell MD, editors: *Enteral and tube feeding*, Philadelphia, 1990, Saunders.

and gluconeogenesis, thus increasing glucose flow from the liver.[108] In the child, glycogen stores for meeting the increased energy demands of the burn are limited. The initiation of protein and lipid catabolism for glycogenesis is accelerated. This prolonged metabolic dysfunction may lead to loss of lean body mass and increased morbidity.[109]

Metabolic rates slowly return to normal with wound closure. However, a reactivation of the hypermetabolic response may occur with sepsis or organ failure.

Hypermetabolism

The hypermetabolic response after burn injury profoundly alters the production and use of nutrients. As a consequence of these phenomena, caloric requirements increase dramatically. Advances in burn care have allowed the performance of indirect calorimetry and assessment of metabolic rate at the bedside. Nutritional support must have an increased metabolic rate factored in (increased by 10% to 20%) because of fluctuations in energy use associated with activity. Current recommendations suggest 1.5 to 2 g protein/kg/day for adults and up to 2.5 to 4 g protein/kg/day for children.[110]

In addition to age, body composition has been found to significantly affect the postburn course. Preexisting obesity in burned children has been associated with longer hospital stay and associated morbidity.[111] However, the heightened nutrient requirements of the burned child preclude a reduction in nutritional support during the acute phase of recovery. Aggressive nutritional therapy is critical to the recovery of these children, and programs designed to achieve ideal body weight should not be instituted until wound healing is achieved.

Metabolism of many micronutrients is greatly affected by burn injury. Micronutrient supplementation is necessary because vitamin and mineral requirements increase with the severity of the burn related to heightened protein synthesis, enhanced caloric expenditure, and increased micronutrient losses. Preburn status also indicates individual vitamin and mineral needs.[85] Hypermetabolism results in a rapid turnover in vitamins and trace minerals important in the wound healing and immune response. A deficiency of specific nutrients interferes with carbohydrate and nucleic acid metabolism, collagen formation, and immune function.

The thermoregulatory response after burn injury results in an elevation in core body temperature. Burned individuals strive for temperatures of about 38°C (100.4°F). Depressed or "normal" temperature may be indicative of overwhelming sepsis, or an exhausted physiologic capability to maintain temperature, and should be viewed as an ominous sign. Routine methods of heat conservation after a major burn injury are inadequate because of excessive heat loss through convection and evaporation.[111] Therapeutic intervention, such as operative procedures and dressing changes, and transport present situations requiring increased diligence to prevent inadvertent cooling. Infants are at increased risk for a precipitous drop in core body temperature caused by an inability to regulate heat loss by shivering. Heat is also lost because of evaporation of water from damaged skin surfaces. Infants and children are especially vulnerable because of the large surface area relative to metabolically active tissue.[98]

Nutritional Support

The heightened metabolic demands after burn injury combined with a poor appetite often necessitate supplementation of oral intake. Children with burns in excess of 20% of TBSA often require supplementation with tube feeding. Feeding does not need to be delayed pending resolution of paralytic ileus and the resumption of bowel sounds because the small bowel maintains motility and absorptive capability. A small-bore feeding tube placed in the duodenum provides a safe route for the delivery of essential nutrients. Parenteral hyperalimentation is reserved for those children who are unable to tolerate enteral support because of attendant risks of catheter sepsis and loss of intestinal integrity. Early enteral supplementation preserves gut mucosal integrity and improves intestinal blood flow, as well as motility.[112] Early initiation of enteral supplementation along with aggressive management of complications permits successful enteral alimentation in most burned children, which plays a key role in blunting the metabolic response to burn injury but is insufficient by itself. Severe burn injury causes exaggerated muscle protein catabolism, contributing to weakness and delayed healing. Several pharmacologic therapies have been identified that counteract this catabolic state, which include nonspecific beta blockade with propranolol, oxandrolone (anabolic steroid analog of testosterone), and recombinant human growth hormone (rhGH). These pharmacologic therapies reverse muscle-protein catabolism and reduce muscle resting energy expenditure.[109] Outpatient follow-up should include regular weighing of the child and nutritional assessment to identify children at risk for further weight loss.

Wound Management

The goals of wound management include prevention of infection, removal of devitalized tissue, and closure of the wound (see *What's New?* Advances in Burn Wound Care). Burns that are clearly deep dermal or full-thickness injuries are surgically excised as soon as the child is hemodynamically stable after resuscitation. Early excision reduces the incidence of wound

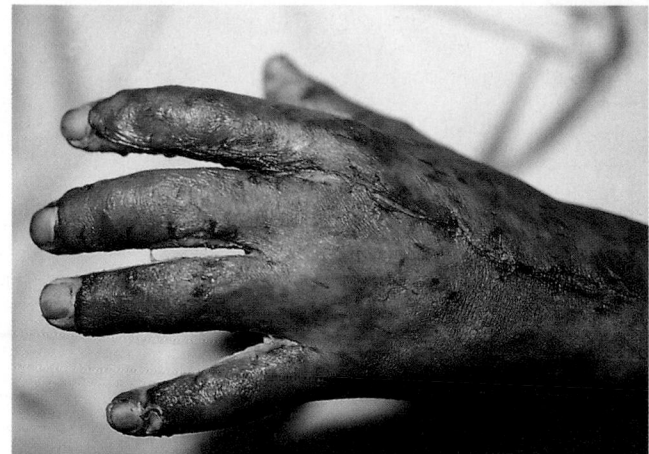

FIGURE 50.11 Split-Thickness Sheet Graft.

WHAT'S NEW?

Advances in Burn Wound Care

Skin substitutes for treating extensive burns can provide a temporary or permanent covering to facilitate repair and regeneration, restoring the functional properties of the skin. Two different types exist: synthetic skin substitutes (those made up of acellular materials) and natural, or tissue-engineered, substitutes (made of cultured epidermal cells, those with only dermal components, and those containing both epidermal and dermal components). Tissue-engineered skin substitute contains epidermal and dermal components that lie in an extracellular matrix (ECM) that helps to bind and support the cells. Advances in tissue-engineered skin substitutes have led to advantages such as decreased donor sites and decreased length of hospital stay. A large number of these cells facilitate rapid re-formation of the skin barrier in both regeneration and functionality, thus decreasing morbidity and mortality. Although commercial products are readily available, most share problems of extremely high cost, subnormal skin microstructure, and inconsistent engraftment, particularly in full-thickness burns. Use of the individual's own skin still provides the best graft.

Data from Chua AW et al: *Burns Trauma* 4:3, 2016; Varkey M, Ding J, Tredget EE: *J Funct Biomater.* 6(3):547-563, 2015.

infection and systemic sepsis.[113-115] Coverage of the excised wound is necessary to achieve wound closure. The choice of a coverage technique depends on the availability of donor skin.

Split-thickness sheet grafts are selected for areas of maximal functional and cosmetic results (Fig. 50.11). Children with very large burn injuries often do not have sufficient unburned skin available to facilitate use of the sheet graft. In these cases the surgeon uses a meshing technique to expand the available skin and increase the size of the graft. The pattern created heals by migration of epithelium from the meshed edges. Scar formation is increased, and the mesh pattern remains clearly visible (Fig. 50.12). The color, texture, vascularity, thickness, and hair-bearing nature of the skin vary from one area to another. Site selection and depth of donor sites require careful consideration. Skin grafts for the face should be taken, if possible, from above the nipple line for best color match and "blush" ability.[114]

Scar Maturation

In normal epidermal healing, minimal disruption in skin color, texture, and thickness occurs. However, burn wounds that extend into the dermis

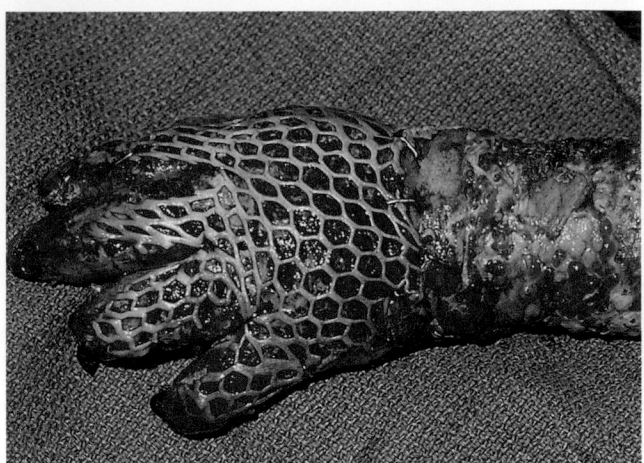

FIGURE 50.12 Meshed Autograft.

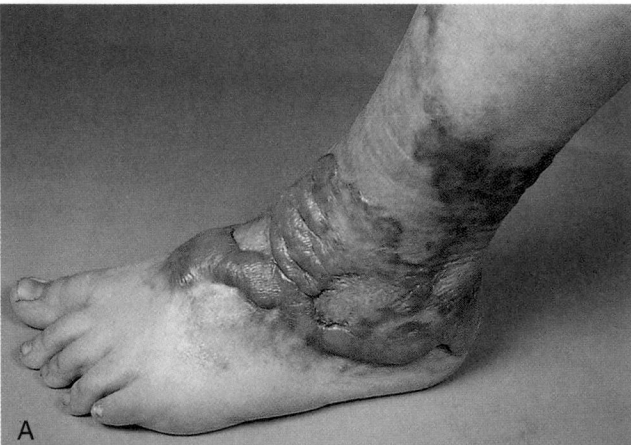

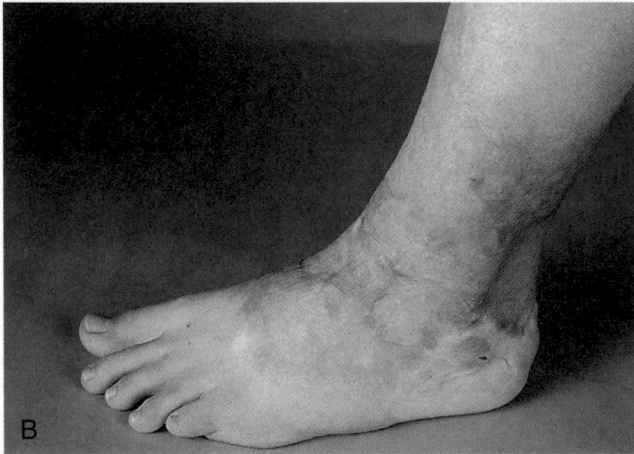

FIGURE 50.13 Scar Maturation. **A,** Immature hypertrophic scar. **B,** Flat, mature scar after pressure therapy.

are repaired through scar formation and may result in an overgrowth of dermal constituents (Fig. 50.13, *A*). Accelerated collagen synthesis most likely begins with high levels of activity in granulation tissue. The hypertrophic scar consists of hypercellular and disorganized connective tissue that is erythematous, raised, and pruritic. Normal dermis contains thick fibers and fiber bundles running parallel to the surface. In the hypertrophic scar, the collagen is arranged in whorls and nodules that account for its inelasticity and increased turgor.[115] As the hypertrophic

scar matures, collagen begins to orient in a more parallel fashion, and vascularity decreases (see Fig. 50.13, *B*). Collagen synthesis is very active soon after wound closure, and alteration of the scar can be accomplished before strong cross-linking of the collagen is established.

Although duration of wound healing varies among individuals, the length of time required to achieve wound closure is the most reliable predictor of hypertrophic scarring. Deeper burns demonstrate increased scarring caused by the formation of granulation tissue and prolonged healing time. Generally, darker-pigmented races are more susceptible to hypertrophic scarring.[115,116] Although age has not been found to be a predictor of hypertrophic scar formation, younger individuals are more susceptible to trauma and have greater skin tension and an accelerated rate of collagen synthesis. Increased tension with resultant trauma stimulates inflammation, which in turn results in the formation of additional collagen.

Scar tissue is metabolically active and highly vascular. Collagen is deposited in random patterns, and contraction of the scar can result in disabling deformities. The scar is active as long as it is raised, red, and firm. Scar maturation requires 1 to 2 years and depends on individual differences and compliance with the rehabilitation program. The mature scar is characterized by increased suppleness, flattening, and pigmented color.

Scar tissue does not grow and expand like normal tissue. Although massage therapy offers some benefit in stretching, functional limitation may develop as the child grows. This is particularly evident over joints. Reconstructive surgery is often necessary to restore anatomic integrity and to promote independent function.

Itching may occur at any time during burn wound healing. As a complication, healed skin may be scratched away in an effort to obtain relief. The combination of H_1 and H_2 antagonists may be used to control itching.[117]

Comfort Management

Pain management presents a significant challenge in the pediatric population. Burns can be extremely painful. In addition to procedural pain, there is a component of background pain that is present without activity. Pain perception also is affected by the degree of emotional overlay, anxiety, or affective experience. Anxiety and poor pain management can contribute to a delay in wound healing.[118] Both pharmacologic and nonpharmacologic interventions are important in treating patients with burns. The measurement of pain is particularly challenging in young infants, who lack the language skills to express pain. A variety of tools, from physiologic monitors to behavioral analyses and analog scales, have been developed to measure pediatric pain. The quality of pain control in burn centers has improved along with the ability to assess pain in the pediatric population.

Recovery from Burn Injury

Rehabilitation becomes the major focus of care once wound coverage has been achieved and continues until all reconstructive procedures have been completed. This phase may extend over many years in the pediatric population. Children require specialized management to ensure optimal functional and cosmetic results. Scar and contracture management is necessary for prolonged periods because of changes in body composition as the child grows and matures. Very young children present unique challenges because the small body size can be difficult to fit with pressure garments and splints, growth is rapid, and cooperation with the rehabilitation program is limited.

Infant skin is thinner, and the epidermis is more loosely connected to the dermis. This increases the risk of blistering, chafing, and rash formation. The infant also produces less sebum and sweat, which further exacerbates the propensity to skin irritation. Because scar tissue contains no sweat glands, these characteristics of the skin in growing children compound the difficulty in maintaining pressure on maturing scars while cooling the body.

Positioning and splinting to prevent contracture formation, as well as rehabilitative aspects of therapy, are instituted on admission and continue throughout the hospitalization. Physical therapy and occupational therapy provide exercise to maintain range of motion and function. Psychosocial support is very important for the child and the family. The information provided should be consistent and honest to allow clarification of concerns. In addition to the functional aspects of rehabilitation, attention must be directed to psychosocial needs and community reintegration.

A method to facilitate the transition from the hospital to the community is a school reentry program offered by many burn centers. These programs provide education for teachers and peers about the injury, appearance, and abilities of the returning child.

SUMMARY REVIEW

Shock and Multiple Organ Dysfunction Syndrome

1. Shock in children is present when there are signs of poor systemic perfusion, regardless of blood pressure.
2. Hypovolemic shock is the most common type of shock in children and most frequently results from dehydration and trauma. Hypovolemic shock also may result from expansion of the vascular space, producing inadequate intravascular volume relative to the vascular space.
3. Hypotension is a sign of severe (preterminal), decompensated shock, referred to as *hypotensive shock.*
4. Clinical manifestations of hypovolemic shock include inadequate systemic perfusion associated with intravascular fluid loss. Adrenergic compensatory mechanisms can produce tachycardia, redistribution of blood flow, peripheral vasoconstriction, cool extremities, delayed capillary refill, and oliguria.
5. Neurogenic shock is caused by a loss of vasomotor tone after severe injury to the spinal cord.
6. Clinical manifestations of neurogenic shock include warm skin, hypotension with a low diastolic blood pressure, and poor systemic perfusion. Tachycardia is not present.
7. Cardiogenic shock, with decreased cardiac output, is observed most commonly after cardiovascular surgery or with inflammatory diseases of the heart, such as cardiomyopathy and myocarditis. It is also found in children with obstructive congenital heart disease and those with drug toxicity or severe electrolyte or acid-base imbalances.
8. Clinical manifestations of cardiogenic shock include inadequate systemic perfusion despite adequate intravascular volume. Cardiac output is typically low. Adrenergic compensatory mechanisms, including peripheral vasoconstriction and decreased urine volume, are similar to those found in hypovolemic shock.
9. Once septic shock is present, immediate treatment is urgently needed. Therapy in the first hour includes aggressive fluid resuscitation (typically 60 to 80 mL/kg administered in the first hour of therapy, and approximately 200 to 240 mL/kg in the first 8 hours of therapy). If the child does not respond to volume administration alone, vasoactive support must be initiated within the first hour of treatment. Antibiotics also must be administered within the first hour. Goals of therapy are to rapidly normalize the heart rate and blood pressure for age and to normalize capillary refill to less than 2 seconds. The child's shock index (heart rate/systolic blood pressure) should fall during the first hour of management if therapy is effective. Fluid and vasoactive therapy should support high cardiac output and oxygen delivery, maintaining the $S\overline{v}O_2$ at approximately 70%.
10. Sepsis is a systemic response to infection. It is present when manifestations of SIRS are observed. SIRS is present when the child demonstrates two or more of the following as an acute change from baseline values: altered temperature, altered heart rate, altered respiratory rate, and alteration in the WBC count. The newborn often develops hypothermia rather than fever as a sign of infection and may develop bradycardia instead of tachycardia.
11. Severe sepsis is present when there is evidence of SIRS and signs of organ dysfunction, hypoperfusion, or hypotension.
12. The development of septic shock is heralded when the child with severe sepsis develops signs of cardiovascular dysfunction. The child may become hypotensive despite adequate fluid resuscitation or require vasopressors to maintain blood pressure.
13. Reperfusion and inflammatory injury stimulate free oxygen radicals that can damage cell membranes, denature proteins, and disrupt chromosomes. This process likely affects endothelial cells and the microvasculature, causing MODS.
14. Lactic acidosis (i.e., rise in serum lactate) may be the most sensitive indicator of inadequate systemic perfusion in children; effective shock therapy should eliminate lactic acidosis.
15. The general goals of treatment for shock are maximization of oxygen delivery and minimization of oxygen demand. This requires support of airway, oxygenation, and ventilation. Support of cardiovascular function requires support of appropriate heart rate and rhythm, adequate intravascular volume, good myocardial function, and appropriate vascular resistance and distribution of blood flow. The child should be kept warm, but fever must be treated promptly.
16. The signs of shock should lessen or disappear if management of shock is effective. The warmth of the child's extremities, briskness of capillary refill, quality of peripheral pulses, level of consciousness and responsiveness, urine volume, oxygenation, ventilation, and acid-base status should improve throughout shock therapy.

Burns

1. Burns in children are often the result of inadequate supervision, curiosity, inability to escape the burning agent, or nonaccidental trauma.
2. Scald injuries are commonly seen in young children and result from exposure to hot water, grease, or other hot liquids, whereas flame burns are more prevalent among older children.
3. A child's skin is thinner and thus more susceptible to injury than adult skin. The kitchen and bathroom are common sites of burn injury.
4. Approximately 8% to 12% of all forms of child abuse cases in the United States result from burn injury.
5. Flame burns involving flammable liquids, most notably gasoline, are more common in older children. Risk-taking behaviors in young males can lead to electrical burns. Children may be exposed to chemical injury by swallowing caustic agents at home.
6. Use of the standard Rule of Nines results in inaccurate calculation of the percentage of TBSA in children. A modified Rule of Nines deducts 1% from the head and adds 0.5% to each leg for each year of life after 2 years of age.

SUMMARY REVIEW—cont'd

7. Major burn trauma involves all body systems, and the consequences of injury include shock, infection, hypermetabolism, organ failure, and functional limitations. These effects can be magnified in the pediatric population as a result of physiologic immaturity and age-related variation in treatment modalities.

8. Infection, trauma, or applying ice to the burn area may convert a partial-thickness injury to a full-thickness one, especially in young children, who have thinner, more delicate skin.

9. Marked reduction in cardiac output occurs immediately after injury and is accompanied by an initial increase in systemic vascular resistance. The inefficient and labile peripheral circulation of the infant complicates management of the burn shock phase of treatment. A higher risk of chest constriction and impairment of respiratory excursion may result because of the increased pliability of the rib cage, especially in very young children. Younger children are also more susceptible to increased intraabdominal pressure.

10. The leading cause of death in children after burn injury, as in adults, is inhalation injury.

11. Children require fluid resuscitation for smaller burns than does the adult population as a result of limited physiologic reserves. Colloid replacement, although controversial, may be required in the very young child who fails to respond to fluid replacement.

12. Children younger than 2 years lack the ability to concentrate urine because of the immaturity of the renal system and are therefore at increased risk for dehydration. Because children have a relatively larger body surface area in relation to weight than adults, they require proportionately increased fluid during burn shock resuscitation to compensate for evaporative water losses.

13. Some children exhibit immunosuppression for a prolonged period after wound closure.

14. A biphasic pattern of physiologic responses is evident in the burn-injured child. The initial ebb phase occurs during the immediate postburn period and continues for 3 to 5 days. This phase is characterized by reduced oxygen consumption, impaired circulation, and cellular shock. After this phase and the restoration of volume, the metabolic response shifts to a catabolic, or flow, phase. This phase is characterized by hypermetabolism with an increased oxygen consumption and elevation of catecholamines, glucocorticoids, and glucagon.

15. Glycogen stores are limited in children, making it hard for them to meet the increased energy demands of the burn. This prolonged metabolic dysfunction may lead to loss of lean body mass and increased morbidity.

16. Although age was not found to be a predictor of hypertrophic scarring, children have greater skin tension and an accelerated rate of collagen synthesis.

17. Children require specialized management to ensure optimal functional and cosmetic results. Long-term scar and contracture management is necessary because of changes in body composition as the child grows and matures.

KEY TERMS

Bradycardia, 1573
Cardiogenic shock, 1577
Catabolic (flow) phase, 1592
Chemical burn, 1587
Child abuse, 1587
Cold shock, 1582
Colloid, 1583
Colloid replacement, 1590
Compensated shock, 1572
Contact burn, 1588
Crystalloid, 1583
Depth of injury, 1588
Dermal ischemia, 1589
Ebb phase, 1592
Electrical burn, 1587
Eschar, 1589
Evaporative fluid loss, 1591
Flame burn, 1587

Fluid resuscitation, 1591
Hemoconcentration, 1589
Hypermetabolism, 1592
Hypertrophic scar, 1594
Hypotensive shock, 1572
Hypovolemia, 1590
Hypovolemic shock, 1575
Hypoxia, 1572
Intraabdominal pressure, 1589
Intraosseous cannulation, 1590
Ischemia, 1572
Maintenance fluid, 1590
Multiple organ dysfunction syndrome (MODS), 1572
Myoglobin, 1591
Neurogenic shock, 1579
New or progressive MODS (NPMODS), 1572
Obstructive shock, 1582

Rehabilitation, 1594
Reperfusion (reoxygenation) injury, 1582
Scald injury, 1587
Scar formation, 1594
Scar maturation, 1594
Sepsis, 1579
Septic shock, 1581
Severe sepsis, 1581
Shock, 1572
Split-thickness sheet graft, 1593
Systemic inflammatory response syndrome (SIRS), 1581
Tachycardia, 1573
Thermoregulatory response, 1593
"Third spacing" of fluids, 1576
Warm shock, 1582

REFERENCES

1. Haque IU, Zaritsky AL: Analysis of the evidence for the lower limit of systolic and mean arterial blood pressure in children. *Pediatr Crit Care* 8:138–144, 2007.

2. Perkin RM, et al: Shock, cardiac arrest and resuscitation. In Hazinski MF, editor: *Nursing care of the critically ill child*, ed 3, St Louis, 2013, Mosby.

3. Samson RA, et al: *Pediatric advanced life support provider manual*, Dallas, 2016, American Heart Association.

4. Lin JC, et al: New or progressive multiple organ dysfunction syndrome in pediatric severe sepsis: a sepsis phenotype with higher morbidity and mortality. *Pediatr Crit Care Med* 18(1):8–16, 2017.

5. Goldstein B, Giroir B, Randolph A: International Pediatric Sepsis Consensus Conference: definitions for sepsis and organ dysfunction in pediatrics. *Pediatr Crit Care Med* 6:2–8, 2005.

6. Proulx F, et al: The pediatric multiple organ dysfunction syndrome. *Pediatr Crit Care Med* 10:12–22, 2009.

7. Upperman JS, et al: Specific etiologies associated with the multiple organ dysfunction syndrome in children, part 1. *Pediatr Crit Care Med* 18: S50–S57, 2017.

8. Upperman JS, et al: Specific etiologies associated with the multiple organ dysfunction syndrome in children, part 2. *Pediatr Crit Care Med* 18: S58–S66, 2017.

9. Watson RS, et al: Epidemiology and outcomes of pediatric multiple organ dysfunction syndrome. *Pediatr Crit Care Med* 18:S4–S16, 2017.

10. Typpo KV, Lacroix JR: Monitoring severity of multiple organ dysfunction syndrome: new and progressive multiple organ dysfunction syndrome, scoring systems. *Pediatr Crit Care Med* 18: S17–S23, 2017.

11. Hazinski MF: Children are different. In Hazinski MF, editor: *Nursing care of the critically ill child*, ed 3, St Louis, 2013, Mosby.

12. Otieno H, et al: Are bedside features of shock reproducible between different observers? *Arch Dis Child* 89(10):977–979, 2004.

13. Samson RA, et al: Recognition of arrhythmias. In Samson RA, et al, editors: *Pediatric advanced life support provider manual*, Dallas, 2016, American Heart Association.

14. Samson RA, et al: Management of arrhythmias. In Samson RA, et al, editors: *Pediatric advanced life support provider manual*, Dallas, 2016, American Heart Association.

15. Rudolph AM: *Congenital diseases of the heart*, Chicago, 1974, Year Book Medical.

16. Wynn JL, et al: Time for a neonatal-specific consensus definition for sepsis. *Pediatr Crit Care Med* 15:523–528, 2014.

17. Pike NA, Klee LA, Zemetra BA: Mechanical support of cardiopulmonary function: extracorporeal membrane oxygenation, ventricular assist devices, and the intraaortic balloon pump. In Hazinski MF, editor: *Nursing care of the critically ill child*, ed 3, Saint Louis, 2013, Mosby.

18. Roberts KE: Fluid, electrolyte and endocrine problems. In Hazinski MF, editor: *Nursing care of the critically ill child*, ed 3, St Louis, 2013, Mosby.

19. Doctor A, et al: Pediatric multiple organ dysfunction syndrome: promising therapies. *Pediatr Crit Care Med* 18:S67–S82, 2017.

20. Nayak PP, et al: Early change in blood glucose concentration is an indicator of mortality in critically ill children. *Intensive Care Med* 39(1): 123–128, 2012.

21. Bhutia TD, Lodha R, Kabra SK: Abnormalities in glucose homeostasis in critically ill children. *Pediatr Crit Care Med* 14(1):e16–e25, 2013.

22. Samson RA, et al: Recognition of shock. In Samson RA, et al, editors: *Pediatric advanced life support provider manual*, Dallas, 2016, American Heart Association.

23. American College of Surgeons: *Advanced trauma life support student manual*, ed 9, Chicago, 2012, Author.

24. Armstrong A, Unni P, Pietsch JB: Pediatric trauma. In Hazinski MF, editor: *Nursing care of the critically ill child*, ed 3, St Louis, 2013, Mosby.

25. Ulate KP, et al: An elevated low cardiac output syndrome score is associated with morbidity in infants after congenital heart surgery. *Pediatr Crit Care Med* 18:26–33, 2017.

26. Hartman ME, et al: Trends in the epidemiology of pediatric severe sepsis. *Pediatr Crit Care Med* 14:686–693, 2013.

27. Ruth A, et al: Pediatric severe sepsis: current trends and outcomes from the pediatric health information systems database. *Pediatr Crit Care Med* 15:828–838, 2014.

28. Weiss SL, et al: Global epidemiology of pediatric severe sepsis: the sepsis prevalence outcomes, and therapies study. *Am J Resp Crit Care Med* 191(10): 1147–1157, 2015.

29. Trimarchi T: Fundamentals of patient safety and quality improvement. In Hazinski MF, editor: *Nursing care of the critically ill child*, ed 3, St Louis, 2013, Mosby.

30. Wheeler DS, et al: Sepsis in the pediatric cardiac intensive care unit. *World J Pediatr Congenit Heart Surg* 2:393–399, 2011.

31. Nadel S: Severe pediatric sepsis. *Expert Rev Anti Infect Ther* 10(2):111–114, 2012.

32. Wong HR: Genetics and genomics in pediatric septic shock. *Crit Care Med* 40:2012, 1618-1626.

33. Brandtzaeg P, van Deuren M: Classification and pathogenesis of meningococcal infections. *Methods Molec Biol* 799:21–35, 2012.

34. Aneja RK, Carcillo JA: Differences between adult and pediatric septic shock. *Minerva Anesthesiol* 77:986–992, 2011.

35. Haley M, et al: Activated protein C in sepsis: emerging insights regarding its mechanism of action and clinical effectiveness. *Curr Opin Infect Dis* 17(3):205–211, 2004.

36. Bernard GR, et al: Efficacy and safety of recombinant human activated protein C for severe sepsis. *N Engl J Med* 344(10):699–709, 2001.

37. Martí-Carvajal AJ, et al: Human recombinant protein C for severe sepsis and septic shock in adult and paediatric patients. *Cochrane Database Syst Rev* (12):CD004388, 2012.

38. Carcillo JA, et al: A systemic inflammation mortality risk assessment contingency table for severe sepsis. *Pediatr Crit Care Med* 18:143–150, 2017.

39. Batzofin BM, Sprung CL, Weiss YG: The use of steroids in the treatment of severe sepsis and septic shock. *Best Pract Res Clin Endocrinol Metab* 25(5):735–743, 2011.

40. Hebbar KB, Petrillo T, Fortenberry JD: Adrenal insufficiency and response to corticosteroids in hypotensive critically ill children with cancer. *J Crit Care* 27(5):480–487, 2012.

41. Karaguzel G, et al: The effects of three specific conditions related to the critical care on adrenal function in children. *Intensive Care Med* 38(10): 1689–1696, 2012.

42. Davis AL, et al: American College of Critical Care Medicine clinical practice parameters for hemodynamic support of pediatric and neonatal septic shock. *Crit Care Med* 45(6):1061–1093, 2017.

43. Singer M, et al: The third international consensus definitions for sepsis and septic shock (sepsis-3). *JAMA* 315:801–810, 2016.

44. Kissoon N, Orr RA, Carcillo JA: Updated American College of Critical Care Medicine-Pediatric advanced life support guidelines for management of pediatric and neonatal septic shock: relevance to the emergency care clinician. *Pediatr Emerg Care* 26(11):867–869, 2010.

45. Saini SS, Kumar P, Kumar RM: Hemodynamic changes in preterm neonates with septic shock: a prospective observational study. *Pediatr Crit Care Med* 15:443–450, 2014.

46. Yasaka Y, Khemani RG, Markovitz BP: Is shock index associated with outcome in children with sepsis/septic shock? *Pediatr Crit Care Med* 14: e372–e379, 2013.

47. Rousseaux J, et al: Prognostic value of shock index in children with septic shock. *Pediatr Emerg Care* 29:1055–1059, 2013.

48. Banz Y, Rieben R: Role of complement and perspectives for intervention in ischemia-reperfusion damage. *Ann Med* 44:205–217, 2012.

49. Franciscketti I, et al: Leukocytes and the inflammatory response in ischemia-reperfusion injury. *Rev Bras Cir Cardiovasc* 25(4):575–584, 2010.

50. Lacroix J, Cotting J, for the Pediatric Acute Lung Injury and Sepsis Investigators (PALISI) Network: Severity of illness and organ dysfunction scoring in children. *Pediatr Crit Care Med* 6(Suppl 3):S126–S134, 2005.

51. Bestati N, et al: Differences in organ dysfunctions between neonates and older children: a prospective, observational, multicenter study. *Crit Care* 14:R202, 2010.

52. Leteurtre S, et al: Daily estimation of the severity of multiple organ dysfunction syndrome in critically ill children. *CMAJ* 182(11):1181–1187, 2010.

53. Hutton P, et al: An assessment of the Dinamap 845. *Anesthesiology* 39:261, 1984.

54. Davis JW, et al: Are automated blood pressure measurements accurate in trauma patients? *J Trauma* 55(5):860–863, 2003.

55. Vlasselaers D, et al: Intensive insulin therapy for patients in paediatric intensive care: a prospective, randomised controlled study. *Lancet* 373:547–556, 2009.

56. Agus MSD, et al: Tight glycemic control in critically ill children. *N Engl J Med* 376:729–741, 2017.

57. Samson RA, et al: Management of shock. In Samson RA, et al, editors: *Pediatric advanced life support provider manual*, Dallas, 2016, American Heart Association.

58. Lacroix J, et al: Transfusion strategies for patients in pediatric intensive care units. *N Engl J Med* 356:2007, 1609-1619.

59. Lacroix J, Demaret P, Tucci M: Red blood cell transfusion: decision making in pediatric intensive care units. *Semin Perinatol* 36:225–231, 2012.

60. Burke ML, Salani D: Hematologic and oncologic emergencies requiring critical care. In Hazinski MF, editor: *Nursing care of the critically ill child*, ed 3, St Louis, 2013, Mosby.

61. Carcillo JA, Davis AL, Zaritsky A: Role of early fluid resuscitation in pediatric septic shock. *JAMA* 266(9):1242–1245, 1991.

62. de Oliveira CE, et al: ACCM/PALS haemodynamic support guidelines for paediatric septic shock: an outcomes comparison with and without monitoring central venous oxygen saturation. *Intensive Care Med* 34:1065–1075, 2008.

63. de Caen AR, et al: Part 12: pediatric advanced life support; 2015 American Heart Association guidelines update for cardiopulmonary resuscitation and emergency cardiovascular care. *Circulation* 132(18 Suppl 2):S526–S542, 2015.

64. Ventura AM, et al: Double-blind prospective randomized controlled trial of dopamine versus epinephrine as first-line vasoactive drugs in pediatric septic shock. *Crit Care Med* 43: 2292–2302, 2015.

65. Tømte O, et al: Strong and weak aspects of an established post-resuscitation treatment protocol—a five-year observational study. *Resuscitation* 82:1186–1193, 2011.

66. Samson RA, et al: Post-cardiac arrest care. In Samson RA, et al, editors: *Pediatric advanced life support provider manual*, Dallas, 2016, American Heart Association.

67. Bembea MM, et al: Temperature patterns in the early postresuscitation period after pediatric in-hospital arrest. *Pediatr Crit Care Med* 11(6): 723–730, 2010.

68. Pietrini D, et al: Neuroprotection and hypothermia in infants and children. *Curr Drug Targets* 13(7):925–935, 2012.

69. Polderman KH: Mechanisms of action, physiological effects, and complications of hypothermia. *Crit Care Med* 37(Suppl):S186–S202, 2009.

70. Shankaran S, et al: Whole body hypothermia for neonates with hypoxic-ischemic encephalopathy. *N Engl J Med* 353:1574–1584, 2005.

71. Hypothermia After Cardiac Arrest Study Group: Mild therapeutic hypothermia to improve the neurologic outcome after cardiac arrest. *N Engl J Med* 346(8):549–556, 2002.

72. Nielsen N, et al: Targeted temperature management at 33°C versus 36°C after cardiac arrest. *N Engl J Med* 369:2197–2206, 2013.

73. Moler FW, et al: Therapeutic hypothermia after out-of-hospital cardiac arrest in children. *N Engl J Med* 372(20):908–2015, 1898.

74. Moler FW, et al: Therapeutic hypothermia after in-hospital cardiac arrest in children. *N Engl J Med* 376(4):318–329, 2017.

75. Typpo KV, et al: Monitoring severity of multiple organ dysfunction syndrome: new technologies. *Pediatr Crit Care Med* 18:S24–S31, 2017.

76. Committee on Trauma: *Resource for optimal care of the injured patient [pamphlet]*, Chicago IL, 2014, American College of Surgeons.

77. Safe Kids Worldwide (SKW): *Burn and scalds safety, 2015*. Available at: http://www.safekids.org/fact-sheet/burns-and-fire-safety-fact-sheet-2015-pdf.

78. American Burn Association: *Pediatric burn injuries*. Advanced burn life support provider manual *2016 update*, Chicago IL, 2016, Author.

79. Fujii TK, Schwartz SJ, Phillips BJ: Inhalation injury. In Phillips BJ, editor: *Pediatric burns*, Amherst, 2012, Cambria.

80. Wibbenmeyer L, et al: Factors related to child maltreatment in children presenting with burn injuries. *J Burn Care Rehabil* 35(5):374–381, 2014.

81. Paul AR, Adamo MA: Non-accidental trauma in pediatric patients: a review of epidemiology, pathophysiology, diagnosis and treatment. *Transl Pediatr* 3(3):195–207, 2014.

82. Knox BL, Starling SP: *Medical evaluation of burn injuries, National Center for Prosecution of Child Abuse Update 22 (Number 2&3)*, 2009. Available at: www.ndaa.org/pdf/update_22_2and3.pdf.

83. Greenhalgh DG: Burn-related child abuse. In Phillips BJ, editor: *Pediatric burns*, Amherst, 2012, Cambria.

84. Sheridan RL, Tompkins RG: Alternative wound coverings. In Herndon DN, editor: *Total burn care*, Philadelphia, 2012, Saunders.

85. Nordlund MJ, Pham TN, Gibran NS: Micronutrients after burn injury: a review. *J Burn Care Rehabil* 35(2):121–133, 2014.

86. Helvig E: Pediatric burn injuries. *AACN Clin Issues Crit Care Nurs* 4(2):433–442, 1993.

87. Strang SG, et al: A systematic review on intra-abdominal pressure in severely burned patients. *Burns* 40:9–16, 2014.

88. Peng D, Huang W: Etiology of immune dysfunction in thermal injuries. In Phillips BJ, editor: *Pediatric burns*, Amherst, 2012, Cambria.

89. Walker PF, et al: Diagnosis and management of inhalation injury: an updated review. *Crit Care* 19:351, 2015.

90. Conrardy PA, et al: Alteration of endotracheal tube position. *Crit Care Med* 4(2):8, 1976.

91. Sharar SR: Endotracheal tube tip position in an infant with severe burns. *J Burn Care Rehabil* 16(6):654, 1995.

92. Trout S, et al: Influence of head and neck position on endotracheal tube tip position on chest x-ray examination: a potential problem in the infant undergoing intubation. *J Burn Care Rehabil* 15(5):405–407, 1994.

93. Palmieri TL: What's new in critical care of the burn-injured patient? *Clin Plast Surg* 36(4):607–615, 2009.

94. Greathouse ST, et al: High-frequency oscillatory ventilators in burn patients: experience of Riley Hospital for Children. *J Burn Care Res* 33(3):425–435, 2012.

95. Phillips BJ: Pediatric burn resuscitation. In Phillips BJ, editor: *Pediatric burns*, Amherst, 2012, Cambria.

96. Tintinalli JE, et al: *Emergency medicine: a comprehensive study guide*, New York, 2004, McGraw-Hill.

97. Lee JO, Herndon DH, Norbury WB: Special considerations of age: the pediatric burn patient. In Herndon DH, editor: *Total burn care*, Philadelphia, 2012, Saunders.

98. Saffle JR: The phenomenon of "fluid creep" in acute burn resuscitation. *J Burn Care Res* 28(5):382–395, 2007.

99. Colon NC, Schlegel C, Chung DH: Surgical management of complications of burn injury. In Herndon DH, editor: *Total burn care*, Philadelphia, 2012, Saunders.

100. Deitch EA: Nutritional support of the burn patient. *Crit Care Med* 11(3):735, 1995.

101. Supple KG: Physiologic response to burn injury. *Crit Care Nurs Clin North Am* 16(1):119, 2004.

102. Stratta RJ, et al: Immunologic parameters in burned patients: effect of therapeutic interventions. *J Trauma* 26(1):7, 1986.

103. Murphey ED, Sherwood ER, Tolliver-Kinsky T: The immunological response and strategies for intervention. In Herndon DN, editor: *Total burn care*, Philadelphia, 2012, Saunders.

104. Klein GL: Disruption of bone and skeletal muscle in severe burns. *Bone Res* 3:15002, 2015.

105. Phillips BJ, Carter MJ: Changes to the hypothalamic-pituitary-adrenal axis in burns and the use of steroids. In Phillips BJ, editor: *Pediatric burns*, Amherst, 2012, Cambria.

106. Gallagher JJ, et al: Treatment of infection in burns. In Herndon DN, editor: *Total burn care*, Philadelphia, 2012, Saunders.

107. Wilmore DW: Nutrition and metabolism following thermal injury. *Clin Plast Surg* 1(4):603–619, 1974.

108. Jensen AR, Hughes WB, Grewal H: Secondary abdominal compartment syndrome in children with burns and trauma: a potentially lethal complication. *J Burn Care Res* 27(2):242–246, 2006.

109. Mandell SP, Gibran NS: Early enteral nutrition for burn injury. *Adv Wound Care (New Rochelle)* 3(1):64–70, 2014.

110. Rodriguez NA, et al: Nutrition in burns: Galveston contributions. *J Parenter Enteral Nutr* 35(6):704–714, 2011.

111. Saffle JR, Graves C, Cochran A: Nutritional support of the burned patient. In Herndon DN, editor: *Total burn care*, Philadelphia, 2012, Saunders.

112. Gottschlich MM, Mays T: Nutrition for the burned pediatric patients. In Samour PQ, King K, editors: *Pediatric nutrition*, Sudbury, MA, 2012, Jones & Bartlett.

113. Petersen SR, Umphred E, Warden GD: The incidence of bacteremia following burn wound excision. *J Trauma* 22(4):274–279, 1982.

114. Lee JO, et al: Operative wound management. In Herndon DN, editor: *Total burn care*, Philadelphia, 2012, Saunders.

115. Kwan P, Desmoulière A, Tredget EE: Molecular and cellular basis of hypertrophic scarring. In Herndon DN, editor: *Total burn care*, Philadelphia, 2012, Saunders.

116. Hawkins HK, Finnerty CC: Pathophysiology of the burn scar. In Herndon DN, editor: *Total burn care*, Philadelphia, 2012, Saunders.

117. Baker RU, et al: Burn wound itch control using H1 and H2 antagonists. *J Burn Care Rehabil* 22(4):263, 2001.

118. Brown NJ, et al: Predictors of re-epithelialization in pediatric burn. *Burns* 40:751, 2014.

A

Absolute polycythemia excessive red blood cell production; a physiologic response resulting from increased erythropoietin secretion in response to chronic hypoxia or as a symptom of polycythemia vera.

Absorption atelectasis see Atelectasis.

Acid maltase deficiency (glycogen storage disease type II or Pompe disease) an autosomal recessive metabolic disorder that damages muscle and nerve cells throughout the body by an accumulation of glycogen in the lysosome attributable to deficiency of the lysosomal acid α-glucosidase enzyme. The buildup of glycogen causes progressive muscle weakness (myopathy) throughout the body and affects various body tissues, particularly in the heart, skeletal muscles, liver, and nervous system.

Acne a common skin disease characterized by pimples on the face, chest, and back. It occurs when the pores of the skin become clogged with oil, dead skin cells, and bacteria.

Acne conglobata severe cystic acne characterized by cystic lesions, abscesses, communicating sinuses, and thickened, nodular scars; usually does not affect the face.

Acne rosacea a chronic form of dermatitis of the face in which the middle portion of the face appears red with small red lines caused by dilation of capillaries.

Acne vulgaris an inflammatory eruption of the sebaceous follicles usually occurring on the face, upper back, and chest that consists of blackheads, cysts, papules, and pustules.

Noninflammatory acne open comedones caused by the enlargement and dilation of a plug resulting from the accumulation of oil and dead skin cells inside the hair follicle and by closed comedones that form if the hair follicle pore remains closed; they appear as a tiny, sometimes pink bump in the skin.

Acquired immunodeficiency syndrome (AIDS) see Immune deficiency.

Acquired sideroblastic anemia see Anemia.

ACTH deficiency a condition characterized by decreased or absent production of adrenocorticotropic hormone (ACTH) by the pituitary gland, resulting in a reduction in the secretion of adrenal hormones and subsequent weight loss, lack of appetite, weakness, nausea, vomiting, and low blood pressure.

Actinic keratosis a condition in which a premalignant small, reddish, rough spot appears on skin chronically exposed to the sun.

Acute chest syndrome a syndrome occurring in association with sickle cell disease defined by a new infiltrate on chest radiograph; associated with one or more new symptoms: fever, cough, sputum production, dyspnea, or hypoxia. It occurs most commonly in the 2- to 4-year-old age group and declines in incidence with age.

Acute colonic pseudo-obstruction (Ogilvie syndrome) a massive dilation of the large bowel that occurs in critically ill patients and immobilized older adults. It is characterized by significant dilation of the cecum and absence of mechanical obstruction, and is related to excessive sympathetic motor input or decreased parasympathetic motor input.

Acute confusional state (ACS) a form of delirium caused by interference with the metabolic or other biochemical processes essential for normal brain functioning. Symptoms may include disturbances in cognition and levels of awareness, short-term memory deficit, retrograde and anterograde amnesia, and disturbances in orientation, accompanied by restlessness, apprehension, irritability, and apathy. The condition may be associated with an acute physiologic state, delirium, toxic psychosis, or acute brain syndrome.

Acute coronary syndrome a classification encompassing clinical presentations ranging from unstable angina through infarction.

Acute cystitis an inflammation of the bladder, which is the most common site of urinary tract infection.

Acute epiglottitis an infection that causes inflammation of the epiglottis and surrounding tissues and may lead to upper airway blockage.

Acute gastritis an inflammatory disorder of the gastric mucosa, usually caused by injury of the protective mucosal barrier by drugs, chemicals, or *Helicobacter pylori* infection.

Acute glomerulonephritis see Glomerulonephritis.

Acute gouty arthritis an abrupt pain of a joint, most often the great toe, which is swollen, hot, and shiny secondary to an attack of gout.

Acute idiopathic thrombotic thrombocytopenic purpura (TTP) see Thrombocytopenia.

Acute leukemia see Leukemia.

Acute liver failure (fulminant liver failure) a rare clinical syndrome resulting from severe impairment or necrosis of liver cells without pre-existing liver disease or cirrhosis. Acetaminophen overdose is the leading cause.

Acute lung injury (ALI)/acute respiratory distress syndrome (ARDS) a spectrum of acute lung inflammation and diffuse alveolocapillary injury.

Acute lymphoblastic leukemia (ALL) see Leukemia.

Acute mesenteric ischemia caused by acute occlusion of the mesenteric artery that results in a significant reduction in mucosal blood flow to the large and small intestines. Aortic aneurysms, arterial thrombi, or emboli can be causes.

Acute mountain sickness (AMS) the presence of a combination of nonspecific symptoms that appear within a few hours after ascent to altitude, and may include headache, loss of appetite, nausea, vomiting, weakness, lassitude, dizziness, and difficulty sleeping.

Acute myelogenous leukemia (AML) see Leukemia.

Acute orthostatic hypotension an abnormal decrease in blood pressure when a person stands. This may lead to fainting.

Acute otitis media (AOM) an infection of the middle ear space, behind the eardrum (tympanic membrane); characterized by pain, dizziness, and partial loss of hearing.

Acute pancreatitis inflammation of the pancreas resulting from obstruction to the outflow of pancreatic digestive enzymes caused by bile duct or pancreatic duct obstruction (e.g., gallstones). Usually a mild disease and resolves spontaneously.

Acute poststreptococcal glomerulonephritis (PSGN) see Glomerulonephritis.

Acute pyelonephritis acute inflammation of the renal parenchyma and pelvis characterized by small cortical abscesses and yellowish streaks in the medulla resulting from the accumulation of pus in the collecting tubules and interstitial tissue.

Acute renal failure (acute renal injury) a sudden decline in kidney function with a decrease in glomerular filtration and accumulation of nitrogenous waste products in the blood as demonstrated by an elevation in plasma creatinine and blood urea nitrogen levels.

Acute respiratory distress syndrome (ARDS) capillaries or alveoli of the lungs are damaged as a result of infection, injury, blood loss, or inhalation injury causing fluid to leak from the capillaries into the alveoli, resulting in pulmonary edema and collapse of some alveoli.

Acute tubular necrosis (ATN) the kidney undergoes ischemic or nephrotoxic injury because of severe hypotension, aminoglycosides, or radiocontrast agents and produces granular and epithelial cell casts in urine.

Acute urethral syndrome the bladder is irritated and the typical symptoms of a urinary tract infection are present in the absence of an infection.

Adenocarcinoma tumor arising from epithelial cells with a glandular or glandlike pattern.

Adenocystic tumor (cylindroma) rare bronchial gland tumors that arise predominantly in the trachea or large airways and cause obstruction.

Adenomyosis the presence of islands of endometrial glands surrounded by benign endometrial stroma within the uterine myometrium.

Adenosine deaminase (ADA) deficiency see Immune deficiency.

Adrenarche growth of axillary and pubic hair and other physiologic changes induced by hyperactivity of the suprarenal cortex and adrenocortical secretion of androgenic hormones in early puberty.

Agammaglobulinemia see Immune deficiency.

Ageusia loss of the sense of taste.

Agoraphobia a mental disorder characterized by an irrational fear of leaving the familiar setting of home, or venturing into the open; it is so pervasive that a large number of external life situations are entered into reluctantly or are avoided; often associated with panic attacks.

Agranulocytosis see Immune deficiency.

Akinesia slowness or loss of normal motor function resulting in impaired muscle movement.

Akinetic mutism (AM) a syndrome characterized by the inability to speak, loss of voluntary movement, and apparent loss of emotional feeling. It is related to lesions of the upper brainstem.

Albright syndrome (Albright-McCune-Sternberg syndrome) a syndrome characterized by polyostotic fibrous dysplasia, patchy dermal pigmentation, and endocrine dysfunction.

Alcoholic cirrhosis see Cirrhosis.

Alcoholic fatty liver (steatosis) the mildest form of alcoholic liver disease; can be caused by chronic ingestion of relatively small amounts of alcohol, may be asymptomatic, and is reversible with cessation of drinking.

Alcoholic hepatitis (steatohepatitis) a precursor of cirrhosis characterized by inflammation; degeneration and necrosis of hepatocytes; infiltration of neutrophils, macrophages, and lymphocytes; immunologic alterations; and lipid peroxidation.

Algor mortis postmortem reduction of body temperature.

Alkaline reflux gastritis inflammation of the stomach caused by reflux of bile and alkaline pancreatic secretions that contain proteolytic enzymes and disrupt the mucosal barrier in the remnant stomach.

Allergic contact dermatitis contact dermatitis attributable to allergic sensitization.

Allodynia a condition in which pain arises from a stimulus that would not normally be experienced as painful.

Allostasis long-term or chronic exaggerated responses to stress.

Alogia inability to speak because of mental deficiency, mental confusion, or aphasia.

Alopecia loss of hair.

Alopecia areata an autoimmune T-cell–mediated chronic inflammatory disease directed at hair follicles that results in baldness, usually in round patches.

Alpha-thalassemia major see Anemia.

Alpha-thalassemia minor see Anemia.

Alzheimer disease (dementia of Alzheimer type [DAT], senile disease complex) a degenerative disease characterized by amyloid plaques and fibrillary tangles in the cortex and atrophy and widened sulci in the frontal and temporal lobes.

Amblyopia poor vision caused by abnormal development of visual areas of the brain in response to abnormal visual stimulation during early development.

Amenorrhea lack of menstruation; most common causes (aside from pregnancy) are chromosomal abnormalities, hypothalamic dysfunction, polycystic ovarian syndrome, hyperprolactinemia, hypothyroidism, malnutrition, and ovarian failure.

Amyotrophic lateral sclerosis (ALS) (sporadic motor system disease, sporadic motor neuron disease, motor neuron disease, Lou Gehrig disease) a disease that breaks down tissues in the nervous system (a neurodegenerative disease); it is of unknown cause and affects the nerves responsible for movement.

Anaphylactic shock a state of shock caused by a severe allergic reaction that lowers blood pressure and results in urticaria, breathing difficulties, and possibly death.

Anaphylactoid purpura (allergic purpura, Henoch-Schönlein purpura) nonthrombocytopenic purpura attributable to immune hypersensitivity to foods, drugs, and insect bites.

Anemia hemoglobin concentration is less than normal because of a deficiency in red blood cells, a low level of hemoglobin in cells, or both; it manifests as pallor of the skin and mucous membranes, weakness, dizziness, easy fatigability, and drowsiness caused by oxygen deficiency.

Congenital hemolytic anemias

Alpha-thalassemia major thalassemia in which all four α chains of hemoglobin are defective, resulting in a fatal condition because oxygen cannot be released to the tissues.

Alpha-thalassemia minor thalassemia in which two α chains of hemoglobin are defective.

Beta-thalassemia major (Cooley anemia) thalassemia in which α-chain synthesis and β-chain synthesis are uncoupled; β-chain production is depressed moderately in the heterozygous form, beta-thalassemia minor, and severely in the homozygous form, beta-thalassemia major, resulting in erythrocytes that have a reduced amount of hemoglobin and accumulations of free α chains.

Beta-thalassemia minor see above.

Glucose-6-phosphate dehydrogenase (G6PD) deficiency an inherited condition that is asymptomatic in the absence of exposure to particular substances such as certain medicines, mothballs, or severe infections; with exposure the red blood cells undergo destruction, producing excessive bilirubin that overloads the liver and causes jaundice.

Hemoglobin H disease a form of alpha-thalassemia in which a hemoglobin H gene is expressed but cannot bind oxygen.

Hereditary spherocytosis (congenital hemolytic anemia, congenital acholuric jaundice) a defect in the cell membrane of red blood cells that causes thickened, fragile red blood cells that are susceptible to spontaneous hemolysis and results in chronic anemia, jaundice, fever, and abdominal pain.

Sickle cell anemia (sickle cell disease [SCD]) an inherited autosomal recessive disorder of the blood caused by abnormal hemoglobin that distorts red blood cells and makes them fragile and prone to rupture and can cause anemia, joint pain, fever, leg ulcers, and jaundice.

Sickle cell–Hb C disease a heterozygous form in which the child simultaneously inherits a hemoglobin C gene from another parent.

Sickle cell–thalassemia disease a heterozygous form in which the child simultaneously inherits a thalassemia gene from another parent.

Sickle cell trait an inherited condition in which an individual carries only one gene for sickle cell disease and is without symptoms.

Thalassemia a potentially fatal genetic disorder in which hemoglobin molecules are abnormal, resulting in severe anemia; enlarged heart, liver, and spleen; and skeletal deformation.

Macrocytic anemia (megaloblastic anemia) a condition characterized by erythrocytes that are larger than normal; associated with deficiency of vitamin B_{12} or folic acid caused by inadequate intake or insufficient absorption secondary to alcoholism or drugs that inhibit DNA replication.

Pernicious anemia an autoimmune disorder that causes a deficiency in intrinsic factor, resulting in the inability to absorb vitamin B_{12} and a subsequent increase in the production of abnormal erythrocytes.

Microcytic-hypochromic anemia a condition in which red blood cells are smaller than normal as a result of iron deficiency.

Acquired sideroblastic anemia a heterogeneous group of disorders characterized by anemia of varying severity caused by a defect in mitochondrial heme synthesis; occurs as a primary disorder with no known cause (idiopathic) or is associated with other myeloproliferative or myelodysplastic disorders.

Hereditary sideroblastic anemia heterogeneous group of rare disorders characterized by anemia of varying severity caused by a defect in mitochondrial heme synthesis; occurs almost exclusively in males, suggesting a predominant recessive X-linked transmission.

Hypoplastic anemia a condition in which anemia results from greatly depressed, inadequately functioning bone marrow and smaller-than-normal erythrocytes.

Iron deficiency anemia (IDA) an insufficient dietary intake or absorption of iron, resulting in decreased incorporation of hemoglobin into red blood cells and subsequent feelings of fatigue, weakness, and shortness of breath as well as pale earlobes, palms, and conjunctivae.

Reversible sideroblastic anemia associated with alcoholism; results from nutritional deficiencies of folate.

Sideroblastic anemia (SA) refractory anemia of varying severity that is caused by altered mitochondrial metabolism and is marked by sideroblasts in the bone marrow.

Normocytic-normochromic anemia (NNA) erythrocytes are of normal size and hemoglobin content but of insufficient number; usually caused by hereditary spherocytosis, drug-induced anemia, and anemia secondary to malignancies.

Anemia of chronic disease (ACD) a mild to moderate anemia resulting from decreased erythropoiesis in individuals with conditions of chronic systemic disease or inflammation.

Aplastic anemia decreased bone marrow production of adequate amounts of new red blood cells; results from an autoimmune disorder or exposure to radiation or substances such as benzene or certain drugs.

Aplastic crisis temporary loss of bone marrow causes erythropoiesis, resulting in an acute fall in hemoglobin levels and subsequent anemia.

Atrial septal defect (ASD) an abnormal communication between the atria; isolated ASD occurs in about 5% to 10% of all congenital cardiac defects.

Autoimmune hemolytic anemia (AIHA) a form of hemolytic anemia involving auto-antibodies against red blood cell antigens.

Cold agglutinin autoimmune hemolytic anemia acquired disorder caused by autoantibodies against antigens normally on the surface of erythrocytes; mediated by immunoglobulin M (IgM) antibodies that optimally bind to and agglutinate erythrocytes in colder portions of the body (e.g., fingers, toes), and occurs less often than warm antibody hemolysis, affecting mostly middle-aged and older adults.

Cold hemolysin autoimmune hemolytic anemia (paroxysmal cold hemoglobinuria) a disorder in which exposure to cold initiates acute and severe intravascular hemolysis that, unlike cold agglutinin anemia, results in hemoglobinuria. The chronic form of this anemia is extremely rare, but an acute form of paroxysmal cold hemoglobinuria is frequently observed in autoimmune hemolytic anemia of childhood.

Drug-induced hemolytic anemia a form of immune hemolytic anemia usually resulting from an allergic reaction against foreign antigens (e.g., antibiotics) that have attached to the surface of red blood cells.

Fanconi anemia a genetic disease affecting bone marrow that is characterized by pancytopenia, hypoplasia of the bone marrow, congenital anomalies, and pigment changes of the skin and that predisposes the individual to myelodysplasia and to acute myeloid leukemia or cancers of the mouth, esophagus, intestinal and urinary tracts, and reproductive organs.

Hemolytic anemia a condition in which red blood cells are destroyed in response to certain toxic or infectious agents or in certain inherited blood disorders and the rate of breakdown exceeds the body's ability to compensate.

Hemolytic disease of the newborn (HDN) (erythroblastosis fetalis) a condition that affects a fetus or newborn in which red blood cells break down because of antibodies made by the mother that are directed against the infant's red cells, potentially resulting in anemia, heart failure, jaundice, and brain damage.

Posthemorrhagic anemia a type of normocytic-normochromic anemia that is caused by sudden blood loss in an individual with normal iron stores and triggers a compensatory response in which water and electrolytes from tissues and interstitial spaces are used to expand plasma volume and accelerate the formation and development of blood cells.

Warm autoimmune hemolytic anemia the most common form of autoimmune hemolytic anemia; caused by IgG that binds to erythrocytes at normal body temperature; often secondary to other diseases, especially lymphomas, chronic lymphocytic leukemia, other neoplastic disorders, or systemic lupus erythematosus (SLE).

Anencephaly anomaly in which the soft, bony component of the skull and much of the brain are missing.

Angelman syndrome (happy puppet syndrome) an inherited syndrome of jerky puppet like movements, frequent laughter, mental and motor retardation, peculiar open-mouthed facies, and seizures.

Angina pectoris chest pain caused by reduced cardiac blood flow and myocardial ischemia.

Anhedonia absence of pleasure from the performance of acts that would ordinarily be pleasurable.

Ankylosing spondylitis (AS, spondyloarthritis) chronic inflammation of the spine and sacroiliac joints with gradual fusion of the vertebrae that immobilizes the spine.

Anorexia nervosa (AN) a disorder with both psychologic and physiologic components that begins with dieting to lose weight and manifests into an inappropriate self-control behavior; continued restrictive eating may lead to starvation and eventually death.

Anorgasmia (orgasmic dysfunction) the inability of the woman to reach or achieve orgasm.

Anuria urine output less than 50 mL/day.

Anxiety disorder a group of disorders involving various manifestations of anxiety that are grouped together and include panic disorder, specific phobia, social phobia, obsessive-compulsive disorder (OCD), posttraumatic stress disorder (PTSD), acute stress disorder, generalized anxiety disorder (GAD), and anxiety disorders secondary to medical conditions or substance-induced or not otherwise specified.

Aplastic anemia see Anemia.

Aplastic crisis see Anemia.

Appendicitis inflammation of the appendix as a result of blockage of the opening from the appendix into the cecum; the appendix wall becomes infected and ruptures, allowing the infection to spread throughout the abdomen and cause pain, anorexia, fever, nausea, vomiting, and diarrhea.

Apraxia a disorder of voluntary movement consisting of impairment of the performance of skilled or purposeful movements; results from acquired cerebral disease.

Arcus senilis a gray to white ring at the periphery of the cornea; caused by deposits of cholesterol in the cornea or hyaline degeneration and occurs primarily in older persons.

Areflexia absence of reflexes.

Arterial ischemic stroke (pediatric arterial ischemic stroke) a rare disorder in children resulting from embolism, arteriopathy, or, rarely, sinovenous thrombosis and leading to a decreased flow of blood and oxygen to areas of the brain.

Asbestosis pulmonary inflammation and fibrosis resulting from inhalation of hydrous silicates of various metals in fibrous form.

Aseptic meningitis a form of inflammation of the meninges and subarachnoid space surrounding the brain and spinal cord without evidence of bacterial infection; may be associated with viral infection, systemic disease, or drugs.

Aspiration pneumonitis a condition caused by the abnormal entry of fluids, particulate matter, or secretions into the lower airways that can lead to chemical pneumonitis from entry of toxic material such as gastric acid, from bacterial infection, or by mechanical obstruction of the lower airways.

Asthma a chronic inflammatory disorder of the airways involving bronchial hyperresponsiveness and airway obstruction marked by periodic attacks of wheezing, shortness of breath, a tight feeling in the chest, and a cough that produces mucus because of an allergic reaction triggered by certain drugs, irritants, viral infection, exercise, or emotional stress.

Asymptomatic bacteriuria the presence of bacteria in the urine without evidence of infection.

Ataxia-telangiectasia (AT) see Immune deficiency.

Ataxic cerebral palsy a form of cerebral palsy associated with damage to the cerebellum and resulting in gait disturbances and instability; at birth the infant may have hypotonia, but develops stiffness of the trunk muscles later in infancy.

Atelectasis part of or an entire lung collapses and the alveoli deflate as a result of surgery, smoking, or blockage of a bronchiole.

Absorption atelectasis collapse of lung tissue resulting from gradual absorption of air from obstructed or hypoventilated alveoli or from inhalation of concentrated oxygen or anesthetic agents.

Compression atelectasis air pressure in the pleural space pushes against the already recoiled lung, causing compression atelectasis, and against the mediastinum, compressing and displacing the heart and great vessels.

Surfactant impairment decreased production or inactivation of surfactant, which is necessary to reduce surface tension in the alveoli and causes lung collapse during expiration; can occur because of premature birth, acute respiratory distress syndrome, anesthesia, or mechanical ventilation.

Atherosclerosis a type of arteriosclerosis in which the inflammatory changes of thickening and hardening of the walls of large- and medium-sized arteries are caused by an atheroma or plaque of lipids, cells, and connective tissue in the tunica intima.

Atopic dermatitis (AD) (allergic dermatitis) a chronic hereditary skin disease characterized by intense itching and inflamed skin that causes redness, swelling, cracking, crusting, and scaling.

Atrial septal defect (ASD) a congenital heart disease involving the interatrial septum of the heart that separates the right and left atria, which results in misdirected blood flow between the two sides of the heart.

Atrioventricular canal (AVC) defect a large hole is present in the center of the heart where the wall between the atria joins the wall between the ventricles, and the tricuspid and mitral valves are formed into a single large valve that crosses the defect.

Atypical ductal hyperplasia (ADH) abnormal proliferating cells in breast ducts.

Atypical hyperplasia increased number of cells with some variation in cellular structure but without sufficient qualitative or quantitative features of carcinoma.

Atypical lobular hyperplasia (ALH) abnormal proliferating cells in breast lobules.

Autoimmune hemolytic anemia (AIHA) see Anemia.

Autoimmune neonatal thrombocytopenia see Thrombocytopenia.

Autoimmune vascular purpura (allergic purpura) purpura caused by antibody-mediated injury of blood vessel walls, typically arterioles and capillaries. The reaction is directed to foreign proteins or chemicals in the blood (microorganisms, drugs, or other chemicals) that deposit on the vessel walls.

Autonomic hyperreflexia (dysreflexia) a syndrome resulting from afferent stimuli that cause intense sympathetic discharge originating with spinal cord injury above the major splanchnic outflow; characterized by hypertension, bradycardia, sweating of the forehead, severe headache, and piloerection on distention of the bladder and rectum.

Autosomal agammaglobulinemia see Immune deficiency.

Autosomal dominant polycystic kidney disease (ADPKD) a progressive disease characterized by formation of multiple cysts of varying size scattered diffusely throughout both kidneys, resulting in compression and destruction of renal parenchyma, usually with hypertension, gross hematuria, and uremia leading to progressive renal failure.

Autosomal hyper-IgM syndrome see Immune deficiency.

Azotemia kidney dysfunction characterized by increased serum urea levels and frequently associated with increased creatinine levels.

B

Bacterial pneumonia an acute or chronic disease marked by inflammation of the lungs caused by bacterial infection.

Bacterial tracheitis a condition in which the larynx, trachea, and bronchi are inflamed and present with signs similar to those of epiglottitis and croup; may result in airway obstruction secondary to subglottic edema or sloughing of the epithelial lining or the mucopurulent membrane within the trachea.

Bacterial vaginosis (BV) a condition caused by an overgrowth of normal vaginal bacteria, causing vaginal discharge with a foul odor.

Balanitis inflammation of the glans penis caused by irritation by environmental substances, physical trauma, or infection.

Bare lymphocyte syndrome see Immune deficiency.

Barrett esophagus chronic peptic ulceration of the esophagus; formation of precancerous lesions with possible progression to adenocarcinoma.

Bartholinitis (Bartholin cyst) inflammation of one or both of the ducts that lead from the introitus (vaginal opening) to the Bartholin/greater vestibular glands.

Basal cell carcinoma a surface epithelial tumor of the skin originating from undifferentiated basal or germinative cells.

B-cell neoplasm see Lymphoma.

Becker muscular dystrophy a general term for a number of late-onset X-linked recessive hereditary, progressive degenerative disorders affecting skeletal muscles, and often other organ systems.

Beckwith-Wiedemann syndrome an inherited disorder characterized by exomphalos, macroglossia, and gigantism; often associated with visceromegaly, adrenocortical cytomegaly, and dysplasia of the renal medulla.

Benign breast disease (BBD) a spectrum of noncancerous changes in ducts and lobules of the breast, including irregular lumps, cysts, sensitive nipples, and itching.

Benign prostatic hyperplasia (BPH) enlargement of the prostate gland, which may press against the urethra and bladder, interfering with urine flow.

Beta-thalassemia major (Cooley anemia) see Anemia.

Beta-thalassemia minor see Anemia.

Biliary atresia a condition in newborn children in which the biliary tract is blocked or absent, causing bile accumulation and progressive liver failure.

Biliary cirrhosis see Cirrhosis.

Bipolar disorder psychiatric disorder characterized by alternating mania or hypomania and depression, often with periods of normal mood in between, and changes in energy and behavior according to mood.

Blast injury tissue damage from compressive waves of air against the body followed by waves of decreased pressure.

Blepharitis inflammation of the eyelids.

B-lymphocyte deficiency see Immune deficiency.

Bradycardia an abnormally low heart rate, which can cause a fall in cardiac output or can be a symptom of deterioration.

Bradykinesia decreased spontaneity and movement; a feature of extrapyramidal disorders, such as Parkinson disease.

Brainstem gliomas a group of tumors located in the brainstem that are usually classified as high grade and result in the sudden onset of symptoms including headaches, vomiting, and visual disturbances.

Bronchial carcinoid tumor an obstructing tumor of the trachea or large bronchi that may cause paraneoplastic symptoms.

Bronchiectasis dilation of the bronchi in response to obstruction, necrotizing pneumonias, cystic fibrosis, or Kartagener syndrome (a hereditary syndrome consisting of dextrocardia, bronchiectasis, and sinusitis).

Bronchiolitis inflammation of the bronchioles usually caused by viral infection.

Bronchiolitis obliterans partial or complete obliteration of bronchioles and some bronchi by granulation and fibrotic tissue masses.

Bronchiolitis obliterans with organizing pneumonia (BOOP) obstruction of the bronchioles and alveolar ducts by fibrous granulation tissue that is further complicated by the development of pneumonia.

Bronchopulmonary dysplasia (BPD) a condition most often found in premature infants in which chronic pulmonary insufficiency occurs because of long-term artificial pulmonary ventilation.

Bruton agammaglobulinemia see Immune deficiency.

Bulbar palsy a form of palsy resulting from impaired function of the cranial nerves from degeneration of the motor neurons of primarily the brainstem; manifested as weakness and wasting of the various bulbar muscles, resulting in difficulty articulating words (dysarthria) and difficulty swallowing (dysphagia); fluid regurgitation is a major symptom and can cause aspiration.

Bullous pemphigoid (BP) a more benign autoimmune disease than pemphigus vulgaris, with blistering of the subepidermal skin layer.

Burkitt lymphoma see Lymphoma.

Burn shock a phenomenon consisting of both a hypovolemic cardiovascular component and a cellular component; results from massive fluid losses from the circulating blood volume.

Bursitis a trauma or overuse injury that can cause painful inflammation in the bursal sacs.

C

C1 deficiency see Immune deficiency.

C2 deficiency see Immune deficiency.

C3 deficiency see Immune deficiency.

C3 receptor deficiency see Immune deficiency.

C4 deficiency see Immune deficiency.

C9 deficiency see Immune deficiency.

Cachexia illness and malnutrition seen in individuals with cancer that results in wasting and eventual death.

Calculi or urinary stone (urolithiasis) masses of crystals, protein, or other substances that are a common cause of urinary tract obstruction in adults.

Candidiasis a fungal infection caused by an overgrowth of normal *Candida albicans* found in the skin and mucous membranes of the mouth, respiratory tract, or vagina.

Caplan syndrome formation in coal workers of intrapulmonary nodules in pneumoconiosis that are histologically similar to subcutaneous rheumatoid nodules associated with rheumatoid arthritis.

Carbuncles a condition in which a bacterial infection of the hair follicle or sebaceous gland ducts becomes painful and discharges pus through various openings.

Carcinoma epithelial cell tumor.

Carcinoma in situ (CIS) preinvasive epithelial malignant tumors of glandular or squamous cell origin.

Cardiogenic shock a condition resulting from decreased cardiac output caused by heart disease in which the heart is unable to pump blood through the body, usually because of myocardial infarction.

Cardiomyopathy(ies) a diverse group of diseases primarily affecting the myocardium and resulting from tissue remodeling caused by myocardial and neurohumoral responses to ischemic and hypertensive alterations.

Cavernous (congenital) hemangioma a birthmark that is similar to the strawberry hemangioma but is more deeply rooted and may appear as a red-blue spongy mass of tissue filled with blood.

Cellulitis an infection of the dermis and subcutaneous tissue usually caused by *Staphylococcus*, CA-MRSA, or group B streptococci.

Central core disease (CCD) an autosomal dominant congenital myopathy characterized by hypotonia, delay of motor development in infancy, and nonprogressive or slowly progressive muscle weakness; on biopsy the central core of muscle fibers stains abnormally, myofibrils are abnormally compact, and there is virtual absence of mitochondria and sarcoplasmic reticulum; histochemically, the cores are devoid of oxidative enzyme, phosphorylase, and ATPase activity.

Central precocious puberty a condition in which puberty begins prematurely with normal changes in the hypothalamus-pituitary-gonad (HPG) axis and with premature development of secondary sexual characteristics and premature closure of the epiphysis of long bones, resulting in lifelong short stature.

Centriacinar emphysema see Emphysema.

Cerebellar astrocytoma brain tumor of the right or left cerebellar hemisphere that causes motor symptoms on the same side as the tumor.

Cerebral palsy (CP) a developmental brain injury that occurs before or shortly after birth and causes muscular impairment affecting motor function and also may alter speech and learning abilities.

Cerebrovascular accidents (CVAs) the leading cause of disability, the third leading cause of death in women, and the fifth leading cause of death in men in the United States; classified pathophysiologically as ischemic, hemorrhagic, or cryptogenic.

Cervical dysplasia (cervical intraepithelial neoplasia [CIN]) a condition characterized by the appearance of abnormal cervical cells that are considered precancerous.

Cervicitis inflammation of the mucous membrane of the uterine cervix caused by infection, typically by chlamydia, genital herpes, or gonorrhea.

Chediak-Higashi syndrome see Immune deficiency.

Cheyne-Stokes respiration an abnormal pattern of breathing in which tidal volume gradually increases followed by a gradual decrease and a period of apnea before returning to a normal respiratory pattern.

Chickenpox an infectious viral disease that is spread by direct contact or through the air by coughing or sneezing; it causes a blister-like rash that first affects the face and trunk and then can spread over the rest of the body; symptoms include severe itching, fatigue, and fever.

Childhood absence epilepsy (petit mal seizures, nonconvulsive epilepsy) a type of generalized epilepsy; age of onset is 4 to 10 years.

Chlamydia a sexually transmitted bacterial infection that can cause infertility and blindness.

Choking asphyxiation obstruction of the internal airways.

Cholangiocellular carcinoma (cholangiocarcinoma) primary carcinomas of the liver that develop in the bile ducts.

Cholecystitis inflammation of the gallbladder commonly caused by impaction of a gallstone that causes right upper quadrant pain and possibly a rupture and abscess in the gallbladder.

Cholelithiasis the presence or formation of gallstones in the gallbladder or bile ducts.

Chondrosarcoma a cancer of the cartilage that usually occurs in the pelvic bones, shoulder bones, and the upper part of the arms and legs.

Chronic active hepatitis the persistence of clinical manifestations and liver inflammation after the acute stages with consistently abnormal liver function tests and persistent hepatitis B surface antigen (HBsAg) creating a predisposition to cirrhosis and primary hepatocellular carcinoma.

Chronic bronchitis particularly as a cause of chronic cough in smokers.

Chronic gastritis tends to occur in older adults with chronic inflammation, mucosal atrophy, and epithelial metaplasia; may be immune (fundal) or nonimmune (antral), depending on the pathogenesis and location of the lesions.

Chronic glomerulonephritis see Glomerulonephritis.

Chronic granulomatous disease (CGD) see Immune deficiency.

Chronic kidney disease (CKD) progressive loss of renal function associated with systemic diseases such as hypertension, diabetes mellitus, systemic lupus erythematosus, or intrinsic kidney disease, including kidney stones, acute kidney injury, chronic glomerulonephritis, chronic pyelonephritis, obstructive uropathies, or vascular disorders.

Chronic leukemia see Leukemia.

Chronic lymphocytic leukemia (CLL) see Leukemia.

Chronic mesenteric ischemia development of regions of compromised blood flow in the mesenterium secondary to atherosclerosis (most common), congestive heart failure, dysrhythmias, hemorrhage, thrombus formation, aortic aneurysm, or any condition that decreases arterial blood flow. Chronic occlusion is often accompanied by formation of collateral circulation that may be able to nourish the resting intestine.

Chronic mucocutaneous candidiasis see Immune deficiency.

Chronic myelogenous leukemia (CML) see Leukemia.

Chronic obstructive pulmonary disease (COPD) any of a group of irreversible respiratory diseases (chronic bronchitis, emphysema, α_1-antitrypsin deficiency) that are characterized by airflow obstruction or limitation.

Chronic pancreatitis inflammation of the pancreas resulting from repeated exacerbations of acute pancreatitis that lead to chronic changes; associated with obstruction from gallstones, autoimmune disease, gene mutations, smoking, occupational chemical exposure, and obesity.

Chronic pyelonephritis persistent or recurrent infection of the kidney leading to scarring.

Chronic relapsing thrombotic thrombocytopenic purpura (TTP) see Thrombocytopenia.

Chronic venous insufficiency (CVI) persistent ambulatory lower extremity venous hypertension.

Cirrhosis degeneration of liver tissue resulting in fibrosis with nodule and scar formation that compromises liver function.

> **Alcoholic cirrhosis** destructive inflammation of the liver caused by the toxic effects of alcohol metabolism, immunologic processes, lipid peroxidation, and malnutrition.
>
> **Biliary cirrhosis** a form of alcoholic cirrhosis in which damage and inflammation leading to cirrhosis begin in bile canaliculi and bile ducts, rather than in the hepatocytes.
>
> **Primary biliary cirrhosis** a T-lymphocyte- and antibody-mediated destruction of the small intrahepatic bile ducts.

Cloacal exstrophy family of congenital anomalies with two exstrophied bladder units separated by an exstrophied segment of intestine, which is usually cecum, receiving the ileum superiorly and continuing distally to a blind ending microcolon.

Clubfoot describes a range of foot deformities in which the foot turns inward and downward.

Cluster headache one of a group of rare disorders referred to as *trigeminal autonomic cephalagia*; they occur in clusters (up to eight attacks per day) on one side of the head primarily, with pain that is severe, stabbing, and throbbing.

Coal worker pneumoconiosis (coal miner lung, black lung) mild to severe pneumoconiosis (pulmonary fibrosis) caused by coal dust (coal, silica, quartz) deposits in the lung; symptoms initially present as a productive cough and wheezing, but may advance to chronic bronchitis and emphysema.

Coarctation of the aorta (COA) a condition in which the aorta narrows in the area where the ductus arteriosus inserts; narrowing usually occurs preductal in children and postductal in adults.

Cold agglutinin autoimmune hemolytic anemia see Anemia.

Cold hemolysin autoimmune hemolytic anemia (paroxysmal cold hemoglobinuria) see Anemia.

Combined T- and B-lymphocyte deficiency see Immune deficiency.

Common variable immune deficiency see Immune deficiency.

Communicating (extraventricular) hydrocephalus a disorder in which the cerebrospinal fluid pathways are intact but cerebrospinal fluid absorption is impaired.

Community-acquired pneumonia (CAP) a major cause of morbidity and mortality in children, particularly in developing countries.

Complement deficiency see Immune deficiency.

Complete precocious puberty refers to the early onset and progression of all pubertal features (i.e., thelarche, pubarche, and menarche).

Complex febrile seizure seizures with characteristic features similar to those of simple febrile seizure with a longer duration and focal characteristics; occur more than once in a 24-hour period.

Complex regional pain syndrome (CRPS) diffuse persistent pain usually in an extremity often associated with vasomotor disturbances, trophic changes, and limitation or immobility of joints; frequently follows a local injury.

Compression atelectasis see Atelectasis.

Compressive syndrome (sensorimotor syndrome; crush syndrome) a shocklike state that follows release of a limb (or limbs) or the trunk and pelvis after a prolonged period of compression, such as by a heavy weight; characterized by suppression of renal function, probably the result of damage to the renal tubules by myoglobin from the damaged muscles.

Congenital adrenal hyperplasia a group of autosomal recessively inherited disorders associated with a deficiency of one of the enzymes involved in cortisol biosynthesis, resulting in elevation of ACTH levels and overproduction and accumulation of cortisol precursors proximal to the block; androgens are produced in excess, causing virilization. The most common disorder is the 21-hydroxylase deficiency, caused by mutation in the cytochrome P450 21-hydroxylase gene (*CYP21*) on chromosome 6p.

Congenital aganglionic megacolon (Hirschsprung disease) a congenital defect in which the nerves that innervate the anus through the wall of the bowel are absent, resulting in enlargement of the bowel superior to the point where the nerves are missing and a subsequent decrease in peristalsis that results in chronic constipation.

Congenital hydrocephalus excessive accumulation of cerebrospinal fluid present at birth and characterized by increased intracranial pressure (ICP). This increase may be caused by a blockage within the ventricular system in which the CSF flows, an imbalance in the production of CSF, or a reduced reabsorption of CSF that results in ventricular enlargement and increased ICP.

Congenital hypothyroidism lack of secretion of thyroid hormone.

Congenital (infantile) nephrotic syndrome (Finnish type) a very rare form of nephrotic syndrome caused by a defect in a kidney protein resulting in excessive amounts of protein excreted in the urine.

Congestive splenomegaly enlargement of the spleen accompanied by ascites, portal hypertension, and esophageal varices; most commonly seen in those with hepatic cirrhosis.

Consumptive thrombohemorrhagic disorders heterogeneous group of conditions that demonstrate the entire range of hemorrhagic and thrombotic pathologic conditions.

Contact dermatitis an allergic response to an environmental antigen binding to specific carrier proteins contained in an individual's skin.

Contrecoup injury brain injury resulting from the brain hitting the inside of the skull on the side opposite the site of blunt force trauma.

Cor pulmonale right-sided heart failure caused by prolonged pulmonary hypertension.

Coronary artery disease (CAD) narrowing of the lumen of one or more of the coronary arteries, usually attributable to atherosclerosis, leading to myocardial ischemia; can cause congestive heart failure, angina pectoris, or myocardial infarction.

Craniopharyngioma a brain tumor that develops in the pituitary gland and most often affects children, causing headache, seizure, diabetes insipidus, early onset of puberty, and delayed growth.

Craniosynostosis (craniostenosis) (see Syndromic craniosynostosis) premature ossification of the skull and closure of the sutures, resulting in abnormal skull expansion and asymmetrical skull growth.

Cri du chat syndrome a hereditary congenital syndrome characterized by hypertelorism, microcephaly, severe mental deficiency, and a plaintive catlike cry; caused by deletion of the short arm of chromosome 5.

Crohn disease (CD) an autoimmune condition in which the intestines and possibly other regions of the digestive system are chronically inflamed and ulcerated, causing chronic diarrhea, disrupted digestion, and subsequent difficulty eating and digesting food.

Croup a viral infection that involves the larynx, trachea, and the airways leading to the lungs and that can result in serious breathing difficulties, hoarseness, sore throat, and a hacking cough.

Cryptorchidism the scrotum of one or both testes is absent because of failure of the testis to descend from the abdominal position during fetal development.

Curling ulcer ischemic ulcers of the stomach and duodenal mucosa that develop within hours after an event, such as hemorrhage, multisystem trauma, severe burns, heart failure, or sepsis.

Cushing disease adrenal hyperplasia caused by an ACTH-secreting basophil adenoma of the pituitary.

Cushing syndrome increased synthesis and secretion of cortisol from a tumor of the adrenal cortex; caused by administration of glucocorticoid drugs or by the presence of an ACTH-secreting tumor of the anterior lobe of the pituitary gland (Cushing disease), resulting in weight gain, glucose intolerance, and muscle wasting.

Cushing ulcer a stress ulcer associated with severe head trauma or brain surgery.

Cyclic neutropenia see Immune deficiency.

Cylindrical bronchiectasis a reversible bronchial dilation with symmetrically dilated airways, as can be seen after pneumonia.

Cystic fibrosis (CF) a genetic disorder of the exocrine glands caused by a mutation in the CF transmembrane regulator gene, resulting in impairment in chloride transfer across cell membranes and subsequent chloride and water accumulation in organs and in thickened secretions that block ducts and form cysts.

Cystitis a condition characterized by acute or chronic inflammation of the urinary bladder, usually caused by bacterial infection of the urethra; symptoms include frequent burning on urination, blood in the urine, pain in the pubic area, chills and fever, back pain, and nausea. See Painful bladder syndrome/interstitial cystitis (PBS/IC) for further information.

D

Dandy-Walker malformation congenital defect of midline cerebellar structures and the fourth ventricle in which hydrocephalus is caused by atresia of the foramina of Luschka or Magendie, which normally allow the fourth ventricle to empty into the areas surrounding the brain, leading the ventricular flow of CSF into a "blind pouch."

Dawn phenomenon abrupt increases in fasting levels of plasma glucose between 5 and 9 AM, in the absence of antecedent hypoglycemia; occurs in diabetic patients receiving insulin therapy.

Decompression sickness (DCS) (caisson disease) gas embolism created when a person under water returns to the surface too quickly, resulting in cellular hypoxia, joint and muscle pain, and tissue necrosis.

Deep venous thrombosis (DVT) a blood clot or thrombus in a deep vein, usually of the leg.

Degenerative disk disease (DDD) intervertebral disk tissue is replaced by fibrocartilage during aging; functional capacity is rarely altered.

Demyelinating polyneuropathy a type of polyneuropathy in which the peripheral nerve myelin is primarily affected; can be familial (Charcot-Marie-Tooth disease, type 1) or acquired (Guillain-Barré syndrome); motor nerve conduction is slowed or blocked.

Dermatitis herpetiformis pruritic chronic dermatitis with successive groups of symmetrical, erythematous, papular, vesicular, eczematous, or bullous lesions; usually associated with asymptomatic gluten-sensitive enteropathy.

Detrusor areflexia a lower motor neuron disorder that results in underactive, hypotonic, or atonic bladder function with retention of urine and distention.

Detrusor hyperreflexia (uninhibited or reflex bladder) upper motor neuron disorders in which the bladder empties automatically when it becomes full and the external sphincter functions normally.

Developmental dysplasia of the hip (DDH) a condition in which the hip joint of babies or young children is malformed, with the ball being completely out of the socket or the socket being too shallow to support the ball.

Diabetes diseases having in common the triad of symptoms of polyuria, weight loss, and significant glucosuria.

Diabetes insipidus a disease caused by a deficiency in or resistance to antidiuretic hormone that is characterized by excretion of large amounts of dilute urine because of a decrease in water reabsorption in the kidney.

Gestational diabetes mellitus (GDM) carbohydrate intolerance of variable severity with onset during pregnancy.

Type 1 diabetes mellitus a disorder of carbohydrate metabolism characterized by a decrease in insulin production, resulting in hyperglycemia, ketoacidosis, and eventually renal failure and coronary artery disease.

Type 2 diabetes mellitus a condition of glucose intolerance that normally appears first in adulthood and is exacerbated by obesity and an inactive lifestyle.

Maturity-onset diabetes of youth (MODY) a non–insulin-requiring diabetes in lean individuals typically younger than 25 with evidence of autosomal dominant inheritance.

Diabetic nephropathy a progressive kidney disease caused by diabetes-induced angiopathy of capillaries in the glomeruli that causes nodular glomerulosclerosis.

Diabetic neuropathy combined sensory and motor disorder often seen in older diabetic patients as a result of microvascular injury involving small blood vessels that supply nerves.

Diabetic retinopathy damage to the retina caused by an overaccumulation of glucose or fructose that damages the blood vessels in the retina; in advanced stages, lack of oxygen in the retina causes fragile blood vessels to grow along the retina and in the vitreous fluid of the eye that may bleed and cause blurred vision.

Diaper dermatitis a type of dermatitis characterized by inflammation of the skin in the diaper area in infants caused by exposure of the skin to feces and urine.

Diastolic heart failure a condition in which heart contractions are normal but the ventricle does not relax completely; therefore less blood enters the heart.

Diffuse brain injury (diffuse axonal injury) injury to neuronal axons in many areas of the brain caused by stretching and shearing forces received during brain injury.

DiGeorge syndrome see Immune deficiency.

Dilated cardiomyopathy (congestive cardiomyopathy) a condition in which all four chambers of the heart are enlarged and weakened, resulting in progressive congestive heart failure and the need for heart transplantation.

Discoid (cutaneous) lupus erythematosus (DLE) see Lupus erythematosus.

Dislocation the temporary displacement of a bone from its normal position in a joint.

Disorders of desire (hypoactive sexual desire, decreased libido) the most common sexual dysfunction in women; prevalence increases with age and may be a biologic manifestation of depression, alcohol or other substance abuse, prolactin-secreting pituitary tumors, or testosterone deficiency.

Disseminated intravascular coagulation (DIC) an acquired clinical syndrome characterized by widespread activation of coagulation resulting in formation of fibrin clots in medium and small vessels (microvasculature) throughout the body.

Distal intestinal obstruction syndrome (DIOS) a syndrome seen in cystic fibrosis secondary to impaction with feces and inspissated mucus.

Diverticulitis inflammation of the herniations or saclike outpouchings of mucosa through the muscle layers of the colon wall.

Diverticulosis the presence of multiple bulging sacs pushing outward from the wall of the large intestine that may become infected and rupture, causing abdominal pain, tenderness, and fever.

Down syndrome trisomy or translocation of chromosome 21, resulting in intellectual disability; distinctive facial appearance with a low nasal bridge, epicanthal folds, protruding tongue, and flat, low-set ears; poor muscle tone (hypotonia); and short stature. Congenital heart defects, reduced ability to resist respiratory tract infections, and increased risk for leukemia are common.

Drug-induced hemolytic anemia see Anemia.

Duchenne muscular dystrophy (DMD) an X-linked genetic disorder in which fat and fibrous tissue infiltrate and weaken muscle tissues such as in the legs and pelvis, lungs, and heart; usually results in death before adulthood.

Dumping syndrome rapid emptying of hypertonic chyme from a surgically created residual stomach causing nausea, vomiting, bleeding, and diarrhea about 20 minutes after a meal.

Duodenal ulcer most common type of peptic ulcer; usually associated with altered mucosal defenses, rapid gastric emptying, elevated serum gastrin levels, or acid production stimulated by smoking.

Dysfunctional uterine bleeding (DUB) heavy or irregular bleeding in the absence of organic disease, such as submucous fibroids, endometrial polyps, blood dyscrasias, pregnancy, infection, or systemic disease.

Dyskinetic cerebral palsy extreme difficulty in fine motor coordination and purposeful movements resulting from injury to the basal ganglia or thalamus.

Dysphoric mood mood of general dissatisfaction, restlessness, depression, and anxiety; a feeling of unpleasantness or discomfort.

Dysplasia (atypical hyperplasia) abnormal changes in the size, shape, and organization of mature cells; considered a form of atypical hyperplasia.

Dyspraxia the partial inability to perform purposeful or skilled motor acts in the absence of paralysis, sensory loss, abnormal posture and tone, abnormal involuntary movement, incoordination, or inattentiveness.

Dysrhythmias (arrhythmias) disturbances of cardiac rhythm and the most common complication of acute MI.

Dyssynergia development of lesions in the upper motor neurons of the brain and spinal cord; results in loss of coordinated neuromuscular contraction and overactive or hyperreflexive bladder function.

E

Eczema most common inflammatory disorder of the skin; generally characterized by pruritus, lesions with indistinct borders, and epidermal changes.

Eisenmenger syndrome a progressively developing condition in which a congenital heart defect such as ventricular septal defect is left untreated and causes a reversed right-to-left shunt secondary to increased pressures on the right side of the heart because of pulmonary hypertension.

Embryonic tumor a tumor originating in the gestational period that contains predominantly immature blast cells that cannot differentiate into mature functional cells.

Emphysema pulmonary inflammation resulting in increased work of breathing or physiologic dead space and abnormal permanent enlargement of gas-exchange airways (acini) accompanied by destruction of alveolar walls without obvious fibrosis.

Centriacinar emphysema diminished pulmonary function resulting from septal destruction in the respiratory bronchioles and alveolar ducts, usually in the upper lobes of the lung.

Panacinar emphysema destruction of the entire acinus, with damage more randomly distributed and involving the lower lobes of the lung. It tends to occur in older adults and in those with α_1-antitrypsin deficiency.

Empyema (infected pleural effusion) a condition in which purulent fluid is persistently discharged into the pleural space as a result of complications of bacterial infections.

Encephalitis inflammation of the brain usually caused by a virus.

Endometriosis a condition that is common in women of reproductive age in which the tissue lining the uterus is found outside of the uterus, resulting in pain and infertility.

End-stage kidney disease (ESKD) a condition in which there is significant loss of renal function; usually less than 10% of renal function remains.

Eosinophilic esophagitis rare, idiopathic inflammatory disease of the esophagus characterized by infiltration of eosinophils; associated with atopic disease, including asthma and food allergies.

Ependymoma intracranial tumor that is most commonly found in children and typically arises from the inner lining of the fourth ventricle and the spinal canal.

Epididymitis a painful condition in which the epididymis becomes inflamed, usually as a result of a secondary bacterial infection that is triggered by a variety of underlying conditions such as urinary tract or sexually transmitted infections.

Epilepsy a group of chronic neurologic disorders with paroxysmal brain dysfunction from excessive neuronal discharge; symptoms vary widely from complex behavioral abnormalities to focal convulsions, to momentary spells of impaired consciousness.

Epispadias a birth defect in which the urethra opens on the upper penile surface.

Erysipelas a highly contagious bacterial infection that produces shiny, red, swollen areas and fever and can lead to blood poisoning and pneumonia.

Erythema multiforme a skin disease that is caused by allergies, seasonal changes, or drug sensitivities, resulting in the formation of red macules, papules, or subdermal vesicles on the skin and mucous membranes.

Erythema toxicum neonatorum a temporary eruption of redness of the skin, small papules, and occasionally pustules in newborns that is associated with contact dermatitis or hypersensitivity to milk or other allergens.

Erythrodermic (exfoliative) psoriasis see Psoriasis.

Erythromyalgia chronic disorder characterized by warmth, pain, and redness, occurring primarily in the feet and lower legs.

Essential (primary) thrombocythemia (ET) excessive production of platelets (platelet count greater than 400,000/mm^3 of blood); may be primary or secondary (reactive) and is usually asymptomatic until the count exceeds 1 million/mm^3 of blood when intravascular clot formation (thrombosis), hemorrhage, or other abnormalities can occur.

Ewing sarcoma a malignant neoplasm of bone, primarily those of the extremities, including the shoulder girdle, with a predilection for the metaphysis; histologically presents as conspicuous foci of necrosis in association with irregular masses of small, regular, rounded, or ovoid cells.

Exstrophy of the bladder a congenital defect in which the lower abdominal wall is malformed and ruptures.

Extrapyramidal/nonspecific cerebral palsy any of a group of clinical disorders considered to be due to malfunction in the extrapyramidal system and marked by abnormal involuntary movements; included are parkinsonism, athetosis, and chorea.

F

Facioscapulohumeral muscular dystrophy (FSHD) an autosomal dominant genetic disorder that begins in childhood and causes muscle wasting and weakness, primarily in the face, shoulder, and arms.

Factor H deficiency see Immune deficiency.

Factor I deficiency see Immune deficiency.

Failure to thrive (FTT) also called *growth faltering*, it is a physical sign demonstrating that a child is receiving inadequate nutrition for optimal growth and development. FTT is manifested as a deceleration in weight gain, a low weight/height ratio, a low weight/height/head circumference ratio, or a low body mass index (BMI).

Fanconi anemia see Anemia.

Fetal alcohol syndrome (FAS) a syndrome of altered prenatal growth and morphogenesis that occurs in infants born to women who were chronically alcoholic during pregnancy; it includes maxillary hypoplasia, prominence of the forehead and mandible, short palpebral fissures, microphthalmia, epicanthal folds, severe growth retardation, intellectual disability, and microcephaly.

Fibromyalgia a condition in which muscles, tendons, and joints are painful, stiff, and tender; often accompanied by restless sleep, fatigue, anxiety, depression, and disturbances in bowel function.

Fibrosarcoma a malignant tumor of fibrous connective tissue that usually is derived from immature proliferating fibroblasts.

Fibrous dysplasia (FD) a genetic disorder in which tumor-like growths or lesions form in one or more bones and replace the medullary bone with fibrous tissue, resulting in expansion and weakening of the bone.

Florid hyperplasia rapid and unexpected cell growth in the lining of the breast ducts.

Focal segmental glomerulosclerosis (FSGS) a condition in which glomerular capillaries with thickened basement membranes and increased mesangial matrix collapse in segments. Usually presents as nephrotic syndrome.

Frontotemporal dementia (FTD) (Pick disease) progressive circumscribed cerebral atrophy; a rare type of cerebrodegenerative disorder manifested primarily as dementia, in which there is striking atrophy of portions of the frontal and temporal lobes.

FSH deficiency a condition characterized by decreased or absent production of follicle-stimulating hormone (FSH), resulting in a decline in spermatogenesis/oogenesis and associated infertility.

Furuncles a staphylococcal infection produces painful pus-filled inflamed hair follicles and involves surrounding skin and subcutaneous tissue.

Fusiform aneurysm (giant aneurysm) a large aneurysm that stretches to affect the entire circumference of the arterial wall.

G

Galactorrhea (inappropriate lactation) a condition in which milk-like fluid is secreted from the breast because of hormonal alterations that are not associated with childbirth or nursing.

Ganglioneuroblastoma an embryonal aggressive tumor of intermediate cellular differentiation that originates outside the CNS in the developing sympathetic nervous system.

Ganglioneuroma a benign neoplasm composed of mature ganglionic neurons scattered within a stroma of neurofibrils and collagenous fibers.

Gangliosidosis any disease characterized by abnormal accumulation of specific gangliosides within the nervous system (e.g., Tay-Sachs disease).

Gastroesophageal reflux disease (GERD) the reflux of acid and pepsin from the stomach to the esophagus that causes esophagitis.

General adaptation syndrome (GAS) the sum of all nonspecific reactions of the body to prolonged systemic stress, comprising alarm, resistance, and exhaustion.

Generalized anxiety disorder (GAD) an anxiety disorder characterized by an excessively anxious mood lasting at least 1 month that interferes with daily functioning and may be accompanied by jitteriness, sweating, feelings of catastrophe concerning one's family or self, and irritability.

Generalized neuropathy a functional disturbance or pathologic change in the cell body of one type of peripheral neuron.

Genital herpes a sexually transmitted viral infection that is caused primarily by herpes simplex virus type 2 and is characterized by painful lesions in the genital and anal regions.

Gestational diabetes mellitus (GDM) see Diabetes.

GH deficiency a condition characterized by decreased or absent production of growth hormone (GH), resulting in a decline in insulin-like growth factor 1 and dwarfism if the deficiency is prepubertal.

Glaucoma a disease of the eye characterized by increased intraocular pressure, excavation, and atrophy of the optic nerve; produces defects in the field of vision and eventual blindness.

Glomerulonephritis inflammation of the renal glomeruli that may not produce symptoms or may present with hematuria and proteinuria.

Acute glomerulonephritis an inflammatory disease of both kidneys predominantly affecting children from ages 2 to 12.

Acute poststreptococcal glomerulonephritis (PSGN) a kidney disease secondary to infection with *Streptococci* in which bacterial antigens complex with antibodies in the blood, deposit in the kidneys, and initiate an immune complex–mediated hypersensitivity reaction.

Chronic glomerulonephritis a slowly progressive glomerulonephritis most often associated with other systemic disease, including diabetes, malaria, hepatitis, or systemic lupus erythematosus, that generally leads to irreversible renal failure.

Membranoproliferative glomerulonephritis (MPGN) a chronic, slowly progressive glomerulonephritis in which the glomeruli are enlarged as a result of proliferation of mesangial cells and irregular thickening of the capillary walls, which narrows the capillary lumina.

Membranous glomerulonephritis a slowly progressive disease of unknown origin or that occurs secondary to autoimmune conditions, infections, specific drugs, or malignant tumors that is caused by immune complexes formed from the binding of antibodies to antigens of the glomerular basement membrane (GBM) or antigens transported from the systemic circulation and implanted in the GBM.

Membranous nephropathy (membranous glomerulonephritis) membranous nephropathy is caused by subepithelial deposition of antibodies (IgG4 subclass) to antigens (M-type phospholipase A_2 receptor [PLA2R] protein) located on glomerular podocytes and activation of complement-mediated inflammation with injury and release of inflammatory mediators by mesangial and epithelial cells, resulting in increased membrane permeability, thickening of the glomerular membrane, and ultimately glomerular sclerosis.

Mesangial proliferative glomerulonephritis deposition of immune complexes in the mesangium with mesangial cell proliferation and expansion reducing blood flow and altering filtration membrane permeability with development of hematuria, proteinuria, hypertension, and uremia (nephritic syndrome); associated with IgA nephropathy, lupus nephritis, or early diabetic nephropathy.

Rapidly progressive (crescentic) glomerulonephritis (RPGN) (subacute or extracapillary glomerulonephritis) develops over days to weeks, primarily affects adults in their fifties and sixties, and may be idiopathic or associated with a proliferative glomerular disease (diffuse proliferation of extracapillary cells), such as lupus or poststreptococcal glomerulonephritis.

Glucose-6-phosphate dehydrogenase (G6PD) deficiency see Anemia.

Gluten-sensitive enteropathy (celiac sprue) a condition characterized by mucosal inflammation and villous atrophy in the gastrointestinal tract formed in response to a genetic predisposition for an immune response to gluten and similar proteins.

Gonorrhea a sexually transmitted disease caused by the bacteria gonococci that invade the mucous membranes of the genitals and urinary tract and in women the cervix, fallopian tubes, and ovaries, causing chronic pelvic pain or infertility.

Gout a disorder of uric acid metabolism that causes painful inflammation of the joints, commonly the big toe, and arthritic attacks resulting from elevated levels of uric acid in the blood and the deposition of negatively birefringent urate crystals around the joints.

Gouty arthritis inflammation of the joints in gout.

Graft rejection immunologic rejection of transplanted tissue or organs based on antigen differences between the donor and recipient.

Acute graft rejection cell-mediated immune rejection that occurs within days to months after transplantation; immune response is usually against unmatched HLA antigens and develops after transplantation.

Chronic graft rejection slow, progressive organ failure after a period of months or years of normal function by a developing weak cell-mediated immune response against minor histocompatibility antigens on the endothelial cells lining the blood vessels of the grafted tissue.

Hyperacute graft rejection immediate rejection of a graft because of preexisting antibodies against antigens expressed on the grafted tissue or organ.

Graft-versus-host disease (GVHD) condition in which mature T cells in a transplanted graft (e.g., transfused blood) are capable of a destructive cell-mediated reaction against unmatched histocompatibility antigens on the tissues in the graft recipient.

Granuloma inguinale a bacterial-induced disease, also called *donovanosis*, that is thought to be transmitted primarily by anal rather than vaginal intercourse and causes painless genital ulcers like syphilis but progresses to destroy the internal and external genital tissue.

Graves disease autoimmune hyperthyroidism caused by antibodies that continuously activate TSH receptors, resulting in uncontrolled production of thyroxine and characterized by an enlarged thyroid gland, protrusion of eyeballs, a rapid heartbeat, and nervous excitability.

Guillain-Barré syndrome (GBS) (Landry-Guillain-Barré syndrome, idiopathic polyneuritis, acute inflammatory polyradiculopathy, acute autoimmune neuropathy) an acute, immune-mediated disorder of peripheral nerves, spinal roots, and cranial nerves that commonly presents as a rapidly progressive, areflexic, relatively symmetrical ascending weakness of the limb, truncal, respiratory, pharyngeal, and facial musculature, with variable sensory and autonomic dysfunction; typically reaches its peak activity within 2 to 3 weeks, followed by a plateau period of similar duration, and gradual but complete recovery in most cases; often preceded by a respiratory tract or gastrointestinal tract infection and is associated with albuminocytologic dissociation of the cerebrospinal fluid.

Guttate psoriasis see Psoriasis.

Gynecomastia abnormal breast tissue development on adolescent boys or men as a result of an imbalance in hormones.

H

Heat exhaustion occurs when sufficient salt and water loss results in hemoconcentration with hypotension occurring secondary to fluid loss (hypovolemia), and the individual feels weak, is nauseated, and can suddenly collapse.

Heat stroke a life-threatening condition associated with high environmental temperatures and humidity causing core body temperature to rise as a result of thermoregulatory failure.

Hematemesis accumulation of blood in the gastrointestinal tract causing irritation, increased peristalsis, and vomiting.

Hematochezia rapid bleeding from the upper GI tract producing bright red stools.

Hemochromatosis disorder of iron metabolism characterized by excessive absorption of ingested iron, saturation of iron-binding protein, and deposition of hemosiderin in tissue, particularly in the liver, pancreas, and skin; cirrhosis of the liver, diabetes (bronze diabetes), bronze pigmentation of the skin, and eventually heart failure may occur; also can result from administration of large amounts of iron orally, by injection, or in forms of blood transfusion therapy.

Hemoglobin H disease see Anemia.

Hemolytic anemia see Anemia.

Hemolytic disease of the newborn (HDN) (erythroblastosis fetalis) see Anemia.

Hemolytic jaundice (prehepatic jaundice, nonobstructive jaundice) jaundice resulting from excessive hemolysis of red blood cells.

Hemolytic-uremic syndrome (HUS) a condition in which platelets aggregate within the kidney's small blood vessels, resulting in reduced blood flow to the kidney and subsequent kidney failure and destruction of the red blood cells; occurs usually after exposure to Shiga-like toxin from a strain of *E. coli*.

Hemophilia A (classic hemophilia) a genetic disorder in which a mutation in factor VIII causes prolonged clotting time, decreased formation of thromboplastin, and diminished conversion of prothrombin.

Hemophilia B (Christmas disease) a genetic disorder similar to hemophilia A in terms of symptoms but with a mutation in the factor IX gene.

Hemophilia C (factor XI deficiency) a genetic disorder characterized by a deficiency in factor XI, resulting in a mild form of hemophilia.

Hemorrhagic stroke (spontaneous intracranial hemorrhage) stroke usually caused by hypertension that results in bleeding in the brain and typically increases intracranial pressure and may lead to death.

Henoch-Schönlein purpura nephritis inflammation of the blood vessels causing bleeding into the skin, mucous membranes, internal organs, and other tissues; pain and inflammation in the joints; abdominal pain; gastrointestinal bleeding; inflammation of the kidneys; subcutaneous edema; encephalopathy; and inflammation of the testis.

Heparin-induced thrombocytopenia (HIT) see Thrombocytopenia.

Hepatic encephalopathy a condition that is usually caused by liver cirrhosis and portal hypertension in which toxins produced by the gut pass into the systemic circulation and damage brain cells, resulting in impaired cognition, tremor, and a decreased level of consciousness.

Hepatitis B virus one of six types of hepatitis virus that cause liver infection; it is most commonly sexually transmitted.

Hepatocellular carcinoma (hepatocarcinoma; HCC) primary carcinoma of the liver developing in hepatocytes.

Hepatopulmonary syndrome intrapulmonary vasodilation, intrapulmonary shunting, and hypoxia and portopulmonary hypertension (pulmonary vasoconstriction and vascular remodeling) are common respiratory complications of advanced liver disease and portal hypertension.

Hepatorenal syndrome (HRS) acute renal failure occurs because of a decrease in renal blood flow secondary to liver disease.

Hereditary angioedema an inherited, autosomal dominant disease characterized by episodic appearance of nonpitting edema, most often affecting the limbs, but capable of involving other parts of the body, including mucosal surfaces such as those of the intestine (causing abdominal pain) or respiratory tract (causing asphyxia); associated with deficiency of inhibitor of the first component of complement pathway (C1 esterase inhibitor).

Hereditary hemochromatosis (HH) autosomal recessive chronic liver disease caused by excessive intestinal absorption of elemental iron; characterized by elevated serum iron saturation, transferrin, and ferritin levels; improves with phlebotomy; increased risk of developing cirrhosis, liver cancer, and liver failure.

Hereditary sideroblastic anemia see Anemia.

Hereditary spherocytosis see Anemia.

Hiatal hernia an anatomic abnormality in which the esophageal hiatus is larger than normal, causing part of the stomach to protrude through the diaphragm and up into the esophagus or chest.

High altitude cerebral edema (HACE) an increase in severity of symptoms or signs of neurologic dysfunction, such as ataxia or altered consciousness, related to high altitude.

High altitude pulmonary edema (HAPE) a noncardiogenic pulmonary edema associated with pulmonary hypertension and elevated capillary pressure related to high altitude illness.

Hirsutism abnormal growth and distribution of androgen-sensitive hair growth on the face, body, and pubic area in a male pattern that occurs in women.

Hodgkin lymphoma (HL) see Lymphoma.

Hormonal hyperplasia growth of cellular layers chiefly in estrogen-dependent organs, such as the uterus and breast. After ovulation, for example, estrogen stimulates the endometrium to grow and thicken for reception of the fertilized ovum.

Huntington disease (HD) an autosomal dominant disease causing a progressive increase in involuntary, jerky, dyskinetic movements; mental deterioration; and premature death.

Hyaline membrane disease (HMD) a type of respiratory distress syndrome of the newborn in which there is formation of a hyaline-like membrane lining the terminal respiratory passages; extensive atelectasis is attributed to lack of surfactant.

Hydrocele a collection of fluid within the tunica vaginalis that is the most common cause of scrotal swelling.

Hydrocephalus ex vacuo hydrocephalus attributable to loss or atrophy of brain tissue; less commonly associated with raised intracranial pressure and dilation of the cerebral ventricles.

Hydrops fetalis edema formation in the fetal subcutaneous tissue because of an enzyme deficiency or any one of several other disorders.

Hyperosmolar hyperglycemic nonketotic syndrome (HHNKS) a complication seen in diabetes mellitus in which very marked hyperglycemia occurs, causing osmotic shifts in water in brain cells, and resulting in coma. It can be fatal or lead to permanent neurologic damage.

Hypersensitive pneumonitis (extrinsic allergic alveolitis) an allergic, inflammatory disease of the lungs caused by inhalation of organic particles or fumes.

Hypertrophic cardiomyopathy a genetic disorder caused by various mutations that thicken the heart muscle, possibly leading to obstruction of blood flow and heart dysfunction; this is a common cause of sudden death in young athletes.

Hypogammaglobulinemia see Immune deficiency.

Hypoplastic anemia see Anemia.

Hypoplastic left heart syndrome (HLHS) a condition in which the left side of the heart, including the aorta, aortic valve, left ventricle, and mitral valve, is underdeveloped and blood returning from the lungs flows through an opening in the atrial septum and the right ventricle pumps the blood into the pulmonary artery and then into the aorta.

Hypospadias a birth defect in which the urethral opening is abnormally placed, opening anywhere from the tip of the glans penis, to the shaft, or to the junction of the penis and scrotum or perineum in males; usually opens in the vagina in females.

Hypotonia decreased muscle tone; a condition in which passive movement of a muscle occurs with little or no resistance. A symptom of cerebellar and pure pyramidal tract damage, it is thought to be caused by decreased muscle spindle activity secondary to decreased excitability of neurons.

Hypovolemic shock caused by loss of whole blood (hemorrhage), plasma (burns), or interstitial fluid (diaphoresis, diabetes mellitus, diabetes insipidus, emesis, or diuresis) in large amounts.

Hypoxemia reduced oxygen levels in the blood, which contributes to cardiovascular dysfunction by causing dilation of arterioles, capillaries, and venules and leads to decreased vascular resistance and increased flow.

I

Iatrogenic pneumothorax see Pneumothorax.

Icterus neonatorum (neonatal jaundice) jaundice in newborn infants caused by functional immaturity of the liver; usually subsides within the first few days of life.

Idiopathic pulmonary fibrosis (IPF) an excessive amount of fibrous or connective tissue in the lung.

Idiopathic thrombocytopenic purpura (ITP) (autoimmune or primary thrombocytopenic purpura) see Thrombocytopenia.

IgA nephropathy (Berger disease) the most common form of idiopathic acute glomerulonephritis in developed countries, especially Asia; cause is unknown.

IgA pemphigus the most benign form of pemphigus characterized by tissue-bound and circulating IgA antibodies targeting desmosomal or nondesmosomal cell surface components in the basement membrane of the epidermis.

IgG subclass deficiency see Immune deficiency.

IL-7 receptor deficiency see Immune deficiency.

Immune deficiency a group of disorders in which one or more components of the immune or inflammatory response is impaired, resulting in increased susceptibility to infections. **Primary (congenital) immune deficiencies** result from genetic defects, and secondary immune deficiencies result from nongenetic factors, such as infections and other physiologic or pathophysiologic conditions. Primary immune deficiencies include:

B-lymphocyte deficiency a group of disorders in which B-cell development is defective, resulting in lower levels of circulating immunoglobulins and increased susceptibility to infections in which antibodies are the primary protective mechanism. These include:

Agammaglobulinemia a condition in which no antibodies are produced.

Autosomal agammaglobulinemia an autosomal recessive form of agammaglobulinemia resulting from mutations in the B-cell receptor.

Autosomal hyper-IgM syndrome inability to class-switch resulting from mutations in CD40 on B cells.

Bruton agammaglobulinemia a defect in B-cell development results in lower levels of circulating immunoglobulins and increased susceptibility to infections in which antibodies are the primary protective mechanism.

Common variable immune deficiency the most commonly diagnosed immune deficiency; hypogammaglobulinemia of IgG and other antibody classes; normal numbers of B cells, with or without associated T-cell defects.

Hypogammaglobulinemia a condition in which immunoglobulin levels are much lower than normal.

IgG subclass deficiency deficiencies in certain subclasses of antibody.

Selective IgA deficiency failure to produce IgA, with or without diminished production of other classes of antibody.

X-linked hyper-IgM syndrome inability to class-switch resulting from a defect in activation-induced cytidine deaminase (AICD).

Combined T- and B-lymphocyte deficiency a group of immune deficiencies in which both T and B lymphocytes are defective. The most severe of these deficiencies is called *severe combined immune deficiency (SCID)*. These include:

Adenosine deaminase (ADA) deficiency a form of SCID caused by an autosomal recessive mutation in the enzyme ADA, leading to death of rapidly dividing cells, particularly lymphocytes.

Ataxia-telangiectasia (AT) an autosomal recessive disorder resulting from a large variety of sporadic mutations in the *ATM* gene; often associated with ataxia (unsteady gait), telangiectasia (dilation of capillaries), and variable effects on both B and T cells.

Bare lymphocyte syndrome forms of SCID characterized by an inability of lymphocytes and macrophages to present antigen because of defects in class I (MHC class I deficiency) or class II (MHC class II deficiency) MHC antigen expression.

IL-7 receptor deficiency a form of SCID resulting from mutations in the IL-7 receptor, which is necessary for maturation of T cells.

JAK3 deficiency a form of SCID resulting from mutations in JAK3, which encodes an enzyme (a tyrosine kinase) associated with the receptor for IL-2.

Purine nucleoside phosphorylase (PNP) deficiency a form of SCID resulting from a mutation in the enzyme PNP.

RAG-1 and RAG-2 deficiencies autosomal recessive mutations in recombination-activating gene (RAG-1 or RAG-2) enzymes that are necessary for genetic rearrangement of antibody and T-cell receptor variable regions.

Reticular dysgenesis the most severe form of SCID in which a common stem cell for all white blood cells is absent; therefore T cells, B cells, and phagocytic cells never develop.

Wiskott-Aldrich syndrome (WAS) an X-linked recessive trait resulting in chronic eczema with chronic suppurative otitis media, anemia, thrombocytopenic purpura, poor antibody response to polysaccharide antigens, and dysfunctions of cell-mediated immunity.

X-linked SCID a form of SCID with arrested maturation of T and natural killer (NK) cells and the production of immature B cells as a result of a defect in the IL-2 receptor gamma chain (IL-2Rγ), which is shared with many other cytokine receptors.

Complement deficiency a group of conditions in which specific proteins of the complement system are absent or suboptimal, resulting in diminished complement activity. These include:

C1 deficiency a deficiency of the first component of the classical pathway.

C2 deficiency a deficiency with an increased risk for recurrent respiratory tract infections with encapsulated bacteria and a systemic lupus erythematosus–like syndrome that may be complicated by kidney disease (glomerulonephritis).

C3 deficiency the most severe complement defect; an associated deficit of C3b, which is a major opsonin, results in a risk for recurrent life-threatening infections with encapsulated bacteria.

C3 receptor deficiency deficiencies in the complement receptor for C3 result in recurrent bacterial infections, particularly of the skin.

C4 deficiency results in an increased risk for recurrent respiratory tract infections with encapsulated bacteria and a systemic lupus erythematosus–like syndrome that may be complicated by kidney disease (glomerulonephritis).

C9 deficiency the most common terminal pathway defect and generally asymptomatic.

Factor H deficiency a deficiency of complement factor H resulting in increased destruction of C3 and a secondary C3 deficiency.

Factor I deficiency a deficiency of complement factor I resulting in increased destruction of C3 and a secondary C3 deficiency.

Mannose-binding lectin (MBL) deficiency a defect of the lectin pathway of complement activation resulting in an increased risk of infection with microorganisms that have polysaccharide capsules rich in mannose.

Properdin deficiency an X-linked defect in the alternative pathway of complement activation resulting in recurrent meningococcal infections.

Phagocytic deficiency a group of conditions in which phagocytes are diminished, resulting in increased bacterial infections. These include:

Chediak-Higashi syndrome a lethal, progressive, autosomal recessive, systemic disorder associated with oculocutaneous albinism, massive leukocyte inclusions (giant lysosomes), histiocytic infiltration of multiple body organs, development of pancytopenia, hepatosplenomegaly, and recurrent or persistent bacterial infections.

Chronic granulomatous disease (CGD) both X-linked and autosomal forms of mutations of the NADPH oxidase complex, resulting in diminished production of hydrogen peroxide and other oxygen products necessary for the bactericidal activity of myeloperoxidase.

Cyclic neutropenia an autosomal dominant mutation in the *ELA2* gene resulting in periods of neutropenia lasting a few days to weeks.

Severe congenital neutropenia inadequate numbers of neutrophils resulting in a variety of recurrent and severe bacterial infections beginning early in life.

Secondary immune deficiencies

Acquired immunodeficiency syndrome (AIDS) an epidemic, transmissible retroviral disease caused by infection with the human immunodeficiency virus (HIV), resulting in destruction of T-helper cells, suppression of both antibody and cellular immune responses, and development of life-threatening infections with opportunistic organisms.

Agranulocytosis complete absence of granulocytes in the blood is usually secondary to arrested hematopoiesis in the bone marrow or massive cell destruction in the circulation.

Qualitative leukocyte disorder a group of conditions with various disruptions of leukocyte function.

Quantitative leukocyte disorder a group of conditions, frequently associated with infections and leukemias, with decreased production of leukocytes in the bone marrow or accelerated destruction of leukocytes in the circulation.

Transient hypogammaglobulinemia of infancy a period at 6 to 8 months when the newborn may not have produced adequate amounts of antibody to replace maternal antibody; in some infants this may lead to a period of increased susceptibility to infections.

T-lymphocyte deficiency a group of disorders in which T-cell development is defective, resulting in lower levels of cellular immunity. Diminished T-helper cell function may also decrease the production of antibody. These include:

Chronic mucocutaneous candidiasis a primary defect of T-lymphocyte response to a specific infectious agent, the yeast *C. albicans*.

DiGeorge syndrome a genetic disorder caused by deletion of a piece of chromosome 22 that results in cardiac defects, abnormal facies, thymic aplasia, cleft palate, and hypocalcemia.

Immune thrombocytopenic purpura (ITP) see Thrombocytopenia.

Imperforate anus a congenital defect in which the anal opening is absent because of the presence of a membranous septum or complete absence of the anal canal.

Impetigo a contagious bacterial infection that produces superficial red blisters that rupture and produce thick yellow crusts that commonly occur on the face but can spread to other regions of the body easily.

Infectious mononucleosis (IM) a disease caused by the Epstein-Barr virus or the cytomegalovirus that is transmitted by exchanging saliva or blood or by coughing and sneezing and acts by infecting the B cells and atypical T cells, resulting in fever, sore throat, and fatigue.

Infective endocarditis (IE) a general term used to describe infection and inflammation of the endocardium, especially the cardiac valves.

Infertility the inability to conceive after 1 year of unprotected intercourse with the same, opposite-sex partner.

Intracerebral hematoma (intraparenchymal hemorrhage) blood accumulation that partially clots inside the brain, usually in the frontal and temporal lobes.

Intraductal papilloma array of papillary cells that grow from the wall of a cyst into the lumen of the duct; growth occurs within a dilated duct often near or beside the nipple, causing benign nipple discharge.

Intrarenal (intrinsic) acute kidney injury (AKI) a sudden decline in kidney function with a decrease in glomerular filtration and an accumulation of nitrogenous waste products in the blood (elevation in plasma creatinine and blood urea nitrogen levels); may result from ischemic acute tubular necrosis (ATN), nephrotoxic ATN (i.e., exposure to radiocontrast media or antibiotics), acute glomerulonephritis, vascular disease (malignant hypertension, disseminated intravascular coagulation, and renal vasculitis), allograft rejection, or interstitial disease (drug allergy, infection, tumor growth).

Invasive breast carcinoma a malignant invasive epithelial lesion derived from the terminal duct lobular area.

Invasive carcinoma of the cervix invasion of cervical carcinoma into adjacent tissues, such as ureters and structures of the lateral pelvic wall, the vaginal stroma and epithelium, and the lower uterine segment and myometrium.

Inverse psoriasis see Psoriasis.

Iron deficiency anemia (IDA) see Anemia.

Irritable bowel syndrome (IBS) a chronic noninflammatory disease with a psychophysiologic basis; characterized by abdominal pain, diarrhea or constipation, or both; no detectable pathologic change.

Irritative syndrome (radicular syndrome) a combination of changes usually seen with compromise of a spinal root within the intraspinal canal; these include neck or back pain and, in the affected root distribution, dermatomal pain, paresthesias, or both; decreased deep tendon reflexes; and occasionally myotomal weakness.

Isolated systolic hypertension loss of elasticity of the arteries resulting in an increase in cardiac output or stroke volume, a systolic blood pressure consistently greater than 160 mmHg, and a diastolic pressure less than 90 mmHg.

J

JAK3 deficiency see Immune deficiency.

Jaundice (icterus) yellowish brown staining of the skin and the conjunctivae caused by high bilirubin levels in blood secondary to excessive erythrocyte breakdown, obstruction in or around the liver, or liver disease.

Juvenile idiopathic arthritis (JIA) chronic pauciarticular arthritis and destruction of joints beginning in childhood and often going into remission at puberty.

Juvenile myoclonic epilepsy a type of epilepsy that occurs in adolescents and young adults, usually on awakening, and is characterized by jerks of the neck, shoulders, and arms and by clonic-tonic seizures.

K

Kaposi sarcoma (KS) a rare cancer of connective tissue caused by herpesvirus 8 (HHV8) in which many bluish red nodules appear on the skin, especially skin of the lower extremities; occurs in a particularly virulent form in individuals with AIDS.

Kawasaki disease a vascular disease characterized by an inflamed heart and vessels; a coronary artery aneurysm, thickening, and stenosis; a fever that lasts at least 5 days; and at least four of the following: inflammation with reddening of the whites of the eyes; red, swollen hands or feet or peeling skin; rash; swollen lymph glands in the neck; inflamed lips or throat; or red "strawberry" tongue.

Klinefelter syndrome smallness of testes with fibrosis and hyalinization of seminiferous tubules, variable degrees of masculinization, azoospermia, infertility, and increased levels of urinary gonadotropins; associated typically with an XXY chromosome complement although variants include XXYY, XXXY, and XXXXY.

Kwashiorkor a condition in which children do not receive enough protein in their diet, resulting in a swollen and severely bloated abdomen secondary to decreased albumin levels in the blood, skin changes resulting in a reddish discoloration of the hair and skin in dark-skinned children, severe diarrhea, fatty liver, muscle atrophy, and restricted development.

L

Lactase deficiency a condition in which insufficient lactase is present in the small intestine to digest lactose, resulting in lactose intolerance characterized by diarrhea, bloating, and gas in response to exposure to lactose.

Lactose intolerance a condition caused by lactase deficiency in which lactose is not metabolized, making it impossible for the small intestine to absorb it and causing excessive gas production and diarrhea when exposed to lactose-containing foods.

Lambert-Eaton myasthenic syndrome a generalized disorder of neuromuscular transmission caused by a defect in the release of acetylcholine from the presynaptic nerve terminals; often associated with small cell carcinoma of the lung, particularly in elderly men with a long history of cigarette smoking; weakness tends to affect solely axial muscles, girdle muscles, and less often the limb muscles; autonomic disturbances, dry mouth, and impotence are common; the deep tendon reflexes are unelicitable; caused by loss of voltage-sensitive calcium channels located on the presynaptic motor nerve terminal.

Laryngomalacia a congenital anomaly caused by a developmental delay in the laryngeal cartilage and supporting structures of the larynx that causes the cartilage to be floppy and fold in on itself during inspiration, producing high-pitched, coarse, and low-pitched sounds.

Left heart failure (congestive heart failure) inability of the left ventricle to maintain its circulatory load, with a corresponding rise in pressure in the pulmonary circulation usually with pulmonary congestion and ultimately pulmonary edema.

Legg-Calvé-Perthes disease blood supply to the head of the femur near the hip joint is interrupted, resulting in osteonecrosis of the corresponding epiphysis.

Lennox-Gastaut syndrome a generalized myoclonic epilepsy that occurs in children between 1 and 5 years of age as a result of various cerebral afflictions such as perinatal hypoxia, hemorrhage, encephalitis, and metabolic disorders of the brain; it is characterized by mental retardation, personality disorders, and generalized tonic seizures.

Leukemia a clonal malignant disorder of leukocytes in the bone marrow and usually, but not always of the blood; uncontrolled proliferation of malignant leukocytes, causing an overcrowding of bone marrow and decreased production and function of normal hematopoietic cells.

Acute leukemia characterized by undifferentiated or immature cells, usually a blast cell, and the onset of disease is abrupt and rapid.

Acute lymphoblastic/lymphocytic leukemia (ALL) excessive production and proliferation of malignant and immature white blood cells (lymphoblasts) in the bone marrow that progresses rapidly if left untreated.

Acute myelogenous leukemia (AML) excessive number of immature myeloid cells (myeloblasts) in the blood and bone marrow, overcrowding the marrow and decreasing the function of other cells.

Chronic leukemia Slow-growing cancer with many immature lymphocytes in the blood and bone marrow; the predominant cell is more differentiated but does not function normally.

Chronic lymphocytic leukemia (CLL) malignant transformation and progressive accumulation in the marrow of monoclonal B lymphocytes; rarely are CLL malignancies of T-cell origin.

Chronic myelogenous leukemia (CML) production of heterogeneous myeloid cells in the bone marrow, the majority of which express the Philadelphia chromosome; CML is considered a myeloproliferative disorder.

Leukocytosis a leukocyte count that is higher than normal.

LH deficiency a condition characterized by decreased or absent production of luteinizing hormone (LH), resulting in a decline in sex steroid production in testes/ovaries and associated infertility.

Lichen planus a recurrent rash of small, flat-topped bumps and rough scaly patches appearing on the skin, in the lining of the mouth, and in the vagina in response to inflammation or an allergy to a specific medication.

Localized scleroderma (morphea) rare and idiopathic sclerosis of the skin, usually with childhood onset.

Locked-in syndrome quadriplegia and mutism with intact consciousness and preservation of some eye movements; usually results from a vascular lesion of the anterior pons.

Lupus erythematosus any of a group of autoimmune connective tissue disorders that commonly produce red scaly lesions and are accompanied by fever, malaise, myalgia, fatigue, and weight loss.

Discoid (cutaneous) lupus erythematosus (DLE) lupus erythematosus limited to the skin; can progress to systemic lupus erythematosus (SLE).

Systematic lupus erythematosus (SLE) a chronic, multisystem, inflammatory disease; is one of the most common, complex, and serious of the autoimmune disorders.

Lyme disease (borreliosis) tick-borne spirochete bacterial infection that is characterized by a rash in the area of the bite, headache, neck stiffness, chills, fever, myalgia, arthralgia, malaise, fatigue, and possible development of arthritis in large joints.

Lymphadenopathy an alteration of lymphoid function characterized by enlarged lymph nodes.

Lymphoblastic lymphoma (LL) see Lymphoma.

Lymphogranuloma venereum (LGV) a sexually transmitted bacterial infection that enters the body through breaks in the skin or across the epithelial cell layer of mucous membranes and primarily targets the lymphatics and lymph nodes.

Lymphoma Diverse group of neoplasms arising from cell proliferation in lymphoid tissue.

B-cell neoplasm a group of lymphomas including myelomas that originate from B cells at various stages of differentiation; previously part of non-Hodgkin lymphoma.

Burkitt lymphoma an aggressive malignancy of the B lymphocytes characterized by a large osteolytic lesion in the facial bones and associated with Epstein-Barr virus infection.

Hodgkin lymphoma (HL) a neoplasm of lymphoid tissue that progresses from one group of lymph nodes to another; the lymph nodes, spleen, and liver become enlarged with the presence of Reed-Sternberg cells and is often accompanied by anemia, fever, and eventually death if not treated at an early stage; also referred to as *Hodgkin disease*.

Lymphoblastic lymphoma (LL) a progressive neoplasm arising in the thymus; most are of T-cell origin; a variant of acute lymphoblastic leukemia; common cause of non-Hodgkin lymphoma (NHL) in children.

Lymphoplasmacytic lymphoma also called *Waldenström macroglobulinemia*.

Mucosa-associated lymphoid tissue (MALT) lymphoma a low-grade B-cell lymphoma linked to infection with *H. pylori*.

Mycosis fungoides most common cutaneous T-cell lymphoma; present as focal or widespread erythematous patches or plaques, follicular papules, comedone-like lesions, and tumors.

NK-cell neoplasm a group of lymphomas that originate from natural killer (NK) cells at various stages of differentiation; previously part of non-Hodgkin lymphoma.

Non-Hodgkin lymphoma (NHL) a group of malignancies of lymphoid tissue reclassified as B-cell, T-cell, and NK-cell lymphomas with varied biologic and clinical features.

T-cell neoplasm a variety of lymphomas that originate from T cells at various stages of differentiation; previously part of non-Hodgkin lymphoma.

Waldenström macroglobulinemia a rare type of slow-growing plasma cell tumor that secretes a monoclonal IgM molecule; also called *lymphoplasmacytic lymphoma*.

Lymphoplasmacytic lymphoma see Lymphoma.

Lysosomal storage diseases a group of more than 30 disorders that result from impaired lysosomal function, leading to mucopolysaccharidoses, lipid storage disorders, mucolipidoses, leukodystrophies, and glycoprotein storage disorders.

M

Macrocytic anemia (megaloblastic anemia) see Anemia.

Major (unipolar) depression severely depressed mood and loss of pleasure that may begin suddenly or slowly; it persists for at least 2 weeks and may recur throughout life.

Malignant hyperthermia an inherited life-threatening disorder that causes muscle rigidity, a hypermetabolic state, tachycardia, and increased body temperature in response to administration of general anesthesia.

Malnutrition lack of nourishment from inadequate amounts of calories, protein, vitamins, or minerals; caused by improper diet, alterations in digestion or absorption, chronic disease, or a combination of these factors.

Mannose-binding lectin (MBL) deficiency see Immune deficiency.

Marasmus a childhood disorder characterized by protein and energy malnutrition, resulting in dry skin, loss of adipose tissue from normal areas of fat deposits such as buttocks and thighs, and behavior that is fretful and irritable.

Maturity-onset diabetes of youth (MODY) see Diabetes mellitus.

McArdle disease a metabolic disorder involving an enzyme defect that causes deficiency of muscle phosphorylase, which helps break down glycogen, and consequently this disorder causes an energy deficit in the muscles, resulting in muscle pain and cramping.

Meconium ileus obstruction with thickened meconium in the intestine of a newborn child as a result of a lack of trypsin and associated with cystic fibrosis of the pancreas.

Medulloblastoma a malignant cerebellar tumor near the fourth ventricle that is most often found in children and consists of neoplastic cells that resemble the undifferentiated cells of the neural tube.

Melanoma a malignant tumor of the skin originating from the transformation of melanocytes.

Membranoproliferative glomerulonephritis (MPGN) see Glomerulonephritis.

Membranous glomerulonephritis see Glomerulonephritis.

Membranous nephropathy (membranous glomerulonephritis) see Glomerulonephritis.

Ménière disease (endolymphatic hydrops) dilation of the membranous labyrinth of the inner ear that is thought to be due to impaired absorption of endolymph in the endolymphatic sac; the pathologic finding in Ménière disease.

Ménière syndrome an affliction characterized clinically by vertigo, nausea, vomiting, tinnitus, and fluctuating and progressive sensory hearing loss associated with endolymphatic hydrops.

Meningioma a slow-growing mass of the meninges that is usually benign but increases intracranial pressure.

Meningocele neural tube defect in the skull or spinal column that forms a cyst filled with cerebrospinal fluid through which the meninges of the brain protrude.

Mesangial proliferative glomerulonephritis see Glomerulonephritis.

Mesenteric venous thrombosis a condition in which a blood clot obstructs one of the mesenteric veins and compromises the intestinal blood supply; can result in intestinal gangrene and tissue death.

Mesothelioma a type of cancer that is usually associated with previous exposure to asbestos, which affects the pleura, the lining of the abdominal cavity, the pericardium, and most internal organ coverings.

Metabolic acidosis a condition in which the concentration of non–carbonic acids increases or bicarbonate (base) is lost from the extracellular fluid or cannot be regenerated by the kidney.

Metabolic syndrome a condition of unknown cause that presents with symptoms of insulin resistance, obesity, hypertension, dyslipidemia, and systemic inflammation.

Metatarsus adductus a foot deformity in which the front half of the foot bends inward, possibly because of the infant's position in the uterus.

Methicillin-resistant *Staphylococcus aureus* (MRSA) an infection that carries the extrachromosomal gene *mecA* for resistance to methicillin and has less sensitivity to inhibition by antibiotics.

MHC class I deficiency see Immune deficiency.

MHC class II deficiency see Immune deficiency.

Microcephaly a defect in which failure of normal brain growth causes delayed skull growth and production of a small head.

Microcytic-hypochromic anemia see Anemia.

Microscopic colitis a relatively common cause of diarrhea; occurs primarily in females and older adults.

Migraine headache a headache that usually begins in the temporal region unilaterally after vascular changes of cranial arteries and may cause irritability, nausea, vomiting, constipation or diarrhea, and photophobia.

Mild concussion (mild traumatic brain injury) temporary axonal disturbances without the loss of consciousness in response to a violent blow, jarring, shaking, or other closed-head injury.

Miliaria a skin disease caused by partially obstructed sweat glands that results in small and itchy rashes usually located in skinfolds and on areas of the body that may rub against clothing, such as the back, chest, and stomach.

Minimal change nephropathy (MCN) the foot processes of the renal capillary basement membrane are fused and deformed because of a T-cell disorder that reduces the anion component of the basement membrane and allows proteins to leak into the renal tubule.

Minimally conscious state (MCS) a condition in which a severely brain-damaged patient is capable of deliberate behavior distinguishable from unconscious reflexive actions.

Mitral valve prolapse syndrome the mitral valve cannot close properly because of one or both flaps being too large, possibly resulting in mitral valve regurgitation.

Mixed precocious puberty development of some secondary sex characteristics of the opposite sex (virilization of a girl or feminization of a boy); usually evident at birth and rare in older children.

Molluscum contagiosum a viral infection of the skin occurring in young children that affects the body, arms, and legs; it is spread through direct contact, saliva, or shared articles of clothing and is considered a sexually transmitted disease in adults, affecting the genitals, lower abdomen, buttocks, and inner thighs.

Monoclonal gammopathy of undetermined significance (MGUS) production of monoclonal antibodies by noncancerous plasma cells that accumulate in the blood.

Motility diarrhea diarrhea caused by excessive motility decreases transit time, mucosal surface contact, and fluid absorption secondary to resection of the small intestine (short bowel syndrome), surgical bypass of an area of the intestine, fistula formation between loops of intestine, irritable bowel syndrome–diarrhea predominant, diabetic neuropathy, hyperthyroidism, and laxative abuse.

Moyamoya disease an abnormality of the blood vessels that supply the frontal region of the brain in which vessels constrict or become completely occluded, resulting in diminished blood flow. The body attempts to compensate by growing new vessels at the base of the brain, which appear as a puff of smoke on angiography.

Mucoepidermoid carcinoma a tumor of the main or lobar bronchi lumen that may extend into the peribronchial tissue.

Mucolipidosis (ML) accumulation of both carbohydrates and lipids.

Mucopolysaccharidosis carbohydrate excess disorders.

Mucopurulent cervicitis (MPC) inflammation of the cervix with purulent endocervical exudate that may be asymptomatic or cause abnormal vaginal discharge and vaginal bleeding.

Mucosa-associated lymphoid tissue (MALT) lymphoma see Lymphoma.

Multiple myeloma (MM) most common and most aggressive plasma cell tumor; a clonal plasma cell cancer characterized by the slow proliferation of malignant cells as tumor cells form masses in the bone marrow that usually result in destruction of the bone; most secrete large amounts of monoclonal proteins that resemble intact immunoglobulins.

Multiple organ dysfunction syndrome (MODS) progressive disease often involving the ultimate failure of two or more organ systems after a severe illness or injury; disease process is initiated and perpetuated by uncontrolled systemic inflammatory and stress responses and is characterized by a hypermetabolic and hyperdynamic state that persists as organ dysfunction develops.

Multiple papilloma (diffuse papillomatosis) a minimum of five papillomas within a localized segment of breast tissue.

Multiple sclerosis (MS) chronic demyelinating disease of the central nervous system that causes inflammation and scarring of myelin sheaths.

Muscular dystrophy a general term for a number of hereditary, progressive degenerative disorders affecting skeletal muscles, and often other organ systems.

Myasthenia gravis neuromuscular disorder caused by an autoimmune response in which antibodies to acetylcholine receptors impair neuromuscular transmission.

Mycosis fungoides see Lymphoma.

Myelodysplastic syndrome (MDS) a group of hematologic conditions characterized by ineffective production of blood cells, resulting in anemia that requires chronic blood transfusion.

Myoadenylate deaminase deficiency (MDD) a genetic disorder in which an enzyme deficiency prevents the conversion of adenosine monophosphate (AMP) to inosine monophosphate, resulting in increased AMP loss and the inability to synthesize adenosine triphosphate for energy.

Myocardial infarction a heart condition of sudden onset in which muscle tissue dies because of a lack of blood flow, resulting in varying degrees of chest pain or discomfort, weakness, sweating, nausea and vomiting, and possibly loss of consciousness.

Myositis inflammation of a muscle, usually a voluntary muscle, resulting in pain, tenderness, and sometimes spasm in the affected area.

Myositis ossificans a condition in which bone is deposited in muscle tissue, causing pain and swelling.

Myxedema cutaneous edema caused by deposition of connective tissue (e.g., glycosaminoglycans and hyaluronic acid) and associated with hypothyroidism and Graves disease; characterized by dry skin, pretibial myxedema, swelling around the lips and nose, mental deterioration, and a decrease in basal metabolic rate.

N

Necrotizing enterocolitis (NEC) a condition of extensive ulceration and necrosis of the ileum and colon in premature infants during the neonatal period.

Necrotizing fasciitis a rare, rapidly spreading inflammation starting in the fascia, muscles, and subcutaneous fat with subsequent necrosis of the overlying skin; it is initiated by bacterial infection and treated with antibiotics; often requires surgical débridement.

Neonatal alloimmune thrombocytopenic purpura (NATP) see Thrombocytopenia.

Neonatal purpura fulminans a fatal syndrome found in neonates who are homozygous or double heterozygous for types I and II protein deficiency.

Nephritic syndrome a disorder of the glomerular filtration membrane in which plasma proteins and red blood cells pass into the urine, resulting in mild proteinuria, hematuria, and mild hypertension.

Nephroblastoma (Wilms tumor) a malignant renal tumor of young children that compresses the normal kidney parenchyma, causing an abdominal mass, blood in the urine, and fever and may be associated with anorexia, vomiting, and malaise; often inherited as an autosomal dominant trait.

Nephrotic syndrome a disorder of the glomerular filtration membrane that permits proteins to pass into the urine, resulting in proteinuria, hypoalbuminemia, hyperlipidemia, and systemic edema.

Neural tube defect (NTD) lack of closure of the neural groove caused by an arrest of the normal development of the brain and spinal cord during the first month of embryonic development.

Neuroblastoma a malignant tumor containing neuroblast cells that originate in the autonomic nervous system or the adrenal medulla; is most common in infants and young children.

Neurogenic shock (vasogenic shock) a type of shock caused by the sudden loss of the sympathetic nervous system signals to the smooth muscle in vessel walls, causing the vessels to relax and a decrease in peripheral vascular resistance and blood pressure.

Neuroleptic malignant syndrome hyperthermia with autonomic and extrapyramidal side effects caused by the administration of neuroleptic drugs.

NK-cell neoplasm see Lymphoma.

Nonalcoholic fatty liver disease (NAFLD) accumulation of fat in hepatocytes, primarily in the form of triglycerides, occurring either in the absence of alcohol or with little alcohol intake; causes progressive inflammation and scarring that is usually asymptomatic for years.

Nonalcoholic steatohepatitis (NASH) a more serious form of nonalcoholic fatty liver disease resulting from hepatocellular injury, inflammation, and fibrosis; this condition is difficult to distinguish from alcohol-induced liver fibrosis; may progress to cirrhosis, end-stage liver disease, and an increased risk for hepatocellular carcinoma.

Nonbacterial infectious cystitis see Painful bladder syndrome/interstitial cystitis (PBS/IC).

Nonbacterial prostatitis prostatitis causes chronic pain that disappears and returns without warning but shows no signs of bacterial infection in the prostatic fluid even though the semen and other fluids from the prostate contain immune cells that the body produces in response to infection.

Non-Hodgkin lymphoma (NHL) see Lymphoma.

Noninfectious cystitis see Painful bladder syndrome/interstitial cystitis (PBS/IC).

Noninflammatory acne see Acne.

Noninflammatory joint disease a disease in which alterations in the structure or mechanics of the joint result in pain during motion.

Nonoliguric renal failure excretion of more than 500 mL/day of urine concurrent with renal failure; although adequate volume of urine is excreted, renal tubules have impaired reabsorption and concentration and dilution function so that filtration is defective, resulting in accumulation of uremic toxins in the blood.

Nonossifying fibroma (fibrous cortical deficit) a benign fibrous tissue tumor forms in the metaphysis of any of the long bones but usually occurs in the thigh and shin bones in children and adolescents.

Nonpuerperal hyperprolactinemia the presence of excessive amounts of prolactin (the pituitary hormone that stimulates milk production) in the blood not related to pregnancy or childbirth; most common cause of galactorrhea.

Nonsyndromic craniosynostosis (see Craniosynostosis) the premature closure of one or more of the cranial sutures during the first 18 to 20 months of an infant's life, but an isolated defect unrelated to syndrome.

Normocytic-normochromic anemia (NNA) see Anemia.

O

Obesity hypoventilation syndrome (pickwickian syndrome) a condition of severely overweight individuals related to the inability to breathe rapidly or deeply enough to maintain adequate blood oxygen levels; characterized by obstructive sleep apnea, somnolence, hypoventilation, erythrocytosis, and heart failure.

Obsessive-compulsive disorder (OCD) an anxiety disorder characterized by obsessive thoughts and repetitive compulsive actions, such as cleaning, checking, or counting.

Obstructive jaundice jaundice related to extrahepatic or intrahepatic obstruction.

Obstructive pulmonary disease airway obstruction that is worse with expiration so that more force or more time is required to expire a given volume of air and emptying of the lungs is slowed; characterized by shortness of breath (dyspnea) and wheezing.

Obstructive sleep apnea syndrome (OSAS) a disorder of sleep characterized by airway obstruction and episodes of apnea accompanied by snoring.

Obstructive uropathy the blockage of urine flow, often by ureteral or kidney stones, resulting in the reflux of urine and subsequent injury to kidneys.

Onychomycosis a fungal infection of the fingernails or toenails that causes thickening, roughness, and splitting of the nails.

Oophoritis inflammation of the ovaries.

Open pneumothorax (communicating pneumothorax) see Pneumothorax.

Optic glioma tumor originating from glial cells in the brain that affects the optic nerve; commonly seen in children with neurofibromatosis.

Organic brain syndrome a constellation of physical brain disorders with psychologic or behavioral signs and symptoms and grouped according to symptoms rather than etiology.

Orthopnea shortness of breath (dyspnea) that occurs when an individual lies flat and is common in individuals with heart failure.

Orthostatic (postural) hypotension a sudden drop in blood pressure when a person assumes a standing position, resulting in dizziness, lightheadedness, blurred vision, and temporary loss of consciousness.

Osmotic diarrhea nonabsorbable substance in the intestine draws water into the lumen by osmosis, resulting in large-volume diarrhea; caused by drinking solutions with excessive sugars, salt, or vitamin C; maldigestion syndromes.

Osteoarthritis (OA) inflammatory degenerative joint disease in which synthesis and degradation of the articular cartilage in the movable joints are altered, resulting in wearing and destruction of cartilage.

Osteochondrosis (Osgood-Schlatter disease) a condition in children that results from the tendons pulling on the epiphysis of long bones, causing pain just below the knee, irritation and swelling, and possibly abnormal bone growth.

Osteogenesis imperfecta (brittle bone disease) a genetic disease in which collagen production is deficient, making the bones abnormally fragile and causing recurring fractures with only minimal trauma, deformity of long bones, a bluish coloration of the sclerae, and often the development of otosclerosis.

Osteoid osteoma a benign tumor in one of the bones of the lower extremities that is painful and is characterized by vascularized connective tissue and osteoid material that is surrounded by a large zone of thickened bone.

Osteomalacia a disease in which vitamin D or calcium deficiency or excessive renal phosphate loss causes a softening of the bones with accompanying pain and weakness.

Osteomyelitis a bacterial infection of the bone and bone marrow that occurs through open fractures, penetrating wounds, surgical operations, or by infiltration of the bloodstream; causes pain, high fever, and formation of an abscess at the site of infection.

Osteoporosis a disease in which the bones become porous and weakened, making bones easily fracture and slow to heal.

Overactive bladder syndrome (OAB) a chronic syndrome of overactivity of the detrusor muscle; characterized by urgency with involuntary detrusor contractions during the bladder filling phase.

Oxygen toxicity an iatrogenic inflammatory condition caused by prolonged exposure to high concentrations of supplemental oxygen resulting from damage to alveolocapillary membranes, disruption of surfactant production, and interstitial and alveolar edema; caused by oxygen free radicals.

P

Paget disease of bone (PDB or osteitis deformans) a bone disorder in which excessive bone remodeling causes enlarged, deformed bones that can weaken the bone integrity and result in bone pain, arthritis, deformities, or fractures.

Painful bladder syndrome/interstitial cystitis (PBS/IC) (see Cystitis) a condition occurring in women ages 20 to 40 years who have symptoms of cystitis, such as frequency, urgency, dysuria, and nocturia, for more than 6 weeks' duration; usually related to bacterial infection.

Nonbacterial infectious cystitis cystitis with negative urine cultures and no other known etiology; most common in immunocompromised individuals and related to viral, mycobacterial, chlamydial, or fungal infection.

Noninfectious cystitis cystitis without evidence of infection; usually autoimmune or related to exposure to radiation or chemotherapy treatment for pelvic or urogenital cancers.

Panacinar emphysema see Emphysema.

Pancreatic insufficiency a condition in which the pancreas does not secrete enough hormones and digestive enzymes for normal digestion to occur, resulting in malabsorption, malnutrition, vitamin deficiencies, and weight loss.

Pancreatitis inflammation of the pancreas, usually resulting in abdominal pain.

Panhypopituitarism a condition in which the secretion of all anterior pituitary hormones is inadequate or absent; caused by a variety of disorders that result in destruction or loss of function of all or most of the anterior pituitary gland.

Panic disorder a psychologic disorder that is characterized by recurrent attacks of anxiety or terror and usually results in the development of one or more phobias.

Papulosquamous disorder collective reference to inflammatory disorders characterized by papules, scales, plaques, and erythema, including psoriasis, pityriasis rosea, and lichen planus.

Paraesophageal hiatal hernia herniation of the greater curvature of the stomach through a secondary opening in the diaphragm.

Paralytic ileus also known as *functional obstruction*, it is a failure of motility after intestinal or abdominal surgery, acute pancreatitis, or hypokalemia.

Paraneoplastic pemphigus see Pemphigus.

Paraphimosis a condition in which the foreskin becomes trapped behind the glans penis and cannot return to its normal flaccid position covering the glans penis.

Parkinson disease degeneration of the basal ganglia dopaminergic nigrostriatal pathway that causes hypokinesia, tremor, and muscular rigidity.

Parkinsonism (Parkinson syndrome, parkinsonian syndrome) a neurologic condition characterized by tremors, rigidity, hypokinesia, and postural instability as a result of degeneration of the corpus striatum or substantia nigra caused by Parkinson disease and other conditions related to toxins or metabolic conditions.

Paronychia an acute or chronic infection of the cuticle. One or more fingers or toes may be involved.

Paroxysmal nocturnal dyspnea (PND) attacks of breathing discomfort, shortness of breath, and coughing that occur at night with varying intensity so that individuals must sit up or stand to relieve dyspnea; may occur in individuals with heart failure or lung disease.

Partial obstruction of the bladder outlet or urethra partial obstruction related to deposition of collagen within the smooth muscle bundles of the detrusor muscle; causes an increase in the force of detrusor contraction.

Partial precocious puberty the partial development of appropriate secondary sex characteristics alone or in combination.

Pediculosis pubis a contagious condition, also known as *crabs* or *crab lice,* that is an infestation of the pubic hair in which the louse feeds on human blood and multiplies rapidly.

Pelvic inflammatory disease (PID) inflammation of the female genital tract caused by microorganisms, typically those that are sexually transmitted such as chlamydia and gonococci; characterized by severe abdominal pain, high fever, vaginal discharge, and possibly infertility.

Pelvic organ prolapse (POP) bladder outlet obstruction in women caused most commonly by a cystocele (the downward protrusion of the bladder into the vagina) that descends below the level of the urethral outlet.

Pemphigus a category of autoimmune skin diseases marked by groups of itching blisters and raw sores on the skin and mucous membranes.

Paraneoplastic pemphigus the most severe form of pemphigus; is associated with lymphoproliferative neoplasms and affects internal organs, including lungs, thyroid, kidney, smooth muscle, and gastrointestinal tract.

Pemphigus foliaceus a milder form of pemphigus involving loss of cell-to-cell adhesion (acantholysis) at the subcorneal level with blistering, erosions, scaling, crusting, and erythema usually of the face and chest.

Pemphigus vulgaris the most common form of pemphigus with acantholysis at the suprabasal level and initiated by IgG autoantibodies against the desmoglein adhesion molecules, resulting in acantholysis in the epidermis with fluid accumulation and blister formation; oral lesions precede the onset of skin blistering.

Pericarditis the pericardium is infected by a virus, bacteria, parasite, or fungus and becomes inflamed, resulting in pain and fluid and blood components entering into the pericardial space.

Perihepatitis (Fitz-Hugh–Curtis syndrome) a complication of pelvic inflammatory disease secondary to gonococci bacteria traveling up the peritoneum to the upper abdomen and causing inflammation.

Periodic paralysis one of a group of diseases in which muscular weakness or flaccid paralysis occurs without loss of consciousness, speech, or sensation.

Peripheral artery disease (PAD) any of a group of diseases caused by the obstruction of large peripheral arteries secondary to atherosclerosis, inflammatory processes, embolism, or thrombus formation that causes ischemia.

Pernicious anemia see Anemia.

Pes planus (flatfoot) a condition in which the arch of the foot never develops or it collapses and contacts the ground.

Peyronie disease (bent nail syndrome) a condition in which fibrous plaques grow in the soft tissue of the penis because of injury of the internal cavity of the penis that is accompanied by bleeding and scar tissue formation at the tunica albuginea of the corpora cavernosa.

Phagocytic deficiency see Immune deficiency.

Phenylketonuria (PKU) a genetic disorder in which the body lacks the enzyme necessary to metabolize the amino acid phenylalanine to tyrosine, resulting in accumulation of phenylalanine and subsequent brain damage and progressive mental retardation.

Pheochromocytoma a tumor of the adrenal medulla that causes the chromaffin cells to secrete increased amounts of epinephrine or norepinephrine.

Phimosis the foreskin of the penis of an uncircumcised male cannot be fully retracted.

Pick disease progressive atrophy of the cerebral convolutions in a limited area (lobe) of the brain, with clinical manifestations and course similar to those of Alzheimer disease.

Pityriasis rosea a skin disorder, thought to be caused by a virus, in which patches of ovular pink rash appear primarily on the trunk and extremities.

Plaque psoriasis see Psoriasis.

Pneumoconiosis a chronic disease of the lungs typically seen in miners, sandblasters, and metal grinders that is caused by repeated inhalation of dust particles, including iron oxides, silicates, and carbonates, that collect in the lungs and become sites for the formation of fibrous nodules that eventually replace lung tissue.

Pneumonia an infection of one or both lungs caused by a bacterium, virus, fungus, or other organism that enters the body through respiratory passages and causes high fever, chills, chest pain, difficulty breathing, cough with sputum, and possibly bluish skin from insufficiently oxygenated blood.

Pneumothorax the collapse of a lung and subsequent escape of air into the pleural cavity between the lung and the chest wall that is caused by trauma, environmental factors, or spontaneous occurrence and results in a sudden pain in the chest.

Iatrogenic pneumothorax the presence of air or gas in the pleural space caused by a rupture in the visceral pleura (which surrounds the lungs) or the parietal pleura and chest wall; is most commonly caused by transthoracic needle aspiration.

Open pneumothorax (communicating pneumothorax) spontaneous and traumatic pneumothorax in which air pressure in the pleural space equals barometric pressure because air that is drawn into the pleural space during inspiration (through the damaged chest wall and parietal pleura or through the lungs and damaged visceral pleura) is forced out during expiration.

Primary (spontaneous) pneumothorax occurs unexpectedly in healthy individuals (usually men) between ages 20 and 40 years; is most often caused by the spontaneous rupture of blebs on the visceral pleura.

Secondary (traumatic) pneumothorax spontaneous or secondary pneumothorax beginning with sudden pleural pain, tachypnea, and possibly mild dyspnea.

Tension pneumothorax the site of pleural rupture acts as a one-way valve, permitting air to enter on inspiration, but preventing its escape by closing during expiration and leading to air pressure in the pneumothorax exceeding barometric pressure.

Polycystic ovary syndrome (PCOS) a hormonal condition in which multiple ovarian cysts form because of elevated levels of androgens, resulting in hirsutism, obesity, menstrual abnormalities, infertility, and enlarged ovaries.

Polycythemia vera a chronic, progressive disease that is characterized by overgrowth of the bone marrow, excessive red blood cell production, and an enlarged spleen and causes headache, inability to concentrate, and pain in the fingers and toes.

Pompe disease see Acid maltase deficiency.

Port-wine (nevus flammeus) stain a birthmark caused by superficial and deep dilated capillaries in the skin that produce a reddish to purplish discoloration of the skin, usually on the face, but can occur anywhere on the body.

Postconcussive syndrome physical and personality changes that may occur after concussion of the brain, including amnesia, headache, dizziness, tinnitus, irritability, fatigability, sweating, heart palpitations, insomnia, and difficulty concentrating.

Posthemorrhagic anemia see Anemia.

Postobstructive pulmonary edema (POPE) (negative pressure pulmonary edema) a rare life-threatening complication that can occur after relief of upper airway obstruction (e.g., postextubation laryngospasm after anesthesia induction, epiglottitis, laryngeal tumor, or obstructive tonsils).

Postrenal acute kidney injury rare complication of urinary tract obstruction that affects the kidneys bilaterally (e.g., bilateral ureteral obstruction, bladder outlet obstruction–prostatic hypertrophy, tumors or neurogenic bladder, and urethral obstruction); obstruction causes an increase in intraluminal pressure upstream from the site of obstruction.

Postthrombotic syndrome (PTS) a syndrome that follows a vascular thrombosis, such as persistent edema.

Posttraumatic stress disorder (PTSD) a psychologic disorder that may develop in individuals who have experienced or witnessed traumatic events; is characterized by recurrent flashbacks of the traumatic event, nightmares, irritability, anxiety, fatigue, forgetfulness, and social withdrawal.

Potter syndrome a syndrome of renal agenesis with hypoplastic lungs and associated neonatal respiratory distress, hemodynamic instability, acidosis, cyanosis, edema, and characteristic (Potter) facies; death usually occurs from respiratory insufficiency, which develops before uremia.

Poverty of content a disorder, also called *poverty of speech content,* that is characterized by disorganized speech that conveys little information and may be vague or contain repetitive or obscure phrases.

Prader-Willi syndrome a rare genetic disorder caused by gene deletions on paternal chromosome 15 that result in short stature, hypotonia, small hands and feet, obesity, mild to moderate mental retardation, and hypogonadism.

Precocious puberty a condition in which a boy or girl undergoes the changes associated with puberty at an unexpectedly early age; often caused by a pathologic process that increases the secretion of estrogens or androgens.

Premenstrual dysphoric disorder (PMDD) recurrence in the luteal phase of the menstrual cycle of distressing physical, psychologic, or behavioral changes that impair interpersonal relationships or interfere with usual activities.

Premenstrual syndrome (PMS) a group of symptoms that occur in many women from 2 to 14 days before menstruation begins, including abdominal bloating, breast tenderness, headache, fatigue, irritability, depression, and emotional distress.

Prerenal acute kidney injury rapid development of renal hypoperfusion with elevation of serum creatinine and urea levels.

Presbyopia a form of farsightedness usually accompanying advanced age in which the lens loses elasticity and becomes unable to accommodate and focus light for near vision.

Priapism a painful condition in which the erect penis maintains an erection in the absence of physical and psychologic stimulation.

Primary accidental hypothermia unintentional drop in core body temperature below 35°C (95°F) of a previously healthy person attributable to the changes that occur with cold temperatures.

Primary adrenal insufficiency (Addison disease) adrenal hypofunction resulting in bronzelike pigmentation of the skin, severe prostration, progressive anemia, low blood pressure, diarrhea, and digestive disturbance.

Primary amenorrhea continued absence of menarche and menstrual function by 14 years of age without the development of secondary sex characteristics or by age 16 years if these changes have occurred.

Primary biliary cirrhosis see Cirrhosis.

Primary (congenital) immune deficiency see Immune deficiency.

Primary dysmenorrhea painful menstruation because of a functional disturbance rather than because of inflammation, growths, or anatomic factors.

Primary gout acute episodes of urate crystal–induced synovitis resulting from abnormality of purine metabolism; lower-than-normal urinary excretion of urate leads to hyperuricemia and acute episodes of joint inflammation.

Primary hyperaldosteronism (Conn disease, primary aldosteronism) an adrenocortical disorder caused by excessive secretion of aldosterone and characterized by headaches, nocturia, polyuria, fatigue, hypertension, potassium depletion, hypokalemic alkalosis, hypervolemia, and decreased plasma renin activity; may be associated with small benign adrenocortical adenomas.

Primary hyperparathyroidism usually the result of a benign parathyroid tumor that secretes parathyroid hormone and increases circulating calcium levels; this condition is accompanied by hypercalcemia, nausea, vomiting, lethargy, depression, muscular weakness, and an altered mental state.

Primary hypertension (essential hypertension, idiopathic hypertension) elevated blood pressure of unknown etiology accompanied by increased total peripheral vascular resistance as a result of vasoconstriction, increased cardiac output, or both.

Primary multiple organ dysfunction syndrome (MODS) multiple organ injury directly associated with a specific insult, most often ischemia or impaired perfusion from an episode of shock or trauma, thermal injury, soft tissue necrosis, or invasive infection with decreased local perfusion in the injured organs.

Primary (spontaneous) pneumothorax see Pneumothorax.

Primary syphilis a stage of syphilis infection that occurs after an incubation period of 10 to 90 days and is characterized by a primary sore or chancre that develops at the point of initial exposure and lasts 4 to 6 weeks.

Prinzmetal angina a form of angina pectoris characterized by pain that is not precipitated by cardiac work; it is of longer duration and usually more severe, and is associated with unusual electrocardiographic results including elevated ST segments.

Progressive bulbar palsy (see Bulbar palsy) a slowly progressive neurodegenerative disorder of the motor neurons of the cerebral cortex, spinal cord, and brainstem, resulting in progressive symptoms of bulbar palsy that may advance to loss of ability to manipulate food in the mouth, inability to swallow, choking, and emotional changes; may lead to aspiration of food and fluid and death from pneumonia.

Progressive spinal muscular atrophy a progressive degenerative disorder of the motor neurons of the spinal cord causing muscular weakness and wasting, typically beginning in the distal portions of the limbs and spreading proximally.

Prolactinoma the most common type of anterior pituitary tumor; produces visual disturbances and prolactin excess that results in infertility and changes in menstruation in females and in impotence, loss of libido, and infertility in males.

Properdin deficiency see Immune deficiency.

Prostatitis inflammation of the prostate gland caused by urinary tract infection.

Protein C deficiency a disorder characterized by a lack of anticoagulant activity and an increased tendency to form blood clots because of decreased degradation of factor Va and factor VIIIa secondary to thrombosis, deep vein thrombosis, pulmonary embolism, thrombophlebitis, neonatal purpura fulminans, and disseminated intravascular coagulation.

Protein S deficiency a disorder characterized by a lack of anticoagulant activity and an increased tendency to form blood clots because of decreased degradation of factor Va and factor VIIIa.

Pseudothrombocytopenia see Thrombocytopenia.

Psoriasis a noncontagious autoimmune skin disorder in which the skin becomes scaly and inflamed when cells in the outer layer of skin reproduce faster than normal and accumulate as plaques on the skin surface.

Erythrodermic (exfoliative) psoriasis widespread red, scaling lesions that cover a large body surface area; often accompanied by itching or pain associated with constitutional symptoms (fever, chills, fatigue) and skin infections.

Guttate psoriasis sudden appearance of small papules on the trunk and extremities, occasionally after a streptococcal respiratory tract infection in children.

Inverse psoriasis rare development of large, smooth, dry, and deep red lesions in skinfolds (i.e., axilla or groin).

Plaque psoriasis most common form of psoriasis; begins with well-demarcated, thick, silvery, scaly erythematosus inflammatory lesions with epidermal hyperproliferation and the presence of activated T lymphocytes that may become mild, moderate, or severe, depending on the size, distribution, and inflammation of the lesions.

Pustular psoriasis blisters of noninfectious pus that develop over areas of plaque psoriasis.

Pulmonary artery hypertension (PAH) increased blood pressure in the pulmonary artery attributable to vasoconstriction that may eventually lead to fibrosis, increased workload, hypertrophy of the right ventricle, and right heart failure; etiology may be idiopathic, familial, or associated with other diseases.

Pulmonary embolism (PE) dislodgement of a blood clot from its site of origin and embolization to the arterial blood supply of one of the lungs, resulting in shortness of breath and difficulty breathing, rapid breathing that is painful, cough, and (in severe cases) hypotension, shock, loss of consciousness, and death.

Pulmonary stenosis a condition in which the opening into the pulmonary artery from the right ventricle narrows.

Pure red cell aplasia (PRCA) an acquired or congenital condition in which the bone marrow lacks red blood cell precursors even though megakaryocytes and white blood cell precursors are usually present at normal levels.

Purine nucleoside phosphorylase (PNP) deficiency see Immune deficiency.

Pustular psoriasis see Psoriasis.

Pyloric stenosis a congenital abnormality in which the pylorus is narrow, resulting in poor feeding, weight loss, and progressively worsening vomiting.

Pyramidal/spastic cerebral palsy palsy resulting from damage or defects in the brain's corticospinal pathways (upper motor neuron) in either one or both hemispheres.

Q

Qualitative leukocyte disorder see Immune deficiency.

Quantitative leukocyte disorder see Immune deficiency.

R

RAG-1/RAG-2 deficiencies see Immune deficiency.

Rapidly progressive (crescentic) glomerulonephritis (RPGN) see Glomerulonephritis.

Raynaud disease a condition in which the blood vessels spasm because of inadequate blood supply, resulting in discoloration of the fingers and/or toes after exposure to changes in temperature or emotional events.

Raynaud phenomenon a condition caused by the temperature-dependent deposition of immune complexes in the capillary beds of the peripheral circulation, which blocks the circulation and causes localized pallor and numbness, followed by cyanosis and eventually gangrene if the circulation is not restored.

Rectocele a condition caused by childbirth or hysterectomy in which the region between the rectum and vagina bulges toward the vagina, resulting in a sense of pressure or protrusion within the vagina, the feeling of incomplete emptying of the rectum, difficulty passing stool, discomfort or pain during evacuation or intercourse, constipation, vaginal bleeding, fecal incontinence, prolapse of the bulge through the opening of the vagina, or rectal prolapse through the anus.

Refeeding syndrome metabolic disturbances that occur upon initiating parenteral or enteral nutritional therapy to individuals who are severely malnourished; starvation results in movement of phosphate, magnesium, and potassium ions out of the cells and into the plasma and refeeding increases insulin levels and stimulates movement of glucose and these ions back into the cells, resulting in dangerously low levels in the plasma (hypophosphatemia, hypomagnesemia, hypokalemia, hyponatremia, hypocalcemia, and vitamin deficiency) and other potentially fatal metabolic complications.

Relative polycythemia a relative increase in the number of red blood cells caused by loss of the fluid portion of the blood.

Renal agenesis only one functional kidney is present at birth.

Renal calculi (nephrolithiasis) also called *urinary stones (urolithiasis)*; masses of crystals, protein, or other substances that can be located in the kidneys, ureters, and urinary bladder and are a common cause of urinary tract obstruction in adults.

Renal cell carcinoma (RCC) the most common renal neoplasm (approximately 80% of all renal neoplasms).

Renal dysplasia abnormal tissue development in one or both kidneys.

Respiratory acidosis occurs when there is alveolar hypoventilation. Carbon dioxide is retained, increasing $[H^+]$ (as H_2CO_3), thus decreasing the ratio of HCO_3^- to P_{CO_2} and producing acidosis.

Respiratory alkalosis occurs when there is alveolar hyperventilation and decreased concentration of plasma carbon dioxide (termed *hypocapnia*), thus increasing the ratio of HCO_3^- to P_{CO_2} (H_2CO_3).

Respiratory distress syndrome (RDS) of the newborn a condition, also known as *hyaline membrane disease (HMD)*, that is a type of respiratory distress in newborns, most often in prematurely born infants, those born by cesarean section, or those having a diabetic mother; the immature lungs do not produce enough surfactant to retain air so the air spaces empty completely and collapse after exhalation.

Reticular dysgenesis see Immune deficiency.

Retinoblastoma an autosomal dominant or sporadic disorder in which a malignant tumor forms in the retina of one or both eyes; typically found in infants.

Reversible sideroblastic anemia see Anemia.

Rhabdomyolysis a potentially fatal condition in which skeletal muscle breaks down as a result of injury such as physical damage to the muscle, high fever, metabolic disorders, excessive exertion, convulsions, or anoxia of the muscle for several hours; large amounts of myoglobin are usually excreted.

Rheumatic fever an inflammatory disease that is associated with recent streptococcal infection and causes inflammation of the joints, fever, jerky movements, nodules under the skin, and skin rash and often is followed by serious heart damage or disease secondary to antibodies that react both with streptococcal antigens and with those of the heart valve.

Rheumatic heart disease (RHD) sequela to rheumatic fever in which heart valves are repeatedly inflamed, developing fibrosis and thickening that can result in valve deformities, stenosis, or regurgitation.

Rheumatoid arthritis an autoimmune disease that causes chronic inflammation of the joints and the tissue around the joints and other organs.

Rickets a bone disease that is caused by a deficiency of vitamin D or calcium and manifests in children as softening of bones, abnormal growth of bones, and enlargement of cartilage at the ends of long bones.

Ringed sideroblast an erythroblast in which one-third or more of the nucleus is encircled by 10 or more siderotic granules that may be caused by antituberculous drugs and alcohol abuse.

Roseola a viral disease in infants and young children that causes fever and a spotty rash that appears shortly after the fever has subsided.

Rotavirus a viral infection seen in young children that causes diarrhea by attacking the lining of the small intestine, resulting in the inability to absorb fluid and electrolytes.

Rubella an infectious viral disease of children and young adults that is spread by a droplet spray from the respiratory tract of an infected individual; the disease causes a rash that lasts about 3 days with tender and swollen lymph nodes behind the ears.

Rubeola an infectious viral disease of young children, also known as *measles*, that is spread by a droplet spray from the nose, mouth, and throat of individuals in the infective stage and causes a rash, white spots in the mouth, a rash on the face that spreads to the rest of the body, and fever.

Russell-Silver syndrome (Russell-Silver dwarfism) a growth disorder manifesting as retardation, proportionate short stature, leg length discrepancy, and a small, triangular-shaped face.

S

Saccular aneurysm (berry aneurysm) a localized, progressively growing sac that affects only a portion of the circumference of the arterial wall and may be the result of congenital anomalies or degeneration.

Saccular bronchiectasis (see Bronchiectasis) bronchiectasis resulting in dilated bronchi that become balloon-like.

Salmon patches (nevus simplex) patches, also known as *stork bites*, of small, pink, flat spots that are small, dilated blood vessels visible through the skin and are usually found on the forehead, eyelids, and upper lip; between the eyebrows; and on the back of the neck.

Salpingitis inflammation of one of the two fallopian tubes caused by infection spreading from the vagina or uterus.

Sarcoma tumor of the connective tissue cells.

Sarcopenia age-related loss in skeletal muscle, which is a direct cause of the age-related decrease in muscle strength.

Scabies skin infestation with the itch mite, *Sarcoptes scabiei*, acquired through close contact with an infected person or contaminated clothing that produces intense itching.

Schizophrenia a psychotic disorder characterized by delusions, hallucinations, loosening of associations, disturbances in mood and sense of self and relationship to the external world, and bizarre, purposeless behavior.

Sclerosing adenosis a condition in which the number of acini per terminal duct is more than twice the number of normal terminal ducts and is associated with a significantly increased risk of subsequent breast carcinoma.

Scoliosis a condition in which the spine is curved sideways to varying degrees; occurs because of either physiologic curvature or functional curvature in which contraction of the paraspinal muscles of the back creates a vertebral curve.

Seborrheic dermatitis scaly, flaky, itchy, and red skin on the scalp, face, and trunk because of a yeast infection.

Seborrheic keratosis a benign proliferation of cutaneous basal cells that produces smooth or warty elevated lesions; seen primarily in older people and presents as multiple lesions on the chest, back, and face.

Secondary amenorrhea menstruation begins at puberty but then is subsequently suppressed for three or more cycles or for 6 months in women who previously menstruated.

Secondary dysmenorrhea altered menstruation because of inflammation, infection, tumor, or anatomic factors.

Secondary generalization the process by which a simple partial seizure involving one hemisphere becomes a generalized seizure involving the second hemisphere.

Secondary hyperparathyroidism a condition of elevated levels of parathyroid hormone resulting from disease such as renal failure in which parathyroid hormone concentration is elevated in response to vitamin D deficiency.

Secondary hypertension a condition of elevated blood pressure that is associated with other conditions, primarily with renal disease by a renin-dependent mechanism or a fluid volume–dependent mechanism.

Secondary hypothermia depressed body temperature as a consequence of a serious systemic disorder, for example, endocrine disorders.

Secondary (acquired) immune deficiency see Immune deficiency.

Secondary MODS the result of an excessive inflammatory reaction, after a latent period following the initial injury, in organs distant from the site of the original injury. It is postulated that the resulting organ trauma is caused by the host response to a second insult rather than being a direct result of the primary injury.

Secondary (traumatic) pneumothorax see Pneumothorax.

Secondary septic arthritis a bacterial infection in the joints, causing them to become inflamed and the bacteria to proliferate.

Secondary syphilis the most contagious stage of syphilis infection; characterized by a skin rash that appears on the trunk and extremities 1 to 6 months after the primary infection and possibly mucous patches on the genitals or inside the mouth.

Selective IgA deficiency see Immune deficiency.

Sepsis severe physiologic stress typically caused by an infection; its complications result from activation of biochemical and physiologic cascades that lead to the formation or activation of cytokines and other mediators that produce vasodilation, increased capillary permeability, maldistribution of blood flow, and cardiovascular and cellular dysfunction.

Septic shock a condition caused by systemic infection that results in decreased tissue perfusion and oxygenation and can lead to multiple organ dysfunction syndrome and death.

Serum sickness a form of hypersensitivity caused by injection of soluble antigen such as antiserum, which activates a type III hypersensitivity response (formation of soluble circulating antigen-antibody [IgG or IgM] complexes) that activates the complement system.

Severe combined immune deficiency (SCID) see Immune deficiency.

Severe congenital neutropenia see Immune deficiency.

Shock a condition in which the circulatory system is unable to provide adequate circulation to the body tissues because of inadequate pumping by the heart, a reduction in blood volume, or a reduction in blood pressure; it results in slowing of vital functions and possibly death.

Short bowel syndrome a group of malabsorption conditions resulting from massive resection of the small bowel, the degree and kind of malabsorption depending on the site and extent of the resection; it is characterized by diarrhea, steatorrhea, and malnutrition.

Sickle cell anemia   see Anemia.

Sickle cell disease (SCD)   see Anemia.

Sickle cell–Hb C disease   see Anemia.

Sickle cell–thalassemia disease   see Anemia.

Sickle cell trait   see Anemia.

Sideroblastic anemia (SA)   see Anemia.

Silicosis   inflammation of the lung resulting from the inhalation of free silica (silicon dioxide) and silica-containing compounds, which occurs in mining and related industries.

Simple febrile seizure   benign and most common form of childhood seizure.

Simple fibroadenoma   benign solid tumors composed of both fibrous and glandular tissue.

Sliding hiatal hernia   the most common type of hernia, occurring when the proximal portion of the stomach moves into the thoracic cavity through the esophageal hiatus, an opening in the diaphragm for the esophagus and vagus nerves.

Small cell lung carcinoma (SCLS)   the most common type of neuroendocrine lung tumor; mostly arise from the central part of the lung.

Smallpox (variola)   an infectious viral disease that is caused by a poxvirus and result in high fever, aches, and widespread eruption of large sores that leave scars.

Smoldering myeloma   a condition in which abnormal plasma cells produce a monoclonal protein, but no symptoms or complications of myeloma are present and may not be present for several years.

Solitary plasmacytoma   a solitary tumor of malignant plasma cells that may result in a single lytic bone lesion or may be in the tissues (extramedullary plasmacytoma).

Spina bifida occulta   the mildest form of congenital disorder of incomplete closure of the embryonic neural tube; the outer part of some vertebrae may not be completely closed, but the defect is not apparent to the unaided eye and usually causes no serious neurologic dysfunctions.

Spinal stenosis   narrowing of the spinal canal as a result of congenital anomaly or spinal degeneration, resulting in pain, paresthesias, and neurogenic claudication.

Spondylolisthesis   forward displacement of one of the lower lumbar vertebrae over the vertebra below it or over the sacrum.

Sprain   a ligament tear, which occurs most commonly in the wrist, ankle, elbow, and knee joints.

Squamous cell carcinoma (SCC)   a tumor of the epidermis and the second most common human cancer.

Stable angina   a condition in which ischemic attacks occur at predictable frequencies and duration after activities that increase myocardial oxygen demands such as exercise and stress.

Staphylococcal scalded-skin syndrome (SSSS)   a disease in infants that is caused by a staphylococcal infection with release of an exfoliative toxin that results in peeling of large areas of skin.

Stevens-Johnson syndrome   an inflammatory eruption of circular lesions that can cover the majority of the skin and mucous membranes and usually occurs after a respiratory tract infection or as an allergic reaction to drugs or other substances.

Strabismus   the deviation of one eye from the other when a person is looking at an object; it results in failure of the two eyes to simultaneously focus on the same image and therefore loss of binocular vision.

Strawberry hemangioma   a red birthmark caused by densely packed blood vessels that usually appears on the face, scalp, back, and chest and disappears during childhood.

Stress ulcer   acute peptic ulcer that occurs in association with various other pathologic conditions, including burns, cor pulmonale, intracranial lesions, and surgical operations.

Structural scoliosis   a side-to-side curvature of the spine.

Subacute thyroiditis (subacute granulomatous thyroiditis, de Quervain thyroiditis)   a painful inflammation of the thyroid that develops suddenly in a patient who has had a viral infection, such as mumps or an upper respiratory tract illness. Pain radiates throughout the neck and patients feel ill and feverish.

Subglottic stenosis   narrowing of the airway below the larynx caused by a congenital anomaly or acquired narrowing secondary to injury, possibly resulting in respiratory distress, cyanotic episodes, or recurrent lung infections.

Subluxation   an injury in which the contact between two joint surfaces is only partially lost.

Sudden infant death syndrome (SIDS)   a syndrome, also known as *crib death,* that is characterized by the sudden, unexpected, and unexplained death of an apparently healthy infant less than 1 year of age.

Superior vena cava syndrome (SVCS)   restriction of the blood flow through the superior vena cava secondary to compression by malignancies or lymphadenopathy.

Sydenham chorea (St. Vitus dance)   a postinfectious chorea appearing several months after a streptococcal infection with subsequent rheumatic fever. The chorea typically involves the distal limbs and is associated with hypotonia and emotional lability.

Symphysis   fibrocartilaginous joint; a type of joint in which the apposed bony surfaces are firmly united by a plate of fibrocartilage.

Synchondrosis   a cartilaginous joint creating a union between two immovable bones, such as the synchondroses of the cranium, the pubic symphysis, the sternum, and the manubrium.

Syndesmosis   a fibrous union in which two bones are connected by interosseous ligaments, such as the anterior and the posterior ligaments in the radioulnar and tibiofibular articulations; is usually converted into bone before adult life.

Syndrome of inappropriate antidiuretic hormone (ADH) secretion (SIADH)   a condition in which the release of ADH from the posterior pituitary is elevated relative to serum sodium levels, resulting in increased water reabsorption by the kidneys and fluid overload.

Syndromic craniosynostosis (see Craniosynostosis)   synostosis that occurs as part of a genetic syndrome; usually associated with various dysmorphisms involving the face, skeleton, and nervous system and usually accompanied by developmental delay.

Syphilis   a chronic infectious disease that is transmitted by direct contact, usually in sexual intercourse, or passed from mother to child in utero, and progresses through three stages characterized by chancres, ulcerous skin eruptions, and systemic infection that leads to damage to the cardiovascular and nervous systems.

Systemic inflammatory response syndrome (SIRS)   a generalized inflammatory response that may lead to depressed cardiac function and decreased organ perfusion.

Systemic lupus erythematosus (SLE) (see Lupus erythematosus)   a chronic, multisystem, inflammatory disease and one of the most common, complex, and serious of the autoimmune disorders.

Systolic heart failure   a condition in which the heart muscle contracts so weakly that insufficient oxygenated blood is pumped throughout the body.

T

Tay-Sachs disease (GM2 gangliosidosis)   a fatal autosomal recessive lysosomal storage disorder in which the lysosomal enzyme hexosaminidase A (HexA) is deficient, leading to accumulation of gangliosides in the brain and nerve tissue, mental retardation, convulsions, blindness, and premature death.

T-cell neoplasm   see Lymphoma.

Tension pneumothorax   see Pneumothorax.

Tertiary syphilis   the most severe stage of syphilis, which can begin as early as 1 year after the initial infection but can take up to 10 years to manifest and is characterized by gummas—soft, tumor-like growths found in the skin and mucous membranes and often in the skeleton—joint deformity, neurosyphilis, and cardiovascular syphilis.

Tethered cord syndrome   a group of neurologic disorders related to malformation of the spinal cord in which the cord becomes abnormally attached or tethered as a result of scar tissue that develops as the cord transcends the vertebral canal with growth; tethering may decrease blood flow.

Tetralogy of Fallot   a congenital condition that is characterized by four malformations including ventricular septal defect, misplacement of the origin of the aorta, narrowing of the pulmonary artery, and enlargement of the right ventricle.

Thalassemia   see Anemia.

Thromboangiitis obliterans (Buerger disease)   inflammation of the medium-sized arteries and veins because of thrombotic occlusion, resulting in ischemia and gangrene.

Thrombocythemia   a chronic disorder of sustained megakaryocyte proliferation that increases the number of circulating platelets and results in megakaryocytic hyperplasia, splenomegaly, and complications by hemorrhagic and thrombotic episodes.

Thrombocytopenia   a reduced number of circulating platelets.

Acute idiopathic thrombotic thrombocytopenic purpura   a form of thrombocytopenic purpura (TTP) characterized by thrombotic microangiopathy in which platelets aggregate and cause occlusion of arterioles and capillaries within the microcirculation, leading to increased platelet consumption and organ ischemia.

Autoimmune neonatal thrombocytopenia destruction of platelets in a fetus/neonate by antiplatelet antibodies produced in the mother against her own platelet antigens (autoimmune) that are shared with the child, and the antibodies are transported across the placenta and destroy the child's platelets.

Chronic relapsing thrombotic thrombocytopenic purpura a rare familial form of TTP characterized by recurring episodes of thrombocytopenia; usually seen in children.

Heparin-induced thrombocytopenia (HIT) a form of drug-induced thrombocytopenia caused by IgG antibodies against the heparin–platelet factor 4 complex leading to platelet activation and thrombocytopenia.

Idiopathic thrombocytopenic purpura (ITP) (autoimmune or primary thrombocytopenic purpura) the most common cause of thrombocytopenia, secondary to increased immune-mediated platelet destruction; can be acute or chronic.

Immune thrombocytopenic purpura (ITP) a condition in which the number of platelets in the blood is reduced by the production of antibodies against platelets, resulting in ecchymoses and hemorrhage from mucous membranes, anemia, and extreme weakness.

Neonatal alloimmune thrombocytopenic purpura (NATP) a condition in which fetal platelets have an antigen from the father that is absent in the mother, and the mother forms antibodies that cross the placenta and destroy the fetal platelets.

Pseudothrombocytopenia an artificially low platelet count in anticoagulated blood caused by cooling of the blood and autoagglutination of platelets.

Thrombotic thrombocytopenic purpura (TTP) altered blood coagulation caused by an enzymatic deficiency that is characterized by a reduced number of platelets in the blood, the formation of blood clots in tissue arterioles and capillaries, and neurologic damage.

Thrombophilia genetic or acquired abnormality of the coagulation system with an increased risk for thrombosis.

Thrombotic thrombocytopenic purpura (TTP) see Thrombocytopenia.

Thrush a yeast infection of the mouth and throat that presents as creamy white curdlike patches on the tongue, inside the mouth, and on the back of the throat and that is commonly associated with yeast infection of the esophagus.

Thyrotoxicosis excessive concentrations of thyroid hormones in the body that are marked by increased metabolic rate, heat intolerance, goiter, reproductive disorders, excessive sweating, and other alterations in systemic function.

Tinea capitis fungal infections of the skin classified according to their location on the body.

Tinea corporis (ringworm) a fungal infection of the scalp; much more common in children than in adults.

Tinea infection one of a group of fungal skin infections that include athlete's foot, folliculitis, jock itch, ringworm, and pityriasis versicolor.

Tinea pedis chronic, superficial fungal infection of the skin of the foot common in adults.

Tinea unguium a fungal infection of the nails.

Tinnitus a condition in which the person hears ringing, buzzing, or other sounds without an external cause.

T-lymphocyte deficiency see Immune deficiency.

Tophaceous gout a form of purine metabolism disorder characterized by formation of chalky deposits of sodium biurate under the skin and in the joints.

Toxic epidermal necrolysis (TEN) a rare adverse reaction to certain drugs in which a large portion of the skin becomes intensely red, may develop blisters, and exfoliates.

Toxoplasmosis a protazoan infection that is the most common opportunistic infection and occurs in one-third of persons with HIV.

Tracheomalacia (tracheobronchomalacia) a congenital or acquired condition characterized by weakness of the tracheal support cartilage, resulting in tracheal collapse when increased airflow is needed.

Trachoma (granular conjunctivitis or Egyptian ophthalmia) a contagious, chronic inflammation of the mucous membranes of the eyes, caused by *Chlamydia trachomatis*.

Transcortical dysphasia (transcortical sensory dysphasia, mixed transcortical dysphasia, isolated speech center) a type of aphasia with poor comprehension, but fluent grammatically correct speech. Patients can communicate well and are capable of good repetition.

Transient hypogammaglobulinemia of infancy see Immune deficiency.

Transient ischemic attack (TIA) a brief episode in which the brain receives insufficient blood supply; symptoms depend on the site of the blockage.

Transposition of the great arteries (TGAs) the aorta arises from the right ventricle and the pulmonary artery arises from the left ventricle.

Traumatic (dissecting) aneurysm aneurysm caused by weakening of arterial walls, by a penetrating missile, or after neurosurgery or neuroimaging following an injury.

Trichomoniasis a sexually transmitted bacterial infection of the urethra in males and the vagina in females that can cause urethral and bladder infection in males and urinary tract infection and painful, malodorous vaginitis in women.

Tricuspid atresia congenital absence of the tricuspid orifice, circulation being made possible by the presence of an atrial septal defect.

True aneurysm localized dilation of an artery with an expanded lumen lined by stretched remnants of the arterial wall.

Truncus arteriosus a congenital defect in which a large great vessel arises from a ventricular septal defect and does not divide into the aorta and pulmonary artery, resulting in one vessel carrying blood both to the body and to the lungs.

TSH deficiency a condition characterized by decreased or absent production of thyroid-stimulating hormone (TSH), resulting in a decline in thyroid hormone level and subsequent symptoms such as fatigue, cold intolerance, weakness, depression, muscle aches, weight gain, and constipation.

Tuberculosis (TB) an infectious disease of humans caused by *Mycobacterium tuberculosis* that results in the formation of tubercles on the lungs and other tissues of the body.

Tuberous sclerosis complex (TSC) an inherited disease caused by mutation of the *hamartin* and *tuberin* genes and resulting in malformation of the brain, retina, and viscera and development of epileptic seizures, mental retardation, and skin nodules on the face.

Turner syndrome gonadal dysgenesis with short stature, undifferentiated (streak) gonads, and variable abnormalities such as webbing of the neck, low posterior hair line, increased carrying angle of elbow, cubitus valgus, and cardiac defects. The genotype is XO (45, X) or X/XX or X/XXX mosaic. The phenotype is female.

Type 1 diabetes mellitus see Diabetes.

Type 2 diabetes mellitus see Diabetes.

U

Ulcerative colitis chronically inflamed and ulcerated mucosal and submucosal lining of the large intestine, resulting in abdominal pain, diarrhea, and rectal bleeding.

Unclassified epileptic seizure seizure disorders that do not fit neatly into a classified grouping. These seizures characteristically have a wide variety of abnormal clinical activity. Examples of this activity include rhythmic eye movements, chewing, and swimming movements. These activities are commonly seen in neonatal seizures.

Undifferentiated large cell anaplastic cancer a cancer of epithelial origin that has lost all evidence of differentiation and may have arisen from a stem cell.

Unilateral neglect syndrome hemiapraxia with failure to pay attention to body grooming and stimuli on one side but not the other; usually caused by a lesion in the central nervous system.

Unstable angina a condition in which unprovoked ischemic attacks occur at unpredictable frequencies and may increase in severity.

Upper airway obstruction (UAO) infections, foreign body aspiration, angioedema, obstructive sleep apnea, and trauma in children.

Uremia syndrome of renal failure resulting in elevated blood urea and creatinine levels.

Uremic syndrome a complex of symptoms resulting from the accumulation of urea and other nitrogenous compounds and toxins in the blood, leading to alterations in levels of fluid and electrolytes, metabolic acidosis, anemia, hyperphosphatemia, and hypocalcemia; symptoms include hypertension, anorexia, nausea, vomiting, diarrhea or constipation, malnutrition and weight loss, pruritus, edema, anemia, and neurologic, cardiovascular disease, and skeletal changes.

Ureterohydronephrosis dilation of both the ureter and the pelvicaliceal system.

Ureteropelvic junction (UPJ) obstruction an impediment to the drainage of urine from the kidney, usually attributable to partial or intermittent blockage of the renal collecting system at the junction of the renal pelvis and ureter.

Urethral atresia congenital absence or closure of a normal body opening or tubular structure; congenital imperforation of the urethra.

Urothelial (transitional cell) carcinoma the most common bladder malignancy, appearing on the inner lining of the bladder.

Urticaria hives; a dermal (skin) manifestation of type I allergic reactions.

Usual ductal hyperplasia (UDH) description of normal hyperplasia of cells that line the ducts in the normal breast; additional layers of benign cells are present, but with normal cellular structure and arrangement.

Uterine prolapse descent or herniation of the uterus into or beyond the vagina because of weakness of the pelvic musculature, ligaments, and fascia or obstetric trauma and lacerations sustained during labor and delivery.

V

Vacuolar myelopathy HIV-induced loss of myelin and spongy degeneration of the spinal cord that may cause spastic paraparesis, sensory ataxia in lower limbs, and unsteady gait.

Vaginismus a form of sexual dysfunction that is caused by a psychologic disorder or vaginal inflammation in which the muscles at the entrance to vagina contract and prevent sexual intercourse.

Vaginitis infection of the vagina usually caused by a fungus that may cause itching or burning and a discharge.

Vaginosis vaginal irritation without white blood cells or other indication of infection.

Varicocele a painful condition in which the veins in the scrotum that develop in the spermatic cord enlarge, and if the valves that regulate blood flow from these veins become dysfunctional, blood does not leave the testis, thereby causing swelling in the veins above and behind the testis.

Varicose bronchiectasis a condition in which the bronchi become large and balloon-like.

Venous angioma abnormal veins, usually near the ventricular wall, that form as a congenital anomaly.

Venous stasis ulcer a condition affecting the lower leg in which leaky valves, obstructions, or regurgitation in veins impairs blood flow back to the heart, resulting in pooling of blood in the lower leg and subsequent tissue damage.

Ventricular septal defect (VSD) a congenital malformation in which the wall between the left and right ventricles has a hole that allows blood to travel between the left and right ventricles, potentially leading to congestive heart failure.

Vesicoureteral reflux (VUR) reflux of urine from the bladder into the ureter.

Vestibular nystagmus involuntary rapid movement of the eyeball that is due to disturbance of the vestibular system; eye movements are rhythmic, with slow and fast components.

Vitiligo an autoimmune-related loss of melanocytes resulting in the depigmentation of patches of skin.

von Willebrand disease an inherited disease in which the von Willebrand factor proteins that are made in the blood vessel walls and function to control platelet activity are abnormal or absent, resulting in a tendency to hemorrhage.

Vulvodynia also referred to as *vulvitis, vestibulitis,* or *vulvovestibulitis*; chronic pain and inflammation of the vulva or vestibule, or both.

W

Waldenström macroglobulinemia see Lymphoma.

Wallerian degeneration the degeneration of a nerve fiber that has been separated from its nutritive center by injury or disease; characterized by segmentation of the myelin and resulting in atrophy and destruction of the axon.

Warm autoimmune hemolytic anemia see Anemia.

Wilms tumor see Nephroblastoma.

Wilson disease a genetic disease in which the ability to metabolize copper is impaired, resulting in an accumulation of copper deposits in organs such as the brain, liver, and kidneys and subsequent organ dysfunction and failure.

Wiskott-Aldrich syndrome (WAS) see Immune deficiency.

X

Xanthelasma a planar xanthoma involving the eyelid(s).

X-linked hyper-IgM syndrome see Immune deficiency.

X-linked SCID see Immune deficiency.

Z

Zika virus a single-stranded RNA virus from the Flaviviridae family, genus *Flavivirus*, that is predominantly transmitted through bites from infected mosquitos; infection during pregnancy has been associated with severe fetal infection and associated CNS abnormalities.

Zollinger-Ellison syndrome the association of atypical, intractable, sometimes fulminating peptic ulcers with extreme gastric hyperacidity and benign or malignant gastrinomas in the pancreas.

INDEX

Page numbers followed by *f*, indicate figures, *t*, tables, or *b*, boxes respectively. Syndromes and disorders appear in boldface.

COMMON LABORATORY VALUES

CONSTITUENT	NORMAL MEAN VALUE AND SOME RANGES	NORMAL RANGE IN SI UNITS
Electrolytes	Total, 1% of plasma weight	
Na^+	135–145 mEq/L	135–145 mmol/L
K^+	3.5–5 mEq/L	3.5–5 mmol/L
Ca^{++} (serum)	8.4–10.6 mg/dL	2.1–2.65 mmol/L
Mg^{++}	1.3–2.1 mg/dL	0.65–1.05 mmol/L
Cl^-	96–106 mEq/L	96–106 mmol/L
HCO_3^- (venous)	23–29 mEq/L	23–29 mmol/L
Phosphate (mostly HPO_4^-)	3–4.5 mg/L	1–1.5 mmol/L
SO_4^-	1 mEq/L	0.25–0.75 mmol/L
Proteins	6–8 g/dL	60–80 g/L
Albumin	3.3–5.5 g/dL	33–55 g/L
Gamma globulin	0.7–1.7 g/dL	7–17 g/L
Globulins	2–4 g/dL	20–40 g/L
Fibrinogen	200–400 mg/dL	2–4 g/L
Troponin I	0.05–0.5 ng/mL	0.05–0.5 ng/mL
Blood Gases		
pH (arterial)	7.35–7.45	7.35–7.45
CO_2 content (arterial)	35–45 mmHg	35–45 mmHg
O_2 content (arterial)	80–100 mmHg	80–100 mmHg
Bicarbonate (arterial)	21–27 mEq/L	21–27 mmol/L
Nutrients		
Glucose (fasting)	75–110 mg/dL	3.85–6.05 nmol/L
Total proteins	6–8 g/dL	—
Total lipids	400–800 mg/dL	4–8 g/L
Cholesterol (total)	<200 mg/dL	<5.20 mmol/L
Triglycerides (after 12 hr fast)	<150 mg/dL	0.45–1.81 mmol/L (males)
		0.40–1.52 mmol/L (females)
Phospholipids	150–380 mg/dL	1.5–3.8 mmol/L
Free fatty acids	9–15 mM/L	9–15 mM/L
Waste Products		
Urea (BUN)	24–49 mg/dL	4–8.2 nmol/L
Uric acid (serum)	2.2–8 mg/dL	130–476 µmol/L
Creatinine	0.6–1.2 mg/dL	53–106 µmol/L
Creatinine clearance	107–139 mL/min	1.78–2.32 mmol/L
Bilirubin (conjugated)	0.1–0.4 mg/dL	1.7–6.8 µmol/L
Bilirubin (total)	0.3–1.1 mg/dL	5.1–19 µmol/L
Individual Hormones		
Prolactin	<20 ng/mL	<20 µg/L
Thyroid tests		
Thyroxine (T_4)	4–11 µg/mL	58–154 nmol/L
T_4 expressed as iodine	3.2–7.2 ng/dL	253–569 nmol/L
T_3	75–220 ng/dL	975 nmol/L
Free thyroxine (T_4)	0.9–2.1 ng/dL	12–27 pmol/L
TSH	0.4–4.8 µIU/mL	0.4–4.8 µIU/L
Hematology Values		
Erythrocyte (red blood cell count)	4.2–6.2 million/mm^3	$4.2–6.2 \times 10^{12}$/L
Leukocyte (white blood cell count)	4500–11,000/mm^3	$4.5–11.2 \times 10^9$/L
Lymphocyte	25%–33% of leukocyte differential	$1500–3000 \times 10^6$/L
Monocyte and macrophage	3%–7% of leukocyte differential	$300–500 \times 10^6$/L
Eosinophil	1%–3% of leukocyte differential	$50–250 \times 10^6$/L
Neutrophil (segmented)	54%–62% of leukocyte differential	$3000–5800 \times 10^6$/L

Continued